Unit VIII   The Hematologic System

25   Structure and Function of the Hematologic System, 952
26   Alterations of Erythrocyte Function, 989
27   Alterations of Leukocyte, Lymphoid, and Hemostatic Function, 1014
28   Alterations of Hematologic Function in Children, 1062

Unit IX   The Cardiovascular and Lymphatic Systems

29   Structure and Function of the Cardiovascular and Lymphatic Systems, 1091
30   Alterations of Cardiovascular Function, 1142
31   Alterations of Cardiovascular Function in Children, 1209

Unit X   The Pulmonary System

32   Structure and Function of the Pulmonary System, 1242
33   Alterations of Pulmonary Function, 1266
34   Alterations of Pulmonary Function in Children, 1310

Unit XI   The Renal and Urologic Systems

35   Structure and Function of the Renal and Urologic Systems, 1344
36   Alterations of Renal and Urinary Tract Function, 1365
37   Alterations of Renal and Urinary Tract Function in Children, 1402

Unit XII   The Digestive System

38   Structure and Function of the Digestive System, 1420
39   Alterations of Digestive Function, 1452
40   Alterations of Digestive Function in Children, 1516

Unit XIII   The Musculoskeletal System

41   Structure and Function of the Musculoskeletal System, 1540
42   Alterations of Musculoskeletal Function, 1568
43   Alterations of Musculoskeletal Function in Children, 1618

Unit XIV   The Integumentary System

44   Structure, Function, and Disorders of the Integument, 1644
45   Alterations of the Integument in Children, 1680

Unit XV   Multiple Interacting Systems

46   Shock, Multiple Organ Dysfunction Syndrome, and Burns in Adults, 1696
47   Shock, Multiple Organ Dysfunction Syndrome, and Burns in Children, 1727

Glossary, 1755

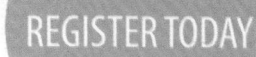

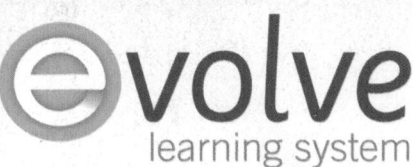
evolve
learning system

To access your Student Resources, visit:

http://evolve.elsevier.com/McCance

Register today and gain access to:

- **Review Questions**
  Provides more than 775 questions with rationales for both correct and incorrect options

- **25 Archie Animations**
  Offers another tool for understanding difficult material

- **Audio Glossary**
  Enables students to confirm their pronunciation of important terminology

- **WebLinks**
  Links you to hundreds of websites carefully chosen to supplement the content of your textbook. The WebLinks are regularly updated, with new links added as they develop.

- **Key Points**
  Includes chapter summaries available in downloadable PDF and audio for on-the-go review.

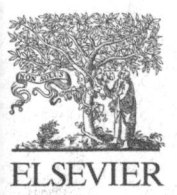
ELSEVIER

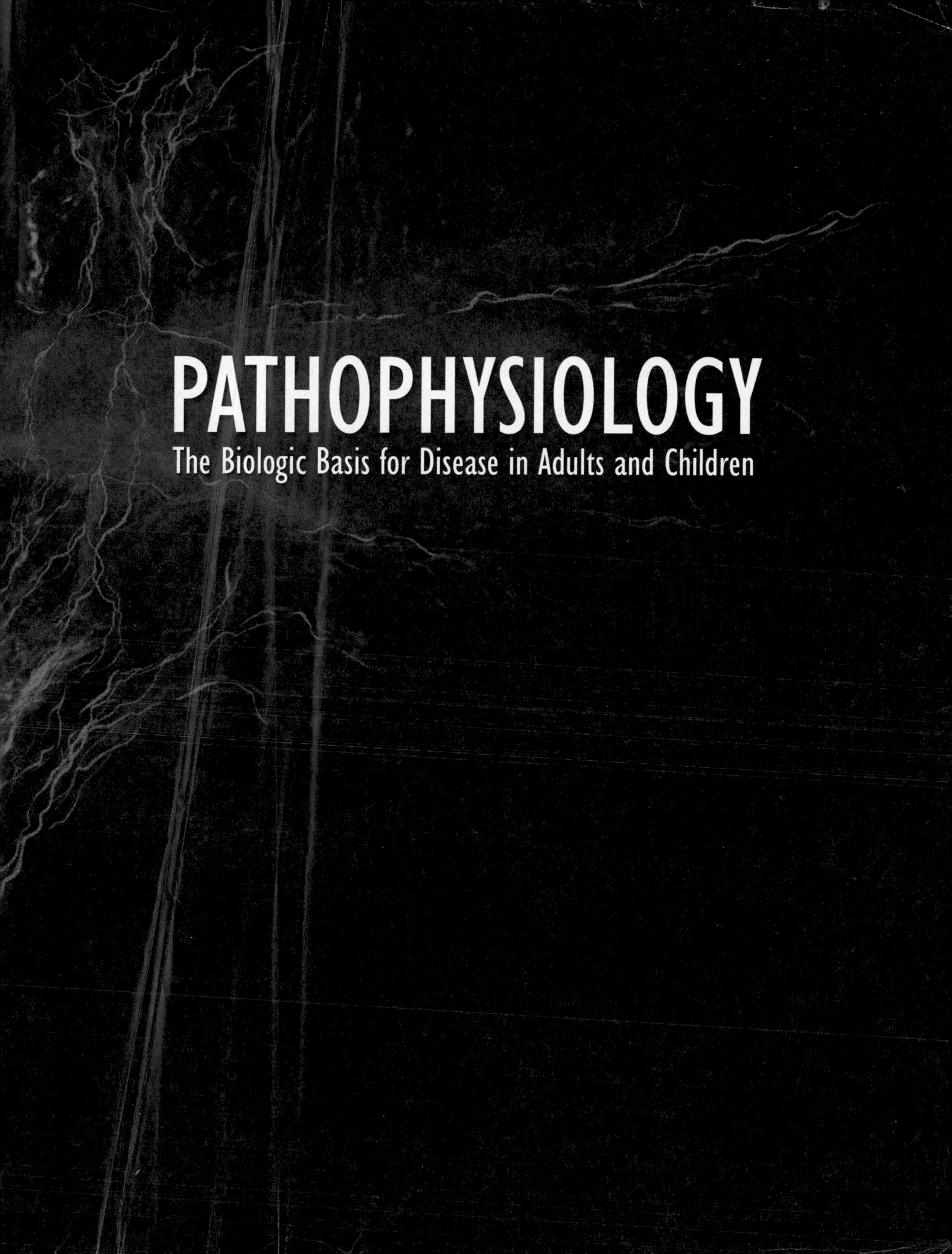

PATHOPHYSIOLOGY
The Biologic Basis for Disease in Adults and Children

ABOUT THE COVER

Selected Topics in Carcinogenesis—The book cover illustration includes important findings in cancer biology. There is compelling evidence that cancer is a tissue-based disease involving abnormal aberrant wound healing and an inflammatory stromal component. In many human cancers the disrupted stroma or microenvironment is correlated with invasive cancer and a poorer prognosis. Early alterations in the stroma that occur with wound healing and inflammation include activation of mesenchymal cells including fibroblasts, endothelial cells, and immune cells, for example, macrophages.

The background of the cover is normal stromal tissue from a photomicrograph of a terminal end bud (TEB, mouse) of a mammary gland. Red are the macrophages, green collagen fibrils, and blue cells. Macrophages release cytokines and growth factors that stimulate local cell proliferation and new blood vessel growth to promote wound healing. The resultant stromal changes can promote tumor invasion and tumor cell migration. This stunning photomicrograph was taken by Dr. Jeffrey W Pollard. Another concept featured on the cover includes the fibroblast—large purple cell—which is associated with cancer cells at all stages. This is actually a common "footprint" or "signature" as an independent marker of local cancer recurrence. This somewhat haunting and beautiful image was taken by Dennis Kunkel. The cover also features a wispy red floating-like cell at the top that is a schematic of a standard fibroblast cell from the 3T3 cell line. Studies using these cells have been important for understanding the cancer characteristic of immortality or indefinite growth. The final major cover image is the green image on the right that is a human lung carcinoma cell—a common cause of cancer fatalities in men and women.

SIXTH EDITION

PATHOPHYSIOLOGY

The Biologic Basis for Disease in Adults and Children

Kathryn L. McCance, RN, PhD
Professor
College of Nursing
University of Utah
Salt Lake City, Utah

Sue E. Huether, RN, PhD
Professor Emeritus

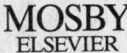

MOSBY
ELSEVIER

3251 Riverport Lane
Maryland Heights, Missouri 63043

PATHOPHYSIOLOGY: THE BIOLOGIC BASIS FOR DISEASE IN ADULTS AND CHILDREN, ed 6   ISBN: 978-0-323-06584-9
Copyright © 2010, 2006, 2002, 1998, 1994, 1990 by Mosby, Inc.

Notice

ISBN: 978-0-323-06584-9

Library of Congress Cataloging-in-Publication Data
Pathophysiology: the biologic basis for disease in adults and children / [edited by]
Kathryn L. McCance, Sue E. Huether; section editors, Valentina L. Brashers, Neal S. Rote
-- 6th ed.
         p. ; cm.
    Includes bibliographical references and index.
    ISBN 978-0-323-06584-9 (hardcover: alk. paper) 1. Physiology, Pathological. 2. Nursing.
I. McCance, Kathryn L. II. Huether, Sue E.
    [DNLM: 1. Pathology--Nurses' Instruction. 2. Disease--Nurses' Instruction. 3. Physiological
Phenomena--Nurses' Istruction. QZ 4 P3027 2010]
    RB113.M35 2010

Senior Editor: Sandra Clark
Senior Developmental Editor (Student Evolve Website): Cindi Crismon Jones
Developmental Editor: Charlene Ketchum
Editorial Assistant: Brooke Bagwill
Publishing Services Manager: Jeffrey Patterson
Project Manager: Jeanne Genz
Design Direction: Margaret Reid
Cover Designer: Jeanne Robertson and Margaret Reid
Multimedia Producer: Sarah Spalding-Eichorn

CONTRIBUTORS*

Rose A. Urdiales Baker, PhD(c), MSN, PMHCNS-BC, RN
Adjunct Faculty
College of Nursing
Kent State University
Kent, Ohio

Barbara J. Boss, PhD, APRN, FNP-BC, APN-BC
Professor of Nursing
University of Mississippi Medical Center
Jackson, Mississippi

Valentina L. Brashers, MD
Professor of Nursing and Attending Physician in
Internal Medicine
University of Virginia
Charlottesville, Virginia

Kristen Lee Carroll, MD
Associate Professor
Department of Orthopedics
University of Utah
Salt Lake City, Utah
Shriners Hospital for Children Intermountain
Salt Lake City, Utah

Dennis J. Cheek, RN, PhD, FAHA
Abell-Hanger Professor of Gerontological Nursing
Harris College of Nursing and Health Sciences
Texas Christian University
Fort Worth, Texas

Margaret F. Clayton, PhD, FNP-BC
Assistant Professor
College of Nursing
University of Utah
Salt Lake City, Utah

Christy L. Crowther-Radulewicz, MS, CRNP
Nurse Practitioner
Anne Arundel Orthopaedic Surgeons
Annapolis, Maryland

Angela Deneris, CNM, PhD
Associate Professor,
Clinical College of Nursing
University of Utah
Salt Lake City, Utah

Beth A. Forshee, PhD
Assistant Professor of Physiology
Lake Erie College of Osteopathic Medicine
Erie, Pennsylvania

Deborah K. Froh, MD
Associate Professor of Pediatrics
University of Virginia
Charlottesville, Virginia

Kristi Gott, MSN, RN, PNP-BC
Instructor of Nursing
School of Nursing
University of Virginia
Charlottesville, Virginia

Todd Cameron Grey, MD
Chief Medical Examiner
State of Utah
Adjunct Associate Professor of Pathology
School of Medicine
University of Utah
Salt Lake City, Utah

Mary Fran Hazinski, RN, MSN, FAAN, FAHA
Professor
School of Nursing
Vanderbilt University
Nashville, Tennessee
Clinical Nurse Specialist
Vanderbilt Children's Hospital
Nashville, Tennessee

Robert E. Jones MD, FACP, FACE
Professor of Medicine (Clinical)
School of Medicine
University of Utah
Salt Lake City, Utah
Medical Director
Utah Diabetes Center
Salt Lake City, Utah

Lynn B. Jorde, PhD
H.A. and Edna Benning Presidential Professor
Department of Human Genetics
School of Medicine
University of Utah
Salt Lake City, Utah

*The authors would also like to thank the previous edition
contributors.

Lisa Kaloczi, CNM, MSN
Clinical Instructor
College of Nursing
University of Utah
Salt Lake City, Utah

Nancy E. Kline, PhD, RN, CPNP, FAAN
Director, Evidence-Based Practice and Research
Memorial Sloan-Kettering Cancer Center
New York, New York

Gwen A. Latendresse, CNM, PhD
Assistant Professor
College of Nursing
University of Utah
Salt Lake City, Utah

Linda L. Martin, RN, DNP, C-FNP
Clinical Professor
College of Nursing and Health Sciences
Texas Christian University–Harris
Fort Worth, Texas

Nancy L. McDaniel, MD
Associate Professor of Pediatrics
Department of Pediatrics
University of Virginia
Charlottesville, Virginia

Mary A. Mondozzi, MSN, APRN-BC
Burn Center Education/Outreach Coordinator
Akron Children's Hospital
The Paul and Carol David Foundation Burn Institute
Akron, Ohio

Katherine Morgan, MSN, WHNP, ANP
Associate Clinical Professor
University of Utah
College of Nursing
Salt Lake City, Utah

Stephen E. Morris, MD
Associate Professor of Surgery
University of Utah Burn Center
Salt Lake City, Utah

Noreen Heer Nicol, MS, RN, FNP
Affiliate—National Jewish Health
Clinical Senior Instructor
University of Colorado
Denver, Colorado

Neal S. Rote, PhD
William H. Weir, MD Professor of Reproductive Biology
    and Professor of Pathology
Case Western Reserve School of Medicine
and Vice-Chair for Academic Affairs and
Director, Research Division
Department of Obstetrics and Gynecology
University Hospitals of Cleveland
Case Medical Center
Cleveland, Ohio

Richard A. Sugerman, PhD
Assistant Vice President for Academic Program
Development
Professor of Anatomy
College of Osteopathic Medicine of the Pacific
Western University of Health Sciences
Pomona, California

Lorey K. Takahashi, PhD
Professor of Psychology
University of Hawaii at Manoa
Honolulu, Hawaii

David M. Virshup, MD
Professor and Director
Program in Cancer and Stem Cell Biology
Duke-NUS Graduate Medical School
Singapore
Professor of Pediatrics
Duke University School of Medicine
Durham, North Carolina

REVIEWERS

Deborah Dawn Hutchinson Allen, RN, MSN, CNS, FNP-BC, AOCNP
Oncology Clinical Nurse Specialist
Duke Brain Tumor Center Nurse Practitioner
Comprehensive Cancer Center
Duke University Medical Center
Durham, North Carolina

Nancy D. Blasdell, RN, PhD
Assistant Professor
School of Nursing
Rhode Island College
Providence, Rhode Island

Mandi Counters, RN, MSN, CNRN
Assistant Professor
Nursing Department
Mercy College of Health Sciences
Des Moines, Iowa

David J. Derrico, RN, MSN
Assistant Clinical Professor
Department of Adult and Elderly Nursing
University of Florida College of Nursing
Gainesville, Florida

Benjamin Djulbegovic, MD, PhD
Professor of Medicine and Oncology
Clinical Translational Science Institute, and
Department of Hematological Malignancies
University of South Florida, H. Lee Moffit Cancer Center
Tampa, Florida

Jennifer J. Donwerth, MSN, RN, ANP-BC, GNP-BC
Faculty
Department of Nursing
Tarleton State University
Stephenville, Texas

Nancy Evans, BS
Health Science Consultant
Self-Employed
San Francisco, California

Judith L. Myers, MSN, RN
Assistant Professor of Nursing
Grand View College
Des Moines, Iowa

Jo A. Voss, PhD, RN, CNS
Associate Professor
West River Department of Nursing
South Dakota State University
Rapid City, South Dakota

Diane Young, PhD, CNE, RN
Professor
Nursing Department
Allen College
Waterloo, Iowa

PREFACE

Pathophysiology incorporates basic, translational, and clinical research to advance understandings of disease and dysfunction. The study of pathophysiology involves many biomedical sciences and a wide range of research activities. Multiple aspects of cellular physiology are progressing rapidly, generating vast amounts of data to understand molecular, cellular, and tissue level interactions. The information expansion involves a greater understanding of the behavior of individual cells, their neighboring microenvironment, and of the molecules that not only make up those cells but also communicate with their surroundings. Fascinating is the idea that the cell is at once a crowded structural and chemical space and surrounded by a fragile "soft" space subjected to molecular and physical forces that create structural rearrangements and pathologic states. These new findings are creating the need for an integrative approach among numerous sciences to the study of pathophysiology.

Although these advancements have created an ever-increasing state of excitement, they have also created the problem of how students, teachers, and clinicians can cope with the expanding new information. Compressing these data into simplified discussions for students and clinicians is challenging. Our approach in this book has been to emphasize this emergence by explaining new concepts in greater detail than perhaps is usual and by giving extra emphasis to important but difficult content. The primary focus is on pathophysiology, and there is less emphasis on the evaluation and treatment that is found in clinical management textbooks. In this edition are some major new chapters and several extensively rewritten previous chapters with new art.

As in previous editions, our specific goals for the textbook are to:

- Draw attention to differences in etiology, epidemiology, and pathophysiology, according to gender and age
- Include major difference in clinical manifestations and treatment by gender and age
- Pay careful attention to presentations of emerging new data on controversial topics
- Integrate health promotion and disease prevention by updating risk factors, explaining certain relationships between nutrition and disease, and noting screening recommendations and other therapeutic approaches

ORGANIZATION AND CONTENT: WHAT'S NEW IN THE SIXTH EDITION

The book is organized into two parts. The application of the principles and concepts in Part One determines the learner's ability to grasp the cellular and tissue responses to the most common diseases presented in Part Two. All content has been reviewed with extensive new references.

Part One: Central Concepts of Pathophysiology: Cells and Tissues

Part One begins with an in-depth study of the cell and progresses to cover the underlying processes of disease. Concepts covered include cell signaling and cell communication processes; genes and common genetic diseases; fluid electrolyte and acid-base balance; inflammation, cytokines and their biologic functions, normal and altered immunity; infection, stress, coping, and immunity; tumor biology, and epidemiology of cancer. Particularly important revisions and additions to Part One include the following:

- Updated content on cellular organelles, cell signaling, and communication (Chapter 1)
- Updated content on oxidative stress, types of cell death, apoptosis, and aging (Chapter 2)
- Updated content on normal innate and adaptive immunity (Chapters 6 and 7)
- Updated content on alterations of immunity and inflammation (Chapter 8)
- Extensively revised chapter on infection (Chapter 9)
- Reorganization and updated content on stress and disease (Chapter 10)
- Extensive revisions and reorganization of tumor biology and invasion and metastases (Chapter 11)
- Extensive revisions and reorganization of epidemiology of cancer (Chapter 12)

Part Two: Pathophysiologic Alterations: Organs and Systems

Part Two is a systematic survey of diseases within body systems. Each unit focuses on a specific body system and begins with an anatomy and physiology chapter to provide a basis of comparison for understanding the alterations brought about by disease. A brief summary of normal aging is included at the end of the section on anatomy and physiology. The discussion of each disease in the alterations chapters is developed in a logical manner that begins with an introductory paragraph on etiology and epidemiology, followed by pathophysiology, clinical manifestations, and evaluation and treatment. Separate chapters are dedicated to pediatric pathophysiology, and sensitivity is paid to gender and age. Especially significant revisions and additions to Part Two include the following:

- New information on pain modulation, chronic pain syndromes, and classification of sleep disorders (Chapter 15)

- Updated content on concepts of altered cognition and coma, seizures, mechanisms of dementia, and alterations in motor function (Chapter 16)
- Rewritten content on secondary and tertiary responses to brain injury and chronic neurologic disorders including immune mechanisms associated with multiple sclerosis (Chapter 17)
- Updated content on schizophrenia, mood disorders, and anxiety (Chapter 18)
- Updates on genes and brain defects in children, brain infection, and brain tumors (Chapter 19)
- New content on neuroregulation of hormone responses and hormonal immune system interaction (Chapter 20)
- Extensive updates on the genetics of hormone disorders, pituitary and thyroid disorders, immune mechanisms of diabetes mellitus, the pathophysiology of insulin resistance, gestational diabetes, and the chronic complications of diabetes (Chapter 21)
- Extensively rewritten material on reproductive disorders, benign breast diseases, breast cancer, and prostate cancer (Chapter 23)
- Reorganized and updated content on normal blood cells, hemostasis, platelet function, and coagulation (Chapter 25)
- Extensively revised and updated content on alterations of leukocyte, lymphoid, and hemostatic function (Chapter 27)
- Reorganized and updated content on the anatomy and physiology of the cardiovascular system (Chapter 29)
- Extensively updated coverage of atherosclerosis, endothelial injury and dysfunction, coronary artery disease, myocardial infarction, and heart failure (Chapter 30)
- Major revisions of the signs and symptoms of respiratory disease and disorders of the chest wall. Updates in gene-environment interaction and the role of cytokines in the pathophysiology of asthma; pulmonary hypertension, pulmonary embolism, and lung cancers (Chapters 33)
- Major revisions in upper airway disorders in children, childhood obstructive sleep apnea syndrome, respiratory distress syndrome, lung infections, and asthma (Chapter 34)
- Major reorganization and updates on urinary tract and renal disorders including obstructive uropathies, glomerulopathies, and chronic renal failure (Chapter 36)
- New information for inherited disorders of renal function, infection and urinary tract disease, and renal failure in children (Chapter 37)
- Major revisions and new content on peptic ulcer disease, irritable bowel syndrome, inflammatory bowel disease, intestinal obstruction, obesity, and liver disease (Chapter 39)
- New information on esophageal reflux and esophagitis, necrotizing enterocolitis, and infections of the intestine in children (Chapter 40)
- Updated content on alterations of musculoskeletal system (Chapter 42)

- Updated content on allergic and autoimmune diseases of the skin, skin infections, and skin cancer (Chapter 44)
- Updated content on atopic dermatitis and immune reactions to skin infections and drug treatment in children (Chapter 45)
- Updated content on septic shock, multiple organ dysfunction syndrome, and burns for adults and children (Chapters 46 and 47)

FEATURES TO PROMOTE LEARNING

Ease of learning has been enhanced by designing a number of features that guide and support understanding, including:
- Each chapter opener notes the corresponding module in the Online Review Course. The course is available as a separate purchase.
- *Chapter Outlines* for each chapter
- *Special Headings* to underscore the consistent treatment of each disease—Pathophysiology, Clinical Manifestations, and Evaluation and Treatment
- More than 80 *What's New?* boxes review the most current research and clinical developments
- *Nutrition & Disease* boxes to emphasize nutrition as a health promotion strategy that may alter disease risk or pathogenesis
- End-of-chapter *Summary Review* sections summarize the content in each chapter and serve as built-in content review guides
- Boldface *Key Terms* with end-of-chapter term lists and page numbers for rapid access
- A comprehensive *Glossary* of more than 1000 terms on **Evolve** helps students with the often-difficult terminology related to pathophysiology; a brief version is included at the back of this book

ART PROGRAM

The art program was carefully crafted. More than 300 new full-color illustrations and photographs were created and strategically placed throughout the textbook. The art program received as much attention as the narrative. Also included are many new high-quality, full-color photographs of clinical manifestations, pathologic specimens, and clinical imaging techniques. The combination of illustrations, algorithms, photographs, and use of color for tables and boxes allows clarification for complex concepts and the emergence of easily recognized essential information.

ANCILLARIES

For Students

On **Evolve**, students may register for **free** access to 775 review questions, a comprehensive glossary, an audio glossary, 25 animations to help students master the text content, downloadable audio chapter Key Points, and updated WebLinks, which are carefully chosen Internet sites related to each chapter in the text.

The **Study Guide** includes learning objectives, special *Memory Check!* boxes, concise summaries of key concepts, and a practice examination for each chapter. Each of the disease chapters also includes a case study with a critical thinking question. Answers are found in the back.

For Instructors

The **Evolve Instructor Resources** for this textbook provide the following teaching aids:

- Teaching Difficult Concepts tool for each chapter
- Audience Response Questions (iClicker) for each chapter (141 total)
- Critical Thinking Exercises for each chapter (231 total)
- Test Bank in ExamView and Word with more than 2300 questions (in true/false, multiple choice, matching, and completion formats) with answers and textbook page references

- Image Collection with approximately 1100 key figures from the text
- Lecture Slides on PowerPoint for every chapter
- Chapter Summaries

Evolve is an Internet-based learning environment that works in coordination with the text. This resource enables you to publish your class syllabus, outline, and lecture notes; set up "virtual office hours" and e-mail communication; share important dates and information through the online class calendar; and encourage student participation through chat rooms and discussion boards. Free with qualified adoption. Contact your sales representative or visit http://evolve.elsevier.com for more information about integrating **Evolve** into your curriculum.

ACKNOWLEDGMENTS

The enormous task of keeping this book current and readable greatly depends on our contributors. We thank them for their knowledge and tremendous labor of reviewing relevant literature, synthesizing it, and writing and revising chapters to make them highly readable for others. Several chapters were completely rewritten for this edition. We have a special appreciation for Dr. Neal Rote and Dr. Tina Brashers, section editors, for their tireless editing, writing, and development of new art. Dr. Rote managed the immunity, infection, and hematology chapters. His ability to integrate, simplify, and illustrate this complex content is exceptional. Always motivated to *really* help students and clinicians–Neal, we thank you. Dr. Brashers managed the endocrine, pulmonary, and cardiovascular chapters. Tina has unsurpassed energy. She contributes major effort and tedious detail–all with an amazing sense of humor and support to contributing authors. Thank you, Tina. In addition, Dr. Brashers, Susanna Cunningham, Annette Rivera, Marie O' Toole, Linda Turchin, and Diane Young developed modules for the Online Review Course. There were also many faculty and clinicians who provided reviews for content revision and we are grateful for their insight and recommendations.

We are also grateful to those who contributed to the book supplements. Textbook contributor Beth Forshee also wrote the glossary. Dr. Linda Edelman wrote the review questions for the Student Evolve website. Drs. Nancy Blasdell, Diane Young, Margaret Clayton, and Beth Forshee updated and developed new material for the Evolve Instructor Resources including the critical thinking exercises, teaching difficult concepts, PowerPoint lecture slides, and Test Bank. Susan Frazier created the audience response questions. We would also like to acknowledge Dr. Kraig Chugg for his previous contributions to the instructor material and PowerPoint slides and Dr. Susan Wilson for her previous work on the test bank. Thank you all for your help.

The process of completing this book is dependent on the "behind the scenes work" of numerous people. Manuscript management and final word processing is a huge and complex effort and was completed by Sue Meeks who has worked with us for 26 years. Her unwavering dedication to excellence and detail keeps us sane and on track. It seems like every edition is monumental work—and she retypes and recounts endlessly—and unruffled. As always, thanks for your continuing skill and patience.

Our developmental editor at Elsevier is Charlene Ketchum. This job is key. Charlene is organized, practical, and kept this project on target. Easy to work with and unflappable, even at times with remarkable restraint, she managed this project with a reassuring and professional style. Thank you Charlene. Senior editor Sandra Clark, solid and serious, provided wise counsel and continued encouragement. Thank you, Sandra. Brooke Bagwill, conscientious and skillful, coordinated reviewer projects and ensured that we had all of the resources we needed.

The project manager for a book of this size and complexity of content has an enormous responsibility. The project manager was Jeanne Genz. She is exacting and a gem to work with. A woman of few but critical words she orchestrated numerous changes despite shifting work locations. Thank you, Jeanne. Our book designer Margaret Reid did an outstanding job designing the interior portion of the book—we are especially pleased with the dynamic colors and presentation of pedagogy. Thank you, Margaret.

Much of the new art program with spectacular renderings and colors was done by Jeanne Robertson. Despite our terminally clumsy and complex drawings, Jeanne interpreted, redrew, and produced the illustrations. Margaret Reid and Jeanne Robertson worked together to create the awesome and contemporary cover design. For the cover, Dennis Kunkel provided the fibroblast slide and Dr. Jeffrey Pollard provided the TEB micrograph of mammary stromal tissue. We also thank the Department of Dermatology at the University of Utah School of Medicine, which provided numerous photos of skin lesions. Thanks to Dr. Arthur R. Brothman, University of Utah School of Medicine, for the *N-myc* gene amplification slides used to illustrate the discussion of neuroblastoma and to Dr. John Hoffman for the PET scan images of non–small cell lung cancer.

We are grateful to the many colleagues and friends at the University of Utah College of Nursing, School of Medicine, College of Pharmacy, and Eccles Medical Library for their assistance with references and consultation on content. Thanks for the outstanding extra help—Nancy Evans and Ruth Weinberg—when it was needed the most. To Bobbie Cleave, Margaret Smith, Caroline Gaudy, Kelly Wade, and Harrison Berry, your kindness and skill in a time of need is much appreciated. Thanks to physical therapists Lauren Hatchell and Andie Lewis for the gifted, unique, and not teeth-clenching therapy—it has hastened the completion of this book. Thanks to the trauma team at University of Utah School of Medicine for smart, swift, and kind care, especially Erik Kubiak, MD.

Special thanks are given to students, particularly nursing and other health science students for the e-mails and phone calls we receive. Your questions and suggestions are inspiring and guide us in our efforts to prepare a clear and up to date manuscript with much visual punctuation.

Love and thanks to our families for their continued support and "hands on help," especially to you John, my trusted in-house researcher and cook.

INTRODUCTION TO PATHOPHYSIOLOGY

The word root "patho" is derived from the Greek word *pathos*, which means suffering. The Greek word root "logos" means discourse or more commonly, system of formal study, and "physio" pertains to functions of organisms. Generally, pathophysiology is the systematic study of the functional changes in cells, tissues, and organs altered by disease and/or injury. Important, however, is the inextricable component of suffering.

Knowledge of cellular biology as well as anatomy and physiology and the various organ systems of the body is an essential foundation for the study of pathophysiology. To understand pathophysiology the student must also use principles, concepts, and basic knowledge from other fields of study, including pathology, genetics, immunology, and epidemiology. A number of terms are used to focus the discussion of pathophysiology; they may be used interchangeably at times, but that does not necessarily indicate that they have the same meaning. These terms are reviewed in Table I-1.

Pathophysiology is one of the most important bridging sciences between preclinical and clinical courses for students in the health sciences and it requires in-depth study at an early stage in the curriculum. The definitions or conceptual models of pathophysiology that we carry in our minds influence what we do with our observations and what rationale we provide for our actions. Therefore, the clinician must understand that although pathophysiology is a science, it also designates suffering in people; the clinician should never lose sight of this aspect of its definition.

As students study clinically related sciences, they learn to recognize and categorize disease. From the formulation of a differential diagnosis one understands the different *clinical manifestations*, the signs, and the symptoms of certain pathologies. These understandings structure further investigations, treatment plans, and evaluation. The interaction of these activities determines clinical outcomes and treatment success. Still, the concept of disease can be inherently ambiguous and elusive; many pathologies remain hidden and resist easy classification. One should appreciate that the naming and diagnosing of diseases involve evaluative judgments as well as scientific fact, and that the process is as much a social endeavor as it is a scientific one. Some diseases, such as tuberculosis, identify a highly specific causative or etiologic agent or process. Others, such as Alzheimer disease or arthritis, indicate pathologic changes of unclear cause. In addition, syndromes and functional disorders simply describe multiple symptoms and signs that frequently occur together. Does commonality exist in all of these labels?

The answer is yes and no and depends on our conception of health and disease. In the strictest sense, objective scientific facts help us know if an individual is healthy or suffering from disease. However, the individual's conception of disease is based on personal beliefs and histories, professional and lay healers who interact with that individual, and society at large. Each idea or construct has the power to influence other ideas and constructs, and each relationship has the ability to shape the way disease is understood and experienced.[1] In short, defining and understanding disease is tremendously ambiguous. Perhaps the most important and desirable trait for the new student of pathophysiology is an open and tolerant mind. To believe that science alone can overcome ignorance and that clinical training and technology can overcome ineptitude only encourages arrogance and undermines the scientific purpose.

Table I-1	Terms and Definitions Related to Pathophysiology
Pathology	Study of structural alterations in cells, tissues and organs that help to identify the cause of disease
Pathogenesis	Pattern of tissue changes associated with the development of disease
Etiology	Study of the cause(s) of disease and/or injury
Idiopathic	Diseases with no identifiable cause
Iatrogenic	Diseases and/or injury as a result of medical intervention
Clinical manifestations	Signs and symptoms
Nosocomial	Diseases acquired as a consequence of being in a hospital environment
Diagnosis	Naming or identification of disease
Prognosis	Expected outcome of a disease
Acute disease	Sudden appearance of signs and symptoms lasting a short time
Chronic disease	Develops more slowly lasting a long time or a lifetime
Remissions	Periods when clinical manifestations disappear or diminish significantly
Exacerbations	Periods when clinical manifestations become worse or more severe
Sequelae	Any abnormal conditions that follow and are the result of a disease, treatment, or injury

Pathophysiology has had great success in explaining the mechanisms and clinical manifestations associated with infectious diseases. Syndromes of unclear etiology such as headache and fibromyalgia have proven to be troublesome. Even more difficult are multifactorial conditions, such as atherosclerosis or type 2 diabetes mellitus, in which several interacting factors contribute to the etiology. Learning how interacting factors relate to one another to increase morbidity or actually cause disease contributes to an appreciation of how emerging concepts revolutionize current understandings. For example, for many years the bacterial forms seen in gastric biopsies were interpreted as contaminants. It took several decades to understand the bacterial origin of gastritis, peptic ulcer disease, and even gastric carcinoma. Such findings are a major revolution in thought. One revolution in thought that has driven intensive research is that low levels of chronic inflammation cause or contribute to many diseases.

The language that clinicians use to discuss diseases and their manifestations is powerful. Lives are altered by a few words uttered by a clinician in a white coat or uniform. "AIDS," "cancer," and "heart attack" have become culturally ingrained symbols that portend an individual's future. Although some futures are determined by scientific evidence, others are determined by subjective experience.[2] For example, a person diagnosed with a familial disease may ask, "Will I suffer like my mother did?" This questioning influences individuals' suffering.

In conclusion, pathophysiology—the understanding of disease—requires descriptive evidence as well as an evaluative component regarding suffering and the language we use to describe it. Combining objective and subjective perspectives requires new conceptual models that take into account the complex interactions among the body, mind, environment, and spirit.

REFERENCES

1. Magid C: Developing tolerance for ambiguity, *JAMA* 285(1):88, 2001.
2. Goldstein J: In the twilight: life in the margins between sick and well, *JAMA* 285(1):92, 2001.

CONTENTS

PART ONE   CENTRAL CONCEPTS OF PATHOPHYSIOLOGY: CELLS AND TISSUES

UNIT I   The Cell

Chapter 1   Cellular Biology, 1
Kathyrn L. McCance

Prokaryotes and Eukaryotes, 1
Cellular Functions, 2
Structure and Function of Cellular Components, 2
  Nucleus, 2
  Cytoplasmic Organelles, 4
  Plasma Membranes, 10
  Cellular Receptors, 13
Cell-to-Cell Adhesions, 15
  Extracellular Matrix, 15
  Specialized Cell Junctions, 16
Cellular Communication and Signal Transduction, 18
  Signal Transduction, 19
  Extracellular Messengers and Channel Regulation, 20
  Second Messengers, 20
Cellular Metabolism, 21
  Role of Adenosine Triphosphate, 22
  Food and Production of Cellular Energy, 23
  Oxidative Phosphorylation, 24
Membrane Transport: Cellular Intake and Output, 25
  Movement of Water and Solutes, 26
  Transport by Vesicle Formation, 30
  Movement of Electrical Impulses: Membrane
    Potentials, 32
Cellular Reproduction: The Cell Cycle, 33
  Phases of Mitosis and Cytokinesis, 34
  Rates of Cellular Division, 35
  Growth Factors, 35
Tissues, 35
  Tissue Formation, 35
  Types of Tissues, 36

Chapter 2   Altered Cellular and Tissue Biology, 46
Kathryn L. McCance and Todd Cameron Grey

Cellular Adaption, 47
  Atrophy, 47
  Hypertrophy, 47
  Hyperplasia, 48
  Dysplasia: Not a True Adaptive Change, 49
  Metaplasia, 50

Cellular Injury, 50
  General Mechanisms of Cell Injury, 52
  Hypoxic Injury, 52
  Free Radicals and Reactive Oxygen Species, 54
  Chemical Injury, 55
  Unintentional and Intentional Injuries, 62
  Infectious Injury, 69
  Immunologic and Inflammatory Injury, 69
  Injurious Genetic Factors, 69
  Injurious Nutritional Imbalances, 69
  Injurious Physical Agents, 71
Manifestations of Cellular Injury, 76
  Cellular Manifestations: Accumulations, 76
  Systemic Manifestations, 81
Cellular Death, 81
  Necrosis, 81
  Apoptosis, 84
Aging and Altered Cellular and Tissue Biology, 86
  Normal Life Span, 86
Somatic Death, 90

Chapter 3   The Cellular Environment: Fluids and Electrolytes, Acids and Bases, 96
Sue E. Huether

Distribution of Body Fluids, 96
Aging and Distribution of Body Fluids, 97
  Water Movement Between ICF and ECF, 97
  Water Movement Between Plasma and Interstitial Fluid, 98
Alterations in Water Movement, 98
  Edema, 98
Sodium, Chloride, and Water Balance, 101
  Sodium and Chloride Balance, 101
  Water Balance, 102
Alterations in Sodium, Chloride, and Water Balance, 102
  Isotonic Alterations, 102
  Hypertonic Alterations, 103
  Hypotonic Alterations, 104
Alterations in Potassium, Calcium, Phosphate, and Magnesium Balance, 106
  Potassium, 106
  Calcium and Phosphate, 111
  Magnesium, 114
Acid-Base Balance, 114
  Hydrogen Ion and pH, 114
  Buffer Systems, 115
  Acid-Base Imbalances, 117

UNIT II   Genes and Gene-Environment Interaction

Chapter 4   Genes and Genetic Diseases, 126
Lynn B. Jorde

DNA, RNA, and Proteins: Heredity at the Molecular Level, 129
DNA, 129
From Genes to Proteins, 132
Chromosomes, 134
Chromosome Aberrations and Associated Diseases, 135
Elements of Formal Genetics, 143
Phenotype and Genotype, 145
Dominance and Recessiveness, 145
Transmission of Genetic Diseases, 145
Autosomal Dominant Inheritance, 146
Autosomal Recessive Inheritance, 151
X-Linked Inheritance, 152
Evaluation of Pedigrees, 155
Linkage Analysis and Gene Mapping, 155
Classical Pedigree Analysis, 155
Assigning Loci to Specific Chromosomes, 157
Complete Human Gene Map: Prospects and Benefits, 157

Chapter 5   Genes, Environment, and Common Diseases, 164
Lynn B. Jorde

Factors Influencing Incidence of Disease in Populations, 164
Concepts of Incidence and Prevalence, 164
Analysis of Risk Factors, 165
Principles of Multifactorial Inheritance, 165
Basic Model, 165
Threshold Model, 166
Recurrence Risks and Transmission Patterns, 167
Nature and Nurture: Disentangling the Effects of Genes and Environment, 169
Twin Studies, 170
Adoption Studies, 170
Genetics of Common Diseases, 172
Congenital Malformations, 172
Multifactorial Disorders in the Adult Population, 172

UNIT III   Mechanisms of Self-Defense

Chapter 6   Innate Immunity: Inflammation, 183
Neal S. Rote and Sue E. Huether

Human Defense Mechanisms, 184
First Line of Defense: Physical, Mechanical, and Biochemical Barriers, 184
Physical and Mechanical Barriers, 184
Biochemical Barriers, 184
Second Line of Defense: The Inflammatory Response, 186
Vascular Response, 186

Plasma Protein Systems, 187
Cellular Mediators of Inflammation, 192
Cellular Products, 203
Local Manifestations of Inflammation, 205
Systemic Manifestations of Acute Inflammation, 205
Fever, 206
Leukocytosis, 206
Plasma Protein Synthesis, 206
Chronic Inflammation, 206
Resolution and Repair, 208
Reconstructive Phase, 208
Maturation Phase, 210
Dysfunctional Wound Healing, 211
Pediatrics and Mechanisms of Self-Defense, 212
Aging and Mechanisms of Self-Defense, 213

Chapter 7   Adaptive Immunity, 217
Neal S. Rote

General Characteristics of Adaptive Immunity, 217
Humoral and Cell-Mediated Immunity, 219
Active vs. Passive Immunity, 220
Recognition and Response, 220
Antigens and Immunogens, 221
Molecules That Recognize Antigen, 222
Molecules That Present Antigen, 226
Molecules That Hold Cells Together, 228
Cytokines and Their Receptors, 228
Generation of Clonal Diversity, 229
T-Cell Maturation, 230
B-Cell Maturation, 233
Induction of an Immune Response: Clonal Selection, 235
Secondary Lymphoid Organs, 235
Antigen Processing and Presentation, 235
Helper T Lymphocytes, 237
B-Cell Activation: The Humoral Immune Response, 240
T-Cell Activation: The Cellular Immune Response, 243
Effector Mechanisms, 244
Antibody Function, 244
T-Lymphocyte Function, 247
Fetal and Neonatal Immune Function, 250
Aging and Immune Function, 251

Chapter 8   Alterations in Immunity and Inflammation, 256
Neal S. Rote

Hypersensitivity: Allergy, Autoimmunity, and Alloimmunity, 256
Mechanisms of Hypersensitivity, 258
Antigenic Targets of Hypersensitivity Reactions, 264
Autoimmune and Alloimmune Disease, 271
Deficiencies in Immunity, 275
Initial Clinical Presentation, 275
Primary Immune Deficiencies, 275
Secondary Immune Deficiencies, 284

Clinical Evaluation of Immunity, *286*
Replacement Therapies for Immune Deficiencies, *287*

Chapter 9   Infection, 293
Neal S. Rote and Sue E. Huether

Microorganisms and Humans: A Dynamic Relationship,
295
Microorganisms and Infections, *295*
Process of Infection, *295*
Clinical Infectious Disease, *296*
Classes of Infectious Microorganisms, *297*
Acquired Immunodeficiency Syndrome (AIDS), *318*
Transmission, *318*
Pathogenesis, *319*
Clinical Manifestations, *321*
Treatment and Prevention, *322*
Pediatric AIDS and Central Nervous System
Involvement, *324*
Countermeasures Against Pathogens, *326*
Infection Control Measures, *326*
Antimicrobials, *327*
Active Immunization: Vaccines, *329*
Passive Immunotherapy, *332*

Chapter 10   Stress and Disease, 336
Beth A. Forshee, Margaret F. Clayton,
and Kathryn L. McCance

Concepts of Stress, *337*
General Adaptation Syndrome, *338*
Psychologic Mediators and Specificity, *338*
Psychoneuroimmunologic Mediators of Stress, *339*
Stress Response, *339*
Central Stress Response, *339*
Stress and the Immune System, *347*
Stress, Personality, Coping, and Illness, *352*
Aging and Stress: Stress-Age Syndrome, 355

UNIT IV   Cellular Proliferation: Cancer

Chapter 11   Biology, Clinical Manifestations, and
Treatment of Cancer, 360
David M. Virshup

Cancer Characteristics and Terminology, *360*
Tumor Classification and Nomenclature, *361*
The Biology of Cancer Cells, *362*
Tumor Markers, *367*
The Genetic Basis of Cancer, *367*
Cancer-Causing Mutations in Genes, *367*
Types of Genes Misregulated in Cancer, *368*
Oncogenes and Tumor-Suppressor Genes: Accelerators
and Brakes, *370*
Guardians of the Genome, *375*
Inflammation, Immunity, and Cancer, *377*
The Immune System Protects Us Against Viral-
Associated Cancers, *378*

Viral Causes of Cancer, *378*
Bacterial Cause of Cancer, *380*
Cancer Invasion and Metastasis, *381*
Only Rare Cells in a Cancer are Able to Metastasize, *382*
Detachment and Invasion, *382*
Survival and Spread in the Circulation, *382*
Selective Adherence in Favorable Sites, *383*
Escape from the Circulation and Development of a New
Microenvironment, *384*
Clinical Manifestations and Treatment of Cancer, *384*
Clinical Manifestations of Cancer, *384*
Cancer Treatment, *387*

Chapter 12   Cancer Epidemiology, 396
Kathryn L. McCance

Genes, Environmental-Lifestyle Factors, and Risk
Factors, *396*
Epigenetics and Genetics, *401*
Tobacco Use, *404*
Diet, *404*
Alcohol Consumption, *415*
Ionizing Radiation, *416*
Ultraviolet Radiation, *422*
Electromagnetic Radiation, *424*
Sexual and Reproductive Behavior: Human
Papillomaviruses, *425*
Other Viruses and Microorganisms, *425*
Physical Activity, *425*
Chemicals and Occupational Hazards as Carcinogens,
426
Air Pollution, *426*

Chapter 13   Cancer in Children, 436
Nancy E. Kline

Incidence and Types of Cancer, *436*
Etiology, *437*
Genetic Factors, *438*
Environmental Factors, *439*
Prognosis, *440*

PART TWO   PATHOPHYSIOLOGIC
ALTERATIONS: ORGANS AND
SYSTEMS

UNIT V   The Neurologic System

Chapter 14   Structure and Function of the
Neurologic System, 442
Richard A. Sugerman

Overview and Organization of the Nervous System, *442*
Cells of the Nervous System, *443*
Neuron, *443*
Neuroglia and Schwann Cells, *444*
Nerve Injury and Regeneration, *445*

Nerve Impulse, 446
Synapses, 446
Neurotransmitters, 447
Central Nervous System, 449
Brain, 449
Spinal Cord, 456
Motor Pathways, 458
Sensory Pathways, 458
Protective Structures, 459
Blood Supply, 462
Peripheral Nervous System, 465
Autonomic Nervous System, 467
Anatomy of the Sympathetic Nervous System, 467
Anatomy of the Parasympathetic Nervous System, 467
Functions of the Autonomic Nervous System, 470
Aging and the Nervous System, 471
Tests of Nervous System Function, 474
Skull and Spine Roentgenograms, 474
Computed Tomography, 474
Magnetic Resonance Imaging, 474
Magnetic Resonance Angiography, 475
Positron-Emission Tomography Scan, 475
Brain Scan, 475
Cerebral Angiography, 476
Myelography, 476
Echoencephalography (Ultrasound), 476
Electroencephalography, 476
Evoke Potentials, 476
Cerebrospinal Fluid Analysis, 476

Chapter 15   Pain, Temperature Regulation, Sleep, and Sensory Function, 481
Sue E. Huether

Pain, 482
Theories of Pain, 482
Neuroanatomy of Pain, 482
Neuromodulation of Pain, 486
Clinical Description of Pain, 490
Pediatrics and Perception of Pain, 495
Aging and Perception of Pain, 495
Temperature Regulation, 496
Hypothalamic Control of Temperature, 496
Pediatrics and Changes in Temperature Regulation, 498
Aging and Changes in Temperature Regulation, 498
Pathogenesis of Fever, 498
Benefits of Fever, 498
Disorders of Temperature Regulation, 500
Sleep, 502
Non–Rapid Eye Movement (NREM) Sleep, 503
Pediatrics and Sleep Patterns, 504
Aging and Sleep Patterns, 504
Sleep Disorders, 504
Sleep Disorders Associated with Mental, Neurologic, or Medical Disorders, 505
Special Senses, 506
Vision, 506
Aging and Vision, 508

Hearing, 512
Aging and Hearing, 514
Olfaction and Taste, 515
Aging and Olfaction and Taste, 516
Somatosensory Function, 517
Touch, 517
Proprioception, 517

Chapter 16   Alterations in Cognitive Systems, Cerebral Hemodynamics, and Motor Function, 525
Barbara J. Boss

Alterations in Cognitive Systems, 525
Coma, 528
Seizures, 536
Alterations in Awareness, 542
Data Processing Deficits, 546
Alterations in Cerebral Hemodynamics, 557
Cerebral Hemodynamics, 557
Increased Intracranial Pressure, 557
Herniation Syndromes, 559
Cerebral Edema, 559
Hydrocephalus, 560
Alterations in Motor Function, 561
Alterations in Muscle Tone, 562
Alterations in Movement, 564
Alterations in Complex Motor Performance, 575
Extrapyramidal Motor Syndromes, 577

Chapter 17   Disorders of the Central and Peripheral Nervous Systems and the Neuromuscular Junction, 583
Barbara J. Boss

Central Nervous System Disorders, 583
Trauma, 583
Degenerative Disorders of the Spine, 596
Cerebrovascular Disorders, 600
Headache, 609
Tumors of the Central Nervous System, 611
Infection and Inflammation of the Central Nervous System, 620
Demyelinating Disorders, 630
Neurodegenerative Disorders, 633
Peripheral Nervous System and Neuromuscular Junction Disorders, 635
Peripheral Nervous System Disorders, 635
Neuromuscular Junction Disorders, 638

Chapter 18   Neurobiology of Schizophrenia, Mood Disorders, and Anxiety Disorders, 646
Lorey K. Takahashi

Schizophrenia, 647
Etiology and Pathophysiology, 647
Clinical Manifestations, 650
Treatment, 651

Mood Disorders: Depression and Bipolar Disorder, *652*
  Etiology and Pathophysiology, *652*
  Clinical Manifestations, *655*
  Treatment, *657*
Anxiety Disorders, *658*
  Panic Disorder, *659*
  Generalized Anxiety Disorder, *660*
  Posttraumatic Stress Disorder, *660*
  Obsessive-Compulsive Disorder, *661*

Chapter 19   Alterations of Neurologic Function in Children, 665
Barbara J. Boss and Sue E. Huether

Structure and Function of the Nervous System in Children, *665*
  Myelin Sheath, *667*
  Normal Growth and Development, *668*
Structural Malformations, *668*
  Defects of Neural Tube Closure, *668*
Encephalopathies, *675*
  Statis Encephalopathies, *675*
  Acute Encephalopathies, *681*
  Human Immunodeficiency Virus Encephalopathy, *684*
Cerebrovascular Disease in Children, *684*
  Occlusive Cerebrovascular Disease, *685*
  Hemorrhagic Cerebrovascular Disease, *685*
Childhood Tumors, *685*
  Brain Tumors, *685*
  Embryonal Tumors, *688*

UNIT VI   The Endocrine System

Chapter 20   Mechanisms of Hormonal Regulation, 696
Valentina L. Brashers and Robert E. Jones

Mechanisms of Hormonal Regulation, *696*
  Regulation of Hormone Release, *697*
  Hormone Transport, *698*
  Cellular Mechanisms of Hormone Action, *699*
Structure and Function of the Endocrine Glands, *703*
  Hypothalamic-Pituitary Axis, *703*
  Thyroid and Parathyroid Glands, *708*
  Endocrine Pancreas, *712*
  Adrenal Glands, *715*
  Neuroendocrine Response to Stressors, *720*
  Tests of Endocrine Function, *720*
Aging and the Endocrine System, *720*

Chapter 21   Alterations of Hormonal Regulation, 727
Robert E. Jones, Valentina L. Brashers, and Sue E. Huether

Mechanisms of Hormonal Alterations, *727*
Alterations of the Hypothalamic-Pituitary System, *728*
  Diseases of the Posterior Pituitary, *728*
  Disease of the Anterior Pituitary, *731*

Alterations of Thyroid Function, *736*
  Hyperthyroidism, *736*
  Hypothyroidism, *739*
Alterations of Parathyroid Function, *742*
  Hyperparathyroidism, *742*
  Hypoparathyroidism, *744*
Dysfunction of the Endocrine Pancreas: Diabetes Mellitus, *745*
  Types of Diabetes Mellitus, *745*
  Acute Complications of Diabetes Mellitus, *754*
  Chronic Complications of Diabetes Mellitus, *758*
Alterations of Adrenal Function, *765*
  Disorders of the Adrenal Cortex, *765*
  Disorders of the Adrenal Medulla, *772*

UNIT VII   The Reproductive Systems

Chapter 22   Structure and Function of the Reproductive Systems, 781
Angela Deneris and Sue E. Huether

Development of the Reproductive Systems, *781*
  Sexual Differentiation and Hormone Production in Utero, *781*
  Puberty, *784*
The Female Reproductive System, *784*
  External Genitalia, *784*
  Internal Genitalia, *786*
  Female Sex Hormones, *790*
  The Menstrual Cycle, *792*
The Male Reproductive System, *796*
  External Genitalia, *796*
  Internal Genitalia, *799*
  Spermatogenesis, *800*
  Male Sex Hormones, *800*
Structure and Function of the Breast, *802*
  The Female Breast, *802*
  The Male Breast, *805*
Tests of Reproductive Function, *805*
  Infection and Cancer Tests, *805*
  Fertility Tests, *807*
Aging and Reproduction Function, *807*
  Aging and the Female Reproductive System, *807*
  Aging and the Male Reproductive System, *811*

Chapter 23   Alterations of the Reproductive Systems, 816
Gwen A. Latendresse, Kathryn L. McCance, and Katherine Morgan

Alterations of Sexual Maturation, *816*
  Delayed Puberty, *817*
  Precocious Puberty, *818*
Disorders of the Female Reproductive System, *819*
  Hormonal and Menstrual Alterations, *819*
  Infection and Inflammation, *828*
  Pelvic Organ Prolapse (POP), *833*
  Benign Growths and Proliferative Conditions, *836*

Cancer, 841
Sexual Dysfunction, 848
Impaired Fertility, 849
Disorders of the Male Reproductive System, 850
Disorders of the Urethra, 850
Disorders of the Penis, 850
Disorders of the Scrotum, Testis, and Epididymis, 854
Disorders of the Prostate Gland, 860
Sexual Dysfunction, 869
Impairment of Sperm Production and Quality, 870
Disorders of the Breast, 871
Disorders of the Female Breast, 871
Disorders of the Male Breast, 909

Chapter 24   Sexually Transmitted Infections, 923
*Lisa Kaloczi, Gwen Latendresse, and
Katherine Morgan*

Sexually Transmitted Urogenital Infections, 924
Bacterial Infections, 924
Chlamydia Infections, 935
Viral Infections, 938
Parasitic Infections, 942
**Sexually Transmitted Infections of Other Body Systems,
946**
Gastrointestinal Infections, 946
Systemic Diseases, 947

UNIT VIII   The Hematologic System

**Chapter 25   Structure and Function of the
Hematologic System, 952**
Neal S. Rote and Kathryn L. McCance

Components of the Hematologic System, 952
Composition of the Blood, 952
Lymphoid Organs, 957
Development of Blood Cells, 961
Hematopoiesis, 961
Development of Erythrocytes, 965
Development of Leukocytes, 971
Development of Platelets, 971
Mechanisms of Hemostasis, 972
Function of Blood Vessels, 972
Function of Platelets, 972
Function of Clotting Factors, 976
Control of Hemostatic Mechanisms, 977
Lysis of Blood Clots, 979
Clinical Evaluation of the Hematologic System, 980
Tests of Bone Marrow Function, 980
Blood Tests, 982
Pediatrics and the Hematologic System, 982
Aging and the Hematologic System, 982

**Chapter 26   Alterations of Erythrocyte Function,
989**
Neal S. Rote and Kathyrn L. McCance

Anemia, 989
Classification, 989
Macrocytic-Normochromic Anemias, 990
Microcytic-Hypochromic Anemias, 995
Normocytic-Normochromic Anemias, 1000
**Myeloproliferative Red Blood Cell Disorders
(Polycythemia), 1008**

**Chapter 27   Alterations of Leukocyte, Lymphoid,
and Hemostatic Function, 1014**
Neal S. Rote and Kathyrn L. McCance

Alterations of Leukocyte Function, 1014
Quantitative Alterations of Leukocytes, 1014
Infectious Mononucleosis, 1017
Leukemias, 1019
Alterations of Lymphoid Function, 1030
Lymphadenopathy, 1030
Malignant Lymphomas, 1030
Plasma Cell Malignancies, 1037
Alterations of Splenic Function, 1042
Alterations of Platelets and Coagulation, 1044
Disorders of Platelets, 1044
Disorders of Coagulation, 1049

**Chapter 28   Alterations of Hematologic Function
in Children, 1062**
Nancy E. Kline

Fetal and Neonatal Hematopoiesis, 1062
Postnatal Changes in the Blood, 1063
Erythrocytes, 1064
Leukocytes and Platelets, 1064
Disorders of Erythrocytes, 1065
Acquired Disorders, 1065
Inherited Disorders, 1068
Disorders of Coagulation and Platelets, 1078
Inherited Hemorrhagic Disease, 1078
Antibody-Mediated Hemorrhagic Disease, 1081
Leukemia and Lymphoma, 1083
Leukemia, 1083
Lymphomas, 1086

**UNIT IX   The Cardiovascular and Lymphatic
Systems**

**Chapter 29   Structure and Function of the
Cardiovascular and Lymphatic
Systems, 1091**
Valentina L. Brashers and Kathryn L. McCance

Circulatory System, 1091
The Heart, 1093
Structures That Direct Circulation Through the Heart,
1093

Structures That Support Cardiac Metabolism: The
    Coronary Vessels, 1096
Structures that Control Heart Action, 1099
Factors Affecting Cardiac Output, 1109
System Circulation, 1113
Structure of Blood Vessels, 1113
Factors Affecting Blood Flow, 1117
Regulation of Blood Pressure (Arterial Pressure), 1122
Regulation of Coronary Circulation, 1130
Lymphatic System, 1131
Tests of Cardiovascular Function, 1133
Cardiac and Coronary Artery Evaluation, 1133
Systemic Vascular Evaluation, 1135
Aging and the Cardiovascular System, 1136

**Chapter 30   Alterations of Cardiovascular
                Function, 1142**
                Valentina L. Brashers

Diseases of the Veins, 1142
Varicose Veins and Chronic Venous Insufficiency, 1142
Thrombus Formation in Veins, 1143
Superior Vena Cava Syndrome, 1144
Diseases of the Arteries, 1144
Aneurysm, 1144
Thrombus Formation, 1147
Embolism, 1147
Peripheral Arterial Diseases, 1148
Hypertension, 1149
Orthostatic (Postural) Hypotension, 1156
Atherosclerosis, 1157
Peripheral Artery Disease, 1160
Coronary Artery Disease, Myocardial Ischemia, and
    Acute Coronary Syndromes, 1160
Disorders of the Heart Wall, 1176
Disorders of the Pericardium, 1176
Disorders of the Myocardium: The Cardiomyopathies,
    1178
Disorders of the Endocardium, 1181
Cardiac Complications in Acquired Immunodeficiency
    Syndrome, 1189
Manifestations of Heart Disease, 1189
Heart Failure, 1189
Dysrhythmias, 1196

**Chapter 31   Alterations of Cardiovascular
                Function in Children, 1209**
                Nancy L. McDaniel

Development of the Cardiovascular System, 1209
Developmental Anatomy, 1209
Transitional Circulation, 1211
Postnatal Development, 1213
Congenital Heart Defects, 1213
Classification of Congenital Heart Defects and
    Associated Conditions, 1215
Hypoxemia, 1217
Defects Increasing Pulmonary Blood Flow, 1218

Defects Decreasing Pulmonary Blood Flow, 1223
Obstructive Defects, 1226
Mixing Defects, 1230
Acquired Cardiovascular Disorders, 1234
Kawasaki Disease, 1234
Systemic Hypertension, 1235
Childhood Obesity, 1237

UNIT X   The Pulmonary System

**Chapter 32   Structure and Function of the
                Pulmonary System, 1242**
                Valentina L. Brashers

Structures of the Pulmonary System, 1242
Conducting Airways, 1242
Gas-Exchange Airways, 1244
Pulmonary and Bronchial Circulation, 1247
Chest Wall and Pleura, 1249
Functions of the Pulmonary System, 1249
Ventilation, 1249
Gas Transport, 1255
Control of the Pulmonary Circulation, 1260
Tests of Pulmonary Function, 1261
Aging and the Pulmonary System, 1263

**Chapter 33   Alterations of Pulmonary Function,
                1266**
                Valentina L. Brashers

Clinical Manifestations of Pulmonary Alterations, 1266
Signs and Symptoms of Pulmonary Disease, 1266
Conditions Caused by Pulmonary Disease or Injury,
    1269
Disorders of the Chest Wall and Pleura, 1271
Disorders of the Chest Wall, 1271
Pleural Abnormalities, 1272
Pulmonary Disorders, 1274
Restrictive Lung Disorders, 1274
Obstructive Pulmonary Disease, 1282
Respiratory Tract Infections, 1290
Pulmonary Vascular Disease, 1294
Malignancies of the Respiratory Tract, 1298

**Chapter 34   Alterations of Pulmonary Function
                in Children, 1310**
                Kristi Gott and Deborah K. Froh

Structure and Function, 1310
Upper Airway, 1310
Lower Airways and Lung Parenchyma, 1310
Chest Wall Dynamics, 1311
Metabolic Characteristics, 1312
Immunologic Incompetence, 1312
Physiologic Control of Respiration, 1312
Pulmonary Disorders, 1313
Disorders of the Upper Airways, 1313
Disorders of the Lower Airways, 1320
Sudden Infant Death Syndrome, 1339

UNIT XI   The Renal and Urologic Systems

Chapter 35   Structure and Function of the Renal and Urologic Systems, 1344
Sue E. Huether

Structures of the Renal System, 1344
Structures of the Kidney, 1344
Urinary Structures, 1350
Renal Blood Flow, 1351
Autoregulation, 1351
Neural Regulation, 1351
Hormones and Other Factors, 1352
Kidney Function, 1352
Nephron Function, 1352
Concentration and Dilution of Urine, 1357
Renal Hormones, 1358
Tests of Renal Function, 1360
The Concept of Clearance, 1360
Blood Tests, 1360
Urinalysis, 1361
Aging and Renal Function, 1362

Chapter 36   Alterations of Renal and Urinary Tract Function, 1365
Sue E. Huether and Beth A. Forshee

Urinary Tract Obstruction, 1365
Upper Urinary Tract Obstruction, 1365
Lower Urinary Tract Obstruction, 1369
Tumors, 1372
Urinary Tract Infection, 1373
Causes of Urinary Tract Infection, 1373
Glomerular Disorders, 1378
Glomerulonephritis, 1379
Nephrotic Syndrome, 1384
Acute Kidney Injury, 1386
Classification of Kidney Dysfunction, 1386
Acute Kidney Injury, 1386
Chronic Kidney Disease, 1389
Creatinine and Urea Clearance, 1393
Fluid and Electrolyte Balance, 1393
Calcium, Phosphate, and Bone, 1394

Chapter 37   Alterations of Renal and Urinary Tract Function in Children, 1402
Sue E. Huether

Structure and Function of the Urinary System in Children, 1402
Development of the Urinary System, 1402
Fluid and Electrolyte Balance in Children, 1404
Alterations in Renal and Bladder Function in Children, 1404
Congenital Abnormalities, 1404
Glomerular Disorders, 1407
Renal Injury, 1411
Bladder Disorders, 1411
Wilms Tumor, 1413
Enuresis, 1414

UNIT XII   The Digestive System

Chapter 38   Structure and Function of the Digestive System, 1420
Sue E. Huether

The Gastrointestinal Tract, 1421
Mouth and Esophagus, 1421
Stomach, 1423
Small Intestine, 1428
Large Intestine, 1435
Intestinal Bacteria, 1437
Accessory Organs of Digestion, 1437
Liver, 1438
Gallbladder, 1442
Exocrine Pancreas, 1443
Tests of Digestive Function, 1444
Gastrointestinal Tract, 1444
Liver, 1446
Gallbladder, 1446
Exocrine Pancreas, 1446
Aging and the Gastrointestinal System, 1447

Chapter 39   Alterations of Digestive Function, 1452
Sue E. Huether

Disorders of the Gastrointestinal Tract, 1452
Clinical Manifestations of Gastrointestinal Dysfunction, 1452
Disorders of Motility, 1456
Gastritis, 1463
Peptic Ulcer Disease, 1464
Malabsorption Syndromes, 1470
Inflammatory Bowel Disease, 1471
Appendicitis, 1475
Vascular Insufficiency, 1477
Disorders of Nutrition, 1477
Disorders of the Accessory Organs of Digestion, 1482
Clinical Manifestations of Liver Disorders, 1482
Disorders of the Liver, 1488
Disorders of the Gallbladder, 1494
Disorders of the Pancreas, 1495
Cancer of the Digestive System, 1498
Cancer of the Gastrointestinal Tract, 1498
Cancer of the Accessory Organs of Digestion, 1503

Chapter 40   Alterations of Digestive Function in Children, 1516
Sue E. Huether

Disorders of the Gastrointestinal Tract, 1516
Congenital Impairment of Motility, 1516
Esophageal Malformations, 1518
Acquired Impairment of Motility, 1522
Impairment of Digestion, Absorption, and Nutrition, 1524
Diarrhea, 1530
Disorders of the Liver, 1531
Disorders of Biliary Metabolism and Transport, 1531

Inflammatory Disorders, *1532*
Portal Hypertension, *1533*
Metabolic Disorders, *1534*

UNIT XIII   The Musculoskeletal System

Chapter 41   Structure and Function of the Musculoskeletal System, 1540
Christy L. Crowther-Radulewicz

Structure and Function of Bones, *1540*
Elements of Bone Tissue, *1540*
Types of Bone Tissue, *1545*
Characteristics of Bone, *1546*
Maintenance of Bone Integrity, *1547*
Structure and Function of Joints, *1548*
Fibrous Joints, *1549*
Cartilaginous Joints, *1549*
Synovial Joints, *1550*
Structure and Function of Skeletal Muscles, *1554*
Whole Muscle, *1555*
Components of Muscle Function, *1561*
Tests of Musculoskeletal Function, *1563*
Tests of Bone Function, *1563*
Tests of Joint Function, *1563*
Tests of Muscular Function, *1563*
Aging and the Musculoskeletal System, *1564*
Aging of Bones, *1564*
Aging of Joints, *1564*
Aging of Muscles, *1564*

Chapter 42   Alterations of Musculoskeletal Function, 1568
Christy L. Crowther-Radulewicz and Kathryn L. McCance

Musculoskeletal Injuries, *1568*
Skeletal Trauma, *1568*
Support Structures, *1573*
Disorders of Bones, *1576*
Metabolic Bone Diseases, *1576*
Infectious Bone Disease: Osteomyelitis, *1586*
Bone Tumors, *1588*
Disorders of Joints, *1592*
Osteoarthritis, *1592*
Classic Inflammatory Joint Disease, *1596*
Disorders of Skeletal Muscle, *1606*
Secondary Muscular Dysfunction, *1606*
Muscle Membrane Abnormalities, *1609*
Metabolic Muscle Diseases, *1610*
Inflammatory Muscle Diseases: Myositis, *1611*
Myopathy, *1612*
Muscle Tumors, *1613*

Chapter 43   Alterations of Musculoskeletal Function in Children, 1618
Kristen Lee Carroll

Musculoskeletal Development in Children, *1618*
Bone Formation, *1618*
Bone Growth, *1619*
Skeletal Development, *1620*
Muscle Growth, *1620*
Musculoskeletal Alterations in Children, *1620*
Congenital Defects, *1620*
Abnormal Density of Modeling of the Skeleton, *1624*
Bone Infection: Osteomyelitis, *1628*
Juvenile Rheumatoid Arthritis, *1630*
Avascular Diseases of the Bone: Osteochondrosis, *1631*
Cerebral Palsy, *1632*
Muscular Dystrophy, *1633*
Musculoskeletal Tumors in Children, *1637*
Nonaccidental Trauma, *1640*

UNIT XIV   The Integumentary System

Chapter 44   Structure, Function, and Disorders of the Integument, 1644
Noreen Heer Nicol and Sue E. Huether

Structure and Function of the Skin, *1644*
Layers of the Skin, *1644*
Subcutaneous Layer, *1645*
Aging and Skin Integrity, *1646*
Tests of Skin Function, *1647*
Clinical Manifestations of Skin Dysfunction, *1647*
Disorders of the Skin, *1655*
Inflammatory Disorders, *1655*
Papulosquamous Disorders, *1657*
Vesiculobullous Disorders, *1660*
Infections, *1662*
Vascular Disorders, *1665*
Insect Bites, *1667*
Benign Tumors, *1668*
Cancer, *1669*
Frostbite, *1673*
Disorders of the Hair, *1673*
Alopecia, *1673*
Hirsutism, *1674*
Disorders of the Nail, *1674*
Paronychia, *1674*
Onychomycosis, *1674*

Chapter 45   Alterations of the Integument in Children, 1680
Noreen Heer Nicol and Sue E. Huether

Acne Vulgaris, *1680*
Dermatitis, *1681*
Atopic Dermatitis, *1681*
Diaper Dermatitis, *1682*
Infections of the Skin, *1683*
Bacterial Infections, *1683*

Fungal Infections, *1684*
Viral Infections, *1685*

Insect Bites and Parasites, *1688*
Scabies, *1688*
Pediculosis (Lice Infestation), *1689*
Fleas, *1689*
Bedbugs, *1689*

Hemangiomas and Vascular Malformations, *1690*
Hemangiomas, *1690*
Vascular Malformations, *1691*

Other Skin Disorders, *1692*
Miliaria, *1692*
Erythema Toxicum Neonatorum, *1692*
Toxic Epidermal Necrolysis and Stevens-Johnson
Syndrome, *1692*

UNIT XV   Multiple Interacting Systems

**Chapter 46   Shock, Multiple Organ Dysfunction
Syndrome, and Burns in Adults, 1696**
*Dennis J. Cheek, Linda L. Martin, and
Stephen E. Morris*

Shock, *1696*
Cellular Alterations, *1697*
Impairment of Cellular Metabolism, *1697*
Types of Shock, *1699*
Treatment for Shock, *1707*

Multiple Organ Dysfunction Syndrome, *1707*
Burns, *1714*
Epidemiology and Etiology, *1714*
Burn Wound Depth, *1714*

**Chapter 47   Shock, Multiple Organ Dysfunction,
and Burns in Children, 1727**
*Mary Fran Hazinski, Mary A. Mondozzi,
and Rose A. Urdiales Baker*

Shock and Multiple Organ Dysfunction, *1727*
Types of Shock, *1728*
Reperfusion and Inflammatory Injury, *1737*
Evaluation and Treatment of Shock, *1737*
Burns, *1741*
Severity of Injury, *1742*

Glossary, 1755

Index, 1778

CELLULAR BIOLOGY

KATHRYN L. McCANCE

MEDIA RESOURCES

CHAPTER OUTLINE

PROKARYOTES AND EUKARYOTES
CELLULAR FUNCTIONS
STRUCTURE AND FUNCTION OF CELLULAR
  COMPONENTS
  Nucleus
  Cytoplasmic Organelles
  Plasma Membranes
  Cellular Receptors
CELL-TO-CELL ADHESIONS
  Extracellular Matrix
  Specialized Cell Junctions
CELLULAR COMMUNICATION AND SIGNAL
  TRANSDUCTION
  Signal Transduction
  Extracellular Messengers and Channel Regulation
  Second Messengers

CELLULAR METABOLISM
  Role of Adenosine Triphosphate
  Food and Production of Cellular Energy
  Oxidative Phosphorylation
MEMBRANE TRANSPORT: CELLULAR INTAKE AND
  OUTPUT
  Movement of Water and Solutes
  Transport by Vesicle Formation
  Movement of Electrical Impulses: Membrane Potentials
CELLULAR REPRODUCTION: THE CELL CYCLE
  Phases of Mitosis and Cytokinesis
  Rates of Cellular Division
  Growth Factors
TISSUES
  Tissue Formation
  Types of Tissues

All body functions depend on the integrity of cells. Therefore, an understanding of cellular biology is intrinsically necessary for an understanding of disease. An overwhelming amount of information is revealing how cells behave as a multicellular "social" organism. At the heart of cellular biology is cellular communication ("cellular crosstalk")—how messages originate and are transmitted, received, interpreted, and used by the cell. Fossil records suggest that unicellular organisms resembling bacteria were present on earth 3.5 billion years ago, yet it took another 2.5 billion years for the first multicellular organisms to appear. This delay was seemingly slow because elaborate signaling mechanisms had to evolve that would allow cells to crosstalk. This streamlined conversation between, among, and within cells maintains cellular function. Intercellular signals allow each cell to determine its position and specialized role. Cells must demonstrate a "chemical fondness" for other cells and their surrounding environment to maintain the integrity of the entire organism. When they no longer tolerate this fondness, the conversation breaks down and cells either adapt (sometimes altering function) or become vulnerable to isolation, injury, or disease.

PROKARYOTES AND EUKARYOTES

Living cells generally are divided into two major classes—eukaryotes and prokaryotes. The cells of higher animals and plants are eukaryotes, as are the single-celled organisms fungi, protozoa, and most algae. Prokaryotes include cyanobacteria (blue-green algae), bacteria, and rickettsiae. Prokaryotes traditionally were studied as core subjects of molecular biology. Current emphasis is on the eukaryotic cell; much of its structure and function has no counterpart in bacterial cells.

Eukaryotes (*eu* = good; *karyon* = nucleus) are larger and have more extensive intracellular anatomy and organization than do prokaryotes. Eukaryotic cells have a characteristic set of membrane-bound intracellular compartments, called *organelles*, that includes a well-defined nucleus. **Prokaryotes** contain no organelles, and their nuclear material is not encased by a nuclear membrane. Prokaryotic cells are characterized by lack of a distinct nucleus.

In addition to having structural differences, prokaryotic and eukaryotic cells differ in chemical composition and biochemical activity. The *nuclei* of prokaryotic cells carry genetic information in a single circular chromosome, and they lack a class of proteins called *histones,* which in eukaryotic cells bind with deoxyribonucleic acid (DNA) and are involved in the supercoiling of DNA (see Figure 1-2). Eukaryotic cells have several chromosomes. Protein production, or synthesis, in the two classes of cells also differs because of major structural differences in ribonucleic acid (RNA) protein complexes. Other distinctions include differences in mechanisms of transport across the outer cellular membrane and differences in enzyme content.

CELLULAR FUNCTIONS

Cells become specialized through the process of **differentiation,** or maturation, so that some cells eventually perform one kind of function and other cells perform other functions. Highly developed functions, such as movement, are often associated with the absence of some other property, such as hormone production, which is more highly developed in some other type of specialized cell. The eight chief cellular functions follow:

1. *Movement.* Muscle cells can generate forces that produce motion. Muscles that are attached to bones produce limb movements, whereas those that enclose hollow tubes or cavities move or empty contents when they contract. For example, the contraction of smooth muscle cells surrounding blood vessels changes the diameter of the vessels; the contraction of muscles in walls of the urinary bladder expels urine.
2. *Conductivity.* Conduction as a response to a stimulus is manifested by a wave of excitation, an electrical potential, that passes along the surface of the cell to reach its other parts. Conductivity is the chief function of nerve cells.
3. *Metabolic absorption.* All cells take in and use nutrients and other substances from their surroundings. Cells of the intestine and the kidney are specialized to carry out absorption. Cells of the kidney tubules reabsorb fluids and synthesize proteins. Intestinal epithelial cells reabsorb fluids and synthesize protein enzymes.
4. *Secretion.* Certain cells, such as mucous gland cells, can synthesize new substances from substances they absorb and then secrete the new substances to serve as needed elsewhere. Cells of the adrenal gland, testis, and ovary can secrete hormonal steroids.
5. *Excretion.* All cells can rid themselves of waste products resulting from the metabolic breakdown of nutrients. Membrane-bound sacs (lysosomes) within cells contain enzymes that break down, or digest, large molecules, turning them into waste products that are released from the cell.
6. *Respiration.* Cells absorb oxygen, which is used to transform nutrients into energy in the form of adenosine triphosphate (ATP). Cellular respiration, or oxidation, occurs in organelles called *mitochondria.*
7. *Reproduction.* Tissue growth occurs as cells enlarge and reproduce themselves. Even without growth, tissue maintenance requires that new cells be produced to replace cells that are lost normally through cellular death. Not all cells are capable of continuous division (see Chapter 2).
8. *Communication.* Communication is critical for all the other functions above that enable the survival of the society of cells. Pancreatic cells, for instance, secrete and release insulin to tell muscle cells to take up sugar from the blood for energy. Constant communication allows the maintenance of a dynamic steady state.

STRUCTURE AND FUNCTION OF CELLULAR COMPONENTS

Figure 1-1 shows a "typical" eukaryotic cell. It consists of three components: an outer membrane called the *plasma membrane,* or *plasmalemma;* a fluid filling called **cytoplasm;** and the "organs" of the cell-membrane–bound intracellular organelles, among them the nucleus.

Nucleus

The **nucleus,** which is surrounded by the cytoplasm and generally is located in the center of the cell, is the largest membrane-bound organelle. Two membranes comprise the **nuclear envelope** (Figure 1-2, *A*). The outer membrane is continuous with membranes of the endoplasmic reticulum. The nucleus contains the **nucleolus,** a small dense structure composed largely of RNA; most of the cellular DNA; and the DNA-binding proteins, the histones, that regulate its activity. The DNA chain in eukaryotic cells is so extensive that the risk of breakage is high. Therefore, the histones that bind to DNA cause the folding of DNA into chromosomes (Figure 1-2, *C*). The wrapping of DNA into tight packages of chromosomes is essential for cell division in eukaryotes.

The primary functions of the nucleus are cell division and control of genetic information. Other functions include the replication and repair of DNA and the transcription of the information stored in DNA. Genetic information is transcribed into RNA, which can be processed into messenger, transport, and ribosomal RNA and introduced into the cytoplasm, where it directs cellular activities. Most of the processing of

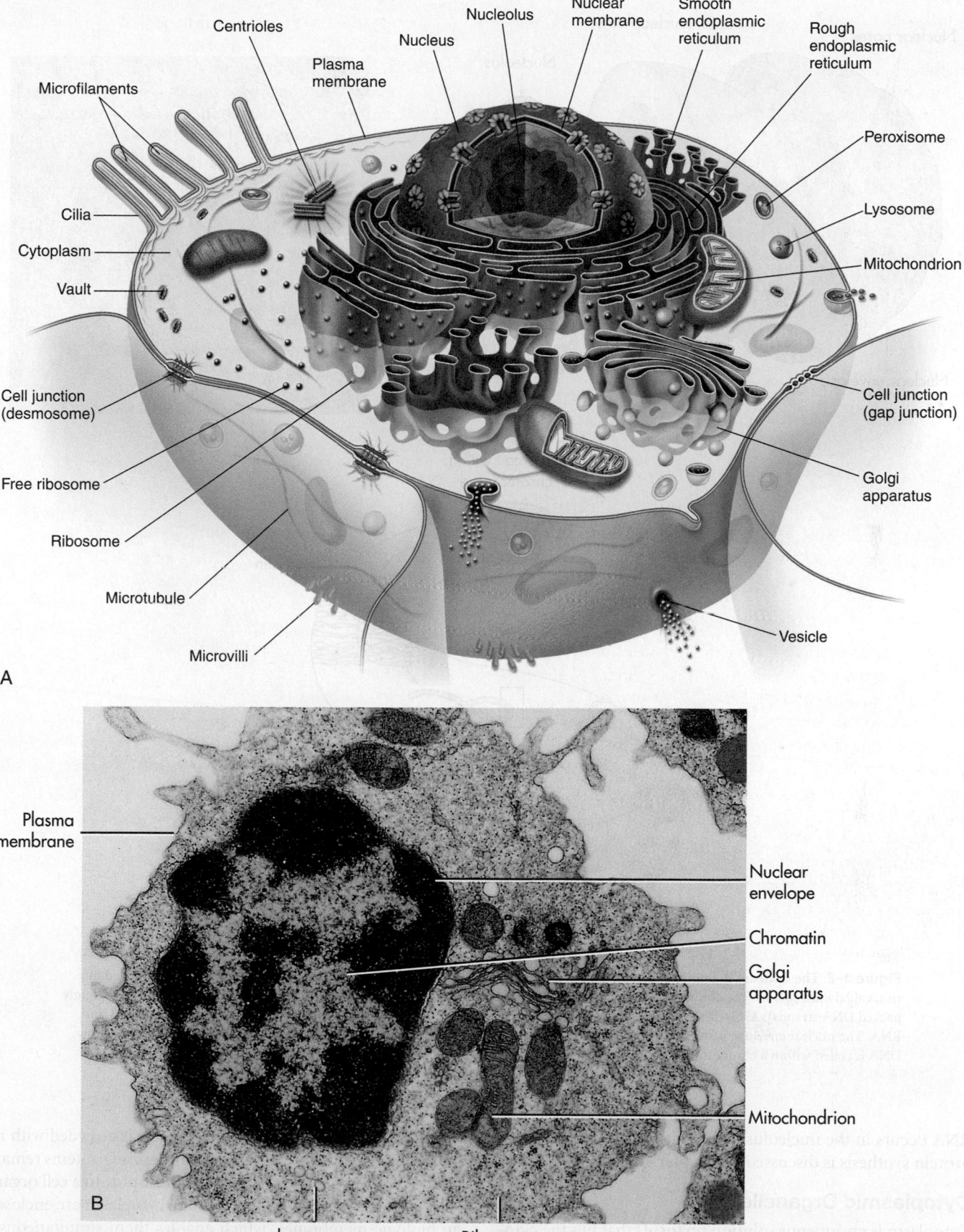

Figure 1-1 **Typical or composite cell. A,** Artist's interpretation of cell structure. **B,** Color-enhanced electron micrograph of a cell. Both show the many mitochondria known as the "power plants of the cell." Note, too, the innumerable dots bordering the endoplasmic reticulum. These are ribosomes, the cell's "protein factories." (**B** from Thibodeau GA, Patton KT: *Anatomy & physiology*, ed 5, St Louis, 2003, Mosby.)

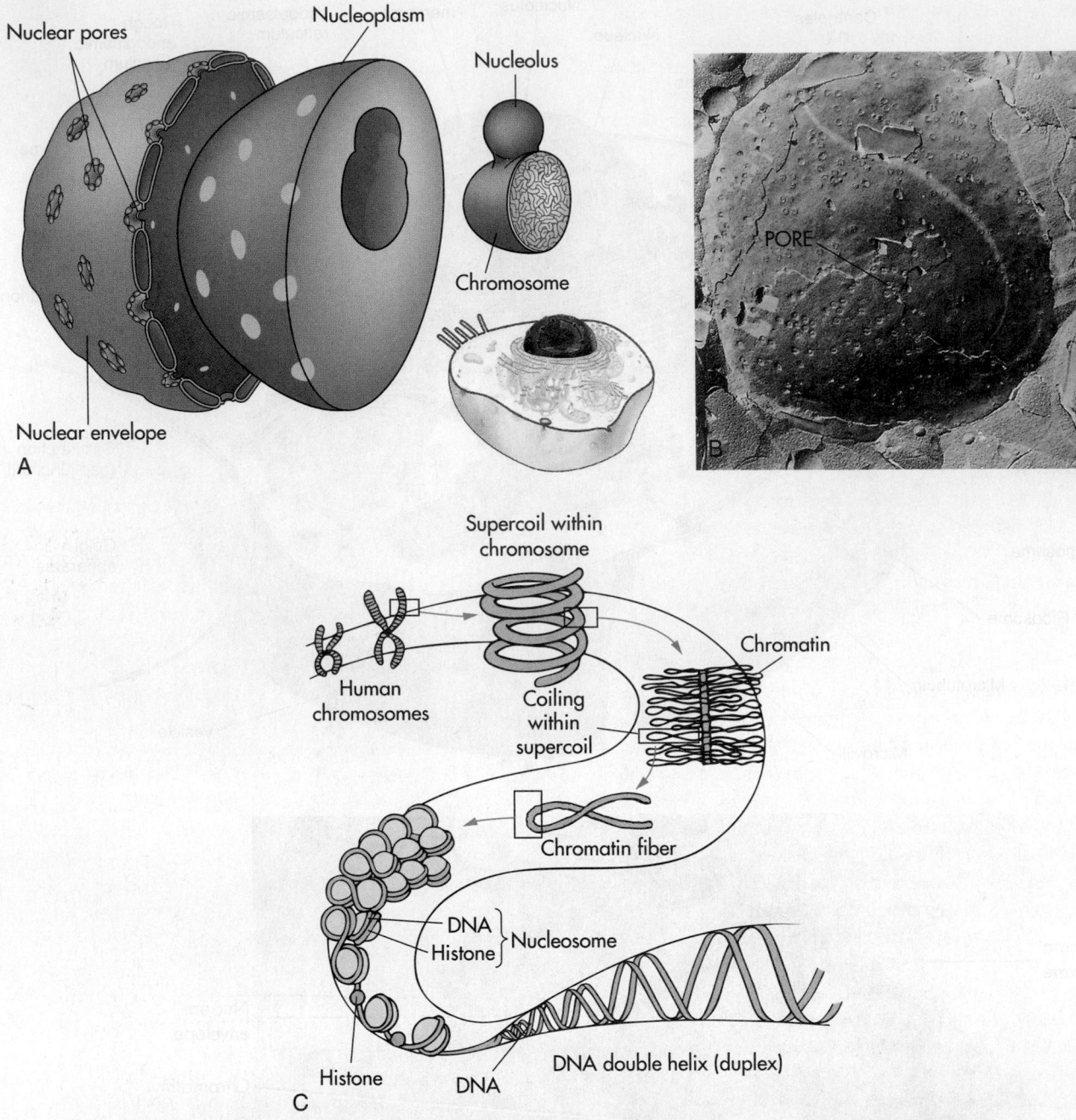

Figure 1-2 **The nucleus.** The nucleus is composed of a double membrane, called a *nuclear envelope,* that encloses the fluid-filled interior, called *nucleoplasm.* The chromosomes are suspended in the nucleoplasm (shown here much larger than real size to show the tightly packed DNA strands). **A,** Swelling at one or more points of the chromosome occurs at a nucleolus, where genes are being copied into RNA. The nuclear envelope is studded with pores. **B,** The pores are visible as dimples in this freeze etch of a nuclear envelope. **C,** How DNA is coiled within a chromosome. (**B** from Raven PH, Johnson GB: *Biology,* St Louis, 1992, Mosby.)

RNA occurs in the nucleolus. (The role of DNA and RNA in protein synthesis is discussed in Chapter 4.)

Cytoplasmic Organelles

Cytoplasm is an aqueous solution (**cytosol**) that fills the **cytoplasmic matrix**—the space between the nuclear envelope and the plasma membrane. The cytosol represents about half the volume of a eukaryotic cell. It contains thousands of enzymes

involved in intermediate metabolism and is crowded with ribosomes making proteins. Newly synthesized proteins remain in the cytosol if they lack a signal for transport to a cell organelle.[1] The organelles suspended in the cytoplasm are enclosed in biologic membranes, which enables them simultaneously to carry out functions that require different biochemical environments. These functions, many of which are directed by coded messages carried from the nucleus by RNA, include synthesis of proteins and hormones and their transport out of the cell, isolation and elimination of waste products from the cell, metabolic processes, breakdown and disposal of cellular debris and foreign proteins (antigens), and maintenance of cellular structure and motility. Also the cytosol functions as a storage unit for fat, carbohydrate, and secretory vesicles.

Ribosomes

Ribosomes are RNA-protein complexes (nucleoproteins) that are synthesized in the nucleolus and secreted into the cytoplasm, possibly through pores in the nuclear envelope. These tiny organelles may float free in the cytoplasm or attach themselves to the outer membranes of the endoplasmic reticulum (see Figure 1-1). Their chief function is to provide sites for cellular protein synthesis. Newly formed ribosomes synthesize a "recognition sequence," or signal, like an address on a letter. Signal recognition particles (SRPs) in the cytosol bind to the ribosome after recognizing the SRP. Ribophorins, receiver proteins found on the rough sections of the endoplasmic reticulum (ER), act as the "address" site or binding sites. The developing protein threads its way through the ER membrane into the lumen. The SRP is removed and the new protein chain is folded into its final conformation.

Endoplasmic Reticulum

The **endoplasmic reticulum** (*endo* = within; *plasma* = cytoplasm; *reticulum* = network) is a membrane factory that specializes in the synthesis and transport of the protein and lipid components of most of the cell's organelles. It consists of a network of tubular or saclike channels (cisternae) that extend throughout the cytoplasm and are continuous with the outer nuclear membrane (Figure 1-3). The folded membranes that form the cisternae of the endoplasmic reticulum may be *rough* (granular) or *smooth* (agranular). The **rough endoplasmic reticulum** is rough because ribosomes and ribonucleoprotein particles are attached to it (see Figure 1-3). Some of the proteins synthesized by these ribosomes remain in the endoplasmic reticulum, and others are used to construct membranes of other organelles (the Golgi complex, lysosomes, peroxisomes, nucleus) and of the cell itself.

Smooth endoplasmic reticulum does not contain ribosomes or ribonucleoprotein particles (see Figure 1-1). Rather, membranous surfaces of the smooth endoplasmic reticulum contain enzymes involved in the synthesis of steroid hormones and are responsible for a variety of reactions required to remove toxic substances from the cell. The endoplasmic reticulum communicates with the Golgi complex and interacts with other organelles, particularly lysosomes and peroxisomes.

Golgi Complex

The **Golgi complex** (or **Golgi apparatus**) is a network of flattened, smooth membranes and vesicles frequently located near the nucleus of the cell (Figure 1-4). Proteins from the endoplasmic reticulum are processed and packaged into small membrane-bound sacs or vesicles called **secretory vesicles,** which collect at the end of the membranous folds of the Golgi bodies—called **cisternae.** The secretory vesicles then break off from the Golgi complex and migrate to a variety of intracellular and extracellular destinations, including the plasma membrane. The vesicles fuse with the plasma membrane, and their contents are released from the cell. The best known vesicles are those that have coats made largely of the protein **clathrin** and are called *clathrin-coated vesicles.* They bud from the Golgi complex on the outward secretory pathway and from the plasma membrane on the inward endocytotic pathway (see p. 30). Many molecules, including lipids, proteins, glycoproteins, and enzymes of lysosomes, pass through the Golgi complex at some stage in their maturation. The Golgi complex is a refining plant and directs traffic (e.g., protein, polynucleotide, polysaccharide molecules) in the cell[1] (Figure 1-5).

Lysosomes

Lysosomes (*lyso* = dissolution; *soma* = body) are saclike structures that originate from the Golgi complex (see Figure 1-1). They contain more than 40 digestive enzymes called **hydrolases,** which catalyze bonds in proteins, lipids, nucleic acids, and carbohydrates. Lysosomes function as the intracellular digestive system (Figure 1-6). Lysosomal enzymes are capable of digesting most cellular constituents down to their basic forms, such as amino acids, fatty acids, and sugars.

The lysosomal membrane acts as a protective shield between the powerful digestive enzymes within the lysosome and the cytoplasm, preventing their leakage into the cytoplasmic matrix. Disruption of the membrane by various treatments or cellular injury leads to a release of the lysosomal enzymes, which can then react with their specific substrates, causing *cellular self-digestion.* Lysosomal abnormalities are involved in a number of conditions that involve cellular injury and death.

Lysosomal storage diseases may be the result of a genetic defect or lack of one or more lysosomal enzymes. For example, the lack of lysosomal α-1,4-glucosidase leads to an accumulation of glycogen in lysosomes known as *Pompe disease.* Tay-Sachs disease is characterized by an accumulation of GM2 ganglioside (a lipid) in lysosomes as a result of the deficiency or absence of lysosomal hexosaminidase A. In gout, undigested uric acid accumulates within lysosomes, damaging the lysosomal membrane. Subsequent enzyme leakage results in cell death and tissue injury.

Lysosomes are necessary for normal digestion of cellular nutrients, intracellular debris, and potentially harmful extracellular substances that must be removed from the body. Extracellular substances are taken into the cell and encapsulated in a membrane-bound vesicle (see discussion on endocytosis, p. 30). Lysosomes merge with the vesicle to form a digestive vacuole. Lysosomes remain fully active by maintaining a low internal pH. They do this by pumping hydrogen ions into their interiors. The hydrolytic enzymes are only maximally active at acid pH values. Lysosomes that are not active do not maintain such an acid internal pH. Lysosomes in this "holding pattern" are called **primary lysosomes.** When a primary lysosome fuses with a vacuole or other organelle, its pH falls and the

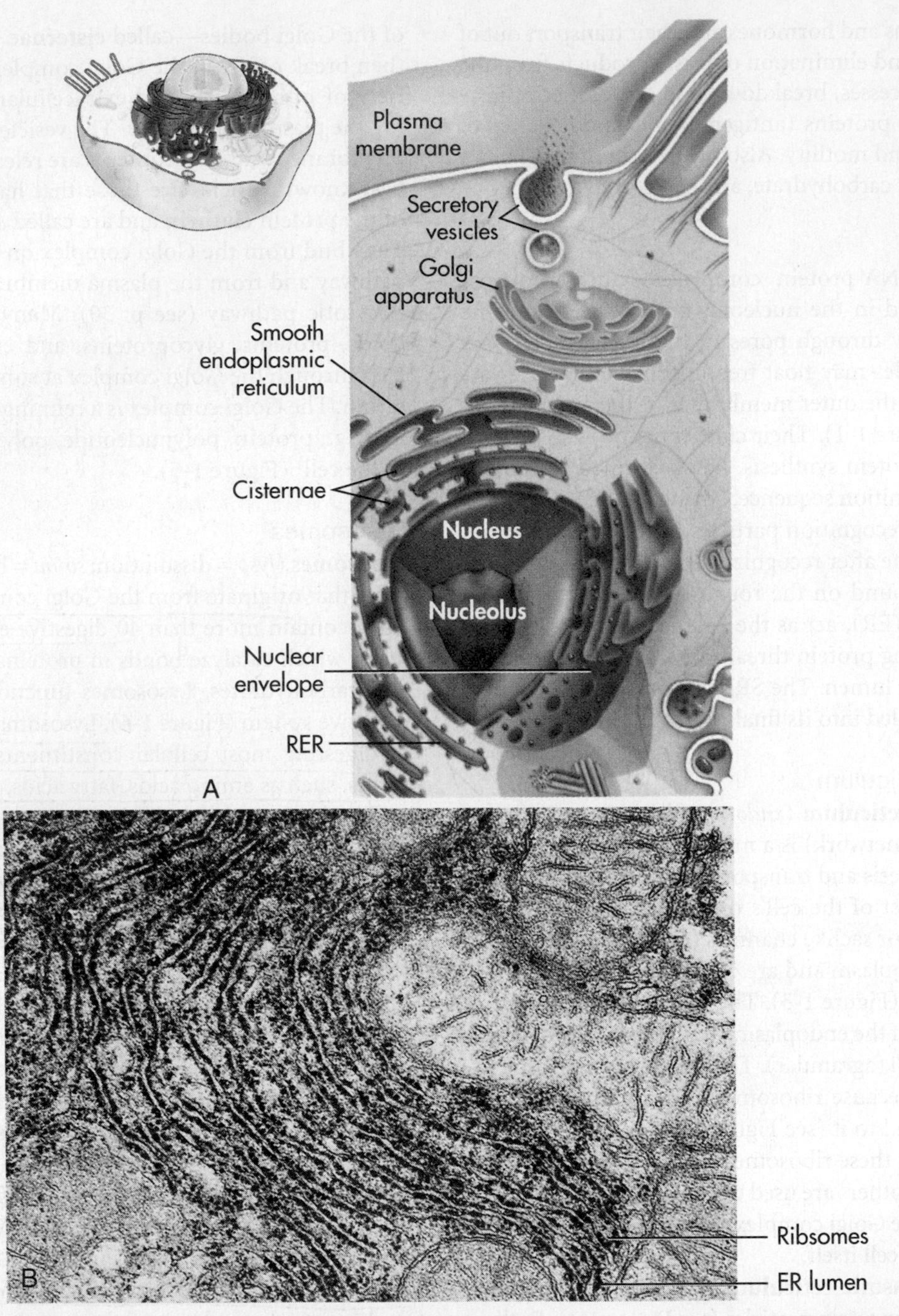

Figure 1-3 Endoplasmic reticulum (ER). **A**, The ER consists of rough endoplasmic reticulum (RER) arranged into ribosome-coated cisternae and vesicles of smooth endoplasmic reticulum (SER). **B**, Electron micrograph of rough and smooth ER. (**B** courtesy Kelloes C and Farmer M, Center for Advanced Ultrastructural Research, University of Georgia. From Lindsay DT: *Functional human anatomy*, St Louis, 1996, Mosby.)

hydrolytic enzymes become activated. When it becomes active, it is called a **secondary lysosome,** or **heterophagosome.**

As cells complete their life span and die, lysosomes digest the resultant cellular debris. Lysosomes involved in this process, which is called **autodigestion,** are called **autolysosomes,** or **autophagosomes.** In living cells, cellular debris is encapsulated within a vesicle that reacts with a lysosome to complete its degradation. This process is called **autophagy.** Autophagy also occurs during starvation, enabling the cell to use a part of its own substance for fuel without doing itself irreparable harm.

Products of autophagy (and of phagocytosis, the ingestion of harmful foreign substances; see Chapter 6) pass out of the lysosome and are reused by the cell. Indigestible material is stored in vesicles called **residual bodies,** whose contents are actively expelled from the cell (see Figure 1-6). High concentrations of lipids may accumulate within the residual bodies and remain there for a long time. The lipids are eventually oxidized,

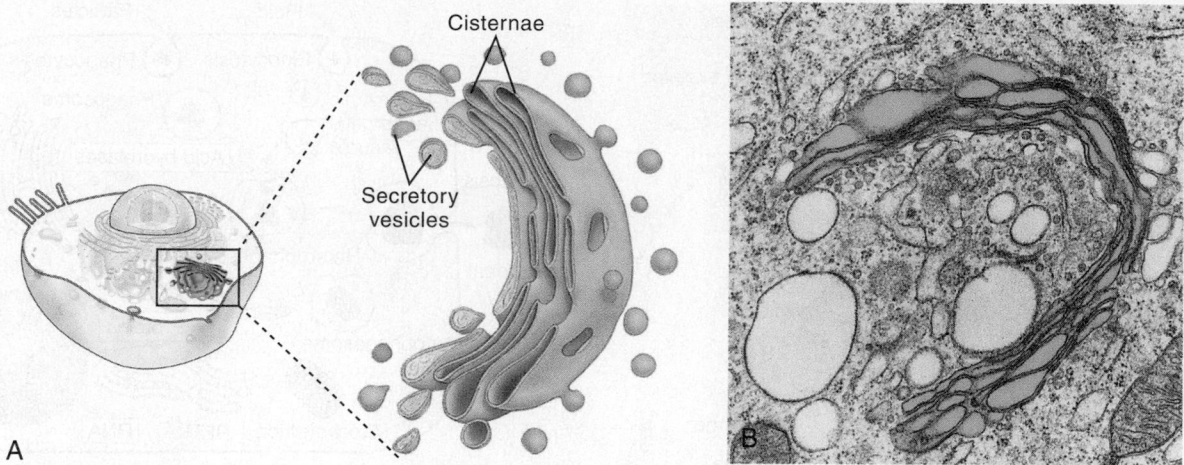

Figure 1-4 Golgi complex. **A,** Schematic representation of the Golgi complex showing a stack of flattened sacs, or cisternae, and numerous small membranous bubbles, or secretory vesicles. **B,** Transmission electron micrograph showing the Golgi complex highlighted with color. (From Thibodeau GA, Patton KT: *Anatomy & physiology,* ed 6, St Louis, 2007, Mosby.)

and a pigmented substance containing polyunsaturated fatty acids and proteins accumulates in the cell. This pigmented substance, termed *lipofuscin,* is often called "age pigment" or "age spots," and is noted in older individuals (see Chapter 2).

Peroxisomes

Peroxisomes (microbodies) are similar to lysosomes in microscopic appearance, but they are larger and oval or irregular in shape. Peroxisomes contain several oxidative enzymes, such as *catalase* and *urate oxidase.* Like mitochondria, peroxisomes are major sites of oxygen utilization. Peroxisomes are so named because they usually contain enzymes that use oxygen to remove hydrogen atoms from specific substrates in an oxidative reaction that produces hydrogen peroxide (H_2O_2). Hydrogen peroxide is a powerful oxidant, potentially destructive if it accumulates or escapes from peroxisomes. Catalase, an antioxidant enzyme, uses the H_2O_2 to oxidize a variety of other substrates—phenols, formic acid, formaldehyde, and alcohol—by the peroxidative reaction:

$$H_2O_2 + R^1H_2 \rightarrow R^1 + 2H_2O$$

Thus the reaction of H_2O_2 breaks down to H_2O and O_2 (see discussion of free radicals in Chapter 2). Peroxisomes also have an important role in the synthesis of specialized phospholipids necessary for nerve cell myelination. Such reactions are important in detoxifying various wastes within the cell or foreign components that enter the cell, such as ethanol.

Mitochondria

Mitochondria (*mito* = thread; *chondros* = granule) are of much interest because of their role in cellular energy metabolism (see p. 21). These cytoplasmic organelles appear as spheres, rods, or filamentous bodies that are bound by a double membrane (Figure 1-7). The **outer membrane** is smooth and surrounds the mitochondrion itself; the inner membrane is convoluted in the mitochondrial matrix to form partitions called **cristae.**

The **inner membrane** contains the enzymes of the respiratory chain—the name given to the electron transport chain. These enzymes are essential to the process of oxidative phosphorylation that generates most of the cell's ATP. Metabolic pathways involved in the metabolism of carbohydrates, lipids, and amino acids and special pathways involving urea and heme synthesis are located in the mitochondrial matrix.

The outer membrane is permeable (passable) to many substances, but the inner membrane is highly selective and contains many transmembranous transport systems. The inner membrane contains a transporter to move electrically charged calcium (calcium ions). (Membrane transport is discussed on p. 25.)

Vaults

Vaults are cytoplasmic ribonucleoproteins, much larger than ribosomes, and shaped like octagonal barrels (Figure 1-8). Their name comes from their multiple arches, which reminded their discoverers of vaulted or cathedral ceilings. A single cell can contain thousands of vaults. Vaults were identified only recently because of changes in staining techniques. The function of vaults may be related to their octagonal shape. Similarly, the pores in the membrane surrounding the nucleus (see Figure 1-2, *B*) are also octagonally shaped and the same size as vaults, leading to speculation that vaults may be cellular "trucks." Further, vaults would dock at nuclear pores, pick up molecules synthesized in the nucleus, and deliver their load elsewhere in the cell. Because at any given time about 5% of the vaults are localized near the nuclear pores, it is thought that vaults may be carrying messenger RNA (mRNA) from the nucleus to the ribosomal sites of protein synthesis within the cytoplasm. Investigators suggest that vaults transport several copies of untranslated RNA and that they are transported along cytoskeletal-based cellular tracks—much like an assembly line.[2] Researchers are investigating the role of vaults in cancer cells' resistance to drug therapy. Perhaps transporting chemotherapy drugs to sites for exocytosis from the cancer cell increases the drugs'

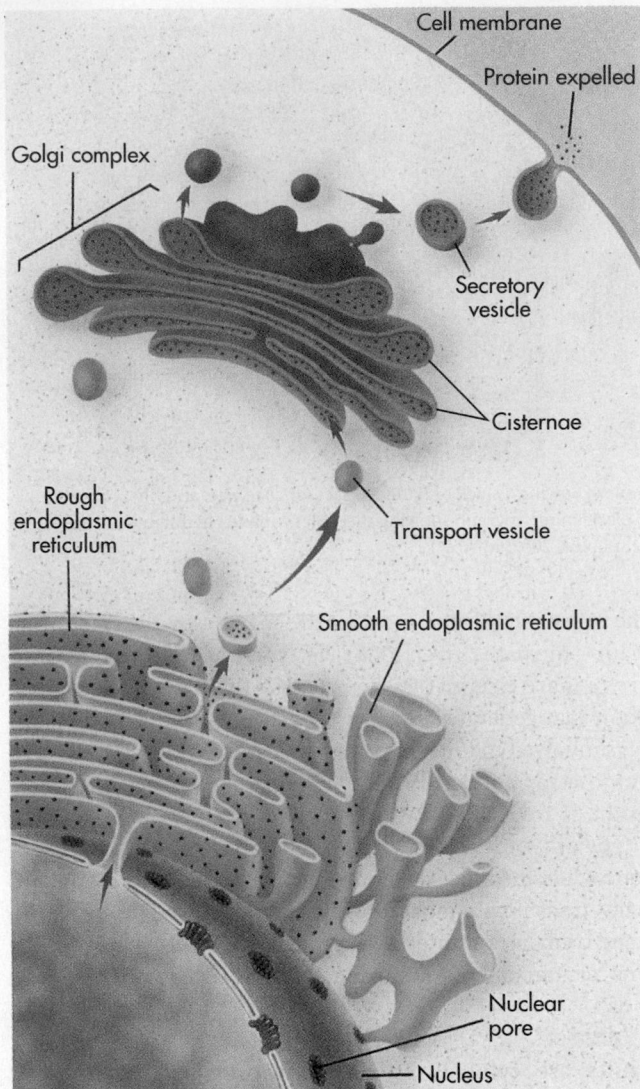

Figure 1-5 How the internal membrane system of a cell packages a protein for export. The instructions for making a protein that is destined for export from a cell, such as a digestive enzyme made by a pancreas cell, are first transcribed from DNA by RNA in the nucleus. The RNA then leaves the nucleus through a nuclear pore and proceeds to a ribosome located on the rough endoplasmic reticulum (ER). There it provides instructions for the correct sequence of amino acids for synthesizing that particular digestive enzyme. When enzyme synthesis is complete, the enzyme travels through the ER and is then encapsulated in a transport vesicle. The transport vesicle fuses with a Golgi body, releasing the enzyme. In the Golgi complex the enzyme is further modified and is then shunted to the ends of the Golgi complex, or cisternae. There the enzyme waits for a secretory vesicle, which will carry it to the perimeter of the cell, the cell membrane. The secretory vesicle membrane then fuses with the cell membrane, and the enzyme is released outside the cell. (From Raven PH, Johnson GB: *Understanding biology*, ed 3, Dubuque, IA, 1995, Brown.)

elimination, or vaults may mediate multidrug resistance by transporting drugs away from their intracellular targets, for example, the nucleous.[3] Although the normal cellular function of the vault is as yet undetermined, the structure of the vault is consistent with a role in either subcellular transport or sequestering large nuclear protein assemblies.[4]

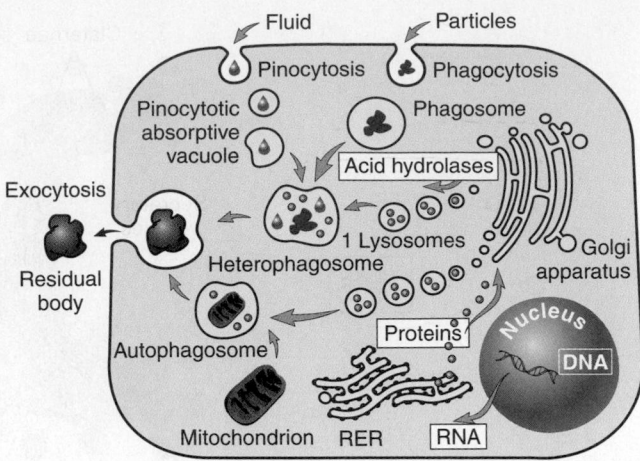

Figure 1-6 Lysosomes. Primary (1) lysosomes, which originate from the Golgi apparatus, give rise to heterophagosomes and autophagosomes. Undigested material in phagosomes is extruded from the cell or remains in the cytoplasm as lipofuscin-rich residual bodies. *RER*, Rough endoplasmic reticulum. (From Damjanov I: *Pathology for the health-related professionals*, ed 3, Philadelphia, 2006, Saunders.)

soluble proteins are created in the cell. The cytoplasm's cytomembranes, also known collectively as the *endoplasmic reticulum*, and is used in the synthesis of various cell molecules.

Cytosol

Cytosol is the gelatinous, semiliquid portion of the cytoplasm accounting for about 55% of the total cell volume. Functions of the cytosol include intermediary metabolism involving enzymatic biochemical reactions; ribosomal protein synthesis; and storage of carbohydrates, fat, and secretory vesicles.

Intermediary metabolism refers to the intracellular chemical reactions that include synthesis, degradation, and transformation of small organic molecules (e.g., simple sugars, fatty acids, and amino acids). All intermediary metabolism occurs in the cytoplasm or that portion of the cell interior not occupied by the nucleus—with most of the metabolism being accomplished in the cytosol. These reactions enable energy to be used for cellular activities and for providing substrates to maintain cell integrity.

Ribosomal protein synthesis takes place in free ribosomes in the cytosol. Cytosolic ribosomes that synthesize identical proteins are collected together in "factories" known as **polyribosomes.**

Storage of excess nutrients not immediately used for ATP production is converted in the cytosol into storage forms; for example, excess glucose is stored as glycogen. These temporary masses are known as *inclusions* (see Chapter 2). Secretory vesicles that have been processed and packaged by the endoplasmic reticulum and Golgi complex also remain in the cytosol. By means of signaling, the vesicles transport and empty their contents to the outside.

Cytoskeleton

All eukaryotic cells contain elaborate and specialized internal structures in the cytosol that provide the "bones and muscles" of the cell—the **cytoskeleton.** The cytoskeleton maintains the cell's shape and internal organization, and it permits movement of substances within the cell and movement of external

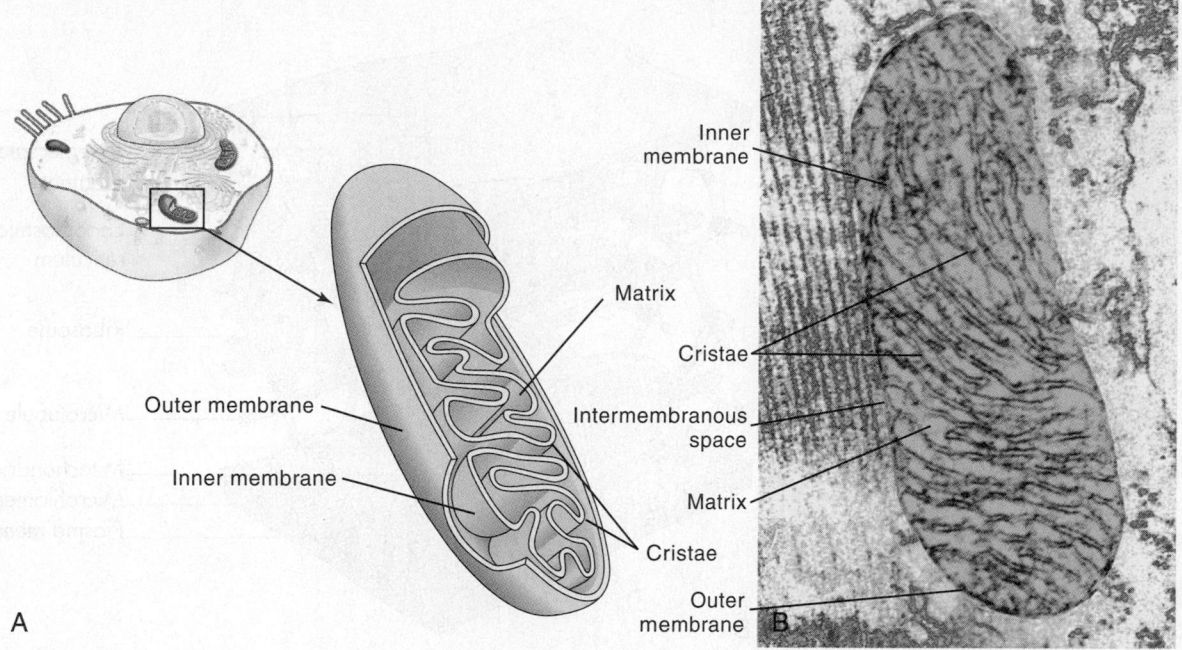

A

B

Figure 1-7 Mitochondrion. **A,** Cutaway sketch showing outer and inner membranes. Note the many folds (cristae) of the inner membrane. **B,** Transmission electron micrograph of a mitochondrion. Although some mitochondria have the capsule shape shown here, many are round or oval. (From Thibodeau GA, Patton KT: *Anatomy & physiology,* ed 6, St Louis, 2007, Mosby.)

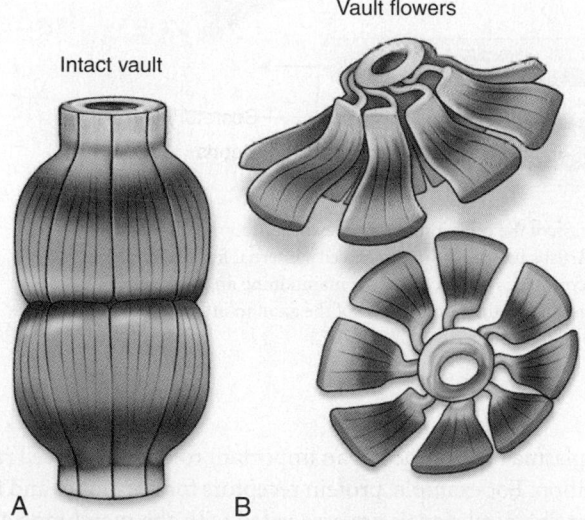

Figure 1-8 Vaults. **A,** Schematic three-dimensional representation of a vault, an octagonal barrel-shaped organelle believed to transport messenger RNA from the nucleus to the cytoplasmic ribosomes. **B,** Schematic representation of an opened vault, showing its octagonal structure.

projections (cilia or microvilli; flagella in sperm) outside the plasma membrane. The internal skeleton is composed of a network of protein filaments; two of the most important are microtubules and actin filaments, or microfilaments.

Microtubules are small, hollow, cylindric, unbranched tubules made of protein. When found together, microtubules exhibit rigidity, unlike the rest of the cytoplasm. Microtubules thus add strength to the cell's structure (Figure 1-9, *A*). Within the cell, microtubules support and move organelles from one part of the cytoplasm to another, facilitate transport of impulses along nerve cells, and have roles in the inflammatory and immune responses and hormone secretion. Microtubules are also involved in external movement, or motility, of some cells.

Microtubules are arranged in the thickened base, or basal body, of a protrusion from the cell's plasma membrane. This arrangement occurs in the basal bodies of sperm flagella and the cilia of certain other cells. The long, whiplike flagella enable sperm cells to move. Cilia usually move substances past the cell, which remains stationary. For example, cilia on cells lining the respiratory tract move together to "beat" mucus toward the throat so it can be removed by coughing.

While the cell is not in the process of division, only a few microtubules are assembled; cellular division (mitosis) or defense (phagocytosis) does, however, induce a cycle of rapid assembly and disassembly. Microtubules involved in cellular division are arranged in a **centriole.** Centrioles always consist of nine bundles containing three microtubules each. During division the pairs of centrioles split and migrate to opposite poles of the cell (see p. 34).

Alterations of microtubular function are implicated in disease processes. For example, alterations in actin microfilament act as a driving force for cell extension during cancer spread.[5]

Actin filaments (microfilaments) are smaller fibrils that generally occur in bundles rather than singly (Figure 1-9, *C*). Like microtubules, actin filaments are associated with cellular locomotion and maintenance of cell and tissue shape.[5]

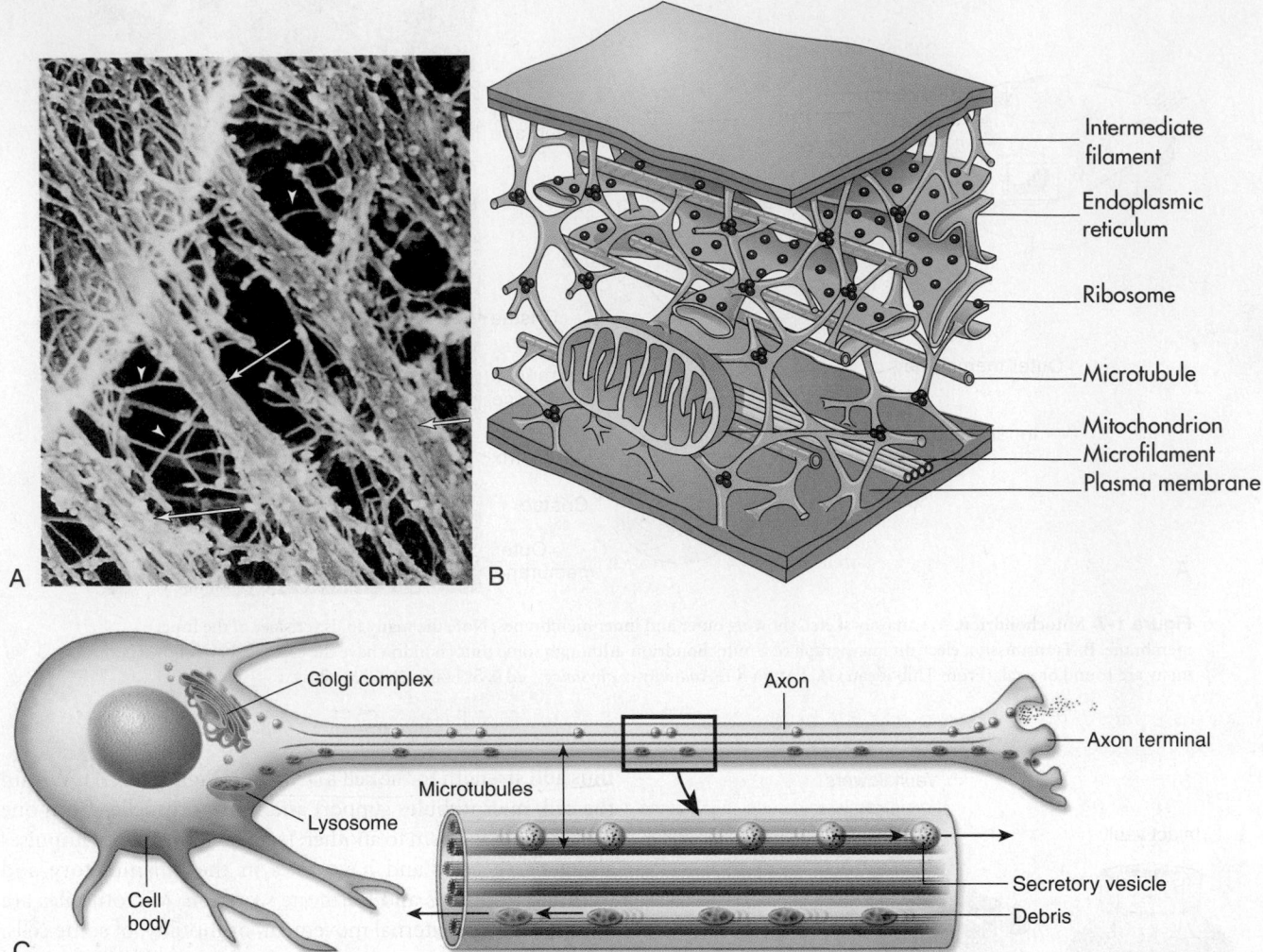

Figure 1-9 Cytoskeleton. **A,** Color-enhanced electron micrograph of a portion of the cell's internal framework. Arrowheads mark the intermediate filaments, and the complete arrows mark the microtubules. **B,** Artist's interpretation of the cell's internal framework. Note that the "free" ribosomes and other organelles are not really free at all. **C,** Microtubules are necessary for maintaining an asymmetric cell shape, such as that of a nerve cell. In addition, specific chemicals are released from the terminal end of the axon to influence neural transmission. (**A** and **B** from Thibodeau GA, Patton KT: *Anatomy & physiology,* ed 6, St Louis, 2007, Mosby.)

In addition, microfilaments are necessary for regulating cell growth.[6] Cellular locomotion depends on contractile properties that involve both microtubules and actin filaments. Anesthetic drugs can affect both structures, disrupting intracellular movement and cellular motility.

Plasma Membranes

Whether they surround the cell or enclose an intracellular organelle, membranes are exceedingly important to normal physiologic function because they control the composition of the space, or compartment, they enclose. Membranes can allow or exclude various molecules, and because of selective transport systems, they can move molecules into or out of the space (Figure 1-10). By controlling the movement of substances from one compartment to another, membranes exert a powerful influence on metabolic pathways. In addition to these functions,

the plasma membrane has an important role in cell-to-cell recognition. For example, protein receptors for hormones and for other chemical signals are associated with the membrane and act as markers that identify a cell to its neighbors. Other functions of the plasma membrane include cellular mobility and the maintenance of cellular shape (Table 1-1).

Membrane Composition

The outer surface of the plasma membrane is not smooth but dimpled with cavelike indentations known as caveolae ("tiny caves"). Caveolae were not thought to be functionally significant until the mid-1990s, when evidence suggested that they (1) serve as a repository for some receptors, (2) provide a new route for transport into the cell, and (3) act as the initiator for relaying signals from several extracellular chemical messengers into the cell's interior[7] (see p. 32).

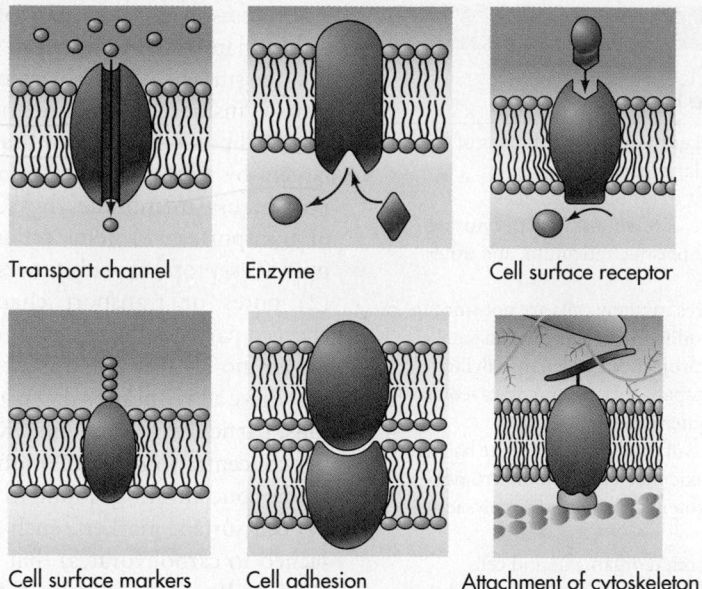

Transport channel   Enzyme   Cell surface receptor

Cell surface markers   Cell adhesion   Attachment of cytoskeleton

Figure 1-10 Functions of plasma membrane proteins. The plasma membrane proteins illustrated here show a variety of functions performed by the different types of plasma membranes. (From Raven PH, Johnson GB: *Understanding biology,* ed 3, Dubuque, IA, 1995, Brown.)

The major chemical components of all membranes are lipids and proteins, but the percentage of each varies among different membranes. Lipid molecules are the most abundant, but the protein molecules are so large that in total mass these two constituents are roughly equal. The structure of a plasma membrane is shown in Figure 1-11. Intracellular membranes have a higher percentage of proteins than do plasma membranes, presumably because most enzymatic activity occurs within organelles. Carbohydrates are mainly associated with plasma membranes, where they are combined chemically with lipids, forming glycolipids, and with proteins, forming glycoproteins.

Lipids

The basic component of the plasma membrane is a bilayer of lipid molecules—phospholipids, glycolipids, and cholesterol (respective ratios 70:5:25). The lipids are responsible for the structural integrity of the membrane. Each lipid molecule is said to be polar, or amphipathic. An **amphipathic molecule** is one in which one part is **hydrophobic** (uncharged, or "water hating") and another part is **hydrophilic** (charged, or "water loving") (see Figure 1-11). The membrane spontaneously organizes itself into a bilayer because of these two incompatible solubilities. The hydrophobic region (hydrophobic tail) of each lipid molecule is protected from water, whereas the hydrophilic region (hydrophilic head) is immersed in it. The bilayer's structure accounts for one of the essential functions of the plasma membrane: it is impermeable to most water-soluble molecules (molecules that dissolve in water) because they are insoluble in the oily core region. The bilayer serves as a barrier to the diffusion of water and hydrophilic substances while allowing lipid-soluble molecules, such as oxygen (O_2) and carbon dioxide (CO_2), to diffuse through it readily.

Because the bilayer is fluid at temperatures above freezing, components of the cellular environment move slowly and selectively across the membrane all the time. (Components of the cellular environment are also discussed in Chapter 3.)

Proteins

Research suggests two ways to classify membrane proteins. One way is classification as peripheral or integral proteins. **Integral membrane proteins** are those embedded in the lipid bilayer linked to either *phosphatidylinositol*, a minor phospholipid, or a fatty acid chain. The integral proteins can be removed from the membrane only by detergents that solubilize (dissolve) the liquid. **Peripheral membrane proteins** are not embedded in the bilayer but reside at one surface or the other, bound to an integral protein.

Although the classification of membrane proteins as peripheral or integral is commonly used, it does not describe how proteins are associated with the bilayer. The second mode of classification does so by taking into account the membrane-spanning, or transmembranous, nature of membrane proteins[1] (see Figure 1-13). According to this classification, proteins are associated with the lipid bilayer in four ways:

1. Some proteins, called **transmembrane proteins,** extend across the bilayer and are exposed to an aqueous environment on both sides of it.
2. Some intracellular proteins extend their polypeptide chain partially through the bilayer by means of a fatty acid chain.
3. Some cell-surface proteins are attached to the bilayer by a covalent linkage (i.e., a specific oligosaccharide).
4. Some proteins do not extend even partially through the bilayer but are bound to the membrane by noncovalent linkages with other membrane proteins.

Table 1-1	Plasma Membrane Functions

Cellular Mechanism	Membrane Functions
Structure	Usually thicker than the membranes of intracellular organelles
	Containment of cellular organelles
	Maintenance of relationship with cytoskeleton, endoplasmic reticulum, and other organelles
	Outer surfaces in many cells are not smooth but are studded with cilia or even smaller cylindric projections called microvilli; both are capable of movement; caveolae are also outer indentations
	Maintenance of fluid and electrolyte balance
Protection	Barrier to toxic molecules and macromolecules (proteins, nucleic acid, polysaccharides)
	Barrier to foreign organisms and cells
Activation of cell	Hormones (regulation of cellular activity)
	Mitogens (cellular division, see Chapter 4)
	Antigens (antibody synthesis, see Chapter 7)
	Growth factors (proliferation and differentiation)
Transport	Diffusion and exchange diffusion
	Endocytosis (pinocytosis and phagocytosis); receptor-mediated endocytosis
	Exocytosis (secretion)
	Active transport
Cell-to-cell interaction	Communication and attachment at junctional complexes
	Symbiotic nutritive relationships
	Release of enzymes and antibodies to extracellular environment
	Relationships with extracellular matrix

Modified from King DW, Fenoglio CM, Lefkowitch JH: *General pathology: principles and dynamics,* Philadelphia, 1983, Lea & Febiger.

Proteins exist in densely folded molecular configurations rather than straight chains, so an excess of hydrophilic units is at the surface of the molecule and an excess of hydrophobic units is inside. Although membrane structure is determined by the lipid bilayer, membrane functions are determined largely by proteins. For example, proteins facilitate transport across membranes by serving as receptors, enzymes, or transporters. Proteins act as (1) recognition and binding units (receptors) for substances moving in and out of the cell; (2) pores or transport channels for various electrically charged particles called *ions* or *electrolytes* and specific carriers for amino acids and monosaccharides; (3) specific enzymes that drive active pumps that promote concentration of certain ions, particularly potassium (K^+), within the cell while keeping concentrations of other ions, for example, sodium (Na^+), below concentrations found in the extracellular environment; (4) cell surface markers, such as **glycoproteins** (proteins attached to carbohydrates) that identify a cell to its neighbor; (5) **cell adhesion molecules (CAMs)** or proteins that allow cells to hook together and form attachments to the cytoskeleton for maintaining cellular shape; and (6) catalysts of chemical reactions, for example, conversion of lactose to glucose (see Figure 1-10). (Membrane transport is discussed on p. 25.)

The interaction of plasma membrane proteins with lipids is complex and is currently the subject of much research. The role of proteins in the onset and progression of disease is important because of their enzymatic, transport, and recognition-receptor functions in cellular physiology.

Proteolytic Cascades

About 500 human genes encode proteases.[8] Proteases are involved in the physiologic regulation of essential processes by participating in a tightly orchestrated sequence of events termed a **proteolytic cascade.** Four major proteolytic cascades with disease relevance are candidates for treatment modalities including (1) cell death or caspase-mediated apoptosis, (2) blood coagulation cascade, (3) degrading membrane enzymes or matrix

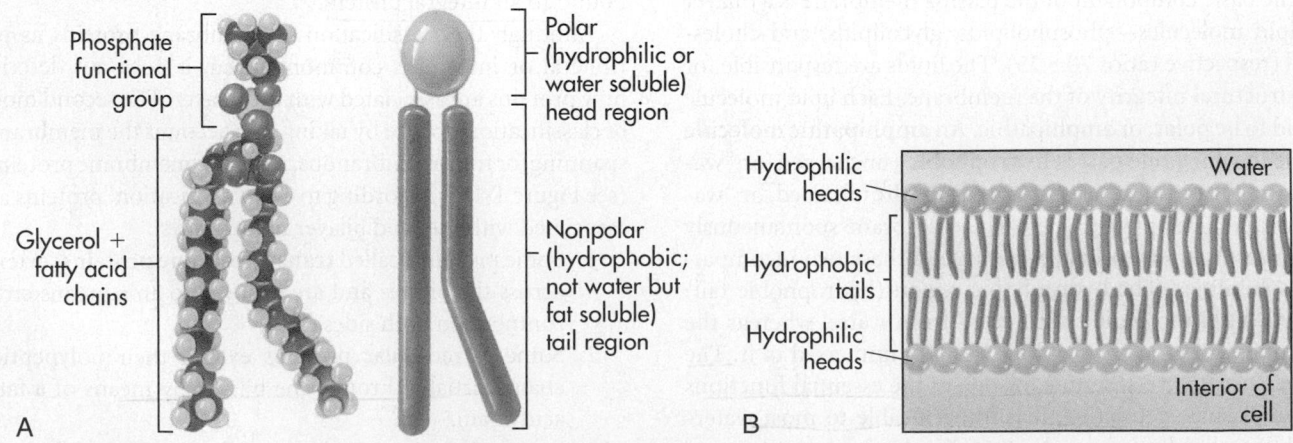

Figure 1-11 Structure of a phospholipid molecule. **A,** Each phospholipid molecule consists of a phosphate functional group and two fatty acid chains attached to a glycerol molecule. **B,** The fatty acid chains and glycerol form nonpolar, hydrophobic "tails," and the phosphate functional group forms the polar, hydrophilic "head" of the phospholipid molecule. When placed in water, the hydrophobic tails of the molecule face inward, away from the water, and the hydrophilic head faces outward, toward the water. (From Raven PH, Johnson GB: *Understanding biology,* ed 3, Dubuque, IA, 1995, Brown.)

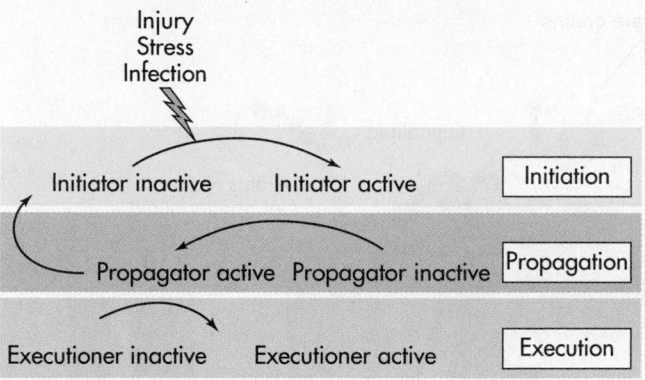

Figure 1-12 Schematic representation of a prototype proteolytic cascade. In the initiation phase, the cascade is triggered by an external stimulus, such as injury, stress, or infection. During the propagation phase, the initiator converts a downstream propagator into its active form by proteolysis. In the execution phase, the propagator will activate an executor. The process of coagulation is the best known proteolytic cascade. (Redrawn with permission from Amour A et al: General considerations for proteolytic cascades, *Biochem Soc Trans* 32:15-16, 2004. © the Biochemical Society.)

metalloproteinase cascade, and (4) the complement cascade. Some proteases within a proteolytic cascade act as initiators, others are involved in amplification and propagation and execution (Figure 1-12). Understanding the various steps involved is crucial for designing drug interventions. Dysregulation of proteases features prominently in many human diseases, including cancer, autoimmunity, and neurodegenerative disorders.[9-11]

Carbohydrates

A significant amount of carbohydrate is contained within the plasma membrane in the form of glycoprotein. Intercellular recognition, which is required for tissue formation, is an important function of membrane glycoproteins. Abnormal surface carbohydrate markers have been identified in certain tumor cells, leading investigators to claim that these markers are involved in tissue growth. Cells do not normally "trespass" their boundaries and overgrow their own territory.

Membrane Fluidity: The Fluid Mosaic Model

In the 1960s GL Nicholson and SJ Singer proposed the popular fluid mosaic model for biologic membranes (Figure 1-13). The model, which is continually being modified, presents integral proteins as pieces of a mosaic that float singly or as aggregates in the fluid lipid bilayer. The protein molecules serve to (1) transport other molecules into and out of the cell; (2) facilitate (catalyze) membrane reactions; (3) receive messages, thus acting as receptors for extracellular and intracellular signals; and (4) create structural linkages between the external and internal cellular environments. The fluid mosaic model accounts for the flexibility of cellular membranes, their self-sealing properties, and their impermeability to many substances.

New revisions of the model now state that most membrane proteins do not enjoy unrestricted, lateral movement. Instead, multiple modes of diffusion and transport indicate a mix or heterogeneity in the membrane. Thus *some* proteins may randomly diffuse, others are confined or static, and still others

are tethered to the cytoskeleton. The degree of a membrane's fluidity depends on temperature. At lower temperatures the lipids are in a gel crystalline state, and at higher temperatures they become highly fluid. These properties are critical for cellular growth, division, and receptor function. Because some proteins are free to move within the plasma membranes (like floating icebergs), certain foreign proteins (antigens) may become buried in the bilayer, emerging at the surface only after injury and then attracting antibodies (proteins produced by the immune system), which attack host cells. Antigens and antibodies, which are the cause and effect of the immune response, are discussed in Chapter 7. The burial and reemergence of antigens may be one cause of autoimmune disease, described in Chapter 8.

In the fluid mosaic model, cellular membranes are dynamic. Not only do some lipids and proteins move laterally on the membrane, but also ions and other molecules move through it. Cells, however, do have ways of immobilizing specific membrane proteins in a specific region of the membrane. Confinement may be necessary for certain functions to occur, for example, formation of intercellular junctions by proteins. The fluid mosaic model is logical in that it describes the membrane as existing in a state of change and modulation, which allows the cell to protect itself actively against injurious agents. Hormones, bacteria, viruses, drugs, antibodies, chemicals that transmit nerve impulses (neurotransmitters), and other substances attach to the plasma membrane by means of receptor molecules on its outer layer. The number of receptors present may vary at different times, and the cell is capable of modulating the effects of injurious agents by altering receptor number and pattern.[12] This aspect of the fluid mosaic model has drastically modified previously held concepts concerning the onset of disease.

The concentration of cholesterol in the plasma membrane affects membrane fluidity. Increased concentration results in less fluidity on the membrane's hydrophilic outer surface and more fluidity at its hydrophobic core. Changes in cholesterol content are factors in some diseases. In cirrhosis of the liver, for example, the cholesterol content of the red blood cell's plasma membrane increases. This causes an overall decrease in membrane fluidity that seriously affects the cell's ability to transport oxygen.

Stiff groupings of membrane molecules, often cholesterol rich, form loglike **rafts.** Rafts are noted as raised groupings of membranes (see Figure 13, *B*) that help organize components of a membrane.

Cellular Receptors

Cellular receptors are protein molecules (proteins are discussed on p. 11) on the plasma membrane, in the cytoplasm, or in the nucleus that are capable of recognizing and binding with specific smaller molecules called **ligands.** Hormones, for example, are ligands. Recognition and binding depend on the chemical configuration of the receptor and its smaller ligand, which must fit together somewhat like pieces of a jigsaw puzzle (see Chapter 20). New data reveal that activation of a receptor also may depend on differences in *movement* and *binding* of the extracellular face of the receptor.[13]

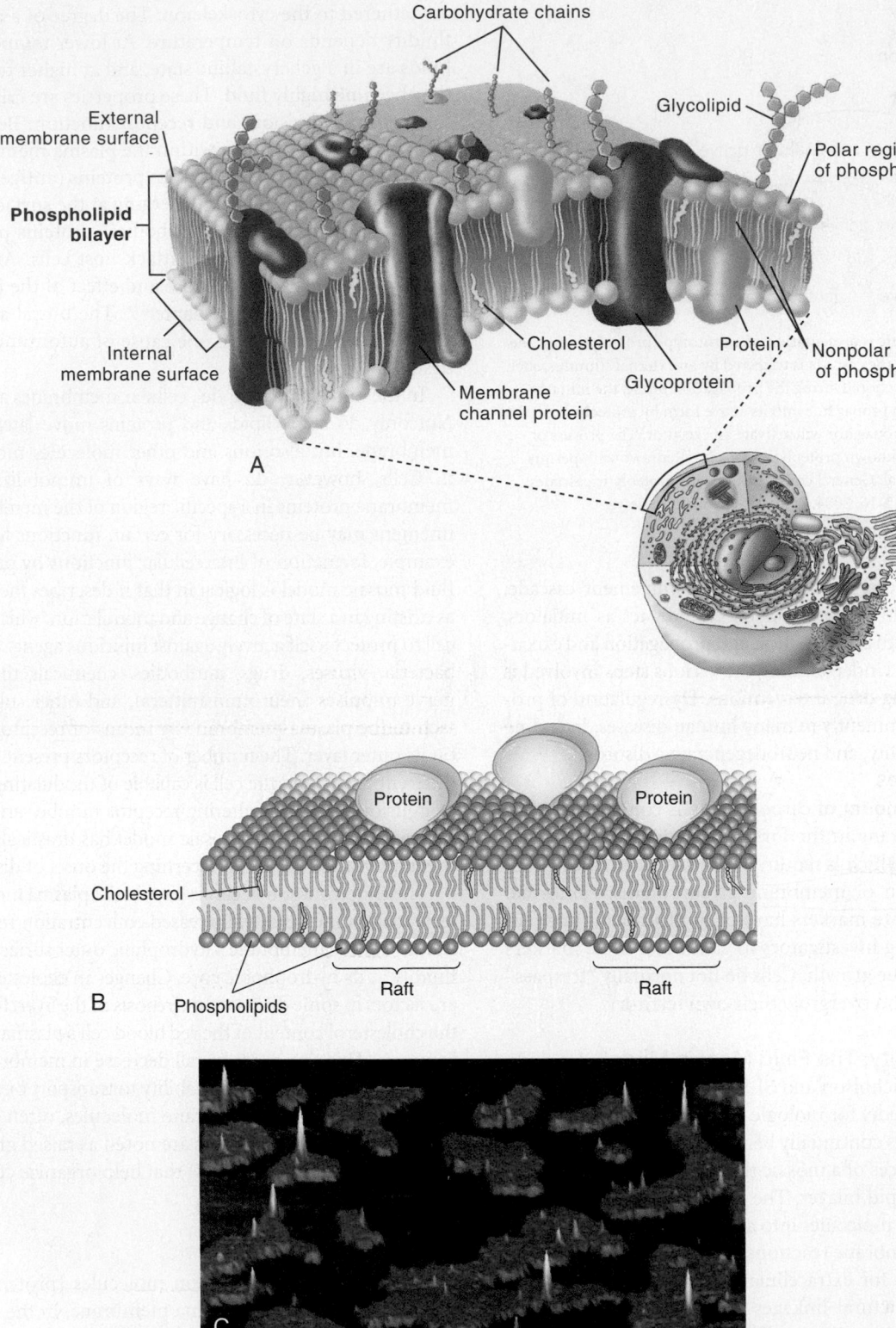

Figure 1-13 Fluid mosaic model and rafts. A, Schematic, three-dimensional view of the fluid mosaic model of membrane structure. The lipid bilayer provides the basic structure and serves as a relatively impermeable barrier to most water-soluble molecules. **B,** Diagram showing the basic structure of a membrane with rafts. The raft phospholipids have a richer supply of cholesterol than surrounding regions do and, along with attached proteins, form rather rigid floating platforms in the surface of the membrane. Rafts help organize functions at the surfaces of cells and organelles. **C,** Atomic force micrograph (AFM) in which an extremely fine-tipped needle drags over the surface of a cell membrane to reveal detailed surface features. Rafts are seen here as raised red-orange areas surrounded by black areas of less rigid phospholipid structure. (Modified from Thibodeau GA, Patton KT: *Anatomy & physiology,* ed 6, St Louis, 2007, Mosby.)

Table 1-2	Classes of Plasma Membrane Receptors

Type of Receptor	Description
Channel linked	Also called ligand-gated channels; involve rapid synaptic signaling between electrically excitable cells. Channels open and close briefly in response to neurotransmitters changing ion permeability of plasma membrane of postsynaptic cell.
Catalytic	Once activated by ligands, function directly as enzymes. Composed of transmembrane proteins that function intracellularly as tyrosine-specific protein kinases.
G-protein linked	Indirectly activate or inactivate plasma membrane enzyme or ion channel; interaction mediated by guanosine triphosphate (GTP)–binding regulatory protein (G protein). When activated, a chain of reactions occurs that alters concentration of intracellular messengers, such as cyclic adenosine monophosphate (cAMP) and calcium, or signaling molecules. Other target proteins' behavior also altered. May also interact with inositol phospholipids, which are significant in cell signaling, and molecules involved in the inositol-phospholipid transduction pathway. A G protein–linked receptor activates the enzyme phosphoinositide-specific phospholipase, which in turn generates two intracellular messengers: (1) inositol triphosphate (InP_3) releases Ca^{++}, and (2) diacylglycerol remains in the plasma membrane and activates protein kinase C. Protein kinase C further activates various cell proteins. Several different plasma membrane receptors are known to use the inositol-phospholipid transduction pathway.

Data from Alberts B et al: *Molecular biology of the cell,* ed 4, New York, 2001, Garland.

Plasma membrane receptors are particularly important for cellular uptake of ligands (Table 1-2). They protrude from or are exposed at the external surface of the membrane and often are attached to integral proteins. Some of these recognition units have all the mobile properties related to membrane fluidity. The ligands that bind with membrane receptors include hormones, neurotransmitters, antigens, complement components, lipoproteins, infectious agents, drugs, and metabolites. The past several years have brought many new discoveries concerning the specific interactions of cellular receptors with their respective ligands. In many instances this information has provided a basis for understanding disease.

Although the chemical nature of both ligands and the receptors to which they bind differs, receptors are classified on the basis of their location and function (see Cellular Communication and Signal Transduction, p. 18). Cellular type determines overall cellular function, but plasma membrane receptors determine which ligands a cell will bind with and how the cell will respond to binding with each. For example, the ability of a hormone or a neurotransmitter to stimulate a cell is regulated by the specificity and number of receptors present on the plasma membrane. Specific processes also control intracellular mechanisms. Hormone binding, for example, depends on special messenger molecules that regulate protein synthesis within the cell (see Chapter 20). Neurotransmitters (discussed in Chapter 14) also operate by causing special messengers to react with specific receptors.

Receptors for different drugs are found on the plasma membrane, in the cytoplasm, and in the nucleus. Membrane receptors have been found for certain anesthetics, opiates, endorphins, enkephalins, antibiotics, cancer chemotherapeutic agents, digitalis, and other drugs. Membrane receptors for endorphins, which are opiate-like peptides isolated from the pituitary gland, are found in large quantities in pain pathways of the nervous system (see Chapters 14 and 15). With binding, the endorphins (or drugs like morphine) change the cell's permeability to ions, increase the concentration of molecules that regulate intracellular protein synthesis, and initiate molecular events that modulate pain perception.

Receptors for infectious microorganisms, or antigen receptors, bind bacteria, viruses, and parasites. Antigen receptors on white blood cells (lymphocytes, monocytes, macrophages, granulocytes) recognize and bind with antigenic microorganisms and activate the immune and inflammatory responses (see Chapters 6 and 7).

CELL-TO-CELL ADHESIONS

Cells are small and squishy, not at all like bricks. They are enclosed only by a flimsy membrane, yet the cell depends on the integrity of this membrane for its survival. How can cells be formed together strongly, with their membranes intact, to form a muscle that can lift this textbook? Plasma membranes not only serve as the outer boundaries of all cells but also allow groups of cells to be held together robustly, in **cell-to-cell adhesions,** to form tissues and organs. Once arranged, cells are held together by three different means: the extracellular matrix, cell adhesion molecules in the cell's plasma membrane, and specialized cell junctions.

Extracellular Matrix

Cells can be bound together by attachment to one another or via the **extracellular matrix** (also including the **basement membrane**), which the cells secrete around themselves. The extracellular matrix is an intricate meshwork of fibrous proteins embedded in a watery, gel-like substance composed of complex carbohydrates (Figure 1-14). The matrix is like glue; however, it does provide a pathway for diffusion of nutrients, wastes, and other water-soluble traffic between the blood and tissue cells. Interwoven within the matrix are three groups of **macromolecules:** (1) fibrous structural proteins, including collagen and elastin; (2) a diverse group of adhesive

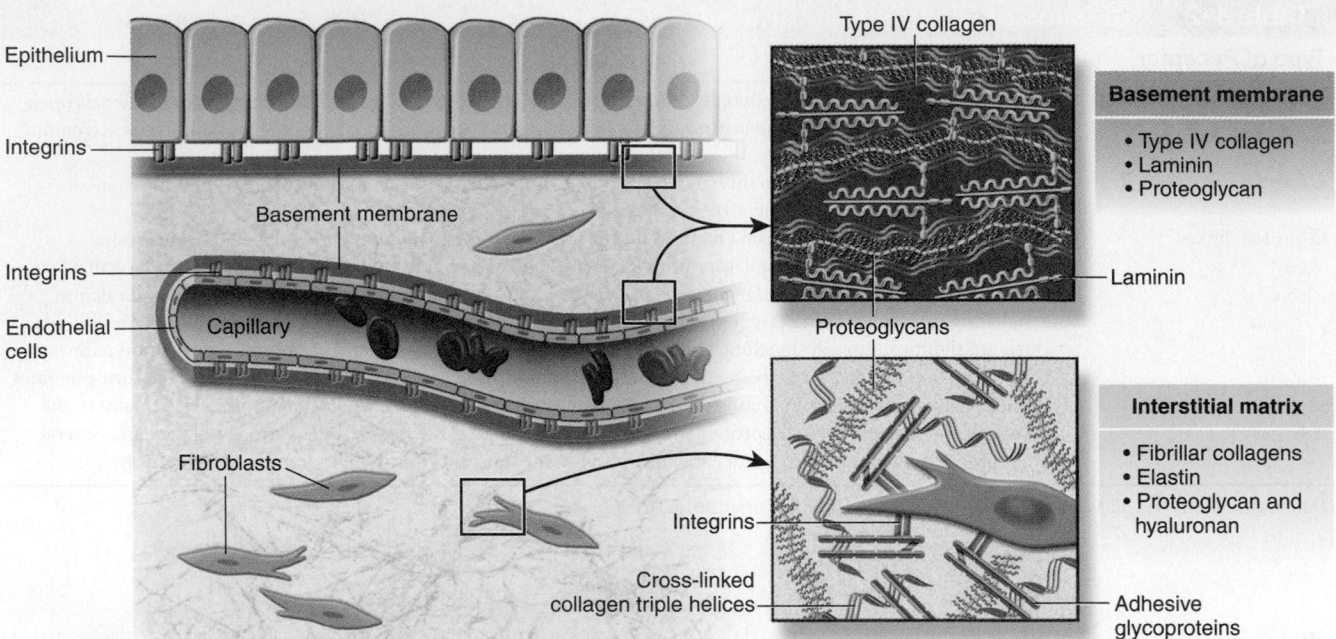

Epithelium

Integrins

Basement membrane

Integrins

Endothelial cells   Capillary

Fibroblasts

Type IV collagen

Basement membrane
- Type IV collagen
- Laminin
- Proteoglycan

Laminin

Proteoglycans

Interstitial matrix
- Fibrillar collagens
- Elastin
- Proteoglycan and hyaluronan

Integrins

Cross-linked collagen triple helices

Adhesive glycoproteins

Figure 1-14 **Extracellular matrix.** Tissues are not just cells but also extracellular space. The extracellular space is an intricate network of macromolecules called the *extracellular matrix (ECM)*. The macromolecules that constitute the ECM are secreted locally (by mostly fibroblasts) and assembled into a meshwork in close association with the surface of the cell that produced them. Two main classes of macromolecules include proteoglycans, which are bound to polysaccharide chains called *glycosaminoglycans,* and fibrous proteins (e.g., collagen, elastin, fibronectin, and laminin), which have structural and adhesive properties. Together the proteogylcan molecules form a gel-like ground substance in which the fibrous proteins are embedded. The gel permits rapid diffusion of nutrients, metabolites, and hormones between the blood and the tissue cells. Matrix proteins modulate cell-matrix interactions including normal tissue remodeling (which can become abnormal, for example, with chronic inflammation), embryogenesis, wound healing, and angiogenesis. Disruption of this balance results in serious diseases such as arthritis, tumor growth, and others. (Modified from Kumar V, Abbas A, Fausto N: *Robbins and Cotran pathologic basis of disease,* ed 7, Philadelphia, 2005, Saunders.)

glycoproteins, such as fibronectin; and (3) proteoglycans and hyaluronic acid.

Collagen forms cable-like fibers or sheets that provide tensile strength or resistance to longitudinal stress. Collagen breakdown, such as occurs in osteoarthritis, destroys the fibrils that give cartilage its tensile strength.

Elastin is a rubber-like protein fiber most abundant in tissue that must be capable of stretching and recoiling, such as the lungs.

Fibronectin, a large glycoprotein, promotes cell adhesion and cell anchorage. Reduced amounts have been found in certain types of cancerous cells; this allows cancer cells to travel or metastasize to other parts of the body.

All of these macromolecules occur in intercellular junctions and cell surfaces and may assemble into two different components: interstitial matrix and basement membrane (BM)[14] (see Figure 1-14).

The extracellular matrix is secreted by **fibroblasts** ("fiber formers"), local cells that are present in the matrix. The matrix and the cells within it are known collectively as *connective tissue* because they connect cells together to form tissue and organs. Human connective tissues are enormously varied. They can be hard and dense, like bone; flexible, like tendons or the dermis of the skin; resilient and shock-absorbing, like

cartilage; or soft and transparent, like the jelly that fills the eye. In all these examples, the majority of the tissue is composed of extracellular matrix, and the cells that produce the matrix are scattered within it like raisins in a pudding[15] (see Figure 1-14).

The matrix is not just a passive scaffolding for cellular attachment; it also helps regulate the functions of the cells within which it interacts. The matrix helps regulate cell growth, movement, and differentiation.

Specialized Cell Junctions

Cells in direct physical contact with neighboring cells are often linked together at specialized regions of their plasma membranes called **cell junctions.** Cell junctions have two main functions: (1) to hold cells together and (2) to allow small molecules to pass from cell to cell, allowing coordination of the activities of cells that form tissues. The three main types of cell junctions are (1) desmosomes (adhering junctions, or macula adherens), (2) tight junctions (impermeable junctions, or zonula occludens), and (3) gap junctions (adhering [communicating] junctions) (Figure 1-15). Together they form the **junctional complex. Desmosomes** hold cells together by forming either continuous bands or belts of epithelial sheets or button-like points of contact.

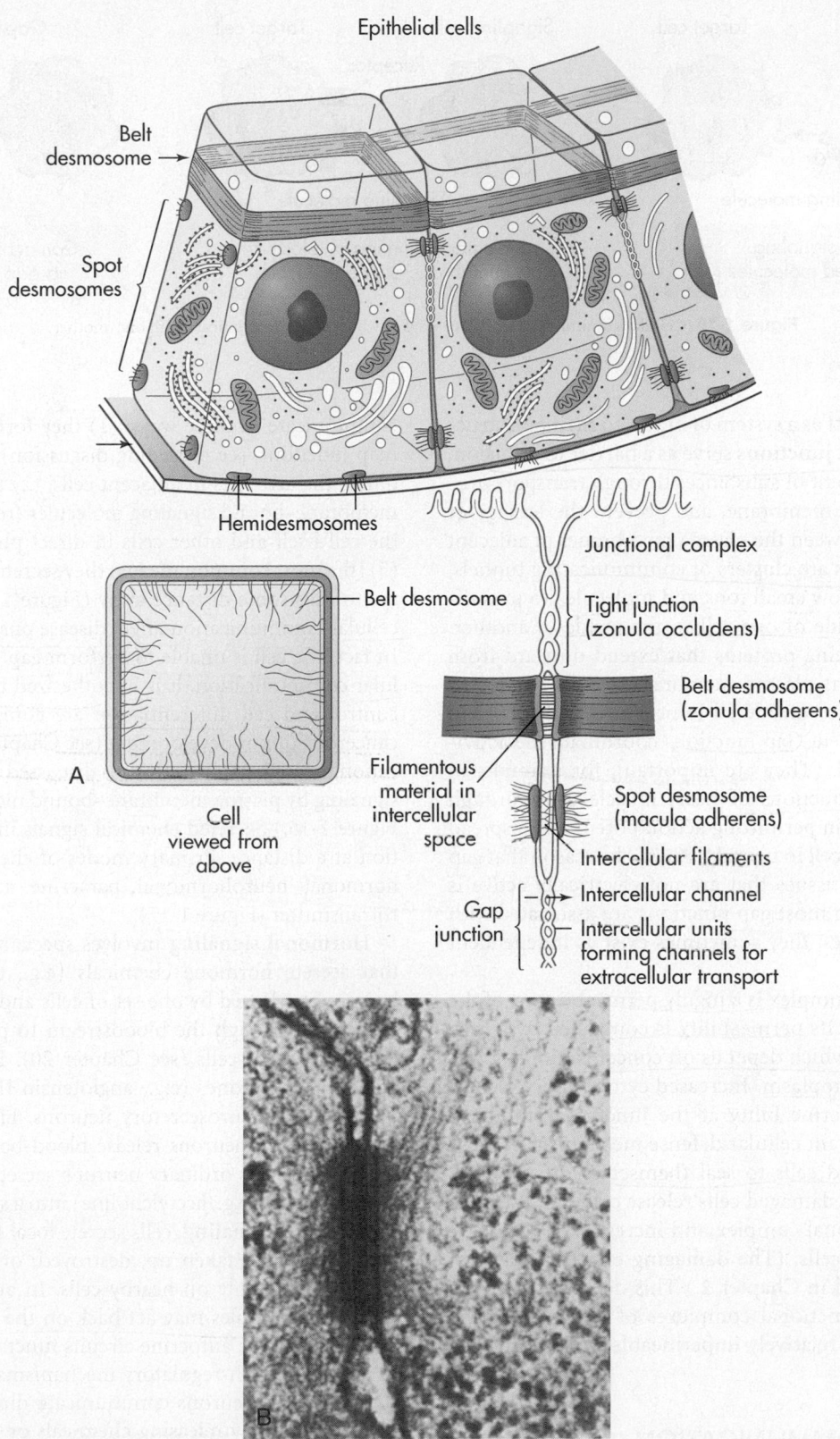

Figure 1-15 Types of cell connections. **A,** Schematic drawing of a belt desmosome between epithelial cells. This junction, also called *zonula adherens,* encircles each interacting cell. The spot desmosomes and hemidesmosomes, like the belt desmosomes, are adhering junctions. This tight junction is an impermeable junction that holds cells together but seals them in such a way that molecules cannot leak between them. The gap junction, as a communicating junction, mediates the passage of small molecules from one interacting cell to the other. **B,** Electron micrograph of desmosomes. (From Raven PH, Johnson GB: *Biology,* St Louis, 1992, Mosby.)

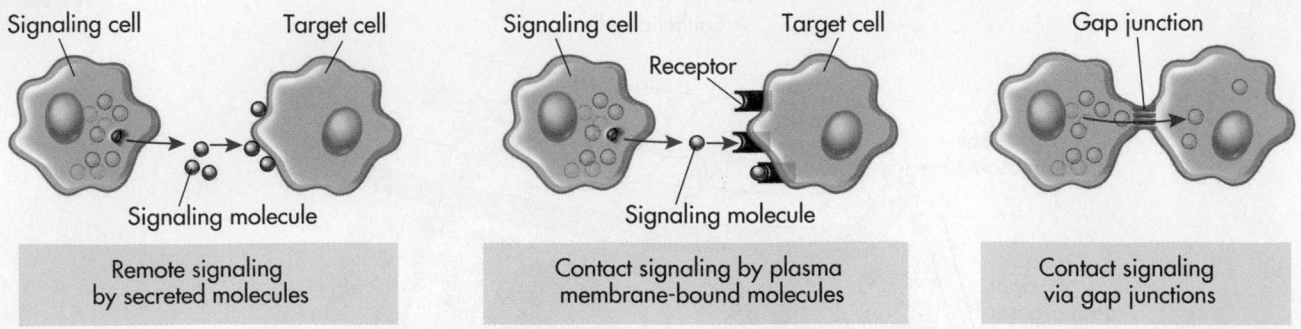

Signaling cell   Target cell

Signaling molecule

Remote signaling by secreted molecules

Signaling cell   Target cell

Receptor

Signaling molecule

Contact signaling by plasma membrane-bound molecules

Gap junction

Contact signaling via gap junctions

Figure 1-16 **Cellular communication.** Three ways in which cells communicate with one another.

Desmosomes also act as a system of braces to maintain structural stability. **Tight junctions** serve as a barrier to diffusion, prevent the movement of substances through transport proteins in the plasma membrane, and prevent the leakage of small molecules between the plasma membranes of adjacent cells. **Gap junctions** are clusters of communicating tunnels, **connexons,** that allow small ions and molecules to pass directly from the inside of one cell to the inside of another. Connexons are joining proteins that extend outward from each of the adjacent plasma membranes. Cells connected by gap junctions are considered ionically (electrically) and metabolically coupled. Gap junctions coordinate the activities of adjacent cells. They are important, for example, in synchronizing contractions of heart muscle cells through ionic coupling and in permitting action potentials to spread rapidly from cell to cell in neural tissues. The reason that gap junctions occur in tissues that are not electrically active is unknown. Although most gap junctions are associated with junctional complexes, they sometimes exist as independent structures.

The junctional complex is a highly permeable part of the plasma membrane. Its permeability is controlled by a process called **gating,** which depends on concentrations of calcium ions in the cytoplasm. Increased cytoplasmic calcium causes decreased permeability at the junctional complex. Gating is an important cellular defense mechanism because it enables uninjured cells to seal themselves off from injured neighbors. As damaged cells release calcium, it travels through the junctional complex and increases calcium levels in neighboring cells. (The damaging effects of calcium influx are described in Chapter 2.) This decreases the permeability of the junctional complexes of the neighboring cells, which form a relatively impermeable wall around the injured area.

CELLULAR COMMUNICATION AND SIGNAL TRANSDUCTON

Cells need to communicate with each other to maintain a stable internal environment, or **homeostasis;** to regulate their growth and division and their development and organization into tissues; and to coordinate their functions. Cells communicate in three ways: (1) they form protein channels (gap junctions, see preceding discussion) that directly coordinate the activities of adjacent cells; (2) they display plasma membrane–bound signaling molecules (receptors) that affect the cell itself and other cells in direct physical contact; and (3) (the most common means) they secrete chemicals that signal to cells some distance away (Figure 1-16). Alterations in cellular communication affect disease onset and progression. In fact, if a cell is unable to perform gap junctional intercellular communication, it is hypothesized that normal growth control and cell differentiation are compromised, favoring cancerous tumor development (see Chapter 11). (Communication through gap junctions is discussed earlier, and contact signaling by plasma membrane–bound molecules is shown in Figure 1-16.) Secreted chemical signals involve communication at a distance. Primary modes of chemical signaling are hormonal, neurohormonal, paracrine, autocrine, and neurotransmitter (Figure 1-17).

Hormonal signaling involves specialized endocrine cells that secrete hormone chemicals (e.g., thyroid-stimulating hormone) released by one set of cells and travel through the tissue and through the bloodstream to produce a response in other sets of cells (see Chapter 20). In **neurohormonal signaling,** hormones (e.g., angiotensin II) are released into the blood by neurosecretory neurons. Like endocrine cells, neurosecretory neurons release blood-borne chemical messengers, whereas ordinary neurons secrete short-range neurotransmitters (e.g., acetylcholine) into a small discrete space. In **paracrine signaling,** cells secrete local chemical mediators that are quickly taken up, destroyed, or immobilized. The mediators act only on nearby cells. In **autocrine signaling,** signaling molecules may act back on the cells of *origin* (i.e., *autostimulation*); autocrine circuits function as a component of normal growth-regulatory mechanisms in many adult tissue types.[16,17] Neurons communicate directly with the cells they innervate by releasing chemicals or **neurotransmitters** at specialized junctions called **chemical synapses;** the neurotransmitter diffuses across the synaptic cleft and acts on the postsynaptic target cell (Figure 1-17). In each type of chemical signaling, the target cell receives the signal by first attaching to its receptors. Many of these same signaling molecules are receptors used in hormonal, neurohormonal, paracrine,

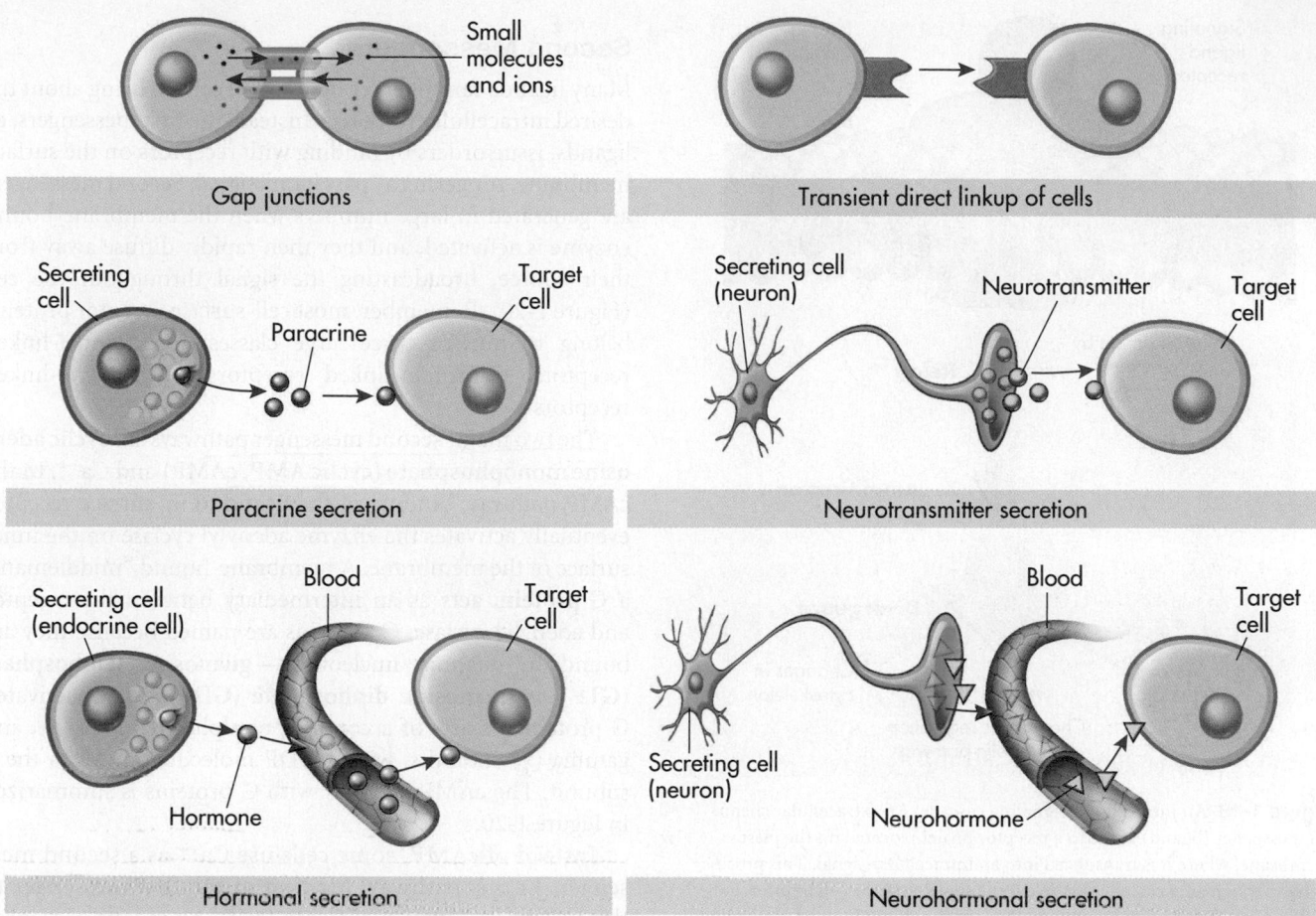

Figure 1-17 Modes of chemical signaling and cell communication. Paracrines, neurotransmitters, hormones, and neurohormones are all intercellular chemical messengers that accomplish communication between cells. Gap junctions provide the most intimate means of intercellular communication where small molecules and ions are exchanged between interacting cells without even entering the extracellular fluid. Autocrine stimulation (not illustrated) occurs when the secreting cell targets itself.

and autocrine signaling. The important differences lie in the speed and selectivity with which the signals are delivered to their targets.[1]

Plasma membrane receptors belong to one of three classes that are defined by the signaling (transduction) mechanism used. Table 1-2 summarizes these receptors.

Signal Transduction

Signal transduction involves incoming signals or instructions from extracellular chemical messengers (ligands) that are conveyed to the cell's interior for execution. Within the outer surface of the plasma membrane, specialized protein receptors bind with the selected chemical messengers. This combination of messenger with receptor triggers a cascade of cellular events important to the maintenance of homeostasis, such as membrane transport, cell division and differentiation, movement, secretion, and metabolism. Some types of altered cell behavior, such as increased cell growth and division, involve changes in gene expression and the synthesis of new proteins and therefore occur slowly. Others, such as changes in cell movement, secretion, or metabolism, do not

involve the nuclear machinery and therefore occur more rapidly. If deprived of appropriate signals, most cells undergo a form of cell suicide known as *programmed cell death*, or *apoptosis* (see p. 84).

Signaling cascades, or relay chains, of intercellular signaling molecules have several important functions (see Figure 1-18):

1. They physically *transfer* the signal from the place at which it is received to some other part of the cell where the response is expected.
2. They *amplify* the signal received, making it stronger; this is caused by a multiplying effect in the pathways; for example, binding of one ligand molecule to a receptor activates a number of adenylyl cyclase molecules.
3. They *distribute* the signal so that it influences several processes in parallel; at any step in the pathway, the signal can *diverge* and be relayed to several different intracellular targets, creating branches in the flow and causing a complex response (Figure 1-19).
4. Last, the signal can be *modulated* by other interfering factors prevailing inside or outside the cell.

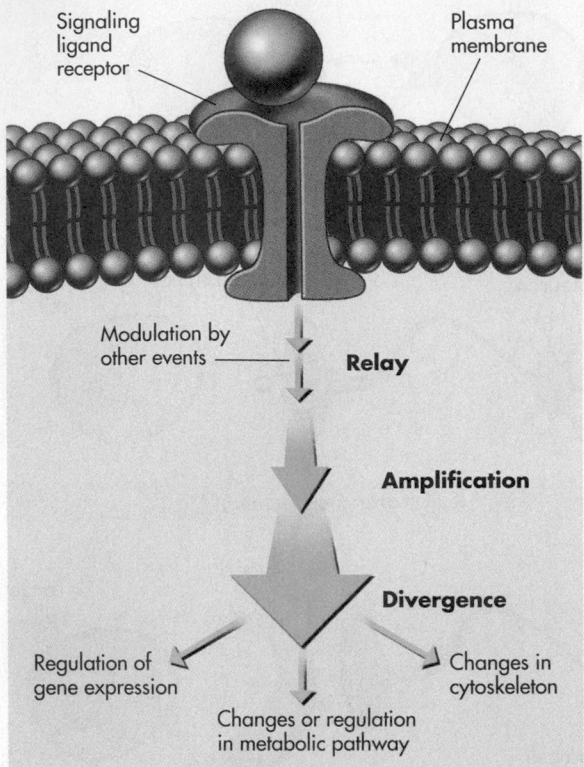

Figure 1-18 An intracellular signaling cascade. An extracellular chemical messenger (ligand) binds to a receptor protein located on the plasma membrane, where it is transduced into an intracellular signal. This process initiates a signaling cascade that relays the signal into the cell interior, amplifying and distributing it en route. Steps in the cascade can be modulated by other events in the cell.

Two general responses from binding of the extracellular chemical messenger, or **first messenger,** to the membrane receptors occur: (1) opening or closing specific channels in the membrane to regulate the movement of ions into or out of the cell, and (2) transferring the signal to an intracellular messenger, or **second messenger,** which in turn triggers a cascade of biochemical events within the cell.

Extracellular Messengers and Channel Regulation

Membrane channels, or "gates," can open and close depending on the circumstances of the first messenger. Opening and closing occur because of conformational changes (shaping) of the proteins that form the channels—blocking the channel (closing) or permitting passage through it (opening). Channel opening and closing can be initiated in one of three ways: (1) by binding of a ligand to a specific membrane receptor that is closely associated with the channel (for example, G proteins); (2) by changes in electric current in the plasma membrane, altering flow of Na$^+$ and K$^+$; and (3) by stretching or other chemical deformation of the channel. Figure 1-19 summarizes ways by which extracellular messengers regulate channel function for the other two methods of controlling channels (see p. 28).

Second Messengers

Many ligands cannot enter their target cells to bring about the desired intracellular response. Instead, the first messengers, or ligands, issue orders by binding with receptors on the surface membrane, triggering a "pass it on" signal. Second messengers are generated in large numbers when the membrane-bound enzyme is activated, and they then rapidly diffuse away from their source, broadcasting the signal throughout the cell (Figure 1-20). Remember, most cell-surface receptor proteins belong to one of three large classes: ion-channel-linked receptors, G-protein-linked receptors, or enzyme-linked receptors.

The two major second messenger pathways are **cyclic adenosine monophosphate (cyclic AMP, cAMP)** and Ca^{++}. In the cAMP pathway, binding of the ligand to its surface receptor eventually activates the enzyme adenylyl cyclase on the inner surface of the membrane. A membrane-bound "middleman," a **G protein,** acts as an intermediary between the receptor and adenylyl cyclase. G proteins are named because they are bound to guanine nucleotides—**guanosine triphosphate (GTP)** or **guanosine diphosphate (GDP).** An unactivated G protein consists of a complex of alpha (α), beta (β), and gamma (γ) subunits, with a GDP molecule bound to the α subunit. The cAMP pathway with G proteins is summarized in Figure 1-20.

Instead of cAMP, some cells use Ca^{++} as a second messenger. In this pathway, binding of the first messenger to the surface receptor eventually leads, by means of G proteins, to activation of the enzyme phospholipase C, an enzyme protein effector (an ion channel for an enzyme) that is bound to the inner side of the membrane. Figure 1-21 summarizes the Ca^{++} second messenger pathway. The cAMP and Ca^{++} pathways frequently overlap in bringing about a specific cellular response. For example, cAMP and Ca^{++} can influence each other. Calcium-activated calmodulin can regulate adenylyl cyclase and thus influence cAMP; conversely, cAMP-dependent kinase may phosphorylate and thereby change the activity of Ca^{++} channels or carriers. In some instances, both Ca^{++} and cAMP regulate the same intracellular protein. In a few cells, **cyclic guanosine monophosphate (cyclic GMP, cGMP)** serves as a second messenger similar to the cAMP pathway. For example, cGMP is the signal transduction pathway involved in vision. Some cellular responses mediated by cAMP and phospholipase C are summarized in Table 1-3. Major types of receptors and signal transduction pathways are contained in Table 1-4.

A large number of human disorders involve problematic signaling in cells. Cancer, for example, results from genetic mutations leading to the overactivity of proteins in signal relaying pathways that normally induce the cells to divide. Affected proteins cause cells to behave as if other cells were constantly telling them to reproduce, even when no such orders were sent.[18] Signal blockers are already in use against breast cancer.

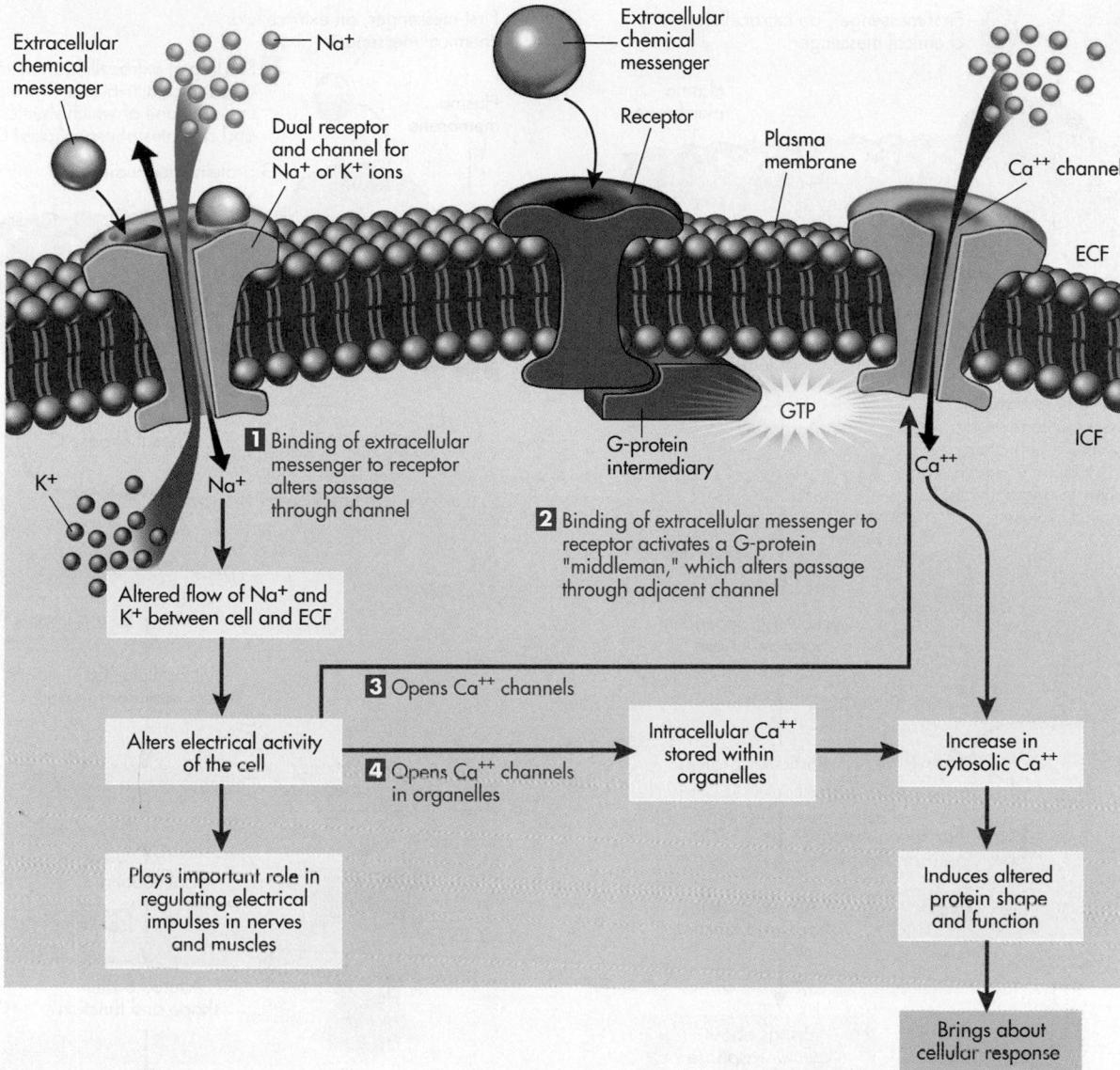

Figure 1-19 How extracellular messengers regulate channel function. Binding of an extracellular messenger to a dual receptor/channel brings about a quick opening or closing of ion channels, such as Na^+ or K^+ channels, which generates electrical impulses (1). A transient opening of membrane Ca^{++} channels occurs when binding of an extracellular messenger to a receptor activates a G-protein intermediary, which alters a nearby ion channel, such as a Ca^{++} channel (2). A transient opening of Ca^{++} channels also occurs indirectly in response to electrical impulses produced by extracellular messenger-induced changes in Na^+ and K^+ channels (3). Release of Ca^{++} from intracellular stores results when Ca^{++} channels in organelles open in response to electrical impulses (4). An increase in cytosolic Ca^{++} arising from pathways 2, 3, or 4 causes change in the shape and function of specific intracellular proteins to produce the desired cellular response. *ECF*, Extracellular fluid; *GTP*, guanosine triphosphate; *ICF*, intracellular fluid. (Redrawn with permission from Sherwood L: *Human physiology*, ed 3. © 1997 Brooks/Cole, a part of Cengage Learning, Inc. Reproduced by permission. www.cengage.com/permissions.)

CELLULAR METABOLISM

All the chemical tasks of maintaining essential cellular functions are referred to as **cellular metabolism.** The energy-using process of metabolism is called **anabolism** (*ana* = upward), and the energy-releasing process is known as **catabolism** (*cata* = downward). Metabolism provides the cell with the energy it needs to synthesize (produce) cellular structures.

Dietary proteins, fats, and starches are hydrolyzed in the intestinal tract into amino acids, fatty acids, and glucose. These constituents are then absorbed, circulated, and taken up by the cell, where they may be used for various vital cellular processes, including the production of ATP. The process by which ATP is produced is one example of a series of reactions called a **metabolic pathway.** A metabolic pathway involves several intermediate steps whose end products are not always detectable. A key feature of cellular metabolism is the directing of biochemical reactions by protein catalysts, or enzymes. Most biochemical reactions in a pathway are catalyzed by a specific enzyme. Each enzyme has a high affinity for a **substrate**—a specific substance that is converted to a product of the reaction.

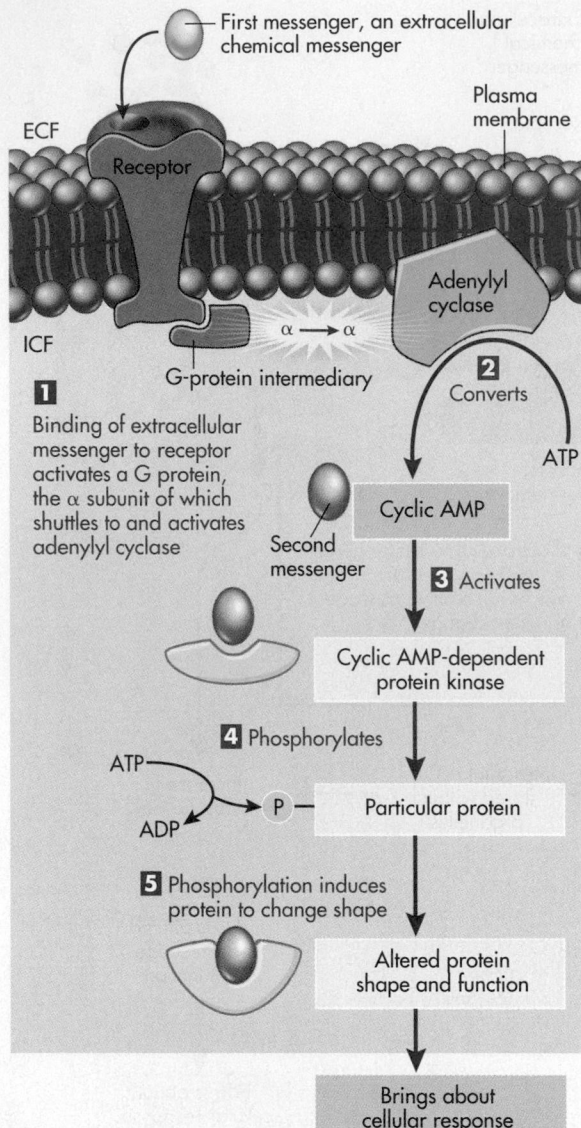

Figure 1-20 Extracellular messenger and activation of the cAMP second messenger system. The first messenger, or binding of an extracellular chemical messenger to a surface membrane receptor, activates the membrane-bound enzyme adenylyl cyclase by means of a G-protein intermediary (1), which in turn converts intracellular ATP into cAMP (2). cAMP is an intracellular second messenger, triggering the cellular response by activating the cAMP-dependent protein kinase (3), which in turn phosphorylates (4), and therefore modifies (5) a specific intracellular protein. The altered protein then directs the cellular response dictated by the extracellular messenger. *ADP,* adenosine diphosphate; *AMP,* adenosine monophosphate; *ATP,* adenosine triphosphate; *ECF,* Extracellular fluid; *ICF,* intracellular fluid. (Redrawn with permission from Sherwood L: *Human physiology,* ed 3. © 1997 Brooks/Cole, a part of Cengage Learning, Inc. Reproduced by permission. www.cengage.com/permissions.)

Role of Adenosine Triphosphate

For a cell to function it must be able to extract and use the chemical energy contained within the structure of organic molecules. When 1 mole of glucose is metabolically broken down in the presence of oxygen into carbon dioxide (CO_2) and water (H_2O), 686 kilocalories (kcal) of energy are

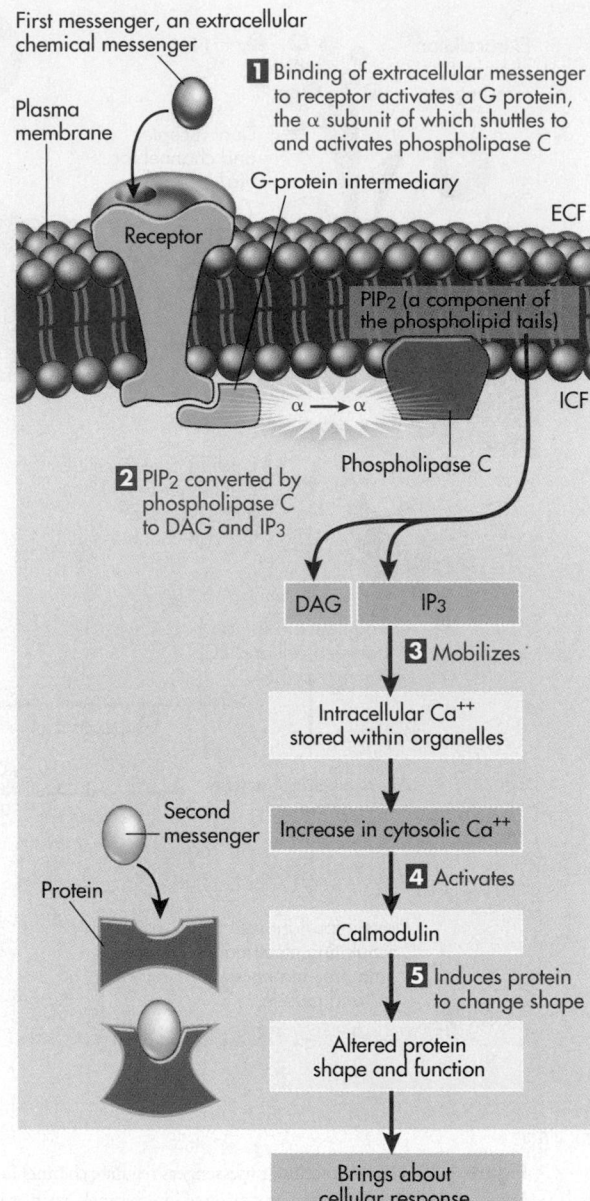

Figure 1-21 Extracellular messenger and activation of the calcium second messenger system. Binding of an extracellular messenger to a membrane receptor activates the membrane-bound enzyme phospholipase C by means of a G-protein intermediary (1). Phospholipase C converts phosphatidylinositol biphosphate (PIP_2) into diacylglycerol (DAG) and inositol triphosphate (IP_3) (2). IP_3 then mobilizes Ca^{++} stored within organelles (3). Ca^{++}, as a second messenger, activates calmodulin (4), causing a change in the shape and function of a specific intracellular protein to produce the cellular response (5). *ECF,* Extracellular fluid; *ICF,* intracellular fluid. (Redrawn with permission from Sherwood L: *Human physiology,* ed 3. © 1997 Brooks/Cole, a part of Cengage Learning, Inc. Reproduced by permission. www.cengage.com/permissions.)

released. In a test tube this energy is released as heat. Because a cell cannot transform heat into work, chemical energy, rather than heat, is created by metabolism. The chemical energy lost by one molecule is transferred to the chemical structure of another molecule by an energy-carrying or transferring

Table 1-3	Hormone-Induced Cell Responses Mediated by cAMP	
Signaling Ligands	Target Tissue	Major Response
Epinephrine	Heart	Increase in heart rate and force of contraction
Epinephrine, ACTH	Muscle	Glycogen breakdown
Glucagon	Fat	Fat breakdown
ACTH	Adrenal gland	Cortisol secretion
Antidiuretic hormone	Liver	Glycogen breakdown
Acetylcholine	Pancreas; smooth muscle	Amylase secretion; contraction
Antigen	Mast cells	Histamine secretion
Thrombin	Blood platelets	Serotonin and platelet-derived growth factor secretion; platelet aggregation

ACTH, Adrenocorticotropic hormone; cAMP, Cyclic adenosine monophosphate.

Table 1-4	Major Types of Receptors and Signaling Transduction Pathways
Receptor and Signaling Pathway	Ligands
Receptors with Intrinsic Tyrosine Kinase Activity	
P13 kinase pathway, MAP-kinase pathway, IP$_3$ pathway	Signaling ligands include most growth factors (EGF, TGF-α, HGF, PDGF, VEGF, FGF), stem cell factor, insulin
Receptors Lacking Intrinsic Tyrosine Kinase Activity	
JAK/STAT pathway	Several cytokines including IL-2, IL-3, others; interferons α, β, and γ; erythropoietin; G-CSF; growth hormone; and prolactin
G-Protein–Coupled Receptors	
cAMP pathway	ADH, serotonin, histamine, epinephrine, norepinephrine, calcitonin, glucagon, parathyroid hormone, corticotropin, rhodopsin, and many drugs
Steroid Hormone Receptors	
Includes steroid hormone receptors as well as a group called *peroxisome proliferator-activated receptors (PPARs)*	Many steroid hormones, thyroid hormone, vitamin D, and retinoids

ADH, Antidiuretic hormone; cAMP, cyclic adenosine monophosphate; EGF, epidermal growth factor; FGF, fibroblast growth factor; G-CSF, granulocyte colony-stimulating factor; HGF, hepatocyte growth factor; IL-2, IL-3, interleukin-2 and interleukin-3; IP$_3$, inositol triphosphate; JAK/STAT, Janus kinase-signal transducers and activators of transcription; MAP-kinase, mitogen activated protein kinase; PDGF, platelet-derived growth factor; TGF-α, transforming growth factor-alpha; VEGF, vascular endothelial growth factor.

molecule, such as ATP. The energy stored in ATP can be used in a variety of energy-requiring reactions and in the process is generally converted to adenosine diphosphate (ADP) and inorganic phosphate (Pi). The energy available as a result of this reaction is about 7 kcal/mol of ATP. In addition to its use in synthesis (anabolism) of organic molecules, ATP is used by the cell for muscle contraction and active transport of molecules across cellular membranes. The function of ATP is not only to *store* energy but also to *transfer* it from one molecule to another. Energy is stored by molecules of carbohydrate, lipid, and protein, which, when catabolized, transfer energy to ATP.

Food and Production of Cellular Energy

The process of catabolism of the proteins, lipids, and polysaccharides found in food can be divided into three phases (Figure 1-22). In phase 1, large molecules are broken down into their smaller subunits—proteins into amino acids, polysaccharides into simple sugars, and fats into fatty acids and glycerol. These processes are called **digestion** and occur outside the cell by the action of secreted enzymes.

In phase 2 the small molecules enter cells and are further broken down in the cytoplasm. Most of the sugars are converted into pyruvate. Pyruvate then enters mitochondria and is converted to the acetyl groups of acetyl coenzyme A (acetyl CoA). Acetyl CoA, like ATP, releases energy when it is hydrolyzed. The most important part of phase 2 is the lysis (splitting) of glucose, known as **glycolysis** (Figure 1-23). Glycolysis produces a net of two molecules of ATP per glucose molecule through the process of **oxidation,** or the removal and transfer of a pair of electrons. This process, often called **oxidative cellular metabolism,** involves 10 biochemical reactions. In reactions 1 through 5, glucose is converted to two, three-carbon aldehyde (glyceraldehyde-3-phosphate [G3P]), which requires energy in the form of ATP. The next five reactions convert G3P molecules into pyruvate molecules and generate four molecules of ATP for each two molecules of G3P. In addition, two molecules of nicotinamide adenine dinucleotide (NAD) are further oxidized to produce four more molecules of ATP. After subtracting two molecules of ATP to drive the reactions, the net yield is six ATP molecules for each molecule of glucose.

Phase 3 occurs when the acetyl group of acetyl CoA is completely degraded to CO_2 and H_2O. It is in this final phase that most of the ATP is generated. Phase 3 begins with the **citric acid cycle** (also called the **Krebs cycle** or the **tricarboxylic acid cycle**) and ends with oxidative phosphorylation. The citric acid cycle accounts for approximately two thirds of the total oxidation of carbon compounds in most cells. Its major end products are CO_2 and two dinucleotides, reduced NADH, and the reduced form of flavin adenine dinucleotide

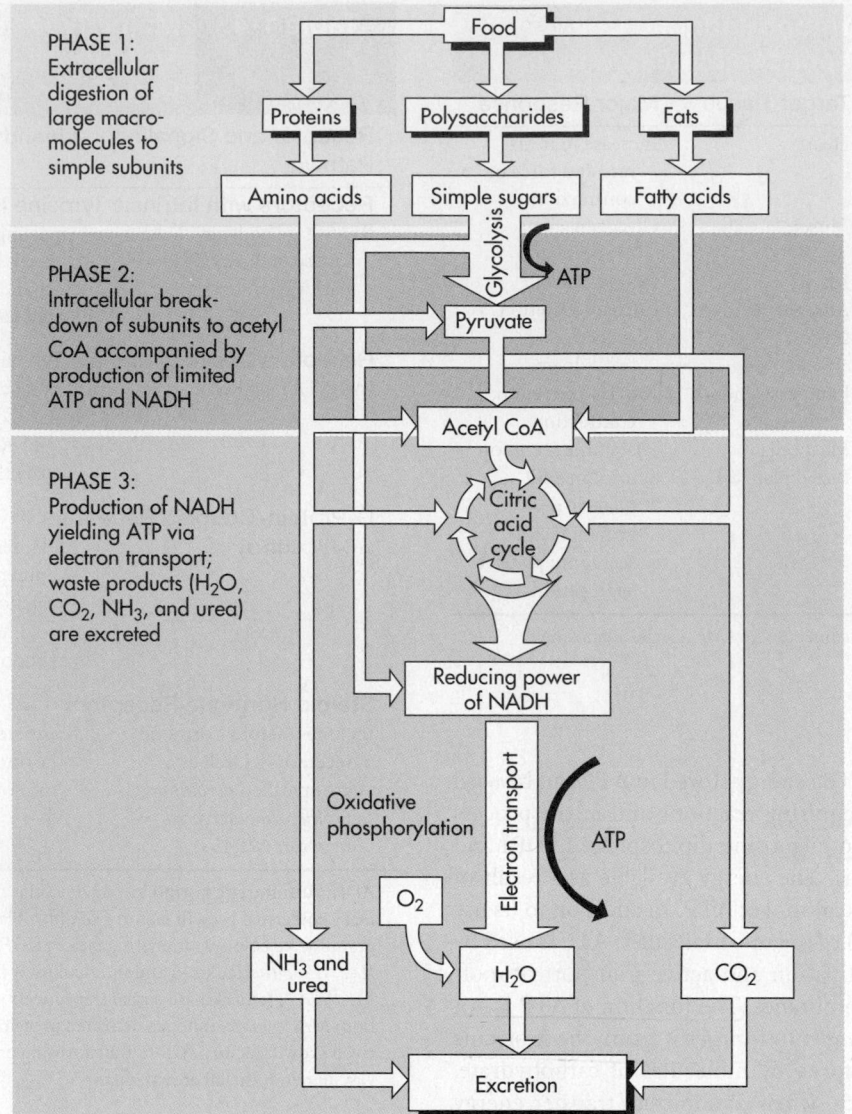

PHASE 1:
Extracellular
digestion of
large macro-
molecules to
simple subunits

PHASE 2:
Intracellular break-
down of subunits to acetyl
CoA accompanied by
production of limited
ATP and NADH

PHASE 3:
Production of NADH
yielding ATP via
electron transport;
waste products (H_2O,
CO_2, NH_3, and urea)
are excreted

Figure 1-22 Three phases of catabolism, which leads from food to waste products. These reactions produce ATP, which is used to drive other processes in the cell.

($FADH_2$), which transfer their electrons into the electron-transport chain.

Oxidative Phosphorylation

Oxidative phosphorylation occurs in the mitochondria and is the mechanism by which the energy produced from carbohydrates, fats, and proteins is transferred to ATP. During the breakdown (catabolism) of foods, many of the reactions involve the removal of electrons from various intermediates. These reactions generally require a coenzyme (a nonprotein carrier molecule), such as nicotinamide adenine dinucleotide (NAD), to transfer the electrons and thus are called **transfer reactions.**

In oxidative phosphorylation, molecules of NAD and flavin adenine dinucleotide (FAD) transfer electrons they have gained from the oxidation of substrates to molecular oxygen,

O_2. The electrons from reduced NAD and FAD, NADH and $FADH_2$, are transferred to a series of carrier molecules (the **electron-transport chain**) on the inner surfaces of the mitochondria with the release of hydrogen ions. Some of the carrier molecules are a group of brightly colored iron-containing proteins known as **cytochromes** that accept a pair of electrons. After passing through a sequence of different cytochromes, these electrons are eventually combined with molecular oxygen. If oxygen is not available to the electron-transport chain, ATP will not be formed by the mitochondria. Instead, an anaerobic (without oxygen) metabolic pathway synthesizes ATP. This process, called *substrate phosphorylation,* or **anaerobic glycolysis,** does not take place in the mitochondria and is linked to the breakdown (glycolysis) of carbohydrate (Figure 1-24).

Because glycolysis occurs in the cytoplasm of the cell, it provides energy for cells that lack mitochondria. However, as

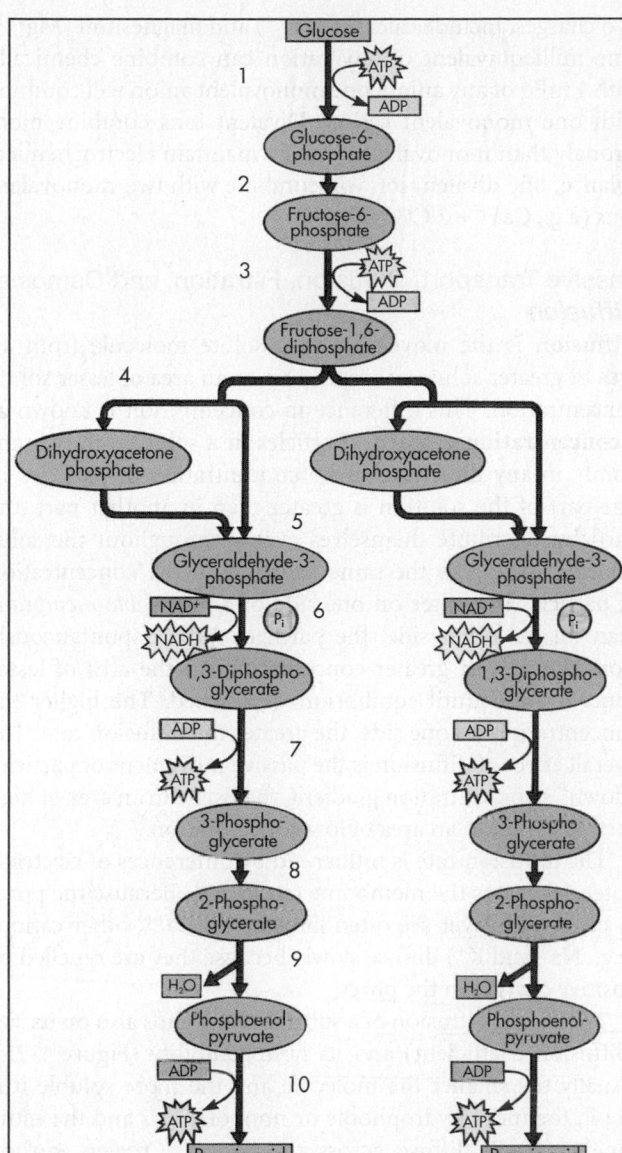

Figure 1-23 Glycolysis. Each of the numbered reactions is catalyzed by a different enzyme. At step 4, a six-carbon sugar is broken down to give two three-carbon sugars, so that the number of molecules at every step after this is doubled. Reactions 5 and 6 are the reactions responsible for the net synthesis of adenosine triphosphate (ATP) and reduced nicotinamide adenine dinucleotide (NADH) molecules. (Modified from Thibodeau GA, Patton KT: *Anatomy & physiology,* ed 6, St Louis, 2007, Mosby.)

noted, glycolysis also provides energy to the cell when oxygen delivery is insufficient or delayed (e.g., with strenuous exercise). The reactions in anaerobic glycolysis involve the conversion of glucose to pyruvic acid (pyruvate) with the simultaneous production of ATP. With the glycolysis of one molecule of glucose, two ATP molecules and two molecules of pyruvate are liberated. If oxygen is present, the two molecules of pyruvate move into the mitochondria, where they enter the citric acid cycle. If oxygen is absent, pyruvate is converted to lactic acid, which is released into the extracellular fluid (see Figure 1-24). The conversion of pyruvic acid to lactic acid is

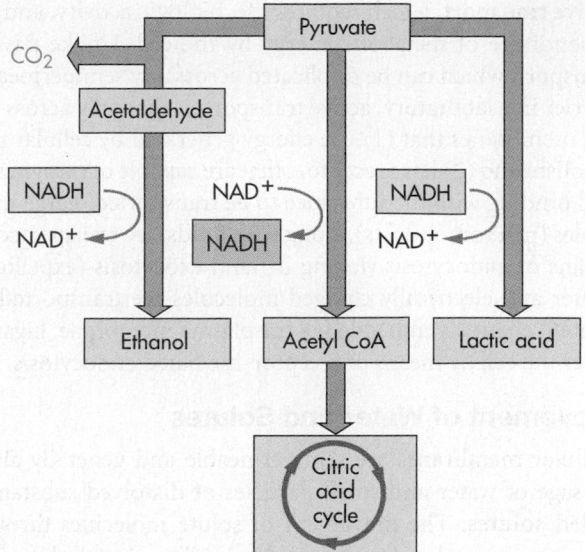

Figure 1-24 What happens to pyruvate, the product of glycolysis? In the presence of oxygen, pyruvate is oxidized to acetyl coenzyme A (CoA) and enters the citric acid cycle. In the absence of oxygen, pyruvate instead is reduced, accepting the electrons extracted during glycolysis and carried by reduced nicotinamide adenine dinucleotide (NADH). When pyruvate is reduced directly, as it is in muscle, the product is lactic acid. When CO_2 is first removed from pyruvate and the remainder reduced, as it is in yeasts, the product is ethanol.

reversible; therefore, once oxygen is restored, lactic acid is quickly converted back to either pyruvic acid or glucose. The anaerobic generation of ATP from glucose, through the reactions of glycolysis, is not as efficient as the aerobic generation of ATP. The addition of an oxygen-requiring stage to the catabolic process (stage 3) provides cells with a much more powerful method for extracting energy from food molecules.

MEMBRANE TRANSPORT: CELLULAR INTAKE AND OUTPUT

Cells continually take in nutrients, fluids, and chemical messengers from the extracellular environment and expel metabolites or the products of metabolism and end products of lysosomal digestion. Intake and output, or transport, occur by different mechanisms, depending on the characteristics of the substance to be transported. Water and small electrically uncharged molecules move easily through pores in the plasma membrane's lipid bilayer. This process, called **passive transport**, will occur naturally through any semipermeable barrier. It is driven by osmosis, hydrostatic pressure, and diffusion, all of which depend on the laws of physics and do not require life. The process is passive in that it does not require any expenditure of energy by the cell.

Other molecules cannot be driven across the plasma membrane solely by forces of diffusion, hydrostatic pressure, or osmosis because they are too large or are ligands that have bound with receptors on the cell's plasma membrane. Some of these molecules are moved into the cell by mechanisms of

active transport, which requires life, biologic activity, and the expenditure of metabolic energy by the cell. Unlike passive transport, which can be duplicated across any semipermeable barrier in a laboratory, active transport occurs only across living membranes that (1) use energy generated by cellular metabolism and (2) have receptors that are capable of recognizing and binding with the substance to be transported. Large molecules (macromolecules), along with fluids, are transported by means of endocytosis (taking in) and exocytosis (expelling). Water and electrically charged molecules are transported by protein channels embedded in the plasma membrane. Ligands enter the cell by means of receptor-mediated endocytosis.

Movement of Water and Solutes

Cellular membranes are semipermeable and generally allow passage of water and small particles of dissolved substances called **solutes.** The movement of solute molecules through membranes is related to their size, solubility, electrical properties, and concentration on either side of the membrane. Small lipid-soluble particles, such as oxygen, carbon dioxide, and urea, can readily pass through the lipid bilayers of the plasma membrane. Larger, water-soluble particles may pass through pores in the membranes. Although large protein molecules, such as albumin and globulin, pass through membranes by endocytosis, they influence the movement of water by exerting an osmotic effect (see p. 27).

Body fluids are composed of two types of solutes: **electrolytes,** which are electrically charged and dissociate into constituent **ions** when placed in solution; and nonelectrolytes, such as glucose, urea, and creatinine, which do not dissociate. Electrolytes account for approximately 95% of the solute molecules in body water. Electrolytes exhibit **polarity** by orienting themselves toward the positive or negative pole. Ions with a positive charge are known as **cations** and migrate toward the negative pole, or cathode, if an electrical current is passed through the electrolyte solution. **Anions** carry a negative charge and migrate toward the positive pole, or anode, in the presence of electrical current. Anions and cations are located in both the intracellular fluid (ICF) and extracellular fluid (ECF) compartments, although concentration of particular ions varies depending on their location. (Fluid and electrolyte balance between body compartments is discussed in Chapter 3.) For example, Na^+ is the predominant extracellular cation, and K^+ is the principal intracellular cation. The difference in ICF and ECF concentrations of these ions is important to the transmission of electrical impulses across the plasma membranes of nerve and muscle cells.

Electrolytes are measured in milliequivalents per liter (mEq/L) or milligrams per deciliter (mg/dl). Milliequivalents per liter indicate the number of electrical charges per unit volume of fluid. The term *milliequivalent* thus indicates the chemical-combining activity of an ion, which depends on the electrical charge, or valence, of its ions. In abbreviations, valence is indicated by the number of plus or minus signs. Monovalent ions, or ions with one charge, include sodium (Na^+), chloride (Cl^-), and potassium (K^+). Divalent ions, which have two charges, include calcium (Ca^{++}) and magnesium (Mg^{++}). One milliequivalent of any cation can combine chemically with 1 mEq of any anion: one monovalent anion will combine with one monovalent cation. Divalent ions combine more strongly than monovalent ions. To maintain electrochemical balance, one divalent ion will combine with two monovalent ions (e.g., $Ca^{++} + 2\ Cl^- = CaCl_2$).

Passive Transport: Diffusion, Filtration, and Osmosis
Diffusion

Diffusion is the movement of a solute molecule from an area of greater solute concentration to an area of lesser solute concentration. This difference in concentration is known as a **concentration gradient.** Particles in a solution move randomly in any direction. If the concentration of particles in one part of the solution is greater than in another part, the particles distribute themselves evenly throughout the solution. According to the same principle, if the concentration of particles is greater on one side of a *permeable membrane* than on the other side, the particles diffuse spontaneously from the area of greater concentration to the area of lesser concentration until equilibrium is reached. The higher the concentration on one side, the greater the diffusion rate. The overall effect of diffusion is the passive movement of particles "down" a concentration gradient, that is, from an area of high concentration to an area of low concentration.

The diffusion rate is influenced by differences of electrical potential across the membrane (see p. 33). Because the pores in the lipid bilayer are often linked with Ca^{++}, other cations (e.g., Na^+ and K^+) diffuse slowly because they are repelled by positive charges in the pores.

The rate of diffusion of a substance depends also on its size (diffusion coefficient) and its lipid solubility (Figure 1-25). Usually the smaller the molecule and the more soluble it is in oil, the more hydrophobic or nonpolar it is and the more rapidly it will diffuse across the bilayer. Oxygen, carbon dioxide, and the steroid hormones are all examples of nonpolar molecules. Water-soluble substances, such as sugars and inorganic ions, diffuse very slowly, whereas uncharged lipophilic ("lipid-loving") molecules, such as fatty acids and steroids, diffuse rapidly. Ions and other polar molecules generally diffuse across cellular membranes more slowly than lipid-soluble substances.

Water readily diffuses through biologic membranes because water molecules are small and uncharged. Although the mechanism is not known with certainty, the dipolar structure of water allows it to cross rapidly the regions of the bilayer containing the lipid head groups. Lipid head groups constitute the two outer regions of the lipid bilayer.

Filtration: Hydrostatic Pressure

Filtration is the movement of water and solutes through a membrane because of a greater pushing pressure (force) on one side of the membrane than on the other side. **Hydrostatic pressure** is the mechanical force of water pushing against cellular membranes. In the vascular system, hydrostatic pressure is the *blood pressure* generated in vessels by the contraction of

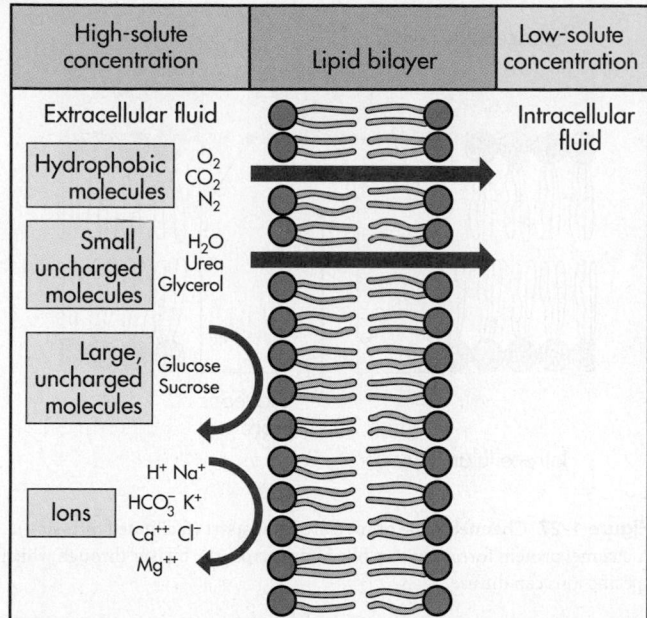

Figure 1-25 Passive diffusion of solute molecules across plasma membrane. Oxygen, nitrogen, water, urea, glycerol, and carbon dioxide can diffuse readily down the concentration gradient. Macromolecules are too large to diffuse through pores in the plasma membrane. Ions may be repelled if the pores contain substances with identical charges. If the pores are lined with cations, for example, other cations will have difficulty diffusing because the positive charges will repel one another. Diffusion can still occur, but it occurs more slowly.

the heart. Blood reaching the capillary bed has a hydrostatic pressure of 25 to 30 mmHg, which is sufficient force to push water across the thin capillary membranes into the interstitial space. Hydrostatic pressure is partially balanced by osmotic pressure, whereby water moving *out* of the capillaries is partially balanced by osmotic forces that tend to *pull* water *into* the capillaries. Water that is not osmotically attracted back into the capillaries moves into the lymph system (see discussion of Starling forces in Chapter 3).

Osmosis

Osmosis is the movement of water "down" a concentration gradient, that is, across a semipermeable membrane from a region of higher water concentration to a lower water concentration. For osmosis to occur, the membrane must be more permeable to water than to solutes and the concentration of solutes must be greater so that water moves more easily. Osmosis is directly related to both hydrostatic pressure and solute concentration but *not* to particle size or weight. For example, particles of the plasma protein albumin are small but more concentrated in body fluids than the larger and heavier particles of globulin. Therefore, albumin exerts a greater osmotic force than globulin.

Osmolality controls distribution and movement of water between body compartments. The terms *osmolality* and *osmolarity* are often used interchangeably in reference to osmotic activity, but they define different measurements. **Osmolality** is a measure of the number of milliosmoles per kilogram of water, or the concentration of molecules per *weight* of water.

Osmolarity is a measure of the number of milliosmoles per liter of solution, or the concentration of molecules per *volume* of solution. When solute is added to water, the volume is expanded and includes the original liter of water plus the volume occupied by the solute particles. In measuring osmolarity, the volume of water is therefore reduced by an amount equal to the volume of added solute.

In solutions that contain only dissociable substances, such as Na^+ and Cl^-, the difference between the two measurements is negligible. In considering all the different solutes in plasma (e.g., proteins, glucose, lipids), however, the difference between osmolality and osmolarity becomes more significant. In plasma, less of the plasma weight is water and the overall concentration of particles is therefore greater. The osmolality will be greater than the osmolarity because of the smaller proportion of water. Osmolality is thus the preferred measure of osmotic activity in clinical assessment of individuals.

The normal osmolality of body fluids is 280 to 294 mOsm/kg (milliosmoles per kilogram). The osmolality of intracellular and extracellular fluid tends to equalize and so provides a measure of body fluid concentration and thus the body's hydration status (see Chapter 3). Hydration is also affected by hydrostatic pressure because the movement of water by osmosis can be opposed by an equal amount of hydrostatic pressure. The amount of hydrostatic pressure required to oppose the osmotic movement of water is called the **osmotic pressure** of the solution. Factors that determine osmotic pressure are the type and thickness of the plasma membrane, the size of the molecules, the concentration of molecules or the concentration gradient, and the solubility of molecules within the membrane. Examples of movement of water in relation to hydrostatic and osmotic forces occur in the glomerulus in the kidney (see Chapter 35) and in the capillaries of the microcirculation (see Chapter 29).

Effective osmolality is sustained osmotic activity and depends on the concentration of solutes remaining on one side of a permeable membrane. If the solutes penetrate the membrane and equilibrate with the solution on the other side of the membrane, the osmotic effect will be diminished or lost. For example, urea is a small solute that readily diffuses across cellular membranes. Solutions containing urea rapidly lose their effective osmolality because they rapidly equilibrate. Solutes too large to pass through the membrane thus sustain an effective osmolality, meaning that they enhance osmotic activity. Plasma proteins are examples of molecules that provide effective osmolality because they normally do not cross cellular membranes.

Plasma proteins also influence osmolality because they have a negative charge. The principle by which the plasma protein charge influences osmolality is known as *Gibbs-Donnan equilibrium*, and it affects the distribution of ions across cellular membranes. Gibbs-Donnan equilibrium occurs when fluid in one compartment contains small diffusible ions such as Na^+ and Cl^-, together with large, nondiffusible charged particles, such as plasma proteins. Because the body tends to maintain an electrical equilibrium, the nondiffusible protein molecules cause asymmetry in the distribution of

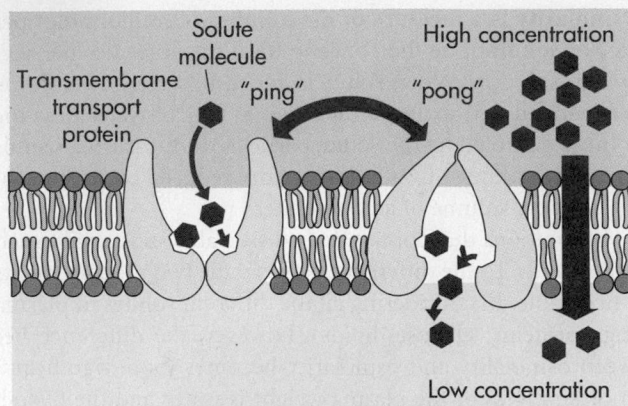

Figure 1-26 Conformational-change model of mediated transport (facilitated diffusion). The transporter protein has two states, "ping" and "pong." In the ping state, sites for molecules of a specific solute are exposed on the outside of the bilayer. In the pong state, the sites are exposed to the inner side of the bilayer.

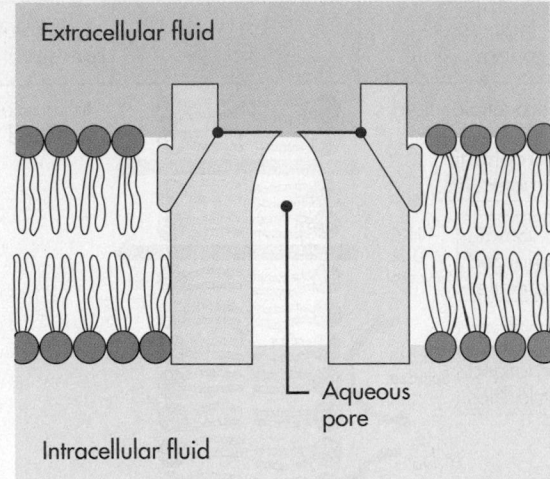

Figure 1-27 Channel mode of mediated transport (facilitated diffusion). A channel protein forms a water-filled pore across the bilayer through which specific ions can diffuse.

small ions. Anions such as Cl⁻ are thus driven out of the cell or plasma, and cations such as Na⁺ are attracted. The protein-containing compartment will maintain a state of electroneutrality, but the osmolality will be higher. The overall osmotic effect of colloids, such as plasma proteins, is called the **oncotic pressure,** or **colloid osmotic pressure.**

Tonicity describes the effective osmolality of a solution. (The terms *osmolality* and *tonicity* may be used interchangeably; also see Chapter 3.) Solutions, then, have relative degrees of tonicity. An **isotonic solution** (or isoosmotic solution) has the same osmolality or concentration of particles (285 mOsm/kg) as the ICF or ECF. Diarrhea, for example, is loss of isoosmotic fluid from the gastrointestinal tract. As a result, ECF volume decreases but there is no change in ECF osmolarity. Examples of isotonic solutions include 5% dextrose in water and normal (0.9%) saline solution. A **hypotonic solution** has a lower concentration and is thus more dilute than body fluids. Water is a hypotonic solution. Consequently, water is osmotically pulled into the cells, causing them to swell or burst. A **hypertonic solution** has a concentration of more than 285 to 294 mOsm/kg. An example of a hypertonic solution is 3% saline solution. Water can be pulled out of the cells by a hypertonic solution, so the cells shrink. The concept of tonicity is important when correcting water and solute imbalances by administering different types of replacement solutions.

Mediated and Active Transport
Mediated Transport
Mediated transport (passive and active) involves integral or transmembrane proteins with receptors having a high degree of specificity for the substance being transported. Inorganic anions and cations (e.g., Na⁺, K⁺, Ca⁺⁺, Cl⁻, HCO₃⁻) and charged and uncharged organic compounds (e.g., amino acids, sugars) require specific transport systems to facilitate movement through different cellular membranes. Rates at which substances are moved by mediated transport

mechanisms have often been measured, yet the specific membrane proteins involved have not been identified. Mediated transport is much faster than simple diffusion.

A **transport protein** (carrier protein) is a transmembrane or integral protein that binds with and transfers a specific solute molecule across the lipid bilayer. (Proteins are discussed on p. 11.) Each transport protein, or transporter, has receptors for a specific solute. When the transporter is saturated—that is, when all receptor sites are occupied by solute molecules—the rate of transport is maximal. Solute binding can be blocked by **competitive inhibitors** that compete for the same receptor site and may or may not be transported by the transport protein. Noncompetitive inhibitors bind elsewhere but can alter the structure of the transporter.

The transporter protein is a multipass transmembrane protein; that is, its polypeptide chain crosses the lipid bilayer multiple times. This chain forms a continuous pathway enabling solutes to pass across the membrane without coming into direct contact with the hydrophobic interior of the lipid bilayer (Figure 1-26). (Transmembrane proteins are illustrated in Figure 1-13.)

Another mechanism of mediated transport is the channel protein. The protein transporter creates a water-filled pore or channel across the bilayer through which specific ions can diffuse. These channels are sometimes called *ion channels,* and because they are permeable mainly to K⁺, they are also called K⁺ *leak channels* (Figure 1-27). The channel is controlled by a gate mechanism that determines which receptor-bound solutes can move into the channel that is created after receptor-solute contact. Binding stimulates conformational changes in the protein transporter that move the solute through the channel short distances at a time until it reaches the other side of the membrane. Ion channels are responsible for the electrical excitability of nerve and muscle cells and play a critical role in the membrane potential.

Mediated transport systems can move solute molecules singly or two at a time. Two molecules can be moved

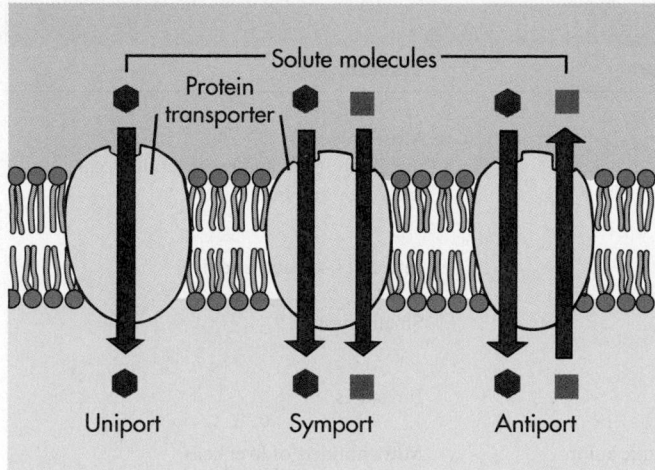

Figure 1-28 Mediated transport. Simultaneous movement of a single solute molecule in one direction (uniport), of two different solute molecules in one direction (symport), and of two different solute molecules in opposite directions (antiport).

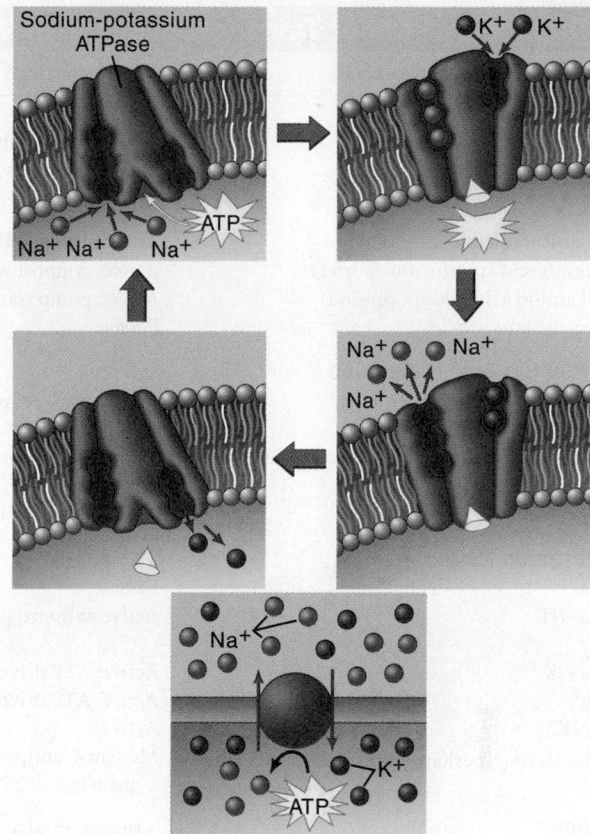

Figure 1-29 Active transport and the sodium-potassium pump. Three Na$^+$ ions bind to sodium-binding sites on the carrier's inner face. At the same time an energy-containing adenosine triphosphate (ATP) molecule produced by the cell's mitochondria binds to the carrier. The ATP breaks apart, transferring its stored energy to the carrier. The carrier then changes shape, releases the three Na$^+$ ions to the outside of the cell, and attracts two K$^+$ ions to its potassium-binding sites. The carrier then returns to its original shape, releasing the two K$^+$ ions and the remnant of the ATP molecule to the inside of the cell. The carrier is now ready for another pumping cycle. (From Thibodeau GA, Patton KT: *Anatomy & physiology*, ed 6, St Louis, 2007, Mosby.)

simultaneously in one direction (a process called **symport**) or in opposite directions (called **antiport**), or a single molecule can be moved in one direction (called **uniport**) (Figure 1-28).

In **passive mediated transport**, also called **facilitated diffusion**, the protein transporter moves solute molecules through cellular membranes without expending metabolic energy. The direction of movement is the same as in simple diffusion—down the concentration gradient. Perhaps the most widely referred to passive transport system is that for glucose in erythrocytes (red blood cells). Glucose is transported by a uniport mechanism and demonstrates saturation kinetics; that is, the transport system is saturated when all the glucose-specific receptors on the membrane are occupied and operating at their maximal capacity.

The anions Cl$^-$ and bicarbonate HCO$_3^-$ also undergo passive mediated transport in the erythrocyte. This antiport mechanism allows Cl$^-$ movement in one direction and simultaneous HCO$_3^-$ movement in the opposite direction. The directions of movement depend on the concentration gradients of the ions across the membrane.

In **active mediated transport**, also called **active transport**, the protein transporter moves molecules against, or up, the concentration gradient. Unlike passive mediated transport, active mediated transport requires the expenditure of energy. Many active mediated transport systems, or pumps, have ATP as their primary energy source, but not all. Some use the electrochemical gradient of Na$^+$ across the membrane (Figure 1-29). Energy in the form of ATP, however, is required for activation of the Na$^+$ gradient.

A "carrier" mechanism in the plasma membrane mediates the transport of ions, such as Na$^+$, K$^+$, H$^+$, Cl$^-$, and HCO$_3^-$, and of nutrients, such as glucose and amino acids. Energy supplied by ATP is required to pump ions against a concentration gradient. The best-known pump is the Na$^+$-K$^+$–dependent ATPase pump. It continuously regulates the

cells' volume by controlling leaks through pores or protein channels and maintains the ionic concentration gradient necessary for cellular excitation and membrane conductivity (see p. 33). The maintenance of intracellular K$^+$ concentrations is also required for enzyme activity, including that of enzymes involved in protein synthesis.

Active Transport of Na$^+$ and K$^+$

The active transport system for Na$^+$ and K$^+$ is found in virtually all mammalian cells. The Na$^+$-K$^+$ antiport system (Na$^+$ moving out of and K$^+$ moving into the cell) uses the direct energy of ATP to move these cations. The transporter protein is an enzyme, ATPase. ATPase has a requirement for Na$^+$, K$^+$, and Mg^{++} ions. The concentration of ATPase in plasma membranes is directly related to Na$^+$-K$^+$ transport activity. Approximately 60% to 70% of the ATP synthesized by cells, especially muscle and nerve cells, is used to maintain the Na$^+$-K$^+$ transport system. Excitable tissues (e.g., muscle and nerve tissues) have a high concentration of Na$^+$-K$^+$ ATPase, as

Table 1-5   Major Transport Systems in Mammalian Cells

Substance Transported	Mechanism of Transport	Tissues
Sugars		
Glucose	Passive protein channel	Most tissues
Fructose	Active: symport with Na$^+$	Small intestines and renal tubular cells
	Passive	Intestines and liver
Amino Acids	Coupled channels	
Amino acid specific transporters	Active: symport with Na$^+$	Intestines, kidney, and liver
All amino acids except proline	Active: group translocation	Liver
Specific amino acids	Passive	Small intestine
Other Organic Molecules		
Cholic acid, deoxycholic acid, and taurocholic acid	Active: symport with Na$^+$	Intestines
Organic anions, e.g., malate, α-ketoglutarate, glutamate	Antiport with counter-organic anion	Mitochondria of liver cells
ATP-ADP	Antiport transport of nucleotides; can be active	Mitochondria of liver cells
Inorganic Ions		
Na$^+$	Passive	Distal renal tubular cells
Na+/H$^+$	Active antiport, proton pump	Proximal renal tubular cells and small intestines
Na+/K$^+$	Active: ATP driven, protein channel	Plasma membrane of most cells
Ca^{++}	Active: ATP driven, antiport with Na$^+$	All cells, antiporter in red cells
H$^+$/K$^+$	Active	Parietal cells of gastric cells secreting H$^+$
Cl$^-$/ HCO$_3^-$ (perhaps other anions)	Mediated: antiport (anion transporter–band 3 protein)	Erythrocytes and many other cells
Water	Osmosis passive	All tissues

Data from Alberts B et al: *Molecular biology of the cell,* ed 4, New York, 2001, Garland; Devlin TM, editor: *Textbook of biochemistry: with clinical correlations,* ed 3, New York, 1992, Wiley; Raven PH, Johnson GB: *Understanding biology,* ed 3, Dubuque, IA, 1995, Brown.

NOTE: The known transport systems are listed here; others have been proposed. Most transport systems have been studied in only a few tissues, and their sites of activity may be more limited than indicated.

ADP, Adenosine diphosphate; *ATP,* adenosine triphosphate.

do other tissues that transport significant amounts of Na$^+$, for example, kidneys and salivary glands. For every ATP molecule hydrolyzed, three molecules of Na$^+$ are transported out of the cell, whereas only two molecules of K$^+$ move into the cell. The process leads to an electrical potential and is called *electrogenic,* with the inside of the cell more negative than the outside. The exact mechanism for transport of Na$^+$ and K$^+$ across the membrane is uncertain. One proposal is that ATPase induces the transporter protein to undergo several conformational changes, causing Na$^+$ and K$^+$ to move short distances (see Figure 1-29). The conformational change creates a lowering affinity for Na$^+$ and K$^+$ to the ATPase transporter, resulting in the release of the cations after transport.

The sarcoplasmic reticulum of heart muscle and skeletal muscle has an ATP-dependent Ca^{++} active transport system that regulates the Ca^{++} levels in the cell's cytoplasm, which in turn regulates muscle contraction and relaxation cycles (see Chapter 29). The Ca^{++} transport system depends on ATPase activity and is similar to that of Na$^+$-K$^+$ ATPase.

The transport of sugars and amino acids across the plasma membrane depends on the simultaneous movement (symport) of Na$^+$ or Na$^+$-dependent transport (see Figure 1-28). Na$^+$-dependent symport occurs primarily in the plasma membrane of epithelial cells of the kidney tubules and intestines. The transport of glucose is not directly dependent on the hydrolysis of ATP; however, the Na$^+$ gradient is ATP dependent, and thus ATP is indirectly involved in glucose transport.

The epithelial cells that line the intestines depend on Na$^+$ to transport various amino acids. Similarly, the uptake of Cl$^-$ by the small intestine depends on Na$^+$ symport and antiport mechanisms for the secretion of Ca^{++} from the cell.

Table 1-5 summarizes the major mechanisms of transport through pores and protein transporters in the plasma membranes. Many disease states are caused or manifested by loss of these membrane transport systems.

Transport by Vesicle Formation

Endocytosis and Exocytosis

The active transport mechanisms by which the cells move large proteins, polynucleotides, or polysaccharides (macromolecules) across the plasma membrane are very different from those that mediate small solute and ion transport. Transport of macromolecules involves the sequential formation and fusion of membrane-bound vesicles.

In **endocytosis** a section of the plasma membrane enfolds substances from outside the cell, invaginates (folds inward), and separates from the plasma membrane, forming

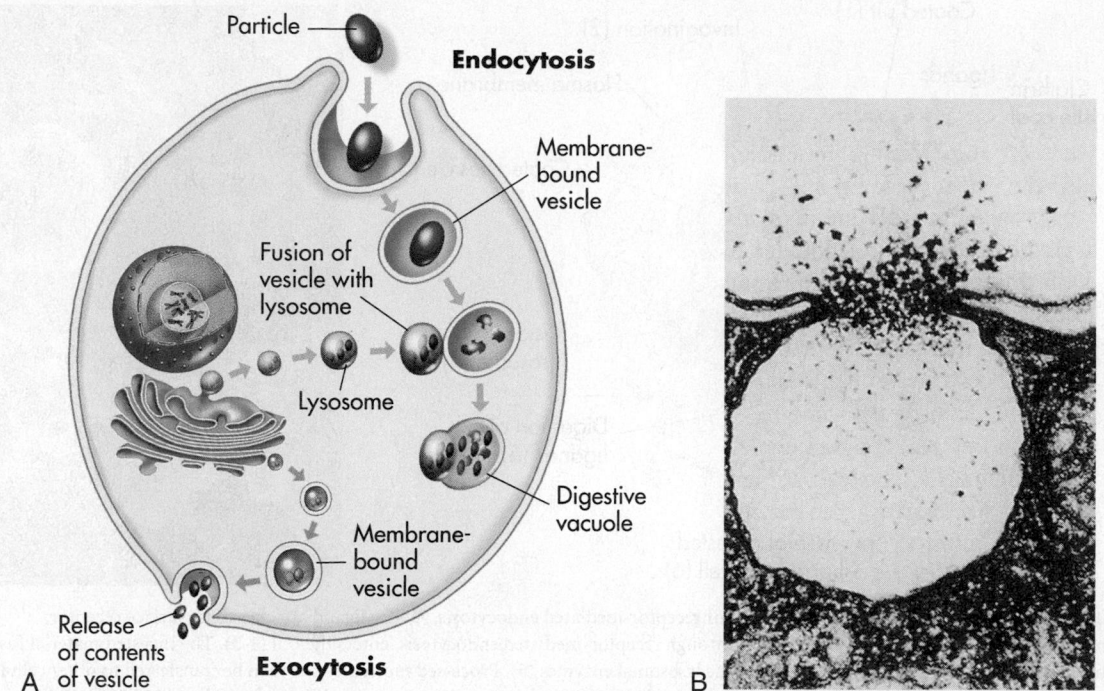

Figure 1-30 Endocytosis and exocytosis. **A,** Endocytosis and fusion with lysosome and exocytosis. **B,** Electron micrograph of exocytosis. (**B** from Raven PH, Johnson GB: *Biology,* ed 5, New York, 1999, McGraw-Hill.)

a vesicle that moves into the inside of the cell (Figure 1-30, *A*). Two types of endocytosis are designated based on the size of the vesicle formed. **Pinocytosis** (cell drinking) involves the ingestion of fluids and solute molecules through formation of small vesicles, and **phagocytosis** (cell eating) involves the ingestion of large particles, such as bacteria, through formation of large vesicles (also called *vacuoles*).

Because most cells continually ingest fluid and solutes by pinocytosis, the terms *pinocytosis* and *endocytosis* are often used interchangeably. In pinocytosis the vesicle containing fluids, solutes, or both fuses with a lysosome, and lysosomal enzymes digest them for use by the cell. In phagocytosis the large molecular substances are engulfed by the plasma membrane and enter the cell so that they can be isolated and destroyed by lysosomal enzymes (see Chapter 6). Substances that are not degraded by lysosomes are isolated in residual bodies and released by the cell by exocytosis. Both pinocytosis and phagocytosis require metabolic energy and often involve binding of the substance with plasma membrane receptors before membrane invagination and fusion with lysosomes in the cell.

In eukaryotic cells, secretion of macromolecules almost always occurs by exocytosis (see Figure 1-30, *B*). **Exocytosis** is the discharge or secretion of material from the intracellular vesicles at the cell surface. For example, to secrete macromolecules of insulin across plasma membranes, insulin-producing cells store and package insulin molecules in intracellular vesicles, which fuse with the plasma membrane and open to the extracellular space, or matrix, releasing the insulin. Not all secreted substances are secreted into the extracellular matrix. Some adhere to the plasma membrane

and are thought to replace segments of the membrane lost through endocytosis or diffuse into the blood to nourish or signal other cells. Recent findings suggest membrane lipids may be a regulator of exocytosis.[19] Exocytosis has two main functions: (1) replacement of portions of the plasma membrane that have been removed by endocytosis, and (2) release of molecules synthesized by the cells into the extracellular matrix.

Receptor-Mediated Endocytosis

Ligand binding to *some* plasma membrane receptors leads to clustering, aggregation, and immobilization of the receptors in specialized areas of the membrane called **coated pits** (Figure 1-31). The pits, which are coated with bristle-like structures (clathrin), deepen and enfold (invaginate), internalizing ligand-receptor complexes and forming a coated vesicle. The clathrin coat or bristles are thought to be responsible for trapping membrane receptors in coated pits. This internalization process, called **receptor-mediated endocytosis (ligand internalization),** is rapid and enables the cell to ingest large amounts of specific ligands without ingesting large volumes of extracellular fluid. Inside the cell, the ingested material is processed by lysosomal enzymes.

The cellular uptake of cholesterol, for example, depends on receptor-mediated endocytosis. Cholesterol (a ligand) is carried primarily in blood plasma attached to an acceptor protein. This cholesterol-protein complex is called *low-density lipoprotein (LDL).* LDL receptors, which bind LDL to the plasma membrane, control the rate at which cholesterol is transferred into the cell (see Chapter 30).

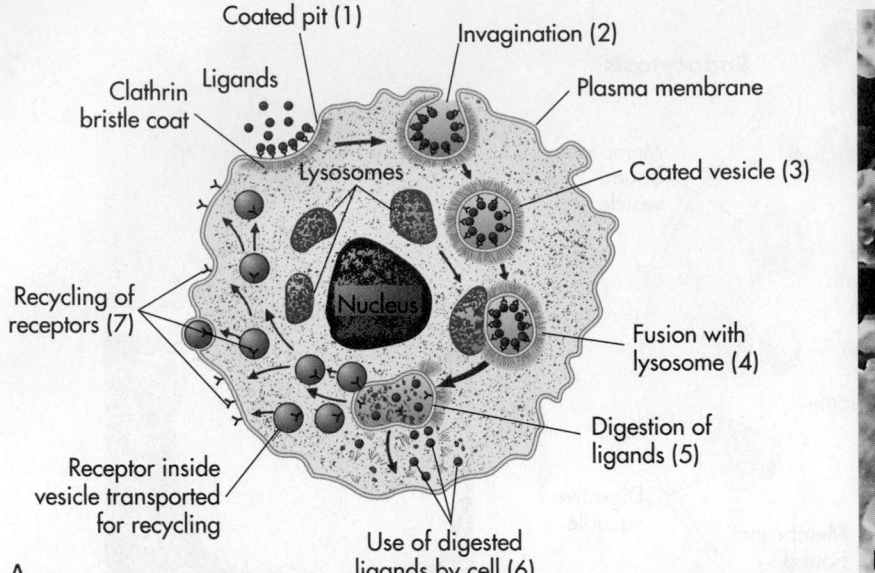

Figure 1-31 Ligand internalization by means of receptor-mediated endocytosis. **A,** The ligand attaches to its surface receptor (through the bristle coat or clathrin coat) and, through receptor-mediated endocytosis, enters the cell (1-3). The ingested material fuses with a lysosome (4) and is processed by hydrolytic lysosomal enzymes (5). Processed molecules can then be transferred to other cellular components (6 or **recycled** 7). **B,** Electron micrograph of a coated pit showing different sizes of filaments of the (×382,000). (**B** from Erlandsen SL, Magney JE: *Color atlas of histology,* St Louis, 1992, Mosby.)

Caveolae

The outer surface of the plasma membrane is dimpled with tiny flask-shaped pits (cavelike) called caveolae. Caveolae are also called **microdomains. Caveolae** are cholesterol-rich domains where protein caveolin are involved in several processes, including clathrin-independent endocytosis, the regulation and transport of cellular cholesterol, and cell communication.[20] Many proteins, including a variety of receptors, cluster in these tiny chambers. Some of these receptors appear to be important in a new form of cellular uptake of small molecules and ions, for example, the cellular uptake of the B vitamin folic acid. When folic acid binds with its receptors, which are concentrated in the caveolae, the extracellular openings of these tiny caves close off. Closure of the caveolar indentation facilitates the movement of this vitamin across the caveolar membrane into the cytoplasm. Cellular uptake through the opening and closing of caveolae is called **potocytosis.** Potocytosis is thought to be an uptake mechanism for a variety of small molecules and ions, in contrast to receptor-mediated endocytosis, which transports selected large molecules into the cell. In potocytosis the caveolae are thought to *remain* attached to the plasma membrane and not form a membrane-enclosed vesicle such as occurs with endocytosis.

Caveolae not only function as uptake vesicles but also are important sites for signal transduction, a tedious process in which extracellular chemical messages or *signals* are communicated to the cell's interior for execution (see p. 18). For example, strong evidence exists that plasma membrane estrogen receptors localize in caveolae and crosstalk with estradiol causing several intracellular functions, including cell growth and survival, migration, and new blood vessel formation.[21-23]

Movement of Electrical Impulses: Membrane Potentials

All body cells are electrically polarized, with the inside of the cell more negatively charged than the outside. The difference in electrical charge, or voltage, is known as the **resting membrane potential** and is about −70 to −85 millivolts. The difference in voltage across the plasma membrane is a result of the differences in ionic composition of ICF and ECF. Sodium ions have a greater concentration in the ECF, and potassium ions have a greater concentration in the ICF. The concentration difference is maintained by the active transport of Na^+ and K^+ (the sodium-potassium pump), which transports sodium outward and potassium inward (Figure 1-32). Because the resting plasma membrane is more permeable to K^+ than to Na^+, K^+ can diffuse easily from its area of higher concentration in the ICF to its area of lower concentration in the ECF. Because Na^+ and K^+ are both cations, the net result is an excess of anions inside the cell, resulting in the resting membrane potential.

Nerve and muscle cells are excitable and can change their resting membrane potential in response to electrochemical stimuli. Changes in resting membrane potential convey messages from cell to cell. When a nerve or muscle cell receives a stimulus that exceeds the membrane threshold value, there is a rapid change in the resting membrane potential known as the **action potential.** The action potential carries signals along the nerve or muscle cell and conveys information from one cell to another. (Nerve impulses are described in Chapter 14.) When a resting cell is stimulated through voltage-regulated channels, the cell membranes become more permeable to sodium. There is a net movement of sodium into the cell, and the membrane potential decreases, or "moves forward," from

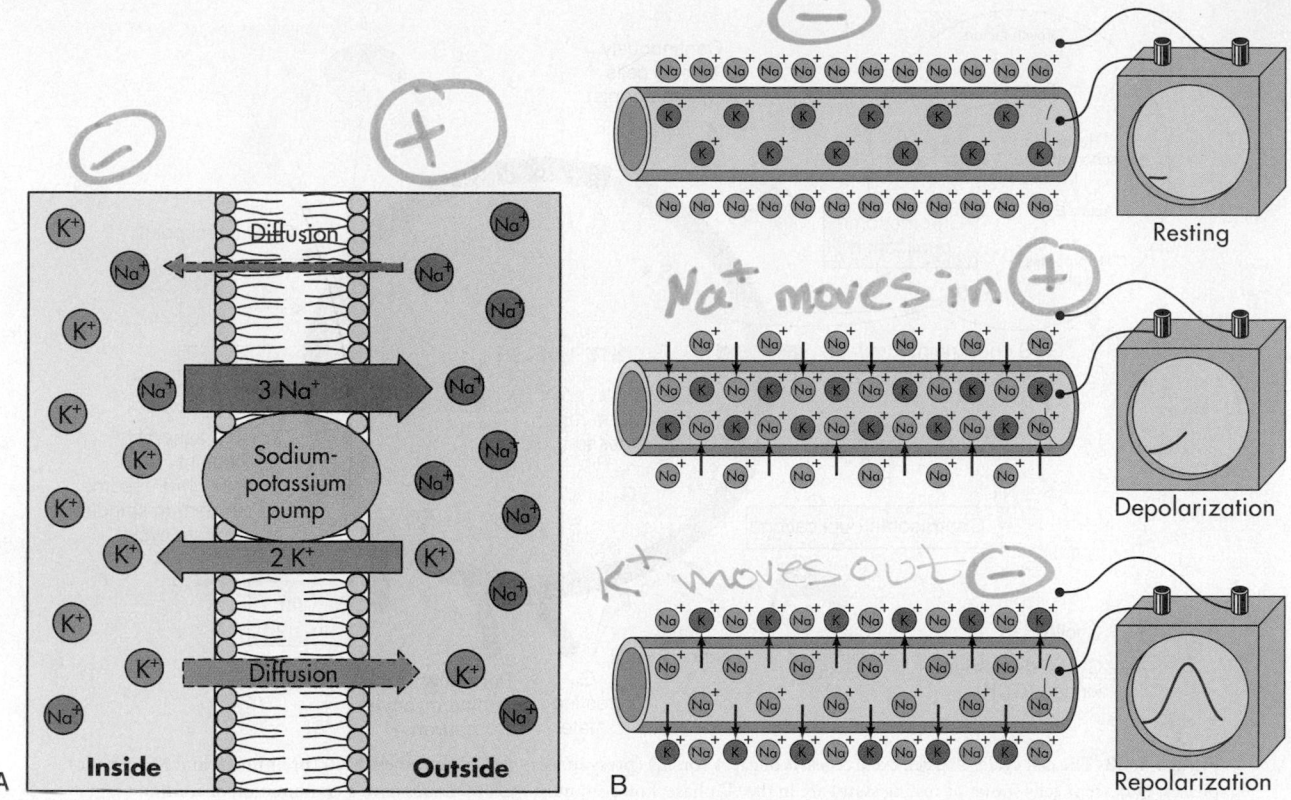

Figure 1-32 Sodium-potassium pump and propagation of an action potential. **A,** Concentration difference of Na+ and K+ intracellularly and extracellularly. The direction of active transport by the sodium-potassium pump is also shown. **B,** Top diagram represents the polarized state of a neuronal membrane when at rest. The lower diagrams represent changes in sodium and potassium membrane permeabilities with depolarization and repolarization. (From Thibodeau GA, Patton KT: *Anatomy & physiology*, ed 6, St Louis, 2007, Mosby.)

a negative value (in millivolts) to zero. This decrease is known as **depolarization.** The depolarized cell is more positively charged, and its polarity is neutralized.

To generate an action potential and the resulting depolarization, a critical value known as the **threshold potential** must be reached. Generally this occurs when the cell has depolarized by 15 to 20 millivolts. When the threshold is reached, the cell will continue to depolarize with no further stimulation. The sodium gates open, and sodium rushes into the cell, causing the membrane potential to reduce to zero and then become positive (depolarization). The rapid reversal in polarity results in the action potential.

During **repolarization** the negative polarity of the resting membrane potential is reestablished. As the voltage-gated sodium channels begin to close, voltage-gated potassium channels open. Membrane permeability to sodium decreases, and potassium permeability increases, with an outward movement of potassium ions. The sodium gates close, and with the outward movement of potassium, the membrane potential becomes more negative. The Na+-K+ pump then returns the membrane to the resting potential by pumping potassium back into the cell and sodium out of the cell.

During most of the action potential, the plasma membrane cannot respond to an additional stimulus. This time is known as the **absolute refractory period** and is related to changes in permeability to sodium. During the latter phase of the action potential, when permeability to potassium increases, a stronger-than-normal stimulus can evoke an action potential known as the **relative refractory period.**

When the membrane potential is more negative than normal, the cell is in a *hyperpolarized* (less excitable) state. A larger-than-normal stimulus is then required to reach the threshold potential and generate an action potential. When the membrane potential is more positive than normal, the cell is in a *hypopolarized* (more excitable than normal) state, and a smaller-than-normal stimulus is required to reach the threshold potential. Changes in the intracellular and extracellular concentration of ions or a change in membrane permeability can cause these alterations in membrane excitability.

CELLULAR REPRODUCTION: THE CELL CYCLE

Human cells are subject to wear and tear, and most do not last for the lifetime of the individual. In almost all tissues, new cells are created as fast as old ones die. Cellular reproduction is therefore necessary for the maintenance of life. Reproduction of gametes (sperm and egg cells) occurs through a process called *meiosis,* described in Chapter 4. The reproduction, or division, of other body cells (somatic cells) involves two sequential phases: **mitosis,** or nuclear division, and **cytokinesis,** or cytoplasmic division. These two phases occur in

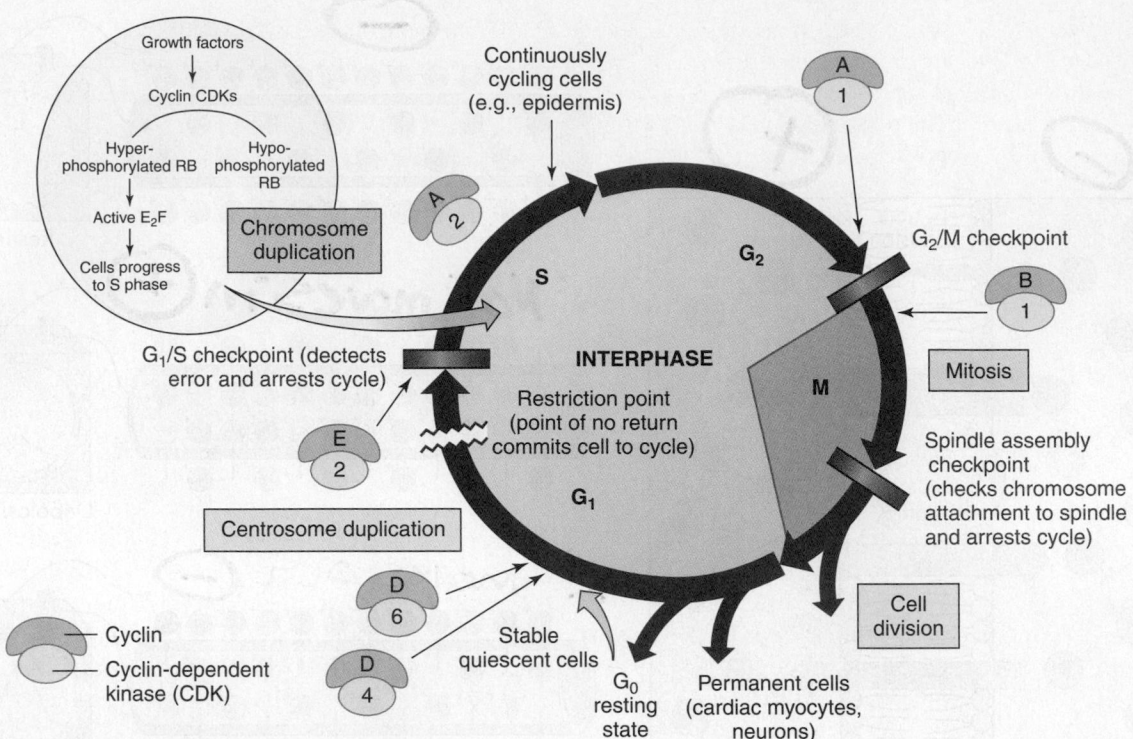

Figure 1-33 The cell cycle. The cell cycle consists of gap 1 (or G_1) (presynthesis), S (DNA synthesis), G_2 (premitotic) and M (mitotic) phases. Quiescent cells (quiet or resting state) are in the G_0 phase; however, most mature tissues have a combination of continuously dividing cells, terminally differentiated cells, stems cells, and some quiescent cells that infrequently enter the cell cycle. Continuously dividing cells replace those that are destroyed (e.g., epithelia of the oral cavity, skin). Quiescent or stable tissues exhibit a low level of replication; however, these cells can undergo rapid division in response to stimuli such as growth factors (e.g., EGF, TGF-α). Cyclins increase and activate cyclin-dependent protein kinase (CDK) complexes at the G_1/S restriction point, causing phosphorylation (addition of phosphate group) of the molecular ON-OFF switch, the retinoblastoma susceptibility protein (RB). In its hypophosphorylated state, RB prevents cells from replicating by forming a tight inactive complex with the transcription factor E_2F. Phosphorylation of RB eliminates the "brakes" to cell cycle progression and promotes cell replication. The orderly progression of cells through the phases of the cell cycle is regulated by cyclins, CDKs, and their inhibitors. Cyclin levels rise and fall (thus the name cyclin) during the cell cycle, periodically activating CDKs. Unless CDKs are bound to cyclins, they have no protein kinase activity. Cyclin-CDK complexes trigger cell cycle events. Each complex phosphorylates a different set of proteins that then promote advancement to the next phase (G_1, S, G_2, M, G_0). After completion of the task, cyclin levels decline rapidly. The activity of cyclin-CDK complexes is regulated by CDK inhibitors including Cip/Kip and the 7NK4/ARF.

close succession, with cytokinesis beginning toward the end of mitosis. Before a cell can divide, however, it must double its mass and duplicate all its contents. Most of the work of preparing for division occurs during the growth phase, called **interphase.** The alternation between mitosis and interphase in all tissues with cellular turnover is known as the **cell cycle.**

Most of the early work on the cell cycle was limited to microscopic observation of mitosis and cytokinesis. Interphase was considered the "resting stage" of the cell. With recent technologic advances a considerable amount has been learned about the interphase part of the cell cycle. During interphase many important processes are taking place as the cell produces DNA, RNA, protein, lipids, and other substances, and each pair of **chromosomes** (paired organelles that carry genetic information) makes exact copies of themselves.

The four designated phases of the cell cycle are (1) the G_1 phase (G = gap), which is the period between the M phase and the start of DNA synthesis; (2) the S phase (S = synthesis), in which DNA is synthesized in the cell nucleus; (3) the G_2

phase, in which RNA and protein synthesis occurs, the period between the completion of DNA synthesis and the next phase (M); and (4) the M phase (M = mitosis), which includes both nuclear and cytoplasmic division (Figure 1-33).

Phases of Mitosis and Cytokinesis

Interphase (the G_1, S, and G_2 phases) is the longest phase of the cell cycle. During interphase the chromatin consists of very long, slender rods that are jumbled together in the nucleus. Late in interphase, strands of **chromatin** (the substance that gives the nucleus its granular appearance) begin to coil, causing them to shorten and thicken.

The M phase of the cell cycle, mitosis and cytokinesis, begins with **prophase,** the first appearance of chromosomes. As the phase proceeds, each chromosome is seen as two identical halves called **chromatids,** which lie together and are attached at some point by a spindle attachment site called a **centromere.** (The two chromatids of each chromosome, which are genetically identical, are sometimes called *sister chromatids.*)

The nuclear membrane, which surrounds the nucleus, disappears. Spindle fibers are microtubules formed in the cytoplasm. **Spindle fibers** radiate from two centrioles located at opposite poles of the cell. The role of the spindle fibers is to pull the chromosomes to opposite sides of the cell.

During **metaphase,** the next phase of mitosis and cytokinesis, the spindle fibers begin to pull the centromeres of the chromosomes. The centromeres become aligned in the middle of the spindle, which is called the **equatorial plate** (or **metaphase plate**) of the cell. In this stage chromosomes are easiest to observe microscopically because they are highly condensed and arranged in a relatively organized fashion in the two-dimensional equatorial plate.

Anaphase begins when the centromeres split and the sister chromatids are pulled apart. The spindle fibers shorten, causing the sister chromatids to be pulled, centromere first, toward opposite sides of the cell. When the sister chromatids are separated, each is considered to be a chromosome. Thus the cell has 92 chromosomes during this stage. By the end of anaphase, 46 chromosomes are lying at each side of the cell. Barring mitotic errors, each of the two groups of 46 chromosomes is identical to the original 46 chromosomes present at the start of the cell cycle.

During **telophase,** the final stage, a new nuclear membrane is formed around each group of 46 chromosomes, the spindle fibers disappear, and the chromosomes begin to uncoil. Cytokinesis causes the cytoplasm to divide into roughly equal parts during this phase. At the end of telophase, two identical diploid cells, called *daughter cells,* have been formed from the original cell.

Rates of Cellular Division

Although the complete cell cycle lasts 12 to 24 hours, about 1 hour is generally required for the four stages of mitosis and cytokinesis. All types of cells undergo mitosis during formation of the embryo, but many adult cells, such as nerve cells, lens cells of the eye, and muscle cells, lose their ability to replicate and divide. The cells of other tissues, particularly epithelial cells (e.g., of the intestine, lung, skin), divide continuously and rapidly, completing the entire cell cycle in less than 10 hours.

The difference between cells that divide slowly and cells that divide rapidly is the length of time spent in the G_1 phase of the cell cycle. Some cells that divide very slowly remain in the G_1 phase for days or even years. Once the S phase begins, however, progression through mitosis takes a relatively constant amount of time. Once a cell has progressed out of the G_1 phase, there is no turning back; it is committed to completing the S, G_2, and M phases. Times associated with the four successive phases differ.

The mechanisms that control cell division depend on "social control genes" and protein growth factors. Individual cells are members of a complex cellular society in which survival of the *entire organism* is key and not survival or proliferation of just the *individual cells.* To grow and divide, a cell must receive specific positive signals from other cells. Many of these signals *are* protein growth factors that act by overriding intracellular negative controls that block progress of the cell cycle.[1]

When a need arises for new cells, as in repair of injured cells, previously nondividing cells must be rapidly triggered to reenter the cell cycle. With continual wear and tear, the cell birth rate and the cell death rate must be kept in balance. Therefore, cell-division controls must govern this balance. Protein growth factors governing the proliferation of different cell types and genes involved in the social control of cell division are currently being identified.[1]

The best model for understanding disruption of cell division and study of these so-called social control genes is tumor biology. Current emphasis in locating and identifying these genes is to study tumor cells that have presumably originated because of mutations to these genes, or proto-oncogenes. Proto-oncogenes are thought to encode key components of the normal system of social controls of cell division[1]; that is, the mechanisms by which signals from a cell's neighbors can impel it to divide, differentiate, or die. Some proto-oncogenes code for growth factors, some for growth factor receptors, some for intracellular regulatory proteins that are involved in cell adhesion, and some for proteins that help relay signals for cell division to the cell nucleus.[1] Although more than 50 proto-oncogenes have been identified, many more are yet to be discovered (see Chapter 11).

Growth Factors

Growth factors, also called *cytokines*, are peptides that transmit signals within and between cells. They have a major role in the regulation of tissue growth and development (Table 1-6). Having nutrients is not enough for a cell to proliferate; it must also receive stimulatory chemical signals (growth factors) from other cells, usually its neighbors. These signals act to overcome intracellular braking mechanisms that tend to restrain cell growth and block progress through the cell cycle.

Different types of cells require different factors; for example, **platelet-derived growth factor** (**PDGF**) stimulates the production of connective tissue cells. Table 1-6 summarizes the most significant growth factors. Cells that respond to a particular growth factor have specific receptors for the growth factor in their plasma membrane. Recent evidence shows that some growth factors are also regulators of other cell processes, such as cellular differentiation. In addition to growth factors that stimulate cellular processes, there are factors that inhibit functions; these factors are not well understood. Cells that are starved of growth factors come to a halt after mitosis and enter the **arrested,** or **G_0, state** of the cell cycle[1] (see p. 33 for cell cycle).

TISSUES

The body is made up of four levels of organization: cells, tissues, organs, and systems. Cells of common structure and function are organized into **tissues,** of which there are four primary types: *muscle, neural, epithelial,* and *connective* tissue.

Tissue Formation

To form tissues cells must exhibit intercellular recognition and adhesion. Specialized cells are thought to form a tissue in one of two ways. First and simplest is mitosis of one or

Table 1-6	Examples of Growth Factors and Their Actions
Growth Factor	**Physiologic Actions**
Platelet-derived growth factor (PDGF)	Stimulates proliferation of connective tissue cells and neuroglial cells
Epidermal growth factor (EGF)	Stimulates proliferation of epidermal cells and other cell types
Insulin-like growth factor I (IGF-I)	Collaborates with PDGF and EGF; stimulates proliferation of fat cells and connective tissue cells
Insulin-like growth factor II (IGF-II)	Collaborates with PDGF and EGF; stimulates proliferation of fat cells and connective tissue cells
Transforming growth factor β (TGF-β)	Stimulates or inhibits response of most cells to other growth factors; regulates differentiation of some cell types (e.g., cartilage)
Fibroblast growth factor (FGF)	Stimulates proliferation of fibroblasts, endothelial cells, myoblasts, and other cell types
Interleukin-2 (IL-2)	Stimulates proliferation of T lymphocytes
Nerve growth factor (NGF)	Promotes axon growth and survival of sympathetic and some sensory and CNS neurons
Hematopoietic cell growth factors (IL-3, GM-CSF, M-CSF, G-CSF, erythropoietin)	See Chapter 25

CNS, Central nervous system; *CSF,* colony-stimulating factor; *G,* granulocyte; *GM,* granulocyte-macrophage; *M,* macrophage.

more **founder cells** (the most basic precursor cell). Founder cells are prevented from "wandering away" by macromolecules in the extracellular matrix and by adherence to one another at specialized junctions on their plasma membranes. Mitosis of founder cells forms, for example, epithelial cell sheets (Figure 1-34).

The second way in which specialized cells form tissues involves their migration to and subsequent assembly at the site of tissue formation. During embryonic development, for example, cells from the neural crest migrate to several different regions, where they differentiate and assemble into a variety of tissues, including those of the peripheral nervous system. Migrant cells are thought to arrive at the site of tissue formation through chemotaxis or contact guidance. **Chemotaxis** is movement along a chemical gradient caused by chemical attraction (see Chapter 6). Cells at the migrant cells' destination secrete a chemical, called *chemotactic factor,* that attracts specific migrant cells. **Contact guidance** is movement along a pathway, or "pavement," in the extracellular matrix.[1]

Tissues are not randomly arranged into organs. No matter how tissue is formed, staying together in groups means that cells must recognize each other and remain distinct from the cells of surrounding tissues. Little is known about the mechanisms involved in these processes.

Types of Tissues

Epithelial Tissue

Epithelial tissue covers most internal and external surfaces of the body. Epithelial cells are closely joined and are attached to a basement membrane or lamina (extracellular matrix), which provides a supporting layer and separates the epithelium from underlying connective tissue (see Figure 1-14). Because of its variety of locations, epithelial tissue has several diverse functions, including protection, absorption, secretion, and excretion. For example, the epidermis provides a protective barrier between the host and the outside environment, and the linings of the internal body organs help absorb substances into the body, excrete waste products, and secrete substances into body cavities.

Epithelial cell surfaces differ according to their location and function. Epithelial cells that line body cavities and blood vessels are smooth, whereas other epithelial cells have tiny cytoplasmic projections called **microvilli** on their free surfaces. Microvilli considerably increase a cell's surface area and are found on cells whose main functions are absorption and secretion, such as the epithelial cells lining the digestive tract. **Cilia,** which are hairlike projections that propel mucus, pus, and dust particles out of the body, characterize cells lining the respiratory passages.

Epithelial tissue is classified in two ways: (1) according to the number and arrangement of cell layers, and (2) according to cell shape. Epithelium that is formed by a single layer of cells, all of which are in contact with the basement membrane, is called **simple epithelium. Stratified epithelium** has two or more layers of cells, and only the deepest layer is in contact with the basement membrane. Tissue that appears to consist of several cellular layers but is actually a single layer with all cells contacting the basement membrane is called **pseudostratified epithelium.**

Three basic cell shapes are found in epithelium: squamous, cuboidal, and columnar. **Squamous cells** are flat and thin; **cuboidal cells** are as high as they are wide and thus appear square in vertical sections; and **columnar cells** are taller than they are wide and appear rectangular in vertical sections. Overall classifications of epithelial tissue, which take into account both the number of cell layers and cell shape, are summarized in Table 1-7.

Connective Tissue

Connective tissue varies considerably in structure and function but is most common as the framework on which epithelial cells cluster to form organs. Other functions include binding various tissues and organs together, supporting them in their locations, and serving as storage sites for excess nutrients.

In contrast to epithelial tissue, connective tissue is characterized by an abundant extracellular matrix that surrounds few cells. The extracellular matrix is composed of ground substance and fibers. **Ground substance** is a homogeneous mass that varies in consistency from fluid to semisolid gel. Fibers are produced by connective tissue cells (fibroblasts) found within the ground substance. The three types of fibers are collagenous (white), elastic (yellow), and reticular. **Collagenous fibers** are formed of bundles of smaller fibers appearing as wavy bands

Mitosis

Founder cell

Mitosis

Recognition and adherence
at specialized cell junction

Basement membrane

Epithelial
cell
sheet

A

Migration

Chemotaxis

Chemotactic factor at site
of tissue formation

Specialized migrant cells

Contact guidance

Site of tissue
formation

Specialized
migrant
cells

Pathway in extracellular
matrix

Recognition, adherence, aggregation, and differentiation into tissue

Neural crest

Neural tube

B

Figure 1-34 **Tissue formation by mitosis and migration. A,** Tissue formation by mitosis. Founder cells are kept in place by extracellular matrix and recognition and adherence at cell junctions. **B,** Tissue formation by migration. Specialized cells are attracted to the site of tissue formation by chemotaxis or contact guidance; then they aggregate and differentiate into organized tissue.

Table 1-7	Some Types of Epithelial Tissue with Location and Function	
Type of Epithelial Tissue	**Location**	**Function**
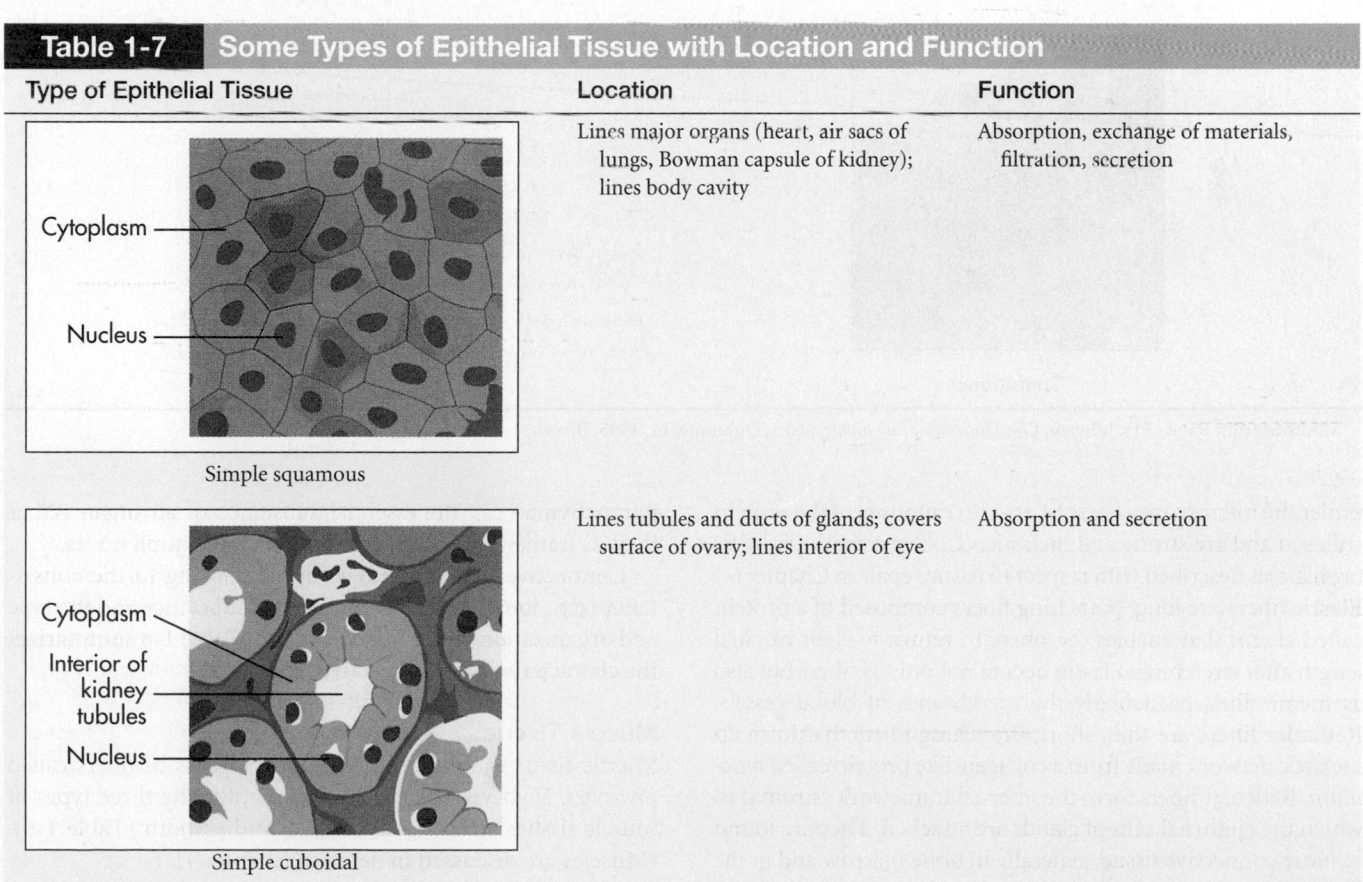 Cytoplasm — Nucleus — Simple squamous	Lines major organs (heart, air sacs of lungs, Bowman capsule of kidney); lines body cavity	Absorption, exchange of materials, filtration, secretion
Cytoplasm — Interior of kidney tubules — Nucleus — Simple cuboidal	Lines tubules and ducts of glands; covers surface of ovary; lines interior of eye	Absorption and secretion

Continued

Table 1-7   Some Types of Epithelial Tissue with Location and Function—cont'd

Type of Epithelial Tissue	Location	Function
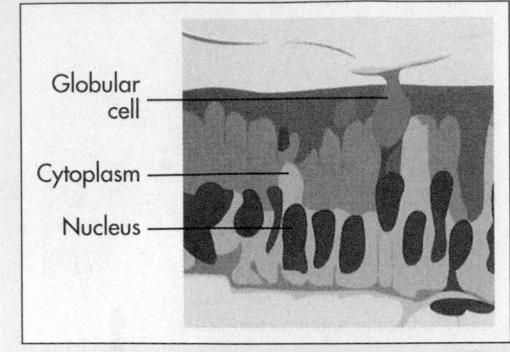 Simple columnar	Lines gastrointestinal tract	Secretion from special goblet cells of materials, absorption
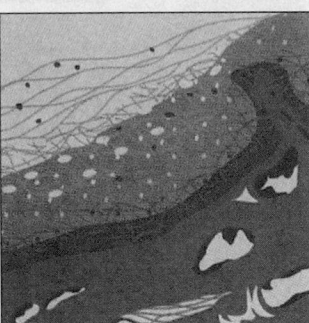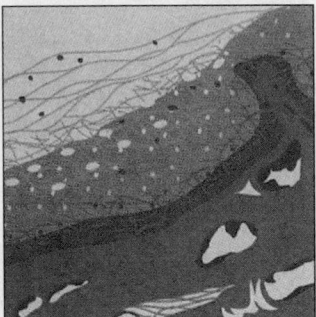 Stratified squamous	Lines interior of mouth, tongue, esophagus, vagina	Protection
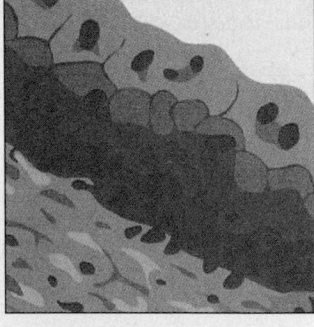 Transitional	Lines urinary bladder	Permits stretching

Labels in first image: Globular cell, Cytoplasm, Nucleus

Modified from Raven PH, Johnson GB: *Understanding biology,* ed 3, Dubuque, IA, 1995, Brown.

under the microscope. These fibers are composed of the protein collagen and are strong and inelastic. (Collagen synthesis by fibroblasts is described with respect to tissue repair in Chapter 6.) **Elastic fibers** are long, branching fibers composed of a protein called *elastin* that enables the fibers to return to their original length after stretching. Elastin occurs not only as fibers but also as membranes, particularly the membranes of blood vessels. **Reticular fibers** are thin, short, branching fibers that form an inelastic network made from a collagen-like protein called *reticulum*. Reticular fibers form the internal framework (stroma) to which the epithelial cells of glands are attached. They are found in loose connective tissue, generally in bone marrow and in the

parenchyma (i.e., the essential substance of an organ rather than its framework) of the liver, spleen, and lymph nodes.

Connective tissues are classified according to the consistency (e.g., loose, dense) of the ground substance and the type and organization of the fibers within it. Table 1-8 summarizes the characteristics of connective tissues.

Muscle Tissue

Muscle tissue is composed of long, thin cells or fibers called *myocytes*. Myocytes are highly contractile. The three types of muscle tissues are skeletal, cardiac, and smooth (Table 1-9). (Muscles are discussed in detail in Chapter 41.)

Table 1-8   Types of Connective Tissue with Location and Function

Type of Connective Tissue	Location	Function
 Loose connective tissue	Deep layers of skin, blood vessels, nerves, body organs	Support, elasticity
 Dense connective tissue	Tendons, ligaments	Attaches structures to one another; provides great strength
 Elastic connective tissue	Lungs, arteries, trachea, vocal chords	Provides elasticity
 Reticular connective tissue	Spleen, liver, lymph nodes	Provides internal scaffold for soft organs

Continued

Table 1-8	Types of Connective Tissue with Location and Function—cont'd

Type of Connective Tissue	Location	Function
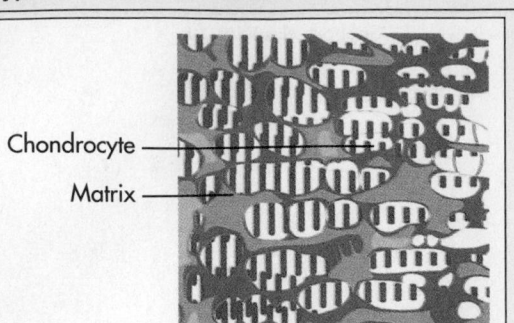 Cartilage	Ends of long bones; tip of nose; parts of larynx, trachea	Provides flexibility and support
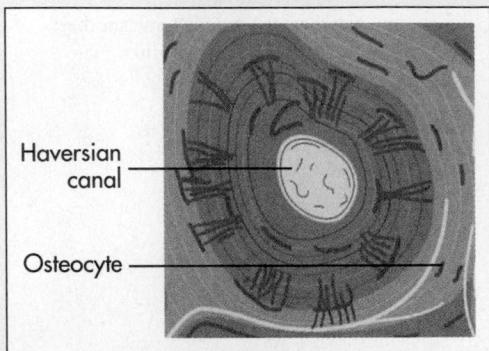 Bone	Bones	Protection, support, muscle attachment
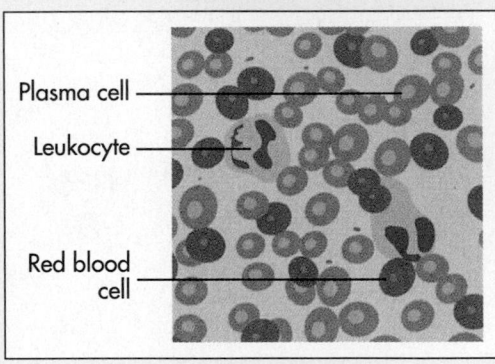 Vascular connective tissue	Within blood vessels	Transport oxygen and carbon dioxide; immune response; blood clotting
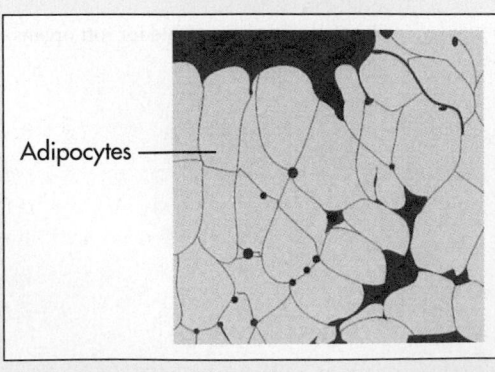 Adipose tissue	Deep layers of skin; surrounds heart and kidneys; padding around joints; paracrine hormones	Support, protection, heat conservation, energy source

Modified from Raven PH, Johnson GB: *Understanding biology,* ed 3, Dubuque, IA, 1995, Brown.

Table 1-9   Types of Muscle Tissue with Location and Function

Type of Muscle Tissue	Location	Function
Smooth muscle	Gastrointestinal tract, uterus, urinary bladder, blood vessels	Propulsion of materials
Cardiac muscle	Heart	Contraction
Skeletal muscle	Attached to bones	Movement

Modified from Raven PH, Johnson GB: *Understanding biology,* ed 3, Dubuque, IA, 1995, Brown.

Neural Tissue

Neural tissue is composed of highly specialized cells called *neurons,* which receive and transmit electrical impulses very rapidly across junctions called synapses. **Synapses** are points of functional contact between neurons. At synapses, impulses pass from neuron to neuron or from a neuron to a muscle cell as chemical messengers called *neurotransmitters* are released (see Chapter 14). The total number of neurons is fixed at birth, and replacement is impossible thereafter.

Different types of neurons have special characteristics that depend on their distribution and function within the nervous system. All neurons, however, are composed of the following parts: (1) a cell body, (2) a single axon, and (3) one or more dendrites (see Figure 14-1 on p. 444). The cell body contains special cytoplasmic structures, as well as microtubules, actin filaments, Golgi complex, lysosomes, and lipofuscin. The axons and dendrites can be very long. Generally, the axon conducts nerve impulses away from the cell body, and dendrites conduct nerve impulses toward the cell body. (Neuronal transmission is discussed in Chapter 14.)

SUMMARY REVIEW

Cellular Functions

1. Cells become specialized through the process of differentiation, or maturation.
2. The eight specialized cellular functions are movement, conductivity, metabolic absorption, secretion, excretion, respiration, reproduction, and communication.

Structure and Function of Cellular Components

1. The eukaryotic cell consists of three general components: the plasma membrane, the cytoplasm, and the intracellular organelles.
2. The nucleus is the largest membrane-bound organelle and is usually found in the cell's center. The chief functions of the nucleus are cell division and control of genetic information.
3. Cytoplasm, or the cytoplasmic matrix, is an aqueous solution (cytosol) that fills the space between the nucleus and the plasma membrane.
4. The organelles are suspended in the cytoplasm and are enclosed in biologic membranes.
5. The endoplasmic reticulum is a network of tubular channels (cisternae) that extend throughout the outer nuclear membrane. It specializes in the synthesis and transport of protein and lipid components of most of the organelles.
6. The Golgi complex is a network of smooth membranes and vesicles located near the nucleus. The Golgi complex is responsible for processing and packaging proteins into secretory vesicles that break away from the Golgi complex and migrate to a variety of intracellular and extracellular destinations, including the plasma membrane.
7. Lysosomes are saclike structures that originate from the Golgi complex and contain digestive enzymes. These enzymes are responsible for digesting most cellular substances down to their basic form, such as amino acids, fatty acids, and sugars.
8. Cellular injury leads to a release of the lysosomal enzymes, causing cellular self-digestion.
9. Peroxisomes are similar to lysosomes but contain several enzymes that either produce or use hydrogen peroxide.
10. Mitochondria contain the metabolic machinery necessary for cellular energy metabolism. The enzymes of the respiratory chain (electron transport chain), found in the inner membrane of the mitochondria, generate most of the cell's ATP.
11. Vaults are newly discovered ribonucleoproteins thought to function as cellular "trucks" carrying mRNA from the nucleus to the ribosomal sites of protein synthesis.
12. The cytoskeleton is the "bone and muscle" of the cell. The internal skeleton is composed of a network of protein filaments including microtubules and actin filaments (microfilaments).
13. The plasma membrane encloses the cell and, by controlling the movement of substances across it, exerts a powerful influence on metabolic pathways.
14. The plasma membrane is a bilayer of lipids (phospholipids, glycolipids) and cholesterol, which gives the membrane its structural integrity.
15. Membrane functions are determined largely by proteins. These functions include (a) recognition and binding units (receptors) for substances moving in and out of the cell; (b) pores or transport channels; (c) enzymes that drive active pumps; (d) cell surface markers, such as glycoproteins; (e) cell adhesion molecules; and (f) catalysts of chemical reactions.
16. The fluid mosaic model accounts for the fluidity of the lipid bilayer and the flexibility, self-sealing properties, and selective impermeability of the plasma membrane.
17. Cellular receptors are protein molecules on the plasma membrane, in the cytoplasm, or in the nucleus, capable of recognizing and binding smaller molecules, called *ligands*.
18. The dynamic nature of the fluid plasma membrane enables it to vary the number of receptors on its surface. The cell is therefore capable of "hiding" from injurious agents by altering receptor number and pattern.
19. The ligand-receptor complex initiates a series of protein interactions, causing adenylyl cyclase to catalyze the transformation of cellular ATP to messenger molecules that stimulate specific responses within the cell.

Cell-to-Cell Adhesions

1. Cell-to-cell adhesions are formed on plasma membranes, thereby allowing the formation of tissues and organs. Cells are held together by three different means: (a) the extracellular membrane, (b) cell adhesion molecules in the cell's plasma membrane, and (c) specialized cell junctions.
2. The extracellular matrix includes three types of protein fibers: collagen, elastin, and fibronectin. The matrix helps regulate cell growth and differentiation.
3. The three main types of cell junctions are desmosomes, tight junctions, and gap junctions.

Cellular Communication and Signal Transduction

1. Cells communicate in three ways: (a) they form protein channels (gap junctions); (b) they display receptors that affect intracellular processes or other cells in direct physical contact; and (c) they secrete signals for long-distance communication.
2. Primary modes of chemical signaling include hormonal, neurohormonal, paracrine, autocrine, and neurotransmitter.
3. Signal transduction involves signals or instructions from extracellular chemical messengers that are conveyed to the cell's interior for execution.
4. Signaling cascades, or relay chains, have several important functions, including physically transferring the signal around the cell, amplifying the signal, distributing the signal, and modulating the signal.
5. Two important second messenger pathways are cAMP and Ca^{++}.
6. G protein is an intermediary between the receptor and adenylyl cyclase.
7. Phospholipase C, an enzyme protein effector, is bound to the inner side of the membrane.

Cellular Metabolism

1. The chemical tasks of maintaining essential cellular functions are referred to as *cellular metabolism*. Anabolism is the energy-using process of metabolism, whereas catabolism is the energy-releasing process.
2. ATP functions as an energy-transferring molecule. Energy is stored by molecules of carbohydrate, lipid, and protein, which, when catabolized, transfer energy to ATP.
3. Oxidative phosphorylation occurs in the mitochondria and is the mechanism by which the energy produced from carbohydrates, fats, and proteins is transferred to ATP.

Membrane Transport: Cellular Intake and Output

1. Water and small, electrically uncharged molecules move through pores in the plasma membrane's lipid bilayer in the process called *passive transport*.
2. Passive transport does not require the expenditure of energy; rather, it is driven by the physical effects of osmosis, hydrostatic pressure, and diffusion.
3. Larger molecules and molecular complexes (e.g., ligand-receptor complexes) are moved into the cell by active transport, which requires expenditure of energy (by means of ATP) by the cell.
4. The largest molecules (macromolecules) and fluids are transported by the processes of endocytosis (ingestion) and exocytosis (expulsion).

5. Two types of solutes exist in body fluids: electrolytes and nonelectrolytes. Electrolytes are electrically charged and dissociate into constituent ions when placed in solution. Nonelectrolytes do not dissociate when placed in solution.

6. Diffusion is the passive movement of a solute from an area of higher solute concentration to an area of lower solute concentration.

7. Hydrostatic pressure is the mechanical force of water pushing against cellular membranes.

8. Osmosis is the movement of water across a semipermeable membrane from a region of lower solute concentration to a region of higher solute concentration.

9. The amount of hydrostatic pressure required to oppose the osmotic movement of water is called the *osmotic pressure* of the solution.

10. The overall osmotic effect of colloids, such as plasma proteins, is called the *oncotic pressure* or *colloid osmotic pressure.*

11. Mediated transport can be passive or active. Mediated transport includes the movement of two molecules simultaneously in one direction (symport), or in opposite directions (antiport), or the movement of a single molecule in one direction (uniport).

12. Passive mediated transport is also called *facilitated diffusion.* It does not require the expenditure of metabolic energy.

13. Active mediated transport requires metabolic energy (ATP) to move molecules against the concentration gradient.

14. Active transport also occurs by endocytosis, or vesicle formation, in which the substance to be transported is engulfed by a segment of the plasma membrane, forming a vesicle that moves into the cell.

15. Pinocytosis is a type of endocytosis in which fluids and solute molecules are ingested through formation of small vesicles.

16. Phagocytosis is a type of endocytosis in which large particles, such as bacteria, are ingested through formation of large vesicles, called *vacuoles.*

17. In receptor-mediated endocytosis, the plasma membrane receptors are clustered, along with bristle-like structures, in specialized areas called *coated pits.*

18. Endocytosis occurs when coated pits invaginate, internalizing ligand-receptor complexes in coated vesicles.

19. Inside the cell, material ingested by endocytosis is processed and digested by lysosomal enzymes.

20. Caveolae are tiny flask-shaped pits on the outer surface of the plasma membrane. Cellular uptake through the opening and closing of caveolae is called *potocytosis.*

21. All body cells are electrically polarized, with the inside of the cell more negatively charged than the outside. The difference in voltage across the plasma membrane is the resting membrane potential.

22. When an excitable (nerve or muscle) cell receives an electrochemical stimulus, cations enter the cell, causing a rapid change in the resting membrane potential known as the *action potential.* The action potential "moves" along the cell's plasma membrane and is transmitted to an adjacent cell. This is how electrochemical signals convey information from cell to cell.

Cellular Reproduction: The Cell Cycle

1. Cellular reproduction in body tissues involves mitosis (nuclear division) and cytokinesis (cytoplasmic division).

2. Only mature cells are capable of division. Maturation occurs during a stage of cellular life called *interphase* (growth phase).

3. The cell cycle is the reproductive process that begins after interphase in all tissues with cellular turnover. The four phases of the cell cycle are (a) the S phase, during which DNA synthesis takes place in the cell nucleus; (b) the G_2 phase, the period between the completion of DNA synthesis and the next phase (M); (c) the M phase, which involves both nuclear (mitotic) and cytoplasmic (cytokinetic) division; and (d) the G_1 phase (growth phase, or interphase), after which the cycle begins again.

4. The M phase (mitosis) involves four stages: prophase, metaphase, anaphase, and telophase.

5. The mechanisms that control cell division depend on "social control genes" and protein growth factors.

6. Cyclin-CDK complexes trigger cell cycle events.

Tissues

1. Cells of one or more types are organized into tissues, and different types of tissues compose organs. Organs are organized to function as tracts or systems.

2. Specialized cells are thought to form tissue by mitosis of one or more founder cells or by migration of founder cells and their subsequent assembly at the site of tissue formation.

3. The four basic types of tissues are epithelial, muscle, neural, and connective tissues.

4. Epithelial tissue covers most internal and external surfaces of the body. The functions of epithelial tissue include protection, absorption, secretion, and excretion.

5. Connective tissue binds various tissues and organs together, supporting them in their locations and serving as storage sites for excess nutrients.

6. Muscle tissue is composed of long, thin, highly contractile cells or fibers called *myocytes.* Muscle tissue that is attached to bones enables voluntary movement. Muscle tissues in internal organs enable involuntary movement, such as the heartbeat.

7. Neural tissue is composed of highly specialized cells called *neurons* that receive and transmit electric impulses very rapidly across junctions called *synapses.*

KEY TERMS

Absolute refractory period, 33
Actin filament (microfilament), 9
Action potential, 32
Active mediated transport (active transport), 26, 29
Active transport, 29
Amphipathic molecule, 11
Anabolism, 21
Anaerobic glycolysis, 24
Anaphase, 35

Anions, 26
Antiport, 29
Arrested (G_0) state, 35
Autocrine signaling, 18
Autodigestion, 6
Autolysosome (autophagosome), 6
Autophagy, 6
Basement membrane, 15
Catabolism, 21
Cation, 26

Caveolae, 32
Cell adhesion molecule (CAM), 12
Cell cycle, 34
Cell junction, 16
Cell-to-cell adhesion, 15
Cellular metabolism, 21
Cellular receptor, 13
Centriole, 9
Centromere, 34
Chemical synapse, 18

KEY TERMS—cont'd

Chemotaxis, 36
Chromatid, 34
Chromatin, 34
Chromosome, 34
Cilia, 36
Cisternae, 5
Citric acid cycle (Krebs cycle, tricarboxylic acid cycle), 23
Clathrin, 5
Coated pit, 31
Collagen, 16
Collagenous fiber, 36
Columnar cell, 36
Competitive inhibitor, 28
Concentration gradient, 26
Connexon, 18
Contact guidance, 36
Cristae, 7
Cuboidal cell, 36
Cyclic adenosine monophosphate (cyclic AMP, cAMP), 20
Cyclic guanosine monophosphate (cyclic GMP, cGMP), 20
Cytochrome, 24
Cytokinesis, 33
Cytoplasm, 2
Cytoplasmic matrix, 4
Cytoskeleton, 8
Cytosol, 4
Depolarization, 33
Desmosome, 16
Differentiation, 2
Diffusion, 26
Digestion, 23
Effective osmolality, 27
Elastic fiber, 38
Elastin, 16
Electrolyte, 26
Electron-transport chain, 24
Endocytosis, 30
Endoplasmic reticulum, 5
Equatorial plate (metaphase plate), 35
Eukaryote, 2
Exocytosis, 31
Extracellular matrix (basement membrane), 15
Fibroblast, 16
Fibronectin, 16
Filtration, 26
First messenger, 20
Founder cell, 36
G protein, 20

Gap junction, 18
Gating, 18
Glycolysis, 23
Glycoprotein, 12
Golgi complex (Golgi apparatus), 5
Ground substance, 36
Growth factor, 35
Guanosine diphosphate (GDP), 20
Guanosine triphosphate (GTP), 20
Homeostasis, 18
Hormonal signaling, 18
Hydrolases, 5
Hydrophilic, 11
Hydrophobic, 11
Hydrostatic pressure, 26
Hypertonic solution, 28
Inner membrane, 7
Integral membrane protein, 11
Intermediary metabolism, 8
Interphase, 34
Ion, 26
Isotonic solution, 28
Junctional complex, 16
Ligand, 13
Lysosome, 5
Macromolecule, 15
Mediated transport, 28
Metabolic pathway, 21
Metaphase, 35
Microdomain, 32
Microtubule, 9
Microvilli, 36
Mitochondria, 7
Mitosis, 33
Neurohormonal signaling, 18
Neurotransmitter, 18
Nuclear envelope, 2
Nucleolus, 2
Nucleus, 2
Oncotic pressure (colloid osmotic pressure), 28
Osmolality, 27
Osmolarity, 27
Osmosis, 27
Osmotic pressure, 27
Outer membrane, 7
Oxidation, 23
Oxidative cellular metabolism, 23
Oxidative phosphorylation, 24
Paracrine signaling, 18
Parenchyma, 38

Passive mediated transport (facilitated diffusion), 29
Passive transport, 25
Peripheral membrane protein, 11
Peroxisome (microbody), 7
Phagocytosis, 31
Pinocytosis, 31
Plasma membrane receptor, 15
Platelet-derived growth factor (PDGF), 35
Polarity, 26
Polyribosome, 8
Potocytosis, 32
Primary lysosome, 5
Prokaryote, 2
Prophase, 34
Proteolytic cascade, 12
Pseudostratified epithelium, 36
Raft, 13
Receptor-mediated endocytosis (ligand internalization), 31
Relative refractory period, 33
Repolarization, 33
Residual body, 6
Resting membrane potential, 32
Reticular fiber, 38
Ribosomal protein synthesis, 8
Ribosome, 5
Rough endoplasmic reticulum, 5
Second messenger, 20
Secondary lysosome (heterophagosome), 6
Secretory vesicle, 5
Signal transduction, 19
Simple epithelium, 36
Smooth endoplasmic reticulum, 5
Solute, 26
Spindle fiber, 35
Squamous cell, 36
Stratified epithelium, 36
Substrate, 21
Symport, 29
Synapses, 41
Telophase, 35
Threshold potential, 33
Tight junction, 18
Tissue, 35
Tonicity, 28
Transfer reaction, 24
Transmembrane protein, 11
Transport protein, 28
Uniport, 29
Vault, 7

REFERENCES

1. Alberts B et al: *Molecular biology of the cell*, ed 5, New York, 2008, Garland.
2. van Zon A et al: Vault mobility depends in part on microtubules and vaults can be recruited to the nuclear envelope, *Exp Cell Res* 312(3):245-255, 2006.
3. Steiner E et al: Cellular functions of vaults and their involvement in multidrug resistance, *Cult Drug Targets* 7(8):923–934, 2006 review.
4. Anderson DH et al: Draft crystal structure of the vault shell at 9-A resolution, *Plos Biol* 5(11):e318, 2007.
5. Mooney DJ, Mikos AG: Growing new organs, *Sci Am* 280(4):60-65, 1999.
6. Fasshauer M, Iwig M, Glaesser D: Synthesis of proto-oncogene proteins and cyclins depends on intact microfilaments, *Eur J Cell Biol* 77(3):188-195, 1998.
7. Lofthouse RA et al: Identification of caveolae and detection of caveolin in normal human osteoblasts, *J Bone Joint Surg Br* 83(1):124-129, 2001.
8. Southan C: Drug discovery, *Today* 6:681-688, 2001.
9. Amour A et al. General considerations for proteolytic cascades, *Biochem Soc Trans* 32(Pt 1):15-16, 2004.
10. Logue SE, Martin SJ: Caspase activation cascades in apoptosis, *Biochem Soc Trans* 36(Pt 1):1-9, 2008.

11. Chang HY, Yang X: Proteases for cell suicide: functions and regulations of caspases, *Microbiol Mol Biol Rev* 64(4):821-846, 2000.

12. Catt KJ et al: Hormonal regulation of peptide receptors and target cell responses, *Nature* 280(5718):109-116, 1979.

13. LaPorte SL et al: Molecular and structural basis of cytokine receptor pleiotropy in the interleukin-4/13 system, *Cell* 132:259-272, 2008.

14. Kumar V, Abbas A, Fausto N: *Robbins and Cotran pathologic basis of disease*, ed 7, Philadelphia, 2005, Saunders.

15. Alberts B et al: *Essential cell biology*, New York, 1998, Garland.

16. Baserga R, Morrione A: Differentiation and malignant transformation: two roads diverge in a wood, *J Cell Biochem Suppl* 32-33:68-75, 1999.

17. Singh AB, Harris RC: Autocrine, paracrine, and juxtacrine signaling by EGFR ligands, *Cell Signal* 17(10):1183-1193, 2005.

18. Scott JD, Pawson T: Cell communication: the inside story, *Sci Am* 282(6):72-79, 2000.

19. He B et al: Exo 70 interacts with phospholipids and mediates the targeting of the exocyst to the plasma membrane, *EMBO* 26(18):4053-4065, 2007.

20. Schwencke C et al: Caveolae and cavolin in transmembrane signaling: implications for human disease, *Cardiovasc Res* 70(1):42-49, 2006.

21. Levin ER, Pietras RJ: Estrogen receptors outside the nucleus in breast cancer, *Breast Cancer Res Treat* 108(3):351-361, 2008.

22. Li L, Haynes MP, Bender JR: Plasma membrane localization and function of the estrogen receptor alpha variant (ER46) in human endothelial cells, *Proc Natl Acad Sci U S A* 100(8):4807-4812, 2003.

23. Mineo C, Shaul PW: Circulating cardiovascular disease risk factors and signaling in endothelial cell caveolae, *Cardiovasc Res* 70(1):31-41, 2006.

ALTERED CELLULAR AND TISSUE BIOLOGY

KATHRYN L. McCANCE • TODD CAMERON GREY

MEDIA RESOURCES

 Evolve Website (http://evolve.elsevier.com/McCance/)
- Review Questions and Answers
- Animations
- Glossary (with audio pronunciation for selected terms)
- WebLinks

OnLine Course
- Module 1

CHAPTER OUTLINE

CELLULAR ADAPTATION
  Atrophy
  Hypertrophy
  Hyperplasia
  Dysplasia: Not a True Adaptive Change
  Metaplasia
CELLULAR INJURY
  General Mechanisms of Cell Injury
  Hypoxic Injury
  Free Radicals and Reactive Oxygen Species
  Chemical Injury
  Unintentional and Intentional Injuries
  Infectious Injury

Immunologic and Inflammatory Injury
Injurious Genetic Factors
Injurious Nutritional Imbalances
Injurious Physical Agents
MANIFESTATIONS OF CELLULAR INJURY
  Cellular Manifestations: Accumulations
  Systemic Manifestations
CELLULAR DEATH
  Necrosis
  Apoptosis
    Aging and Altered Cellular and Tissue Biology
  Normal Life Span
SOMATIC DEATH

Knowledge of the structural and functional reactions of cells and tissues to injurious agents, including genetic defects, is key to understanding disease processes. Diseases are now defined and interpreted in molecular terms and not just in general descriptions of altered structure. Altered cellular and tissue biology can be the result of adaptation, injury, neoplasia, aging, or death. (Neoplasia is discussed in Chapters 11 through 13.) Adaptation occurs in response to both normal, or physiologic, conditions and adverse, or pathologic, conditions. For example, the uterus adapts to pregnancy—a normal physiologic state—by enlarging. Enlargement occurs because of an increase in the size and number of uterine cells. In response to physiologic stressors or pathologic adaptations, such as high blood pressure, myocardial cells are stimulated to enlarge by the increased work of pumping. Like most of the body's adaptive mechanisms, however, cellular adaptations to adverse conditions are usually only temporarily

successful. Severe or long-term stressors overwhelm adaptive processes, and cellular injury or death ensues.

Cellular injury can be caused by any factor that disrupts cellular structures or deprives the cell of oxygen and nutrients required for survival. Injury may be reversible *(sublethal)* or irreversible *(lethal)* and is classified broadly as chemical, hypoxic (lack of sufficient oxygen), free radical, unintentional or intentional, and immunologic or inflammatory. Cellular injuries from various causes have different clinical and pathophysiologic manifestations.

Cellular death is confirmed by structural changes seen when cells are stained and examined with a microscope. The most important changes are nuclear changes; clearly, without a healthy nucleus, the cell cannot survive.

Cellular aging causes structural and functional changes that eventually lead to cellular death or a decreased capacity to recover from injury. Mechanisms explaining how and why cells age are not known, and distinguishing between pathologic changes and physiologic changes that occur with aging is often difficult. Aging clearly causes alterations in cellular structure and function, yet *senescence*—growing old is both inevitable and normal.

CELLULAR ADAPTATION

Cells adapt to their environment to escape and protect themselves from injury. An adapted cell is neither normal nor injured—its condition lies somewhere between these two states. Cellular adaptations, however, are a common and central part of many disease states. In the early stages of a successful adaptive response, cells may have enhanced function; thus it is hard to know what is a pathologic response vs. an extreme adaptation to an excessive functional demand. The most significant adaptive changes in cells include atrophy (decrease in cell size), hypertrophy (increase in cell size), hyperplasia (increase in cell number), and metaplasia (reversible replacement of one mature cell type by another less mature cell type). Dysplasia (deranged cellular growth) is not considered a true cellular adaptation but rather an atypical hyperplasia. These changes are shown in Figure 2-1.

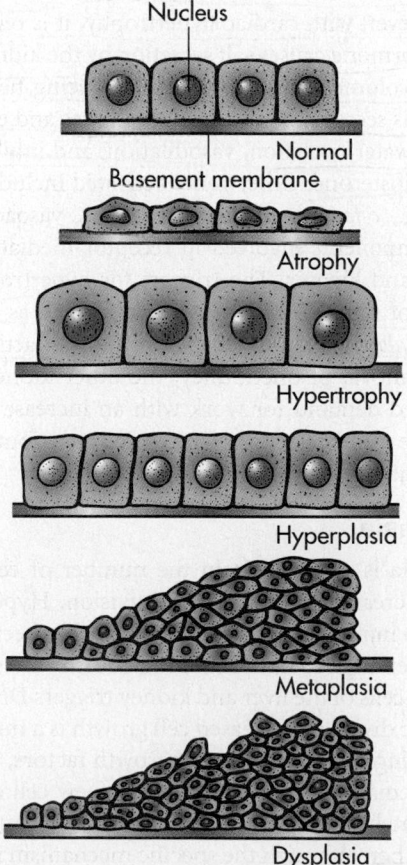

Nucleus

Normal

Basement membrane

Atrophy

Hypertrophy

Hyperplasia

Metaplasia

Dysplasia

Figure 2-1 Adaptive alterations in simple cuboidal epithelial cells. (From Lewis SM, Heitkemper MM, Dirksen SR: *Medical-surgical nursing: assessment and management of clinical problems,* ed 6, St Louis, 2004, Mosby.)

Atrophy

Atrophy is a decrease or shrinkage in cellular size. If atrophy occurs in a sufficient number of an organ's cells, the entire organ shrinks or becomes atrophic. Atrophy can affect any organ, but it is most common in skeletal muscle, the heart, secondary sex organs, and the brain (Figure 2-2). Atrophy can be classified as *physiologic* or *pathologic*. **Physiologic atrophy** occurs with early development. For example, the thymus gland undergoes physiologic atrophy during childhood. **Pathologic atrophy** occurs as a result of decreases in workload, use, pressure, blood supply, nutrition, hormonal stimulation, and nervous stimulation. Individuals immobilized in bed for a prolonged time exhibit a type of skeletal muscle atrophy called *disuse atrophy*. Aging causes brain cells to become atrophic and endocrine-dependent organs, such as the gonads, to shrink as hormonal stimulation decreases. Whether atrophy is caused by normal physiologic conditions or by pathologic conditions, atrophic cells exhibit the same basic changes.

The atrophic muscle cell contains less endoplasmic reticulum and fewer mitochondria and myofilaments (part of the muscle fiber that controls contraction) than does the normal cell. In muscular atrophy caused by nerve loss, oxygen consumption and amino acid uptake are rapidly reduced. The biochemical changes of atrophy are just beginning to be understood. The mechanisms probably include decreased protein synthesis, increased protein catabolism, or both. The primary pathway of protein catabolism is the **ubiquitin-proteasome pathway,** and **up-regulation of proteasome** (protein degrading complex) activity is characteristic of atrophic muscle changes.[1] Proteins degraded in this pathway are first conjugated to *ubiquitin* (another small protein) and then degraded by proteaosomes.

Atrophy as a result of chronic malnutrition is often accompanied by a "self-eating" process called *autophagy* creating **autophagic vacuoles.** These vacuoles are membrane-bound vesicles within the cell that contain cellular debris—small fragments of mitochondria and endoplasmic reticulum—and hydrolytic enzymes. Atrophic change causes a rapid increase in hydrolytic enzymes, which are isolated in autophagic vacuoles to prevent uncontrolled cellular destruction. Thus the vacuoles proliferate as needed to protect the uninjured organelles from the injured organelles and are eventually taken up and destroyed by lysosomes (see p. 5). Certain contents of the autophagic vacuole may resist destruction by lysosomal enzymes and persist in membrane-bound residual bodies. An example of this is granules that contain **lipofuscin,** the yellow-brown age pigment. Lipofuscin accumulates primarily in liver cells, myocardial cells, and atrophic cells.

Hypertrophy

Hypertrophy is an increase in the size of cells and consequently in the size of the affected organ. The cells of the heart and kidneys are particularly responsive to enlargement. The increase in cellular size is associated with an increased accumulation of protein in the cellular components (plasma

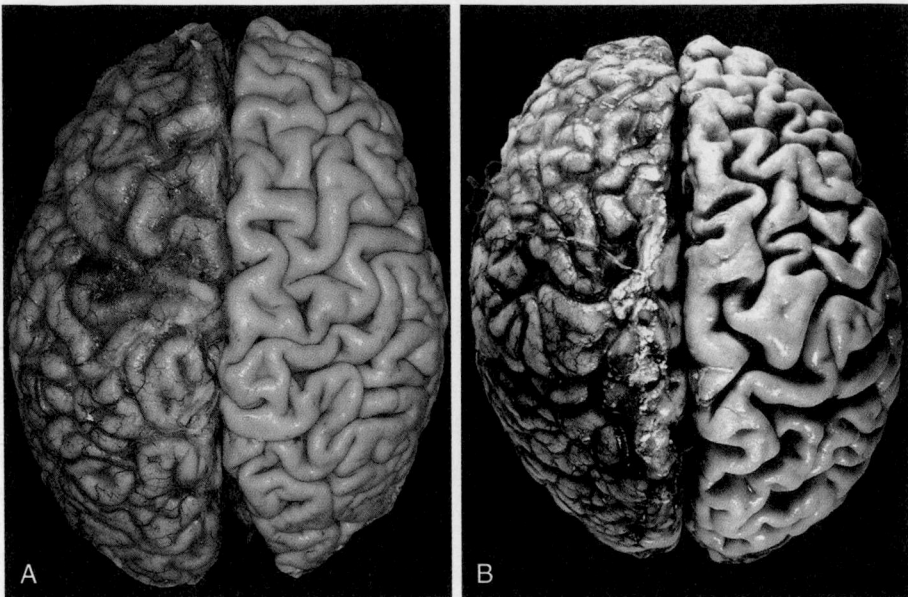

Figure 2-2 Atrophy. **A,** Normal brain of a young adult. **B,** Atrophy of the brain in an 82-year-old male with atherosclerotic disease. Atrophy of the brain is because of aging and reduced blood supply. Note that loss of brain substance narrows the gyri and widens the sulci. The meninges have been stripped from the right half of each specimen to reveal the surface of the brain. (From Kumar V, Abbas A, Fausto N: *Robbins and Cotran pathologic basis of disease,* ed 8, Philadelphia, 2007, Saunders.)

membrane, endoplasmic reticulum, myofilaments, mitochondria) and *not* with an increase in cellular fluid. Hypertrophy can be *physiologic* or *pathologic* and is caused by specific hormone stimulation or by increased functional demand. For example, physiologic hypertrophy during pregnancy is hormone induced and involves both hypertrophy and hyperplasia. Hypertrophy as an adaptive response—muscular enlargement—occurs in the striated muscle cells of both the heart and skeletal muscles. These cells cannot adapt to increased metabolic demands by mitotic division and production of new cells to share the work. Thus they enlarge and the stimulus appears to be an increased workload. In the heart, pathologic hypertrophy is secondary to hypertension or problem valves. In skeletal muscle, physiologic hypertrophy occurs in response to heavy work. Muscular hypertrophy tends to diminish if the excessive workload diminishes.

In myocardial hypertrophy, initial enlargement is caused by dilation of the cardiac chambers, but this is short lived and is followed by increased synthesis of cardiac muscle proteins, allowing muscle fibers to do more work. The nucleus is also hypertrophic and exhibits increased synthesis of deoxyribonucleic acid (DNA).[2] Although fully matured (e.g., terminally differentiated) muscle cells are unable to undergo further mitosis, they are capable of increased DNA synthesis. Why cardiac muscle cells are unable to progress through the cell cycle to mitosis is unclear[3] (see Chapters 1 and 11). Eventually, however, advanced hypertrophy can lead to myocardial failure (Figure 2-3) (see Chapter 30).

A number of genes are activated during hypertrophy, including the genes for atrial natriuretic peptide (ANP) and brain natriuretic peptide (BNP) also called B-type natriuretic peptide.

The ANP gene is usually expressed only during early development; however, with cardiac hypertrophy, it is reinduced and the ANP hormone causes salt secretion by the kidney, decreasing blood volume and pressure and reducing hemodynamic load. BNP is secreted by the heart ventricles and enhances sodium and water excretion, vasodilation, and inhibition of renin and aldosterone. Other genes activated include regulatory factors (e.g., *c-fos, c-jun*), growth factors, vasoactive agents, certain components involved in receptor-mediated signaling pathways, and kinases. The triggers for hypertrophy include two types of signals: *mechanical signals,* such as stretch, and *trophic signals,* such as growth factors and vasoactive agents.

After removal of one kidney, the other kidney adapts to an increased demand for work with an increase in both the size and the number of cells. The major contribution to renal enlargement is hypertrophy.

Hyperplasia

Hyperplasia is an increase in the number of cells resulting from an increased rate of cellular division. Hyperplasia as a response to injury occurs when the injury has been severe and prolonged enough to have caused cell death.[2] Loss of epithelial cells and cells of the liver and kidney triggers DNA synthesis and mitotic division. Increased cell growth is a multistep process involving the production of growth factors, which stimulate the remaining cells to synthesize new cell components and, ultimately, to divide. Hyperplasia and hypertrophy often occur together, although the specific mechanism is unknown. Hyperplasia and hypertrophy both take place if the cells are capable of synthesizing DNA; however, in *nondividing cells* (e.g., myocardial fibers) only hypertrophy occurs.

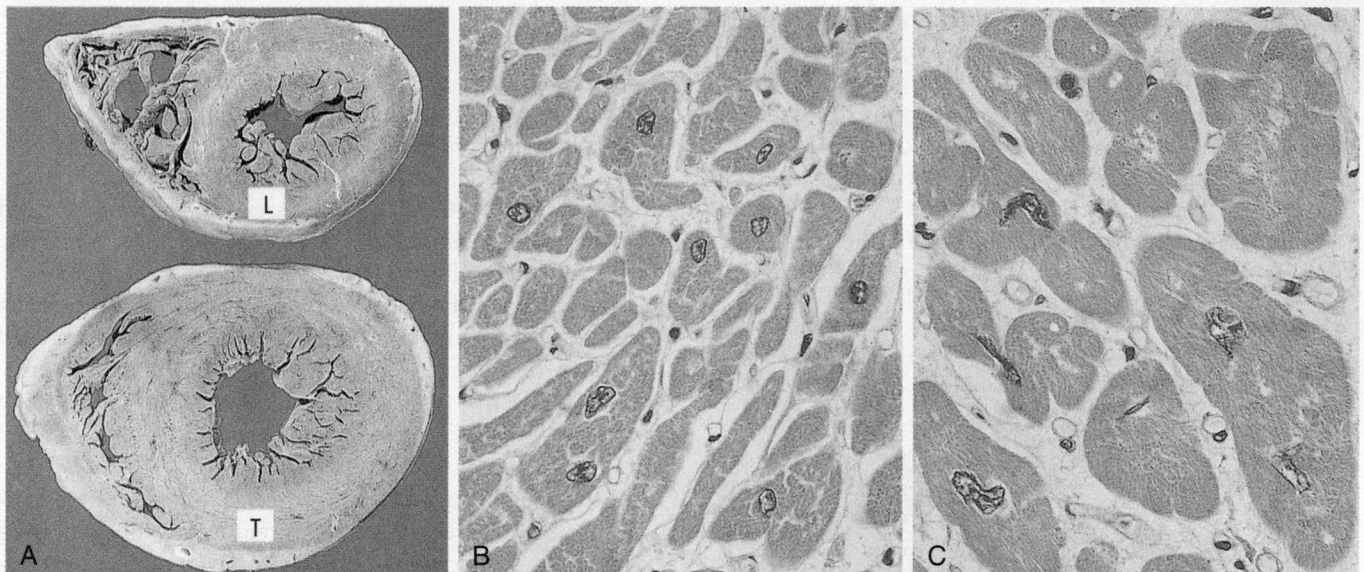

Figure 2-3 Hypertrophy of cardiac muscle in response to valve disease. **A,** Transverse slices of a normal heart and a heart with hypertrophy of the left ventricle. (*L,* Normal thickness of left ventricular wall; *T,* thickened wall from heart in which severe narrowing of aortic valve caused resistance to systolic ventricular emptying.) **B,** Histology of cardiac muscle from a normal heart. **C,** Histology of cardiac muscle from a hypertrophied heart. (From Stevens A, Lowe J: *Pathology,* London, 1995, Mosby.)

Two types of normal, or physiologic, hyperplasia are compensatory hyperplasia and hormonal hyperplasia. **Compensatory hyperplasia** is an adaptive mechanism that enables certain organs to regenerate. For example, removal of part of the liver leads to hyperplasia of the remaining liver cells (hepatocytes) to compensate for the loss. Even with removal of 70% of the liver, regeneration is complete in about 2 weeks. The remarkable regenerating capacity of the liver was even noted by the ancient Greeks. According to one story, Prometheus was chained to a mountain and his liver was eaten daily by a vulture, only to regenerate every night. A protein, **hepatocyte growth factor (HGF),** is thought to be a mediator in vitro of liver regeneration.[4] In addition, other in vitro growth factors and cytokines (cell-signaling proteins) that increase hepatic cell regeneration include transforming growth factor-α (TGF-α), epidermal growth factor (EGF), interleukin-6 (IL-6), and tumor necrosis factor-α (TNF-α).

Not all types of mature cells have the same capacity for compensatory hyperplastic growth. Some cells, such as nerve, skeletal muscle, and myocardial cells and the lens cells of the eye, do not regenerate. Skeletal muscle cells, however, can be made by the fusion of myoblasts.[5] Much research also is being done with the peripheral nervous system (PNS). PNS nerve regeneration enables severed limbs to be reattached and continue growing. Significant compensatory hyperplasia occurs in epidermal and intestinal epithelia, hepatocytes, bone marrow cells, and fibroblasts, and some hyperplasia is noted in bone, cartilage, and smooth muscle cells. An example of compensatory hyperplasia is a **callus,** or thickening, of the skin as a result of hyperplasia of epidermal cells in response to a mechanical stimulus. Another example is the response to wound healing as part of the inflammation process (see Chapter 6).

Hormonal hyperplasia occurs chiefly in estrogen-dependent organs, such as the uterus and breast. After ovulation, for example, estrogen stimulates the endometrium to grow and thicken for reception of the fertilized ovum. If pregnancy occurs, hormonal hyperplasia, as well as hypertrophy, enables the uterus to enlarge. (Hormone function is described in Chapters 20 and 21.)

Pathologic hyperplasia is the abnormal proliferation of normal cells and can occur as a response to excessive hormonal stimulation or the effects of growth factors on target cells (Figure 2-4). Hyperplastic cells are identified by pronounced nuclear enlargement, clumping of chromatin, and one or more enlarged nucleoli. The most common example is pathologic hyperplasia of the endometrium (which is caused by an imbalance between estrogen and progesterone secretion, with oversecretion of estrogen) (see Chapter 23). Pathologic endometrial hyperplasia, which causes excessive menstrual bleeding, is under the influence of regular growth-inhibition controls. If these controls fail, hyperplastic endometrial cells can undergo malignant transformation. (Malignant cell transformation is discussed in Chapter 11.)

Dysplasia: Not a True Adaptive Change

Dysplasia refers to abnormal changes in the size, shape, and organization of mature cells. Dysplasia is not considered a true adaptive process but is related to hyperplasia and is often called **atypical hyperplasia.** Dysplastic changes frequently are encountered in epithelial tissue of the cervix and respiratory tract, where they are strongly associated with common neoplastic growths and often are found adjacent to cancerous cells. Importantly, the term *dysplasia* does *not* indicate cancer and may not progress to cancer.

Dysplasia is often classified as mild, moderate, or severe; however, this subjective scheme has prompted recommendations to use either "low grade" or "high grade." Grading of dysplasia, for example, of the female reproductive tract (i.e., Papanicolaou [Pap] test) is discussed in Chapter 23 (Figure 2-5). Data indicate that atypical hyperplasia is a strong predictor of breast cancer development.[6,7] If the inciting stimulus is removed, dysplastic changes often are reversible.

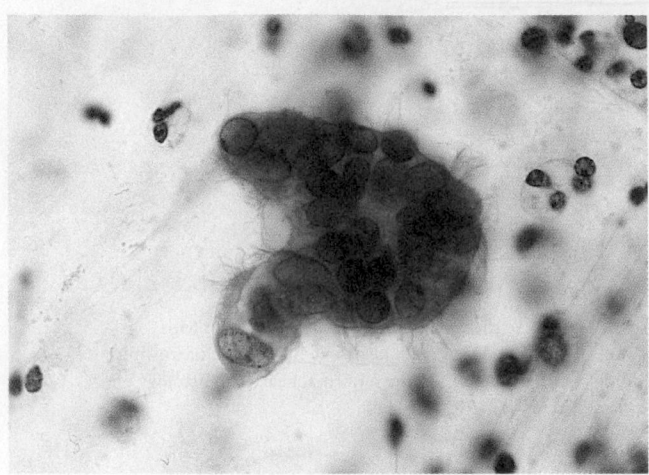

Figure 2-4 Hyperplasia of bronchial epithelium. (Bronchial brush.) (From Damjanov I, Linder J: *Anderson's pathology,* ed 10, St Louis, 1996, Mosby.)

Metaplasia

Metaplasia is the reversible replacement of one mature cell by another, sometimes less differentiated, cell type. The best example of metaplasia is replacement of normal columnar ciliated epithelial cells of the bronchial (airway) lining by stratified squamous epithelial cells (Figure 2-6). The newly formed squamous epithelial cells do not secrete mucus or have cilia, causing loss of a vital protective mechanism.

Metaplasia is thought to develop from a reprogramming of stem cells existing in most epithelia or of undifferentiated mesenchymal (tissue from embryonic mesoderm) cells present in connective tissue. These precursor cells mature along a new pathway because of signals generated by cytokines and growth factors in the cell's environment.

Bronchial metaplasia can be reversed if the inducing stimulus, usually cigarette smoking, is removed. With prolonged exposure to the inducing stimulus, however, cancerous transformation can occur.

CELLULAR INJURY

Most diseases begin with cell injury, and all forms of loss of function derive from cell injury and cell death. Cellular injury occurs if the cell is unable to maintain homeostasis—a normal or adaptive steady state—in the face of injurious stimuli.

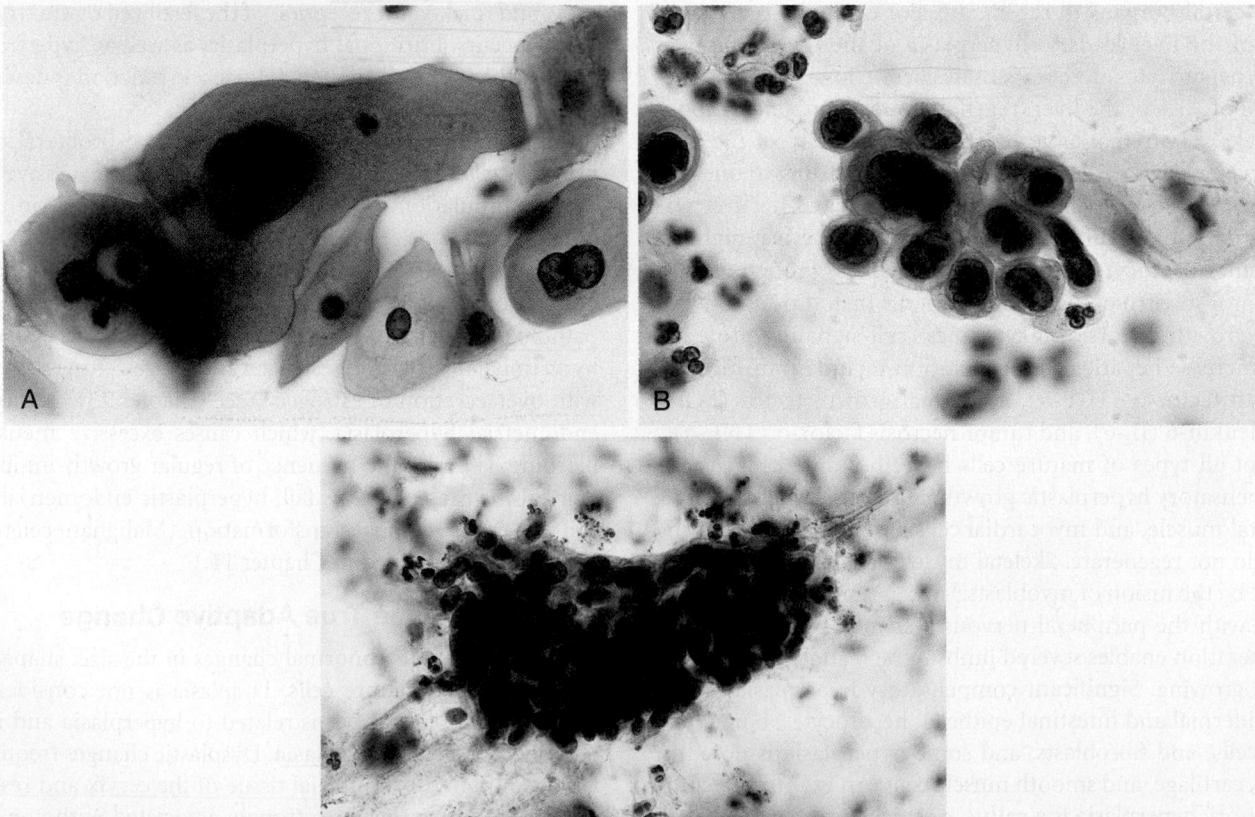

Figure 2-5 Dysplasia of uterine cervix. A, Mild dysplasia. B, Severe dysplasia. C, Carcinoma in situ (see Chapter 11). (From Damjanov I, Linder J: *Anderson's pathology,* ed 10, St Louis, 1996, Mosby.)

Injured cells may recover (**reversible injury**) or die (**irreversible injury**). Injurious stimuli include chemical agents, lack of sufficient oxygen (hypoxia), free radicals, infectious agents, physical and mechanical factors, immunologic reactions, genetic factors, and nutritional imbalances. Types of cellular injury and their responses are summarized in Table 2-1 and Figure 2-7.

Cell injury and cell death often result from exposure to toxic chemicals, infections, and hypoxia. The mechanisms causing chemical and hypoxic injury are perhaps the best understood.

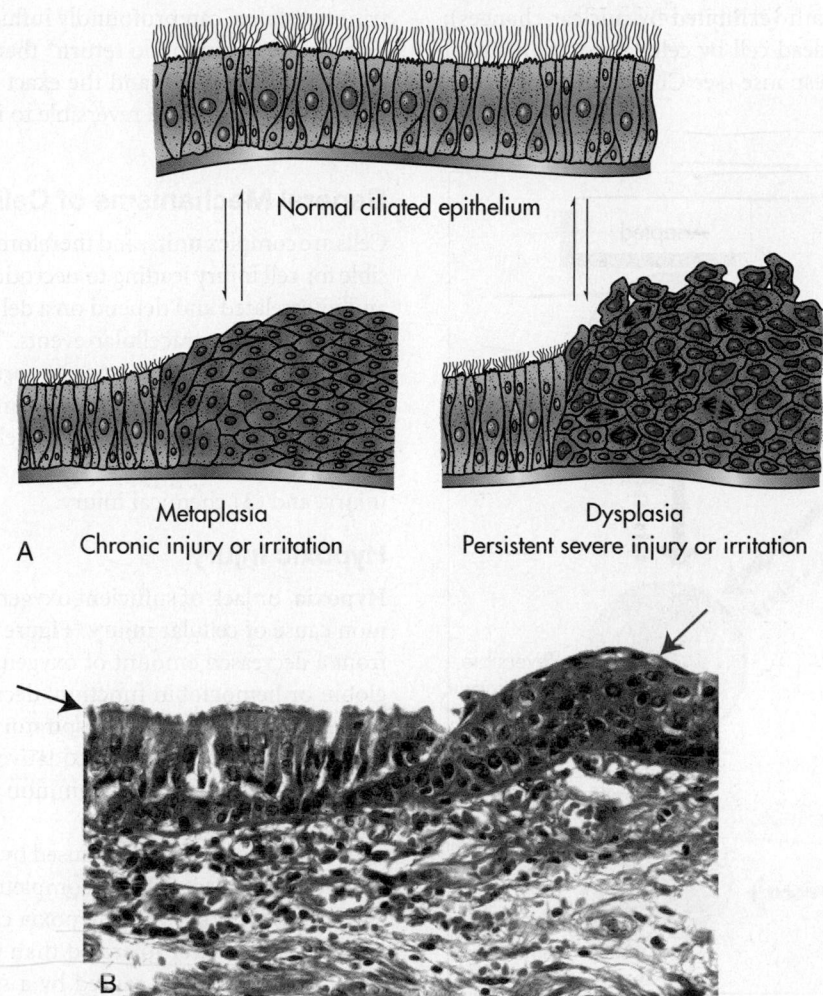

Figure 2-6 Reversible changes in cells lining the bronchi. **A,** Normal ciliated epithelium, metaplasia and dysplasia. **B,** Histological slide with upper left *(black arrow)* normal columnar epithelium and basement membrane, and upper right *(red arrow)* squamous metaplasia. (B from Kumar V, Abbas A, Fausto N: *Robbins and Cotran pathologic basis of disease,* ed 8, Philadelphia, 2007, Saunders.)

Table 2-1	Progressive Types of Cell Injury and Responses
Type	**Responses**
Adaptation	Atrophy, hypertrophy, hyperplasia, metaplasia
Active cell injury	Immediate response of "entire" cell
Reversible	Loss of adenosine triphosphate (ATP), cellular swelling, detachment of ribosomes, autophagy of lysosomes
Irreversible	"Point of no return" structurally when severe vacuolization occurs of the mitochondria and Ca^{++} moves into the cell including the mitochondria membrane damage
Necrosis	Common type of cell death with severe cell swelling and breakdown of organelles
Apoptosis, a type of programmed cell death	Cellular self-destruction for elimination of unwanted cell populations
Chronic cell injury (subcellular alterations)	Persistent stimuli response may involve only specific organelles or cytoskeleton (e.g., phagocytosis of bacteria)
Accumulations or infiltrations	Water, pigments, lipids, glycogen, proteins
Pathologic calcification	Dystrophic and metastatic calcification

(Infections are discussed in Chapter 9.) Both of these mechanisms can lead to disruption of selective permeability (i.e., transport mechanisms) of the plasma membrane; reduction or cessation of cellular metabolism; lack of protein synthesis; damage to lysosomal membranes, with leakage of destructive enzymes into the cytoplasm; enzymatic destruction of cellular organelles; cellular death (exhibited by nuclear changes); and phagocytosis of the dead cell by cellular components of the acute inflammatory response (see Chapter 6). The extent of cellular injury depends on the type, state (including level of cell differentiation and increased susceptibility to fully differentiated cells), and adaptive processes of the cell, as well as the type, severity, and duration of the injurious stimulus. Two individuals exposed to an identical stimulus may incur varying degrees of cellular injury. Modifying factors, such as nutritional status, can profoundly influence the extent of injury. The precise "point of no return" that leads to cellular death is a biochemical puzzle, and the exact mechanisms responsible for the transition from reversible to irreversible cellular damage are being debated.

General Mechanisms of Cell Injury

Cells are complex units, and therefore the mechanisms responsible for cell injury leading to necrotic cell death are numerous and interrelated and depend on a delicate balance between intracellular and extracellular events. There are, however, four common biochemical themes important to cell injury and cell death regardless of the injuring agent (Table 2-2).

The three common forms of cell injury are (1) hypoxic injury, (2) reactive oxygen species and free radical–induced injury, and (3) chemical injury.

Hypoxic Injury

Hypoxia, or lack of sufficient oxygen, is the single most common cause of cellular injury (Figure 2-8). Hypoxia can result from a decreased amount of oxygen in the air, loss of hemoglobin or hemoglobin function, decreased production of red blood cells, diseases of the respiratory and cardiovascular systems, and poisoning of the oxidative enzymes (cytochromes) within the cells. The most common cause of hypoxia is **ischemia** (reduced blood supply).

Ischemic injury is often caused by gradual narrowing of arteries (arteriosclerosis) and complete blockage by blood clots (thrombosis). Progressive hypoxia caused by gradual arterial obstruction is better tolerated than the sudden acute **anoxia** (total lack of oxygen) caused by a sudden obstruction, such as can occur with an embolus (a blood clot or other plug in the circulation). An acute obstruction in a coronary artery can cause myocardial cell death (infarction) within minutes if

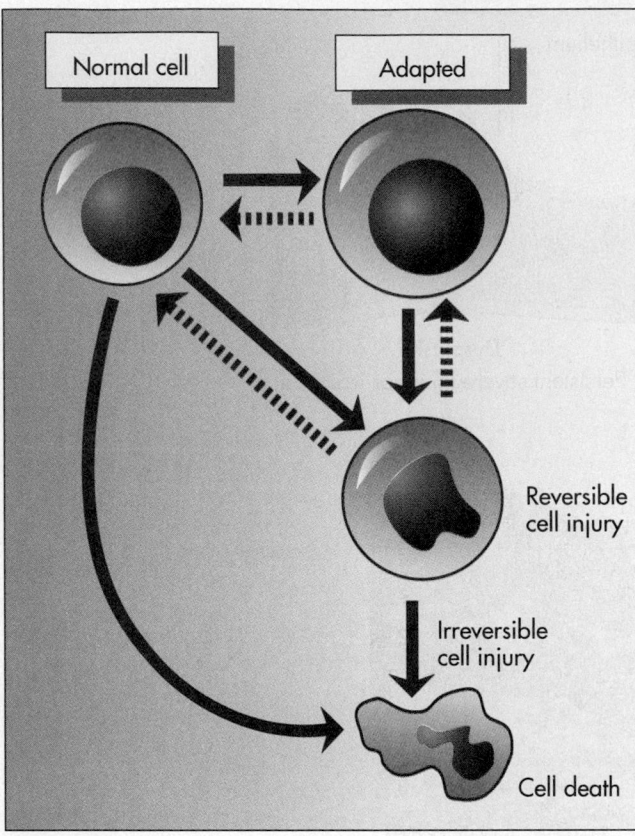

Figure 2-7 Cellular injury and responses. Depicted here is the relationship among normal, adapted (hypertrophy), and reversibly injured cells and cell death of myocardial cells.

Table 2-2	Common Themes in Cell Injury and Cell Death
Theme	**Comments**
ATP depletion	Loss of mitochondrial ATP and decreased ATP synthesis; results include cellular swelling, decreased protein synthesis, decreased membrane transport, and lipogenesis, all changes that contribute to loss of integrity of plasma membrane (see text)
Oxygen and oxygen-derived free radicals	Lack of oxygen is key in progression of cell injury in ischemia (reduced blood supply); activated oxygen species (free radicals, O_2^-, H_2O_2, $OH\cdot$, NO) cause destruction of cell membranes and cell structure
Intracellular calcium and loss of calcium steady state	Normally intracellular cytosolic calcium concentrations are very low; ischemia and certain chemicals cause an increase in cytosolic Ca^{++} concentrations; sustained levels of Ca^{++} continue to increase with damage to plasma membrane; Ca^{++} causes intracellular damage by activating a number of enzymes (see text)
Defects in membrane permeability	Early loss of selective membrane permeability found in all forms of cell injury (see text)

ATP, Adenosine triphosphate.

Reversible Cell Injury   Irreversible Injury (cell death)

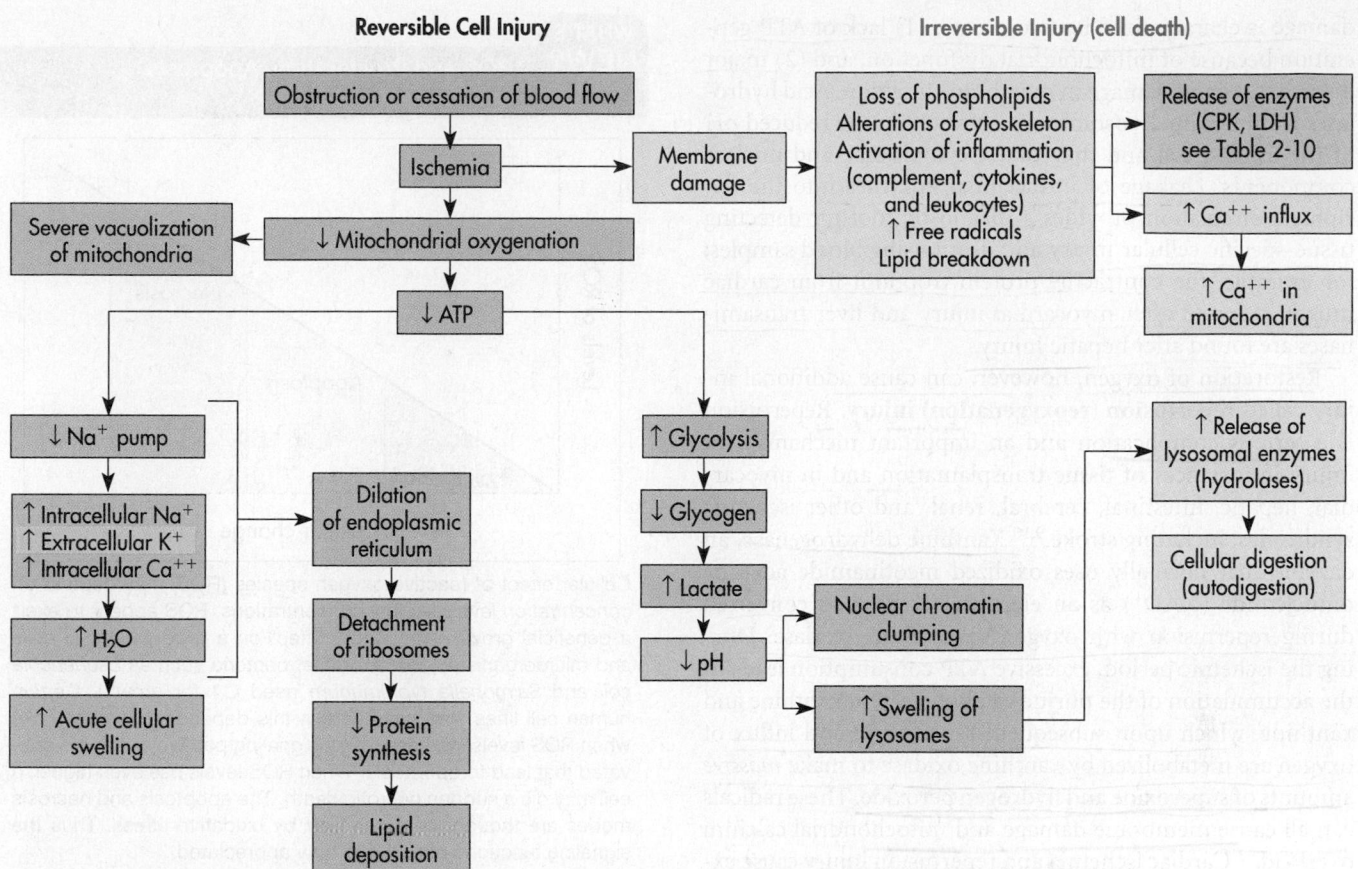

Figure 2-8 Hypoxic injury induced by ischemia. *Purple boxes* involve reversible cell injury, and *light blue boxes* involve irreversible cell death. *Green boxes* are clinical manifestations.

the blood supply is not restored, whereas the gradual onset of ischemia usually results in myocardial adaptation. Myocardial infarction and stroke, which are common causes of death in the United States, generally result from atherosclerosis (a type of arteriosclerosis) and consequent ischemic injury. (Vascular obstruction is discussed in Chapter 30.)

Cellular responses to hypoxic injury have been extensively studied in heart muscle. Within 1 minute after blood supply to the myocardium is interrupted, the heart becomes pale and has difficulty contracting normally. Within 3 to 5 minutes the ischemic portion of the myocardium ceases to contract. The abrupt lack of contraction is caused by a rapid decrease in mitochondrial phosphorylation, which results in insufficient adenosine triphosphate (ATP) production. Lack of ATP leads to an increase in anaerobic metabolism, which generates ATP from glycogen when there is insufficient oxygen. When glycogen stores are depleted, even anaerobic metabolism ceases.

A reduction in ATP levels causes the plasma membrane's sodium-potassium (Na+, K+) pump and sodium-calcium exchange to fail, which leads to an intracellular accumulation of sodium and calcium and diffusion of potassium out of the cell. (The Na+, K+ pump is discussed in Chapter 1.) Sodium and water then can enter the cell freely, and cellular swelling results. Because all cells are bathed in a fluid rich in calcium ions, cell membrane damage allows rapid movement of

calcium intracellularly. The movement of water and ions into the cell causes early dilation of the endoplasmic reticulum. Dilation causes the ribosomes to detach from the rough endoplasmic reticulum, resulting in reduced protein synthesis. With continued hypoxia, the entire cell becomes markedly swollen, with increased concentrations of sodium, water, and chloride and decreased concentrations of potassium. These disruptions are reversible if oxygen is restored. If oxygen is not restored, however, there is **vacuolation** (formation of vacuoles or cytoplasmic small cavity) within the cytoplasm, swelling of lysosomes, and marked swelling of the mitochondria resulting from mitochondrial membrane damage. Continued hypoxic injury with accumulation of calcium subsequently activates multiple enzyme systems, including proteases, nitric oxide synthase, phospholipases, and endonuclease, resulting in cytoskeleton disruption, membrane damage, activation of inflammation, DNA degradation, and eventual cell death (see Figure 2-27). Structurally, with plasma membrane damage, extracellular calcium readily moves into the cell and intracellular calcium stores are released. Intracellular calcium results in the activation of enzymes that can further damage membranes, proteins, ATP, and nucleic acids.[8] The increased permeability of the membrane causes continued loss of proteins, essential coenzymes, and ribonucleic acids. In addition, the substrates necessary to reconstitute ATP are lost. Irreversible damage is characterized by two events: (1) lack of ATP generation because of mitochondrial dysfunction, and (2) major disturbances and damage in membrane function. Acid hydrolases from leaking lysosomes are activated in the reduced pH of the injured cell and they digest cytoplasmic and nuclear components. Leakage of intracellular enzymes into the peripheral circulation provides a diagnostic tool for detecting tissue-specific cellular injury and death using blood samples; for example, the contractile protein troponin from cardiac muscle is found after myocardial injury and liver transaminases are found after hepatic injury.

Restoration of oxygen, however, can cause additional injury called **reperfusion (reoxygenation) injury.** Reperfusion is a serious complication and an important mechanism of injury in instances of tissue transplantation and in myocardial, hepatic, intestinal, cerebral, renal, and other ischemic syndromes, including stroke.[9,10] Xanthine dehydrogenase, an enzyme that normally uses oxidized nicotinamide adenine dinucleotide (NAD^+) as an electron acceptor, is converted during reperfusion with oxygen to xanthine oxidase. During the ischemic period, excessive ATP consumption leads to the accumulation of the purine catabolites hypoxanthine and xanthine, which upon subsequent reperfusion and influx of oxygen are metabolized by xanthine oxidase to make *massive* amounts of superoxide and hydrogen peroxide. These radicals can all cause membrane damage and mitochondrial calcium overload.[11] Cardiac ischemia and reperfusion injury cause excessive reactive oxygen species (ROS) and calcium overload of the mitochondria. These changes lead to the opening of pores on the mitochondrial membrane with massive escape of ATP leading to cell death activation (apoptosis). Interestingly, release of *low* levels of nitric oxide can acutely protect myocardial mitochondria against reperfusion injury[12] (see What's New? ROS and Proliferation, Apoptosis, and Necrosis). Neutrophils are especially affected with reperfusion injury, and neutrophil adhesion to the endothelium enhances the process. Antioxidant treatment reverses both neutrophil adhesion (leukocyte adhesion) and neutrophil (leukocyte) mediated heart injury in the post-ischemic period.[9] Other potential and current treatments include blockage of inflammatory mediators and inhibition of apoptotic pathways.

Free Radicals and Reactive Oxygen Species

An important mechanism of membrane damage is injury induced by free radicals, especially by excess ROS called **oxidative stress.** Oxidative stress occurs when *excess ROS* overwhelms endogenous antioxidant systems. A **free radical** is an electrically uncharged atom or group of atoms having an unpaired electron. Having one unpaired electron makes the molecule unstable; thus to stabilize, it gives up an electron to another molecule or steals one. Therefore, it is capable of injurious chemical bond formation with proteins, lipids, carbohydrates—key molecules in membranes and nucleic acids. Free radicals are difficult to control and initiate chain reactions. Emerging data indicate that ROS play major roles in the initiation and progression of cardiovascular alterations

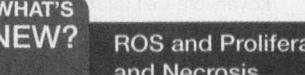

WHAT'S NEW?   ROS and Proliferation, Apoptosis, and Necrosis

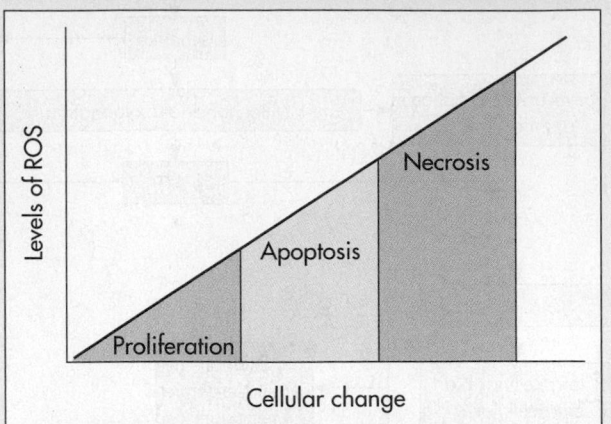

Cellular effect of reactive oxygen species (ROS) may depend on *concentration levels*. At low concentrations, ROS appear to exert a beneficial growth-stimulatory effect on a wide variety of cells and microorganisms. For example, bacteria such as *Escherichia coli* and *Salmonella typhimurium* need O_2^- for growth. Certain human cell lines also have shown this dependency in vitro. Yet when ROS levels increase, other signaling pathways may be activated that lead to apoptosis. When ROS levels rise even higher, a cell may die a sudden necrotic death. The apoptosis and necrosis modes are thought to be caused by oxidative stress. Thus the signaling functions of ROS are now appreciated.

Data from Buetler TM, Krauskopf A, Ruegg UT: *News Physiol Sci* 19:120-123, 2004; Valko M et al: *Int J Biochem Cell Biol* 39(1): 44-84, 2007.

associated with hyperlipidemia, diabetes mellitus, hypertension, ischemic heart disease, and chronic heart failure. ROS produced by migrating inflammatory cells (e.g., neutrophils), as well as vascular cells (endothelial cells, vascular smooth muscle cells, and adventitial fibroblasts) have distinct effects on each cell type.[13] These cell effects are shown in Figure 2-9.

Free radicals may be initiated within cells by (1) the absorption of extreme energy sources (e.g., ultraviolet light, x-rays); (2) endogenous, usually oxidative, reactions that occur during normal metabolic processes (Figure 2-10); or (3) enzymatic metabolism of exogenous chemicals or drugs (e.g., chloromethyl $[CCl_3^-]$, a product of carbon tetrachloride $[CCl_4]$). Table 2-3 describes the most significant free radicals.

Although wide-ranging effects can occur from these reactive species, three are particularly important in regard to cell injury: (1) lipid peroxidation; (2) alterations of proteins causing fragmentation of polypeptide chains; and (3) alterations of DNA, including breakage of single strands. **Lipid peroxidation** is the destruction of unsaturated fatty acids. Fatty acids of lipids in membranes possess double bonds between some of the carbon atoms. Such bonds are vulnerable to attack by oxygen-derived free radicals, especially $OH\cdot$. The lipid-radical interactions themselves yield peroxides. The peroxides set off a chain reaction resulting in membrane, organelle, and cellular

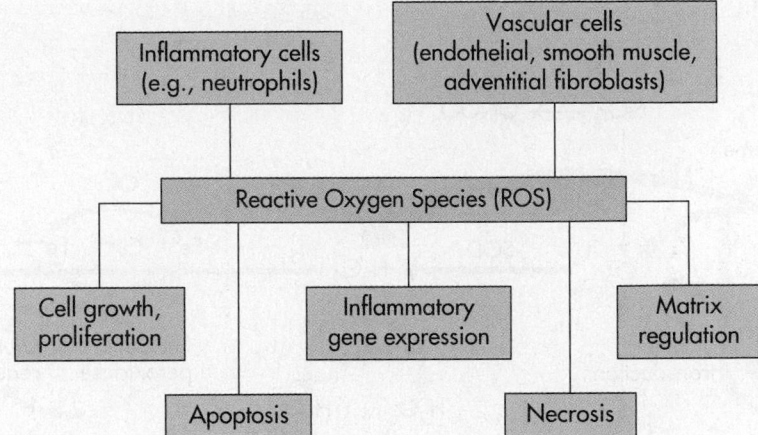

Figure 2-9 ROS can cause distinct functional effects depending on cell type. All cells are capable of making reactive oxygen species (ROS). Emphasis has been on inflammatory and vascular cells because of their widespread disease-causing effect. Some examples include angiotensin II, which can induce vascular smooth muscle cells (VSMC) to hypertrophy; NAD(P)H oxidase-derived ROS has been implicated in the growth response; H_2O_2 has been shown to induce proliferation and migration of endothelial cells; ROS act as mediators of vascular endothelial growth factor, thus modulating angiogenesis; endothelial injury or exposure to O_2^- and H_2O_2 induces apoptosis of endothelial cells. Activity of the extracellular matrix by matrix metalloproteinases (MMPs) can be modulated by ROS. Cytokines play a significant role in the progression of vascular lesions. An important mechanism by which cytokine gene expression is increased is the activation of nuclear factor-κβ (NF-κβ). NF-κβ is a ROS-sensitive transcription factor and has a role in the expression of proinflammatory genes. (Data from Buetler TM, Krauskopf A, Ruegg UT: *News Physiol Sci* 19:120-123, 2004; Dröge W: *Physiol Rev* 82:47-95, 2002; Valko M et al: *Int J Biochem Cell Biol*, 39(1):44-84, 2007.) (Also see What's New? ROS and Proliferation, Apoptosis, and Necrosis.)

destruction. Because of our understanding of free radicals, a growing number of diseases and disorders have been linked either directly or indirectly to these reactive species (Table 2-4).

It is fortunate that the body can sometimes rid itself of free radicals. Superoxide may spontaneously decay into oxygen and hydrogen peroxide. Table 2-5 summarizes other methods that contribute to inactivation or termination of free radicals. The toxicity of certain drugs and chemicals can be attributed to either conversion of these chemicals to free radicals or the formation of oxygen-derived metabolites.[9] This process is discussed in Chemical Injury, which follows.

Chemical Injury

Mechanisms

Chemical injury begins with a biochemical interaction between a toxic substance and the cell's plasma membrane, which is ultimately damaged, leading to increased permeability. Not all the mechanisms causing chemically induced membrane destruction are known; however, the two general mechanisms include (1) direct toxicity by combining with a molecular component of the cell membrane or organelles and (2) reactive free radicals and lipid peroxidation.

Because it has been investigated extensively, carbon tetrachloride (CCl_4) injury is a useful example of chemical injury. Carbon tetrachloride, an agent formerly used in dry cleaning, harms cells because an enzyme system (P-450) in the smooth endoplasmic reticulum of liver cells converts it into chloromethyl (CCl_3^-), a highly toxic free radical.

In CCl_4 injury, newly formed CCl_3^- rapidly destroys the endoplasmic reticulum of the liver cell by way of lipid peroxidation breaking down the reticulum's lipid component. The

lipid molecules accumulate within the cytoplasm, starting within cisternae of the endoplasmic reticulum (Figure 2-11). Fatty liver develops because CCl_4 poisoning blocks the synthesis of **lipid-acceptor proteins (apoproteins)** that normally bind with triglycerides to form lipoproteins, which are transported out of the cell. Blockage of triglyceride (lipoprotein) secretion begins 10 to 15 minutes after CCl_4 exposure. Fat droplets that accumulate in cisternae of the endoplasmic reticulum combine to form larger droplets and fill vacuoles, which in turn fill the entire cytoplasm. Approximately 10 to 12 hours later the liver appears grossly enlarged and pale because of the accumulation of fat. (Accumulation of fat is discussed further on p. 76.)

In the meantime, cellular swelling progresses because of alterations in the selective permeability of the plasma membrane. Cellular swelling becomes severe when the plasma membrane loses its ability to prevent the passive inward diffusion of sodium ions, water, and calcium. The most serious consequence of plasma membrane damage is, as in hypoxic injury, to the mitochondria. An influx of calcium ions from the extracellular compartment activates multiple enzyme systems resulting in cytoskeleton disruption, membrane damage, activation of inflammation, and eventually DNA degradation. Calcium ion accumulation in the mitochondria cause the mitochondria to swell, an occurrence that is associated with irreversible cellular injury. The injured mitochondria can no longer generate ATP, but they do continue to accumulate calcium ions. The influx of calcium into the mitochondria interferes with oxidative metabolism (by uncoupling oxidative phosphorylation).

Decreasing cellular pH (caused by the loss of oxidative phosphorylation and ATP-stimulating glycolysis), together with fluid and electrolyte imbalances (increased sodium,

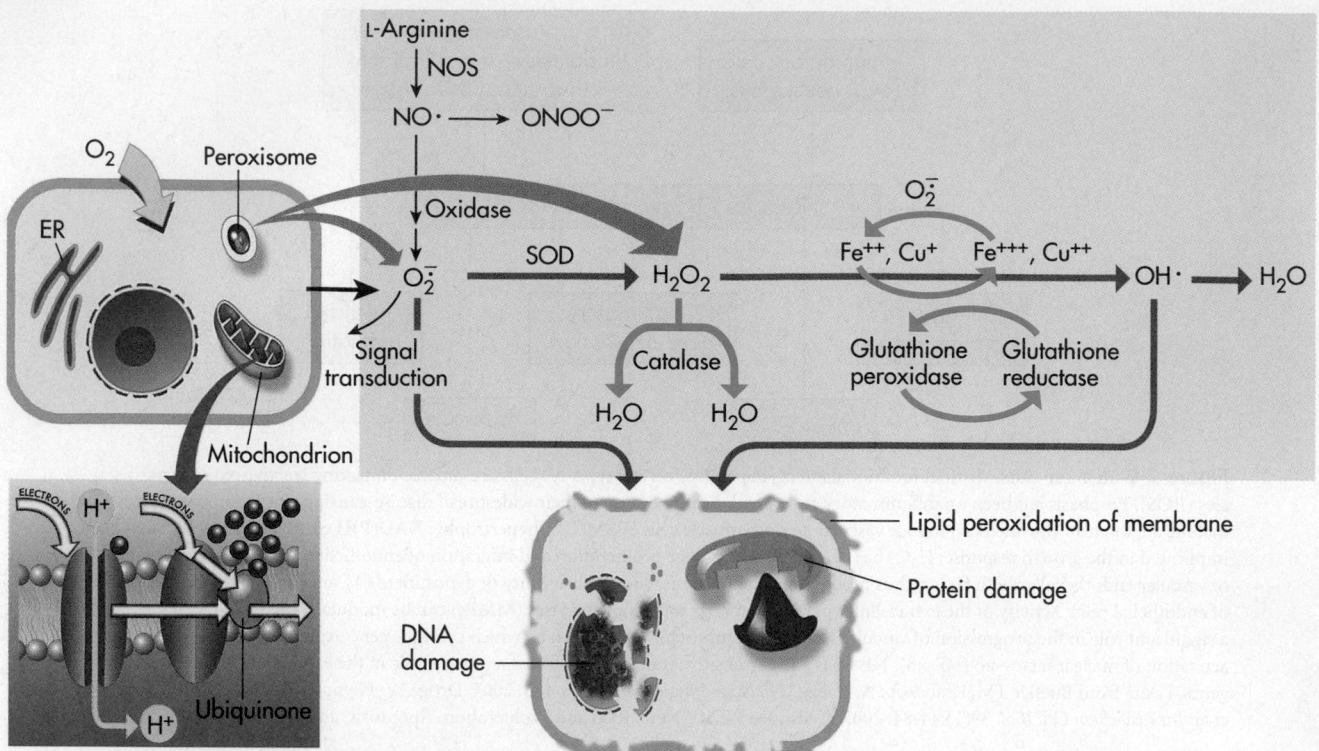

Figure 2-10 Generation of reactive oxygen species (ROS) and antioxidant mechanisms in biologic systems. Mitochondria have four sites of entry for electrons coming into the electron transport system: one for reduced nicotinamide adenine dinucleotide (NADH) and three for reduced form of flavin adenine dinucleotide ($FADH_2$). These pathways meet at the small, lipophilic molecule, ubiquinone (coenzyme Q), at the beginning of the common electron transport pathway. Ubiquinone transfers electrons in the inner membrane, ultimately enabling their interaction with O_2 and H_2 to yield H_2O. In so doing, the transport allows free energy change and the synthesis of one mole of adenosine triphosphate (ATP). With the transport of electrons, free radicals are generated within the mitochondria. ROS (H_2O_2, OH·, and O_2^{-} and nitric oxide [NO]) act as physiologic modulators of some mitochondrial functions but also may cause cell damage. O_2 is converted to superoxide (O_2^{-}) by oxidative enzymes in the mitochondria, endoplasmic reticulum (ER), plasma membrane, peroxisomes, and cytosol. O_2 is converted to H_2O_2 by superoxide dismutase (SOD) and further to OH· by the Cu^{++}/Fe^{++} Fenton reaction. Superoxide catalyzes the reduction of Fe^{++} to Fe^{+++}, thus increasing OH· formation by the Fenton reaction. H_2O_2 is also derived from oxidases in peroxisomes. The NO· (radical) is produced by the oxidation of one of the terminal guanido-nitrogen atoms of L-arginine. Depending on the microenvironment, NO can be converted to other reactive nitrogen species including the highly reactive peroxynitrite ($ONOO^{-}$). Both OH· and $ONOO^{-}$ are very reactive and can modify cellular macromolecules and cause toxicity. The less reactive molecules O_2^{-} and H_2O_2 can serve as cellular signaling molecules. The major antioxidant enzymes include SOD, catalase, and glutathione peroxidase. (Data from Dröge W: *Physiol Rev* 82:47-95, 2002; Buetler TM, Krauskopf A, Ruegg UT: *News Physiol Sci* 19: 120-123, 2004.)

calcium, and water and decreased potassium), leads to lysosomal membrane injury, causing a leakage of lysosomal enzymes into the cytoplasm. Enzymatic digestion of cellular organelles, including the nucleus and nucleolus, ensues, halting synthesis of DNA and ribonucleic acid (RNA). The leakage of lysosomal enzymes apparently occurs late in chemical injury, well after irreversible lipid accumulation, mitochondrial swelling, and ATP loss.

Chemical Agents

Many chemical agents cause cellular injury. Minute amounts of some, such as arsenic and cyanide, can rapidly destroy enough cells to cause death of the individual. Long-term exposure to air pollutants, insecticides, and herbicides can cause cellular injury. Carbon monoxide, carbon tetrachloride, and social drugs, such as alcohol, can significantly alter cellular function and injure cellular structures. Over-the-counter and prescribed drugs also may cause cellular injury,

sometimes leading to death. Acetaminophen (outside the United States is known as paracetamol), commonly used as an analgesic, is one of the most common causes of poisoning worldwide.[14] In 2005, acetaminophen poisoning was responsible for more than 70,000 visits to healthcare clinics and about 300 deaths.[15,16] Drug-induced acute liver failure accounts for about 20% of liver failure in children and a higher percentage in adults[17] (see What's New?, Chapter 39). Accidental or suicidal poisonings by chemical agents cause numerous deaths. The injurious effects of some of these agents—lead, carbon monoxide, ethyl alcohol, and mercury—exemplify common cellular injuries.

Lead. Lead is a heavy metal ubiquitous in the environment. Despite efforts to reduce exposure through government regulation, phasing out production of leaded gasoline, and banning use of lead paint, excessive lead exposure still persists in the environment for many people and lead toxic-

Table 2-3	Biologically Relevant Free Radicals
Free Radical	**Comments**
Reactive oxygen species (ROS) Superoxide $O_2^{\bar{\cdot}}$ $O_2 \rightarrow$ oxidase $O_2^{\bar{\cdot}}$	Generated either (1) directly during autooxidation in mitochondria, or (2) enzymatically by enzymes in the cytoplasm, such as xanthine oxidase or cytochrome P-450; once produced, it can be inactivated spontaneously or more rapidly by the enzyme superoxide dismutase (SOD): $O_2^{\bar{\cdot}}$ + $O_2^{\bar{\cdot}}$ + 2H+ $\rightarrow$ SOD H_2O_2 + O_2 $O_2^{\bar{\cdot}}$, a signaling molecule in growing or differentiating tissue, including hypertrophy, can alter cellular responses to growth factors and vasoconstrictor hormones; increasing levels of $O_2^{\bar{\cdot}}$ may lead to apoptosis (see Figure 2-9)
Hydrogen peroxide (H_2O_2) $O_2^{\bar{\cdot}}$ + $O_2^{\bar{\cdot}}$ + 2H $\rightarrow$ SOD H_2O_2 + O_2 or Oxidases present in peroxisomes O_2 peroxisome $O_2^{\bar{\cdot}} \rightarrow$ SOD H_2O_2	Generated by SOD or directly by oxidases in intracellular peroxisomes; SOD is considered an antioxidant because it converts superoxide to $H_2O_2^{\cdot}$, catalase (another antioxidant) can then decompose H_2O_2 to O_2 + H_2O; H_2O_2 can serve as a cellular signaling molecule
Hydroxyl radicals (OH^-) $H_2O \rightarrow H\cdot + OH\cdot$ or $Fe^{++} + H_2O_2 \rightarrow Fe^{+++} + OH\cdot + OH^-$ or $H_2O_2 + O_2^{\bar{\cdot}} \rightarrow OH\cdot + OH^- + O_2$	Generated by the hydrolysis of water caused by ionizing radiation or by interaction with metals—especially iron (Fe) and copper (Cu); iron is important in toxic oxygen injury because it is required for maximal oxidative cell damage; $OH\cdot$ is highly reactive and can modify cellular macromolecules and cause toxicity
Nitric oxide (NO) $NO\cdot + O_2^{\bar{\cdot}} \rightarrow ONOO^- + H+$ $\uparrow \downarrow$ $OH\cdot + NO_2 \Leftrightarrow ONOOH \rightarrow NO_3^-$	NO by itself is an important mediator that can act as a free radical; it can be converted to another radical—peroxynitrite anion ($ONOO^-$), as well as $NO_2\cdot$ and NO_3^-; NO is formed in neuronal cells, where it modulates neurotransmission; in endothelial cells as a modulator of vessel relaxation; and in neutrophils and macrophages as a factor in vessel relaxation and inactivation of pathogens

Data from Kumar V, Abbas A, Fausto N: *Robbins and Cotran pathologic basis of disease,* ed 7, Philadelphia, 2005, Saunders; Buetler TM, Krauskopf A, Ruegg UT: *News Physiol Sci* 19:120-123, 2004.

Table 2-4	Diseases and Disorders Linked to Oxygen-Derived Free Radicals
Deterioration noted in aging	Iron overload
Atherosclerosis	Lung disorders
Heart disease	Asbestosis
Stroke	Oxygen toxicity
Brain disorders	Emphysema
Ischemic brain injury	Nutritional deficiencies
Aluminum toxicity	Radiation injury
Alzheimer disease	Reperfusion injury
Neurotoxins	Rheumatoid arthritis
AIDS-associated dementia	Skin disorders
Cancer	Solar radiation
Cardiac myopathy	Burns
Chronic granulomatous disease	Contact dermatitis
Diabetes mellitus	Bloom syndrome
Eye disorders	Toxic states
Macular degeneration	Xenobiotics (CCl_4, paraquat, cigarette smoke, etc.)
Cataracts	Metal ions (Ni, Cu, Fe, etc.)
Inflammatory disorders	Amyotrophic lateral sclerosis
Other	Huntington disease?
	Parkinson disease?

AIDS, Acquired immunodeficiency syndrome.
Data from Knight JA: *Ann Clin Lab Sci* 25(2):111, 1995; Bergendi L et al: *Life Sci* 65(18-19): 1865, 1999; Maccarrone M, Ullrich V: *Cell Death Differ* 11:949-952, 2004.

Table 2-5	Methods Contributing to Inactivation or Termination of Free Radicals	
Method	**Process**	
Antioxidants	Endogenous or exogenous; either blocks synthesis or inactivates (e.g., scavenges) free radicals; includes vitamin E, vitamin C, cysteine, glutathione, albumin, ceruloplasmin, transferrin	
Enzymes	Superoxide dismutase,* which converts superoxide to H_2O_2; catalase* (in peroxisomes) decomposes H_2O_2; glutathione peroxidase* decomposes $OH\cdot$ and H_2O_2	

*These enzymes are important in modulating the cellular destructive effects of free radicals, also released in inflammation.

ity is still a primary hazard to children.[18] Particularly worrisome is lead exposure to the fetus during pregnancy because the developing nervous system is especially vulnerable. Developing fetuses and young children absorb lead more easily than adults[18]; however, the exact transport mechanisms have not yet been elucidated. Exposure to lead during neurologic development has significant effects on neurobehavioral and intellectual performance, resulting in learning disorders, hyperactivity, and attention problems.[18]

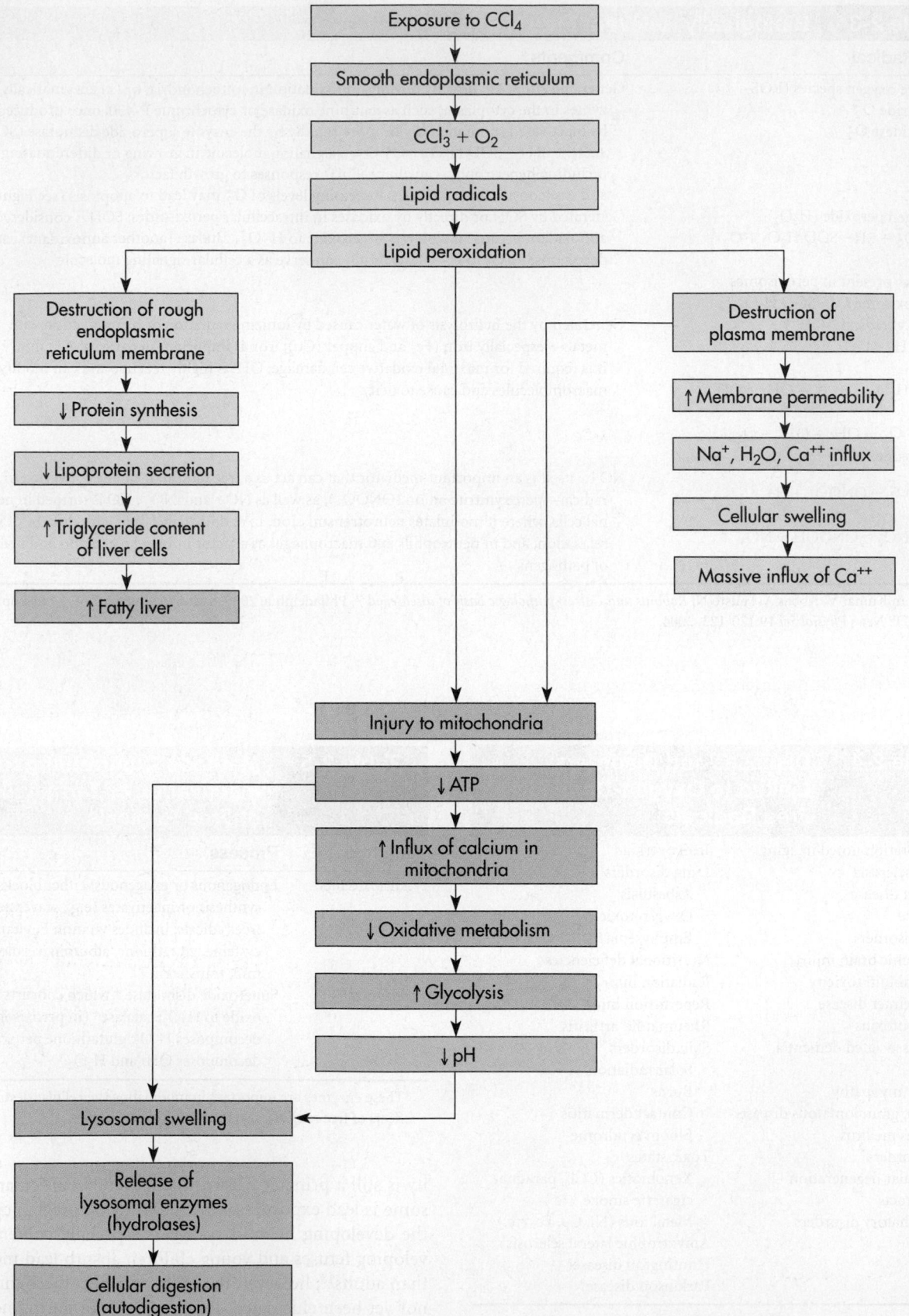

Figure 2-11 Chemical injury of liver cells induced by carbon tetrachloride (CCl_4) poisoning. *Light blue boxes* are mechanisms unique to chemical injury; *purple boxes* involve hypoxic injury. *Green boxes* are clinical manifestations.

Lead-based paint, which has a sweet taste, is often ingested by children when they have access to surfaces painted with it. Other sources of lead in daily life include the dust and soil found in inner-city urban and possibly rural areas, debris from household renovations, baby formula mixed with lead-contaminated tap water, newsprint, water that flows through lead pipes, hair dyes, food stored in soldered tin cans or eaten off of pottery made with lead-based glazes, and contamination from leaded gasoline.[19] If nutrition is compromised, especially if dietary intake of iron, calcium, zinc, and vitamin D is insufficient, lead's toxic effects are enhanced.

The organ systems primarily affected by lead include the nervous system, the hematopoietic system (tissues that produce blood cells), and the kidneys. Lead affects many different biologic activities at the cellular and molecular levels, many of which may be related to its ability to interfere with the functions of calcium.[18] Lead is able to *increase* intracellular calcium concentrations and become a calcium substitute, and some calcium-binding proteins are capable of binding to lead.[18] Very tiny concentrations (subnanomolar) of lead activate protein kinase C (PKC) in a process that is partially dependent on calcium.[13,20] The PKC-mediated lead-induced rise in intracellular free calcium may be the cause of cellular disruption. Lead appears to have its greatest effects during the later stages of brain development, possibly by altering development of synaptic connections (i.e., trimming/pruning) and neuronal death (apoptosis).[18] Alterations in calcium may play a crucial role in the interference with neurotransmitters, which may cause hyperactive behavior and proliferation of capillaries of the white matter and intercerebral arteries.[2,18] Lead inhibits several enzymes involved in hemoglobin synthesis. A significant manifestation of lead toxicity is anemia caused by lysis of red blood cells (hemolysis). Other manifestations of brain involvement include convulsions and delirium and, with peripheral nerve involvement, wrist, finger, and sometimes foot paralysis. Renal lesions can cause tubular dysfunction resulting in glycosuria (glucose in the urine), aminoaciduria (amino acids in the urine), and hyperphosphaturia (excess phosphate in the urine). Gastrointestinal symptoms are less severe and include nausea, loss of appetite, weight loss, and abdominal cramping.

Carbon Monoxide. Gaseous substances can be classified according to their ability to asphyxiate (interrupt respiration) or irritate. Toxic asphyxiants, such as carbon monoxide, hydrogen cyanide, and hydrogen sulfide, directly interfere with cellular respiration. Carbon monoxide is widely available.

Carbon monoxide (CO), a gas, is odorless, colorless, and undetectable unless it is mixed with a visible or odorous pollutant. It is produced by the incomplete combustion of such fuels as gasoline. In dense urban environments, CO produced by incomplete combustion from motor vehicles increases air pollution. Although CO is a chemical agent, the ultimate injury it produces is a hypoxic injury, namely, oxygen deprivation. Normally, oxygen molecules are carried to tissues bound to hemoglobin in red blood cells (see Chapter 29). Because CO's affinity for hemoglobin is 300 times greater than that

of oxygen, it quickly binds with the hemoglobin, preventing oxygen molecules from doing so. Minute amounts of CO can produce significant percentages of **carboxyhemoglobin** (carbon monoxide bound with hemoglobin).

Symptoms related to CO poisoning include headache, giddiness, tinnitus (ringing in the ears), nausea, weakness, and vomiting. At risk for CO exposure are those who: (1) breathe air polluted by gasoline engines or defective furnaces; (2) work in occupations such as coal mining, fire fighting, welding,[21] or engine repair; and (3) smoke cigarettes, cigars, or pipes. The fetus is especially at risk from the effects of carbon monoxide because fetal carboxyhemoglobin levels are likely to be 10% to 15% greater than maternal levels.[22]

Ethanol. Alcohol (**ethanol**) is the number one moodaltering drug used in the United States. Because alcohol is not only a psychoactive drug but also a food, it is considered part of the basic food supply in many societies.

A large intake of alcohol has enormous effects on nutritional status. Major nutritional deficiencies include magnesium, vitamin B$_6$, thiamine, and phosphorus. Liver and nutritional disorders are the most serious consequences of alcohol abuse. New understandings of the mechanisms of ethanol-induced liver injury have emerged through the clarification of a pathway for ethanol oxidation, the microsomal P-450 oxidase pathway (see following).

The major effects of acute alcoholism involve the central nervous system (CNS). After ingestion, alcohol is absorbed, unaltered, into the stomach and small intestine. Fatty foods and milk slow absorption.[23] Alcohol then is distributed to all tissues and fluids of the body in direct proportion to the blood concentration.

Most of the alcohol in the blood is metabolized in the liver through one major and two accessory pathways. The major pathway involves hepatic alcohol dehydrogenase (ADH), an enzyme of the cytosol that catalyzes the conversion of ethanol to acetaldehyde (Figure 2-12).

The microsomal ethanol oxidizing system (MEOS) depends on cytochrome P-450, an enzyme necessary for cellular oxidation.[24] Activation of the MEOS requires a high ethanol concentration and thus is thought to be important in the accelerated ethanol metabolism (i.e., tolerance) noted in people with chronic alcoholism.[24]

Individuals differ in their capability to metabolize alcohol. Genetic differences in metabolism of liver alcohol, including aldehyde dehydrogenases, have been identified.[25] People with chronic alcoholism develop certain levels of tolerance because of enzyme induction, leading to an increased rate of metabolism (e.g., P-450).

Studies conducted since 1997 have contributed to our understanding of the association between alcohol consumption and cardiovascular disease. Consistent results validate the so-called *J-shaped inverse association* between alcohol and cardiovascular disease mortality and morbidity. That is, moderate drinkers exhibiting a decreased risk compared with both heavy drinkers and nondrinkers. Surprisingly, consistent epidemiologic studies show that daily light to moderate alcohol

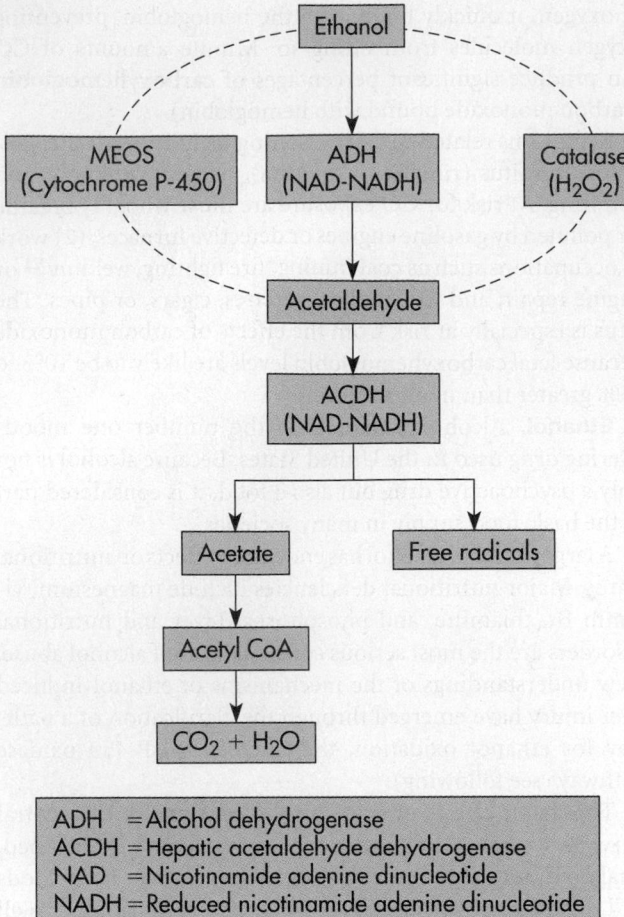

ADH = Alcohol dehydrogenase
ACDH = Hepatic acetaldehyde dehydrogenase
NAD = Nicotinamide adenine dinucleotide
NADH = Reduced nicotinamide adenine dinucleotide
MEOS = Microsomal ethanol oxidizing system

Figure 2-12 Major pathway of metabolism of alcohol in the liver through alcohol dehydrogenase (ADH).

intake reduces the risk of coronary heart disease (CHD) as compared with those who do not drink alcoholic beverages at all. Alcohol possibly reduces the risk of CHD through increases in fibrinolysis[26] and increases in plasma high density lipoprotein-cholesterol (HDL-C) levels.[27] Alcohol also may increase insulin sensitivity.[28] Limited data suggest that the level for optimal benefit may be slightly lower for women. Thus the American Heart Association recommends no more than two drinks per day for men and one drink per day for women.[27]

Acute alcoholism mainly affects the CNS but may induce reversible hepatic and gastric changes. The hepatic changes, initiated from acetaldehyde, include deposition in fat, enlargement of the liver, interruption of microtubular transport of proteins and their secretion, increase in intracellular water, depression of fatty acid oxidation in the mitochondria, increased membrane rigidity, and acute liver cell necrosis (see Chapter 39). In the CNS, alcohol is itself a depressant, initially affecting subcortical structures (probably the brainstem reticular formation).[29] Consequently, motor and intellectual activities become disoriented. Acute alcoholism contributes significantly to motor vehicle fatalities. At higher blood levels,

medullary centers become depressed, affecting respiration. Much investigation is under way to determine the extent of the relationship between alcohol and snoring and obstructive sleep apnea (cessation of breathing).[30,31]

Chronic alcoholism causes structural alterations in practically all organs and tissues in the body, especially the liver and stomach. Much progress has been made in understanding the pathogenesis of alcoholic liver disease, which should increase the likelihood of prevention and successful therapy.[32] Cellular damage is increased by ROS and oxidative stress (see p. 54). New data on the cellular and molecular mechanisms of liver fibrosis are presented in What's New? Cellular Mechanisms of Fibrosis and Reversal. In addition, the activation of methionine, an essential amino acid, to S-adenosyl-L-methionine (SAMe) is decreased in those with alcoholism.[32] Replacement of SAMe in baboons decreased liver mitochondrial lesions, replenished the antioxidant glutathione, and reduced mortality from cirrhosis.[33] Oxidative stress is associated with phospholipid depletion. In baboons, replacement of polyenylphosphatidylcholine (PPC) corrected the phospholipid depletion.[33] Clinical trials with PPC involving individuals with alcoholic liver disease are ongoing. Chronic alcoholism is related to several disorders, including

WHAT'S NEW? Cellular Mechanisms of Fibrosis and Reversal

Historically, fibrosis has been defined by the increased growth and hardening and/or scarring of various tissues. These processes have been attributed to excess deposition of extracellular matrix components (see Figure 1-14), particularly collagen. Current treatments target inflammation; however, accumulating evidence reveals factors involved are different from those regulating inflammation. The key cellular mediator of fibrosis is *myofibroblast* that, when activated, produces collagen. Myofibroblasts are activated by numerous mechanisms, providing many other therapeutic possibilities. Important regulators of fibrosis include cytokines (IL-13, IL-21, TGF-β1), chemokines, angiogenic factors, growth factors, acute phase proteins, and the renin-angiotensin-aldosterone system (ANG-II) (see Chapter 29). Investigators from the University of California at San Diego have shown that liver fibrosis in animals can be stopped and reversed! Their discovery opens new possibilities for curing viral hepatitis, fatty liver disease, cirrhosis, pulmonary fibrosis, scleroderma, and burns. By blocking an enzyme that leads to overproduction of scar tissue the investigators not only stopped the fibrotic progression but also reversed it. Activation of a protein called RSK results in hepatic stellate cell (HSC) activation that is critical for the progression of liver fibrosis. The animals were given an RSK-inhibitory peptide that stopped the HSC from proliferating. RSK-inhibitory peptide also activated apoptotic caspases (cell death), which killed the cells producing liver cirrhosis. Worldwide almost 800,000 people die each year from liver cirrhosis because there is no treatment. These latest findings are important steps for understanding fibrosis and developing therapies.

Data from Buck M, Chojkier M: *Plos One* 2(12):e1372, 2007; Mir AI et al: *Indian J Exp Biol* 45(7):626-629, 2007; Wynn T: *J Pathol* 214(2):199-210, 2008.

an increased tendency for hypertension, a higher incidence of acute and chronic pancreatitis, and regressive changes in skeletal muscle (see Chapter 39). Ethanol is implicated in the onset of a variety of immune defects, including effects on the production of cytokines involved in inflammatory responses. The deleterious effects of prenatal alcohol exposure (e.g., **fetal alcohol syndrome [FAS]**) also have been noted. FAS can lead to growth retardation, cognitive impairment, facial anomalies, and ocular disturbances.[34,35] In some cases, full-blown FAS may not be indicated but CNS defects may *still* be present and are classified as alcohol-related birth defects (ARBDs) and alcohol-related neurodevelopmental disorders (ARNDs).[36]

Autopsies of children with FAS have revealed widespread severe damage, including failure of certain brain regions to develop, malformations of brain tissue, and failure of certain cells to migrate to their necessary location during development.[37] Imaging studies reveal that in addition to an overall reduction in brain size, the corpus callosum is reduced in size or missing, the cerebellum is significantly reduced, and the basal ganglia and caudate nucleus are significantly reduced.[19,38]

Animal studies have shown that ethanol at moderate concentrations inhibits epidermal growth factor–dependent replication of hepatocytes. This finding may account for the growth or development impairment associated with FAS and decreased liver regeneration in those with alcoholic liver disease.[39,40] The wide variety of cellular or biochemical effects of ethanol on fetal tissue is itself a puzzle, reflecting a multifactorial problem. These effects are conceptually connected to membrane structure and function involving transport systems, membrane fluidity, Na^+, K^+ pump expression, and EGF receptor expression.[40] Recent evidence points to oxidative stress as being potentially causative of these membrane-related events.[41] Additionally, ethanol has been shown to increase apoptotic cell death.[42]

Whatever the cause, people with chronic alcoholism have a significantly shortened life span related mainly to damage to the liver, stomach, brain, and heart. Alcohol is a well-known cause of hepatic injury, terminating in cirrhosis (see Chapter 39) (Figure 2-13).

Mercury. Mercury has been used medically and commercially for centuries.[43] In the past it was a common component in medications. Mercury is still present in some thermometers and blood pressure cuffs and in batteries, switches, and fluorescent light bulbs. Large amounts of mercury exist as part of the electrodes formed in the electrolytic production of chlorine and sodium hydroxide from saline. Today people are exposed to mercury from three major sources: fish consumption, dental amalgams, and vaccines. All of these uses give rise to possible accidental and occupational exposures.[43]

Dental Amalgams. Dental amalgams have been used for more than 150 years. They are believed to be more durable and easier to use than other types of fillings, as well as being relatively inexpensive. Amalgams consist of about 50% mercury amalgamated or combined with other metals, such as silver and copper. The controversies and heated debates

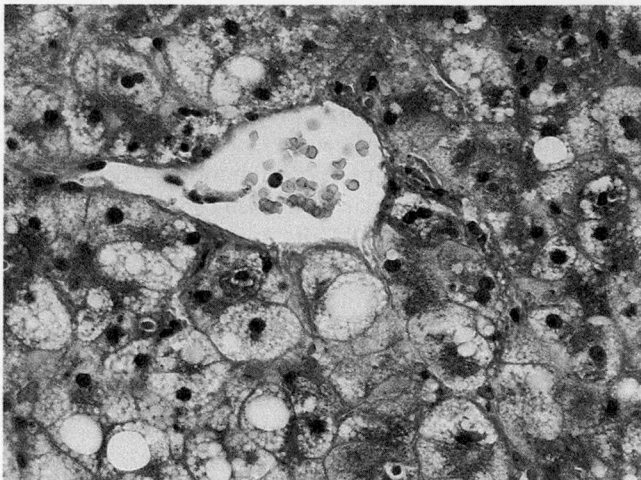

Figure 2-13 Alcoholic hepatitis. Chicken-wire fibrosis extending between hepatocytes. (Mallory trichrome stain.) (From Damjanov I, Linder J: *Anderson's pathology,* ed 10, St Louis, 1996, Mosby.)

concerning amalgams peaked in the 1970s with the discovery that amalgams can release mercury vapors into the mouth in concentrations that are higher than those deemed safe by occupational health guidelines.

Since then it was realized that the actual inhaled dose was small because of the small volume of the oral cavity.[43] Yet, brain, blood, and urinary concentrations correlate with the number of amalgam surfaces present in a person. Removal of amalgam fillings also can cause temporary elevations in blood concentration because the removal transiently increases the amount of mercury vapor inhaled.

Current health risk concerns arise from claims that long-term exposure to low concentrations of mercury vapor either causes or worsens degenerative diseases, such as amyotrophic lateral sclerosis, Alzheimer disease, multiple sclerosis, and Parkinson disease. Concern about the effect of mercury vapor in relation to Alzheimer disease was intensified for a time after a report that the brains of individuals with Alzheimer disease had elevated mercury concentrations. Several epidemiologic investigations, however, failed to provide evidence of a role of dental amalgams in these degenerative diseases; these include a long-term Swedish study,[44] an ongoing Swedish study,[45] and a study of 129 nuns 75 to 102 years of age.[46] Recently, a randomized prospective trial of 507 children failed to show exposure to mercury from amalgams is linked to neurobehavioral or neurologic effects.[47] A difficult problem is that mercury can inhibit various biochemical processes in vitro without having the same effects in vivo. Thus, at present it is unknown whether removal of amalgams reduces risk of certain diseases, especially because removal itself affects blood concentrations of mercury vapor, which will rise before they eventually decline, thereby adding to the controversy.

Fish Consumption. The major source of exposure to methyl mercury is the consumption of fish and sea mammals. Clinical reports of mercury poisoning from fish consumption are those from Japan in the 1950s and 1960s. Environmental

Protection Agency (EPA) guidelines are derived from reports of neuropsychologic changes noted in the Faeroe Islands study, in which subjects had been inadvertently exposed to methyl mercury mainly from whale consumption.[48] A similar study in the United States shows methyl mercury levels to be slightly higher than the EPA guideline for safe consumption.[43] The health risk posed by exposure to mercury from fish consumption is being debated. The U.S. Food and Drug Administration (FDA) has, however, recommended that pregnant women, nursing mothers, and young children avoid eating fish with a high mercury content (>1 part per million [ppm]), such as shark, swordfish, tile fish, king mackerel, and whale meat.[43] Other advocates, however, have published more extensive lists including fish with the lowest levels, e.g., blue crab, croaker, fish sticks, flounder, haddock, trout, salmon (wild), and shrimp.[49]

Vaccines. Thimerosal has been used as a preservative in many vaccines since the 1930s.[43] It contains the ethyl mercury radical ($CH_3CH_2Hg^+$). Earlier toxicology studies and a 2007 study[50] found either no adverse effects or no support for a causal relationship between thimerosal and deficits in neuropyschologic functioning. An earlier reevaluation of thimerosal, however, performed by applying the revised EPA guideline for methyl mercury to ethyl mercury found the usual U.S. program of recommended vaccines caused patients to receive more ethyl mercury than the EPA guidelines (i.e., >1 mcg of mercury per kilogram per day) deemed safe.[51,52] Steps were rapidly taken to remove thimerosal from vaccines by switching to single-dose vials that did not require a preservative. Since 2003 no vaccines contain thimerosal. Recent findings indicate that the half-life of ethyl mercury compared with methyl mercury is shorter.[53] The half-life of methyl mercury in blood, which is used to indicate the total body burden, is assumed to be about 50 days.[54] For children receiving thimerosal in vaccines, however, the half-life of ethyl mercury in blood was 7 to 10 days, or ½ to ⅕ as long as that of methyl mercury.[52,53] Thus in the 2-month periods between vaccinations (at birth and at 2, 4, and 6 months), all of the mercury should be excreted with no accumulation.[43]

Social or Street Drugs. The social or "recreational" use of psychoactive drugs is widespread in many parts of the world. Most popular and dangerous are the drugs methamphetamine ("meth"), marijuana, cocaine, and heroin. Although the prevalence of cocaine use in the general population decreased in 1986, morbidity and mortality related to cocaine increased sharply in the 1990s. Illicit use of drugs is a prevalent risk behavior among adolescents.[55] Table 2-6 summarizes the effects of these drugs.

Unintentional and Intentional Injuries

Unintentional and intentional injuries are an important health problem in the United States. In 2005 there were 173,573 deaths in this category, an injury death rate of 57.76/100,000.[56] Death due to injury is significantly more common for men than women; the overall rate for men is 84.16/100,000 vs. 33.12/100,000 for women. Significant racial differences exist in the death rate, too: whites at 57.42./100,000, blacks at 67.31/100,000, and other racial groups at a combined rate of 35.76/100,000. A bimodal age distribution for injury-related deaths also has been noted, with peaks in the young adult and older adult groups. Unintentional injury is the leading cause of death for people between the ages of 1 and 34 years, with intentional injury (suicide, homicide) ranking between the second and fourth leading causes of death in this age group. A 1999 report published by the Institute of Medicine (IOM) indicated that between 44,000 and 98,000 unnecessary deaths per year occurred in hospitals alone as a result of errors by health care professionals. An accurate account is a tremendous challenge because of disagreements over reported statistics.[57] Statistics on nonfatal injuries are harder to document accurately, but they are known to be a significant cause of morbidity and disability and to cost society billions of dollars annually. The more common terms used to describe and classify unintentional and intentional injuries and brief descriptions of important features of these are discussed here.

Blunt Force Injuries

Blunt force injuries are the result of the application of mechanical energy to the body resulting in the tearing, shearing, or crushing of tissues. They are the most common type of injuries seen in most healthcare settings. Blunt force injury may be caused by blows (a moving object strikes the body), impacts (the moving body strikes a fixed object), or a combination of both. Motor vehicle accidents and falls are the most common causes of these injuries, accounting for 45,520 and 20,426 deaths, respectively, in 2005.

Contusion

A **contusion** (bruise) is bleeding into the skin or underlying tissues as a consequence of a blow that squeezes or crushes the soft tissues and consequently ruptures blood vessels without breaking the skin. It may take several hours after injury before any change in skin color is seen. A bruise will be red-purple initially, eventually becoming blue-black, and then gradually changing to yellow-brown or green before fully disappearing (Figure 2-14). These color changes reflect the progression of tissue damage and healing that develops in the area of underlying injury. The length of time depends on such factors as the extent and location of the injury and the degree of vascularization in the area. Small contusions may resolve in a matter of days, whereas larger ones can take weeks to completely heal. Bruising of soft tissues may sometimes be confined to deeper structures; thus no injury is visible externally. Blood in deeper structures may dissect along fascial planes, so discoloration of the skin may be seen in areas not directly injured by the initiating blow or impact, such as bruising of the thigh occurring with a hip or pelvis fracture or "black eyes" with orbital plate fractures. Contusions also may be seen in internal organs in cases of severe injury.

A collection of blood in soft tissues or an enclosed space also may be referred to as a **hematoma** (see Figures 17-3 and 17-6). A **subdural hematoma** is a collection of blood between the inner surface of the dura mater and the surface of the brain, resulting from the shearing of small veins that bridge the subdural space. Subdural hematomas can result from

Table 2-6	Social or Street Drugs and Their Effects
Type of Drug	**Description and Effects**
Marijuana	Active substance: delta 9-tetrahydrocannabinol (THC), found in resin of the *Cannabis sativa* plant
	With smoking (e.g., "joints"), about 50% is absorbed through the lungs; when ingested only 10% is absorbed; with heavy use the following adverse effects have been reported: alterations of sensory perceptions, cognitive and psychomotor impairment (e.g., inability to judge time, speed, distance); smoking 3 or 4/day is similar to smoking 20 cigarettes/day in regard to frequency of chronic bronchitis and may contribute to lung cancer; data from animal studies only, indicate reproductive changes including reduced fertility, decreased sperm motility, and decreased circulatory testosterone; fetal abnormalities including low birth weight and increased frequency of childhood leukemia; increased frequency of infectious illness is thought to be the result of depressed cell-mediated and humoral immunity
Methamphetamine (meth)	An amine derivation of amphetamine (C10H15N) used as crystalline hydrochloride
	CNS stimulant; in large doses causes irritability, aggressive (violent) behavior, anxiety, excitement, auditory hallucinations, and paranoia (delusions and psychosis); mood changes are common and the abuser can swiftly change from friendly to hostile; paranoiac swings can result in suspiciousness, hyperactive behavior, and dramatic mood swings
	Appeals to abusers because body's metabolism is increased and produces euphoria, alertness, and perception of increased energy
	Stages:
	Low intensity: user is not psychologically addicted and uses methamphetamine by swallowing or snorting
	Binge and high intensity: user has psychologic addiction and smokes or injects to achieve a faster, stronger high
	Tweaking: most dangerous stage; user is continually under the influence, not sleeping for 3 to 15 days, extremely irritated, and paranoid
Cocaine and crack	Extracted from the leaves of the coca plant and sold as a water-soluble powder (cocaine hydrochloride) liberally diluted with talcum powder or other white powders; extraction of pure alkaloid from cocaine hydrochloride is "free-base" called crack because it "cracks" when heated
	Crack is more potent than cocaine; cocaine is widely used as an anesthetic, usually in procedures involving the oral cavity; it is a potent CNS stimulant, blocking reuptake of neurotransmitters norepinephrine, dopamine, and serotonin; also increases synthesis of norepinephrine and dopamine; dopamine induces a sense of euphoria, and norepinephrine causes adrenergic potentiation, including hypertension, tachycardia, and vasoconstriction; cocaine can therefore cause severe coronary artery narrowing and ischemia; not clear why cocaine increases thrombus formation; other cardiovascular effects include dysrhythmias, sudden death, dilated cardiomyopathy, rupture of descending aorta (i.e., secondary to hypertension); effects on the fetus include premature labor, retarded fetal development, stillbirth, hyperirritability
Heroin	An opiate closely related to morphine, methadone, and codeine
	Highly addictive, and withdrawal causes intense fear ("I'll die without it"); sold "cut" with similar-looking white powder; dissolved in water it is often highly contaminated; feeling of tranquility and sedation lasts only a few hours and thus encourages repeated intravenous or subcutaneous injections; acts on the receptors enkephalins, endorphins, and dynorphins, which are widely distributed throughout the body with high affinity to the CNS; effects can include infectious complications, especially *Staphylococcus aureus,* granulomas of the lung, septic embolism, and pulmonary edema—in addition, viral infections from casual exchange of needles and HIV; sudden death is related to overdosage secondary to respiratory depression, decreased cardiac output, and severe pulmonary edema

CNS, Central nervous system; *HIV,* human immunodeficiency virus.

Data from Cotran RS, Kumar V, Colllins T: *Robbins pathologic basis of disease,* ed 7, Philadelphia, 2005, Saunders; Nahas G, Sutin K, Bennett WM: Review of marijuana and medicine, *N Engl J Med* 343(7):514, 2000.

blows, falls, or sudden acceleration/deceleration of the head, as occurs in *shaken baby syndrome.* An **epidural hematoma** is a collection of blood between the inner surface of the skull and the dura. It is caused by a torn artery and is almost always associated with a skull fracture.

Contusions of the brain may result from (1) a blow, or (2) a fall or impact. In blows, when a moving object strikes the stationary head, a cerebral contusion grouped in the portions of the brain underlying the area of scalp and skull injury is known as a *coup* pattern of injury. In falls or impacts, in which the moving head strikes a fixed object, a cerebral contusion seen in the area of the brain opposite the external injury is known as a *contrecoup* pattern of injury (see Figure 17-1). Contrecoup injury results when the head accelerates and the brain lags behind and presses into the areas of the skull directly opposite the direction of motion. When the head suddenly stops, the areas of the brain pressing into the skull are injured. For example, a person who falls directly backward striking the occiput (back of the head) will have cerebral contusions of the frontal and temporal tips (these injuries are discussed further in Chapter 17).

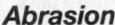

Bruising

↓

Extravasated
red cells

↓

Phagocytosis of
red cells by
macrophages

↓   ↓

Hemosiderin   Iron-free
pigments

Figure 2-14 Hemosiderin accumulation is noted as the color changes in a "black eye."

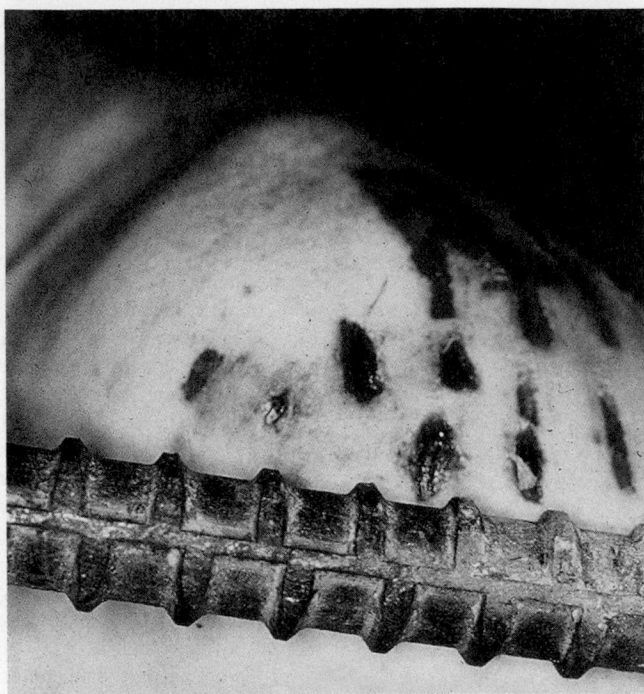

Figure 2-15 Patterned abrasion caused by a piece of rebar. Note the tissue tags at the inferior margins indicating the downward direction of the blow that caused this injury.

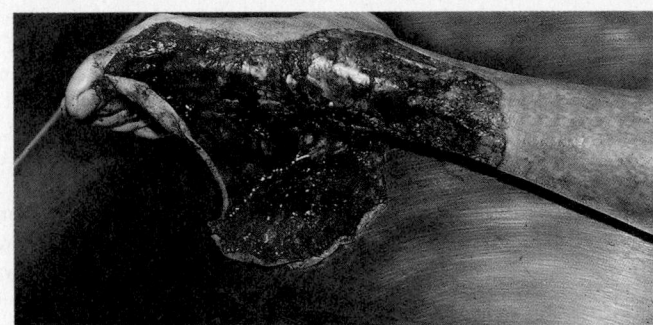

Figure 2-16 Avulsed laceration in motor vehicle accident victim. The victim was the driver and this injury most likely was caused by the brake pedal.

Abrasion

An **abrasion** (scrape) results from removal of the superficial layers of the skin caused by friction between the skin and injuring object. Abrasions vary in size and severity from fine, thin scratches to large denuded areas (road rash). In cases in which force is applied in a tangential, nonperpendicular direction to the skin surface, tags of tissue may be heaped up at the trailing or downstream edge of the abrasion. An abrasion will have a pale, moist, yellow-brown appearance at first. The color darkens to brown or even black as the injury dries. The injury may ooze fluid for 1 or 2 days until it is completely covered by a crust, or scab, which eventually flakes off of the underlying regenerated skin.

Abrasions and contusions may have a patterned appearance that mirrors the shape and features of an injuring object (Figure 2-15). Patterning of injuries can be of crucial importance in cases of automobile accidents, assaults, or homicides by documenting the connection between the victim's injuries and a suspect vehicle or weapon. Bite marks (usually a combination of abrasion and contusion) are another example of a patterned injury that can demonstrate a link between an assailant and victim.

Laceration

A **laceration** is a tear or rip resulting when the tensile strength of the skin or tissue is exceeded. Unlike an incision, in which the tissue is cleanly divided by a sharp edge, a laceration is much more jagged and irregular, and the edges are abraded. The depths of the laceration are irregular, and often tissue "bridges" of small vessels or nerves that have been stretched but not broken are present, crossing from one side of the wound to the other. If the injuring force is applied perpendicularly to the skin, crushing of the surrounding tissue with associated abrasion and contusion will be noted. If force is applied tangentially, undermining of the wound also will occur, with tissues at the trailing edge of the wound being lifted away from the underlying structures, creating a pocket in the direction opposite the blow. An extreme example is an **avulsion** (Figure 2-16), in which a wide area of tissue may be pulled away, creating a large flap. Usually, the shallower the angle of incidence of the blow, the more extensive the undermining.

Lacerations of internal organs are not uncommon in blunt impact injuries. Lacerations of the liver, spleen, kidneys, and bowel may occur in cases of blows to the abdomen, often with no externally visible injury to the abdominal wall. The thoracic aorta may be lacerated in sudden deceleration accidents. This results from the arch of the aorta being freely mobile, whereas the descending portion is attached to the spinal column. Rapid deceleration causes horizontal shearing with either partial or complete transection just below the takeoff of the left subclavian artery. Severe blows or impacts to the chest also may cause rupturing of the heart with lacerations of the atria or ventricles.

Fractures

Blunt force blows or impacts also can cause bone to break or shatter. Fractures are extensively covered in Chapter 42 and are not discussed here.

Sharp Force Injuries

Cutting and piercing injuries accounted for 2795 deaths in 2005. As with all injuries, men have a higher rate (1.43/100,000) than women (0.46/100,000). Here, too, are greater differences among races, with whites at 0.73/100,000, blacks at 2.29/100,000, and other racial groups at 0.80/100,000.

Incised Wounds

An **incised wound** is a cut that is *longer* than it is *deep*. The wound may be straight or jagged, depending on the object used and how the injury occurred; sharp, distinct edges without abrasion. Because the wound is caused by a sharp edge, the tissues are cleanly divided and no tissue bridging or undermining occurs. An incised wound may be thin and narrow or more elliptic and gaping in appearance because of varying lines of tension in the skin, depending on the location and orientation of the wound. Incised wounds tend to produce significant external bleeding with minimal internal hemorrhage. These wounds are often seen in sharp force injury suicides. In most cases, in addition to a deep, lethal cut, multiple superficial incisions are grouped in the surrounding area; these are known as *hesitation marks* (Figure 2-17).

Stab Wounds

A **stab wound** is a penetrating sharp force injury that is *deeper* than it is *long*. Because a sharp instrument is used, the depths of the wound are clean and distinct with no underlying or associated crushing injury. The edges are usually clean but may be abraded if the object is inserted deeply with enough force so that a wider, blunter portion of the instrument (e.g., the hilt of a knife) impacts the skin. Figure 2-18 illustrates this type of wound.

A number of the offending blade's characteristics may be determined from careful examination of the stab wound. If a *single-edge* blade is used, one margin of the wound will be sharp and the other blunt; if a *double-edge* blade causes the wound, both margins will have a sharp appearance. Stab wounds produced by a *serrated-edge* blade are often indistinguishable from those made by a *smooth-edge* blade. If any hesitation marks or scraping of the skin edges by the blade occurs, an interrupted pattern of abrasion may be seen, but this is uncommon. As with incised wounds, skin tension may cause the wound to gape, giving it an elliptic appearance. The edges must be brought into opposition so there is no distortion before trying to determine whether the margins are sharp or blunt. The length of the stab wound may or may not correlate with the width of the blade, depending on whether there was any cutting or twisting when the blade was inserted or withdrawn. Once the edges are in opposition, the thickness of the blade may be estimated from the width of the wound. Depth of the wound may not correlate with the length of the blade because the blade may not have been inserted fully, or as a consequence of compression of tissues caused by a forceful thrust, the wound may be deeper than the length of the blade.

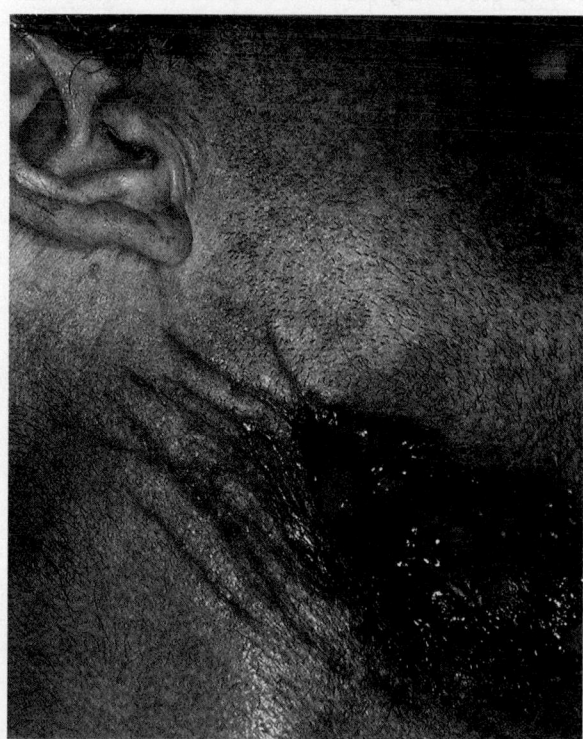

Figure 2-17 Self-inflicted incised wound of the neck with multiple hesitation marks.

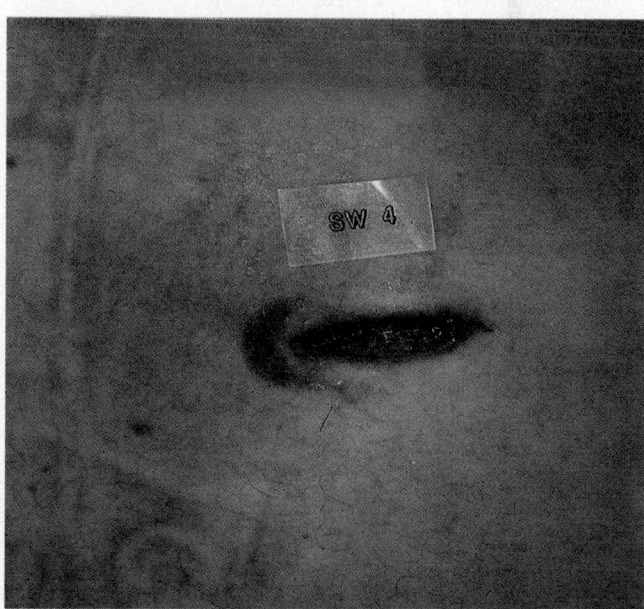

Figure 2-18 Stab wound with associated hilt mark. Note the sharp margin away from the hilt mark with the blunt margin toward it. This wound was caused by a single-edged knife.

Depending on size and location of the stab wound, the amount of external bleeding may be surprisingly small. After an initial spurt, even if a major vessel or the heart is struck, the wound track may be almost completely closed by tissue pressure, allowing only a trickle of visible blood externally despite copious internal bleeding.

Puncture Wounds

Instruments or objects with sharp points but without sharp edges may produce penetrating **puncture wounds.** A classic example is a wound of the foot caused by stepping on a nail. These injuries often will have abrasion of the edges of the wound, are prone to infection, and can be quite deep despite a sometimes innocuous external appearance.

Chopping Wounds

Heavy, edged instruments (axes, hatchets, propeller blades) produce injuries—**chopping wounds**—with a combination of sharp and blunt force characteristics. In addition to cutting, there is usually associated crushing of the wound edges and underlying tissues.

Gunshot Wounds

Injuries caused by gunfire accounted for 30,694 deaths in the United States in 2005. Of these, 17,002 were suicides, 12,682 homicides, 789 unintentional, and 221 classified as undetermined. Men are much more likely to die from gunshot injury than women. The male death rate in 2005 was 18.30/100,000 vs. 2.67/100,000 for women. Black men between the ages of 15 and 24 years have the greatest gunfire injury death rate: 87.07/100,000. To put this statistic into perspective, if this were the rate for the United States as a whole, there would be more than 257,000 gunshot wound deaths per year.

Gunshot wounds may be either penetrating (bullet retained in the body) or perforating (bullet exits the body). In some cases, the bullet may fragment, so pieces of the missile are retained even though there is an exit wound. The most important factors determining the appearance of a gunshot injury are whether it is an entrance or an exit wound and the range of fire.

Entrance Wounds

Although all **entrance wounds** share some common features, the overall appearance is most affected by the range of fire.

Contact range entrance wounds occur when the gun is held so the muzzle rests on or presses into the skin surface, causing a distinctive type of wound. In addition to the hole made by the bullet, there will be searing of the edges of the wound from the flame and hot gases exiting the barrel and soot or smoke deposited on the edges of and in the depths of the wound. In hard contact wounds, where the barrel is firmly pressed into the skin, there may be minimal soot and searing on the outside of the wound but deep penetration of smoke, burning gunpowder fragments, and hot gases into the depths of the injury. In hard contact wounds of the head, where there is only a thin layer of skin and muscle overlying bone, the large amount of gas and explosive energy sent into the wound may cause severe tearing and disruption of the tissues, giving the

wound a large, gaping, and jagged appearance—a phenomenon known as **blow back.** In areas of the body with thicker layers of soft tissue, the blow back may not cause tearing but will forcefully drive the skin back onto the end of the barrel, producing a patterned abrasion that mirrors the features of the weapon, known as a **muzzle imprint** (Figure 2-19).

Intermediate-range entrance wounds are surrounded by gunpowder tattooing or stippling (Figure 2-20). **Tattooing** results from fragments of burning or unburned pieces of gunpowder exiting the barrel and striking the skin surface with enough force to be driven into the epidermis or superficial dermis. **Stippling** results when fragments of powder strike with enough force to abrade the skin but not actually penetrate the surface. This phenomenon can be seen when the

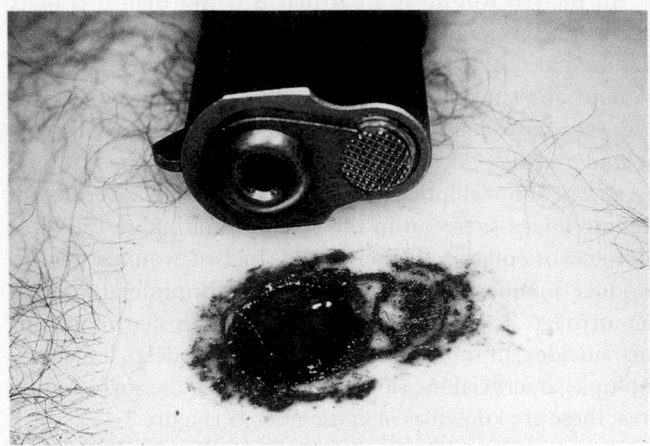

Figure 2-19 Contact range gunshot wound of the chest with a muzzle abrasion.

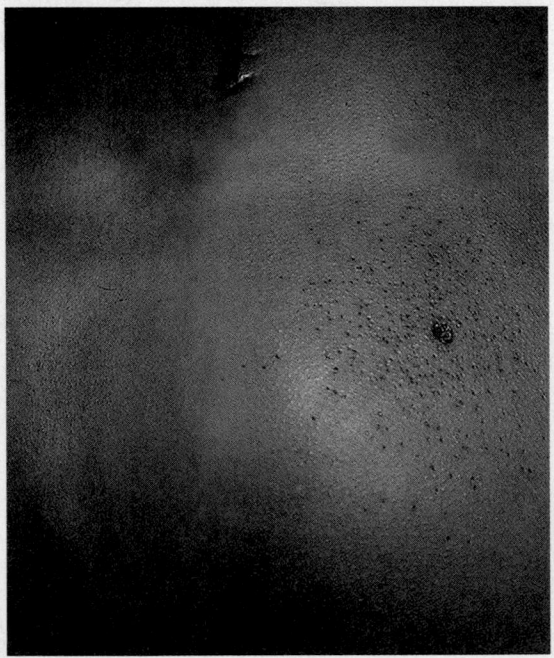

Figure 2-20 Intermediate range gunshot wound with stippling and tattooing.

muzzle-to-target range is less than 48 inches of most handguns. Beyond this distance, pieces of gunpowder disperse and slow down so much that tattooing or stippling cannot occur. The closer the muzzle is to the skin, the tighter the distribution and greater the density of powder fragments will be around the actual entrance hole. Soot also may be deposited.

An **indeterminate-range (distant) entrance wound** occurs when flame, soot, or gunpowder does not reach the skin surface and the only thing striking the body is the bullet. The term *indeterminate* is used rather than *distant* because it does not imply that one can actually determine the range of fire from the appearance of the wound. For example, if an individual is shot through multiple layers of clothing, the entrance wound may have no sooting, searing, or stippling even though the actual range of fire is only a matter of inches; the wound would look the same as if the shot came from a range of 6 meters (20 feet) or more. Indeterminate wounds are characterized by a hole surrounded by a rim of abrasion. The size of the hole can vary according to a number of factors. It is important to remember that one cannot say what caliber of weapon inflicted the wound based solely on the size of the entrance wound. The collar of abrasion results from the fact that the bullet first causes stretching and scraping of the skin before it actually perforates. If the bullet strikes perpendicular to the skin, the margin of the abrasion collar is concentrically disturbed about the defect; if it strikes at an angle, the collar is eccentric, with the wider margin pointing in the direction from which the bullet came (Figure 2-21). If the bullet has struck an intermediary target before hitting the skin, it can be turning and tumbling, producing an irregular abrasion collar.

Exit Wounds

Exit wounds, or where the bullet comes out, have the same general appearance no matter what the range of fire. Their shape can vary from round to slitlike to completely irregular. As with entrance wounds, the size does not correlate very well with the caliber of the projectile making the wound. The most important factors affecting exit wounds are the speed of the projectile and the degree of deformation. A smaller, highly deformed bullet exiting at high speed can produce a large, irregular wound, whereas a larger, intact, slower-moving bullet may only make a small hole. Size *cannot* be used to determine whether the hole is an exit or entrance wound. In most cases, the margins of an exit wound will *not* have an abrasion collar. An exit wound will have clean edges that can often be reapproximated to cover the defect. The exception is when something is pressing against the skin surface at the exit site, such as tight clothing or the back of a chair. In this situation, the bullet will push the skin against the supporting surface causing rubbing and scraping around the exit defect as it comes out, a defect known as a **shored exit wound.**

It is important to remember that because the skin is so elastic and deformable, it is one of the toughest structures for a bullet to go through. It is not uncommon for a bullet to pass entirely through the body and be stopped just beneath the skin on the opposing side of the body. Often no visible injury of the overlying skin is seen; however, careful palpation of the area may allow one to locate the bullet.

Wounding Potential of Firearms

The amount of damage done by a bullet is a function of a number of variables. For the most part, the damage caused is a result of the amount of energy transferred to the tissues impacted. The energy a bullet has is determined by the following formula:

$$KE = 1/2 \, MV^2$$

where KE is the energy, M is the mass, and V is the speed.

Clearly, increasing the speed of a bullet has a much greater effect on its potential to cause damage than increasing its size. As the bullet passes through tissue and slows down, its energy is dissipated into the surrounding structures. This energy transfer causes tissue destruction in a zone that can be much larger than the actual size of the bullet; the zone of destruction may be several inches in diameter with very high-powered bullets. This transfer of energy in head wounds may lead to orbital plate fractures and palpebral ecchymosis (black eyes) or blood draining from the ears even though the path of the bullet does not come near the base of the skull. The amount of damage caused may be exacerbated by the generation of secondary missiles of bone fragments when portions of the skeleton are struck. Some bullets are designed to expand or fragment when they strike an object, thereby increasing the cross-sectional area of the projectile, increasing drag, and enhancing the transfer of energy into the tissues. Hollow-point ammunition is an example of this kind of bullet.

Obviously the lethality of a gunshot injury depends on what structures are damaged. Depending on the extent of damage, even gunshot wounds of the brain may not be lethal; however, they are usually immediately incapacitating and lead to significant long-term disability. It is important to remember that a victim with a "lethal" injury (wound of the heart or aorta) may not be immediately incapacitated and may engage in varying degrees of physical activity after being injured. Just

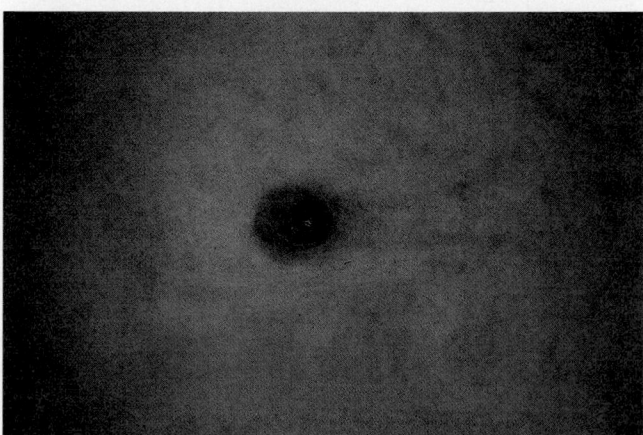

Figure 2-21 Indeterminate-range entrance wound with eccentric collar of abrasion resulting from the bullet striking the skin at an angle.

because the victim is active or even combative when first evaluated does not mean the individual may not have experienced a potentially lethal injury.

Asphyxial Injuries

Asphyxial injuries are caused by a failure of cells to receive or use oxygen. Deprivation of oxygen may be partial *(hypoxia)* or total *(anoxia)*. Asphyxial injuries can be grouped into four general categories: suffocation, strangulation, chemical, and drowning.

Suffocation

Suffocation, or oxygen failing to reach the blood, can result from a lack of oxygen in the environment (entrapment in an enclosed space or filling the environment with a suffocating gas) or blockage of the external airways. Classic examples of these types of asphyxial injuries are a child who is trapped in an abandoned refrigerator or a person who commits suicide by putting a plastic bag over the head. A reduction in the ambient oxygen level to 16% (normal is 21%) is immediately dangerous. If the level is below 5%, death can ensue within a matter of minutes. The diagnosis of these types of asphyxial injuries depends on the history of what happened, because there will be no specific physical findings.

Diagnosis and treatment in **choking asphyxiation** (obstruction of the internal airways) depend on locating and removing the obstructing material. Injury or disease also may cause swelling of the soft tissues of the airway, leading to partial or complete obstruction and subsequent asphyxiation. Suffocation also may result from compression of the chest or abdomen (mechanical or compressional asphyxia), preventing normal respiratory movements. Usual signs and symptoms include florid facial congestion and petechiae (pinpoint hemorrhages) of the eyes and face.

Strangulation

Strangulation is caused by compression and closure of the blood vessels and air passages resulting from external pressure on the neck. This causes cerebral hypoxia or anoxia secondary to the alteration or cessation of blood flow to and from the brain. It is important to remember that the amount of force needed to close the jugular veins (2 kg [4.5 lb]) or carotid arteries (5 kg [11 lb]) is significantly less than that required to crush the trachea (15 kg [33 lb]). It is the alteration of cerebral blood flow in most types of strangulation that causes injury or death—not the lack of airflow. With complete blockage of the carotid arteries, unconsciousness can occur within 10 to 15 seconds.

A noose is placed around the neck, and the weight of the body is used to cause constriction of the noose and compression of the neck in **hanging strangulations.** The body does not need to be completely suspended to produce severe injury or death. Depending on the type of ligature used, there usually is a distinct mark on the neck, an inverted V with the base of the V pointing toward the point of suspension. Internal injuries of the neck are actually quite rare in hangings, and only in judicial hangings, in which the body is weighted and dropped, is significant soft tissue or cervical spinal trauma seen. Petechiae of the eyes or face may be seen, but they are rare.

In **ligature strangulation,** the mark on the neck is horizontal, without the inverted V pattern seen in hangings. Petechiae may be more common because intermittent opening and closure of the blood vessels may occur as a result of the victim's struggles. Internal injuries of the neck are rare.

Variable amounts of external trauma on the neck with contusions and abrasions are noted in **manual strangulation** caused either by the assailant or by the victim clawing at one's own neck in an attempt to remove the assailant's hands. Internal damage can be quite severe, with bruising of deep structures and even fractures of the hyoid bone and tracheal and cricoid cartilages. Petechiae are common.

Chemical Asphyxiants

Chemical asphyxiants either prevent the delivery of oxygen to the tissues or block its use. Carbon monoxide is the most common chemical asphyxiant (see p. 59). **Cyanide** acts as an asphyxiant by combining with the ferric iron atom in cytochrome oxidase, thereby blocking the intracellular use of oxygen. A victim of cyanide poisoning has the same cherry-red appearance as a carbon monoxide intoxication victim because cyanide blocks the use of circulating oxyhemoglobin. An odor of bitter almonds also may be detected. (The ability to smell cyanide is a genetic trait that is absent in a significant portion of the general population.) **Hydrogen sulfide (sewer gas)** is a chemical asphyxiant in which victims of hydrogen cyanide poisoning may have brown-tinged blood in addition to the nonspecific signs of asphyxiation.

Drowning

Drowning is an alteration of oxygen delivery to tissues resulting from the breathing in of fluid, usually water. In 2005 there were 4248 drowning deaths in the United States. Although research done in the 1940s and 1950s indicated that changes in blood electrolyte levels and volume as a result of absorption of fluid from the lungs may be an important factor in some drownings, the major mechanism of injury is hypoxemia (low blood oxygen levels). Even in freshwater drownings, where large amounts of water can pass through the alveolar-capillary interface, there is no evidence that increases in blood volume cause significant electrolyte disturbances or hemolysis, or that the amount of fluid loading is beyond the compensatory capabilities of the kidneys and heart. Airway obstruction is the more important pathologic abnormality, underscored by the fact that in up to 15% of drownings, little or no water enters the lungs because of vagal nerve–mediated laryngospasms. This phenomenon is called *dry-lung drowning.*

No matter what mechanism is involved, cerebral hypoxia leads to unconsciousness in a matter of minutes. Whether this progresses to death depends on a number of factors, including age and health of the individual. One of the most important factors is the temperature of the water. Irreversible injury develops much more rapidly in warm water than it does in cold water. Submersion times of up to 1 hour with subsequent survival have been reported in children retrieved from very cold water. Complete submersion is not necessary for a person to drown. An incapacitated or helpless individual (such as a person with epilepsy or alcoholism or an infant) may drown in only a few inches of water.

It is important to remember that there are no specific or diagnostic findings to *prove* that a person recovered from the water is actually a drowning victim. In cases in which water has entered the lung, there may be large amounts of foam coming from the nose and mouth, although this also can be seen in certain types of drug overdoses. A body recovered from water with signs of prolonged immersion could just as easily be a victim of some other type of injury who has been put in the water to obscure the actual cause of death. When working with a living victim recovered from water, it is essential to keep in mind that an underlying condition may have led to the person's becoming incapacitated and submersed—a condition that also may need to be treated or corrected while correcting hypoxemia and dealing with its sequelae.

Infectious Injury

The pathogenicity (virulence) of microorganisms lies in their ability to survive and proliferate in the human body, where they injure cells and tissues. The disease-producing potential of a microorganism depends on its ability to (1) invade and destroy cells, (2) produce toxins, and (3) produce damaging hypersensitivity reactions (see Chapter 8 for further discussion).

Immunologic and Inflammatory Injury

Cellular membranes are injured by direct contact with cellular and chemical components of the immune and inflammatory responses, such as phagocytic cells (lymphocytes, macrophages) and substances such as histamine, antibodies, lymphokines, complement, and proteases (see Chapter 6). Complement is responsible for many of the membrane alterations that occur during immunologic injury.

Membrane alterations are associated with rapid leakage of potassium (K^+) out of the cell and rapid influx of water. Antibodies can interfere with membrane function by binding to and occupying receptor molecules on the plasma membrane. This type of injury is found in certain forms of diabetes mellitus and in myasthenia gravis. Antibodies also can block or destroy cellular junctions, interfering with intercellular communication (see Chapters 7 and 8).

Injurious Genetic Factors

Genetic disorders may be the result of genetic factors that alter the cell's nucleus and the plasma membrane's structure, shape, receptors, or transport mechanisms. For example, enzymatic genetic defects can lead to abnormalities in membrane transport. Genetic disorders can cause structural alterations of the red blood cell, for example, sickle cell anemia. (Mechanisms causing genetic abnormalities are discussed in Unit II.)

Injurious Nutritional Imbalances

Essential nutrients—proteins, carbohydrates, lipids (fats), vitamins, and minerals—are required for cells to function normally. If these nutrients are not consumed in the diet and transported to the body's cells or if excessive amounts of nutrients are consumed and transported, pathophysiologic cellular effects develop.

Proteins, which consist of chains of amino acids, are the major structural units of the cell and participate in many enzymatic and hormonal functions. Protein deficiency causes a decrease in the intestinal mucosal mass, decreasing the absorptive function. The integrity of the pancreas is also affected, resulting in diminished exocrine secretion. With starvation or malnutrition, the lowered plasma proteins, particularly albumin, cause fluid to move into the interstitium (edema). Protein-calorie malnutrition (PCM) is the predominant worldwide type of malnutrition. Malnourished children are very susceptible to disease and often die of infectious diseases. Even with adequate protein intake, cellular injury can occur if amino acid transport mechanisms fail or are defective. In Fanconi syndrome, for example, renal tubular cells may contain accumulated protein droplets that have been absorbed but cannot be transported.

Glucose is the major carbohydrate obtained from the breakdown of starch (see Chapter 1). **Hyperglycemia** (excessive glucose in the blood) caused by excessive carbohydrate intake may lead to obesity. Deficiencies of glucose result from starvation or from lack of use, as in diabetes. In both conditions the body compensates by metabolizing fat (lipids). (For details on diabetes, see Chapter 21.)

In lipid deficiency, or **hypolipidemia,** the body compensates by mobilizing fatty acids from adipose tissue. This causes an increase in the production and circulation of ketone bodies, which are acidic by-products of lipid metabolism. The excretion of ketone bodies results in loss of water and electrolytes and causes dehydration and thirst. Severe increases in ketone bodies cause ketoacidosis, coma, and death. **Hyperlipidemia,** or an increase in lipoproteins in the blood, results in deposits of fat in the heart, liver, and muscle.

Vitamins are not sources of energy but are necessary for maintaining normal cellular functions. Adequate vitamin intake is necessary because most vitamins are not synthesized by the body. Research from the 1990s resulted in the identification of 13 vitamins as being essential for humans. These include 8 B vitamins (thiamine, niacin, riboflavin, folate, vitamin B_6, vitamin B_{12}, biotin, and pantothenic acid), vitamin C or ascorbic acid, and the fat-soluble vitamins A, D, E, and K. Minerals are discussed in Chapter 3. Vitamins are involved in numerous reactions, including metabolism of visual pigments (vitamin A), calcium and phosphate metabolism (vitamin D), prothrombin synthesis (vitamin K), and antioxidation reactions (vitamins E and C). Pyridoxal (vitamin B_6) affects amino acid transfer reactions; flavin adenine dinucleotide (FAD), flavin mononucleotide (FMN), and NAD help the reaction transfer of electrons (see Chapter 1). Table 2-7 presents vitamins and their association with deficiency-related diseases/disorders. New are the many diseases related to vitamin D deficiency, which may include many common cancers, type 1 diabetes, cardiovascular disease, osteoporosis, and fibromyalgia (Figure 2-22 and see Nutrition & Disease, Vitamin D: Importance for Health Promotion).[58]

Table 2-7	Vitamin Deficiencies and Associated Disorders and Diseases
Vitamin	**Associated Deficiency**
Niacin	Rough skin (pellagra) symptoms include lassitude, anorexia, dermatitis, diarrhea, inflammation of the mouth and other mucous membranes
Riboflavin (vitamin B_2)	Decreased growth; skin lesions; soreness and burning of the lips, mouth, and tongue; burning and itching of the eyes; stomatitis; photophobia; vascularization of the cornea; glossitis; anemia; neuropathy
Thiamine (vitamin B_1)	Beriberi; chronic alcoholism contributes to deficiency; megaloblastic anemia; lactate acidosis; subacute necrotizing encephalomyelopathy; individuals at risk include those undergoing long-term dialysis or intravenous feedings and those with chronic febrile infection
Folate	Defects in DNA synthesis (fast-growing tissue, embryo); megaloblastic anemia; vascular disease (e.g., hyperhomocysteinemia); cancers including colon cancer (see Chapter 12); malabsorption syndromes (tropical and nontropical sprue)
Vitamin B_{12}	Pernicious anemia; neurologic (demyelination and peripheral neuropathy); memory loss and dementia; hyperhomocysteinemia and vascular disease
Vitamin B_6	Seborrheic dermatitis; microcytic anemia; convulsions; depression; confusion
Pantothenic acid (vitamin B_5)	Listlessness, fatigue, and weakness; headaches; personality changes; sleep disturbances; impaired motor coordination; gastrointestinal disturbances
Biotin	Severe ketoacidosis, seizures, ataxia, lethargy, coma at birth; hair loss; skin rashes; hearing loss; optic atrophy
Vitamin C	Scurvy (bleeding under the skin, gums, joint pain, joint effusions, shortness of breath); fatigue; increased risk to infection (decreased immune function)
Vitamin K	Hemorrhagic disease of the newborn; depression of vitamin K–dependent coagulation factors; individuals at risk are those on antibiotic therapy (interferes with synthesis) and those who have osteoporosis
Vitamin E	Status may depend on selenium and sulfur-containing amino acids; necrotizing myopathy (skeletal, heart, smooth muscle); decreased life span of red blood cells and increased risk of hemolysis; neurologic abnormalities; increased susceptibility to effects of oxidizing agents in the environment; decreased immune function, possibly vascular disease and coronary heart disease; possibly certain cancers (head, neck, lung, colorectal)
Vitamin A	Possibly several types of cancer; decreased immune function; fetal malformations; vision abnormalities (including night blindness, cornea changes, drying)
Vitamin D	Rickets; type 1 diabetes; cardiovascular disease, some common cancers, osteoporosis; fibromyalgia; multiple sclerosis; parathyroid disorders, autoimmune disorders

NUTRITION & DISEASE

Vitamin D: Important for Health Promotion

Most tissues in the body have a vitamin D receptor with enzymatic processes that convert vitamin D precursors to its active form. These findings have excited researchers because it is now possible to study vitamin D's role and risk for many chronic diseases, including common cancers, autoimmune diseases, infectious diseases, and cardiovascular disease. It is now known that a diet *high* in oily fish prevents vitamin D deficiency. Solar ultraviolet B radiation penetrates the skin and converts 7-dehydrocholesterol to previtamin D_3, which is quickly converted to vitamin D_3. Few foods are fortified with vitamin D. Vitamin D from the skin and diet is metabolized in the liver to 25-hydroxyvitamin D, which is used to determine an individual's vitamin D status. Although controversial on what is an optimal level of 25-hydroxyvitamin D, vitamin D deficiency is defined by most experts as a level less than 20 ng/ml (50 nmol/L) and a level of 30 ng/ml or greater possibly indicates sufficient vitamin D. Vitamin D intoxication is observed at levels greater than 150 ng/ml (374 nmol/L). With these defined levels, vitamin D deficiency has been estimated to affect 1 billion people worldwide. Estimates from several studies report that 40% to 100% of U.S. and European older adult men

and women have vitamin D deficiency. Importantly, more than 50% of postmenopausal women taking medications for osteoporosis had lower levels of 25-hydroxyvitamin D. Evidence also shows children and young adults (Hispanic, black, and white) are at risk for vitamin D deficiency. People living near the equator *without* sun protection have adequate levels of vitamin D. The recommended intake of vitamin D is now thought to be inadequate. A minimum of 1000 international units is thought to be a minimum (especially at high altitudes with reduced sun exposure) amount required to maintain a healthy concentration of vitamin D (25[OH]D) in the blood.

Vitamin D increases the efficiency of intestinal calcium absorption. Deficiencies of vitamin D in utero may decrease calcium in the skeleton. As vitamin D deficiency continues it can cause secondary hyperparathyroidism. Vitamin D controls more than 200 genes, including those responsible for regulating cellular proliferation, differentiation, apoptosis, and angiogenesis. It increases differentiation of cells, thereby decreasing cancer development. Vitamin D facilitates immune function, inhibits renin synthesis, increases insulin production, and increases myocardial contractibility (see Figure 2-22).

Data from Holick MF: *Am J Clin Nutr* 79(3):362-372, 2004; Zittermann A: *Prog Biophys Mol Biol* 92(1):39-48, 2006.

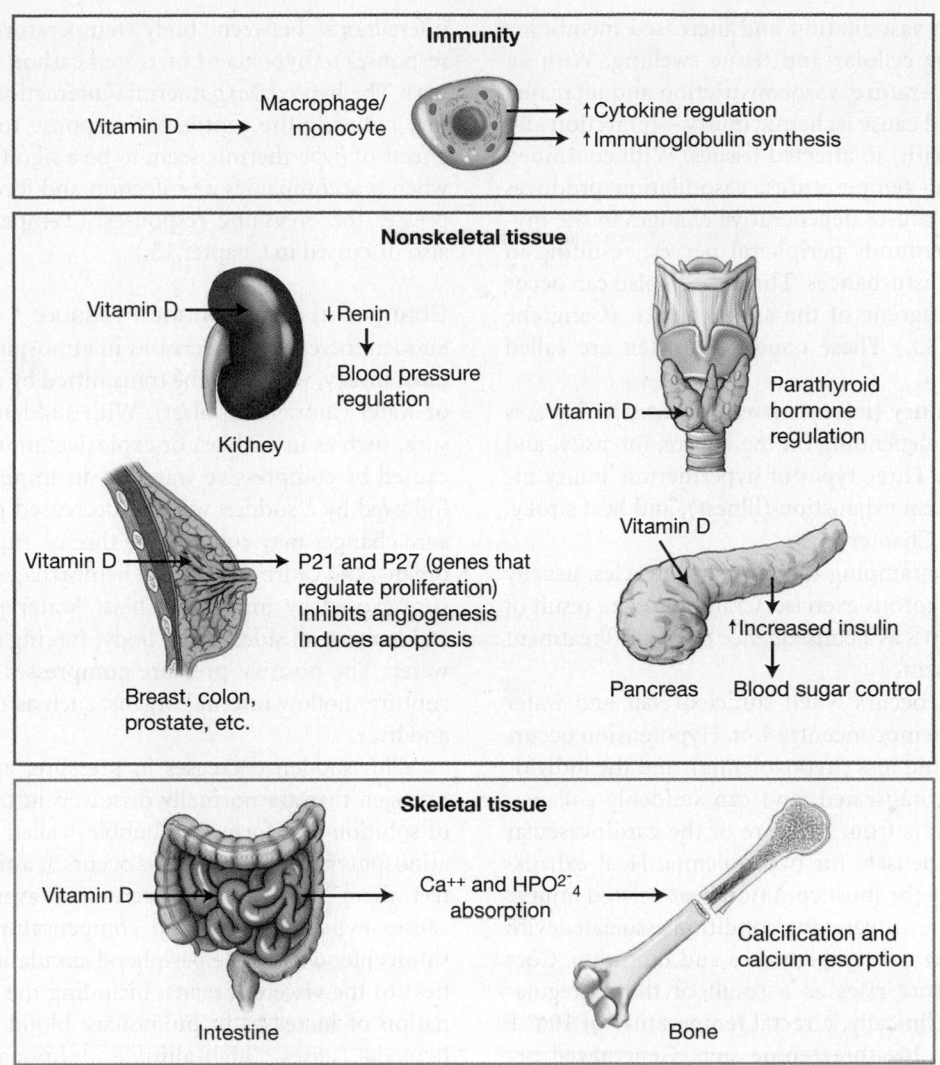

Figure 2-22 The many functions of vitamin D. Most tissues have a vitamin D receptor, thus vitamin D has enormous effects. Vitamin D deficiency is implicated in many chronic diseases including common cancers, autoimmune diseases, infectious diseases, and cardiovascular disease (also see Nutrition & Disease: Vitamin D Importance for Health Promotion, p. 70).

Injurious Physical Agents

Injurious physical agents include temperature extremes, changes in atmospheric pressure, radiation, illumination, mechanical factors, noise, and prolonged vibration. Physical injury can result from excessive exposure to many environmental agents, as well as to agents used for the diagnosis and treatment of illness.

Temperature Extremes

Chilling or freezing of cells causes **hypothermic injury.** Hypothermia has proved to be strongly injurious to a variety of cells. Prolonged exposure to low ambient temperature is a common risk factor found in homeless persons. Hypothermic injury has long been attributed to disturbances of cellular ion balance or homeostasis, especially of sodium balance (i.e., increased intracellular sodium levels). Hypothermia increases intracellular Ca^{++} by slowing the Na^+, K^+-ATPase

pump activity, leading to Na^+ accumulation intracellularly.[59] In recent years, however, a role for ROS has gained importance.[60] In animal studies, hypothermia resulted in cell damage caused by formation of ROS.[61-63] Hypothermic perfusion of the heart increased O_2^- (superoxide, see Table 2-3); in turn O_2^- reacted with nitric oxide (NO) to form another radical peroxynitrate anion ($ONOO^-$).[59]

Therapeutically, hypothermia is widely used to protect cells and tissues against injurious processes. In some cell types, however, such as hepatocytes and liver endothelial cells, hypothermia can cause pronounced cell injury mediated by ROS.[63] During the body's exposure to cold, injury is inhibited by hypoxia and by a number of antioxidants, especially iron chelators.[63]

Indirect forms of injury occur because of changes in small blood vessels (the microcirculation). Slow chilling can cause vasoconstriction followed by paralysis of vasomotor control, resulting in vasodilation and increased membrane permeability causing cellular and tissue swelling. With an abrupt drop in temperature, vasoconstriction and increased viscosity of the blood cause ischemic injury—infarction and necrosis (cellular death) in affected tissues. With continued exposure to freezing temperatures, vasodilation produces severe swelling that causes degenerative changes in the myelin sheath that surrounds peripheral nerves, resulting in sensory and motor disturbances. Thrombosis also can occur and may lead to gangrene of the affected part. (Gangrene is discussed on p. 83.) These conditions often are called *frostbite.*

Hyperthermic injury (injury caused by excessive heat) is common and varies depending on the nature, intensity, and extent of the injury. Three types of hyperthermic injury include heat cramps, heat exhaustion (illness), and heat stroke. (For more detail see Chapter 15.)

Heat cramps are cramping of voluntary muscles, usually as a result of vigorous exercise. Cramps are the result of salt and water loss as a consequence of sweat. Treatment is salt replacement.

Heat exhaustion occurs when sufficient salt and water loss results in hemoconcentration. Hypotension occurs secondary to fluid loss (hypovolemia), and the individual feels weak, nauseated, and can suddenly collapse. Collapsing results from a failure of the cardiovascular system to compensate for hypovolemia. Heat exhaustion is probably the most common heat-related injury.

Heat stroke is a life-threatening condition associated with high environmental temperatures and humidity. Core body temperature rises as a result of thermoregulatory failures. Clinically, a rectal temperature of 106° F is considered a life-threatening sign. Generalized peripheral vasodilation and decreased circulating blood volume are significant. At risk are older adults, athletes, military recruits, and people with cardiovascular disorders.

Burns are caused by local heat injury. A full-thickness burn is an open wound involving skin layers—epidermis, dermis, and subcutaneous layers—and causing extensive loss of fluids and plasma proteins. Cellular regeneration is not possible; therefore, skin from a donor or from the host must be grafted to the site. Partial-thickness burns result in reddening of the area as a result of dilation of small blood vessels and increased permeability of cellular membranes, with loss of protein-rich fluid, resulting in the typical "burn blister." In surface epithelial cells, membrane permeability increases, causing both cytoplasmic and nuclear swelling. Temperature-sensitive enzymes within certain cells respond to heat by increasing cellular metabolism, with detrimental effects. Intense heat also damages the vascular endothelium and causes coagulation of the blood vessels. (Burns are discussed further in Chapter 46.)

Epidemiologic investigators have reported a relationship between overheating in infants; that is overdressing infants in the winter, and sudden infant deaths. Studies suggest interactions between body temperature and respiratory responses to hypoxia or increased carbon dioxide (hypercapnia). The hypoxia/*hypo*thermia interaction depresses breathing, reducing the ventilatory response to hypercapnia. The effects of *hyper*thermia seem to be a significant problem only when it accompanies an infection and fever and alters or depresses the breathing responses. (Temperature changes are also discussed in Chapter 15.)

Changes in Atmospheric Pressure

Sudden increases or decreases in atmospheric pressure cause **blast injury,** which can be transmitted by either air (air blast) or water (immersion blast). With sudden increases in pressure, such as in air blast or explosive injuries, tissue injury is caused by compressive waves of air impinging on the body, followed by a sudden wave of decreased pressure. The pressure changes may collapse the thorax, rupture internal solid organs, and cause widespread hemorrhage. In increased pressure caused by immersion blast, water pressure is applied suddenly to all sides of the body, forcing the body up out of water. The positive pressure compresses the abdomen and ruptures hollow internal organs, such as the spleen, kidneys, and liver.

With sudden decreases in pressure, carbon dioxide and nitrogen that are normally dissolved in the blood come out of solution and form tiny bubbles called *gas emboli.* At low atmospheric pressure, such as occurs at altitudes above 15,000 feet, there is a significant decrease in available oxygen. This causes hypoxic injury, and compensatory vasoconstriction shunts blood from the peripheral circulation (in the extremities) to the visceral organs, including the lungs. The combination of increases in pulmonary blood flow and systemic hypoxia causes "high-altitude pulmonary edema"[64] (see Chapter 33).

Deep-sea divers and underwater construction workers who return to the surface too quickly develop a form of gas embolism called **decompression sickness** or **caisson disease** ("the bends"). If water pressure is reduced too rapidly, the gases dissolved in blood bubble out of solution, forming emboli. Oxygen is quickly redissolved, but nitrogen bubbles may persist and obstruct blood vessels. Ischemia resulting from gas emboli causes cellular hypoxia, particularly in the muscles, joints, and tendons, which are especially susceptible to changes in oxygen supply. Emboli and interstitial gas accumulate around the joints and skeletal muscles, causing the individual to double up in pain. Tissues of the heart and brain also may be affected by emboli, causing necrosis. The gases can be promptly redissolved in blood by raising the atmospheric pressure. This is accomplished by placing the individual in a decompression chamber. First, pressure is increased until it approximates pressure at the depth to which the diver had descended. This redissolves the gas bubbles in the blood. Then the pressure in the chamber is decreased gradually until it equals pressure at the surface of the water. The slow decrease in pressure slows the release of gas bubbles out of solution.

Ionizing Radiation

Ionizing radiation is any form of radiation capable of removing orbital electrons from atoms, resulting in the production of negatively charged free electrons and positively charged ionized atoms. Ionizing radiation is emitted by x-rays, gamma rays, and alpha and beta particles (which are emitted from atomic nuclei in the process of radioactive decay) and from neutrons, deuterons, protons, and pions (all of which are emitted from cobalt or linear accelerators). Ionizing radiation of three types (x-radiation, gamma radiation, and neutrons) was classified as a carcinogen in 2004.[65]

The most abundant source of exposure to ionizing radiation is the environment. This source includes emission from radioactive material inside the body, cosmic rays from outer space, and radiation emitted from such substances as soil and building materials. Environmental radioactivity is emitted primarily by uranium, thorium, and potassium. Other sources are from medical uses (e.g., x-rays, computed tomography [CT] scans, etc.) used for medical diagnosis and treatment, uranium and thorium mines, nuclear weapons, and nuclear reactors that generate electricity. Table 2-8 includes types of ionizing radiation and their magnitude of tissue penetration.

Ionizing radiation (x-radiation and gamma rays) causes a large spectrum of genetic changes including gene mutations, mini-satellite mutations (altered numbers of tandem repeats of DNA sequences), micronucleus formation (sign of chromosome damage or loss), chromosomal aberrations (structural or number), ploidy changes (number of sets of chromosomes), DNA strand breaks, and chromosomal instability.[65] All phases of the cell cycle can be affected by ionizing radiation. Sensitivity of the cell appears to be greatest in G_2, that gap of the cell just before mitosis; irradiation during this phase retards the onset of cell division. Irradiation during mitosis induces chromosomal aberrations. Membrane molecules and enzymes also are damaged by radiation (see Chapter 12). The intensity, duration, and cumulative effects of exposure to ionizing radiation determine the extent of injury. X-radiation and gamma radiation induce genetic alterations in somatic cells and heritable mutations in germ cells (sperm and egg and their precursor cells). DNA may be damaged *directly* or *indirectly* by interaction with reactive products (i.e., free electrons, hydroxyl radicals, hydrogen free radicals) from the degradation of water (Figure 2-23). The observed genetic damage is thought to be the result of DNA repair but also may arise from errors in replication.[65] Epigenetic mechanisms (a change in gene *expression* and not in the DNA sequence) that damage genes may be involved in radiation-induced tumor formation. These mechanisms include genomic instability, mutations by irradiation of the cytoplasm (includes ROS, inflammatory cell signaling pathways, extracellular matrix alterations), "bystander effects" induction of genetic damage in innocent or cells not *directly* irradiated, possibly through cellular gap junctions and signaling pathways (see Chapter 12).

Not all cells and tissues have the same sensitivity to radiation, although all cells can be affected. Radiosensitivity depends on the rate of mitosis and cellular maturity. Because fetal cells are both immature and undergoing rapid cycling, the fetus is at great risk for injury caused by ionizing radiation. Particularly vulnerable are embryonic germ cells, which are precursors of ova and sperm. Throughout life, cells of the bone marrow, intestinal mucosa, testicular seminiferous epithelium, and ovarian follicles are susceptible to injury because they are always undergoing mitosis, which ensures the presence of vulnerable, immature daughter cells. Ioniz-

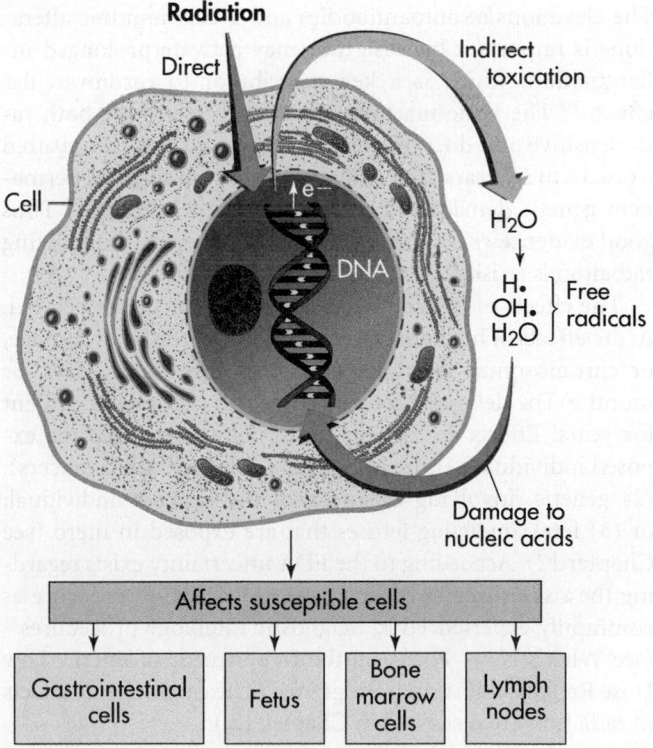

Figure 2-23 Cellular damage caused by ionizing radiation. Radiation can damage macromolecules in two ways: (1) directly, in which the micromolecules are ionized; and (2) indirectly, in which water is ionized and produces free radicals that in turn damage macromolecules. Cells that are particularly susceptible to damage are those of the gastrointestinal tract, bone marrow, lymph nodes, a fetus, and ovarian follicles. (Also see Chapter 18.)

Table 2-8	Types of Ionizing Radiation and Their Tissue Penetration
Type	**Tissue Penetration**
X-rays	High
Gamma (γ) rays	High
Beta (β) particles	Low
Alpha (α) particles	Very low
Protons	Intermediate between α and β
Neutrons	High

Data from Damjanov I, Linder J, editors: *Anderson's pathology*, ed 10, St Louis, 1996, Mosby.

ing radiation is a known human carcinogen. Exposure to x-radiation and gamma radiation is most strongly correlated with leukemia and cancers of the thyroid, breast, and lung; these correlates have been reported at absorbed low levels, less than 0.2 gray (Gy). The risk of developing these cancers may to some extent depend on age at exposure.[65] Two studies suggest that radiation could cause liver cancer.[66,67] Radiation exposure to children may increase the incidence of lymphomas, leukemias, melanomas, breast cancers, and others. At high-treatment radiation doses, the first study[68] of sarcomas added angiosarcoma to the list of radiation-induced cancers.

Studies of A-bomb survivors have found increased mortality from noncancer diseases.[69] The majority of radiation-induced noncancer deaths are cardiovascular problems (i.e., myocardial infarction and stroke). Individuals exposed to radiation at less than 40 years of age revealed an excess relative risk of myocardial infarction of 0.25.[70] In addition, radiation exposure was significantly related to hypertension and elevated total cholesterol.[70] Risk estimates for heart disease and stroke indicated higher susceptibility in women.[70] Studies of the late effects of radiation in A-bomb survivors reveal elevated levels of mediators of inflammation (interleukin (IL)-6 and C-reactive protein [CRP]). Persistent elevations were documented of leukocyte counts, erythrocyte sedimentation rates, immunoglobulins, and sialic acid with radiation exposure. Also elevated were other inflammatory markers (TNF-α, IL-10, immunoglobulin (Ig), IgM, IgA, and interferon (IFN-γ). The elevations of autoantibodies and T cell–immune alterations is important because they may activate prolonged inflammation, which is a key contributor to cardiovascular effects.[70] The bone marrow and thymus gland are both radiosensitive and documented immunologic effects measured from 40 to 50 years after radiation exposure suggests permanent genetic damage to lymphocyte progenitor cells.[70] Thus good evidence exists that at doses of 0.5 sievert (Sv) ionizing radiation is a risk factor for cardiovascular disease.

The effects of ionizing radiation may be acute or delayed. Acute effects of high doses, such as skin redness, skin damage, or chromosomal aberrations, occur within hours, days, or months. The delayed effects of low doses may not be evident for years! Effects are usually (1) somatic, involving the exposed individual's entire body (e.g., leukemia, other cancers); (2) genetic, involving offspring of the exposed individual; or (3) fetal, involving fetuses that are exposed in utero (see Chapter 12). According to the FDA uncertainty exists regarding the risk estimates for low levels of radiation exposure as commonly experienced in diagnostic radiology procedures[71] (see What's New? Focus on the Department of Energy Low Dose Radiation Research Program). (The carcinogenic effects of radiation are discussed in Chapter 12.)

Illumination

The retina is a highly specialized sense organ that is constantly subjected to environmental stresses, including illumination. Focused light rays can increase oxidative stress and is prevented by a wide array of retinal antioxidant mechanisms.[72]

WHAT'S NEW? Focus on the Department of Energy Low Dose Radiation Research Program

The Department of Energy's (DOE) Low Dose Radiation Research Program supports research aimed at informing the development of a national radiation risk policy for the public and workplace. In general, the focus of research is for total radiation doses that are less than 0.1 sievert (10 rem). As of March 2007, more than 400 publications from the program resulted in 52 published papers in 2007.

Solid data from populations receiving high doses at high dose rates (mainly the Japanese A-bomb Survivor Life Span Study) have shown that ionizing radiation increases rates of cancer in human populations at a level of about 5% to 6% per 1 Sv (or 6%/100 rem). Epidemiology, however, has never been able to demonstrate higher cancer risks in humans exposed to lower doses (<0.1 Sv, or 10 rem) or to chronic low-dose rate exposures at slightly higher total doses. Thus mathematical models were needed to determine or estimate health risks from low-dose radiation. Until recently these models assumed independent action of ionization effects in cells and tissues. These models also assumed that an energy ionization event increased the probability of DNA breaks. Historically, measurements of damage (e.g., cell death, chromosome aberrations, etc.) revealed a fairly linear response with dose, but these experiments seldom used doses lower than 0.5 Sv (50 rem).

Research from the DOE challenges these older assumptions. The findings provide "compelling" evidence that ionization effects are biologically different than those of higher levels of radiation and that tissues have surveillance mechanisms that significantly affect the development of cancer and the behavior of cancer cells. This research highlights a *system* response (i.e., crosstalk) in tissue between irradiated cells and nearby nonirradiated cells and not just the initial events within an individual cell. Crosstalk between irradiated cells and "innocent, nonirradiated" bystander cells cannot be explained by the older mathematical models or paradigms. These new data demonstrate the "social" nature of individual cells and their surrounding tissue, that is, they are all connected. The Low Dose Program is therefore key to advancing our understanding of low-dose radiation from cellular and molecular actions within cells to the understanding of cancer as a multicellular disease.

Data available at www.lowdose.energy.gov/about_overview. Accessed 2007.

Antioxidant mechanisms can, however, be overwhelmed by excessive light exposure, particularly of short wavelength, high-frequency blue light, and ultraviolet light. Since fluorescent lighting was introduced to the workplace, complaints of headaches, eyestrain, and eye discomfort have increased.[73] The rapid modulation of light from fluorescent lamps is responsible for eyestrain and headaches.[74] The modulation can be reduced by wearing tinted glasses.[74] The shorter wavelengths in radiant energy in environmental lighting influence the absorption, scattering, and fluorescence, thus obscuring vision.[74]

Vision is obstructed at night by decreased illumination and by disabling glare from oncoming vehicle headlights. High-intensity discharge (HID) headlamps project light farther down roads, thus improving the driver's safety. However, oncoming glare, which is proportional to headlamp brightness, is *not* good for any drivers of oncoming vehicles and even worse for older drivers.[75] Older drivers experience more intraocular light scattering, glare sensitivity, and longer recovery time in reaction to photo stress.[76]

Studies have demonstrated the in vitro toxicity of halogen lamps.[77,78] A pilot study of 12 mice illuminated with varying intensities and durations of halogen exposure resulted in benign forms of skin cancer (papillomas) as well as malignant tumor growth. Fortunately, prevention is simple if commercial models are available with glass or plastic covers.

Mechanical Stresses

Mechanical stimulation of body tissues and cells is constant. For example, gravity as an external force and the pumping of the heart as an internal force are continual. Acutely these forces elicit adaptive responses (to rapidly alter function) chronically; however, the responses may induce tissue remodeling to accommodate load-bearing capabilities.[79] When the mechanical forces exceed unknown thresholds, injury results.[79] Injury can initiate more reparative responses, transient or continuous dysfunction, or progressive degenerative changes that incorporate nearby and surrounding tissue. Cellularly, the structural responses to deformation and strain (e.g., biomechanical) are causing investigators to focus on the cell membrane. Disruption of cell membranes, or **mechanoporation**, is central to the biologic progression. Mechanical injury can progress to cell death involving both cell necrosis and delayed apoptosis.[79] The heterogeneous distribution of atherosclerosis in the vasculature is possibly related to biomechanical factors, that is, certain arteries (e.g., coronary and carotid arteries) are more susceptible to plaque formation than others.[80] Biomechanical forces probably are not systemic and vary with location. Mechanical stimuli include *shear forces* because of blood flow, *strain* from pressure distension of the vessel walls, and strain from *tethering* to a surrounding tissue area (e.g., the heart).[80]

Recent inter age has led investi coronary angioplasty. eter that is advanced alo blocked region of the vessel eter is then inflated, pushing t outward. Sometimes metal tubes, keep the vessel open. Without the ster rowing, or restenosis, often occurs at the ever, the injury causes an adaptive respons of the smooth muscle cells and an increase i activity. The macrophages release cytokines a factors, causing intimal cell proliferation and sub renarrowing.

The major focus of occupational biomechanics is the re sponse of tissue to mechanical stress, especially the prevention of overexertion disorders of the lower back and upper extremities. Many mechanical stresses can cause overt injuries (e.g., a head injury when a worker is struck in the head with a dropped object). Most stresses, however, are subtle and can cause *accumulative* injuries and disorders.[81] Table 2-9 summarizes common types of occupational mechanical stresses and associated types of injury.

Noise

Noise is sound that has the potential for inflicting bodily harm. The most common pathophysiologic effect of noise is hearing impairment. Noise trauma can be caused by acute loud noise, as well as by the cumulative effects of various intensities, frequencies, and durations of noise. Common irritating noise is caused by numerous sources, including lawn care machinery; high-decibel, low-frequency speakers; loud movies; roaring highways; and so on. According to the National Institutes of Health, more than 10 million Americans suffer some permanent noise-associated hearing loss.[82] The largest increase in hearing loss from noise occurs in people 45 to 64 years old. Noise pollution is now considered a public health threat.

Table 2-9	Common Types of Occupational Mechanical Stresses and Associated Types of Injury	
Mechanical Stresses	**Type of Injury**
Forceful exertions (e.g., lifting, pushing, pulling of heavy loads)	Low back pain
Awkward trunk postures (e.g., flexion, lateral bending, axial twisting, prolonged sitting)	Low back pain
Whole body vibration (e.g., vibrating seat or platform)	Low back pain; bone deformities; alteration nerve conduction (carpal tunnel syndrome)
Repetitive or prolonged exposure (e.g., to any of the above)	Low back pain; numbness and tingling of wrists and hands
Extreme reaching	Trauma disorders of upper arms (synovitis, Raynaud phenomenon, bursitis, tendinitis)
Low temperatures (e.g., exposure to cold air, tools, materials)	
Vibration (segmental and whole)	
Forceful exertions (e.g., friction, balance, posture, pace, use of heavy objects)	
Ulnar deviation of the wrist	
Repetitive functions (e.g., walking, climbing stairs, carrying, shoveling, pushing, lifting objects, computer use)	Localized and/or whole body fatigue (shortness of breath, general weakness, hypoxic injury)

st in mechanical injury and blood vessel damage, investigators to study balloon catheterization or Coronary angioplasty involves a catheterization in a blood vessel until it reaches the The balloon section of the catheter walls of the blocked vessel called *stents*, are inserted to ts, however, vessel narrowing of hypertrophy macrophage and growth frequent

associated with PTS, although not fully understood, include intracellular changes in the sensory cells (hair cells) and swelling of the auditory nerve endings.[29] With PTS, cochlear blood flow may be impaired and hair cells are damaged with each exposure. Noise-induced hearing loss is gradual and painless. Symptoms of noise-induced hearing loss include loudness recruitment and tinnitus. In loudness recruitment, soft sounds are not heard but loud sounds are heard normally. Tinnitus is a constant high-pitched ringing that annoys the individual and contributes to loss of sleep.

MANIFESTATIONS OF CELLULAR INJURY

Cellular Manifestations: Accumulations

Cellular accumulations, also known as **infiltrations,** occur as a result of not only sublethal injury sustained by cells but also normal (but inefficient) cell function. Common accumulations consist of substances that are normally present, such as fluids and electrolytes, triglycerides (lipids), glycogen, calcium, uric acid, proteins, melanin, and bilirubin. Abnormal accumulations of these substances can occur in the cytoplasm (frequently in the lysosomes) or in the nucleus if (1) the normal, endogenous substance is produced in excess or at an increased rate; (2) an endogenous substance (normal or abnormal) is not effectively catabolized, usually because of lack of a vital lysosomal enzyme; or (3) harmful exogenous materials, such as heavy metals, mineral dusts, or microorganisms, accumulate because of inhalation, ingestion, or infection.

In all storage diseases the cells attempt to digest, or catabolize, the "stored" substances. As a result, excessive amounts of metabolites (products of catabolism) accumulate in the cells and are expelled into the extracellular matrix, where they are taken up by phagocytic cells called *macrophages* (see Chapter 6). Some of these scavenger cells circulate throughout the body, whereas others remain fixed in certain tissues, such as the liver or spleen. As more and more macrophages

and other phagocytes migrate to tissues that are producing excessive metabolites, the affected tissues begin to swell. This is the mechanism that causes enlargement of the liver (hepatomegaly) or the spleen (splenomegaly). Enlargement of one of these organs is a clinical manifestation of many of the storage diseases.

Water

Cellular swelling, the most common degenerative change, is caused by the shift of extracellular water into the cells. In hypoxic injury, movement of fluid and ions into the cell is associated with acute failure of metabolism and loss of ATP production. Normally, the pump that transports sodium ions out of the cell is maintained by the presence of ATP and ATPase, the active-transport enzyme. In metabolic failure caused by hypoxia, reduced ATP and ATPase permit sodium to accumulate in the cell, whereas potassium diffuses outward. The increase of intracellular sodium increases osmotic pressure, which draws more water into the cell (transport mechanisms are described in Chapter 1). The cisternae of the endoplasmic reticulum become distended, rupture, and coalesce to form large vacuoles that isolate the water from the cytoplasm, a process called vacuolation. Progressive vacuolation results in **oncosis** (which has replaced the old term *hydropic degeneration*) or **vacuolar degeneration** (degeneration by water) (Figure 2-24). If cellular swelling affects all cells in an organ, the organ increases in weight and becomes distended and pale.

Cellular swelling is reversible and is considered to be sublethal. It is, in fact, an early manifestation of almost all types of cellular injury, including severe or lethal cell injury. It is also associated with high fever, hypokalemia (abnormally low concentrations of potassium in the blood; see Chapter 3), and certain infections.

Lipids and Carbohydrates

Certain metabolic disorders result in the abnormal intracellular accumulation of carbohydrates and lipids. These substances may accumulate throughout the body but are found primarily in the cells of the spleen, liver, and CNS. Accumulations in cells of the CNS can cause neurologic dysfunction and severe mental retardation. Lipids accumulate in Tay-Sachs, Niemann-Pick, and Gaucher diseases, whereas in the diseases known as mucopolysaccharidoses, carbohydrates are in excess. The mucopolysaccharidoses are progressive disorders that usually involve multiple organs, including the liver, spleen, heart, and blood vessels. The accumulated mucopolysaccharides are found in reticuloendothelial cells, endothelial cells, intimal smooth muscle cells, and fibroblasts throughout the body. These carbohydrate accumulations can cause clouding of the cornea, joint stiffness, and mental retardation.[2]

Although lipids sometimes accumulate in heart and kidney cells, the most common site of intracellular lipid accumulation, or **fatty change,** is liver cells. Because hepatic metabolism and secretion of lipids are crucial to proper body function,

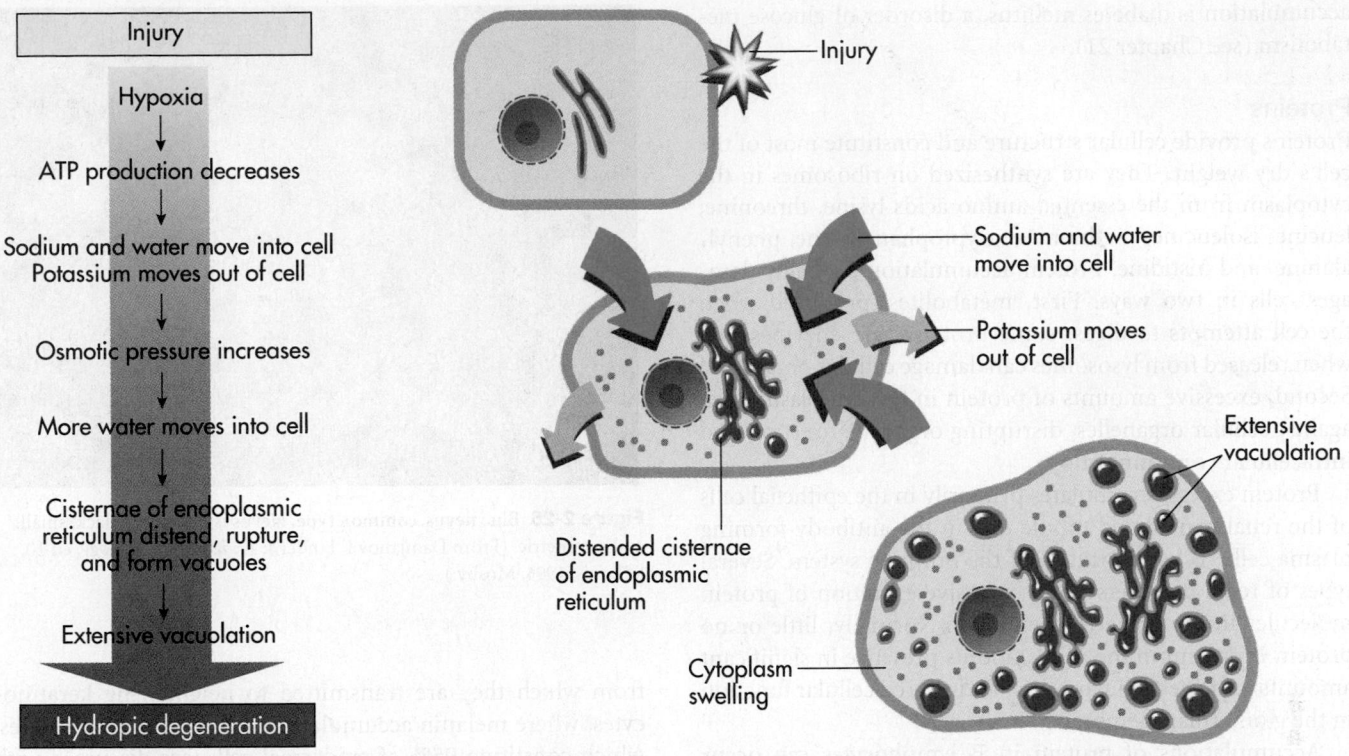

Figure 2-24 The process of oncosis (formerly known as hydropic degeneration). *ATP*, Adenosine triphosphate.

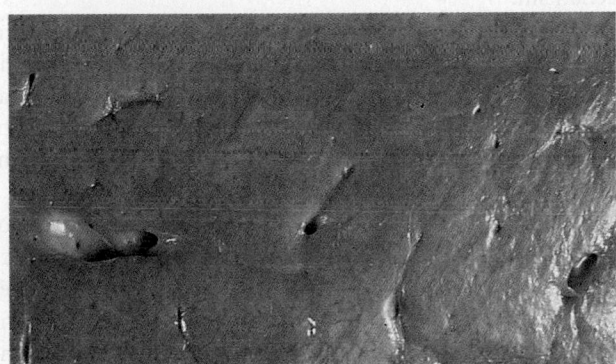

Figure 2-25 Fatty liver. The liver appears yellow. (From Damjanov I, Linder J: *Pathology: a color atlas,* St Louis, 2000, Mosby.)

imbalances and deficiencies in these processes lead to major pathologic changes. Lipid accumulation in liver cells causes an organic condition known as *fatty liver,* or *fatty change* (Figure 2-25). As lipids fill the cells, vacuolation pushes the nucleus and other organelles aside. Grossly, the liver looks yellowish and greasy.

Lipid accumulation in liver cells occurs after cellular injury sets one or more of the following mechanisms in motion:

1. Increased movement of free fatty acids into the liver (starvation, for example, increases breakdown of triglycerides in adipose tissue, releasing fatty acids that subsequently enter liver cells)

2. Failure of the metabolic process that converts fatty acids to phospholipids, resulting in the preferential conversion of the fatty acids to triglycerides

3. Increased synthesis of triglycerides from fatty acids (increases in the enzyme, α-glycerophosphatase, which can accelerate triglyceride synthesis)

4. Decreased synthesis of apoproteins (lipid-acceptor proteins)

5. Failure of lipids to bind with apoproteins and form lipoproteins

6. Failure of mechanisms that transport lipoproteins out of the cell

7. Direct damage to the endoplasmic reticulum by free radicals released by alcohol's toxic effects

Alcohol abuse is one of the most common causes of fatty liver (see Chapter 39). Fatty change caused by alcohol can lead to a form of liver fibrosis called *cirrhosis* (see What's New? Cellular Mechanisms of Fibrosis and Reversal). If alcohol intake ceases, the cirrhotic liver can return to a normal size and function. Fatty change from other causes, notably carbon tetrachloride poisoning, is often irreversible.

Glycogen

Intracellular accumulations of glycogen are seen in genetic disorders called *glycogen storage diseases* and in disorders of glucose and glycogen metabolism. Like water and lipid accumulation, glycogen accumulation results in excessive vacuolation of the cytoplasm. The most common cause of glycogen accumulation is diabetes mellitus, a disorder of glucose metabolism (see Chapter 21).

Proteins

Proteins provide cellular structure and constitute most of the cell's dry weight. They are synthesized on ribosomes in the cytoplasm from the essential amino acids lysine, threonine, leucine, isoleucine, methionine, tryptophan, valine, phenylalanine, and histidine. Protein accumulation probably damages cells in two ways. First, metabolites, produced when the cell attempts to digest some proteins, are enzymes that when released from lysosomes can damage cellular organelles. Second, excessive amounts of protein in the cytoplasm push against cellular organelles, disrupting organelle function and intracellular communication.

Protein excess accumulates primarily in the epithelial cells of the renal convoluted tubule and in the antibody-forming plasma cells (B lymphocytes) of the immune system. Several types of renal disorders cause excessive excretion of protein molecules in the urine (proteinuria). Normally, little or no protein is present in the urine, and its presence in significant amounts indicates cellular injury and altered cellular function in the glomerular membrane.

Accumulations of protein in B lymphocytes can occur during active synthesis of antibodies during the immune response. The excess aggregates of protein are called *Russell bodies*. Russell bodies have been identified in multiple myeloma (plasma cell tumor) (see Chapter 27).

Pigments

Pigment accumulations may be normal or abnormal, endogenous (produced within the body) or exogenous (produced outside the body). Endogenous pigments are derived, for example, from amino acids (e.g., tyrosine, tryptophan). They include melanin and the blood proteins—porphyrins, hemoglobin, and hemosiderin (ferritin). Lipid-rich pigments such as lipofuscin (the aging pigment or spots) give a yellow-brown color to cells undergoing slow, regressive, and often atrophic changes. Exogenous pigments include mineral dusts containing silica and iron particles, lead, silver salts, and dyes for tattoos.

Melanin

Melanin accumulates in epithelial cells (keratinocytes) of the skin and retina. It is an extremely important pigment because it protects the skin against long exposure to sunlight and is considered an essential factor in the prevention of skin cancer (see Chapters 12 and 44). Ultraviolet light (e.g., sunlight) stimulates the synthesis of melanin, which probably absorbs ultraviolet rays during subsequent exposure. Melanin also may protect the skin by trapping the injurious free radicals produced by the action of ultraviolet light on skin.

Melanin is a brown-black pigment derived from the amino acid tyrosine. It is synthesized by epidermal cells called *melanocytes* and is stored in membrane-bound cytoplasmic vesicles called *melanosomes*. Melanosomes are particularly abundant in projections of melanocytic cytoplasm, called *dendrites,*

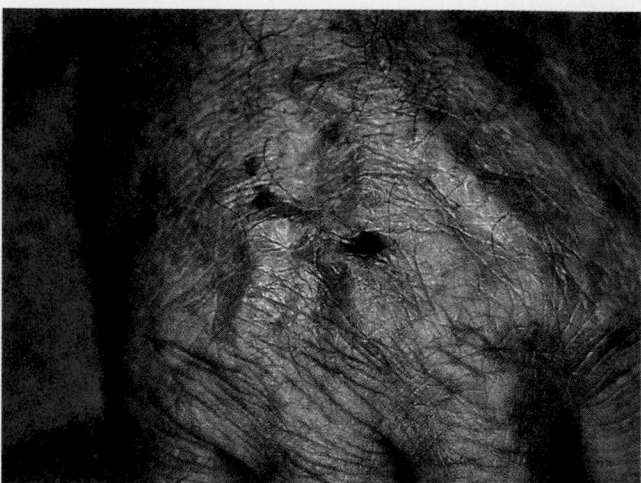

Figure 2-26 *Blue nevus, common type.* Nevus is dark blue-black, small, and symmetric. (From Damjanov I, Linder J: *Anderson's pathology,* ed 10, St Louis, 1996, Mosby.)

from which they are transmitted to neighboring keratinocytes, where melanin accumulation occurs.[10] (Keratinocytes, which constitute 95% of epidermal cells, are discussed with other skin components in Chapter 44.) The dendritic melanocytes form bridges between neighboring keratinocytes and inject melanosomes into the keratinocytes by an unknown mechanism.

Melanin also can accumulate in melanophores (melanin-containing pigment cells), macrophages, or other phagocytic cells in the dermis. Presumably these cells acquire the melanin from nearby melanocytes or from pigment that has been extruded from dying epidermal cells. This is the mechanism that causes freckles.

Although rare, melanin accumulation occurs in the skin of individuals with Addison disease (adrenocortical insufficiency resulting from disorders of the adrenal cortex; see Chapter 21). The increased melaninogenesis (melanin production) seen in Addison disease is caused by the loss of feedback control of adrenocorticotropic hormone (ACTH). Decreased hormonal secretion from the adrenal gland causes increased release of ACTH from the pituitary gland. In Addison disease the increase in melanin occurs presumably because a segment of the ACTH molecule contains the melanin-stimulating hormone (MSH).

An increase in melanin also occurs in the benign form of "pigmented moles" called *nevi* (Figure 2-26) (see Chapter 44). Malignant melanoma is a cancerous skin tumor that contains melanin and invades normal tissue early and widely and often leads to death.

A decrease in melanin production occurs in the inherited disorder of the melanin metabolism called *albinism.* Albinism is often diffuse, involving all the skin, the eyes, and the hair. Albinism is also related to phenylalanine metabolism. In classic types the person with albinism is unable to convert tyrosine to dopa (3,4-dihydroxyphenylalanine), an intermediary in melanin biosynthesis. Melanin-producing cells are present in normal numbers, but they are unable to make melanin. Individuals with albinism are very sensitive to sunlight and quickly become sunburned. They are also at high risk for skin cancer.

Hemoproteins

Hemoproteins are among the most essential of the normal endogenous pigments. They include hemoglobin and the oxidative enzymes, the cytochromes. Central to an understanding of disorders involving these pigments is knowledge of iron uptake, metabolism, excretion, and storage (see Chapter 25). Hemoprotein accumulations in cells are caused by excessive storage of iron, which is transferred to the cells from the bloodstream. Iron enters the blood from three primary sources: (1) tissue stores, (2) the intestinal mucosa, and (3) macrophages that remove and destroy dead or defective red blood cells. The amount of iron in blood plasma also depends on the metabolism of the major iron-transport protein, *transferrin*.

Iron is stored in tissue cells in two forms: as ferritin and, when greater levels of iron are present, as hemosiderin. **Hemosiderin** is a yellow-brown pigment derived from hemoglobin. With pathologic states, excesses of iron cause hemosiderin to accumulate within cells. Accumulation of hemosiderin often occurs in areas of bruising and hemorrhage and in the lungs and spleen after congestion caused by heart failure. With a local hemorrhage, the skin first appears red-blue and then lysis of the escaped red blood cells occur, causing the hemoglobin to be transformed to hemosiderin. The color changes noted in bruising reflect this transformation.

Hemosiderosis is a condition in which excess iron is stored as hemosiderin in the cells of many organs and tissues. This condition is common in individuals who have received repeated blood transfusions or prolonged parenteral administration of iron. Hemosiderosis is also associated with increased absorption of dietary iron, conditions in which iron storage and transport are impaired, and hemolytic anemia. Excessive alcohol ingestion also can lead to hemosiderosis. Normally, absorption of excessive dietary iron is prevented by an iron-absorption process in the intestines. Failure of this process can lead to total-body iron accumulations in the range of 60 to 80 g, compared with normal iron stores of 4.5 to 5 g. Excessive accumulations of iron, such as occur in hemochromatosis (a genetic disorder of iron metabolism and the most severe example of iron overload), are associated with liver and pancreatic cell damage.

Bilirubin is a normal yellow-to-green pigment of bile derived from the porphyrin structure of hemoglobin. Excesses of bilirubin within cells and tissues cause jaundice (icterus), or yellowing of the skin. Jaundice occurs when the bilirubin level exceeds 1.5 to 2 mg/dl of plasma, compared with the normal values of 0.4 to 1 mg/dl. Hyperbilirubinemia occurs with (1) destruction of red blood cells (erythrocytes), such as in hemolytic jaundice; (2) diseases affecting the metabolism and excretion of bilirubin in the liver; and (3) diseases that cause obstruction of the common bile duct, such as gallstones or pancreatic tumors. (For a detailed description of these diseases, see Chapter 39.) Certain drugs, specifically chlorpromazine and other phenothiazine derivatives, estrogenic hormones, and halothane (an anesthetic), can cause the obstruction of normal bile flow through the liver.

Because unconjugated bilirubin is lipid soluble, it can injure the lipid components of the plasma membrane. Albumin, a plasma protein, provides significant protection by binding unconjugated bilirubin in plasma. Unconjugated bilirubin causes two cellular effects: uncoupling of oxidative phosphorylation and a loss of cellular proteins. These two effects could cause structural injury to the various membranes of the cell.

Calcium

Calcium salts accumulate in both injured and dead tissues (Figure 2-27). An important mechanism of cellular calcification is the influx of extracellular calcium in injured mitochondria (see pp. 53 and 80). Another mechanism that causes calcium accumulation in alveoli (gas-exchange airways of the lungs), gastric epithelium, and renal tubules is the excretion of acid at these sites, leading to the local production of hydroxyl ions. Hydroxyl ions result in precipitation of calcium hydroxide ($Ca[OH]_2$) and hydroxyapatite ($3Ca_3[PO_4]_2Ca[OH]_2$), a mixed salt. Damage occurs when calcium salts clump and harden, interfering with normal cellular structure and function.

Pathologic calcification can be dystrophic or metastatic. **Dystrophic calcification** is the calcification of dying and dead tissues and occurs in chronic tuberculosis of the lungs and lymph nodes, in arteries with advanced atherosclerosis (narrowing as a result of plaque accumulation), and often in injured heart valves (Figure 2-28). Calcification of the heart valves interferes with opening and closing of the valves, causing heart murmurs (see Chapter 30). Calcification of the coronary arteries predisposes them to severe narrowing and thrombosis, which can lead to myocardial infarction. Another site of dystrophic calcification is the center of tumors. Over time, the center is deprived of oxygen supply, dies, and becomes calcified. The calcium salts appear as gritty, clumped granules that can become hard as stone. When several layers clump together, they resemble grains of sand and are called **psammoma bodies.**

The exact pathogenic mechanisms responsible for dystrophic calcification are unknown. A popular hypothesis is that with progressive deterioration of dead cells, the exposed denatured (changed) proteins preferentially bind with phosphate ions. The phosphate ions then react with calcium ions to form deposits of phosphate carbonate precipitates and, sometimes, crystalline formations of calcium phosphate. Dystrophic calcification develops slowly and is an explicit marker for the site of dead cells.

Metastatic calcification consists of mineral deposits that occur in undamaged normal tissues as the result of hypercalcemia (excess of calcium in the blood; see Chapter 3). Conditions that cause hypercalcemia include hyperparathyroidism, toxic levels of vitamin D, hyperthyroidism, idiopathic hypercalcemia of infancy, Addison disease (adrenocortical insufficiency), systemic sarcoidosis, milk-alkali syndrome, and the increased

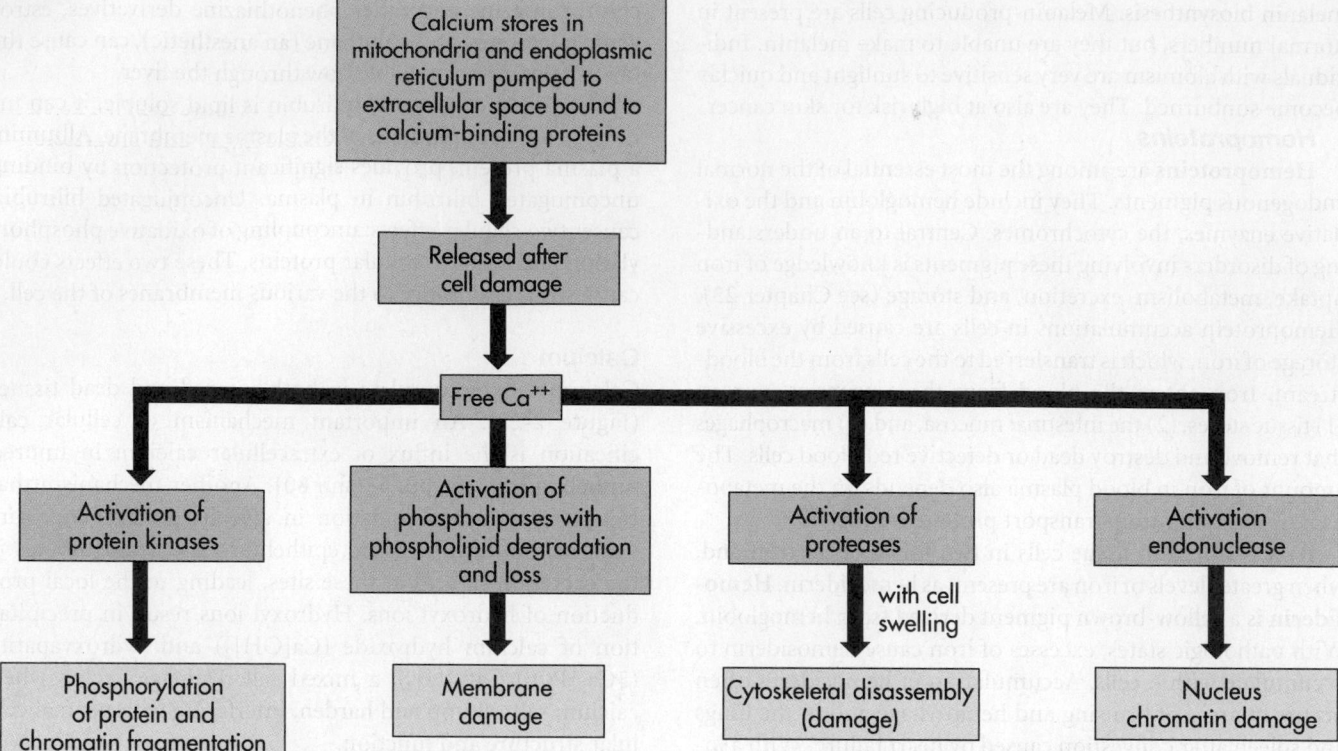

Figure 2-27 Free cytosolic calcium: a destructive agent. Normally calcium is removed from the cytosol by adenosine triphosphate (ATP)–dependent calcium pumps. In normal cells, calcium is bound to buffering proteins, such as calbindin or paralbumin, and is contained in the endoplasmic reticulum and the mitochondria. If there is abnormal permeability of calcium-ion channels, direct damage to membranes, or depletion of ATP (i.e., hypoxic injury), calcium increases in the cytosol. If the free calcium cannot be buffered or pumped out of cells, uncontrolled enzyme activation takes place, causing further damage. Uncontrolled entry of calcium into the cytosol is an important final pathway in many causes of cell death.

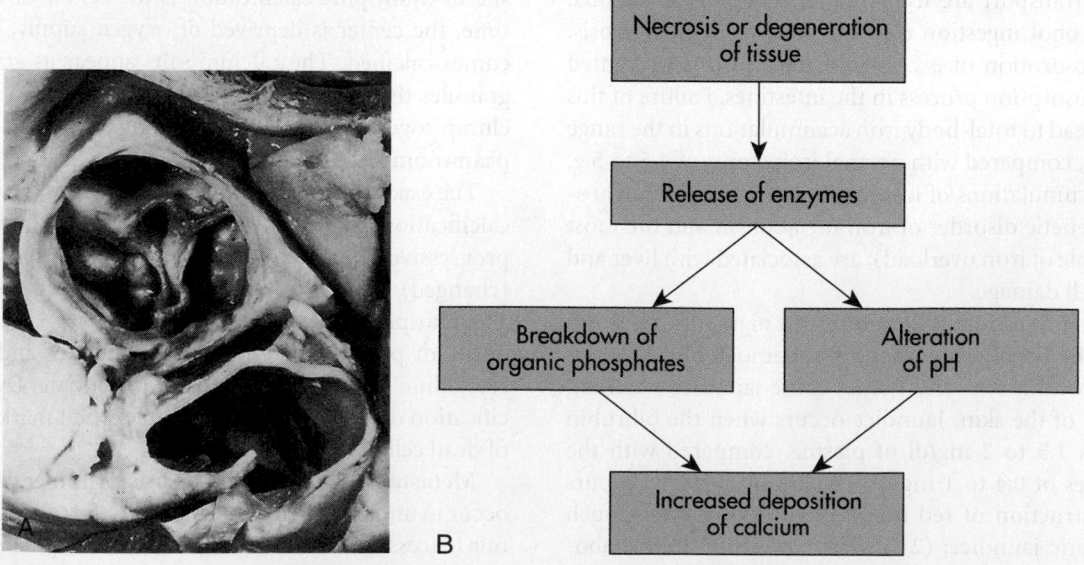

Figure 2-28 Aortic valve calcification. A, This aortic valve was unable to close because of calcification caused by rheumatic heart disease. **B,** Algorithm showing the dystrophic mechanism of calcification. (A from Damjanov I, Linder J, editors: *Anderson's pathology,* ed 10, St Louis, 1996, Mosby.)

bone demineralization that results from bone tumors, leukemia, and disseminated cancers. Hypercalcemia also can occur in some instances of advanced renal failure with phosphate retention, resulting in hyperparathyroidism.[10]

Urate

In humans, uric acid (**urate**) is the major end product of purine catabolism because of the absence of the enzyme urate oxidase. Serum urate concentration is, in general, stable: approximately 5 mg/dl in postpubertal males and 4.1 mg/dl in postpubertal females. Disturbances in maintaining serum urate levels result in hyperuricemia and deposition of sodium urate crystals in the tissues, leading to painful disorders collectively called *gout*. These disorders include acute arthritis, chronic gouty arthritis, tophus (firm nodular subcutaneous deposits of urate crystals surrounded by fibrosis), and nephritis (inflammation of the nephron).

Chronic hyperuricemia results in the deposition of urate in tissues, cell injury, and inflammation. Because urate crystals are not degraded by lysosomal enzymes, they persist in dead cells.

Systemic Manifestations

Systemic manifestations of cellular injury include a general sense of fatigue and malaise, a loss of well-being, and altered appetite. Fever is frequently present because of biochemicals produced during the inflammatory response (see Chapter 6). Table 2-10 summarizes the most significant systemic manifestations of cellular injury.

CELLULAR DEATH

Two main types of cell death are necrosis and apoptosis. Necrosis, or accidental cell death, occurs after severe and sudden injury. Programmed cell death is often referred to as apoptosis, but other forms have been determined with sophisticated ultrastructural studies (see What's New? Programmed Cell Death More Than Apoptosis).

Necrosis

Necrosis is the sum of cellular changes after local cell death and the process of cellular lysis and it provokes an inflammatory reaction in surrounding tissue (Figure 2-29). The structural signs that indicate irreversible injury and progression to necrosis are the dense clumping and progressive disruption of genetic material and disruption of the plasma and organelle membranes. In later stages of necrosis, most organelles are disrupted, and **karyolysis** (nuclear dissolution and lysis of chromatin from the action of hydrolytic enzymes) is under way. In some cells the nucleus shrinks and becomes a small, dense mass of genetic material—a process called nuclear **pyknosis.** The pyknotic nucleus eventually dissolves (by karyolysis) as a result of the action of hydrolytic lysosomal enzymes on DNA. **Karyorrhexis** means fragmentation of the nucleus into smaller particles or "nuclear dust."

WHAT'S NEW?   Programmed Cell Death More Than Apoptosis

With better technologies to study cell death, recent work has revealed at least three distinct forms of cell death. The best studied is apoptosis or type 1 cell death (see p. 84). Type 2 cell death, called autophagic cell death (Greek: *auto,* oneself; *phagy,* to eat), refers to any cellular degradative pathway that delivers cytoplasmic products to the lysosome (see Figure 2-29). In autophagic death, membrane sheets, mostly from the endoplasmic reticulum (ER), form cytoplasmic vacuoles that engulf intracellular organelles and cytoplasmic materials. The vesicles fuse with lysosomes, called autolysosomes, in which the contents are digested. This process is thought to be the cell's major mechanism for degrading organelles and long-lived proteins. Type 3 cell death, the least studied, is characterized by the swelling of intracellular organelles and a non-lysosomal cell death similar to necrosis.

Data from Levine B, Kroemer G: *Cell* 132(1):27-42, 2008.

Table 2-10   Systemic Manifestations of Cellular Injury

Manifestation	Cause
Fever	Release of endogenous pyrogens (interleukin-1, tumor necrosis factor-α (TNF-α), prostaglandins) from bacteria or macrophages; acute inflammatory response
Increased heart rate	Increase in oxidative metabolic processes resulting from fever
Increase in leukocytes (leukocytosis)	Increase in total number of white blood cells because of infection; normal is 5000-9000/mm³ (increase is directly related to the severity of the infection)
Pain	Various mechanisms, such as release of bradykinins, obstruction, pressure
Presence of cellular enzymes in extracellular fluid	Release of enzymes from cells of tissue*
Lactate dehydrogenase (LDH) (LDH isoenzymes)	Release from red blood cells, liver, kidney, skeletal muscle
Creatine kinase (CK) (CK isoenzymes)	Release from skeletal muscle, brain, heart
Aspartate aminotransferase (AST; SGOT)	Release from heart, liver, skeletal muscle, kidney, pancreas
Alanine aminotransferase (ALT; SGPT)	Release from liver, kidney, heart
Alkaline phosphatase (ALP)	Release from liver, bone
Amylase	Release from pancreas
Aldolase	Release from skeletal muscle, heart

*The rapidity of enzyme transfer is a function of the weight of the enzyme and the concentration gradient across the cellular membrane. The specific metabolic and excretory rates of the enzymes determine how long levels of enzymes remain elevated.

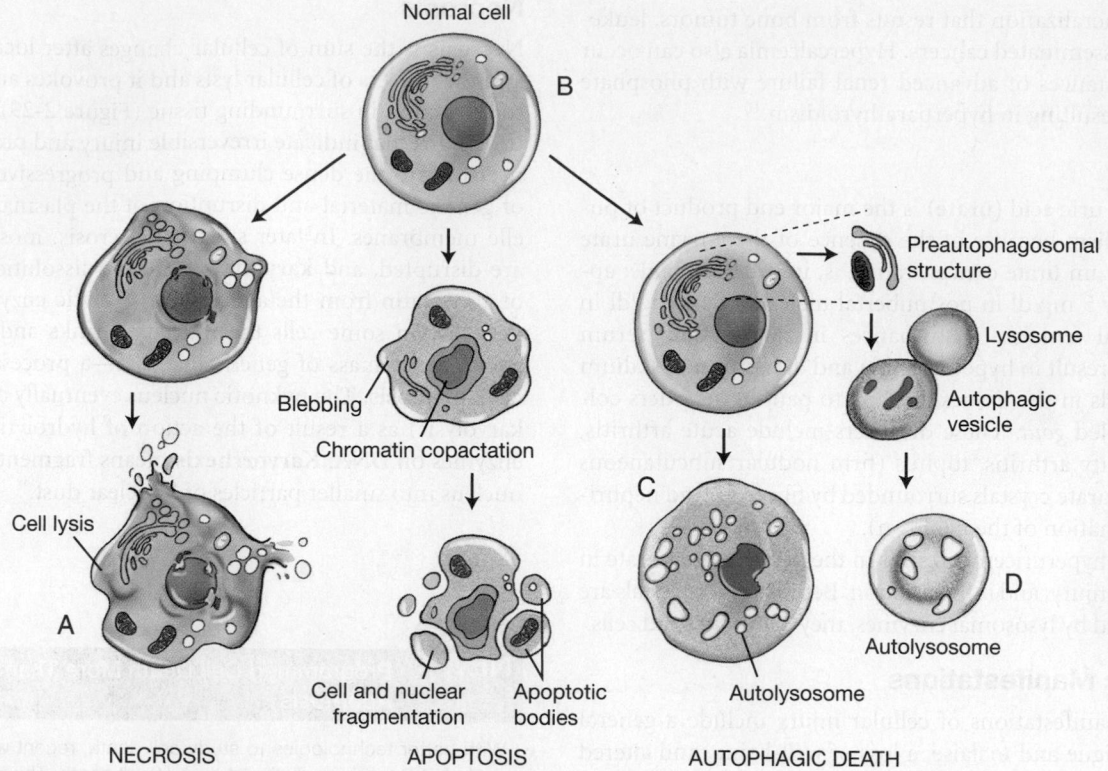

Figure 2-29 Different forms of cell death. **A,** Schematic illustration of structural changes that characterize cell death by necrosis, apoptosis, and autophagic cell death. Whereas necrotic cell death culminates in cell lysis and provokes immediate inflammation, apoptotic cells are packaged into apoptotic bodies that are then engulfed by adjacent cells without an inflammatory response. Autophagic cell death is characterized by the appearance of cytoplasmic vesicles engulfing bulk cytoplasm and organelles. The contents of the vesicles are digested by the lysosomal system of the same cell after the fusion of the autophagic vesicles with lysosomes. *Inset:* Formation of autolysosome by fusion of autophagic vesicle and lysosome with the cell undergoing autophagy. **B-D,** Ultrastructural features of cells undergoing apoptotic and autophagic cell death: **(B)** a normal cell, **(C)** an apoptotic cell, and **(D)** a cell undergoing autophagic cell death are shown. Polyribosomes, mitochondria, and autophagic vacuoles are indicated. Although autophagic vacuoles can be seen in healthy cells and apoptotic cells, they are much more abundant during autophagic cell death. (Redrawn from Bursch et al: *J Cell* Sci 113:1189-1198, 2000, by permission)

Different types of necroses tend to occur in different organs or tissues and sometimes can indicate the mechanism or cause of cellular injury. The four major types of necroses are coagulative, liquefactive, caseous, and fatty. Another type, gangrenous necrosis, is *not* a distinctive type of cell death but refers to larger areas of tissue death.

Coagulative necrosis, which occurs primarily in the kidneys, heart, and adrenal glands, commonly results from hypoxia caused by severe ischemia or hypoxia caused by chemical injury, especially ingestion of mercuric chloride (Figure 2-30). Coagulation is caused by protein denaturation, which causes the protein albumin to change from a gelatinous, transparent state to a firm, opaque state, similar to that of a cooked egg white. The necrotic tissues appear firm and slightly swollen. Recent evidence indicates that an abnormality in intracellular levels of Ca^{++} (e.g., increased) may be a critical event in coagulation necrosis.[3]

Liquefactive necrosis commonly results from ischemic injury to neurons and glial cells in the brain (Figure 2-31). Dead brain tissue is readily affected by liquefactive necrosis because brain cells are rich in the digestive hydrolytic enzymes and lipids, and the brain contains little connective tissue. As the cells are digested by their own hydrolases, the tissue becomes soft, liquefies, and is walled off from healthy tissue, forming cysts. (Cyst formation is described in Chapter 6.)

Liquefactive necrosis can also result from bacterial infection, particularly by staphylococci, streptococci, and *Escherichia coli.* In this case the hydrolases are released from the lysosomes of neutrophils, which are phagocytes attracted to the infected area to kill the bacteria. Liquefaction of bacterial cells and neighboring tissue cells by neutrophilic hydrolases results in the accumulation of pus.

Caseous necrosis, which commonly results from tuberculous pulmonary infection, particularly by *Mycobacterium tuberculosis,* is a combination of coagulative and liquefactive necrosis (Figure 2-32). The dead cells disintegrate, but the debris is not digested completely by hydrolases. Tissues appear soft and granular and resemble clumped cheese, which gives this type of necrosis its name. A granulomatous inflammatory wall encloses areas of caseous necrosis.

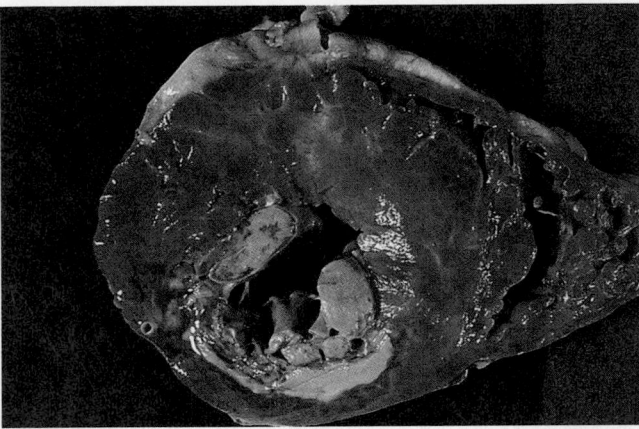

Figure 2-30 Coagulative necrosis of myocardium of posterior wall of left ventricle of heart. A large anemic (white) infarct is readily apparent; note also the necrosis of papillary muscle. (From Damjanov I, Linder J: *Anderson's pathology*, ed 10, St Louis, 1996, Mosby.)

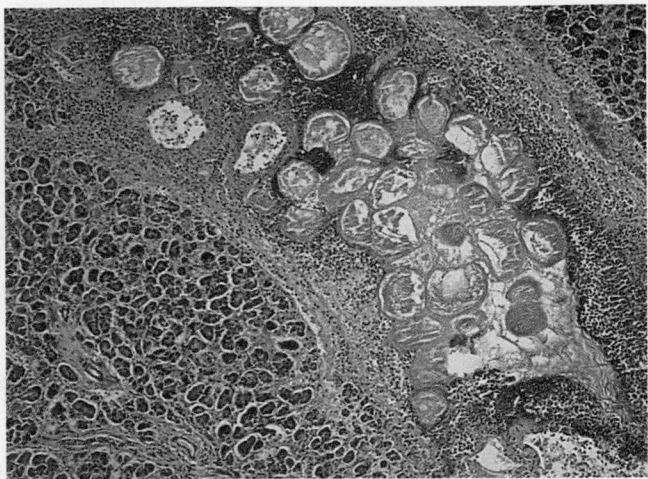

Figure 2-33 Fat necrosis of pancreas. Interlobular adipocytes are necrotic; these are surrounded by acute inflammatory cells. (From Damjanov I, Linder J: *Anderson's pathology*, ed 10, St Louis, 1996, Mosby.)

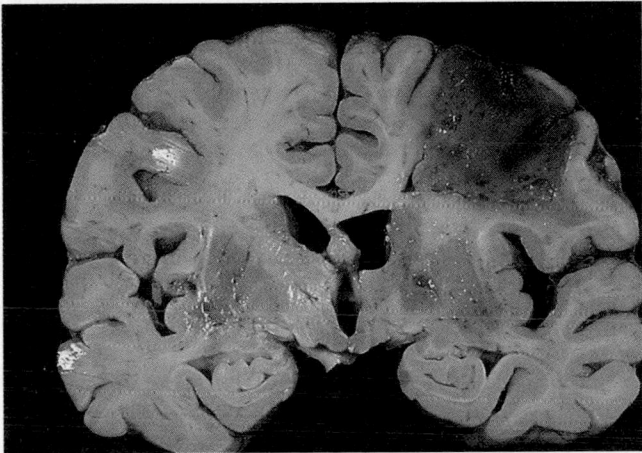

Figure 2-31 Liquefactive necrosis. Liquefactive necrosis of the brain developed at a large cerebral infarct caused by ischemia. (From Damjanov I, Linder J: *Anderson's pathology*, ed 10, St Louis, 1996, Mosby.)

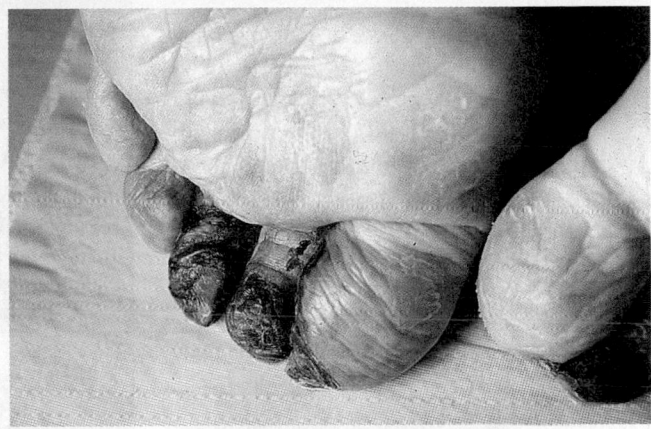

Figure 2-34 Gangrene of toes. Dry gangrene. (From Damjanov I: *Pathology for the health-related professions*, ed 2, Philadelphia, 2000, Saunders.)

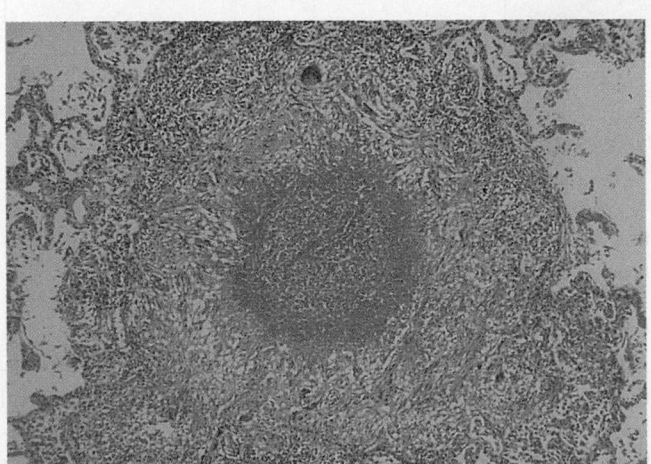

Figure 2-32 Granuloma with central caseous necrosis typical of pulmonary tuberculosis. (From Damjanov I, Linder J: *Anderson's pathology*, ed 10, St Louis, 1996, Mosby.)

Fat necrosis, which occurs in the breast, pancreas, and other abdominal structures, is cellular dissolution caused by powerful enzymes called *lipases* (Figure 2-33). Lipases break down triglycerides, releasing free fatty acids, which then combine with calcium, magnesium, and sodium ions, creating soaps (a process known as *saponification*). The necrotic tissue appears opaque and chalk white.

Gangrenous necrosis, a term commonly used in surgical clinical practice, refers to death of tissue and results from severe hypoxic injury, commonly occurring because of arteriosclerosis, or blockage, of major arteries, especially in the lower leg. With hypoxia and subsequent bacterial invasion, the tissues can undergo necrosis. **Dry gangrene** is usually the result of coagulative necrosis. The skin becomes very dry and shrinks, resulting in wrinkles, and its color changes to dark brown or black (Figure 2-34). **Wet gangrene** develops when neutrophils invade the site, causing liquefactive necrosis. This usually occurs in internal organs, causing the site

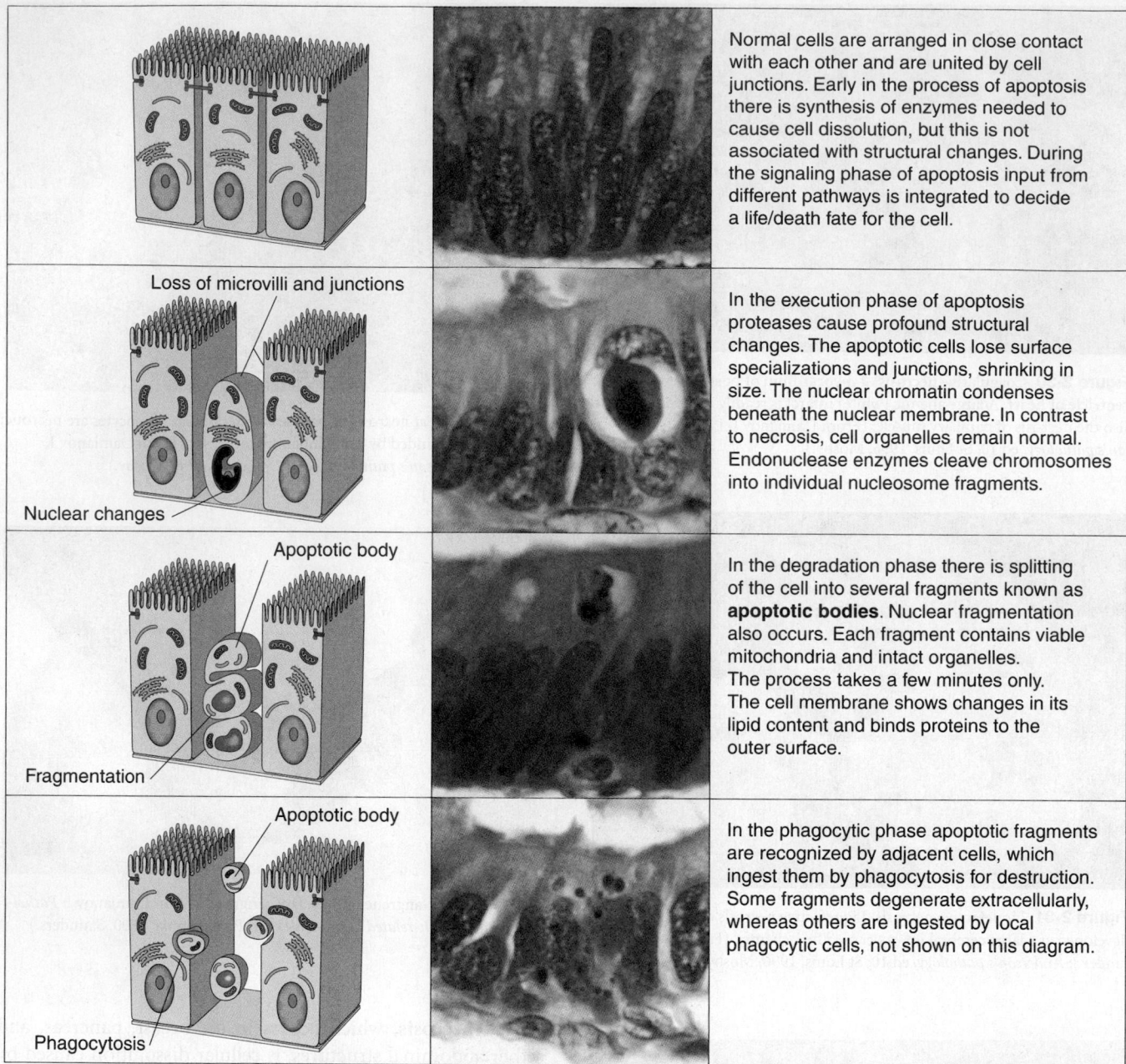

Loss of microvilli and junctions

Nuclear changes

Normal cells are arranged in close contact with each other and are united by cell junctions. Early in the process of apoptosis there is synthesis of enzymes needed to cause cell dissolution, but this is not associated with structural changes. During the signaling phase of apoptosis input from different pathways is integrated to decide a life/death fate for the cell.

In the execution phase of apoptosis proteases cause profound structural changes. The apoptotic cells lose surface specializations and junctions, shrinking in size. The nuclear chromatin condenses beneath the nuclear membrane. In contrast to necrosis, cell organelles remain normal. Endonuclease enzymes cleave chromosomes into individual nucleosome fragments.

Apoptotic body

Fragmentation

In the degradation phase there is splitting of the cell into several fragments known as **apoptotic bodies**. Nuclear fragmentation also occurs. Each fragment contains viable mitochondria and intact organelles. The process takes a few minutes only. The cell membrane shows changes in its lipid content and binds proteins to the outer surface.

Apoptotic body

Phagocytosis

In the phagocytic phase apoptotic fragments are recognized by adjacent cells, which ingest them by phagocytosis for destruction. Some fragments degenerate extracellularly, whereas others are ingested by local phagocytic cells, not shown on this diagram.

Figure 2-35 Apoptosis. Apoptosis of cells is a programmed and energy-dependent process designed specifically to switch cells off and eliminate them. This controlled pattern of cell death, termed *programmed cell death,* is very different from that which occurs as a direct result of acute alterations, for example, trauma. (From Stevens A, Lowe J: *Pathology,* ed 2, London, 2000, Mosby.)

to become cold, swollen, and black. A foul odor is present, produced by pus, and if systemic symptoms become severe, death can ensue.

Gas gangrene, a special type of gangrene, is caused by infection of injured tissue by one of many species of *Clostridium.* These anaerobic bacteria produce hydrolytic enzymes and toxins that destroy connective tissue and cellular membranes and cause bubbles of gas to form in muscle cells. Gas gangrene can be fatal if enzymes lyse the membranes of red blood cells, destroying their oxygen-carrying capacity. Death is the result of shock. The condition is treated with antitoxins

and supplemental oxygen delivered in a hyperbaric (pressurized) chamber.

Apoptosis

Apoptosis (Greek for "dropping off") is an important distinct type of cell death[84] that differs from necrosis in several respects (Figure 2-35). Apoptosis is an active process of cellular self-destruction, called *programmed cell death,* that is implicated in both normal and pathologic tissue changes.[85] Newer sophisticated studies have revealed that programmed cell death includes other forms than just apoptosis (see

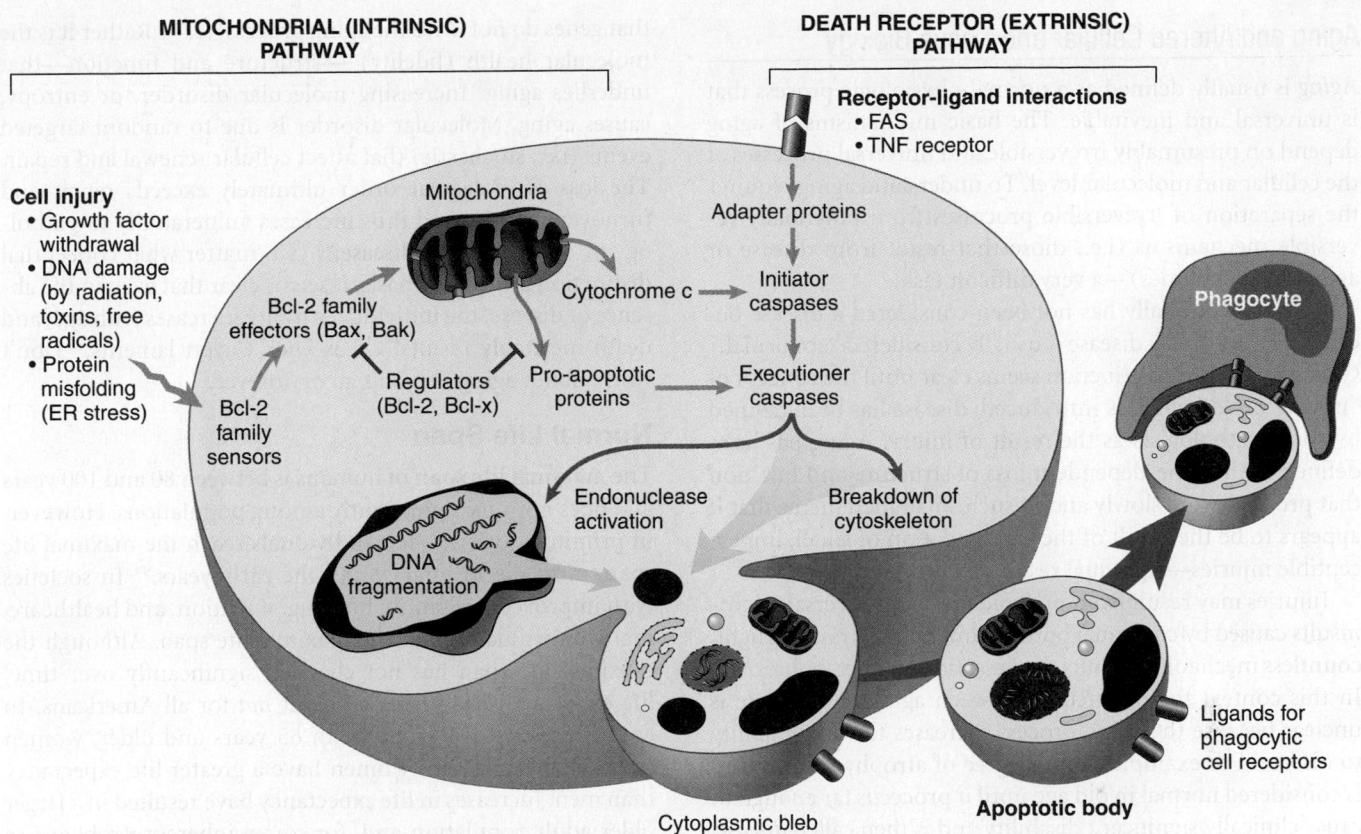

MITOCHONDRIAL (INTRINSIC) PATHWAY

DEATH RECEPTOR (EXTRINSIC) PATHWAY

Receptor-ligand interactions
• FAS
• TNF receptor

Mitochondria

Adapter proteins

Cell injury
• Growth factor withdrawal
• DNA damage (by radiation, toxins, free radicals)
• Protein misfolding (ER stress)

Bcl-2 family effectors (Bax, Bak)

Bcl-2 family sensors

Regulators (Bcl-2, Bcl-x)

Cytochrome c

Initiator caspases

Pro-apoptotic proteins

Executioner caspases

Endonuclease activation

DNA fragmentation

Breakdown of cytoskeleton

Phagocyte

Ligands for phagocytic cell receptors

Cytoplasmic bleb

Apoptotic body

Figure 2-36 Mechanisms of apoptosis. The two pathways of apoptosis differ in their induction and regulation, and both culminate in the activation of "executioner" caspases. The induction of apoptosis is dependent on the balance between pro- and anti-apoptotic signals and intracellular proteins. The figure shows the pathways that induce apoptotic cell death, and the anti-apoptotic proteins that inhibit mitochondrial leakiness and cytochrome c–dependent caspase activation and thus function as regulators of mitochondrial apoptosis. (From from Kumar V, Abbas A, Fausto N: *Robbins and Cotran pathologic basis of disease,* ed 8, Philadelphia, 2007, Saunders.)

What's new? Programmed Cell Death More than Apoptosis). Cells need to die, otherwise endless proliferation would lead to gigantic bodies. Every day an average adult may create 10 billion new cells and kill off the same number. Apoptosis is responsible for local deletion of cells during normal embryonic development, bone cells dying during turnover, lymphocytes dying during receptor repertoire selection, infected cells, and so on. It has been shown to play a major role in endocrine-dependent tissues that are undergoing atrophic change. Apoptosis can occur spontaneously in malignant tumors and in normal, rapidly proliferating cells treated with cancer chemotherapeutic agents and ionizing radiation.[86] Defects in apoptosis can cause cancer.[87] Its significance in aging is unknown; however, apoptosis is required to maintain a balance between cell proliferation and cell death.[87]

Necrosis and apoptosis affect tissues differently. Unlike necrosis, apoptosis affects scattered, single cells. Apoptosis is nuclear, and cytoplasmic shrinkage of a cell (i.e., unlike necrosis, in which cells swell and lyse) is followed by fragmentation into membrane-bound fragments and subsequent phagocytosis by neighboring, healthy cells.[10] Apoptosis depends on a tightly regulated cellular program for its

initiation and execution.[86] Programmed cell death involves enzymes that cut up other proteins (proteases) that are, themselves, activated by proteolytic activity in response to signals that induce apoptosis.[88] These proteases are called **caspases,** a family of aspartic acid–specific proteases. The activated suicide caspases cleave, and thereby activate, other members of the family resulting in an amplifying "suicide" cascade. The activated caspases then cleave other key proteins in the cell, killing it quickly and neatly.[88-90] Two different pathways converge on caspase activation called the *mitochondrial pathway* and the *death receptor pathway* (Figure 2-36). Cells that die by apoptosis release chemical factors that recruit phagocytes that quickly engulf the remains of the dead cell, thus reducing chances of inflammation. With necrosis, cell death is not neat because cells that die as a result of acute injury swell, burst, and spill their contents all over their neighbors, likely causing a damaging inflammatory response.[88] Molecular helpers in apoptosis are present in different subcellular compartments, including the plasma membrane, cytosol, mitochondria, and nucleus. The progression of apoptosis depends on the interplay among these compartments and the exchange of specific signaling molecules.[86]

Aging and Altered Cellular and Tissue Biology

Aging is usually defined as a normal physiologic process that is universal and inevitable. The basic mechanisms of aging depend on presumably irreversible and universal processes at the cellular and molecular level. To understand aging requires the separation of irreversible processes from potentially reversible mechanisms (i.e., those that result from disease or age-related debilities)—a very difficult task!

Aging traditionally has not been considered a disease because it is "normal"; disease is usually considered "abnormal." Conceptually, this distinction seems clear until the concept of "injury" or "damage" is introduced; disease has been defined by some pathologists as the result of injury. Aging has been defined as the time-dependent loss of structure and function that proceeds very slowly and in such small increments that it appears to be the result of the accumulation of small, imperceptible injuries—a gradual result of wear and tear.

Injuries may result from unavoidable and universal microinsults caused by continual bombardment by ultraviolet light, countless mechanical insults, and reactions to metabolites.[91,92] In this context the distinction between aging and disease is unclear because the aging process increases the vulnerability to disease. For example, some degree of atrophy of the brain is considered normal in old age until it proceeds far enough to cause clinically significant disability and is then called *disease*. Likewise, most humans have atherosclerosis, and the plaques progress with age, but at what point in this progression is it considered abnormal? These conceptual distinctions have given rise to two general categories of theories of aging. The first category proposes that aging is the result of the accumulation of random injuries and events. The second category proposes that aging is the result of a genetically controlled developmental program, or built-in self-destructive processes. A classic experiment done by Hayflick[84] demonstrated that fibroblasts are limited to a finite number of generations (40 to 60 doublings). Hayflick himself, however, reports this theory of aging is now losing support. "The weight of evidence indicates

that genes do not *drive* the aging process. ..."[93] Rather it is the molecular health (fidelity) —structure and function—that underlies aging. Increasing molecular disorder, or entropy, causes aging. Molecular disorder is due to random targeted events (i.e., stochastic) that affect cellular renewal and repair. The loss of molecular order ultimately exceeds repair and turnover capacity and thus increases vulnerability to pathology or age-associated disease.[93] (No matter what conceptual distinction is used as a basis, it seems clear that even in the absence of disease, the individual's frailty increases with age, and death inevitably results! Or as Dick Cavett laments, "Don't worry about aging, it won't go on forever."

Normal Life Span

The **maximal life span** of humans is between 80 and 100 years and does not vary significantly among populations. However, in primitive societies, few individuals reach the maximal life span; most die in infancy and the early years.[94] In societies with improved sanitation, housing, nutrition, and healthcare, many individuals attain the maximal life span. Although the maximal life span has not changed significantly over time, life expectancy has increased—but *not* for all Americans. In each successive age group from 65 years and older, women outnumber men; thus women have a greater life expectancy than men. Increases in life expectancy have resulted in a larger older adult population and, for some, inherent problems of disability, disease, and socioeconomic hardship.

Life Expectancy Differences Across America

Life expectancy is the average number of years of life remaining at a given age. Although the slow but steady rise in life expectancy has occurred generally in the United States, disparities exist among various counties. A surprising government-sponsored study by Harvard researchers found life expectancy actually *declined* in a number of counties (e.g., smallest unit of analysis) from 1983 to 1999, particularly for women (see What's New? Decline in Life Expectancy in Some U.S. Counties).

WHAT'S NEW? Decline in Life Expectancy in Some U.S. Counties

Continuing rise in life expectancy for *all* Americans is not happening. Long-term analysis of county trends has revealed startling data.

Between 1961 and 1999, *average* life expectancy in the United States increased from 73.5 to 79.6 years for women and 66.9 to 74.1 years for men. However, the differences in mortality by county between the most disadvantaged populations and those with the most advantages began to *widen* in the early 1980s. Life expectancy between 1961 and 1999 in the male advantaged population (best-off group) rose from 70.5 to 78.7 years and from 76.9 to 83 years for females. In the female disadvantaged populations (worst-off group) starting in the early 1980s, life expectancy remained relatively stable (68.7 years in 1961, 74.5 years in 1983, and only 75.5 years in 1999). The worst-off men had a decline, rising again in the 1990s.

The gains made, particularly for cardiovascular disease, began to level off in the 1980s because of rising mortality from lung cancer,

chronic obstructive pulmonary disease, and diabetes. A major contributor, which peaked later for women than men, is smoking. Smoking is thought to be a significant contributor for women, as well as overweight, obesity, and hypertension. The worst-off counties also showed a rise in HIV/AIDS and homicide in men.

Statistically significant declines for women occurred in 180 of 3141 counties and in 11 counties for men. In addition, 783 counties declined for women and 48 declined for men, but this was not statistically significant. Life expectancy was worse in all southwestern Virginia counties, with a drop over the 16-year period of about 6 years in women and 2.5 years in men. The greatest improvements occurred in western desert counties where life expectancy rose almost 5 years for women and about 7 years for men.

The life expectancy "gap" is *increasing* between rich and poor and high and low educational attainment. This increase is occurring

WHAT'S NEW?   Decline in Life Expectancy in Some U.S. Counties—cont'd

despite the gap between men and women and between blacks and whites. In addition, other indices include geography and community assets.

The analysis of county data demonstrates that the 1980s and 1990s were the beginning of the era of increased inequalities in mortality in the United States. Dividing the United States into eight "Americas," it is now evident that disparities in mortality affect millions of Americans. The gap is enormous. The eight Americas analysis revealed the highest levels of life expectancy on record (to be U.S.-born Asian females (America 1), 3 years higher than that of females in Japan). The next highest group was low-income, white rural populations in Minnesota, the Dakotas, Iowa, Montana, and

Nebraska (America 2) with a life expectancy of 76.2 years for males and 81.8 years for females. Blacks living in high-risk urban areas (America 8) had the lowest life expectancy, with an almost four times' likelihood than the America 1 (Asian) group would die before the age of 60 years and between 3.8 and 4.7 times more likely to die before age 45! The excess young and middle-aged deaths in America 8 were observed to be caused by injuries, cardiovascular disease, liver cirrhosis, diabetes, HIV, and homicide.

In summary, large disparities in life expectancy exist across America because of differences in chronic diseases and injuries with known risk factors, including alcohol use, tobacco smoking, overweight and obesity, elevated blood pressure, cholesterol, and glucose control.

Data from Ezzati M et al: The reversal of fortunes: trends in county mortality and cross-country mortality disparances in the United States, *PLOS Med* 5(4):e66 doi: 10.1371/journal.pmed.0050066; Murray CJL et al: Eight Americas: Investigating mortality disparities across races, counties, and race-counties in the United States, *PLOS Med* 3(9):e260 doi:10.1371/journal.pmed.0030260.

AIDS, Acquired immunodeficiency syndrome; *HIV,* human immunodeficiency virus.

Theories and Mechanisms of Aging

Relatively little "indisputable" knowledge exists on the subject of aging. Gaining support, however, is that aging is the result of cellular damage and molecular disorder. Table 2-11 presents the historical development of aging research. Numerous theories exist about the causes of aging. Many of these theories overlap, interact, and are similar. Some of them have focused on a single mechanism—the so-called magic bullet approach to arrest aging. It is doubtful that a single theory will explain all the mechanisms of aging. Emerging from active investigation are some common mechanisms. These mechanisms are included in the What's New? The Emerging Focus on the Biology of Aging.

WHAT'S NEW?   The Emerging Focus in the Biology of Aging

Areas of primary focus in the biology of aging include endocrine regulation through endocrine signaling pathways, nuclear architecture and genomic instability, decline in cell renewal by adult stem cells, and accumulation of cellular damage related to cancer and aging.

The insulin/insulin-like growth factor-1 (IGF-1) signaling pathway is well established in mammals as an endocrine regulator of aging. Insulin has a role in certain tissues to regulate life span. Insulin-like signaling is necessary for homeostasis, growth, and survival. Reduced insulin signaling in lower animals extends life span. Reduced insulin signaling in higher animals (rodents and mammals) causes glucose intolerance and hyperinsulinemia, progressing to type 2 diabetes mellitus and shortening life span. Investigators recently proposed that the brain is where reduced or inefficient insulin-like signaling can extend life span similarly as in lower animals. Reduced insulin-like signaling can increase antioxidant enzymes and proteins that promote DNA repair. Main factors affected by insulin-like signaling are the transcription factors forkhead box O (FOXO). FOXO controls gene expression that regulates the cell cycle, apoptosis, DNA repair, metabolism, and resistance to oxidative stress. Increased peripheral sensitivity to insulin and reduced circulating insulin can be achieved by calorie restriction (CR), daily exercise, and weight loss. Questionable is whether calorie restriction increases *human* life span—it seems clear that CR does decrease age-related diseases. What is confusing is that some studies reveal *no* correlation between longevity and low body mass index.

Cells vary in shape and size, yet they all seem to age. DNA-protein complexes, or chromatin, stabilize the genome and determine gene expression. Thus the maintenance of chromatin dictates nuclear architecture. DNA damage might lead to significant changes in gene expression to promote human aging. A model, the *epigenetic*

balance hypothesis, is proposed to explain gene expression changes that may occur as a result of chromatin modification. The hypothesis includes the idea that DNA damage mediates remodeling of chromatin and nuclear architecture over a lifetime. These ideas seem consistent with oxidative stress and that DNA damage can accelerate aging. Confusing, however, is that the aging process could *directly* affect chromatin structure through some unknown mechanism that then leads to DNA damage.

Another hot topic is aging and stem cells. Aging might be associated with a decline in replication directed by adult stem cells. Data suggest that as we grow older our stem cells age as a result of mechanisms that suppress the development of cancer (e.g., senescence, apoptosis). Stem cell aging may happen with accumulating DNA damage or other nuclear support mechanisms, or both. Anticancer mechanisms, such as senescence and apoptosis, that depend on chromosome telomere shortening and/or p53 (guardian of the genome) and p16 INK4a (an inhibitor of cell cycle progression) activation are thought to promote aging just as their failure increases cancer risk.

Telomeres, like the plastic ends of shoelaces, form the end of chromosomes. Telomeres are short, repeated sequences of DNA that not only encode only gene product but also are important for ensuring the complete replication of chromosome ends and protecting the end from degradation. Telomeres shorten with each cell division, limiting proliferation of human cells by inducing a nondividing state called *replicative senescence*. Replicative senescence involves incomplete replication with progressive shortening of the telomeres and eventual cell cycle arrest. Telomere capping is necessary to distinguish the chromosome ends from DNA interruptions or breaks within the genome. A DNA break signals cell cycle arrest,

Continued

which can lead to DNA repair or apoptosis. Thus telomeres help maintain chromosome stability, which depends on chromosome telomere length. The lengths of telomeres are maintained by an enzyme called *telomerase*. Telomerase is an RNA-protein complex in which RNA serves as the template for telomere nucleotide synthesis, adding telomere length. Telomerase is active during embryogenesis but is suppressed in most somatic tissues postnatally. In adults, telomerase remains active in germ cells and certain stem cells. Thus as cells age their telomeres shorten, causing cell cycle arrest and an inability to generate new cells to replace damaged cells. Contrarily, telomerase is reactivated and telomeres are not shortened in immortal cancer cells, suggesting that telomere lengthening may be an important step in cancer development (see Chapter 11). The importance of telomeres is actively being investigated and their relationship to both aging and cancer is not now fully elucidated.

Data from Appels CW, Vandenbroucke JP: *N Engl J Med* 355:2699, 2006; Oberdoerffer P, Sinclair DA: *Nat Rev* 8:692-702, 2007; Serrano M, Blasco MA: *Nat Rev* 8:715-722m, 2008; Sharpless NE, DePinho RA: *Nat Rev* 8:703-713, 2008; Taguchi A, White MF: *Ann Rev Physiol* 70:191-212, 2008; Yang D et al: *Obes Rev* 4:9-16, 2003.

Table 2-11	Theories of Aging	
Theory	**Year**	**Proponent**
Waste product theory	1923	Carrell and Ebeling
Wear-and-tear theory	1924	Pearl
Rate of living theory[a]	1928	Pearl
Neuroendocrine theory (including DHEA and melatonin)	1947	Korenchevsky and Jones
Free-radical theory	1955	Harman
Collagen theory[b]	1957	Verzar
Metabolic theory[a]	1957; 1961	Carlson et al; Johnson et al
Somatic mutation theory	1959	Sziliard
Error-catastrophe theory	1963; 1970	Orgel
Cross-linking theory[b]	1968	Bjorksten
Programmed senescence theory	1969	Hayflick
Immunologic theory	1969	Walform
Mitochondrial theory	1972	Harman
Evolution theory	1977	Kirkwood

Data from Schneider EL: Theories of aging: a perspective. In Warner HR et al, editors: *Modern biological theories of aging,* New York, 1987, Raven; Madison HE: Theories of aging. In Lueckenotte A: *Gerontologic nursing,* ed 2, St Louis, 2000, Mosby; Hayflick L: *How and why we age,* New York, 1996, Ballantine Books.

NOTE: Theories with the same superscript may represent the same theory. *DHEA,* Dehydroepiandrosterone.

Degenerative Extracellular Changes

Extracellular factors that affect the aging process include the binding of collagen; the increase in free radicals' effects on cells; the structural alterations of fascia, tendons, ligaments, bones, and joints; and peripheral vascular disease, particularly arteriosclerosis (see Chapter 30).

Aging affects the extracellular matrix with increased cross-linking (e.g., aging collagen becomes more insoluble, chemically stable, but rigid, resulting in a decrease of cell permeability), decreased synthesis, and increased degradation of collagen. These changes, together with the disappearance of elastin and changes in proteoglycans and plasma proteins, cause disorders of the ground substance that result in dehydration and wrinkling of the skin (see Chapter 44). Other age-related defects in the extracellular matrix include skeletal muscle alterations (e.g., atrophy, decreased tone, loss of contractility), cataracts, diverticula, hernias, and rupture of intervertebral disks.

Free radicals of oxygen that result from oxidative cellular metabolism, called oxidative stress (e.g., respiratory chain, phagocytosis, prostaglandin synthesis), are known to damage tissues during the aging process (Figure 2-37). The oxygen radicals produced include superoxide radical, hydroxyl radical, and hydrogen peroxide (see p. 54). These oxygen products are extremely reactive and can damage nucleic acids, destroy polysaccharides, oxidize proteins, peroxidize unsaturated fatty acids, and kill and lyse cells. Oxidant effects on target cells can give rise to malignant transformation, presumably through DNA damage. That progressive and cumulative damage from oxygen radicals may lead to harmful alterations in cellular function is consistent with those alterations of aging. This hypothesis is founded on the wear-and-tear theory of aging, which states that damages accumulate with time, decreasing the organism's ability to maintain a steady state. Because these oxygen-reactive species not only can permanently damage cells but also may lead to cell death, there is new support for their role in the aging process.

Of much interest is the relationship between aging and the disappearance or alteration of extracellular substances important for vessel integrity. With aging, lipid, calcium, and plasma proteins are deposited in vessel walls. These depositions cause serious basement membrane thickening and alterations in smooth muscle functioning, resulting in arteriosclerosis. Arteriosclerosis is a progressive disease that causes serious problems in the aged individual, including stroke, myocardial infarction, renal disease, and peripheral vascular disease.

Cellular Aging

Cellular changes characteristic of aging include atrophy, decreased function, and loss of cells, possibly caused by apoptosis. Loss of cellular function from any of these causes initiates the compensatory mechanisms of hypertrophy and hyperplasia of remaining cells, which can lead to metaplasia, dysplasia, and neoplasia. All these changes can alter receptor

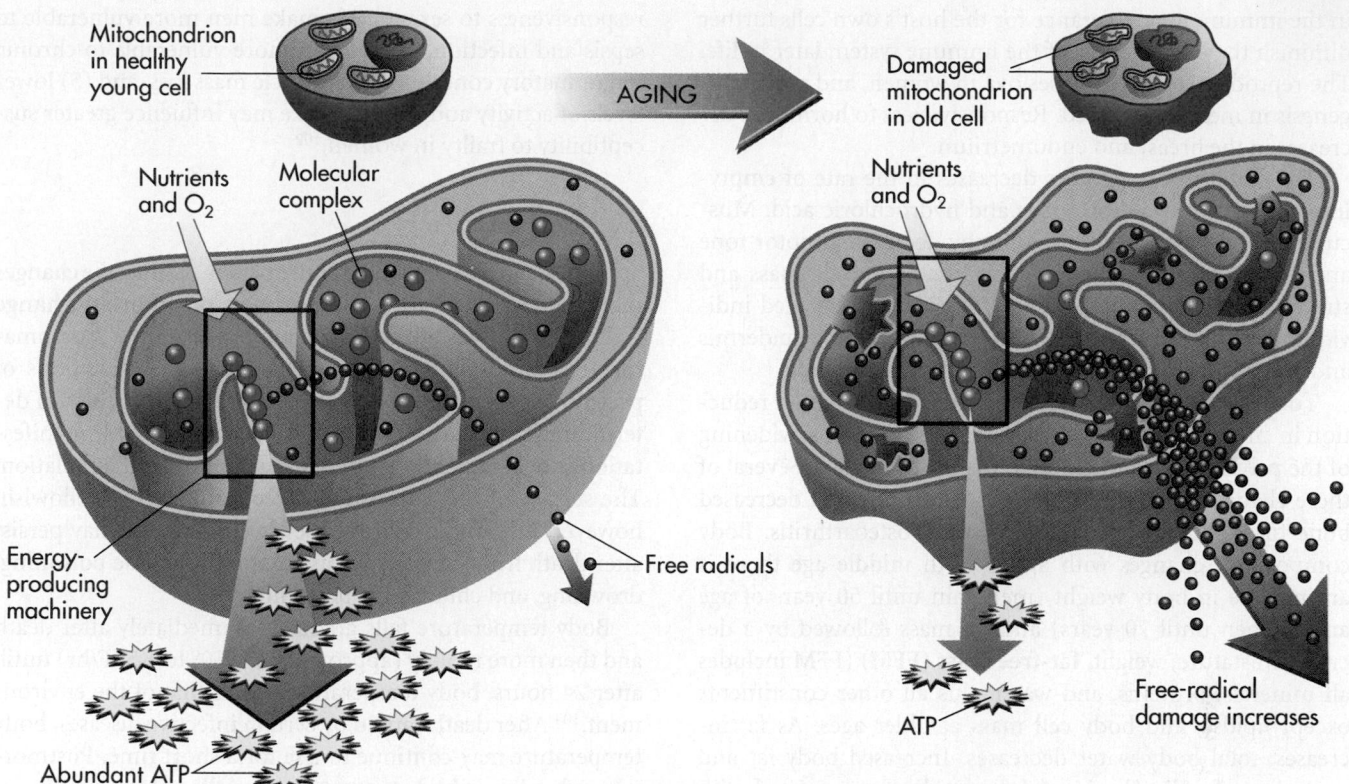

Figure 2-37 Theory of aging: destructive free radicals. *ATP,* Adenosine triphosphate.

placement and function, nutrient pathways, secretion of cellular products, and neuroendocrine control mechanisms. In the aged cell, DNA, RNA, cellular proteins, and membranes are most susceptible to injurious stimuli. DNA is particularly vulnerable to such injuries as breaks, deletions, and additions. Although DNA can repair itself with time, the aged cell's capacity for DNA repair is decreased. Lack of DNA repair increases the cell's susceptibility to mutations that may be lethal or may promote the development of neoplasia (see What's New? The Emerging Focus on the Biology of Aging).

Mitochondria are the organelles responsible for the generation of most of the energy used by eukaryotic cells. Mitochondrial DNA (mtDNA) encodes some of the proteins of the electron transfer chain, the system necessary for the conversion of adenosine diphosphate (ADP) to ATP. Mutations in mtDNA can deprive the cell of ATP, and mutations are correlated with the aging process. The most common age-related mtDNA mutation in humans is a large rearrangement called the *4977 deletion,* or *common deletion,* and is found in humans more than 40 years old. It is a deletion that removes all or part of 7 of the 13 protein-encoding mtDNA genes and 5 of the 22 tRNA genes. Individual cells containing this deletion have a condition known as *heteroplasmy.* Heteroplasmy levels rise with aging and are tissue dependent.[95-97]

The production of ROS under physiologic conditions is associated with activity of the respiratory chain in aerobic ATP production. Therefore, increased mitochondrial activity per

se can be an "oxidative stress" to cells. The production of ROS is markedly increased in many pathologic conditions in which the respiratory chain is impaired. Because mtDNA, which is essential for normal oxidative phosphorylation, is located in proximity to the ROS-generating respiratory chain, it is more oxidatively damaged than is nuclear DNA. Cumulative damage of mtDNA is implicated in the aging process as well as in the progression of such common diseases as diabetes, cancer, and heart failure.

Tissue and Systemic Aging

It is probably safe to say that every physiologic process can be shown to function less efficiently with increasing age. The most characteristic tissue change with age is a progressive stiffness or rigidity that affects many systems, including the arterial, pulmonary, and musculoskeletal systems. A consequence of blood vessel and organ stiffness is a progressive increase in peripheral resistance to blood flow. The movement of intracellular and extracellular substances also usually decreases with age as does the diffusion capacity of the lung. Blood flow through organs decreases; for example, renal plasma flow decreases.

Changes in the endocrine and immune systems include thymus atrophy. Although this occurs at puberty, causing a decreased immune response to T-dependent antigens (foreign proteins), increased autoantibodies and immune complexes (antibodies bound to antigen) and an overall decrease in the immunologic tolerance for the host's own cells further diminish the effectiveness of the immune system later in life. The reproductive system loses ova in women, and spermatogenesis in men is decreased. Responsiveness to hormones decreases in the breast and endometrium.

The stomach experiences decreases in the rate of emptying and secretion of hormones and hydrochloric acid. Muscular atrophy diminishes mobility by decreasing motor tone and contractility. **Sarcopenia,** the loss of muscle mass and strength, can occur into old age. The skin of the aged individual is affected by atrophy and wrinkling of the epidermis and alterations in underlying dermis, fat, and muscle.

Total body changes include a decrease in height; a reduction in circumference of the neck, thighs, and arms; widening of the pelvis; and lengthening of the nose and ears. Several of these changes are the result of tissue atrophy and decreased bone mass caused by osteoporosis and osteoarthritis. Body composition changes with age.[98] With middle age there is an increase in body weight (men gain until 50 years of age and women until 70 years) and fat mass followed by a decrease in stature, weight, **fat-free mass (FFM)** (FFM includes all minerals, proteins, and water plus all other constituents except lipids), and body cell mass at older ages. As fat increases, total body water decreases. Increased body fat and centralized fat distribution (abdominal) are associated with non–insulin-dependent diabetes and heart disease. Total body potassium also decreases because of decreased cellular mass. An increased sodium/potassium ratio suggests that the decreased cellular mass is accompanied by an increased extracellular compartment.

Although some of these alterations are probably inherent in aging, others represent consequences of aging. Advanced age increases susceptibility to disease, and death occurs after an injury or insult because of diminished cellular, tissue, and organic function. To determine that an individual "died of old age" would be a monumental if not impossible task.

Frailty

Frailty is imprecisely defined as a wasting syndrome of aging, leaving a person vulnerable to falls, functional decline, disease, and death.[99] The syndrome is complex, involving decreased protein synthesis, sarcopenia, neuroendocrine and muscular decline, and immune dysfunction. The clinical condition of frailty includes decreased lean body mass (sarcopenia), osteopenia, cognitive impairment, and anemia.[100] The most evident feature is sarcopenia. The altered skeletal muscle mass is associated with fatigue, weakness, imbalance, altered gait, and speed.[101] Recent studies raise the possibility of dysregulated inflammatory processes and ROS as being involved or central to patterns of aging and frailty.[100] Several physiologic gender differences may explain differing levels of frailty: (1) higher baseline levels of muscle mass for men may be protective against frailty, (2) testosterone and growth hormone can provide advantages in muscle mass maintenance, (3) cortisol is more dysregulated in older women than older men, (4) alterations in immune function and immune responsiveness to sex steroids make men more vulnerable to sepsis and infection and women more vulnerable to chronic inflammatory conditions and muscle mass loss, and (5) lower levels of activity and caloric intake may influence greater susceptibility to frailty in women.[102]

SOMATIC DEATH

Somatic death is death of the entire person. Unlike the changes that follow cellular death in a live body, **postmortem change** is diffuse and does not involve components of the inflammatory response. Within minutes of death, manifestations of postmortem change appear, eliminating any difficulty in determining that death has occurred. The most notable manifestations are complete cessation of respiration and circulation. The surface of the skin usually becomes pale and yellowish; however, the lifelike color of the cheeks and lips may persist after death from causes such as carbon monoxide poisoning, drowning, and chloroform poisoning.[103]

Body temperature falls gradually immediately after death and then more rapidly (approximately 1.0° to 1.5° F/hr) until, after 24 hours, body temperature equals that of the environment.[104] After death caused by certain infective diseases, body temperature may continue to rise for a short time. Postmortem reduction of body temperature is called **algor mortis.**

Blood pressure within the retinal vessels decreases, causing muscle tension to decrease and the pupils to become dilated. The face, nose, and chin begin to look "sharp" or "peaked" as blood and fluids drain away.[103] Gravity causes blood to settle in the most dependent, or lowest, tissues, which develop a purple discoloration called **livor mortis.** Incisions at this time usually fail to cause bleeding. The skin loses its elasticity and transparency.

Within 6 hours after death, acidic compounds accumulate within the muscles because of the breakdown of carbohydrate and depletion of ATP. This interferes with ATP-dependent detachment of myosin from actin (contractile proteins), and muscle stiffening, or **rigor mortis,** sets in. The smaller muscles are usually affected first, particularly the muscles of the jaw. Within 12 to 14 hours, rigor mortis usually affects the entire body.

Signs of putrefaction—state of decay with foul-smelling odor—are generally obvious about 24 to 48 hours after death. Rigor mortis gradually diminishes, and the body becomes flaccid in 12 to 14 hours. Putrefactive changes vary depending on the temperature of the environment. The most visible is greenish discoloration of the skin, particularly on the abdomen. The discoloration is thought to be related to the diffusion of hemolyzed blood into the tissues and the production of sulfhemoglobin.[105] Slippage or loosening of the skin from underlying tissues occurs at the same time. After this, swelling or bloating of the body and liquefactive changes occur, sometimes causing opening of the body cavities. At a microscopic level, putrefactive changes are associated with the release of enzymes and lytic dissolution called **postmortem autolysis.**

Cellular Adaptation

1. Cellular adaptation is an alteration that enables the cell to maintain a steady state despite adverse conditions.

2. Atrophy is a decrease in cellular size. The mechanisms probably include decreased protein synthesis, increased protein catabolism, or both.

3. Physiologic atrophy occurs with early development; for example, the thymus gland involutes and atrophies. Pathologic atrophy occurs as a result of decreases in workload, use, pressure, blood supply, nutrition, hormonal stimulation, and nervous stimulation.

4. Aging causes brain cells and endocrine-dependent organs, such as the gonads, to become atrophic.

5. Hypertrophy is an increase in the size of cells by increased work demands or hormonal stimulation. Hypertrophy can be physiologic or pathologic. Amounts of protein in the plasma membrane, endoplasmic reticulum, microfilaments, and mitochondria are increased.

6. Hyperplasia is an increase in the number of cells caused by an increased rate of cellular division. Compensatory hyperplasia enables certain organs to regenerate. Hormonal hyperplasia is stimulated by hormones to replace lost tissue or support new growth, such as during pregnancy.

7. Pathologic hyperplasia is the abnormal proliferation of normal cells in response to excessive hormonal stimulation of growth factors on target cells.

8. Dysplasia, or atypical hyperplasia, is an abnormal change in the size, shape, and organization of mature tissue cells.

9. Metaplasia is the reversible replacement of one mature cell type by another less mature cell type. Metaplasia is thought to develop from a reprogramming of stem cells existing in most epithelia or of undifferentiated mesenchymal cells in connective tissue.

Cellular Injury

1. Most diseases begin with cell injury. Injured cells may recover (reversible injury) or die (irreversible injury).

2. Cellular injury is caused by a lack of oxygen (hypoxia), free radicals, caustic or toxic chemicals, infectious agents, unintentional and intentional injury, inflammatory and immune responses, genetic factors, insufficient nutrients, or physical trauma from many causes.

3. Cell injury can be acute or chronic, and it can be reversible or irreversible. It can involve necrosis, apoptosis (including autophagic cell death), accumulation, or pathologic calcification.

4. Four biochemical themes are important to cell injury: (a) ATP depletion, (b) oxygen and oxygen-derived free radicals, (c) intracellular calcium and loss of calcium steady state, and (d) defects in membrane permeability.

5. The sequence of events leading to cell death is commonly decreased ATP production, failure of active transport mechanisms (the Na^+, K^+ pump), cellular swelling, detachment of ribosomes from the endoplasmic reticulum, cessation of protein synthesis, mitochondrial swelling as a result of calcium accumulation, vacuolation, leakage of digestive enzymes from lysosomes, autodigestion of intracellular structures, lysis of the plasma membrane, and death.

6. The initial insult in hypoxic injury is usually ischemia—the cessation of blood flow into vessels that supply the cell with oxygen and nutrients.

7. An important mechanism of membrane damage is injury caused by free radicals. Free radicals are difficult to control and initiate chain reactions.

8. Free radicals can cause (a) lipid peroxidation or the destruction of unsaturated fatty acids, (b) alterations of proteins, and (c) alterations in DNA.

9. The initial insult in chemical injury is damage or destruction of the plasma membrane. Examples of chemical agents that cause cellular injury include lead, carbon monoxide, ethanol, mercury, and social or street drugs.

10. Unintentional and intentional injuries are an important health problem in the United States. Death caused by injuries is more common in men than women and higher among blacks than whites and other racial groups.

11. Injuries by blunt force are the result of the application of mechanical energy to the body resulting in tearing, shearing, or crushing of tissues. The most common types of blunt force injuries include motor vehicle accidents and falls.

12. A contusion is bleeding into the skin or underlying tissues as a consequence of a blow. A collection of blood in soft tissues or an enclosed space may be referred to as a *hematoma*.

13. An abrasion (scrape) results from removal of the superficial layers of the skin caused by friction between the skin and injuring object. Abrasions and contusions may have a patterned appearance that mirrors the shape and features of an injuring object.

14. A laceration is a tear or rip resulting when the tensile strength of the skin or tissue is exceeded.

15. An incised wound is a cut that is longer than it is deep. A stab wound is a penetrating sharp force injury that is deeper than it is long.

16. Gunshot wounds may be either penetrating (bullet retained in the body) or perforating (bullet exits). The most important factors determining the appearance of a gunshot injury are whether it is an entrance or an exit wound and the range of fire.

17. Asphyxial injuries are caused by a failure of cells to receive or use oxygen. These injuries can be grouped into four general categories: suffocation, strangulation, chemical, and drowning.

18. Injury from microorganisms lies in their ability to survive and proliferate in the human body. Injury depends on the microorganisms' ability to invade and destroy cells, produce toxins, and produce damaging hypersensitivity reactions.

19. Activation of inflammation and immunity, which occurs after cellular injury or infection, involves powerful biochemicals and proteins capable of damaging normal (uninjured and uninfected) cells.

20. Genetic disorders injure cells by altering the nucleus and the plasma membrane's structure, shape, receptors, or transport mechanisms.

21. Deprivation of essential nutrients (proteins, carbohydrates, lipids, vitamins) can cause cellular injury by altering cellular structure and function, particularly of transport mechanisms, chromosomes, the nucleus, and DNA.

22. Injurious physical agents include temperature extremes, changes in atmospheric pressure, ionizing radiation, illumination, mechanical stresses (e.g., repetitive body movements), and noise.

Manifestations of Cellular Injury

1. Cellular manifestations of cellular injury include accumulations of water, lipids, carbohydrates, glycogen, proteins, pigments, hemosiderin, bilirubin, calcium, and urate.

2. Accumulations harm cells by "crowding" the organelles and by causing excessive (and sometimes harmful) metabolites to be produced during their catabolism. The metabolites are released into the cytoplasm or expelled into the extracellular matrix.

Continued

3. Cellular swelling, the accumulation of excessive water in the cell, is caused by the failure of transport mechanisms and is a sign of many types of cellular injury.

4. Accumulations of organic substances—lipids, carbohydrates, glycogen, proteins, and pigments—are caused by disorders in which (a) cellular uptake of the substance exceeds the cell's capacity to catabolize (digest) or use it or (b) cellular anabolism (synthesis) of the substance exceeds the cell's capacity to use or secrete it.

5. Dystrophic calcification (accumulation of calcium salts) is always a sign of pathologic change because it occurs only in injured or dead cells. Free calcium in the cytosol can cause activation of protein kinases, activation of phospholipases and membrane damage, and damage or disassembly of the cytoskeleton. Metastatic calcification, however, can occur in uninjured cells in individuals with hypercalcemia.

6. Disturbances in urate metabolism can result in hyperuricemia and deposition of sodium urate crystals in tissue, leading to a painful disorder called *gout*.

7. Systemic manifestations of cellular injury include fever, leukocytosis, increased heart rate, pain, and serum elevations of enzymes in the plasma.

Cellular Death

1. Two main types of cell death are necrosis and apoptosis. With apoptosis, best studied is type 1 cell death (caspases, etc.) type 2 is called autophagic cell death.

2. Necrosis is the sum of the changes after local cell death and includes the processes of inflammation and cellular lysis.

3. The four major types of necrosis are coagulative, liquefactive, caseous, and fat. Different types of necrosis occur in different tissues.

4. Structural signs that indicate irreversible injury and progression to necrosis are the dense clumping and disruption of genetic material and the disruption of the plasma and organelle membranes.

5. Gangrenous necrosis, or gangrene, is tissue necrosis caused by hypoxia and subsequent bacterial invasion.

6. Apoptosis, a different type of cellular death, is a process of selective cellular self-destruction called programmed cell death. Other forms of programmed cell death (type 2) have been determined, including autophagic ("eat oneself") cell death.

Aging

1. It is difficult to determine the physiologic (normal) from the pathologic changes of aging.

2. Humans have an inherent maximal life span (80 to 100 years) that is dictated by currently unknown intrinsic mechanisms.

3. Although the maximal life span has not changed significantly over time, the average life span, or life expectancy, has increased. However, this increase in life expectancy in the United States is not happening for all Americans.

4. The emerging focus in the biology of aging includes endocrine regulation from endocrine signaling pathways, nuclear architecture and genomic instability, decline in cell renewal by adult stem cells, and accumulated cell damage related to cancer and aging.

5. Frailty is imprecisely defined as a wasting syndrome of aging that leaves a person vulnerable to falls, functional decline, disease, and death. Women have a higher risk of frailty than men.

Somatic Death

1. Somatic death is death of the entire organism. Postmortem change is diffuse and does not involve the inflammatory response.

2. Manifestations of somatic death include cessation of respiration and circulation, gradual lowering of body temperature, pupil dilation, loss of elasticity and transparency in the skin, muscle stiffening (rigor mortis), and skin discoloration (livor mortis). Signs of putrefaction are obvious about 24 to 48 hours after death.

KEY TERMS

Abrasion, 64
Algor mortis, 90
Anoxia, 52
Apoptosis, 84
Asphyxial injury, 68
Atrophy, 47
Atypical hyperplasia, 49
Autophagic vacuole, 47
Avulsion, 64
Bilirubin, 79
Blast injury, 72
Blow back, 66
Blunt force injury, 62
Callus, 49
Carbon monoxide (CO), 59
Carboxyhemoglobin, 59
Caseous necrosis, 82
Caspase, 85
Cellular accumulation (infiltration), 76

Cellular swelling, 76
Chemical asphyxiant, 68
Choking asphyxiation, 68
Chopping wound, 66
Coagulative necrosis, 82
Compensatory hyperplasia, 49
Contact range entrance wound, 66
Contusion, 62
Cyanide, 68
Decompression sickness (caisson disease), 72
Drowning, 68
Dry gangrene, 83
Dysplasia (atypical hyperplasia), 49
Dystrophic calcification, 79
Entrance wound, 66
Epidural hematoma, 63
Ethanol, 59
Exit wound, 67

Fat necrosis, 83
Fat-free mass (FFM), 90
Fatty change, 76
Fetal alcohol syndrome (FAS), 61
Frailty, 90
Free radical, 54
Gangrenous necrosis, 83
Gas gangrene, 84
Hanging strangulation, 68
Heat cramp, 72
Heat exhaustion, 72
Heat stroke, 72
Hematoma, 62
Hemoprotein, 79
Hemosiderin, 79
Hemosiderosis, 79
Hepatocyte growth factor (HGF), 49
Hormonal hyperplasia, 49
Hydrogen sulfide (sewer gas), 68

KEY TERMS—cont'd

Hyperglycemia, 69
Hyperlipidemia, 69
Hyperplasia, 48
Hyperthermic injury, 72
Hypertrophy, 47
Hypolipidemia, 69
Hypothermic injury, 71
Hypoxia, 52
Incised wound, 65
Indeterminate-range (distant) entrance wound, 67
Intermediate-range entrance wound, 66
Ionizing radiation, 73
Irreversible injury, 51
Ischemia, 52
Karyolysis, 81
Karyorrhexis, 81
Laceration, 64
Lead, 56
Life expectancy, 86
Ligature strangulation, 68

Lipid-acceptor protein (apoprotein), 55
Lipid peroxidation, 54
Lipofuscin, 47
Liquefactive necrosis, 82
Livor mortis, 90
Manual strangulation, 68
Maximal life span, 86
Mechanoporation, 75
Melanin, 78
Metaplasia, 50
Metastatic calcification, 79
Muzzle imprint, 66
Necrosis, 81
Noise, 75
Oncosis (vacuolar) degeneration, 76
Oxidative stress, 54
Pathologic atrophy, 47
Pathologic hyperplasia, 49
Physiologic atrophy, 47
Postmortem autolysis, 90
Postmortem change, 90

Psammoma body, 79
Puncture wound, 66
Pyknosis, 81
Reperfusion (reoxygenation) injury, 54
Reversible injury, 51
Rigor mortis, 90
Sarcopenia, 90
Shored exit wound, 67
Somatic death, 90
Stab wound, 65
Stippling, 66
Strangulation, 68
Subdural hematoma, 62
Suffocation, 68
Tattooing, 66
Ubiquitin-proteasome pathway, 47
Up-regulation of proteasome, 47
Urate, 81
Vacuolation, 53
Wet gangrene, 83

REFERENCES

1. Dahlmann B: Role of proteasomes in disease, *BMC Biochem* 8(Suppl):S3, 2007.
2. Damjanov I, Linder J: *Anderson's pathology*, ed 10 , St Louis, 1996, Mosby.
3. Bicknell KA, Coxon CH, Brooks G: Can the cardiomyocyte cell cycle be reprogrammed?, *J Mol Cell Cardiol* 42(4):706-721, 2007.
4. Bottaro DP et al: Identification of the hepatocyte growth factor receptor as the c-met proto-oncogene product, *Science* 251(4995):802-804, 1991.
5. Alberts B, et al: *Molecular biology of the cell*, ed 5, New York, 2008, Garland.
6. Degnim AC et al: Stratification of breast cancer risk in women with atypia: a Mayo cohort study, *J Clin Oncol* 25(19):2672-2677, 2007.
7. Reis-Filho JS, Lakhani SR: The diagnosis and management of pre-invasive breast disease: genetic alterations in pre-invasive lesions, *Breast Cancer Res* 5:313-319, 2004.
8. Kumar V, Abbas A, Fausto N: *Robbins and Cotran pathologic basis of disease*, ed 7 , Philadelphia, 2005, Saunders.
9. Valko M et al: Free radicals and antioxidants in normal physiological functions and human disease, *Int J Biochem Cell Biol* 39(1):44-84, 2007.
10. Li C, Jackson RM: Reactive species mechanisms of cellular hypoxia—reoxygenation injury, *Am J Physiol Cell Physiol* 282:C227-C241, 2002.
11. Murphy E, Steenbergen C: Mechanisms underlying acute protection from cardiac ischemia—reperfusion injury, *Physiol Rev* 88(2):581-609, 2008.
12. Burwell LS, Brookes PS: Mitochondria as a target for the cardioprotective effects of nitric oxide in ischemia-reperfusion injury, *Antioxid Redox Signal* 10(3):579-599, 2008.
13. Papaharalambus CA: Basic mechanisms of oxidative stress and reactive oxygen species in cardiovascular injury, *Trends Cardiovasc Med* 17(2):48-54, 2007.
14. Gunnell D, Murray V, Hawton K: Use of paracetamol (acetaminophen) for suicide and nonfatal poisoning: worldwide patterns of use and misuse, *Suicide Life Threat Behav* 30:313-326, 2000.
15. Lai MW et al: Annual report of the American Association of Poison Control Centers' national poisoning and exposure database, *Clin Toxicol (Phila)* 44(6-7):803-932, 2005:2006.
16. Heard KJ: Acetlycysteine for acetaminophen poisoning, *N Engl J Med* 359(3):285-292, 2008.
17. Murray KF et al: Drug-associated hepatotoxicity and acute liver failure, *J Pediatr Gastroenterol Nutr* 47(5):395-405, 2008.
18. Markel H: Getting the lead out: the Rhode Island Lead Pain Trials and Their Impact on Children's Health, *JAMA* 297(24):2773-2775, 2007.
19. Roberts JW et al: Reducing dust, lead, dust mites, bacteria, and fungi in carpets by vacuuming, *Arch Environ Contam Toxicol* 36(4):477-484, 1999.
20. Schanne FA, Long GJ, Rosen JF: Lead induced rise in intracellular free calcium is mediated through activation of protein kinase C in osteoblastic bone cells, *Biochem Biophys Acta* 1360(3):247 254, 1997.
21. Meo SA, Al-Khlawi T: Health hazards of welding fumes, *Saudi Med J* 24(11):1176-1182, 2003.
22. Holbrook J: Cigarette smoking. In Rom WH, editor: *Environmental and occupational medicine*, Boston, 1993, Little, Brown.
23. Cassel CK, et al: *Geriatric medicine*, ed 2 , New York, 1990, Springer-Verlag.
24. Lieber CS: Microsomal ethanol-oxidizing system (MEOS): the first 30 years (1968-1998)—a review, *Alcohol Clin Exp Res* 23(6):991-1007, 1999: Review.
25. Agarwal DP: Genetic polymorphisms of alcohol metabolizing enzymes, *Pathol Biol (Paris)* 49(9):703-709, 2001:Review.
26. Booyse FM et al: Mechanisms by which alcohol and wine polyphenols affect coronary heart disease risk, *Ann Epidemiol* 17(5 Suppl):S24-S31, 2007.
27. Sesso HD: Alcohol and cardiovascular health: recent findings, *Am J Cardiovasc Drugs* 1(3):167-172, 2001.
28. O'Keefe JH, Bybee KA, Lavie CJ: Alcohol and cardiovascular health: the razor-sharp double-edged sword, *Am J Coll Cardiol* 50(11):1009-1014, 2007.
29. May JJ: Occupational hearing loss, *Am J Ind Med* 37(1):112-120, 2000.
30. Punjabi NM: The epidemiology of adult obstructive sleep apnea, *Proc Am Thorac Soc* 5(2):136-143, 2008.
31. Guilleminault A, Abad VC: Obstructive sleep apnea syndromes, *Med Clin North Am* 88(3):611-630, 2004.
32. Lieber CS: Metabolism of alcohol, *Clin Liver Dis* 9(1):1-35, 2005.
33. Lieber CS: Alcoholic liver disease: new insights in pathogenesis lead to new treatments, *J Hepatol* 32(1 Suppl):113-128, 2000.
34. Clark CM et al: Structural and functional brain integrity of fetal alcohol syndrome in nonretarded cases, *Pediatrics* 105(5):1096, 2000.
35. Saito M et al: Ethanol alters lipid profiles and phosphorylation status of AMP-activated protein kinase in the neonatal mouse brain, *J Neurochem* 103(3):1208-1218, 2007.
36. Stratton K, Howe C, Battaglia F, editors: *Fetal alcohol syndrome: diagnosis, epidemiology, prevention and treatment*, Washington, DC, 1996, National Academy Press.
37. Mattson SN, Riley EP: Brain anomalies in fetal alcohol syndrome. In Abel EA, editor: *Fetal alcohol syndrome: from mechanism to prevention*, Boca Raton, FL, 1996, CRC Press.

38. Cortese BM et al: Magnetic resonance and spectroscopic imaging in prenatal alcohol-exposed children: preliminary findings in the caudate nucleus, *Neurotoxicol Teratol* 28(5):597-606, 2006.

39. Boonstra J et al: The epidermal growth factor, *Cell Biol Int* 19(5):413-430, 1995.

40. Henderson GI et al: Ethanol, oxidative stress, reactive aldehydes, and the fetus, *Front Biosci* 15(4):D541, 1999.

41. Lieber CS: CYP2EI: from ASH to NASH, *Hepatol Res* 28(1):1-11, 2004.

42. Donohue TM Jr. et al: Role of the proteasome in ethanol-induced liver pathology, *Alcohol Clin Exp Res* 31(9):1446-1459, 2007.

43. Clarkson TW, Magos L, Myers GI: The toxicology of mercury—current exposures and clinical manifestations, *N Engl J Med* 349(18):1731-1737, 2003.

44. Ahlquist M et al: Serum mercury concentrations in relation to survival, symptoms, and disease: results from the prospective population study of women in Gothenburg, Sweden, *Acta Odontol Scand* 57:168-174, 1999.

45. Bjorkman L, Pedersen NL, Lichtenstein P: Physical and mental health related to dental amalgam fillings in Swedish twins, *Community Dent Oral Epidemiol* 24(4):260-267, 1996.

46. Saxe SR et al: Dental amalgam and cognitive function in older women: findings from the Nun Study, *J Am Dent Assoc* 126(11):1495-1501, 1995.

47. Lauterbach M et al: Neurological outcomes in children with and without amalgam-related mercury exposure: seven years of longitudinal observations in a randomized trial, *J Am Dent Assoc* 139(2):138-145, 2008.

48. Powell LW, Kerr JFR: Pathology of the liver in hemochromatosis, *Pathobiol Annu* 5:317-337, 1975.

49. Available at www.ewg.org/mercury1. Accessed 2008.

50. Thompson WW et al: Early thimerosal exposure and neuropsychological outcomes at 7 to 10 years, *N Engl J Med* 357(13):1281-1292, 2007.

51. Pichichero ME et al: Mercury concentrations and metabolism in infants receiving vaccines containing thimerosal: a descriptive study, *Lancet* 360(9347):1737-1741, 2002.

52. Smith JC, Farris FF: Methyl mercury pharmacokinetics in man: a reevaluation, *Toxicol Appl Pharmacol* 137(2):254, 1996.

53. Baumgartner RN et al: Age-related changes in sex hormones affect the sex difference in serum leptin independently of changes in body fat, *Metabolism* 48(3):378-384, 1999.

54. Fraker PJ, Lill-Elghanian DA: The many roles of apoptosis in immunity as modified by aging and nutritional status, *J Nutr Health Aging* 8(1):56-63, 2004.

55. Stanton B, Galbraith J: Drug trafficking among African-American early adolescents: prevalence, consequences, and associated behaviors and beliefs, *Pediatrics* 93(6, Pt 2):1039-1043, 1994.

56. Centers for Disease Control and Prevention: *Injury statistics website*, Washington, DC, 2002, Centers for Disease Control and Prevention.

57. Kopec D et al: The state-of-the-art in the reduction of medical errors, *Stud Health Technol Inform* 121:126-137, 2006.

58. Holick MF: Vitamin D: importance in the prevention of cancers, type 1 diabetes, and osteoporosis, *Am J Clin Nutr* 79(3):362-372, 2004.

59. Camara AK et al: Hypothermia augments reactive oxygen species detected in the guinea pig isolated perfused heart, *Am J Physiol Heart Circ Physiol* 286(4):H1289-H1299, 2004.

60. Rauen U, de Groot H: Mammalian cell injury induced by hypothermia—the emerging role for reactive oxygen species, *Biol Chem* 383(3-4):477-488, 2002.

61. Bartels-Stringer M et al: Preserved vascular reactivity of rat renal arteries after cold storage, *Cryobiology* 48(1):95-98, 2004.

62. Osorio RA et al: Reactive oxygen species in pregnant rats: effects of exercise and thermal stress, *Comp Biochem Physiol C Toxicol Pharmacol* 135(1):89-95, 2003.

63. Rauen U et al: Hypothermia: injury/cold-induced apoptosis—evidence of an increase in chelatable iron causing oxidative injury in spite of low O^-_2/H_2O_2 formation, *FASEB J* 14(13):1953-1964, 2000.

64. Roy SB et al: Haemodynamic studies in high altitude pulmonary oedema, *Br Heart J* 31(1):52-58, 1969.

65. U.S. Department of Health and Human Services: *Report on carcinogens*, ed 11, 2004. Available at ntp.nichs.nih.gov/ntp/roc/toc11.html.

66. Cologne JB et al: Effects of radiation on incidence of primary liver cancer among atomic bomb survivors, *Radiat Res* 152(4):364-373, 1999.

67. Gilbert ES et al: Liver cancers in Mayak workers. *Radiat Res* 154(3):246-252, 2000.

68. Yap J et al: Sarcoma as a second malignancy after treatment for breast cancer, *Int J Radiat Oncol Biol Phys* 52(5):1231-1237, 2002.

69. Preston DL, Shimizu Y, Pierce DA: Studies of mortality of atomic bomb survivors. Report 13: solid cancer and noncancer disease mortality. *Radiat Res* 160:381-407, 2003.

70. Hoel DG: Ionizing radiation and cardiovascular disease. *Ann N Y Acad Sci* 1076:309-317, 2006.

71. U.S. Food and Drug Administration: *What are the radiation risks from CT?*, 2002. Available at www.fda.gov/edrh/et/risks.html

72. Siu TL, Morley JW, Coroneo MT: Toxicology of the retina: advances in understanding the defence mechanisms and pathogenesis of drug- and light-induced retinopathy. *Clin Experiment Ophthalmol* 36(2):176-185, 2008.

73. Available at www.ccoks.ca/oshansevers/ergonomics/lighting-flicker.html. Accessed 2008.

74. Wilkins AJ, Wilkinson P: A tint to reduce eye-strain from fluorescent lighting? Preliminary observations, *Ophthalmic Physiol Opt* 11(2):172-175, 1991.

75. Rubin GS et al: A prospective, population-based study of the role of visual impairment in motor vehicle crashes among older drivers: the SEE study, *Invest Ophthalmol Vis Sci* 48(4):1483-1491, 2007.

76. Mainster MA, Timberlake GT: Why HID headlights bother older drivers, *Br J Opthalmol* 87(1):113-117, 2003.

77. De Flora S, D'Agostini F: Halogen lamp carcinogenicity, *Nature* 356:569, 1992.

78. Bloom E et al: Halogen lamp phototoxicity, *Dermatology* 193(3):207-211, 1996.

79. Barbee KA: Mechanical cell injury, *Ann N Y Acad Sci* 1066:67-84, 2005.

80. Van Epps JS, Vorp DA: Mechanopathobiology of atherogenesis: a review, *J Surg Res* 142(1):202-217, 2007.

81. Keyserling WM, Armstrong TJ: Ergonomics. In Last JM, Wallace RB, editors: *Maxey-Roseneau-Last: public health and preventive medicine*, ed 13, Norwalk, Conn, 1992, Appleton & Lange.

82. NIDCD: *Statistics about hearing disorders, ear infections, and deafness*, Washington, DC, 2005, National Institutes of Health. Available at www.nidcd.nih.gov/health/statistics/nearing.asp.

83. Halpern NA et al: Hearing loss in critical care: an unappreciated phenomenon, *Crit Care Med* 27(1):211-219, 1999.

84. Hayflick L: The limited in vitro lifetime of human diploid cell strains, *Exp Cell Res* 37:614-636, 1965.

85. Kerr JFR, Searle J: Apoptosis: its nature and kinetic role. In Meyn RE, Withers HR, editors: *Radiation biology in cancer research*, New York, 1980, Raven.

86. Wyllie AH, Kerr JFR, Currie AR: Cell death: the significance of apoptosis, *Int Rev Cytol* 68:251-306, 1980.

87. Basu A: Involvement of protein kinase C-delta in DNA damage-induced apoptosis, *J Cell Mol Med* 7(4):341-350, 2003.

88. Alberts B, et al: Essential cell biology: an introduction to the molecular biology of the cell, ed 2, New York, 2004, Garland.

89. Amour A et al: General considerations for proteolytic cascades, *Biochem Soc Trans* 32(Pt 1):15-16, 2004.

90. Logue SE, Martin SJ: Caspase activation cascades in apoptosis, *Biochem Soc Trans* 36(Pt 1):1-19, 2008.

91. Johnson HA, editors: Is aging physiological or pathological? In Johnson HA ed: *Relations between normal aging and disease*, New York, 1985, Raven.

92. Vijg J: Somatic mutations and aging: a re-evaluation, *Mutat Res* 447(1):117-135, 2000.

93. Hayflick L: Biological aging is no longer an unsolved problem, *Ann N Y Acad Sci* 1100:1-13, 2007: Review.

94. Poehlman ET et al: Physiological predictors of increasing total and central adiposity in aging men and women, *Arch Intern Med* 155(22):2443-2448, 1995.

95. Butow RA, Avadhani NG: Mitochondrial signaling: the retrograde response, *Mol Cell* 14(1):1-15, 2004.

96. Maassen JA et al: Mitochondrial diabetes: molecular mechanisms and clinical presentation, *Diabetes* 152(Suppl):S103-S109, 2004.

97. Samuels DC: Mitochondrial DNA repeats constrain the life span of mammals, *Trends Genet* 20(5):226-229, 2004.

98. Baumgartner RN et al: Cross-sectional age differences in body composition in persons 60+ years of age, *J Gerontol A Biol Sci Med Sci* 50(6):M307-M316, 1995.

99. Muhlberg W, Sieber C: Sarcopenia and frailty in geriatric patients: implications for training and prevention, *Z Gerontol Geriatr* 37(1):2-8, 2004.

100. Ershler WB: A gripping reality: oxidative stress, inflammation, and the pathway to frailty, *J Appl Physiol* 103:3-5, 2007.

101. Greenlund LJ, Nair KS: Sarcopenia—consequences, mechanisms, and potential therapies, *Mech Ageing Dev* 124:287-299, 2003.

102. Gillick M: Pinning down frailty, *J Gerontol A Biol Sci Med Sci* 56(3):M134-M135, 2001.

103. Shennan T: *Postmortems and morbid anatomy*, ed 3 , Baltimore, 1935, William Wood.

104. Minckler J, Anstall HB, Minckler TM: *Pathobiology: an introduction*, St Louis, 1971, Mosby.

105. Richter C et al: Oxidants in mitochondria: from physiology to diseases, *Biochim Biophys Acta* 1271(1):67-74, 1995.

THE CELLULAR ENVIRONMENT: FLUIDS AND ELECTROLYTES, ACIDS AND BASES

SUE E. HUETHER

MEDIA RESOURCES

evolve **Evolve Website** (http://evolve.elsevier.com/McCance/)
- Review Questions and Answers
- Animations
- Glossary (with audio pronunciation for selected terms)
- WebLinks

 Online Course
- Module 2

CHAPTER OUTLINE

DISTRIBUTION OF BODY FLUIDS
    Aging and Distribution of Body Fluids
  Water Movement Between ICF and ECF
  Water Movement Between Plasma and Interstitial Fluid
ALTERATIONS IN WATER MOVEMENT
  Edema
SODIUM, CHLORIDE, AND WATER BALANCE
  Sodium and Chloride Balance
  Water Balance
ALTERATIONS IN SODIUM, CHLORIDE, AND WATER BALANCE
  Isotonic Alterations
  Hypertonic Alterations
  Hypotonic Alterations

ALTERATIONS IN POTASSIUM, CALCIUM, PHOSPHATE, AND MAGNESIUM BALANCE
  Potassium
  Calcium and Phosphate
  Magnesium
ACID-BASE BALANCE
  Hydrogen Ion and pH
  Buffer Systems
  Acid-Base Imbalances

The cells of the body live in a fluid environment that requires an electrolyte concentration and pH value (measure of the acidity or alkalinity of a solution) that are regulated within a very narrow range. A balance is maintained by an integration of renal, hormonal, and neural functions. Changes in the composition of electrolytes affect electrical potentials of excitatory cells and cause shifts of fluid from one compartment to another. Alterations in pH disrupt the cellular function of enzyme systems. Fluid fluctuations affect blood volume and cellular function. Disturbances in these functions are common and can be life threatening. Understanding how alterations occur and the body's ability to compensate or correct the disturbance is important to understanding many pathophysiologic conditions.

DISTRIBUTION OF BODY FLUIDS

The fluids of the body are distributed among functional compartments, or spaces, and provide a transport medium for cellular and tissue function. Water moves freely among body compartments and is distributed by osmotic and hydrostatic forces. Two thirds of the body's water is **intracellular fluid (ICF)** and one third is in the **extracellular fluid (ECF)** compartments. The two main ECF compartments are the **interstitial fluid** and the **intravascular fluid,** which is the blood plasma. Other ECF compartments include the lymph and the transcellular fluids, such as the synovial, intestinal, biliary, hepatic, pancreatic, and cerebrospinal fluids; sweat; urine; and pleural, synovial, peritoneal, pericardial, and intraocular fluids.

Table 3-1	Distribution of Body Water	
	Percentage of Body Weight	Volume (L)
Intracellular fluid (ICF)	40	28
Extracellular fluid (ECF)	20	14
Interstitial	(15)	(11)
Intravascular	(5)	(3)
Total body water (TBW)	60	42

Table 3-2	Total Body Water in Relation to Body Weight		
Body Build	TBW (%) Adult Male	TBW (%) Adult Female	TBW (%) Infant
Normal	60	50	70
Lean	70	60	80
Obese	50	42	60

NOTE: TBW (total body water) is a percentage of body weight.

Table 3-3	Normal Water Gains and Losses (70-kg Man)		
	Daily Intake (ml)		Daily Output (ml)
Drinking ≈ 60%	1400-1800	Urine ≈ 60%	1400-1800
Water in food ≈ 30%	700-1000	Stool ≈ 2%	100
Water of oxidation ≈ 10%	300-400	Skin ≈ 10%	300-500
		Lungs ≈ 28%	600-800
TOTAL	2400-3200		2400-3200

The sum of fluids within all compartments constitutes the **total body water (TBW)** (Table 3-1). The volume of TBW is usually expressed as a percentage of body weight in kilograms. The standard value for TBW is 60% of the weight of a 70-kg adult male, which is equivalent to 42 L of fluid (Table 3-2). The rest of the body weight is made up of fat and fat-free solids, particularly bone.

Although the amount of fluid within the various compartments is relatively constant, exchange of solutes and water occurs between compartments to maintain their unique compositions. The percentage of TBW varies with the amount of body fat and age. Because fat is water repelling (hydrophobic), very little water is contained in adipose cells. Individuals with more body fat have proportionately less TBW and tend to be more susceptible to fluid imbalances that cause dehydration.

Aging and Distribution of Body Fluids

The distribution and amount of TBW change with age (see Table 3-2). In newborn infants, TBW is about 75% to 80% of body weight because infants store less fat. The percentage of TBW decreases to about 67% of body weight during the first year of life. In the immediate postnatal period, a physiologic loss of body water occurs, which amounts to 5% of body weight, as the infant adjusts to a new environment. Infants are particularly susceptible to significant changes in TBW because of their high metabolic rate and the accelerated turnover of body fluids caused by their greater body surface area in proportion to total body size. Loss of fluids

from diarrhea can represent a significant proportion of body weight. Renal mechanisms that regulate fluid and electrolyte conservation may not be mature enough to counter the losses, so dehydration may develop rapidly.

During childhood TBW slowly decreases to 60% to 65% of body weight. At adolescence the percentage of TBW approaches adult proportions, and gender differences begin to appear. Males eventually have a greater percentage of body water as a function of increasing muscle mass. Females have more body fat and less muscle as a function of estrogens and therefore have less body water.

With increasing age the percentage of TBW declines further still. The decrease is caused in part by an increased amount of fat and a decreased amount of muscle and by a reduced ability to regulate sodium and water balance. With older age the kidney becomes less efficient in producing concentrated urine, and the responses for conserving sodium become sluggish. Thirst perception may be impaired. The normal reduction of TBW in older adults becomes clinically important when the body is under stress, such as development of fever or dehydration from any cause; loss of body fluids at such times can be severe and life threatening.[1]

Although daily fluid intake may fluctuate widely, the body regulates water volume within a relatively narrow range. The primary sources of body water are drinking, ingestion of water in food, and water derived from oxidative metabolism. Normally, the largest amounts of water are lost through renal excretion. Lesser amounts are eliminated through the stool and through vaporization from the skin and lungs (insensible water loss) (Table 3-3).

Water Movement Between ICF and ECF

The movement of water between ICF and ECF compartments is primarily a function of osmotic forces. (Osmosis and other mechanisms of passive transport are discussed in Chapter 1.) Water moves freely by diffusion through the lipid bilayer cell membrane and through **aquaporins**, a family of water channel proteins that provide permeability to water.[2] The osmolality of TBW is normally at equilibrium. Sodium is the most

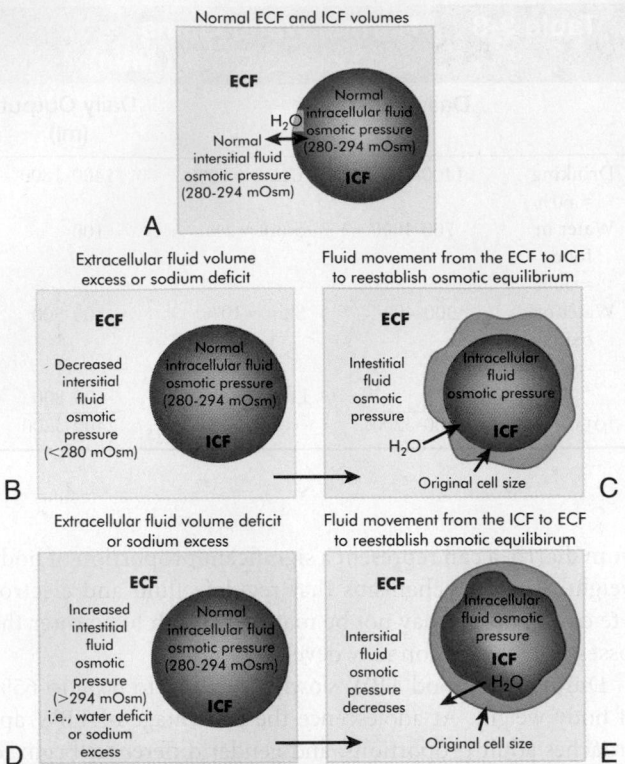

Normal ECF and ICF volumes

A

Extracellular fluid volume excess or sodium deficit

B

Fluid movement from the ECF to ICF to reestablish osmotic equilibrium

C

Extracellular fluid volume deficit or sodium excess

D

Fluid movement from the ICF to ECF to reestablish osmotic equilibrium

E

Figure 3-1 Examples of changes in osmotic equilibrium between ECF and ICF. A, Normal ECF and ICF volumes. Intracellular and extracellular fluid osmotic pressure are equal and water is equally distributed between the compartments. **B,** Extracellular fluid volume excess or sodium deficit. ECF volume excess or sodium deficit decreases the ECF osmotic pressure, and water is attracted to the ICF space (see *C*). **C,** Fluid movement from the ECF to ICF to reestablish osmotic equilibrium. The intracellular osmotic pressure attracts water from the ECF, causing an increase in ICF water volume with a balancing of osmotic forces between the ECF and ICF. The consequence is an increase in ICF volume and cell swelling. **D,** Extracellular fluid volume deficit or sodium excess. ECF volume deficit increases the ECF osmotic pressure, and intracellular water is attracted to the ECF space (see *E*). **E,** Fluid movement from the ICF to the ECF to reestablish osmotic equilibrium. Water from the intracellular space has moved to the extracellular space until the osmotic forces are equal. The consequence is a decrease in ICF water volume and cell size. *ECF,* Extracellular fluid; *ICF,* intracellular fluid.

abundant ECF ion and is responsible for the osmotic balance of the ECF space. Potassium maintains the osmotic balance of the ICF space. The osmotic force of ICF proteins and other nondiffusible substances is balanced by the active transport of ions out of the cell. Normally the ICF is not subject to rapid changes in osmolality, but when there are changes in ECF osmolality, a net transfer of water from one compartment to another occurs until osmotic equilibrium is reestablished. Figure 3-1 shows a model of the maintenance of osmotic equilibrium between the ICF and ECF.

Water Movement Between Plasma and Interstitial Fluid

The distribution of water and the movement of nutrients and waste products among the capillary, plasma, and interstitial spaces occur as a result of changes in hydrostatic pressure and

osmotic forces at the arterial and venous ends of the capillary. Because water, sodium, and glucose readily move across the capillary membrane, the plasma proteins (particularly albumin) maintain the effective osmolality (concentration of solutes per kilogram of solution) by generating plasma oncotic pressure. Osmotic forces within the capillary are balanced by the hydrostatic pressure, which arises from cardiac contraction. The movement of fluid back and forth across the capillary wall is called **net filtration** and is best described by the **Starling hypothesis**:

Net filtration = (Forces favoring filtration) −

(Forces opposing filtration)

The *forces favoring filtration,* or movement of water out of the capillary and into the interstitial space, include the capillary hydrostatic pressure and the interstitial oncotic pressure. The *forces opposing filtration* are the plasma oncotic pressure (pressure of plasma proteins) and the interstitial hydrostatic pressure. Normally the interstitial forces are negligible because only a very small percentage of plasma proteins crosses the capillary membrane and interstitial fluid moves into cells or is drawn back into the plasma. Thus the major forces for filtration are within the capillary.

As the plasma flows from the arterial to the venous end of the capillary, the force of hydrostatic pressure facilitates the movement of water across the capillary membrane. Oncotic pressure remains fairly constant because plasma proteins normally do not cross the capillary membrane. At the arterial end of the capillary, hydrostatic pressure is greater than capillary oncotic pressure and water filters into the interstitial space. Because of oncotic forces, some water moves back into the capillary, but the net effect is loss of water from the capillary. The movement of water from the plasma decreases the hydrostatic pressure within the capillary. Thus at the venous end of the capillary, oncotic pressure exceeds hydrostatic pressure. Fluids then are attracted back into the circulation, balancing the movement of fluids between the plasma and the interstitial space. The overall effect is filtration at the arterial end and reabsorption at the venous end (Figure 3-2). Interstitial hydrostatic pressure promotes the movement of about 10% of the interstitial fluid along with small amounts of protein into the lymphatics, which then returns to the circulation.

An important factor in capillary filtration of fluid is the integrity of the capillary membrane. Changes in membrane permeability may permit the escape of plasma proteins into the interstitial space. The normal relationship defined by the Starling hypothesis is altered with the osmotic movement of water into the interstitial space, causing tissue edema.

ALTERATIONS IN WATER MOVEMENT
Edema

Edema is the excessive accumulation of fluid within the interstitial spaces. It is a problem of fluid distribution and does not necessarily indicate a fluid excess. In some

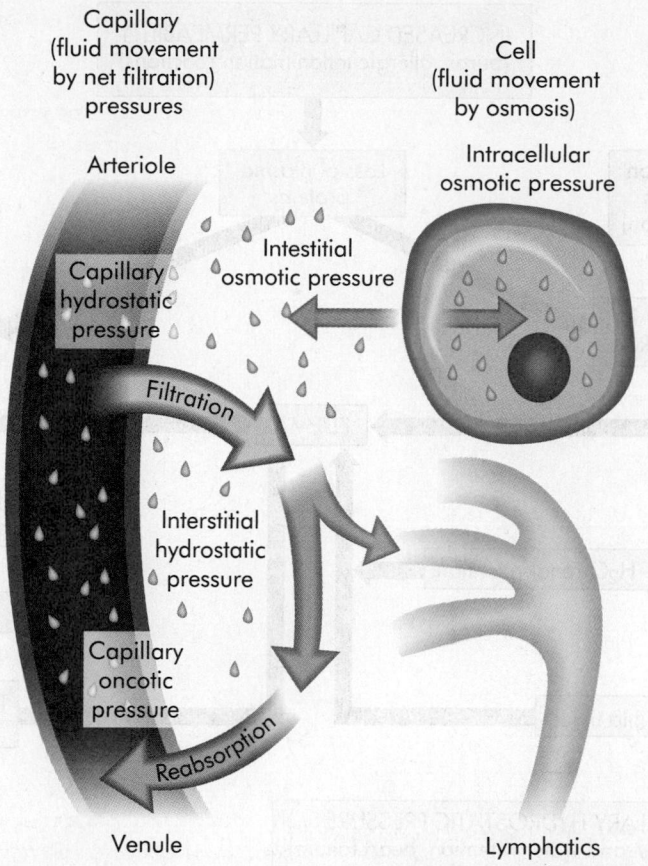

Arterial Capillary Pressures		Venous Capillary Pressures	
Capillary hydrostatic pressure	35 mmHg	Capillary hydrostatic pressure	18 mmHg
Interstitial fluid hydrostatic pressure	2 mmHg	Interstitial fluid hydrostatic pressure	1 mmHg
Net hydrostatic pressure	**33 mmHg**	**Net hydrostatic pressure**	**17 mmHg**
Capillary oncotic pressure	24 mmHg	Capillary oncotic pressure	25 mmHg
Interstitial fluid oncotic pressure	0 mmHg	Interstitial fluid oncotic pressure	0 mmHg
Net oncotic pressure	**24 mmHg**	**Net oncotic pressure**	**25 mmHg**
Net filtration pressure	+9 mmHg	Net filtration pressure	−8 mmHg

Figure 3-2 Capillary filtration forces. Water, electrolytes, and small molecules exchange freely between the vascular compartment and the interstitial space at the site of capillaries and small venules. The rate and amount of exchange are driven by the physical forces of hydrostatic and oncotic pressures and the permeability and surface area of the capillary membranes. The two opposing hydrostatic pressures are capillary hydrostatic pressure and interstitial hydrostatic pressure. The two opposing oncotic pressures are capillary oncotic pressure and interstitial oncotic pressure. The *forces that favor filtration* from the capillary are capillary hydrostatic pressure and interstitial oncotic pressure, and the *forces that oppose filtration* are capillary oncotic pressure and interstitial hydrostatic pressure. The sum of their effects is known as *net filtration pressure* (NFP). In the example of normal exchange above, a small amount of fluid moves to the lymph vessels, which accounts for the net filtration difference between the arterial and venous ends of the capillary.

conditions, sequestered fluids can cause both edema and dehydration. The pathophysiologic process is related to an increase in the forces favoring fluid filtration from the capillaries or lymphatic channels into the tissues. The four most common mechanisms are increased capillary hydrostatic pressure, decreased plasma oncotic pressure, increased capillary membrane permeability, and lymphatic obstruction (Figure 3-3).

PATHOPHYSIOLOGY An *increase in hydrostatic pressure* can result from venous obstruction or salt and water

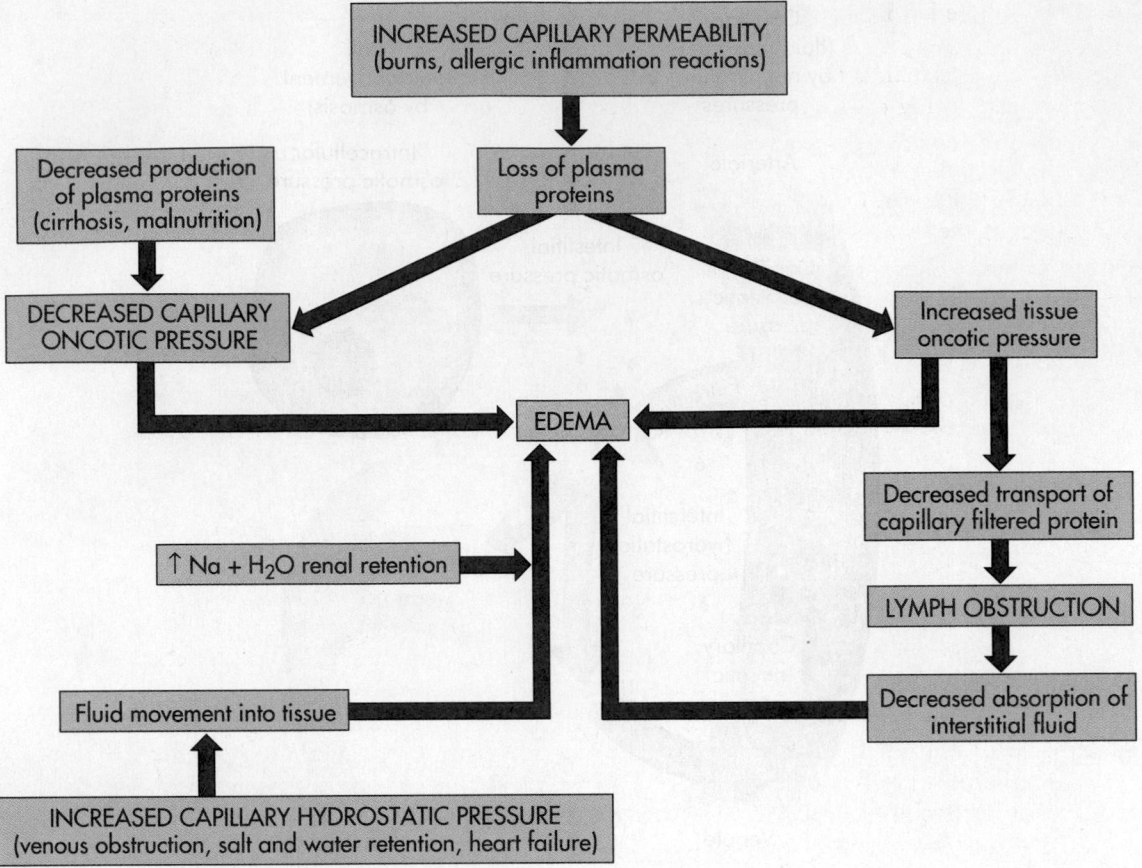

Figure 3-3 Mechanisms of edema formation.

retention. *Venous obstruction* can increase the hydrostatic pressure of fluid within the capillaries enough to cause fluid to escape into the interstitial spaces. Thrombophlebitis, hepatic obstruction, tight clothing around the extremities, and prolonged standing are common causes of venous obstruction. Congestive heart failure, renal failure, and cirrhosis of the liver are conditions associated with excessive salt and water retention, which in turn cause volume overload, increased venous pressure, and edema.

Losses or diminished production of plasma albumin contributes to a decrease in plasma oncotic pressure. Decreased oncotic attraction of fluid within the capillary causes fluid to move into the interstitial space. Decreased production of plasma protein and decreased oncotic pressure may occur with liver disease or protein malnutrition. Losses of plasma proteins occur with glomerular diseases of the kidney (nephrotic syndrome), serous drainage from open wounds, hemorrhage, burns, and cirrhosis of the liver.

Increases in capillary permeability are usually associated with inflammation and the immune response. (Immunity is discussed in Chapters 6, 7 and 8; inflammation is discussed in Chapters 6 and 8.) These responses are often the result of trauma such as burns or crushing injuries, neoplastic disease, and allergic reactions. Proteins escape

from the plasma and produce edema through a loss of capillary oncotic pressure and a gain in interstitial fluid proteins.

The lymphatic system normally absorbs interstitial fluid and the small amount of proteins that normally pass across the capillary membrane. When the lymphatic channels are blocked (because of infection or tumor) or are surgically removed, proteins and fluid accumulate in the interstitial space, causing **lymphedema.** For example, lymphedema of the arm or leg will occur after surgical removal of axillary and femoral lymph nodes for treatment of carcinoma.[3]

CLINICAL MANIFESTATIONS Edema may be localized or generalized. Some localized edema is limited to the site of trauma, as in a sprained finger or within particular organ systems. This includes cerebral edema, pulmonary edema, pleural effusion, pericardial effusion, and ascites (accumulation of fluid in the peritoneal space). Dependent edema, in which fluid accumulates in gravity-dependent areas of the body, might be a sign of more generalized edema. Dependent edema might appear in the feet and legs when standing and in the sacral area and buttocks when supine. Dependent edema can be identified by using the fingers to press away edematous fluid in tissues overlying bony prominences. A pit will be left in the skin; hence the term *pitting edema.*

Edema is usually associated with weight gain, swelling and puffiness, tight-fitting clothes and shoes, limited movement of the affected area, and symptoms associated with the underlying pathologic condition. The accumulation of fluid increases the distance required for nutrients, oxygen, and wastes to move between capillaries and tissues. Increased tissue pressure may diminish capillary blood flow. Therefore, wounds heal more slowly and the risks of infection and formation of pressure sores increase. Edema of specific organs, such as the brain, lung, or larynx, can be life threatening.

Although the accumulation of fluid is excessive, it is trapped in a "third space" (i.e., the interstitial space, pleural space, pericardial space) and is not available for metabolic processes or perfusion. Therefore, a state of dehydration can develop as a result of the sequestering of the edematous fluid. An example of such sequestration occurs with severe burns, in which large amounts of vascular fluid are lost to the interstitial spaces, reducing plasma volume and causing shock (see Chapter 46).

EVALUATION AND TREATMENT Specific conditions causing edema require diagnosis. Edema may be treated symptomatically until the underlying disorder is corrected. Supportive measures include elevating edematous limbs, using compression stockings, avoiding prolonged standing, restricting salt intake, and taking diuretics.

SODIUM, CHLORIDE, AND WATER BALANCE

The kidneys and hormones have a central role in maintaining sodium and water balance. Because water follows the osmotic gradients established by changes in salt concentration, sodium balance and water balance are intimately related. Sodium is regulated by the renal effects of aldosterone from the adrenal cortex and natriuretic peptides Water balance is primarily regulated by antidiuretic hormone (ADH; also known as *arginine-vasopressin*) from the posterior pituitary.

Sodium and Chloride Balance

Sodium accounts for 90% of the ECF cations (positively charged ions). (The distribution of electrolytes in body compartments is summarized in Table 3-4.) As the most abundant ECF cation, along with its constituent anions (negatively charged ions) chloride and bicarbonate, sodium regulates extracellular osmotic forces and therefore regulates water balance. Sodium has many important body functions, including regulation of osmolality (interstitial and intravascular fluid volume), working with potassium and calcium to maintain neuromuscular irritability for conduction of nerve impulses, regulation of acid-base balance (through sodium bicarbonate and sodium phosphate), participation

Table 3-4	Distribution of Electrolytes in Body Compartments	
	Extracellular Fluid (mEq/L)	Intracellular Fluid (mEq/L)
Cations		
Sodium	142	10
Potassium	5	156
Calcium	5	4
Magnesium	2	26
TOTAL	154	196
Anions		
Bicarbonate	24	12
Chloride	104	4
Phosphate	2	40-95
Proteins	16	54
Other anions	8	31-86
TOTAL	154	196 (average)

in cellular chemical reactions, and membrane transport (see Chapter 1).

The concentration of sodium is maintained within a narrow range (136 to 145 mEq/L), primarily by the kidney in conjunction with neural and hormonal mediators. The average dietary intake of sodium ranges from 5 to 6 g/day; the minimal daily requirement of sodium is 500 mg. Sweating depletes sodium and water volume and increases the body's sodium requirement.

The kidney regulates sodium balance primarily through renal tubular reabsorption. Under normal rates of sodium intake, the tubules of the kidney function to reabsorb sodium. With an excess or deficit of sodium in relation to water, a combination of hormonal, neural, and renal mechanisms acts synergistically to control sodium balance.

The hormonal regulation of sodium balance is mediated by **aldosterone,** a mineralocorticoid (steroid) synthesized and secreted from the adrenal cortex (see Chapter 20). Aldosterone secretion is influenced by both plasma concentrations of sodium (Na^+) and potassium (K^+) and circulating blood volume (i.e., aldosterone is secreted when sodium levels are depressed, potassium levels are increased, or renal perfusion is decreased). Aldosterone increases the reabsorption of sodium and secretion of potassium by the distal tubule of the kidney. As a result, sodium concentration of the ECF is enhanced and potassium is excreted with the urine.

When circulating blood volume or blood pressure is reduced, **renin,** an enzyme secreted by the juxtaglomerular cells of the kidney, is released in response to sympathetic nerve stimulation and decreased perfusion of the renal vasculature. Renin stimulates the formation of **angiotensin I,** an inactive polypeptide, which is then converted into **angiotensin II.** Angiotensin II has two major functions: it stimulates the secretion of aldosterone, and it causes vasoconstriction. The aldosterone then promotes sodium and water reabsorption, conserving blood volume. The vasoconstriction elevates the systemic blood pressure and restores renal perfusion. The restoration of sodium levels, fluid volume, and renal perfusion then inhibits further release of renin. This sodium and water regulation mechanism is known as the **renin-angiotensin-aldosterone system** (see Chapter 35).

Natriuretic peptides are hormones that include atrial natriuretic peptide (ANP) produced by the myocardial atria, brain natriuretic peptide (BNP) produced by the myocardial ventricles, and urodilatin within the kidney. Natriuretic peptides decrease blood pressure and increase sodium and water excretion. They are natural antagonists to the renin-angiotensin-aldosterone system. ANP and BNP are released when there is an increase in transmural atrial pressure (increased volume) as may occur with congestive heart failure.[4] Natriuretic peptides are sometimes called a "third factor" in sodium regulation. (Increased glomerular filtration rate is thus the first factor and aldosterone the second factor.)

Chloride is the major anion in the extracellular fluid. It provides electroneutrality, particularly in relation to sodium. The transport of chloride is generally passive and follows the active transport of sodium so that increases or decreases in chloride are proportional to changes in sodium. Because bicarbonate is the other major anion in the ECF, the concentration of chloride tends to vary inversely with changes in bicarbonate concentration.

Water Balance

Water balance is maintained by balancing the amount of water excreted with water intake by ingestion and generated by metabolism. Secretion of ADH and perception of thirst are primary factors in the regulation of water balance. Thirst is a sensation that stimulates water-drinking behavior. Thirst is experienced when water loss equals 2% of an individual's body weight or when there is an increase in osmolality. Dry mouth, hyperosmolality, and plasma volume depletion activate **osmoreceptors** (neurons located in the hypothalamus that are stimulated by increased osmolality). The action of the osmoreceptors then causes thirst. Drinking water restores plasma volume and dilutes the ECF osmolality.

The secretion of ADH is initiated by an increase in plasma osmolality or a decrease in circulating blood volume and a lowered blood pressure. An increase in plasma osmolality occurs with a deficit of water or an excess of sodium in relation to water. The increased osmolality results in decreased extracellular and interstitial fluid volume and stimulates hypothalamic osmoreceptors. In addition to causing thirst, the stimulated osmoreceptors increase the release of ADH. The action of ADH is to increase the permeability of renal tubular cells to water, and water is then reabsorbed into the plasma from the distal tubules and collecting ducts of the kidney. Urine concentration increases, and the reabsorbed water decreases plasma osmolality, returning it toward normal. Like most hormones, ADH is regulated by a feedback mechanism (Figure 3-4).

With volume depletion, such as dehydration from vomiting, diarrhea, or excessive sweating, **volume-sensitive receptors**

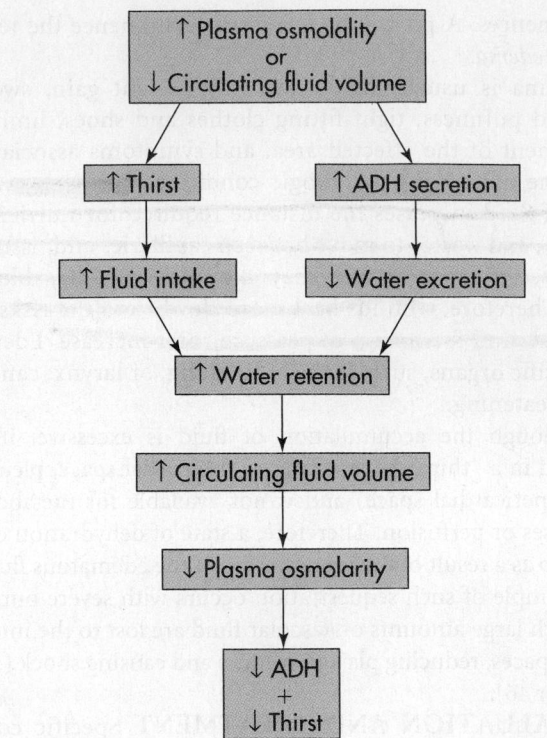

Figure 3-4 Regulation of thirst and antidiuretic hormone (ADH) secretion.

and **baroreceptors** (stretch receptors that are sensitive to changes in volume and pressure) stimulate release of ADH. The volume receptors are located in the right and left atria and thoracic vessels; baroreceptors are in the aorta, pulmonary arteries, and carotid sinus. Secretion of ADH is caused by a decrease in atrial pressure, as occurs with decreased blood volume. The reabsorption of water mediated by ADH then promotes the restoration of plasma volume. When there is an increase in the blood volume returning to the heart from the venous system ADH secretion is inhibited and fluid volume decreases.

ALTERATIONS IN SODIUM, CHLORIDE, AND WATER BALANCE

Alterations in sodium and water balance are closely related. Water imbalances may develop because of changes in osmotic gradients caused by gain or loss of salt. Likewise, sodium imbalances occur with alterations in body water volume (see Figure 3-1). Generally the alterations can be classified as changes in tonicity, or the change in concentration of electrolytes in relation to water (see Chapter 1). Alterations can therefore be classified as isotonic, hypertonic, or hypotonic (Table 3-5).

Isotonic Alterations

Isotonic alterations occur when changes in TBW are accompanied by proportional changes in electrolytes and water. For example, if an individual loses pure plasma or

ECF, fluid volume is depleted but the number and type of electrolytes (i.e., sodium) and the osmolality remain within a normal range. Excessive amounts of isotonic body fluids can result from excessive administration of intravenous normal saline or oversecretion of aldosterone with renal retention of both sodium and water. Losses of isotonic body fluids include hemorrhage, severe wound drainage, excessive diaphoresis (sweating), intestinal losses, and decreased fluid intake.

Isotonic volume depletion causes contraction of the ECF volume with resulting weight loss, dryness of skin and mucous membranes, decreased urine output, and symptoms of hypovolemia. Indicators of hypovolemia include a rapid heart rate, flattened neck veins, and normal or decreased blood pressure. In severe states, hypovolemic shock can occur (see Chapter 46).

Isotonic volume excesses result from excessive administration of intravenous fluids, hypersecretion of aldosterone, the effects of drugs such as cortisone, or renal failure. As the plasma volume expands, symptoms of hypervolemia develop. Weight gain and a decrease in hematocrit and plasma protein concentration caused by the diluting effect of excess plasma volume will occur. The neck veins may distend, and the blood pressure increases. Increased capillary hydrostatic pressure leads to edema formation. If the plasma volume is great enough, pulmonary edema and heart failure develop.

Hypertonic Alterations

Hypertonic fluid alterations develop when the osmolality of the ECF is elevated above normal. The most common causes are an increased concentration of ECF sodium (hypernatremia) or a deficit of ECF free water. In both instances the hypertonicity of the ECF attracts water from the intracellular space, causing ICF dehydration. A primary increase in ECF sodium causes an osmotic attraction of water and symptoms of *hypervolemia*. In contrast, a hypertonic state caused primarily by free water loss leads to *hypovolemia* (Table 3-6).

Table 3-5   Water and Solute Imbalances

Tonicity	Mechanism
Isotonic (isoosmolar) imbalance	Gain or loss of extracellular fluid (ECF) resulting in a concentration equivalent to a 0.9% sodium chloride (salt) solution (normal saline); no shrinking or swelling of cells
Hypertonic (hyperosmolar) imbalance	Imbalances that result in an ECF concentration >0.9% salt solution; i.e., water loss or solute gain; cells shrink in a hypertonic fluid
Hypotonic (hypoosmolar) imbalance	Imbalance that results in an ECF <0.9% salt solution; i.e., water gain or solute loss; cells swell in a hypotonic fluid

TABLE 3-6   Causes and Consequences of Hypertonic Imbalances

Causative Factor	Mechanism	ECF Effects	ICF Effects
Increased sodium (hypernatremia)	Excessive hypertonic salt solutions Intravenous hypertonic sodium Saline-induced abortions Selected infant formulas Hyperaldosteronism Cushing syndrome	Hypervolemia Weight gain Bounding pulse Increased blood pressure Edema Venous distention Neuromuscular symptoms Muscle weakness Seizures	Intracellular dehydration Thirst Fever Decreased urine output Shrinkage of brain cells Csonfusion Coma Cerebral hemorrhage
Water deficit	Water deprivation Confusion or coma Inability to communicate Loss of thirst Water loss Watery diarrhea Diabetes insipidus Excessive diuresis Excessive diaphoresis	Hypovolemia Weight loss Weak pulses Postural hypotension Tachycardia	Intracellular dehydration See above
Other factors	Hyperglycemia	Initial dilutional hyponatremia Polyuria Polydipsia Weight loss Hypovolemia Late hypernatremia	Intracellular dehydration See above

ECF, Extracellular fluid; *ICF,* intracellular fluid.

Hypernatremia

PATHOPHYSIOLOGY Hypernatremia occurs when serum sodium levels exceed 147 mEq/L. Excessive serum sodium may be caused by an acute gain in sodium or a loss of water. Sodium gains cause intracellular dehydration; the movement of water to the ECF may cause hypervolemia. With an accompanying water loss, both ICF dehydration and ECF dehydration occur. Hyperosmolality is a common result of hypernatremia.

High amounts of dietary sodium rarely cause hypernatremia. More commonly, high sodium levels occur because of (1) inadequate free water intake, (2) inappropriate administration of hypertonic saline solution (e.g., as sodium bicarbonate for treatment of acidosis during cardiac arrest), (3) high sodium levels as a result of oversecretion of aldosterone (as in primary hyperaldosteronism), or (4) Cushing syndrome (caused by excess secretion of adrenocorticotropic hormone [ACTH], which also causes increased secretion of aldosterone).[5]

Increased sodium in relation to water deprivation or water loss is associated with fever or respiratory infections, which increase the respiratory rate and enhance water loss from the lungs. Diabetes insipidus (deficiency of ADH), diabetes mellitus, polyuria, profuse sweating, and diarrhea cause water loss in relation to sodium concentration. Infants with severe diarrhea are particularly vulnerable. Insufficient water intake also can cause hypernatremia, particularly in individuals who are comatose, confused, immobilized, or receiving gastric feedings. Those who cannot communicate because of age (infants) or disease also cannot express thirst and are at risk.

CLINICAL MANIFESTATIONS Water is redistributed to the extracellular space, and intracellular dehydration ensues. Seizures, coma, and pulmonary edema are the most serious symptoms. Thirst, fever, dry mucous membranes, hypotension, tachycardia, low jugular venous pressure, and restlessness are associated with hypernatremia as a result of water loss.

EVALUATION AND TREATMENT The serum sodium level is usually more than 147 mEq/L. If there is water loss, urine specific gravity will be greater than 1.030 and hematocrit and plasma proteins will be elevated. The treatment of hypernatremia is to give an isotonic salt-free fluid (5% dextrose in water) until the serum sodium level returns to normal. Hypervolemia and edema require treatment of the underlying clinical condition.

Hyperchloremia

Hyperchloremia occurs when serum chloride levels exceed the normal range of 97 to 105 mEq/L and is often associated with an excess of sodium (hypernatremia) or a deficit of bicarbonate (metabolic acidosis) (see p. 117) Ingestion of excessive chloride infrequently accompanies the use of an ammonium chloride diuretic. No specific symptoms are associated with chloride excess.

Alterations in chloride levels are usually secondary to their pathophysiologic processes. Treatment therefore generally is related to management of the underlying disorder.

Water Deficit

PATHOPHYSIOLOGY Dehydration describes water deficit, but dehydration is also commonly used to indicate both sodium loss and water loss (isotonic or isoosmolar dehydration). Pure **water deficits** (hyperosmolar or hypertonic dehydration) are rare because most people have access to water. Individuals who are comatose or paralyzed continue insensible water losses through the skin and lungs with a minimal obligatory formation of urine. Hyperventilation caused by fever also may precipitate water deficit. The most frequent cause of water loss is increased renal clearance of free water as a result of impaired tubular function or inability to concentrate the urine, as with diabetes insipidus (see Chapter 21).

CLINICAL MANIFESTATIONS Marked water deficit is manifested by symptoms of dehydration: headache, thirst, dry skin and mucous membranes, elevated temperature, weight loss, and decreased or concentrated urine (with the exception of diabetes insipidus). Skin turgor may be normal or decreased. Symptoms of hypovolemia, including tachycardia, weak pulses, and postural hypotension, may be present.

EVALUATION AND TREATMENT An elevated hematocrit and serum sodium concentration are associated with moderate water loss in addition to clinical signs and symptoms.

Treatment is to give water and stop fluid loss. Fluid replacement must be given slowly enough to prevent rapid movement of water into brain cells, which causes cerebral edema, seizures, brain injury, and death. When intravenous replacement is required, 5% dextrose in water should be used because pure water lyses red blood cells.

Hypotonic Alterations

Hypotonic fluid imbalances occur when the osmolality of the ECF is less than normal. The most common causes are sodium deficit (**hyponatremia**) or free water excess (**water intoxication**). Either of these causes leads to an intracellular overhydration (cellular edema) and cell swelling. When there is a sodium deficit, the osmotic pressure of the ECF decreases and water moves into the cell, where the osmotic pressure is greater (see Figure 3-1). The plasma volume then decreases, leading to symptoms of hypovolemia. With free water excess, both the ICF volume and the ECF volume increase, causing symptoms of hypervolemia (Table 3-7) and water intoxication with cerebral and pulmonary edema.[6]

Hyponatremia

PATHOPHYSIOLOGY Hyponatremia develops when the serum sodium concentration decreases to less than 135 mEq/L. Sodium deficits usually cause hypoosmolality with movement of water into cells with cell swelling. Several clinical syndromes may cause hyponatremia. These syndromes may be caused by sodium loss, inadequate sodium intake, or dilution of the body's sodium level.

Table 3-7	Causes and Consequences of Hypotonic Imbalances		
Causative Factor	Mechanism	ECF Effects	ICF Effects
Decreased sodium (hyponatremia)	Inadequate intake Hypoaldosteronism Excessive diuretic therapy 　Furosemide 　Ethacrinic acid 　Thiazides	Extracellular volume contraction and hypovolemia (but may not be if there is water excess)	Increased intracellular water; edema Brain cell swelling, irritability, depression, confusion Systemic cellular edema, including weakness, anorexia, nausea, and diarrhea
Water excess	Excessive pure water intake Excessive administration of hypotonic intravenous solutions Drinking water to replace isotonic fluid losses Tap water enemas 　Psychogenic polydipsia 　Renal water retention 　Syndrome of inappropriate secretion of antidiuretic hormone (SIADH)	Extracellular volume expands with hypervolemia (but may not be if fluid is trapped in intracellular space)	Edema (see above)
Other factors	Isotonic dehydration treated with intravenous D_5W; glucose in D_5W solution is metabolized to water, contributing to hyponatremia Nephrotic syndrome Cirrhosis Cardiac failure	Hypervolemia or hypovolemia	Edema (see above)

ECF, Extracellular fluid; *ICF*, intracellular fluid.

Pure sodium deficits usually are caused by diuretics[7] and extrarenal losses such as vomiting, diarrhea, gastrointestinal suctioning, or burns. **Inadequate intake** of dietary sodium is rare but can occur in individuals on low-sodium diets, particularly among those taking diuretics. **Dilutional hyponatremias** occur when there is an excess of TBW in relation to total body sodium or a shift of water from the ICF to ECF space (e.g., administration of mannitol). Replacement of fluid loss with intravenous 5% dextrose in water also can cause a dilutional hyponatremia because once the glucose is metabolized, a hypotonic solution remains with a diluting effect. Use of excess hypotonic saline (e.g., 0.45 NaCl) may also result in dilution. In addition, excessive sweating may stimulate thirst and intake of large amounts of water, which dilute sodium and may be associated with endurance exercise when there is only pure water replacement.

Hyponatremia also may be hypoosmolar or hypertonic. During acute oliguric renal failure, severe congestive heart failure, or cirrhosis, renal excretion of water is impaired. Both TBW and sodium levels are increased, but TBW exceeds the increase in sodium, producing a **hypotonic hyponatremia.**

Hypertonic hyponatremia develops with the shift of water from the ICF to the ECF as occurs with hyperglycemia, hyperlipidemia, and hyperproteinemia. Plasma increases in glucose, lipids, or proteins displace water volume and decrease sodium concentration. Hyperglycemia increases ECF osmolality and attracts water from the ICF compartment. The osmotic fluid shift to the ECF in turn dilutes the concentration of sodium and other electrolytes.

WHAT'S NEW?   Hospital-Acquired Hyponatremia

Severe hyponatremia (serum sodium <120 mmol/L) is the most common electrolyte abnormality among hospitalized individuals with risk for severe morbidity and mortality. Hyponatremia can be difficult to diagnose because it can develop with euvolemia, hypervolemia, or hypovolemia. In addition to older adults, children and premenopausal women are at particular risk as well as those with cirrhosis with ascites, heart failure syndromes, brain injury, or infection and receiving treatment in intensive care units. Death or brain damage may range from 50% to 83% and is related to cerebral edema, increased intracranial pressure, and cerebral hypoxemia, with symptoms of seizure, respiratory arrest, coma, and death. Postoperative hyponatremia is caused by administration of hypotonic fluids and dysregulation of the secretion of antidiuretic hormone (arginine vasopressin). Treatment with fluid restriction, diuretic treatment, sodium replacement, and urea is effective in less severe cases. Hypertonic sodium chloride is usually safe with acute hyponatremia. Brain myelinolysis is a risk if treatment is given too rapidly. Arginine vasopressin receptor antagonists can provide effective treatment. Frequent monitoring with attention to subtle symptoms and early treatment lead to improved outcomes.

Data from Lien YH, Shapiro JI: Hyponatremia: clinical diagnosis and management, *Am J Med* 120(8):653-658, 2007; Moritz ML, Ayus JC: Hospital-acquired hyponatremia—why are hypotonic parenteral fluids still being used? *Nat Clin Pract Nephrol* 3(7):374-382, 2007; Hoorn EJ, Zietse R: Hyponatremia revisited: translating physiology to practice, *Nephron Physiol* 108(3):46-59, 2008.

CLINICAL MANIFESTATIONS Deficits of sodium alter the ability of cells to depolarize and repolarize normally (see Chapter 1). Behavioral and neurologic changes characteristic of hyponatremia include lethargy, headache, confusion, apprehension, seizures, and coma. Pure sodium losses may be accompanied by loss of ECF, causing an isotonic **hypovolemia** with symptoms of hypotension, tachycardia, and decreased urine output. Weight gain, edema, ascites, and jugular vein distention are characteristic of dilutional hyponatremias.

EVALUATION AND TREATMENT In hyponatremic states, serum sodium concentration falls to less than 135 mEq/L. With pure sodium deficits, the hematocrit and plasma protein levels may be elevated. Urine specific gravity is less than 1.010 when renal function is normal because sodium is maximally conserved.

Treatment of hyponatremia is related to the contributing disorder. Losses of sodium and water volume are calculated from the clinical evaluation, and appropriate solutions then are selected for replacement. Restriction of water intake is required in most cases of dilutional hyponatremia because body sodium levels may be normal or increased even though serum levels are low. Hypertonic saline solutions are used cautiously with severe symptoms, such as seizures.[8]

Hypochloremia

Loss of chloride, or **hypochloremia,** is usually the result of hyponatremia, or elevated bicarbonate concentration, as in metabolic alkalosis (see p. 119). Hypochloremia develops with vomiting and loss of hydrochloric acid. Sodium deficit related to restricted intake or use of diuretics is accompanied by chloride deficiency. Cystic fibrosis, for example, is also characterized by hypochloremia. As with hyperchloremia, treatment of the underlying condition is required.

Water Excess

PATHOPHYSIOLOGY When the body is functioning normally, it is almost impossible to produce an excess of TBW. However, some individuals with psychogenic disorders develop water intoxication from **compulsive water drinking.** Acute renal failure, severe congestive heart failure, and cirrhosis are clinical conditions that can precipitate water excess. **Decreased urine formation** from intrinsic renal disease or decreased renal blood flow contributes to water excess. The overall effect is dilution of the ECF with the movement of water to the intracellular space by osmosis. Water excess produces a hypotonic or hypoosmolar water imbalance and is usually accompanied by hyponatremia.

The **syndrome of inappropriate secretion of ADH (SIADH),** also know as **vasopressin dysregulation,** is another circumstance contributing to excess water.[9] SIADH occurs when factors other than hyperosmolality or hypovolemia stimulate the secretion of or response to ADH. The amount of ADH is inappropriate in relation to serum sodium levels. SIADH is not caused by excess water intake but by increased renal reabsorption of water as a result of inappropriate increases in ADH. Serum sodium and osmolality are reduced by dilution. The kidney continues to excrete sodium, and urine sodium and urine osmolality are elevated; water is reabsorbed, increasing body fluid volume, and urine volume is decreased. Several clinical conditions associated with stress result in SIADH. These include fear; pain; acute infection; brain trauma; surgery; drugs, such as analgesics and anesthetics; and ADH-secreting tumor cells in the lung, pancreas, or other tissues.

CLINICAL MANIFESTATIONS The symptoms of water excess are related to the rate at which water loading has occurred. Acute excesses cause cerebral edema with confusion and convulsions. Weakness, nausea, muscle twitching, headache, and weight gain are common symptoms of chronic water accumulation.

EVALUATION AND TREATMENT Serum sodium concentration can be decreased, but this also can occur with a pure sodium deficit. Serum and urine osmolality are decreased because water will be in excess of sodium. Urine sodium will be reduced. The hematocrit is reduced from the dilutional effect of water excess.

Withholding fluid for 24 hours is effective treatment if there are no convulsions. Small amounts of intravenous hypertonic sodium chloride (i.e., 3% sodium chloride) can be given when neurologic symptoms are severe. Arginine vasopressin receptor antagonists are effective in SIADH cases.[10]

ALTERATIONS IN POTASSIUM, CALCIUM, PHOSPHATE, AND MAGNESIUM BALANCE

Potassium

Potassium (K^+) is the major intracellular electrolyte and is found in most body fluids (Table 3-8). Total body potassium content is about 4000 mEq, with most of it located in the cells. Daily dietary intake of potassium is 40 to 150 mEq/day, with an average of 1.5 mEq/kg body weight. The ICF concentration of K^+ is 150 to 160 mEq/L; the ECF concentration is 3.5 to 4.5 mEq/L.

The difference in the K^+ intracellular to extracellular concentration is maintained by a sodium-potassium active transport system (Na^+, K^+-ATPase pump). The ratio of ICF K^+ to ECF K^+ is the major determinant of the resting membrane potential, which is necessary for the transmission and conduction of nerve impulses, maintenance of normal cardiac rhythms, and skeletal and smooth muscle contraction. (Membrane transport and membrane potentials are discussed in Chapter 1.) The diffusion of positively charged K^+ out of the cell and down its concentration gradient makes the interior of cells electronegative in relation to the ECF. Changes in the ratio of ICF to ECF potassium are responsible for many of the symptoms associated with potassium imbalance.

As the predominant ICF ion, K^+ exerts a major influence in the regulation of ICF osmolality and provides the balance for intracellular electrical neutrality in relation to hydrogen (H^+) and Na^+. Potassium is also necessary for a variety of metabolic functions and is required for glycogen deposition in liver and skeletal muscle cells.

Table 3-8	Approximate Concentration of Electrolytes in Body Fluids			
Fluid	Na$^+$ (mEq/L)	K$^+$ (mEq/L)	Cl$^-$ (mEq/L)	HCO$_3^-$ (mEq/L)
Saliva	33	20	34	0
Gastric juice*	60	9	84	0
Bile	149	5	101	45
Pancreatic juice	141	5	77	92
Ileal fluid	129	11	116	29
Cecal fluid	80	21	48	22
Cerebrospinal fluid	141	3	127	23
Sweat	45	5	58	0

*The Cl$^-$ concentration exceeds the Na$^+$, K$^+$ concentration by 15 mEq/L in gastric juice. This largely represents the secretions of HCl acid by parietal cells.
Cl$^-$, Chloride; *HCO*$_3^-$, bicarbonate; *H*$^+$, hydrogen; *K*$^+$, potassium; *Na*$^+$, sodium.
From Smith LH, Thier SO: *Pathophysiology: the biological principles of disease,* Philadelphia, 1981, Saunders.

The kidney provides the most efficient regulation of potassium balance over time. The amount of K$^+$ excreted varies in proportion to the dietary intake (40 to 120 mEq/day). Potassium is freely filtered by the renal glomerulus, and 90% is reabsorbed by the proximal tubule and loop of Henle. The principal cells in the collecting tubule secrete potassium. The reabsorption of K$^+$ occurs in the adjacent intercalated cell. Dietary potassium intake, aldosterone, and distal tubule urine flow determine the amount of K$^+$ excreted from the body. Unlike sodium, the renal mechanism for conserving K$^+$ is weak, even when total body potassium stores are depleted. However, a low K$^+$ intake also suppresses renal K$^+$ excretion.[11]

Several factors related to passive transport and aldosterone contribute to renal regulation of potassium. These factors include the concentration gradients for potassium at the distal tubule and collecting duct, changes in pH (causing acidosis or alkalosis), changes in electrical potential differences across the distal tubule, and aldosterone levels. (Renal mechanisms are described in more detail in Chapter 35.)

The concentration of potassium in the distal tubular cell is determined primarily by the plasma concentration in the peritubular capillaries. When plasma K$^+$ concentration increases because of increased dietary intake or shifts from the ICF occur, potassium is secreted into the urine by principal cells in the distal tubules. Decreases in plasma potassium result in decreased distal tubular secretion and reabsorption by intercalated cells, although K$^+$ losses of approximately 5 to 15 mEq/day will continue. Changes in the rate of filtrate flow through the distal tubule also influence the concentration gradient for K$^+$ secretion. When the flow rate is high, as occurs with the administration of diuretics, the concentration of potassium in the distal tubular urine is lower, favoring the secretion of potassium.[12]

Changes in pH and thus in hydrogen ion concentration also affect K$^+$ *balance.* Hydrogen ions move from the ECF to the ICF during states of acidosis. During acidosis, when hydrogen is moving into the cell, potassium shifts out of the cell to the ECF to maintain a balance of cations across the cell membrane. This occurs in part because of a decrease in Na$^+$, K$^+$-ATPase pump activity. The decreased ICF K$^+$ results in decreased secretion of K$^+$ into the urine by the distal tubular

cells, contributing to hyperkalemia, although total body potassium may not change. In contrast, intracellular fluid levels of hydrogen are diminished during states of alkalosis. Alkalosis causes potassium to shift into the cell, so the distal tubular cells increase their secretion of K$^+$ into the urine, contributing to hypokalemia. The management of potassium alterations associated with acid-base imbalances require that the acid-base imbalances must be treated before or concurrently with treatment of changes in potassium.

Three hormones (aldosterone, insulin, and epinephrine [β-adrenergic stimulation]) promote movement of potassium from the extracellular to intracellular fluid. Besides acting to conserve sodium, *aldosterone is a major factor in potassium regulation.* When potassium concentration is increased, aldosterone is released, stimulating secretion of potassium into the urine by the distal tubules of the kidney. Aldosterone also increases the secretion of K$^+$ from the sweat glands.

Insulin contributes to the regulation of plasma potassium levels by stimulating the Na$^+$, K$^+$-ATPase pump, thereby promoting the movement of potassium into liver and muscle cells simultaneously with glucose transport after eating. The intracellular movement of potassium prevents an acute hyperkalemia related to food intake. Insulin also can be used to treat hyperkalemia. However, dangerously low levels of plasma potassium can result from the administration of insulin when potassium levels are depressed. Potassium balance is especially significant in the treatment of conditions requiring insulin administration, such as insulin-dependent diabetes mellitus. Glucagon blocks entry of potassium into cells and glucocorticoids promote potassium excretion.

Catecholamines also influence K$^+$ *concentration in ECF.* β$_1$ adrenergics stimulate the movement of K$^+$ into cells, and α-adrenergics shift K$^+$ out of cells.[13]

An interesting aspect of K$^+$ regulation is the ability of the body to adapt to increased levels of potassium intake over time. A sudden increase in potassium may be fatal, but if the intake of potassium is slowly increased by amounts no more than 120 mEq/day, the kidney is able to increase the urinary excretion of potassium and maintain potassium balance. This tolerance to increasing amounts of potassium is known as **potassium adaptation.**

Hypokalemia

PATHOPHYSIOLOGY Potassium deficiency, or **hypokalemia,** develops when the serum potassium concentration decreases to less than 3.5 mEq/L. Because intracellular and total body stores of potassium are difficult to measure, changes in potassium balance are described by the plasma concentration, although changes in total body potassium are not always reflected in the plasma potassium concentration. Generally, lowered serum potassium indicates a loss of total body potassium. Because potassium is lost from the ECF, the change in the concentration gradient favors movement of K^+ from the cell to the ECF. The ICF/ECF concentration ratio is maintained, but total body K^+ is depleted.

ECF hypokalemia can develop without losses of total body potassium, but only when potassium is redistributed between the ICF and ECF. For example, potassium shifts into the cell during states of respiratory or metabolic alkalosis or after administration of insulin. In the event of alkalosis, K^+ shifts into the cell in exchange for H^+ to maintain plasma acid-base balance. Insulin also promotes cellular uptake of K^+ and can cause an ECF potassium deficit, particularly with the intake of high carbohydrate loads.[14]

Plasma K^+ levels may be normal or elevated when total body potassium is depleted. In such instances, potassium shifts from the ICF to the ECF. One of the common causes of this problem is diabetic ketoacidosis, in which the increased hydrogen ion concentration in the ECF causes H^+ to shift into the cell in exchange for potassium. A normal level of potassium is maintained in the plasma, but potassium continues to be lost in the urine, causing a deficit in total body potassium. Severe, even fatal, hypokalemia may occur if insulin is administered without also providing potassium supplements. Thus total body potassium depletion becomes evident when insulin treatment is initiated.

Potassium loss also occurs through normal body functions, but without causing hypokalemia. Average daily losses of potassium are as follows:

Location	Daily Loss (mEq/L)
Stool	5-10
Sweat	0-20
Urine	40-120

Factors contributing to the development of hypokalemia include *reduced intake of potassium, increased entry of potassium into cells,* and *increased losses of body potassium.* Dietary deficiency of potassium is a rare cause of hypokalemia. It may occur in older adults with both low protein intake and inadequate intake of fruits and vegetables and in people with alcoholism or anorexia nervosa. Generally, reduced potassium intake becomes a problem when combined with other causes of potassium depletion.

Shifts of potassium from the extracellular to intracellular space cause apparent deficits in total body potassium. Alkalosis, particularly respiratory alkalosis, is the most common clinical problem. ECF potassium will exchange with ICF hydrogen and correct the alkalosis by decreasing the pH of the ECF. Treatment of pernicious anemia with vitamin B_{12} or folate also may precipitate hypokalemia if the formation of new red blood cells causes enough potassium uptake to effect an extracellular decrease in potassium. **Familial hypokalemic periodic paralysis** is a rare genetically transmitted disease that also causes potassium to shift into the intracellular space.

Losses of potassium from body stores are most commonly caused by gastrointestinal and renal disorders. Diarrhea (from any cause), intestinal drainage tubes or fistulae, and laxative abuse also may result in hypokalemia. Normally, only 5 to 10 mEq of potassium and 100 to 150 ml of water are excreted in the stool each day. With diarrhea, fluid and electrolyte losses can be voluminous, with several liters of fluid and 100 to 200 mEq of potassium lost per day. Vomiting or continuous nasogastric suction frequently is associated with potassium depletion, partly because of the potassium lost from the gastric fluid but principally because of renal compensation for volume depletion and the metabolic alkalosis (elevated bicarbonate levels) that occurs from sodium, chloride, and hydrogen ion losses. The loss of fluid and sodium stimulates the secretion of aldosterone, which in turn causes renal losses of potassium. The elevated flow of bicarbonate at the distal tubule contributes to renal excretion of potassium because of increased tubular lumen electronegativity.

Renal losses of potassium are related to increased secretion of potassium by the distal tubule. Use of diuretics, excessive aldosterone secretion, increased distal tubular flow rate, and low plasma magnesium concentration all may contribute to urinary losses of potassium. Many diuretics, including thiazides, furosemide, ethacrynic acid, and osmotic diuretics, inhibit the reabsorption of sodium chloride, causing the diuretic effect. The distal tubular flow rate then increases, promoting potassium excretion. If sodium loss is severe, the compensating aldosterone secretion (which causes secondary hyperaldosteronism) may further deplete potassium stores. Primary hyperaldosteronism with excessive secretion of aldosterone from an adrenal adenoma also causes potassium wasting. Many kidney diseases result in a reduced ability to conserve sodium. The disordered sodium reabsorption produces a diuretic effect, and the increased distal tubule flow rate favors the secretion of potassium. Magnesium deficits stimulate renin release and hyperaldosteronism, causing hypokalemia. Several antibiotics, including amphotericin B, gentamicin, and carbenicillin, are known to cause hypokalemia.

CLINICAL MANIFESTATIONS A wide range of metabolic dysfunctions may result from potassium deficiency. Carbohydrate metabolism is affected because hypokalemia depresses insulin secretion and alters hepatic and skeletal muscle glycogen synthesis. Renal function is impaired, with a decreased ability to concentrate urine. Polyuria (increased urine) and polydipsia (increased thirst) are associated with decreased responsiveness to ADH. Chronic potassium deficits lasting more than 1 month may damage renal tissue, with resulting interstitial fibrosis and tubular atrophy.

Neuromuscular and cardiac effects of hypokalemia produce the most common symptoms.[15] Neuromuscular excitability is

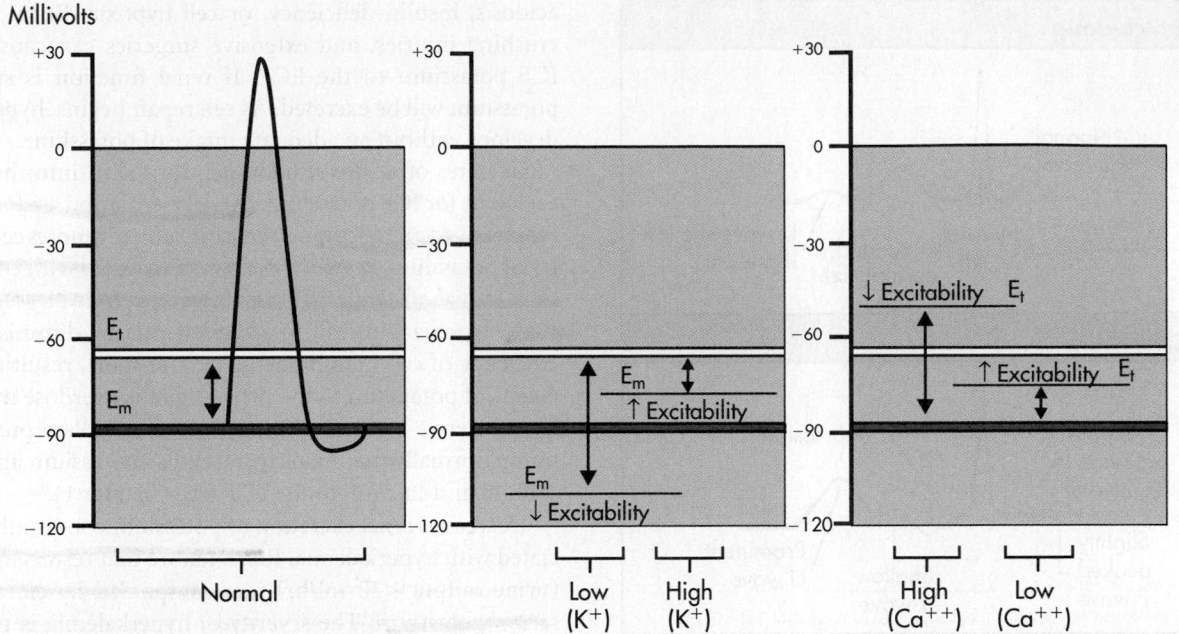

Figure 3-5 Effects of potassium (K^+) and calcium (Ca^{++}) on membrane excitability. *Potassium* affects resting membrane potential (E_m), and calcium affects threshold potential (E_t).

decreased, causing skeletal muscle weakness, smooth muscle atony, and cardiac dysrhythmias. As Chapter 1 describes, the resting membrane potential (E_m) is determined by the *ratio* of extracellular to intracellular potassium ion concentration. Because the concentration of potassium in the ECF is small, only small changes in ECF potassium are required to influence the resting membrane potential and affect neuromuscular excitability (the difference between resting membrane and threshold potentials). When extracellular potassium levels decrease rapidly, intracellular potassium diffuses more readily out of the cell and the resting membrane potential becomes more negative (i.e., from −90 to −100 mV). If the threshold potential (E_t) remains stable, the difference between resting membrane potential and threshold potential increases and the cell membrane becomes **hyperpolarized**, requiring a stronger stimulus to initiate an action potential (decreasing excitability) (Figure 3-5).

Factors such as calcium concentration and pH also contribute to the changes in neuromuscular excitability associated with hypokalemia. Increases in ECF calcium concentration tend to make the threshold potential less negative and decrease membrane excitability, potentiating the neuromuscular effects of hypokalemia.

The onset of symptoms is related to the rate of potassium depletion. Because the body can accommodate slow losses of potassium, the decrease in ECF concentration may be slow enough to allow potassium to shift from the intracellular space. The extracellular to intracellular potassium concentration gradient then is restored toward normal, with less severe neuromuscular changes. With acute losses of potassium, changes in neuromuscular excitability are more profound. Skeletal muscle weakness initially occurs in the larger muscles of the legs and arms and ultimately affects the diaphragm and depresses ventilation. Paralysis and respiratory arrest then can

occur. Loss of smooth muscle tone is manifested by constipation, intestinal distention, anorexia, nausea, vomiting, and paralytic ileus.

The cardiac effects of hypokalemia are related also to changes in membrane excitability (see Figure 3-5). Because potassium contributes to the repolarization phase of the action potential, hypokalemia delays ventricular repolarization and the frequency of action potentials. A variety of dysrhythmias may occur, including sinus bradycardia, atrioventricular block, and paroxysmal atrial tachycardia. The characteristic changes in the electrocardiogram reflect delayed repolarization. For instance, the amplitude of the T wave is decreased; the amplitude of the U wave is increased; and the ST segment is depressed (Figure 3-6). In severe states of hypokalemia, P waves peak and the QRS complex is prolonged. Hypokalemia also increases the risk of digitalis toxicity by slowing the sodium-potassium pump, which augments the action of digitalis in cardiac muscle by excessively increasing intracellular calcium and sodium.

EVALUATION AND TREATMENT The diagnosis of hypokalemia is significantly related to the medical history and the identification of disorders associated with potassium loss or shifts of extracellular potassium to the intracellular space. Treatment involves an estimation of total body potassium losses and correction of acid-base imbalances. Further losses of potassium should be prevented, and the individual should be encouraged to eat foods rich in potassium. The maximal rate of oral replacement is 40 to 80 mEq/day if renal function is normal. A maximal safe rate of intravenous replacement is 20 mEq/hr. Because potassium is irritating to blood vessels, a maximal concentration of 40 mEq/L should be used. Serum potassium values can be monitored until normokalemia is achieved.

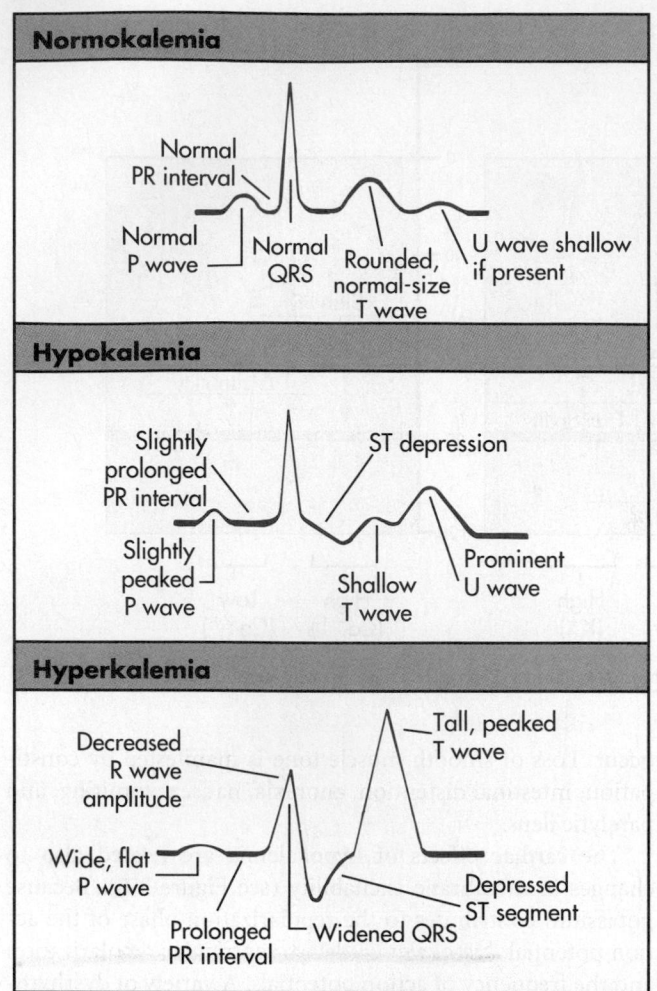

Figure 3-6 Electrocardiogram (ECG) changes with potassium imbalance.

Hyperkalemia

PATHOPHYSIOLOGY An elevation of ECF potassium *above 5.5 mEq/L* constitutes **hyperkalemia.** Because of efficient renal excretion, increases in total body potassium are relatively rare. Acute increases in serum potassium are handled quickly through an increase in cellular uptake and renal excretion of body potassium excesses. Excretion is partially mediated by the secretion of aldosterone because it facilitates excretion of potassium into the urine.

Excesses of serum potassium may be caused by increased intake, a shift of potassium from cells to the ECF, or decreased renal excretion. If renal function is normal, slow, long-term increases in potassium intake are usually well tolerated through potassium adaptation, although acute potassium loading can exceed renal excretion rates. Use of stored whole blood and intravenous boluses of penicillin G or replacement potassium can precipitate hyperkalemia, particularly if renal function is impaired. Dietary excesses of potassium are uncommon, but accidental ingestion of potassium salt substitutes can cause toxicity.

Movement of potassium from the ICF to the ECF occurs with cell trauma or a change in cell membrane permeability,

acidosis, insulin deficiency, or cell hypoxia. Burns, massive crushing injuries, and extensive surgeries can cause loss of ICF potassium to the ECF. If renal function is sustained, potassium will be excreted. As cell repair begins, hypokalemia develops without an adequate intake of potassium.

In states of acidosis, hydrogen ions shift into the cells in exchange for ICF potassium; hyperkalemia and acidosis therefore often occur together. Because insulin promotes cellular entry of potassium, insulin deficits, which occur with conditions such as diabetic ketoacidosis, are accompanied by hyperkalemia. Hypoxia can lead to hyperkalemia by diminishing the efficiency of cell membrane active transport, resulting in the escape of potassium to the ECF. Digitalis overdose may cause hyperkalemia by inhibiting the Na^+, K^+-ATPase pump. This pump normally maintains intracellular potassium and moves sodium and calcium to the ECF (see Chapter 1).

Decreased renal excretion of potassium commonly is associated with hyperkalemia. Renal failure that results in oliguria (urine output <30 ml/hr) is accompanied by elevations of serum potassium. The severity of hyperkalemia is related to the amount of potassium intake, the degree of acidosis, and the rate of renal cell damage. In acute renal failure potassium levels rise more rapidly with more serious consequences than the slower rises associated with chronic renal failure. Decreases in the secretion or renal effects of aldosterone also can cause decreases in the urinary excretion of potassium. For example, Addison disease results in decreased production and secretion of aldosterone and thus contributes to hyperkalemia. Potassium-sparing diuretics (e.g., spironolactone, which inhibits sodium reabsorption and potassium and hydrogen secretion by the distal tubule) also may contribute to hyperkalemia. Frequently, however, these diuretics are used in combination with diuretics that cause potassium wasting in an attempt to balance renal potassium gains and losses.

CLINICAL MANIFESTATIONS Symptoms of hyperkalemia vary, but common characteristics are muscle weakness or paralysis and arrhythmias with changes in the electrocardiogram. During mild attacks, increased neuromuscular irritability may be manifested as tingling of lips and fingers, restlessness, intestinal cramping, and diarrhea. Severe hyperkalemia causes muscle weakness, loss of muscle tone, and paralysis. In mild states of hyperkalemia, the more rapid repolarization is reflected in the electrocardiogram as narrow and taller T waves with a shortened QT interval. Severe hyperkalemia (serum levels ≥6 mEq/L) depresses the ST segment, prolongs the PR interval, and widens the QRS complex (see Figure 3-6). Bradydysrhythmias are common in hyperkalemia, with alterations in cardiac conduction causing ventricular fibrillation or cardiac arrest.

As with hypokalemia, changes in the ratio of intracellular to extracellular potassium concentration contribute to the symptoms of hyperkalemia. If extracellular potassium concentration increases without a significant change in intracellular potassium, the resting membrane potential becomes more positive (i.e., changes from −90 to −80 mV) and the cell membrane is **hypopolarized** (the inside of the cell becomes less negative or partially depolarized [increase excitability]) (Electrical properties of cells are discussed in Chapter 1.) With relatively mild elevations in extracellular potassium, the cell more rapidly repolarizes and becomes more irritable (peaked T waves). An action potential then is initiated more rapidly because the distance between the resting membrane potential and the threshold potential has been shortened. With more severe hyperkalemia, the resting membrane potential approaches or exceeds the threshold potential (wide QRS merging with T wave). In this case the cell is not able to repolarize and therefore does not respond to excitation stimuli. The most serious consequence is cardiac standstill.

Like the effects of hypokalemia, the neuromuscular effects of hyperkalemia are related to the rate of increase in the ECF potassium concentration and the presence of other contributing factors, such as acidosis and calcium balance. Long-term increases in ECF potassium concentration result in shifts of potassium into the cell because the tendency is to maintain a normal ratio of intracellular/extracellular potassium concentrations. Acute elevations of extracellular potassium affect neuromuscular irritability because this ratio is disrupted.[16]

Because calcium influences the threshold potential, changes in extracellular fluid calcium concentration can augment or override the effects of hyperkalemia. With hypocalcemia the threshold potential becomes more negative, enhancing the neuromuscular effects of hyperkalemia. Hypercalcemia causes the threshold potential to become less negative, counteracting the effects of hyperkalemia on resting membrane potential (see Figure 3-5).

EVALUATION AND TREATMENT Hyperkalemia should be investigated when there is a history of renal disease, massive trauma, insulin deficiency, Addison disease, use of potassium salt substitutes, or metabolic acidosis. The acuity of the onset of symptoms may be related to the underlying cause.

Management of hyperkalemia is related to treating the contributing causes and correcting the potassium excess. Normalizing the extracellular potassium concentration can be achieved with a variety of methods; the treatment chosen is related to the cause and severity of the problem. Calcium gluconate can be administered to restore normal neuromuscular irritability when serum potassium levels are dangerously high. Administration of glucose, which readily stimulates insulin secretion, or administration of glucose and insulin for those with diabetes, facilitates cellular entry of potassium. Sodium bicarbonate corrects metabolic acidosis and lowers serum potassium. Oral or rectal administration of cation exchange resins, which exchange sodium for potassium in the intestine, can be effective. Dialysis effectively removes potassium when renal failure has occurred.

Calcium and Phosphate

The total body content of calcium is about 1200 g. Most calcium (99%) is located in bone as hydroxyapatite (an inorganic compound that contributes to bone rigidity), and the remainder is in the plasma and body cells. Of the calcium in the plasma, 50% is bound to plasma proteins (2.5 mEq/L),

and about 40% is in the free or ionized form (2.4 mEq/L). The total fraction of calcium circulating in the blood is small (4.5 to 5.5 mEq/L, or 8.6 to 10.5 mg/dl). Ionized calcium has the most important physiologic functions.

Calcium is a necessary ion for many fundamental metabolic processes. It is the major cation for the structure of bones and teeth. It serves as an enzymatic cofactor for blood clotting and is required for hormone secretion and the function of cell receptors. Plasma membrane stability and permeability are directly related to calcium ions, as is the transmission of nerve impulses and the contraction of muscles. Intracellular calcium is located primarily in the mitochondria.

Phosphate is found primarily in bone (85%), with smaller amounts found within the intracellular and extracellular spaces. In the serum, phosphate exists in phospholipids and phosphate esters and as inorganic phosphate, which is the ionized form. The normal serum levels of inorganic phosphate range from 2.5 to 4.5 mg/dl and may be as high as 6.0 to 7.0 mg/dl in infants and young children. Intracellular phosphate has many metabolic forms, including the high-energy structures creatine phosphate and adenosine triphosphate (ATP). Phosphate acts as an intracellular and extracellular anion buffer in the regulation of acid-base balance; in the form of ATP it provides energy for muscle contraction.

Calcium and phosphate concentrations are rigidly controlled. They are related by the product of calcium (Ca^{++}) and phosphate ($HPO_4^=$), which is a constant (K) [$Ca^{++} \times HPO_4^= = K$]. Thus if the concentration of one ion increases, that of the other decreases.

Calcium and phosphate balance is regulated by three hormones: parathyroid hormone (PTH), vitamin D, and calcitonin. Acting together, these substances determine the amount of dietary calcium and phosphate absorbed from the intestine, the deposition and absorption of calcium and phosphate from the bone, and the renal reabsorption and excretion of calcium and phosphate by the kidney.

The parathyroid glands are sensitive to changes in serum calcium concentrations, and **parathyroid hormone** controls ionized calcium in the blood and extracellular fluids. The parathyroid glands secrete PTH in response to low serum calcium. (The specific actions of PTH in relation to calcium and phosphorus are described in Chapter 20.) The renal regulation of calcium and phosphate balance requires PTH. As PTH secretion is stimulated by low levels of serum calcium, reabsorption of calcium along the distal part of the nephron increases and inhibition of phosphate reabsorption by the proximal segment of the nephron increases. The net result is an increase in serum calcium and urinary excretion of phosphate. Figure 3-7 summarizes hormonal regulation of calcium.

Another hormone important to calcium and phosphate regulation is vitamin D. **Vitamin D** (cholecalciferol) is a fat-soluble steroid ingested in food or synthesized in the skin in the presence of ultraviolet light. Several steps of activation are required before vitamin D can act on target tissues. The first step occurs in the liver; final activation is in the kidney. The renal activation of vitamin D begins when the serum calcium

$\downarrow ADH \rightarrow \uparrow K^+$

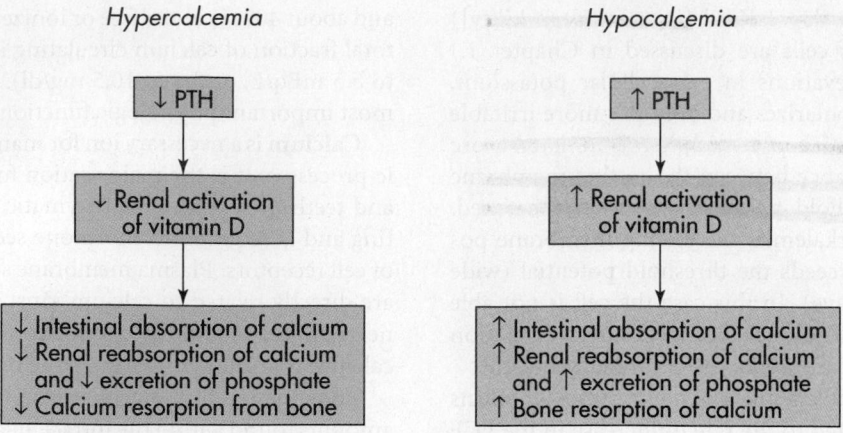

Hypercalcemia   *Hypocalcemia*

↓ PTH   ↑ PTH

↓ Renal activation of vitamin D   ↑ Renal activation of vitamin D

↓ Intestinal absorption of calcium   ↑ Intestinal absorption of calcium
↓ Renal reabsorption of calcium   ↑ Renal reabsorption of calcium
  and ↓ excretion of phosphate   and ↑ excretion of phosphate
↓ Calcium resorption from bone   ↑ Bone resorption of calcium

Figure 3-7 Hormonal regulation of calcium balance. *PTH,* Parathyroid hormone.

level decreases and stimulates secretion of PTH. PTH then acts to increase calcium reabsorption and enhance renal excretion of phosphate, producing decreased phosphate levels. The combination of low calcium, PTH secretion, and low phosphate thus causes the renal activation of vitamin D. The activated vitamin D (vitamin D_3—calcitriol) then circulates in the plasma and acts to increase absorption of calcium in the small intestine, enhance bone absorption of calcium, and increase renal tubular reabsorption of calcium. When renal failure occurs, vitamin D is not activated; serum calcium levels decrease; and phosphate levels increase.

The exchange of calcium and phosphate between serum and bone is regulated also by hormones. When serum calcium levels are low, PTH increases and vitamin D3 stimulates intestinal calcium absorption and renal calcium reabsorption. Osteoclasts are stimulated to resorb bone and release calcium and phosphate into the plasma.

As calcium levels increase, an opposite adaptation occurs, leading to suppression of PTH secretion, decreased renal vitamin D activation, and decreased intestinal calcium absorption and increased renal phosphate reabsorption. **Calcitonin** primarily decreases calcium levels by inhibiting osteoclastic activity in bone.

The fractions of serum calcium that are freely ionized or bound to plasma proteins are influenced by pH. In states of acidosis, levels of ionized calcium increase. When alkalosis develops, with an increase in pH, protein-bound calcium increases and the physiologically active, ionized calcium decreases. The decreased concentration of ionized calcium may be great enough to cause symptoms of hypocalcemia, such as tetany.

Hypocalcemia
PATHOPHYSIOLOGY **Hypocalcemia** occurs when serum calcium concentrations are less than 8.5 mg/dl and ionized levels are less than 4.0 mg/dl. Deficits in calcium are related to inadequate intestinal absorption, deposition of ionized calcium into bone or soft tissue, blood administration, or decreases in PTH and vitamin D.

Nutritional deficiencies of calcium can occur in the instance of inadequate sources of dairy products or green, leafy vegetables. Excessive amounts of dietary phosphorus also bind with calcium, so neither mineral is absorbed when such an excess occurs. Blood transfusions are also a common cause of hypocalcemia because the citrate solution used in storing whole blood binds with calcium. Pancreatitis causes release of lipases into soft tissue spaces, so the free fatty acids that are formed bind calcium, causing a decrease in ionized calcium. Neoplastic bone metastases tend to inhibit bone resorption and increase calcium deposition into bone, thereby decreasing serum calcium levels.

Vitamin D deficiency, which can result from inadequate intake or avoidance of sunlight, causes decreased intestinal absorption of calcium. Malabsorption of fat, including fat-soluble vitamin D, may also contribute to calcium deficiency. Removal of the parathyroid glands with the resulting loss of PTH also causes hypocalcemia. Metabolic or respiratory alkalosis causes symptoms of hypocalcemia because the change in pH enhances protein binding of ionized calcium. Hypoalbuminemia lowers total serum calcium levels by decreasing the amount of bound calcium in the plasma.

CLINICAL MANIFESTATIONS The clinical manifestations of hypocalcemia are caused primarily by an increase in neuromuscular excitability. Calcium deficits cause partial depolarization of nerves and muscle as the threshold potential approaches the resting membrane potential (see Figure 3-5). Therefore, a smaller stimulus is required for initiating the action potential. The symptoms include confusion, paresthesias around the mouth and in the digits, carpopedal spasm (muscle spasms in the hands and feet), and hyperreflexia.

Two clinical signs are Chvostek sign and Trousseau sign. Chvostek sign is elicited by tapping on the facial nerve just below the temple. A positive sign is a twitch of the nose or lip. Trousseau sign is contraction of the hand and fingers when the arterial blood flow in the arm is occluded for 5 minutes.

Severe symptoms include convulsions and *tetany,* a continuous severe muscle spasm that can interfere with breathing and cause death. The characteristic electrocardiogram (ECG) change is a prolonged QT interval, indicating prolonged ventricular depolarization and decreased cardiac contractility. Intestinal cramping and hyperactive bowel sounds also may be present because hypocalcemia affects the smooth muscles of the gastrointestinal tract.

EVALUATION AND TREATMENT The health history may signify underlying pathologic conditions that require further evaluation and treatment. Severe symptoms of hypocalcemia require emergency treatment with intravenous 10% calcium gluconate. Oral calcium replacement should be initiated, and serum calcium levels should be monitored. Decreasing phosphate intake facilitates long-term management of hypocalcemia.

Hypercalcemia

PATHOPHYSIOLOGY Hypercalcemia with serum calcium concentrations exceeding 12 mg/dl can be caused by a number of diseases. The most common among these are hyperparathyroidism; bone metastases with calcium resorption from breast, prostate, cervical cancer, or hematologic malignancy; sarcoidosis; and excess vitamin D. Many tumors produce PTH and elevate the serum calcium levels. Sarcoidosis appears to increase vitamin D levels. Prolonged immobilization can also lead to hypercalcemia from bone resorption. Acidosis decreases serum binding of calcium to albumin, increasing ionized calcium.

CLINICAL MANIFESTATIONS Many symptoms of hypercalcemia are nonspecific. Because serum calcium levels are increased, a greater amount of calcium is also contained inside the cells. The threshold potential becomes more positive, and the cell membrane becomes refractory to depolarization (see Figure 3-5). Thus many of the symptoms are related to loss of cell membrane excitability. (Membrane potentials and membrane excitability are discussed in Chapter 1.) Fatigue, weakness, lethargy, anorexia, nausea, and constipation are common. Behavioral changes may occur. Impaired renal function frequently develops, and kidney stones form as precipitates of calcium salts. A shortened QT segment and depressed widened T waves also may be observed on the ECG, with bradycardia and varying degrees of heart block.

EVALUATION AND TREATMENT With elevated serum calcium levels, often a reciprocal decrease in serum phosphate values occurs. Specific diagnostic procedures to identify the contributing pathologic condition are required.

Treatment is related to severity of symptoms and the underlying disease. When renal function is normal, oral phosphate administration is effective. When acute illness and high calcium levels are present, treatment options include intravenous administration of large amounts of normal saline to enhance renal excretion of calcium, bisphosphonates in the absence of renal failure, and administration of calcitonin. Corticosteroids and the cytotoxic drug mithramycin (for use with malignant disease) also are used to treat hypercalcemia. Ultimately, the underlying pathologic condition must be treated.

Hypophosphatemia

PATHOPHYSIOLOGY Hypophosphatemia is a serum phosphate level less than 2 mg/dl and is usually an indication of phosphate deficiency. In some conditions, total body phosphate is normal but serum volumes are low. The most common causes are intestinal malabsorption and increased renal excretion of phosphate. Inadequate absorption is associated with vitamin D deficiency, use of magnesium- and aluminum-containing antacids (which bind with phosphorus), long-term alcohol abuse, and malabsorption syndromes. Respiratory alkalosis can cause severe hypophosphatemia because of cellular use of phosphorus for an accelerated glucose metabolism. Increased renal excretion of phosphorus is associated with hyperparathyroidism.

CLINICAL MANIFESTATIONS The consequences of phosphate deficiency are not clinically evident until hypophosphatemia is severe. There is reduced capacity for oxygen transport by red blood cells and disturbed energy metabolism. Transport and release of oxygen are associated with 2,3-diphosphoglycerate (2,3-DPG) and ATP. When phosphate is depleted, 2,3-DPG and ATP levels become low and diminish release of oxygen to the tissues. The oxyhemoglobin curve shifts to the left (see Chapter 32), and hypoxia can occur with bradycardia and varying degrees of heart block.

Leukocyte and platelet dysfunctions also are associated with hypophosphatemia. There is a greater risk of infection and blood-clotting impairment, with potential for hemorrhage. Nerve and muscle function can be affected because of derangement in energy metabolism. Muscle weakness may become serious enough to cause respiratory failure, and cardiomyopathies also can develop. Irritability, confusion, numbness, coma, and convulsions develop with severe phosphate losses. In response to low phosphate levels, bone resorption occurs and may lead to rickets or osteomalacia.

EVALUATION AND TREATMENT To correct the condition, the underlying cause must be identified and treated. Although serum phosphate levels are below normal, the administration of phosphate salts is dangerous, and low phosphate levels are usually not considered life threatening.[17]

Hyperphosphatemia

PATHOPHYSIOLOGY Hyperphosphatemia, or an elevated serum phosphate level of more than 4.5 mg/dl, develops with exogenous or endogenous addition of phosphorus to the ECF or with significant loss of glomerular filtration.[18] Because most phosphate is located in cells, the cell destruction associated with treatment of metastatic tumors with chemotherapy can release large amounts of phosphate into the serum. Long-term use of phosphate-containing enemas or laxatives also may lead to hyperphosphatemia. Hypoparathyroidism can cause elevated phosphate by increasing renal tubular reabsorption of phosphate.

High levels of serum phosphate also lower serum calcium levels, and increased amounts of phosphate and calcium are deposited in bone and soft tissues. Serum calcium levels may become low enough to cause symptoms of hypocalcemia, including tetany.

CLINICAL MANIFESTATIONS Symptoms of hyperphosphatemia are related primarily to low serum calcium levels and thus are comparable to symptoms of hypocalcemia.

With prolonged hyperphosphatemia, calcification of soft tissues occurs in the lungs, kidneys, and joints.

EVALUATION AND TREATMENT To correct the condition, the underlying pathologic condition must be identified and treated. Aluminum hydroxide may be administered because it binds phosphate in the gastrointestinal tract and is then eliminated but can deposit in the central nervous system, bone, and hematopoietic cells. New non-aluminum and non–calcium phosphate binders are available.[19] Dialysis is required for management of renal failure.

Magnesium

Magnesium (Mg^{++}) is a major intracellular cation. About 40% to 60% is stored in muscle and bone with 30% in the cells. A small amount (1%) is in the serum. Plasma concentration is 1.8 to 2.4 mEq/L with about one third bound to plasma proteins and the rest in ionized form. Regulation of magnesium metabolism is balanced by the small intestine and kidney. Low serum levels cause renal conservation of magnesium. Magnesium is a cofactor in intracellular enzymatic reactions, protein synthesis, nucleic acid stability, and neuromuscular excitability. Calcium and magnesium often interact in reactions at the cellular level.

Hypomagnesemia occurs when serum magnesium concentration is less than 1.5 mEq/L and increases in neuromuscular excitability and tetany are present. Malnutrition, malabsorption syndromes, alcoholism, renal tubular dysfunction, metabolic acidosis, and loop and thiazide diuretics can cause magnesium losses. Diabetes mellitus is associated with hypomagnesemia partly as a function of osmotic diuresis.[20] Because magnesium inhibits potassium channels, loss of magnesium results in movement of potassium out of the cell, with renal excretion resulting in hypokalemia. Signs and symptoms of hypomagnesemia are similar to those of hypocalcemia. Depression, confusion, irritability, increased reflexes, muscle weakness, ataxia, nystagmus, tetany, convulsions, and tachyarrhythmias may be observed.[21] Treatment is intramuscular or intravenous administration of magnesium sulfate.

Hypermagnesemia, in which magnesium concentration is greater than 2.5 mEq/L, is rare and usually is caused by renal failure. Magnesium-containing antacids (e.g., Gaviscon, Gelusil) can potentiate excess magnesium. Excess magnesium depresses skeletal muscle contraction and nerve function. Signs and symptoms include nausea and vomiting, muscle weakness, hypotension, bradycardia, and respiratory depression.[22] Treatment is avoidance of magnesium-containing substances and removal of magnesium by dialysis.

ACID-BASE BALANCE

Acid-base balance and hydrogen ion concentration must be regulated within a narrow range for the body to function normally. Slight changes in amounts of hydrogen can significantly alter biologic processes in cells and tissues. Hydrogen ion

is necessary to maintain membrane integrity and the speed of enzymatic reactions. Most pathologic conditions disturb acid-base balance, and the degree of severity may be more harmful than the disease process.

Hydrogen Ion and pH

The hydrogen ion concentration $[H^+]$ is commonly expressed as the pH, the negative logarithm of hydrogen ions in solution. The logarithmic value means that as the pH changes one unit (e.g., 7.0 to 6.0), the $[H^+]$ changes tenfold (i.e., 0.0000001 to 0.000001). The relationship is commonly expressed as follows:

$$pH = \log \frac{1}{[H^+]} \text{ or } pH = -\log_{10}[H^+]$$

As the $[H^+]$ increases, the pH decreases; likewise, as the $[H^+]$ decreases, the pH increases. The greater the $[H^+]$, the more acidic the solution and the lower the pH. The lower the $[H^+]$, the more basic the solution and the higher the pH. In biologic fluids, a pH of less than 7.4 is defined as acidic and a pH greater than 7.4 is defined as basic.

Different body fluids have different pH values as follows:

Body Fluid	pH
Gastric juices	1.0-3.0
Urine	5.0-6.0
Arterial blood	7.38-7.42
Venous blood	7.37
Cerebrospinal fluid	7.32
Pancreatic fluid	7.8-8.0

Body acids are formed as end products of cellular metabolism. The average person generates acid in the amount of 50 to 100 mEq/day from the metabolism of protein, carbohydrates, and fats and from loss of base in the stools. To maintain a normal pH, an equal amount of acid therefore must be neutralized or excreted. The lungs, kidneys, and bone are the major organs involved in the regulation of acid-base balance. The systems are interrelated and work together to regulate short- or long-term changes in acid-base status. Body acids exist in two forms: **volatile** (respiratory acids—eliminated as carbon dioxide [CO_2] gas) and **nonvolatile** (metabolic acids—eliminated by the kidney or metabolized by the liver). The volatile acid is carbonic acid (H_2CO_3), which is formed from the hydration of carbon dioxide:

$$\begin{matrix} \text{Regulated by lung} & & \text{Regulated by kidney} \\ CO_2 + H_2O & \longleftrightarrow H_2CO_3 \longleftrightarrow & HCO_3^- + H^+ \end{matrix}$$

Carbonic acid is a weak acid, and in the presence of carbonic anhydrase, it readily dissociates into carbon dioxide. Approximately 12,000 to 15,000 millimoles of CO_2 is produced in the human body per day.[23] The carbon dioxide is then eliminated by pulmonary ventilation. Sulfuric, phosphoric, and other metabolic acids (lactic acid, pyruvic acid, and keto acids associated with diabetes mellitus) are nonvolatile acids

Table 3-9	Buffer Systems			
Buffer Pairs	**Buffer System**	**pK Values**	**Reaction**	**Rate**
HCO_3^-/H_2CO_3	Bicarbonate	6.1	$H^+ + HCO_3^- \gtrless H_2O + CO_2$	Instantaneous
Hb^-/HHb	Hemoglobin	7.3	$HHb \rightleftharpoons H^+ + Hb^-$	Instantaneous
$HPO_4^=/H_2PO_4^-$	Phosphate	6.8	$H_2PO_4^- \rightleftharpoons H^+ + HPO_4^=$	Instantaneous
Pr^-/HPr	Plasma proteins	6.7	$HPr \rightleftharpoons H^+ + Pr^-$	Instantaneous
Organs	**Mechanism**			**Rate**
Lungs	Regulates retention or elimination of CO_2 and therefore H_2CO_3 concentration			Minutes-hours
Ionic shifts	Exchange of intracellular potassium and sodium for hydrogen			2-4 hours
Kidneys	Bicarbonate reabsorption and regeneration, ammonia formation, phosphate buffering			Hours-days
Bone	Exchanges of calcium, phosphate, and release of carbonate			Hours-days

H^+, Hydrogen; HCO_3^-, bicarbonate; H_2CO_3, carbonic acid; Hb^-, hemoglobin; $H_2PO_4^-$, monobasic phosphate; $HPO_4^=$, dibasic phosphate; HPr, hydrogenated protein; HHb, hydrogenated hemoglobin; Pr^-, protein.

produced from the metabolism of proteins, carbohydrates, and fats. (Strong acids are those that readily give up their hydrogen; weak acids do not.) Nonvolatile acids are eliminated by the renal tubules with the regulation of HCO_3^-. Thus the lungs and kidneys, with the help of body buffer systems, are the prime regulators of acid-base balance.

Buffer Systems

Buffering occurs in response to changes in acid-base status. **Buffers** can absorb excessive H^+ (acid) or OH^- (base) without a significant change in pH. The buffer systems are located in both the ICF and ECF compartments, and they function at different rates. Buffer systems exist as buffer pairs, consisting of a weak acid and its conjugate base (Table 3-9). The most important plasma buffer systems are carbonic acid–bicarbonate and hemoglobin. Phosphate and protein are the most important intracellular buffers.

An important factor for effective buffering is a function known as the *pK value*, which represents the pH at which a buffer pair is half dissociated. Buffer pairs can associate and dissociate (see Table 3-9).

The pK provides a rate constant for the chemical reaction. A buffer system is most effective when the pK for the buffer is close to the pH of the fluid in which the buffer is acting. For the bicarbonate–carbonic acid buffer system, the pK is 6.1. This value is not as high as the pK for other buffer systems (see Table 3-9), but this buffer system is still very effective because carbon dioxide is rapidly removed from the blood by the lungs.

The pK value is also a term in the equation used to determine pH. The relationships among pH, pK, and the ratio of bicarbonate to carbonic acid can be expressed as follows by the *Henderson-Hasselbalch equation*:

$$pH = pK + \log \frac{[HCO_3^-]}{[H_2CO_3]}$$

The pH then can be determined when specific values are included in the equation:

$$pH = pK + \log \frac{[HCO_3^-]}{[H_2CO_3]}$$
$$= 6.1 + \log \frac{24}{1.2}$$
$$= 6.1 + \log \frac{20}{1}$$
$$= 6.1 + 1.3$$
$$= 7.40$$

Carbonic Acid–Bicarbonate Buffering

The carbonic acid–bicarbonate buffer pair operates in both the lung and the kidney. The greater the carbon dioxide partial pressure (Pco_2), the more carbonic acid is formed. The relationship that exists between carbonic acid (H_2CO_3) and carbon dioxide (Pco_2) can be expressed as follows:

$$H_2CO_3 = 0.03 \times Pco_2 \text{ (mmHg)}$$

The 0.03 represents the solubility coefficient for carbon dioxide in water. The Pco_2 of arterial blood is normally about 40 mmHg. Therefore the amount of H_2CO_3 is equal to about 1.2 mmol/L (0.03×40). As the amount of carbon dioxide increases or decreases, the amount of H_2CO_3 changes in the same direction.

The relationship between bicarbonate and carbonic acid is usually expressed as a ratio. When the pH is 7.40, this ratio is 20:1 (bicarbonate/carbonic acid). The ratio is defined by the amount of bicarbonate and carbon dioxide (carbonic acid) in the arterial blood. Bicarbonate concentration (HCO_3^-) is normally about 24 mEq/L. Therefore, the 20:1 ratio can be developed as follows:

$$\frac{[HCO_3^-] = 24 \text{ mEq/L}}{[H_2CO_3] = (0.03 \times 40 \text{ mmHg})} = \frac{24}{1.2} = \frac{20}{1}$$

The values for HCO_3^- and Pco_2 (H_2CO_3) can increase or decrease proportionately, but the 20:1 ratio is maintained.

The lungs can decrease the amount of carbonic acid by blowing off CO_2 and leaving water. The kidneys can reabsorb

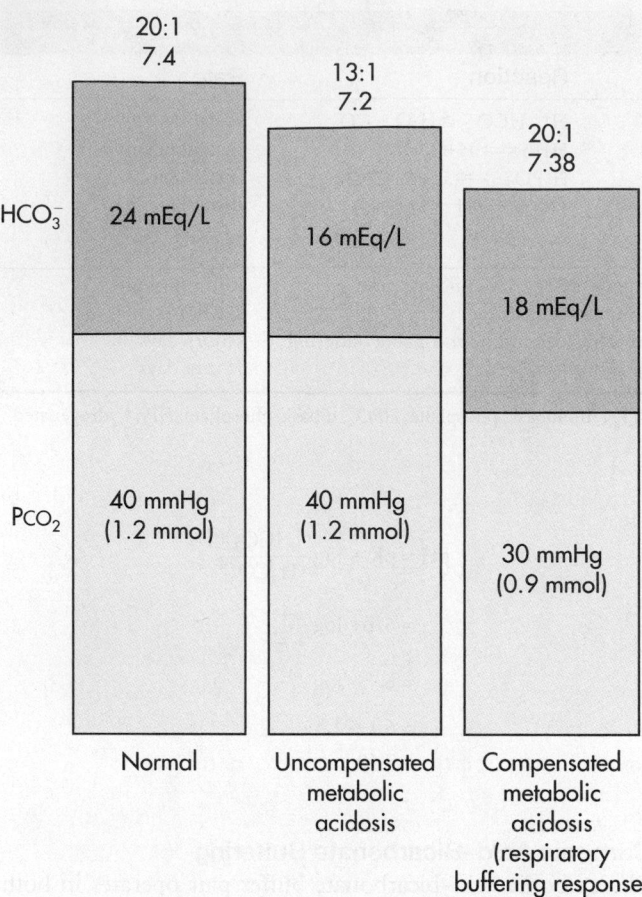

Figure 3-8 Compensated maintenance of HCO_3^-/Pco_2 (H_2CO_3) ratio in metabolic acidosis.

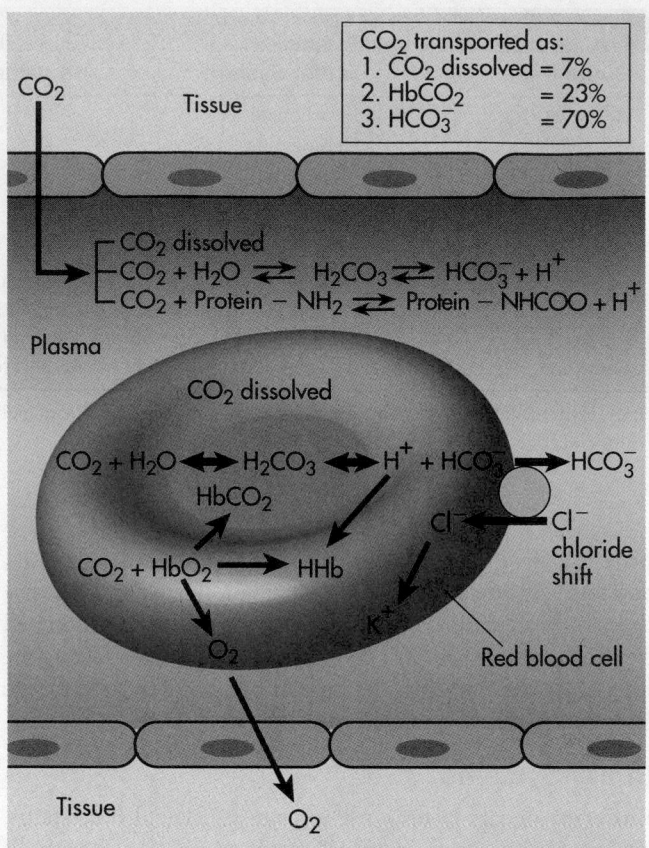

Figure 3-9 Buffering of hydrogen with hemoglobin and carbon dioxide (CO_2) transport. CO_2 is produced in tissue cells and diffuses to plasma, where it is transported as dissolved CO_2, or it combines with water to form carbonic acid (H_2CO_3), or it combines with protein from which hydrogen has been released. Most of the CO_2 diffuses into the red blood cells and combines with water to form H_2CO_3. The H_2CO_3 dissociates to form hydrogen (H^+) and bicarbonate (HCO_3^-). The HCO_3^- shifts into the plasma and chloride (Cl^-) shifts into the red blood cell to maintain electroneutrality. Hydrogen combines with hemoglobin that has released its oxygen to form HHb, which buffers the hydrogen and makes venous blood slightly more acidic than arterial blood.

bicarbonate or regenerate new bicarbonate from CO_2 and water. The renal mechanism does not act as rapidly as the lungs, but the two systems are very effective together because acid concentration can be rapidly adjusted by the lungs and bicarbonate is easily reabsorbed or regenerated by the kidneys. The pH equation can be symbolically expressed as follows:

$$pH = \frac{Base}{Acid} \text{ or } pH = \frac{Renal\ regulation\ (slow)}{Pulmonary\ regulation\ (fast)}$$

or

$$pH = \frac{Metabolic\ acid\text{-}base\ function}{Respiratory\ acid\text{-}base\ function}$$

Changes in either the numerator or the denominator will change the pH. For example, if the amount of bicarbonate is decreased, the pH also decreases, causing a state of acidosis. The pH can be returned to a normal range if the value of the denominator or the amount of carbonic acid also decreases. This type of adjustment in pH is known as **compensation.** With compensation, a 20:1 ratio may be achieved, but the actual values for HCO_3^- and H_2CO_3 are not normal. The respiratory system compensates for changes in pH by increasing or decreasing ventilation. The renal system compensates by producing more acidic or more alkaline urine. **Correction**

occurs when the values for both components of the buffer pair return to normal (Figure 3-8).

Protein Buffering

Both intracellular and extracellular proteins have negative charges and can serve as buffers for H^+, but because most proteins are inside cells, they are primarily an intracellular buffer system. Hemoglobin (Hb) is an excellent intracellular buffer because of its ability to bind with H^+ (forming HHb) and carbon dioxide (forming $HHbCO_2$). Hemoglobin bound to H^+ becomes a weak acid. Less saturated hemoglobin (venous blood) is a better buffer than hemoglobin saturated with oxygen (arterial blood). The hemoglobin buffer system is illustrated in Figure 3-9.

Renal Buffering

The distal tubule of the kidney regulates acid-base balance by secreting hydrogen into the urine and reabsorbing bicarbonate with a maximum urine acidity of about 4.4 to 4.7.

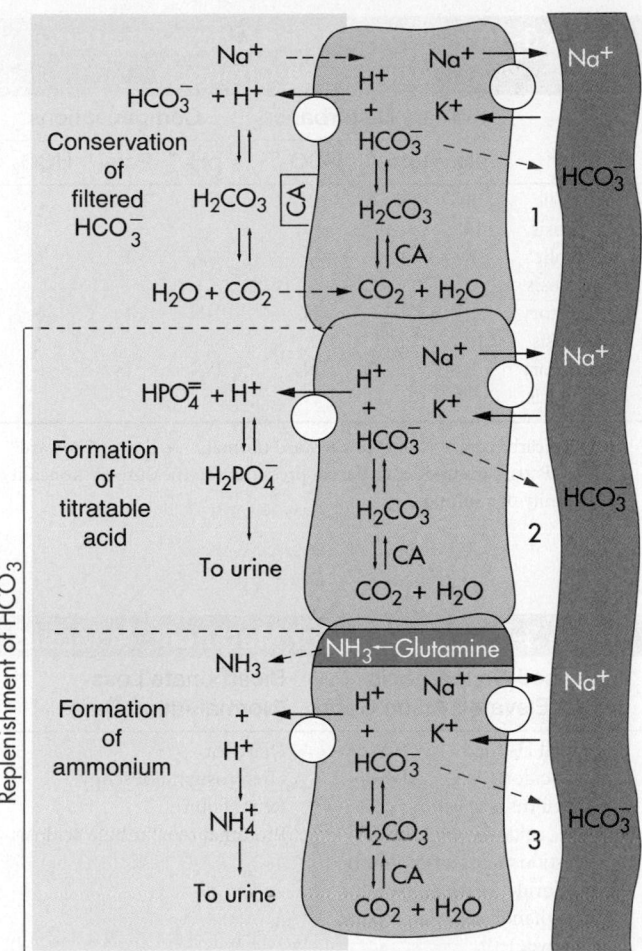

Figure 3-10 Renal excretion of acid. **1,** *Conservation of filtered bicarbonate.* Filtered bicarbonate combines with secreted hydrogen in the presence of carbon anhydrase (CA) to form carbonic acid (H_2CO_3), which then dissociates to water (H_2O) and carbon dioxide (CO_2); both diffuse into the epithelial cell. The CO_2 and H_2O combine to form H_2CO_3 in the presence of CA, and the resulting bicarbonate (HCO_3^-) is reabsorbed into the capillary. **2,** *Formation of titratable acid.* Hydrogen ion is secreted and combines with dibasic phosphate ($HPO_4^=$) to form monobasic phosphate ($H_2PO_4^-$). The secreted hydrogen is formed from the dissociation of H_2CO_3, and the remaining HCO_3^- is reabsorbed into the capillary. **3,** *Formation of ammonium.* Ammonia (NH_3) is produced from glutamine in the epithelial cell and diffuses to the tubular lumen, where it combines with H^+ to form ammonium (NH_4^+). Once NH_4^+ has been formed, it cannot return to the epithelial cell (diffusional trapping), and the bicarbonate remaining in the epithelial cell is reabsorbed into the capillary.

Buffers in the tubular fluid combine with hydrogen ions, allowing more H^+ to be secreted before the limiting pH value is reached. Dibasic phosphate ($HPO_4^=$) and ammonia (NH_3) are two important renal buffers. Dibasic phosphate is filtered at the glomerulus. About 75% is reabsorbed, and the remainder is available for buffering H^+. Secreted H^+ combines with $HPO_4^=$ to form monobasic phosphate ($H_2PO_4^-$). The remaining negative charge on the molecule makes it lipid insoluble, and it cannot diffuse back across the tubular cell and into the blood. Thus it is excreted in the urine (Figure 3-10).

Ammonia (NH_3) is an important renal buffer; it is not ionized (does not carry a charge), and therefore it is lipid soluble

and can cross the cell membrane. The presence of NH_3 in the cell creates a concentration gradient, and it diffuses into the renal tubular fluid, where it combines with hydrogen to form ammonium ion (NH_4^+), which is eliminated in the urine (see Figure 3-10). The renal buffering of hydrogen ions requires the use of CO_2 and H_2O to form H_2CO_3. The enzyme carbonic anhydrase catalyzes the formation of $H^+ + HCO_3^-$. The hydrogen is secreted from the tubular cell and buffered in the lumen by phosphate and ammonia. The bicarbonate is reabsorbed. The end effect is the addition of new bicarbonate, which contributes to the alkalinity of the plasma, because the hydrogen ion is excreted from the body (see Figure 3-10).

Other Buffers

A cellular ion exchange mechanism is also an important buffering system. The best example is the shift of potassium in exchange for hydrogen during states of acidosis or alkalosis. During acidosis, potassium tends to leave the intracellular space in exchange for hydrogen. The reverse occurs during alkalosis. Although the ionic shifts facilitate buffering, the changes in intracellular or extracellular potassium concentrations may have serious consequences.

Acid-Base Imbalances

Pathophysiologic changes in the concentration of hydrogen ion or base in the blood lead to acid-base imbalances. **Acidemia** is a state in which the pH of arterial blood is less than 7.35. A systemic increase in hydrogen ion concentration or loss of base is termed **acidosis. Alkalemia** is a state in which the pH of arterial blood is greater than 7.45. A systemic decrease in hydrogen ion concentration or an excess of base is termed **alkalosis.** Acid-base imbalances may have a metabolic or respiratory etiology or may be of mixed etiology. Figure 3-11 summarizes the relationships among pH, P_{CO_2}, and bicarbonate during different acid-base alterations.

Metabolic Acidosis

PATHOPHYSIOLOGY In **metabolic acidosis,** noncarbonic acids increase or bicarbonate (base) is lost from the extracellular fluid or cannot be regenerated by the kidney (Tables 3-10 and 3-11). This can occur quickly, as in lactic acidosis from poor perfusion or hypoxemia, or more slowly, as in renal failure or diabetic ketoacidosis.

The buffer systems compensate for the excess acid and attempt to maintain the arterial pH within a normal range. Hydrogen ions will move to the intracellular space, and to maintain an ionic balance, potassium will move to the extracellular space (see p. 110). Buffering by bicarbonate lowers the serum value of hydrogen ions and increases the pH. The respiratory system compensates for a metabolic acidosis as the reduced pH stimulates hyperventilation, lowering the $Paco_2$ and the amount of H_2CO_3 circulating in the blood. The kidneys excrete the excess acid as NH_4^+ and titratable acid ($H_2PO_4^-$). When the acidosis is severe, the buffers are unable to compensate for the increasing H^+ load and the pH continues to decrease. The result is a decrease in the 20:1 ratio

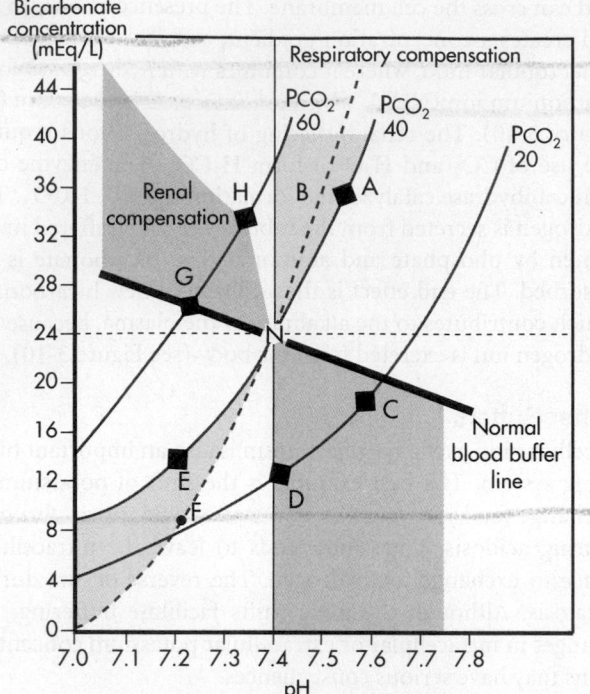

Bicarbonate concentration (mEq/L)

Figure 3-11 Graph of pH, PCO₂, and bicarbonate relationships. *Solid red lines* represent different carbon dioxide partial pressure (PCO₂) values. *Vertical axis* represents bicarbonate concentration, and *horizontal axis* represents acidity or alkalinity (pH) values. Thus for any indicated PCO₂, there is a corresponding pH and bicarbonate concentration. Any point on the graph predicts the required PCO₂, pH, and bicarbonate values. *Dashed horizontal line* shows behavior of bicarbonate as a pure buffer at 24 mEq/L. The *normal blood buffer line* represents values that would be obtained if blood were equilibrated at different CO₂ values. **Point N** represents normal values. **Point A** represents uncompensated metabolic alkalosis, indicated by a normal PCO₂ of 40 and pH greater than 7.4. Respiratory compensation is achieved by hypoventilation, which raises the PCO₂ to **point B** and decreases the pH. Uncompensated respiratory alkalosis is represented by **point C** and reflects hypocapnia (decreased PCO₂). Renal compensation for respiratory alkalosis is increased renal excretion of bicarbonate to normalize pH at **point D**. Uncompensated metabolic acidosis at **point E** represents normal PCO₂ and a decrease in bicarbonate and pH. Respiratory compensation by hyperventilation is indicated by **point F**. Uncompensated respiratory acidosis at **point G** indicates high PCO₂ and low pH values. Renal compensation for chronic high PCO₂ values is indicated by **point H**.

of bicarbonate to carbonic acid (Figure 3-12). In states of ketoacidosis, potassium is redistributed from the intracellular to the extracellular space, and is reabsorbed at the apical membrane of the renal collecting tubule (see p. 110). There is also an increase in levels of ionized calcium as acidosis decreases the amount of calcium bound to albumin (see p. 113).

The evaluation of the **anion gap** can be helpful when used cautiously to distinguish different types of metabolic acidosis.[24] Normally, the concentrations of cations and anions in the plasma are equivalent. Some anions, such as protein, sulfates, phosphates, and organic acids, however, are not measured in the common laboratory evaluations of the blood. Therefore the normal anion gap represents these unmeasured negative ions (sulfate, phosphate, lactate, ketoacids, albumin).

Table 3-10	**Primary and Compensatory Acid-Base Changes**					
	Primary Disturbance			**Compensations**		
	pH	Pco₂	HCO₃⁻	pH	Pco₂	HCO₃⁻
Metabolic acidosis	↓	N	↓	↑-N	↓	↓
Metabolic alkalosis	↑	N	↑	↓-N	↑	↑
Respiratory acidosis	↓	↑	N	↑-N	↑	↑
Respiratory alkalosis	↑	↓	N	↓-N	↓	↓

HCO₃⁻, bicarbonate; *↑-N,* increase toward normal; *↓-N,* decrease toward normal; *Pco₂,* carbon dioxide partial pressure; *pH,* measure of the acidity or alkalinity of a solution.

Table 3-11	**Causes of Metabolic Acidosis**
Increased Noncarbonic Acids (Elevated Anion Gap)	**Bicarbonate Loss (Normal Anion Gap)**
Increased H⁺ load	Diarrhea
Ketoacidosis (e.g., diabetes	Ureterosigmoidoscopy
mellitus, starvation)	Renal failure
Lactic acidosis (e.g., shock)	Proximal renal tubule acidosis
Ingestions (e.g., ammonium	
chloride, ethylene glycol,	
methanol, salicylates, paral-	
dehyde)	
Decreased H⁺ excretion	
Uremia	
Distal renal tubule acidosis	

A convenient measure of the anion gap is the difference between the sum of Na^+ and K^+ and the sum of HCO_3^- and Cl^-, or about 10 to 12 mEq:

$$\text{Anion gap} = [Na^+\,(140) + K^+\,(4.0)] - [HCO_3\,(24) + Cl^=\,(110)] = 10\text{-}12 \text{ mEq/L}$$

In metabolic acidosis a **normal anion gap** is characteristic of conditions related to bicarbonate loss with retention of chloride to maintain an ionic balance. This is called **hyperchloremic metabolic acidosis.** An elevated anion gap is characteristic of acidosis associated with accumulation of anions other than chloride (see Table 3-11).

CLINICAL MANIFESTATIONS Metabolic acidosis is manifested by changes in the neurologic, respiratory, gastrointestinal, and cardiovascular systems. Headache and lethargy are early symptoms, which progress to coma with severe acidosis. Deep, rapid respirations (Kussmaul respirations) are indicative of respiratory compensation. Anorexia, nausea, vomiting, diarrhea, and abdominal discomfort are common. Severe acidosis can compromise ventricular contraction and produce life-threatening dysrhythmias and hypotension.

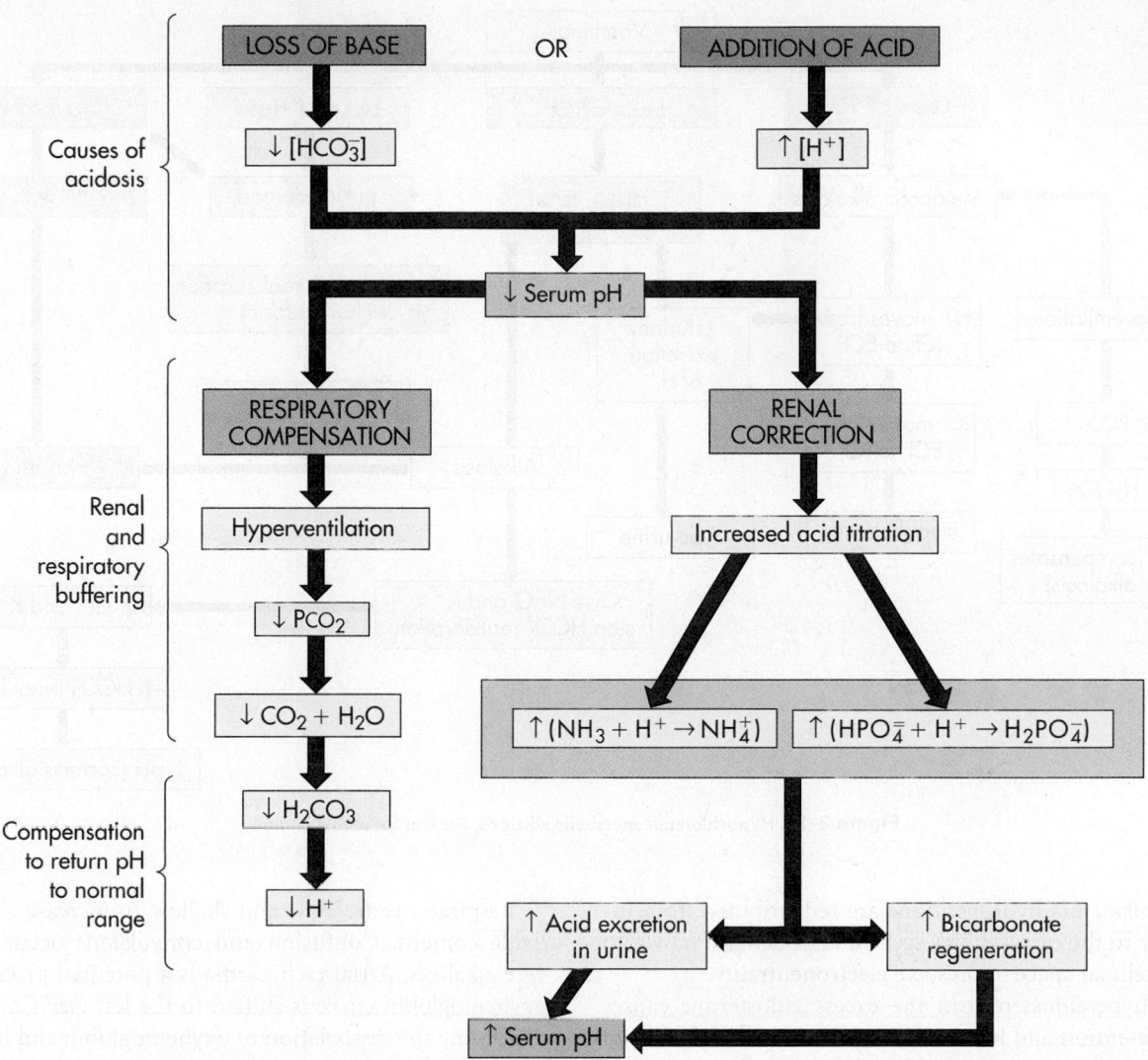

Figure 3-12 Metabolic acidosis with compensation and correction. See text for abbreviations.

EVALUATION AND TREATMENT The diagnosis of metabolic acidosis is established from the health history, clinical symptoms, and laboratory findings. Arterial blood pH is below 7.35, and bicarbonate concentration is less than 24 mEq/L. The anion gap can isolate the specific cause. The underlying condition must be diagnosed to establish effective treatment. During severe acidosis (pH ≤7.1), bicarbonate administration is required to elevate the pH to a safe level, particularly if there is renal failure. Accompanying sodium and water deficits must also be corrected.[25]

Metabolic Alkalosis

PATHOPHYSIOLOGY Metabolic alkalosis is common and occurs when bicarbonate is increased, usually caused by excessive loss of metabolic acids. Among the conditions that can result in metabolic alkalosis are prolonged vomiting, gastrointestinal suctioning, excessive bicarbonate intake, hyperaldosteronism with hypokalemia, and diuretic therapy.[26]

When acid loss is caused by vomiting with depletion of ECF and chloride (**hypochloremic metabolic alkalosis**), renal compensation is not very effective because the volume depletion and loss of electrolytes (Na^+, K^+, H^+, Cl^-) stimulate a paradoxical response by the kidneys. The kidneys increase sodium and bicarbonate reabsorption with excretion of hydrogen. Bicarbonate is reabsorbed to maintain an anionic balance because the ECF chloride concentration is decreased. When the potassium concentration is depleted, hydrogen moves to the intracellular space and is excreted to maintain an electrochemical balance. The urine is acidic, and the reabsorbed bicarbonate prevents correction of the alkalosis (Figure 3-13). Correction is achieved when the ECF is expanded with a solution of sodium chloride and potassium. The volume replacement decreases the renal stimulus to reabsorb Na^+, and chloride as an anion is replaced. Bicarbonate then can be lost in the urine, and hydrogen ion excretion decreases, correcting the pH.

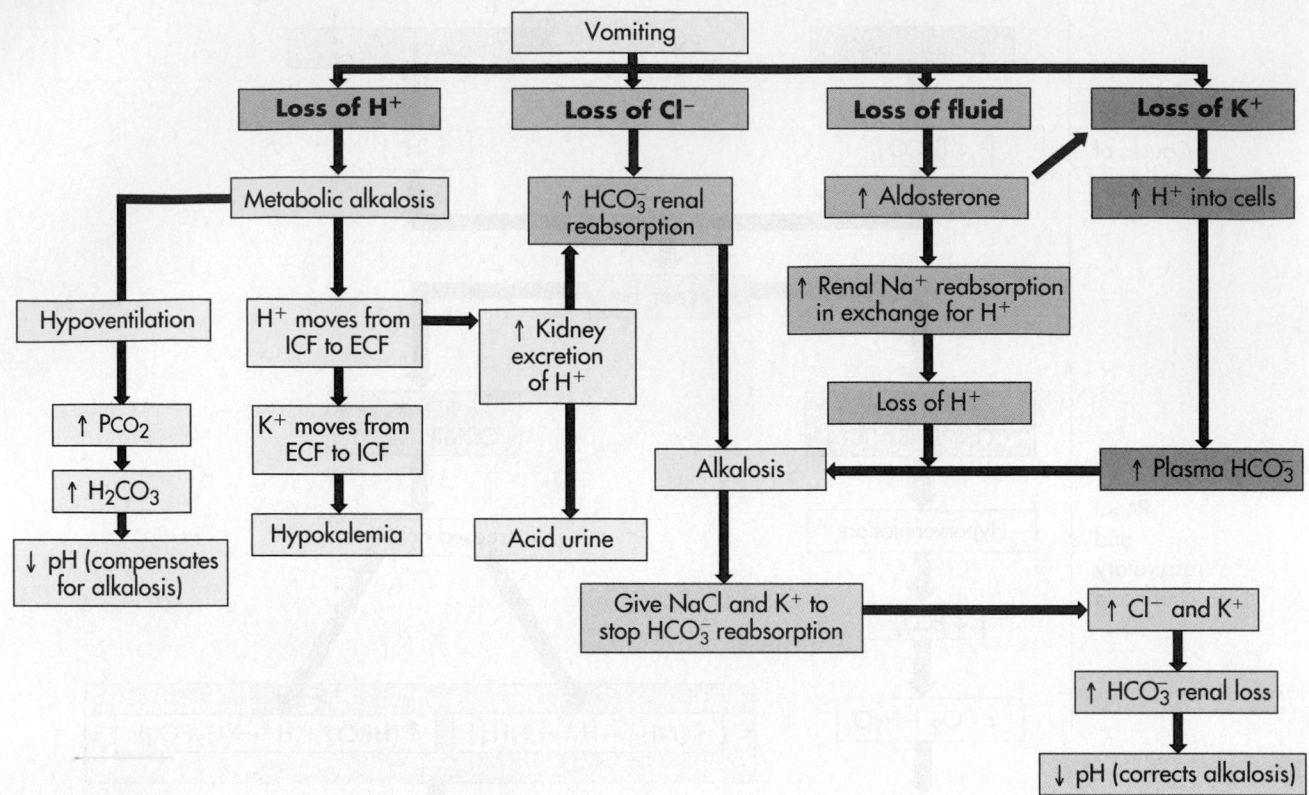

Figure 3-13 Hypochloremic metabolic alkalosis. See text for abbreviations.

With alkalemia hydrogen ions are redistributed from intracellular to the extracellular space and potassium moves to the intracellular space to preserve electroneutrality.

With hyperaldosteronism the excess aldosterone causes sodium retention and loss of hydrogen and potassium. Mild volume expansion ensues, and bicarbonate is retained along with the sodium, thereby causing alkalosis.

Diuretics, such as thiazides, ethacrynic acid, and furosemide, produce mild alkalosis by enhancing sodium, potassium, and chloride excretion more than bicarbonate excretion.

Respiratory compensation for metabolic alkalosis occurs when the elevated pH inhibits the respiratory center. The rate and depth of ventilation are decreased, causing retention of carbon dioxide. The ratio of HCO_3^- to H_2CO_3 is reduced toward normal. Respiratory compensation is not very efficient, however, and chronic or severe metabolic alkalosis requires therapeutic intervention (Figure 3-14).

CLINICAL MANIFESTATIONS Because of the many causes of metabolic alkalosis, the symptoms vary. Some common symptoms, such as weakness, muscle cramps, and hyperactive reflexes, are related to volume depletion and electrolyte losses. Because alkalosis increases binding of Ca^{++} to plasma proteins (albumin), ionized calcium decreases, causing excitable cells to become hypopolarized, which initiates an action potential more easily. Paresthesias, numbness/tingling of the fingertips and perioral area, tetany, and seizures may develop (see Hypocalcemia, p. 112).

Respirations are slow and shallow to increase carbon dioxide content. Confusion and convulsions occur with severe alkalosis. Atrial tachycardia is a potential problem. The oxyhemoglobin curve is shifted to the left (see Chapter 32), decreasing the dissociation of oxyhemoglobin and increasing the risk of dysrhythmias.

EVALUATION AND TREATMENT The health history provides significant clues to the diagnosis of metabolic alkalosis. The arterial pH is greater than 7.45, and bicarbonate levels exceed 26 mEq/L. With respiratory compensation, the Pco_2 rises above 40 mmHg. With hypochloremic alkalosis, serum chloride values are below normal. Serum potassium levels are usually depleted because hydrogen is released from the cells in exchange for potassium to help regulate the pH level. The K^+ is then secreted from renal distal tubule cells into the urine.

With hypochloremic alkalosis or contraction alkalosis with volume depletion, a sodium chloride solution is required for correction. The renal stimulus to increase ECF volume by retaining Na^+ is diminished, and HCO_3^- can be excreted as $NaHCO_3$ in the urine. The administration of potassium corrects alkalosis caused by hyperaldosteronism or hypokalemia. The potassium causes hydrogen to move back into the ECF and decreases loss of hydrogen from the distal tubule.

Respiratory Acidosis

PATHOPHYSIOLOGY Respiratory disorders of acid-base balance are caused by increases or decreases of alveolar ventilation in relation to the metabolic production of carbon

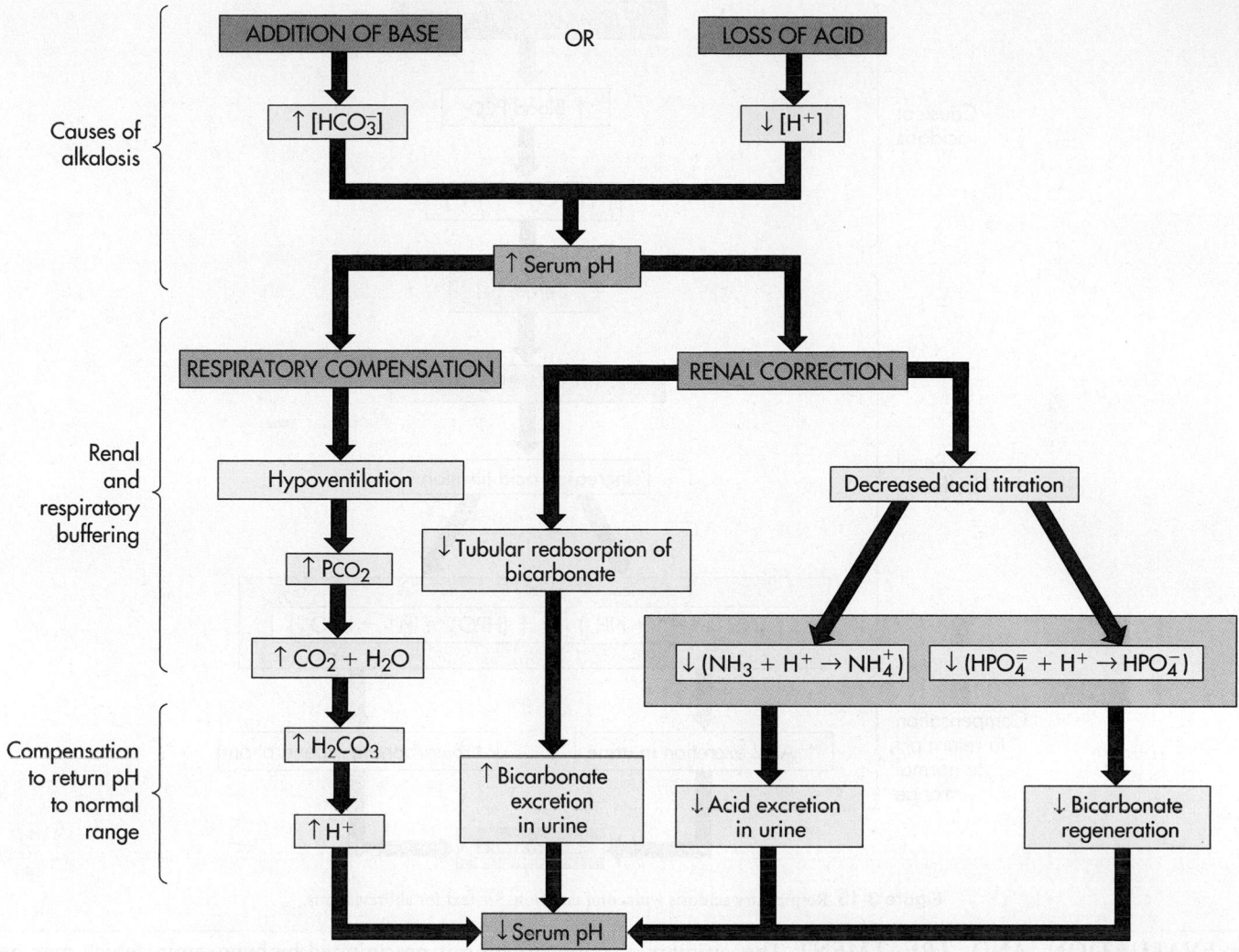

Figure 3-14 Metabolic alkalosis with compensation and correction. See text for abbreviations.

dioxide. **Respiratory acidosis** occurs when there is alveolar hypoventilation. Carbon dioxide is retained, increasing [H+] (as H_2CO_3) and producing acidosis. Carbon dioxide excess is called **hypercapnia**. The common causes include depression of the respiratory center (brainstem trauma, oversedation), respiratory muscle paralysis, disorders of the chest wall (kyphoscoliosis, pickwickian syndrome, flail chest), and disorders of the lung parenchyma (pneumonitis, pulmonary edema, emphysema, asthma, bronchitis).

Respiratory acidosis may be acute or chronic. Airway obstruction is the most common cause of acute respiratory acidosis. Acute compensation for respiratory acidosis is not effective because the renal buffer mechanism takes time to function. Further, the protein buffers provide marginal compensation, and HCO_3^- is not a good buffer for CO_2. Acute uncompensated respiratory acidosis is characterized by decreased arterial pH, elevated P_{CO_2}, and normal or slightly increased bicarbonate.

Chronic respiratory acidosis is commonly associated with chronic obstructive pulmonary disease and deformities of the chest wall or neuromuscular disorders. Renal compensation is effective and is established over several days. The acidosis produced from CO_2 retention stimulates the kidney to secrete hydrogen ions and regenerate bicarbonate. Serum bicarbonate and arterial P_{CO_2} are elevated, and pH is restored toward normal (Figure 3-15).

CLINICAL MANIFESTATIONS The symptoms of respiratory acidosis are related to acuity of onset and severity of P_{CO_2} retention. Initial symptoms include headache, restlessness, blurred vision, and apprehension followed by lethargy, muscle twitching, tremors, convulsions, and coma. Neurologic symptoms are caused by a decrease in the pH of cerebrospinal fluid and vasodilation because CO_2 readily crosses the blood-brain barrier. The respiratory rate is rapid at first and gradually becomes depressed because over time, the respiratory center adapts to increasing levels of CO_2. Cyanosis does not occur unless there is an accompanying hypoxemia, and the skin may instead be pink from vasodilation caused by the elevated CO_2.

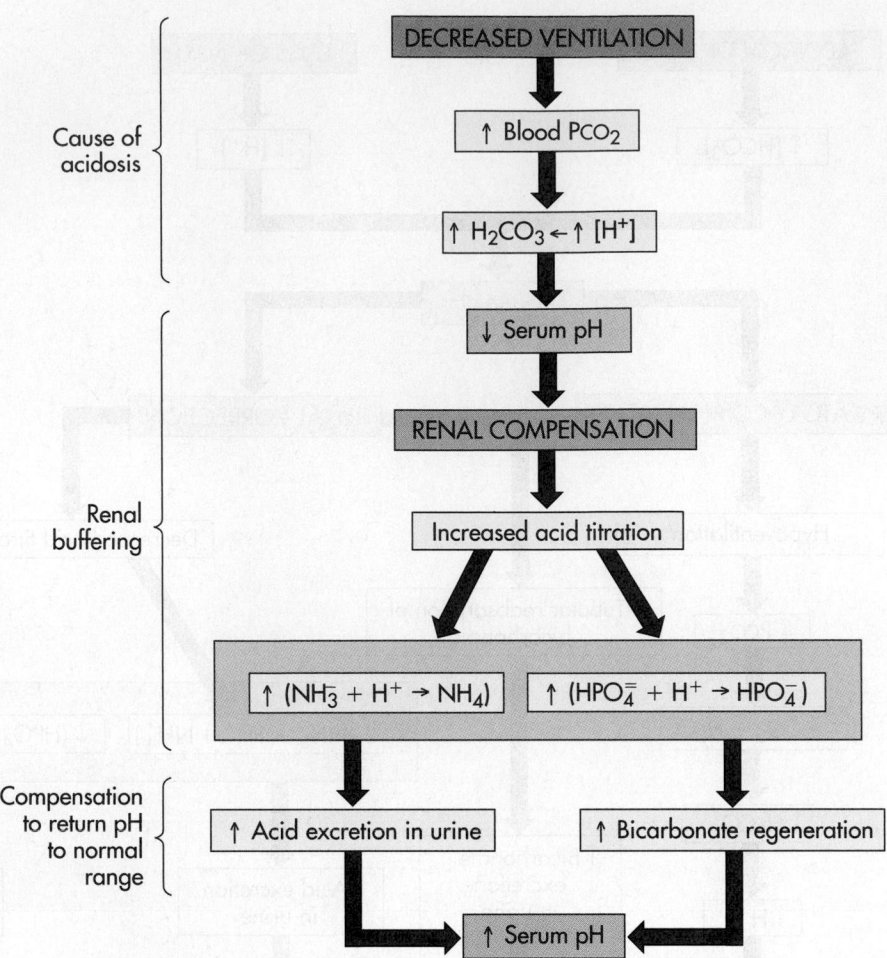

Figure 3-15 Respiratory acidosis with compensation. See text for abbreviations.

EVALUATION AND TREATMENT The primary diagnostic indicators are an arterial pH less than 7.35 and hypercapnia. Acute respiratory acidosis must be distinguished from chronic acidosis; the health history and clinical laboratory data are therefore helpful. With renal compensation, bicarbonate levels are elevated and the pH is restored toward normal.

The restoration of adequate alveolar ventilation removes excess CO_2. If alveolar ventilation cannot be maintained spontaneously because of drug overdose or neuromuscular disorders, mechanical ventilation is required. The arterial pH, P_{CO_2}, P_{O_2}, and HCO_3^- must be carefully monitored. Rapid reduction of P_{CO_2} can cause respiratory alkalosis with seizures and death.

Renal buffering is usually effective in compensating for uncomplicated chronic respiratory acidosis. The underlying diseases are treated to achieve maximal ventilation. In the presence of hypoxemia and hypercapnia, oxygen can function as a respiratory depressant when the respiratory center is no longer stimulated by the lower pH and elevated P_{CO_2}. Therefore, oxygen should be given cautiously.

Respiratory Alkalosis
PATHOPHYSIOLOGY Respiratory alkalosis occurs when there is alveolar hyperventilation and decreased plasma carbon dioxide (termed **hypocapnia**). Stimulation of ventilation is precipitated by hypoxemia, which may be caused by pulmonary disease, congestive heart failure, or high altitudes; hypermetabolic states such as fever, anemia, and thyrotoxicosis; early salicylate intoxication; hysteria; cirrhosis; and gram-negative sepsis. Improper use of mechanical ventilators can cause iatrogenic respiratory alkalosis. Secondary respiratory alkalosis may develop from hyperventilation stimulated by metabolic or respiratory acidosis.

The onset of acute respiratory alkalosis occurs within minutes of hyperventilation. Cellular buffers provide immediate compensation with shifts of H^+ from ICF to ECF. The H^+ shifts are not very effective, however, if P_{CO_2} is significantly decreased. When chronic respiratory alkalosis is present, renal compensation restores pH toward normal by decreasing H^+ excretion and bicarbonate absorption (Figure 3-16).

CLINICAL MANIFESTATIONS Respiratory alkalosis, like metabolic alkalosis, is irritating to the central and peripheral nervous systems. Symptoms include dizziness, confusion, tingling of extremities (paresthesias), convulsions, and coma. Carpopedal spasm and other symptoms of hypocalcemia are similar to those of metabolic alkalosis (see p. 120). Deep and rapid respirations (tachypnea) are primary symptoms that cause respiratory alkalosis.

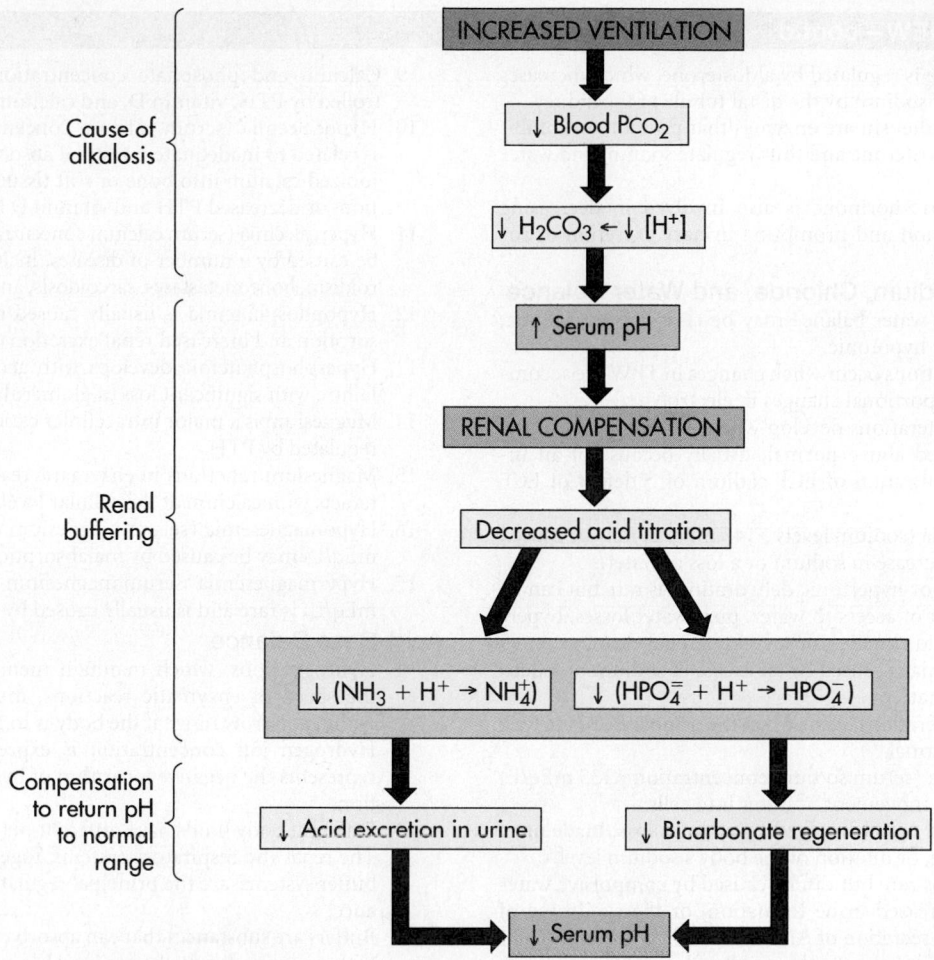

Figure 3-16 Respiratory alkalosis with compensation. See text for abbreviations.

EVALUATION AND TREATMENT The underlying disturbance must be identified. The arterial pH is greater than 7.45, and the Pa_{CO_2} is less than 38 mmHg. In acute states, bicarbonate levels are normal. With chronic respiratory alkalosis, a compensatory decrease in the bicarbonate level occurs and the pH is closer to normal.

Treating the underlying disturbance is the most effective treatment. Hypoxemia must be corrected and hypermetabolic states reversed. Symptoms from hysterical hyperventilation can be corrected by rebreathing from a paper bag, which increases the concentration of inspired carbon dioxide and reverses the respiratory alkalosis.

SUMMARY REVIEW

Distribution of Body Fluids
1. Body fluids are distributed among functional compartments and are classified as ICF or ECF.
2. The sum of all fluids is the TBW, which varies with age and amount of body fat.
3. Water moves between the ICF and ECF compartments principally by osmosis.
4. Water moves between the plasma and interstitial fluid by osmosis and hydrostatic pressure, which occur across the capillary membrane.
5. Movement across the capillary wall is called *net filtration* and is described according to the Starling law.

Alterations in Water Movement
1. Edema is a problem of fluid distribution that results in accumulation of fluid within the interstitial spaces.

2. Edema is caused by arterial dilation, venous or lymphatic obstruction, loss of plasma proteins, increased capillary permeability, and increased vascular volume.
3. The pathophysiologic process that leads to edema is related to an increase in forces favoring fluid filtration from the capillaries or lymphatic channels into the tissues.
4. Edema may be localized or generalized and usually is associated with weight gain, swelling and puffiness, tighter-fitting clothes and shoes, and limited movement of the affected area.

Sodium, Chloride, and Water Balance
1. Sodium and water balance are intimately related; chloride levels are generally proportional to changes in sodium levels.
2. Water balance is regulated by the sensation of thirst and by antidiuretic hormone, which is initiated by an increase in plasma osmolality or a decrease in circulating blood volume.

3. Sodium balance is regulated by aldosterone, which increases reabsorption of sodium by the distal tubule of the kidney.

4. Renin and angiotensin are enzymes that promote or inhibit secretion of aldosterone and thus regulate sodium and water balance.

5. Atrial natriuretic hormone is also involved in decreasing tubular resorption and promoting urinary excretion of sodium.

Alterations in Sodium, Chloride, and Water Balance

1. Alterations in water balance may be classified as isotonic, hypertonic, or hypotonic.

2. Isotonic alterations occur when changes in TBW are accompanied by proportional changes in electrolytes.

3. Hypertonic alterations develop when the osmolality of the ECF is elevated above normal, usually because of an increased concentration of ECF sodium or a deficit of ECF water.

4. Hypernatremia (sodium levels >147 mEq/L) may be caused by an acute increase in sodium or a loss of water.

5. Water deficit, or hypertonic dehydration, is rare but can be caused by lack of access to water, pure water losses, hyperventilation, arid climates, or increased renal clearance.

6. Hyperchloremia is caused by an excess of sodium or a deficit of bicarbonate.

7. Hypotonic alterations occur when the osmolality of the ECF is less than normal.

8. Hyponatremia (serum sodium concentration <135 mEq/L) usually causes movement of water into cells.

9. Hyponatremia may be caused by sodium loss, inadequate sodium intake, or dilution of the body's sodium level.

10. Water excess is rare but can be caused by compulsive water drinking, decreased urine formation, or the syndrome of inappropriate secretion of ADH.

11. Hypochloremia is usually the result of hyponatremia or elevated bicarbonate concentrations.

Alterations in Potassium, Calcium, Phosphate, and Magnesium Balance

1. Potassium is the predominant ICF ion; it functions to regulate ICF osmolality, maintain the resting membrane potential, and deposit glycogen in liver and skeletal muscle cells.

2. Potassium balance is regulated by the kidney, by aldosterone and insulin secretion, and by changes in pH.

3. A mechanism known as *potassium adaptation* allows the body to accommodate slowly to increased levels of potassium intake.

4. Hypokalemia (serum potassium concentration <3.5 mEq/L) indicates loss of total body potassium, although ECF hypokalemia can develop without losses of total body potassium and plasma K^+ levels may be normal or elevated when total body potassium is depleted.

5. Hypokalemia may be caused by reduced potassium intake, increased ICF-to-ECF potassium concentration, loss of potassium from body stores, increased aldosterone secretion (e.g., caused by hypernatremia), and increased renal excretion.

6. Hyperkalemia (potassium levels >5.5 mEq/L) may be caused by increased potassium intake, a shift from ICF to ECF potassium, or decreased renal excretion.

7. Calcium is a necessary ion in the structure of bones and teeth, in blood clotting, in hormone secretion and the function of cell receptors, and in membrane stability.

8. Phosphate acts as a buffer in acid-base regulation and provides energy for muscle contraction.

9. Calcium and phosphate concentrations are rigidly controlled by PTH, vitamin D, and calcitonin.

10. Hypocalcemia (serum calcium concentration <8.5 mg/dl) is related to inadequate intestinal absorption, deposition of ionized calcium into bone or soft tissue, blood administration, or decreased PTH and vitamin D levels.

11. Hypercalcemia (serum calcium concentration >12 mg/dl) can be caused by a number of diseases, including hyperparathyroidism, bone metastases, sarcoidosis, and excess vitamin D.

12. Hypophosphatemia is usually caused by intestinal malabsorption and increased renal excretion of phosphate.

13. Hyperphosphatemia develops with acute or chronic renal failure with significant loss of glomerular filtration.

14. Magnesium is a major intracellular cation and is principally regulated by PTH.

15. Magnesium functions in enzymatic reactions and often interacts with calcium at the cellular level.

16. Hypomagnesemia (serum magnesium concentrations <1.5 mEq/L) may be caused by malabsorption syndromes.

17. Hypermagnesemia (serum magnesium concentrations >2.5 mEq/L) is rare and is usually caused by renal failure.

Acid-Base Balance

1. Hydrogen ions, which maintain membrane integrity and the speed of enzymatic reactions, must be concentrated within a narrow range if the body is to function normally.

2. Hydrogen ion concentration is expressed as pH, which represents the negative logarithm of hydrogen ions in solution.

3. Different body fluids have different pH values.

4. The renal and respiratory systems, together with the body's buffer systems, are the principal regulators of acid-base balance.

5. Buffers are substances that can absorb excessive acid or base without a significant change in pH.

6. Buffers exist as acid-base pairs; the principal plasma buffers are carbonic acid–bicarbonate, protein (hemoglobin), and phosphate.

7. Buffer pairs can associate and dissociate; the pK value is the pH at which a buffer pair is half dissociated.

8. The lungs and kidneys act to compensate for changes in pH by increasing or decreasing ventilation and by producing more acidic or more alkaline urine.

9. Correction is a process different from compensation; correction occurs when the values for both components of the buffer pair are returned to normal.

10. Acid-base imbalances are caused by changes in the concentration of H^+ in the blood; an increase causes acidosis, and a decrease causes alkalosis.

11. An abnormal increase or decrease in bicarbonate concentration causes metabolic acidosis or metabolic alkalosis; changes in the rate of alveolar ventilation produce respiratory acidosis or respiratory alkalosis.

12. Metabolic acidosis is caused by an increase in noncarbonic acids or loss of bicarbonate from the extracellular fluid.

13. Metabolic alkalosis occurs with an increase in bicarbonate usually caused by loss of metabolic acids from conditions such as vomiting, gastrointestinal suctioning, excessive bicarbonate intake, hyperaldosteronism, and diuretic therapy.

14. Respiratory acidosis occurs with a decrease of alveolar ventilation and an increase in levels of carbon dioxide, which in turn causes hypercapnia.

15. Respiratory alkalosis occurs with alveolar hyperventilation and excessive reduction of carbon dioxide, or hypocapnia.

KEY TERMS

Acidemia, 117
Acidosis, 117
Aldosterone, 101
Alkalemia, 117
Alkalosis, 117
Angiotensin I and II, 101
Anion gap, 118
Aquaporins, 97
Baroreceptors, 102
Buffering, 115
Buffers, 115
Calcitonin, 112
Calcium, 111
Chloride, 102
Compensation, 116
Compulsive water drinking, 106
Correction, 116
Decreased urine formation, 106
Dehydration, 104
Dilutional hyponatremia, 105
Edema, 98
Extracellular fluid (ECF), 96
Familial hypokalemic periodic paralysis, 108
Hypercalcemia, 113
Hypercapnia, 121
Hyperchloremia, 106

Hyperchloremic metabolic acidosis, 118
Hyperkalemia, 110
Hypermagnesemia, 114
Hypernatremia, 104
Hyperphosphatemia, 113
Hyperpolarized, 109
Hypertonic hyponatremia, 105
Hypocalcemia, 112
Hypocapnia, 122
Hypochloremia, 106
Hypochloremic metabolic alkalosis, 119
Hypokalemia, 108
Hypomagnesemia, 114
Hyponatremia, 104
Hypophosphatemia, 113
Hypopolarized, 110
Hypotonic hyponatremia, 105
Hypovolemia, 106
Inadequate intake, 105
Interstitial fluid, 98
Intracellular fluid (ICF), 96
Intravascular fluid, 96
Lymphedema, 100
Magnesium, 114
Metabolic acidosis, 117
Metabolic alkalosis, 119

Natriuretic peptides, 102
Net filtration, 98
Nonvolatile, 114
Normal anion gap, 118
Osmoreceptors, 102
Parathyroid hormone, 111
Phosphate, 111
Potassium adaptation, 107
Pure sodium deficits, 105
Renin, 101
Renin-angiotensin-aldosterone system, 102
Respiratory acidosis, 121
Respiratory alkalosis, 122
Sodium, 101
Starling hypothesis, 98
Syndrome of inappropriate secretion of ADH (SIADH), 106
Total body water (TBW), 97
Vasopressin dysregulation, 106
Vitamin D, 111
Volatile, 114
Volume-sensitive receptors, 102
Water deficits, 104
Water intoxication, 104

REFERENCES

1. Allison SP, Lobo DN: Fluid and electrolytes in the elderly, *Curr Opin Clin Nutr Metab Care* 7(1):27-33, 2004.
2. Fu D, Lu M: The structural basis of water permeation and proton exclusion in aquaporins, *Mol Membr Biol* 24(5-6):366-374, 2007.
3. Warren AG et al: Lymphedema: a comprehensive review, *Ann Plast Surg* 59(4):464-472, 2007.
4. Lee CY, Burnett JC Jr: Natriuretic peptides and therapeutic applications, *Heart Fail Rev* 12(2):131-142, 2007.
5. Achinger SG, Moritz ML, Ayus JC: Dysnatremias: why are patients still dying? *South Med J* 99(4):353-362, 2006.
6. Offenstadt G, Das V: Hyponatremia, hypernatremia: a physiological approach, *Minerva Anestesiol* 72(6):353-356, 2006.
7. Yeates KE, Singer M, Morton AR: Salt and water: a simple approach to hyponatremia, *CMAJ* 170(3):365-369, 2004.
8. Decaux G, Soupart A: Treatment of symptomatic hyponatremia, *Am J Med Sci* 326(1):25-30, 2003.
9. Multz AS: Vasopressin dysregulation and hyponatremia in hospitalized patients, *J Intensive Care Med* 22(4):216-223, 2007.
10. Lien YH, Shapiro JI: Hyponatremia: clinical diagnosis and management, *Am J Med* 120(8):653-658, 2007.
11. Wang W: Regulation of renal K transported by dietary K intake, *Annu Rev Physiol* 66:547-569, 2004.
12. Gennari FJ: Disorders of potassium homeostasis, hypokalemia and hyperkalemia, *Crit Care Clin* 18(2):273-288, vi, 2002.
13. Koeppen BM, Stanton BA: *Renal physiology*, Philadelphia, 2007, Mosby, p 116.

14. Alazami M et al: Unusual causes of hypokalaemia and paralysis, *QJM* 99(3):181-192, 2006.
15. Alfonzo AV et al: Potassium disorders—clinical spectrum and emergency management, *Resuscitation* 70(1):10-25, 2006.
16. Parham WA et al: Hyperkalemia revisited, *Tex Heart Inst J* 33(1):40-47, 2006.
17. Brunelli SM, Goldfarb S: Hypophosphatemia: clinical consequences and management, *J Am Soc Nephrol* 18(7):1999-2003, 2007.
18. Albaaj F, Hutchison A: Hyperphosphataemia in renal failure: causes, consequences and current management, *Drugs* 63(6):577-596, 2003.
19. Salusky IB: A new era in phosphate binder therapy: what are the options? *Kidney Int Suppl* (105):S10-S15, 2006.
20. Mouw DR, Latessa RA, Sullo EJ: What are the causes of hypomagnesemia? *J Fam Pract* 54(2), 2005.
21. Laires MH, Monteiro CP, Bicho M: Role of cellular magnesium in health and human disease, *Front Biosci* 9:262-276, 2004.
22. Onishi S, Yoshino S: Cathartic-induced fatal hypermagnesemia in the elderly, *Intern Med* 45(4):207-210, 2006.
23. Rose DB, Post T: *Clinical physiology of acid-base and electrolyte disorders*, ed 5, New York, 2001, McGraw-Hill.
24. Kraut JA, Madias NE: Serum anion gap: its uses and limitations in clinical medicine, *Clin J Am Soc Nephrol* 2(1):162-174, 2006.
25. Adrogué HJ: Metabolic acidosis: pathophysiology, diagnosis and management, *J Nephrol* 19(Suppl 9):S62-S69, 2006.
26. Khanna A, Kurtzman NA: Metabolic alkalosis, *J Nephrol* 19(Suppl 9):S86-S96, 2006.

GENES AND GENETIC DISEASES

CHAPTER

4

LYNN B. JORDE

MEDIA RESOURCES

 Evolve Website (http://evolve.elsevier.com/McCance/)
- Review Questions and Answers
- Animations
- Glossary (with audio pronunciation for selected terms)
- WebLinks

Online Course
- Module 3

CHAPTER OUTLINE

DNA, RNA, AND PROTEINS: HEREDITY AT THE MOLECULAR LEVEL
DNA
From Genes to Proteins
CHROMOSOMES
Chromosome Aberrations and Associated Diseases
ELEMENTS OF FORMAL GENETICS
Phenotype and Genotype
Dominance and Recessiveness

TRANSMISSION OF GENETIC DISEASES
Autosomal Dominant Inheritance
Autosomal Recessive Inheritance
X-Linked Inheritance
Evaluation of Pedigrees
LINKAGE ANALYSIS AND GENE MAPPING
Classical Pedigree Analysis
Assigning Loci to Specific Chromosomes
Complete Human Gene Map: Prospects and Benefits

In the nineteenth century, microscopic studies of cells led scientists to suspect that the nucleus of the cell contained the important mechanisms of inheritance. Scientists found that chromatin, the substance that gives the nucleus a granular appearance, is observable in nondividing cells. Just before the cell divides, the chromatin condenses to form discrete, dark-staining organelles called chromosomes. (Cell division is discussed in Chapter 1.) With the rediscovery of Gregor Mendel's important breeding experiments at the turn of the twentieth century, it soon became apparent that the chromosomes contained **genes**, the basic units of inheritance. Chromosomes were the subject of much study, but because of poorly developed laboratory techniques, progress was slow. Since the mid-1950s, however, technologic advances have permitted a rapid increase in scientific knowledge of the form, composition, and function of chromosomes.

The primary constituent of the chromatin is **deoxyribonucleic acid (DNA).** Genes are composed of sequences of DNA. By serving as the blueprints of proteins in the body, genes ultimately influence all aspects of body structure and function. Estimates suggest that there are approximately 20,000 to 25,000 genes. An error in one of these genes can lead to a recognizable genetic disease.

To date, more than 15,000 genetic conditions have been identified and cataloged.[1] As infectious diseases come under increasingly effective control, the proportion of beds in pediatric hospitals occupied by children with genetic diseases has risen to one third.[2] In addition, many common diseases that affect primarily adults, such as hypertension, coronary heart disease, diabetes, and cancer, are now known to have important genetic components. (These diseases are also affected by environmental factors. The interaction between genetic and environmental components is discussed in Chapter 5.)

Great progress is being made in the diagnosis of genetic diseases and the understanding of genetic mechanisms underlying them. With the huge strides being made in molecular genetics, gene therapy—the direct alteration of genes in cells—has begun. Genetics is now one of the most rapidly advancing fields of medicine (Box 4-1).

| Box 4-1 | Genetic Engineering and Gene Therapy: The "New Genetics" |

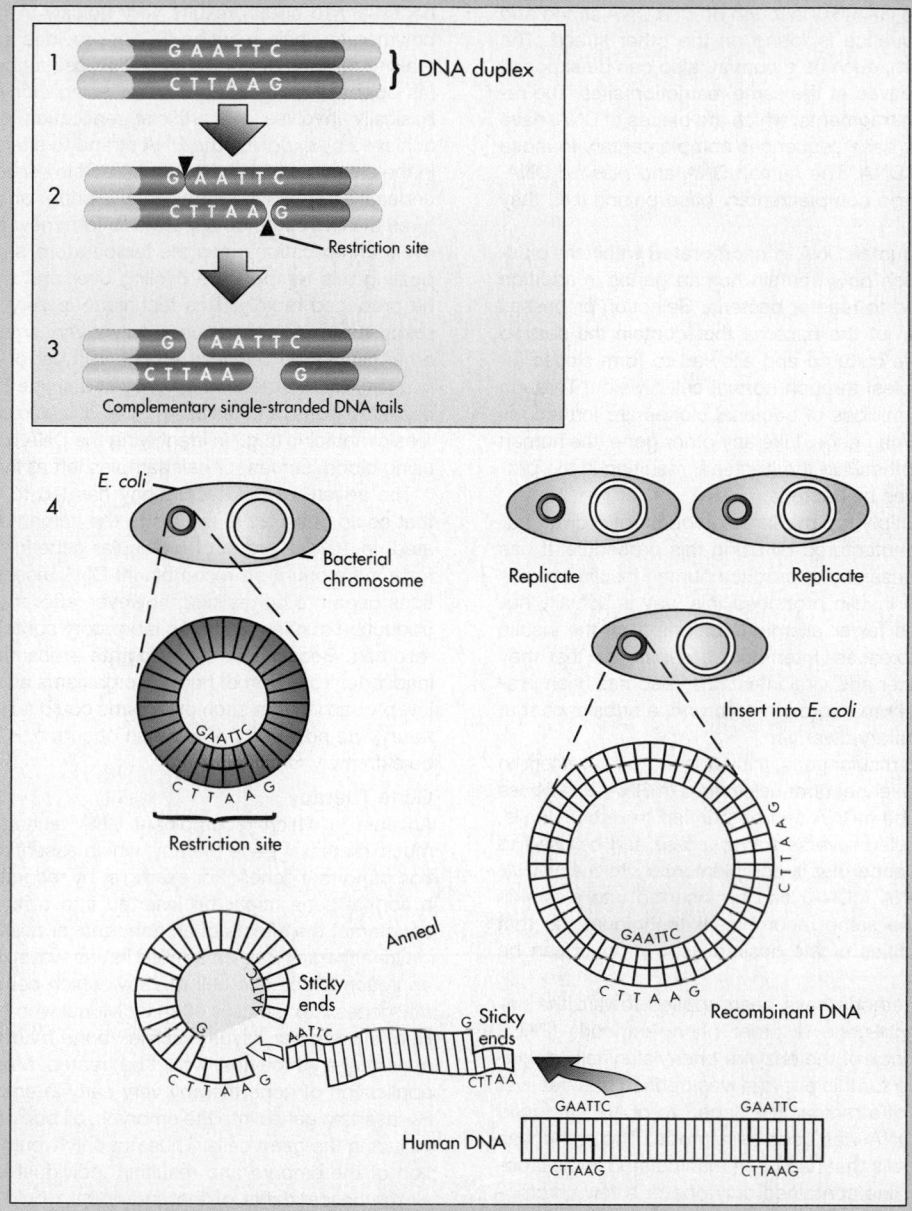

Recombinant DNA technology. Human DNA and circular plasmid DNA are both cleaved by a restriction enzyme, producing sticky ends (1 to 3). This allows the human DNA to anneal and recombine with the plasmid DNA. Inserted into the plasmid DNA, the human DNA is now replicated when plasmid is inserted into the bacterium, such as *E. coli* (4). *G*, Guanine; *A*, adenine; *T*, thymine; *C*, cytosine. (From Jorde LB et al: *Medical genetics*, ed 3, St Louis, 2003, Mosby.)

Terms such as *cloning, genetic engineering,* and *recombinant DNA* have received much exposure in the popular press during the past several years as the news media have recognized the potential importance of these techniques. Indeed they are part of the scientific revolution sometimes known as the *new genetics.*

Recombinant DNA
Genetic engineering refers to laboratory alteration of genes. Most alterations are accomplished by using recombinant DNA techniques, which involve combining the DNA of two or more different organisms. A number of sophisticated methods have been invented to do this; described here is a common approach that is similar in principle to most other approaches.

Among the key components of recombinant DNA research are bacterial plasmids—small, circular pieces of self-replicating DNA that reside in many bacteria but often are not essential to the growth or survival of the bacteria. Plasmids can therefore be extracted from or inserted into bacteria without seriously disrupting bacterial growth or reproduction. Once they are extracted from their bacterial hosts, the plasmids are exposed to restriction endonucleases, which are enzymes that cleave, or cut, the plasmid DNA at a specific nucleotide sequence, called a *restriction site.*

Different restriction endonucleases have different restriction sites. A commonly used restriction endonuclease is called *Eco*RI (from the bacteria that produce it, *Escherichia coli*). *Eco*RI cleaves DNA

Box 4-1   Genetic Engineering and Gene Therapy: The "New Genetics"—cont'd

only when the sequence GAATTC is found on one DNA strand and the complementary sequence is found on the other strand. The DNA of another organism, such as a human, also can be exposed to *Eco*RI and can be cleaved at the same restriction sites. The resulting human restriction fragments, which are pieces of DNA, have exposed ends that have base sequences complementary to those of the cleaved plasmid DNA. The human DNA and plasmid DNA, if mixed together, undergo complementary base pairing (i.e., they recombine).

The result is that the human DNA is incorporated within the plasmid. The plasmids, which now contain human genes in addition to their own, are allowed to reenter bacteria. Selection processes can be applied to pick out the bacteria that contain the desired human genes. These are cultured and allowed to form clones (or genetically identical copies) through normal cell division. Through continued cell division, millions of bacterial clones are formed, all containing the same human gene. Like any other gene, the human gene directs protein synthesis in the bacteria, resulting in the production of human proteins by bacteria.

Because bacteria multiply rapidly, large amounts of a given human protein can be manufactured by using this procedure. It has already been used successfully to produce human insulin in mass quantities. Because the insulin produced this way is actually human insulin, it produces fewer allergic reactions than the insulin taken from animal pancreases. Interferon, a substance that may help the body fight cancer and viral infections, also has been produced this way, as has human growth hormone, a substance that can be used to cure pituitary dwarfism.

In trying to isolate a particular gene, it is often more convenient to begin work with the messenger ribonucleic acid (mRNA) that codes for the gene product. The mRNA can be purified from body cells, and then an enzyme called *reverse transcriptase* can be used to generate the DNA sequence that is complementary to the mRNA. This complementary DNA (cDNA) can be inserted into plasmids and cloned by using the same recombinant techniques, so that virtually unlimited quantities of the desired gene product can be manufactured.

Recombinant DNA methods have been applied toward the understanding of the single-gene disorder phenylketonuria (PKU), which is the result of a lack of the enzyme phenylalanine hydroxylase. First, mRNA coding for this enzyme was purified from rat liver cells. After attachment of a radioactive "label" to cDNA produced from this mRNA, the cDNA was used as a probe. The probe was exposed to a series of cells that had been manipulated in the laboratory so that each cell line contained only one or a few chromosomes. When the probe hybridized consistently with only the cells containing chromosome 12, it proved that the gene that produces phenylalanine hydroxylase and thus causes PKU is located on this chromosome. Knowing the chromosome location of a gene is a very important step in the diagnosis and understanding of a genetic disease. Ultimately, therapeutic techniques might be developed to correct such disorders by replacing or repairing the abnormal gene.

The use of recombinant DNA techniques to clone DNA sequences has been (and continues to be) of great importance in genetics. However, the cloning process can take a great deal of time, even for well-studied genes. When doing genetic diagnoses, it is often

necessary to obtain results very quickly. A newer technique, the polymerase chain reaction (PCR), provides a very rapid means of making millions of copies of a DNA sequence in only a few hours (as opposed to 1 week or more using cloning techniques). PCR basically involves the artificial replication of a DNA sequence, achieved by exposing the DNA strand to alterations in temperature in the presence of free DNA bases. At lower temperatures the DNA undergoes complementary base pairing, and at higher temperatures the DNA strands separate to form new templates for another cycle of replication when the temperature is again lowered. By repeating this temperature cycling over and over, DNA copies can be produced rapidly. This technique is very useful for diagnostic purposes because it requires only a very small sample of blood or other tissue and because a large number of copies can be made in a very short time. In theory, even a single DNA molecule can be copied millions of times using PCR. It is also used extensively in forensic medicine (e.g., in identifying the DNA of criminal suspects by using blood, semen, or hair samples left at the scene of a crime).

The advent of this technology has led to fears that organisms that could pose grave threats to the human species might be created. In 1974 a group of molecular geneticists themselves called for a moratorium on recombinant DNA research when its implications began to be realized; however, after much study and the introduction of rules regarding laboratory containment, research was resumed. Because of the elaborate precautions taken to prevent inadvertent creation of harmful organisms and because of the very low probability that such organisms could survive outside the laboratory, the possibility of such an occurrence is now considered to be extremely remote.

Gene Therapy

An area in which recombinant DNA techniques have generated much interest is gene therapy, which essentially involves the insertion of normal genes. For example, by recombinant DNA methods, a normal gene might be inserted into a human chromosome to counteract the effects of an abnormal or missing gene.

Gene therapy can be applied in two ways. The less controversial approach is somatic cell therapy, which consists of inserting normal genes into the cells of an individual who has a genetic disease. Here a particular tissue, such as bone marrow cells that produce abnormal erythrocytes, would be treated. More controversial is the application of gene therapy very early in embryonic development. By inserting genes into the embryos, all body cells could be altered, including the germ cells. Thus not only would the genetic constitution of the embryo and resulting individual be changed, but also all the descendants of that individual would have altered genetic constitutions. This procedure is sometimes referred to as *germ cell therapy*.

Somatic cell therapy has now been initiated for a number of human diseases, including hemophilia, cystic fibrosis, familial hypercholesterolemia, and several types of cancer.* More than 1300 somatic cell gene therapy protocols are being tested. Although significant setbacks have occurred, considerable technologic progress is being made and somatic cell therapy is beginning to demonstrate therapeutic effects for some diseases. Because of several important technical and ethical considerations, germline therapy will not be attempted in humans in the foreseeable future.

---

*Kootstra NA, Verma IM: *Annu Rev Pharmacol Toxicol* 43:413-439, 2003; Thomas CE, Ehrhardt A, Kay MA: *Nat Rev Genet* 4:346-358, 2003.

DNA, RNA, AND PROTEINS: HEREDITY AT THE MOLECULAR LEVEL

DNA

Composition and Structure

Genes are composed of DNA, which has three basic components: the pentose sugar molecule, deoxyribose; a phosphate molecule; and four types of nitrogenous bases (Figure 4-1). Two of the bases, **cytosine** and **thymine,** are single carbon-nitrogen rings called **pyrimidines.** The other two bases, **adenine** and **guanine,** are double carbon-nitrogen rings called **purines.** The four bases are commonly represented by their first letters: A, C, T, and G.

One of Watson and Crick's contributions was to demonstrate how these molecules are physically assembled together as DNA. They proposed the now-famous **double-helix** model, in which DNA can be envisioned as a twisted ladder with chemical bonds as its rungs (see Figure 4-1). The two sides of the ladder are composed of the sugar and phosphate molecules, held together by strong phosphodiester bonds. Projecting from each side of the ladder, at regular intervals, are the nitrogenous bases. The base projecting from one side is bound to the base projecting from the other by a weak hydrogen bond. Therefore, the nitrogenous bases form the rungs of the ladder; adenine pairs with thymine, and guanine pairs with cytosine. Each DNA subunit—consisting of one deoxyribose molecule, one phosphate group, and one base—is called a **nucleotide.**

DNA as the Genetic Code

To serve as the basis of genetic inheritance DNA must be able to direct the synthesis of all the body's proteins. Proteins are composed of one or more **polypeptides** (intermediate protein compounds), which are in turn composed of sequences of **amino acids** (organic acids containing NH_2). The body contains 20 different types of amino acids, and the amino acid sequences that make up polypeptides must in some way be specified by the DNA molecule.

Because there are 20 possible amino acids and only four possible bases, each single nucleotide cannot specify an amino acid. Similarly, the amino acids cannot be specified by couplets of bases (e.g., adenine-guanine, thymine-guanine, guanine-cytosine) because there are only 4×4, or 16, possible couplets. If series of three bases are translated into amino acids, however, there are $4 \times 4 \times 4$, or 64, possible combinations—more than enough to specify each different amino acid. By manufacturing synthetic nucleotide sequences and allowing them to direct the formation of amino acids in the laboratory, it was proved that amino acids were specified by these triplets of bases, or **codons.**

Of the 64 possible codons, three signal the end of a gene and are known as **termination,** or **nonsense, codons.** The remaining 61 all specify amino acids, which means that most amino acids can be specified by more than one codon. The genetic code is thus said to be redundant, although each codon can specify only one amino acid.

Another significant feature of the genetic code is that it is universal: all living organisms use precisely the same DNA codes to specify proteins. The one known exception to this rule occurs in mitochondria—cytoplasmic organelles that are the sites of cellular respiration (see Chapter 1). The mitochondria have their own extranuclear DNA. Several codons of mitochondrial DNA encode different amino acids than do the same nuclear DNA codons.

Replication

In addition to having the ability to specify amino acid sequences, DNA must be able to replicate itself accurately during cell division if it is to serve as the basic genetic material. DNA replication consists of the breaking of the weak hydrogen bonds between the bases, leaving a single strand with each base unpaired. The consistent pairing of adenine with thymine and of guanine with cytosine, known as **complementary base pairing,** is the key to accurate replication. The principle of complementary base pairing dictates that the unpaired base will attract a free nucleotide only if the nucleotide has the proper complementary base. Thus a portion of a single strand with a sequence of bases labeled ATTGCT will bond with a series of free nucleotides with the bases TAACGA. When replication is complete, a new double-stranded molecule identical to the original is formed (Figure 4-2, *A*). The single strand is said to be a **template,** or molecule on which a complementary molecule is built, and is the basis for synthesizing the new double strand.

Several different proteins are involved in DNA replication. One protein unwinds the double helix, one holds the strands apart, and others perform different distinct functions. The most important of these proteins is an enzyme known as **DNA polymerase.** This enzyme travels along the single DNA strand, adding the correct nucleotides to the free end of the new strand (see Figure 4-2, *B*). Besides adding the new nucleotides, the DNA polymerase performs a proofreading procedure. After the new nucleotide has been added to the chain, the DNA polymerase checks to make sure that its base is actually complementary to the template base. If it is not, the incorrect nucleotide is excised and replaced with a correct one. This procedure, one of the mechanisms of DNA repair, substantially enhances the accuracy of DNA replication.

Mutation

A **mutation** is any inherited alteration of genetic material. Chromosome aberrations that cause congenital defects are examples of mutations. Other mutations are subtle and are not observable as chromosome aberrations. One such mutation is the **base pair substitution,** in which one base pair is replaced by another. This mutation is sometimes called **missense mutation** as the "sense" of the codon produced after transcription of the mutant gene is altered (Figure 4-3). This substitution sometimes results in a change in amino acid sequence, but because of the redundancy of the genetic code, it may have no consequence. If an amino acid change does not

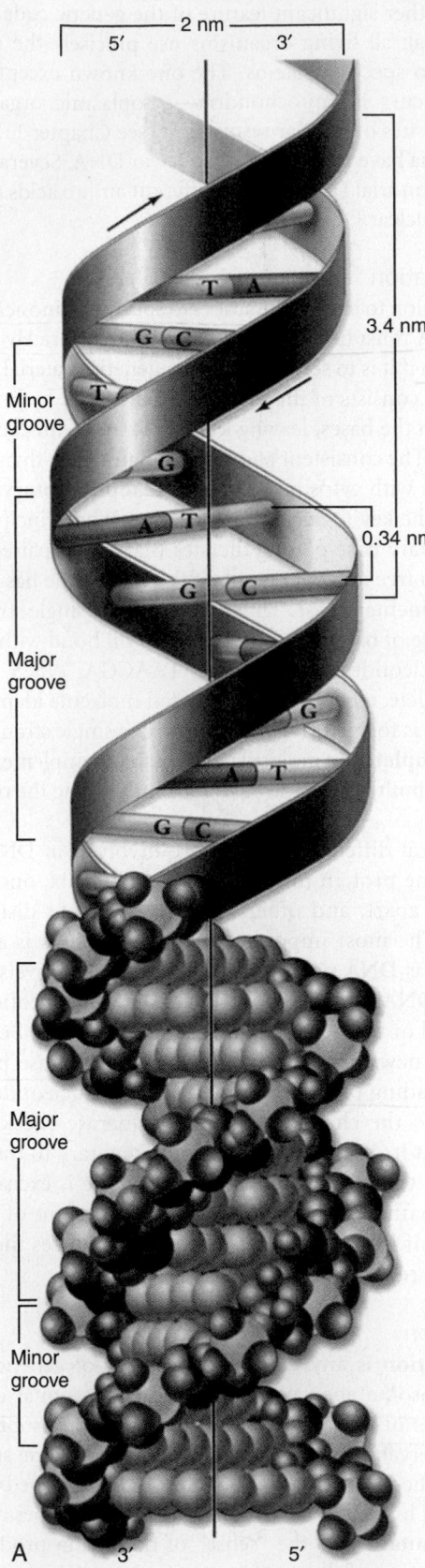

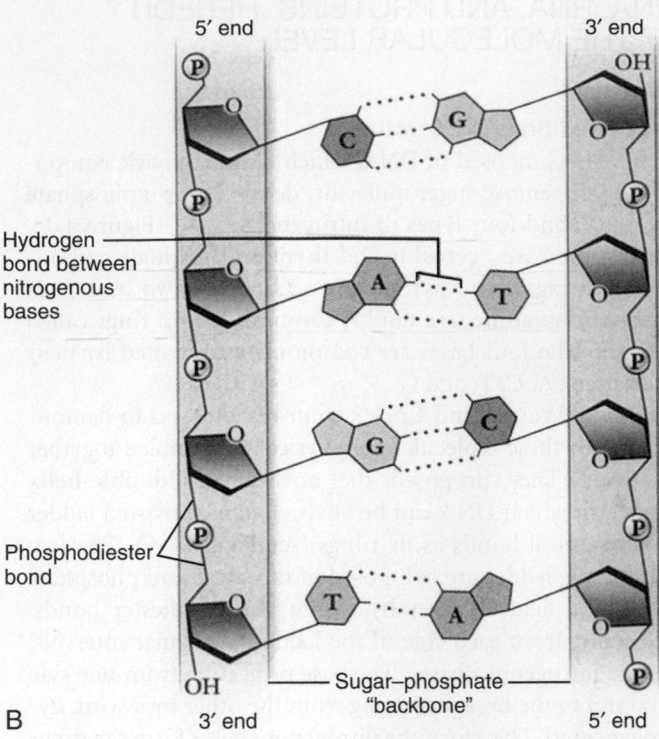

Figure 4-1 Structure of DNA. **A,** Double helix. Shown with the phosphodiester backbone as a ribbon on top and a space-filling model on the bottom. The bases protrude into the interior of the helix where they hold it together by base pairing. The backbone forms two grooves, the larger major groove and the smaller minor groove. **B,** Base pairing holds strands together. The H-bonds that form between A and T and between G and C are shown with dashed lines. These produce AT and GC base pairs that hold the two strands together. This always pairs a purine with a pyrimidine, keeping the diameter of the double helix constant. (From Raven PH et al: *Biology*, ed 8, New York, 2008, McGraw-Hill.)

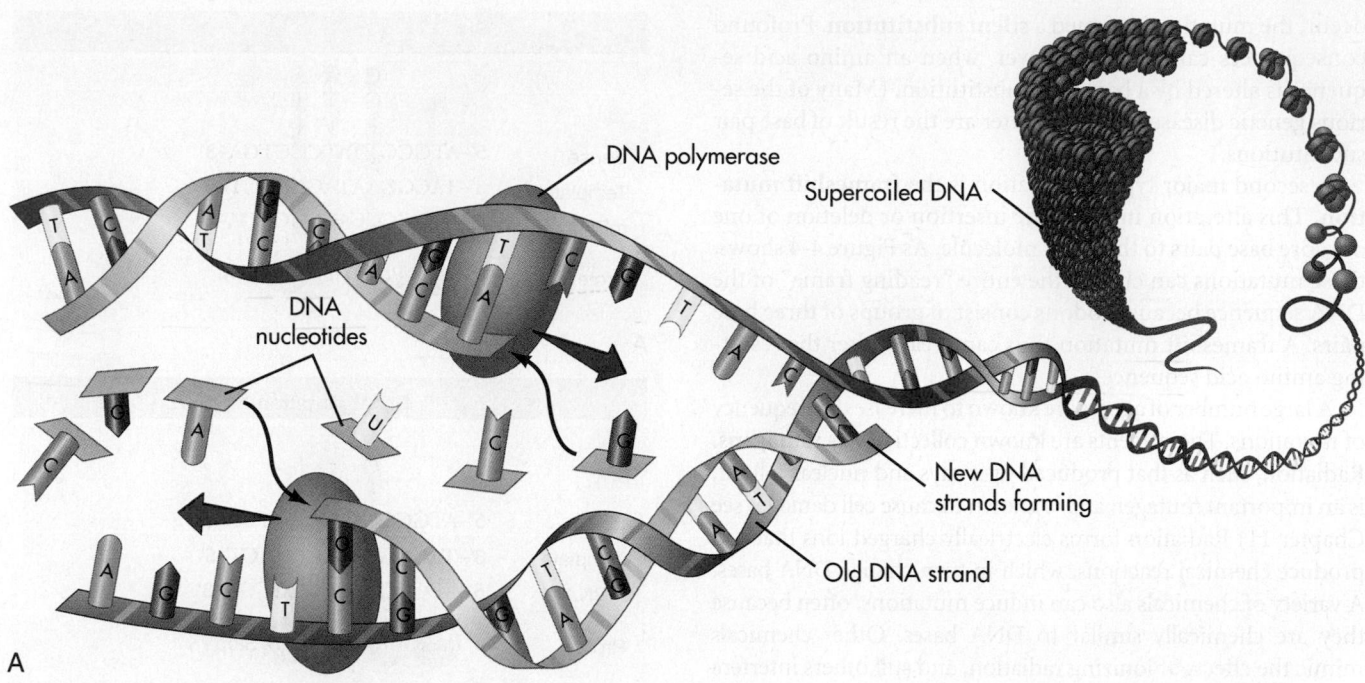

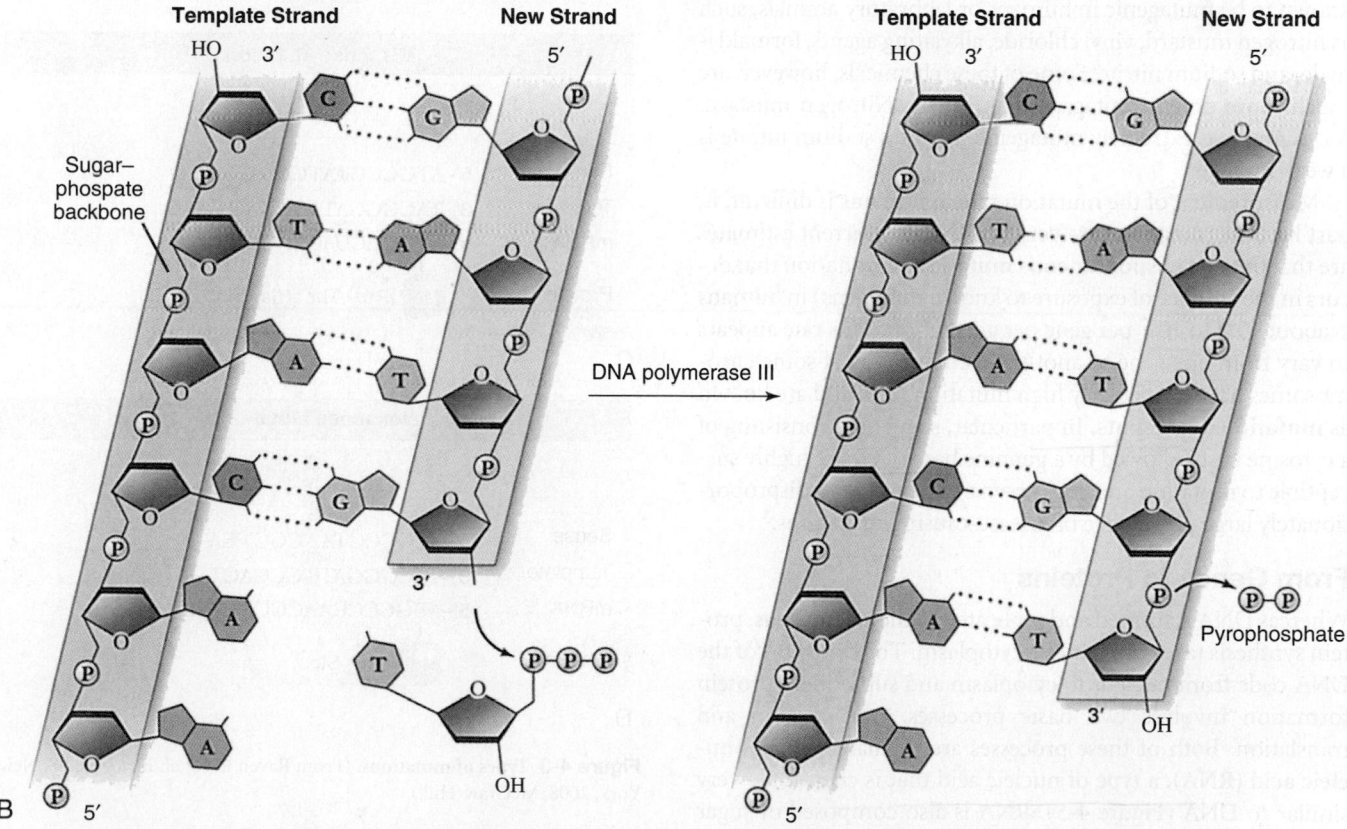

Figure 4-2 Replication and action of DNA. A, Replication of DNA. **B,** Action of DNA polymerase. DNA polymerases add nucleotides to the 3' end of a growing chain. The nucleotide added depends on the base that is in the template strand. Each new base must be complementary to the base in the template strand. With the addition of each new nucleotide, triphosphate, two of its phosphates are cleaved off as pyrophosphate. *A,* Adenine; *T,* thymine; *G,* guanine; *C,* cytosine. (A from Thibodeau GA, Patton KT: *Anatomy & physiology,* ed 6, St Louis, 2007, Mosby; B adapted from Raven PH et al: *Biology,* ed 8, New York, 2008, McGraw-Hill.)

occur, the mutation is termed a **silent substitution.** Profound consequences can result, however, when an amino acid sequence is altered by a base pair substitution. (Many of the serious genetic diseases discussed later are the result of base pair substitutions.)

A second major type of mutation is the **frameshift mutation.** This alteration involves the insertion or deletion of one or more base pairs to the DNA molecule. As Figure 4-4 shows, these mutations can change the entire "reading frame" of the DNA sequence because codons consist of groups of three base pairs. A frameshift mutation thus can greatly alter the resulting amino acid sequence.

A large number of agents are known to increase the frequency of mutations. These agents are known collectively as **mutagens.** Radiation, such as that produced by x-rays and nuclear fallout, is an important mutagen and is known to cause cell damage (see Chapter 11) Radiation forms electrically charged ions that can produce chemical reactions, which in turn change DNA bases. A variety of chemicals also can induce mutations, often because they are chemically similar to DNA bases. Other chemicals mimic the effects of ionizing radiation, and still others interfere with the process of base pairing. Hundreds of chemicals are now known to be mutagenic in humans or laboratory animals, such as nitrogen mustard, vinyl chloride, alkylating agents, formaldehyde, and sodium nitrite. Some of these chemicals, however, are much more potent mutagens than others. Nitrogen mustard, for example, is extremely mutagenic, whereas sodium nitrate is a weak mutagen.

Measurement of the mutation rate in humans is difficult, in part because mutations are very rare events. Current estimates are that the rate of **spontaneous mutation** (a mutation that occurs in the absence of exposure to known mutagens) in humans is about 10^{-4} to 10^{-7} per gene per generation. This rate appears to vary from one gene to another. Certain areas of some chromosomes have particularly high mutation rates and are known as **mutational hot spots.** In particular, sequences consisting of a cytosine base followed by a guanine base (CG) are highly susceptible to mutation and are known to account for a disproportionately large percentage of disease-causing mutations.[3]

From Genes to Proteins

Whereas DNA is formed and replicated in the cell nucleus, protein synthesis takes place in the cytoplasm. The transport of the DNA code from nucleus to cytoplasm and subsequent protein formation involves two basic processes: transcription and translation. Both of these processes are mediated by **ribonucleic acid (RNA),** a type of nucleic acid that is chemically very similar to DNA (Figure 4-5). RNA is also composed of sugar molecules, phosphate groups, and nitrogenous bases. RNA differs from DNA in that the sugar molecule is ribose rather than deoxyribose and that uracil rather than thymine is one of the four bases. The other bases of RNA, as in DNA, are adenine, cytosine, and guanine. Uracil is structurally very similar to thymine, so it also can pair with adenine. The final difference between RNA and DNA is that whereas DNA usually occurs as a double strand, RNA usually occurs as a single strand.

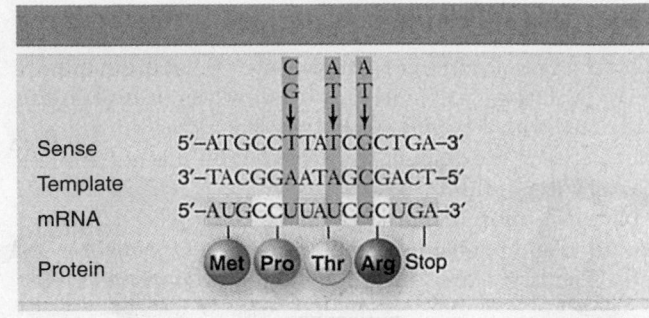

A

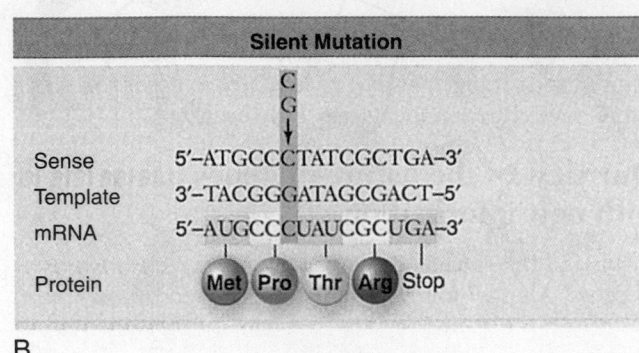

B

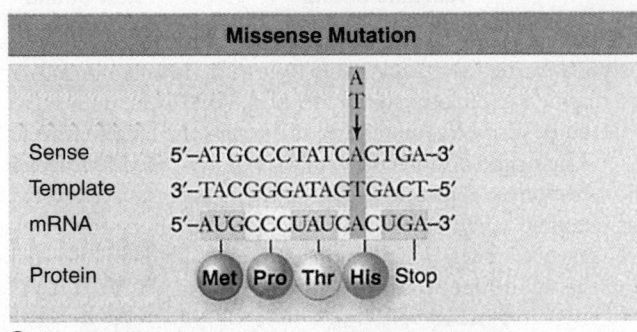

C

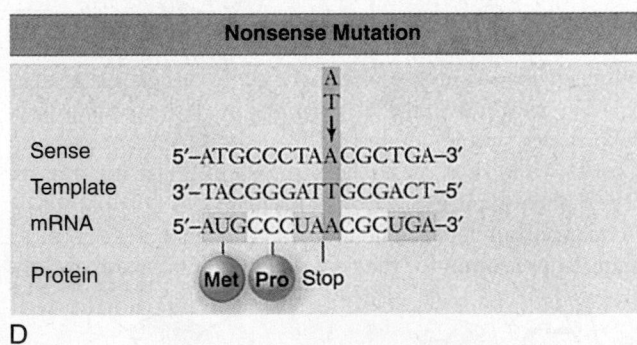

D

Figure 4-3 Types of mutations. (From Raven PH et al: *Biology,* ed 8, New York, 2008, McGraw-Hill.)

Transcription

Transcription is the process by which RNA is synthesized from a DNA template. The result is the formation of **messenger RNA (mRNA)** from the base sequence specified by the DNA molecule. An enzyme called *DNA-dependent RNA polymerase,* or **RNA polymerase,** binds to a **promoter site** on the DNA. A promoter site is a sequence of DNA that specifies the

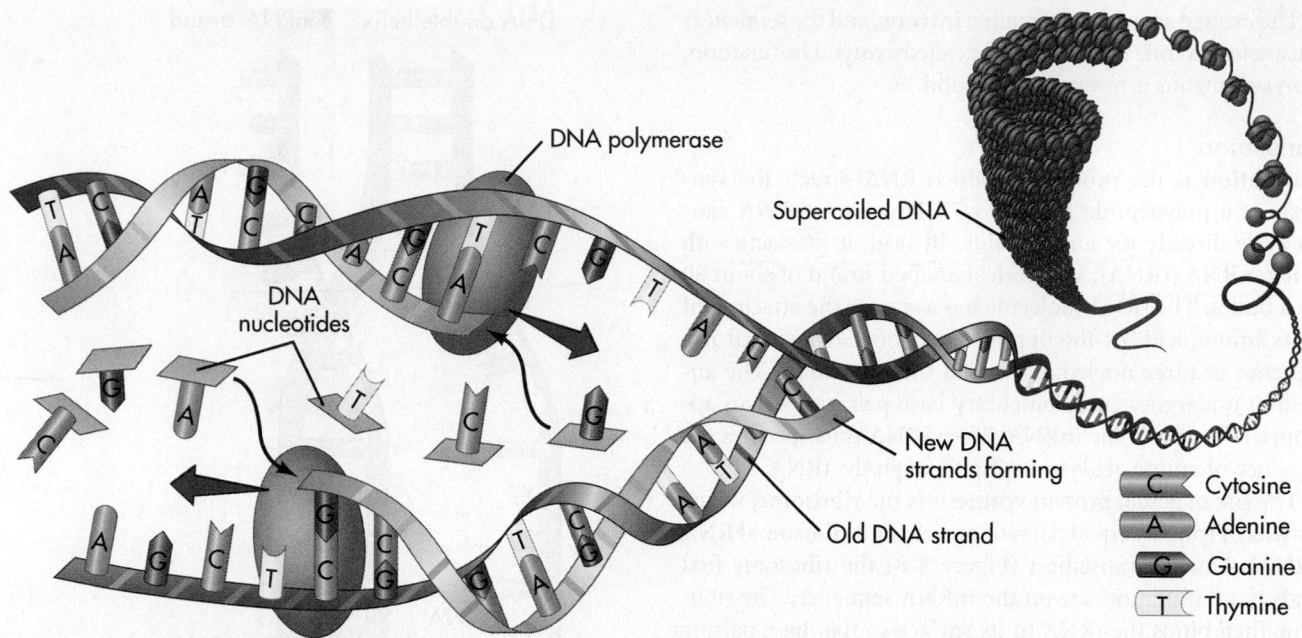

Figure 4-4 Different kinds of mutations. (From Patton KT, Thibodeau GA: *Anatomy & Physiology,* ed 7, 2010, St Louis Mosby.)

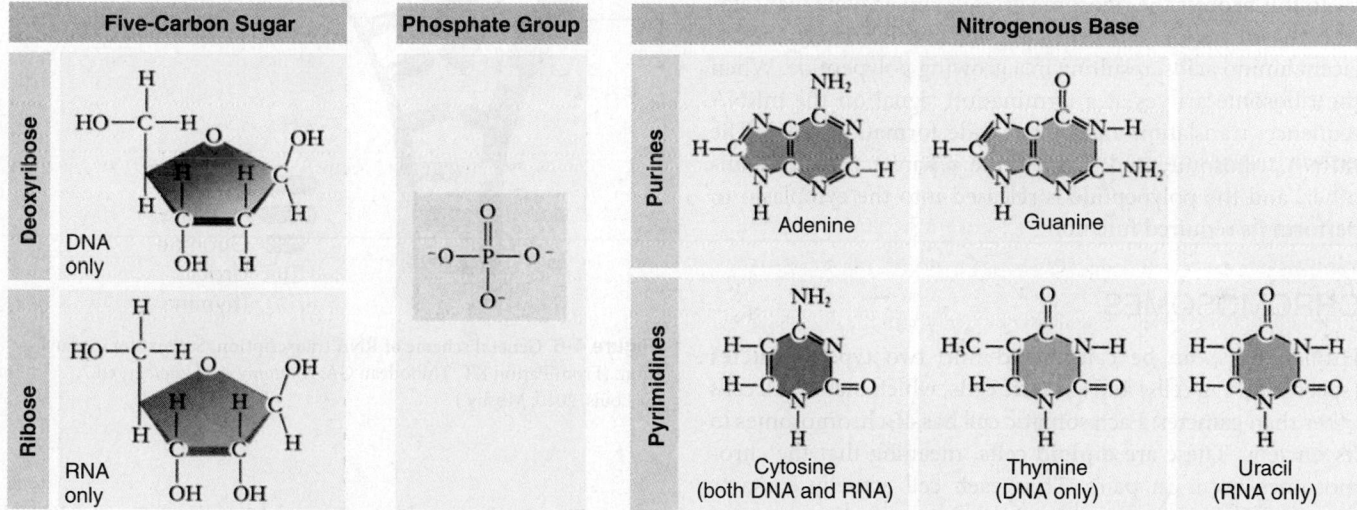

Figure 4-5 Nucleotide subunits of DNA and RNA. (From Raven PH et al: *Biology,* ed 8, New York, 2008, McGraw-Hill.)

beginning of a gene. The RNA polymerase then pulls a portion of the DNA strands apart from one another, allowing unattached DNA bases to be exposed. One of the DNA strands then provides the template for the sequence of mRNA nucleotides.

The sequence of bases in the mRNA is thus complementary to that of the template strand, and with the exception of the presence of uracil instead of thymine, the mRNA sequence is identical to that of the other DNA strand. Transcription continues until a DNA sequence called a **termination sequence** is reached. Then the RNA polymerase detaches from the DNA, and the transcribed mRNA is freed to move out of the nucleus and into the cytoplasm. Figure 4-6 summarizes the process of transcription.

Gene Splicing

After the mRNA first has been transcribed from the DNA template, it reflects exactly the base sequence of the DNA. The RNA in this state is sometimes called **heterogeneous nuclear RNA (hnRNA).** In eukaryotes an important step takes place before this RNA leaves the nucleus. Many of the RNA sequences are removed by nuclear enzymes, and the remaining sequences are spliced together to form the functional mRNA that will migrate to the cytoplasm.

The excised sequences are called **introns**, and the sequences that are left to code for proteins are called **exons**. The function, if any, of introns is not yet understood.

Translation

Translation is the process by which RNA directs the synthesis of a polypeptide (Figure 4-7). However, mRNA cannot code directly for amino acids. Instead, it interacts with **transfer RNA (tRNA)**, a cloverleaf-shaped strand of about 80 nucleotides. The tRNA molecule has a site for the attachment of an amino acid. At the opposite side of the cloverleaf is a sequence of three nucleotides called the **anticodon**. The anticodon undergoes complementary base pairing with an appropriate codon in the mRNA. The mRNA thus specifies the sequence of amino acids by acting through the tRNA.

The site of actual protein synthesis is the **ribosome**, which consists of roughly equal parts of protein and **ribosomal RNA (rRNA)**. During translation (Figure 4-8) the ribosome first binds to an initiation site on the mRNA sequence. The ribosome then binds the tRNA to its surface so that base pairing can occur between tRNA and mRNA. The ribosome then moves along the mRNA sequence, codon by codon. As each codon is processed, an amino acid is translated by the interaction of mRNA and tRNA.

In this process the ribosome provides an enzyme that catalyzes the formation of covalent peptide bonds between the adjacent amino acids, resulting in a growing polypeptide. When the ribosome arrives at a termination signal on the mRNA sequence, translation and polypeptide formation cease. The mRNA, ribosome, and polypeptide separate from one another, and the polypeptide is released into the cytoplasm to perform its required function.

CHROMOSOMES

Human cells can be categorized into two types: **gametes** (sperm and egg cells) and **somatic cells,** which include all cells other than gametes. Each somatic cell has 46 chromosomes in its nucleus. These are **diploid cells,** meaning that the chromosomes occur in pairs. Thus each cell actually contains 23 pairs of chromosomes. One member of each pair comes from an individual's mother, and one comes from the father. New somatic cells are formed through mitosis and cytokinesis, through which the cell nucleus and cytoplasm are replicated. (The division process that creates new copies of somatic cells is described in Chapter 1.) Gametes are **haploid cells:** they have only one member of each chromosome pair, giving them a total of 23 chromosomes. The process by which these haploid cells are formed from diploid cells is called **meiosis** (Figure 4-9).

In 22 of the 23 chromosome pairs, the two members of each pair are virtually identical in microscopic appearance and are thus said to be **homologous** to one another. These 22 chromosome pairs are homologous in both males and females and are termed **autosomes.** The remaining pair of chromosomes, the **sex chromosomes,** consists of two homologous X

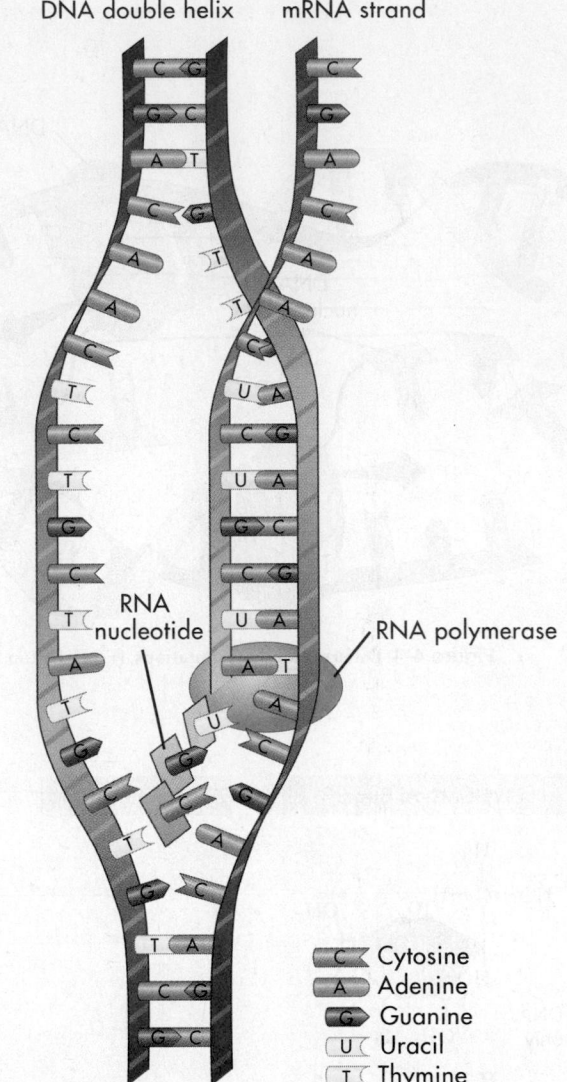

DNA double helix   mRNA strand

RNA nucleotide

RNA polymerase

C Cytosine
A Adenine
G Guanine
U Uracil
T Thymine

Figure 4-6 General scheme of RNA transcription. See text for explanation. (From Patton KT, Thibodeau GA: *Anatomy & physiology*, ed 7, St Louis, 2010, Mosby.)

chromosomes in females and a nonhomologous pair, X and Y, in males.

Figure 4-10, *A*, illustrates a **metaphase spread,** which is a photograph of the chromosomes as they appear in the nucleus of a somatic cell during metaphase. (Chromosomes are easiest to visualize during this stage of mitosis.) A **karyotype** is an ordered display of chromosomes. In Figure 4-10, *B*, the chromosomes are arranged according to size, with the **homologous chromosomes** paired together. The 22 autosomes are numbered according to length, with chromosome 1 as the longest and chromosome 22 as the shortest. Some natural variation in relative chromosome length can be expected from person to person, however, so it is not always possible to distinguish each chromosome by its length. Therefore, the position of the centromere is also used to classify the chromosomes (Figure 4-11).

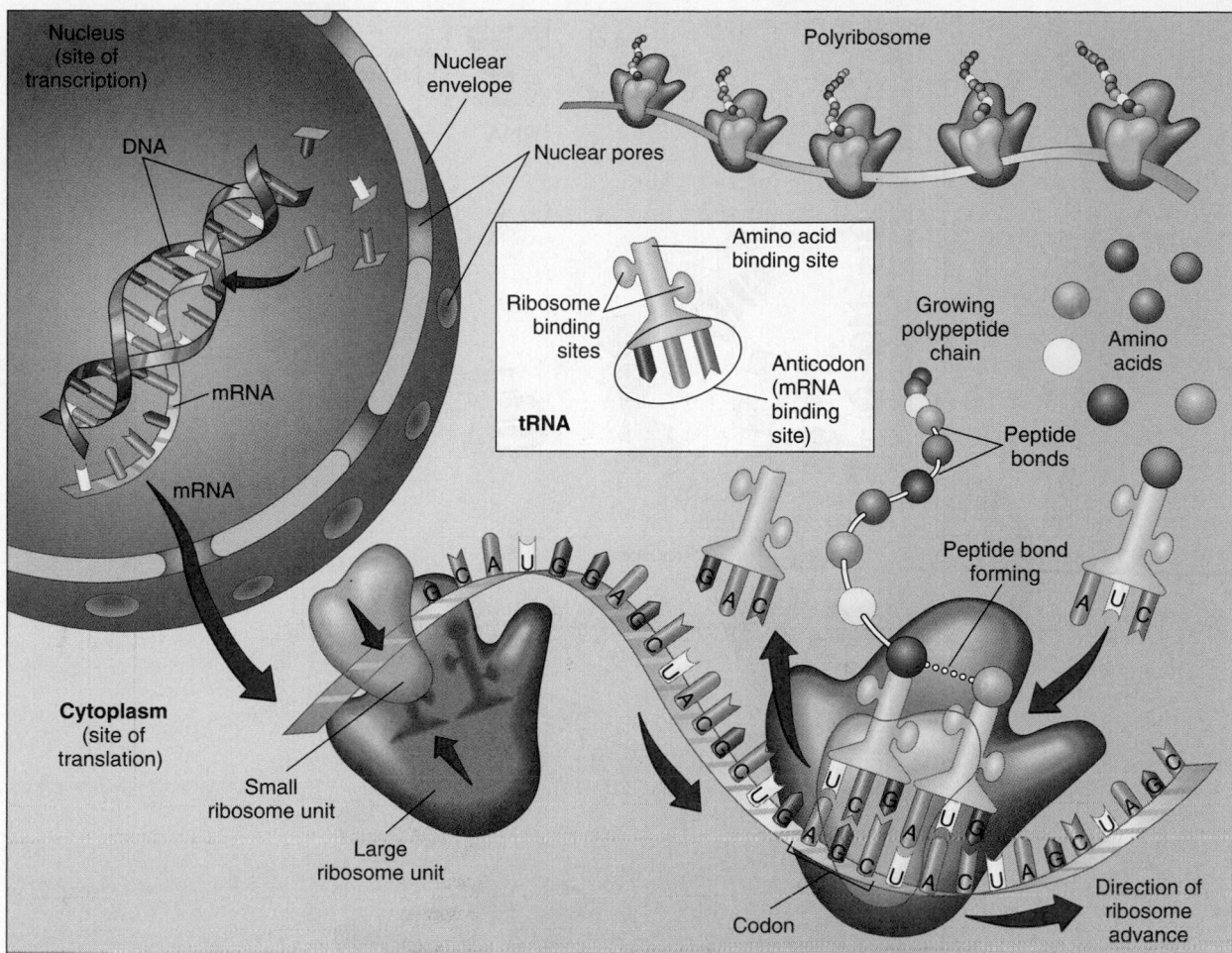

Figure 4-7 Protein synthesis. Protein synthesis begins with *transcription,* a process in which an mRNA molecule forms along one gene sequence of a DNA molecule within the cell's nucleus. As it is formed, the mRNA molecule separates from the DNA molecule and leaves the nucleus through the large nuclear pores. Outside the nucleus, ribosome subunits attach to the beginning of the mRNA molecule and begin the process of *translation.* In translation, transfer RNA (tRNA) molecules bring specific amino acids—encoded by each mRNA codon—into place at the ribosome site. As the amino acids are brought into the proper sequence, they are joined together by peptide bonds to form long strands called *polypeptides.* Several polypeptide chains may be needed to make a complete protein molecule. *A,* Adenine; *C,* cytosine; *G,* guanine; *U,* uracil. (From Thibodeau GA, Patton KT: *Anatomy & Physiology,* ed 6, St Louis, 2007, Mosby.)

The chromosomes in Figure 4-10, *A,* were stained with a substance that penetrates all areas of the chromosome (a "solid stain"). In the late 1960s and early 1970s, several staining materials were found to bind preferentially to certain areas of chromosomes. The resulting distinctive **chromosome bands** are evident in various patterns in the different chromosomes so that each chromosome can be distinguished easily. One of the most commonly used stains is **Giemsa stain.** By using banding techniques, chromosomes can be unambiguously numbered, and individual variation in chromosome composition can be studied. Missing or duplicated portions of chromosomes, which often result in serious diseases, also can be readily identified.

Chromosome Aberrations and Associated Diseases

Chromosome abnormalities are the leading known cause of mental retardation and miscarriage. Estimates indicate that a major chromosome aberration occurs in at least 1 in 12 conceptions. Most of these fetuses do not survive to term; in fact, about 50% of all recovered first-trimester spontaneous abortuses have major chromosomal aberrations.[4] The number of live births affected by these abnormalities is significant; about 1 in 150 has a major diagnosable chromosome abnormality[5] (Box 4-2).

Polyploidy

Cells that have a multiple of the normal number of chromosomes are said to be **euploid cells** (Greek *eu* = good or true). Because normal gametes are haploid and most normal somatic cells are diploid, they are both euploid forms. When a euploid cell has more than the diploid number of chromosomes, it is said to be a **polyploid cell.** Several types of body tissues, including some liver, bronchial, and epithelial tissues, are normally polyploid. A zygote having three copies of each chromosome, rather than the usual two, has a form of polyploidy called **triploidy. Tetraploidy,** a condition

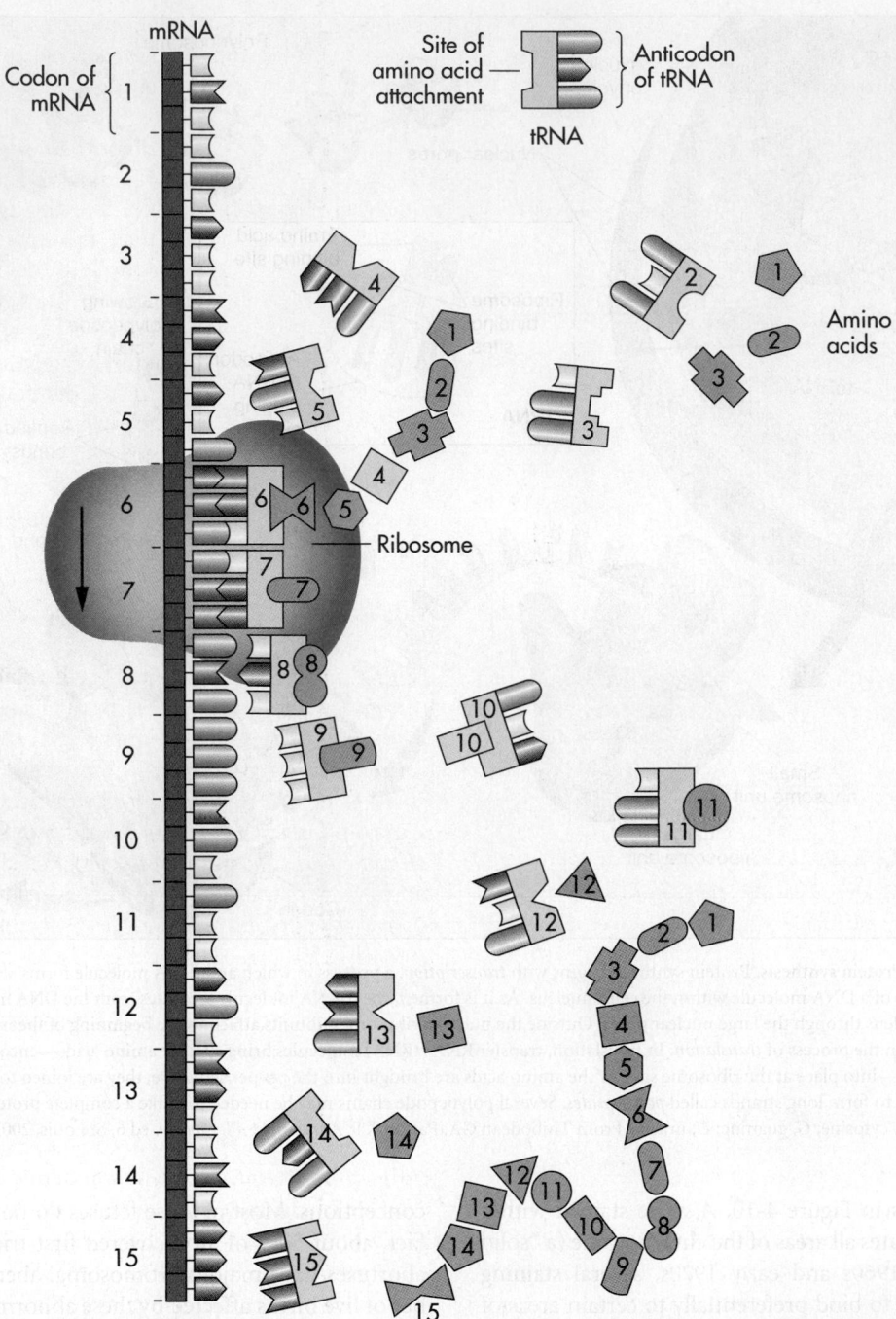

Figure 4-8 A ribosome "reading" the code of mRNA and assembling a polypeptide chain.

in which euploid cells have 92 chromosomes, also has been observed. Both of these conditions are incompatible with postnatal survival. Nearly all triploid fetuses are spontaneously aborted or stillborn. A few have survived to term but have died shortly after birth. Tetraploidy has been found primarily in early abortuses, although occasionally affected infants have been born alive. Like triploid infants, however, they do not survive. Triploidy and tetraploidy are relatively common conditions, accounting for approximately 10% of all known miscarriages.[4]

Aneuploidy

A somatic cell that does not contain a multiple of 23 chromosomes is an **aneuploid cell.** A cell containing three copies of one chromosome is said to be trisomic (a condition termed **trisomy**) and is aneuploid. **Monosomy,** the presence of only one copy of a given chromosome in a diploid cell, is the other common form of aneuploidy. Among the autosomes, monosomy of any chromosome is lethal, but newborns with trisomy of some chromosomes can survive. This difference illustrates an important principle: in general, loss

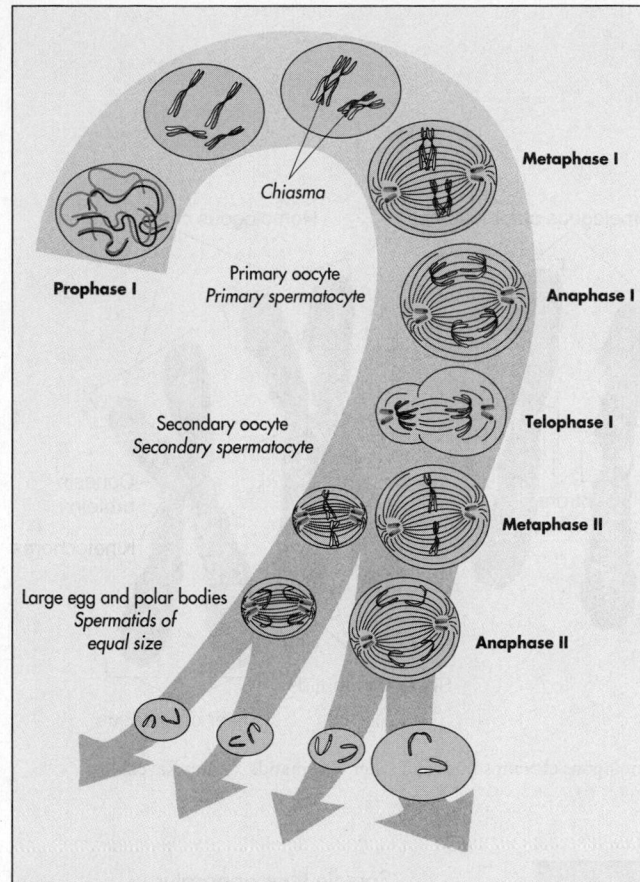

Figure 4-9 Stages of meiosis. From these stages, haploid gametes are formed from a diploid stem cell. For brevity, prophase II and telophase II are not shown. Note the relationship between meiosis and spermatogenesis and oogenesis. (From Jorde LB et al: *Medical genetics,* ed 3, St Louis, 2003, Mosby.)

of chromosome material has more serious consequences than duplication of chromosome material.

Aneuploidy of the sex chromosomes is less serious than that of the autosomes. For the Y chromosome, this is true because very little genetic material is located on this chromosome. For the X chromosome, inactivation of extra chromosomes largely diminishes their effect. A zygote bearing *no* X chromosome, however, will not survive.

Aneuploidy is usually the result of **nondisjunction,** an error in which homologous chromosomes or sister chromatids fail to separate normally during meiosis or mitosis (Figure 4-12). Nondisjunction during either stage of meiosis produces some gametes that have two copies of a given chromosome and others that have no copies of the chromosome. When such gametes unite with normal haploid gametes, the resulting zygote is monosomic or trisomic for that chromosome. Occasionally a cell can be monosomic or trisomic for more than one chromosome.

Autosomal Aneuploidy

Trisomy can occur for any chromosome, but the only forms seen with an appreciable frequency in live births are trisomies of the thirteenth, eighteenth, or twenty-first chromosome.

Fetuses with most other chromosomal trisomies do not survive to term. Trisomy 16, for example, is the most commonly known trisomy among abortuses, but it is not seen in live births.[4]

Partial trisomy, in which only an extra portion of a chromosome is present in each cell, also can occur. The consequences of partial trisomies are not as severe as those of complete trisomies. Trisomies also may occur in only some cells of the body. Individuals thus affected are said to be **chromosomal mosaics,** meaning that the body has two or more different cell lines, each of which has a different karyotype. Mosaics are usually formed by early mitotic nondisjunction occurring in one embryo cell but not in others.

The best-known example of aneuploidy in an autosome is trisomy of the twenty-first chromosome, which causes **Down syndrome** (named after J. Langdon Down, who first described the disease in 1866). Down syndrome was formerly called *mongolism,* but this inappropriate term is no longer used. Down syndrome is seen in 1 in 800 live births.[4] Individuals with this disease are mentally retarded, with IQs usually ranging from 25 to 70. The facial appearance is distinctive (Figure 4-13), with a low nasal bridge, epicanthal folds (which produce a superficially Asian appearance), protruding tongue, and flat, low-set ears. Poor muscle tone (hypotonia) and short stature are both characteristic. Congenital heart defects affect about one third to one half of live-born children with Down syndrome; a reduced ability to fight respiratory infections and an increased susceptibility to leukemia also contribute to reduced survival rate. By 40 years of age, individuals with Down syndrome virtually always develop symptoms that are nearly identical to those of Alzheimer disease. About three fourths of fetuses known to have Down syndrome are spontaneously aborted or stillborn. About 20% of infants born with Down syndrome die during their first 10 years of life. For those who survive beyond 10 years, average life expectancy is now about 60 years.

About 97% of Down syndrome cases are caused by nondisjunction during the formation of one of the parent's gametes or during early embryonic development. The remaining 3% result from translocations (discussed later). In approximately 90% to 95% of cases, the nondisjunction occurs in the formation of the mother's egg cell. Paternal nondisjunction is responsible for the remaining cases. Among individuals with Down syndrome, about 1% are known to be mosaics. Because mosaics have a large number of normal cells, the effects of the trisomic cells are attenuated and symptoms are often less severe.

The risk of having a child with Down syndrome increases greatly with maternal age. As Figure 4-14 demonstrates, women younger than 30 years have a risk ranging from about 1 in 1000 births to 1 in 2000 births. The risk begins to rise substantially after 35 years of age, and it reaches 3% to 5% for women older than 45 years of age. This dramatic increase in risk may be caused by the age of maternal egg cells, which are held in an arrested state of prophase I from the time they are formed in the female embryo until they are shed in ovulation.

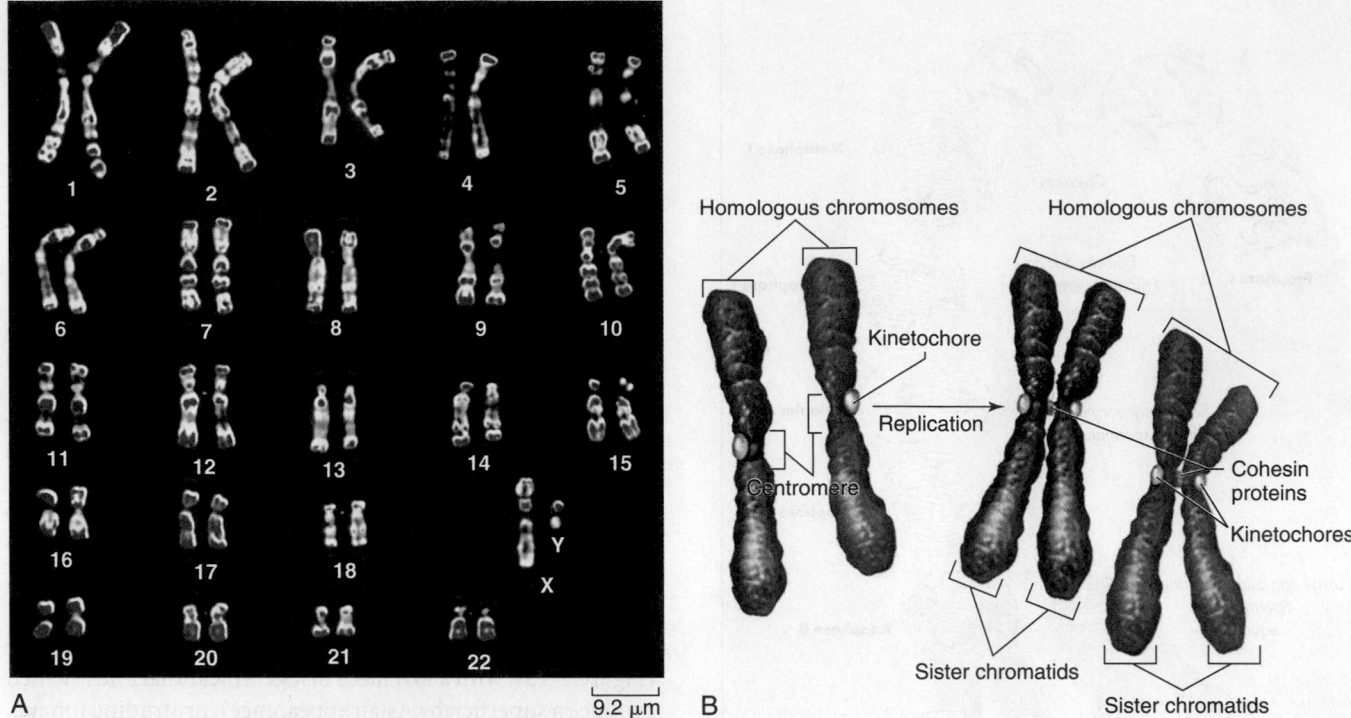

Figure 4-10 Karyotype of chromosomes. **A,** Human karyotype. **B,** Homologous chromosomes and sister chromatids. (From Raven PH et al: *Biology,* ed 8, New York, 2008, McGraw-Hill.)

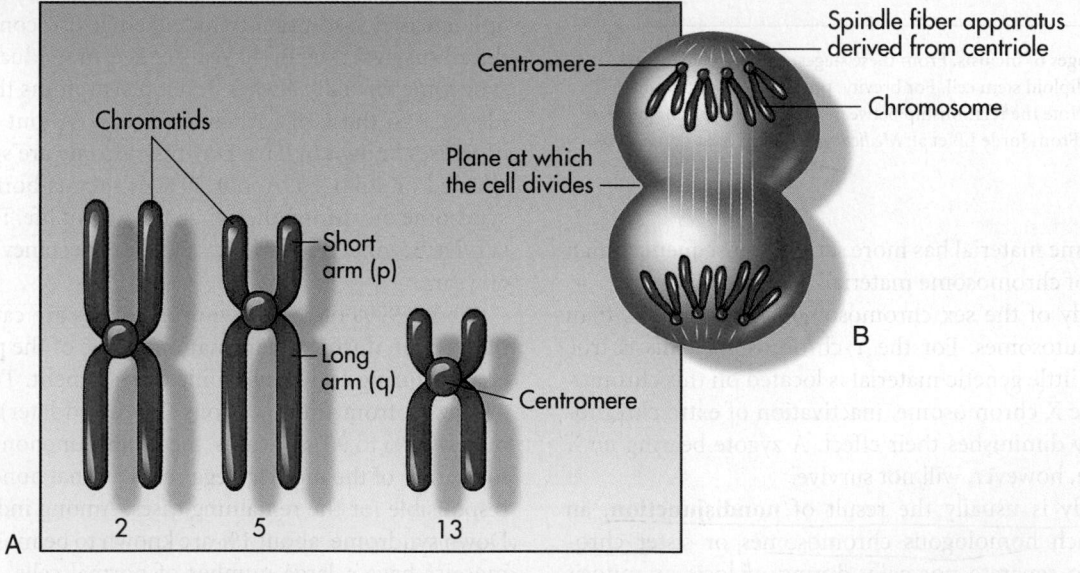

Figure 4-11 Structure of chromosomes. **A,** Human chromosomes 2, 5, and 13. Each is replicated and consists of two chromatids. Chromosome 1 is a metacentric chromosome because the centromere is close to middle; chromosome 5 is submetacentric because the centromere is set off from middle; chromosome 13 is acrocentric because the centromere is at or very near the end. **B,** During mitosis, the centromere divides and chromosomes move to opposite poles of the cell. At the time of centromere division, the chromatids are designated chromosomes.

Thus an egg cell formed by a 45-year-old woman is itself 45 years old. This long suspended state may allow for the accumulation of errors leading to nondisjunction. The risk of Down syndrome, as well as other trisomies, does not appear to increase with paternal age.[6]

Sex Chromosome Aneuploidy

Among live births, about 1 in 400 males and 1 in 650 females have a form of sex chromosome aneuploidy.[7] Because these conditions are generally less severe than autosomal aneuploidies, all forms except complete absence

| Box 4-2 | Prenatal Diagnosis of Chromosome Abnormalities |

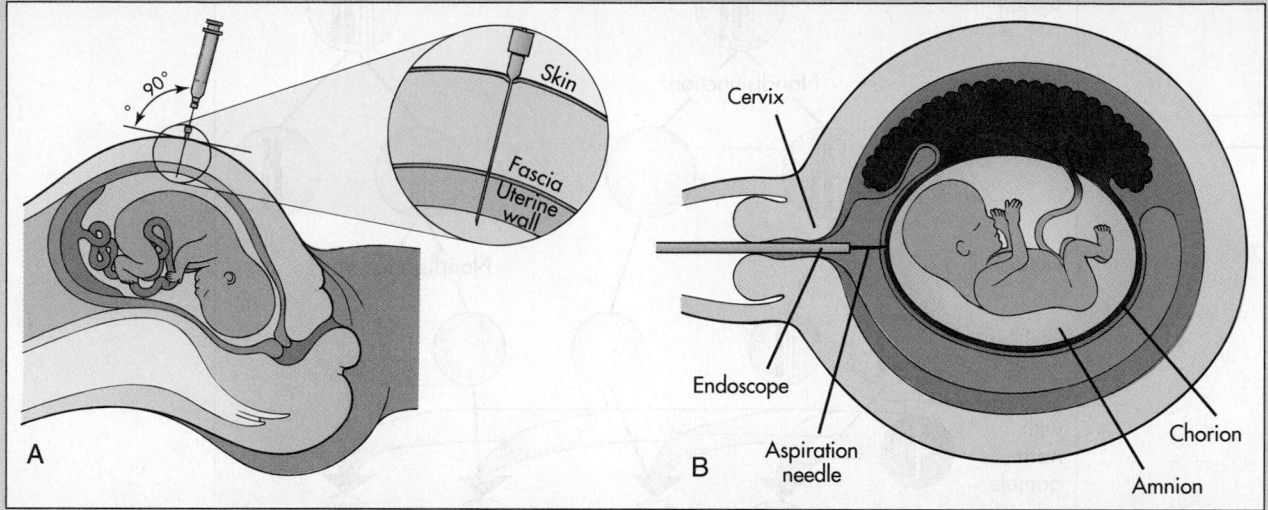

All the chromosome abnormalities discussed here can be detected prenatally, using a procedure called *amniocentesis* **(A)**. At about the sixteenth week of gestation, a sufficient amount of amniotic fluid is available to enable the withdrawal of a small amount of fluid (2 to 20 ml). This fluid contains live skin cells (fibroblasts) shed by the fetus. These cells can be cultured and karyotyped, and chromosome abnormalities can be detected.

Other disorders can be detected with this procedure. These include most neural tube defects, which cause an elevation of α-fetoprotein in the amniotic fluid, and hundreds of diseases caused by mutations of single genes. The procedure involves a risk of losing the fetus, estimated to be about 0.5% or less. Thus amniocentesis is recommended only for pregnancies known to have an elevated risk for a genetic disease. These include pregnancies of women older than 35 years, in which the risk for Down syndrome and other aneuploidies is elevated, and pregnancies in which parents are known to carry translocations or certain disease genes.

One problem with prenatal diagnosis by amniocentesis is that by the time the sixteenth week of gestation is reached and another 2 or 3 weeks to culture the fibroblasts and test for genetic disease elapse, the mother is near the twentieth week of pregnancy. Pregnancy termination of an affected fetus at this stage can present serious emotional and personal dilemmas as well as some medical risk. For many parents, abortion would be more acceptable for a fetus at an earlier gestational age. A newer technique, *chorionic villus sampling* **(B)**, consists of extracting a small amount of villous tissue directly from the chorion. This procedure can be performed at 10 weeks' gestation and does not require in vitro culturing of cells because sufficient numbers are directly available in the extracted tissue. Thus the procedure allows prenatal diagnosis at about 3 months' gestation rather than at nearly 5 months' gestation. Chorionic villus sampling involves a slightly higher fetal loss rate than amniocentesis, approximately 1%.

Data from Wang BT et al: *Am J Med Genet* 53:307, 1994; illustrations from Pagana KD, Pagana TJ: *Mosby's manual of diagnostic and laboratory tests,* ed 2, St Louis, 2002, Mosby.

of an X chromosome allow at least some individuals to survive.

One of the most common sex chromosome aneuploidies, affecting about 1 in 1000 newborn females, is trisomy X. Instead of two X chromosomes, these females have three X chromosomes in each cell. Most of them have no overt physical abnormalities, although sterility, menstrual irregularity, or mental retardation is sometimes seen. Some females have four X chromosomes, and they are more often mentally retarded. Those with five or more X chromosomes generally have more severe mental retardation and various physical defects.

A condition that leads to somewhat more serious problems is the presence of a single X chromosome and no homologous X or Y chromosome, so the individual has a total of 45 chromosomes. The karyotype is designated 45,X, and it causes a set of symptoms known as **Turner syndrome** (Figure 4-15). Because they have no Y chromosomes, people with Turner

syndrome are females. They are usually sterile, however, and have gonadal streaks rather than ovaries. These streaks of connective tissue are susceptible to cancer in mosaics who have some cells containing a Y chromosome. Other features of the disorder include short stature, webbing of the neck in about half of cases, widely spaced nipples, coarctation (narrowing) of the aorta (in 15% to 20% of cases), edema of the feet in newborns, reduced carrying angle at the elbow (cubitus valgus), and sparse body hair. They are not considered retarded, although evidence indicates some impairment of spatial and mathematical reasoning ability. About three fourths of recognized 45,X conceptions inherit their X chromosome from the mother. Thus most cases are caused by a loss of the paternal X chromosome.

The frequency of Turner syndrome is low compared with that of other sex chromosome aneuploidies: only about 1 in 3000 newborn females is affected.[8] About half of individuals

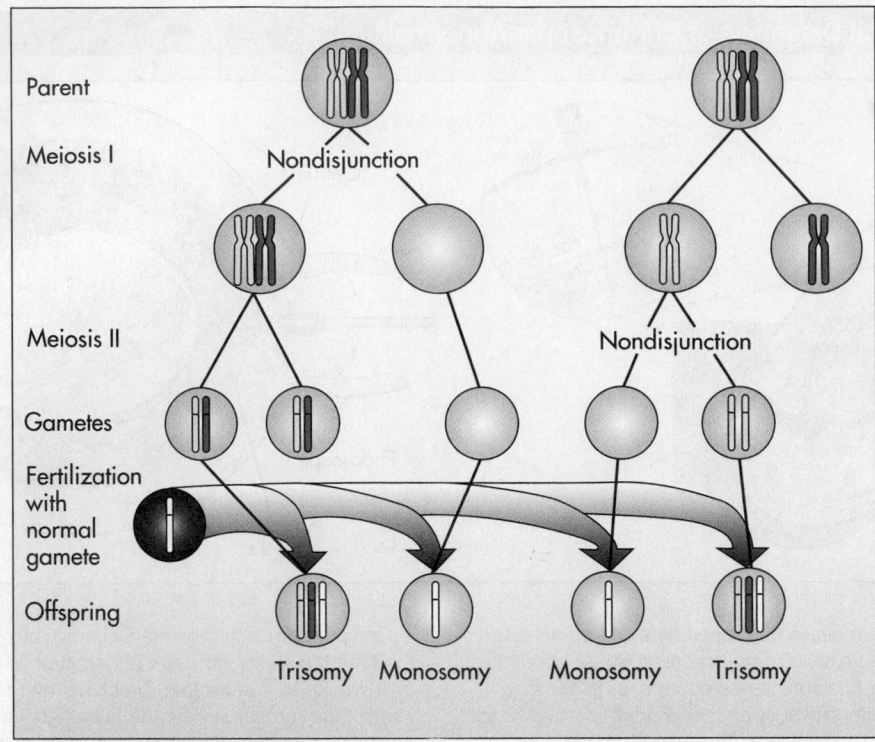

Figure 4-12 Nondisjunction causes aneuploidy when chromosomes or sister chromatids fail to divide properly. (From Jorde LB et al: *Medical genetics,* ed 3, St Louis, 2003, Mosby.)

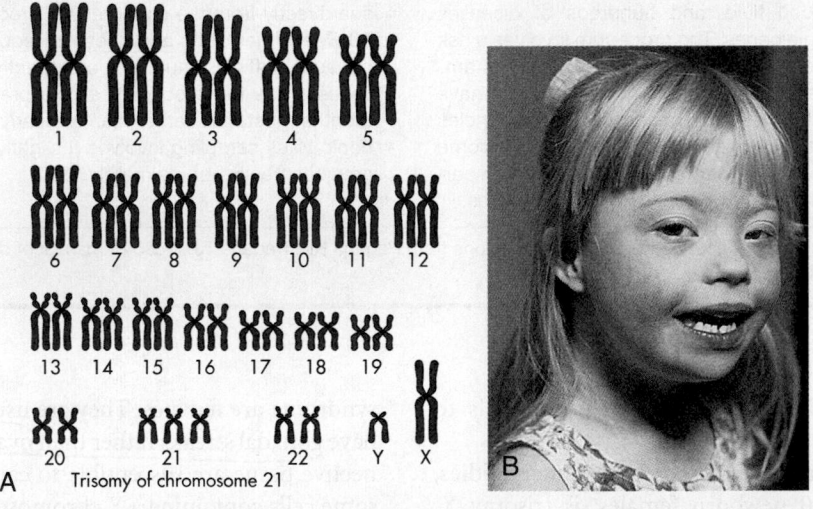

Figure 4-13 Down syndrome. A, The karyotype of Down syndrome consists of 47 chromosomes and shows trisomy 21. B, A child with Down syndrome. (A from Damjanov I: *Pathology for the health-related professions,* ed 3, Philadelphia, 2006, Saunders; B courtesy Olney A and MacDonald M, University of Nebraska Medical Center, Omaha.)

with Turner syndrome have simple monosomy of the X chromosome; others have one of several more complex X chromosome abnormalities. The 45,X karyotype is more common among conceptions, however, and about 15% to 20% of spontaneous abortions with chromosome abnormalities have this karyotype, making it one of the most common single-chromosome aberrations. Thus the condition is highly lethal during gestation: less than 1% of 45,X conceptions survive to term. Most fetuses that survive to term are mosaics, with

combinations of 45,X cells and XX, XXX, or XY cells. It is likely that the presence of some normal cells in mosaic fetuses enhances fetal survival.

Teenagers with Turner syndrome are typically treated with estrogen to promote the development of secondary sexual characteristics. The dose is then continued at a reduced level to maintain these characteristics and to help avoid osteoporosis. Human growth hormone is sometimes administered to increase stature.

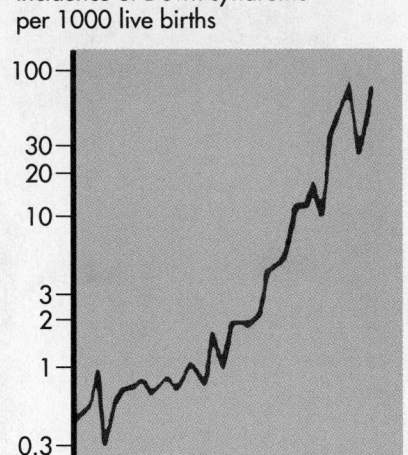

Incidence of Down syndrome per 1000 live births

Maternal age (yr)

Figure 4-14 **Down syndrome increases with maternal age.** Rate is per 1000 live births related to maternal age.

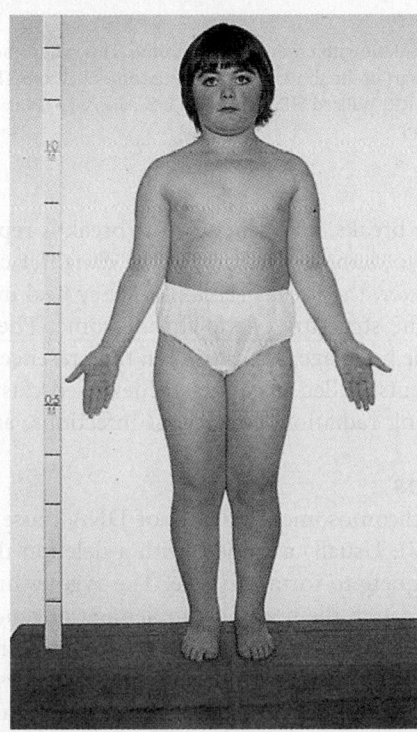

Figure 4-15 **Turner syndrome.** A sex chromosome is missing, and the person's chromosomes are 45,X. Characteristic signs are short stature, female genitalia, webbed neck, shieldlike chest with underdeveloped breasts and widely spaced nipples, and imperfectly developed ovaries. (From Patton KT, Thibodeau GA: *Anatomy & physiology,* ed 7, St Louis, 2010, Mosby.)

Individuals with at least two X chromosomes and a Y chromosome in each cell (47,XXY karyotype) have a disorder known as **Klinefelter syndrome** (Figure 4-16). Because of the presence of a Y chromosome, these individuals have a male appearance, but they are usually sterile, and about half develop

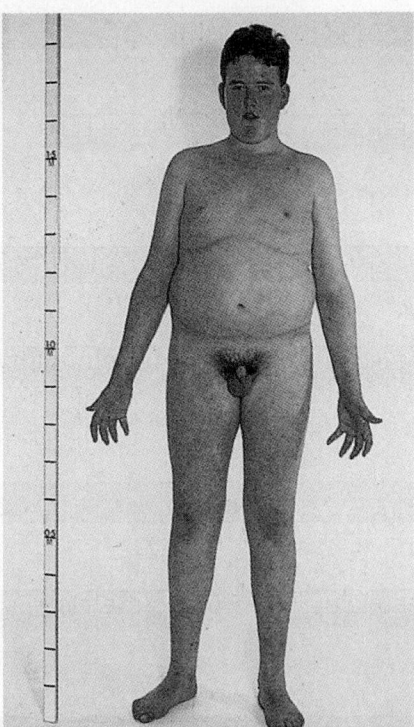

Figure 4-16 **Klinefelter syndrome.** This young man exhibits many characteristics of Klinefelter syndrome: small testes, some development of the breasts, sparse body hair, and long limbs. This syndrome results from the presence of two or more X chromosomes with one Y chromosome (genotypes XXY or XXXY, for example). (From Patton KT, Thibodeau GA: *Anatomy & physiology,* ed 7, St Louis, 2010, Mosby.)

female-like breasts (a condition called *gynecomastia*). The testes are small, body hair is sparse, the voice is often somewhat high pitched, stature is elevated, and a moderate degree of mental impairment may be present. Klinefelter syndrome is found in about 1 in 1000 male births. About two thirds of the cases are caused by nondisjunction of the X chromosomes in the mother, and the frequency of the disorder rises with maternal age. Individuals with the XXXY and XXXXY karyotypes also are considered to have Klinefelter syndrome, and the degree of physical and mental impairment increases with each additional X chromosome. Regardless of the number of X chromosomes, however, these individuals have a male appearance. The presence of a single Y chromosome, which causes the undifferentiated gonads to become testes, always produces a male. Mosaicism is sometimes seen in Klinefelter syndrome and results in less severe disease; the most prevalent combination is XXY and XY cells.

The other sex chromosome aneuploidy that affects males is the 47,XYY karyotype. Individuals with this karyotype tend to be taller than average, and they have a 10- to 15-point reduction in average IQ. This condition, which causes few serious physical problems, achieved notoriety when it was found that its incidence in prison populations was about 1 in 30 (compared with 1 in 1000 in the general male population). This discovery led to the suggestion that this chromosome might predispose affected individuals to violent, criminal behavior. Several dozen studies have addressed this issue, and they have

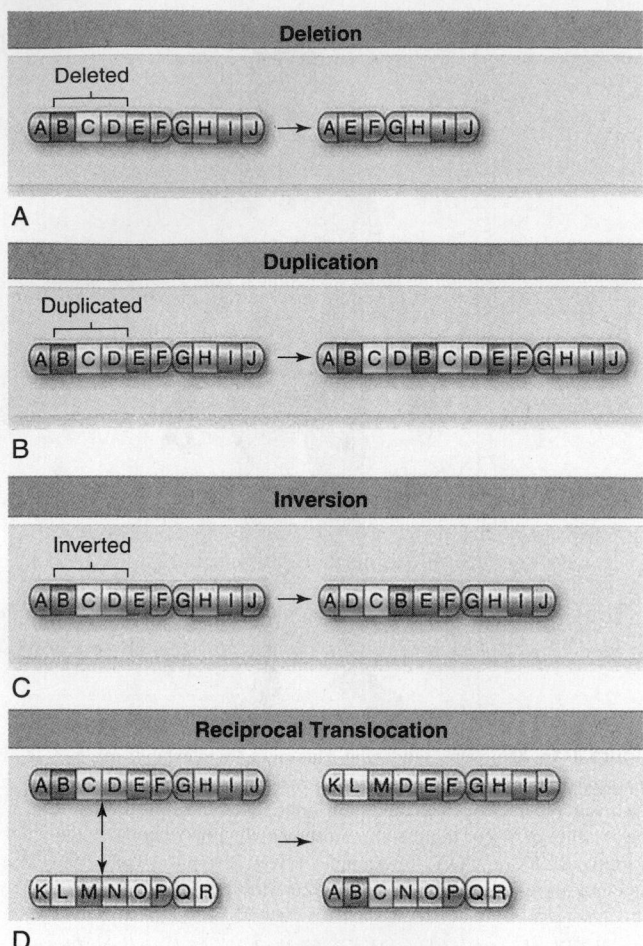

Figure 4-17 Chromosomal mutations. Larger-scale changes in chromosomes are also possible. Material can be deleted (**A**), duplicated (**B**), and inverted (**C**). Translocations occur when one chromosome is broken and becomes part of another chromosome. This often occurs where both chromosomes are broken and exchange material, an event called a reciprocal translocation (**D**). (From Raven PH et al: *Biology*, ed 8, New York, 2008, McGraw-Hill.)

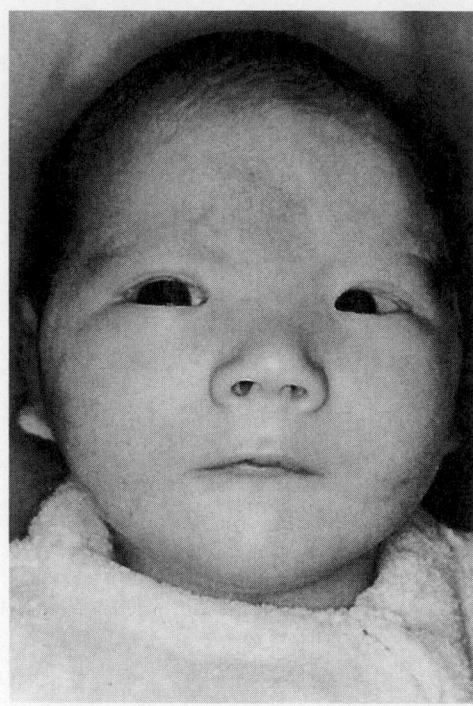

Figure 4-18 Infant with cri du chat syndrome. This syndrome is caused by deletion of part of the short arm of chromosome 5. (From Thompson MW, McInnes RR, Willard HF: *Genetics in medicine*, ed 5, Philadelphia, 1991, Saunders.)

shown that 47,XYY males are not inclined to commit violent crimes. However, even after adjusting for the effects of decreased IQ, some evidence exists for an increased incidence of behavioral disorders.

Abnormalities of Chromosome Structure

In addition to the loss or gain of whole chromosomes, parts of chromosomes can be lost or duplicated as gametes are formed, and the arrangement of genes on chromosomes can be altered. Unlike aneuploidy and polyploidy, these changes sometimes do not have serious consequences for an individual's health. Some of them can even go entirely unnoticed, especially when very small pieces of chromosomes are involved. Nevertheless, abnormalities of chromosome structure also can produce serious disease in individuals or their offspring.

During meiosis and mitosis, chromosomes usually maintain their structural integrity very well, but **chromosome breakage** occasionally does occur. Mechanisms exist to "heal" these breaks, and generally the break is repaired perfectly with no damage resulting to the daughter cell. Sometimes, however, the breaks remain, or they heal in a fashion that alters the structure of the chromosome. The extent of chromosome breakage is increased in the presence of certain harmful agents, called **clastogens.** Identified clastogens include ionizing radiation, some viral infections, and certain chemicals.

Deletions

Broken chromosomes and loss of DNA cause **deletions** (Figure 4-17). Usually a gamete with a deletion unites with a normal gamete to form a zygote. The zygote thus has one chromosome with the normal complement of genes and one with some missing genes. Because a fairly large number of genes can be lost in a deletion, serious consequences can result even though one copy of the chromosome is normal. An often cited example of a disease caused by a chromosomal deletion is the **cri du chat syndrome** (Figure 4-18). The term, which literally means "cry of the cat," describes the characteristic cry of the affected child. Other symptoms include low birth weight, severe mental retardation, microcephaly (smaller than normal head size), heart defects, and the typical facial appearance shown in Figure 4-18. The disease is caused by a deletion of part of the short arm of chromosome 5.

Duplications

Duplications of chromosome material are, like deletions, a form of chromosome aberration (see Figure 4-17). Because a deficiency of genetic material is more harmful than an excess, duplications usually have less serious consequences than deletions. For example, a deletion of a region of chromosome 5 causes cri du chat syndrome, but a duplication of the same region causes less severe disease.

Inversions

An **inversion** is the occurrence of two breaks on a chromosome, followed by the reinsertion of the missing fragment at its original site but in inverted order (see Figure 4-17). Thus a chromosome symbolized as ABCDEFG might become ABEDCFG after an inversion.

Unlike deletions and duplications, inversions result in no loss or gain of genetic material. They are thus said to be a "balanced" alteration of chromosome structure, and they often have no apparent physical effect. Genes are sometimes influenced by neighboring DNA sequences, however, and this **position effect,** a change in a gene's expression caused by its position, does sometimes result in physical defects in persons with inversions.

The serious problems caused by inversions usually occur in the offspring of individuals carrying the inversion. Because chromosomes must line up in perfect order during prophase I, a chromosome with an inversion must form a loop to line up with its normal homolog. Crossing over within this loop can result in duplications or deletions in the chromosomes of daughter cells. Thus the offspring of individuals who carry inversions often have chromosome deletions or duplications.

Translocations

The interchanging of genetic material between nonhomologous chromosomes is called **translocation.** The clinically most important type of translocation is termed a **Robertsonian translocation.** In this translocation the long arms of two nonhomologous chromosomes fuse at the centromere, forming a single chromosome (Figure 4-19). Robertsonian translocations are confined to chromosomes 13, 14, 15, 21, and 22 because the short arms of these chromosomes are very small and contain no essential genetic material. When a Robertsonian translocation takes place, the short arms are usually lost during subsequent cell divisions. Because the carriers of Robertsonian translocations lose no important genetic material, they are normal, although they have only 45 chromosomes in each cell. Their offspring, however, may have serious deletions or duplications (see Figure 4-19). For example, a common Robertsonian translocation involves the fusion of the long arms of chromosomes 21 and 14. An offspring who inherits a gamete carrying the fused chromosome receives an extra copy of the long arm of chromosome 21 and thus develops Down syndrome. Robertsonian translocations are responsible for approximately 3% to 5% of Down syndrome cases. Parents who carry a Robertsonian translocation involving chromosome 21 have an increased risk for producing multiple offspring with Down syndrome.

A **reciprocal translocation** occurs when breaks take place in two different chromosomes and the material is exchanged (see Figure 4-17). As with Robertsonian translocations, the carrier of a reciprocal translocation is usually normal because the individual has a normal complement of genetic material. However, the carrier's gametes can be normal, can carry the translocation, or can have duplications and deletions.

Fragile Sites

For reasons not yet fully understood, a number of areas on chromosomes develop distinctive breaks and gaps (observable microscopically) when the cells are cultured in a folate-deficient medium. Most of these **fragile sites** have no apparent relationship to disease. However, one fragile site, located on the long arm of the X chromosome, is associated with a disorder of considerable importance, both clinically and genetically. This disorder is known as the *fragile X syndrome.* The most important feature of this syndrome is mental retardation. With a relatively high population prevalence (affecting approximately 1 in 4000 males and 1 in 8000 females), the fragile X syndrome is the second most common genetic cause of mental retardation (after Down syndrome).

Fragile X syndrome involves a puzzling pattern of inheritance. In particular, males who inherit the mutation do not necessarily express the disease condition but they can pass it on to descendants who do express it. Ordinarily, a male who inherits a disease gene on the X chromosome expresses the condition because he has only one X chromosome. Another uncommon feature of this disease is that about one third of carrier females are affected, although less severely than males. Many mechanisms have been proposed to account for the complex mode of inheritance of the fragile X syndrome. It has been shown that unaffected transmitting males have an elevated number (more than about 50) of repeated DNA sequences in the first exon of the fragile X gene. These "repeats" consist of CGG sequences that are duplicated again and again. Affected males have a much larger number of these repeats—200 or more[9] (Figure 4-20). An increase in the number of these repeated sequences in successive generations can lead to expression of the fragile X syndrome. More than 20 other genetic diseases also are caused by this mechanism.[10,11]

ELEMENTS OF FORMAL GENETICS

The mechanisms by which an individual's set of paired chromosomes produces traits are the principles of genetic inheritance. Mendel's work with garden peas first defined these principles. Later geneticists have refined Mendel's work to explain patterns of inheritance for traits and diseases that appear in families.

Analysis of traits that occur with defined, predictable patterns has helped geneticists link the pieces of the human gene map. Research focuses on assigning genes to specific locations on chromosomes. Eventually, diseases and defects caused by single genes can be traced, and therapies to prevent and treat such diseases can be developed.

Many traits are caused by single genes and are often called *mendelian traits* (after Gregor Mendel). Each gene occupies a position along a chromosome known as a **locus.** The genes at a particular locus can take different forms (i.e., they can

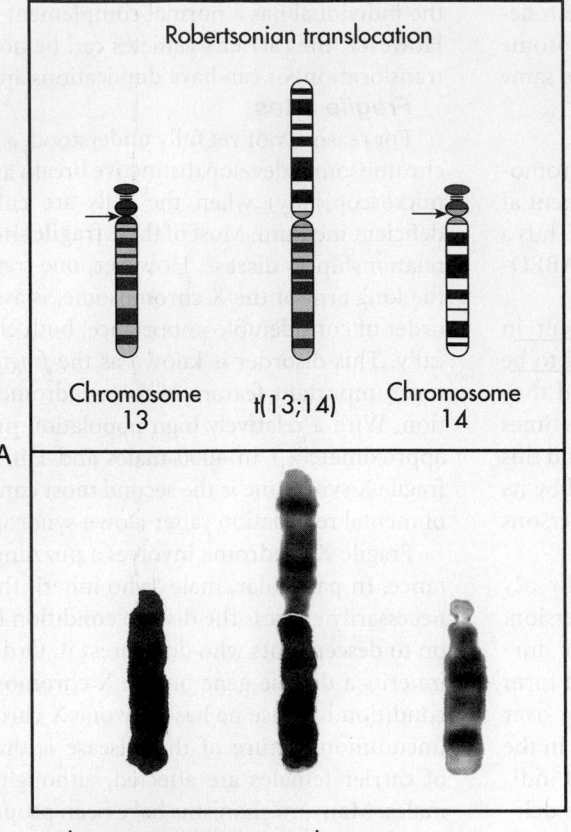

Robertsonian translocation

Chromosome 13   t(13;14)   Chromosome 14

A

Figure 4-19 Translocation. A, In a Robertsonian translocation, shown here, the long arms of two acrocentric chromosomes (13 and 14) fuse, forming a single chromosome. **B,** The possible segregation patterns for gametes formed by a carrier of a Robertsonian translocation. Alternate segregation (quadrant **a** alone, or quadrant **b** with quadrant **c**) produces either a normal chromosome constitution or a translocation carrier with a normal phenotype. Adjacent segregation (quadrant **a** with **c**, quadrant **c** alone, quadrant **a** with **b**, or quadrant **b** alone) produces unbalanced gametes and results in conceptions with translocation Down syndrome, monosomy 21, trisomy 14, or monosomy 14, respectively. For example, monosomy 14 is produced when the parent who carries the translocation transmits a copy of chromosome 21 but does not transmit a copy of chromosome 14 (as in the lower right corner). (From Jorde LB et al: *Medical genetics,* ed 3, St. Louis, 2003, Mosby.)

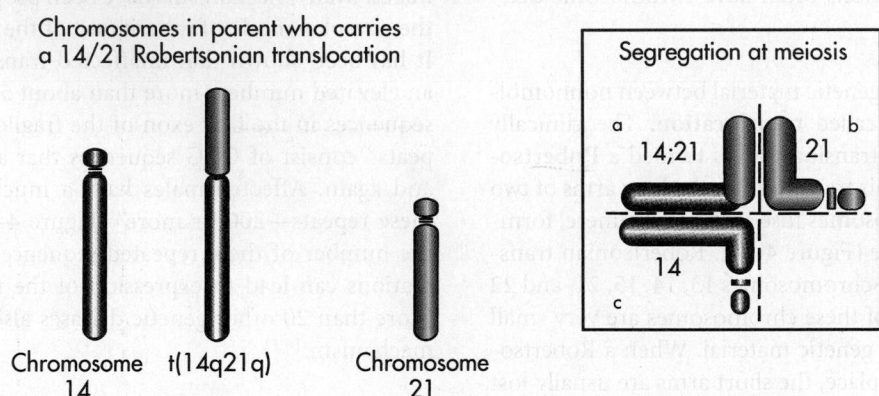

Chromosomes in parent who carries
a 14/21 Robertsonian translocation

Chromosome 14   t(14q21q)   Chromosome 21

Segregation at meiosis

a   14;21   21   b

14   c

B

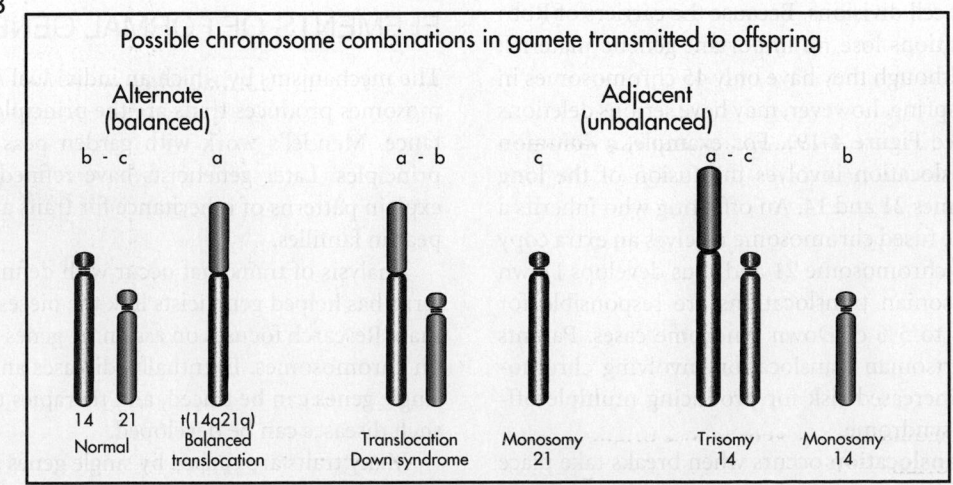

Possible chromosome combinations in gamete transmitted to offspring

Alternate
(balanced)

b - c   a

14 21   t(14q21q)
Normal   Balanced
translocation

Adjacent
(unbalanced)

a - b   c   a - c   b

Translocation   Monosomy   Trisomy   Monosomy
Down syndrome   21   14   14

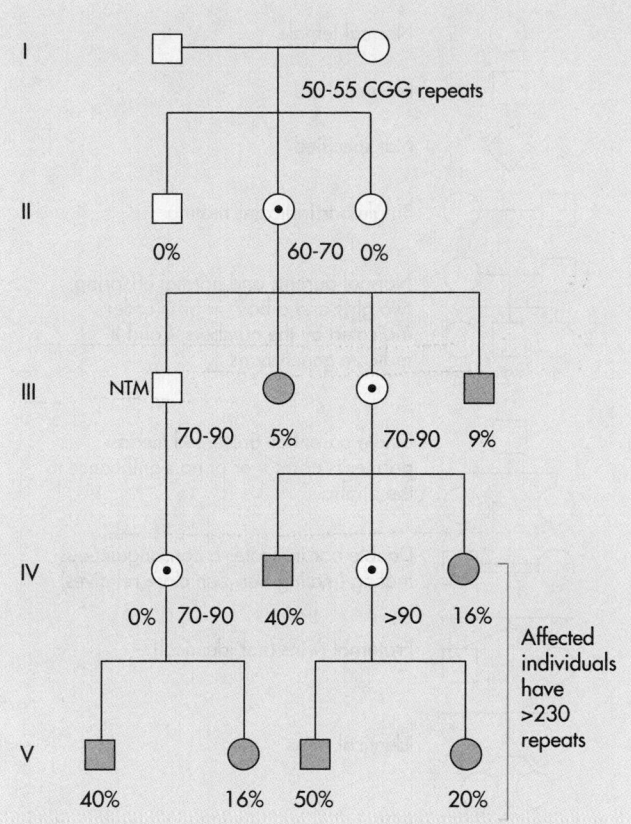

Figure 4-20 A pedigree showing the inheritance of the fragile X syndrome. Females who carry a premutation (50 to 320 CGG repeats) are represented with a ⊙. Affected individuals are represented by solid symbols. A normal transmitting male (NTM), who carries a premutation of 70 to 90 repeats increases each time the mutation is passed through another female. Also, only 5% of the NTM's sisters are affected, and only 9% of his brothers are affected, but 40% of his grandsons and 16% of his granddaughters are affected. This is the Sherman paradox. (From Jorde LB et al: *Medical genetics,* ed 3, St Louis, 2003, Mosby.)

be composed of different nucleotide sequences). These different forms are called **alleles.** For example, most people have a type of hemoglobin known as *hemoglobin A.* A few individuals have an alternative form of hemoglobin, termed *hemoglobin S,* which differs from hemoglobin A by a single amino acid substitution in the beta-globin component of the molecule. The β-globin locus thus has two different alleles, one that encodes hemoglobin A and another that encodes hemoglobin S. A locus that has two or more alleles that occur with an appreciable frequency in a population is said to be **polymorphic** or a **polymorphism.**

Because humans are diploid organisms, each chromosome is represented twice, with one member of the chromosome pair contributed by the father and one by the mother. At a given locus an individual has one gene whose origin is paternal and one whose origin is maternal. When the two genes are identical, the individual is **homozygous** at that locus. When the genes are not identical, the individual is **heterozygous** at the locus.

Phenotype and Genotype

The composition of genes at a given locus is known as the **genotype.** The outward appearance of an individual, which is the result of both genotype and environment, is the **phenotype.** For example, an infant who is born with an inability to metabolize the amino acid phenylalanine has the single-gene disorder known as *phenylketonuria (PKU)* and thus has the PKU genotype. If the condition is left untreated, abnormal metabolites of phenylalanine will begin to accumulate in the infant's brain and irreversible mental retardation will occur. Mental retardation is thus one aspect of the PKU phenotype. By imposing dietary restrictions to limit the intake of food containing phenylalanine, however, retardation can be prevented. Although the child still has the PKU genotype, a modification of the environment (in this case the child's diet) produces an outwardly normal phenotype.

Dominance and Recessiveness

In many loci the effects of one allele mask those of another when the two are found together in a **heterozygote.** The allele whose effects are observable is said to be **dominant.** The allele whose effects are hidden is said to be **recessive** (from the Latin root for "hiding"). Traditionally, for loci having two alleles, the dominant allele is denoted by an uppercase letter and the recessive allele is denoted by a lowercase letter. When one allele is dominant over another, the heterozygote genotype *Aa* has the same phenotype as the dominant homozygote *AA.* For the recessive allele to be expressed, it must exist in the **homozygote** form, *aa.*

When the heterozygote is distinguishable from both homozygotes, the locus is said to exhibit **codominance.** For example, in the MN blood group, both alleles, *M* and *N,* of the heterozygote are detectable and therefore codominant. Another example is the ABO blood group, in which heterozygotes having the *A* and *B* alleles express both of them as A and B antigens on their red cells (forming blood group AB).

A **carrier** is an individual who has a disease gene but is phenotypically normal. Most genes for recessive diseases occur in heterozygotes who carry one copy of the gene but do not express the disease. Because many recessive genes are lethal in the homozygous state, they are eliminated from the population when they occur in homozygotes. By "hiding" in carriers, however, most recessive genes for diseases survive to be passed on to the next generation.

TRANSMISSION OF GENETIC DISEASES

An important aspect of a genetic disease is the pattern in which it is inherited through the generations of a family, or its **mode of inheritance.** Once the mode of inheritance is known, much can be learned about the disease gene itself, and reliable genetic counseling can be given to members of families in which the disease is present.

Modes of inheritance were systematically studied by Mendel, who formulated two basic laws of inheritance. His **principle of segregation** states that homologous genes separate from one another during reproduction and that each reproductive cell carries only one of the homologous genes. Mendel's second law, the **principle of independent assortment,** states that the hereditary transmission of one gene has no effect on the transmission of another. Mendel discovered these laws in the mid-nineteenth century by performing breeding experiments with garden peas. He had no knowledge of chromosomes. Early in the twentieth century geneticists found that the behavior of chromosomes does essentially correspond to Mendel's laws, which now form the basis for the **chromosome theory of inheritance.**

The known single-gene diseases can be classified into four major modes of inheritance: autosomal dominant, autosomal recessive, X-linked dominant, and X-linked recessive. The first two types involve genes known to occur on the 22 pairs of autosomes. The last two types occur on the X chromosome; no good documentation exists of disease genes occurring on the Y chromosome. The number of diseases assigned to each category is growing rapidly. Current catalogs of single-gene traits, which include disease-producing and nonclinical traits (e.g., attached earlobes), list more than 17,000 known autosomal traits and 1027 X-linked traits.[1]

An important tool in the analysis of modes of inheritance is the **pedigree** chart. It summarizes family relationships and shows which members of a family are affected by a genetic disease (Figure 4-21). Generally, the pedigree begins with one individual in the family, the **proband,** also termed the **propositus** (male) or **proposita** (female). This individual is usually the first person in the family diagnosed or seen in a clinic.

Autosomal Dominant Inheritance

Characteristics of Pedigrees

Diseases caused by autosomal dominant genes are rare. The most common occur in fewer than 1 in 500 individuals, so it is uncommon for two individuals both affected by the same autosomal dominant disease to produce offspring together. Figure 4-22, A, illustrates this unusual pattern. More often, affected offspring are produced by the union of a normal parent with an affected heterozygous parent. The diagram (Punnett square) in Figure 4-22 illustrates this mating. The affected parent can pass either a disease gene or a normal gene to his or her children. Each event has a probability of 0.5; thus on the average, half of the children will be heterozygous and will express the disease and half will be normal.

Figure 4-23, A, is a typical pedigree showing the transmission of an autosomal dominant gene. The gene shown here causes achondroplasia (Figure 4-23, B). Several important characteristics of this pedigree support the conclusion that the trait is caused by an autosomal dominant gene:

1. The two sexes exhibit the trait in approximately equal proportions, and males and females are equally likely to transmit the trait to their offspring.

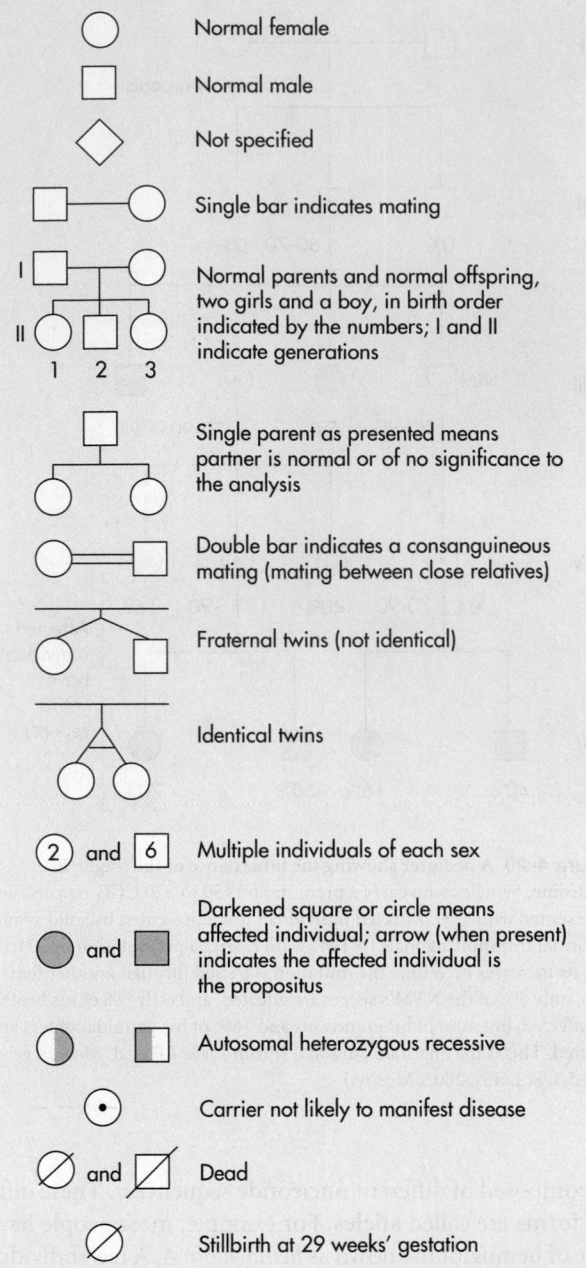

Figure 4-21 Symbols commonly used in pedigrees.

Normal female

Normal male

Not specified

Single bar indicates mating

Normal parents and normal offspring, two girls and a boy, in birth order indicated by the numbers; I and II indicate generations

Single parent as presented means partner is normal or of no significance to the analysis

Double bar indicates a consanguineous mating (mating between close relatives)

Fraternal twins (not identical)

Identical twins

Multiple individuals of each sex

Darkened square or circle means affected individual; arrow (when present) indicates the affected individual is the propositus

Autosomal heterozygous recessive

Carrier not likely to manifest disease

Dead

Stillbirth at 29 weeks' gestation

2. There is no skipping of generations. If an individual has achondroplasia, one parent must also have it. If neither parent has the trait, none of the children has it (with the exception of new mutations, as discussed later).

3. Affected heterozygous individuals transmit the trait to approximately half of their children, but because gamete transmission is subject to chance fluctuations, it is possible that all or none of the children of an affected parent may have the trait. When large numbers of matings of this type are studied, however, the proportion of affected children will closely approach one half.

Affected parent

	D	d
D	DD Homozygous affected (usually rare)	Dd Heterozygous affected
d	Dd Heterozygous affected	dd Homozygous normal

Affected parent

A

Normal parent

	d	d
D	Dd Heterozygous affected	Dd Heterozygous affected
d	dd Homozygous normal	dd Homozygous normal

Affected parent

B

Figure 4-22 **Punnett square and autosomal dominant traits.** A, Punnett square for the mating of two individuals with an autosomal dominant gene. Here both parents are affected by the trait. B, Punnett square for the mating of a normal individual with a carrier for an autosomal dominant gene.

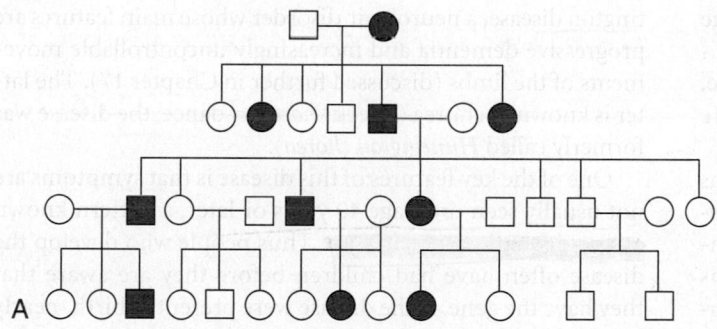

A

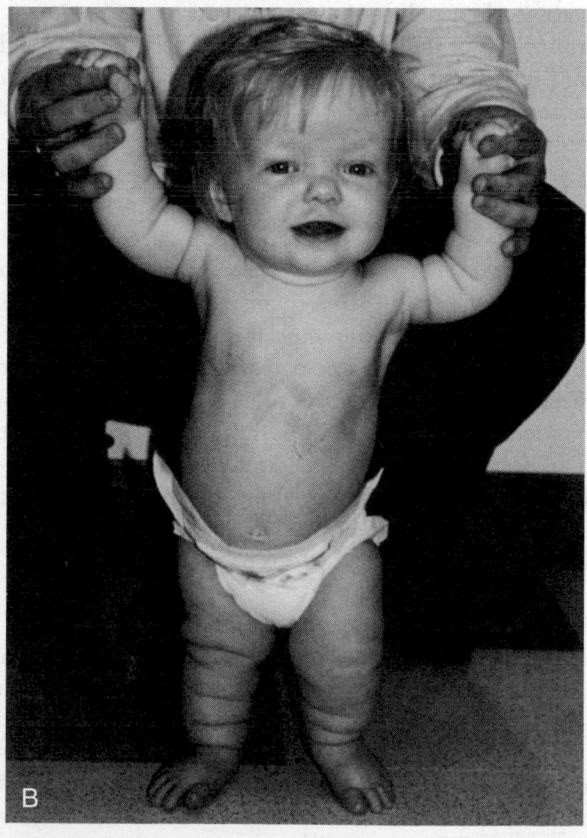

B

Figure 4-23 **Pedigree for achondroplasia.** A, Pedigree showing the transmission of an autosomal dominant disease. B, Achondroplasia. This girl has short limbs relative to trunk length. She also has a prominent forehead, low nasal root, and redundant skin folds in the arms and legs. (B from Jorde LB et al: *Medical genetics,* ed 3, St Louis, 2003, Mosby.)

Recurrence Risks

Parents at risk for producing children with a genetic disease nearly always ask the question, "What is the *chance* that our child will have this disease?" When one child has already been born with a genetic disease, the parents can be given a **recurrence risk,** which is the probability that subsequent children also will have the disease. When one parent is affected by an autosomal dominant disease (and is a heterozygote) and the other is normal, the recurrence risks for each child are one half.

An important principle is that each birth is an independent event, much like a coin toss. Thus, even though parents may already have had a child with the disease, their recurrence risk remains one half. If they have had several children, all affected (or all unaffected) by the disease, the law of independence dictates that the probability that their next child will have the disease is still one half. Parents' misunderstanding of this principle is a common problem encountered in genetic counseling.

If a child has been born with an autosomal dominant disease and there is no history of the disease in the family, the child is probably the product of a new mutation. The gene transmitted by one of the parents has thus undergone a mutation from a normal to a disease-causing allele. The genes at this locus in most of the parent's other germ cells would still be normal. In this situation the recurrence risk for the parent's subsequent offspring is not greater than that of the general population. The offspring of the affected child, however, will have an occurrence risk of one half. Because these diseases often reduce the potential for reproduction, a large proportion of the observed cases of many autosomal dominant diseases are the result of new mutations. For example, approximately seven eighths of all cases of achondroplasia are caused by new mutations.

Occasionally, two or more offspring will present symptoms of an autosomal dominant disease when there is no family history of the disease. Because mutation is a rare event, it is unlikely that this disease would be a result of multiple mutations in the same family. The mechanism most likely to be responsible is termed **germline mosaicism.** During the embryonic development of one of the parents, a mutation occurred that affected all or part of the germline but few or none of the somatic cells of the embryo. Thus the parent carries the mutation in his or her germline but does not actually express the disease. As a result, the unaffected parent can transmit the mutation to multiple offspring. This phenomenon, although relatively rare, can have significant effects on recurrence risks.[12]

Penetrance and Expressivity

An important variation seen in some autosomal dominant diseases is incomplete penetrance. The **penetrance** of a trait is the percentage of individuals with a specific genotype who also exhibit the expected phenotype. Incomplete penetrance means that individuals who have the gene for a disease may not exhibit the disease phenotype at all, even though the gene and the associated disease may be transmitted to the next generation. A pedigree illustrating the transmission of an autosomal

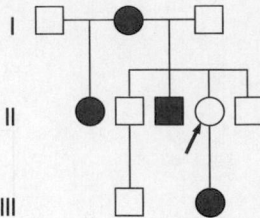

Figure 4-24 Pedigree for retinoblastoma showing incomplete penetrance. The female with marked arrow in line II must be heterozygous, but she does not express the trait.

dominant gene with incomplete penetrance is given in Figure 4-24. Retinoblastoma, the most common malignant eye tumor affecting children, is one disease that typically exhibits incomplete penetrance. About 10% of the individuals who are **obligate carriers** of the gene (i.e., those who have an affected parent and affected children and therefore must themselves carry the gene) do not have the disease. The penetrance of the gene is then said to be 90%.

The gene responsible for retinoblastoma has been mapped to the long arm of chromosome 13, and its DNA sequence has been studied extensively. This gene is known as a **tumor-suppressor gene:** the normal function of its protein product is to regulate the cell cycle so that cells do not grow uncontrollably. When a mutation alters the protein, its tumor-suppressing capacity is lost and a tumor can form[13,14] (see Chapters 11 and 19).

Another well-known autosomal dominant diseases is Huntington disease, a neurologic disorder whose main features are progressive dementia and increasingly uncontrollable movements of the limbs (discussed further in Chapter 17). The latter is known as chorea (Greek *khoreia* = dance; the disease was formerly called *Huntington chorea*).

One of the key features of this disease is that symptoms are not usually seen until age 40 years or later, a pattern known as **age-dependent** penetrance. Thus people who develop the disease often have had children before they are aware that they have the gene. If the disease were present at birth, nearly all those affected would die before reaching reproductive age, and the occurrence of the gene in the population would be much lower. From the gene's "point of view," a delayed age of onset is quite advantageous. An individual whose parent has the disease has a 50% chance of developing it during middle age. He or she is thus confronted with a torturous question: "Should I have children, knowing that there is a 50-50 chance that I may have this disease gene and pass it to half my children?" Age-dependent penetrance characterizes a number of important genetic diseases, including familial breast cancer, hemochromatosis, and polycystic kidney disease.

Most genetic diseases exhibit variable expressivity. **Expressivity** is the extent of variation in phenotype associated with a particular genotype. If expressivity of a disease is variable, the penetrance may be complete but the severity of the disease can vary greatly. A well-known example of variable expressivity in an autosomal dominant disease is type 1 neurofibromatosis, or von Recklinghausen disease. The gene that causes neurofibromatosis has been mapped to the long arm of chromosome 17, and studies of its DNA sequence indicate that it, like the retinoblastoma gene, is a tumor-suppressor gene.[15] The expression of this gene can vary from a few harmless café-au-lait spots ("coffee with milk," describing the light brown color) on the skin to numerous malignant neurofibromas, scoliosis, seizures, gliomas, neuromas, hypertension, and learning disabilities (Figure 4-25).

A parent with mild expression of the disease—so mild that he or she is not aware of it—can transmit the gene to a child, who can then exhibit severe expression of the disease. As with incomplete penetrance, variable expressivity provides a mechanism by which autosomal dominant genes can be maintained at higher prevalence rates in populations.

Several factors can cause variation in expressivity. Genes at other loci can sometimes modify the expression of a disease gene (these are termed *modifier genes*). Environmental factors also can influence the expression of a disease gene. Finally, different types of mutations at a locus can cause variation in severity. For example, a base substitution resulting in a single amino acid change usually produces a mild form of the clotting disorder hemophilia A (Box 4-3). A base substitution resulting in a "stop" codon (and thus premature termination of translation) usually produces a more severe form of hemophilia A.

Epigenetics and Genomic Imprinting

Although the emphasis of this chapter is on DNA sequence variation and its consequence for disease, there is increasing evidence that the same DNA sequence can produce dramatically different phenotypes, depending on chemical modifications that alter the expression of genes (these modifications are collectively termed **epigenetic**). An important example of such a modification is **DNA methylation,** the attachment of methyl groups to cytosine bases in the DNA sequence (Figure 4-26). When the DNA sequence near a gene becomes heavily methylated, the DNA is less likely to be transcribed into mRNA. In other words, the gene becomes **transcriptionally inactive** or **silenced** (also see Chapters 11 and 12). A study showed that identical (monozygotic) twins accumulate different methylation patterns in the DNA sequences of their somatic cells as they age, causing increasing numbers of phenotypic differences. Intriguingly, twins with more differences in their lifestyles (e.g., smoking versus nonsmoking) accumulated larger numbers of differences in their methylation patterns. The twins, despite having identical DNA sequences, become more and more different as a result of epigenetic changes, which in turn affect the expression of genes.

Epigenetic alteration of gene activity can have important disease consequences. For example, a major cause of one form of inherited colon cancer (termed hereditary nonpolyposis colorectal cancer, or HNPCC) is the methylation of a gene whose protein product repairs damaged DNA. When this gene becomes inactive, damaged DNA accumulates, resulting eventually in colon tumors.

Approximately 100 human genes are thought to be methylated differentially, depending on which parent transmits the gene. This epigenetic modification, characterized by methylation and other changes, is termed **genomic imprinting.** For

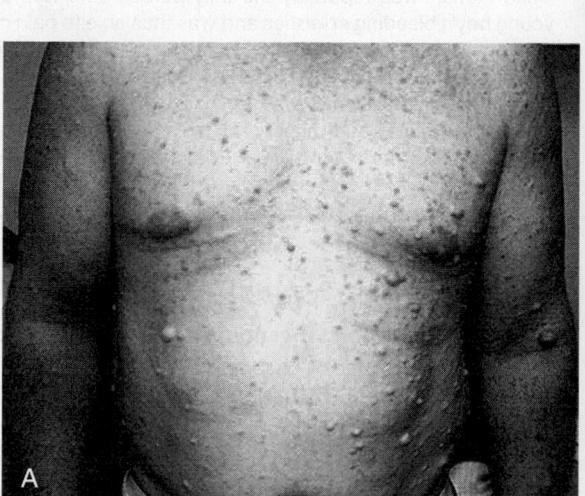
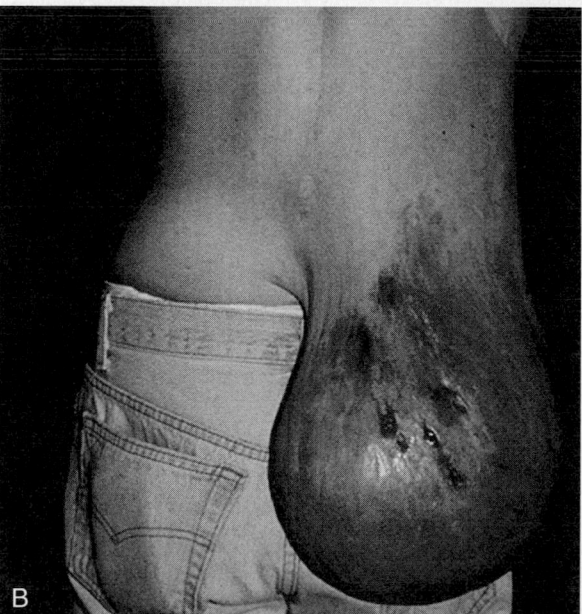

Figure 4-25 Neurofibromatosis. **A,** Young adult with multiple dermal neurofibromas of the trunk. **B,** Individual has a large plexiform neurofibroma hanging from lower right back, causing considerable inconvenience and discomfort (substantially improved by surgical removal of tumor). (From Jorde LB et al: *Medical genetics,* ed 3, St Louis, 2003, Mosby. **B** courtesy Dr. D. Viskochil, University of Utah Health Sciences Center.)

Box 4-3   Hemophilia A and the Russian Revolution

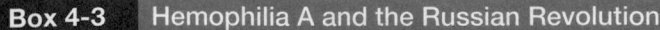

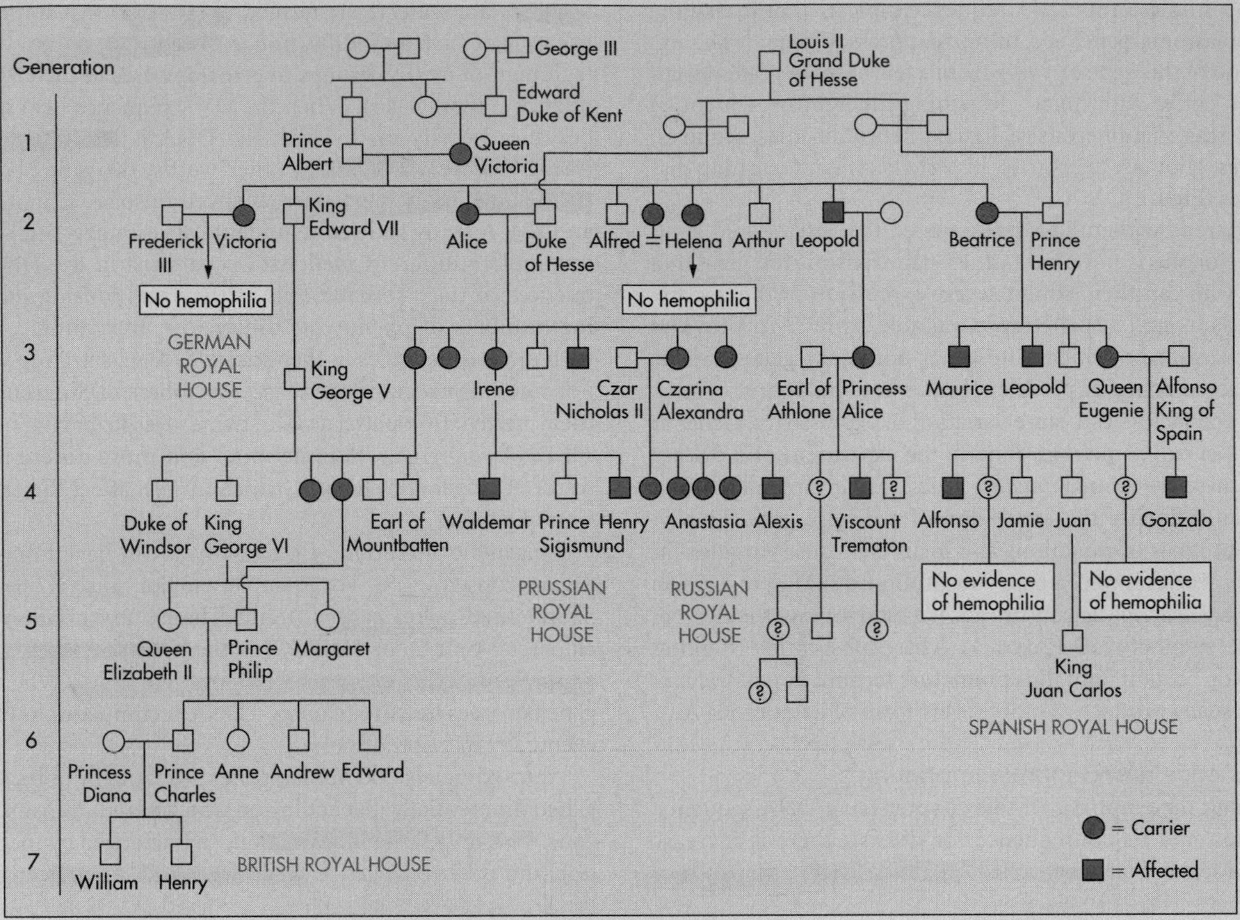

Partial pedigree for descendants of Queen Victoria, showing appearance of hemophilia A in one of her sons and in his descendants and in descendants of her daughters and granddaughters. Royal families of Prussia, Hesse, Battenberg (Mountbatten), Russia, and Spain were thus affected with the disease. The present royal family of England, however, is free of the disease, in spite of inbreeding.

The figure (partial pedigree for descendants of Queen Victoria) is one of the best-known disease pedigrees in existence. It shows the transmission of hemophilia A in the European royal families. This disease, often called a *bleeder syndrome,* is caused by a defect in one of the blood-clotting factors, factor VIII, and can cause severe hemorrhages. In this pedigree Queen Victoria of England was the first known carrier of the disease, and several of her male descendants were affected by it. One of the most historically significant consequences of this pedigree involves the hemophiliac Czarevich

Alexis, son of Czar Nicholas II of Russia. Gregori Rasputin, the "mad monk," was reputedly the only person able to prevent the young boy's bleeding episodes and was thus able to gain considerable power over the royal family. Rasputin's destabilizing influence is thought to have hastened the 1917 Bolshevik revolution.

The Russian royal family was again touched by genetics. Modern DNA "fingerprints" and mitochondrial DNA sequences were used to prove that a mass burial near Ekaterinburg, Russia, contained the remains of most of the executed members of the czar's family.

each of these genes, one of the parents "imprints" the gene (inactivates it) when it is transmitted to the offspring. An example is the insulin-like growth factor 2 gene (*IGF-II*) on chromosome 11, which is transmitted by both parents. But the copy inherited from the mother is normally methylated and inactivated (imprinted). Thus, only one copy of IGF-II is active in normal individuals. However, the maternal "imprint" is occasionally lost, resulting in two active copies of IGF-II. This causes excess fetal growth and a condition known as Beckwith-Wiedemann syndrome.

A second example of genomic imprinting is a deletion of part of the long arm of chromosome 15 (15q11-q13) which, when inherited from the father, causes the offspring to manifest a disease known as *Prader-Willi syndrome* (short stature, obesity, hypogonadism). When the same deletion is inherited from the mother, the offspring develop *Angelman syndrome* (mental retardation, seizures, ataxic gait). The two different phenotypes reflect the fact that different genes are normally active in the maternally and paternally transmitted copies of this region of chromosome 15.

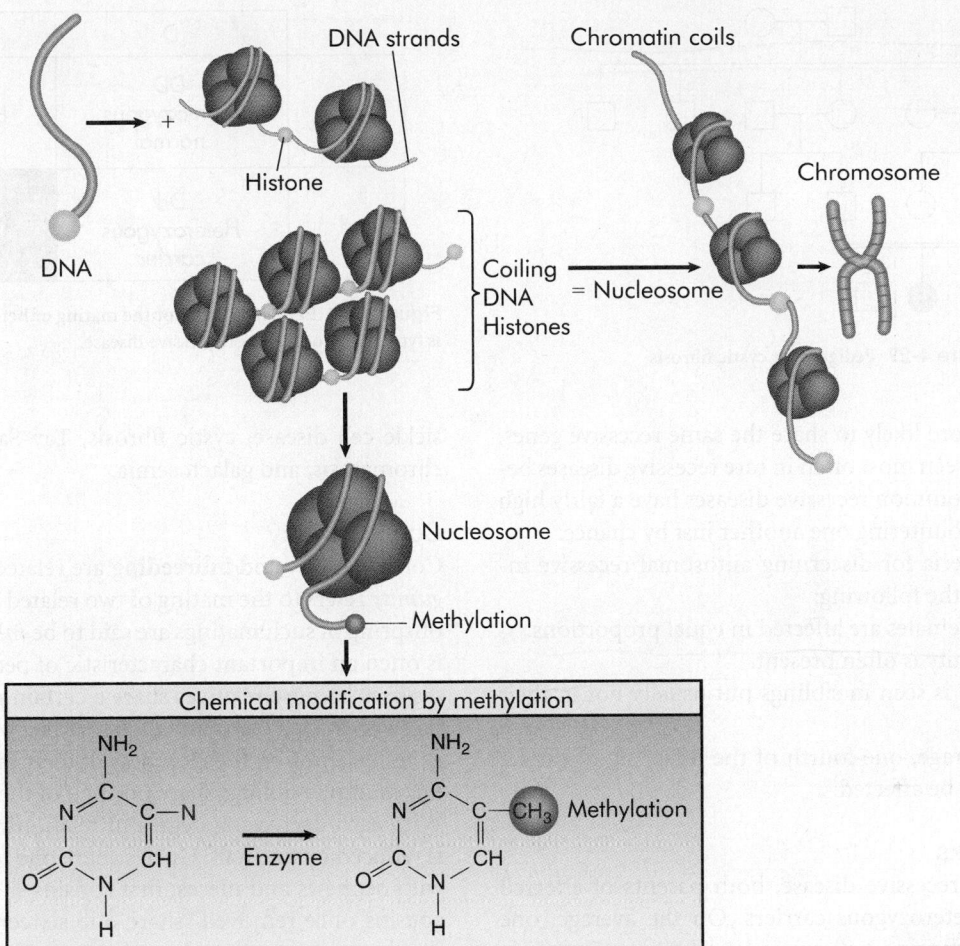

Figure 4-26 Epigenetic modifications. Because DNA is a long molecule, it needs packaging to fit into the tiny nucleus. Packaging involves coiling of the DNA in a "left-handed" spiral around spools, made of four pairs of proteins individually known as histones and collectively as the histone octamer. The entire spool is called a nucleosome. Nucleosomes are organized into chromatin, the repeating building blocks of a chromosome. Histone modifications are correlated with methylation, are reversible, and occur at multiple sites. Methylation occurs at the 5 position of cytosine and provides a "footprint" or signature as a unique epigenetic alteration (red). When genes are expressed, chromatin is open or active; however, when chromatin is condensed because of methylation and histone modification, genes are inactivated.

Autosomal Recessive Inheritance

Characteristics of Pedigrees

Like autosomal dominant diseases, those caused by autosomal recessive genes are rare in populations, although the number of carriers for recessive diseases can be high. The most common lethal recessive disease in white children, cystic fibrosis, occurs in about 1 in 2500 births. Approximately 1 in 25 whites carries one copy of the gene for cystic fibrosis (see Chapter 34). Because an individual must be homozygous for a recessive gene to express the disease, the carriers are phenotypically normal. Because most genes for recessive diseases are maintained in normal carriers, they are able to survive in the population from one generation to the next. As with many autosomal dominant diseases, many autosomal recessive diseases are characterized by delayed age of onset, incomplete penetrance, and variable expressivity.

Figure 4-27 shows a pedigree for cystic fibrosis. The cystic fibrosis gene, which has been mapped to the long arm of chromosome 7, encodes a protein product that forms chloride channels in the membranes of specialized epithelial cells.[16] Defective transport of chloride ions leads to a salt imbalance that results in secretions of abnormally thick, dehydrated mucus. Some of the digestive organs, particularly the pancreas, become obstructed, causing malnutrition, and the lungs become clogged with mucus, making them highly susceptible to bacterial infections (especially *Pseudomonas*). Death from lung disease or heart failure occurs on average by about 37 years of age. In the pedigree shown, the two affected individuals are the offspring of the marriage of two first cousins. Marriage between related individuals, termed **consanguinity** (from the Latin root meaning "with blood"), is often a factor in producing children with recessive diseases because related

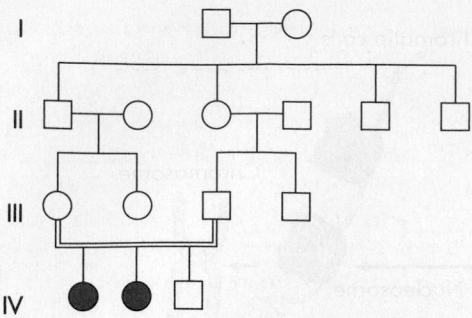

Figure 4-27 Pedigree for cystic fibrosis.

	D	d
D	DD Homozygous normal	Dd Heterozygous carrier
d	Dd Heterozygous carrier	dd Homozygous affected

Figure 4-28 Punnett square for the mating of heterozygous carriers. This is typical of most cases of recessive disease.

individuals are more likely to share the same recessive genes. Consanguinity is seen most often in rare recessive diseases because carriers of common recessive diseases have a fairly high probability of encountering one another just by chance.

Important criteria for discerning autosomal recessive inheritance include the following:

1. Males and females are affected in equal proportions.
2. Consanguinity is often present.
3. The disease is seen in siblings but usually not in their parents.
4. On the average, one fourth of the offspring of carrier parents will be affected.

Recurrence Risks

In most cases of recessive disease, both parents of affected individuals are heterozygous carriers. On the average, one fourth of their offspring will be normal homozygotes, one half will be phenotypically normal carrier heterozygotes, and one fourth will be homozygotes with the disease (Figure 4-28). Thus the recurrence risk for the offspring of carrier parents is 25%. As stated, these are the *average* figures. In any given family, chance fluctuations are likely, but a study of a large number of families would yield figures close to these proportions.

If two parents have a recessive disease, they each must be homozygous for the disease. Therefore, when two parents are affected by a recessive disease, all their children also must be affected. This observation helps to distinguish recessive from dominant inheritance, because two parents both affected by a dominant gene are nearly always both heterozygotes and thus one fourth of their children will be unaffected.

Because carrier parents usually are unaware that they both carry the same recessive gene, they often produce an affected child before knowing of their condition. **Carrier detection tests** can identify heterozygotes by measuring the reduced amount of a critical enzyme available. The critical enzyme is totally lacking in a homozygous recessive individual, but an essentially normal phenotype is seen when it is present in a reduced quantity in the carrier. Often carriers can be detected by direct examination of the disease locus for a mutation. Such testing is especially valuable for siblings of known carriers, who may themselves be carriers. Some recessive diseases for which carrier detection tests are now available are PKU,

sickle cell disease, cystic fibrosis, Tay-Sachs disease, hemochromatosis, and galactosemia.

Consanguinity

Consanguinity and **inbreeding** are related concepts. *Consanguinity* refers to the mating of two related individuals, and the offspring of such matings are said to be *inbred.* Consanguinity is often an important characteristic of pedigrees for recessive diseases because relatives share a certain proportion of genes received from a common ancestor. The proportion of shared genes depends on the closeness of their biologic relationship. For example, siblings share one half of their genes on average. With each decreasing degree of relationship, this proportion is reduced by one half. Uncles share one fourth of their genes with nephews and nieces; first cousins share one eighth; first cousins once removed* share one sixteenth; second cousins share one thirty-second; and so on. With consanguineous matings, recessive disorders are significantly increased. Most empirical studies show that the proportion of offspring of marriages of first cousins who are affected by genetic diseases is approximately double that of the general population.[17] Marriages between first cousins are prohibited in most states of the United States. Marriages between closer relatives (except between double first cousins†) are prohibited throughout the United States.

X-Linked Inheritance

Not all genetic diseases are caused by genes located on the 22 autosomes. Some conditions are instead caused by genes located on the sex chromosomes, and that mode of inheritance is referred to as **sex-linked.** The Y chromosome contains only a few dozen genes, so most sex-linked traits are located on the X chromosome and are said to be X-linked. Only a few diseases are known to be inherited as X-linked dominant traits. Because these diseases are so seldom encountered, only the much more common X-linked recessive diseases are discussed here.

Because females receive two X chromosomes, one from the father and one from the mother, they can be homozygous for

---

*First cousins once removed are the offspring of one's own first cousins.
†Double first cousins share both sets of grandparents; ordinarily first cousins share just one set of grandparents.

a disease allele at a given locus, homozygous for the normal allele at the locus, or heterozygous. Males, having only one X chromosome, are said to be **hemizygous** for genes on this chromosome. A male who inherits a recessive disease gene on the X chromosome will be affected by the disease because the Y chromosome does not carry a normal allele to counteract the effects of the disease gene. Males are always more frequently affected by X-linked recessive diseases, with the difference becoming more pronounced as the disease becomes rarer.

X Inactivation

In the late 1950s Mary Lyon proposed that one X chromosome in the somatic cells of females is permanently inactivated, a process termed *X inactivation*.[18] This proposal, known as the *Lyon hypothesis*, explains why most gene products coded by the X chromosome are present in equal amounts in males and females, even though males have only one X chromosome and females have two X chromosomes. This phenomenon is called **dosage compensation.** The inactivated X chromosomes are observable in many interphase cells as highly condensed intranuclear chromatin bodies, termed **Barr bodies** (after Barr and Bertram, who discovered them in the late 1940s). Normal females have one Barr body in each somatic cell, whereas normal males have no Barr bodies.

The actual process of inactivation occurs very early in embryonic development—approximately 7 to 14 days after fertilization. In each somatic cell one of the two X chromosomes is inactivated. In some cells the X chromosome contributed by the father is inactivated; in others the maternal X chromosome is inactivated. Because the inactivation process is random, the maternal X chromosome is inactivated in approximately half the cells and the paternal X chromosome is inactivated in approximately half the cells. Once the X chromosome has been inactivated in a cell, all the descendants of that cell have the same chromosome inactivated. Thus inactivation is said to be *random* but *fixed.*

Some individuals do not have the normal number of X chromosomes in their somatic cells. For example, males with Klinefelter syndrome typically have two X chromosomes and one Y chromosome. These males *do* have one Barr body in each cell. Females whose cell nuclei have three X chromosomes have two Barr bodies in each cell, and females whose cell nuclei have four X chromosomes have three Barr bodies in each cell. Females with Turner syndrome have only one X chromosome and no Barr bodies. Thus the number of Barr bodies is always one less than the number of X chromosomes in the cell. All but one X chromosome are always inactivated.

People with abnormal numbers of X chromosomes, such as those with Turner syndrome or Klinefelter syndrome, are not physically normal. This situation presents a puzzle because they presumably have only one active X chromosome, just as individuals with normal numbers of chromosomes do. However, the distal portions of the short and long arms of the X chromosome, as well as several other regions on the chromosome, are not inactivated. Thus X inactivation is also known to be *incomplete.*

Although the mechanism underlying X inactivation is still incompletely understood, the gene responsible for initiating X inactivation, *XIST*, has been located.[19] This gene encodes an mRNA that coats one of the X chromosomes, which is then inactivated. Methylation of X chromosome DNA, a process in which DNA is inactivated when cytosine bases are enzymatically converted to 5-methylcytosine, occurs on the inactivated X chromosome. Inactive X chromosomes can be at least partially reactivated in vitro by administering 5-azacytidine, a demethylating agent.

Sex Determination

The process of sexual differentiation, in which the embryonic gonads become either testes or ovaries, begins during the sixth week of gestation. A key principle of sex determination in the human is that one copy of the Y chromosome is sufficient to initiate the process of gonadal differentiation that produces a male fetus (Figure 4-29, *B*). The number of X chromosomes does not alter this process. For example, an individual with two X chromosomes and one Y chromosome in each cell is still phenotypically a male. Thus it is logical that the Y chromosome must contain a gene that begins the process of male gonadal development.

This gene, termed *SRY* (for "sex-determining region on the Y") has been located on the short arm of the Y chromosome.[20,21] The *SRY* gene lies immediately proximal to the distal tip of the Y chromosome, known as the **pseudoautosomal** region (Figure 4-29, *A*). This portion of the Y chromosome is so named because it pairs with the distal tip of the short arm of the X chromosome during meiosis and exchanges genetic material with it (crossover), just as autosomes do. The DNA sequences of these regions on the X and Y chromosomes are highly similar. The remainder of the X and Y chromosomes, however, do not exchange material and are not similar in DNA sequence. An important piece of evidence that supports *SRY* as the male-determining gene is that female mouse embryos injected with this gene develop as phenotypic males.

Although the *SRY* gene is located on the Y chromosome, the other genes that contribute to male differentiation are located on other chromosomes. Thus *SRY* appears to act as a trigger that initiates the action of genes on other chromosomes (e.g., those that control Sertoli cell differentiation or secretion of müllerian-inhibiting substance). This concept is supported by the fact that the *SRY* gene is similar in sequence to other genes that are known to regulate the transcription of DNA (i.e., they turn other genes on and off).

Occasionally the crossover between X and Y occurs closer to the centromere than it should, placing the *SRY* gene on the X chromosome after crossover. This variation can result in offspring with an apparently normal XX karyotype but a male phenotype. Such XX males are seen in about 1 in 20,000 live births and closely resemble males with Klinefelter syndrome, although their stature is normal. Conversely, it is possible to inherit a Y chromosome that has lost the *SRY* gene (because of either a crossover error or a deletion of the gene). This situation produces an XY female. Such females have gonadal

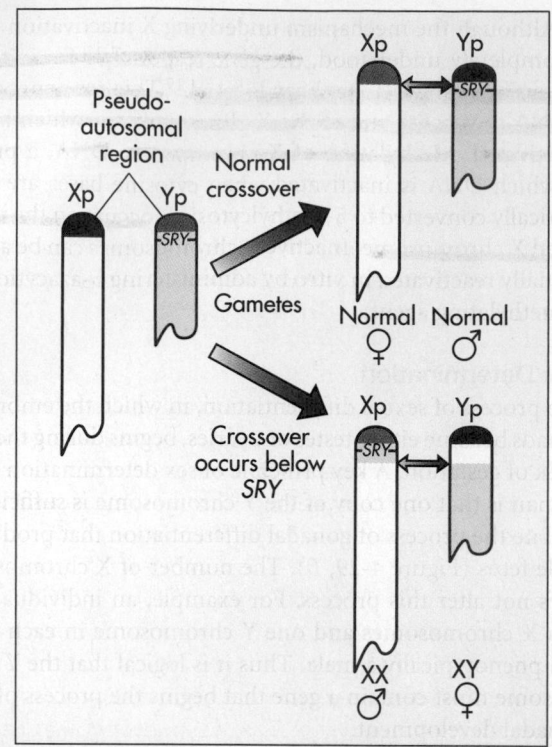

A

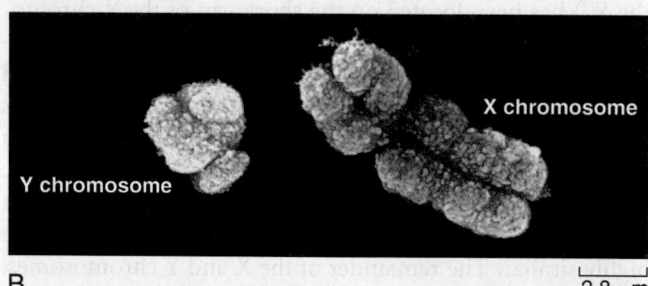

B   2.8 μm

Figure 4-29 The distal short arms of the X and Y chromosomes exchange material during meiosis in the male. **A,** The region of the Y chromosome in which this crossover occurs is called the *pseudoautosomal region.* The *SRY* gene, which triggers the process leading to male gonadal differentiation, is located just outside the pseudoautosomal region. Occasionally, the crossover occurs on the centromeric side of the *SRY* gene, causing it to lie on an X chromosome instead of a Y chromosome. An offspring receiving this X chromosome will be an XX male, and an offspring receiving the Y chromosome will be an XY female. **B,** X and Y chromosomes. (**A** from Jorde LB et al: *Medical genetics,* ed 3, St Louis, 2003, Mosby. **B** from Raven PH et al: *Biology,* ed 8, New York, 2008, McGraw-Hill.)

streaks rather than ovaries and have poorly developed secondary sex characteristics.

Characteristics of Pedigrees
X-linked pedigrees show distinctive modes of inheritance. The most striking characteristic is that females are seldom affected. To express an X-linked recessive trait, a female must be homozygous: either both her parents are affected or her father is affected and her mother is a carrier. Such matings are rare.

An important example of an X-linked recessive disease is hemophilia A. The pedigree shown in Box 4-3 demonstrates the following principles of X-linked recessive inheritance:

1. The trait is seen much more often in males than in females.
2. Because a father can give a son only a Y chromosome, the trait is never transmitted from father to son.
3. The gene can be transmitted through a series of carrier females, causing the appearance of a "skipped generation."
4. The gene is passed from an affected father to all his daughters, who, as phenotypically normal carriers, transmit it to approximately half their sons, who are affected.

The most common and severe of all X-linked recessive disorders is Duchenne muscular dystrophy (DMD), which affects approximately 1 in 3500 males. As its name suggests, this disorder is characterized by progressive muscle degeneration. Affected individuals are usually unable to walk by 10 to 12 years of age. The disease affects the heart and respiratory muscles, and death caused by respiratory or cardiac failure usually occurs before 20 years. Until recently, the underlying pathologic origin of this disorder was a mystery. However, mapping and cloning of the disease gene (on the short arm of the X chromosome) have greatly increased our understanding of the disorder.[22] The *DMD* gene is the largest gene ever found in the human, spanning more than 2 million DNA bases. It encodes a previously undiscovered muscle protein, termed **dystrophin.** Extensive study of dystrophin indicates that it plays an essential role in maintaining the structural integrity of muscle cells: one end of the protein binds to actin filaments in the cytoplasm of the cell, and the other end binds to a group of membrane-spanning proteins known as the *dystrophin-associated glycoproteins.* When dystrophin is absent, as in individuals with DMD, the cell cannot survive, and muscle deterioration ensues.

Most cases of Duchenne muscular dystrophy are caused by deletions of portions of the *DMD* gene. They generally involve frameshift deletions in which all the amino acids following the deletion are altered. It is interesting that an "in frame" deletion (in which a multiple of three bases is deleted, and the amino acids following the deletion are not altered) produces a milder form of muscular dystrophy, the Becker type. These two types of dystrophy are examples of a disease in which different types of mutations at the same locus produce variable expression of the disease.

Recurrence Risks
The most common mating type involving X-linked recessive genes is the combination of a carrier female and a normal male. On the average, the carrier mother will transmit the disease gene to half her sons and half her daughters. As Figure 4-30, *A,* shows, half the daughters in such a mating will be carriers, whereas half will be normal. Half the sons will be normal, whereas half will have the disease. These are probabilities that indicate what risks can be expected on the *average* (see Box 4-3).

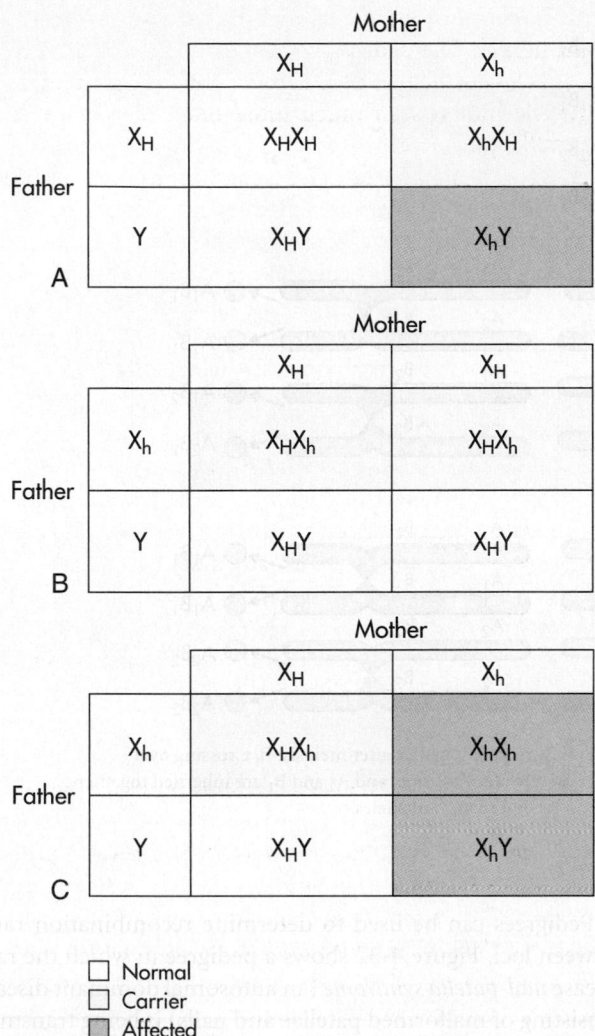

Mother

	X_H	X_h
X_H	X_HX_H	X_hX_H
Y	X_HY	X_hY

A

Mother

	X_H	X_H
X_h	X_HX_h	X_HX_h
Y	X_HY	X_HY

B

Mother

	X_H	X_h
X_h	X_HX_h	X_hX_h
Y	X_HY	X_hY

C

☐ Normal
☐ Carrier
▨ Affected

Figure 4-30 Punnett square and X-linked recessive traits. **A,** Punnett square for the mating of a normal male (X_HY) and a female carrier of an X-linked recessive gene (X_HX_h). **B,** Punnett square for the mating of a normal female (X_HX_H) with a male affected by an X-linked recessive disease (X_hY). **C,** Punnett square for the mating of a female who carries an X-linked recessive gene (X_HX_h) with a male who is affected with the disease caused by the gene (X_hY).

The other common mating type is an affected father and a normal mother (see Figure 4-30, *B*). In this situation all the sons must be normal because the father can transmit only his Y chromosome to them. Because all the daughters must receive the father's X chromosome, they will all be heterozygous carriers. Because the sons *must* receive the Y chromosome and the daughters *must* receive the X with the disease gene, these are predictions and not probabilities. None of the children will express the disease.

The final mating pattern, less common than the other two, involves an affected father and a carrier mother (see Figure 4-30, *C*). With this pattern, on average, half the daughters will be heterozygous carriers and half will be homozygous for the disease gene and thus affected. Half the sons will be normal, and half will be affected. Some X-linked recessive diseases,

such as DMD, are fatal or incapacitating before the affected individual reaches reproductive age, and therefore affected fathers are rare or nonexistent.

Sex-Limited and Sex-Influenced Traits

Confusion sometimes exists regarding the difference between traits that are sex-linked and those that are sex-limited or sex-influenced. A **sex-limited trait** is one that can occur in only one of the sexes, often because of anatomic differences. Inherited uterine and testicular defects are two obvious examples.

A **sex-influenced trait** is one that occurs much more often in one sex than in the other. A good example of a sex-influenced trait is male-pattern baldness, which occurs in both males and females but is much more common in males. Another example is autosomal dominant breast cancer, which is approximately 70 times more common in females than males.

Evaluation of Pedigrees

With complications such as incomplete penetrance, variable expressivity, delayed age of onset, and sex-influenced traits, it is not always possible simply to look at a disease pedigree and determine the mode of inheritance. A sophisticated statistical methodologic approach has evolved to deal with such complications. Incorporated into computer programs, these statistical techniques assess the probability of observing a certain pedigree if a particular mode of inheritance (e.g., autosomal dominant with incomplete penetrance) is in effect.

LINKAGE ANALYSIS AND GENE MAPPING

Locating genes on chromosomes and on specific areas of chromosomes is one of the most important endeavors in human genetics. The location of a gene can tell much about the function of the gene, its interaction with other genes, and the likelihood that certain individuals will develop a genetic disease.

Classical Pedigree Analysis

Mendel's second law, the principle of independent assortment, states that an individual's genes will be transmitted to the next generation independently of one another. This law is only partly true, however, because genes located close together on the same chromosome *do* tend to be transmitted together to the offspring. Thus Mendel's principle of independent assortment holds true for most pairs of genes but not those that occupy the same region of a chromosome. Such loci demonstrate **linkage** and are said to be linked.

During the first meiotic stage, the arms of homologous chromosome pairs intertwine and sometimes exchange portions of their DNA (Figure 4-31) in a process known as **crossing over.** During crossing over, new combinations of alleles can be formed. For example, two loci on a chromosome have alleles *A* and *a* and alleles *B* and *b*. Alleles *A* and *B* are located together on one chromosome arm, and alleles *a* and *b* are located on the other arm. The genotype of this individual is denoted as *AB/ab*.

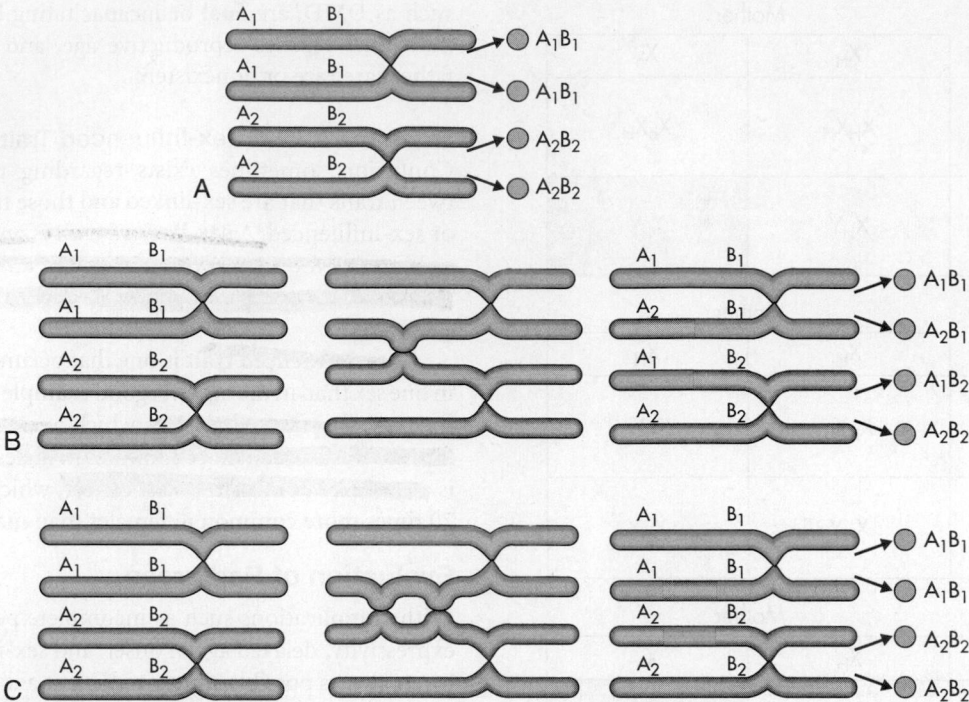

Figure 4-31 The genetic results of crossing over. A, No crossing over: A_1 and B_1 remain together after meiosis. B, Crossing over between A and B results in a recombination: A_1 and B_2 are inherited together on one chromosome, and A_2 and B_1 are inherited together on another chromosome. C, A double crossover between A and B results in no recombination of alleles.

As Figure 4-31, A, shows, the allele pairs *AB* and *ab* would be transmitted together when no crossing over occurs. However, when crossing over does occur (Figure 4-31, B), all four possible pairs of alleles can be transmitted to the offspring: *AB*, *aB*, *Ab*, and *ab*. The process of forming such new arrangements of alleles is called **recombination.** Crossing over does not necessarily lead to recombination, however, because double crossing over between two loci can result in no actual recombination of the alleles at the loci (Figure 4-31, C).

The rate of crossing over can be used to infer the distance between two loci on a chromosome because the probability of crossovers occurring between two loci increases as the loci become more distant. For example, if an individual with genotype *AB/ab* produces recombinant offspring gametes (composition of *Ab* and *aB*) 2% of the time, it is said that the two loci are two map units apart. One **map unit** equals a 1% recombination rate between two loci. When loci on the same chromosome are 50 or more map units apart, they are considered unlinked because their recombination frequency is just as great as it would be if they were on different chromosomes (where the probability of being transmitted together must equal one half). Because they are on the same chromosome, they are said to be unlinked but **syntenic loci.** Recombination frequencies provide a good estimate of actual physical distance between loci at smaller distances, but because of double crossovers, they tend to yield underestimates at larger distances. On average, each map unit is equal to approximately 1 million DNA base pairs.

Pedigrees can be used to determine recombination rates between loci. Figure 4-32 shows a pedigree in which the rare disease *nail-patella syndrome* (an autosomal dominant disease consisting of malformed patellae and nails) is being transmitted. The individuals in this pedigree have been typed for the ABO blood group, whose locus is also located on chromosome 9. Examination of generations I and II shows that the nail-patella gene must be on the same chromosome arm as the gene for blood type A because the mother, whose blood type was B, was unaffected with the disease. The daughter's genotype would then be *AN/Bn*, in which N indicates the disease allele and n indicates the normal allele. The daughter's husband (individual II-1) must have the genotype *On/On*. If the loci for nail-patella syndrome and the ABO blood group are linked, the children of this union who are affected with nail-patella syndrome should have blood type A; those who are unaffected should have blood type B. In six of seven cases we find this to be true. In one case a recombination occurred (individual III-6), indicating a recombination rate of 1 in 7, or 14%. The two loci are therefore 14 map units apart.

In practice, a much larger sample of families would be used to ensure against statistical artifacts. Also, as with the determination of mode of inheritance, the situation is not always as clear as that pictured in Figure 4-32. Elaborate statistical procedures have been devised to evaluate the probabilities that two loci are linked at a given map distance.

Once a close linkage has been established between a disease locus and a **marker locus** (a DNA variant that can easily

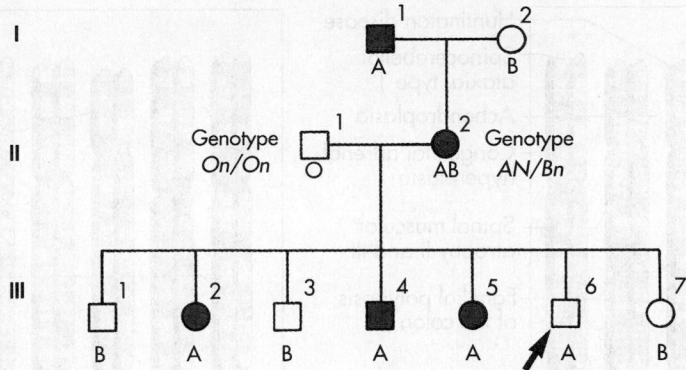

Figure 4-32 The ABO nail-patella linkage in three generations of a family. Letters below symbols indicate ABO blood groups. Individual III-6 shows recombination.

be assayed in the laboratory) and once the alleles of the two loci that are inherited together within a family have been determined, reliable predictions of whether a member of a family will develop the disease can be made. If, for example, the recombination rate between a disease locus and a marker locus, such as the ABO blood group, is less than 1%, family members can simply have their ABO blood type assayed to find out, with 99% or greater certainty, whether each member carries the disease gene.

This capability is especially important for diseases with delayed age of onset. Linkage has been established between several DNA polymorphisms and the gene for Huntington disease. Determining this kind of linkage means that it is possible for offspring of an individual with Huntington disease to know whether they also carry the gene and thus could pass it on to their own children. The difficult decision of whether to have children will be made easier for these individuals, although some individuals may prefer to remain uninformed of their genotypes. Other delayed-onset diseases for which linked markers have been found include adult polycystic kidney disease, familial Alzheimer disease, and two forms of autosomal dominant breast cancer (about 5% of breast cancer cases are caused by an autosomal dominant gene). Pinpointing specific mutations in these genes also has made direct genetic diagnosis possible. The advantage of direct diagnosis is that it is more accurate because it tests for the disease-causing mutation itself.

For some genetic diseases, prophylactic treatment is available if the condition can be diagnosed in time. An example of this is hemochromatosis—a recessive genetic disease in which excess iron is retained, causing degeneration of the heart, liver, brain, and other vital organs. Diagnosis is usually made at about 40 years of age in males, after which most individuals survive only a few years. If earlier tests could determine whether an individual had the disease, preventive treatment, consisting of phlebotomies to remove blood and thus excess iron, could be administered before degeneration began. This has been made easier by mapping the hemochromatosis gene to a specific region of chromosome 6 and subsequently identifying the major disease-causing mutations. Individuals at risk

for developing the disease can be identified by testing for presence of the mutations, and if necessary, preventive therapy can be given, ensuring an ordinary life span. This example is one instance in which genetics contributes to preventive medicine in its best sense.

Assigning Loci to Specific Chromosomes

With completion of the human DNA sequence (see following), computer analysis of the published sequence has become an effective and popular approach for identifying genes. Computerized databases of known DNA sequences play an important role in gene identification. When studying a specific region of DNA to find a gene, it is common to search for similarity between DNA sequences from the region and DNA sequences in the database. The sequences in the database may derive from genes with known function or tissue-specific expression patterns. Suppose, for example, that we have used linkage analysis to identify a region containing a gene that causes a developmental disorder such as a limb malformation. As we evaluate DNA sequences in the region, we would look for similarity between a DNA sequence from this region and a plausible sequence from the database (e.g., sequence from a gene that encodes a protein involved in bone development, such as a fibroblast growth factor). Because genes that encode similar protein products usually have similar DNA sequences, a match between the sequence from our region and a sequence in the database could be a vital clue that this particular DNA sequence is actually part of the gene that causes the limb malformation.

Complete Human Gene Map: Prospects and Benefits

Rapid progress is being made in assigning genes to their chromosomal locations. A number of important genetic diseases have been located on specific areas of individual chromosomes: these include Huntington disease, retinoblastoma, DMD, hemophilia A, cystic fibrosis, PKU, neurofibromatosis, familial breast cancer, and familial Alzheimer disease[23] (Figure 4-33). Table 4-1 contains a partial list of mapped diseases. The development of thousands of new DNA markers is especially

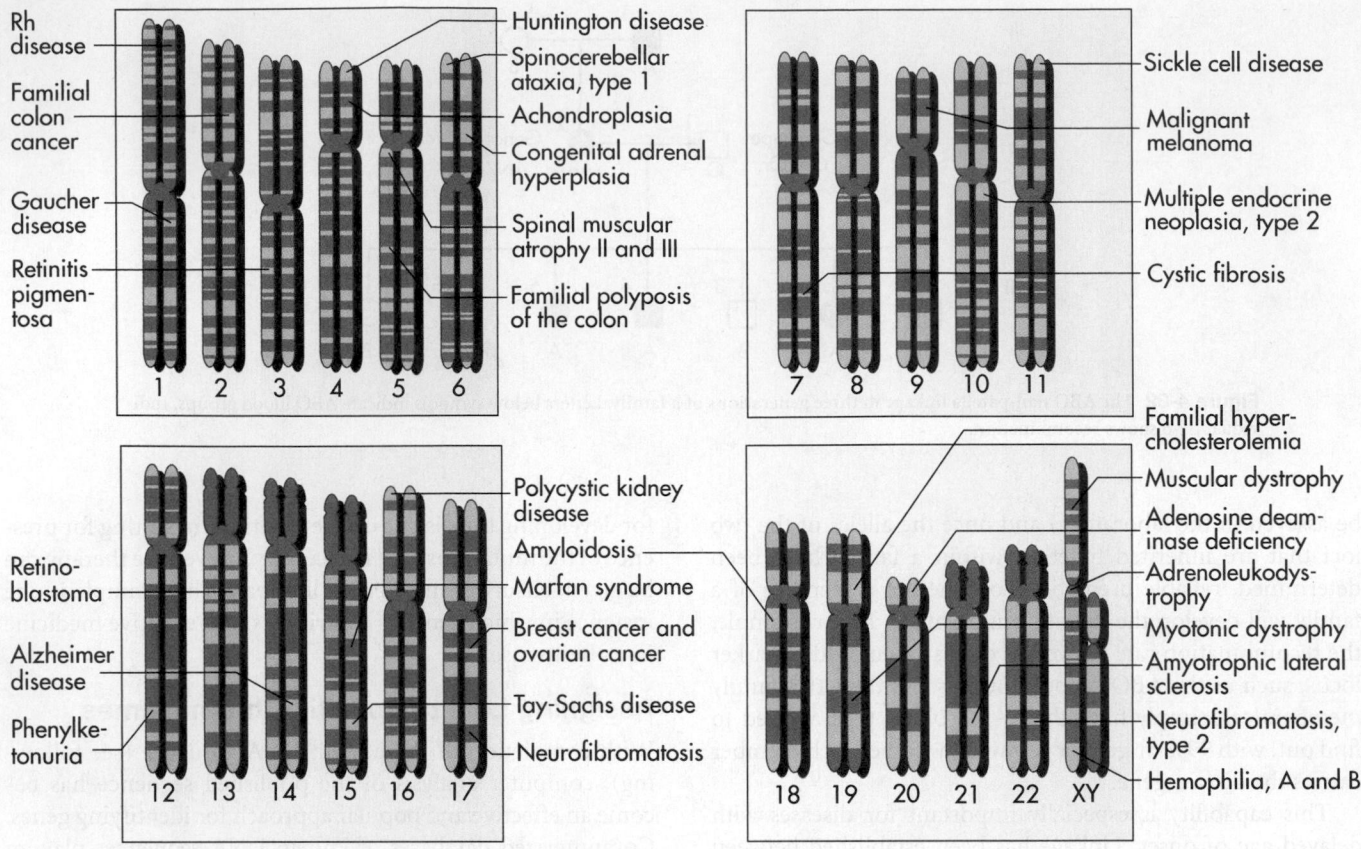

Figure 4-33 Example of diseases: gene map.

Table 4-1	Examples of Disease Genes That Have Been Mapped and Cloned*	
Disease	**Chromosome Location**	**Gene Product**
α_1-Antitrypsin deficiency	14q	Serine protease inhibitor
α-Thalassemia	16p	α-Globin component of hemoglobin
β-Thalassemia	11p	β-Globin component of hemoglobin
Achondroplasia	4p	Fibroblast growth factor receptor 3
Adult polycystic kidney disease	16p	Polycystin-1 membrane protein
Alzheimer disease*	14q	Presenilin 1
	1q	Presenilin 2
	19q	Apolipoprotein E
	21q	α-Amyloid precursor protein
Amyotrophic lateral sclerosis	21q	Superoxide dismutase 1
Ataxia telangiectasia	11q	Cell cycle control protein
Beckwith-Wiedemann syndrome	11p	Insulin-like growth factor II
Breast cancer (familial)	17q	BRCA1 tumor suppressor/DNA repair protein
	13q	BRCA2 tumor suppressor/DNA repair protein
	22q	CHEK2 DNA repair protein
Li-Fraumeni syndrome	17p	p54 Tumor suppressor
Charcot-Marie-Tooth disease (type 1A)*	17p	Peripheral myelin protein 22
Cystic fibrosis	7q	Cystic fibrosis transmembrane regulator (CFTR)
Deafness, nonsyndromic (more than 75 genes	13q	Connexin-26 gap junction protein
identified to date; representative examples	5q	Actin polymerization regulator
shown here)	7q	Pendrin (anion transporter; mutations also found in Pendred syndrome)
	11q	α-Tectorin

Table 4-1	Examples of Disease Genes That Have Been Mapped and Cloned—cont'd	
Disease	**Chromosome Location**	**Gene Product**
Diabetes		
(MODY1)	20q	Hepatocyte nuclear factor-4α
(MODY2)	7p	Glucokinase
(MODY3)	12q	Hepatocyte nuclear factor-1α
(MODY4)	13q	Insulin promoter factor-1
(MODY5)	17q	Hepatic transcription factor-2
(MODY6)	2q	NeuroD transcription factor
Duchenne/Becker muscular dystrophy	Xp	Dystrophin
Ehlers-Danlos syndrome*	2q	Collagen (COL3A1); numerous types of this disorder are known, most of which are produced by mutations in collagen genes
Ellis van Creveld syndrome	4p	Protein with possible leucine zipper domain
Familial polyposis coli	5q	APC tumor suppressor
Fragile X syndrome	Xq	FMR1 RNA-binding protein
Galactosemia	9p	Galactose-1-phosphate-uridyltransferase
Hemochromatosis	6p	Transferrin receptor binding protein
Hemophilia A	Xq	Clotting factor VIII
Hemophilia B	Xq	Clotting factor IX
Hereditary nonpolyposis colorectal cancer	3p	MLH1 DNA mismatch repair protein
Huntington disease	4p	Huntingtin
Hypercholesterolemia (familial)	19p	LDL receptor
Long QT syndrome (LQT1)*	11p	KVLQT1 cardiac potassium channel α subunit
Marfan syndrome	15q	Fibrillin-1
Melanoma (familial)*	9p	Cyclin-dependent kinase inhibitor tumor suppressor
	12q	Cyclin-dependent kinase 4
Myotonic dystrophy	19q	Protein kinase
	3q	Zinc finger protein
Myoclonus epilepsy (Unverricht-Lundborg)	21q	Cystatin B cysteine protease inhibitor
Neurofibromatosis type 1	17q	Neurofibromin tumor suppressor
Neurofibromatosis type 2	22q	Merlin (schwannomin) tumor suppressor
Parkinson disease		
(familial)	4q	α-Synuclein
(autosomal recessive early-onset)	6q	Parkin
Phenylketonuria	12q	Phenylalanine hydroxylase
Retinoblastoma	13q	pRB tumor suppressor
Sickle cell disease	11p	β Globin component of hemoglobin
Tay-Sachs disease	15q	Hexosaminidase A
Wilms tumor*	11p	WT1 zinc finger protein tumor suppressor
Wilson disease	13q	Copper transporting ATPase
Von Willebrand disease	12q	von Willebrand clotting factor

*Additional disease-causing loci have been mapped and/or cloned.
Modified from Jorde LB et al: *Medical genetics*, ed 3, St Louis, 2003, Mosby.

helpful in this effort. A marker map of the human genome has been completed, and completion of the entire sequence of the human genome was announced in April 2003. Achievement of this goal serves several purposes:

1. Markers are available to establish close linkages for genetic diseases. With the establishment of a comprehensive marker map, accurate predictions can be made for the inheritance of most genetic diseases.
2. Knowing the location of genes often yields valuable information about the way genes function and interact with one another. A number of genes with similar functions (e.g., some of the globin genes) are located close to one another on the same chromosome. This

characteristic can have important implications for the diseases caused by these genes.

3. Mapping a disease gene is an important step toward isolating and **cloning** the gene (clones are identical copies of genes). Once a gene can be cloned, its DNA sequence can be studied to determine the nature and function of the protein encoded by the gene. Cloning the genes that cause diseases such as cystic fibrosis and DMD has contributed immensely to our understanding of the pathophysiologic aspect of these disorders. In addition, the ability to clone a gene opens up the possibility of gene therapy for the disorder (Box 4-4).

For a variety of reasons, germline gene therapy is not being undertaken in humans. Nevertheless, it has been noted that germline gene therapy is in many ways technically easier to perform than is somatic cell therapy. Germline therapy also offers (in theory) the possibility of "genetic enhancement," the introduction of favorable genes into the embryo. However, a gene that is favorable in one environment may be quite unfavorable in another (e.g., the sickle cell mutation, which is only advantageous for heterozygotes in a malarial environment). And, because of pleiotropy, the introduction of "favorable" genes may have completely unintended consequences (e.g., a gene thought to enhance one characteristic could negatively affect another). For these reasons, and because germline therapy usually destroys the targeted embryo, neither germline therapy nor genetic enhancement is advocated by the scientific community.

Controversy also surrounds the prospect of cloning humans. A number of species (e.g., sheep, pigs, cattle, goats, mice, and cats) have been successfully cloned by introducing a diploid nucleus from an adult cell into an egg cell from which the original haploid nucleus was removed. The cell is manipulated so that all of its genes can be expressed (recall that most genes in a typical adult cell are transcriptionally silent). This procedure, termed *reproductive cloning* when allowed to proceed through a full-term pregnancy, could likely be used to produce a human being. Some argue that human cloning offers childless couples the opportunity to produce

children to whom they are biologically related or even to "replace" a child who has died. Others respond with the challenge that this method of creating life is too artificial. In any case, it is important to keep in mind that a clone is only a *genetic* copy. The environment of the individual, which also plays a large role in development, cannot be replicated. Furthermore, the great majority of cloning attempts in mammals fail: in most cases the embryo either dies or has gross malformations. Because the consequences of human cloning would almost certainly be similar, reproductive cloning to produce a human is condemned almost universally by scientists.

It is now possible to derive embryonic stem cells from early-stage human embryos. These stem cells can be treated to form many types of differentiated cells (e.g., neurons for individuals with Parkinson disease, myocytes for individuals with heart disease). The combination of embryonic stem cell technology and human cloning offers an interesting possibility: a pre-embryo could in theory be created from an individual's own cell, producing embryonic stem cells that would be a perfect match immunologically for the individual (creating a clone to provide embryonic stem cells has been termed *therapeutic cloning*).

Although these technologies offer the hope of effective treatment for some recalcitrant diseases, they also present thorny ethical issues. Clearly, decisions regarding their use must be guided by constructive input from scientists, legal scholars, philosophers, and others.

SUMMARY REVIEW

DNA, RNA, and Proteins: Heredity at the Molecular Level

1. Genes, the basic units of inheritance, are composed of DNA and are located on the chromosomes.
2. DNA is composed of deoxyribose, a phosphate molecule, and four types of nitrogenous bases. The physical structure of DNA is a double helix.
3. The DNA bases code for amino acids, which in turn make up proteins. The amino acids are specified by triplet codons of nitrogenous bases.
4. DNA replication is based on complementary base pairing, in which a single strand of DNA serves as the template for attracting bases that form a new strand of DNA.
5. DNA polymerase is the primary enzyme involved in replication. It adds bases to the new DNA strand and performs "proofreading" functions.
6. A mutation is an inherited alteration of genetic material (i.e., DNA).
7. Substances that cause mutations are called mutagens.
8. The mutation rate in humans varies from locus to locus and ranges from 10^{-4} to 10^{-7} per gene per generation.
9. Transcription and translation, the two basic processes in which proteins are specified by DNA, both involve RNA. RNA is chemically similar to DNA, but it is single stranded, has a ribose sugar molecule, and has uracil rather than thymine as one of its four nitrogenous bases.
10. Transcription is the process by which DNA specifies a sequence of mRNA.
11. Much of the RNA sequence is spliced from the mRNA before the mRNA leaves the nucleus. The excised sequences are called introns, and those that remain to code for proteins are called exons.
12. Translation is the process by which RNA directs the synthesis of polypeptides. This process takes place in the ribosomes, which consist of proteins and rRNA.
13. During translation, mRNA interacts with tRNA, a molecule that has an attachment site for a specific amino acid.

Chromosomes

1. Human cells consist of diploid somatic cells (body cells) and haploid gametes (sperm and egg cells).
2. Humans have 23 pairs of chromosomes: 22 of these pairs are autosomes. The remaining pair consists of the sex chromosomes. Females have 2 homologous X chromosomes as their sex chromosomes; males have an X and a Y chromosome.
3. A karyotype is an ordered display of chromosomes arranged according to length and the location of the centromere.
4. Various types of stains can be used to make chromosome bands more visible.
5. About 1 in 150 live births has a major diagnosable chromosome abnormality. Chromosome abnormalities are the leading known cause of mental retardation and miscarriage.
6. Polyploidy is a condition in which a euploid cell has some multiple of the normal number of chromosomes. Humans have been observed to have triploidy (three copies of each chromosome) and tetraploidy (four copies of each chromosome); both conditions are lethal.
7. Somatic cells that do not have a multiple of 23 chromosomes are aneuploid. Aneuploidy is usually the result of nondisjunction.
8. Trisomy is a type of aneuploidy in which one chromosome is present in three copies in somatic cells. A partial trisomy is one in which only part of a chromosome is present in three copies.

9. Monosomy is a type of aneuploidy in which one chromosome is present in only one copy in somatic cells.

10. In general, monosomies cause more severe physical defects than do trisomies, illustrating the principle that the loss of chromosome material has more severe consequences than the duplication of chromosome material.

11. Down syndrome, a trisomy of chromosome 21, is the best-known disease caused by a chromosome aberration. It affects 1 in 800 live births and is much more likely to occur in women older than 35 years of age.

12. Most aneuploidies of the sex chromosomes have less severe consequences than those of the autosomes.

13. The most commonly observed sex chromosome aneuploidies are the 47,XXX karyotype, 45,X karyotype (Turner syndrome), 47,XXY karyotype (Klinefelter syndrome), and 47,XYY karyotype.

14. Abnormalities of chromosome structure include deletions, duplications, inversions, and translocations.

Elements of Formal Genetics

1. Mendelian traits are caused by single genes, each of which occupies a position, or locus, on a chromosome.

2. Alleles are different forms of genes located at the same locus on the chromosome.

3. At any given locus in a somatic cell, an individual has two genes, one from each parent. An individual may be homozygous or heterozygous for a locus.

4. An individual's genotype is his or her genetic makeup, and the phenotype reflects the interaction of genotype and environment.

5. At a heterozygous locus, a dominant gene's effects mask those of a recessive gene. The recessive gene is expressed only when it is present in two copies.

Transmission of Genetic Diseases

1. Genetic diseases caused by single genes usually follow autosomal dominant, autosomal recessive, or X-linked recessive modes of inheritance.

2. Pedigree charts are an important tool in the analysis of modes of inheritance.

3. Recurrence risks specify the probability that future offspring will inherit a genetic disease. For single-gene diseases, recurrence risks remain the same for each offspring, regardless of the number of affected or unaffected offspring.

4. The recurrence risk for autosomal dominant diseases is usually 50%.

5. Germline mosaicism can alter recurrence risks for genetic diseases because unaffected parents can produce multiple affected offspring. This situation occurs because the germline of one parent is affected by a mutation but the parent's somatic cells are unaffected.

6. Skipped generations are not seen in classic autosomal dominant pedigrees.

7. Males and females are equally likely to exhibit autosomal dominant diseases and to pass them on to their offspring.

8. A gene that is not always expressed phenotypically is said to have incomplete penetrance.

9. Penetrance may be age-dependent, as in Huntington disease and familial breast cancer.

10. Variable expressivity is a characteristic of many genetic diseases.

11. Evidence is increasing that the same DNA sequence can produce different phenotypes. Chemical modifications can alter the phenotype or expression of genes.

12. Epigenetics is the term used to describe modifications that affect phenotype without altering DNA sequencing.

13. Genomic imprinting, which may involve methylation, results in differing expressions of a disease gene, depending on which parent transmitted the gene.

14. Most commonly, parents of children with autosomal recessive diseases are both heterozygous carriers of the disease gene.

15. The recurrence risk for autosomal recessive diseases is 25%.

16. Males and females are equally likely to be affected by autosomal recessive diseases.

17. Consanguinity is often present in families with autosomal recessive diseases, and it becomes more prevalent with rarer recessive diseases.

18. Carrier detection tests for an increasing number of autosomal recessive diseases are available.

19. The frequency of genetic diseases approximately doubles in the offspring of first-cousin matings.

20. In each normal female somatic cell, one of the two X chromosomes is inactivated early in embryogenesis.

21. X inactivation is random, fixed, and incomplete (i.e., only part of the chromosome is actually inactivated). It may involve methylation.

22. Gender is determined embryonically by the presence of the *SRY* gene on the Y chromosome. Embryos that have a Y chromosome (and thus the *SRY* gene) become males, whereas those lacking the Y chromosome become females. When the Y chromosome lacks the *SRY* gene, an XY female can be produced. Similarly, an X chromosome that contains the *SRY* gene can produce an XX male.

23. X-linked genes are those that are located on the X chromosome. Nearly all known X-linked diseases are caused by X-linked recessive genes.

24. Males are hemizygous for genes on the X chromosome.

25. X linked recessive diseases are seen much more often in males than in females because males need only one copy of the gene to express the disease.

26. Fathers cannot pass X-linked genes to their sons.

27. Skipped generations are often seen in X-linked recessive disease pedigrees because the gene can be transmitted through carrier females.

28. Recurrence risks for X-linked recessive diseases depend on the carrier and affected status of the mother and father.

29. A sex-limited trait is one that occurs in only one of the sexes.

30. A sex-influenced trait is one that occurs more often in one sex than in the other.

Linkage Analysis and Gene Mapping

1. During meiosis I, crossing over occurs and can cause recombinations of alleles located on the same chromosome.

2. The frequency of recombinations can be used to infer the map distance between loci on the same chromosome.

3. Loci that are on the same chromosome are syntenic.

4. A marker locus, when closely linked to a disease-gene locus, can be used to predict whether an individual will develop a genetic disease.

5. A more complete gene map will facilitate marker studies, studies of gene function and interaction, and gene therapy.

KEY TERMS

Adenine, 129
Age-dependent, 148
Allele, 145
Amino acid, 129
Aneuploid cell, 136
Anticodon, 134
Autosome, 134
Barr body, 153
Base pair substitution, 129
Carrier, 145
Carrier detection test, 152
Chromosomal mosaic, 137
Chromosome band, 135
Chromosome breakage, 142
Chromosome theory of inheritance, 146
Clastogen, 142
Cloning, 159
Codominance, 145
Codon, 129
Complementary base pairing, 129
Consanguinity, 151
Cri du chat syndrome, 142
Crossing over, 155
Cytosine, 129
Deoxyribonucleic acid (DNA), 126
Diploid cell, 134
DNA methylation, 149
DNA polymerase, 129
Dominant, 145
Dosage compensation, 153
Double helix, 129
Down syndrome, 137
Duplication, 142
Dystrophin, 154
Epigenetic, 149
Euploid cell, 135
Exon, 134
Expressivity, 148
Fragile site, 143
Frameshift mutation, 132
Gamete, 134

Gene, 126
Genomic imprinting, 149
Genotype, 145
Germline mosaicism, 148
Giemsa stain, 135
Guanine, 129
Haploid cell, 134
Hemizygous, 153
Heterogeneous nuclear RNA (hnRNA), 133
Heterozygote, 145
Heterozygous, 145
Homologous, 134
Homologous chromosome, 134
Homozygote, 145
Homozygous, 145
Inbreeding, 152
Intron, 134
Inversion, 143
Karyotype, 134
Klinefelter syndrome, 141
Linkage, 155
Locus, 143
Map unit, 156
Marker locus, 156
Meiosis, 134
Messenger RNA (mRNA), 132
Metaphase spread, 134
Missense mutation, 129
Mode of inheritance, 145
Monosomy, 136
Mutagen, 132
Mutation, 129
Mutational hot spot, 132
Nondisjunction, 137
Nucleotide, 129
Obligate carrier, 148
Partial trisomy, 137
Pedigree, 146
Penetrance, 148
Phenotype, 145
Polymorphic (polymorphism), 145
Polypeptide, 129

Polyploid cell, 135
Position effect, 143
Principle of independent assortment, 146
Principle of segregation, 146
Proband (propositus/proposita), 146
Promoter site, 132
Pseudoautosomal, 153
Purine, 129
Pyrimidine, 129
Recessive, 145
Reciprocal translocation, 143
Recombination, 156
Recurrence risk, 148
Ribonucleic acid (RNA), 132
Ribosomal RNA (rRNA), 134
Ribosome, 134
RNA polymerase, 132
Robertsonian translocation, 143
Sex chromosome, 134
Sex-influenced trait, 155
Sex-limited trait, 155
Sex-linked (inheritance), 152
Silent substitution, 132
Somatic cell, 134
Spontaneous mutation, 132
Syntenic loci, 156
Template, 129
Termination (nonsense) codon, 129
Termination sequence, 133
Tetraploidy, 135
Thymine, 129
Transcription, 132
Transcriptionally inactive (silenced), 149
Transfer RNA (tRNA), 134
Translation, 134
Translocation, 143
Triploidy, 135
Trisomy, 136
Tumor-suppressor gene, 148
Turner syndrome, 139

REFERENCES

1. Online: Mendelian inheritance in man, available at www.ncbi.nlm.nih.gov/sites/entrez?db=OMIM
2. Hall JG et al: The frequency and financial burden of genetic disease in a pediatric hospital, *Am J Med Genet* 1(1):417-436, 1978.
3. Crow JF: The origins, patterns and implications of human spontaneous mutation, *Nat Rev Genet* 1:40-47, 2000.
4. Hall H, Hunt P, Hassold T: Meiosis and sex chromosome aneuploidy: how meiotic errors cause aneuploidy; how aneuploidy causes meiotic errors, *Curr Opin Genet Dev* 16(3):323-329, 2006.
5. Tolie JL, MacFayden U: Clinical genetics of common autosomal trisomies. In Rimoin DL et al, editors: *Emery and Rimoin's principles and practice of medical genetics*, ed 5, Philadelphia, 2007, Churchill Livingstone, pp 1015-1037.
6. Antonarakis SE, Epstein CJ: The challenge of Down syndrome, *Trends Molec Med* 12(10):473-479, 2006.
7. Jorde LB et al: *Medical genetics*, ed 3, St Louis, 2006, Mosby.

8. Graham GE, Allanson JE, Gerritsen JA: Sex chromosome abnormalities. In Rimoin DL et al, editors: *Emery and Rimoin's principles and practice of medical genetics*, ed 5, Philadelphia, 2007, Churchill Livingstone, pp 1038-1057.
9. Garber KB, Visootsak J, Warren ST: Fragile X syndrome, *Eur J Hum Genet* 16(6):666-672, 2008.
10. Ranum NL, Cooper TA: RNA-mediated neuromuscular disorders, *Annu Rev Neurosci* 29:259-277, 2006.
11. Orr HT, Zoghbi HY: Trinucleotide repeat disorders, *Annu Rev Neurosci* 30:575-621, 2007.
12. Zlotogora J: Germ line mosaicism, *Hum Mol Genet* 102(4):381-386, 1998.
13. Balmain A, Gray J, Ponder B: The genetics and genomics of cancer, *Nat Genet* 33:238-244, 2003.
14. Knudson AG: Cancer genetics, *Am J Med Genet* 111(1):96-102, 2002.
15. Theos A, Korf BR: Pathophysiology of neurofibromatosis type 1, *Ann Intern Med* 144(11):842-849, 2006.
16. Rowe SM, Miller S, Sorscher EJ: Cystic fibrosis, *N Engl J Med* 342(19):1992-2001, 2005.

17. Jorde LB: Inbreeding in human populations. In Dulbecco R, editor: *Encyclopedia of human biology*, vol 5, New York, 1997, Academic Press.

18. Lyon MF: Sex chromatin and gene action in the mammalian X-chromosome, *Am J Hum Genet* 14:135-148, 1962.

19. Wutz A, Gribnau J: X inactivation Xplained, *Curr Opin Genet Dev* 17(5):387-393, 2007.

20. Fleming A, Vilain E: The endless quest for sex determination genes, *Clin Genet* 67(1):15-25, 2005.

21. Ostrer H: Sex determination: lessons from families and embryos, *Clin Genet* 59(4):207-215, 2001.

22. Dalkilic I, Kunkel LM: Muscular dystrophies: genes to pathogenesis, *Curr Opin Genet Dev* 13(3):231-238, 2003. Review.

23. Collins FS, Morgan M, Patrinos A: The Human Genome Project: lessons from large-scale biology, *Science* 300(5617):286-290, 2003.

GENES, ENVIRONMENT, AND COMMON DISEASES

LYNN B. JORDE

MEDIA RESOURCES

 Evolve Website (http://evolve.elsevier.com/McCance/)
- Review Questions and Answers
- Animations
- Glossary (with audio pronunciation for selected terms)
- WebLinks

Online Course
- Module 3

CHAPTER OUTLINE

FACTORS INFLUENCING INCIDENCE OF DISEASE IN POPULATIONS
Concepts of Incidence and Prevalence
Analysis of Risk Factors
PRINCIPLES OF MULTIFACTORIAL INHERITANCE
Basic Model
Threshold Model
Recurrence Risks and Transmission Patterns

NATURE AND NURTURE: DISENTANGLING THE EFFECTS OF GENES AND ENVIRONMENT
Twin Studies
Adoption Studies
GENETICS OF COMMON DISEASES
Congenital Malformations
Multifactorial Disorders in the Adult Population

Chapter 4 focuses on diseases that are caused by single genes or by abnormalities of single chromosomes. Much progress has been made in identifying specific mutations that cause these diseases, leading to better risk estimates and, in some cases, more effective treatment of the disease. However, these conditions form only a small portion of the total burden of human genetic disease. Most congenital malformations are not caused by single genes or chromosome defects. Many common adult diseases, such as cancer, heart disease, and diabetes, have genetic components, but again they are usually not caused by single genes or by chromosomal abnormalities.[1] These diseases, whose treatment collectively occupies the attention of most health care practitioners, are the result of a complex interplay of multiple genetic and environmental* factors.

*In human genetics, it is common practice to use the term "environment" to designate all non-genetic factors, such as diet and lifestyle.

FACTORS INFLUENCING INCIDENCE OF DISEASE IN POPULATIONS

Concepts of Incidence and Prevalence

How common is a given disease, such as diabetes, in a population? Well-established measures are used to answer this question.[2] The **incidence rate** is the number of new cases of a disease reported during a specific period (typically 1 year) divided by the number of individuals in the population. The denominator is often expressed as *person-years*. The incidence rate can be contrasted with the **prevalence rate,** which is the proportion of the population affected by a disease at a specific point in time. Prevalence is thus determined by both the incidence rate and the length of the survival period in affected individuals. For example, the prevalence rate of acquired immunodeficiency syndrome (AIDS) is larger than the yearly incidence rate because most people with AIDS survive for several years after diagnosis.

Many diseases vary in prevalence from one population to another. Cystic fibrosis is relatively common among Europeans, occurring about once in every 2500 births. In contrast, it is quite rare in Asians, occurring only once in every 90,000 births. Similarly, sickle cell disease affects approximately 1 in 600 American blacks, but it is rarely seen in whites. Both of these diseases are single-gene disorders, and they vary among populations because disease-causing mutations are more or less common in different populations. (This is in turn the result of differences in the evolutionary history of these populations.) Nongenetic (environmental) factors have little influence on the current prevalence of these diseases.

The picture often becomes more complex with the common diseases of adulthood. For example, colon cancer was until recently relatively rare in Japan, but it is the second most common cancer in the United States. Stomach cancer, on the other hand, is common in Japan but relatively rare in the United States. These statistics, in themselves, cannot distinguish environmental from genetic influences in the two populations. However, because large numbers of Japanese emigrated first to Hawaii and then to the U.S. mainland, we can observe what happens to the rates of stomach and colon cancer among the migrants. It is important that the Japanese émigrés have maintained a genetic identity, marrying largely among themselves. Among first-generation Japanese in Hawaii, the frequency of colon cancer rose several-fold—not yet as high as in the U.S. mainland but higher than in Japan. Among second-generation Japanese on the U.S. mainland, colon cancer rates rose to 5%, equal to the U.S. average. At the same time, stomach cancer has become relatively rare among Japanese-Americans.

These observations strongly indicate an important role for environmental factors in the etiology of cancers of the colon and stomach. In each case, diet is a likely culprit—a high-fat, low-fiber diet in the United States is thought to increase the risk of colon cancer, whereas techniques used to preserve and season the fish commonly eaten in Japan are thought to increase the risk of stomach cancer. It is interesting that the incidence of colon cancer in Japan has increased dramatically during the past several decades as the Japanese population has adopted a more "Western" diet. These results do not, however, rule out the potential contribution of genetic factors in common cancers. Genes also play a role in the etiology of colon and other cancers.

Analysis of Risk Factors

The comparison just discussed is one example of the analysis of risk factors (in this case, diet) and their influence on the prevalence of disease in populations. A common measure of the effect of a specific risk factor is the **relative risk.** This quantity is expressed as a ratio:

$$\frac{\text{Incidence rate of the disease among individuals exposed to a risk factor}}{\text{Incidence rate of the disease among individuals } not \text{ exposed to a risk factor}}$$

A classic example of a relative risk analysis was carried out in a sample of more than 40,000 British physicians to determine the relationship between cigarette smoking and lung cancer.

This study compared the incidence of death from lung cancer in physicians who smoked with those who did not. The incidence of death from lung cancer was 1.66 (per 1000 person-years) in heavy smokers (more than 25 cigarettes daily), but it was only 0.07 in the nonsmokers. The ratio of these two incidence rates is 1.66/0.07, which yields a relative risk of 23.7 deaths. We can thus conclude that the risk of dying from lung cancer increased by about 24-fold in heavy smokers compared with nonsmokers. Many other studies have obtained similar risk figures.

Although cigarette smoking clearly increases one's risk of developing lung cancer (as well as heart disease, as we will see later), it is equally clear that *most* smokers do not develop lung cancer. Other lifestyle factors are likely to contribute to one's risk of developing this disease (e.g., exposure to cancer-causing substances in the air, such as asbestos fibers). In addition, differences in genetic background may be involved. Some studies have suggested that mutations in a gene called *FHIT* may make some individuals more sensitive to the carcinogenic effects of tobacco smoke.

Many factors can influence the risk of acquiring a common disease such as cancer, diabetes, or high blood pressure. These include age, gender, diet, exercise, and family history of the disease. Usually, complex interactions occur among these genetic and nongenetic factors. The effects of each factor can be quantified in terms of relative risks. The following discussion demonstrates how genetic and environmental factors contribute to the risk of developing common diseases.

PRINCIPLES OF MULTIFACTORIAL INHERITANCE

Basic Model

Traits in which variation is thought to be caused by the combined effects of multiple genes are **polygenic** ("many genes"). When environmental factors are also believed to cause variation in the trait, which is usually the case, the term **multifactorial trait** is used.[3] Many **quantitative traits** (those, such as blood pressure, that are measured on a continuous numeric scale) are multifactorial. Because they are caused by the additive effects of many genetic and environmental factors, these traits tend to follow a normal, or bell-shaped, distribution in populations.

An example illustrates this concept. To begin with the simplest case, suppose (unrealistically) that height is determined by a single gene with two alleles, A and a. Allele A tends to make people tall, whereas allele a tends to make them short. If there is no dominance at this locus, then the three possible genotypes (AA, Aa, aa) will produce three phenotypes: tall, intermediate, and short. Assume that the gene frequencies of A and a are each 0.50. If we look at a population of individuals, we will observe the height distribution depicted in Figure 5-1, A.

Now suppose, a bit more realistically, that height is determined by two loci instead of one. The second locus also has two alleles, B (tall) and b (short), and they affect height in exactly the same way as alleles A and a. There are now nine possible genotypes in our population: aabb, aaBb, aaBB,

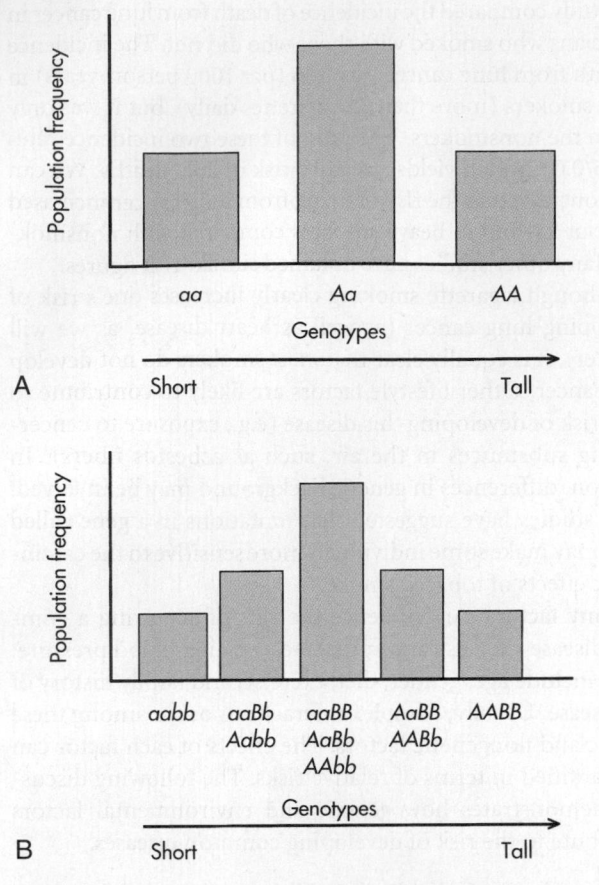

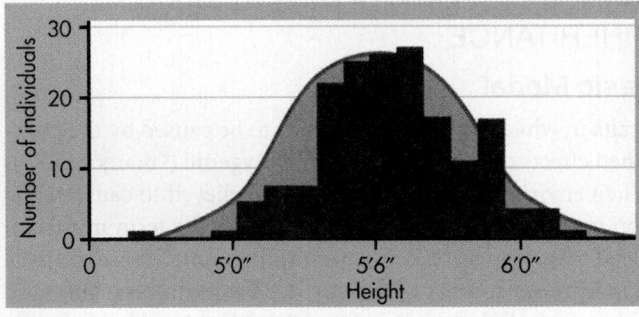

C

Figure 5-1 Distribution of height. **A,** Distribution of height in a population, assuming that height is controlled by a single locus with genotypes *AA, Aa,* and *aa.* **B,** Distribution of height, assuming that height is controlled by two loci. Five distinct genotypes are shown instead of three, and the distribution begins to look more like the normal distribution. **C,** Height is portrayed, realistically, as a trait with a continuous statistical distribution. Because many genes contribute height and tend to segregate independently of one another, the cumulative contribution of different combinations of alleles to height forms a continuous distribution of possible heights, in which the extremes are much rarer than the intermediate values. Variation also can be due to environmental factors such as nutrition. (A and B from Jorde LB et al: *Medical genetics,* ed 3, St Louis, 2003, Mosby; C from Raven PH et al: *Biology,* ed 8, New York, 2008, McGraw-Hill.)

Aabb, AaBb, AaBB, AAbb, AABb, and *AABB.* An individual may have zero, one, two, three, or four "tall" alleles, so now five distinct phenotypes are possible (Figure 5-1, *B*). Although the height distribution in our fictional population is still not normal compared with an actual population, it approaches a normal distribution more closely than in the single-gene case just described.

We now extend our example so that *many* genes and environmental factors influence height, each having a small effect. Then many phenotypes are possible, each differing slightly from the others, and the height distribution of the population approaches the bell-shaped curve shown in Figure 5-1, *C*.

It should be emphasized that the individual genes underlying a multifactorial trait such as height follow the mendelian principles of segregation and independent assortment, just like any other gene. The only difference is that many of them *act together* to influence the trait.

Blood pressure is another example of a multifactorial trait. A correlation exists between parents' blood pressures (systolic and diastolic) and those of their children. The evidence is good that this correlation is partially caused by genes, but blood pressure is also influenced by environmental factors, such as diet, exercise, and stress. Two goals of genetic research are the identification and measurement of the relative roles of genes and environment in the causation of multifactorial diseases.

Threshold Model

A number of diseases do not follow the bell-shaped distribution. Instead, they appear to be either present or absent in individuals, yet they do not follow the inheritance patterns expected of single-gene diseases. A commonly used explanation for such diseases is that there is an underlying **liability distribution** for the disease in a population (Figure 5-2). Those individuals who are on the "low" end of the distribution have little chance of developing the disease in question (i.e., they have few of the alleles or environmental factors that would cause the disease). Individuals who are closer to the "high" end of the distribution have more of the disease-causing genes and environmental factors and are more likely to develop the disease. For diseases that are either present or absent, it is thought that a **threshold of liability** must be crossed before the disease is expressed. Below the threshold, an individual appears normal; above it, he or she is affected by the disease.

A disease that is thought to correspond to this threshold model is *pyloric stenosis,* a disorder that presents shortly after birth and is caused by a narrowing or obstruction of the pylorus, the area between the stomach and intestine. Chronic vomiting, constipation, weight loss, and electrolyte imbalance result from the condition, but it sometimes resolves spontaneously or can be corrected by surgery. The prevalence of pyloric stenosis is about 3 per 1000 live births in whites. It is much more common in males than females, affecting 1 of 200 males and 1 of 1000 females. It is thought that this difference in prevalence reflects two thresholds in the liability distribution—a lower one in males and a higher one in females (see Figure 5-2).

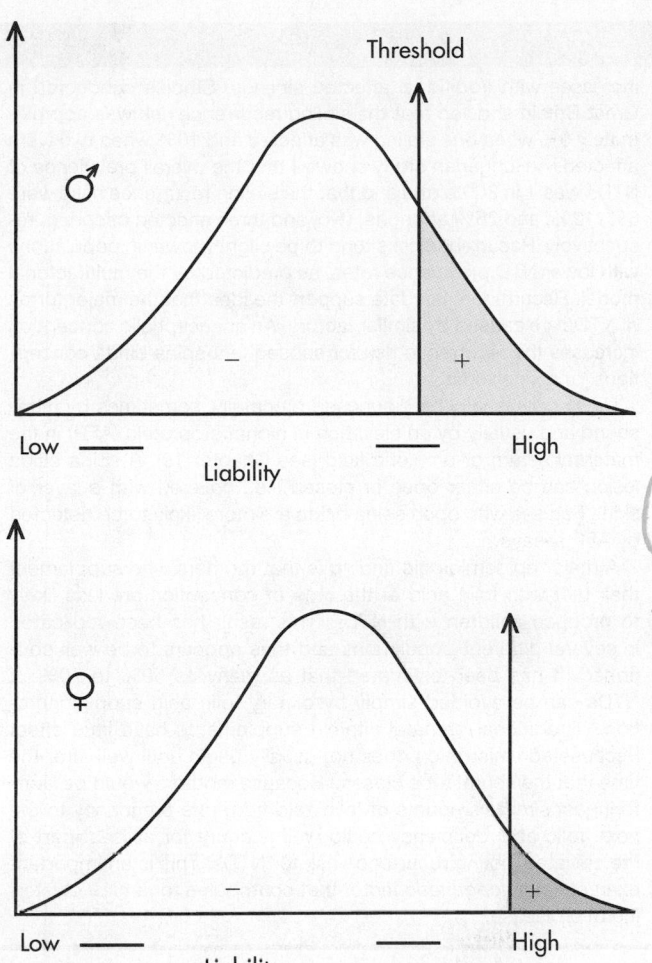

Figure 5-2 A liability distribution in a population for a multifactorial disease. To be affected with the disease, an individual must exceed the threshold on the liability distribution. This figure shows two thresholds, a lower one for males and a higher one for females (as in pyloric stenosis; see text). (From Jorde LB et al: *Medical genetics,* ed 3, St Louis, 2003, Mosby.)

A lower male threshold implies that fewer disease-causing factors are required to generate the disorder in males.

The liability threshold concept may explain the pattern of recurrence risks for pyloric stenosis seen in Table 5-1. Note that males, having a lower threshold, always have a higher risk than females. However, the sibling risk also depends on the gender of the proband (i.e., the individual from which the pedigree begins). It is higher when the proband is female than when the proband is male. This reflects the concept that females, having a higher liability threshold, must be exposed to more disease-causing factors than males to develop the disease. Thus a family with an affected female must have more genetic and environmental risk factors, producing a higher recurrence risk for pyloric stenosis in future offspring. It would be expected that the highest risk category would be *male* relatives of *female* probands; Table 5-1 shows that this is the case.

A similar pattern has been observed in a study of *infantile autism,* a behavioral disorder in which the male/female ratio is

Table 5-1	Recurrence Risks (%) for Pyloric Stenosis, Subdivided by Genders of Affected Probands and Relatives[*]			
	Male Probands		Female Probands	
Relatives	London	Belfast	London	Belfast
Brothers	3.8	9.6	9.2	12.5
Sisters	2.7	3	3.8	3.8

[*]Note that the risks differ somewhat between the two populations. Data from Carter CO: *Br Med Bull* 32(1):21-26, 1976.

approximately 4:1. As expected for a multifactorial disorder, the recurrence risks for siblings of male probands (3.5%) is substantially lower than that of siblings of female probands (7%). When the sex ratio for a disease is reversed (i.e., more affected females than males), one would expect a higher recurrence risk when the proband is male.

A number of other congenital malformations are thought to correspond to this model. They include isolated *cleft lip and/or cleft palate (CL/P), neural tube defects (anencephaly, spina bifida), clubfoot (talipes),* and some forms of congenital heart disease. In this context, isolated means that this is the only observed disease feature (i.e., the feature is not part of a larger constellation of findings, as in CL/P secondary to trisomy 13). In addition, many common adult diseases, such as *hypertension, coronary heart disease, stroke, diabetes mellitus* (types 1 and 2), and some cancers, are caused by complex genetic and environmental factors and can thus be considered multifactorial diseases.

Recurrence Risks and Transmission Patterns

Whereas recurrence risks can be given with confidence for single-gene diseases (e.g., 50% for typical autosomal dominant diseases, 25% for autosomal recessive diseases), the situation is more complicated for multifactorial diseases. This is because the number of genes contributing to the disease is usually not known, the precise allelic constitution of the parents is not known, and the extent of environmental effects can vary substantially. For most multifactorial diseases, **empirical risks** (i.e., risks based on direct observation of data) have been derived. To estimate empirical risks, a large series of families is examined in which one child has developed the disease (the proband). Then the siblings of each proband are surveyed to calculate the percentage who also have developed the disease. For example, in the United States about 3% of siblings of individuals with neural tube defects also have neural tube defects (Box 5-1). Thus the recurrence risk for parents who have had one child with a neural tube defect is 3% in the United States. For conditions such as CL/P that are not lethal or severely debilitating, recurrence risks also can be estimated for the offspring of affected parents. Empirical recurrence risks are, of course, specific for each multifactorial disease.

Box 5-1   Neural Tube Defects

Neural tube defects (NTDs), which include *anencephaly, spina bifida,* and *encephalocele* (as well as several other less common forms), are one of the most important classes of birth defects, with a birth prevalence of 1 to 3 per 1000.[4] The prevalence of NTDs among different populations varies considerably, with an especially high rate among some northern Chinese populations (as high as 6 or more per 1000 births). For reasons that are not fully known, the prevalence of NTDs has been decreasing in many parts of the United States and Europe during the past 2½ decades.

Normally the neural tube closes at about the fourth week of gestation. A defect in closure, or a subsequent reopening of the neural tube, results in a neural tube defect. Spina bifida (Figure 5-3, *A*) is the most commonly observed NTD and consists of a protrusion of spinal tissue through the vertebral column (the tissue usually includes meninges, spinal cord, and nerve roots). About 75% of individuals with spina bifida have secondary hydrocephalus, which sometimes in turn produces mental retardation. Paralysis or muscle weakness, lack of sphincter control, and clubfeet are often observed. A study conducted in British Columbia showed that survival rates for people with spina bifida have improved dramatically over the past several decades. Less than 30% of people born between 1952 and 1969 survived to 10 years of age, whereas 65% of those born between 1970 and 1986 survived to this age. Anencephaly (see Figure 5-3, *B*) is characterized by partial or complete absence of the cranial vault and calvarium and partial or complete absence of the cerebral hemispheres. At least two thirds of newborns with anencephaly are stillborn; term deliveries do not survive more than a few hours or days.

NTDs are thought to arise from a combination of genetic environmental factors. In most populations surveyed thus far, empirical recurrence risks for siblings of affected people range from 2% to 5%. Consistent with a multifactorial model, the recurrence risk increases with additional affected siblings. Studies conducted in Great Britain showed that the sibling recurrence risk was approximately 5% when one sibling was affected and 10% when two were affected. A Hungarian study showed that the overall prevalence of NTDs was 1 in 300 births and that the sibling recurrence risks were 3%, 12%, and 25% after one, two, and three affected offspring, respectively. Recurrence risks tend to be slightly lower in populations with lower NTD prevalence rates, as predicted by the multifactorial model. Recurrence risk data support the idea that the major forms of NTDs are caused by similar factors. An anencephalic conception increases the recurrence risk for subsequent spina bifida conceptions, and vice versa.

NTDs can usually be diagnosed prenatally, sometimes by ultrasound and usually by an elevation in alpha fetoprotein (AFP) in the maternal serum or amniotic fluid (see Chapter 19). A spina bifida lesion can be either open or closed (i.e., covered with a layer of skin). Fetuses with open spina bifida are more likely to be detected by AFP assays.

A major epidemiologic finding is that mothers who supplement their diet with folic acid at the time of conception are less likely to produce children with NTDs. This result has been replicated in several different populations and thus appears to be well confirmed. It has been estimated that as many as 50% to 70% of NTDs can be avoided simply by dietary folic acid supplementation.[5] (Traditional prenatal vitamin supplements have little effect because administration does not usually begin until well after the time that the neural tube closes.) Because mothers would be likely to ingest similar amounts of folic acid from one pregnancy to the next, folic acid deficiency could well account for at least part of the elevated sibling recurrence risk for NTDs. This is an important example of a *nongenetic* factor that contributes to familial clustering of a disease.

In contrast to most single-gene diseases, recurrence risks for multifactorial diseases can change substantially from one population to another because gene frequencies as well as environmental factors can differ among populations (note the differences between the London and Belfast populations in Table 5-1).

It is sometimes difficult to distinguish polygenic or multifactorial diseases from single-gene diseases that have reduced penetrance or variable expression. Large data sets and good epidemiologic data are necessary to make the distinction. Several criteria are commonly used to define multifactorial inheritance.

First, *the recurrence risk becomes higher if more than one family member is affected.* For example, the sibling recurrence risk for a *ventricular septal defect* (VSD), a type of congenital heart defect) is 3% if one sibling has had a VSD but increases to approximately 10% if two siblings have had VSDs.[6] In contrast, the recurrence risk for single-gene diseases remains the same regardless of the number of affected siblings. It should be emphasized that this increase does not mean that the family's risk has actually *changed.* Rather, it means that we now have more information about the family's true risk: because they have had two affected children, they are probably located higher on the liability distribution than a family with only one affected child. In other words, they have more risk factors (genetic or environmental) and are more likely to produce an affected child.

Second, *if the expression of the disease in the proband is more severe, the recurrence risk is higher.* This is again consistent with the liability model because a more severe expression indicates that the affected individual is at the extreme tail end of the liability distribution (see Figure 5-2). His or her relatives are thus at a higher risk for inheriting disease genes. For example, the occurrence of a bilateral (both sides) CL/P confers a higher recurrence risk on family members than does the occurrence of a unilateral (one side) cleft.

Third, *the recurrence risk is higher if the proband is of the less commonly affected sex* (see the preceding discussion of pyloric stenosis). This is because an affected individual of the less susceptible gender is usually at a more extreme position on the liability distribution.

Fourth, *the recurrence risk for the disease usually decreases rapidly in more remotely related relatives* (Table 5-2). Whereas the recurrence risk for single-gene diseases decreases by 50% with each degree of relationship (e.g., an autosomal dominant disease has a 50% recurrence risk for siblings, 25% for uncle-nephew relationships, 12.5% for first cousins), it decreases much more quickly for multifactorial diseases. This reflects the fact that many genes and environmental factors must combine to produce a trait. All the necessary

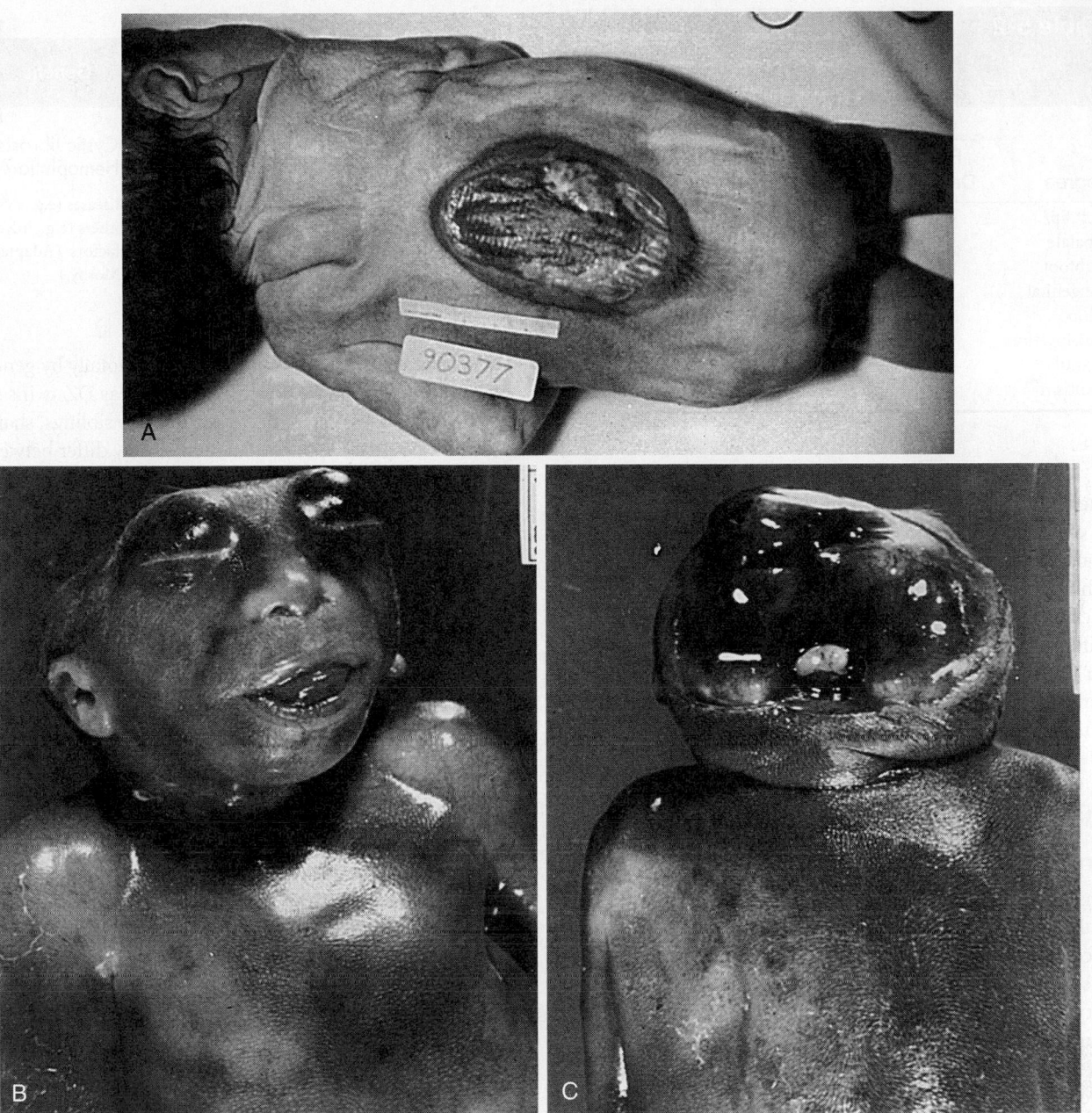

Figure 5-3 Spina bifida and anencephaly. **A,** Spina bifida in a newborn. **B** and **C,** Anencephaly, showing the absence of the cranial vault. (From Jorde LB et al: *Medical genetics,* ed 3, St Louis, 2003, Mosby.)

risk factors are unlikely to be present in less closely related family members.

Finally, *if the prevalence of the disease in a population is f, the risk for offspring and siblings of probands is approximately $\sqrt{f}$*. This does not hold true for single-gene traits because their recurrence risks are independent of population prevalence. It is not an absolute rule for multifactorial traits either, but many such diseases tend to conform to this prediction. Examination of the risks given in Table 5-2 shows that the first three diseases follow the prediction fairly well. However, the observed sibling risk for the fourth disease, infantile autism, is substantially higher than predicted by $\sqrt{f}$.

NATURE AND NURTURE: DISENTANGLING THE EFFECTS OF GENES AND ENVIRONMENT

Family members share genes and a common environment. Family resemblance in traits such as blood pressure reflects both genes and environment ("nature" and "nurture," respectively). For centuries people have debated the relative importance of these two types of factors. It is a mistake, of course, to view them as mutually exclusive. Few traits are influenced only by genes or only by environmental factors. Most are influenced by both. It is useful to try to determine the *relative*

Table 5-2	Recurrence Risks (%) for First-, Second-, and Third-Degree Relatives			
	Risk			
Degree	First Degree	Second Degree	Third Degree	General Population
Cleft lip/ palate	4	0.7	0.3	0.1
Clubfoot	2.5	0.5	0.2	0.1
Congenital hip dislocation	5	0.6	0.4	0.2
Infantile autism	4.5	0.1	0.05	0.04

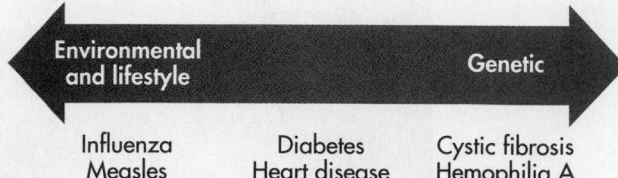

Figure 5-4 **Continuum of genetic diseases.** Some diseases (e.g., cystic fibrosis) are strongly determined by genes, whereas others (e.g., infectious diseases) are strongly determined by environmental factors. (Adapted from Jorde LB et al: *Medical genetics*, ed 3, St Louis, 2003, Mosby.)

influence of genetic and environmental factors (Figure 5-4). This can lead to a better understanding of disease etiology. It can also help in planning public health strategies. A disease in which the genetic influence is relatively small, such as lung cancer, may be prevented most effectively through emphasis on lifestyle changes (avoidance of tobacco). When a disease has a relatively larger genetic component, as in breast cancer, examination of family history should be emphasized in addition to lifestyle modification.

Here, two research strategies are reviewed that often are used to estimate the relative influence of genes and environment: twin studies and adoption studies.

Twin Studies

Twins occur with a frequency of about 1 in 100 births in white populations. They are a bit more common in blacks and a bit less common among Asians. **Monozygotic (MZ, identical) twins** originate when, for unknown reasons, the developing embryo divides to form two separate but identical embryos. Because they are genetically identical, MZ twins are an example of natural clones. **Dizygotic (DZ, fraternal) twins** are the result of a double ovulation followed by the fertilization of each egg by a different sperm. Thus dizygotic twins are genetically no more similar than siblings. Because two different sperm cells are required to fertilize the two eggs, it is possible for each DZ twin to have a different father. Whereas MZ twinning rates are constant across populations, DZ twinning rates vary somewhat. DZ twinning increases with maternal age until about 40 years, after which it declines.

Because MZ twins are genetically identical, any differences between them should be caused only by environmental effects.[7] MZ twins should thus resemble one another very closely for traits that are strongly influenced by genes. DZ twins provide a convenient comparison because their environmental differences should be similar to those of MZ twins, but their genetic differences are as great as those between siblings. Twin studies thus usually consist of comparisons between MZ and DZ twins.[8] If both members of a twin pair share a trait (e.g., a cleft lip), it is said to be a **concordant trait.** If they do not share the trait, it is

a **discordant trait.** For a trait determined totally by genes, MZ twins should always be concordant, whereas DZ twins should be concordant less often, because they, like siblings, share only 50% of their genes. Concordance rates may differ between opposite-sex DZ twin pairs and same-sex DZ pairs for some traits, such as those that have different frequencies in males and females. For such traits, only same-sex DZ twin pairs should be used when comparing MZ and DZ concordance rates, because MZ twins are necessarily of the same sex.

Table 5-3 gives concordance rates for a number of traits. Note that the concordance rates for contagious diseases such as measles are quite similar in MZ and DZ twins. This is expected because a contagious disease is unlikely to be influenced markedly by genes. On the other hand, the concordance rates are quite dissimilar for *schizophrenia* and *bipolar affective disorder,* suggesting a sizable genetic component for these diseases. The MZ correlations for dermatoglyphics (fingerprints), which are determined almost entirely by genes, are close to 1.0.

At one time, twins were thought to provide a perfect "natural laboratory" in which to determine the relative influences of genetics and environment, but several difficulties arise. One of the most important is the assumption that the environments of MZ and DZ twins are equally similar. As one would expect, MZ twins are often treated more similarly than DZ twins. A greater similarity in environment can make MZ twins more concordant for a trait, inflating the apparent influence of genes. In addition, MZ twins may be more likely to seek the same type of environment, further reinforcing environmental similarity. On the other hand, it has been suggested that MZ twins tend to develop personality differences in an attempt to assert their individuality.

Adoption Studies

Studies of adopted children also are used to estimate the genetic contribution to a multifactorial trait. Children born to parents who have a disease but are then subsequently adopted by parents lacking the disease can be studied to find out whether these children develop the disease. In some cases such children develop the disease more often than a comparative control population (i.e., adopted children who were born to parents who do *not* have the disease). This provides some evidence that genes may be involved in the causation of the disease, because the adopted children do not share an environment with their affected natural parents. For example,

Table 5-3	Concordance Rates in MZ and DZ Twins for Selected Traits and Diseases*		
	Concordance Rate		
Trait or Disease	**MZ Twins**	**DZ Twins**	**Heritability**
Affective disorder (bipolar)	0.79	0.24	>1†
Affective disorder (unipolar)	0.54	0.19	0.7
Alcoholism	>0.6	<0.3	0.6
Autism	0.92	0	>1
Blood pressure (diastolic)‡	0.58	0.27	0.62
Blood pressure (systolic)‡	0.55	0.25	0.6
Body fat percentage‡	0.73	0.22	>1
Body mass index‡	0.95	0.53	0.84
Cleft lip/palate	0.38	0.08	0.6
Clubfoot	0.32	0.03	0.58
Dermatoglyphics (finger ridge count)‡	0.95	0.49	0.92
Diabetes mellitus	0.45-0.96	0.03-0.37	>1
Diabetes mellitus (type 1)	0.55	—	—
Diabetes mellitus (type 2)	0.9	—	—
Epilepsy (idiopathic)	0.69	0.14	>1
Height‡	0.94	0.44	1
Intelligence quotient (IQ)‡	0.76	0.51	0.5
Measles	0.95	0.87	0.16
Multiple sclerosis	0.28	0.03	0.5
Myocardial infarction (males)	0.39	0.26	0.26
Myocardial infarction (females)	0.44	0.14	0.6
Schizophrenia	0.47	0.12	0.7
Spina bifida	0.72	0.33	0.78

NOTE: Heritability, which is defined as the proportion of the variation in a trait that is due to genetic factors, can be measured as $2(C_{MZ} - C_{DZ})$, where C_{MZ} and C_{DZ} are the concordance rates for MZ twins and DZ twins, respectively.

*These figures were compiled from a large variety of sources and represent primarily European and U.S. populations.

†Several heritability estimates exceed 1. Because it is impossible for >100% of the variance of a trait to be genetically determined, these values indicate that other factors, such as shared environmental factors, must be operating.

‡Because these are quantitative traits, correlation coefficients are given rather than concordance rates.

DZ, Dizygotic; *MZ*, monozygotic.

about 8% to 10% of adopted children of a schizophrenic parent develop *schizophrenia*, whereas only 1% of adopted children of normal parents develop schizophrenia.

As with twin studies, several precautions must be exercised in interpreting the results of adoption studies. First, prenatal

α_1-Antitrypsin (α_1-AT) deficiency is one of the most common autosomal recessive disorders among whites, affecting approximately 1 in 2500 members of this ethnic group. α_1-AT, synthesized primarily in the liver, is a serine protease inhibitor. It does bind trypsin, as its name suggests. However, α_1-AT binds much more strongly to neutrophil elastase, a protease that is produced by neutrophils (a type of leukocyte) in response to infections and irritants. It carries out its binding and inhibitory role primarily in the lower respiratory tract, where it prevents elastase from digesting the alveolar septi of the lung.

Individuals with less than 10% to 15% of the normal level of α_1-AT activity will experience significant lung damage and typically develop emphysema during their 30s, 40s, or 50s. In addition, at least 10% develop liver cirrhosis as a result of the accumulation of variant α_1-AT molecules in the liver; α_1-AT deficiency accounts for nearly 20% of all nonalcoholic liver cirrhosis in the United States. An important feature of this disease is that cigarette smokers with α_1-AT deficiency develop emphysema much earlier than do nonsmokers. This is because cigarette smoke irritates lung tissue, increasing secretion of neutrophil elastase. At the same time it inactivates α_1-AT, so there is also less inhibition of elastase. One study showed that the median age of survival of nonsmokers with α_1-AT deficiency was 62 years, whereas it was only 40 years for smokers with this disease. Because the combination of cigarette smoking (an environmental factor) and the α_1-AT mutation (a genetic factor) produces more severe disease than either factor alone, it is an example of a gene-environment interaction.

environmental influences could have long-lasting effects on an adopted child. Second, children are sometimes adopted after they are several years old, ensuring that some environmental influence would have been imparted by the natural parents. Finally, adoption agencies sometimes try to match the adoptive parents with the natural parents in terms of background, socioeconomic status, and so on. All of these factors could exaggerate the apparent influence of biologic inheritance.

These reservations, as well as those summarized for twin studies, underscore the need for caution in basing conclusions on twin and adoption studies. These approaches do not provide definitive measures of the role of genes in multifactorial disease nor can they identify specific genes responsible for disease. Instead, they serve a useful purpose in providing a preliminary indication of the extent to which a multifactorial disease may be caused by genetic factors. Sophisticated molecular techniques are being used to identify the specific genes that underlie predisposition to multifactorial diseases.

This discussion should make clear that most common diseases are not the result of either genetics *or* environment. Instead, genetic and nongenetic factors usually interact to influence one's likelihood of developing a common disease. In some cases a genetic predisposition may interact with an environmental factor to increase the risk of disease to a much higher level than would either factor acting alone. A good example of a **gene-environment interaction** is given by α_1-antitrypsin deficiency, a genetic condition that causes pulmonary emphysema and is greatly exacerbated by cigarette smoking (Box 5-2).

GENETICS OF COMMON DISEASES

Some common multifactorial disorders, the congenital malformations, are by definition present at birth. Others, including heart disease, cancer, diabetes, and most psychiatric disorders, are seen primarily in adolescents and adults. Because these disorders are complex, unraveling their genetics is a daunting task. Nonetheless, significant progress is being made.

Congenital Malformations

Congenital diseases are present at birth. Approximately 2% of newborns present with a congenital malformation; most of these are multifactorial in etiology. Table 5-4 lists some more common congenital malformations. In general, sibling recurrence risks for most of these disorders range from 1% to 5%.

Some congenital malformations, such as CL/P and pyloric stenosis, are relatively easy to repair and thus are not considered to be serious problems. Others, such as the neural tube defects, usually have more severe consequences. Although some cases of congenital malformations occur in the absence of any other problems, it is quite common for them to be associated with other disorders. For example, hydrocephaly and clubfoot are often seen secondary to spina bifida, CL/P is often seen in babies with trisomy 13, and congenital heart defects are seen in children with many other disorders, including Down syndrome.

Environmental factors also cause some congenital malformations. An example is thalidomide, a sedative used during pregnancy in the early 1960s. When ingested during early pregnancy this drug often caused **phocomelia** (severely shortened limbs) in babies. Maternal exposure to retinoic acid, which is used to treat acne, can cause congenital defects of the heart, ear, and central nervous system. Maternal rubella infection can cause congenital heart defects.

Multifactorial Disorders in the Adult Population

Until quite recently, very little was known about specific genes responsible for common adult diseases. With the more powerful laboratory and analytic techniques now available, this situation is changing. This section reviews recent progress in understanding the genetics of the major common adult diseases. Table 5-5 gives approximate prevalence figures for these disorders in the United States.

Coronary Heart Disease

It is well known that coronary heart disease (CHD) is the leading killer of Americans, accounting for approximately 25% of all deaths in the United States. It is caused by *atherosclerosis* (narrowing as a result of the formation of lipid-laden lesions) of the coronary arteries. This narrowing impedes blood flow to the heart and can eventually result in a *myocardial infarction* (destruction of heart tissue caused by an inadequate supply of oxygen). When atherosclerosis occurs in arteries supplying blood to the brain, a *stroke* can result. Many risk factors for heart disease have been identified, including obesity, cigarette smoking, hypertension, elevated cholesterol level, and positive family history (usually defined as having one affected first-degree relative). Many studies have examined the role of family history in CHD, and they show that an individual with a positive family history is two to seven times more likely to have heart disease than is an individual with no family history (this would be the relative risk of heart disease as a result of a positive family history). Generally, these studies also show that the risk increases if (1) there are more affected relatives; (2) the affected relative or relatives are female (the less commonly affected sex) rather than male; and (3) age of onset in the

Table 5-4	Prevalence Rates of Common Congenital Malformations in Whites
Disorder	**Prevalence per 1000 Births (Approximate)**
Cleft lip/palate	1
Clubfoot	1
Congenital heart defects	4-8
Hydrocephaly	0.5-2.5
Isolated cleft palate	0.4
Neural tube defects	1-3
Pyloric stenosis	3

Table 5-5	Prevalence of Common Adult Diseases in the United States
Disease	**Number Affected (Approximate)**
Alcoholism	14 million
Alzheimer disease	4 million
Arthritis	43 million
Asthma	17 million
Cancer	8 million
Cardiovascular disease (all forms)	
Coronary artery disease	13 million
Congestive heart failure	5 million
Congenital defects	1 million
Hypertension	50 million
Stroke	5 million
Depression and bipolar disorder	17 million
Diabetes (type 1)	1 million
Diabetes (type 2)	15 million
Epilepsy	2.5 million
Multiple sclerosis	350,000
Obesity*	60 million
Parkinson disease	500,000
Psoriasis	3-5 million
Schizophrenia	2 million

*Body mass index >30.
Data from National Center for Chronic Disease Prevention and Health Promotion; American Heart Association (2002 Heart and Stroke Statistical Update); National Institute on Alcohol Abuse and Alcoholism; Office of the U.S. Surgeon General; American Academy of Allergy, Asthma and Immunology; Cown WM, Kandel ER: *JAMA* 285:594-600, 2001; Flegal et al: *JAMA* 288:1723–1727, 2002.

Box 5-3   Familial Hypercholesterolemia

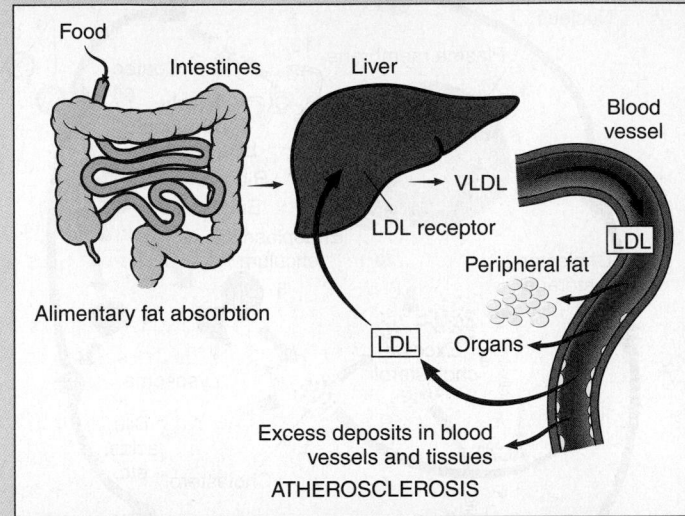

Food

Intestines   Liver

Blood vessel

VLDL

LDL receptor

LDL

Peripheral fat

Alimentary fat absorbtion

LDL   Organs

Excess deposits in blood vessels and tissues
ATHEROSCLEROSIS

Autosomal dominant familial hypercholesterolemia (FH) is an important cause of heart disease, accounting for approximately 5% of myocardial infarctions in individuals less than 60 years of age.[9] FH is one of the most common autosomal dominant disorders: in most populations surveyed to date, about 1 in 500 people is a heterozygote. Plasma cholesterol levels are approximately twice as high as normal (i.e., about 300 to 400 mg/dl), resulting in substantially accelerated atherosclerosis and distinctive cholesterol deposits in skin and tendons (xanthomas, Figure 5-5). Data compiled from five studies showed that approximately 75% of men with FH developed coronary disease and 50% had a fatal myocardial infarction by 60 years. The corresponding percentages for women were lower (45% and 15%) because women generally develop heart disease at a later age than men.

Consistent with Hardy-Weinberg predictions, about 1 in 1 million births is homozygous for the FH gene. Homozygotes are much more severely affected, with cholesterol levels ranging from 600 to 1200 mg/dl. Most experience myocardial infarctions before 20 years of age, and a myocardial infarction at 18 months of age has been reported. If untreated, most FH homozygotes die before 30 years of age.

All cells require cholesterol as a component of their plasma membrane. They can either synthesize their own cholesterol, or, preferably, obtain it from the extracellular environment, where it is carried primarily by low-density lipoprotein (LDL). In a process known as endocytosis, LDL-bound cholesterol is taken into the cell via LDL receptors on the cell's surface (Figure 5-6). FH is caused by a reduction in the number of functional LDL receptors on cell surfaces. Lacking the normal number of LDL receptors, cellular cholesterol uptake is reduced and circulating cholesterol levels increase.

Much of what we know about endocytosis has been learned through the study of LDL receptors. The process of endocytosis and the processing of LDL in the cell are described in detail in Figure 5-6 (endocytosis is discussed in Chapter 1). These processes result in a fine-tuned regulation of cholesterol levels within cells, and they influence the level of circulating cholesterol as well.

The isolation and cloning of the LDL receptor gene in 1984 were critical steps in understanding exactly how LDL receptor defects cause FH. More than 600 different mutations, including missense and nonsense substitutions as well as insertions and deletions, have been identified in the LDL receptor gene. These can be grouped into five broad classes according to their effects on the activity of the receptor.[10] Class 1 mutations result in no detectable protein product. Thus heterozygotes would produce only half the normal number of LDL receptors. Class 2 mutations in the LDL receptor gene result in production of the LDL receptor, but it is altered such that it cannot leave the endoplasmic reticulum. It is eventually degraded. Class 3 mutations produce an LDL receptor that is capable of migrating to the cell surface but incapable of normal binding to LDL. Class 4 mutations, which are comparatively rare, produce receptors that are normal except that they do not migrate specifically to coated pits and thus cannot carry LDL into the cell. The final group of mutations, class 5, produces an LDL receptor that cannot dissociate from the LDL particle after entry into the cell. The receptor cannot return to the cell surface and is degraded. Each class of mutations reduces the number of effective LDL receptors, resulting in decreased LDL uptake and hence elevated levels of circulating cholesterol. The number of effective receptors is reduced by about half in FH heterozygotes, and homozygotes have virtually no functional LDL receptors.

Understanding the defects that lead to FH has helped to develop effective therapies for the disorder. Dietary reduction of cholesterol (primarily through the reduced intake of saturated fats) has only modest effects on cholesterol levels in FH heterozygotes. Because cholesterol is reabsorbed into the gut and then recycled through the liver (where most cholesterol synthesis takes place), serum cholesterol levels can be reduced by the administration of bile acid–absorbing resins, such as cholestyramine. The absorbed cholesterol is then excreted. It is interesting that reduced recirculation from the gut causes the liver cells to form additional LDL receptors, lowering circulating cholesterol levels. However, the decrease in intracellular cholesterol also stimulates cholesterol synthesis by liver cells, so the overall reduction in plasma LDL is only about 15% to 20%. This treatment is much more effective when combined with agents such as lovastatin that reduce cholesterol synthesis by inhibiting 3-hydroxy-3-methylglutaryl coenzyme A (HMG-CoA) reductase. Decreased synthesis leads to further production of LDL receptors. When these therapies are used in combination, serum cholesterol levels in FH heterozygotes can be reduced to approximately normal levels.

The picture is less encouraging for FH homozygotes. The therapies just discussed can enhance cholesterol elimination and reduce its synthesis, but they are largely ineffective because homozygotes have few or no LDL receptors. Liver transplants, which provide hepatocytes that have normal LDL receptors, have been successful in some cases, but this option is often limited by a lack of donors. Plasma exchange, carried out every 1 to 2 weeks, in combination with drug therapy, can reduce cholesterol levels by about 50%. However, this therapy is difficult to continue for long periods. Somatic cell gene therapy, in which hepatocytes carrying normal LDL receptor genes are introduced into the portal circulation, is now being tested. It may eventually prove to be an effective treatment for FH homozygotes.

The FH story illustrates how medical research has made important contributions both to our understanding of basic cell biology and to advances in clinical therapy. The process of receptor-mediated endocytosis, elucidated largely by research on the LDL receptor defects, is of fundamental significance for cellular processes throughout the body. Equally important is that this research, by clarifying how cholesterol synthesis and uptake can be modified, has led to significant improvements in therapy for this important cause of heart disease.

Illustration form Damjanov I: *Pathophysiology for the health-related professions,* ed 2, Philadelphia, 2000, Saunders.

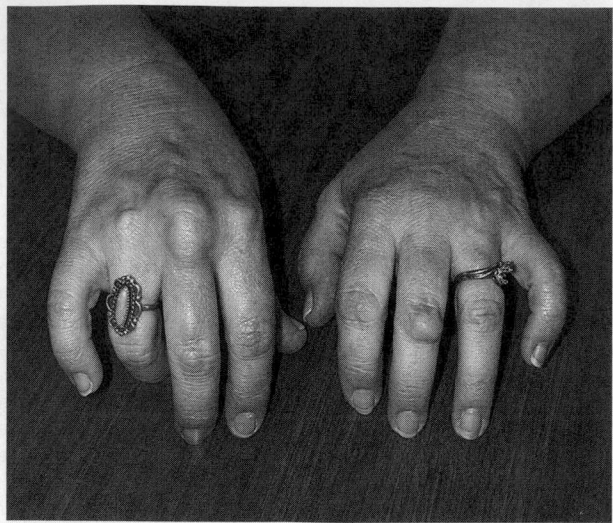

Figure 5-5 Xanthoma. Fatty deposits, referred to as xanthomas as seen here on the knuckles, are often noted in individuals with familial hyper-cholesterolemia. (From Jorde LB et al: *Medical genetics,* ed 3, St Louis, 2003, Mosby.)

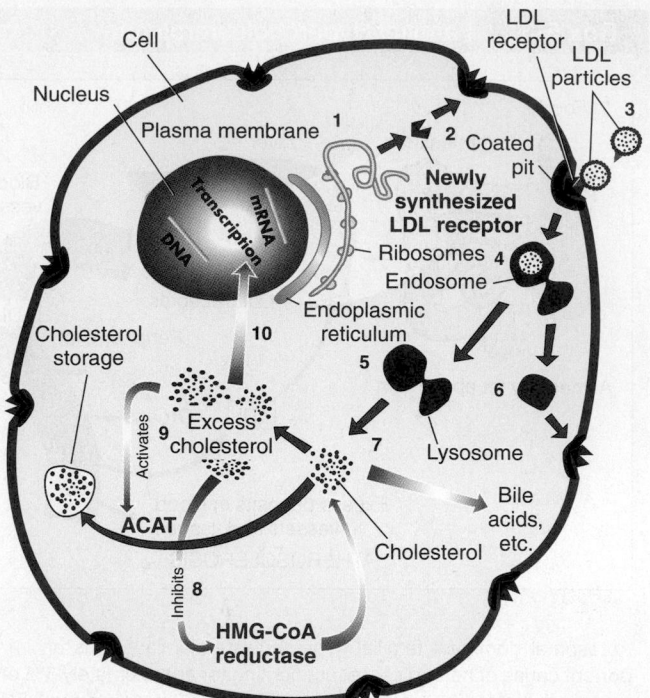

Figure 5-6 Process of receptor-mediated endocytosis. Numbers in parentheses correspond to numbers shown in the figure. (1) The low-density lipoprotein (LDL) receptors, which are glycoproteins, are synthesized in the endoplasmic reticulum of the cell. (2) From here, they pass through the Golgi apparatus to the cell surface, where part of the receptor protrudes outside the cell. (3) The circulating LDL particle is bound by the LDL receptor and localized in cell-surface depressions called *coated pits* (so named because they are coated with a protein called clathrin). (4) The coated pit invaginates, bringing the LDL particle inside the cell. (5) Once inside the cell, the LDL particle is separated from the receptor, taken into a lysosome, and broken down into its constituents by lysosomal enzymes. (6) The LDL receptor is recirculated to the cell surface to bind another LDL particle (each LDL receptor goes through this cycle approximately once every 10 minutes even if it is not occupied by an LDL particle). (7) Free cholesterol is released from the lysosome for incorporation into cell membranes or metabolism into bile acids or steroids. Excess cholesterol can be stored in the cell as a cholesterol ester or removed from the cell by associating with high-density lipoprotein (HDL). (8) As cholesterol levels in the cell rise, cellular cholesterol synthesis is reduced by inhibition of the rate-limiting enzyme HMG-CoA (3-hydroxy-3-methylglutaryl coenzyme A) reductase. (9) Rising cholesterol levels also increase the activity of acyl coenzyme A (acyl CoA): cholesterol acyltransferase (ACAT), an enzyme that modifies cholesterol for storage as cholesterol esters. (10) In addition, the number of LDL receptors is decreased by lowering the transcription rate of the LDL receptor gene itself. This decreases cholesterol uptake. (From Jorde LB et al: *Medical genetics,* ed 3, St Louis, 2003, Mosby.)

affected relative is early (before 55 years). For example, one study showed that men between the ages of 20 and 39 years had a relative risk of 3 for CHD if they had one affected first-degree relative. The relative risk increased to 13 if two first-degree relatives were affected with CHD before 55 years of age.[11]

What part do genes play in the familial clustering of heart disease? Because of the key role of lipids in atherosclerosis, many studies are focusing on the genetic determination of various lipoproteins.[12] An important advance in this area has been the isolation and cloning of the gene for the low-density lipoprotein (LDL)–receptor defects that cause *familial hypercholesterolemia* (see Box 5-3). Many other genes involved in lipid variation, coagulation, and hypertension have been identified, including several genes encoding apolipoproteins (the protein components of lipoproteins) (Table 5-6). Functional analysis of these genes is leading to an increased understanding, and eventually more effective treatment, of CHD.

Environmental factors, many of which are easily modified, are also important causes of CHD. Abundant epidemiologic evidence shows that cigarette smoking and obesity increase the risk of CHD, whereas exercise and a diet low in saturated fats decrease the risk. Indeed, the approximate 50% decline in CHD prevalence in the United States during the past 40 years is usually attributed to a decrease in the proportion of adults who smoke cigarettes, decreased consumption of saturated fats, and an increased emphasis on exercise and a generally healthier lifestyle.

Hypertension

Systemic hypertension, which is seen in at least 15% of the populations of most developed countries, is a key risk factor for heart disease, stroke, and kidney disease. Studies of blood pressure correlations within families indicate that about 20% to 40% of the variation in both systolic and diastolic blood pressure is caused by genetic factors. The fact that this figure is substantially less than 100% indicates that environmental factors also must be important causes of blood pressure variation. The most important environmental risk factors for hypertension are increased sodium intake, decreased physical activity, psychosocial stress, and obesity (but, as discussed later, the latter factor is itself influenced by both genes and environment).

Blood pressure regulation is a highly complex process that is influenced by many physiologic systems, including various

Table 5-6	Lipoprotein Genes Known to Contribute to Coronary Artery Disease Risk	
Gene	**Chromosome Location**	**Function of Protein Product**
Apolipoprotein A-I	11q	HDL component; LCAT cofactor
Apolipoprotein A-IV	11q	Component of chylomicrons and HDL; may influence HDL metabolism
Apolipoprotein C-III	11q	Allelic variation associated with hypertriglyceridemia
Apolipoprotein B	2p	Ligand for LDL receptor; involved in formation of VLDL, LDL, IDL, and chylomicrons
Apolipoprotein D	2p	HDL component
Apolipoprotein C-I	19q	LCAT activation
Apolipoprotein C-II	19q	Lipoprotein lipase activation
Apolipoprotein E	19q	Ligand for LDL receptor
Apolipoprotein A-II	1p	HDL component
LDL receptor	19p	Uptake of circulating LDL particles
Lipoprotein (a)	6q	Cholesterol transport
Lipoprotein lipase	8p	Hydrolysis of lipoprotein lipids
Hepatic triglyceride lipase	15q	Hydrolysis of lipoprotein lipids
LCAT	16q	Cholesterol esterification
Cholesterol ester transfer protein	16q	Facilitates transfer of cholesterol esters and phospholipids between lipoproteins

HDL, High-density lipoprotein; *IDL,* intermediate-density lipoprotein; *LCAT,* lecithin cholesterol acyltransferase; *LDL,* low-density lipoprotein; *VLDL,* very-low-density lipoprotein.

Adapted in part from King RA, Rotter JI, editors: *The genetic basis of common diseases,* ed 2, New York, 2002, Oxford University Press.

aspects of kidney function, cellular ion transport, and heart function. Because of this complexity, it is unlikely that family studies of simple blood pressure will reveal much about genes responsible for hypertension. For this reason most research now focuses on specific components that may influence blood pressure variation, such as angiotensin, angiotensinogen, urinary kallikrein, and sodium-lithium countertransport[13] (Figure 5-7). These factors are more likely to be under the control of smaller numbers of genes. For example, studies have implicated the angiotensinogen gene in the causation of both hypertension and preeclampsia (a form of pregnancy-induced hypertension).

Cancer

Cancer is the second leading cause of death in the United States. It is well established that many major types of cancer (e.g., breast, colon, prostate, ovarian) cluster strongly in families. This is caused by both shared genes and shared environmental factors. Although numerous cancer genes are being isolated,[14] environmental factors also play an important role in causing cancer. In particular, tobacco use is estimated to account for one third of all cancer cases in the United States, making it the most important known cause of cancer.[15]

Breast Cancer

Breast cancer is the most common cancer among women, affecting approximately 12% of American women who live to 85 years or more. Formerly the leading cause of cancer death among women, it has been surpassed by lung cancer. Breast cancer aggregates strongly in families. If a woman has one affected first-degree relative, her risk of developing breast cancer doubles. This risk increases if the age of onset in the affected relative is early and if the cancer is bilateral (tumors in both breasts).

An autosomal dominant form of breast cancer accounts for approximately 5% of breast cancer cases in the United

States. Genes responsible for this form of breast cancer have been mapped to chromosomes 17 *(BRCA1)* and 13 *(BRCA2).* Each of these genes has been cloned, and it is possible to test them for cancer-causing mutations.[16] Women who inherit a mutation in *BRCA1* or *BRCA2* experience a 50% to 80% lifetime risk of developing breast cancer. *BRCA1* mutations also increase the risk of ovarian cancer among women (20% to 50% lifetime risk), and they confer a modestly increased risk of prostate and colon cancers. *BRCA2* mutations also confer an increased risk of ovarian cancer (10% to 20% lifetime prevalence). Approximately 6% of males who inherit a *BRCA2* mutation will develop breast cancer; this represents a 100-fold increase over the risk in the general male population. The evaluation of the *BRCA1* and *BRCA2* gene products, which are both involved in deoxyribonucleic acid (DNA) repair, is yielding valuable evidence on the etiology of breast cancer in general.

Although *BRCA1* and *BRCA2* mutations are the most common known causes of inherited breast cancer, this disease also can be caused by inherited mutations in several other tumor suppressor genes (e.g., the *CHK2* and *TP53* genes). Germline mutations in a tumor suppressor gene called *PTEN* are responsible for Cowden disease, which is characterized by multiple benign tumors and an increased susceptibility to breast cancer.

Colorectal Cancer

Colorectal cancer is second only to lung cancer in the number of cases occurring annually in the United States, with nearly 154,000 new cases in 2007.[17] Approximately 1 in 20 Americans will develop colorectal cancer. Like breast cancer, it clusters in families (in fact, familial clustering of this form of cancer was reported in the medical literature as early as 1881). The risk of colorectal cancer in people with one affected first-degree relative is two to three times higher than in the general population.

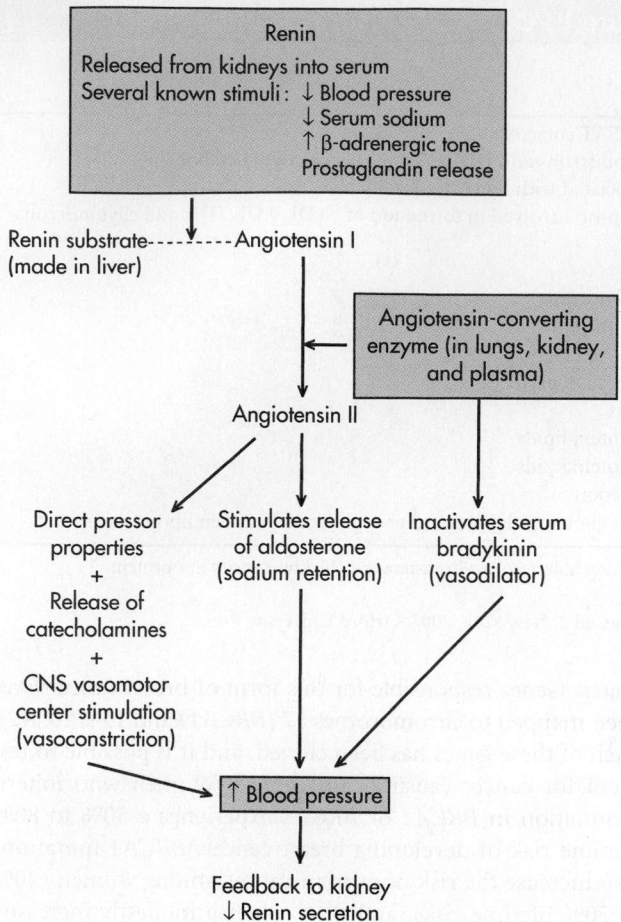

Renin
Released from kidneys into serum
Several known stimuli : ↓ Blood pressure
↓ Serum sodium
↑ β-adrenergic tone
Prostaglandin release

Renin substrate- - - - - - - Angiotensin I
(made in liver)

Angiotensin-converting enzyme (in lungs, kidney, and plasma)

Angiotensin II

Direct pressor properties
+
Release of catecholamines
+
CNS vasomotor center stimulation (vasoconstriction)

Stimulates release of aldosterone (sodium retention)

Inactivates serum bradykinin (vasodilator)

↑ Blood pressure

Feedback to kidney
↓ Renin secretion

Figure 5-7 Renin-angiotensin-aldosterone system. *CNS,* Central nervous system. (From Jorde LB et al: *Medical genetics,* ed 3, St Louis, 2003, Mosby.)

This familial aggregation is caused in part by subsets of colorectal cancer cases that are inherited as single-gene traits. *Familial adenomatous polyposis* occurs in approximately 1 in 8000 whites. The gene responsible for this disorder, *APC,* was mapped to chromosome 5, and the gene itself was subsequently cloned.[18] Identification of the protein product of this gene showed that it functions as a tumor suppressor. Importantly, somatic mutations of *APC* are found in at least 85% of all colon tumors. Thus although inherited *APC* mutations play a vital role in relatively rare familial adenomatous polyposis, somatic mutations are involved in the great majority of all common colon cancers.

Hereditary nonpolyposis colorectal cancer, which may account for as many as 5% of colorectal cancer cases, is caused by mutations in any of six genes.[19] Cloning of these genes has shown that all of them are involved in the vital process of DNA repair. When this function is compromised, cancer-causing mutations can persist in cells, leading eventually to growth of a tumor.

Other colorectal cancer cases are likely to be caused by a complex interaction of multiple genes. In addition,

environmental factors, such as a high-fat, low-fiber diet, are thought to increase the risk of colorectal cancer.

Other Cancers

The genetic basis of various other cancers, including retinoblastoma, has been discussed. Although each of these cancers is relatively rare, study of the causative genes has provided many important insights into the nature of carcinogenesis in general. This will lead to more effective treatment and prevention of all cancers.

Diabetes Mellitus

Like the other disorders discussed in this chapter, the etiology of diabetes mellitus is complex and not fully understood. Nevertheless, progress is being made in understanding the genetic basis of this disorder, which is a leading cause of blindness, heart disease, and kidney failure.[20,21] An important advance has been the recognition that diabetes is actually a heterogeneous group of disorders, all characterized by elevated blood sugar. The focus here is on the two major types of diabetes: type 1 (insulin-dependent diabetes mellitus [IDDM]) and type 2 (non–insulin-dependent diabetes mellitus [NIDDM]).

Type 1 Diabetes

Type 1 diabetes, which is characterized by T-cell infiltration of the pancreas and destruction of the insulin-producing beta cells, usually (though not always) presents before age 40. Individuals with type 1 diabetes must receive exogenous insulin to survive. In addition to T-cell infiltration of the pancreas, autoantibodies are formed against pancreatic cells; the latter can be observed long before clinical symptoms occur. These findings, along with a strong association between type 1 diabetes and the presence of several human leukocyte antigen (HLA) class II alleles, indicate that this is an autoimmune disease.

Siblings of individuals with type 1 diabetes face a substantial elevation in risk: approximately 6%, as opposed to a risk of about 0.3% to 0.5% in the general population. The recurrence risk is also elevated when there is a diabetic parent, although this risk varies with the sex of the affected parent. The risk for offspring of diabetic mothers is only 1% to 3%, whereas it is 4% to 6% for the offspring of diabetic fathers (because type 1 diabetes affects males and females in roughly equal proportions in the general population, this risk difference is inconsistent with the sex-specific threshold model for multifactorial traits). Twin studies show that the empirical risks for identical twins of people with type 1 diabetes range from 30% to 50%. In contrast, the concordance rates for dizygotic twins are 5% to 10%. The fact that type 1 diabetes is not 100% concordant among identical twins indicates that genetic factors are not solely responsible for the disorder. There is good evidence that specific viral infections contribute to the causation of type 1 diabetes in at least some individuals, possibly by activating an autoimmune response.

The association of specific HLA class II alleles (see Chapter 21) and type 1 diabetes has been studied extensively, and it is estimated that the HLA system accounts for about 40% of the familial clustering of type 1 diabetes. Approximately 95% of whites with type 1 diabetes have the HLA DR3 and/or DR4 alleles, whereas only about 50% of the general white population has either of these alleles. If an affected proband and a sibling are heterozygous for the DR3 and DR4 alleles, the sibling's risk of developing type 1 diabetes is nearly 20% (i.e., about 40 times higher than the risk in the general population). In addition, the presence of aspartic acid at position 57 of the DQ chain is strongly associated with resistance to type 1 diabetes. In fact, those who do not have this amino acid at position 57 (and instead are homozygous for a different amino acid) are 100 times more likely to develop type 1 diabetes. The aspartic acid substitution alters the shape of the HLA class II molecule and thus its ability to bind and present peptides to T cells. Altered T-cell recognition may help protect individuals with the aspartic acid substitution from an autoimmune episode.

The insulin gene, which is located on the short arm of chromosome 11, is another logical candidate for type 1 diabetes susceptibility. Polymorphisms within and near this gene have been tested for association with type 1 diabetes. It is estimated that inherited genetic variation in the insulin region accounts for approximately 10% of the familial clustering of type 1 diabetes.

Within the past several years, additional genes have been shown to be associated with susceptibility to type 1 diabetes. The most significant of these are cytotoxic lymphocyte associated-4 (CTLA4), which encodes a protein involved in the regulation of T-cell proliferation, and PTPN22, which encodes a lymphoid specific tyrosine phosphatase that negatively regulates T-cell activation. It is interesting that variation in the latter gene has been associated with several other autoimmune diseases, including systemic lupus erythematosus (SLE), rheumatoid arthritis, and autoimmune thyroid disease.

Type 2 Diabetes

Type 2 diabetes accounts for more than 90% of all diabetes cases and affects 10% to 20% of the adult populations of many developed countries. A number of features distinguish it from type 1 diabetes. There is nearly always some endogenous insulin production in people with type 2 diabetes, and the disease can often be treated successfully with dietary modification and/or oral drugs. People with type 2 diabetes suffer from insulin resistance (i.e., their cells have difficulty in using insulin). This disease typically occurs among people older than age 40 and, in contrast to type 1 diabetes, is seen more commonly among the obese. The incidence of type 2 diabetes is rising dramatically among adolescents and young adults in developed countries, however, and is strongly correlated with an increased incidence of obesity. Neither HLA associations nor autoantibodies are seen commonly in this form of diabetes. Monozygotic twin concordance rates are substantially higher than in type 1 diabetes, often exceeding 90% (because of age dependence, the concordance rate increases if older subjects are studied). The empirical recurrence risks for first-degree relatives of type 2 diabetes cases are higher than those for type 1, generally ranging from 10% to 15%. The differences between type 1 and type 2 diabetes are summarized in Table 5-7.

Table 5-7	Comparison of Major Features of Types 1 and 2 Diabetes Mellitus	
Feature	Type 1 Diabetes	Type 2 Diabetes
Age of onset	Usually <40 yr	Usually >40 yr (except maturity-onset diabetes of the young [MODY])
Insulin production	None	Partial
Insulin resistance	No	Yes
Autoimmunity	Yes	No
Obesity	Not common	Common
Monozygotic (MZ) twin concordance	0.55	0.90
Sibling recurrence risk	1%-6%	10%-15%

A significant association has been observed between type 2 diabetes and a common allele of the gene that encodes peroxisome proliferator–activated receptor-γ (PPAR-γ), a transcription factor that is involved in adipocyte differentiation and glucose metabolism. Although this allele confers only a 25% increase in the risk of developing type 2 diabetes, it is found in more than 75% of individuals of European descent. Thus it may help account for a significant proportion of type 2 diabetes cases. Other genes that are significantly associated with type 2 diabetes susceptibility are TCF7L2, which encodes a transcription factor associated with blood glucose homeostasis, and KCNJ11, which encodes a potassium channel that is essential for the regulation of insulin secretion by pancreatic beta cells.

The two most important risk factors for type 2 diabetes are positive family history and obesity; the latter increases insulin resistance. The disease tends to rise in prevalence when populations adopt a diet and exercise pattern typical of U.S. and European populations. Increases have been seen, for example, among Japanese immigrants to the United States and among some native populations of the South Pacific, Australia, and the Americas. Several studies, conducted on male and female subjects, have shown that regular exercise can substantially lower one's risk of developing type 2 diabetes, even among individuals with a family history of the disease. This is partly because exercise reduces obesity. However, even in the absence of weight loss, exercise increases insulin sensitivity and improves glucose tolerance.

Because of the dramatic increase in obesity in the United States and other developed countries, the prevalence of type 2 diabetes is also rising rapidly, and the average age of onset is decreasing. A small proportion of type 2 diabetes cases occurs early in life, typically before 25 years of age, and typically exhibits autosomal dominant inheritance (unlike most type 2 diabetes). This subset is termed maturity-onset diabetes of the young (MODY). Studies of MODY pedigrees have shown that about half of cases of the disease are caused by mutations in the glucokinase gene. Glucokinase converts glucose to glucose-6-phosphate in the pancreas. In addition to the glucokinase gene, five other genes, all of which are involved in pancreatic development or insulin regulation, have now been shown to be causes of MODY.

Obesity

Obesity is most commonly defined as a body mass index (BMI) greater than 30.* Using this criterion, a survey published in 2006 showed that approximately 32% of American adults are obese, and an additional 35% are overweight (BMI greater than 25 but less than 30). The proportion of obese adults and children continues to increase rapidly. Although obesity itself is not a "disease," it is an important risk factor for several common diseases, including heart disease, stroke, hypertension, and type 2 diabetes.

As one might expect, there is a strong correlation between obesity in parents and their children. This could easily be ascribed to common environmental effects: parents and children usually share similar dietary and exercise habits. However, there is good evidence for genetic components as well. Four adoption studies each showed that the body weights of adopted individuals correlated significantly with their natural parents' body weights but not with those of their adoptive parents. Twin studies also provide evidence for a genetic effect on body weight, with most studies yielding heritability estimates between 0.60 and 0.80.

Research, aided substantially by mouse models, has shown that several genes each play a role in human obesity. Important among these are the genes that encode leptin (Greek, "thin") and its receptor. The leptin hormone is secreted by adipocytes (fat storage cells) and binds to receptors in the hypothalamus, the site of the body's appetite control center. Cloning of the human leptin gene and its receptor led to optimistic predictions that leptin could be a key to weight loss in humans (without the perceived unpleasantness of dieting and exercise). Although mutations in the human leptin gene and its receptor have been identified in a few humans with severe obesity (BMI >40), they both appear to be extremely rare. Clinical trials using recombinant leptin have demonstrated moderate weight loss in a subset of obese individuals. In addition, leptin participates in important interactions with other components of appetite control, such as neuropeptide Y and α–melanocyte-stimulating hormone and its receptor, the melanocortin-4 receptor (MC4R). Mutations in the gene that encodes MCR4 have been found in 3% to 5% of severely obese individuals. Recently, homozygosity for a DNA variant in the *FTO* gene (which is seen in 16% of whites) has been associated with 40% and 70% increases in the risks of overweight and obesity, respectively. Identification of these human genes is leading to a better understanding of natural weight control in the human, and it could eventually lead to effective treatments for some cases of obesity.

Alzheimer Disease

Alzheimer disease (AD), which is responsible for 60% to 70% of cases of progressive cognitive impairment among older adults, affects approximately 5% to 10% of the population older than 65 years of age and 40% of the population older than 85 years of age. Because of the aging of the population, the number of Americans with AD is predicted to increase substantially during the coming decade. AD is characterized by progressive dementia and memory loss and by the formation of amyloid plaques and neurofibrillary tangles in the brain, particularly in the cerebral cortex and hippocampus. The plaques and tangles lead to progressive neuronal loss, and death usually occurs within 7 to 10 years after the first appearance of symptoms.

The risk of developing AD doubles in individuals who have an affected first-degree relative. Although most cases do not appear to be caused by single loci, approximately 10% follow an autosomal dominant mode of transmission. About 3% to 5% of AD cases occur before age 65 and are considered early onset; these are much more likely to be inherited in autosomal dominant fashion.[22]

AD is a genetically heterogeneous disorder. Approximately half of early-onset cases can be attributed to mutations in any of three genes, all of which affect amyloid-β deposition.[23] Two of the genes, presenilin 1 *(PS1)* and presenilin 2 *(PS2),* are very similar to one another, and their protein products are involved in cleavage of the amyloid-β precursor protein (APP). When APP is not cleaved normally, a long form of it accumulates excessively and is deposited in the brain. This is thought to be a primary cause of AD. Mutations in *PS1* typically result in especially early onset of AD, with the first occurrence of symptoms in the fifth decade of life.

A small number of cases of early-onset AD are caused by mutations of the gene that encodes APP itself, which is located on chromosome 21. These mutations disrupt normal cleavage sites in APP, again leading to the accumulation of the longer protein product. It is interesting that this gene is present in three copies in trisomy 21 individuals, in which the extra gene copy leads to amyloid deposition and the occurrence of AD in those with Down syndrome (see Chapter 4).

An important risk factor for the more common late-onset form of AD is allelic variation in the apolipoprotein E *(APOE)* locus, which has three major alleles: *ε2, ε3,* and *ε4.* Studies conducted in diverse populations have shown that persons who have one copy of the *ε4* allele are at least 2 to 5 times more likely to develop AD, whereas those with two copies of this allele are at least 5 to 10 times more likely to develop AD. The risk varies somewhat by population, with higher *ε4*-associated risks in Europeans and Japanese and relatively lower risks in Hispanics and blacks. Despite the strong association between *ε4* and AD, approximately half of individuals who develop late-onset AD do not have a copy of the *ε4* allele, and many who are homozygous for *ε4* remain free of AD even at

---

*BMI is defined as W/H², in which W is weight in kilograms and H is height in meters.

advanced age. The apolipoprotein E protein product is not involved in cleavage of APP but instead appears to be associated with clearance of amyloid from the brain.

Alcoholism

At some point, alcoholism is diagnosed in approximately 10% of adult males and 3% to 5% of adult females in the United States. The national cost of alcoholism, in terms of lost productivity and direct medical costs, is approximately $200 billion per year. More than 100 studies have shown that this disease clusters in families.[24] The risk of developing alcoholism among individuals with one affected parent is three to five times higher than for those with unaffected parents.

Most twin studies have yielded concordance rates for DZ twins less than 30% and concordance rates for MZ twins in excess of 60%. Adoption studies have shown that the offspring of an alcoholic parent, even when raised by nonalcoholic parents, have a fourfold increased risk of developing the disorder. To control for possible prenatal effects in an alcoholic mother, some studies have included only the offspring of alcoholic fathers. The results have remained the same. One study showed that the offspring of nonalcoholic parents, when reared by alcoholics, did *not* have an increased risk of developing alcoholism. These data argue that there may be genes that predispose some people to alcoholism.

It has long been known that an individual's physiologic response to alcohol can be influenced by variation in the key enzymes responsible for alcohol metabolism (alcohol dehydrogenases [ADH]), which convert ethanol to acetaldehyde, and aldehyde dehydrogenases (ALDH), which convert acetaldehyde to acetate. In particular, an allele of the *ALDH2* gene *(ALDH2*2)* results in excessive accumulation of acetaldehyde and thus in facial flushing, nausea, palpitations, and lightheadedness. Because of these unpleasant effects, individuals who have the *ALDH2*2* allele are much less likely to become alcoholics. This "protective" allele is common in some Asian populations but is rare in other populations.

More recently genetic studies have implicated genes that encode gamma-aminobutyric acid (GABA) receptors. Because GABA is the brain's primary inhibitory neurotransmitter, GABA receptor genes are important potential contributors to a genetic susceptibility to alcoholism.

It should be underscored that genes may increase one's *susceptibility* to alcoholism. Obviously this is a disease that requires an environmental component, regardless of genetic constitution.

Psychiatric Disorders

The major psychiatric diseases, schizophrenia and affective disorder, have been the subjects of numerous genetic studies.[25] Twin, adoption, and family studies have shown that both disorders aggregate in families.

Schizophrenia

Schizophrenia is a severe emotional disorder characterized by delusions, hallucinations, retreat from reality, and bizarre, withdrawn, or inappropriate behavior. (Contrary to popular

Table 5-8	Recurrence Risks for Relatives of Schizophrenic Probands*
Relationship to Proband	Recurrence Risk (%)
Monozygotic twin	44.3
Dizygotic twin	12.1
Offspring	9.4
Sibling	7.3
Niece/nephew	2.7
Grandchild	2.8
First cousin	1.6
Spouse	1

*Figures are based on multiple studies of Western European populations.
Data from McGue M, Gottesman II, Rao DC: *Behav Genet* 16(1):75-87, 1986.

belief, schizophrenia is not a "split personality" disorder.) The lifetime recurrence risk for schizophrenia among the offspring of one affected parent is approximately 8% to 10%, which is about 10 times higher than the risk in the general population.[26] As one might expect, the empirical risks increase when more relatives are affected. For example, an individual with an affected sibling and an affected parent has a risk of about 17%, and an individual with two affected parents has a risk of 46%. The risks decrease when the affected family member is a second- or third-degree relative. Details are given in Table 5-8. On inspection of Table 5-8, it may seem puzzling that the proportion of schizophrenic probands who have a schizophrenic parent is only about 5%, which is substantially lower than the risk for other first-degree relatives (e.g., siblings, affected parents, their offspring). This can be explained by the fact that people with schizophrenia are less likely to marry and produce children than are other individuals. Thus substantial selection against schizophrenia occurs in the population.

Twin and adoption studies also indicate that genetic factors are likely to be involved in schizophrenia. Data pooled from five different twin studies show a 47% concordance rate for MZ twins, compared with a concordance rate of only 12% for DZ twins. When the offspring of a schizophrenic parent are adopted by normal parents, their risk of developing the disease is about 10%, which is approximately the same as the risk when raised by a schizophrenic biologic parent. Although no schizophrenia gene has yet been conclusively identified, promising associations have been uncovered between schizophrenia and several brain-expressed genes whose products interact with glutamate receptors. These include dysbindin 1 (chromosome 6p), neuregulin 1 (chromosome 8p), and G72 (chromosome 13q). Each of these associations has been identified in specific populations, and further studies in other populations will be needed to replicate these findings.

Bipolar Affective Disorder

Bipolar affective disorder, also known as *manic-depressive disorder,* is a form of psychosis with extreme mood swings and emotional instability. The incidence of the disorder in the general population is approximately 0.5%, but it rises to

5% to 10% among those with an affected first-degree relative. A study using the Danish twin registry yielded concordance rates of 79% and 24% for MZ and DZ twins, respectively.[27] The corresponding concordance rates for unipolar disorder (major depression) were 54% and 19%. In general, it appears that bipolar disorder is more strongly influenced by genetic factors than is unipolar disorder.

Comments on Psychiatric Disorders

Large-scale linkage studies involving hundreds of polymorphisms throughout the genome have been carried out for both schizophrenia and bipolar affective disorder. Most of these studies have produced negative results, although a few recent large-scale studies have yielded promising findings. A number of candidate genes have been tested for linkage or association with both diseases. Most of these candidates were chosen on the basis of the known involvement of certain neurotransmitters, receptors, or neurotransmitter-related enzymes in each disease (e.g., schizophrenia can be treated by drugs that block dopamine receptors, and bipolar affective disorder is sometimes treated with lithium). None of the candidate genes tested thus far, including those for sodium-lithium countertransport, various components of the dopaminergic system, and several neurotransmitter-related enzymes (e.g., monoamine oxidase, dopamine-β-hydroxylase, tyrosine hydroxylase), has been shown unequivocally to be linked or associated with either disease.

These results reflect some of the difficulties encountered in doing genetic studies of psychiatric disorders. These disorders are undoubtedly heterogeneous, reflecting the influence of numerous genetic and environmental factors. Also, definition of the phenotype is not always straightforward and it may change through time, significantly complicating genetic analysis.

Other Complex Disorders

The disorders discussed in this chapter represent some of the most common multifactorial disorders and those for which significant progress has been made in identifying genes. Many other multifactorial disorders are being studied as well, and in some cases specific susceptibility genes have been identified. These include, for example, Parkinson disease, hearing loss, multiple sclerosis, amyotrophic lateral sclerosis, epilepsy, asthma, inflammatory bowel disease, and some forms of blindness.

Some General Principles and Conclusions

Some general principles can be deduced from the results obtained thus far on the genetics of complex disorders. First, the more strongly inherited forms of complex disorders generally have an earlier age of onset (e.g., breast cancer, AD, heart disease). Often these represent subsets of cases in which there is single-gene inheritance. Second, when laterality is a component, the bilateral forms are more likely to cluster strongly in families (e.g., breast cancer, CL/P). Third, although the sex-specific threshold model fits some of the complex disorders (e.g., pyloric stenosis, CL/P, autism, heart disease), it fails to fit others (e.g., type 1 diabetes).

A tendency exists, particularly among the lay public, to assume that the presence of a genetic component means that the course of a disease cannot be altered. *This is incorrect.* Most of the diseases discussed in this chapter have both genetic and environmental components. Thus lifestyle modification (e.g., diet, exercise, stress reduction) often can reduce risk significantly. Such modification may be especially important for individuals with a family history of a disease because they are likely to develop the disease earlier in life. Those with a family history of heart disease, for example, can often add many years of productive living with relatively minor lifestyle alterations. By targeting those who can benefit most from intervention, genetics helps to serve the goal of preventive medicine.

In addition, it should be stressed that the identification of a specific genetic lesion can lead to more effective prevention and treatment of the disease. Identification of mutations that cause autosomal dominant breast cancer may enable early screening and prevention of metastasis. Pinpointing a gene responsible for a neurotransmitter defect in a behavioral disorder such as schizophrenia could lead to the development of more effective drug treatments. In some cases, such as those with familial hypercholesterolemia, gene therapy may prove to be useful in treating the disease. It is important for healthcare practitioners to help individuals understand these facts.

Although the genetics of common disorders is complex and often confusing, the community health effect of these diseases, together with the evidence for hereditary factors in their etiology, demands that genetic studies be pursued. Substantial progress is already being made. The next decade will undoubtedly witness many further advances in the understanding and treatment of these disorders.

SUMMARY REVIEW

Factors Influencing Incidence of Disease in Populations

1. The incidence rate is the number of new cases of a disease reported during a specific period (typically 1 year) divided by the number of individuals in the population.
2. The prevalence rate is the proportion of the population affected by a disease at a specific point in time. This rate, and the incidence rate, can be used to compare population variations in disease frequency.
3. Relative risk is a common measure of the effect of a specific risk factor. It is expressed as a ratio of the incidence rate of the disease among individuals exposed to a risk factor divided by the incidence of the disease among individuals *not* exposed to a risk factor.
4. Many factors can influence the risk of acquiring a common disease, such as cancer, diabetes, or hypertension. The factors can include age, gender, diet, exercise, and family history of the disease.

Principles of Multifactorial Inheritance

1. Traits in which variation is thought to be caused by the combined effects of multiple genes are polygenic.
2. The term *multifactorial* is used when environmental factors also are believed to cause variation in the trait.
3. Many quantitative traits (e.g., blood pressure) are multifactorial.
4. Because traits are caused by the additive effects of many genetic and environmental factors, they tend to follow a normal or bell-shaped distribution in populations.
5. Those diseases, however, that do not follow a bell-shaped distribution appear to be either present or absent in individuals. They do not follow the inheritance patterns of single-gene disease. Instead, such diseases may follow an underlying liability distribution. It is thought that a threshold of liability must be crossed before the disease is expressed.
6. Examples of diseases that correspond to the liability model include pyloric stenosis, neural tube defects, CL/P, and some forms of congenital heart disease.
7. Many of the common adult diseases, such as hypertension, coronary heart disease, stroke, diabetes mellitus (types 1 and 2), and some cancers, are caused by complex genetic and environmental factors and are thus multifactorial diseases.
8. For most multifactorial diseases, empirical risks (risks based on direct observation of data) have been derived.
9. In contrast to most single-gene diseases, recurrence risks for multifactorial diseases can change significantly from one population to another because gene frequencies, as well as environmental factors, can differ among populations.

10. Several criteria are used to define multifactorial inheritance: (a) the recurrence risk becomes higher if more than one family member is affected; (b) if the expression of the disease in a proband is more severe, the recurrence risk is higher; (c) the recurrence risk is higher if the proband is of the less commonly affected sex; (d) the recurrence risk for the disease usually decreases rapidly in more remotely related relatives; and (e) if the prevalence of the disease in a population is f, the risk for offspring and siblings of probands is approximately $\sqrt{f}$.

Nature and Nurture: Disentangling the Effects of Genes and Environment

1. Family members share genes and a common environment; therefore, resemblance in traits, such as high blood pressure, reflects both genetic and environmental factors (nature and nurture, respectively).
2. Few traits are influenced *only* by genes or *only* by environment. Most are influenced by both.
3. When a disease has a relatively larger genetic component, as in breast cancer, examination of family history should be emphasized in addition to lifestyle modification.
4. Two research strategies often are used to estimate the relative influence of genes and environment-lifestyle: twin studies and adoption studies.
5. Monozygotic twins originate when the developing embryo divides to form two separate but identical embryos.
6. Dizygotic twins are the result of a double ovulation followed by the fertilization of each egg by a different sperm.
7. If both members of a twin pair share a trait, they are said to be *concordant*. If they do not share the same trait, they are *discordant*.
8. Studies of adopted children also are used to estimate the genetic contribution to a multifactorial trait.
9. A genetic predisposition may interact with an environmental-lifestyle factor to increase the risk of disease; this is called a *gene-environment interaction*.

Genetics of Common Diseases

1. Congenital diseases are those present at birth. Most of these diseases are multifactorial in etiology.
2. Multifactorial diseases in adults include coronary heart disease, hypertension, breast cancer, colon cancer, diabetes mellitus, obesity, AD, alcoholism, schizophrenia, and bipolar affective disorder.
3. It is incorrect to assume that the presence of a genetic component means that the course of a disease cannot be altered—most diseases have *both* genetic and environmental aspects.

KEY TERMS

Concordant trait, 170
Congenital disease, 172
Discordant trait, 170
Dizygotic (DZ, fraternal) twin, 170
Empirical risk, 167
Gene-environment interaction, 171

Incidence rate, 164
Liability distribution, 166
Monozygotic (MZ, identical) twin, 170
Multifactorial trait, 165
Phocomelia, 172
Polygenic, 165

Prevalence rate, 164
Quantitative trait, 165
Relative risk, 165
Threshold of liability, 166

REFERENCES

1. King RA, Rotter JI, Motulsky AG: *The genetic basis of common diseases,* ed 2, Oxford, 2002, Oxford University Press.
2. Rothman KJ: *Modern epidemiology,* New York, 1998, Lippincott.
3. Tiwari HK et al: Multifactorial inheritance and complex diseases. In Rimoin DL et al, editors: *Emery and Rimoin's principles and practice of medical genetics,* ed 5, Philadelphia, 2007, Churchill Livingstone, pp 299-306.
4. Kibar Z, Capra V, Gros P: Toward understanding the genetic basis of neural tube defects, *Clin Genet* 71(4):295-310, 2007.
5. Daly LE, et al: Folate levels and neural tube defects: implications for prevention, *JAMA* 274(21):1698-1702, 1995.
6. Harper PS: *Practical genetic counseling,* ed 5, Oxford, 1998, Butterworth Heinemann.
7. Boomsma D, Busjahn A, Peltonen L: Classical twin studies and beyond. *Nat Rev Genet* 3(11):872-882, 2002.
8. Neale MC, Cardon LR: *Methodology for genetic studies of twins and families,* Dordrecht, The Netherlands, 1992, Kluwer.
9. Marks D et al: A review on the diagnosis, natural history, and treatment of familial hypercholesterolaemia, *Atherosclerosis* 168(1):1-14, 2003.
10. Jansen AC, et al: Phenotypic variability in familial hypercholesterolaemia: an update, *Curr Opin Lipidol* 13(2):165-171, 2002.
11. Hunt SC, Williams RR, Barlow GK: A comparison of positive family history definitions for defining risk of future disease, *J Chron Dis* 39(10):809-821, 1986.
12. Lusis AJ, Mar R, Pajukanta P: Genetics of atherosclerosis, *Annu Rev Genomics Hum Genet* 5(1):189-218, 2004.
13. Jeunemaitre X, et al: Molecular basis of human hypertension. In Rimoin DL et al, editors: *Emery and Rimoin's principles and practice of medical genetics,* ed 5, Philadelphia, 2007, Churchill Livingstone, pp 1283-1300.
14. Vogelstein B, Kinzler KW: *The genetic basis of human cancer,* ed 2, New York, 2002, McGraw-Hill.
15. Peto J: Cancer epidemiology in the last century and the next decade, *Nature* 411(6835):390-395, 2001.
16. Robson M, Offit K: Management of an inherited predisposition to breast cancer, *N Engl J Med* 357(2):154-162, 2007.
17. American Cancer Society: Cancer statistics, website: www.cancer.org/docroot/STT/stt_0.asp.
18. Galiatsatos P, Foulkes WD: Familial adenomatous polyposis, *Am J Gastroenterol* 101(2):385-398, 2006.
19. Rowley PT: Inherited susceptibility to colorectal cancer, *Annu Rev Med* 56:539-554, 2005.
20. Owen KR, McCarthy MI: Genetics of type 2 diabetes, *Curr Opin Genet Dev* 17(3):239-244, 2007.
21. Daneman D: Type 1 diabetes, *Lancet* 367(9513):847-858, 2006.
22. Bird TD: Genetic factors in Alzheimer's disease, *N Engl J Med* 352(9):862-864, 2005.
23. Blennow K, de Leon MJ, Zetterberg H: Alzheimer's disease, *Lancet* 368(9533):387-403, 2006.
24. Edenberg HJ, Foroud T: The genetics of alcoholism: identifying specific genes through family studies, *Addict Biol* 11(3-4):386-396, 2006.
25. Farmer A, Elkin A, McGuffin P: The genetics of bipolar affective disorder, *Curr Opin Psychiatry* 20(1):8-12, 2007.
26. Norton N, Williams HJ, Owen MJ: An update on the genetics of schizophrenia, *Curr Opin Psychiatry* 19(2):158-164, 2006.
27. Bertelsen A, Harvald B, Hauge M: A Danish twin study of manic-depressive disorders, *Br J Psychiatry* 130:330-351, 1977.

INNATE IMMUNITY: INFLAMMATION

NEAL S. ROTE • SUE E. HUETHER

MEDIA RESOURCES

 Evolve Website (http://evolve.elsevier.com/McCance/)
- Review Questions and Answers
- Animations
- Glossary (with audio pronunciation for selected terms)
- WebLinks

Online Course
- Module 4

CHAPTER OUTLINE

HUMAN DEFENSE MECHANISMS
FIRST LINE OF DEFENSE: PHYSICAL, MECHANICAL, AND BIOCHEMICAL BARRIERS
  Physical and Mechanical Barriers
  Biochemical Barriers
SECOND LINE OF DEFENSE: THE INFLAMMATORY RESPONSE
  Vascular Response
  Plasma Protein Systems
  Cellular Mediators of Inflammation
  Cellular Products
LOCAL MANIFESTATIONS OF INFLAMMATION

SYSTEMIC MANIFESTATIONS OF ACUTE INFLAMMATION
  Fever
  Leukocytosis
  Plasma Protein Synthesis
CHRONIC INFLAMMATION
RESOLUTION AND REPAIR
  Reconstructive Phase
  Maturation Phase
  Dysfunctional Wound Healing
    Pediatrics and Mechanisms of Self-Defense
    Aging and Mechanisms of Self-Defense

People are exposed daily to an environment containing a large variety of toxic substances and potentially infectious and disease-causing microorganisms. Without an efficient system of protection most individuals would succumb to these hazards early in life. That system consists of multiple complementary and interdependent layers. An outer layer of specialized epithelium, including the skin and mucosal surfaces, is relatively resistant to most environmental hazards and resists infection with disease-causing microorganisms.[1] If the epithelial barrier is damaged, a highly efficient local and systemic response **(inflammation)** is mobilized to limit the extent of damage, protect against infection, and initiate repair of the damaged tissue. The natural epithelial barrier and inflammation confer innate resistance and protection, commonly referred to as **innate, native,** or **natural immunity.** Inflammation associated with infection usually initiates an adaptive process that results in a long-term and very effective immunity to the infecting microorganism, referred to as **adaptive, acquired,** or *specific immunity.* Adaptive immunity is relatively slow to develop but has memory and more rapidly targets and eradicates a second infection with a particular disease-causing microorganism.

The information presented in this chapter introduces the components and processes of innate immunity and sets the stage for Chapter 7, which discusses adaptive immunity. Although inflammation and acquired immunity provide protection, either genetic or acquired aberrations in these processes can lead to disease. Diminution of innate or acquired immunity may lead to critically decreased resistance to infection. Excessive inflammation or acquired immunity may lead to damage to normal tissue or organs. Both may result in severe and potentially fatal disease, examples of which are discussed in Chapter 8. Many microorganisms that cause disease have developed methods of bypassing our protective systems. These are discussed in Chapter 9. Each chapter is designed to render an overview and is not intended to be all-inclusive. Protective mechanisms consist of a very large number of soluble factors and cells and would require many more pages to discuss in adequate detail. Different classes or groups of molecules and cells will be discussed, but only a few examples will be described in detail. Some components directly participate in the protective response, whereas others are designed to limit the extent of the response.

HUMAN DEFENSE MECHANISMS

Innate immunity includes two lines of defense: natural barriers and inflammation (Table 6-1). **Natural barriers** are physical, mechanical, and biochemical barriers at the body's surfaces and are in place at birth to prevent damage by substances in the environment and thwart infection by pathogenic microorganisms. If the surface barriers are breached, the second line of defense, the **inflammatory response,** is activated to protect the body from further injury, prevent infection of the injured tissue, and promote healing. The inflammatory response is a rapid activation of biochemical and cellular processes that is relatively nonspecific, with similar responses being initiated against a wide variety of causes of tissue damage.

FIRST LINE OF DEFENSE: PHYSICAL, MECHANICAL, AND BIOCHEMICAL BARRIERS

Physical and Mechanical Barriers

The physical barriers that protect against damage and infection are composed of tightly associated epithelial cells including those of the skin and of the membranous sheets lining the gastrointestinal, genitourinary, and respiratory tracts (Figure 6-1).[2] The mucosal epithelial cells are highly interconnected

junctions that prohibit the passage of microorganisms. The normal turnover of the cells in these sites as well as mechanisms for "washing" the surfaces may mechanically remove many infectious microorganisms and prevent their residence on the epithelial surfaces. For instance, the routine sloughing off and replacement of dead skin cells also removes adherent bacteria. Mechanical cleansing of the surfaces includes vomiting and urination. Goblet cells of the upper respiratory tract produce mucus that coats the epithelial surface and traps microorganisms that are removed by hairlike cilia that mechanically move the mucus upward to be expelled by coughing or sneezing. Additionally, the low temperature on the skin generally inhibits microorganisms, most of which prefer temperatures near 37° C for more efficient growth.

Biochemical Barriers

Epithelial surfaces also provide biochemical barriers by synthesizing and secreting substances meant to trap or destroy microorganisms. Mucus, perspiration (or sweat), saliva, tears, and earwax are all examples of biochemical secretions that can trap potential disease-causing microorganisms and contain substances that will kill the microorganisms. Sebaceous glands in the skin also secrete antibacterial and antifungal fatty acids and lactic acid. Perspiration, tears, and saliva contain an enzyme (lysozyme) that attacks the cell walls of gram-positive bacteria. These glandular secretions result in an acidic skin surface (pH 3 to 5), making it an inhospitable environment for most bacteria.

Table 6-1	Overview of Human Defenses		
	Innate Immunity		
Characteristics	**Barriers**	**Inflammatory Response**	**Adaptive (Acquired) Immunity**
Level of defense	First line of defense against infection and tissue injury	Second line of defense; occurs as a response to tissue injury or infection	Third line of defense; initiated when innate immune system signals the cells of adaptive immunity
Timing of defense	Constant	Immediate response	Delay between primary exposure to antigen and maximum response; immediate against secondary exposure to antigen
Specificity	Broadly specific	Broadly specific	Response is very specific toward "antigen"
Cells	Epithelial cells	Mast cells, granulocytes (neutrophils, eosinophils, basophils), monocytes/macrophages, natural killer (NK) cells, platelets, endothelial cells	T lymphocytes, B lymphocytes, macrophages, dendritic cells
Memory	No memory involved	No memory involved	Specific immunologic memory by T and B lymphocytes
Peptides	Defensins, cathelicidins, collectins, lactoferrin, bacterial toxins	Complement, clotting factors, kinins	Antibodies, complement
Protection	Protection includes anatomic barriers (i.e., skin and mucous membranes), cells and secretory molecules or cytokines (e.g., lysozymes, low pH of stomach and urine) and ciliary activity	Protection includes vascular responses, cellular components (e.g., mast cells, neutrophils, macrophages), secretory molecules or cytokines, and activation of plasma protein systems	Protection includes activated T and B lymphocytes, cytokines, and antibodies

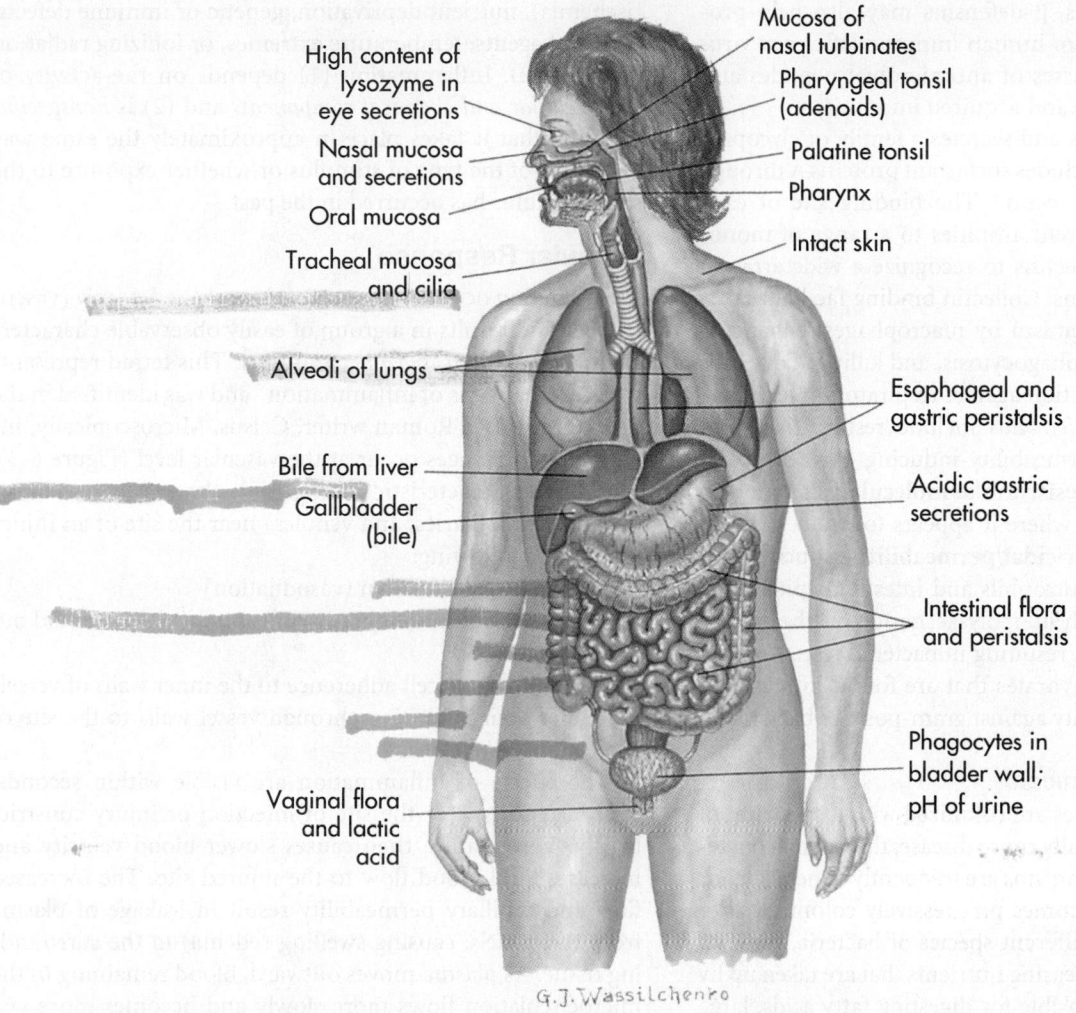

Figure 6-1 The closed barrier. The digestive, respiratory, and genitourinary tracts and skin form closed barriers between the internal organs and the environment. (From Grimes DE: *Infectious diseases*, St Louis, 1991, Mosby.)

In addition, the body has a complex array of proteins that function to destroy pathogens before they can colonize a human host. Some of these proteins function on the surface of the same epithelial sheets that provide the physical barrier. Others, however, are meant to defeat microorganisms that have already crossed the physical barrier.

Epithelial-Derived Chemicals

Epithelial cells secrete small-molecular-weight **antimicrobial peptides.** These are generally positively charged polypeptides of approximately 15 to 95 amino acids and can be divided into two classes—cathelicidins and defensins—based on their three-dimensional structures. Both classes are in very high local concentrations and are toxic to several bacteria, fungi, and viruses.[3-5] **Cathelicidins** have a linear α-helical shape, and only one is currently known to function in humans. In contrast, about 50 different defensins have been identified thus far. All are triple-stranded β-sheet structures. **Defensin** molecules contain three intrachain disulfide bonds and can be further subdivided into α (at least 6 identified in humans)

and β types (at least 10 identified, but perhaps up to 40 different molecules), depending on how the cysteine residues are connected during formation of the disulfide linkages. The α-defensins often require activation by proteolytic enzymes, whereas the β-defensins are synthesized in active forms. Bacteria have cholesterol-free cell membranes, which may allow cathelicidins to insert into and disrupt their membranes. Given the similarity in their chemical charges, defensins may kill bacteria in the same way. These same chemicals also may contribute to other means of protection because they are also produced by monocytes, macrophages, and neutrophils, which are components of the inflammatory response. Cathelicidin is stored in neutrophils, mast cells, and a variety of epithelial cells. The α-defensins are particularly rich in the granules of neutrophils and may contribute to the killing of bacteria by those cells. They are also found in Paneth cells lining the small intestine, where they protect against a variety of disease-causing microorganisms. The β-defensins are found in a variety of epithelial cells lining the respiratory, urinary, and intestinal tracts, as well as in the skin. In addition to antibacterial properties, β-defensins may also help protect epithelial surfaces from human immunodeficiency virus (HIV) infection. Both classes of antimicrobial peptides also can activate cells of innate and acquired immunity.

The lung also produces and secretes a family of glycoproteins, **collectins,** which includes surfactant proteins A through D and mannose-binding lectin.[6] The binding site of each collectin reacts with different affinities to a range of monosaccharides, enabling collectins to recognize a wide array of pathogenic microorganisms. Collectin binding facilitates recognition of the microorganism by macrophages, enhancing macrophage attachment, phagocytosis, and killing. Collectins play a major role in protection against respiratory infections.[7]

Other *epithelial antimicrobials* include resistin-like molecule β, bactericidal/permeability-inducing protein, and antimicrobial lectins.[2,8] **Resistin-like molecule β** is found in the intestinal goblet cells, where it appears to protect against helminth infections. **Bactericidal/permeability-inducing protein (BPI)** is stored in neutrophils and intestinal epithelium. BPI specifically reacts with lipopolysaccharide on the surface of gram-negative bacteria, resulting in bacterial lysis. **Antimicrobial lectins** are carbohydrates that are found in intestinal epithelium and have activity against gram-positive bacteria.

Bacteria-Derived Chemicals

Many of the body's surfaces are colonized with a spectrum of bacteria that do not normally cause disease, the **normal bacterial flora.** These microorganisms are frequently beneficial. For instance, the intestine becomes progressively colonized after birth with hundreds of different species of bacteria, some of which help digest food, releasing nutrients that are taken up by the body. They are responsible for digesting fatty acids, large polysaccharides, and other dietary substances, producing vitamin K, and assisting in the absorption of various ions, such as calcium, iron, and magnesium. The normal flora also contributes to our innate protection by producing several chemicals (e.g., ammonia, phenols, indols) that inhibit colonization by disease-causing microorganisms.[9] The normal intestinal flora can be altered by prolonged antibiotic treatment, decreasing its protective activity, and leading to overgrowth of other microorganisms, such as the yeast *Candida albicans* or the bacterium *Clostridium difficile.* The bacterium *Lactobacillus* is a major constituent of the normal vaginal flora in healthy women. This microorganism produces a variety of chemicals (e.g., hydrogen peroxide, lactic acid, bacteriocins) that help prevent infections of the vagina and urinary tract by other bacteria and yeast. Prolonged antibiotic treatment can also diminish colonization with *Lactobacillus* and increase the risk for urologic or vaginal infections, such as toxic shock syndrome.

SECOND LINE OF DEFENSE: THE INFLAMMATORY RESPONSE

If cells and tissues are damaged the **inflammatory response** is usually activated. Injury can have a variety of causes including infection, mechanical damage, oxygen deprivation (ischemia), nutrient deprivation, genetic or immune defects, chemical agents, temperature extremes, or ionizing radiation (Figure 6-2). Inflammation (1) depends on the activity of both *cellular and chemical components* and (2) is *nonspecific,* meaning that it takes place in approximately the same way regardless of the type of stimulus or whether exposure to the same stimulus has occurred in the past.

Vascular Response

Inflammation occurs in tissue that has a blood supply (vascularized) and results in a group of easily observable characteristics: *redness, heat, swelling,* and *pain.* This tetrad represents the "cardinal signs of inflammation" and was identified in the first century by a Roman writer, Celsus. Microscopically, inflammatory changes occur at the vascular level (Figure 6-3). The three characteristic changes in the microcirculation (arterioles, capillaries, and venules) near the site of an injury include the following:

1. Blood vessel dilation (vasodilation)
2. Increased vascular permeability and leakage of fluid out of the vessel
3. White blood cell adherence to the inner walls of vessels and their migration through vessel walls to the site of injury (diapedesis)

The effects of inflammation are visible within seconds. First, arterioles near the site of infection or injury constrict briefly. Vasodilation then causes slower blood velocity and increases local blood flow to the injured site. The increased flow and capillary permeability result in leakage of plasma from the vessels, causing swelling (edema) in the surrounding tissue. As plasma moves outward, blood remaining in the microcirculation flows more slowly and becomes more viscous. The increased blood flow and increasing concentration of red cells at the site of inflammation cause locally increased warmth and redness. Leukocytes adhere to vessel walls. At the same time, biochemical mediators (e.g., histamine, bradykinins, leukotrienes, prostaglandins) stimulate the endothelial cells that line capillaries and venules to retract, creating spaces at junctions between the cells, allowing leukocytes and plasma to enter the surrounding tissue (intercellular junctions are described in Chapter 1).

Each of the characteristic changes associated with inflammation is the direct result of the activities and interactions of a host of chemicals and cellular components found in the blood and tissues. The vascular changes deliver leukocytes, plasma proteins, and other biochemical mediators to the site of injury. Once in the tissues, the cells and chemicals associated with the inflammatory response act in concert to do the following:

1. Prevent infection and further damage by contaminating microorganisms through the influx of fluid to dilute toxins produced by bacteria and released from dying cells, the influx and activation of plasma protein systems that help destroy and contain bacteria (e.g., complement system, clotting system), and the influx of cells (e.g., neutrophils, macrophages) that "eat" and destroy cellular debris and infectious agents.

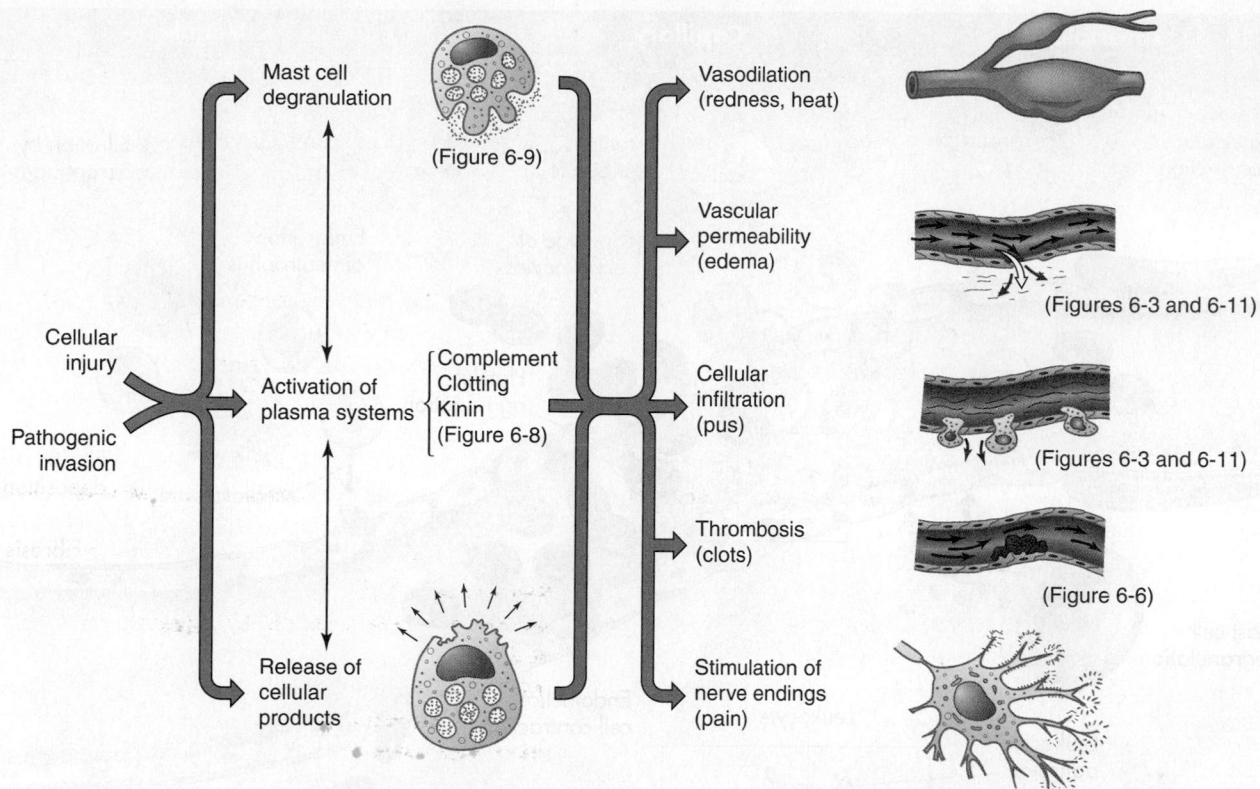

Figure 6-2 **Acute inflammatory response.** Inflammation is usually initiated by cellular injury, which results in mast cell degranulation, the activation of three plasma systems, and the release of subcellular components from the damaged cells. These systems are interdependent, so that induction of one (e.g., mast cell degranulation) can result in activation of the other two. The result is the development of microscopic changes in the inflamed site, as well as characteristic clinical manifestations. The figure numbers refer to those in which more detailed information may be found on that portion of the response.

2. Limit and control the inflammatory process through the influx of plasma protein systems (e.g., clotting system), plasma enzymes, and cells (e.g., eosinophils) that prevent the inflammatory response from spreading to areas of healthy tissue.

3. Interact with components of the adaptive immune system to elicit a more specific response to contaminating pathogen(s) through the influx of macrophages and lymphocytes.[10]

4. Prepare the area of injury for healing through removal of bacterial products, dead cells, and other products of inflammation (e.g., by way of channels through the epithelium or drainage by lymphatic vessels) and initiation of mechanisms of healing and repair.

Fluid and debris that accumulate at an inflamed site are drained by lymphatic vessels. This process also facilitates the development of acquired immunity because microbial antigens in lymphatic fluid pass through the lymph nodes, where they activate both B and T lymphocytes. (This process is discussed in Chapter 7, and the lymphatic system is described in Chapter 25.)

Inflammation and repair can be divided into several phases (Figure 6-4). The characteristics of the early (i.e., acute) inflammatory response differ from those of the later (i.e., chronic) response, and each phase involves different biochemical mediators and cells that function together. The acute inflammatory response is of short duration, that is, it continues only until the immediate threat to the host is eliminated. This usually takes 8 to 10 days from onset to healing. The acute inflammatory response begins immediately after cellular injury or infection occurs (see Figure 6-4) and involves a vascular response, activation of plasma protein systems, and activation of a variety of cells. (Mechanisms of cellular injury are described in Chapter 2.)

Plasma Protein Systems

Three key **plasma protein systems** are essential to an effective inflammatory response. These are the complement system, the clotting system, and the kinin system (see Figures 6-5, 6-6, and 6-7). Although each system has a unique role in inflammation, they also have many similarities. Each system consists of multiple proteins in the blood. To prevent activation in unnecessary situations, each protein is normally in an inactive form. Several of the proteins are enzymes that circulate in inactive forms as **proenzymes.** Each system contains a few proteins that can be activated by products of tissue damage or infection. Activation of the first component of a system results in sequential activation of other components, leading

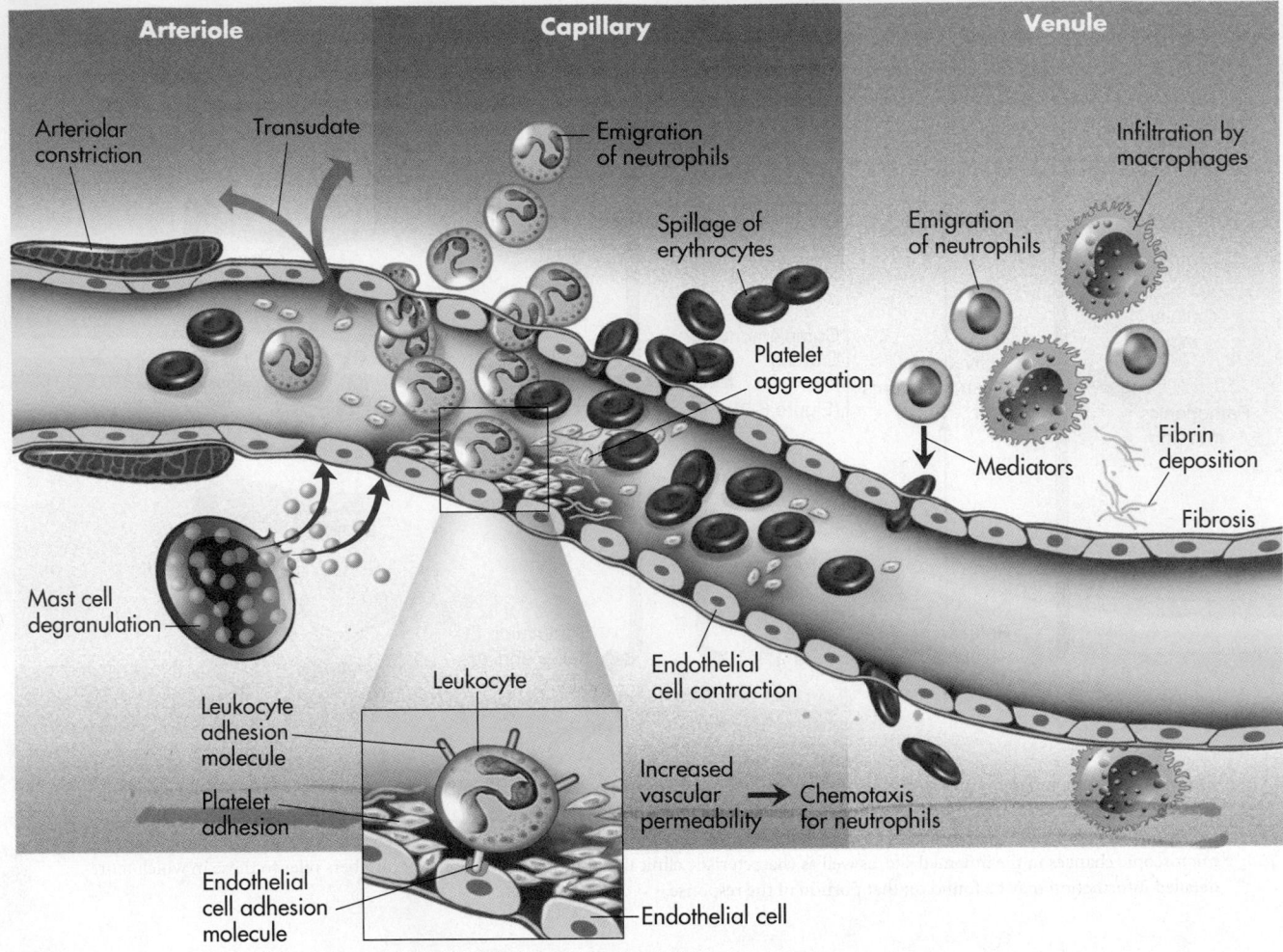

Figure 6-3 Sequence of events in the acute inflammatory response. See text for details.

to a biologic function that helps protect the individual. This sequential activation is referred to as a *cascade*. Thus, we refer to the complement cascade, the clotting cascade, or the kinin cascade. In some cases, activation of a protein may require that it be enzymatically cut into two pieces or fragments of different size. Usually the larger fragment continues the cascade by activating the next component, and the smaller fragment frequently has potent biologic activities to promote inflammation.

Complement System

The complement system consists of several plasma proteins (sometimes called *complement components*) that together constitute about 10% of the total circulating serum protein.[11] The complement system is extremely important because activation of the **complement cascade** may destroy pathogens directly and can activate or collaborate with virtually every other component of the inflammatory response.[12,13] For these reasons, proteins of the complement system are among the body's most potent defenders against bacterial infection.

Activation of the complement system can be accomplished in three different pathways or cascades, all of which converge at the third component (C3) of the pathway:

1. **Classical pathway:** activated by proteins of the acquired immune system (antibodies) bound to their specific targets (antigen)
2. **Lectin pathway:** activated by certain bacterial carbohydrates
3. **Alternative pathway:** activated by gram-negative bacterial and fungal cell wall polysaccharides

The principal routes by which the complement cascade may be activated are shown in Figures 6-5.

Activation of the *classical pathway* begins with the activation of protein C1 and is preceded by formation of a complex between an antigen and an antibody to form an **antigen-antibody complex (immune complex)** (discussed in Chapter 7).[14] The antigen may be a unique chemical component of the surface of a bacterium or other microorganism. Most pathogens express multiple antigens; therefore, multiple antibodies are usually bound in the complex. The first component of the classical complement cascade, C1, has six sites that can bind

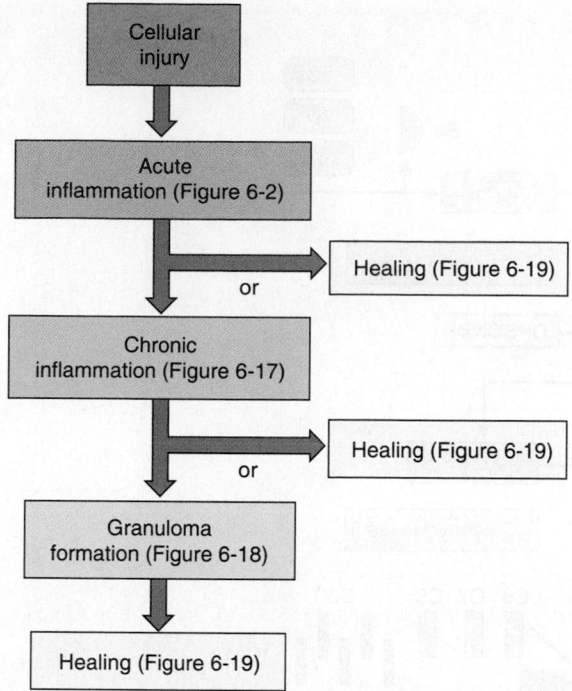

Figure 6-4 **Inflammatory phases.** Cellular injury leads to acute inflammation and may result in resolution and healing of the injured site or progress into chronic inflammation. Chronic inflammation in turn may result in healing or progress to development of a granuloma. The final step of the inflammatory process is usually healing and reconstruction of the damaged tissue. The figure numbers refer to those in which more detailed information on that portion of the process may be found.

to antibodies, and efficient activation of the complement cascade usually requires concurrent binding of C1 to at least two antibody molecules.[15] The complex formed by antigen-antibody-complement binding is shown in Figure 6-5. C1 is a macromolecular complex consisting of C1q and two molecules each of C1r and C1s. A conformational change in C1 results in an enzymatically active molecule whose substrates are C4 and C2. The resultant complex formed by the interaction of C1, C4, and C2 uses C3 as a substrate resulting in the production of C3a and C3b. A complex that has C3 as a substrate is generally referred to as a **C3 convertase.** The complex formed by the activation of C3 then has C5 as a substrate, resulting in the conversion of C5 to C5a and C5b. A complex that has C5 as a substrate is generally called a **C5 convertase.** Thus activation of C1 initiates the sequential enzymatic activation of all other components of the classic pathway, ultimately resulting in the activation of C5. The classical pathway also can be activated to a lesser degree by biologic molecules other than antibody, including heparin (a charged molecule that prevents clotting), deoxyribonucleic acid (DNA) or ribonucleic acid (RNA), and C-reactive protein, which is increased in the blood during inflammation.

Even under normal conditions small amounts of circulating C3 are spontaneously broken down into C3b and C3a by a number of naturally occurring enzymes in the blood. The rate of C3 spontaneous activation is generally very low, and C3b is

usually readily inactivated by complement regulator proteins in the blood (e.g., factor H and factor I). However, materials produced by some infectious microorganisms (e.g., lipopolysaccharides [endotoxin] on the bacterial surface, yeast cell wall carbohydrates [zymosan]) can bind the naturally produced C3b and protect it from inactivation. This will initiate activation of the *alternative complement pathway.*[16] The C3b bound to bacterial products can react with another normally occurring component, factor B. The complex of C3b and factor B is recognized by an enzyme, factor D, which activates factor B, producing factor Bb. The resultant C3b/Bb complex is very unstable unless it binds to properdin (P). The C3b/Bb/P complex is a C3 convertase that produces further C3b, resulting in a C3b/Bb/P/C3b complex that is a C5 convertase, which activates C5.

The *lectin pathway* is similar to the classical pathway but is antibody independent. It is activated by a plasma protein called *mannose-binding lectin (MBL).*[17] MBL is similar to C1q and binds to bacterial polysaccharides containing the carbohydrate mannose. MBL-associated serine proteases (MASP-1 and MASP-2) substitute for C1r and C1s and activate C4 and C2 to create a C3 convertase.

After activation of C5, the cascade continues through the terminal components C6, C7, C8, and C9. Components C5b through C9 assemble to form complexes (*membrane attack complex,* or *MAC*) capable of creating pores in cell membranes and permitting the influx of water and ions and may ultimately result in **cell lysis.**

The most important result of complement activation is the production of fragments during the activation of C4, C2, C3, and C5. The fragments C4a, C2b, C3a, and C5a are soluble and of low-molecular-weight that contribute in other ways to the inflammatory response. C2b affects smooth muscle, causing vasodilation and increased vascular permeability. C3a, C5a, and to a limited extent C4a, are **anaphylatoxins,** that is, they induce rapid **mast cell degranulation** (release of granular contents) and the release of histamine (see Figure 6-9) causing vasodilation and increased capillary permeability.[18] C5a is the major chemotactic factor for neutrophils. C3a is approximately 100 times less potent in chemotactic and anaphylatoxic activity. A **chemotactic factor** is a biochemical substance that attracts leukocytes to the site of inflammation.

The dual functions of a chemotactic factor and an anaphylatoxin are not needed simultaneously or to the same degree. Anaphylatoxic activity is necessary early in inflammation and occurs close to the inflammatory site to induce local mast cell degranulation and to increase the number of soluble mediators available to enhance vascular permeability and vasodilation. Chemotactic activity, on the other hand, is required for a much longer period and occurs distal to the inflammatory site to attract leukocytes from the circulation. Thus it is beneficial to an effective inflammatory response to limit the range of anaphylatoxic activity while allowing widespread chemotactic activity. A plasma enzyme, a **carboxypeptidase,** removes a terminal arginine on both C3a and C5a peptides, thereby

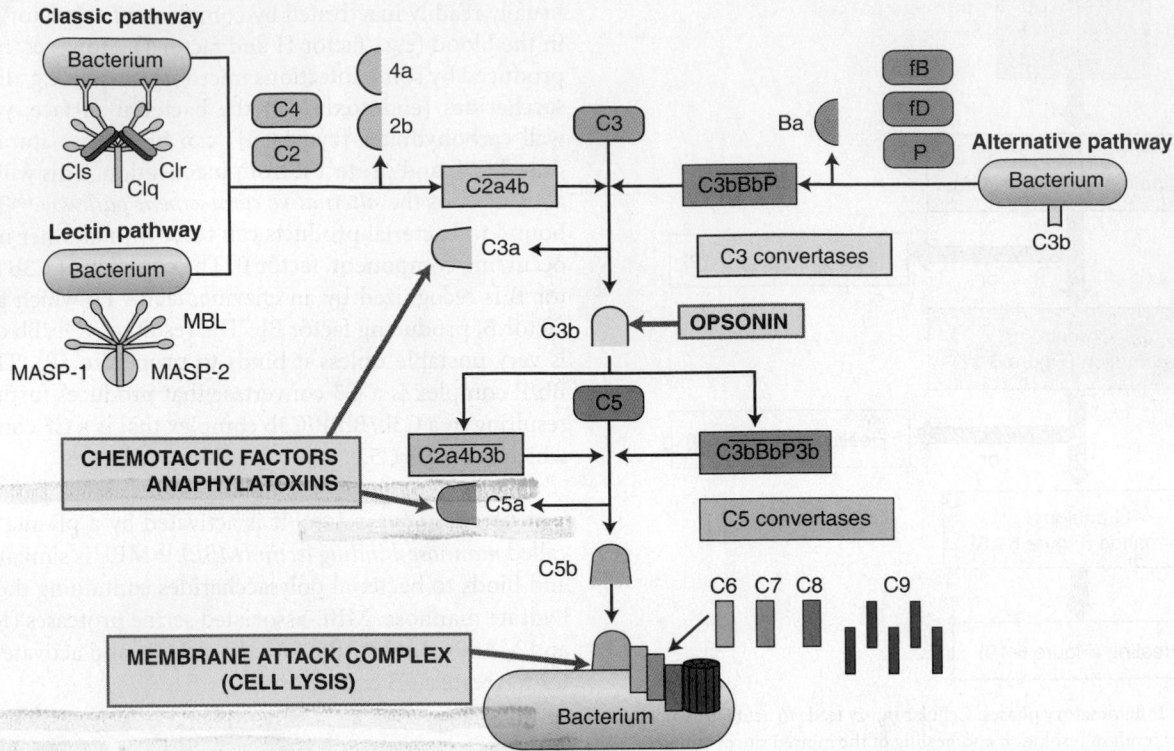

Figure 6-5 Pathways of complement cascade activation. The complement system is activated by three pathways: the classic pathway, the lectin pathway, and the alternative pathway. During activation, many complement components are cleaved into fragments (2b, 4a, Ba, 3a, and 5a). The smaller fragments frequently have potent biologic activities and may serve as chemotactic factors and anaphylatoxins. The larger activated fragments are usually converted into active enzymes (indicated by the bar above the names) and form complexes with additional components in the cascade. The **classic pathway** is usually activated by antigen-antibody complexes through component C1, which consists of C1q and two C1r and C1s molecules. As indicated, the C1q must simultaneously bind to two antibody molecules (indicated by Y-shaped structures). The **lectin pathway** is activated by mannose-binding lectin (MBL), which binds to two mannose-rich pathogen-associated molecular patterns on the surface of a bacterium. MBL contains two associated enzymes, MASP-1 and MASP-2, and functions in a manner similar to C1. C1 and MBL each activate complement components C4 and C2. The **alternative pathway** is activated by many agents, such as bacterial polysaccharides, which bind and stabilize C3b, which is produced by normal breakdown of C3 in the blood. The C3b forms the site of binding of factor B (fB), which is activated by factor D (fD) into Bb and the small fragment Ba. Properdin (P) helps stabilize the complex. Each pathway produces C3 and C5 convertases, which are enzymatically active complexes that activate C3 and C5, respectively. C3b produced by the C3 convertase can function as an opsonin. C5b initiates assemblage of the membrane attack complex (MAC), which results in multiple C9 molecules forming a pore in the bacterial membrane.

producing "C3a desArg" and "C5a desArg," which are inactive as anaphylatoxins but retain chemotactic activity. Thus chemotactic activity is retained, while not inducing distal mast cell degranulation that would result in considerable enlargement of the inflammatory response to the detriment of surrounding healthy tissue.

C3b adheres to the surface of a pathogenic microorganism and serves as an efficient opsonin. **Opsonins** are molecules that "tag" microorganisms for destruction by cells of the inflammatory system (primarily neutrophils and macrophages [see p. 190]). C3b on the cell surface also can be broken down by several enzymes in the blood into inactive fragments (e.g., iC3b), which retain opsonic activity.

In summary, the complement cascade can be activated by at least three different means, and its products have four functions: (1) anaphylatoxic activity resulting in mast cell degranulation, (2) leukocyte chemotaxis, (3) opsonization, and (4) cell lysis.

Clotting System

The clotting (coagulation) system is a group of plasma proteins that form a fibrinous meshwork at an injured or inflamed site.[19] This (1) prevents the spread of infection to adjacent tissues, (2) traps microorganisms and foreign bodies at the site of inflammation for removal by infiltrating cells (e.g., neutrophils and macrophages), (3) forms a clot that stops bleeding, and (4) provides a framework for future repair and healing. The main substance in this fibrinous mesh is an insoluble protein called *fibrin* that is the end product of the **coagulation cascade.**

Like the complement cascade, the coagulation cascade can be activated through different convergent pathways (see Figure 6-6). The coagulation cascade consists of the **extrinsic pathway** and the **intrinsic pathway** that converge at factor X.[20] From that point on, a common pathway leads to formation of a fibrin clot. The coagulation cascade is discussed in more detail and illustrated again in Chapter 25.

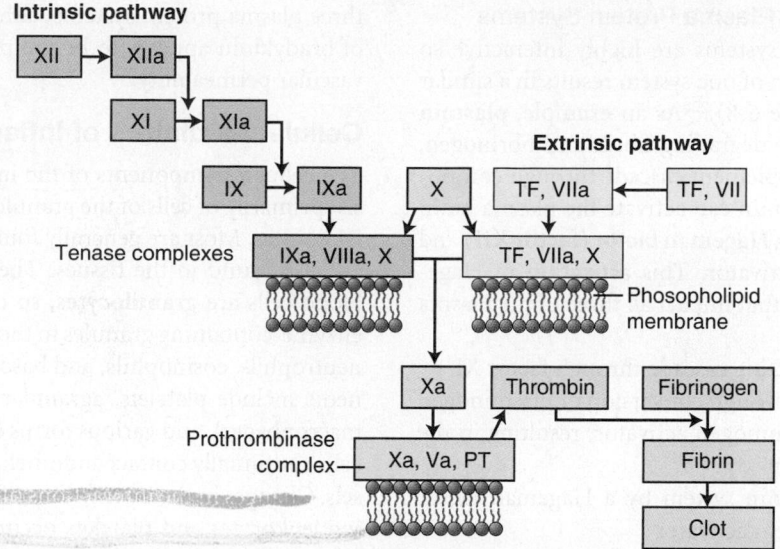

Intrinsic pathway

Extrinsic pathway

Tenase complexes

Phosopholipid membrane

Prothrombinase complex

Figure 6-6 Coagulation cascade. Clotting is activated through two pathways: the intrinsic pathway and the extrinsic pathway. The intrinsic pathway is initiated by the activation of Hageman factor (XII) into XIIa (activated factors are enzymes and are indicated by a lowercase a). The sequential activation of other intrinsic pathway components results in formation of a complex of IXa, VIIIa, and X. The extrinsic pathway is activated by exposure of tissue factor (TF) during tissue damage. TF complexes with factor VII, which is activated (VIIa) and forms a complex with factor X (TF, VIIa, X). Both the intrinsic and extrinsic pathway complexes are dependent on calcium, form on phospholipid membranes that are rich in phosphatidylserine, and have "tenase" activity (can activate factor X into Xa). Factor X begins a common pathway in which Xa complexes with Va and prothrombin (PT), with calcium and phospholipid membranes, to form an active prothrombinase (activates prothrombin into thrombin). Thrombin is an enzyme the cuts high-molecular-weight fibrinogen into fibrin molecules. Fibrin polymerizes to form a clot.

The clotting system can be activated by many substances that are released during tissue destruction and infection, including collagen, proteinases, kallikrein, and plasmin, as well as by bacterial products such as endotoxins. As with the complement cascade, activation of the clotting cascade produces fragments that enhance the inflammatory response. Two low-molecular-weight fibrinopeptides, A and B, are released from fibrinogen when fibrin is produced. Both fibrinopeptides (especially fibrinopeptide B) are chemotactic for neutrophils and increase vascular permeability by enhancing the effects of bradykinin (formed from the kinin system).

Kinin System

The third plasma protein system, the **kinin system,** augments inflammation in several ways.[21] The primary kinin produced from the kinin system is **bradykinin,** which causes dilation of blood vessels, acts with prostaglandins to stimulate nerve endings and induce pain, causes smooth muscle cell contraction, increases vascular permeability, and may increase leukocyte chemotaxis (see Figure 6-2). Bradykinin induces smooth muscle contraction more slowly than histamine and, along with prostaglandins of the E series, is probably responsible for endothelial cell retraction and increased vascular permeability in the later phases of inflammation (endothelial cell retraction is shown in Figures 6-3 and 6-11).

The kinin system is activated by stimulation of the **plasma kinin cascade** (see Figure 6-7). The conversion of plasma prekallikrein to kallikrein is induced by *prekallikrein activator,*

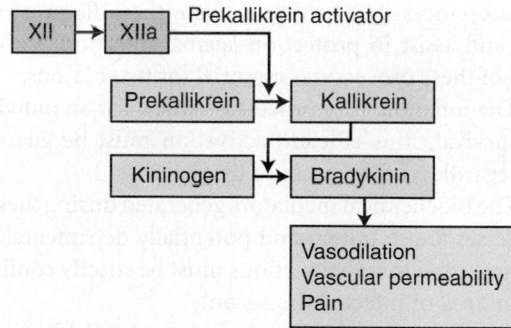

Prekallikrein activator

Figure 6-7 Plasma kinin cascade. The kinin pathway is activated by factor XIIa from the clotting system, which functions as an enzyme (prekallikrein activator) to convert prekallikrein into kallikrein. Enzymatically active kallikrein converts kininogen into bradykinin.

which is identical to factor XIIa (the product that results from activation of Hageman factor—factor XII) of the clotting cascade. Kallikrein then converts kininogen to bradykinin. Although the plasma kinin cascade is one pathway that leads to the production of bradykinin, tissue kallikreins in saliva, sweat, tears, urine, and feces provide another source for this inflammatory mediator. These tissue kallikreins convert serum kininogens to kallidin, also known as *Lys-bradykinin,* which may be converted to bradykinin by plasma aminopeptidase. In order to control the extent of inflammation, kinins are rapidly degraded by **kininases,** enzymes present in plasma and tissues.

Interactions Among the Plasma Protein Systems

The three plasma protein systems are highly interactive so that activation or regulation of one system results in a similar effect on the others (Figure 6-8).[22] As an example, **plasmin** regulates clot formation by degrading fibrin and fibrinogen, and it can activate the complement cascade through components C1, C3, and C5. Plasmin can activate the plasma kinin cascade as well by activating **Hageman factor (factor XII)** and producing prekallikrein activator. This activation of Hageman factor has four effects that impact all three of the plasma protein systems:

1. Activation of the clotting cascade through factor XI
2. Control of clotting through conversion of plasminogen proactivator to plasminogen activator, resulting in the generation of plasmin
3. Activation of the kinin system by a Hageman factor fragment, prekallikrein activator
4. Activation of C1 in the complement cascade

The activity of plasmin itself is also regulated because it is synthesized as a proenzyme, plasminogen. Plasminogen is converted to plasmin by several factors, including plasminogen activator generated from the kallikrein system, thrombin generated from the clotting system, bacterial factors such as streptokinase produced by hemolytic streptococci, plasminogen activators produced by endothelial cells, and several cellular enzymes released during tissue destruction.

Activation of any of the plasma protein systems results in production of a large number of very potent, biologically active substances that further activate the inflammatory response and assist in protection against infection. Very tight control of these processes is essential for two reasons:

1. The inflammatory process is critical for an individual's survival, thus efficient activation must be guaranteed regardless of the cause of tissue injury.
2. The biochemical mediators generated during these processes are so potent and potentially detrimental to the host itself that their actions must be strictly confined to injured or infected tissues only.

Therefore, multiple mechanisms are available to either *activate* or *inactivate (regulate)* these plasma protein systems.

As mentioned, many enzymes from the plasma regulate the activity of these pathways, such as carboxypeptidase inactivating the anaphylatoxic activities of C3a and C5a and kininases degrading kinins. Many other natural inhibitors are present, including enzymes that degrade histamine (histaminase), activated complement components, kallikrein, and plasmin. Another example of a common regulator is **C1 esterase inhibitor (C1 inh).**[23] C1 inh inhibits complement activation through reactivity with C1 (classic pathway), MASP-2 (lectin pathway), and C3b (alternative pathway). It is also a major inhibitor of the clotting and kinin pathways (e.g., kallikrein, activated Hageman factor XIIa). A genetic defect in C1 inh (C1 inh deficiency) results in **hereditary angioedema,** which is a self-limiting edema of cutaneous and mucosal layers resulting from stress, illness, or relative minor or unapparent trauma. The disease is characterized by hyperactivation of all three plasma protein systems, although excessive production of bradykinin appears to be the principal cause of increased vascular permeability.

Cellular Mediators of Inflammation

The cellular components of the inflammatory response consist primarily of cells of the granulocytic or monocytic lines of leukocytes. Most are generally found in the blood, but several are also found in the tissues. The primary circulating white blood cells are **granulocytes,** so called because of the many enzyme-containing granules in their cytoplasm. These include neutrophils, eosinophils, and basophils. Other blood components include platelets, agranular monocytes (precursors of macrophages), and various forms of lymphocytes. Circulating cells continually contact endothelial cells lining the blood vessels. Changes in the interactions of endothelium with circulating leukocytes and platelets occur during inflammation and account for several of the characteristics of the inflammatory response. Other cellular members of the inflammatory system are found in various tissues and organs. These include mast cells and cells derived from the monocytes/macrophage lineage. Lymphoid-derived natural killer cells are found in the circulation and tissues and can recognize and destroy cells that have been altered by viral infection or malignancy.

The cells of the inflammatory system secrete and respond to biochemical mediators. Thus most of these cells are recruited and activated by products of the plasma protein systems and by biochemicals released during cell destruction, secreted by other inflammatory cells, or produced by microbes. All of these inflammatory cells and protein systems, along with the substances they produce, preferably act at the site of tissue injury to confine the extent of damage, kill microorganisms, and remove the debris of "battle" in preparation for healing: tissue regeneration or repair (processes known as *resolution*).

Inappropriate or exaggerated inflammatory processes have deleterious effects on the host. Even appropriate inflammation can be painful and harm healthy tissues. Because inflammation is complex, is nonspecific, and can be triggered and maintained by a great variety of stimuli, it is often difficult to control with drugs.

Cellular Receptors

Cells of both innate and acquired immunity must recognize and respond to their environment, whether to products of damaged cells or to potential pathogenic microorganisms. Each cell has receptors on the cell surface that specifically bind soluble substances produced during tissue damage or infection. Receptor binding results in activation of intracellular signaling pathways and activation of the cell itself. As will be discussed in Chapter 7, B and T lymphocytes of the acquired immune system have evolved surface receptors (i.e., the T-cell receptor, or TCR, and the B-cell receptor, or BCR) that bind a large spectrum of antigens. Cells involved in innate resistance have evolved a different set of receptors that recognize a much more limited array of specific molecules. These are referred to as **pattern recognition receptors (PRRs),** and they recognize

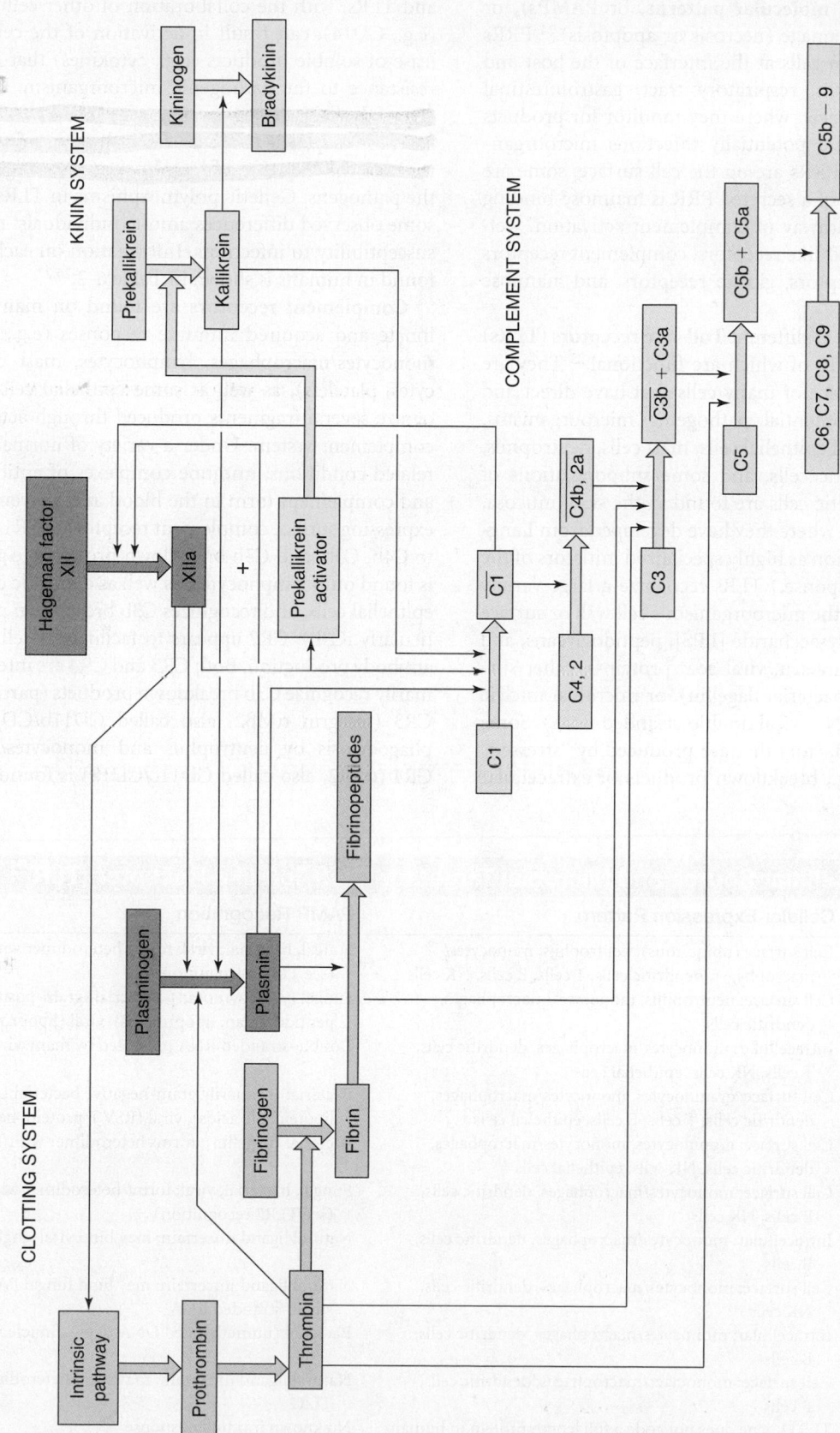

Figure 6-8 Interactions between the complement, clotting, kinin, and fibrinolytic (plasmin) systems. *Thick colored arrows* denote where a particular factor activates another system. *Thin arrows* denote the activation of factors within a system.

molecular "patterns" on infectious agents or their products (**pathogen-associated molecular patterns, or PAMPs),** or products of cellular damage (necrosis or apoptosis).[24] PRRs are generally found on cells at the interface of the host and environment (i.e., skin, respiratory tract, gastrointestinal tract, genitourinary tract), where they monitor for products of cellular damage and potentially infectious microorganisms. Although most PRRs are on the cell surface, some are secreted. An example of a secreted PRR is mannose-binding lectin of the lectin pathway of complement activation. Cellular PRRs include Toll-like receptors, complement receptors (CRs), scavenger receptors, glucan receptors, and mannose receptors.

In humans, at least 11 different **Toll-like receptors (TLRs)** have been described, 10 of which are functional.[25] They are expressed on the surface of many cells that have direct and early contact with potential pathogenic microorganisms. These include mucosal epithelial cells, mast cells, neutrophils, macrophages, dendritic cells, and some subpopulations of lymphocytes. (Dendritic cells are found in the skin, mucosa, and lymphoid tissues, where they have developed from Langerhans cells and function as highly specialized initiators of the acquired immune response.) TLRs recognize a large variety of PAMPs located on the microorganism's cell wall or surface (e.g., bacterial lipopolysaccharide [LPS], peptidoglycans, and lipoproteins, yeast zymosan, viral coat proteins), other surface structures (e.g., bacterial flagellin), or microbial nucleic acid (e.g., bacterial DNA, viral double-stranded RNA). Some TLRs recognize host factors that are produced by "stressed" or damaged cells (e.g., breakdown products of extracellular

matrix proteins, chromatin). Interactions between PAMPs and TLRs, with the collaboration of other cellular receptors (e.g., CD14), can result in activation of the cell and the release of soluble products (e.g., cytokines) that increase local resistance to the pathogenic microorganism. TLRs are also one of the bridges between innate resistance and the acquired immune response through the induction of cytokines that increase the response of lymphocytes to foreign antigens on the pathogens. Genetic polymorphisms in TLRs may explain some observed differences among individuals' resistance and susceptibility to infections. Information on each of the TLRs found in humans is shown in Table 6-2.[26,27]

Complement receptors are found on many cells of the innate and acquired immune responses (e.g., granulocytes, monocytes/macrophages, lymphocytes, mast cells, erythrocytes, platelets), as well as some epithelial cells.[28] They recognize several fragments produced through activation of the complement system. Under a variety of normal and disease-related conditions, immune complexes of antibody, antigen, and complement form in the blood and are removed by cells expressing surface complement receptor-1 (CR1), which binds to C4b, C3b, and C3b breakdown products (e.g., iC3b). CR2 is found on B lymphocytes, as well as dendritic cells and some epithelial cells, and recognizes C3b breakdown products (particularly iC3b). CR2 appears to facilitate B-cell function and antibody production. Both CR3 and CR4 are integrins that primarily recognize C3b breakdown products (particularly iC3b). CR3 (integrin αMβ2, also called CD11b/CD18) facilitates phagocytosis by neutrophils and monocytes/macrophages. CR4 (αXβ2, also called CD11c/CD18) is found primarily on

Table 6-2	Cellular Source and Microbial Target for Each Toll-like Receptor (TLR)	
Receptor	**Cellular Expression Pattern**	**PAMP Recognition**
TLR1	Cell surface (ubiquitous): neutrophils, monocytes/macrophages, dendritic cells, T cells, B cells, NK cells	Fungal, bacterial, viral; forms heterodimer with TLR2 (see TLR2 recognition)
TLR2	Cell surface: neutrophils, monocytes/macrophages, dendritic cells	Fungal (yeast zymosan), bacterial (gram-positive bacterial peptidoglycan, lipoproteins), viral (lipoproteins)
TLR3	Intracellular: monocytes/macrophages, dendritic cells, T cells, NK cells, epithelial cells	Double-stranded RNA produced by many viruses
TLR4	Cell surface: granulocytes, monocytes/macrophages, dendritic cells, T cells, B cells, epithelial cells	Bacterial (primarily gram-negative bacterial LPS, lipoteichoic acids), viral (RSV F protein, hepatitis C)
TLR5	Cell surface: granulocytes, monocytes/macrophages, dendritic cells, NK cells, epithelial cells	Bacterial (flagellin); forms heterodimer with TLR4
TLR6	Cell surface: monocytes/macrophages, dendritic cells, B cells, NK cells	Fungal, bacterial, viral; forms heterodimer with TLR2 (see TLR2 recognition)
TLR7	Intracellular: monocytes/macrophages, dendritic cells, B cells	Natural ligand uncertain; may bind viral single-strand RNA
TLR8	Cell surface: monocytes/macrophages, dendritic cells, NK cells	Natural ligand uncertain; may bind fungal PAMPs or viral single-stranded RNA
TLR9	Intracellular: monocytes/macrophages, dendritic cells, B cells	Bacterial (unmethylated DNA [CpG dinucleotides])
TLR10	Cell surface: monocytes/macrophages, dendritic cells, B cells	Natural ligand uncertain; may form heterodimers with TLR2
TLR11	TLR11 gene does not code a full length protein in humans	No known immune response

DNA, Deoxyribonucleic acid; *LPS,* lipopolysaccharide; *NK,* natural killer; *PAMPs,* pathogen-associated molecular patterns; *RNA,* ribonucleic acid; *RSV,* respiratory syncytial virus.

platelets. (**Integrins** are cell surface receptors that have a role in cell adhesion and attachment and mediate intracellular signaling within the extracellular matrix [see Figure 1-14]).

Scavenger receptors are primarily expressed on macrophages and facilitate recognition and phagocytosis of bacterial pathogens, as well as damaged cells and altered soluble lipoproteins associated with vascular damage (e.g., HDL, acetylated LDL, oxidized LDL). More than eight receptors have been identified. Some scavenger receptors (e.g., SR-PSOX) recognize the cell membrane phospholipid phosphatidylserine (PS). PS is normally sequestered on the cytoplasmic surface of the cell membrane, but is externalized under a very limited variety of conditions, including erythrocyte senescence and cellular apoptosis. Thus macrophages, through this receptor, can identify and remove old red blood cells and cells undergoing apoptosis. Another important scavenger receptor is CD14, which recognizes the complex of LPS and LPS-binding protein. LPS-binding

protein is up-regulated during inflammation by the cytokines interleukin-6 (IL-6) and IL-1 and helps remove bacterial lipopolysaccharide (endotoxin) from the circulation.[29-31]

Mast Cells

A central cell in inflammation is the mast cell.[32] **Mast cells,** first described by Paul Ehrlich in 1877,[33] are cellular bags of granules located in the loose connective tissues close to blood vessels (Figure 6-9). They are found in large numbers in areas directly exposed to the environment including the skin and lining the gastrointestinal and respiratory tracts. A great number of stimuli cause mast cells to become activated, resulting in initiation of the inflammatory response. Typical causes of mast cell activation include (1) physical injury (e.g., heat, mechanical trauma, ultraviolet light, and x-rays), (2) chemical agents (e.g., toxins, snake and bee venoms, proteolytic enzymes, and antimicrobial peptides),

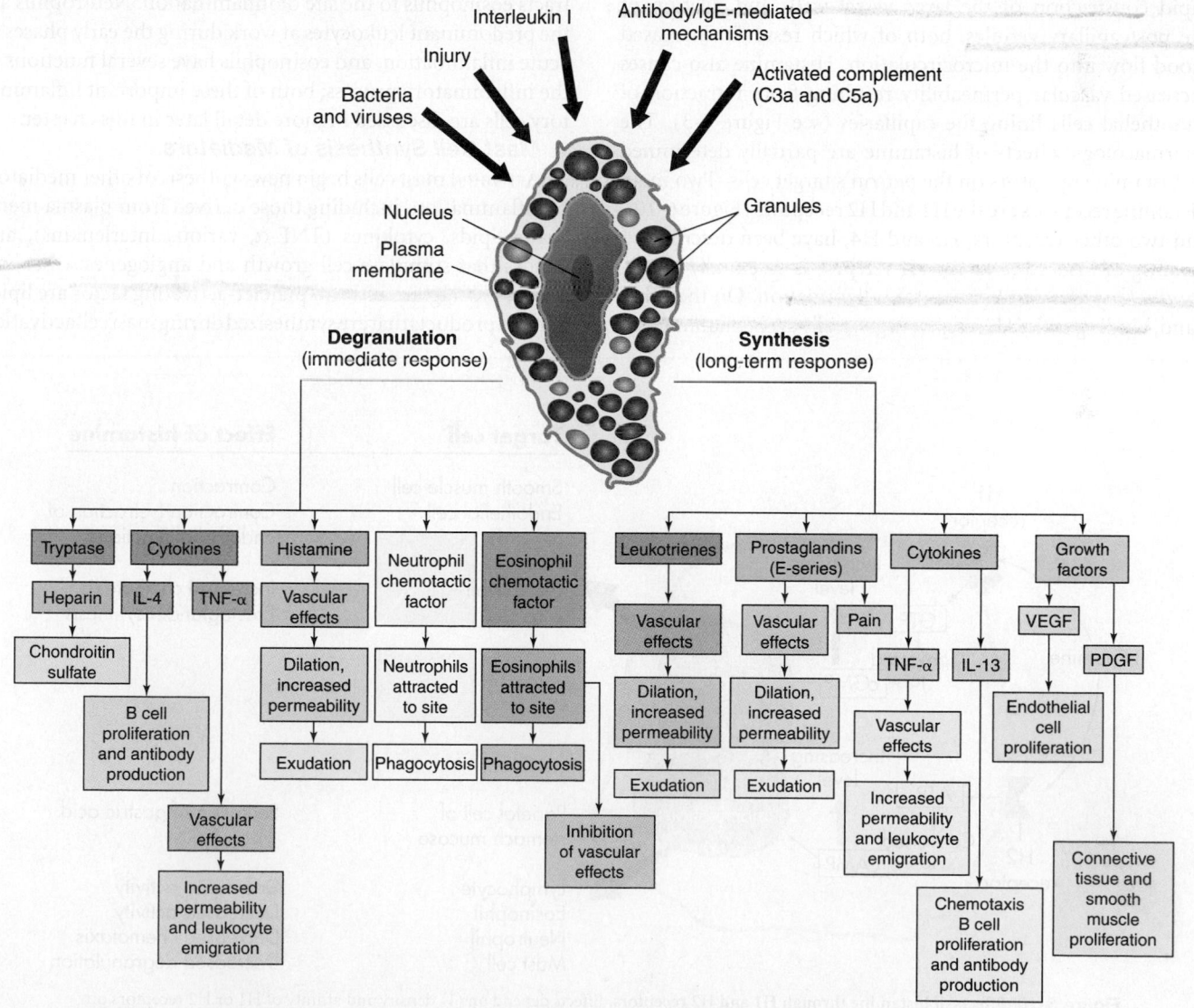

Figure 6-9 Effects of degranulation *(left)* and synthesis *(right)* by mast cells. The depiction of a tissue mast cell shows darkly stained granules in the cytoplasm. *PDGF,* Platelet-derived growth factor; *VEGF,* vascular endothelial growth factor.

(3) immunologic means (e.g., anaphylatoxins released during activation of complement components or particular types of antibody [e.g., immunoglobulin E (IgE)] produced by cells of the acquired immune response [see Chapter 7]), and (4) activation of TLRs by bacteria and viruses.[34,35] Soluble and extremely potent chemicals from the mast cell are responsible for its effects on inflammation. These are released in two ways: by release of the contents of their preformed granules (*degranulation*) and by new synthesis of lipid-derived inflammatory mediators. Mast cells are also involved in initiating many allergic responses (discussed in Chapters 7 and 8).

Mast Cell Degranulation

In response to a stimulus, biochemical mediators in the mast cell granules, including histamine, chemotactic factors (e.g., neutrophil chemotactic factor, **eosinophil chemotactic factor of anaphylaxis** or **ECF-A**), and cytokines (e.g., tumor necrosis factor-alpha [TNF-α], IL-4) are released within seconds and exert their effects immediately (see Figure 6-9).

Histamine is a vasoactive amine that causes temporary, rapid constriction of the large vessel walls and dilation of the postcapillary venules, both of which result in increased blood flow into the microcirculation. Histamine also causes increased vascular permeability resulting from retraction of endothelial cells lining the capillaries (see Figure 6-3). The pharmacologic effects of histamine are partially determined by histamine receptors on the person's target cells. Two main histamine receptors are the H1 and H2 receptors (Figure 6-10), and two other receptors, H3 and H4, have been described.[36] Binding of histamine to the *H1 receptor* is essentially proinflammatory, that is, it promotes inflammation. On the other hand, binding to the *H2 receptor* is generally anti-inflammatory

because it results in suppression of leukocyte function. The H1 receptor is present on smooth muscle cells, especially those of the bronchi, and causes bronchial smooth muscle to contract (bronchoconstriction) when stimulated. Both types of receptors are distributed among many different cells and are often present on the same cells and may act in an antagonistic fashion. For instance, neutrophils express both types of receptors, with stimulation of H1 receptors resulting in the augmentation of neutrophil chemotaxis, and H2 stimulation resulting in its inhibition. The H2 receptor is especially abundant on parietal cells of the stomach mucosa and induces the secretion of gastric acid as part of the normal physiology of the stomach. The role of H1 and H2 receptors is discussed further in Chapter 8.

Two chemotactic factors, neutrophil chemotactic factor and ECF-A, are also released during mast cell degranulation. **Chemotaxis** is directional movement of cells along a chemical gradient formed by a chemotactic factor (Figure 6-11). **Neutrophil chemotactic factor** attracts neutrophils, and ECF-A attracts eosinophils to the site of inflammation. Neutrophils are the predominant leukocytes at work during the early phases of acute inflammation, and eosinophils have several functions in the inflammatory process; both of these important inflammatory cells are discussed in more detail later in this chapter.

Mast Cell Synthesis of Mediators

Activated mast cells begin new synthesis of other mediators of inflammation, including those derived from plasma membrane lipids, cytokines (TNF-α, various interleukins), and factors that stimulate cell growth and angiogenesis. Leukotrienes, prostaglandins, and platelet-activating factor are lipid-derived products that are synthesized during mast cell activation

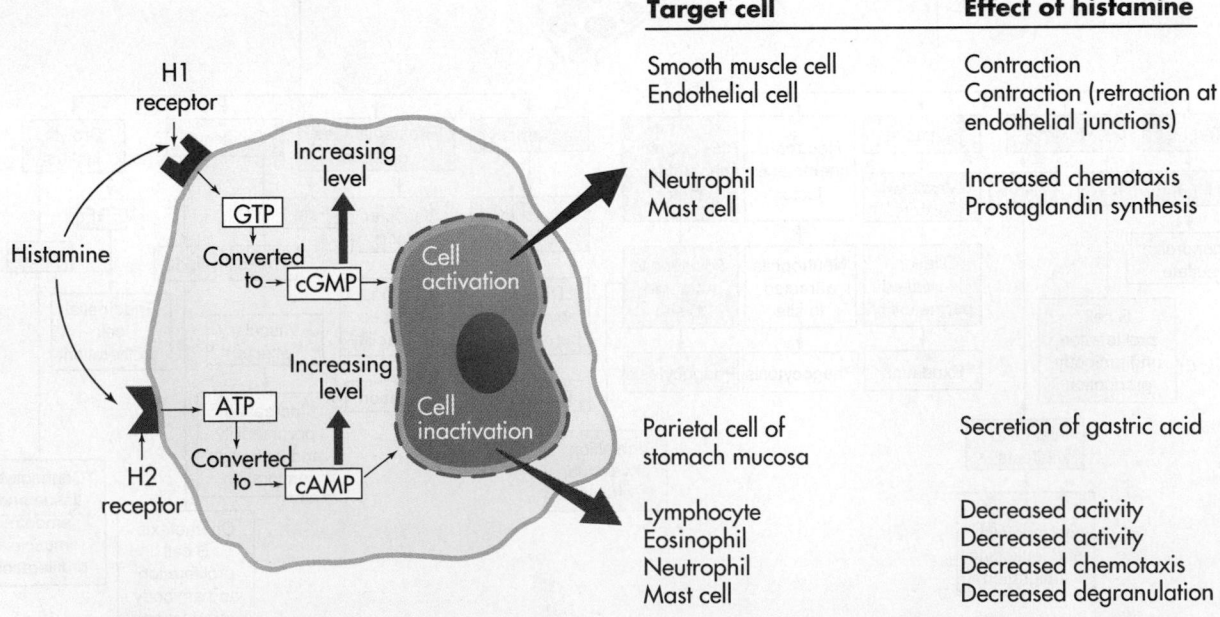

Target cell	Effect of histamine
Smooth muscle cell	Contraction
Endothelial cell	Contraction (retraction at endothelial junctions)
Neutrophil	Increased chemotaxis
Mast cell	Prostaglandin synthesis
Parietal cell of stomach mucosa	Secretion of gastric acid
Lymphocyte	Decreased activity
Eosinophil	Decreased activity
Neutrophil	Decreased chemotaxis
Mast cell	Decreased degranulation

Figure 6-10 Effects of histamine through H1 and H2 receptors. Effects depend on (1) density and affinity of H1 or H2 receptors on the target cell and (2) the identity of the target cell. *ATP,* Adenosine triphosphate; *cAMP,* cyclic adenosine monophosphate; *cGMP,* cyclic guanosine monophosphate; *GTP,* guanosine triphosphate.

A. Tissue

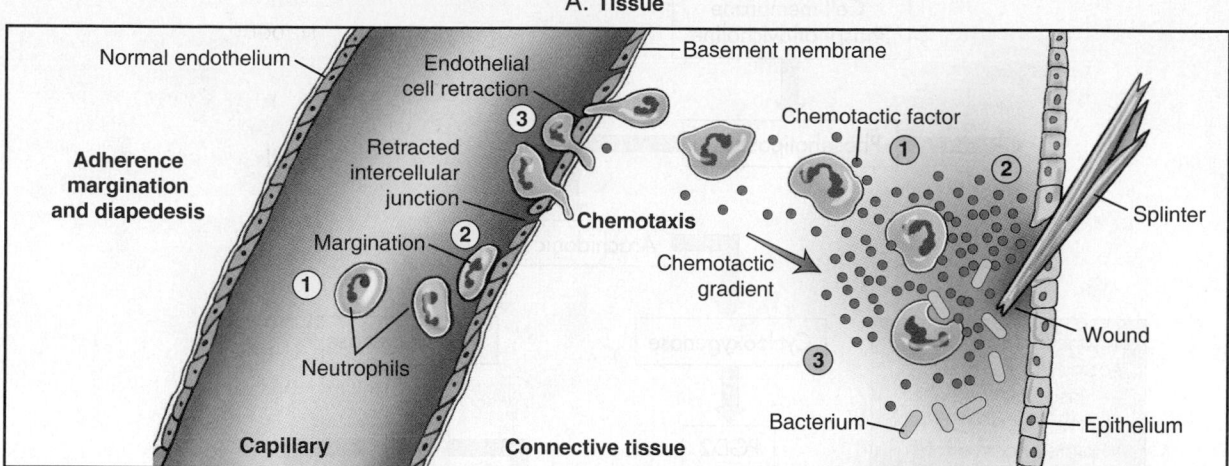

B. Recognition and attachment   C. Phagocytosis

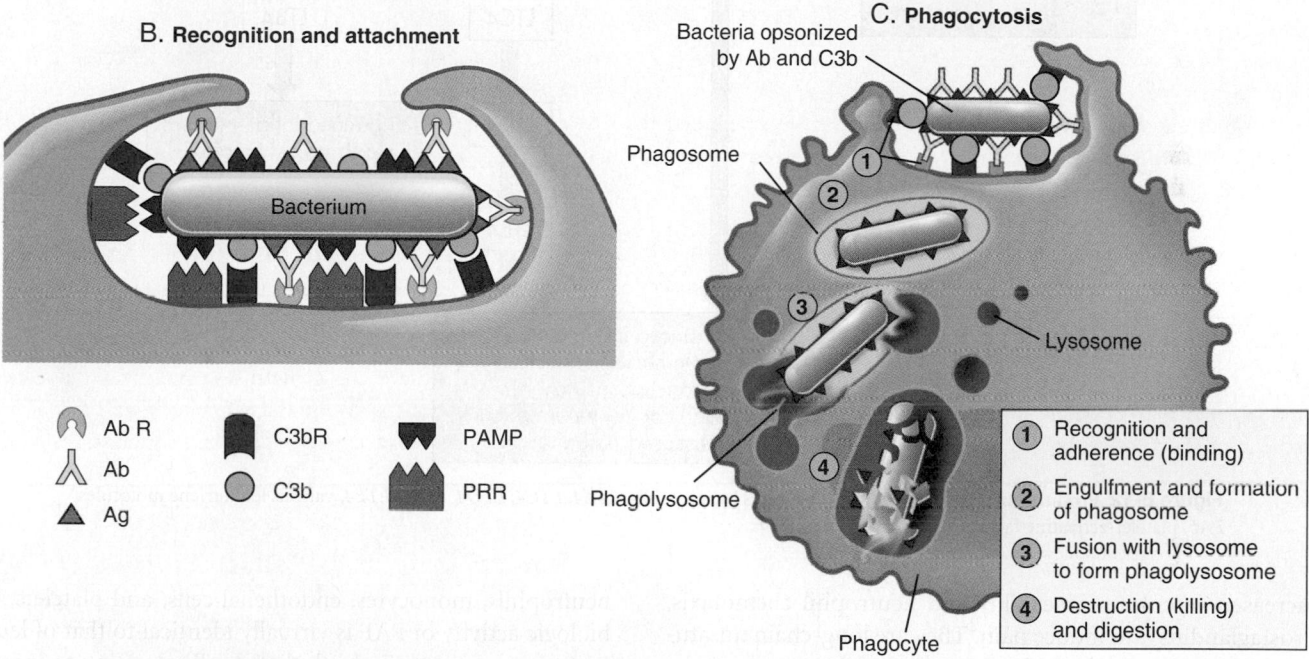

Ab R	
Ab	
Ag	
C3bR	
C3b	
PAMP	
PRR	

1. Recognition and adherence (binding)
2. Engulfment and formation of phagosome
3. Fusion with lysosome to form phagolysosome
4. Destruction (killing) and digestion

Figure 6-11 **Process of phagocytosis.** The process that results in phagocytosis is characterized by three interrelated steps: adherence and diapedesis, tissue invasion by chemotaxis, and phagocytosis. **A,** *Adherence, margination, diapedesis,* and *chemotaxis.* The primary phagocyte in the blood is the neutrophil, which usually moves freely within the vessel (**1**). At sites of inflammation, the neutrophil progressively develops increased adherence to the endothelium, leading to accumulation along the vessel wall (margination or pavementing) (**2**). At sites of endothelial cell retraction the neutrophil exits the blood by means of diapedesis (**3**). *Chemotaxis:* In the tissues, the neutrophil detects chemotactic factor gradients through surface receptors (**1**) and migrates towards higher concentrations of the factors (**2**). The high concentration of chemotactic factors at the site of inflammation immobilizes the neutrophil (**3**). **B,** *Specific receptors for recognition and attachment.* **C,** *Phagocytosis.* Opsonized microorganisms bind to the surface of a phagocyte through specific receptors (**1**). The microorganism is engulfed (ingested) into a phagocytic vacuole, or phagosome (**2**). Lysosomes fuse with the phagosome, resulting in the formation of a phagolysosome (**3**). During this process the microorganism is exposed to products of the lysosomes, including a variety of enzymes and products of the hexose-monophosphate-shunt (e.g., H_2O_2, O_2^-). The microorganism is killed and digested (**4**). *Ab,* Antibody; *AbR,* antibody receptor; *C3b,* complement component C3b; *C3bR,* complement C3b receptor; *PAMP,* pathogen-associated molecular pattern; *PRR,* pattern recognition receptor.

(Figure 6-12). Leukotrienes are a product of another lipid, arachidonic acid, which is released from mast cell membranes by an intracellular phospholipase that acts on membrane phospholipids.[37] **Leukotrienes** are acidic, sulfur-containing lipids that produce effects similar to those of histamine, namely, smooth muscle contraction, increased vascular permeability,

and perhaps neutrophil and eosinophil chemotaxis. Leukotrienes appear to be important in the later stages of the inflammatory response because they stimulate slower and more prolonged responses than do histamines.

The mast cell also synthesizes **prostaglandins,** which, like leukotrienes, are a product of arachidonic acid and cause

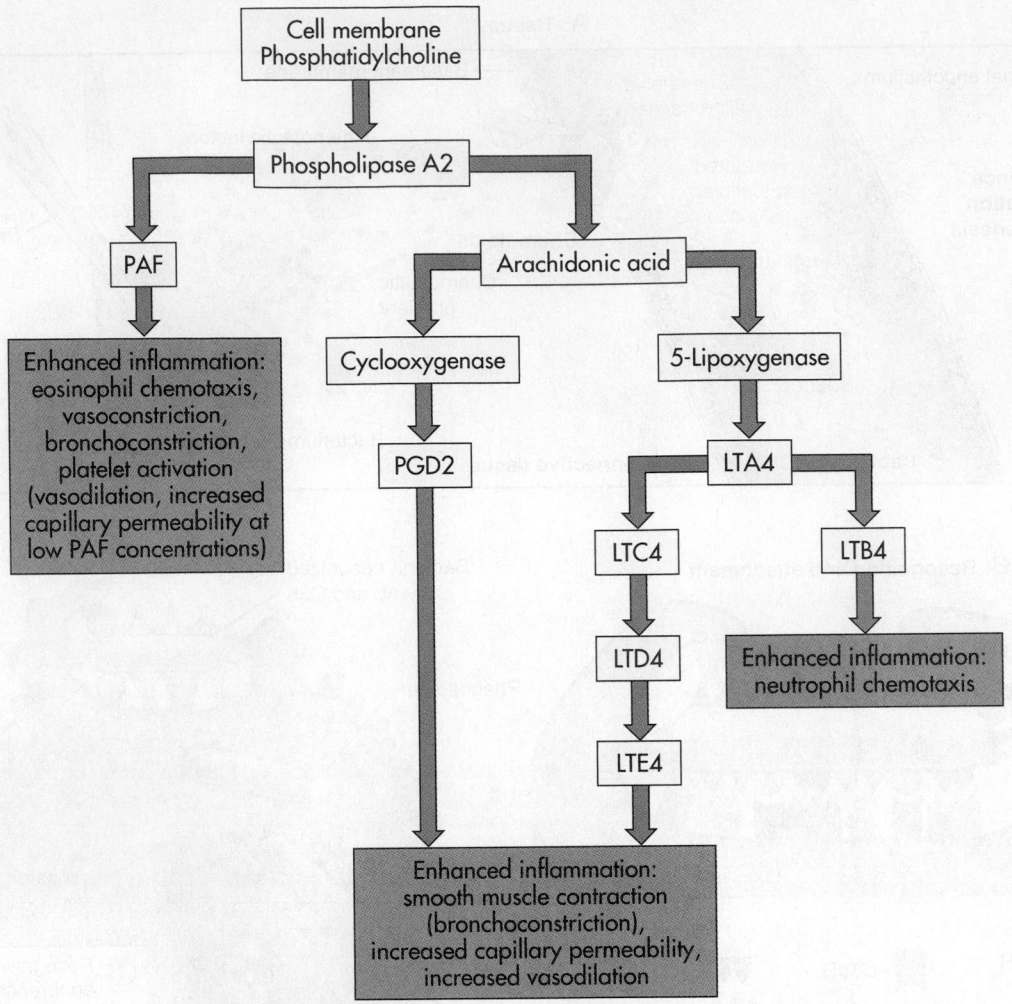

Figure 6-12 Production of lipid vasoactive substances by mast cells. *LTA4, LTC4, LTD4, LTE4, LTB4,* various leukotriene molecules; *PAF,* platelet-activating factor; *PGD2,* prostaglandin D2.

increased vascular permeability and neutrophil chemotaxis. Prostaglandins also induce pain. They are long-chain unsaturated fatty acids produced by the action of the enzyme *cyclooxygenase* and are classified into groups (E, D, A, F, and B) according to their structure. Prostaglandins E_1 and E_2 cause increased vascular permeability and smooth muscle contraction, apparently acting directly on postcapillary venules. They can inhibit some aspects of inflammation by suppressing both the release of histamine from mast cells and the release of lysosomal enzymes (enzymes responsible for killing and digesting microorganisms) from neutrophils. Enhancement or suppression of the inflammatory response may be related to the concentration of prostaglandins. Aspirin and some other nonsteroidal anti-inflammatory drugs (NSAIDs) block the synthesis of prostaglandins of the E series and other arachidonic acid derivatives, thereby inhibiting inflammation.

Platelet-activating factor (PAF), another mast cell–derived lipid, is produced by removal of a fatty acid from the plasma membrane phospholipid phosphatidylcholine by phospholipase A_2. Although mast cells are a major source of PAF, this molecule also can be produced during inflammation by neutrophils, monocytes, endothelial cells, and platelets. The biologic activity of PAF is virtually identical to that of leukotrienes, namely causing endothelial cell retraction to increase vascular permeability, leukocyte adhesion to endothelial cells, and platelet activation.

Phagocytosis

Phagocytosis is the process by which a cell ingests and disposes of damaged cells and foreign material, including microorganisms (see Figure 6-11). Because most phagocytes are circulating in the blood, they must leave the bloodstream and migrate to the site of inflammation before initiating phagocytosis. Under normal conditions, the circulation in the capillaries and venules is rapidly moving with red blood cells in the main stream and neutrophils and other leukocytes tending to flow more slowly along the vessel's periphery. Many of the biochemical products produced early at inflammatory sites (e.g., histamine, TNF-α, bradykinin, leukotrienes, prostaglandins) diffuse to the vessels and affect both leukocytes and endothelial cells. Both cell populations respond by producing new **adhesion molecules (selectins and integrins)**

NUTRITION & DISEASE

Essential Fatty Acids and Inflammation

Both omega-3 and omega-6 polyunsaturated fatty acids are essential fatty acids available only in the diet. They are essential because human physiology cannot add the necessary double bonds to the carbon chains. Omega-6 fatty acids are contained in vegetable oils, and most are linolenic acid. Omega-3 essential fatty acids are found in green leafy vegetables, walnuts, flaxseed, and canola oil and are mostly alpha-linolenic acid. The metabolic products of alpha-linolenic acid are eicosapentaenoic acid (EPA) and docosahexaenoic acid (DHA), and the richest source of these acids is in the oils of deep-sea cold-water fish. Both the omega-3 and omega-6 fatty acids use the same enzymes to produce their metabolic products, and they compete for this enzyme, delta-5-desaturase. *Delta-5-desaturase* converts EPA into anti-inflammatory prostaglandins (PG) of the PGE3 series. The omega-6 fatty acid, dihomogamma-linolenic acid (DGLA), can be converted to either anti-inflammatory PG1 or into arachidonic acid (AA), a precursor of inflammatory PG2 and leukotrienes. Conversion of DGLA into PG1 does not require any enzymes, but conversion of DGLA into AA requires the enzymes delta-6- and delta-5-desaturase. When the diet is high in omega-3 fatty acids, most of the delta-5-desaturase will be used in the omega-3 pathway and the production of anti-inflammatory prostaglandins. Little delta-5-desaturase will be available to convert DGLA into arachidonic acid, and subsequently inflammatory mediators. DGLA ends up being converted into the anti-inflammatory PG1 and overall, inflammation is decreased. The resulting anti-inflammatory effects of omega-3 essential fatty acids decreases the risk for cardiovascular disease, cancer, and other conditions associated with inflammation. Omega-3 fatty acids have been shown to decrease blood triglyceride concentrations; decrease production of chemoattractants, growth factors, and adhesion molecules; lower blood pressure; increase nitric oxide production and endothelial relaxation and vascular compliance; decrease thrombosis and cardiac dysrhythmias; and stabilize atherosclerotic plaque. The American diet tends to be high in saturated and omega-6 fatty acids and deficient in omega-3 fatty acids, with a ratio estimated at about 15:1. The Mediterranean-style diet has more whole grains, fish, olive oil, fresh fruits and vegetables, and a more balanced ratio of omega-6 to omega-3 fatty acids estimated at about 3-4:1. Increasing omega-3 fatty acids in the diet may significantly improve health and reduce the risk of cardiovascular disease and cancer.

Data from Berquin IM et al: *Cancer Lett* 269(2):363-377, 2008; Calder PC: *Clin Sci (Lond)* 107(1):1-11, 2004; Chrysohoou C et al: *J Am Coll Cardiol* 44(1):152-158, 2004; Das UN: *Lipids Health Dis* 7:37, 2008; Esposito K et al: *JAMA* 292(12):1440-1446, 2004; Sijben JW and Calder PC: *Proc Nutr Soc* 66(2):237-259, 2007.

Table 6-3 Examples of Cellular Adhesion Molecules (CAMs) Involved in Leukocyte Interaction with Endothelial Cells

	Activity of Leukocyte		
	"Rolling" Low Affinity	"Margination" Firm Attachment	"Diapedesis"
Leukocyte adhesion molecule	L-selectin	Integrin α4β1 (VLA-4) Integrin α4β7	Integrin αLβ2 (LFA-1) Integrin αMβ2 (MAC-1) PCAM-1
Endothelial adhesion molecule	P-selectin E-selectin	VCAM-1	ICAM-1 ICAM-2 PCAM-1

Selectins (lectin-like molecules): *L-selectin*, leukocyte selectin; *P-selectin*, platelet selectin; *E-selectin*, endothelial selectin.
Integrins (noncovalent heterodimers of alpha [α] and beta [β] subunits): *VLA-4*, very late antigen-4; *LFA-1*, lymphocyte function antigen-1; *MAC-1*, macrophage antigen-1.
Immunoglobulin-like molecules: *VCAM-1*, vascular cell adhesion molecule-1; *ICAM-1, ICAM-2*, immunoglobulin-like molecules-1 and 2; *PCAM-1*, platelet-endothelial cell adhesion molecule-1.

on their surfaces (Table 6-3).[38] (See page 195 for integrins). **Selectins** are adhesion molecules that bind carbohydrate ligands. The reciprocal change in adhesion molecules on leukocytes, as well as platelets, promotes their interaction with the endothelial cells.[39] The initial change of surface molecules increases the adhesion, or stickiness, between leukocytes and endothelial cells, causing the leukocytes to adhere more avidly to the walls of the capillaries and venules in a process called **margination,** or **pavementing.**[40,41] Adhesion molecules that

are expressed later lead to **diapedesis,** or emigration of the cells through the endothelial junctions that have retracted in response to the same mediators (see Figure 6-11). The leukocytes digest the basement membrane and migrate into the surrounding tissues.

Additionally, **endothelial cells** release nitric oxide (NO), a gas that under normal conditions maintains vascular tone. Inflammation induces additional endothelial nitric oxide synthase, increasing the amount of NO production.[42] Effects of NO on inflammation include vasodilation by inducing relaxation of vascular smooth muscle, a response that is local and short-lived, and suppression of mast cell function as well as platelet adhesion and aggregation.

Once inside the connective tissue in the perivascular space, leukocytes migrate to the inflammatory site by means of chemotaxis. They detect chemotactic factors in the environment through chemoreceptors at multiple locations on their plasma membranes and migrate in the direction of highest concentration (see Figure 6-11). The primary chemotactic factors include many bacterial products, complement fragments C3a and C5a, kallikrein, plasminogen activator, products of fibrin degradation, and chemokines. Eosinophils and neutrophils also respond to chemotactic factors released from mast cells. Monocytes are attracted toward a factor (monocyte chemotactic factor) that has been released by neutrophils already at the site of injury. And although histamine is not itself chemotactic, it may facilitate the chemotactic effects of other factors.

Once the phagocytic cell enters the inflammatory site, the process of phagocytosis involves five steps: (1) *opsonization, recognition* of the target and *adherence* of the phagocyte to it, (2) *engulfment* (ingestion or endocytosis) and formation of *phagosome*, (3) *fusion* with lysosomal granules within the phagocyte (phagolysosome), and (4) *destruction* of the target (see Figure 6-11) (lysosomes are described in Chapter 1). Throughout the process, both the target and digestive enzymes are isolated within membrane-bound vesicles. Isolation protects the phagocyte itself from the harmful effects of the target microorganisms, as well as its own enzymes.

Most phagocytes can trap and engulf bacteria using cellular PRRs and PAMPs normally expressed on the bacterial surface (see Figure 6-11). However, that process is slow and inefficient. Opsonization, usually by antibody or complement component C3b, greatly enhances both recognition and adherence. Phagocytosis of an opsonized (antibody and/or complement-protein coated) red blood cell is illustrated in Figure 6-13. Opsonins function as "glue" between the phagocyte and the target cell because receptors on the phagocyte are specific for sites on the opsonin (Fc receptors for antibody,

C3b receptors for C3b). This enables the phagocyte to bind an opsonized target very tightly to its surface. Antibody forms a stronger attachment, but C3b facilitates phagocytosis to a greater extent.

Although the inflammatory response is considered to be nonspecific, opsonins and other recognition molecules add a degree of specificity to efficient phagocytosis. Antibodies on the surface of bacteria are directed against antigens that are highly specific to that particular microorganism. If the complement fragment C3b serves as an opsonin, those bacteria with certain polysaccharide coatings are particularly sensitive to activation of the alternative and lectin pathways of complement activation.

Engulfment (endocytosis) is carried out by small pseudopods that extend from the plasma membrane and surround the adherent microorganism (see Figures 6-11 and 6-13) forming an intracellular phagocytic vacuole, or **phagosome**.[43] The membrane that surrounds the phagosome consists of inverted plasma membrane. After the formation of the phagosome,

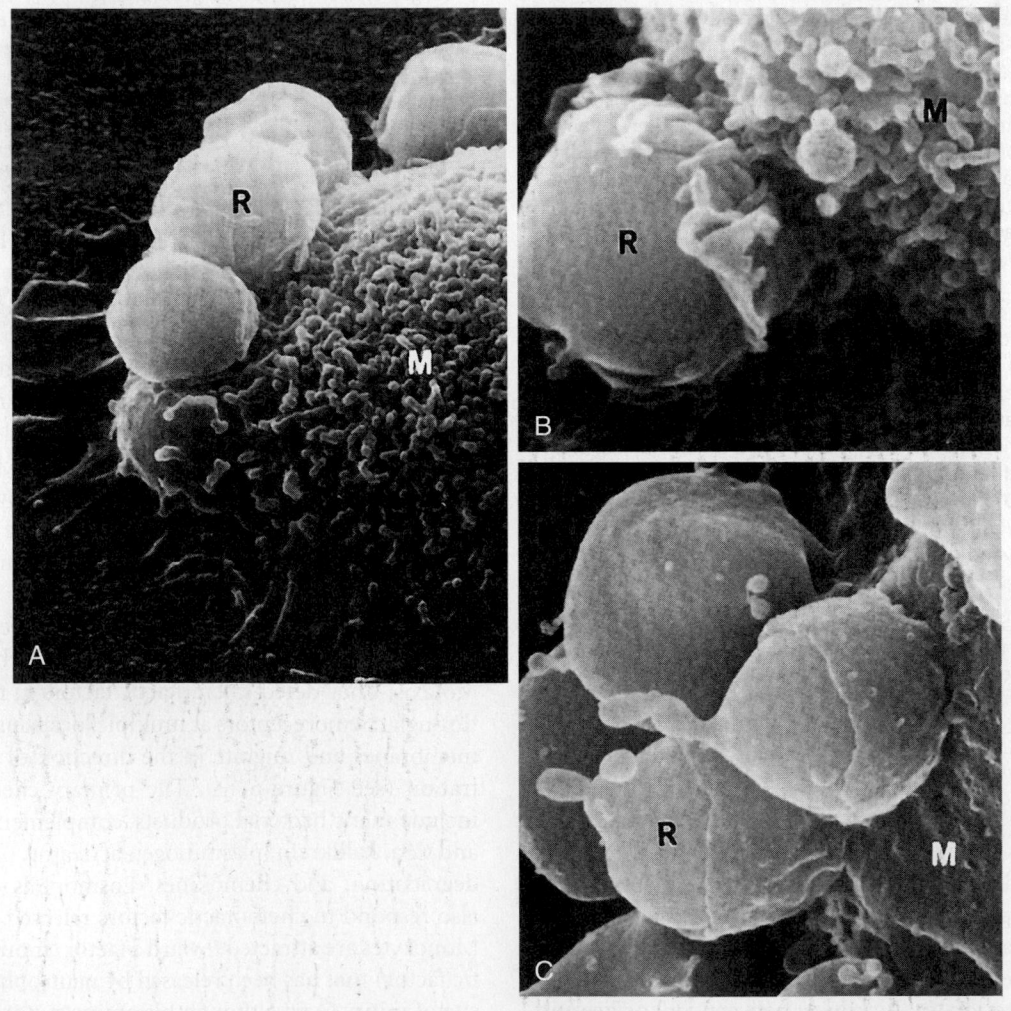

Figure 6-13 Steps in phagocytosis. This scanning electron micrograph shows the progressive steps in phagocytosis. **A,** Red blood cells *(R)* attach to the surface of a macrophage *(M)*. **B,** Part of macrophage *(M)* membrane starts to enclose the red cell *(R)*. **C,** The red blood cells are almost totally engulfed by the macrophage. (From King DW, Fenoglio CM, Lefwitch JH: *General pathology: principles and dynamics,* Philadelphia, 1983, Lea & Febiger.)

lysosomes converge, fuse with the phagosome, and discharge their contents, creating a **phagolysosome.** The **primary lysosomal granules** *(azurophilic granules)* contain a variety of bactericidal molecules, including myeloperoxidase, lysozyme, defensins, acid hydrolases, elastase, and others. Most phagocytes also contain **secondary granules** *(specific granules)* with molecules that are bactericidal and involved in remodeling the surrounding tissue, including lysozyme, collagenase, lactoferrin, and other proteases. Destruction of the bacterium takes place within the phagolysosome and is accomplished by both oxygen-dependent and oxygen-independent mechanisms.[44]

Phagocytosis is accompanied by a burst of oxygen uptake by the phagocyte, termed the "respiratory burst," which results from a shift in much of the cell's glucose metabolism to the hexose-monophosphate shunt. The nicotinamide adenine dinucleotide phosphate (NADPH) that is produced because of this shift is used by a membrane-associated enzyme, NADPH oxidase, to generate superoxide, a reactive oxygen intermediate that is converted to hydrogen peroxide and other reactive oxygen species.[45] These steps comprise the *oxygen-dependent killing mechanism.* Many of the reactive oxygen species are directly toxic to the microorganism. Hydrogen peroxide also can collaborate with the lysosomal enzyme *myeloperoxidase* and halide anions (Cl^- and Br^-) to form acids, such as hypochlorous (HClO) and hypobromous (HBrO) acids. These acids probably kill bacteria and fungi by adding Cl^- or Br^- to the surface of these cells. *Oxygen-independent mechanisms* of microbial killing are likely the result of (1) the acidic pH (3.5 to 4.0) of the phagolysosome caused by lactic acid production; (2) cationic proteins, such as defensins and cathelicidins, that bind to and damage target cell membranes; (3) enzymatic attack of the mucopeptides in the target cell wall by lysozyme and elastase; and (4) inhibition of bacterial growth by lactoferrin binding of iron.

When a phagocyte dies at an inflammatory site, it frequently lyses (breaks open) and releases its cytoplasmic contents, including the lysosomal enzymes, into the tissue. Enzymes released from lysosomes can digest the connective tissue matrix, causing much of the tissue destruction associated with inflammation. The destructive effects of many enzymes released by dying phagocytes are minimized by natural inhibitors found in the blood, such as α_1-**antitrypsin,** a plasma protein produced by the liver. An inherited deficiency of α_1-antitrypsin often results in chronic lung damage and emphysema as a result of inflammation. (The pulmonary effects of α_1-antitrypsin deficiency are described in Chapter 33.) Released lysosomal products also may contribute to inflammation by increasing vascular permeability, attracting additional monocytes, and activating the complement and kinin systems.

Neutrophils

The **neutrophil,** or **polymorphonuclear neutrophil (PMN),** is a member of the granulocytic series and is named for the characteristic staining pattern of its granules as well as its multilobed nucleus.[46] Neutrophils are the predominant **phagocytes** in the early inflammatory site, arriving within 6 to 12 hours after the initial injury, where they ingest (phagocytose) bacteria, dead cells, and cellular debris. Several inflammatory mediators (e.g., some bacterial proteins, complement fragments C3a and C5a, and mast cell neutrophil chemotactic factor) specifically attract neutrophils from the circulation and activate them. Macrophages and lymphocytes, on the other hand, enter the site later, usually after 24 hours, and gradually replace the neutrophils.

Because the neutrophil is a mature cell incapable of division and sensitive to the acidic environment of inflammatory lesions, it is short lived at the inflammatory site and becomes a component of the purulent exudate, or *pus,* which is removed from the body through the epithelium or via the lymphatic system. (The lymphatic system is described in Chapter 25) The primary roles of the neutrophil are removal of debris in sterile lesions, such as burns, and phagocytosis of bacteria in nonsterile lesions.

Monocytes and Macrophages

The next phagocytes on the scene are monocytes and macrophages, which perform many of the same functions as neutrophils but for a longer time and in a later stage of the inflammatory response.[47,48] **Monocytes** are the largest normal blood cells (14 to 20 μm in diameter) and have a nucleus that is often indented or horseshoe shaped. Monocytes are produced in the bone marrow, enter the circulation, and migrate to the inflammatory site, where they develop into macrophages. Monocytes also appear to be the precursors of macrophages that are found in tissues (tissue macrophages, discussed in Chapter 7), including Kupffer cells in the liver, alveolar macrophages in the lungs, and microglia in the brain. **Macrophages** are generally larger (20 to 40 μm) and are more active as phagocytes than their monocytic precursors. Macrophages, particularly those residing in the tissues, are often important cellular initiators of the inflammatory response (Figure 6-14).

Monocyte-derived macrophages from the circulation may appear at the inflammatory site as soon as 24 hours after the initial neutrophil infiltration, but usually arrive 3 to 7 days

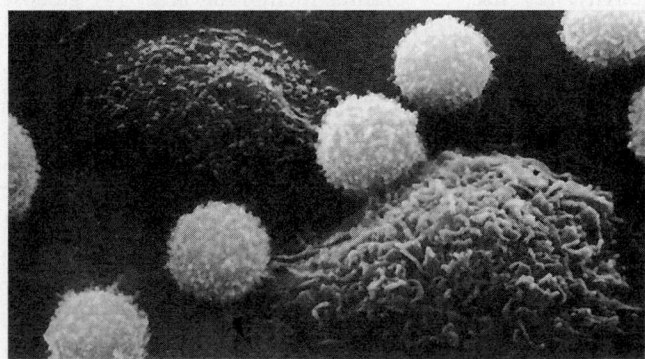

Figure 6-14 Scanning electron micrograph of lymphocytes and macrophages. The lymphocytes are small and spherical; the macrophages are larger and more irregular in shape. (From Raven PH, Johnson GB: *Biology,* St Louis, 1992, Mosby.)

later. They migrate to the site more slowly than neutrophils because they move more sluggishly and also because many of the chemotactic factors that attract them, such as macrophage chemotactic factor, must first be released by neutrophils. Macrophages are better suited than neutrophils to long-term defense against infectious agents because macrophages can survive and divide in the acidic inflammatory site or where there is low oxygen tension.

Neutrophils and monocytes/macrophages differ chiefly in the following ways:

1. *Speed:* Neutrophils arrive at the injury site first.
2. *Active life span:* Macrophages survive and divide in the inflammatory site, whereas neutrophils cannot.
3. *Chemotactic factors:* Neutrophils and macrophages are not attracted by the same factors.
4. *Enzymatic content of their lysosomes, or digestive vacuoles*
5. *Role in the immune response:* Macrophages, but not neutrophils, are involved in activation of the adaptive immune system.
6. *Role in wound repair:* Macrophages are the primary cells that infiltrate tissue in wounds, remove cells and cellular debris, and produce cytokines that suppress further inflammation and initiate healing.

Macrophage Activation

Several bacteria are resistant to killing by granulocytes and can even survive inside macrophages. Microorganisms such as *Mycobacterium tuberculosis* (tuberculosis), *Mycobacterium leprae* (leprosy), *Salmonella typhi* (typhoid fever), *Brucella abortus* (brucellosis), and *Listeria monocytogenes* (listeriosis) can remain dormant or even multiply inside the phagolysosomes of macrophages. However, the bactericidal activity of macrophages can be markedly increased with the help of inflammatory **cytokines** produced by cells of the acquired immune system (subsets of T lymphocytes) or cells activated through Toll-like receptors. (Cytokines are discussed in detail later in this chapter.) Macrophages have cell surface receptors for these cytokines and are further activated to become more effective killers of infectious microorganisms.

Macrophage activation results in increased (1) phagocytic activity, (2) size, (3) plasma membrane area, (4) glucose metabolism, and (5) number of lysosomes.[49] Activated macrophages also secrete factors that stimulate the growth, differentiation, and activation of additional inflammatory cells as well as control the initiation of healing processes. These include granulocyte colony-stimulating factor (G-CSF), gamma interferon (IFN-γ), interleukin-1 (IL-1β), angiogenic factor, fibroblast activating factor, and growth factors that promote regrowth of damaged tissues. Macrophages are also the primary cells that infiltrate wounds to remove cellular debris and initiate the regenerative process.[50] In some cases, inadequate macrophage activation results from defects in acquired immune responses and deficits in the production of appropriate cytokines. For example, a form of leprosy called *lepromatous leprosy* is characterized by the survival of phagocytosed *M. leprae* bacteria in macrophage phagolysosomes.

In individuals with lepromatous leprosy, cells of the acquired immune system have failed to secrete the cytokines necessary to transform macrophages into highly efficient killing cells.

Eosinophils

Another population of granulocytes is the **eosinophil.** Although eosinophils are only mildly phagocytic, they have two specific functions: (1) they serve as the body's primary defense against parasites and (2) they help regulate vascular mediators released from mast cells.[51] Their role in resistance to parasites occurs in collaboration with specific antibodies produced by the acquired immune system and will be discussed in Chapter 7.

The second function, regulation of mast cell-derived inflammatory mediators, is a critical function of eosinophils. As with most defense systems of the body, the acute inflammatory response is usually needed only in a circumscribed area and for a limited time. Therefore, control mechanisms are necessary to prevent biochemical mediators from evoking more inflammation than is needed. Mast cells produce ECF-A, which attracts eosinophils to the site of inflammation. Eosinophil lysosomes contain several enzymes that degrade vasoactive molecules, thereby controlling the vascular effects of inflammation. These enzymes include histaminase, which mediates the degradation of histamine, and arylsulfatase B, which mediates the degradation of some of the lipid-derived mediators produced by mast cells.

Basophils

The **basophil** is the least prevalent granulocyte in the blood. It is very similar to mast cells in the content of its granules and, in addition, is an important source of the cytokine IL-4, which is a key regulator of the acquired immune response.[52] Although often associated with allergies and asthma, its primary role is yet unknown.

Natural Killer Cells

The main function of **natural killer (NK) cells** is recognition and elimination of cells infected with viruses, although they are also somewhat effective at elimination of other abnormal host cells, specifically cancer cells. NK cells seem to be more efficient in this role when they encounter an infected cell within the circulatory system as opposed to within tissues.[53] Along with TLRs, NK cells have additional inhibitory and activating receptors that allow differentiation between infected or tumor cells and normal cells. If the NK cell binds to a target cell through activating receptors, it produces several cytokines and toxic molecules that can kill the target. (Mechanisms of cell to cell killing by NK cells and T cells are discussed further in Chapter 7.)

Platelets

Platelets (thrombocytes) are cellular fragments formed from megakaryocytes. They circulate in the bloodstream until vascular injury occurs. After injury, platelets can be activated by many products of both the innate and adaptive immune responses, including collagen, thrombin, thromboxane, PAF, and antigen-antibody complexes. Activation results in (1) their interaction with components of the coagulation cascade to stop bleeding and (2) degranulation. Platelets contain alpha (α) granules and dense granules. *Alpha granules* generally contain polypeptides that affect inflammation, including coagulation proteins (e.g., fibrinogen, factor V), soluble adhesion molecules (e.g., von Willebrand factor, vitronectin), growth factors (e.g., platelet-derived growth factor, epidermal growth factor), protease inhibitors (e.g., plasminogen activator inhibitor-1, α2-antiplasmin), and membrane adhesion molecules (e.g., P-selectin, αIIbβ3). *Dense granules* contain several small molecules, including adenosine diphosphate (ADP), serotonin, calcium, and magnesium. Serotonin is a vasoactive amine with vascular effects similar to those of histamine. (Platelet function is described in detail in Chapter 25.)

Cellular Products

To elicit an effective inflammatory (or acquired immune) response, it is necessary that many different kinds of cells cooperate. Many cells secrete soluble factors that contribute to the regulation of innate or acquired resistance by affecting other neighboring cells (Figure 6-15). These factors are referred to as *chemokines* or *cytokines* and are either *pro-inflammatory* or *anti-inflammatory* in nature, depending on whether they tend to induce or inhibit the inflammatory response.[54] These molecules usually diffuse over short distances, bind to the appropriate target cells, and affect the function of the target cell. Some effects occur over long distances, such as the systemic induction of fever by some cytokines (i.e., endogenous pyrogens) that are produced at an inflammatory site. The binding of chemokines or cytokines to a target cell often induces synthesis of additional cellular products. For example, binding of the cytokine TNF-α to a cell may result in synthesis and release of IL-1. Chemokine and cytokine binding is mediated through specific cell-surface receptors that are themselves sometimes under the regulation of secreted cellular products.

The actions of chemokines and cytokines are *pleiotropic*, indicating that the same molecule may have a large variety of different biologic activities depending on the particular target cell to which it binds. In addition, the same molecule may be

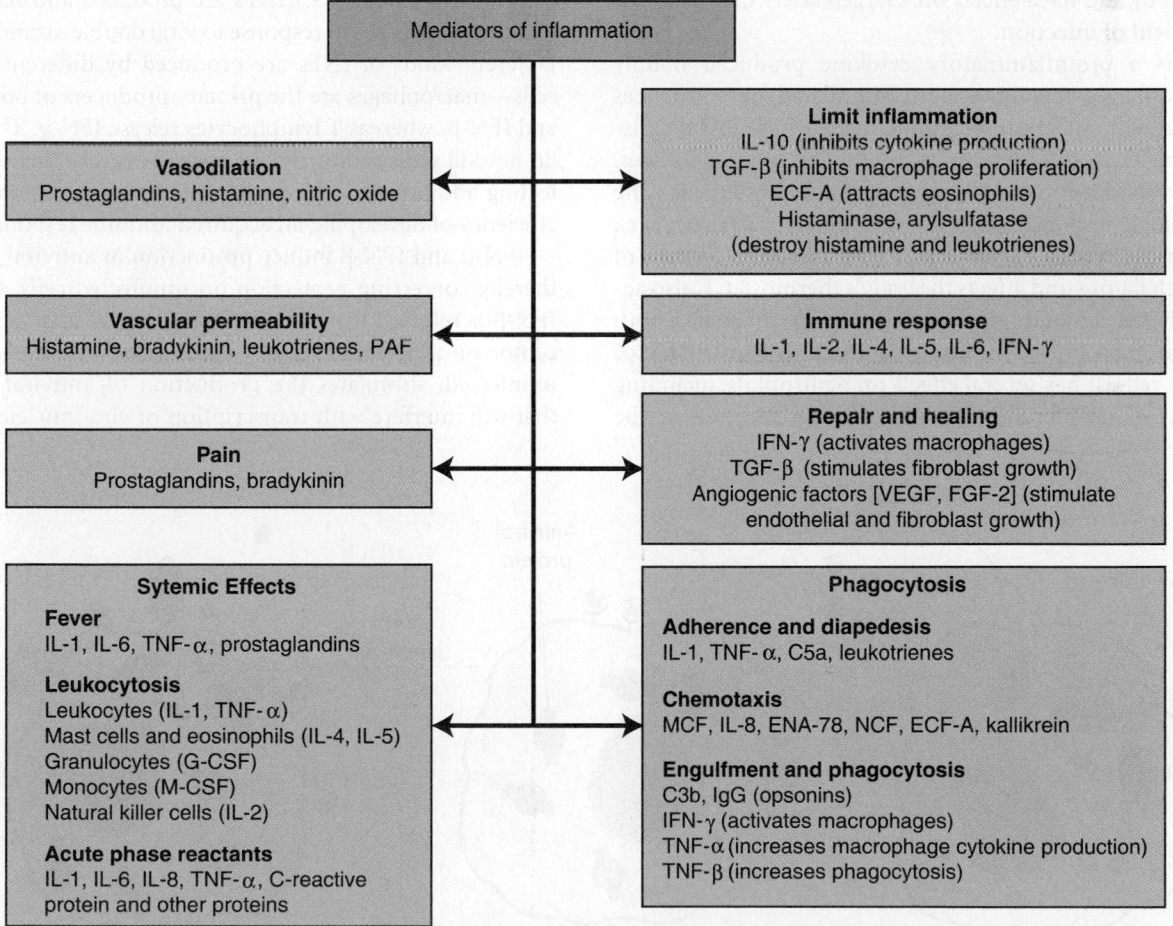

Figure 6-15 **Principal mediators of inflammation.** *C3b,* Large fragment produced from complement component C3; *C5a,* small fragment produced from complement component C5; *ECF-A,* eosinophil chemotactic factor of anaphylaxis; *ENA,* epithelial-dermoid neutrophil attractant; *FGF,* fibroblast growth factor; *G-CSF,* granulocyte colony-stimulating factor; *IFN,* interferon; *IgG,* immunoglobulin G (predominant class of antibody in the blood); *IL,* interleukin; *MCF,* monocyte chemotactic factor; *M-CSF,* monocyte colony-stimulating factor; *NCF,* neutrophil chemotactic factor; *PAF,* platelet-activating factor; *TGF,* T-cell growth factor; *TNF,* tumor necrosis factor; *VEGF,* vascular endothelial growth factor.

produced by a large spectrum of cells, many of which are not part of inflammation or the immune system. These molecules may be *synergistic,* so that their combined activity exceeds the sum of their individual activities, or have *antagonistic* properties that cause them to inhibit each other. (A partial list of relevant cytokines is provided in Chapter 7, Table 7-5.)

Cytokines

The majority of important cytokines are classified as ILs or IFNs. Other critical cytokines, however, are not classified as either. Many of these same cytokines are produced by cells of the acquired immune system in response to specific antigens and are discussed further in Chapter 7.

Interleukins

The **interleukins (ILs)** are biochemical messengers produced predominantly by macrophages and lymphocytes in response to their recognition of a microorganism or stimulation by other products of inflammation. One important function of this class of cytokines is enhancement of the acquired immune response against pathogenic microorganisms and other foreign substances. Interleukins, however, are both produced by and have effects on a large variety of cells, often independent of infection.

IL-1 is a proinflammatory cytokine produced mainly by macrophages that have been stimulated by substances associated with infection, including many of the PAMPs discussed earlier in this chapter, as well as by other cytokines. IL-1 is synthesized in two forms, α and β that often elicit the same biologic responses. IL-1 is an endogenous pyrogen (i.e., fever-causing cytokine) that reacts with receptors on cells of the hypothalamus and affects the body's thermostat. It also activates phagocytes and lymphocytes, thereby enhancing both the innate and acquired immunity, and acts as a growth factor for many cells. It has several effects on neutrophils, including induction of proliferation (resulting in an increase in the

number of circulating neutrophils), chemotaxis, increased cellular respiration, and increased lysosomal enzyme activity.

IL-10 is an example of an anti-inflammatory cytokine and is primarily produced by lymphocytes to down-regulate both the inflammatory and acquired immune responses. IL-10 suppresses growth of lymphocytes and production of proinflammatory cytokines by macrophages.

More than 30 human interleukins have been identified, although the functions of several have not yet been defined. Their varied effects include the following:

1. Alteration of adhesion molecule expression on many types of cells
2. Induction of leukocyte chemotaxis
3. Induction of proliferation and maturation of leukocytes in the bone marrow
4. General enhancement or suppression of inflammation (see Table 7-5)

Interferons

Interferons (INFs) are low-molecular-weight proteins that primarily protect against viral infections and modulate the inflammatory response. (Mechanisms of viral infection are described in Chapter 9.) INFs are produced and released by virally infected cells in response to viral double-stranded RNA. Different kinds of INFs are produced by different types of cells—macrophages are the primary producers of both IFN-α and IFN-β, whereas T lymphocytes release IFN-γ. These INFs do not kill viruses directly but instead prevent them from infecting additional healthy cells. Interferons also enhance the efficiency of developing an acquired immune response.

IFN-α and IFN-β induce production of antiviral proteins, thereby conferring protection on uninfected cells. IFN-α or IFN-β is released from virally infected cells, attaches to a receptor on a neighboring cell, and if the neighboring cell is uninfected, stimulates the production of antiviral proteins that will interfere with transcription of viral nucleic acids or

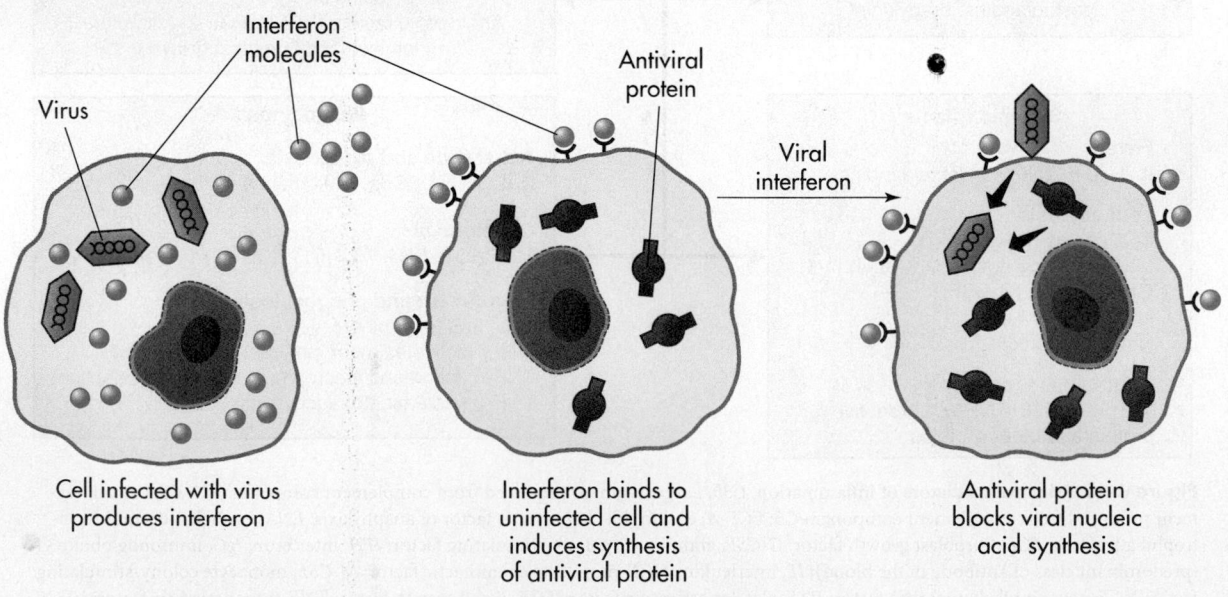

| Cell infected with virus produces interferon | Interferon binds to uninfected cell and induces synthesis of antiviral protein | Antiviral protein blocks viral nucleic acid synthesis |

Figure 6-16 The action of interferon.

with viral replication (Figure 6-16). These interferons have no effect on cells that have already been virally infected. IFN-γ enhances the inflammatory response by increasing the microbicidal activity of macrophages. This cytokine also facilitates development of the acquired immune response against viral antigens on infected cells. Interferons are species specific, meaning that human interferon is effective only in humans; however, these cytokines are not virus specific, meaning that they are effective against almost all viruses.

Other Cytokines

Despite the numerous interleukins and interferons, other essential cytokines are needed to mount an efficient inflammatory response. One of the most important of these is **tumor necrosis factor-alpha (TNF-α)**. Macrophages secrete TNF-α in response to recognition of PAMPs by TLRs. Other cells, such as mast cells, are additional and crucial sources of this proinflammatory cytokine.[55] TNF-α is initially synthesized as a membrane-spanning protein, which is cleaved into a soluble form by a membrane-associated protease, TNF-converting enzyme (TACE). Soluble TNF-α induces a multitude of proinflammatory effects, including enhancement of endothelial cell adhesion molecule expression and induction of chemokine production by both endothelial cells and macrophages. When secreted in large amounts, TNF-α has systemic effects as well:

1. Induces fever by acting as an endogenous pyrogen
2. Causes increased synthesis of proinflammatory proteins by the liver
3. Causes muscle wasting (cachexia) and intravascular thrombosis as a consequence of prolonged production in cases of severe infection or cancer

Chemokines

Chemokines are members of a family of low-molecular-weight (8 to 10 kDa) peptides that function primarily to induce leukocyte chemotaxis.[56] This response can be elicited either by soluble chemokines or by chemokines that are bound to extracellular glycosaminoglycan carbohydrates. Chemokines can be synthesized by multiple cell types, including macrophages, fibroblasts, and endothelial cells, in response to pro-inflammatory cytokines. Macrophages can be stimulated to produce chemokines by recognition of either infectious microorganisms or a β-defensin (both through TLR-4). To date, more than 40 different human chemokines have been described, the vast majority of which are classified as either CC-chemokines (β-chemokines) or CXC-chemokines (α-chemokines), depending on the arrangement of cysteine amino acids in the protein.[57] This amino acid arrangement also determines which target cell(s) will respond to a given chemokine. CC-chemokines affect mainly monocytes, lymphocytes, and eosinophils, whereas CXC-chemokines generally affect neutrophils. Examples of CC-chemokines include RANTES (regulated on activation, normal T expressed and secreted), monocyte/macrophage chemotactic proteins (MCP-1, MCP-2, and MCP-3), and macrophage inflammatory proteins (MIP-1α and MIP-1β). CXC-chemokines include IL-8 and epithelial-dermoid neutrophil attractant (ENA-78).

LOCAL MANIFESTATIONS OF INFLAMMATION

The cells and plasma protein systems described previously interact to produce all the characteristics of inflammation, whether local or systemic, as well as determine the duration of inflammation, either acute or chronic. Local inflammation accompanies all types of cellular and tissue injury, whether infected or sterile, from fractures or strains of the musculoskeletal system to burn injuries (see Chapter 2) and is responsible for initiating healing.

All the *local* manifestations of acute inflammation (i.e., swelling, pain, heat, and redness) result from vascular changes and the subsequent leakage of circulating components into the tissue. **Heat** and **redness** are the result of vasodilation and increased blood flow through the injured site. **Swelling** occurs as exudate (fluid and cells) accumulates. Swelling is usually accompanied by **pain** caused by pressure exerted by exudate accumulation, as well as the presence of soluble biochemical mediators such as prostaglandins and bradykinin. Loss of function may be associated with these manifestations.

Exudate varies in composition, depending on the stage of the inflammatory response and, to some extent, the injurious stimulus. In early or mild inflammation, the exudate is watery (**serous**) with very few plasma proteins or leukocytes. An example of serous exudate is the fluid in a blister. In more severe or advanced inflammation, the exudate may be thick and clotted (**fibrinous exudate**), such as in the lungs of individuals with pneumonia. If a large number of leukocytes accumulate, as in persistent bacterial infections, the exudate consists of pus and is called a **purulent (suppurative) exudate.** Purulent exudate is characteristic of walled-off lesions (**cysts** or **abscesses**). If bleeding occurs, the exudate is filled with erythrocytes and is described as a **hemorrhagic exudate.**

Although the local manifestations of inflammation can affect all vascularized tissues, lesions vary depending on the organ or tissue involved. The lesion resulting from widespread cellular death (necrosis), for example, differs in myocardial (heart muscle), brain, and hepatic (liver) tissues. Cellular death resulting from myocardial infarction (deprivation of oxygen caused by cessation of blood flow) causes a response that proceeds to replacement of the dead tissue with a fibrinous scar. The same injury to brain tissue is more likely to result in the formation of an abscess filled with necrotic tissue (types of necrosis are described in Chapter 2). Destruction of liver tissue stimulates the regrowth, or regeneration, of liver cells.

SYSTEMIC MANIFESTATIONS OF ACUTE INFLAMMATION

The three primary *systemic* changes associated with the acute inflammatory response are fever, leukocytosis (a transient increase in circulating leukocytes), and increased levels in circulating plasma proteins.

Fever

An early systemic response is **fever,** which is partially induced by specific cytokines, for example, IL-1 released from neutrophils and macrophages.[58] These fever-causing cytokines are known as **endogenous pyrogens** to differentiate them from pathogen-produced *exogenous pyrogens.* Pyrogens act directly on the hypothalamus, the portion of the brain that controls the body's thermostat. The release of endogenous pyrogens by inflammatory cells occurs after phagocytosis, after exposure to bacterial endotoxin, or after exposure to antigen-antibody complexes. (Mechanisms of temperature regulation are discussed in Chapter 15.)

The generation of a febrile response can be beneficial because the microorganisms that cause some conditions (e.g., syphilis, gonococcal urethritis) are highly sensitive to small increases in body temperature. On the other hand, fever may have some harmful side effects because it may enhance the person's susceptibility to the effects of endotoxins associated with gram-negative bacterial infections (bacterial toxins are described in Chapter 2).

Leukocytosis

Another systemic change associated with acute inflammation is **leukocytosis.** During many infections, numbers of circulating leukocytes, primarily neutrophils, increase. This increase is usually accompanied by a "left shift" in the ratio of immature to mature neutrophils, so that the more immature forms of neutrophils, such as band cells, metamyelocytes, and occasionally myelocytes, are present in relatively greater than normal proportions. (Chapter 25 discusses the development and maturation of blood cells.) Production of immature leukocytes increases primarily because proliferation and release of granulocyte and monocyte precursors in the bone marrow are stimulated by several products of inflammation, including complement product C3a and G-CSF.

Plasma Protein Synthesis

The synthesis of many plasma proteins, most of which are products of the liver, is increased during the primary stages of inflammation. These proteins, which can be either pro- or anti-inflammatory in nature, are referred to as **acute-phase reactants** (Table 6-4). Acute-phase reactants reach maximal circulating levels within 10 to 40 hours of initial infection. In addition to inducing fever, IL-1 also indirectly induces the synthesis of acute-phase reactants. IL-1 up-regulates release of IL-6, which then increases synthesis of acute-phase reactants directly by stimulating liver cells. Administration of IL-1 into animals leads to both fever and elevation of most acute-phase reactants, including fibrinogen, C-reactive protein, haptoglobin, amyloid A, α_1-antitrypsin, and ceruloplasmin.

Acute inflammation can be verified by a series of hematologic tests, which are described in detail in Chapter 25. For example, an increase in blood levels of acute-phase reactants, primarily fibrinogen, is usually associated with an increased erythrocyte sedimentation rate. The alteration in

Table 6-4	Circulating Levels of Acute-Phase Reactants During Inflammation	
Function	**Increased**	**Decreased**
Coagulation components	Fibrinogen Prothrombin Factor VIII Plasminogen	None
Protease inhibitors	α_1-Antitrypsin α_1-Antichymotrypsin	Inter-α-antitrypsin
Transport proteins	Haptoglobin Hemopexin Ceruloplasmin Ferritin	Transferrin
Complement components	C1s, C2, C3, C4, C5, C9, factor B, C1 inhibitor	Properdin
Miscellaneous proteins	α_1-Acid glycoprotein Fibronectin Serum amyloid A (SAA) C-reactive protein (CRP)	Albumin Prealbumin α_1-Lipoprotein β-Lipoprotein

plasma proteins probably leads to an enhanced erythrocyte rouleaux formation (stacking of erythrocytes, as in a stack of coins) and thereby an increased rate of sedimentation. Although increased erythrocyte sedimentation is a nonspecific reaction, it is considered a good indicator of an acute inflammatory response. Other symptoms of acute inflammation include somnolence (drowsiness), malaise (generalized feeling of discomfort or illness), anorexia (lack of desire to eat), and muscle aching.

CHRONIC INFLAMMATION

Superficially, the difference between acute and chronic inflammation is purely one of duration, in that chronic inflammation lasts 2 weeks or longer, regardless of cause. Characteristic histologic and mechanistic differences also may be present (Figure 6-17). Chronic inflammation is sometimes preceded by an unsuccessful acute inflammatory response. For example, if bacterial contamination or foreign objects (e.g., dirt, wood splinter, glass) persist in a traumatic wound, an acute response may be prolonged beyond 2 weeks. Pus formation, suppuration (purulent discharge), and incomplete wound healing may characterize this type of chronic inflammation.

Chronic inflammation can occur also as a distinct process without much previous acute inflammation. Some microorganisms (e.g., mycobacteria that cause tuberculosis) have cell walls with a very high lipid and wax content, making them relatively insensitive to degradation by phagocytes and therefore relatively resistant to clearance in an acute inflammatory response. Other microorganisms, such as those that cause

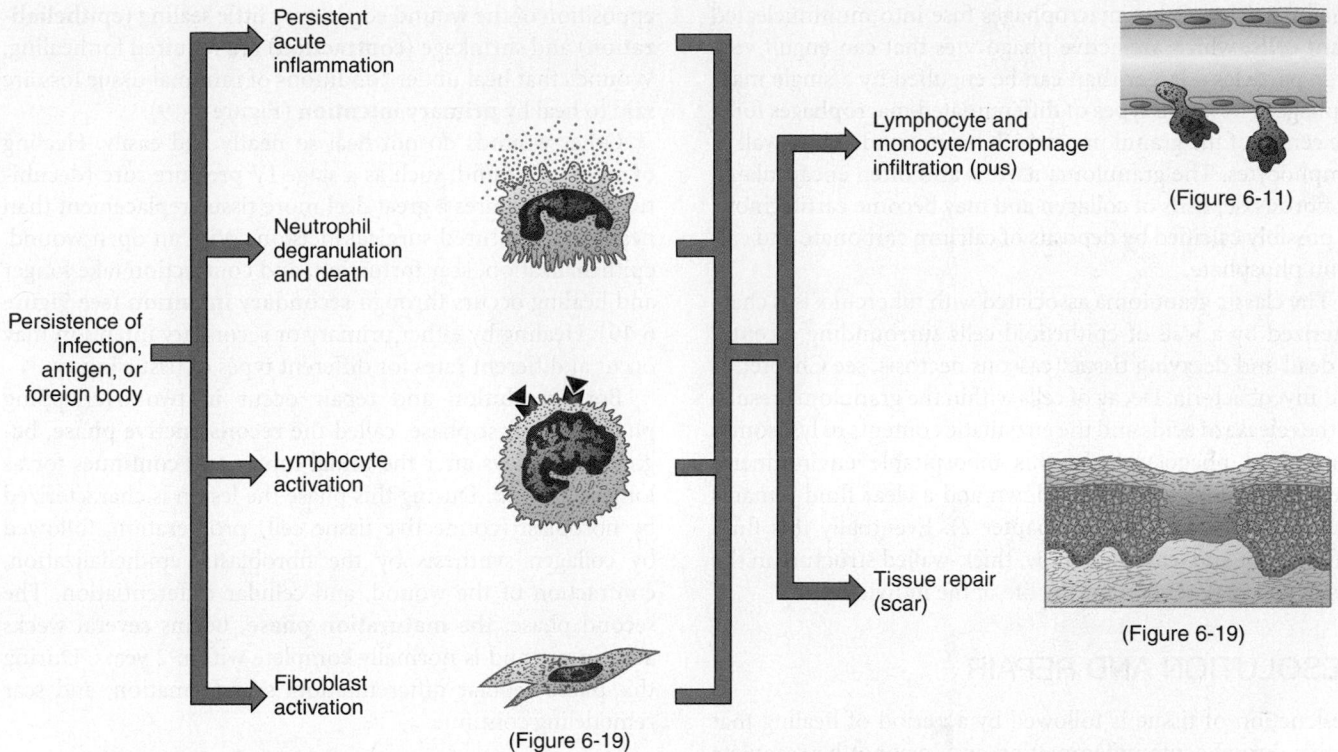

Figure 6-17 The chronic inflammatory response. Inflammation usually becomes chronic because of the persistence of an infection, an antibody, or a foreign body in the wound. Chronic inflammation is characterized by the persistence of many of the processes of acute inflammation. In addition, large amounts of neutrophil degranulation and death, the activation of lymphocytes, and the concurrent activation of fibroblasts result in the release of mediators that induce the infiltration of more lymphocytes and monocytes/macrophages and the beginning of wound healing and tissue repair.

leprosy, syphilis, and brucellosis, can survive within the macrophage and thereby also avoid clearance by the acute inflammatory response. In addition, some microorganisms produce toxins that stimulate tissue-damaging reactions even after they themselves are killed. Persistent inflammation can result from prolonged irritation by these toxins. Finally, chemicals, particulate matter, or physical irritants (e.g., inhaled dusts, wood splinters, and suture material) also can cause an inflammatory response that lasts longer than 2 weeks.

Chronic inflammation is characterized by a dense infiltration of lymphocytes and macrophages. If macrophages are unable to limit the tissue damage or infection, the body attempts to wall off and isolate the infected area, thus forming a **granuloma** (Figure 6-18). Granulomas may form if neutrophils and macrophages are unable to destroy microorganisms during the acute inflammatory response. For example, infections caused by some bacteria (*Listeria* sp., *Brucella* sp.), fungi (histoplasmosis, coccidioidomycosis) and parasites (leishmaniasis, schistosomiasis, toxoplasmosis) can result in granuloma formation. Large antigen-antibody complexes such as those present in rheumatoid arthritis also can result in the formation of these structures. The process of granuloma formation begins when some of the macrophages differentiate into large **epithelioid cells,** cells that are incapable of phagocytosing large bacteria but are capable of taking up debris and other

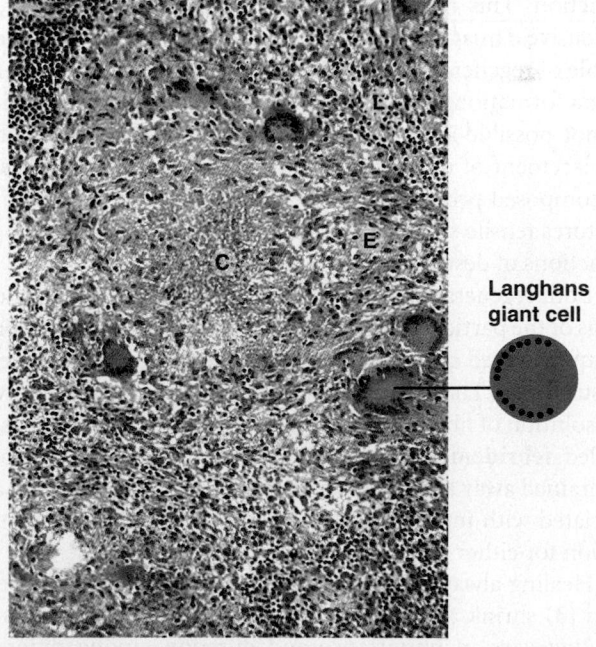

Figure 6-18 Tuberculous granuloma. A central area of amorphous caseous necrosis (C) is surrounded by a zone of lymphocytes (L) and enlarged epithelioid cells (E). Activated macrophages frequently fuse to form multinucleated cells (Langhans giant cells). In tuberculoid granulomas the nuclei of the giant cells move to the cellular margins in a horseshoe-like formation.

small particles. Other macrophages fuse into multinucleated **giant cells,** which are active phagocytes that can engulf very large particles—larger than can be engulfed by a single macrophage. These two types of differentiated macrophages form the center of the granuloma, which is surrounded by a wall of lymphocytes. The granuloma itself is also often encapsulated by fibrous deposits of collagen and may become cartilaginous or possibly calcified by deposits of calcium carbonate and calcium phosphate.

The classic granuloma associated with tuberculosis is characterized by a wall of epithelioid cells surrounding a center of dead and decaying tissue (caseous necrosis, see Chapter 2) and mycobacteria. Decay of cells within the granuloma results in the release of acids and the enzymatic contents of lysosomes from dead phagocytes. In this inhospitable environment, the cellular debris is broken down and a clear fluid remains (liquefaction necrosis, see Chapter 2). Eventually this fluid diffuses out and leaves a hollow, thick-walled structure in the tissue that may remain for the life of the individual.

RESOLUTION AND REPAIR

Destruction of tissue is followed by a period of healing that begins during acute inflammation and may not be complete for as long as 2 years.[59] The most favorable outcome of healing is tissue **regeneration** with complete return to normal structure and function. This is an ideal that is often not possible, particularly in adults. However, if damage is minor, no complications occur, and destroyed tissues are capable of regeneration, it is possible to return injured tissues to an approximation of their original structure and physiologic function. This restoration is called **resolution.** However, if extensive damage is present, if injury occurs in tissues not capable of regeneration, if infection results in abscess or granuloma formation, or if fibrin persists in the lesion, resolution is not possible and repair takes place instead. **Repair** is the replacement of destroyed tissue with scar tissue. **Scar tissue** is composed primarily of collagen that fills in the lesion and restores tensile strength but cannot carry out the physiologic functions of destroyed tissue.

Both regeneration and repair actually begin with phagocytosis of the particulate matter found at the site of injury (fibrin from dissolved clots, microorganisms, erythrocytes, and dead tissue cells). This cleanup of the lesion, which also involves dissolution of fibrin clots (or scabs) by fibrinolytic enzymes, is called **débridement.** After débridement, the remaining debris is drained away and the vascular dilation and permeability associated with inflammation are reversed, thus preparing the lesion for either regeneration or repair.

Healing always involves processes that (1) fill in, (2) seal, and (3) shrink the wound. These common denominators of healing vary in importance and duration among different types of wounds. A clean incision, such as a paper cut or a sutured surgical wound, heals primarily through the process of collagen synthesis. Because sealing of this type of wound has already been facilitated by minimal tissue loss and close apposition of the wound edges, very little sealing (**epithelialization**) and shrinkage (**contraction**) are required for healing. Wounds that heal under conditions of minimal tissue loss are said to heal by **primary intention** (Figure 6-19).

Other wounds do not heal so neatly and easily. Healing of an open wound, such as a stage IV pressure sore (decubitus ulcer), requires a great deal more tissue replacement than healing of a sutured surgical incision. With an open wound, epithelialization, scar formation, and contraction take longer and healing occurs through **secondary intention** (see Figure 6-19). Healing by either primary or secondary intention may occur at different rates for different types of tissue injury.

Both resolution and repair occur in two overlapping phases. The first phase, called the **reconstructive phase,** begins 3 to 4 days after the initial injury and continues for as long as 2 weeks. During this phase the lesion is characterized by fibroblast (connective tissue cell) proliferation, followed by collagen synthesis by the fibroblasts, epithelialization, contraction of the wound, and cellular differentiation. The second phase, the **maturation phase,** begins several weeks after injury and is normally complete within 2 years. During this phase cellular differentiation, scar formation, and scar remodeling continue.

Reconstructive Phase

Because surgical wounds exhibit both the reconstructive and maturation phases, they are useful models of both normal and abnormal (dysfunctional) healing. Such wounds are initially sealed off by a blood clot containing fibrin and trapped cells. The cross-linked mesh of fibrin is created by activation of the coagulation cascade and initially traps platelets to form a platelet plug that further seals damaged vessels (see Chapter 25). Most surgical wounds are completely sealed with platelet plugs within hours after closure. This sealing helps unite the wound edges and acts to create a physical barrier to bacterial invasion, although pathogenic invasion is not always prevented. The fibrin mesh ultimately acts as a scaffold for the collagen or regenerated tissue cells that ultimately fill the wound.

For healing to proceed, the fibrin clot must be dissolved and then replaced by normal tissue (for resolution) or scar tissue (for repair).[60] Enzymatic digestion of the clot usually occurs after activation of the plasma fibrinolytic system (plasmin generation, see Chapter 25) or release of lysosomal enzymes from dead neutrophils. Macrophages invade the dissolving clot and, by phagocytosis, clear away debris and dead cells. Débridement by macrophages and remaining neutrophils is followed by regeneration of destroyed cells (resolution) or, if regeneration is not possible, by repair (see Figure 6-19).

The process of healing begins as **granulation tissue** grows inward from surrounding healthy connective tissue. Granulation tissue is filled with new capillaries (angiogenesis) that give it a red, granular appearance and is surrounded by fibroblasts and macrophages. First, capillary buds sprout from vascular endothelial cells around the wound and extend into the débrided areas. Loops form when the young capillaries join (*anastomose*). The loops are more fragile and permeable

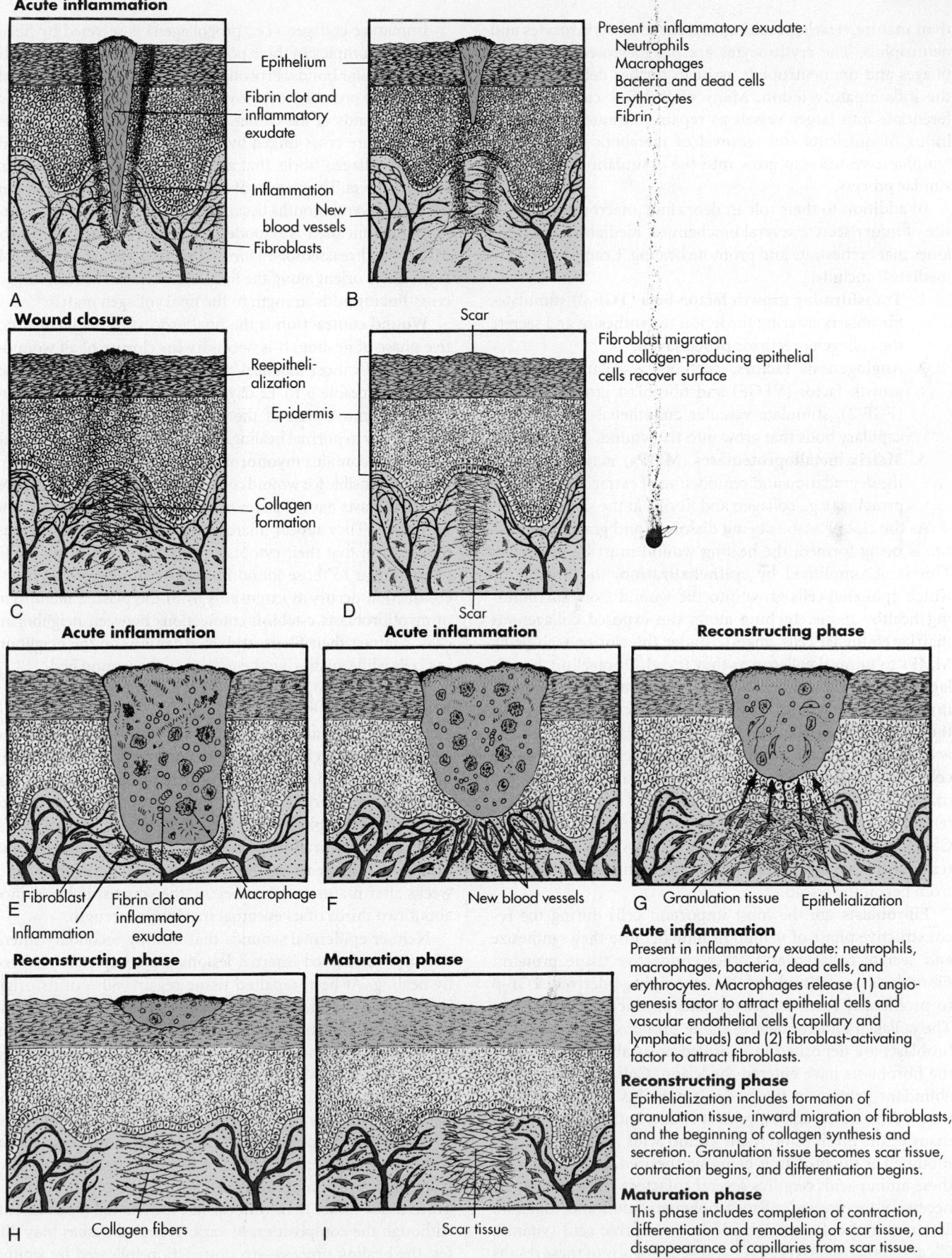

Acute inflammation

A — Epithelium, Fibrin clot and inflammatory exudate, Inflammation, New blood vessels, Fibroblasts

B — Present in inflammatory exudate:
- Neutrophils
- Macrophages
- Bacteria and dead cells
- Erythrocytes
- Fibrin

Wound closure

C — Reepithelialization, Epidermis, Collagen formation

D — Scar, Fibroblast migration and collagen-producing epithelial cells recover surface, Scar

Acute inflammation

E — Fibroblast, Fibrin clot and inflammatory exudate, Macrophage, Inflammation

Acute inflammation

F — New blood vessels

Reconstructing phase

G — Granulation tissue, Epithelialization

Acute inflammation

Present in inflammatory exudate: neutrophils, macrophages, bacteria, dead cells, and erythrocytes. Macrophages release (1) angiogenesis factor to attract epithelial cells and vascular endothelial cells (capillary and lymphatic buds) and (2) fibroblast-activating factor to attract fibroblasts.

Reconstructing phase

Epithelialization includes formation of granulation tissue, inward migration of fibroblasts, and the beginning of collagen synthesis and secretion. Granulation tissue becomes scar tissue, contraction begins, and differentiation begins.

Maturation phase

This phase includes completion of contraction, differentiation and remodeling of scar tissue, and disappearance of capillaries from scar tissue.

Reconstructing phase

H — Collagen fibers

Maturation phase

I — Scar tissue

Figure 6-19 Wound repair by primary or secondary intention. A to D, Healing by primary intention. E to I, Healing by secondary intention.

than mature vessels, resulting in leakage of erythrocytes and neutrophils. The erythrocytes are phagocytosed by macrophages and the neutrophils assist in further débridement of the inflammatory lesion. Many of the new capillaries differentiate into larger vessels as repair continues promoting influx of nutrients and removal of metabolic wastes. New lymphatic vessels also grow into the granulation tissue by a similar process.

In addition to their role in débriding, macrophages at the site of injury secrete several biochemical mediators and cytokines that orchestrate and promote healing. Examples of these mediators include:

1. **Transforming growth factor-beta (TGF-β)** stimulates fibroblasts entering the lesion to synthesize and secrete the collagen precursor **procollagen.**
2. **Angiogenesis factors,** such as vascular endothelial growth factor (VEGF) and fibroblast growth factor-2 (FGF-2), stimulate vascular endothelial cells to form capillary buds that grow into the wound.
3. **Matrix metalloproteinases (MMPs)** may function in the degradation and remodeling of extracellular matrix proteins (e.g., collagen and fibrin) at the site of injury.

As the clot or scab is being dissolved and granulation tissue is being formed, the healing wound must be protected. This is accomplished by **epithelialization,** the process by which epithelial cells grow into the wound from surrounding healthy tissue. Inching along the exposed collagenous matrix, epithelial cells migrate under the clot or scab using MMPs to unravel collagen as they travel. Unraveling the collagen enables the epithelial cells to move rather than remain immobile (see Figure 6-19); the intact collagen ahead of them provides a pathway on which they can maneuver forward. Eventually the migrating epithelial cells contact similar cells from all sides of the wound and seal it, thereby halting migration and proliferation. The epithelial cells undergo differentiation to give rise to the various epidermal layers (see Chapter 44). Epithelialization of a skin wound can be hastened if the wound is kept moist, preventing the fibrin clot from becoming a scab.

Fibroblasts are the most important cells during the reconstructive phase of wound healing because they synthesize and secrete collagen and other connective tissue proteins. Fibroblasts are stimulated by macrophage-derived TGF-β to proliferate, enter the lesion, and produce these proteins. The collagen and connective tissue proteins produced by fibroblasts are deposited in débrided areas about 6 days after the fibroblasts have entered the lesion. **Collagen** is the most abundant protein in the body. It contains high concentrations of the amino acids glycine, proline, and lysine, although many of the proline and lysine amino acids are enzymatically modified as the protein is being synthesized. Modification of these amino acids requires several cofactors and is absolutely necessary for proper collagen polymerization and function. The required cofactors include iron, ascorbic acid (vitamin C), and molecular oxygen (O_2); absence of any of these results in incomplete or impaired wound healing.

Immature collagen (i.e., procollagen) is secreted by fibroblasts as a complex of three polypeptide chains cross-linked by intermolecular bonds. Procollagen is converted to mature collagen by the proteolytic removal of small polypeptide sequences at both ends of the trimer. As healing progresses, collagen molecules are cross-linked by intramolecular covalent bonds to form collagen fibrils that are further cross-linked to form collagen fibers. The process of complete collagen matrix assembly takes several months because collagen is initially deposited randomly but then is remodeled by repeated dissolution (by MMPs) and reassembly. During this remodeling period, collagen fibers orient along the lines of mechanical stress; further cross-linking adds strength to the final collagen matrix.

Wound contraction is the final process of the reconstructive phase of healing. It is necessary for closure of all wounds, but especially those that heal by secondary intention. Contraction is noticeable 6 to 12 days after injury and may amount to inward movement of the wound edge by approximately 0.5 mm/day in normal healing. The granulation tissue of a healing wound contains **myofibroblasts**—specialized cells that are likely responsible for wound contraction. As their name implies, myofibroblasts have features of both smooth muscle cells and fibroblasts. They appear microscopically similar to fibroblasts, but differ in that their cytoplasm contains bundles of parallel fibers similar to those found in smooth muscle cells. Wound contraction occurs as extensions from the plasma membrane of myofibroblasts establish connections between neighboring cells, contract their fibers, and exert tension on the neighboring cells while anchoring themselves to the wound bed.

Maturation Phase

Collagen matrix assembly, tissue regeneration, and wound contraction all *begin* during the reconstructive phase but are not yet completed when the reconstructive phase ends, about 2 weeks after injury. Therefore, these processes continue into the **maturation phase**—a phase that can persist for years. During the maturation phase scar tissue is remodeled and capillaries disappear, leaving the scar avascular. Within 2 to 3 weeks after maturation has begun, the scar tissue has gained about two thirds of its eventual maximum strength.

Neither epidermal wounds that heal by secondary intention nor unsutured internal lesions are completely restored by healing. At best, repaired tissue regains 80% of its original tensile strength. Only epithelial, hepatic (liver), and bone marrow cells are capable of the complete mitotic regeneration known as *compensatory hyperplasia* (hyperplasia is described in Chapter 2). In fibrous connective tissue such as joints and ligaments, normal healing results in replacement of the original tissue with new tissue that does not have exactly the same structure or function as that of the original. Some tissues heal without replacement of cells. For example, damage resulting from myocardial infarction heals with a scar composed of fibrous tissue rather than with cardiac muscle cell replacement. Although the composition of various healed tissues may differ, the healing process—reconstruction followed by wound maturation—is essentially the same for all wounds.

Dysfunctional Wound Healing

Dysfunctional wound healing may occur if any of the involved processes occurs abnormally. This can include abnormalities in the inflammatory response itself, insufficient or excessive repair, or if a wound is reinfected. Abnormalities may result from a predisposing disease, such as diabetes mellitus, or from an acquired condition, such as hypoxemia (insufficient oxygen in arterial blood). Numerous drugs and nutrients can affect wound healing as well.

Dysfunction During Inflammatory Response

Healing may be prolonged if bleeding is not stopped during acute inflammation. *Hemorrhage* in a damaged area delays healing for several reasons. Initially the excess blood cells that accumulate at the site of injury must be cleared—a process that requires additional time. In addition to the cellular accumulation caused by excessive bleeding, formation of a clot increases the amount of space that granulation tissue has to fill and serves as a mechanical barrier to oxygen diffusion. The great amount of fibrin that is released during hemorrhage also must eventually be reabsorbed in order to prevent its organization into *fibrous adhesions*. Once formed, these **adhesions** can bind organs together by fibrous bands; with time, shrinkage of these bands can distort or strangulate nearby organs. This is clinically significant, particularly if they form within the pleural, pericardial, or abdominal cavities.

Accumulated blood as a result of hemorrhage also serves as an excellent culture medium for bacteria, promoting continued *infection* and prolonging inflammation by increasing purulent exudate formation. Prolonged infection can promote *excess scar formation* or even prevent healing completely. Continued infection of a wound, termed *wound sepsis*, can be clinically treated in several ways. Most important is the débridement of necrotic tissue and foreign bodies. This removal is accomplished either through surgery or through the use of absorbent dressings. Wound irrigation and antibiotic therapy also may assist in combating continued infection.

Although local hemorrhage during the inflammatory process can pose a huge impediment to healing, many additional factors, both physiologic and pharmacologic, also may adversely affect the healing of an inflamed tissue. *Hypovolemia*—decreased blood volume—hinders inflammation. The physiologic response to hypovolemia is vessel constriction rather than the dilation required to deliver inflammatory cells to the site of injury. Optimal nutrition is important during all phases of healing because metabolic needs are increased. The most essential nutrients for healing are glucose, oxygen, and amino acids. Because leukocytes need glucose to produce the energy needed for chemotaxis, phagocytosis, and intercellular killing, the wounds of persons with diabetes who receive insufficient insulin heal poorly, mainly due to a prolonging of infection. Persons with diabetes are also at risk for ischemic wounds because they are likely to have both small-vessel diseases that impair the microcirculation and altered (glycosylated) hemoglobin, which has an increased affinity for oxygen and thus does not readily release oxygen in tissues.[61] (Hemoglobin's function as the oxygen-carrying component of blood is described in Chapter 25.) Oxygen delivery is also compromised by hypoxemic states because ischemic tissue is susceptible to infection. *Hypoproteinemia* prolongs inflammation because the associated decrease in available amino acids is an impediment to fibroblast proliferation. Finally, anti-inflammatory steroids can have an impact upon wound healing. These drugs prevent macrophages from migrating to the site of injury and inhibit their release of collagenase and plasminogen activator. *Anti-inflammatory steroids* also inhibit fibroblast migration into the wound during the reconstructive phase of healing and impair angiogenesis, wound contraction, and reepithelialization.

Dysfunction During Reconstructive Phase of Healing

Three of the essential processes that occur during the reconstructive phase are assembly and remodeling of the collagen matrix, epithelialization of the wound bed, and contraction of the wound. Dysfunctional wound healing can result from the impairment of any of these processes.

Impaired Collagen Matrix Assembly

A number of factors may interfere with the production of collagen in healing tissues, most being nutritional. Scurvy, for example, is a condition caused by a deficiency in ascorbic acid, one of the cofactors required for the amino acid modification that is necessary for proper collagen matrix assembly. The complication of scurvy is a poorly formed collagen matrix and, therefore, greatly impaired wound healing. Other nutrients, including iron, copper, and calcium, play additional roles in the enzymatic reactions required for collagen modification and assembly. Usually, however, such minute amounts of these substances are required that deficiencies are not clinically significant. Nutritionally, appropriate protein intake is also essential for collagen synthesis. The amino acid methionine that is found in proteins is converted to cysteine, the role of which in collagen synthesis is twofold: (1) it functions as an important cofactor in the enzymatic reactions required for collagen synthesis; and (2) it contains sulfur, which contributes to formation of the strong covalent bonds in cross-linked collagen fibrils.

Dysfunctional healing also may result from excessive production of collagen. Overproduction of collagen causes surface overhealing, which is manifested in the skin by formation of a keloid or a hypertrophic scar (Figure 6-20). A **keloid** is a raised scar that extends beyond the original boundaries of the wound. It invades surrounding tissue and is likely to recur after surgical removal. A familial tendency toward keloid formation has been observed, with a greater incidence in blacks relative to whites. Similar to a keloid, a **hypertrophic scar** is also raised but differs in that it remains within the original boundaries of the wound. Hypertrophic scars tend to regress over time, whereas keloids do not. Both keloids and hypertrophic scars are caused by an imbalance between collagen synthesis and collagen degradation in which synthesis is increased relative to degradation. Although the precise mechanism of

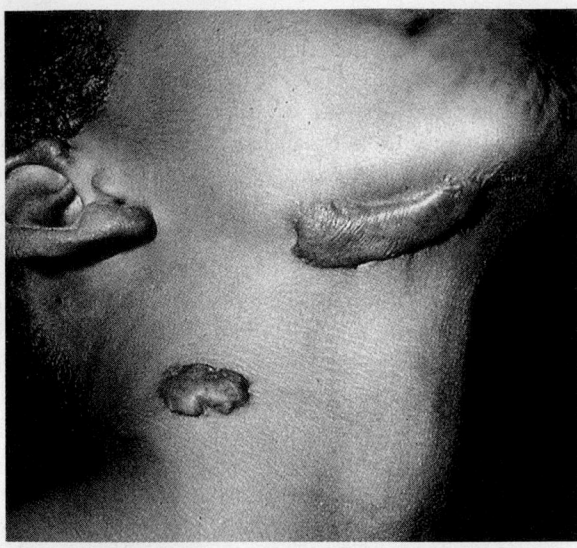

Figure 6-20 Keloids. (From Damjanov I, Linder J: *Anderson's pathology,* ed 10, St Louis, 1996, Mosby.)

this imbalance is unknown, recent evidence suggests that keloid fibroblasts have lower rates of apoptosis and an inability to respond to normal suppressive feedback.[62]

Impaired Epithelialization

The process of epithelialization is suppressed by anti-inflammatory steroids, hypoxemia, and nutritional deficiencies. Anti-inflammatory steroids inhibit phagocyte production of the biochemical mediators required for epithelialization, hypoxemia deprives cells of the energy required for the process, and dietary zinc is necessary for the MMP activity that is crucial to cellular migration.

Wound care techniques also may greatly influence epithelial cell migration. External wounds that are draining or healing by secondary intention often are clinically débrided and protected with dressings. The ideal dressing is one that absorbs some drainage without being incorporated into the clot or granulation tissue. Because epithelial cells must migrate across the wound during healing, dressings that débride healthy epithelial cells along with necrotic tissue prolong epithelialization. Many solutions that traditionally have been used to clean or irrigate wounds are now known to be deleterious to the fragile new cells in the wound bed. Normal saline is the most innocuous solution that can be used to cleanse or irrigate a wound that is healing primarily by epithelialization. Solutions such as povidone-iodine and hydrogen peroxide are desiccating (drying) and, as such, inhibit rather than promote epithelial cell migration.

Impaired Contraction

Excessive wound contraction may result in a deformity or **contracture.** Burn wounds are especially susceptible to the development of contractures. Internal contractures may occur as well, and are common in cirrhosis of the liver. Internally, scar tissue that becomes contracted constricts blood flow that may contribute to the development of portal hypertension and esophageal varices. Other types of internal contraction deformity include duodenal strictures caused by dysfunctional healing of an ulcer and esophageal strictures caused by chemical burns.

Proper positioning and range-of-motion exercises, as well as surgery, are among the physical means used to overcome the excessive myofibroblast-derived tension that results in contractures. Clinical use of pharmacologic methods for control of wound contracture is still largely experimental, but includes control of myofibroblast contraction by the administration of smooth muscle cell inhibitors such as colchicine and inhibition of proper collagen matrix assembly with drugs that prevent either collagen cross-linking or MMP activity. These latter treatments are based on the knowledge that myofibroblast binding to collagen can "lock" contracted cells into position.

Wound Disruption

Finally, a potential complication in the healing of wounds that are sutured closed is **dehiscence,** in which the wound pulls apart at the suture line. The greatest incidence of dehiscence occurs 5 to 12 days after suturing, paradoxically at the time when collagen synthesis is at its peak. Approximately 50% of dehiscence occurrences are associated with wound sepsis, although dehiscence also may occur when sutures break as a result of excessive strain. Obesity increases the risk of suture breakage because adipose tissue is difficult to suture. Wound dehiscence usually is heralded by an increase in serous drainage from the wound. In addition, patients may report a feeling that "something gave way." Prompt surgical attention is required.

Pediatrics and Mechanisms of Self-Defense

Neonates commonly have transiently depressed inflammatory and immune function. For example, neutrophils and perhaps monocytes may not be capable of efficient chemotaxis. Insufficient response to chemotactic factors appears to be caused by lack of fluidity in the phagocyte's plasma membrane so that pseudopod formation and migration are impaired. Neonates are prone to infections associated with chemotactic defects, including cutaneous abscesses caused by staphylococci and cutaneous candidiasis. Further, neutrophils in neonates who were stressed by in utero infection or respiratory insufficiency have diminished oxidative and bacterial responses. (Acquired phagocytic defects, which may be induced by a variety of infections, metabolic disorders, nutrition deficiencies, or drugs, are described in Chapter 8.)

Neonates also are partially deficient in complement, especially components of the alternative pathway. They tend to have a relative deficiency of factor B and to develop severe, overwhelming sepsis and meningitis when infected with bacteria against which there is no transferred maternal antibody. Low levels of mannose-binding lectin increase the risk for neonatal hospital-acquired sepsis.[63] Neonates also may be deficient in some of the collectins and collectin-like proteins. This is especially true of preterm neonates.[64] Some preterm infants with respiratory distress syndrome are deficient in at least one collectin, which provides innate defense against respiratory infections.

Aging and Mechanisms of Self-Defense

The older adult population is also at risk for impaired inflammation and wound healing. In some cases, impaired healing is not directly associated with aging in general but can instead be linked to a chronic illness such as cardiovascular disease or diabetes mellitus. In addition, many older adults require medications such as anti-inflammatory steroids that can interfere with the healing process.

Older adults have increased susceptibility to bacterial infections of the lungs, urinary tract, and skin. Because of impaired sensation or mobility and physiologic changes in the skin, older adults are at increased risk for sustaining various wounds. With aging, subcutaneous fat is lost, diminishing a layer of protection. Collagen fibers become thicker and a certain percentage of elastin is lost, further contributing to loss of protection. The regenerative capability of the skin is maintained with aging, but the epidermis undergoes age-associated changes that include atrophy of the underlying capillaries. The consequent decrease of perfusion makes older adults more susceptible than others to the adverse effects of hypoxia in the wound bed. In addition, aging fibroblasts may have a slower rate of proliferation and therefore wound healing is attenuated.[65]

Infections of other organ systems in older adults may be due to a diminished natural ability to ward off infection. Several cellular components of innate resistance are deficient in number (e.g., alveolar macrophages) or have diminished activity (e.g., neutrophil chemotaxis, degranulation, and phagocytosis). One explanation for this diminished inflammatory cellular activity is an age-related decrease in expression and function of several, if not all, TLRs.

SUMMARY REVIEW

Human Defense Mechanisms

1. There are two types of human defense mechanisms: innate resistance or immunity conferred by natural barriers and the inflammatory response, and the adaptive (acquired) immune system.

First Line of Defense: Physical, Mechanical, and Biochemical Barriers

1. Physical and mechanical barriers are the first lines of defense encountered by invading pathogens; these include the skin and mucous membranes.
2. Antibacterial peptides in mucous secretions, perspiration, saliva, tears, and other secretions provide a biochemical barrier against invading pathogens in the extracellular space.
3. Cathelicidins and defensins are two classes of antimicrobial peptides produced by epithelial cells.
4. The normal bacterial flora provide protection by inhibiting colonization by pathogens and by releasing chemicals that prevent infection.

Second Line of Defense: The Inflammatory Response

1. The inflammatory response, our body's second line of defense against invading microorganisms, is nonspecific, rapidly initiated, and has no memory cells.
2. The vascular response in acute inflammation includes vasodilation, increased capillary permeability, and white blood cell adherence to inner vessel walls and their migration through vessel walls.
3. Three plasma protein systems provide a biochemical barrier against invading pathogens in the circulation. These include the complement system, the clotting system, and the kinin system.
4. The plasma protein systems work with each other as well as with antimicrobial peptides and the cellular component of the innate immune system to prevent microbial infection.
5. The complement proteins can be activated in three pathways: the classical pathway, the alternative pathway, and the lectin pathway.
6. Activation of the complement pathways results in opsonization, activation of anaphylatoxins, cell lysis, and leukocyte chemotaxis.
7. The clotting (coagulation) cascade prevents spread of microorganisms, contains microorganisms and foreign bodies at the site of greatest inflammatory cell activity, and provides a framework for repair and healing.
8. The kinin system proteins promote vasodilation and increased capillary permeability and induce pain.
9. Plasmin and Hageman factor (factor XII) interact to activate the clotting cascade, the complement system, and the kinin proteins.
10. The plasma proteins are finely regulated to prevent injury to host tissue and to guarantee activation when needed. Some of the inhibitors in the plasma protein systems include carboxypeptidase, histaminases, kinases, and C1 esterase inhibitor.
11. Many different types of cells are involved in the inflammatory process including mast cells, neutrophils, monocytes/macrophages, eosinophils, NK cells, platelets, and nonleukocytic cells.
12. The cells of the innate immune system secrete many biochemical mediators that are responsible for the vascular changes associated with inflammation and for modulating the localization and activities of other inflammatory cells. The mediators include histamine, chemotactic factors, leukotrienes, prostaglandins, and platelet-activating factor.
13. The inflammatory response is initiated upon tissue injury or when PAMPs are recognized by PRRs on cells of the innate immune system.
14. The PRRs include TLRs, complement, scavenger, glycan, and mannose receptors.
15. TLRs recognize PAMPs, complement receptors recognize complement fragments, and scavenger receptors promote phagocytosis.
16. Most cells are central cells of inflammation and release histamine chemotactic factors, cytokines, leukotrienes, prostaglandins, growth factors, and other mediators.
17. H1-histamine receptors promote inflammation, and H2-histamine receptors inhibit the inflammatory response.
18. Phagocytosis is the destruction of microorganisms and cellular debris.
19. The stages of phagocytosis include recognition and adherence, engulfment, lysosomal fusion, and destruction.

SUMMARY REVIEW—cont'd

20. Phagocytic killing can be oxygen-dependent with the production of reactive oxygen intermediates or oxygen-independent with lysosomal enzymes.

21. Neutrophils are the predominant phagocyte of early inflammation. They are attracted to the inflammatory site by chemotactic factors.

22. Monocytes and macrophages arrive at the inflammatory site later than neutrophils and remain longer to clean up debris and promote wound healing.

23. Eosinophils help control mast cell vascular mediators and defend against parasite infection.

24. Basophils are granulocytes that are very similar to mast cells.

25. NK cells recognize and eliminate viruses, cancer cells, and other abnormal cells.

26. Platelets interact with the coagulation cascade to stop bleeding and release a number of mediators that promote and control inflammation.

27. Cytokines are soluble factors that regulate the inflammatory response and include interleukins, interferons, and tumor necrosis factor.

28. ILs are biochemical messengers primarily produced by macrophages and lymphocytes and significantly help regulate the inflammatory response.

29. IFNs provide protection from viral infection in uninfected cells.

30. Tumor necrosis factor is primarily produced by macrophages and promotes inflammation with both local and systemic effects.

31. Chemokines are synthesized by a number of different cells and induce leukocyte chemotaxis, and are classified as either CC or CXC, depending on their amino acid arrangement. CC chemokines affect monocytes, lymphocytes, and eosinophils. CXC chemokines generally affect neutrophils.

Local Manifestations of Inflammation

1. Local manifestations of inflammation are the result of the vascular changes associated with the inflammatory process, including vasodilation and increased capillary permeability. The symptoms include redness, heat, swelling, and pain.

2. The functions of the vascular changes are to dilute toxins, carry plasma proteins and leukocytes to the injury site, and carry bacterial toxins and debris away from the site.

Systemic Manifestations of Acute Inflammation

1. The three primary systemic effects of inflammation are fever, leukocytosis, and increase in levels of circulating plasma proteins.

2. Acute phase reactants are proteins produced by the liver during acute inflammation and include fibrinogen, C-reactive protein, haptoglobin, amyloid A, α_1-antitrypsin, and ceruloplasmin.

Chronic Inflammation

1. Chronic inflammation can be a continuation of acute inflammation that lasts 2 weeks or longer. It also can occur as a distinct process without much preceding acute inflammation.

2. Chronic inflammation is characterized by a dense infiltration of lymphocytes and macrophages. The body may wall off and isolate the infection to protect against tissue damage by formation of a granuloma.

Resolution and Repair

1. Resolution (regeneration) is the return of tissue to nearly normal structure and function. Repair is healing by scar tissue formation.

2. Inflammatory lesions proceed to resolution, meaning that original tissue structure and function have been restored if little tissue has been lost or injured tissue is capable of regeneration. This is called *healing by primary intention*.

3. Inflammatory lesions that involve extensive damage or tissues incapable of regeneration heal by the process of repair that results in the formation of a scar. This is called *healing by secondary intention*.

4. Resolution and repair occur in two separate phases: the *reconstructive phase*, in which the wound begins to heal, and the *maturation phase*, in which the healed wound is remodeled.

5. Dysfunctional wound healing can occur as a result of abnormalities in either the inflammatory response or in the reconstructive phase of resolution and repair.

Pediatrics and Mechanisms of Self-Defense

1. Neonates commonly have transiently depressed inflammatory function.

2. Infants often have deficiencies in complement and in a number of collectins, making them more susceptible to bacterial infection.

Aging and Mechanisms of Self-Defense

1. Older adults are at risk for impaired wound healing, often because of underlying illnesses.

2. Diminished immune function may interfere with an older adult's natural ability to ward off infection.

KEY TERMS

α_1-antitrypsin, 201
Abscess, 205
Acute-phase reactant, 206
Acquired immunity, 183
Adaptive immunity, 183
Adhesion molecule, 198
Adhesions, 211
Alternative pathway, 188
Anaphylatoxin, 189
Angiogenesis factor, 210

Antigen-antibody complex (immune complex), 188
Antimicrobial lectin, 186
Antimicrobial peptide, 185
Bactericidal/permeability-inducing protein, 186
Basophil, 202
Bradykinin, 191
C1 esterase inhibitor (C1 inh), 192
C3 convertase, 189

C5 convertase, 189
Carboxypeptidase, 189
Cathelicidin, 185
Cell lysis, 189
Chemokine, 205
Chemotactic factor, 189
Chemotaxis, 196
Classical pathway, 188
Coagulation cascade, 190
Collagen, 210

KEY TERMS—cont'd

Collectin, 186
Complement cascade, 188
Complement receptor, 194
Contraction, 208
Contracture, 212
Cyst, 205
Cytokine, 202
Débridement, 208
Defensin, 185
Dehiscence, 212
Diapedesis, 199
Endogenous pyrogen, 206
Endothelial cell, 199
Eosinophil, 202
Eosinophil chemotactic factor of
    anaphylaxis (ECF-A), 196
Epithelialization, 208, 210
Epithelioid cell, 207
Extrinsic pathway, 190
Exudate, 205
Fever, 206
Fibrinous exudate, 205
Fibroblast, 210
Giant cell, 208
Granulation tissue, 208
Granulocyte, 192
Granuloma, 207
Hageman factor (factor XII), 192
Heat, 205
Hemorrhagic exudate, 205
Hereditary angioedema, 192
Histamine, 196
Hypertrophic scar, 211
Inflammation, 183

Inflammatory response, 184, 186
Innate immunity, 183
Integrins, 195
Interferon (INF), 204
Interleukin (IL), 204
Intrinsic pathway, 190
Keloid, 211
Kinin system, 191
Kininase, 191
Lectin pathway, 188
Leukocytosis, 206
Leukotriene, 197
Macrophage, 201
Margination (pavementing), 199
Mast cell, 195
Mast cell degranulation, 189
Matrix metalloproteinase (MMP), 210
Maturation phase, 208, 210
Monocyte, 201
Myofibroblast, 210
Native immunity, 183
Natural barrier, 184
Natural immunity, 183
Natural killer (NK) cell, 202
Neutrophil, 201
Neutrophil chemotactic factor, 196
Normal bacterial flora, 186
Opsonin, 190
Pain, 205
Pathogen-associated molecular pattern
    (PAMP), 194
Pattern recognition receptor (PRR), 192
Phagocyte, 201
Phagocytosis, 198

Phagolysosome, 201
Phagosome, 200
Plasma kinin cascade, 191
Plasma protein system, 187
Plasmin, 192
Platelet, 202
Platelet-activating factor (PAF), 198
Polymorphonuclear neutrophil
    (PMN), 201
Primary intention, 208
Primary lysosomal granule, 201
Procollagen, 210
Proenzyme, 187
Prostaglandin, 197
Purulent (suppurative) exudate, 205
Reconstructive phase, 208
Redness, 205
Regeneration, 208
Repair, 208
Resistin-like molecule β, 186
Resolution, 208
Scar tissue, 208
Scavenger receptor, 195
Secondary granule, 201
Secondary intention, 208
Selectins, 199
Serous, 205
Swelling, 205
Toll-like receptor (TLR), 194
Transforming growth factor-beta
    (TGF-β), 210
Tumor necrosis factor-alpha
    (TNF-α), 205
Wound contraction, 210

REFERENCES

1. Tosi MF: Innate immune responses to infection, *J Allergy Clin Immunol* 116(2):241-249, 2005.
2. Dann SM, Eckmann L: Innate immune defenses in the intestinal tract, *Curr Opin Gastroenterol* 23(2):115-120, 2007.
3. Braff MH, Gallo RL: Antimicrobial peptides: an essential component of the skin defensive barrier, *Curr Top Microbiol Immunol* 306:91-110, 2006.
4. Yamasaki K, Gallo RL: Antimicrobial peptides in human skin disease, *Eur J Dermatol* 18(1):11-21, 2008.
5. Ooi EH, Wormald PJ, Tan LW: Innate immunity in the paranasal sinuses: a review of nasal host defenses, *Am J Rhinol* 22(1):9-13, 2008.
6. Holmskov U, Theil S, Jensenius JC: Collections and ficolins: humoral lectins of the innate immune defense, *Ann Rev Immunol* 21:547-578, 2004.
7. Kuroki Y, Takahashi M, Nishitani C: Pulmonary collectins in innate immunity in the lung, *Cell Microbiol* 9(8):1871-1879, 2007.
8. Wershil BK, Furuta GT: Gastrointestinal mucosal immunity, *J Allergy Clin Immunol* 121(2 Suppl):S380-S383, 2008.
9. Magalhaes JF, Tattoli I, Girardin SE: The intestinal epithelial barrier: how to distinguish between the microbial flora and pathogens, *Semin Immunol* 19(2):106-115, 2007.
10. Dempsey PW, Vaidya SA, Cheng G: The art of war: innate and adaptive immune responses, *Cell Mol Life Sci* 60(12):2604-2621, 2003.
11. Goldfarb RD, Parrillo JE: Complement, *Crit Care Med* 33(12):S482-S484, 2005.

12. Markiewski MM, Lambris JD: The role of complement in inflammatory diseases from behind the scenes into the spotlight, *Am J Pathol* 171(3):715-727, 2007.
13. Wills-Karp M: Complement activation pathways: a bridge between innate and adaptive immune responses in asthma, *Proc Am Thorac Soc* 4(3):247-251, 2007.
14. Lutz HU, Jelezarova E: Complement amplification revisited, *Mol Immunol* 43(1-2):2-12, 2006.
15. Gros P, Milder FJ, Janssen BJC: Complement driven by conformational changes, *Nat Rev Immunol* 8(1):48-58, 2008.
16. Thurman JM, Holers VM: The central role of the alternative complement pathway in human disease, *J Immunol* 176(3):1305-1310, 2006.
17. Degn SE, Thiel S, Jensenius JC: New perspectives on mannan-binding lectin-mediated complement activation, *Immunobiol* 212(4-5):301-311, 2007.
18. Haas P-J, van Strijp J: Anaphylatoxins: their role in bacterial infection and inflammation, *Immunol Res* 37(3):161-175, 2007.
19. Aird WC: Coagulation, *Crit Care Med* 33(12 Suppl):S485-S487, 2005.
20. Lwaleed BA et al: Tissue factor: a critical role in inflammation and cancer, *Biol Res Nurs* 9(2):97-107, 2007.
21. Schmaier AH, McCrae KR: The plasma kallikrein-kinin system: its evolution from contact activation, *J Thromb Haemost* 5(12):2323-2329, 2007.
22. Markiewski MM et al: Complement and coagulation: strangers or partners in crime? *Trends Immunol* 28(4):184-192, 2007.
23. Cicardi M, Zingale LC: The deficiency of C1 inhibitor and its treatment, *Immunobiol* 212(4-5):325-331, 2007.

24. Kawai T, Akira S: Pathogen recognition and Toll-like receptors, *Curr Opin Immunol* 17(4):338-344, 2005.

25. Kawai T, Akira S: TLR signaling, *Semin Immunol* 19(1):24-32, 2007.

26. Uematsu S, Akira S: Toll-Like receptors (TLRs) and their ligands, *Handb Exp Pharmacol* 183:1-20, 2008.

27. Arancibia SA et al: Toll-like receptors are key participants in innate immune responses, *Biol Res* 40(2):97-112, 2007.

28. Hawlisch H, Kohl J: Complement and Toll-like receptors: key regulators of adaptive immune responses, *Mol Immunol* 43(1-2):13-21, 2006.

29. Azhar S, Leers-Sucheta S, Reaven E: Cholesterol uptake in adrenal and gonadal tissues: the SR-BI and "selective" pathway connection, *Front Biosci* 8:S998-S1029, 2003.

30. Horiuchi S, Sakamoto Y, Sakai M: Scavenger receptors for oxidized and glycated proteins, *Amino Acids* 25(3-4):283-292, 2003.

31. Rhainds D, Brissette L: The role of scavenger receptor class B type I (SR-B1) in lipid trafficking: defining the rules for lipid traders, *Int J Biochem Cell Biol* 36(1):39-77, 2004.

32. Vliagoftis H, Befus AD: Mast cells at mucosal frontiers, *Curr Mol Med* 5(6):573-589, 2005.

33. Ehrlich P: Dietbage zur Kenntnis der Anilinsfarb und Ihrer Verwendung nin ungen der Mikroskopichen technik, *Arch Mikr Anat* 13:263, 1877.

34. Galli SJ, Tsai M: Mast cells: versatile regulators of inflammation, tissue remodeling, host defenses and homeostasis, *J Dermatol Sci* 49(1):7-19, 2007.

35. Hide M, Yanase Y, Greaves MW: Cutaneous mast cell receptors, *Dermatol Clin* 25(4):563-575, 2007.

36. Huang JF, Thurmond RL: The new biology of histamine receptors, *Curr Allergy Asthma Rep* 8(1):7-21, 2008.

37. Peters-Golden M, Henderson WR Jr: Leukotrienes, *N Engl J Med* 357(18):1841-1854, 2007.

38. Garrood T, Lee L, Pitzalis C: Molecular mechanisms of cell recruitment to inflammatory sites: general and tissue-specific pathways, *Rheumatol* 45(3):250-260, 2006.

39. Pober JS, Sessa WC: Evolving functions of endothelial cells in inflammation, *Nat Rev Immunol* 7(10):803-815, 2007.

40. Ley K et al: Getting to the site of inflammation: the leukocyte adhesion cascade updated, *Nat Rev Immunol* 7(9):678-689, 2007.

41. Woodfin A, Voisin M-B, Nourshargh S: PECAM-1: a multi-functional molecule in inflammation and vascular biology, *Arterioscler Thromb Vasc Biol* 27(12):2514-2523, 2007.

42. Stephens C, Fawcett TN: Nitric oxide and nursing: a review, *J Clin Nurs* 16(1):67-76, 2007.

43. Nauseef WM: How human neutrophils kill and degrade microbes: an integrated view, *Immunol Rev* 219(1):88-102, 2007.

44. Segal AW: How neutrophils kill microbes, *Ann Rev Immunol* 23:197-223, 2005.

45. Babior BM: NADPH oxidase, *Curr Opin Immunol* 16(1):42-47, 2004.

46. Marshall JS, King CA, McCurdy JD: Mast cell cytokine and chemokine responses to bacterial and viral infection, *Curr Pharm Des* 9(1):11-24, 2003.

47. Cavaillon J-M, Adib-Conquy M: Monocytes/macrophages and sepsis, *Crit Care Med* 33(12 Suppl):S506-S509, 2005.

48. Gordon S: The macrophage: past, present and future, *Eur J Immunol* 37(Suppl1):S9-S17, 2007.

49. Ma J et al: Regulation of macrophage activation, *Cell Mol Life Sci* 60(11):2334-2346, 2003.

50. Zhang X, Mosser DM: Macrophage activation by endogenous danger signals, *J Pathol* 214(2):161-178, 2008.

51. Hogan SP et al: Eosinophils: biological properties and role in health and disease, *Clin Exp Allergy* 38(5):709-750, 2008.

52. Min B, Paul WE: Basophils and type 2 immunity, *Curr Opin Hematol* 15(1):59-63, 2008.

53. Vivier E et al: Functions of natural killer cells, *Nat Immunol* 9(5):503-510, 2008.

54. Steinke JW, Borish L: Cytokines and chemokines, *J Allergy Clin Immunol* 117(2 Suppl Mini-Primer):S441-S445, 2006.

55. Galli SJ, Nakae S: Mast cells to the defense, *Nat Immunol* 4(12):1160-1162, 2003.

56. Allen SJ, Crown SE, Handel TM: Chemokine: receptor structure, interactions, and antagonism, *Annu Rev Immunol* 25:787-820, 2007.

57. Rot A, von Andrian UH: Chemokines in innate and adaptive host defense: basic chemokinese grammar for immune cells, *Ann Rev Immunol* 22:891-928, 2004.

58. Thompson HJ: Fever, a concept analysis, *J Adv Nurs* 51(5):484-492, 2005.

59. Broughton G 2nd, Janis JE, Attinger CE: Wound healing: an overview, *Plast Reconstr Surg* 117(7 Suppl):1e-S-32e-S, 2006.

60. Broughton G 2nd, Janis JE, Attinger CE: The basic science of wound healing, *Plast Reconstr Surg* 117(7 Suppl):12S-34S, 2006.

61. Sweitzer SM et al: What is the future of diabetic wound care? *Diabetes Educ* 32(2):198-210, 2006.

62. Robles DT, Berg D: Abnormal wound healing: keloids, *Clin Dermatol* 25(1):26-32, 2007.

63. de Benedetti F et al: Low serum levels of mannose binding lectin are a risk for neonatal sepsis, *Pediatr Res* 61(3):325-328, 2007.

64. Awasthi S et al: Deficiencies in lung surfactant proteins A and D are associated with lung infection in very premature neonatal baboons, *Am J Respir Crit Care Med* 163(2):389-397, 2001.

65. Renshaw M et al: Cutting edge: impaired Toll-like receptor expression and function in aging, *J Immunol* 169(9):4697-4701, 2002.

ADAPTIVE IMMUNITY

NEAL S. ROTE

MEDIA RESOURCES

 Evolve Website (http://evolve.elsevier.com/McCance/)
- Review Questions and Answers
- Animations
- Glossary (with audio pronunciation for selected terms)
- WebLinks

Online Course
- Module 5

CHAPTER OUTLINE

GENERAL CHARACTERISTICS OF ADAPTIVE IMMUNITY
   Humoral and Cell-Mediated Immunity
   Active vs. Passive Immunity
RECOGNITION AND RESPONSE
   Antigens and Immunogens
   Molecules That Recognize Antigen
   Molecules That Present Antigen
   Molecules That Hold Cells Together
   Cytokines and Their Receptors
GENERATION OF CLONAL DIVERSITY
   T-Cell Maturation
   B-Cell Maturation

INDUCTION OF AN IMMUNE RESPONSE: CLONAL SELECTION
   Secondary Lymphoid Organs
   Antigen Processing and Presentation
   Helper T Lymphocytes
   B-Cell Activation: The Humoral Immune Response
   T-Cell Activation: The Cellular Immune Response
EFFECTOR MECHANISMS
   Antibody Function
   T-Lymphocyte Function
      Fetal and Neonatal Immune Function
      Aging and Immune Function

The third line of defense in the human body is **adaptive (acquired) immunity,** often called the **immune response,** or **immunity.** Once external barriers have been compromised and inflammation (see Chapter 6) has been activated, the adaptive immune response is called into action. The molecules and cells of the immune response are closely integrated with those of the innate response. Many components of the innate response facilitate the development of the adaptive immune response. Conversely, products of the adaptive immune response use many components of the inflammatory response. Thus both systems are essential for complete protection against infectious disease: inflammation is relatively rapid, nonspecific, and short-lived, whereas adaptive immunity is slower acting, specific, and very long-lived. Because many inflammatory processes are triggered or affected by immune processes and vice versa, an understanding of both systems is necessary for a complete appreciation of how pathogenic infections are combated. Chapter 8 discusses medically relevant aberrations in both inflammation and

immunity, including allergies, diseases that involve unwanted immunologic destruction of healthy tissue, and diseases that are caused by a deficiency in the normal immune or inflammatory responses. Chapter 9 presents an overview of infection and Chapter 10 discusses the connection between stress and disease and the interrelatedness of the immune, nervous, and endocrine systems.

GENERAL CHARACTERISTICS OF ADAPTIVE IMMUNITY

The immune system of the normal adult is continually challenged by a spectrum of substances that it may recognize as foreign, or "non-self." These substances, called **antigens,** are often associated with pathogens such as viruses, bacteria, fungi, or parasites, although they are also found on noninfectious environmental agents such as pollens, foods, and bee venom, and still others are associated with clinically derived drugs, vaccines, transfusions, and transplanted tissues (Table 7-1). Unlike inflammation, which is nonspecifically activated by cellular damage as well as pathogenic microorganisms, the immune response is primarily designed to afford long-term specific protection (i.e., immunity) against particular invading microorganisms, that is, it has a "memory" function.[1] The products of the adaptive immune response include a type of serum protein—**immunoglobulins,** or **antibodies**—and a type of blood cell—**lymphocytes** (Figure 7-1).

Specificity and memory are the primary characteristics that differentiate the immune response from other protective mechanisms. This chapter first discusses the nature of that specificity by defining the various types of antigens that may be seen by the immune system, how they are recognized by antibodies and lymphocytes, and the specific intercellular recognition molecules that are necessary for effective immune responses. After the recognition molecules are defined, the development of the immune response is discussed. An immune response can be divided into two phases (Figure 7-2). Before birth, humans produce a large population of **T lymphocytes (T cells)** and **B lymphocytes (B cells)** that have the capacity to recognize almost any foreign antigen found in the environment. Each individual T or B cell, however, specifically recognizes only one particular antigen, but the sum of the population of lymphocyte specificities may represent millions of foreign antigens. This process is called the *generation of clonal diversity* and occurs in specialized (primary) lymphoid organs; the thymus for T cells and the bone marrow for B cells. While passing through these tissues, the lymphocytes mature and undergo changes that commit them to becoming either B or T cells. Lymphocytes are released from these organs into the circulation as immature cells that have the capacity to react with antigen (**immunocompetent**). These cells migrate to other (secondary) lymphoid organs in the body in preparation for exposure to antigen (Figure 7-3).

The lymphocytes remain dormant until antigen initiates the second phase of the immune response, *clonal selection*. This process involves a complex interaction among cells. To

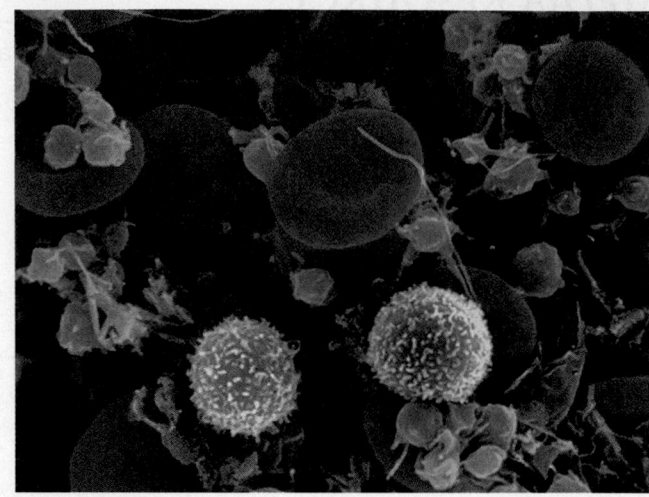

Figure 7-1 Scanning electron micrograph showing lymphocytes (yellow), red blood cells, and platelets. (Copyright Dennis Kunkel Microscopy, Inc.)

Table 7-1	Clinical Use of Antigen or Antibody			
	Use of Antigen or Antibody			
Antigen Source	**Protection: Combat Active Disease**	**Protection: Vaccination**	**Diagnosis**	**Therapy**
Infectious agents	Neutralize or destroy pathogenic microorganisms (e.g., antibody response against viral infections)	Induce safe and protective immune response (e.g., recommended childhood vaccines)	Measure circulating antigen from infectious agent or antibody (e.g., diagnosis of hepatitis B infection)	Passive treatment with antibody to treat or prevent infection (e.g., administration of antibody against hepatitis A)
Cancers	Prevent tumor growth or spread (e.g., immune surveillance to prevent early cancers)	Prevent cancer growth or spread (e.g., vaccination with cancer antigens)	Measure circulating antigen (e.g., circulating PSA for diagnosis of prostate cancer)	Immunotherapy (e.g., treatment of cancer with antibodies against cancer antigens)
Environmental substances	Prevent entrance into body (e.g., secretory IgA limits systemic exposure to potential allergens)	No clear example	Measure circulating antigen or antibody (e.g., diagnosis of allergy by measuring circulating IgE)	Immunotherapy (e.g., administration of antigen for desensitization of individuals with severe allergies)
Self-antigens	Immune system tolerance to self-antigens, which may be altered by an infectious agent leading to autoimmune disease (see Chapter 8)	Some cases of vaccination alter tolerance to self-antigens leading to autoimmune disease	Measure circulating antibody against self-antigen for diagnosis of autoimmune disease (see Chapter 8)	No clear example

PSA, Prostate-specific antigen.

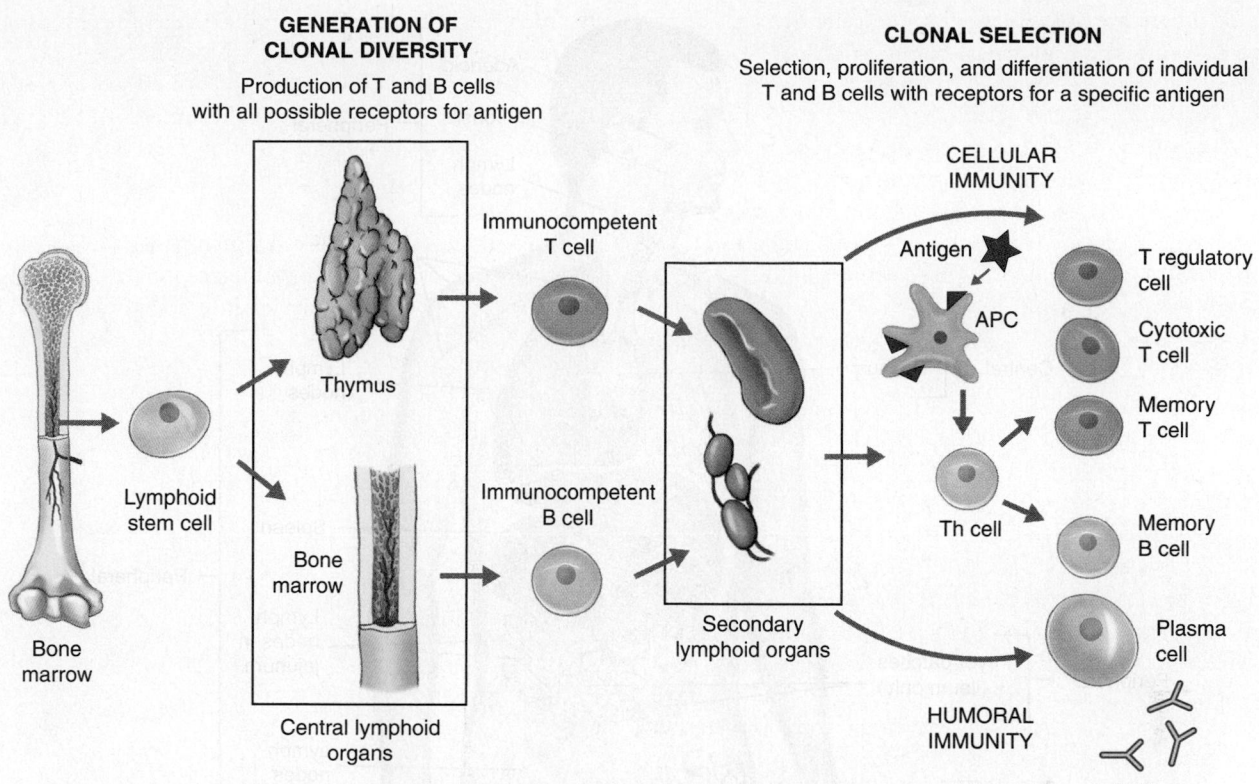

GENERATION OF CLONAL DIVERSITY

Production of T and B cells with all possible receptors for antigen

CLONAL SELECTION

Selection, proliferation, and differentiation of individual T and B cells with receptors for a specific antigen

Figure 7-2 Overview of immune response. The immune response can be separated into two phases: the *generation of clonal diversity* and *clonal selection*. During the generation of clonal diversity, lymphoid stem cells from the bone marrow migrate to the central lymphoid organs (the thymus or regions of the bone marrow), where they undergo a series of cellular division and differentiation stages resulting in either immunocompetent T cells from the thymus or immunocompetent B cells from the bone marrow. (This process is outlined in more detail in Figures 7-10 and 7-12.) These cells are still naive in that they have never encountered foreign antigen. The immunocompetent cells enter the circulation and migrate to the secondary lymphoid organs (e.g., spleen and lymph nodes), where they take up residence in B- and T-cell–rich areas. The clonal selection phase is initiated by exposure to foreign antigen. The antigen is usually processed by antigen-presenting cells (APCs) for presentation to helper T cells (Th cells) (more detail in Figure 7-16). The intercellular cooperation among APCs, Th cells, and immunocompetent T and B cells results in a second stage of cellular proliferation and differentiation (more details in Figures 7-19 and 7-22). Because antigen has "selected" those T and B cells with compatible antigen receptors, only a small population of T and B cells undergo this process at one time. The result is an active cellular immunity or humoral immunity, or both. Cellular immunity is mediated by a population of "effector" T cells that can kill targets (cytotoxic T cells) or regulate the immune response (T regulatory cells), as well as a population of memory cells (memory T cells) that can respond more quickly to a second challenge with the same antigen. Humoral immunity is mediated by a population of soluble proteins (antibodies) produced by plasma cells and by a population of memory B cells that can produce more antibody rapidly to a second challenge with the same antigen.

initiate an effective immune response, most antigens must be "processed" because they cannot react directly with cells of the immune system but must be shown or "presented" to the immune cells in a very specific manner. This is the job of antigen-processing (antigen-presenting) cells, generally referred to as APCs. In general, three groups of cells must cooperate to make an immune response. The APCs interact with subpopulations of T cells that facilitate immune responses (**helper T cells**), and immunocompetent B or T cells, resulting in differentiation of B cells into active antibody-producing cells (plasma cells) and T cells into effector cells, such as cytotoxic T cells. The last portion of this chapter discusses how these products (antibody and T cells) protect against infection, including how they interact with components of the inflammatory process.

Humoral and Cell-Mediated Immunity

The immune response has two arms: antibody and T cells, both of which protect against infection. Antibody circulates in the blood and binds to antigens on infectious agents. This interaction can result in direct inactivation of the microorganism or activation of a variety of inflammatory mediators (e.g., complement, phagocytes) that will destroy the pathogen. Antibody is primarily responsible for protection against many bacteria and viruses. This arm of the immune response is termed **humoral immunity.**

T cells also undergo differentiation during an immune response and develop into several subpopulations of cells that react directly with antigen on the surface of infectious agents. Some develop into T cells that can stimulate the activities of other leukocytes via cell-to-cell contact or through the

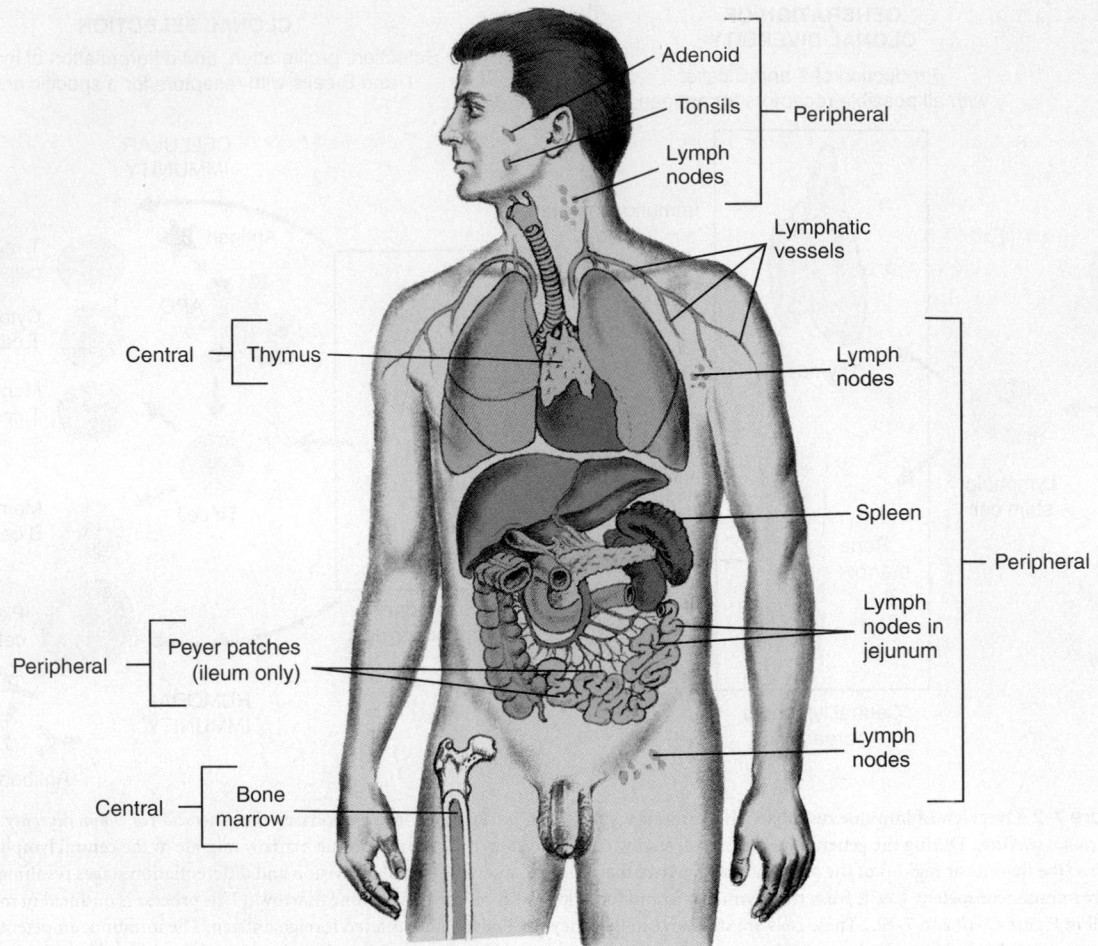

Figure 7-3 Lymphoid tissues: sites of B-cell and T-cell differentiation. Immature lymphocytes migrate through central (primary) lymphoid tissues: the bone marrow (central lymphoid tissue for B lymphocytes) and the thymus (central lymphoid tissue for T lymphocytes). Mature lymphocytes later reside in the T- and B-lymphocyte–rich areas of the peripheral (secondary) lymphoid tissues.

secretion of cytokines. Others develop into cytotoxic T cells (Tc cells) that attack and kill targets directly. Targets for Tc cells include cells infected by a variety of viruses, as well as cells that have become cancerous. This arm of the immune response is termed **cellular immunity.** As discussed in this chapter, the humoral and cellular immune responses are interdependent at many levels. In the end, the success of an acquired immune response depends on the functions of both the humoral and cellular responses, as well as the appropriate interactions between them. Additionally, both arms produce specialized subpopulations of **memory cells** that are long-lived and capable of "remembering" the antigen and responding more rapidly and efficiently on subsequent exposure to the same antigen.[2] On reexposure, memory cells do not require much further differentiation and will therefore rapidly become new plasma cells or effector T cells.

Active vs. Passive Immunity

Adaptive immunity can be either active or passive, depending on whether the antibodies or T cells are produced by the individual in response to antigen or are administered directly.

Active acquired immunity (active immunity) is produced by an individual after either natural exposure to an antigen or after immunization, whereas **passive acquired immunity (passive immunity)** does not involve the host's immune response at all. Rather, passive immunity occurs when preformed antibodies or T lymphocytes are transferred from a donor to the recipient. This can occur naturally, as in the passage of maternal antibodies across the placenta to the fetus, or artificially, as in a clinic using immunotherapy for a specific disease.[3] Unvaccinated individuals who are exposed to particular infectious agents (e.g., hepatitis A virus, rabies virus) often will be given immunoglobulins that are prepared from individuals who already have antibodies against that particular pathogen. Whereas active acquired immunity is long-lived, passive immunity is only temporary because the donor's antibodies or T cells are eventually destroyed.

RECOGNITION AND RESPONSE

The foundation of any successful immune response is the specific recognition of antigen by antibody or receptors on the surface of B or T cells, followed by a set of complex intercellular communications among a variety of antigen-presenting cells and lymphocytes. To fully understand the immune response, it is necessary to initially understand the basis for that recognition. Many of the molecules discussed in this chapter are part of a nomenclature that uses the prefix "CD" followed by a number (e.g., CD1 or CD2) (Table 7-2). The definition of the **CD (cluster of differentiation)** format has changed over time. It was originally used to describe proteins found on the surface of lymphocytes. Currently, CD is the accepted format for labeling a very large family of proteins found on the surface of many cells. Many have alternative names, which may be used in this chapter. The list of identified molecules is constantly increasing (the number of molecules with a CD designation is probably in excess of 250). In a similar fashion, the list of known cytokines is continually growing, with more than 100 having been identified so far. A large number of CD molecules and cytokines contribute to the acquired immune response. We have attempted to focus on a small number of highly important examples to illustrate the immensely complicated, but highly effective, interactions that take place to produce a protective immune response.

Antigens and Immunogens

An **antigen** is a molecule that can *react with* antibodies or antigen receptors on B and T cells. Most, but not all, antigens are also **immunogens.** An antigen that is **immunogenic** will induce an immune response resulting in the production of antibodies or functional T cells. Although the terms *antigen* and *immunogen* commonly are used as synonyms, there are some differences between the two, so a substance may be antigenic yet not be immunogenic.

To function as an antigen, at least a portion of a molecule's chemical structure must be recognized by and bound to an antibody and/or to specific receptors on a lymphocyte. The precise portion of the antigen that is configured for recognition

and binding is called its **antigenic determinant,** or **epitope.** The matching portion on the antibody or the lymphocyte receptor is sometimes referred to as the *antigen-binding site,* or **paratope.** The size of an antigenic determinant is relatively small, perhaps just a few amino acids or sugar residues on the surface of a large molecule (Figure 7-4). Therefore, macromolecules (e.g., proteins, polysaccharides, nucleic acids)

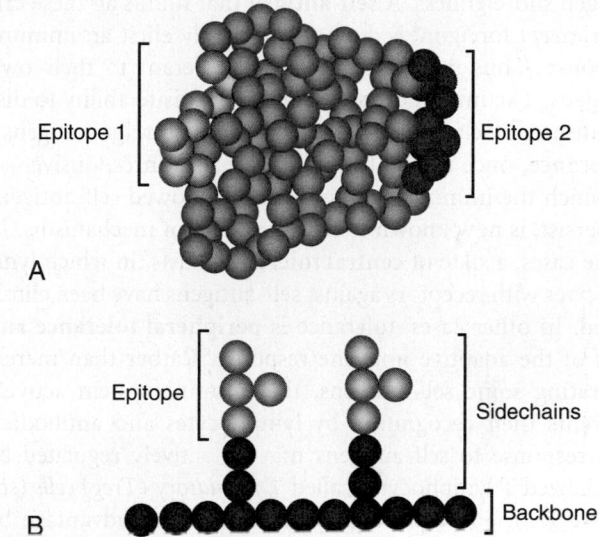

Figure 7-4 Antigenic determinants (epitopes). Shown are generic examples of epitopes on protein (**A**) and polysaccharide (**B**) molecules. In **A**, an antigenic protein may have multiple different epitopes (epitopes 1 and 2) that react with different antibodies. Each sphere represents an amino acid with the yellow spheres representing epitope 1 and the red spheres representing epitope 2. Individual epitopes may consist of 8 or 9 amino acids. In **B**, a polysaccharide is constructed of a backbone with branched side chains. Each sphere represents an individual carbohydrate with the yellow spheres representing the carbohydrates that form the epitope. In this example, two identical epitopes are shown that would bind two identical antibodies.

Table 7-2	Select CD Molecules and Their Functions	
CD Molecules	**Primary Location**	**Functions**
CD1	APCs	Presents lipid antigens
CD2	All T cells, NK cells	T-cell marker; adhesion molecule that binds to CD58 (LFA-3) and provides a co-stimulatory signal
CD3	All T cells	Associated with TCR and provides intracellular signaling
CD4	Th cells	Binds to MHC class II as co-receptor with the TCR
CD8	Tc cells	Binds to MHC class I as co-receptor with the TCR
CD19	B cells	Complexes with CD21 to form a co-receptor for B cells
CD20	B cells	Major regulator of B-cell function
CD21	B cells	A receptor for complement that complexes with CD19 to form a co-receptor for B cells
CD25	Activated T cells	α-chain of IL-2 receptor
CD28	T cells	Adhesion molecule that binds to CD80 to provide co-stimulatory signal for Tc cells
CD40	B cells, macrophages	Adhesion molecule that binds to CD154 to provide co-stimulatory signal for B cells
CD45	All lymphocytes	Has multiple types; augments antigen signal
CD58 (LFA-3)	Most cells	Adhesion molecule that binds to CD2 to provide a co-stimulatory signal
CD80 (B7-1)	APCs	Adhesion molecule that binds to CD28 to provide a co-stimulatory signal
CD154 (CD40L)	Th2 cells	Adhesion molecule that binds to CD40 to provide a co-stimulatory signal

APCs, Antigen-presenting cells; *IL,* interleukin; *MHC,* major histocompatibility complex; *NK,* natural killer; *Tc,* cytotoxic; *TCR,* T-cell receptor; *Th,* helper T cell.

usually contain multiple and diverse antigenic determinants, and the immune response against the macromolecule will usually consist of a mixture of specific antibodies against several of these determinants.

Certain criteria influence the degree to which an antigen is immunogenic. These include (1) foreignness to the host, (2) appropriateness in size, (3) having an adequate chemical complexity, and (4) being present in a sufficient quantity.

Foremost among the criteria for immunogenicity is the antigen's foreignness. A **self-antigen** that fulfills all these criteria *except* foreignness does not normally elicit an immune response. Thus most individuals are tolerant to their own antigens. The immune system has an exquisite ability to distinguish self (self-antigens) from non-self (foreign antigens). **Tolerance,** once thought to be a state of nonresponsiveness in which the immune system passively allowed self-antigens to persist, is now known to have a variety of mechanisms. In some cases, a state of **central tolerance** exists, in which lymphocytes with receptors against self-antigens have been eliminated. In other cases, tolerance is **peripheral tolerance** and part of the adaptive immune response. Rather than merely tolerating some self-antigens, the immune system actively prevents their recognition by lymphocytes and antibodies. The response to self-antigens may be actively regulated by specialized T lymphocytes called *T regulatory (Treg) cells* (see Figure 7-2). Some pathogens have a survival advantage by their capacity to mimic self-antigens and avoid inducing an immune response.

Molecular size also contributes to an antigen's immunogenicity. In general, large molecules (those bigger than 10,000 daltons), such as proteins, polysaccharides, and nucleic acids, are most immunogenic. Low-molecular-weight molecules such as amino acids, monosaccharides, fatty acids, and the purine and pyrimidine bases, tend to be unable to induce an immune response. Many small molecules can function as **haptens:** antigens that are too small to be immunogens by themselves but become immunogenic in combination with larger molecules that function as **carriers** for the hapten. For example, the antigens of penicillin and poison ivy are haptens, but they initiate allergic responses only after binding to large-molecular-weight proteins in the allergic individual's blood or skin. Antigens that induce an allergic response are also called **allergens.**

Chemical complexity affects immunogenicity. The best immunogens contain a diversity of chemically different components. For instance, a large synthetic protein consisting only of alanine amino acids would not be very immunogenic, despite its size and foreignness. However, if other amino acids, such as tyrosine, tryptophan, or phenylalanine, were inserted into the structure, the degree of immunogenicity would increase greatly.

Finally, antigens that are present in extremely small or large quantities may be unable to elicit an immune response and therefore by definition are also nonimmunogenic. In many cases, high or low extremes of antigen quantities may induce a state of tolerance rather than immunity.

Even if an antigen fulfills all these criteria, the quality and intensity of the immune response may still be affected by a variety of additional factors. For example, the route and vehicle of antigenic entry or administration are critical to the immunogenicity of some antigens. This has important clinical implications. The most common routes for clinical administration of antigen, such as vaccines, are intravenous, intraperitoneal, subcutaneous, intranasal, and oral. Each route preferentially stimulates a different set of lymphocyte-containing (lymphoid) tissues and therefore results in the induction of different types of cell-mediated or humoral immune responses. For some vaccines, the route may affect the protectiveness of the immune response so that the individual is protected if immunized by one route, but may remain susceptible to infection if administered through a different route. Immunogenicity of an antigen also may be altered by being delivered along with substances that stimulate the immune response; these substances are known as *adjuvants.* Finally, the genetic makeup of a host can play a critical role in the immune system's ability to respond to many antigens; some individuals appear to be unable to respond to immunization with a particular antigen, whereas they respond well to other antigens. For instance, a small percentage of the population fails to produce a measurable immune response to the most common vaccines, despite multiple injections. Many other factors can modulate the immune response. These include the individual's age, nutritional status, genetic background, and reproductive status, as well as exposure to traumatic injury, concurrent disease, or the use of immunosuppressive medications.

Molecules That Recognize Antigen

Antigen is directly recognized by three molecules: circulating antibody and antigen receptors on the surface of B lymphocytes (**B-cell receptor**, or **BCR**) and T lymphocytes (**T-cell receptor**, or **TCR**) (Figure 7-5).

Antibody

An **antibody,** or immunoglobulin, is a serum glycoprotein produced by plasma cells in response to a challenge by an immunogen. The term *immunoglobulin* is used to denote all molecules that are known to have specificity for antigen, whereas the term *antibody* is generally used to denote one particular set of immunoglobulins with specificity against a known antigen. There are five molecular classes of immunoglobulins (IgG, IgA, IgM, IgE, and IgD) that are characterized by antigenic, structural, and functional differences (Figure 7-6). Within two of the immunoglobulin classes are several distinct subclasses including four subclasses of IgG and two subclasses of IgA.

Classes

IgG is the most abundant class of immunoglobulins; they constitute 80% to 85% of those circulating in the body and account for most of the protective activity against infections (Tables 7-3 and 7-4). As a result of selective transport across the placenta, maternal IgG is also the major class of antibody found in blood of the fetus and newborn. Four subclasses of IgG have been described: IgG1, IgG2, IgG3, and IgG4.

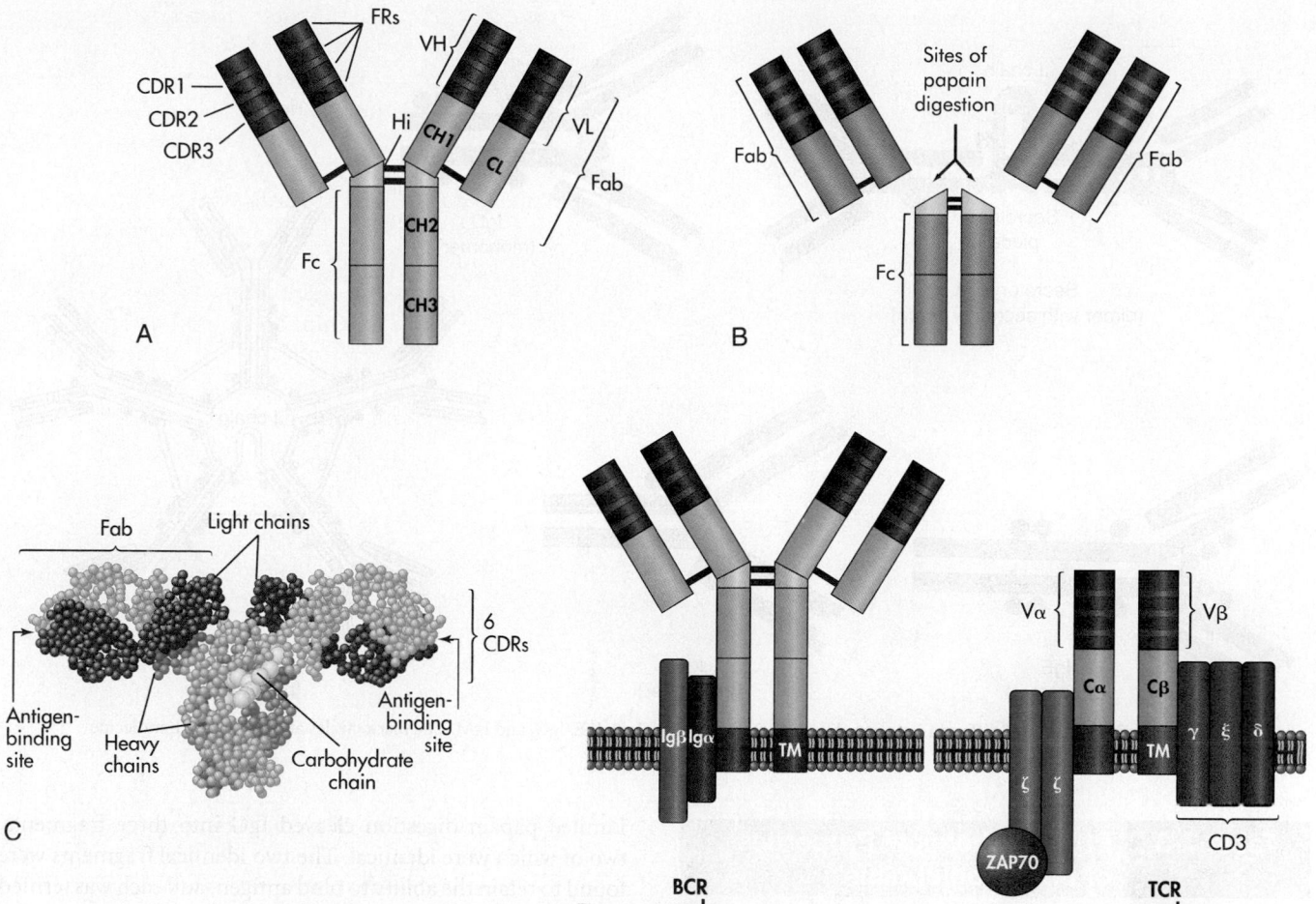

Figure 7-5 Antigen-binding molecules. Antigen-binding molecules include soluble antibody (A, B, C) and cell-surface receptors (D). A, The typical antibody molecule consists of two identical heavy chains and two identical light chains connected by interchain disulfide bonds (– between chains in the figure). Each heavy chain is divided into three regions with relatively constant amino acid sequences (CH1, CH2, and CH3) and a region with a variable amino acid sequence (VH). Each light chain is divided into a constant region (CL) and a variable region (VL). The hinge region (Hi) provides flexibility in some classes of antibody. Within each variable region are three highly variable complementary-determining regions (CDR1, CDR2, CDR3) separated by relatively constant framework regions (FRs) B, Fragmentation of the antibody molecule by limited digestion with the enzyme papain has identified three important portions of the molecule: an Fc and two identical Fab fragments. Both Fab fragments bind antigen. As the antibody folds (C), the CDRs are placed in proximity to form the antigen-binding site. D, The antigen receptor on the surface of B cells (BCR complex) is a monomeric antibody with a structure similar to circulating antibody, with an additional hydrophobic transmembrane region (TM) that anchors the molecule to the cell surface. The active BCR complex contains molecules (Igα and Igβ) that are responsible for intracellular signaling after the receptor has bound antigen. The T-cell receptor (TCR) consists of an α- and a β-chain joined by a disulfide bond. Each chain consists of a constant region (Cα and Cβ) and a variable region (Vα and Vβ). Each variable region contains CDRs and FRs in a structure similar to that of antibody. The active TCR is associated with several molecules that are responsible for intracellular signaling. These include CD3, which is a complex of γ (gamma), ε (epsilon), and δ (delta) subunits and a complex of two ζ (zeta) molecules. The ζ molecules are attached to a cytoplasmic protein kinase (ZAP70) that is critical to intracellular signaling. (C from Patton KT, Thibodeau GA: *Anatomy & physiology*, ed 7, St Louis, 2010, Mosby.)

IgA can be divided into two subclasses, IgA1 and IgA2. IgA1 molecules are found predominantly in the blood, whereas IgA2 is the predominant class of antibody found in normal body secretions. The IgA molecules found in bodily secretions are dimers anchored together through a J chain and "secretory piece." This secretory piece is attached to the IgAs inside mucosal epithelial cells and may function to protect these immunoglobulins against degradation by enzymes also found in the secretions.

IgM is the largest of the immunoglobulins and usually exists as a pentamer that is stabilized by a J (joining) chain. It is the first antibody produced during the initial, or primary, response to antigen. IgM is synthesized early in neonatal life, and its synthesis may be increased as a response to infection in utero.

Information on the role of IgD is limited. This class of immunoglobulins is found in very low concentrations in the blood, where they do not appear to have a known function.

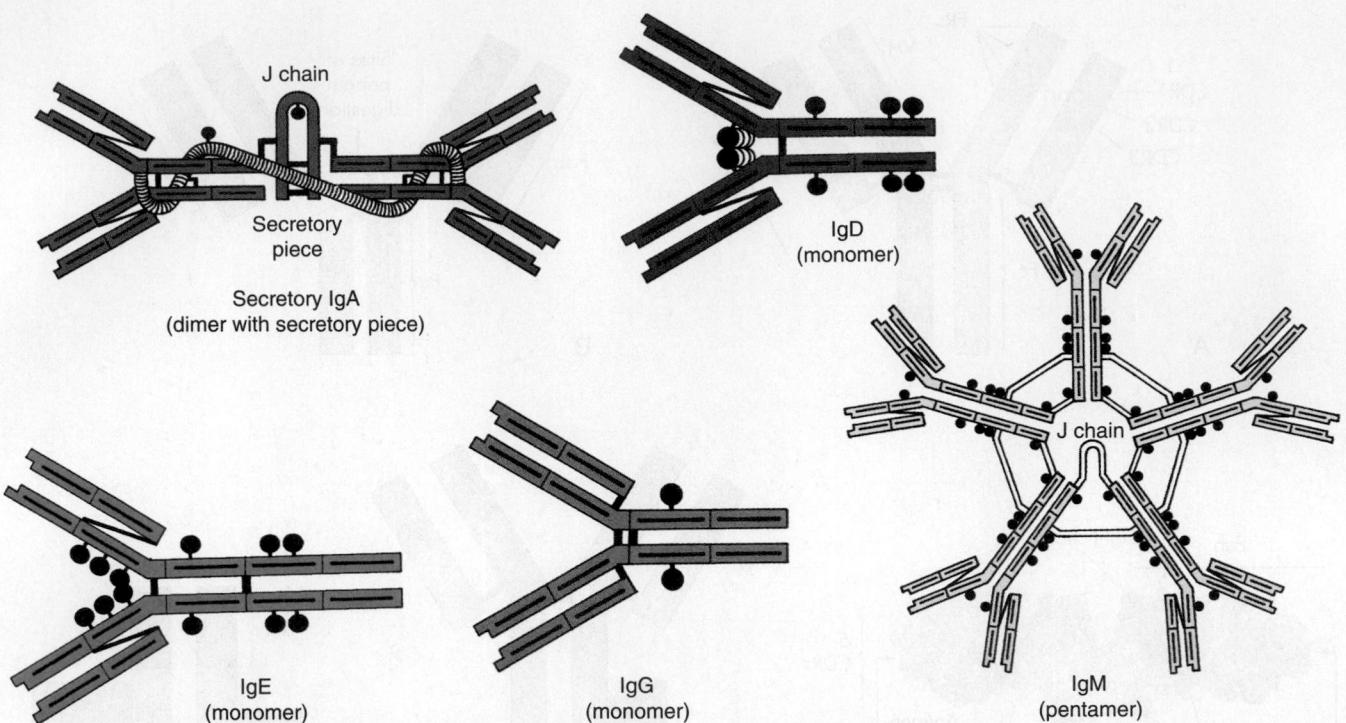

Figure 7-6 Structure of different immunoglobulins. Secretory IgA, IgD, IgE, IgG, and IgM. The black circles attached to each molecule represent carbohydrate residues.

Table 7-3	Physicochemical Properties of Immunoglobulins			
Class	Subclass	Heavy Chain	Molecular Weight (daltons)	Adult Serum Levels (mg/dl)
IgG	IgG1	(γ_1)	146,000	800-900
	IgG2	(γ_2)	146,000	280-300
	IgG3	(γ_3)	165,000	90-100
	IgG4	(γ_4)	146,000	50
IgM	IgM	(μ)	970,000	120-150
IgA	IgA1	(α_1)	160,000	280-300
	IgA2	(α_2)		50
	sIgA	(α_1, α_2)	385,000	5
IgD	IgD	(δ)	184,000	3
IgE	IgE	(ε)	190,000	0.03

Ig, Immunoglobulin; *s,* secretory.

IgD is located primarily on the surface of developing B lymphocytes, where they function as one type of B-cell antigen receptors.

IgE is the least concentrated of any of the immunoglobulin classes in the circulation. It appears to have very specialized functions as a mediator of many common allergic responses (see Chapter 8) and in the defense against parasitic infections.

Molecular Structure

Structural analysis of immunoglobulins began with Porter's early studies on the effects of the enzyme papain on IgG.[4] The nomenclature of antibody structure originated from that work.

Limited papain digestion cleaved IgG into three fragments, two of which were identical. The two identical fragments were found to retain the ability to bind antigen, and each was termed an **antigen-binding fragment (Fab)**. The third fragment crystallized when separated from the Fab portions and was termed the **crystalline fragment (Fc)** (see Figure 7-5).

What Porter learned about the structure of IgG still applies not only to this class of immunoglobulins but also to each of the other classes. The Fab portions of an immunoglobulin contain the recognition sites (receptors) for antigenic determinants and confer the molecule's specificity toward a particular antigen. The Fc portion is responsible for most of the biologic functions of antibodies, including activation of the complement cascade and opsonization by binding to Fc receptors on the surface of the cells of the innate immune system.

The basic structure of the antibody molecule consists of four polypeptide chains—two identical light (L) chains and two identical heavy (H) chains (see Figure 7-5). Within the same molecule, the two heavy chains are identical and the two light chains are identical. The class of antibody is determined by which heavy chain is used: gamma (IgG), mu (IgM), alpha (IgA), epsilon (IgE), or delta (IgD). The light chains of an antibody molecule are of either the kappa (κ) or lambda (λ) type. The light and heavy chains are held together by two major forces: noncovalent bonds and disulfide linkages. A set of disulfide linkages between the heavy chains occurs in the **hinge region** and in some instances lends a degree of molecular flexibility at that site so that the Fab regions can move.

Light and heavy chains are further subdivided into constant (C) and variable (V) regions. The constant regions have

Table 7-4	Biologic Properties of Immunoglobulins								
	Complement Activation		Binding to Fc Receptors on				Placental Transfer	Presence in Secretions	Induction of Agglutination
Subclass	Classic	Alternate	Macrophages	PMNs	Mast Cells	Platelets			
IgG1	++	−	+	+	−	+	+++	±	+
IgG2	+	−	−	−	−	+	+	±	+
IgG3	+++	−	+	+	−	+	+++	±	+
IgG4	−	−	−	±	+	+	++	±	+
IgM	++++	−	−	−	−	−	−	+	+++
IgA1	−	+	±	±	−	−	−	+	−
IgA2	−	+	−	±	−	−	−	+	−
sIgA	−	−	−	−	−	−	−	++++	−
IgD	−	±	−	−	−	−	−	−	−
IgE	−	±	?	−	+++	−	−	+	−

Fc, Crystalline fragment; *Ig*, immunoglobulin; *PMN*, polymorphonuclear neutrophil; *sIgA*, secretory immunoglobulin A; −, lack of activity; +, relative degree of activity.

relatively stable amino acid sequences within a particular immunoglobulin class or subclass. Thus the amino acid sequence of the constant region of one IgG1 should be almost identical with the sequence of the same region of another IgG1, even if they react with different antigens. Conversely, among different antibodies, the sequences of the variable regions are characterized by a large number of amino acid differences. Therefore, two IgG1 molecules against different antigens may have many differences in the amino acid sequence of their variable regions. The variable region can be further subdivided because most of the region's viability in amino acid sequence is localized into three areas of the variable region. These three areas were once called *hypervariable regions*, but are now called **complementary-determining regions (CDRs)**. The four regions separating the CDRs have relatively stable amino acid sequences and are called **framework regions (FRs)**.

Antigen Binding

The combined amino acid sequences of the variable regions of both the heavy (V_H) and light (V_L) chains determine the conformation of the antigen-binding site and therefore the antigenic specificity of the immunoglobulin molecule.[5] Most proteins will naturally fold and take on secondary or tertiary structures. As the immunoglobulin molecules fold, the FRs control the accuracy of folding in the variable region, and the CDRs in both variable regions are moved into proximity, resulting in an antigen-binding site formed by the three CDRs of the heavy chain and the three CDRs of the light chain. The chemical nature of the particular amino acids in those sites, as well as the topography of the site, determine specificity toward a particular antigen. The antigen that will bind most strongly must have complementary chemistry and topography with the binding site formed by the antibody. The antigen fits into this binding site with the specificity of a key into a lock and is held there by noncovalent chemical interactions (Figure 7-7). In some cases the substitution of a single critical amino acid in a CDR may have a significant effect on the shape of the binding site and thus the specificity of the antibody molecule.

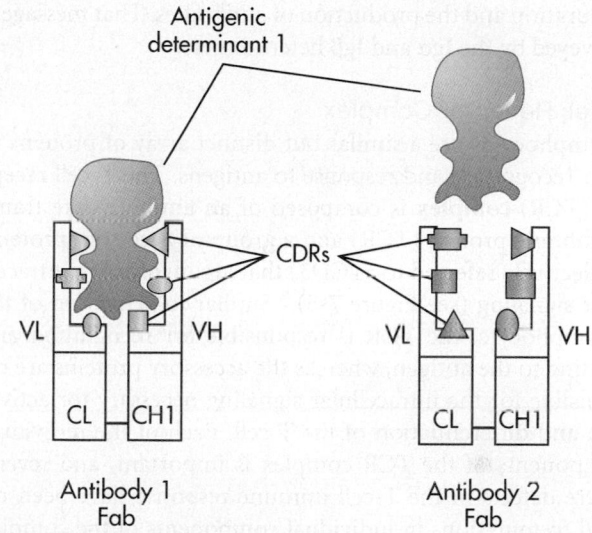

Figure 7-7 Antigen-antibody binding. The specificity required for antibody binding with an antigen is determined by the shape and chemistry of the six complementary-determining regions (CDRs) in the combining site on the variable region of the antibody. This figure indicates two different antibodies (Fab portions of antibody 1 and antibody 2) that have different sets of CDRs and therefore different specificities. As indicated, the antigenic determinant that reacts well with antibody 1 is unable to react with antibody 2 because of differences in the antibody combining site. *Fab*, Antigen-binding fragment.

Because the heavy and light chains are identical within the same antibody molecule, the two binding sites are also identical and have specificity for the same antigen. The number of functional binding sites is called the antibody's **valence.** Most antibody classes (i.e., IgG, IgE, IgD, and circulating IgA) have a valence of 2, but secretory IgA has a valence of 4. IgM, being a pentamer, has a theoretical valence of 10, but can simultaneously use only about five binding sites because a large antigen binding to one site blocks antigen binding to another site.

B-Cell Receptor Complex

The **B-cell receptor (BCR) complex** is located on the surface of B lymphocytes (see Figure 7-5). Its role is to recognize antigen, but unlike circulating antibody, the receptor must communicate that information to the cell's nucleus.[6] Therefore, the BCR complex consists of antigen-recognition molecules and accessory molecules involved in intracellular signaling (Igα and Igβ). BCRs on the surface of immunocompetent B cells are membrane-associated IgM and IgD immunoglobulins that are produced from the same genes that are used by plasma cells to produce soluble antibodies. As a BCR, however, IgM is a monomer rather than the pentamer primarily found in the blood.

The BCR signaling complex consists of two Igα and Igβ heterodimers that are closely associated with the BCR and contain tyrosine kinase signaling activity. The antibody portion of the BCR complex is responsible for recognition and binding to an antigen, but by itself cannot provide the intracellular signals required to activate the B cell and complete its maturation and the production of antibodies. That message is conveyed by the Igα and Igβ heterodimers.

T-Cell Receptor Complex

T lymphocytes use a similar but distinct array of proteins in their recognition and response to antigens. The **T-cell receptor (TCR) complex** is composed of an antibody-like transmembrane protein (TCR) and a group of accessory proteins (collectively referred to as CD3) that are involved in intracellular signaling (see Figure 7-5).[7] Similar to activation of the B lymphocyte, the TCR is responsible for recognition and binding to the antigen, whereas the accessory proteins are responsible for the intracellular signaling necessary for activation and differentiation of the T cell. Each of the individual components of the TCR complex is important, and several severe defects in the T-cell immune response have been related to mutations in individual components of the complex (see Chapter 8).

Molecules That Present Antigen

For an effective immune response, most antigens must be processed within cells and expressed on the surface of those cells in a very specific manner. Some types of antigen are managed only by highly specialized cells: **antigen-presenting cells,** or **APCs**. Other types of antigens can be processed and presented by almost any type of cell. Several sets of cell-surface molecules have the responsibility for appropriately presenting antigen. These molecules are described below.

Major Histocompatibility Complex

An essential set of recognition molecules are members of the **major histocompatibility complex (MHC)**. Most antibody and cellular immune responses are dependent on antigen presentation by APCs. Additionally, the role of cytotoxic T cells in killing virally infected cells depends on presentation of the viral antigen on the infected cell's surface. **Antigen presentation** is the primary role of molecules of the MHC.[8]

MHC molecules are glycoproteins found on the surface of all human cells except red blood cells. They are divided into two general classes, class I and class II, based on their molecular structure, distribution among cell populations, and function in antigen presentation. MHC class I molecules are heterodimers composed of a large α-chain along with a smaller chain called β₂ *microglobulin*. MHC class II molecules are also heterodimers with both α- and β-chains. The general properties of each of the MHC classes are summarized in Figure 7-8.

Molecules of the two MHC classes are encoded from different genetic loci that are located as a large complex of genes on the short arm of human chromosome 6 (see Figure 7-8). The MHC also contains other genes that control the quality and quantity of an immune response, which are commonly referred to as class III MHC genes. The primary **MHC class I genes** consist of three closely linked loci on this chromosome labeled A, B, and C. The primary **MHC class II genes** are located within the D region, which actually consists of three separate and independent loci, DR, DP, and DQ.

The class I and class II MHC loci are the most genetically diverse (polymorphic) of any human genetic loci. Within the human population, the numbers of possible different alleles (i.e., forms of the gene) expressed by each locus is astounding: 649 at the A locus, 1029 at the B locus, 350 at the C locus, 643 at the DR locus (α and β), 125 at the DQ locus (α and β), and 154 at the DP locus (α and β). These numbers are based on the polymorphism of observed DNA sequences and may not reflect differences in function. Clearly, not every allele is expressed in the same individual. Humans have two copies of each MHC locus (one inherited from each parent) that are codominant so that molecules encoded by each parent's genes are expressed on the cell surface. Within an individual, each locus will be expressing only one allele. For instance, each person will have only two different A proteins (one from each parent). However, with the tremendous number of possible alleles that can be expressed, it is likely that any two unrelated individuals will have different sets of MHC molecules on their cell surfaces so that each of us is distinct.

Transplantation

The diversity of MHC molecules becomes clinically relevant during organ transplantation. Cells in transplanted tissue or organs from one individual will have a different set of MHC surface antigens than those of the recipient; therefore, the recipient can mount an immune response against the foreign MHC antigens, resulting in rejection of the transplanted tissue. As a result of studies of transplantation, the human MHC molecules are also referred to as **human leukocyte antigens (HLAs)**, and the different MHC genetic loci are commonly called HLA-A, HLA-B, HLA-C, HLA-DR, HLA-DQ, and HLA-DP. To minimize the chance of tissue rejection, the donor and recipient are often *tissue typed* beforehand to identify differences in HLA antigens.[9] The more similar two individuals are in their HLA tissue type, the more likely a transplant from one to the other will be successful.

Although a large number of alleles exist at the molecular level, the diversity is considerably less at the antigenic

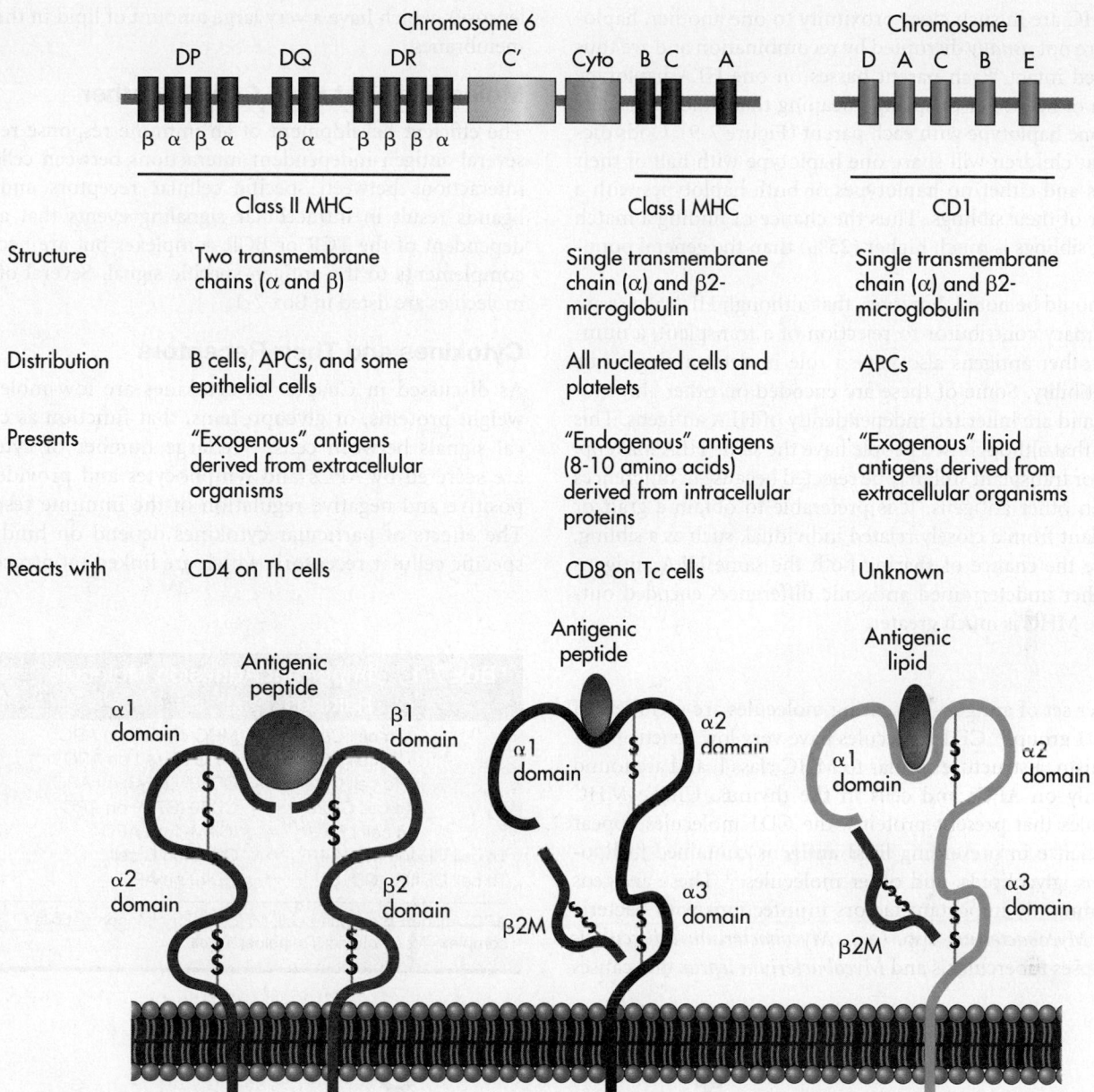

Figure 7-8 Genetics and structure of antigen-presenting molecules. Three sets of molecules are primarily responsible for antigen presentation: MHC class I, MHC class II, and CD1. The MHC molecules are encoded from the MHC region on chromosome 6, which contains information for class I and class II molecules, as well as for several other molecules that participate in the innate or immune responses. These include several complement proteins (C′) and cytokines (cyto), which are referred to as MHC class III molecules. Three principal class I molecules, HLA-A, HLA-B, and HLA-C, are presented here, but this region contains information for the α-chains of several other molecules, including HLA-E, HLA-F, and HLA-G. The MHC class I products complex with β2-microglobulin, which is encoded by a gene on chromosome 15. The MHC class I molecules present small peptide antigens in a pocket formed by the α1 and α2 domains of the α-chain. The conformation of the molecule is stabilized by β2-microglobulin as well as by intrachain disulfide bonds (-S-S-). The α- and β-chains of class II molecules are also encoded in this region: HLA-DR, HLA-DP, and HLA-DQ. In some cases, multiple genes for α- and β-chains are available. The MHC class II molecules present peptide antigens in a pocket formed by the α1 domain of the α-chain and β1 domain of the β-chain. The genes for CD1 molecules are encoded on chromosome 1, which contains genes for five α-chains (CD1A-E), and the α-chains complex with β2-microglobulin to present lipid antigens in a pocket formed by the α1 and α2 domains. All three sets of antigen-presenting molecules are anchored to the plasma membrane by hydrophobic regions on the ends of the α- and β-chains. *MHC,* major histocompatibility complex.

level: there are approximately 67 different HLA-A antigens, 149 HLA-B antigens, and 39 HLA-C antigens. Because of the large number of different alleles, it is highly unlikely that a perfect "match" can be found in the general population between a potential donor and the recipient.

The specific combination of alleles at the six major HLA loci on one chromosome (A, B, C, DR, DQ, and DP) is termed a **haplotype.** Each individual has two HLA haplotypes, one from the paternal chromosome 6 and another from the maternal chromosome. Because the different HLA loci within the MHC are in such close proximity to one another, haplotypes are not *usually* disrupted by recombination and are thus inherited intact. Each parent passes on one HLA haplotype to each of his or her offspring, meaning that children usually share one haplotype with each parent (Figure 7-9). Odds dictate that children will share one haplotype with half of their siblings and either no haplotypes or both haplotypes with a quarter of their siblings. Thus the chance of finding a match among siblings is much higher (25%) than the general population.

It should be noted, however, that although HLA alleles are the primary contributor to rejection of a transplant, a number of other antigens also have a role in determining tissue compatibility. Some of these are encoded on other chromosomes and are inherited independently of HLA antigens. This means that although two people have the same HLA makeup, a graft or transplant still may be rejected because of differences between other antigens. It is preferable to obtain a graft or transplant from a closely related individual, such as a sibling, because the chance of sharing both the same HLA antigens and other undetermined antigenic differences encoded outside the MHC is much greater.

CD1

Another set of antigen-presenting molecules are members of the CD1 group.[10] CD1 molecules have very low genetic polymorphism, a structure similar to MHC class I, and are found primarily on APCs and cells in the thymus. Unlike MHC molecules that present proteins, the CD1 molecules appear to specialize in presenting lipid antigens contained in lipoproteins, glycolipids, and other molecules.[11] These antigens are commonly important factors in infections with bacteria of the *Mycobacterium* spp. (e.g., *Mycobacterium tuberculosis* that causes tuberculosis and *Mycobacterium leprae* that causes

leprosy), which have a very large amount of lipid in their cell membranes.

Molecules That Hold Cells Together

The efficient development of an immune response requires several antigen-independent interactions between cells. The interactions between specific cellular receptors and their ligands result in intracellular signaling events that are independent of the TCR or BCR complexes but are necessary complements to the antigen-specific signal. Several of these molecules are listed in Box 7-1.

Cytokines and Their Receptors

As discussed in Chapter 6, cytokines are low-molecular-weight proteins, or glycoproteins, that function as chemical signals between cells.[12] A large number of cytokines are secreted by APCs and lymphocytes and provide both positive and negative regulation of the immune response. The effects of particular cytokines depend on binding to specific cellular receptors, which are linked to intracellular

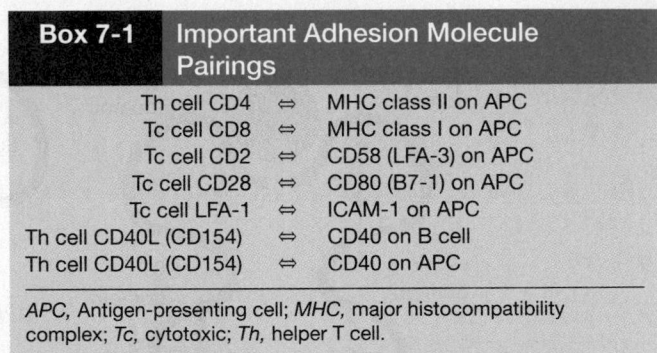

Box 7-1	**Important Adhesion Molecule Pairings**
Th cell CD4 ⇔	MHC class II on APC
Tc cell CD8 ⇔	MHC class I on APC
Tc cell CD2 ⇔	CD58 (LFA-3) on APC
Tc cell CD28 ⇔	CD80 (B7-1) on APC
Tc cell LFA-1 ⇔	ICAM-1 on APC
Th cell CD40L (CD154) ⇔	CD40 on B cell
Th cell CD40L (CD154) ⇔	CD40 on APC

APC, Antigen-presenting cell; *MHC,* major histocompatibility complex; *Tc,* cytotoxic; *Th,* helper T cell.

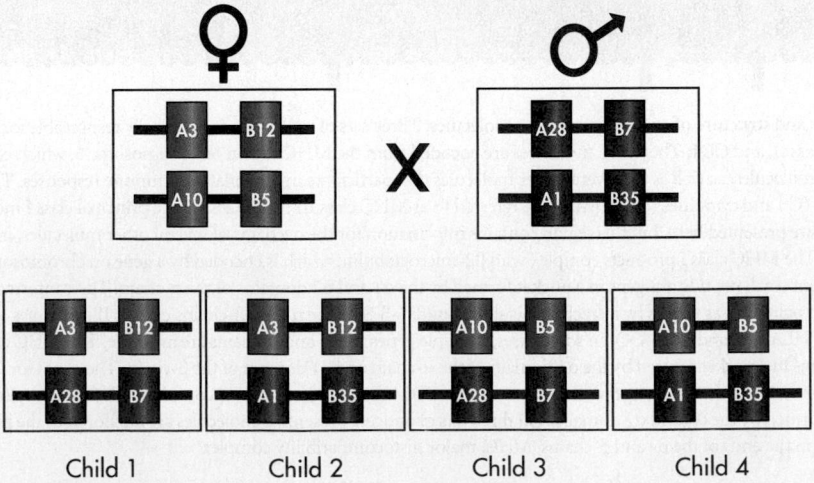

Figure 7-9 Inheritance of HLA. HLA alleles are inherited in a codominant fashion so that both maternal and paternal antigens are expressed. Specific HLA alleles are commonly given numbers to indicate different antigens. In this example, the mother has linked genes for HLA-A3 and HLA-B12 on one chromosome 6 and genes for HLA-A10 and HLA-B5 on the second chromosome 6. The father has HLA-A28 and HLA-B7 on one chromosome and HLA-A1 and HLA-B35 on the second chromosome. On one particular chromosome, the HLA antigens are firmly linked, with crossovers occurring in only 1% of individuals. The children from this pairing may have one of four possible combinations of maternal and paternal HLA. *HLA,* Human leukocyte antigen.

signaling pathways. The lymphocyte may respond in many ways. One of the most common responses is an increase in the production of proteins, many of which are other cytokines or cytokine receptors. Many cytokines also cause a lymphocyte to proliferate and differentiate. The participation of cytokines is essential to the development of an adequate immune response, and in general, the precise combination of cytokines influences the ultimate response of a given cell. Specific deficiencies in the immune response that result from genetic mutations that lead to defective cytokine production or defective cytokine receptors are discussed in Chapter 8. Table 7-5 provides information about key cytokines and receptors that are known to influence the immune response.

GENERATION OF CLONAL DIVERSITY

It has been suggested that more than 10^8 different antigenic determinants may be recognized by receptors on an individual's immunocompetent B cells. A similar number may be recognized by T-cell receptors. However, each T or B cell has only a single receptor specificity that recognizes only one antigen, and each is present before that individual is ever exposed to foreign antigen. Thus before the individual is exposed to

Table 7-5	Key Cytokines and Receptors That Influence the Immune Response	
Cytokine	**Primary Source**	**Primary Function**
Interleukin (IL)		
IL-1	APCs	Stimulates T cells to proliferation and differentiation; induces acute phase proteins in inflammatory response; endogenous pyrogen
IL-2	Th1 cells, NK cells	Stimulates proliferation and differentiation of T cells and NK cells
IL-4	Th2 cells, mast cells	Induces B-cell proliferation and differentiation; up-regulates MHC class II expression; induces class-switch to IgE
IL-5	Th2 cells, mast cells	Induces eosinophil proliferation and differentiation; induces B-cell proliferation and differentiation
IL-6	Th2 cells, APCs	Induces B-cell proliferation and differentiation into plasma cells; induces acute phase proteins in inflammatory response
IL-7	Thymic epithelial cells, bone marrow stromal cells	Major cytokine for induction of B- and T-cell proliferation and differentiation in the central lymphoid organs
IL-8	Macrophages	Chemotactic factor for neutrophils
IL-10	Th cells, B cells	Inhibits cytokine production; activator of B cells
IL-12	B cells, APCs	Induces NK-cell proliferation; increases production of IFN-γ
IL-13	Th2 cells	IL-4–like properties; decreases inflammatory responses
IL-17	Th17 cells	Increases inflammation; increased influx of neutrophils and macrophages; increased epithelial cell chemokine production
IL-22	Th17 cells	Increases inflammation; increased epithelial cell production of antimicrobial peptides
Interferon (IFN)		
IFN-α, IFN-β	Macrophages, some virally infected cells	Antiviral; increases expression of MHC class I; activates NK cells
IFN-γ	Th1 cells, NK cells, Tc cells	Increases expression of MHC class II; activates macrophages and NK cells
Tumor Necrosis Factor (TNF)		
TNF-α (cachectin)	Macrophages	IL-1–like properties; induces cellular proliferation
TNF-β (lymphotoxin)	Tc cells	Kills some cells; increases phagocytosis by macrophages and neutrophils
Transforming Growth Factor (TGF)		
TGF-β	Lymphocytes, Macrophages, fibroblasts	Chemotactic for macrophages; increases macrophage IL-1 production; stimulates wound healing
Cytokine Receptors: Type of Receptor	**Ligand**	**Additional Information**
Class I receptors dimers (α- and β-chains)	IL-3, IL-5, IL-6, IL-11, IL-12, IL-13	IL-3 and IL-5 share a common α-chain; IL-6 and IL-11 share a common β-chain
Trimers (α-,β-, and γ-chains)	IL-2, IL-4, IL-7, IL-9, IL-15	All share a common γ- chain
Class II receptors	IFNα, β, and γ	Two chains
TNF receptors	TNF-α, TNF-β, CD40, Fas	Single chain
Immunoglobulin-like receptors	IL-1	Single chain with immunoglobulin-like characteristics

APCs, Antigen-presenting cells; *MHC,* major histocompatibility complex; *NK,* natural killer; *Tc,* cytotoxic; *Th,* helper T cells.

any foreign antigen, millions of different T- and B-cell antigen receptors must be constructed to recognize *any* potential antigenic determinant.

Several theories were proposed to explain how such a great diversity of recognition could be produced. The process occurs in two phases: the **generation of clonal diversity,** during which all the necessary receptor specificities are produced, and **clonal selection,** during which antigen selects those lymphocytes with compatible receptors, expands their population, and causes differentiation into antibody-secreting plasma cells or mature T cells (Table 7-6).[13,14] The generation of clonal diversity takes place in the **primary (central) lymphoid organs** (i.e., thymus and bone marrow), is driven by hormones, does not require foreign antigen, and results in the generation of immature but immunocompetent T and B cells with receptors that can recognize virtually any antigenic molecule. Both T and B cells are derived from common precursor cells (**lymphoid stem cells**) that arise in either the liver (in the fetus) or in the bone marrow (of a child or adult). These precursor cells are distinct from the precursor cells that give rise to cells of the innate immune system. The immunocompetent T and B cells migrate from the primary lymphoid organs to **secondary (peripheral) lymphoid organs** (e.g., spleen, lymph nodes, adenoids, tonsils, Peyer patches), where they await antigen. Clonal selection is initiated by antigen and results in a mature and specific immune response against that antigen.

Although generation of clonal diversity primarily occurs in the fetus, it probably continues to a low degree throughout most of adult life. Clonal selection usually begins at birth and proceeds throughout the life of the individual as new antigens are encountered, although it can begin as early as the eighth week of gestation in humans.

As a result of this process, T and B lymphocytes have the capacity to react against virtually any antigen found in nature. This endless array of possible antibodies and TCRs certainly cannot be constructed from the amount of DNA that is in the nucleus of a human lymphocyte. The enormous repertoire of specificities is instead made possible by rearrangement of existing deoxyribonucleic acid (DNA) during T and B cell development in the primary lymphoid organs. Loci in the DNA that encode for the variable regions of immunoglobulins and TCRs are recombined in a unique way to generate receptors that collectively can recognize and bind to any possible antigen. The DNA in the nucleus of a developing T and B cell is actually cut and spliced (repaired), a process known as **somatic recombination,** so that after this manipulation, the progeny of a single lymphocyte will synthesize identical immunoglobulins or TCRs. Those variable regions, however, are cut and spliced differently from those of another lymphocyte, making each cell unique and therefore able to react with different antigens. The particular process for B and T cells is discussed following.

T-Cell Maturation

Central Lymphoid Organ

The central lymphoid organ for T-cell development is the thymus, which is an organ located near the heart. Precursor cells (lymphoid stem cells) arise in early embryonic life from the yolk sac and fetal liver and later from the bone marrow. They migrate to the thymus and enter in the subcapsular region.[15-17] As the cells move through the thymic cortex to the medulla, they are instructed by interactions with various thymic cells (epithelial cells, macrophages, and dendritic cells) and thymic hormones to undergo proliferation and progressive development of the characteristics of immunocompetent T cells (Figure 7-10).[18] Changes include the development of the T-cell receptor complex and expression of characteristic surface molecules. Many T cells randomly develop TCRs against self-antigens, but are deleted during this process. The final antigen-reactive T cells are released into the blood and take up residence in the secondary lymphoid organs to await antigen.

Table 7-6	Generation of Clonal Diversity vs. Clonal Selection	
	Generation of Clonal Diversity	**Clonal Selection**
Purpose?	To produce large numbers of T and B lymphocytes with the maximum diversity of antigen receptors	Select, expand, and differentiate clones of T and B cells against a specific antigen
When does it occur?	Primarily in the fetus	Primarily after birth and throughout life
Where does it occur?	Central lymphoid organs: thymus for T cells, bone marrow for B cells	Peripheral lymphoid organs, including lymph nodes, spleen, and other lymphoid tissues
Is foreign antigen involved?	No	Yes, antigen determines which clones of cells will be selected
What hormones/cytokines are involved?	Thymic hormones, IL-7, others	Many cytokines produced by Th cells and APCs
Is tolerance induced?	Central tolerance induced as autoreactive cells are deleted	Peripheral tolerance induced as autoreactive cells are regulated
Final product?	Immunocompetent T and B cells that can react with antigen but have not seen antigen, and migrate to the secondary lymphoid organs	Plasma cells that produce antibody, effector T cells that help (Th), kill targets (Tc), or regulate immune responses (Treg); memory B and T cells

APCs, Antigen-presenting cells; *IL,* interleukin; *Tc,* cytotoxic T cells; *Th,* helper T cells; *Treg,* regulatory T cells.

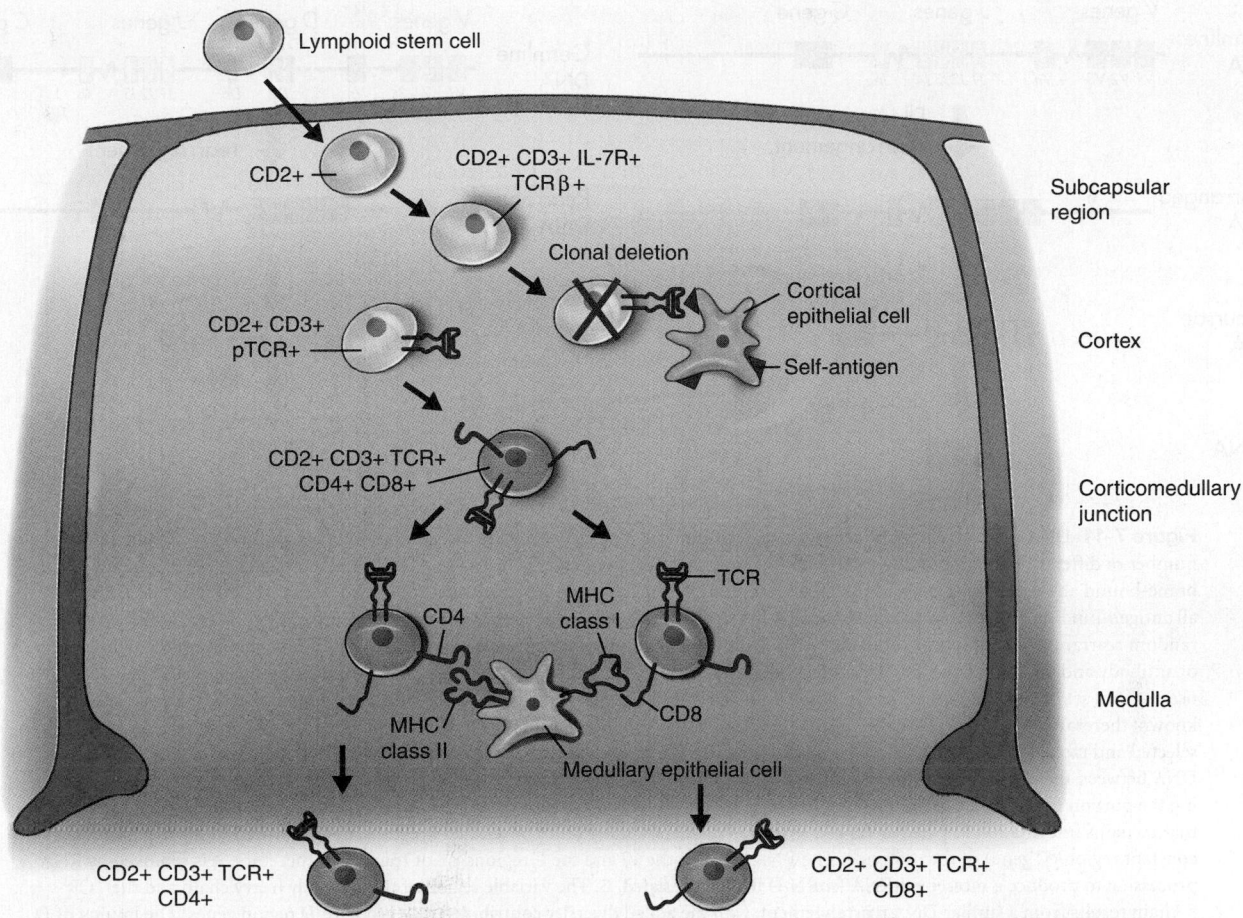

Figure 7-10 T-cell development in the thymus. During the generation of clonal diversity in the fetus, lymphoid stem cells undergo several stages of cellular division and differentiation in a central lymphoid organ (the thymus) under the control of hormones but without the influence of foreign antigen. A simplified scheme for that process is presented here. The differentiation process is characterized by the up-regulation of many important surface molecules (only some of which are shown) and the random development of a huge number of different T-cell receptors against all possible antigens that the adult may encounter. The lymphoid stem cell enters the subcapsular region of the thymus, where it begins to undergo differentiation. One of the first surface changes is the appearance of the molecule CD2, which is a marker for all T cells. In the cortex of the thymus, the developing cell encounters epithelial cells that guide most of the early differentiation process. The pre–T cell begins expressing the surface receptor for the cytokine IL-7, which is produced by the epithelial cell along with other thymic hormones to drive the T-cell differentiation process. At this stage the T cell begins constructing the T-cell receptor (TCR) by first rearranging and expressing the TCR β-chain (more detail is provided in Figure 7-11) and expressing CD3 molecules. Although the TCR α-chain has not yet been produced, the β-chain is expressed on the surface as a pre-TCR (pTCR) using a protein that acts as a surrogate for the α-chain. Because of the randomness of the process, some pTCRs are produced with specificities toward self-antigens. Many of these undergo negative selection and are deleted (clonal deletion) by apoptosis induced through interactions with self-antigens presented by the epithelial cells. Survivors of negative selection move toward the thymic cortex and begin expressing the TCR α-chain, the normal TCR, and both CD4 and CD8 on their surfaces. These CD4+, CD8+ "double-positive" cells encounter medullary epithelial cells that express both MHC class I and class II molecules. The phenotype of the developing T cell is positively selected so that interaction between CD4 and MHC class II selects for retention of CD4 expression, whereas interaction between CD8 and MHC class I favors the CD8 phenotype. Thus two populations of "single-positive" immunocompetent T cells leave the thymus: one cell is CD4+, CD8− (destined to be a helper T [Th] cell) and the other is CD4−, CD8+ (destined to be a cytotoxic T [Tc] cell).

Production of the T-Cell Receptor

Like antibody, the TCR reacts with antigen (see Figure 7-5). Although the structure of the TCR closely resembles a Fab portion of antibody, the TCR uses different protein chains than are used for antibody. The most common TCR contains α- and β-chains, each of which has a variable region and a constant region. Within each variable region are three CDR regions separated by FR regions.

The great amount of variable region diversity necessary for identifying the huge number of antigens found in nature is produced by random recombination of multiple genes to encode the variable regions of both the α- and β-chains. In the germline genes, the information for the amino acid sequence of the α-chain variable region is found on chromosome 14 in two separated, but closely associated, locations: a set of *V* region genes and a set of *J* region genes (Figure 7-11). The

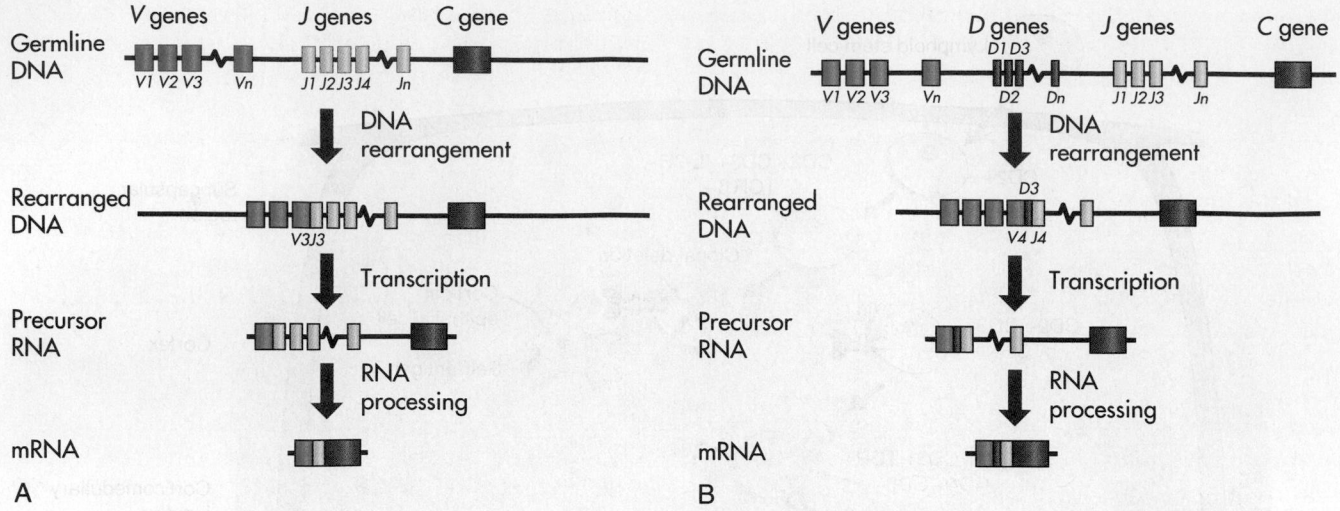

Figure 7-11 DNA rearrangement of genes for antigen-binding molecules. During the generation of clonal diversity, a tremendous number of different antigen-binding molecules are produced. These include the B-cell receptor (BCR), which consists of a membrane-bound antibody molecule, and the T-cell receptor (TCR). The process by which receptor diversity is created is identical for all antigen-binding molecules and is summarized in this figure. Maximum diversity with minimum use of DNA is accomplished by random rearrangement of sets of genes that encode different portions of the variable regions. **A,** The variable regions of the light chain of antibody and the α-chain of the TCR independently rearrange two sets of genes: *V* region genes and *J* region genes. The light chain uses its own set of genes, and the α-chain uses a completely different set. In neither case is the exact number of *V* or *J* region genes known; therefore, in this figure they are numbered from 1 to an unknown value *(n)*. In a particular cell's DNA, one *V* gene is randomly selected and moved to a position immediately adjacent to a randomly selected *J* gene. In this example, *V3* and *J3* were selected. The DNA between the selected genes is enzymatically removed and the DNA repaired, so that the rearranged DNA in this example is missing the portion found in the germline DNA between *V3* and *J3*. This product is transcribed into a precursor ribonucleic acid (RNA) that contains information for the rearranged *VJ* pair, a span containing other unselected *J* regions, and information for the appropriate constant region (*C* gene) of the molecule. The RNA between the *VJ* and the *C* regions is not translated; therefore, it is removed by RNA processing to produce a messenger RNA (mRNA) that is translated. **B,** The variable region of the antibody heavy chain and the TCR β-chain results from a similar DNA rearrangement, with the added diversity contributed by a group of *D* region genes. The joining of *D* and *J* occurs first, with the removal of intervening DNA. In this example, *D3* and *J4* were chosen. This is followed by rearrangement of the *V* gene (e.g., *V4*) and formation of a *VDJ* region in the rearranged DNA. The precursor RNA contains information for the *VDJ*, the intervening portion of DNA, and the appropriate constant region. After RNA processing, an mRNA is formed for the intact antibody heavy chain or the TCR β-chain. Once the DNA is rearranged and spliced in a given B or T cell, all of the antigen receptors produced by that cell employ the same *V, D,* and *J* segments and have the same specificity.

TCR α-chain locus has multiple (at least 50) *V* genes and multiple (at least 50) *J* genes. During somatic recombination in a developing T cell, one of the possible *V* genes is randomly selected and spliced to one of the *J* genes, with the intervening DNA being removed. This DNA rearrangement process is controlled by two enzymes produced by the genes *RAG-1* and *RAG-2* (recombination activating genes). These enzymes cut double-stranded DNA at specific recognition sites (recombinant signal sequences); then repair the break resulting in excision of the DNA between the selected *V* and *J* genes. At transcription, the genetic information for the α-chain variable region is still separated from the gene for the α-chain constant region. This product is transcribed into messenger ribonucleic acid (mRNA) that contains information for the variable region *(VJ)* separated by a span of RNA from the information for the α-chain constant region. An RNA-processing step removes the intervening span, bringing the message for the variable and constant regions together into a final mRNA product that is translated into the intact α-chain protein. The random selection and pairing of 50 *V* and 50 *J* genes by a large number of developing T cells can result in more than 2500 possible α-chains.

In a similar fashion, the TCR β-chain locus on chromosome 7 has three sets of genes that rearrange to encode the variable region of that chain: at least 20 *V* genes, 13 *J* genes, and 2 intervening and relatively short *D* genes that add further diversity. Using the RAG-1 and RAG-2 enzymes, a developing T cell randomly selects a set of *V, D,* and *J* genes for DNA recombination. The *VDJ* rearranged segment is transcribed with a β-chain constant region, the intervening RNA is removed during processing, and the final mRNA is translated into an intact β-chain.

The α- and β-chains are joined by that cell and inserted into the membrane to make an antigen-specific TCR. The enormous number of possible combinations of α-chain *V* and *J* regions along with the β-chain *V, D,* and *J* regions enables the generation of a population of T cells with a large diversity of TCRs (estimated at 1.3×10^5 possible combinations). For both chains, the *V* region genes encode the amino acid sequences that include CDR1 and CDR2 and their appropriate FR regions. The *J* regions contain information for CDR3 and FR4. The TCR β-chain *D* regions encode a short amino acid sequence found in the CDR3 and greatly increases the diversity of the β-chain CDR3. Imprecise joining increases the diversity of the CDR3 regions of both the α- and β-chains even further. For example, the sites of *VJ* and *VDJ* joining may shift slightly resulting in an amino acid being inserted or deleted from the protein.

Although the αβ TCR is the preferred antigen receptor, some T cells use alternative genes: gamma (γ) (chromosome 7) and delta (δ) (chromosome 14, in the middle of α-chain genes). T cells with γδ TCRs appear to migrate to unique areas of the body (the epithelial areas in the skin, reproductive tract, intestine, respiratory tract) and have different and less well understood functions than the T cells with αβ TCRs.

Changes in Characteristic Surface Markers

Differentiation of T cells in the thymus also results in changes in a variety of important surface molecules. As the developing T cells move through the thymic cortex, they initiate the expression of the molecule CD2 on the cell surface. CD2 is a marker for T cells and is expressed on virtually every subpopulation of cells that have undergone development in the thymus. Within the cortex, the cells begin rearranging the variable region genes necessary for forming a functional T-cell receptor. The T-cell receptor undergoes several stepwise changes until the final αβ TCR is formed. Concurrently, the TCR accessory molecules (collectively called CD3) are expressed. The cell also begins making two important surface proteins, CD4 and CD8, which are concurrently expressed on the developing cell's surface at this stage. These CD4+, CD8+ cells are often called "double-positive" cells. Much of T-cell development is controlled by hormones and cytokines in the thymus, and an early step in maturation is expression of the receptor for interleukin (IL)-7 (IL-7R), which is a major cytokine that drives the differentiation process. After entering the medulla of the thymus, the double-positive cells become "single-positive." That is, some of the cells suppress production of the CD8 molecule and remain only CD4+, whereas others suppress CD4 production and remain CD8+. This branch in the differentiation pathway leads to two groups of cells with different functional characteristics: CD4 cells tend to recognize antigen presented by MHC class II molecules and develop into helpers in the later clonal selection process (helper T cells), whereas CD8 cells recognize antigen presented by MHC class I molecules and become mediators of cell-mediated immunity and kill other cells directly (cytotoxic T cells).

Central Tolerance

During the random rearrangement of *VJ* and *VDJ* genes to produce the T-cell receptor, some combinations result in specificities that recognize self-antigens. If some of these *autoreactive* T cells were allowed to progress further in development and leave the thymus, a severe immunologic reaction against the individual's own tissues could result. One stage at which tolerance for self-antigens is maintained is the deletion of autoreactive T cells in the thymus, which is referred to as central tolerance.

A variety of self-antigens are expressed by thymic cells. Many thymic cells express MHC class I or MHC class II molecules. During the T cell's double-positive stage, if a TCR strongly reacts with MHC class I or class II, the T cell will undergo apoptosis, referred to as *clonal deletion*. A large spectrum of other self-antigens is expressed on the surface of thymic macrophages, dendritic cells, and especially epithelial cells. If a developing T cell's TCR binds strongly with a self-antigen, it is deleted. Although this process of *negative selection* induces more than 95% of T cells to undergo apoptosis in the thymus, a limited number of autoreactive clones persist and must be controlled by other means in the peripheral lymphoid organs (**peripheral tolerance**).

The destiny of the double-positive cells with TCRs specific for foreign antigens (which are not expressed in the thymus) is determined by their interaction in the thymus with MHC antigens. If their surface CD4 molecules bind to MHC class II molecules on the thymic cells, the T cell will become CD4 single-positive. However, if their surface CD8 reacts with MHC class I molecules, the cells will become CD8 single-positive. This *positive selection* process results in about 60% of immunocompetent T cells being CD4+ and 40% being CD8+ when they leave the thymus.

B-Cell Maturation

Central Lymphoid Organ

Although the thymus is the central lymphoid organ for T-cell development, humans do not appear to have a discrete organ for B-cell development. In chickens, B lymphocytes undergo differentiation in an organ called the *bursa of Fabricius*. In humans, portions of the bone marrow function as a bursal-equivalent tissue for B cell development.[19]

Regardless of the lack of a discrete organ, B-cell differentiation undergoes a very similar process to that described above for T cells. Lymphoid stem cells in the bone marrow interact with stromal cells through a variety of intercellular adhesion molecules (Figure 7-12). As the stem cell begins to mature, it progressively develops a variety of necessary surface markers, the earliest being CD45R and the IL-7 receptor. IL-7, produced by the stromal cells, is critical in driving the further differentiation and proliferation of the B cell. The next stage in development is formation of the B-cell receptor.

Production of the B-Cell Receptor

The BCR is an antibody that is anchored to the plasma membrane. The process by which BCR diversity is generated is virtually identical to the process in T cells and also requires the genetic rearrangement of *V*, *D*, and *J* genes.[20] The segments of DNA that encode either kappa (κ) (chromosome 2) or lambda (λ) (chromosome 22) light chains contain about 70 *V* and 5 *J* segments, whereas the heavy chain locus on chromosome 14 contains about 80 *V*, 30 *D*, and 6 *J* regions. The locus for the antibody heavy chain also contains multiple sequential regions for different constant regions, with the gene for the mu (μ) constant region being closest to the VDJ region, and the delta (δ) constant region gene being next in sequence (Figure 7-13). These are followed by the constant region genes for other classes and subclasses. In the developing B cell, the

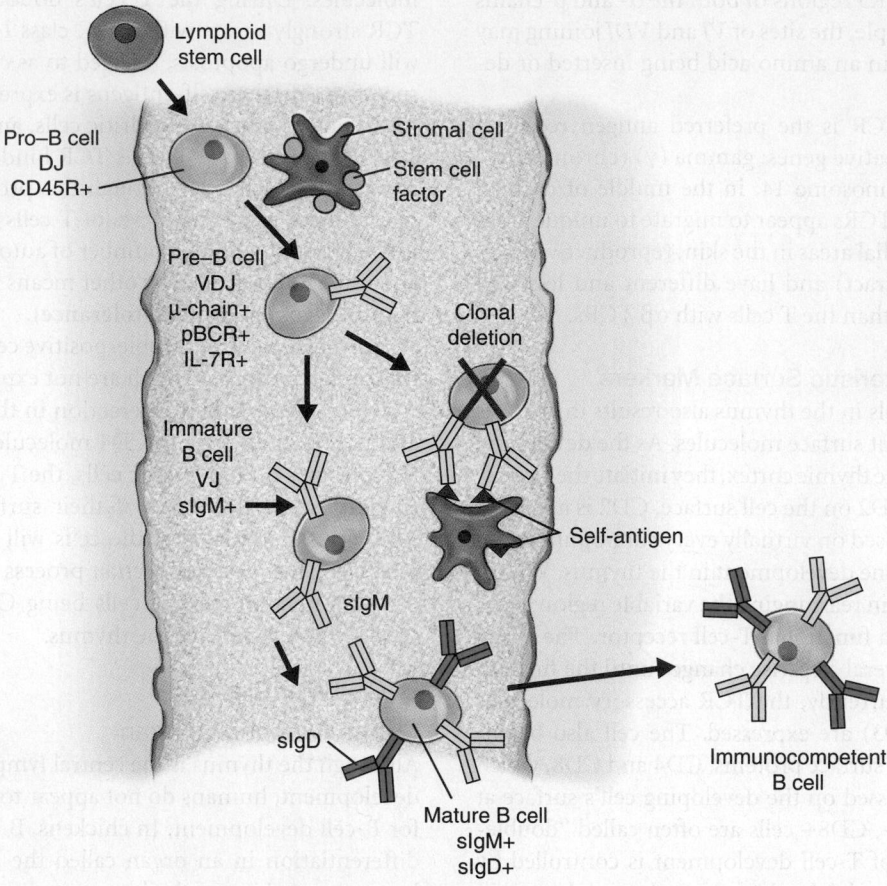

Figure 7-12 B-cell development in the bone marrow. During the generation of clonal diversity, lymphoid stem cells enter portions of the bone marrow that serve as the central lymph organ for B-cell development. Interactions with a series of bone marrow stromal cells guide the proliferation and differentiation process through direct cell-to-cell contact and the production of cytokines and hormones by the stromal cells, but without the presence of foreign antigen. A simplified scheme for that process is presented here. As with T-cell development, the differentiation process of B cells is characterized by the up-regulation of many important surface molecules (only some of which are shown) and the random development of a huge number of different B-cell receptors. The early B cell (pro–B cell) binds to a membrane-bound cytokine (stem cell factor) on the stromal cell and initiates expression of the surface molecule CD45R and begins to rearrange the *DJ* regions of the antibody heavy-chain gene. As the cell progresses to the pre–B-cell stage, it concludes DNA rearrangement of the heavy chain *(VDJ)* and begins expressing cytoplasmic mu (μ) heavy chain. The μ- chain is incorporated into a pre–B-cell receptor (pBCR) using a surrogate protein in place of the light chain. The cell also up-regulates the IL-7 receptor (IL-7R), which interacts with IL-7 produced by the stromal cells to drive the remaining steps in differentiation. Some pBCRs have specificities toward self-antigen. Many of these encounter self-antigen expressed on the stromal cells and undergo negative selection (clonal deletion). The surviving cells (immature B cells) rearrange the light chain DNA *(VJ)* and express a BCR consisting of light chain and the μ-heavy chain (surface IgM [sIgM]). In the mature B cell, changes in processing of the heavy-chain precursor RNA results in co-expression of sIgM and IgD (sIgD) (see Figure 7-13 for more details).

initial RNA transcript contains information for the *VDJ* recombination, the μ constant region, and the δ constant region. Transcription is signaled to stop immediately after the δ constant region. During the following RNA processing step to form a final mRNA product, the cell can alternatively process one mRNA to retain the μ constant region only or process another mRNA molecule to remove the μ constant region and retain the δ constant region. Thus one cell can use multiple mRNA molecules and alternative RNA processing to simultaneously produce two different heavy chains, μ and δ, both of which have the same variable region.

The developing B cell rearranges and expresses the heavy chain, which is followed by the rearrangement of either the κ or λ light chain so that only one type is produced. The light

chains are assembled with two μ heavy chains to form a monomeric IgM antibody or with two δ chains to form an IgD antibody. Because each heavy chain used the same VDJ rearrangement and the same light chain, the variable regions and therefore the specificities of the IgM and IgD are identical. At this stage of B-cell development, both antibodies have hydrophobic, or sticky, "tails" that results in insertion into the plasma membrane and the co-expression of IgM and IgD receptors on the cell surface.

Changes in Characteristic Surface Markers

As with T cells, B-cell differentiation is also characterized by the development of a variety of important surface molecules. These include CD21 (a complement receptor) and

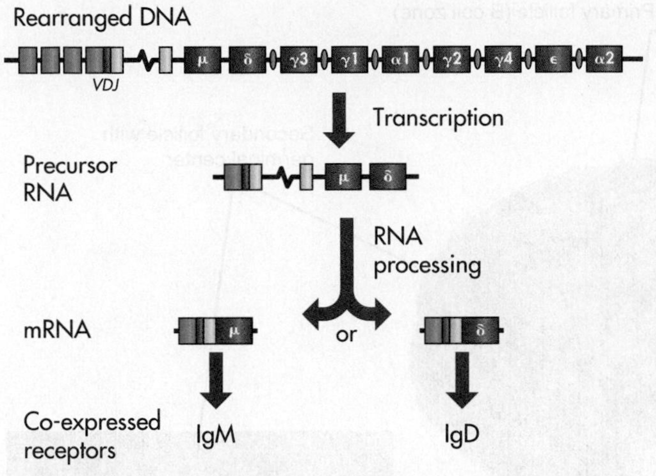

Figure 7-13 Genetics of the B-cell receptor. Most mature immunocompetent B cells express both surface IgM and IgD as the B-cell receptor. In the germline DNA, the heavy chain gene complex consists of a series of V, D, J, and constant region genes. In humans, each class and subclass of antibody has a unique constant region gene arranged in the indicated order. Switch regions occur preceding every constant region gene, except mu (μ) (IgM) and delta (δ) (IgD). After successful DNA rearrangement of the VDJ regions, a ribonucleic acid (RNA) molecule is transcribed that contains the information from the VDJ, intervening DNA, the μ constant region, and the δ constant region. Precursor RNA molecules are alternatively processed to produce messenger RNAs (mRNAs) containing either μ or δ. Initially, RNA processing favors the μ chain and production of surface IgM (see Figure 7-12), but as the B cell matures, both mRNA molecules are produced.

CD40 (adhesion molecule required for later interactions with Th).

Central Tolerance

During formation of the BCR in the bone marrow, a large number of autoreactive B cells are eliminated if exposed to self-antigen.[21] It is estimated that more than 90% of developing B cells are induced to undergo apoptosis.

INDUCTION OF AN IMMUNE RESPONSE: CLONAL SELECTION

As described in the previous chapter, successful invasion by a pathogen will initially elicit an inflammatory response as a host attempts to destroy and clear the invading microorganism. In addition to carrying out their roles as inflammatory effector cells, some of the cells involved in innate immunity are responsible for communicating with immature B and T lymphocytes to initiate specific and longer-acting acquired immunity. This intercellular communication occurs via direct cellular contact in peripheral lymphoid tissues and is essential for the specificity of the adaptive immune response.

Secondary Lymphoid Organs

The secondary lymphoid organs include the spleen, lymph nodes, adenoids, tonsils, Peyer patches (intestines), and the appendix (see Figure 7-3). Immunocompetent lymphocytes enter the secondary lymphoid organs through the blood and enter specialized small veins, called **high endothelial venules (HEVs)**, where they bind to the endothelium through a family of adhesion molecules.[22] The lymphocytes migrate from the vessels into the lymphoid tissues, which contain B- and T-cell–rich areas. B lymphocytes that encounter antigen in the secondary lymph organs usually undergo a process of differentiation and proliferation that results in the formation of specialized germinal centers in these organs (Figure 7-14).[23]

Antigen Processing and Presentation

Most antigens do not react directly with T or B cells, but require processing and presentation in the appropriate fashion.[24] This is the duty of APCs.

Pathogens that penetrate the external barriers and enter the tissues or bloodstream encounter a variety of phagocytic cells and are therefore likely to be ingested and destroyed. If the infectious agent is in the tissues, they may elicit an inflammatory response that results in the infiltration of macrophages into the site. Additionally, the infectious agent or fragments of the microorganism may be removed by the lymphatics, which drain to the lymph nodes. The lymph nodes are extremely rich in dendritic cells and macrophages, which phagocytose the material and function as APCs for T and B lymphocytes in the lymph nodes. Pathogens entering through the blood stream may be removed by phagocytic cells in the spleen and other lymphoid tissues. In either case, the phagocytic cells that digest invading pathogens are also responsible for processing antigens from the pathogen and displaying or presenting those antigens on the phagocyte's surface to neighboring lymphocytes in order to initiate the adaptive immune response against that specific pathogen.

Many cells have the capacity to present antigen to some degree, but dendritic cells, macrophages, and B lymphocytes are so efficient at antigen presentation that they are considered "professional" APCs. Each of these three APCs is responsible for the presentation of antigens of different types and from different sources. B cells present antigen to Th cells that facilitate development of the humoral immune response. Macrophages are very effective in presenting antigen to memory Th cells in order to initiate a rapid response to antigens (i.e., secondary immune response). The dendritic cells are perhaps the most effective in presenting antigen to naive immunocompetent Th cells.[25] Dendritic cells develop from bone marrow precursor cells, either of myeloid or lymphoid lineage (at least two populations of dendritic cells have been described). They migrate to the peripheral tissues (e.g., skin, intestinal tract) and to the secondary lymphoid organs. Immature dendritic cells at a site of inflammation function as phagocytes, and the process of phagocytosis can initiate differentiation and directed migration to the secondary lymphoid organs, particularly the lymph nodes (Figure 7-15). Thus dendritic cells can carry processed antigen from a site of inflammation to the T-cell–rich areas of the lymph nodes.

Both antigen processing and presentation are necessary for an adaptive immune response to occur. Although B and T lymphocytes are immunocompetent before they have "seen"

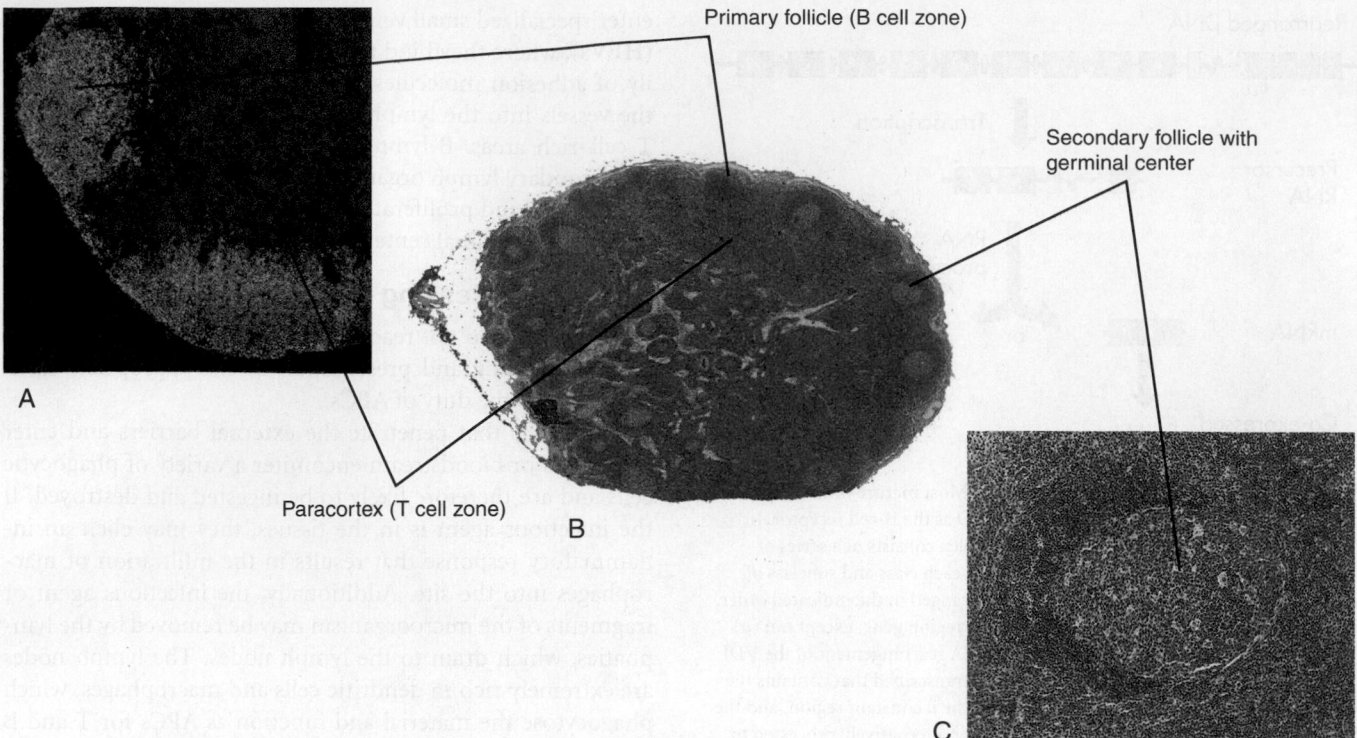

Primary follicle (B cell zone)

Secondary follicle with germinal center

Paracortex (T cell zone)

A

B

C

Figure 7-14 Histology of a secondary lymphoid organ. **A,** The lymph node contains areas (primary follicles) that are rich in immunocompetent B cells *(stained green)*, and T cells *(stained red)* in the paracortex. **B,** A lymph node is organized into an outer cortex and an inner medulla. **C,** In response to antigen, B cells undergo proliferation, resulting in the formation of secondary follicles with germinal centers. (Modified from Kumar V, Abbas A, Fausto N: *Robbins and Cotran pathologic basis of disease,* ed 7, Philadelphia, 2005, Saunders.)

an antigen on the surface of an APC, they are considered "naive" until they have actually done so. The processing and presentation of antigens to naive lymphocytes result in activation of an acquired immune response only if (1) the antigen is of the appropriate type; (2) the lymphocytes are prepared to recognize the presented antigen; and (3) the antigen is presented appropriately.

Pathways of Antigen Processing

In general, the immune system responds to two types of antigens: exogenous and endogenous.[26] Using infection as a model, exogenous antigens are carried on microorganisms that are trapped and killed by phagocytic cells; therefore, they come from outside the cell. Endogenous antigens are synthesized within a cell. These include viral antigens because viruses infect cells and use the normal cellular protein-synthesizing machinery to translate the viral genes into viral proteins. Endogenous antigens also may include those uniquely produced by cancerous cells. When many cells undergo malignant change, they begin producing unique proteins that are specific to cancer cells and are presented as foreign antigens on the cell surface.

Exogenous and endogenous antigens are preferentially presented by different classes of MHC molecules: class I MHC molecules generally present endogenous antigens, and class II molecules prefer exogenous antigens (Figure 7-16). Because

class I MHC molecules are expressed on all cells, except red blood cells, any change in that cell due to viral infection or malignancy may result in foreign antigen being presented by MHC class I on that cell's surface. Class II MHC molecules are co-expressed with MHC class I on a more limited number of cells that have APC function, including macrophages, dendritic cells, B lymphocytes, activated T lymphocytes, and some endothelial cells.

Thus the term **antigen processing** relates to the process by which exogenous and endogenous antigens are linked with the appropriate MHC molecules. Endogenous antigens are usually components of proteins synthesized in the cytosol. They are degraded in the cytosol by proteasomes into small peptides and transported by TAP (transporter associated with antigen processing) proteins (TAP-1 and TAP-2) into the endoplasmic reticulum, where MHC class I and class II molecules are assembled.[27] The class I MHC molecules have open antigen-binding sites so that antigen, the class I MHC α-chain, and a β2-microglobulin molecule form a stable complex that is transported through the Golgi apparatus to the plasma membrane. The antigenic peptides presented by class I MHC are usually very small, 8 to 10 amino acids in length.

MHC class II molecules are also assembled in the endoplasmic reticulum but do not bind with endogenous antigen because the antigen-binding site is blocked by a small protein called **invariant chain.** Exogenous antigens are internalized

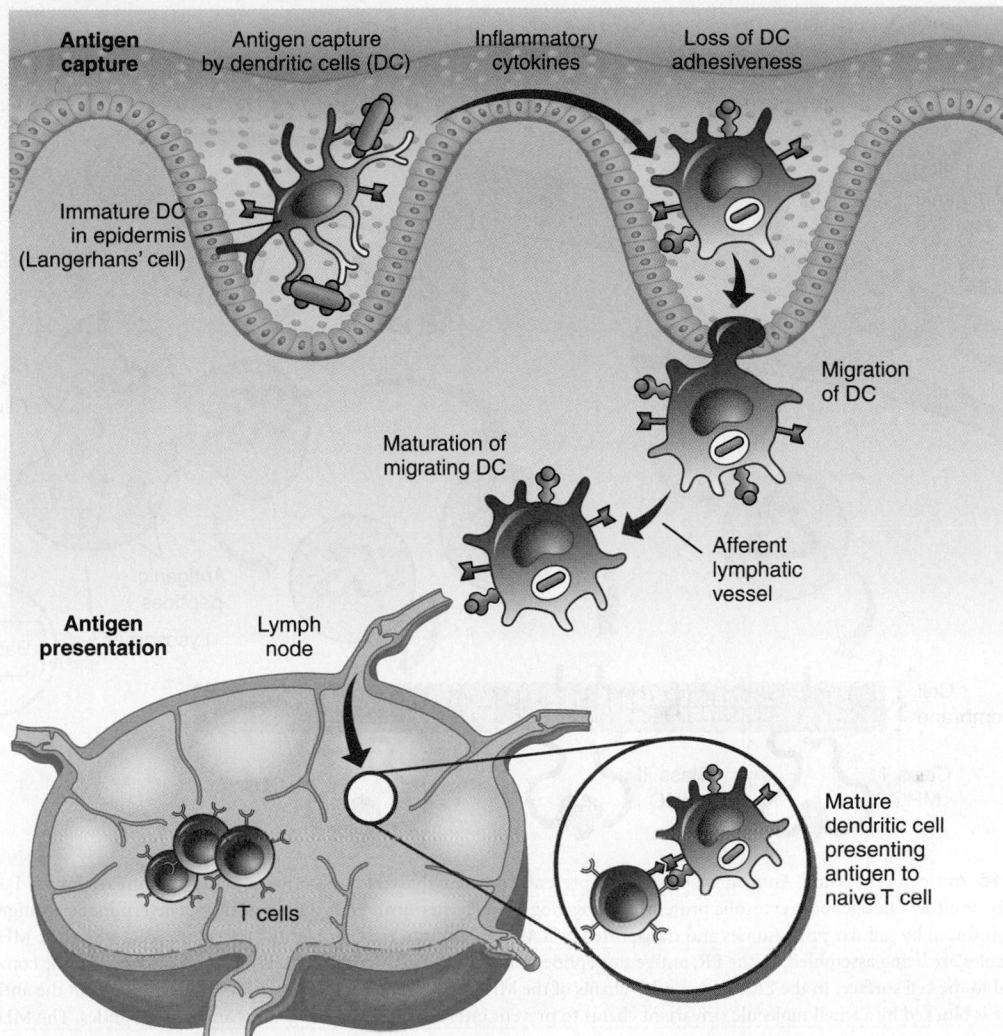

Figure 7-15 The role of the dendritic cell in capturing antigen. Immature dendritic cells in the tissues encounter and phagocytose antigen, which results in the production of inflammatory cytokines and a loss of adhesive interactions with neighboring cells. The maturing dendritic cell migrates through the lymphatic vessels to a regional lymph node, where it presents the antigen to immunocompetent T cells to initiate the clonal selection process. (Redrawn from Kumar V, Abbas A, Fausto N: *Robbins and Cotran pathologic basis of disease,* ed 7, Philadelphia, 2005, Saunders.)

by phagocytosis and small antigenic molecules produced by digestion in the lysosomes. The MHC class II complexes of the class II α- and β-chains, with invariant chain, are transported to the lysosomes containing exogenous antigens. In the lysosomal environment, the invariant chain is digested and replaced by antigenic molecules that are usually slightly larger (in excess of 12 amino acids in length) than those presented by MHC class I.

CD1 presents a variety of lipid-containing antigens that are usually derived from phagocytosis and digestion of infectious microorganisms with very high lipid content in their cell membranes. Therefore, CD1 complexes with antigen in the lysosomes, in a fashion similar to MHC class II. The "pocket" that holds antigen for presentation by CD1 is generally more narrow and deeper than described for MHC molecules, and it is lined with many hydrophobic amino acids that interact with lipid.

Helper T Lymphocytes

Regardless of whether an antigen primarily induces a cellular or humoral immune response, a subpopulation of T lymphocytes, **helper T cells (Th cells),** is usually necessary for the process.[28],[29] As indicated by the name, this group of T cells *helps* the antigen-driven maturation of both B and T cells. They perform this task by facilitating and magnifying the interaction between APCs and the immunocompetent lymphocytes. This extremely important role involves three distinct steps: (1) the Th cell directly interacts with the APC through a variety of antigen-specific and antigen-independent receptors; (2) the Th cell undergoes a differentiation process during which a variety of cytokine genes are activated; and (3) depending on the pattern of cytokines expressed, the mature Th cell interacts with either immunocompetent B or T cells to enhance their response to antigen, which results in differentiation into either plasma cells or effector T cells, such as cytotoxic

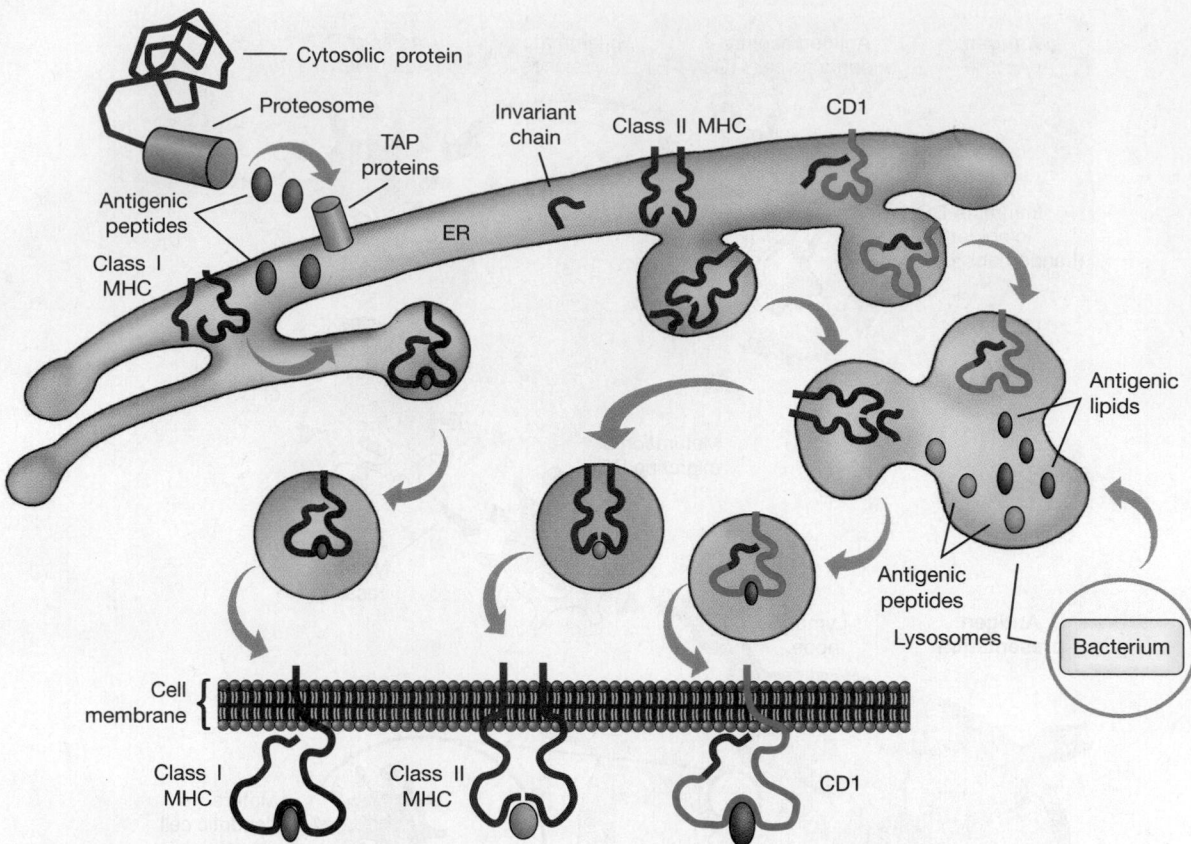

Figure 7-16 Antigen processing. Antigen processing and presentation are required for initiation of most immune responses. Foreign antigen may be either endogenous (cytosolic protein) or exogenous (e.g., bacterium). Endogenous antigenic determinants (antigenic peptides) are produced by cellular proteasomes and transported by TAP proteins into the endoplasmic reticulum (ER) where the MHC and CD1 molecules are being assembled. In the ER, antigenic peptides bind to the α-chains of the MHC class I molecule, and the complex is transported to the cell surface. In the ER, the α- and β-chains of the MHC class II molecules are also being assembled, but the antigen-binding site is blocked by a small molecule (invariant chain) to prevent interactions with endogenous antigenic peptides. The MHC class II–invariant chain complex is transported to lysosomes, where exogenous antigenic fragments have been generated as a result of phagocytosis. In the lysosomes the invariant chain is digested and replaced by exogenous antigenic peptides, after which the MHC class II–antigen complex is inserted into the cell membrane. CD1 is also assembled in the ER, but its antigen-binding site is specific for lipid antigenic determinants and does not bind endogenous antigenic peptides. The CD1 molecule is transported to the lysosomes and may encounter and bind antigenic lipids produced by phagocytic digestion of engulfed bacteria. The CD1-antigen complex is transported to the cell membrane and presents lipid antigens. *MHC,* Major histocompatibility complex; *TAP,* transporter associated with antigen processing.

T cells. Th cells are critical to most immune responses, and a variety of major Th-cell defects that lead to severely diminished immune responses are discussed in later chapters.

APC-Th Cooperation

Cells that are destined to become Th cells emerge from the thymus with characteristic cell surface markers. They have a functional αβ TCR complex and express the surface molecule CD4 and lack CD8. These are generally referred to as precursor Th cells, or sometimes Thp cells (Figure 7-17). As described previously, the TCR recognizes antigen, and the CD4 molecule confines antigen presentation to MHC class II molecules, thus CD4+ cells are *class II restricted*. In order to undergo maturation, the Th cell must receive three independent signals; antigen binding through the combined interaction of the TCR complex and CD4, co-stimulatory signals through a variety of intercellular adhesion molecules, and activation

of specific cytokine receptors.[30] If the appropriate signaling pathways are activated, the cell will differentiate through multiple intermediate stages into functional Th cells.

The complex of an antigenic peptide presented by an MHC class II molecule is recognized by multiple molecules on the Th-cell surface. The TCR binds directly to the antigen, whereas CD4 independently binds to a different site on the MHC class II β-chain. This co-recognition of the MHC/antigen complex by the TCR and CD4 brings CD4 into proximity with the CD3 components of the TCR complex, which initiates a series of enzymatic interactions among other molecules associated with the cytoplasmic portions of CD3 and CD4, such as the protein kinases p56[lck] and ZAP-70. These molecules activate a signaling pathway from the TCR to the Th-cell nucleus.

The antigenic signal alone is inadequate and may even inactivate the Th cell if co-stimulatory signals are not present. Co-stimulatory molecules are necessary for proper differentiation

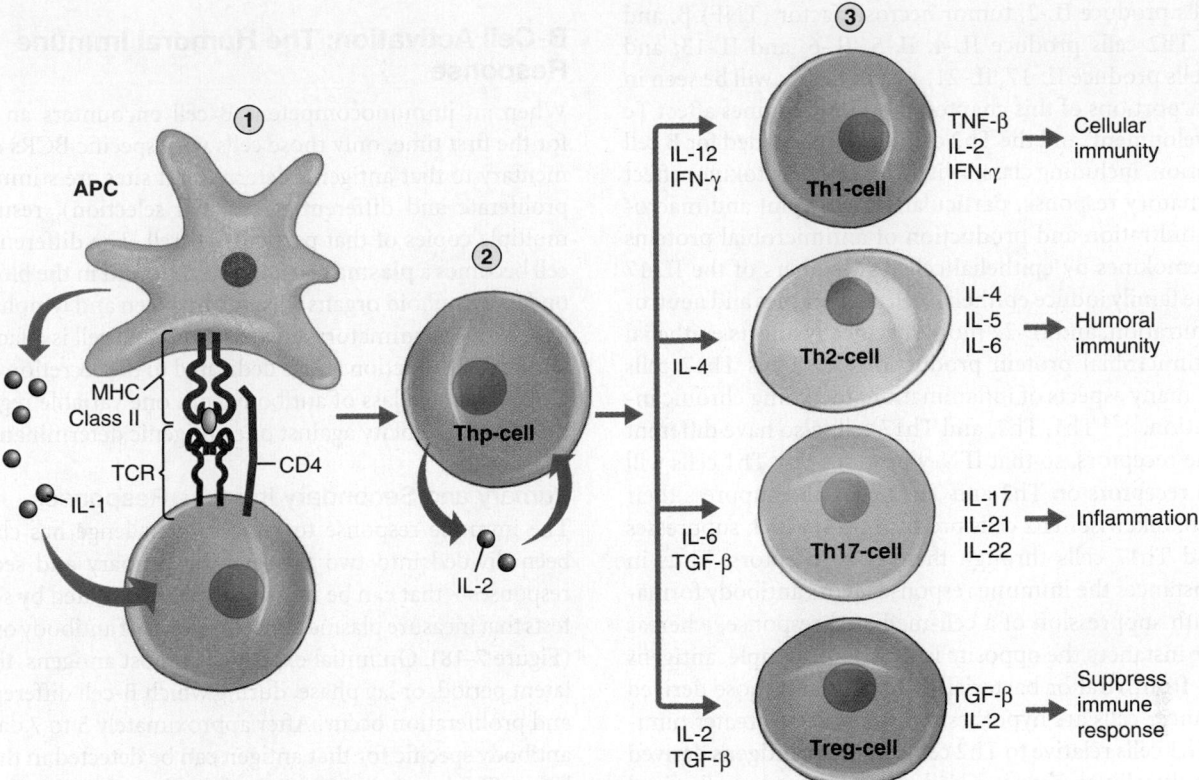

Figure 7-17 Development of T-cell subsets. The most important step in clonal selection is the production of populations of helper T (Th) cells (Th1, Th2, and Th17) and regulatory T (Treg) cells that are necessary for the development of cellular and humoral immune responses. In this model, APCs (probably multiple populations) may influence whether a precursor Th cell (Thp cell) will differentiate into a Th1, Th2, Th17, or Treg cell. Differentiation of the Thp cell is initiated by three signaling events. The antigen signal is produced by the interaction of the T-cell receptor (TCR) and CD4 with antigen presented by MHC class II molecules. A set of co-stimulatory signals is produced from interactions between adhesion molecules (e.g., CD80 and CD28) (not shown). A third signal is produced by the interactions of cytokines (particularly interleukin [IL]-1) with appropriate cytokine receptors (IL-1R) on the Thp cell. The Thp cell up-regulates IL-2 production and expression of the IL-2 receptor (IL-2R), which act in an autocrine fashion to accelerate Thp-cell differentiation and proliferation. Commitment to a particular phenotype results from the relative concentrations of other cytokines. IL-12 and IFN-γ produced by some populations of APCs favor differentiation into the Th1-cell phenotype; IL-4, which is produced by a variety of cells, favors differentiation into the Th2-cell phenotype; IL-6 and TGF-β (T-cell growth factor) facilitate differentiation into Th17 cells; IL-2 and TGF-β induce differentiation into Treg cells. The Th1 cell is characterized by the production of cytokines that assist in the differentiation of cytotoxic T (Tc) cells, leading to cellular immunity, whereas the Th2 cell produces cytokines that favor B-cell differentiation and humoral immunity. Th1 and Th2 cells affect each other through the production of inhibitory cytokines: IFN-γ will inhibit development of Th2 cells, and IL-4 will inhibit the development of Th1 cells. Th17 cells produce cytokines that affect phagocytes and increase inflammation. Treg cells produce immunosuppressive cytokines that prevent the immune response from being excessive. *APC,* Antigen presenting cell; *IFN,* interferon; *MHC,* major histocompatibility complex; *TGF,* transforming growth factor.

to occur. A variety of molecular interactions have been described, but the most critical appears to involve B7 on the APC and CD28 on the Th cell. Other interactions occur between CD48 on the APC and CD2 on the Th cell and between a variety of other adhesion molecules. In each case, the Th-cell molecule sends an activation signal to the nucleus. An additional signal is provided by cytokine. At this early stage of Th-cell differentiation, IL-1 secreted by the APC provides this signal through interaction with the IL-1 receptor on the Th cell.

The initial differentiation response by the Th cell includes the production of the cytokine IL-2 and up-regulation of IL-2 receptors. IL-2 is secreted and acts in an autocrine (self-stimulating) fashion to induce further maturation and proliferation of the Th cell. Without IL-2 production, the Th

cell cannot efficiently mature into a functional helper cell. At this point, Th cells undergo one of several different differentiation pathways into Th subsets.

Th Subsets

The most clearly characterized Th-cell subsets are **Th1** and **Th2 cells**, and the newly described **Th17 cells** (see Figure 7-17). These subsets have different functions: Th1 cells help develop cellular immunity, Th2 cells help develop humoral immunity, and Th17 cells increase the inflammatory response. A fourth subset, Treg cells, is discussed later in this chapter. The Th subsets differ considerably in the spectrum of cytokines produced by each, as well as the expression of surface cytokine receptors and intercellular adhesion molecules.

Th1 cells produce IL-2, tumor necrosis factor (TNF)-β, and IFN-γ; Th2 cells produce IL-4, IL-5, IL-6, and IL-13; and Th17 cells produce IL-17, IL-21, and IL-22. As will be seen in the next portions of this chapter, the Th1 cytokines affect Tc cell development, and the Th2 cytokines are needed for B cell maturation, including class-switch. Th17 cell cytokines affect inflammatory response, particularly neutrophil and macrophage infiltration and production of antimicrobial proteins and chemokines by epithelial cells.[31] Members of the IL-17 cytokine family induce epithelial cell chemokines and neutrophil infiltration, and IL-22 more specifically affects epithelial cell antimicrobial protein production.[29,32] Thus Th17 cells control many aspects of inflammation, including chronic inflammation.[33,34] Th1, Th2, and Th17 cells also have different cytokine receptors, so that IFN-γ produced by Th1 cells will bind to receptors on Th2 and Th17 cells and suppress their function. Likewise, Th2 cells produce IL-4, which suppresses Th1 and Th17 cells through their IL-4 receptors. Thus in some instances the immune response favors antibody formation, with suppression of a cell-mediated response, whereas in other instances the opposite is true. For example, antigens derived from viral or bacterial pathogens and those derived from cancer cells are hypothesized to induce a greater number of Th1 cells relative to Th2 cells, whereas antigens derived from multicellular parasites and allergens are hypothesized to result in production of more Th2 cells.[29] Many antigens (e.g., tetanus vaccine), however, produce excellent humoral and cell-mediated responses simultaneously.

How a Th cell is guided into becoming a Th1, Th2, or Th17 cell is not fully known. Some evidence indicates that different subpopulations of APCs influence the choice by secreting different profiles of cytokines that may favor one route of differentiation over another (see Figure 7-17).[29]

B-Cell Activation: The Humoral Immune Response

When an immunocompetent B cell encounters an antigen for the first time, only those cells with specific BCRs complementary to that antigen's determinant sites are stimulated to proliferate and differentiate (clonal selection), resulting in multiple copies of that particular B cell. The differentiated B cell becomes a **plasma cell** and can be found in the blood, secondary lymphoid organs (primarily spleen and lymph nodes), and some inflammatory sites. Each plasma cell is a factory for antibody production and is dedicated to the secretion of a single class or subclass of antibody with one variable region and therefore specificity against one antigenic determinant.

Primary and Secondary Immune Responses

The immune response to antigenic challenge has classically been divided into two phases—the primary and secondary responses—that can be most easily demonstrated by serologic tests that measure plasma concentrations of antibody over time (Figure 7-18). On initial exposure to most antigens, there is a latent period, or lag phase, during which B-cell differentiation and proliferation occur. After approximately 5 to 7 days, IgM antibody specific for that antigen can be detected in the circulation. The lag phase is a result of the time necessary for clonal selection, including antigen processing and presentation, induction of Th cells, interactions between immunocompetent B cells and Th cells, and the maturation and proliferation of the B cells into plasma cells and memory cells.

This is the initial response, or **primary immune response.** Typically, IgM will be produced first, followed by IgG against the same antigen. The quantity of IgG may be about equal to or less than the amount of IgM production. If no further

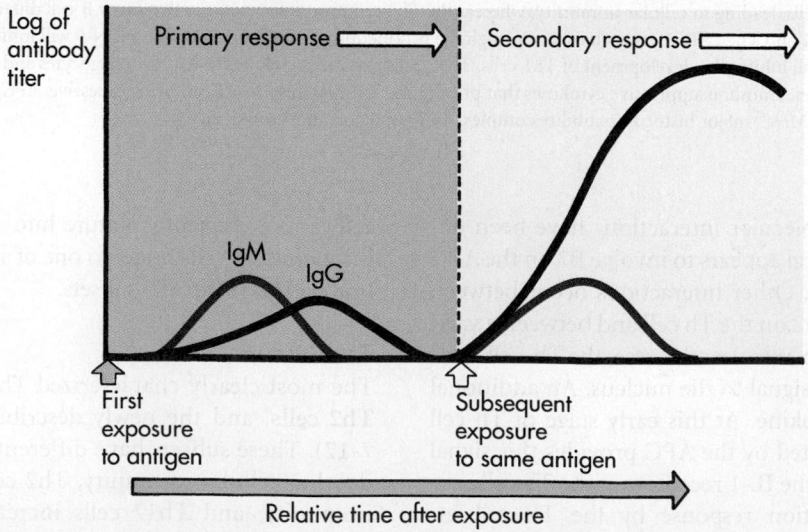

Figure 7-18 Primary and secondary immune responses. Antigen responses are dominated by two classes of immunoglobulins, IgM and IgG. IgM predominates on initial exposure to the antigen in the primary response, with IgG appearing later. After the host's immune system is primed, another challenge by the same antigen induces the secondary response in which some IgM and larger amounts of IgG are produced.

exposure to the antigen occurs, the circulating antibody is catabolized (broken down) and measurable quantities fall. The individual's immune system, however, has been primed. A second challenge by the same antigen results in the **secondary (anamnestic) immune response,** which is characterized by the more rapid production of a larger amount of antibody than the primary response. The rapidity of the secondary immune response is the result of the presence of memory cells that do not require further differentiation. IgM may be transiently produced in the secondary response and the quantity may be about the same as that produced in the primary response. IgG production is increased considerably, making it the predominant antibody class of the secondary response. It is often present in concentrations several times larger than those of IgM, and levels of circulating IgG specific for that antigen may remain elevated for an extended period of time. If the antigenic challenge is in the form of a vaccine or occurs through natural infection, the level of protective IgG may remain elevated for decades.

The existence of a prolonged and protective secondary immune response explains how vaccinations provide protection against certain pathogenic microorganisms. Edward Jenner, an English physician of the late eighteenth century, performed the first well-documented vaccine trial.[35,36] Although some of the stories about Jenner's experiments are fanciful, it is known that Jenner recognized that milkmaids were protected from the deadly smallpox virus if they had previously developed cowpox, a bovine equivalent of smallpox that causes only mild disease in humans. Jenner took material from a cowpox pustule on the hand of an infected milkmaid and injected it into the arm of an 8-year-old boy. After the boy's initial inflammatory reaction to the injection subsided, Jenner injected him again, this time with material from a smallpox pustule. Fortunately, the experiment was a success because Jenner is reported to have reinjected smallpox virus into the boy at least 20 times without the child becoming ill. In Jenner's experiment, the antigens on the cowpox virus and the smallpox virus were sufficiently similar that the cowpox antigen functioned as an altered or attenuated smallpox antigen. The antibodies and lymphocytes that recognized and destroyed cowpox also were able to recognize the smallpox virus, thereby protecting the immunized child against smallpox. In 1798, Jenner used the term *vaccination* (*vacca* = cow) to describe his technique.

Cellular Interactions

As with most aspects of immunity, a sequence of cellular interactions is required to produce an effective antibody response (Figure 7-19).[37] The immunocompetent B cell is also an APC and expresses surface IgM and IgD BCRs. Unlike the T-cell

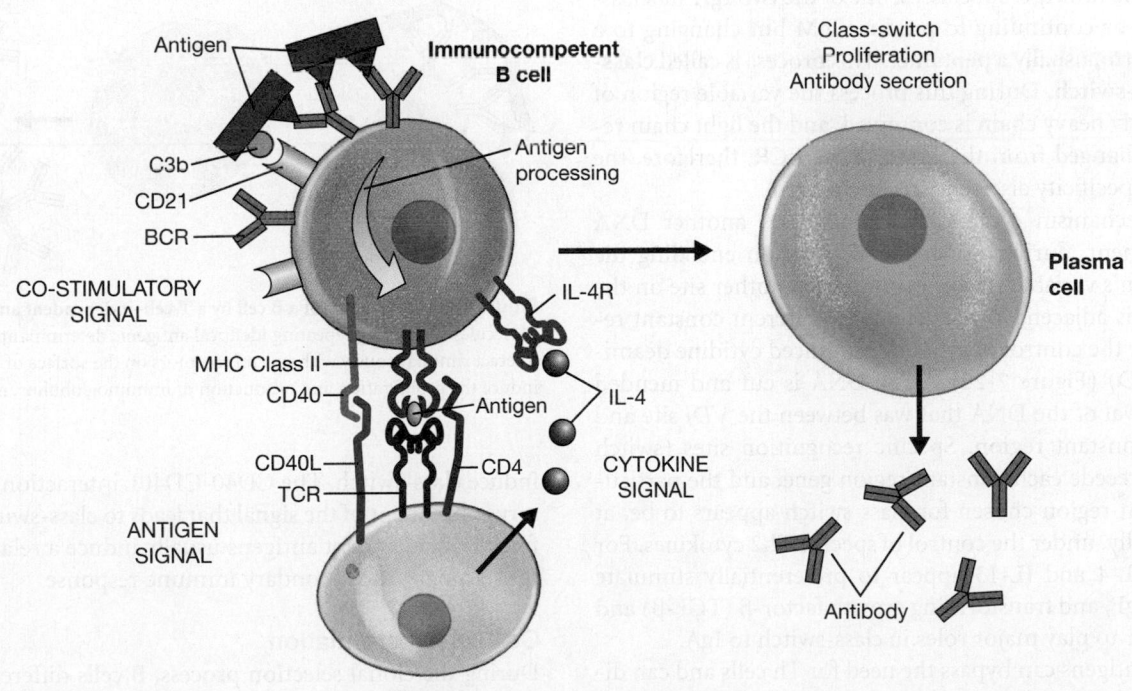

Figure 7-19 B-cell clonal selection. Immunocompetent B cells undergo proliferation and differentiation into antibody-secreting plasma cells. Three signals are necessary. The antigen signal is provided by the B cell itself. A B cell can recognize soluble antigen directly through the B-cell receptor and co-receptors, such as complement receptors (CD21), which usually involve accessory molecules such as CD19 (not shown). Antigen is internalized and processed for presentation by MHC class II molecules, which interact with the T-cell receptor (TCR) and CD4 on Th2 cells. Co-stimulatory signals are provided through adhesion molecules, particularly CD40 and CD40L (CD154). The cytokine signal is provided by Th2 cytokines (particularly IL-4) binding to appropriate cytokine receptors (IL-4R) on the B cell. Additional cytokines influence switch to particular classes or subclasses of antibody. *MHC,* Major histocompatibility complex.

receptor that can only "see" processed and presented antigen, the BCR can react with soluble antigen. Antigen binding to the BCR complex activates intracellular kinases, in a fashion similar to the TCR receptor complex. In many instances, circulating antigen, either on macromolecules or the surface of a pathogen, will have activated the complement system through the alternative or lectin pathways. Thus complement receptors on the B cell, such as CD19 and CD21, act as co-receptors to bind antigen. As a result of signaling from the BCR complex and other surface co-receptors, the antigen-bearing macromolecule is internalized, broken down in the lysosomes, and complexes with MHC class II molecules for presentation on the cell surface, where it is recognized by a Th2 cell through the TCR and CD4. The intercellular bridge created through antigen induces the Th2 cell to up-regulate additional surface receptors and secrete cytokines. Direct interaction between CD40 on the B-cell surface and the CD40 ligand (CD40L, also called CD154) on the Th2 cell, as well as the interaction of B7 on the B cell and CD28 on the Th cell and exposure of the B cell to Th2-cell cytokines (particularly IL-4) induces proliferation of the B cell and maturation into a plasma cell. A major component of maturation is class switch.

Class-Switch

The immunocompetent B cell uses IgM and IgD as receptors. During the clonal selection process, however, each B cell has the option of changing the class of antibody to a secreted form of one of the four IgG subclasses, one of the two IgA subclasses, or IgE, or continuing to produce IgM but changing to a secreted form, usually a pentamer. This process is called **class-** or **isotype-switch.** During this process the variable region of the antibody heavy chain is conserved, and the light chain remains unchanged from that used in the BCR; therefore, the antigenic specificity also remains unchanged.

The mechanism of class-switch involves another DNA rearrangement, during which the *VDJ* region encoding the heavy chain's variable region is moved to another site on the DNA that is adjacent to the gene for a different constant region under the control of activation-induced cytidine deaminase (AICD) (Figure 7-20).[38] The DNA is cut and mended with removal of the DNA that was between the *VDJ* site and the new constant region. Specific recognition sites (switch regions) precede each constant region gene, and the particular constant region chosen for class-switch appears to be, at least partially, under the control of specific Th2 cytokines. For instance, IL-4 and IL-13 appear to preferentially stimulate switch to IgE, and transforming growth factor-β (TGF-β) and IL-5 appear to play major roles in class-switch to IgA.

A few antigens can bypass the need for Th cells and can directly stimulate B-cell maturation and proliferation. These are called *T-independent antigens* (Figure 7-21). They are mostly bacterial products that are large and are likely to have repeating antigenic determinants (multiple identical antigenic determinant sites) that bind and crosslink several B-cell receptors. The accumulated intracellular signal is adequate to induce differentiation to a plasma cell but is not adequate to

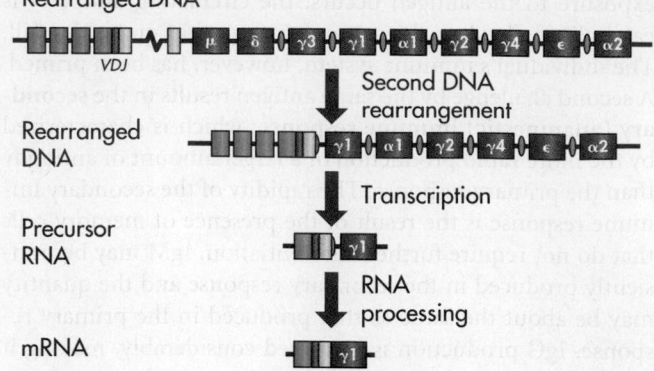

Figure 7-20 Genetics of class-switch. During clonal selection, most B cells switch from expression of surface IgM and IgD to a different class or subclass of antibody. A first set of DNA rearrangements during the generation of clonal diversity resulted in formation of the *VDJ* region. The class-switch process involves a second DNA rearrangement during which the *VDJ* region is moved to a switch region (orange ovals) immediately preceding the new class/subclass of antibody. In this example, the B cell undergoes class-switch to a γ1 heavy chain and secretion of an IgG1 antibody. The intervening DNA between the *VDJ* and the selected switch region is excised, and the DNA is repaired (DNA after second rearrangement) and transcribed into a precursor ribonucleic acid (RNA). The RNA is processed to a messenger RNA (mRNA) with information for the new heavy chain.

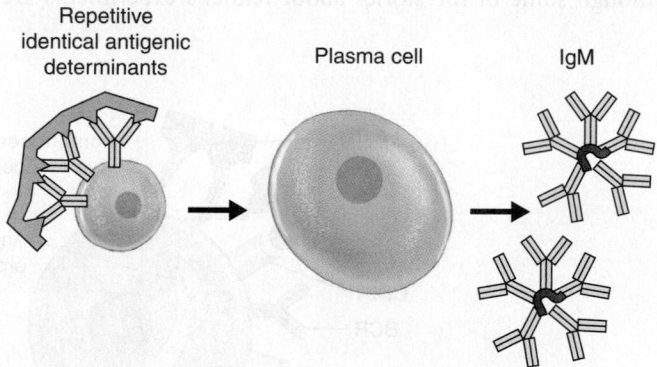

Figure 7-21 Activation of a B cell by a T-cell–independent antigen. Molecules containing repeating identical antigenic determinants may interact simultaneously with several receptors on the surface of the B cell and induce the proliferation and production of immunoglobulins, mainly IgM.

induce class-switch. The CD40-CD40L interaction is a necessary component of the signal that leads to class-switch. Therefore, T-independent antigens usually induce a relatively pure IgM primary and secondary immune response.

Cellular Differentiation

During the clonal selection process, B cells differentiate into antibody-producing plasma cells and into a set of long-lived memory cells. During B cells' differentiation into plasma cells, the CDR portions of the antibody variable region are prone to somatic point mutations that lead to changes in single amino acids. Some of these changes produce better antibodies that bind more strongly (higher affinity) to the antigen. The presence of antigen creates a positive selective pressure toward the developing B cells that express the higher-affinity antibody, which results in a process called *affinity maturation,* in which the quality of the circulating antibody improves over time.

The memory cells remain inactive until subsequent exposure to the same antigen. On reexposure, these memory cells do not require much further differentiation and will therefore differentiate rapidly into new plasma cells.[39]

T-Cell Activation: The Cellular Immune Response

Activation of the cell-mediated arm of the immune response begins with the binding of antigen to specific T-cell receptors. Through a variety of intercellular collaborations that are mediated by specific cellular receptors and cytokines, the naive T cell proliferates and differentiates into a functional (effector) T cell. The two main effector functions of activated T cells are (1) direct killing of foreign and/or abnormal cells and (2) assistance and/or activation of other cells, such as macrophages. The first function is carried out by a subclass of T cells termed cytotoxic T lymphocytes (Tc cells, or CTLs). Activation of macrophages is performed by a special subset of Th cells. Additional T cells develop into cells that regulate the immune response in order to avoid inadvertently attacking self-antigens or to avoid overactivation of the immune response.

This mixed population of cells is termed **T regulatory (Treg) cells.** Finally, **memory T cells** are also produced to help induce secondary cell-mediated immune responses.

Cellular Interactions

During the clonal selection phase of the cell-mediated immune response, immunocompetent T cells in the peripheral lymphoid organs must recognize antigen that has been processed and presented by MHC class I molecules (Figure 7-22).[40] The antigen is usually an endogenous antigen expressed on the surface of cells infected with a virus or that have become malignant. The T cells have a functional αβ TCR complex and express the surface molecule CD8, rather than CD4. The presence of the CD8 molecule confines antigen recognition to MHC class I molecules, therefore CD8+ T cells are *class I restricted.* The TCR binds directly to the antigenic peptide, whereas CD8 independently binds to a different site on the MHC class I α-chain. This co-recognition of the MHC/antigen complex by the TCR and CD8 brings CD8 into proximity with the CD3 components of the TCR complex, which initiates a series of enzymatic interactions among other molecules associated with the cytoplasmic portions of CD3 and CD4, as was described for Th-cell activation. These molecules activate a signaling pathway from the TCR to the T-cell nucleus.

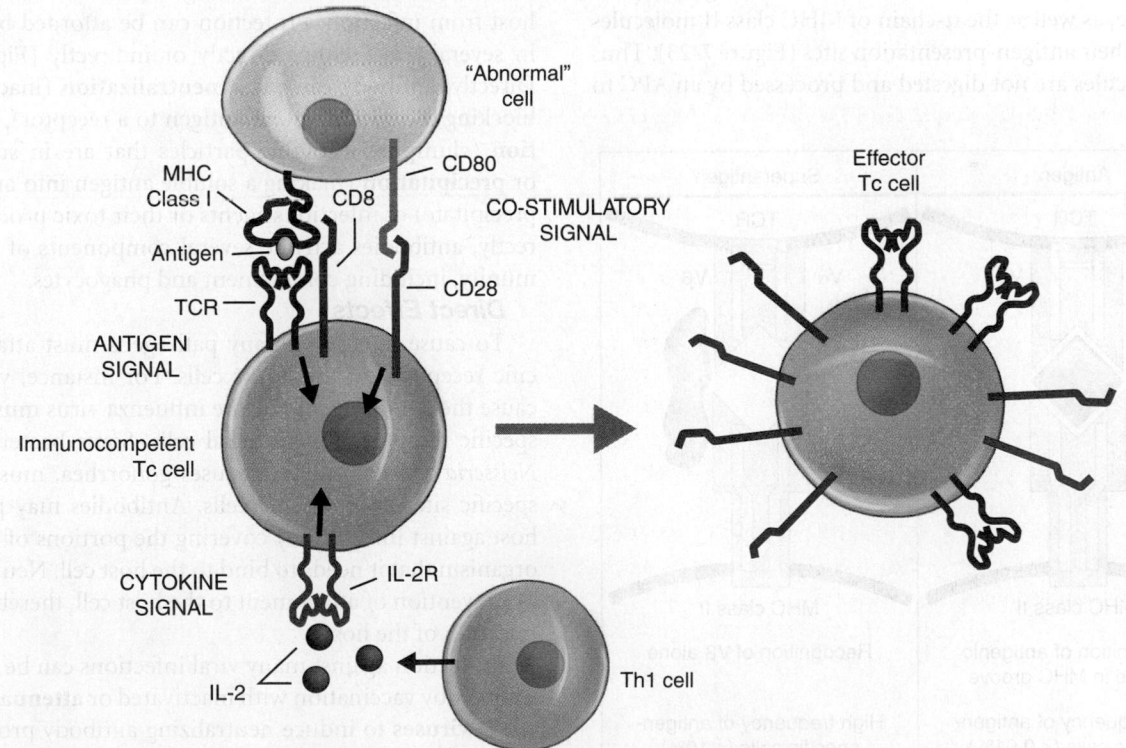

Figure 7-22 Tc-cell clonal selection. The development of effector cytotoxic T (Tc) cells during clonal selection results from three cooperative signaling events provided by antigen, co-stimulatory adhesion molecules, and cytokines. The immunocompetent Tc cell "sees" antigen presented by MHC class I molecules on the surface of a virally infected or cancerous "abnormal" cell. The antigen–MHC class I complex is recognized simultaneously by the T-cell receptor (TCR), which binds to antigen, and CD8, which binds to the MHC class I molecule. The proximity of signaling molecules associated with the cytoplasmic portions of CD8 and the TCR result in intracellular signaling. A separate signal results from the interaction of several groups of adhesion molecules (e.g., CD80 and CD28 in this example). The third signal is provided by the interaction of cytokine, particularly IL-2 from Th1 cells, and the appropriate receptor. *MHC,* Major histocompatibility complex.

To undergo maturation, the T cell must receive independent signals from a variety of co-stimulatory intercellular adhesion molecules and specific cytokine receptors. If the appropriate signaling pathways are activated, the cell will proliferate and differentiate through multiple intermediate stages into functional Tc cells. The co-stimulatory signals for Tc-cell maturation are virtually the same as has been described for Th-cell maturation: B7 on the cell-presenting antigen and CD28 on the T cell, CD48 on the antigen-presenting cell and CD2 on the T cell, and a variety of other adhesion molecules. Development of Tc cells also requires cytokines, especially IL-2, produced by the Th1 cell.

Cellular Differentiation

The result of these cellular interactions is the production of active Tc cells with the capacity to identify antigens on the surface of infected or malignant cells and then to destroy those cells. As with B cells, some of the T cells that become activated in response to antigen presentation will not become effectors that destroy infected targets, but instead develops into a population of memory T cells. These cells have the capacity to rapidly respond to further exposure to the same antigen.

Superantigens

A group of molecules has the ability to bind the variable portion of the TCR β-chain outside of its normal antigen-specific binding site, as well as the α-chain of MHC class II molecules outside of their antigen-presentation sites (Figure 7-23). Thus these molecules are not digested and processed by an APC to be presented to an immune cell. This binding results in adherence of the TCR and MHC class II molecules, independent of antigen recognition, and provides an activation signal for Th-cell activation and proliferation. The normal antigen-specific recognition between Th cells and APCs results in activation of relatively few cells: only those cells with specific TCRs against that antigen. The type of binding described here results in activation of large populations of T lymphocytes, regardless of antigen specificity.[41,42] Thus these molecules have been referred to as **superantigens (SAGs).**

SAGs induce an excessive production of cytokines, including IL-2, IFN-γ and TNF-α.[41,42] The overproduction of inflammatory cytokines results in symptoms of a systemic inflammatory reaction, including fever, low blood pressure, and potentially, fatal shock. Some examples of SAGs are the bacterial toxins produced by *Staphylococcus aureus* and *Streptococcus pyogenes* (including the superantigens that cause toxic shock syndrome and food poisoning).[43] Some viruses are also able to produce superantigens, although the exact nature of these antigens is unclear.

EFFECTOR MECHANISMS

Antibody Function

Protection Against Infection

The chief function of circulating antibodies is to protect the host from infection. Protection can be afforded by antibody in several ways, either directly or indirectly (Figure 7-24). Directly, antibody can cause **neutralization** (inactivating or blocking the binding of an antigen to a receptor), **agglutination** (clumping insoluble particles that are in suspension), or **precipitation** (making a soluble antigen into an insoluble precipitate) of infectious agents or their toxic products. Indirectly, antibodies activate several components of innate immunity, including complement and phagocytes.

Direct Effects

To cause infection, many pathogens must attach to specific receptors on the host's cells. For instance, viruses that cause the common cold or the influenza virus must attach to specific receptors on epithelial cells. Some bacteria, such as *Neisseria gonorrhoeae* that causes gonorrhea, must attach to specific sites on epithelial cells. Antibodies may protect the host against infection by covering the portions of the microorganism that it needs to bind to the host cell. Neutralization, or prevention of attachment to the host cell, thereby prevents infection of the host.

Protection against many viral infections can be elicited effectively by vaccination with inactivated or **attenuated** (weakened) **viruses** to induce neutralizing antibody production at the site of typical viral entrance into the body. A good indication of the degree of protection against viral infection is the level of circulating antibodies found in the blood. The level of circulating antibodies is referred to as an **antibody titer.** However, many viruses (e.g., measles, herpes) are inaccessible to antibodies after initial infection because they do not circulate in the bloodstream but instead remain inside infected

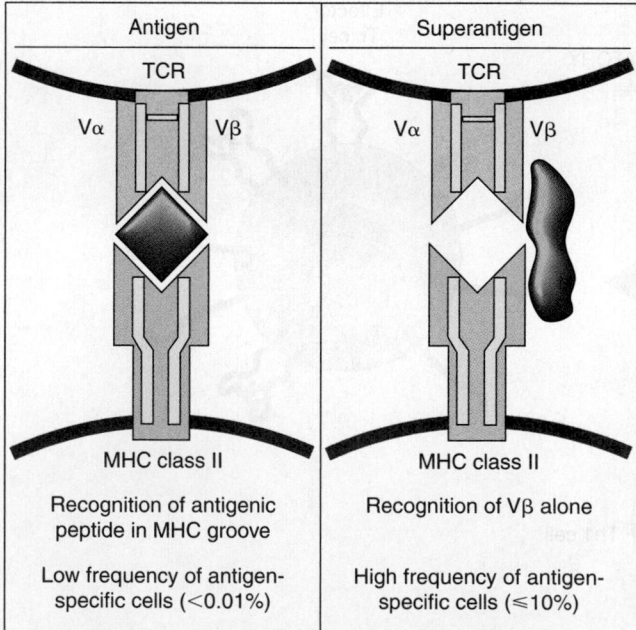

Figure 7-23 Superantigens. The T-cell receptor (TCR) and an MHC class II molecule normally simultaneously interact with a processed antigen to induce T-cell differentiation. Superantigens, such as some bacterial toxins, bind directly to the TCR and the MHC class II molecules. Superantigens activate Th cells independently of TCR antigen specificity. *MHC,* Major histocompatibility complex.

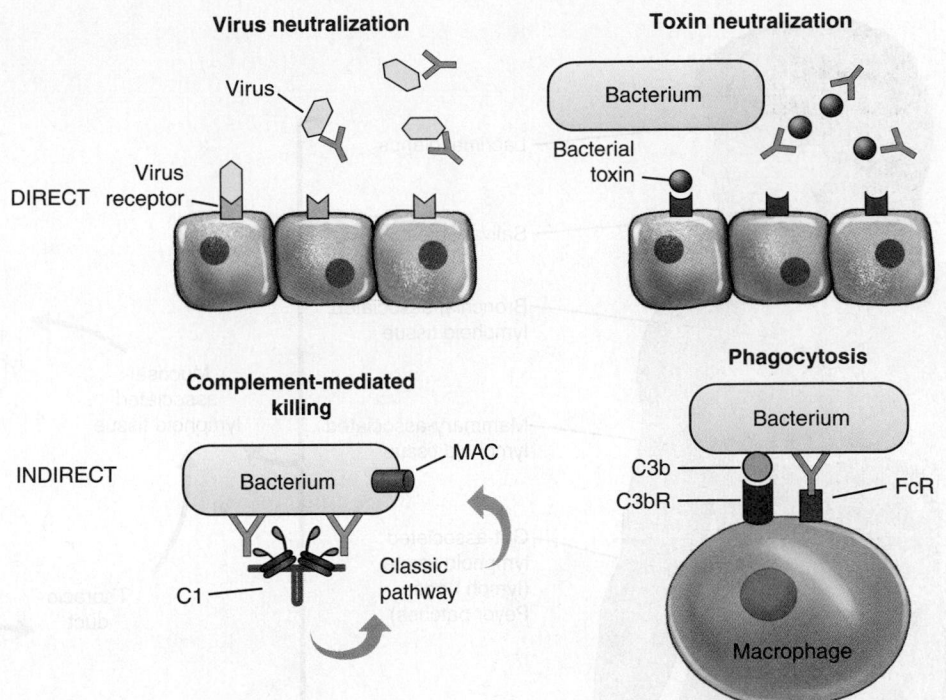

Figure 7-24 Direct and indirect functions of antibody. Protective activities of antibodies can be direct (through the action of antibody alone) or indirect (requiring activation of other components of the innate immune response, usually through the Fc region). Direct means include neutralization of viruses or bacterial toxins before they bind to receptors on the surface of the host's cells. Indirect means include activation of the classical complement pathway through C1, resulting in formation of the membrane-attack complex (MAC) or by increased phagocytosis of bacteria opsonized with antibody and complement components bound to appropriate surface receptors (FcR and C3bR).

cells, spreading by direct cell-to-cell contact. Neutralizing antibodies against this type of virus are most effective in preventing the initial infection. Other viruses, such as polio and influenza, spread through the blood, are more susceptible to the effects of circulating antibodies, and can be controlled by antibodies even after the initial infection.

The symptoms of some infectious diseases result directly from toxins produced by infecting bacteria. For instance, the symptoms of tetanus or diphtheria are mediated by specific toxins. To cause disease, most toxins must bind to surface molecules on the individual's cells. Protective antibodies can bind to the toxins, prevent their interaction with cells, and neutralize their biologic effects. Detection of the presence of an antibody response against a specific toxin (antibodies referred to as *antitoxins*) can aid in the diagnosis of diseases. For example, laboratory tests that detect antistreptolysin O also can be very useful in diagnosing group A streptococcal infections. Antibodies that neutralize bacterial toxins can be induced to confer immunity against bacterial pathogens by means of immunization. To prevent harming the recipient of immunization, bacterial toxins are chemically inactivated so that they have lost most of their harmful properties but still retain their immunogenicity. These are referred to as *toxoids*. Examples of bacterial pathogens for which immunization with toxoids can provide immunologic protection include those that cause diphtheria and tetanus.

A new therapeutic application of antibodies uses their normal properties to treat human disease (see What's New? Antibodies as Drugs).

WHAT'S NEW?   Antibodies as Drugs

A development in clinical treatment is the use of laboratory-produced immunoglobulins as drugs. Two such drugs commercially available are infliximab (Remicade) and rituximab (Rituxan). Infliximab, a recombinant chimeric antibody directed against tumor necrosis factor (TNF), is used in the treatment of inflammatory bowel diseases, such as Crohn disease, and autoimmune diseases, such as rheumatoid arthritis. Intravenous administration of infliximab is intended to decrease inflammation by neutralization of the proinflammatory cytokine TNF. Rituximab is a recombinant antibody that recognizes a glycoprotein on the surface of B lymphocytes (CD20). Administration of rituximab results in antibody binding to CD20 and subsequent immunoglobulin- and complement-mediated killing of CD20-positive B cells. Depletion of B cells is effective in the treatment of lymphoproliferative disorders, such as non-Hodgkin lymphoma, and autoimmune diseases, such as hemolytic anemia.

Data from Joyce RM et al: *Ann Oncol* 14(Suppl 1):i21-27, 2003; Moreland LW: *Pharmacoeconomics* 22(2 Suppl):39-53, 2004; Nagajothi N et al: *Leuk Lymphoma* 45(4):795-799, 2004; Stio M et al: *Dig Dis Sci* 49(2):328-335, 2004; Wakim M et al: *Am J Hematol* 76(2):152-155, 2004.

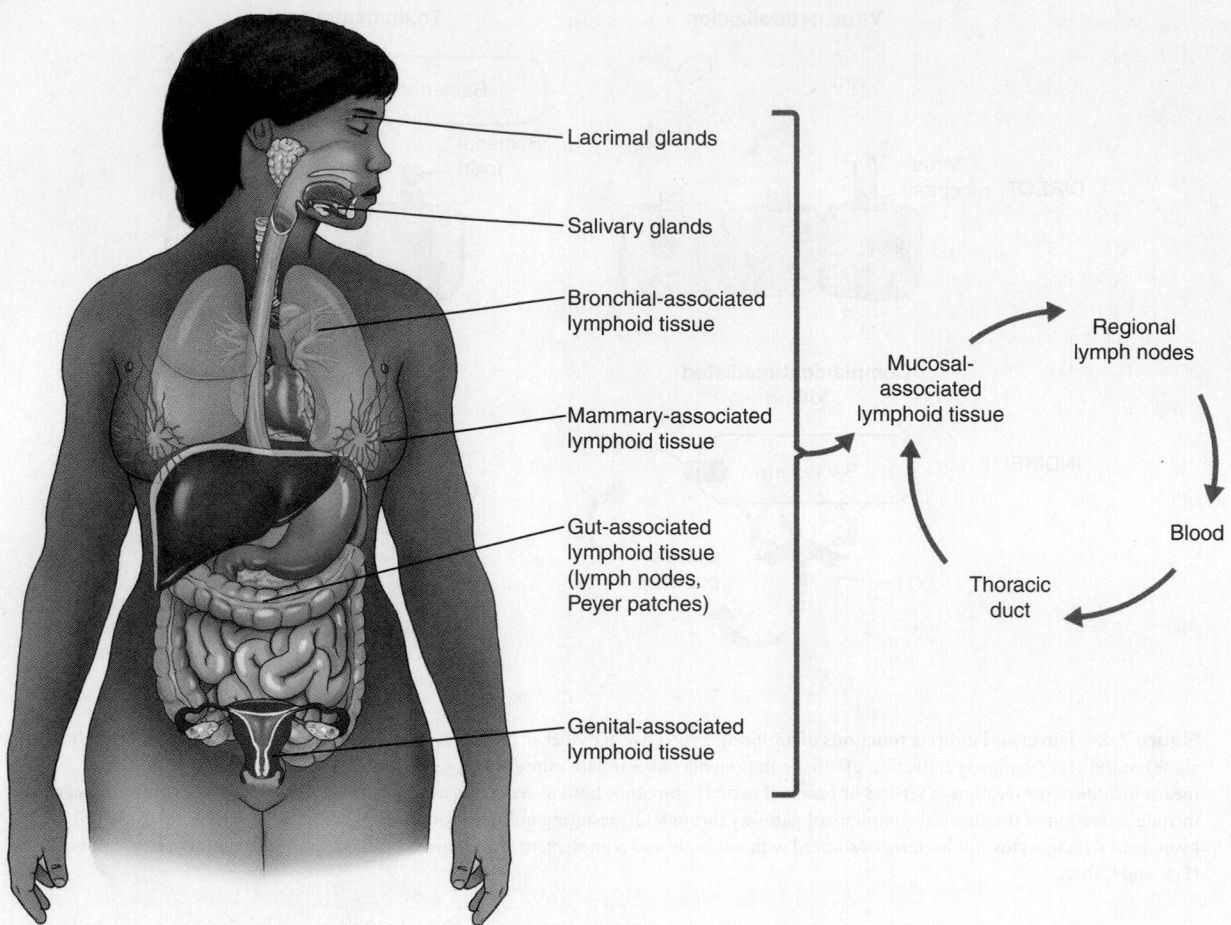

Lacrimal glands

Salivary glands

Bronchial-associated
lymphoid tissue

Mammary-associated
lymphoid tissue

Gut-associated
lymphoid tissue
(lymph nodes,
Peyer patches)

Genital-associated
lymphoid tissue

Mucosal-
associated
lymphoid tissue

Regional
lymph nodes

Blood

Thoracic
duct

Figure 7-25 Secretory immune system. Lymphocytes from the mucosal-associated lymphoid tissues circulate throughout the body in a pattern separate from other lymphocytes. For example, lymphocytes from the gut-associated lymphoid tissue circulate through the regional lymph nodes, the thoracic duct, and the blood and return to other mucosal-associated lymphoid tissues rather than to lymphoid tissue of the systemic immune system.

Indirect Effects

Antibody can be protective by interacting with or activating components of nonspecific inflammation. Indirect effects are mediated by the Fc portion of the antibody molecule and include opsonic activity leading to enhanced phagocytosis and activation of the complement system that may lead to complement-mediated destruction of the pathogen or increased opsonic activity through deposition of C3b.[44,45]

In their role as **opsonins,** antibody and C3b make the pathogen more susceptible to phagocytosis through binding to Fc or C3b receptors on the phagocyte's surface. **Opsonization** is often necessary for efficient bacterial clearance because many bacteria have an outer capsule that deters recognition by phagocytes unless it is coated with an antibody or complement protein. Bacterial surface molecules are usually complex and have multiple accessible antigenic determinants, enabling them to bind several different antibodies simultaneously. When an antigen reacts with the Fab regions of antibody, the Fc portion of that antibody is recognized and binds to Fc receptors on the surfaces of inflammatory cells. Engagement of Fc receptors results in their activation, making phagocytosis of the opsonized

bacterium more efficient.[46] The clustering of Fc regions has the added effect of more efficient complement activation.

Secretory Immune Response

The immune response that protects the entire body is produced by the **systemic immune system.** A distinct set of lymphoid tissues makes up another, partially independent, immune system at the external surfaces of the body. This system is called the **secretory (mucosal) immune system** (Figure 7-25). Most humoral immune responses occur when antibodies or B cells encounter antigens in the blood, but sometimes this encounter occurs in other body fluids. Antibodies are present in bodily secretions such as tears, sweat, saliva, mucus, and breast milk, where they can protect the body against antigens that have not yet penetrated the skin or mucous membranes.

Antibodies in secretions are produced by plasma cells of the secretory (mucosal) immune system.[47] The B cells of these two systems follow a different pattern of migration after they leave the bone marrow. B lymphocytes of the systemic immune system travel through the spleen and most lymph nodes, whereas those of the secretory immune system travel through a different group of lymphoid tissues including the lacrimal and salivary glands and the lymphoid tissues of the breasts, bronchi, intestines, and genitourinary tract. Immunoglobulins that are secreted at these sites are called **secretory immunoglobulins** and act locally rather than systemically.

Local protection is necessary to combat antigens (chiefly infectious microorganisms) that are inhaled, swallowed, or otherwise come into contact with external body surfaces. Once they have taken up residence in the external layers of the body, harmful microorganisms can cause local disease or possibly penetrate the barriers described in Chapter 6 to cause systemic disease. Alternatively, the microorganisms may fail to cause disease in the individual, either because the microorganisms are passed out of the body without any ill effects or because the infection is thwarted by the systemic immune system. In the latter case the individual may continue to "carry" the infectious agent in the mucosal areas, thereby enabling its spread to other individuals. The major function of the secretory immune system is to halt viral and bacterial invasion before local or systemic disease can develop and to prevent a carrier state that may result in spread of the infection to others.

IgA is the dominant secretory immunoglobulin, although IgM and IgG also are present in secretions. The primary role of IgA is to prevent the attachment and invasion of pathogens through mucosal membranes, such as those of the gastrointestinal, pulmonary, and genitourinary tracts. To induce protective immunity against some pathogens that enter through these routes, local immunization seems to be preferable to inducing only systemic immunity. For instance, two different vaccines have been used against polio. The Sabin vaccine was administered orally as an attenuated (i.e., inactivated so as to render relatively harmless) live virus. This route caused a transient, limited infection and induced effective systemic immunity and secretory immunity, preventing both the disease and the establishment of a carrier state. The Salk vaccine, on the other hand, consisted of killed viruses that were administered intradermally. It induced adequate systemic protection but did not generally prevent an intestinal carrier state.

Because B lymphocytes of the secretory/mucosal immune system travel through breast-associated lymphoid tissue, most antigens to which the mother has been exposed gastrointestinally (e.g., poliovirus) induce secretion of specific IgAs, IgMs, and IgGs into the breast milk. Antibodies in the milk may provide protection against these infectious disease agents to the nursing newborn. Although colostral antibodies (i.e., found in colostrum of breast milk) provide the newborn with passive immunity against gastrointestinal infections, they do not provide systemic immunity because they do not cross the newborn's gut into the bloodstream after the first 24 hours of life. Passive systemic immunity is provided by maternal antibodies that passed across the placenta into the fetus before birth.

The mechanisms and functions of antigen-antibody binding are the same in the secretory immune system as they are in the systemic immune systems; that is, binding neutralizes or opsonizes the antigen, preventing it from harming the host. The major differences between the two systems include (1) the order of utilization—the secretory immune response is part of the body's first-line defense, whereas the systemic response is the body's final defense; (2) the lymphocytes of each system follow different paths of migration and pass through different secondary lymphoid tissues; and (3) the secretory response occurs locally and externally (in body secretions), whereas the systemic response occurs systemically and internally (in blood and tissues).

IgE

IgE is a special class of antibody that is designed to help protect the individual from infection with large parasitic worms.[48] However, when IgE is produced against relatively innocuous environmental antigens, it is also the primary cause of common allergies (e.g., hay fever, dust allergies, bee stings). The role of IgE in allergies is discussed in Chapter 8.

Large multicellular parasites usually invade mucosal tissues (Figure 7-26). In response to parasitic antigens, a variety of different antibody classes are produced with many B cells class-switching to IgE-secreting plasma cells under the direction of Th2 cells primarily producing IL-4 and IL-13. IgG, IgM, and IgA bind to the surface of parasites, activate complement, generate chemotactic factors for neutrophils and macrophages, and serve as opsonins for those phagocytic cells. The influx of neutrophils and macrophages progressively leads to development of a granulomatous response around the parasite.[49] Unique to parasitic infections, the eosinophil is a primary cell in the granuloma. The influx of eosinophils results from IgE-triggered mast cell degranulation. Mast cells in the tissues have very high affinity Fc receptors for IgE, which rapidly bind IgE to the mast cell surface. Soluble macromolecules with multiple antigenic determinants are released from the parasite, react with the IgE-Fc receptors, and initiate mast cell degranulation (see Chapter 6). Eosinophil chemotactic factor of anaphylaxis (ECF-A) is released from mast cell granules and attracts eosinophils to the site of infection, as well as up-regulates surface receptors for IgG and complement component C3b. Eosinophil attachment to the parasite results in degranulation, releasing a variety of very toxic proteins that are at unusually high concentrations in eosinophilic granules, *major basic protein* (binds to heparin sulfate proteoglycans), *eosinophil cationic protein* (a member of the RNase A family), and others. These can cause extensive damage to the parasite if an adequate number of eosinophils are involved.

T-Lymphocyte Function

Killing Abnormal Cells

Cytotoxic T Lymphocytes

Cytotoxic T lymphocytes (Tc cells or **CTLs)** are responsible for the cell-mediated destruction of such targets as tumor cells or cells infected with viruses.[50] To perform this function, the Tc cell must directly adhere to the target cell through antigen

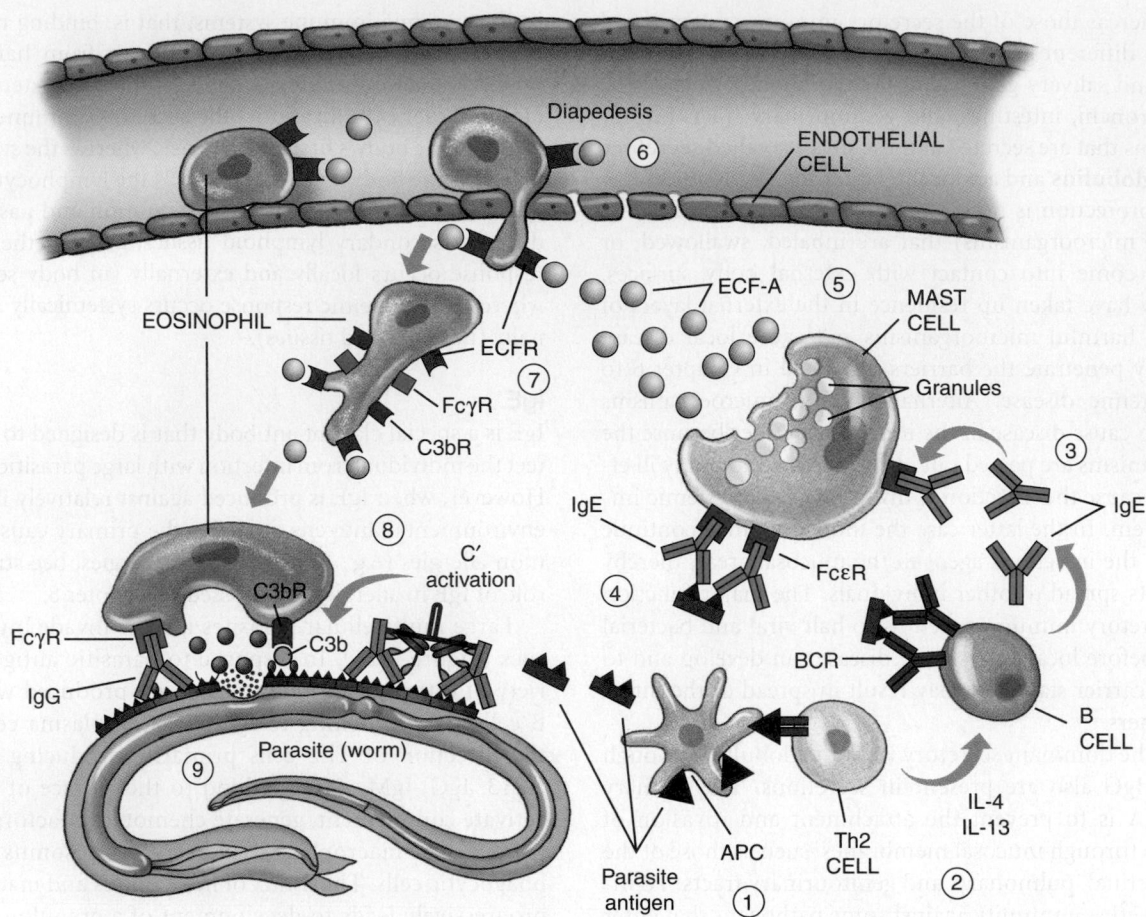

Figure 7-26 IgE function. Soluble antigens from a parasitic infection are processed by local antigen-presenting cells (APCs) and presented to Th2 cells (1), which respond by producing cytokines that favor class-switch to IgE production (2). B cells bind soluble parasite antigen, and some switch to producing IgG, whereas others switch to IgE. The secreted IgE molecules bind to IgE-specific receptors (FcεR) on the mast cell surface (3). Additional soluble parasite antigen crosslinks IgE-FcεR complexes on the mast cell surface (4), leading to mast cell degranulation and release of many proinflammatory products, including eosinophil chemotactic factor of anaphylaxis (ECF-A) (5). Eosinophils have receptors for ECF-A (ECFR) and are stimulated to increase adherence to the vessel walls and initiate diapedesis (6) and invasion of the surrounding tissue. The eosinophil also responds by increasing the density of surface receptors for IgG (FcγR) and complement component C3b (C3bR) (7). IgG had previously attached to the antigens on the parasite's surface and activated the complement cascade (C′ activation) in a failed attempt to damage the parasite. The eosinophil attaches to the parasite's surface through Fc and C3b receptors (8). Once bound to the parasite, the eosinophil releases its lysosomal enzymes onto the parasite, damaging its outer membrane (9).

presentation in association with MHC class I molecules and appropriate adhesion molecules (Figure 7-27). Most Tc-cell killing requires the αβ TCR complex and CD8 and is therefore *class I restricted.* Because of the cellular distribution of MHC class I molecules, Tc cells can recognize antigen on the surface of almost any type of cell that has been infected by a virus or has become cancerous.

After attachment to a target cell, killing can occur by at least two different mechanisms that induce apoptosis: through the actions of perforin and granzyme or direct receptor interactions. Perforins and granzymes are contained in the Tc-cell lysosomal granules, which are released onto the surface of the target cell. Perforin acts in a fashion similar to C9 of the complement cascade and penetrates, polymerizes, and

forms pores in the target cell's plasma membrane. The granzymes enter the target cell through the perforin-lined pores and activate cellular enzymes (caspases) that are involved in apoptosis, resulting in death of the target. Additionally, target cell apoptosis can be induced directly through the stimulation of specific receptors on the cell surface. For instance, Tc cells express a surface molecule called *Fas ligand,* which is very similar to TNF-α and reacts with a protein called *Fas* (CD95) on the target cell surface. Activation of Fas signals the target cell to undergo apoptosis.

Other Cells That Kill Abnormal Cells

A variety of other cells kill targets in a fashion similar to Tc lymphocytes. Prominent among these cells are natural killer (NK) cells (see Chapter 6). In many ways, NK cells complement

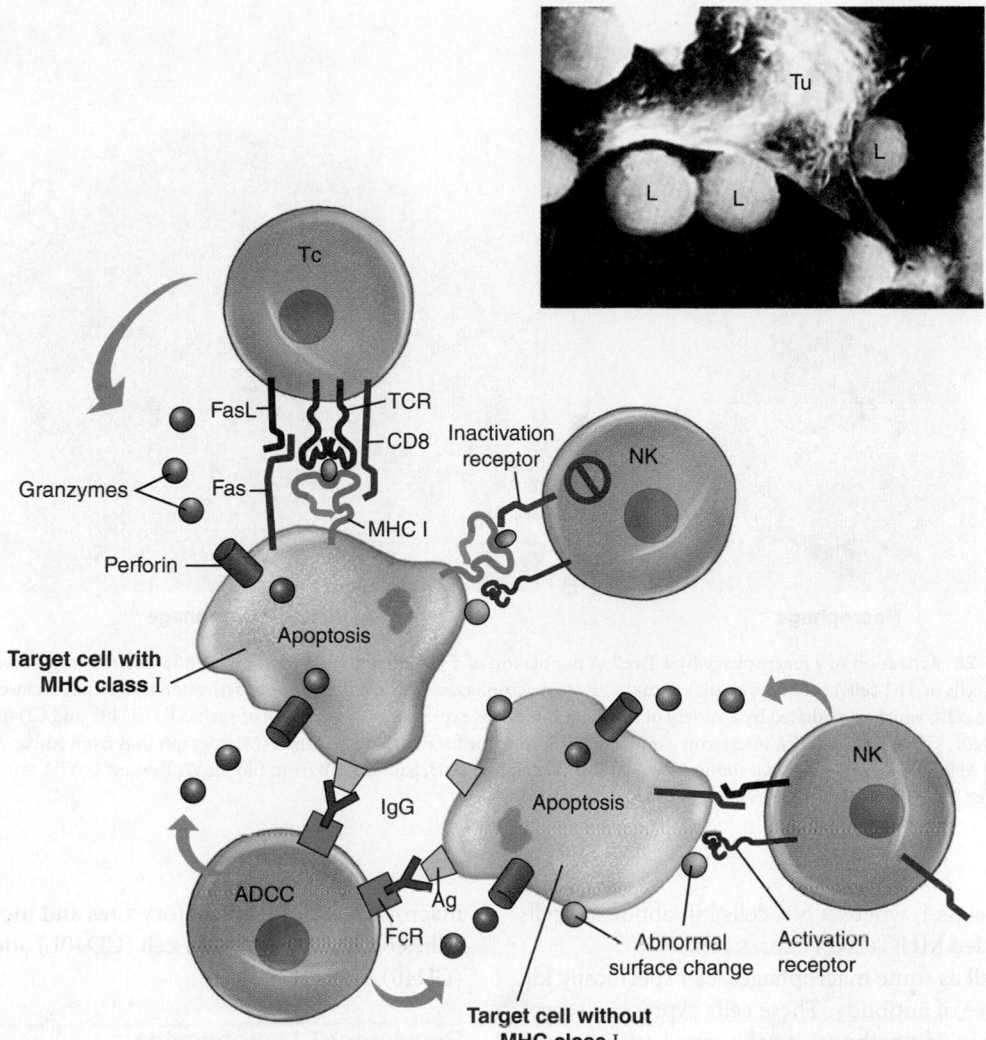

Figure 7-27 **Cell killing mechanisms.** Several cells have the capacity to kill abnormal (e.g., virally infected, cancerous) target cells. Cytotoxic T (Tc) cells recognized endogenous antigen presented by MHC class I molecules *(cell on upper left).* The intercellular interaction is enhanced through a variety of co-stimulatory adhesion molecules (not shown). The Tc cell mobilizes multiple killing mechanisms that induce apoptosis of the target cell, including the secretion of perforin that creates pores for the entrance of granzymes into the target cell and stimulation of Fas molecules on the target cell surface by Fas ligand (FasL) on the Tc cell. Natural killer (NK) cells *(cells on right)* use the same mechanisms to kill target cells through activation receptors that recognize "abnormal surface changes." NK cells specifically kill targets that have down-regulated expression of surface MHC class I molecules. Targets expressing MHC class I molecules inactivate NK cells through a variety of inactivation receptors *(cell on upper right).* Several cells, including macrophages and NK cells, can kill by antibody-dependent cellular cytotoxicity (ADCC). IgG antibody binds to foreign antigen on the target cell. Cells involved in ADCC *(cell on lower left)* bind IgG through Fc receptors (FcRs) and initiate killing. The insert is a scanning electron microscopic view of Tc cells (L) attacking a much larger tumor cell (Tu). *MHC,* Major histocompatibility complex. (From Thibodeau GA, Patton KT: *Anatomy & physiology,* ed 5, St Louis, 2003, Mosby).

the effects of Tc cells.[51] In some instances, a virally infected or cancerous cell will "protect" itself by down-regulating MHC class I molecule expression. Without surface MHC class I molecules, a cell becomes resistant to Tc-cell recognition and killing. NK cells are a special group of lymphoid cells that are similar to T cells but do not undergo maturation in the thymus and lack antigen-specific receptors.[52] Instead, they express Fc receptors (CD16) for IgG and a variety of NK-specific cell surface receptors (similar to pattern recognition receptors, see Chapter 6) that identify protein changes on the surface of cells

that have been infected or are in other ways abnormal. After attachment, the NK cell kills its target in a manner similar to that of Tc cells. However, NK cells also express another set of receptors, inhibitory receptors, that bind to MHC class I molecules.[53] If the target cell continues to express MHC class I, the NK cell will bind to the class I molecule, and an inhibitory signal will result. Thus NK cells do not inadvertently kill MHC class I–bearing cells. If these cells are infected or malignant, yet still express MHC class I, they remain sensitive to Tc-cell killing. Thus Tc cells kill abnormal cells that continue

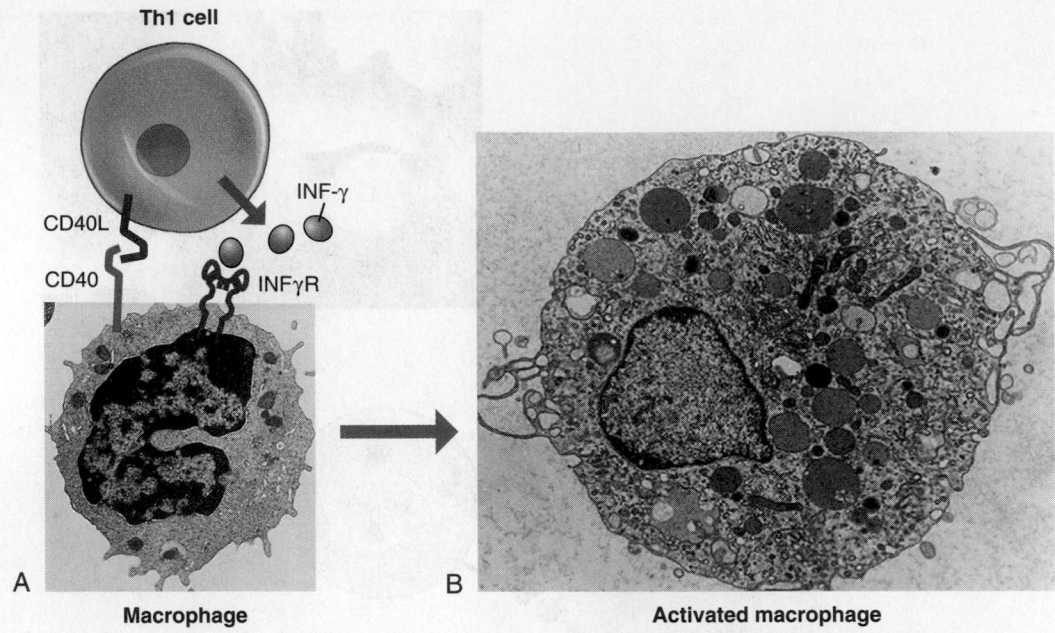

Figure 7-28 Activation of a macrophage by a T cell. A population of T cells that helps immune and inflammatory responses (helper T cells or Th1 cells) produces cytokines that activate macrophages. Optimal macrophage activation also requires close contact among the cells, which is mediated by a variety of adhesion molecules expressed on the surface of each cell (CD40L and CD40 shown here). *CD40L*, CD40 ligand; *INFγ*, interferon gamma; *INFγR*, receptor for interferon gamma. (Micrograph in **A** from Abbas AK, Lichtman AH: *Cellular and molecular immunology*, ed 5, Philadelphia, 2003, Saunders; **B** from Bloom W, Fawcett DW: *A textbook of histology*, ed 11, Philadelphia, 1986, Saunders.)

to express MHC class I, whereas NK cells kill abnormal cells that have suppressed MHC class I expression.

NK cells, as well as some macrophages, can specifically kill targets through use of antibody. These cells express Fc receptors on their surface. If a pathogen or abnormal cell expresses a foreign antigen that elicits IgG antibody, which binds to the antigen, the NK cell can attach to the IgG through Fc receptors and activate its normal killing mechanisms. This is referred to as **antibody-dependent cell-mediated cytotoxicity (ADCC)** (see Figure 7-27).

Another population of NK-like cells has been identified, NK-T cells. NK-T cells are produced in the thymus and more closely resemble Tc cells. However, they express TCRs that have very limited variability and recognize antigens presented by CD1.

T Cells That Activate Macrophages

Under conditions of chronic inflammation, T cells produce cytokines that activate macrophages (see Chapter 6). Macrophage activation is usually accomplished by Th1 cells that recognize antigen and produce cytokines (particularly IFN-γ) that, in cooperation with microbial products (e.g., LPS), stimulate the macrophage to become a more efficient phagocyte and increase production of proteolytic enzymes and other antimicrobial substances (Figure 7-28).[54,55] IFN-γ-induced macrophage activation also achieved by NK cells and CD8+ T cytotoxic cells. Additional signals (e.g., the CXC chemokine macrophage migration inhibitory factor) retain

macrophages at inflammatory sites and increase intercellular adhesion between the Th1 cell (CD40L) and the macrophage (CD40).[56]

Regulatory T Lymphocytes

One form of peripheral tolerance to self-antigens occurs in Treg cells, a subpopulation of CD4+ T cells (see Figure 7-17).[33,57-59] As with Th cells, Treg cells are activated by antigen presented in the context of class II MHC and differentiation under the control of specific cytokines, primarily TGF-β and IL-2, during which they express CD25 (the α-chain of the IL-2 receptor) and are frequently designated CD4+, CD25+ Treg cells. The role of Treg cells is to control or limit the immune response to protect the host's own tissues against autoimmune reactions.[60] Treg produce very high levels of TGF-β and IL-10, an immunosuppressive cytokine, which generally decrease Th1 and Th2 activity and suppress antigen recognition and Th cell proliferation. The role of Treg cells and other regulatory cells (e.g., CD25-cells, CD8+ regulatory cells, and Breg cells) is under intense investigation to determine the degree of their heterogeneity of derivation, function, and specificity.

Fetal and Neonatal Immune Function

The normal human infant is immunologically immature at birth. Although cell-mediated immunologic capabilities begin developing early in gestation and probably are completely

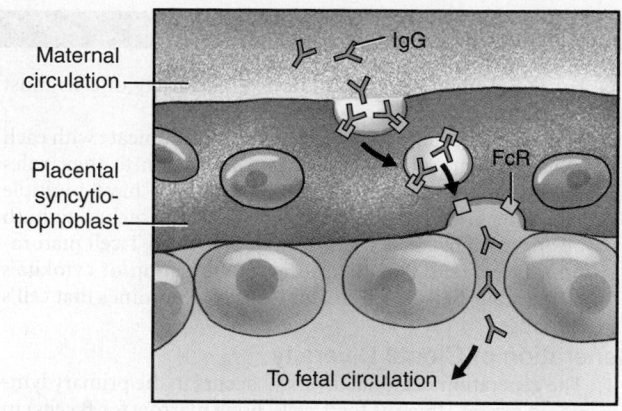

Figure 7-29 Transport of IgG across the syncytiotrophoblast. The human placenta is covered with a specialized multinucleated cell, the syncytiotrophoblast. Transport of maternal IgG across the syncytiotrophoblast and into the fetal circulation is an active process. Maternal IgG binds to Fc receptors on the surface of the syncytiotrophoblast and is internalized by the process of endocytosis. Receptors on the syncytiotrophoblast are specific for the Fc portion of IgG and do not bind other classes of immunoglobulins. Interaction of IgG with Fc receptors protects the antibody from lysosomal digestion during transport of the vacuole across the cell (i.e., transcytosis). On the fetal side of the syncytiotrophoblast, IgG is released by exocytosis (see Chapter 1).

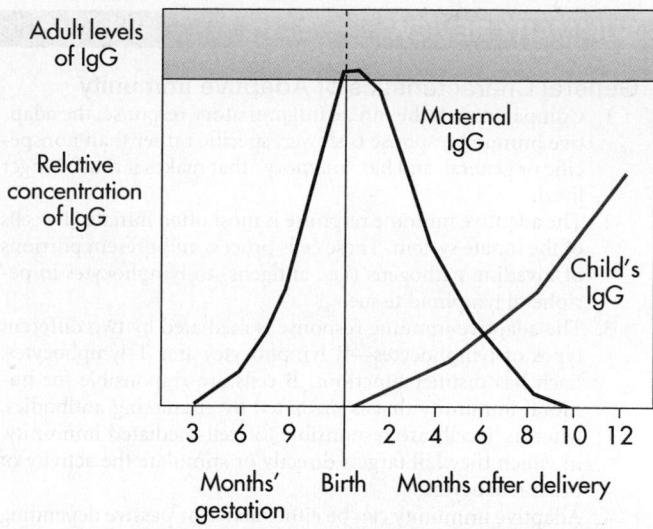

Figure 7-30 Antibody levels in umbilical cord blood and in neonatal circulation. Early in gestation maternal IgG begins crossing the placenta and enters the fetal circulation as shown in Figure 7-29. At birth, the fetal circulation may contain nearly adult levels of IgG, which is almost exclusively from the maternal source. The fetal immune system has the capacity to produce IgM and small amounts of IgA before birth (not shown). After delivery, maternal IgG is rapidly catabolized and neonatal IgG production increases.

functional at birth, antibody production is clearly deficient. In the last trimester, the fetus appears capable of producing a primary immune response (almost entirely IgM) to antigenic challenge in utero but is unable to produce a significant IgG response. Although some IgA can be detected, the capacity to produce IgA is underdeveloped.

To protect the child against infectious agents both in utero and during the first few postnatal months, a system of active transport facilitates the passage of maternal antibodies into the fetal circulation (Figure 7-29).[61] In the placenta, maternal and fetal blood is separated by a layer of specialized cells termed *trophoblasts*. Immunoglobulins are too large to diffuse across this cellular layer so the trophoblastic cells actively transport immunoglobulins from the maternal to the fetal circulation. Active transport of maternal IgG is mediated by surface receptors that are specific for the Fc portion of free IgG but not for IgM, IgE, or IgA. Active transport sometimes results in higher antibody titers in umbilical cord blood than in maternal blood. (Active transport mechanisms are discussed in Chapter 1.)

At birth, total IgG levels in the umbilical cord are near adult levels (Figure 7-30). When the source of maternal antibodies is severed at birth, antibody titers in the newborn begin to drop as maternal antibody is catabolized. Thus antibody titers drop rapidly as the neonate's production of IgG is beginning to rise. The rate of catabolism is usually more rapid than the rate of production so that the total immunoglobulin

levels reach a minimum at 5 to 6 months in the normal child, occasionally causing transient hypogammaglobulinemia (insufficient quantities of circulating immunoglobulins). Many normal infants experience recurrent mild respiratory tract infections at this age.

Aging and Immune Function

Immune function decreases in old age as a result of changes in both lymphocyte function and relative lymphocyte populations. Individuals older than 60 years of age generally exhibit decreased T cell activity as demonstrated by laboratory assays of T-cell function,[62] as well as in vivo reductions in cell-mediated responses to infections. The thymus, where T cells begin their development, reaches its maximum size at sexual maturity and then begins involuting until thymic size is only 15% of its maximum by middle age. Thymic capacity to mediate T-cell differentiation decreases with this atrophy. Although the total number of circulating T cells does not decrease with age, there is a shift in the populations of T-cell subtypes.

B-cell function is also altered with age as shown by decreases in specific antibody production in response to antigenic challenge, with concomitant increases in circulating immune complexes and in circulating autoantibodies (antibodies against self-antigens). A decrease in the number of circulating memory B cells is also observed.

SUMMARY REVIEW

General Characteristics of Adaptive Immunity

1. Compared with the innate inflammatory response, the adaptive immune response is slower, specific rather than nonspecific or general, and has "memory" that makes it much longer lived.
2. The adaptive immune response is most often initiated by cells of the innate system. These cells process and present portions of invading pathogens (i.e., antigens) to lymphocytes in peripheral lymphoid tissue.
3. The adaptive immune response is mediated by two different types of lymphocytes—B lymphocytes and T lymphocytes. Each has distinct functions. B cells are responsible for humoral immunity that is mediated by circulating antibodies, whereas T cells are responsible for cell-mediated immunity, in which they kill targets directly or stimulate the activity of other leukocytes.
4. Adaptive immunity can be either active or passive depending on whether immune response components originated in the host or came from a donor.

Recognition and Response

1. Antigens are the molecules that can react with components of the adaptive immune system, including antibodies and lymphocyte surface receptors. Immunogens are antigens that can initiate the adaptive immune response. To be immunogenic, an antigen must be of the correct type, size, and complexity and be present in sufficient quantities. Haptens are small-molecular-weight antigens that are not themselves immunogenic.
2. Both B and T lymphocytes bind antigen through cognate receptor complexes on their surfaces. These receptor complexes (i.e., the BCR and TCR complexes, respectively) work in conjunction with accessory proteins to produce lymphocyte activation.
3. The antigen-binding molecule of the BCR is antibody. Antibodies are composed of four polypeptide chains—two identical heavy chains and two identical light chains—held together by disulfide bonds. Each heavy chain has a variable region and a large constant region. Each light chain has a variable region and a short constant region. The class of antibody is determined by which constant regions make up their heavy chains, giving each class a slightly different molecular structure. The classes include IgG (the most prevalent), IgA (mostly in secretions), IgE (the most rare), IgD, and IgM (the first and largest immunoglobulin produced). The parts of antibody that bind antigen are called the Fab, and the part that reacts with cells and molecules of the innate system is called the Fc. Antigen binds to hypervariable regions (complementary determining regions, or CDRs) of both the heavy and light chains.
4. For most antigens to elicit an immune response, they must be presented to lymphocytes by molecules on the surface of antigen-presenting cells. Endogenous protein antigens are presented by class I molecules of MHC. Exogenous protein antigens are presented by class II MHC molecules. Lipid antigens are presented by CD1.
5. The MHC is a cluster of genes found on human chromosome 6. The products of these genes are also called *HLA antigens*. The MHC genes are highly polymorphic, having many different possible alleles. An individual will carry only two alleles at each locus, one from each parent. The particular combination of alleles a given individual carries defines his or her MHC haplotype.
6. For an immune response to develop, a variety of cells must interact through surface adhesion molecules.
7. During their interactions, cells must communicate with each other through soluble cytokines. In addition to their roles in the innate immune response, cytokines have multiple functions in the adaptive immune response including both positive and negative regulation of B cell and T cell maturation. In general, it is the precise combination of cytokines influencing a given cell that ultimately determines that cell's response.

Generation of Clonal Diversity

1. The generation of clonal diversity occurs in the primary lymphoid organs (thymus for T cells, bone marrow for B cells) in the fetus.
2. An individual's population of T cells and B cells has the collective ability to respond to virtually any antigen. This ability results from genetic rearrangement of various genes to form the variable regions for the TCR and BCR. Rearrangement of V and J genes results in the variable regions of the TCR α- chain and the BCR light chain, and rearrangement of V, D, and J genes result in the variable regions of the TCR β-chain and the BCR heavy chain.
3. Differentiation of B cells and T cells in the primary lymphoid organs results in expression of several characteristic surface markers, such as CD4 on helper T cells, CD8 on cytotoxic T cells, and CD21 and CD40 on B cells.
4. During generation of clonal diversity, B cells and T cells that produce receptors against self-antigens are eliminated by a process of central tolerance.
5. Cells leaving the primary lymphoid organs are immunocompetent (capable of reacting to antigen) and enter the circulation and secondary lymphoid organs.

Induction of an Immune Response: Clonal Selection

1. Clonal selection is the process by which antigen selects lymphocytes with complementary TCRs or BCRs and induces an immune response with the production of specific antibody or cytotoxic T cells, or both.
2. For lymphocyte activation, most antigens must be processed and presented by an APC in the context of the appropriate molecule, either MHC class I, MHC class II, or CD1 molecules.
3. Most immune responses require helper T cells (Th cells). Precursor Th cells interact with APCs through the TCR/CD4 complex, a variety of adhesion molecules, and cytokines, especially IL-1, and develop into either Th1 or Th2 subsets. Th1 cells are responsible for helping to activate macrophages and cytotoxic T cells, whereas Th2 cells are responsible for helping to activate B cells.
4. Another set of Th cells, Th17 cells, provides help in developing inflammation, particularly attraction of neutrophils and macrophages and induction of chemokine and antimicrobial protein production by epithelial cells.
5. B cell activation results from recognition of soluble antigen by the BCR, processing of the antigen, and presentation by MHC class II antigens to Th2 cells. Interactions between the B cells and Th2 cells through adhesion molecules (e.g., CD40 and CD40L) are also required. Depending on the particular combination of cytokines produced by the Th2 cell, the B cells can undergo class-switch from making IgM antibody to making and secreting either IgA, IgE, or IgG.

6. The humoral immune response is divided into two phases, primary and secondary. These differ in the relative amounts of IgG produced—the secondary response having a much higher proportion of IgG relative to IgM. The two responses also differ in the speed with which each occurs after antigen challenge—the secondary response being much more rapid than the primary response because of the presence of memory cells in the secondary phase.

7. B cells become activated upon recognition of a particular antigen to proliferate and differentiate into plasma cells that function as factories for the synthesis of large amounts of antibody that is specific for the recognized antigen or into memory B cells.

8. T cell activation results from recognition by the TCR and CD8 of antigen presented by MHC class I. Appropriate intercellular adhesion molecules and cytokines, such as IL-2 from Th1 cells, are also necessary for efficient differentiation. T cells become CTLs or memory T cells.

9. Superantigens are molecules produced by infectious agents that can bind to the Th cell's TCR outside the normal antigen-binding site and to class II MHC on the APCs, resulting in activation of a large number of Th cells and excessive production of proinflammatory cytokines that may cause shock and death of the patient. Examples of these antigens, called *superantigens*, include the bacterial toxins that can cause toxic shock syndrome and food poisoning.

Effector Mechanisms

1. The antibodies that are produced by B cells affect antigens by several different mechanisms that can be categorized as either direct or indirect. Direct mechanisms are mediated by the antigen-binding portions of antibodies (the Fab portions containing the variable regions). This binding results in neutralization of the biologic activity of antigens and possibly removal of the antigen by agglutination or precipitation. Indirect mechanisms depend on both the Fab and the nonantigen-binding portion of antibodies (the Fc portions containing the constant regions), which interact with components of innate immunity.

2. Antibodies of the systemic immune system function throughout the body, whereas antibodies of the secretory (mucosal) immune system—primarily immunoglobulins of the IgA class—are associated with bodily secretions and function to prevent pathogenic infection on epithelial surfaces.

3. Cytotoxic T cells (Tc cells) adhere directly to antigen presented by MHC class I on target cells (virus-infected cells or cancer cells) through the TCR, CD8, and a variety of adhesion proteins. This contact results in killing of the target by apoptosis through the release of perforin and granzymes and/or direct stimulation of apoptotic receptors on the target (e.g., Fas).

4. NK cells kill targets in a fashion similar to that of Tc cells. However, NK cells recognize target cells that do not express MHC class I.

5. With infections that are resistant to cells of innate immunity, some Th1 cells produce cytokines that activate macrophages to become more efficient phagocytes.

6. Treg cells control (suppress) immune responses and prevent overreaction against foreign and self-antigens.

Fetal and Neonatal Immune Function

1. The human neonate has a poorly developed immune response, particularly in the production of IgG. The fetus and neonate are protected in utero and during the first few postnatal months by maternal antibody that was actively transported across the placenta.

2. The maternal antibodies are slowly catabolized after birth until they disappear altogether by about 10 months of age. The neonate begins producing IgG at birth, and the child's antibodies reach protective levels after about 6 months of age.

Aging and Immune Function

1. T-cell activity is deficient in older adults, and a shift in the balance of T cell subsets is observed. These changes may result in increased susceptibility to infection.

2. Antibody production to specific antigens is inferior, although older adults tend to have increased levels of circulating autoantibodies.

KEY TERMS

Active acquired immunity (active immunity), 220
Adaptive (acquired) immunity (immune response), 217
Agglutination, 244
Allergen, 222
Antibody, 218, 222
Antibody-dependent cell-mediated cytotoxicity (ADCC), 250
Antibody titer, 244
Antigen, 217, 221
Antigen-binding fragment (Fab), 224
Antigen presentation, 226
Antigen-presenting cell (APC), 226
Antigen processing, 236
Antigenic determinant, 221
Attenuated virus, 244
B lymphocyte (B cell), 218
B-cell receptor (BCR), 222
B-cell receptor (BCR) complex, 226
Carrier, 222
CD (cluster of differentiation), 221
Cellular immunity, 220
Central tolerance, 222
Class-switch, 242
Clonal selection, 230
Complementary-determining region (CDR), 225

Crystalline fragment (Fc), 224
Cytotoxic T lymphocyte (Tc cell or CTL), 247
Epitope, 221
Framework region (FR), 225
Generation of clonal diversity, 230
Haplotype, 227
Hapten, 222
Helper T cell (Th cell), 219, 237
Hinge region, 224
High endothelial venule (HEV), 235
Human leukocyte antigen (HLA), 226
Humoral immunity, 219
Immunity, 217
Immunocompetent, 218
Immunogen, 221
Immunogenic, 221
Immunoglobulin, 218
Invariant chain, 236
Isotype-switch, 242
Lymphocyte, 218
Lymphoid stem cell, 230
Major histocompatibility complex (MHC), 226
MHC class I gene, 226
MHC class II gene, 226
Memory cell, 220
Memory T cell, 243
Neutralization, 244

Opsonin, 246
Opsonization, 246
Paratope, 221
Passive acquired immunity (passive immunity), 220
Plasma cell, 240
Peripheral tolerance, 222
Precipitation, 244
Primary (central) lymphoid organ, 230
Primary immune response, 241
Secondary (anamnestic) immune response, 241
Secondary (peripheral) lymphoid organ, 230
Secretory (mucosal) immune system, 246
Secretory immunoglobulin, 247
Self-antigen, 222
Somatic recombination, 230
Superantigen (SAG), 244
Systemic immune system, 246
T-cell receptor (TCR), 222
T-cell receptor (TCR) complex, 226
T lymphocyte (T cell), 218
Th1 cell, 239
Th2 cell, 239
Th17 cell, 239
T regulatory (Treg) cells, 243
Tolerance, 222
Valence, 225

REFERENCES

1. Chaplin DD: Overview of the human immune response, *J Allergy Clin Immunol* 117(2 Suppl Mini-Primer):S430-S435, 2006.
2. Kalia V et al: Differentiation of memory B and T cells, *Curr Opin Immunol* 18(3):255-264, 2006.
3. Casadevall A, Dadachova E, Pirofski LA: Passive antibody therapy for infectious diseases, *Nat Rev Microbiol* 2(9):695-703, 2004.
4. Porter RR: The hydrolysis of rabbit γ-globulin and antibodies with crystalline papain, *Biochem J* 73:119-126, 1959.
5. Vargas-Madrazo E, Paz-Garcia E: An improved model of association for VH-VL immunoglobulin domains: asymmetries between VH and VL in the packing of some interface residues, *J Mol Recognit* 16(3):113-120, 2003.
6. Dal Porto JM et al: B cell antigen receptor signaling 101, *Mol Immunol* 41(6-7):599-613, 2004.
7. Krogsgaard M, Davis MM: How T cells "see" antigen, *Nat Immunol* 6(3):239-245, 2005.
8. Morris CR et al: Association of intracellular proteins with folded major histocompatibility complex class I molecules, *Immunol Res* 30(2):171-179, 2004.
9. *Immunogenetics database.* Available at www.ebi.ac.uk/imgt/hla/stats. html. Accessed June 11, 2008.
10. Lawton AP, Kronenberg M: The third way: progress on pathways of antigen processing and presentation by CD1, *Immunol Cell Biol* 82(3):295-306, 2004.
11. Barral DC, Brenner MB: CD1 antigen presentation: how it works, *Nat Rev Immunol* 7(12):929-941, 2007.
12. Metcalf D: Hematopoietic cytokines, *Blood* 111(2):485-491, 2008.
13. Jerne NK: The natural-selection theory of antibody formation, *Proc Natl Acad Sci U S A* 41:849-857, 1955.
14. Burnet FM: *The clonal selection theory of acquired immunity*, London, 1959, Cambridge University Press.
15. Kyewski B, Derbinski J: Self-representation in the thymus: an extended view, *Nat Rev Immunol* 4(9):688-698, 2004.
16. von Boehmer H: Selection of the T-cell repertoire: receptor-controlled checkpoints in T-cell development, *Adv Immunol* 84:201-238, 2004.

17. Bosselut R: CD4/CD8-lineage differentiation in the thymus: from nuclear effectors to membrane signals, *Nat Rev Immunol* 4(7):529-540, 2004.
18. Ciofani M, Zúñiga-Pflücker JC: A survival guide to early T cell development, *Immunol Res* 34(2):117-132, 2006.
19. Fuentes-Panana EM, Bannish G, Monroe JG: Basal B-cell receptor signaling in B lymphocytes: mechanisms of regulation and role in positive selection, differentiation, and peripheral survival, *Immunol Rev* 197:26-40, 2004.
20. Chowdhury D, Sen R: Regulation of immunoglobulin heavy-chain gene rearrangements, *Immunol Rev* 200:182-196, 2004.
21. Verkoczy LK, Martensson AS, Nemazee D: The scope of receptor editing and its association with autoimmunity, *Curr Opin Immunol* 16(6):808-814, 2004.
22. Pabst O et al: Elucidating the functional anatomy of secondary lymphoid organs, *Curr Opin Immunol* 16(4):394-399, 2004.
23. Klein U, Dalla-Favera R: Germinal centres: role in B-cell physiology and malignancy, *Nat Rev Immunol* 8(1):22-33, 2008.
24. Trombetta ES, Mellman I: Cell biology of antigen processing in vitro and in vivo, *Ann Rev Immunol* 23:975-1028, 2005.
25. Steinman RM: Dendritic cells: understanding immunogenicity, *Eur J Immunol* 37(Suppl 1):S53-S60, 2007.
26. Watts C: The exogenous pathway for antigen presentation on major histocompatibility complex class II and CD1 molecules, *Nat Immunol* 5(7):685-692, 2004.
27. Savina A, Amigorena S: Phagocytosis and antigen presentation in dendritic cells, *Immunol Rev* 219:143-156, 2007.
28. Jiang H, Chess L: Regulation of immune responses by T cells, *N Engl J Med* 354(11):1166-1176, 2006.
29. Kidd P: Th1/Th2 balance: the hypothesis, its limitations, and implications for health and disease, *Altern Med Rev* 8(3):223-246, 2003.
30. Ochoa JB, Makarenkova V: T lymphocytes, *Crit Care Med* 33(12 Suppl):S510-S513, 2005.
31. McGeachy MJ, Cua DJ: Th17 cell differentiation: the long and winding road, *Immunity* 28(4):445-453, 2008.
32. Ouyang W, Kools JK, Zheng Y: The biological functions of T helper 17 cell effector cytokines in inflammation, *Immunity* 28(4):454-467, 2008.

33. Sigal LH: CD4+ T-cell subsets of probable clinical consequence, *J Clin Rheum* 13(4):229-233, 2007.

34. Dong C: T$_H$17 cells in development: an updated view of their molecular identity and genetic programming, *Nat Rev Immunol* 8(5):337-348, 2008.

35. Jenner E: An inquiry into the causes and effects of the variolae vaccinae: a disease discovered in some of the western counties of England, particularly Gloucestershire, and known by the name of the cow pox, London, 1798, Sampson Low.

36. Eyler JM: Smallpox in history: the birth, death, and impact of a dread disease, *J Lab Clin Med* 142(4):216-220, 2003.

37. MacConmara M, Lederer JA: B cells, *Crit Care Med* 33(12 Suppl):S514-S516, 2005.

38. Chaudhuri J, Alt FW: Class-switch recombination: interplay of transcription, DNA deamination and DNA repair, *Nat Rev Immunol* 4(7):541-552, 2004.

39. Cerutti A: The regulation of IgA class switching, *Nat Rev Immunol* 8(6):421-434, 2008.

40. van der Merwe PA, Davis SJ: Molecular interactions mediating T cell antigen recognition, *Ann Rev Immunol* 21:659-684, 2003.

41. Petersson K, Forsberg G, Walse B: Interplay between superantigens and immunoreceptors, *Scand J Immunol* 59(4):345-355, 2004.

42. Baker MD, Acharya KR: Superantigens: structure-function relationships, *Int J Med Microbiol* 293(7-8):529-537, 2004.

43. Silverman GJ, Goodyear CS: Confounding B cell defenses: lessons from a staphylococcal superantigen, *Nat Rev Immunol* 6(6):465-475, 2006.

44. Delves PJ, Roitt IM: The immune system. I, *N Engl J Med* 343(1):37-49, 2000.

45. Delves PJ, Roitt IM: The immune system. II, *N Engl J Med* 343(1):108-117, 2000.

46. Nimmerjahn F, Ravetch JV: Fcγ receptors as regulators of immune responses, *Nature Rev Immunol* 8(1):34-47, 2008.

47. Brandtzaeg P: Induction of secretory immunity and memory at mucosal surfaces, *Vaccine* 25(30):5467-5484, 2007.

48. Zacharia B, Sherman P: Atopy, helminths, and cancer, *Med Hypotheses* 60(1):1-5, 2003.

49. Anthony RM et al: Protective immune mechanisms in helminth infection, *Nat Rev Immunol* 7(12):975-987, 2007.

50. Waterhouse NJ et al: Cytotoxic lymphocytes; instigators of dramatic target cell death, *Biochem Pharmacol* 68(6):1033-1040, 2004.

51. Bottino C et al: Learning how to discriminate between friends and enemies, a lesson from natural killer cells, *Mol Immunol* 41(6-7):569-575, 2004.

52. Vivier E et al: Functions of natural killer cells, *Nat Immunol* 9(5):503-510, 2008.

53. Lanier LL: NK cell recognition. *Ann Rev Immunol* 23:225-274, 2005.

54. Martinez FO et al: Macrophage activation and polarization, *Front Biosci* 13:453-461, 2008.

55. Egen JG et al: Macrophage and T cell dynamics during the development and disintegration of mycobacterial granulomas, *Immunity* 28(2):271-284, 2008.

56. Bernhagen J et al: MIF is a noncognate ligand of CXC chemokine receptors in inflammatory and artherogenic cell recruitment, *Nat Med* 13(5):587-596, 2007.

57. Sakaguchi S, Wing K, Miyara M: Regulatory T cells—a brief history and perspective, *Eur J Immunol* 37(Suppl 1):S116-S123, 2007.

58. Matarese G, De Rosa V, La Cava A: Regulatory CD4 T cells: sensing the environment, *Trends Immunol* 29(1):12-17, 2008.

59. TretJiang H, Chess L: An integrated view of suppressor T cell subsets in immunoregulation, *J Clin Invest* 114(9):1198-1208, 2004.

60. D'Ambrosio D: Regulatory T cells: how do they find their space in the immunological arena? *Semin Cancer Biol* 16(2):91-97, 2006.

61. Simister NE: Placental transport of immunoglobulin G, *Vaccine* 21(24):3365-3369, 2003.

62. Hakim FT et al: Aging, immunity and cancer, *Curr Opin Immunol* 16(2):151-156, 2004.

ALTERATIONS IN IMMUNITY AND INFLAMMATION

NEAL S. ROTE

MEDIA RESOURCES

 Evolve Website (http://evolve.elsevier.com/McCance/)
- Review Questions and Answers
- Animations
- Glossary (with audio pronunciation for selected terms)
- WebLlinks

Online Course
- Module 6

CHAPTER OUTLINE

HYPERSENSITIVITY: ALLERGY, AUTOIMMUNITY, AND ALLOIMMUNITY
Mechanisms of Hypersensitivity
Antigenic Targets of Hypersensitivity Reactions
Autoimmune and Alloimmune Diseases

DEFICIENCIES IN IMMUNITY
Initial Clinical Presentation
Primary Immune Deficiencies
Secondary Immune Deficiencies
Clinical Evaluation of Immunity
Replacement Therapies for Immune Deficiencies

The immune system is a finely tuned network that protects the host against foreign antigens, particularly infectious agents. Sometimes this network breaks down, causing the immune system to react inappropriately. Inappropriate immune responses may be (1) exaggerated against environmental antigens (allergy); (2) misdirected against the host's own cells (autoimmunity); (3) directed against beneficial foreign tissues, such as transfusions or transplants (alloimmunity); or (4) insufficient to protect the host (immune deficiency). All of these can be serious or life threatening. Exaggerated immune responses (allergy) are the most common, but usually the least life threatening.

HYPERSENSITIVITY: ALLERGY, AUTOIMMUNITY, AND ALLOIMMUNITY

Hypersensitivity is an altered immunologic response to an antigen that results in disease or damage to the host. *Hypersensitivity reactions* can classified in two ways: by the source of the antigen that the immune system is attacking (allergy, autoimmunity, alloimmunity; Table 8-1) and by the

mechanism that causes disease (types I, II, III, IV; see Table 8-3). The term **allergy** originally denoted both facets of the immune response: immunity, which is beneficial, and hypersensitivity, which is harmful. Allergy has now come to mean the deleterious effects of hypersensitivity to environmental (exogenous) antigens, and immunity means the protective responses to antigens expressed by disease-causing agents.

Autoimmunity is a disturbance in the immunologic tolerance of self-antigens. The immune system normally does not strongly recognize the individual's own antigens. Healthy individuals of all ages, but particularly older adults, may produce low quantities of antibodies against their own antigens *(autoantibodies)*, without development of overt autoimmune disease. Therefore, the presence of low quantities of autoantibodies does not necessarily indicate a disease state. Autoimmune diseases occur when the immune system reacts against self-antigens to such a degree that the person's own tissues are damaged by autoantibodies or autoreactive T cells. Many clinical disorders are associated with autoimmunity and are collectively referred to as **autoimmune diseases** (Table 8-2).

Alloimmunity (also termed *isoimmunity*) occurs when the immune system of one individual produces an immunologic reaction against tissues of another individual. Alloimmunity

Table 8-1   Relative Incidences and Examples of Hypersensitivity Reactions*

	Mechanism			
Target Antigen	Type I (Immunoglobulin E–[IgE] Mediated)	Type II (Tissue Specific)	Type III (Immune Complex)	Type IV (Cell Mediated)
Allergy	++++	+	+	++
Environmental antigens	Hay fever	Hemolysis in drug allergies	Gluten (wheat) allergy	Poison ivy allergy
Autoimmunity	±	++	+++	+
Self-antigens	May contribute to some type III reactions	Autoimmune thrombocytopenia	Systemic lupus erythematosus	Hashimoto thyroiditis
Alloimmunity	±	++	+	++
Another person's antigens	May contribute to some type III reactions	Hemolytic disease of the newborn	Anaphylaxis to IgA in IV gamma globulin	Graft rejection

*The frequency of each reaction is indicated in a range from rare (±) to very common (++++). An example of each reaction is given.

Table 8-2   Disorders Associated with Autoimmunity

System Disease	Organ or Tissue	Probable Self-Antigen
Endocrine System		
Hyperthyroidism (Graves disease)	Thyroid gland	Receptors for thyroid-stimulating hormone on plasma membrane of thyroid cells
Autoimmune thyroiditis	Thyroid gland	Thyroglobulin; microsomes
Primary myxedema	Thyroid gland	Microsomes
Insulin-dependent diabetes	Pancreas	Islet cells, insulin, insulin receptors on pancreatic cells
Addison disease	Adrenal gland	Surface antigens on steroid-producing cells; microsomes of adrenal cortex
Premature gonadal failure	Ovary	Interstitial cells; corpus luteum
Male infertility	Testis	Surface antigens on spermatozoa
Orchitis	Testis	Germinal epithelium
Female infertility	Ovary	Zona pellucida
Idiopathic hypoparathyroidism	Parathyroid gland	Surface antigens on chief cells (epithelial cells of gland)
Partial pituitary deficiency	Pituitary gland	Prolactin-producing cells; growth hormone–producing cells
Skin		
Pemphigus vulgaris	Skin	Intercellular substances in stratified squamous epithelium
Bullous pemphigoid	Skin	Basement membrane
Dermatitis herpetiformis	Skin	Basement membrane (immunoglobulin A[IgA])
Vitiligo	Skin	Surface antigens on melanocytes (melanin-producing cells)
Neuromuscular Tissue		
Polymyositis (dermatomyositis)	Muscle	Nuclear materials; myosin
Multiple sclerosis	Neural tissue	Unknown
Myasthenia gravis	Neuromuscular junction	Acetylcholine receptors; striations of skeletal and cardiac muscle
Polyneuritis	Nerve cell	Peripheral myelin
Rheumatic fever	Heart	Cardiac tissue (subsarcolemmal membrane); cross reaction with group A streptococcal antigen
Cardiomyopathy	Heart	Cardiac muscle
Postvaccinal or postinfectious encephalitis	Central nervous system	Central nervous system myelin or basic protein
Gastrointestinal System		
Celiac disease (gluten-sensitive enteropathy)	Intestine	Gluten
Ulcerative colitis	Colon	Mucosal cells
Crohn disease	Ileum	Unknown
Pernicious anemia	Stomach	Surface antigens of parietal cells; intrinsic factor
Atrophic gastritis	Stomach	Parietal cells
Primary biliary cirrhosis	Liver	Mitochondria; cells of bile duct

Continued

Table 8-2	Disorders Associated with Autoimmunity—cont'd	
System Disease	**Organ or Tissue**	**Probable Self-Antigen**
Chronic active hepatitis	Liver	Surface antigens, nuclei, microsomes, mitochondria or hepatocytes; smooth muscle
Eye		
Sjögren syndrome	Lacrimal gland	Antigens of lacrimal gland, salivary gland, thyroid, and nuclei of cells; immunoglobulin G (IgG)
Uveitis	Uveal structures	Antigens of the iris, ciliary body, and choroid
Connective Tissue		
Ankylosing spondylitis	Joints	Sacroiliac and spinal apophyseal joint
Rheumatoid arthritis	Joints	IgG, collagen
Systemic lupus erythematosus	Multiple sites	Numerous antigens in nuclei, organelles, and extracellular matrix
Mixed connective tissue disease	Multiple sites	Ribonucleoprotein and numerous other nucleoproteins
Polyarteritis nodosa (necrotizing vasculitis)	Arterioles (small arteries)	Unknown
Scleroderma (progressive systemic sclerosis)	Multiple organs	Nuclear antigens; IgG
Felty syndrome	Joints	IgG
Antiphospholipid antibody syndrome	Platelets, endothelial cells, trophoblast of placenta	Membrane phospholipids, especially phosphatidylserine
Renal System		
Immune complex glomerulonephritis	Kidney	Numerous immune complexes
Goodpasture disease	Kidney	Glomerular basement membrane
Hematologic System		
Idiopathic neutropenia	Neutrophil	Surface antigens on polymorphonuclear neutrophils
Idiopathic lymphopenia	Lymphocytes	Surface antigens on lymphocytes
Autoimmune hemolytic anemia	Erythrocytes	Surface antigens on erythrocytes
Autoimmune thrombocytopenic purpura	Platelets	Surface antigens on platelets
Respiratory System		
Goodpasture disease	Lung	Septal membrane of alveolus

can be observed during immunologic reactions against transfusions, transplanted tissue, or the fetus during pregnancy.

The mechanism that initiates the onset of hypersensitivity, whether it consists of allergy, autoimmunity, or alloimmunity, is not completely understood. It is generally accepted that genetic, infectious, and possibly environmental factors contribute to hypersensitivity. Most diseases caused by hypersensitivity develop because of the interactions of at least three variables: (1) an original "insult," which alters **immunologic homeostasis** (a steady state of tolerance to self-antigens or lack of immune reaction against environmental antigens); (2) the individual's genetic makeup, which determines the degree of the resultant immune response from the effects of the insult; and (3) an immunologic process that causes the symptoms of the disease.

Mechanisms of Hypersensitivity

Diseases caused by hypersensitivity reactions can be characterized also by the particular immune mechanism that results in the disease (see Table 8-1). These mechanisms are apparent in most hypersensitivity reactions and have been divided into four distinct types: **type I (immunoglobulin E [IgE]–mediated) hypersensitivity reactions**, **type II (tissue-specific) hypersensitivity reactions**, **type III (immune complex–mediated) hypersensitivity reactions**, and **type IV (cell-mediated) hypersensitivity reactions** (Table 8-3).[1] This classification is artificial and seldom is a particular disease associated with only a single mechanism. The four mechanisms are interrelated, and in most hypersensitivity reactions, several mechanisms can be at work simultaneously or sequentially. Some of the mechanisms are secondary to the disease and not directly involved in the pathologic process, whereas others are the primary cause of tissue destruction.

Hypersensitivity reactions require *sensitization* against a particular antigen that results in primary and secondary immune responses. An individual is sensitized when an adequate amount of antibodies or T cells is available to cause a noticeable reaction on reexposure to the antigen. Some individuals become sensitized quite rapidly (after an apparent single exposure to the antigen), whereas others require multiple exposures that may occur over years. After sensitization has been achieved, hypersensitivity reactions can be immediate or delayed, depending on the time between exposure to the antigen and the onset of clinical symptoms. Reactions that occur within minutes to a few hours are termed **immediate hypersensitivity reactions. Delayed hypersensitivity reactions** may take several hours to appear and are at maximum severity days after reexposure to the antigen.

| Table 8-3 | Immunologic Mechanisms of Tissue Destruction | | | | | |

Type	Name	Rate of Development	Class of Antibody Involved	Principal Effector Cells Involved	Complement Participation	Examples of Disorders
I	IgE-mediated reaction	Immediate	IgE	Mast cells	No	Seasonal allergic rhinitis
II	Tissue-specific reaction	Immediate	IgG IgM	Macrophages in tissues	Frequently	Autoimmune thrombocytopenic purpura, Graves disease, autoimmune hemolytic anemia
III	Immune complex–mediated reaction	Immediate	IgG IgM	Neutrophils	Yes	Systemic lupus erythematosus
IV	Cell-mediated reaction	Delayed	None	Lymphocytes, macrophages	No	Contact sensitivity to poison ivy and metals (jewelry)

Ig, Immunoglobulin.

The most rapid and severe immediate hypersensitivity reaction is **anaphylaxis.**[2] Anaphylaxis occurs within minutes of reexposure to the antigen and can be either systemic (generalized) or cutaneous (localized).[3] Symptoms of systemic anaphylaxis include itching, erythema, headaches, vomiting, abdominal cramps, diarrhea, and breathing difficulties. In severe cases, contraction of bronchial smooth muscle, laryngeal edema, and vascular collapse may result in respiratory distress, decreased blood pressure, shock, and death. Examples of systemic anaphylaxis are allergic reactions to bee stings, peanuts, and fish.[4] Cutaneous anaphylaxis causes the less severe symptoms of local inflammation.

Type I: IgE-Mediated Hypersensitivity Reactions

Type I reactions are mediated by antigen-specific IgE and the products of tissue mast cells (Figure 8-1).[5] Most common allergies (e.g., pollen allergies) are type I reactions. In addition, most type I reactions occur against environmental antigens and are therefore allergic. Because of this strong association, many healthcare professionals use the term *allergy* to indicate only IgE-mediated reactions. However, IgE can contribute to a few autoimmune and alloimmune diseases, and many common allergies (e.g., poison ivy) are not mediated by IgE.

In some individuals, exposure to an environmental antigen causes primarily IgE production.[6] Repeated exposure to the antigen usually is required to elicit enough IgE so that the person becomes "sensitized." IgE has a relatively short life span in the blood because it rapidly binds to very-high-affinity Fc receptors on the plasma membranes of mast cells (see Figure 8-1).[7] The subclass IgG4 also has specific receptors on the mast cell and may contribute to the type I mechanism. Antibody that binds to mast cells is termed **cytotropic antibody** (able to bind to cell surfaces) or **reagin** (skin-sensitizing antibody). Unlike Fc receptors on phagocytes, which bind IgG that has reacted with antigen, the Fc receptors on mast cells bind with IgE that has not previously interacted with antigen.

If further exposure of a sensitized individual to the antigen occurs, one molecule of antigen may bind simultaneously to two molecules of IgE-Fc receptor complexes on the mast cell's surface (cross-link) resulting in activation of intracellular signaling pathways and mast cell degranulation (see Figure 8-1, *B,* and Chapter 6). The antigen that triggers cross-linking must have at least two antigenic determinants on the same molecule. Sometimes an IgE-mediated response is beneficial to the host, as is the case of some immune reactions against parasites. (This mechanism is described in Chapter 7 and illustrated in Figure 7-26.)

The products of mast cell degranulation can modulate almost all aspects of an acute inflammatory response.[8] (The effects of biochemical mediators released by mast cells are illustrated in Figure 6-9). The most potent mediator is histamine, which affects several key target cells.[9] Acting through the H1 receptors, histamine contracts bronchial smooth muscles, causing bronchial constriction; increases vascular permeability, causing edema; and causes vasodilation, increasing blood flow into the affected area (see Figures 6-3 and 6-10). The interaction of histamine with H2 receptors results in increased gastric acid secretion and a decrease of histamine released from mast cells and basophils. The action of histamine through H2 receptors suggests an important negative-feedback mechanism that stops degranulation. That is, the released histamine inhibits release of additional histamine by interacting with H2 receptors on the mast cells. Histamine also may affect control of the immune response through H2 receptors on most cells of the immune system.[10] Another important activity of histamine is enhancement of the chemotactic activity of other factors, such as eosinophil chemotactic factor of anaphylaxis (ECF-A), which attracts eosinophils into sites of allergic inflammatory reactions and prevents them from migrating out of the inflammatory site. (The role of the eosinophil in inflammation is discussed in Chapter 6.)

Type II: Tissue-Specific Hypersensitivity Reactions

Type II hypersensitivity reactions are generally characterized by a specific cell or tissue being the target of an immune response. In addition to major histocompatibility locus antigens (HLAs; discussed in Chapter 7), most cells have other antigens on their surfaces. Some of these other antigens are called **tissue-specific antigens** because they are expressed on the plasma membranes of only certain cells in specific tissues. Platelets, for example, have groups of antigens that are found on no other cells of the body. The symptoms of many type II diseases are determined by which tissue or organ expresses the particular antigen. Environmental antigens (e.g., drugs or their metabolites) may bind to the plasma membranes of specific cells (especially erythrocytes and platelets) and function as targets of type II reactions.

The five general mechanisms by which type II hypersensitivity reactions can affect cells are shown in Figure 8-2. All of these mechanisms begin with antibody binding to tissue-specific antigens or antigens that have attached to particular tissues. First, the cell can be destroyed by antibody (IgG or IgM) and activation of the complement cascade through the classical pathway. Formation of the membrane attack complex (C5-9) damages the membrane and may result in lysis of the cell (see Figure 8-2, *A*). For example, erythrocytes are destroyed by complement-mediated lysis in individuals with autoimmune hemolytic anemia (see Chapter 26) or as a result of an alloimmune reaction to ABO-mismatched transfused blood cells.

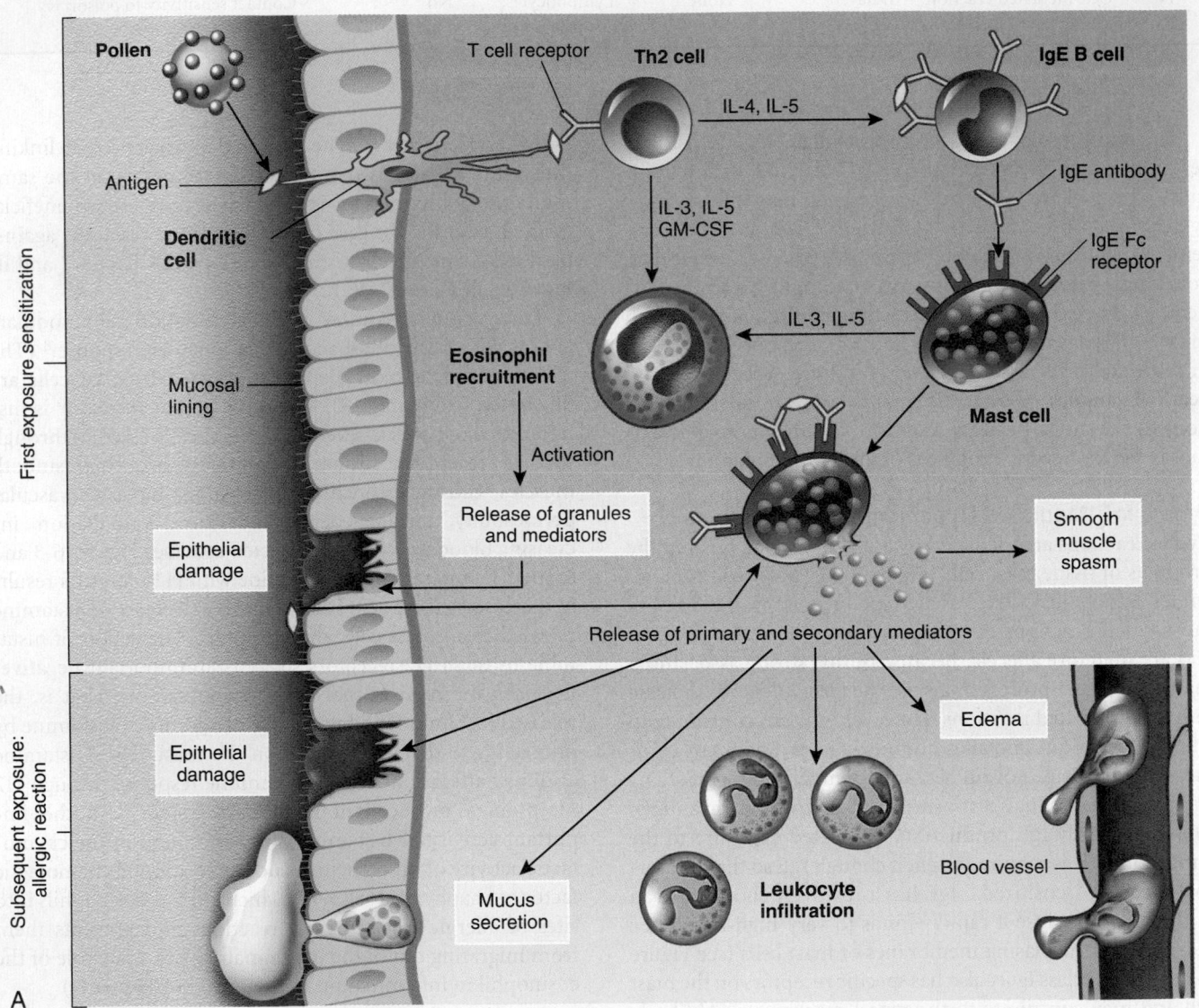

Figure 8-1 Mechanism of type I IgE–mediated reactions. A, Th2 cells are activated by antigen-presenting dendritic cells to produce cytokines, including IL-3, IL-4, IL-5, and granulocyte-macrophage colony-stimulating factor (GM-CSF). IL-3, IL-5, and GM-CSF attract and promote the survival of eosinophils. Other cytokines (e.g., IL-4) induce B cells to class-switch to IgE-producing plasma cells. The IgE coats the surface of the mast cell by binding with IgE-specific Fc receptors on the mast cell's plasma membrane (sensitization). Further exposure to the same allergen cross-links the surface-bound IgE and activates signals from the cytoplasmic portion of the IgE Fc receptors. These signals initiate two parallel and interdependent processes: mast cell degranulation and discharge of preformed mediators (e.g., histamine, eosinophil-chemotactic factor of anaphylaxis) and production of newly formed mediators such as arachidonic metabolites (leukotrienes, prostaglandins). Many local type I hypersensitivity reactions have two well-defined phases. The *initial phase* is characterized by vasodilation, vascular leakage, and depending on the location, smooth muscle spasm or glandular secretions. These changes usually become evident within 5 to 30 minutes after exposure to the antigen. The *late phase* occurs 2 to 8 hours later without additional exposure to the antigen. The late phase has more intense infiltration of tissues with eosinophils, neutrophils, basophils, monocytes, and Th cells and tissue destruction in the form of mucosal epithelial cell damage.

Second, antibody may cause cell destruction through phagocytosis by macrophages. IgG, as well as C3b of the complement system, are opsonins that bind to receptors on the macrophage (see Figure 8-2, *B*). Phagocytosis of the target cell follows. (Phagocytosis is illustrated in Figures 6-11 and 6-13.) For example, antibodies against platelet-specific antigens or against red blood cell antigens of the Rh system coat those cells at low density, resulting in their preferential removal by phagocytosis in the spleen, rather than by complement-mediated lysis.

Third, antibody and complement may attract neutrophils. Either antigen expressed normally on the vessel walls or soluble antigen in the circulation (e.g., released from cells within the body or from infectious agents or by way of drugs or medications) that has been deposited on the surface of endothelial cells may bind antibody (see Figure 8-2, *C*). The antibody initiates the complement cascade, resulting in the release of C3a and C5a, which are chemotactic for neutrophils, and deposition of complement component C3b. Neutrophils bind to the tissues through receptors for the Fc portion of antibody (Fc receptor) or for C3b and attempt to phagocytose the tissue. Because the tissue is large, phagocytosis cannot be completed; even so, neutrophils release their granules onto the healthy tissue. The components of neutrophil granules, as well as the several toxic oxygen products produced by these cells, will damage the tissue.

The fourth mechanism is **antibody-dependent cell-mediated cytotoxicity (ADCC)** (see Figure 8-2, *D*). This mechanism involves a subpopulation of cytotoxic cells that are not antigen specific (natural killer [NK] cells). Antibody on the target cell is recognized by Fc receptors on the NK cells, which release toxic substances that destroy the target cell.

The fifth mechanism does not destroy the target cell, but rather causes it to malfunction. In this mechanism of type II injury, the antibody is usually directed against antigenic determinants associated with specific cell-surface receptors, and the symptoms of the disease are a result of a direct effect of antibody binding alone (see Figure 8-2, *E*).[11] The antibody reacts with the receptors on the target cell surface and modulates the function of the receptor by preventing interactions with their normal ligands, replacing the ligand and inappropriately stimulating the receptor, or destroying the receptor. For example, in the hyperthyroidism (excessive thyroid activity) of Graves' disease, autoantibody binds to and activates receptors for thyroid-stimulating hormone (TSH) (a pituitary hormone that controls the production of the hormone *thyroxine* by the thyroid).[12] In this way the antibody stimulates the thyroid cells to produce thyroxine. Under normal conditions, the increasing levels of thyroxine in the blood would signal the pituitary to decrease TSH production, which would result in less stimulation of the TSH receptor in the thyroid and a concomitant decrease in thyroxine production. Because the level of anti-TSH receptor antibody is not controlled by the pituitary, increasing amounts of thyroxine in the blood have no effect on antibody levels, and thyroxine production continues to increase despite decreasing amounts of TSH (see Chapter 21).[13]

Type III: Immune Complex–Mediated Hypersensitivity Reactions

Mechanisms of Type III Hypersensitivity

Most type III hypersensitivity diseases are caused by antigen-antibody (immune) complexes that are formed in the circulation and deposited later in vessel walls or extravascular tissues (Figure 8-3).[14] The primary difference between type II and type III mechanisms is that in type II hypersensitivity antibody binds to the antigen on the cell surface, whereas in type III the antibody binds to soluble antigen that was released into the blood or body fluids, and the complex is then deposited in the tissues. Type III reactions are not organ specific, and symptoms have little to do with the particular antigenic target of the antibody. The harmful effects of immune complex deposition are caused by complement activation, particularly through the generation of chemotactic factors for neutrophils. The neutrophils bind to antibody and C3b contained in the complexes and attempt to ingest the immune complexes.

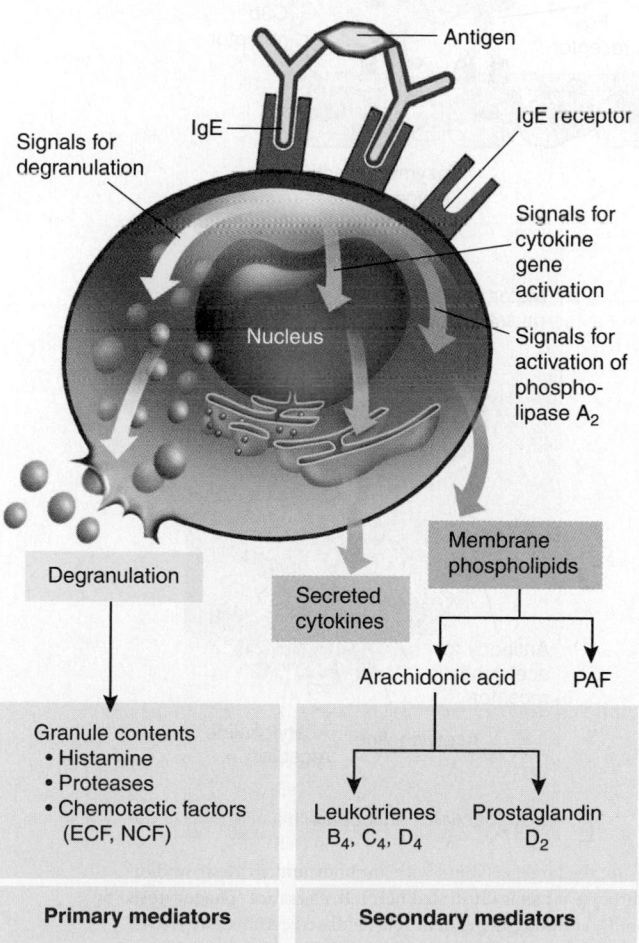

Figure 8-1, cont'd B, Activation of mast cells leading to degranulation of preformed mediators (primary mediators) and synthesis of newly formed (de novo) mediators (secondary mediators). *ECF,* Eosinophilic chemotactic factor; *NCF,* neutrophil chemotactic factor; *PAF,* platelet-activating factor.

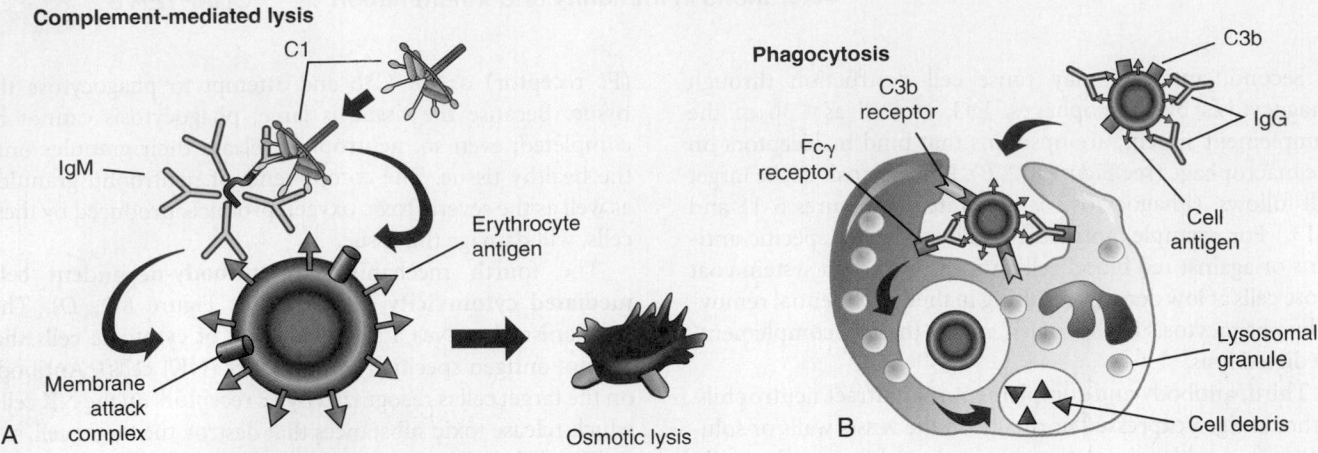

Complement-mediated lysis

C1

IgM

Erythrocyte
antigen

Membrane
attack
complex

Osmotic lysis

A

Phagocytosis

C3b

C3b
receptor

Fcγ
receptor

IgG

Cell
antigen

Lysosomal
granule

Cell debris

B

Neutrophil-mediated damage

3. Complement
activated

2. Antibody
binds

1. Antigen
deposits
in tissues

Antigen

IgG

C1

C3b

4. Neutrophil
chemotaxis

Lysosomal
granule

C5a

Fcγ
receptor

5. Neutrophil
adherence and
degranulation

C3b
receptor

Enzymes, reactive
oxygen species

C

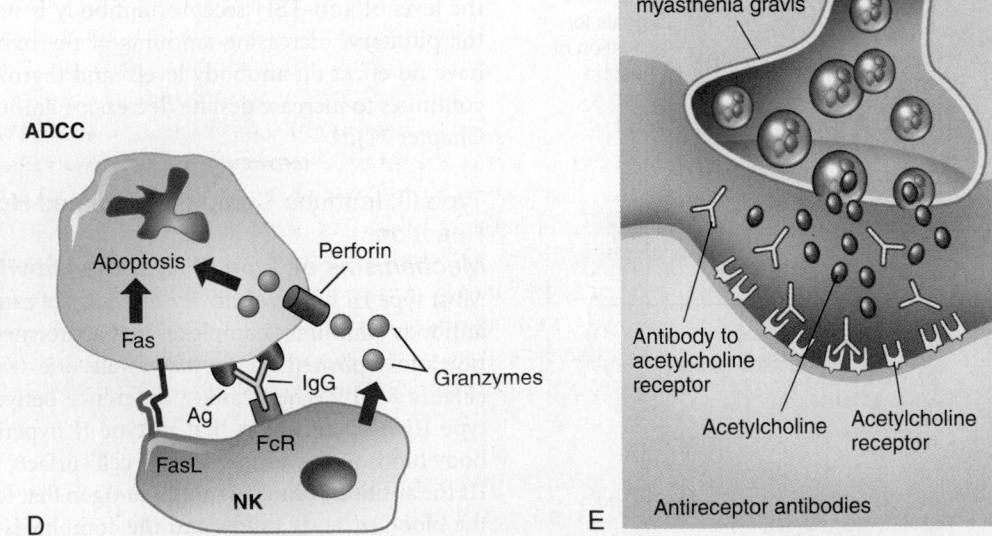

ADCC

Apoptosis

Perforin

Fas

Granzymes

Ag

IgG

FcR

FasL

NK

D

Motor end-plate in
myasthenia gravis

Antibody to
acetylcholine
receptor

Acetylcholine

Acetylcholine
receptor

Antireceptor antibodies

E

Figure 8-2 Mechanisms of type II, tissue-specific, reactions. Antigens on the target cell bind with antibody and are destroyed or prevented from functioning by **A,** complement-mediated lysis (an erythrocyte target is illustrated here); **B,** clearance (phagocytosis) by macrophages in the tissue; **C,** neutrophil-mediated immune destruction; **D,** antibody-dependent cell-mediated cytotoxicity (ADCC) (apoptosis of target cells is induced by granzymes and perforin produced by natural killer [NK] cells and interactions of Fas ligand [FasL] on the surface of NK cells with Fas on the surface of target cells); or **E,** modulation or blocking the normal function of receptors by antireceptor antibody. This example of mechanism E depicts myasthenia gravis in which acetylcholine receptor antibodies block acetylcholine from attaching to its receptors on the motor end plates of skeletal muscle, thereby impairing neuromuscular transmission and causing muscle weakness. *C1,* Complement component C1; *C3b,* complement fragment produced from C3, which acts as an opsonin; *C5a,* complement fragment produced from C5, which acts as a chemotactic factor for neutrophils; *Fcγ receptor,* cellular receptor for the Fc portion of IgG; *FcR,* Fc receptor.

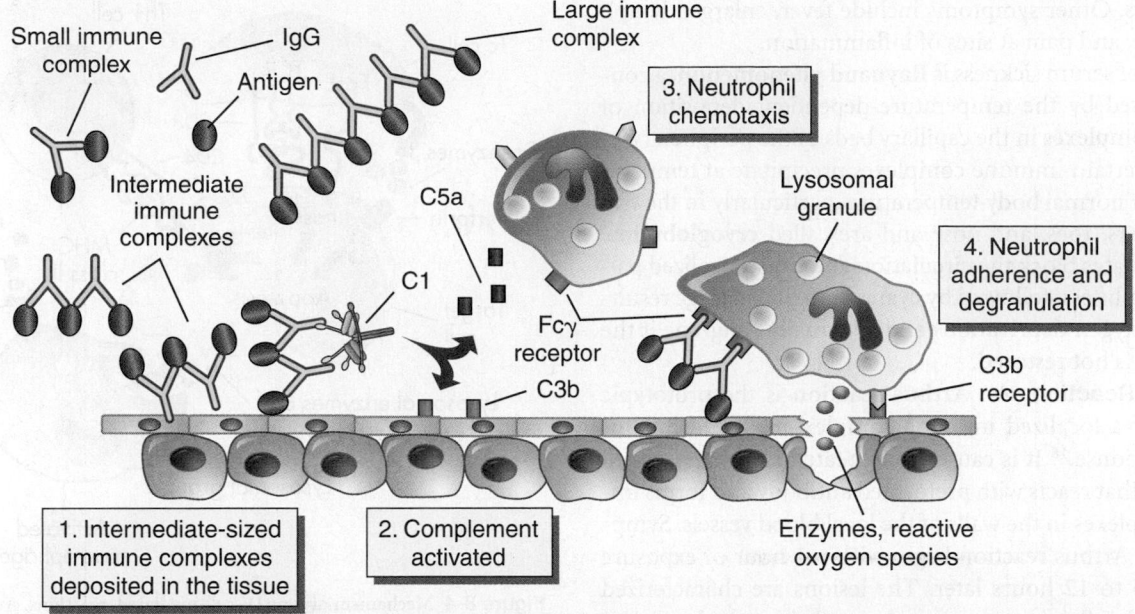

Figure 8-3 Mechanism of type III, immune complex–mediated reactions. Immune complexes form in the blood from circulating antigen and antibody. Both small and large immune complexes are removed successfully from the circulation and do not cause tissue damage. Intermediate-sized complexes are deposited in certain target tissues in which the circulation is slow or filtration of the blood occurs. The complexes activate the complement cascade through C1 and generate fragments including C5a and C3b. C5a is chemotactic for neutrophils, which migrate into the inflamed area and attach to the IgG and C3b in the immune complexes. The neutrophils attempt unsuccessfully to phagocytose the tissue and in the process release a variety of degradative enzymes that destroy the healthy tissues. Fcγ receptor is the cellular receptor for the Fc portion of IgG.

They are often unsuccessful because the complexes are bound to large areas of tissue. During the attempted phagocytosis, large quantities of lysosomal enzymes are released into the inflammatory site instead of into phagolysosomes. The attraction of neutrophils and the subsequent release of lysosomal enzymes cause most of the resulting tissue damage.

Immune complexes can be of various sizes, depending on the relative amounts of antigen and antibody. Fairly large immune complexes are cleared rapidly from the circulation by tissue macrophages, whereas very small complexes eventually are filtered from blood through the kidneys, without any pathologic consequences. Intermediate-sized immune complexes (formed at a ratio of antigen to antibody that has a slight excess of antigen) are likely to be deposited in certain target tissues, where they have severe pathologic consequences, such as inflammation in the kidneys (glomerulonephritis), the vessels (vasculitis), or the joints (arthritis or degenerative joint disease).

Immune Complex Disease

The nature of the immune complexes may change during the progression of the disease, with resultant changes in the severity of the symptoms. Immune complex formation is dynamic as variations in the ratio of antigen to antibody, the class and subclass of antibody, and the quantity and quality of circulating antigen occur. Thus complexes formed early in a disease process may differ from those formed later, and several types of immune complexes may be present simultaneously. With the tremendous potential heterogeneity of immune complexes, it is not surprising that immune-complex diseases are characterized by a variety of symptoms and periods of remission or exacerbation of symptoms.

Because many immune complexes activate complement very effectively, complement levels in the blood may decrease during active disease. At times the individual's blood may become **hypocomplementemic** (i.e., contains below normal amounts of complement activity). During type I, II, or IV hypersensitivity reactions, complement levels are unaffected, or some components of the complement cascade, such as C3, may even be increased.

Two prototypic models of type III hypersensitivity help explain the variety of diseases in this category. Serum sickness is a model of systemic type III hypersensitivities, and the Arthus reaction is a model of localized or cutaneous reactions.

Serum Sickness. The systemic prototype of immune complex–mediated disease is called **serum sickness** because it was initially described as being caused by the therapeutic administration of foreign serum, such as horse serum that contained antibody against tetanus toxin.[15] Foreign serum generally is not administered to individuals today, although serum sickness reactions can be caused by the repeated intravenous administration of other antigens, such as drugs, and the characteristics of serum sickness are observed in systemic type III autoimmune diseases. Serum sickness–type reactions are caused by the formation of immune complexes in the blood and their subsequent generalized deposition in target tissues. Typically affected tissues are the blood vessels, joints, and kidneys. Other symptoms include fever, enlarged lymph nodes, rash, and pain at sites of inflammation.

A form of serum sickness is **Raynaud phenomenon,** a condition caused by the temperature-dependent deposition of immune complexes in the capillary beds of the peripheral circulation. Certain immune complexes precipitate at temperatures below normal body temperature, particularly in the tips of the fingers, toes, and nose and are called **cryoglobulins.** The precipitates block the circulation and cause localized pallor and numbness, followed by cyanosis (a bluish tinge resulting from oxygen deprivation) and eventually gangrene if the circulation is not restored.

Arthus Reaction. An **Arthus reaction** is the prototypic example of a localized immune complex–mediated inflammatory response.[16] It is caused by repeated local exposure to an antigen that reacts with preformed antibody and forms immune complexes in the walls of the local blood vessels. Symptoms of an Arthus reaction begin within 1 hour of exposure and peak 6 to 12 hours later. The lesions are characterized by a typical inflammatory reaction, with increased vascular permeability, an accumulation of neutrophils, edema, hemorrhage, clotting, and tissue damage.

Type IV: Cell-Mediated Hypersensitivity Reactions

Whereas types I, II, and III hypersensitivity reactions are mediated by antibody, type IV reactions are mediated by T lymphocytes and do not involve antibody (Figure 8-4). Type IV mechanisms occur through either cytotoxic T lymphocytes (Tc cells) or lymphokine-producing Th1 cells.[17] Tc cells attack and destroy cellular targets directly. Th1 cells produce cytokines that recruit and activate phagocytic cells, especially macrophages. Destruction of the tissue is usually caused by direct killing by toxins from Tc cells or the release of soluble factors, such as lysosomal enzymes and toxic reactive oxygen species (ROS), from activated macrophages.

Clinical examples of type IV hypersensitivity reactions include graft rejection and allergic reactions resulting from contact with such substances as poison ivy and metals. A type IV component also may be present in many autoimmune diseases. For example, T cells against type II collagen (a protein present in joint tissues) contribute to the destruction of joints in rheumatoid arthritis; T cells against a thyroid cell surface antigen contribute to the destruction of the thyroid in autoimmune thyroiditis (Hashimoto disease); and T cells against an antigen on the surface of pancreatic beta cells (the cell that normally produces insulin) are responsible for beta-cell destruction in insulin-dependent (type 1) diabetes mellitus.

A type IV hypersensitivity reaction in the skin was thoroughly described first by Ehrlich in 1891 and led to the development of a diagnostic skin test for tuberculosis.[18] The reaction follows an intradermal injection of tuberculin antigen into a suitably sensitized individual and is called a *delayed hypersensitivity skin test* because of its slow onset—24 to 72 hours to reach maximum intensity. The reaction site is infiltrated with T lymphocytes and macrophages, resulting in a clear hard center (induration) and a reddish surrounding area (erythema).

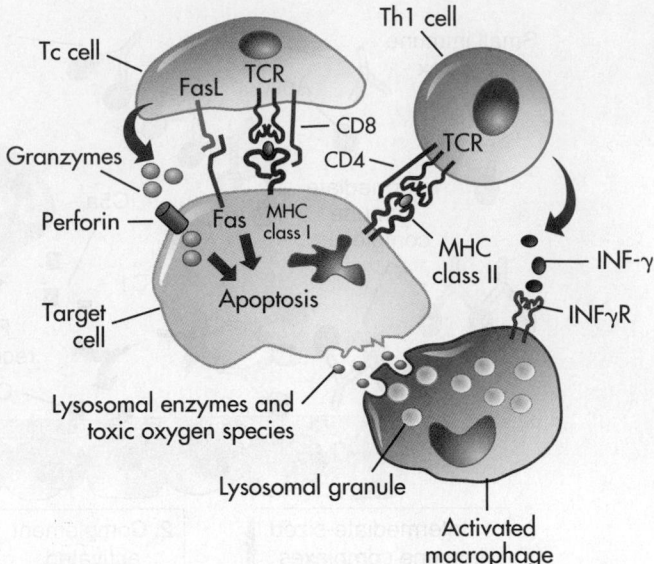

Figure 8-4 Mechanism of type IV, cell-mediated, reactions. Antigens from target cells stimulate T cells to differentiate into cytotoxic T cells (Tc cells), which have direct cytotoxic activity, and helper T cells (Th1 cells) involved in delayed hypersensitivity. The Th1 cells produce lymphokines (especially interferon-γ [IFN-γ]) that activate the macrophage through specific receptors (e.g., IFN-γ receptor [IFNγR]). The macrophages can attach to targets and release enzymes and reactive oxygen species that are responsible for most of the tissue destruction.

Antigenic Targets of Hypersensitivity Reactions

Allergy

Allergy is a hypersensitivity response against an environmental antigen **(allergen).** Although the most common allergies are type I hypersensitivities, any of the other three mechanisms may cause allergic responses.[19]

Typical allergens that induce type I hypersensitivity include pollens (e.g., ragweed), molds and fungi (e.g., *Penicillium notatum*), foods (e.g., milk, eggs, fish), animals (e.g., cat dander, dog dander), cigarette smoke, components of house dust (e.g., fecal pellets of house mites), and almost anything else we may encounter in our environment. Allergens that primarily elicit type IV allergic hypersensitivities include plant resins (e.g., poison ivy, poison oak), metals (e.g., nickel, chromium), acetylates and chemicals in rubber, cosmetics, detergents, and topical antibiotics (e.g., neomycin). Type II and type III allergic hypersensitivities are relatively rare but may include antibiotics (e.g., penicillin, sulfonamides) and soluble antigens produced by infectious agents (e.g., hepatitis B).

Usually a sensitization process involving multiple exposures to the allergen occurs before adequate amounts of antibody or T cells are available to elicit a hypersensitivity response. In some instances, exposure to a particular allergen may not be apparent in the case of allergens that are drugs, additives, or preservatives in food. For example, milk may contain trace amounts of penicillin used for treating cows for mastitis. Thus, the first therapeutic exposure to penicillin may cause an unexpected hypersensitivity reaction. Additionally, penicillin shares a β-lactam structure with cephalosporin, so that one antibiotic may be sensitive against another.[20]

Genetic Predisposition

Certain individuals are genetically predisposed to develop allergies, particularly type I allergies, and are called **atopic**.[21,22] In families in which one parent has an allergy, allergies develop in about 40% of the offspring. If both parents have allergies, the incidence in the offspring may be as high as 80%.[23] (Principles of genetic inheritance are discussed in Chapter 4.)

Atopic individuals tend to produce higher quantities of IgE and to have more Fc receptors for IgE on their mast cells. The airways and the skin of atopic individuals are also more responsive to a wide variety of both specific and nonspecific stimuli than are the airways and skin of individuals who are not atopic. Multiple genes have been associated with the atopic state, including polymorphisms in a large variety of cytokines that regulate IgE synthesis (e.g., interleukin [IL]-4, IL-5, IL-12, IL-13) and cellular receptors.

Clinical Symptoms of Type I Allergies

The clinical manifestations of type I reactions are attributable mostly to the biologic effects of histamine.[24] Tissues most commonly affected contain large numbers of mast cells and are sensitive to the effects of histamine released from them.[25] These tissues are found in the gastrointestinal tract, the skin, and the respiratory tract (Figure 8-5 and Table 8-4). The particular symptoms frequently reflect the main portal of entry for the allergen. For instance, pollens and other airborne allergens usually cause respiratory symptoms.

Effects of allergens on the mucosa of the eyes, nose, and respiratory tract include conjunctivitis (inflammation of the membranes lining the eyelids), rhinitis (inflammation of the mucous membranes of the nose), and asthma (constriction of the bronchi). Symptoms are caused by vasodilation, hypersecretion of mucus, edema, and swelling of the respiratory mucosa. Because the mucous membranes lining the respiratory tract (accessory sinuses, nasopharynx, and upper and lower respiratory tract) are continuous, they are all adversely affected. The degree to which each is affected determines the symptoms of the disease.

Gastrointestinal allergies are caused primarily by allergens that enter through the mouth—usually foods or medicines. Symptoms include vomiting, diarrhea, or abdominal pain and may be severe enough to result in malabsorption or protein-losing enteropathy, if the reactions are prolonged or recurrent. Foods most often implicated in gastrointestinal allergies are milk, chocolate, citrus fruits, eggs, wheat, nuts, peanut butter, and fish. When food is the allergen, the active immunogen may be a product of food breakdown by digestive enzymes.

Urticaria, or **hives,** is a dermal (skin) manifestation of type I allergic reactions (see Figure 8-5). The underlying mechanism is the localized release of histamine and increased vascular permeability, resulting in limited areas of edema. Urticaria is characterized by white fluid-filled blisters (wheals) surrounded by areas of redness (flares). The **wheal and flare reaction** is usually accompanied by itching. Not all urticarial symptoms are caused by allergic (immunologic) reactions. Some, termed *nonimmunologic urticaria,* result from exposure to cold temperatures, emotional stress, medications, systemic diseases, hyperthyroidism, or malignancies (e.g., lymphomas).

If possible, avoidance of the allergen is the best method to limit allergic responses. Approximately 30% of laboratory animal handlers have allergies to animal dander and must use face masks or other devices to avoid contact.[26]

Although some type I allergic responses can be controlled by blocking histamine receptors with antihistamines, the primary mechanism of control is the autonomic nervous system. The autonomic nervous system includes biochemical mediators (e.g., epinephrine, acetylcholine) that, like the mediators of the inflammatory response, have profound effects on cells. These mediators bind to appropriate receptors on mast cells and the target cells of inflammation (e.g., smooth muscle), thereby controlling (1) release of inflammatory mediators from mast cells and (2) the degree to which target cells respond to inflammatory mediators (see Chapter 6).

Allergic Disease: Bee Sting Allergy

An example of a life-threatening allergy is an anaphylactic reaction to a bee sting. Bee venoms contain a mixture of enzymes and other proteins that may serve as allergens. About 1% of children may have an anaphylactic reaction to bee venom. Within minutes they may develop excessive swelling (edema) at the bee sting site, followed by generalized hives, itching, and swelling in areas distal from the sting (e.g., eyes, lips), and other systemic symptoms including flushing, sweating, dizziness, and headache. The most severe symptoms may include gastrointestinal (e.g., stomach cramps, vomiting), respiratory (e.g., tightness in the throat, wheezing, difficulties breathing), and vascular (e.g., low blood pressure, shock) reactions. Severe respiratory and vascular reactions may lead to death.

If a child has had a previous anaphylactic reaction to bee stings, the chance of having another is about 60%. During the reaction the administration of antihistamines has little effect because histamine has already bound H1 receptors and initiated severe bronchial smooth muscle contraction. Most individuals carry self-injectable epinephrine. Autonomic nervous system mediators, such as epinephrine, bind to specific receptors on smooth muscle and reverse the effects of histamine and result in muscle relaxation. Similar anaphylactic reactions have been described against peanuts and other nuts, shellfish, fish, milk, eggs, and some medications.

Tests of IgE-Mediated Allergy

Allergic reactions can be life threatening; therefore, it is essential that severely allergic individuals be made aware of the specific allergen against which they are sensitized and instructed to avoid contact with that material. Several tests are available, including food challenges, skin tests with allergens, and laboratory tests for total IgE and allergen-specific IgE in the blood.

Reactivity to a particular food allergen may be tested by controlled administration of small doses of the suspected

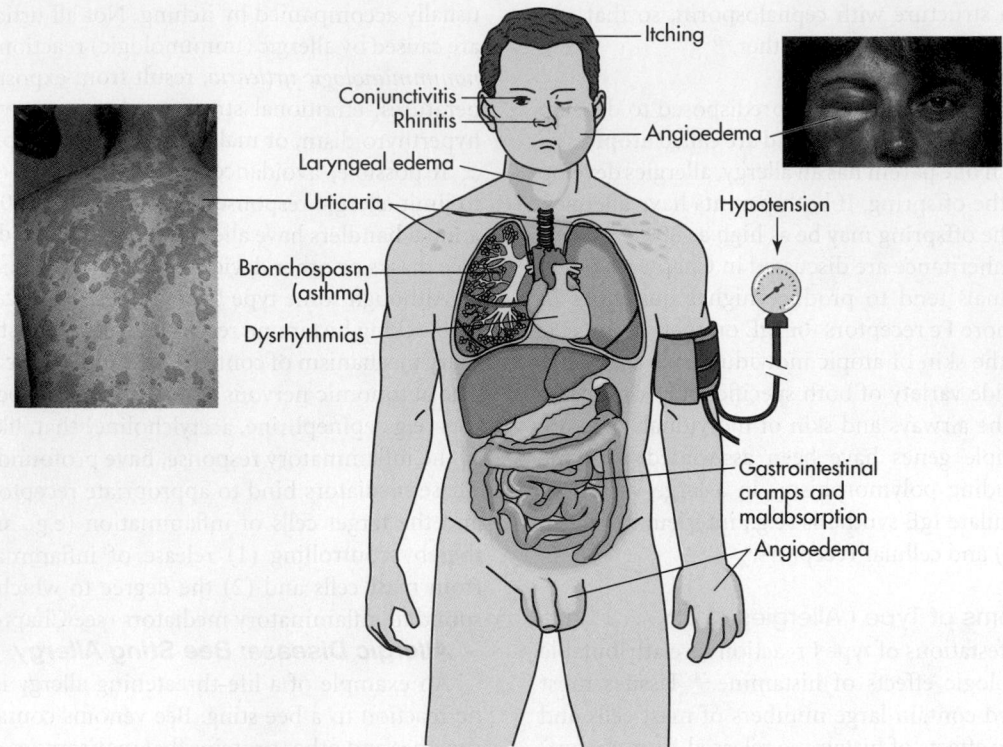

Figure 8-5 Type I hypersensitivity reactions. Manifestations of allergic reactions as a result of type I hypersensitivity include itching, angioedema (swelling caused by exudation), edema of the larynx, urticaria (hives), bronchospasm (constriction of airways in the lungs), hypotension (low blood pressure) and dysrhythmias (irregular heartbeat) because of anaphylactic shock, and gastrointestinal cramping caused by inflammation of the gastrointestinal mucosa. Photographic inserts show a diffuse allergic-like eye and skin reaction on an individual. The skin lesions have raised edges and develop within minutes or hours, with resolution occurring after about 12 hours. (From Roitt I, Brostoff J, Male D: *Immunology,* ed 6, St. Louis, 2001, Mosby.)

Table 8-4	Causes of Clinical Manifestations of Allergy	
Typical Allergen	**Mechanism of Hypersensitivity**	**Clinical Manifestation**
Ingestants		
Foods	Type I	Gastrointestinal allergy
Drugs	Types I, II, III	Urticaria, immediate drug reaction, hemolytic anemia, serum sickness
Inhalants		
Pollens, dust, molds	Type I	Allergic rhinitis, bronchial asthma
Aspergillus fumigatus	Types, I, III	Allergic bronchopulmonary aspergillosis
Thermophilic actinomycetes*	Types III, IV	Extrinsic allergic alveolitis
Injectants		
Drugs	Types, I, II, III	Immediate drug reaction, hemolytic anemia, serum sickness
Bee venom	Type I	Anaphylaxis
Vaccines	Type III	Localized Arthus reaction
Serum	Types I, III	Anaphylaxis, serum sickness
Contactants		
Poison ivy, metals	Type IV	Contact dermatitis

*An order of fungi that is stimulated by warmth to grow and proliferate.
Modified from Bellanti JA: *Immunology III,* Philadelphia, 1985, Saunders.

allergen in order to evoke a mild allergic response. This approach can be dangerous if the individual has a history of anaphylactic responses. A safer approach is injection of an allergen into (intradermal) or onto (epicutaneous or prick test) the skin. If the individual is allergic to a particular allergen,

a local wheal and flare reaction may occur within a few minutes at the site of injection. The diameter of the flare reaction is usually indicative of the individual's degree of sensitivity to that allergen.[27] In the most severely allergic individuals, even the extremely small amounts of allergen used for the skin test may evoke a systemic anaphylaxis. Skin test is also contraindicated if the patient is using medications that may affect the test or has diffuse dermatitis, which would make the reaction difficult to interpret.[28]

A variety of laboratory tests can detect IgE antibodies in serum. These assays have various commercial acronyms, depending on whether they are radioimmunoassays (RIAs; reactivity detected by measuring a radioactive reagent) or enzyme immunoassays (EIAs or ELISA [enzyme-linked immunosorbent assay]; reactivity detected by measuring a color change caused by an enzyme-labeled reagent). One set of assays measures circulating levels of total IgE, with atopic individuals usually having elevated levels. Other assays are capable of measuring circulating levels of specific IgE antibodies against selected allergens. The amount of IgE against a specific allergen correlates well with the degree of skin test reactivity and the severity of clinical symptoms related to the same allergen, although the laboratory text is less sensitive.

Desensitization

Clinical **desensitization** to allergens can be achieved in some individuals.[29] Minute quantities of the allergen are injected in increasing doses over a prolonged period. The procedure may reduce the severity of the allergic reaction in the treated individual. However, this form of therapy is associated with a risk of systemic anaphylaxis, which can be severe and life threatening. This approach works best for allergies against some food allergens and with biting insect allergies (80% to 90% rate of desensitization over 5 years of treatment).[30]

The mechanisms by which desensitization occurs may be several, one of which is the production of large amounts of so-called blocking antibodies, usually circulating IgG. A **blocking antibody** presumably competes in the tissues or in the circulation for binding with antigenic determinants on the allergen so that the allergen is "neutralized" and is unable to bind with IgE on mast cells. Sublingual desensitization (another approach that works best with some food allergies) produces sIgA and circulating IgG that may prevent the allergen from accessing mast cells. Desensitization injections also may stimulate the generation of clones of regulatory T lymphocytes, which inhibit hypersensitivity by suppressing the production of IgE or modifying the Th1/Th2 interactions in favor of production of anti-inflammatory cytokines.

Other approaches to suppressing type I allergic responses have been tested, with some preliminary success. An example is injection of anti-IgE antibody directed against the Fc portion of the IgG in order to decrease binding of IgE to mast cells.

Type IV Allergic Hypersensitivities

The allergens that induce a type IV allergic reaction are mostly haptens that react with normal self-proteins in the skin. When presented in this fashion, these antigens induce a cell-mediated response. The primary result is an allergic **contact dermatitis** that is confined to the area of contact with the allergen. The best-known example is poison ivy (Figure 8-6). The antigen in that instance is a plant catechol, *urushiol,* that reacts with normal skin proteins and evokes a cell-mediated immune response.

As noted, type I hypersensitivity reactions may result in a skin reaction (e.g., hives formed during an allergic reaction to a particular food).[31] The distribution of the lesions may suggest whether the reaction is caused by immediate (type I) or delayed (type IV) hypersensitivity mechanisms. Immediate hypersensitivity reactions, termed **atopic dermatitis,** are usually characterized by widely distributed lesions, whereas contact dermatitis (delayed hypersensitivity) consists of lesions only at the site of contact with the allergen, such as a metal allergy to jewelry (see Figure 8-6).

Types II and III Allergic Hypersensitivities

Type II allergic hypersensitivities are usually against allergic haptens that bind to the surface of cells and elicit an IgG or IgM response. For instance, allergic reactions against many drugs (e.g., penicillin, sulfonamides) occur after the drug binds to proteins on the plasma membranes of a person's cells and becomes immunogenic.[32] The immune system attacks the allergen on the cell membrane and destroys the cell as well. In allergic reactions to penicillin, the immunogenic antigen is a metabolite of penicillin catabolism that binds to the plasma membranes of erythrocytes or platelets and induces an antibody response that destroys the cells (type II hypersensitivity), causing anemia or thrombocytopenia. Type II allergic reactions also can occur against antigens of infectious diseases. For instance, encephalitis secondary to a rubella infection may result from damage to cells of the nervous system by an immune response against rubella virus antigen on the cell's plasma membrane.

Type III allergic reactions occur after the formation of immune complexes containing soluble allergens. For instance, Arthus reactions may be observed after injection, ingestion, or inhalation of allergens. Skin reactions can follow subcutaneous or intradermal inoculation with drugs, fungal extracts, or antigens used in skin tests. Gastrointestinal reactions, such as gluten-sensitive enteropathy (celiac disease), follow ingestion of antigen, usually gluten from wheat products (see Chapter 39). Allergic alveolitis is a type III acute hemorrhagic inflammation of the air sacs (alveoli) of the lungs resulting from inhalation of fungal antigens, usually particles from moldy hay (farmer's lung) or pigeon feces (pigeon breeder's disease) (see Chapter 33). Circulating drugs (e.g., penicillin) or antigens produced from infectious diseases (e.g., hepatitis B, streptococcal infection) may form circulating immune complexes that are deposited in the circulation (vasculitis) or the kidneys (glomerulonephritis).

Autoimmunity

Breakdown of Tolerance

Self-antigens are usually in a state of tolerance, or immunologic homeostasis, with the host's own immune system.[33] *Central tolerance* develops in humans during the embryonic period as autoreactive lymphocytes are either eliminated or suppressed in the primary lymphoid organs during differentiation and proliferation of immature T or B lymphocytes

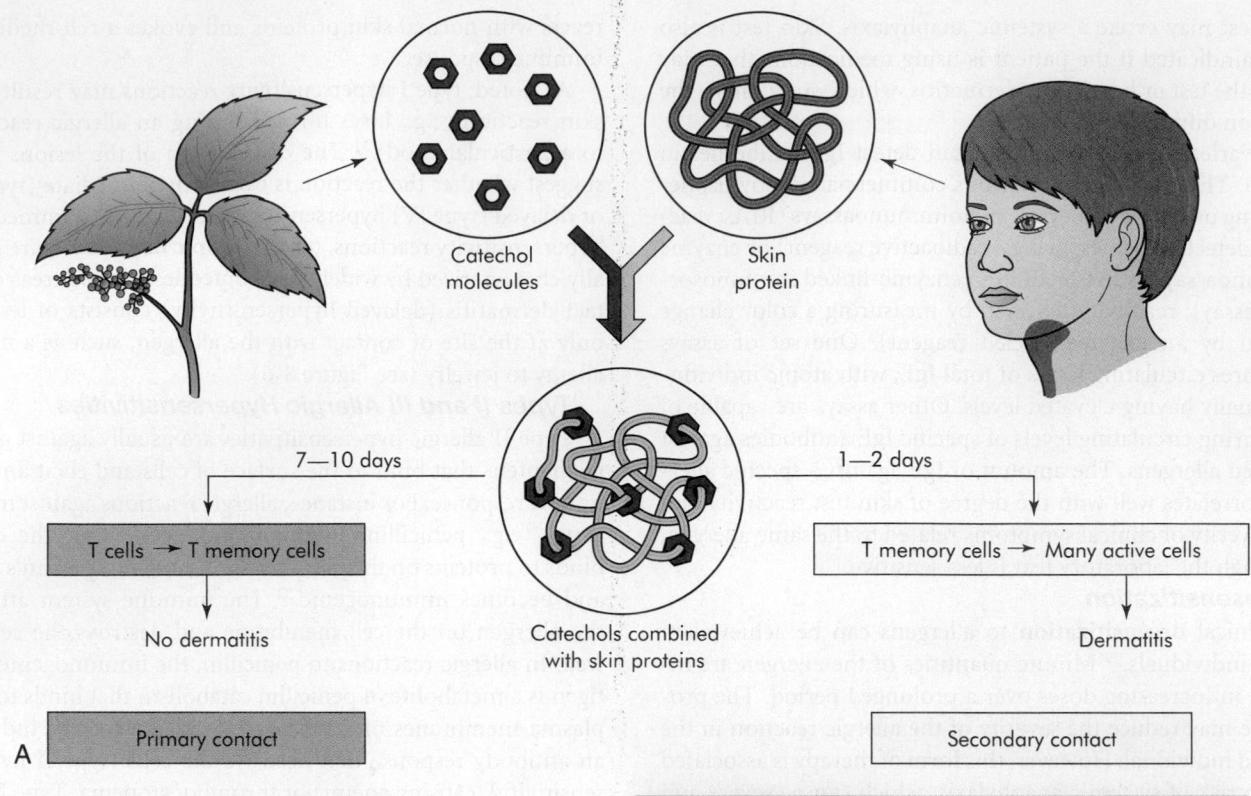

Catechol molecules

Skin protein

7—10 days

1—2 days

T cells → T memory cells

No dermatitis

Catechols combined with skin proteins

T memory cells → Many active cells

Dermatitis

A   Primary contact

Secondary contact

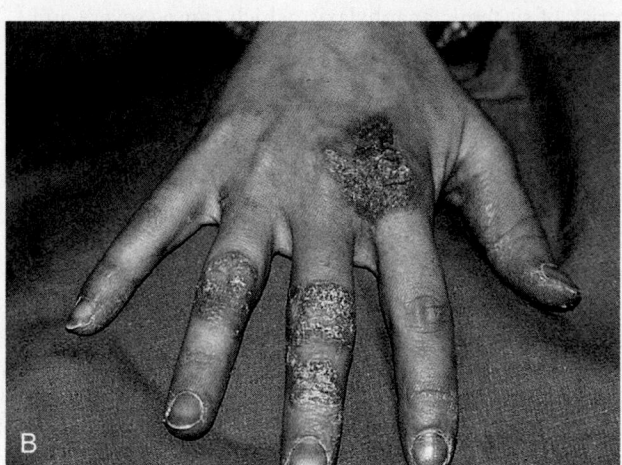

B

Figure 8-6 Development of allergic contact dermatitis, a delayed hypersensitivity reaction. **A,** Shown here is the development of allergy to catechols from poison ivy. No dermatitis results from the primary contact because the antigens (catechols) are sensitizing the immune response and producing memory T cells. Secondary contact, however, quickly activates a type IV, cell-mediated reaction that causes dermatitis. **B,** This contact dermatitis was caused by a delayed hypersensitivity reaction that led to vesicles and scaling at the sites of contact. (From Damjanov I, Linder J: *Anderson's pathology*, ed 10, St Louis, 1996, Mosby.)

(see Figures 7-10 and 7-12). Clones of cells with antigen receptors for self-antigens are deleted. *Peripheral tolerance* is maintained in the secondary lymphoid organs through the action of regulatory T lymphocytes or antigen-presenting dendritic cells. **Autoimmunity** is a breakdown of tolerance in which the body's immune system begins to recognize self-antigens as foreign.[34] In most autoimmune conditions the mechanism of tolerance breakdown is unknown, although several potential mechanisms have been suggested.

Sequestered Antigen. The induction of central tolerance requires that the self-antigen be present in the fetus and exposed to the developing fetal immune system. Some self-antigens may not normally encounter the immune system in either fetal or adult life, but are sequestered or hidden from the immune system in **immunologically privileged sites,** so named because foreign tissues can be transplanted into these sites with less chance of immunologic rejection. For example, several sites (e.g., anterior chamber of the eye, the brain) are separated from the circulation by barriers (blood-ocular and blood-brain barriers) that offer protection against many immune cells and to lead to relatively poor lymphatic drainage. Lymphocytes that enter these sites encounter tissue that expresses Fas ligand (FasL) and tumor necrosis factor (TNF)–related apoptosis-inducing ligand (TRAIL).[35] These molecules induce the lymphocytes to undergo apoptosis, thus protecting the tissue. Self-antigens in these sites are not normally seen by the immune system and are therefore not immunogenic. However, if the barriers are damaged, antigenic sensitization can occur, and the resultant antibodies and lymphocytes can enter the site and cause additional damage to the tissue. For instance, physical trauma to one eye may result in release of sequestered antigen into the blood or lymphatics, resulting in immunologic injury to the other eye (sympathetic uveitis).

Infectious Disease. A long-standing hypothesis is that foreign antigens from infectious microorganisms can initiate autoimmune disease through a process of **molecular mimicry.**[36] Some antigens of infectious agents so closely resemble (mimic) a particular self-antigen that antibodies or T cells produced to protect against the infection also recognize the self-antigen as foreign (**cross-reactive antibody** or **T cell**). Although the relationship between many autoimmune diseases and predisposing infections is being investigated, the only clearly defined example so far is acute rheumatic fever that may occur after a group A streptococcal sore throat (see following).

Neoantigen. In certain situations a neoantigen that induces an allergic reaction may lead also to autoimmunity. Many **neoantigens** (new antigens) are haptens, which become immunogenic after binding to self-proteins. The immune reaction against the neoantigen may lead to an immunologic reaction against normal antigenic determinants on the protein. Many experimental autoimmune diseases (e.g., experimental autoimmune thyroiditis) can be initiated by this mechanism.

Forbidden Clone. During differentiation and proliferation of lymphoid stem cells into immature T and B lymphocytes (see Figures 7-10 and 7-12), some lymphocytes produce receptors that react with self-antigens. Many autoreactive lymphocytes interact with self-antigens and other co-stimulatory molecules on the surface of thymic epithelial cells and are induced to undergo clonal deletion by a process of apoptosis.[37] Thus lymphocytes reactive against self-antigen are prevented, or "forbidden," from maturing. Autoimmunity may result from the survival of a **forbidden clone** and its proliferation later in life.

Defective Peripheral Tolerance. Tolerance to some self-antigens is controlled in the secondary lymphoid organs. This process is controlled by a variety of cells, including antigen-presenting dendritic cells and members of a family of regulatory T lymphocytes (Treg cells) that normally suppress immune responses against self. Defects in particular regulatory cells may result in expansion of clones of autoreactive cells and the development of autoimmune disease. Systemic lupus erythematosus, which is characterized by the production of a large array of autoantibodies, may be caused by a general breakdown in the regulatory network.

Original Insult

Although many theories exist, the initial cause of most autoimmune diseases is unknown (see What's New? Maternal Microchimerism and Autoimmune Disease). It is suspected that some autoimmune diseases are initiated by infections that have resolved without leaving evidence that would lead to identification of the particular infectious agent. The evidence for an infectious causation is clear for only one autoimmune disease: acute rheumatic fever.[38] In a small number of individuals with group A streptococcal sore throats, the M proteins in the bacterial capsule induce antibodies that also react with proteins in the heart valve, damaging the valve.

Additionally, some streptococcal skin or throat infections result in the release of bacterial antigens into the blood and the formation of circulating immune complexes. The complexes

---

WHAT'S NEW?

Maternal Microchimerism and Autoimmune Disease

Half of the genes of a child are from its father. Therefore, fetal cells express antigens that are foreign to the mother. The placenta was once considered an immunologic "barrier" that protected the fetus from the mother's immune rejection. New understandings, however, reveal the barrier is porous. Both maternal and fetal cells routinely cross the placenta so that fetal cells can be found in the mother's blood, and maternal cells can be found in the child's blood. The possible long-term implications of that exchange have only recently been described. It now seems that the child's cells can take up long-term residence in the mother's tissues and develop a state of **microchimerism** (mixing of cells of different origins).

Microchimerism is documented usually by the presence of male (Y chromosome) deoxyribonucleic acid (DNA) or male cells in the mother's blood or tissues. Using fluorescent probes that are specific for markers on the X or Y chromosome, male cells can be detected in about 90% of a woman's blood and tissues for decades after her last pregnancy with a male child.[39] Maternal cells also cross the placenta and can persist in the child into adulthood.[40] Because the techniques used in these studies differentiate between cells with or without the Y chromosome, there is no clear information on the degree of microchimerism resulting from carrying a female child.

Increased amounts of male DNA or cells are linked to several autoimmune diseases, such as scleroderma, dermatomyositis, Sjögren's syndrome, thyroiditis, primary biliary cirrhosis, and systemic lupus erythematosus. Healthy individuals have low levels of fetal microchimerism. In a study of systemic sclerosis, the level of male DNA in the circulation was much higher in patients with sclerosis than in healthy controls.[41] Elevated levels of male DNA were also found in skin lesions in patients with this disease.[42]

Maternal microchimerism in the offspring also may increase their risk for autoimmune disease. Increased levels of maternal cells in the child's blood have been reported in cases of juvenile inflammatory myopathy and neonatal lupus syndrome.[43]

Alternatively, fetal cells may benefit the mother by providing a source of pluripotent stem cells for tissue regeneration.[44] Several chimeric cell types have been detected, including liver cells, epithelial cells, lymphocytes, and others.[45] Many of these cell types may originate from stem cells that cross the placenta, take up residence in various organs, and differentiate into cells characteristic of that organ.

The primary question is the significance of microchimerism. To date, increased indications of microchimerism have been associated with autoimmune disease in the mother and the child. However, it cannot yet be determined whether the foreign cells are initiators of autoimmune damage or whether injury to the tissue results in their increased proliferation. Thus these observations remain intriguing but of unknown significance.

may deposit in the kidneys and initiate an immune complex glomerulonephritis (inflammation of the kidney). Thus capsular antigens of the group A *Streptococcus* may mimic *(antigenic mimicry)* normal heart antigens resulting in a type II autoimmune hypersensitivity (rheumatic fever), whereas in another person this infection may release bacterial antigen (an environmental antigen) into the blood, resulting in a type III allergic hypersensitivity (poststreptococcal glomerulonephritis).

Genetic Factors

Genetic factors that contribute to autoimmunity are easier to identify than the original insult that initiates the disease.[46] It is fairly well established that autoimmune diseases can be familial. Affected family members may not all develop the same disease, but several members may have different disorders characterized by a variety of hypersensitivity reactions, including autoimmune and allergic.

Associations with particular autoimmune diseases have been identified for a variety of major histocompatibility complex (MHC) alleles (see Chapter 7) or non-MHC genes. The specific HLA alleles of susceptible and resistant individuals have been analyzed for almost every known disease, and almost universally individuals with certain diseases are more likely than the general population to have a specific HLA allele or set of alleles. Some associations are strong; others are more tenuous (Table 8-5). The reason some HLA alleles are associated with inappropriate immune function is unclear, but it may directly involve the ability of particular HLA molecules to present antigen or the use of particular HLAs as receptors for disease-causing microorganisms. These genes may determine an individual's susceptibility to specific infectious agents or the capacity of that individual to mount an immune response against specific antigens. Therefore, an individual of a specific HLA type may have inappropriate or exaggerated immune responses against a microorganism, resulting in a hypersensitivity reaction.

A large variety of non-MHC genes also have been identified as risk factors for the development of specific autoimmune diseases. Most of these genes encode for inflammatory cytokines or co-stimulatory molecules found on the cell surface.

Alloimmunity

Alloimmunity occurs when an individual's immune system reacts against antigens on the tissues of other members of the same species. The two clinically relevant examples of this reactivity are (1) several transient neonatal diseases (in which the maternal immune system becomes sensitized against antigens expressed by the fetus) and (2) transplant rejection and transfusion reactions (in which the immune system of a recipient of an organ transplant or blood transfusion reacts against antigens on the donor cells).

Transient Neonatal Alloimmunity

Because the fetus is a hybrid between the mother and father, it expresses paternal antigens that are not found in the mother. Occasionally these fetal antigens cross the placenta

Table 8-5	Examples of Associations Between Specific HLA Alleles and Disease

Disease	HLA Allele	RR
Acute anterior uveitis	B27	14
Addison disease	DR3	6
Ankylosing spondylitis	B27	90
Behçet syndrome	B51	4
Celiac disease	DR3	11
Chronic active hepatitis	DR3	13
Dermatitis herpetiformis	DR3	16
Diabetes (type 1)	DR3	5
	DR4	6
	DR3/DR4	20
Goodpasture syndrome	DR2	16
Graves disease	DR3	4
Hashimoto disease	DR11	3
Multiple sclerosis	DR2	4
Myasthenia gravis	DR3	3
Pemphigus vulgaris	DR4	13
Postgonococcal arthritis	B27	14
Reiter syndrome	B27	37
Rheumatoid arthritis	DR4	4
Sjögren syndrome	DR3	9
Systemic lupus erythematosus	DR3	6

HLA, Human leukocyte antigen; *RR,* the approximate relative risk, which is the frequency of a disease in individuals with the particular HLA allele compared with individuals without that allele.

and elicit an immune response in the mother (e.g., production of alloantibodies against the fetal antigens). The maternal alloantibody may be transported across the placenta into the fetal circulation, bind to the fetal cells, and produce alloimmune disease in the fetus and neonate. The mother's immune system produces the antibody, but because her cells do not express the target antigen, she has no symptoms of the disease.

Neonatal alloimmune disease may be secondary to maternal autoimmune diseases in which the mother produces an IgG autoantibody specific for maternal self-antigens that are found on fetal cells as well. Therefore, symptoms of the same autoimmune disease may affect mother and child, even though the autoantibody is being produced only by the mother's immune system. This form of disease usually occurs only in association with type II (tissue-specific) hypersensitivity reactions. It does not occur in association with IgE-mediated (type I) reactions, immune complex–mediated (type III) reactions, or cell-mediated (type IV) reactions because the immunologic factors (IgE, immune complexes, T cells) that cause these reactions do not readily cross the placenta and enter the fetal circulation in sufficient quantity.

Symptoms of the alloimmune disease may be present in utero or immediately after birth and may be fatal to the fetus or neonate. At birth, maternal circulating antibody can no longer enter the child, and if symptoms are successfully treated, the disease will disappear as the maternal antibody is catabolized.

Examples of maternal immunologic hypersensitivity diseases in which the child can be affected include the following antibody-mediated diseases:

1. *Graves disease*—an autoimmune disease in which maternal antibody against the receptor for TSH causes neonatal hyperthyroidism
2. *Myasthenia gravis*—an autoimmune disease in which maternal antibody binds with receptors for neural transmitters on muscle cells (acetylcholine receptors), causing neonatal muscular weakness (see Chapter 17)
3. *Immune thrombocytopenic purpura*—both autoimmune and alloimmune variants in which maternal antiplatelet antibody destroys platelets in the fetus and neonate (see Chapter 27)
4. *Alloimmune neutropenia*—in which maternal antibody against neutrophils destroys neutrophils in the neonate
5. *Systemic lupus erythematosus*—autoimmune disease in which diverse maternal autoantibodies induce anomalies (e.g., congenital heart defects) in the fetus or cause pregnancy loss
6. *Rh and ABO alloimmunization (e.g., erythroblastosis fetalis)*—in which maternal antibody against erythrocyte antigens induces anemia in the child (see Chapter 28).

Autoimmune and Alloimmune Diseases

Many examples of autoimmune or **alloimmune diseases** have been described. Several basic principles are exemplified by two examples, systemic lupus erythematosus (an autoimmune disease) and tissue rejection (i.e., transplant rejection or transfusion reaction) (an alloimmune phenomenon). Most of the classic autoimmune diseases, including disorders of the endocrine system (autoimmune thyroiditis and Graves disease), hematologic system (the hemolytic and pernicious anemias), nervous system (myasthenia gravis), and connective tissue in joints (rheumatoid arthritis), are discussed in Unit II of this book.

Systemic Lupus Erythematosus

Systemic lupus erythematosus (SLE) is a chronic, multisystem, inflammatory disease and is one of the most common, complex, and serious of the autoimmune disorders.[47,48] SLE is characterized by the production of a large variety of autoantibodies against nucleic acids, erythrocytes, coagulation proteins, phospholipids, lymphocytes, platelets, and many other self-components.[49] The most characteristic autoantibodies produced in SLE are against nucleic acids (e.g., single-stranded deoxyribonucleic acid [DNA], double-stranded DNA), histones, ribonucleoproteins, and other nuclear materials.

Deposition of circulating immune complexes containing antibody against DNA produces tissue damage in individuals with SLE. DNA and DNA-containing immune complexes have a high affinity for glomerular basement membranes and therefore may be selectively deposited in the glomerulus (Figure 8-7). (Kidney structures are described in Chapter 35.) The presence of DNA in the circulation increases from cellular damage in response to trauma, drugs, or infections and is

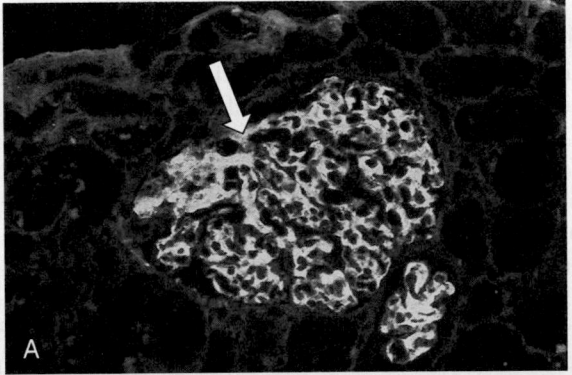

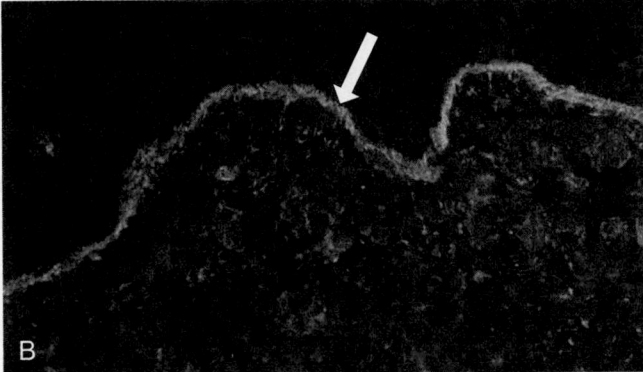

Figure 8-7 Deposition of IgG in the kidney and skin of individuals with lupus. These photographs of tissue were obtained from individuals with lupus and stained with fluorescent anti-IgG. **A,** Section from a kidney showing a glomerulus with deposits of IgG (*arrow,* indicating bright areas of staining). **B,** Section of the skin showing deposition of IgG along the dermal-epidermal junction (*arrow,* indicating bright green staining). (A courtesy of Dr. Helmut Rennke, Department of Pathology, Brigham and Women's Hospital, Boston; B courtesy of Dr. Richard Sontheimer, Department of Dermatology, University of Texas Southwestern Medical School, Dallas. Modified from Kumar V, Abbas A, Fausto N: *Robbins and Cotran pathologic basis of disease,* ed 7, Philadelphia, 2005, Saunders.)

usually removed in the liver. Removal of circulating DNA is slowed in the presence of immune complexes, thereby increasing the potential for deposition in the kidney. (The liver's role in removing waste products from the blood is discussed in Chapter 35.) Deposition of immune complexes composed of DNA and antibody also causes inflammatory lesions in the renal tubular basement membranes, brain (choroid plexus), heart, spleen, lung, gastrointestinal tract, skin (see Figure 8-7), and peritoneum.

SLE, as with most autoimmune diseases, occurs more often in women (approximately a 10:1 predominance of females), especially in the 20- to 40-year-old age group. Blacks are affected more often than whites (about an eightfold increased risk). A genetic predisposition for the disease has been implicated on the basis of increased incidence in twins and the existence of autoimmune disease in the families of individuals with SLE.[50]

A transient lupus-like syndrome that is indistinguishable both clinically and in the laboratory from spontaneously occurring SLE can develop from the prolonged use of drugs. The drugs most often implicated are hydralazine (an antihypertensive agent) and procainamide (an antidysrhythmic drug). In genetically susceptible individuals, certain environmental agents, such as ultraviolet light, and several infectious agents may trigger lupus-like immune reactions.

Clinical manifestations of SLE include arthralgias or arthritis (90% of individuals), vasculitis and rash (70% to 80% of individuals), renal disease (40% to 50% of individuals), hematologic abnormalities (50% of individuals, with anemia being the most common complication), and cardiovascular diseases (30% to 50% of individuals). As with most autoimmune diseases, the disease process develops slowly (up to 10 years from occurrence of the first autoantibody until diagnosis)[51] and is characterized by frequent remissions and exacerbations. Because the signs and symptoms affect almost every body system and tend to come and go, SLE is extremely difficult to diagnose. This has led to the development of a list of 11 common clinical findings. The serial or simultaneous presence of at least four of them indicates that the individual has SLE.[52]

1. Facial rash confined to the cheeks (malar rash)
2. Discoid rash (raised patches, scaling)
3. Photosensitivity (skin rash developed as a result of exposure to sunlight)
4. Oral or nasopharyngeal ulcers
5. Nonerosive arthritis of at least two peripheral joints
6. Serositis (pleurisy, pericarditis)
7. Renal disorder (proteinuria of 0.5 g/day or cellular casts)
8. Neurologic disorders (seizures or psychosis)
9. Hematologic disorders (hemolytic anemia, leukopenia, lymphopenia, or thrombocytopenia)
10. Immunologic disorders (positive lupus erythematosus [LE] cell preparation, anti–double-stranded DNA, anti-Smith [Sm] antigen, false-positive serologic test for syphilis, or antiphospholipid antibodies [anticardiolipin antibody or lupus anticoagulant])
11. Presence of antinuclear antibody (ANA)

There is no cure for SLE or most other autoimmune diseases. The goals of treatment are to control symptoms and prevent further damage by suppressing the autoimmune response. Nonsteroidal anti-inflammatory drugs, such as aspirin, ibuprofen, or naproxen, reduce inflammation and relieve pain. Corticosteroids are often prescribed for more serious active disease. Immunosuppressive drugs (e.g., methotrexate, azathioprine, or cyclophosphamide) are used to treat severe symptoms involving internal organs. Ultraviolet light can worsen symptoms (known as flares), and protection from sun exposure is helpful. Prolonged use of certain drugs can cause transient SLE-like symptoms, and the medication history is important for diagnostic evaluation. Improved outcomes may be available in the future with the continued advances in medical research and the use of stem cell treatments.[53]

Transfusion Reactions

Red blood cells (erythrocytes) express several important surface antigens, known collectively as the **blood group antigens,** which can be targets of alloimmune reactions.[54] More than 80 different red cell antigens are grouped into several dozen blood group systems, each determined by a different locus or set of loci. The most important of these, because they provoke the strongest humoral alloimmune response, are the ABO and Rh systems.

ABO System

Human blood transfusions were carried out as early as 1818, but they were often unsuccessful. Sometimes after a transfusion, the recipient's red blood cells would clump together, thereby blocking the capillaries and causing death in some instances. In 1901, Karl Landsteiner reported that this reaction was related to the ABO antigens located on the surface of erythrocytes.

The **ABO blood group** consists of two major carbohydrate antigens, labeled A and B (Figure 8-8). These two carbohydrate antigens are codominant, which means that both A and B can be simultaneously expressed, resulting in an individual having any one of four different blood types. The erythrocytes of persons with blood type A have the type A carbohydrate antigen (i.e., carry the A antigen), those with blood type B carry the B antigen, those with blood type AB carry both A and B antigens, and those of blood type O carry neither the A nor the B antigen. A person with type A blood also has circulating antibodies to the B carbohydrate antigen. If this person receives blood containing B antigens (i.e., blood from a type AB or B individual), a severe transfusion reaction occurs and the transfused erythrocytes are destroyed by agglutination (Figure 8-9) or complement-mediated lysis. Similarly, a type B individual (whose blood contains anti-A antibodies) cannot receive blood from a type A or AB donor. Type O individuals, who have neither A or B antigen but have both anti-A and anti-B antibodies, cannot accept blood from any of the other three types. These naturally occurring antibodies, called **isohemagglutinins,** are immunoglobulins of the IgM class and are induced by similar antigens expressed on naturally occurring bacteria in the intestinal tract.

Because individuals with type O blood lack both types of antigens, they are considered **universal donors,** meaning that anyone can accept their red blood cells. Similarly, type AB individuals are considered **universal recipients** because they lack both anti-A and anti-B antibodies and can be transfused with any ABO blood type. When large volumes of *whole blood* (i.e., cells plus plasma) are transfused, however, antibodies in the *donor's* blood can bind to antigenic determinants on the *recipient's* erythrocytes, causing agglutination of the recipient's own cells. Agglutination and lysis cause harmful transfusion reactions that can be prevented only by complete and careful ABO matching between donor and recipient.

Rh System

The **Rh blood group** is the most polymorphic system of red cell antigens, consisting of at least 50 separate antigens.[55] At least five major antigens and a large number of rare variants have been identified and are expressed primarily on erythrocytes. The major antigens are contained on two proteins encoded from two closely linked genes, *RHD* and *RHCE.* The RhD protein expresses the dominant antigen,

Blood Type

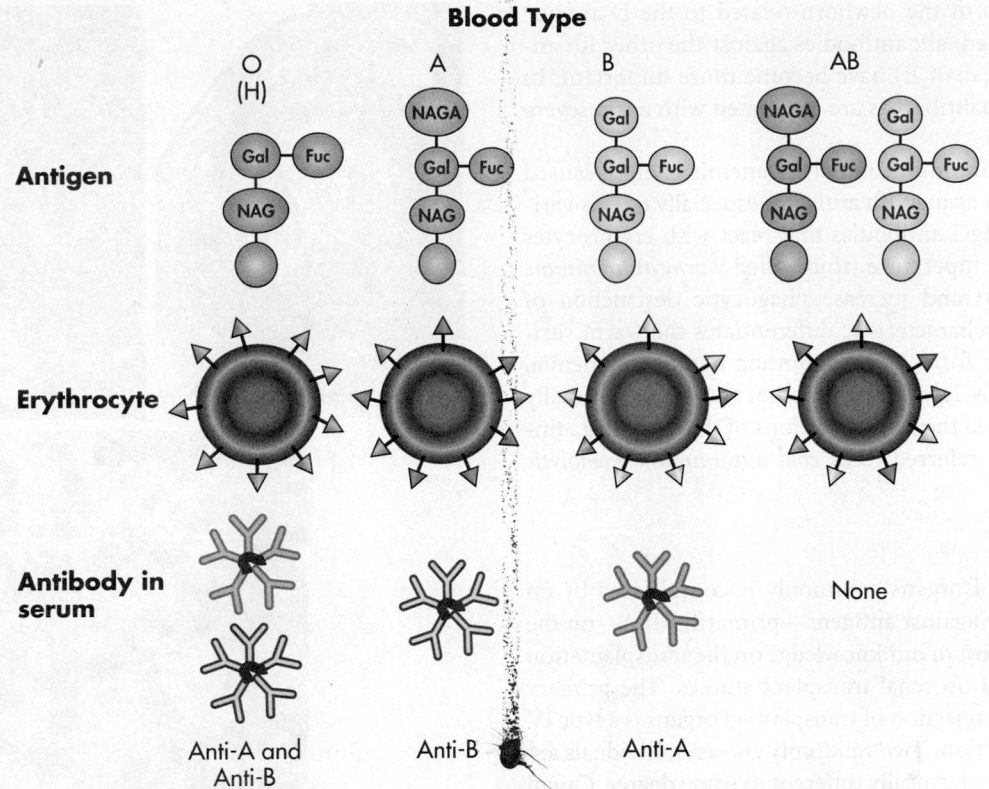

Figure 8-8 ABO blood types. This figure shows the antigens and antibodies associated with the ABO blood groups. The surfaces of erythrocytes of individuals with blood group O have the core H antigenic carbohydrate. Their sera contain IgM antibodies against both A and B carbohydrates. In individuals of the blood group A, some of the H antigens have been modified into A antigens by the addition of N-acetylgalactosamine (NAGA). The sera of these individuals have IgM antibodies against the B antigen. In individuals with blood group B, some of the H antigens have been modified into B antigens by the addition of galactose (Gal). These individuals have IgM antibodies against the A antigen in their sera. In individuals of the blood group AB, some of the H antigens have been modified into both the A and B antigens. These individuals do not have antibody to either A or B antigens. *NAG,* N-acetylglucosamine; *Fuc,* fucose.

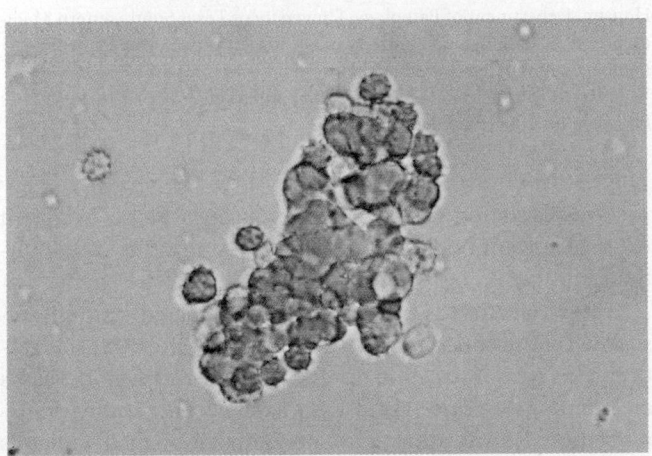

Figure 8-9 Mismatched transfused blood cells. Agglutination of erythrocytes caused by anti-A blood-typing serum. (Copyright Ed Reschke.)

which determines whether an individual is Rh-positive or Rh-negative. Individuals who express the D antigen on the RhD protein are Rh-positive, whereas individuals who do not express the D antigen are Rh-negative. The letter *d* is used to indicate lack of D. Rh-positive individuals can have either a *DD* or *Dd* genotype, whereas Rh-negative individuals have the *dd* genotype. About 15% of North American whites are Rh-negative, whereas the Rh-negative genotype is much less common among members of other ethnic groups. Rh-negative individuals can make anti-D if exposed to Rh-positive erythrocytes, but because the letter *d* is used to indicate the lack of the D antigen and does not represent a different antigen, Rh-positive individuals do not produce an antibody against *d*. The second protein, RhCE, expresses two different antigens, C and E, each of which has two different alleles (C or c, E or e). Therefore, four potential haplotypes of C and E antigens are commonly observed: *CE, Ce, cE,* and *ce*).

IgG anti-D alloantibody produced by Rh-negative mothers against erythrocytes of their Rh-positive fetuses was the primary cause of Rh maternal-fetal incompatibility and the resulting hemolytic disease of the newborn (see Chapter 28). However, over the past several decades, the incidence of mothers with high titers of anti-D antibody has decreased dramatically because of the use of prophylactic anti-D immunoglobulin. By mechanisms that are still not completely understood, administration of anti-D antibody within a few days of exposure to RhD-positive erythrocytes completely prevents sensitization against the D antigen. Because hemolytic disease of the newborn related to the D antigen has been controlled, alloantibodies against the other Rh antigens (usually C, c, or E) have become more important. In general, these alloantibodies are associated with a less severe hemolytic disease.

A form of autoimmune hemolytic anemia is often caused by autoantibodies against Rh antigens, especially e. This variant is caused by IgG antibodies that react with erythrocytes at normal body temperature (thus called *warm autoimmune hemolytic anemia*) and increase phagocytic destruction of the red cell. This characteristic differentiates the warm variant from another form of autoimmune hemolytic anemia, which is caused by IgM autoantibodies that react optimally with erythrocytes in the cooler portions of the body (e.g., fingers, toes) and is referred to as *cold autoimmune hemolytic anemia*.

Graft Rejection

Transplantation of organs commonly is complicated by an immune response against antigens—primarily HLA—on the donated tissue. Most of our knowledge on the transplantation of organs is based on renal transplant studies. The primary mechanism of the rejection of transplanted organs is a type IV cell-mediated reaction. Two randomly chosen individuals are almost certainly antigenically different to some degree. Organ transplants between them could be rejected in approximately 2 weeks without the extensive use of immunosuppressive drugs.

After the donor and recipient are matched for ABO antigens, HLAs are the principal targets of the rejection reaction; HLA matching of donor and recipient enhances the probability of acceptance of the graft.[56] Not all HLA loci are equally important; matching at the HLA-DR locus appears to be the most critical for graft acceptance, and matching at HLA-A and HLA-B of slightly lesser importance. (These loci are discussed in Chapter 7.)

Transplant rejection may be classified as hyperacute, acute, or chronic, depending on the amount of time that elapses between transplantation and rejection. **Hyperacute rejection** is immediate and rare. When the circulation is reestablished to the grafted area, the graft may immediately turn white (the so-called *white graft*) instead of a normal pink. Hyperacute rejection usually occurs in recipients with preexisting antibody to antigens in the graft. The antibodies may have resulted from rejection of a previous graft or from prior blood transfusions that contained platelets and white blood cells with foreign HLA. Additionally, about half of women who have had multiple pregnancies have circulating antibodies against their husband's HLA antigens. As the circulation to the graft is established, antibodies bind to the vascular endothelial cells in the grafted tissue and activate the inflammatory response, including the coagulation cascade, which results in stasis of blood flow into the tissue (Figure 8-10). (Coagulation is described in Chapters 6 and 25.) Biopsies of the graft often show deposits of antibody (IgG and IgM), complement, and neutrophils. This condition is rare because of effective

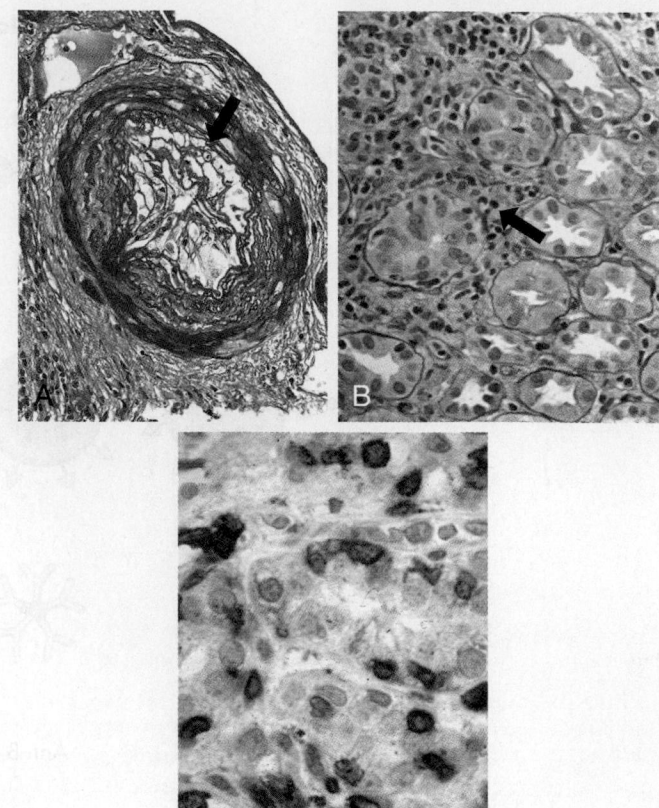

Figure 8-10 Examples of hyperacute and acute rejection of renal allografts. **A,** Hyperacute antibody-mediated damage to the blood vessel of a renal allograft. The blood vessel is thickened, and the lumen *(arrow)* is obstructed by proliferating fibroblasts and macrophages. **B,** Acute cellular rejection of a renal allograft with intense mononuclear cell infiltrate *(arrow).* **C,** Acute cellular rejection stained with immunoperoxidase reagent (brown) against T cells, which are infiltrating the tissue. (**A** courtesy of Dr. Ihsan Housini, Department of Pathology, University of Texas Southwestern Medical School, Dallas; **B** and **C** courtesy of Dr. Robert Colvin, Department of Pathology, Massachusetts General Hospital, Boston. Modified from Kumar V, Abbas A, Fausto N: *Robbins and Cotran pathologic basis of disease,* ed 7, Philadelphia, 2005, Saunders.)

pretransplantation cross-matching during which a recipient is tested for antibodies against the HLA antigens of the potential donor.

Acute rejection is primarily a cell-mediated immune response that occurs within days to months after transplantation. This type of rejection occurs when the recipient develops an immune response against unmatched HLAs after transplantation. Sensitization is usually initiated by the recipient's lymphocytes interacting with the donor's dendritic cells within the transplanted tissue, resulting in induction of recipient Th1 and Tc cells against the donor's antigens. The Th1 cells release cytokines that activate infiltrating macrophages, and the Tc cells directly attack the endothelial cells in the transplanted tissue. A biopsy of the rejected organ usually shows an infiltration of lymphocytes and macrophages characteristic of a type IV reaction. Immunosuppressive drugs may delay or lessen the intensity of acute rejection.

Another form of acute rejection, *acute antibody-mediated rejection*, has recently been recognized and accounts for about 10% of acute rejections.[57] This form of rejection is mediated by antibody and complement. The predominant antibodies are against HLA antigens or, on occasion, autoantigens in the graft (e.g., vimentin, angiotensin receptor), but, unlike those antibodies that cause hyperacute rejection, are not present at the time of transplantation. Sensitization takes 2 weeks or longer and results in the accumulation of antibody, complement, neutrophils, and thrombi in the vasculature of the graft (a type II hypersensitivity reaction).

Chronic rejection may occur after a period of months or years of normal function. It is characterized by slow, progressive organ failure. Chronic rejection may be caused by inflammatory damage to endothelial cells lining blood vessels as a result of a weak cell-mediated immunologic reaction against minor histocompatibility antigens on the grafted tissue.

DEFICIENCIES IN IMMUNITY

Disorders resulting from immune deficiency are the clinical sequelae (results) of impaired function of one or more components of the immune or inflammatory response, including B cells, T cells, phagocytes, and complement (Table 8-6). An **immune deficiency** is the failure of these mechanisms of self-defense to function at their normal capacity, resulting in increased susceptibility to infections. **Primary (congenital) immune deficiency** is caused by a genetic anomaly, whereas **secondary (acquired) immune deficiency** is caused by another illness, such as cancer or viral infection, or by normal physiologic changes, such as aging. Acquired forms of immune deficiency are far more common than the congenital forms.

Initial Clinical Presentation

The clinical hallmark of immune deficiency is a tendency to develop unusual or recurrent, severe infections. Preschool and school-age children normally may have 6 to 12 infections per year, of which 3 or 4 are ear infections, and adults may have 2 to 4 infections per year. Most of these are not severe and are limited to viral infections of the upper respiratory tract, recurrent streptococcal pharyngitis, or mild otitis media.

Potential immune deficiencies are considered if the individual has had severe, documented bouts of pneumonia, otitis media, sinusitis, bronchitis, septicemia, or meningitis or infections with opportunistic microorganisms that normally are not pathogenic or usually confined to one site (e.g., *Pneumocystis jirovecii*, disseminated *Candida* infection, cytomegalovirus [CMV]). Infections are generally recurrent with only short intervals of relative health, and multiple simultaneous infections are common. Individuals with primary immune deficiencies often have eight or more ear infections, two or more serious sinus infections, and two or more pneumonias, recurrent abscesses or infections in unusual sites, or persistent fungal infections (particularly thrush in an individual at least 1 year old) within a year. Recurrent internal infections, such as meningitis, osteomyelitis, or sepsis, are common. Prolonged antibiotic use is commonly ineffective by oral or injected routes and may necessitate intravenous administration. Additional symptoms may include failure to thrive and chronic diarrhea. A familial history of immune deficiency may be found in some types of primary deficiency.

The type of recurrent infections that manifest may indicate the type of immune defect. Deficiencies in T-cell immune responses are suggested when recurrent infections are caused by certain viruses (e.g., varicella, vaccinia, herpes, cytomegalovirus), fungi and yeasts (e.g., *Candida*, *Histoplasma*), or certain atypical microorganisms (e.g., *P. jirovecii*). B-cell deficiencies and phagocyte deficiencies, however, are suggested if the individual has documented, recurrent infections with microorganisms that require opsonization (e.g., encapsulated bacteria) or viruses against which humoral immunity is normally effective (e.g., rubella). Some complement deficiencies resemble defects in antibody or phagocyte function, but others are commonly associated with disseminated infections with bacteria of the genus *Neisseria* (*Neisseria meningitidis* and *Neisseria gonorrhoeae*).

Much of our current understanding of the development of the immune system and the interactions of the cells in the immune response was developed by studying congenital and acquired immune deficiencies or, as they have been called, "experiments of nature." Many immune deficiencies result from selective altering or removal of one component of the immune system. We can understand the importance of that component by observing the effect of its removal on the remainder of the immune response.

Primary Immune Deficiencies

Most primary immune deficiencies are the result of a single gene defect[58] (Figure 8-11). Generally, the mutations are sporadic and not inherited: a family history exists in only about 25% of individuals. The sporadic mutations occur before birth, but the onset of symptoms may be early or later, depending on the particular syndrome. In approximately 60% of the cases symptoms of immune deficiency appear within the first 2 years of life, whereas other immune deficiencies are progressive, with the onset of symptoms appearing in the second or third decade of life. The most common symptoms include sinusitis (68% of individuals), pneumonia (51%), ear infections (51%), diarrhea (30%), and bronchitis (55%), with the incidence varying depending on the specific syndrome.

Many immune deficiencies also are associated with other characteristic defects; some of which appear to be unrelated to the immune system yet may be life threatening in themselves. Examples include eczema and thrombocytopenia (in Wiskott-Aldrich syndrome); cardiac anomalies, low levels of calcium in the blood, and structural anomalies of the face (in DiGeorge syndrome); or a severe lack of muscular coordination and dilation of the small blood vessels (in ataxia-telangiectasia). These associated symptoms can be useful diagnostically. For instance, the principal immunologic defect in **DiGeorge syndrome** is the partial or complete absence of T-cell immunity.

Table 8-6   Classes of Primary Immune Deficiencies

Classification*	Example	Mutation	Immune Deficiency
B-Cell Defects			
B-cell receptor signaling	Bruton's/X-linked agammaglobulinemia	Btk	Little or no B-cell maturation or antibody
	Autosomal agammaglobulinemia	IgMμ chain	
Class-switch: hyper-IgM	X-linked hyper-IgM syndrome	CD40 ligand	Little or no class-switch to IgG or IgA, with overproduction of IgM
	Autosomal hyper-IgM syndrome	CD40	
	AICD deficiency	AICD	
Class-switch: selective	IgG subclass deficiency	Unknown	Defective switch to an IgG subclass
	Selective IgA deficiency	Unknown	Defective switch to IgA
	Common variable immune deficiency	Multiple	Defective switch to ≥1 antibody class
T-Cell Defects			
Defective primary lymphoid organ for T-cell development	DiGeorge syndrome	Development of 3rd and 4th pharyngeal pouches	Little or no T-cell maturation
Antigen specific response	Chronic mucocutaneous candidiasis	Unknown	Little or no response to *Candida*
Combined T- and B-Cell Defects			
SCID: No WBC stem cells	Reticular dysgenesis	Unknown	Complete; lack of white blood cells
SCID: Enzyme defects	Adenosine deaminase deficiency	ADA	Complete; few or no T, B, or NK cells
	Purine nucleoside phosphorylase deficiency	PNP	Partial; few T or NK cells
SCID: cytokine receptor defects	X-linked SCID	IL-2Rγ	Partial; little or no maturation of Th or NK cells
	IL-7 receptor deficiency	IL-7Rα	
	JAK3 deficiency	JAK3	
SCID: TCR/BCR defects	RAG-1 or RAG-2 deficiency	RAG-1/RAG-2	Complete; little or no maturation of T or B cells; normal NK cells
SCID: TCR defects S	CD45 deficiency	CD45	Partial; incomplete T-cell maturation, normal B and NK cells
	CD3 deficiency	CD3 γ, δ, or ε chains	
	ZAP-70 deficiency	ZAP-70	
Antigen presentation defects	MHC class I deficiency	TAP1 or TAP2	Abnormal cytotoxic T cell activity
	MHC class II deficiency	Multiple	Abnormal helper T cell activity
Cytoskeletal defect	Wiskott-Aldrich syndrome	WASP	Altered T and B cells; decreased IgM
DNA repair defect	Ataxia-telangiectasia	ATM	Altered T and B cells; absent IgA
Complement Defects			
Classical pathway	C1q,r,s, C4, or C2 deficiency	C1q,r, or s, C4, or C2	Defective classical pathway, intact alternative pathway
Lectin pathway	Mannose-binding lectin deficiency	MBL	Defective lectin pathway
Alternative pathway	Properdin, factor D or B deficiency	Properdin, factor D or B	Defective alternative pathway
	Factor H, factor I deficiency	Factor H, factor I	Secondary C3 deficiency
C3	C3 deficiency	C3	Entire complement cascade blocked
Terminal pathway	C5, C6, C7, C8, or C9 deficiency	C5, C6, C7, C8, or C9	Membrane attack complex blocked, normal opsonization and chemotaxis
Phagocyte Defects			
Quantitative defects	Severe congenital neutropenia	ELA2, WASP	Inadequate numbers of neutrophils
	Cyclic neutropenia	ELA2	
Adhesion defects	Leukocyte adhesion defect (LAD)–1	CD18	Decreased phagocyte adhesion to endothelium
	LAD-2	Transport enzymes for fucose	
Phagocytosis defects	C3 receptor deficiency	C3R	Defective opsonization
Bacterial killing defects	Chédiak-Higashi syndrome	CHS1	Defective lysosomal granules
	Myeloperoxidase deficiency	MPO	Lack of myeloperoxidase
	Chronic granulomatous disease	NADPH oxidase	Defective production of H_2O_2

AICD, Activation-induced cytidine deaminase; *SCID*, severe combined immune deficiency; *TCR/BCR*, T-cell receptor/B-cell receptor; *MHC*, major histocompatibility complex; *NADPH*, nicotinamide adenine dinucleotide phosphate; *NK*, natural killer; *RAG*, recombination activating; *ZAP*, zeta chain associated protein.

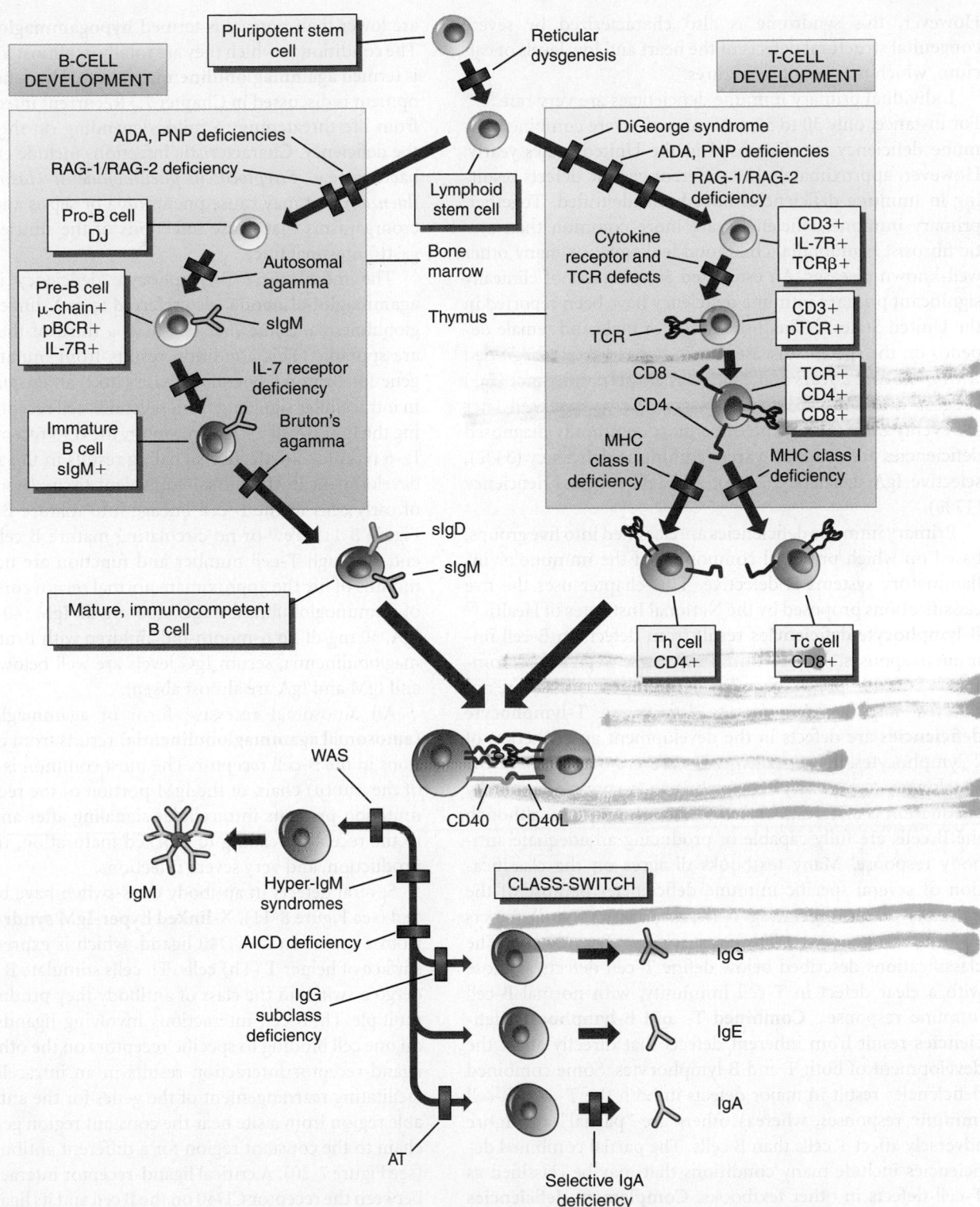

Figure 8-11 Lymphocyte development defects. This diagram shows defects in lymphocyte development that may account for congenital (primary) immune deficiencies. See the text and refer to Figures 7-10 through 7-12 for more detailed information. Pluripotent stem cell indicates the common stem cells for lymphocytic, granulocytic, and monocytic lineages. Cytokine receptor defects include X-linked severe combined immunodeficiency (SCID) (IL-2 receptor defect), JAK3 defects, and IL-7 receptor defects. T-cell receptor (TCR) defects include defects in CD3, CD45, and ZAP-70. Neither common variable immune deficiency nor chronic mucocutaneous candidiasis is included in this figure because the cause of these defects remains unknown. See Table 8-6 for further information on each defect. *ADA,* Adenosine deaminase deficiency; *Agamma,* Agammaglobulinemia; *AICD* deficiency, activation-induced cytidine deaminase deficiency; *AT,* ataxia-telangiectasia; *PNP,* purine nucleoside phosphorylase deficiency; *sIgM* and *sIgD,* Surface IgM and IgD. *WAS,* Wiskott-Aldrich syndrome.

However, this syndrome is also characterized by severe congenital structural defects of the heart and low levels of calcium, which may result in seizures.

Individual primary immune deficiencies are very rare.[59,60] For instance, only 30 to 50 new cases of severe combined immune deficiency are diagnosed in the United States yearly. However, approximately 150 different genetic defects resulting in immune deficiencies have been identified. Together, primary immune deficiencies are more common than cystic fibrosis, hemophilia, childhood leukemia, or many other well-known diseases. An estimated 50,000 cases of clinically significant primary immune deficiency have been reported in the United States.[61] The distribution of male and female depends on the specific disease, but in general those diagnosed within the first 2 years of life have a male preponderance (5:1) because many are X-linked, whereas those diagnosed later are evenly distributed. The three most commonly diagnosed deficiencies are common variable immune deficiency (34%), selective IgA deficiency (24%), and IgG subclass deficiency (17%).

Primary immune deficiencies are classified into five groups, based on which principal component of the immune or inflammatory systems is defective. This chapter uses the five classifications proposed by the National Institutes of Health.[62] **B-lymphocyte deficiencies** result from defects in B-cell immune responses.[63] T-cell immunity rarely depends on competent B-cell responses, thus T-cell immune responses are not affected in pure B-lymphocyte deficiencies. **T-lymphocyte deficiencies** are defects in the development and function of T lymphocytes. Because helper T cells are obligatory in the development of many B-lymphocyte responses, antibody production is often diminished in these conditions, although the B cells are fully capable of producing an adequate antibody response. Many textbooks disagree on the classification of several specific immune deficiencies because of the difficulty in distinguishing between primary B-cell defects and those that are secondary to a primary T-cell defect. The classifications described below define T-cell defects as those with a clear defect in T-cell immunity, with normal B-cell immune responses. **Combined T- and B-lymphocyte deficiencies** result from inherent defects that directly affect the development of both T and B lymphocytes. Some combined deficiencies result in major defects in both the T- and B-cell immune responses, whereas others are "partial" and more adversely affect T cells than B cells. The partial combined deficiencies include many conditions that may be classified as T-cell defects in other textbooks. **Complement deficiencies** and **phagocytic deficiencies** frequently present like antibody deficiencies because of the close interactions among antibody, complement, and phagocytes.

B-Lymphocyte Deficiencies

A defect in B-cell development results in lower levels of circulating immunoglobulins and increased susceptibility to infections in which antibodies are the primary protective mechanism.[64] The condition in which immunoglobulin levels are lower than normal is termed **hypogammaglobulinemia.** The condition in which they are totally or almost totally absent is termed **agammaglobulinemia.** (Normal lymphocyte development is discussed in Chapter 7.) Recurrent infections range from life threatening to mild, depending on the severity of the deficiency. Characteristic infections include encapsulated bacteria (e.g., *Streptococcus pneumoniae* or *Haemophilus influenzae*) that may cause pneumonia or sepsis and other microorganisms that cause infections of the sinuses, ears, and gastrointestinal tract.

The most severe B-lymphocyte deficiency is **Bruton's agammaglobulinemia,** also referred to as X-linked agammaglobulinemia. Somewhat less than a third of the mutations are sporadic. This condition results from mutations in the gene for Bruton's tyrosine kinase (Btk); an enzyme involved in intracellular signaling from several B-cell receptors, including the IgM B-cell antigen receptor, the IL-5 receptor, and the IL-6 receptor. Ineffective signaling results in the arrest of the development in the bursal-equivalent tissue (bone marrow) of early cells in the B-cell lineage into mature B cells[65] (see Figure 8-11). Few or no circulating mature B cells are present, although T-cell number and function are normal. At 6 months of life the approximate normal serum concentrations of immunoglobulins are IgG, 400 mg/dl; IgM, 40 mg/dl; and IgA, 30 mg/dl. In 6-month-old children with Bruton's agammaglobulinemia, serum IgG levels are well below 100 mg/dl and IgM and IgA are almost absent.

An autosomal recessive form of agammaglobulinemia (**autosomal agammaglobulinemia**) results from other mutations in the B-cell receptor. The most common is a mutation of the mu (μ) chain of the IgM portion of the receptor. This mutation prevents intracellular signaling after antigen binds to the receptor, leading to blocked maturation, no antibody production, and very severe infections.

Several defects in antibody class-switch have been identified (see Figure 8-11). **X-linked hyper-IgM syndrome** results from a mutation in CD40 ligand, which is expressed on the surface of helper T (Th) cells. Th cells stimulate B cells to undergo a switch in the class of antibody they produce through multiple Th–B cell interactions involving ligands expressed on one cell binding to specific receptors on the other cell. The ligand-receptor interaction results in an intracellular signal facilitating rearrangement of the genes for the antibody variable region from a site near the constant region gene for the μ chain to the constant region for a different antibody H chain (see Figure 7-20). A critical ligand-receptor interaction occurs between the receptor CD40 on the B cell and its ligand (CD154 or CD40L) on the Th cell. A mutation in CD40L results in **defective class-switch,** decreased or absent production of IgG and IgA, poor development of memory B cells, and overproduction of IgM, which does not require class-switch. T-cell immunity is not affected.[66]

Defects in other components of Th–B-cell interaction result in **autosomal hyper-IgM syndrome.** Mutations in CD40 on B cells result in a similar effect to that described above. A defect in a DNA editing enzyme (activation-induced cytidine deaminase; AICD) also inhibits class-switch. During class-switch and movement of the H chain genetic information for the variable region to a different constant region gene, the double-stranded DNA must be cut and mended. This enzyme is responsible for cutting and mending the DNA.

Deficiencies in certain subclasses of antibody (**IgG subclass deficiency**), particularly IgG2, may result from a defect in switch to a particular subclass constant region (see Figure 8-11). The IgG2 subclass is often increased in response to polysaccharide antigens such as those on the surface of encapsulated bacteria. Low levels of IgG2 may be responsible for recurrent risk for pneumonias caused by these bacteria. Whether IgG subclass deficiencies are unique immune deficiency conditions is unclear because many are apparently early indications of the development of common variable immune deficiency (see following) or are secondary to selective IgA deficiency.

One of the most common primary immune deficiencies is a **selective IgA deficiency.** Because many affected individuals are asymptomatic, the true incidence is uncertain, although estimates of 1 person in 300 to 1 in 3000 have been made. Individuals with selective IgA deficiency are able to produce other classes of immunoglobulins but fail to produce IgA (see Figure 8-11). Many will have B cells that have undergone class-switch to IgA, but for unknown reasons, cannot undergo the terminal steps of differentiation to IgA-secreting plasma cells. Although many individuals are asymptomatic, others present with a history of severe recurring sinus, lung, and gastrointestinal infections. They commonly also have chronic intestinal candidiasis (infection with *Candida albicans*). (The secretory, or mucosal, immune system is described in Chapter 7.)

Complications of IgA deficiency include severe atopic disease and autoimmune diseases; selective IgA deficiency is two or three times more common in atopic individuals than in others. Secretory IgA normally may prevent the uptake of allergens from the environment so that IgA deficiency may lead to increased allergen uptake and a more intense challenge to the immune system because of prolonged exposure to environmental antigens. One of the most severe complications of IgA deficiency is an anaphylactic reaction that can follow administration of blood products that contain IgA. Serious anaphylactic reactions can occur in individuals totally lacking IgA because the immune system recognizes donor IgA as a foreign antigen. Initial sensitization can occur in fetal life through exposure to maternal IgA that leaks across the placenta or later through the ingestion of maternal IgA in breast milk or bovine IgA in cow's milk. Sensitization also can occur with initial administration of blood products containing IgA. The individual's primed immune system then acts against donor IgA on subsequent exposure.

Common variable immune deficiency is the most commonly diagnosed immune deficiency. As the name implies, the presentation is very heterogeneous. It is characterized by hypogammaglobulinemia, but the particular class of antibody that is decreased varies: most have low amounts of IgG, which may or may not be accompanied by decreased levels of IgA or IgM, or both, with normal numbers of B cells. Some may have accompanying T-cell defects. Multiple genetic defects in terminal differentiation account for this condition, although the specific defects have not been identified in most patients. The age of onset of symptoms, such as recurrent bacterial respiratory tract infections, is generally later than most primary immune deficiencies (late 20s). Secondary complications include arthritis (infectious and noninfectious), gastrointestinal symptoms (malabsorption, chronic diarrhea) autoimmune disease (anemia, thrombocytopenia, endocrine diseases), and cancer (of the lymphoid system, skin, and gastrointestinal tract).

T-Lymphocyte Deficiencies

Two well-studied examples of T-lymphocyte defects that represent different ends of the T-cell differentiation process include DiGeorge syndrome and chronic mucocutaneous candidiasis. Lymphoid stem cells begin maturing into functional T lymphocytes in the thymus. DiGeorge syndrome (congenital thymic aplasia or hypoplasia) is caused by the lack, or more commonly partial lack, of the thymus, resulting in greatly decreased T-cell numbers and function and in life-threatening viral, fungal, and intracellular bacterial infections[67,68] (see Figure 8-11). The defect is attributed usually to deletions on chromosome 22 (some deletions also have been identified on chromosome 10); about 25% of which are inherited. The deleted region encodes information for formation of organs that originate from the third and fourth pharyngeal pouches during the twelfth week of gestation. In addition to the lack of thymus development, the individual may present with a partial or complete absence of the parathyroid gland (resulting in decreased blood calcium levels), major structural defects in the heart and the aorta (resulting in inadequate blood flow and inadequate oxygenation of the tissues), and abnormal facial characteristics (e.g., underdeveloped chin, low-set ears, shortened structure of the upper lip) (Figure 8-12).

Chronic mucocutaneous candidiasis is a primary defect of T lymphocytes in response to a specific infectious agent, the yeast *C. albicans*. At least seven variants of this condition have been described. All are characterized by mild to extremely severe chronic mucocutaneous candidiasis: *Candida* infections that involve the mucous membranes, nails, and skin. Invasive candidiasis is extremely rare. Although most B- and T-cell immune responses may be normal, most individuals with this defect cannot react to antigens from *Candida*. The cause of this defect is unknown.

Combined T- and B-Lymphocyte Deficiencies

The most severe deficiencies usually occur when both the B- and T-cell immune responses are affected. A great deal of knowledge about the evolution of bone marrow stem cells into functional B- and T-cell effectors came from studying children with the most severe immune deficiency, **severe combined immune deficiency (SCID).**[69] The most severe form of SCID is **reticular dysgenesis** (failure of blood cells to develop), in which a common stem cell for all white blood cells is

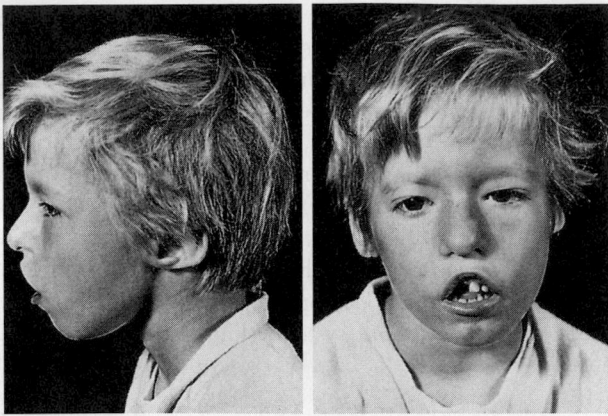

Figure 8-12 Facial anomalies associated with DiGeorge syndrome. Note the wide-set eyes, low-set ears, and shortened structure of the upper lip. (From Roitt I, Brostoff J, Male D: *Immunology,* ed 6, St Louis, 2001, Mosby.)

absent; therefore T cells, B cells, and phagocytic cells never develop (see Figure 8-11). Most children with reticular dysgenesis die in utero or very soon after birth. More typically, a defect occurs after some stem cells become committed to developing into lymphocytes (lymphoid stem cells); therefore, most individuals with SCID are deficient in lymphocyte development, but have normal numbers of all other white blood cells. SCID often results in few or absent T and B lymphocytes in the circulation and secondary lymphoid organs (spleen, lymph nodes). The thymus is usually hypoplastic (underdeveloped) because of the absence of T cells. Immunoglobulin levels, especially of IgM and IgA, are absent or greatly reduced, although IgG levels may be almost normal in the first months of life because of the presence of maternal antibodies. In the most severe defects, death occurs at about 1 year of life.

At least 20 different forms of SCID have been identified. Depending on the specific genetic mutation, the defect may involve T cells, B cells, and NK cells or may suppress more severely the function of one cell type, with relatively minor effects on the others. All three cells are adversely affected (T–, B–, NK–) in SCID resulting from a deficiency of adenosine deaminase (**adenosine deaminase [ADA] deficiency**), which is an enzyme involved in purine metabolism[69] (see Figure 8-11). This defect is autosomal recessive and results in the accumulation of toxic purine metabolites to which rapidly dividing cells, such as lymphocytes, are especially sensitive. ADA deficiency accounts for about 16% of all persons with SCID. The development of T cells, B cells, and NK cells is arrested very early, and very few lymphocytic cells are found in the blood. In some forms of SCID, the defect resides in receptors for cytokines that are necessary for maturation of lymphocytes (see Figure 8-11). T cells and NK cells are preferentially affected (T–, B+, NK–), but often the defect results in the production of immature B cells that cannot respond well to antigen because of the lack of Th cells. The most common (44% of those with SCID) is an **X-linked SCID** resulting from a defect in the IL-2 receptor gamma (γ)-chain (IL-2Rγ). This protein is

a component of several receptors for cytokines, including IL-2, IL-4, IL-7, IL-9, IL-15, and IL-21. These cytokines participate in the early development of immunocytes, particularly T and NK cells. Defective IL-2Rγ results in arrested maturation of T and NK cells and the production of immature B cells. A similar deficiency occurs with mutation in JAK3 (**JAK3 deficiency**), which is an enzyme (a tyrosine kinase) that associates with IL-2Rγ in normal cells and communicates information from the receptor to the nucleus. Thus cells with defects in JAK3 cannot respond to cytokines that bind to these receptors on the cell surface. An autosomal form results from mutations of one of the protein chains (α-chain) of the IL-7 receptor (**IL-7 receptor deficiency**). IL-7 appears to be necessary for the maturation of T cells, so that this deficiency has relatively normal levels of B cells and NK cells.

Mutations in another purine metabolism enzyme, purine nucleoside phosphorylase (**purine nucleoside phosphorylase [PNP] deficiency**) are less severe than ADA deficiency (see Figure 8-11). T cells and NK cells appear to be more susceptible to mutations in PNP so that B-cell function can be relatively normal.

Another form of SCID preferentially affects T cells and B cells (T–, B–, NK+). T and B lymphocytes possess receptors for antigen, whereas NK cells do not. Those receptors result from a process of genetic rearrangement of *V* and *J* genes to form the variable regions of the L chain (B-cell receptor [BCR]) and the α-chain (T-cell receptor [TCR]) and the *V, D,* and *J* genes to form the variable regions of the H chain (BCR) and β-chain (TCR). Successful rearrangement is controlled by two recombination activating enzymes (RAG-1 and RAG-2). RAG enzymes cut and repair double-stranded breaks in DNA that are necessary for genetic rearrangement. **RAG-1** or **RAG-2 deficiencies** are autosomal recessive and result in arrested lymphocyte development from blocked recombination of variable regions of B-cell and T-cell receptors (see Figure 8-11).

Forms of partial SCID, with the defect being primarily of T cells, arise from mutations in several components of the TCR complex (see Figure 8-11). Defects in the TCR result in inadequate maturation of T cells, with normal B and NK cells. Antibody production may be depressed because of the lack of Th cells. The TCR is a complex organization of proteins that react with antigen (α- and β-chains), then provide an intracellular signal to the nucleus (γ-, δ-, and ε-chains [collectively called CD3] and the associated molecules CD45 and ZAP-70). Examples of these deficiencies include mutations in CD3, CD45, or ZAP-70. The T-cell defect in each can range from mild to severe in nature, with normal B lymphocytes.

Even if nearly adequate numbers of B and T cells are produced, their ability to process and present antigen may be defective. The **bare lymphocyte syndrome** is a group of immune deficiencies characterized by an inability of lymphocytes and macrophages to present antigen because of defects in class I or class II MHC antigen expression (see Figure 8-11). **MHC class I deficiency** results from mutations in the genes for TAP1 or TAP2, which control the transport of antigenic protein fragments across the endoplasmic reticulum and the formation of MHC class I/antigen complexes for transportation to the cell surface (see Figure 7-16). Because MHC class I molecules preferentially present antigen to CD8+ Tc cells, the resultant deficiency is of CD8+ cytotoxic cells, with normal levels of CD4+ helper cells and normal antibody production. **MHC class II deficiency** is more severe. A variety of mutations prevent normal production of MHC class II molecules, which present antigen to CD4+ helper cells. Because of defective recruitment of helper T cells, normal antibody responses are greatly suppressed. Children with this deficiency develop life-threatening infections and usually die before age 5 years.

Some combined immune deficiencies are secondary to mutations that affect a variety of cells other than immunocytes. For instance, **Wiskott-Aldrich syndrome** (WAS; an X-linked recessive disorder) results from sporadic mutations in the WAS protein (WASP), which is involved in intracellular signaling and regulation of the organization of the cell's actin cytoskeleton[70] (see Figure 8-11). The defects in the cytoskeleton lead to the classic symptoms of thrombocytopenia (with resultant bleeding disorders), scaly eczema, and defective T and B cells. IgA and IgG levels are usually normal, but IgM responses are highly depressed. Antibody responses against antigens that elicit primarily an IgM response, such as polysaccharide antigens from bacterial cell walls (e.g., of *Pseudomonas aeruginosa, S. pneumoniae, H. influenzae,* and other microorganisms with polysaccharide outer capsules), are deficient. Persons with WAS have a very high risk of lymphoid malignancies (leukemias and lymphomas).

Ataxia-telangiectasia (AT) is an autosomal recessive disorder resulting from a large variety of sporadic mutations in the *ATM* gene, which encodes a protein involved in repair of double-stranded breaks in DNA. Affected infants often develop ataxia (unsteady gait), which usually becomes apparent when the child is learning to walk. The neurologic defect may eventually lead to confinement in a wheelchair. Telangiectasia (dilation of capillaries) can occur in the eyes and skin, especially on the ears, neck, and extremities. Both B and T cells are variably affected and unrepaired double-stranded DNA breaks are commonly observed in the regions encoding the T-cell and B-cell receptors. About 70% of those with AT are IgA deficient, occasionally accompanied by deficiencies in IgG (see Figure 8-11). Individuals with AT are at high risk for developing leukemias and lymphomas.

Complement Deficiencies

Complement activation is a necessary component of protection against many infectious agents. As a result, some defects in the complement cascade often resemble antibody deficiencies, with recurrent infections with encapsulated bacteria (e.g., *H. influenzae* and *S. pneumoniae*).[71] Additionally, the Fc portion of IgG and some activated complement components, such as C3b, function as opsonins and facilitate phagocytosis by neutrophils and macrophages. In addition to recurrent infections, deficiencies in the classical pathway commonly lead to a SLE-like syndrome. As noted, excessive levels of circulating complexes of antibody, antigen, and complement may

lead to type III hypersensitivity diseases (immune complex diseases). However, healthy individuals release small amounts of soluble intracellular antigens into the blood during normal cell turnover. Low levels of naturally occurring autoantibodies and limited activation of the classical pathway of the complement system through C3 facilitate the removal of this debris by phagocytes. Thus some complement defects may slow the clearance from the blood of natural immune complexes, leading to SLE-like symptoms.

C3 deficiency is the most severe complement defect (Figure 8-13). C3 is the component that unites all pathways of complement activation, and complement component C3b is a major opsonin. Persons with C3 deficiency are at risk for recurrent life-threatening infections with encapsulated bacteria at an early age, as well as a SLE-like syndrome that may be complicated by kidney disease (glomerulonephritis).[72] **C2 deficiency,** more so than **C1** or **C4 deficiencies,** also has an increased risk for recurrent respiratory infections with encapsulated bacteria (e.g., *S. pneumoniae, H. influenzae*).

Mannose-binding lectin (MBL) deficiency is the primary defect of the lectin pathway of complement activation. The defect results in increased risk of infection with microorganisms that have polysaccharide capsules rich in mannose, particularly the yeast *Saccharomyces cerevisiae* and encapsulated bacteria such as *N. meningitidis* and *S. pneumoniae.*

Deficiencies in the alternative pathway also result in recurrent infections with encapsulated bacteria. **Properdin deficiency** is associated with recurrent meningococcal infections and is X-linked, whereas all other complement deficiencies are autosomal recessive. Symptoms generally appear in the second decade of life. Factor I and factor H are major regulators of the complement cascade and control the level of spontaneous activation of C3. **Factor I deficiency** and **factor H deficiency** can be severe because they lead to increased spontaneous destruction of C3 and a secondary C3 deficiency.

Deficiencies of components of the terminal portion of the complement cascade (C5, C6, C7, C8, or C9 deficiencies) are associated with increased infections with only one group of bacteria; those of the genus *Neisseria* (*N. meningitidis* or *N. gonorrhoeae*). *Neisseria* usually cause localized infections (meningitis or gonorrhea), but those individuals with terminal pathway defects have more than an 8000-fold increased risk for systemic infections with atypical strains of these microorganisms. **C9 deficiency** is the most common terminal pathway defect, appears primarily in Japanese populations, and is generally asymptomatic. The other deficiencies of the terminal pathway are extremely rare, but are characterized by more aggressive infections. The risk for systemic infections with *Neisseria* is also increased in those with deficiencies of C2, factor D, factor B, and properdin.

Phagocytic Deficiencies

Phagocytosis is generally aided by bacterial opsonization with IgG or C3b; therefore, defects in phagocytic killing usually result in recurrent infections with the same group of microorganisms (encapsulated bacteria) associated with antibody and

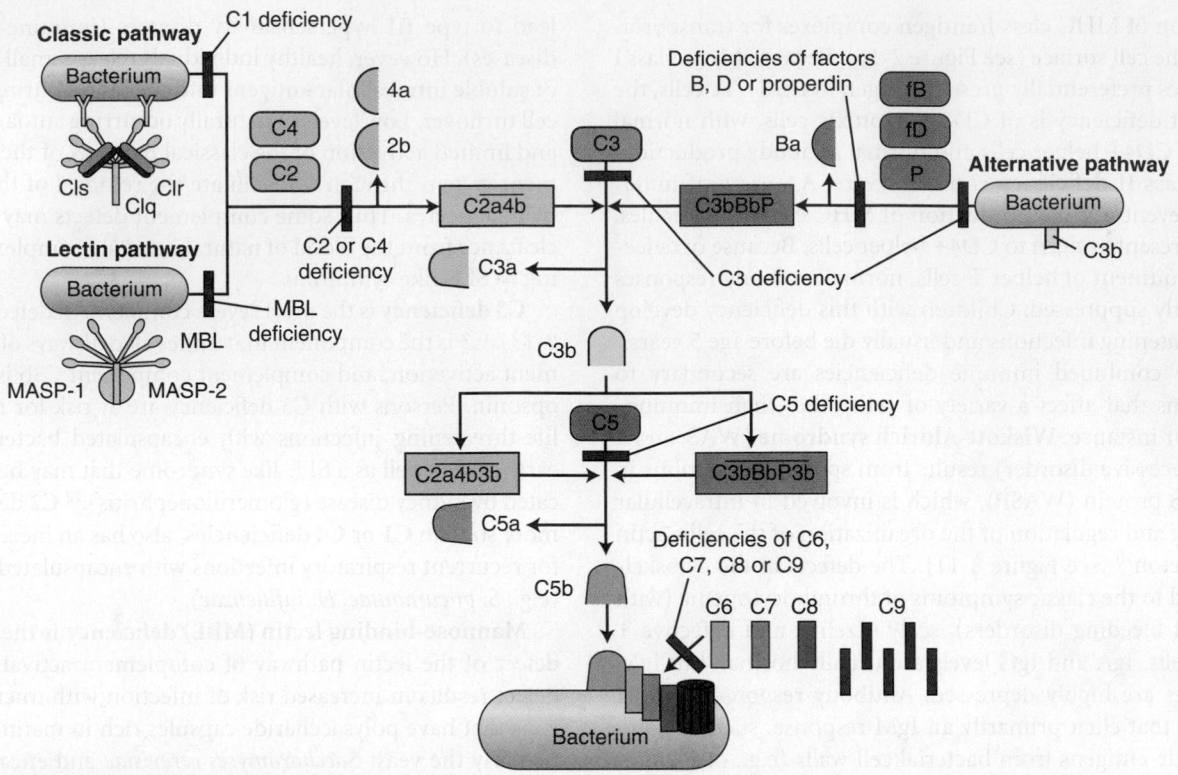

Figure 8-13 Complement defects. The complement cascade is initiated through three pathways: the classical pathway, the lectin pathway, and the alternative pathway. Each of the three pathways produces a C3 convertase, which activates C3 leading to the formation of a C5 convertase. The activation of C5 initiates formation of the membrane attack complex (MAC). For more details, see the text and Figure 6-5. The most severe defect is a C3 deficiency because it blocks all three pathways. *MASP,* MBL-associated serine protease; *MBL,* Mannose-binding lectin.

complement deficiencies. Phagocytosis is a multistep process that involves initial adhesion between circulating phagocytes and the endothelial cells lining the circulation (see Figure 6-11). The phagocytes exit the circulation and move to a site of infection by a chemotactic process in response to soluble chemotactic factors released by the infection. The process of phagocytosis itself begins with attachment of the phagocyte to the targeted bacteria through the interaction of opsonins on the microorganism and matched receptors on the phagocyte's surface. Phagocytic engulfment results in internalization of the infectious agent and activation of a variety of oxygen-dependent and oxygen-independent killing mechanisms. Deficiencies can arise from mutations that affect one or more of these steps (Figure 8-14).

Inadequate numbers of phagocytes, particularly neutrophils **(severe congenital neutropenias),** result in a variety of recurrent and severe bacterial infections beginning early in life. Approximately 50% of these patients have a mutation in the neutrophil elastase gene *(ELA2)*. Other mutations have been identified (e.g., *WAS* gene) in the other 50%. A milder form, **cyclic neutropenia,** is autosomal dominant with almost 100% of affected individuals having a mutation in the *ELA2* gene. Changes in neutrophil levels are cyclic and may remain at or near normal for 2 to 3 weeks, followed by periods of neutropenia lasting a few days to weeks. During the neutropenia,

the individual has increased susceptibility to recurrent bacterial infections.

Near sites of inflammation, soluble mediators diffuse into the circulation and induce expression of a variety of adhesion molecules on the phagocyte surface, which interact with complementary molecules on the endothelial cells to increase adherence between the phagocyte and the vessel wall and allow for margination and diapedesis to occur.[73] **Leukocyte adhesion deficiencies (LAD)** result from mutations in various phagocyte adhesion molecules (see Table 6-3). Leukocyte adhesion deficiency, type 1 (LAD-1) results from an autosomal recessive mutation in CD18, which is a β_2 integrin chain that is shared by several different receptors. LAD-2 results from a defect in adding the monosaccharide fucose to carbohydrates on the phagocyte surface. Surface carbohydrates with fucose are ligands for selectins on the endothelial and leukocyte. These and other defects in leukocyte adhesion molecules usually result in increased levels of neutrophils in the blood (leukocytosis) because they cannot leave the circulation and in increased recurrent bacterial and fungal infections.

Additional deficiencies diminish the leukocyte's recognition of opsonins of the complement cascade (e.g., C3b). Deficiencies in the complement receptor for C3 **(C3 receptor deficiency)** result in recurrent bacterial infections, particularly of the skin.

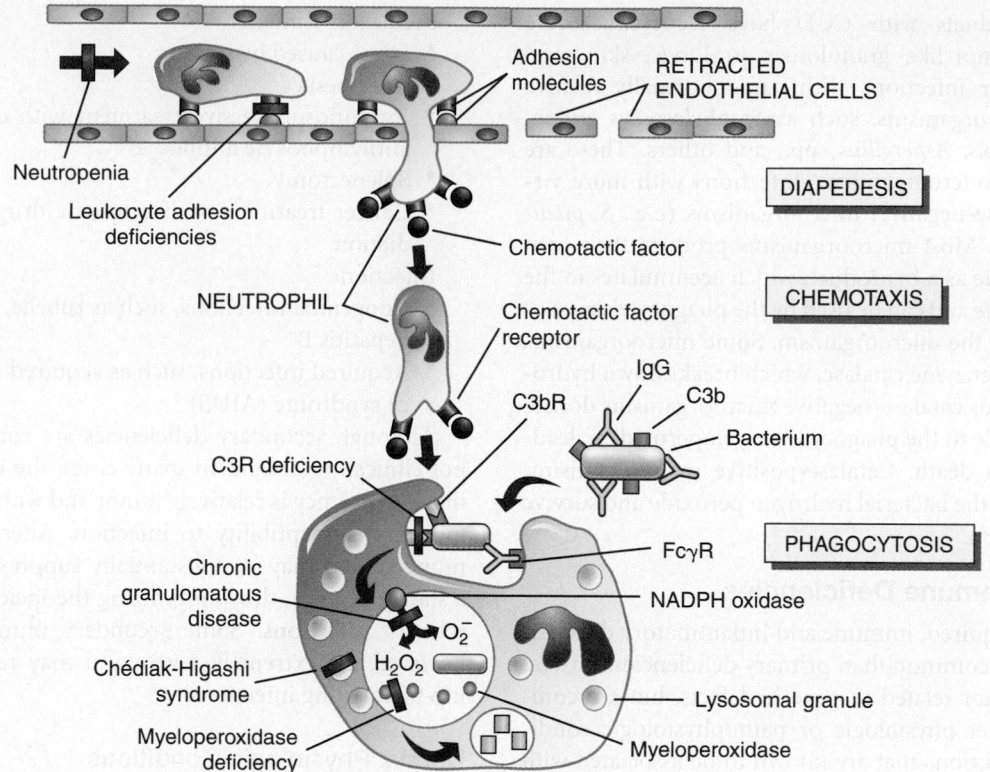

Figure 8-14 Phagocytic defects. Several genetic defects in the process leading up to and including phagocytosis result in increased susceptibility to bacterial infections. See the text and refer to Figure 6-11 and Table 6-3 for more detailed information. The phagocyte leaves the bloodstream and enters the tissue through interactions between leukocyte and endothelial adhesion molecules and the process of diapedesis. The cell is attracted to the inflammatory site by chemotaxis, where it encounters opsonized bacteria, and attaches to and engulfs the microorganism. Inside the phagocyte the bacteria are killed and broken down by the combination of lysosomal granule constituents and reactive oxygen products of the hexose-monophosphate shunt and nicotinamide adenine dinucleotide phosphate (NADPH) oxidase. *C3R*, C3 receptor, which includes the C3b receptor (C3bR); *FcγR*, receptor for the Fc portion of IgG; H_2O_2, hydrogen peroxide; O_2^-, reactive oxygen.

A variety of defects in killing of microorganisms have been described. **Chédiak-Higashi syndrome** results from a defect in cytoplasmic granules from an autosomal recessive mutation in the lysosomal trafficking regulator gene *(CHS1)*. The CHS1 protein helps control movement of granules to cellular membranes in preparation for degranulation. As a result of these mutations, the granules remain in the cytoplasm and form large aggregates that are readily apparent microscopically. Leukocytes from individuals with Chédiak-Higashi syndrome have decreased chemotaxis, granular fusion, and bacterial killing. Platelet granules also may be affected, resulting in prolonged bleeding, and partial albinism can occur because of defects in melanocyte granules. Affected children develop recurrent infections of the skin, respiratory tract, and mucous membranes, especially with gram-positive bacteria.

The enzyme myeloperoxidase participates in a major mechanism of bacterial killing in phagocytes. Myeloperoxidase is found in primary granules and catalyzes the formation of acids from halides (e.g., chloride ion) and hydrogen peroxide (H_2O_2). As a result of phagocytosis, neutrophils and other phagocytes switch much of their glucose metabolism to the hexose-monophosphate shunt. A byproduct of this

pathway is the conversion of molecular oxygen by nicotinamide adenine dinucleotide phosphate (NADPH) oxidase and other enzymes into highly reactive and toxic oxygen derivatives, including hydrogen peroxide. Two deficiencies in the myeloperoxidase–hydrogen peroxide killing process have been extensively studied. **Myeloperoxidase deficiency** is a relatively mild disorder characterized by a complete or partial deficiency in myeloperoxidase. Individuals do not have severe recurrent infections because most infectious bacteria are sensitive to direct killing by many of the toxic oxygen molecules produced by NADPH oxidase. The exception is the person with concurrent diabetes, who may have recurrent disseminated candidiasis.

Chronic granulomatous disease (CGD) is a more severe defect in the myeloperoxidase–hydrogen peroxide system. Several forms of the disease have been characterized, both X-linked (about 70% of the individuals) and autosomal recessive, with the X-linked being more severe. CGD results from a variety of mutations (at least four have been identified) in portions of the NADPH oxidase complex, resulting in deficiencies in the production of hydrogen peroxide and other oxygen products. Thus individuals have adequate myeloperoxidase and chloride but lack the necessary hydrogen peroxide. Individuals with CGD have recurrent severe pneumonias; tumor-like granulomas in lungs, skin, and bones; and other infections with some normally relative innocuous microorganisms, such as *Staphylococcus aureus*, *Serratia marcescens, Aspergillus* spp., and others. These are catalase-positive microorganisms. Infections with more virulent, but catalase-negative, microorganisms (e.g., *S. pneumoniae*) are rare. Most microorganisms produce their own hydrogen peroxide as a byproduct, which accumulates in the phagocytic vacuole and can be used by the phagocyte's myeloperoxidase to kill the microorganism. Some microorganisms also produce the enzyme catalase, which breaks down hydrogen peroxide. Thus catalase-negative microorganisms donate hydrogen peroxide to the phagocyte's myeloperoxidase, leading to their own death. Catalase-positive microorganisms, however, destroy the bacterial hydrogen peroxide and survive and cause infection.

Secondary Immune Deficiencies

Secondary, or acquired, immune and inflammatory deficiencies are far more common than primary deficiencies.[74] These deficiencies are not related to genetic defects, but are complications of other physiologic or pathophysiologic conditions. Some conditions that are known to be associated with acquired deficiencies include:

Normal physiologic conditions
- Pregnancy
- Infancy
- Aging

Psychologic stress
- Emotional trauma
- Eating disorders

Dietary insufficiencies
- Malnutrition caused by insufficient intake of large categories of nutrients, such as protein or calories
- Insufficient intake of specific nutrients, such as vitamins, iron, or zinc

Malignancies
- Malignancies of lymphoid tissues, such as Hodgkin disease, acute or chronic leukemia, or myeloma
- Malignancies of nonlymphoid tissues, such as sarcomas and carcinomas

Metabolic diseases or genetic syndromes
- Diabetes
- Cystic fibrosis
- Alcoholic cirrhosis
- Sickle cell disease
- SLE
- Chromosome abnormalities, such as trisomy 21 (Down syndrome)

Environmental
- Ultraviolet (UV) light
- Ionizing radiation
- Chronic hypoxia

Physical trauma
- Burns

Medical treatments
- Stress caused by surgery
- Anesthesia
- Immunosuppressive treatment with corticosteroids or antilymphocyte antibodies
- Splenectomy
- Cancer treatment with cytotoxic drugs or ionizing radiation

Infections
- Congenital infections, such as rubella, cytomegalovirus, hepatitis B
- Acquired infections, such as acquired immunodeficiency syndrome (AIDS)

Although secondary deficiencies are common, many are not clinically relevant. In many cases, the degree of the immune deficiency is relatively minor and without any apparent increased susceptibility to infection. Alternatively, the immune system may be substantially suppressed, but only for a short duration, thus minimizing the incidence of clinically relevant infections. Some secondary immune deficiencies, however, are extremely severe and may result in recurrent life-threatening infections.

Normal Physiologic Conditions

The competence of an individual's immune system varies throughout life. Pregnancy itself is considered by many to be an immunocompromised condition. Pregnant women may have decreased reactivity or altered results in several tests of the immune system, including skin tests against various antigens, circulating numbers of T lymphocytes, and other very general tests. Pregnancy itself, however, is not associated with a marked change in infections, suggesting that the mother's immune system is not severely altered.

The newborn child is immunologically immature. Although T-cell immune responses may be normal or near normal, other components of the immune system (especially antibody production) are just beginning to mature. Beginning at about 32 weeks of pregnancy, the placenta transports maternal antibodies into the fetal blood to protect the child during the first months of life (see Figure 7-30). After the delivery, the level of the mother's antibodies slowly decreases in the newborn so that maternal antibodies no longer protect the child by about 6 months of life. By 6 to 8 months, the newborn should be efficiently protected by antibodies produced by its own B cells. In some infants, the development of antibody production is delayed, and a transient low level of antibody may persist for several months (**transient hypogammaglobulinemia of infancy**), during which the child has increased susceptibility to infections. Premature infants are particularly immunologically immature and are at increased risk for neonatal infections. The blood of infants born before 32 weeks' gestation is generally devoid of maternal antibody.

Aging is also associated with a progressive depression in immune responses.[75,76] Older adults generally have more severe bacterial and fungal infections, greater difficulty resolving those infections, and lower responses to vaccination.

Several meaningful changes occur during aging, although variations in the degree of change and a corresponding increased susceptibility to infection can be considerable among individuals. The thymus involutes over time, resulting in decreased production of fresh T cells. A concurrent depletion of memory T cells results in depressed responses to both new and "recall" antigens. A shift toward Th2 cells also may occur with a resultant decrease in Th1 cytokines. Total numbers of B cells may decrease. Numbers of NK cells may remain normal, although their activity is decreased. Similarly, neutrophil numbers may remain normal, with decreased phagocytosis and killing.

Psychologic Stress

The relationship between emotional stress and depressed immune function has become an area of intense clinical and research interest. For many decades anecdotal reports have suggested that increased incidences of infection and malignancy are associated with periods of both intense stress (e.g., the loss of a loved one, divorce) and relatively minor stress (e.g., final examination periods at colleges and universities). In addition, early studies showed that immune function, as demonstrated by delayed hypersensitivity skin test results, could be depressed through posthypnotic suggestion.

We are now beginning to understand the mechanisms of the relationship between emotional stress and the immune system. Many lymphoid organs are innervated and can be affected by nerve stimulation. In addition, lymphocytes have receptors for many hormones (e.g., sex hormones, neurotransmitters, and neuropeptides) and can respond to changing levels of these chemicals with increased or decreased function. For instance, stress-induced catecholamines affect the expression of adhesion molecules and movement of lymphocytes among lymphoid organs. (Further discussion of the effects of stress on susceptibility to disease is the subject of Chapter 10.)

Dietary Insufficiencies

Nutritional status can have a profound effect on immune function, and malnutrition is the predominant cause of secondary immune deficiencies worldwide. Severe deficits in calorie or protein intake lead to deficiencies in T-cell function and numbers. The humoral immune response is less affected by starvation, although complement activity, neutrophil chemotaxis, and bacterial killing within neutrophils often are depressed, resulting in infections with microorganisms that are normally destroyed by opsonization and phagocytosis.

Deficient zinc intake can profoundly depress both T- and B-cell function. Zinc is required as a cofactor for at least 70 different enzymes, some of which are found in lymphocytes and are necessary for their function. Secondary zinc deficiencies may be associated with malabsorption syndrome (failure to absorb zinc), chronic renal disease (loss of zinc in the urine), chronic diarrhea (loss of zinc through the gut), or burns or severe psoriasis (loss of zinc through the skin). Deficiencies of other enzyme cofactors, such as vitamins (e.g., pyridoxine, pantothenic acid, folic acid, vitamins A, C, E, and B_{12}), also may result in severe depressions of B- and T-cell function, phagocytosis, and complement activity.

Malignancies

Many malignancies are complicated by a wasting syndrome (cachexia) in the later stages, which can suppress the immune system secondary to the resultant malnutrition. Additionally, a very close relationship exists between the immune system and the development of malignancies. It is generally accepted that successful malignancies have developed mechanisms to avoid rejection by the individual's immune system. Persons with primary immune deficiencies are usually at greater risk for developing malignancies, particularly malignancies of lymphoid tissues, such as leukemias or lymphomas. Malignancies aggressively depress the individual's immune system. The effect is commonly nonspecific, resulting in a generalized deficiency of the immune response and a greatly increased susceptibility to developing life-threatening infections. In fact, many people with malignancies die from infection rather than from direct effects of the tumor.

Malignancies of lymphoid tissues, such as Hodgkin disease, acute or chronic leukemia, or myeloma, result in depletion of normal lymphocytes and their replacement by the malignant cells. Thus the number of B or T cells capable of responding to infections is depleted. Many malignancies, even those of nonlymphoid tissues, produce cytokines (e.g., transforming growth factor-beta [TGF-β] and vascular endothelial growth factor [VEGF]) that nonspecifically suppress the immune responses.

Metabolic Diseases or Genetic Syndromes

Diabetes suppresses many aspects of the immune and inflammatory responses, including phagocytosis and chemotaxis, lymphocyte proliferation, and glucose metabolism. The effects of trisomy 21 are less severe, but primarily include diminished neutrophil function. Patients with cystic fibrosis have decreased airway clearance of bacteria, thus increasing the probability of major respiratory tract infections.

Environmental

Individuals are constantly exposed to environmental agents that affect the immune system. UV light from sun exposure or tanning salons induces apoptosis of lymphoid stem cells, increases production of Treg cells that suppress defenses against cancer, and increases the production of anti-inflammatory cytokines. Ionizing radiation affects rapidly dividing cells, including those of the immune system. At very high doses, the entire immune system can be depleted.

Physical Trauma

Trauma that compromises the epithelial barrier also predisposes an individual to infection. Burn victims are susceptible to severe bacterial infections. Thermal burns appear to be associated with suppressed neutrophil function (especially chemotaxis), complement levels, cell-mediated immunity, and primary humoral responses, although secondary humoral responses are normal. The mechanism of this immunosuppression may be twofold. Blood from burned individuals contains nonspecific immunosuppressive factors (all immune responses are suppressed, regardless of the antigen involved). In addition, burn victims also have increased regulatory T-cell function, which may increase antigen-specific suppression.

Medical Treatments

Medical treatments themselves may produce suppression of immune responses. Depression of B- and T-cell formation is manifested as a progressive increase in infections with opportunistic microorganisms (especially *P. jirovecii*, cytomegalovirus, *C. albicans*, and other fungi), the extent and location of which are unusual.

Many drugs that are used to fight cancer (e.g., cancer chemotherapeutic agents) are not specific for cancer cells, but are designed to attack cells in susceptible stages in their cell cycles or rapidly proliferating cells, which includes cells of the immune system as well as malignant cells. The immunosuppressive effects of chemotherapeutic drugs are exacerbated by concurrent treatment with ionizing radiation (x-rays), which also affect cells that are rapidly making new DNA. Therefore, a person's immune response can be profoundly depressed as a result of the therapy. Other drugs, such as corticosteroids, are intentionally used to suppress the immune system and control hypersensitivity diseases (especially autoimmune disease) or prevent rejection of transplants. Because of their nonspecific activity, however, immune responses against infectious agents also can be suppressed, increasing an individual's susceptibility to infection. The list of drugs that affect the immune response is ever increasing and includes analgesics, antithyroid medications, anticonvulsants, antihistamines, antimicrobial agents, antilymphocyte antibodies, and tranquilizers.

Surgery and anesthesia also can suppress T- and B-cell function. Transient, severe lymphopenia is a common postoperative condition that can last as long as 1 month. Surgery to remove the spleen (splenectomy) can result in a depressed humoral response against encapsulated bacteria (especially *S. pneumoniae, H. influenzae, S. aureus,* group A streptococci, and *N. meningitidis*), depressed serum IgM levels, and decreased levels of opsonins.

Infections

Many infectious microorganisms are successful at invading the human body because they have evolved mechanisms for fighting off specific immune/inflammatory responses against themselves (discussed in Chapter 9). However, some infectious agents (e.g., human immunodeficiency virus [HIV], Epstein-Barr virus [EBV], CMV, herpes simplex virus type 6, measles) can generally suppress the immune response. HIV is one of the few microorganisms that directly attacks the central processes involved in the development of an immune response (discussed in detail in Chapter 9). It infects and destroys the T-helper cell, which is necessary to provide help for the maturation of both plasma cells and cytotoxic T cells. Therefore, HIV suppresses the immune response against

itself and secondarily creates a generalized immune deficiency by suppressing the development of immune responses against other pathogens and opportunistic microorganisms.

Several viruses (e.g., hepatitis B, rubella, CMV) can establish congenital infections through transmission from an infected mother to her child at birth when the child's immune system is immature. These children may have suppressed immune responses, although the degree of the deficiency is not usually severe, but as the child's immune system develops, the viral antigens may be partially seen as "self" so that a chronic infection is established.

Clinical Evaluation of Immunity

Evaluation and Care of Those with Immune Deficiency

Routine care of individuals with immune deficiencies must be tempered with the knowledge that the immune system may be totally ineffective.[61] Administration of conventional immunizing agents or blood products to these individuals may be unsafe because of the risk that the immunizing agent will cause an uncontrolled infection. Attenuated vaccines contain live but weakened microorganisms (e.g., live polio vaccine, vaccines against measles, mumps, and rubella) that can cause disseminated infection. Although the vaccine virus is attenuated enough to be destroyed by a normal immune system, it can survive, multiply, and cause severe disease in an immune-deficient recipient. Additionally, even healthy recipients of vaccines containing live microorganisms can shed those microorganisms for a short time, increasing the risk of infection to family members or other close associates who are immune deficient. Even simple procedures, such as penetrating the skin for routine blood tests, may lead to fatal septicemia (bacterial infection of the blood) in the immune-deficient person.

Individuals with immune deficiencies are also at risk for **graft-versus-host disease (GVHD)**.[77] Mature T cells in a transplanted graft (e.g., transfused blood) are capable of a destructive cell-mediated reaction against unmatched histocompatibility antigens on the tissues in the graft recipient. Symptoms of an acute graft-versus-host reaction usually appear within 10 to 30 days after the transplant. The primary targets for GVHD are the skin (e.g., rash, loss or increase of pigment, thickening of skin), liver (e.g., damage to bile duct, hepatomegaly), mouth (e.g., dry mouth, ulcers, infections), eyes (e.g., burning, irritation, dryness), and gastrointestinal tract (e.g., severe diarrhea) and may lead to death from infections.

GVHD is not a problem when the recipient is immunocompetent, that is, has an immune system that can control the donor's lymphocytes. If, however, the recipient's immune system is deficient, the grafted T cells remain unchecked and attack the recipient's tissues. Most GVHD is prevented by treating whole blood with irradiation to kill white blood cells before transfusion.

The most common presenting symptom of immune deficiencies is recurrent severe infections. Significant information concerning the nature of the specific immune deficiency can be obtained by noting the types of infection, as well as certain

Table 8-7	Laboratory Evaluation of Immunodeficiencies	
Function Tested	**Laboratory Test**	**Interpretation of Test**
Tests of Humoral Immune Function		
Antibody production	Total immunoglobulin levels	Presence of antibody-producing B cells
	Levels of isohemagglutinins	Capacity to produce specific IgM antibodies
	Levels of antibodies against vaccines—especially diphtheria and tetanus toxoids	Capacity to produce specific IgG antibodies
B-cell numbers	Numbers of lymphocytes with surface immunoglobulin	Presence of circulating B cells
Tests of Cellular Immune Function		
Delayed hypersensitivity	Skin test reaction against previously encountered antigens—especially *Candida albicans* or tetanus toxoid	Presence of antigen-responsive T cells and skin test cellular interactions (e.g., lymphokine activity and macrophage function)
T-cell numbers	Numbers of T cells forming rosettes with sheep erythrocytes or expressing membrane CD3 or CD11 antigen	Presence of circulating T cells
T-cell proliferation in vitro	Proliferative response to nonspecific mitogens (e.g., phytohemagglutinin)	Capacity of all T cells to divide in response to nonspecific stimulation (mitogens)
	Proliferative response to antigens (e.g., tetanus toxoid)	Capacity of antigen-reactive T cells to respond to antigen

characteristics of the affected individual, including gender, age of disease onset, the presence of any associated anomalies, family history, and risk factors associated with secondary immune deficiencies.[78] Humoral deficiencies are generally characterized by recurrent sinopulmonary infections with encapsulated bacteria, gastrointestinal malabsorption, and poor growth. T-cell defects generally present with failure to thrive, chronic diarrhea, persistent thrush, and opportunistic infections (e.g., *Mycobacterium, Pneumocystis, Candida,* and certain viruses). Phagocytic defects are usually associated with recurrent abscesses, oral ulcers, and infections with specific bacteria (e.g., catalase-positive bacteria). Complement defects may be linked to SLE-like disease and recurrent and disseminated infections with *Neisseria* spp.

A variety of laboratory tests are available to evaluate specific immune deficiencies (Table 8-7). The choice of which particular tests to perform is determined on the characteristics described previously. A basic screening test is a **complete blood count (CBC)** with a differential. The CBC provides information on the numbers of red cells, white cells, and platelets, and the differential indicates the quantities of lymphocytes, granulocytes, and monocytes in the blood. Quantitative determination of immunoglobulins (IgG, IgM, IgA) is a screening test for antibody production, and an assay for total complement (total hemolytic complement, CH_{50}) is useful if a complement defect is suspected.

If the nature of the immune deficiency remains uncertain after the screening tests, additional relatively common tests can be performed. For instance, subpopulations of lymphocytes (T or B) or antibodies (IgG, IgM, IgA) can be quantified. The proportion of B and T lymphocytes can be determined using characteristic surface markers, such as surface immunoglobulin for B cells and CD3 for T cells. T-cell populations

can be further subdivided using additional surface markers, such as CD4 (helper T cells) or CD8 (cytotoxic T cells). For antibodies, routine assays are available to quantify subclasses of IgG, such as IgG2.

An additional level of testing would include determination of immune responses against specific antigens. Determination of isohemagglutinins is informative about antigen-specific IgM production. Antibody responses to vaccines (e.g., tetanus, pertussis, measles, diphtheria, hepatitis B) are usually indicative of IgG responses. T-cell immunity against specific antigens can be measured by skin tests against antigens to which the individual had been exposed: "recall antigens." These include antigens from vaccines (e.g., mumps, tetanus) or from microorganisms with which the person had a previous active infection (e.g., *Candida*). An adequate T-cell immunity results in a positive delayed hypersensitivity skin test reaction.

If the tests do not identify the immune deficiency, more esoteric tests are offered by reference laboratories or research laboratories. These include quantification of individual complement components, in vitro proliferation (mitogenic response) of T or B cells to antigens or nonspecific mitogens, and a variety of tests of phagocyte function (e.g., nitroblue tetrazolium test [NBT] for hexose-monophosphate shunt activity, specific tests for phagocytosis, chemotaxis, or bacterial killing).

Replacement Therapies for Immune Deficiencies

Gamma-Globulin Therapy
Individuals with B-cell deficiencies that cause hypogammaglobulinemia or agammaglobulinemia usually can be treated successfully with administration of gamma globulins, which

are antibody-rich fractions prepared from plasma pooled from large numbers of donors. Administration of gamma globulin temporarily replaces the individual's antibodies. Antibodies from these preparations are removed slowly from the person's blood, with half of the antibodies being removed by 3 to 4 weeks. Thus individuals must be treated repeatedly to maintain a protective level of antibodies in the blood.

Commercial gamma-globulin preparations are usually administered intramuscularly or by intravenous (IV) infusion. The dosage varies among individuals and is primarily determined by body weight. The schedule and dosage are also determined according to titers of circulating immunoglobulins and the incidence of infections in the individual. Commercial gamma-globulin preparations usually contain small amounts of IgM and IgA. Individuals with selective IgA deficiency occasionally develop allergic reactions to IgA in gamma-globulin preparations.

Individuals who need larger amounts of IgM or IgA can be given fresh frozen plasma in monthly IV infusions. Complications associated with plasma therapy include the potential transmission of hepatitis or AIDS. The plasma is irradiated to destroy immunocompetent T cells and to avoid GVHD in individuals with accompanying T-cell deficiencies. Administration of fresh frozen plasma is successful in individuals with WAS (IgM deficient), AT (IgA deficient), or complement component deficiencies.

Transplantation and Transfusion

Several primary immune deficiencies originate from defects in lymphoid stem cells that interfere with their development in the primary lymphoid organs. Some of these (e.g., SCID, WAS, leukocyte adhesion defect) have benefited from replacement of stem cells through transplantation of bone marrow, umbilical cord cells, or other cell populations that are rich in stem cells.[79]

The source of donor cells, particularly bone marrow, may contain a mixed population of stem cells and more mature T lymphocytes. In order to avoid GVHD, the preferred donor would be matched with the recipient for HLA antigens. Several other diseases involving depletion of the bone marrow (i.e., aplastic anemia, leukemia requiring eradication of tumor cells in the marrow) also are treated by bone marrow transplantation. At least 75% of bone marrow transplants between individuals who are matched for HLA-A, HLA-B, HLA-C, and HLA-DR are accepted. In immunocompetent recipients, most rejections of HLA-matched transplants occur because of recognition of minor histocompatibility antigens by individuals who have received multiple blood transfusions and are, as a result, sensitized against those antigens, which are not evaluated in tissue typing. For stem cell transplants, differences in minor histocompatibility antigens may lead to GVHD. Because HLA antigens are inherited in a codominant fashion, the preferred donor would be a relative, especially a sibling. Although the donor is not tested for minor histocompatibility antigens, the use of a close relative also would minimize differences at those loci.

Chronic GVHD appears in 30% to 50% of transplants between HLA-matched siblings and 60% to 70% of transplants between unrelated donors. Symptoms may appear about 4 to 7 months after the transplant, but may begin much earlier or later. Depletion of T cells from bone marrow before transplantation significantly lowers the incidence of both acute and chronic GVHD. One method of doing this is to infuse the graft with monoclonal antibody against plasma membrane antigens found only on mature T cells. Another is to use fetal tissue as the graft. For example, fetal liver, which contains stem cells but not immunocompetent lymphocytes, is sometimes grafted in place of bone marrow if an HLA-matched donor cannot be found.

One therapy for deficiency diseases in which the individual lacks a thymus or thymic function (e.g., DiGeorge syndrome, ataxia-telangiectasia, or chronic mucocutaneous candidiasis) is reconstitution of thymic function. The procedure is to transplant fetal thymus tissue, which lacks immunocompetent T cells, or thymic epithelial cells (the cells that produce the thymic hormones) from which mature T cells have been removed. In some individuals transplantation increases the number of circulating mature T cells, but in most cases improvement is only temporary.

Enzymatic defects that cause SCID (e.g., adenosine deaminase deficiency) have been treated successfully with transfusions of glycerol frozen-packed erythrocytes. The donor erythrocytes contain the needed enzyme and can, at least temporarily, provide sufficient enzyme for normal lymphocyte function. An alternative method is administration of purified adenosine deaminase that has been stabilized with polyethylene glycol (PEG).

Treatment with Soluble Immune Modulators

The administration of soluble materials that affect lymphocyte function can restore T-cell function, especially in individuals with WAS or chronic mucocutaneous candidiasis. Successful for some individuals is the use of transfer factor, a low-molecular-weight nucleoprotein prepared from lymphocyte lysates, which can confer specific reactivity against certain antigens. Thymosin, a thymic hormone, also has been used, although with limited success. Cytokine therapy also has been effective in some cases of chronic granulomatous disease.

Gene Therapy

The first successful therapeutic replacement of defective genes was performed in two girls with SCID caused by an ADA deficiency.[80,81] The normal gene for ADA was cloned and inserted into a retroviral vector. The gene for ADA replaced some retroviral genes, resulting in a virus that carried the normal human gene but did not cause disease. The virus was used to infect bone marrow stem cells from these children. The retrovirus inserted the normal ADA gene into the individuals' genetic material. The genetically altered stem cells were infused into the children, resulting in reconstitution of their immune systems.

SUMMARY REVIEW

Hypersensitivity: Allergy, Autoimmunity, and Alloimmunity

1. Inappropriate immune responses are misdirected against the host's own tissues (autoimmunity); directed against beneficial foreign tissues, such as transfusions or transplants (alloimmunity); exaggerated responses against environmental antigens (allergy); or insufficient to protect the host (immune deficiency).

2. Allergy, autoimmunity, and alloimmunity are collectively known as *hypersensitivity reactions*.

3. Mechanisms of hypersensitivity are classified as type I (IgE-mediated) reactions, type II (tissue-specific) reactions, type III (immune complex–mediated) reactions, and type IV (cell-mediated) reactions.

4. Hypersensitivity reactions can be immediate (developing within minutes to a few hours) or delayed (developing within several hours or days).

5. Anaphylaxis, the most rapid immediate hypersensitivity reaction, is an explosive reaction that occurs within minutes of reexposure to the antigen and can lead to cardiovascular shock.

6. Allergens are antigens that cause allergic responses.

7. Type I (IgE-mediated) reactions are mediated through the binding of IgE to Fc receptors on mast cells and cross-linking of IgE by antigens that bind to the Fab portions of IgE. Cross-linking causes mast cell degranulation and the release of histamine (the most potent mediator) and other inflammatory substances.

8. Histamine enhances the chemotaxis of eosinophils into sites of type I allergic reactions

9. Atopic individuals tend to produce higher quantities of IgE and to have more Fc receptors for IgE on their mast cells.

10. Type II (tissue-specific) reactions are caused by five possible mechanisms: complement-mediated lysis, opsonization and phagocytosis, neutrophil-mediated tissue damage, antibody-dependent cell-mediated cytotoxicity, and modulation of cellular function.

11. Type III (immune complex–mediated) reactions are caused by the formation of immune complexes that are deposited in target tissues, where they activate the complement cascade, generating chemotactic fragments that attract neutrophils into the inflammatory site. Neutrophils release lysosomal enzymes that result in tissue damage.

12. Intermediate-sized immune complexes are the most likely to have severe pathologic consequences.

13. Immune complex disease can be a systemic reaction, such as serum sickness, or localized, such as the Arthus reaction.

14. Type IV (cell-mediated) reactions are caused by either cytotoxic T lymphocytes (Tc cells) or lymphokine-producing Th1 cells.

15. Typical allergens include pollen, molds and fungi, certain foods (milk, eggs, fish), animals, certain drugs, cigarette smoke, and house dust.

16. Clinical manifestations of allergic reactions usually are confined to the areas of initial intake or contact with the allergen. Ingested allergens induce gastrointestinal symptoms, airborne allergens induce respiratory or skin manifestations, and contact allergens induce allergic responses at the site of contact.

17. Autoimmunity is a breakdown of immunologic homeostasis, the immune system's tolerance of self-antigens. Central tolerance develops during the embryonic period. Peripheral tolerance is maintained in secondary lymphoid organs by regulatory T lymphocytes or antigen-presenting dendritic cells.

18. Autoimmune disease can be caused by the exposure of a previously sequestered antigen, the development of a neoantigen, the complications of infectious disease, the emergence of a forbidden clone of lymphocytes, or ineffective peripheral tolerance.

19. Alloimmunity is the immune system's reaction against antigens on the tissues of other members of the same species.

20. Alloimmune disorders include transient neonatal disease, in which the maternal immune system becomes sensitized against antigens expressed by the fetus, transplant rejection, and transfusion reactions, in which the immune system of the recipient of an organ transplant or blood transfusion reacts against foreign antigens on the donor's cells.

21. SLE is a chronic, multisystem, inflammatory disease and is one of the most serious of the autoimmune disorders. SLE is characterized by the production of a large variety of autoantibodies.

22. Hyperacute graft rejection (preexisting antibody) is immediate and rare, acute rejection is cell mediated and occurs days to months after transplantation, and chronic rejection is caused by inflammatory damage to endothelial cells as a result of a weak cell-mediated reaction.

23. Red blood cell antigens may be the targets of autoimmune or alloimmune reactions. The most important of these, because they provoke the strongest humoral immune response, are the ABO and Rh systems.

Deficiencies in Immunity

1. Disorders resulting from immune deficiency are the clinical sequelae of impaired function of components of the immune or inflammatory response, phagocytes, or complement.

2. Immune deficiency is the failure of mechanisms of self-defense to function in their normal capacity.

3. Immune deficiencies are either congenital (primary) or acquired (secondary). Primary immune deficiencies are caused by genetic defects that disrupt lymphocyte development, whereas secondary immune deficiencies are secondary to disease or other physiologic alterations.

4. The clinical hallmark of immune deficiency is a propensity to unusual or recurrent severe infections. The type of infection usually reflects the immune system defect.

5. The most common infections in individuals with defects of cell-mediated immune response are fungal and viral, whereas infections in individuals with defects of the humoral immune response or complement function are primarily bacterial.

6. Defects in B-cell function are diverse, ranging from a complete lack of the human bursal equivalent function, the lymphoid organs required for B-cell maturation (as in Bruton's agammaglobulinemia), to deficiencies in a single class of immunoglobulins (e.g., selective IgA deficiency).

7. DiGeorge syndrome (congenital thymic aplasia or hypoplasia) is characterized by complete or partial lack of the thymus (resulting in depressed T-cell immunity) and the parathyroid glands (resulting in hypocalcemia) and the presence of cardiac anomalies.

8. SCID is a total lack of T-cell function and a severe (either partial or total) lack of B-cell function. SCID can result from mutations in critical enzymes (ADA deficiency, PNP deficiency), in cytokine receptors (X-linked SCID, JAK3 deficiency, IL-7 receptor deficiency), or in antigen receptors (RAG-1/RAG-2 deficiencies, CD45 deficiency, CD3 deficiency, ZAP-70 deficiency). Other combined defects may result from deficiencies in antigen-presenting molecules (bare lymphocyte syndrome), cytoskeletal proteins (WAS), or DNA repair (ataxia-telangiectasia).

SUMMARY REVIEW—cont'd

9. Almost any portion of the complement cascade may be defective. The most severe defect is C3 deficiency, which results in recurrent life-threatening bacterial infections. Defects in proteins of the membrane-attack complex usually result in unusual disseminated infections with bacteria of the *Neisseria* spp.

10. Defects in phagocyte function, which include insufficient numbers of phagocytes or defects of chemotaxis, phagocytosis, or killing, can result in recurrent life-threatening infections such as septicemia and disseminated pyogenic lesions.

11. Acquired immunodeficiencies are caused by superimposed conditions, such as aging, malnutrition, infections, malignancies, physical or psychologic trauma, environmental factors, some medical treatments, or other diseases.

12. Deficiencies in immunity usually are treated by replacement therapy. Deficient antibody production is treated by replacement of missing immunoglobulins with commercial gamma-globulin preparations. Lymphocyte deficiencies are treated with the replacement of host lymphocytes with transplants of bone marrow, fetal liver, or fetal thymus from a donor.

KEY TERMS

ABO blood group, 272
Acute rejection, 274
Adenosine deaminase (ADA) deficiency, 280
Agammaglobulinemia, 278
Allergen, 264
Allergy, 256
Alloimmune disease, 271
Alloimmunity, 256, 270
Anaphylaxis, 259
Antibody-dependent cell-mediated cytotoxicity (ADCC), 261
Arthus reaction, 264
Ataxia-telangiectasia (AT), 281
Atopic, 265
Atopic dermatitis, 267
Autoimmune disease, 256
Autoimmunity, 256, 258
Autosomal agammaglobulinemia, 278
Autosomal hyper-IgM syndrome, 278
Bare lymphocyte syndrome, 280
Blocking antibody, 267
Blood group antigen, 272
B-lymphocyte deficiency, 278
Bruton's agammaglobulinemia, 278
C1 deficiency, 281
C2 deficiency, 281
C3 deficiency, 281
C4 deficiency, 281
C9 deficiency, 281
C3 receptor deficiency, 282
Chédiak-Higashi syndrome, 283
Chronic granulomatous disease (CGD), 283
Chronic mucocutaneous candidiasis, 279
Chronic rejection, 275
Combined T- and B-lymphocyte deficiency, 278
Common variable immune deficiency, 279

Complement deficiency, 278
Complete blood count (CBC), 287
Contact dermatitis, 267
Cross-reactive antibody (T cell), 269
Cryoglobulin, 264
Cyclic neutropenia, 282
Cytotropic antibody, 259
Defective class-switch, 278
Delayed hypersensitivity reaction, 258
Desensitization, 267
DiGeorge syndrome, 275
Factor H deficiency, 281
Factor I deficiency, 281
Forbidden clone, 269
Graft-versus-host disease (GVHD), 286
Hyperacute rejection, 274
Hypersensitivity, 256
Hypocomplementemic, 263
Hypogammaglobulinemia, 278
IgG subclass deficiency, 279
IL-7 receptor deficiency, 280
Immediate hypersensitivity reaction, 258
Immune deficiency, 275
Immunologic homeostasis, 258
Immunologically privileged site, 268
Isohemagglutinin, 272
JAK3 deficiency, 280
Leukocyte adhesion deficiency (LAD), 282
Mannose-binding lectin (MBL) deficiency, 281
MHC class I deficiency, 280
MHC class II deficiency, 281
Microchimerism, 269
Molecular mimicry, 269
Myeloperoxidase deficiency, 280
Neoantigen, 269
Phagocytic deficiency, 278

Primary (congenital) immune deficiency, 275
Properdin deficiency, 281
Purine nucleoside phosphorylase (PNP) deficiency, 280
RAG-1 deficiency, 280
RAG-2 deficiency, 280
Raynaud phenomenon, 264
Reagin, 259
Reticular dysgenesis, 279
Rh blood group, 272
Secondary (acquired) immune deficiency, 275
Selective IgA deficiency, 279
Serum sickness, 263
Severe combined immune deficiency (SCID), 279
Severe congenital neutropenia, 282
Systemic lupus erythematosus (SLE), 271
Tissue-specific antigen, 259
T-lymphocyte deficiency, 278
Transient hypogammaglobulinemia of infancy, 284
Type I (IgE-mediated) hypersensitivity reaction, 258
Type II (tissue-specific) hypersensitivity reaction, 258
Type III (immune complex-mediated) hypersensitivity reaction, 258
Type IV (cell-mediated) hypersensitivity reaction, 258
Universal donor, 272
Universal recipient, 272
Urticaria (hives), 265
Wheal and flare reaction, 265
Wiskott-Aldrich syndrome (WAS), 281
X-linked hyper-IgM syndrome, 278
X-linked SCID, 280

REFERENCES

1. Gell PGH, Coombs RRA, Lachman PT: *Clinical aspects of immunology,* Oxford, England, 1975, Blackwell Scientific.
2. Simons FER: Anaphylaxis, *J Allergy Clin Immunol* 121(2 Suppl):S402-S407, 2008.
3. Portier P, Richet C: De l'action anaphylactique de certains venins, *Comptes Rendus Societie Biologie (Paris)* 54:170, 1902.
4. Roberts G: Anaphylaxis to foods, *Pediatr Allergy Immunol* 18(6): 543-548, 2007.
5. Prussin C, Metcalfe DD: IgE, mast cells, basophils, and eosinophils, *J Allergy Clin Immunol* 117(2 Suppl):S450-S456, 2006.
6. Saini SS, MacGlashan D: How IgE upregulates the allergic response, *Curr Opin Immunol* 14(6):694-697, 2002.
7. Gould HJ, Sutton BJ: IgE in allergy and asthma today, *Nature Rev Immunol* 8(3):205-217, 2008.
8. Robbie-Ryan M, Brown MA: The role of the mast cells in allergy and autoimmunity, *Curr Opin Immunol* 14(6):728-733, 2002.
9. Nelson HS: Allergen immunotherapy: where is it now? *J Allergy Clin Immunol* 119(4):769-779, 2007.

10. Jutel M et al: Immune regulation by histamine, *Curr Opin Immunol* 14(6):735-740, 2002.

11. Romi F, Gilhus NE, Aarli JA: Myasthenia gravis: clinical, immunologic, and therapeutic advances, *Acta Neurol Scand* 111(2):134-141, 2005.

12. Rapoport B, McLachian SM: The thyrotropin receptor in Graves' disease, *Thyroid* 17(10):911-922, 2007.

13. Reid JR, Wheeler SF: Hyperthyroidism: diagnosis and treatment, *Am Fam Physician* 72(4):635-636, 2005.

14. Jancar S, Crespo MS: Immune complex-mediated tissue injury: a multistep paradigm, *Trends Immunol* 26(1):48-55, 2005.

15. Pirquet C, Schick B: *Serum sickness*, Leipzig, Germany, 1905, Franz Denticke.

16. Arthus M, Breton M: Lésions cutanées produites par les injections de sérum, *Comptes Rendus Societe de Biologie* 55:817, 1903.

17. Blanco P et al: Cytotoxic T lymphocytes and autoimmunity, *Curr Opin Rheumatol* 17(6):731-734, 2005.

18. Koch R: Fortsetzung der mitteilungen, ber ein heilmittel gegen tuberkulose, *Deutsche Med Wochenschr* 9:101, 1891.

19. Sicherer SH, Leung DYM: Advances in allergic skin disease, anaphylaxis, and hypersensitivity reactions to foods, drugs, and insects, *J Allergy Clin Immunol* 119(6):1462-1469, 2007.

20. Thien FCK: Drug hypersensitivity, *Med J Aust* 185(6):333-338, 2006.

21. Geha RS: Allergy and hypersensitivity: nature versus nurture in allergy and hypersensitivity, *Curr Opin Immunol* 15(6):603-608, 2003.

22. Akbari O et al: Role of regulatory T cells in allergy and asthma, *Curr Opin Immunol* 15(6):627-633, 2003.

23. Vercelli D: Discovering susceptibility genes for asthma and allergy, *Nat Rev Immunol* 8(3):169-182, 2008.

24. Kinet J-P: Allergy and hypersensitivity, *Curr Opin Immunol* 14(6):685-687, 2002.

25. Brown JM, Wilson TM, Metcalfe DD: The mast cell and allergic diseases: role in pathogenesis and implications for therapy, *Clin Exp Allergy* 38(1):4-18, 2007.

26. Bardana EJ Jr: Occupational asthma, *J Allergy Clin Immunol* 121(2 Suppl):S408-S411, 2008.

27. Haydon RC: Allergic rhinitis—current approaches to skin and in vitro testing, *Otolaryngol Clin North Am* 41(2):331-346, 2008.

28. Ahlstedt S, Murray CS: In vitro diagnosis of allergy: how to interpret IgE antibody results in clinical practice, *Primary Care Resp J* 15(4):228-236, 2006.

29. Douglass JA, O'Hehir RE: Diagnosis, treatment and prevention of allergic disease: the basics, *Med J Aust* 185(4):228-233, 2006.

30. Burks AW, Laubach S, Jones SM: Oral tolerance, food allergy, and immunotherapy: implications for future treatment, *J Allergy Clin Immunol* 121(6):1344-1350, 2008.

31. Bieber T: Atopic dermatitis, *N Engl J Med* 358(14):1483-1494, 2008.

32. Averbeck M et al: Immunologic principles of allergic disease, *J Dtsch Dermatol Ges* 5(11):1015-1028, 2007.

33. Schwartz RS: Shattuck lecture: diversity of the immune repertoire and immunoregulation, *N Engl J Med* 348(11):1017-1026, 2003.

34. Ohashi PS, DeFranco AL: Making and breaking tolerance, *Curr Opin Immunol* 14(6):744-759, 2002.

35. Ferguson TA, Griffith TS: A vision of cell death: Fas ligand and immune privilege 10 years later, *Immunol Rev* 213(1):228-238, 2006.

36. Fourneau JM et al: The elusive case for a role of mimicry in autoimmune diseases, *Mol Immunol* 40(14-15):1095-1102, 2004.

37. Venanzi ES, Benoist C, Mathis D: Good riddance: thymocyte clonal deletion prevents autoimmunity, *Curr Opin Immunol* 16(2):197-202, 2004.

38. Cunningham MW: Pathogenesis of group A streptococcal infections and their sequelae, *Adv Exp Med Biol* 609:29-42, 2000.

39. Adams KM, Nelson JL: Microchimerism: an investigative frontier in autoimmunity and transplantation, *JAMA* 291(9):1127-1131, 2004.

40. Maloney S et al: Microchimerism of maternal origin persists into adult life, *J Clin Invest* 104(1):41-47, 1999.

41. Nelson JL et al: Microchimerism and HLA-compatible relationships of pregnancy in scleroderma, *Lancet* 351(9102):559-562, 1998.

42. Ohtsuka T et al: Quantitative analysis of microchimerism in systemic sclerosis skin tissue, *Arch Dermatol Res* 293(8):387-391, 2001.

43. Artlett CM et al: Chimeric cells of maternal origin in juvenile idiopathic inflammatory myopathies, *Lancet* 356(9248):2155-2156, 2000.

44. Lissauer D et al: Persistence of fetal cells in the mother: friend or foe? *Brit J Obstet Gynecol* 114(11):1321-1325, 2007.

45. Khosrotehrani K et al: Transfer of fetal cells with multilineage potential to maternal tissue, *JAMA* 292(1):75-80, 2004.

46. Morahan G, Morel L: Genetics of autoimmune diseases in humans and in animal models, *Curr Opin Immunol* 14(6):803-811, 2002.

47. Shmerling RH: Autoantibodies in systemic lupus erythematosus—there before you know it, *N Engl J Med* 349(16):1499-1500, 2003.

48. Rahman A, Isenberg DA: Systemic lupus erythematosus, *N Engl J Med* 358(9):929-939, 2008.

49. Riemekasten G, Hahn BH: Key autoantigens in SLE, *Rheumatol* 44(8):975-982, 2005.

50. Perdriger A, Werner-Leyval S, Rollot-Elamrani K: The genetic basis for systemic lupus erythematosus, *Joint Bone Spine* 70(2):103-108, 2003.

51. Arbuckle MR et al: Development of autoantibodies before the clinical onset of systemic lupus erythematosus, *N Engl J Med* 349(16):1526-1533, 2003.

52. American College of Rheumatology 2004 systemic lupus erythematosus. Available at www.rheumatology.org/public/factsheets/lupus.asp?aud=pat#4.

53. Burt RK et al: Clinical applications of blood-derived and marrow-derived stem cells for nonmalignant diseases, *JAMA* 299(8):925-936, 2008.

54. Nydegger UE et al: Histo-blood group antigens as allo- and autoantigens, *Ann N Y Acad Sci* 1050:40-51, 2005.

55. Westhoff CM: The structure and function of the Rh antigen complex, *Semin Hematol* 44(1):42-50, 2007.

56. Sheldon S, Poulton K: HLA typing and its influence on organ transplantation, *Methods Mol Biol* 333:157-174, 2006.

57. Truong LD et al: Acute antibody-mediated rejection of renal transplant: pathogenetic and diagnostic considerations, *Arch Pathol Lab Med* 131(8):1200-1208, 2007.

58. Cooper MA, Pommering TL, Koranyi K: Primary immunodeficiencies, *Am Fam Physician* 68(10):2001-2008, 2003.

59. Fischer A: Human primary immunodeficiency diseases, *Immunity* 27(12):835-845, 2007.

60. Fleisher TA: Primary immune deficiencies: windows into the immune system, *Pediatr Rev* 27(10):363-372, 2006.

61. Verbsky JW, Grossman WJ: Cellular and genetic basis of primary immune deficiencies, *Pediatr Clin North Am* 53(4):649-684, 2006.

62. Primary Immunodeficiency. National Institute of Child Health and Human Development, NIH, DHHS, Washington D.C., Government Printing Office. Available at www.nichd.nih.gov/publications/pubs/primary_immuo.cfm, updated 04/07/2008.

63. Simonte SJ, Cunningham-Rundles C: Update on primary immunodeficiency: defects of lymphocytes, *Clin Immunol* 109(2):109-118, 2003.

64. Cunningham-Rundles C, Ponda PP: Molecular defects in T- and B-cell primary immunodeficiency diseases, *Nature Rev Immunol* 5(11):880-892, 2005.

65. Bruton OC: Agammaglobulinemia. *Pediatrics* 9(6):722-728, 1952.

66. Notarangelo LD et al: Defects in class-switch recombination, *J Allergy Clin Immunol* 117(4):855-864, 2006.

67. Demczuk S, Aurias A: DiGeorge syndrome and related syndromes associated with 22q11.2 deletions, *Annales Genetique* 38:59, 1995.

68. DiGeorge AM: Congenital absence of the thymus and its immunologic consequences. In Bergsma D, McKusick FA, editors: *Immunologic deficiency diseases in man*, National Foundation—March of Dimes original article series, Baltimore, 1968, Williams & Wilkins.

69. Fischer A: Have we seen the last variant of severe combined immunodeficiency? *N Engl J Med* 349(19):1789-1792, 2003.

70. Notarangelo LD, Miao CH, Ochs HD: Wiskott-Aldrich syndrome, *Curr Opin Hematol* 15(1):30-36, 2008.

71. Sjöholm AG et al: Complement deficiency and disease: an update, *Mol Immunol* 43(1-2):78-85, 2006.

72. Lewis MJ, Botto M: Complement deficiencies in humans and animals: links to autoimmunity, *Autoimmunity* 39(5):367-378, 2006.

73. Smith CW: Adhesion molecules and receptors, *J Allergy Clin Immunol* 121(2 Suppl):S375-S379, 2008.

74. Chinen J, Shearer WT: Secondary immunodeficiencies, including HIV infection, *J Allergy Clin Immunol* 121(2 Suppl):S388-S392, 2008.

75. Schroder AK, Rink L: Neutrophil immunity of the elderly, *Mech Ageing Dev* 124(4):419-425, 2003.

76. Hakim FT et al: Aging, immunity and cancer, *Curr Opin Immunol* 16(2):151-156, 2004.

77. Bhushan V, Collins RH Jr: Chronic graft-vs-host disease, *JAMA* 290(19):2599-2603, 2003.

78. Buckley RH: Primary immunodeficiency or not? Making the correct diagnosis, *J Allergy Clin Immunol* 117(4):756-758, 2006.

79. Buckley RH: Molecular defects in human severe combined immunodeficiency and approaches to immune reconstitution, *Ann Rev Immunol* 22(1):625-655, 2004.

80. Blaese RM: Development of gene therapy for immunodeficiency: adenosine deaminase deficiency, *Pediatr Res* 33(1 Suppl):S49-S53, 1993.

81. Onodera M et al: Gene therapy for severe combined immunodeficiency caused by adenosine deaminase deficiency: improved retroviral vectors for clinical trials, *Acta Haematol* 101(2):89-96, 1999.

INFECTION

NEAL S. ROTE • SUE E. HUETHER

CHAPTER OUTLINE

MICROORGANISMS AND HUMANS: A DYNAMIC
RELATIONSHIP
MICROORGANISMS AND INFECTIONS
  Process of Infection
  Clinical Infectious Disease
  Classes of Infectious Microorganisms
ACQUIRED IMMUNODEFICIENCY SYNDROME (AIDS)
  Transmission
  Pathogenesis

  Clinical Manifestations
  Treatment and Prevention
  Pediatric AIDS and Central Nervous System Involvement
COUNTERMEASURES AGAINST PATHOGENS
  Infection Control Measures
  Antimicrobials
  Active Immunization: Vaccines
  Passive Immunotherapy

Modern healthcare has shown great progress in preventing and treating infectious diseases through the success of public health initiatives, vaccination programs, and the use of antibiotics. In developed countries death from infections is most common among those with debilitating diseases, nutritional deficiencies, or immunosuppression. Death from influenza and pneumonia and from sepsis were the eighth and tenth leading causes of death in the United States in 2006 estimates (see Table 30-1). Infectious disease remains a significant threat to life in many parts of the world, including India, Africa, and Southeast Asia (Table 9-1), although the advent of sanitary living conditions, clean water, uncontaminated food, vaccinations, and antimicrobials had improved the health of many. As a result of these initiatives, smallpox has been eradicated from the globe (the last reported case was in 1975 in Somalia), measles is almost eradicated in the Western Hemisphere, and many diseaes, such as tuberculosis and polio, are on the decline.

Despite the widescale implementation of progressive public health and immunization policies infectious disease remains a significant cause of morbidity and mortality because of the emergence of previously unknown infections, the re-emergence of old infections that were thought to be under control, and the development of infectious agents that are resistant to multiple antibiotics.[1] The causes for these occurences are numerous and include the following:

- Vast and rapid urbanization in many areas of the world, resulting in a breakdown in public health programs and a more rapid spread of infection
- Poverty and social inequality
- War and famine
- Global travel, allowing more rapid spread of disease from isolated areas to virtually any point around the world in a few hours
- Globalization of the food supply
- Human encroachment into wilderness areas, resulting in contact with previously sequestered infectious agents
- Antibiotics that are prescribed excessively, that are not taken for a complete course of therapy, or that, even when appropriately used, result in the selection of antibiotic-resistant microorganisms
- Decreases in federal research budgets to study infectious disease
- Denial of a problem by governments, allowing infections to spread in an uncontrolled way

- Diminished use of effective insecticides
- Increased global warming, allowing insect vectors to spread into and breed in areas that were previously too cool for them

---

The emergence of previously unknown infections is not a new event in human history. However, the current rate may be unprecedented. Within one generation, more than 40 previously unknown infections have arisen and some examples are presented in Table 9-2. Several have extremely high mortality rates of more than 50% including severe acute respiratory syndrome (SARS) (in those older than 65 years), Ebola virus, Marburg virus, "mad cow" disease, Nipah virus (up to 75%), and acquired immunodeficiency syndrome (AIDS) (almost 100% in untreated persons). But most either spread very slowly (e.g., AIDS) or initially break out in relatively isolated areas and are effectively controlled by quarantine (e.g., Ebola virus). Although none of these infections has developed into the worldwide scourges portrayed in movies "*Andromeda Strain*" and "*I Am Legend*," the potential of reversion to more rapidly spreading variants is a concen of public health agencies worldwide.

Concurrently, the incidence and spread of at least 20 previously known infections are increasing. A new strain of cholera that arose in Indonesia in 1961 has spread to Africa and in 1991 to South America. Malaria, dengue fever, and yellow fever are reemerging in areas where they had been eliminated or were unknown. The incidence of tuberculosis is increasing in countries that had reported declines and has risen by almost one third between the mid-1980s and early 1990s. Diphtheria has reemerged as a major health issue in Russia. In 1994 plague was reported in India after being dormant for a generation. War has led to outbreaks of Marburg hemorrhagic fever during civil war in Angola during 1975-2002 and cholera in the Democratic Republic of the Congo among Rwandan refugees in 1994; about 50,000 refugees died from a combination of cholera and shigella dysentery. The spread of cholera, yellow fever, and epidemic meningococcal disease has rebounded. Decreased insect control programs that were previously successful have led to spread of vector-borne diseases: African trypanosomiasis, dengue hemorrhagic fever, and malaria. Although the United States is relatively free of most of these diseases, the effects of global warming and relaxed control of vectors may result in resurgence. It should not be forgotten that in 1793 a yellow fever outbreak in Philadelphia killed 2000 of the city's 55,000 inhabitants and forced the U.S. government to abandon the city until the outbreak ceased.

Many common and reemerging infections have become antibiotic and drug resistant. *Streptococcus pneumoniae*, a common cause of otitis media, pneumonia, and bacteremia, has been treated routinely and successfully with penicillin. Now at least 25% of isolates are penicillin resistant, and some are resistant to multiple antibiotics. Multiple antibiotic-resistant forms of *Staphylococcus aureus*, a primary cause of infections of wounds, surgical incisions, and catheters, are endemic in some hospitals. Some forms of this microorganism once were sensitive only to a single antibiotic, vancomycin, and now

have become vancomycin-resistant. Antimicrobial resistance is now routinely observed in tuberculosis, diarrheal diseases, hospital-acquired infections, malaria, meningitis, respiratory tract infections, sexually transmitted infections (STIs), and human immunodeficiency virus (HIV).

Added to this collage of microbiologic dangers is the rising risk of bioterrorism. Agents such as smallpox, anthrax, and plague are continuing threats to public health and safety. All healthcare providers should have information about the

Table 9-1	Estimated Annual Number of Deaths by Cause Worldwide	
Cause of Death	**Number**	**%**
Communicable diseases*	**18,324,000**	**32.1**
Infectious and parasitic diseases	10,904,000	19.1
HIV/AIDS[†]	2,777,000	
Diarrheal diseases	1,798,000	
Tuberculosis	1,566,000	
Malaria	1,272,000	
Childhood diseases	1,124,000	
Sexually transmitted infections (excluding AIDS)	180,000	
Meningitis	173,000	
Hepatitis	157,000	
Tropical diseases	129,000	
Others	51,000	
Respiratory infections	3,963,000	6.9
Perinatal conditions	2,462,000	4.3
Maternal conditions	510,000	0.9
Nutritional deficiencies	485,000	0.9
Noncommunicable Diseases	**33,537,000**	**58.8**
Cardiovascular diseases	16,733,000	29.3
Malignant neoplasms	7,121,000	12.5
Respiratory diseases	3,702,000	6.5
Digestive diseases	1,968,000	3.5
Neuropsychiatric disorders	1,112,000	1.9
Diabetes mellitus	988,000	1.7
Genitourinary diseases	848,000	1.5
Congenital abnormalities	493,000	0.9
Nutritional/endocrine disorders	243,000	0.4
Other neoplasms	149,000	0.3
Musculoskeletal diseases	106,000	0.2
Others	74,000	0.2
Injuries	**5,168,000**	**9.1**
Unintentional	3,551,000	6.2
Intentional	1,618,000	2.8

From World Health Organization: The World Health Report 2004. Death by cause, sex, and mortality stratum in WHO regions, estimates for 2002, Annex Table 2. Available at www.who.int/whr/2004/annex/topic/en/annex_2_en.pdf.
*Communicable diseases, maternal and perinatal conditions and nutritional deficiencies
[†]Global data for human immunodeficiency syndrome/acquired immunodeficiency syndrome (HIV/AIDS) cases reported remain highly distorted for three reasons: (1) there are wide intercountry and interregional differences in the completeness of AIDS case detection and reporting, (2) reporting of AIDS cases to public health authorities and recognition of its importance have occurred in different countries at different times, and (3) pediatric AIDS remains substantially underrecognized and underreported.

Table 9-2	Examples of Emergent Infections		
Year	Disease	Causative Agent	Site of Discovery
1955	Orally transmitted non-A, non-B infectious hepatitis	Hepatitis E virus	India
1967	Viral hemorrhagic fever	Marburg virus	Germany
1969	Lassa fever	Lassa virus	Nigeria
1976	Ebola hemorrhagic fever	Ebola virus	Zaire and Sudan
1976	Legionnaires disease	*Legionella pneumophila*	United States
1978	Toxic shock syndrome	Toxin-producing strains of *Staphylococcus* spp.	United States
1981	Acquired immunodeficiency syndrome (AIDS)	Human immunodeficiency virus	United States
1982	Lyme disease	*Borrelia burgdorferi*	Northeast United States
1982	Hemolytic-uremic syndrome, bloody diarrhea	*Escherichia coli* 0157:H7	United States, Japan
1983	Peptic ulcer disease	*Helicobacter pylori*	Australia
1986	Roseola	Human herpesvirus 6	United States
1989	Non-A, non-B infectious hepatitis, hepatocellular carcinoma	Hepatitis C virus	United States
1992	Cholera	*Vibrio cholerae* 0139	Indonesia
1993	Hemorrhagic fever with renal syndrome	Hantavirus	Korea
1994	Kaposi sarcoma	Human herpesvirus 8	United States
1994	Encephalitis transmitted from horses to humans	Hendra virus	Australia
1995	Bovine spongiform encephalopathy (BSE or "mad cow" disease)	Prion, variant of Creutzfeldt-Jakob disease agent	United Kingdom
1999	Encephalitis transmitted from pigs to humans	Nipah virus	Malaysia
2003	SARS (severe acute respiratory syndrome)	SARS-associated coronavirus	China

characteristics and clinical manifestations of these biologic agents. The theoretical threat of bioterrorism became real in 2001 when letters containing anthrax were mailed; 22 individuals became infected and 5 died.

MICROORGANISMS AND HUMANS: A DYNAMIC RELATIONSHIP

For many microorganisms the human body is a hospitable site in which to grow and flourish because of its sufficient nutrients and appropriate conditions of temperature and humidity. In many cases a symbiotic relationship exists, in which both humans and microorganisms benefit (Box 9-1). These microorganisms make up the *normal flora*—the resident microorganisms found in different parts of the body, including the skin, mouth, gastrointestinal tract, respiratory tract, and genital tract.[2] For instance, the normal bacterial flora of the human gut are provided with nutrients from ingested food and in exchange produce enzymes that facilitate the digestion and use of many of the more complex molecules found in the human diet, produce antibacterial factors (e.g., bacteriocins, colicins) that prevent colonization by pathogenic microorganisms, and produce usable metabolites (e.g., vitamin K, B vitamins). This beneficial homeostasis is normally maintained through the physical integrity of the gut and other mechanisms that sequester these microorganisms on the mucosal surface.

MICROORGANISMS AND INFECTIONS

Process of Infection

The symbiotic relationship with the normal flora can be breached as a result of injury that compromises the physical

BOX 9-1	The Many Relationships Between Humans and Organisms

Symbiosis: Benefits only the human; no harm to the organism
Mutualism: Benefits the human and the organism
Commensalism: Benefits only the organism; no harm to the human
Pathogenicity: Benefits the organism; harms the human
Opportunism: A situation in which benign human organisms become pathogenic because of decreased human host resistance

protective barriers. Damage to the intestinal tract releases intestinal bacteria into the bloodstream, potentially leading to sepsis, shock, and death. Cuts in the skin may allow normally noninfectious bacteria (e.g., *S. aureus*) to cause local infections (e.g., abscesses, boils) and invade further and infect various organs. Symbiosis is also maintained by the immune and inflammatory systems. If those systems are compromised, many microorganisms will leave their normal sites and cause infection elsewhere in the body. Individuals with immune deficiencies easily become infected with *opportunistic microorganisms*, which normally would not cause disease but seize the opportunity to do so when a person's defensive systems are weakened or suppressed (see Chapter 8).

Unlike opportunistic infectious agents, *true pathogens* have devised means to circumvent the individual's defenses (discussed in Chapters 6 and 7) and directly cause infection. Successful infection with theses agents is usually dependent on adequate numbers of microorganisms rather than compromise of the host's defenses.

From the perspective of the microorganisms that cause disease, the infectious process undergoes four separate stages of progression: colonization, invasion, multiplication, and spread.

Colonization

Infectious microorganisms usually exist in reservoirs, such as the environment (e.g., contaminated water, soil), animals, or another human who is infected or in a noninfectious state within the individual's normal flora. An individual may obtain an infectious microorganism from a reservoir by several means.

Infections contracted from animal reservoirs (zoonotic infections) may be transmitted by direct contact (e.g., transmission of the rabies virus through bites) or indirectly by means of vectors (e.g., insects). Mechanical vectors (e.g., housefly) passively transfer microorganisms from a contaminated site to an individual.[3] Biologic vectors (e.g., fleas, lice, mosquitoes, ticks) transmit infectious microorganisms through bites and stings. Individuals can also become infected by direct exposure to contaminated materials, such as fecal-oral transmission through food or water (e.g., salmonella food poisoning, cholera, hepatitis A infection, polio, rotavirus infection) or soil (e.g., tetanus).

Human-to-human transmission may occur through aerosolized microorganisms in droplets (e.g., produced by coughing or sneezing), which is the primary means of transmission for respiratory infections (e.g., agents that cause the common cold, influenza, streptococcal sore throat, bacterial meningitis). Other infectious agents require physical contact (e.g., sexual, blood transfusion, direct contact with contaminated clothes or bandages, entrance through wounds or openings in the skin). Direct contact is usually required for transmission of STIs, hepatitis B virus, cytomegalovirus (CMV), herpes simplex virus, or warts. Some microorganisms have the capacity to spread from mother to child across the placenta (e.g., *Treponema pallidum, Listeria monocytogenes*, cytomegalovirus [CMV], *Toxoplasma gondii*), ascending the birth canal or during delivery (e.g., group B *Streptococcus, Escherichia coli, Chlamydia trachomatis, Neisseria gonorrhoeae*, hepatitis B virus, HIV, *Candida albicans*), or through the breast milk (e.g., *S. aureus*). This is classified as *vertical transmission*, whereas spread from one person to another is *horizontal transmission*. In a very few instances, the infectious agent may develop airborne transmission.[4] Effective *airborne transmission* may occur by prolonged presence of aerosolized droplets released by respiration, exercise, or other bodily activity and has been observed with SARS, tuberculosis, Norovirus, and smallpox.[5]

After deposition in receptive environments for colonization, the microorganism stabilizes the adherence to the tissue through specific surface receptors.[6] For instance, infectious agents that cause respiratory infections specifically bind to molecules found on respiratory epithelium. Adherence helps protect the microorganism from removal by mechanical nonspecific forces, such as coughing of respiratory mucus. The specificity of adherence results in a particular microorganism being limited to where infections can occur (**tissue tropism**) such as the confinement of common cold viruses to producing respiratory infections.

Invasion

Once colonization has occurred the infectious agent can invade the surrounding tissue and, in many cases, other sites in the individual. Successful infectious agents have developed mechanisms to penetrate the tissues and evade the host's nonspecific and specific defenses (inflammation and immunity). Many of these are discussed throughout this chapter.

Multiplication

Within the warm and nutrient-filled environment of human tissue most microorganisms undergo rapid multiplication with production of many new infectious progeny. Viral pathogens replicate within infected cells, and some bacteria are intracellular pathogens and replicate in macrophages and other cells. Many extracellular bacteria and fungi form multicellular masses called **biofilms**, which provides an optimal environment for growth.[7]

Spread

Many successful pathogens produce localized infections without spread to other regions of the body (e.g., *Vibrio cholerae*). Others, however, are highly invasive and may enter the lymphatics, blood, and internal organs. Successful spread relies on a variety of virulence factors, including adhesion molecules, toxins, and protection against the individual's inflammatory and immune systems. Fungi, in particular, are opportunistic. In an individual with an intact immune system, the microorganism remains localized, whereas the infection may rapidly spread if the individual's immune or inflammatory systems are compromised.

Clinical Infectious Disease

From the perspective of the individual who is infected, the clinical process occurs in four distinct stages:

- *Incubation period*—the period from initial exposure to the infectious agent and the onset of the first symptoms, during which the microorganism has entered the individual, undergone initial colonization, and begun multiplying, but is yet in insufficient numbers to cause symptoms; this period may last from several hours to years
- *Prodromal stage*—the occurrence of initial symptoms, which are often very mild and include a feeling of discomfort and tiredness
- *Invasion period*—the pathogen is multiplying rapidly, invading farther and affecting the tissues at the site of initial colonization as well as other areas; the immune and inflammatory responses are being triggered; development of symptoms specifically related to the pathogen and symptoms related to the ongoing protective inflammatory response
- *Convalescence*—in most instances, the individual's immune and inflammatory systems have successfully removed the infectious agent, and symptoms decline; alternatively the disease may be fatal or may enter a latency phase with resolution of symptoms until reactivation at a later time

Clinical manifestations of infectious disease vary, depending on the pathogen, the organ system affected, and the severity. Effects of infection may be acute, chronic, secondary to the immune and inflammatory responses, or a consequence of bacterial toxins or viral injury. Manifestations can arise directly from the infecting microorganism or its products; however, the majority of manifestations result from the host's inflammatory and immune responses. Infectious diseases typically begin with the nonspecific or general symptoms of fatigue, malaise, weakness, and loss of concentration. Generalized aching and loss of appetite are common complaints. However, the hallmark of most infectious diseases is fever.

Fever is not failure of the body to regulate temperature; rather, body temperature is being regulated at a higher level than normal. Body temperature is regulated by nervous system feedback to the hypothalamus, which functions as a central thermostat (see Chapter 15). A large number of agents (pyrogens) can produce fever. In current classification, those pyrogens derived from outside the host are termed **exogenous pyrogens** and those produced by the individual are termed **endogenous pyrogens.** There is little evidence that exogenous pyrogens cause fever directly. Such pyrogens indirectly affect the hypothalamus through endogenous pyrogens released by cells of the host. A number of cytokines have been identified as endogenous pyrogens. They are interleukins 1 and 6 (IL-1 and IL-6), interferon (IFN), tumor necrosis factor (TNF), and others (see Figure 15-8). These cytokines seem to raise the thermoregulatory set point through stimulation of prostaglandin synthesis and turnover in both thermoregulatory (brain) and non-thermoregulatory (peripheral) tissue. These mechanisms are discussed in detail in Chapter 15. Although it is generally believed that fever has a beneficial value in infection, the molecular mechanism behind the beneficial effects has not been established. Many investigators, however, consider fever as an adaptive host-defense response.

Several factors influence the capacity of a pathogen to cause disease.

- *Communicability:* The ability to spread from one individual to others and cause disease: measles and pertussis spread very easily, HIV is of lower communicability
- *Immunogenicity:* The ability of pathogens to induce an immune response
- *Infectivity:* The ability of the pathogen to invade and multiply in the host

- *Mechanism of action:* How the microorganism damages tissue
- *Pathogenicity:* The ability of an agent to produce disease—success depends on communicability, infectivity, extent of tissue damage, and virulence
- *Portal of entry:* Route by which a pathogenic microorganism infects the host: direct contact, inhalation, ingestion, or bites of an animal or insect
- *Toxigenicity:* The ability to produce soluble toxins or endotoxins, factors that greatly influence the pathogen's degree of virulence
- *Virulence:* Capacity of a pathogen to cause severe disease—for example, measles virus is of low virulence; rabies virus is highly virulent

Infectious diseases are also classified by their prevalence and spread within the community.

- *Endemic:* Diseases with relatively high, but constant, rates of infection in a particular population
- *Epidemic:* The number of new infections in a particular population greatly exceeds the number usually observed
- *Pandemic:* An epidemic that spreads over a large area, such as a continent or worldwide (Table 9-3)

Classes of Infectious Microorganisms

Infectious disease can be caused by microorganisms that range in size from 20 nm (poliovirus) to 10 m (tapeworm). Classes of pathogenic microorganisms and their characteristics are summarized in Table 9-4 and discussed in detail in the following sections.

Bacterial Infection

Bacteria are prokaryotic unicellular microorganisms with no nuclei, mitochondria, or membrane-bound organelles. They are generally divided into several groups.

- "*True bacteria*" divide by binary fission and may have a variety of morphologies, including cocci (spherical), bacilli (rod shaped), vibrios (comma-shaped rods), or spirilla (twisted, rod shaped). Most disease-causing bacteria fall into this classification.
- *Filamentous bacteria* may have branching, mycelium-like structures that resemble fungi. Examples include the mycobacteria (*Mycobacterium tuberculosis, Mycobacterium leprae*) that cause tuberculosis and leprosy.

Table 9-3	Historic Examples of Pandemics		
Year	**Cause**	**Site**	**Estimated Deaths**
1347-1352	Bubonic plague (black death) (70% mortality rate)	Europe (worldwide)	50 million (a third of Europe's population); up to 100 million worldwide
1775-1782	Smallpox (35% mortality rate)	North America	>150,000
1829-1851	Cholera	Europe	Several hundred thousands
1914-1918	Typhus (*Rickettsia prowazekii*), spread by body lice, 40% mortality rate	Europe during WWI	9 million
1916	Polio	United States	6000
1918-1919	Influenza (Spanish flu)	United States, became worldwide	20-40 million
1981-?	AIDS	Worldwide	>25 million

Table 9-4	Classes of Organisms Infectious to Humans		
Class	Size	Site of Reproduction	Example
Virus	20-300 nm	Intracellular	Poliomyelitis
Chlamydiae	200-1000 nm	Intracellular	Urethritis
Rickettsiae	300-1200 nm	Intracellular	Rocky Mountain spotted fever
Mycoplasma	125-350 nm	Extracellular	Atypical pneumonia
Bacteria	0.8-15 mcg	Skin	Staphylococcal wound infection
		Mucous membranes	Cholera
		Extracellular	Streptococcal pneumonia
		Intracellular	Tuberculosis
Fungi	2-200 mcg	Skin	Tinea pedis (athlete's foot)
		Mucous membranes	Candida (e.g., thrush)
		Extracellular	Sporotrichosis
		Intracellular	Histoplasmosis
Protozoa	1-50 mm	Mucosal	Giardiasis
		Extracellular	Sleeping sickness
Helminths	3 mm to 10 m	Intracellular	Trichinosis
		Extracellular	Filariasis

- *Spirochetes* are flexible spiral filaments that are motile. Most are anaerobic. Pertinent examples include *Borrelia recurrentis* (relapsing fever), *T. pallidum* (syphilis), and *Borrelia burgdorferi* (Lyme disease).
- *Mycoplasma* lack a rigid cell wall and are small and pleomorphic. They are the smallest and most simple members of the bacteria. *Mycoplasma pneumoniae* causes atypical pneumonia, and *Mycoplasma genitalium* is a suspected cause of urethritis and pelvic inflammatory disease.
- *Rickettsia* are strict intracellular parasites that can be rod-shaped, spherical, or pleomorphic. They are typically spread by insect vectors and cause Rocky Mountain spotted fever *(Rickettsia rickettsii)* and typhus *(Rickettsia prowazekii)*.
- *Chlamydia* are also strict intracellular parasites, but with more complex intracellular life cycles. The primary chlamydial pathogen is *Chlamydia trachomatis*, which causes the most the most common bacterial sexual transmitted infection (pelvic inflammatory disease) and eye infections (conjunctivitis).

Bacteria are also categorized as gram-negative or gram-positive. Gram-negative bacteria do not retain crystal violet dye in the gram-staining process whereas gram-positive bacteria do retain crystal violet dye. Gram-negative bacteria also have a lipopolysaccharide (LPS) coat in the outer membrane which consists of lipid A, a core polysaccharide and O antigen. The LPS coat is also known as endotoxin (See Figure 9-1 and further discussion on page 301.)

Common bacterial pathogens are listed in Table 9-5.

Transmission and Colonization

Transmission of bacterial infections occurs through the same routes generally described above. Many pathogenic bacteria normally reside in humans without causing disease. For instance, *Streptococcus pyogenes* (pharyngitis), *S. pneumoniae* (pneumonia, meningitis), *Neisseria meningitidis* (meningitis), and *Haemophilus influenzae* type b (meningitis). In most cases

they are either present in inadequate numbers to cause disease or are effectively controlled by local protective mechanisms. Others reside in nature and cause infection after being ingested or entering wounds (e.g., *V. cholerae* [cholera] in contaminated water or *Clostridium tetani* [tetanus] in contaminated soil).

A large number require human-to-human contact, including several that are unstable on environmental surfaces (e.g., *Bordetella pertussis* [whooping cough], *N. gonorrhoeae* [gonorrhea], *T. pallidum* [syphilis]). Even the human-to-human spread of infectious bacteria contracted initially from environmental reservoirs can be facilitated by certain aspects of the disease, e.g., the explosive diarrhea of cholera. Chlamydia, which may be contracted as an STI, can spread from the mother to child during childbirth and may establish long-term intracellular persistence in the newborn.

The establishment of stable colonization requires adhesion.[6] Many bacteria attach through **pili** (also called **fimbriae**), which are thin rod-like projections from the bacterial surface (see Figure 9-1 and Figure 9-2). Pathogenic strains of *Escherichia coli* involved in urinary tract infections have a variety of different specific pili-associated adhesion molecules, including mannose-binding protein that binds with glycoproteins specifically expressed on the bladder epithelium and PapG (pyelonephritis-associated protein) adhesin the binds to galactoses of the human P blood group. PapG is a specific adhesion for urinary tract epithelium, but PapG variants are specific for other cell types so that the particular PapG expressed will determine the preferred site of infection with *E. coli*. The particular adhesin may vary depending on growth conditions under which bacteria may undergo a "phase change" and shift from one type to another.

Neisseria spp. bind to urinary tract epithelial cell membrane-associated cofactor protein (CD46), which is a receptor that regulates complement and protects cells by helping inactivate C3b and C4b. Several other microorganisms (e.g., *B. pertussis*, *Legionella pneumophila*, *Mycobacterium tuberculosis*) bind to the

| Table 9-5 | Common Bacterial Infections | | |

Microoorganism	Gram Stain	Respiratory Pathway	Intracellular or Extracellular
Respiratory Infections			
Upper Respiratory Tract Infections			
Corynebacterium diphtheriae (diphtheria)	Gram +	Facultative anaerobic	Extracellular
Haemophilus influenzae	Gram −	Facultative anaerobic	Extracellular
Streptococcus pyogenes (group A)	Gram +	Facultative anaerobic	Extracellular
Otitis Media			
Haemophilus influenzae	Gram −	Facultative anaerobic	Extracellular
Moraxella catarrhalis	Gram −	Aerobic	Extracellular
Streptococcus pneumoniae	Gram +	Facultative anaerobic	Extracellular
Lower Respiratory Tract Infections			
Bacillus anthracis (pulmonary anthrax)	Gram +	Facultative anaerobic	Extracellular
Bordetella pertussis (whooping cough)	Gram −	Aerobic	Extracellular
Chlamydia pneumoniae	Not stainable	Aerobic	Obligate intracellular
Escherichia coli	Gram −	Facultative anaerobic	Extracellular
Haemophilus influenzae	Gram −	Facultative anaerobic	Extracellular
Klebsiella pneumoniae	Gram −	Facultative anaerobic	Extracellular
Legionella pneumophila	Gram −	Aerobic	Facultative intracellular
Mycobacterium tuberculosis	Weak gram +	Aerobic	Extracellular
Mycoplasma pneumoniae	Not stainable	Aerobic	Extracellular
Neisseria meningitidis (develops into meningitis)	Gram −	Aerobic	Extracellular
Pseudomonas aeruginosa	Gram −	Aerobic	Extracellular
Streptococcus agalactiae (group B; develops into meningitis)	Gram +	Facultative anaerobic	Extracellular
Streptococcus pneumoniae	Gram +	Facultative anaerobic	Extracellular
Yersinia pestis (plague)	Gram −	Facultative anaerobic	Extracellular
Gastrointestinal Infections			
Inflammatory Gastrointestinal Infections			
Bacillus anthracis (gastrointestinal anthrax)	Gram +	Facultative anaerobic	Extracellular
Clostridium difficile	Gram +	Anaerobic	Extracellular
Escherichia coli 0157:H7	Gram −	Facultative anaerobic	Extracellular
Vibrio cholerae	Gram −	Facultative anaerobic	Extracellular
Vibrio parahaemolyticus	Gram −	Facultative anaerobic	Extracellular
Invasive Gastrointestinal Infections			
Brucella abortus (brucellosis, undulant fever leading to sepsis, heart infection)	Gram −	Aerobic	Intracellular
Campylobacter jejuni	Gram −	Microaerophilic	Extracellular
Francisella tularensis	Gram −	Strict anaerobic	Facultative intracellular
Helicobacter pylori (gastritis and peptic ulcers)	Gram −	Microaerophilic	Extracellular
Listeria monocytogenes (leading to sepsis and meningitis)	Gram +	Aerobic	Intracellular
Salmonella typhi (typhoid fever)	Gram −	Anaerobic	Extracellular
Shigella sonnei	Gram −	Facultative anaerobic	Extracellular
Food Poisoning			
Bacillus cereus	Gram +	Facultative anaerobic	Extracellular
Clostridium botulinum	Gram +	Anaerobic	Extracellular
Clostridium perfringens	Gram +	Anaerobic	Extracellular
Staphylococcus aureus	Gram +	Facultative anaerobic	Extracellular

Continued

Table 9-5   Common Bacterial Infections—cont'd

Microoorganism	Gram Stain	Respiratory Pathway	Intracellular or Extracellular
Sexually Transmitted Infections			
Chlamydia trachomatis (pelvic inflammatory disease)	Not stainable	Aerobic	Intracellular
Neisseria gonorrhoeae (urethritis)	Gram −	Aerobic	Facultative intracellular
Treponema pallidum (spirochete; syphilis)	Gram −	Aerobic	Extracellular
Skin and Wound Infections			
Bacillus anthracis (cutaneous anthrax)	Gram +	Facultative anaerobic	Extracellular
Borrelia burgdorferi (Lyme disease; spirochete)	Gram −	Aerobic	Extracellular
Clostridium tetani (tetanus)	Gram +	Anaerobic	Extracellular
Clostridium perfringens (gas gangrene)	Gram +	Anaerobic	Extracellular
Mycobaterium leprae (leprosy)	Gram + (weakly)	Aerobic	Extracellular
Pseudomonas aeruginosa	Gram −	Aerobic	Extracellular
Rickettsia prowazekii (rickettsia; typhus)	Gram −	Aerobic	Obligate intracellular
Staphylococcus aureus	Gram +	Facultative anaerobic	Extracellular
Streptococcus pyogenes (group A)	Gram +	Facultative anaerobic	Extracellular
Eye Infections			
Chlamydia trachomatis (conjunctivitis)	Not stainable	Aerobic	Obligate intracellular
Haemophilus aegyptus (pink eye)	Gram −	Facultative anaerobic	Extracellular
Zoonotic Infections			
Bacillus anthracis (anthrax)	Gram +	Facultative anaerobic	Extracellular
Brucella abortus (brucellosis, also called undulant fever)	Gram −	Aerobic	Intracellular
Borrelia burgdorferi (spirochete; Lyme disease)	Gram −	Aerobic	Extracellular
Listeria monocytogenes	Gram +	Aerobic	Intracellular
Rickettsia rickettsii (rickettsia; Rocky Mountain spotted fever)	Gram −	Aerobic	Obligate intracellular
Rickettsia prowazekii (rickettsia; typhus)	Gram −	Aerobic	Obligate intracellular
Yersinia pestis (plague)	Gram −	Facultative anaerobic	Extracellular
Nosocomial Infections			
Enterococcus faecalis	Gram +	Facultative anaerobic	Extracellular
Enterococcus faecium	Gram +	Facultative anaerobic	Extracellular
Escherichia coli (cystitis)	Gram −	Facultative anaerobic	Extracellular
Pseudomonas aeruginosa	Gram −	Obligate anaerobic	Extracellular
Staphylococcus aureus	Gram +	Facultative anaerobic	Extracellular
Staphylococcus epidermidis	Gram +	Facultative anaerobic	Extracellular

CR3 complement receptor (a receptor for C3b and C3b breakdown products) on the surface of monocytes/macrophages. *B. pertussis* expresses a surface hemagglutinin that recognizes CR3, whereas *L. pneumophila* and *M. tuberculosis* initially absorb inactivated C3b (C3bi) for use as an adhesin for CR3.

A variety of proteins and carbohydrates not associated with pili function as adhesion molecules. Flagella (used for motion) act as adhesions in *V. cholerae*. Hemagglutinins on *B. pertussis*, *Salmonella* spp., and *Helicobacter pylori* bind to erythrocyte surface molecules. Fibronectin is a common component of mucosal cell surfaces and is frequently used as a receptor. Several bacteria (*S. pyogenes*, *S. aureus*, *T. pallidum*) have developed specific adhesion molecules that recognize a particular amino acid sequence (Arg-Gly-Asp) in fibronectin.

Many other bacteria have developed adhesion molecules that bind to collagen, laminin, and vitronectin, which are plentiful in connective tissue. A surface polysaccharide (poly-N-acetylglucosamine) is on nonencapsulated *Staphylococcus* spp., *E. coli* that infect the urinary system. *Yersinia pestis*, which causes plague, mediates adherence to the material in catheters and prosthetic devices, thus increasing the risk of infection of joint replacements and other implanted materials.

Invasion and Evasion

Invasion results in direct confrontation with the individual's primary defense mechanisms against bacteria, which include the complement system, antibodies, and phagocytes, such as neutrophils and macrophages (see Chapters 6, 7, and 8). Bacterial survival and growth depend on the effectiveness of the body's defenses and on the bacterium's capacity to resist those defenses and obtain nutrients and multiply. Evasion of the body's defense mechanisms may result in infectious microorganisms being transported in the blood (**bacteremia**) to infect other organs or even multiplying in the blood (**sepsis**).[8]

Efficient pathogens produce a variety of toxic molecules that may kill the individual's cells, disrupt tissue, and protect against inflammation. **Exotoxins** are proteins released during bacterial growth. They are usually enzymes and have highly specific effects; they include cytotoxins, neurotoxins, pneumotoxins, enterotoxins, and hemolysins. Exotoxins can damage cell membranes, activate second messengers, and inhibit protein synthesis. For instance, a key component of invasion by *N. meningitidis* is a toxin that weakens intercellular adhesion between epithelial cells, thus allowing penetration into the underlying tissue. Pathogenic strains of streptococci and staphylococci produce hyaluronidase, lipases, and hemolysins that break down cells and intercellular matrix. Exotoxins are immunogenic and elicit the production of antibodies known as **antitoxins.** Consequently, vaccines are available for many of the exotoxins (i.e., tetanus, diphtheria, and pertussis).

Endotoxins are **lipopolysaccharides (LPSs)** contained in the cell walls of gram-negative bacteria and released during lysis (or destruction) of the bacteria (see Figure 9-1). The innermost part of the lipopolysaccharide, *lipid A,* is made of polysaccharides and fatty acids and is responsible for the substance's toxic effects. Bacteria that produce endotoxins are called *pyrogenic bacteria* because they stimulate the release of inflammatory mediators, produce fever and the local and systemic effects of inflammation including septic shock (Figure 9-3).[8] Endotoxin also may be released from the membrane of the bacteria, either during bacterial growth or during treatment with antibiotics. Therefore, antibiotics cannot prevent the toxic effects of the endotoxin.

Evasion of the individual's immune and inflammatory systems is multifaceted, and the most successful pathogens incorporate several mechanisms (Table 9-6).[9]

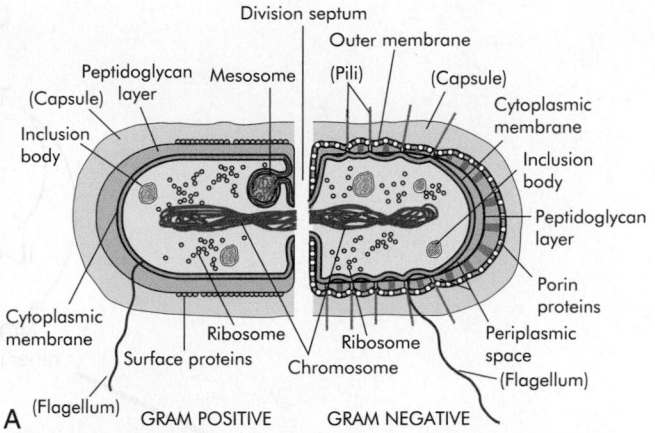

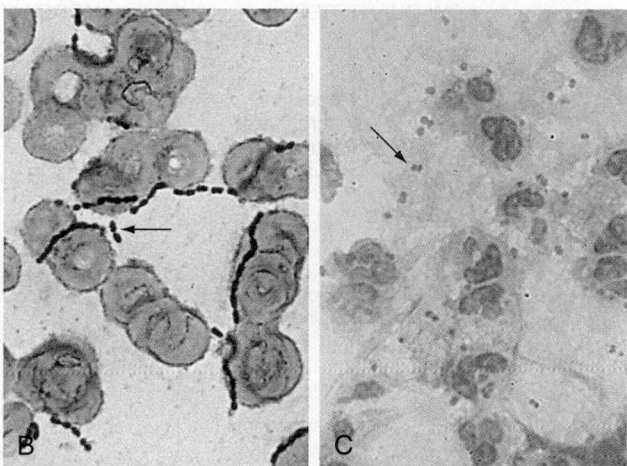

Figure 9-1 **Gram-positive and gram-negative bacteria. A,** The structure of the bacterial cell wall determines its staining characteristics with Gram stain. Gram-positive bacteria have a thick layer of peptidoglycan *(left).* Gram-negative bacteria have a thin peptidoglycan layer and an outer membrane of lipopolysaccharide (LPS) *(right).* **B,** Example of a gram-positive (darkly stained microorganisms, *arrow*) group A *Streptococcus.* This microorganism consists of cocci that frequently form chains. **C,** Example of a gram-negative (pink microorganisms, *arrow*) *Neisseria meningitidis* in cerebrospinal fluid. *Neisseria* form complexes of two cocci (diplococci).

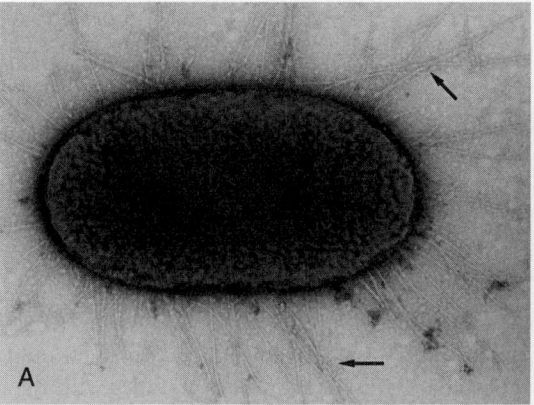

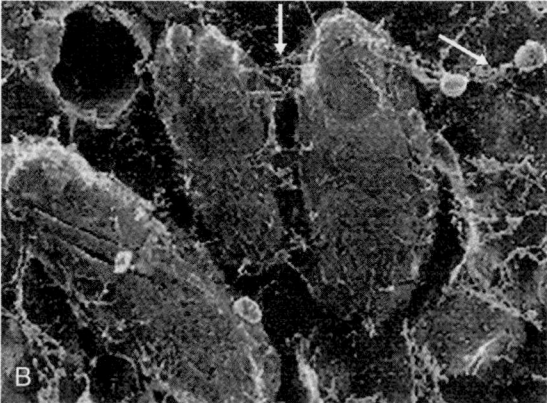

Figure 9-2 Attachment of *Escherichia coli* through pili. **A,** Transmission electron micrograph showing pili *(arrows)* of pathogenic *E. coli.* **B,** Scanning electron micrograph of *E. coli* (yellow) attached by pili *(arrows)* to bladder epithelium (blue). (A from Mandell G, Bennett J, Dolin R: *Principles and practice of infectious diseases,* ed 6, Philadelphia, 2005, Churchill Livingstone; **B** modified from Wein A et al: *Campbell-Walsh urology,* ed 9, Philadelphia, 2007, Saunders.)

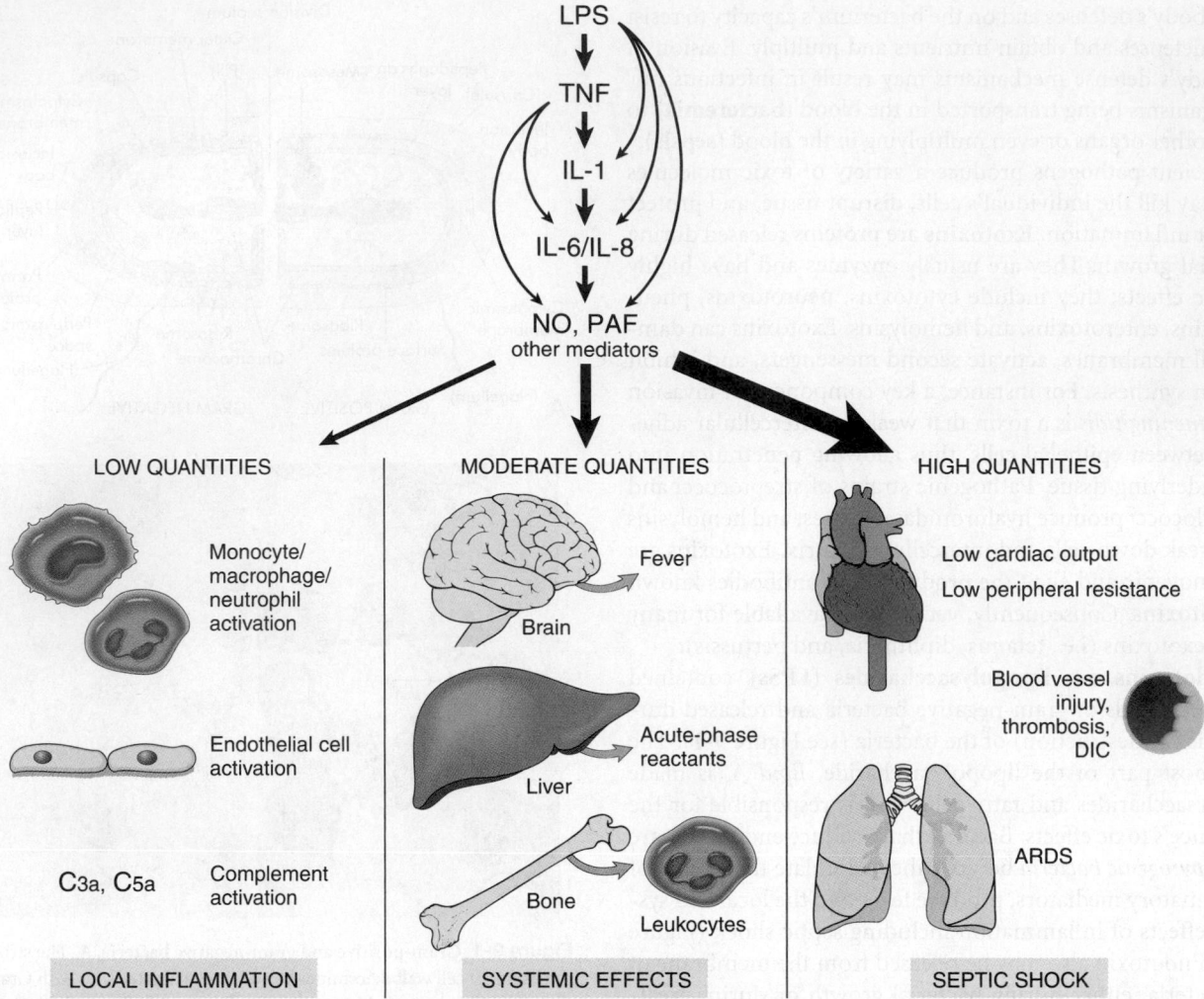

Figure 9-3 **The many activities of lipopolysaccharide (LPS).** Bacterial endotoxin (LPS) activates almost every aspect of inflammation. The release of LPS from gram-negative bacteria triggers successive waves of cytokine production, including tumor necrosis factor (TNF), interleukin-1 (IL-1), interleukin-6 (IL-6), and interleukin-8 (IL-8), and secondary mediators of inflammation, such as nitric oxide (NO) and platelet-activating factor (PAF). At low levels of LPS the effect is local. Moderate levels of LPS cause more systemic inflammatory responses. High levels of LPS may lead to septic shock and death. *DIC*, Disseminated intravascular coagulation; *ARDS*, acute respiratory distress syndrome. (From Kumar V, Abbas A, Fausto N: *Robbins and Cotran pathologic basis of disease*, ed 7, Philadelphia, 2005, Saunders.)

Rapid Division. Because the primary immune response may take 3 to 5 days to reach protective levels, some pathogens proliferate at rates that surpass the development of the immune system. Cholera causes severe vomiting and watery diarrhea, has a 60% mortality rate, and develops within 2 to 3 days of ingestion of the bacteria. Some strains of toxin-producing group A streptococci cause destructive skin infections and pneumonia that may kill an individual within 2 days. Group B streptococci from the maternal vagina may ascend the birth canal, penetrate fetal membranes, and infect the fluid surrounding the fetus. This microorganism may have already established an active infection of the child's lungs by the time of birth, resulting in a pneumonia (50% mortality rate in newborns) that is too advanced to be treated successfully by antibiotics.

Intracellular Survival. Bacteria may hide from the immune response by growth in sites that are relatively poorly protected by immune cells, for example, *V. cholerae* in the gastrointestinal (GI) tract, and *Salmonella typhi* in the intestinal tract and biliary tract (gallbladder). Even asymptomatic people may undergo prolonged local colonization and shed infectious microorganisms in urine and feces, thus creating a *carrier state.*

Survival within cells *(intracellular bacteria)* affords a distinct advantage to some bacteria.[10] Many intracellular bacteria can survive and even multiply in macrophages *(Brucella, Listeria, M. leprae, M. tuberculosis)* or in other cells *(Yersinia, Shigella, Listeria, E. coli).* Normally a macrophage would efficiently kill bacteria by fusing lysosomal granules with the phagosome to produce a phagolysosome and using oxygen-dependent and oxygen-independent mechanisms. Successful intracellular bacteria may block killing in several ways. Several microorganisms are resistant to killing and survive in the phagolysosome.

Table 9-6	Mechanisms Used by Microorganisms to Defend Against Inflammation and Immunity			
Strategy	**Bacterial Mechanism**	**Fungal Mechanism**	**Parasite/Protozoan Mechanism**	**Viral Mechanism**
Rapid division	Initial proliferation in protective environment	NA	NA	Rapid proliferation of viruses with small genomes
Intracellular survival	Intracellular bacteria block granule fusion, survive in phagolysosomes, enter and multiply in cytoplasm	Multiplication in phagosomes, inhibition of lysosomal enzymes	Resistance to lysosomal enzymes, block granule fusion, enter and multiply in cytoplasm	Obligative intracellular life cycle, latency (e.g., herpes simplex virus in dorsal root ganglia)
Protection against phagocytosis	Capsules with antiphagocytic and anticomplement activities, toxins to kill phagocytes (e.g., α-toxin and leukocidin)	Polysaccharide capsule, toxins that inhibit phagocytosis	Glycocalyx, toxins that inhibit phagocytosis	NA
Coating with self	Adsorption of fibronectin or IgG (e.g., protein A), sialic acid capsule	NA	Adsorption of IgG by Fc receptor	Enveloped viruses with plasma membrane
Antigenic variation	Large diversity of surface molecules, phase changes in pili or membrane proteins, strain-to-strain serotype differences	Changes in surface antigens	Changing morphologic forms during life cycle, antigen switching	Viral enzymes that produce translational errors, antigen shift and drift, diversity of serotypes
Degrade immune molecules	Proteases for IgA and IgG, degrade complement, defensins, and cathelicidins	NA	IgG and IgA proteases	
Neutralization of immune molecules	Shedding of surface antigens	NA	Shedding of surface antigens	Secretion of viral proteins to neutralize antibody, molecules to neutralize cytokines
Complement evasion	Proteases degrade complement (e.g., C3b, C5a), capsules that prevent complement deposition, inhibitors of complement components and convertases	NA	Degrade or inactivate C3b, C3a, and C5a, break down C3 convertase	Cellular complement inhibitors in envelope
Immune suppression	Induction of anergy, direct suppression of Th cell development	Stimulation of anti-inflammatory cytokines, inhibition of proinflammatory cytokines	Release of soluble antigens that induce "tolerance," polyclonal B-cell activation, induction of anti-inflammatory cytokines, cytotoxic molecules	Infect and kill immune cells, inhibit Tc and natural killer (NK) recognition of major histocompatibility complex (MHC), inhibit antigen presentation

NA, Not applicable.

Species of *Salmonella* secrete products that alter the environment of the phagolysosome. Production of catalase and superoxide dismutase *(N. gonorrhoeae, Brucella abortus, S. aureus)* destroys toxic oxygen products produced by the hexose-monophosphate-shunt. *S. aureus* also produces a cell-bound pigment (carotenoid) that "quenches" singlet oxygen. A second means of avoiding killing is escape from the phagosome. Several bacteria secrete lysins (e.g., hemolysin of *Shigella*, listeriolysin O and phospholipase C of *L. monocytogenes*, phospholipase A of

Rickettsia spp.) that break down the phagosome membrane, and the bacteria are released into the cytoplasm, where they multiply.[11] A third means of avoiding killing is by prevention of phagosome-lysosome fusion. *M. tuberculosis* and *T. gondii* produce toxins that prevent fusion so that the environment in the phagosome remains relatively nontoxic.

Protection Against Phagocytosis. Bacteria produce a large variety of toxins and extracellular enzymes, some of which kill phagocytic cells (e.g., *Pseudomonas aeruginosa*

exotoxin A).[12] Staphylococcal hemolysins and toxins from *Bacillus anthracis* and *B. pertussis* decrease phagocytic and chemotactic activities and may be toxic. Streptococcal products, such as streptolysin O, bind to cholesterol in the phagocyte's plasma membrane and initiate destruction through the internal release of enzymes in lysosomal granules.[13]

Antiphagocytic **capsules** are expressed by most bacterial pathogens involved in pneumonia and meningitis (Figure 9-4). Capsules are mostly polysaccharide, although some very important proteins may be capsular components, which inhibit complement activation and phagocytosis. Such coatings inhibit phagocytosis and include the thick polysaccharide covering of the pneumococcus (*S. pneumoniae*), the waxy capsule surrounding the tubercle bacillus *(M. tuberculosis),* the polysaccharide "slime" capsule of *P. aeruginosa,* and the M protein of *S. pyogenes.* The M protein binds fibrinogen and fibrin and functions as an adhesin.

Coating with Self-Protein. Some bacterial surface proteins (protein A of *S. aureus,* protein G of *S. pyogenes*) bind the Fc portion of the individual's antibody, thus forming a protective coat of "self" protein. Binding through the Fc holds the antibody in an orientation that does not allow complement activation or phagocytosis. *S. aureus* produces a surface coagulase that induces fibrin clotting on the bacterial surface. *T. pallidum* coats itself with fibronectin. Capsules are produced that contain sialic acid (*E. coli* K-12), which closely

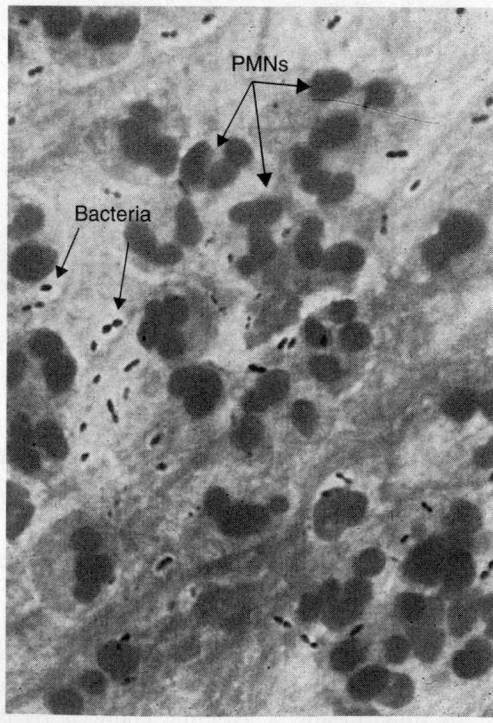

Figure 9-4 **Bacterial capsule.** Gram stain of a sputum sample from an individual with pneumococcal pneumonia (×1000 magnification). The sputum is rich in polymorphonuclear (PMN) cells (see arrow) and slightly elongated, gram-negative cocci (*Streptococcus pneumoniae*). Clear areas *(arrows)* around the bacteria indicate capsules. (Modified from Mandell G, Bennett J, Dolin R: *Principles and practice of infectious diseases,* ed 6, Philadelphia, 2005, Churchill Livingstone.)

resembles the sialic acid on the surface of most human cells, and hyaluronic acid (group A streptococci), which is the basic substance in connective tissue.

Antigenic Variation. **Antigenic variation** allows the pathogen to alter surface molecules that express antigens that are the targets of protective immune responses. Thus as the individual develops protective levels of antibodies, the pathogen responds by changing antigens and becoming resistant. The three primary mechanisms of antigenic variation are *mutation, recombination,* and *gene switching.* Antigenic variation can occur during the course of an infection in the host or during the spread of infection through the environment.

Neisseria use pili to adhere to epithelium, and antibody against these antigens can abrogate adherence. *Neisseria* undergoes *phase shifts* during which pilar antigens are changed by progressive silencing of one set of 10 or 11 available pili genes and activation of others that express different antigens. The spirochete *B. recurrentis* (relapsing fever) repeatedly relapses with spiking fevers as a result of as many as 10 episodes of antigenic changes over weeks or months. Many other bacteria have a large number of different antigenic types (serotypes) across the species. At least 80 different strains of group A *S. pyogenes* express different serotypes of the capsular M protein. *S. pneumoniae* has at least 100 different serotypes based on capsular polysaccharides. Multiple serotypes are also found in *V. cholerae, S. aureus, E. coli, N. gonorrhoeae,* and others. Although the particular serotype is stable on that bacterium, an immune response against one serotype will result in increased growth of a different serotype. Some gram-negative bacteria can revert to "rough" forms in which serotype-specific carbohydrates are deleted, thus becoming resistant to antibody and activation of complement.

Degradation of Immune Molecules. Protection is afforded by the breakdown of molecules of the immune or inflammatory system. An **IgA protease** produced by meningitis-causing microorganisms and other related bacteria *(N. gonorrhoeae, N. meningitidis, H. influenzae, S. pneumoniae)* cleaves IgA at the hinge region into ineffective Fc and Fab'$_2$ regions. A staphylokinase produced by *Staphylococcus* spp. activates plasmin (resulting in the breakdown of clots) and degrades IgG and C3b of the complement system. *Pseudomonas* produces elastase (breakdown C3 of the complement system) and a 56-kDa protease (breaks down C5a).

Salmonella membrane protease degrades nonspecific antimicrobial molecules like defensins and cathelicidins. *Salmonella* can also alter surface lipid A by changing its fatty acid content to become resistant to small-molecular-weight antimicrobials.

Neutralization of Immune Molecules. Bacteria may spontaneously release surface molecules that bind to and neutralize antibody. These include endotoxin from gram-negative bacteria, capsular antigens from *S. pneumoniae* and *N. meningitidis,* and protein A from *S. aureus.* During infection the blood may contain high levels of complexes between antibody and bacterial antigen. At certain antigen-antibody ratios the complexes will deposit in the kidney, joints, and other target organs and initiate type III hypersensitivity reactions (Chapter 8).

Complement Evasion. Complement is a major component of the defense against bacterial infection through production of opsonin (C3b) and chemotactic factors (C3a, C5a) for neutrophils. Teichoic acid in the Gram-positive cell wall provides resistance against complement-mediated lysis.[14] *Staphylococcus* produces proteins that inhibit complement activity, including C3 and C5 convertases, C5, C2, and the C5a receptor that mediates complement-induced chemotaxis.[15] Bacterial regulatory proteins (e.g., *Borrelia* complement-regulator-acquiring protein, *Neisseria* porins, and members of the *Streptococcus* M protein family) affect complement activation, including destabilization of the C3 convertase complex or degradation of the opsonin C3b.

Immune Suppression. Although more prominent in viral infections, some bacterial pathogens can broadly suppress immune responses against their own antigens as well as other antigens unrelated to the infectious agent. Chronic bacterial infections, like leprosy *(M. leprae)* and tuberculosis *(M. tuberculosis)* induce anergy (suppressed response to multiple antigens) in infected hosts. *H. pylori* can release LPS that binds to dendritic cells and blocks development of Th1 cells, as well as produce toxins that block the T cell IL-2 receptor signaling pathway, thus inhibiting maturation of Th cells. *N. gonorrhoeae* pili antigens bind to adhesion molecules on CD4+ cells and prevent their activation.

Tissue Damage

Bacterial infections damage tissue either directly by means of bacterial products or indirectly as a result of inflammation.[12] Many toxins break down tissue directly. These include a large variety of proteases, lipases, hyaluronidase, hemolysins, and many others discussed above. Some bacterial diseases arise completely from the systemic effects of toxins. Diphtheria is a respiratory tract infection *(Corynebacterium diphtheriae)* with systemic complications caused by toxin that inhibits messenger ribonucleic acid (mRNA) translation and causes low blood pressure, necrosis in the heart and liver, degeneration of myelin sheaths, and death. Gastrointestinal pathogens *(V. cholerae, Salmonella, Shigella, E. coli)* may produce enterotoxins that are cytotoxic and alter the permeability of intestinal cells leading to diarrheal diseases.

Clostridia are anaerobic bacteria that produce some of the most powerful toxins known. One type of food poisoning is caused by *Clostridium botulinum* that produces a paralytic neurotoxin (botulinum toxin) that blocks the release of acetylcholine at nerve-muscle synapses and results in flaccid paralysis. Infection of deep wounds with *C. tetani* results in release of a neurotoxin that causes severe muscle spasms, spastic paralysis of the voluntary muscles, and potentially death. *C. perfringens* produces multiple toxins that cause gas gangrene. One of these, alpha toxin, is a lecithinase that destroys the infected tissue by digesting cellular plasma membranes. Infection of the colon with *Clostridium difficile* results in watery diarrhea from toxins that damage the mucosa.

Bacterial superantigens are toxins that increase the adherence between major histocompatibilitiy complex (MHC) class II proteins on antigen-presenting cells and the T-cell receptor. Because the effect is independent of antigen, a large population of T cells is activated and overproduces proinflammatory cytokines, such as IL-1, IL-6, and TNF-α. Superantigens are responsible for several diseases, including food poisoning (enterotoxins of *S. aureus* and *C. perfringens*), toxic shock syndrome (toxic shock syndrome toxin [TSST] of *S. aureus*), and scarlet fever (erythrogenic toxin of *S. pyogenes*).

Inflammation is the body's initial response to the presence of the bacteria.[16] Vascular permeability is increased, allowing blood-borne substances (e.g., the complement system) involved in bacterial destruction to access the site of infection. The release of anaphylatoxins (C5a and C3a) of the complement cascade may increase the inflammatory response and lead to an increase in capillary permeability sufficient to permit the escape of large volumes of plasma, contributing to hypotension and, in severe cases, cardiovascular shock (see Chapter 46). Many persistent bacterial infections (e.g., *M. tuberculosis*) may lead to formation of *granulomas,* which diminishes the function of the affected organ (e.g., the lung).[17]

The release of a sufficient amount of endotoxin can lead to fatal **endotoxic shock (septic shock),** which is one of the leading causes of death in intensive care units.[18] The usual cause is proliferation of gram-negative bacteria, although shock may be caused by a few gram-positive bacteria and fungi. Once in the blood, endotoxins cause the release of vasoactive peptides and cytokines that affect blood vessels, producing vasodilation, which reduces blood pressure, causes decreased oxygen delivery, and produces subsequent cardiovascular shock (see Figure 9-3 and Chapter 46). Endotoxin can activate the coagulation cascade, leading to the syndrome of disseminated (or diffuse) intravascular coagulation (see Chapter 27). Additionally, endotoxin induces the release of TNF-α (cachectin) by macrophages. TNF is a potent proinflammatory cytokine that is also called *cachectin* because of its role in promoting cachexia in individuals with cancer. (Cachexia is discussed in Chapter 11; cytokines are discussed in Chapters 6 and 7.)

Example of Bacterial Pathogenesis

S. aureus has become a major cause of hospital-acquired (nosocomial) infections.[19] This microorganism is a common commensal inhabitant of normal skin and nasal passages (about 30% of individuals are nasal carriers) and can be transmitted by direct skin-to-skin contact or contact with shared items or surfaces that have become contaminated from someone else's infection (e.g., towels, used bandages).

Skin infections may occur at sites of trauma, such as cuts and abrasions, and at areas of the body covered by hair (e.g., back of neck, groin, buttock, armpit, beard area of men). Most infections are relatively mild and localized, appearing as red and swollen pustules on the skin, containing pus or other drainage (Figure 9-5). They can develop into abscesses, boils, carbuncles, cellulitis, or furunculosis. Invasive disease may originate from wound infections (e.g., trauma, surgical wounds, indwelling medical devices, prosthetic

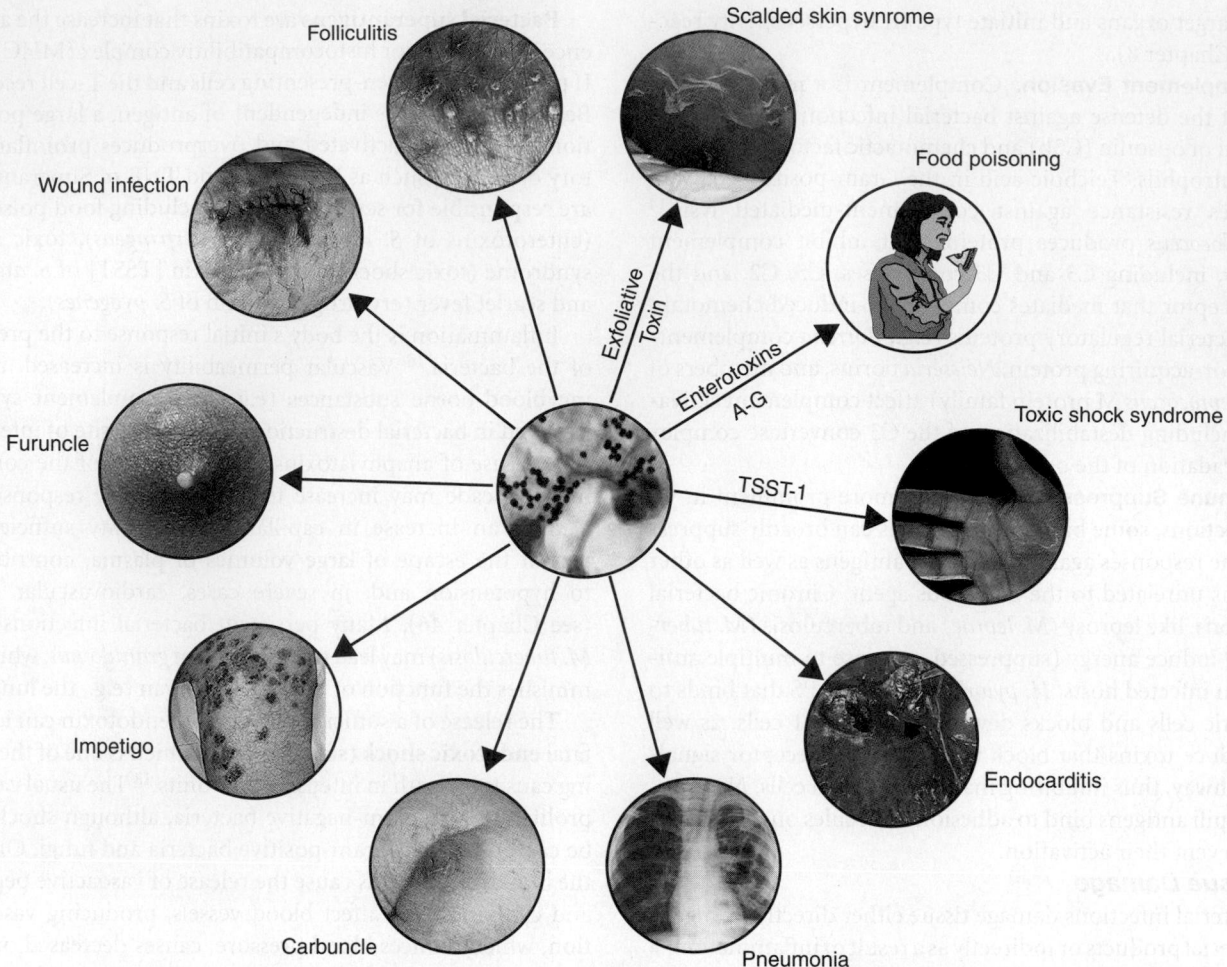

Figure 9-5 Staphylococcus aureus infections. Different strains of *S. aureus* (gram-positive cocci in sputum from an individual with pneumonia *[center photograph]*) cause a variety of infections. The particular infection may depend on the toxin produced: exfoliative toxin (scalded skin syndrome), enterotoxins A-G (food poisoning), or toxic-shock syndrome toxin-1 (TSST-1; Toxic shock syndrome, carbuncle, impetigo, and wound infection photos from Cohen J and Powderly WG: *Infectious diseases,* ed 2, St. Louis, 2004, Mosby. Folliculitis photo from Goldman L and Ausiello D: *Cecil medicine,* ed 23, Philadelphia, 2008, Saunders. Center photo and photos of food poisoning and endocarditis from Kumar V et al: *Robbins & Cotran Pathologic basis of disease,* ed 7, Philadelphia, 2005, Saunders. Furuncle photo from Long S et al: *Principles and practice of pediatric infectious diseases,* ed 3, Philadelphia, 2009, Saunders. Scalded skin syndrome and pneumonia photos from Mandell G et al: *Principles and practice of infectious diseases,* ed 6, Philadelphia, 2005, Churchill Livingstone.)

joints) and lead to fatal septicemia and abscesses in internal organs (e.g., lungs, kidney, bones, skeletal muscle, meninges, or heart).

Adherence to tissue is mediated by surface proteins that attach to connective tissue (laminin, fibrin, fibronectin) and endothelium. Attachment to collagen occurs in osteomyelitis and septic arthritis-causing strains, and capsular polysaccharide mediate attachment to prosthetic devices.

Staphylococci also produce very effective polysaccharide capsules that protect against phagocytosis as well as surface protein A that binds IgG by the Fc portion and masks Sbacterial antigens under a surface of self-proteins.[20] Many pathogenic strains have increased resistance to intracellular oxidative killing when engulfed by a phagocyte.

Invasion is mediated by a variety of toxins, including membrane-damaging toxins (α-toxin, which forms pores

in membranes; hemolysin, which destroys erythrocytes; β-toxin, which is a sphingomyelinase; δ-toxin, a detergent-like toxin; leukocidin, which lyses phagocytes), coagulase (causes clots), staphylokinase (breaks down of clots), exfoliatin toxins (causes separation of epidermis resulting in scalded skin syndrome), lipase (degrades lipids on skin surface; facilitates abscess formation), and a variety of enterotoxins.[21] Many of the enterotoxins are superantigens that are responsible for staphylococcal food poisoning with diarrhea and vomiting and toxic shock syndrome. Each infectious strain of *S. aureus* produces a few of these toxins so that strains may differ in their capacities to cause particular diseases, thus different strains can cause purulent dermal infections, food poisoning, or toxic shock syndrome.

Antibiotic resistance has become a major problem with *S. aureus*.[19] For several decades pathogenic strains have commonly produced β-**lactamase,** an enzyme that destroys penicillin. More recently staphylococci have developed resistance (methicillin-resistant *Staphylococcus aureus* [MRSA]) to broad spectrum antibiotics, including methicillin-like antibiotics, which were widely used to treat penicillin-resistant microorganisms.

Fungal Infections

Fungi are eukaryotic microorganisms with thick rigid cell walls and the capacity to form a variety of complex structures (Figure 9-6). Fungi may grow as a **mold** with branched filaments or a meshwork mycelium structure (e.g., *Aspergillus* spp., causing aspergillosis), **yeast** with ovoid or spherical shapes (*C. albicans*, which causes candidiasis), or **dimorphic** with a yeastlike appearance in tissue and mycelium in culture (e.g., *Histoplasma capsulatum*, which causes histoplasmosis, a systemic respiratory disease). The cell wall is composed of polysaccharides that differ from the peptidoglycans of bacteria and are thus are resistant to bacterial cell wall inhibitors such as penicillin and cephalosporin. In contrast to bacteria, the cytosol of fungi contains organelles: mitochondria, Golgi apparatus, microtubules, microvesicles, endoplasmic reticulum, and nuclei. Molds are aerobic, and yeasts are facultative anaerobes. Common pathologic fungi are summarized in Table 9-7.

Fungi are diagnosed by microscopic observation of specimens treated with potassium hydroxide and stained to enhance visualization of spheres and filaments. Specimens also can be cultured. Skin tests are available for species of *Aspergillus*. Many of the antifungal drugs (e.g., amphotericin B, ketoconazole, fluconazole) used to treat deep or systemic infections are toxic to the host because the fungal cell composition is similar to the human cell.

Transmission and Colonization

Infection with a fungus is called **mycosis.** Most pathogenic fungi (e.g., *H. capsulatum*, *Coccidioides immitis*, *Blastomyces dermatitidis*) grow as saprophytes in the environment and are transmitted by inhalation or contamination of wounds. The majority of medically relevant fungi either exist as human commensals or cause relatively mild infections (superficial mycoses) of the skin, nails, hair, and mucous membranes of the mouth and vagina. These include dermatophytes (e.g., tineas, which refers to several skin mycoses including ringworm, athlete's foot, and others) or yeasts (e.g., *Candida*, *Aspergillus*, *Cryptococcus*).

Human-to-human transmission is only a concern with dermatophyte infections. Systemic mycosis caused by pathogenic fungi generally results from inhalation of spores present in a contaminated environment and initially presents as a pulmonary infection. Infection that disseminates to other

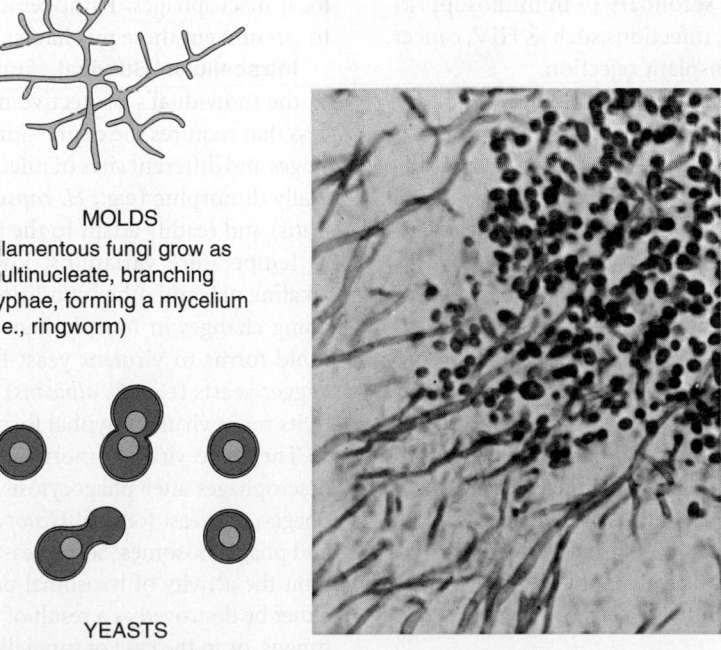

MOLDS
Filamentous fungi grow as multinucleate, branching hyphae, forming a mycelium (i.e., ringworm)

YEASTS
Yeasts grow as ovoid or spherical; single cells multiply by budding and division (i.e., *Histoplasma*)

Figure 9-6 Morphology of fungi. Fungi may be either mold or yeast forms, or dimorphic. The photograph shows *Candida albicans* with both the mycelial and the yeast forms. (A from Mims CA et al: *Medical microbiology,* ed 3, London, 2004, Mosby; B from Townsend C et al: *Sabiston textbook of surgery,* ed 18, Philadelphia, 2008, Saunders.)

Table 9-7	Common Pathogenic Fungi		
Primary Site of Infection	**Fungus**	**Disease (Primary)**	**Symptoms**
Superficial (no tissue invasion, little inflammation)	*Malassezia furfur*	Tinea versicolor, seborrheic dermatitis, dandruff	Red rash on body
Cutaneous (no tissue invasion, inflammatory response)	Dermatophytes		
	Trichophyton mentagrophytes	Tinea pedis (athlete's foot)	Scaling, fissures, itching
	Trichophyton rubrum	Tinea cruris (jock itch)	Rash, itching
	Microsporum canis	Tinea corporis (ringworm)	Lesion, raised border, scaling.
	Candida albicans	Cutaneous candidiasis	Lesions in most areas of skin, mucous membranes, thrush, vaginal infection
Subcutaneous (tissue invasion)	*Sporothrix schenckii*	Sporotrichosis	Ulcers or abscesses on skin and other organ systems
Systemic (dimorphic; causes disease in healthy individuals)	*Stachybotrys chartarum* or "black mold"	Black mold disease	Rash, headaches, nausea, pains
	Coccidioides immitis	Coccidioidomycosis	Valley fever, flulike symptoms
	Histoplasma capsulatum	Histoplasmosis	Lung, flulike symptoms, disseminates to multiple organs, eye
	Blastomyces dermatitidis	Blastomycosis	Flulike symptoms, chest pains
Systemic (opportunistic)	*Aspergillus fumigatus, Aspergillus flavus*	Aspergillosis	Invasive to lungs and other organs
	Pneumocystis jiroveci	Pneumocystis pneumonia (PCP)	Pneumonia
	Cryptococcus neoformans	Cryptococcosis	Pneumonia-like illness, skin lesions, disseminates to brain, meningitis
	Candidia albicans	Systemic candidiasis	Sepsis, endocarditis, meningitis

organs can be life threatening. Systemic mycosis caused by opportunistic fungi is usually secondary to immunosuppression caused by genetic defects, infections such as HIV, cancer, and drugs used to prevent transplant rejection.

Specific adherence to epithelium is provided by several polysaccharides on the fungal surface. Glucan, mannan, glycoprotein, and chitin molecules adhere with host receptors, including Toll-like receptors (TLRs), mannose receptors, dectin-1, and cadherins, respectively. A cell wall adhesion molecule, agglutinin-like sequence (ALS3), on several fungi (e.g., *C. albicans*) promotes adherence to epithelial cells as well as silicone, thus facilitating infection of implants and other medical devices.

In 2006, the opportunist pathogen *Pneumocystis carinii* was reclassified as a fungus, and the specific variant that infects humans was renamed *Pneumocystis jiroveci*.[22] Despite the official change in nomenclature, much of the literature will continue to use *P. carinii* for some time. As with many fungi and protozoa, *Pneumocystis* has two life-cycle forms: a trophic form and the cyst form. Two surface proteins, glycoprotein A (gpA) and major surface glycoprotein (MSG), mediate attachment to alveolar epithelial cells.

Invasion and Evasion

The host defense against fungal infection includes the fungistatic properties of neutrophils and macrophages. T lymphocytes are crucial in limiting the extent of infection and producing cytokines to further activate macrophages. Human host defense against the inhaled spores begins with the mucous layer and the ciliary action in the respiratory tract,

which then remove the fungus or facilitate phagocytosis by local macrophages. Pathogenic fungi have developed means to circumvent these mechanisms (see Table 9-6).

Intracellular Survival. Fungal virulence and resistance to the individual's protective mechanisms is a complex process that requires the expression of multiple genes at different stages and different sites of infection. Pathologic fungi are generally dimorphic (e.g., *H. capsulatum, B. dermatitidis, C. immitis*) and readily adapt to the host environment, responding to temperature variations, low oxygen environment, more alkaline pH, and other conditions in the host tissue by undergoing changes in morphology and switching from avirulent mold forms to virulent yeast forms. Similar conditions also trigger yeasts (e.g., *C. albicans*) to switch from the yeast form to its more virulent hyphal form.

The more virulent morphologies allow fungi to survive in macrophages after phagocytosis. After phagocytosis by macrophages, the yeast form of *Histoplasma* replicates in phagosomes and phagolysosomes. Some yeast may produce proteins that inhibit the activity of lysosomal proteases. The macrophage may either be destroyed as a result of membrane modification by the fungus, or in the case of fungi like *Histoplasma,* harbor the fungus in granulomas. Breakdown of the granulomas over time may result in release of viable fungi and recurrence of the infection.

Protection Against Phagocytosis. Encapsulated yeast cells (e.g., *Cryptococcus neoformans*) are more resistant to phagocytosis than unencapsulated yeast. The cryptococcal polysaccharide capsule is antiphagocytic by blocking recognition by macrophages and may also be immunosuppressive by inhibiting migration of leukocytes into the site of fungal infection. *Aspergillus fumigatus* and many other fungi produce toxic metabolites (e.g., gliotoxin) that inhibit macrophage and neutrophil phagocytosis. Molecules like gliotoxin may also be immunosuppressive, including suppression of mast cell activation, degranulation, and secretion of leukotrienes and cytokines.

Antigenic Variation. Altered antigen expression affords protection against the developing immune responses, although this defense strategy is rarely used by fungal pathogens. *Pneumocystis* contains approximately 80 different gpA and MSG genes, only one of which is expressed at a time.[23] Modulation of these antigens may provide resistance against immune destruction.

Immunosuppression. Several yeasts stimulate the production of immunosuppressive cytokines, resulting in downregulation of some aspects of the host's immune response. The yeast *C. neoformans* suppresses inflammation by inhibiting production of the proinflammatory cytokines TNF-α and IL-12 and inducing production of the anti-inflammatory cytokine IL-10. The overall result is suppression of macrophage function and protection against killing.

Tissue Damage

Fungal infections damage tissue directly by secretion of enzymes and indirectly by initiating an inflammatory response. Secreted enzymes, such as proteases, phospholipases, and elastases, damage cells and intercellular matrix, leading to necrosis. Many molds secrete mycotoxins when grown in environmental locations, such as on nuts, beans, and grains. Ingestion of this toxin affects muscle coordination, causes tremors, and may be fatal. Some fungal toxins may cause cancer; aflatoxins produced by some *Aspergillus* are especially carcinogenic.[24]

The typical immune and inflammatory reaction against fungal infections involves a cell-mediated response with infiltration of T cells and macrophages, as well as neutrophils.[16] The inflammatory site is rich in proinflammatory cytokines. Fungal infections can be very difficult for these systems to eradicate, leading to progressively increasing production of cytokines. Thus, as the host's response increases so do the destructive effects on surrounding healthy tissue. In cases of persistent infection, granulomas form and compromise the normal function of the infected tissue.

Example of Fungal Pathogenesis

Candida albicans is the most common cause of fungal infections in humans. It is an opportunistic yeast that is a commensal in the normal flora of many healthy individuals, residing in the skin, gastrointestinal tract, mouth (30% to 55% of healthy individuals), and vagina (20% of healthy women) and normally under the control of local defense mechanisms, including members of the bacterial flora that produce antifungal agents.[25] In healthy individuals, particularly those whose normal flora has been disturbed by antibiotic therapy (e.g., diminished levels of *Lactobacillus* in the vaginal flora), *Candida* overgrowth may occur resulting in vaginitis or oropharyngeal infection (thrush). In those with an intact immune system the infection remains localized.

In immunocompromised individuals, particularly those with diminished levels of neutrophils (neutropenia), disseminated infection may occur.[26] *Candida* is the most common fungal infection in people with cancer (particularly acute leukemia and other hematologic cancers), transplantation (bone marrow and solid organ), and HIV/AIDS. Almost 90% of people with AIDS have *Candida* at least one time during the disease, although infection is usually contained locally (thrush or vaginitis) because of adequate numbers of neutrophils (Figure 9-7). Invasive candidiasis may also be secondary to indwelling catheters, intravenous lines, or peritoneal dialysis, which provides direct entrance into the blood.

Disseminated candidiasis may involve several internal organs, including abscesses in the kidney, brain, liver, and heart, and is characterized by persistent or recurrent fever, gram-negative shocklike symptoms (hypotension, tachycardia), disseminated intravascular coagulation (DIC), and death.[27] The mortality rates of sepsis or disseminated candidiasis are in the range of 30% to 40%.

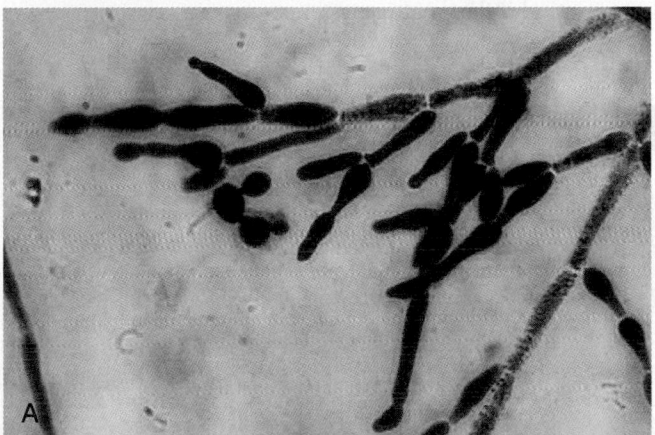

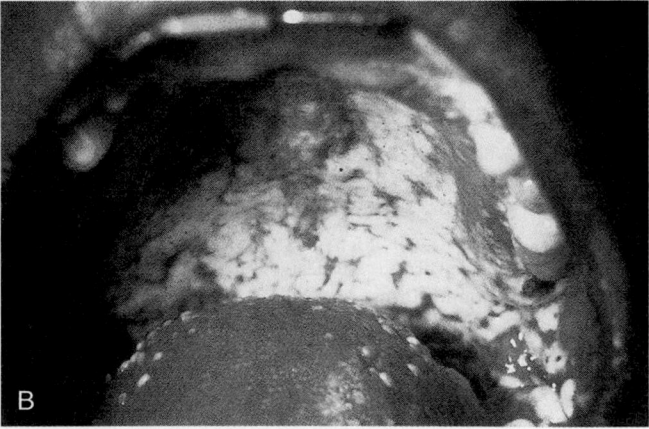

Figure 9-7 *Candida albicans.* Gram stain *(upper photograph)* of sputum showing chains of elongated budding yeasts of *C. albicans* producing pseudohyphae (×1000). Oral candidiasis (thrush) *(lower photograph).* (A from McPherson R, Pincus M: *Henry's clinical diagnosis and management by laboratory methods,* ed 21, Philadelphia, 2006, Saunders; B from Mandell G, Bennett J, Dolin R: *Principles and practice of infectious diseases,* ed 6, Philadelphia, 2005, Churchill Livingstone.)

Like most pathogenic yeasts, *Candida* undergoes morphologic changes from unicellular yeast to filamentous hyphal forms under conditions of neutral to alkaline pH, elevated temperature, and host serum factors. Switching of morphology results in altered profiles of surface antigens and increased resistance to immunologic destruction as well as altered tissue adhesion specificity.[28] *Candida* expresses diverse surface adhesion molecules that permit adherence to materials in implants, epithelium, extracellular matrix (fibronectin, laminin, collagen), and leukocytes and facilitate invasion into tissue. One surface adherence molecule is a glycoprotein, INT1p (integrator complex subunit 1), which specifically binds to integrins. EAP1 (enhanced adhesion to plastic) is a glycoprotein that permits *Candida* to bind to epithelial cells and a variety of synthetic materials found in implants.

Candida secretes several enzymes that function as virulence factors and contribute to tissue destruction.[27] Acid proteases and phospholipases damage the cell membrane and enhance invasive capacity. Secreted aspartic proteinases (Saps) increase the virulence of *Candida* by destroying cell membranes and removing surface molecules, including from cells of the immune and inflammatory systems.

Candida may suppress the host's immune system. Production of the cytokine granulocyte-monocyte colony-stimulating factor (GM-CSF), suppresses monocyte/macrophage function, including the production of components of the complement cascade. Decreased production of C3 results in less opsonization (C3b) and production of chemotactic activity (C3a) for phagocytes.

Parasitic and Protozoan Infections

Parasitic organisms establish symbiosis with another species in which the parasite benefits at the expense of the other species. Parasites range from unicellular protozoan to large worms. Parasitic worms (helminths) include intestinal and tissue nematodes (e.g., hookworm, roundworm), flukes (e.g., liver fluke, lung fluke), and tapeworms. A protozoan is a eukaryotic, unicellular microorganism with a nucleus and cytoplasm. Pathogenic protozoa include malaria *(Plasmodium)*, amoebae (e.g., *Entamoeba histolytica*, which causes amoebic dysentery), and flagellates (e.g., *Giardia lamblia,* which causes diarrhea; *Trypanosoma*, which causes sleeping sickness). Although less common in the United States, parasites and protozoa are common causes of infections worldwide, with a significant effect on the mortality and morbidity of individuals in developing countries. Important parasites of humans are listed in Table 9-8.

Table 9-8	Parasites That Are Important in Humans			
Category	Subgroup	Species	Disease	Organs Affected/Symptoms
Protozoa	Amoeboid	*Entamoeba histolytica*	Amebiasis	Dysentary, liver abscess
	Flagellate	*Giardia lamblia*	Giardiasis*	Diarrhea
		Leishmania donovani, L. tropica	Leishmaniasis	Sores on skin, progression to liver, spleen
		Trichomonas vaginalis	Trichomoniasis	Inflammation of reproductive organs
		Trypanosoma cruzi, T. brucei	Chagas disease: African sleeping sickness	Generalized, blood, lymph nodes, progressing to cardiac and central nervous system (CNS)
	Ciliate	*Balantidium coli*	Balantidiasis	Small intestines, invasion of colon, diarrhea
	Sporozoa (nonmotile)	*Cryptosporidium parvum, C. hominis*	Cryptosporidiosis*	Intestine, diarrhea
		Plasmodium spp.	Malaria	Blood, liver
		Toxoplasma gondii	Toxoplasmosis*	Intestine, eyes, blood, heart, liver
Helminths	Flukes (trematodes)	*Fasciola hepatica*	Fasciolosis	Liver destruction
		Paragonimus westermani	Lung fluke disease	Granuloma in lung, spinal cord
		Schistosoma mansoni	Schistosomiasis	Blood, diarrhea, bladder, generalized symptoms
	Tapeworms (cestodes)	*Taenia solium*	Pork tapeworm	Encysts in muscle, brain, liver
	Roundworms (nematodes)	*Ascaris lumbricoides*	Ascariasis	Intestinal obstruction, bile duct obstruction
		Necator americanus (hookworm)	Hookworm disease	Intestinal parasite
		Trichuris trichiura (whipworm)	Trichuriasis	Diarrhea
		Trichinella spiralis	Trichinosis*	Intestine, diarrhea, muscle, CNS, death
		Wuchereria bancrofti	Filariasis, elephantiasis	Lymphatics
		Enterobius vermicularis (pinworm)	Pinworm infection	Intestines
		Strongyloides stercoralis (threadworm)	Strongyloidiasis	Intestinal parasite, skin infection
		Onchocerca volvulus	Onchocerciasis	Blindness, dermatitis

*Most common in the United States.

Transmission and Colonization

Parasitic and protozoal infections are rarely transmitted from human to human. The predominant means is through vectors in which the organism spends part of its life cycle. Examples include the transmission of malaria (*Plasmodium* spp.) by mosquitoes, trypanosomes (*Trypanosoma cruzi*, which causes Chagas disease in South America; *Trypanosoma brucei*, which causes sleeping sickness in Africa) by the tsetse fly, and *Leishmania* spp. by sand fleas. Many of the protozoal infectious agents (e.g., *E. histolytica*, *G. lamblia*) are encountered in contaminated water or food and transmission is by ingestion.

The initial attachment depends on whether the microorganism is injected into the bloodstream by a vector or whether entrance is through the gastrointestinal tract. Microorganisms in the bloodstream frequently have surface lectins that react with carbohydrates on specific cells. Malarial parasites attach to erythrocytes that express Duffy blood group antigens. Thus Duffy-negative individuals are resistant to malaria. *T. cruzi* can infect both CD4- and CD8-postive T cells through a T-cell surface receptor. Several parasites express surface glycoproteins that facilitate preferential entrance into monocytes/macrophages using various receptors, including the receptors for complement component C3b (*Leishmania* spp.). *Leishmania* expresses a surface glycoprotein (gp63) that is necessary for its entrance into macrophages. The gp63 molecule binds complement components (C3b, C3bi) and uses the macrophage complement receptors. *E. histolytica* expresses two surface proteins that react with the disaccharide galactose/*N*-acetylgalactosamine on epithelium.

Invasion and Evasion

An effective immune response varies depending on the particular parasite or protozoan. Intercellular pathogens are susceptible to cell-mediated immunity and activation of macrophages by T cells. Other organisms are more sensitive to antibody, particularly used in antibody-dependent cell-mediated cytotoxicity (ADCC) by macrophages and natural killer (NK) cells. Many helminth infections are sensitive to damage by eosinophils, which are attracted by IgE-mediated mast cell degranulation and release of eosinophil chemotactic factor of anaphylaxis (ECF-A). Evasion of the individual's defenses is accomplished by several means (see Table 9-6).[29]

Intracellular Survival. *Leishmania* spp. are obligative intracellular parasites of monocytes/macrophages.[30] They are protected from being killed in the phagosome and phagolysosome in which they multiply. Protection may be afforded by a surface protein that inhibits fusion of lysosomes to the phagosome, thus decreasing the amount of degradative enzymes within the phagolysosome. *Toxoplasma* spp. may be protected by entrance into a variety of cells, including macrophages.[31] The probability of survival is increased by inhibiting fusion of lysosomes with the phagosome. Many of the intracellular organisms are sensitive to macrophage activation by T cells. *T. cruzi* bypasses the effects of macrophage activation by escaping from the phagosome and growing in the macrophage cytoplasm.

Protection Against Phagocytosis. Because many unicellular parasites survive within macrophages, the development of antiphagocytic capsules does not seem to be a major protective strategy. In some cases, a surface glycocalyx may function in a similar fashion as capsules to mask surface antigens from binding antibody. Some organisms produce toxins to protect themselves against phagocytosis; *E. histolytica* releases phospholipase and pore-forming proteins that disrupt the phagocyte's plasma membrane.

Coating with Self-Proteins. Pathogens that coat themselves with human proteins may be disguised and "fool" the immune system. Schistosomes and trypanosomes mask their antigens by absorbing IgG by the Fc portion of the molecule.

Antigenic Variation. In general, those organisms that undergo part of their life cycle in humans or may assume multiple morphologic forms will also undergo antigenic changes related to the stage in the life cycle or morphology. Some protozoa have developed very complex alterations in surface antigens using **gene switching**. Infection with African trypanosomes may lead to fatal neurologic disease. During infection protective antibody is produced against surface antigens called variable surface glycoproteins (VSGs). An IgG or IgM response will successfully kill most of protozoa. However, a small percentage will undergo a gene shift that results in a change in VSG. The existing antibodies will not recognize the new VSG, and the level of schistosomes will rebound, causing recurrent disease. The schistosome has genetic information (about 10% of the genome) for hundreds of variations in VSG, which are expressed one at a time. Thus the organism undergoes periodic shifts in VSG expression, resulting in periodicity of parasites in the blood. A similar process occurs in some helminths (*Trichinella spiralis*).

Degradation of Immune Molecules. If a microorganism is sensitive to a particular component of the immune or inflammatory system, a survival advantage is obtained by production of enzymes that specifically degrade that component. Schistosomes secrete an enzyme that diminishes the effectiveness of IgG by specifically removing a critical peptide. *E. histolytica* secretes a protease that can degrade IgG and IgA.

Neutralization of Immune Molecules. Large parasitic organisms may release large amount of soluble antigen to neutralize antibody.

Complement Evasion. Complement activation is effective against several parasites.[14] Some parasites (e.g., *Echinococcus* spp., *Leishmania* spp.) produce complement regulatory proteins that affect complement function by destabilizing C3 convertase or promoting degradation of C3b. Trypanosomes produce complement regulatory factors, including a surface gp63-like molecule, that confer resistance to complement. *E. histolytica* produces complement regulatory factors that inactivate C3a and C5a, thus inhibiting phagocyte chemotaxis activity.

Immune Suppression. Parasites may produce both pathogen-specific and nonspecific immune suppression.[32] The release of large amounts of soluble antigen may induce specific tolerance to the pathogen as well as induce dysfunctional macrophage antigen processing. The function of immune cells is directly blocked by secretion of cytotoxic molecules *(T. spiralis)*, selective inhibitors of T-cell function (schistosomes), or inducers of polyclonal B-cell activation (B-cell mitogen released by trypanosomes).

E. histolytica induces T-cell hyporesponsiveness by induction of IL-4 and IL-10 that down-regulate maturation of Th cells. The VSG molecules of African trypanosomes stimulate macrophages to overproduce TNF-α and CD8-positive cells to secrete high levels of IFN-γ, which impairs T-cell responses. *Leishmania* has developed an interesting approach to circumventing antigen processing by macrophages. This pathogen adsorbs IgG, which binds to the macrophage Fc receptor, resulting in the hyperproduction of IL-10 and suppression of IL-12 from infected macrophages. IL-10 prevents macrophage responses to IFN-γ, allowing the parasites to survive even in the immunologically intact individual.

Tissue Damage

Tissue damage may result directly by parasitic infestation in the tissue or be secondary to the individual's immune and inflammatory responses. The particular process depends a great deal on burden of parasites infesting the site and sensitivity of the particular site to damage. Large infestations may lead to physical loss of function in a tissue or organ. For instance, a large number of intestinal parasites (e.g., the roundworm *Ascaris lumbricoides*, tapeworms, *Giardia* spp.) compete for and prevent uptake of nutrients, leading to various forms of malabsorption, blocked uptake of fats, or anemia from malabsorption of B_{12} or from large amounts of blood loss. Filarial parasites (e.g., *Wuchereria bancrofti* and *Brugia malayi*, which causes elephantiasis) block the lymphatics and cause accumulation of lymph in tissues. The larvae of tapeworms (e.g., *Taenia solium*) encyst in and prevent normal function of organs (e.g., muscle, liver, eye), which is particularly dangerous in the human brain.

Toxins released from the parasite may cause significant irreversible organ damage. Proteolytic enzymes from *E. histolytica* are very cytolytic leading to ulceration of intestinal walls, bloody diarrhea, amoebic dysentery, dehydration, and death in infants and young children. *T. cruzi* secretes a neurotoxin that affects the anatomic nervous system, a small-molecular-weight toxin that causes fever, and proteases and phospholipases, leading to tissue destruction.

The infected individual's immune and inflammatory responses result in considerable histopathology.[33] Schistosomiasis results in the deposition of eggs in organs (e.g., the liver), which leads to formation of granulomas and tissue destruction through fibrosis. Some parasitic products (*T. brucei*, malarial parasites) activate macrophages to overproduce cytokines, which leads to exacerbated inflammation.[34] The IgE produced against parasitic worms is protective, but can also stimulate excessive degranulation of mast cells and even anaphylactic shock. Polyclonal B-cell activation leads to broad spectrum of autoantibodies that may precipitate autoimmune diseases. Overproduction of antigens by some pathogens (e.g., malaria, trypanosomiasis, schistosomiasis) may lead to excessive levels of pathogenic circulating immune complexes and initiation of type III hypersensitivity reactions (Chapter 8) in the kidneys and vasculature.

Example of Parasitic Pathogenesis

Malaria is one of the most common infections worldwide.[35] Yearly an estimated 400 million cases occur, with about 1 million deaths. Four species infect humans: *Plasmodium falciparum* (accounts for most fatalities), *Plasmodium vivax*, *Plasmodium ovale* (both of which are more benign), and *Plasmodium malariae*. The four strains differ in disease severity and incidence of fever. Infection with *P. falciparum*, the most severe form, results in severe chills, high fever, sweating, headache, muscle pains, vomiting, severe anemia, pulmonary edema, and many other complications. Neurologic complications may result from infected red blood cells (RBCs) adhering to endothelium in capillaries of the brain. The individual may develop cardiovascular collapse, shock, coma, and death.

Transmission is through the bite of an infected female *Anopheles* mosquito, where the microorganism grows in the salivary gland. The infectious form enters the bloodstream, survives in the liver and invades parenchymal cells. After several rounds of division, the liver cell ruptures, and several thousand parasites enter the blood, where they infect red blood cells (Figure 9-8).[36] Multiplication occurs in RBCs,

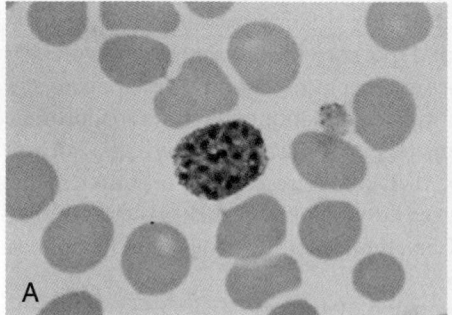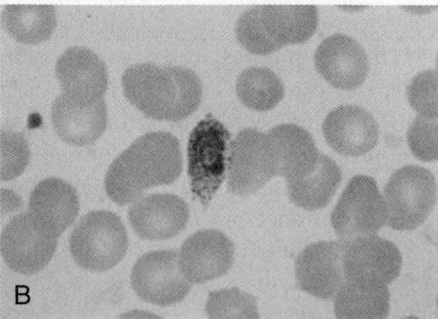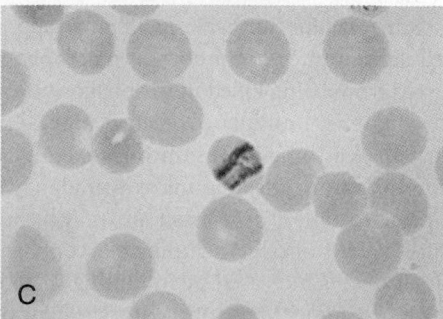

Figure 9-8 Malaria. Giemsa-stained smears. **A,** *Plasmodium vivax* schizont. **B,** *Plasmodium ovale* trophozoite. **C,** Characteristic band from trophozoite of *Plasmodium malariae* containing intracellular pigment hemozoin. (From Kliegman R et al: *Nelson textbook of pediatrics,* ed 18, St Louis, 2007, Saunders.)

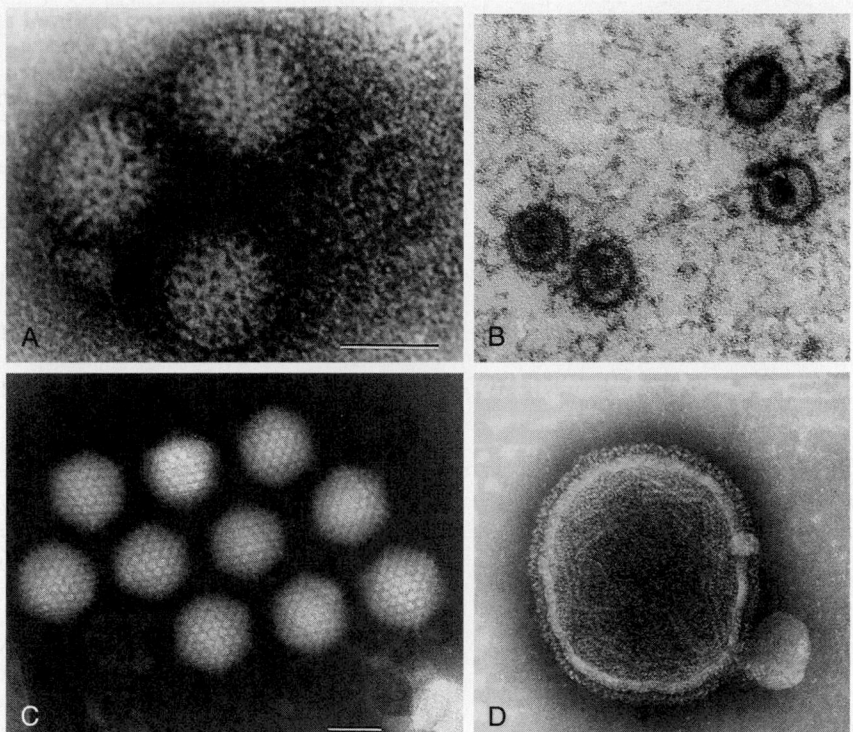

Figure 9-9 Electron micrographs of representative viral structures. **A,** Rotavirus: particles with a double shell and a characteristic "wheel-and-spoke" appearance. **B,** Epstein-Barr virus: icosahedral enveloped DNA virus. **C,** Adenovirus: particles with characteristic icosahedral structures. **D,** Paramyxovirus: spherical enveloped RNA virus. RNA is seen spilling out of the disrupted virus. (**A** and **C** from Kumar V et al: *Robbins and Cotran pathologic basis of disease,* ed 7, Philadelphia, 2005, Saunders; **B** and **D** from Long S, Pickering L, Prober C: *Principles and practice of pediatric infectious diseases,* ed 3, Philadelphia, 2008, Churchill Livingstone.)

resulting in the release of daughter parasites that reinfect other erythrocytes.

P. vivax and *P. ovale* malaria can remain dormant in the liver for years, protected from the immune system by intracellular residence. The parasite in the blood avoids destruction by phagocytes in the spleen by expressing adhesion proteins that cause adherence and sequestration along the walls of the small vessels. Additionally, *P. falciparum* undergoes gene switching among about 60 different antigenic variants of antigens expressed on the surface of infected erythrocytes (*P. falciparum* erythrocyte membrane protein, *Pf*EMP).[37] Malaria induces a form of immune suppression. CD4 and CD8 T cells are diminished and lymphocytes from individuals infected with *P. falciparum* do not proliferate in the presence of *Pf*EMP antigen in vitro.

Viral Infection and Injury

Viruses are extremely simple microorganisms and do not possess any of the metabolic organelles found in prokaryotes (e.g., bacteria) or eukaryotes (e.g., human cells). The basic viral structure (virion) consists of nucleic acid protected by a protein shell, the capsid. The capsid may take many characteristic shapes; helical, icosahedral, or large pleiomorphic (poxvirus) (Figure 9-9). Some viruses also have a protective envelope surrounding the capsid, which consists of the plasma membrane from the previously infected cell.

Viruses are classified by the format of nucleic acid in the virion, which may be RNA or deoxyribonucleic acid (DNA), and either single-stranded (ss) or double-stranded (ds), and whether the virus uses the enzyme reverse transcriptase (RT) for replication. Thus seven classifications are used: ds-DNA (e.g., herpesvirus, smallpox virus), ssDNA (parvovirus), dsRNA (rotavirus), ssRNA +sense (+sense functions as mRNA) (e.g., hepatitis A and C viruses, SARS virus, poliovirus, rhinovirus), ssRNA −sense (e.g., Ebola virus, Marburg virus, Nipah, influenza virus, and viruses that cause measles, mumps, and rabies, hantavirus, Lassa virus), ssRNA +sense with RT (e.g., HIV), and dsDNA with RT (e.g., hepatitis B virus).

Viral diseases are the most common afflictions of humans and include the common cold, the "cold sore" of herpes simplex virus, several forms of hepatitis, HIV, and several types of cancer. Examples of human diseases caused by specific viruses are listed in Table 9-9.

Transmission and Colonization

Viruses are obligatory intracellular parasites, thus transmission is usually from one infected individual to an uninfected individual or from an animal reservoir (**zoonotic infection**). Transmission may be direct or through a vector, such as mosquitoes. Human-to-human transmission may take many forms, including aerosols of respiratory fluids, contact with infected blood, or sexual contact.

Table 9-9   Human Diseases Caused by Specific Viruses

Baltimore Classification	Family	Virus	Envelope	Main Route of Transmission	Disease
dsDNA	Adenoviruses	Adenovirus	No	Droplet contact	Acute febrile pharyngitis
	Herpesviruses	Herpes simplex type 1 (HSV-1)	Yes	Direct contact with saliva or lesions	Lesions in mouth, pharynx, conjunctivitis
		Herpes simplex type 2 (HSV-2)	Yes	Sexually, contact with lesions during birth	Sores on labia, meningitis in children
		Herpes simplex type 8 (HSV-8)	Yes	Sexually?, body fluids	Kaposi sarcoma
		Epstein-Barr virus (EBV)	Yes	Saliva	Mononucleosis, Burkitt lymphoma
		Cytomegalovirus (CMV)	Yes	Body fluids, mother's milk, transplacental	Mononucleosis, congenital infection
		Varicella-zoster virus (VZV)	Yes	Droplet contact	Chickenpox, shingles
ssDNA	Papovaviruses	Papillomavirus	No	Direct contact	Warts, cervical carcinoma
dsRNA	Reoviruses	Rotavirus	No	Fecal-oral	Severe diarrhea
ssRNA+	Picornaviruses	Coxsackievirus	No	Fecal-oral, droplet contact	Nonspecific febrile illness, conjunctivitis, meningitis
		Hepatitis A virus	No	Fecal-oral	Acute hepatitis
		Poliovirus	No	Fecal-oral	Poliomyelitis
		Rhinovirus	No	Droplet contact	Common cold
	Flaviviruses	Hepatitis C virus	Yes	Blood, sexually	Acute or chronic hepatitis, hepatocellular carcinoma
		Yellow fever virus	Yes	Mosquito vector	Yellow fever
		Dengue virus	Yes	Mosquito vector	Dengue fever
		West Nile virus	Yes	Mosquito vector	Meningitis, encephalitis
	Togaviruses	Rubella virus	Yes	Droplet contact, transplacental	Acute or congenital rubella
	Coronaviruses	SARS	Yes	Droplets in aerosol or direct contact	Severe respiratory disease
	Caliciviruses	Norovirus	No	Fecal-oral	Gastroenteritis
ssRNA−	Orthomyxoviruses	Influenzavirus	Yes	Droplet contact	Influenza
	Paramyxoviruses	Measles virus	Yes	Droplet contact	Measles
		Mumps virus	Yes	Droplet contact	Mumps
		Parainfluenza virus	Yes	Droplet contact	Croup, pneumonia, common cold
		Respiratory syncytial virus (RSV)	Yes	Droplet contact, hand-to-mouth	Pneumonia, influenza-like syndrome
	Rhabdoviruses	Rabies virus	Yes	Animal bite, droplet contact	Rabies
	Bunyaviruses	Hantavirus	Yes	Aerosolized animal fecal material	Viral hemorrhagic fever
	Filoviruses	Ebola virus	Yes	Direct contact with body fluids	Viral hemorrhagic fever
		Marburg virus	Yes	Direct contact with body fluids	Viral hemorrhagic fever
	Arenavirus	Lassa virus	Yes	Aerosolized animal fecal material	Viral hemorrhagic fever
ssRNA+ with RT	Retroviruses	HIV	Yes	Sexually, blood products	AIDS
dsDNA with RT	Hepadnaviruses	Hepatitis B virus	Yes	All body fluids	Acute or chronic hepatitis, hepatocellular carcinoma

AIDS, Acquired immunodeficiency syndrome; *DNA,* deoxyribonucleic acid; *ds,* double-stranded; *HIV,* human immunodeficiency virus; *RNA,* ribonucleic acid; *RT,* reverse transcriptase; *SARS,* severe acute respiratory syndrome; *ss;* single-stranded.

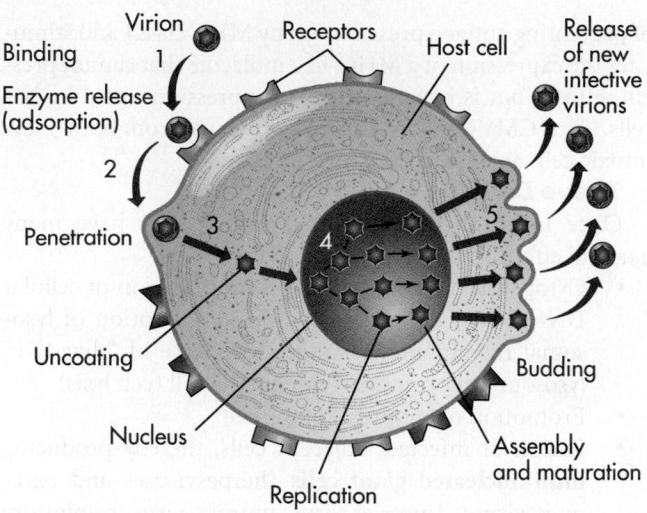

Figure 9-10 Stages of viral infection of an infected cell.

The viral life cycle is completely intracellular and involves several steps: *attachment* to the target cell (determines host range and tropism), *penetration* (by endocytosis or membrane fusion), *uncoating* (release of viral nucleic acid from the viral capsid by viral or host enzymes), *replication* (synthesis of viral proteins and mRNA), *assembly* (formation of new virions), and *release* (by lysis, budding) (Figure 9-10).

Attachment involves specific interactions between surface proteins on the virus and receptors on the cell to be infected.[38] The specificity of the virus for these receptors and the distribution of receptors throughout the individual's tissues dictate the range of host cells that a particular virus can infect. For example, HIV has a glycoprotein (gp120) that attaches to the CD4 molecule expressed on helper T cells, monocytes, and microglia. Rotavirus recognizes sialic acid and other constituents of epithelial junctions. Epstein-Barr virus (EBV, which causes mononucleosis) binds to complement receptor 2 (CR2) on B lymphocytes.

Once bound, the virion penetrates the plasma membrane by receptor-mediated endocytosis, by envelope fusion with the plasma membrane, or by directly crossing the plasma membrane.[39] Within the cytoplasm the virus uncoats the protective nucleocapsid and releases viral genetic information. Most RNA viruses directly produce mRNA, which is translated into viral proteins, and genomic RNA, which is eventually packaged into new viruses. One particular family of viruses, retroviruses (e.g., HIV) carries an enzyme *reverse transcriptase* that creates a double-stranded DNA version of the virus. The DNA "provirus" enters the cell's nucleus, where it becomes integrated into the host cell's chromosomal DNA. DNA viruses also enter the nucleus and are transcribed into mRNA before protein translation. Some DNA viruses also may integrate into the infected cell's chromosomal DNA.

The translation of viral-specific mRNA results in viral proteins that self-assemble. New virions are released from the cell for transmission of the viral infection to neighboring uninfected cells. Enveloped viruses are released through *budding*, in which shed viral particles are enveloped in the plasma membrane from the surface of the infected cell. Nonenveloped viruses commonly are released in large numbers concurrent with the destruction of the cell. Viral DNA that has become integrated with host DNA is transmitted to the daughter cells during mitosis. By this process, viral genes can become part of the genetic information of the cell and its progeny.

Invasion and Evasion

The primary defense mechanisms against viruses include antibody that prevents viral entrance into a cell and cellular immunity that recognizes antigenic changes on the surface of infected cells. Nonspecific defense includes production of α- and β-interferons that block intracellular viral replication. However, many viruses are highly successful pathogens and have developed a variety of mechanisms for bypassing immune rejection (see Table 9-6).[9]

Rapid Division. Some viruses, particularly those with small genomes, rapidly proliferate after the initial infection and by doing so produce a large number of virions more quickly than the immune system can develop. Norovirus virus and rotavirus (causes of severe diarrhea and vomiting) and Ebola virus, Marburg virus, and hantavirus (causes of hemorrhagic fever) have very short incubation periods. By the development of an effective adaptive immune response in 4 or 5 days, the virus has spread and caused severe clinical disease.

Intracellular Survival. As obligative intracellular pathogens, viruses hide within cells and away from normal inflammatory or immune responses. Viral agents that spread from cell to cell after the initial infection must encounter the immune response, which in most cases cures the infection. Thus most viral infections are self-limiting.

If a symbiotic relationship is maintained between the cell and the virus, persistent unapparent infection may result (latency). The infected cell will be functional, and the virus persists until it is activated to replicate (e.g., the recurrent coldsores of herpes simplex virus infection). Latent viruses usually possess latency-associated transcript (LAT) genes that control persistence indefinitely. Reactivation usually results from expression of lytic genes that lead to increased viral expression and destruction of the infected cell. Latency is characteristic of several chronic viral infections (e.g., HIV, hepatitis B and C viruses).

Coat with Self-Proteins. Enveloped viruses are the prime examples of how this mechanism may succeed. The viral capsid is completely surrounded by a cellular plasma membrane that is highly similar to that of an uninfected cell. Only a few critical differences exist. In order to infect another cell the viron expresses envelope proteins (SU and TM proteins) that are critical for the intercellular fusion process. These proteins are virus-specific and targets for protective immune responses.

Antigenic Variation. One of the classic examples of antigenic variation is influenza. This virus undergoes frequent antigen shifts and drifts, which are described in detail within the Example of Viral Pathogenesis section, later. Other viruses (e.g., HIV) add antigenic diversity by incorporating frequent functional translational errors. Some viral enzymes are designed to create small errors in reading mRNA leading to minor changes in the viral proteins. These changes are not at functionally critical sites, but may provide resistance to specific and nonspecific defense mechanisms.

In a manner similar to bacteria, some viruses have multiple stable antigenic serotypes. A person who recovers from an infection with one serotype may not have protective immunity against other serotypes of the same virus. At least 100 serotypes of rhinovirus can cause the "common cold," which explains why individuals can catch many colds throughout their lives. HIV and hepatitis C virus also have multiple serotypes.

Neutralization of Immune Molecules. As with other pathogens, the secretion of large amounts of soluble viral antigen may lead to neutralization of antibody and formation of immune complexes. In infection such as hepatitis B significant levels of circulating immune complexes may form and be deposited in target tissues, such as the kidneys.

Some viruses also have the capacity to neutralize cytokines, such as IL-1 and TNF-α. Cells infected with vaccinia virus produce a protein that can bind to IL-1. These molecules are frequently called cytokine decoys.

Complement Evasion. Several viruses induce expression of regulators of complement activation.[14] Cellular complement inhibitors are incorporated into the envelope of some viruses (e.g., HIV-1, vaccinia).[15] Cytomegalovirus (CMV) induces complement inhibitors on the surface of infected cells. Herpes simplex virus expresses a cell surface protein (glycoprotein C-1) that binds and inhibits C3b, as well blocks the membrane attack complex.

Immune Suppression. HIV and other viruses have developed the capacity to infect and kill immune cells, thus protecting themselves, but also leading to a broad immunosuppression against other antigens. This process is discussed more thoroughly in the section on AIDS.

Some viruses have developed mechanisms for interfering with antigen processing and presentation by MHC class I molecules.[40] Endogenous antigens, such as viral antigens, are normally degraded by proteasomes, transported by TAP proteins into the endoplasmic reticulum, and complexed with MHC class I molecules for expression on the cell surface and presentation to appropriate cells of the immune response (see Chapter 7). Many of the herpesviruses and retroviruses prevent steps in this process. For instance, Epstein-Barr virus inhibits degradation by the proteasomes. Herpes simplex virus can prevent binding of the antigenic peptide to MHC class I. Inhibition of antigen presentation by MHC class I prevents the generation of effective T-cell immune responses.

Human CMV has developed a unique modification of affecting MHC processing. NK cells are the principal defenders against tumor cells or virally infected cells that have down-regulated MHC expression and are therefore not recognized by T-cytotoxic cells. NK cell function is suppressed by targets with surface class I MHC molecules. CMV is capable of preventing antigen presentation by MHC class I and stimulates the expression of a MHC-like molecule that cannot present antigen but is recognized as a suppression signal by NK cells. Thus CMV-infected cells are protected from both T-cytotoxic cells and NK cell killing.

Tissue Damage
Once inside the infected cell, viruses may have many harmful effects, including the following:
- Cytopathic effects resulting from inhibition of cellular DNA, RNA, or protein synthesis, disruption of lysosomal membranes, resulting in release of "digestive" lysosomal enzymes that can kill the cell (cell lysis)
- Promotion of apoptosis of the cell
- Fusion of infected, adjacent cells, thereby producing **multinucleated giant cells** (herpesviruses and paramyxoviruses [measles virus, mumps virus, respiratory syncytial virus])
- Transformation of infected cell into cancerous cells, resulting in uninhibited and unregulated growth
- Alteration of the antigenic properties, or "identity," of the infected cell, causing the immune system to attack the cell as if it were foreign[16]

Example of Viral Pathogenesis
Influenza is an ssRNA (−strand) with a segmented genome (seven or eight pieces of ssRNA) (Figure 9-11).[4] It is transmitted through aerosols or body fluids and is highly infectious. The virions attach to respiratory epithelial cells and enter by endocytosis. Symptoms begin 1 to 4 days after infection and may include chills, fever, sore throat, muscle aches, severe headaches, coughing, weakness, generalized discomfort, nausea, and vomiting, and may lead to pneumonia; it can be fatal, particularly in young children and older adults.[41] The normal rate of infectivity is about 5% to 15%, with a mortality rate of about 0.1%, and in most cases recovery occurs in 1 to 2 weeks. Yearly seasonal influenza outbreaks result in about 250,000 to 500,000 deaths worldwide.

The influenza virion expresses two surface proteins that are essential to virulence.[41,42] The hemagglutinin (HA) protein is a glycoprotein that is necessary for entrance into cells by binding to glycan receptors, which are richly expressed on the surface of respiratory epithelium. The surface neuraminidase (NA) is an enzyme that is necessary for release of new virions from infected cells by cleaving cellular sialic acids (a common component of mammalian cell membranes).

Antibodies against the HA and NA antigens are responsible for protection against influenza infection. Infections are seasonal and protection gained from 1 year's infection does not totally protect against influenza in the following year because the HA and NA antigens undergo yearly change.[43] Usually antigenic variation is relatively minor (**antigenic drift**) and results from **mutations.** Individuals frequently have partial protection resulting from the previous year's infection, which lessens the effects of the disease. Two groups of influenza virus, influenza A and influenza B, infect humans, and the yearly vaccine against it is a trivalent mixture of inactivated proteins from two influenza A subtypes and one influenza

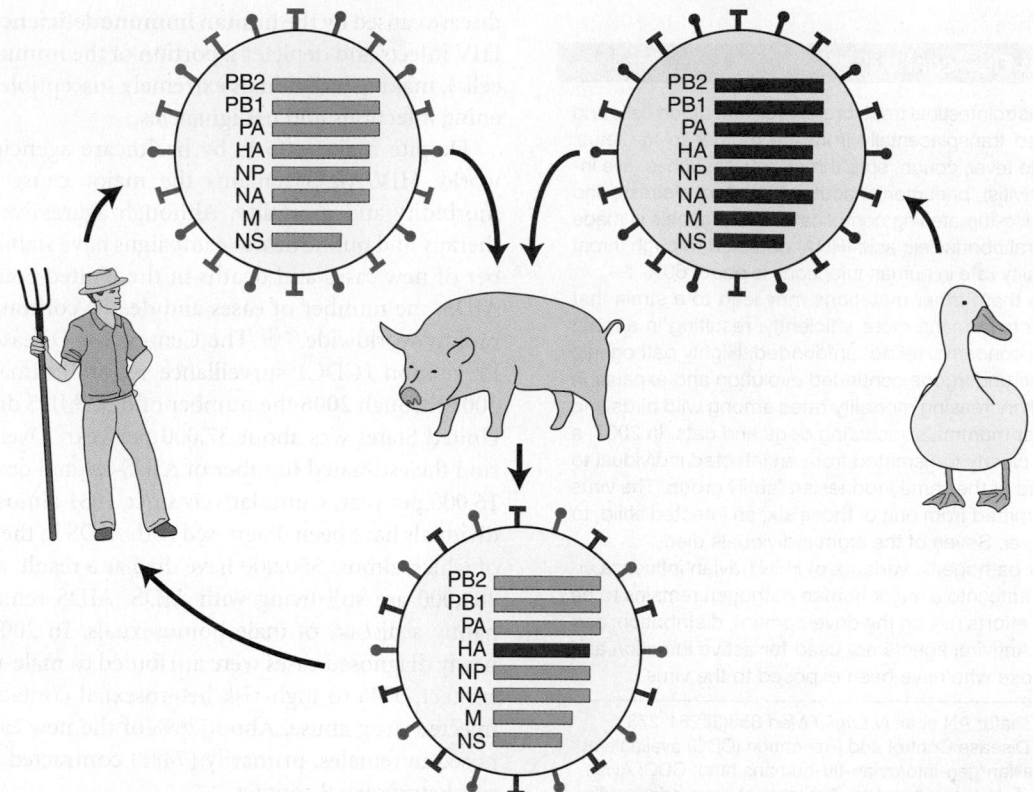

Figure 9-11 Antigenic shifts in influenza virus. One theory proposes that antigenic shifts occur when a human influenza virus (blue) and an avian influenza virus (red) coinfect a species that is permissive for both. The 8 ssRNA strands are co-expressed in the same infected cell, resulting in mixing of the strands so that a hybrid virus can be produced. The hybrid virus indicated here contains all the genetic information of the original virus that infected humans, but contains a new hemagglutinin (HA)-containing stand from the avian virus. This virus expresses a new HA antigen and will be less susceptible to residual immunity that normally provides partial protection against yearly influenza infections.

B subtype. Influenza B almost exclusively infects humans, mutates at a much lower rate than influenza A, and has reduced rate of antigenic change. Influenza B, however, has antigenically distinct subtypes based on HA (16 forms) and NA (9 forms) antigens and is infectious to birds and mammals. Currently subtypes H1N1, H1N2, and H3N2 are the primary causes of influenza worldwide.

Periodically influenza B undergoes major antigenic changes (**antigenic shifts**) (see Figure 9-11).[41] Shifts occur in animals coinfected by a human and an avian strain of influenza. Because the genome is segmented, the segments can undergo **recombination** during which the human virus obtains a new HA or NA antigen. When such changes occur, previous protection may not exist, resulting in a major pandemic and much more severe disease. In 1918 an antigenic shift occurred in the western United States (first reported in Fort Riley, Kansas) resulting in an influenza A virus with an H1N1 serotype (called Spanish flu). The virus spread worldwide throughout 1918 and 1919. Symptoms were unusually severe, resulted from excessive production of cytokines, and included deaths from secondary bacterial pneumonia, massive hemorrhages, and pulmonary edema.[44] Spanish flu possessed an extremely high rate of infectivity (up to 50%) and mortality (killed 20%

WHAT'S NEW?   Avian Flu

Influenza viruses infect a wide variety of species, including humans, different strains of birds, and swine. The species specificity of a particular variant of influenza is determined by the amino acid sequence of the hemagglutinin (HA) molecule on the viral surface. Influenza viruses have a relatively high mutation rate that can result in minor changes in the HA and change the species specificity. As a result, an influenza virus strain that primarily infects birds may, after a mutation, become efficiently infectious for humans.

Various strains of a highly pathogenic avian influenza A (H5N1) have arisen in the past few years. These strains were first reported in 1996 in China. The most pathogenic variants have a near 100% mortality rate in domestic poultry and have spread globally, killing tens of millions of birds. The global spread may be a result of collateral nonfatal infection of wild migrating birds, such as ducks and geese.

In 1997, the first human infections with the H5N1 avian virus were reported in Hong Kong involving 18 cases, 6 of whom died. As of September 10, 2008, 387 individuals have become infected, with 245 deaths. So far, human infections occur primarily in those individuals who have been in close contact with infected birds (especially whose who have handled sick or dead poultry). No cases have been identified among short-term travelers visiting countries affected by outbreaks. The H5N1 strain infects the lungs and targets type 2 alveolar pneumocytes and macrophages. It also passes throughout

Continued

the body to the gastrointestinal tract, brain, liver, and blood cells and can be transmitted transplacentally from the mother to the fetus. Symptoms include fever, cough, sore throat, muscle aches, eye infections (conjunctivitis), pneumonia, acute respiratory distress, and other severe and life-threatening complications. Diagnosis is made by detection of viral ribonucleic acid (RNA) obtained through throat swabs. The mortality rate in human infections is about 60%.

The concern is that further mutations may lead to a strain that spreads and infects humans more efficiently, resulting in a rapid pandemic. These concerns are not unfounded. Highly pathogenic H5N1 strains have undergone continued evolution and expansion of host range with increasing mortality rates among wild birds and infectivity for other mammals, including dogs and cats. In 2007, a H5N1 strain was clearly transmitted from an infected individual to six other members of the same Indonesian family group. The virus was further transmitted from one of those six, an infected child, to the child's caregiver. Seven of the eight individuals died.

Whether highly pathogenic variants of H5N1 avian influenza virus eventually mutate into a major human pathogen remains to be seen. Prevention efforts rely on the development, distribution, and use of vaccines. Antiviral agents are used for active infection and prophylaxis of those who have been exposed to the virus.

Data from Abdel-Ghafar AN et al: *N Engl J Med* 358(3):261-273, 2008; Centers for Disease Control and Prevention (CDC) available at www.cdc.gov/flu/avian/gen-info/avian-flu-humans.html; CDC: *Avian influenza: a virus infections of humans.* Available at www.cdc.gov/flu/avian/gen-info/avian-flu-humans.htm, last modified on May 23, 2008; CDC: *Avian influenza: current H5N1 situation.* Available at www.cdc.gov/flu/avian/outbreaks/current.htm, last modified on October 27, 2008; CDC: *Key facts about avian influenza (bird flu) and avian influenza A (H5N1) virus.* Available at www.cdc.gov/flu/avian/gen-info/facts.htm, last modified on May 7, 2007; World Health Organization (WHO): *Cumulative number of confirmed human cases of avian influenza A/(H5N1).* Available at www.who.int/csr/disease/avian_influenza/country/cases_table_2008_09_10/en/index.htm, last updated on September 10, 2008; WHO: *H5N1 avian influenza: timeline of major events.* Available at www.who.int/csr/disease/avian_influenza/Timeline_08%2009%2023.pdf, last updated on September 23, 2008; WHO: available at www.who.int/csr/disease/avian-influenza/en/index.html; Writing Committee of the Second World Health Organization Consultation on Clinical Aspects of Human Infection with Avian Influenza A (H5N1) Virus.

or more of those infected) and resulted in an estimated 40 million deaths worldwide. Strain variations due to antigenic drift occur within both HA and NA, and some may further affect virulence of that virus. The 1918 H1N1 serotype also possessed several mutations in the HA that resulted in a far greater virulence than the currently circulating H1N1 type. Studies have demonstrated that survivors of the 1918 pandemic still have protective levels of antibodies against that particular virus, confirming that protection against a particular influenza strain may be lifelong.

ACQUIRED IMMUNODEFICIENCY SYNDROME (AIDS)

The most notable form of secondary or acquired immune deficiency caused by an infectious agent is **acquired immunodeficiency syndrome (AIDS)**.[45] AIDS is a viral disease caused by the **human immunodeficiency virus (HIV)**. HIV infects and depletes a portion of the immune system (Th cells), making individuals extremely susceptible to life-threatening infections and malignancies.

Despite major efforts by healthcare agencies around the world, HIV/AIDS remains the major cause of worldwide morbidity and mortality. Although aggressive antiretroviral therapy and public health campaigns have stabilized the number of new cases and deaths in the United States from HIV/AIDS, the number of cases and deaths continues to increase rapidly worldwide.[46,47] The Centers for Disease Control and Prevention (CDC) surveillance report estimates that from 2002 through 2006 the number of new AIDS diagnoses in the United States was about 37,000 per year. Over the same period the estimated number of AIDS-related deaths was about 16,000 per year. Cumulatively since 1981 almost a million individuals have been diagnosed with AIDS in the United States, of which almost 550,000 have died as a result, and more than 400,000 are still living with AIDS. AIDS remains predominantly a disease of male homosexuals. In 2006, 50% of the newly diagnosed cases were attributed to male-to-male sexual contact, 33% to high-risk heterosexual contact, and 13% to injected drug abuse. About 26% of the new cases were diagnosed in females, primarily (74%) contracted through high-risk heterosexual contact.

Sub-Saharan Africa is still the epicenter of the AIDS pandemic. In 2007, the World Health Organization (WHO) estimated that 32% of newly diagnosed cases of HIV infection and AIDS-related deaths occurred in this region. In some areas AIDS is having a devastating effect. The United Nations (UN) AIDS program estimated that in 2006 from 4.9 million to 6.1 million people were HIV infected in South Africa, which has a total population of 48 million (national incidence of HIV infection is 10.8%). Women have the highest risk of infection: 13% of females are HIV infected, 90% of the newly diagnosed HIV infections are in 15- to 24-year-old women, and 29% of pregnant women are HIV infected. It is estimated that AIDS is responsible for almost 50% of all deaths in South Africa and 71% of deaths among individuals in the 15- to 40-year age group. As a result, the average life expectancy is now 54 years, whereas it would be at least 64 without AIDS. More than half of the current 15-year-olds are not expected to live to age 60.

The effects of AIDS are not limited to South Africa. In five countries in Africa the prevalence of HIV-infected adults exceeds 15%. In 2006, in Swaziland 26% of adults, 44% of men between the ages of 30 and 39, and 49% of pregnant women between the ages of 20 and 34 were HIV infected.

Transmission

HIV is a blood-borne pathogen present in body fluids (e.g., blood, vaginal fluid, semen, breast milk) with the typical routes of transmission: blood or blood products, intravenous drug abuse, heterosexual and homosexual activity, and maternal-child transmission before or during birth. As of the end of 2006, an estimated 8508 children in the United States developed AIDS after contracting HIV infection from their mothers across the placenta, through contact with infected blood during delivery, or through the milk during breast-feeding. Without treatment, symptoms usually develop within 6 months of life, and life expectancy is generally less than 3 years.

As with all blood-borne infections, healthcare providers are at increased risk of contracting the infection from an individual's blood.[48] The first reported case of occupational HIV infection was an emergency department nurse who became infected in 1986. The route of infection was probably through cuts in her hand that came into contact with contaminated blood through a gauze pad she was holding on a person's open wound. Tens of thousands of healthcare workers have become infected with HIV, but as of January 2007, only 57 cases of confirmed HIV/AIDS and 140 possible cases were contracted by occupational exposure.[49] Since initiation of widespread educational programs on universal precautions published by the CDC only 3 new cases have been reported. Nurses (42% of total cases) and clinical laboratory technicians (28% of cases) are by far the most commonly exposed healthcare workers.

Pathogenesis

HIV-1 was initially isolated by researchers at the Pasteur Institute as the lymphadenopathy/AIDS virus (LAV); a discovery for which they received the 2008 Nobel Prize in Medicine.[50] A second major and less virulent variant, HIV-2, was identified later and is found mostly in western Africa. HIV is a member of the retrovirus family, which carries genetic information in the form of two copies of RNA (Figure 9-12). Retroviruses use a viral enzyme, **reverse transcriptase,** to convert RNA into double-stranded DNA (Figure 9-13). Using a second viral enzyme, an **integrase,** the new DNA is inserted into the infected cell's genetic material, where it may remain dormant. If the cell is activated, translation of the viral information may be initiated, resulting in the formation of new virions, lysis and death of the infected cell, and shedding of infectious HIV particles. If, however, the cell remains relatively dormant, the viral genetic material may remain latent for years, and is probably present for the life of the individual.

The primary surface receptor on HIV is the envelope glycoprotein gp120, which binds to the molecule CD4, found primarily on the surface of helper T cells (see Figure 9-13).[51] Several other necessary co-receptors have been identified on the target cells, particularly the chemokine receptors CXCR4 and CCR5. Different strains of HIV-1 are selective for the CXCR4 or CCR5 co-receptors, which influences the tropism for different target cells. Strains that prefer the CXCR4 co-receptor tend to be T-cell tropic, usually found later in an infection, and cause infected cells to fuse and form a multinucleate **syncytium.** Strains that react better with the co-receptor CCR5 are macrophage-tropic, usually cause the primary HIV infection, and do not cause syncytium formation.

The primary cellular targets for HIV include the following:

- CD4-positive Th cells
- Dendritic cells (depending on the level of chemokine receptors the cell expresses)
- Macrophages (express low levels of CD4, but high amounts of heparin sulfate proteoglycans [syndecan] and other molecules [CCR5] that bind to gp120 and adsorb HIV)
- CD8-positive Tc cells (low rate of infection, but CD4 can be expressed by activated CD8-positive Tc cells)
- Double positive thymic cells (express CD4 and CD8 simultaneously)
- NK cells (some are CD4+, CCR5+)
- Neural cells of monocyte origin (macrophages and microglial cells)

Initially, the lymphoid areas of the mucosal surfaces are the primary sites of infection (Figure 9-14). Dendritic cells and mucosal T cells probably spread the infection to other peripheral lymphoid organs (especially follicular dendritic cells in the lymph nodes, which infect T cells). Infection also may involve the thymus and bone marrow, including the bone marrow stromal cells. Cells in the central nervous system (CNS) may act as a reservoir in which HIV can be relatively protected from antiviral drugs. The virus is also found in T cells and macrophages in semen and in the renal epithelium.

The major immunologic finding in AIDS is the striking decrease in the number of CD4+ Th cells (Figure 9-15). Individuals who are not HIV infected typically have 800 to 1000 CD4+ cells/μL of blood, with a range from 600 to 1200/μL. Numbers of CD8+ T cells are usually normal or slightly elevated. The decrease in CD4+ cell numbers results in a reversal of the normal CD4/CD8 T-cell ratio (normally about 1.9) to lower than 0.9 and often near zero.

HIV causes destruction of Th cells by a variety of means. Production of new HIV virions can be directly cytopathic to the infected cell, causing lysis (breakdown of the cell) or inducing apoptosis. Additionally, HIV-infected cells express new surface antigens and are targets for Tc-mediated lysis.

However, it is not unusual for a large majority (>98%) of peripheral CD4+ T cells to *not* be infected with HIV-1, although a significant amount (10% to 50%) show signs of apoptosis. Therefore, HIV-1 killing is probably an indirect rather than direct effect. HIV-infected cells shed soluble viral envelope protein, gp120, which can induce apoptotic cell death of uninfected T lymphocytes, neurons, and monocytes through interaction with cell surface receptors. The interaction between viral envelope protein on the surface of infected cells and its receptors on neighboring uninfected cells also can result in intercellular fusion and syncytium formation. The syncytia undergo apoptosis after a phase of latency. Envelope protein present on the surface of HIV-1–infected cells also can create partial fusion (hemifusion, membrane damage) that results in death of the uninfected cell. The presence of HIV virions and soluble viral antigen can result in a chronic activation of uninfected T cells with HIV-specific T-cell receptors (TCRs). Because activated T cells more efficiently support HIV replication, the most susceptible cells are those with TCRs against HIV, which undergo antigen-driven activation and infection. This observation may not bode well

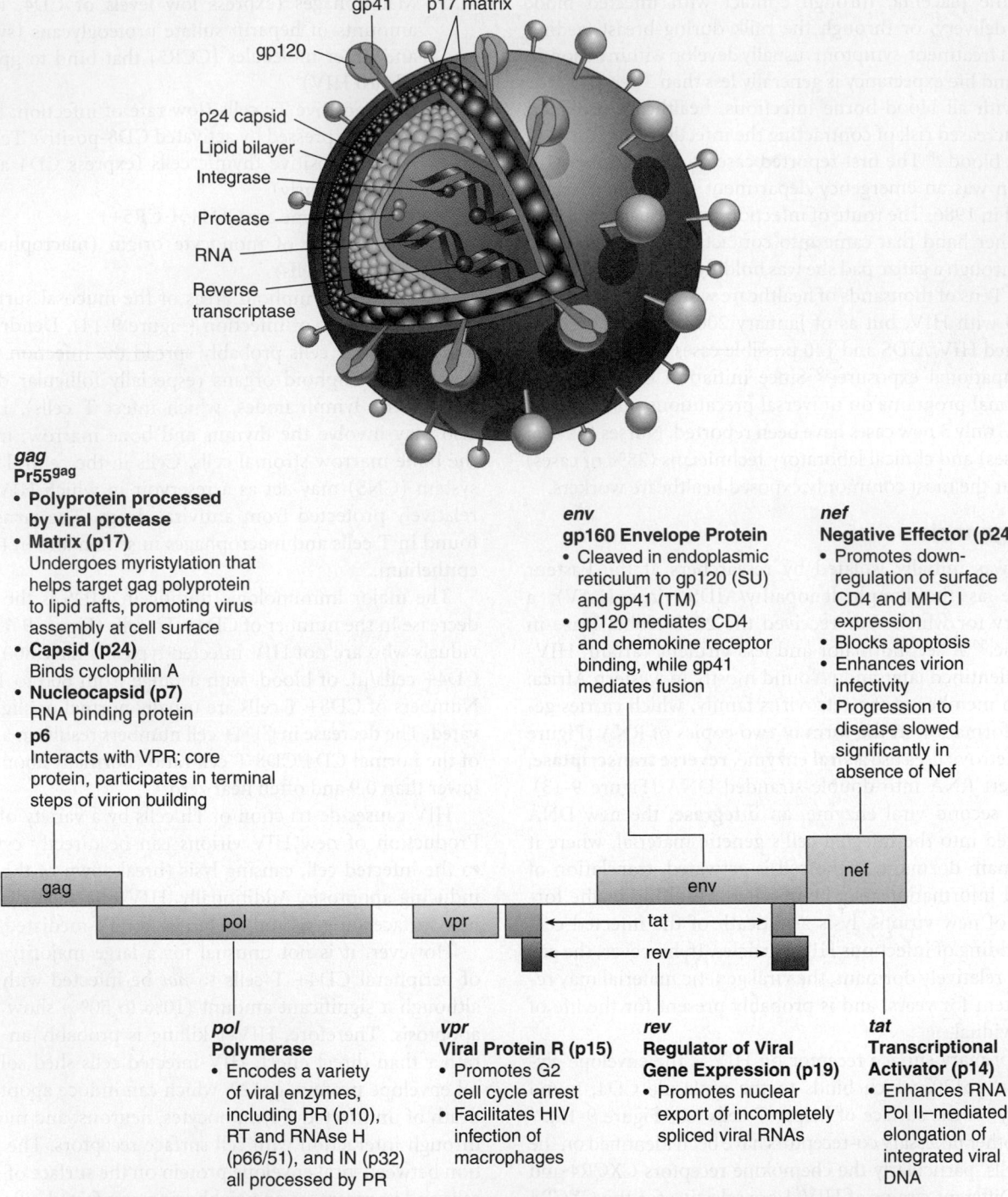

gp41   p17 matrix
gp120
p24 capsid
Lipid bilayer
Integrase
Protease
RNA
Reverse
transcriptase

gag
Pr55^gag
- **Polyprotein processed by viral protease**
- **Matrix (p17)**
  Undergoes myristylation that helps target gag polyprotein to lipid rafts, promoting virus assembly at cell surface
- **Capsid (p24)**
  Binds cyclophilin A
- **Nucleocapsid (p7)**
  RNA binding protein
- **p6**
  Interacts with VPR; core protein, participates in terminal steps of virion building

env
gp160 Envelope Protein
- Cleaved in endoplasmic reticulum to gp120 (SU) and gp41 (TM)
- gp120 mediates CD4 and chemokine receptor binding, while gp41 mediates fusion

nef
Negative Effector (p24)
- Promotes down-regulation of surface CD4 and MHC I expression
- Blocks apoptosis
- Enhances virion infectivity
- Progression to disease slowed significantly in absence of Nef

gag

pol

vpr

env   nef

tat

rev

pol
Polymerase
- Encodes a variety of viral enzymes, including PR (p10), RT and RNAse H (p66/51), and IN (p32) all processed by PR

vpr
Viral Protein R (p15)
- Promotes G2 cell cycle arrest
- Facilitates HIV infection of macrophages

rev
Regulator of Viral Gene Expression (p19)
- Promotes nuclear export of incompletely spliced viral RNAs

tat
Transcriptional Activator (p14)
- Enhances RNA Pol II–mediated elongation of integrated viral DNA

Figure 9-12 The structure and genetic map of HIV-1. The HIV-1 virion consists of a core of two identical strands of viral RNA molecules of viral enzymes (reverse transcriptase [RT], protease [PR], integrase [IN]), encoated in a core capsid structure consisting primarily of the structural viral protein p24. The capsid is further encased in a matrix consisting primarily of a viral protein, p17. The outer surface is an envelope consisting of the plasma membrane of the cell from which the virus budded (lipid bilayer) and two viral glycoproteins: a transmembrane gp41 and a noncovalently attached surface protein, gp120. The HIV-1 genome contains regions that encode the structural proteins (*gag*), the viral enzymes (*pol*), and the envelope proteins (*env*). The *gag* region is translated into a large precursor (Pr55^gag) that is cut by the HIV protease into smaller proteins that construct the capsid and matrix. The *env* region is translated into a gp160 precursor protein that is cut by a host-cell protease into the gp120 and gp41 envelope proteins. The genome of complex retroviruses, like HIV-1, often contain a variety of small regions that regulate expression of the virus. (Modified from Kumar V, Abbas A, Fausto N: *Robbins and Cotran pathologic basis of disease*, ed 7, Philadelphia, 2005, Saunders.)

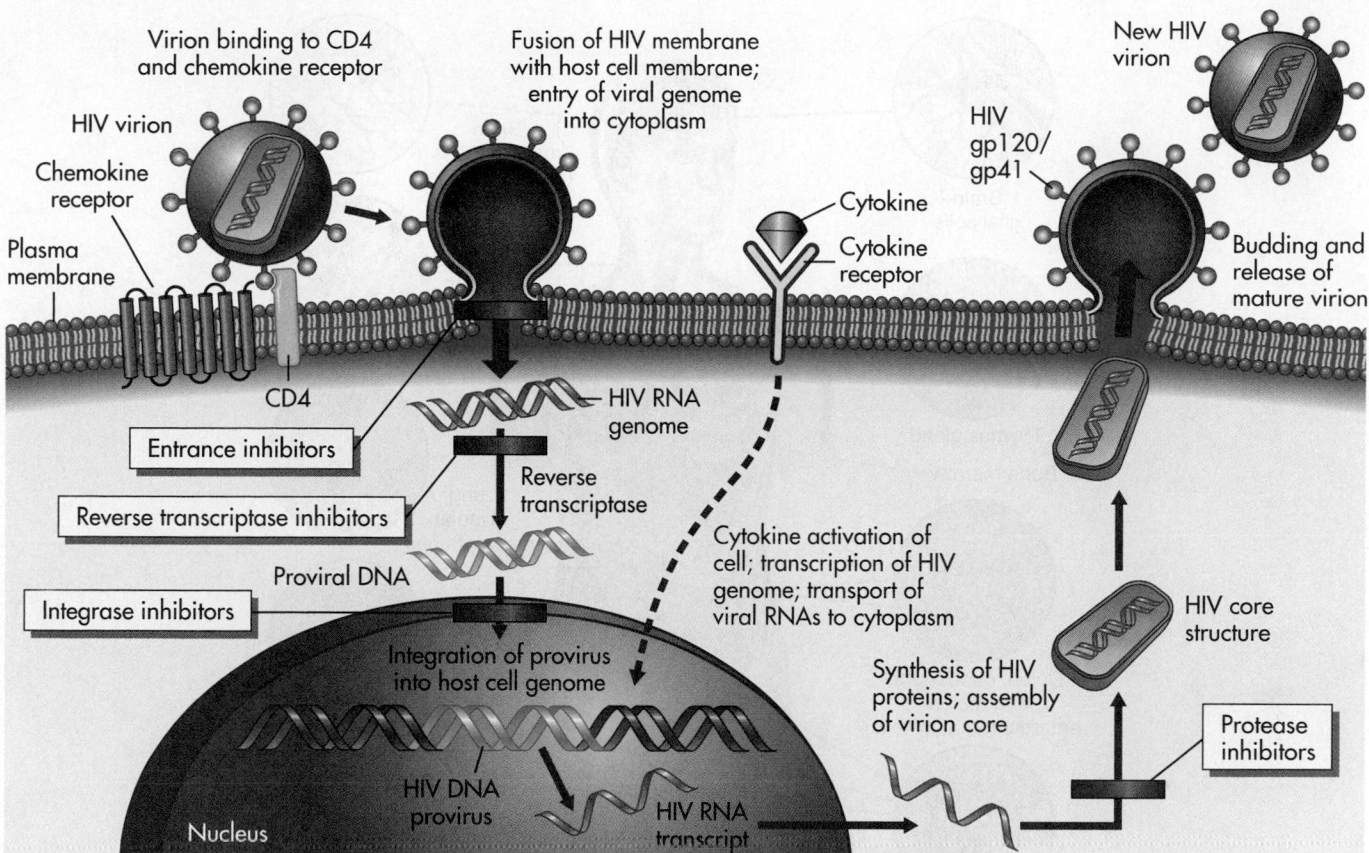

Figure 9-13 Life cycle and possible sites of therapeutic intervention of HIV-1. HIV infection begins when a virion, or virus particle, binds to CD4 and chemokine co-receptors on a susceptible cell. The HIV virion has viral proteins gp41 and gp120 on its surface (envelope), which interact with CD4 and the CCR5 co-receptor and initiate fusion between the viral envelope and the plasma membrane, resulting in the core of the virus being injected into the cytoplasm. Uncoating occurs in the cytoplasm, during which the core proteins are removed, and the viral RNA is released into the infected cell's cytoplasm. The viral RNA is converted to a double-stranded DNA provirus by the action of the viral reverse transcriptase. The provirus migrates into the nucleus and is integrated into the cell's own DNA. The provirus may remain latent. If the infected cell is activated (e.g., by cytokines), the provirus may be transcribed and translated into viral protein precursors. The precursor proteins are modified by viral (gag proteins) and cellular (env proteins) proteases into smaller proteins that are used to package the viral RNA into new virions that bud from the cell. The HIV-1 life cycle is susceptible to blockage at several sites. Some agents could block the attachment and entrance of the virus (entrance inhibitors). Reverse transcriptase inhibitors (e.g., azidothymidine [AZT]) prevent the reverse transcription of viral RNA into DNA. Drugs also may be able to inhibit the viral integrase (integrase inhibitors) and prevent insertion of the provirus into the host's chromosomes. Protease inhibitors specifically inhibit the viral protease and prevent the processing of the gp160 into viral capsid and matrix proteins. (Modified from Kumar V, Abbas A, Fausto N: *Robbins and Cotran pathologic basis of disease*, ed 7, Philadelphia, 2005, Saunders.)

for successful vaccine development if the induced and supposedly protective CD4+ cells are also the most susceptible targets for HIV.

As a result of these processes the level of T cells decreases (particularly memory T cells, which seem more susceptible to HIV infection), thymic production of new T cells is decreased, and the secondary lymphoid organs (particularly the lymph nodes) are damaged.

Clinical Manifestations

Depletion of CD4+ cells has a profound effect on the immune system, causing a severely diminished response to a wide array of infectious pathogens and malignant tumors (Box 9-2).

At the time of diagnosis, the individual may manifest one of several different conditions: serologically negative (no detectable antibody), serologically positive (positive for antibody against HIV) but asymptomatic, early stages of HIV disease, or AIDS (see Figure 9-15).

The presence of circulating antibody against the HIV indicates infection by the virus, although many of these individuals are asymptomatic. Antibody appears rather rapidly after infection through blood products, usually within 4 to 7 weeks. After sexual transmission, however, the individual can be infected yet seronegative for 6 to 14 months or, in at least one case, for years. In addition, in the late stages of the disease, some individuals become seronegative because of a deficient immune system.

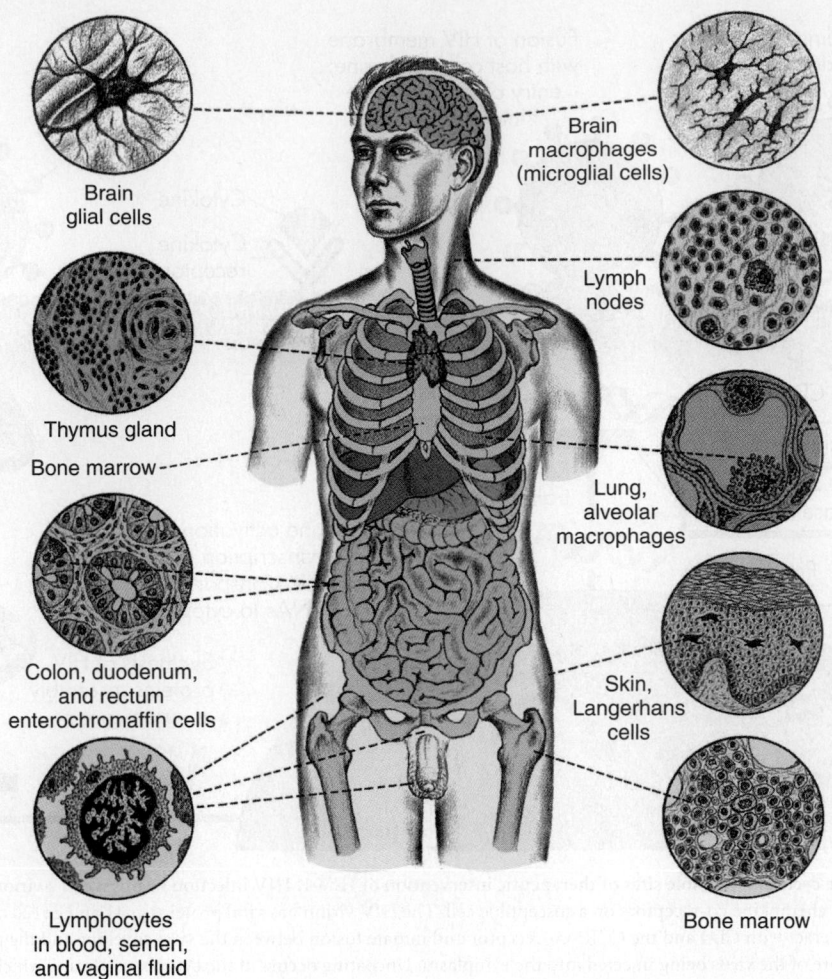

Figure 9-14 Distribution of tissues that can be infected by the HIV. Infection is closely linked to the presence of CD4 receptors or chemokine co-receptors on host tissue, particularly T cells and macrophages. (Modified from Weber JN, Weiss RA: *HIV infection: the cellular picture, in the science of AIDS: readings from Scientific American,* New York, 1989, Freeman.)

The period between infection and the appearance of antibody is referred to as the **window period** (see Figure 9-15). Although the individual may not have antibody, he or she may have virus growing, have virus in the blood and body fluids, and be infectious to others. Early symptoms are relatively nonspecific to HIV and include fatigue, fever, muscle aches, and headaches.

Those with the early stages of HIV disease *(early stage disease* or *clinical latency)* are usually asymptomatic. The early stage may last as long as 10 years in untreated people, during which viral load increases and numbers of CD4+ cells progressively decrease. Some estimates are that approximately 99% of untreated HIV-infected individuals would eventually progress to AIDS.

The currently accepted definition of AIDS relies on both laboratory tests and clinical symptoms. The most common laboratory test is for antibodies against HIV proteins (particularly p24). If the individual is seropositive, the diagnosis of

AIDS is made in association with various clinical symptoms (see Box 9-2). The symptoms include atypical or opportunistic infections and cancers, as well as indications of debilitating chronic disease (e.g., wasting syndrome, recurrent fevers) (Figure 9-16). Most commonly, new cases of AIDS are diagnosed initially by decreased CD4+ T-cell numbers at or below 200 cells/μL.

Treatment and Prevention

The current regimen for treatment of HIV infection is a combination of drugs, termed **highly active antiretroviral therapy (HAART)**.[52] The combination includes at least three drugs from at least two classes of antiretroviral agents, including nucleoside reverse transcriptase inhibitors combined with a viral **protease inhibitor** or a non-nucleoside **reverse transcriptase inhibitor** (see Figure 9-13). Death from AIDS-related diseases has been reduced significantly since the introduction of HAART; without treatment an individual may

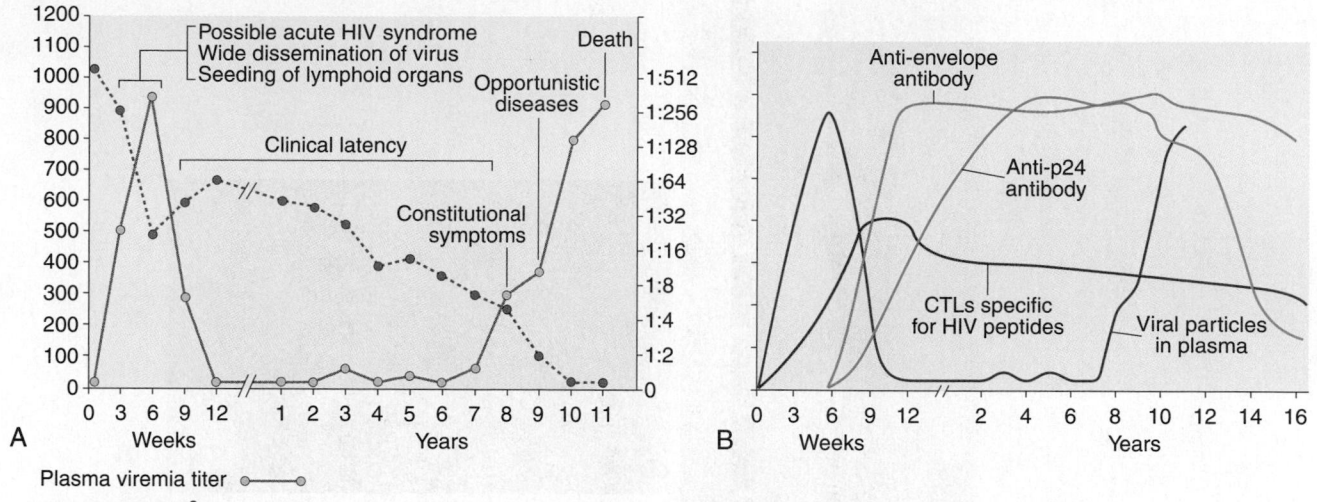

Figure 9-15 **Typical course of progression from HIV infection to AIDS in untreated persons. A,** Within weeks after infection, the person may experience symptoms of acute HIV syndrome. During this early period the virus progressively infects mucosal T cells and dendritic cells, propagates, and spreads to the lymphoid organs, with a sharp decrease in circulating CD4+ T cells. The resulting immune response usually induces a period of clinical latency, during which viral replication and T-cell destruction continue in the lymph nodes, although the individual is generally asymptomatic. As the disease progresses, the person may develop HIV-related disease (constitutional symptoms)—a variety of symptoms of acute viral infection that do not involve opportunistic infections or malignancies. When the number of CD4+ cells is critically suppressed, the person becomes susceptible to a variety of opportunistic infections and cancers. The length of time for progression from HIV infection to AIDS may vary considerably from person to person. **B,** Antibody and Tc cell (cytotoxic T lymphocytes [CTLs]) levels change during the progression to AIDS. During the initial phase antibodies against HIV-1 are not yet detectable (window period), but viral products, including p24 antigen, viral RNA, and infectious virus, may be detectable in the blood a few weeks after infection. Most antibodies produced against envelope proteins in the early phase are absorbed onto viral particles in the blood and are not detectable by most routine assays. During the latent phase of infection antibody levels against p24 and other viral proteins, as well as HIV-specific CTLs, generally increase, then remain constant until the development of AIDS. As the immune system becomes severely depressed and excess viral antigen is released into the blood, measurable antibody levels decrease. Disease progression usually ends in the death of the untreated individual. (**A** redrawn from Fauci AS, Lane HC: Human immunodeficiency virus disease: AIDS and related conditions. In Fauci AS et al, editors: *Harrison's principles of internal medicine,* ed 14, New York, 1997, McGraw-Hill; **B** from Kumar V, Abbas A, Fausto N: *Robbins and Cotran pathologic basis of disease,* ed 7, Philadelphia, 2005, Saunders.)

BOX 9-2   AIDS-Defining Opportunistic Infections and Neoplasms Found in Individuals with HIV Infection

Infections
Protozoal and helminthic infections
  Cryptosporidiosis or isosporiasis (enteritis)
  Pneumocystosis (pneumonia or disseminated infection)
  Toxoplasmosis (pneumonia or central nervous system [CNS] infection)
Fungal Infections
  Candidiasis (esophageal, tracheal, or pulmonary)
  Cryptococcosis (CNS infection)
  Coccidioidomycosis (disseminated)
  Histoplasmosis (disseminated)
Bacterial Infections
  Mycobacteriosis (atypical, e.g., *Mycobacterium avium-intracellulare,* disseminated or extrapulmonary; *Mycobacterium tuberculosis,* pulmonary or extrapulmonary)

Nocardiosis (pneumonia, meningitis, disseminated)
Salmonella infections (disseminated)
Viral infections
  Cytomegalovirus (pulmonary, intestinal, retinitis, or CNS infections)
  Herpes simplex virus (localized or disseminated)
  Varicella-zoster virus (localized or disseminated)
  Progressive multifocal (leukoencephalopathy)
Neoplasms
  Kaposi sarcoma
  B-cell non-Hodgkin lymphomas
  Primary lymphoma of the brain
  Invasive cancer of the uterine cervix

From Kumar V, Abbas A, Fausto N: *Robbins and Cotran pathologic basis of disease,* ed 7, Philadelphia, 2005, Saunders.

live only 9 to 10 months after diagnosis of AIDS, whereas those who respond well to HAART may survive for several decades. However, many people do not respond to HAART therapy, those who do respond are not "cured", and resistant variants to these drugs have been identified.[53]

Drug therapy for AIDS is difficult because, like most retroviruses, the AIDS virus incorporates into the genetic material of the host and may never be removed by antimicrobial therapy. Therefore, drug administration to control the virus may have to continue for the lifetime of

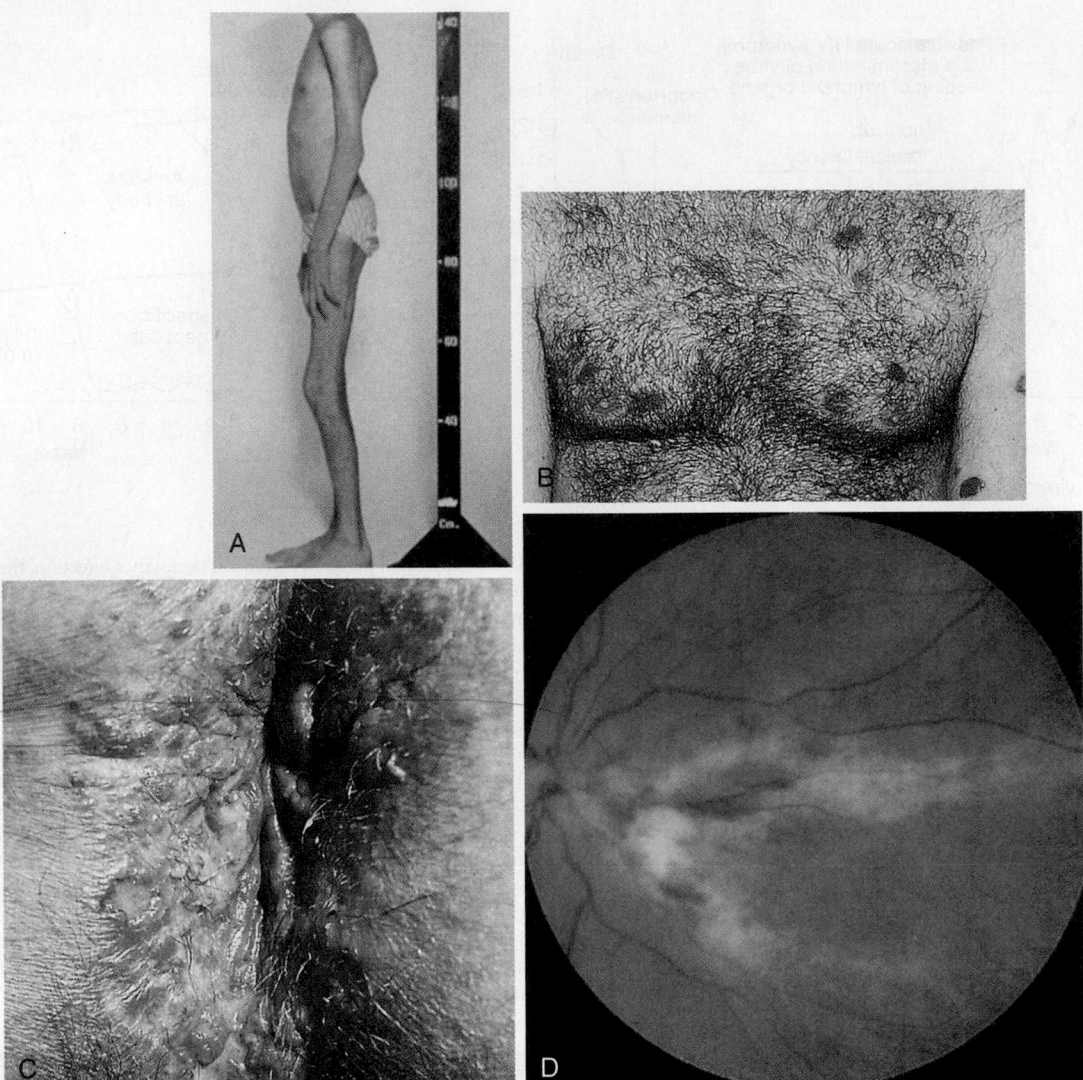

Figure 9-16 Clinical symptoms of AIDS. **A,** Severe weight loss and anorexia. **B,** Biopsy-proven Kaposi sarcoma lesions. **C,** Perianal vesicular and ulcerative lesions of herpes simplex infection. **D,** Deterioration of vision from cytomegalovirus retinitis leading to areas of infection; unless treated the progressive impairment will lead to blindness. (A and D from Taylor PK: *Diagnostic picture tests in sexually transmitted diseases,* London, 1995, Mosby; B and C from Morse SA et al editors: *Atlas of sexually transmitted diseases and AIDS,* ed 3, London, 2003, Mosby.)

the individual. Additionally, HIV may persist in regions where the antiviral drugs are not as effective, such as the CNS. Inhibitors of the initial viral entrance into the target cell (**entrance inhibitors**) may provide benefit for those who HAART does not benefit. Entrance inhibitors include the natural or modified ligands for the co-receptors (CXCR4 and CCR5) and can block infection and inhibit cell membrane fusion. Inhibitors of the viral integrase (**integrase inhibitors**) have undergone clinical trials and eventually may be added to the combination.

To date the development of an effective vaccine is the only hope for preventing the spread of HIV infection. Most common antiviral vaccines (e.g., rubella, mumps, influenza) induce protective antibodies that block the initial infection. Only one vaccine (rabies) is used after the infection has occurred. That approach is successful because the

rabies virus proliferates and spreads very slowly. Whether an HIV vaccine would be effective in either preventing or treating HIV infection is problematic, and the results of a recent vaccine trial have for the moment dampened enthusiasm.

Pediatric AIDS and Central Nervous System Involvement

The clinical diagnosis of HIV in children is very often a difficult task. The CDC revised the classification in 1994 for HIV infection in children younger than 13 years (Box 9-3). The HIV infection may be identified by viral culture of blood or tissue, and the diagnosis is confirmed by the presence of specific antibodies to the virus. However, the presence of passive maternal antibody limits the use of HIV antibody testing in infants in the high-risk category up to 15 months of age.

WHAT'S NEW? HIV Vaccine Trials

Very soon after the discovery in 1983 of the virus that causes AIDS, knowledgeable scientists and public officials predicted that an effective vaccine would be marketed within a few years. The prediction was not viewed as overly optimistic because vaccines had been produced against many other viral diseases, and the technology was available to swiftly purify, test, and manufacture viral antigens. In 2008, 25 years after the discovery of HIV, the chances of producing vaccine protection against AIDS appear more bleak than ever before.

The goal of an AIDS vaccine is to either prevent the initial infection or enhance the immune response of an infected individual to reduce viral load, or both. There was a great deal of interest in a recent trial (the STEP Study) of vaccine V520, produced by Merck. V520 was designed to produce a T-cell response because a considerable amount of data supported the role of T cells in controlling HIV infection. The immunization protocol was very complex and elicited an immune response against several HIV antigens, including products of HIV *env*, *gag*, *pol*, and *nef* genes expressed in an altered adenovirus, which would normally cause a common cold. The trial was prematurely stopped in September of 2007 because the initial analysis indicated that the vaccine neither prevented HIV infection nor lowered virus in the blood of those who became infected. The vaccine was suspected of increasing the risk for HIV infection in some recipients. Of 741 individuals who received at least one dose of the vaccine, 24 became infected during the trial, compared with 21 who became infected of the 762 who received the sham control vaccine.

Since the first large scale vaccine trial that used recombinant HIV gp120 envelope protein, no trial has shown protection against HIV infection, although HIV-specific antibody or T cells have been induced. Despite optimistic predictions for vaccine success, several major caveats had been discussed. The scale of genetic diversity of HIV envelope proteins is more like influenza virus, which requires a new vaccine yearly, than other viral infections, such as measles, mumps, and others that express stable antigens. However, unlike influenza, which changes antigens yearly, HIV undergoes antigenic change during infection of each individual. HIV also remains latent within infected cells, and no vaccine has been developed to rid the individual of other latent viruses. Perhaps the most overlooked concern is that an antibody response to HIV may actually facilitate infection. T cells and macrophages express surface receptors for the Fc portion of IgG and for complement components, thus an HIV virion coated with IgG or C3b may rapidly enter the very target cells that support infection.

Thus, with the recurrent failure of AIDS vaccine trials, the only effective means to limit the spread of HIV are behavioral changes. In Africa in particular, the rate of HIV infection has been reduced by education about appropriate condom use, increased application of male circumcision, and reductions in multiple sexual partnerships. However, these approaches only diminish the spread of HIV; therefore, vaccination remains the only probable means of completely preventing transmission of HIV.

Data from Johnston MI, Fauci AS: *N Engl J Med* 356(20):2073-2081, 2007; Johnston MI, Fauci AS: *N Engl J Med* 359(9):888-890, 2008; Potts M et al: *Science* 320(5877):749-750, 2008; Steinbrook R: *N Engl J Med* 357(26):2653-2655, 2007; Walker BD, Burton DR: *Science* 320(5877):760-764, 2008; Patterson S et al: *Handb Exp Pharmacol* 188:275-293, 2009.

Therefore, two definitions of infection in children are necessary: one for prenatally exposed infants up to 15 months of age and one for older children.

HIV directly invades most major organ systems, including the CNS. Therefore, the clinical manifestations vary greatly from child to child. The initial signs and symptoms may be nonspecific and subtle, and they may progress slowly or rapidly to an acute, life-threatening condition. A definite diagnosis of HIV is made by personal history, viral culture, and clinical manifestations. Monitoring CD8+ T lymphocytes and monocytes, in addition to CD4+ T lymphocytes, has been suggested for predicting risk for progressive encephalopathy. Decreases in CD8+ T lymphocytes diminish defenses against viral infection and facilitate infected monocytes to cross the blood-brain barrier.

A particularly vulnerable site of HIV infection in infants and children is the CNS. HIV encephalopathy is more common in the advanced stages. Because survival of children with HIV has been prolonged with effective treatment, the incidence of progressive encephalopathy has increased. The 1994 classification from the CDC[54] requires one of the following progressing findings to be present for at least 2 months, in the absence of a concurrent illness other than HIV that could explain the following findings:

- Failure to attain or loss of developmental milestones, or loss of intellectual ability, verified by standard developmental scale or neuropsychologic tests
- Impaired brain growth or acquired microcephaly demonstrated by head circumference measurements or brain atrophy demonstrated by computed tomography (CT) or magnetic resonance imaging (MRI) with serial imaging required in children less than 2 years of age
- Acquired symmetric motor deficits manifested by affecting a child 1 month of age or older

The onset of progressive encephalopathy may be a prognostic indicator of a poor outcome.

It may be difficult to completely differentiate the effect of HIV infection on the CNS from the effect of prenatal and perinatal exposure. In addition, other insults may accompany HIV in a young child and affect growth and development, such as drug exposure, prematurity, chronic illness, and a chaotic social atmosphere. The pathogenesis of HIV encephalopathy in children is poorly understood, but the presence of inflammatory mediators may be a contributing factor.

A growing number of investigational protocols are available for treatment of children with HIV. In general, treatment is focused on the preservation and maintenance of the immune system, aggressive response to opportunistic infections, and support and relief of symptomatic occurrences and administration of HAART.

BOX 9-3 Pediatric Human Immunodeficiency Virus (HIV) Classification

Immunologic Categories	N: No Signs/ Symptoms	A: Mild Signs/ Symptoms	B: Moderate Signs/ Symptoms	C: Severe Signs/ Symptoms
1. No evidence	N1	A1	B1	C1
2. Evidence of moderate suppression	N2	A2	B2	C2
3. Severe suppression	N3	A3	B3	C3

Clinical Categories for Children with HIV Infection

Category N: not symptomatic
Children who have no signs or symptoms considered to be the result of HIV infection or who have only one of the conditions listed in Category A

Category A: mildly symptomatic
Children with two or more of the conditions listed below but none of the conditions listed in Category B or C:
Lymphadenopathy
Hepatomegaly
Splenomegaly
Dermatitis
Parotitis
Recurrent or persistent upper respiratory infection, sinusitis, or otitis media

Category B: moderately symptomatic
Children who have symptomatic conditions other than those listed for Category A or C that are attributed to HIV infection; examples of conditions in clinical Category B include but are not limited to:
Anemia (≤8 g/dl), neutropenia (≤1000mm³), or thrombocytopenia (≤100,000mm³) persisting ≥30 days
Bacterial meningitis, pneumonia, or sepsis (single episode)
Candidiasis or oropharyngeal (thrush) persisting (≥2 months) in children ≥6 months of age
Cardiomyopathy
Cytomegalovirus infection with onset before 1 month of age
Diarrhea, recurrent or chronic
Hepatitis
Herpes simplex virus (HSV), recurrent stomatitis (more than two episodes within 1 year)
HSV bronchitis, pneumonitis, or esophagitis with onset before 1 month of age
Herpes zoster (shingles) involving at least two distinct episodes or more than 1 dermatome
Leiomyosarcoma
Lymphoid interstitial pneumonia (LIP) or pulmonary lymphoid hyperplasia complex
Neuropathy
Nocardiosis
Persistent fever (lasting ≥1 month)
Toxoplasmosis, onset before 1 month of age
Varicella, disseminated (complicated chickenpox)

Category C: severely symptomatic
Children who have any condition listed in the 1987 surveillance case definition of acquired immunodeficiency with the exception of LIP.

Data from Centers for Disease Control and Prevention: *MMWR Morb Mortal Wkly Rep* 43(12):1, 1994.

COUNTERMEASURES AGAINST PATHOGENS

An extremely effective means of countering infectious microorganisms is rigorous use of environmental infection control measures, including control of insect vector populations, modern sanitation facilities, providing clean water and uncontaminated food supplies, and other measures. Additionally, prophylactic or interventive procedures have been developed to prevent pathogens from initiating disease (vaccines) or to subdue the pathogen once the disease process has started (antimicrobials). Vaccine development has focused successfully on preventing the most severe and common infections (Table 9-10). With the initial success of antibiotic therapy, there was no perceived need for vaccination against many common and non–life-threatening infections. The increasing problem of antibiotic-resistant pathogens, however, forced a reappraisal of that strategy, and a greater emphasis is being placed on the development of new vaccines.

Infection Control Measures

Although effective means of safeguarding populations from exposure to infectious disease are well known, lack of implementation or breakdowns in application of these initiatives has led to the reemergence of some infectious diseases.

John Snow, a British physician, is considered the "father of epidemiology."[55] Industrialization in England in the nineteenth century resulted in rapid expansion of London's population that outgrew city services. An outbreak of cholera in the Soho area of London in 1854 resulted in more than 600 deaths. Snow discovered that the outbreak centered around one particular public water pump, which got water from a well

Table 9-10	Reduction in Vaccine-Preventable Diseases in the United States		
Disease	Baseline 20th Century Annual Cases*	2006 Cases	% Reduction
Diphtheria	175,885	0	100
Measles	503,282	55	99.9
Mumps	152,209	6584	95.7
Pertussis	147,271	15,632	89.4
Smallpox	48,164	0	100
Polio	16,316	0	100
Rubella	47,745	11	99.9
Tetanus	1,314	41	96.9
Haemophilus influenzae type b, invasive	20,000	29	99.9

From National Institute of Allergy and Infectious Disease, National Institutes of Health: Vaccine, Vaccine Benefits available at www3.niaid.nih.gov/topics/vaccines/understanding/vaccineBenefits.htm. Accessed February 15, 2009.

*Average number of reported cases over multiple years before initiation of vaccine (Centers for Disease Control and Prevention: *MMWR Morb Mortal Wkly Rep* 48[12]:243-248, 1999, *Morb Mortal Wkly Rep* 57[11]:289-291, 2008.)

that had been dug 3 feet from a cesspool (open sewage was common in London at that time). After the pump was closed, the rate of new cholera cases rapidly diminished. Snow's observation stimulated the development of the construction of clean water supplies and sewers throughout the city.

Sewage removal and other public health initiatives (e.g., routine trash collection, disposal of garbage by incineration or in landfills) are now the expected norm in developed countries. The quality of water and food, as well as disposal of human and animal waste, remains poor in many developing countries. Rapid urbanization as well as other problems (e.g., poverty, overcrowding, mass relocation of people due to war, rapid destruction of forests) has put pressure on already inadequate systems.[56] A 1991 outbreak of cholera in Peru resulted in an estimated 10,000 deaths and was attributed to inadequate sanitation.

Additionally, previously successful programs designed to control the breeding of insect vectors have been reversed. Despite an international emphasis on draining standing water that provides breeding grounds for mosquitoes, large unmanaged areas still abound. A very successful international mosquito eradication program resulted in decreasing incidence of mosquito-borne diseases. Some regions were declared "free" of mosquito-borne diseases. However, since the international ban on DDT for agricultural work and limitation of its use for control of disease vectors, mosquitoes and mosquito-related diseases have rebounded in previously disease-free areas. In northern India, heavy rains in the 1990s resulted in an increase in standing water that was not drained because of the lack of government-provided public health information and inadequate insecticides to control mosquitoes. Since 1996, recurrent and increasingly severe outbreaks of dengue fever (caused by dengue virus, which is related to yellow fever virus and West Nile virus) have occurred in this region. In the 2006 outbreak 10,344 cases were reported, with 162 deaths. This problem is exacerbated by the development of insecticide-resistant mosquitoes.

Antimicrobials

Since the first use of penicillin during World War II, antibiotics have had the greatest effect on controlling infection. Antibiotics are natural products of fungi, bacteria, and related

microorganisms and kill or inhibit the growth of other microorganisms. Numerous chemicals or antimicrobials have been identified that either prevent the growth of microorganisms or directly destroy them. Antibiotics generally act by preventing the function of enzymes or cell structures that are unique to the infecting agent. Because viruses use the enzymes of the host's cells, there has been far less success in developing antiviral antibiotics.

Immediately after antibiotics became widely used, microorganisms mutated and developed resistance.[57] By 1944 an adequate supply of penicillin allowed its widespread use to treat infections. In 1946 a hospital in Britain reported that 14% of all *S. aureus* were penicillin resistant. By 1950 the same hospital reported an increase to 59% and to greater than 89% in the 1990s. Over the past few decades healthcare providers have observed increasing incidences of drug-resistant malaria, tuberculosis, gonorrhea, salmonellosis, shigellosis, and staphylococcal infections. *S. pneumoniae,* which causes pneumonia, meningitis, and acute otitis media (ear infections), was once routinely susceptible to penicillin. Since the 1980s, however, the incidence of penicillin-resistant microorganisms has risen to greater than 30% in some populations.

The goal of antibiotic therapy is elimination of the pathogenic microorganism. Some antibacterial antibiotics are **bactericidal** (kill the organism), whereas others are **bacteriostatic** (inhibit growth until the organism is destroyed by the individual's own protective mechanisms). The mechanisms of action of most antibiotics are (1) inhibition of the function or production of the cell wall, (2) prevention of protein synthesis, (3) blockage of DNA replication, or (4) interference with folic acid metabolism.

Antibiotic resistance is usually a result of genetic mutations that can be transmitted directly to neighboring microorganisms by plasmid exchange. Microorganisms commonly develop the capacity to inactivate antibiotics. Penicillin resistance, for example, results from the production of an enzyme (β-lactamase) that breaks down the structure of the antibiotic. Other forms of resistance result from modification of the target molecule. Azidothymidine (AZT) is a family of antivirals that suppresses the enzymatic activity of reverse transcriptase,

WHAT'S
NEW?   Phage Therapy

The rapid spread of infections caused by antibiotic-resistant bacteria has outpaced the development of new antibiotics and vaccines. Scientists and healthcare providers are seriously considering alternative forms of antibacterial therapy. Considerable excitement has arisen concerning phage therapy. Phages (i.e., bacteriophages) are viruses that specifically attach to bacteria and inject their nucleic acid (most phages have dsDNA genomes). The infected bacteria produce many daughter phages (in excess of 100 progeny per infected bacterium), which are released from the bacteria by lysis.

As it turns out, phage therapy was actually "rediscovered" in the United States and Western Europe. In the 1920s scientists in the Republic of Georgia, then part of the Soviet Union, began to study the use of phages to treat infection. Similar studies were being performed in the West but interest disappeared with the development of antibiotics in the 1940s. In the Soviet Union, however, phage therapy was used extensively during WWII with reportedly good success rates, particularly in preventing gas gangrene caused by *Clostridium perfringens*. Although research and clinical applications of phage therapy continued until today, Western scientists and clinicians remained relatively uninformed of the progress because most of the studies were published in Russian or in local journals in Georgian or Ukrainian.

Phages have several advantages over antibiotics. Because phages do not infect human cells there are none of the side effects associated with antibiotic use. Usually only a single dose is necessary because of the multiplicative effect of phage propagation in the bacteria. They are more specific than drugs, thus do not alter the normal flora.

The greater specificity may also be a disadvantage because one phage may only react with a particular serotype of a bacterium, and considerable time would be needed to identify the infecting bacteria and match it with a particular phage. This problem has been overcome by using mixtures of phages against most of the common pathogenic bacteria. Gastrointestinal infections have been successfully treated by oral administration of mixtures of phages (as many as 30 different phages) with reactivities against *Salmonella* spp., *Escherichia coli*, *Shigella*, and *Vibrio*. Wound infections have been prevented using dressings containing a mixture of phages against *Staphylococcus aureus*, *Streptococcus* spp., *Pseudomonas aeruginosa*, *Proteus* spp., and *E. coli*. To minimize the complexity of phage mixtures, reagents with broader specificity are under development. For example, a highly virulent and specific phage has been developed that is active against about 80% to 95% of *Staphylococcus aureus* strains, including methicillin-resistant *Staphylococcus aureus* (MRSA).

A potential disadvantage is related to the rapid release of endotoxin and other bacterial toxins from infected cells undergoing lysis. A rapid surge in circulating endotoxin could induce a fatal endotoxic shock. Several nonlytic variants of phages, which kill bacteria without lysis, are under development. However, without lysis the number of phages would not increase because of proliferation, and an increase in the dose or number of injections may be necessary.

Studies in experimental animals have confirmed the therapeutic and prophylactic potential of phage therapy against *S. aureus* abscesses and infection of burns with *P. aeruginosa*. Phages also can be administered systemically and can access several sites (e.g., the brain) that are difficult to treat with antibiotics. Tests in animal models with disseminated bacterial infections (e.g., *E. coli*) confirm that phages may be more effective than antibiotics.

Several companies are testing phage therapy in phase I and II clinical trials in Europe and the United States. Although the medical use of phage therapy may be years away in the United States, this technology is being applied in the food industry. In 2006 the U.S. Food and Drug Administration (FDA) approved the use of a phage cocktail to spray ready-to-eat meat products to eliminate contaminating *Listeria monocytogenes*. Additional testing is being performed using phages to eliminate *Campylobacter jejuni* (a major cause of diarrhea from eating contaminated chicken) from food products.

Data from Fischetti VA, Nelson D, Schuch R: *Nat Biotech* 24(12):1508-1511, 2006; Hanlon GW: *Int J Antimicrob Agents* 30(2):118-128, 2007; Mann NH: *Res Microbiol* 159(5):400-405, 2008; Mattey M, Spencer J: *Curr Opin Biotechnol*, 2008, Nov 4 [Epub ahead of print]; Thiel K: *Biotech* 22(1):31-36, 2004.

a viral-specific enzyme responsible for the replication of viral RNA and production of a DNA copy. HIV frequently mutates and produces an AZT-resistant reverse transcriptase. A third mechanism of resistance is mediated by multidrug transporters in the microorganism's membrane. These transporters affect the rate of intracellular accumulation of the antimicrobial by preventing entrance or, more commonly, increasing active efflux of the antibiotic. Antibiotic-resistant strains of *M. tuberculosis* are protected from aminoglycosides and tetracycline by the Tap protein (a mycobacterial multidrug efflux pump).

Many microorganisms are now resistant to multiple antibiotics. **Methicillin-resistant *Staphylococcus aureus* (MRSA)** incorporates several different mechanisms of resistance. MRSA produces a β-lactamase (penicillinase). Penicillinase-resistant antibiotics (e.g., methicillin) can be used as a substitute, but MRSA carrying the gene *mecA*, is also methicillin resistant because of a lower affinity for β-lactams. Resistance to the glycopeptide antibiotic vancomycin is controlled by the gene *vanA*, that results in alterations in peptidoglycans and loss of the vancomycin binding site.[58]

Why have multiple antibiotic–resistant microorganisms appeared? Overuse of antibiotics can lead to the destruction of the normal flora, allowing the selective overgrowth of antibiotic-resistant strains or pathogens that had previously been kept under control.[59] For example, after treatment with the antibiotic clindamycin, the normal intestinal flora can become compromised, allowing the overgrowth of *C. difficile* and the development of pseudomembranous colitis. Also, lack of compliance concerning the necessity of completing the therapeutic regimen with antibiotics allows the selective resurgence of microorganisms that are more relatively resistant to the antibiotic.

With the development of multiple antibiotic–resistant strains, creativity in addressing this challenge must be rekindled. New antibiotics may solve a portion of the problem or may exacerbate it further as pathogens develop resistance to new antibiotics as well. Available antibiotics that prove to be no longer effective must be replaced with alternative forms of therapy, including the increased development and use of vaccines and other therapies.

| Table 9-11 | Recommended Adult Immunization Schedule by Vaccine and Age Group—United States, October 2007 to September 2008 |

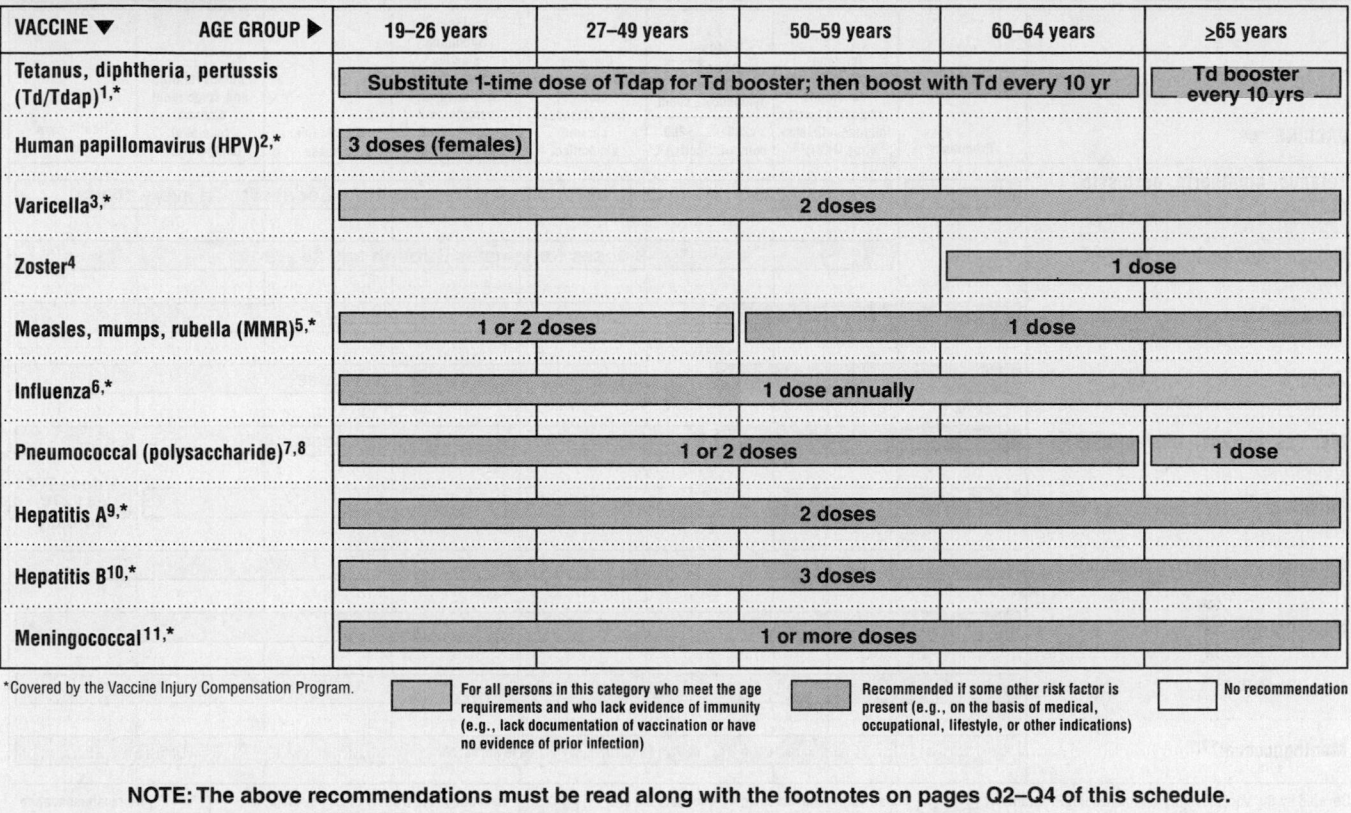

VACCINE ▼ AGE GROUP ▶	19–26 years	27–49 years	50–59 years	60–64 years	≥65 years
Tetanus, diphtheria, pertussis (Td/Tdap)[1],*	Substitute 1-time dose of Tdap for Td booster; then boost with Td every 10 yr				Td booster every 10 yrs
Human papillomavirus (HPV)[2],*	3 doses (females)				
Varicella[3],*	2 doses				
Zoster[4]				1 dose	
Measles, mumps, rubella (MMR)[5],*	1 or 2 doses		1 dose		
Influenza[6],*	1 dose annually				
Pneumococcal (polysaccharide)[7],[8]	1 or 2 doses				1 dose
Hepatitis A[9],*	2 doses				
Hepatitis B[10],*	3 doses				
Meningococcal[11],*	1 or more doses				

*Covered by the Vaccine Injury Compensation Program.

For all persons in this category who meet the age requirements and who lack evidence of immunity (e.g., lack documentation of vaccination or have no evidence of prior infection)

Recommended if some other risk factor is present (e.g., on the basis of medical, occupational, lifestyle, or other indications)

No recommendation

NOTE: The above recommendations must be read along with the footnotes on pages Q2–Q4 of this schedule.

From the Centers for Disease Control and Prevention. Available at www.cdc.gov/vaccines/recs/schedules/default.htm.

Active Immunization: Vaccines

Contracting and surviving an infectious disease is the most effective means of developing lifelong immunity against a particular pathogen. However, some infections cause a great deal of morbidity and mortality. The purpose of vaccination is to induce active immunologic protection before exposure to the risks of infection. For each vaccine an initial immunization protocol is developed to produce large numbers of memory cells and a sustained protective secondary immune response in the greatest number of individuals. In general, vaccine-induced protection does not persist as long as infection-induced immunity, thus booster injections may be necessary to maintain protection throughout life.

Common vaccines used in the United States and their abbreviations, as noted in Tables 9-11 and 9-12, are as follows:

- Diphtheria (D): A bacterial infection of the throat; produces a toxin that can lead to heart failure or paralysis; the vaccine is an inactivated form of diphtheria toxin (toxoid); part of DTaP combined vaccine
- *H. influenzae* type b (Hib): A bacterial infection that is commonly contracted by children younger than 5 years and infects the blood, joints, bones, and membrane covering the heart; most common cause of serious bacterial meningitis in children; the vaccine is an extracted bacterial antigen conjugated to a protein carrier

- Hepatitis A virus: A virus that causes liver disease; recommended in selected states and regions; vaccine is an inactivated virus
- Hepatitis B virus: Causes cirrhosis of the liver and liver cancer; the vaccine is a recombinant viral protein
- Influenza: a virus that causes severe upper respiratory tract infections; the most common vaccine is an injected inactivated virus
- Measles and mumps (MM): Viruses that cause fever and rash (measles) or inflammation of the salivary glands (mumps); mumps also may cause meningitis; both vaccines are attenuated live viruses; part of MMR combined vaccine
- Meningococcal: *N. meningitidis* is a major bacterial cause of meningitis, particularly in young adults; the vaccine contains four different extracted capsular polysaccharides
- Pertussis (acellular pertussis [aP]), or whooping cough: A bacterial infection that causes severe coughing in children younger than 5 years; the vaccine is an inactivated toxin and other bacterial antigens; part of DTaP combined vaccine
- Pneumococcal: *S. pneumoniae* causes pneumonia, particularly in older adults; the childhood vaccine is a protein conjugate with 7 different capsular antigens; the adult vaccine is a mixture of 10 extracted capsular polysaccharides

Table 9-12	Recommended Immunization Schedule for Persons Ages 0 to 6 Years—United States 2008

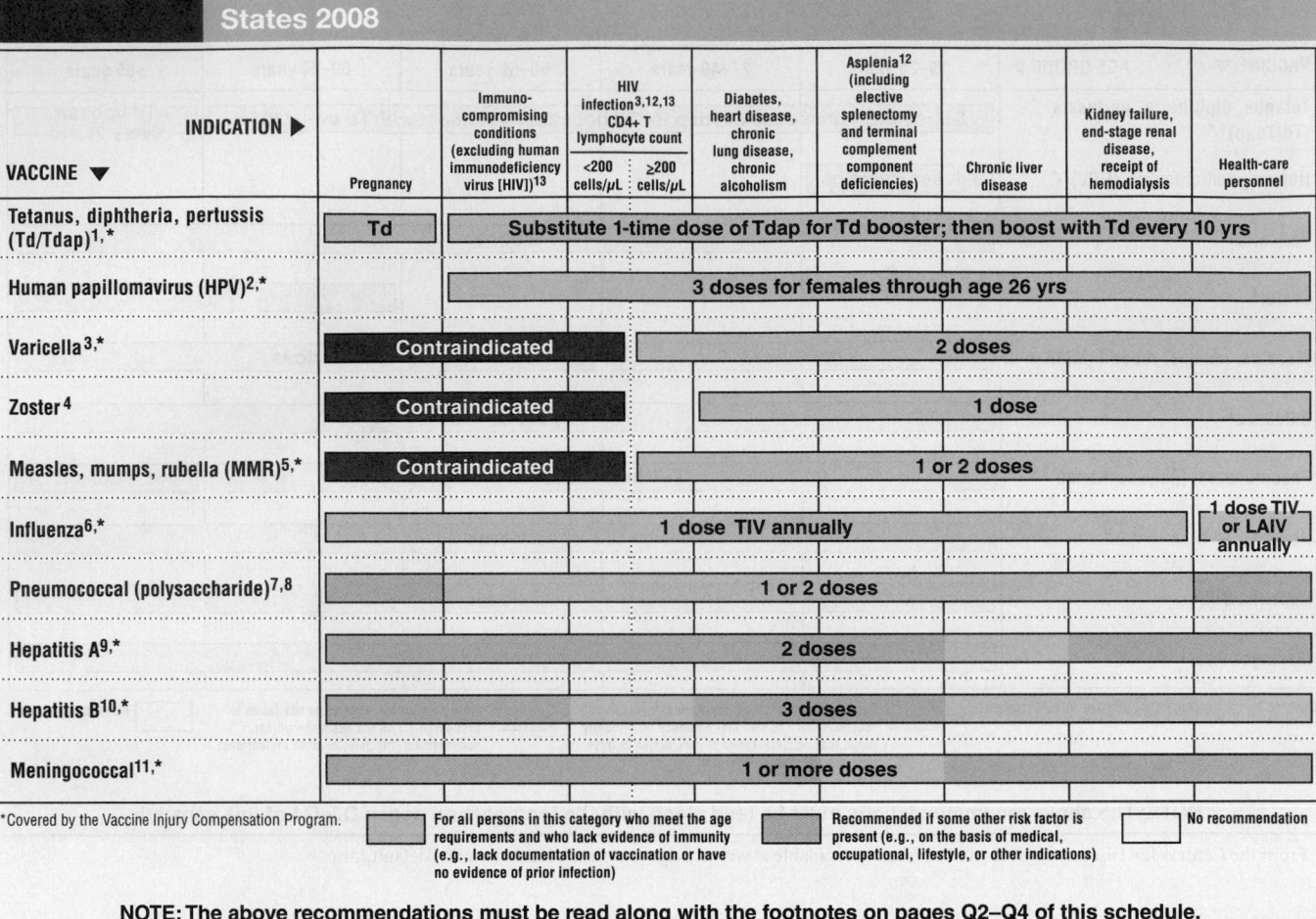

VACCINE ▼ INDICATION ▶	Pregnancy	Immuno-compromising conditions (excluding human immunodeficiency virus [HIV])[13]	HIV infection[3,12,13] CD4+ T lymphocyte count <200 cells/μL	HIV infection[3,12,13] CD4+ T lymphocyte count ≥200 cells/μL	Diabetes, heart disease, chronic lung disease, chronic alcoholism	Asplenia[12] (including elective splenectomy and terminal complement component deficiencies)	Chronic liver disease	Kidney failure, end-stage renal disease, receipt of hemodialysis	Health-care personnel
Tetanus, diphtheria, pertussis (Td/Tdap)[1,*]	Td	Substitute 1-time dose of Tdap for Td booster; then boost with Td every 10 yrs							
Human papillomavirus (HPV)[2,*]		3 doses for females through age 26 yrs							
Varicella[3,*]	Contraindicated			2 doses					
Zoster[4]	Contraindicated				1 dose				
Measles, mumps, rubella (MMR)[5,*]	Contraindicated			1 or 2 doses					
Influenza[6,*]	1 dose TIV annually								1 dose TIV or LAIV annually
Pneumococcal (polysaccharide)[7,8]	1 or 2 doses								
Hepatitis A[9,*]	2 doses								
Hepatitis B[10,*]	3 doses								
Meningococcal[11,*]	1 or more doses								

*Covered by the Vaccine Injury Compensation Program.

For all persons in this category who meet the age requirements and who lack evidence of immunity (e.g., lack documentation of vaccination or have no evidence of prior infection)

Recommended if some other risk factor is present (e.g., on the basis of medical, occupational, lifestyle, or other indications)

No recommendation

NOTE: The above recommendations must be read along with the footnotes on pages Q2–Q4 of this schedule.

From the Centers for Disease Control and Prevention. Available at www.cdc.gov/vaccines/recs/schedules/default.htm.

- Polio: Polio is a viral infection that causes paralysis and death; the vaccine is an inactivated virus
- Rotavirus: A viral infection that causes severe diarrhea primarily in babies and young children; the vaccine is an attenuated live virus
- Rubella (R), or German measles: A viral infection that causes fever and rash; may cause severe birth defects in pregnant women infected in the first trimester; part of MMR combined vaccine
- Tetanus (T): A bacterial infection that produces a toxin that attacks the nervous system and may cause death; the vaccine is an inactivated form of the tetanus toxin (toxoid); part of DTaP combined vaccine
- Varicella-zoster (varicella): A virus that causes chickenpox; vaccine is an attenuated live virus

Mass vaccination programs have led to major changes in the health of the world's population. In the early 1950s an estimated 50 million cases of smallpox occurred each year, with about 15 million deaths. The World Health Organization (WHO) conducted a smallpox immunization campaign from 1967 to 1977 that resulted in the global eradication of smallpox by 1979. The 1988 immunization initiative against polio resulted in a 99% decrease in that disease. In 1960, 2525 cases of paralytic polio were reported in the United States, but no cases of naturally acquired polio have been reported since 1979. In 1994, polio was declared officially eradicated in all the Americas. The goal of the WHO is to eradicate polio worldwide in the next few years (Figure 9-17). Similar trends occurred for each disease against which an effective vaccine has been developed.

Development of a successful vaccine depends on many factors. These include characterizing the desired protective immune response (e.g., antibody, T cell), identifying the appropriate antigen to induce that response (i.e., immune responses against some antigens on an infectious agent are ineffective or even increase the risk for infection), determining the most effective route of administration (e.g., injected, oral, inhaled), optimizing the number and timing of vaccine doses to induce protective immunity in a large proportion of the at-risk population, and deciding the most effective, yet safe, form in which to administer the vaccine. For instance, most vaccines against viral infections (e.g., measles, mumps,

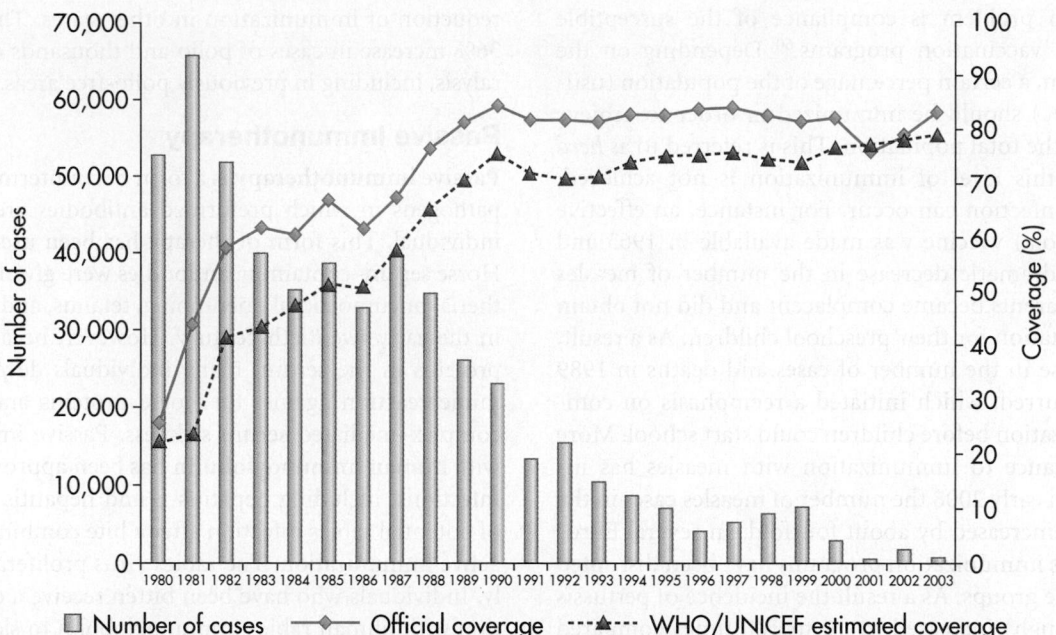

Figure 9-17 Effect of immunization on the global reported cases of polio, 1980 to 2003. The number of global cases of polio has progressively decreased in an inverse relationship to the extent of vaccination. The "official coverage" is the percent of the world's population that has been reported to the World Health Organization (WHO) by 192 member countries as being immunized. The "WHO/UNICEF estimated coverage" indicates the best estimate of the real percentage of the population that has been immunized. (From World Health Organization: *WHO vaccine-preventable diseases: monitoring system, 2003 global summary*, Geneva, Switzerland, 2003. Additional information is available at www.who.int/vaccines-documents.)

rubella, varicella [chickenpox], rotavirus) contain live viruses that are weakened (**attenuated**) to continue expressing the appropriate antigens but are unable to establish more than a limited and easily controlled infection. The limited proliferative capacity of attenuated live viruses appears to afford better long-term protection than using purified viral antigen. Two exceptions are the vaccines against hepatitis B, which uses a recombinant viral protein, and hepatitis A, which is an inactivated (killed) virus.

Even attenuated viruses can, however, establish life-threatening infections in vaccine recipients whose immune system is congenitally deficient or suppressed (see Chapter 8). Two different vaccines were developed against polio. The Sabin vaccine is an attenuated virus that is administered orally. It provides systemic protection and induces a secretory immune response to prevent growth of the poliovirus in the intestinal tract. The live attenuated vaccine causes polio in some children who have unsuspected immune deficiencies (about 1 case in 2.4 million doses). The Salk vaccine is a completely inactivated virus administered by injection. It induces protective systemic immunity but does not provide adequate secretory immunity. Therefore, even if the individual is protected from systemic infection the "wild-type" poliovirus can transiently infect the intestinal mucosa, be shed, and spread to others. When polio was epidemic, the live oral vaccine was preferred; however, about eight cases of paralytic polio per year in the United States resulted from the vaccine strain proliferating in individuals with inadequate immune systems. As

a result, the CDC currently recommends vaccination with the killed virus.

Some common bacterial vaccines are killed microorganisms or extracts of bacterial antigens. The vaccine against pneumococcal pneumonia consists of a mixture of capsular polysaccharides from 10 strains of *S. pneumoniae*. Of the more than 90 known strains of this microorganism, only these 10 cause the most severe illnesses. However, the capsular vaccine is not very immunogenic in young children. A "conjugated" vaccine is available that contains capsular polysaccharides from 7 strains that are conjugated to carrier proteins in order to increase immunogenicity. A similar vaccine is available for Hib.

Some bacterial diseases are caused by potent toxins that act locally or systemically. These include diphtheria, cholera, and tetanus. Vaccination against the toxins is achieved using **toxoids**—purified toxins that have been chemically detoxified without loss of immunogenicity. Pertussis (whooping cough) vaccine was changed from a killed whole cell vaccine to an acellular vaccine that contained the pertussis toxin and additional bacterial antigens.

With so many available vaccines there has been an effort to mix vaccines in order to minimize the number of required injections. One of the first licensed vaccine mixtures was DPT, which now usually contains diphtheria (D) and tetanus (T) toxoids and acellular pertussis vaccine (aP). More recent mixtures include DTaP with inactivated poliovirus, with either Hib conjugate to tetanus toxoid or with hepatitis B vaccine.

A common problem is compliance of the susceptible population in vaccination programs.[60] Depending on the microorganism, a certain percentage of the population (usually about 85%) should be immunized in order to achieve protection of the total population. This is referred to as *herd immunity*. If this level of immunization is not achieved, outbreaks of infection can occur. For instance, an effective measles (rubeola) vaccine was made available in 1963 and resulted in a dramatic decrease in the number of measles cases. Many parents became complacent and did not obtain measles vaccination for their preschool children. As a result, a large increase in the number of cases and deaths in 1989 and 1990 occurred, which initiated a reemphasis on complete immunization before children could start school. More recently resistance to immunization with measles has increased, and in early 2008 the number of measles cases in the United States increased by about fourfold. In several European countries immunization programs have been disrupted by anti-vaccine groups. As a result the incidence of pertussis (whooping cough) increased by 10 to 100 times compared with neighboring countries that maintained a high incidence of immunization.

The refusal to vaccinate has generally been based on potential vaccine dangers. As with any medicine, complications can arise. In the case of vaccines, these include pain and redness at the injection site, fever, allergic reactions to vaccine ingredients, infection associated with attenuated viruses in immunodeficient individuals, and others. For instance, a rotavirus vaccine approved a decade ago was found to increase the risk for a life-threatening bowel obstruction resulting from twisting of the intestines, and the vaccine was recalled.[61] A commonly discussed fear is related to the presence of the preservative thimerosal in vaccines. Thimerosal is a mercury-containing compound that has been used as a preservative since the 1930s. Although no cases of mercury toxicity have been reported secondary to vaccination, thimerosal was removed from all vaccines in 2001, with the exception of inactivated influenza vaccines.[62] In 2003, groups in northern Nigeria claimed that the oral polio vaccine was unsafe, which led to suspension of polio immunization in two states and reduction of immunization in other states. The result was a 36% increase in cases of polio and thousands of cases of paralysis, including in previously polio-free areas.

Passive Immunotherapy

Passive immunotherapy is a form of countermeasure against pathogens in which preformed antibodies are given to the individual. This form of therapy has been used for decades. Horse serum–containing antibodies were given to treat diphtheria, pneumococcal pneumonia, tetanus, and other diseases in the early twentieth century. However, because of foreign proteins in the serum, many individuals developed an immune reaction against the horse proteins and an immune complex–mediated serum sickness. Passive immunotherapy with **human immunoglobulin** has been approved for several infections, including hepatitis B and hepatitis A. Treatment of potential rabies infection after a bite combines passive and active immunization. The rabies virus proliferates very slowly. Individuals who have been bitten receive a onetime injection with human rabies immunoglobulin to slow down viral proliferation further, followed by multiple injections with a killed viral vaccine to induce greater protective immunity. For several diseases more specific therapy with monoclonal antibodies is being evaluated, and a monoclonal antibody against respiratory syncytial virus has been approved for therapy.

In the past, vaccines and therapeutic antibodies were developed for only the most deadly pathogens. With the increase in antibiotic-resistant microorganisms, the development and widespread use of new vaccines and antibodies against these microorganisms must be considered. For example, otitis media, a purulent ear infection, is caused primarily by *Streptococcus, Haemophilus,* and *Staphylococcus.* This infection routinely has been treated successfully with antibiotics; however, the increase in multiple antibiotic–resistant microorganisms may force a reevaluation of the use of childhood immunization as an alternative to preventing this disease. Other vaccines used now only to a limited degree may be used more widely in the future, and others may be developed soon, including vaccines against cholera, typhoid, malaria, West Nile virus, hantavirus, SARS, and several other diseases.

SUMMARY REVIEW

1. Death from infections are the eighth (influenza and pneumonia) and tenth (sepsis) leading causes of death in the United States and account for about one third of deaths worldwide.
2. Infectious disease is a significant cause of death and morbidity because of the reemergence of old infections thought to be controlled, emergence of previously unknown infections, and infections resistant to multiple antibiotics.
3. The current rate of emergence of previously unknown infections may be unprecedented. More than 40 unknown infections have arisen within one generation.
4. Although most infections are controlled, some uncontrolled infections have high mortality rates including SARS, Ebola virus, Marburg virus, "mad cow disease," Nipah virus, and AIDS.
5. Many common and reemerging infections have become antibiotic and drug resistant. At least 25% of *S. pneumoniae* are penicillin resistant and some are resistant to multiple antibiotics.
6. Resistant forms of *S. aureus,* a primary cause of infections of wounds, surgical incisions, and catheters, are endemic in some hospitals.
7. Antimicrobial resistance is routinely observed in tuberculosis, diarrheal diseases, hospital-acquired infections, malaria, meningitis, respiratory tract infections, STIs, and HIV.

Microorganisms and Humans: A Dynamic Relationship

1. The human body is a hospitable site for microorganisms to grow and flourish. These microorganisms make up the *normal flora* of the body.
2. The beneficial homeostasis between humans and microorganisms is maintained through the physical integrity of the gut and other mechanisms that sequester these microorganisms on the mucosal surface.

Microorganisms and Infections

1. The symbiotic relationship with the normal flora can be altered by injury, compromising protective barriers.
2. Cuts in the skin and compromised immunity can increase infections.
3. Damage to the intestinal track releases intestinal bacteria into the bloodstream, potentially leading to sepsis, shock, and death.
4. When an individual's immune system is deficient, the person can become infected with opportunistic infections.
5. Unlike opportunistic infectious agents, true pathogens can circumvent an individual's defenses and directly cause infection. Successful infection with these agents usually requires adequate numbers of microorganisms rather than compromised immune defenses.
6. The process of infection includes colonization, invasion, multiplication, and spread.
7. Infectious microorganisms usually exist in reservoirs (e.g., contaminated soil, contaminated water, breast milk), animals, or another human.
8. As part of colonization, the microorganism stabilizes the adherence to tissue through surface receptors. Once colonization occurs, the infectious agent can invade surrounding tissue.
9. Because tissue is warm and nutrient rich, most microorganisms undergo *rapid* multiplication. Viral pathogens replicate within infected cells and some bacteria are intracellular pathogens and replicate in macrophages and other cells.
10. Many pathogens produce only localized infections. Others are, however, highly invasive.
11. Successful spreading requires a variety of virulence factors, including adhesion molecules, toxins, and the ability to evade immunity.
12. Clinical infectious disease occurs in four distinct stages: (1) incubation period, (2) prodromal state, (3) invasion period, and (4) convalescence.
13. The hallmark of most infectious diseases is fever. Body temperature is regulated at a higher than normal level.
14. A large number of agents (pyrogens) can produce fever. Current classifications include endogenous (e.g., cytokines) and exogenous agents. However, the evidence for exogenous agents is limited and they indirectly affect the hypothalamus through endogenous pyrogens.
15. Several factors influence the capacity of a pathogen to cause disease, including communicability, immunogenicity, infectivity, mechanisms of action, pathogenicity, entry portal, toxigenicity, and virulence.
16. Infectious diseases also are classified by their prevalence and spread as endemic, epidemic, and pandemic.
17. Classes of infectious microorganisms include bacterial, fungal, parasitic, protozoal, and viral.
18. Bacteria are divided into several groups: "true bacteria," filamentous, spirochetes, mycoplasma, rickettsia, and chlamydia.
19. Stable colonization of bacteria requires adhesion. Many bacteria attach through pili, also called fimbriae.
20. Invasion by bacteria results in direct confrontation with an individual's defense mechanisms, including complement, antibodies, and phagocytes (neutrophils, macrophages). Evasion of these defenses can result in bacteremia and sepsis.
21. Efficient pathogens can produce a variety of toxic molecules that may kill the individual's cells, disrupt tissue, and protect themselves against inflammation. Exotoxins are released by bacteria during bacterial growth and can damage cell membranes, activate second messengers, and inhibit protein synthesis.
22. Endotoxins are contained in the cell walls of gram-negative bacteria and released during lysis of the bacteria. Bacteria that produce endotoxins are called *pyrogenic bacteria* because they activate inflammation and produce fever.
23. Bacteria can protect against phagocytosis by producing toxins and extracellular enzymes that destroy phagocytic cells.
24. Some bacteria can coat the Fc portion of an individual's antibody, preventing complement activation or phagocytosis.
25. Antigenic variation allows the pathogen to alter surface molecules that express antigens that are the targets of protective immune responses. The pathogen thus becomes resistant.
26. Other self-protective mechanisms for bacteria and other pathogens include degrading immune molecules, neutralization of immune molecules, complement evasion, and immune suppression.
27. Tissue damage from bacterial infections is either directly by bacterial products or indirectly from infection.
28. *S. aureus* has become a major cause of hospital-acquired (nosocomial) infections. Antibiotic resistance also has become a major problem with *S. aureus*.
29. Fungal infection is called mycosis. Most pathologic fungi are from the environment and transmitted by inhalation or contamination of wounds.
30. In 2006, the opportunistic pathogen *P. carinii* was reclassified as a fungus and the specific variant that infects humans was renamed *P. jiroveci*.
31. *C. albicans* is the most common cause of fungal infections in humans. It resides in the skin, gastrointestinal tract, mouth, and vagina. Local defense mechanisms, including members of the bacterial flora, produce antifungal agents. The infection remains localized in individuals with an intact immune system.
32. Parasitic organisms establish a symbiosis with another species, whereby the parasite benefits. They range from unicellular protozoa to large worms. Although less common in the United States, parasites and protozoa are common causes of infection worldwide.
33. Parasitic and protozoal infections are rarely transmitted from human to human. Infection mainly spreads through vectors and includes malaria by mosquito bites, trypanosomes by the tsetse fly, and *Leishmania* spp. by sand fleas. Others are found in contaminated water or food (e.g., *G. lamblia*).
34. Malaria is one of the most common infections worldwide. It is transmitted through the bite of an infected *Anopheles* mosquito. The parasite enters the bloodstream, survives in the liver, and invades parenchymal cells. After several rounds of division, the liver cell ruptures and thousands of parasites enter the blood, infecting red blood cells.

Continued

35. Viruses are classified by the format of nucleic acid in the virion (RNA or DNA), either single stranded (ss) or double stranded (ds), and whether it uses the enzyme RT for replication.

36. Viral diseases are the most common affliction of humans and include the common cold, the "coldsore," hepatitis, HIV, and several types of cancer.

37. Viruses are intracellular parasites. The viral life cycle is completely intracellular and involves several stages: attachment, penetration, uncoating, replication, assembly, and release. New virions are released from the cell for transmission of the viral infection to neighboring, uninfected cells.

38. The primary defense mechanisms against viruses include antibody and cellular immunity. Nonspecific defenses include α- and β-interferons that block intracellular replication.

39. Successful viruses use a variety of mechanisms for bypassing immune rejection, including rapid division, intracellular survival, coating with self proteins, antigenic variation, neutralization, complement evasion, and immune suppression.

40. Viruses inside the infected cell have several harmful effects, including inhibition of DNA, RNA, or protein synthesis; disruption of lysosomal membranes result in lytic enzyme release; promotion of cell apoptosis; fusion of adjacent cells (i.e., giant cells); transformation into a neoplastic cell; and alteration of antigenic properties (i.e., decreasing immune effectiveness).

Acquired Immunodeficiency Syndrome (AIDS)

1. AIDS is a viral disease caused by HIV.

2. HIV infects and depletes a portion of the immune system (Th cells) making individuals susceptible to life-threatening infections and malignancies.

3. HIV/AIDS remains a major cause of death worldwide.

4. Aggressive antiretroviral therapy and public health campaigns have stabilized the number of new cases and deaths in the United States from HIV/AIDS, but the cases and deaths continue to increase rapidly worldwide.

5. In 2006, 50% of newly diagnosed cases were attributed to male-to-male sexual contact, 33% to high-risk heterosexual contact, and 13% to injected drug abuse. About 26% of newly diagnosed cases were female, with about 74% contracted through high-risk heterosexual contact.

6. The epicenter of the AIDS pandemic is Sub-Saharan Africa. Women have the highest risk of infection. The life expectancy with AIDS has dropped from 64 years to 54 years.

7. HIV is a blood-borne pathogen present in body fluids (e.g., blood, vaginal fluid, semen, breast milk) with typical routes of transmission: blood or blood products, intravenous drug abuse, heterosexual and homosexual activity, and maternal-child transmission before or during birth.

8. At the end of 2006, an estimated 8508 children in the United States developed AIDS after contracting HIV infection from their mothers (e.g., across the placenta, through contact with infected blood during delivery, or breast milk)

9. Healthcare providers are at increased risk of contracting infections from another person's blood. However, as of January 2007, only 57 cases of confirmed HIV/AIDS and 140 possible cases were contracted by occupational exposure.

10. HIV is a member of the *retrovirus* family, which carries genetic information in the form of two copies of RNA. An enzyme, RT, converts RNA into a double-stranded DNA. Another enzyme, an *integrase*, inserts the new DNA into the infected cell's genetic material. On activation, translation of the viral information may be initiated, forming new virions, resulting in lysis and death of the infected cell, and shedding infectious HIV particles.

11. The primary surface receptor on HIV is the envelope glycoprotein gp120, which binds to the CD4 molecule found mostly on the surface of helper T cells. Several other important co-receptors have been identified.

12. The major immunologic finding in AIDS is the striking decrease in the number of CD4 Th cells.

13. The presence of circulating antibody against HIV indicates infection by the virus, although many individuals are asymptomatic.

14. The current treatment for HIV infection is a combination of drugs called HAART.

Countermeasures Against Pathogens

1. Effective means of countering infectious microorganisms is rigorous use of environmental infection control measures, including insect control, modern sanitation facilities, and clean water and food. Prophylactic or interventive procedures include vaccines and antimicrobials.

2. With antibiotic-resistant pathogens, a greater emphasis is placed on the development of new vaccines.

KEY TERMS

Acquired immunodeficiency syndrome (AIDS), 318
Antibiotic resistance, 306
Antigenic drift, 316
Antigenic shift, 317
Antigenic variation, 304
Antitoxin, 301
Attenuated, 331
Bacteremia, 301
Bacterial superantigens, 305
Bactericidal, 327
Bacteriostatic, 327
β-Lactamase, 307
Biofilms, 296
Capsule, 304
Dimorphic, 307
Endogenous pyrogen, 297

Endotoxic shock (septic shock), 305
Endotoxin, 301
Entrance inhibitor, 324
Exogenous pyrogen, 297
Exotoxin, 301
Gene switching, 311
Highly active antiretroviral therapy (HAART), 322
Human immunodeficiency virus (HIV), 318
Human immunoglobulin, 332
IgA protease, 304
Integrase, 319
Integrase inhibitor, 324
Lipopolysaccharide (LPS), 301
Methicillin-resistant *Staphylococcus aureus* (MRSA), 328
Mold, 307

Multinucleated giant cell, 316
Mutation, 316
Mycosis, 307
Passive immunotherapy, 332
Pili (fimbriae), 298
Protease inhibitor, 322
Recombination, 317
Reverse transcriptase, 319
Reverse transcriptase inhibitor, 322
Sepsis, 301
Syncytium, 319
Tissue tropism, 296
Toxoid, 331
Window period, 322
Yeast, 307
Zoonotic infection, 313

REFERENCES

1. Fauci AS, Touchette NA, Folkers GK: Emerging infectious diseases: a 10-year perspective from the National Institutes of Allergy and Infectious Disease, *Emerg Infect Dis* 11(4):519-525, 2005.
2. Hull MW, Chow AW: Indigenous microflora and innate immunity of the head and neck, *Infect Dis Clin North Am* 21(2):265-282, 2007.
3. Greger M: The human/animal interface: emergence and resurgence of zoonotic infectious diseases, *Crit Rev Microbiol* 33(4):243-299, 2007.
4. Gillim-Ross L, Subbarao K: Emerging respiratory viruses: challenges and vaccine strategies, *Clin Microbiol Rev* 19(4):614-636, 2006.
5. Rothman RE, Hsieh YH, Yang S: Communicable respiratory threats in the ED: tuberculosis, SARS, and other aerosolized infections, *Emerg Med Clin North Am* 24(4):989-1017, 2006.
6. Pizarro-Cerda J, Cossart P: Bacterial adhesion and entry into host cells, *Cell* 124(4):715-727, 2006.
7. Otto M: Staphylococcal biofilms. *Curr Top Microbiol Immunol* 322(1):207-228, 2008.
8. Kleinpell RM, Graves BT, Ackerman MH: Incidence, pathogenesis, and management of sepsis: an overview, *AACN Adv Crit Care* 17(4):385-393, 2006.
9. Finlay BB, McFadden G: Anti-immunology: evasion of the host immune system by bacterial and viral pathogens, *Cell* 124(4):767-782, 2006.
10. Hybiske K, Stephens RS: Exit strategies of intracellular pathogens, *Nat Rev Microbiol* 6(2):99-110, 2008.
11. Pizarro-Cerda J, Cossart P: Subversion of cellular functions by *Listeria monocytogenes*, *J Pathol* 208(2):215-223, 2006.
12. Labbe K, Saleh M: Cell death in the host response to infection, *Cell Death Differ* 15(9):1339-1349, 2008.
13. Kwinn LA, Nizer V: How group A *Streptococcus* circumvents host phagocyte defenses, *Future Med* 2(1):75-84, 2007.
14. Lambris JD, Ricklin D, Geisbrecht BV: Complement evasion by human pathogens, *Nat Rev Microbiol* 6(2):132-142, 2008.
15. Zipfel PF, Wurzner R, Skerka C: Complement evasion of pathogens: common strategies are shared by diverse organisms, *Mol Immunol* 44(16):3850-3857, 2007.
16. Mizgerd JP: Acute lower respiratory tract infection, *N Engl J Med* 358(7):716-727, 2008.
17. Karin M, Lawrence T, Nizet V: Innate immunity gone awry: linking microbial infections to chronic inflammation and cancer, *Cell* 124(4):823-835, 2006.
18. Gao H, Evans TW, Finney SJ: Bench-to-bedside review: sepsis, severe sepsis, and septic shock—does the nature of the infecting organism matter? *Crit Care* 12(3):213, 2008.
19. Gordon RJ, Lowy FD: Pathogenesis of methicillin-resistant *Staphylococcus aureus* infection, *Clin Infect Dis* 46(Suppl 5):S350-S359, 2008.
20. Kraus D, Peschel A: *Staphylococcus aureus* evasion of innate antimicrobial defense, *Future Microbiol* 3(4):437-451, 2008.
21. Diep BA, Otto M: The role of virulence determinants in community-associated MRSA pathogenesis, *Trends Microbiol* 16(8):361-369, 2008.
22. D'Avignon LC, Schofield CM, Hospenthal DR: *Pneumocystis* pneumonia, *Semin Respir Crit Care Med* 29(2):132-140, 2008.
23. Stringer JR: Antigenic variation in *Pneumocystis*, *J Eukaryot Microbiol* 54(1):8-13, 2007.
24. Ferguson LR, Philpott M: Nutrition and mutagenesis, *Ann Rev Nutr* 28(1):313-329, 2008.
25. Netea MG et al. An integrated model of the recognition of *Candida albicans* by the innate immune system, *Nat Rev Microbiol* 6(1):67-78, 2008.
26. Marodi L, Johnston RB Jr: Invasive *Candida* species disease in infants and children: occurrence, risk factors, management, and innate host, *Curr Opin Pediatr* 19(6):693-697, 2007.
27. Mavor AL, Thewes S, Hube B: Systemic fungal infections caused by *Candida* species: epidemiology, infection process and virulence attributes, *Curr Drug Targets* 6(8):863-874, 2005.
28. Calderone RA, Fonzi WA: Virulence factors of *Candida albicans*, *Trends Microbiol* 9(7):327-335, 2001.
29. Zambrano-Villa S et al: How protozoan parasites evade the immune response, *Trends Parasitol* 18(6):272-278, 2002.
30. Mosser DM, Miles SA: Avoidance of innate immune mechanisms by the protozoan parasite, *Leishmania spp.* In Denkers E, Gazzinelli R, editors: *Protozoans in macrophages*, pp 118-129, Austin, TX, 2007, Landes Bioscience.
31. Alves MJ, Colli W: *Trypanosoma cruzi*: adhesion to the host cells and intracellular survival, *IUBMB Life* 59(4-5):274-279, 2007.
32. van Riet E, Hartgers FC, Yazdanbakhsh M: Chronic helminth infections induce immunomodulation: consequences and mechanisms, *Immunobiol* 212(6):475-490, 2007.
33. Raes G et al: Alternatively activated macrophages in protozoan infections, *Curr Opin Immunol* 19(4):454-459, 2007.
34. Stijlemans B et al: African trypanosomosis: from immune escape and immunopathology to immune intervention, *Vet Parasitol* 148(1):3-13, 2007.
35. Greenwood BM et al: Malaria: progress, perils, and prospects for eradication, *J Clin Invest* 118(4):1266-1276, 2008.
36. Cowman AF, Crabb BS: Invasion of red blood cells by malaria parasites, *Cell* 124(4):755-766, 2006.
37. Dzikowski R, Templeton TJ, Deitsch K: Variant antigen gene expression in malaria, *Cell Microbiol* 8(9):1371-1381, 2006.
38. Stewart PL, Nemerow GR: Cell integrins: commonly used receptors for diverse viral pathogens, *Trends Microbiol* 15(11):500-507, 2007.
39. Marsh M, Helenius A: Virus entry: open sesame, *Cell* 124(4):729-740, 2006.
40. Loch S, Tampe R: Viral evasion of the MHC class I antigen-processing machinery, *Eur J Physiol* 451(3):409-417, 2005.
41. Taubenberger JK, Morens DM: The pathology of influenza virus infections, *Annu Rev Pathol* 3(1):499-522, 2008.
42. Beigel JH: Influenza, *Crit Care Med* 36(9):2660-2666, 2008.
43. Boni MF: Vaccination and antigenic drift in influenza, *Vaccine* 26(Suppl 3):C8-C14, 2008.
44. Perrone LA, Tumpey TM: Reconstruction of the 1918 pandemic influenza virus, *Infect Disord Drug Targets* 7(4):294-303, 2007.
45. Chinen J, Shearer WT: Secondary immunodeficiencies, including HIV infection, *J Allergy Clin Immunol* 121(2):S388-S392, 2008.
46. Merson MH et al: The history and challenge of HIV prevention, *Lancet* 372(9637):475-488, 2008.
47. Padian NS et al: Biomedical interventions to prevent HIV infection: evidence, challenges, and way forward, *Lancet* 372(9638):585-599, 2008.
48. Do AN et al: Occupationally acquired human immunodeficiency virus (HIV) infection: national case surveillance data during 20 years of the HIV epidemic in the United States, *Infect Control Hosp Epidemiol* 24(2):86-96, 2003.
49. Centers for Disease Control and Prevention: *Fact sheet: surveillance of occupationally acquired HIV/AIDS in healthcare personnel, as of December 2006.* Available at www.cdc.gov/ncidod/dhqp/bp_hcp_w_hiv.html. Updated September, 2007.
50. Barre-Sinoussi F et al: Isolation of a T-lymphotropic retrovirus from a patient at risk for acquired immune deficiency syndrome (AIDS), *Science* 220(4599):868-871, 1983.
51. Goff SP: Host factors exploited by retroviruses, *Nat Rev Microbiol* 5(4):253-263, 2007.
52. Panel on Antiretroviral Guidelines for Adults and Adolescents: *Guidelines for the use of antiretroviral agents in HIV-1-infected adults and adolescents,* pp 1-139, Washington, DC, 2008 November 3, Department of Health and Human Services. Available at www.aidsinfo.nih.gov/ContentFiles/AdultandAdolescentGL.pdf. Accessed November 14, 2008.
53. Daar ES: Emerging resistance profiles of newly approved antiretroviral drugs, *Top HIV Med* 16(4):110-116, 2008.
54. Caldwell MB et al: 1994 revised classification system for human immunodeficiency virus infection in children less than 13 years of age, *MMWR Morb Mortal Wkly Rep* 43(RR-12):1-10, 1994.
55. Snow SJ: John Snow: the making of a hero? *Lancet* 372(9632):22-23, 2008.
56. de Waal A: On famine crimes and tragedies, *Lancet* 372(9649):1538-1539, 2008.
57. Hawkey PM: The growing burden of antimicrobial resistance, *J Antimicrob Chemother* 62(Suppl 1):i1-i9, 2008.
58. Werner G, Strommenger B, Witte W: Acquired vancomycin resistance in clinically relevant pathogens, *Future Micro* 3(5):547-562, 2008.
59. Gould IM: Who's winning the war? *J Antimicrob Chemother* 62(Suppl 3):iii3-iii6, 2008.
60. Feikin DR et al: Individual and community risks of measles and pertussis associated with personal exemptions to immunization, *JAMA* 284(24):3145-3150, 2000.
61. Centers for Disease Control and Prevention (CDC): Intussusception among recipients of rotavirus vaccine—United States, 1998-1999, *MMWR Morb Mortal Wkly Rep* 48(27):577-581, 1999.
62. Schecter R, Grether JK: Continuing increases in autism reported to California's developmental services system: mercury in retrograde, *Arch Gen Psych* 65(1):19-24, 2008.

STRESS AND DISEASE

BETH A. FORSHEE • MARGARET F. CLAYTON •
KATHRYN L. McCANCE

MEDIA RESOURCES

evolve **Evolve Website** (http://evolve.elsevier.com/McCance/)
- Review Questions and Answers
- Animations
- Glossary (with audio pronunciation for selected terms)
- WebLinks

CHAPTER OUTLINE

CONCEPTS OF STRESS
    General Adaptation Syndrome
    Psychologic Mediators and Specificity
    Psychoneuroimmunologic Mediators of Stress
STRESS RESPONSE
    Central Stress Response
    Stress and the Immune System

STRESS, PERSONALITY, COPING, AND ILLNESS
    Aging and Stress: Stress-Age Syndrome

Modern society is full of stress. As a culture, Westerners are champions of the work ethic, a Protestant philosophy originating in the sixteenth century that views idleness as taboo. In *Poor Richard's Almanac,* Ben Franklin counseled people not to waste time. Driven by this perspective, Westerners have devoted time and energy to inventing time-saving devices such as cell phones and portable internet access. These inventions have fueled the drive of the "workaholic" American and, despite our prosperity, have not resulted in more leisure hours. The pressure to remain in contact despite illness, travel, vacation, and other events that used to provide socially acceptable absences is now customary in American, and indeed global, culture. This prevalent assumption of constant availability is a newly identified stressor contributing to the more global and better studied stressors of work related and relationship stressors. Tensions may be created due to the need to balance work and leisure time. When added to other well identified stressors such as financial problems, the result may be potential suffering from the so-called *stress-related disorders.*

It is often reported that use of the term stress in a biologic sense began with Hans Selye in 1946. Selye defined physiologic stress as a chemical or physical disturbance in the cells or tissue fluid produced by a change, either in the external environment or within the body itself, that requires a response.[1] In 1914, however, Walter B. Cannon used the term in both a physiologic and a psychologic sense in a paper reporting psychoendocrine studies. In his report Cannon used such phrases as "great emotional stress" and "times of stress."[1] In 1935 Cannon published another paper called "Stresses and Strains of Homeostasis." In it he applied the engineering concept of stress and strain in a physiologic context.[2] Cannon thought also that stress involved psychologic factors; his paper stated that physical as well as emotional stimuli can cause stress. The *popularization* of the term, however, began with Selye's work.

In the past decade it was been demonstrated that the interactions among social, psychologic, biologic, and behavioral factors are inherent in the causes and courses of many diseases. Molecular biologists, immunologists, neurologists, clinicians, and behavioral scientists began exploring the role of the neglected half of the mind-body (dualistic) model—that is, the mind. What is now emerging is a more holistic and complex model of health and disease states. This model involves the biochemical relationships of the central and autonomic nervous systems, the endocrine system, and the immune system and their relationships to stress-elicited coping behaviors, such as smoking and poor diet, that can also modify the integrity of the immune system. Discoveries of these complex links have led to the creation of the field of psychoneuroimmunology.

CONCEPTS OF STRESS

Psychologic stress may cause or exacerbate (worsen) several disease states, including many of the diseases implicated as the leading causes of death in the United States, such as cardiovascular disease and infectious diseases.[3,4] (Table 10-1). Important effects of acute emotional stress, such as the death of a loved one, on the heart include three areas: (1) left ventricular contractile dysfunction, (2) myocardial ischemia, and (3) disturbances of heart rhythm (see What's New? Acute Emotional Stress and Adverse Heart Effects). Evidence implicates stress as a *precipitating* factor for some diseases and conditions and *worsens* symptoms and outcomes in a number of others, including irritable bowel syndrome, ulcers, asthma, autoimmune disorders, delayed wound healing, reproductive dysfunction, diabetes, and depression.[5,6] Effects of stress on inflammatory and immune processes influence coronary artery disease, depression, autoimmune disorders (e.g., rheumatoid arthritis, lupus, multiple sclerosis) and some cancers

(e.g., virally mediated).[7] Evidence published since 2000 has generally supported a role for stress on human immunodeficiency virus (HIV) progression.[8] Moreover, stress has been linked to the recurrence of genital herpes virus in women with HIV.[8] Further, stress-induced, chronic inflammation is suggested as being important in the functional decline that leads to frailty, disability, and untimely death.[9,10] As evidence has mounted concerning the important role that stress plays in certain disease processes, research has focused on the mechanisms responsible for these mind-body interactions. Along with a greater understanding of the relationship between the human stress response and disease, new strategies for treatment of stress-related disorders are emerging. This chapter describes definitions of stress, the history of stress research, and recent findings on the role of stress in disease.

The term *stress* has been used persistently and widely in specialties such as biology, health sciences, and social sciences despite numerous disagreements over its definition. Nevertheless, in recent years **stress** has been more usefully defined as a *transactional* or *interactional concept*. Transactionally, stress is viewed as the state of affairs arising when a person relates to (i.e., interacts or transacts with) situations in certain ways. People are not disturbed by situations per se but by the ways they appraise and react to situations. In general, a person experiences stress when a demand *exceeds* a person's coping abilities, resulting in reactions such as disturbances of cognition, emotion, and behavior that can adversely affect well-being.

Table 10-1	Examples of Stress-Related Diseases and Conditions
Target Organ or System	**Disease or Condition**
Cardiovascular system	Coronary artery disease
	Hypertension
	Stroke
	Disturbances of heart rhythm
Muscle	Tension headaches
	Muscle contraction (backache)
Connective tissues	Rheumatoid arthritis (autoimmune disease)
	Related inflammatory diseases of connective tissue
Immune system	Asthma (hypersensitivity reaction)
	Hay fever (hypersensitivity reaction)
	Immunosuppression or deficiency
	Autoimmune diseases
Gastrointestinal system	Ulcer
	Irritable bowel syndrome
	Diarrhea
	Nausea and vomiting
	Ulcerative colitis
Genitourinary system	Diuresis
	Impotence
	Frigidity
Skin	Eczema
	Neurodermatitis
	Acne
Endocrine system	Type 2 diabetes mellitus
	Amenorrhea
Central nervous system	Fatigue and lethargy
	Type A behavior
	Overeating
	Depression
	Insomnia
	Impaired learning and memory

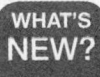

WHAT'S NEW?   Acute Emotional Stress and Adverse Heart Effects

Myocardial Ischemia

Individuals with coronary heart disease may develop myocardial ischemia during mental or acute emotional stress even though their exercise results are negative.

Systemic vascular resistance increases during periods of mental or acute emotional stress with concomitant increased myocardial oxygen demand.

Left Ventricular Dysfunction

More evidence in older women

After acute emotional stress or trauma, there is an increase in sudden chest pain and shortness of breath.

Left ventricular dysfunction is more common in the cardiac apex.

Alterations possibly because of increases in catecholamines

Ventricular Dysrhythmias

Intense or unusual acute stress precipitates about 20% of serious ventricular dysrhythmias or sudden cardiac death.

Altered brain activity may lead to changes in ventricular repolarization and electrical instability of the cardiac muscle.

Data from Critchley HD et al: *Brain* 128(pt 1):75-85, 2005; Ramachandruni S et al: *J Am Coll Cardiol* 47(5):987-991, 2006; Soufer R: *Circulation* 110(13):1710-1713, 2004; Wittstein IS et al: *N Engl J Med* 352(6):539-548, 2005; Ziegelstein RC: *JAMA* 298(3):324-329, 2007.

General Adaptation Syndrome

Selye[11] originally sought to discover a new sex hormone when he discovered the biologic syndrome of stress. In his attempts to discover the new hormone, Selye injected crude ovarian extracts into rats. Repeatedly, he found that the following triad of structural changes occurred: (1) enlargement of the cortex of the adrenal gland, (2) atrophy of the thymus gland and other lymphoid structures, and (3) development of bleeding ulcers of the stomach and duodenal lining. Selye soon discovered that this triad of manifestations was not specific for his ovarian extracts but also occurred after he exposed the rats to other noxious stimuli, such as cold, surgical injury, and restraint. He called these stimuli **stressors**. Selye concluded that this triad or syndrome of manifestations represented a nonspecific response to noxious stimuli. Because many diverse agents caused the same syndrome, Selye suggested that it be called the **general adaptation syndrome (GAS).**

Selye later defined three successive stages in development of the GAS: (1) the **alarm stage,** in which the central nervous system (CNS) is aroused and the body's defenses are mobilized (i.e., flight or fight); (2) the **stage of resistance or adaptation,** during which mobilization contributes to flight or fight; and (3) the **stage of exhaustion,** in which continuous stress causes the progressive breakdown of compensatory mechanisms (acquired adaptations) and homeostasis. The stage of exhaustion, Selye believed, marked the onset of certain diseases he called **diseases of adaptation.**

The nonspecific physiologic response identified by Selye consists of interaction among the sympathetic branch of the autonomic nervous system (ANS) (see Chapter 14) and other neural signals that activate the endocrine system, known as the **hypothalamic-pituitary-adrenal (HPA) axis,** or interactions among the hypothalamus, pituitary gland, and the adrenal gland. The alarm phase of the GAS begins when a stressor triggers the actions of the hypothalamus and the sympathetic nervous system (SNS) (Figure 10-1). The resistance or adaptation phase begins with the actions of the adrenal hormones cortisol, norepinephrine, and epinephrine. Exhaustion occurs if stress continues and adaptation is not successful, ultimately causing impairment of the immune response, heart failure, and kidney failure, leading to death.

Selye defined **physiologic stress** as a chemical or physical disturbance in the cells or tissue fluid produced by a change, either in the external environment or within the body itself, that requires a response (i.e., begins the GAS) to counteract the disturbance. Selye identified three components of physiologic stress: (1) the exogenous or endogenous stressor initiating the disturbance, (2) the chemical or physical disturbance produced by the stressor, and (3) the body's counteracting (adaptational) response to the disturbance.[11]

Psychologic Mediators and Specificity

Although Selye's identification of the GAS is regarded as tremendously important and the cornerstone of stress research, the idea that stress is a purely physiologic response is oversimplified. In the mid-1950s, studies showed that activation of the adrenal cortex occurred in humans in response to psychologic stressors[12]; in monkeys with conditioned emotional responses[13]; and in humans subjected to a stressful interview technique.[14] In the early 1960s, researchers found that plasma cortisol levels in groups of subjects increased while they watched war movies and decreased while they viewed Disney nature films.[15,16] Later, Mason[17] demonstrated in a series of experiments that occurrence of the GAS depended on psychologic factors surrounding the stressors. Mason demonstrated that several factors, including degrees of discomfort, unpleasantness, or suddenness of the stress, could account for the presence or absence of the physiologic stress response.

Selye believed that stressors cause a general or nonspecific response. However, research in the past 30 years has shown the remarkable sensitivity of the central nervous system and endocrine system to psychologic influences (emotion is included in psychologic and social stress and acts through psychologic mechanisms).

As with a physically mediated stress response, psychologic stressors can elicit a reactive stress response. The **reactive response** is a physiologic response derived from psychologic stressors. For example, the stress of taking an examination may produce an increased heart rate and dry mouth in the unprepared student. Although no physical stressor is involved, the psychologic effect of taking an examination elicits a reactive physiologic response in the body.[18]

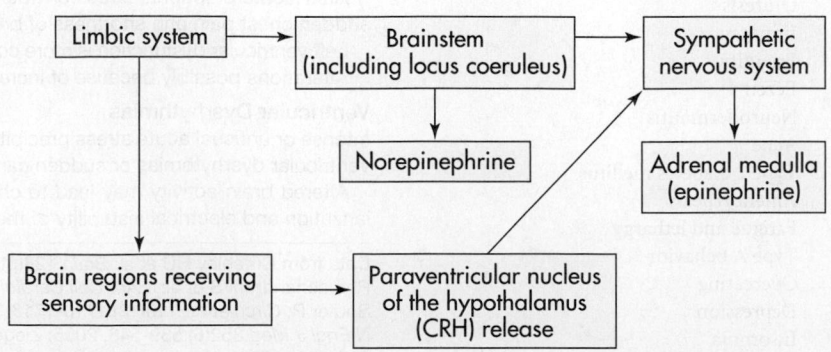

Figure 10-1 Neural recognition and response to real or predicted stressors.

Another type of psychologic-mediated stress response is the **anticipatory response.** Rather than reacting to an obvious stressor, the body mounts a physiologic stress response in anticipation of disruption of the optimal steady-state, also known as **homeostasis.** These anticipatory responses can be generated either by species-specific innate programs, such as reacting to the presence of predators and unfamiliar situations, or by experience-dependent memory programs created by conditioning.[18] In a **conditional response** the organism learns that specific stimuli (i.e, objects or situational context) are associated with danger, and anticipation of subsequent encounters with the stimulus produces a physiologic stress response. For example, a child that is abused by a parent may experience a physiologic stress response in anticipation of further abuse when the parent enters the room. Under some circumstances these memory programs may become so strong that psychologic disorders, such as phobias, develop. In a similar fashion, some persons develop **post-traumatic stress disorder (PTSD)** in response to the memory as opposed to the anticipation of traumatic events, characterized by flashback memories, sleep disturbances, depression, and other symptoms. These symptoms often render a person incapable of employment and frequently disrupt personal relationships.

Anticipatory responses are learned responses under fine control by brain regions located in the limbic system. These regions are those most frequently associated with learning and memory and include the hippocampus, amygdala, and prefrontal cortex. In order for these regions to elicit a stress response, the paraventricular nucleus (PVN) of the hypothalamus must be stimulated (see Chapter 20). The limbic structures rarely interact directly with the PVN and are believed to influence the stress response through intermediary neurons, some of which are primarily used for the reactive response.

Psychoneuroimmunologic Mediators of Stress

Psychoneuroimmunology (PNI) is the study of the interaction of consciousness *(psycho),* brain and spinal cord *(neuro),* and the body's defense against external infection and abnormal cell division *(immunology).* Psychoneuroimmunology assumes that all immune-related disease is multifactorial, or the result of interrelationships among psychosocial, emotional, genetic, neurologic, endocrine, and immune systems and behavioral factors.[19,20] The immune system is integrated with other physiologic processes and is sensitive to changes in CNS and endocrine functioning, such as those that accompany psychologic states. Stressors can elicit the stress response or stress system through the action of the nervous and endocrine systems. Stressors include, but are not limited to, infection, noise, decreased oxygen supply, pain, malnutrition, heat, cold, trauma, prolonged exertion, radiation, responses to life events (including anxiety, depression, anger, fear, and excitement), obesity, old age, drugs, disease, surgery, and medical treatment. The volume of psychoneuroimmunologic research is growing rapidly and represents a substantial presence in the psychosomatic literature. Sufficient data now exist to conclude that immune modulation by psychosocial stressors or interventions leads directly to health outcomes. The strongest support for the link between psychosocial stressors and health outcomes is found in studies of infectious disease and wound healing.[21-26]

STRESS RESPONSE

The **stress response** is initiated by the central nervous system and endocrine system (see Figure 10-1). Specifically, **corticotropin-releasing hormone (CRH)** is released from the hypothalamus, the sympathetic nervous system, the pituitary gland, and the adrenal gland (Figure 10-2). CRH is also released peripherally at inflammatory sites called **peripheral, or immune, CRH.** The activation of these systems redirects adaptive energy to the CNS and stressed body sites.

Where the stress response begins depends on whether the stressor is perceived or real. Perceived stressors elicit an anticipatory response that usually begins in the limbic system of the brain, the area responsible for emotions and cognition. The limbic system indirectly elicits an endocrine stress response by stimulating neural pathways responsible for receiving sensory information and a central response by directly stimulating the locus coeruleus (LC) to release norepinephrine (Figure 10-1). Norepinephrine release promotes arousal, increased vigilance, increased anxiety, and other protective emotional responses. Real stressors elicit a reactive response that can begin either in the limbic system or in regions of the brain receiving specific sensory information (see Figure 10-1). This information is then relayed to the PVN. The PVN stimulates the LC and both central and endocrine stress responses.

Central Stress Response

The sympathetic nervous system (SNS) is aroused during the stress response and causes the medulla of the adrenal gland to release catecholamines (80% epinephrine and 20% norepinephrine) into the bloodstream. The adrenal medulla is actually an extension of the SNS because preganglionic fibers from the splanchnic nerve terminate in the medulla, where they innervate the chromaffin cells that produce the catecholamine hormones. Simultaneously, hypothalamic CRH stimulates the pituitary gland to release a variety of hormones, including antidiuretic hormone and oxytocin from the posterior pituitary gland, and prolactin, endorphins, growth hormone (GH), and adrenocorticotropic hormone (ACTH) from the anterior pituitary gland. ACTH stimulates the cortex of the adrenal gland to release cortisol.

Catecholamines

In response to stress, the chromaffin cells of the adrenal medulla produce large quantities of epinephrine and small amounts of norepinephrine. Once released, catecholamines circulate bound to the plasma protein albumin. Epinephrine is rapidly transported to and acts on several organs, but it is

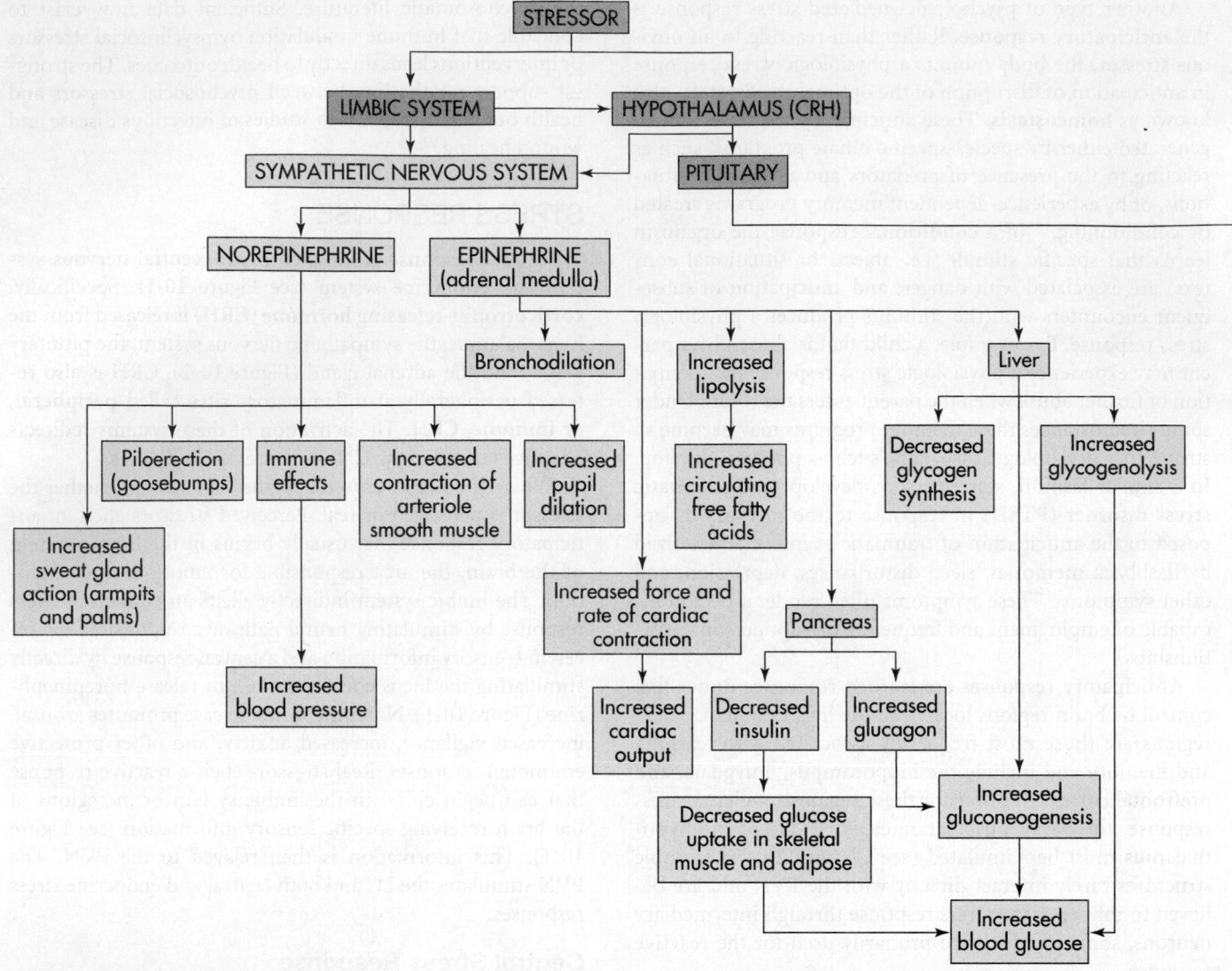

Figure 10-2 The stress response. *ACTH,* Adrenocorticotropic hormone; *CRH,* corticotropin-releasing hormone; *ADH,* antidiuretic hormone; *IGF-1,* insulin-like growth factor-1; *PMNs,* polymorphonuclear leukocytes; *RNA,* ribonucleic acid. See text for explanation of hormone functions. (*See p. 344 for immune effects. †Explained in text.)

metabolized quickly making it short acting. Further, very little adrenal norepinephrine reaches distal tissue; thus, the effects caused by norepinephrine during the stress response are primarily elicited from the SNS.[27,28]

The catecholamines stimulate two major classes of receptors: α-adrenergic receptors and β-adrenergic receptors. These two classes are divided further into two subclasses: (1) α_1 and α_2 and (2) β_1 and β_2. Table 10-2 summarizes the actions of the two subclasses of adrenergic receptors. (A thorough discussion of receptors can be found in Chapters 1, 20, and 29.) Epinephrine binds to and activates both α- and β-adrenergic receptors. Norepinephrine at physiologic concentrations binds primarily to α-adrenergic receptors.[29]

The circulating catecholamines essentially mimic direct sympathetic stimulation. (Sympathetic function is described in Chapter 14.) Norepinephrine regulates blood pressure

by constricting smooth muscle in all blood vessels. During stress, norepinephrine raises blood pressure by constricting peripheral vessels; it dilates the pupils of the eye, causes piloerection, and increases sweat gland action in the armpits and palms (see Figure 10-2).

Epinephrine has a greater influence on cardiac action and is the principal catecholamine involved in metabolic regulation. Epinephrine enhances myocardial contractility (inotropic effect), increases the heart rate (chronotropic effect), and increases venous return to the heart, all of which increase cardiac output and blood pressure. Epinephrine dilates blood vessels of skeletal muscle, allowing for greater oxygenation. Metabolically, epinephrine causes transient hyperglycemia (high blood sugar) by activating enzymes whose actions promote glucose formation (gluconeogenesis) and glycogen breakdown (glycogenolysis) in the liver while inhibiting

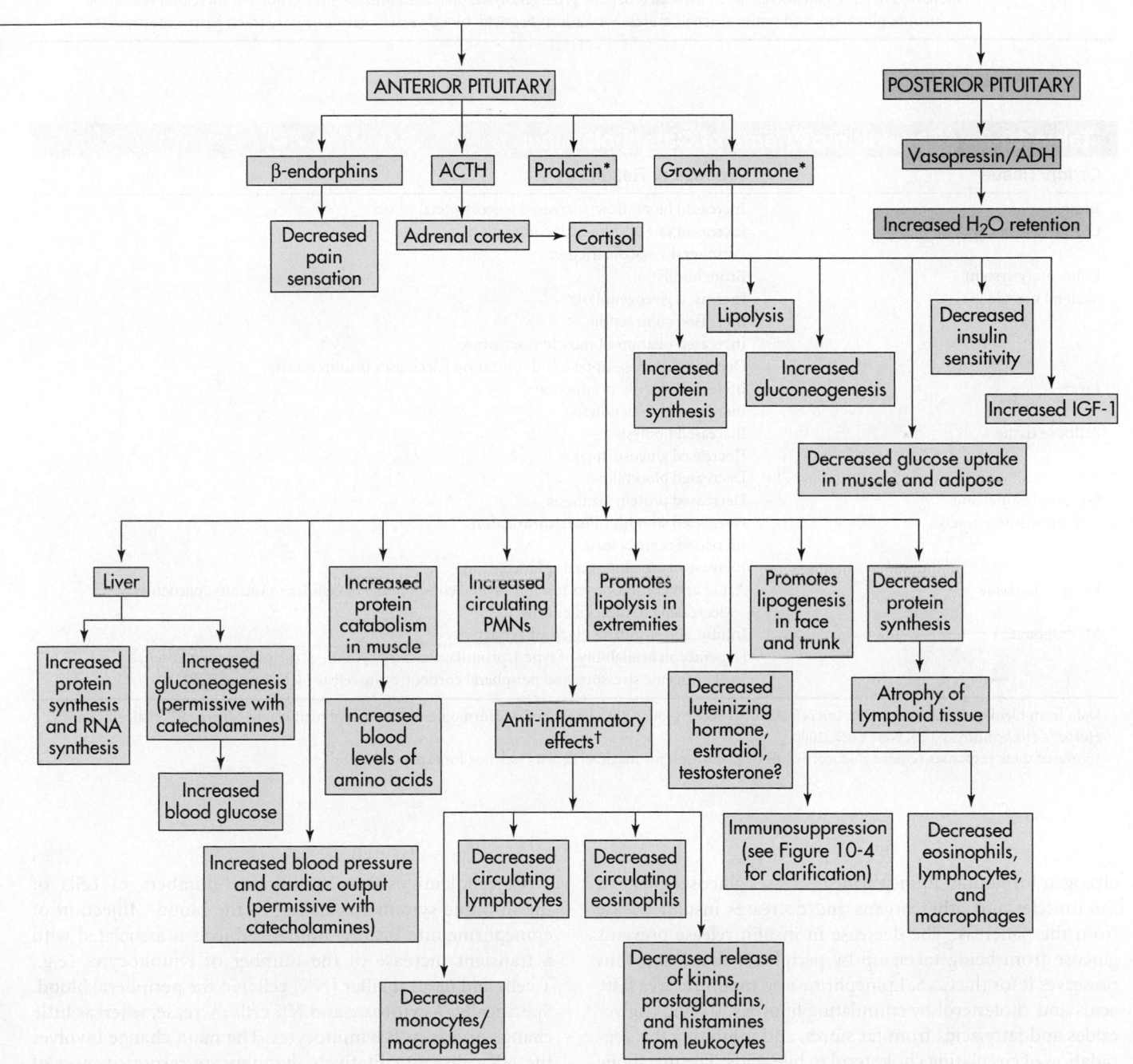

Figure 10-2—cont'd The stress response.

Table 10-2	Physiologic Actions of α- and β-Adrenergic Receptors
Receptor	**Physiologic Actions**
α_1	Increased glycogenolysis; smooth muscle contraction (blood vessels, genitourinary tract)
α_2	Smooth muscle relaxation (gastrointestinal tract); smooth muscle contraction (some vascular beds); inhibition of lipolysis, renin release, platelet aggregation, and insulin secretion
β_1	Stimulation of lipolysis; myocardial contraction (increased rate, increased force of contraction)
β_2	Increased hepatic gluconeogenesis; increased hepatic glycogenolysis; increased muscle glycogenolysis; increased release of insulin, glucagon, and renin; smooth muscle relaxation (bronchi, blood vessels, genitourinary tract, gastrointestinal tract)

Table 10-3	Physiologic Effects of Catecholamines*
Organ/Tissue	**Process or Result**
Brain	Increased blood flow; increased glucose metabolism
Cardiovascular system	Increased rate and force of contraction
	Peripheral vasoconstriction
Pulmonary system	Bronchodilation
Skeletal muscle	Increased glycogenolysis
	Increased contraction
	Increased dilation of muscle vasculature
	Decreased glucose uptake and utilization (decreases insulin release)
Liver	Increased glucose production
	Increased glycogenolysis
Adipose tissue	Increased lipolysis
	Decreased glucose uptake
Skin	Decreased blood flow
Gastrointestinal and	Decreased protein synthesis
genitourinary tracts	Decreased smooth muscle contraction
	Increased renin release
	Increased gastrointestinal sphincter tone
Lymphoid tissue	Acute and chronic stress inhibits several components of cellular immunity, particularly decreasing natural killer cells
Macrophages	Inhibit and stimulate macrophage activity
	Depends on availability of type 1/proinflammatory cytokines, the presence or absence of antigenic stressors, and peripheral corticotropin-releasing hormone (CRH)

Data from Elenkov IJ, Chrousos GP: *Ann N Y Acad Sci* 966:290-303, 2002; Granner DK: Hormones of the adrenal medulla. In Murray RK et al, editors: *Harper's biochemistry,* ed 25, New York, 2000.

*Some of these responses require glucocorticoids (e.g., cortisol) for maximal activity (see text for explanation).

glycogen formation. Epinephrine decreases glucose uptake in the muscles and other organs and decreases insulin release from the pancreas. The decrease in insulin release prevents glucose from being taken up by peripheral tissue and thus preserves it for the CNS. Epinephrine also mobilizes free fatty acids and cholesterol by stimulating lipolysis, freeing triglycerides and fatty acids from fat stores, and inhibiting the degradation of circulating cholesterol to bile acids. The metabolic actions of epinephrine aid the metabolic actions of cortisol, which are similar. Table 10-3 summarizes other well-known effects of adrenal catecholamines. All of these effects prepare the body to take physical action: to fight or flee. Stressors commonly associated with catecholamine release by the adrenal medulla include exercise, thermal changes, and acute emotional states.

Catecholamines can modify the numbers of cells of the immune system circulating in the blood.[1] Injection of epinephrine into healthy human subjects is associated with a transient increase of the number of lymphocytes (e.g., T cells and natural killer [NK] cells) in the peripheral blood. Specifically, T cytotoxic and NK cells increase, whereas little change occurs in B lymphocytes. The main change involves the NK cells.[1] Qualitatively, lymphocyte responsiveness of T and B lymphocytes is reduced. Similar quantitative and qualitative changes are found 5 to 6 minutes after exposure to a psychologic or physical stressor.[30] The effects of acute elevation of catecholamines on the alteration of lymphocyte function are short lived, lasting only about 2 hours.[2] However, a study of stress duration and susceptibility to infection[22] found that chronic elevation of catecholamines is immunosuppressive, but it is unclear whether the increase in lymphocytes comes from the bone marrow or the peripheral tissues.

Cortisol

The adrenal cortex is activated during stress by ACTH (see Figure 10-1), which increases adrenocortical secretion of glucocorticoid hormones, primarily cortisol (a synthetically produced but chemically identical version of cortisol known also as *hydrocortisone*). Cortisol circulates in the plasma, both protein bound and free. The main plasma-binding protein is called **transcortin** or **corticosteroid-binding globulin.** The unbound, or free, fraction is approximately 8% of the total plasma cortisol and is biologically active.[29] Cortisol mobilizes substances needed for cellular metabolism. One of the primary effects of cortisol is the stimulation of gluconeogenesis, or the formation of glucose from noncarbohydrate sources, such as amino or free fatty acids in the liver. In addition, cortisol enhances the elevation of blood glucose promoted by other hormones, such as epinephrine, glucagon, and growth hormone. This action by cortisol is said to be *permissive* for the actions of other hormones. Cortisol also inhibits the uptake and oxidation of glucose by many body cells. The overall action of cortisol increases blood glucose, thereby enabling the body to combat the stressor. The physiologic effects of cortisol are summarized in Table 10-4.

Cortisol also affects protein metabolism. It has an anabolic effect, that is, it increases the rate of synthesis of proteins and ribonucleic acid (RNA) in liver. The anabolic effect of cortisol, however, is countered by its catabolic effect on protein stores in other tissues. Protein catabolism acts to increase circulating amino acids, and chronic exposure to excess cortisol can severely deplete protein stores in muscle, bone, connective tissue, and skin. Further, cortisol acts to reduce protein synthesis in nonhepatic tissues, a loss for which dietary protein cannot compensate. Some evidence suggests that cortisol depresses transport of amino acids into muscle cells while enhancing their uptake into the liver.

Cortisol also has a powerful effect that reverses the insulin-induced suppression of hepatic gluconeogenesis, and basal levels of cortisol stimulate the activity of hepatic enzymes responsible for glycogen and glucose production. The increased amino acid uptake into liver and glucose-producing enzymes favors the production of glucose. Although diseases of excess cortisol secretion, such as Cushing disease, produce characteristics of type 2 (non-insulin dependent) diabetes mellitus, recent studies found that chronic stress also may facilitate the development of type 2 diabetes[31,32] (see What's New? Glucocorticoids, Insulin, Inflammation, and Obesity). The mechanism for this action is under investigation, but it is believed that the development of diabetes is secondary to cortisol-induced obesity. Cortisol promotes lipogenesis in certain regions of the body and to a lesser extent promotes lipolysis in other regions by increasing the actions of lipolytic hormones, such as catecholamines and growth hormone. Chronic cortisol excess induces lipogenesis in the abdomen, trunk, and face resulting in central obesity.

Table 10-4	Physiologic Effects of Cortisol
Functions Affected	**Physiologic Effects**
Carbohydrate and lipid metabolism	Diminishes peripheral uptake and use of glucose; promotes gluconeogenesis in liver cells; enhances the gluconeogenic response to other hormones; promotes lipolysis in adipose tissue
Protein metabolism	Increases protein synthesis in the liver and decreased protein synthesis (including immunoglobulin synthesis) in muscle, lymphoid tissue, adipose tissue, skin, and bone; increases plasma level of amino acids; stimulates deamination in the liver
Anti-inflammatory effects (systemic effects)	High levels of cortisol used in drug therapy suppress the inflammatory response; inhibits proinflammatory activity of many growth factors and cytokines; however, over time some patients may develop tolerance to glucocorticoids, causing an increased susceptibility to inflammatory and autoimmune diseases
Proinflammatory effects (possible local effects)	Cortisol levels released during the stress response may increase proinflammatory effects (this very complex physiology is reviewed on p. 344).
Lipid metabolism	Lipolysis in the extremities and lipogenesis in the face and trunk
Immune effects	Immunosuppression of T-cell or cellular immunity at therapeutic levels; nontherapeutic levels, such as those seen with stress, can suppress cellular (Th1) and increase humoral (Th2) immunity—the so-called Th2 shift
Digestive function	Promotes gastric secretion
Urinary function	Enhances excretion of calcium
Connective tissue function	Decreases proliferation of fibroblasts in connective tissue (thus delaying healing)
Muscle function	Maintains normal contractility and maximal work output for skeletal and cardiac muscle
Bone function	Decreases bone formation
Vascular system and myocardial function	Maintains normal blood pressure; permits increased responsiveness of arterioles to the constrictive action of adrenergic stimulation; optimizes myocardial performance
Central nervous system function	Modulates perceptual and emotional functioning, essential for normal arousal and initiation of daytime activity
Possible synergism with estrogen in pregnancy?	Suppresses maternal immune system to prevent rejection of fetus?

The signs and symptoms of Cushing syndrome (e.g., excess glucocorticoids [GCs]) include truncal obesity, relatively thin extremities, a "moon face," and a "buffalo [neck] hump." In such individuals the possibility of associated hypertension is high as well as increased risk of infection and metabolic syndrome or frank type 2 diabetes. In addition, the likelihood of an elevated ratio of intra-abdominal subcutaneous fat mass to nonabdominal fat mass is high because the glucocorticoids mediate the redistribution of stored calories into the abdominal region. The specific increase in abdominal fat stores is a consequence of elevated glucocorticoids combined with increased insulin action. However, the increased glucocorticoids need not be present in the circulation, but can be generated locally in fat through conversion of inactive cortisone to active cortisol through the action of the isoenzyme 11-β-hydroxysteroid dehydrogenase (11-β-HSD) type-1. This conversion is referred to as "pre-receptor" metabolism of cortisol. The active steroid is secreted directly to the liver through the portal vein. In vitro insulin synthesis and secretion from the pancreas are inhibited by the glucocorticoids. However, increasing glucocorticoids in vivo are associated with increasing insulin secretion possibly because of an anti-insulin effect on the liver, which appears to be vulnerable to the negative effects of glucocorticoids on insulin action. Hepatic insulin resistance is strongly associated with abdominal obesity.

Recent data reveal that the plasma concentration of inflammatory mediators, such as tumor necrosis factor-α (TNF-α) and interleukin-6 (IL-6), is increased in the insulin-resistant states of obesity and type 2 diabetes. Two mechanisms might be involved in the pathogenesis of inflammation: (1) glucose and macronutrient intake (i.e., which can be mediated through chronic stress) causes oxidative stress; and (2) the increased concentrations of TNF-α and IL-6 associated with obesity and type 2 diabetes might interfere with insulin signal transduction. This interference might promote inflammation. Chronic overnutrition (obesity) might thus be a proinflammatory state with oxidative stress.

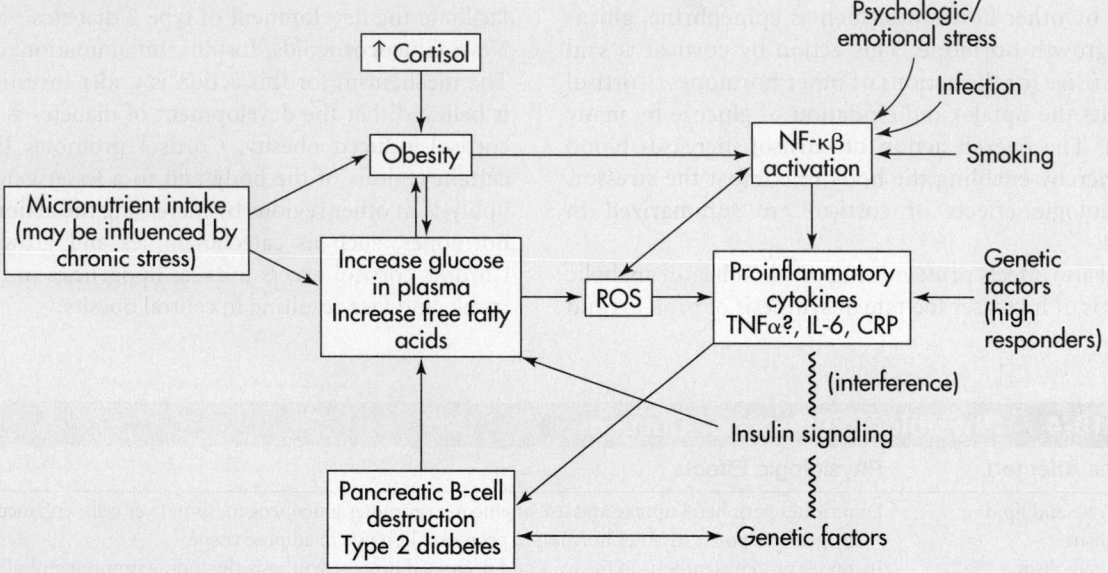

Stress, inflammation, obesity, and type 2 diabetes. The induction of reactive oxygen species (ROS) generation and inflammation through the proinflammatory transcription factor, NF-kβ, activates most proinflammatory genes. Macronutrient intake, obesity, free fatty acids, infection, smoking, psychologic stress, and genetic factors increase the production of ROS. Interference with insulin signaling (insulin resistance) leads to hyperglycemia and proinflammatory changes. Proinflammatory changes increase TNF-α, increase IL-6, and also lead to the inhibition of insulin signaling and insulin resistance. Inflammation in pancreatic B cells leads to B-cell dysfunction, which in combination with insulin resistance leads to type 2 diabetes. *CRP,* C-reactive protein.

Data from Dallman MF et al: *Endocrinology* 145(6):2633-2638, 2004; Dandona P, Aljada A, Brandyopadhyay A: *Trends Immunol* 25(1):4-7, 2004; Kim SP et al: *Diabetes* 52:2453-2460, 2003; Masuzaki H et al: *Science* 94:2166-2170, 2001; Padgett DA, Glaser R: *Trends Immunol* 24(8):444-448, 2003; Strack AM et al: *Am J Physiol* 268:R142-R149, 1995; Thakore JH et al: *Biol Psychiatry* 47:1140-1142, 1998; Wagen Knecht LE et al: *Diabetes* 52:2490-2496, 2003.

In the gastrointestinal tract, cortisol promotes gastric secretion. This effect is opposite that of norepinephrine, which reduces gastric secretion. Excessive cortisol may stimulate gastric secretion enough to cause ulceration of the gastric mucosa. This could account for the gastrointestinal ulceration observed by Selye.

Cortisol and the Immune System

Stress hormones, especially glucocorticoids (cortisol), have been used therapeutically as powerful anti-inflammatory/immunosuppressive agents. Data suggest, however, that glucocorticoids and catecholamines (epinephrine and norepinephrine) at concentration levels reached during stress may paradoxically result in decreased cellular immunity and increased autoimmune (humoral) responses. These data may help explain the seemingly contradictory response to stress of immunosuppression and increased risk of infection (decreased cellular immunity) and a heightened antibody response and autoimmune disease (increased humoral immunity).

As discussed in Chapters 6 and 7, immune responses are regulated by cells of *innate immunity* called *antigen-presenting cells (APCs),* such as monocytes/macrophages, dendritic cells, and other phagocytic cells, and by cells of adaptive immunity, such as lymphocyte subclasses T-helper 1 (Th1) and T-helper 2 (Th2) cells. These cells regulate the immune system by the secretion of chemicals called cytokines. Cytokines are a group of chemicals such as interferons, interleukins, and tumor necrosis factors that can stimulate or inhibit various components of the immune system. APCs release cytokines that induce T cells to differentiate into Th1 cells. Th1 cells and APC cytokines work together to stimulate the immune activity of cytotoxic T cells, NK cells, and activated macrophages—the major components of cellular immunity. These cytokines also stimulate the synthesis of nitric oxide and other inflammatory mediators that increase chronic delayed-type inflammatory responses. Because of this effect, these cytokines are considered to be the major proinflammatory cytokines.[32-35] The cytokines secreted by the Th2 cells act to inhibit Th1 cells and can promote humoral immunity by stimulating growth and activation of mast cells and eosinophils, as well as the differentiation of B-cell immunoglobulins. Thus these cytokines are considered to be the major anti-inflammatory cytokines[33] (Figure 10-3).

Stress influences immunity by stimulating cortisol and epinephrine secretion from the adrenal glands and norepinephrine from the sympathetic nervous system. Cortisol acts to suppress the activity of Th1 cells, which leads to a decrease in cellular immunity and to the proinflammatory response. Cortisol also stimulates the activity of the Th2 cells, which leads to an increase in adaptive humoral immunity and the anti-inflammatory response. Epinephrine and norepinephrine have a similar effect: the decrease in Th1 activity and the increase in Th2 activity. This decrease in Th1 activity and increase in Th2 activity is sometimes called a **Th1 to Th2 shift.** Individuals experiencing a Th1 to Th2 shift are more likely to experience allergic responses, infections and temporary worsening of autoimmune conditions such as arthritis.

The above description of the effect of stress hormones on the Th1-Th2 balance may not be accurate for certain local responses.[33] It has been documented that the release of catecholamines (epinephrine and norepinephrine) can cause certain epithelial cells of the lung to release cytokines that promote recruitment of leukocytes potentially enhancing inflammation and worsening lung function. This paradoxical stress-induced potentiation of inflammation in the lungs may explain why "acute respiratory distress syndrome" often develops in individuals with major infections associated with profound activity of the stress response.[36]

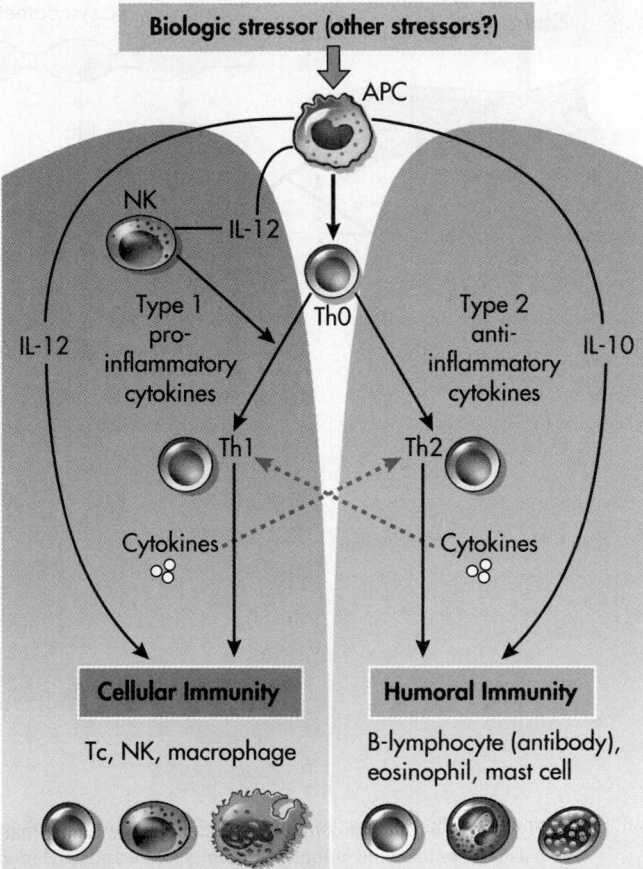

Figure 10-3 Role of Th1 and Th2 cells in the regulation of cellular and humoral immunity. Humoral immunity provides protection against multicellular parasites, extracellular bacteria, some viruses, soluble toxins, and allergens. Cellular immunity provides protection against intracellular bacteria, fungi, protozoa, and several viruses. Type 1 cytokines or proinflammatory cytokines include IL-12, interferon-gamma (IFN-γ), and tumor necrosis factor-alpha (TNF-α). Type 2 cytokines or anti-inflammatory cytokines include IL-10 and IL-4. Solid lines *(black)* represent stimulation, whereas dashed lines *(blue)* represent inhibition (i.e., Th1 and Th2 are mutually inhibitory, IL-12 and IFN-γ inhibit Th2, and vice versa; IL-4 and IL-10 inhibit Th1 responses). *APC,* Antigen-presenting cell; *B,* B cell; *IL,* interleukin; *NK,* natural killer cell; *Th,* T-helper cell; *Tc,* cytotoxic T cell. (Redrawn from: Elenkov IJ, Chrousos GP: *Trends Endocrinol Metab* 10[9]:359-368, 1999.)

CRH influences the immune system indirectly by the activation of cortisol (glucocorticoids) and catecholamines. CRH is secreted by the hypothalamus and also peripherally at inflammatory sites.[33,37,38] Peripheral (immune) CRH is proinflammatory, causing an increase in vasodilation and vascular permeability.[39] Therefore, it appears that mast cells are the target of peripheral CRH. Mast cells release histamine, which is a well-known mediator of acute inflammation and allergic reactions (Figure 10-4). Recent evidence has indicated that immune cells may have histamine receptors and that histamine may have an effect similar to catecholamines. This finding suggests that histamine induces acute inflammation and allergic reactions while suppressing Th1 activity (decreasing cellular immunity) and promoting Th2 activity (increasing humoral immunity).[39-42]

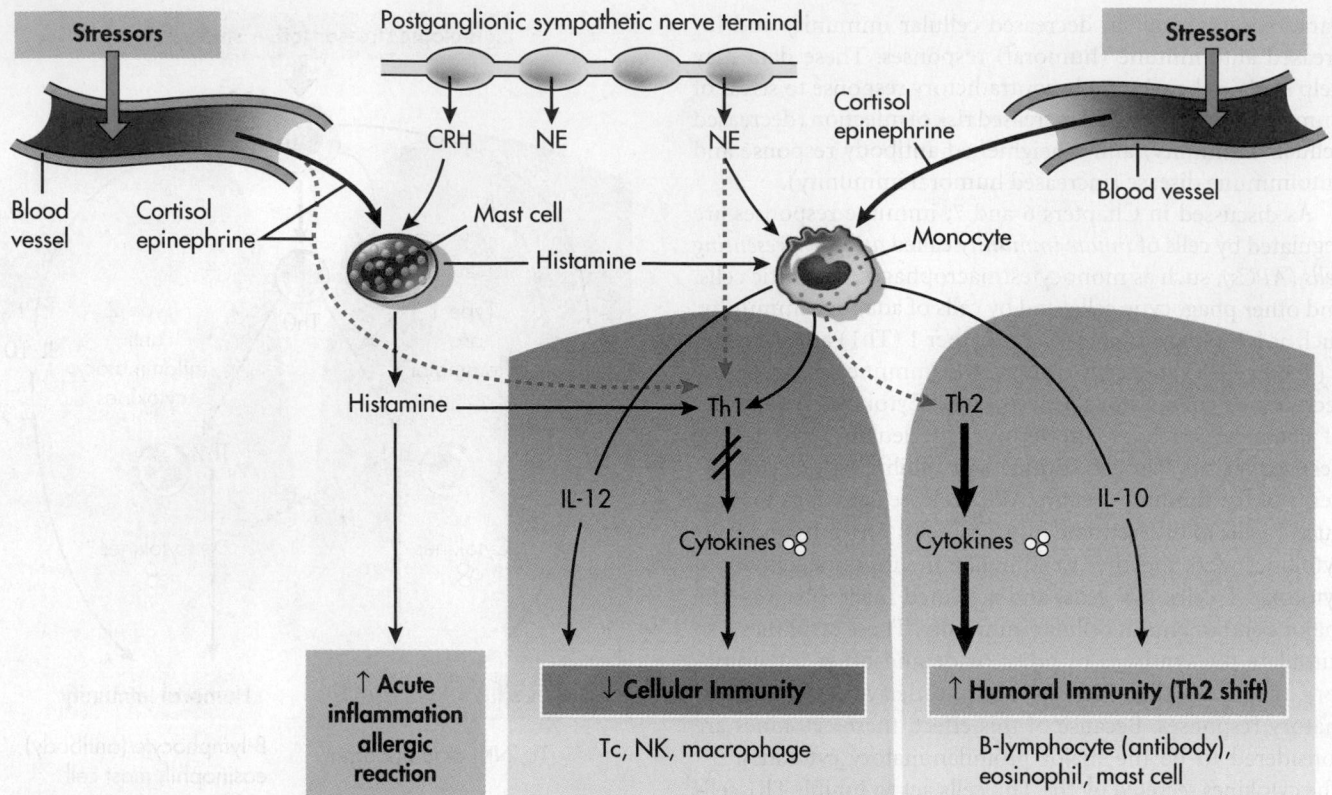

Figure 10-4 Effect of corticotropin-releasing hormone—mast cell—histamine axis, cortisol, and catecholamines on the Th1/Th2 balance—cellular and humoral immunity. Stress and CRH modulate inflammatory/immune and allergic responses by stimulating cortisol (glucocorticoid), catecholamines, and peripheral (immune) CRH secretion and by changing the production of regulatory cytokines and histamines. Solid lines *(black)* represent stimulation, and dashed lines *(blue)* represent inhibition. *B,* B cell; *CRH* (peripheral, immune), corticotropin-releasing hormone; *NE,* norepinephrine; *Th,* T-helper cell; *IL,* interleukin; *Tc,* cytotoxic T cell; *NK,* natural killer cell; ↓ decreased (inhibited); ↑ increased (stimulation). (Redrawn from Elenkov IJ, Chrousos GP: Stress hormones, Th1/Th2 patterns, pro-/anti-inflammatory cytokines and susceptibility to disease, *Trends Endocrinol Metab* 10[9]:359-368, 1999.)

In summary, stress can activate an excessive immune response and, through cortisol and catecholamines, suppress the Th1 response and cause a Th2 shift. Locally, stress can exert proinflammatory or anti-inflammatory effects depending on what chemicals are released in the local environment and how the cells of the local environment respond to those chemicals. Finally, recent evidence indicates that responses to stressful events can be considered variable and may even be specific.[25] Moreover, different types of stressors may have variable effects on the immune response. Thus *systemic responses to stress* may cause a decrease in cellular immunity and enhance humoral immunity, whereas *local responses to stress,* under certain conditions, can induce proinflammatory activities that may influence the onset and cause of infection, autoimmune/inflammatory, allergic, and neoplastic disease.

Therapeutic levels of glucocorticoids inhibit the accumulation of leukocytes at the site of inflammation and inhibit the release of substances involved in the inflammatory response (i.e., kinins, plasminogen-activating factor, prostaglandins, and histamine) from the leukocytes. Glucocorticoids inhibit fibroblast proliferation and function at the site of an inflammatory response. This inhibition accounts for the poor wound healing, increased susceptibility to infection, and decreased inflammatory response that often are noted in individuals with chronic glucocorticoid excess.

It is not entirely clear why cortisol secretion during stress is beneficial. It has been suggested that gluconeogenesis promoted by cortisol ensures an adequate source of glucose (energy) for body tissues, and nerve cells in particular. The pooling of amino acids from catabolized proteins may ensure amino acid availability for protein synthesis in certain cells. The redistribution of protein to sites where replacement is critical, such as muscle or cells of damaged tissue, would be beneficial. Short-term, cortisol-induced alterations in immune cell distribution (e.g., traffic) patterns may be adaptive, with a decrease in peripheral blood cell numbers as effector cells locate to sites of injury or inflammation. In addition, with high concentrations of cortisol, decreased immune-cell activity (both T cell and B cell) prevents immune-mediated tissue damage by prolonged cell exposure to high levels of certain cytokines.[43] Whether cortisol-induced effects are adaptive or destructive may depend on the intensity, type, and duration of the stressor, and the subsequent concentration and length of cortisol exposure that target cells of the individual experience.

Stress and the Immune System

Many immune-related conditions and diseases are associated with stress. Several conditions with variable pathophysiologic characteristics appear to have a common origin[44,45] relating to chronic inflammatory processes. These conditions include

The link between stress and coronary heart disease was proposed as early as the 1970s; however, it was only recently that conclusive evidence and proposed mechanisms for development of the disease were identified. Much work continues to focus on elucidating the interaction between stress and cardiovascular disease.

One of the primary risk factors for coronary heart disease is hypertension. A designation of prehypertension was recently created and found to be a good predictor for future cardiovascular events. Prehypertension is defined as a systolic blood pressure of 120 to 139 mmHg or a diastolic blood pressure of 80 to 89 mmHg. Individuals with prehypertension are much more likely to develop frank hypertension and eventually coronary heart disease.

Studies show that people with highly reactive personality types, who experience high levels of anxiety with stress, are much more likely to progress from prehypertension to hypertension then to develop cardiac disease, specifically coronary heart disease, than those who have better coping abilities. Further long-term psychologic stress, such as experienced in a strained marriage or an unhappy work environment, was shown to not only speed the progression of hypertension and coronary heart disease but also to be correlated with higher mortality rates from coronary heart disease.

Trait anger, defined as a stable personality trait characterized by frequency, intensity, and duration of anger, also was shown to be a factor in the development of coronary heart disease at higher rates than the general population. Individuals with trait anger also experienced more strokes.

One popular mechanism for the interaction between psychosocial stress and cardiovascular disease suggests that stress triggers an inflammatory response that over time increases the chances of developing coronary heart disease. The primary mechanisms proposed are chronically elevated cortisol levels and dysregulation of the circadian rhythm for cortisol release. Further, chronic stress alters hypothalamic-pituitary-adrenal (HPA) function, resulting in an abnormal stress response pattern. This alteration in HPA activity was found in persons with coronary heart disease along with increased inflammatory markers. The elevation in inflammatory markers seen with chronic stress is important because these markers were shown to interact with lipids, specifically low-density lipoproteins (LDLs), to increase the production of atherosclerotic plaques.

Because coronary heart disease is one of the major killers in industrialized countries, development of successful interventional programs is of high priority. Programs in which dietary changes, exercise, stress management, and positive support systems are implemented continue to show positive results for slowing the progression of heart disease and decreasing the risk factors for disease development. Further, individuals in these programs experience improvement in depression, stress, and overall mental health.

Data from Nijm J et al: *J Int Med* 262(3):375-384, 2007; Player MS et al: *Ann Fam Med* 5(5):403-411, 2007; Shamaei-Tousi A et al: *Cell Stress Chaperones* 12(4):384-392, 2007; Vizza J et al: *J Cardiopulm Rehabil Prev* 27(6):376-383, 2007.

cardiovascular disease, osteoporosis, arthritis, type 2 diabetes mellitus, chronic obstructive pulmonary disease (COPD), other diseases associated with aging, and some cancers; all are characterized by the prolonged presence of proinflammatory cytokines.[44,46] (Inflammation is discussed in Chapter 6.) Stress and negative emotions are associated directly with the production of increased levels of proinflammatory cytokines, providing a possible link between stress, immune function, and disease (see What's New? Psychosocial Stress and Progression to Coronary Heart Disease). The specific stress-induced mechanisms causing these illnesses are not clearly defined. Research is focused on the regulatory interactions between the immune system and the nervous and endocrine systems, which may represent mechanistic pathways for stress-associated immune-mediated diseases (see Table 10-1).

The immune, nervous, and endocrine systems communicate through similar pathways involving hormones, neurotransmitters, neuropeptides, and immune cell products. Immune system responses are potentially affected by all known neuroendocrine-produced factors involved in the stress reaction. Conversely, immune cell–derived cytokines and other products have effects on neurocrine and endocrine cells[47,48] (see Table 7-4). Several pathways regulate communication among these systems with both direct and indirect patterned effects (Figure 10-5).

The stress response directly influences the immune system through hypothalamic and pituitary peptides and through products of the sympathetic branch of the ANS. These factors include CRH, ACTH, endorphins, substance P, epinephrine, norepinephrine, dopamine, serotonin, histamine, GH, vasoactive intestinal polypeptide (VIP), β-endorphin, methionine-enkephalin, leucine-enkephalin, and somatostatin[49-52] (Table 10-5). Direct suppressive effects of CRH have been reported also on two immune cell types possessing CRH receptors—the

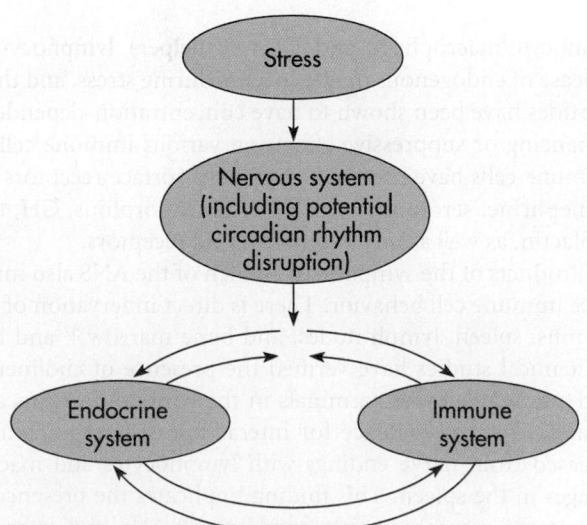

Figure 10-5 Nervous system—endocrine system—immune system interactions. Interconnections of pathways of communication among the immune, nervous, and endocrine systems.

Table 10-5   Other Hormones that Probably Influence the Stress Response

Hormone	Source	Comments
Melatonin	Produced by pineal gland	Increases during the stress response; release is suppressed by light and increased in the dark; receptors have been identified on lymphoid cells, possibly higher density of receptors on T cells than B cells; suppression of lymphocyte function by trauma was reversed by melatonin (Maestroni, 1999)
Somatostatin (SOM)	Produced by sensory nerve terminals found in and released from lymphoid cells and hypothalamus	Natural killer (NK) cell function and immunoglobulin synthesis is decreased by SOM; growth hormone secretion decreased by SOM
Vasoactive intestinal peptide (VIP)	Found in neurons of the central nervous system (CNS) and in peripheral nerves	VIP increases during stress; VIP-containing nerves are located in primary and secondary lymphoid tissues, around blood vessels, and the gastrointestinal tract; VIP receptors are on T and B cells; VIP may influence lymphocyte maturation; cytokine production by T cells is modified by VIP; B-cell and antibody production is influenced by VIP
Calcitonin gene–related peptide (CGRP)	Found in spinal cord motor neurons and in sensory neurons near dendritic cells of the skin and in primary and secondary lymphoid tissues	CGRP receptors are present on T and B lymphocytes, thus it is likely that CGRP can modulate immune function; CGRP may enhance the acute inflammatory response because it is a vasodilator; maturation of immune B lymphocytes is inhibited by CGRP; IL-1 is inhibited by CGRP, which is important for the activation of T cells; it has been shown to interfere with lymphocyte activation
Neuropeptide Y (NPY)	Present in the neurons of the CNS and in neurons throughout the body; co-localized in nerve terminals in lymphatic tissues with norepinephrine	Lymphocytes have receptors for NPY and thus may modulate their function (Pettito et al, 1994); several lines of evidence suggest that NPY is a neurotransmitter and neurohormone involved in the stress response; increased levels of NPY occur in plasma in response to severe or prolonged stress; it may be responsible for stress-induced regional vasoconstriction (splanchnic, coronary, and cerebral); it may also increase platelet aggregation (Rabin, 1999)
Substance P (SP)	Produced by a neuropeptide classified as a tachykinin (increases heart rate subsequent to lowering blood pressure) found in the brain, as well as nerves innervating secondary lymphoid tissues	SP increases in response to stress; receptors for SP are found on the membrane of T and B cells, mononuclear phagocytic cells, and mast cells; proinflammatory activity induces the release of histamine from mast cells during the stress response; causes smooth muscle contraction; causes macrophages and T cells to release cytokines, and increases antibody production

Data from Maestroni GJ: *Adv Exp Med Biol* 460:396, 1999; Pettito JM et al: *J Neuro Immunol* 54:81, 1994; Rabin BS: The nervous system—immune system connection. In Rabin BS: *Stress, immune function, and health: the connection,* Wiley-Liss, 1999, New York.

monocyte/macrophage and CD4 (T helper) lymphocyte.[53] Release of endogenous opiates occurs during stress, and these peptides have been shown to have concentration-dependent, enhancing or suppressive effects on various immune cells.[49] Immune cells have been shown to have surface receptors for epinephrine, serotonin, ACTH, CRH, endorphins, GH, and prolactin, as well as intracellular steroid receptors.

Products of the sympathetic branch of the ANS also influence immune cell behavior. There is direct innervation of the thymus, spleen, lymph nodes, and bone marrow,[52] and histochemical studies have verified the presence of cholinergic and adrenergic nerve terminals in the lymphoid organs and tissues. There is evidence for interaction of norepinephrine released from nerve endings with lymphocytes and macrophages in the spleen. This finding implicates the presence of a route of communication between the ANS and immune system through direct delivery of chemical mediators that alter immune cell behavior in a paracrine (cell to adjacent cell) fashion in the microenvironment of the lymphoid organ.

The pineal gland regulates the immune response and mediates the apparent effects of circadian rhythm on immunity. Blockage of production of melatonin (by continuous light or by pharmacologic means) results in suppression of immune response, whereas administration of melatonin reverses these effects.[54] This immunomodulation pathway may affect immune changes found with dysregulation of circadian rhythm, a common occurrence among older adults, acutely ill, and stressed individuals.[55] Melatonin also modulates seasonal changes in immune function and affects tumor development.[56]

The HPA axis may produce indirect effects on the CNS that modulate immune responses. This is the most extensively studied pathway, with original interest stemming from early studies showing profound effects of prolonged severe stress on immunologic structures.[57] It was noted that the adrenal gland enlarged with simultaneous involution of the thymus and lymph nodes. Increased levels of GCSs may be an important mechanism in stress-related immune structure alterations and in suppression of immune responses.[57] The GCS level increases are attributable to pituitary ACTH production—a result of increased hypothalamic CRH. A number of stress factors initiate CRH production, including high levels of interleukin-1 (IL-1) and IL-6. Increased CRH secretion results in an increase in cortisol secretion. Cortisol feeds back to inhibit further cytokine release by macrophages and monocytes.

The observation that IL-1 can elicit changes in the nervous and endocrine systems by stimulating CRH production in the hypothalamus is part of a growing body of evidence demonstrating immune-induced regulation of the CNS. The release of immune inflammatory mediators IL-6, tumor necrosis factor-beta (TNF-α), and interferon is triggered by bacterial or viral infections, cancer, and tissue injury that in turn initiate a stress response through the HPA pathway described previously. Enhanced systemic production of these cytokines also induces other CNS and behavior changes seen frequently during the acute phase of an infectious episode, acting either directly in a distant systemic "endocrine" way or through the mediation of neuropeptides.[47,58-60] These effects include pyrogenesis (fever), induction of slow wave sleep, and anorexia, all of which are adaptive responses to infection and possibly cancer. Slow wave sleep is associated with enhanced release of GH and a reduction in levels of cortisol, which is beneficial for tissue repair and enhanced immune response.[61] Normal and predictive changes in sleep occur in response to infections, and these changes appear to be of important recuperative value to the individual.[62]

Lymphocytes also are known to produce ACTH and endorphins in small amounts, which probably influence immune response in an autocrine or a paracrine manner in the local microenvironment of an ongoing immune response.[63] The T-cell growth factor (IL-2) can up-regulate pituitary ACTH. Immune-derived cytokines have significant influence on neuroendocrine function, with evidence for direct and indirect cytokine effects on nervous and adrenal cell functions. Thus the immune system has an adaptive role as a "signal" organ to alert other systems of inner threatening stimuli (e.g., infection, tissue damage, tumor cells) that may upset the dynamic steady state.

Neuropeptides and hormones have a significant effect on the immune response. Whether this effect on immune function is suppressive or potentiating depends on the type of factor secreted, with some factors enhancing, some suppressing activities, and some doing both, depending on the concentration and length of exposure, the target cell, and the specific immune function studied.[48] Neuropeptides and neuroendocrine hormones may directly control biochemical events affecting cell proliferation, differentiation, and function or may indirectly control immune cell behavior by affecting the production or activity of cytokines.[48]

In summary, a significant body of evidence supports a link among the nervous, endocrine, and immune systems. The bidirectional communication among these systems involves common use of signal molecules and their receptors, which in turn regulates the behavior of cells in each system. Thus

the most recent findings are that (1) there are direct effects of CNS neuropeptides on immune cells; (2) stress-induced endocrine products influence immune cell and neurologic cell function; and (3) immune cell products (cytokines) affect nervous and endocrine cell function through direct and indirect pathways.

Stress-Induced Hormonal Alterations

Elevation of glucocorticoid concentration associated with psychologic stress or physical exercise is not as high as that achieved by pharmacologic means.[1] Stress produces changes in levels of hormones other than glucocorticoids; the interaction of these various hormones in modifying the function of other physiologic systems still needs investigation.

Female Reproductive System

Cortisol exerts inhibiting effects by suppressing levels of luteinizing hormone (LH), estradiol, progesterone, and possibly testosterone.[64,65] The HPA axis exerts powerful, multilevel effects on the female reproductive system. Stress generally inhibits the female reproductive system (Figure 10-6), primarily through the HPA axis by (1) suppression of hypothalamic gonadotropin-releasing hormone (GnRH) secretion by CRH and CRH stimulation of β-endorphin release; (2) inhibition of GnRH, pituitary LH, and ovarian estradiol (E_2) secretion by cortisol; and (3) cortisol-induced target tissue resistance by estradiol.[65,66] The locus coeruleus-norepinephrine (LC/NE) system (see Figure 10-6) provides positive input to the reproductive system, which is frequently altered by the stress-activated HPA axis. Sexual stimulation and GnRH neuron activation, however, may cause the gonadal axis to be resistant to suppression by the HPA axis. Through estradiol, the reproductive system provides positive input to both components of the stress system by stimulating CRH secretion and inhibiting reuptake and catabolism of catecholamines. Table 10-6 presents potential pathologic effects of central and peripheral CRH in women.

Estrogen stimulates the HPA axis. Compared with controls, pregnant women and women receiving high-dose estrogen therapy had elevated levels of cortisol in morning and evening plasma samples.[67] In addition, it appears that the HPA axis responsiveness is greater in women than men.[68] Estrogen directly stimulates the CRH gene promoter and the central noradrenergic (norepinephrine) system, which may help explain adult women's slight hypercortisolism, increases in affective anxiety and eating disorders, mood cycles, and vulnerability to autoimmune and inflammatory disease, all of which follow estradiol fluctuations. Estradiol down-regulates glucocorticoid receptor binding in the anterior pituitary, hypothalamus, and hippocampus—this tends to *increase* HPA activity by interfering with glucocorticoid-negative feedback, whereas progesterone opposes these effects.[69] Thus alterations in estradiol during normal menses, perimenopause (including increases as well as decreases), and menopause alter the regulatory feedback loop, and adaptations over time develop as a new equilibrium is established in the relation as shown in Figure 10-6. Over time, these changes increase the incidence

Table 10-6	Potential Pathologic Effects of Central and Peripheral Corticotropin-Releasing Hormone (CRH) in Women	
Changes		**Alterations**
Central CRH		
Increased secretion		Hypercortisolism
		Melancholic depression
		Eating disorders
		Chronic active alcoholism
		Chronic active exercise
		Consequences: osteoporosis, visceral obesity, infertility
Decreased secretion		Atypical depression
		Seasonal affective disorder
		Chronic fatigue and fibromyalgia syndromes
		Rheumatoid arthritis
		Postpartum blues, depression, and autoimmunity
		Premenstrual tension syndrome
		Menopausal depression
Peripheral CRH		
Increased secretion of immune CRH		Inflammatory disorders
Increased secretion of placental CRH		Premature labor
Decreased secretion of placental CRH		Delayed labor
Decreased secretion of ovarian CRH		Ovarian dysfunction
		Anovulation
		Defective corpus luteum function
Increased secretion of ovarian CRH		Early menopause
Decreased secretion of endometrial CRH		Infertility
		Early spontaneous abortion

Data from Chrousos GP et al: *Ann Intern Med* 129(3):229-240; Kalantaridou SN et al: *J Reprod Immunol* 62(1-2):61-68, 2004.

of mood alterations, eating disorders, anxiety, depression, weight alterations, and inflammatory and immune disorders.

The adipocyte-derived peptide hormone leptin interacts directly and indirectly with the adrenal and gonadal axes; leptin levels are higher in women than in men. Leptin regulates appetite (satiety) and energy balance. It also inhibits the HPA axis at both hyopothalamic and adrenocortical levels. In addition, leptin positively influences the female reproductive axis by inhibition of the HPA axis and arcuate proopiomelanocortin (POMC) neuronal system and through activation of the LC/NE system. By promoting satiety and sympathetic system outflow, leptin is thought to provide the peripheral signal to a central mechanism regulating the size of body fat stores.[70] Thus leptin may be significant in control of the onset of puberty because of its relationship to the amount of fat mass, in the adaptive activation of the HPA axis, and in inhibition of gonadal function that takes place in cases of starvation and anorexia nervosa.[71-73]

Endorphins and Enkephalins

Endorphins and enkephalins (endogenous opiates) are released into the blood as part of the response to stressful stimuli. They are proteins found in the brain that have pain-relieving capabilities. Stressful stimuli include traumatic injury and an acute, intense stress situation, such as first-time parachute jumping. In inflamed tissue, immune cell–derived endorphins activate endorphin receptors on peripheral sensory nerves, leading to pain relief or analgesia.[74] Hemorrhage increases β-endorphin levels that appear to inhibit blood pressure increase or delay compensatory changes that would increase blood pressure.[75] Thus endogenous opiates modulate blood pressure instability and neuroendocrine and cytokine responses to blood losses.[76,77]

The secretion of ACTH and β-endorphin is stimulated by CRH; β-endorphins are released from the pituitary gland.[78] Enkephalin is released from the adrenal medulla. Evidence is accumulating that β-endorphins can modulate ACTH secretion and, with ACTH, inhibit hypothalamic CRH secretion, a possible down-regulation pathway of the stress response.[79]

In a number of conditions or activities in which endogenous opiate activity is increased, subjects not only experience insensitivity to pain but also report increased feelings of excitement, positive well-being, or euphoria. In addition, cells of the immune system synthesize and release opioids when the lymphoid cells are activated.[80] T and B lymphocytes and mononuclear phagocytic cells have receptors for opioids.[1] Endorphins may play a role in the excitement and exhilaration produced by dancing, contact sports, and combat. There is little direct evidence, however, documenting the endorphin system in most of these activities.

Growth Hormone (Somatotropin)

GH is synthesized from the anterior pituitary gland and is produced by lymphocytes and mononuclear phagocytic cells.[81] GH affects protein, lipid, and carbohydrate metabolism

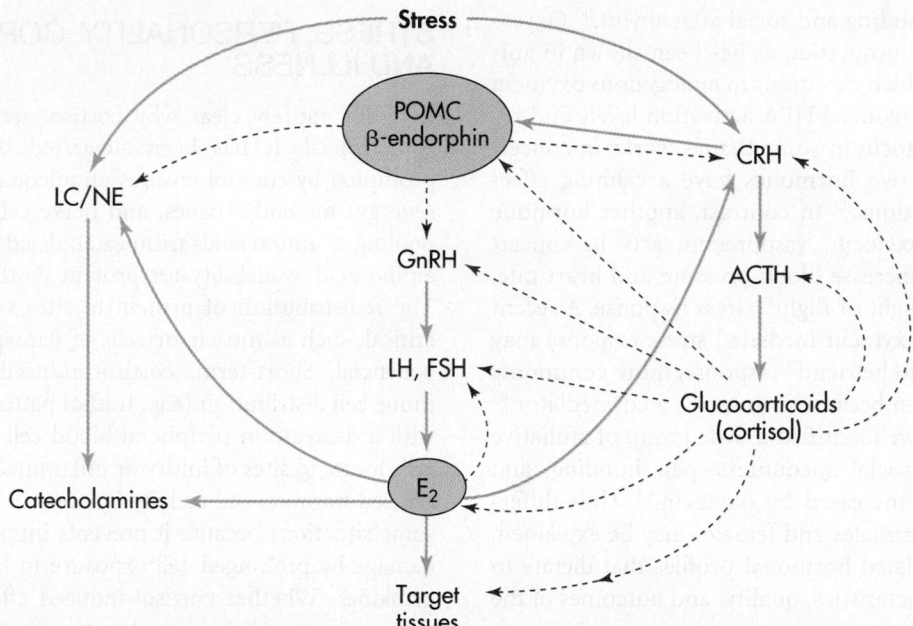

Figure 10-6 Stress and the female reproductive system. Interactions of the reproductive system with the hypothalamic-pituitary-adrenal (HPA) axis and locus coeruleus–norepinephrine system (LC/NE). Corticotrophic cells of the pituitary gland express proopiomelanocortin (POMC) peptides. Stress generally inhibits the female reproductive system primarily through the HPA by (1) suppressing hypothalamic gonadotropin-releasing hormone (GnRH) secretion by corticotropin-releasing hormone (CRH) and CRH-induced β-endorphins; (2) inhibiting GnRH, pituitary luteinizing hormone (LH), and ovarian estradiol (E₂) secretion by cortisol; and (3) cortisol-induced target tissue resistance to estradiol. The LC/NE system provides positive input to the reproductive system, which can be overridden by the stress-activated HPA. Estradiol can cause the reproductive system to stimulate the stress system by stimulating CRH secretion and inhibiting reuptake and catabolism of catecholamines. *ACTH,* Adrenocorticotropic hormone; *FSH,* follicle-stimulating hormone. Dashed lines refer to inhibitory pathways. Solid lines refer to direct stimulatory pathways. (Adapted from Chrousos GP et al: Interactions between the hypothalamic-pituitary-adrenal axis and the female reproductive system, *Ann Intern Med* 129[3]:229-240, 1998.)

and counters the effects of insulin. It is involved in tissue repair and may participate in the growth and function of the immune system.[1] Receptors for GH are present on lymphoid cells.[82] This finding suggests a role for GH in regulating phagocytic function and possibly antigen presentation.[1] GH appears to have enhancing effects on immune function.[1] GH levels increase in the blood after a variety of acutely stressful stimuli, such as cardiac catheterization, electroshock therapy, gastroscopy, surgery, fever, and physical exercise. Psychologic stimuli associated with increased levels of GH include taking examinations, viewing of violent or sexually arousing films, anticipation of exhausting exercise, and certain psychologic performance tests. However, prolonged activation of the stress response (chronic stress) leads to suppression of GH and other growth factor effects on target tissues.[83] (This is not to be confused with a congenital GH deficiency which leads to short stature, decreased muscular strength and bone density problems.) When under stress, chronic glucocorticoid stimulation decreases the release of GH from the pituitary gland, resulting in potentially decreased skeletal muscle, bone catabolism, reduced oxygen uptake, increased fat production, worsening sleep patterns, decreased force of cardiac contractions, decreased thyroid function, and poorer mood state. In other words, glucocorticoids antagonize the beneficial actions of GH.[84]

Prolactin

Prolactin is released from the anterior pituitary gland as well as numerous extrapituitary tissue sites.[85] It is necessary for lactation and breast development.[86] Prolactin receptors are present in many different tissues, including the liver, kidney, intestine, and adrenals. Prolactin is also produced by lymphoid cells.[1,87] Prolactin levels in plasma increase as a result of a variety of stressful stimuli, including gastroscopy, proctoscopy, pelvic examination, and surgery.[88] The level of prolactin also rises during parachute jumping, during motion sickness, after taking examinations, and after receiving various sexual stimuli, for example, stimulation of the nipple or areola in women. Unlike GH, prolactin levels show little change after exercise. Like GH, however, a prolactin increase appears to require more intense stimuli than those leading to increases in catecholamine or cortisol levels. Immune cells also are influenced by prolactin. Prolactin acts as a second messenger for IL-2 and is known to have a positive influence on B-cell activation and differentiation.[89] Several classes of lymphocytes have receptors for prolactin, suggesting a direct effect of prolactin on immune function.

Oxytocin

Oxytocin is well known as a hormone produced in high levels by the hypothalamus during childbirth and lactation. It is also produced during orgasm in both sexes and has been shown to promote bonding and social attachment.[90] Oxytocin also has antistress properties, as has been shown in animal experiments in which elevations in endogenous oxytocin were associated with reduced HPA activation levels and reduced anxiety.[91] Oxytocin in some tissues works in concert with estrogen; these two hormones have a calming effect during stressful situations.[92] In contrast, another hormone closely resembling oxytocin, vasopressin, acts in concert with testosterone to increase blood pressure and heart rate, thus enhancing the "fight or flight" stress response. A recent proposal is that the oxytocin-mediated stress response may promote the "tend and befriend" response, more commonly experienced by women because estrogen is a co-mediator.[93] Studies in animals have identified a wide group of affiliative behaviors involving social encounters, pair bonding, and attachment as being increased by oxytocin.[94] Thus different effects of stress on males and females may be explained, in part, by gender-related hormonal profiles that dictate to some extent the characteristics, quality, and outcomes of the stress response.

Testosterone

Testosterone, a hormone secreted by Leydig cells, regulates male secondary sex characteristics and libido. Testosterone levels decrease after stressful stimuli. The decrease in testosterone occurs after stimuli such as ether or anesthesia, surgery, marathon running, and mountain climbing.[95] The mechanism causing decreased levels of testosterone is thought to be exerted by cortisol and β-endorphin.

Psychologic stimuli also lead to a decrease in testosterone levels. Men engaged in rigorous combat training and those engaged in the first several weeks of officer candidate school experience significant drops in testosterone levels.[96,97] However, recent data indicate that the psychologic stress associated with some types of competition (e.g., pistol shooting) *increases* both testosterone and cortisol, especially in athletes older than 45 years.[98] Individuals with acute illness, such as respiratory failure, burns, and congestive heart failure, show a marked reduction in plasma testosterone.[99]

The direct immunologic effects of sex hormones contribute to the sexual dimorphism seen in the incidence of autoimmune disease[100] and the greater susceptibility to sepsis and mortality in males following injury.[101] Estrogens generally are associated with a depression of T-cell–dependent immune function and enhancement of B-cell functions, and androgens suppress both T- and B-cell responses.[99] In injury, however, males produce greater amounts of proinflammatory cytokines, a profile that is associated with poor outcome.[102] Additionally, androgens appear to induce a greater degree of immune cell apoptosis following injury, a mechanism that may elicit a greater immunosuppression in injured males versus females.[103] (See Table 10-5 for other hormones, including melatonin, substance P, neuropeptide Y, calcitonin gene–related peptide, somatostatin, and vasoactive intestinal peptide.)

STRESS, PERSONALITY, COPING, AND ILLNESS

It is not entirely clear why cortisol secretion during stress is beneficial. It has been suggested that gluconeogenesis prompted by cortisol ensures an adequate source of glucose (energy) for body tissues, and nerve cells in particular. The pooling of amino acids from catabolized proteins may ensure amino acid availability for protein synthesis in certain cells. The redistribution of protein to sites where replacement is critical, such as muscle or cells of damaged tissue, would be beneficial. Short-term, cortisol-induced alterations in immune cell distribution (e.g., traffic) patterns may be adaptive, with a decrease in peripheral blood cell numbers as effector cells locate to sites of injury or inflammation. In addition, decreased immune cell activity by cortisol may be beneficial in some situations because it prevents immune-mediated tissue damage by prolonged cell exposure to high levels of certain cytokines. Whether cortisol-induced effects are adaptive or destructive may depend on the intensity, type, and duration of the stressor, and the subsequent concentration and length of cortisol exposure that target cells of the individual experience.

Extreme physiologic stressors, such as severe burn injury, represent a predictable stimulus for the stress responses described previously. A less severe and defined event or situation, however, can be a stressor for one person and not for another. Many stressors, such as fasting or temperature changes, do not necessarily cause a physiologic stress response if psychologic factors are minimized. Stress itself is not an independent entity but a system of interdependent processes that are moderated by the nature, intensity, and duration of the stressor and the perception, appraisal, and coping efficacy of the affected individual, all of which in turn mediate the psychologic and physiologic response to stress. Further, adjustment to repetitive stressors is known to be individualized, based on a person's appraisal of a situation.[104] Illustrating the influence of an individualized stress appraisal on physiologic processes, a meta-analysis of the relationships between stressors and immunity found that a higher *perception* of stress was associated with reduced T-cytotoxic (Tc)-cell cytotoxicity although not with levels of circulating Th or Tc lymphocytes.[105]

Psychosocial distress may be predictive of psychologic and physical health outcomes. In **psychologic distress** the individual feels a general state of unpleasant arousal after life events that manifests as physiologic, emotional, cognitive, and behavioral changes.[106] Periods of depression and emotional upheaval often are associated with adverse life events and place the affected individual at risk for immunologic deficits, increasing the risk of ill health.[107] A meta-analysis of studies shows a relationship between depression and reduction in lymphocyte proliferation and NK cell activity.[108] Multiple moderating factors may be important in immune modulation in depressed individuals, including comorbidities such as alcoholism. Examples of triggering mechanisms include bereavement, academic and job-related pressures, life events (positive and negative changes),[107] and aging. Adverse life events having the most negative effect on immunity are characterized as uncontrollable, undesirable, and overtaxing the individual's ability to cope.[109,110]

Studies have strengthened the association of stress with potential for illness in humans. One study examined medical students who were immunized with hepatitis B vaccine on the third day of a stressful examination period; the time to seroconversion and level of antibody titer to the vaccine were measured later. The students with the most rapid seroconversion and the highest titers also reported being less stressed and had a good social support system (which may reduce stress).[111] Even more convincing is a study in which the psychologic stress status was determined in healthy individuals after experimentally controlled exposure to respiratory virus by nasal inoculation. Individuals reporting more stress had an increased incidence of clinical cold and respiratory symptoms compared with subjects reporting less stress, and other infections, including HIV, were shown to be potentially influenced by psychosocial factors.[112-115]

Evidence also suggests adverse changes in immune function following intense exercise, with increased cortisol levels, changes in lymphocyte counts, and alterations in cytokine production.[116] Some of these immune changes could be reduced by administration of carbohydrate beverages to endurance athletes, implying that dehydration and decreased tissue perfusion were catalysts for the exercise stress–induced immune changes.

Animal studies have found that stress contributes to the initiation, growth, and metastasis of certain tumors.[7,117] Studies of mechanisms in humans reveal stress affects important processes in cancer including antiviral responses, deoxyribonucleic acid (DNA) repair, and aspects of cellular aging.[117] But the overall evidence is mixed from prospective studies linking stress with cancer incidence. Stress may be more likely to influence progression and recurrence of cancer; however, the critical prospective studies have been mostly unsupportive.[7] Studies examining impairments in antiviral immunity and chronic activation of hormonal responses (e.g., HIV-related tumors, hepatocellular carcinoma, and cervical cancer) may be more successful designs for defining the stress-related mechanisms.[117]

Evidence is showing a relationship between immune stimulation and heart disease.[118] The relationship between stress and cardiovascular health may be mediated by stress-induced changes in immune function, which may potentiate proinflammatory processes and permit alterations that lead to heart disease[119] (see What's New? Acute Emotional Stress and Adverse Heart Effects, p. 337, and What's New? Psychosocial Stress and Progression to Coronary Heart Disease, p. 347).

In the past decade a significant amount of evidence has accumulated linking severe psychosocial stress resulting from negative life events to a chronic syndrome with mental and physical consequences. Posttraumatic stress disorder (PTSD) has been described in many populations.[120-122] A cascade model has been proposed to describe the pathogenesis and clinical course illustrating the clinical, epidemiologic, neurobiologic, and psychosocial components of PTSD.[123] The study of PTSD has contributed to the knowledge concerning mechanisms involved in the chronic stress and disease relationship. Recently an appreciation of the association of chronic stress with high levels of cortisol production and paradoxical biounavailability (i.e., bound to plasma protein and therefore not bioavailable) of cortisol has been gained.[124]

The interaction with healthcare providers in a clinical setting, the diagnosis of a major illness, and various clinical procedures (e.g., blood draws, injections, examinations, surgical procedures) also may represent significant negative life events to many individuals (Figure 10-7). For example, mammography and the activation of the HPA axis.

The influence of repetitive but episodic stress on cancer survivors demonstrates a connection between events such as mammography and activation of the HPA axis. Early research with breast cancer survivors by Cordova and colleagues[125] demonstrated a link between sympathetic activity and HPA axis activation, noting that some women reported symptoms of PTSD (heart palpitations, panic, shakiness, nausea) during thoughts of recurrence triggered by events such as finding themselves near the hospital where they received initial treatment.[125] HPA axis activation also influences organs and tissues that enable bidirectional communication processes (feedback loops) between neuroendocrine and immune processes.[126] For example, among breast cancer survivors 3 to 5 years post diagnosis, elevated baseline cortisol levels and blunted cortisol reactivity were reported in response to the anticipation of a real, regularly scheduled mammogram, and alterations in cortisol and heart rate variability were reported in women simulating the threat of cancer with a controlled laboratory stressor.[127,128] Further, Ma and colleagues[127] reported that the threat of cancer recurrence (using a simulated mammography event as a stressor to elicit thoughts of cancer recurrence) elicited greater alterations in heart rate variability when compared with another simulated controlled stressor. These studies suggest activation of the autonomic nervous system to events, such as mammography, that occur repeatedly throughout breast cancer survivorship, although the timing of onset of these autonomic activation responses to a stressor is unclear. Similar ANS activation may occur in association with events particular to the management of many other types of chronic illnesses as well as interactions with the healthcare system.

These additional stresses may affect the course of illness as well as interfere with the efficacy of the medical intervention. Identifying and reducing stress in the clinical setting have particular applicability in both disease prevention and illness management. In addition to medical procedures, patient-provider communication also provides an important area for future research. Recent studies of cancer communication and patient-provider interaction have demonstrated a link between communication events and emotional outcomes, such as uncertainty and mood state in breast cancer survivors.[129,130] Although a logical extension, it remains to be seen if these emotional outcomes affect physiologically-based health outcomes caused by activation of the HPA axis and subsequent immune processes.

POTENTIAL EFFECTS IN HEALTHY INDIVIDUALS

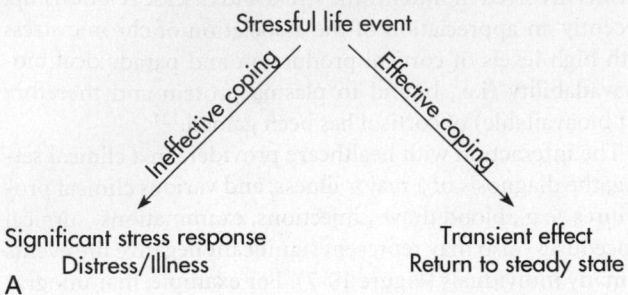

POTENTIAL EFFECTS IN SYMPTOMATIC INDIVIDUALS

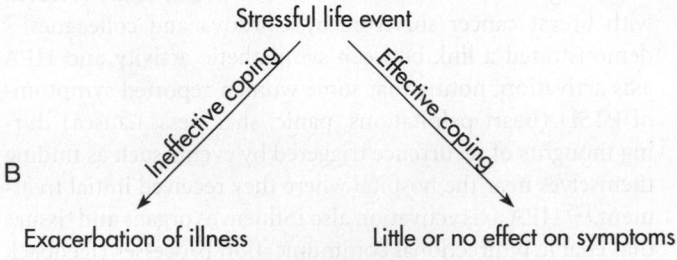

POTENTIAL EFFECTS DURING MEDICAL INTERVENTION

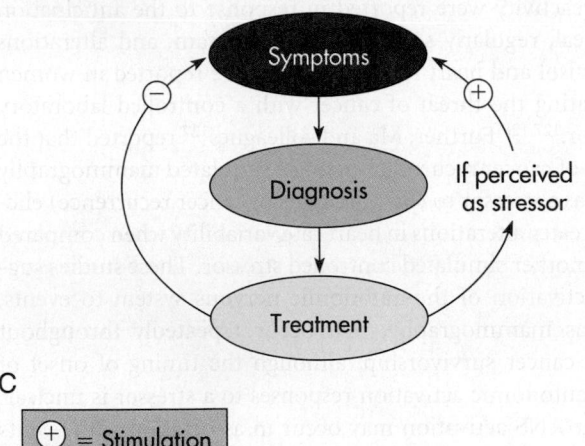

Figure 10-7 Health outcome determination in stressful life situations is moderated by numerous factors. Whether a life-challenged individual experiences distress or illness depends on the subject's appraisal of the event and the coping strategies used during the stressful period. A and B reflect possible outcomes in stressed healthy and symptomatic individuals. C illustrates the dynamic clinical setting in which the diagnosis of a serious illness and subsequent medical interventions may be perceived as stressful challenges and have potentially detrimental influences on physical outcome.

Personality characteristics are associated with individual differences in appraisal and response to stressors.[131] The coping response of individuals may exaggerate or moderate physical consequences of the stress response. **Coping** is

defined as the process of managing stressful demands and challenges that are appraised as taxing or exceeding the resources of the person.[132] One response may be a negative change in behavior resulting in potentially adverse health effects (e.g., increased smoking, change in eating habits). Serious disturbances of the sleep-wake cycle are observed in many people under stress and in many clinical settings. Further, sleep disturbances may exacerbate the pathophysiologic status of certain patient populations.[133-135] Investigators have reported that sleep deprivation and circadian disruption, even in young, otherwise healthy individuals, have detrimental influences on respiratory and immune system function. Even partial sleep deprivation was associated with reduced NK cell activity in healthy subjects, and only recently have seriously ill patients been assessed for adequacy and structure of sleep during recovery.[133]

Adaptive coping strategies, especially those that are problem focused and those that encourage seeking social support, are beneficial during stressful experiences. The extent to which an individual responds to distress, using effective positive coping strategies, determines the degree of successful moderation of the stress challenge. Conversely, ineffective negative coping attempts may exacerbate the effects of distress on health, thus augmenting the potential for illness. Mediating factors that may influence stress susceptibility or resilience include age, socioeconomic status, gender, social support status, personality and lifestyle, self-esteem, genetics, life events, past experiences, and current health status.[136] Evidence suggests that effective intervention may result in greater stress resilience and improved psychologic and physiologic outcomes. In a study of nursing home residents randomly assigned to control or social support intervention groups, improved psychologic measures and immune function (NK cell activity) were observed in the experimental group at 6 weeks.[137] In another study, women with recurrent metastatic breast cancer were given either routine follow-up (routine care) or weekly support group sessions. Survival in the support treatment group was an average of 19 months longer than in the routine care group, suggesting a mediating influence of additional support for these women.[32,138]

The importance of social support for seriously ill individuals has focused attention on the health and well-being of family members who function as caregivers. Significant stress manifested as depression, anxiety, and fatigue has been noted in family caregivers of those with cancer, Alzheimer disease, and burn trauma. Individuals and caretakers exhibited suppression of various measures of immune function, with improved function associated with better perceived social support.[139-141] Gender-based coping differences may be attributed, in part, to the hormonal milieu of the individual, with females more likely to offer social support, a behavior with an oxytocin/estrogen association.[92]

Interventions to prevent or manage stress-related psychologic or physical problems include both short- and long-term coping strategies. Stress management consists of educational components specific to the individual's problems and relaxation techniques, which may include meditation, imagery, massage, and biofeedback. These approaches may be used on an individual or a support group basis. Incorporation of these approaches into clinical training facilitates their use in the clinical arena. Research should focus on the efficacy of such approaches with various populations.

Aging and Stress: Stress-Age Syndrome

With aging, sometimes a set of neurohormonal and immune alterations, as well as tissue and cellular changes, develops. These changes, which recently have been defined as stress-age syndrome, include the following[136,142]:

- Irregular excitability of structures of the limbic system influencing the relationship with the hypothalamus

- Rise of the blood concentration of catecholamines, antidiuretic hormone (ADH), ACTH, and cortisol
- Decrease of testosterone, thyroxine, and other hormones
- Alterations in opioid peptide concentration
- Immunodepression
- Alterations in lipoproteins
- Hypercoagulation of the blood
- Free radical damage of cells

Some of the alterations are adaptational, whereas others are potentially damaging. These stress-related alterations of aging can influence the course of developing stress reactions and lower adaptive reserve and coping.

SUMMARY REVIEW

Concepts of Stress
1. Modern society is full of stress.
2. Psychologic stress may cause or exacerbate (worsen) several disease states. Stress is related to the severity of symptoms and outcomes of diseases and conditions. Research is focused on the mechanisms responsible for these mind-body interactions.
3. Stress has been defined as the state of affairs arising when a person relates to (i.e., interacts or transacts with) situations in a certain way. Important is how he or she appraises and reacts to situations.
4. In general, a person experiences stress when a demand exceeds a person's coping abilities.
5. Hans Selye identified three structural changes in rats subjected repeatedly to noxious stimuli (stressors): enlargement of the cortex of the adrenal gland, atrophy of the thymus gland and other lymphoid tissues, and gastrointestinal ulceration.
6. Selye believed that the three changes were caused by a nonspecific physiologic response to any long-term stressor. He called this response the GAS.
7. The GAS occurs in three stages: the alarm stage, the stage of resistance or adaptation, and the stage of exhaustion. Diseases of adaptation develop if the stage of resistance or adaptation does not restore homeostasis.
8. Selye identified three components of physiologic stress: the stressor, the physiologic or chemical disturbance produced by the stressor, and the body's adaptational response to the stressor.
9. The nonspecific physiologic response consists of interaction among the sympathetic branch of the ANS and other neural signals that activate the endocrine system known as the HPA axis.
10. The nonspecific physiologic response is a common residual response and can be elicited with diverse agents such as cold, heat, x-rays, adrenaline, insulin, tubercle bacilli, and muscular exercise. Although the reactions of these stages are nonspecific, evidence supports the coexistence of highly specific, adaptive reactions to any of these agents.
11. As with a physically mediated stress response, psychologic stressors can elicit a reactive stress response, that is, a physiologic response derived from psychologic stressors.

12. Another type of psychologic-mediated stress response is the anticipatory response.
13. In a conditioned response, the organism learns that specific stimuli are associated with danger and anticipation of subsequent encounters with that particular stimulus produces a physiologic stress response.
14. Psychoneuroimmunology is the study of the interaction of consciousness (psycho), brain and spinal cord (neuro), and the body's defense against external infection and abnormal cell division (immunology).
15. Psychoneuroimmunology assumes that all immune-related disease is multifactorial. The immune system is integrated with other physiologic processes and is sensitive to changes in CNS and endocrine functioning, such as those that accompany psychologic states.
16. CRH is released centrally from the brain and peripherally at inflammatory sites.

Stress Response
1. The stress response is initiated by the CNS and endocrine system. Where the stress response begins depends on whether the stressor is perceived or real.
2. Perceived stressors elicit an anticipatory response that usually begins in the limbic system of the brain. The limbic system elicits an endocrine stress response indirectly by stimulating neural pathways responsible for receiving sensory information and elicits a central response directly by stimulating the LC to release LC/NE.
3. Real stressors elicit a reactive response that can begin either in the limbic system or in the brain in response to specific sensory information. This information is then relayed to the PVN. The PVN stimulates the LC and both central and endocrine stress responses.
4. The neuroendocrine response to stress consists of sympathetic stimulation of the adrenal medulla to secrete catecholamines (norepinephrine and epinephrine) and stressor-induced stimulation of the hypothalamus to secrete CRH, which in turn stimulates the pituitary to secrete ACTH, which then stimulates the adrenal cortex to secrete steroid hormones, particularly cortisol.
5. In general, the catecholamines prepare the body to act, and cortisol mobilizes energy (glucose) and other substances needed to fuel the action.

Continued

SUMMARY REVIEW—cont'd

6. Epinephrine exerts its chief effects on the cardiovascular system. Epinephrine increases cardiac output and increases blood flow to the heart, brain, and skeletal muscles by dilating vessels that supply these organs. It also dilates the airways, thereby increasing delivery of oxygen to the bloodstream.

7. Norepinephrine's chief effects complement those of epinephrine. Norepinephrine constricts blood vessels of the viscera and skin; this has the effect of shifting blood flow to the vessels dilated by epinephrine. Norepinephrine also increases mental alertness.

8. CRH influences the immune system indirectly by the activation of glucocorticoids (cortisol) and catecholamines. Peripheral CRH is proinflammatory, causing vasodilation and vascular permeability. It appears that the mast cells are the target of peripheral CRH.

9. Cortisol's chief effects involve metabolic processes. By inhibiting the use of metabolic substances while promoting their formation, cortisol mobilizes glucose, amino acids, lipids, and fatty acids and delivers them to the bloodstream. Cortisol's effect on the immune system is concentration and location dependent and may include either stimulation or inhibition of the immune system.

10. The nervous, endocrine, and immune systems communicate through the common use of signal molecules and their receptors, which in turn regulate the behavior of cells in each system during stress challenge.

11. There are direct and indirect pathways of influence among the nervous, endocrine, and immune systems. Neuropeptides have direct effects on immune cells, as well as indirect influences through neuromediated endocrine modulation of immune function. Endocrine products (cortisol) also influence nerve cell behavior. Immune cell products affect both nerve and endocrine cell function, reflecting an adaptive role for the immune system as a "signal" organ to alert other systems of threatening stimuli.

12. Other hormones are affected by the stress response and include increased circulating levels of β-endorphins, growth hormone, and prolactin and a decrease in antidiuretic hormone with extreme stress. Luteinizing hormone, estradiol, progesterone, and possibly testosterone decrease during the stress response.

Stress, Personality, Coping, and Illness

1. Stress is a system of interdependent processes that are moderated by the nature, intensity, and duration of the stressor and the coping efficacy of the affected individual, all of which in turn mediate the psychologic and physiologic response to stress.

2. Many studies have linked psychologic distress with altered immune function, and evidence strengthens the association of stress with potential for illness in humans.

3. Adaptive coping strategies, especially those that are problem focused and those that encourage seeking social support, are beneficial during stressful experiences.

Aging and Stress: Stress-Age Syndrome

1. With aging, sometimes a set of neurohormonal and immune alterations develop; these changes have been defined recently as stress-age syndrome.

2. These stress-related alterations of aging can influence the course of developing stress reactions and lower adaptive reserve and coping.

KEY TERMS

Alarm stage, 338
Anticipatory response, 339
Conditional response, 339
Coping, 354
Corticosteroid-binding globulin, 343
Corticotropin-releasing hormone (CRH), 339
Disease of adaptation, 338
General adaptation syndrome (GAS), 338

Homeostasis, 339
Hypothalamic-pituitary-adrenal (HPA) axis, 338
Peripheral (immune) CRH, 339
Physiologic stress, 338
Post-traumatic stress disorder (PTSD), 339
Psychologic distress, 352
Psychoneuroimmunology (PNI), 339

Reactive response, 338
Stage of exhaustion, 338
Stage of resistance or adaptation, 338
Stress, 337
Stress response, 339
Stressor, 338
Th2 shift, 345
Transcortin, 343

REFERENCES

1. Rabin BS: The nervous system—immune system connection. In Rabin BS: *Stress, immune function, and health: the connection*, New York, 1999, Wiley-Liss.

2. Kapcala LP et al: The protective role of the hypothalamic-pituitary-adrenal axis against lethality produced by immune, infections, and inflammatory stress, *Ann N Y Acad Sci* 771:419-437, 1995.

3. Black PH, Garbutt LD: Stress, inflammation and cardiovascular disease, *J Psychosom Res* 52(1):1-23, 2002.

4. Kiecolt-Glaser JK et al: Psychoneuroimmunology: psychological influences on immune function and health, *J Consult Clin Psychol* 70(3):537-547, 2002.

5. Liu LY et al: School examinations enhance airway inflammation to antigen challenge, *Am J Respir Crit Care Med* 165(8):1062-1067, 2002.

6. Cohen S, Janicki-Deverts D, Miller GE: Psychological stress and disease, *JAMA* 298(14):1685-1687, 2007.

7. Vedhara K, Irwin M, editors: *Human pyschoimmunology*, Oxford, England, 2005, Oxford University Press.

8. Pereira DB et al: Stress as a predictor of symptomatic genital herpes virus recurrence in women with human immunodeficiency virus, *J Psychosom Res* 54(3):237-244, 2003.

9. Hamerman D: Toward an understanding of frailty, *Ann Intern Med* 130(11):945-950, 1999.

10. Taaffe DR et al: Cross-sectional and prospective relationships of interleukin-6 and C-reactive protein with physical performance in elderly persons: MacArthur studies of successful aging, *J Gerontol A Biol Sci Med Sci* 55(12):M709-M715, 2000.

11. Selye H: The general adaptation syndrome and the diseases of adaptation, *J Clin Endocrinol Metab* 6:117, 1946.

12. Hill SR et al: Studies on adrenocortical and psychological responses to stress in man, *Arch Intern Med* 97:269, 1956.

13. Mason JW, Brady JV: Plasma 17-hydroxycortico-steroid changes related to reserpine effects on emotional behaviors, *Science* 124:983, 1956.

14. Hetzel BS et al: Changes in urinary 17-hydroxycorticosteroid excretion during stressful life experiences in man, *J Clin Endocrinol Metab* 15(9):1057-1068, 1955.

15. Handlon JH et al: Psychological factors lowering plasma 17-hydroxycorticosteroid concentration, *Psychosom Med* 24:535-541, 1962.

16. Wadeson RW et al: Plasma and urinary 17-OHCS responses to motion pictures, *Arch Gen Psychiatry* 14:146-156, 1963.

17. Mason JW: Organization of psychoendocrine mechanisms: a review and reconsideration of research. In Greenfield NS, Steinbach RA, editors: *Handbook of psychophysiology*, New York, 1972, Holt, Rinehart, & Winston.

18. Herman JP et al: Central mechanisms of stress integration: hierarchical circuitry controlling hypothalmo-pituitary-adrenocortical responsiveness, *Front Neuroendocrinol* 24(3):151-158, 2003.

19. Bauer-Wu SM: Psychoneuroimmunology. Part I: Physiology. *Clin J Oncol Nurs* 6(3):167-170, 2002.

20. Bauer-Wu SM: Psychoneuroimmunology. Part II: Mind-body interventions, *Clin J Oncol Nurs* 6(4):243-246, 2002.

21. Cohen S et al: Types of stressors that increase susceptibility to the common cold in healthy adults, *Health Psychol* 17(3):214-223, 1998.

22. McCain NL et al: A randomized clinical trial of alternative stress management interventions in persons with HIV infection, *J Consult Clin Psychol* 76(3):431-441, 2008.

23. Glaser R et al: Chronic stress modulates the immune response to a pneumococcal pneumonia vaccine, *Psychosom Med* 62(6):804-807, 2000.

24. Marucha PT, Kiecolt-Glaser JK, Favagehi M: Mucosal wound healing is impaired by examination stress, *Psychosom Med* 60(3):362-365, 1998.

25. Pacak K et al: Heterogeneous neurochemical responses to different stressors: a test of Selye's doctrine of nonspecificity, *Am J Physiol* 275(4Pt2):R1247-R1255, 1998.

26. Repka-Ramirez MS, Baraniuk JN: Histamine in health and disease, *Clin Allergy Immunol* 17:1-25, 2002.

27. Dimsdale JE, Ziegler MG: What do plasma and urinary measures of catecholamines tell us about human response to stressors? *Circulation* 83(4 Suppl):II36-II42, 1991.

28. Herd JA: Cardiovascular response to stress. *Physiol Rev* 71(1):305-330, 1991.

29. Sapolsky RM, Romero LM, Munck AU: How do glucocorticoids influence stress responses? Integrating permissive, suppressive, stimulatory, and preparative actions, *Endocr Rev* 21(1):55-89, 2000.

30. Moyna NM et al: The effects of incremental submaximal exercise on circulating leukocytes in physically active and sedentary males and females, *Eur J Appl Physiol Occup Physiol* 74(3):211-218, 1996.

31. Drapeau V et al: Is visceral obesity a physiological adaptation to stress? *Panminerva Medica* 45(3):189-195, 2003.

32. Rosmond R: Stress induced disturbances of the HPA axis: a pathway to type 2 diabetes? *Med Sci Monit* 9(2):):RA35-RA39, 2003.

33. Elenkov IJ, Chrousos GP: Stress hormones, proinflammatory and antiinflammatory cytokines, and autoimmunity, *Ann N Y Acad Sci* 966:290-303, 2002.

34. Fearon DT, Locksley RM: The instructive role of innate immunity in the acquired immune response, *Science* 272(5258):50-53, 1996 review.

35. Mosmann TR, Sad S: The expanding universe of T-cell subsets: Th1, Th2, and more, *Immunol Today* 17(3):138-146, 1996 (review).

36. Meduri GU, Chrousos GP: Duration of glucocorticoid treatment and outcome in sepsis: is the right drug used the wrong way? *Chest* 114(2):355-360, 1998.

37. Chrousos GP: The hypothalamic-pituitary-adrenal axis and immune-mediated inflammation, *N Engl J Med* 332(20):1351-1362, 1995.

38. Karalis K et al: Autocrine or paracrine inflammatory actions of corticotropin-releasing hormone in vivo, *Science* 254(5030):421-423, 1991.

39. Chrousos GP, Elenkov IJ: Interactions of the endocrine and immune systems. In DeGroot LG, Jameson JL, editors: *Endocrinology*, ed 4, Philadelphia, 2001, Saunders.

40. Elenkov IJ: Glucocorticoids and the Th1/Th2 balance, *Ann N Y Acad Sci* 1024:138-146, review, 2004.

41. Lagier B et al: Different modulation by histamine of IL-4 and interferon-gamma (IFN-gamma) release according to the phenotype of human Th0, Th1, and Th2 clones, *Clin Exp Immunol* 108(3):545-551, 1997.

42. Rocklin RE, editor: *Histamine and H₂ antagonists in inflammation and immunodeficiency*, New York, 1990, Marcel Dekker.

43. Kiecolt-Glaser JK et al: Chronic stress and age-related increases in the proinflammatory cytokine IL-6, *Proc Natl Acad Sci U S A* 100(15):9090-9095, 2003.

44. Rohleder N et al: Age and sex steroid-related changes in glucocorticoid sensitivity of proinflammatory cytokine production after psychosocial stress, *J Neuroimmunol* 126(1-2):69-77, 2002.

45. Bone RC: Toward an epidemiology and natural history of SIRS (systemic inflammatory response syndrome), *JAMA* 268(24):3452-3455, 1992.

46. Poynter ME, Daynes RA: Peroxisome proliferator–activated receptor alpha activation modulates cellular redox status, represses nuclear factor-kappaB signaling, and reduces inflammatory cytokine production in aging, *J Biol Chem* 273(49):32833-32841, 1998.

47. Aoki N, Ohno Y, Imamura M: Physiological interactions between the immune and endocrine systems: are cytokines hormones? *Med Sci Res* 18:195-201, 1990.

48. Khansari DN, Murgo AJ, Faith RE: Effects of stress on the immune system, *Immunol Today* 11(5):170-175, 1990.

49. Dunn AJ: Psychoneuroimmunology for the psychoneuro-endocrinologist: a review of animal studies of nervous system-immune system interactions, *Psychoneuroendocrinology* 14(4):251-274, 1989.

50. Friedman EM, Irwin MR: A role for CRH and the sympathetic nervous system in stress-induced immunosuppression, *Ann N Y Acad Sci* 771:396-418, 1995.

51. Jankovic BD: Neuroimmunomodulation: facts and dilemmas, *Immunol Lett* 21(2):101-118, 1989.

52. Rabin BS et al: Bidirectional interaction between the central nervous system and the immune system, *Clin Rev Immunol* 9(4):279-312, 1989.

53. Jain R et al: Corticotropin-releasing factor modulating the immune response to stress in the rat, *Endocrinology* 128(3):1329-1336, 1991.

54. Maestroni GJ, Conti A: Anti-stress role of the immuno-opioid network: evidence for a physiological mechanism involving T cell–derived, immunoreactive beta-endorphin and MET-enkephalin binding to thymic opioid receptors, *Int J Neurosci* 61(3-4):289-298, 1991.

55. Schwab RJ: Disturbances of sleep in the intensive care unit, *Crit Care Clin* 10(4):681-694, 1994.

56. Nelson RJ, Drazen DL: Melatonin mediates seasonal adjustment in immune function, *Reprod Nutr Dev* 39(3):383-398, 1999.

57. Ader R, Felten D, Cohen N: Interactions between the brain and the immune system, *Annu Rev Pharmacol Toxicol* 30:561-602, 1990.

58. Busbridge NJ, Grossman AB: Stress and the single cytokine: interleukin modulation of the pituitary-adrenal axis, *Mol Cell Endocrinol* 82(2-3):C209-214, 1991.

59. Hori T et al: Immune cytokines and regulation of body temperature, food intake, and cellular immunity, *Brain Res Bull* 27(3-4):309-313, 1991.

60. Navarra P et al: Interleukins-1 and -6 stimulate the release of corticotropin-releasing hormone-41 from rat hypothalamus in vitro via the eicosanoid cyclooxygenase pathway, *Endocrinology* 128(1):37-44, 1991.

61. Hall NRS, O'Grady MP: Regulation of pituitary peptides by the immune system, *BioEssays* 11(5):141-144, 1989.

62. Krueger JM et al: Sleep, microbes, and cytokines, *Neuroimmunomodulation* 1(2):100-109, 1994.

63. Weigent DA, Carr DJ, Blalock JE: Bidirectional communication between the neuroendocrine and immune systems: common hormones and hormone receptors, *Ann N Y Acad Sci* 579:17-27, 1990.

64. Chrousos GP, Gold PW: The concepts of stress and stress system disorders: overview of physical and behavioral homeostasis, *JAMA* 267(9):1244-1252, 1992.

65. Chrousos GP et al: Interactions between the hypothalamic-pituitary-adrenal axis and the female reproductive system, *Ann Intern Med* 129(3):229-240, 1998.

66. Kalantaridou SN et al: Stress and the female reproductive system. Review, *J Reprod Immunol* 62(1-2):61-68, 2004.

67. Lindholm J, Schultz-Moller N: Plasma and urinary cortisol in pregnancy and during estrogen-gestagen treatment, *Scand J Clin Lab Invest* 31(1):119-122, 1973.

68. Gallucci WT et al: Sex differences in sensitivity of the hypothalamic-pituitary-adrenal axis, *Health Psychol* 12(5):420-425, 1993.
69. Peiffer A, Lapointe B, Barden H: Hormonal regulation of type II glucocorticoid receptor messenger ribonucleic acid in rat brain, *Endocrinology* 129(4):2166-2174, 1991.
70. Caro JF et al: Leptin: the tale of an obesity gene, *Diabetes* 45(11):1455-1462, 1996.
71. Ahima RS et al: Role of leptin in the neuroendocrine response to fasting, *Nature* 382(6588):250-252, 1996.
72. Boden G et al: Effect of fasting on serum leptin in normal human subjects, *J Clin Endocrinol Metab* 81(9):3419-3423, 1996.
73. Grinspoon S et al: Serum leptin levels in women with anorexia nervosa, *J Clin Endocrinol Metab* 81(11):3861-3863, 1996.
74. Machelska H et al: Opioid control of inflammatory pain regulated by intercellular adhesion molecule-1, *J Neurosci* 22(13):5588-5596, 2002.
75. Molina PE: Stress-specific opioid modulation of haemodynamic counter-regulation, *Clin Exp Pharmacol Physiol* 29(3):248-253, 2002.
76. Jochem J, Josko J, Gwozdz B: Endogenous opioid peptides system in haemorrhagic shock—central cardiovascular regulation, *Med Sci Monit* 7(3):545-549, 2001.
77. Molina PE: Opiate modulation of hemodynamic, hormonal, and cytokine responses to hemorrhage, *Shock* 15(6):471-478, 2001.
78. Curtis AL et al: Previous stress alters corticotropin-releasing factor neurotransmission in the locus coeruleus, *Neuroscience* 65(2):541-550, 1995.
79. Calogero AE et al: Multiple feedback regulatory loops in hypothalamic corticotropin-releasing hormone secretion: potential clinical implications, *J Clin Invest* 82(3):767-774, 1988.
80. Cabot PJ et al: Immune cell-derived beta-endorphin: Production, release, and control of inflammatory pain in rats, *J Clin Invest* 100(1):142-148, 1997.
81. Weigent DA et al: Characterization of the promoter-directing expression of growth hormone in a monocyte cell line, *Neuroimmunomodulation* 7(3):126-134, 2000.
82. Kelly PA et al: The prolactin/growth hormone receptor family, *Endocr Rev* 12(3):235-251, 1991.
83. Burguera B et al: Dual and selective actions of glucocorticoid upon basal and stimulated growth hormone release in man, *Neuroendocrinology* 51(1):51-58, 1990.
84. Tsigos C, Chrousos GP: Hypothalamic-pituitary-adrenal axis, neuroendocrine factors and stress, *J Psychosom Res* 53(4):865-871, 2002.
85. Ben-Jonathan N et al: Extrapituitary prolactin: distribution, regulation, functions, and clinical aspects, *Endocr Rev* 17(6):639-669, 1996. Review.
86. Shiu RP, Friesen HG: Mechanisms of action of prolactin in the control of mammary gland function, *Annu Rev Physiol* 42:83-96, 1980.
87. Van De Weerdt C et al: Far upstream sequences regulate the human prolactin promoter transcription, *Neuroendocrinology* 71(2):124-137, 2000.
88. Noel GL et al: Human prolactin and growth hormone release during surgery and other conditions of stress, *J Clin Endocrinol Metab* 35(6):840-851, 1972.
89. Prystowsky MB, Clevenger CV: Prolactin as a second messenger for interleukin 2, *Immunomethods* 5(1):49-55, 1994.
90. Anderson-Hunt M, Dennerstein L: Oxytocin and female sexuality, *Gynecol Obstet Invest* 40(4):217-221, 1995.
91. Neumann ID: Alterations in behavioral and neuroendocrine stress coping strategies in pregnant, parturient, and lactating rats, *Prog Brain Res* 133:143-152, 2001.
92. Liu Y et al: Differential expression of vasopressin, oxytocin, and corticotrophin-releasing hormone messenger RNA in the paraventricular nucleus of the prairie vole brain following stress, *J Neuroendocrinol* 13(12):1059-1065, 2001.
93. Taylor SE et al: Biobehavioral responses to stress in females: tend-and-befriend, not fight-or-flight, *Psychol Rev* 107(3):411-429, 2000.
94. Insel TR: A neurobiological basis of social attachment, *Am J Psychiatry* 154(6):726-736, 1997.
95. Matsumoto K et al: Plasma testosterone levels following surgical stress in male patients, *Acta Endocrinol* 65(1):11-17, 1970.
96. Aakvaag A et al: Testosterone and testosterone-binding globulin (TeBG) in young men during prolonged stress, *Int J Androl* 1:22, 1978.
97. Kreuz LE, Rose RM, Jennings JR: Suppression of plasma testosterone levels and psychological stress: a longitudinal study of young men in Officer Candidate School, *Arch Gen Psychiatry* 26(5):479-482, 1972.
98. Guezennec CY et al: Effect of competition stress on tests used to assess testosterone administration in athletes, *Int J Sports Med* 16(6):368-372, 1995.
99. Rose RM: Psychoendocrinology. In Wilson JD, Foster DW, editors: *Williams textbook of endocrinology*, ed 7 , Philadelphia, 1985, Saunders.
100. Da Silva JA: Sex hormones and glucocorticoids: interactions with the immune system, *Ann N Y Acad Sci* 876:102-117, 1999.
101. Offner PJ, Moore EE, Biffl WL: Male gender is a risk factor for major infections after surgery, *Arch Surg* 134(9):935-938, 1999.
102. Angele MK et al: Sex steroids regulate pro- and anti-inflammatory cytokine release by macrophages after trauma-hemorrhage, *Am J Physiol* 277(1Pt1):C35-42, 1999.
103. Angele MK et al: Gender dimorphism in trauma-hemorrhage–induced thymocyte apoptosis, *Shock* 12(4):316-322, 1999.
104. McEwen BS: Protective and damaging effects of stress mediators, *N Engl J Med* 338(3):171-179, 1998.
105. Segerstrom SC, Miller GE: Psychological stress and the human immune system: a meta-analytic study of 30 years of inquiry, *Psychol Bull* 130(4):601-630, 2004.
106. Thoits PA: Dimensions of life events that influence psychological distress: an evaluation and synthesis of the literature. In Kaplan HB, editor: *Psychosocial stress: trends in theory and research*, Orlando, FL, 1983, Academic Press.
107. Rozlog LA et al: Stress and immunity: implications for viral disease and wound healing, *J Periodontol* 70(7):786-792, 1999.
108. Irwin M: Immune correlates of depression, *Adv Exp Med Biol* 461:1-24, 1999.
109. Irwin M et al: Impaired natural killer activity during bereavement, *Brain Behav Immun* 1:98, 1988.
110. Kiecolt-Glaser J et al: Modulation of cellular immunity in medical students, *J Behav Med* 9(1):5-21, 1986.
111. Glaser R et al: Stress-induced modulation of the immune response to recombinant hepatitis B vaccine, *Psychosom Med* 54(1):22-29, 1992.
112. Cohen S: Psychosocial stress and susceptibility to upper respiratory infections, *Am J Respir Crit Care Med* 152(4Pt2):S53-58, 1995.
113. Evans DL et al: Stress-associated reductions of cytotoxic T lymphocytes and natural killer cells in asymptomatic HIV infection, *Am J Psychiatry* 152(4):543-550, 1995.
114. Nott KH, Vedhara K, Spickett GP: Psychology, immunology and HIV, *Psychoneuroendocrinology* 20(5):451-474, 1995.
115. Sheridan JF et al: Psychoneuroimmunology: stress effects on pathogenesis and immunity during infection, *Clin Microbiol Rev* 7(2):200-212, 1994.
116. Nieman DC: Nutrition, exercise, and immune system function, *Clin Sports Med* 18(3):537-548, 1999.
117. Antoni MH et al: The influence of bio-behavioral factors on tumor biology: pathways and mechanisms, *Nat Rev Cancer* 6(3):240-248, 2006.
118. Sharma R, Coats AJ, Anker SD: The role of inflammatory mediators in chronic heart failure: cytokines, nitric oxide, and endothelin-1, *Int J Cardiol* 72(2):175-186, 2000.
119. Sher L: Effects of psychological factors on the development of cardiovascular pathology: role of the immune system and infection, *Med Hypotheses* 53(2):112-113, 1999.
120. Bremner JD et al: Neural correlates of memories of childhood sexual abuse in women with and without posttraumatic stress disorder, *Am J Psychiatry* 156(11):1787-1795, 1999.
121. Clohessy S, Ehlers A: PTSD symptoms, response to intrusive memories and coping in ambulance service workers, *Br J Clin Psychol* 38(pt 3):251-265, 1999.
122. Donnelly CL, Amaya-Jackson L, March JS: Psychopharmacology of pediatric posttraumatic stress disorder, *J Child Adolesc Psychopharmacol* 9(3):203-220, 1999.
123. Heim C, Ehlert U, Hellhammer DH: The potential role of hypocortisolism in the pathophysiology of stress-related bodily disorders, *Psychoneuroendocrinology* 25(1):1-35, 2000.
124. Alarcon RD, Glover SG, Deering CG: The cascade model: an alternative to comorbidity in the pathogenesis of posttraumatic stress disorder, *Psychiatry* 62(2):114-124, 1999.
125. Cordova MJ et al: Frequency and correlates of posttraumatic-stress-disorder-like symptoms after treatment for breast cancer, *J Consult Clin Psychol* 63(6):981-986, 1995.
126. Reiche EM, Nunes SO, Morimoto HK: Stress, depression, the immune system, and cancer, *Lancet Oncol* 5(10):617-625, 2004.

127. Ma Z, Faber A, Dube L: Exploring women's psychoneuroendocrine responses to cancer threat: insights from a computer-based guided imagery task, *Can J Nurs Res* 39(1):98-115, 2007.

128. Porter LS et al: Cortisol levels and responses to mammography screening in breast cancer survivors: a pilot study, *Psychosom Med* 65(5):842-848, 2003.

129. Clayton MF, Dudley WN, Musters A: Communication with breast cancer survivors, *Health Commun* 23(3):207-221, 2008.

130. Clayton MF, Mishel MH, Belyea M: Testing a model of symptoms, communication, uncertainty, and well-being, in older breast cancer survivors, *Res Nurs Health* 29(1):18-39, 2006.

131. Kiecolt-Glaser JK et al: Psychoneuroimmunology and psychosomatic medicine: back to the future, *Psychosom Med* 64(1):15-28, 2002. Review.

132. Folkman S, Lazarus RS: The relationship between coping and emotion: implications for theory and research, *Soc Sci Med* 26(3):309-317, 1988.

133. Irwin M et al: Partial sleep deprivation reduces natural killer cell activity in humans, *Psychosom Med* 56(6):493-498, 1994.

134. Pollmacher T et al: Influence of host defense activation on sleep in humans, *Adv Neuroimmunol* 5(2):155-169, 1995.

135. White D et al: Sleep deprivation and the control of ventilation, *Am Rev Respir Dis* 128(6):984-986, 1983.

136. Frolkis VV: Stress-age syndrome, *Mech Aging Dev* 69(1-2):93-107, 1993.

137. Kiecolt-Glaser J et al: Psychosocial enhancement of immunocompetence in a geriatric population, *Health Psychol* 4(1):25-41, 1985.

138. Spiegel D: Psychosocial intervention in cancer, *J Natl Cancer Inst* 85(15):1198-1205, 1993.

139. Baron RS et al: Social support and immune function among spouses of cancer patients, *J Pers Soc Psychol* 59(2):344-352, 1990.

140. Kiecolt-Glaser J et al: Chronic stress and immune function in family caregivers of Alzheimer's disease victims, *Psychosom Med* 45(5):523, 1987.

141. Shelby J et al: Severe burn injury: effects on psychologic and immunologic function in noninjured close relatives, *J Burn Care Rehabil* 13(1):58-63, 1992.

142. Mazzeo RS: Aging, immune function, and exercise: hormonal regulation, *Int J Sports Med* 21(Suppl 1):S10-S13, 2000. Review.

BIOLOGY, CLINICAL MANIFESTATIONS, AND TREATMENT OF CANCER

DAVID M. VIRSHUP

MEDIA RESOURCES

CHAPTER OUTLINE

CANCER CHARACTERISTICS AND TERMINOLOGY
Tumor Classification and Nomenclature
The Biology of Cancer Cells
Tumor Markers
THE GENETIC BASIS OF CANCER
Cancer-Causing Mutations in Genes
Types of Genes Misregulated in Cancer
Oncogenes and Tumor-Suppressor Genes: Accelerators
    and Brakes
Guardians of the Genome
Inflammation, Immunity, and Cancer
The Immune System Protects Us Against Viral-Associated
    Cancers

Viral Causes of Cancer
Bacterial Cause of Cancer
CANCER INVASION AND METASTASIS
Only Rare Cells in a Cancer Are Able to Metastasize
Detachment and Invasion
Survival and Spread in the Circulation
Selective Adherence in Favorable Sites
Escape from the Circulation and Development of a New
    Microenvironment
**CLINICAL MANIFESTATIONS AND TREATMENT
OF CANCER**
Clinical Manifestations of Cancer
Cancer Treatment

Cancer is a leading disease, cause of death, and source of morbidity of adults in the Western world. The incidence of cancer increases markedly with advancing age and is strongly affected by gender, lifestyle, ethnicity, infection, and genetics. Over the past 35 years intensive research has led to a significantly enhanced understanding of this complex and frightening disease. We now understand that cancer is a collection of many different diseases, caused by an accumulation of genetic and epigenetic alterations. Environment, heredity, and behavior interact to modify the risk of developing cancer and the response to treatment. Improvements in treatment strategies and supportive care, coupled with new, often individualized therapies based on advances in our fundamental understanding of the basic pathophysiology of malignancy, have contributed to an increasing number of effective options for these diverse, often lethal, disorders collectively called *cancer*.

CANCER CHARACTERISTICS AND TERMINOLOGY

Any discussion of cancer must start with a definition of what it is and what it is not. Although most readers may have an intuitive understanding of this disorder, composing an exact definition that encompasses this broad category is more challenging. A definition from 1922 may summarize cancer as well as any:

> The most generally accepted definition of a tumor is that it is a tissue overgrowth which is independent of the laws governing the remainder of the body. It is usual to add as a qualifying phrase to separate tumors from reparative processes, such as bone callus, that the neoplasm overgrowth serves no useful purpose to the organism.[1]

The term *cancer* derives from the Greek word for crab, *karkinoma,* which the physician Hippocrates used to describe the appendage-like projections extending from tumors. The word **tumor** originally referred to any swelling that was caused by inflammation, but is now generally reserved for describing a new growth, or **neoplasm.** Not all tumors or neoplasms, however, are cancer. The term **cancer** refers to a *malignant* tumor and is not used to refer to *benign* growths such as lipomas or hypertrophy of an organ. Yet it is important to recognize that benign neoplasms also can be life threatening if they enlarge in critical locations. For example, a benign meningioma at the base of the skull may cause symptoms by compressing adjacent normal brain tissue. The definitions of benign versus malignant are presented in the following text and in Table 11-1. Box 11-1 contains information on the diagnosis and clinical staging of cancer.

Tumor Classification and Nomenclature

Proper identification of a cancer is important for many reasons. Different lesions will have different causes, different rates and patterns of progression, and different responses to treatment. Cancer classification starts with knowing the site of origin and microscopic appearance of the lesion, but can extend to a detailed description of critical genetic changes in the cancer.

Benign tumors, which are not referred to as cancers, are usually encapsulated and well differentiated. They retain some normal tissue structure and do not invade the capsules surrounding them or spread to regional lymph nodes or distant locations. Benign tumors are generally named according to the tissues from which they arise, and include the suffix "-oma." For example, a benign tumor of the smooth muscle of the uterus is a *leiomyoma,* and a benign tumor of fat cells is a *lipoma.*

Some tumors initially described as benign can progress to cancer and then are referred to as **malignant tumors.** These tumors are distinguished from benign tumors by their more rapid growth rates and specific microscopic alterations, including loss of differentiation and absence of normal tissue organization. One of the hallmarks of cancer cells, as seen under the microscope, is **anaplasia,** the loss of cellular differentiation, irregularities of the size and shape of the nucleus, and loss of normal tissue structure. Malignant tumors lack a capsule and grow to invade nearby blood vessels, lymphatics, and surrounding structures. The most important and most deadly characteristic of malignant tumors is their ability to spread far beyond the tissue of origin, a process known as *metastasis* (Figures 11-1 and 11-2; see Table 11-1).

In general, cancers are named according to the cell type from which they originate. Cancers arising in epithelial tissue are called **carcinomas,** and if they arise from or form ductal or glandular structures are named **adenocarcinomas.** Hence, a malignant tumor arising from breast glandular tissue is a mammary adenocarcinoma. Cancers arising from connective tissue usually have the suffix **sarcoma.** For example, malignant cancers of skeletal muscle are known as rhabdomyosarcomas. Cancers of lymphatic tissue are called **lymphomas,** whereas cancers of blood-forming cells are called **leukemias.** However, many cancers, such as Hodgkin disease and Ewing

Table 11-1	Characteristics of Benign versus Malignant Tumors
Benign Tumors	**Malignant Tumors**
Grow slowly	Grow rapidly
Have a well-defined capsule	Are not encapsulated
Are not invasive	Invade local structures and tissues
Well differentiated; looks like the tissue from which it arises	Poorly differentiated; may not be able to tell from what tissue it arose
Have a low mitotic index; dividing cells are rare	High mitotic index; many dividing cells
Do not metastasize	Can spread distantly, often through blood vessels and lymphatics

sarcoma, are named for historical reasons that do not follow this naming convention. Table 11-2 presents the nomenclature and classification of selected tumors.

Classification of Tumors—Classical Histology and Modern Genetics

Carcinoma in situ (often abbreviated **CIS**) refers to preinvasive epithelial malignant tumors of glandular or squamous cell origin. These early stage cancers are localized to the epithelium and have not broken through the local basement membrane or invaded the surrounding stroma (see Figure 11-1). *Carcinoma in situ* is recognized in a number of sites, including the cervix, skin, oral cavity, esophagus, and bronchus. In glandular epithelium, in situ lesions occur in the stomach, endometrium, breast, and large bowel. In the breast, ductal carcinoma in situ (DCIS) fills the mammary ducts but has not progressed to local tissue invasion. DCIS lesions are readily treatable, although the optimal therapeutic approach is controversial. The time that such preinvasive lesions remain in situ before becoming invasive is unknown.[2] Some carcinomas of the cervix appear as preinvasive lesions in situ for several years before they progress to invasive carcinoma and metastatic tumors (see Figure 11-1).

As our knowledge about the molecular alterations that cause cancer increases, it becomes increasingly important for clinicians to gather extensive information about each cancer. The classification of cancers was originally based on gross and light microscopic appearance, but this is now often aided by additional immunohistochemical analysis of protein expression. In selected cases, this is supplemented by extensive molecular analysis of the tumors. Sometimes a single gene is examined (for example, to determine if there is a characteristic translocation diagnostic of chronic myelogenous leukemia [CML]), and sometimes a panel of genes and proteins are examined (e.g., in breast cancer) to determine if the tumor expresses estrogen receptor, progesterone receptor, and the epidermal growth factor (EGF) receptor HER2. In a research setting, panels of gene expression analysis are measured using microarray technology, in which the expression levels of a very large number of genes are measured. This analysis can

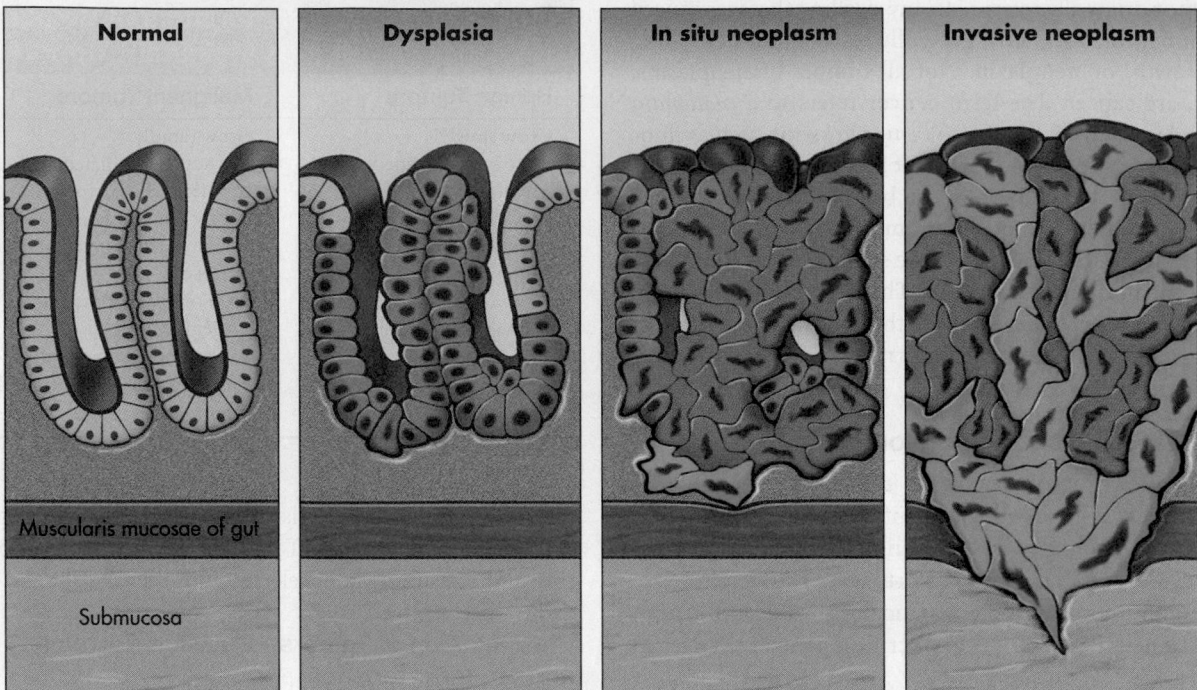

| Normal | Dysplasia | In situ neoplasm | Invasive neoplasm |

Muscularis mucosae of gut

Submucosa

Figure 11-1 Progression from normal to neoplasm. A sequence of cellular and tissue changes progressing from dysplasia to carcinoma in situ and then to invasive cancer is seen often in the development of cancer. In clinical specimens, distinguishing between dysplasia and in situ cancer is difficult. The presence of anaplastic cells and loss of normal tissue architecture signify the development of cancer. This sequence of changes is most easily seen in the squamous epithelium of the uterine cervix, the epidermis of sun-exposed skin, and colonic and gastric mucosa after long-standing inflammation. The high rate of cell division, local mutagens, and inflammatory mediators all contribute to the accumulation of genetic abnormalities that lead to cancer. (Modified from Stevens A, Lowe J: *Pathology*, ed 2, London, 2000, Mosby.)

be used to classify tumors more precisely and may predict what the most effective therapy will be. This detailed analysis of each tumor is a form of **personalized medicine** offering therapy based on a very detailed knowledge of individuals' characteristics and their specific cancer.[3]

The Biology of Cancer Cells

Transformation and Differentiation

Cancer cells behave differently than normal cells in several important ways. **Transformation** refers to the process by which a normal cell becomes a cancer cell. **Autonomy** refers to the cancer cell's independence from normal cellular controls and is part of the transformational process. These differences are most readily seen in specialized laboratory assays, especially those examining the growth patterns of normal and cancerous cells in laboratory incubators. Transformed cells lack many of the normal "social controls" seen in nontransformed cells. Normal cells cease to divide when they fill a Petri (or tissue culture) dish, whereas transformed cells continue to crowd and eventually pile up on each other (Figure 11-3). Normal cells usually will not grow unless they are attached to a firm surface (like a Petri dish). However, cancer cells are often **anchorage independent,** that is, they continue to divide even when suspended in a soft agar gel. Cancerous cells can be assayed in mice as well; normal human

cells when injected into a special type of mouse (genetically engineered to lack an immune system to prevent rejection of human cells) will not grow. However, cancerous cells from humans can continue to grow and even metastasize in these mice. Normal cells have a limited life span in the laboratory; they may divide in a Petri dish 10 or 50 times, but then they cease growing. Cancer cells usually are **immortal** in that they seem to have an unlimited life span and will continue to divide for years under appropriate laboratory conditions. One of the most commonly used laboratory cell lines, HeLa cells, was derived from a cervical cancer specimen obtained in 1951 that continues to grow and divide in laboratories around the world.[4]

Cancer cells often show defects in the normal process of differentiation, that is, the process of acquiring a specialized function and organization, such as evolving into a muscle cell (see Chapter 41) or a nerve cell (see Chapter 14). **Anaplasia** is the absence of differentiation (see Figures 11-2 and 11-4) and means literally "without form." In clinical specimens, *anaplasia* is recognized by a loss of organization and a marked increase in nuclear size with evidence of ongoing proliferation. In contrast to normal cells, which are uniform in size and shape, *anaplastic* cells are of variable size and shape, or **pleomorphic.** For example, a benign muscle tumor (benign myoma) will retain the ability to make muscle,

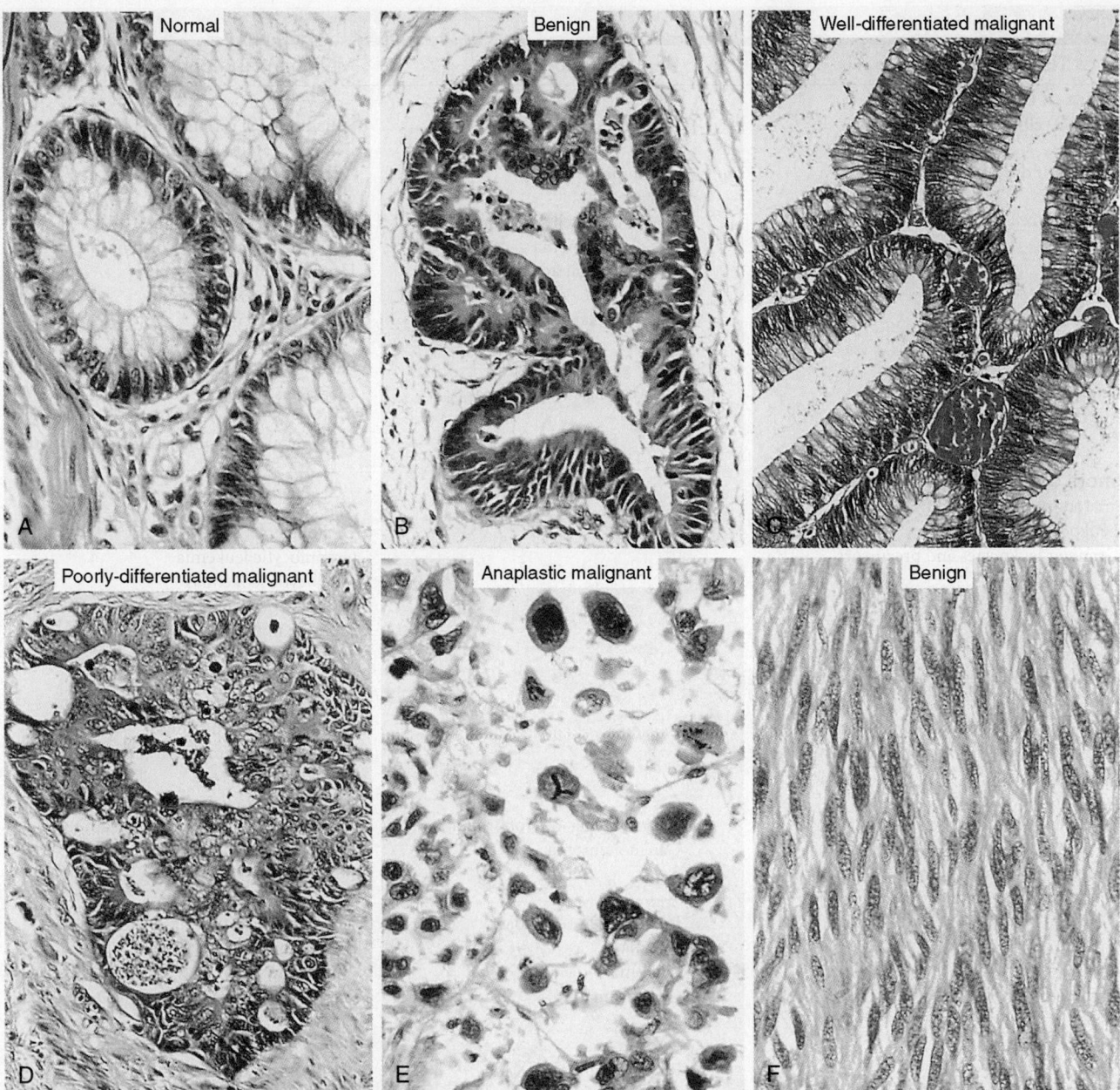

Figure 11-2 Loss of cellular and tissue differentiation during the development of cancer. The cells of a benign neoplasm (B) resemble those of the normal colonic epithelium (A), in that they are columnar and have an orderly arrangement. Loss of some degree of differentiation is evident in that the neoplastic cells do not show much mucin vacuolization. Cells of the well-differentiated malignant neoplasm (C) of the colon have a haphazard arrangement and although gland lumina are formed, they are architecturally abnormal and irregular. Nuclei vary in shape and size, especially when compared with A. Cells in the poorly differentiated malignant neoplasm (D) have an even more haphazard arrangement, with very poor formation of gland lumina. Nuclei show greater variation in shape and size compared with the well-differentiated malignant neoplasm in C. Cells in anaplastic malignant neoplasms (E) bear no relation to the normal epithelium, with no recognizable gland formation. Tremendous variation is found in the size of cells and their nuclei, with very intense staining (hyperchromatic nuclei). Not knowing the site of origin would make it impossible to tell what sort of tumor this is by microscopic appearance alone. Well-differentiated tumors often resemble their cell of origin, as shown in the example of a benign tumor of smooth muscles (F). (From Stevens A, Lowe J: *Pathology,* ed 2, London, 2000, Mosby.)

whereas in a malignant muscle tumor (rhabdomyosarcoma), new muscle formation is seen only rarely, and even then appears highly disorganized. Thus the muscle cancer cells appear undifferentiated (see Figure 11-4). The most malignant tumors tend to have the most *anaplasia* and be the least differentiated.

Cancer Stem Cells

Many tissues, most notably the skin, intestines, and blood-forming cells, continuously renew themselves. The human gut sheds and replaces hundreds of grams of cells each day. This ongoing proliferation of these tissues with a high turnover rate depends on their regeneration from a small fraction

Table 11-2	Nomenclature and Classification of Benign and Malignant Tumors*	
Cell or Tissue of Origin	**Benign Tumor**	**Malignant Tumor**
Tumors of Epithelial Origin		
Squamous cells	Squamous cell papilloma	Squamous cell carcinoma
Basal cells	—	Basal cell carcinoma
Glandular or ductal epithelium	Adenoma	Adenocarcinoma
	Cystadenoma	Cystadenocarcinoma
Transitional cells	Transitional cell papilloma	Transitional cell carcinoma
Bile duct	Bile duct adenoma	Bile duct carcinoma (cholangiocarcinoma)
Liver cells	Hepatocellular adenoma	Hepatocellular carcinoma
Melanocytes	Nevus	Malignant melanoma
Renal epithelium	Renal tubular adenoma	Renal cell carcinoma
Skin adnexal glands		
Sweat glands	Sweat gland adenoma	Sweat gland carcinoma
Sebaceous glands	Sebaceous gland adenoma	Sebaceous gland carcinoma
Germ cells (testis and ovary)	—	Seminoma (dysgerminoma)
		Embryonal carcinoma, yolk sac carcinoma
Tumors of Mesenchymal Origin		
Hematopoietic/lymphoid tissue		
Leukocytes		Leukemias
Granular leukocytes and precursors		Granulocytic leukemia
		Myelocytic leukemias
		Myelogenous leukemias
Plasma cells		Multiple myeloma
Lymphoid		
Nongranular leukocytes and prelymphocytes		Lymphomas
Proliferating lymphocytes and monocytes		Lymphocytic leukemia
Proliferating immature precursor monocytes		Lymphoblastic leukemia
Solid tumors of lymph tissue (thymus, spleen, lymph nodes)		Lymphoma or lymphosarcoma
Neural and retinal tissue		
Nerve sheath	Neurilemoma, neurofibroma	Malignant peripheral nerve sheath tumor
Nerve cells	Ganglioneuroma	Neuroblastoma
Retinal cells (cones)	—	Retinoblastoma
Connective tissue		
Fibrous tissue	Fibromatosis (desmoid)	Fibrosarcoma
Fat	Lipoma	Liposarcoma
Bone	Osteoma	Osteogenic sarcoma
Cartilage	Chondroma	Chrondrosarcoma
Muscle		
Smooth muscle	Leiomyoma	Leiomyosarcoma
Striated muscle	Rhabdomyoma	Rhabdomyosarcoma
Endothelial and related tissues		
Blood vessels	Hemangioma	Angiosarcoma
		Kaposi sarcoma
Lymph vessels	Lymphangioma	Lymphangiosarcoma
Synovium	—	Synovial sarcoma
Mesothelium	—	Malignant mesothelioma
Meninges	Meningioma	Malignant meningioma
Tumors of Uncertain Origin	—	Ewing tumor

Modified from Murphy GP et al: *American Cancer Society's textbook of clinical oncology,* ed 2, New York, 1995, American Cancer Society.
*This list is intended to provide only an introduction to tumor nomenclature.

of cells known as **adult stem cells.** Adult stem cells have two essential characteristics: first, they self-renew (that is, some fraction of the cell divisions create new stem cells) and second, they are **multipotent,** or have the ability to differentiate into multiple different cell types. In the bone marrow, it is estimated that only 0.05% (1 in 20,000) of the blood-forming cells are stem cells, yet this small pool of stem cells can be stimulated to divide and to repopulate all the mature bone marrow–derived cells in approximately 2 weeks after bone marrow transplantation. As few as 10 stem cells are sufficient to entirely repopulate the entire bone marrow of a mouse in bone marrow transplantation experiments. Similarly, the

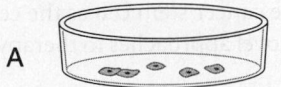
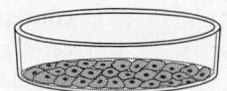
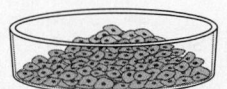

A   Non-cancerous cells are anchorage-dependant and only proliferate when attached to a surface.   When these cells form a complete monolayer, they stop dividing due to contact inhibition.   Cancer cells do not exhibit contact inhibition, and continue to divide, piling up on each other.

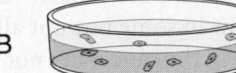
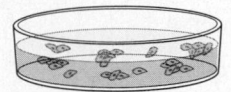

B   Normal cells suspended in soft agar cannot attach and therefore cannot proliferate.   Cancer cells are anchorage-independant and can proliferate suspended in soft agar.

Figure 11-3 Cancerous cells show abnormal growth in the laboratory. Cancer cells, unlike most normal cells, (**A**) usually continue to grow and pile on top of one another after they have formed a confluent monolayer in culture (loss of contact inhibition) and (**B**) can grow without being attached to a surface, called anchorage independence.

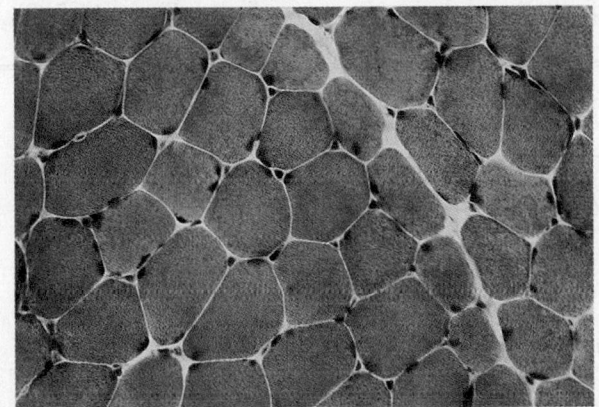
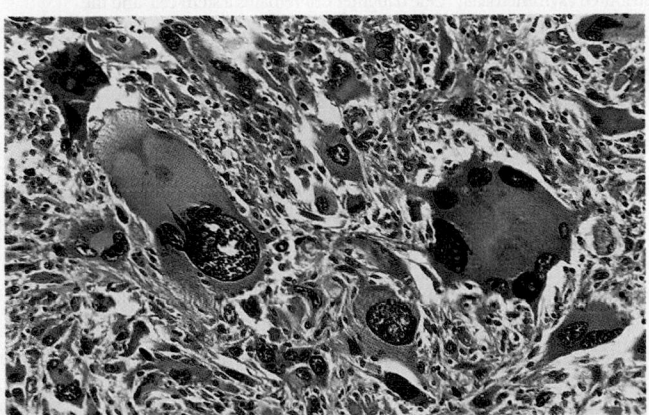

A   B

Figure 11-4 Normal and anaplastic skeletal muscle cells. **A,** Normal skeletal muscle cells. **B,** Anaplastic tumor of the skeletal muscle (rhabdomyosarcoma). Note the marked cellular and nuclear pleomorphism (cellular and nuclear variation in size and shape), hyperchromatic nuclei, and tumor giant cells. The prominent cell in the center field has an abnormal tripolar spindle. Often the tissue of origin of an anaplastic tumor can be established only by the use of molecular markers, such as immunohistochemical stains and chromosome analysis. (A from Damjanov I, Linder J, editors: *Anderson's pathology,* ed 10, St Louis, 1996, Mosby; B from Kumar V, Abbas AK, Fausto N: *Pathologic basis of disease,* ed 7, Philadelphia, 2005, Saunders; courtesy of Dr. Trace Worrell, Department of Pathology, University of Texas Southwestern Medical School.)

absorptive and goblet cells lining the intestine have a life span of less than 1 week, after which they undergo cell death, or apoptosis, and slough into the intestinal lumen. They too must be replenished by ongoing proliferation of intestinal stem cells. A key feature of stem cells is that they can divide asymmetrically; they can give rise to another stem cell and one daughter cell that ultimately terminally differentiates into diverse cell types, depending on the needs of the tissue (Figures 11-5 and 11-6). Multipotent bone marrow stem cells can self-renew and differentiate into all types of bone marrow–derived cells, such as red cells, lymphocytes, and neutrophils. Certain adult stem cells have a broader range of potential fates. For example, mesenchymal stem cells are able to differentiate into multiple types of cells, such as blood

vessels, neurons, and muscle cells (see Figure 11-6). Theoretically, such a stem cell might be able to give rise to all cell types in the body, and as such, could be useful in regeneration of diseased tissues.

Just as normal tissues in adults can arise from a rare tissue stem cell, cancers may arise from cancer stem cells. First shown in acute myeloid leukemias,[5] rare cells capable of transmitting the cancer have been demonstrated in many other cancers[6] as well (Figure 11-7, *A*). These studies[6,7] show that only a small subset of cancer cells have the ability to divide indefinitely and give rise to full-blown cancer. For example, only a small fraction of cells from a breast cancer are able to divide indefinitely and generate a full-blown breast cancer when transplanted into experimental animals. This emerging

Stem cell
Asymmetric distribution of cytoplasmic determinants
Different daughter cells
Terminally differentiated cells

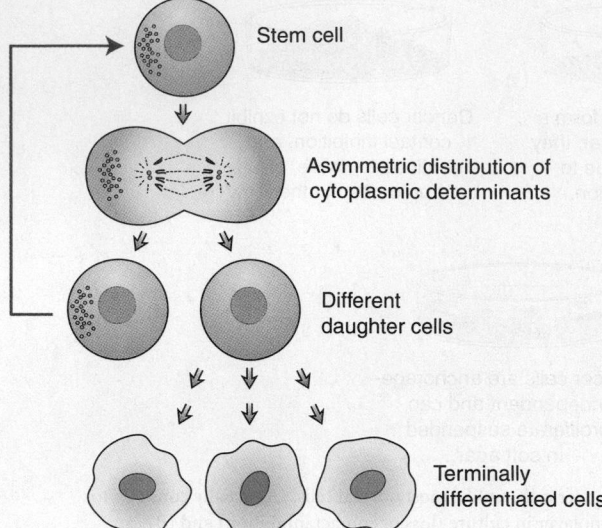

Figure 11-5 Asymmetric division is a requirement for stem cell proliferation. When a stem cell undergoes asymmetric division, cellular contents and cell fates are distributed asymmetrically. One daughter cell remains a stem cell, and the other goes into an amplification pathway that ends in terminal differentiation.

concept of the cancer stem cell as the central problem in cancer suggests novel approaches to therapy targeting this specific population.

In a typical cancer stem cell experiment, up to 100,000 unselected breast cancer cells must be injected into a laboratory mouse to transmit breast cancer, whereas after laboratory procedures (such as cell sorting) to enrich for the cancer stem cells and remove the other cells, it takes only 100 cells or less to transmit the cancer.[6] One strong conclusion of this work is that in some but not all tumors,[6] greater than 99% of the cells in the cancer are not capable of propagating the cancer, and that the most important cell in the cancer may be a rare "tumor initiating cell" or "cancer stem cell." An important implication of this work is that current cancer treatments were not designed to kill the rare cancer stem cell. Current treatments that effectively shrink tumors by killing 99% of cancer cells appear relatively ineffective at killing the cancer stem cells.[8] Consequently, therapies may shrink cancers but when the cancer stem cell is not killed, the cancer can grow back. This has led to major efforts to find therapies that specifically target the cancer stem cells (see Figure 11-7, *B*).

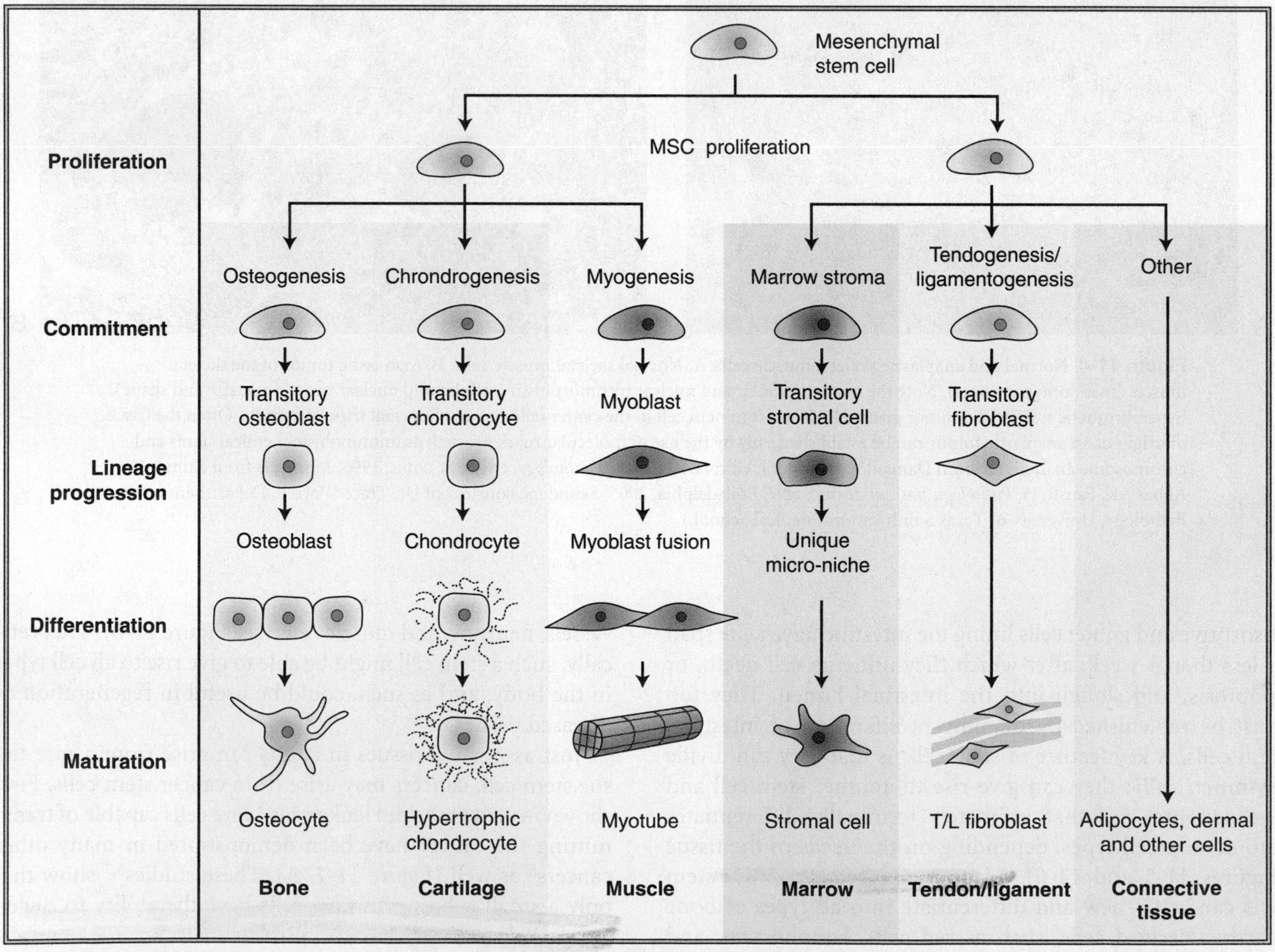

Mesenchymal stem cell
MSC proliferation
Proliferation
Commitment
Lineage progression
Differentiation
Maturation
Osteogenesis
Chrondrogenesis
Myogenesis
Marrow stroma
Tendogenesis/ ligamentogenesis
Other
Transitory osteoblast
Transitory chondrocyte
Myoblast
Transitory stromal cell
Transitory fibroblast
Osteoblast
Chondrocyte
Myoblast fusion
Unique micro-niche
Osteocyte
Hypertrophic chondrocyte
Myotube
Stromal cell
T/L fibroblast
Adipocytes, dermal and other cells
Bone
Cartilage
Muscle
Marrow
Tendon/ligament
Connective tissue

Figure 11-6 Postulated multiple lineage-specific differentiation of mesenchymal stem cells. Differentiation occurs progressively as the offspring of stem cells commit to various lineages. Mesenchymal stem cells can renew themselves and give rise to multiple tissue types. (Modified from Caplan A, Bruder S: Mesenchymal stem cells: Building blocks for molecular medicine in the 21st century, *Trends Mol Med* 7(6):259-264, 2001.)

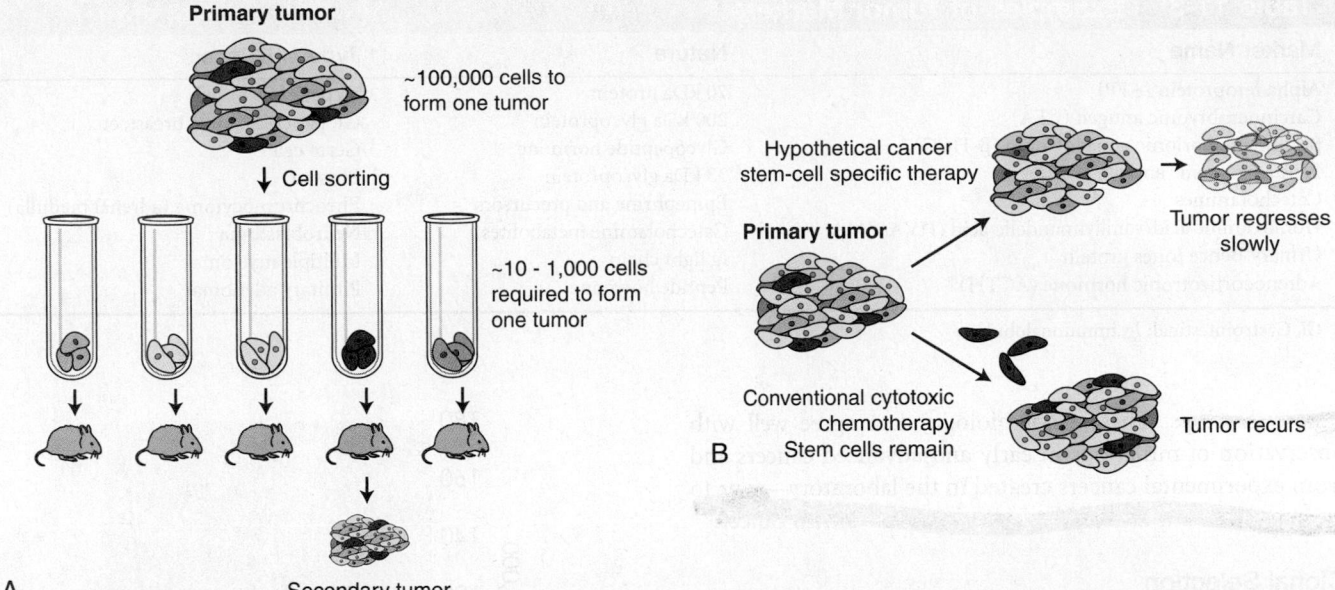

Figure 11-7 The concept of cancer stem cells. **A,** Only rare cells within a cancer can initiate cancer regrowth. In laboratory experiments it takes as many as 100,000 breast cancer cells injected into a mouse mammary fat pad to form a new cancer. If the breast cancer cells are sorted, one rare subtype *(shown here in red)* is much more proficient at forming new cancers. **B,** Conventional chemotherapy can destroy the bulk of a cancer. However, if the cancer stem cells *(red cells)* are not destroyed, the cancer may regrow. If therapies can be devised that kill the cancer stem cells, then durable long-term responses may be achieved.

Tumor Markers

Tumor markers (biologic markers) are substances produced by cancer cells that are found either in or on the tumor cells or in the blood, spinal fluid, or urine (Table 11-3). Some tumor markers have been known for many decades. For diseases associated with a tumor marker, there is indeed a "blood test for cancer." Tumor markers include hormones, enzymes, genes, antigens, and antibodies. For example, the adrenal medulla normally secretes the catecholamine epinephrine (adrenaline). Benign tumors of the adrenal medulla can produce catecholamines in vast excess, leading to rapid pulse, high blood pressure, sweats, and tremors. Elevated blood or urine levels of catecholamines in someone with this set of symptoms strongly suggest the presence of an adrenal medullary tumor (pheochromocytoma). Liver and germ cell tumors secrete a protein known as *alpha fetoprotein* (AFP) into the blood, and prostate tumors secrete *prostate specific antigen* (PSA) into the blood. These tumor markers can be used in three ways: (1) to screen and identify individuals at high risk for cancer; (2) to help diagnose the specific type of tumor in individuals with clinical manifestations relating to cancer, as in adrenal tumors; and (3) to follow the clinical course of cancer. For example, a falling PSA after therapy for prostate cancer indicates successful treatment, and a later rise in the PSA may indicate a recurrence.

A significant problem in diagnosing cancer using tumor marker assays is that nonmalignant conditions also can produce tumor markers. The presence of an elevated tumor marker therefore may suggest a specific diagnosis, but it is not used alone as a definitive diagnostic test. Identification of ideal sensitive and specific tumor markers that are elevated early in the course of common cancers remains a high priority because the early detection of cancer often improves the treatment outcome.

THE GENETIC BASIS OF CANCER

Cancer-Causing Mutations in Genes

Prior to the advent of modern molecular biology, many different causes of cancer were postulated, based on epidemiologic studies, studies of carcinogens, and studies of viruses. We now understand that changes in the genes of the cancer cell cause the cell to become cancerous. As our knowledge of cancer biology continues to increase so too does our understanding of the many ways that heritable changes in cells can contribute to cancer. These changes include deoxyribonucleic acid (DNA) mutations, but also include changes in DNA and histone chemical modification (epigenetic changes), and, most recently recognized, changes in micro-ribonucleic acid (miRNA) expression (also see Chapters 4 and 12). Although the word *mutation* is used extensively here, it can also refer to heritable changes in gene expression (**epigenetics**) that do not involve changes in DNA sequence.

Cancer is predominantly a disease of aging. Perhaps the most telling epidemiologic data are presented in Figure 11-8. The incidence of cancer, that is, the fraction of individuals in each age group who develop cancer, increases dramatically with age. The best explanation for this epidemiologic data is that each individual acquires a number of genetic "hits" or mutations over time. When sufficient mutations have occurred,

Table 11-3	Examples of Tumor Markers	
Marker Name	**Nature**	**Type of Cancer**
Alpha fetoprotein (AFP)	70 kDa protein	Hepatic, germ cell
Carcinoembryonic antigen (CEA)	200 kDa glycoprotein	GI, pancreas, lung, breast, etc.
β-Human chorionic gonadotropin (β-HCG)	Glycopeptide hormone	Germ cell
Prostate-specific antigen (PSA)	33 kDa glycoprotein	Prostate
Catecholamines	Epinephrine and precursors	Pheochromocytoma (adrenal medulla)
Homovanillic acid/vanillylmandelic acid (HVA/VMA)	Catecholamine metabolites	Neuroblastoma
Urinary Bence Jones protein	Ig light chain	Multiple myeloma
Adrenocorticotropic hormone (ACTH)	Peptide hormone	Pituitary adenomas

GI, Gastrointestinal; *Ig,* immunoglobulin.

cancer develops. These epidemiologic data agree well with observation of mutations in early and advanced cancers and from experimental cancers created in the laboratory—four to seven specific hits are required to cause a full-blown cancer.[9]

Clonal Selection

As a cell accumulates specific mutations, it can acquire, step by step, the characteristics of a cancer cell, for example, increased growth rate or, alternatively, decreased apoptosis, or death rate. That mutant cell may then have a selective advantage over its neighbors; its progeny can accumulate faster than its nonmutant neighbors. This is referred to as **clonal proliferation** or **clonal expansion** (Figure 11-9). As a clone with a mutation proliferates, it may become an early stage tumor, for example, a carcinoma in situ or a benign colonic polyp. Additional heritable changes can occur in these early lesions that permit progression to more advanced tumors. The process of tumor development is a form of darwinian evolution; cells with a genetic change that confers a survival advantage out-compete their neighbors. The progressive accumulation of distinct advantageous (from the point of view of the cancer cell, not the individual!) mutations leads from normal cells to fully malignant cancers.

One organ in which this correlation of genetic and clinical progression has been especially well studied is the colon.[10] The colon is accessible to inspection with a colonoscope, and so neoplastic lesions of varying size can readily be detected and removed. Intestinal polyps are benign neoplasms and the first stage in development of colon cancer. Small polyps tend to have only a few detectable mutations. Large polyps have more mutations, whereas frank colon cancers have even more mutations. This type of genetic information provided the framework for the now widely accepted concept that it is the *stepwise accumulation* of alterations in specific genes that is required for the development of cancer (see Figure 11-9).

Types of Genes Misregulated in Cancer

Alterations in Progrowth and Antigrowth Signals

We now understand that multiple genetic hits are required for the evolution of full-blown cancer. One key question is, what types of genes must be altered to cause a cancer? In 2000, a highly influential paper by Hanahan and Weinberg[11] proposed six specific pathways that must be misregulated for cancer to develop (see Figures 11-9 and 11-10). First, cancer

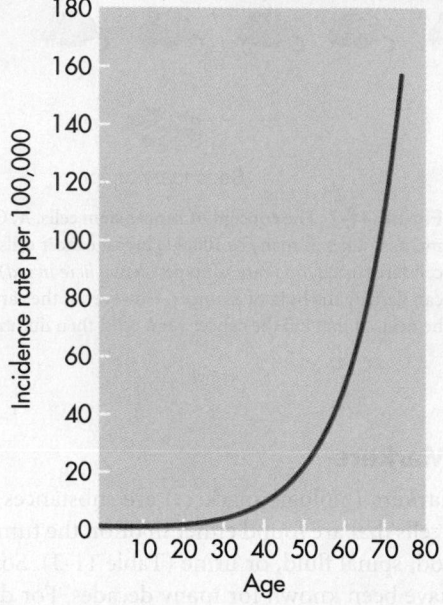

Figure 11-8 Marked increases in cancer with age. The graph depicts the number of cases of colon cancer diagnosed per 100,000 women in England and Wales in 1 year. The incidence of cancer increases dramatically with advancing age. These data suggest that accumulation of genetic and epigenetic alterations over time increases the risk of developing cancer. The slope of the curve suggests that five to seven mutations must occur before full-blown cancer develops. (Modified from Alberts B et al: *Molecular biology of the cell,* ed 4, New York, 2002, Garland.)

cells must have mutations that enable them to proliferate in the absence of external growth signals. To achieve this, some cancers acquire the ability to secrete growth factors that stimulate their own growth, a process known as **autocrine stimulation** (also see Chapter 1). Other cancers have an increase in growth factor receptors; for example, in breast cancer, the epidermal growth factor (EGF) receptor HER2/neu is up-regulated, and likely sends growth signals into the cell even when growth factors are at very low levels. Inhibitors of HER2 and other EGF receptors that block this pathway are effective in treating selected breast and lung cancers.[12] Alternatively, the signal cascade from the cell surface receptor to the nucleus may be mutated in the "on" position. Up to one third of all cancers have an activating mutation in the gene for an intracellular signaling protein called **RAS**. This mutant RAS stimulates cell growth even when growth factors are missing (Figure 11-11).

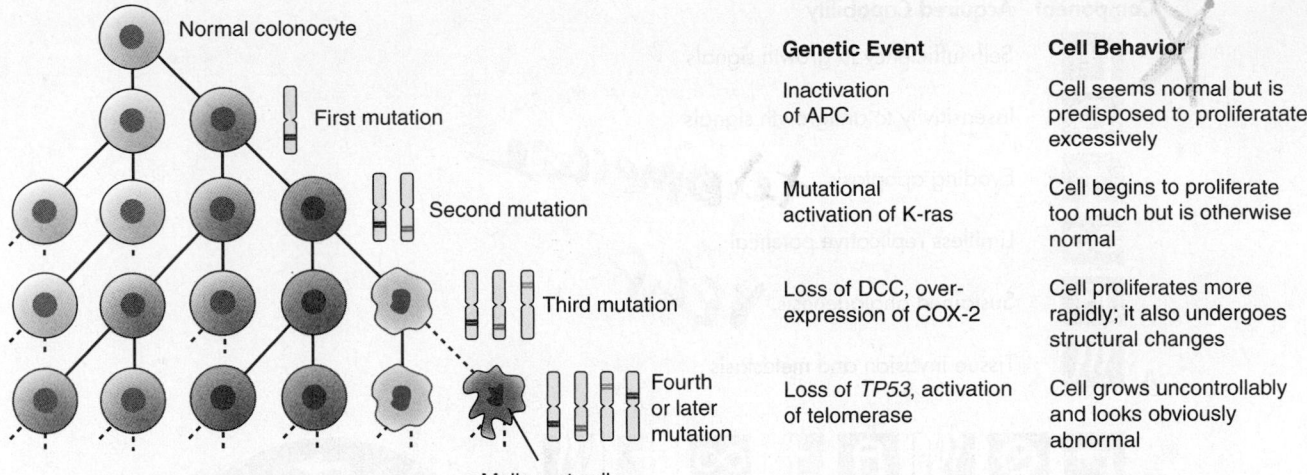

Figure 11-9 Clonal proliferation model of neoplastic progression. During clonal proliferation, progressively altered populations of cells arise over time. As genetic and epigenetic changes occur, different subclones (indicated by different color cells) coexist for a time. Clones that grow the fastest out-compete other clones, producing ever-more malignant, and abnormal-appearing, growths. The sequential accumulation of mutations has been well studied in the progression from a normal colon cell to a benign intestinal polyp to a malignant colon cancer. One of the earliest mutations in colon cancer is loss of the tumor suppressor gene *APC*. Additional mutations, often in the oncogene *ras*, activation of COX-2, and loss of the tumor suppressors DCC and *TP53* occur as the lesion progresses from a benign polyp to an invasive carcinoma. *APC*, Adenomatous polyposis coli; *DCC*, deleted in colon cancer; *COX-2*, cyclooxygenase-2. (Modified from Mendelsohn I et al: *The molecular basis of cancer*, ed 2, Philadelphia, 2001, Saunders; Kumar V, Cotran RS, Robbins SL: *Basic pathology*, ed 6, Philadelphia, 1997, Saunders.)

Cells also usually receive diverse "antigrowth" signals from their normal milieu. Contact with other cells, with basement membranes, and with soluble factors all normally signal cells to stop proliferating. These mechanisms can put a halt to unregulated cell growth. In addition, this normal antigrowth signal must be inactivated or ignored. Common mutations that subvert the antigrowth signal include inactivation of the tumor suppressor *retinoblastoma* or, conversely, activation of the protein kinases that drive the cell cycle, the *cyclin-dependent kinases* (see Chapter 1). Next, cells have a mechanism that causes them to self-destruct when growth is excessive and cell cycle checkpoints have been ignored. This self-destruct mechanism, called **apoptosis,** is triggered by diverse stimuli, including normal development and excessive growth (see Chapter 2). The pathway to apoptosis is disabled in advanced cancers. The most common mutations conferring resistance to apoptosis occur in the *TP53* gene.

Angiogenesis

If cancers are to grow larger than a millimeter in diameter, they need their own blood supply to deliver oxygen and nutrients. However, in adults new blood vessel growth is normally limited to areas of wound healing and to the uterus during the proliferative phase of the menstrual cycle. Tiny cancers lack the ability to grow new blood vessels and may never grow larger than a grain of sand. More advanced cancers can, however, secrete multiple factors that stimulate new blood vessel growth (called neovascularization or **angiogenesis**). The **angiogenic factors,** such as *vascular endothelial growth factor* (*VEGF*), *platelet-derived growth factor* (*PDGF*), and *basic fibroblast growth factor* (*bFGF*), by recruiting new vascular endothelial cells and initiating the proliferation of existing blood vessel cells, allow small cancers to become large cancers.[13] Therapies directed against new vessel growth are in clinical use; these agents include bevacizumab, a monoclonal antibody that inhibits VEGF; erlotinib, sorafenib, and sunitinib, inhibitors of the VEGF and PDGF receptor tyrosine kinases; and thalidomide, which decreases vascular proliferation (Figure 11-12).[14]

Telomeres and Immortality

A hallmark of cancer cells is their immortality. Usually the only cells in the body that are "immortal" are germ cells (those that generate sperm and eggs) and stem cells. Other cells in the body are not immortal and can divide only a limited number of times (known as the Hayflick limit) before they cease dividing. One major block to unlimited cell division (i.e., immortality) is the size of a specialized structure called the *telomere*. **Telomeres** are protective ends, or caps, on each chromosome and are placed and maintained by a specialized enzyme called **telomerase** (Figure 11-13). As you might expect, telomerase is usually active only in germ cells (in ovaries and testes) and in stem cells. All other cells of the body lack telomerase. Therefore, when nongerm cells begin to proliferate abnormally, their telomere caps become smaller and smaller with each cell division. Short telomeres normally signal the cell to cease cell division. If the telomeres become critically small, the chromosomes become unstable and fragment, and then the cells die. Cancer cells, when they reach a critical age, activate telomerase somehow in order to restore and maintain their telomeres and thereby make it possible to divide over and over again.[15] Because telomerase is specifically

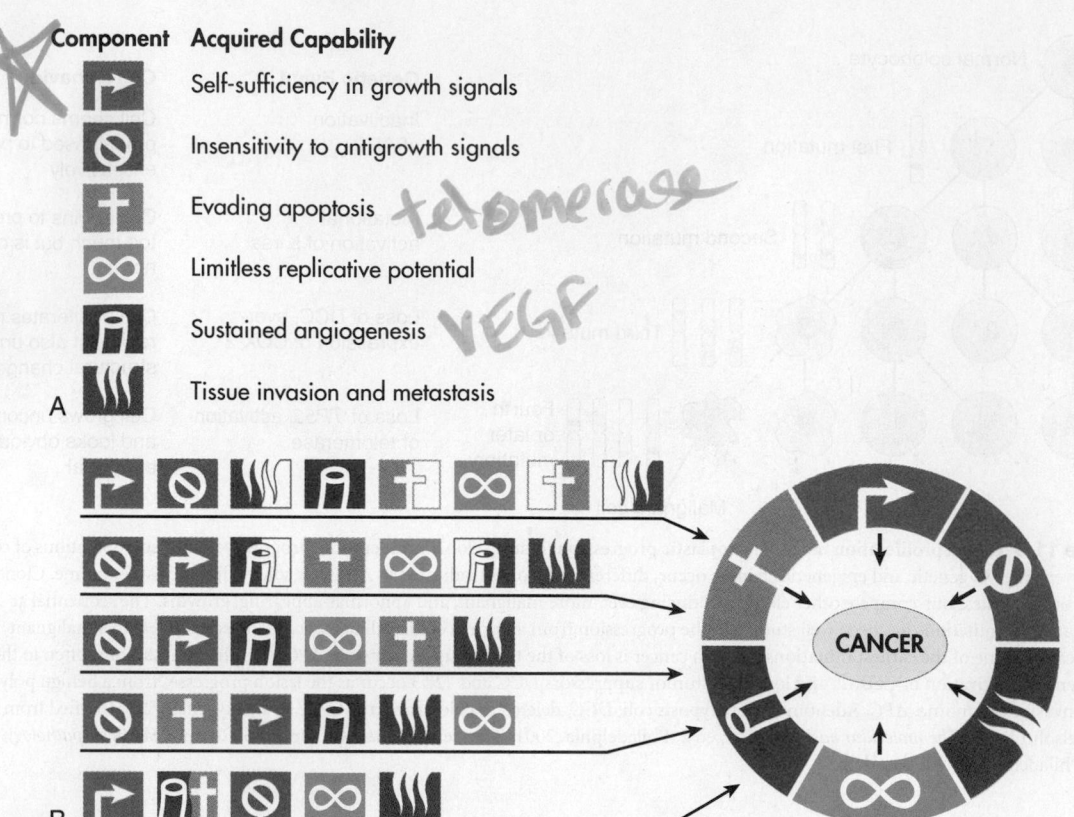

Component   Acquired Capability

Self-sufficiency in growth signals

Insensitivity to antigrowth signals

Evading apoptosis   *telomerase*

Limitless replicative potential

Sustained angiogenesis   *VEGF*

Tissue invasion and metastasis

A

B

Figure 11-10 Six hallmarks of cancer. **A,** Most cancers acquire mutations in six distinct areas of cell control during their development. **B,** Multiple pathways of carcinogenesis. All cancers must acquire mutations in the six areas, but their means of doing so varies mechanistically and chronologically. As shown, the order in which these capabilities are acquired is variable across different cancers. In some tumors, a particular mutation may confer several capabilities simultaneously, decreasing the number of intermediate mutational steps required for full development. Loss of the *p53* tumor suppressor gene may facilitate resistance to apoptosis and angiogenesis (e.g., in the five-step pathway shown [bottom pathway]). In other tumors, by comparison, a collaboration of two or more distinct genetic changes may be needed to acquire a given trait. In the eight-step model (top pathway), invasion metastasis and resistance to apoptosis are each acquired in two steps. (Modified from Hanahan D, Weinberg RA: The hallmarks of cancer, *Cell* 100[1]:57-70, 2000.)

activated in cancer cells, and potentially in cancer stem cells, it is an attractive therapeutic target.[16]

Finally, it appears genetic differences exist between cells that successfully metastasize and those that do not.[17] Specific genes regulate the ability to metastasize. Decreased cell-to-cell adhesion, the secretion of various proteases that digest surrounding barriers, and the ability to grow in new locations, all contribute to successful metastasis[18] (discussed later in this chapter).

Oncogenes and Tumor-Suppressor Genes: Accelerators and Brakes

The previous discussion refers to the activating and inactivating of various genes as being key in the development of cancer. Just what types of changes in genes actually occur in cancer? First, it is useful to distinguish between oncogenes and tumor-suppressor genes. Table 11-4 compares the two types of cancer genes. **Oncogenes** are mutant genes that in their normal non-mutant state direct synthesis of proteins that positively regulate (accelerate) proliferation. Conversely, **tumor-suppressor genes** encode proteins that in their normal state negatively regulate (halt, or "put the brakes on") proliferation. Hence, they also have been referred to as anti-oncogenes.

In its normal, nonmutant state, an oncogene is referred to as a **proto-oncogene.** An example of a proto-oncogene would be a growth factor (e.g., epidermal growth factor), or a growth factor receptor (e.g., epidermal growth factor receptor). Other positive regulators of proliferation are in the signal transduction pathway that transmits the signal from the growth factor receptor to the cell nucleus. Normally, *ras* is a proto-oncogene (see Figure 11-11). *pg 368 RAS*

Mutation of Normal Genes into Oncogenes
Point Mutations
Several types of genetic events can activate oncogenes (Box 11-1 and Figure 11-14). Perhaps the most common events are small scale changes in DNA such as **point mutations,** the alteration of one or a few nucleotide base pairs (see Chapter 4). This type of mutation can have profound effects on the activity of proteins. A point mutation in the *ras* gene converts it from a regulated proto-oncogene to an unregulated oncogene, an accelerator of cellular proliferation. Activating point mutations in *ras* are found in many cancers, especially pancreatic and colorectal cancer.[19] Specialized tests, such as direct DNA sequencing, can detect such point mutations in clinical samples.

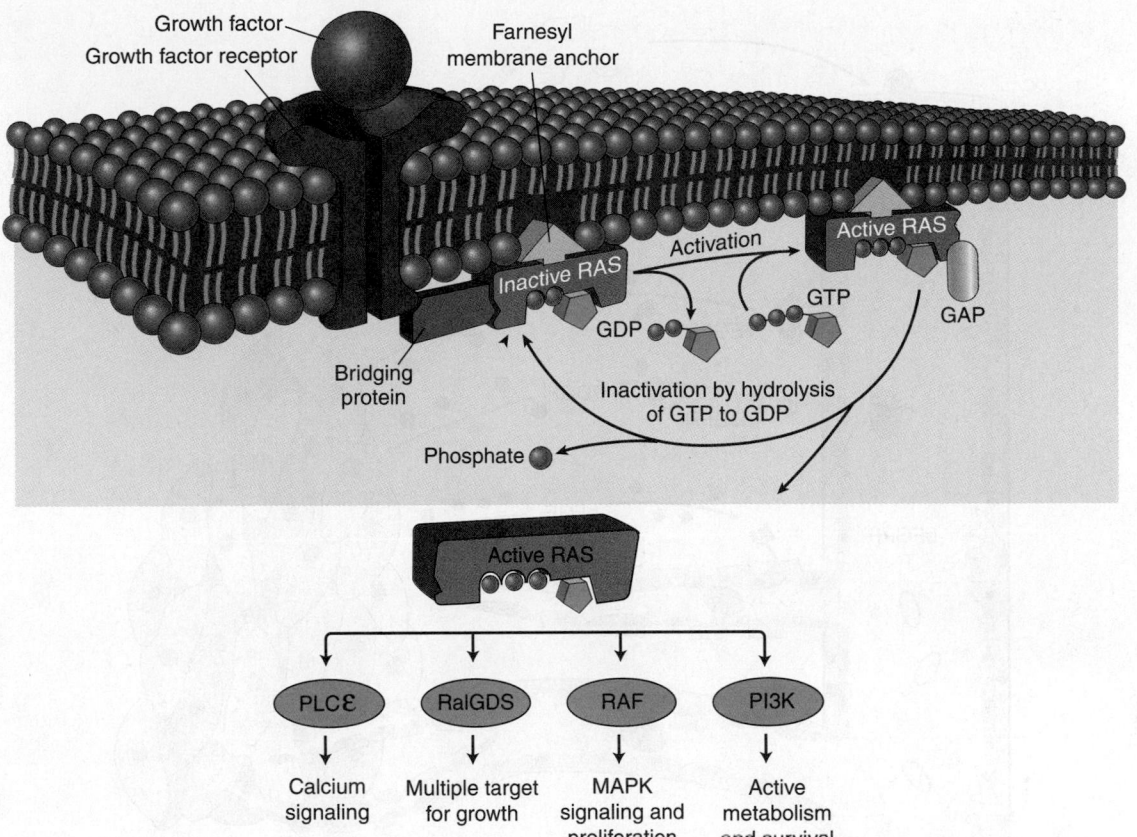

Figure 11-11 Many growth factors signal through the RAS protein. When a normal cell is stimulated through a growth factor binding to its receptor, inactive RAS exchanges GDP for GTP, becoming active. Active (GTP-bound) RAS sends growth signals throughout the cell by interacting with a number of signaling proteins, including RalGDS, RAF, PLCε, and PI3K. RAS is normally inactivated when it hydrolyzes GTP to GDP. Oncogenic Ras has a mutation that blocks hydrolysis of GTP, thereby locking RAS in the active configuration. *GDP,* guanosine diphosphate; *GTP,* guanosine triphosphate; *MAP,* mitogen-activated protein; PI3K, Phosphoinositide-I3 kinase; PLCε, phospholipase C; RalGDS, Ral guanine nucleotide dissociation stimulator; *ras,* oncogene; *ras,* protein. (Adapted from Kumar V, Abbas A, Fausto N, Mitchell R: *Basic pathology,* ed 8, Philadelphia, 2007, Saunders.)

Box 11-1	Types of Genetic Lesions in Cancer

1. Point mutations
2. Subtle alterations (insertions, deletions)
3. Chromosome changes (aneuploidy and loss of heterozygosity)
4. Amplifications
5. Gene silencing (DNA methylation, histone modification, microRNAs)
6. Exogenous sequences (tumor viruses)

Chromosome Translocations

Chromosome translocations, in which a piece of one chromosome is translocated to another chromosome, can activate oncogenes by way of either of two distinct mechanisms. First, a translocation can cause excess and inappropriate production of a proliferation factor. One of the best examples is the t(8;14) translocation found in many Burkitt lymphomas[20]; t(8;14) designates a chromosome that has a piece of chromosome 8 fused to a piece of chromosome 14 (see Chapter 27). Burkitt lymphoma is an aggressive cancer of B lymphocytes. The *myc* proto-oncogene found on chromosome 8 is normally turned on at low levels in proliferating lymphocytes and is turned off in mature lymphocytes. The **MYC protein** is part of the positive signal for cell proliferation. If an accidental formation of the t(8;14) translocation occurs, the *myc* gene is aberrantly placed under the control of a B cell immunoglobulin *(Ig)* gene present on chromosome 14. The *Ig* gene is very active in maturing B lymphocytes. The t(8;14) alters the control of *myc*; its normal low level is switched to high levels, as directed by an *Ig* gene promoter. MYC, when inappropriately high, drives proliferation and blocks differentiation. Hence, the t(8;14) translocation causes cancer of maturing B cells (see Figure 11-14, *C*).

Chromosome translocations also can lead to production of novel proteins with growth-promoting properties. In a different type of leukemia, CML, a specific chromosome translocation is almost always present. This translocation, t(9;22), was first identified in association with CML in Philadelphia in 1960 and so is often referred to as the Philadelphia chromosome.[21] This translocation fuses two chromosomes right in the middle of two genes, *bcr* on chromosome 9 and *abl* on chromosome 22. The result is production of a BCR-ABL fusion protein containing the first half of BCR and the second half of ABL. BCR-ABL is a misregulated protein tyrosine kinase that promotes growth of myeloid cells. Imatinib,

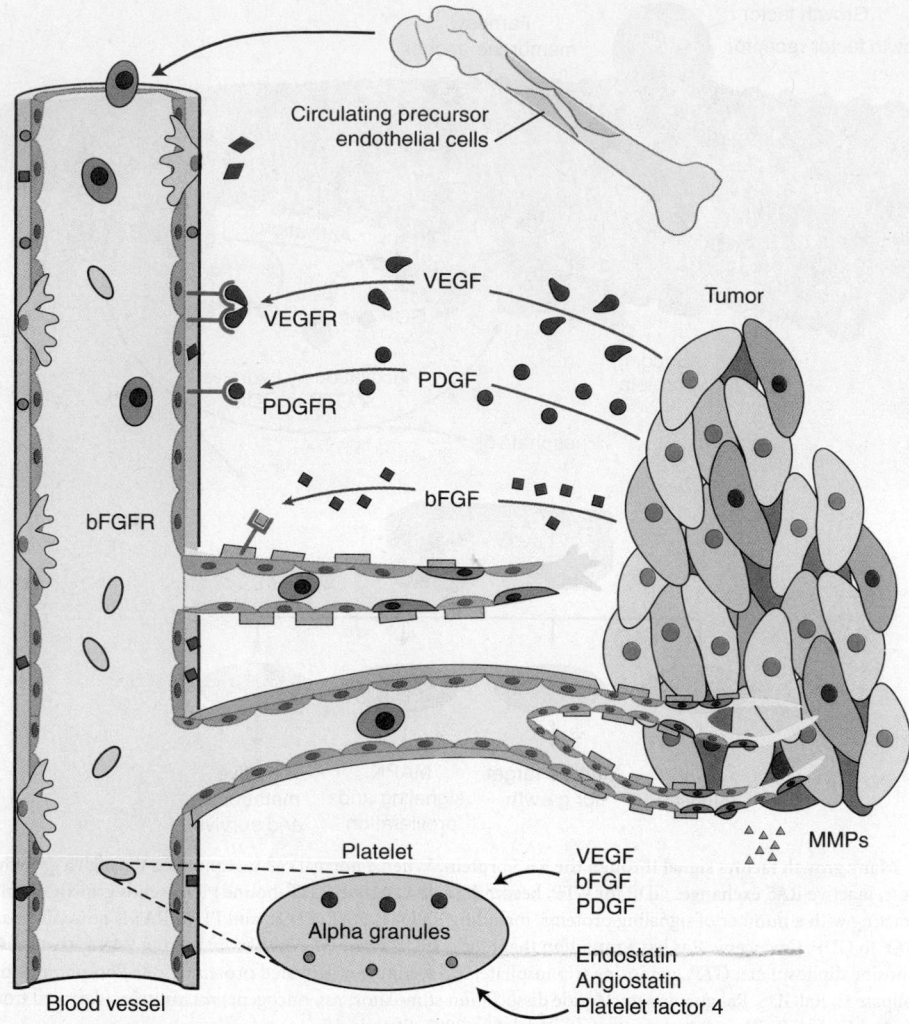

Figure 11-12 Tumor-induced angiogenesis. Malignant tumors secrete angiogenic factors and tissue-remodeling matrix metalloproteinases (MMPs) that actively induce formation of new blood vessels. New blood vessels are formed from both local endothelial cells and circulating precursor cells recruited from the bone marrow. Circulating platelets can also release regulatory proteins into the tumor. *MMPs*, matrix metalloproteases; *PDGF* and *PDGFR*, platelet-derived growth factor and its receptor; *VEGF* and *VEGFR*, vascular endothelial growth factor and its receptor; *bFGF* and *bFGFR*, basic fibroblast growth factor and its receptor. (Adapted from Folkman J: Angiogenesis: an organizing principle for drug discovery? *Nat Rev Drug Discov* 6[4]:273-826, 2007.)

a drug that specifically targets this tyrosine kinase, represents the first successful chemotherapy targeted against the product of a specific oncogenic mutation. Imatinib and related drugs are highly effective in CML and, because of their specificity, lack the toxic side effects noted with nonspecific anticancer drugs.[22] These drugs are not effective in those who do not have the t(9;22) translocation or related mutations. In modern personalized cancer therapy, knowing the specific genetic alteration can predict which drugs are best for the individual.

Gene Amplification

Another type of genetic abnormality that turns on oncogenes is **gene amplification** (see Figures 11-14, *B* and 11-15). Amplifications are the result of duplication of a small piece of a chromosome over and over again, so that instead of the normal two copies of a gene, tens or even hundreds of copies are present (see Chapter 4). Gene amplification results in

increased expression of an oncogene, or in some cases, drug resistance genes. The *N-myc* oncogene is amplified in 25% of childhood neuroblastoma cases and confers a poor prognosis.[23] The epidermal growth factor receptor *erbB2* is amplified in 20% of breast cancers.[24] Individuals whose cancers have erbB2 amplification respond well to drugs specifically targeted to this oncogene.[12]

Tumor-Suppressor Genes

Tumor suppressor genes are genes whose major function is to negatively regulate cell growth and prevent mutations. Tumor suppressors may normally slow the cell cycle, inhibit proliferation resulting from growth signals, or stop cell division when cells are damaged. Examples of several tumor suppressors are given in Table 11-5. One of the first discovered tumor suppressor genes, the **retinoblastoma** *(Rb)* **gene,** normally strongly inhibits the cell division cycle (see Chapter 1). When it is inactivated, the cell division cycle can proceed unchecked. *Rb* is mutated in childhood retinoblastoma, and in many lung, breast, and bone cancers as well.

Whereas oncogenes are activated in cancers, tumor suppressors must be inactivated to allow cancer to occur (see Table 11-5 and Figure 11-16). A single genetic event can activate an oncogene because it can act in a dominant manner in the cell. However, we have two copies, or alleles, of each gene, one from each parent. It therefore takes two hits to inactivate the two alleles of a tumor-suppressor gene. The first allele of a tumor suppressor is often inactivated by point mutations. For example, the *Rb* gene may be inactivated on one chromosome by a point mutation (e.g., the copy inherited from the father). Because the other copy of the retinoblastoma gene

(in this example, the one from the mother) is intact, a functional RB protein can still be made and therefore the cell division cycle can be regulated appropriately. If the remaining gene is mutated or silenced, then all RB function is lost and another step toward cancer occurs (see Chapter 5).

Loss of Heterozygosity

For the function of a tumor suppressor to be lost, both chromosomal copies (alleles) of the gene must be inactivated. This is because they act in a recessive manner at the level of the cell. Although it may seem intuitive that simple inactivating mutations might disrupt both alleles, in fact this is not what usually happens.[25] Instead, the first allele (in the preceding example, the paternal copy) is inactivated by simple mutation, but the second allele (in this example, the maternal copy) is lost because entire regions of the maternal chromosome are epigenetically silenced or a piece of the chromosome can be simply lost (see Figure 11-16, *A*). Because you have two chromosomes, one from each parent, you can be *heterozygous* for nearby genetic markers; loss of a chromosome region in a tumor is referred to as **loss of heterozygosity,** or **LOH.** Loss of heterozygosity, like silencing, unmasks inactivating mutations in recessive tumor suppressor genes. For example, the *Rb* gene resides on chromosome 13, in a region referred to as q14 (13q14). Most individuals with *Rb* mutations have a subtle mutation in one allele and have lost the other copy of *Rb* through loss of the 13q14 chromosome region on the other chromosome.

Cancer Epigenetics—Turning Off Genes Without Mutation

Abnormal gene silencing is emerging as a major cause of cancer. Gene expression can be regulated in a heritable manner (i.e., passed from a parent to a child or from a single cell to its progeny) by an "epigenetic" mechanism called **silencing** that is passed from mother to daughter cells during cell division and does not require mutations or changes in DNA sequence (also see Chapter 4). More simply, the same DNA sequence can produce dramatically different phenotypes depending on chemical modifications that alter the expression of genes. Epigenetic silencing is caused by reversible chemical modification (methylation, addition of methyl group; acetylation, addition of acetyl group) of histones and related chromatin components, as well as methylation of cytosine residues in DNA known as **DNA methylation** (see Figure 11-16, Figure 4-26 and Chapter 12). Whole regions of chromosomes are normally shut off by silencing, so that the pattern of gene expression is different than in other cells with the same genes. In

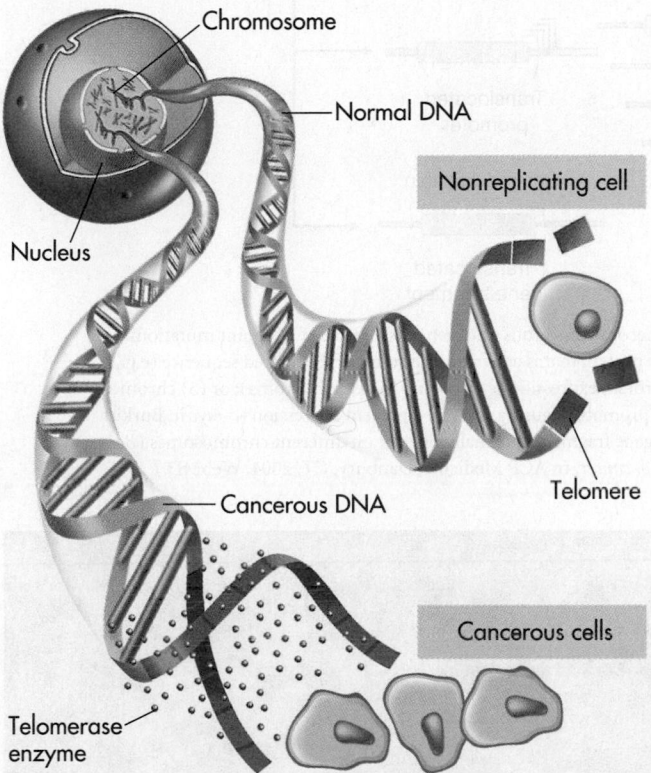

Figure 11-13 Control of immortality: telomeres and telomerase. Normal cells cannot divide indefinitely because the ends of their chromosomes are capped by telomeres. In the absence of the telomerase enzyme, telomeres get shorter and shorter with each division until, when they are critically short, they signal to the cell to stop dividing. In cancer cells the telomerase gene is "switched on," producing an enzyme that rebuilds the telomeres. Thus the cancer cell becomes immortal and able to divide indefinitely without losing its telomeres.

Table 11-4	Comparison of Cancer Gene Types	
Gene Type	**Normal Function**	**Mutation Effect**
Dominant oncogenes*	Encode proteins that promote growth (e.g., growth factors)	Overexpression, amplification, gain of function
Tumor suppressors (recessive oncogenes)	Encode proteins that inhibit proliferation and prevent or repair mutations	Loss of function of both alleles

*Nonmutant state referred to as proto-oncogene.

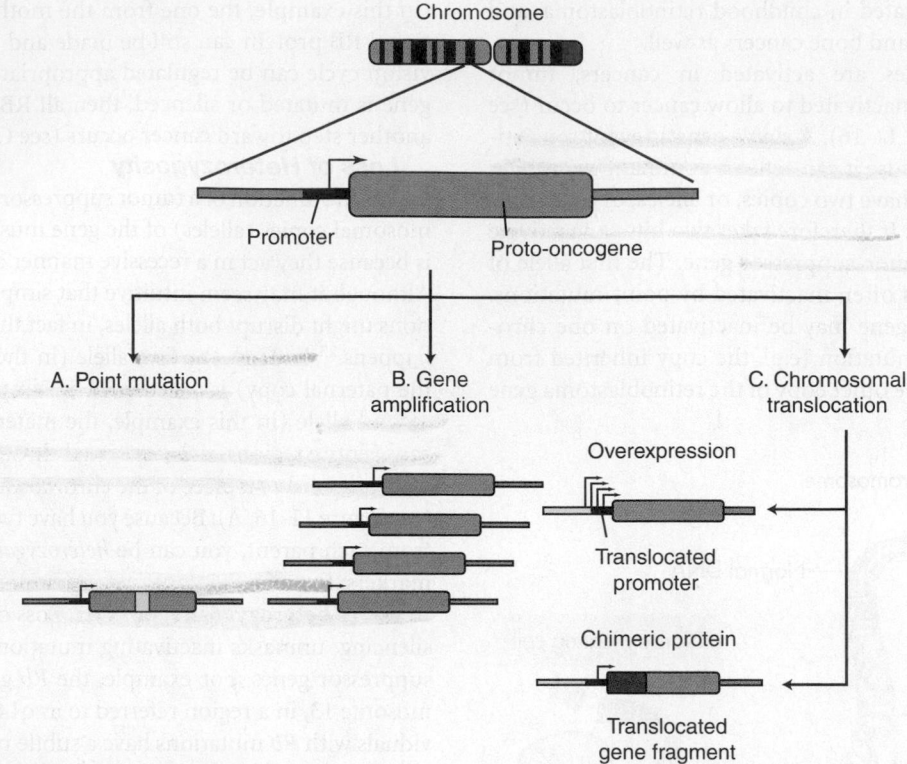

Figure 11-14 Oncogene activation mechanisms. Cellular genes may become cancerous oncogenes as a result of (1) point mutations that alter one or a few nucleotide base pairs, causing the production of a protein that is activated as a result of the altered sequence (e.g., *ras*); (2) amplification of the cellular gene, resulting in higher levels of protein expression (e.g., *N-myc* in neuroblastoma); or (3) chromosomal translocations that either (a) lead to the juxtaposition of a strong promoter, causing increased protein expression (*c-myc* in Burkitt lymphoma), or (b) produce a novel fusion protein that is derived from gene fragments normally present on different chromosomes (*Bcr-Abl* in chronic myeloid leukemia). (From Haber DA: *Molecular genetics of cancer.* In ACP Medicine, Danbury, CT, 2004, WebMD.)

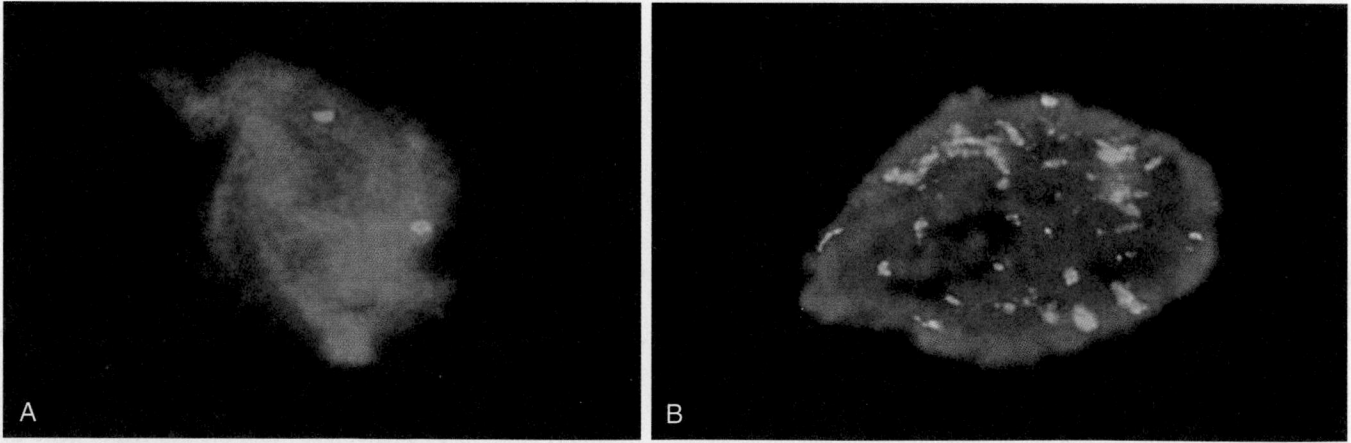

Figure 11-15 *N-myc* **gene amplification in neuroblastoma.** The *N-myc* gene is detected in human neuroblastoma cells using a technique called FISH (fluorescent in situ hybridization) **A,** A single pair of *N-myc* genes are detected in normal cells and in low-grade neuroblastoma. **B,** Multiple, amplified copies of the *N-myc* gene are detected in some cases of neuroblastoma. Amplification of the *N-myc* gene strongly associated with a poor prognosis in childhood neuroblastoma. (Courtesy of Arthur R. Brothman, PhD, FACMG, University of Utah School of Medicine.)

this way, the progeny of liver cells remain liver cells, and skin cells remain skin cells. Notably, *global* changes in epigenetic silencing can turn these cells back into stem cells.[26]

Changes in gene silencing contribute to the development of cancer.[27] Many cancers have increased methylation of

DNA in the promoter region of tumor suppressor genes (in CpG islands or C-cytosine and G-guanine, p-phosphodiester bond, rich sequences that are often located near promoter regions; see Chapters 4 and 12). They also have associated changes in the modification of histones in the chromatin,

Table 11-5	Some Familial Cancer Syndromes Caused by Tumor-Suppressor Gene Function Loss
Syndrome	**Gene**
Retinoblastoma	*Rb*
Li-Fraumeni syndrome	*TP53*
Familial melanoma	*p16^{INK4a}*
Neurofibromatosis	Neurofibromin
Familial adenomatous polyps	*APC*
Breast cancer	*BRCA1*

including methylation of lysines 9 and 27 in histone H3. In addition, overexpression of chromosome silencing proteins known as the polycomb complex, and loss of expression of histone deacetylases (enzymes that remove acetyl groups from histone proteins) SIRT1 is seen in human cancers. These changes in chromatin-modifying genes alter the promoter regions of genes leading to their silencing. The boundaries of the normally silenced regions can also spread in cancer cells, thereby shutting off previously active genes. In either case, silencing can shut off critical tumor suppressor genes in the absence of mutations in the gene. Early in the development of cancer, these changes in gene expression can lead to a selective advantage for affected cells, perhaps leading to their immortalization and clonal expansion. Silencing of tumor suppressors may be a faster way to create cancer cells than mutational or genetic loss of tumor suppressors.[28] Conversely, loss of silencing can contribute to inappropriate expression of oncogenes. Chemotherapeutic drugs that can regulate gene silencing, including histone deacetylase (HDAC) inhibitors and 5 azacytidine (which reverses the effects of DNA methyltransferases (DNMTs), have proven effective in reactivating silenced tumor-suppressor genes in the treatment of selected cancers[29,30] (see Figure 11-16).

Guardians of the Genome

The previous discussion of mutations leads naturally to the question of how mutations occur in the first place. The integrity of genetic information can be compromised at several points: during each round of DNA synthesis, during each mitosis when chromosomes are segregated to daughter cells, and when external mutagens (e.g., chemicals and radiation) alter or disrupt DNA. Multiple mechanisms have evolved to protect and repair the genome.[31] These repair mechanisms are directed by **caretaker genes,** genes that are responsible for the maintenance of genomic integrity. Caretaker genes encode proteins that are involved in repairing damaged DNA, such as occurs with errors in DNA replication, mutations caused by ultraviolet or ionizing radiation, and mutations caused by chemicals and drugs. Loss of function of caretaker genes leads to increased mutation rates. If DNA damage is severe, the cell undergoes programmed cell death, or apoptosis, rather than simply dividing with damaged DNA.

Inherited mutations can disrupt the caretaker genes that protect the integrity of the genome. Examples include the disorder xeroderma pigmentosum (XP); affected individuals have defects in the repair of ultraviolet light–induced DNA damage and should avoid direct sunlight exposure. They have a very high incidence of skin cancer. Hereditary nonpolyposis colorectal cancer (HNPCC) results from an inherited defect in repairing DNA base pair mismatches that occur from time to time during DNA replication. Affected individuals have an increased rate of small insertions and deletions in DNA, leading to a high rate of colon and other cancers.[32] Finally, there are inherited mutations that threaten the integrity of entire chromosomes. Bloom syndrome and Fanconi aplastic anemia are two autosomal recessive disorders in which affected individuals demonstrate marked chromosomal instability. Chromosome breaks, aberrant fusions, and chromosome loss are common. As a consequence, these individuals have a high risk of developing cancer at an early age.

The rate of individual gene mutation is probably too low to account for the acquisition of many new mutations during the evolution of a malignant cancer clone. In addition to abnormal epigenetic silencing, **chromosome instability** (often referred to as CIN) also appears to be increased in malignant cells.[33] The underlying mechanism of this instability is not clear but may be caused by malfunctions in the cellular machinery that regulates chromosome segregation at mitosis.[34] Chromosome instability results in a high rate of chromosome loss, as well as loss of heterozygosity and chromosome amplification. Each of these events can accelerate the loss of tumor-suppressor genes and the overexpression of oncogenes.

Genetics and Cancer-Prone Families

Genetic events are the primary basis of carcinogenesis.[35] Most of the genetic and epigenetic alterations that cause cancer occur during the lifetime of the individual within the somatic tissues. As discussed, the frequency of genetic changes can be increased by exposure to **mutagens,** that is, agents causing mutations, and by defects in DNA repair. Because these genetic events occur in somatic cells as opposed to germ cells, they are not transmitted to future generations. Even though they are genetic events they are not inherited! It is possible, however, for cancer-predisposing mutations to occur in germline cells (cells that produce gametes) (Figure 11-17). Mutations present in germline cells result in the transmission of cancer-causing genes from one generation to the next, producing families with a high incidence of specific cancers. These inherited mutations that predispose to cancer are almost invariably found in tumor-suppressor genes (see Table 11-5).

Although rare, such "cancer families" demonstrate that inheritance of a mutated gene can cause cancer (Figure 11-18). In these families, inheritance of one mutant allele predisposes a person to a specific form of cancer: individuals who inherit the germline mutant allele will inevitably suffer loss of the normal allele by loss of heterozygosity (LOH) or **epigenetic silencing** (see Figure 11-16) in some cells and go on to develop the tumor. Examples of human cancers that

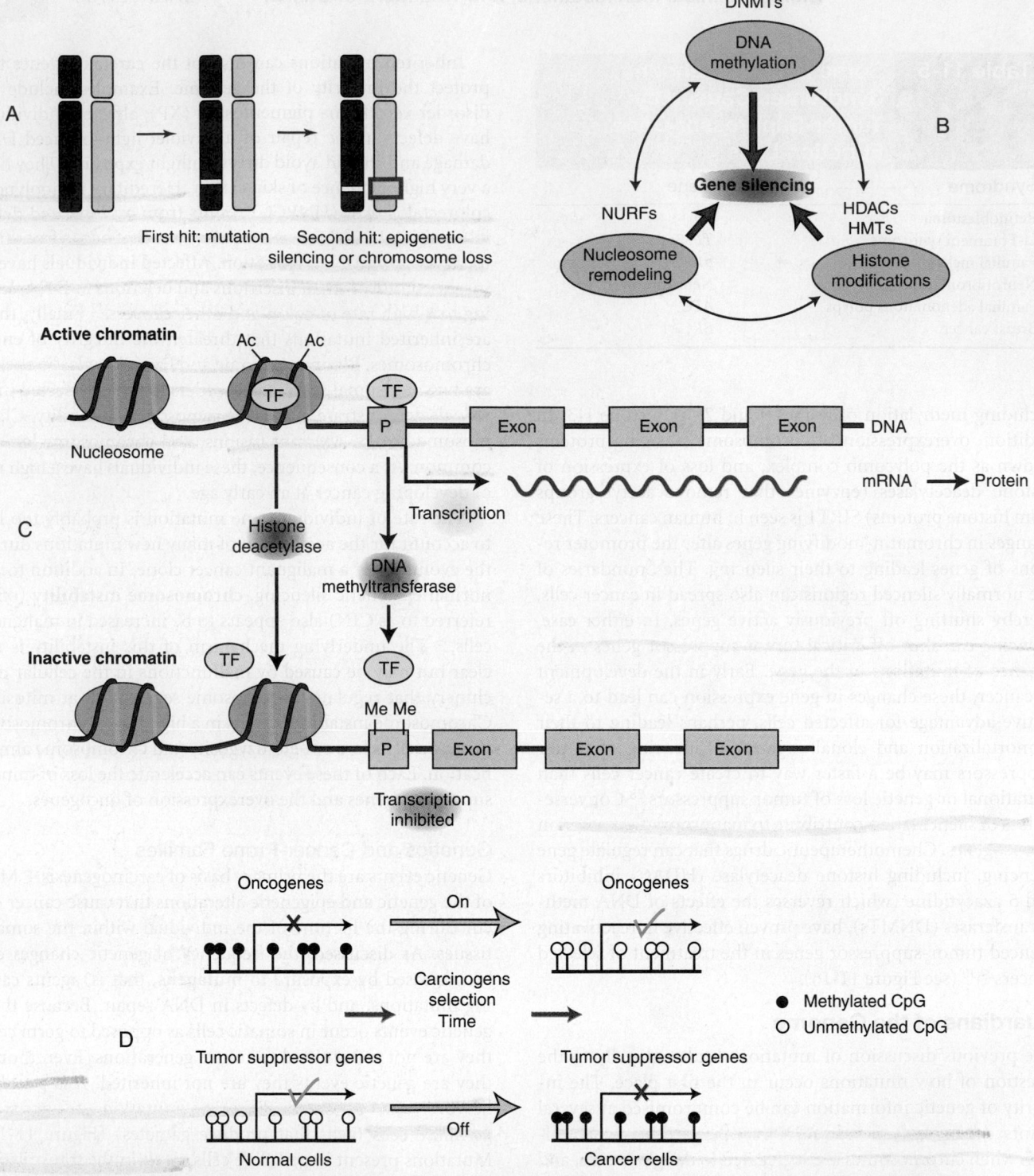

Figure 11-16 Silencing tumor-suppressor genes by epigenetic alterations. Tumor suppressor genes can be turned off by a variety of mechanisms. **A,** In this example, the first hit is a point mutation in a tumor suppressor gene (white box), followed by either epigenetic silencing or chromosome loss of the second allele (red box). **B,** Genes can normally be silenced by a variety of interacting processes including DNA methylation, histone modifications, nucleosomal remodeling, and microRNAs (not shown). A number of cellular enzymes contribute to these modifications, including DNA methyltransferases (DNMTs), histone deacetylases (HDACs), histone methyltransferases (HMTs), and complex nucleosomal remodeling factors (NURFs). Gene silencing is essential for normal development and differentiation. **C,** Histone modification and promoter methylation regulate gene expression. Genes are transcribed when chromatin is modified by addition of acetyl (Ac) groups to specific lysine groups in histones. Gene expression can be turned off when specific acetyl groups are removed (by histone deacetylase (HDACs)) or when the CpG-rich promoter regions of genes are modified by direct DNA methylation (by DNA methyltransferase). In addition, small endogenous RNA molecules (microRNAs or miRNA) can bind to mRNA and reduce gene expression. **D,** Changes in promoter methylation turn cancer genes off and on. Oncogenes can be turned on by promoter hypomethylation, and tumor suppressor genes can be turned off by promoter hypermethylation. Each of these changes can produce selective growth and survival advantage for the cancer cell. (B adapted from Jones PA, Baylin SB: The epigenomics of cancer, *Cell* 128:683-692, 2007. C from Gluckman PD et al: *N Engl J Med* 359[1]:66, 2008; D from Shames DS, Minna JF, Gazdar AF: DNA methylation in health, disease, and cancer, *Curr Mol Med* 7:85-102, 2007.)

can be inherited are retinoblastoma, a childhood cancer of the eye that can be caused by germline mutations in one allele of the *Rb* gene; Wilms tumor, a childhood cancer of the kidney *(Wt1)*; neurofibromatosis *(Nf1)*; inherited breast cancer *(BRCA1)*; and familial polyposis coli or adenomas of the colon *(APC)*. A specific tumor-suppressor gene has been found in each of these cancers. In many cases, these tumor-suppressor genes also are inactivated in sporadic (as opposed to inherited) cancers. For example, inherited mutations in the *APC* gene are rare and account for only a few percent of all colon cancers. However, 85% of sporadic colon cancers also have acquired mutations of *APC*, mutations that occurred over time

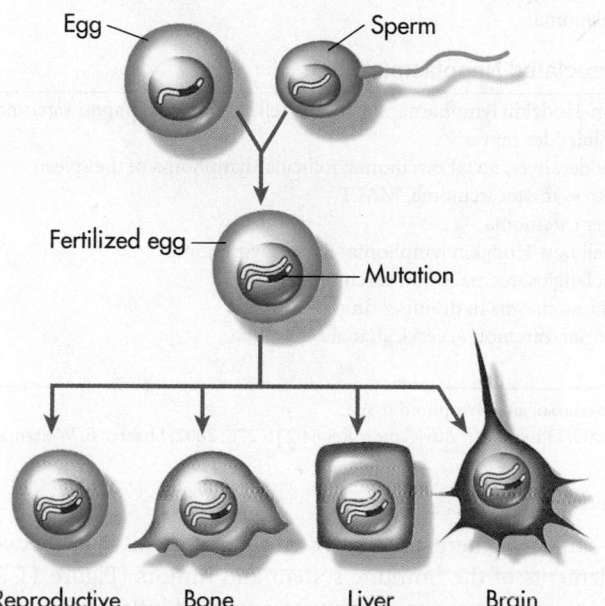

Figure 11-17 Germline mutation. Inherited mutations are carried in the deoxyribonucleic acid (DNA) of reproductive cells. When reproductive cells containing mutations combine to produce offspring, the mutation will be present in all of the offspring's body cells. (Modified with permission from Lea DN, Jenkins JF, Francomano CA: *Genetics in clinical practice*, Jones and Bartlett Publishers, 1998. www.jbpub.com.)

in the individual. Characterization of cancer-causing genes and other genetic factors helps identify individuals prone to developing cancer (see Figure 11-18) and contributes to our understanding of sporadic cancers. Individuals known to carry mutations in tumor-suppressor genes (for example, women with a germline *BRCA1* mutation) are offered targeted cancer screening to facilitate early cancer detection and therapy.[36]

Inflammation, Immunity, and Cancer

Chronic inflammation has been recognized for close to 150 years as being an important factor in the development of cancer.[37,38] Epidemiologic studies strongly support the conclusion that the active immune response in chronic inflammation predisposes to cancer. Individuals who have suffered with ulcerative colitis for 10 years or more have up to a 30-fold increase in the risk of developing colon cancer. Chronic viral hepatitis caused by hepatitis B virus (HBV) or hepatitis C virus (HCV) infection markedly increases the risk of liver cancer. A large study found a 66% increase in risk of lung cancer among women with chronic asthma, an inflammatory disease of the airways.[39] Table 11-6 details the various inflammatory conditions and infectious agents associated with cancer.

The reasons for the association of inflammation and cancer are complex and differ from site to site. After injury and during infection, inflammatory cells, including neutrophils, lymphocytes, and macrophages release cytokines and growth and survival factors that stimulate local cell proliferation and new blood vessel growth to promote wound healing by tissue remodeling (see Chapter 6). These factors combine in chronic inflammation to promote continued proliferation (Figures 11-19 and 11-20). In addition, inflammatory cells release compounds such as reactive oxygen species (ROS), and other reactive molecules that can promote mutations and block the cellular response to DNA damage. Notably, increased abundance of the enzyme cyclooxygenase-2 (COX-2), which generates prostaglandins during acute inflammation, has been associated with colon and some other cancers. Nonsteroidal

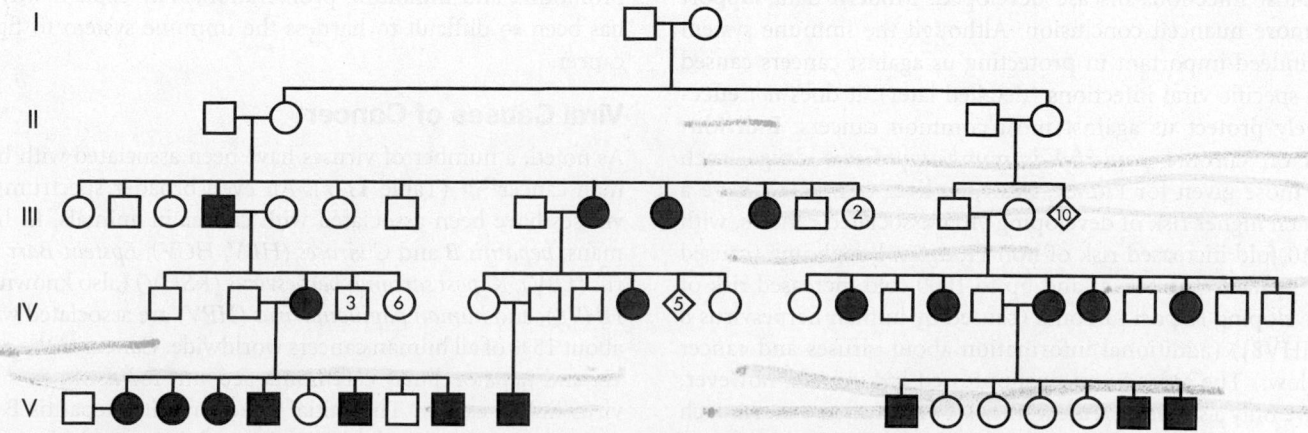

Figure 11-18 A familial colon cancer pedigree. Darkened symbols represent individuals diagnosed with colon cancer. One of the individuals in the first generation must have carried a mutation in the APC gene. (From Jorde LB et al: *Medical genetics*, ed 3, St Louis, 2003, Mosby.)

Table 11-6	Chronic Inflammatory Conditions and Infectious Agents Associated with Neoplasms

Inflammatory Condition	Associated Neoplasm(s)
Asbestosis, silicosis	Mesothelioma, lung carcinoma
Bronchitis	Lung carcinoma
Cystitis, bladder inflammation	Bladder carcinoma
Gingivitis, lichen planus	Oral squamous cell carcinoma
Inflammatory bowel disease, Crohn disease, chronic ulcerative colitis	Colorectal carcinoma
Lichen sclerosus	Vulvar squamous cell carcinoma
Chronic pancreatitis, hereditary pancreatitis	Pancreatic carcinoma
Reflux esophagitis, Barrett esophagus	Esophageal carcinoma
Sialadenitis	Salivary gland carcinoma
Sjögren syndrome, Hashimoto thyroiditis	MALT lymphoma
Skin inflammation	Melanoma

Infectious Agent	Associated Neoplasm(s)
AIDS (HIV, herpesvirus type 8)	Non-Hodgkin lymphoma, squamous cell carcinomas, Kaposi sarcoma
Chronic cholecystitis	Gallbladder cancer
Chronic cystitis (schistosomiasis)	Bladder, liver, rectal carcinoma; follicular lymphoma of the spleen
Gastritis, gastric ulcers (*Helicobacter pylori*)	Gastric adenocarcinoma, MALT
Hepatitis	Liver carcinoma
Mononucleosis (Epstein-Barr virus)	B cell non-Hodgkin lymphoma, Burkitt lymphoma
Opisthorchis, cholangitis (liver flukes, bile acids)	Cholangiosarcoma, colon carcinoma
Osteomyelitis	Skin carcinoma in draining sinuses
Pelvic inflammatory disease, chronic cervicitis (HPV, gonorrhea, chlamydia)	Ovarian carcinoma, cervical/anal carcinoma

HIV, Human immunodeficiency virus; *HPV,* human papillomavirus; *MALT,* mucosa-associated lymphoid tissue.
Modified from Coussens LM, Werb Z: *Nature* 420(6917):860-867, 2002; Dalgleish AG, O'Byrne KJ: *Adv Cancer Res* 84:231-276, 2002; Shacter E, Weitzman SA: *Oncology* 16(2):217-226, 229, 2002.

anti-inflammatory drugs (NSAIDs), such as aspirin. that inhibit COX-2 can reduce the risk of colon cancer by as much as 20% (see Chapter 5).[40]

The Immune System Protects Us Against Viral-Associated Cancers

It is a popular belief that damage to the immune system may lead to development of common cancers. This idea arose decades ago as our understanding of the immune response against infectious disease developed. Modern data support a more nuanced conclusion. Although the immune system is indeed important in protecting us against cancers caused by specific viral infections (detailed later), it does *not* effectively protect us against most common cancers. Individuals on chronic powerful immunosuppressive drugs, such as those given for kidney, heart, or liver transplant, have a much higher risk of developing viral-associated cancers, with a 10-fold increased risk of non-Hodgkin lymphoma (caused by Epstein-Barr virus) and up to 1000-fold increased risk of developing Kaposi sarcoma (caused by human herpesvirus 8 [HHV8]) (additional information about viruses and cancer below.) The same immunosuppressed individuals, however, have only a slight increase in the risk of common cancers such as lung and colon cancer (and this could well be because of increased inflammation at those sites) and no increase in the risk of breast or prostate cancer.[41,42]

In fact, there are many complex interactions between elements of the immune system and tumors (Figure 11-20). Tumors activate surrounding stromal and inflammatory cells, including tumor-infiltrating lymphocytes and macrophages, to secrete multiple cytokines that support tumor growth and spread. In parallel, various cells of the immune system can exert antitumor effects through factors such as TNF-related apoptosis-inducing ligand (TRAIL), interleukin (IL)-10 and IL-12. The double-edged effects of the immune cells, both promoting and inhibiting proliferation, may explain why it has been so difficult to harness the immune system to fight cancer.

Viral Causes of Cancer

As noted, a number of viruses have been associated with human cancer[43,44] (Table 11-7). An even broader spectrum of viruses have been associated with cancer in animals. In humans, *hepatitis B* and *C viruses (HBV, HCV), Epstein-Barr virus (EBV), Kaposi sarcoma herpesvirus (KSHV)* (also known as *HHV8*), and *human papillomavirus (HPV)* are associated with about 15% of all human cancers worldwide. Cancer of the cervix and hepatocellular carcinoma account for about 80% of virus-linked cancer. The initial infection with hepatitis B or C is not associated with cancer; instead, it is acquisition of a chronic viral hepatitis that markedly increases cancer risk (also see Inflammation, Immunity and Cancer). Chronic hepatitis

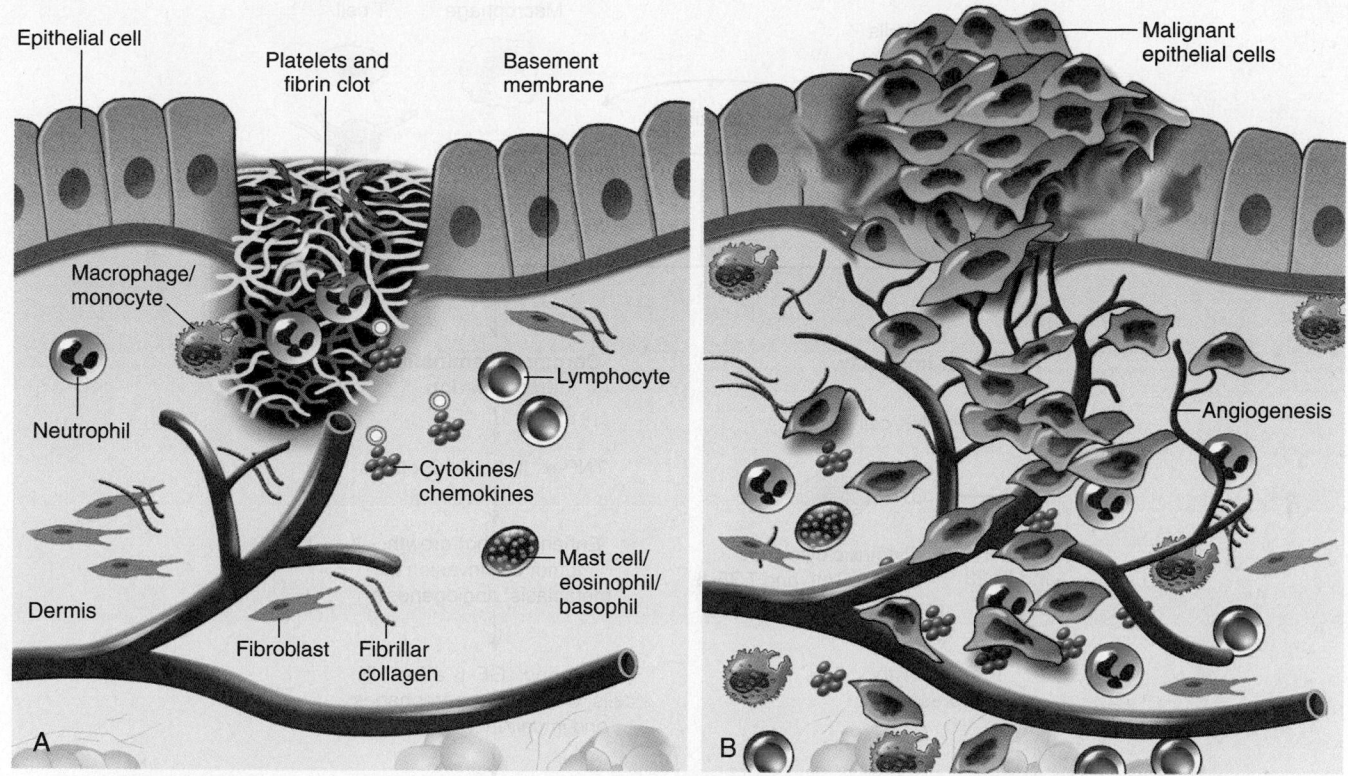

Figure 11-19 Wound healing versus invasive tumor growth. **A,** Wounds simulate a local inflammatory response. With tissue injury, a blood clot with activated platelets forms, releasing multiple factors that stimulate wound healing. Chemotactic factors such as transforming growth factor-beta and platelet-derived growth factor, derived from activated platelets, initiate granulation tissue formation, activation of fibroblasts, and secretion of proteolytic enzymes (including matrix metalloproteinases) necessary for remodeling of the extracellular matrix. Signaling from many cell types in the wound, including stromal cells, facilitates healing. Once the wound is healed, the signals presumably stop. **B,** Invasive carcinomas act as disorganized wounds. Neoplastic cells produce angiogenic factors, cytokines and chemokines that are mitogenic and/or chemoattractants for numerous cells. In return, activated fibroblasts and infiltrating inflammatory cells also secrete proteolytic enzymes, cytokines, and chemokines, which are mitogenic for neoplastic cells as well as for endothelial cells involved in neoangiogenesis. These factors, which in the normal situation promote wound healing, now can stimulate tumor growth and angiogenesis, induce fibroblast migration and maturation, and promote metastatic spread through the venous or lymphatic networks. (Adapted from Coussens LM, Werb Z: *Nature* 420[6917]:860-867, 2002.)

B infections are common in parts of Asia and Sub-Saharan Africa and confer up to a 200-fold increased risk of developing liver cancer. Chronic hepatitis C infections have become increasingly recognized in Western countries. Up to 80% of liver cancer worldwide is associated with chronic hepatitis caused either by HBV or HCV. In both cases, it appears that a lifetime of chronic liver inflammation predisposes to the development of hepatocellular carcinoma. Widespread use of the HBV vaccine is expected to significantly decrease the incidence of chronic hepatitis B and hence hepatocellular carcinoma. Unfortunately, a vaccine for HCV is not yet available.

Virtually all cervical cancer is caused by infection with specific subtypes of HPV, which infects basal skin cells and commonly causes warts. There are more than 100 HPV subtypes, but only a few (HPV16, 18, 31, 45, and a few others) are associated with cervical, anogenital, and penile cancer (see Chapters 12 and 23). HPV causes cancer when the viral DNA becomes accidentally integrated into the genomic DNA of the infected basal cell of the cervix and directs the persistent production of viral oncogenes. Early oncogenic HPV infection is readily detected by the Papanicolaou (Pap) test, an examination of cervical epithelia scrapings. Early detection of cellular atypia in a Pap test alerts healthcare providers to the possibility of cervical carcinoma in situ, which can be effectively treated. The Pap test is probably the most effective cancer screening test developed to date. Most recently, vaccines protecting against two or four common oncogenic HPV subtypes have been approved for clinical use; if widely given to young women prior to initial HPV infection, these vaccines can prevent many cases of cervical cancer.[45]

EBV and HHV8 are members of the herpesviridae family.[43] EBV, the cause of infectious mononucleosis, infects B lymphocytes and stimulates their proliferation. In individuals who are immunosuppressed because of HIV infection or because of drugs given for an organ transplant, persistent EBV infection can lead to the development of B-cell lymphomas. This development in those with organ transplants is known as **post-transplant lymphoproliferative disorder (PTLD)**.[46]

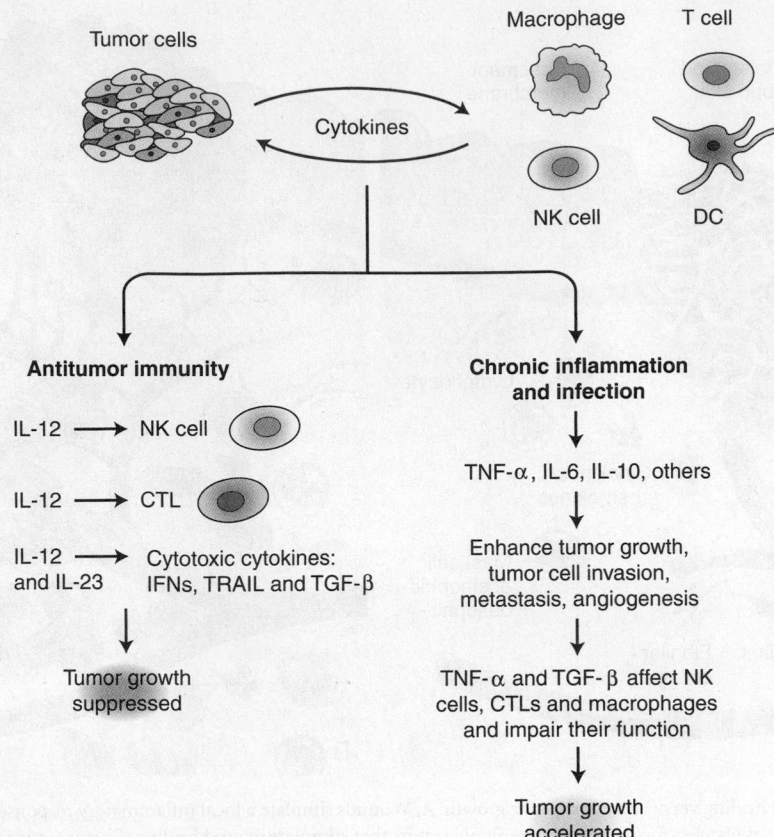

Figure 11-20 Cytokines link innate immunity, inflammation, and cancer. Tumor and immune cells both secrete cytokines that influence tumor growth. Some cytokines (interferons, TRAIL, TGF-β) have antitumor activity, while others stimulate NK and CTL cells to attack the tumor. Balancing the antitumor immunity, however, TNF-α and several interleukins accelerate tumor progression by multiple mechanisms, including growth stimulation, promotion of angiogenesis and by suppressing the activity of infiltrating immune cells. *CTL*, cytotoxic T lymphocyte; *DC*, dendritic cell; *IFN*, interferon; *IL*, Interleukin; NK, natural killer cells; *TGF-β*, transforming growth factor beta; *TNF*, tumor necrosis factor. (Adapted from Lin W, Karin M: *J Clin Invest* 117[5]:1175-1183.)

One effective therapy for PTLD is, if possible, to decrease or stop immunosuppressant drugs and allow the immune system to attack the virus. EBV infection also is associated with Burkitt lymphoma in areas of endemic malaria and with nasopharyngeal carcinoma, a cancer endemic in Chinese populations in Southeast Asia.[47] HHV8 is linked to the development of Kaposi sarcoma, a cancer that occurs in older adult men and in a markedly more virulent form in immunocompromised individuals, especially those infected with HIV. HHV8 also has been linked to several rare lymphomas.

Human T-cell leukemia-lymphoma virus (HTLV) is an oncogenic retrovirus linked to the development of adult T-cell leukemia and lymphoma (ATLL).[44] HTLV is transmitted vertically, that is, inherited by children from infected parents, and horizontally, by breast-feeding, sexual intercourse, blood transfusions, and exposure to infected needles. Infection with HTLV may be asymptomatic, and only a small fraction of infected individuals develop ATLL, often many years after acquiring the virus. It is clear that infection by an oncogenic virus is far from sufficient to cause cancer. For example, in some industrialized regions, Epstein-Barr virus

can infect 90% of the adolescent and young adult population, yet only a very small percentage of these individuals develop EBV-related cancer. For each of these infections, important cofactors increase the risk that an infection will develop into cancer.

Bacterial Cause of Cancer

Helicobacter pylori is a bacterium that infects more than half of the world's population. Chronic infection with *H. pylori* is an important cause of peptic ulcer disease and is strongly associated with gastric carcinoma, a leading cause of cancer deaths worldwide. It is also associated with a less common cancer, gastric mucosa–associated lymphoid tissue (MALT) lymphomas.[48] *H. pylori* infection is often acquired in childhood and disproportionately affects lower socioeconomic classes. Although most infections are asymptomatic, prolonged chronic inflammation can lead to atrophic gastritis that can, in a small fraction of individuals, progress to dysplastic changes and finally frank gastric adenocarcinoma. Recent data have shown that *H. pylori* infection induces methylation of specific genes in the gastric mucosa.[49] Eradication of *H. pylori* from infected individuals prior to the development of dysplasia may prevent the development of cancer.[50] However, there is no expert consensus on the value of population screening and treatment strategies.[51] The MALT lymphomas associated with chronic *H. pylori* infections may depend on chronic inflammation and antigenic stimulation associated with infections, and therefore treatment with antibiotics may be useful even in cases of early lymphoma.[52]

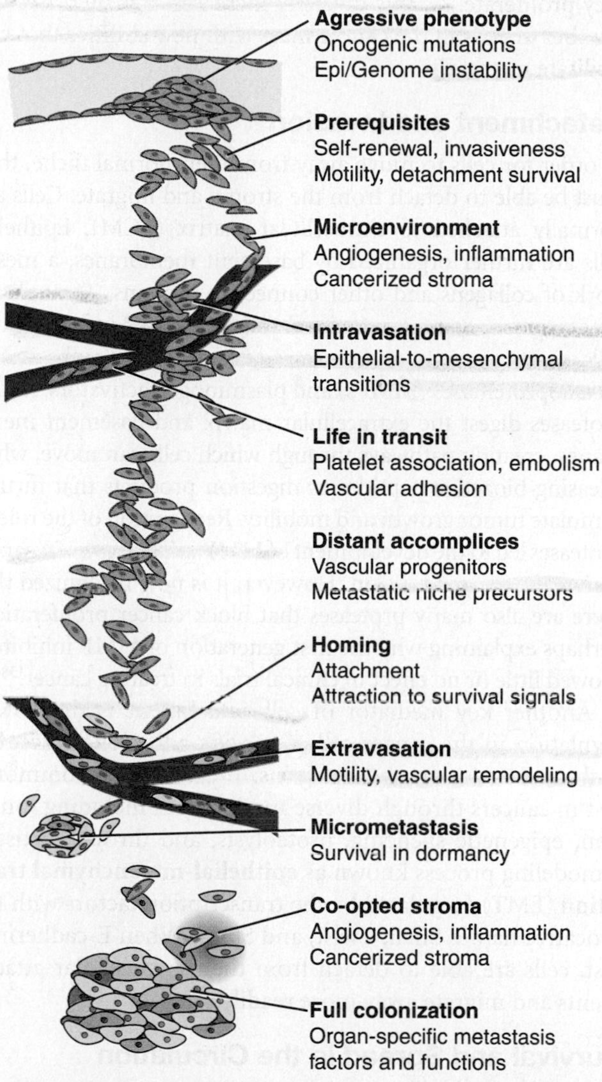

CANCER INVASION AND METASTASIS

Metastasis is the spread of cancer cells from the site of the original tumor to distant tissues and organs through the body. Metastasis is a defining characteristic of cancer, contributes significantly to the pain and suffering from cancer, and is the major cause of death from cancer. When localized, low-stage cancer can often be cured by a combination of surgery, chemotherapy, and radiation. These same therapies are frequently ineffective against cancer that has metastasized. For example, in appropriately treated women with low-stage breast cancer, the 5-year survival rate is often greater than 90%.[53] Tragically, less than 30% of women with metastatic breast cancer are alive 5 years after diagnosis.[54] A growing body of basic and clinical research is defining the biologic principles of metastasis, with the hope that this improved understanding will lead to novel diagnostic approaches and better therapies to prevent and treat metastatic cancers.[55]

Invasion, or local spread, is a prerequisite for metastasis and is the first step in the metastatic process. In its earliest stages local invasion may occur by direct tumor extension.[56] Eventually, however, cells migrate away from the primary tumor and invade the surrounding tissues. Mechanisms important in local invasion include (1) ongoing cancer proliferation; (2) digestion of connective tissue capsules and other structural barriers by secreted proteases; (3) changes in cell-to-cell adhesion, often by changes in expression of cell adhesion molecules, such as cadherins and integrins, making the cancer cells more slippery and mobile; and (4) increased motility of individual tumor cells (Figure 11-22). To transition from local to distant metastasis, the cancer cells must also be able to invade local blood and lymphatic vessels, a task facilitated by stimulation of neoangiogenesis and lymphangiogenesis by factors such as VEGF. Finally, a successful metastatic cell must be able to survive in the circulation, attach in an appropriate new microenvironment, and multiply to produce an entire new tumor, similar to the characteristics of a cancer stem cell. Because metastasis requires successful completion of each and every step, there may be many opportunities to interrupt this potentially lethal pathway.

Agressive phenotype
Oncogenic mutations
Epi/Genome instability

Prerequisites
Self-renewal, invasiveness
Motility, detachment survival

Microenvironment
Angiogenesis, inflammation
Cancerized stroma

Intravasation
Epithelial-to-mesenchymal transitions

Life in transit
Platelet association, embolism
Vascular adhesion

Distant accomplices
Vascular progenitors
Metastatic niche precursors

Homing
Attachment
Attraction to survival signals

Extravasation
Motility, vascular remodeling

Micrometastasis
Survival in dormancy

Co-opted stroma
Angiogenesis, inflammation
Cancerized stroma

Full colonization
Organ-specific metastasis
factors and functions

Figure 11-21 Multistep nature of metastasis. (From Gupta GP, Massagué J: Cancer metastasis: building a framework, *Cell* 127[4]:697-708, 2006.)

Table 11-7	Human Viruses Associated with Cancer		
Virus Family	Type	Human Cancer	Cofactors
Hepatitis viruses	Hepatitis B	Hepatocellular carcinoma	Alcohol, smoking, aflatoxins
	Hepatitis C	Hepatocellular carcinoma	Alcohol
Herpesviruses	Epstein-Barr	Burkitt lymphoma, nasopharyngeal carcinoma	Malaria
	KSHV/HHV-8 Immunodeficiency	Kaposi sarcoma	
Papillomaviruses	HPV-16, HPV-18, HPV-31, HPV-33, other	Cervical, anogenital	Smoking, oral contraceptives
Retroviruses	HTLV-1	Adult T-cell leukemia/lymphoma	Unknown

KSHV/HHV-8, Kaposi sarcoma–associated herpesvirus/human herpesvirus-8; *HPV*, human papillomavirus; *HTLV-1*, human T-cell leukemia/lymphoma virus-1.
Modified from Mendelsohn J et al, editors: *The molecular basis of cancer*, ed 2, Philadelphia, 2001, Saunders.

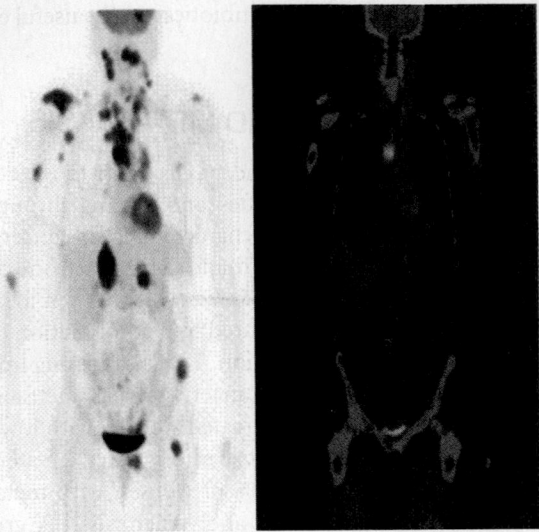

Figure 11-22 Metastatic non-small cell lung cancer. This 54-year-old woman had a non-small cell lung cancer (NSCLC) resected from the left upper lobe. Five years later, these studies were obtained. The positron emission tomography (PET) scan using 18-fluoro-deoxyglucose shows metastatic lesions in the brain, right shoulder, mediastinal and cervical lymph nodes, as well as the liver, left pelvis, and proximal femur. *(Left)* PET whole-body image. *(Right)* Representative coronal image from the whole body FDG-PET/CT–fused image of the same patient. The fused image consists of the CT image with the metabolic information superimposed in color. The pattern of spread is most likely from the primary tumor to the large mediastinal lymph nodes, followed by lymphatic spread to cervical nodes. Blood-borne spread produced the bone, brain, and liver metastases. Normally, only the heart, brain, and bladder show strong signal in PET scan. *CT,* Computed tomography; *FDG,* fluorodeoxyglucose. (Images courtesy John Hoffman, MD, Huntsman Cancer Institute, Salt Lake City, Utah.)

Only Rare Cells in a Cancer Are Able to Metastasize

Metastasis is a highly inefficient process. A landmark clinical review examined a group of women with advanced ovarian cancer.[57] These unfortunate women had accumulated a large amount of peritoneal fluid filled with malignant ovarian cancer cells (malignant ascites). To relieve the pressure caused by the ascites, the fluid was surgically shunted into the venous circulation. This palliative procedure relieved the abdominal pressure but had the side effect of moving millions of ovarian cancer cells an hour directly into the bloodstream. Despite this direct injection of billions of cancer cells into the circulation, these women unexpectedly had no increased number of metastases when they died. The conclusion from this clinical study, that most cancer cells cannot successfully cause metastases, has been supported by many other clinical and laboratory studies as well.[56] The reason lies both in the seed and the soil. Cancer cells (the seeds) must surmount multiple physical and physiologic barriers in order to spread, survive, and proliferate in distant locations, and the destination (the soil) must be receptive to the growth of the cancer. It has been suggested that the metastatic cell must, like a decathlon champion, be successful in every event to allow a cancer to spread.[56]

How do cancer cells develop the ability to metastasize? As cancers grow, they develop increasing heterogeneity. This reflects the genetic instability of cancer and aberrant differentiation of subclones of the malignant cells. The same changes that happen in cells to cause the primary cancer, including gene mutations, deletions, translocations, and epigenetic silencing, all work to provide genetic heterogeneity in the tumor cells as they proliferate. As this diversity increases, this increases the number of cells in the cancer mass with new abilities that can facilitate metastasis.

Detachment and Invasion

In order for cells to move away from their normal niche, they must be able to detach from the stroma and migrate. Cells are normally attached to extracellular matrix (ECM). Epithelial cells are further organized by basement membranes, a meshwork of collagens and other connective proteins. To facilitate cancer spread, many tumors and their associated inflammatory cells secrete proteases and protease activators, such as the matrix metalloproteinases (MMPs) and plasminogen activators. Active proteases digest the extracellular matrix and basement membranes, creating pathways through which cells can move, while releasing bioactive peptides as digestion products that further stimulate tumor growth and mobility. Recognition of the role of proteases led to the development of MMP inhibitors as a weapon against cancer progression. However, it is now recognized that there are also many proteases that block cancer proliferation, perhaps explaining why the first generation of MMP inhibitors showed little or no effect in clinical trials in treating cancer.[58]

Another key mediator of cell detachment is the down-regulation in the cancer cell of specific adhesion molecules, such as E-cadherin and integrins. E-cadherin is commonly lost in cancers through diverse mechanisms including mutation, epigenetic silencing, proteolysis, and through a tissue remodeling process known as **epithelial-mesenchymal transition (EMT)** (regulated by the transcription factors with the evocative names Snail, Twist, and Slug). When E-cadherin is lost, cells are able to detach from their extracellular attachments and migrate away more readily.

Survival and Spread in the Circulation

Normal cells, when separated from their ECM, undergo *anoikis*, a form of apoptosis. In contrast, tumor cells that have already adapted to a hypoxic environment have already been selected for resistance to apoptosis, often by loss of normal cell death pathways. For example, neuroblastomas with loss of the proapoptotic caspase 8 genes are able to avoid apoptosis after loss of integrins, and are more able to metastasize than the same cells with normal levels of caspase 8. Accordingly, individuals whose neuroblastomas have low levels of caspase 8 have a poor prognosis.[59] (See Chapter 2.)

Selective Adherence in Favorable Sites

After release from the ECM and digestion of basement membranes, cancer cells gain access to the circulation through new tumor-associated blood vessel growth or angiogenesis

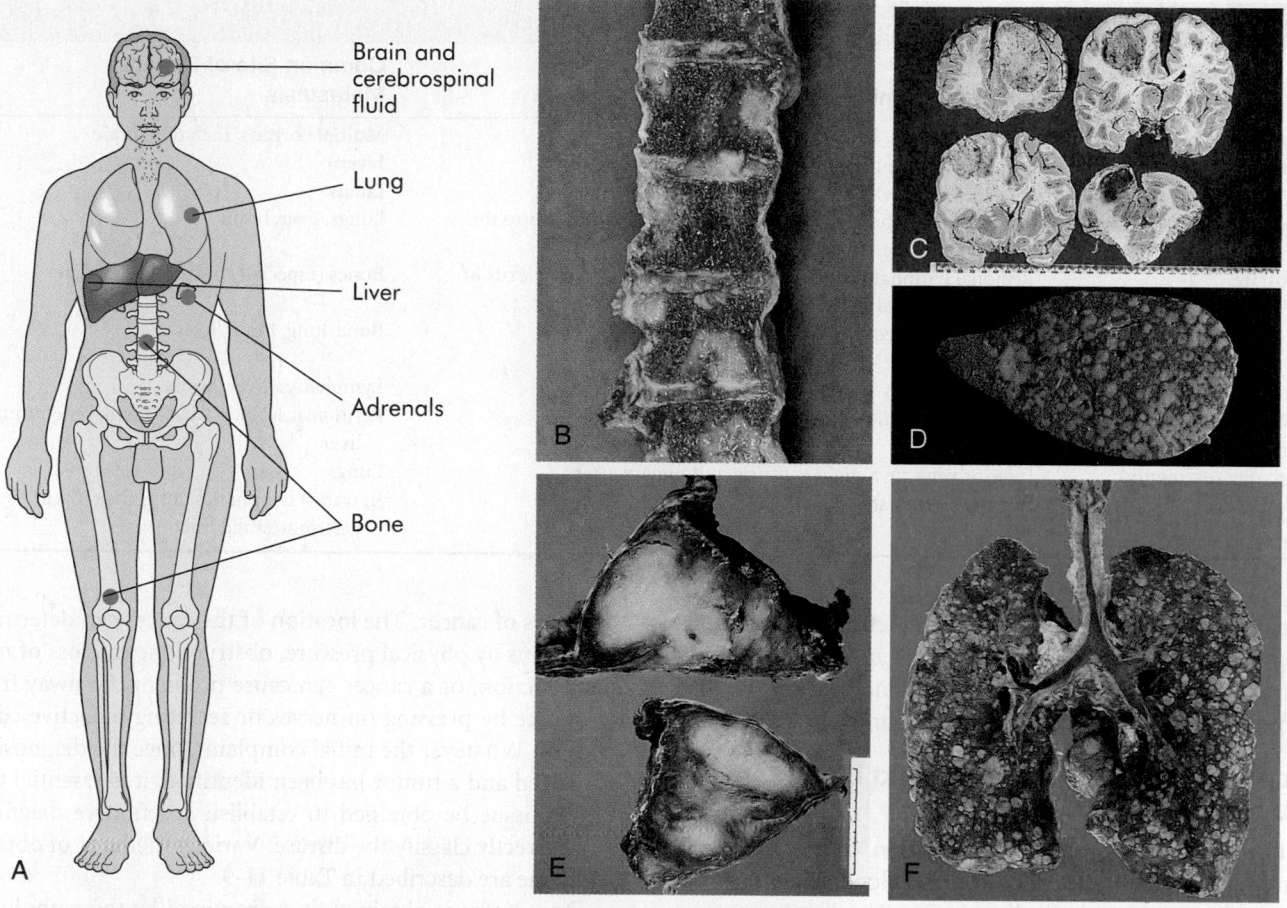

Figure 11-23 Patterns of metastatic spread. **A,** Sites of hematogenous metastasis. Blood-borne tumor metastasis leads to growth of secondary tumors in several main sites. The macroscopic appearance of bone metastasis are shown in **B,** where lesions are seen in vertebrae. **C,** Numerous metastases from a neoplasm of the stomach are seen in the brain in **D,** The liver is the most common site for metastases from tumors in the gastrointestinal tract which arose from a colonic neoplasm. **E,** Metastatic tumor has replaced both adrenal glands, as is commonly seen with spread from lung and breast tumors. **F,** The lung is the most common site for blood-borne metastases from tumors outside the spinal tract, particularly mesenchymal tumors.

(described earlier), also known as neovascularization. Mobile tumor cells are able to enter the circulation, perhaps facilitated by the leaky newly made vessels and attraction of the cells because of chemoattractants coming from these new vessels. Once in the circulation, metastatic cells must be able to withstand the physiologic stresses of travel in the blood and lymphatic circulation, including high shear rates and exposure to immune cells. One mechanism is for tumor cells to bind to blood platelets, giving them a protective coat of nonmalignant blood cells that both shields the tumor cells and creates a small tumor embolus, or cancer clot, that can promote cancer cell survival in distant locations.

The patterns of metastasis are dictated by the interaction between the cancer cells and the microenvironments in which they land. Two distinct mechanisms give rise to patterns of distant spread. First, cancer cells spread through vascular and lymphatic pathways, as well as natural tissue planes. The **neovascularization** of a cancer offers malignant cells direct access into the venous blood, and draining lymphatics can carry malignant cells to regional lymph nodes. Single cells, clumps,

and even tumor fragments can disseminate by these routes. Anatomic patterns of lymphatic and venous blood flow help determine how colon cancers spread to the liver, liver cancers spread through the portal vein to the lungs, lung cancers spread through the systemic circulation to the brain, and breast cancer spreads through lymphatics to axillary lymph nodes (Figure 11-23). There is also a major yet poorly understood selectivity of different cancers for different sites. Thus metastatic breast cancer often spreads through the bloodstream to bones but rarely to kidney or spleen, whereas lymphomas often spread to the spleen but uncommonly spread to bone. In a key study, Schackert and Fidler[60] injected different types of cancer cells into the carotid artery of mice. Despite identical blood flow–mediated distribution of the cancer cells, each cancer cell type produced cancers in very different parts of the brain. This tissue selectivity is likely caused by specific interactions between the cancer cells and specific receptors on the small blood vessels in different organs (Table 11-8). Experimental metastasis studies in mice are beginning to reveal additional molecular reasons for this tissue specificity

Table 11-8	Common Sites of Metastasis	
Primary Tumor	Major Anatomic Pathway	Common Site of Distant Metastasis
Lung	Pulmonary vein, left ventricle	Multiple organs, including brain
Colorectal	Mesenteric lymphatics, portal venous system	Liver
	Inferior vena cava, right ventricle, pulmonary artery	Lungs
Testicular	Lymphatics to the periaortic area to the subclavian veins to the right ventricle	Lungs, liver, brain
Prostate	Regional lymphatics and veins, which drain to Batson plexus of presacral veins	Bones (especially lumbar spine), liver
Breast	Axillary, transpectoral, and internal mammary lymphatics	Bone, lung, brain, liver
Head and neck	Direct extension	Lymphatics, liver, bones
Ovarian	Direct extension, peritoneal seeding, mesenteric veins	Peritoneal surfaces, diaphragm, omentum, liver
Sarcoma (extremity)	Inferior vena cava, right ventricle, pulmonary artery	Lungs
Melanoma	Regional lymphatics	In transit lymphatics, lung, liver, brain, gastrointestinal tract

(Figure 11-24). Examples include interaction between α3β1 integrins binding to laminin-5 receptors in the lung, and the chemokine receptor CXCR4 on breast cancer cells promoting homing to lung tissues expressing the ligand CXCL12.[55]

Escape from the Circulation and Development of a New Microenvironment

As the study with women with ovarian cancer illustrates, pumping millions of cancer cells in the bloodstream does not necessarily cause metastatic disease. Cancer cells may arrive in a new location and survive but not proliferate to form a clinically relevant metastasis. The tumor cells that do not make the transition from simple survival to robust proliferation in a new location are said to be in a state of *dormancy*. This dormancy may account for the observation that solitary tumor cells can be detected in the blood years after a complete clinical remission in individuals, and that many people with detectable micrometastases will not develop clinically obvious metastases.[61,62] One of the factors that allow proliferation of cancer cells in the new environment may be cancer's recruitment of normal cells from local and circulating bone marrow stem cells. One developing concept is that successful metastatic tumor cells secrete factors that recruit circulating mesenchymal stem cells to the metastatic site (see Figure 11-12). These newly recruited stem cells then differentiate into tumor-supporting stroma and new blood vessels. One area of research is aimed at understanding why some micrometastases remain dormant; new therapies might block their progression to clinically important disease.

CLINICAL MANIFESTATIONS AND TREATMENT OF CANCER

Clinical Manifestations of Cancer

Diagnosis and Staging

Cancer can be discovered in many ways: after screening tests, routine exams, and after investigation of symptoms (see Box 11-2). The symptoms a cancer produces are as diverse as the types of cancer. The location of the cancer can determine symptoms by physical pressure, obstruction, and loss of normal function, or a cancer can cause problems far away from its source by pressing on nerves or secreting bioactive compounds. Whatever the initial complaint, once the diagnosis is suspected and a tumor has been identified, it is essential that tumor tissue be obtained to establish a definitive diagnosis and correctly classify the disease. Various methods of obtaining tissue are described in Table 11-9.

Once tissue is obtained, it is examined by the pathologist under the microscope for the histologic hallmarks of cancer detailed in the beginning of the chapter. The classification of the cancer can be further facilitated by a variety of clinically available tests, including immunohistochemical stains, flow cytometry, electron microscopy, chromosome analysis, and nucleic acid–based molecular studies.

If the diagnosis of cancer is established, it is critical to establish if the cancer has spread, known as the **stage** of the cancer. Staging initially involves determining the size of the tumor, the degree to which it has locally invaded, and the extent to which it has spread (metastasized) (Figure 11-25). Specific molecular tests are increasingly used in staging as well. Diverse schemes are used for staging different tumors. In general, a four-stage system is used, with carcinoma in situ regarded as a special case. Cancer confined to the organ of origin is stage 1, cancer that is locally invasive is stage 2, cancer that has spread to regional structures, such as lymph nodes, is stage 3, and cancer that has spread to distant sites, such as a liver cancer spreading to the lung or a prostate cancer spreading to bone, is stage 4. One common scheme for standardizing staging is the World Health Organization's TNM system: *T* for tumor spread, *N* for node involvement, and *M* indicating the presence of distant metastasis (see Figure 11-25). The prognosis generally worsens with increasing tumor size, lymph node involvement, and metastasis (Table 11-10). Staging also may alter the choice of therapy, with more aggressive therapy being delivered to more invasive disease.

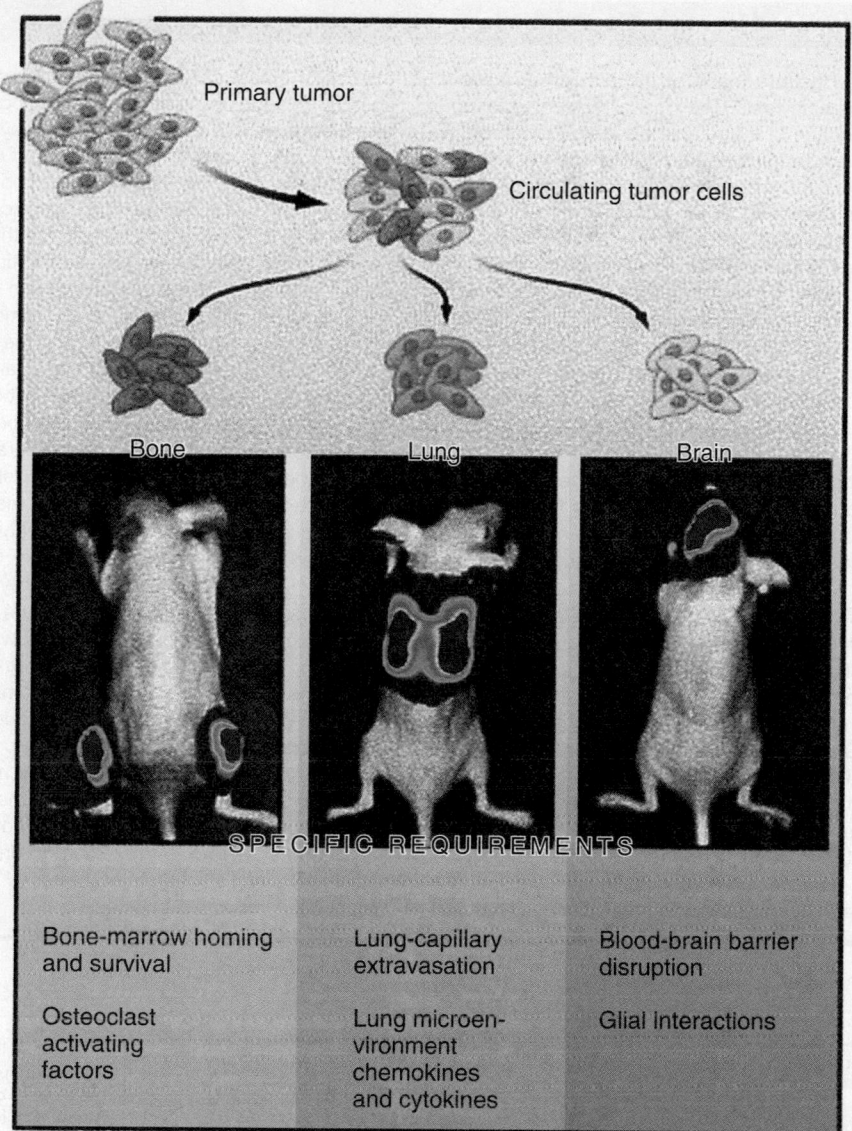

Figure 11-24 Clues as to how the patterns of metastatic spread are determined. Different cancer cells from the same cancer can spread to different locations. This is because tumors are heterogeneous mixtures of cells, with variations in the genes that are turned on and off. Different anatomic locations favor different types of cells. Studies with mice illustrated here show that expression of specific factors such as adhesion molecules, chemokines, and host factors such as blood-brain barrier disruption can favor the spread of specific cancer cells to different locations. In this example, cancer cells were visualized by genetically tagging cells with firefly luciferase for bioluminescent imaging. (From Gupta GP, Massagué J: Cancer metastasis: building a framework, *Cell* 127[4]:679-695, 2006.)

Table 11-9	Obtaining Tissue—The Biopsy	
Procedure	**Purpose**	**Example**
Excisional biopsy	Complete removal, usually with a margin of normal tissue	Full resection, e.g., mastectomy, partial colectomy
Incisional biopsy	Removal of a portion of a lesion	Lymph node biopsy, muscle mass biopsy
Core needle biopsy	Often performed with direct vision, or guided with ultrasound or computed tomography (CT)	Needle biopsy of prostate or liver mass
Fine needle aspiration	Obtains dissociated cells for cytology but does not preserve tissue structure	Thyroid, breast mass
Exfoliative cytology	Cells shed from the surface, for example, from cervix, sputum (lung) or urine.	Brushings from lung or colon endoscopy

Box 11-2   Screening Mammograms: Far from Perfect

Screening mammograms illustrate many of the difficulties faced by population-based screening tests. The goal of screening tests is early and accurate detection of a treatable disease. Professionals want screening tests not to miss disease (to have a low false-negative rate), and to avoid a lot of false alarms (a low false-positive rate). Ideally tests will not detect as abnormal, conditions that do not need treatment (overdiagnosis). Several large studies suggest that screening mammograms can prevent 15% to 20% of deaths from breast cancer when they are routinely performed in women ages 50 and older.[63-66] Screening mammograms may be valuable in younger women with a higher than average risk of breast cancer, for example, those with positive family histories. However, women with genetic predispositions may be more susceptible to the damaging effects of ionizing radiation. Screening methods have a significant downside.

The screening mammogram is far from a perfect test. Routine mammography might reduce the *relative* risk of dying from breast cancer by 15% to 20%, but because most women die of other diseases, the *absolute* reduction in risk of death from all causes is much lower, as low as 0.05% (i.e., 1 in 2000). Even this statistic is not absolute. In the combined Canadian National Breast Cancer studies following almost 90,000 women ages 40 to 59, mammography did not decrease deaths from breast cancer when added to routine physical and breast examinations.[67,68] Screening mammograms might miss 25% or more of breast cancers (the false-negative rate). In a subset of the same Canadian studies, screening approximately 32,000 women identified 45 cancers but missed another 39 that were found clinically within the next 12 months.[69] Screening mammograms also have a remarkably high false-positive rate: in the United States, 9 out of 10 suspicious mammograms interpreted as abnormal turn out not to be cancer.[70] Screening tens of thousands of healthy women annually delivers radiation that itself increases the risk of breast cancer, especially if screening starts at younger ages.[71] In addition, screening mammograms lead to significant **overdiagnosis** and **overtreatment**—they detect ductal carcinoma in situ (DCIS), a condition that might, but often does not, become a malignant disease. The problem with finding DCIS is that because some women with DCIS get cancer, once it is found, it is usually treated with lumpectomy and radiation therapy. The added unnecessary radiation therapy may cause additional health problems. This accumulation of findings, summarized in a recent Cochrane meta-analysis, found that screening 2000 women over 10 years can prevent one breast cancer fatality but at the same time unnecessarily turn 10 healthy women with DCIS into cancer patients.[65] The same authors have generated a fair amount of controversy by concluding: "It is thus not clear whether screening does more good than harm." Women considering screening mammography should be aware that not all experts agree on its value, especially for younger women.[65]

What to recommend? Because the more common the disease, the more effective the screening becomes, it makes sense to recommend screening to women older than 50, especially those with risk factors such as strong family histories of breast and ovarian cancer. Screening has the least benefit and the greatest risks among women younger than 50 with a negative family history. Good lifestyle choices, careful regular breast examinations, and improved analysis of targeted mammograms might do more to reduce breast cancer deaths than routine screening of the general population. From a public health perspective, the resources allocated to screening mammography might be better spent on primary prevention, delivering proven therapies to women without insurance, and more research on the root causes and early detection of breast cancer. Women need to understand the limited benefits and the often understated harms of screening mammography to make truly informed choices.

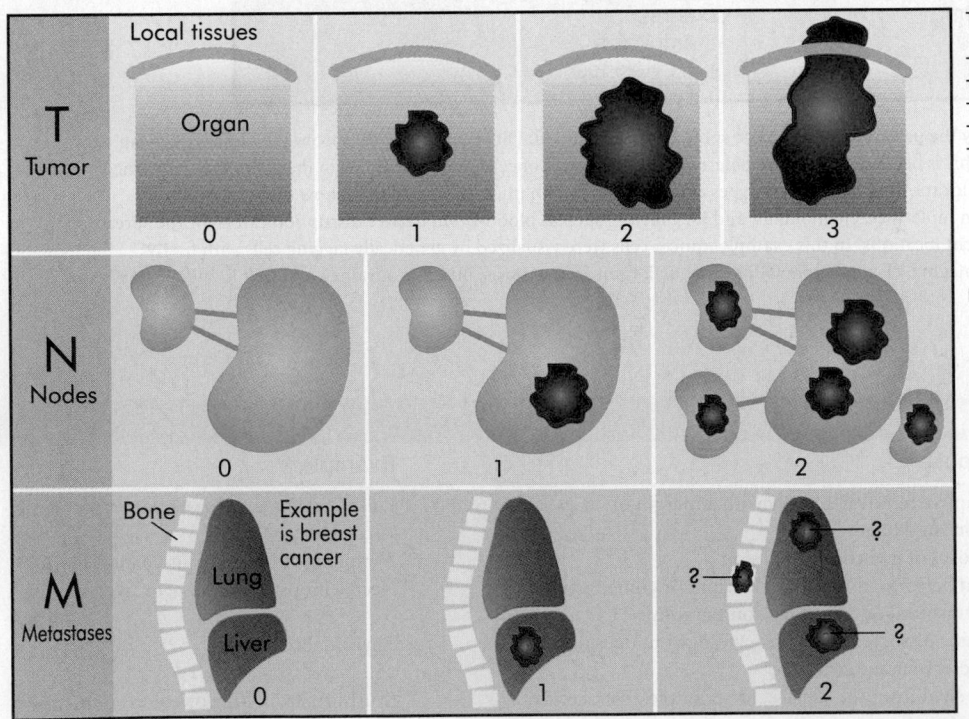

T = Primary tumor; the number equals size of tumor and its local extent. The number can vary according to site.
T0 = Breast free of tumor
T1 = Lesion <2 cm in size
T2 = Lesion 2-5 cm
T3 = Skin and/or chest wall involved by invasion

N = Lymph node involvement; a higher number means more nodes are involved.
N0 = No axillary nodes involved
N1 = Mobile nodes involved
N2 = Fixed nodes involved

M = Extent of distant metastases.
M0 = No metastases
M1 = Demonstrable metastases
M2 = Suspected metastases

Figure 11-25 Tumor staging by the TNM system. Example of staging for breast cancer.

Table 11-10   Cancer Survival Depends on Tumor Type and Stage of Disease

Disease	Stage			
	I	II	III	IV
Colon cancer	>90	75	50	<10
Hodgkin disease	99	95	85	70
Pancreatic cancer	37	26	10	1

Comment: Estimated percentage of individuals surviving 5 years for selected tumors, by stage at diagnosis. Additional factors such as age, molecular lesions, histologic subtypes, and type of treatment modify the outcome as well.

Cancer Treatment

The diagnosis of cancer has a profound effect on individuals and their families. Responses range from depression to resigned fatalism to aggressive no-holds-barred pursuit of therapy. The decision as to what type of therapy to follow should be based on a full consideration by the individual, the family, and the medical team of the individual's diagnosis, prognosis, and therapeutic options. Many types of cancer can be effectively treated with chemotherapy, radiotherapy, surgery, and combinations of these modalities. Caregivers must recognize that many individuals seek additional nonscience-based explanations and therapies and often use alternative therapies, either concurrently or sequentially. Alternative therapies can be biologically harmless or harmful; rarely is there any evidence they are medically effective and in the worst cases they can be expensive, delay the use of effective therapies, and produce unknown side effects. A challenge for the medical team is to provide the same level of psychosocial comfort and support that alternative therapies can provide, while also providing scientifically rational evidence-based therapies.

Chemotherapy

The era of modern chemotherapy began with the observation in World War II that mustard gas exposure caused suppression of the bone marrow. Related compounds, such as nitrogen mustard and cyclophosphamide, were then tested and produced clinical responses in hematologic malignancies, including lymphomas. Also in the late 1940s, based on the remarkable clinical observation that the vitamin folic acid could *increase* leukemia growth, antifolate drugs were developed (leading ultimately to methotrexate) that produced remissions in previously untreatable leukemias.[72]

All chemotherapeutic agents take advantage of specific vulnerabilities in target cancer cells. Antimetabolites, such as methotrexate and L-asparaginase, block normal growth pathways in all cells, but leukemia and other cancer cells are exquisitely sensitive to folic acid and asparagine deprivation, whereas nonmalignant cells are far less sensitive. Similarly, some cancer cells are highly sensitive to DNA-damaging agents, such as cyclophosphamide and anthracyclines, because of the oncogenic mutations that accelerate the cell cycle and DNA synthesis. Cellular checkpoints prevent normal cells treated with microtubule-directed drugs, such as vincristine and the taxanes, from going through mitosis, whereas cancer cells treated with these agents lack normal checkpoints, continue through mitosis, and undergo mitotic catastrophe (see Chapter 1).

Single chemotherapeutic agents often shrink cancers, but these drugs given alone rarely if ever provide a cure. Hence, chemotherapy drugs are usually given in combinations designed to attack a cancer from many different weaknesses at the same time and to limit the dose and therefore the toxicity of any single agent. Cancers contain a very large number of cells, and commonly a small fraction of those cells may be resistant to a particular drug. However, those cells are likely to be sensitive to the second or third drug in a chemotherapy cocktail. Scheduling of drug administration is also very important, with many studies showing cancers are more likely to develop drug resistance if there are significant delays between planned courses of chemotherapy.

The newest highly targeted agents used to treat cancer exploit specific vulnerabilities uncovered by molecular analysis in specific diseases (Table 11-11). These new drugs are still used in combination with conventional chemotherapy and, to be effective, they must be used in diseases in which the

Table 11-11   Examples of Molecular-Era Anticancer Drugs

Drug (Trade Name)	Type of Drug	Molecular Target	Disease
Imatinib (Gleevec)	Small-molecule kinase inhibitor	BCR-ABl tyrosine kinase, FGF receptor tyrosine kinase	Chronic myeloid leukemia (CML), gastrointestinal stromal tumor (GIST)
Erlotinib (Tarceva)	Small-molecule kinase inhibitor	EGF receptor tyrosine kinase	Subset of lung cancer
Trastuzumab (Herceptin)	Monoclonal antibody	HER2 receptor tyrosine kinase	HER2-positive breast cancer
Bevacizumab (Avastin)	Monoclonal antibody	VEGF receptor	Advanced colorectal cancer
Rituximab (Rituxau)	Monoclonal antibody	CD20 antigen on B lymphocytes	B-cell malignancies

EGF, Epidermal growth factor; *FGF,* Fibroblast growth factor; *EGF,* Vascular endothelial growth factor.

molecular target is present. Imatinib is highly effect in treating CML and gastrointestinal stromal tumor (GIST) but ineffective in virtually all other cancers. Fortunately, because these drugs are so tightly targeted they have much less toxicity than conventional chemotherapies that have targets in virtually all cells.

Chemotherapy can be used for several distinct purposes. **Induction chemotherapy** seeks to cause shrinkage or disappearance of tumors. In Hodgkin disease, chemotherapy alone can be used in some cases to cure the disease. In other settings, chemotherapy may shrink the tumor and improve symptoms without ultimately providing a cure. **Adjuvant chemotherapy** is given after surgical excision of a cancer with the goal of eliminating micrometastases. **Neoadjuvant chemotherapy** is given prior to localized (surgical or radiation) treatment of a cancer. As with induction chemotherapy, the effectiveness, or lack thereof, of neoadjuvant therapy can be measured, with follow-up scans. Neoadjuvant therapy can shrink a cancer so that surgery may spare more normal tissue. In the bone cancer *osteogenic sarcoma*, neoadjuvant therapy often converts a large tumor mass into a much smaller mass, allowing the surgeon to perform a limb-sparing excision rather than an amputation.

Radiation Therapy

Radiation therapy is used to kill cancer cells while minimizing damage to normal structures. Ionizing radiation damages cells by imparting enough energy to cause molecular damage, especially to DNA. The damage may be lethal, in which the cell is killed by radiation; potentially lethal, in which the cell is so severely affected by radiation that modifications in its environment will cause it to die; or sublethal, in which the cell can subsequently repair itself. Cellular compartments with rapidly renewing cells are, in general, more radiosensitive. Effective cell killing by radiation also requires good local delivery of oxygen, something not always present in large cancers. Radiation produces slow changes in most cancers and irreversible changes in normal tissues as well. Because of these irreversible changes, each tissue has a maximum lifetime dose of radiation it can tolerate. Radiation is well suited to treat localized disease in areas that are hard to reach surgically, overused in the brain and pelvis. A number of radiation delivery methods are available, with external beam being the most common. Radiation sources, such as small ^{125}iodine capsules (also called seeds), can also be temporarily placed into body cavities, a delivery method termed **brachytherapy.** Brachytherapy is useful in the treatment of cervical, prostate, and head and neck cancers.

Surgery

Surgery plays many roles in the care of individuals with cancer. The multiple approaches to obtaining tissue for diagnosis have been discussed. Surgery is often the definitive treatment of cancers that do not spread beyond the limits of surgical excision. It is also indicated for the relief of symptoms, such as those caused by tumor mass obstruction. In selected high-risk diseases, surgery plays a role in the prevention of cancer. Individuals with familial adenomatous polyposis have close to a 100% lifetime risk of colon cancer because of germline mutations of the *APC* gene, so a prophylactic colectomy is indicated. The role of prophylactic mastectomy in women with *BRCA1* mutations is more controversial.

Key principles apply specifically to cancer surgery, including obtaining adequate surgical margins during a resection to prevent local recurrences, placing needle tracks and biopsy incision scars (that may be contaminated with cancer cells) carefully so they can be removed in subsequent incisions, avoidance of the spread of cancer cells during surgical procedures through careful technique, and attention to obtaining adequate tissue specimens during biopsies so that the pathologist can be confident of the diagnosis. Additionally, the surgeon provides critical staging information by inspection, sampling, and removal of local and regional lymph nodes during procedures.

Complications of Cancer and Its Therapy

Paraneoplastic Syndromes

Paraneoplastic syndromes are symptom complexes that are triggered by a cancer but are not caused by direct local effects of the tumor mass. They are most commonly caused by biologic substances released from the tumor (e.g., hormones) or an immune response set off by the tumor. A small fraction of carcinoid tumors release hormones, including serotonin, into the bloodstream that cause flushing, diarrhea, wheezing, and rapid heartbeat. A number of cancers trigger an antibody response that attacks the nervous system, causing a variety of neurologic disorders that can precede other symptoms of cancer by months.[73]

Although infrequent, paraneoplastic syndromes are significant because they may be the earliest symptom of an unknown cancer and, in affected individuals, can be serious, often irreversible, and sometimes life threatening. Table 11-12 presents the classifications of paraneoplastic syndromes.

Pain

Pain is one of the most feared complications of advanced cancer. Although pain can be one of the presenting symptoms of cancer, most commonly there is little or no pain during the early stages of malignant disease. Significant pain, however, occurs in a large fraction of those individuals who are terminally ill with cancer. Pain is strongly influenced by fear, anxiety, sleep loss, fatigue, and overall physical deterioration. It occurs through an interaction among physiologic, cultural, and psychologic components.[30,74] (The neurophysiology of pain is discussed in Chapter 15.)

Cancer-associated pain can arise from a variety of direct and indirect mechanisms. Direct pressure, obstruction, invasion of a sensitive structure, stretching of visceral surfaces, tissue destruction, infection, and inflammation all can cause pain. Pain can occur at the site of the primary tumor or because of a distant metastatic lesion. Furthermore, pain may be referred away from the involved site and manifest, for example, as back pain.

Specific sites are more prone to cancer-associated pain. Bone metastases, common in advanced breast and prostate cancer, can cause significant pain because of periosteal irritation, medullary pressure, vertebral collapse, and pathologic fractures. Brain tumors (primary or metastatic) can, depending on the location, cause headache, seizures, or neurologic deficits. Pain in the abdomen may be caused by bowel obstruction, or inflammation and infection. Hepatic malignancies can stretch the liver, resulting in a dull pain or a feeling of fullness over the right upper abdominal quadrant. Mucosal surfaces can develop painful ulcerative lesions from the cancer, chemotherapy, and radiation or leukopenia, or both.

The diagnosis and treatment of pain are the primary responsibilities of the health care team. The individual's perception and, hence, reporting of pain can vary widely and be affected by such factors as age and cultural background. The first priority of treatment is to control pain rapidly and completely as judged by the individual.[30] The second priority

Table 11-12 Paraneoplastic Syndromes

Clinical Syndromes	Major Forms of Underlying Cancer	Causal Mechanism
Endocrinopathies		
Cushing syndrome	Small cell carcinoma of lung	ACTH or ACTH-like substance
	Pancreatic carcinoma	
	Neural tumors	
Syndrome of inappropriate antidiuretic hormone (SIADH) secretion	Small cell carcinoma of lung; intracranial neoplasms	Antidiuretic hormone or atrial natriuretic hormones
Hypercalcemia	Squamous cell carcinoma of lung	Parathyroid hormone–related protein (PTHRP), TGF-α, TNF, IL-1
	Breast carcinoma	
	Renal carcinoma	
	Adult T-cell leukemia/lymphoma	
	Ovarian carcinoma	
	Fibrosarcoma	
Hypoglycemia	Other mesenchymal sarcomas	Insulin or insulin-like substance
	Hepatocellular carcinoma	
	Bronchial adenoma (carcinoid)	
Carcinoid syndrome	Pancreatic carcinoma	Serotonin, bradykinin
	Gastric carcinoma	
	Renal carcinoma	
Polycythemia	Cerebellar hemangioma	Erythropoietin
	Hepatocellular carcinoma	
Nerve and Muscle Syndromes		
Myasthenia	Bronchogenic carcinoma	Immunologic
Disorders of the central and peripheral nervous systems	Breast carcinoma	
Dermatologic Disorders		
Acanthosis nigricans	Gastric carcinoma	Immunologic; secretion of epidermal growth factor
	Lung carcinoma	
	Uterine carcinoma	
	Bronchogenic, breast carcinoma	
Dermatomyositis		Immunologic
Osseous, Articular, and Soft Tissue Changes		
Hypertrophic osteoarthropathy and clubbing of the fingers	Bronchogenic carcinoma	Unknown
Vascular and Hematologic Changes		
Venous thrombosis (Trousseau phenomenon)	Pancreatic carcinoma	Tumor products (mucins that activate clotting)
	Bronchogenic carcinoma	
	Other cancers	
	Advanced cancers	
Nonbacterial thrombotic endocarditis	Thymic neoplasms	Hypercoagulability
Anemia		Unknown
Others		
Nephrotic syndrome	Various cancers	Tumor antigens, immune complexes

ACTH, Adrenocorticotropic hormone; *IL,* interleukin; *TGF,* transforming growth factor; *TNF,* tumor necrosis factor.
From Kumar V, Abbas AK, Fausto N: *Pathologic basis of disease,* ed 7, Philadelphia, 2005, Saunders.

is to prevent recurrence of pain. Objective measurements of pain are increasingly being included along with the reporting of more traditional vital signs. Many institutions are using specialized pain management teams that are trained to recognize different types of acute and chronic pain, as well as the individual's response to that pain. Many modalities are available to treat pain, ranging from combinations of NSAIDs and narcotics to palliative surgery and radiation therapy. Individual-controlled analgesia provides many benefits, not the least of which is regaining some control over one's own body. Although cancer pain is a complex problem arising from multiple sources, individuals should be assured that suffering is not inevitable and that relief is attainable.[75]

Fatigue

Fatigue is the most frequently reported symptom of cancer and cancer treatment. The exact mechanisms that produce fatigue are poorly understood.[76] Suggested causes include sleep disturbances, various biochemical changes secondary to disease and treatment, numerous psychosocial factors, level of activity, nutritional status, and other environmental and physical factors.[77]

The physiologic understanding of fatigue probably includes mechanisms for decreased muscle contractility. Overall, studies of muscle function suggest that some individuals with cancer may lose portions of muscle function needed to perform normal physical activities. Other areas of research include muscle function consequences from metabolic products of cancer treatment and associated muscle loss from circulating cytokines (e.g., tumor necrosis factor [TNF] and IL-1) (Figure 11-26). Similar to pain, fatigue is a subjective clinical manifestation. Fatigue is described by individuals with cancer as tiredness, weakness, lack of energy, exhaustion, lethargy, inability to concentrate, depression, sleepiness, boredom, lack of motivation, and decreased mental status. Some of these symptoms have been termed "chemo brain," or mild cognitive impairment. The changes in cognitive function can be caused by the cancer itself or the stress associated with the diagnosis of cancer, however, because symptoms similar to "chemo brain" also occur in individuals who have not received chemotherapy.[78]

Cachexia

The syndrome of **cachexia** includes a constellation of symptoms including anorexia, early satiety (filling), weight loss, anemia, asthenia (marked weakness), taste alterations, and altered protein, lipid, and carbohydrate metabolism. Cachexia is the most severe form of malnutrition associated with cancer and results in wasting, emaciation, and decreased quality of life (Figure 11-27).[79] Cachexia occurs in the face of seemingly adequate calorie intake because metabolic disturbances, including insulin resistance, hypertriglyceridemia, muscle wasting, and general increased derangement of metabolism, lead to significant inefficiency of energy usage. Anorexia, or loss of appetite, frequently worsens the weight loss associated with this abnormal metabolic state. Anorexia, itself, can be caused by pain, depression, chemotherapy, and/or radiotherapy. Alterations in taste by the same causes also

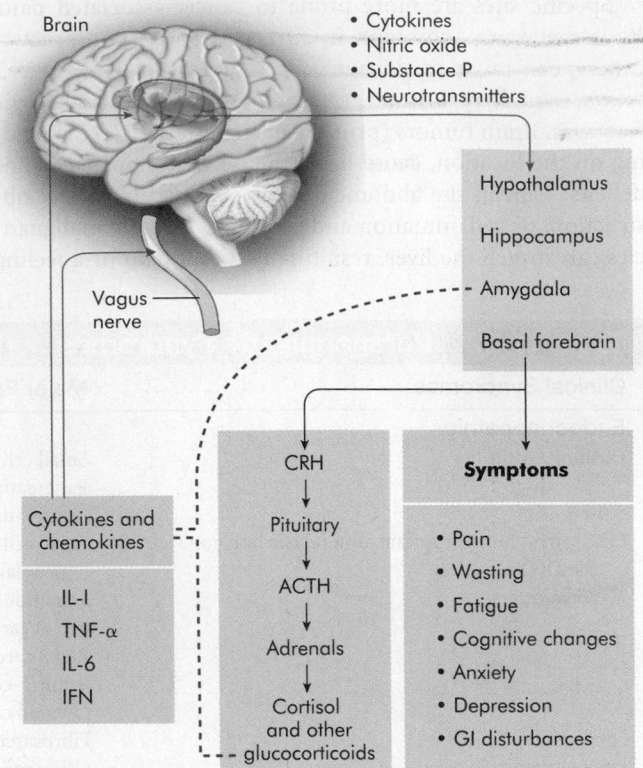

Figure 11-26 Theoretic framework for cytokine-induced cancer symptoms. Proinflammatory cytokines and chemokines (IL-1, TNF-α, IL-6, IFN) *(solid blue lines)* are released by immune cells. They exert their effects on peripheral nerves and the brain. Neurotransmitter responses by the brain are affected. The hypothalamic-pituitary-adrenal axis is activated with increased release of corticosteroids, which provide feedback *(dotted red lines)* to decrease cytokine production. *IL,* Interleukin; *IFN,* interferon; *TNF,* tumor necrosis factor. (Adapted from Cleeland CS et al: *Cancer* 97[11]:2919-2925, 2003.)

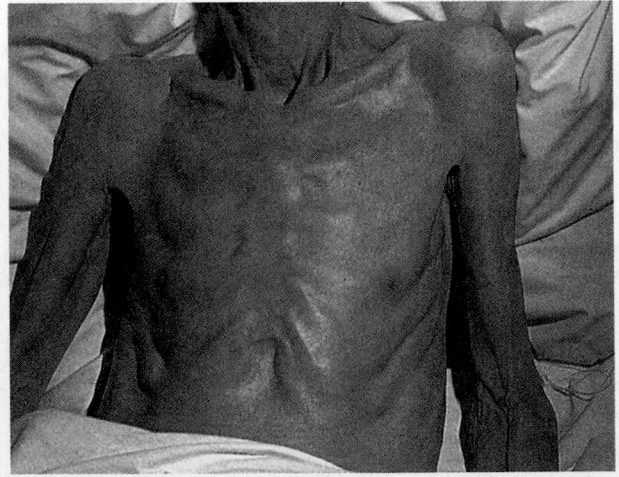

Figure 11-27 Cachexia. This severe form of malnutrition results in wasting and extensive loss of adipose tissue. (From Kamal A, Brockelhurst JC: *Color atlas of geriatric medicine,* ed 2, St Louis, 1991, Mosby.)

can account for the anorexia in people with cancer by making foods seem bland or distasteful.

Altered carbohydrate metabolism causes a syndrome resembling diabetes mellitus. Individuals show hyperinsulinemia, insulin resistance, hyperglycemia, and abnormal glucose tolerance test results. These disturbances cause increased gluconeogenesis, which produces glucose from amino acids. In starvation, protein usually is spared to protect vital structures, but in cancer, protein and fatty acids are used to meet energy needs.

An unusual and frustrating component of cancer care is the person's early satiety, or a sense of being full after only a few mouthfuls of food. Cytokines, including TNF-α, IL-6, and IFN-γ, appear to cause the metabolic alterations associated with tissue loss in cancer wasting. Tumor metabolites may also contribute to a cachectic state. For example, a factor found in the urine of some people with cancer induces the catabolism of muscle. This factor, originally called proteolysis-inducing factor, is a partial fragment of an antimicrobial peptide, dermcidin, normally expressed in the skin.[80] (Cytokines are discussed in detail in Chapter 6.)

Anemia

Anemia is commonly associated with malignancy, with 20% of patients having hemoglobin concentrations below 9 g/dl (normal value = 15 g/dl). Mechanisms that cause anemia in people with cancer include chronic bleeding resulting in iron deficiency, severe malnutrition, cytotoxic chemotherapy, and malignancy in blood-forming organs. Chronic bleeding and iron deficiency can accompany colorectal or genitourinary malignancy. Iron also is malabsorbed in individuals with gastric, pancreatic, or upper intestinal cancer. Often there is a defect in the reutilization of iron because of lack of transfer of iron from the storage pool to blood cell precursors. This defect may be caused by increased secretion of IL-6 and hepcidin.[81] Defects in erythropoietin production and shortened red cell survival have also been documented. In addition, anorexia can cause iron and folate deficiency. Megaloblastic (large red cell) anemias also may develop after methotrexate treatment.

Administration of erythropoietin, which stimulates production of erythrocytes, has been effective in correcting anemia in people with cancer; fewer red blood cell transfusions were required in most of the studied subjects. In addition, anemias occurring after chemotherapy or radiotherapy have been treated successfully with erythropoietin. However, studies have shown that aggressive use of erythropoietin increases the risk of blood clots and may worsen cancer survival, suggesting it should be reserved only for significant cancer-related anemia.[82]

Leukopenia and Thrombocytopenia

Direct tumor invasion of the bone marrow causes both leukopenia (decreased total white blood cell count) and thrombocytopenia (decreased number of platelets). More commonly, many chemotherapeutic drugs are toxic to the bone marrow, often causing granulocytopenia and thrombocytopenia. Granulocytopenia also can result from radiation therapy if it encompasses significant areas of the bone marrow. The duration of granulocytopenia and hence the risk of serious infection can be lessened by treatment with recombinant human granulocyte colony-stimulating factor (rhG-CSF, filgrastim).[83] rhG-CSF stimulates white blood cell precursors in the marrow to proliferate and differentiate rapidly. Thrombocytopenia is a major cause of hemorrhage in people with cancer and is often treated with platelet transfusions. Thrombocytopenia also is an accompanying disorder of disseminated intravascular coagulation that occurs in individuals with acute promyelocytic leukemia (see Chapter 20) and severe infections (see Chapter 25).

Infection

Infection is the most significant cause of complications and death in patients with malignant disease. When the absolute granulocyte count falls below 500 cells per μL, the risk of serious microbial (bacterial and fungal) infection increases. People with cancer also have debility with advanced disease, and immunosuppression from the underlying cancer and the radiotherapy and chemotherapy used to treat it. (Factors that predispose individuals with cancer to infection are summarized in Table 11-13.) Surgery also can lower resistance to infection because removal of large quantities of tissue, together with hemorrhage, dead spaces, and poor tissue perfusion can create favorable sites for infection. Hospital-acquired (nosocomial) infections increase because of indwelling medical devices, inadequate wound care, and the introduction of microorganisms from visitors and other individuals.

Gastrointestinal Tract

The entire gastrointestinal (GI) tract relies on rapidly growing cells to produce an effective barrier to trauma and infection and to provide an absorptive surface for nutrients. Chemotherapy and radiation therapy may cause a decreased cell turnover, thereby leading to oral ulcers (stomatitis), malabsorption, and diarrhea. The disruption of barrier defenses also increases the risk for infection, especially invasion by a person's own GI flora. Therapy-induced nausea, thought to be caused by an agent's direct action on the central nervous system's vomiting centers, historically has been a major obstacle in therapy.

Aggressive antinausea (antiemetic) therapy, including the centrally acting serotonin 5-HT3 antagonists such as ondansetron or dolasetron, have allowed better tolerance of highly emetogenic protocols. Other popular antiemetics include steroids and phenothiazines. Synthetic cannabinoids, the active ingredients in marijuana, increase appetite in addition to having antinausea properties. Analgesia often includes opiate agents, vital in treating severe cases of mucosal lesions. Supplemental nutrition through enteral or parenteral routes may be needed to combat malnutrition. Good oral care and close attention to hygiene may help prevent complications arising from mucosal membrane breakdown.

Hair and Skin

Alopecia (hair loss) results from chemotherapy effects on hair follicles. Alopecia is usually temporary, although hair may grow back with a different texture initially. Not all chemotherapeutic agents cause alopecia. Decreased renewal rates of the epidermal layers in the skin may lead to skin breakdown and dryness, altering the normal barrier protection

Table 11-13	Factors Predisposing Individuals with Cancer to Infection
Factor	**Basis**
Age	Many common malignancies occur mostly in older age.
	Immunologic functions decline with age.
	General debility reduces immunocompetence.
	Immobility predisposes to infection.
	Far-advanced cancer often results in immobility and general debility that worsens with age.
	Older adults are predisposed to nutritional inadequacies.
	Malnutrition impairs immunocompetence.
Tumor	Nutritional derangements can result.
	Sites and circumstances favorable to growth of microorganisms (obstruction, serous or blood effusion, ulceration) can be created.
	Far-advanced disease predisposes patients to debility and immobility.
	Humoral or cellular immune defects may result.
	Metastasis to bone marrow may cause leukopenia or other defects in immunity.
Leukemias	Inadequate granulocyte production (impaired phagocytosis) results.
	Thrombocytopenia (bleeding, breaks in skin integrity) can occur.
	Late effect: Chronic lung disease from *Pneumocystis jiroveci* pneumonia can develop during therapy.
Lymphomas and other mononuclear phagocyte malignancies	Humoral and cellular immune defects (anergy, altered immunoglobulin production) result.
	Late effect: splenectomy in children can cause increased susceptibility to infection.
Surgical treatment	Invasive procedure interrupts first lines of defense.
	Radical nature of surgery (removal of large blocks of tissue in lengthy procedures) causes hemorrhage, decreased tissue perfusion, creation of dead spaces, devitalization of tissues.
	Procedure may be "dirty" surgery (bowel, infected or contaminated areas).
	Surgery patients are often older and at poor risk.
	Long preoperative hospitalization often precedes surgery.
	Patients may have had previous adrenocorticosteroid therapy.
	Patients may have infections at sites remote from operative area.
	Nutritional derangements (especially important in head and neck surgery) may result.
	Lymph node dissection may predispose patient to local infection and impair containment to area.
	Gynecologic surgery may result in fistulas.
	Lung surgery may cause bronchopleural fistulas.
	Debility and immobility may result.

Data from Donovan MI, Girton SF: *Cancer care nursing*, ed 2, New York, 1984, Appleton-Century-Crofts; Murphy GP, Lawrence W, Lenhard RE: *Clinical oncology*, ed 2, New York, 1994, American Cancer Society.

against infection. Radiation therapy may cause skin erythema (redness) and contribute to breakdown.

Reproductive Tract

Radiation therapy and chemotherapy may affect the gametes, leading to varying degrees of decreased fertility and premature menopause. These effects are dose and age dependent, with the prepubertal gonad thought to be more resistant to damage. The potential for harm also is dependent on the agent used, with the alkylating category of chemotherapies carrying

the greatest risk. Craniospinal irradiation for central nervous system tumors also may affect the hypothalamus or pituitary gland, with subsequent secondary gonadal failure because of lack of production of gonadotropin-releasing hormone, luteinizing hormone, and follicle-stimulating hormone. The potential for reproductive harm should be addressed before therapy, if possible, with provisions made for sperm or embryo banking.

SUMMARY REVIEW

Cancer Characteristics and Terminology

1. Benign tumors are usually encapsulated and well differentiated and do not spread to distant locations.
2. Malignant tumors, compared with benign tumors, have more rapid growth rates, specific microscopic alterations (anaplasia, loss of differentiation), absence of normal tissue organization, and no capsule; they invade blood vessels and lymphatics and have distant spread.
3. Carcinomas arise from epithelial tissue, and leukemias are cancers of blood-forming cells. CIS refers to preinvasive epithelial tumors of glandular or squamous cell origin.
4. Localized cancer is considered low stage, whereas cancers that have spread regionally or distantly are termed *stage 3* and *stage 4*, respectively.
5. Cancer cells are characterized by anaplasia, or loss of differentiation, and autonomy, or independence, from normal cellular controls.
6. In the adult, undifferentiated cells not committed to a specific function are known as pluripotent cells, precursor cells, or adult stem cells. Cancerous growth depends on derangements of cell differentiation.
7. Tumor markers are substances (i.e., hormones, enzymes, genes, antigens, antibodies) found in cancer cells and in blood, spinal fluid, or urine. They are used to screen and identify individuals at high risk for cancer, to help diagnose specific types of tumors, and to follow the clinical course of cancer.

The Genetic Basis of Cancer

1. Genetic events are the primary basis of carcinogenesis. Mutations in cancer-causing genes accumulate with age, causing the increasing risk of cancer with advanced age.
2. Epidemiologic and molecular data suggest it takes five or six distinct mutations in different signaling pathways to produce cancer. Mutations activate growth-promotion pathways, block antigrowth signals, prevent apoptosis, turn on telomerase and new blood vessel growth, and allow tissue invasion and distant metastasis.
3. In rare families, cancer is inherited in an autosomal dominant fashion as a result of mutations in tumor suppressor genes such as *TP53*, *Rb*, and *BRCA1*.
4. Proto-oncogenes encode for growth factors (e.g., PDGF), growth-factor receptors (e.g., HER2), signal transducers (e.g., RAS), and nuclear growth-promoting proteins (e.g., MYC).
5. Three key genetic mechanisms have a role in human carcinogenesis: (1) activation of proto-oncogenes resulting in hyperactivity of growth-related gene products (such genes are called *oncogenes*); (2) mutation of genes resulting in loss or inactivity of gene products that normally would inhibit growth (such genes are called *tumor-suppressor genes*); and (3) mutation of genes resulting in overexpression of products that prevent normal cell death, or apoptosis, thus allowing continued growth of tumors.
6. Tumor-suppressor genes encode for proteins that act as inhibitors of growth-factor stimulation. Tumor-suppressor gene proteins block specific phases of the cell cycle, induce end-stage (e.g., terminal) differentiation, and stimulate cell senescence or death.
7. Carcinogenesis, or the development of cancer, involves both inactivation of tumor-suppressor genes (usually by loss of heterozygosity, or by "silencing") and activation of oncogenes.
8. Epigenetic changes in genes by DNA methylation and covalent histone modification can mimic mutation by heritably turning tumor-suppressor genes off.
9. Like many normal adult tissues, cancers can contain rare stem cells. To fully eradicate a cancer, it may be necessary to target the cancer stem cell.
10. Caretaker genes are responsible for maintaining genomic integrity. Inherited mutations can disrupt caretaker genes and cause chromosome instability.
11. A number of viruses can cause cancer. Human cervical cancer is caused by papillomavirus infection. Kaposi sarcoma is caused by infection with HHV8, a member of the herpesviridae family. Chronic hepatitis infection with HBV or HCV is the leading cause of liver cancer.
12. Defects in the immune system increase the risk of viral-associated cancers but have a minimal effect on the risk of other cancers.
13. Active inflammation predisposes to cancer by stimulating a wound-healing response that includes proliferation and new blood vessel growth.
14. Vaccinations can prevent hepatitis B–associated liver cancer and many human papillomavirus-caused cervical cancers
15. Chronic *H. pylori* causes stomach cancer and a rare lymphoma.
16. Metastasis is the major cause of death from cancer.
17. Cancers metastasize by several routes, including direct invasion and spread through lymphatics and veins.
18. Metastasis is a complex process that requires cells to have many new abilities, including the ability to invade, survive, and proliferate in a new environment and recruit new blood vessel growth.

Clinical Manifestations

1. The diagnosis of cancer requires a biopsy and examination of tumor tissue by a pathologist. Cancer classification is established by a variety of tests.
2. Tumor staging involves the size of the tumor, the degree to which it has locally invaded, and the extent to which it has spread. A standard scheme for staging is the T (tumor spread), N (node involvement), and M (metastasis) system.
3. Paraneoplastic syndromes are rare symptom complexes often caused by release of active substances from or stimulation of an immune response by a cancer that causes symptoms not directly caused by the local effects of the cancer.

Cancer Treatment

1. Cancer is treated with surgery, radiation therapy, chemotherapy, and combinations of these modalities.
2. The theoretic basis of chemotherapy is the vulnerability of tumor cells in various stages of the cell cycle. The goal of chemotherapy is to eradicate enough tumor cells so the body's natural defenses can eradicate remaining cells.
3. Modern chemotherapy uses combinations of drugs with different targets and different toxicities.
4. A new generation of specific targeted drugs attacks targets identified by the molecular analysis of cancers.
5. Ionizing radiation causes cell damage, so the goal of radiation therapy is to damage the tumor without causing excessive toxicity or damage to undiseased structures.
6. Surgical therapy is used for nonmetastatic disease, for which cure is possible by removing the tumor, and as a palliative measure to alleviate symptoms.
7. Clinical manifestations of cancer include pain, cachexia, anemia, leukopenia, thrombocytopenia, and infection.
8. Pain is generally associated with the late stages of cancer. It can be caused by pressure, obstruction, invasion of a structure sensitive to pain, stretching, tissue destruction, and inflammation.
9. Fatigue is the most frequently reported symptom of cancer and cancer treatment.

Continued

SUMMARY REVIEW—cont'd

10. Cachexia (loss of appetite, early satiety, weakness, inability to maintain weight, taste alterations, altered metabolism) leads to protein-calorie malnutrition and progressive wasting.

11. Anemia associated with cancer usually occurs because of malnutrition, chronic bleeding and resultant iron deficiency, chemotherapy, radiation, and malignancies in the blood-forming organs.

12. Leukopenia is usually a result of chemotherapy (which is toxic to bone marrow) or radiation (which kills circulating leukocytes).

13. Thrombocytopenia is usually the result of chemotherapy or malignancy in the bone marrow.

14. Infection may be caused by leukopenia, immunosuppression, or debility associated with advanced disease. It is the most significant cause of complications and death.

KEY TERMS

Adenocarcinoma, 361
Adjuvant chemotherapy, 383
Adult stem cell, 364
Anaplasia, 361, 362
Anchorage independent, 362
Angiogenesis, 369
Angiogenic factor, 369
Apoptosis, 369
Autocrine stimulation, 368
Autonomy, 362
Benign tumor, 361
Brachytherapy, 388
Cachexia, 390
Cancer, 361
Carcinoma, 361
Carcinoma in situ (CIS), 361
Caretaker gene, 375
Chromosome instability, 375
Chromosome translocation, 371
Clonal expansion, 368
Clonal proliferation, 368
DNA methylation, 373

Epigenetic change, 367
Epigenetic silencing, 375
Epigenetics, 367
Epithelial-mesenchymal transition (EMT), 382
Gene amplification, 372
Human T-cell leukemia-lymphoma virus (HTLV), 380
Immortal, 362
Induction chemotherapy, 388
Leukemia, 361
Loss of heterozygosity (LOH), 373
Lymphoma, 361
Malignant tumor, 361
Metastasis, 381
Multipotent, 364
Mutagen, 375
MYC protein, 370
Neoadjuvant chemotherapy, 383
Neoplasm, 361
Neovascularization, 383
Oncogene, 370

Overdiagnosis, 386
Overtreatment, 386
Paraneoplastic syndrome, 388
Personalized medicine, 362
Pleomorphic, 362
Point mutation, 370
Post-transplant lymphoproliferative disorder, (PTLD), 379
Proto-oncogene, 370
ras, 370
RAS, 368
Retinoblastoma (Rb) gene, 372
Sarcoma, 361
Silencing, 373
Stage, 384
Telomerase, 369
Telomere, 369
Transformation, 362
Tumor, 361
Tumor marker, 367
Tumor-suppressor gene, 370

REFERENCES

1. Kern SE: Progressive genetic abnormalities in human neoplasia. In Mendelsohn J et al: *The molecular basis of cancer*, Philadelphia, 2001, Saunders.
2. Morrow M, O'Sullivan MJ: The dilemma of DCIS. *Breast* 16(Suppl 2):S59-S62, 2007.
3. van't Veer LJ, Bernards R: Enabling personalized cancer medicine through analysis of gene-expression patterns, *Nature* 452(7187):564-570, 2008.
4. Skloot R: Henrietta's dance, *Johns Hopkins Magazine*, April 2000. Available at www.jhu.edu/~jhumag/0400web/01.html.
5. Reya T et al: Stem cells, cancer, and cancer stem cells, *Nature* 414(6859):105-111, 2001.
6. Al-Hajj M et al: Prospective identification of tumorigenic breast cancer cells, *Proc Natl Acad Sci U S A* 100(7):3983-3988, 2003.
7. Lapidot T et al: A cell initiating human acute myeloid leukaemia after transplantation into SCID mice, *Nature* 367(6464):645-648, 1994.
8. Bao S et al: Glioma stem cells promote radioresistance by preferential activation of the DNA damage response, *Nature* 444:756-760, 2006.
9. Armitage P, Doll R: The age distribution of cancer and a multi-stage theory of carcinogenesis, *Br J Cancer* 91(12):1983-1989, 2004.
10. Kinzler KW, Vogelstein B: Lessons from hereditary colorectal cancer. *Cell* 87(2):159-170, 1996.
11. Hanahan D, Weinberg RA: The hallmarks of cancer, *Cell* 100(1):57-70, 2000.
12. Ciardiello F, Tortora G: EGFR antagonists in cancer treatment, *N Engl J Med* 358(11):1160-1174, 2008.
13. Folkman J: Angiogenesis, *Annu Rev Med* 57:1-18, 2006.
14. Folkman J: Angiogenesis: an organizing principle for drug discovery? *Nat Rev Drug Discov* 6(4):273-286, 2007.

15. Mathon NF, Lloyd AC: Cell senescence and cancer, *Nat Rev Cancer* 1(3):203-213, 2001.
16. Shay et al: Targeting telomerase for cancer therapeutics, *Br J Cancer* 98(4):677-683, 2008.
17. van't Veer LJ et al: Gene expression profiling predicts clinical outcome of breast cancer, *Nature* 415(6871):530-536, 2002.
18. Kang Y et al: A multigenic program mediating breast cancer metastasis to bone, *Cancer Cell* 3(6):537-549, 2003.
19. Bos JL: *ras* oncogenes in human cancer: a review. *Cancer Res* 49(17):4682-4689, 1989.
20. Goldsby RE, Carroll WL: The molecular biology of pediatric lymphomas, *J Pediatr Hematol Oncol* 20(4):282-296, 1998.
21. Nowell P, Hungerford D: A minute chromosome in human granulocytic leukemia, *Science* 132:1497, 1960.
22. Druker BJ et al: Efficacy and safety of a specific inhibitor of the BCR-ABL tyrosine kinase in chronic myeloid leukemia, *N Engl J Med* 344(14):1031-1037, 2001.
23. Brodeur GM et al: Amplification of N-myc in untreated human neuroblastomas correlates with advanced disease stage, *Science* 224(4653):1121-1124, 1984.
24. Berns EM et al: Prevalence of amplification of the oncogenes c-myc, HER2/neu, and int-2 in one thousand human breast tumours: correlation with steroid receptors, *Eur J Cancer* 28(2-3):697-700, 1992.
25. Cavenee WK et al: Expression of recessive alleles by chromosomal mechanisms in retinoblastoma, *Nature* 305(5937):779-784, 1983.
26. Takahashi K, Yamanaka S: Induction of pluripotent stem cells from mouse embryonic and adult fibroblast cultures by defined factors, *Cell* 126(4):663-676, 2006.

27. Jones PA, Baylin SB: The epigenomics of cancer, *Cell* 128(4):683-692, 2007.

28. Baylin SB, Ohm JE: Epigenetic gene silencing in cancer—a mechanism for early oncogenic pathway addiction? *Nat Rev Cancer* 6(2):107-116, 2006.

29. Dokmanovic M, Clarke C, Marks PA: Histone deacetylase inhibitors: overview and perspectives, *Mol Cancer Res* 5(10):981-989, 2007.

30. Karpf AR, Jones DA: Reactivating the expression of methylation silenced genes in human cancer, *Oncogene* 21(35):5496-5503, 2002.

31. Rouse J, Jackson SP: Interfaces between the detection, signaling, and repair of DNA damage, *Science* 297(5581):547-551, 2002.

32. Liu B et al: Analysis of mismatch repair genes in hereditary non-polyposis colorectal cancer patients, *Nat Med* 2(2):169-174, 1996.

33. Lengauer C, Kinzler KW, Vogelstein B: Genetic instability in colorectal cancers, *Nature* 386(6625):623-627, 1997.

34. Weaver BA et al: Aneuploidy: instigator and inhibitor of tumororigenesis instability, *Cancer Res* 67(21):10103-10105, 2007.

35. Jorde LB et al: *Medical genetics*, ed 3 , St. Louis, 2005, Mosby.

36. Schneider K: *Counseling about cancer: strategies for genetic counseling*, ed 2 , Hoboken, NJ, 2001, Wiley.

37. Coussens LM, Werb Z: Inflammation and cancer, *Nature* 420(6917):860-867, 2002.

38. Fitzpatrick FA: Inflammation, carcinogenesis and cancer, *Int Immunopharmacol* 1(9-10):1651-1667, 2001.

39. Vesterinen E et al: Cancer incidence among 78,000 asthmatic patients, *Int J Epidemiol* 22(6):976-982, 1993.

40. Dubé C et al: The use of aspirin for primary prevention of colorectal cancer: a systematic review prepared for the U.S. Preventive Services Task Force, *Ann Int Med* 146(5):365-375, 2007.

41. Stewart T et al: Incidence of de-novo breast cancer in women chronically immunosuppressed after organ transplantation, *Lancet* 346(8978):796-798, 1995.

42. Vajdic CM et al: Cancer incidence before and after kidney transplantation, *JAMA* 296(23):2823-2831, 2006.

43. Howley PM, Ganem D, Kieff E: Etiology of cancer: DNA viruses. In DeVita VT, et al: *Cancer: principles and practice of oncology*, ed 8 , Philadelphia, 2008, Lippincott Williams & Wilkins.

44. Poeschla EM et al: Etiology of cancer: RNA viruses. In DeVita VT et al: *Cancer: principles and practice of oncology*, ed 8 , Philadelphia, 2008, Lippincott Williams & Wilkins.

45. Paavonen J, Lehtinen M: Introducing human papillomavirus vaccines—questions remain, *Ann Med* 40(3):162-166, 2008.

46. Buell JF et al: Malignancy in pediatric transplant recipients, *Semin Pediatr Surg* 15(3):179-187, 2006.

47. Yang XR et al: Evaluation of risk factors for nasopharyngeal carcinoma in high-risk nasopharyngeal carcinoma families in Taiwan, *Cancer Epidemiol Biomarkers Prev* 14(4):900-905, 2005.

48. *Helicobacter* and Cancer Collaborative Group: Gastric cancer and *Helicobacter pylori*: a combined analysis of 12 case control studies nested within prospective cohorts, *Gut* 49(3):347-353, review, 2001.

49. Ushijima T: Epigenetic field for cancerization, *J Biochem Mol Biol* 40(2):142-150, 2007.

50. Wong BC et al: *Helicobacter pylori* eradication to prevent gastric cancer in a high-risk region of China: a randomized controlled trial, *JAMA* 291(2):187-194, 2004.

51. Correa P, Houghton J: Carcinogenesis of *Helicobacter pylori*, *Gastroenterol* 133(2):659-672, 2007.

52. Isaacson PG, Du MQ: MALT lymphoma: from morphology to molecules, *Nat Rev Cancer* 4(8):644-653, 2004.

53. Fyles AW et al: Tamoxifen with or without breast irradiation in women 50 years of age or older with early breast cancer, *N Engl J Med* 351:963-970, 2004.

54. Carrick S et al: Single agent versus combination chemotherapy for metastatic breast cancer, *Cochrane Database Syst Rev* (2) CD003372, 2005.

55. Gupta GP, Massagué J: Cancer metastasis: building a framework, *Cell* 127(4):697-708, 2006.

56. Fidler IJ: The pathogenesis of cancer metastasis: the "seed and soil" hypothesis revisited, *Nat Rev Cancer* 3:453-458, 2003.

57. Tarin D et al: Clinicopathological observations on metastasis in man studied in patients treated with peritoneovenous shunts, *BMJ* 288(6419):749-751, 1984.

58. López-Otín C, Matrisian LM: Emerging roles of proteases in tumour suppression, *Nat Rev Cancer* 7(10):800-808, 2007.

59. Dwayne G et al: Potentiation of neuroblastoma metastasis by loss of caspase-8, *Nature* 439(7072):95-99, 2006.

60. Schackert G, Fidler IJ: Site-specific metastasis of mouse melanomas and a fibrosarcoma in the brain or meninges of syngeneic animals, *Cancer Res* 48:3478-3484, 1998.

61. Aguirre-Ghiso JA: Models, mechanisms and clinical evidence for cancer dormancy, *Nat Rev Cancer* 7(11):834-846, 2007.

62. Meng S et al: Circulating tumor cells in patients with breast cancer dormancy, *Clin Cancer Res* 10(24):8152-8162, 2004.

63. Armstrong K et al: Screening mammography in women 40 to 49 years of age: a systematic review for the American College of Physicians, *Ann Intern Med* (146):516-526, 2007.

64. Fletcher SW, Elmore JG: Clinical practice: Mammographic screening for breast cancer, *N Engl J Med* (348):1672-1680, 2003.

65. Gøtzsche PC, Nielsen M: Screening for breast cancer with mammography, *Cochrane database of systematic reviews (Online)* CD001877, 2006.

66. Qaseem et al: Screening mammography for women 40 to 49 years of age: a clinical practice guideline from the American College of Physicians, *Ann Intern Med* (146):511-515, 2007.

67. Miller AB et al: Canadian National Breast Screening Study-2: 13-year results of a randomized trial in women aged 50-59 years, *J Natl Cancer Inst* (92):1490-1499, 2000.

68. Miller AB et al: The Canadian National Breast Screening Study-1: breast cancer mortality after 11 to 16 years of follow-up. A randomized screening trial of mammography in women age 40 to 49 years, *Ann Intern Med* (137):305-312, 2002.

69. Baines et al: Impact of menstrual phase on false-negative mammograms in the Canadian National Breast Screening Study, *Cancer* (80):720-724, 1997.

70. Elmore JG et al: International Variation in Screening Mammography Interpretations in Community-Based Programs, *J Natl Cancer Inst* 95(18):1384-1395.

71. Berrington de González A, Reeves G: Mammographic screening before age 50 years in the UK: comparison of the radiation risks with the mortality benefits, *Br J Cancer* (93):590-596, 2005.

72. Chu E, DeVita VT Jr: In DeVita VT, et al: editors: *Cancer: Principles and practice of oncology*, ed 8, Philadelphia, 2008, Lippincott Williams & Wilkins.

73. Darnell RB, Posner JB: Paraneoplastic syndromes involving the nervous system, *N Engl J Med* 349:1543-1554, 2003.

74. Esteller M et al: A gene hypermethylation profile of human cancer, *Cancer Res* 61(8):3225-3229, 2001.

75. Dy SM et al: Evidence-based standards for cancer pain management, *J Clin Oncol* 26(23):3879-3885, 2008.

76. Ryan JL et al: Mechanisms of cancer-related fatigue, *Oncologist* 12(Suppl 1):22-34, 2007.

77. Miller AH et al: Neuroendocrine-immune mechanisms of behavioral comorbidities in patients with cancer, *J Clin Oncol* 26(6):971-982, 2008.

78. Hess LM, Insel KC: Chemotherapy-related change in cognitive function: a conceptual model, *Oncol Nurs Forum* 34(5):981-994, 2007.

79. Baracos VE: Cancer-associated cachexia and underlying biological mechanisms, *Annu Rev Nutr* 26:435-461, review, 2006.

80. Porter D et al: A neural survival factor is a candidate oncogene in breast cancer, *Proc Natl Acad Sci* 100(10):10931-10936, 2003.

81. Nemeth E et al: IL-6 mediates hypoferremia of inflammation by inducing the synthesis of the iron regulatory hormone hepcidin, *J Clin Invest* 113(9):1271-1276, 2004.

82. Kelly AM, Khuri FR: Unraveling the mystery of erythropoietin-stimulating agents in cancer promotion, *Can Res* 68:4013-4017, 2008.

83. Bhana N: Granulocyte colony-stimulating factors in the management of chemotherapy-induced neutropenia: evidence based review, *Curr Opin Oncol* 19(4):328-335, 2007.

CANCER EPIDEMIOLOGY

KATHRYN L. McCANCE

MEDIA RESOURCES

CHAPTER OUTLINE

GENES, ENVIRONMENTAL-LIFESTYLE FACTORS,
    AND RISK FACTORS
    Epigenetics and Genetics
    Tobacco Use
    Diet
    Alcohol Consumption
    Ionizing Radiation
    Ultraviolet Radiation

Electromagnetic Radiation
Sexual and Reproductive Behavior: Human
    Papillomaviruses
Other Viruses and Microorganisms
Physical Activity
Chemicals and Occupational Hazards
    as Carcinogens
Air Pollution

Although cancer arises from a complicated and an interacting web of multiple causes, preventing exposures to **individual carcinogens**, or cancer-causing substances, may prevent many cancers. Research has shown that environmental-lifestyle factors and occupational exposure fuels the number of cancer cases and deaths.[1-3] Widespread general exposure to pollutants from water; air; the work environment; personal lifestyle choices (such as smoking, excessive alcohol, and poor diet) and involuntary or unknowing exposures to carcinogens in the air, water, and occupational environments are major contributors to cancer. The National Cancer Institute (NCI) and the National Institute for Environmental Health Sciences (NIEHS) notes in the document titled "Cancer and the Environment" that two thirds of all cancers are caused by environmental-lifestyle factors.[3]

GENES, ENVIRONMENTAL-LIFESTYLE FACTORS, AND RISK FACTORS

Cancers are caused by environmental-lifestyle and genetic factors. At the level of the cell, cancer is genetic. Although complex, investigators are struggling to connect the complex web between genotype, phenotype, and the environment to understand a person's chances of developing cancer. Environmental-lifestyle factors include cigarette smoking, excessive alcohol consumption, poor diet, lack of exercise, excessive sunlight exposure, and sexual behavior that increases exposure to certain viruses. Additional factors include exposure to radiation, hormones, medical drugs, viruses, bacteria, pesticides, and other environmental chemicals present in air, water, food, soil, and the workplace. Investigations of occupational groups with high exposure to chemicals have identified numerous chemicals as carcinogens (Table 12-1).

Studies of gene-environmental interactions whereby individuals with particular genetic predispositions may be more susceptible to the biologic effects of environmental exposures cannot explain the increased cancer risk in studies of exposed groups. More simply, it appears that the majority of cancers are caused by carcinogen exposure, rather than by rare genetic conditions.[2] For example, for women who have mutated cancer susceptibility genes, *BRCA1* or *BRCA2*, the risk of having breast cancer at age 50 is 24% for those born before 1940 but 67% for those born later.[4] The implication here is related to lifestyle factors that changed from 1940 (i.e., hormone therapy, later age at first pregnancy, increased

Text continued on p 401.

Table 12-1	Summary of Environmental and Occupational Links with Cancer			
Category	Carcinogenic Agent	Source/Uses	Strong*	Suspected†
Aromatic amines	Benzidine, 1-naphylamine, 4,4'-methlyenebis 2-choloraniline (MOCA), chlornaphazine heterocyclic aromatic amines	Antioxidants in the production of rubber and cutting oils, intermediates in azo dye manufacturing, and as pesticides. Contaminant in chemical and mechanic industries and aluminum transformation and an air contaminant from tobacco smoking. Used widely in the textile industry and as hair dyes.	Bladder (benzidine, 2-naphylamine, 4,4'-methylenebis, 2-choloraniline (MOCA), chlornaphazine)	Prostate (heterocyclic aromatic amines)
Chlorination byproducts	Trihalomethanes	Chloroform, bromodichloromethane, chlorodibromomethane, and bromoform. Result from the interaction of chlorine with organic chemicals. Several halogenated compounds may form from these reactions although trihalomethanes are the most common. Brominated byproducts are also formed from the reaction of chlorinated byproducts with low levels of bromide in drinking water.		Bladder, rectal
Environmental tobacco smoke	Contains more than 50 known carcinogens	Environmental tobacco smoke (ETS, also known as passive smoke), is a combination of smoke emitted from the burning end of a cigarette, cigar, or pipe and smoke exhaled by the smoker.	Lung; breast	
Metals	Arsenic	A byproduct of nonferrous metal production, mostly from copper production, comprising greater than 10% of dust content in some smelter operations. Inorganic arsenic is commonly used to preserve wood but also as a pesticide on cotton plants.	Bladder, lung, skin, soft tissue sarcoma (angiosarcoma of the liver)	Brain/CNS, kidney, liver and biliary, prostate, soft tissue sarcoma
	Beryllium	Nuclear, aircraft, and medical devices industry. An alloy or in specialty ceramics for electrical and electronic applications. Found as a contaminant in the combustion of coal and fuel oil.	Lung	
	Cadmium	Occurs naturally in ores together with zinc, lead and copper. Used as stabilizers in PVC products, color pigment, several alloys and now most commonly in rechargeable nickel-cadmium batteries. Also present as a pollutant in phosphate fertilizers.	Lung	Pancreatic, kidney, prostate
	Chromium	Chromium is used in steel and other alloy production. Chromium III and chromium VI are used in chrome plating, the manufacture of dyes and pigments, leather tanning, and wood preserving.	Lung, nasal and nasopharynx	
	Lead	Used primarily in the production of batteries, ammunition, metal products such as solder and pipes, and devices to shield x-rays. Lead is also found in gasoline, paints, ceramic products, caulking, and pipe solder, but has been reduced dramatically in the United States.		Brain/CNS, kidney, stomach
	Nickel	Used primarily as an alloy in stainless steel. Also used in nickel plating and battery production.	Lung, nasal and nasopharynx	Laryngeal, pancreatic, stomach

Continued

Table 12-1 Summary of Environmental and Occupational Links with Cancer—cont'd

Category	Carcinogenic Agent	Source/Uses	Strong	Suspected†
Metalworking fluids and/or mineral oils	Straight oils, soluble oils, synthetic and semisynthetic fluids	Used in a variety of industries including metal machining, print press operating, and cotton and jute spinning.	Bladder, laryngeal, lung, nasal and nasopharynx (mineral oils), rectal, skin, stomach	Esophageal; pancreatic; prostate
Natural fibers/dust	Asbestos	An inorganic naturally occurring fibrous silicate particle used primarily in acoustical and thermal insulation. Asbestos fibers can be divided into two groups: chrysolite (most widely used) and amphibole which include amosite, crocidolite, anthophyllite, actinolite, and tremolite fibers.	Laryngeal, lung, mesothelioma	
	Silica	An inorganic particle used in foundries, brick-making and sandblasting.	Lung	
	Talc containing asbestiform fibers	A mineral used in the manufacture of pottery, paper, paint, and cosmetics.	Lung	
	Wood dust	Used primarily in carpentry, joinery, and in furniture and cabinetry making.	Lung, nasal and nasopharynx	Laryngeal
Pesticides	Herbicides, fungicides, and insecticides	Used for preventing, destroying, repelling, or mitigating any pest or in use as a plant regulator, defoliant, or desiccant. The majority of pesticides as registered with the U.S. EPA are used in agricultural applications, although residential application is also an important source.		Brain/CNS, breast, colon, Hodgkin lymphoma, leukemia, lung, multiple myeloma, non-Hodgkin lymphoma, ovarian, pancreatic, kidney, soft tissue sarcoma, stomach, testicular
Petrochemicals and combustion byproducts	Petroleum products, motor vehicle exhaust (including diesel), polycyclic aromatic hydrocarbons (PAHs), soot, and dioxins	Petrochemicals are derived from natural gas or petroleum and used to produce a variety of other chemicals and materials including pesticides, plastics, medicines, and dyes. Substances can be produced as the building blocks for other products, but mainly result from the incomplete combustion of burning coal, oil, gas (diesel exhaust), household waste, tobacco, and other organic substances. Dioxins are a class of chemical that are the byproducts of combustion processes containing chlorine and carbon-based chemicals such as polyvinyl chloride (PVC) plastics. Dioxins are also created during the chlorine-bleaching processes for whitening paper and wood pulp.	Lung (PAHs, air pollution including diesel exhaust, soot, dioxin), NHL (dioxin), soft tissue sarcoma (dioxin), skin (PAHs)	Bladder (PAHs), breast (dioxin), esophageal (soot), laryngeal (PAHs), multiple myeloma (dioxin), prostate (dioxin and PAHs)
Radiation	Ionizing radiation	Any one of several types of particles and rays given off by radioactive material, high-voltage equipment, nuclear reactions, and stars. Alpha and beta particles, x-rays and γ-rays are radiation particles of concern to human health.	Bone, brain and CNS, breast, leukemia, liver and biliary, lung, multiple myelomas, soft tissue sarcoma, skin, thyroid	Bladder, colon, nasal and nasopharynx, ovarian, stomach
	Nonionizing	Composed of microwaves and electromagnetic frequencies including radio waves and extremely low-frequency electromagnetic fields.		Brain, breast, leukemia
	Ultraviolet radiation	Ultraviolet radiation is part of the solar radiation emitted by the sun.	Skin	

	Agent	Description		
Reactive chemicals	Butadiene	Used in the production of polymers for the manufacture of styrene-butadiene rubber for tires; nitrile rubber for hoses, gaskets, adhesives and footwear; acrylonitrile-butadiene-styrene polymers for parts, pipes, and various appliances; and styrene-butadiene latexes for paints and carpet backing.		Leukemia
	Ethylene oxide	Used as a sterilant, disinfectant, and pesticide. It is also used as a raw ingredient in making resins, films, and antifreeze.	Leukemia	Breast
	Formaldehyde	Primary use is in the production of urea, phenol, or melamine resins for molded products such as appliances, electric controls, and telephones; in particle-board, plywood, and surface coatings.		Nasal and nasopharynx
	Mustard gas	Produced and used primarily in World War I as a chemical warfare agent.	Lung	Laryngeal
	Vinyl chloride	Vinyl chloride is used in polyvinyl resins for the production of plastic pipes, floor coverings, and in electrical and transportation applications.	Liver and biliary, soft tissue sarcoma (angiosarcoma of the liver)	
	Sulfuric acid	Used widely in industry for the production of isopropanol, ethanol; treatment of metals; and the manufacture of soaps; detergents; and batteries.	Laryngeal	Lung
	Benzene	Used as an intermediate in the production of plastics, resins, and some synthetic and nylon fibers. Also used to make some types of rubbers, lubricants, dyes, detergents, drugs, and pesticides. Is also found in crude oil, gasoline, and cigarette smoke.	Leukemia, NHL	Brain/CNS, lung, nasal and nasopharynx, multiple myeloma
Solvents	Carbon tetrachloride	Used primarily in various industrial applications. Before being banned, it was also used in the production of refrigeration fluid and propellants for aerosol cans, as a pesticide, as a cleaning fluid and degreasing agent, in fire extinguishers, and in spot removers.		Leukemia
	Methylene chloride	Used primarily as a solvent in industrial applications and as a paint stripper. It may also be found in some aerosol and pesticide products and in the production of photographic film.		Brain/CNS, liver and biliary
	Styrene	Used in the production of rubber, plastic, insulation, fiberglass, pipes, automobile parts, food containers, and carpet backing.		NHL
	Toluene	Used in the production of paints, paint thinners, fingernail polish, lacquers, adhesives, and rubber. Also used in some printing and leather-tanning processes.		Brain/CNS, lung, rectal
	Trichloroethylene (TCE)	Mainly used for degreasing metal parts. Previous use as a dry cleaning agent. TCE may be found in printing inks, varnishes, adhesives, paints, and lacquers. Important contaminant in the general environment as a result of emissions and leakage from industrial settings.	Liver and biliary, kidney	Cervical, Hodgkin lymphoma, leukemia, NHL, kidney
	Tetrachloroethylene (PCE)	Used to degrease metal parts and as a solvent in a variety of industrial applications. Since the 1930s it was used by an increasingly large percentage of U.S. dry-cleaning operations.		Bladder, cervical, esophageal, NHL, kidney
	Xylene(s)	Used as a cleaning agent, a thinner for paint, and in paint and varnishes; in printing rubber and leather industries; and found in small amounts in gasoline and airplane fuel.		Brain/CNS, rectal

Continued

Table 12-1 Summary of Environmental and Occupational Links with Cancer—cont'd

Category	Carcinogenic Agent	Source/Uses	Strong*	Suspected†
Other	Creosotes	Includes coal tar and coal tar pitch formed by high-temperature treatment of wood or coal or from the resin of the creosote bush. Wood creosote was historically used as a disinfectant, laxative, and cough treatment. Coal tar products are used in medicine, animal and bird repellents, and pesticides. Coal tar, coal tar pitch, and coal tar pitch volatiles are used in roofing, road paving, aluminum smelting, and coking.	Bladder (coal tars), lung, skin	
	Endocrine disruptors	A number of chemicals capable of mimicking the body's natural hormones. See: www.ourstolenfuture.org/Basics/chemlist.htm.	Breast (DES); cervical (DES)	Breast, prostate, testicular
	Hair dyes	Coloring products used on hair. Hair dyes usually fall into one of four categories: temporary, semipermanent, demi, and permanent. Chemical agents used in dyes are specific to the color and the degree of permanency.		Bladder, brain/CNS, leukemia, multiple myeloma, NHL
	Nitrosamines and N-nitroso compounds	A class of chemicals that forms as a result when anines and nitrosating agents chemically react. Found in the rubber, metal, and agricultural industries, and in cosmetics and foods such as fried bacon and cured meats.		Brain/CNS
	Polychlorinated biphenyls (PCBs)	Used as coolants and lubricants in transformers, capacitors, and other electrical equipment. PCBs were banned in the United States in 1997.	Liver and biliary	Breast, NHL

*Strong causal evidence of a causal link is based primarily on a Group 1 designation by the International Agency for Research on Cancer.
†Suspected evidence of a causal link is based on our assessment that results of epidemiologic studies is mixed, yet positive findings from well-designed and conducted studies warrant precautionary action and additional scientific investigation.
CNS, Central nervous system; DES, diethylstilbestrol; EPA, Environmental Protection Agency; NHL, non-Hodgkin lymphoma.
From Clapp RW, Jacobs MM, Loechler EL: Environmental and occupational causes of cancer: new evidence, 2005-2007. Lowell Center for Sustainable Production, Lowell, MA. Cancer working Group of the Collaborative on Health and the Environment.

nulliparity, etc.). Investigations of more complex gene-gene environment interactions and proteomics may or may not alter these conclusions.

Strong evidence suggests that certain environmental-lifestyle and occupational exposures are associated with bladder cancer, bone, brain and central nervous system (CNS) cancer, breast cancer, Ewing sarcoma, liver cancer, laryngeal cancer, melanoma, mesothelioma, non-Hodgkin lymphoma (NHL), renal cancer, scrotal cancer, skin cancer, soft tissue sarcoma, and thyroid cancer (see Table 12-1).

Although tobacco smoke remains the single most preventable cause of cancer, it is not linked to the majority of cancers that have increased substantially in the United States. These cancers include melanoma, non-Hodgkin lymphoma, testicular, brain, and thyroid.[2] For example, testicular cancer affects men mostly in their 20s and 30s. Incidence rates in these age groups in the United States increased about 75% from the 1970s to the 1980s and remain about 11 to 12/100,000. This increase is *not* attributed to improved diagnostic methods and cancer registration rates.[5] Among all population groups, brain and nervous system cancers increased from 10 in 1973 to 20.9 in 1992—an astounding 109% increase.[2,6]

Lung cancer rates have risen and fallen paralleling the prevalence of smoking. Meanwhile, stomach cancer in the United States dropped dramatically over the past century.[2] The decrease may be caused by lifestyle factors or decreasing or controlling bacterial infection from *Helicobacter pylori*, or both.

Compelling is the role of environmental-lifestyle contributions to cancer from studies comparing different populations around the world. Breast cancer, for example, is prevalent among northern Europeans and Americans but is relatively rare among women in developing countries. If ethnicity played a major role, then immigrants should retain the cancer incidence rates of their country of origin. Instead, immigrants acquire the same cancer rates of where they move within one or two generations.[7,8] A particularly instructive group of studies has been the Multiethnic Cohort (MEC) study. These studies are focused on ethnic and migrant populations in Hawaii, which has large populations of ethnic groups that assist with interethnic comparisons and disentangling the effects of genes, the environment, and lifestyle on cancer rates. These results and others support the claim that cancer risk is substantially influenced by environmental factors (Box 12-1).

Elevated cancer rates are more common in cities, in farming locations, near hazardous waste sites, downwind of industrial and radiation activities, and near contaminated water wells. In addition, cancers are associated with areas of high pesticide use, toxic work exposures, waste incinerators, and other sources of pollution.[9,10]

Farmers have increased death rates from brain, multiple myeloma, prostate cancer, Hodgkin lymphoma, leukemia, non-Hodgkin lymphoma, and lip and stomach cancers.[11] Migrant farmers also experience elevated rates of some of these cancers.[2]

Box 12-1	Established Environmental-Lifestyle Factors and Risk of Cancer

Tobacco use
Dietary items (fruits, vegetables, fat, fiber, alcohol)
Obesity
Reproductive/menstrual traits (age at menarche, age at menopause, parity, age at first birth, lactation)
Sun exposure
Ionizing radiation
Viruses (hepatitis B and C viruses, human papillomaviruses, Epstein-Barr virus)
Bacteria (*Helicobacter pylori*)
Occupational exposures (asbestos, rubber, others [see p. 397])
Population-wide screening activities (prostate-specific antigen [PSA]), mammography, Pap smears*

Data from Kolonel LN, Altshuler D, Henderson BE: *Nat Rev Cancer* 4(7):519-527, 2004.
*Not a risk factor per se but increases the rates of cancer in the short term and in the long term can actually increase the number of cancer cases diagnosed by detecting latent, potentially noninvasive, but histopathologically apparent cancer.

A new paradigm shift suggests that susceptibility to disease is set in utero or neonatally as the result of nutrition and exposures to environmental toxins or stressors, or both.[12] Children also may be affected by prenatal exposures, parental exposures prior to conception, and breast milk. Epidemiologic studies have linked higher risks of childhood leukemia and brain and CNS cancers with parental and childhood exposure to particular solvents, pesticides, petrochemicals, dioxins, and polycyclic aromatic hydrocarbons.[13]

Environmental-lifestyle factors play important roles in cancer development, but there are major gaps in our knowledge of how these factors affect our individual resistances to cancer-causing agents. Research needed for shaping public policy concerning environmental exposures should focus on (1) the relationship between the timing of exposure (periods of vulnerability), multiple exposures, and chronic exposures; (2) risks among racial groups and gender; (3) human contamination (biomonitoring); and (4) scrutinization of unexplained patterns of risk. In addition, public health advocates have argued for mandating that producers of environmental hazards (chemicals, tobacco, drugs, radiologic products, etc.) assess health, safety, and environmental effects before introducing them to the marketplace and making that information publicly available. Table 12-2 summarizes the estimated new cases and deaths caused by cancer, by gender, for specified sites.

Epigenetics and Genetics

The idea that increased risk of disease originates from interactions among genes and environmental-lifestyle factors, in fact, *may* not be driven by the genetic code. A hot debate has been the relative importance of genetic versus epigenetic processes. Although it is clear that inherited variation in deoxyribonucleic acid (DNA) sequence influences individual risk of cancer, this occurs in only a small percentage of the

Table12-2 **Estimated New Cancer Cases and Deaths by Sex, U.S., 2009***

	Estimated New Cases			Estimated Deaths		
	Both Sexes	**Male**	**Female**	**Both Sexes**	**Male**	**Female**
All sites	1,479,350	766,130	713,220	562,340	292,540	269,800
Oral cavity & pharynx	35,720	25,240	10,480	7,600	5,240	2,360
Tongue	10,530	7,470	3,060	1,910	1,240	670
Mouth	10,750	6,450	4,300	1,810	1,110	700
Pharynx	12,610	10,020	2,590	2,230	1,640	590
Other oral cavity	1,830	1,300	530	1,650	1,250	400
Digestive system	275,720	150,020	125,700	135,830	76,020	59,810
Esophagus	16,470	12,940	3,530	14,530	11,490	3,040
Stomach	21,130	12,820	8,310	10,620	6,320	4,300
Small intestine	6,230	3,240	2,990	1,110	580	530
Colon†	106,100	52,010	54,090	49,920	25,240	24,680
Rectum	40,870	23,580	17,290			
Anus, anal canal, & anorectum	5,290	2,100	3,190	710	260	450
Liver & intrahepatic bile duct	22,620	16,410	6,210	18,160	12,090	6,070
Gallbladder & other biliary	9,760	4,320	5,440	3,370	1,250	2,120
Pancreas	42,470	21,050	21,420	35,240	18,030	17,210
Other digestive organs	4,780	1,550	3,230	2,170	760	1,410
Respiratory system	236,990	129,710	107,280	163,790	92,240	71,550
Larynx	12,290	9,920	2,370	3,660	2,900	760
Lung & bronchus	219,440	116,090	103,350	159,390	88,900	70,490
Other respiratory organs	5,260	3,700	1,560	740	440	300
Bones & joints	2,570	1,430	1,140	1,470	800	670
Soft tissue (including heart)	10,660	5,780	4,880	3,820	1,960	1,860
Skin (excluding basal & squamous)	74,610	42,920	31,690	11,590	7,670	3,920
Melanoma	68,720	39,080	29,640	8,650	5,550	3,100
Other non-epithelial skin	5,890	3,840	2,050	2,940	2,120	820
Breast	194,280	1,910	192,370	40,610	440	40,170
Genital system	282,690	201,970	80,720	56,160	28,040	28,120
Uterine cervix	11,270		11,270	4,070		4,070
Uterine corpus	42,160		42,160	7,780		7,780
Ovary	21,550		21,550	14,600		14,600
Vulva	3,580		3,580	900		900
Vagina & other genital, female	2,160		2,160	770		770
Prostate	192,280	192,280		27,360	27,360	
Testis	8,400	8,400		380	380	
Penis & other genital, male	1,290	1,290		300	300	
Urinary system	131,010	89,640	41,370	28,100	18,800	9,300
Urinary bladder	70,980	52,810	18,170	14,330	10,180	4,150
Kidney & renal pelvis	57,760	35,430	22,330	12,980	8,160	4,820
Ureater & other urinary organs	2,270	1,400	870	790	460	330
Eye & orbit	2,350	1,200	1,150	230	120	110
Brain & other nervous system	22,070	12,010	10,060	12,920	7,330	5,590
Endocrine system	39,330	11,070	28,260	2,470	1,100	1,370
Thyroid	37,200	10,000	27,200	1,630	690	940
Other endocrine	2,130	1,070	1,060	840	410	430
Lymphoma	74,490	40,630	33,860	20,790	10,630	10,160
Hodgkin lymphoma	8,510	4,640	3,870	1,290	800	490
Non-Hodgkin lymphoma	65,980	35,990	29,990	19,500	9,830	9,670
Myeloma	20,580	11,680	8,900	10,580	5,640	4,940
Leukemia	44,790	25,630	19,160	21,870	12,590	9,280
Acute lymphocytic leukemia	5,760	3,350	2,410	1,400	740	660
Chronic lymphocytic leukemia	15,490	9,200	6,290	4,390	2,630	1,760
Acute myeloid leukemia	12,810	6,920	5,890	9,000	5,170	3,830
Chronic myeloid leukemia	5,050	2,930	2,120	470	220	250
Other leukemia‡	5,680	3,230	2,450	6,610	3,830	2,780
Other & unspecified primary sites‡	31,490	15,290	16,200	44,510	23,920	20,590

*Rounded to the nearest 10; estimated new cases exclude basal and squamous cell skin cancers and in situ carcinomas except urinary bladder. About 62,280 female carcinoma in situ of the breast and 53,120 melanoma in situ will be newly diagnosed in 2009. †Estimated deaths for colon and rectum cancers are combined.

‡More deaths than cases suggests lack of specificity in recording underlying causes of death on death certificates.

Source: Estimated new cases are based on 1995-2005 incidence rates from 41 states and the District of Columbia as reported by the North American Association of Central Cancer Registries (NAACCR), representing about 85% of the US population. Estimated deaths are based on data from US Mortality Data, 1969-2006, National Center for Health Statistics, Centers for Disease Control and Prevention, 2009. © 2009, American Cancer Society. *Cancer Facts and Figures 2009.* Atlanta: American Cancer Society, Inc.

population.[14] In addition, how structural variation of the genome increases cancer risk is unknown. An explosion of data now indicates the importance of epigenetic processes, especially those with resultant gene silencing of *key* regulatory genes (see Chapter 11). Epigenetic changes collaborate with genetic changes and environmental-lifestyle factors to *cause* the development of cancer. These changes are mitotically and meiotically heritable.[15,16]

The three major areas of epigenetics are (1) methylation (the addition of methyl group [CH_3] to cytosine ring) (see Figure 11-16); aberrant methylation, which can lead to silencing of tumor-suppressor genes; (2) histone modifications (histone acetylation, alterations in chromatin); and (3) micro-ribonucleic acids (miRNAs), small RNA molecules that can target gene expression post-transcriptionally. The expression of miRNAs has been linked to carcinogenesis because they can act as either oncogenes or tumor-suppressor genes.[17] An important feature of epigenetic mechanisms and their role in development and disease is that epigenetic processes can be modified by lifestyle, particularly diet and the environment, pharmacologic interventions, or both.[18] Data on aging also have shown to affect DNA methylation in many cell types in various organisms.[19-21] Significant evidence for environment-lifestyle as the major contributor to these age-related effects on the "epigenome" involves a recent study of monozygotic (MZ) twins. Cell types and patterns of DNA methylation across the genome were similar in young MZ twins, but the patterns diverged in older twins.[22] These data suggest that environmental-lifestyle factors act on individuals throughout life, changing gene expression through epigenetic mechanisms with subsequent implications for health.

Nutrition has become a major focus because it influences DNA methylation in several ways (see p. 405). Biologically active food components modify DNA methylation directly (see p. 406). Nutrition influences metabolic effects associated with energy balance. Because adipose tissue is endocrine tissue, obese individuals accumulate macrophages that secrete various proinflammatory signaling molecules and cytokines (see p. 414). Inflammation is strongly associated with cancer development, and inflammatory bowel disease is related to methylation in the colon.[23] The role of nutrition and diet is discussed on p. 405.

In Utero and Early Life Conditions

From studies of the etiology of certain cancers, it is widely accepted that a long latency period precedes the onset of adult cancers. Accumulating data suggest early life events influence later susceptibility to certain chronic diseases.[24] **Developmental plasticity** is the degree to which an organism's development is contingent on its environment. It requires stable gene expression that in part appears to be modulated by epigenetic processes such as DNA methylation and histone modification (Figure 12-1).[24] Sensitivity to environmental-lifestyle factors influences the mature phenotype and is dependent on the interactions of both the genome and epigenome.

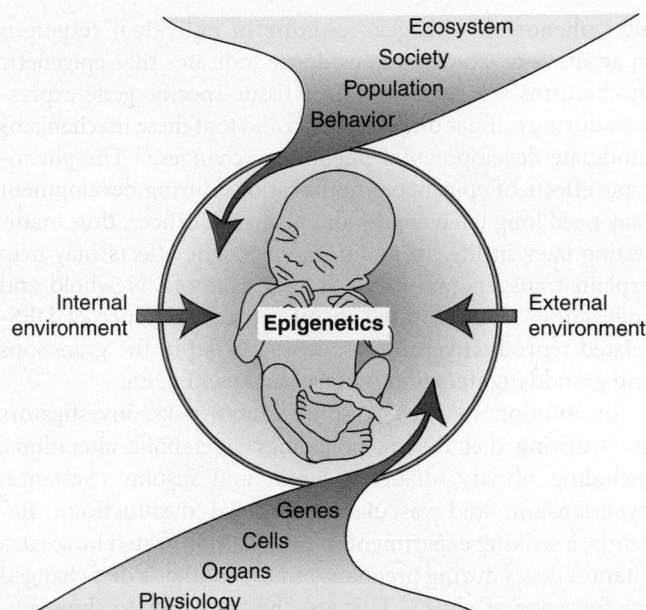

Figure 12-1 Fetal vulnerability to external and internal environments. The fetus is particularly vulnerable to changes in the external and internal environments, which can have immediate and lifelong consequences. Such environmentally induced changes can occur at multiple levels, including molecular and behavioral. Ultimately these alterations may be epigenetic, inducing mitotically heritable alterations in gene expression without changing the DNA. (Adapted from Crews E, McLachlan JA: *Endocrinology* 147[6 Suppl]: S4-S10, 2006.)

Perhaps one of the best examples of early life events and future cancer is the chemical exposure to diethylstilbestrol (DES), a synthetic estrogen. This medication was prescribed between 1938 and 1971 to attempt to prevent multiple pregnancy-related problems, such as miscarriage, premature birth, and abnormal bleeding.[25] In 1953, a clinical study found that DES did not reduce the risk of miscarriage, and by the 1950s it became clear that DES interfered with the *development* of the reproductive system in the fetus. Recent data suggest that DES-associated increase in clear cell adenocarcinoma is elevated throughout a woman's reproductive years.[26] More recent studies have revealed that daughters of women who took DES during pregnancy may have a slight increased risk of breast cancer before age 40 (i.e., 1.9 times the risk compared with unexposed women at age 40).[27] For every 1000 DES-exposed women ages 45 to 49 it is estimated that 4 will be diagnosed with breast cancer.

Research from animal studies has demonstrated a relationship between DES exposure and an increased rate of a rare type of testicular cancer (rete testis) and prostate cancer.[28,29] In terms of in utero exposures, testicular cancer has been linked to exposure to abnormal levels of estrogen,[30] and testicular cancer is a risk factor for men with undescended testicles, a factor in some studies correlated with DES exposure. However, studies in humans for risk of testicular or prostate cancer and DES exposure are unclear and continuing.[31]

In summary, epidemiologic and animal studies reveal that small changes in the developmental environment can alter phenotypic changes, resulting in individual responses in adulthood. Continuing evidence indicates that epigenetic mechanisms are responsible for tissue-specific gene expression during cellular differentiation and that these mechanisms modulate developmental phenotypic changes.[24] The phenotypic effects of epigenetic modifications during development may need long latency periods, such as in cancer, thus manifesting later in life. In addition, epigenetic effects may help explain transgeneration effects. For example, Newbold and colleagues[29] demonstrated in mice the occurrence of DES-related reproductive cancers also occurred in the grandsons and granddaughters of mothers treated with DES!

In addition to altering some cancer risks, investigators are studying diet during pregnancy (metabolic alterations, including obesity, diabetes, leptin and insulin resistance; hypertension; and vascular endothelial dysfunction). Recently, a striking experiment in mice demonstrated how extra vitamin doses during pregnancy in the mother's diet changed the fur color of pups.[32] This was the first study to show maternal nutrition and subsequent phenotype and disease. The nutrients (B_{12}, folic acid, choline, and betaine) silenced the gene that rendered mice fat and yellow but did not alter its DNA sequence. Silencing, or switching the gene off, linked prenatal diet to such diseases as diabetes, obesity, and cancer. These concepts are defining the hypothesis of disease onset called the developmental basis of health and disease. Subsequently the focus of disease prevention and intervention needs to include the decades prior to onset—that is, in utero and neonatal periods.

Tobacco Use

Cigarette smoking is carcinogenic and remains the most important cause of cancer. The risk is greatest in those who begin to smoke when young and continue throughout life.[33] Globally, tobacco use is greatest in developing countries, where 84% of 1.3 billion current smokers live.[34] The World Health Organization (WHO) World Cancer Report[35] reports that in the twentieth century approximately 100 million people died worldwide from tobacco-associated diseases (cancer, chronic lung disease, cardiovascular disease, and stroke). About 50% of regular smokers are killed by the habit. About 25% of smokers will die prematurely during middle age (35 to 69 years).[35]

Cigarette smoking accounts for 1 of every 5 deaths each year in the United States.[36] About 21% of all U.S. adults smoke cigarettes. Estimates of cigarette smoking by age are 23.6% ages 18 to 24, 23.8% ages 25 to 44, 22.4% ages 45 to 64, and 8.8% ages 65 and older.[37] Cigarette smoking is more common among men (23.9%) than women (18.5%), and the prevalence of cigarette smoking is highest among Native Americans/Native Alaskans (32.4%) than whites (22.2%), blacks (20.2%), Hispanics (15%), and Asians (10.4%).[37] It is more common among adults living below the poverty level (30.6%) than those at or above the poverty level (20.4%).[37]

Overall, cigarette smoking in developed countries is responsible for 30% of all cancer deaths, and an epidemic of cancer deaths is expected in developing countries.[35] Tobacco use is associated primarily with squamous and small cell adenocarcinomas. In addition, smoking causes *even more* deaths from vascular, respiratory, and other diseases than from cancer. Smoking tobacco is linked to cancers of the lower urinary tract (renal, penis, and bladder), upper aerodigestive tract (oral cavity, pharynx, larynx, nasal cavity, paranasal sinuses, esophagus, and stomach), liver, kidney, pancreas, cervix, and uterus, as well as myeloid leukemia.[38] Evidence is *lacking* that smoking causes breast, prostate, or endometrial cancer of the uterus.[35] However, tobacco smoke is known to cause mammary tumors in animals. In 2005, Japanese researchers reported that both active and passive smoking increased the risk of breast cancer in pre-menopausal women.[38a]

Secondhand smoke, also called **environmental tobacco smoke (ETS)**, is the combination of sidestream smoke (burning end of a cigarette, cigar, or pipe) and mainstream smoke (exhaled by the smoker). More than 4000 chemicals have been identified in mainstream tobacco smoke (250 chemicals as toxic)[39] of which 60 are considered carcinogenic.[40] Measuring secondhand smoke is difficult. Nonsmokers who live with smokers are at greatest risk for lung cancer as well as numerous noncancerous conditions.[40]

Cigar or pipe smoking, or both, is strongly and causally related to cancers of the oral cavity, oropharynx, hypopharynx, larynx, esophagus, and lung. Cigar smokers who inhale deeply may be at increased risk for developing coronary heart disease and chronic obstructive pulmonary disease.[41] Pipe smokers have a lower risk of dying from tobacco than cigarette smokers, but it is as harmful as and perhaps more harmful than cigar smoking.[42] Bidi smoking, a small amount of tobacco wrapped in the leaf of another plant (used in South Asia), delivers higher amounts of nicotine per gram of tobacco and comparable or greater amounts of tar compared with cigarettes.[38] Case-controlled studies indicate bidi smoking can cause cancers of the respiratory and digestive sites. Epidemiologic data from the United States and Asia reveal an increased risk of oral cancer with smokeless tobacco products.[43] These data, however, are not confirmed in northern European studies.[43]

Measures that prevent young adults from starting smoking would substantially avoid future disease burden. A public health approach is therefore needed that *prevents* young people from *starting* smoking and helps others *stop* smoking.

Diet

Understanding dietary factors that increase the risk for cancer can be difficult. The ways in which diet affects one's likelihood of developing cancer are complicated by the variety of foods consumed, the many constituents of foods, the metabolic consequences of eating, and the temporal changes in the patterns of food use. Cancer risks in older adults may depend as much on diet in early life as on current eating practices.[33,44] In addition, studies in humans targeting diet and disease associations face a variety of challenges including measurements of specific nutrients, food types, and dietary patterns.

Humans are constantly exposed to a variety of compounds termed **xenobiotics** (Greek *xenos,* "foreign"; *bios,* "life") that include toxic, mutagenic, and carcinogenic chemicals. Many of these chemicals are found in the human diet. Most xenobiotics are transported in the blood by lipoproteins and penetrate lipid membranes. These chemicals can react with cellular macromolecules, such as proteins and DNA, or can react directly with cell structures to cause cell damage.[45] The body has two defense systems for counteracting these effects: (1) detoxification enzymes and (2) antioxidant systems (see Chapter 2). Enzymes that activate xenobiotics are called **phase I activation enzymes** and are represented by the multigene cytochrome P-450 family, aldehyde oxidase, xanthine oxidases, and peroxidases. **Phase II detoxification enzymes** then protect further against a large array of reactive intermediates and nonactivated xenobiotics.[45] These enzymes are located predominantly in the liver and provide clearance of compounds through the portal circulation, thereby preventing the potentially carcinogenic agent(s) from entering the body through the gastrointestinal tract and portal circulation. These enzymes also occur in the skin epithelia and can be induced in other extrahepatic tissue, such as the lung.

Dietary sources of carcinogenic substances include compounds produced in the cooking of fat, meat, or protein, and naturally occurring carcinogens associated with plant food substances, such as alkaloids or mold byproducts.[45] The most studied and most relevant carcinogens produced by cooking are the polycyclic aromatic hydrocarbons benzo[a]pyrene and heterocyclic aromatic amines generated by meat protein. The greatest levels are found in well-done charbroiled beef. People, likewise, ingest xenobiotics that are found in environmental or industrial contaminants (e.g., particulate matter of diesel exhaust, contaminating pesticides in food and water supplies) and in certain prescribed and over-the-counter medicines.

Nutrition may directly influence epigenetic factors that silence genes that should be active or activate genes that should be silent.[46] Dietary components can act directly as mutagens or interfere with mutagen elimination. Nutritional factors may alter cellular environments by modulating hormonal axes or influencing cellular proliferation, or both.[46] Importantly, specific nutrients may directly affect the phenotype or expression of key genes, for example, epigenetically through abnormalities of methylation of the promoter regions of genes or histones. These alterations can affect DNA structure and mRNA for transcription.[46] Clearly, epigenetic events are susceptible to change, thus offering potential explanations of *how* environmental factors (e.g., diet) may modify cancer risk and tumor behavior. DNA methylation—the attachment of a methyl group to the 5-position of cytosine within cytosine guanine dinucleotides (CpGs)—is one of several epigenetic changes important in gene regulation and expression (Figure 12-2). CpGs are distributed evenly throughout the genome and remain in short stretches, or clusters, called CpG islands. These islands are located in the promoter region of genes found in half of all human genes.[47] DNA is also susceptible to hypomethylation, which can cause overexpression of transcription of proto-oncogenes, increased recombination and mutation (i.e., oncogenes), and failure to imprint. These alterations can all promote cancer.[48] Aberrant DNA methylation patterns occur in several cancers (colon, lung, prostate, and breast). Dietary factors may be related to DNA methylation in four ways:

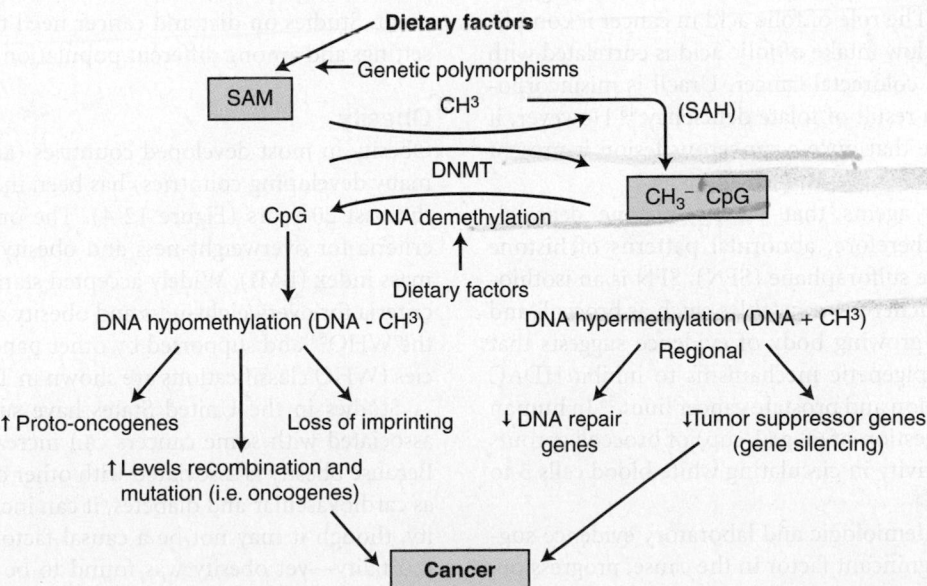

Figure 12-2 Dietary factors, DNA methylation, and cancer. Certain dietary factors (see Table 12-5) may supply methyl groups (+CH3) that can be donated through S-adenosylmethonine (SAM) to many acceptors in the cell (DNA, proteins, lipids, and metabolites). Donation and removal (demethylation) are affected by numerous enzymes, including DNA methyltransferase (DNMT). Increased DNMT activity is known to occur in many tumor cells. Hypermethylation can inhibit or silence tumor-suppressor genes (see Chapter 11) and DNA methylation inhibitors as anticancer agents can block DNMT and, thus, reactivate tumor-suppressor genes. DNA hypomethylation can reactivate and mutate genes, including cancer-causing oncogenes. *SAH,* S-adenolyhomocysteine.

(1) they may influence the *supply* of methyl groups for the formation of S-adenosylhomocysteine (SAM) (see p. 411); (2) they may modify the *use* of methyl groups, e.g., by shifts in an important enzyme, DNA methyltransferase (DNMT) (see p. 411); (3) they may *reduce* methyl groups called demethylation; and (4) DNA methylation patterns may influence the *response* to a dietary factor.[49]

Specific nutritional factors seem to influence susceptibility to cancer. Continuing studies are determining whether certain deficiencies, such as vitamin D and compounds found in fruits and vegetables, can increase cancer incidence.[48] Excess intake of alcohol can promote cancer (see p. 415). Aflatoxin (produced by mold) can contaminate corn, peanuts, and rice stored in hot, humid environments, and Chinese-style salted fish are known to cause cancer. With emphasis on epigenetic and aberrant methylation (Figure 12-3) the role of folic acid in cancer is prominent. The methyl group of 5-methylenetetrahydrofolate is the precursor of methyl group of methionine and eventually SAM (see Table 12-5, p. 410). Cancer cells reveal *both* genome overall (global) hypomethylation and regional hypermethylation (see Figure 12-2). Global hypomethylation in cancer is widely observed and can lead to genomic instability.[50] Regional hypermethylation has been observed in various cancers and when it involves tumor methylation can cause their inactivation or silencing (see Figure 12-2). Low intake of folate combined with high intake of alcohol is associated with global hypomethylation and colorectal cancer. Aberrant folate metabolism leading to DNA methylation is prevalent in the highly aggressive HER2/neu-positive breast cancers.[51] Regional hypermethylation and gene silencing are found in the majority of invasive breast lobular carcinomas.[52] Aberrant methylation is progressively acquired in the early stages of colorectal cancer.[53] The role of folic acid in cancer is complicated. For example, low intake of folic acid is correlated with an increased risk of colorectal cancer. Uracil is misincorporated into DNA as a result of folate deficiency.[48] However, it is important to note that once a cancerous lesion is present folate intake may *increase* tumor growth.[54]

Selective dietary agents that inhibit histone deacetylase (HDAC) and, therefore, abnormal patterns of histone modification include sulforaphane (SFN). SFN is an isothiocyanate found in cruciferous vegetables, such as broccoli and broccoli sprouts. A growing body of evidence suggests that SFN acts through epigenetic mechanisms to inhibit HDAC activity in human colon and prostate cancer lines.[55] In human subjects, a single ingestion of 68 g (1 cup) of broccoli sprouts inhibited HDAC activity in circulating white blood cells 3 to 6 hours after eating.[56]

In summary, epidemiologic and laboratory evidence suggests that diet is a significant factor in the cause, progression, and prevention of cancer (Table 12-3). Diet affects many pathways to cancer including cell cycle control, differentiation, DNA repair, gene silencing, inflammation, apoptosis, and carcinogen metabolism. Many of these processes are likely influenced, if not regulated, by DNA methylation, an epigenetic mechanism that affects gene function. Imbalances

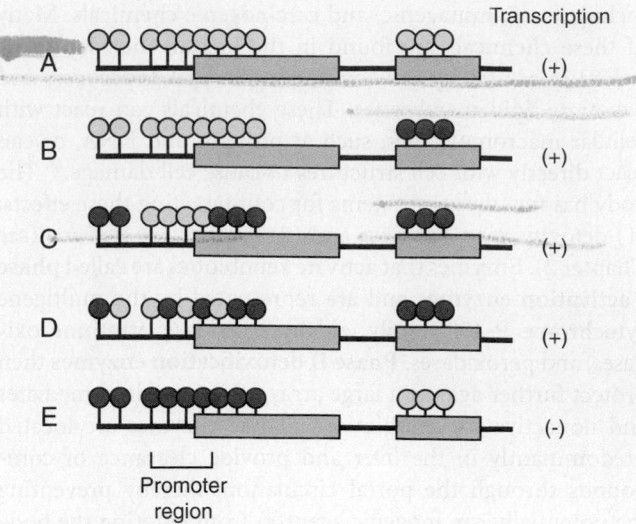

Figure 12-3 Methylation of a gene region and its effect on gene transcription. Green circles, unmethylated cytosine guanine dinuceotide (CpG) sites; (**A**) and dark circles, methylated CpG sites. Methylation of exons (**B, C**) does not block gene transcription. Mosaic methylation of promoter CpG island also does not block transcription (**D**). However, dense methylation of promoter CpG islands completely blocks transcription, and is often associated with hypomethylation of downstream regions (**E**). (From Ushijima T: *J Biochem Mol Biol* 40[2]:143, 2007.)

of nutrients can lead to global hypomethylation, and there is reason to believe that diet can affect gene-specific hypomethylation or hypermethylation, or both.[49] Much more research is needed to identify how specific nutrients can alter DNA methylation and restore gene function as well as other pathways (i.e., apoptosis, etc.) that can prevent tumor development. Studies on diet and cancer need testing in a variety of settings and among different population groups.

Obesity

Obesity in most developed countries (and in urban areas of many developing countries) has been increasing rapidly over the past 20 years (Figure 12-4). The only globally accepted criteria for overweight-ness and obesity are based on body-mass index (BMI). Widely accepted standards based on BMI criteria for overweight-ness and obesity are recommended by the WHO[54] and supported by other panels and federal agencies (WHO classifications are shown in Table 12-4).

Studies in the United States have suggested that obesity associated with some cancers can increase mortality rates.[57] Because obesity is associated with other chronic diseases such as cardiovascular and diabetes, it can increase overall mortality, though it may not be a causal factor involved in cancer mortality—yet obesity was found to be related to increased incidence of several cancer types. A recent hypothesis states that the observed increased incidence of such cancers as breast, endometrium, colon, liver, kidney, and the esophagus may be associated with obesity.[58,59]

A large prospective study of 900,000 American adults showed obesity is linked to cancer. Starting with a mean age

Table 12-3 Relationship of Dietary Factors with Risk of Major Cancers[a]

Diet	Colorectal	Breast	Prostate	Lung	Stomach	Esophageal	Oral	Pancreatic	Bladder	Kidney	Endometrial	Cervical
Micronutrients/Energy Balance												
Obesity												
GI/GL,[c] IGF, height, or metabolic syndrome	↑↑	↑↑	↑		↑[b]	↑[b]		↑		↑	↑↑	
Animal fat		↑	↑							↑	↑	
Nutrients												
Folic acid	↓↓	↓[f]						↑				
Defects methionine pathway (folic acid, vitamin B₁₂ deficiency)						↑↑						
Alcohol		↑↑		↑↑[e]		↑↑	↑					
Calcium	↓		↑									
Vitamin D	↓		↑									
β-carotene supplements			↑		↓							
Lycopene-containing foods			↓	↓??								
Vitamin C			↓?									
Vitamin E			↓?	↓??								
Selenium			↓?									
Foods												
Red or processed meat	↑		↑		↑		→					
Fruits[d]	↓	↓	→	↓	↓	↓	→		↓		↓	
Vegetables[d]	↓		→	↓	↓	↓	→				↓	
Other												
Grilled meat	↑	↑	↑									
Western diet pattern	↑											
High-fiber diet	↓											
Salt, preserved foods					↑		↑					
Hot beverages						↑						

From Koushik A et al: *J Natl Cancer Inst* 99(19):1471-1483, 2007; McCullough ML, Giovannucci EL: *Oncogene* 23(38):6349-6364, 2004; Zhang SM et al: *Cancer Epidemiol Biomarkers Prev* 14(8):2004-2008, 2005.

[a]Two arrows indicate more consistent evidence.
[b]Cancers of the gastric cardia.
[c]GI/GL, glycemic index/glycemic load.
[d]Evidence for a potential benefit from some components of fruits and vegetables (not necessarily blanket effect).
[e]Increased risk limited to smokers.
[f]Data support hypothesis that higher folate intake reduces estrogen receptor–breast cancer, particularly important with alcohol consumption.
IGF, Insulin-like growth factor.
?: SELECT TRIAL.
??: VITAL TRIAL.

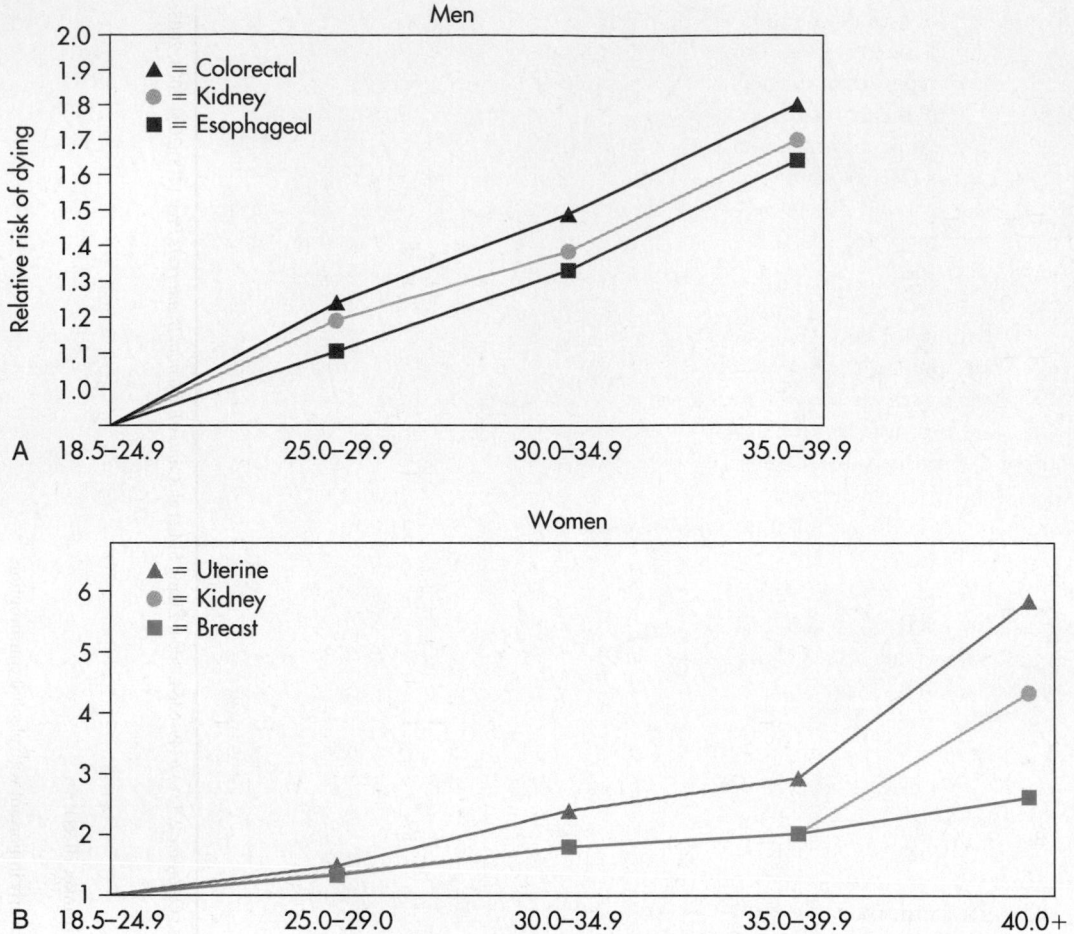

Figure 12-4 Weight and risk of dying from cancer. A, As a man's body mass index (BMI) rises above the normal range (18.5 to 24.9), his risk of dying of colorectal, esophageal, kidney, and other cancers also rises. For example, the risk of dying of colorectal cancer is 10% higher for men who are overweight (BMI 25 to 29.9) than for men of normal or lower BMI. For the most obese men (BMI 35 or higher) the risk is almost double (84%). **B,** As a woman's BMI rises above the normal range (18.5 to 24.9), her risk of dying of breast, kidney, uterine, and other cancers rises. For example, the risk of dying of breast cancer is 34% higher for women who are overweight. For the most obese women (BMI >40), the risk of dying of breast cancer is double. The risk of kidney disease is almost five times higher, and the risk of uterine cancer is six times higher. (Data from Calle EE et al: *N Engl J Med* 348:1625-1638, 2003.)

Table 12-4	WHO Classification of Body Mass Index (BMI)	
BMI (kg/m²)*	**WHO Classification**	**Other Descriptions**
<18.5	Underweight	Thin
18.5-24.9	Normal range	"Healthy," "normal," or "acceptable" weight
25-29.9	Grade 1 overweight	Overweight
30-39.9	Grade 2 overweight	Obesity
≥40	Grade 3 overweight	Morbidly overweight

*The cutoffs are somewhat arbitrary, although they are derived from epidemiologic studies of BMI and overall mortality. It is important to understand that within each category of BMI there can be substantial individual variation in total and visceral adiposity and in related metabolic factors. These variations are also true for the normal range BMI.
WHO, World Health Organization.

of 57 years, individuals were followed for 16 years and cancer mortality data were collected during that interval.[57] Compared with men whose BMI was in the normal range (18.5 to 24.9), men with substantial obesity (BMI ≥40) showed significant increases in cancer mortality. Women had a similar risk. Although significant, people with lesser degrees of obesity had slighter increases in cancer mortality. In men with higher BMI, there were higher rates of death from esophageal, stomach, colorectal, liver, gallbladder, pancreatic, prostate, and kidney cancers and non-Hodgkin lymphoma, multiple myeloma, and leukemia.[57] Among women, high BMI correlated to greater morbidity from colorectal, liver, gallbladder, pancreatic, breast, uterine, cervical, ovarian, and kidney cancers and from non-Hodgkin lymphoma and multiple myeloma.

The mechanisms of obesity-associated cancer risks are unclear and may vary by type of tumor and distribution of body fat. Abdominal obesity, as defined by waist circumference or waist/hip ratio, has been shown to be more strongly related to some tumor types than obesity as defined by BMI.[58] Possible associated mechanisms include insulin resistance and resultant chronic hyperinsulinemia, increased insulin-like growth factors (IGFs), or increased steroid hormones, increased tissue-derived hormones, and cytokines (adipokines) or inflammatory mediators.[58]

Endogenous Hormones

Three mechanisms involve how adiposity influences the synthesis and bioavailability of endogenous sex steroids, the estrogens, progesterone, and androgens (see Figure 12-6):

1. Adipose tissue expresses various sex-steroid metabolizing enzymes that promote the formation of estrogens from androgenic precursors (secreted by the gonads and adrenal glands).

2. Adipose cells increase the circulating levels of insulin and increase IGF-1 biologic activity. This results in reduced liver synthesis and blood levels of sex hormone–binding globulin (SHBG), a binding hormone with affinity for estradiol and testosterone. The adiposity-related decrease in SHBG increases bioavailable estradiol in men and women. In women, decreased SHBG also leads to increased levels of testosterone; in men, contrarily, decreases in SHBG generally lead to reduction in total testicular testosterone production and *no* increase in bioavailable testosterone.

3. High insulin levels can increase ovarian and, possibly, adrenal androgen synthesis and in some genetically susceptible premenopausal women cause the development of polycystic ovary syndrome (PCOS).[60] PCOS is characterized by ovarian hyperandrogenism, chronic anovulation, and progesterone deficiency. PCOS is relatively common with an estimated prevalence of 4% to 6%.[61]

Epidemiologic evidence shows that adiposity-induced alterations in blood levels of sex steroids could explain the correlation noted between indices of excess weight and risks of breast cancer (postmenopausal only) and endometrial cancer (both pre- and postmenopausal).[61]

For breast and endometrial cancers, estrogen and progesterone play a central role, as established by a large body of experimental and clinical evidence. These sex steroids are important regulators of cellular proliferation, differentiation, and apoptosis. Further evidence that increased endogenous estrogen levels might drive the association between BMI and breast cancer comes from studies of hormone replacement therapy (HRT). BMI is more strongly related to breast cancer incidence among postmenopausal women who have *never* received HRT compared with women who have.[62-64] Possibly, only in women whose levels of estrogen are low (after menopause with no HRT) does increased adiposity and, therefore, an increase in peripheral aromatase activity by androgenous activity and androgenous estrogen production, lead to an increase in breast cancer risk. In addition, mortality is higher among heavier women than among leaner women.[61,65]

Several case-control and prospective studies have reported increased risks among pre- and postmenopausal women who have lower blood levels of SHBG and thus high levels of androgens and testosterone. Among postmenopausal women, risk is also correlated to levels of estrone and total bioavailable (free) estradiol.[66]

Among men, prostate carcinogenesis is thought to be related to endogenous hormone metabolism, including androgen production and, possibly, estrogens. Yet excess weight does not appear to be a prominent risk factor except with advanced disease.[67] Other dietary factors and the outcome of studies for cancer risk are presented in Table 12-5. Hormones and cancer are discussed in Chapter 23.

Biologic Mechanisms

Although hypothetical, the role of obesity and cancer may involve alterations in the hormonal milieu. Adipose tissue is active endocrine and metabolic tissue and can have greater effects on the physiology of other tissue (see Chapter 39). In response to endocrine and metabolic signals from other organs, adipose tissue responds by increasing or decreasing the release of free fatty acids—fuel for skeletal muscle and other tissues. When triglycerides, the main storage lipid, are metabolically hydrolyzed, they release free fatty acids into the blood. Abdominal visceral adipocytes are more metabolically active than abdominal subcutaneous adipocytes and because visceral adipocytes have high lipolytic activity and release large amounts of free fatty acids, accurate measurements of adiposity must consider the amount and the site of deposition of the adipose tissue. Adipose tissue is very important in the regulation of energy balance and lipid metabolism through the release of peptide hormones, including leptin, adiponectin, resistin, and tumor necrosis factor-gamma (TNF-γ) (Figure 12-5). Increased release of free fatty acids, resistin, and TNF-γ by adipose tissue and reduced release of adiponectin give rise to insulin resistance—a state characterized by the reduced metabolic response of tissues (muscle, liver, adipose tissue) to insulin and to compensatory hyperinsulinemia[61] (Figure 12-5). Involvement of signaling pathways (i.e., AKT, JAK/STAT) and other inflammatory cascades (i.e., nuclear factor kappa beta [NF-κβ]) has been linked with obesity and cancer.[116] Adipose tissue cells also produce various steroid-hormone-metabolizing enzymes and are an important source of circulating estrogens in postmenopausal women (see Figure 12-6).

Excess weight, increased plasma triglyceride levels, low levels of physical activity, and certain dietary factors can contribute to chronic hyperinsulinemia. Chronically increased insulin levels have been correlated with the development of colon, breast, pancreatic, and endometrial cancers[67,117,118] (see Figure 12-6). These pathogenic effects of insulin might be mediated by insulin receptors in the preneoplastic or neoplastic target cells or could be due to alterations in endogenous hormone metabolism secondary to hyperinsulinemia. For example, insulin promotes the synthesis and biologic activity of the growth factor **insulin-like growth factor-1 (IGF-1)**. IGF-1 is a peptide hormone with a molecular

Text continued on p. 414.

Table 12-5	Studies of Dietary Factors and Associated Cancer Risk
Dietary Factor	**Study Results**
Fat	Results are inconsistent
	Hypothesized to modulate sex hormone levels for breast and prostate cancers and to increase colon cancer risk by stimulating mutagenic activity secondary to bile acid secretion
	Confirming a role for fat independent of calories and other constituents of meat and dairy foods has been difficult
	Case-controlled, prospective, or intervention studies have not shown any consistent findings
	Inconsistencies may be resolved through use of biomarkers instead of questionnaires; however, markers are subject to recent intakes and interindividual variation
	Evidence is the strongest for animal fats in prostate cancer but correlations seem to vary by the type of fat and study design
	Marine fatty acids and their sources (fish) may reduce breast and prostate cancer risk although findings are inconsistent[68]
Carbohydrates	Carbohydrates include starches, nonstarch polysaccharides, and sugars
	Because high glycemic index carbohydrates are correlated with higher postprandial blood glucose and insulin levels and higher fasting insulin levels in insulin-resistant states, they are hypothesized to increase cancer risk; epidemiologic studies have not supported this relationship to date
	Nonetheless, abnormal glucose and insulin metabolism is important in carcinogenesis, especially in obese individuals and sedentary individuals
Meat	Evidence for meat consumption in increasing cancer risk, especially of the colon, rectum, and prostate, has fairly consistent data over time and across study designs
	Countries with higher meat consumption have a higher incidence of colon cancer than those with lower meat consumption
	A meta-analysis with 14 prospective studies reported a significant (12% to 17%) increase in risk with each daily 100-g increment of all meat or red meat intake (>3 oz) and a 49% increased risk for each 25-g increment of processed meats (about 1 slice)[69]
	The increased risk of colon cancer associated with red and processed meats has several cancer-related hypotheses:
	1. Heterocyclic amines (HCAs)
	2. Polycyclic aromatic hydrocarbons (PAHs) formed at high temperatures or over an open flame
	3. Mutagenic N-nitroso compounds (NOCs)
	4. Meat components on hormone metabolism (and possibly hormones in meat)
	5. Diets high in red meat may be low in vegetables[68]
Dairy	Recent studies suggest a lower risk of cancer with higher intakes of low-fat dairy products and a higher risk of breast cancer with high-fat dairy intakes[70]
	Some studies have shown dairy products associated with higher risk of prostate and ovarian cancers[71]
	Their overall influence, however, remains inconsistent
Vitamin D	Experimental data show a protective role for 1,25(OH)$_2$D (the active form of vitamin D) on growth regulation and cell differentiation (also see Chapter 2)
	Populations with greater exposure to ultraviolet (UV) light generally have lower risks of breast, colon, and prostate cancer
	Vitamin D is synthesized in the skin after exposure to UV radiation and is obtained from fortified milk products, breakfast cereals, fatty fish, and multivitamin supplements
Calcium	Calcium has been shown to influence cancer risk in a complex way
	It has been inversely related to the risk of colorectal cancer and adenoma recurrence, but high amounts also have been associated with other cancers, particularly prostate[72-74]
	Calcium has been hypothesized to protect against colorectal cancer by binding secondary bile acids and ionized fatty acids in the colon, forming insoluble soaps and reducing proliferative stimuli on the mucosa[73,75]
	Calcium also may cause terminal differentiation[76]
	Prospective studies of colon cancer suggest that total calcium intake >1000 mg may not confer any additional benefit
	Case-control studies of calcium and prostate and breast cancer have been inconsistent
	One hypothesis of how high levels of calcium may increase the risk of prostate cancer is by down-regulating production of 1,25(OH)$_2$D, the active form of vitamin D
	In vitro, vitamin D reduces cell proliferation and induces cell differentiation; these functions are thought to be mediated by the vitamin D receptor (VDR)
Folate	Diet may influence carcinogenesis through its effects on DNA synthesis and methylation (see illustration on p. 411 and Figure 12-2)
	Folate is essentially for the transfer of methyl groups. Folate relationship to cancers is complex.
	Low folate (as 5-methyltetrahydrofolate, see figure on p. 411) reduces intracellular S-adenosylmethionine (SAM), altering cytosine methylation in DNA and potentially causing inappropriate activation of proto-oncogenes[77] or inactivation of tumor-suppressor genes; folate is involved in the synthesis of nucleotides needed for proliferating cancer cells
	Low-folate metabolites can lead to misincorporation of uracil for thymidine, which occurs during DNA synthesis,[78,79] increasing the need for DNA repair[80]; these alterations can be reversed with folic acid supplementation
	Low folate intake has been associated with several cancers, most notably colorectal,[81] breast, and cervical[82]
	Folate is obtained from fruits, vegetables, and legumes and is now available in grains; however, reviews of both observational and experimental studies suggest limited evidence that foods containing folate protect against colon cancer.[73] With 1 mg supplement, folate was related to an increase in high-grade colon adenomas.[82a]

Table 12-5	Studies of Dietary Factors and Associated Cancer Risk—cont'd
Dietary Factor	**Study Results**

	Long-term use of folate-containing supplements has been correlated with a 30% to 75% reduction in risk of colon cancer; however, once colon cancer occurs folate may increase risk (see p. 406)[83]
	Alcohol interferes with folate absorption and transport
	Several studies report lower risk of breast cancer with higher folate intake[82,84,85]; however the Prostate, Lung, Colorectal, and Ovarian (PLCO) Cancer Screening trial reported a potential harmful effect of high folate intake ≥400 mcg/day on breast cancer risk[86]
	Interactions of folate and folate metabolites with MTHFR (see figure below)
	Polymorphisms add additional evidence for a causal role of folate in carcinogenesis[68]

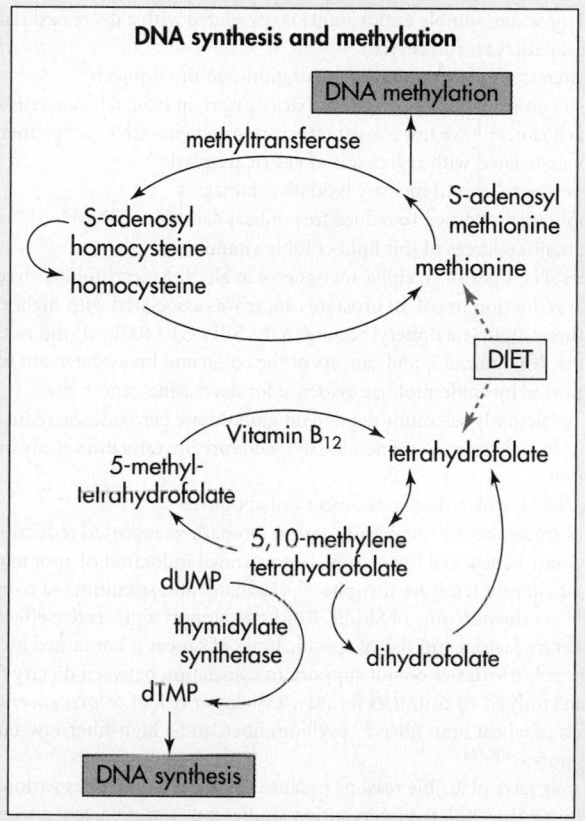

Carotenoids, including lycopene	More than 500 carotenoids are present in nature, but only 20 have been identified in human serum and only 5 are abundant (β-carotene, α-carotene, lycopene, lutein/zeaxanthin, β-cryptoxanthin[87]; they are not synthesized in animals, thus the sources are fruits and vegetables
	They act as antioxidants, pro-oxidants, and nuclear transcription factors (those with provitamin activity) and can reduce tumor formation by blocking the insulin-like growth factor (IGF)[87]
	More data are available on β-carotene and lycopene
	Prospective studies show β-carotene, and others, associated with reduced risk of lung cancer
	Studies of breast cancer are inconsistent[88]
	Intervention studies, however, have *not* isolated β-carotene as protective, and in two large chemoprevention trials found unexpected increased risk of lung cancer with larger than typical doses of β-carotene as supplements in smokers[89]
	When data were reevaluated, only alcohol consumers of more than 11 g/day developed lung cancer under β-carotene supplementation[90]
	Alcohol-induced cytochrome P-450 2E1 (CYP2E1) metabolized ethanol to acetaldehyde and generates toxic and carcinogenic metabolites from retinol (i.e., β-carotene supplementation)
	β-carotene supplementation did not increase the risk of lung cancer in nonsmoking men and women
	Cigarette smoke can oxidize β-carotene in vitro, which may increase cytochrome P-450 breakdown of retinoic acid, thus increasing metaplastic potential[91]
	β-Carotene supplements were shown to reduce colorectal adenomas by 44% in individuals who did smoke or consume alcohol but doubled the risk among those who smoked and drank more than one drink per day[92]
	Data from the Alpha-Tocopherol Beta Carotene (ATBC) Prevention Study showed that baseline dietary intakes, as well as baseline serum β-carotene and serum retinol, were correlated with *decreased* lung cancer risk over 14 years[89]

Continued

Table 12-5	Studies of Dietary Factors and Associated Cancer Risk—cont'd
Dietary Factor	**Study Results**
Antioxidants: vitamins C and E and selenium	Lycopene from food (tomatoes, tomato products, watermelon, pink grapefruit) is related to a decreased risk of some cancers, but no long-term trials of supplementation have been done
	Lycopene is not converted to vitamin A and therefore may be completely available for other metabolic functions, such as antioxidation
	In some population studies, lycopene came from tomato sources, thus other protective components may be responsible or assist, including lutein and zeaxanthin[93]
	Oxidant metabolites (see Chapter 2) can damage DNA, protein, and lipids
	Antioxidants influence cancer risk in complicated processes
	They neutralize free radicals that can damage DNA
	Vitamin C (a major water-soluble antioxidant) is correlated with a decreased risk for cancer of the mouth, esophagus, stomach, lungs, pancreas, and cervix
	Vitamin C can interrupt the formation of nitrosamines in the stomach
	Interaction with a common bacterium, *Helicobacter pylori*, in stomach cancer is suggested as significant,[94] yet prevention trials of stomach cancer have not consistently supported vitamin C supplements; multiple antioxidant nutrients, however, were associated with regression of gastric dysplasia[95]
	Vitamin C interacts with iron to increase oxidative damage[94]
	Vitamin E (tocopherol) is known to reduce free radical damage to DNA[68]
	Fats and oils are major sources of this lipid-soluble vitamin
	Gamma-tocopherol is superior to alpha-tocopherol in altering electrophilic (free radical) oxides such as nitrogen oxides
	A very significant reduction in risk of prostate cancer was associated with higher levels of serum gamma-tocopherol[96] however, synthetic alpha-tocopheryl acetate in the SELECT (400Iu/d) did not prevent prostate cancer [97]
	Intervention studies of vitamin E and cancers of the colon and breast have not found a significant benefit[98]
	Selenium is supported by epidemiologic evidence for decreasing cancer risk
	Selenoproteins, particularly selenium-dependent glutathione peroxidases, reduce production of oxidative free radicals
	Selenium content in soil can vary tremendously; therefore, investigators study biochemical markers of intake or selenium supplementation
	Selenium targets *TP53*, which increases cancer cell apoptosis
	Two case-control studies of the toenail and serum biomarkers reported reduction in risk of prostate cancer[99,100]
	The SELECT prostate cancer cell lines study demonstrated induction of apoptosis of prostate cancer cells with a combination of vitamin E (alpha-tocopherol succinate) and selenium—a combination perhaps more effective than either alone,[101] yet the outcome of SELECT did not support a protective effect (see above)[97]
	A summary of dietary factors and risk of specific types of cancer is contained in Table 12-3
Fiber	Most prospective cohort studies do not support an association between dietary fiber and colon cancer risk,[68] yet a recent large European study of 10 countries found a 25% lower risk of colon cancer associated with high fiber[102]
	Intervention trials of wheat bran fiber,[103] psyllium fiber, and a high-fiber/low-fat diet failed to reduce the risk of recurrent adenomatous polyps[104,105]
	Inconsistencies may have plausible reasons because dietary fiber includes various nondigestible components with different physiologic effects; thus isolated intervention studies may not represent a true test
	Confounding by other nutrients with potential anticarcinogenic activity is problematic; for example, a high-fiber diet is correlated with other nutrients, such as folate
	Burkitt's original hypothesis that fiber may be responsible for the lower rates of colon cancer in African men, compared with men living in developed countries, also emphasized that refined grains and sugars were deleterious,[106] thus other metabolic effects such as sugar-induced insulin changes also may be operating
Fruits and vegetables	Case-control studies reveal subjects who consume diets high in certain fruits and/or vegetables have lower risk of some but not all cancers[68]; the problem with case-control studies is recall bias; prospective studies of fruits and/or vegetables in stomach, breast, and colorectal cancer have weaker results[107,108,109]
	An AARP Diet and Health Study found lower intake of meat and potatoes and higher intake of fruit, vegetables, and low fat foods decreased the risk of colon cancer[110]
	Intervention study of fruits and vegetables on recurrence of colorectal adenoma did not find a reduction in risk[105]; combining fruits and vegetables in analyses may "hide" strong protective effects of phytochemical or botanic substances; numerous substances with potential anticarcinogenic activity include folate, carotenoids, flavonoids, vitamins, isothiocyanates, dithiolthiones, glucosinolates, allium compounds, and limonene; potential protective mechanisms include modulation of DNA methylation,[77] prevention of DNA adduct formation[111]; induction of phase II carcinogen-metabolizing enzymes[112]; alteration of hormone levels[113]; and inhibition of nitrosamine formation[114]
	National Cancer Institute and the American Institute for Cancer Research recommend eating five to nine servings/day to improve health outcomes
	Improved health outcomes may be greater by maximizing fruits and vegetables by color code:
	Red-purple: red apples, grapes, berries, and wine all contain anthocyanins (antioxidants)
	Orange: carrots, mangos, etc., contain β-carotene

Table 12-5	Studies of Dietary Factors and Associated Cancer Risk—cont'd
Dietary Factor	**Study Results**
	Orange-yellow: oranges, lemons, etc., contain citrus flavonoids that may induce cell-cycle arrest and apoptosis, induce detoxification enzymes, and prevent oxidation
	Green: broccoli, Brussels sprouts, etc., contain glucosinolates that influence detoxification enzymes
	White-green: onions, garlic, etc., contain allylic sulfides and induce glutathione transferase to increase antioxidants
	One serving of each meets the minimum recommendations
Nitrates	Strongest data in animals causing cancer of glandular stomach; dietary salts enhance metabolism to other nitrosable compounds; Chinese populations have high rates of gastric cancer and ingest large quantities of nitrates
Polyunsaturated fatty acids (PFAs)	PFAs are oxidized to yield free radicals and peroxidases) that can be toxic to cells and increase tumor development
	Omega-6 fatty acids (e.g., polyunsaturated vegetable oils, etc.), promote cancer more effectively than saturated fats; however, omega-3 fatty acids (e.g., fatty fish, cod liver oil) appear to decrease the number and size of tumors and increase the time before tumors appear
	Protective effects may be caused by enzyme and protein activity related to intracellular signaling and, ultimately, cell-to-cell proliferation or by a decrease in angiogenesis, and inflammation
	Destruction of toxic peroxides or radicals also may depend on selenium-containing enzymes
Conclusions	Substantial progress has been made since the early reports from Doll and Peto[115]
	Hypotheses have been tested, clarified, refuted, and altered, for example, a decade ago, leading hypotheses included total calories; factors in fruits and vegetables (β-carotene, fiber); fat; and vitamins A, E, and C
	The hypothesis for fat has weakened; strengthened for energy balance and obesity
	Specific phytonutrients (e.g., lycopene, folate, flavonoids, fiber) continue to be actively studied, although studies are difficult to execute (i.e., recall bias, confounding variables, extensive time requirements, expense) and identifying *the* biologic element in plant foods is daunting
	Supplemental nutrients may have different health effects than nutrients in food, and other lifestyle factors can interfere, such as alcohol ingestion or smoking
	In addition, varying genotypes, for example, folate metabolizing enzymes, represent complex biologic challenges
	Biologically driven hypotheses are necessary to understand diet and cancer, for example, the importance of active vitamin D (1,25[OH]$_2$D) in tumor development led to studies of calcium and vitamin D, and understanding DNA methylation led to analyses of folate nutrition
	In summary, a combination of multiple exposures will be necessary to move our understanding forward, such as dietary intake, energy balance (obesity), and exercise, because they influence growth factors (e.g., IGF) in a complex and integrative fashion

IGF, Insulin-like growth factor; *MTHFR,* 5,10-methylene tetrahydrofolate reductase.

NUTRITION & DISEASE

Components of a Cancer-Prevention Diet

Some foods increase the risk of cancer, whereas other foods decrease the risk. Observing the following dietary guidelines might reduce the risk of cancer.

Increase

- Fruits and vegetables (especially broccoli, cauliflower, cabbage, spinach, onions, garlic, bok choy, brussels sprouts, kale, chard, collard greens, chicory, romaine, blueberries, and grapes)
- Fiber (limiting glycemic index)
- Foods containing vitamins A, C, D, and E; mineral selenium (not to exceed 200 mcg/day)
- Vitamin B$_6$ (grains, beans, liver, avocados)
- Vitamin D (see Chapter 2)
- Vitamin C (complicated, see Table 12-5)
- Foods containing folate (fruits, vegetables [asparagus, broccoli], legumes, grains*)

- Epigallocatechin gallate (found in green tea)
- Spices (curcumin [turmeric], garlic, cloves, capascin, ginger, coriander, fennel, fenugreek)
- Whole grains instead of refined grains (wheat, rice, maize)
- Lycopene (tomatoes, tomato paste, watermelon)†
- Legumes (lentils, peas)
- Nuts

Decrease

- Fat (especially large amounts of omega-6 fatty acids)
- High-glycemic-index carbohydrates
- Foods with high amounts of preservatives
- Alcohol
- Grilled, blackened foods
- Fried foods
- High levels of calcium ($\geq$2000 mg)
- Refined grain products

Data from Ingraham BA et al: *Curr Med Res Opin* 24:139-149, 2008; Lee KW et al: *Am J Clin Nutr* 78:1074-1078, 2003.
*Whole grains.
†Recent data of inhibition of AK-signaling pathway.

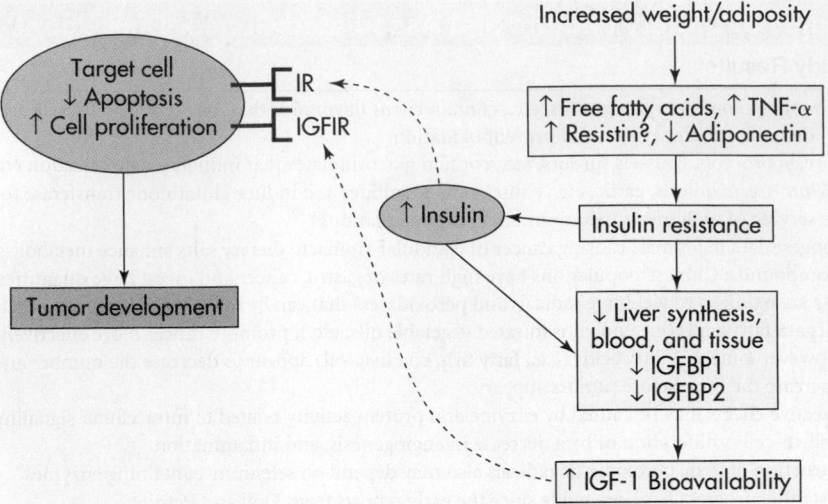

Figure 12-5 Energy balance, lipid metabolism, and insulin sensitivity and tumor development. In obesity, increased release from adipose tissue of free fatty acids (FFAs), tumor necrosis factor-alpha (TNF-α) and resistin, and reduced release of adiponectin lead to insulin resistance and compensatory chronic hyperinsulinemia. Increased insulin levels ultimately lead to decreased liver synthesis and blood levels of insulin-like growth factor–binding protein-1 (IGFBP1) and, theoretically, also decrease IGFBP1 synthesis locally in other tissues. Increased fasting levels of insulin in plasma are also correlated with decreased levels of IGFBP2 in the blood, leading to increased levels of bioavailable IGF-1. Insulin and IGF-1 signal through the insulin receptors (IRs) and IGF-1 receptor (IGF1R) to stimulate cellular proliferation and inhibit apoptosis in many tissue types. These effects could promote tumor development. (Adapted from Calle EE, Kaaks R: *Nat Rev Cancer* 4[8]:579-591, 2004.)

structure similar to insulin that regulates cellular proliferation in response to available energy and nutrients from diet and body constituents (see Figure 12-6).[119] Insulin also can promote the synthesis and biologic availability of the male and female sex hormones, including estrogens, progesterone, and androgens[61] (see Figure 12-6).

In vitro studies have established that insulin and IGF-1 act as growth factors that promote cell proliferation and inhibit apoptosis.[120-123] Epidemiologic evidence supports the hypothesis that chronic hyperinsulinemia increases cancer risk. Type 2 diabetes mellitus associated with insulin resistance and increased pancreatic insulin secretion for long periods before and after disease onset is associated with increased risks of cancer of the colon, endometrium, kidney, and pancreas.[67,118,124,125] Prospective cohort studies have shown increased risk of cancers of the colon or colorectum among individuals with increased prediagnostic blood levels of **C-peptide** (a marker for pancreatic insulin secretion), fasting glucose levels, or insulin measured 2 hours after absorption of a standard oral dose of glucose.[126] Similar data have found a direct relationship between cancer risk and prediagnostic C-peptide levels for endometrial cancer.[66] The study also found inverse relationships between cancer risk and blood levels of IGF-binding protein 1 (IGFBP1) and IGF-binding protein 2 (IGFBP2),[66] which reduce the amount of bioavailable IGF-1. However, a case-control study nested within the European Prospective Investigation found the C-peptide risk association was substantially decreased after adjustment for free estradiol in postmenopausal women.[127] The Physicians Health Study reported the first association between plasma insulin levels or C-peptide *before prostate cancer diagnosis*

(prediagnostic) and the *risk of prostate cancer mortality*.[128] This finding suggests excess body weight and a high plasma level of C-peptide predispose men to the development of prostate cancer and to an increased likelihood of dying from their disease. More studies are needed to confirm these findings.

The IGFBPs regulate the availability of IGF-1 because they stabilize the large pool of IGF-1 in the circulation, the efflux of IGF-1 from this circulation pool toward target tissues and binding of IGF-1 to its receptor.[61] IGFBP3 increases tissue apoptosis, so decreased amounts may contribute to carcinogenesis.

More than 80% of IGF-1 is provided by growth hormone (GH). In overnourished states and in individuals with type 2 diabetes mellitus, endogenous insulin levels and liver GH-receptor levels are high and large amounts of IGF-1 are produced.[61] Contrarily, however, obese individuals have lower blood levels of IGF-1 than normal weight individuals.[129] A compelling explanation for the lower levels of IGF-1 in obese individuals, despite increased GH sensitivity of liver and other tissues, is that reduction in IGFBP1 and IGFBP2 levels leads to increased negative feedback by free IGF-1 (unbound to IGFBPs) on pituitary gland secretion of GH. Overall, this feedback results in reduced synthesis of IGF-1 and reduced plasma IGF-1 concentrations.

IGF-1 has been shown to promote proliferation of normal epithelial breast cells.[119] The IGF-signaling pathway has been linked to breast carcinogenesis in animal studies,[130] and previous epidemiologic studies have reported increased blood levels of IGF-1 as directly related to different forms of cancer. These studies reported that high levels of IGF-1 and low levels of IGFBP3 are correlated with increased risk of premenopausal

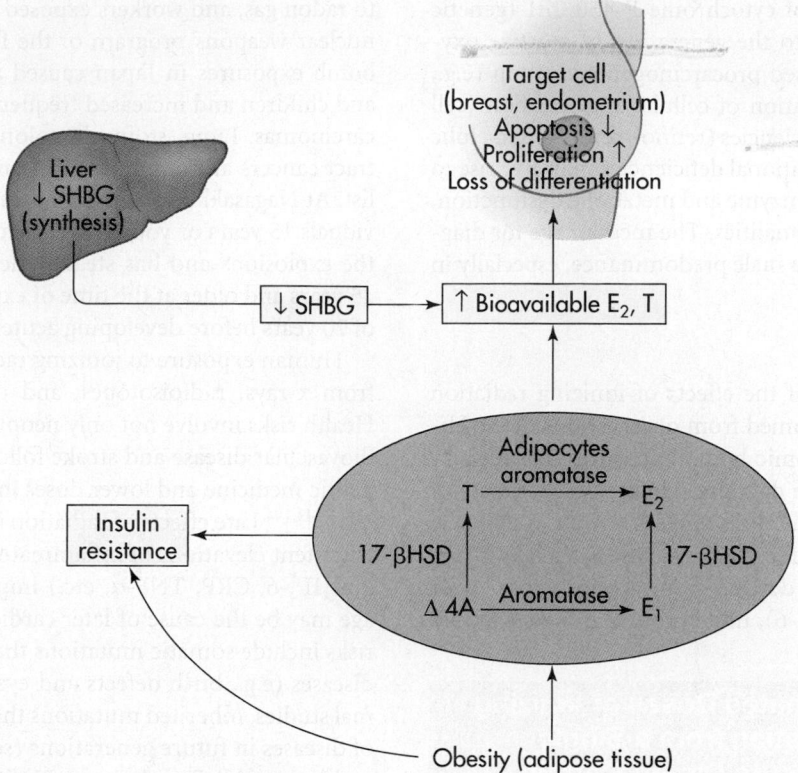

Figure 12-6 Effects of obesity on hormone alterations. Adipose tissue produces the enzymes aromatase and 17-beta hydroxysteroid dehydrogenase (17-βHSD). In obese persons, therefore, there is an increased conversion of the androgens Δ4-androstenedione (Δ4A) and testosterone (T) into the estrogens estrone (E_1) and estradiol (E_2), respectively, by the enzyme aromatase. The important enzyme 17-βHSD converts the less biologically active hormones Δ4A and E_1 into the more active hormones T and E_2, respectively. In parallel, obesity leads to hyperinsulinemia, which causes a decrease in the liver synthesis and blood circulating levels of sex hormone-binding globulin (SHBG). The combined effect of increased synthesis of estrone and testosterone, along with reduced levels of SHBG (their transporter), leads to an increase in the bioavailablity (or free fractions) of E_2 and T that can diffuse to target tissue, where they bind to estrogen and androgen receptors. Binding to their respective receptors in some tissue (e.g., breast and endometrium) promotes cellular proliferation and inhibits apoptosis. Thus they can increase tumor development. In both men and women, adiposity-related decreases in SHBG generally increase the fraction of bioavailable or free estradiol. In contrast, decreases of SHBG in men only generally lead to reductions in testicular production of testosterone and no increase in bioavailable testosterone. (Adapted from Calle EE, Kaaks R: *Nat Rev Cancer* 4[8]:579-591, 2004.)

breast cancer.[131,132] Similar risks were reported for cancers of the prostate and colorectum.[133-136] An analysis for the Breast and Prostate Cancer Cohort Consortium (BPC3) from six large cohorts found no association between common genetic variations in the IGF-1, IGFBP1, and IGFBP3 genes in relation to circulating levels of IGF-1 and IGFBP3 and breast cancer risk (also no effect by menopausal status).

From the epidemiologic studies, breast and prostate cancer showed no clear relationship with BMI or other indices of adiposity. Colon cancer, however, did show positive relationships with BMI and other indices of adiposity. In addition, there was no clear linear relationship between circulating levels of IGF-1 and the degree of adiposity.[61]

Alcohol Consumption

Chronic alcohol consumption is a strong risk factor for cancer of the oral cavity, pharynx, hypopharynx, larynx, esophagus, and liver.[137] Although evidence is inconsistent, alcohol consumption is less strongly related to breast cancer and colorectal cancer; however, it is known to increase cell growth of human breast cancer cells in vitro.[138] In addition, although the risk is lower, breast carcinogenesis can be enhanced with relatively low daily amounts of alcohol.[137] A meta-analysis showed no consistent relationship between alcohol and cancers of the pancreas, lung, prostate, or bladder.[139] Alcohol interacts with smoke, increasing the risk of malignant tumors, possibly by acting as a solvent for the carcinogenic chemicals in smoke products. In individuals who have never smoked, substantial alcohol consumption (i.e., three or more drinks per day) has been associated with head and neck cancers.[140] Inherited factors also put some individuals at increased risk in the ability to repair DNA, carcinogen metabolism, and cell cycle control.[141] The strongest genetic associations to alcoholism are those with alcohol dehydrogenase (ADH) and mitochondrial aldehyde dehydrogenase (ALDH2). Specifically, individuals having the genes encoding 32-ADH or the dominant negative allele for ALDH2 are at reduced risk of alcoholism, despite being at much higher risk for oropharyngeal cancer.[142]

Mechanisms involved in alcohol-related carcinogenesis include the effect of acetaldehyde, the first metabolite of ethanol oxidation; the induction of cytochrome P-450 2E1 (genetic variant CYP2E1) leading to the generation of reactive oxygen species (ROS); increased procarcinogen activation (e.g., nitrosamines) and modulation of cellular regeneration (cell cycle); and nutritional deficiencies (retinol, retinyl esters, folic acid, other vitamins). Nutritional deficiencies may give rise to altered mucosal integrity, enzyme and metabolic dysfunction, and other structural abnormalities. The median age for diagnosis is the early 60s, with a male predominance, especially in laryngeal cancer.[140]

Ionizing Radiation

Much of the knowledge of the effects of ionizing radiation on human cancer has stemmed from observations of the Hiroshima and Nagasaki atomic bomb exposures, particularly the Life Span Study. These data provide the best estimate of human cancer risk over the dose range from 20 to 250 cGy for low linear energy transfer (LET) radiation, such as x-rays or γ-rays. Other data are derived from groups exposed for medical reasons (Table 12-6), underground miners exposed

Table 12-6	Estimated Doses of Ionizing Radiation from a Single Exposure During Certain Diagnostic Procedures

Procedure	Effective Dose mSv (mrem)
Chest examination (lateral [LAT])	0.04
Chest examination (anteroposterior [AP])	0.02
Skull (AP)	0.03
Skull (LAT)	0.01
Pelvis (LAT)	0.07
Thoracic spine (AP)	0.4
Lumbar spine (AP)	0.7
Mammogram (4 views)	0.7
Abdomen	1.2
Hip	0.8
Hand or foot	0.005
DEXA (whole body)	0.0004
Dental (LAT)	0.02
Dental (panoramic)	0.09
Pyelogram (IV, kidneys; 6 films)	2.5
Barium swallow (24 images, fluoroscopy)	1.5
Barium enema (10 images, fluoroscopy)	7
CT head	2
CT chest	8
CT abdomen	10
CT pelvis	10
Angioplasty (heart study)	7.5-57
Coronary angiogram	4.6-15.8
Brain (PET)	1
Various PET studies (FFDG)	14
Air travel from Athens to New York	0.06
Background annual dose (sea level)	1

Data from Health Physics Society: *Diagnostic imaging procedures.* Available at www.hps.org/documents/mediaimaging.pdf. Accessed June 2008.

CT, Computed tomography (CAT scan); *FFDG,* nuclear medicine with F-fluorodeoxyglucose; *IV,* intravenous; *PET,* positron-emission tomography.

to radon gas, and workers exposed to high doses while in the nuclear weapons program of the former USSR. The atomic bomb exposures in Japan caused acute leukemias in adults and children and increased frequencies of thyroid and breast carcinomas. Lung, stomach, colon, esophageal, and urinary tract cancers and multiple myeloma have been added to the list. At Nagasaki and Hiroshima, leukemia incidence in individuals 15 years or younger reached its peak 6 to 7 years after the explosions and has steadily declined since 1952. People 45 years and older at the time of exposure had a latent period of 20 years before developing acute leukemia.

Human exposure to ionizing radiation includes emissions from x-rays, radioisotopes, and other radioactive sources. Health risks involve not only neoplastic diseases but also cardiovascular disease and stroke following high doses in therapeutic medicine and lower doses in A-bomb survivors (BEIR VII).[143,144] Late effects of radiation in A-bomb survivors show persistent elevations of inflammatory markers (e.g., interleukin [IL]-6, CRP, TNF-α, etc.) implying immunologic damage may be the cause of later cardiovascular effects.[145] Other risks include somatic mutations that may contribute to other diseases (e.g., birth defects and eye maladies) and from animal studies, inherited mutations that may affect the incidence of diseases in future generations (see What's New? Radiation and Vulnerable Populations). Heritable mutations are of particular concern for women because the number of oocytes are presumably fixed at birth and mutations, if not repaired, are cumulative (see p. 421).[146] An important summary point in BEIR VII[143] is the concern from high-dose medical exposure, for example computed tomography (CT) (see What's New? Increasing Use of Computed Tomography Scans and Risks). In 2009, the National Council on Radiation Protection and Measurements[147] reported Americans were exposed to more than seven times as much ionizing radiation from medical procedures compared to the 1980s (Figure 12-7).

The risks of low-dose radiation are being debated among radiobiologists, geneticists, physicists, and others because of the potential effect on the health of current and future generations.[146] Two opposing hypotheses have emerged: (1) there is no dose of radiation considered safe and the use of radiation must always be considered on the basis of risk versus benefit and (2) the health risks of diagnostic doses less than 10 cGy are not now measurable and may be nonexistent. Limiting is that general findings on the health risks of low-dose radiation are made by analyses of data on the risk of cancer alone.[146] The expression of radiation-induced damage depends not only on dose, fractionation, and protraction but also on repair mechanisms, bystander effects, radioprotective substances such as antioxidants, and how it is delivered.[146]

Radiation-Induced Cancer

Ionizing radiation (IR) is a mutagen and carcinogen and can penetrate cells and tissues and deposit energy in tissues at random in the form of ionizations (e.g., excitation or removal of an electron from the target atom). These ionizations can lead to irreversible or indirect damage from formation and

WHAT'S NEW? **Radiation and Vulnerable Populations: Pregnant Women, Embryos, Fetus, and Children**

Protection of pregnant females against ionizing radiation is unique because of the high fetal radiosensitivity during various gestational stages. The main adverse effects to the embryo and fetus include malformations, mental retardation, induced cancer, hereditary effects, and death. These effects differ by absorbed dose, gestational period and exposure, and type of radiation. All of these concerns have demanded better radiation dosimetry (e.g., standards) for pregnant women. Although setting standards is extremely complex, models of pregnant women have, until very recently, been based on the same methodology developed 40 years ago. These models were developed by the Oak Ridge National Laboratory (ORNL) for the Medical Internal Radiation Dose (MIRD) Committee of the Society of Nuclear Medicine. Today the only published data on fetal doses for external neutron exposure are those by Chen and Taranenko and Xu. The 2008 report by Taranenko and Xu noted that comparison with previously published data showed deviations from 100% to 150% for the fetal doses at 50 keV. The only previous data available of coefficients for photons were based on stylized models of simplified anatomy. To improve these earlier models, a new set of models, called RPI-P series, represent a pregnant female with the fetus at 3, 6, and 9 months' gestation. The deviations in data points are attributed to the differences in anatomic models. In 2003 the American Academic of Pediatrics Committee on Environmental Health brought attention to the issue of radiation and children with the policy statement "Radiation Disasters and Children" (see *Pediatrics* 111[6 Pt 1]:1455-1466, 2003). The following statements summarize the risks of children from radiation:

Children have a number of vulnerabilities that place them at greater risk of harm after radiation exposure. Because they have a relatively greater minute ventilation compared with adults, children are likely to have greater exposure to radioactive gases (e.g., those emitted from a nuclear power plant disaster). Nuclear fallout quickly settles to the ground, resulting in a higher concentration of radioactive material in the space where children most commonly live and breathe. Studies of airborne pollutants are needed to test the long-held belief that the short stature of children brings them into greater contact than adults with fallout as it settles to earth. Radioactive iodine is transmitted to human breast milk, contaminating this valuable source of nutrition to infants. Cow milk, a staple in the diet of most children, can also be quickly contaminated if radioactive material settles onto grazing areas.

In utero exposure to radiation also has important clinical effects, depending on the dose and form of the radiation; transmission of radionuclides across the placenta may occur, depending on the agent…

Radiation-induced cancers occur more often in children than in adults exposed to the same dose. Finally, children also have mental health vulnerabilities after any type of disaster, with a greater risk of long-term behavioral disturbances.

Radiation risks to infants and children per unit of exposure are far greater than they are to adults. In addition, a higher cancer risk is noted in females for most cancers.

Data from Chen J: *Health Phys* 86.285-295, 2004; Chen J: *Health Phys* 90:223-231, 2006; Chen J: *Radiat Prot Dosimetry* 126(1-4): 567-671, 2007; International Commission on Radiological Protection: *Ann ICRP* 30(1):iii-viii, 1-43, 2000; International Commission on Radiological Protection: *Ann ICRP* 31(1-3):19-515, 2001; International Commission on Radiological Protection: *Ann ICRP* 33(1-2):5-206, 2003; Suárez RC et al: *Radiat Prot Dosimetry* 127(1-4):19-22, 2007; Taranenko V, Xu XG: *Phys Med Biol* 53:1425-1445, 2008.

WHAT'S NEW? **Increasing Use of Computed Tomography Scans and Risks**

A review article in the *New England Journal of Medicine* on computed tomography (CT) and radiation exposure has received much media attention. The article was written by radiology researchers at Columbia University. In short, the numbers of CT scans have greatly increased in the United States. This increase has occurred in both diagnostic treatment for individuals with symptoms and in those without symptoms for heart, lung, colon, and whole-body screening. Faster scanning times are partly responsible for increased CT use in pediatric populations. Typical doses are larger from CT scans than a conventional examination (e.g., 50 times more radiation to stomach than an x-ray). Based on data correlations from Japanese survivors of atomic bombs, the authors estimated that 1.5% to 2.0% of cancers in the United States might be attributable to CT radiation. The authors note that CT scans are sometimes ordered excessively and repeated unnecessarily because of defensive medicine. They also include three ways to reduce radiation exposure from CT: (1) reduce radiation doses in individual studies (i.e., use modern scanners), (2) substitute ultrasonography with magnetic resonance imaging (MRI) for CT when possible, and (3) order CT scans only when absolutely necessary.

Data from Brenner DJ, Hall EJ: *N Engl J Med* 357:2277, 2007; Brett AS: *J Watch* 28(1):3, 2008.

attack by water-based free radicals (radiolysis).[148] IR affects many cell processes, including gene expression, disruption of mitochondrial function, cell cycle arrest, and cell death. IR is a potent DNA damaging agent causing cross-linking, nucleotide base damage, and single- and double-strand breaks (Figure 12-8).[149] Damage to DNA and disrupted cellular regulation processes can lead to carcinogenesis.[149-151] The double-strand break (DSB) (see Figure 12-8) is considered the characteristic lesion observed for the effects of IR. In certain experimental systems, a single DSB may lead to cell cycle arrest and possible further repair. Yet many DSBs appear to result from *clustered damage*, a consequence of the pattern of distribution of ionizations with DNA. These patterns of clustered damage may be more difficult to accurately repair.[148] Importantly, DSBs are mostly repaired by the nonhomologous end joining (NHEJ) pathway. This pathway is efficient for joining the DNA broken ends; however, errors can occur. Irradiated human cells unable to execute the NHEJ are supersensitive to the introduction of large-scale mutations and chromosomal aberrations.[148]

A long-held assumption is that cellular alterations—mutations and malignant transformation—occur only in cells *directly* radiated. It is now known that radiation may induce a type of *genomic instability* to the progeny of the directly

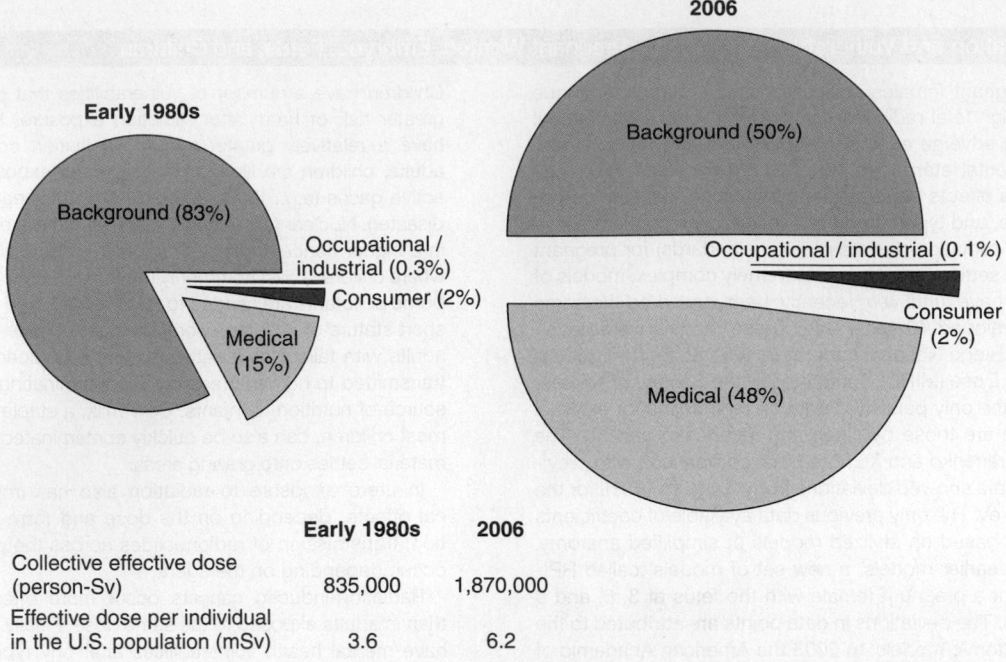

	Early 1980s	2006
Collective effective dose (person-Sv)	835,000	1,870,000
Effective dose per individual in the U.S. population (mSv)	3.6	6.2

Figure 12-7 Ionizing radiation exposure of the population of the United States. (NCRP report no. 160.)

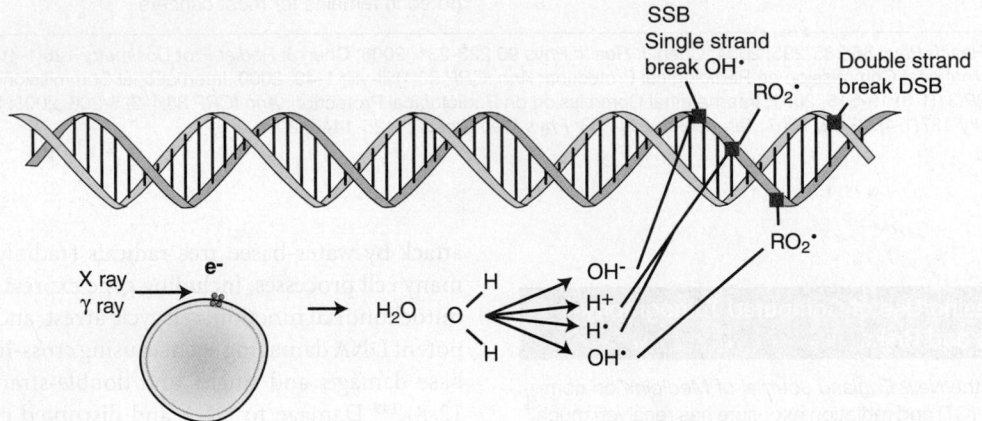

Figure 12-8 Free radicals. Free radicals formed by water nearby and around DNA cause indirect effects. These effects have a short life of single free radicals. Oxygen can modify reaction, enabling longer lifetimes of oxidative free radicals.

irradiated cells over many generations of cell radiation, leading to an *increased* rate at which the genetic effects (i.e., mutations/chromosomal aberrations) arise in these distant progeny called **transgeneration effects.** The directly irradiated cells also can lead to genetic effects in so-called bystander cells or innocent cells (called *bystander effects*) even though they themselves received no direct radiation exposure.[148] For example, using an in vivo mouse model, investigators found that localized radiation to the head led to induced bystander effects in the lead-shielded distant spleen tissue.[152] The vast majority of bystander effects have been described in cell-culture systems. In vivo (i.e., in an organism) was reported in lead shielded mouse heads after radiation exposure of the remainder of the body (Mancuso et al 2008).[153] These mice

showed unexpected enhancement of medulloblastoma in cerebellum of radiosensitive *Patched-1 (Ptch1)* heterozygous mice. Both double-strand DNA breaks and apoptotic cell death were induced by bystander effects supporting the role of gap-junctional intercellular communication (GJIC, see p. 423). The bystander and genomic instability effects also have been termed **"nontargeted" effects** (see pp. 420-422). Although bystander and transgeneration IR effects are associated with induced genomic instability leading to chromosome aberrations, gene mutations, late cell death, and aneuploidy, all of these effects may be epigenetically mediated (see p. 401). The epigenetic changes include DNA methylation, histone modification, and RNA-associated silencing (see p. 403 and Chapter 11).[152]

Radiation-induced cancer in humans seems to have long latent periods; 10 years for leukemia and more than 30 years for solid tumors.[154] This implies that radiation-induced gene mutations or chromosomal alterations that can be detected early (within 24 hours of radiation exposure) are not *solely* responsible for tumor development in normal human cells. Such mutations, however, provide a critical hit or induce *genetic instability* that makes cells more susceptible to accumulation of genetic alterations caused by other spontaneous or induced mutations. The accumulation of mutations leads to full transformation and cancer.[148]

The majority of evidence on radiation-induced human cancer risk is from epidemiologic studies of exposed populations. For example, an increase of total cancers after the Chernobyl radioactive fallout was reported in Sweden.[155] Most direct data, however, are available only at relatively high doses (greater than 0.1 Gy) from mainly low-LET radiation (x- and γ-rays). Data, however, from cell-culture systems and in vivo mouse studies are emerging for low dose radiation. Radiation-induced cancers include some leukemias and lymphomas, thyroid cancers, some sarcomas, skin cancers, and some lung and breast carcinomas.

Constant debate involves risk estimates for human exposure at low-dose, low-LET ionizing radiation (0 to 100 mSv or less than 0.1 Gy). The problem is complicated because setting regulation levels at which levels of interest are so low that data endpoints—mutations and cancer—become difficult to measure with statistical significance[144]; thus theoretic models are used to estimate response curves. Several models include the **linear no-threshold (LNT) relationship,** in which *any* dose, including very low doses, has the potential to cause mutations (Figure 12-9). The **threshold model** proposes a threshold dose below which radiation may not cause cancer in humans. Proponents of this model argue that such thresholds derive,

for example, from the ability to repair damage caused by lower doses of radiation. Another model, the **linear-quadratic relationship,** proposes there is a risk mathematical term that is directly proportional to the dose (linear term) and another proportional to the square of the dose (quadratic term) (see Figure 12-9). There is some evidence that low doses may actually produce a *higher* level of risk per unit of dose called the **supra-linear hypothesis** (see Figure 12-9).[154] Currently, the shape of the response curve for the low-dose region is really unknown.[144] In 1990, the Fifth Biological Effects of Ionizing Radiation Panel (BEIR V) estimated that the risk of radiation was considerably higher than prior official studies.[154] It supported the LNT relationship for solid cancers and included estimates of cancer risk.

Recent data, however, show that the LNT model underestimates the risk from low radiation.[156] The researchers used a precision microbeam device to fire alpha particles into nuclei of human-hamster hybrid cells in Petri dishes. When the researchers irradiated the nuclei with just *one* alpha particle each, 98 mutations of a particular gene occurred per 100,000 surviving cells. Zapping only 5% of the nuclei produced 57 such mutations per 100,000 cells, rather than the 5 mutations that a linear model predicts. These data suggest that the relevant target for radiation-induced mutagenesis is larger than an individual cell and thus supports the need to reconsider the validity of the linear extrapolation model.[156]

An important conclusion from BEIR VII was **hormesis,** or proposed adaptive/stimulatory (beneficial) effects of low doses of ionizing radiation, that exceeds detrimental effects; it is *unwarranted* at this time and not addressed further.[144] A summary of the BEIR VII estimates of cancer risk from low-level radiation changed from BEIR V and is included in Table 12-7. The risk to women is now estimated to be considerably higher.[157] BEIR VII also has provided both estimates of risk of

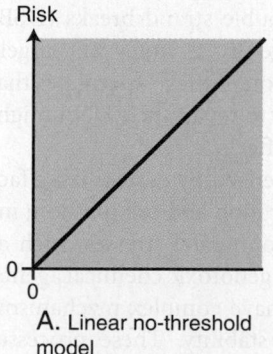

A. Linear no-threshold model

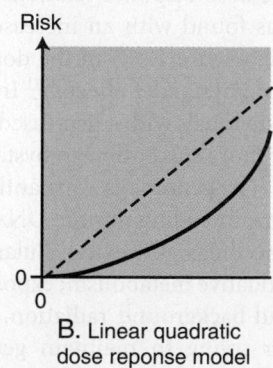

B. Linear quadratic dose reponse model

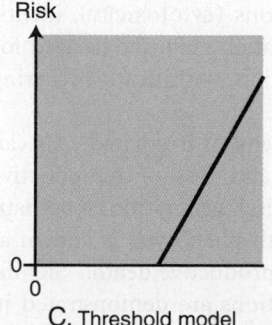

C. Threshold model

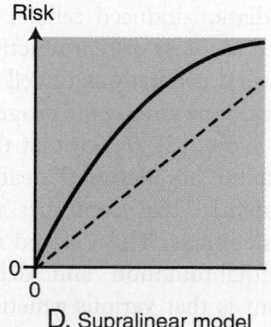

D. Supralinear model

Figure 12-9 **Theoretic models for estimating risk of low-dose ionizing radiation.** Collective population dose is expressed as a person-rem (roentgen equivalent man) (see Table 12-7). Estimating a collective dose then enables an application of a "constant risk factor" to get a statistical estimate of the number of additional cancers (above background radiation) resulting from that exposure. These computations apply to low doses—low-dose rates only (**A**). Many propose the best fit is the Linear No-Threshold (LNT) model (**B**). The most common alternative to the LNT Model is the Linear-Quadratic Model. The quadratic term is the square of the dose. The linear term is equal to zero (**C**). The threshold model is a threshold below which there is *no* increase in cancer risk. Proponents of this model argue that some toxic chemicals/materials exhibit such thresholds and that radiation must, too. Their arguments are related to repair of the radiation damage caused by lower doses of radiation (**D**). Some evidence exists that low levels of radiation produce a higher level of risk per unit dose called the Supra-linear Model. (From Makhijani A, Smith B, Thorne MC: *Science for the vulnerable: setting radiation and multiple exposure environmental health standards to protect those at most risk,* IEER, Takoma Park, Maryland, 2006.)

Table 12-7	Cancer Incidence and Fatality (BEIR VII) Estimates of Low-Level Radiation per Gender					
	Solid Cancers		Leukemia		All Cancers	
	Males	Females	Males	Females	Males	Females
Incidence	800 (400-1600)*	1300 (690-2500)*	100 (30-300)*	70 (20-250)*	900	1370
Fatal cancers only	410 (200-830)*	610 (300-1200)*	70 (20-220)*	50 (10-90)*	480	660

*Estimates correspond to 95% confidence interval in parenthesis.
Estimated number of cancer cases and deaths expected to result in 100,000 persons.

cancer incidence in addition to fatal cancer risk. The risks also have estimated the cancer risk by age.

Carcinogenesis: Genomic Instability

Genomic instability is an increased tendency of the genome to acquire mutations when various processes involved in maintaining and replicating the genome are dysfunctional. Biologic consequences of exposure to ionizing radiation include cell death, gene mutations, and chromosome aberrations. Conventional dogma attributes these effects to alterations resulting from the deposition of energy to the DNA of an irradiated cell. Eventually the cell is presumed repaired by DNA enzymatic mechanisms that also can occur during DNA replication. It was widely accepted that most of these changes took place immediately after exposure. Thus if the damage were faithfully repaired, the descendants of an irradiated cell would be normal (Figure 12-10, *A*). If misrepaired, however, the descendants would be expected to pass on radiation-induced genetic change and all cells derived from such a cell would have the identical genetic alteration, or, more simply, the effect would be clonal (Figure 12-10, *B*). Yet many in vitro studies have demonstrated nonclonal chromosome aberrations and mutations in the clonal progeny of irradiated cells.[158] Furthermore, it has been known for many years that radiation-induced cellular alterations (cytotoxicity), identified as a loss of reproductive potential, might be delayed for several generations of cell replication, with death occurring randomly among the progeny cells.[158]

Now it is known that the progeny of irradiated cells can exhibit an increased death rate and loss of reproductive potential that continues for several generations—perhaps indefinitely. This delayed cell death phenotype is known as "lethal mutation" and "delayed reproductive death." Significant is that various genetic alterations are demonstrated in cells that are *not* themselves irradiated, but in so-called *innocent cells* that are referred to as bystander effects and are considered manifestations of a radiation-induced genomic instability (see following and Figure 12-10, *C*). This instability is similar to inherited chromosome instability syndromes with spontaneously high levels of chromosomal alterations and mutations.[159] Why is radiation-induced genomic instability relevant to low-dose exposure? Little[160] provides a hypothetical model for multistep carcinogenesis incorporating radiation induced genomic instability (RIGI). As part of the multistep model, it is proposed that a number of mutations in individual genes must accumulate in a given group of cells to give rise to an invasive tumor. Thus hypothetically, radiation might act at an initial stage of carcinogenesis but could act at any time in later stages after one or more initiating mutations have occurred.[160] Radiation may induce or increase genomic instability by facilitating new mutations in later generations. This effect may also be mediated by a nontargeted bystander mechanism. Little[160] includes these important summary characteristics of RIGI relevant to low doses:

- RIGI is a "high-frequency" event occurring in 10% or more cells in an irradiated population.
- The biologic effects are manifested *later* after many rounds of cell division, making it possible that RIGI induced in germinal cells could be passed on to the offspring possibly conferring genetic effects including cancer in these children.

Induction of genetic changes in bystander cells, as well as those directly radiated, could lead to a "hyperlinearity" response; that is, a higher level of risk per unit dose, also called the supralinear model of the dose response curve for low dose (low particle fluences) (see Figure 12-9, *D*, p. 419) when only a small number of the cells are irradiated.[160] Direct evidence of the dose-response relationship of a supra-linear relationship was found with an increase in double strand breaks (DSB) (see Figure 12-8) in the dose range of 1.2-5mGy was largely from bystander effects.[161] In addition, Little[160] speculates that individuals with a decreased ability to repair their DNA might be more susceptible to bystander effects.

The genome is constantly challenged by destabilizing factors, including normal DNA replication and cell division; intracellular and extracellular environmental stresses, such as oxidative metabolism; exposure to genotoxic chemical agents; and background radiation. Cells have complex mechanisms for trying to maintain genomic stability. These processes include proofreading of DNA replication, enzymatic repair of DNA damage, and checkpoints monitoring progression through the cell cycle. Failure of any of these processes can result in destabilization of the genome, deleterious mutations, and alterations in cell proliferation.

Although similar to alterations to the chromosome instability syndromes, the radiation-induced genomic instability seems to reflect epigenetic phenomena rather than mutation of genome genes.[149] Experiments have shown that

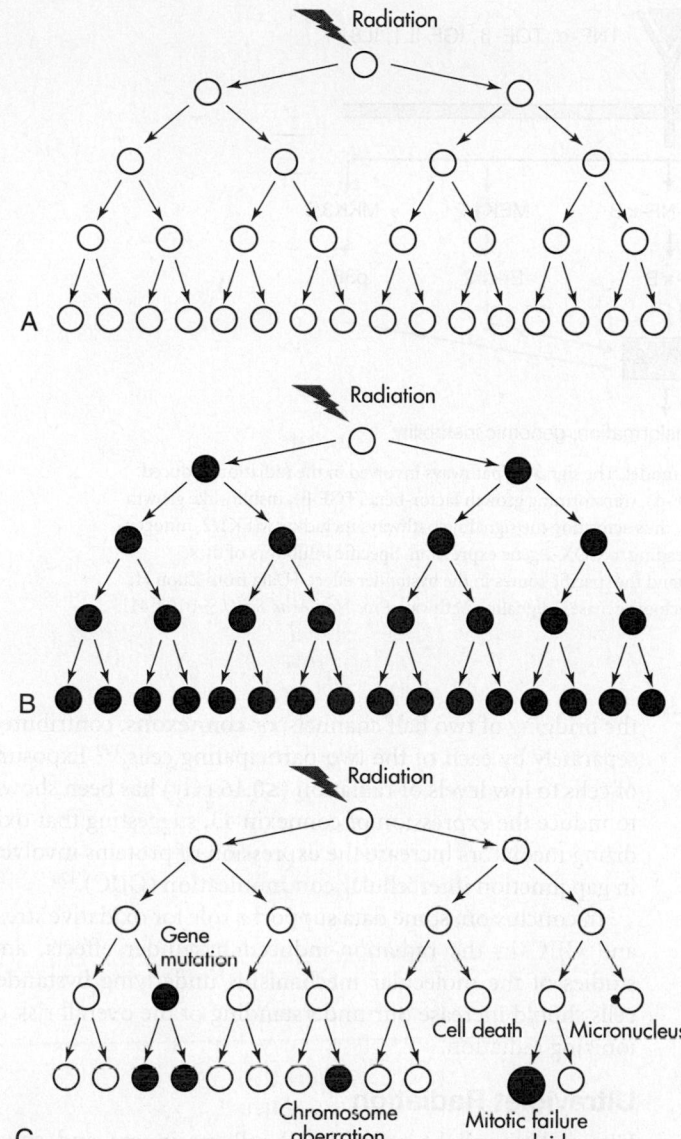

Figure 12-10 Models of the responses of clonogenic cells to ionizing radiation. Mutations and/or chromosomal aberrations are shown as filled circles and apparently normal cells as open circles. **A,** If a cell faithfully repairs DNA damage, then its clonal descendents will appear normal. **B,** If a cell is directly mutated by radiation, then all of its descendants will express the same mutation. **C,** Radiation-induced genomic instability is characterized by nonclonal effects in descendant cells. (From Lorimore SA, Coates PJ, Wright EG: *Oncogene* 22[45]:7058-7069, 2003.)

irradiation can induce growth factors and extracellular matrix (microenvironment) remodeling. A major function of the microenvironment is to control cell differentiation and proliferation, and its disruption is required for the establishment of cancer.[162] These data suggest that such epigenetic events after radiation, including alterations in pathways affecting cell adhesion, extracellular matrix interactions, and cell-to-cell communication, may override the positive or repairing influence of tissue signaling and architecture that inhibits neoplastic progression.[162] The chromosomal instability noted in mouse hematopoietic tissue[163] and mouse mammary epithelium[164] is, however, strongly influenced by genetic factors, with some genotypes being more susceptible than others.

Bystander Effects

In vivo and in vitro culture experiments performed over the past two decades indicate that low-dose ionizing radiation causes significantly divergent biologic responses from high-dose radiation. Two important findings concerning the biologic effects of a low dose (or low fluences) of radiation occur in the irradiated cells and in cells that are not themselves radiated—the so-called **bystander effect:** (1) radiation-induced genomic instability occurs in the descendant cells of the irradiated cell after several generations of cell division, and (2) radiation-induced bystander effects are caused as a consequence of damage signals transmitted from neighboring irradiated cells whereby transmission may be mediated by either direct or intercellular communication through gap junctions or by factors released into the surrounding medium.[165] Bystander effects occur in a wide variety of cell types.[166] The biologic effects may be associated with oxidative stress and the generation of ROS (e.g., superoxide, hydrogen peroxide, COX-2) (Figure 12-11). Nitric oxide, however, may initiate intercellular signaling pathways that influence the bystander effect.[165,167] The first "proof-of-principle" in vivo experiment suggested that COX-2 (e.g., inflammatory/oxidative stress)

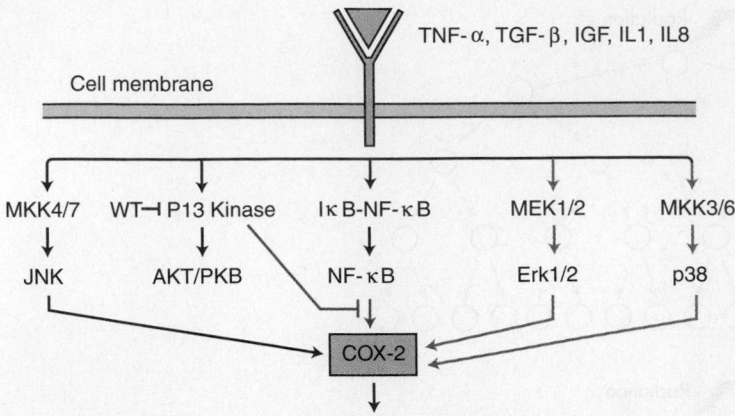

Figure 12-11 Bystander effect and signaling pathways: a working model. The signaling pathways involved in the radiation-induced bystander effect include binding of tumor necrosis factor-alpha (TNF-α), transforming growth factor-beta (TGF-β), insulin-like growth factor (IGF), interleukin-1 (IL-1), and IL-8 ligands to their receptors, thus activating the signaling pathways including MEK1/2, mitogen-activated protein kinase (MKK3/6), and p38 kinase *(purple arrows)* leading to COX-2 gene expression. Specific inhibitors of these pathways, such as Wortmannin (WT), can help investigators understand the specific routes in the bystander effect. (Data from Zhou H, et al: Mechanism of radiation-induced bystander effect: role of the cyclooxygenase-2 signaling pathway, *Proc Natl Acad Sci U S A* 102[41]: 14641-14646, 2005.)

did *not* influence the bystander damage and investigators speculated the role of connexin (gap junction) proteins.[153] Numerous intercellular and intracellular signaling pathways are implicated in the bystander response, and effects have been shown to be transmitted to their descendants (see Figure 12-11). Bystander effects include mutations, sister chromatid exchanges, chromosomal aberrations, neoplastic transformation, and cell death, proliferation, and differentiation.[166]

In vivo experiments also have shown that inflammatory-type responses occur after exposure to ionizing radiation.[168,169] Theses studies revealed that activation of macrophages and neutrophil accumulations were not *direct effects* of irradiation but were instead a consequence of the recognition and phagocytosis of radiation-induced apoptotic cells. The phagocytotic mechanism is suggested for the interactions between irradiated and nonirradiated (i.e., bystander effects) hematopoietic cells, both in vivo and in vitro.[169] Persistent activation of these inflammatory-type responses is implicated as a contributory bystander mechanism for causing delayed DNA damage (see Figure 12-12).[168] Oxidative-stress mediators also have been implicated in the cytotoxic effects observed in solid tumors located at distinct sites away from those receiving radiation.[170] Genes responsible for oxidative stress have been identified.[171] Direct evidence of how these oxidative events occur is, however, lacking; also unclear is the source of the oxidants—are they strictly derived from cytoplasmic membranes or from the mitochondria?

Gap Junction Intercellular Communication

Confluent cell cultures respond as an integrated whole rather than as separate individual cells that have been irradiated, indicating a critical role for cell-to-cell communication in mediating the bystander effect. This mediation could be controlled by gap junctions. Gap junctions consist of a cell-to-cell channel spanning two plasma membranes; they result from

the bridging of two half channels, or **connexons**, contributed separately by each of the two participating cells.[172] Exposure of cells to low levels of radiation (≤0.16 cGy) has been shown to induce the expression of connexin 43, suggesting that oxidizing mediators increase the expression of proteins involved in gap junction intercellular communication (GJIC).[171]

In conclusion, some data support a role for oxidative stress and GJIC in the radiation-induced bystander effects, and studies of the molecular mechanisms underlying bystander cells should increase our understanding of the overall risk of ionizing radiation.

Ultraviolet Radiation

Ultraviolet sunlight *causes* basal cell carcinoma and squamous cell carcinoma (i.e., photocarcinogenesis), two common skin cancers found in white individuals. Exposure to ultraviolet radiation (UVR) can emanate from natural and artificial sources; however, the principal source of exposure for most people is sunlight. With further depletion of the stratospheric ozone layer, people and the environment will be exposed to higher intensities of UVR. The degree of damage in skin depends on the intensity and wavelength content (i.e., ultraviolet A [UVA] or ultraviolet B [UVB]) and the depth of penetration. UV radiation is known to cause specific gene mutations; for example, squamous cell carcinoma involves mutation in the *TP53* gene, basal cell carcinoma in the *patched* gene, and melanoma in the *p16* gene.[173] In addition, UV light induces the release of TNF-α in the epidermis, which may reduce immune surveillance against skin cancer.[174]

Skin exposure to UVR and ionizing radiation, as well as chemical (xenobiotic) agents/drugs, produces ROS in large quantities that can overwhelm tissue antioxidants and other oxygen-degrading pathways.[175] Uncontrolled release of ROS is an important contributor to skin carcinogenesis.[175]

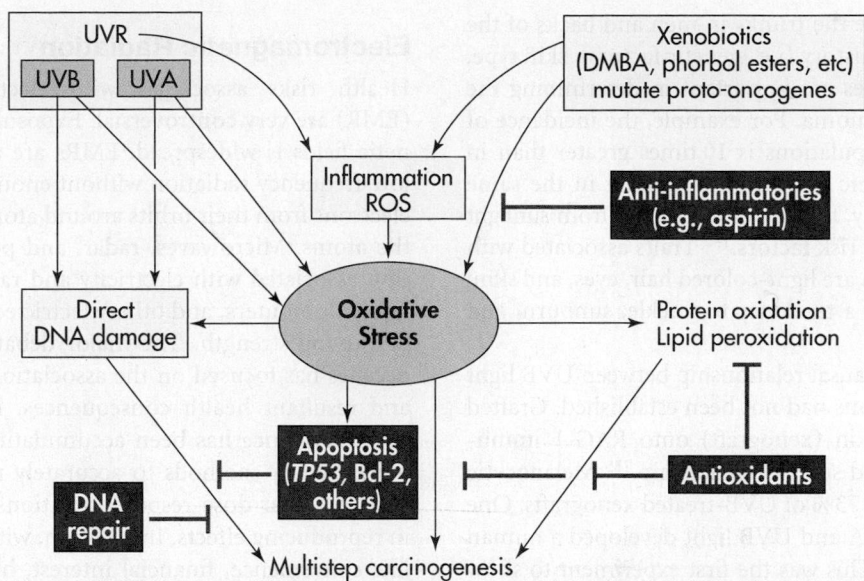

Figure 12-12 Theoretic scheme of multistep skin carcinogenesis. Ultraviolet radiation (UVR), inflammation, and xenobiotics (see p. 405) lead to oxidative stress, resulting in direct DNA damage, protein oxidation, lipid peroxidation, and apoptosis. The protective mechanisms shown in *red* include apoptosis, DNA repair, and antioxidants. *DMBA*, Dimethylbenzene anthracene; *ROS*, reactive oxygen species; *UVA*, ultraviolet A; *UVB*, ultraviolet B. (Adapted from Sander CD et al: *Intl J Dermatol* 43[5]: 326-340, 2004.)

Imbalances in ROS and antioxidants can lead to oxidative stress, tissue injury, and direct DNA damage (see Figure 12-12). ROS can induce a number of transcription factors (e.g., activator protein-1 [AP-1] and NF-κβ).[176] In addition, UVA radiation of skin fibroblast releases iron, which is involved in activation of the transcription factor NF-κβ and other free radicals important in regulating genes that induce inflammation.[175,177] Inflammation is a critical component of tumor progression.

Healthy genes are needed to coordinate the levels of antioxidants and decrease harmful ROS. Antioxidants decrease ROS and oxidative stress and other protective mechanisms including DNA repair and apoptosis (see Figure 12-12). The genetic alterations in proto-oncogenes and tumor-suppressor genes may make epidermal cells resistant to signals for terminal differentiation.[177] With oxidative stress, DNA damage occurs and calcium-dependent enzymes (endonucleases) are activated that produce DNA strand breaks.[177] In addition, ROS are involved in the activation of procarcinogens, such as polycyclic aromatic hydrocarbons including 7,12-dimethyl-benzene(a)anthracene (DMBA). DMBA is capable of initiating a point mutation in the *ras* proto-oncogene, which is evidenced to be the triggering event in mouse carcinogenesis.[178] The essential step appears to be the activation of DMBA by nicotinamide adenine dinucleotide dehydrogenase (NADH) and cytochrome P-450–dependent oxidases.[179] The pathophysiology of skin carcinogenesis is discussed further in Chapter 44.

Basal cell carcinoma commonly occurs on the head and neck. Individuals with these tumors generally have light complexions, light eyes, and fair hair. They tend to sunburn rather than tan and live in areas of high sunlight exposure. Usually these cancers arise on areas of the body that receive the greatest sun exposure, although they are not necessarily restricted to these skin sites. Squamous cell carcinoma is found more commonly in men who work outdoors. These tumors are distributed over the head, neck, and exposed areas of the upper extremities (see Chapter 44).

The incidence of melanoma has been increasing annually at rates of 2% to 7% for white populations.[180] The steady rise in incidence has resulted in an alarming 165% increase in mortality rate.[181] Sun exposure and the risk of melanoma, a malignant pigmented mole, remain complex. Melanomas can appear suddenly without warning but can arise from or near a mole (melanocytic nevus). When detected in the early stages, melanoma is highly curable.[181] About 20% of melanomas, however, are diagnosed at nonlocalized and advanced stages.[181] The pathogenesis of melanoma is complex, involving genetic and environmental factors. The genetic factors can be inherited, for example, in high-susceptibility genes (i.e., cyclin-dependent kinase inhibitor 2A [CDKN2A]) or in low-susceptibility genes (i.e., melanocortin-1). Epidemiologic and case-control studies suggest that UVR exposure is the most significant factor for the development of melanoma. Other evidence, however, reports rates of melanoma are uncommon in persons with outdoor occupations.[182] Although non-melanoma skin cancers are related to cumulative exposure to UV radiation, melanoma is related to episodes of intense, intermittent exposure (measured as history of sunburn).[183] Melanomas more commonly occur in areas less continually exposed to sunlight, like the trunks in men and backs of the legs in women. Family history (i.e., genetic factors), skin type, and the density of moles are important in determining the risk of developing melanoma. For example, the incidence of melanoma in white populations is 10 times greater than in black, Asian, or Hispanic populations residing in the same area.[182] Most importantly, the risk of melanoma from sunlight is certainly modified by risk factors.[182] Traits associated with a high risk of melanoma are light-colored hair, eyes, and skin; an inability to tan; and a tendency to freckle, sunburn, and develop nevi.[184]

Until 1998 a direct causal relationship between UVB light and melanoma in humans had not been established. Grafted newborn human foreskin (xenograft) onto RAG-1 immunodeficient mice showed such a relationship.[185] Melanocytic hyperplasia occurred in 73% of UVB-treated xenografts. One graft treated with DMBA and UVB light developed a human malignant melanoma. This was the first experiment to show that UVB light and an exogenous carcinogen could result in a new malignant melanoma.

A similar study using UVB light and overexpression of an endogenous growth factor, basic fibroblast growth factor (bFGF), also induced human melanoma.[186] Numerous local factors may result in increased cytokine production, including trauma, infection, diet, obesity, hormones, and other causes of inflammation. Sunburn reflects an overdose of UV light, triggering inflammation with an increase in cytokine production.

A very significant finding in 2002 jolted the melanoma field. Davies and colleagues[179] detected an activating point mutation in the *B-raf* (BRAF) proto-oncogene (i.e., somatic, not germline, mutation) in 60% to 70% of malignant melanomas. This mutation results in a marked increase in BRAF kinase activity, leading to activation of the mitogen-activated protein kinase (MAPK) pathway (see Table 1-4). This BRAF mutation and others have recently been linked to sun exposure.[187] Activation of MAPK in melanoma can occur through several mechanisms: (1) mutation in the *B-raf* gene, (2) stimulation of fibroblast growth factor (FGF) and hepatocyte growth factor (HGF), (3) exogenous stimulation by IGF-1, and (4) by adhesion molecule receptor signaling. The development of melanoma is associated with the loss of E-cadherin and the appearance of N-cadherin adhesion molecules. **Cadherins** are cell surface glycoproteins that promote calcium-dependent cell-to-cell adhesion. The major adhesion molecule between keratinocytes and normal melanocytes is E-cadherin, which disappears during melanoma progression,[188] and is expressed in melanoma cells, allowing them to adhere to fibroblasts and endothelial cells. Thus N-cadherin allows the melanoma cells to survive as they migrate through the dermis.[189] (For further discussion, see Chapter 44.)

Increased knowledge of the intricate cellular interactions in melanoma will increase knowledge of melanoma etiology and pathogenesis. This knowledge is essential for early detection and treatment.

Electromagnetic Radiation

Health risks associated with electromagnetic radiation (EMR) are very controversial. Exposure to electric and magnetic fields is widespread. EMRs are a type of nonionizing, low-frequency radiation without enough energy to break off electrons from their orbits around atoms and ionize (charge) the atoms. Microwaves, radar, and power frequency radiation associated with electricity and radio waves, fluorescent lights, computers, and other electric equipment create EMRs of varying strength. The major debate for more than four decades has focused on the association of exposure to EMR and resultant health consequences, including cancer. Scientific evidence has been accumulating slowly because it is hampered by methods to accurately measure exposure, the lack of a clear dose-response relationship, and the difficulty in reproducing effects. In addition, with competing priorities like convenience, financial interest, health necessity, a consensus of the risk/benefit ratio of EMR exposure may be difficult to achieve.[190] A recent case-control study in Japan linked high EMR exposure with a significantly higher risk of childhood leukemia.[191] Other recent studies report the *apparent* link between cordless and cellular phone use with lymphoma and benign and malignant brain tumors.[192-195] Another case-control study reported a link between childhood leukemia and prenatal proximity to high-voltage powerlines.[196] Data from Sweden show adverse EMR has the potential to induce certain skin abnormalities and is a positive factor in the development of melanoma.[197,198] Yet another recent study denied an association between EMR exposure and female breast cancer.[199] A recent population-based study ($N = 5400$ women) linked residential EMR exposure from high voltage power lines to a 60% increased risk of breast cancer in Norwegian women of all ages.[200] In 1998, however, a National Institute of Environmental Health Sciences Electric and Magnetic Fields Working Group recommended that low-frequency electromagnetic fields (EMFs) be classified as possible carcinogens.[201] Sweden has officially categorized electrohypersensitivity as a functional impairment.[202] The United Kingdom Childhood Cancer Study published in 1999 and updated in 2000[203,204] did not support a link between EMR exposure and childhood cancer. A pooled analysis from Europe showed no risk of childhood cancers with *average* exposures (less than 0.1 micro T), no increased risk at *intermediate* exposures, but at the *highest* average exposures (greater than 0.3 micro T American studies or 0.4 micro T European study) increased risk affecting few children (1.4%) with a significant relative risk of 2.[205] In response to public concern, the WHO requested further studies in high-exposure areas like Japan. Thus a case-control study from Japan ($N = 312$ children) found acute lymphocytic leukemia (ALL) cases in the *highest* exposure category above 0.4 micro T.[191]

The controversy about potential health hazards associated with the exposure to EMFs has been stimulated by the increased use of mobile telecommunication devices and emissions from cell towers. Cell phones emit electromagnetic radiation in the range of 800 to 2000 MHz, which is in the microwave range (300 MHz to 300 GHz).

EMR from a cell phone can penetrate the skull and deposit energy 4 to 6 cm into the brain.[206] This energy can result in thermal heating of the tissue. The debate therefore has been whether these thermal effects could induce carcinogenesis. One thermal mechanism proposed is change in protein phosphorylation.[207,208] Exposure of human peripheral blood lymphocytes to EMR associated with cell phones found a linear increase in chromosome 17 aneuploidy.[209] Control experiments (without EMR) involving temperature changes from 24.5° to 38.5° C (76° to 101.3° F) showed that elevated temperature is not associated with genetic or epigenetic alterations. Thus these findings indicated a genotoxic effect of the EMRs is not elicited by a thermal pathway.[209] Increasing evidence indicates that the mechanism of harm from EMR is induction of cell stress and damage of intracellular components (e.g., free radical formation and altered protein conformation).[210] Adverse EMR has been reported to affect DNA synthesis, alter cell division, alter electrical charge of ions, and alter molecules within cells.[211,212] Interference with cellular electrical charges may modify ionic structures, disturbing movement of ions across the membrane, including calcium ions.[188,213]

In 2007, a meta-analysis of cell phones and brain tumors concluded that studies of individuals using cell phones for more than 10 years "give a consistent pattern of an increased risk for acoustic neuroma and glioma."[193] The risk of a tumor is highest on the same side of the head that the phone is used. The studies reported are international including Sweden, Finland, the United Kingdom, Germany, Japan, and the United States. There are no studies of adults who have used cell phones as children or adolescents. Concern is for children in whom the effects may be compounded because of increased vulnerability to radiation and their longer use of cell phones into adulthood. Ongoing unbiased research is desperately needed. Absolute proof of causation may be hindered because of the ethical questions of exposing individuals to potentially harmful interventions.[189]

Sexual and Reproductive Behavior: Human Papillomaviruses

The past decade has demonstrated that sexually transmitted infection with carcinogenic types of human papillomavirus (HPV), referred to as *high-risk types of HPV*, is required for the development of most cervical cancers. In addition, HPV is a newly identified causal factor for squamous cell carcinoma of the head and neck (SCCHN).[140] HPV infections, however, are very common in sexually active women, and the majority of these infections will resolve or only cause transient, minor problems.[214] Eighty HPV types have been sequenced—30 of these types infect the female and male genital tract and two thirds of these are classified as high-risk types. HPV-16, in most countries, accounts for 50% to 60% of cervical cancer cases, followed by HPV-18 (10% to 12%) and HPV-31 and HPV-45 (4% to 5% each).[215,216] HPV types correlated with genital warts, HPV-6 and HPV-11, are called *low risk* because they are rarely associated with cancer.[216] HPV-16 is directly mutagenic by inducing the viral genes *E6* and *E7*. Persistence of infection with high-risk HPV is a prerequisite for the development of cervical intraepithelial neoplasia (CIN) (see Figure 23-17) lesions and invasive cervical cancers.[215] Biologic factors that determine persistence are not understood; controversial risk factors include long-term use of oral contraceptives and smoking.[217] Newer risk factors being studied include drug addiction and reproductive factors (i.e., age at menarche and menopause). In fact, it has been shown that a second peak of high-risk HPV prevalence occurs in postmenopausal women.[217] Smoking has been implicated in acquiring high-risk HPV (HR-HPV) but not as an independent risk factor for high-grade CIN.[218] Earlier reported risk factors, for example, number of sexual partners, are probably indicators of HPV exposure rather than independent risk factors. HPV can be transmitted by genital contact (oral, touching, or sexual intercourse); therefore, condoms are not necessarily protective (see Chapter 23).

About 500,000 cases of invasive cervical cancer are diagnosed each year worldwide—the majority in developing countries. Although HPV is the most prevalent sexually transmitted infection in the United States, less than one third of women and men in the general population have heard of it, and awareness is low among women in high school and college settings.[219] Cervical cancer mortality has decreased over the past five decades in the United States by more than 70%, probably due to screening with the Papanicolaou (Pap) test.[214] HPV vaccination programs have made it possible to eliminate about 70% of all invasive cervical cancers worldwide (see Chapter 23).[219] Human immunodeficiency virus (HIV)–infected individuals have demonstrated an increase in oral and anogenital pathologic conditions because of HPV infection.[220]

The incidence of invasive cervical cancer is substantially higher in women of low socioeconomic standing and is more common in Central and South America, eastern Africa, and the Caribbean.[221] Consensus is that newborn babies can be exposed to cervical HPV infection of the mother. The possible modes of transmission in children, however, are controversial.[222]

Other Viruses and Microorganisms

A discussion on viruses and bacteria and cancer is contained in Chapter 11. Other microorganisms include particular parasites, such as *Opisthorchis viverrini* and *Schistosoma haematobium*. Their specific roles in carcinogenesis are thought to be related to cofactors or carcinogens, or both.

Physical Activity

Physical activity reduces the risk of breast and colon cancers and may reduce the risk of other cancers. Several biologic mechanisms causing this effect have been proposed and include decreasing insulin and IGF levels; decreasing obesity; increasing free radical scavenger systems; altering inflammatory mediators; decreasing circulating sex hormones and metabolic hormones; improving immune function; enhancing cytochrome P-450, thus modifying carcinogen activation; and increasing gut motility.[222-226] For colon cancer, physical activity increases gut motility, which reduces the length of time (transit time) that the bowel lining is exposed to potential mutagens.[227] For breast cancer, vigorous physical activity may decrease exposure of breast tissue to ovarian hormones, insulin, and IGF. A randomized trial found that after 12 months of moderate-intensity exercise, postmenopausal women had significantly decreased serum estrogens.[228] Physical activity also helps prevent type 2 diabetes, which has been associated with risk of cancer of the colon and pancreas.[228,229]

Many questions are unanswered regarding frequency, intensity, and duration of exercise. Much of the literature suggests that between 3.5 and 4 hours of vigorous activity per week are necessary to optimize protection for colon cancer.[226] There is likely a dose-response relationship for colon cancer and breast cancer, and 30 to 60 minutes per day of moderate to vigorous intensity is proposed to decrease breast cancer risk.[230] A randomized controlled trial (12 months) recently supported the Institute of Medicine and Department of Agriculture guidelines of 60 minutes per day of moderate to vigorous physical activity for decreasing weight, BMI, body fat, and intra-abdominal fat.[231]

Chemicals and Occupational Hazards as Carcinogens

An estimated 80,000 synthetic chemicals are used in the United States. Of those, only about 7% have been tested for their health effects.[232] Disturbing is that another 1000 are added each year. Exposure to chemicals occurs everyday — they are present in air, soil, food, water, household products, toys, personal care products, workplaces, and homes. Table 12-1 provides a summary of the chemicals according to strong and suspected links to various types of cancer. Box 12-2 identifies known occupational carcinogenic agents classified by the International Agency for Research on Cancer (IARC), and Box 12-3 identifies probable occupational carcinogenic agents classified by the IARC. A substantial percentage of cancers of the upper respiratory passages, lung, bladder, and peritoneum are attributed to occupational factors; however, fewer studies of nonsmokers exist.[233] One notable occupational factor is **asbestos,** which increases the risk of mesothelioma and lung cancer. Asbestos was used in homes and buildings built before the 1970s to insulate ceiling tiles, flooring, and pipe covers. In western Europe, the epidemic of mesothelioma in building workers and other workers born after 1940 did not become apparent until the 1990s because of long latency. Carcinoma of the bladder has been linked with the manufacture of dyes, rubber, paint, and aromatic amines, especially β-naphthylamine and benzidine. Benzol inhalation is linked to leukemia in shoemakers and in workers in the rubber cement, explosives, and dyeing industries. Other notable occupational hazards include heavy metals (e.g., high-nickel alloy,

chromium VI compounds, inorganic arsenic), silica, polycyclic aromatic hydrocarbons, sulfuric acid, and chloromethyl ether. Studies of occupational exposure to diesel exhaust indicate an increased risk of lung cancer.[234] Disentangling data related to lung cancer, air pollution, and occupational risks is complex, especially in combination with active and passive smoking and the interplay of environmental factors and genetic polymorphisms at multiple loci.

Air Pollution

A person inhales about 20,000 L of air every day; thus even modest contamination of the atmosphere can result in inhalation of appreciable doses of pollutants. Contaminants include outdoor and indoor air pollutants. Concerns include industrial emissions, including arsenicals, benzene, chloroform, formaldehyde, sulfuric acid, mustard gas, vinyl chloride, and acrylonitrile.[235] Living close to certain industries is a recognized cancer risk factor, although it is difficult to determine cancer risk from outdoor pollution *alone* because investigators must accurately control for smoking and radon. Studies that controlled or stratified for smoking demonstrated associations between excess lung cancer rates and heavy metal and aromatic hydrocarbon emissions in polluted air. Evidence for cancers, other than lung cancer and childhood cancer, is inconsistent.[236]

Indoor pollution generally is considered worse than outdoor pollution, partly because of cigarette smoke. Environmental tobacco smoke (ETS; passive smoking) can cause the formation of reactive oxygen free radicals and thus DNA damage. The IARC has classified ETS as a human carcinogen. Another significant indoor air pollutant is radon gas. **Radon** is a natural radioactive gas derived from the radioactive decay of uranium that is ubiquitous in rock and soil; it can become trapped in houses and gives rise to radioactive decay products known to be carcinogenic to humans. The most hazardous houses can be identified by testing and then by being modified to prevent further radon contamination. Exposure levels are greater from underground mines than from houses. Most of the lung cancers associated with radon are bronchogenic; however, small cell carcinoma does occur with greater frequency in underground miners. Radon increases the risk of lung cancer in underground miners whether they smoke or not.

In China, some regions report very high levels of lung cancer in women who spend much of their time indoors. Exposures from heating and cooking combustion sources (e.g., oil vapors) are identified as risk factors for lung cancer.[237] In addition, domestic coal use and ETS increase the risk of lung cancer in women and men.[238]

Inorganic arsenic (known as a carcinogen since the late 1960s), found principally in underground water (from 1000 to 4000 mcg/L), is found in many regions of the world. According to the IARC, strong evidence indicates an increased risk of bladder, skin, and lung cancers following consumption of water with high levels of arsenic (generally greater than 200 mcg/L).[239] Evidence for cancers of the liver, colon,

Box 12-2   Known Carcinogenic Agents Classified by the International Agency for Research on Cancer (IARC)

Agents or Group of Agents

4-Aminobiphenyl
Arsenic and arsenic compounds
Asbestos
Azathioprine
Benzene
Benzidine
Benzo[a]pyrene
Beryllium and beryllium compounds
N,N-Bis(2-chloromethyl)-2-naphthylanine ether and chloromethyl methyl ether*
1,3-Butadiene
1,4-Butanediol dimethanesulfonate (busulphan; Myleran)
Cadmium and cadmium compounds
Chlorambucil
1-(2-chloroethy)-3-(4-methylcyclohexyl)-1-nitrosourea (methyl-CCNU; semustine)
Chromium [IV] compounds
Cyclosporine
Cyclophosphamide
Diethylstilbestrol
Dyes metabolized to benzidine
Epstein-Barr virus
Eronite
Estrogen-progestogen menopausal therapy (combined)
Estrogen-progestogen oral contraceptives (combined)
Estrogens, nonsteroidal
Estrogens, steroidal
Estrogen therapy, postmenopausal
Ethanol
Ethylene oxide
Etoposide
Formaldehyde
Gallium arsenide
Gamma radiation: see x- and gamma (γ) radiation
Helicobacter pylori (infection with)
Hepatitis B virus (chronic infection with)
Hepatitis C virus (chronic infection with)
Human immunodeficiency virus type 1 (infection with)
Human papillomavirus types 16, 18, 31, 33, 35, 39, 45, 51, 52, 56, 58, 59, and 66
Human T-cell lymphotropic virus type I
Melphalan
8-Methoxypsoralen (methoxsalen)
4,4'-Methylenebis (chloroaniline) (MBOCA)
MOPP and other combined chemotherapy including alkylating agents
Mustard gas (sulfur gas)
2-Naphthylamine
Nickel compounds
N'-Nitrosonornicotine (NNN)
Oestrogen: see Estrogen
Opisthorchis viverrini (infection with)
Oral contraceptives, combined estrogen-progestogen: see Estrogen-progestogen oral contraceptives (combined)
Oral contraceptives, sequential
Ortho-toluidine
Phosphorus-32, as phosphate
Plutonium-239 and its decay products (may contain plutonium-240 and other isotopes) as aerosols
Radioiodines, short-lived isotopes, including iodine-131, from atomic reactor accidents and nuclear weapons detonation (exposure during childhood)

Radionuclides, α-particle-emitting, internally deposited
Radionuclides, β-particle-emitting, internally deposited
Radium-224 and its decay products
Radium-226 and its decay products
Radium-228 and its decay products
Radon-222 and its decay products
Schistosoma haematobium (infection with)
Silica, crystalline (inhaled in the form of quartz or cristobalite from occupational sources)
Solar radiation
Talc containing asbestiform fibers
Tamoxifen
2,3,7,8-Tetrachlorodibenzo-para-dioxin
Thiotepa
Thorium-232 and its decay products, administered intravenously as a colloidal dispersion of thorium-232 dioxide
Treosulfan
Vinyl chloride
X- and gamma (γ) radiation

Mixtures

Aflatoxins (naturally occurring mixtures of)
Alcoholic beverages
Areca nut
Betel quid with tobacco
Betel quid without tobacco
Coal-tar pitches
Coal-tars
Herbal remedies containing plant species of the genus Aristolochia
Household combustion of coal, indoor emissions from
Mineral oils, untreated or mildly treated
Phenacetin, analgesic mixtures containing
Salted fish (Chinese-style)
Shale-oils
Soots
Tobacco, smokeless
Wood dust

Exposure Circumstances

Aluminum production
Arsenic in drinking water
Auramine production
Boot and shoe manufacture and repair
Chimney sweeping
Coal gasification
Coal-tar distillation
Coke production
Furniture and cabinet making
Hematite mining (underground) with exposure to radon
Involuntary smoking (exposure to secondhand or "environmental" tobacco smoke)
Iron and steel founding
Isopropyl alcohol manufacture (strong-acid process)
Magenta production
Painter (as occupational exposure)
Paving and roofing with coal-tar pitch
Rubber industry
Strong inorganic-acid mists containing sulfuric acid (occupational exposure to)
Tobacco smoking and tobacco smoke

| Box 12-3 | Probable Carcinogenic Agents Classified by the IARC |

Agents and Group of Agents
Acrylamide
Adriamycin
Androgenic (anabolic) steroids
Aristolochic acids (naturally occurring mixtures of)
Azacitidine
Bischloroethyl nitrosourea (BCNU)
Captafol
Chloramphenicol
α-Chlorinated toluenes (benzal chloride, benzotrichloride, benzyl chloride, and benzoyl chloride) (combined exposures)
1-(2-chloroethyl)-3-cyclohexyl-1-nitrosourea (CCNU)
4-Chloro-ortho-toluidine
Chlorozotocin
Cisplatin
Clonorchis sinensis (infection with)
Cyclopeneta[cd]pyrene
Dibenz[a,i]anthracene
Dibenz[a,l]pyrene
Diethyl sulfate
Dimethylcarbamoyl chloride
1,2-Dimethylhydrazine
Dimethyl sulfate
Epichlorohydrin
Ethyl carbamate (urethane)
Ethylene dibromide
N-Ethyl-N-nitrosourea
Etoposide
Glycidol
Indium phosphide
IQ (2-Amino-3-Methylimidaso[4,5-f]quinoline)
Kaposi sarcoma herpesvirus/human herpesvirus B
Lead compounds, inorganic
5-Methoxypsoralen
Methyl methanesulfonate
N-Methyl-N'-nitro-N-nitrosoguanidine (MNNG)
N-Methyl-N-nitrosourea

Nitrate or nitrite (ingested) under conditions that result in endogenous nitrosation
Nitrogen mustard
N-Nitrosodiethylamine
N-Nitrosodimethylamine
Phenacetin
Procarbazine hydrochloride
Styrene-7,8-oxide
Teniposide
Tetrachloroethylene
Trichloropropane
1,2,3-Trichloropropane
Tris(2,3-dibromoprophyl) phosphate
Ultraviolet radiation A
Ultraviolet radiation B
Ultraviolet radiation C
(Urethane: see Ethyl carbamate)
Vinyl bromide
Vinyl fluoride

Mixtures
Creosotes
Diesel engine exhaust
High-temperature frying, emissions from
Hot mate
Household combustion of biomass fuel (primarily wood), indoor emissions from
Nonarsenical insecticides (occupational exposures to spraying and application of)
Polychlorinated biphenyls

Exposure Circumstances
Art glass, glass container, and pressed ware (manufacture of)
Carbon electrode manufacture
Cobalt metal with tungsten carbide
Hairdresser and barber (occupational exposure as)
Petroleum refining (occupational exposure as)
Shiftwork that involves circadian disruption
Sunlamps and sunbeds

IARC, International Agency for Research on Cancer.

and kidney is weaker. Other sources of inorganic arsenic are related to occupational exposures (see Box 12-2).

The central hypothesis, based on rat studies, for the mechanisms related to particle-induced lung carcinogenesis is that insoluble particles cause pulmonary inflammation (e.g., cytokine release, ROS), which leads to genotoxic stress, proliferative response, and tissue remodeling progressing toward fibrosis and tumor development. Additional research is needed to understand the surface chemistry and lung tissue remodeling in relation to insoluble particles, lung carcinogenesis, and other respiratory problems.[240,241]

SUMMARY REVIEW

Genes, Environmental-Lifestyle Factors, and Risk Factors

1. Environmental-lifestyle factors and occupational exposures are increasing the number of cancer cases and deaths.
2. Cancers are caused by environmental-lifestyle and genetic factors. Investigators are connecting the complex web between genotype, phenotype, and the environment and carcinogenesis.
3. Studies of individuals with particular genetic predispositions who may be more susceptible to the biologic effects of environmental exposures cannot explain the increased cancer risk in exposed groups.
4. It appears that the majority of cancers are caused by carcinogen exposure rather than by rare genetic conditions.
5. The cancers increasing substantially in the United States include melanoma, non-Hodgkin lymphoma, testicular, brain, and thyroid. These cancers are *not* linked to cigarette smoking.
6. Statistics have shown that immigrants acquire the cancer incidence rates of the country where they move within one or two generations, thus ethnicity or their country of origin may not be as important as their immediate environment
7. A new paradigm shift suggests that susceptibility to disease may be set in utero or neonatally.

Epigenetics and Genetics

1. An explosion of data has been the relative importance of genetic versus epigenetic processes.
2. The importance of epigenetic processes includes gene silencing of key regulatory genes.
3. Epigenetic changes collaborate with the genetic changes and environmental-lifestyle factors to cause the development of cancer.
4. Developmental plasticity is the degree to which an organism's development is contingent on its environment. It requires stable gene expression that in part appears to be modulated by epigenetic processes such as DNA methylation, histone modification, and micro-RNAs.
5. Epidemiologic and animal studies reveal that small changes in the developmental environment can alter phenotypic changes resulting in individual responses in adulthood.

Tobacco Use

1. Cigarette smoking is carcinogenic and the most important cause of cancer. The risk is greatest in those who begin to smoke when young and continue throughout life.
2. Cigarette smoking accounts for one of every five deaths each year in the United States. Overall, it accounts for 30% of all cancer deaths in developed countries, and an epidemic is expected in developing countries.
3. In addition, smoking causes even more deaths from vascular, respiratory and other diseases than from cancer.
4. Smoking tobacco is linked to cancers of the lung, lower urinary tract, upper aerodigestive tract, liver, kidney, pancreas, cervix, uterus, and myeloid leukemia.
5. Environmental tobacco smoke (ETS) is the combination of sidestream and mainstream smoke.
6. Over 60 chemicals in tobacco smoke are considered carcinogenic. Nonsmokers who live with smokers are at greatest risk for lung cancer as well as other non-cancerous conditions.
7. Cigar or pipe smoking is strongly and causally related to cancers of the oral cavity, esophagus, and lung. Cigar smokers who inhale deeply may have other disease risks. Bidi smoking can cause cancers of the respiratory and digestive sites.

Diet

1. Diet can expose individuals to xenobiotics.
2. Carcinogenic substances from diet can include cooking of fat (e.g., heterocyclic aromatic amines) and naturally occurring compounds associated with plant foods.
3. Nutrition may directly influence epigenetic factors that silence genes that should be active or activate genes that should be silent.
4. Dietary components can act directly as mutagens or interfere with their elimination.
5. Dietary factors may alter hormonal axes, influence cellular proliferation, and affect phenotype or expression of key genes, for example, epigenetically.
6. Diet affects pathways to cancer including cell cycle control, differentiation, DNA repair, gene silencing, inflammation, apoptosis, and carcinogenic metabolism.

Obesity

1. Obesity has been increasing in developed countries and in urban areas of developing countries. Studies in the United States have suggested obesity is associated with some cancers, though it may not be a causal factor in cancer mortality.
2. A recent hypothesis is obesity may be associated with the incidence of cancers of the breast, endometrium, colon, liver, kidney, and the esophagus.
3. Biologic mechanisms of the association of obesity with cancer include insulin resistance, hyperinsulinemia, increased IGFs, increased steroid hormones, increased tissue-derived hormones, cytokines and/or inflammatory mediators.
4. Adipose tissue is active endocrine and metabolic tissue. Increased release of free fatty acids, resistin, TNF-α, and reduced release of adiponectin give rise to insulin resistance. Adipose tissue cells produce steroid-hormone-metabolizing enzymes and are an important source of estrogens in postmenopausal women. IGF-1 regulates cell proliferation and inhibits apoptosis and the synthesis and biologic availability of female and male sex hormones.
5. Numerous dietary factors are discussed in association with cancer risk. Table 12-5 summarizes major findings.

Alcohol Consumption

1. Chronic alcohol consumption is a *strong* risk factor for cancer of the oral cavity, pharynx, hypopharynx, larynx, esophagus, and liver.
2. Alcohol consumption is *less strongly* but consistently related to breast cancer and colorectal cancer. Also, it is known to increase cell growth of human breast cancer cells in vitro.

Ionizing Radiation

1. Human exposures to ionizing radiation includes background radiation from soil, rocks, radon gas seeping into homes and other buildings, surrounding space and sources within the human body.
2. Also exposures to ionizing radiation include emissions from x-rays, radioisotopes, and other radioactive sources. From the NCRP, concern is from the increased exposure from medical procedures, particularly CT scans and nuclear medicine procedures.
3. The risks from low dose radiation are being debated among radiobiologists, geneticists, physicists, and others because of the potential effect on the health of current and future generations.
4. Ionizing radiation (IR) is a mutagen and carcinogen and can penetrate cells and tissues and deposit energy in tissues at random in the form of ionizations.

Continued

5. IR affects many cellular processes, including gene expression, disruption of mitochondrial function, nucleotide base damage, and single-and double-DNA strand breaks. These changes can lead to carcinogenesis.
6. A long held assumption is that cellular alterations—mutations and malignant transformation—occur only in cells directly radiated. It is now known that radiation may induce a type of genomic instability to the progeny of the directly irradiated cells over many generations of cell radiation and can affect so-called innocent bystander cells.
7. Epigenetic events after radiation include alterations in pathways affecting cell adhesion, extracellular matrix interactions, and cell-to-cell communication.

Ultraviolet Radiation

1. Ultraviolet radiation (UVR) causes basal cell carcinoma and squamous cell carcinoma. The principal source of UVR is sunlight.
2. The degree of damage in skin depends on the intensity and wavelength content—ultavioletA (UVA) or ultraviolet B (UVB).
3. UVR is known to cause specific gene mutations: for example, squamous cell carcinoma involves mutation in the *TP53* gene, basal cell carcinoma in the *patched* gene and melanoma in the *p16 gene.*
4. Skin exposure to UVR produces ROS in large quantities that can overwhelm tissue antioxidants and other oxygen-degrading pathways. Imbalances in ROS can lead to oxidative stress, tissue injury, and direct DNA damage.
5. UVA radiation of skin fibroblast releases iron which is involved in activation of the transcription factor NF-ϰβ and other free radicals important in regulating genes that induce inflammation. Inflammation is a critical component of tumor progression.
6. Melanoma has been increasing annually at rates of 2% to 7% for white populations. The steady rise in incidence has resulted in an alarming 165% increase in mortality rate. The pathogenesis of melanoma is complex including genetic and environmental factors.

Electromagnetic Radiation

1. Health risks associated with electromagnetic radiation (EMR) are controversial. Exposure to electric and magnetic fields is widespread. EMRs are a type of nonionizing and low-frequency radiation.
2. EMRs of varying strength include microwaves, radar, power frequency radiation associated with electricity and radio waves, fluorescent lights, computers, electric equipment, cell and cordless phones, and others.
3. Data has been slow because of methods to accurately measure exposure, the lack of clear dose-response relationships, reproducing effects, financial interests, and other priorities like convenience.
4. Studies differ on findings, however, a pooled analysis with low and high exposures showed at the highest average exposures increased risks affecting few children with childhood cancer. The WHO requested studies in high-exposure areas like Japan and found (case-control study) acute lymphocytic leukemia in children in the highest exposure category.
5. A recent meta-analysis found a consistent pattern of an increased risk for acoustic neuroma and glioma in those using cell phones for more than 10 years. The concern is more for children.

Sexual and Reproductive Behavior

1. High-risk types of HPV is required for the development of most cervical cancers. High-risk types include HPV-16 (50%-60% of cervical cancer cases), HPV-18 (10%-12%), and HPV-31 and HPV-45 (4% to 5% each).
2. Biologic factors that may interact with HPV to promote persistent infection include oral contraceptives and smoking. Newer risk factors include drug addiction and reproductive factors such as age at menarche and menopause. In fact, a second peak of high-risk HPV prevalence occurs in postmenopausal women.
3. HPV may be transmitted by genital contact (oral, touching, or sexual intercourse), therefore condoms are not necessarily protective.
4. HPV vaccination programs have made it possible to eliminate about 70% of all invasive cervical cancer worldwide.

Physical Activity

1. Physical activity reduces the risk for breast and colon cancers and may reduce the risk for others.
2. Biologic mechanisms for the protective effects include decreasing insulin and IGF levels, decreasing obesity, increasing free radical scavenger systems, altering inflammatory mediators, decreasing circulating sex hormones and metabolic hormones improving immune function, enhancing cytochrome P-450, thus modifying carcinogen activation, and increasing gut motility.
3. Physical activity may prevent type 2 diabetes which has been associated with cancer of the pancreas and colon.
4. Many unanswered questions remain regarding frequency of exercise, intensity, and duration.
5. Recent data supports 60 minutes of vigorous activity for decreasing BMI, body fat, and intra-abdominal fat.

Chemicals and Occupational Hazards

1. The International Agency for Research on Cancer (IARC) has classified carcinogenic agents as known and probable.
2. An estimated 80,000 synthetic chemicals are used in the United States. Only 7% have been fully tested for their impact on health and another 1000 are added each year.
3. Chemicals are present in air, soil, food, water, personal care products, toys, household products, medications, workplaces and homes. Table 12-1 is a summary of environmental and occupational links to cancer.
4. Chemicals can persist in the environment and accumulate in body fat and remain there indefinitely. Mechanisms of carcinogenesis for chemicals include direct carcinogenic action, hormonal disruptors, interference with cell signaling pathways and other unknown effects.
5. A substantial percentage of cancers of the upper respiratory passages, lung, bladder, and peritoneum are attributed to occupational factors.
6. Disentangling data related to lung cancer, air pollution, and occupational factors is complex especially in combination with active and passive smoking, environmental factors, and multiple interacting genes.
7. Air pollution is a concern in regard to cancer because of inhalation of emissions, including arsenicals, benzene, chloroform, vinyl chloride, and acrylonitrile. Indoor pollution is considered worse than outdoor pollution because of cigarette smoke and possibly radon gas.

KEY TERMS

Asbestos, 426
Bystander effect, 421
Cadherin, 424
C-peptide, 414
Connexon, 422
Developmental plasticity, 403
Environmental tobacco smoke
    (ETS), 404

Genomic instability, 420
Hormesis, 419
Individual carcinogen, 396
Insulin-like growth factor-1 (IGF-1), 409
Linear no-threshold (LNT) relationship, 419
Linear-quadratic relationship, 419
Nontargeted effect, 418

Phase I activation enzyme, 405
Phase II detoxification enzyme, 405
Radon, 426
Supra-linear hypothesis, 419
Threshold model, 419
Transgeneration effect, 418
Xenobiotics, 404

REFERENCES

1. Clapp RW et al: Environmental and occupational causes of cancer; new evidence 2005-2007, *Rev Environ Health* 23(1):1-37, 2008.
2. Clapp RW, Howe GK, Jacobs MM: Environmental and occupational causes of cancer: a call to act on what we know, *Biomed Pharmacother* 61(10):631-639, 2007.
3. National Cancer Institute: *Cancer and the environment: what you need to know, what you can do,* U.S. Department of Health and Human Services, 2004. Available at www.nci.nih.gov/newscenter/benchmarks-vol4-issue3.
4. King MC, Marks JH, Mandell JB: New York breast cancer study group: breast and ovarian cancer risks due to inherited mutations in BRCA1 and BRCA2, *Science* 302:643-646, 2002.
5. Bergstrom HO et al: Increase in testicular cancer incidence in six European countries: a birth cohort phenomenon, *J Natl Cancer Inst* 88(11):727, 1996.
6. National Cancer Institute DCCPS Surveillance Research Program Cancer Statistics Branch: *Surveillance, epidemiology, and end results (SEER) program.* Available at http://.seer.cancer.gov SEER* Stat Database: Incidence-SEER 9 Regs Public-Use, Nov 2005 Sub (1973-2003), SEER Cancer Query Systems, released April 2006. http://seer.cancer.gov/canques. Accessed July 2008.
7. Flood DM et al: Colorectal cancer incidence in Asian migrants to the United States and their descendants, *Cancer Causes Control* 11(5):403, 2000.
8. Liao KA et al: Endometrial cancer in Asian migrants to the United States and their descendants,. *Cancer Causes Control* 11(5):357, 2003.
9. Knox EG: Childhood cancers, birthplaces, incinerators, and landfill sites, *Int J Epidemiol* 29:391, 2000.
10. Litt JS, Tran NL, Burke TA: Examining urban brownfields through the public health "macroscope," *Environ Health Perspect* 110(Suppl 2):183, 2002.
11. Davis DL, Blair A, Hoel DG: Agricultural exposures and cancer trends in developed countries, *Environ Health Perspect* 100:39, 1992.
12. Heindel JJ et al: Animal models for probing the developmental basis of disease and dysfunction paradigm, *Basic Clin Pharmacol Toxicol* 102(2):76-81, 2008.
13. Gouveia-Vigeant T, Tickner J: *Toxic chemicals and childhood cancer: a review of the evidence,* Lowell Center for Sustainable Production, 2003, University of Massachusetts at Lowell. Available at www.sustainableproduction.org.
14. Kolonel LN, Altshuler D, Henderson BE: The multiethnic cohort study: exploring genes, lifestyle and cancer risk, *Nat Rev Cancer* 4(7):519-527, 2004.
15. Chuang JC, Jones PA: Epigenetics and microRNAs, *Pediatr Res* 61(5 Pt 2):24R-29R, 2007.
16. Sasaki H, Matsui Y: Epigenetic events in mammalian germ-cell development: reprogramming and beyond, *Nat Rev Genet* 9(2):129-140, 2008.
17. Lu J et al: Micro RNA expression of profiles classify human cancers, *Nature* 435:834-838, 2005.
18. Johnson IT, Belshaw NJ: Environment, diet and CpG methylation: epigenetic signals in gastrointestinal neoplasia, *Food Chem Toxicol* 46(4):1346-1359, 2007.
19. Issa JP: CpG-island methylation in aging and cancer, *Curr Top Microbiol Immunol* 249:101-118, 2000.
20. Liu L et al: Aging, cancer and nutrition: the DNA methylation connection, *Mech Ageing Dev* 124:989-998, 2003.
21. Richardson B: Impact of aging on DNA methylation, *Ageing Res Rev* 2:243-261, 2003.
22. Fraga MF et al: Epigenetic differences arise during the lifetime of monzygotic twins, *Proc Natl Acad Sci U S A* 102:10604-10609, 2005.
23. Issa JP et al: Accelerated age-related CpG island methylation in ulcerative colitis, *Cancer Res* 61:3573-3577, 2001.
24. Gluckman PD et al: Effect of in utero and early-life conditions on adult health and disease, *N Engl J Med* 359(1):61-73, 2008.
25. Rubin MM: Antenatal exposure to DES: lesions learned…future concerns, *Obstet Gynecol Surv* 62(8):548–444, 2007.
26. Triosi R, Potischman N, Hoover RN: Exploring the underlying hormonal mechanisms of prenatal risk factors for breast cancer: a review and commentary, *Cancer Epidemiol Biomarkers Prev* 16(9):1700-1712, 2007.
27. Palmer JR et al: Prenatal diethylstilbestrol exposure and risk of breast cancer, *Cancer Epidemiol Biomarkers Prev* 15(8):1509-1514, 2006.
28. McLachlan JA: Commentary: prenatal exposure to diethylstilbestrol (DES): a continuing story, *Int J Epidemiol* 35(4):868-870, 2006.
29. Newbold RR et al: Proliferative lesions and reproductive tract tumors in male descendents of mice exposed developmentally to diethylstilbestrol, *Carcinogenesis* 21:1355-1363, 2000.
30. Petridou E et al: Baldness and other correlates of sex hormones in relation to testicular cancer, *Int J Cancer* 71(6):982-985, 1997.
31. Strohsnitter WC et al: Cancer risk in men exposed in utero to diethylstilbestrol, *J Natl Cancer Inst* 93(7):545-551, 2001.
32. Waterland RA, Jirtle RL: Transposable elements: targets for early nutritional effects on epigenetic gene regulation, *Mol Cell Biol* 23:5293-5300, 2003.
33. Peto J: Cancer epidemiology in the last century and the next decade, *Nature* 411(6835):390-395, 2001.
34. Centers for Disease Control and Prevention: Global youth tobacco surveillance, 2000-2007. *MMWR Morb Mortal Wkly Rep* 57(5501):1-21, 2008.
35. WHO World Cancer Report: *Global cancer rates could increase by 50% to 15 million by 2020.* Available at www.WHO.int/mediacentre/news/release/2003/pr27/en/. Accessed July 2008.
36. Centers for Disease Control and Prevention: Cigarette smoking among adults—United States, 2004, *MMWR Morb Mortal Wkly Rep* 54(44):1121-1124, 2005.
37. Centers for Disease Control and Prevention: Cigarette smoking among adults—United States, 2006, *MMWR Morb Mortal Wkly Rep* 56(44):1157-1161, 2007.
38. Vineis P et al: Tobacco and cancer: recent epidemiological evidence, *J Natl Cancer Inst* 96(2):99-106, 2004.
38a. Hanaoka T et al: Active and passive smoking and breast cancer risk in middle-aged Japanese women, *Int J Cancer* 114:317-322, 2005.
39. Centers for Disease Control and Prevention: *Smoking and tobacco use, fact sheet September 2006.* Available at www.CDC.gov/tobacco/data_statistics/factsheets/secondhandsmoke.htm.
40. National Cancer Institute: *Secondhand smoke: questions and answers.* Available at www.cancer.gov/cancertopics/factsheet/tobacco/ETS, 2005. Accessed July 2008.
41. Centers for Disease Control and Prevention: *Cigars, fact sheet March 2007.* Available at www.CDC.gov/tobacco/data_statistics/factsheets/secondhandsmoke.htm. Accessed July 2008.

42. Henley SJ et al: Association between exclusive pipe smoking and mortality from cancer and other diseases, *J Natl Cancer Inst* 96(11):853-861, 2004.

43. Boffetta P et al: Smokeless tobacco and cancer, *Lancet Oncol* 9(7): 667-675, 2008.

44. *Working Group on Diet and Cancer of the Committee on Medical Aspects of Food and Nutrition Policy: Nutritional aspects of the development of cancer*, London, 1998, Department of Health Rep Health Social Subjects 48, The Stationery Office.

45. Jones DP, Delong MJ: Detoxification and protective functions of nutrients. In Stipanuk M, editor: *Biochemical and physiological aspects of nutrition*, Philadelphia, 2000, Saunders.

46. Wiseman M: The second World Cancer Research Fund/American Institute for Cancer Research expert report. Food, nutrition, physical activity, and the prevention of cancer: a global perspective, *Proc Nutr Soc* 67(3):253-256. Epub 2008 May 1.

47. Baylin SB: DNA methylation and gene silencing in cancer, *Nat Clin Pract Oncol* 2(Suppl 1):S4-S11, review, 2005.

48. Agrawal A, Murphy RF, Agrawal DK: DNA methylation in breast and colorectal cancers, *Mod Pathol* 20(7):711-721, review, 2007.

49. Ross SA: Diet and DNA methylation interactions in cancer prevention. *Ann N Y Acad Sci* 983:197-207, review, 2003.

50. Ushijima T: Epigenetic field for cancerization, *J Biochem Mol Biol* 40(2):142-150, 2007.

51. Ross JS et al: Breast cancer biomarkers and molecular medicine, *Expert Rev Mol Diagn* 3:573-585, 2003.

52. Droufakou S et al: Multiple ways of silencing E-cadherin gene expression in lobular carcinoma of the breast, *Int J Cancer* 92:404-408, 2001.

53. Shames DS et al: DNA methylation in health, disease, cancer, *Curr Mol Med* 7:85-102, 2007.

54. World Health Organization (WHO): Global strategy on diet, physical activity, and health (online), 2004. Available at www.who.int/dietphysicalactivity/strategy/eb11344/en/.

55. Dashwood RH, Ho E: Dietary histone deacetylase inhibitors: from cells to mice to man, *Sem Cancer Biol* 17:363-369, 2007.

56. Myzak MC et al: Sulforaphane retards the growth of human PC-3 xenografts and inhibits HDAC activity in human subjects, *Exp Biol Med* 232:227-234, 2007.

57. Calle EE et al: Overweight, obesity, and mortality from cancer in a prospectively studied cohort of U.S. adults, *N Engl J Med* 348(17):1625-1638, 2003.

58. Pischon T, Nöthlings U, Boeing H: Obesity and cancer, *Proc Nutr Soc* 67(2):128-145, 2008.

59. World Cancer Research Fund: *Food, nutrition, and the prevention of cancer: a global perspective*, pp 371–373, Washington, DC, 1997, American institute for Cancer Research.

60. Dunaif A: Insulin resistance and the polycystic ovary syndrome: mechanism and implications for pathogenesis, *Endocr Rev* 18(6): 774-800, 1997.

61. Calle EE, Kaaks R: Overweight, obesity and cancer: epidemiological evidence and proposed mechanisms, *Nat Rev Cancer* 4(8):579-591, 2004.

62. Collaborative Group on Hormonal Factors in Breast Cancer: Breast cancer and hormone replacement therapy: collaborative reanalysis of data from 51 epidemiological studies of 52,705 women with breast cancer and 108,411 women without breast cancer, *Lancet* 350(9084):1047-1059, 1997.

63. Feigelson HS et al: Weight gain, body mass index, hormone replacement therapy, and postmenopausal breast cancer in a large prospective study, *Cancer Epidemiol Biomarkers Prev* 13(2):220-224, 2004.

64. Schairer C et al: Menopausal estrogen and estrogen-progestin replacement therapy and breast cancer risk, *JAMA* 283(4):485-491, 2000.

65. Coates RJ: Race, nutritional status, and survival from breast cancer, *J Natl Cancer Inst* 82(21):1684-1692, 1990.

66. Lukanova A et al: Prediagnostic levels of C-peptide, IGF-I, IGFBP-1, -2, and -3, and risk of endometrial cancer, *Int J Cancer* 108(2): 262-268, 2004.

67. Giovannucci E: Insulin and colon cancer, *Cancer Causes Control* 6(2):164-179, 1995.

68. McCullough ML, Giovannacci EL: Diet and cancer prevention, *Oncogene* 23(38):6349-6364, 2004.

69. Sandhu MS, White IR, McPherson K: Systematic review of the prospective cohort studies on meat consumption and colorectal cancer risk: a meta-analytical approach, *Cancer Epidemiol Biomarkers Prev* 10(5):439-446, 2001.

70. Cho E et al: Premenopausal dietary carbohydrate, glycemic index, glycemic load, and fiber in relation to risk of breast cancer, *Cancer Epidemiol Biomarkers Prev* 12(11 Pt 1):1153-1158, 2003.

71. Cramer DW et al: A case-control study of galactose consumption and metabolism in relation to ovarian cancer, *Cancer Epidemiol Biomarkers Prev* 9(1):95-101, 2000.

72. Baron JA et al: Calcium supplements for the prevention of colorectal adenomas, Calcium Polyp Prevention Study Group, *N Engl J Med* 340(2):101-107, 1999.

73. Martinez ME, Marshall JR, Giovannucci E: Diet and cancer prevention: the roles of observation and experimentation, *Nat Rev Cancer* 8(9):694-703, 2008.

74. Rodriguez C et al: Calcium, dairy products, and risk of prostate cancer in a prospective cohort of United States men, *Cancer Epidemiol Biomarkers Prev* 12(7):597-603, 2003.

75. McMichael AJ, Potter JD: Dietary influences upon colon carcinogenesis, *Princess Takamatsu Symp* 16:275-290, 1985.

76. Lamprecht SA, Lipkin M: Cellular mechanisms of calcium and vitamin D in the inhibition of colorectal carcinogenesis, *Ann N Y Acad Sci* 952:73-87, 2001.

77. Duthie SJ: Folic acid deficiency and cancer: mechanisms of DNA instability, *Br Med Bull* 55(3):578-592, 1999.

78. Blount BC et al: Folate deficiency causes uracil misincorporation into human DNA and chromosome breakage: implications for cancer and neuronal damage, *Proc Natl Acad Sci U S A* 94(7): 3290-3295, 1997.

79. Wickramasinghe SN, Fida S: Bone marrow cells form vitamin B_{12}- and folate-deficient patients misincorporate uracil into DNA, *Blood* 83(6):1656-1661, 1994.

80. Duthie SJ et al: Folate deficiency in vitro induces uracil misincorporation and DNA hypomethylation and inhibits DNA excision repair in immortalized normal human colon epithelial cells, *Nutr Cancer* 37(2):245-251, 2000.

81. Giovannucci E: Epidemiologic studies of folate and colorectal neoplasia: a review, *J Nutr* 132(Suppl):2350S-2355S, 2002.

82. Eichholzer M et al: Folate and the risk of colorectal, breast, and cervix cancer: the epidemiological evidence, *Swiss Med Wkly* 131(37-38): 539-549, 2001.

82a. Figuerido J et al: Folic acid and risk of prostate cancer: results from a randomized clinical trial, *J Natl Cancer Inst* 101:432, 2009.

83. Jacobs EJ et al: Multivitamin use and colon cancer mortality in the Cancer Prevention Study II cohort (United States), *Cancer Causes Control* 12(10):927-934, 2001.

84. Feigelson HS et al: Alcohol, folate, methionine, and risk of incident breast cancer in the American Cancer Society Cancer Prevention Study II Nutrition Cohort, *Cancer Epidemiol Biomarkers Prev* 12(2):161-164, 2003.

85. Zhang SM et al: Plasma folate, vitamin B_6, vitamin B_{12}, homocysteine, and risk of breast cancer, *J Natl Cancer Inst* 95(5):373-380, 2003.

86. Kim YI: Does high folate intake increase the risk of breast cancer? *Nutr Rev* 64(10 Pt 1):468-475, 2006.

87. Arab L, Steck-Scott S, Bowen P: Participation of lycopene and beta-carotene in carcinogenesis: defenders, aggressors, or passive bystanders? *Epidemiol Rev* 23(2):211-230, 2001.

88. Toniolo P et al: Serum carotenoids and breast cancer, *Am J Epidemiol* 153(12):1142-1147, 2001.

89. Blumberg J, Block G: The Alpha-Tocopherol Beta-Carotene Cancer Prevention Study in Finland, *Nutr Rev* 52(7):242-245, 1994.

90. Albanes D et al: Alpha-tocopherol and beta-carotene supplements and lung cancer incidence in the alpha-tocopherol, beta-carotene cancer prevention study: effects of base-line characteristics and study compliance, *J Natl Cancer Inst* 88(21):1560-1570, 1996.

91. Liu C, Russel RM, Wang XD: Alpha-tocopherol and ascorbic acid decrease the production of beta-apo-carotenals and increase the formation of retinoids from beta-carotene in the lung tissues of cigarette smoke-exposed ferrets in vitro, *J Nutr* 134(2):426-430, 2004.

92. Baron JA et al: Neoplastic and antineoplastic effects of beta-carotene on colorectal adenoma recurrence: results of a randomized trial, *J Natl Cancer Inst* 95(10):717-722, 2003.

93. Mares-Perlman JA et al: The body of evidence to support a protective role for lutein and zeaxanthin in delaying chronic disease. Overview, *J Nutr* 132(3):518S-524S, 2002.

94. Jacob RA: The role of micronutrients in DNA synthesis and maintenance, *Adv Exp Med Biol* 472:101-113, 1999.

95. Correa P et al: Chemoprevention of gastric dysplasia: randomized trial of antioxidant supplements and anti-*Helicobacter pylori* therapy, *J Natl Cancer Inst* 92(23):1881-1888, 2000.

96. Helzlsouer KJ et al: Association between alpha-tocopherol, gamma-tocopherol, selenium, and subsequent prostate cancer, *J Natl Cancer Inst* 92(24):2018-2023, 2000.

97. Lippman SM: Effect of selenium and Vitamin E on risk of prostate cancer and other cancers: the selenium and Vitamin E cancer prevention trial (SELECT), *JAMA* 301(1):39-51, 2008.

98. Pryor WA: Vitamin E and heart disease: basic science to clinical intervention, *Free Radic Biol Med* 28(1):141-164, 2000.

99. Nomura AM et al: Serum selenium and subsequent risk of prostate cancer, *Cancer Epidemiol Biomarkers Prev* 9(9):883-887, 2000.

100. Yoshizawa K et al: Study of prediagnostic selenium level in toenails and the risk of advanced prostate cancer, *J Natl Cancer Inst* 90(16):1219-1224, 1998.

101. Reagan-Shaw S et al: Combination of vitamin E and selenium causes an induction of apoptosis of human prostate cancer cells by enhancing Bax/Bcl-2 ratio, *Prostate* 68(15):1624-1634, 2008.

102. Bingham SA et al: Dietary fibre in food and protection against colorectal cancer in the European Prospective Investigation into Cancer and Nutrition (EPIC): an observational study, *Lancet* 361(9368):1496-1501, 2003.

103. Alberts DS et al: Lack of effect of a high-fiber cereal supplement on the recurrence of colorectal adenomas. Phoenix Colon Cancer Prevention Physicians' Network, *N Engl J Med* 342(16):1156-1162, 2000.

104. Bonithon-Kopp C et al: Calcium and fibre supplementation in prevention of colorectal adenoma recurrence: a randomised intervention trial. European Cancer Prevention Organisation Study Group, *Lancet* 356(9238):1300-1306, 2000.

105. Schatzkin A: Going against the grain? Current status of the dietary fiber-colorectal cancer hypothesis. *Biofactors* 12(1-4):305-311, 2000.

106. Burkitt DP: Epidemiology of cancer of the colon and rectum, *Cancer* 28(1):3-13, 1971.

107. *International Agency for Research on Cancer (IARC): Cancer epidemiology*, Lyon, France, 2004, IARC Press.

108. Smith-Warner SA et al: Intake of fruits and vegetables and risk of breast cancer: a pooled analysis of cohort studies, *JAMA* 285(6):769-776, 2001.

109. Terry P et al: Prospective study of major dietary patterns and colorectal cancer risk in women, *Am J Epidemiol* 154(12):1143-1149, 2001:2001.

110. Flood A et al: Dietary patterns as identified by factor analysis and colorectal cancer among middle-aged Americans, *Am J Clin Nutr* 88(1):176-184, 2008.

111. Ames BN, Gold LS, Willett WC: The causes and prevention of cancer, *Proc Natl Acad Sci U S A* 92(12):5258-5265, 1995.

112. Lampe JW et al: Modulation of human glutathione S-transferases by botanically defined vegetable diets, *Cancer Epidemiol Biomarkers Prev* 9(8):787-793, 2000.

113. Aldercreutz H: Phyto-oestrogens and cancer, *Lancet Oncol* 3(6):364-373, 2002.

114. Steinmetz KA, Potter JD: Vegetables, fruit, and cancer. I. Epidemiology, *Cancer Causes Control* 2(5):325-357, 1991.

115. Doll R, Peto R: The causes of cancer: quantitative estimates of avoidable risks of cancer in the United States today, *J Natl Cancer Inst* 66(6):1191-1308, 1981.

116. Bond VP, Benary V, Sondhaus CA: A different perception of the linear, nonthreshold hypothesis for low-dose irradiation, *Proc Natl Acad Sci U S A* 88(19):8666-8670, 1991.

117. Kaaks R, Lukanova A, Kurzer MS: Obesity, endogenous hormones, and endometrial cancer risk: a synthetic review, *Cancer Epidemiol Biomarks Prev* 11(12):1531-1542, 2002.

118. Weiderpass E et al: Occurrence, trends, and environment etiology of pancreatic cancer, *Scand J Work Environ Health* 24(3):165-174, 1998.

119. Patel AV et al: IGF-I, IGFBP-1, and IGFBP-3 polymorphisms predict circulating IGF levels but not breast cancer risk: findings from the Breast and Prostate Cancer Cohort Consortium (BPC3), *PLos ONE* 3(7):e2578, 2008.

120. Khandwala HM et al: The effects of insulin-like growth factors on tumorigenesis and neoplastic growth, *Endocr Rev* 21(3):215-244, 2000.

121. Lawlor MA, Alessi DR: PKB/Akt: a key mediator of cell proliferation, survival, and insulin responses? *J Cell Sci* 114(Pt 16):2903-2910, 2001.

122. Le Roith D: Regulation of proliferation and apoptosis by the insulin-like growth factor I receptor, *Growth Horm IGF Res* 10(Suppl A):S12-S13, 2000.

123. Prisco M et al: Insulin and IGF-I receptors signaling in protection from apoptosis, *Horm Metab Res* 31(2-3):80-89, 1999.

124. Everhart J, Wright D: Diabetes mellitus as a risk factor for pancreatic cancer. A meta-analysis, *JAMA* 273(20):1605-1609, 1995.

125. Lindblad P et al: The role of diabetes mellitus in the aetiology of renal cell cancer, *Diabetologia* 42(1):107-112, 1999.

126. Schoen RE, et al: Increased blood glucose and insulin, body size, and incident colorectal cancer, *J Natl Cancer Inst* 9(13)1:1147-1154, 1999.

127. Cust AE et al: Serum levels of C-peptide, IGFBP-1 and IGFBP-2 and endometrial cancer risk; results from the European prospective investigation into cancer and nutrition, *Int J Cancer* 120(12):2656-2664, 2007.

128. Ma J et al: Prediagnostic body-mass index, plasma C-peptide concentration, and prostate cancer-specific mortality in men with prostate cancer: a long-term survival analysis, *Lancet Oncol 2008 Oct 3* [Epub ahead of print].

129. Kaaks R, Lukanova A: Energy balance and cancer: the role of insulin and insulin-like growth factor I. *Proc Nutr Soc* 60(1):91-106, 2001.

130. Hadsell DL, Bonnette SG: IGF and insulin action in the mammary gland and in breast cancer, *J Mammary Gland Biol Neoplasia* 5(1):19-30, 2000.

131. Allen Ne et al: A prospective study of serum insulin-like growth factor-I (IGF-I), IGF-II, IGF-binding protein-3 and breast cancer risk, *Br J Cancer* 92(7):1283-1287, 2005.

132. Fletcher O et al: Polymorphisms and circulating levels in the insulin-like growth factor system and risk of breast cancer: a systematic review, *Cancer Epidemiol Biomarkers Prev* 14(1):2-19, 2005.

133. Chan JM et al: Plasma insulin-like growth factor-I and prostate cancer risk: a prospective study, *Science* 279(5350):563-566, 1998.

134. Kaaks R et al: Serum C-peptide, insulin-like growth factor IGF-I, IGF binding proteins, and colorectal cancer risk in women, *J Natl Cancer Inst* 92(19):1592-1600, 2000.

135. Palmqvist R et al: Plasma insulin-like growth factor 1, insulin-like growth factor binding protein 3, and risk of colorectal cancer: a prospective study in northern Sweden, *Gut* 50(5):642-646, 2002.

136. Stattin P et al: Plasma insulin-like growth factor-I, insulin-like growth factor-binding proteins, and prostate cancer risk: a prospective study, *J Natl Cancer Inst* 92(2):1910-1917, 2000.

137. Poschl G, Seitz HK: Alcohol and cancer, *Alcohol Alcohol* 39(3):155-165, 2004.

138. Izevbigie EB et al: Ethanol modulates the growth of human breast cancer cells in vitro, *Exp Biol Med* 227(4):260-265, 2002.

139. Bagnardi V et al: A meta-analysis of alcohol drinking and cancer risk, *Br J Cancer* 85(11):1700-1705, 2001.

140. Argiris A et al: Head and neck cancer, *Lancet* 9625(371):1695-1709, 2008.

141. Sturgis EM, Wei Q: Genetic susceptibility—molecular epidemiology of head and neck cancer, *Curr Opin Oncol* 14(3):310-317, 2002.

142. Crabb DW et al: Overview of the role of alcohol dehydrogenese and aldehyde dehydrogenase and their variants in the genesis of alcohol-related pathology, *Proc Nutr Soc* 63(1):49-63, 2004.

143. Committee on the Biological Effects of Ionizing Radiation: *Health risks from exposure to low levels of ionizing radiation, BEIR VII Phase 2*, Washington DC, 2006, National Academies Press.

144. Preston DL et al: Studies of mortality of atomic bomb survivors. Report 13: solid cancer and noncancer disease mortality: 1950-1997, *Rad Res* 160:381-407, 2003.

145. Hoel DG: Ionizing radiation and cardiovascular disease, *Ann N Y Acad Sci* 1076:309-317, 2006.

146. Prasad KN, Cole WC, Hasse GM: Health risks of low dose ionizing radiation in humans: a review, *Exp Biol Med* 229(5):378-382, 2004.

147. NCRP 1929-2009 Medical Radiation Exposure of the U.S. Population Greatly Increased Since the Early 1980s. March, 2009 http://NCRPonline,org.

148. Little JB: Cellular radiation effects and the bystander response, *Mutat Res* 597:113-118, 2006.

149. Kovalchuk O, Baulch JE: Epigenetic changes and nontargeted radiation effects—is there a link? *Environ Mol Mutagen* 49(1):16-25, 2008.

150. Barcellos-Hoff MH: Integrative radiation carcinogenesis: interactions between cell and tissue responses to DNA damage, *Semin Cancer Biol* 15:138-148, 2005.

151. Sowa M et al: Effects of ionizing radiation on cellular structures, induced instability and carcinogenesis, *EXS* 96:293-301, 2006.

152. Koturbash I et al: In vivo bystander effects: cranial x-irradiation leads to elevated DNA damage, altered cellular proliferation and apoptosis, and increased p53 levels in shielded spleen, *Int J Radiat Oncol Bio Phys* 70(2):554-562, 2008.

153. Mancuso M et al: Oncogenic bystander radiation effects in *Patched heterozygous mouse cerebellum*, *PNAS* 105(34):12445-12450, 2008.

154. *Committee on the Biological Effects of Ionizing Radiation: Biological effects of ionizing radiation BEIR V*, Washington, DC, 1990, National Academy Press.

155. Tondel M et al: Increased incidence of malignancies in Sweden after the Chernobyl accident—a promoting effect? *Am J Ind Med* 49(3):159-168, 2006.

156. Zhou H et al: Induction of a bystander mutagenic effect of alpha particles in mammalian cells, *Proc Natl Acad Sci U S A* 97(5): 2099-2104, 2000.

157. Makhijani A, Smith B, Thorne MC: *Science for the vulnerable setting radiation and multiple exposure environmental health standards to protect those at most risk,* IEER, Takoma Park, Maryland, 2006.

158. Lorimore SA, Coates PJ, Wright EG: Radiation-induced genomic instability and bystander effects: inter-related nontargeted effects of exposure to ionizing radiation, *Oncogene* 22(45):7058-7069, 2003.

159. Futaki M, Liu JM: Chromosomal breakage syndromes and the BRCA1 genome surveillance complex, *Trends Mol Med* 7(12):560-565, 2001.

160. Little JB: Lauriston S. Taylor lecture: nontargeted effects of radiation: implications for low dose exposures, *Health Phys* 91(5):416-426, 2006.

161. Ojima M, Ban N, Kai M: DNA double-strand breaks induced by very low x-ray doses are largely due to bystander effects, *Radiat Res* 170(3):365-371, 2008.

162. Park CC et al: Ionizing radiation induces heritable disruption of epithelial cell interactions, *Proc Natl Acad Sci USA* 100(19): 10728-10733, 2003.

163. Watson GE et al: In vivo chromosomal instability and transmissible aberrations in the progeny of haemopoietic stem cells induced by high- and low-LET radiations, *Int J Radiat Biol* 77(4):409-417, 2001.

164. Ponnaiya B, Cornforth MN, Ullrich RL: Radiation-induced chromosomal instability in BALB/c and C57BL/6 mice: the difference is as clear as black and white, *Radiat Res* 147(2):121-125, 1997.

165. Little JB: Genomic instability and bystander effects: a historical perspective, *Oncogene* 22(45):6978-6987, 2003.

166. Hamada N et al: Intercellular and intracellular signaling pathways mediating ionizing radiation-induced bystander effects, *J Radiat Res (Tokyo)* 48(2):87-95, review, 2007.

167. Shao C et al: Targeted cytoplasmic irradiation induces bystander responses, *Proc Natl Acad Sci U S A* 101(37):13495-13500, 2004.

168. Coates PJ et al: Ongoing activation of p53 pathway is a long-term consequence of radiation exposure in vivo and associates with altered macrophage activities, *J Pathol* 214(5):610-616, 2008.

169. Lorimore SA et al: Inflammatory-type responses after exposure to ionizing radiation in vivo: a mechanism for radiation-induced bystander effects? *Oncogene* 20(48):7085-7095, 2001.

170. Ohba K et al: Primary biliary cirrhosis among atomic bomb survivors in Nagasaki, Japan, *J Clin Epidemiol* 54(8):845-850, 2001.

171. Azzam EI, de Toldeo SM, Little JB: Oxidative metabolism, gap junctions, and the ionizing radiation-induced bystander effect, *Oncogene* 22(45):7050-7057, 2003.

172. Spitz DR et al: Metabolic oxidation/reduction reactions and cellular responses to ionizing radiation: a unifying concept in stress response biology, *Cancer Metastasis Rev* 23(3-4):311-322, 2004.

173. Cleaver JE, Crowley E: UV damage, DNA repair, and skin carcinogenesis, *Front Biosci* 7:d1024-d1043, 2002.

174. Streilein JW et al: Immune surveillance and sunlight-induced skin cancer, *Immunol Today* 15(4):174-179, 1994.

175. Bickers DR, Ather M: Oxidative stress in the pathogenesis of skin disease, *J Invest Dermatol* 126:2562-2575, 2006.

176. Dhar A, Young MR, Colburn NH: The role of AP-1, NF-kappaB, and ROS/NOS in skin carcinogenesis: The JB6 model is predictive, *Mol Cell Biochem* 234-125(1-2):185-193, 2002.

177. Sander CD et al: Role of oxidative stress and the antioxidant network in cutaneous carcinogenesis, *Intl J Dermatol* 43(5):326-335, 2004.

178. Wei S et al: Incidence of *p53* and *ras* gene mutations in DMBA-induced rat leukemias, *J Exp Clin Cancer Res* 21(3):389-396, 2002.

179. Davies H et al: Mutations of the BRAF gene in human cancer, *Nature* 417(6892):949-954, 2002.

180. Lin J et al: Genetics of melanoma, *Br J Dermatol* 159(2):286-291, 2008.

181. Heymann WR: Screening for melanoma, *J Am Acad Dermatol* 56(1):144-145, 2007.

182. Polsky D et al: Molecular biology of melanoma. In Mendelsohn J, et al: *The molecular basis of cancer*, ed 2, Philadelphia, 2001, Saunders.

183. Perlis C, Herlyn M: Recent advances in melanoma biology, *Oncologist* 9(2):182-187, 2004.

184. Rees JL: The melanocortin 1 receptor (MC1R): more than just red hair, *Pigment Cell Res* 13(3):135-140, 2000.

185. Berking C et al: Basic fibroblast growth factor and ultraviolet B transform melanocytes in human skin, *Am J Pathol* 158(3):943-953, 1998.

186. Berking C et al: Basic fibroblast growth factor and ultraviolet B transform melanocytes in human skin, *Am J Pathol* 158:943-954, 2002.

187. Besaratinia A, Pfeifer GP: Sunlight ultraviolet irradiation and BRAF V600 mutagenesis in human melanoma, *Hum Mutat* 29(8):983-1991, 2008.

188. Tang A et al: E-cadherin is the major mediator of human melanocyte adhesion to keratinocytes in vitro, *J Cell Sci* 107(pt 4):983-992, 1994.

189. Li G, Satayamoorthy K, Herlyn M: N-cadherin-mediated intercellular interactions promote survival and migration of melanoma cells, *Cancer Res* 61(9):3819-3825, 2001.

190. Genuis SJ: Fielding a current idea: exploring the public health impact of electromagnetic radiation, *Public Health* 122(2):113-124, 2008.

191. Kabuto M et al: Childhood leukemia and magnetic fields in Japan: a case-control study of childhood leukemia and residential power-frequency magnetic fields in Japan, *Int J Cancer* 119:643-650, 2006.

192. Hardell L, Carlberg M, Hansson Mild K: Use of cellular telephones and brain tumour risk in urban and rural areas, *Occup Environ Health* 62(6):390-394, 2005.

193. Hardell L et al: Long-term use of cellular phones and brain tumours: increased risk associated with use for >or =10 years, *Occup Environ Med* 64(9):626-632, 2007, Review.

194. Hardell L, Sage C: Biological effects from electromagnetic field exposure and public exposure standards,. *Biomed Pharmacother* 62(2):104-109, review, 2008.

195. Hardell L et al: Meta-analysis of long-term phone use and the association with brain tumours,. *Int J Oncol* 32(5):1097-1103, 2008.

196. Draper G et al: Childhood cancer in relation to distance from high voltage power lines in England and Wales: a case-control study, *BMJ* 330:1290, 2005.

197. Hallberg O, Johansson O: Melanoma incidence and frequency modulation (FM) broadcasting, *Arch Environ Health* 57:32-40, 2002.

198. Hallberg O, Johansson O: Maligant melanomas of the skin—not a sunshine story! *Med Sci Monit* 10:CR336-CR340, 2004.

199. Feychting M, Forssén U: Electromagnetic fields and female breast cancer, *Cancer Causes Control* 17(4):553-558, review, 2006.

200. Kliukiene J, Tynes T, Andersen A: Residential and occupational exposure to 50-Hz magnetic fields and breast cancer in women: a population-based study, *Am J Epidemiol* 159(9):852-861, 2004.

201. National Institute of Environmental Health Sciences (NIEHS) Working Group Report: *Assessment of health effects from exposure to power-line frequency electric and magnetic fields*, Washington, DC, 1998, US Government Printing Office.

202. Johansson O: Electrohypersensitivity: state-of-art of a functional impairment, *Electroman Biol Med* 25(4):245-258, review, 2006.

203. UK Childhood Cancer Study Investigators: Exposure to power-frequency magnetic fields and the risk of childhood cancer, *Lancet* 354(9194):1925-1931, 1999.

204. UK Childhood Cancer Study Investigators: Childhood cancer and residential proximity to power lines, *Br J Cancer* 83(11):1573-1580, 2000.

205. Ahlbom A et al: A pooled analysis of magnetic fields and childhood leukaemia, *Br J Cancer* 83(5):692-698, 2000.

206. Christensen HC et al: Cellular telephone use and risk of acoustic neuroma, *Am J Epidemiol* 159(3):277-283, 2004.

207. Independent Expert Group on Mobile Phones: Mobile phones and health (the Stewart report). Didcot, Oxon, United Kingdom, 2000, National Radiological Protection Board. Available at www.iegmp.org.uk/report/text.htm.
208. Repacholi MH: Radiofrequency field exposure and cancer: what do the laboratory studies suggest? *Environ Health Perspect* 105(Suppl 6):1565-1568, 1997.
209. Mashevich M et al: Exposure of human peripheral blood lymphocytes to electromagnetic fields associated with cellular phones leads to chromosomal instability, *Bioelectromagnetics* 24(2):82-90, 2003.
210. World Health Organization (WHO): Sensitivity of children to EMF exposure. Proceedings of a symposium sponsored by the WHO International EMF Project, June 9-10, 2004, Istanbul, Turkey, *Bioelectromagnetics* (Suppl 7):S1-S160 Erratum 27(5):430, 2006.
211. Cherry N: World conference on breast cancer—Ottawa, Canada, July 26-31, 1999. Lincoln: New Zealand Lincoln University; 2002. Available at: www.neilcherry.com/cart/specific+health+effect+review?mode=show_category.
212. Havas M: Biological effects of non-ionizing electromagnetic energy: a critical review of the reports by the US National Research Council and the US National Institute of Environment Health Sciences as they relate to the broad realm of EMF bioeffects, *Environ Rev* 89:173-253, 2000.
213. Blackman CF, Benane SG, House DE: The influence of temperature during electric- and magnetic-field-induced alteration of calcium-ion release from in vitro brain tissue, *Bioelectromagnetics* 12(3):173-182, 1991.
214. Anhang R, Goodman A, Goldie SJ: HPV communication: review of existing research and recommendation for patient education, *CA Cancer J Clin* 54(5):248-259, 2004.
215. Bosch FX, de Sanjose S: Human papillomavirus and cervical cancer—burden and assessment of causality, *J Natl Cancer Inst Monogr* 31:3-13, 2003.
216. Stanley M: Immunobiology of HPV and HPV vaccines, *Gynecol Oncol* 109(2 Supp):S15-S21, review, 2008.
217. Syrjänen K et al: New concepts on risk factors of HPV and novel screening strategies for cervical cancer precursors, *Eur J Gynaecol Oncol* 29(3):205-221, 2008.
218. Syrjänen K et al: Smoking is an independent risk factor for oncogenic human papillomavirus (HPV) infections but not for high-grade CIN, *Eur J Epidemiol* 22(10):723-735, 2007.
219. Herzog TJ et al: Initial lessons learned in HPV vaccination, *Gynecol Oncol* 109(2 Suppl):S4-S11, 2008.
220. Hagensee ME et al: Human papillomavirus infection and disease in HIV-infected individuals, *Am J Med Sci* 328(1):57-63, 2004.
221. Stuver S: Adami H-O: Cervical cancer. In Adami H, Hunter D, Trichopoulos D, editors: *Textbook of cancer epidemiology*, Oxford, 2002, Oxford University Press.
222. Syrjanen S, Puranen M: Human papillomavirus infections in children: the potential role of maternal transmission, *Crit Rev Oral Biol Med* 11(2):259-274, 2000.
223. Eyre H et al: Preventing cancer, cardiovascular disease, and diabetes: a common agenda for the American Cancer Society, the American Diabetes Association, and the American Heart Association, *Stroke* 35(8):1999-2010, 2004.
224. McTiernan A: Mechanisms linking physical activity with cancer, *Nat Rev Cancer* 8(3):205-211, 2008.
225. Rogers CJ et al: Physical activity and cancer prevention: pathways and targets for intervention, *Sports Med* 38(4):271-296, 2008.
226. Slattery ML: Physical activity and colorectal cancer, *Sports Med* 34(4):239-252, 2004.
227. McTiernan A et al: Physical activity and cancer etiology: associations and mechanisms, *Cancer Causes Control* 9(5):487-509, review, 1998.
228. McTiernan A et al: Effect of exercise on serum estrogens in postmenopausal women: a 12-month randomized clinical trial, *Cancer Res* 64(8):2923-2928, 2004.
229. Calle EE et al: Diabetes mellitus and pancreatic cancer mortality in a prospective cohort of United States Adults, *Cancer Causes Control* 9(4):403-410, 1998.
230. Lee IM: Physical activity and cancer prevention…data from epidemiologic studies, *Med Sci Sports Exerc* 35(11):1823-1827, 2003.
231. McTiernan A et al: Exercise effect on weight and body fat in men and women, *Obesity* 15(6):1496-1512, 2007.
232. Gray J: State of the Evidence2008: The connection between breast cancer and the environment, Breast Cancer Fund, San Francisco.
233. Neuberger JS, Field RW: Occupation and lung cancer in nonsmokers, *Rev Environ Health* 18(4):251-267, review, 2003.
234. Vineis P et al: Outdoor air pollution and lung cancer: recent epidemiologic evidence, *Int J Cancer* 111(5):647-652, 2004.
235. Blair A, Kazerouni N: Reactive chemicals and cancer, *Cancer Causes Control* 8(3):473-490, 1997.
236. Boffetta P et al: Mortality among workers employed in the titanium dioxide production industry in Europe, *Cancer Causes Control* 15(7):697-706, 2004.
237. Boffetta P: Involuntary smoking and lung cancer, *Scand J Work Environ Health* 28(Suppl 2):30-40, 2002.
238. Zhao Y et al: Air pollution and lung cancer risks in China—meta-analysis, *Sci Total Environ* 366(2 3):500 513, 2006.
239. Borm PJ, Schins RP, Albrecht C: Inhaled particles and lung cancer, part B: paradigms and risk assessment, *Int J Cancer* 110(1):3-14, 2004.
240. Holguin F: Traffic, outdoor air pollution, and asthma, *Immunol Allergy Clin North Am* 28:577-588, 2008.

CANCER IN CHILDREN

NANCY E. KLINE

CHAPTER OUTLINE

INCIDENCE AND TYPES OF CANCER
ETIOLOGY
    Genetic Factors
    Environmental Factors
PROGNOSIS

Cancer in children is rare, but is still the leading cause of death from disease. Survival rates in children with cancer have dramatically improved in the past 30 years. Some of the factors leading to improved cure rates in children with cancer include the use of combination chemotherapy, clinical trials, and multimodal treatment for childhood solid tumors.

INCIDENCE AND TYPES OF CANCER

In 2004 the mortality rates of children with cancer were 2.4 per 100,000 in children ages 1 to 4 years and 2.5 per 100,000 in children ages 5 to 14 years. In comparison, cancer is the second leading cause of death from disease in adults (second to heart disease), with an overall mortality rate of 187.4 per 100,000 individuals.[1]

The types of malignancies in children are vastly different from those that affect adults. The most common types of cancer among adults include prostate, breast, lung, and colon. Children tend to develop leukemias, brain tumors, and sarcomas. Although many adult cancers have associated lifestyle factors that could theoretically be avoided, such as smoking and exposure to sun, very few environmental factors have been linked to pediatric malignancies. Yet more data are emerging that the developing child may be affected by parental exposures prior to conception, exposures in utero, and the contents of breast milk (see What's New? Increased Emphasis on Child Health and Environmental Contaminants).[2,3]

Most recently, cancer incidence and treatment in adolescents and young adults have become of interest and concern in pediatric oncology. The incidence of cancer among adolescents and young adults represents only 2% of all invasive cancers. However, the malignancy rate in this age group (15- to 29-year-olds) is three times higher than that in children younger than 15 years. The most common cancers among the 15- to 19-year-old population in the United States are Hodgkin lymphoma, germ cell tumors, central nervous system (CNS) tumors, non-Hodgkin lymphoma, thyroid cancer, malignant melanoma, and acute lymphocytic leukemia (ALL). This pattern is different than in younger as well as older populations. Many of the common malignancies in children younger than 5 years of age are virtually absent in the 15- to 19-year-old group.[4] Similarly, cancers that predominate in adults are unusual among adolescents.

WHAT'S
NEW?   Increased Emphasis on Child Health
and Environmental Contaminants

Several publications from epidemiologic and toxicologic studies have suggested increased health risks in adults from in utero and childhood exposures. Children however may be affected differently than adults because of their metabolism, physiology, and behavioral characteristics (e.g., pica).

In 2004, the U.S. Surgeon General concluded there is suggestive evidence of a causal relationship between maternal smoking and preterm delivery, shortened gestation, and oral clefts. Several recent cohort studies have consistently reported significant associations between stillbirth and prenatal elevated maternal diastolic blood pressure (DBP) and between fetal growth deficit and maternal lead exposure. There has been limited evidence for an association between fetal growth deficit and ambient air pollutant levels.

Reviewers found limited evidence for an association between birth defects, especially neural tube defects and cardiac defects, and maternal prenatal residential proximity to hazardous waste disposal sites. Reviewers concluded that neural tube defects also were associated with maternal first-trimester occupational exposure to glycol ethers and paternal occupational solvent exposure.

Early childhood exposure to tobacco smoke is associated with childhood asthma, serious lower respiratory tract infection in children younger than 6 years of age, and acute and chronic childhood middle ear infections. Air pollution from automobile exhaust also increases the risk of developing asthma during childhood.

A review of 21 studies found that the results of 15 of these studies reported statistically significant increased risks between childhood cancer and parental occupational or childhood pesticide exposure. The authors concluded there is an association between pesticide exposure and childhood cancer but the epidemiologic evidence is insufficient to prove a cause-effect relationship. Three other publications suggested an association between childhood leukemia and pesticide exposure, with the greatest risks being childhood exposure to household insecticides and parental exposure to pesticides before or during pregnancy.

The Surgeon General suggested evidence of a causal relationship between childhood leukemia, lymphoma, and brain tumors and prenatal or postnatal environmental tobacco smoke exposure. An expert group found sufficient evidence of a causal association between breast cancer and environmental tobacco smoke exposure, particularly among premenopausal women and those exposed early in life. The Surgeon General concluded that environmental tobacco smoke causes adult lung cancer. Therefore, childhood environmental tobacco smoke exposure contributes to lifetime exposure and risk of adult breast and lung cancer.

Wigle DT et al: J Toxicol Environ Health B Crit Rev
11(5-6):373-517, 2008.

Most childhood cancers originate from the **mesodermal germ layer** that gives rise to connective tissue, bone cartilage, muscle, blood, blood vessels, gonads, kidney, and the lymphatic system. Thus the more common childhood cancers are leukemias, sarcomas, and embryonic tumors. **Embryonic tumors** originate during intrauterine life. These tumors contain abnormal cells that appear to be immature embryonic tissue, unable to mature or differentiate into fully developed functional cells. Embryonic tumors are diagnosed early in life (usually before 5 years of age). Embryonic tumors often contain the term **blast cell** in their name, which refers to the immature nature of the cells.

Leukemia is the most common malignancy in children and the most common type of leukemia is ALL, which represents three fourths of all pediatric leukemia cases. Although the presenting signs of the various types of leukemia may be similar, the treatment and response to treatment of childhood leukemias vary greatly.

CNS tumors are the most common types of solid tumors in children. Not all brain tumors are malignant by histology, but even a benign tumor can have devastating effects on a child. The treatment for brain tumors in children often presents difficulties because therapies, such as radiation, may have debilitating effects on the developing brain.

Lymphoma, including non-Hodgkin lymphoma and Hodgkin lymphoma, is a malignancy common in children and adults. However, the subtypes of lymphoma and treatments in the two populations often differ.

Many pediatric solid tumors usually develop only in the pediatric population but, in rare instances, may occur in adults. These tumors include neuroblastoma, Wilms tumor, rhabdomyosarcoma, retinoblastoma, osteosarcoma, and Ewing sarcoma.

Childhood cancers are most often diagnosed during peak times of physical growth. In general, they are extremely fast growing, with 80% having distant spread (metastases) at diagnosis. Overall, cancer is 10% to 25% more common in white than in black children. Boys are more likely to develop cancer than girls.

ETIOLOGY

The causes of cancer in children are largely unknown. A few environmental factors are known to predispose a child to cancer, but causal factors have not been established for most childhood cancers. A number of host factors, many of which are genetic risk factors or congenital conditions, have been implicated in the development of childhood cancer (Table 13-1). Because the cell types often identified in tumors in children closely resemble undifferentiated cells noted during normal development, it is hypothesized that these genetic changes alter such cells' ability to fully differentiate.[5] It is probably the interaction of many factors that produces cancer, a concept referred to as multiple causation or **multifactorial etiology.** In this view, cancer develops because of the predisposing characteristics of the person who is interacting with the environment.

The **multiple causation** concept is useful when the results of epidemiologic studies are interpreted. For example, laboratory and epidemiologic studies may indicate that exposure to a certain chemical can cause leukemia, but not all children exposed to that chemical will develop leukemia. Additional studies will be needed to determine what other factors must interact with chemical exposure to cause the disease.

Table 13-1   Congenital Factors Associated with Childhood Cancer

Syndrome	Associated Childhood Cancer
Chromosome Alterations	
Down syndrome	Acute leukemia
13q syndrome	Retinoblastoma
Chromosome Instability	
Ataxia-telangiectasia	Lymphoma
Bloom syndrome	Acute leukemia, lymphoma, Wilms tumor
Fanconi anemia	Nonlymphocytic leukemia, myelodysplastic syndrome, hepatic tumors
Hereditary Syndromes	
Beckwith-Wiedemann syndrome	Wilms tumor, sarcoma, brain tumors, neuroblastoma, hepatoblastoma
Neurofibromatosis type I	Brain tumors, sarcomas, neuroblastomas, Wilms tumor, nonlymphocytic leukemia
Neurofibromatosis type II	Meningioma (malignant or benign), acoustic neuroma/schwannoma, gliomas, ependymomas
Tuberous sclerosis	Glial tumors
Li-Fraumeni syndrome	Sarcoma, adrenocortical carcinoma
Von Hippel-Lindau disease	Cerebellar hemangioblastoma, retinal angioma, renal cell carcinoma, pheochromocytomas
Ataxia-telangiectasia	Leukemia, lymphoma, brain tumors
Gorlin syndrome	Medulloblastoma, skin tumors
Immune Deficiency Disorders	
Congenital	
Agammaglobulinemia	Lymphoma, leukemia, brain tumors
Immunoglobulin A (IgA) deficiency	Lymphoma, leukemia, brain tumors
Wiskott-Aldrich syndrome	Leukemia, lymphoma
Acquired	
Aplastic anemia	Leukemia
Organ transplantation	Leukemia, lymphoma
Congenital Malformation Syndromes	
Aniridia, hemihypertrophy, hamartoma, genitourinary anomalies	Wilms tumor
Cryptorchidism	Testicular tumor
Gonadal dysgenesis	Gonadoblastoma
Family Susceptibility	
Twin or sibling with leukemia	Leukemia

Genetic Factors

Oncogenes and tumor-suppressor genes have been associated with childhood malignancies (Table 13-2; also see Chapter 11). **Proto-oncogenes** have a role in normal cell division and growth through a signaling process that orchestrates the cell cycle. If they are mutated, proto-oncogenes become carcinogenic oncogenes. Changes produced by specific oncogenes cause the cell cycle to go out of control. An example of an oncogene in pediatric cancer is *N-myc*, which is involved in neuroblastoma and glioblastoma. Tumor-suppressor genes arise from genes that normally suppress cancer cell proliferation but have lost their suppressor function, thus leading to uncontrolled growth. Some childhood cancers identified with tumor-suppressor genes include osteosarcoma, leukemia, rhabdomyosarcoma, retinoblastoma, and Wilms tumor.[6]

Other genetic factors involve chromosome aberrations or single-gene defects. These chromosome abnormalities include aneuploidy, amplifications, deletions, translocations, and fragility. A well-known chromosomal abnormality is the Philadelphia chromosome found in chronic and acute myelogenous leukemias.[7] Chromosomal deletions are often observed in retinoblastoma and osteosarcoma.

Some congenital malformations herald the onset of pediatric malignancies. For example, certain syndromes involve easily diagnosed abnormalities and the child can then be followed closely and screened for tumor development.

Trisomy 21 (Down syndrome) is the most common genetic defect linked to the development of acute leukemia. Children with Down syndrome have a 10- to 20-fold increased risk of developing acute lymphoblastic and myelogenous

Table 13-2	Selected Oncogenes and Tumor-Suppressor Genes Associated with Childhood Cancer
Gene	**Associated Pediatric Tumor**
Oncogenes	
bcr-abl	Acute lymphoblastic leukemia
N-myc	Neuroblastoma
c-myb	Neural tumors, leukemia, lymphoma, rhabdomyosarcoma, Wilms tumor, neuroblastoma
erb B	Glioblastomas
N-ras	Neuroblastoma, leukemia
H/K-ras	Neuroblastoma, rhabdomyosarcoma, leukemia
ATM	Lymphoma, leukemia
Tumor-Suppressor Genes	
Rb1	Retinoblastoma, sarcoma
WT1, WT2	Wilms tumor, leukemia
WTC	Wilms tumor
NF-1	Sarcoma, primitive neuroectodermal tumor, juvenile chronic myelocytic leukemia
NF-2	Brain tumors, melanoma, meningiomas
p16	Brain tumors, leukemia
TP53	Sarcoma, leukemia, brain tumors, lymphoma
DCC	Ewing sarcoma, rhabdomyosarcoma
p16^{INK4a}	Glioma, leukemia
p15^{ARF}	Glioblastoma, T-cell ALL
CDC2L1	Non-Hodgkin lymphoma, neuroblastoma

ALL, Acute lymphocytic leukemia.
Data from Dome JS, Coppes MS: *Curr Opin Pediat* 14(1):5-11, 2002; Linblom A, Nordenskjold M: *Sem Cancer Biol* 10(4):251-254, 2000; Tischkowitz M, Rosser E: *Eur J Cancer* 40:2459-2470, 2004; Look A, Kirsch IR: Molecular basis of childhood cancer. In Pizzo PA, Poplack DG, editors: *Principles and practices of pediatric oncology*, ed 4, Philadelphia, 2002, Lippincott Williams & Wilkins.

leukemia and a higher risk for developing acute megakaryocytic leukemia. The risk is highest between 1 and 4 years of age.[8] Wilms timor is associated with several congenial syndromes; aniridia, or congenital absence of the iris of the eye; ambiguous genitalia and mental retardation (AGR), neurofibromatosis, and Beckwith-Wiedemann syndrome.[9] Retinoblastoma, a malignant embryonic tumor of the eye, occurs as an inherited defect or as an acquired mutation (see Chapter 19).

Several single-gene defects have been associated with the subsequent development of childhood cancers. Fanconi anemia and Bloom syndrome, two autosomal recessive conditions, are risk factors for the development of ALL.

Although not determined to be genetically transmitted, a child who has a sibling with leukemia has a risk for the development of leukemia that is two to four times greater than for children with healthy siblings. The occurrence of leukemia in monozygous twins is estimated as being as high as 25%.

In families with Li-Fraumeni syndrome (LFS) (an autosomal dominant disorder involving the *TP53* tumor-suppressor gene), the risk of developing cancer as a child or adult is significantly higher than the unaffected population. Children and adults in Li-Fraumeni families are at risk for soft-tissue sarcoma, breast cancer, leukemia, osteosarcoma, melanoma, and cancer of the colon, pancreas, adrenal cortex, and brain. Individuals with LFS are at increased risk for developing multiple primary cancers.[10]

Environmental Factors

Although many adult cancers are associated with environmental agents, few childhood tumors share a similar strong association. Because of the lengthy latency period required between exposure and development of cancer; presumably early exposure to carcinogens does not result in cancer until the child is an adult.

Prenatal Exposure

Prenatal exposure to some drugs and to ionizing radiation has been linked to childhood cancers. The most well-described drug is diethylstilbestrol (DES), which was prescribed by physicians to prevent spontaneous miscarriage (in women with previous miscarriage). In 1971, DES was identified as a transplacental chemical carcinogen because a small percentage of the daughters of the women who took DES developed adenocarcinomas of the vagina. Since then, other studies have attempted to identify other drugs taken by pregnant women that may cause cancer in their offspring, but no other drugs have been found. Prior research suggested an association between antenatal x ray exposure and childhood cancer but have not been replicated or supported in recent literature.

Childhood Exposure

Childhood exposure to ionizing radiation, drugs, or viruses has been associated with the risk of developing cancer. Retrospective research has shown a significant correlation between radiation-induced malignancies from radiotherapy (cancer treatment) or from radiation exposure from diagnostic imaging.[11] In addition to the drug and environmental agents that are known to cause cancer in adults and therefore also are risks for exposure during childhood, a few drugs may particularly increase cancer risk during childhood (Table 13-3).

The relationship between childhood cancer and electromagnetic fields, small appliances, radon, and so on, has been the focus of many epidemiologic studies, yet no conclusive evidence has been observed.[11]

The strongest association between viruses and the development of cancer in children has been the Epstein-Barr virus (EBV), Burkitt lymphoma, nasopharyngeal carcinoma, and Hodgkin disease. Children with acquired immunodeficiency syndrome (AIDS) have an increased risk of developing non-Hodgkin lymphoma and Kaposi sarcoma. However, with the use of highly active antiretroviral therapy in the developed world, the incidence of AIDS-related malignancies has declined dramatically.[12]

Table 13-3	Drugs That May Increase Risk of Childhood Cancer	
Drug Class	**Uses**	**Cancer Risk**
Anabolic androgenic steroids	Stimulate bone growth and appetite Induce puberty Increase muscle mass and physical strength	Hepatocellular carcinoma
Cytotoxic chemotherapy	Cancer treatment	Leukemia
Immunosuppressive agents	Prevent organ rejection following transplantation surgery	Lymphoma

PROGNOSIS

More than 70% of children diagnosed with cancer are cured. Survival rates for children younger than 15 years of age have increased at a rate of 1.5% per year. Similar improvements have been noted in the survival rates of adults older than 50 years of age. However, adolescents and young adults between 15 and 24 years of age have experienced increases in survival of less than 0.5% per year.[4] A partial explanation for the relative lack of progress in curing the adolescent population at the same rate as that realized in the younger pediatric population is the lack of participation in clinical trials. Between 1997 and 2003, the rate of 15- to 19-year-olds with cancer participating in clinical trials was estimated at 10% to 15%. This rate is roughly one fourth the clinical trial participation rate of children younger than 15 years of age.[4] The National Cancer Institute (NCI) and pediatric and adult cooperative groups sponsored by the NCI have launched a national initiative to increase the numbers of adolescents and young adults in clinical trials.

NUTRITION & DISEASE

Preventing Malnutrition in Children with Cancer

Nutritional assessment and support are essential to prevent malnutrition in children with cancer. Specific childhood cancers associated with the poorest prognoses (e.g., brain tumors, neuroblastoma, acute myelogenous leukemia [AML]) tend to have the most intense oncologic treatment regimens and the greatest association with malnutrition. Clinicians can anticipate that treatment (i.e., surgery, radiation, chemotherapy, and bone marrow transplantation) will cause sensory changes and thus decrease adequate intake required to maintain or restore a child's nutritional status.

During illness a child's protein needs increase, and children receiving chemotherapy may require more calories for tissue healing and energy. The recommended dietary allowance (RDA) is used to determine estimated calorie and protein needs. Because the RDAs were developed as recommendations for healthy populations, adjustments are usually necessary to maintain appropriate growth in sick children. The allowances may need to be increased 15% to 50% to compensate for their previous weight losses, malnutrition, or metabolic changes.

SUMMARY REVIEW

Incidence and Types
1. Cancer in children is rare, but is still the leading cause of death from disease.
2. Childhood cancers are extremely fast growing, with 80% having distant spread (metastases) at diagnosis.
3. Children tend to develop leukemias, brain tumors, and sarcomas.

Etiology
1. A number of host factors, many of which are genetic risk factors or congenital conditions, have been implicated in the development of childhood cancer
2. Oncogenes and tumor-suppressor genes have been associated with childhood malignancies.

3. Chromosome aberrations or single-gene defects including aneuploidy, amplifications, deletions, translocations, and fragility are associated with the development of childhood cancer.
4. Wilms tumor and retinoblastoma are pediatric malignancies that are linked in a familial manner.
5. Childhood exposure to ionizing radiation, drugs, or viruses has been associated with the risk of developing cancer.

Prognosis
1. More than 70% of children diagnosed with cancer are cured.
2. Young children are particularly prone to long-term sequelae of cancer therapy. It is imperative that more effective, targeted therapies with fewer side effects be found.

KEY TERMS

Blast cell, 437
Embryonic tumors, 437
Mesodermal germ layer, 437

Multifactorial etiology, 437
Multiple causation, 437
Proto-oncogenes, 438

Some of the factors leading to improved cure rates in pediatric oncology include the use of combination chemotherapy, multimodal treatment for childhood solid tumors, improvements in nursing and supportive care, development of research centers for comprehensive childhood cancer treatment, cooperation among treatment institutions and the development of cooperative study groups, recognition of the psychologic effects of cancer treatment, and continued follow-up to track trends in the late effects of cancer treatment. Young children are particularly prone to long-term sequelae of cancer therapy. It is imperative that more effective, targeted therapies with fewer side effects be found.

REFERENCES

1. Miniño AM, Heron MP, Smith BL: *Deaths: preliminary data for 2004. National vital statistics reports.* Available at www.cdc.gov/nchs/data/nvsr/nvsr54/nvsr54_19.pdf Retrieved July 14, 2008.
2. Clapp RW, Howe GK, Jacobs MM: Environmental and occupational causes of cancer: a call to act on what we know, *Biomed Pharmacother* 61(10):631-639, 2007.
3. Wigle DT et a: Epidemiologic evidence of relationships between reproductive and child health outcomes and environmental chemical contaminants, *J Toxicol Environ Health B Crit Rev* 11(5-6):373-517, 2008.
4. Bleyer A, Budd T, Montello M: Adolescents and young adults with cancer: the scope of the problem and criticality of clinical trials, *Cancer* 107(7 Suppl):1645-1655, 2006.
5. Look AT, Aplan PD: Molecular and genetic basis of childhood cancer. In Pizzo PA, Poplack DG, editors: *Principles and practice of pediatric oncology*, ed 5, pp 38-85, Philadelphia, 2006, Lippincott Williams & Wilkins.
6. Plon SE, Malkin D: Childhood cancer and heredity. In Pizzo PA, Poplack DG, editors: *Principles and practice of pediatric oncology,* ed 5, pp 14-37, Philadelphia, 2006, Lippincott Williams & Wilkins.
7. Soupir CP et al: Philadelphia chromosome-positive acute myeloid leukemia: a rare aggressive leukemia with clinicopathologic features distinct from chronic myeloid leukemia in myeloid blast crisis. *Am J Clin Pathol* 127(4):642-650, 2007.
8. Margolin JF, Steuber CP, Poplack DG: Acute lymphoblastic leukemia In Pizzo PA, Poplack DG, editors: *Principles and practice of pediatric oncology*, ed 5, pp 538-590, Philadelphia, 2006, Lippincott Williams & Wilkins.
9. Dome JS et al: Childhood cancer and heredity. In Pizzo PA, Poplack DG, editors: *Principles and practice of pediatric oncology,* ed 5, pp 905-932, Philadelphia, 2006, Lippincott Williams & Wilkins.
10. Tabori U, Malkin D: Risk stratification in cancer predisposition syndromes: lessons learned from novel molecular developments in Li-Fraumeni syndrome, *Cancer Res* 68(7):2053-2057, 2008.
11. Buka I, Koranteng S, Osomio Vargas AR: Trends in childhood cancer incidence: review of environmental linkages, *Pediatr Clin North Am* 54(1):177-203, 2007.
12. Powles T et al: Head and neck cancer in patients with human immunodeficiency virus-1 infection: incidence, outcome and association with Epstein-Barr virus, *J Laryngol Otol* 118(3):207-212, 2004.

STRUCTURE AND FUNCTION OF THE NEUROLOGIC SYSTEM

RICHARD A. SUGERMAN

MEDIA RESOURCES

evolve **Evolve Website** (http://evolve.elsevier.com/McCance/)
- Review Questions and Answers
- Animations
- Glossary (with audio pronunciation for selected terms)
- WebLinks

CHAPTER OUTLINE

OVERVIEW AND ORGANIZATION OF THE NERVOUS SYSTEM
CELLS OF THE NERVOUS SYSTEM
  Neurons
  Neuroglia and Schwann Cells
  Nerve Injury and Regeneration
NERVE IMPULSES
  Synapses
  Neurotransmitters
CENTRAL NERVOUS SYSTEM
  Brain
  Spinal Cord
  Motor Pathways
  Sensory Pathways
  Protective Structures
  Blood Supply
PERIPHERAL NERVOUS SYSTEM
AUTONOMIC NERVOUS SYSTEM
  Anatomy of the Sympathetic Nervous System
  Anatomy of the Parasympathetic Nervous System
  Functions of the Autonomic Nervous System

Aging and the Nervous System
TESTS OF NERVOUS SYSTEM FUNCTION
  Skull and Spine Roentgenograms
  Computed Tomography
  Magnetic Resonance Imaging
  Magnetic Resonance Angiography
  Positron-Emission Tomography Scan
  Brain Scan
  Cerebral Angiography
  Myelography
  Echoencephalography (Ultrasound)
  Electroencephalography
  Evoked Potentials
  Cerebrospinal Fluid Analysis

The human nervous system is a remarkable structure that is responsible for the body's ability to reciprocally interact with the environment and for the regulation of activities involving internal organs. The nervous system *drives* the other systems of the body. It is a network composed of complex structures that transmit electrical and chemical signals between the body's many organs and tissues and the brain.

OVERVIEW AND ORGANIZATION OF THE NERVOUS SYSTEM

Although the nervous system functions as a unified whole, structures and functions of the nervous system have been divided to facilitate understanding. Structurally, the nervous system is divided into the central nervous system and the peripheral nervous system. The **central nervous system (CNS)** consists of the brain and spinal cord, enclosed within the protective cranial vault and vertebrae, respectively. The **peripheral nervous system (PNS)** is composed of the **cranial nerves,** which project from the brain and pass through foramina (openings) in the skull, and the **spinal nerves,** which project from the spinal cord and pass through intervertebral foramina of the vertebrae. Peripheral nerve pathways are differentiated into **afferent pathways (ascending pathways)** that carry sensory impulses toward the CNS and **efferent pathways (descending pathways)** that innervate **effector organs,** such as skeletal, cardiac, and smooth muscle, as well as glands, by transmitting motor impulses away from the CNS. Organs innervated by specific components of the nervous system are called *effector organs*. Cranial nerves are viewed most correctly as modified spinal nerves. Some cranial nerves function similarly to spinal nerves, whereas others have specialized sensory tasks, such as smell, taste, sight, and hearing.

Functionally the PNS can be divided into the somatic nervous system and the autonomic nervous system. The **somatic nervous system** consists of motor and sensory pathways regulating voluntary motor control of skeletal muscle. The **autonomic nervous system (ANS)** also consists of motor and sensory components and is involved with regulation of the body's internal environment (viscera) through involuntary control of organ systems. The ANS is further divided into sympathetic and parasympathetic divisions. Today we understand that some aspects of the ANS can be controlled through mental practice with or without biofeedback techniques.

CELLS OF THE NERVOUS SYSTEM

The two basic types of cells that make up nervous tissue are neurons and neuroglial cells. The neuron is the primary information/communication cell of the nervous system. Working in parallel systems, neurons can scan the environment, integrate many systems at higher cognitive levels, and initiate body responses to maintain homeostasis. The **neuroglial cells** are found in the CNS and PNS and can provide structural support and nutrition for neurons, remove debris, increase the speed of nerve impulses, and play a significant role, along with neurons, in processing and storing information (i.e., memory).[1]

Neurons

Neuronal structure varies considerably throughout the CNS. Neurons vary in size from micrometers to several meters long and have from one to many cell processes. Even the shapes and complexity of the processes can vary considerably. **Neurons** are specialized cells that share many of the same metabolic activities and constituents as other types of cells. The fuel source for the neuron is predominantly glucose; insulin, however, is not required for cellular glucose uptake in the CNS. Neurons contain many cellular constituents, namely, microtubules, neurofibrils, microfilaments, and Nissl substances. **Microfilaments** and **neurofibrils** are composed of structural proteins and are responsible for structural support within the cell and movement of neuron processes, as seen in amoebas

and white blood cells. **Microtubules** also are made of protein and are believed to be involved in the transport of cellular products. **Nissl substances** consist of endoplasmic reticulum and ribosomes and are involved in protein synthesis. The CNS starts out with more neurons than it needs, and those neurons that do not become involved in functional systems die. Some neurons continue to divide after birth. Olfactory neurons in the nose continue to divide throughout life.

A neuron (Figure 14-1) has three components: a cell body (soma) and the thin processes of the cell—the dendrites and axons. Most cell bodies are located within the CNS. Dense, packed cell bodies in the CNS are called **nuclei.** Cell bodies in the PNS are usually found in groups called **ganglia** or **plexuses.** The **dendrites** are extensions that carry nerve impulses *toward* the cell body. The **dendritic zone** is the receptive portion of a neuron that receives a stimulus and continues further conduction. **Axons** are long, conductive projections from the cell body that carry nerve impulses *away* from the cell body. The **axon hillock** is the cone-shaped, Nissl-free area where the axon leaves the cell body. In large nerves, axons are bundled together as **fascicles.** The initial segment of the axon has the lowest threshold for stimulation, and as a result, action potentials begin there.

A typical neuron has only one axon, which may be covered with a segmented layer of lipid material called **myelin,** which acts as an insulating substance. This entire membrane is referred to as the **myelin sheath;** the thin membrane between the myelin sheath and the **endoneurium,** a delicate connective tissue around each axon in the PNS (see Figure 14-23, *B*), is the **neurilemma (Schwann sheath).** The neurilemma and the myelin sheath are interrupted at regular intervals by the **nodes of Ranvier.** The **Schwann cell** forms and maintains the myelin sheath, and the nodes of Ranvier form the spaces on either side of the Schwann cell. If the myelin layer is tightly wrapped many times around the axon forming nodes of Ranvier, it increases conduction velocity and the neuron is referred to as *myelinated* (see Figure 14-1).

Myelin acts as an insulator that allows ions to flow between segments rather than along the entire length of the membrane, resulting in increased velocity. This mechanism is referred to as **saltatory conduction.** If the Schwann cells are loosely wrapped around the axon, it is referred to as *unmyelinated,* and conduction velocity is not increased. Axons are capable of extensive branching, which occurs at the nodes of Ranvier. Two major principles of information processing in the nervous system are *divergence* and *convergence.* **Divergence** refers to the ability of these branching axons to influence many different neurons. **Convergence** is the term applied to branches of numerous neurons converging on and influencing one or a few neurons. Disorders of the myelin sheath (demyelinating diseases), such as multiple sclerosis and Guillain-Barré syndrome, demonstrate the important role myelin plays in nerve function (see Chapter 17). Besides depending on the myelin coating, conduction velocities also depend on the diameter of the axon. Larger axons transmit impulses at a faster rate.

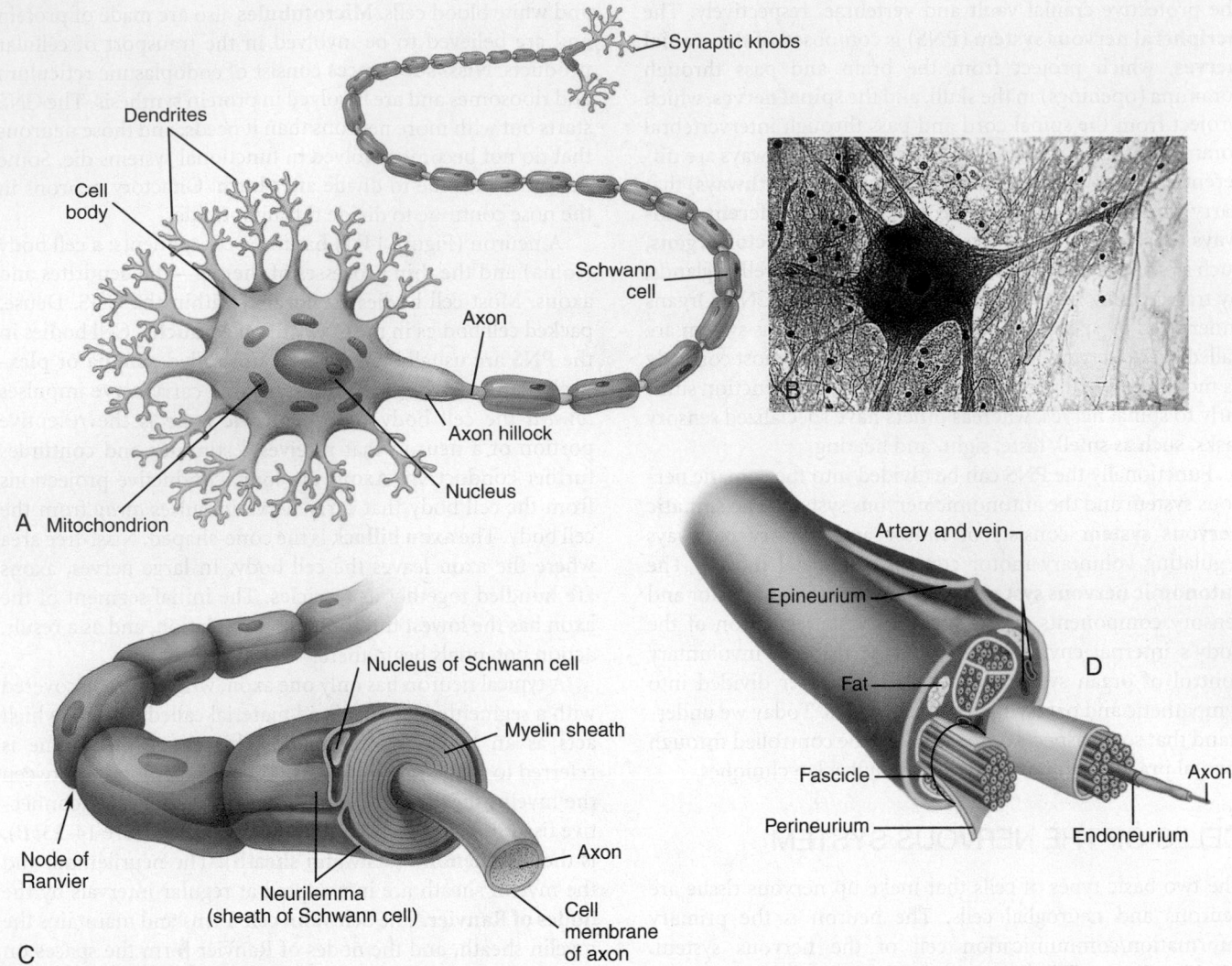

Figure 14-1 Structure of a typical neuron. **A,** Many dendrites carry nerve impulses to the cell body, which then send the nerve impulses along a single, long axon. Long axons are encased at intervals by a myelin sheath. **B,** Photomicrograph of a neuron. **C,** A segment of myelinated fiber in cross section, showing myelin sheath composed of several layers of myelin, which insulate the axon. **D,** Axons bundled into fascicles. (A and C from Thibodeau GA, Patton KT: *Structure and function of the human body,* ed 12, St Louis, 2004, Mosby; B, copyright Edward Reschke; D from Patton KT, Thibodeau GA: *Anatomy & physiology,* ed 7, St Louis, 2010, Mosby.)

Neurons are structurally classified on the basis of the number of processes (projections) extending from the cell body. There are four basic types of cell configuration: (1) unipolar, (2) pseudounipolar, (3) bipolar, and (4) multipolar (Figure 14-2). **Unipolar neurons** have one process that branches shortly after leaving the cell body. One example is found in the retina. **Pseudounipolar neurons** (some authors call them *unipolar*) have one process that has its dendritic portion extending away from the CNS and its axon portion projecting into the CNS (see Figure 14-2). The configuration is typical of sensory neurons in both cranial and spinal nerves. **Bipolar neurons** have two distinct processes arising from the cell body. This type of neuron connects to rod and cone cells of the retina. **Multipolar neurons** are the most common and have multiple processes capable of extensive branching. A motor neuron is typically multipolar.

Functionally there are three types of neurons (with their direction of transmission and typical configuration noted in parentheses): (1) sensory (afferent, mostly pseudounipolar), (2) associational (interneurons, multipolar), and (3) motor (efferent, multipolar). **Sensory neurons** carry impulses from peripheral sensory receptors to the CNS (Box 14-1). **Associational neurons (interneurons)** transmit impulses from neuron to neuron, for example, from sensory to motor neurons, and are also involved in cognitive function. **Motor neurons** transmit impulses away from the CNS to an effector organ. In skeletal muscle the end processes form a complex neuromuscular (myoneural) junction.

Neuroglia and Schwann Cells

Neuroglia ("nerve glue") comprise the general classification of cells that support the neurons of the CNS. They make up approximately half of the total brain and spinal cord volume

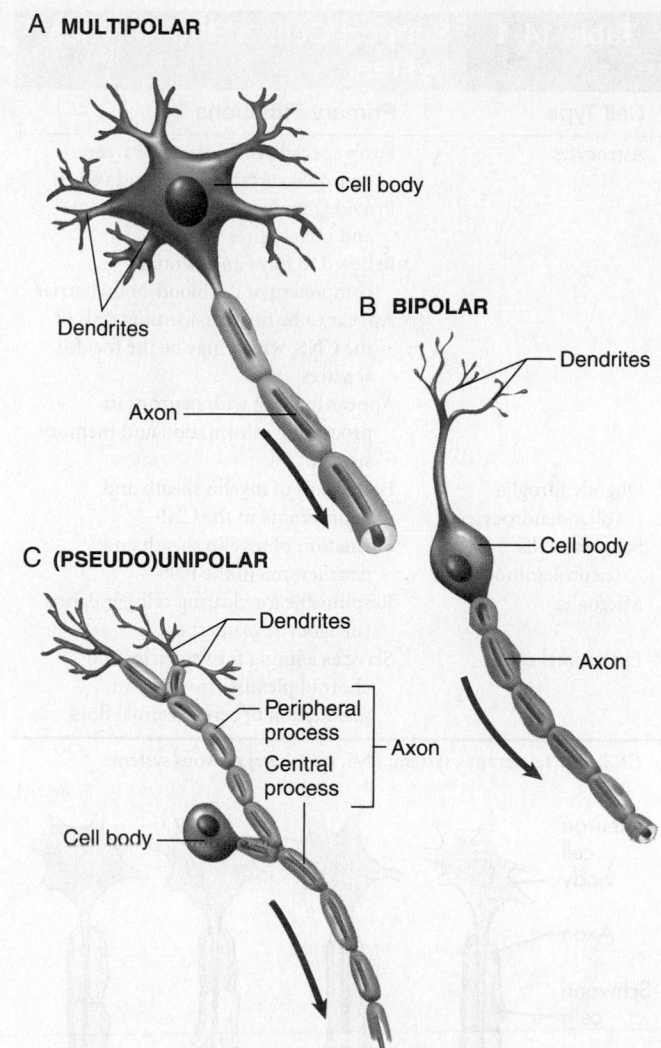

Figure 14-2 Structural classification of neurons. (From Patton KT, Thibodeau GA: *Anatomy & physiology*, ed 7, St Louis, 2010, Mosby.)

A MULTIPOLAR

Cell body
Dendrites
Axon

B BIPOLAR

Dendrites
Cell body
Axon

C (PSEUDO)UNIPOLAR

Dendrites
Peripheral process
Central process
Axon
Cell body

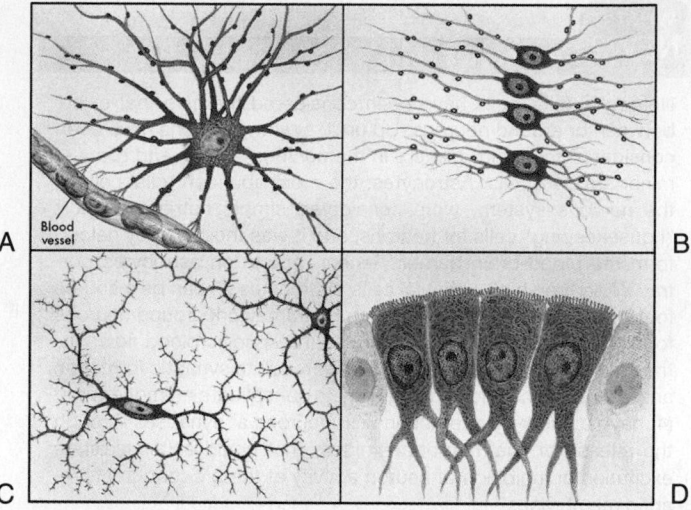

Figure 14-3 Types of neuroglial cells. A, Fibrous astrocyte; B, oligodendrocytes; C, microglial cells; D, ependymal cells. (Modified from Chipps E, Clanin N, Campbell V: *Neurologic disorders*, St Louis, 1992, Mosby.)

Blood vessel

A   B   C   D

Box 14-1	Major Types of Sensory Receptors

Nociceptors (pain)
Mechanoreceptors (touch, pressure, and mechanical deformation or encapsulated endings)
Photochemical (light on the retina)
Chemoreceptors (flavors, odors, oxygen levels, osmolarity of body fluids, and carbon dioxide levels in the blood)
Thermoreceptors (heat and cold)
Proprioception (sensing location of body parts)
Audition and balance (sound and positional movement)

---

and are 5 to 10 times more numerous than neurons. Different types of neuroglia serve different functions. **Astrocytes,** for example, fill the spaces between neurons and surround blood vessels in the CNS; **oligodendroglia (oligodendrocytes)** function to deposit myelin within the CNS. Oligodendroglia are the CNS counterpart of the Schwann cells. **Ependymal cells** line the cerebrospinal fluid (CSF)–filled cavities of the CNS.

Microglia remove debris (phagocytosis) in the CNS. Characteristics of neuroglia and Schwann cells are summarized in Figure 14-3 and Table 14-1.

Nerve Injury and Regeneration

When an axon is severed, a typical sequence of events, known as **wallerian degeneration,** occurs in the portion of the axon distal to the cut: (1) a characteristic swelling appears, (2) the neurofilaments hypertrophy, (3) the myelin sheath shrinks and disintegrates, and (4) this axon portion degenerates and disappears. The myelin sheaths reform into Schwann cells that line up in a column between the cut and the effector organ.

At the proximal end of the injured axon, similar changes occur, but only back as far as the next node of Ranvier. The cell body responds to trauma by swelling and then dispersing the Nissl substance (chromatolysis). During the repair process the cell increases in metabolic activity, protein synthesis, and mitochondrial activity. Approximately 7 to 14 days after the injury, new terminal sprouts project from the proximal segment and may enter the remaining Schwann cell pathway. (Figure 14-4 contains a more detailed representation of these events.) This process, however, is limited to myelinated fibers and generally occurs only in the PNS. The regeneration of axonal constituents in the CNS is limited by increased scar formation and the different nature of myelin formation by the oligodendrocyte.

Nerve regeneration depends on many factors, such as location of the injury, type of injury, the inflammatory responses, and the process of scarring. The closer to the cell body of the nerve, the greater the chances that the nerve cell will die and not regenerate. A crushing injury allows recovery more fully than does a cut injury. Crushed nerves sometimes recover fully, whereas cut nerves often form connective tissue scars that block or slow regenerating axonal branches.

WHAT'S NEW? Astrocytes

Neuroglial (glia) cells have been considered the *glue* that exists between or around neurons. Up until recently, neurons have been considered the major players in the nervous system and glia just minor support cells. Astrocytes, the most abundant glial cells in the nervous system, were considered simple nutrient support "housekeeping" cells for neurons, and it was thought they helped form the blood-brain barrier. Recent reports on astrocytes portray a "partnership" with glial cells. Astrocytes (1) can be a source for new neurons, (2) build a structural framework around neurons forming gliavascular units to provide the specific blood flow (nutrients) that a neuron requires, (3) may regulate synaptic formation and maintenance and in doing so help consolidate memories, and (4) have a two-way interaction with neurons at synapses through the release of glial neurotransmitters that could either facilitate excitation or inhibition of neuron activity at the pre- and postsynaptic membranes.

Data from Fellin T: *J Neurochem* 108(3):533-544, 2009; Wang DD, Bordey A: *Prog Neurobiol* 86(4):342-367, 2008; Seth P, Koul N: *J Biosci* 33(3):405-421, 2008; Araque A: *Neuron Glia Biol* 4(1):3-10, 2008.

WHAT'S NEW? Brain Synthesis of Neurosteroids

Although the brain is a target site for peripheral steroids, the brain glial cells, cerebellar Purkinje, and other cells also synthesize steroids from cholesterol, such as progesterone, pregnenolone, and dehydroepiandrosterone. These steroids are called *neurosteroids* and have diverse functions, including modulation of neurotransmitters (e.g., gamma-aminobutyric acid [GABA-A] and the glutamate and cholinergic systems). Beneficial effects have been shown for memory, learning, stress, depression, regulation of myelination, and neuroprotection and growth of axons and dendrites. Research is advancing potential pharmacologic use of neurosteroids to treat neuropathologies and support normal aging.

Data from VanLandigham JW et al: *J Cereb Blood Flow Metab* 28(11):1786-1794, 2008; Brinton RD et al: *Front Neuroendocrinol* 29(2):313-339, 2008; Sedlácek M et al: *Physiol Res* 57 (Suppl 3): S49-57, 2008.

NERVE IMPULSE

Neurons generate and conduct electrical and chemical impulses by selectively changing the electrical portion of their plasma membranes and influencing other nearby neurons by the release of chemicals (neurotransmitters). A neuron in its unexcited state maintains a resting membrane potential (see Chapter 1). When the membrane potential is raised sufficiently, an action potential is generated (see Figure 1-32), and the nerve impulse then flows to all parts of the neuron. The action potential response occurs only when the stimulus is strong enough; if it is too weak, the membrane remains unexcited. This property is sometimes termed the *all-or-none response*.

Table 14-1	Support Cells of the Nervous System
Cell Type	**Primary Functions**
Astrocytes	Form specialized contacts between neuronal surfaces and blood vessels
	Provide rapid transport for nutrients and metabolites
	Believed to form an essential component of the blood-brain barrier
	Appear to be the scar-forming cells of the CNS, which may be the foci for seizures
	Appear to work with neurons in processing information and memory storage
Oligodendroglia (oligodendrocytes)	Formation of myelin sheath and neurilemma in the CNS
Schwann cells (neurolemmocytes)	Formation of myelin sheath and neurilemma in the PNS
Microglia	Responsible for clearing cellular debris (phagocytic properties)
Ependymal cells	Serve as a lining for ventricles and choroid plexuses involved in production of cerebrospinal fluid

CNS, Central nervous system; *PNS*, peripheral nervous system.

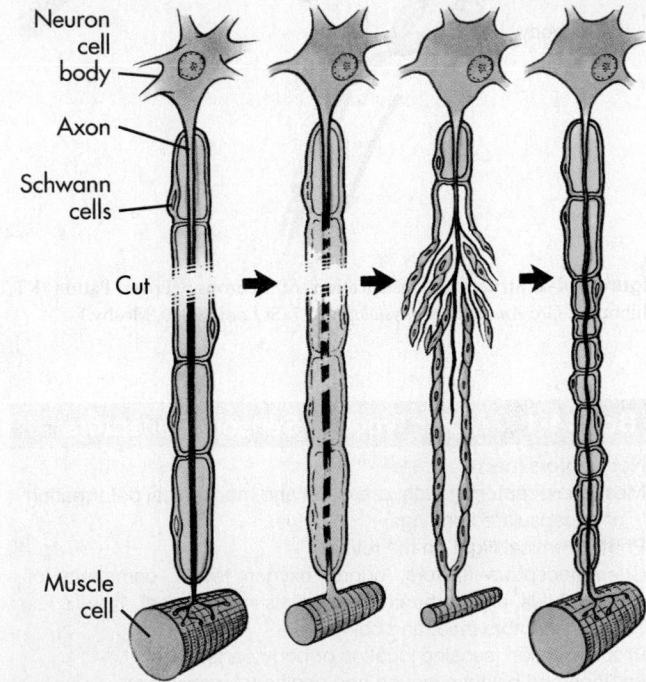

Neuron cell body
Axon
Schwann cells
Cut
Muscle cell

Figure 14-4 Repair of a peripheral nerve fiber. When cut, a damaged motor axon can regrow to its distal connection only if the neurilemma remains intact (to form a guiding tunnel) and if scar tissue does not block its way.

Synapses

Neurons are not physically continuous with one another. The region between adjacent neurons is called a **synapse.** Impulses are transmitted across the synapse by chemical (see Figures 14-5 and 14-14) and electrical conduction (Chapter 1); only chemical

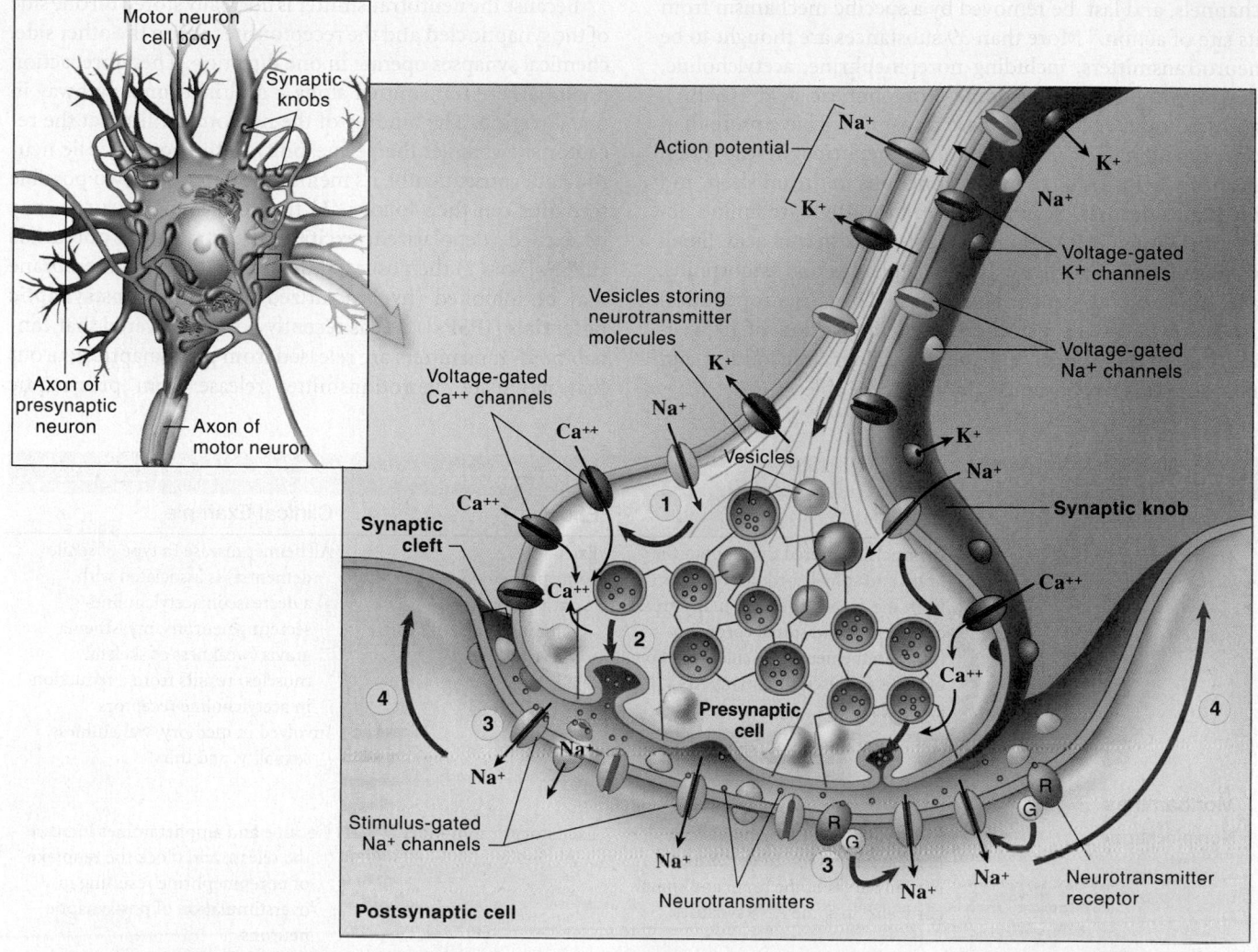

Figure 14-5 **Neuronal transmission and synaptic cleft.** Electrical impulse travels along axon of first neuron to synapse at synaptic knobs. Chemical transmitter is secreted into synaptic space to depolarize membrane (dendrite or cell body) of the next neuron in pathway. Details illustrate the synaptic knob (axon terminal) of a presynaptic neuron, the plasma membrane of a postsynaptic neuron, and a synaptic cleft. At step (1) the arrival of an action potential at the synaptic knob, voltage-gated Ca++ channels open and allow extracellular Ca++ to diffuse into the presynaptic cell. At step (2) the Ca++ triggers the rapid exocytosis of neurotransmitter molecules from vesicles in the knob. At step (3) neurotransmitter diffuses into the synaptic cleft and binds to receptor molecules in the plasma membrane of the postsynaptic neuron. The postsynaptic receptors directly or indirectly trigger the opening of stimulus-gated ion channels, initiating a local potential in the postsynaptic neuron. At step (4) the local potential may move toward the axon, where an action potential may begin. (From Patton KT, Thibodeau GA: *Anatomy & physiology*, ed 7, St Louis, 2010, Mosby.)

conduction is discussed here. The neurons that conduct a nerve impulse are named according to whether they relay impulses *toward* the synapse (**presynaptic neurons**) or *away* from the synapse (**postsynaptic neurons**). Four basic types of connections occur in regions of contact between the presynaptic and postsynaptic neurons. These are between axons (axoaxonic), from axon to cell body (axosomatic), from axon to dendrite (axodendritic), and from dendrite to dendrite (dendrodendritic).

Impulses are transmitted across the synapse by chemical conduction. The conducting substance is called a **neurotransmitter,** and it is often formed in the **synaptic knobs (boutons)** of the presynaptic neuron's axon and stored in synaptic vesicles within the knobs. Action potentials in the presynaptic neuron cause the synaptic vesicles to release their

neurotransmitter or neurotransmitters through the plasma membrane into the **synaptic cleft** (the space between the neurons), where they bind to receptor sites on the plasma membrane of the postsynaptic neuron (see Figure 14-5). Neurons can synthesize more than one neurotransmitter, and postsynaptic membranes can contain more than one type of transmitter-specific receptor.

Neurotransmitters

A neurotransmitter is defined as a chemical that "must be synthesized in the neuron, become localized in the presynaptic terminal [synaptic bouton], be released into the synaptic cleft, bind to a receptor site [binding site] on the postsynaptic membrane of another neuron or effector where it affects ion channels, and last, be removed by a specific mechanism from its site of action." More than 39 substances are thought to be neurotransmitters, including norepinephrine, acetylcholine, dopamine, histamine, gamma-aminobutyric acid (GABA), and serotonin.[2,3] Many of these transmitters have more than one function. For example, norepinephrine in the brain probably helps regulate mood, functions in dream sleep, and maintains arousal. Several neurotransmitters are amino acids, including GABA, glutamic acid, and aspartic acid. Small chains of amino acids, such as enkephalins and endorphins, also function as neurotransmitters. They (neuropeptides) are involved in the perception and integration of pain, as well as in emotional experiences. Neurotransmitter and neuromodulator substances are listed in Table 14-2.

Because the neurotransmitter is normally stored on one side of the synaptic cleft and the receptor sites are on the other side, chemical synapses operate in one direction. Therefore, action potentials are transmitted along a multineuronal pathway in one direction. The binding of the neurotransmitter at the receptor site changes the permeability of the postsynaptic neuron and, consequently, its membrane potential. Two possible scenarios can then follow: (1) the postsynaptic neuron may be excited (depolarized; **excitatory postsynaptic potentials [EPSPs]**) or (2) the postsynaptic neuron's plasma membrane may be inhibited (hyperpolarized; **inhibitory postsynaptic potentials [IPSPs]**). It has recently been discovered that cannabinoid transmitters are released from postsynaptic neurons that modulate neurotransmitter release from presynaptic

Table 14-2	Neurotransmitter and/or Neuromodulator Substances		
Substance	**Location**	**Effect**	**Clinical Example**
Acetylcholine	Many nuclei scattered throughout the brain and spinal cord; nerve tracts from the nuclei extend to many areas of the brain and spinal cord; also found in the neuromuscular junction of skeletal muscle and many ANS synapses	Excitatory Some peripheral parasympathetic inhibition (i.e., of heart via vagus nerve)	Alzheimer disease (a type of senile dementia) is associated with a decrease in acetylcholine-secreting neurons; myasthenia gravis (weakness of skeletal muscles) results from a reduction in acetylcholine receptors Involved in memory, wakefulness, sexuality, and thirst
Monoamines			
Norepinephrine	A few small nuclei in the brainstem; nerve tracts extend from the nuclei to many areas of the brain and spinal cord; also in some ANS synapses	Excitatory or inhibitory	Cocaine and amphetamines increase the release and block the reuptake of norepinephrine resulting in overstimulation of postsynaptic neurons
Serotonin (5-hydroxytryptamine [5-HT])	A few small nuclei in the brainstem; nerve tracts extend from the nuclei to many areas of the brain and spinal cord	Generally inhibitory	Involved with mood, anxiety, and sleep induction; levels of serotonin elevated in schizophrenia (delusions, hallucinations, and withdrawal)
Dopamine	Neurons originating in substantia nigra	Inhibitory in the basal ganglia; may be excitatory in other parts of the brain	Parkinson disease (depression of voluntary motor control) results from destruction of dopamine-secreting neurons; drugs used to increase dopamine production induce vomiting and schizophrenia
Histamine	Hypothalamus, with nerve tracts to many parts of the brain and spinal cord	Generally inhibitory	No clear indication of histamine-associated neuropathologic conditions; histamine apparently is involved with arousal from sleep, pituitary hormone secretion, control of cerebral circulation, and thermoregulation
Amino Acids			
Gamma-aminobutyric acid (GABA)	GABA-secreting neurons mostly control activities in their own area and are not usually involved with transmission from one part of the CNS to another; most neurons of the CNS have GABA receptors	Majority of postsynaptic inhibition in the brain; some presynaptic inhibition in the spinal cord	Drugs that increase GABA function have been used to treat epilepsy (excessive discharge of neurons)

Table 14-2	Neurotransmitter and/or Neuromodulator Substances—cont'd		
Substance	Location	Effect	Clinical Example
Glycine	Spinal cord and brain; like GABA, glycine predominantly produces local effects	Most postsynaptic inhibition in the spinal cord	Glycine receptors are inhibited by the poison strychnine; strychnine increases the excitability of certain neurons by blocking their inhibition; strychnine poisoning results in powerful muscle contractions and convulsions; tetanus of respiratory muscles can cause death
Glutamate and aspartate	Widespread in the brain and spinal cord, especially in nerve tracts that ascend or descend the spinal cord or in tracts that project from one part of the brain to another	Excitatory	Drugs that block glutamate or aspartate are under development; these drugs might prevent seizures and neural degeneration from overexcitation
Nitric Oxide	Brain, spinal cord, adrenal gland, intramural plexus, nerves to penis	Excitatory	Blocking nitric oxide production may prevent stroke damage; stimulating nitric oxide release is used to treat impotence
Neuropeptides			
Endorphins and enkephalins	Widely distributed in the CNS and PNS	Generally inhibitory	The opiates morphine and heroin bind to endorphin and enkephalin receptors on presynaptic neurons and reduce pain by blocking the release of a neurotransmitter, such as substance P
Substance P	Spinal cord, brain, and sensory neurons associated with pain	Generally excitatory	Substance P is a neurotransmitter in pain transmission pathways; blocking its release by morphine reduces pain

ANS, Autonomic nervous system; *CNS*, central nervous system; *PNS*, peripheral nervous system.
From Seeley R, Stephens TD, Tate P: *Anatomy & physiology*, ed 6, St Louis, 2003, Mosby.

neurons.[4,5] (Chapter 1 contains a review of electrical impulses and membrane potentials.)

Usually, a single EPSP cannot induce a neuron's action potential and the propagation of the nerve impulse. Whether an action potential occurs depends on the number and frequency of potentials the postsynaptic neuron receives—a concept known as **summation. Temporal summation** (time relationship) refers to the effects of successive, rapid impulses received from a single neuron on the same synapse. **Spatial summation** (spacing effect) is the combined effects of impulses from a number of neurons on a single synapse at the same time. **Facilitation** refers to the effect of EPSPs on the plasma membrane potential. The plasma membrane is facilitated when summation brings the membrane closer to the threshold potential and decreases the stimulus required to induce an action potential. The effect that a neurotransmitter has on the plasma membrane potential depends on the balance of these effects. The mechanisms of convergence, divergence, summation, and facilitation allow for the integrative processes of the nervous system.

Two points could be helpful in understanding the complexity of brain physiology. First, the aforementioned neuromodulators appear to function to raise or lower the membrane potentials of neurons. These chemicals facilitate or inhibit the effect of neurotransmitters. Second, reciprocal synapses between dendrites—that is, one dendrite being able to depolarize or hyperpolarize the membrane potential of another dendrite through the use of neurotransmitters—demonstrate that the interactions between neurons are far more complicated than postulated by simple on-off models of brain function.

CENTRAL NERVOUS SYSTEM

Brain

The human brain enables individuals to reason, function intellectually, express personality and mood, and interact with the environment. The brain is a pinkish gray organ that weighs approximately 3 pounds and has the consistency of tofu or custard. It receives approximately 15% to 20% of the total cardiac output. The three major divisions of the brain, based on embryologic origin, are (1) the forebrain, formed by the two cerebral hemispheres; (2) the midbrain, which includes the corpora quadrigemina, tegmentum, and cerebral peduncles; and (3) the hindbrain, which includes the cerebellum, pons, and medulla

(Table 14-3). The midbrain, medulla oblongata, and pons make up the **brainstem,** which connects the hemispheres of the brain, cerebellum, and spinal cord. A collection of nuclei (nerve cell bodies) within the brainstem collectively constitute the **reticular formation** (Figure 14-6). The reticular formation is a large network of connected tissue nuclei that regulate vital reflexes, such as cardiovascular function and respiration. The reticular formation is essential for maintaining wakefulness and in conjunction with the cerebral cortex is referred to as the **reticular activating system.** Some nuclei within the reticular formation are involved in motor movements.[1]

In general, many major divisions of the brain are associated with specific functions, such as the occipital lobe and vision, but attributing specific functions to definite regions of the brain is not entirely accurate. Many activities, such as motor movements and memory, may actually be performed in several regions. Understanding functional specificity is very useful to clinical personnel, especially when attempting to localize pathologic conditions in the nervous system. A neurologist often can localize the site of a tumor, stroke, or bullet wound in an individual just by performing a neurologic examination.

Many attempts have been made to ascribe function to various regions of the cerebral cortex. A German neuropsychiatrist, Korbinian Brodmann (1868-1918), is credited with postulating the correlation of various activities to many regions of the cerebral cortex. (Figure 14-7, *B* and *C,* illustrates these regions and identifies some functional areas.) Another basic CNS principle, **plasticity,** holds that the CNS is capable of change. For example, children with brain damage may experience "relocation" of some functional areas to other parts of the brain. This propensity

Table 14-3	Divisions of the Central Nervous System	
Primary Vesicles	**Secondary Vesicles**	**Associated Structures**
Forebrain (prosencephalon)	Telencephalon	Cerebral hemispheres
		Cerebral cortex
		Rhinencephalon
		Basal ganglia
	Diencephalon	Epithalamus
		Thalamus
		Hypothalamus
		Subthalamus
Midbrain (mesencephalon)	Mesencephalon	Corpora quadrigemina
		Tegmentum
		Cerebral peduncles
Hindbrain (rhombencephalon)	Metencephalon	Cerebellum
		Pons
	Myelencephalon	Medulla oblongata
Spinal cord	Spinal cord	Spinal cord

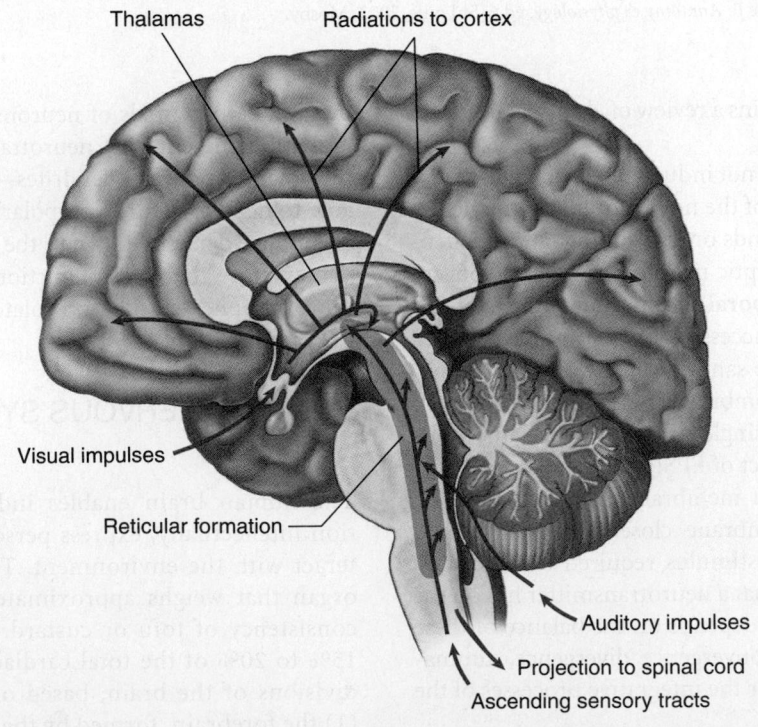

Thalamas   Radiations to cortex

Visual impulses

Reticular formation

Auditory impulses

Projection to spinal cord

Ascending sensory tracts

Figure 14-6 **Reticular activating system.** System consists of nuclei in the brainstem reticular formation plus fibers (axons) that conduct to the nuclei from below and fibers that conduct from the nuclei to widespread areas of the cerebral cortex. Functioning of the reticular activating system is essential for consciousness. (From Patton KT, Thibodeau GA: *Anatomy & physiology,* ed 7, St Louis, 2010, Mosby.)

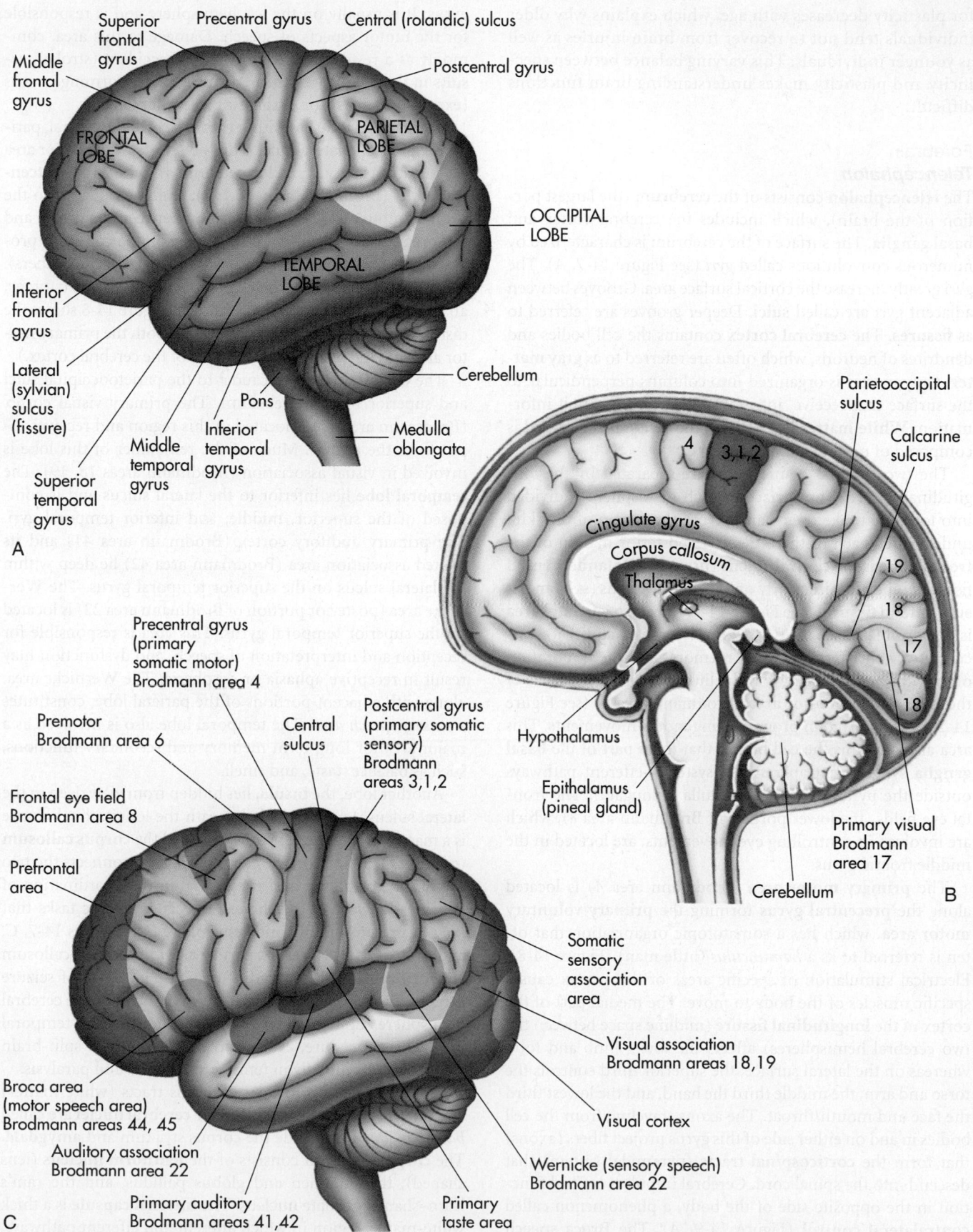

Figure 14-7 Cerebral hemispheres. **A,** Left hemisphere of cerebrum, lateral view. **B,** Functional areas of the cerebral cortex, midsagittal view. **C,** Functional areas of the cerebral cortex, lateral view.

Superior frontal gyrus
Middle frontal gyrus
Precentral gyrus
Central (rolandic) sulcus
Postcentral gyrus
FRONTAL LOBE
PARIETAL LOBE
OCCIPITAL LOBE
TEMPORAL LOBE
Inferior frontal gyrus
Lateral (sylvian) sulcus (fissure)
Superior temporal gyrus
Middle temporal gyrus
Inferior temporal gyrus
Pons
Cerebellum
Medulla oblongata

A

4
3,1,2
Cingulate gyrus
Corpus callosum
Thalamus
Hypothalamus
Epithalamus (pineal gland)
Cerebellum
Parietooccipital sulcus
Calcarine sulcus
19
18
17
18
Primary visual Brodmann area 17

B

Precentral gyrus (primary somatic motor) Brodmann area 4
Premotor Brodmann area 6
Frontal eye field Brodmann area 8
Prefrontal area
Central sulcus
Postcentral gyrus (primary somatic sensory) Brodmann areas 3,1,2
Somatic sensory association area
Visual association Brodmann areas 18,19
Visual cortex
Wernicke (sensory speech) Brodmann area 22
Primary taste area
Broca area (motor speech area) Brodmann areas 44, 45
Auditory association Brodmann area 22
Primary auditory Brodmann areas 41,42

C

for plasticity decreases with age, which explains why older individuals tend not to recover from brain injuries as well as younger individuals. This varying balance between specificity and plasticity makes understanding brain functions difficult.

Forebrain

Telencephalon

The **telencephalon** consists of the **cerebrum** (the largest portion of the brain), which includes the cerebral cortex and **basal ganglia.** The surface of the cerebrum is characterized by numerous convolutions called *gyri* (see Figure 14-7, *A*). The gyri greatly increase the cortical surface area. Grooves between adjacent gyri are called **sulci.** Deeper grooves are referred to as **fissures.** The **cerebral cortex** contains the cell bodies and dendrites of neurons, which often are referred to as **gray matter.** Gray matter is organized into columns perpendicular to the surface that receive, integrate, store, and transmit information. **White matter** lies beneath the cerebral cortex and is composed of myelinated nerve fibers.

The two cerebral hemispheres are separated by the longitudinal fissure. The surface of each hemisphere is divided into lobes that take their names from the region of the skull under which each of them lies. The posterior margin of the **frontal lobe** is the **central sulcus (fissure of Rolando,** central fissure); it borders inferiorly on the **lateral sulcus (sylvian fissure, lateral fissure)** (see Figure 14-7, *A*). The **prefrontal area** is responsible for goal-oriented behavior (i.e., ability to concentrate), short-term or recall memory, and the elaboration of thought and inhibition on the limbic (emotional) areas of the CNS. The **premotor area** (Brodmann area 6) (see Figure 14-7, *C*) is involved in programming motor movements. This area also contains the cell bodies that form part of the **basal ganglia system** (extrapyramidal system—efferent pathways outside the pyramids of the medulla oblongata). The frontal eye fields (the lower portion of Brodmann area 8), which are involved in controlling eye movements, are located in the middle frontal gyrus.

The **primary motor area** (Brodmann area 4) is located along the **precentral gyrus** forming the **primary voluntary motor area,** which has a somatotopic organization that often is referred to as a *homunculus* (little man) (Figure 14-8). Electrical stimulation of specific areas of this cortex causes specific muscles of the body to move. The medial part of the cortex in the **longitudinal fissure** (midline space between the two cerebral hemispheres) affects the lower limb and foot, whereas on the lateral surface, the superior third controls the torso and arm, the middle third the hand, and the lowest third the face and mouth/throat. The axons traveling from the cell bodies in and on either side of this gyrus project fibers (axons) that form the **corticospinal tracts** (pyramidal system) that descend into the spinal cord. Cerebral impulses control function in the opposite side of the body, a phenomenon called **contralateral control** (Figure 14-9, *A*). The **Broca speech area** (Brodmann areas 44, 45) is rostral to the inferior edge of the premotor area (Brodmann area 6) on the inferior frontal gyrus. It is usually on the left hemisphere and is responsible for the motor aspects of speech. Damage to this area, commonly as a result of a cerebrovascular accident (stroke), results in the inability to form, or difficulty in forming, words (expressive aphasia or dysphasia) (see Chapter 17).

The **parietal lobe** lies within the borders of the central, parietooccipital, and lateral sulci. This lobe contains the major area for somatic sensory input, located primarily along the **postcentral gyrus** (Brodmann areas 3, 1, 2), which is adjacent to the primary motor area. Communication between the motor and sensory areas (and among other regions in the cortex) is provided by **association fibers** (i.e., axons from association fibers). Much of this region is involved in sensory association (storage, analysis, and interpretation of stimuli). (Figure 14-8 shows the distribution of functions associated with both the primary motor area and the primary sensory area of the cerebral cortex.)

The **occipital lobe** lies caudal to the parietooccipital sulci and superior to the cerebellum. The primary visual cortex (Brodmann area 17) is located in this region and receives input from the retinas. Much of the remainder of this lobe is involved in visual association (Brodmann areas 18, 19). The **temporal lobe** lies inferior to the lateral sulcus and is composed of the superior, middle, and inferior temporal gyri. The primary auditory cortex (Brodmann area 41) and its related association area (Brodmann area 42) lie deep within the lateral sulcus on the superior temporal gyrus. The **Wernicke area** (posterior portion of Brodmann area 22) is located on the superior temporal gyrus. This area is responsible for reception and interpretation of speech, and dysfunction may result in receptive aphasia or dysphasia. The Wernicke area, along with adjacent portions of the parietal lobe, constitutes a *sensory speech area.* The temporal lobe also is involved as a major area for long-term memory and secondary functions, such as balance, taste, and smell.

Another lobe, the **insula,** lies hidden from view deep in the lateral sulcus. Lying directly beneath the longitudinal fissure is a massive white matter pathway called the **corpus callosum (commissural fibers).** The corpus callosum connects the two cerebral hemispheres and is essential in the coordination of activities between hemispheres, especially specific tasks that may be present in only one hemisphere (see Figures 14-7, *C,* and 14-15). As a last resort, part or all of the corpus callosum is cut to prevent the spread of epileptic loci (site of seizure activity) through the corpus callosum to the opposite cerebral hemisphere. Epileptic loci often are found in the temporal lobe. This procedure, evolved in the well-known split-brain studies, results initially in temporary aphasia and paralysis.

Inside the cerebrum are numerous tracts (white matter) and nuclei (gray matter). The major **cerebral nuclei** are called *basal ganglia* and include the corpus striatum and **amygdala.** The **corpus striatum** consists of the **lentiform nucleus** (lens shaped), the putamen and globus pallidus, and the ram's horn–shaped caudate nucleus. The **internal capsule** is a thick white-matter region in which afferent and efferent pathways, to and from the cerebral cortex, pass through the center of the cerebral hemispheres. The corpus striatum appears striped because of the rostral connections between its gray matter and the white matter of the internal capsule.

Functionally, the basal ganglia include, in addition to the corpus striatum, the subthalamic nucleus of the diencephalon and the substantia nigra of the mesencephalon. The basal ganglia plus their interconnections with the thalamus, premotor cortex, red nucleus, reticular formation, and spinal cord are part of the basal ganglia system (extrapyramidal system). The basal ganglia system is believed to exert a fine-tuning effect on motor movements. Parkinson disease and Huntington disease are conditions associated with defects of the basal ganglia (Box 14-2). They are characterized by various involuntary or exaggerated motor movements (see Chapter 16).

The **limbic system,** first described in 1878 by Broca, is composed of the **Papez circuit** (amygdala, parahippocampal gyrus, **hippocampus,** fornix, mamillary body of the hypothalamus, thalamus, and cingulate gyrus), septal area, habenula, other portions of the hypothalamus, and related autonomic nuclei. It is an extension or modification of the olfactory system. Its principal effects are believed to be involved with primitive behavioral responses, visceral reaction to emotion, feeding behaviors, biologic rhythms, and the sense of smell. Expression of affect (emotional and behavioral states) is mediated by extensive connections with the limbic system and prefrontal cortex. Interestingly, the Papez circuit, first postulated in 1937, appears to have as one of its major functions the consolidation of memory through a reverberating circuit.

Diencephalon

The **diencephalon,** surrounded by the cerebrum, is made up of four divisions: **epithalamus, thalamus, hypothalamus,** and **subthalamus** (see Table 14-3 and Figure 14-7, B). The epithalamus (pineal gland) forms the roof of the third ventricle (a brain cavity) and composes the most superior portion of the diencephalon. It has connections and functions closely associated with those of the limbic system. For example, the hormones of the pineal body have been shown to influence reproductive ability, and the secretion of melatonin is associated with circadian rhythms (see Chapters 10 and 20).

The largest component of the diencephalon is the thalamus. It is approximately the size and volume of the thumb from the tip to the first joint. It borders and surrounds the third ventricle, and it is a major integrating center for afferent impulses to the cerebral cortex, except for olfaction. The perception of various sensations occurs at this level but requires cortical processing for interpretation. The thalamus also serves as a relay center for sensory aspects of motor information from the basal ganglia and cerebellum to appropriate cortical motor areas. Cerebral cortical information also projects to the thalamus, creating reverberating circuits.

The hypothalamus forms the base of the diencephalon. Hypothalamic function falls into two major areas: (1) maintenance of a constant internal environment and (2) implementation of behavioral patterns. Integrative centers control ANS function, regulation of body temperature, endocrine function, and regulation of emotional expression. (Temperature regulation is discussed in Chapter 15.) The hypothalamus exerts

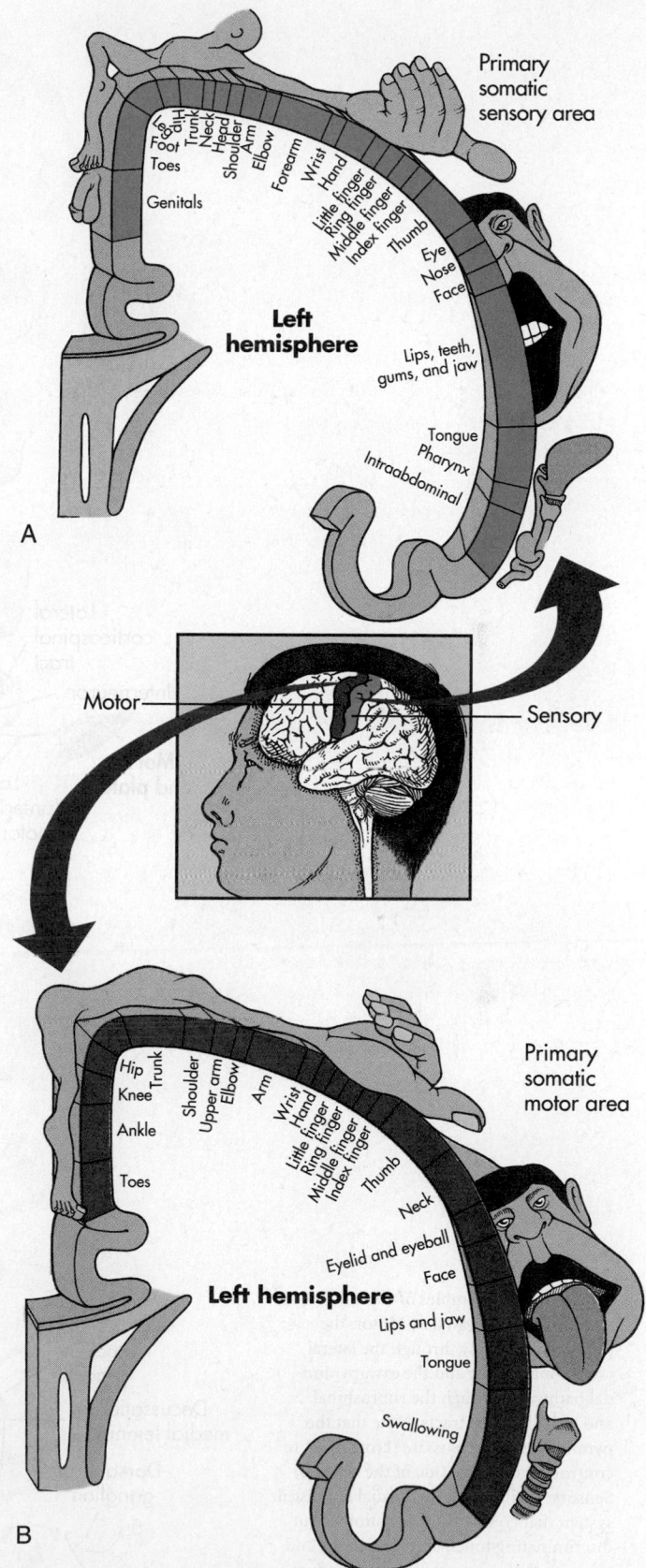

Figure 14-8 Primary somatic sensory (A) and motor (B) areas of the cortex. (From Thibodeau GA, Patton KT: *Anatomy & physiology,* ed 6, St Louis, 2007, Mosby.)

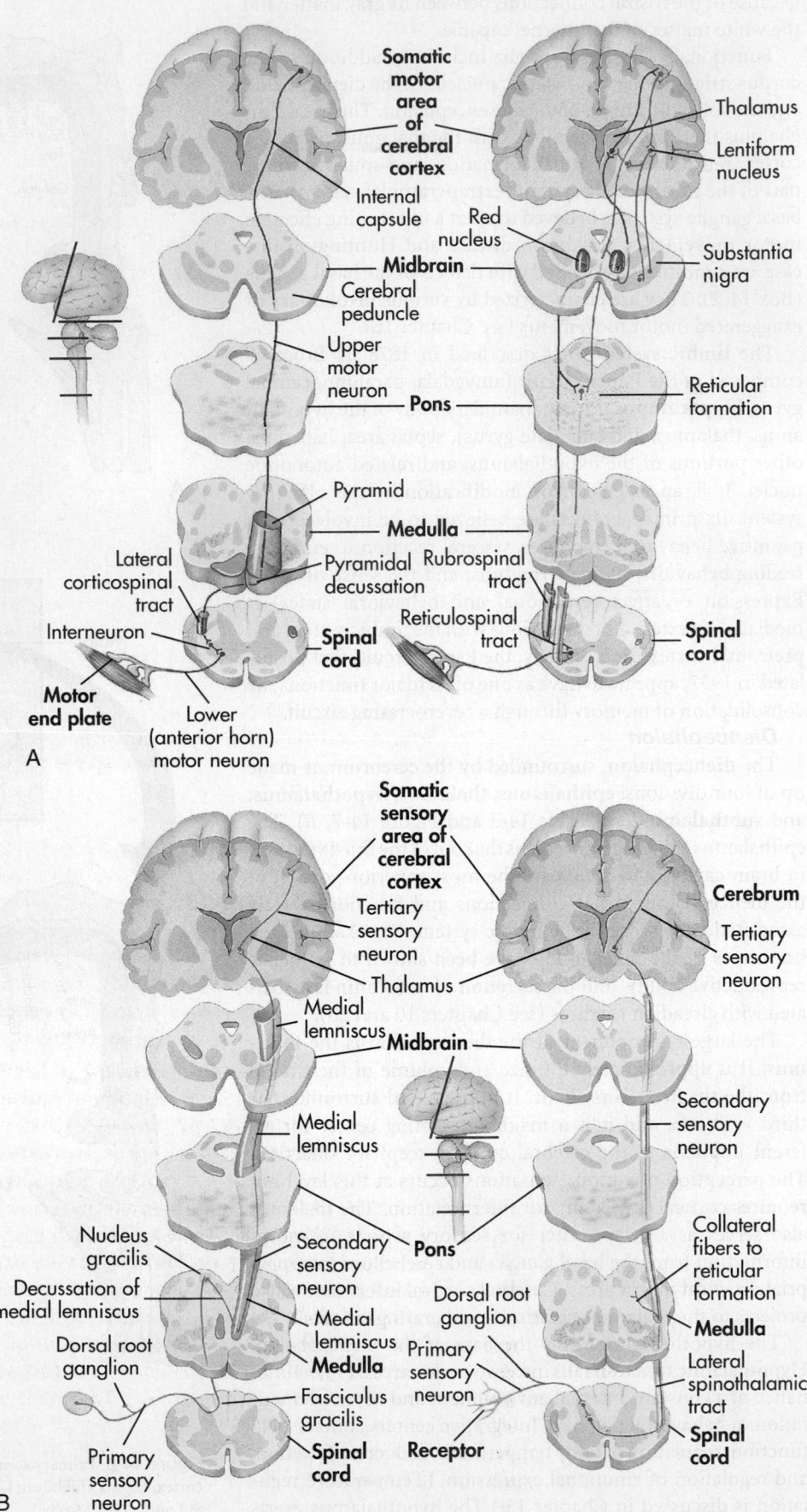

Figure 14-9 Examples of somatic motor and sensory pathways. **A,** Motor: the pyramidal pathway through the lateral corticospinal tract and the extrapyramidal pathways through the rubrospinal and reticulospinal tracts. Note that the pyramidal tracts decussate (cross over) to control the opposite side of the body. **B,** Sensory: pathways of the medial lemniscal system that conducts information about discriminating touch and kinesthesis and the spinothalamic pathway that conducts information about pain and temperature. (From Thibodeau GA, Patton KT: *Anatomy & physiology,* ed 6, St Louis, 2007, Mosby.)

Box 14-2	Invasive Treatments for Parkinson Disease

Surgical treatment can provide gratifying relief from the disabling symptoms of Parkinson disease (PD) when pharmaceutical therapies are no longer effective. The forms of surgical intervention include deep brain stimulation (thalamus, globus pallidus pars internalis, and subthalamic nucleus), ablation (thalamotomy, pallidotomy, and subthalamotomy), cell grafts, and gene therapy (mainly of the striatum). Deep brain stimulation with electrodes is currently the gold standard of treating PD because there is symptom control with minimal tissue destruction. However, an ablation technique can be the preferable option for a particular individual. Stem cell grafts of dopamine neurons are being studied, but a number of problems still remain to be resolved, including poor cell survival of the grafted neurons and reinnervation into the host striatum. Gene therapy strategies include having dopamine synthesizing enzyme genes activated in the subthalamic nucleus. Limited human studies are showing some promise.

Data from Benabid AI et al: *Lancet Neurol* 8(1):67-81, 2009; Fahn S: *Ann Neurol* 64 Suppl 2:S56-64, 2008; Deierborg T et al: *Prog Neurobiol* 85(4):407-432, 2008; Remple MS et al: *Expert Rev Neurother* 8(6):897-906, 2008.

Box 14-3	Functions of the Hypothalamus

Visceral and somatic responses
Affectual responses
Hormone synthesis
Sympathetic and parasympathetic activity
Temperature regulation
Feeding responses
Physical expression of emotions
Sexual behavior
Pleasure-punishment centers
Level of arousal or wakefulness

its influence through the endocrine system, as well as through neural pathways (Box 14-3). (For endocrine functions of the hypothalamus and pituitary, see Chapter 20.)

The subthalamus flanks the hypothalamus laterally. The subthalamus contains the **subthalamic nucleus,** which is part of the basal ganglia system.

Midbrain

The **midbrain (mesencephalon)** is composed of three structures: the **corpora quadrigemina,** or **tectum** (composed of the superior and inferior colliculi); the **tegmentum** (containing the red nucleus and substantia nigra); and the basis pedunculi. (The tegmentum and basis pedunculi are collectively the cerebral peduncles.)

The **superior colliculi** are involved with voluntary and involuntary visual motor movements (e.g., the ability of the eyes to *track* moving objects in the visual field). The **inferior colliculi** accomplish similar motor activities but involve movements affecting the auditory system (e.g., positioning the head to improve hearing). The inferior colliculus is also a major relay center along the auditory pathway. The **red nucleus** is a major motor output center that is influenced by the cerebellum. The inferior-most portion of the basal ganglia is the **substantia nigra,** which synthesizes **dopamine,** a neurotransmitter and precursor of norepinephrine. Its dysfunction is associated with Parkinson disease (see Chapter 16). The **basis pedunculi** are made up of efferent fibers of the corticospinal, corticobulbar, and corticopontocerebellar tracts.

Other notable structures of this region are the nuclei and tracts of the third and fourth cranial nerves. The **cerebral aqueduct (aqueduct of Sylvius),** which carries CSF, also traverses this structure. The plugging of this aqueduct is often the cause of hydrocephalus.

Hindbrain

Metencephalon

The major structures of the **metencephalon** are the cerebellum and the pons. The **cerebellum** (see Figure 14-7, *A* and *B*) is composed of two cerebellar hemispheres covered with small convolutions called *folia.* Each hemisphere is divided by the primary fissure into two lobes (anterior and posterior) that are connected by a midline structure called the **vermis,** meaning worm.

The cerebellum is responsible for conscious and unconscious muscle synergy and for maintaining balance and posture. This is accomplished through extensive neural connections from the spinal cord and medulla oblongata through the inferior cerebellar peduncle and with the midbrain and higher structures through the superior cerebellar peduncle. The two cerebellar hemispheres receive massive cerebral cortical input through the middle cerebellar pedunculi. These connections allow extensive sampling of visual, vestibular, and proprioceptive data from other regions of the CNS and periphery. Damage to the cerebellum is characterized by ipsilateral (same side) loss of equilibrium, balance, and motor coordination. The cerebellum has ipsilateral control of the body, in contrast to the cerebral cortex, which has contralateral (opposite side) control of the body.

The **pons** (bridge) is easily recognized by its bulging appearance below the midbrain and above the medulla oblongata. Primarily, it transmits information from the cerebellum to the brainstem nuclei and relays motor information from the cerebral cortex to the contralateral cerebellar hemisphere. The pons is an important center for the control of respiration (i.e., rate and relationship of inspiration to expiration). The nuclei of cranial nerves V through VIII are located in this structure.

Myelencephalon

The **medulla oblongata** makes up the **myelencephalon** and is the lowest portion of the brainstem. Reflex activities, such as heart rate, respiration, blood pressure, coughing, sneezing, swallowing, and vomiting, are controlled in this area. The nuclei of cranial nerves IX through XII (see Table 14-6 for discussion) are located in this region. The lowest portion of the reticular formation is found here as well.

A major portion of the descending motor pathways (i.e., corticospinal tracts) crosses to the contralateral side, or decussate, at the inferior medulla oblongata (see Figure 14-9, *A*). These pathways, together with other areas of decussation in the CNS, are the basis for the phenomenon of contralateral control.

Spinal Cord

The **spinal cord** is the portion of the CNS that lies within the vertebral canal and is surrounded and protected by the vertebral column. The spinal cord has many functions, which include being a long nerve cable that connects the brain and body, conducting somatic and autonomic reflexes, providing motor pattern control centers, and serving as a sensory and motor modulation center. It continues from the medulla oblongata and ends at the level of the first or second lumbar vertebra in adults (Figure 14-10). The end of the spinal cord, the **conus medullaris,** is cone shaped. Spinal nerves continue from the end of the spinal cord and form a nerve bundle called the **cauda equina**. The filament anchor from the conus medullaris to the coccyx is the **filum terminale** (see Figure 14-10).

Grossly, the spinal cord is divided into sections (8 cervical, 12 thoracic, 5 lumbar, 5 sacral, and 1 coccygeal) that correspond to paired nerves (see Figure 14-10). A cross section of the spinal cord (Figure 14-11) is characterized by a butterfly-shaped inner core of gray matter (containing nerve cell bodies). The **central canal** lies in the center of this region

and extends through the spinal cord from its origin in the fourth ventricle. The gray matter of the spinal cord is divided into three regions with specific functional characteristics. These regions include the **posterior horn (dorsal horn),** which is composed primarily of interneurons and axons from sensory neurons whose cell bodies lie in the **sensory ganglion (dorsal root ganglion).** At the tip of the posterior horn is the **substantia gelatinosa,** a structure involved in pain transmission (see Chapter 15). The **intermediolateral gray (lateral horn)** contains cell bodies involved with the ANS. The **anterior horn (ventral horn)** contains the nerve cell bodies for efferent pathways leaving the spinal cord by way of spinal nerves. The terms *anterior* and *posterior* are preferred by many authors for describing human spinal cord anatomy, whereas *dorsal* and *ventral* are the common zoologic ("cat and dog") terms.

Surrounding the gray matter is white matter that forms ascending and descending pathways called **spinal tracts** and short ascending and descending integrative pathways. Spinal tracts are named to denote their beginning and ending points. For example, the **spinothalamic tract** carries nerve impulses from the spinal cord to the thalamus in the diencephalon. The white matter is subdivided into columns. These consist of the **anterior column (ventral column), lateral column,** and **posterior column (dorsal column),** that is, the fasciculus gracilis

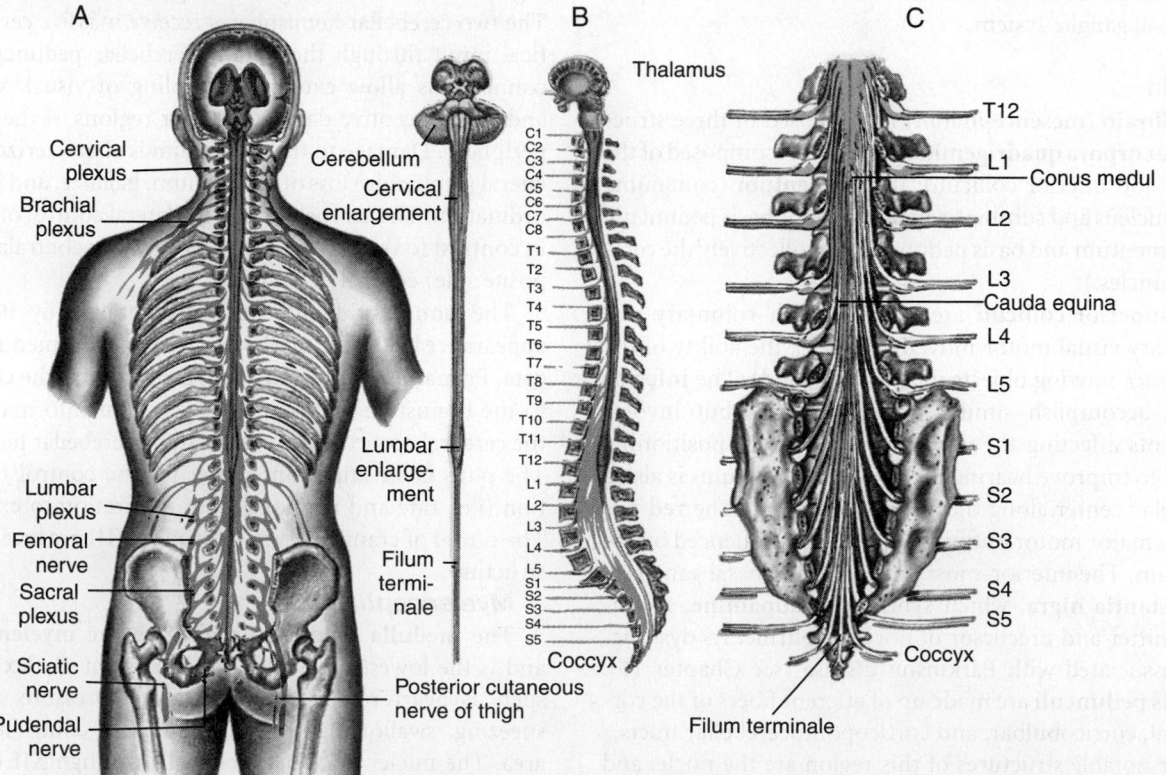

Figure 14-10 Spinal cord within vertebral canal and exiting spinal nerves. A, Posterior view of brainstem and spinal cord in situ with spinal nerves and plexus. **B,** Anterior view of brainstem and spinal cord. **C,** Enlargement of caudal area showing termination of spinal cord (conus medullaris) and group of nerve fibers constituting the cauda equina. (From Rudy EB, editor: *Advanced neurological and neurosurgical nursing,* St Louis, 1984, Mosby.)

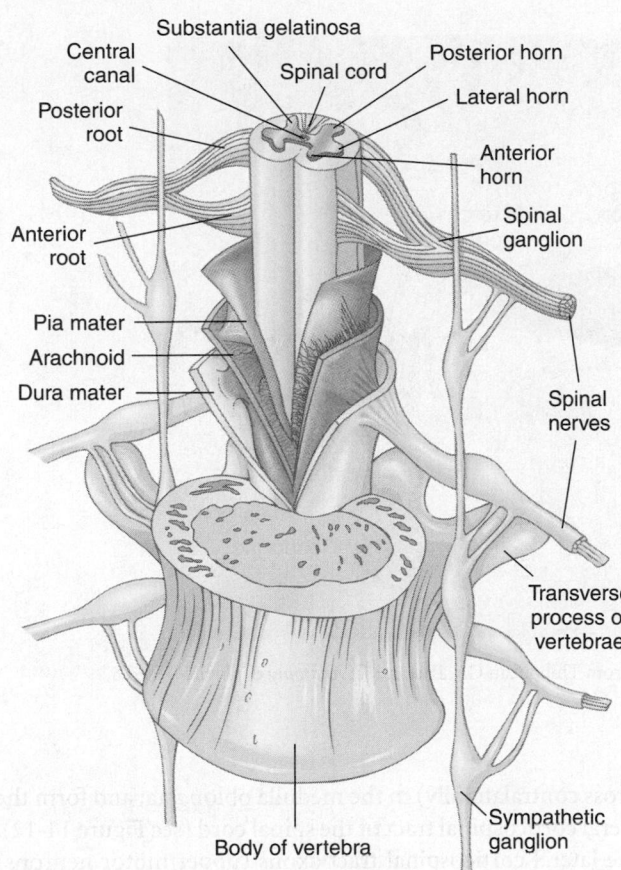

Figure 14-11 Coverings of the spinal cord. Note how the dura mater extends to cover the spinal nerve roots and nerves. The arachnoid is highlighted in *blue* and the pia mater in *pink*. (Modified from Thibodeau GA, Patton KT: *Structure and function of the body,* ed 12, St Louis, 2004, Mosby.)

and fasciculus cuneatus. (Figure 14-12 identifies the location and principal activities of the major spinal tracts.)

Neural circuits in the spinal cord, when activated, display specific sets of motor responses. **Reflex arcs** form basic units that respond to stimuli and provide protective circuitry for motor output. Structures mandatory for a reflex arc are a receptor, an **afferent (sensory) neuron,** an **efferent (motor) neuron,** and an effector muscle or gland. The afferent neuron is a pseudounipolar neuron, with its cell body in the sensory ganglion. A simple reflex arc may contain only two neurons. (Figure 14-13 illustrates a simple reflex arc.) Most reflex arcs consist of three neurons that include an interneuron or association neuron between the afferent and efferent neurons. Transmission time for three-neuron reflexes is slower than in simple reflexes because there are two synaptic delays, rather than one, as well as the delay involved in crossing the interneuron. The afferent neuron of the reflex arc simultaneously sends sensory information to the effector organ and to higher CNS centers (see Figure 14-9, *B*, and Figure 15-3). The motor effects from reflex arcs generally occur before perception of the event in the higher centers of the brain. Much of the regulation of the internal environment is mediated by ANS reflexes.

Afferent pathways transmit information from peripheral receptors and eventually terminate in the cerebral or cerebellar cortex or both. Efferent pathways primarily relay information from the cerebrum to the brainstem or spinal cord (see Figure 14-9, *A*). **Upper motor neurons** (i.e., corticospinal tract) are the classification of motor pathways completely contained within the CNS. Their primary roles include directing, influencing, and modifying reflex arcs, lower-level control

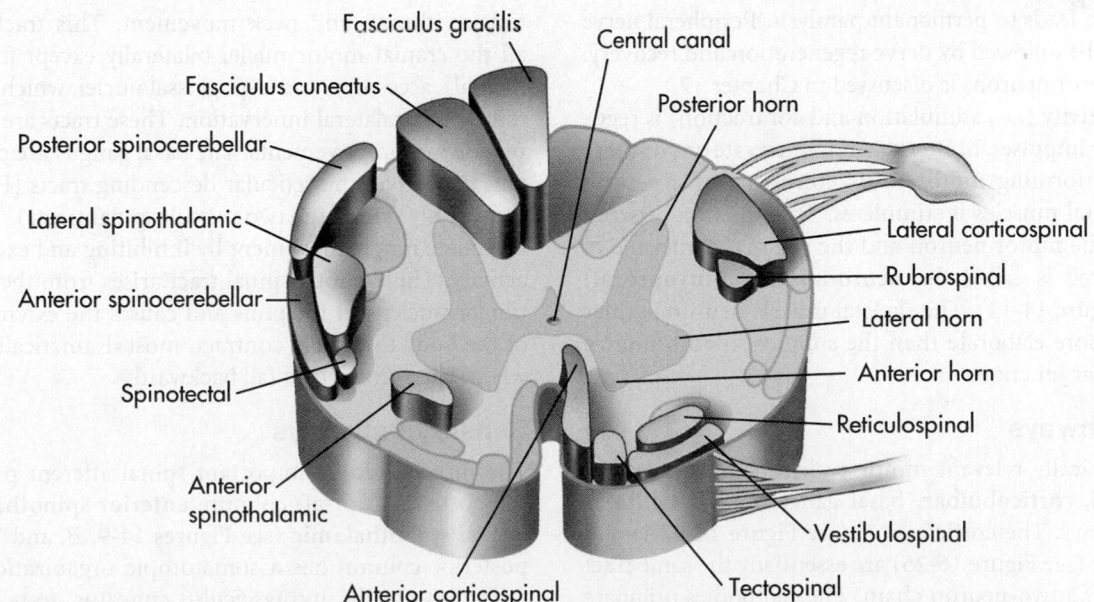

Figure 14-12 Major tracts of the spinal cord. The major ascending (sensory) tracts, shown only on the left here, are highlighted in *blue*. The major descending (motor) tracts, shown only on the right, are highlighted in *red*. (From Thibodeau GA, Patton KT: *Anatomy & physiology,* ed 6, St Louis, 2007, Mosby.)

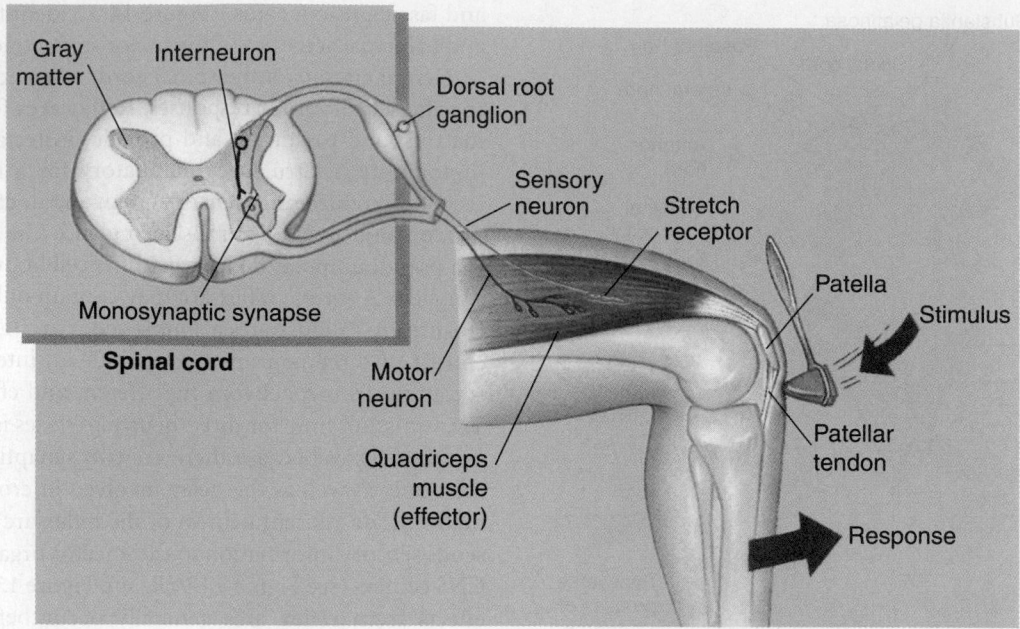

Figure 14-13 Cross section of spinal cord showing simple reflex arc. (From Thibodeau GA, Patton KT: *Anatomy & physiology*, ed 6, St Louis, 2007, Mosby.)

centers, and motor (and some sensory) neurons. Generally, upper motor neurons form synapses with interneurons, which then form synapses with lower motor neurons before projecting into the periphery. **Lower motor neurons** (i.e., cranial and spinal efferent neurons) are responsible for direct influence on muscles. Their cell bodies lie in the gray matter of the spinal cord, but their processes extend into the PNS (see Figure 16-26). Destruction of upper motor neurons usually results in initial paralysis followed within days or weeks by partial recovery, whereas destruction of the lower motor neurons often leads to permanent paralysis. Peripheral nerve damage may be followed by nerve regeneration and recovery. (Injury to motor neurons is discussed in Chapter 17.)

Muscle activity (i.e., stimulation and contraction) is regulated by nerve impulses. Motor neurons innervate one or more muscle cells, forming **motor units** consisting of a neuron and the skeletal muscles it stimulates. The junction between the axon of the motor neuron and the plasma membrane of the muscle cell is called the **neuromuscular (myoneural) junction** (Figure 14-14). The skeletal muscle neuromuscular junction is more elaborate than the simpler smooth muscle neuromuscular junction.

Motor Pathways

The four clinically relevant motor pathways are the **lateral corticospinal, corticobulbar,** basal ganglia, and **vestibulospinal** pathways. The corticospinal (see Figure 14-9, *A*) and corticobulbar (see Figure 16-25) are essentially the same tract and consist of a two-neuron chain. The cell bodies originate in and around the precentral gyrus; pass through the corona radiata of the cerebrum, the internal capsule, middle three fifths of the basis pedunculus, pons, and pyramid; decussate

(cross contralaterally) in the medulla oblongata; and form the lateral corticospinal tract of the spinal cord (see Figure 14-12). The lateral corticospinal tract axons (upper motor neurons) leave the tract to go to specific interneurons or motor neurons in the anterior horn. The lateral corticospinal tract has the same somatotopic organization as the body. These spinal motor neurons project to specific motor units and are lower motor neurons. The corticobulbar (bulbar refers to brainstem) tract can be thought of as the part of the corticospinal tract that innervates the cranial motor nuclei for eye, face, tongue, throat, and neck movement. This tract innervates all the cranial motor nuclei bilaterally except for the facial (spinal), accessory, and hypoglossal nuclei, which receive primarily contralateral innervation. These tracts are involved in precise motor movements. The basal ganglia are part of a system that drives the reticular descending tracts (Figure 14-12 shows only one of the two reticulospinal tracts). These tracts modulate motor movement by inhibiting and exciting spinal activity. The vestibulospinal tract arises from the lateral vestibular nucleus in the pons and causes the extensor muscles of the body to rapidly contract, most dramatically witnessed when a person starts to fall backward.

Sensory Pathways

The three clinically important spinal afferent pathways are the posterior (dorsal) column, **anterior spinothalamic,** and **lateral spinothalamic** (see Figures 14-9, *B*, and 14-12). The posterior column has a somatotopic organization with the fasciculus gracilis and fasciculus cuneatus, respectively, carrying lower body and upper body fine touch, two-point discrimination, and proprioceptive information (i.e., **epicritic**). The posterior column is formed by a three-neuron chain. The

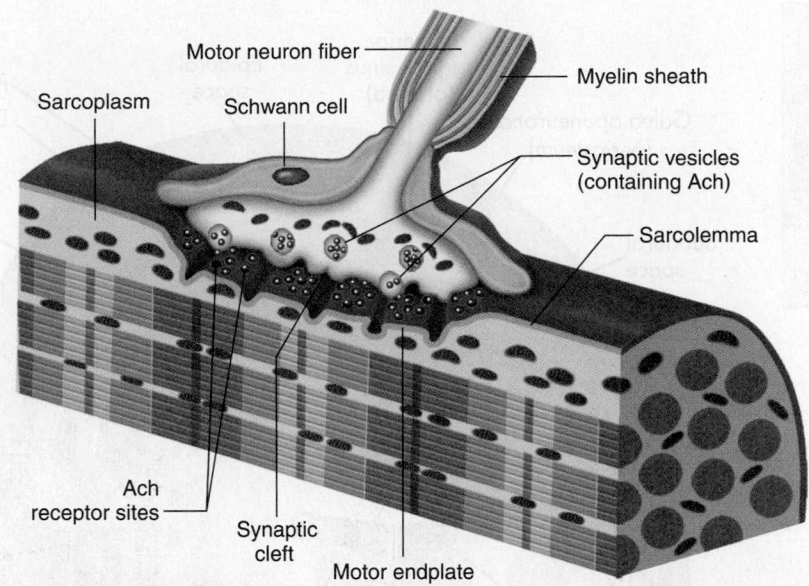

Figure 14-14 Neuromuscular junction. This figure shows how the distal end of a motor neuron fiber forms a synapse, or "chemical junction," with an adjacent muscle fiber. Neurotransmitters (specifically, acetylcholine) are released from the neuron's synaptic vesicles and diffuse across the synaptic cleft where they stimulate receptors in the motor end-plate region of the sarcolemma. (From Patton KT, Thibodeau GA: *Anatomy & physiology*, ed 7, St Louis, 2010, Mosby)

first neuron of the chain is the primary afferent neuron. It is also the sensory neuron of the reflex arc. After entering the spinal cord it sends its axon ipsilaterally up the spinal cord in a specific part of the posterior funiculus and synapses in one of three posterior column nuclei in the hindbrain. A basketball center has primary afferent neurons that run from the great toe up to the pons, which could be more than 6 feet long. The second-order neuron has its cell body in one of the posterior column nuclei and sends its axon contralaterally and ascends to a specific nucleus of the thalamus and synapses. The third-order neuron, originating in the thalamus, continues the tract into the internal capsule, corona radiata, and postcentral gyrus (Brodmann areas 3, 1, 2) (see Figure 14-7, *C*). The anterior and lateral spinothalamic tracts are responsible for vague touch and pain and temperature, respectively (see Figure 14-9, *B*). These modalities are referred to as **protopathic.**

Today the anterior and lateral spinothalamic tracts are combined by many neuroanatomists into the anterolateral system because these modalities are difficult to localize into finite tracts in the spinal cord. These tracts also form a three-neuron chain. However, the primary afferent neurons synapse in the posterior horn of the spinal cord, not just at the level they enter the intervertebral foramen but in a number of spinal segments above and below their point of entry. This is an example of divergence. The second-order neurons in the posterior horn cross to the contralateral side in the spinal cord and ascend to the same thalamic nucleus as the posterior column pathway and continue on with the posterior column pathway to the postcentral gyrus.

Protective Structures

Cranium

The cranium is composed of eight bones. The cranial vault functions to enclose and protect the brain and its associated structures. The **galea aponeurotica,** which is a thick, fibrous band of tissue overlying the cranium between the frontal and occipital muscles, affords added protection to the bony structure of the skull. The subgaleal space has venous connections with the dural sinuses, and with increased intracranial pressure, blood can be shunted to the space, thus reducing pressure in the intracranial cavity. The subgaleal space is also a common site for wound drains to be placed after intracranial surgery.

The floor of the cranial vault is irregular and contains many foramina (openings) for cranial nerves, blood vessels, and the spinal cord to exit. The cranial floor is divided into three fossae (depressions). The frontal lobes lie in the **anterior fossa;** temporal lobes and base of the diencephalon lie in the **middle fossa (temporal fossa);** and the cerebellum lies in the **posterior fossa.** These terms are commonly used anatomic landmarks to describe the location of intracranial lesions.

Meninges

Surrounding the brain and spinal cord are three protective membranes: the dura mater, the arachnoid, and the pia mater. Collectively they are called the **meninges** (Figure 14-15). The **dura mater** (meaning literally "hard mother") is composed of two layers, with the venous sinuses formed between them. The outermost layer forms the **periosteum (endosteal layer)** of the skull, and the **inner dura,** or **meningeal layer,**

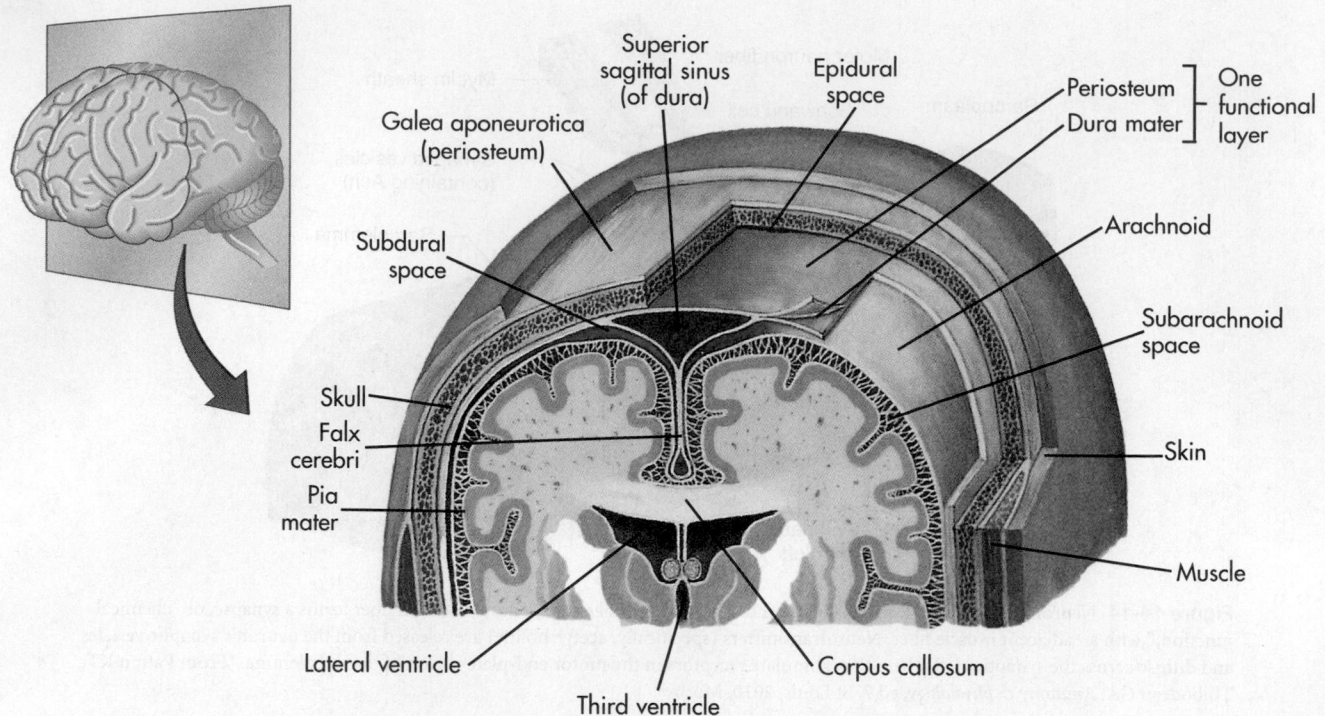

Figure 14-15 Coverings of the brain. Frontal section of the superior portion of the head, as viewed from the front. The bony and the membranous coverings of the brain can be seen. (From Thibodeau GA, Patton KT: *Anatomy & physiology*, ed 6, St Louis, 2007, Mosby.)

is responsible for the formation of rigid, double-thickness membranous plates that serve to support and separate various brain structures.

One of these membranous plates (see Figure 14-15), the **falx cerebri,** dips between the two cerebral hemispheres along the longitudinal fissure. The falx cerebri is anchored anteriorly to the base of the brain at the crista galli of the ethmoid bone. The **tentorium cerebelli** is a membrane that separates the cerebellum below from the cerebral structures above. The tentorium may become involved during periods of increased intracranial pressure caused by an injury to the brain. An injury within the cranial cavity tends to shift intracranial contents, and as structures shift, they tend to be compressed against these rigid membranes, resulting in damage or destruction. A common example is tentorial herniation.

Below the dura mater lies the **arachnoid membrane,** characterized by its filmy, weblike structure. It loosely follows the contours of the cerebral structures but goes over the sulci.

The **subdural space** lies between the dura and arachnoid. Many small bridging veins that have little support traverse the subdural space. Their disruption results in a subdural hematoma (see Chapter 17). The **subarachnoid space,** which contains CSF, lies between the arachnoid and the pia mater (see Figure 14-15). Damage to intracranial vessels can lead to a condition called *subarachnoid hemorrhage,* which frequently results in signs of meningeal irritation, such as neck stiffness, Kernig sign, and low back pain.

Unlike the dura mater and arachnoid, the delicate **pia mater** (see Figure 14-15) closely adheres to the surface of the brain and spinal cord and even follows the sulci and fissures. It provides support for blood vessels serving brain tissue. The **choroid plexuses,** structures that produce CSF, arise from the pia mater. The spinal cord is anchored to the vertebrae by extensions of the meninges called **denticulate ligaments.** The meninges continue beyond the end of the spinal cord to the lower portion of the sacrum. CSF, contained within the subarachnoid space, also circulates down to the large **lumbar cistern,** which extends from the second lumbar vertebra to the second sacral vertebra. Cisterns are expanded areas of the subarachnoid space. The **cerebellomedullary cistern (cisterna magna)** and the pontine cisterns are two other important cisterns.

The meninges form potential and real spaces important to understanding functional and pathologic mechanisms. For example, between the dura mater and skull lies a potential space termed the **epidural space** (see Figure 14-15). In the spinal canal is a real epidural space filled with fatty tissue and a venous plexus. The arterial supply to the meninges consists of blood vessels that lie within grooves in the skull. As a result of trauma, the skull can be fractured and the blood vessels disrupted. The ruptured vessels can lead to an accumulation of blood within the epidural space, called an *epidural hematoma* (see Chapter 17). Persons with alcoholism often fall and injure their head, resulting in an epidural hematoma. An inflammation of the meninges (meningitis) also can have life-threatening implications because of the relative proximity to the brain. (Disorders of the CNS are discussed in Chapter 17.)

Cerebrospinal Fluid and the Ventricular System

Cerebrospinal fluid (CSF) is a clear, colorless fluid similar to blood plasma and interstitial fluid. The intracranial and spinal cord structures float in CSF and are thereby protected from jolts and blows. The buoyant properties of the CSF also prevent the brain from tugging on meninges, nerve roots, and blood vessels. (Constituents of CSF are listed in Table 14-4.) Between 125 and 150 ml of CSF, approximately the quantity of a small cup of coffee, is circulating within the **ventricles** (small cavities) and subarachnoid space at any given time. Approximately 600 ml of CSF is produced daily.

The choroid plexuses in the lateral, third, and fourth ventricles produce the major portion of CSF. (Ventricles are illustrated in Figure 14-15.) These plexuses are characterized by a rich network of blood vessels, supplied by the pia mater, that lie in close contact with the ependymal cells of the ventricles.

The CSF exerts pressure within the brain and spinal cord. When a person is lying down, CSF pressure is approximately 120 to 180 mm of water pressure, or approximately 9 to 14 mmHg pressure. CSF flow is a result of a pressure gradient between the arterial system and the CSF-filled cavities. Beginning in the lateral ventricles, the CSF flows through the **interventricular foramen (foramen of Monro)** into the third ventricle and then passes through the cerebral aqueduct (aqueduct of Sylvius) into the fourth ventricle. From the fourth ventricle, the CSF may pass through either the paired **lateral apertures (foramina of Luschka)** into the pontine cisterns, located along the basal pons, or the midline **median aperture (foramen of Magendie)** into the cerebellomedullary cistern before communicating with the subarachnoid spaces of the brain and spinal cord. The CSF does not, however, accumulate. Instead, it is reabsorbed into the venous circulation through the arachnoid villi, primarily located superior to the

falx cerebri in the **superior sagittal sinus.** The **arachnoid villi** protrude from the arachnoid space, through the dura mater, and lie within the blood flow of the venous sinuses. CSF is reabsorbed by means of a pressure gradient between the arachnoid villi and the cerebral venous sinuses. The villi function as one-way valves directing CSF outflow into the blood but preventing blood flow into the subarachnoid space. Thus CSF is derived from the blood, and after circulating throughout the CNS, it returns to the blood.

Samples of CSF are withdrawn for diagnostic purposes either (1) by inserting a needle between the third and fourth lumbar vertebrae into the lumbar cistern (subarachnoid space)—a procedure called **lumbar puncture**—or (2) from an intraventricular catheter. Spinal anesthesias (blocks) are administered in a manner similar to the lumbar puncture.

Vertebral Column

The **vertebral column** (Figure 14-16) is composed of 33 vertebrae: 7 cervical, 12 thoracic, 5 lumbar, 5 fused sacral, and 4 fused coccygeal. Between each interspace (except the fused sacral and coccygeal vertebrae) is an **intervertebral disk** (Figure 14-17). At the center of the intervertebral disk is the **nucleus pulposus,** a pulpy mass of elastic fibers. The intervertebral disk functions to absorb shocks, preventing damage to the vertebrae. The intervertebral disk is also a common source of back problems. If too much stress is applied to the vertebral column, the disk contents may rupture and protrude into the

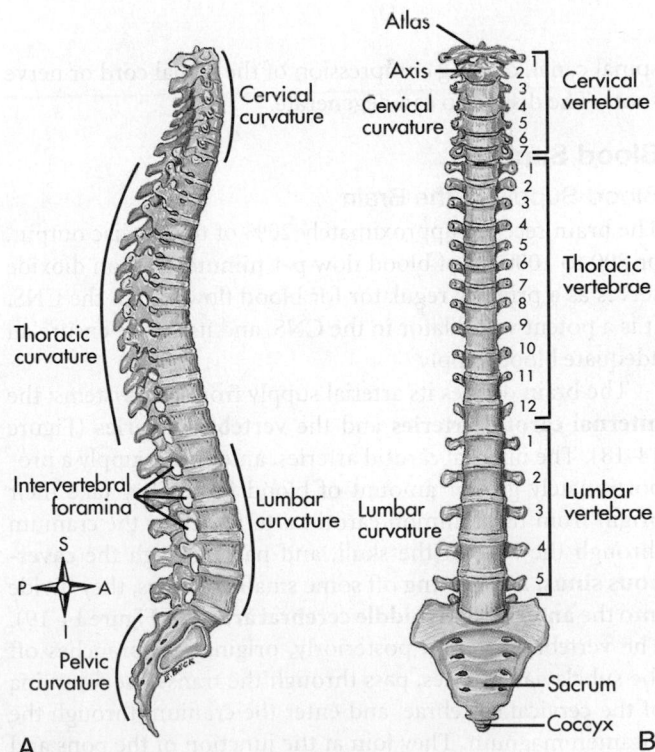

Figure 14-16 Vertebral column. A, Right lateral view. B, Anterior view. (From Thibodeau GA, Patton KT: *Anatomy & physiology,* ed 6, St Louis, 2007, Mosby.)

Table 14-4	Composition of Cerebrospinal Fluid
Constituent	**Normal Value**
Na+	148 mM
K+	2.9 mM
Cl−	125 mM
HCO₃⁻	22.9 mM
Glucose (fasting)	50-75 mg/dl (60% of serum glucose)
Ph	7.3
Protein	15-45 mg/dl
Albumin	80%
Gamma globulin	6%-10%
Cells	
White (lymphocytes)	0-6/mm³
Red (red blood cell [RBC])	0/mm³

Cl⁻, Chloride; *HCO₃⁻,* bicarbonate; *K⁺,* potassium; *Na⁺,* sodium.

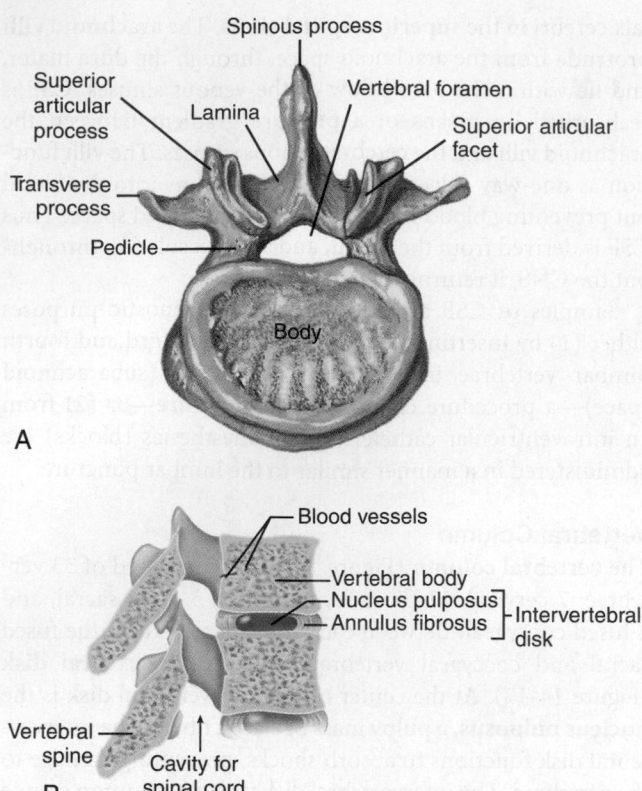

Figure 14-17 A, Lumbar vertebra, superior view; B, Intervertebral disk. (A from Thibodeau GA, Patton KT: *Anatomy & physiology*, ed 6, St Louis, 2007, Mosby; B from Patton KT, Thibodeau GA: *Anatomy & physiology*, ed 7, St Louis, 2010, Mosby.)

spinal canal, causing compression of the spinal cord or nerve roots. The disks also can degenerate.

Blood Supply

Blood Supply to the Brain

The brain receives approximately 20% of the cardiac output, or 800 to 1000 ml of blood flow per minute. Carbon dioxide serves as a primary regulator for blood flow within the CNS. It is a potent vasodilator in the CNS, and its effects ensure an adequate blood supply.

The brain derives its arterial supply from two systems: the **internal carotid arteries** and the **vertebral arteries** (Figure 14-18). The internal carotid arteries, anteriorly, supply a proportionately greater amount of blood flow. They take their origin from the common carotid arteries, enter the cranium through the base of the skull, and pass through the **cavernous sinus.** After giving off some small branches, they divide into the **anterior** and **middle cerebral arteries** (Figure 14-19). The vertebral arteries, posteriorly, originate as branches off the subclavian arteries, pass through the transverse foramina of the cervical vertebrae, and enter the cranium through the foramen magnum. They join at the junction of the pons and medulla oblongata to form the **basilar artery.** The basilar artery divides at the level of the midbrain to form paired **posterior cerebral arteries.** Three major paired arteries perfuse the

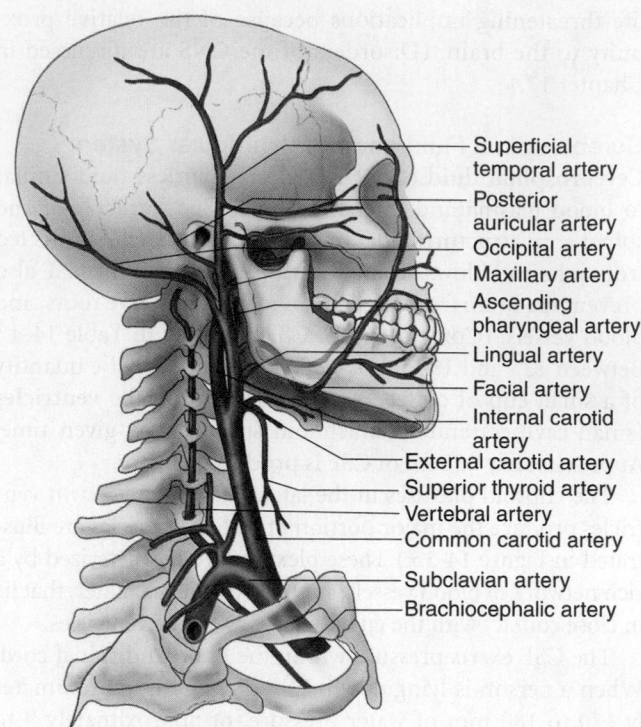

Figure 14-18 Major arteries of the head and neck. (From Patton KT, Thibodeau GA: *Anatomy & physiology*, ed 7, St Louis, 2010, Mosby.)

cerebellum and brainstem and originate from the posterior arterial supply: the posterior inferior cerebellar artery, off the vertebral artery; and the anterior inferior cerebellar and superior cerebellar arteries, off the basilar artery. The basilar artery also gives rise to small pontine arteries. The large arteries on the surface of the brain and their branches are called **superficial arteries (conducting arteries).** The small branches that project into the brain are termed **projecting arteries (nutrient arteries).** Occluding any of these vessels can cause neurologic signs and symptoms that are often diagnostically unique.

The **arterial circle (circle of Willis)** (see Figure 14-19) is a structure credited with the ability to compensate for reduced blood flow from any one of the major contributors (collateral blood flow). The arterial circle is formed by the posterior cerebral arteries, posterior communicating arteries, internal carotid arteries, anterior cerebral arteries, and anterior communicating artery. The anterior cerebral, middle cerebral, and posterior cerebral arteries leave the arterial circle and extend to various brain structures. (Table 14-5 and Figure 14-20 illustrate structures served, functional relationships, and pathologic considerations related to occlusion of cerebral arteries.)

Cerebral venous drainage does not parallel (lie side by side) its arterial supply, whereas the venous drainage of the brainstem and cerebellum does parallel the arterial supply of the structures. The cerebral veins are classified as superficial veins and deep cerebral veins. The veins drain into venous plexuses and dural sinuses (formed between the dural layers) and eventually join the internal jugular veins at the base of the

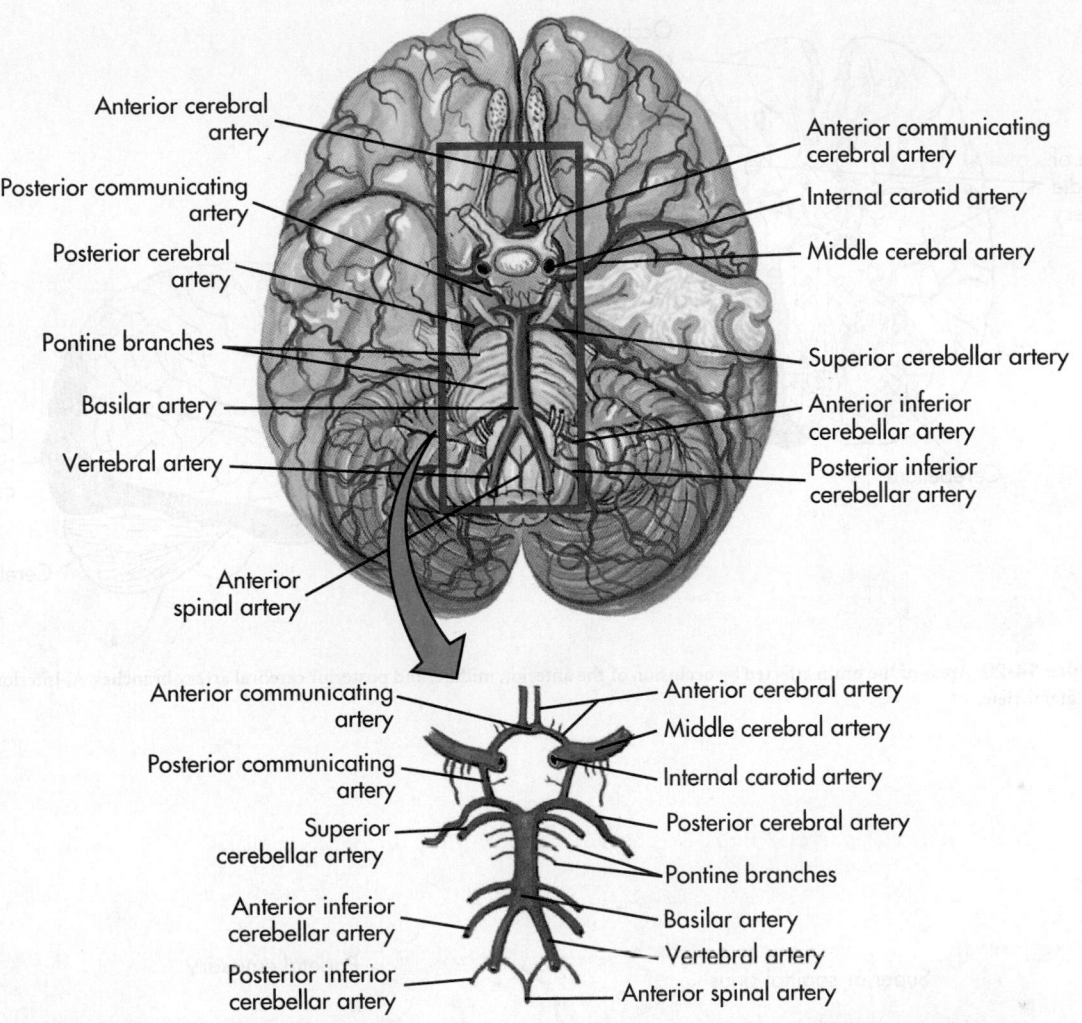

Figure 14-19 Arteries at the base of the brain. The arteries that compose the circle of Willis are the two anterior cerebral arteries, joined to each other by the anterior communicating two short segments of the internal carotids, off of which the posterior communicating arteries connect to the posterior cerebral arteries. (Modified from Thibodeau GA, Patton KT: *Anatomy & physiology*, ed 6, St Louis, 2007, Mosby.)

Table 14-5	Arterial Systems Supplying the Brain	
Arterial Origin	**Structures Served**	**Conditions Caused by Occlusion**
Anterior cerebral artery	Basal ganglia; corpus callosum; medial surface of cerebral hemispheres; superior surface of frontal and parietal lobes	Hemiplegia on contralateral side of body, greater in lower than in upper extremities
Middle cerebral artery	Frontal lobe; parietal lobe; temporal lobe (primarily cortical surfaces)	Aphasia in dominant hemisphere and contralateral hemiplegia (see Chapter 16)
Posterior cerebral artery	Part of diencephalon and temporal lobe; occipital lobe	Visual loss; sensory loss; contralateral hemiplegia if cerebral peduncle affected

skull (Figure 14-21). Adequacy of venous outflow can have a significant effect on intracranial pressure. For example, in individuals with head injury, turning or letting the head fall to the side partially occludes venous return and can increase intracranial pressure because of decreased flow through the jugular veins.

The blood-brain barrier is discussed in Box 14-4.

Blood Supply to the Spinal Cord

The spinal cord derives its blood supply from branches off the vertebral arteries and from branches from various regions of the aorta (Figure 14-22). The **anterior spinal arteries** and the paired **posterior spinal arteries** branch off the vertebral artery at the base of the cranium and descend alongside the spinal cord. Arterial branches from vessels exterior to the

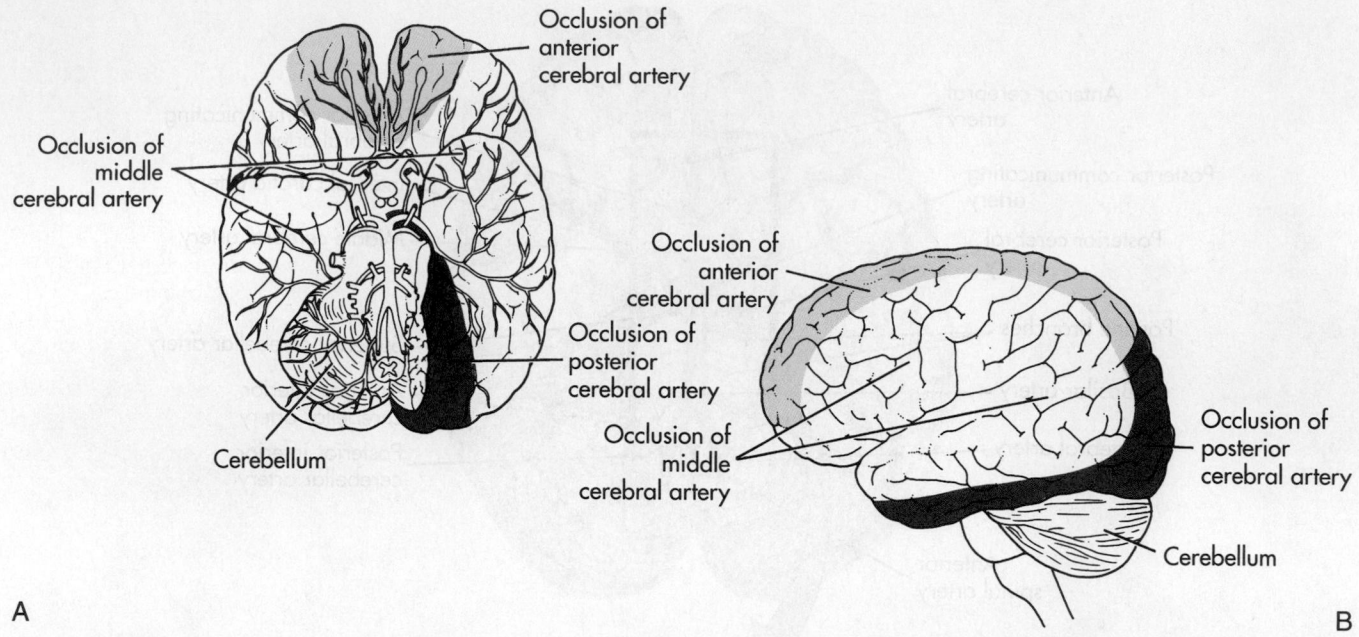

Figure 14-20 Areas of the brain affected by occlusion of the anterior, middle, and posterior cerebral artery branches. A, Inferior view. B, Lateral view.

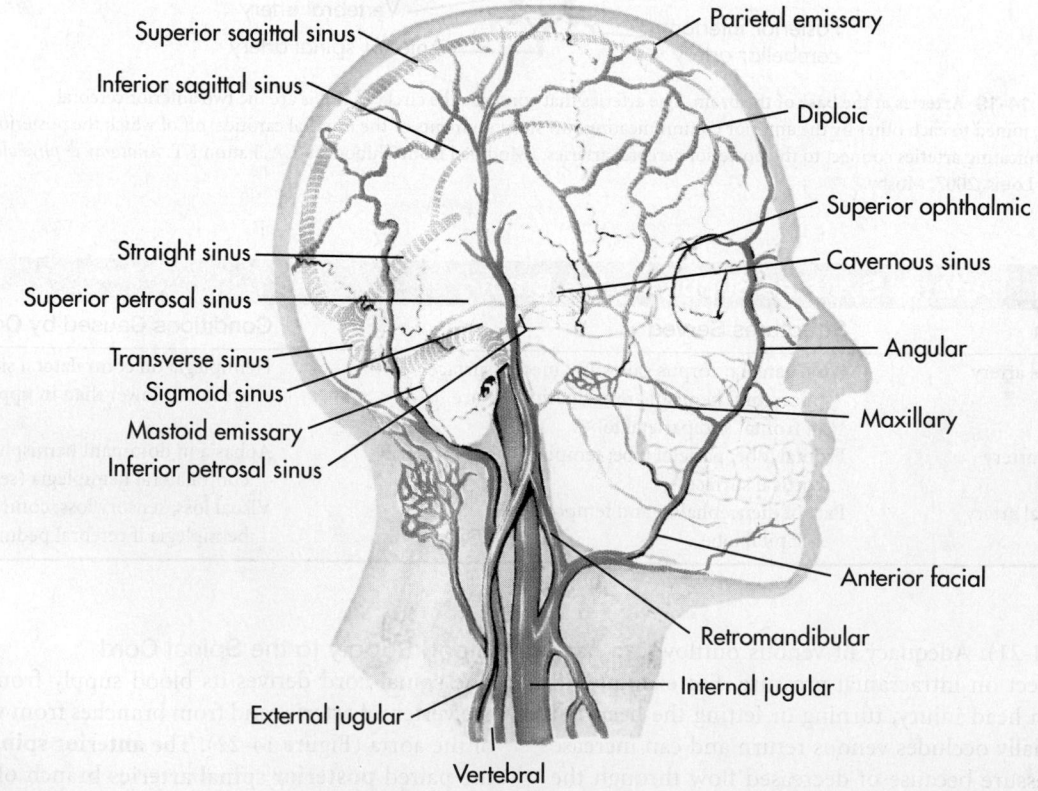

Figure 14-21 Large veins of the head. Deep veins and dural sinuses are projected on the skull. Note connections (emissary veins) between the superficial and deep veins. (From Rudy EB, editor: *Advanced neurological and neurosurgical nursing,* St Louis, 1984, Mosby.)

spinal cord follow the spinal nerve through the intervertebral foramina, pass through the dura, and divide into the anterior and posterior radicular arteries.

The radicular arteries eventually reconnect to the spinal arteries. Branches from the radicular and spinal arteries form plexuses whose branches penetrate the spinal cord, supplying the deeper tissues. Venous drainage parallels the arterial supply closely and drains into venous sinuses located between the dura and periosteum of the vertebrae.

Box 14-4   The Blood-Brain Barrier

The **blood-brain barrier** is a term used to describe cellular structures that selectively inhibit certain substances in the blood from entering the interstitial spaces of the brain or cerebrospinal fluid (CSF). This term emphasizes the impermeability of the nervous system to large and potentially harmful molecules. It is thought that the supporting cells (neuroglia), particularly the astrocytes, and tight junctions between endothelial cells (see Chapter 1) are involved in the formation of the blood-brain barrier. It appears that certain metabolites, electrolytes, and chemicals have differing abilities to cross the blood-brain barrier. This has substantial implications for drug therapy because certain types of antibiotics and chemotherapeutic drugs show a greater propensity than others for crossing the barrier. The permeability of the blood-brain barrier can be affected by hormones and neurotransmitters. Inhibiting these endogenous chemicals with drug therapy may reduce brain edema and slow Alzheimer onset.

Data from Donahue JE, Johanson CE: *J Neuropathol Exp Neurol*, 2008 (Epub); Wolberg H et al: *Cell Tissue Res* 335(1):75-96, 2009.

PERIPHERAL NERVOUS SYSTEM

The cranial and spinal nerves, including their branches and ganglia, constitute the PNS. A peripheral nerve (cranial or spinal) is composed of individual axons/dendrites, with most wrapped in a myelin sheath. These individual fibers are arranged in bundles called **fascicles** (see Figure 14-1 and Figure 14-23, *B*). The coverings supply structural support, a blood supply, and interstitial compartments necessary for the supply of essential electrolytes to support nerve impulse conduction.

The 31 pairs of spinal nerves derive their names from the vertebral level from which they exit. There are eight cervical spinal nerves. The first cervical nerve exits above the first cervical vertebra, and the rest of the spinal nerves exit below their corresponding vertebrae. From the thoracic region (and inferiorly) nerves correspond to the vertebral level above their exit (see Figure 14-10).

Spinal nerves contain both sensory and motor neurons and are called **mixed nerves.** They arise as rootlets from the anterior and posterior horn cells of the spinal cord. These two spinal nerve roots converge in the region of the intervertebral foramen to form the spinal nerve (see Figure 14-11). Shortly after converging, the spinal nerve divides into anterior and posterior rami (branches). The anterior rami (except the thoracic) initially form plexuses (networks of nerve fibers), which then branch into the peripheral nerves. Instead of forming plexuses, the thoracic nerves pass through the intercostal spaces and innervate regions of the thorax.

The main spinal nerve plexuses innervate the skin and the underlying muscles of the limbs. The **brachial plexus,**

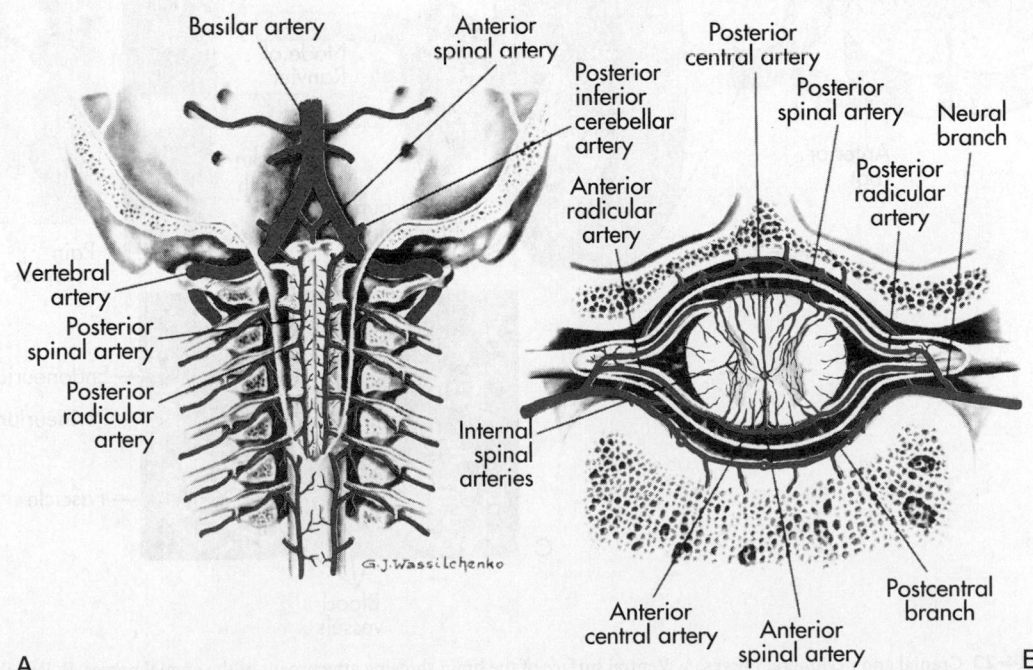

Figure 14-22 Arteries of the spinal cord. **A,** Arteries of cervical cord exposed, posterior view. **B,** Arteries of spinal cord diagrammatically shown in horizontal section. (From Rudy EB, editor: *Advanced neurological and neurosurgical nursing,* St Louis, 1984, Mosby.)

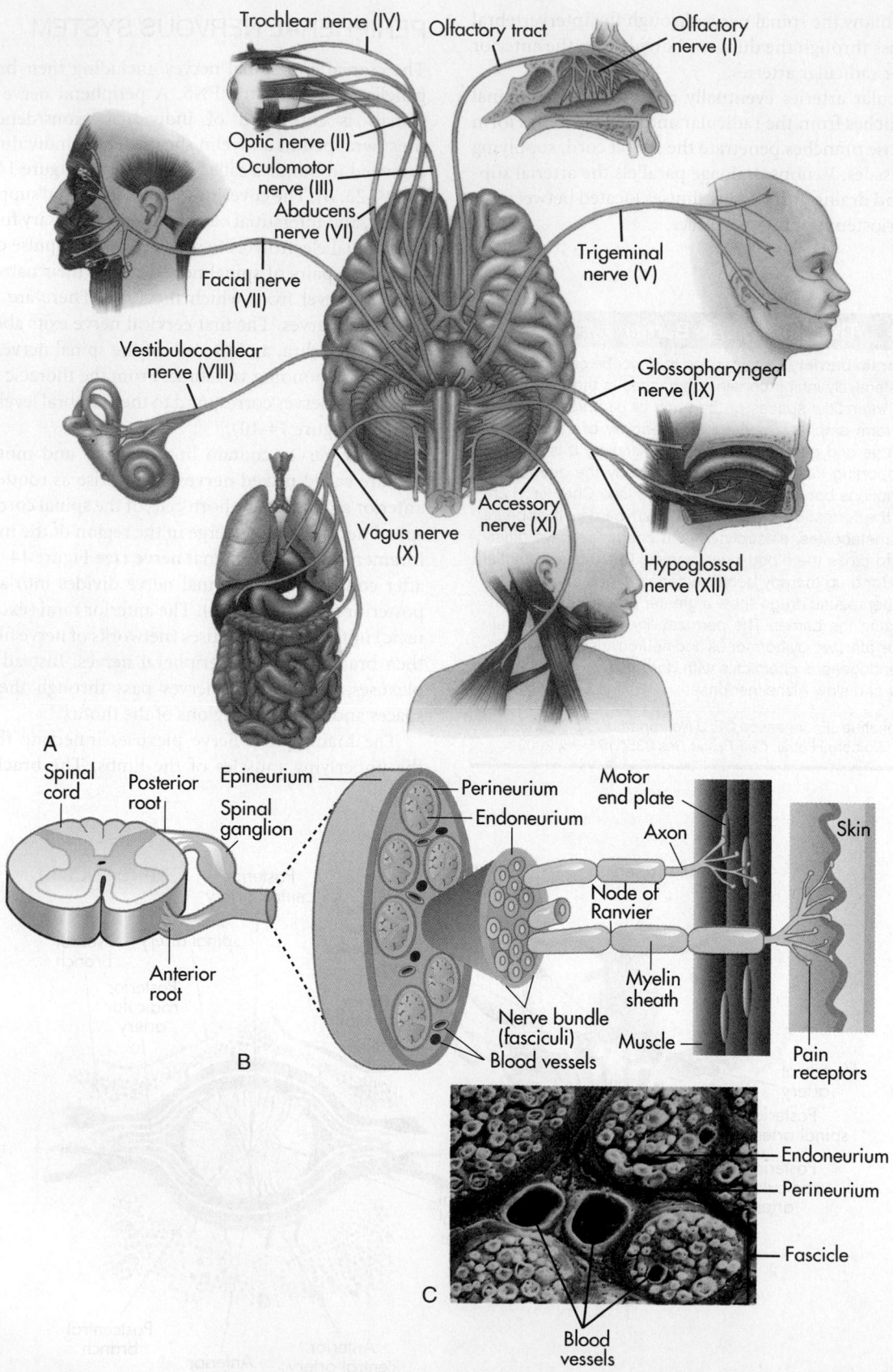

Figure 14-23 Cranial and peripheral nerves. **A,** Ventral surface of the brain showing attachment of the cranial nerves. **B,** Peripheral nerve trunk and coverings. **C,** Scanning electron micrograph of a freeze-fractured preparation of peripheral nerve. (A and C from Thibodeau GA, Patton KT: *Anatomy & physiology,* ed 6, St Louis, 2007, Mosby.)

for example, is formed by the last four cervical nerves (C5-C8) and the first thoracic nerve (T1). The brachial plexus innervates the nerves of the arm, wrist, and hand. The **lumbar plexus** (L2-L4) and **sacral plexus** (L5-S5) contain nerves that innervate the anterior and posterior portions of the lower body, respectively.

The posterior rami of each spinal nerve, with their many processes, are distributed to a specific area in the body. Sensory signals thus arise from specific sites associated with a specific spinal cord segment. Specific areas of cutaneous (skin) innervation at these spinal cord segments are called **dermatomes.** The dermatomes of various spinal nerves are distributed in a fairly regular pattern, although adjacent regions between dermatomes can be innervated by more than one spinal nerve.

Like spinal nerves, cranial nerves are categorized as peripheral nerves. Most of these are mixed nerves (like the spinal nerves), although some are purely sensory or motor. Cranial nerves arise from nuclei in the brain and brainstem. (Figure 14-23, *A*, illustrates their location, and Table 14-6 describes structural and functional characteristics.)

AUTONOMIC NERVOUS SYSTEM

Components of the ANS are located in both the CNS and PNS; however, the ANS is considered part of the efferent division of the PNS, even though visceral afferent neurons are an important part of this system. Many neurons of the ANS travel in spinal nerves and certain cranial nerves. The widespread activity of this system indicates that its components are distributed all over the body. The peripheral autonomic nerves carry mainly efferent fibers. The motor component of the ANS is a two-neuron system consisting of **preganglionic neurons** (myelinated) and **postganglionic neurons** (unmyelinated). This arrangement contrasts with the somatic nervous system, in which a single motor neuron travels from the CNS to the innervated structure. Visceral afferent neurons have their cell bodies in some sensory and cranial ganglia and their fiber processes traveling in peripheral nerves. The CNS has autonomic areas in the intermediolateral horns of the spinal cord, cardiovascular and respiratory centers in the reticular formation, and both sympathetic and parasympathetic areas in the hypothalamus. CNS pathways interconnect all these areas.

The ANS coordinates and maintains a steady-state among visceral (internal) organs, such as regulation of cardiac muscle, smooth muscle, and the glands of the body. This system is considered an involuntary system because one generally cannot *will* these functions to happen. The ANS is separated structurally and functionally into two divisions: (1) the **sympathetic nervous system** (Figure 14-24) and (2) the **parasympathetic nervous system** (Figure 14-25).

Anatomy of the Sympathetic Nervous System

The sympathetic nervous system functions to mobilize energy stores in times of need (e.g., in the fight-or-flight response) (see Figure 10-2; see also Chapter 10). The sympathetic division receives its innervation from cell bodies located from the first thoracic (T1) through the second lumbar (L2) regions of the spinal cord and is therefore called the **thoracolumbar division.** The preganglionic axons of the sympathetic division form synapses shortly after leaving the cord in the **sympathetic (paravertebral) ganglia.** At this point the impulse may travel several ways: (1) directly across the same ganglion level and form a synapse with the cell bodies of the postganglionic neuron, (2) up or down the sympathetic chain before forming synapses with a higher or lower postganglionic neuron (divergence), or (3) through the chain ganglion without synapsing (see Figure 14-24). Some preganglionic axons form pathways called **splanchnic nerves,** which lead to **collateral ganglia** surrounding the abdominal aorta. The collateral ganglia are named according to the branches of the aorta nearest them, namely, the **celiac, superior mesenteric,** and **inferior mesenteric.** The preganglionic neurons synapse with postganglionic neurons within the collateral ganglia. These postganglionic neurons leave the collateral ganglia and innervate the viscera below the diaphragm.

Preganglionic sympathetic neurons that innervate the adrenal medulla also travel in the splanchnic nerves and do not synapse before reaching the gland. The secretory cells in the adrenal medulla are considered modified postganglionic neurons. Because preganglionic sympathetic fibers are all myelinated, travel to the adrenal medulla is quick, and innervation causes the rapid release of epinephrine and norepinephrine. Epinephrine and norepinephrine are mediators of the fight-or-flight response (see Chapter 10).

Anatomy of the Parasympathetic Nervous System

The parasympathetic nervous system functions to conserve and restore energy. The nerve cell bodies of this division are located in the cranial nerve nuclei and in the sacral region of the spinal cord and therefore constitute the **craniosacral division.** Unlike the sympathetic division, the preganglionic fibers in the parasympathetic division travel to ganglia close to the organs they innervate before forming synapses with the relatively short postganglionic neurons (see Figure 14-25). Parasympathetic nerves arising from nuclei in the brainstem travel to the viscera of the head, thorax, and abdomen within cranial nerves—including the oculomotor (III), facial (VII), glossopharyngeal (IX), and vagus (X) nerves.

Preganglionic parasympathetic nerves that originate from the sacral region of the spinal cord run either separately or together with some spinal nerves. The preganglionic axons join to form the **pelvic nerve,** which innervates the viscera of the pelvic cavity. These preganglionic axons synapse with postganglionic neurons in terminal ganglia located close to the organs they innervate.

Neurotransmitters and Neuroreceptors

Sympathetic preganglionic fibers and parasympathetic preganglionic and postganglionic fibers release **acetylcholine**—the same neurotransmitter released by somatic efferent neurons (Figure 14-26; also see Figure 14-23). These fibers are

Table 14-6　The Cranial Nerves

Number and Name	Origin and Course	Function	How Tested
I. Olfactory	Fibers arise from nasal olfactory epithelium and form synapses with olfactory bulbs that transmit impulses to temporal lobe	Purely sensory; carries impulses for sense of smell	Person is asked to sniff aromatic substances, such as oil of cloves and vanilla, and to identify them
II. Optic	Fibers arise from retina of eye to form optic nerve, which passes through sphenoid bone; two optic nerves then form optic chiasma (with partial crossover of fibers) and eventually end in occipital cortex	Purely sensory; carries impulses for vision	Vision and visual field tested with an eye chart and by testing point at which person first sees an object (finger) moving into visual field; inside of eye is viewed with ophthalmoscope to observe blood vessels of eye interior
III. Oculomotor	Fibers emerge from midbrain and exit from skull and extend to eye	Contains motor fibers to inferior oblique, superior, inferior, and medial rectus extraocular muscles that direct eyeball; levator muscles of eyelid; smooth muscles of iris and ciliary body; and proprioception (sensory) to brain from extraocular muscles	Pupils examined for size, shape, and equality; pupillary reflex tested with a penlight (pupils should constrict when illuminated); ability to follow moving objects
IV. Trochlear	Fibers emerge from posterior midbrain and exit from skull to run to eye	Proprioceptor and motor fibers for superior oblique muscle of eye (extraocular muscle)	Tested in common with cranial nerve III relative to ability to follow moving objects
V. Trigeminal	Fibers emerge from pons and form three divisions that exit from skull and run to face and cranial dura mater	Both motor and sensory for face; conducts sensory impulses from mouth, nose, surface of eye, and dura mater; also contains motor fibers that stimulate chewing muscles	Sensations of pain, touch, and temperature tested with safety pin and hot and cold objects; corneal reflex tested with a wisp of cotton; motor branch tested by asking subject to clench teeth, open mouth against resistance, and move jaw from side to side
VI. Abducens	Fibers leave inferior pons and exit from skull and extend to eye	Contains motor fibers to lateral rectus muscle and proprioceptor fibers from same muscle to brain	Tested in common with cranial nerve III relative to ability to move each eye laterally
VII. Facial	Fibers leave pons and travel through temporal bone and extend to face	Mixed: (1) supplies motor fibers to muscles of facial expression and to lacrimal and salivary glands and (2) carries sensory fibers from taste buds of anterior part of tongue	Anterior two thirds of tongue tested for ability to taste sweet (sugar), salty, sour (vinegar), and bitter (quinine) substances; symmetry of face checked; subject asked to close eyes, smile, whistle, and so on; tearing tested with ammonia fumes
VIII. Vestibulocochlear (acoustic)	Fibers run from inner ear (hearing and equilibrium receptors in temporal bone) to enter brainstem just below pons	Purely sensory; vestibular branch transmits impulses for sense of equilibrium; cochlear branch transmits impulses for sense of hearing	Hearing checked by air and bone conduction by use of a tuning fork; vestibular tests: Bárány and caloric tests
IX. Glossopharyngeal	Fibers emerge from midbrain and leave skull and extend to pharynx, salivary glands, and tongue	Mixed: (1) motor fibers serve pharynx (throat) and salivary glands, and (2) sensory fibers carry impulses from pharynx, posterior tongue (taste buds), and pressure receptors of carotid artery	Gag and swallow reflexes checked; subject asked to speak and cough; posterior one third of tongue may be tested for taste
X. Vagus	Fibers emerge from medulla, pass through skull, and descend through neck region into thorax and abdominal region	Fibers carry sensory and motor impulses for pharynx; a large part of this nerve is parasympathetic motor fibers, which supply smooth muscles of abdominal organs; receives sensory impulses from viscera	Same as for cranial nerve IX (IX and X are tested in common) because they both serve muscles of the throat
XI. Spinal accessory	Fibers arise from medulla and superior spinal cord and extend to muscles of neck and back	Provides sensory and motor fibers for sternocleidomastoid and trapezius muscles and muscles of soft palate, pharynx, and larynx	Sternocleidomastoid and trapezius muscles checked for strength by asking subject to rotate head and shrug shoulders against resistance
XII. Hypoglossal	Fibers arise from medulla and exit from skull and extend to tongue	Carries motor fibers to muscles of tongue and sensory impulses from tongue to brain	Subject asked to stick out tongue, and any position abnormalities are noted

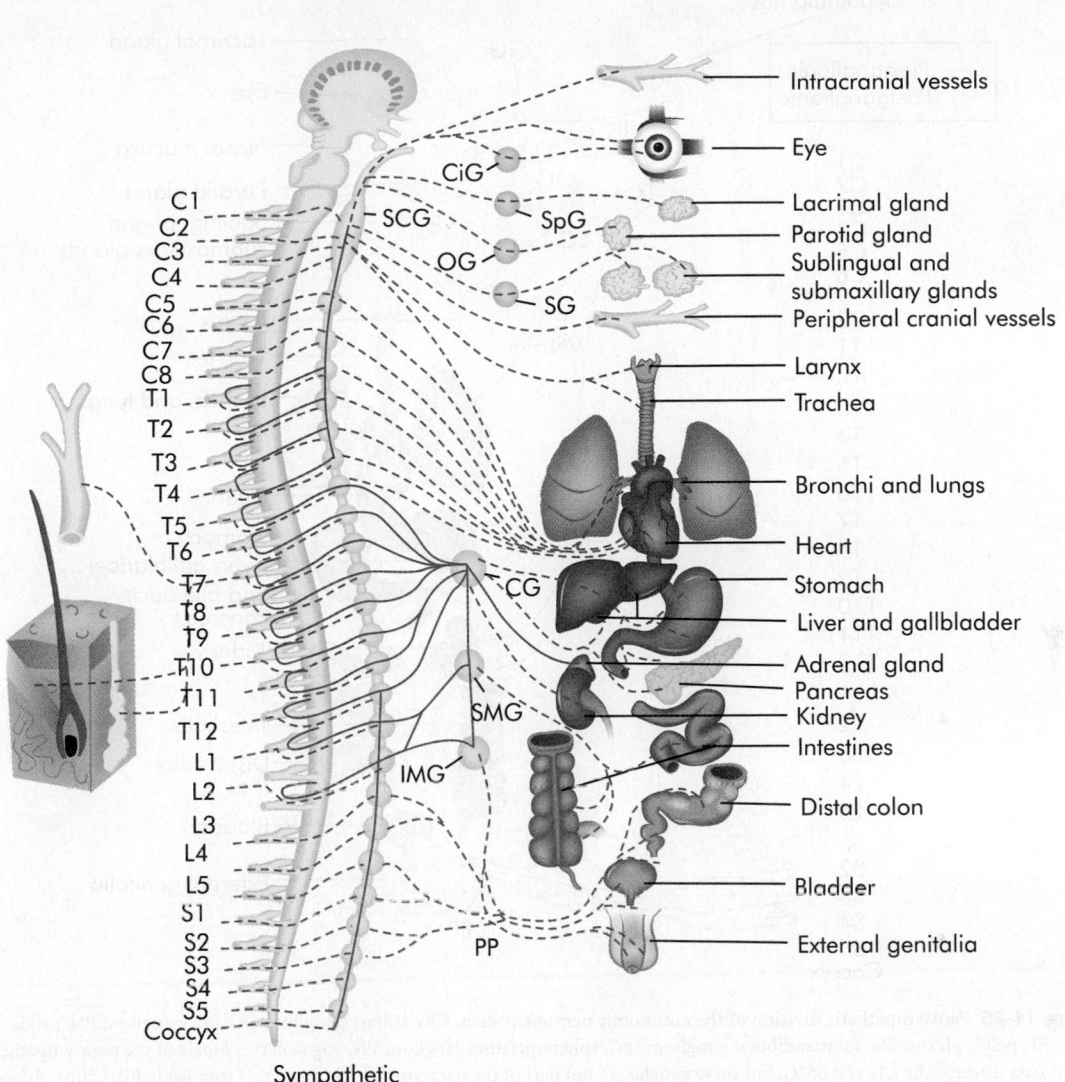

——— Preganglionic neuron
------- Postganglionic neuron

C1
C2
C3
C4
C5
C6
C7
C8
T1
T2
T3
T4
T5
T6
T7
T8
T9
T10
T11
T12
L1
L2
L3
L4
L5
S1
S2
S3
S4
S5
Coccyx

CiG
SCG
SpG
OG
SG
CG
SMG
IMG
PP

Sympathetic
chain

Intracranial vessels
Eye
Lacrimal gland
Parotid gland
Sublingual and
submaxillary glands
Peripheral cranial vessels
Larynx
Trachea
Bronchi and lungs
Heart
Stomach
Liver and gallbladder
Adrenal gland
Pancreas
Kidney
Intestines
Distal colon
Bladder
External genitalia

Figure 14-24 Sympathetic division of the autonomic nervous system. Fibers of the parasympathetic system pass through the CG and SMG, but these ganglia are not part of the parasympathetic system. *CG,* Celiac ganglion; *CiG,* ciliary ganglion; *IMG,* inferior mesenteric ganglion; *OG,* otic ganglion; *PP,* pelvic plexus; *SCG,* superior cervical ganglion; *SG,* submandibular ganglion; *SMG,* superior mesenteric ganglion; *SpG,* sphenopalatine ganglion. (Redrawn from Rudy EB, editor: *Advanced neurological and neurosurgical nursing,* St Louis, 1984, Mosby.)

characterized by **cholinergic transmission.** Most postganglionic sympathetic fibers release **norepinephrine** (adrenaline) and thus are considered to function by **adrenergic transmission.** A few postganglionic sympathetic fibers, such as those that innervate the sweat glands, release acetylcholine.

The action of catecholamines (epinephrine, norepinephrine, dopa) varies with the type of neuroreceptor stimulated. It should be remembered that catecholamines also are released by the adrenal medulla gland that physiologically and biochemically resembles the sympathetic nervous system. Two types of adrenergic receptors exist: α- and β-adrenergic receptors. Cells of the effector organs may have only one or both types of adrenergic receptors. The α-**adrenergic receptors**

have been further subdivided according to the action produced: α_1-adrenergic activity is associated mostly with excitation or stimulation; α_2-adrenergic activity is associated with relaxation or inhibition. Most of the α-adrenergic receptors on effector organs belong to the α_1-adrenergic class. The β-**adrenergic receptors** are classified as β_1-adrenergic receptors (which facilitate increased heart rate and contractility and cause the release of renin from the kidney) and β_2-adrenergic receptors (which facilitate all of the remaining effects attributed to β-adrenergic receptors).[6] Norepinephrine stimulates all α-adrenergic and β_1-adrenergic receptors and only certain β_2-adrenergic receptors. The primary response from norepinephrine, however, is stimulation of the α_1-adrenergic

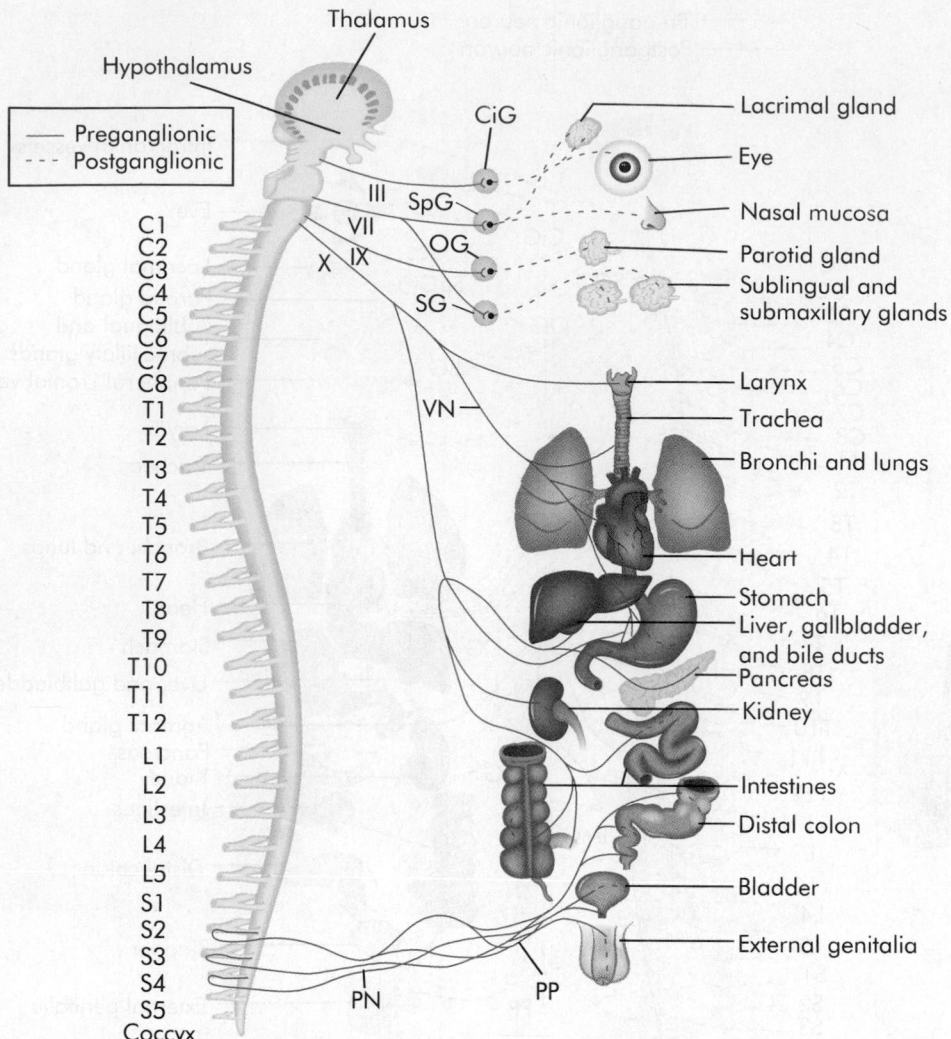

Figure 14-25 **Parasympathetic division of the autonomic nervous system.** *CiG,* Ciliary ganglion; *OG,* otic ganglion; *PN,* pelvic nerve; *PP,* pelvic plexus; *SG,* submandibular ganglion; *SpG,* sphenopalatine ganglion; *VN,* vagus nerve. Fibers of the parasympathetic system pass through the CG and SMG, but these ganglia are not part of the parasympathetic system. (From Rudy EB, editor: *Advanced neurological and neurosurgical nursing,* St Louis, 1984, Mosby.)

receptors that cause vasoconstriction. Epinephrine strongly stimulates all four types of receptors and induces general vasodilation because of the predominance of β-adrenergic receptors in muscle vasculatures. (Table 14-7 summarizes the effects of neuroreceptors on their effector organs.)

Functions of the Autonomic Nervous System

Many body organs are innervated by the sympathetic and parasympathetic nervous systems. The two divisions frequently cause opposite responses; for example, sympathetic stimulation of the gastrointestinal (GI) tract causes decreased peristalsis, whereas parasympathetic stimulation of the GI tract increases peristalsis. In general, sympathetic stimulation promotes responses that are concerned with the protection of the individual. For example, sympathetic activity increases blood sugar levels and temperature and raises blood pressure. In emergency situations a generalized and widespread discharge

of the sympathetic system occurs. This is accomplished by an increased firing frequency of sympathetic fibers and by activation of sympathetic fibers normally silent and at rest (fibers to the sweat glands, pilomotor muscles, and the adrenal medulla, as well as vasodilator fibers to muscle). Regulation of vasomotor tone is considered the single most important function of the sympathetic nervous system. (Figure 14-27 illustrates some of the most important functions of the sympathetic nervous system; also see Figure 10-2.)

Increased parasympathetic activity promotes rest and tranquility and is characterized by reduced heart rate and enhanced visceral functions leading to digestion. Stimulation of the vagus nerve in the GI tract increases peristalsis and secretion, as well as relaxation of sphincters. Activation of parasympathetic fibers in the head, provided by cranial nerves III, VII, and IX, causes constriction of the pupil, tear secretion, and increased salivary secretion. Stimulation of the sacral division

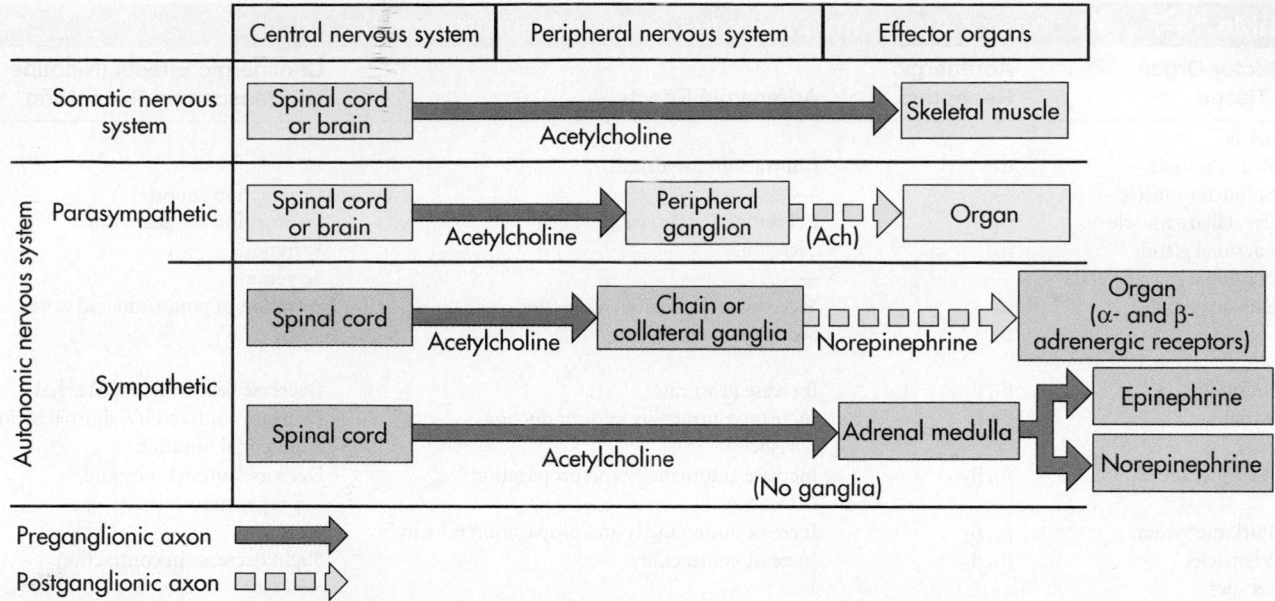

Figure 14-26 The autonomic nervous system and the type of neurotransmitters secreted by preganglionic and postganglionic fibers. Note that all preganglionic fibers are cholinergic (Ach). A somatic nerve is used for comparison.

of the parasympathetic system contracts the urinary bladder and facilitates the process of genital erection.

The parasympathetic system lacks the generalized and widespread response of the sympathetic system. Specific parasympathetic fibers are activated to regulate particular functions. Although the actions of the parasympathetic and sympathetic systems usually are antagonistic, there are exceptions. Changes in the shape of the lens (for near vision) require only oculomotor parasympathetic activity. Most of the blood vessels involved in the control of blood pressure are innervated by sympathetic nerves. Peripheral vascular resistance is increased and decreased by the relative activity of the sympathetic division without a counteracting parasympathetic component. To decrease blood pressure, therefore, it is more important to block or paralyze the continuous (tonic) discharge of the sympathetic system than to promote parasympathetic activity.

Aging and the Nervous System

The CNS mechanisms involved in the aging process are extremely complex, and many questions concerning the neurologic effects of aging have yet to be answered. Some of the identified mechanisms associated with aging are pathologic, but the distinction between these mechanisms and those that are a part of the normal aging process remains somewhat cloudy.

Structural Changes with Aging

The CNS demonstrates many structural changes during the aging process. The primary mechanism responsible for most of these structural changes is a decrease in the number of neurons. Predominant external features of the aging brain include decreased brain weight and size (primarily the frontal hemispheres), increased adherence of the dura mater to the skull, fibrosis and thickening of the meninges, narrowed gyri, and widened sulci with a corresponding increase in the size of the subarachnoid space. The basal ganglia and ventricular system are internal structures that commonly reveal changes with aging. The basal ganglia reveal aberrations in vascular structures, and the ventricles (primarily the lateral and third ventricles) are enlarged, probably because they occupy much of the space left by dead neurons.

Cellular Changes with Aging

Practically every cell type within the CNS reflects specific responses to aging. A decrease in the number of neurons characterizes aging. Although neuronal cell loss is a general feature of aging, the effects are not consistent with deteriorating mental function or age of the individual.[7,8] Controversy regarding the effects of neuronal cell loss is ongoing.

Principal cellular changes associated with aging include dendrite structure, lipofuscin deposition, and the presence of neurofibrillary tangles, senile plaques, and Lewy bodies. Kelly and colleagues[9] described a decreased number of dendritic processes and their multiple synaptic connections. Lipofuscin, a yellow-brown fatty pigment, is found to be deposited intracellularly in increased amounts with age. Controversy still exists concerning whether increasing intracellular quantities of lipofuscin in aging brains and neuropathologic conditions cause these changes leading to cell death or if they are a result of some other underlying factors.[10] For example, decreased circulation, genetic predisposition, or disruption of protein synthesis might be associated factors.

Senile plaques (areas of nerve degeneration) are found in the interstitial spaces of the cerebral cortex associated with tissue degeneration. **Neurofibrillary tangles** involve degenerative changes in neural protein fibers. These entities also

Table 14-7   Actions of Autonomic Nervous System Neuroreceptors

Effector Organ or Tissue	Adrenergic Receptors	Adrenergic Effects	Cholinergic Effects (Nicotine and Muscarinic Receptors)
Eye, iris			
Radial muscle	α_1	Contraction (mydriasis)	—
Sphincter muscle	—	—	Contraction (miosis)
Eye, ciliary muscle	β_2	Relaxation for far vision	Contraction for near vision
Lacrimal glands	α_1	Secretion	Secretion
Nasopharyngeal glands	—	—	Secretion
Salivary glands	α_1	Secretion of potassium and water	Secretion of potassium and water
	β	Secretion of amylase	—
Heart			
SA node	β_1, β_2	Increase heart rate	Decrease heart rate; vagus arrest
Atrial	β_1, β_2	Increase contractility and conduction velocity	Decrease contractility; shorten action potential duration
AV junction	β_1, β_2	Increase automaticity and propagation velocity	Decrease automaticity and propagation velocity
Purkinje system	β_1, β_2	Increase automaticity and propagation velocity	—
Ventricles	β_1, β_2	Increase contractility	Slight decrease in contraction
Arterioles			
Coronary	$\alpha_1, \alpha_2, \beta_2$	Constriction, dilation	Dilation
Skin and mucosa	α_1, α_2	Constriction	Dilation
Skeletal muscle	α, β_2	Constriction, dilation	Dilation
Cerebral	α_1	Constriction (slight)	—
Pulmonary	α_1, β_2	Constriction, dilation	—
Mesenteric	α_1	Constriction	—
Renal	$\alpha_1, \beta_1, \beta_2$	Constriction, dilation	—
Salivary glands	α_1, α_2	Constriction	Dilation
Veins, systemic	α_1, β_2	Constriction, dilation	
Lung			
Bronchial muscle	β_2	Relaxation	Contraction
Bronchial glands	α_1, β_2	Decreased secretion; increased secretion	Stimulation
Stomach			
Motility	$\alpha_1, \alpha_2, \beta_2$	Decrease (usually)	Increase
Sphincters	α_1	Contraction (usually)	Relaxation (usually)
Secretion	—	Inhibition (?)	Stimulation
Liver	α_1, β_2	Glycogenolysis and gluconeogenesis	Glycogen synthesis
Gallbladder and ducts	—	Relaxation	Contraction
Pancreas			
Acini	α	Decrease secretion	Secretion
Islet cells	α_2, β_2	Decreased secretion; increased secretion	—
Intestine			
Motility and tone	$\alpha_1, \alpha_2, \beta_1, \beta_2$	Decrease	Increase
Sphincters	α_1	Contraction (usually)	Relaxation (usually)
Secretion	α_2	Inhibition (?)	Stimulation
Adrenal medulla	—	Secretion of epinephrine and norepinephrine (nicotinic effect)	
Kidney			
Renin secretion	α_1, β_1	Decrease; increase	—
Ureter			
Motility and tone	α_1	Increase	Increase
Urinary bladder			
Detrusor	β_2	Relaxation (usually)	Contraction
Trigone and sphincter	α_1	Contraction	Relaxation
Sex organs, male	α_1	Ejaculation	Erection
Skin			
Pilomotor muscles	α_1	Contraction	—
Sweat glands	α_1	Localized secretion	Generalized secretion
Fat cells	$\alpha_2, \beta_1, \beta_2$	Inhibition of lipolysis; stimulation of lipolysis	—
Pineal gland	β	Melatonin synthesis	—

AV, Atrioventricular; *SA,* sinoatrical.

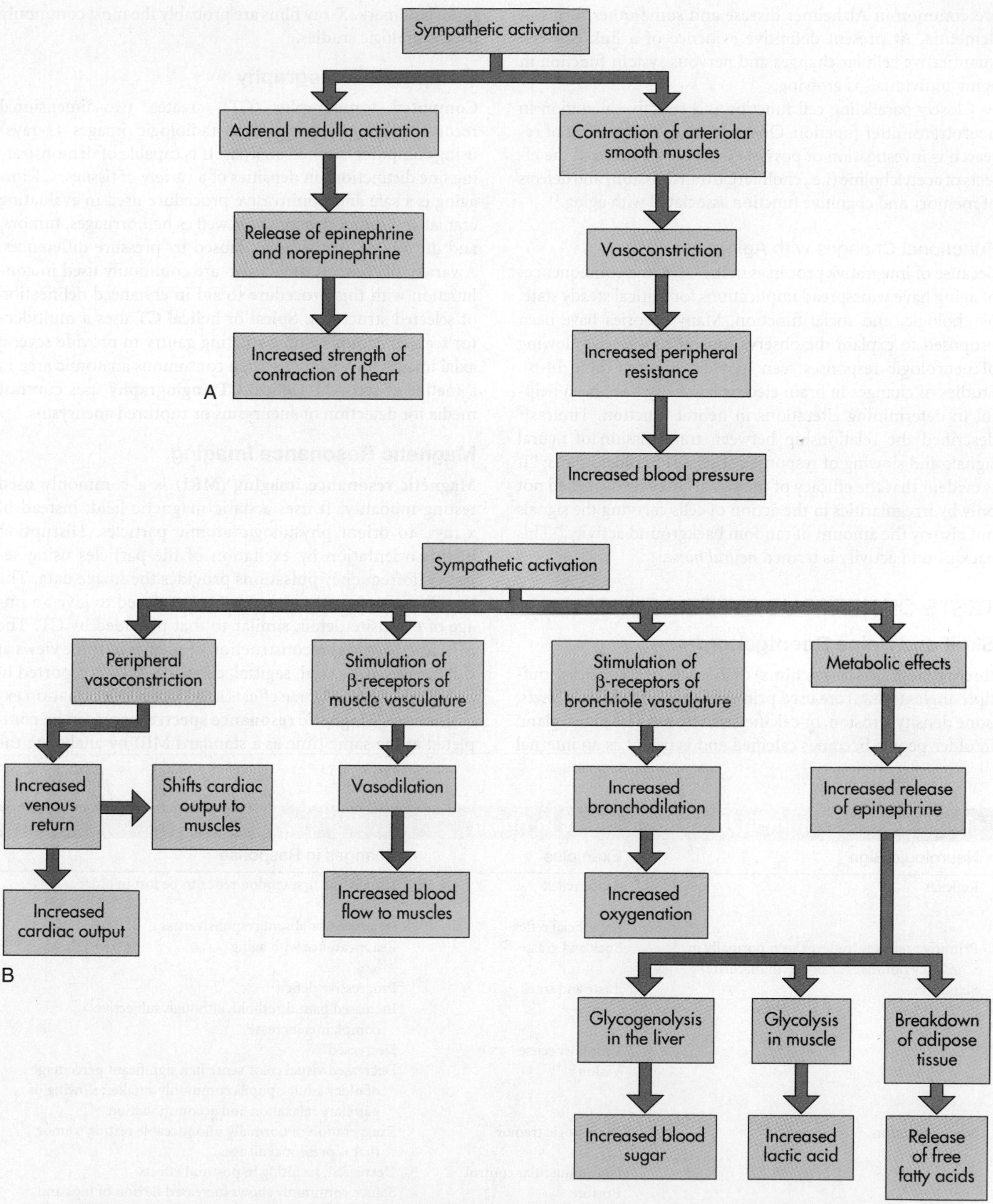

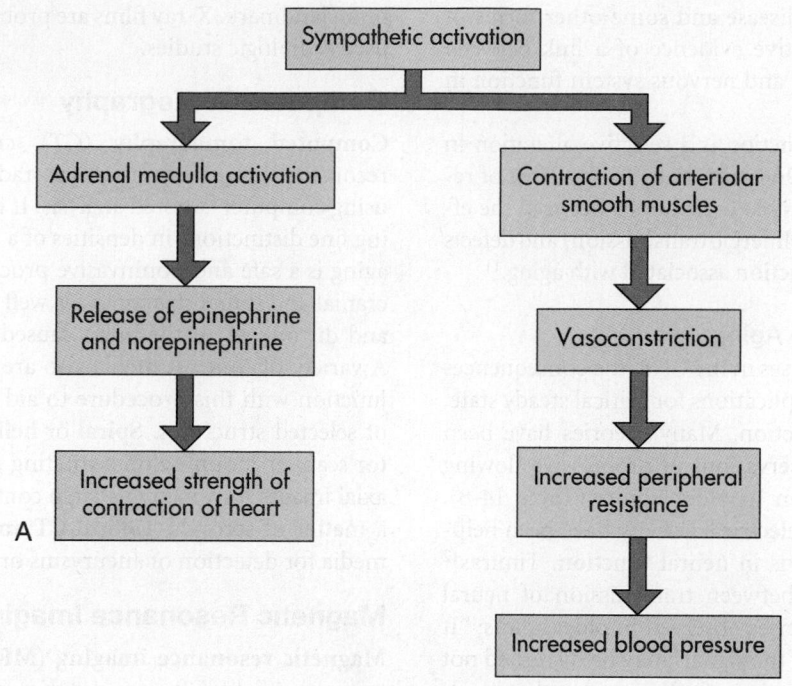

Figure 14-27 Some important functions of the sympathetic nervous system. A, Regulation of vasomotor tone. B, Regulation of strenuous muscular exercise (fight-or-flight response). (See also Chapter 10 and Figure 10-2 for more detail of the stress response.)

are common in Alzheimer disease and some other forms of dementia. At present definitive evidence of a link between quantitative cellular changes and nervous system function in aging individuals is growing.

Closely paralleling cell function is a selective alteration in neurotransmitter function. One potentially fruitful area of research is investigation of possible correlations between the effects of acetylcholine (i.e., cholinergic transmission) and defects of memory and cognitive function associated with aging.[11]

Functional Changes with Aging

Because of integrative processes in the CNS, the consequences of aging have widespread implications for critical steady state, psychologic, and social function. Many theories have been proposed to explain the observations of progressive slowing of neurologic responses seen in older adults (Table 14-8). Studies of changes in brain electrical activity have been helpful in determining alterations in neural function. Timiras[12] described the relationship between transmission of neural signals and slowing of responses observed in older adults: "It is evident that the efficacy of the signals may be disturbed not only by irregularities in the action of cells carrying the signals but also by the amount of random background activity." This background activity is termed *neural noise*.

TESTS OF NERVOUS SYSTEM FUNCTION

Skull and Spine Roentgenograms

Roentgenograms (x-ray films) of the skull or spine from multiple angles (views) are used primarily to localize bony defects, bone density, erosion, or calcified structures. The pineal gland in older people becomes calcified and is useful as an internal brain landmark. X-ray films are probably the most commonly used radiologic studies.

Computed Tomography

Computed tomography (CT) creates two-dimensional reconstructions from multiple radiologic images (x-rays) using computer-assisted analysis. It is capable of demonstrating fine distinctions in densities of a variety of tissues. CT imaging is a safe and noninvasive procedure used in evaluating cranial and spinal structures, as well as hemorrhages, tumors, and distortions in the brain caused by pressure differences. A variety of contrast media also are commonly used in conjunction with this procedure to aid in enhanced delineation of selected structures. **Spiral** or **helical CT** uses a multidector scanner mounted on a rotating gantry to provide several axial images for imaging a large continuous anatomic area in a matter of seconds. **Helical CT angiography** uses contrast media for detection of aneurysms or ruptured aneurysms.

Magnetic Resonance Imaging

Magnetic resonance imaging (MRI) is a commonly used testing modality. It uses a static magnetic field, instead of x-rays, to orient physiologic atomic particles. Disruption of this orientation by excitation of the particles using serial radiofrequency pulsations provides the image data. The specific tissue reaction is computer analyzed to give an image of exquisite detail, similar to that provided by CT. The MRI also provides reconstruction of images in three views at right angles (i.e., axial, sagittal, coronal). MRI is reported to have none of the adverse effects associated with radiation examinations. **Magnetic resonance spectroscopy** can be completed at the same time as a standard MRI by analyzing the

Table 14-8	Common Neurologic Signs in Aging	
Neurologic Sign	**Examples**	**Changes in Response**
Reflexes	Ankle reflex	Usually the first tendon reflex to be lost in older adults
	Superficial reflex	Decreased or absent responsiveness
Primitive reflexes (reflexes seen normally in infancy but that subside with maturity)	Suck and grasp	Reappearance with aging
Sensation	Taste and smell	Progressive deficit
	Pain	Increased pain threshold, although subjective complaints increase
	Vibratory sense	Decreased
	Vision	Decreased visual color sense in a significant percentage of older adults; pupils commonly smaller; slowing of papillary relaxation and accommodation
Motor function	Physiologic tremor	Exaggeration of normally unnoticeable resting tremor that is present at all ages
	Neuromuscular control	Decreased, resulting in postural effects
	Posture	Stance commonly shows increased flexion of hips and knees; swaying motion while standing in one position more common
	Gait	Shuffling or shortened stride; loss of arm movement with walking
	Muscular atrophy	Age-associated loss of muscle fibers

Reinforcement Center (Nucleus Accumbens)

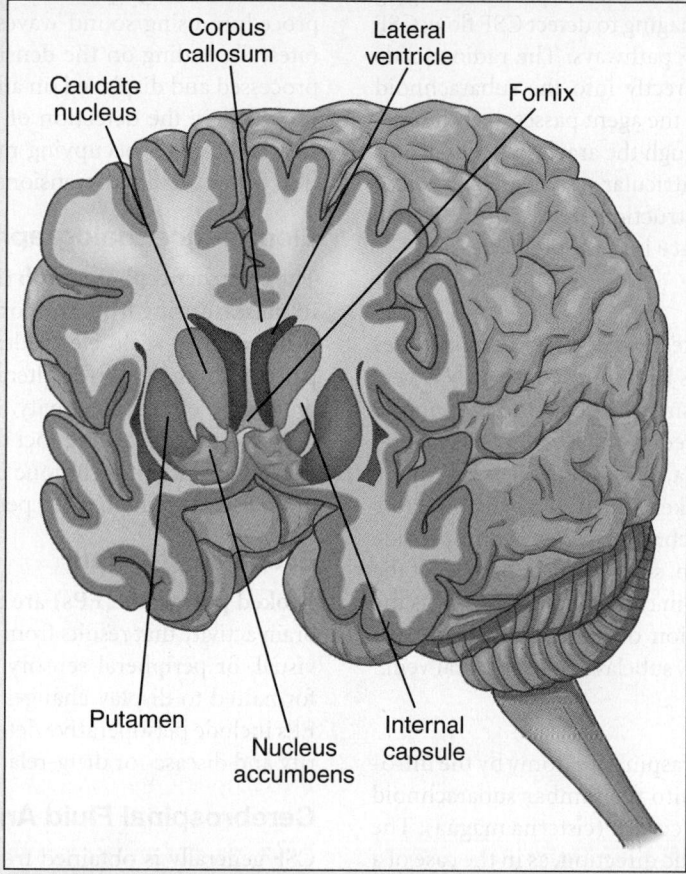

A small nucleus (see accompanying figure) in the septal area of the frontal lobe has become a center of intense research. The nucleus accumbens is considered to be the principal site of action for addictive drugs and the anatomic basis of positive reinforcement. The nucleus accumbens has input from the mesencephalon (ventral tegmental area) and many other neural areas. Mesencephalon neurons project dopamine to the nucleus accumbens and can affect its activity. Other neurotransmitters involved in this positive feedback system are gamma-aminobutyric acid (GABA), serotonin, and glutamate. Opiates can interfere with this system by allowing too much dopamine to go to the nucleus accumbens. The nucleus accumbens is involved in drug craving and withdrawal symptoms and therefore is clinically important.

Data from Wheeler RA, Carelli RM: *Neuropharmacology* 56 (Suppl 1):149-159, 2009; Goto Y, Grace AA: *Trends Neurosci* 31(11):552-558, 2008; Everitt BJ et al: *Philos Trans R Soc Lond B Biol Sci* 363(1507):3125-3135, 2008.

chemical composition of proton (hydrogen) or phosphorus-based molecules and is useful for evaluating the chemical composition and function of various regions of the brain.

Magnetic Resonance Angiography

A newer addition to MRI is **magnetic resonance angiography (MRA).** Special imaging techniques allow the visualization of blood vessels in great detail. MRA is likely to become indispensable, alone or in conjunction with cerebral angiography, in detecting and localizing pathologic lesions of the circulatory system of the brain.

Positron-Emission Tomography Scan

The **positron-emission tomography (PET) scan** uses CT imaging to detect the emission of positive electrons from radioactive substances. These substances are injected into the bloodstream or administered as inhaled gases. As they are distributed in tissues, they display characteristic patterns that indicate physiologic and metabolic processes, for example, glucose and oxygen uptake, cerebral blood flow, neural and neurotransmitter function, and the effects of drugs. As a research tool, PET is being used to visualize the specific brain sites that are involved in the processing of information in the brain.

Brain Scan

The **brain scan** images radionuclide substances (technetium [^{99m}Tc]) that have been introduced into the bloodstream. For example, visualization of tissue uptake of the radioactive agent provides an indication of blood-brain barrier integrity (increased uptake of the agent indicates disruption). This scanning technique also can identify abnormalities in blood flow dynamics and cellular metabolic function. The brain scan is particularly helpful in detecting abnormal vascularity resulting from neoplasms, abscesses, and vascular lesions.

Isotope cisternography is another radionuclide imaging technique that uses brain scan imaging to detect CSF flow, CSF resorption, and integrity of CSF pathways. The radionuclide agent in this case is injected directly into the subarachnoid space. Under normal conditions the agent passes over the cortical surface and is resorbed through the arachnoid villi. Demonstration of the agent in the ventricular system after a specific period of time indicates CSF obstruction; that is, the CSF back flows from the subarachnoid space into the ventricles.

Cerebral Angiography

Angiography is a radiologic technique that demonstrates cerebrovascular blood flow. This technique commonly is performed by the introduction of a small catheter into the femoral artery. The catheter is then passed to the level of the cerebral circulation and through the aorta, and a contrast dye is injected. Serial x-ray films are then taken. These films demonstrate flow of the dye through the cerebral vasculature and provide information on patency, location, size, and flow pattern of the vessels. Another technique used in cerebral angiography is the retrograde (reverse flow) injection of the dye through catheterization of a brachial, axillary, subclavian, or femoral vein.

Myelography

A **myelogram** demonstrates intraspinal anatomy by the introduction of a radiographic dye into the lumbar subarachnoid space or the cerebellomedullary cistern (cisterna magna). The dye is allowed to flow in a cephalic direction, as in the case of a lumbar injection, or inferiorly in a cerebellomedullary cistern puncture. X-ray films are then obtained. The distribution of the dye delineates spinal cord and nerve root structure and integrity.

Echoencephalography (Ultrasound)

Echoencephalography, or **ultrasound,** is a safe, noninvasive procedure using sound waves that are deflected at differing rates, depending on the density of the tissue. Information is processed and displayed on an oscilloscope screen. It is useful primarily in the detection of structural characteristics of intracranial space–occupying mass lesions and the determination of ventricular dimensions, especially in newborns.

Electroencephalography

The **electroencephalograph (EEG)** is a recording of electrical impulses, arising from the cortical surface of the brain, which is detected by scalp electrodes. The recording of brain wave patterns is analyzed for alterations or localization (or both) of specific electrical activity. This test is especially useful in detecting and localizing foci that initiate seizure activity. It is also an important technique in determining, from a person's brain activity, whether the person is legally "brain dead."

Evoked Potentials

Evoked potentials (EPs) are a method of detecting electrical brain activity that results from a stimulus—primarily auditory, visual, or peripheral sensory. Electrical activity is computer formatted to display changes in trends. The primary uses of EPs include perioperative detection of sensory pathway integrity and disease- or drug-related sensory dysfunction.

Cerebrospinal Fluid Analysis

CSF generally is obtained from the lumbar or cisternal subarachnoid space by means of a hollow needle that allows passive flow. The lumbar puncture is performed most often at the L3-L4 interspace (below the level of the spinal cord at L1-L2). Cisternal puncture is performed by the insertion of a needle into the cerebellomedullary cistern using an approach from the back of the neck in the region of the foramen magnum. CSF pressure is commonly measured during these procedures. The CSF can be analyzed also for gross characteristics and constituents (color, blood cells, electrolytes, and protein) and cultured for microorganisms (Table 14-9).

Table 14-9	Cerebrospinal Fluid Analysis		
Parameters	**Normal**	**Abnormal**	**Possible Cause**
Pressure (initial readings)	120-180 mm H$_2$O (9-14 mmHg)	<60 mm H$_2$O	Faulty needle placement Dehydration Spinal block along subarachnoid space Block of foramen magnum
		>200 mm H$_2$O	Muscle tension Abdominal compression Brain tumor Subdural hematoma Brain abscess Brain cyst Cerebral edema (any cause) Hydrocephalus

Table 14-9	Cerebrospinal Fluid Analysis—cont'd		
Parameters	**Normal**	**Abnormal**	**Possible Cause**
Color	Clear, colorless	Cloudy	Increased cell count
			Increased microorganisms
		Yellow	Xanthochromic (caused by red blood cell [RBC] pigments)
			High protein content
		Smoky	Presence of RBCs
Red blood cells	None	Blood-tinged	Traumatic tap
		Grossly bloody	Traumatic tap
			Subarachnoid hemorrhage
White blood cells	0-6/mm³	>10/mm³ (cell counts range from <100 to many thousands depending on causative factor; all are abnormal findings.)	Occurs in many conditions:
			Bacterial infections of meninges
			Viral infections of meninges
			Neurosyphilis
			Tuberculous meningitis
			Metastatic neoplastic lesions
			Parasitic infections
			Acute demyelinating diseases
			Following introduction of air or blood into subarachnoid space
Protein*	15-45 mg/dl (1% of serum protein)	<10 mg/dl	Little clinical significance
		>60 mg/dl	Occurs in many conditions:
			Complete spinal block
			Guillain-Barré syndrome
			Carcinomatosis of meninges
			Tumors close to pial or ependymal surfaces or in cerebellopontine angle
			Acute and chronic meningitis
			Meningeal hemorrhage
			Demyelinating disorders
			Degenerative diseases
Glucose	50-75 mg/dl (approximately 60% of blood glucose level)	<40 mg/dl	Acute bacterial meningitis
			Tuberculous meningitis
			Meningeal carcinomatosis
		>100 mg/dl	Diabetes
Chloride	700-750 mg/dl 116-130 mEq/L	<625 mg/dl	Hypochloremia
		<110 mEq/L	Tuberculous meningitis
		>800 mg/dl	Not of neurologic significance; correlates with blood levels of chloride

Data from Rudy EB, editor: *Advanced neurological and neurosurgical nursing,* St Louis, 1984, Mosby.
*NOTE: If CSF contains blood, this will raise the protein level.

SUMMARY REVIEW

Overview and Organization of the Nervous System
1. The divisions of the nervous system have been categorized as either structural (CNS and PNS) or functional (somatic nervous system and ANS).
2. The CNS is contained within the brain and spinal cord.
3. The PNS is composed of cranial and spinal nerves that carry impulses toward the CNS (afferent) and away from the CNS (efferent) to target organs or skeletal muscle.

Cells of the Nervous System
1. The neuron and neuroglial cells make up nervous tissue. The neuron is specialized to transmit and receive electrical and chemical impulses, and the neuroglial cell provides supportive functions. The neuron is further divided into unipolar, pseudounipolar, bipolar, and multipolar categories, according to structure and particular mechanics of impulse transmission.
2. The neuron is composed of a cell body, one or more dendrites, and an axon. A myelin sheath around selected axons forms an insulation that allows quicker nerve impulse conduction, referred to as *saltatory conduction.*
3. Neurons have four basic types of cell configuration: (1) unipolar, (2) pseudounipolar, (3) bipolar, and (4) multipolar. The three function types of neurons are sensory, associational, and motor.
4. Neuroglial cells ("nerve glue") support the CNS and make up approximately half of the total brain and spinal cord volume.

SUMMARY REVIEW—cont'd

5. Nerve injury triggers a sequence of events known as *wallerian degeneration*. The degree of nerve regeneration that occurs depends on many factors.

Nerve Impulse

1. The region between adjacent neurons is the synapse, and the region between the neuron and muscle is the myoneural junction.
2. Neurotransmitters are responsible for chemical conduction across the synapse and myoneural junction. Nerve impulse is predominantly regulated by a balance of IPSPs and EPSPs, temporal and spatial summation, and convergence and divergence.

Central Nervous System

1. The brain is contained within the cranial vault and is divided into three distinct regions: (a) forebrain, (b) midbrain, and (c) hindbrain.
2. The forebrain comprises the two cerebral hemispheres and allows conscious perception of internal and external stimuli, thought and memory processes, and voluntary control of skeletal muscles. The deep portion of the forebrain is termed the *diencephalon* and processes incoming sensory data. The center for voluntary control of skeletal muscle movements is located along the precentral gyrus in the frontal lobe, whereas the center for perception is along the postcentral gyrus in the parietal lobe. The Broca area (rostral to the postcentral gyrus) and the Wernicke area (superoposterior temporal lobe) are major speech centers.
3. The midbrain is primarily a relay center for motor and sensory tracts, as well as a center for auditory and visual reflexes.
4. The hindbrain allows sampling and comparison of sensory data from the periphery and motor impulses from the cerebral hemispheres for the purpose of coordination and refinement of skeletal muscle movement.
5. The spinal cord contains the majority of nerve fibers connecting the brain with the periphery. Reflex arcs are completed in the spinal cord and influenced by the higher centers in the brain.
6. The four clinically relevant motor pathways are the lateral corticospinal, corticobulbar, basal ganglia, and vestibulospinal.
7. The three clinically important afferent pathways are the posterior column, anterior spinothalamic, and lateral spinothalamic.

8. The CNS is protected by the scalp, bony cranium, meninges, vertebral column, and CSF. The CSF is formed from blood components in the choroid plexuses of the ventricles and is reabsorbed in the arachnoid villi (located in the dural venous sinuses) after circulating through the brain and spinal cord.
9. The paired carotid and vertebral arteries supply blood to the brain and connect to form the circle of Willis. The major branches projecting from the circle of Willis are the anterior, middle, and posterior cerebral arteries. Drainage of blood from the brain is accomplished through the venous sinuses and jugular veins.
10. Blood supply to the spinal cord originates from the vertebral arteries and branches arising from the aorta.

Peripheral Nervous System

1. The PNS functions to relay information from the CNS to muscle and effector organs through cranial and spinal nerve tracts arranged in fascicles (multiple fascicles bound together form the peripheral nerve).
2. The 31 pairs of spinal nerves contain sensory and motor neurons.

Autonomic Nervous System

1. The ANS is responsible for the maintenance of a steady-state in the internal environment. Two opposing systems make up the ANS: (1) the sympathetic nervous system responds to stress by mobilizing energy stores and prepares the body to defend itself, and (2) the parasympathetic nervous system conserves energy and the body's resources.

Aging and the Nervous System

1. Major structural changes with aging include a decrease in number of neurons and a decrease in brain weight and size.
2. Deposition of lipofuscin and the presence of senile plaques, multiple neurofibrillary tangles, and Lewy bodies are common cellular changes with aging.
3. A progressive slowing of neurologic function occurs with advancing age.

Tests of Nervous System Function

1. Tests of nervous system function include x-ray films, CT, MRI and MRA, PET, brain scan, cerebral angiography, myelography, echoencephalography, electroencephalography, EPs potentials, and analysis of the CSF.

KEY TERMS

α-Adrenergic receptor, 469
β-Adrenergic receptor, 469
Acetylcholine, 467
Adrenergic transmission, 469
Afferent pathway (ascending pathway), 443
Afferent (sensory) neuron, 457
Amygdala, 452
Angiography, 476
Anterior cerebral artery, 462
Anterior column (ventral column), 456
Anterior fossa, 459
Anterior horn (ventral horn), 456
Anterior spinal artery, 463
Anterior spinothalamic, 458
Arachnoid membrane, 460
Arachnoid villi, 461

Arterial circle (circle of Willis), 462
Association fiber, 452
Associational neuron (interneuron), 444
Astrocyte, 445
Autonomic nervous system (ANS), 443
Axon, 443
Axon hillock, 443
Basal ganglia, 452
Basal ganglia system, 452
Basilar artery, 462
Basis pedunculi, 455
Bipolar neuron, 444
Brachial plexus, 465
Brain scan, 475
Brainstem, 450
Broca speech area, 452

Cauda equina, 456
Cavernous sinus, 462
Celiac branch of aorta, 467
Central canal, 456
Central nervous system (CNS), 442
Central sulcus (fissure of Rolando), 452
Cerebellomedullary cistern (cisterna magna), 460
Cerebellum, 455
Cerebral aqueduct (aqueduct of Sylvius), 455
Cerebral cortex, 452
Cerebral nuclei, 452
Cerebrospinal fluid (CSF), 461
Cerebrum, 452
Cholinergic transmission, 469

KEY TERMS—cont'd

Choroid plexus, 460
Collateral ganglia, 467
Computed tomography (CT), 474
Contralateral control, 452
Conus medullaris, 456
Convergence, 443
Corpora quadrigemina (tectum), 455
Corpus callosum (commissural fiber), 452
Corpus striatum, 452
Corticobulbar, 458
Corticospinal tract, 452
Cranial nerves, 443
Craniosacral division, 467
Dendrite, 443
Dendritic zone, 443
Denticulate ligament, 460
Dermatome, 467
Diencephalon, 453
Divergence, 443
Dopamine, 455
Dura mater, 459
Echoencephalography (ultrasound), 476
Effector organ, 443
Efferent (motor) neuron, 457
Efferent pathway (descending pathway), 443
Electroencephalograph (EEG), 476
Endoneurium, 443
Ependymal cells, 445
Epicritic, 458
Epidural space, 460
Epithalamus, 453
Evoked potential (EP), 476
Excitatory postsynaptic potential (EPSP), 448
Facilitation, 449
Falx cerebri, 460
Fascicle, 443
Filum terminale, 456
Fissure, 452
Frontal lobe, 452
Galea aponeurotica, 459
Ganglia, 443
Gray matter, 452
Helical CT angiography, 474
Hippocampus, 453
Hypothalamus, 453
Inferior colliculi, 455
Inferior mesenteric branch of aorta, 467
Inhibitory postsynaptic potential (IPSP), 448
Inner dura (meningeal layer), 459
Insula, 452
Intermediolateral gray (lateral horn), 456
Internal capsule, 452
Internal carotid artery, 462
Interventricular foramen (foramen of Monro), 461
Intervertebral disk, 461
Lateral aperture (foramen [pl., foramina] of Luschka), 461
Lateral column, 456
Lateral corticospinal, 458
Lateral spinothalamic, 458
Lateral sulcus (sylvian fissure, lateral fissure), 452

Lentiform nucleus, 452
Limbic system, 453
Longitudinal fissure, 452
Lower motor neuron, 458
Lumbar cistern, 460
Lumbar plexus, 467
Lumbar puncture, 461
Magnetic resonance angiography (MRA), 475
Magnetic resonance imaging (MRI), 474
Magnetic resonance spectroscopy, 474
Median aperture (foramen of Magendie), 461
Medulla oblongata, 455
Meninges, 459
Metencephalon, 455
Microfilament, 443
Microglia, 445
Microtubule, 443
Midbrain (mesencephalon), 455
Middle cerebral artery, 462
Middle fossa (temporal fossa), 459
Mixed nerve, 465
Motor neuron, 444
Motor unit, 458
Multipolar neuron, 444
Myelencephalon, 455
Myelin, 443
Myelin sheath, 443
Myelogram, 476
Neurilemma (Schwann sheath), 443
Neurofibril, 443
Neurofibrillary tangle, 471
Neuroglia, 444
Neuroglial cell, 443
Neuromuscular (myoneural) junction, 458
Neuron, 443
Neurotransmitter, 447
Nissl substance, 443
Nodes of Ranvier, 443
Norepinephrine, 469
Nucleus (pl., nuclei), 443
Nucleus pulposus, 461
Occipital lobe, 452
Oligodendroglia (oligodendrocyte), 445
Papez circuit, 453
Parasympathetic nervous system, 467
Parietal lobe, 452
Pelvic nerve, 467
Periosteum (endosteal layer), 459
Peripheral nervous system (PNS), 443
Pia mater, 460
Plasticity, 450
Plexus (pl., plexuses), 443
Pons, 455
Positron-emission tomography (PET) scan, 475
Postcentral gyrus, 452
Posterior cerebral artery, 462
Posterior column (dorsal column), 456
Posterior fossa, 459
Posterior horn (dorsal horn), 456
Posterior spinal artery, 463
Postganglionic neuron, 467

Postsynaptic neuron, 447
Precentral gyrus, 452
Prefrontal area, 452
Preganglionic neuron, 467
Premotor area, 452
Presynaptic neuron, 447
Primary motor area, 452
Primary voluntary motor area, 452
Projecting artery (nutrient artery), 462
Protopathic, 459
Pseudounipolar neuron, 444
Red nucleus, 455
Reflex arc, 457
Reticular activating system, 450
Reticular formation, 450
Roentgenogram (x-ray film), 474
Sacral plexus, 467
Saltatory conduction, 443
Schwann cell, 443
Senile plaque, 471
Sensory ganglion (dorsal root ganglion), 456
Sensory neuron, 457
Somatic nervous system, 443
Spatial summation, 449
Spinal cord, 456
Spinal nerve, 443
Spinal tract, 456
Spinothalamic tract, 456
Spiral (helical) CT, 474
Splanchnic nerve, 467
Subarachnoid space, 460
Subdural space, 460
Substantia gelatinosa, 456
Substantia nigra, 455
Subthalamic nucleus, 455
Subthalamus, 453
Sulci, 452
Summation, 449
Superficial artery (conducting artery), 462
Superior colliculi, 455
Superior mesenteric branch of aorta, 467
Superior sagittal sinus, 461
Sympathetic nervous system, 467
Sympathetic (paravertebral) ganglia, 467
Synapse, 446
Synaptic bouton, 447
Synaptic cleft, 447
Tegmentum, 455
Telencephalon, 452
Temporal lobe, 452
Temporal summation, 449
Tentorium cerebelli, 460
Thalamus, 453
Thoracolumbar division, 467
Unipolar neuron, 444
Upper motor neuron, 457
Ventricle, 461
Vermis, 455
Vertebral artery, 462
Vertebral column, 456, 461
Vestibulospinal, 458
Wallerian degeneration, 445
Wernicke area, 452
White matter, 452

REFERENCES

1. Haines DE: *Fundamental neuroscience for basic and clinical applications*, ed 3, Philadelphia, 2006, Churchill Livingstone.
2. Kandel ER et al, editors: *Principles of neural science*, ed 4, New York, 2000, McGraw-Hill.
3. Purves D et al: *Neuroscience*, ed 4, Sunderland, 2008, Sinauer Associates.
4. Kolb B, Whishaw IQ: *An introduction to brain and behavior*, ed 2, New York, 2006, Worth.
5. Szabo B, Schicker E: Effects of cannabinoids on neurotransmission, *Handb Exp Pharmacol* (168):327-365, 2005.
6. Benarroch EE et al: *Medical neurosciences: An Approach to Anatomy, Pathology, and Physiology by Systems and Levels*, ed 5, Philadelphia, 2008, Lippincott Williams & Wilkins.
7. Brodal P: *The central nervous system, structure and function*, ed 3, New York, 2004, Oxford University Press.
8. Whitehouse PJ, George D: *The myth of Alzheimer's: what you aren't being told about today's most dreaded diagnosis*, New York, 2008, St. Martin's Press.
9. Kelly et al: The neurobiology of aging, *Epilepsy Res* 68(Suppl 1):S5-S20, 2006.
10. Keller JN: Age related neuropathology, cognitive decline and Alzheimer's disease. *Ageing Res Rev* 5(1):1-13, 2006.
11. Schliebs R, Arendt T: The significance of the cholinergic system in the brain during aging in Alzheimer's disease, *J Neural Transm* 113(11):1625-1644, 2006.
12. Timiras PS, editor: *Physiologic basis of aging and geriatrics*, ed 3, Boca Raton, FL, 2003, CRC Press.

PAIN, TEMPERATURE REGULATION, SLEEP, AND SENSORY FUNCTION

SUE E. HUETHER

MEDIA RESOURCES

Evolve Website (http://evolve.elsevier.com/McCance/)
- Review Questions and Answers
- Animations
- Glossary (with audio pronunciation for selected terms)
- WebLinks

CHAPTER OUTLINE

PAIN
- Theories of Pain
- Neuroanatomy of Pain
- Neuromodulation of Pain
- Clinical Description of Pain
  - Pediatrics and Perception of Pain
  - Aging and Perception of Pain

TEMPERATURE REGULATION
- Hypothalamic Control of Temperature
  - Pediatrics and Changes in Temperature Regulation
  - Aging and Changes in Temperature Regulation
- Pathogenesis of Fever
- Benefits of Fever
- Disorders of Temperature Regulation

SLEEP
- Non–Rapid Eye Movement (NREM) Sleep
- Rapid Eye Movement Sleep
  - Pediatrics and Sleep Patterns
  - Aging and Sleep Patterns

- Sleep Disorders
- Sleep Disorders Associated with Mental, Neurologic, or Medical Disorders

SPECIAL SENSES
- Vision
  - Aging and Vision
- Hearing
  - Aging and Hearing
- Olfaction and Taste
  - Aging and Olfaction and Taste

SOMATOSENSORY FUNCTION
- Touch
- Proprioception

Alterations in sensory function may involve dysfunctions of the general or the special senses. Dysfunctions of the general senses include chronic pain, abnormal temperature regulation, tactile dysfunction, and proprioceptive dysfunction. Dysfunctions of the special senses include visual, auditory, vestibular, olfactory, and gustatory (taste).

Pain is a unique sensory experience that although universally described as unpleasant, is nonetheless essential to our survival. Pain provides protection by signaling the presence of disease or injury. Unlike pain, which need not be a part of everyday life, temperature is carefully monitored and regulated within clearly defined normal limits. Like pain, however, variations in temperature can signal disease. Fever is a

common manifestation of dysfunction and is often the first symptom observed in an infectious or inflammatory condition. If the body's temperature regulatory mechanism is out of balance, the result may be death.

Sleep is a normal, cyclic process that restores the body's energy and maintains normal functioning. Sleep is so essential to physiologic and psychologic function that sleep deprivation causes a wide range of clinical manifestations. Prolonged deprivation or disruption of sleep ultimately leads to serious dysfunction.

The special senses of vision, hearing, touch, smell, and taste are the means by which individuals perceive stimuli that are essential for interacting with the environment. Special sensory receptors are connected to specific areas of the brain through the afferent pathways of the peripheral and central nervous system (CNS). Each of the special senses thus involves a connected system of organs and tissues that receives stimuli and sends sensory messages to areas of the CNS, where they are processed and guide behavior.

PAIN

Pain is one of the body's most important adaptive and protective mechanisms and all definitions suggest it is a complex phenomenon and cannot be characterized as only a response to injury. A widely accepted definition of pain is that drafted by the International Association for the Study of Pain (IASP) and accepted by the American Pain Society and the World Health Organization: "Pain is an unpleasant sensory and emotional experience associated with actual or potential tissue damage or described in terms of such damage."[1] McCaffery maintains that "pain is whatever the experiencing person says it is, existing whenever he says it does."[2] Waddell defines pain as "a symptom, not a clinical sign, diagnosis or disease...."[3] A clear understanding of the complexities of the pain experience—specifically one that encompasses an individual's emotions, cognition, motivation, prior history, and even issues of secondary gain—is needed to manage pain and to further understanding the pain processes.

Theories of Pain

In the seventeenth century, the French philosopher and mathematician René Descartes proposed that the body works like a machine that can be studied by scientific methods and that injury activates specific pain receptors and fibers that project to the brain. He further postulated that the *intensity of pain* is directly related to the amount of associated tissue injury. For instance, pricking one's finger with a needle would cause minimal pain, whereas cutting one's hand with a knife would produce more pain. This theory—the **specificity theory**—is generally accurate when applied to certain types of injuries and the acute pain associated with them. But the specificity theory did not allow for psychologic contributions, such as attention to pain, prior experience, and the emotions involved in the "meaning" of the situation.[4] Nevertheless, it was this theory of pain, with some modification, that was still operational entering the twentieth century.

The **gate control theory,** proposed in 1965 by Melzack and Wall, provided the first cohesive explanation for the emerging complexities of pain phenomena, particularly chronic pain, and this has had a powerful effect on pain research and therapy.[5] According to this theory, pain transmission is modulated by a balance of impulses transmitted to the spinal cord by large A-delta (Aδ) and small C fibers. These fibers terminate on inhibitory interneurons in the substantia gelatinosa (laminae in the dorsal horn of the spinal cord). Cells in the substantia gelatinosa function as a gate, regulating transmission of impulses to the CNS. Stimulation of nonnociceptive larger A fibers such as touch, vibration or thermal stimuli, cause the cells in the substantia gelatinosa to "close the pain gate" which diminishes pain perception. Small fiber input inhibits cells in the substantia gelatinosa and "opens the pain gate", enhancing pain perception. The CNS, through efferent pathways, may also close, partially close, or open the gate. The gate control theory is inadequate to explain some chronic pain problems such as phantom limb pain, and the neuromatrix theory was proposed to explain such pain (see p. 494). Over the past 20 years exceptional progress has been made in strengthening the gate control theory of pain by elucidating the neuroanatomy and neuropharmacology of pain pathways in the peripheral and central nervous systems.

Neuroanatomy of Pain

The perception of pain is called **nociception** and depends on specifically dedicated receptors and afferent pathways that detect and transmit noxious or damaging or potentially damaging stimuli. The gate control theory describes these pathways in great detail, and explains the experience of pain by emphasizing the activation of non-nociceptive afferent input coming into the dorsal horn of the spinal cord to inhibit pain signals as well as the dynamic role of the brain in modulating pain processes.

Nociceptors

Nociceptive impulses arising from skin, muscle, joints, arteries, and the viscera are transmitted from unspecialized, bare sensory nerve endings called **nociceptors** that respond to chemical, mechanical, and thermal stimuli (Table 15-1). The variable nature and distribution of nociceptors affects relative sensitivity to pain in different areas of the body. For example, fingertips have more nociceptors than the skin of the back, and all skin has many more nociceptors than the internal organs. Unlike sensory neurons of the special senses of vision, gustation, and olfaction (discussed later), which are required to detect only one type of sensory stimulus (e.g., light for the sense of vision), primary nociceptive afferents have the remarkable ability to detect a wide range of stimuli. To do this nociceptors are equipped with an array of transduction channels that can sense different forms of noxious stimulation and at different intensities. In addition to the previously well studied voltage-gated potassium, sodium, and calcium channels, research has delineated the presence of up to seven other types of transmembrane receptors (called *transient receptor potential* [*TRP*] *channels*), which reside on "naked nerve endings" and respond to a variety of physical, chemical, and thermal stimuli.[6]

Nociceptors are categorized according to the stimulus to which they respond and by the properties of the axons associated with them. Severe mechanical deformation excites *mechanonociceptors*, whereas *mechanothermal nociceptors* are stimulated by mechanical deformation and/or extremes of temperature. These two receptors are associated with lightly myelinated, medium-sized Aδ fibers. Other types of

Table 15-1	Stimuli That Activate Nociceptors (Pain Receptors)
Location of Receptor	**Provoking Stimuli**
Skin	Pricking, cutting, crushing, burning, freezing
Gastrointestinal tract	Engorged or inflamed mucosa, distention or spasm of smooth muscle, traction on mesenteric attachment
Skeletal muscle	Ischemia, injuries of connective tissue sheaths, necrosis, hemorrhage, prolonged contraction, injection of irritating solutions
Bone	Periosteal injury, inflammation, fractures, tumors
Joints	Synovial membrane inflammation
Arteries	Piercing, inflammation
Head	Traction, inflammation, or displacement of arteries, meningeal structures, and sinuses; prolonged muscle contraction
Heart	Ischemia and inflammation

mechanical, thermal, and chemical nociception are transmitted by excitation of polymodal nociceptors and are carried on small, unmyelinated C fibers.

The nerve action potentials generated by excitation of any of these nociceptors travel along these two fiber types to reach the spinal cord. Nociceptive transmission through the larger Aδ fibers occurs more quickly than it does through C fibers. **Aδ fibers** carry well-localized, sharp pain sensations and are important in initiating rapid reactions to stimuli (fast pain). The small **unmyelinated C polymodal nociceptors** are responsible for the transmission of the diffuse burning or aching sensations that follow (slow pain) (Figure 15-1).

Pathways of Nociception

The cell bodies of *primary-order neurons* or pain-transmitting neurons reside in the dorsal root ganglia just lateral to the spine along the sensory pathways that penetrate the posterior part of the cord. Once the axons of the primary afferents (Aδ and C fibers) enter the cord (Figure 15-2), they synapse with second-order neurons that may branch into ascending or descending collaterals for one or two cord segments in neuronal projections called the *dorsolateral tract of Lissauer* (named after the German neurologist who first described it in the late nineteenth century). Eventually all of the primary afferents

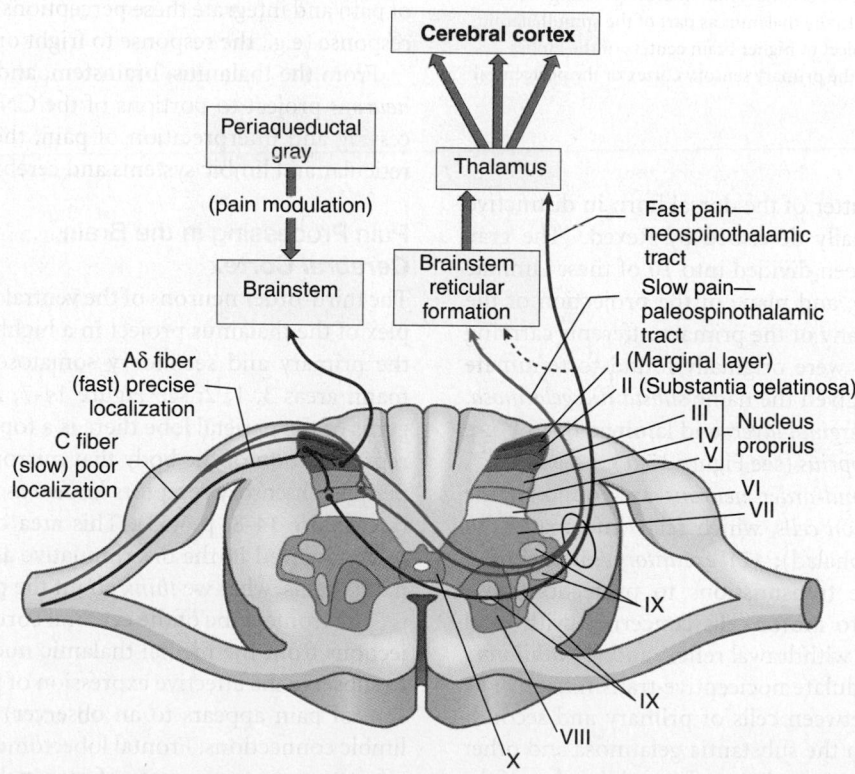

Figure 15-1 Pain fibers that terminate primarily in laminated II and V of the dorsal horn. The myelinated Aδ fibers (fast localized pain) synapse on a second set of neurons that carry the signal to the thalamus via the neospinothalamic tracts. The C fibers (slow pain) synapse on laminae II and V interneurons that connect with neurons in laminae II, IV, and V and carry the pain signal to the reticular formation and midbrain via the paleospinothalamic tract. The axons of the spinothalamic tracts cross over the spinal cord to ascend in the anterior and lateral spinal cord white matter.

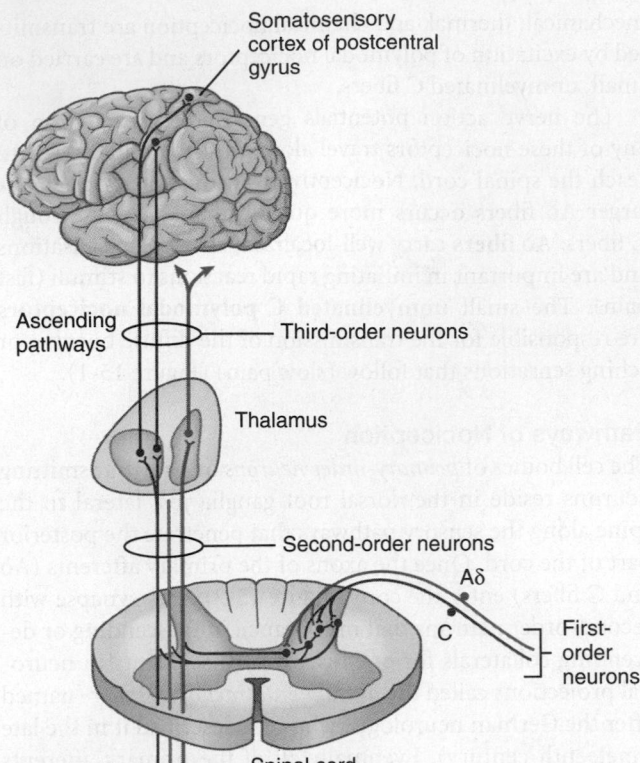

Somatosensory
cortex of postcentral
gyrus

Ascending
pathways

Third-order neurons

Thalamus

Second-order neurons

Aδ

C

First-
order
neurons

Spinal cord

Figure 15-2 Nociception pathways. Aδ and C fibers comprise the primary, first-order sensory afferents coming into the gate at the posterior part of the spinal cord. Here we see second-order neurons crossing the cord ("decussating") and ascending to the thalamus as part of the spinothalamic tract. Third-order afferents project to higher brain centers of the limbic system, the frontal cortex, and the primary sensory cortex of the postcentral gyrus of the parietal lobe.

terminate in the gray matter of the dorsal horn in distinctive layers or *laminae* originally described by Rexed.[7] The gray matter of the cord has been divided into 10 of these laminae based on the size, shape, and plane of the projection of the neurons found there. Many of the primary afferents carrying nociceptive information were originally found to terminate in lamina II, which was given the name *substantia gelatinosa.* Lamina I is called the *marginal layer,* and laminae III to V are known as the *nucleus proprius* (see Figure 15-1).

Three classes of *second-order neurons* are found in the dorsal horn: (1) *projection cells,* which relay information to higher brain areas (cephalad); (2) *excitatory interneurons,* which relay nociceptive transmissions to projection cells, other interneurons, or to motor cells concerned with local reflexes such as the pain withdrawal reflex; and (3) *inhibitory interneurons,* which modulate nociceptive transmission. The synaptic connections between cells of primary and second-order neurons located in the substantia gelatinosa and other Rexed laminae function as a "pain gate," providing one of the major tenets advanced by the gate control theory. This "gate" in the spinal cord regulates the transmission of pain impulses that ascend to the brain for further processing and interpretation (see p. 482).

From the gate in the dorsal horn, nociception continues on the axons of the second-order neurons as they cross the midline of the cord and ascend to various areas of the brain. These ascending fibers are organized into tracts or funiculi that are found in the white matter of the spinal cord, and are named according to their location in the cord and to where they project—either to the higher cord and brainstem or to the diencephalon (thalamus and hypothalamus) and limbic structures. Most nociceptive information travels by means of ascending columns in the lateral spinothalamic tract (also called the anterolateral funiculus). Other bits of nociceptive signals travel in the posterior columns of the cord to the dorsal column nuclei of the medulla, and from there ascend in the medial lemniscus to the lateral thalamus. Several other spinal cord projection systems convey nociceptive information directly or indirectly to the reticular formation of the brainstem and the periaqueductal gray (PAG) matter of the midbrain. These include the postsynaptic dorsal column, and the spinocervical, spinoreticular, spinomesencephalic, spinoparabrachial, spinohypothalamic, and other spinolimbic pathways[8] (Figure 15-3).

Although the organization of all of the ascending tracts is complex, the principal target for nociceptive afferents is the thalamus (the major relay station of sensory information in general). The thalamus is divided into medial and lateral groups by a band of fibers called the internal medullary lamina. The ventral posterior lateral (VPL) and ventral posterior medial (VPM) nuclei of the thalamus facilitate the localization of pain and integrate these perceptions into a neuroendocrine response (e.g., the response to fright or to surgical stress).[9,10]

From the thalamus, brainstem, and midbrain, *third-order neurons* project to portions of the CNS involved in the processing and interpretation of pain, the chief areas being the reticular and limbic systems and cerebral cortex.

Pain Processing in the Brain
Cerebral Cortex
The third-order neurons of the ventral posterior nuclear complex of the thalamus project in a highly organized manner to the primary and secondary somatosensory cortex[11] (Brodmann areas 3, 1, 2; see Figure 14-7, *B*). On the postcentral gyrus of the parietal lobe there is a topographically organized representation of the body that mirrors the concentration of peripheral sensory receptors known as the *sensory homunculus* (see Figure 14-8, p. 453). This area of the brain is thought to be involved in the discriminative and cognitive aspects of pain; that is, what we *think* about the pain.[12]

The frontal lobe of the cerebral cortex receives diffuse projections from the medial thalamic nuclei, which are thought to subserve the affective expression of pain (how your expression of pain appears to an observer) through their frontal-limbic connections. Frontal lobectomies were once used in an effort to treat some cases of intractable pain. Postsurgically individuals continued to report pain if questioned, but they seldom asked for medications and no longer seemed to care about their pain. This response is also observed in bilateral thalamic lesions.[13]

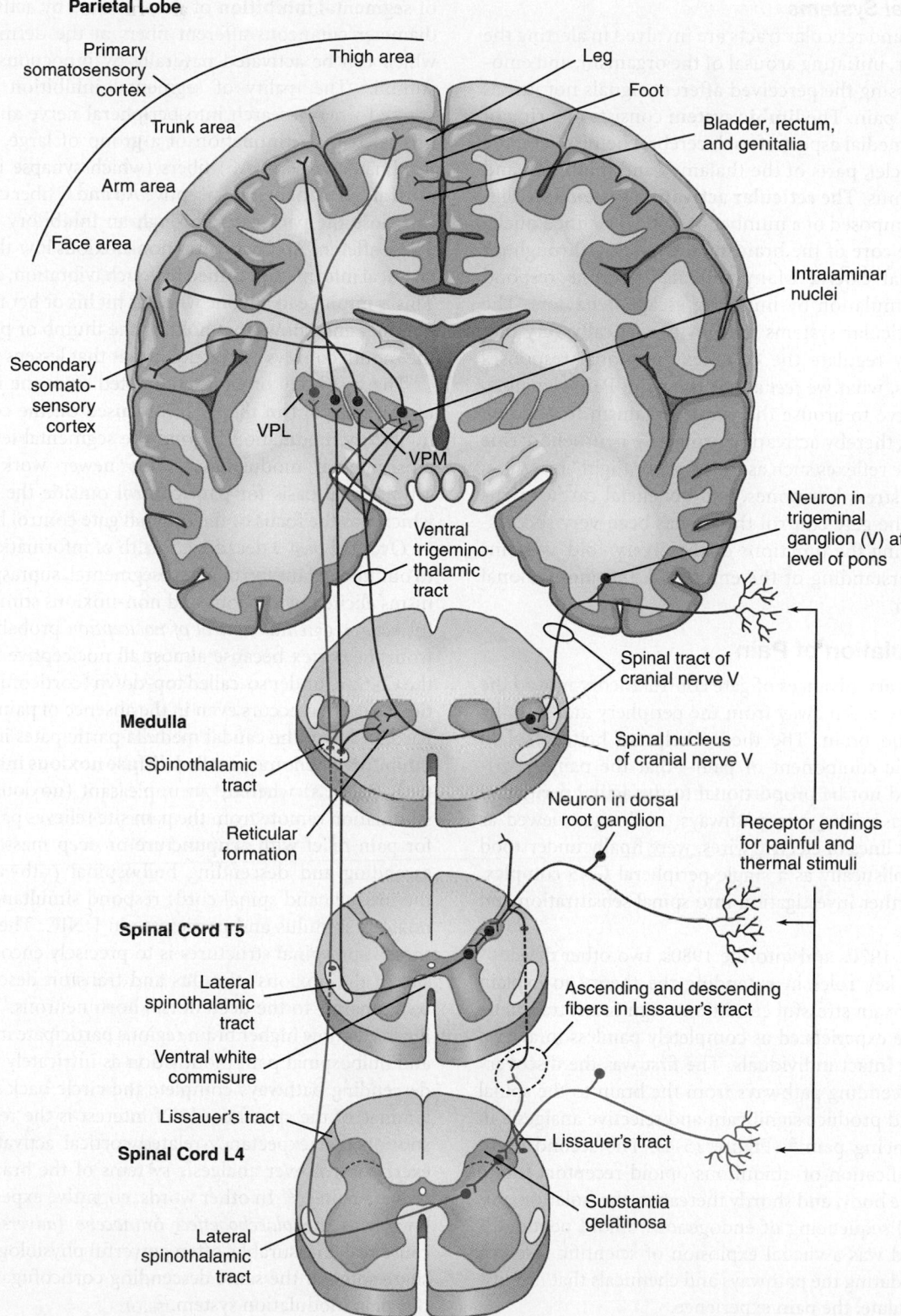

Figure 15-3 Central nervous system pathways that mediate the sensations of pain and temperature. *VPM,* Ventral posterior medial thalamic nuclei; *VPL,* ventral posterior lateral thalamic nuclei.

Subcortical Systems

The limbic and reticular tracts are involved in alerting the body to danger, initiating arousal of the organism, and emotionally processing the perceived afferent signals not just as stimuli, but as pain. The **limbic system** consists of a ring of cortex on the medial aspect of each cerebral hemisphere, the subcortical nuclei, parts of the thalamus and midbrain, and the hypothalamus. The **reticular activating system** (see Figure 14-6) is composed of a number of vaguely defined nuclei situated in the core of the brainstem extending throughout its rostrocaudal extent. Many reticular neurons respond to noxious stimulation by initiating escape behaviors. The limbic and reticular systems are phylogenetically very old. Together, they regulate the complex emotional responses to pain; that is, what we *feel* about the pain. Pain signals to these areas serve to arouse the whole organism to ongoing tissue damage, thereby activating protective neuroendocrine and autonomic reflexes such as the "fight or flight" response, the release of stress hormones, and beneficial cardiovascular changes. The gate control theory has been very successful in integrating the functions of these very "old" systems into our understanding of the emotional and motivational aspects of pain.

Neuromodulation of Pain

The extraordinary advances of gate control theory moved the focus of pain research away from the periphery and into the spinal cord and brain. The theory helps to better explain the psychologic component of pain—that the pain experience itself need not be proportional to the actual peripheral injury or disease. The pain pathways, no longer viewed as merely labeled lines of electric wires, were finally understood to function holistically as a single peripheral CNS complex, promoting further investigation into spinal sensitization and CNS plasticity.

By the mid-1970s and into the 1980s, two other developments played key roles in extending the theory to explain how, under certain stressful conditions, significant traumatic injuries can be experienced as completely painless in awake, neurologically intact individuals. The first was the discovery of specific descending pathways from the brain to the spinal cord that could produce significant and selective analgesia in those experiencing pain[14] (Figure 15-4). The second event was the identification of ubiquitous opioid receptors found throughout the body, and shortly thereafter, the isolation, purification, and sequencing of endogenous opioid peptides.[15] What followed was a virtual explosion of scientific research aimed at elucidating the pathways and chemicals that modify, or neuromodulate, the pain experience.

Pathways of Neuromodulation

How does central processing, including memory and interpretation of pain in the brain, lead to changes in how much algogenic (pain related) information passes through the spinal cord gate? When Melzack and Wall originally proposed the gate control theory, they described the possibility of **segmental inhibition** of pain, elicited by activity in large-diameter cutaneous afferent fibers at the dermatome level, which can be activated naturally by innocuous mechanical stimuli.[4] The reality of segmental inhibition was quickly verified when research into peripheral nerve anatomy demonstrated that stimulation of a group of large, fast, heavily myelinated A-beta (Aβ) fibers (which synapse in the dorsal horn along with their nociceptive Aδ and C fiber counterparts) can close the pain gates through an inhibitory interneuron. These afferent Aβ fibers carry non-noxious low-threshold mechanical information gained by touch, vibration, and pressure. This is intuitive to anyone who has hit his or her thumb with a hammer and knows that holding the thumb or putting it into the mouth conveys distraction input that lessens the pain.

The vast body of work completed since the inauguration of the gate control theory has focused on the complexity of inhibitory modulation beyond the segmental level (i.e., heterosegmental modulation). This newer work emphasizes a functional basis for pain control outside the dorsal horn, which was the focus of the original gate control hypothesis.

Over the past 3 decades a wealth of information has added to our understanding of heterosegmental, supraspinal mechanisms elicited by noxious and non-noxious stimuli.[16] Powerful *heterosegmental control of nociception* probably originates from the cortex because almost all nociceptive relays within the CNS are under so-called top-down (corticofugal) modulation that often occurs even in the absence of painful stimuli.[17] Farther down, the caudal medulla participates in widespread inhibitory phenomena called **diffuse noxious inhibitory controls (DNICs)** whereby an unpleasant (noxious) peripheral stimulation remote from the pain site relieves pain—the basis for pain relief with acupuncture or deep massage.[18] Several ascending and descending bulbospinal pathways (between the medulla and spinal cord) respond simultaneously to the noxious stimulus and participate in DNIC. The net effect of these supraspinal structures is to precisely encode the intensity of the noxious stimulus and transmit descending feedback, mainly to the deep dorsal horn neurons.[19] Figure 15-4 illustrates how higher brain regions participate in corticofugal and bulbospinal pain modulation as intricately incorporated descending pathways complete the circle back to the Rexed laminae of the spinal cord. Of interest is the recent demonstration that expectancy-related cortical activation also can exert control over analgesic systems of the brainstem to attenuate pain.[20,21] In other words, cognitive expectations (also known as the *placebo effect* or *nocebo [adverse] effect*) can cause real, measurable, often powerful physiologic effects that share some of the same descending corticofugal pathways as our pain modulation system.[22]

The entire complex of pathways now can be visualized as an integration of peripheral sensory axon terminals, spinal interneurons, and top-down control pathways that converge on the spinal dorsal horns. The result is to modify, dampen, or augment nociceptive transmission, depending on the many factors existing both within and without the organism.

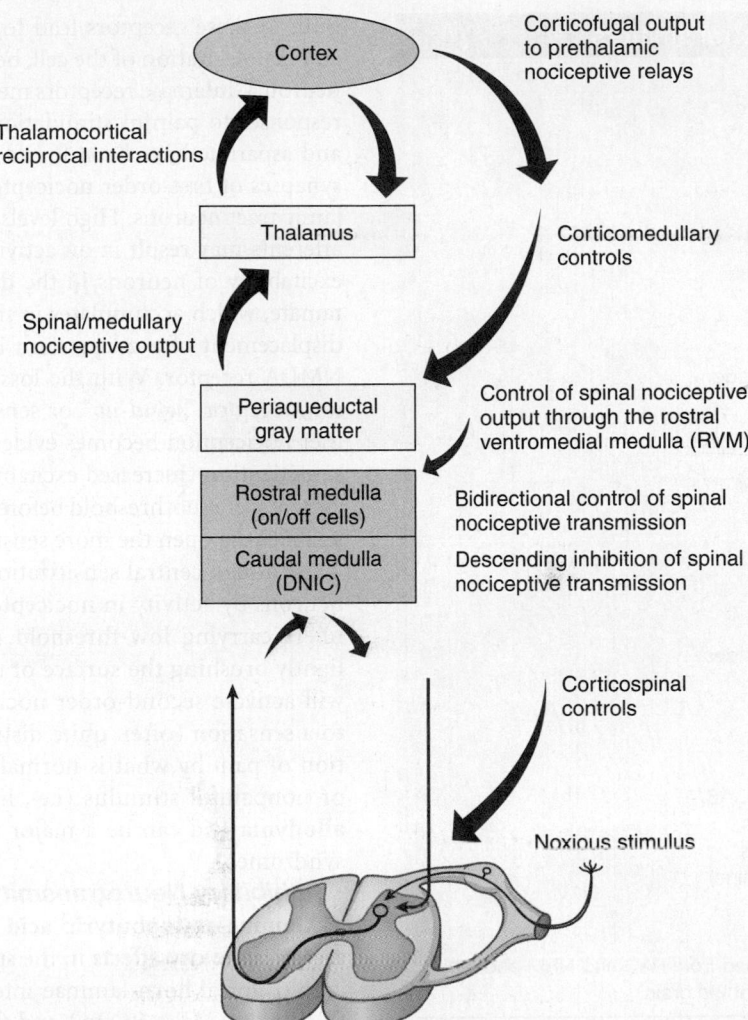

Figure 15-4 Diagram representing the central mechanisms of pain modulation. A noxious peripheral stimulus activates both segmental and bulbospinal heterosegmental modulatory mechanisms, which either accentuate or inhibit afferent pain transmission to the brain. The most important and widespread source of top-down (corticofugal) modulation arises from the cortex. Both thalamic and prethalamic nociceptive relays are under the influence of this corticofugal control. The dorsal horn of the spine is also under the influence of the caudal medulla through diffuse noxious inhibitory control (DNIC). (Modified from Villanueva L, Fields HL: *The pain system in normal and pathological states: a primer for clinicians,* Seattle, 2004, IASP Press.)

Neurotransmitters of Neuromodulation

Many neurotransmitters mediate the transmission of pain in the periphery, the spinal cord, and the brain. In the periphery, local injury and inflammation can result in direct or indirect excitation of nociceptors. Pain neurotransmitters can be classified as inflammatory, pain excitatory, or pain inhibitory (Box 15-1).

Direct excitation occurs when nociceptors respond with a threshold depolarization initiated by the application of heat, radiation, toxic chemicals, or tissue trauma. *Indirect excitation* occurs through the release of inflammatory mediators after the tissue is injured. The tissue injury results in inflammation and the release of prostaglandins such as PGE_2 and PGI_2, tumor necrosis factor-alpha (TNF-α), nitric oxide, bradykinins, and histamine (see Chapter 6). For example, it has been shown that lymphokines released in chronic lymphocytic

inflammatory lesions contribute to some types of chronic pain. In addition, activity within the nociceptors causes them to release peptides and neurotransmitters such as substance P, neurokinin A, calcitonin gene-related peptide (CGRP), and adenosine triphosphate (ATP), which promote the spread of pain locally and further contribute to vasodilation, increased vascular permeability, and degranulation of even more mast cell cytokines. The resultant "inflammatory soup" serves to lower the threshold for nociceptive depolarization resulting in **peripheral sensitization** and pain augmentation—**hyperalgesia**. This is readily recognized by anyone who has suffered a bad sunburn and then notices the resulting extrasensitivity of the skin to stimuli (such as mild heat or touch) that normally would be considered non-noxious. Normally peripheral sensitization phenomena extinguish themselves as the tissue heals and inflammation subsides. However, when

Box 15-1   Pain Neurotransmitters

Inflammatory Mediators
Bradykinin
Leukotrienes
Prostaglandins
Serotonin
Substance P
Interleukins
Tumor necrosis factor-alpha
Nitric oxide
ATP
Neurokinins
Calcitonin gene-related peptide

Excitatory Transmitters
Glutamate (fast pain)
NMDA
AMPA
Tachykinins
Neurokinin A
Neurokinin B
Substance P
Other receptors
Calcitonin gene-related peptides
Somatostatins
Bombesins
Cholecystokinins

Inhibitory Transmitters
Gamma-aminobutyric acid (GABA)
Descending pain modulators
Norepinephrine–α_2-receptors
Serotonin (5-hydroxytryptamine)
Opioids (μ, δ, κ receptors)
　Endorphins
　Enkephalins ⎫ Released from PAG and NRM and other
　Dynorphins ⎭ areas of the brain

ATP, Adenosine triphosphate; *NMDA, N*-methyl-D-aspartate; *AMPA,* alpha-amino-3-hydroxy-5-methyl-4-isoxazole-propionate; *NRM,* nucleus raphes magnus; *PAG,* periaqueductal gray.

primary afferent function is altered in an enduring way by injury or disease of the nervous system, hyperalgesia may persist and be highly resistant to treatment.

In the spinal cord and brain, a wide variety of biogenic amines and other neurotransmitters act to modulate control over the transmission of pain impulses. Serotonin, norepinephrine, glutamate, aspartate, glycine, gamma-aminobutyric acid, and an array of endogenous opioids have been found to stimulate or inhibit interneurons in the CNS. This in turn may serve to stimulate or inhibit the pain gate and the primary nociceptive tracts.

Excitatory Neurotransmitters

Glutamate and aspartate, amino acid precursors, are the most common excitatory neurotransmitters in the brain and spinal cord. **Glutamate** activates two different kinds of receptors: AMPA/kinate (alpha-amino-3-hydroxy-5-methyl-4-isoxazole propionate) receptors, which are very fast, and *N*-methyl-D-aspartate (NMDA) receptors, which are implicated in memory and long-term potentiation of synapses.

Both of these receptors lead to excitation of the membrane and depolarization of the cell, be it an inhibitory or excitatory neuron. Glutamate receptors mediate many spinal and central responses to painful stimulation.[23] High levels of glutamate and aspartate have been found in the PAG as well as at the synapses of first-order nociceptors with ascending spinothalamic tract neurons. High levels of activity in the nociceptive afferents may result in an activity-dependent increase in the excitability of neurons in the dorsal horn of the cord. Glutamate, which accumulates in the dorsal horn, results in the displacement of a magnesium ion that serves to inhibit the NMDA receptor. With the loss of the blocking magnesium ion, receptor *"wind-up"* or sensitization in the CNS to further nociception becomes evident. As a result of this **central sensitization** (increased excitability of neurons), activity levels that were subthreshold before the sensitizing event become sufficient to open the more sensitive pain gate.

Although central sensitization is triggered in dorsal horn neurons by activity in nociceptors, innocuous activation of fibers carrying low-threshold mechanoreception (such as lightly brushing the surface of the skin with a cotton swab) will activate second-order nociceptive neurons, giving rise to a sensation (often quite distressing) of pain. The induction of pain by what is normally considered an innocuous or nonpainful stimulus (i.e., light touch) is referred to as **allodynia** and can be a major feature of neuropathic pain syndromes.

Inhibitory Neurotransmitters

Gamma-aminobutyric acid (GABA) and **glycine** have major inhibitory effects in the spinal cord and brain. For example, dorsal horn laminae interneurons are rich in GABA (GABA-A, GABA-B, etc.) and function to inhibit release of pain neurotransmitters. Norepinephrine and 5-hydroxytryptamine (serotonin) contribute to pain modulation (inhibition) in the medulla and pons.

Endogenous opioids are a family of morphine-like neuropeptides that inhibit transmission of pain impulses in the spinal cord, brain, and periphery.[24] There are four types of opioid neuropeptides: (1) *enkephalins,* (2) *endorphins,* (3) *dynorphins,* and (4) *endomorphins.* These substances are neurohormones that act as neurotransmitters by binding to one or more G-protein–coupled opioid receptors. Three distinct types of **opioid receptors** are found in the body: mu (μ) (with subtypes μ_{-1} and μ_{-2}), kappa (κ), and delta (δ). Each receptor type binds differently with the various types of opioids.

Agonist activity at the opioid receptors by endogenous opioids inhibits the release of excitatory neurotransmitters such as substance P in the dorsal horn (blocking the transmission of the painful stimulus) or in other areas of the brain such as the PAG or the rostral ventromedial nuclei in the brainstem[25] (Figure 15-5). Opioids from the midbrain release adrenergic and serotonergic descending pathways from GABAergic inhibition and decrease pain. Leukocytes release opioids and participate in peripheral pain control[26] (see What's New? Opioid-Producing Leukocytes and Pain Control).

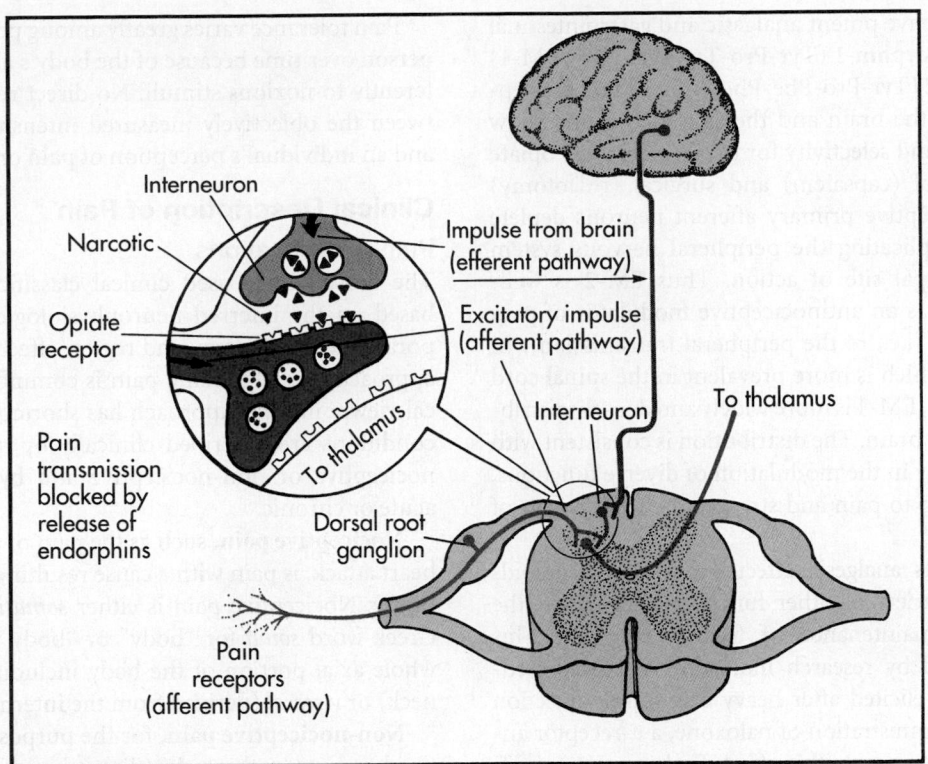

Figure 15-5 Descending pathway and endorphin response. The biologic receptors of the enkephalins and endorphins are located close to known pain receptors in the periphery and ascending and descending pain pathways.

WHAT'S NEW?
Opioid-Producing Leukocytes and Pain Control

At sites of peripheral inflammation, leukocytes release inflammatory mediators that cause pain. However, infiltrating leukocytes also produce anti-inflammatory cytokines and opioid peptides that produce analgesia. Inflammation in peripheral tissue results in up-regulation of opioid receptors at peripheral sensory nerve terminals with enhanced peripheral efficacy of opioids. Opioid-containing immune cells migrate to inflamed tissues using chemokines and adhesion molecules. Under stressful conditions or in response to releasing agents such as corticotropin-releasing factor, cytokines, chemokines, and catecholamines, leukocytes secrete opioids. Once released opioid peptides activate peripheral opioid receptors and produce analgesia by inhibiting the excitability of sensory nerves and/or the release of excitatory neuropeptides. Of clinical significance, these effects occur *without central untoward side effects* such as respiratory depression, somnolence, clouding of consciousness, or addiction. Future pain management strategies include the selective targeting of opioid-containing leukocytes and peripheral endogenous opioid systems to achieve analgesia with few side effects.

Data from: Smith HS: *Pain Physician* 11(2 Suppl):S121-S132, 2008; Machelska H: *Neuropeptides* 41(6):355-363, 2007; Rittner HL et al: *Br J Anaesth* 101(1):40-44, 2008.

Perhaps the best known and the most prevalent of these natural opioids are the **enkephalins.** There are two types of enkephalins, *methionine enkephalin* (met-enkephalin) and *leucine enkephalin* (leu-enkephalin), and their ratio is 4:1, respectively. They were the first endogenous opioids extracted in research. Enkephalins, which like the other endogenous opioids can be identified immunohistochemically, are found concentrated in the hypothalamus, the PAG matter, the nucleus raphe magnus of the medulla, and the dorsal horns of the spine.

Endorphins were first discovered in the human PAG in 1979, β-endorphin being the best studied of the group. The synthesis and activity of β-endorphin is concentrated in the hypothalamus and the pituitary gland; β-endorphin is purported to produce a greater sense of exhilaration, or "high," than all of the other endorphin types. It is a strong μ-receptor agonist and is generally believed to provide substantial natural pain relief.

Dynorphins (the most potent of these endogenous neurohormones) are found in the hypothalamus, the brainstem PAG rostral ventromedial medulla (PAG-RVM) system, and the spine. Dynorphins, which bind strongly to κ receptors located in the dorsal horn of the spinal cord, generally serve to impede pain signals but can, in certain areas, incite pain by activation of bradykinin receptors.[27,28]

Endomorphins have potent analgesic and gastrointestinal (GI) effects. Endomorphin-1 (Tyr-Pro-Trp-Phe-NH$_2$, EM-1) and endomorphin-2 (Tyr-Pro-Phe-Phe-NH$_2$, EM-2) are peptides isolated from the brain and the spinal cord and show the highest affinity and selectivity for the μ *(morphine)* opiate receptor.[29] Chemical (capsaicin) and surgical (rhizotomy) disruption of nociceptive primary afferent neurons deplete levels of EM-2, implicating the peripheral nervous system as being the principal site of action. Thus EM-2 is well-positioned to serve as an antinociceptive modulator of pain in its earliest stages (i.e., in the peripheral transmission). In contrast to EM-2, which is more prevalent in the spinal cord and lower brainstem, EM-1 is more widely and densely distributed throughout the brain. The distribution is consistent with the role peptides play in the modulation of diverse functions, including adaptation to pain and stress and enhancement of reward perceptions.

In addition to its analgesic effects, endogenous opioids are involved in a variety of other functions throughout the body—one being maintenance of feeding behavior. This finding is supported by research indicating enhanced feeding responses being elicited after heavy exertion or injection of β-endorphin. Administration of naloxone, a μ-receptor antagonist, was found to negate this effect. Endogenous opioids also have been linked to moderation of drinking behavior and cough suppression. Stress, excessive physical exertion, acupuncture, intercourse, and other factors increase the levels of circulating endogenous opioids—serotonin, norepinephrine, and other neurotransmitters—and consequently raise the pain threshold.[29] Endogenous opioids of one type or another are found to bind to almost all tissues in the body and may be responsible for general sensations of well-being or lack thereof.[24]

Pain Threshold and Pain Tolerance

The **pain threshold** is the point at which a stimulus is perceived as pain. The threshold does not vary significantly among people or in the same person over time. Intense pain at one location, however, may cause an increase in the threshold in another location. For example, a person with severe pain in one knee is less likely to experience chronic back pain that is less intense. This phenomenon is called **perceptual dominance.** Because of perceptual dominance, an individual with many painful sites may report only the most painful one. After the dominant pain is diminished, the individual may then identify other painful areas.[4]

Pain tolerance is the duration of time or the intensity of pain that an individual will endure before initiating overt pain responses. It is the amount of pain the person will tolerate before outwardly responding to it. Pain tolerance is influenced by the person's cultural perceptions, expectations, role behaviors, and physical and mental health. Pain tolerance generally is decreased with repeated exposure to pain. Tolerance is decreased also by fatigue, anger, boredom, apprehension, and sleep deprivation. Tolerance may be increased by alcohol consumption, persistent use of pain medication, hypnosis, warmth, distracting activities, and strong beliefs or faith.

Pain tolerance varies greatly among people and in the same person over time because of the body's ability to respond differently to noxious stimuli. No direct relationship exists between the objectively measured intensity of painful stimuli and an individual's perception of pain or response to pain.

Clinical Description of Pain

Pain Classifications

The most widely used clinical classifications for pain are based on the inferred neurophysiologic mechanisms, temporal aspects, etiology, and region affected. The mechanistic approach to categorizing pain is common, but from a clinical viewpoint, this approach has shortcomings. Usually pain conditions are described clinically by mechanism as either nociceptive or non-nociceptive and by duration as either acute or chronic.

Nociceptive pain, such as the pain of a crushed finger or a heart attack, is pain with a cause resulting from normal tissue injury. Nociceptive pain is either *somatic* (derived from the Greek word *soma* for "body" or "body wall"—meaning the whole axial portion of the body including trunk, head, and neck) or *visceral* (derived from the internal organs).

Non-nociceptive pain, for the purposes of this text, is defined as neuropathic pain (discussion of psychogenic pain is not covered in this chapter). Neuropathic pain is subdivided into peripheral and central categories (see page 493).

Additionally, somatic, visceral, and neuropathic pains can all occur as acute or chronic presentations. These broad categories have been summarized in Box 15-2. Some of the most common clinical pain presentations are detailed below.

Acute Pain

Acute pain is a protective mechanism that alerts the individual to a condition or experience that is immediately harmful to the body. The onset of acute pain is sudden, and usually dissipates after the stimulus is removed and the tissues have healed. A direct one-to-one relationship between physical signs of disease and accompanying symptoms is almost always present. Peripheral and central sensitization, that is, wind-up (see p. 486), is not evident. Anxiety is common in acute pain states and is usually apparent in the alterations of vital signs. Tachycardia, hypertension, fever, diaphoresis, dilated pupils, and outward pain behavior such as moaning, touching, or rocking motions are discernible to an observer. Other physical manifestations include elevation of blood sugar levels, decreases in gastric acid secretion and intestinal motility, and a general decrease in blood flow to the viscera and skin. Nausea occasionally occurs.

The signs, symptoms, and behaviors of acute pain are a predictable response to the threat inherent in the painful experience, including issues surrounding the cause of pain, its treatment, and prognosis (Table 15-2). Individuals often psychologically respond to acute pain with fear (e.g., fear of diagnosis, fear of continued pain), anxiety, and a general sense of unpleasantness or unease. The stress of fear itself may in turn contribute to the physiologic signs of pain. Some individuals are reluctant to discuss or report their pain,[30] although hope of recovery is usually present.

Acute pain arises from cutaneous and deep somatic tissue, or from visceral organs and can be classified as (1) acute somatic, (2) acute visceral, and (3) referred.

Box 15-2   Categories of Pain

I. Neurophysiologic pain
  A. Nociceptive pain
    1. Somatic
    2. Visceral
  B. Neuropathic (non-nociceptive)
    1. Central pain (lesion in brain or spinal cord)
    2. Peripheral pain (lesion in peripheral nervous system [PNS])
II. Neurogenic pain
  A. Neuralgia (pain in the distribution of a nerve)
  B. Constant
    1. Sympathetically independent
    2. Sympathetically dependent
III. Temporal pain (time related)
  A. Acute pain
    1. Somatic
    2. Visceral
  B. Chronic
IV. Regional pain
  A. Abdominal pain
  B. Chest pain
  C. Headache
  D. Low back pain
  E. Orofacial pain
  F. Pelvic pain
V. Etiologic pain
  A. Cancer pain
  B. Dental pain
  C. Inflammatory pain
  D. Ischemic pain
  E. Vascular pain

Adapted from Derasari MD: Taxonomy of pain syndromes: classification of chronic pain syndromes. In Raj PP, editor: *Practical management of pain,* ed 3, St Louis, 2000, Mosby.

Somatic pain arises from connective tissue, muscle or bone, and skin and is either sharp and well localized (especially fast pain carried by Aδ fibers) or dull, aching, and poorly localized pain as seen in polymodal C fiber transmissions.

Visceral pain refers to pain in internal organs and the abdomen and is transmitted by sympathetic afferents. It is poorly localized because of the lesser number of nociceptors in the visceral structures, which often can be cauterized or cut without any sensation of pain being felt. However, any stretching or distention of internal organs or the abdomen will elicit a violent response.

Visceral pain is associated with nausea and vomiting, hypotension, restlessness, and, in some cases, shock. It often radiates (spreads away from the actual site of the pain) or is referred. Visceral pain that is primarily nociceptive and not referred is carried by second-order neurons that travel in the dorsal column pathway to the gracilis nucleus of the medulla and then in contralateral pathways of the medial lemniscus to finally synapse in the thalamus.[31]

Referred pain is pain that is present in an area removed or distant from its point of origin. Referred pain usually, but not always, originates from the viscera and so is discussed here. The most familiar examples are pain in the shoulder from myocardial infarction, pain in the back from pancreatic or renal disease, and pain in the right shoulder from an inflamed gallbladder. Referred visceral pain is carried by second-order neurons that travel in the contralateral spinothalamic tracts. The area of referred pain is supplied by the same spinal segment as the actual site of pain because impulses from many cutaneous and visceral neurons converge. The presumed mechanism is one of afferent fibers from this conjoint area in the spinal cord, relaying the mistaken perception that the pain arises from the referral site. Because the skin has more receptors, the painful sensation is more often experienced there instead of at the site of origin.[32] (Common areas of referred pain and their associated sites of origin appear in Figure 15-6.)

Table 15-2   Comparison of Acute and Chronic Pain

Characteristic	Acute Pain	Chronic Pain
Experience	An event	A situation; state of existence
Source	External agent or internal disease usually known	Unknown; if known, treatment is prolonged or ineffective
Onset	Usually sudden	May be sudden or develop insidiously
Duration	Transient (up to 6 months)	Prolonged and persistent (months to years)
Pain identification	Painful and nonpainful areas generally well identified	Painful and nonpainful areas less easily differentiated: change in sensations becomes more difficult to evaluate
Clinical signs	Typical response pattern with more visible signs	Response patterns vary; fewer overt signs (adaptation)
Significance	Significant (informs person something is wrong)	Person looks for significance
Pattern	Self-limiting or readily corrected	Continuous or intermittent; intensity may vary or remain constant
Course	Suffering usually decreases over time	Suffering usually increases over time
Actions	Leads to actions to relieve pain	Leads to actions to modify pain experience
Prognosis	Likelihood of eventual complete relief	Complete relief usually not possible

Data from Black RG: *Surg Clin North Am* 55(4):999, 1975.

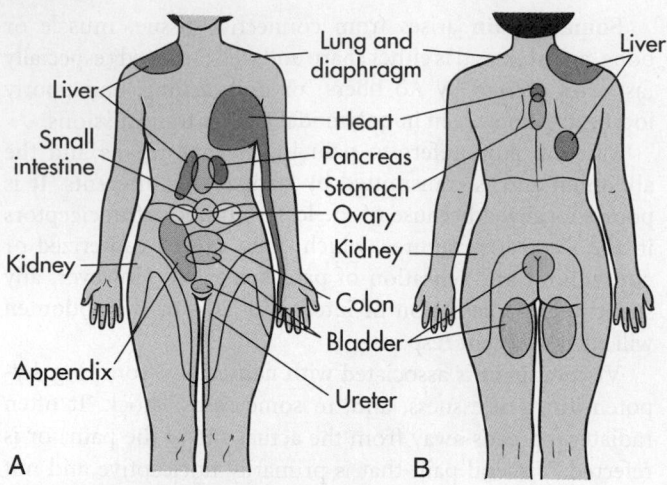

Figure 15-6 Sites of referred pain. A, Front. B, Back.

Chronic Pain

Chronic pain also can be nociceptive, but it is prolonged—usually defined as lasting at least 3 months. Perhaps even more important than the duration of the pain are the attendant physical and emotional issues that often appear to be way out of proportion to any observable tissue injury. Thus the cause of chronic pain often is unknown, and even if the cause is known or suspected, the pain does not respond to usual therapy. Chronic pain may be persistent as in chronic low back pain or occur intermittently as seen in migraine or muscle tension–migraine variant headache syndromes. The onset may be sudden, but chronic pain often develops insidiously so that the individual generally experiences more suffering over time. Individual behavior is adaptive and directed toward modifying the pain. Chronic pain is often associated with a sense of hopelessness and helplessness as relief becomes more elusive and the timeframe more protracted. The pain is perceived as meaningless, and depression is often a concomitant finding, as either a result of the chronic pain state or as a contributor to its development. It is significantly more difficult to manage than acute pain, and complete relief usually is never obtained (see Table 15-2).

Physiologic responses to chronic pain depend on whether it is persistent or intermittent. Intermittent pain produces a physiologic response similar to that of acute pain (i.e., tachycardia, diaphoresis, elevated blood pressure, etc). Persistent, chronic pain, however, allows for physiologic adaptation so that a person with chronic pain may have normal heart and respiratory rates and normal blood pressure. The absence of acute physiologic responses has led many to mistakenly assume that people in chronic pain are malingering because they do not appear to be in pain.

Chronic pain produces significant behavioral and psychologic changes.[33] Individuals with chronic pain often are depressed, have difficulty sleeping and eating, and may become preoccupied with the pain.[34] Living with chronic pain requires constant attention to the earliest signs of pain so that the pain-provoking stimuli can be identified and avoided. People with chronic pain generally attempt to keep pain-related behavior to a minimum so that they appear as normal as possible. A desire for the validation of the pain and the need to hide the pain are usually conflicting drives for those with chronic pain. They tend not to report pain for fear of being labeled complainers. They often deny pain and sometimes engage in activities that provoke pain in an effort to keep up with others. Even in learning to pace themselves throughout the day's activities, they may inadvertently aggravate the pain.[35]

Chronic pain states are thought to arise from a misinterpretation of nociceptive input—an imbalance of neuromodulation controls such as might occur with a decreased level of endorphins or a predominance of C-neuron stimulation[36,37] (Table 15-3). The following mechanisms have been implicated in the initiation and entrenchment of chronic pain states[38,39]:

- Changes in sensitivity of neurons—lower threshold with peripheral and central sensitization
- Spontaneous impulses from regenerating peripheral nerves
- Alterations in the dorsal root ganglion in response to peripheral nerve injury and neurotransmitters—reorganization of nociceptive neurons (deafferentation pain)
- Loss of pain inhibition in the spinal cord
- Up-regulation of chemokines and their receptors

The most common chronic, disabling pain condition in the United States is persistent *low back pain*, which became a medical disaster in the twentieth century. Over the past few decades much has been learned about back pain—where back pain fits into the pain spectrum and how people react to and are affected by it. Predictions that chronic low back pain (and the disability arising from it) would be reducing are unfounded; instead both the report of low back pain and the accompanying disability are on the rise. Recent figures estimate that 7% to 14% of adults in the United States have some disability related to back pain, and 1% to 2% of the population are totally disabled by back pain at any given time.[40,41]

Myofascial pain syndrome (MPS) is associated with injury to muscle, fascia and tendons and include myositis, fibrositis, myofibrositis, myalgia, and muscle strain. These conditions involve myofascial trigger points within a taut band of skeletal muscle.[42] The pain may be the result of low-threshold mechanosensitive afferents projecting to sensitized dorsal horn neurons.[43] Compression of the trigger point causes referred pain, motor dysfunction, and autonomic responses. During the early stages of the disorder the pain is localized, but as the disorder progresses it becomes deep, aching, and more generalized. These, like many other chronic conditions, begin as a result of poor muscle tone, inactivity, muscle or tendon strain, or sudden vigorous exercise and can evolve into a chronic pain state.

Chronic postoperative pain occurs in some individuals and includes complex regional pain syndrome, phantom limb pain, chronic donor site pain, post-thoracotomy pain syndrome, postmastectomy pain syndrome, and joint arthroplasty pain. Plastic changes in the peripheral nervous system (PNS)

Table 15-3   Common Chronic Pain Conditions

Condition	Description
Persistent low back pain	Most common chronic pain condition
	Results from poor muscle tone, inactivity, muscle strain, or sudden, vigorous exercise
Myofascial pain syndromes	Second most common chronic pain condition
	Pain results from muscle spasm, tenderness, and stiffness
	Examples include myositis, fibrositis, myofibrositis, myalgia, and muscle strain—conditions that involve injury to the muscle and fascia
	As disorder progresses, pain becomes increasingly generalized
Chronic postoperative pain	Chronic pain that can occur with disruption or cutting of sensory nerves
Cancer pain	Can be pain attributed to advance of disease, associated with treatment, or attributed to coexisting disease entities
Deafferentation pain	Painful condition resulting from damage to a peripheral nerve
	Common types include severe burning pain triggered by various stimuli, such as cold, light touch, or sound, and reflex sympathetic dystrophies (occur after peripheral nerve injury and are characterized by continuous, severe, burning pain associated with vasomotor changes and muscle wasting)
Hyperesthesias	Increased sensitivity and decreased pain threshold to tactile and painful stimuli
	Pain is diffuse, modified by fatigue and emotion and mixed with other sensations
	May result from chronic irritations of central nervous system areas
Hemiagnosia	Loss of ability to identify source of pain on one side of the body
	Painful stimuli on that side produce discomfort, anxiety, moaning, agitation, and distress but no attempt to withdraw from the stimulus
	Associated with stroke
Phantom limb pain	Pain experienced in amputated limb after stump has completely healed; may be immediate or occur months later
	Influenced by emotions or sympathetic stimulation
	Trigger points—small hypersensitive regions in muscle or connective tissues that, when stimulated, produce pain in a specific area

and CNS contribute to pain development, and multimodal approaches to analgesia are needed for pain management.[44,45]

Cancer pain is often chronic and associated with neuropathies. Studies done at Memorial Sloan-Kettering Cancer Center indicate three major categories of pain syndromes that result in chronic pain in the individual with cancer.[46] The categories are (1) pain attributed to the advance of the disease, (2) pain associated with treatment of the disease, and (3) pain attributed to coexisting entities (e.g., osteoarthritis) that are unrelated to the disease. Cancer pain is by far the most common cause of chronic pain attributed to the advance of an identifiable disease.[46] Pain can be caused by infection and inflammation, increasing pressure of a growing tumor on nerve endings, tissue destruction, stretching of visceral surfaces, or obstruction of ducts and intestine. Therapeutic approaches to the management of cancer pain have advanced significantly in recent years, particularly in palliative care and hospice programs.[47] Frequent pain assessment, management of breakthrough pain and implementation of therapeutic strategies including pharmacotherapy, anesthetic, neurosurgical, psychologic, and rehabilitation techniques and frequent evaluations are essential to optimal cancer pain management.[48-50]

Neuropathic Pain

Neuropathic pain is the result of trauma or disease of nerves and leads to long term plastic changes along somatosensory pathways from the periphery to cortex and abnormal processing of sensory information by the PNS and CNS.[51] Most neuropathic pain seen commonly in clinical practice is chronic. Chronic neuropathic pain syndromes can be divided into two groups based on a central or peripheral location of the nervous system lesion.[52] Examples of peripheral causes of neuropathic pain include trauma, diabetic or alcohol abuse–induced neuropathy, carcinoma, and human immunodeficiency virus (HIV). Examples of central causes of neuropathic pain include brain or spinal cord trauma, tumors, vascular lesions, multiple sclerosis, postherpetic neuralgia (PHN), phantom limb pain, and reflex sympathetic dystrophy. Diabetic neuropathy (PDN) and post herpetic neuralgia are both significant causes of neuropathic pain.[53] Neuropathic pain is often paroxysmal with paresthesias (tingling sensations of pins and needles), burning, shooting, or stabbing sensations. Neuropathic pain is often described as "gnawing" and miserable. Pain sensation can occur in the absence of a stimulus, be evoked by movement (*incident pain*), and hypersensitivity and/or allodynia may be present in the involved body part. No single diagnostic test for neuropathic pain (or for pain in general) is available, and differentiating some neuropathies from other chronic somatic pain syndromes can be difficult.[54] When injured nerves become hyperexcitable, they generate ectopic discharges, resulting in spontaneous firing of some neurons with low thresholds for mechanical, chemical, or thermal stimuli.[55,56] Injury resulting in a permanent loss of sensory input from a part of the body is called *deafferentation*, and differentiates peripheral neuropathic pain syndromes from central forms of the disease.

Deafferentation pain results from trauma or chemical injury to the peripheral nervous system; tumor infiltration of nerve tissue; or damage from radiation, chemotherapy, or surgical sectioning of a nerve with loss of sensory input to the CNS. It is associated with hyperactivity of the somatosensory thalamus and cortex.[57] Deafferentation pain, which is poorly controlled by many analgesics, is usually described as a constant, dull, viselike ache, accompanied by paroxysms of burning or electric shock-like sensations.[58,59]

Central pain is neuropathic and is caused by a lesion or dysfunction in the CNS (brain or spinal cord) and may be related to alterations in thalamocortical transmission.[60] The lesions of central pain can include infarction, hemorrhage, abscess, degeneration, tumors, or traumatic injury and can develop in diseases such as Parkinson disease and multiple sclerosis. The pain may manifest over a large and diffuse area or be well defined and circumscribed. It is usually irritating and constant, can be difficult to treat, and can cause considerable suffering. *Hemiagnosia pain* is one form of central pain associated with stroke that produces paralysis and a hypersensitivity/allodynia on one half of the body. In this painful condition, often a concomitant loss of ability to identify the source of pain through normal sensory pathways occurs. The result is a confusing picture in which even mild stimulation of the affected side of the body produces discomfort, anxiety, moaning, agitation, and distress, with a diminished ability to withdraw from the offending stimulus. *Thalamic pain* is another form of central pain that involves lesions in the thalamus.

Phantom limb pain is pain that an individual feels in an amputated limb after the stump has completely healed. Nonpainful phantom limb sensations occur in almost all amputees, but the sensations usually fade with time. This is distinguished from the syndrome of phantom limb pain, a chronic pain occurring in 80% to 100% of amputees.[61,62] It is more likely to appear in individuals who experienced pain in the limb before amputation. Theories about the cause of phantom limb pain include regeneration or activity of injured or cut peripheral nerves, scar tissue or neuroma formation in the cut peripheral nerves, spinal cord deafferentation, and alterations in the thalamus and cortex. It has been proposed that CNS integration, including reorganization and plastic changes of the somatosensory cortex, results in the perception of pain from receptors associated with the amputated limb even though the limb itself is no longer present[63,64] (see What's New? The Concept of a Neuromatrix and Pain). The cause is likely multifactorial, contributing to the difficulty of prevention or effective treatment.

Sympathetically maintained pain (SMP) is another type of neuropathic pain that occurs after peripheral nerve or extremity injury and is characterized as continuous and severe with a burning quality. Sympathetically maintained pain is often associated with vasospasm and vasomotor changes in the affected limb. The diseases formerly called *reflex sympathetic dystrophy* and *causalgia*, both thought to arise from sympathetic nervous system imbalance, are now called **complex regional pain syndromes (CRPSs)**, types I and II. CRPS develops 1 to 2 weeks after an extremity injury (i.e., a fracture without identifiable nerve injury) (type I—reflex sympathetic dystrophy) or injury to the brachial plexus, the median, sciatic, or other peripheral nerves (type II—causalgia). The exact pathophysiology is unclear, but a combination of injury and the presence of inflammatory cytokines and neuropeptides may lead to peripheral nociceptive sensitization and physiologic change in pain transmission and autonomic and motor systems.[65] The severe, diffuse, and persistent pain occurs in the extremity supplied by the injured nerve. Discoloration and changes in the texture of the skin may appear in the affected area. Vasomotor changes usually begin with vasodilation and are followed by vasoconstriction and cool, cyanotic, and edematous extremities. Excessive nail growth may be noted, and swelling and stiffness of proximate joints may occur. Hair loss is usually noted, and allodynia is often prominent, disabling, and difficult to treat.[66-68]

In the evaluation and management of neuropathic pain, as well as all other chronic pain states, psychologic components (e.g., depression or anxiety), sleep disturbances,

---

WHAT'S NEW?   The Concept of a Neuromatrix and Pain

Ronald Melzack proposes a neuromatrix theory of chronic pain that amends the gate control theory and provides new directions for pain research. Chronic pain is theorized to be a multidimensional experience produced by patterns of nerve impulses known as *neurosignatures*. These nerve impulses are generated in the brain by a widely distributed network known as the *body-self neuromatrix*. The *body-self* represents the unique distinction of the self with unity of feeling, experiences, and genetic predisposition. It is multidimensional, including sensory, cognitive, affective, postural, evaluative, and other components. The *neuromatrix* is composed of centers and loops of neurons in the brain whose links and synapses are initially determined genetically but can be changed and modified by sensory inputs. The neurosignature patterns may be triggered by sensory inputs from the body or may originate in the brain independently of peripheral sensory input. It is the output, not input, of the widely distributed neuromatrix that generates the neurosignature pattern of pain. This explains most types of chronic pain in which there is no discernible cause or correlation between pathology and pain (e.g., phantom limb pain and neuropathies). The neuromatrix theory also provides a rationale for various alternative approaches to pain management. In summary, neuromatrix theory suggests that the brain can detect and analyze inputs and generate perceptual experience when no external input is evoked by injury, inflammation, or other pathology. It is representative of the nervous system's plasticity. Neuromatrix theory provides a wholistic, integrated, dynamic consideration of pain.

Data from Giummarra MJ et al: *Brain Res Rev* 54(1):219-232, 2007; Melzack R: Toward a new concept of pain for the new millennium. In Waldman SD, editor: *Interventional pain management*, ed 2, Philadelphia, 2001, Saunders; Moseley GL: *Man Ther* 8(3):130-140, 2003; Trout KK: *J Midwifery Womens Health* 49(6):482-488, 2004; Yoo SS et al: *Neuroimage* 22(2):932-940.

work-related issues of impairment and disability, treatment expectations, the availability of social support from family and friends (or lack thereof) and legal compensation should not be overlooked.[69]

Pediatrics and Perception of Pain

Children and infants have the anatomic and functional ability to perceive pain. Pain pathways and cortical and subcortical centers for pain perception, as well as neurochemicals associated with pain transmission and modulation, are functional in preterm and newborn infants.[70] The nociceptor system is functional in fetuses by 20 to 24 weeks of gestation although the cortical experience may be minimal.[71] Repetitive, painful experiences and prolonged exposure to analgesic drugs in infants during the neonatal period may permanently alter synaptic and neuronal organization,[72] and fetal pain may have an enduring effect on behavior and pain perception.[73]

Facial expression, crying, body movements, and lack of consolability are the most consistent expressions of pain in infants. The painful facial expression includes lowered brows drawn together; presence of a vertical bulge and furrows in the forehead between the brows; broadened nasal root; tightly closed, scourged eye fissures; and angular, squarish mouth and chin quiver (Figure 15-7). Physiologic responses include increases in heart rate, blood pressure, and respiratory rate. There may be flushing or pallor, sweating, and decreased oxygen saturation.[74] Toddlers also express pain with crying, facial expression, and body

language (tensed body, guarding, and hands holding body). Older children, between ages 5 and 18 years, tend to have a lower pain threshold than do adults. Children, like adults, have highly individual responses to pain. Any pain must be carefully and accurately assessed [75] and adequately treated for children of all ages.[76]

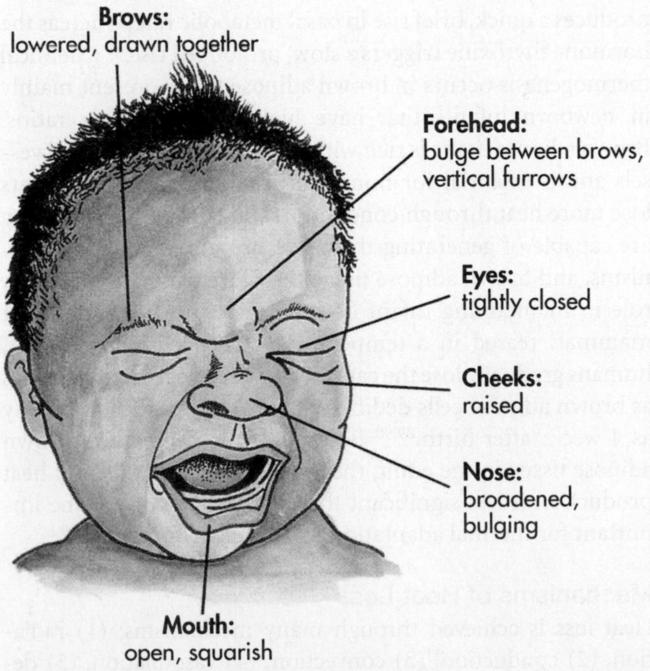

Aging and Perception of Pain

Studies on pain perception in the older adult population have yielded conflicting evidence. Some studies show an increase in pain threshold with aging; others show no change.[77,78] The varied results are probably a function of independent variation in the sensory-discriminative, motivational-affective, and cognitive-evaluative components of the pain experience. In general, studies confirm that an increase in the pain threshold occurs in some older adults. This change may be caused by peripheral neuropathies and changes in the thickness of the skin.[79] (Neuropathies are discussed in Chapter 17.) A decrease in pain tolerance is also evident in some older adults, and women appear to be more sensitive to pain than are men[80] (see What's New? Pain and Gender). Pain in the older adult is also influenced by liver and renal function, including alterations in metabolism of drugs and metabolites and age-associated brain changes. Pain must be accurately assessed in relation to its effect on cognitive function, coexisting disease, drug interactions, other reactions to treatment, and an individual's ability to express pain.[81] Poorly managed pain can result in depression, inactivity, and failure to maintain activities of daily living.[82-84]

Figure 15-7 Painful facial expression of infants. (From Hockenberry MJ: *Wong's nursing care of infants and children,* ed 7, St Louis, 2003, Mosby.)

Brows: lowered, drawn together

Forehead: bulge between brows, vertical furrows

Eyes: tightly closed

Cheeks: raised

Nose: broadened, bulging

Mouth: open, squarish

WHAT'S NEW?   Pain and Gender

Gender and sex differences in the experience of pain and response to analgesics have been documented in both animal and human research. Women report higher pain levels or have less tolerance for pain stimulus intensities, or both. Gender differences exist also in the prevalence of painful diseases; for example, women are more affected by intestinal cystitis, fibromyalgia, and rheumatoid arthritis, and men are more affected by cluster headache. Pain symptoms differ for men and women for diseases such as coronary artery disease, irritable bowel syndrome, appendicitis, and cancer. Sex hormones are known to have an effect on the mechanisms and outcomes of opiate analgesia, and in rodents, morphine analgesia is greater in males than in females. Pain sensitivities in women also vary across the phases of the menstrual cycle. A recent human study now suggests that κ-opioid receptor analgesia is greater in women than in men and may reflect a difference in endogenous pain circuits activated by different opiate receptor subtypes. Gender differences with respect to pain also are influenced by role socialization, cognitive factors, and culture. Continuing research is needed to further understanding of gender differences in the operation of pain mechanisms and the development of more specific pain management strategies.

Data from Craft RM: *Pain* 132(Suppl 1):S3-S12, 2007; Dahan A et al: *Anesth Analg* 107(1):83-95, 2008; Greenspan JD et al: *Pain* 132 (Suppl 1):S26-S45, 2007; Hurley RW, Adams MC: *Anesth Analg* 107(1):4-5, 2008; Wiesenfeld-Hallin Z: *Gender Med* 2(3)137-145, 2005.

TEMPERATURE REGULATION

In all homeothermic animals, temperature regulation is achieved through precise balancing of heat production, heat conservation, and heat loss. In humans, body temperature is maintained around 37° C (98.6° F) and rarely exceeds 41° C. The normal range is 36.2° to 37.7° C (97.2° to 99.9° F), but all parts of the body do not have the same temperature. The extremities, for example, are generally cooler than the trunk. The temperature at the core of the body (as measured by rectal temperature) is generally 0.5° C higher than at the surface (as measured by oral temperature) and has minimal fluctuations. The internal temperature varies normally in response to activity, environmental temperature, and daily fluctuation of **circadian rhythm** (the pattern of each 24-hour day). Oral temperatures generally fluctuate within 0.2° to 0.5° C over a 24-hour period. Women tend to have wider fluctuations that follow the menstrual cycle, with a sharp rise in temperature just before ovulation. In both sexes the daily fluctuating temperature peaks around 6 PM and is at its lowest during sleep.[85] Maintenance of body temperature within the normal range is necessary for life.

Hypothalamic Control of Temperature

Temperature regulation is mediated by thermoregulatory centers in the hypothalamus.[86] Peripheral thermoreceptors in the skin and central thermoreceptors in the hypothalamus, spinal cord, abdominal organs, and other central locations provide the hypothalamus with information about skin and core temperatures. If these temperatures are low or high, the hypothalamus responds by triggering heat production, heat conservation, or heat loss mechanisms.

Increased **heat production** is initiated by a series of hormonal mechanisms involving the hypothalamus and its connections with the endocrine system (see Chapter 20). The heat-producing mechanism begins with a hypothalamic hormone, thyroid-stimulating hormone-releasing hormone (TSH-RH). In turn, TSH-RH stimulates the anterior pituitary to release TSH, which acts on the thyroid gland, stimulating release of thyroxine (T_4), one of the thyroid hormones. This hormone then acts on the adrenal medulla, causing the release of epinephrine (a catecholamine and vasopressive hormone) into the bloodstream (see Chapter 20). Epinephrine causes vasoconstriction, stimulates glycolysis, and increases metabolic rates, thus increasing heat production.

The hypothalamus also triggers heat conservation. The mechanisms of heat conservation involve stimulating the sympathetic nervous system, which is responsible for stimulating the adrenal cortex, increasing skeletal muscle tone, initiating the shivering response, and producing vasoconstriction. The hypothalamus also functions in raising body temperatures by relaying information to the cerebral cortex. Awareness of cold provokes voluntary responses such as increased body movement and adding protective clothing.

The hypothalamus responds to warmer core and peripheral temperatures by reversing the same mechanisms. The TSH-RH pathway is shut down. The sympathetic pathway is prompted to produce cutaneous vasodilation, decreased muscle tone, and increased sweat production. Hypothalamic stimulation of the cerebral cortex provokes voluntary measures to reduce heat production and promote heat loss.

Mechanisms of Heat Production

Body heat is produced by the chemical reactions of metabolism, skeletal muscle tone and contraction, and chemical thermogenesis. Heat is distributed by the circulatory system.

Chemical Reactions of Metabolism

The chemical reactions that occur during the ingestion and metabolism of food and those required to maintain the body at rest (basal metabolism) require energy and give off heat. These processes occur in the body core (primarily the liver) and are in part responsible for the maintenance of core temperature.

Skeletal Muscle Contraction

Skeletal muscles produce heat through two mechanisms: (1) gradual increase in muscle tone and (2) rapid muscle oscillations (shivering—which does not occur in neonates). Both increasing muscle tone and *shivering* are controlled by the posterior hypothalamus and occur in response to cold. As peripheral temperature drops, muscle tone increases and shivering begins. Shivering is a fairly effective method for increasing heat production because no work is performed and all the energy produced is retained as heat.[87]

Chemical Thermogenesis

Chemical thermogenesis, also called *nonshivering thermogenesis* or *adrenergic thermogenesis,* results from the release of epinephrine and norepinephrine. Epinephrine and norepinephrine produce a rapid, transient increase in heat production by raising the body's basal metabolic rate. Chemical thermogenesis seems to be different from hormone-triggered increases in the basal metabolic rate. Chemical thermogenesis produces a quick, brief rise in basal metabolic rate, whereas the hormone thyroxine triggers a slow, prolonged rise.[88] Chemical thermogenesis occurs in brown adipose tissue present mainly in newborn infants that have high surface:volume ratios. Brown adipose tissue is rich with mitochondria and blood vessels and is essential for nonshivering thermogenesis. Infants lose more heat through conduction and convection than they are capable of generating through normal metabolic mechanisms, and brown adipose tissue therefore plays an important role in maintaining infant body temperature. As with most mammals reared in a temperature-controlled environment, humans gradually lose the capacity for chemical thermogenesis as brown adipose cells dedifferentiate. This can occur as early as 4 weeks after birth.[89,90] Because of the decrease in brown adipose tissue in the adult, the role of this mechanism of heat production is less significant than in infants, but may be important for thermal adaptation in cold environments.[91,92]

Mechanisms of Heat Loss

Heat loss is achieved through many mechanisms: (1) radiation, (2) conduction, (3) convection, (4) vasodilation, (5) decreased muscle tone, (6) evaporation, (7) increased respiration, (8) voluntary measures, and (9) adaptation to warmer climates.

Radiation

Radiation refers to heat loss through electromagnetic waves. These waves emanate from surfaces with temperatures higher than the surrounding air. Thus if the temperature of the skin is higher than that of the air, the skin and therefore the body lose heat to the air.

Conduction

Conduction refers to heat loss by direct molecule-to-molecule transfer from one surface to another. Through conduction, the warmer surface loses heat to the cooler surface. Thus the skin loses heat through direct contact with cooler air, water, or another surface. In the same manner, the core of the body loses heat to the cooler body surface.

Convection

Convection is the transfer of heat through currents of gases or liquids. It greatly aids heat loss through conduction by exchanging warmer air at the surface of the body with cooler air in the surrounding space. Convection occurs passively as warmer air at the surface of the body rises away from the body and is replaced by cooler air, but the process may be aided by fans or wind. (The combined effect of conduction and convection by wind is conventionally measured as the *windchill factor*.)

Vasodilation

Peripheral vasodilation increases heat loss by diverting core-warmed blood to the surface of the body. As the core-warmed blood passes through the periphery, heat is transferred by conduction to the skin surface and from the skin to the surrounding environment. Because heat loss through conduction depends on the surrounding temperature, it is minimal to nonexistent if the surrounding air or water is warmer than the body surface.

Vasodilation occurs in response to autonomic stimulation under the control of the hypothalamus. It is useful in instances of moderate temperature elevation. As core temperature increases, vasodilation increases until maximal dilation is achieved. At that point the body must use additional heat loss mechanisms.

Decreased Muscle Tone

To decrease heat production, muscle tone may be moderately reduced and voluntary muscle activity curtailed. These mechanisms explain in part the "washed-out" feeling associated with high temperatures and warm weather. Decreased muscle tone and reduced activity have a limited effect on decreasing heat production; however, because muscle tone and heat production cannot be reduced below basal body requirements.

Evaporation

Evaporation of body water from the surface of the skin and the linings of the mucous membranes is a major source of heat reduction. Insensible water loss (in the absence of perceptible sweating) accounts for a loss of about 600 ml of water per day. Heat is lost as surface fluid is converted to gas, so that heat loss by evaporation is increased if more fluids are available at the body surface. To speed this process, fluids are actively secreted through the sweat glands.

As much as 2.2 L of fluid per hour may be lost by sweating. Electrolytes are lost with the water. Therefore, loss of large volumes through sweating may result in decreased plasma volume, decreased blood pressure, weakness, and fainting. (Alterations in fluid balance are discussed in Chapter 3.)

Like other heat reduction mechanisms, stimulation of sweating occurs in response to sympathetic neural activity and depends on a favorable temperature difference between the body and the environment. In addition, heat loss through evaporation is affected by the relative humidity of the air. If the humidity is low, sweat evaporates quickly, but if the humidity is high, sweat does not evaporate and instead remains on the skin or drips off.

Increased Pulmonary Ventilation

Exchanging air with the environment through the normal pulmonary ventilation provides some heat loss, although it is minimal in humans. As air is inhaled, the air draws heat from the upper respiratory tract. The air is further warmed in the alveoli by blood in the microcirculation. This warmed air then is exhaled into the environment. This normal process occurs faster at higher body temperatures through an increase in ventilatory rates. Thus hyperventilation is associated with hyperthermia. (Normal pulmonary function is discussed in Chapter 32.)

Voluntary Mechanisms

In response to high body temperatures, people physically "stretch out," thereby increasing the body surface area available for heat loss. They also "slow down" or "take it easy," thereby decreasing skeletal muscle work, and they "dress for warm weather" with light-colored, loose-fitting garments to reflect heat and promote convection, conduction, and evaporation.

Adaptation to Warmer Climates

The body of an individual who moves from a cooler to a much warmer climate undergoes a period of adjustment, a process that takes several days to weeks. At first the individual experiences feelings of lassitude, weakness, and faintness with even moderate activity. Body temperatures rise with any work. Within several days, however, the individual experiences an earlier onset of sweating, the volume of sweat is increased, and the sodium content is lowered. Heart rate is decreased and stroke volume increased so that cardiac output remains unchanged. Extracellular fluid volume increases, as does plasma volume. These physiologic adaptations result in improved warm weather functioning and decreased symptoms of heat intolerance. People's work output, endurance, and coordination increase, and their subjective feelings of discomfort decrease.[93]

Mechanisms of Heat Conservation

The body conserves heat and protects core temperature through two important mechanisms: (1) involuntary vasoconstriction mediated by the sympathetic nervous system and (2) voluntary mechanisms.[94] To preserve core temperature, the skin and periphery are used as an insulating cover.[93]

Vasoconstriction

By constricting peripheral blood vessels, centrally warmed blood is shunted away from the periphery (where radiation, conduction, and convection would allow heat loss) to the core of the body, where heat can be retained. This mechanism takes advantage of the insulating layers of the skin and subcutaneous fat to protect core temperature.

Voluntary Mechanisms

In response to lower body temperatures, individuals typically "bundle up," "keep moving," or "curl up in a ball." Bundling up involves dressing with several layers of clothes that allow air to be trapped between the skin and the clothing, thus providing an additional layer of insulation. Keeping moving, stamping feet, clapping hands, jogging, and other types of physical activity increase skeletal muscle activity and thus promote heat production. Curling up in a ball decreases the amount of skin surface available for heat loss through radiation, convection, and conduction.

Pediatrics and Changes in Temperature Regulation

Infants and older adults require special attention to maintenance of body temperature. Infants produce sufficient body heat but are unable to efficiently conserve it. This poor heat conservation is caused by the infant's small body size and greater ratio of body surface to body weight, which gives the infant more surface area for heat loss. Infants also have a very thin layer of subcutaneous fat and thus are not as well insulated as adults.[95]

Aging and Changes in Temperature Regulation

Older adults have poor responses to environmental temperature extremes as a result of slowed blood circulation, structural and functional changes in the skin, and an overall decrease in heat-producing activities. Other factors affecting thermal regulation in the older adult population include decreased shivering response (delayed onset and decreased effectiveness), slowed metabolic rate, sedentary lifestyle, decreased vasoconstrictor and vasodilator responses, diminished or absent sweating, desynchronization of circadian rhythm, undernutrition, and decreased perception of heat and cold.[96,97]

Pathogenesis of Fever

Fever is part of the acute phase response to infection or inflammation (see Chapter 9). Fever is a complex, integrated cascade of behavioral, neurologic, and endocrine responses to an immune challenge initiated by endogenous pyrogens or disorders of the hypothalamus. It is a normal adaptive response to cytokines and prostaglandin E_2 (PGE_2).[98] The thermoregulatory mechanisms of the hypothalamus and brainstem adjust heat production, conservation, and loss to maintain body core temperature at a normal level. During fever this level is raised so that the thermoregulatory centers adjust heat production, conservation, and loss to maintain the core temperature at the new, higher temperature, which functions as a new balance point or set point.[86,98]

The pathophysiology of fever begins with the introduction of **exogenous pyrogens** (i.e., endotoxins from gram-negative bacteria) (Figure 15-8). The most frequently encountered exogenous pyrogens are the lipopolysaccharide complex in the cell wall of gram-positive bacteria and viruses.[99] **Endogenous pyrogens**, including PGE_2, interleukin-1 (IL-1), IL-6, TNF-α), and interferon-γ, are produced by phagocytic cells as they destroy microorganisms within the host.[100] The endogenous pyrogens act on the preoptic nucleus of the hypothalamus to produce the late phases of fever. An integrated behavioral, endocrine, and autonomic nervous system response is then initiated. Centers in the hypothalamus and brainstem signal an increase in heat production and heat conservation to raise body temperature to the new set point. Peripheral vasoconstriction occurs with shunting of blood from the skin to the body core. Epinephrine release increases metabolic rate, and muscle tone increases. Decreased release of vasopressin reduces the volume of body fluid to be heated. Shivering also may occur. The individual dresses more warmly, decreases body surface area by curling up, and may go to bed in an effort to get warm. Body temperature is maintained at the new level until the fever "breaks."

During fever, arginine vasopressin (AVP), α-melanocyte-stimulating hormone (α-MSH), and corticotropin-releasing factor are released from the brain, and systemic anti-inflammatory cytokines (i.e., IL-1 receptor agonist and IL-10) can act as **endogenous cryogens** or **antipyretics** to help diminish the febrile response.[101] This antipyretic effect constitutes a negative-feedback loop (see Figure 15-8). The antipyretic effect may help explain fluctuations in the febrile response. When the fever breaks, the set point is returned to normal. The hypothalamus responds by signaling a decrease in heat production and an increase in heat-reduction mechanisms. The result is decreased muscle tone, peripheral vasodilation, flushed skin, and sweating. The individual feels very warm, replaces warm clothing with cooler clothes, throws off the covers, and stretches out. Once the body has returned to a normal temperature, the individual feels more comfortable and the hypothalamus adjusts thermoregulatory mechanisms to maintain the new temperature.

Benefits of Fever

Fever production aids responses to infectious processes through several mechanisms.[102] A raised body temperature kills many microorganisms and has adverse effects on the growth and replication of others. Higher body temperatures decrease serum levels of iron, zinc, and copper, all of which are needed for bacterial replication. The body switches from burning glucose to a metabolism based on lipolysis and proteolysis, thereby depriving bacteria of a food source. Anorexia and somnolence reduce the demand for muscle glucose.[103] Increased temperature also causes lysosomal breakdown and autodestruction of cells, thus preventing viral replication in infected cells. Acute-phase proteins produced by the liver

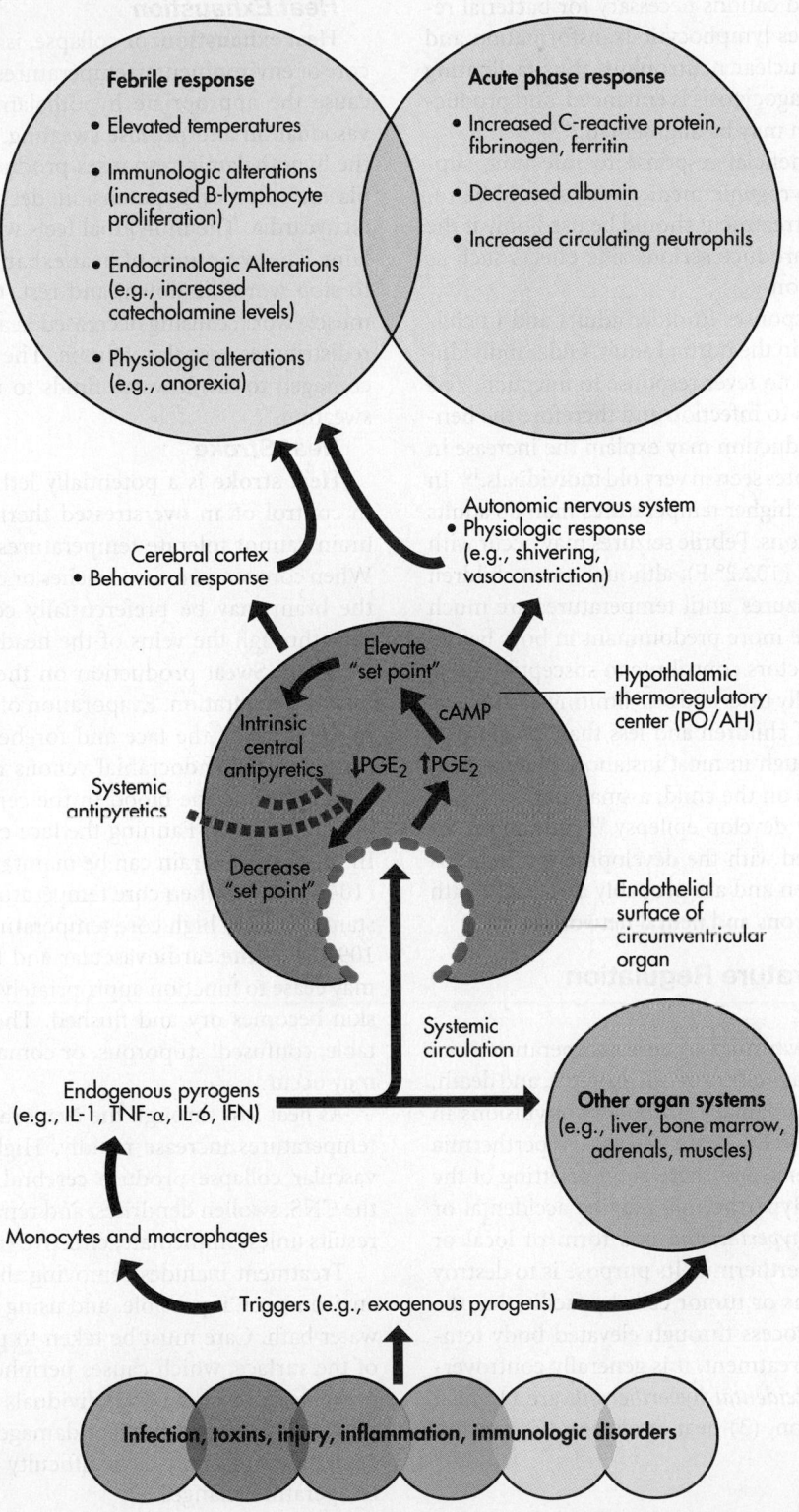

Figure 15-8 Pathogenesis of fever and acute-phase response. Certain disease states, through the elaboration of exogenous pyrogens, stimulate monocytes and macrophages to produce endogenous pyrogens such as IL-1, IL-6, TNF-α, and interferon-γ. These pyrogenic cytokines act at the endothelial surface of the circumventricular organ of the preoptic area of the anterior hypothalamus (PO/AH) to induce the production of PGE₂, which elevates the body's thermal set point. Physiologic and behavioral responses may be invoked to raise body temperature to a new set point. This febrile response must be considered in the context of an overlapping acute-phase response as a global nonspecific response to the original insult. Intrinsic central antipyretics and systemic antipyretics exert their effects by decreasing levels of PGE₂, decreasing the "set point" and lowering body temperature. The red dotted line represents a negative feedback response. *cAMP,* Cyclic adenosine monophosphate; *IFN,* interferon; *IL-1, IL-6,* interleukin-1, interleukin-6; *PGE₂,* prostaglandin E₂, *TNF-α,* tumor necrosis factor-alpha. (Modified from Armstrong D, Cohen J: *Infectious diseases,* 2nd ed, St Louis, 2004, Mosby.)

during inflammation bind cations necessary for bacterial reproduction. Heat increases lymphocytic transformation and motility of polymorphonuclear neutrophils, thus facilitating the immune response. Phagocytosis is enhanced, and production of antiviral interferon may be augmented.[104,105]

Because fever is a beneficial response to infection, suppressing fever with antipyrogenic medications should be reviewed carefully.[106] Such treatment should be used only if the fever is high enough to produce serious side effects such as nerve damage or convulsion.

Infection and fever responses in older adults and in children may vary from those in the normal adult. Older individuals may have decreased or no fever response to infection. The absence of fever responses to infection and therefore the beneficial aspects of fever production may explain the increase in morbidity and mortality rates seen in very old individuals.[107] In contrast, children develop higher temperatures than do adults for relatively minor infections. Febrile seizures may occur with temperatures above 39° C (102.2° F), although most children do not develop febrile seizures until temperatures are much higher. Febrile seizures are more predominant in boys before age 5 years, and genetic factors contribute to susceptibility.[108] Febrile seizures are generally brief and self-limiting, lasting less than 5 minutes in 40% of children and less than 20 minutes in 75% of children. Although in most instances there appear to be no long-term effects on the child, a small percentage of children (1% to 2%) may develop epilepsy.[109] Prolonged febrile seizures are associated with the development of temporal lobe epilepsy in children and are probably associated with functional changes in neurons and neural networks.[110]

Disorders of Temperature Regulation

Hyperthermia

Hyperthermia (marked warming of core temperature) can produce nerve damage, coagulation of cell proteins, and death. At 41° C (105.8° F), nerve damage produces convulsions in the adult. At 43° C (109.4° F), death results. Hyperthermia is not mediated by pyrogens, and there is no resetting of the hypothalamic set point. Hyperthermia may be accidental or therapeutic. *Therapeutic hyperthermia* is a form of local or general body-induced hyperthermia. Its purpose is to destroy pathologic microorganisms or tumor cells by facilitating the host's natural immune process through elevated body temperature.[111] As a form of treatment, it is generally controversial. The four forms of *accidental hyperthermia* are (1) heat cramps, (2) heat exhaustion, (3) heat stroke, and (4) malignant hyperthermia.[112]

Heat Cramps

Heat cramps are severe spasmodic cramps in the abdomen and extremities that follow prolonged sweating and associated sodium loss. Heat cramps usually appear in individuals who are not accustomed to heat or in those who are performing strenuous work in very warm climates. Fever, rapid pulse, and increased blood pressure often accompany the cramps. Treatment involves administration of dilute salt solutions through oral or parenteral routes.

Heat Exhaustion

Heat exhaustion, or collapse, is a result of prolonged high core or environmental temperatures. These high temperatures cause the appropriate hypothalamic response of profound vasodilation and profuse sweating. Over a prolonged period the hypothalamic responses produce dehydration, decreased plasma volumes, hypotension, decreased cardiac output, and tachycardia. The individual feels weak, dizzy, nauseated, and faint. The symptoms of heat exhaustion cause the individual to stop work, lie down, and rest. Ceasing activity decreases muscle work, causing decreased heat production. Lying down redistributes vascular volume. The individual should be encouraged to drink warm fluids to replace fluid lost through sweating.

Heat Stroke

Heat stroke is a potentially lethal result of a breakdown in control of an overstressed thermoregulatory center. The brain cannot tolerate temperatures over 40.5° C (104.9° F). When core temperature reaches or exceeds 40.5° C (104.9° F), the brain may be preferentially cooled by maximal blood flow through the veins of the head and face, specifically the forehead. Sweat production on the face is maintained even during dehydration. Evaporation of the sweat cools the blood in the veins of the face and forehead; the blood then is returned to the endocranial venous network and sinus cavernosus, cooling the blood in the cerebral arterial vessels that lie in proximity. Fanning the face enhances this mechanism. In this way the brain can be maintained temporarily at 40° C (104° F), even when core temperatures are higher.[93,113] In instances of very high core temperatures (40° to 43° C [104° to 109.4° F]), the cardiovascular and thermoregulatory centers may cease to function appropriately. Sweating ceases, and the skin becomes dry and flushed. The individual may be irritable, confused, stuporous, or comatose. Visual disturbances may occur.

As heat loss through the evaporation of sweat ceases, core temperatures increase rapidly. High core temperatures and vascular collapse produce cerebral edema, degeneration of the CNS, swollen dendrites, and renal tubular necrosis. Death results unless immediate, effective treatment is initiated.[114]

Treatment includes removing the person from the warm environment, if possible, and using a cooling blanket or cool water bath. Care must be taken to prevent too rapid cooling of the surface, which causes peripheral vasoconstriction and prevents core cooling. Individuals who recover from heat stroke may have permanent damage to the thermoregulatory center and thus may have difficulty tolerating environmental temperature changes.[115]

Children are more susceptible to heat stroke than adults because (1) they produce more metabolic heat when exercising, (2) they have a greater surface area:mass ratio, and (3) their sweating capacity is less than that of adults.[116]

Malignant Hyperthermia

Malignant hyperthermia is a potentially lethal complication of a rare inherited muscle disorder. The condition is precipitated by the administration of volatile anesthetics and neuromuscular-blocking agents. About 1 in 200 individuals may be at risk for the muscle disorder. Malignant hyperthermia is caused by either increased calcium release or decreased calcium uptake with muscle contraction. This allows intracellular calcium levels to rise, producing sustained, uncoordinated muscle contractions, which in turn increase muscle work, oxygen consumption, and lactic acid production. As a result of these contractions, acidosis develops and temperature rises (body temperature may rise 1° C [1.8° F] every 5 minutes); approximately 5% of those who develop malignant hyperthermia do not survive.[117] Malignant hyperthermia occurs most often in children and young adults immediately after the induction of anesthesia. Sympathetic responses and acidosis produce tachycardia and cardiac dysrhythmias, followed by hypotension, decreased cardiac output, and eventually, cardiac arrest. Increasing temperature, acidosis, hyperkalemia, and hypoxia produce coma-like symptoms in the CNS (including unconsciousness, absent reflexes, fixed pupils, apnea, and sometimes a flat electroencephalogram [EEG]). Oliguria and anuria are common, probably resulting from shock, ischemia, and low cardiac output.[118]

Treatment includes withdrawal of the provoking agents and administration of dantrolene sodium (a skeletal relaxant that inhibits calcium release during muscle contraction). Procainamide (Pronestyl) is used to treat cardiac dysrhythmias. Sodium bicarbonate also may be used. Body temperature can be decreased through use of ice bags, a cooling blanket, and iced saline lavage.[119]

Hypothermia

Hypothermia (core body temperature less than 35° C [95° F]) is caused by prolonged exposure to cold—from 1999 to 2002 there were 4607 deaths reported in the United States.[120] Hypothermia produces vasoconstriction, shivering, alterations in microcirculation, coagulation, and ischemic tissue damage. In a controlled situation, such as a surgical procedure, most tissues can tolerate temperatures as low as 33° C (91.4° F). In severe hypothermia (less than 28° C [82.4° F]), ice crystals forming on the inside of the cell cause cells to rupture and die. Tissue hypothermia slows the rate of chemical reactions (tissue metabolism), increases the viscosity of the blood, slows blood flow through the microcirculation, facilitates blood coagulation, and stimulates profound vasoconstriction. Hypothermia may be accidental or therapeutic. In accidental hypothermia, high energy phosphates (e.g., ATP) are depleted and in therapeutic hypothermia, ATP storage is preserved.[121]

Accidental Hypothermia

Accidental hypothermia (temperature below 35° C [95° F]) is generally the result of sudden immersion in cold water or prolonged exposure to cold environments.[122] At particular risk for accidental hypothermia are young persons and older adults, because thermoregulatory mechanisms are altered in these two groups.[123] Also at risk are individuals with conditions that diminish the ability to generate heat. Such conditions include hypothyroidism, hypopituitarism, decreased

liver function, malnutrition, Parkinson disease, and rheumatoid arthritis. Other risk factors include chronic increased vasodilation and decreased thermoregulatory control caused by cerebral injuries, ketoacidosis, uremia, and drug overdoses.[124,125] In acute hypothermia, peripheral vasoconstriction shunts blood away from the cooler skin to the core in an effort to decrease heat loss, which produces peripheral tissue ischemia. Intermittent reperfusion of the extremities (the Lewis phenomenon) helps preserve peripheral oxygenation. Intermittent peripheral perfusion continues until core temperatures drop dramatically.

The hypothalamic center stimulates **shivering** in an effort to increase heat production. Severe shivering occurs at core temperatures of 35° C (95° F) and continues until core temperature drops to about 30° to 32° C (86° to 89.6° F). Prolonged shivering can lead to exhaustion of liver glycogen stores. Thinking becomes sluggish and coordination is decreased at 34° C (93.2° F). As hypothermia deepens, paradoxical undressing may occur as hypothalamic control of vasoconstriction is lost and vasodilation occurs with loss of core heat to the periphery. The hypothermic individual therefore feels suddenly warm and begins to remove clothing.[126]

At 30° C (86° F), the individual becomes stuporous; heart rate and respiratory rate decline; and cardiac output is diminished. Cerebral blood flow is decreased. Metabolic rate declines, further decreasing core temperature. Sinus node depression occurs with slowing of conduction through the atrioventricular node. In severe hypothermia (core temperature of 26° to 28° C [78.8° to 82.4° F]), pulse and respirations may be undetectable. Acidosis is moderate to severe. Ventricular fibrillation and asystole are common.[124] Surface cooling may cause frostbite and fat necrosis.

If hypothermia is mild, passive rewarming may be sufficient. Passive rewarming includes provision of warm, dry clothes and warm drinks and performance of isometric exercises to increase heat production and minimize heat loss. Core temperature should be checked as soon as possible.[127,128]

If core temperature is greater than 30° C (86° F), active rewarming also may be required. Active rewarming uses warm-water baths, warm blankets, heating pads, and warm oral fluids when the individual is fully alert. Active core rewarming is performed when core temperatures have dropped below 30° C (86° F) or when severe cardiovascular abnormalities appear. Core rewarming may be accomplished through administration of warm intravenous (IV) solutions, warm gastric lavage, warm peritoneal lavage, inhalation of warmed gases, and, in extreme cases, exchange transfusions, warming blood in a pump oxygenator circuit, and mediastinal lavage.[129,130]

Rewarming generally should proceed no faster than a few degrees per hour. (Short-term complications of rewarming are listed in Table 15-4.) Long-term complications include congestive heart failure, hepatic and renal failure, abnormal erythropoiesis, myocardial infarction, pancreatitis, and neurologic dysfunctions.

Table 15-4   Accidental Hypothermia: Complications of Rewarming

Complication	Mechanism
Acidosis	Rewarming stimulates peripheral vasodilation; peripheral blood, returning to the core from the ischemic peripheral tissues, causes a reduction in the pH of core blood
Rewarming shock	As rewarming and vasodilation progress, the body is unable to maintain blood pressure because of reduced fluid volume (from "cold diuresis"), catecholamine depletion (prolonged shivering), and myocardial injury
Deep-ended hypothermia	As colder surface blood is returned to the core, core temperature may drop; this is also referred to as "after fall" or "after drop"
Dysrhythmia	Rewarming places an additional stress on an already severely stressed myocardium

Therapeutic Hypothermia

Therapeutic hypothermia is used to slow metabolism and preserve ischemic tissue after brain trauma or during brain surgery, after cardiac arrest, and in neonatal hypoxic encephalopathy. Hypothermia protects the brain by reduction in metabolic rate, ATP consumption and oxidative stress, reduction of the critical threshold for oxygen delivery, modulation of excitotoxic neurotransmitters, calcium antagonism, preservation of protein synthesis, preservation of the blood-brain barrier and decreased edema formation, and modulation of the inflammatory response.[131] Survival from accidental hypothermia has been reported in individuals with core temperatures at 16° C (60.8° F) and from therapeutic hypothermia with temperatures at 9° C (48.2° F).[132-135]

Trauma

Major body trauma has varying effects on temperature regulation, depending on the body systems involved. Five types of traumatic injury that usually affect temperature regulation are (1) CNS trauma (discussed in Chapter 17), (2) accidental injury, (3) hemorrhagic shock, (4) major surgery, and (5) thermal burns.

Central Nervous System Trauma

CNS trauma that causes CNS damage, inflammation, increased intracranial pressures, or intracranial bleeding typically produces a fever greater than 39° C (102.2° F). This temperature, often referred to as *neurogenic fever,* appears with or without relative bradycardia and is not caused by infection. The temperature is sustained, does not induce sweating, and is highly resistant to antipyretic therapy.[136]

Accidental Injuries

Mild accidental injuries may produce a slight elevation in core temperature. Moderate to severe injuries result in peripheral vasoconstriction with decreased surface and core temperatures. Core temperature is thought to be inversely related to the severity of the injury and may be a result of decreased oxygen transport to the tissues. In severe injuries, shivering is absent and some alteration in thermoregulation is evident.[137]

Hemorrhagic Shock

Loss of blood volume in hemorrhage triggers peripheral vasoconstriction and hypoxia contributing to hypothermia.[138] Risk for subsequent decreases in core temperature

occurs when hemorrhagic shock is treated with unwarmed, volume-expanding solutions and surgery. Volume expansion with warmed solutions is recommended to prevent the deleterious effects of hypothermia on cardiac output, cardiac rhythm, and the immune system.

Major Surgery

Major surgery often induces significant hypothermia through exposure of body cavities to the relatively cool operating room environment, irrigation of body cavities with room temperature solutions, infusion of room temperature intravenous solutions, use of drugs that impair thermoregulatory mechanisms, and inhalation of unwarmed anesthetic agents. Anesthesia induces hypothermia, reduces platelet function, and impairs the coagulation cascade contributing to transfusion requirements and postoperative complications.[139] Use of warmed irrigating and intravenous solutions and perioperative forced air and other warming procedures reduces intraoperative hypothermia and postoperative complications.[140,141]

Thermal Burns

Large burn injuries produce significant hypothermia because of the loss of the skin barrier to fluid evaporation and the loss of control of the microcirculation in the skin. Severe burns also compromise the normal insulation of the skin and subcutaneous tissues. (Burns are discussed in Chapter 46.)

SLEEP

Sleep is an active, multiphase, complex brain process that provides restorative functions and promotes memory consolidation. Several areas of the brain are associated with sleep and sleep-wake cycles. A small group of hypothalamic nerve cells, the **suprachiasmatic nucleus (SCN)**, controls the timing of the sleep-wake cycle and coordinates this cycle with circadian rhythms (24-hour rhythm cycles) in other areas of the brain and other tissues.[142]

Normal sleep has two phases that can be documented by EEG: rapid eye movement (REM) sleep and non-REM (NREM), or slow-wave, sleep. REM and NREM sleep succeed each other in 90- to 110-minute intervals in a predictable pattern.[143] Four to six cycles occur during a normal sleep period. NREM sleep is divided into four stages based on changes in the EEG pattern (Figure 15-9):

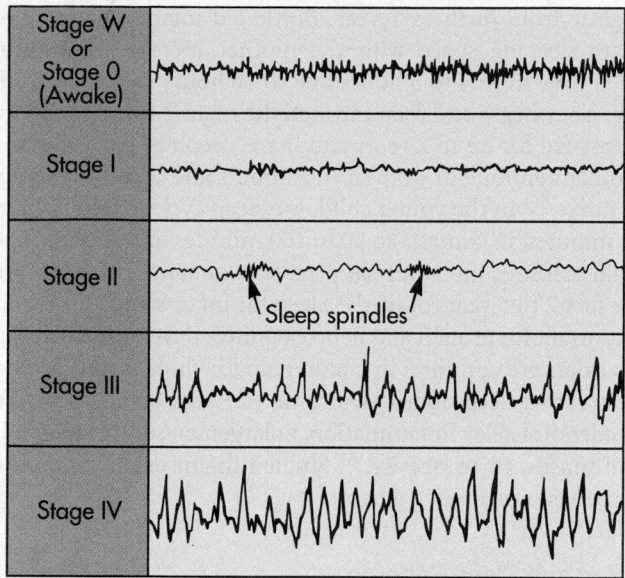

Figure 15-9 Electroencephalogram (EEG) stages of wakefulness and NREM sleep. *Stage W or stage 0 awake,* low-voltage fast activity; *stage I,* falling asleep; *stage II,* light sleep with sleep spindles; *stage III,* moderately deep sleep; *stage IV,* deep sleep with slow delta waves. Rapid eye movement (REM) sleep looks similar to awake and stage I.

Stage W or stage 0—Wakefulness with eyes closed and predominated by alpha waves (8 to 25 Hz).

Stage I—Light sleep, with alpha waves (6 to 8 Hz) interspersed with low-frequency theta waves; slow eye movements (3% to 8% of sleep time)

Stage II—Further slowing of the EEG (4 to 7 Hz) with the presence of sleep spindles and slow eye movements (45% to 55% of sleep time)

Stage III—Low-frequency (1 to 3 Hz) high-amplitude delta waves with occasional sleep spindles—also known as *slow-wave sleep;* no slow eye movements (15% to 20% of sleep time)

Stage IV—Delta waves, slow-wave sleep (15% to 20% of sleep time)

Non–Rapid Eye Movement (NREM) Sleep

NREM (slow-wave) sleep accounts for 75% to 80% of sleep time and is initiated by the withdrawal of neurotransmitters from the reticular formation and by the inhibition of arousal mechanisms in the cerebral cortex. During NREM sleep, respiration is controlled by metabolic processes.[144] The basal metabolic rate is decreased by 10% to 15%. Temperature is decreased 0.5° to 1° C (0.9° to 1.8° F). Heart rate decreases by 10 to 30 beats per minute. Respiration, blood pressure, and muscle tone all decrease. Knee-jerk reflexes are absent. Pupils are constricted. During stages I and II, cerebral blood flow to the brainstem and cerebellum is decreased. During stages III and IV, cerebral blood flow to the cortex is decreased.[145,146] Growth hormone is released during stage IV, and levels of corticosteroids and catecholamines are depressed.

Rapid Eye Movement Sleep

Rapid eye movement (REM) sleep accounts for 20% to 25% of sleep time and is characterized by desynchronized, low-voltage, fast activity that occurs for 5 to 60 minutes about every 90 minutes beginning after 1 to 2 hours of NREM sleep. The brain is quite active in REM sleep with vivid dreaming. REM sleep is also known as *paradoxic sleep* because the EEG pattern is similar to the normal awake pattern. Alternating periods of REM and NREM sleep occur throughout the night, with lengthening intervals of REM sleep and fewer intervals of deeper stages of NREM sleep toward morning. REM sleep is characterized by bursts of conjugate rapid eye movement; atonia of antigravity muscles; suppressed temperature regulation; alteration in heart rate, blood pressure,[147] and respiration; penile erection in men and clitoral engorgement in women; and a high rate of memorable dreams. Steroids are released in short bursts. During REM sleep, respiratory control is thought to be largely independent of metabolic requirements and oxygen variation. Loss of normal voluntary muscle control in the tongue and upper pharynx may produce some respiratory obstruction. Cerebral blood flow to both hemispheres is increased. REM sleep is controlled by the pontine reticular formation.

An individual progresses through REM and NREM sleep in a predictable cycle while asleep. The first cycle of the night begins with stage I. The individual then progresses through stages II, III, IV, and REM sleep (Stage V). A new cycle, beginning with stage II, follows each REM sleep. With each successive cycle, the amount of time spent in stage IV sleep decreases and the amount of time spent in REM sleep (Stage V) increases (Figure 15-10). The individual who is awakened begins the next cycle with stage I.

The hypothalamus as a major sleep center secretes hypocretins (orexins), neuropeptides that promote wakefulness and REM sleep as well as appetite, energy consumption, and pleasure or reward. In addition to the hypocretins, acetylcholine and glutamate are important waking factors. The preoptic area of the hypothalamus promotes sleep through inhibitory modulation of multiple arousal systems with involvement of the inhibitory neurotransmitter GABA.[148] The reticular formation is primarily responsible for generating REM sleep and projections from the reticular formation and other areas of the mesencephalon and brainstem produce NREM sleep.[149]

Many neurotransmitters are associated with excitatory and inhibitory sleep mechanisms. Sleep-promoting neurotransmitters include prostaglandin D$_2$, L-tryptophan, serotonin, adenosine, melatonin, GABA, and growth hormones.[150-152] Awake-promoting neurotransmitters include hypocretin (orexin), acetylcholine, and glutamate.[153] Their mechanism of action is complex and not clearly understood. Growth hormone is associated with initiation of sleep, and cortisol rises in the morning just before waking.[154] Acetylcholine and somatostatin play a role in stages of sleep transition. Forced awakenings in the middle of the night may result in increased difficulty returning to sleep or may alter the normal

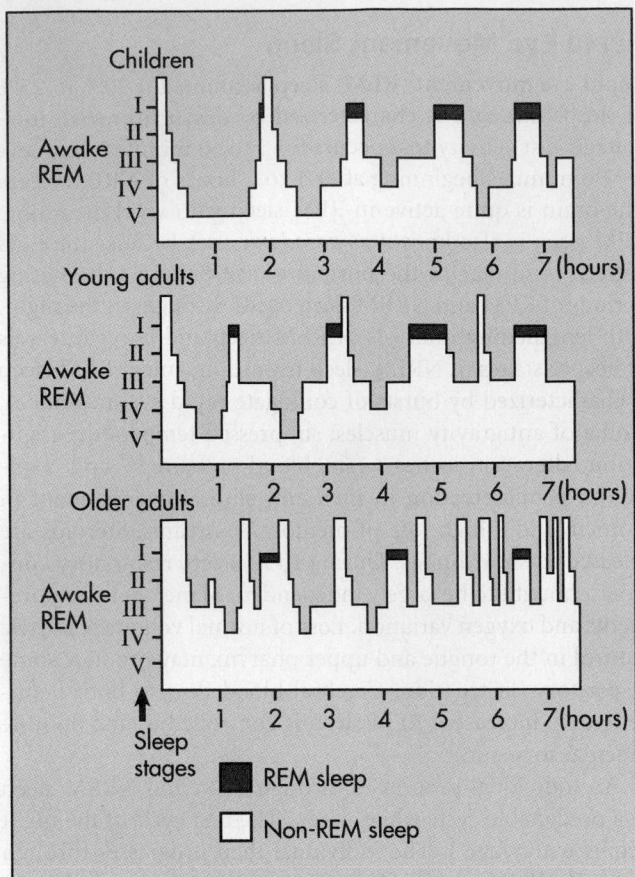

Figure 15-10 Normal sleep cycles. Rapid eye movement (REM) sleep (Stage V) occurs cyclically throughout the night at intervals of approximately 90 minutes in all age groups. REM sleep shows little variation in the different age groups, whereas stage IV sleep decreases with age. In addition, older adults awaken frequently and show a marked increase in total time awake.

progression of sleep, or both.[155,156] The purpose of sleep is unknown, although restorative processes, particularly neuronal repair and generation of new neural pathways, have been proposed. Loss of REM sleep impairs learning and memory. Sleep is important enough that people spend about one third of their life sleeping.

Pediatrics and Sleep Patterns

The sleep patterns of the newborn and young child vary from those of the adult in total sleep time, cycle length, and percentage of time spent in each sleep cycle.[157] Newborns sleep about 16 to 17 hours per day. About 53% of that time is spent in active sleep (REM sleep), 23% in quiet sleep (NREM sleep), and the remainder in an indeterminate phase. The infant sleep cycle is approximately 50 to 60 minutes long, with 20 minutes of NREM sleep and 10 to 45 minutes of REM sleep, in contrast to the adult sleep cycle. Newborns enter REM sleep immediately on falling asleep.[158,159] At about 1 year of age, an infant spends approximately 45% of total sleep time in quiet sleep and 41% in REM sleep. Total sleep time decreases

slightly from birth to 1 year. Bottle-fed infants that do not share sleeping space with the mother increase maximum sleep time from 4 to 5 hours to 8 to 10 hours by 4 months of age. They begin to "sleep through the night." Infants that are breast-fed for up to 2 years and share sleeping space with the mother continue to sleep in short bouts and wake frequently to nurse.[160] In the young child, the sleep cycle length is 45 to 60 minutes, in contrast to 90 to 100 minutes in the adult. The child assumes the adult sleep pattern at some point during the first 2 to 5 years of life.[161] Sleep for infants and children is important for growth and neurocognitive development. Sleep disorders are common in children and include insomnia and obstructive sleep apnea syndrome (OSAS). OSAS is related to adenotonsillar inflammation, enlargement of the adenoids and tonsils, or to obesity.[162] Sudden infant death syndrome (SIDS) is presented in Chapter 34.

Aging and Sleep Patterns

The sleep pattern of the older adult differs from that of the younger adult or child. Total sleep time is decreased, and the older individual takes longer to fall asleep. Older adults tend to go to sleep earlier in the evening and awaken more frequently during the night and earlier in the morning. REM and slow-wave sleep decreases. On EEG, the spindle indicating stage II sleep is less well formed.[163,164] Changes in the older adult's sleep pattern may be associated with changes in lifestyle, chronic disease, lack of daily routine, desynchronization of circadian rhythm, and use of sedatives. Growth hormone and cortisol are diminished in the older adult and may affect sleep patterns.[165] The alteration in sleep pattern typically appears about 10 years later in women than in men. Older adults are less able than younger individuals to tolerate sleep deprivation.[163]

Sleep Disorders

The classification of sleep disorders is complex and a system has been produced by the American Academy of Sleep Medicine[166] that includes four general classifications: (1) dyssomnias (intrinsic and extrinsic sleep disorders and circadian rhythm sleep disorders); (2) parasomnias (arousal and sleep-wake transition disorders and REM sleep disorders); (3) sleep disorders associated with mental, neurologic, or other medical disorder; and (4) proposed sleep disorders. The most common dyssomnias and parasomnias are presented here.

Common Dyssomnias

The **dyssomnias** are sleep disorders related to difficulty in initiating or maintaining sleep or excessive sleepiness. The most common dyssomnias include insomnia, obstructive sleep apnea syndrome, restless leg syndrome, circadian rhythm disorder, and hypersomnia.

Insomnia is the inability to fall or stay asleep and is more common in women.[167] Primary insomnia may be transient, lasting a few days, and related to travel across time zones, disrupted sleep schedules, or acute stress. Secondary insomnia is associated with drug or alcohol abuse, chronic pain disorders, or chronic depression, obesity, and aging.[168] Drugs known to produce insomnia include amphetamines, steroids, central adrenergic blockers, bronchodilating agents, and caffeine.[169]

Obstructive sleep apnea syndrome (OSAS) is a disorder of breathing during sleep related to upper airway obstruction that is associated with reduced blood oxygen saturation and hypercapnia. Risk factors include obesity, male gender, and age.[170] Premenstrual women may be protected from sleep-disordered breathing because the female hormone progesterone is a respiratory stimulant.[171,172] The longer pharyngeal airway in males also may contribute to increased risk for OSAS. Obese individuals often have a short, thick neck; impaired respiratory mechanics; and depressed respiratory control, particularly during sleep. **Obesity hypoventilation syndrome** may be related to leptin resistance because leptin is also a respiratory stimulant.

OSAS is characterized by repetitive increases in resistance to airflow within the upper airway with loud snoring, gasping, intervals of apnea lasting from 10 to 30 seconds, fragmented sleep, and chronic daytime sleepiness. The obstruction is caused by the soft palate or base of the tongue, or both, collapsing against the pharyngeal walls because of decreased muscle tone especially during REM sleep. In the supine position, the tongue may fall farther back, obstructing the airway. The level of negative intrathoracic pressure is the most likely stimulus for arousal, possibly mediated by mechanoreceptors in the upper airway. Potentially fatal systemic illnesses often associated with OSAS include hypertension, pulmonary hypertension, heart failure, nocturnal cardiac dysrhythmias, myocardial infarction, and ischemic stroke.[173] The combination of intermittent hypoxia and hypercapnia, arousals, increased sympathetic tone, altered baroreflex control during sleep, and cardiovascular changes induced by increased negative intrathoracic pressure contribute to these complications. Many individuals are not aware of their heavy snoring and nocturnal arousals and may remain undiagnosed. Fatigue, decline in cognitive function, car accidents, and poor work performance are common.

Diagnosis of OSAS is confirmed with polysomnography. Treatments include continuous positive airway pressure, dental devices that modify the position of the tongue or jaw, upper airway surgical reconstruction, and weight reduction.[174]

Restless leg syndrome (RLS) is a common sensorimotor disorder associated with unpleasant sensations (prickling, tingling, crawling) that occurs at rest and is worse in the evening or at night. There is a compelling urge to move the legs for relief, with a significant effect on sleep and quality of life. The disorder is more common in women, older adults, and individuals with iron deficiency. RLS has a familial tendency and is associated with a circadian fluctuation of dopamine in the substantia nigra. Iron is a cofactor in dopamine production, and some individuals respond to iron administration as well as dopamine agonists.[175-177]

Hypersomnia is excessive daytime sleepiness and is commonly associated with voluntary sleep deprivation. There may also be an underlying sleep disorder such as OSAS or narcolepsy. Individuals may fall asleep while driving, working, or even conversing with significant concerns for safety. Treatment is symptomatic with reinforcement of good sleeping habits.

Narcolepsy is characterized by hypersomnia, cataplexy (brief spells of muscle weakness), hallucinations, and sleep paralysis. The disorder is associated with hypothalamic hypocretin (orexin) deficiency and may be related to immune-mediated destruction of hypocretin-secreting cells. There is a genetic component to the disorder in animals.[178]

Circadian rhythm sleep disorders are common disorders of the sleep-wake schedule and include rapid time-zone change (jet-lag syndrome), changing sleep schedule with an advance or a delay of 3 hours or more in sleep time, or a change in total sleep time from day to day. These changes in the timing of established sleep schedules have been shown to desynchronize circadian rhythm. Degree of vigilance, performance of psychomotor tasks, and subjective reports of levels of arousal are markedly depressed after alterations in the sleep-wake schedule. Individuals may experience short sleep episodes called *microsleeps* without being aware of decreased vigilance.[179,180]

It is well established that industrial shift workers exhibit a decrease in accuracy and increased accident proneness.[181] For similar reasons, people suffering from jet lag require several days to adapt to a new time zone. Travel across time zones requires 2 days to adjust the sleep-wake schedule, 5 days to adjust the body temperature cycle, and 8 days to adjust cortisol secretion. Transmeridian travel requires up to 10 days to adjust the body clock when traveling from east to west. Czeisler's experiments with timed bright-light stimulation have had some success in retiming or resetting the body clock before or after time-zone shifts.[182]

Common Parasomnias

Parasomnias are complex behaviors related to awakening from REM sleep or partial arousal from NREM sleep and disorders of sleep stage transitions. Three types of parasomnias include *arousal disorders* such as confusional arousals, sleepwalking (somnambulism), night terrors (dream anxiety attacks), rearranging furniture, eating food, violent behavior, bruxism (teeth grinding), and sleep enuresis; *sleep-wake transition disorders* such as rhythmic movements (head banging), sleep talking, and nocturnal leg cramps; and *disorders associated with REM sleep* such as sleep paralysis and nightmares, sleep apnea, and SIDS. SIDS affects children primarily in the first 2 years of life and may be related to central sleep apnea (a disorder of thalamic breathing control) episodes (see Chapter 34). Parasomnias are more common in children and may be familial.[183]

Sleep Disorders Associated with Mental, Neurologic, or Medical Disorders

Many mental and physical disorders are associated with alterations in sleep (secondary sleep disorders). Many disorders produce alterations in the quantity and quality of sleep or affect sleep stages including mental disorders (i.e., depression and anxiety), disorders of neurocognitive function (i.e., dementia or Parkinson disease), and physical disorders (i.e., alterations in thyroid hormone, pain, and many acute and chronic diseases). In other instances, sleep stages may contribute to disease (sleep-provoked disorders) such as chronic obstructive pulmonary disease (COPD), asthma, cardiac ischemia diabetes mellitus, and gastroesophageal reflux.

REM sleep behavior disorder is loss of normal skeletal muscle atonia during REM sleep and may cause injury from acting out of dreams. It is more common in older adult men and is associated with Parkinson disease and other neurodegenerative diseases.[184]

Individuals who are depressed have difficulty falling asleep and exhibit less slow-wave sleep, less time spent in REM sleep, early awakening, and less total sleep time. In addition, depressed individuals move through the sleep stages more quickly than do individuals who are not depressed. The same neurotransmitters that may be disturbed in depression also regulate sleep.[185]

Coronary artery disease is most affected during REM sleep. During REM, dreams may provoke nocturnal angina, increased heart rate, and electrocardiogram (ECG) changes. In adults, attacks of bronchial asthma may occur at any time during the night. The attacks cause the individual to spend more of the sleep period awake and thus cause a decrease in stage IV sleep. In children, bronchial asthma attacks are uncommon during the first one third of the night, when stage IV sleep predominates, and occur more frequently during the final two thirds of the night. Stage IV sleep is decreased overall in the child with bronchial asthma. In addition to these changes, asthmatic individuals may experience bronchial spasm during REM sleep.[186]

People with COPD experience significantly lowered oxygen tension and increases in carbon dioxide retention during sleep. The lowered oxygen tension is most significant in the tonic phase of REM sleep when voluntary neuromuscular control, including intercostal muscle function, is depressed. Pulmonary spasm and transient pulmonary hypertension result. These changes are particularly evident in the "blue bloater" individual and may contribute to early pulmonary hypertension and cor pulmonale in these people.[187]

Because blood glucose levels vary during sleep, individuals with uncontrolled diabetes may need to pay careful attention to blood sugar levels. Studies show that people with duodenal ulcers secrete 3 to 20 times more gastric acid during REM sleep than do people without duodenal ulcers. This increased gastric acid secretion often produces nocturnal epigastric pain.

SPECIAL SENSES

Vision

The eyes are complex sense organs responsible for vision. Within a protective casing, each eye has receptors, a lens system for focusing light on the receptors, and a system of nerves for conducting impulses from the receptors to the brain. Visual dysfunction may be caused by abnormal ocular movements or alterations in visual acuity, refraction, color vision, or accommodation. Visual dysfunction also may be the secondary effect of another neurologic disorder.

External Eye Structures

The external structures protecting the eye include the eyelids (palpebrae), conjunctivae, and lacrimal apparatus (Figure 15-11). Infection and inflammatory responses are the most common conditions affecting the supporting structures of the eyes. **Blepharitis** is an inflammation of the eyelids caused by *Staphylococcus* or seborrheic dermatitis. Redness, edema, and itching are common symptoms. A **hordeolum (stye)** is an infection of the sebaceous glands of the eyelids, and a **chalazion** is an infection of the meibomian (oil-secreting) gland. These conditions are treated symptomatically.[188]

Conjunctivitis

Conjunctivitis is an inflammation of the conjunctiva (mucous membrane covering the front part of the eyeball). Conjunctivitis may be caused by bacteria, viruses, allergies, or chemical irritations. The inflammatory response produces redness, edema, pain, and lacrimation. Treatment is related to cause.[189]

Acute bacterial conjunctivitis (pinkeye) is highly contagious and often is caused by gram-positive organisms (*Staphylococcus, Haemophilus, Proteus*), although other bacteria may be involved. The onset is acute, characterized by mucopurulent drainage from one or both eyes. Preventing spread of the

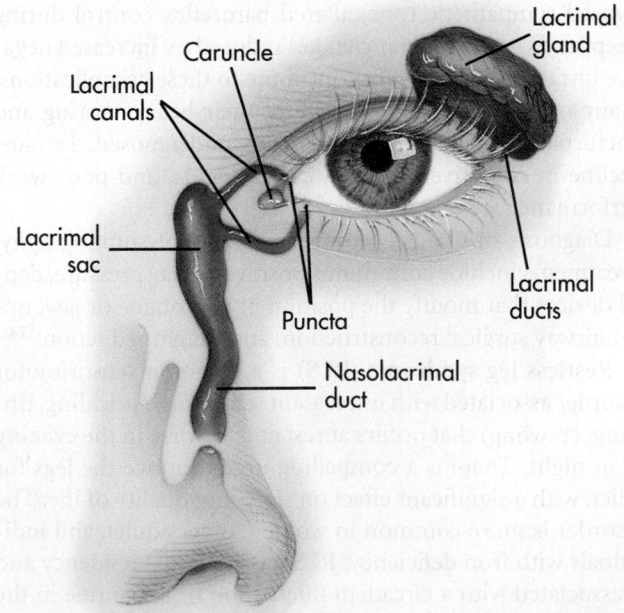

Figure 15-11 Lacrimal apparatus. Fluid produced by lacrimal glands (tears) streams across the eye surface, enters the canals, and then passes through the nasolacrimal duct to enter the nose. (From Patton KT, Thibodeau GA: *Anatomy & physiology*, ed 7, St Louis, 2010, Mosby.)

organism with meticulous handwashing and use of separate towels is important. The disease often is self-limiting and resolves spontaneously in 10 to 14 days. Antibiotic eyedrops usually are effective.

Viral conjunctivitis is caused by an adenovirus. Symptoms vary from mild to severe. Some strains of virus cause conjunctivitis and pharyngitis (pharyngoconjunctival fever), and others cause keratoconjunctivitis. Both diseases are contagious, with watering, redness, and photophobia. Treatment is symptomatic.

Allergic conjunctivitis is associated with a variety of antigens, including pollens. Ocular itching is associated with photophobia, burning, and gritty sensations in the eye. Treatment is symptomatic and may include antihistamines, steroids, and vasoconstrictors.

Chronic conjunctivitis is the result of any persistent conjunctivitis. The cause requires identification for effective treatment.

Trachoma (chlamydial conjunctivitis) is caused by *Chlamydia trachomatis*. It often is associated with poor hygiene and is the leading cause of preventable blindness in the world. The severity of the disease varies, but it can involve inflammation with scarring of the conjunctiva and eyelids causing distorted lashes to abrade the cornea leading to corneal scarring and blindness. Chlamydial organisms are sensitive to local or systemic antibiotics. The World Health Organization aims to eliminate trachoma as a public health problem by 2020 using the SAFE Strategy: Surgery for inturned lashes, Antibiotics, Facial cleanliness, and Environmental improvement.[190]

Keratitis

Keratitis is an infection of the cornea that can be caused by bacteria or viruses. Bacterial infections often cause corneal ulceration and require intensive antibiotic treatment. Type I herpes simplex virus can involve the cornea and conjunctiva. Common symptoms include photophobia, pain, and lacrimation. Severe ulcerations with residual scarring require corneal transplantation.

The Eye

The wall of the eye is formed of three layers: sclera, choroid, and retina (Figure 15-12). The **sclera** is the thick, white, outermost layer. It becomes transparent at the **cornea,** the portion of the sclera in the central anterior region that allows light to enter the eye. The **choroid** is the deeply pigmented middle layer that prevents light from scattering inside the eye. The **iris,** part of the choroid, has a round opening, the **pupil,** through which light passes. Smooth muscle fibers control the size of the pupil so that in close vision and bright light the pupil constricts and in distant vision and dim light the pupil dilates.

The innermost layer of the eye, the **retina,** contains millions of **rods** and **cones,** special photoreceptors that convert light energy into nerve impulses. In the retina, rods mediate peripheral and dim light vision and are densest at the periphery. Cones, densest in the center of the retina, are color and detail receptors. The photoreceptive rods and cones are distributed over the entire retina, except where the optic nerve leaves the eyeball. Lack of rods and cones in this area results in the **optic disc,** or blind spot. Lateral to each optic disc is the **fovea centralis,** a tiny area that contains only cones and provides the greatest visual acuity (see Figure 15-12).

As shown in Figure 15-13, nerve impulses pass through the optic nerves after leaving the retinas. At the optic chiasm the fibers from the inner (nasal) halves of the retinas cross to the opposite side, where they join fibers from the

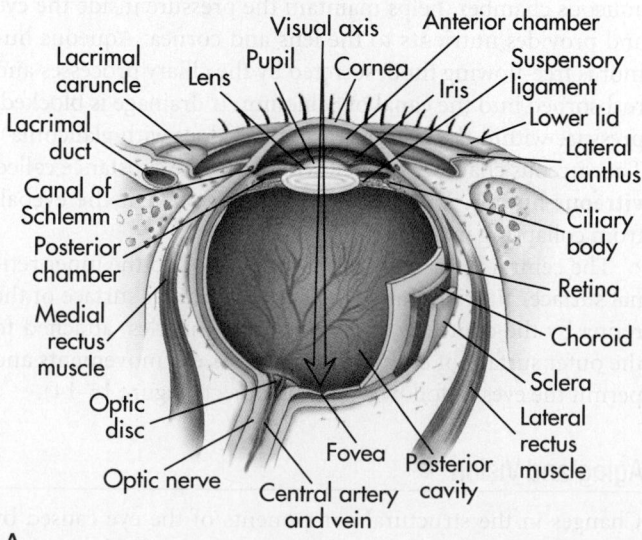

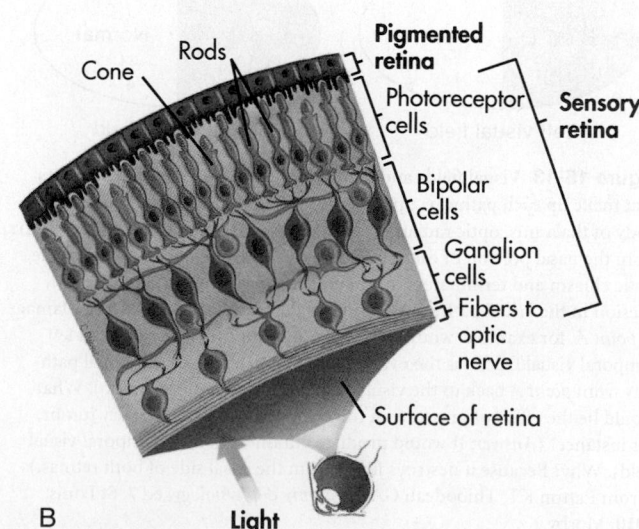

Figure 15-12 Structure of the eyeball and cell layers of the retina. **A,** Horizontal section through the left eyeball. The eye is viewed from above. **B,** Pigmented and sensory layers of the retina. (From Patton KT, Thibodeau GA: *Anatomy & physiology,* ed 7, St Louis, 2010, Mosby.)

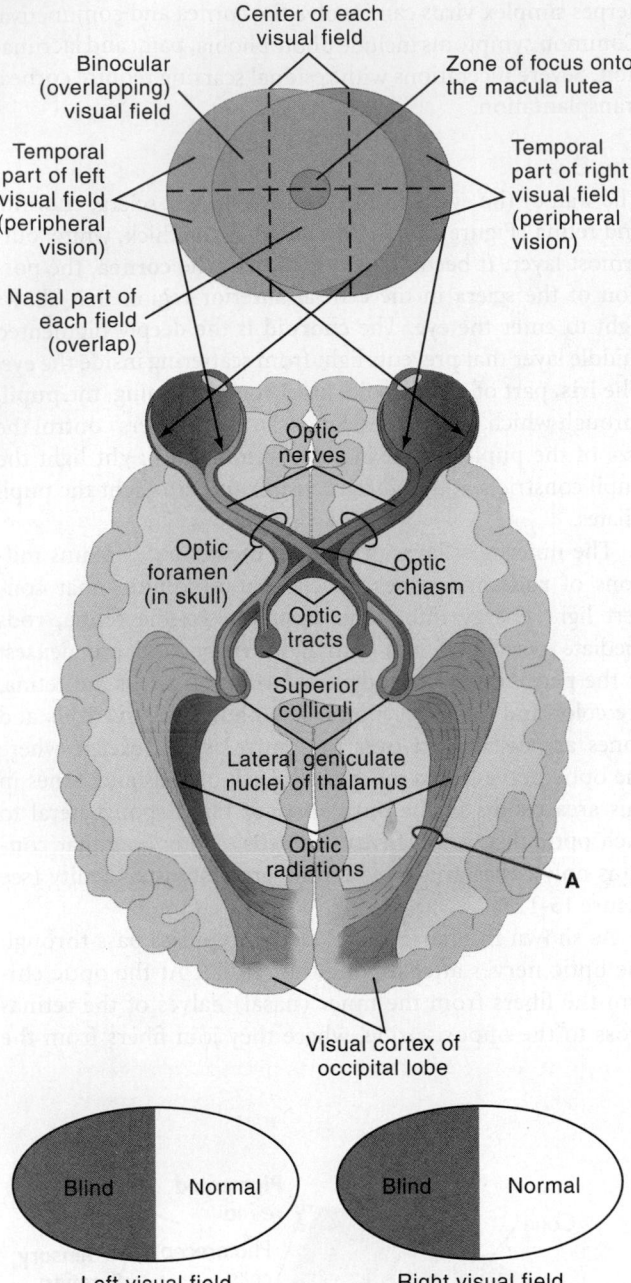

Figure 15-13 Visual fields and neuronal pathways. Note the structures that make up each pathway: optic nerve, optic chiasm, lateral geniculate body of thalamus, optic radiations, and visual cortex of occipital lobe. Fibers from the nasal portion of each retina cross over to the opposite side at the optic chiasm and terminate in the lateral geniculate nuclei. Location of a lesion in the visual pathway determines the resulting visual defect. Damage at *point A*, for example, would cause blindness in the right nasal and left temporal visual fields (as the ovals beneath indicate; trace the visual pathway from *point A* back to the visual field map to see why this is so). What would be the effect of pressure on the optic chiasm, by a pituitary tumor, for instance? (*Answer*: It would produce blindness in both temporal visual fields. Why? Because it destroys fibers from the nasal side of both retinas.) (From Patton KT, Thibodeau GA: *Anatomy & physiology*, ed 7, St Louis, 2010, Mosby.)

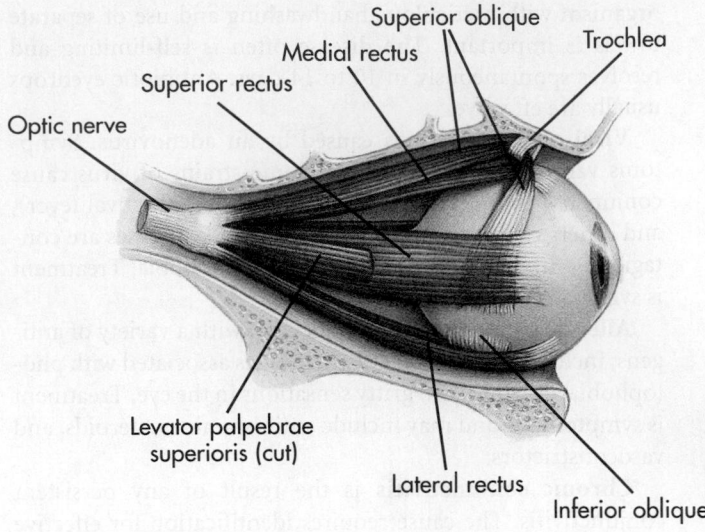

Figure 15-14 Extrinsic muscles of the right eye, superior view. (From Patton KT, Thibodeau GA: *Anatomy & physiology*, ed 7, St Louis, 2010, Mosby.)

outer (temporal) halves of the retinas to form the optic tracts. The fibers of the optic tracts synapse in the dorsal lateral geniculate nucleus, and from there the geniculocalcarine fibers pass by way of the optic radiation (or geniculo-calcarine tract) to the primary visual cortex in the occipital lobe of the brain.

Light entering the eye is focused on the retina by the **lens**—a flexible, biconvex, crystal-like structure. In youth the lens is transparent and has the consistency of hardened jelly. With age the lens becomes increasingly hard and opaque. The lens divides the anterior chamber into (1) the aqueous chamber and (2) the vitreous chamber. **Aqueous humor,** which fills the aqueous chamber, helps maintain the pressure inside the eye and provides nutrients to the lens and cornea. Aqueous humor is free-flowing fluid, secreted by the ciliary processes and reabsorbed into the canal of Schlemm. If drainage is blocked, pressure within the eye increases (as it does with glaucoma). The vitreous chamber is filled with a gel-like substance called **vitreous humor.** Vitreous humor helps prevent the eyeball from collapsing inward.

The central retinal artery provides blood to the inner retinal surface. Nutrients are supplied to the outer surface of the retina by the choroid. Six extrinsic eye muscles, attached to the outer surface of each eye, allow gross eye movements and permit the eyes to follow a moving object (Figure 15-14).

Aging and Vision

Changes in the structural components of the eye caused by aging begin at an early age, particularly in the lens of the eye. Changes caused by aging are summarized in Table 15-5. Structural changes combined with chronic diseases including diabetes mellitus result in a decline in visual acuity.[191]

Table 15-5	Changes in the Eye Caused by Aging	
Structure	Change	Consequence
Cornea	Thicker and less curved	Increase in astigmatism
	Formation of a gray ring at the edge of cornea (arcus senilis)	Not detrimental to vision
Anterior chamber	Decrease in size and volume caused by thickening of lens	Occasionally exerts pressure on Schlemm canal and may lead to increased intraocular pressure and glaucoma
Lens	Increase in opacity	Decrease in refraction with increased light scattering and decreased color vision (green and blue); can lead to cataracts
Ciliary muscles	Reduction in pupil diameter, atrophy of radial dilation muscles	Persistent constriction (senile miosis); decrease in critical flicker frequency*
Retina	Reduction in number of rods at periphery, loss of rods and associated nerve cells	Increase in the minimum amount of light necessary to see an object

*The rate at which consecutive visual stimuli can be presented and still be perceived as separate.

Visual Dysfunction

Alterations in Ocular Movements

Abnormal ocular movements occur as a result of oculomotor, trochlear, or abducens cranial nerve dysfunction (see Table 14-6). The three types of eye movement disorders are (1) strabismus, (2) nystagmus, and (3) paralysis of individual extraocular muscles.

Strabismus is the deviation of one eye from the other when a person is looking at an object resulting in failure of the two eyes to simultaneously focus on the same image with loss of binocular vision. It is caused by weak or hypertonic muscle in one of the eyes. The deviation may be upward, downward, inward, or outward. Strabismus in children requires early intervention to prevent the development of amblyopia (reduced vision in the affected eye without ocular pathology and with full optical correction). Treatment of amblyopia is patching. The primary symptom of strabismus is **diplopia** (double vision). Strabismus may be caused by a neuromuscular disorder of the eye muscle, diseases involving the cerebral hemispheres, or thyroid disease.[192,193]

Nystagmus is an involuntary unilateral or bilateral rhythmic movement of the eyes and can occur in infants (congenital) or adults (acquired). It may be present at rest, or it may occur with eye movement. The two major forms of nystagmus are pendular nystagmus and jerk nystagmus. **Pendular nystagmus** is characterized by a regular to-and-fro movement of the eyes in which both phases of the movement are equal in length. In **jerk nystagmus** one phase of the eye movement is faster than the other. Nystagmus may be caused by an imbalance in the normally coordinated reflex activity of the inner ear, vestibular nuclei (connecting the vestibular nerve with vestibulospinal tracts), cerebellum, medial longitudinal fascicle (connecting the mesencephalon with the upper portion of the spinal cord), or nuclei of the oculomotor, trochlear, and abducens cranial nerves (see Table 14-6). Drugs, retinal disease, and diseases involving the cervical cord also may produce nystagmus. Acquired untreated nystagmus can lead to loss of visual acuity.[194]

Paralysis of specific extraocular muscles may cause a variety of abnormalities, including limited abduction, abnormal closure of the eyelid, ptosis (drooping of the eyelid), and diplopia. The abnormalities occur as a result of unopposed muscle activity. Trauma or pressure in the area of the cranial nerves may cause paralysis of specific extraocular muscles. Diseases such as diabetes mellitus and myasthenia gravis also may affect specific extraocular muscles.

Alterations in Visual Acuity

Visual acuity is the ability to see objects in sharp detail. With advancing age the eye's lens becomes less flexible and less adjustable. In addition, the sclera changes shape, causing light to fall on the **macula** (an opaque portion of the cornea). Thus visual acuity declines with age. Visual acuity also may change or diminish for many other reasons. Specific causes of visual acuity changes include (1) amblyopia, (2) scotoma, (3) cataracts, (4) papilledema, (5) dark adaptation, (6) glaucoma, (7) retinal detachment, and (8) macular degeneration.

Amblyopia is a reduction or dimness of vision for unknown reasons. It does not result from a change in refraction (i.e., deviation of light rays) or from any visible changes in the eye. Amblyopia is associated with strabismus and anisometropia (refractive error in one eye differs from the other eye) and diseases such as diabetes mellitus, renal failure, and malaria and with toxic substances such as alcohol and tobacco. Amblyopia is the most common cause of vision loss in children and is usually treated by patching the unaffected eye for extended times to ensure a period of use of the affected eye or with atropine drops.[195] Refractive errors are treated with corrective lenses.

A **scotoma** is a circumscribed defect of the central field of vision. It is most often a sequel to demyelinating optic neuritis, an inflammatory lesion of the optic nerve frequently associated with multiple sclerosis (see Chapter 17). Less common causes include the compression of one optic nerve by a retroorbital tumor, neuromyelitis optica (autoantibody-related inflammation of the optic nerve and spinal cord), pernicious anemia, and toxic or metabolic causes such as methyl alcohol poisoning and use of tobacco. The precise mechanisms for these conditions causing a scotoma are uncertain, but the result is always a serious impairment in visual acuity.[196]

A **cataract** is a cloudy or opaque area in the ocular lens. The incidence of cataracts increases with age as the lens enlarges. Cataracts develop because of alterations of metabolism and transport of nutrients within the lens. Although the most common form of cataract is degenerative, cataracts also may occur congenitally or as a result of infection, radiation, trauma, drugs, or diabetes mellitus. Cataracts cause decreased visual acuity, blurred vision, glare, and decreased color perception. Cataracts are treated by removal of the entire lens and replacement with an intraocular artificial lens.[197]

Papilledema is edema and inflammation of the optic nerve at its point of entrance into the eyeball. Generally, papilledema is caused by some obstruction to the venous return from the retina. An early sign is distention of the retinal vein. Obliteration of the physiologic cup (a bright area normally located in the center of the optic disc) follows. Later the optic disc becomes raised above the level of the surrounding retina, and the margins become blurred and indistinct. With severe swelling, hemorrhage and patches of white exudate develop around the disc margins. The three principal causes of papilledema are (1) increased intracranial pressure, (2) retrobulbar neuritis, and (3) changes in the retinal blood vessels. Retinal blood vessel changes are especially prevalent in individuals with diabetes mellitus or hypertension. Such changes account for a large percentage of individuals newly affected with blindness each year. Typically the blood vessels narrow, and hemorrhages and white exudate appear. Ultimately papilledema occurs.

Dark adaptation also affects visual acuity. Low illumination causes impaired visual acuity, particularly in older adults. The average 80-year-old needs more than twice as much light as a 20-year-old to see equally well. Changes in the quantity and quality of rhodopsin, a substance found in the rods and responsible for low-light vision, are thought to be responsible for reduced dark adaptation in older adults.[198] Vitamin A deficiencies can cause the same phenomenon in individuals of any age.

Glaucoma is a leading cause of visual impairment and blindness. It is characterized by intraocular pressures above the normal pressures of 12 to 20 mmHg maintained by the aqueous fluid. Family history is a risk factor, and glaucoma can be inherited.[199] The types of glaucoma are summarized in Table 15-6 and Figure 15-15. Chronic increased intraocular pressure causes death of retinal ganglions and optic nerve degeneration with loss of peripheral vision, followed by central vision impairment and blindness.[200] Extremely high pressures can cause blindness within days or hours. Loss of visual acuity results from pressure on the optic nerve, which is believed to block the flow of cytoplasm from neuronal bodies in the retina to peripheral optic nerve fibers entering the brain. Lack of nutrients, ischemia, cytotoxic factors, and altered immune mechanisms may lead to death of the involved neurons.[201] Acute pain may result. Early detection and treatment prevent optic neuropathy and visual impairment. Glaucoma often is treated with pharmaceutical eyedrops to reduce secretion or increase absorption of aqueous humor. Surgery may be needed to open the spaces of the trabeculae and reduce intraocular pressure. Neuroprotective therapies are being evaluated.[202]

Retinal detachment is a common cause of visual impairment and blindness. Risk factors include retinal holes and vitreoretinal traction. Fluid (exudate, hemorrhage, or liquid vitreous) separates the photoreceptors from the retinal pigment epithelium. The separation deprives the outer retina of oxygen and nutrients because the diffusion distance is increased. Communication is also disrupted between the pigment epithelium and photoreceptors. **Rhegmatogenous retinal detachment** (retinal breaks caused by vitreoretinal traction) is the most common form of retinal detachment. Causes include intracapsular cataract extraction, severe myopia, lattice degeneration, vitreoretinal traction, and trauma. Contraction of fibrous membranes can cause tractional separation of the retinal layers as occurs in proliferative diabetic retinopathy. Treatment involves surgical retinal reattachment.[203]

Age-related macular degeneration (AMD), loss of central vision, is the major cause of vision loss in individuals older than 60 years. Hypertension, cigarette smoking, diabetes mellitus, and genetic predisposition are risk factors that contribute to oxidative stress and capillary injury.[204] The *atropic or dry form* of AMD is most prevalent and involves loss of retinal pigment epithelium and photoreceptors with overall atrophy of cells. The *wet exudative form* (neovascular AMD) is the more severe form and involves proliferation of abnormal choroidal vessels, which leak and bleed, causing retinal detachment.[205] Symptoms include blurred vision, loss of central

Table 15-6	Types of Glaucoma
Type	**Mechanism of Increased Pressure**
Open-angle	Obstruction of outflow of aqueous humor at trabecular meshwork or Schlemm canal; myopia may be a risk factor
Normal or low tension	A form of open-angle glaucoma with symptomless damage to the optic nerve and gradual vision loss when intraocular pressure is within normal range (12-20 mmHg)
Narrow-angle (angle closure)	Forward displacement of iris toward cornea with narrowing of iridocorneal angle and obstruction to outflow of aqueous humor from anterior chamber
Acute-angle closure	Acute closure of iridocorneal angle with a sudden rise in intraocular pressure, producing pain, redness, and visual disturbances
Chronic-angle closure	Progressive, permanent closure of anterior chamber angle
Secondary	Open or closed angle obstruction caused by, for example, uveitis, hemorrhage, rupture of lens or tumors
Congenital glaucoma	Malformation of trabecular meshwork and excess extracellular matrix in outer meshwork.

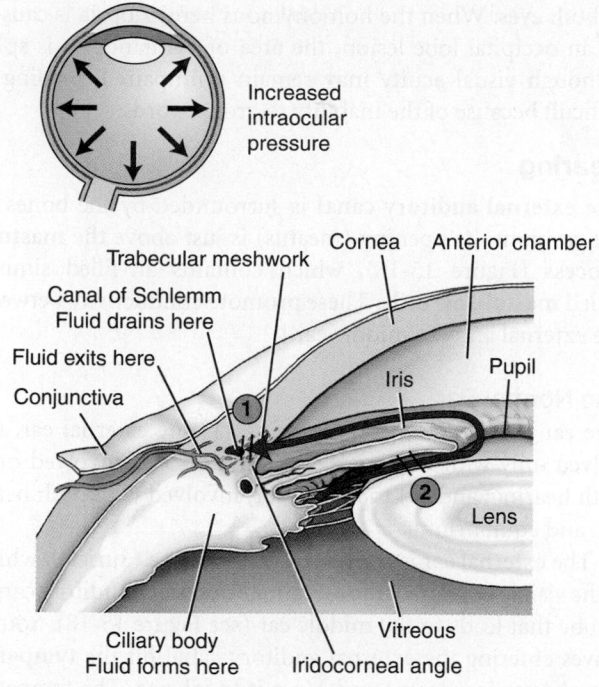

Figure 15-15 Glaucoma. 1, Open-angle glaucoma. The obstruction to aqueous flow lies in the trabecular meshwork. 2, Closed-angle glaucoma. The trabecular meshwork is covered by the root of the iris.

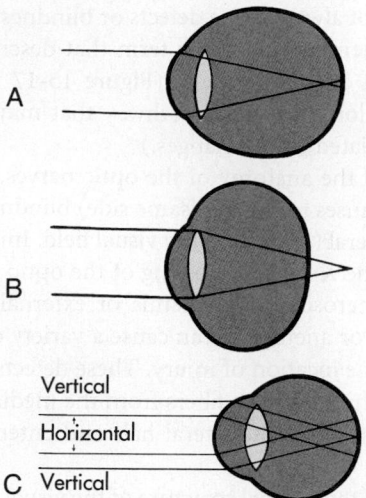

Figure 15-16 Alterations in refraction. **A,** Myopic eye. Parallel rays of light are brought to a focus in front of the retina. **B,** Hyperopic eye. Parallel rays of light come to a focus behind the retina in the unaccommodative eye. **C,** Simple myopic astigmatism. The vertical bundle of rays is focused on the retina; the horizontal rays are focused in front of the retina. (From Stein HA, Slatt BJ, Stein RM: *The ophthalmic assistant: fundamentals in clinical practice,* St Louis, 1988, Mosby.)

vision, difficulty reading, and poor night vision. Progress is being made in antiangiogenic treatments and in understanding genetic factors contributing to AMD.[206]

Alterations in Accommodation

Accommodation is the process whereby the thickness of the lens changes. Accommodation is needed for clear vision and is mediated through the oculomotor nerve. Pressure, inflammation, and disease of the oculomotor nerve may alter accommodation. Symptoms include diplopia, blurred vision, and headache. Accommodation is affected also by the decreased flexibility of the lens that occurs with aging. By 60 years of age the lens has become so inelastic that accommodation is not possible.

Loss of accommodation in older adults is termed **presbyopia**, a condition in which the ocular lens becomes larger, firmer, and less elastic. The major symptom is reduced near vision, causing the individual to hold reading material at arm's length. Correction is accomplished through reading glasses or bifocal lenses, accommodative intraocular lenses, or surgical treatment.[207,208]

Alterations in Refraction

Alterations in refraction are the most common visual problem. Errors in refraction are caused by irregularities of the corneal curvature, the focusing power of the lens, and the length of the eye. The major symptoms of refraction alterations are blurred vision and headache. Three types of refraction alterations are myopia, hyperopia, and astigmatism (Figure 15-16).

In **myopia** (nearsightedness), light rays are focused in front of the retina when a person is looking at a distant object, resulting in burred vision. A concave lens is needed for correction. Myopia requires frequent changes of eyeglasses while the eyeball is lengthening in childhood. Myopia is a risk factor for retinal detachment.

In **hyperopia** (farsightedness), light rays are focused behind the retina when a person is looking at a near object. Hyperopia is corrected with a convex lens. **Astigmatism** is caused by an unequal curvature of the cornea. In astigmatism, light rays are bent unevenly and do not come to a single focus on the retina. Astigmatism may coexist with myopia, hyperopia, or presbyopia. Correction is accomplished with a cylinder lens.

Alterations in Color Vision

Normal sensitivity to color diminishes with age because of the progressive yellowing of the lens that occurs with aging. All colors become less intense, although color discrimination for blue and green is most greatly affected. Color vision deteriorates more rapidly for individuals with diabetes mellitus than for the general population. The deterioration is thought to be an accelerated version of senile color vision deterioration.

Abnormal color vision also may be caused by **color blindness,** an inherited trait. Color blindness is generally an X-linked recessive characteristic affecting 8% of the male population and 0.5% of the female population. Although many forms of color blindness exist, most commonly the affected individual cannot distinguish red from green.[209,210]

Neurologic Disorders Causing Visual Dysfunction

Various neurologic disorders may cause visual dysfunction. Vision may be disrupted at many points along the visual pathway, causing a variety of defects in fields of vision. Visual changes do not always cause defects or blindness in the entire visual field; **hemianopia** is the term that describes defective vision in half of a visual field. (Figure 15-17 illustrates the many areas along the visual pathway that may be damaged and the associated visual changes.)

Because of the anatomy of the optic nerves, injury to the optic nerve causes ipsilateral (same side) blindness but a normal contralateral (opposite side) visual field. Injury to the **optic chiasm** (the X-shaped crossing of the optic nerves), often caused by atherosclerotic ischemia or external compression from trauma or aneurysm, can cause a variety of defects, depending on the location of injury. These defects vary because at the optic chiasm, nerve fibers from the medial half of each retina separate from the lateral half and enter the opposite optic tract.

Because of the normal structure of the visual pathways, destruction of one optic tract causes **homonymous hemianopsia** (complete loss of vision in the inner half of one eye and the outer half of the other). Thus, if an injury to the left optic tract occurs, the individual is blind in the right eye's medial (inner) field and the left eye's lateral (outer) field. If the compression of the optic tract is asymmetric, an incongruous (or uneven) homonymous defect results. Injury to one optic radiation (an ocular pathway in the internal capsule, temporal lobe, or occipital lobe) also causes a homonymous (same field) defect. A major injury in the optic radiation causes homonymous hemianopsia. A lesser injury may cause an upper quadrant homonymous defect. Generally the defects are the same size

in both eyes. When the homonymous hemianopsia is caused by an occipital lobe lesion, the area of hemianopsia is split. Although visual acuity may remain unimpaired, reading is difficult because of the inability to group words.

Hearing

The **external auditory canal** is surrounded by the bones of the cranium. Its opening (meatus) is just above the **mastoid process** (Figure 15-18), which contains air-filled sinuses called **mastoid air cells.** These promote conductivity between the external and the middle ear.

The Normal Ear

The ear is divided into three areas: (1) the external ear, involved only with hearing; (2) the middle ear, involved only with hearing; and (3) the inner ear, involved with both hearing and equilibrium.

The external ear is composed of the **pinna** (auricle), which is the visible portion of the ear, and the external auditory canal, a tube that leads to the middle ear (see Figure 15-18). Sound waves entering the external auditory canal hit the **tympanic membrane** (eardrum) and cause it to vibrate. The tympanic membrane separates the external ear from the middle ear.

The middle ear is composed of the **tympanic cavity,** a small chamber in the temporal bone. Three ossicles (small bones) transmit the vibration of the tympanic membrane to the inner ear. The three ossicles are termed the **malleus (hammer), incus (anvil),** and **stapes (stirrup).** When the tympanic

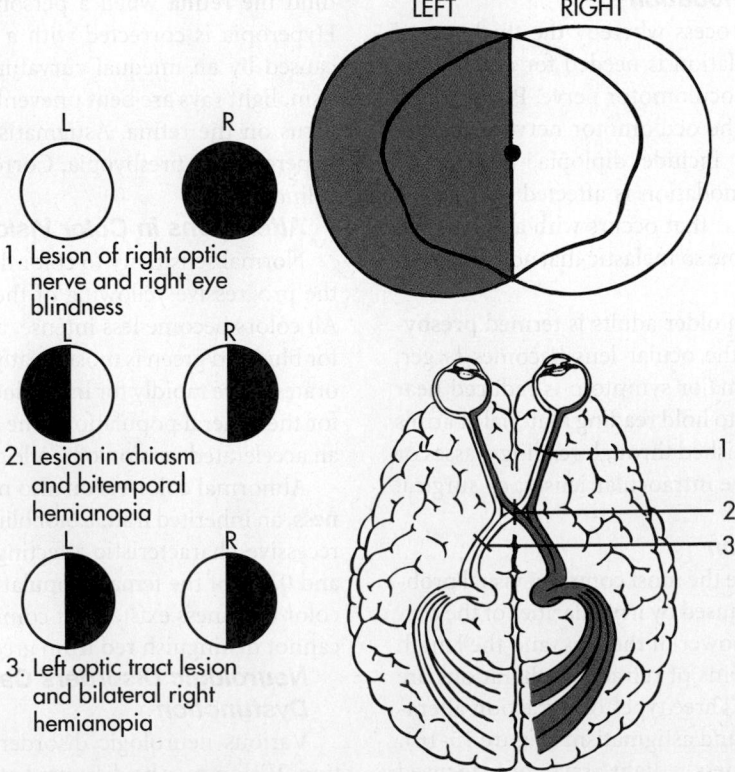

1. Lesion of right optic nerve and right eye blindness

2. Lesion in chiasm and bitemporal hemianopia

3. Left optic tract lesion and bilateral right hemianopia

Figure 15-17 Visual pathway defects. (From Thompson JM et al: *Mosby's clinical nursing,* ed 5, St Louis, 2002, Mosby.)

membrane moves, the malleus moves with it and transfers the vibration to the incus, which passes it on to the stapes. The stapes presses against the **oval window,** a small membrane of the inner ear. The movement of the oval window sets the fluids of the inner ear in motion (Figure 15-19).

The **eustachian (pharyngotympanic) tube** connects the middle ear with the thorax. Normally flat and closed, the eustachian tube opens briefly when a person swallows or yawns, and it equalizes the pressure in the middle ear with atmospheric pressure. Equalized pressure permits the tympanic

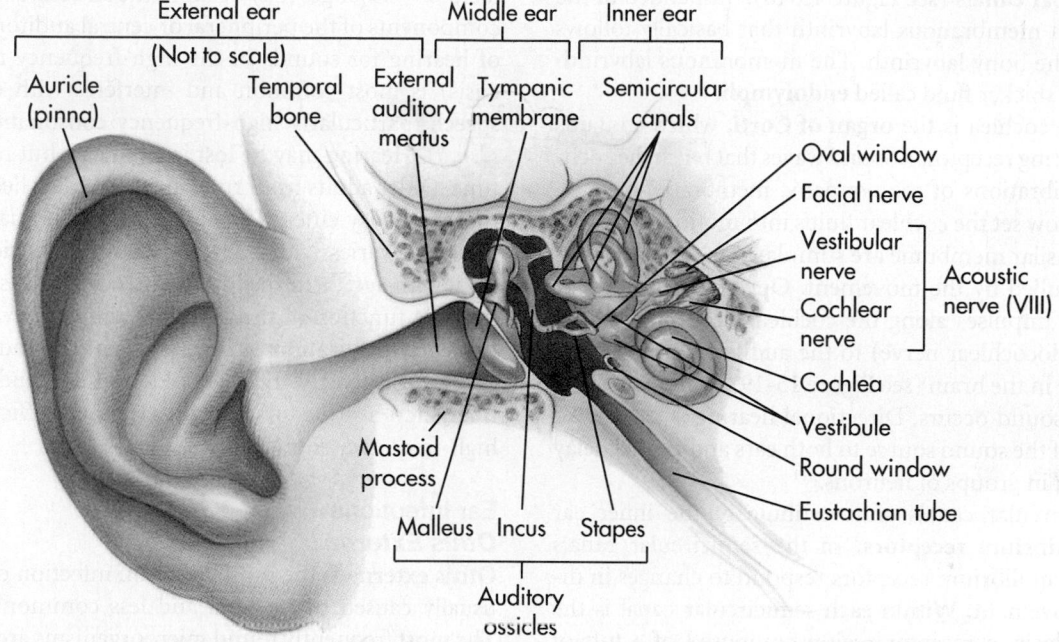

Figure 15-18 The ear. External, middle, and inner ear structures. (Anatomic structures are not drawn to scale. Middle and inner ears enlarged for better visualization here.) (From Patton KT, Thibodeau GA: *Anatomy & physiology,* ed 7, St Louis, 2010, Mosby.)

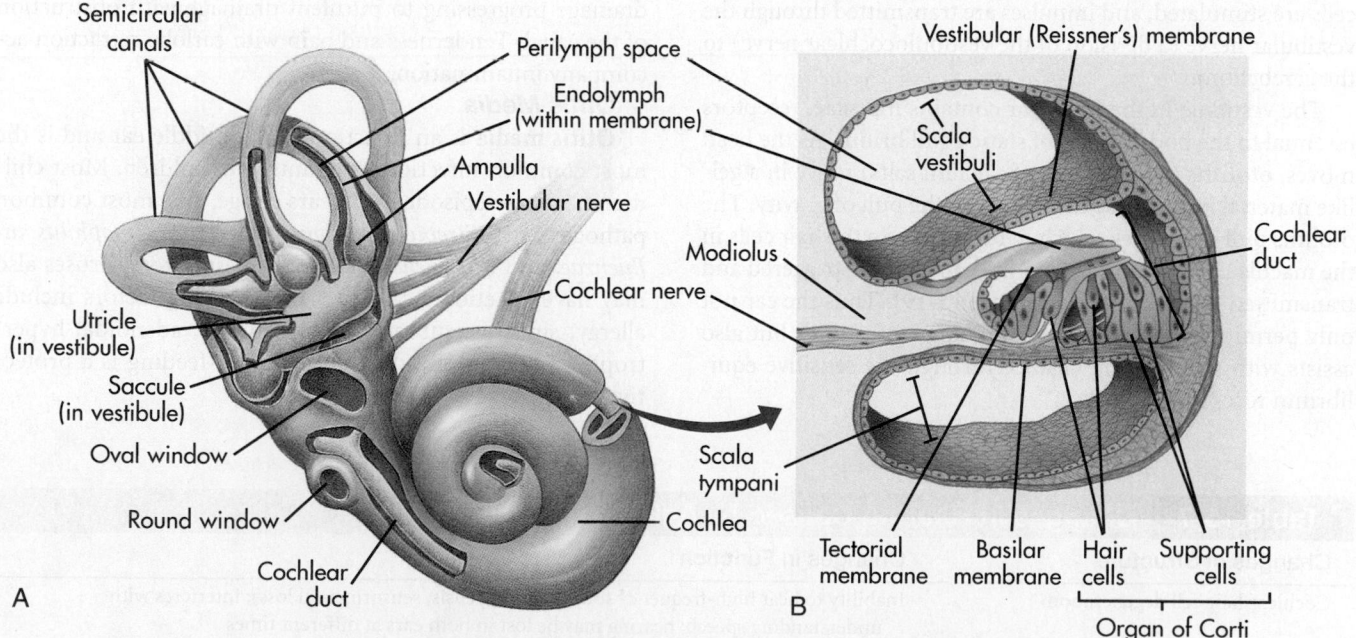

Figure 15-19 The inner ear. A, The bony labyrinth *(orange)* is the hard outer wall of the entire inner ear and includes semicircular canals, vestibule, and cochlea. Within the bony labyrinth is the membranous labyrinth *(purple),* which is surrounded by perilymph and filled with endolymph. Each ampulla in the vestibule contains a crista ampullaris that detects changes in head position and sends sensory impulses through the vestibular nerve to the brain. B, The inset shows a section of the membranous cochlea. Hair cells in the organ of Corti detect sound and send the information through the cochlear nerve. The vestibular and cochlear nerves join to form the eighth cranial nerve. (From Patton KT, Thibodeau GA: *Anatomy & physiology,* ed 7, St Louis, 2010, Mosby.)

membrane to vibrate freely. Through the eustachian tube the mucosa of the middle ear is contiguous with the mucosal lining of the throat.

The inner ear is a system of osseous labyrinths (bony, mazelike chambers) filled with a fluid called **perilymph.** The bony labyrinth is divided into the **cochlea,** the **vestibule,** and the **semicircular canals** (see Figure 15-18). Suspended in the perilymph is a membranous labyrinth that basically follows the shape of the bony labyrinth. The membranous labyrinth is filled with a thicker fluid called **endolymph.**

Within the cochlea is the **organ of Corti,** which contains **hair cells** (hearing receptors). Sound waves that reach the cochlea through vibrations of the tympanic membrane, ossicles, and oval window set the cochlear fluids into motion. Receptor cells on the basilar membrane are stimulated when their hairs are bent or pulled by the movement. Once stimulated, hair cells transmit impulses along the cochlear nerve (a division of the vestibulocochlear nerve) to the auditory cortex of the temporal lobe in the brain (see Figure 15-19), where interpretation of the sound occurs. Directional hearing is controlled by the angle of the sound source to both ears and axonal delay in conduction in groups of neurons.[211]

The semicircular canals and vestibule of the inner ear contain **equilibrium receptors.** In the semicircular canals the dynamic equilibrium receptors respond to changes in direction of movement. Within each semicircular canal is the **crista ampullaris,** a receptor region composed of a tuft of hair cells covered by a gelatinous cupula. When the head is rotated, the endolymph in the canal lags behind and moves in the direction opposite to the head's movement. The hair cells are stimulated, and impulses are transmitted through the vestibular nerve (a division of the vestibulocochlear nerve) to the cerebellum.

The vestibule in the inner ear contains maculae, receptors essential to the body's sense of static equilibrium. As the head moves, **otoliths** (small pieces of calcium salts) move in a gel-like material in response to changes in the pull of gravity. The otoliths pull on the gel, which in turn pulls on the hair cells in the maculae. Nerve impulses in the hair cells are triggered and transmitted to the brain (see Figure 15-19). Thus the ear not only permits the hearing of a large range of sounds but also assists with maintaining balance through the sensitive equilibrium receptors.

Aging and Hearing

Auditory changes caused by aging are common and incremental. Changes in hearing with aging are summarized in Table 15-7. Approximately one third of people older than 65 years have hearing loss caused by genetic and environmental factors.[212] Changes may occur in the structural and functional components of the peripheral or central auditory system. Loss of hearing for sounds in the high-frequency range (presbycusis) is most common and interferes with understanding speech, particularly high-frequency consonant sounds (e.g., s, sh, f). Hearing may be lost in both ears but not at the same time. Older adults from rural areas have less hearing loss than those in noisy cities. The ability to discriminate localization of sound varies with high and low frequencies and diminishes with age.[213] In the low-frequency range, sound localization is a function of the timing of sound arrival between the two ears; localization of high-frequency sounds is a function of sound intensity. Because older adults tend to lose high-frequency hearing first, they may have difficulty localizing high-frequency sounds.

Ear Infections
Otitis Externa
Otitis externa is the most common infection of the outer ear usually caused by bacteria and less commonly a fungus.[214] The most frequently found microorganisms are *Pseudomonas, Escherichia coli,* and *Staphylococcus aureus.* Infection usually follows prolonged exposure to moisture (swimmer's ear). The earliest symptoms are inflammation with swelling and clear drainage progressing to purulent drainage with obstruction of the canal. Tenderness and pain with earlobe retraction accompany inflammation.

Otitis Media
Otitis media is an infection of the middle ear and is the most common infection of infants and children. Most children have one episode by 3 years of age. The most common pathogens are *Streptococcus pneumoniae, Haemophilus influenzae,* and *Moraxella catarrhalis.* Respiratory viruses also may have an etiologic role.[215] Predisposing factors include allergy, sinusitis, submucous cleft palate, adenoidal hypertrophy, and immune deficiency. Breast-feeding is a protective factor.

Table 15-7	Changes in Hearing Caused by Aging	
Changes in Structure	**Changes in Function**
Cochlear hair cell degeneration	Inability to hear high-frequency sounds (presbycusis, sensorineural loss); interferes with understanding speech; hearing may be lost in both ears at different times
Loss of auditory neurons in spiral ganglia of organ of Corti	Inability to hear high-frequency sounds (presbycusis, sensorineural loss); interferes with understanding speech; hearing may be lost in both ears at different times
Degeneration of basilar (cochlear) conductive membrane of cochlea	Inability to hear at all frequencies, but more pronounced at higher frequencies (cochlear conductive loss)
Decreased vascularity of cochlea	Equal loss of hearing at all frequencies (strial loss); inability to disseminate localization of sound
Loss of cortical auditory neurons	Equal loss of hearing at all frequencies (strial loss); inability to disseminate localization of sound

Acute otitis media (AOM) is associated with ear pain, fever, irritability, inflamed tympanic membrane, and fluid in the middle ear. The tympanic membrane progresses from erythema to opaqueness with bulging as fluid accumulates. An increasing prevalence of AOM is caused by methicillin-resistant microorganisms. Otitis media with effusion (OME) is the presence of fluid in the middle ear without symptoms of acute infection. Treatment includes antimicrobial therapy for AOM, particularly in infants 2 years and younger.

Chronic otitis media is persistent or recurring infection of the middle ear. Placement of tympanostomy tubes is considered when bilateral effusion persists for 3 months and for significant hearing loss.[216] Mastoidectomy combined with tympanostomy tubes may be required when there is cholesteatoma (skin growth into the middle ear associated with perforation of the eardrum).[217] Complications include mastoiditis, brain abscess, meningitis, and chronic otitis media with hearing loss. Speech, language, and cognitive disabilities may be affected by persistent middle ear effusions.[218]

Auditory Dysfunction

Between 5% and 10% of the general population have a hearing impairment. The major categories of auditory dysfunction are conductive hearing loss, sensorineural hearing loss, mixed hearing loss, and functional hearing loss.

Conductive Hearing Loss

Conductive hearing loss occurs when a change in the outer or middle ear impairs sound from being conducted from the outer to the inner ear. Conductive hearing loss occurs when there is interference in air conduction. Conditions that commonly cause a conductive hearing loss include impacted cerumen, foreign bodies lodged in the ear canal, benign tumors of the middle ear, carcinoma of the external auditory canal or middle ear, eustachian tube dysfunction, otitis media, acute viral otitis media, chronic suppurative otitis media, cholesteatoma, and otosclerosis.

Symptoms of conductive hearing loss include diminished hearing and soft speaking voice. The voice is soft because often the individual hears his or her voice, conducted by bone, as loud. In addition, although the cause is unknown, the individual often hears better in a noisy environment than in a quiet one (a condition called *paracusia willisiana*). Treatment of the underlying cause generally improves hearing.[219] A hearing aid is used if the hearing loss is between 40 and 50 decibels.

Sensorineural Hearing Loss

A **sensorineural hearing loss** is caused by impairment of the organ of Corti or its central connections. The hearing loss may be gradual or sudden. Conditions that commonly cause sensorineural hearing loss include congenital and hereditary factors, noise exposure, aging, Ménière disease, ototoxicity, and systemic disease (syphilis, Paget disease, collagen diseases, diabetes mellitus). Congenital and neonatal sensorineural hearing loss may be caused by maternal rubella, ototoxic drugs, prematurity, traumatic delivery, erythroblastosis fetalis, and congenital hereditary malfunction. Diagnosis often is made when delayed speech development is noted.

Presbycusis is age-related hearing loss usually in the high frequencies. It is the most common form of sensorineural hearing loss and is especially common in older adutls.[220] Presbycusis may occur because of atrophy of the basal end of the organ of Corti, a loss in the number of auditory receptors, vascular changes, or stiffening of the basilar membranes. Because of the slow progression of hearing loss, onset of symptoms is gradual. In addition, drug ototoxicities (drugs that cause destruction of auditory function) have been observed after exposure to a variety of chemicals, for example, antibiotics such as streptomycin, neomycin, gentamicin, and vancomycin; diuretics such as ethacrynic acid and furosemide; and chemicals such as salicylate, quinine, carbon monoxide, nitrogen mustard, arsenic, mercury, gold, tobacco, and alcohol. Because of increased concentrations of antibiotics in the endolymph, these drugs generally cause damage to the cells of the cristae and maculae (located in the inner ear) or the cells of the organ of Corti. The increased concentration of drugs in the endolymph is preferentially toxic to the cells.

Diuretics affect hearing primarily by altering the sodium-potassium balance, causing extracellular fluid accumulation and changes in the microstructure of secretory cells. Quinine, mercury, and lead affect the neural pathways of hearing, including the spinal ganglia, the eighth cranial nerve, and the cochlear nucleus. The site of action for the other chemicals, including alcohol and tobacco, has not yet been determined. In most instances the drugs and chemicals listed previously initially cause **tinnitus** (ringing in the ear), followed by a progressive high-tone sensorineural hearing loss. Care is aimed at prevention of further hearing loss because the loss is usually permanent.

Mixed Hearing Loss

A **mixed hearing loss** is caused by a combination of conductive and sensorineural losses.

Functional Hearing Loss

A **functional hearing loss** occurs for no organic reason. The individual does not respond to voice and appears not to hear. Functional hearing loss is thought to be caused by emotional or psychologic factors. It occurs only rarely.

Olfaction and Taste

Olfaction is a function of cranial nerve I and part of cranial nerve V. Taste is a function of multiple nerves in the tongue, soft palate, uvula, pharynx, and upper esophagus, including cranial nerves VII and IX. Olfaction (smell) dysfunction and taste (gustation) dysfunction may occur separately or jointly. The strong relationship between smell and taste creates the sensation of flavor. If either sensation is impaired, the perception of flavor is altered. (Olfactory structures are illustrated in Figure 15-20.)

Olfactory cells, which are located in the olfactory epithelium, are the receptor cells for smell. Seven primary classes of olfactory stimulants have been identified: (1) camphoraceous, (2) musky, (3) floral, (4) peppermint, (5) ethereal, (6) pungent, and (7) putrid. The primary sensations of taste

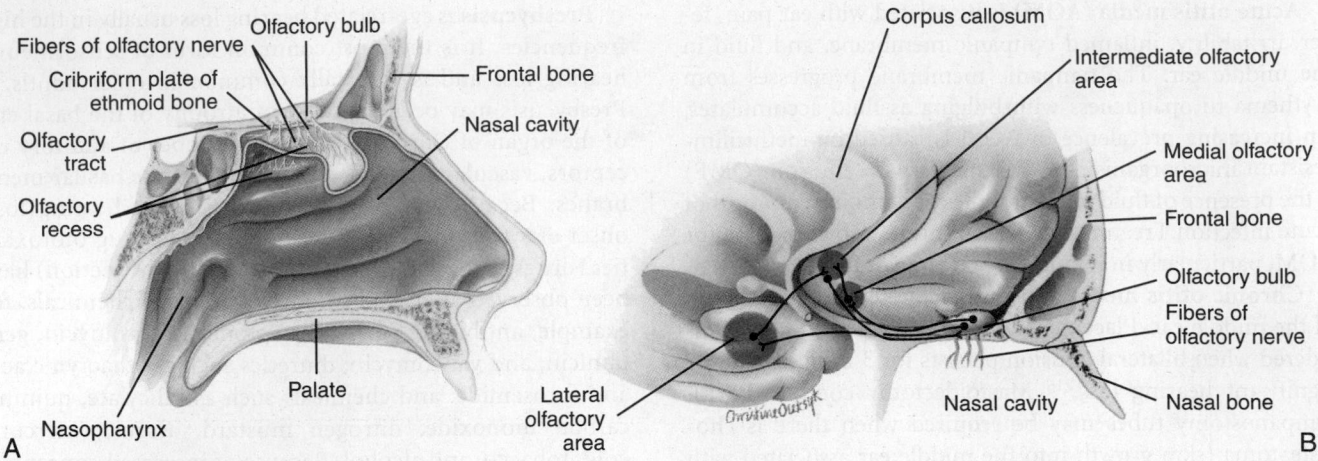

Figure 15-20 Olfaction. Location of olfactory epithelium, olfactory bulb, and neuronal pathways involved in olfaction. A, Midsagittal section of the nasal area shows the locations of major olfactory sensory structures. B, Major olfactory integration centers of the brain. (Modified from Patton KT, Thibodeau GA: *Anatomy & physiology,* ed 7, St Louis, 2010, Mosby.)

are sour, salty, sweet, and bitter. Taste buds sensitive to each of the primary sensations are located in specific areas of the tongue.[221]

Aging and Olfaction and Taste

Olfaction

Sensitivity to odors declines steadily with aging.[222] A study of odor identification indicates an increasing ability from childhood to adolescence and then a decline after 60 years of age. The most significant impairments develop after 80 years.[223] Women generally have better olfactory abilities than men, but the patterns of decline are similar.[224]

The sense of smell begins to degenerate with loss of olfactory sensory neurons and loss of cells from the olfactory bulbs.[225,226] Loss of olfactory sensitivity and odor identification may diminish appetite and food selection and thus may lead to malnutrition. Safety also may be compromised by an inability to smell toxic or hazardous gases.

Taste

The decline in taste sensation is more gradual than that of smell and may be associated with loss of olfaction. Higher concentrations of flavors are required, and older adults have difficulty differentiating combinations of flavors.[227] The best-known change with aging is the decline in the number of fungiform papillae on the tongue, which decrease by 50% by about 50 years of age.[227] Taste also may be affected by decreased salivary gland secretion. Amylase, contained in saliva, facilitates perception of sweet sensations and also is reduced with aging.

Olfactory Dysfunction

Olfactory dysfunctions include hyposmia, anosmia, hallucinations, and parosmia. **Hyposmia** is the impaired sense of smell, and **anosmia** is the complete loss of smell. Both conditions are associated with aging, neurodegenerative and nasal/sinus disorders and head trauma.[228] When hyposmia or anosmia occurs bilaterally, it is usually the result of rhinitis (inflammation of nasal mucosa), sinusitis, nasal polyps, or excessive smoking.[229] Unilateral hyposmia or anosmia may indicate compression of one olfactory bulb (a bulblike portion of the olfactory nerves) or nerve tract (olfactory nerve pathway), possibly by tumor or head trauma. **Olfactory hallucinations** arise from hyperactivity in cortical neurons and involve smelling odors that are not really present. They are associated with temporal lobe seizures and rarely with schizophrenia. **Parosmia,** an abnormal or perverted sense of smell, may occur with severe depression.[230]

Taste Dysfunction

The sense of taste can be impaired by injury, medications, oral infections, or aging. An alteration in taste also may be attributable to impairment of smell associated with injury near the hippocampus.

Hypogeusia is decrease in taste sensation, and **ageusia** is the absence of taste. Ageusia affecting the entire tongue may follow head injury. Damage to the glossopharyngeal nerve (cranial nerve IX, which innervates the posterior one third of the tongue) causes the loss of the ability to detect bitterness. This loss occurs because the receptors for bitter are located on the base of the tongue. Damage to the facial nerve (cranial nerve VII, which innervates the anterior two thirds of the tongue) causes loss of the ability to detect sour, sweet, and salty tastes. Only bitter tastes can be detected. These losses occur because sour, sweet, and salt receptors are located on the anterior portion of the tongue. **Parageusia** is a perversion of taste in which substances possess an unpleasant flavor. Parageusia occasionally develops for no apparent reason in older adults and is common in individuals receiving chemotherapy for cancer. In both cases, parageusia often leads to anorexia and malnutrition.

SOMATOSENSORY FUNCTION

Touch

Touch is not a uniform sensory experience. The sensation of touch involves the fusion of several qualities, including modality, intensity, location, and duration of the sensory stimulus. Receptors sensitive to touch are present in the skin. Meissner and pacinian corpuscles are rapidly adapting receptors, whereas Merkel disks and Ruffini endings are slowly adapting touch receptors. Touch receptors are most numerous in the skin of the fingers and lips and are more scarce in the skin of the trunk. Specific sensory input is carried to the higher levels of the CNS by the dorsal column of the spinal cord and the anterior spinothalamic tract.

Much of the development of the cutaneous senses takes place before birth, but structural growth of the cutaneous senses continues into early adulthood at a reduced rate. Then a gradual decline occurs.[231] Studies have documented loss in tactile sensitivity with advancing age.[232,233] This occurs simultaneously with an increase in the size of pacinian corpuscles and a decrease in the number of corpuscles.

Abnormal tactile perception may be caused by alterations at any level of the nervous system, from the receptor to the cerebral cortex. Any factor that interrupts or impairs reception, transmission, perception, or interpretation of touch also alters tactile sensation. Trauma, tumor, infection, metabolic changes, vascular changes, and degenerative diseases thus may cause tactile dysfunction, which may involve heightened or diminished tactile perceptions.

In addition, most tactile sensations evoke affective responses that determine whether the sensation is unpleasant, pleasant, or neutral. Cerebral and hypothalamic centers influence this response. Sedative drugs and prefrontal injury, which interrupt connections between the prefrontal cortex and subcortical centers, diminish the interpretation of tactile sensations.

Proprioception

Perception and awareness of the position of the body and its parts depend on impulses from the inner ear and from receptors in joints and ligaments. The role of muscle, tendon, and cutaneous receptors is indefinite. Sensory data are transmitted to higher centers, primarily through the dorsal columns and the spinocerebellar tracts, with some data passing through the medial lemnisci and thalamic radiations to the cortex. These stimuli are necessary for the coordination of movements, the grading of muscular contraction, and the maintenance of equilibrium.

A progressive loss of proprioception has been reported in older adults.[233] Proprioceptive dysfunction may be caused by alterations at any level of the nervous system. As with tactile dysfunction, any factor that interrupts or impairs the reception, transmission, perception, or interpretation of proprioceptive stimuli also alters proprioception. Two common causes of proprioceptive dysfunction are vestibular dysfunction and neuropathy.

Specific vestibular dysfunctions are vestibular nystagmus and vertigo. **Vestibular nystagmus** is the constant, involuntary movement of the eyeball caused by ear disturbances. This condition occurs when the semicircular canal system is overstimulated. **Vertigo** is the sensation of spinning that occurs with inflammation of the semicircular canals in the ear. The individual may feel either that he or she is moving in space or that the world is revolving. Vertigo often causes loss of balance. Vertigo and nystagmus may occur in a variety of conditions, including labyrinthitis, vestibular neuritis, acute toxic labyrinthitis, benign paroxysmal positional vertigo, migrainous vertigo, and Ménière disease.[234]

Ménière disease is an idiopathic vestibular disorder that can cause proprioceptive dysfunction. The individual with Ménière disease also can experience vertigo, hearing loss, or tinnitus, and standing or walking may be impossible.

Peripheral neuropathies also can cause proprioceptive dysfunctions. Neuropathies may be caused by a variety of conditions and commonly are associated with renal disease and diabetes mellitus. Although the exact sequence of events is unknown, neuropathies are thought to be caused by a metabolic disturbance of the neuron itself. The result is a diminished or absent sense of body position or position of body parts. Gait changes often occur. (Neuropathies are further discussed in Chapter 17.)

SUMMARY REVIEW

Pain

1. Pain is protective and a complex phenomenon composed of sensory experiences (time, space, intensity) and emotion, cognition, and motivation.
2. The gate control theory of pain describes the modulation of pain in the dorsal horn of the spinal cord by sensory afferent stimulation and central descending impulses that influence the "pain gate" within the substantia gelatinosa of the spinal cord.
3. The portions of the nervous system responsible for the sensation and perception of pain may be divided into three areas: (1) the afferent fibers, (2) the afferent pathways, and (3) the CNS.
4. The afferent system is composed of nociceptors, Aδ and C fibers (first-order neurons), the dorsal horn of the spinal column (second-order neurons), and afferent neurons in the spinothalamic tract (third-order neurons).
5. Nociceptors detect a wide range of stimuli and respond to chemical, mechanical, and thermal stimulation.
6. Myelinated Aδ receptor transmission is fast and conveys mechanical and thermal, sharp, localized pain. Unmyelinated polymodal C fiber transmission is slower and conveys diffuse burning and aching sensations. These primary-order neurons terminate on second-order neurons.

Continued

7. Three classes of second-order neurons modulate pain transmission: projection cells, excitatory interneurons, and inhibitory interneurons. The second-order neurons are located in the spinal cord laminae and function as a pain gate to regulate pain transmission.

8. Second-order neurons cross over the cord and ascend primarily in the lateral spinothalamic tract to projection centers including the thalamus reticular formation, and PAG matter.

9. Third-order neurons carry information to the sensory cortex and reticular and limbic systems for pain processing and interpretation.

10. Efferent pathways from the PAG are responsible for modulation or inhibition of afferent pain signals. The thalamus, cortex, and postcentral gyrus perceive, describe, and localize pain. The reticular formation and limbic system control the emotional and affective response to pain.

11. Pain can be modulated by segmental inhibition, which is the peripheral stimulation of nociceptors by touch, vibration, or pressure resulting in closure of the spinal cord pain gate. The higher brain center also can influence painful stimuli (heterosegmental control of nociception) as well as inhibition from the caudal medulla (diffuse noxious inhibitory controls). Thus pain can be modulated with stimulation from the periphery or by descending impulses from the brain.

12. Pain neurotransmitters can be classified as inflammatory, excitatory, and inhibitory modulators of pain. Inflammatory neurotransmitters include prostaglandins, nitric oxide, bradykinins, and histamine. Glutamate, aspartate, and amino acid precursors are excitatory neurotransmitters. GABA and glycine are inhibitory neurotransmitters. Endogenous opioids including enkephalins, endorphins, dynorphins and endomorphins inhibit pain transmission and are present in varying concentrations in the neurons of the brain, spinal cord, and GI tract. Serotonin, norepinephrine aspartate, and glycine also can modulate pain processing.

13. Pain threshold is the point at which pain is perceived. Pain threshold does not vary significantly among people or within the same person over time.

14. Pain tolerance is the duration of time or the intensity of pain that an individual will endure before initiating overt pain response. Tolerance varies widely among individuals and in the same individual over time.

15. Classifications of pain include nociceptive pain (with a known physiologic cause), non-nociceptive pain (neuropathic pain), acute pain (signal to the person of a harmful stimulus), and chronic pain (persistence of pain of unknown cause or unusual response to therapy).

16. Acute pain may be (1) somatic (superficial), (2) visceral (internal), or (3) referred (present in an area distant from its origin).

17. Somatic pain arises from connective tissue, muscle, bone, and skin and is sharp and localized.

18. Visceral pain is transmitted by sympathetic afferents and is poorly localized.

19. Referred pain usually arises from the viscera and terminates in an area of the spinal cord that is conjoined with fibers originating in the skin and other areas and thereby produces the perception of pain at the referred site.

20. Physiologic responses to acute pain include increased heart rate, respiratory rate, and blood pressure; pallor or flushing; dilated pupils; and diaphoresis. Blood sugar is elevated; gastric secretion and motility are decreased; and blood flow to the viscera and skin is decreased.

21. Chronic pain generally lasts at least 3 months and may be persistent, for example, low back pain or intermittent migraine headache.

22. Chronic pain conditions include myofascial pain syndromes, chronic postoperative pain, low back pain, and chronic pain associated with cancer.

23. Neuropathic pain is usually chronic, results from nerve trauma or disease, and leads to abnormal peripheral and central pain processing. Types of neuropathic pain include deafferentation pain, sympathetically maintained pain, central pain, and phantom pain.

24. Newborns and young children have the anatomic and functional ability to perceive pain. Pain experienced by infants may have prolonged effects on brain organization and responses to pain.

25. Older individuals may or may not have an increased pain threshold. In all age groups, women appear to be more sensitive to pain than are men.

26. Pain in older adults is influenced by liver and renal function, including alterations in metabolism of drugs and metabolites.

Temperature Regulation

1. Temperature regulation is achieved through precise balancing of heat production, heat conservation, and heat loss. Body temperature is maintained around 37° C (98.6° F).

2. Temperature regulation is mediated by the hypothalamus. Peripheral thermoreceptors in the skin and central thermoreceptors in the hypothalamus, spinal cord, and abdominal organs provide the hypothalamus with information about skin and core temperatures.

3. Heat is produced through chemical reactions of metabolism, skeletal muscle contraction (shivering), and chemical thermogenesis.

4. Heat is lost through radiation, conduction, convection, vasodilation, decreased muscle tone, evaporation of sweat, increased ventilation, and voluntary mechanisms.

5. Heat conservation is accomplished through vasoconstriction and voluntary mechanisms.

6. Fever is triggered by the release of pyrogens from leukocytes and other cells involved in the immune response (endogenous pyrogens) and bacteria (exogenous pyrogens). Fever is both a symptom of a disease and a normal immunologic mechanism.

7. Fever involves resetting the hypothalamic thermostat to a higher level. When a fever breaks, the set point is returned to normal.

8. Fever production aids responses to infectious processes. Higher temperatures kill many microorganisms and decrease serum levels of iron, zinc, and copper that are needed for bacterial replication.

9. Infants and older adults require special attention to maintenance of body temperature. Because of their greater body surface:mass ratio and decreased subcutaneous fat, infants do not conserve heat well. Older individuals have poor responses to environmental temperature extremes as a result of slowed blood circulation, structural and functional changes in skin, and an overall decrease in heat-producing activities.

10. Hyperthermia (marked warming of core temperature) can produce nerve damage, coagulation of cell proteins, and death. Forms of accidental hyperthermia include heat cramps, heat exhaustion, heat stroke, and malignant hyperthermia. Heat stroke and malignant hyperthermia are potentially lethal developments.

SUMMARY REVIEW—cont'd

11. Hypothermia (marked cooling of core temperature) slows the rate of chemical reaction (tissue metabolism), increases the viscosity of the blood, slows blood flow through the microcirculation, facilitates blood coagulation, and stimulates profound vasoconstriction. Hypothermia may be accidental or therapeutic.

Sleep

1. Sleep may be divided into REM and NREM stages, each of which has its own series of stages. While asleep, an individual progresses through the four stages of NREM (slow-wave) sleep and REM sleep in a predictable cycle.
2. NREM sleep is initiated by the withdrawal of neurotransmitters from the afferent formation and by the inhibition of arousal mechanisms in the cerebral cortex. REM sleep is controlled by mechanisms in the hypothalamus and pontine reticular formation.
3. During sleep the body is actively engaged in restoring and repairing itself. Sleep deprivation can cause profound changes in personality and functioning.
4. The restorative, reparative, and growth processes occur during slow-wave sleep.
5. The sleep patterns of the newborn and young child vary from those of the adult in total sleep time, cycle length, and percentage of time spent in each sleep cycle. Older adults experience a total decrease in sleep time.
6. Sleep disorders include (1) dyssomnias (2) parasomnias, (3) sleep disorders associated with mental, neurologic or other medical disorder, and (4) proposed sleep disorders.
7. Common dyssomnias include insomnia, OSAS, RLS, circadian rhythm disorder, and hypersomnia.
8. Common parasomnias include arousal disorders, sleep-wake transition disorder, and disorders associated with REM sleep.
9. Sleep and disease are interrelated. Some diseases may produce alterations in the quantity and quality of sleep or affect sleep stages. These are referred to as *secondary sleep disorders*. In some instances sleep stages produce alterations in certain disease states. These are referred to as *sleep-provoked disorders*.

Special Senses

Vision

1. The eyelids, conjunctivae, and lacrimal apparatus protect the eye. Infections are the most common disorders; they include blepharitis, conjunctivitis, chalazion, and hordeolum.
2. Conjunctivitis can be acute or chronic, bacterial, viral, or allergic. Redness, edema, pain, and lacrimation are common symptoms. Trachoma (chlamydial conjunctivitis) is the leading cause of blindness in the world and is associated with poor sanitary conditions.
3. Keratitis is a bacterial or viral infection of the cornea that can lead to corneal ulceration. Photophobia, pain, and tearing are common symptoms.
4. The wall of the eye has three layers: sclera, choroid, and retina. The retina contains millions of photoreceptors known as rods and cones that receive light through the lens and then convey signals to the optic nerve and subsequently to the visual cortex of the brain.
5. The eye is filled with vitreous and aqueous humor, which prevent it from collapsing.
6. Structural eye changes caused by aging or chronic disease result in decreased visual acuity.
7. The major alterations in ocular movement include strabismus, nystagmus, and paralysis of the extraocular muscles.

8. Alterations in visual acuity can be caused by amblyopia, scotoma, cataracts, papilledema, macular degeneration, retinal detachment, glaucoma, and macular degeneration.
9. Alterations in accommodation develop with increased intraocular pressure, inflammation, and disease of the oculomotor nerve. Presbyopia is loss of accommodation caused by loss of lens elasticity with aging.
10. Alterations in refraction, including myopia, hyperopia, and astigmatism, are the most common visual disorders.
11. Alterations in color vision occur with disorders of the cornea and the inherited trait of color blindness.
12. Trauma or disease of the optic nerve pathways or optic radiations, can cause blindness in the visual fields. Homonymous hemianopsia is caused by damage of one optic tract.

Hearing

1. The ear is composed of external, middle, and inner structures. The external structures are the pinna, auditory canal, and tympanic membrane. The tympanic cavity (containing three bones: malleus, incus, and stapes), oval window, eustachian tube, and fluid comprise the middle ear and transmit sound vibrations to the inner ear.
2. The inner ear includes the bony and membranous labyrinths that transmit sound waves through the cochlea to the division of the eighth cranial nerve. The semicircular canals and vestibule help maintain balance through the equilibrium receptors.
3. Approximately one third of all people older than 65 years have hearing loss.
4. Otitis externa is an infection of the outer ear. Otitis media, an infection of the middle ear, is common in children and can be acute or chronic.
5. Acute otitis media is an infection of the middle ear associated with ear pain, fever, an inflamed tympanic membrane and fluid in the middle ear.
6. Chronic otitis media is persistent or recurrent middle ear infection.
7. Hearing loss can be classified as conductive, sensorineural, mixed, or functional.
8. Conductive hearing loss occurs when sound waves cannot be conducted through the middle ear.
9. Sensorineural hearing loss develops with impairment of the organ of Corti or its central connections. Presbycusis is age-related hearing loss and is the most common form of sensorineural hearing loss.
10. A combination of conductive and sensorineural loss is a mixed hearing loss.
11. Loss of hearing with no known organic cause is a functional hearing loss.

Olfaction and Taste

1. The perception of flavor is altered if olfaction or taste dysfunctions occur. Sensitivity to odor and taste decreases with aging.
2. Hyposmia is a decrease in the sense of smell, and anosmia is the complete loss of smell. Inflammation of the nasal mucosa and trauma or tumors of the olfactory nerve lead to a diminished sense of smell.
3. Hypogeusia is a decrease in taste sensation, and ageusia is the absence of taste. Loss of taste buds or trauma to the facial or glossopharyngeal nerves decreases taste sensation.

Somatosensory Function

1. The sensation of touch involves the fusion of several qualities, including modality, intensity, location, and duration of the sensory stimulus.

Continued

SUMMARY REVIEW—cont'd

2. Receptors sensitive to touch are present in the skin; these include Meissner and pacinian corpuscles and Merkel disks and Ruffini endings. The sensory response is conducted to the brain through the dorsal column and anterior spinothalamic tract.

3. Abnormal tactile perception may be caused by alterations at any level of the nervous system, from the receptor to the cerebral cortex.

4. Proprioception is the position and location of the body and its parts. Proprioceptors are located in the inner ear, joints, and ligaments. Proprioceptive stimuli are necessary for balance, coordinated movement, and grading of muscular contraction.

5. Disorders of proprioception can be caused by alterations at any level of the nervous system. Two common causes of proprioceptive dysfunction are vestibular dysfunction and neuropathy.

KEY TERMS

Acute bacterial conjunctivitis (pinkeye), 506
Aδ fiber, 483
Acute otitis media (AOM), 515
Acute pain, 490
Age-related macular degeneration (AMD), 510
Ageusia, 516
Allergic conjunctivitis, 507
Allodynia, 488
Amblyopia, 509
Anosmia, 516
Antipyretic, 498
Aqueous humor, 508
Astigmatism, 511
Blepharitis, 506
Cancer pain, 493
Cataract, 509
Central pain, 494
Central sensitization, 488
Chalazion, 506
Choroid, 507
Chronic conjunctivitis, 507
Chronic otitis media, 515
Chronic pain, 492
Chronic postoperative pain, 492
Circadian rhythm, 496
Circadian rhythm sleep disorder, 505
Cochlea, 514
Color blindness, 511
Complex regional pain syndrome (CRPS), 494
Conduction, 497
Conductive hearing loss, 515
Cone, 507
Convection, 497
Cornea, 507
Crista ampullaris, 514
Dark adaptation, 510
Deafferentation pain, 494
Diffuse noxious inhibitory controls (DNICs), 486
Diplopia, 509
Dynorphin, 489
Dyssomnia, 504
Endogenous cryogen, 498
Endogenous opioid, 488
Endogenous pyrogen, 498
Endolymph, 514
Endomorphin, 490
Endorphin, 489
Enkephalin, 489
Equilibrium receptor, 514
Eustachian (pharyngotympanic) tube, 513
Exogenous pyrogen, 498

External auditory canal, 512
Fovea centralis, 507
Functional hearing loss, 515
Gamma-aminobutyric acid (GABA), 488
Gate control theory, 482
Glaucoma, 510
Glutamate, 488
Glycine, 488
Hair cells, 514
Heat cramps, 500
Heat exhaustion, 500
Heat production, 496
Heat stroke, 500
Hemianopia, 512
Homonymous hemianopsia, 512
Hordeolum (stye), 506
Hyperalgesia, 487
Hyperopia, 511
Hypersomnia, 505
Hyperthermia, 501
Hypogeusia, 516
Hyposmia, 516
Hypothermia, 501
Incus (anvil), 512
Insomnia, 504
Iris, 507
Jerk nystagmus, 509
Lens, 508
Limbic system, 486
Macula, 509
Malignant hyperthermia, 500
Malleus (hammer), 512
Mastoid air cell, 512
Mastoid process, 512
Ménière disease, 517
Mixed hearing loss, 515
Myofascial pain syndrome (MPS), 492
Myopia, 511
Narcolepsy, 505
Neuropathic pain, 493
Nociception, 482
Nociceptive pain, 490
Nociceptor, 482
Non-nociceptive pain, 490
NREM (slow-wave) sleep, 503
Nystagmus, 509
Obesity hypoventilation syndrome 505
Obstructive sleep apnea syndrome (OSAS), 505
Olfactory hallucination, 516
Opioid receptor, 488
Optic chiasm, 510
Optic disc, 507

Organ of Corti, 514
Otitis externa, 514
Otitis media, 514
Otoliths, 514
Oval window, 513
Pain threshold, 490
Pain tolerance, 490
Papilledema, 510
Parageusia, 516
Parasomnia, 505
Parosmia, 516
Pendular nystagmus, 509
Perceptual dominance, 490
Perilymph, 514
Peripheral sensitization, 487
Phantom limb pain, 494
Pinna, 512
Presbycusis, 515
Presbyopia, 511
Pupil, 507
Radiation, 497
Rapid eye movement (REM) sleep, 503
Referred pain, 491
Restless leg syndrome (RLS), 505
Reticular activating system, 486
Retina, 507
Retinal detachment, 510
Rhegmatogenous retinal detachment, 510
Rods, 507
Sclera, 507
Scotoma, 509
Segmental inhibition, 486
Semicircular canal, 514
Sensorineural hearing loss, 515
Shivering, 501
Sleep, 502
Somatic pain, 491
Specificity theory, 482
Stapes (stirrup), 512
Strabismus, 509
Suprachiasmatic nucleus (SCN), 502
Sympathetically maintained pain (SMP), 494
Tinnitus, 515
Trachoma, 507
Tympanic cavity, 512
Tympanic membrane, 512
Unmyelinated C polymodal nociceptor, 483
Vertigo, 517
Vestibular nystagmus, 517
Vestibule, 514
Viral conjunctivitis, 507
Visceral pain, 491
Vitreous humor, 508

REFERENCES

1. American Pain Society: www.ampainsoc.org/ce/npc/I/b_definitions. htm. Accessed July 24, 2004.
2. McCaffery M: Understanding your patient's pain, *Nursing* 10(9):26-31, 1980.
3. Waddell G: *The back pain revolution*, ed 2 , London, 2004, Churchill Livingstone.
4. Melzack R, Wall PD: Pain mechanisms: a new theory, *Science* 150:971, 1965.
5. Melzack R, Wall PD: Pain mechanisms: a new theory, *Science* 150:971-979, 1965.
6. Tominaga M: Nociception and TRP channels, *Handb Exp Pharmacol* (179):489-505, 2007.
7. Rexed B: A cytoarchitectural atlas of the spinal cord in the cat, *J Comp Neurol* 100:297, 1954.
8. Willis WD, Coggeshall RE: *Sensory mechanisms of the spinal cord*, ed 3 , New York, 2004, Kluwer.
9. Romanelli P, Esposito V: The functional anatomy of neuropathic pain, *Neurosurg Clin North Am* 15(3):257-268, 2004.
10. Herrero MT, Barcia C, Navarro JM: Functional anatomy of thalamus and basal ganglia, *Childs Nerv Syst* 18(8):386-404, 2002.
11. Partridge LD: *Nervous system actions and interactions: concepts in neurophysiology*, Boston, 2003, Kluwer.
12. Villemure C, Bushnell MC: Cognitive modulation of pain: how do attention and emotion influence pain processing? *Pain* 95(3):195-199, 2002.
13. Mayer DJ, Price DD: Central nervous system mechanisms of analgesia, *Pain* 2(4):379-404, 1976.
14. Ruda MA, Bennett GJ, Dubner R: Neurochemistry and neurocircuitry in the dorsal horn, *Prog Brain Res* 66:219-268, 1986.
15. Hughes J et al: Identification of two related pentapeptides from the brain with potent opiate agonist activity, *Nature* 258(5536):577-579, 1975.
16. Calvino B, Grilo RM: Central pain control, *Joint Bone Spine* 73(1):10-16, 2006.
17. Rainville P: Brain mechanisms of pain affect and pain modulation, *Curr Opin Neurobiol* 12(2):195-204, 2002.
18. Villenueva L, Le Bars D: The activation of bulbospinal controls by peripheral nociceptive inputs: diffuse noxious inhibitory controls (DNIC), *Biol Res* 28:113-125, 1995.
19. Fields HL, Basbuam AI, Heinricher MM: Central nervous system mechanisms of pain modulation. In McMahon S, Koltzenburg M, editors: *Wall and Melzack's textbook of pain*, ed 5 , Edinburgh, Scotland, 2005, Churchill Livingstone.
20. Ploghaus A et al: Neural circuitry underlying pain modulation: expectation, hypnosis, placebo, *Trends Cogn Sci* 7(5):197-200, 2003.
21. Petrovic P et al: Placebo and opioid analgesia—imaging a shared neuronal network, *Science* 295:1737-1740, 2002.
22. Scott DJ et al: Placebo and nocebo effects are defined by opposite opioid and dopaminergic responses, *Arch Gen Psychiatry* 65(2):220-231, 2008.
23. Bleakman D, Alt A, Nisenbaus ES: Glutamate receptors and pain, *Semin Cell Dev Biol* 17(5):592-604, 2006.
24. Bodnar RJ: Endogenous opiates and behavior, 2006, *Peptides* 28(12):2435-2513, 2007.
25. von Zastrow M: Opioid receptor regulation, *Neuromolec Med* 5(1):51-58, 2004.
26. Rittner HL, Brack A, Stein C: Pain and the immune system, *Br J Anaesth* 101(1):40-44, 2008.
27. Wollemann M, Benyhe S: Non-opioid actions of opioid peptides, *Life Sci* 75(3):257-270, 2004.
28. Lai J et al: Pronociceptive actions of dynorphin via bradykinin receptors, *Neurosci Lett* 437(3):175-179, 2008.
29. Fichna J et al: The endomorphin system and its evolving neurophysiological role, *Pharmacol Rev* 59(1):88-123, 2007.
30. Coward DD, Wilkie DJ: Metastatic bone pain: meanings associated with self-report and self-management decision making, *Cancer Nurs* 23(2):101-108, 2000.
31. Purves D et al: *Neuroscience*, ed 3, Sunderland, MA, 2004, Sinauer.
32. Thibodeau GA, Patton KT: *Anatomy & physiology*, ed 5 , St Louis, 2003, Mosby.
33. Turk DC: The role of psychological factors in pain management, *Acta Anaesthesiol Scand* 43(9):885-888, 1999.
34. Turk DC, Okifuji A: Psychological factors in chronic pain: evolution and revolution, *J Consult Clin Psychol* 70(3):678-690, 2002.
35. Miles A et al: Managing constraint: the experience of people with chronic pain, *Soc Sci Med* 61(2):431-441, 2005.
36. Almay BG et al: Relationships between CSF levels of endorphins and monoamine metabolites in chronic pain patients, *Psychopharmacology* 67(2):139-142, 1980.
37. Schaible HG, Richter F: Pathophysiology of pain, *Langenbecks Arch Surg* 389(4):237-243, 2004.
38. Whitehead W III, Kuhn WF: Chronic pain: an overview. In Miller TW, editor: *Chronic pain,* vol 1, Madison, WI, 1990, International Universities.
39. White FA, Jung H, Miller RJ: Chemokines and the pathophysiology of neuropathic pain, *Proc Natl Acad Sci U S A* 104(51):20151-20158, 2007.
40. Jones GT, Macfarlane GJ: Epidemiology of low back pain in children and adolescents, *Arch Dis Child* 90(3):312-316, 2005.
41. Ehrlich GE: Back pain, *J Rheumatol* 67(Suppl):26-31, 2003.
42. Lavelle ED, Lavelle W, Smith HS: Myofascial trigger points, *Med Clin North Am* 91(2):229-239, 2007.
43. Cummings M, Baldry P: Regional myofascial pain: diagnosis and management, *Best Pract Res Clin Rheumatol* 21(2):367-387, 2007.
44. Kehlet H, Jensen TS, Woolf CJ: Persistent postsurgical pain: risk factors and prevention, *Lancet* 367(9522):1618-1625, 2006.
45. Macrae WA: Chronic post-surgical pain: 10 years on, *Br J Anaesth* 101(1):77-86, 2008.
46. Goudas LC et al: The epidemiology of cancer pain, *Cancer Invest* 23(2):182-190, 2005.
47. Seymour J, Clark D, Winslow M: Pain and palliative care: the emergence of new specialties, *J Pain Symptom Manage* 29(1):2-13, 2005.
48. Cherny NI: The pharmacologic management of cancer pain, *Oncology (Huntingt)* 18(12):1499-1515, 2004.
49. De Leon-Casasola OA: Current developments in opioid therapy for management of cancer pain, *Clin J Pain* 24(Suppl 10):S3-S7, 2008.
50. Dy SM et al: Evidence-based standards for cancer pain management, *J Clin Oncol* 26(23):3879-3885, 2008.
51. Zhuo M: Neuronal mechanism for neuropathic pain, *Mol Pain* 3:14, 2007.
52. Schaible HG: Peripheral and central mechanisms of pain generation, *Handb Exp Pharmacol* (177):3-28, 2007.
53. Edwards JL et al: Diabetic neuropathy: mechanisms, to management, *Pharmacol Ther* 120(1):1-34, 2008.
54. Horowitz SH: The diagnostic workup of patients with neuropathic pain, *Anesthesiol Clin* 25(4):699-708, 2007.
55. Aurillo C et al: Ionic channels and neuropathic pain: physiopathology and applications, *J Cell Physiol* 215(1):8-14, 2008.
56. Ji RR, Strichartz G: Cell signaling and the genesis of neuropathic pain, *Sci STKE* (252):reE14, 2004.
57. De Ridder D et al: Somatosensory cortex stimulation for deafferentation pain, *Acta Neurochir Suppl* 297(Pt 2):67-74, 2007.
58. Backonja MM, Serra J: Pharmacologic management part 2: lesser-studied neuropathic pain diseases, *Pain Med* 5(Suppl 1):S48-S59, 2004.
59. Payne R: Anatomy, physiology, and neuropharmacology of cancer pain, *Med Clin North Am* 71(2):153-167, 1987.
60. Canavero S, Bonicalzi V: Central pain syndrome: elucidation of genesis and treatment, *Expert Rev Neurother* 7(11):1485-1497, 2007.
61. Chahine L, Kanazi G: Phantom limb syndrome: a review, *Middle East J Anesthesiol* 19(2):345-355, 2007.
62. Woodhouse A: Phantom limb sensation, *Clin Exp Pharmacol Physiol* 32(1-2):132-134, 2005.
63. Flor H: Cortical reorganization and chronic pain: implications for rehabilitation, *J Rehabil Med* (41 Suppl):66-72, 2003.
64. Guimmarra MJ et al: Central mechanisms in phantom limb perception: the past, present and future, *Brain Res Rev* 54(1):219-232, 2007.
65. Schwartzman RJ, Alexander GM, Grothusen J: Pathophysiology of complex regional pain syndrome, *Expert Rev Neurother* 6(5):669-681, 2006.
66. Baron R: Mechanistic and clinical aspects of complex regional pain syndrome (CRPS), *Novartis Found Symp* 261:220-233, 2004.
67. Littlejohn G: Regional pain syndrome: clinical characteristics, mechanisms and management, *Nat Clin Pract Rheumatol* 3(9):504-511, 2007.
68. Akbazaz R, Wong YT, Homer-Vanniasinkam S: Complex regional pain syndrome: a review, *Ann Vasc Surg* 22(2):297-306, 2008.

69. Tunks ER, Crook J, Weir R: Epidemiology of chronic pain with psychological comorbidity: prevalence, risk, course, and prognosis, *Can J Psychiatry* 53(4):224-234, 2008.

70. Gupta A, Giordano J: On the nature, assessment, and treatment of fetal pain: neurobiological bases, pragmatic issues, and ethical concerns, *Pain Physician* 10(4):525-532, 2007.

71. Lowery CL et al: Neurodevelopmental changes of fetal pain, *Semin Perinatol* 31(5):275-282, 2007.

72. Grunau RE, Holsti L, Peters JW: Long-term consequences of pain in humans and neonates, *Semin Fetal Neonatal Med* 11(4):268-275, 2006.

73. Van de Velde M et al: Fetal pain perception and pain management, *Semin Fetal Neonatal Med* 11(4):232-236, 2006.

74. Hummel P, van Dijk M: Pain assessment: current status and challenges, *Semin Fetal Neonatal Med* 11(4):237-245, 2006.

75. Duhn JL, Medves JM: A systematic integrative review of infant pain assessment tools, *Adv Neonatal Care* 4(3):126-140, 2004.

76. Golianu B et al: Pediatric acute pain management, *Pediatr Clin North Am* 47(3):559-587, 2000.

77. Gibson SJ, Farrell M: A review of age differences in the neurophysiology of nociception and the perceptual experience of pain, *Clin J Pain* 20(4):227-239, 2004.

78. Zheng Z et al: Age-related differences in the time course of capsaicin-induced hyperalgesia, *Pain* 85(1-2):51-58, 2000.

79. Gibson SJ, Farrell M: A review of age differences in the neurophysiology of nociception and the perceptual experience of pain, *Clin J Pain* 20(4):227-239, 2004.

80. Woodrow KM et al: Pain tolerance: differences according to age, sex, and race, *Psychosom Med* 34(6):548-556, 1972.

81. Karp JF et al: Advances in understanding the mechanisms and management of persistent pain in older adults, *Br J Anaesth* 101(1):111-120, 2008.

82. McCleane G: Pharmacological pain management in the elderly patient, *Clin Interv Aging* 2(4):637-643, 2007.

83. McCleane G: Pain perception in the elderly patient, *Clin Geriatr Med* 24(2):203-211, V, 2008.

84. Weiner DK: Office management of chronic pain in the elderly, *Am J Med* 120(4):306-315, 2007.

85. Dinarello CA, Wolff SM: Pathogenesis of fever in man, *N Engl J Med* 298(11):607-612, 1978.

86. Boulant JA: Role of the preoptic-anterior hypothalamus in thermoregulation and fever, *Clin Infect Dis* 31(Suppl 5):S157-S161, 2000.

87. Mahmood MA, Zweifler RM: Progress in shivering control, *J Neurol Sci* 15:261(1-2):218-227, 2007.

88. Himms-Hagen J: Current status of nonshivering thermogenesis, In Ross Laboratories: *Assessment of energy metabolism in health and disease: a report of the first Ross conference in medical research*, Columbus, OH, 1980, Ross Laboratories.

89. Sell H, Deshaies Y, Richard D: The brown adipocyte: update on its metabolic role, *Int J Biochem Cell Biol* 36(11):2098-2104, 2004.

90. Asakura H: Fetal and neonatal thermoregulation, *J Nippon Med Sch* 71(6):360-370, 2004.

91. Nedergaard J, Bengtsson T, Cannon B: Unexpected evidence for active brown adipose tissue in adult humans, *Am J Physiol Endocrinol Metab* 293(2):E444-E452, 2007.

92. Steegmann AT Jr: Human cold adaptation: an unfinished agenda, *Am J Hum Biol* 19(2):218-227, 2007.

93. Yousef MK: Effects of climatic stresses on thermoregulatory processes in man, *Experientia* 43(1):14-19, 1987.

94. Rintamaki H: Human responses to cold, *Alaska Med* 49(2 Suppl):29-31, 2007.

95. Sherman TI et al: Optimizing the neonatal thermal environment, *Neonatal Netw* 25(4):251-260, 2006.

96. Holowatz LA et al: Altered mechanisms of vasodilation in aged human skin, *Exerc Sport Sci Rev* 35(3):119-125, 2007.

97. Degroot DW, Kenney WL: Impaired defense of core temperature in aged humans during mild cold stress, *Am J Physiol Regul Integr Comp Physiol* 292(1):R99-R102, 2007.

98. Roth J et al: Molecular aspects of fever and hyperthermia, *Neurol Clin* 24(3):421-439, 2006.

99. Steiner AA, Branco LG: Fever and anapyrexia in systemic inflammation: intracellular signaling by cyclic nucleotides, *Front Biosci* 8:s1398-s1408, 2003.

100. Blatteis CM: The onset of fever: new insights into its mechanism, *Prog Brain Res* 162:3-14, 2007.

101. Roth J: Endogenous antipyretics, *Clin Chim Acta* 371(1-2):13-24, 2006.

102. Gregson AL, Mackowiak PA: *Pathogenesis of fever*. In Cohen J, Powderly WG, editors: *Infectious diseases*, vol 1, St Louis, 2004, Mosby.

103. Luheshi G, Rothwell N: Cytokines and fever, *Int Arch Allergy Immunol* 109(4):301-307, 1996.

104. Dinarello CA, Wolff SM: Molecular basis of fever in humans, *Am J Med* 72(5):799-819, 1982.

105. Kluger MS: The adaptive value of fever. In Mackowiak PA, editor: *Fever: basic mechanisms and management*, New York, 1991, Raven.

106. Griesman LA, Mackowiak PA: Fever: beneficial and detrimental effects of antipyretics, *Curr Opin Infect Dis* 15(3):241-245, 2002.

107. Yoshikawa TT, Norman DC: Approach to fever and infection in the nursing home, *J Am Geriatr Soc* 44(1):74-82, 1996.

108. Nakayama J, Arinami T: Molecular genetics of febrile seizures, *Epilepsy Res* 70(Suppl 1):S190-S198, 2006.

109. Fruthaler GJ: Fever in children: phobia vs. facts, *Hosp Pract* 20(11A):49-53, 1985.

110. Dubé CM et al: Fever, febrile seizures and epilepsy, *Trends Neurosci* 30(10):490-496, 2007.

111. Roti Roti JL: Cellular responses to hyperthermia (40-46 degrees C): cell killing and molecular events, *Int J Hyperthermia* 24(1):3-15, 2008.

112. Cleary M: Predisposing risk factors on susceptibility to exertional heat illness: clinical decision-making considerations, *J Sports Rehabil* 16(3):204-214, 2007.

113. Cabanac M, Brinnel H: The pathology of human temperature regulation: thermiatrics, *Experientia* 43(1):19-27, 1987.

114. Bouchama A, Dehbi M, Chaves-Carballe E: Cooling and hemodynamic management in heatstroke: practical recommendations, *Crit Care* 11(3):R54, 2007.

115. Glazer JL: Management of heatstroke and heat exhaustion, *Am Fam Physician* 71(11):2133-2140, 2005.

116. Bytomski JR, Squire DL: Heat illness in children, *Curr Sports Med Rep* 2(6):320-324, 2003.

117. Rosenberg H et al: Malignant hyperthermia, *Orphanet J Rare Dis* 2:21, 2007.

118. Wappler F: Malignant hyperthermia, *Eur J Anaesthesiol* 18(10):632-652, 2001.

119. Ali SZ, Taguchi A, Rosenberg H: Malignant hyperthermia, *Best Pract Res Clin Anaesthesiol* 17(4):519-533, 2003.

120. Centers for Disease Control and Prevention: Hypothermia-related deaths—United States 2003-2004. *MMWR Morb Mortal Wkly Rep* 54(7):173-175, 2004.

121. Hildebrand F et al: Pathophysiologic changes and effects of hypothermia on outcome in elective surgery and trauma patients, *Am J Surg* 187(3):363-371, 2004.

122. Antretter H, Dapunto OE, Bonatti J: Management of profound hypothermia, *Br J Hosp Med* 54(5):215-220, 1995.

123. Reuler JB: Hypothermia: pathophysiology, clinical settings, and management, *Ann Intern Med* 89(4):519-527, 1978.

124. Aslam AF et al: Hypothermia: evaluation, electrocardiographic manifestations, and management, *Am J Med* 119(4):297-301, 2006.

125. Long WB 3rd, et al: Cold injuries, *J Long Term Eff Med Implants* 15(1):7-78, 2005.

126. DeLapp TD: Accidental hypothermia, *Am J Nurs* 83(1):62-67, 1983.

127. Wittmers LE Jr: Pathophysiology of cold exposure, *Minn Med* 84(11):30-36, 2001.

128. Lee-Chiong TL Jr, Stitt JT: Accidental hypothermia: when thermoregulation is overwhelmed, *Postgrad Med* 99(1):7780, 83-84, 87-88, 1996.

129. Jurkovich GJ: Environmental cold-induced injury, *Surg Clin North Am* 87(1):247-267, viii, 2007.

130. McCullough L, Arora S: Diagnosis and treatment of hypothermia, *Am Fam Physician* 70(12):2325-2332, 2004.

131. Sahuquillo J, Vilalta A: Cooling the injured brain: how does moderate hypothermia influence the pathophysiology of traumatic brain injury, *Curr Pharm Des* 13(22):2310-2322, 2007.

132. Axelrod YK, Diringer MN: Temperature management in acute neurologic disorders, *Crit Care Clin* 22(4):767-785, 2006.

133. Azzopardi D, Edwards AD: Hypothermia, *Semin Fetal Neonatal Med* 12(4):303-310, 2007.

134. Cushman L, Warren ML, Livesay S: Bringing research to the bedside: the role of induced hypothermia in cardiac arrest, *Crit Care Nurs Q* 30(2):143-153, 2007.

135. Kabon B, Bacher A, Spiss CK: Therapeutic hypothermia, *Best Pract Res Clin Anaesthesiol* 17(4):551-568, 2003.

136. Agrawal A, Timothy J, Thapa A: Neurogenic fever, *Singapore Med J* 48(6):492-494, 2007.

137. Little RA, Stoner HB: Body temperature after accidental injury, *Br J Surg* 68(4):221-224, 1981.

138. Saski H et al: Is there a self-preserving hypothermic mechanism in shock? *Shock* 27(4):354-357, 2007.

139. Rajagopalan S et al: The effects of mild perioperative hypothermia on blood loss and transfusion requirement, *Anesthesiology* 108(1):71-77, 2008.

140. Okeke LI: Effect of warm intravenous and irrigating fluids on body temperature during transurethral resection of the prostate gland, *BMC Urol* 7:15, 2007.

141. Scott EM, Buckland R: A systematic review of intraoperative warming to prevent postoperative complications, *AORN J* 83(5):1090-1104, 2006:1107–1113.

142. Moore RY: Suprachiasmatic nucleus in sleep-wake regulation, *Sleep Med* 8(Suppl 3):27-33, 2007.

143. Voss U: Functions of sleep architecture and the concept of protective fields, *Rev Neurosci* 15(1):33-46, 2004.

144. Phillipson EA: State-of-the-art control of breathing during sleep, *Am Rev Respir Dis* 118:909, 1978.

145. Sakai F et al: Normal human sleep: regional cerebral hemodynamics, *Ann Neurol* 7(5):471, 1980.

146. Meadows GE et al: Cerebral blood flow response to isocapnic hypoxia during slow-wave sleep and wakefulness, *J Appl Physiol* 97(4):1343-1348, 2004.

147. Silvania A: Physiological sleep-dependent changes in arterial blood pressure: central autonomic commands and baroreflex control, *Clin Exp Pharmacol Physiol* 35(9):987-994, 2008.

148. Ganjavi H, Shapiro CM: Hypocretin/Orexin: a molecular link between sleep, energy regulation, and pleasure, *J Neuropsychiatry Clin Neurosci* 19(4):413-419, 2007.

149. Siegel JM: Mechanisms of sleep control, *J Clin Neurophysiol* 7(1):49-65, 1990.

150. Dugovic C: Role of serotonin in sleep mechanisms, *Rev Neurol (Paris)* 157(11 Pt 2):S16-S19, 2001.

151. Siegel JM: Hypocretin (orexin): role in normal behavior and neuropathology, *Annu Rev Psychol* 55:125-148, 2004.

152. Sutcliffe JG, de Lecea L: The hypocretins: setting the arousal threshold, *Nat Rev Neurosci* 3(5):339-349, 2002.

153. Siegel JM: The neurotransmitters of sleep, *J Clin Psychiatry* 65(Suppl 16):4-7, 2004.

154. Steiger A: Neurochemical regulation of sleep, *J Psychiatr Res* 41(7):537-552, 2007.

155. Campbell SS: Evolution of sleep structure following brief intervals of wakefulness, *Electroencephalogr Clin Neurophysiol* 66(2):175-184, 1987.

156. Kedas A, Lux W, Amodeo S: A critical review of aging and sleep research, *West J Nurs Res* 11(2):196-206, 1989.

157. Meltzer LJ, Mindell JA: Sleep and sleep disorders in children and adolescents, *Psychiatr Clin North Am* 29(4):1059-1076, 2006.

158. Anders TF, Keener M: Developmental course of nighttime sleep-wake patterns in full-term and premature infants during the first year of life, *Sleep* 8(3):173, 1985.

159. Keefe MR: Comparison of neonatal nighttime sleep-wake patterns in nursing versus rooming-in environments, *Nurs Res* 36(3):140, 1987.

160. Elias MF et al: Sleep/wake patterns of breast-fed infants in the first 2 years of life, *Pediatrics* 77(3):322, 1986.

161. Leo G: Parasomnias, *WMJ* 102(1):32-35, 2003.

162. Ivanhoe JR, Lefebvre CA, Stockstill JW: Sleep disordered breathing in infants and children: a review of the literature, *Pediatr Dent* 29(3):193-200, 2007.

163. Espiritu JR: Aging-related sleep changes, *Clin Geriatr Med* 24(1):1-14, v, 2008.

164. Harrington J, Lee-Chiong T Jr: Sleep and older patients, *Clin Chest Med* 28(4):673-684, 2007.

165. Kern W et al: Changes in cortisol and growth hormone secretion during nocturnal sleep in the course of aging, *J Gerontol A Biol Sci Med Sci* 51(1):M3-M9, 1996.

166. American Academy of Sleep Medicine: Diagnostic Classification Steering Committee: *International classification of sleep disorders, revised: diagnostic and coding manual*, Westchester, IL, 2005, American Academy of Sleep Medicine.

167. Voderh olzer U et al: Are gender differences in objective and subjective sleep measures? A study of insomniacs and healthy controls, *Depress Anxiety* 17(3):162-172, 2003.

168. Ancoli-Israel S: Insomnia in the elderly: a review for the primary care practitioner, *Sleep* 23(Suppl 1):S23-S30, discussion S36-S38, 2000.

169. Rigndahl EN, Pereira SL, Delzell JE Jr: Treatment of primary insomnia, *J Am Board Fam Pract* 17(3):212-219, 2004.

170. Patil SP et al: Adult obstructive sleep apnea: pathophysiology and diagnosis, *Chest* 132(1):325-337, 2007.

171. Netzer NC, Eliasson AH, Strohl KP: Women with sleep apnea have lower levels of sex hormones, *Sleep Breath* 7(1):25-29, 2003.

172. Saaresranta T et al: Effect of medroxyprogesterone on inspiratory flow shapes during sleep in postmenopausal women, *Respir Physiol Neurobiol* 134(2):131-143, 2003.

173. Bradley TE, Floras JS: Obstructive sleep apnoea and its cardiovascular consequences, *Lancet* 373(9657):82-93, 2008.

174. Ballard RD: Management of patients with obstructive sleep apnea, *J Fam Pract* 57(8 Suppl):S24-S30, 2008.

175. Lohmann-Hedrich K et al: Evidence for linkage of restless legs syndrome to chromosome 9p: are there two distinct loci? *Neurology* 70(9):686-694, epub: 2007.

176. Patrick LR: Restless legs syndrome: pathophysiology and the role of iron and folate, *Altern Med Rev* 12(2):101-112, 2007.

177. Paulus W et al: Pathophysiological concepts of restless legs syndrome, *Mov Disord* 22(10):1451-1456, 2007.

178. Nishino S: Clinical and neurobiological aspects of narcolepsy, *Sleep Med* 8(4):373-399, 2007.

179. Monk TH: Shift work. In Kryger MH, Roth T, Dement WC, editors: *Principles and practice of sleep medicine*, ed 4, Philadelphia, 2005, Saunders.

180. Sack RL et al: Circadian rhythm sleep disorders: part I, basic principles, shift work and jet lag disorders, An American Academy of Sleep Medicine review, *Sleep* 30(11):1460-1483, review: 2007.

181. Taub JM, Berger RJ: The effects of changing the phase and duration of sleep, *J Exp Psychol Human Percept Perform* 2(1):30, 1976.

182. Eastman CI et al: Advancing circadian rhythms before eastward flight: a strategy to prevent or reduce jet lag, *Sleep* 28(1):33-44, 2005.

183. Sheldon SH: Parasomnias in childhood, *Pediatr Clin North Am* 51(1):69-88, vi: 2004.

184. Gugger JJ, Wagner ML: Rapid eye movement sleep behavior disorder, *Ann Pharmacother* 41(11):1833-1841, 2007.

185. Modell S, Lauer CJ: Rapid eye movement (REM) sleep: an endophenotype for depression, *Curr Psychiatry Rep* 9(6):480-485, 2007.

186. Lewis DA: Sleep in patients with respiratory disease, *Respir Care Clin North Am* 5(3):447-460, ix, 1999.

187. McNicholas WT: Impact of sleep on COPD, *Chest* 117(2 Suppl):48S-53S, 2000.

188. Papier A, Tuttle DJ, Mahar TJ: Differential diagnosis of the swollen red eyelid, *Am Fam Physician* 76(12):1815-1824, 2007.

189. Rao SK et al: The itching, burning eye: diagnostic algorithm and management options, *Compr Ophthalmol Update* 7(4):157-167, 2006.

190. Wright HR, Turner A, Taylor HR: Trachoma, *Lancet* 371(9628):1945-1954, 2008.

191. Rosenberg EA, Sperazza LC: The visually impaired patient, *Am Fam Physician* 77(10):1431-1436, 2008.

192. Doshi NR, Rodriquez ML: Amblyopia, *Am Fam Physician* 74(3):361-367, 2007.

193. Ticho BH: Strabismus, *Pediatr Clin North Am* 50(1):173-188, 2003.

194. Rucker JC: An update on acquired nystagmus, *Semin Ophthalmol* 23(2):91-97, 2008.

195. Shotton K, Elliott S: Interventions for strabismic amblyopia, *Cochrane Database Syst Rev* (2):CD006461, 2008.

196. Brass SD, Zivadinov R, Bakshi R: Acute demyelinating optic neuritis: a review, *Front Biosci* 13:2376-2390, 2008.

197. West S: Epidemiology of cataract: accomplishments over 25 years and future directions, *Ophthalmic Epidemiol* 14(4):173-178, 2007.

198. Jackson RG, Owsley C, McGwin G Jr: Aging and dark adaptation, *Vision Res* 39(23):3975-3982, 1999.

199. Wiggs JL: Genetic etiologies of glaucoma, *Arch Ophthalmol* 125(1):30-37, 2007.

200. Legrun-Julien F, Di Polo A: Molecular and cell-based approaches for neuroprotection in glaucoma, *Optom Vis Sci* 85(6):417-424, 2008.

201. Terzel G, Yang J, Wax MB: Heat shock proteins, immunity and glaucoma, *Brain Res Bull* 62(6):473-480, 2004.

202. Chidlow G, Wood JP, Casson RJ: Pharmacological neuroprotection for glaucoma, *Drugs* 67(5):725-759, 2007.

203. Sodhi A et al: Recent trends in the management of rhegmatogenous retinal detachment, *Surv Ophthalmol* 53(1):50-67, 2008.

204. Montezuma SR, Sobrin L, Seddon JM: Review of genetics in age related macular degeneration, *Semin Ophthalmol* 22(4):229-240, 2007.

205. Zayit-Soudry S, Moroz I, Loewenstein A: Retinal pigment epithelial detachment, *Surv Ophthalmol* 52(3):227-243, 2007.

206. Gohel PS et al: Age-related macular degeneration: an update on treatment, *Ann J Med* 121(4):279-281, 2008.

207. Beiko G: Status of accommodative intraocular lenses, *Curr Opin Ophthalmol* 18(1):74-79, 2007.

208. Callina T, Reynolds TP: Traditional methods for the treatment of presbyopia: spectacles, contact lenses, bifocal contact lenses, *Ophthalmol Clin North Am* 19(1):25-33, 2006.

209. Deeb SS, Kohl S: Genetics of color vision deficiencies, *Dev Ophthalmol* 37:170-187, 2003.

210. Swanson WH, Cohen JM: Color vision, *Ophthalmol Clin North Am* 16(2):179-203, 2003.

211. Javer AR, Schwartz DW: Plasticity in human directional hearing, *J Otolaryngol* 24(2):111-117, 1995.

212. Timiras PS: *Physiological basis of aging and geriatrics*, ed 3, Boca Raton, FL, 2003, CRC Press.

213. Liu XZ, Yan D: Ageing and hearing loss, *J Pathol* 211(2):188-197, 2007.

214. Osguthorpe JD, Nielsen DR: Otitis externa: review and clinical update, *Am Fam Physician* 74(9):1510-1516, 2006.

215. Cripps AW, Otczyk DC: Prospects for a vaccine against otitis media, *Expert Rev Vaccines* 5(4):517-534, 2006.

216. Smith JA, Danner CJ: Complications of chronic otitis media and cholesteatoma, *Otolaryngol Clin North Am* 39(6):1237-1255, 2006.

217. Yoon TH et al: Tympanoplasty, with or without mastoidectomy, is highly effective for treatment of chronic otitis media in children, *Acta Otolaryngol Suppl* (558):44-48, 2007.

218. Paradise JL et al: Tympanostomy tubes and developmental outcomes at 9 to 11 years of age, *N Engl J Med* 356(3):248-261, 2007.

219. De la Cruz A, Angeli S, Slattery WH: Stapedectomy in children, *Otolaryngol Head Neck Surg* 120(4):487-492, 1999.

220. Liu XZ, Yan D: Ageing and hearing loss, *J Pathol* 211(2):188-197, 2007.

221. Temple EC et al: Taste development: differential growth rates of tongue regions in humans, *Brain Res Dev Brain Res* 135(1-2):65-70, 2002.

222. Boyce JM, Shone GR: Effects of ageing on smell and taste, *Postgrad Med J* 82(966):239-241, 2006.

223. Doty RL: Influence of age and age-related diseases on olfactory function, *Ann N Y Acad Sci* 561:76-86, 1989.

224. Cain WS, Reid F, Stevens JC: Missing ingredients: aging and the discrimination of flavor, *J Nutr Elderly* 9(3):3, 1990.

225. Seiberling KA, Conley DB: Aging and olfactory and taste function, *Otolaryngol Clin North Am* 37(6):1209-1228, vii, 2004.

226. Kovacs T: Mechanisms of olfactory dysfunction in aging and neurodegenerative disorders, *Ageing Res Rev* 3(2):215-232, 2004.

227. Winkler S et al: Depressed taste and smell in geriatric patients, *J Am Dent Assoc* 130(12):1759-1765, 1999.

228. Nordin S, Bramerson A: Complaints of olfactory disorders: epidemiology, assessment and clinical implications, *Curr Opin Allergy Clin Immunol* 8(1):10-15, 2008.

229. Bromley SM: Smell and taste disorders: a primary care approach, *Am Fam Physician* 61(2):427-438, 2000.

230. Strous RD, Shoenfeld Y: To smell the immune system: olfaction, autoimmunity and brain development, *Autoimmun Rev* 6(1):54-60, 2006.

231. Besne I, Descombes C, Breton L: Effect of age and anatomical site on density of sensory innervation in human epidermis, *Arch Dermatol* 138(11):1445-1450, 2002.

232. Stevens JC: Age and spatial acuity of touch, *J Gerontol* 47(1):P35-P40, 1992.

233. Shaffer SW, Harrison AL: Aging of the somatosensory system: a translational perspective, *Phys Ther* 87(2):193-207, 2007.

234. Neuhauser HK: Epidemiology of vertigo, *Curr Opin Neurol* 20(1):40-46, 2007.

ALTERATIONS IN COGNITIVE SYSTEMS, CEREBRAL HEMODYNAMICS, AND MOTOR FUNCTION

BARBARA J. BOSS

MEDIA RESOURCES

Evolve Website (http://evolve.elsevier.com/McCance/)
- Review Questions and Answers
- Animations
- Glossary (with audio pronunciation for selected terms)
- WebLinks

CHAPTER OUTLINE

ALTERATIONS IN COGNITIVE SYSTEMS
- Coma
- Seizures
- Alterations in Awareness
- Data Processing Deficits

ALTERATIONS IN CEREBRAL HEMODYNAMICS
- Cerebral Hemodynamics
- Increased Intracranial Pressure

- Herniation Syndromes
- Cerebral Edema
- Hydrocephalus

ALTERATIONS IN MOTOR FUNCTION
- Alterations in Muscle Tone
- Alterations in Movement
- Alterations in Complex Motor Performance
- Extrapyramidal Motor Syndromes

A person achieves functional adequacy (competence) through complex integrated processes. Three major neural systems account for this functional adequacy: cognitive systems, sensory systems, and motor systems. Alterations in any or all of these affect functional adequacy. Alterations in cognitive and sensory systems and motor function are associated with many central and peripheral nervous system injuries and pathologies. The purpose of this chapter is to present the concepts and processes of these alterations as an approach to understanding the manifestation of neurologic dysfunction. Some specific diseases are also presented (i.e., Parkinson and Huntington disease) because they fit best here. The manifestations of these concepts and processes are integrated with specific central and peripheral nervous system disorders and are presented in Chapter 17. Alterations in sensory function are presented in Chapter 15.

The neural systems essential to the cognitive sphere are (1) attentional systems that provide arousal and maintenance of attention over time; and (2) memory and language systems by which information is communicated. These core systems are fundamental to the processes of abstract thinking and reasoning. The products of abstraction and reasoning are organized and made operational through the executive system.

The normal functioning of these systems manifests through the motor system in a behavioral array viewed by others as being appropriate to human activity and successful living.

Genetics and the genetic basis of disease are becoming increasingly important in the study of pathophysiology; selected neurologic disorders that have a genetic basis are presented in Table 16-1.

ALTERATIONS IN COGNITIVE SYSTEMS

Full consciousness, in its broadest sense, is a state of awareness both of oneself and the environment and a set of responses to that environment. Full consciousness implies that the individual responds to external stimuli with a wide array of responses. Any decrease in this state of awareness and varied responses is thus a decrease in consciousness.

Consciousness often is viewed as having two distinct components: arousal and awareness. Arousal, an attentional system, is the state of awakeness that an individual exhibits. Level of arousal is mediated by the reticular activating system,

Table 16-1	Selected Neurologic Disorders with a Genetic Basis		
Syndrome/Disorders	Currently Known Genetic Components	Pathophysiology	Major Neurologic Features
Alterations in Cognitive Systems			
Familial Alzheimer Disease			
Early onset	Autosomal dominant	Three clinically indistinguishable subtypes: AD1: mutations in amyloid precursor protein (*APP* gene) (chromosome 12) AD3: mutations in presenilin 1 (*PSEN1*) gene (chromosome 14) AD4: mutations in *PSEN2* gene (chromosome 1)	Adult onset progressive dementia—onset before age 60-65, often before 55
Late onset	Having 1 or 2 copies of apoE4 suggests an increased risk but is not predictive of Alzheimer	Mutations in *apoE4* gene (chromosome 19); codes a cholesterol processing protein; is a susceptibility gene; several other unidentified genes and environments are thought to influence	Adult onset progressive dementia—onset after age 65
Angelman syndrome	Chromosome 15; transmission maternal deletion, paternal UPD, imprinting center mutation, UBE3A (ubiquitin protein ligase) mutation clinical	Genetic alteration affects the maternal expression of the *UBE3A* gene (expresses the enzyme ubiquitin protein ligase E3A); UBE3A thought to have great importance in degradation of proteins in the brain	Little to no verbal language, mental retardation, seizure disorder, sleep disorder, movement/balance disorder
Batten disease	Autosomal recessive; chromosome 16	Lysosomal storage defect resulting in abnormal storage of cerebral lipofuscins	Develops normally until 6 months to 2 years of age when progressive brain disease becomes apparent; seizures, mental retardation, blindness, and death
Branched-chain ketoaciduria (maple syrup urine disease)	Autosomal recessive; most common type is classic caused by defect in the *BCKDHA* gene on chromosome 19	All types result in inability to metabolize three amino acids; these acids accumulate and are toxic at high levels	Without early diagnosis and treatment, mental retardation seizures, and death
Cri du chat syndrome	Chromosome 5	Deletion on the short arm; deletion of multiple genes responsible for phenotype; evidence that deletion of telomerase reverse transcriptase gene contributes to phenotype	High-pitched cry; mental retardation, microcephaly, low birth weight, failure to thrive; widely spaced eyes (ocular hypertelorism), unusually small jaw (micrognathia)
Lesch-Nyhan syndrome	X-linked recessive	Metabolism disturbance of purines	Mental retardation, progressive neurologic disorder, compulsively bitten lips and fingers
Neurofibromatosis	Autosomal dominant	Variable expressivity	Multiple café-au-lait spots, neurofibromas, learning disability, seizure disorder
NF1 (von Recklinghausen disease)	Chromosome 17	*NF1* gene produces a large, complex protein called *neurofibromin*; scientists theorize this protein acts as a switch to regulate cell growth; mutation may lessen or inhibit the normal output of this protein and allow irregular cell growth that may lead to tumor development	
NF2 (bilateral acoustic NF)	Chromosome 22	*NF2* gene produces a tumor suppressor protein (termed *merlin* or *schwannomin*)	Multiple tumors on cranial and spinal nerves, acoustic neuromas, hearing loss

Table 16-1   Selected Neurologic Disorders with a Genetic Basis—cont'd

Syndrome/Disorders	Currently Known Genetic Components	Pathophysiology	Major Neurologic Features
Progressive myoclonus epilepsy Unverricht-Lundborg disease	Autosomal recessive; chromosome 21	The missing gene codes for the protein cystatin B; this protein regulates enzymes that break down other proteins	Onset at age 6-15 years, severe incapacitating stimulus-sensitive progressive myoclonus, tonic-clonic epileptic seizures and characteristic abnormalities on electroencephalogram; may also develop other neurologic symptoms such as ataxia, incoordination, dysarthria
Lafora disease	Autosomal recessive; chromosome 6	Mutation in the Laforin gene; concentric amyloid (Lafora) bodies found in neurons, liver, skin, bone, and muscle	Grand mal seizures and/or myoclonus at about age 15; rapid and severe motor and coordination impairments, rapid mental deterioration, often with psychotic features; survival is short, less than 10 years after onset
Rett syndrome	X-linked dominant; appears to occur only in girls; defective *MeCP2* gene on the x-chromosome	Caused by defects in the protein MeCP2 involved in regulation of gene expression; defects in this gene allow other genes to come on or stay on at inappropriate times in development	Progressive neurologic disorder; develops normally in first year of life, then loss of mental capacity and motor skills begins; loss of purposeful hand movements; stereotypical hand wringing and flapping
Tay-Sachs disease	Autosomal recessive; chromosome 15	Caused by a deficiency of hexosaminidase, an enzyme, which results in accumulation of a material that damages the brain	Failure to thrive, blindness, seizures, progressive paralysis; usually death by age 4
Tuberous sclerosis	Autosomal dominant; caused by mutation of either the *TSC1* gene (chromosome 9) or *TSC2* gene (chromosome 16)	*TSC1* produces the protein hamartin, *TCS2* produces the protein tuberin; these proteins act as tumor growth suppressors	Develops in early childhood; seizures, mental retardation, skin and eye lesions; multiple benign tumors in brain and other vital organs

Alterations in Motor Function

Syndrome/Disorders	Currently Known Genetic Components	Pathophysiology	Major Neurologic Features
Duchenne muscular dystrophy	X-linked recessive	Mutation of the dystrophin gene results in down-regulation or absence of dystrophin, a protein with an important structural role in muscle	Generalized weakness and muscle wasting affecting limb and trunk muscles first, then progresses to respiratory system; progressive and fatal
Huntington disease	Autosomal dominant; chromosome 4	Mutation of the Huntington gene, a protein that is not well understood, results in neuron destruction in the brain	Jerky uncontrolled movements of the limbs, trunk and face (chorea); progressive loss of mental abilities; development of psychiatric disorders
Parkinson disease (early onset)	Two transmissions: Autosomal dominant—mutation in alpha-synuclein gene (chromosome 4) Autosomal recessive—mutation in the parkin gene (chromosome 6)	Too much of a normal form of the alpha-synuclein gene results in protein buildup Loss of the parkin gene causes buildup of defective proteins	Onset before age 40; tremor, increased muscle tone, bradykinesia

NF, Neurofibromatosis.

which extends from the medulla to the diencephalon. The reticular activating system provides arousal to the cerebral hemispheres (see Figure 14-6). Severe alterations in arousal can occur with brain injury, both in the acute phase of injury and on a long-term basis. Approximately 30% to 40% of survivors of severe brain injury remain in prolonged states of severely reduced consciousness. Awareness encompasses all cognitive functions that embody awareness of self, environment, and affective states (i.e., moods). **Content of thought** is mediated by attentional systems, memory systems, language systems, and executive systems.

Coma

Possible causes of an altered level of arousal with acute onset may be separated into three major groups: structural, metabolic, and psychogenic arousal alterations. Structural causes are divided according to original location of the pathologic condition or lesion: supratentorial (above the tentorium cerebelli), infratentorial (subtentorial, below the tentorium cerebelli), subdural (below the dura mater), extracerebral (outside the brain tissue), and intracerebral (within the brain tissue). Metabolic causes may be further divided into interruption in delivery of energy substrates (hypoglycemia, ischemia, hypoxia) or alteration in neuronal excitability (drug and alcohol intoxication, anesthesia, and epilepsy).[1] All the systemic diseases that eventually produce nervous system dysfunction are part of this metabolic category. Causes of altered level of arousal also are grouped according to pathologic process: infectious, vascular, neoplastic, traumatic, congenital (developmental), degenerative, polygenic, and metabolic.

PATHOPHYSIOLOGY Coma is produced by either (1) bilateral hemisphere damage or suppression by means of metabolic derangement, such as hypoxia, hypoglycemia, uremia, or toxins, such as ammonia from liver failure; or (2) a brainstem lesion or metabolic derangement that damages or suppresses the reticular activating system (RAS/thalamocortical alerting system) or its projections.[2,3] *Supratentorial disorders* produce a decreased level of arousal by one of three mechanisms: (1) diffuse bilateral cortical dysfunction, (2) bilateral subcortical dysfunction, or (3) localized hemispheric dysfunction. Disease processes may produce diffuse bilateral cortical dysfunction (e.g., encephalitis) and actually may occur in either the cerebral cortex or the underlying subcortical white matter. Bilateral subcortical dysfunction involves destructive disease that compromises the RAS (e.g., brainstem trauma or cerebrovascular accident) and probably surrounding structures as well. Localized hemispheric dysfunction generally is caused by masses that directly impinge on deep diencephalic structures or that secondarily compress these structures in the process of herniation. Such localized destructive processes directly impair function of the thalamic or hypothalamic activating systems.

Extracerebral disorders also can produce diffuse bilateral cortical dysfunction. Extracerebral disorders include neoplasms, closed-head trauma with subsequent bleeding, and subdural empyema (accumulation of pus). Intracerebral

disorders (those within the brain substance) function primarily as masses. These disorders include bleeding, infarcts and emboli, and tumors.

Infratentorial disorders produce a reduction in arousal in one of two ways: (1) there may be direct destruction of the RAS and its pathways, or (2) the brainstem may be destroyed either by direct invasion or by indirect impairment of its blood supply. The most common cause of direct destruction is cerebrovascular disease, but demyelinating diseases, neoplasms, granulomas, abscesses, and head injury also may cause brainstem destruction. In addition, decreased level of consciousness may result from compression of the RAS by a disease process. This compression may occur because of (1) direct pressure on the pons and midbrain, producing ischemia and edema of the neurons of the RAS; (2) upward herniation of the cerebellum through the tentorial notch, thus compressing the upper midbrain and diencephalon; or (3) downward herniation of the cerebellum through the foramen magnum, compressing and displacing the medulla oblongata. Specific causes of compression of the brainstem include hematomas, hemorrhage, and aneurysm; cerebellar hemorrhage, infarcts, abscesses, and neoplasms; and demyelinating disorders.

A wide spectrum of diseases may produce a metabolically induced alteration in arousal. In encephalopathic conditions, widespread direct or indirect interference with neuronal metabolism occurs throughout much of the brain, such as occurs with liver failure (hepatic encephalopathy) and renal failure. *Psychogenic unresponsiveness*, although uncommon, may signal general psychiatric disorders. Despite apparent unconsciousness, the person actually is physiologically awake and the neurologic examination reflects normal response.

EVALUATION Evaluating and treating an altered level of arousal requires distinguishing between organic and functional causes. A further distinction between metabolic and structural causes is made because the treatments are different and disease progression can be rapid (Table 16-2). If the cause is structural, the pathologic condition must be localized.

CLINICAL MANIFESTATIONS Patterns of clinical manifestations and their evolution have been identified. The patterns of clinical manifestation are important because they help in determining the extent of brain dysfunction and they serve as indexes for identifying increasing or decreasing central nervous system (CNS) function. The specific clusters of manifestations of abnormal function and their evolution suggest whether the cause of the altered arousal state is supratentorial, infratentorial, metabolic, or psychogenic (Table 16-3). Five categories of neurologic function are critical to the evaluation process: (1) level of consciousness, (2) pattern of breathing, (3) size and reactivity of pupils, (4) eye position and reflexive responses, and (5) skeletal muscle motor responses.

Level of Consciousness

Level of consciousness is the most critical clinical index of nervous system function or dysfunction. An alteration in consciousness indicates either improvement or deterioration of

Table 16-2   Clinical Manifestations of Metabolic and Structural Causes of Comas

Manifestation	Metabolically Induced Coma	Structurally Induced Coma
Blink to threat (cranial nerves II, VII)	Equal	Asymmetric
Discs (cranial nerve II)	Flat, good pulsation	Papilledema
Extraocular movement (cranial nerves III, IV, VI)	Roving eye movements; normal doll's eyes and calorics	Gaze paresis, nerve III palsy, medial longitudinal fasciculus (MLF) syndrome (internuclear ophthalmoplegia)
Pupils (cranial nerves II, III)	Equal and reactive, may be large (e.g., atropine), pinpoint (e.g., opiates), or midposition and fixed (e.g., glutethimide [Doriden])	Asymmetric and/or nonreactive; may be midposition (midbrain injury), pinpoint (pons injury), large (tectal injury)
Corneal reflex (cranial nerve V, VII)	Symmetric response	Asymmetric response
Grimace to pain (cranial nerve VII)	Symmetric response	Asymmetric response
Motor function movement	Symmetric	Asymmetric
Tone	Symmetric	Paratonic, spastic, flaccid, especially if asymmetric
Posture	Symmetric	Decorticate, especially if symmetric; decerebrate, especially if asymmetric
Deep tendon reflexes	Symmetric	Asymmetric
Babinski sign	Absent or symmetric response	Present
Sensation	Symmetric	Asymmetric

Table 16-3   Differential Characteristics of Disorders Causing Coma

Mechanism	Manifestations
Supratentorial mass lesions compressing or displacing diencephalons or brainstem	Initiating signs usually of focal cerebral dysfunction
	Signs of dysfunction progress rostral to caudal
	Neurologic signs at any given time point to one anatomic area (e.g., diencephalon, mesencephalon, medulla)
	Motor signs often asymmetric
Infratentorial mass of destruction, causing coma	History of preceding brainstem dysfunction or sudden onset of coma
	Localizing brainstem signs precede or accompany onset of coma and always include oculovestibular abnormality
	Cranial nerve palsies; usually manifest "bizarre" respiratory patterns that appear at onset
Metabolic coma	Confusion and stupor commonly precede motor signs
Exogenous toxins (drugs)	Motor signs usually are symmetric
Endogenous toxins (organ system failure)	Pupillary reactions usually are preserved
	Asterixis, myoclonus, tremor, and seizures are common
	Acid-base imbalance with hyperventilation or hypoventilation is common
Psychiatric unresponsiveness	Lids close actively
	Pupils reactive or dilated (cycloplegics)
	Oculocephalic reflexes are unpredictable; oculovestibular reflexes are physiologic (nystagmus is present)
	Motor tone is inconsistent or normal
	Eupnea or hyperventilation is usual
	No pathologic reflexes are present
	Electroencephalogram (EEG) is normal

the individual's condition. A person who is alert and oriented to self, others, place, and time is considered to be functioning at the highest level of consciousness, which implies full use of all the person's cognitive capacities.

Because many different terms are used to indicate level of consciousness, definition becomes necessary. The term *unconscious*, for example, has no specific clinical definition and signifies different things to different people. From the normal alert state, levels of consciousness diminish in stages, each of which is clinically defined in Table 16-4.

Pattern of Breathing

Several characteristic respiratory patterns are helpful in evaluating level of brain dysfunction and level of coma. Among these characteristics are rate, rhythm, and pattern of breathing. The breathing patterns can be categorized as hemispheric or brainstem breathing patterns (Table 16-5 and Figure 16-1).

With normal breathing, a neural center believed to be located in the forebrain (cerebrum) produces a rhythmic breathing pattern despite lowered arterial carbon dioxide

Table 16-4	Levels of Acute Coma
State	**Definition**
Confusion	Loss of ability to think rapidly and clearly; impaired judgment and decision making
Disorientation	Beginning loss of consciousness; disorientation to time followed by disorientation to place and impaired memory; lost last is recognition of self
Lethargy	Limited spontaneous movement or speech; easy arousal with normal speech or touch; may not be oriented to time, place, or person
Obtundation	Mild to moderate reduction in arousal (awakeness) with limited response to the environment; falls asleep unless stimulated verbally or tactilely; answers questions with minimum response
Stupor	A condition of deep sleep or unresponsiveness from which the person may be aroused or caused to open eyes only by vigorous and repeated stimulation; response is often withdrawal or grabbing at stimulus
Coma	No verbal response to the external environment or to any stimuli; noxious stimuli such as deep pain or suctioning yields motor movement
Light coma	Associated with purposeful movement on stimulation
Coma	Associated with nonpurposeful movement only on stimulation
Deep coma	Associated with unresponsiveness or no response to any stimulus

Table 16-5	Patterns of Breathing	
Breathing Pattern	**Description**	**Location of Injury**
Hemispheric Breathing Patterns		
Normal	After a period of hyperventilation that lowers the arterial carbon dioxide pressure ($Paco_2$), the individual continues to breathe regularly but with a reduced depth.	Response of the nervous system to an external stressor—not associated with injury to the CNS
Posthyperventilation apnea	Respirations stop after hyperventilation has lowered the Pco_2 level below normal. Rhythmic breathing returns when the Pco_2 level returns to normal. (Usually an intact cerebral cortex will trigger breathing within 10 seconds regardless of Pco_2.)	Associated with diffuse bilateral metabolic or structural disease of the cerebrum
Cheyne-Stokes respirations	The breathing pattern has a smooth increase (crescendo) in the rate and depth of breathing (hyperpnea), which peaks and is followed by a gradual smooth decrease (decrescendo) in the rate and depth of breathing to the point of apnea when the cycle repeats itself. The hyperpneic phase lasts longer than the apneic phase (represents an amplitude change).	Bilateral dysfunction of the deep cerebral or diencephalic structures, seen with supratentorial injury and metabolically induced coma states unrelated to neurologic dysfunction, may see also in CHF
Brainstem Breathing Patterns		
Central reflex hyperpnea (central neurogenic hyperventilation)	A sustained deep rapid but regular pattern (hyperpnea) occurs, with a decreased $Paco_2$ and a corresponding increase in pH and increased Po_2.	May result from CNS damage or disease that involves the lower midbrain and upper pons; seen after increased intracranial pressure and blunt head trauma
Apneusis	A prolonged inspiratory cramp (a pause at full inspiration) occurs. A common variant of this is a brief end-inspiratory pause of 2 or 3 seconds, often alternating with an end-expiratory pause.	Indicates damage to the respiratory control mechanism located at the pontine level; most commonly associated with pontine infarction but documented with hypoglycemia, anoxia, and meningitis
Cluster breathing	A cluster of breaths has a disordered sequence with irregular pauses between breaths.	Dysfunction in the lower pontine and high medullary areas
Ataxic breathing	Completely irregular breathing occurs, with random shallow and deep breaths and irregular pauses. Often the rate is slow.	Originates from a primary dysfunction of the lower pons or upper medulla
Gasping breathing pattern (agonal gasps)	A pattern of deep "all-or-none" breaths is accompanied by a slow respiratory rate.	Indicative of a failing medullary respiratory center

CHF, Congestive heart failure; *CNS,* central nervous system.

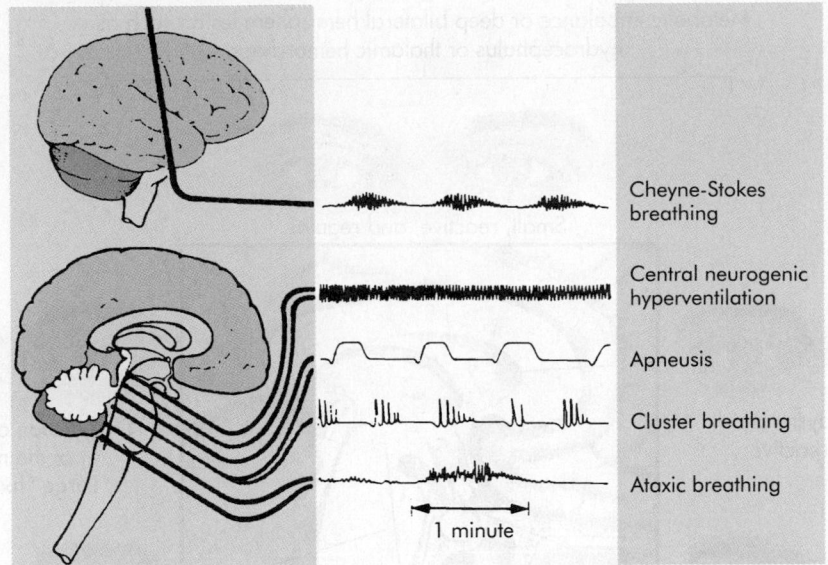

Figure 16-1 Abnormal respiratory patterns with corresponding level of central nervous system activity.

pressure (Paco$_2$). When neural control at this center is lost as consciousness decreases, the lower brainstem centers regulate the breathing pattern by responding only to changes in Paco$_2$ levels. The result is the irregular breathing associated with **posthyperventilation apnea (PHVA)**.

Cheyne-Stokes respiration is an abnormal rhythm of breathing (periodic breathing) that alternates between hyperventilation and apnea. The pathophysiology of Cheyne-Stokes respiration involves a hyperventilatory response to carbon dioxide stimulation. In the damaged brain higher levels of Paco$_2$ (hypercapnia) are required to stimulate ventilation, and the response is hyperventilation. As a result, the Paco$_2$ level decreases to below normal and breathing stops (PHVA) until the carbon dioxide reaccumulates and stimulates hyperventilation. In cases of opiate or sedative drug overdose, the respiratory center is depressed and the rate of breathing gradually decreases until respiratory failure occurs.

Certain motor activities related to breathing signify the level of brain dysfunction. Yawning, vomiting, and hiccups are complex reflex-like motor responses that are integrated by neural mechanisms in the lower brainstem. These responses may be produced by compression or diseases that involve tissues in the medulla oblongata. Such disorders include infection, neoplasm, or infarct. Similar responses are produced by dysfunction in the lower brainstem through direct stimulation.

Most CNS disorders produce nausea and vomiting. *Vomiting* with no associated nausea indicates direct involvement of the central neural mechanism. Vomiting is associated particularly with CNS injuries that (1) involve the vestibular nuclei (located in the lower pons and medulla oblongata) or their immediate projections, particularly when double vision (diplopia) also is present; (2) impinge directly on the floor of the fourth ventricle; or (3) produce brainstem compression secondary to increased intracranial pressure.

Pupillary Changes

Anatomically, brainstem areas that control arousal are adjacent to areas that control pupils. Pupillary changes thus are a valuable guide to evaluating the presence and level of brainstem dysfunction (Figure 16-2).

Certain drugs that affect pupils must be considered in the evaluation of pupillary response in comatose states. Atropine, scopolamine, amphetamines, mydriatics, and cycloplegics in large concentrations fully dilate and fix pupils. Glutethimide in amounts sufficient to produce a coma causes the pupils to become midposition or moderately dilated (4 to 5 mm in diameter), unequal, and frequently fixed to light. Opiates (heroin and morphine) and barbiturates, as well as extensive pontine damage, cause pinhole pupils (1 mm). Severe barbiturate intoxication may produce fixed pupils.

Severe ischemia and hypoxia produce bilaterally wide (5 mm) and fixed pupils in most instances caused by severe midbrain damage. Occasionally the pupils remain small (1 to 2.5 mm) or midposition even in the presence of profound hypoxia. Hypothermia also may cause fixed pupils.

Oculomotor Responses

Resting, spontaneous, and reflexive eye movements (oculocephalic [doll's head, doll's eyes] and oculovestibular [caloric] reflexes) undergo change at various levels of brain dysfunction (Table 16-6). Persons with metabolically induced coma, except in cases of barbiturate-hypnotic and phenytoin (Dilantin) poisoning, generally do retain ocular reflexes, however, even when other signs of brainstem damage, such as central neurogenic hyperventilation, are present.

The presence of brisk oculocephalic reflexes and roving eye movements, as well as the failure to elicit nystagmus with instillation of cold or warm water into the external ear canal, indicates a decrease in consciousness (loss of cortical influence) but an intact brainstem (Figures 16-3 and 16-4).

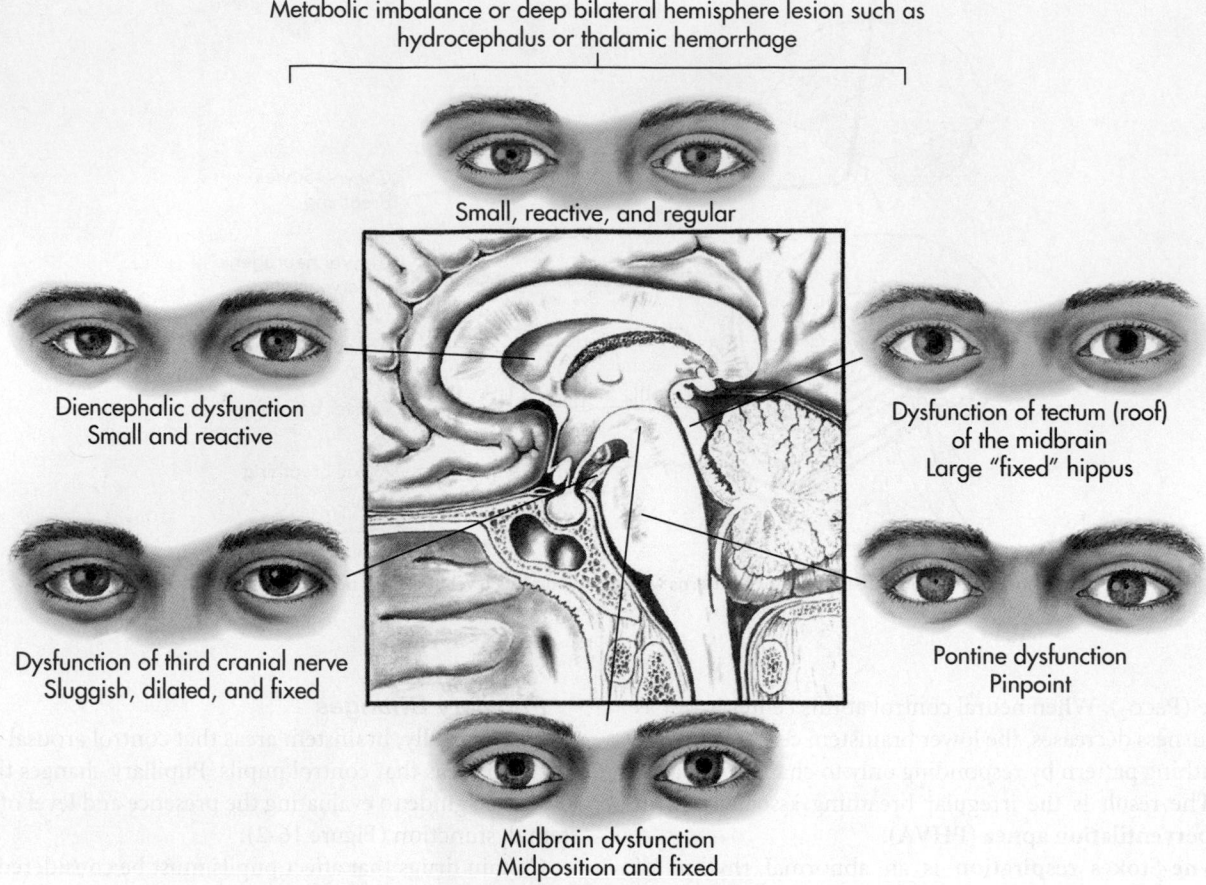

Metabolic imbalance or deep bilateral hemisphere lesion such as hydrocephalus or thalamic hemorrhage

Small, reactive, and regular

Diencephalic dysfunction
Small and reactive

Dysfunction of tectum (roof)
of the midbrain
Large "fixed" hippus

Dysfunction of third cranial nerve
Sluggish, dilated, and fixed

Pontine dysfunction
Pinpoint

Midbrain dysfunction
Midposition and fixed

Figure 16-2 Appearance of pupils at different levels of consciousness.

Destructive or compressive injury to the brainstem causes specific abnormalities of the oculocephalic and oculovestibular reflexes. For example, a skewed deviation, in which one eye diverges downward and the other looks upward, indicates brainstem dysfunction. Destructive or compressive disease processes that involve an oculomotor nucleus or nerve cause the involved eye to deviate outward, producing a resting disconjugate lateral position of the eyes (each eye diverges laterally). Unilateral abducens paralysis (paralysis of cranial nerve VI) results in an upward deviation of the ipsilateral eye. With bilateral abducens paralysis, the eyes come together (converge). Reflexive eye movements may be suppressed by drugs, most commonly phenytoin, tricyclics, and barbiturates. Occasionally alcohol, phenothiazines, and diazepam may alter reflex eye movements.

Motor Responses

Motor responses contribute to evaluating the level of brain dysfunction and determining the side of the brain that is maximally damaged. The pattern of response is described as (1) purposeful (a defensive or withdrawal movement of limbs to noxious stimuli); (2) inappropriate, or not purposeful (generalized motor movement, posturing, grimacing, or groaning); or (3) not present (unresponsive, no motor response). Purposeful movement requires an intact corticospinal system. Nonpurposeful movement is evidence of severe dysfunction of the corticospinal system.

Motor signs indicating loss of cortical inhibition that are commonly associated with decreased consciousness include contralateral or bilateral (depending on whether the process is localized or diffuse) reflex grasping, reflex sucking, snout reflex, palmomental reflex, and rigidity (paratonia) (Figure 16-5). Abnormal flexor and extensor responses in the upper and lower extremities are defined in Table 16-7 and illustrated in Figure 16-6.

Outcomes

Categories of prognostic indicators related to outcome of coma include demographic variables, severity indices, neurologic signs, neuroimaging studies, neuromedical markers, psychologic ratings, and outcome scale scores.[4,5] Outcome domains fall into two divisions—mortality and extent of disability (morbidity). For coma, the extent of disability division has four domains—recovery of consciousness, residual cognitive dysfunction, psychosocial (functional) domain, and vocational domain. These coma outcomes differ depending on the etiology of the injury—traumatic brain injury (TBI) or nontraumatic brain injury (NTBI). The pathophysiology underlying TBI is focal or diffuse trauma-induced injury (see Chapter 17 for further discussion). The pathophysiology of NTBIs is one of hypoxia and ischemia. This may be due, for example, to vascular insult, tumor, hydrocephalus, infection, or anorexia.

Table 16-6	Changes in Oculomotor Responses	
State	Resting and Spontaneous Eye Movements	Reflexive Eye Movements
Full consciousness	Eyes at rest, still (cortical gaze centers inhibit spontaneous roving eye movements)	Eyes move as the head turns Oculocephalic responses not elicited or inconsistently elicited (frontal gaze centers inhibit brainstem reflexes that fix gaze straight ahead) Oculovestibular (caloric) stimulation produces nystagmus
Cortical dysfunction or disruption of efferent pathways	Conjugate, horizontal, roving eye movements may well be present (cortical gaze centers no longer inhibit these brainstem-generated roving eye movements)	Gaze fixed straight ahead regardless of head position—positive doll's eyes reaction (normal oculocephalic reflexes are no longer inhibited by frontal gaze centers)
Diffuse anoxic damage to cortex	"Ocular dipping"—slow, dysrhythmic downward movement followed by faster, upward movement	Nystagmus is no longer induced by caloric stimulation (normally a cold-water stimulus produces deviation of the eyes opposite the irrigated ear; a warm-water stimulus deviates the eyes to the same [ipsilateral] side) With an injury that depresses cortical gaze center function, the eyes (and often the entire head) deviate or appear to look toward the side of the injured hemisphere With an injury that irritates (stimulates) the neurons of the cortical gaze center, the eyes (and often the entire head) deviate away from the injured hemisphere (all fibers from the frontal gaze centers decussate and therefore control the function of the contralateral pontine gaze center, which moves the eyes in the ipsilateral direction)
Mesencephalon dysfunction	Roving eye movements cease and the eyes become immobile and directed ahead (roving eye movements require an intact brainstem) Eyes may turn down and inward	Oculovestibular reflexes become inconsistent and abnormal Loss of Bell phenomenon (upward deviation of eyes on stimulation) (requires intact eye movement pathways from the mesencephalon to pons)
Pontine dysfunction	Loss of spontaneous blinking (requires an intact pons) "Ocular bobbing"—brisk, conjugate, downward movement of eyes with loss of horizontal eye movements	

Table 16-7	Abnormal Motor Responses with Decreased Responsiveness	
Motor Response	Description of Motor Responses	Location of Injury
Decorticate posturing/rigidity: upper extremity flexion, lower extremity extension	Slowly developing flexion of the arm, wrist, and fingers with abduction in the upper extremity and extension, internal rotation, and plantar flexion of the lower extremity	Hemispheric damage above midbrain releasing medullary and pontine reticulospinal systems
Decerebrate posturing/rigidity: upper and lower extremity extensor responses	Opisthotonos (hyperextension of the vertebral column) with clenching of the teeth; extension, abduction, and hyperpronation of the arms; and extension of the lower extremities	Associated with severe damage involving midbrain or upper pons
	In acute brain injury, shivering and hyperpnea may accompany unelicited recurrent decerebrate spasms	Acute brain injury may cause limb extension regardless of location
Extensor responses in the upper extremities accompanied by flexion in the lower extremities		Pons
Flaccid state with little or no motor response to stimuli		Lower pons and upper medulla

Data from Goetz CG: *Textbook of clinical neurology*, ed 3, Philadelphia, 2007 Saunders; Nadeau SE et al: *Medical neuroscience*, Philadelphia, 2004, Saunders.

Related to mortality, two forms of neurologic death—brain death (brainstem death) and cerebral death—may result from severe TBI and NTBI. **Brain death (brainstem death)** occurs when irreversible brain damage is so extensive that the brain has no potential for recovery and no longer can maintain the body's internal homeostasis. Destruction of the neuronal contents of the intracranial cavity includes the brainstem and cerebellum. On postmortem examination the brain is autolyzing (self-digesting) or already autolyzed.

Clinical criteria for brain death include the absence of discernible evidence of cerebral hemisphere function or function of the brainstem's vital centers for an extended period. There is no detectable function above the level of the foramen magnum so there is whole brain death.[6-8] In addition, the abnormality of brain function must result from structural or known metabolic disease and *not* be caused by a depressant drug, alcohol poisoning, neuromuscular blockage, or hypothermia. An isoelectric, or flat, electroencephalogram (EEG) (electrocerebral silence) for a period of 6 to 12 hours in a person who is not hypothermic and has not ingested depressant drugs indicates that no mental recovery is possible and usually means that the brain is already dead. A task force to determine brain death in children recommended the same criteria as for adults[9] but with a longer observation period.

The following summary of medical criteria determines brain death[2,3,6,10]:

1. Completion of all appropriate and therapeutic procedures
2. Unresponsive coma (absence of motor and reflex movements)
3. No spontaneous respiration (apnea)—a Pa_{CO_2} that rises above 60 mmHg without breathing efforts, providing evidence of a nonfunctioning respiratory center (apnea challenge)
4. Absent cephalic reflexes (no ocular responses to head turning or caloric stimulation) with dilated, fixed pupils
5. Isoelectric (flat) EEG (electrocerebral silence)
6. Persistence of these signs for 30 minutes to 1 hour and for 6 hours after onset of coma and apnea
7. Confirming test indicating absence of cerebral circulation (optional)

Cerebral death (irreversible coma) is death of the cerebral hemispheres exclusive of the brainstem and cerebellum. Brain damage is permanent and sufficiently severe that the individual is unable to ever respond behaviorally in any significant way to the environment. The brain, however, may

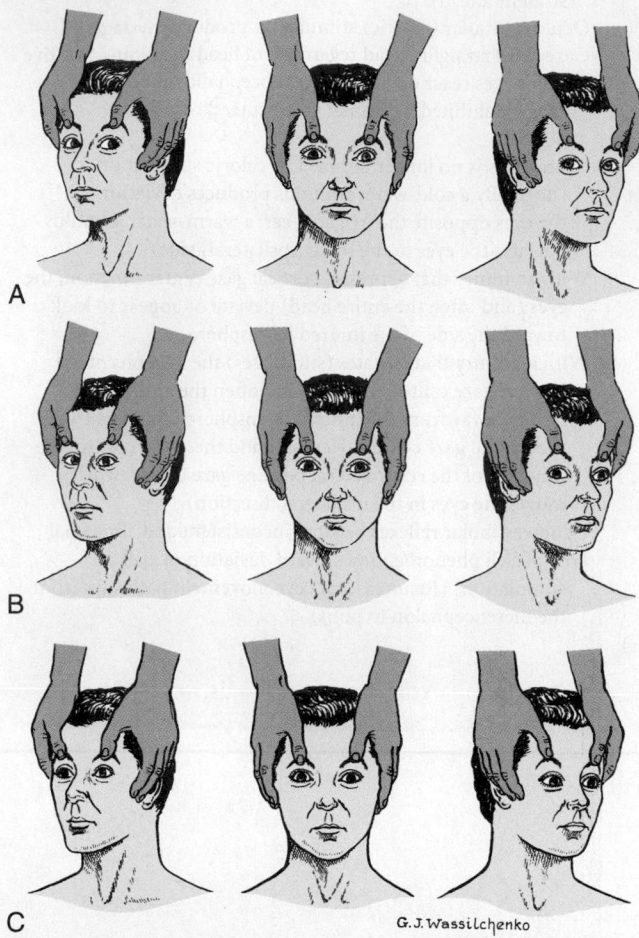

G. J. Wassilchenko

Figure 16-3 Test for oculocephalic reflex response (doll's eyes phenomenon). **A,** Normal response—eyes turn together to side opposite from turn of head. **B,** Abnormal response—eyes do not turn in conjugate manner. **C,** Absent response—eyes do not turn as head position changes. (**A** and **C** from Rudy EB: *Advanced neurological and neurosurgical nursing,* St Louis, 1984, Mosby.)

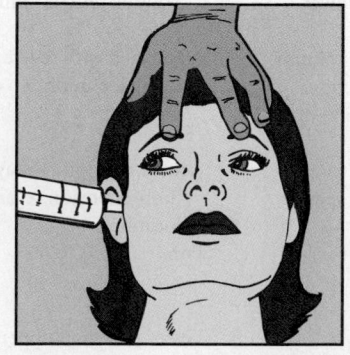 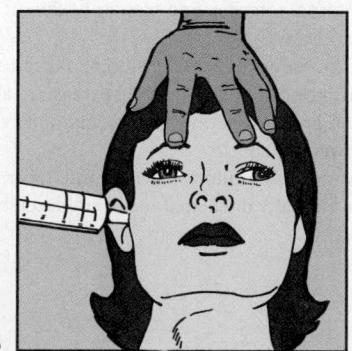 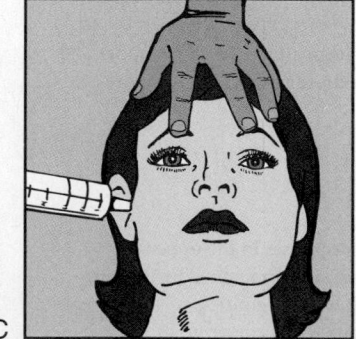

Figure 16-4 Test for oculovestibular reflex (caloric ice-water test). **A,** Normal response—conjugate eye movements. **B,** Abnormal response—dysconjugate or asymmetric eye movements. **C,** Absent response—no eye movements.

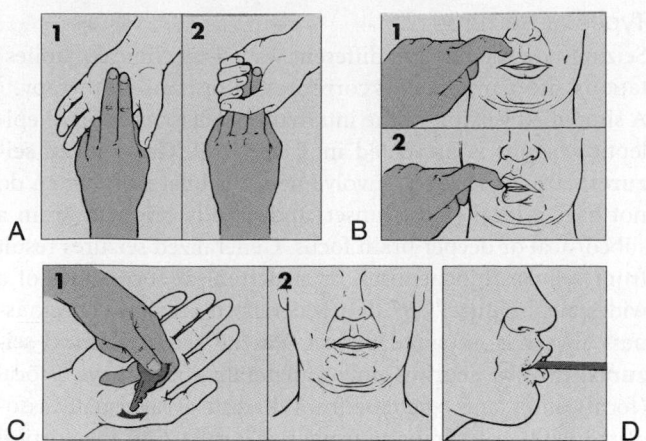

Figure 16-5 Pathologic reflexes. **A**, Grasp reflex. **B**, Snout reflex. **C**, Palmomental reflex. **D**, Suck reflex.

continue to maintain internal homeostasis (normal respiratory and cardiovascular functions, normal temperature control, and normal gastrointestinal function).

Prognosis in coma is related to the extent of disability—the recovery spectrum of neurobehavioral manifestations (in diagnostic terms, clinical states) after severe brain injury include (1) coma, (2) vegetative state, (3) akinetic mutism, (4) minimally conscious state, and (5) locked-in syndrome (Table 16-8).

The survivor of cerebral death may remain in a coma or emerge into a vegetative state. In coma, a state of unarousable neurobehavioral unresponsiveness, the eyes are usually closed with no evidence of eye opening either spontaneously or in response to external stimuli. The person does not follow commands, does not verbalize or mouth words, and has no goal-directed or volitional behavior. There is no sustained visual pursuit movements beyond a 45-degree arc.

A **vegetative state (VS)** has been called a wakeful unconscious state. The Multi-Society Task Force on Persistent Vegetative States (MSTF) identified the diagnostic criteria for VS as (1) periods of eye opening (spontaneous or following stimulation); (2) the potential for subcortical responses to external stimuli, including generalized physiologic responses to pain, such as posturing, tachycardia, and diaphoresis, and subcortical motor responses, such as grasp reflex; (3) return of so-called vegetative (autonomic) functions, including sleep-wake cycles and normalization of respiratory and digestive system functions; and (4) occasional roving eye movements without concomitant visual tracking ability.[11] The person's eyes open spontaneously or following stimulation, or both. There may be random hand, extremity, or head movements. The individual maintains blood pressure and breathing without support. Brainstem reflexes (pupillary, oculocephalic, chewing, swallowing) are intact. No discrete localizing motor responses are present, and the individual does not speak any comprehensible words or follow commands. There is no awareness of self or the environment.[12]

Some survivors of coma progress to a minimally conscious state. The term **minimally conscious state (MCS)** was first used by the International Working Party on Vegetative States and supported by the Brain Injury Interdisciplinary Special Interest Group of the American Congress of Rehabilitation Medicine (ACRM). ACRM defined MCS as a condition of severely altered consciousness in which the person demonstrates minimal but defined behavioral evidence of self or environmental awareness.[11,13] The clinical features include (1) following simple commands, (2) manipulation of objects, (3) gestural or verbal "yes/no" responses, (4) intelligible verbalization, and (5) stereotypic movements (e.g., blinking, smiling) that occur in a meaningful relationship to the eliciting stimulus and are not attributable to reflexive activity.

Akinetic mutism (AM) is a neurobehavioral state characterized by a severe disturbance in behavioral drive (motivation). Generally, these individuals evidence eye opening with visual tracking and have little or no spontaneous speech or following of commands. Little movement is present. This is not attributable to decreased wakefulness or motor weakness or impairment. The pathology involves damage to the frontal lobe or cingulate gyrus.[14]

With **locked-in syndrome** there is injury to the ventral pons. Both the content of thought and level of arousal are intact, but the efferent pathways are disrupted with quadriplegia and anarthria.[15] Thus the individual cannot communicate either through speech or through body movement but is fully conscious, with intact cognitive function. The upper cranial nerves (I through IV) often are preserved, however, so that the person possesses vertical eye movement and blinking as a means of communication.

Prognostic Indicators for Emergence from Coma. To date, no indicators except those of brain death predict outcome of coma. Etiology of injury and time since onset of coma are currently the best prognostic indicators of recovery of consciousness or functional outcome. In NTBI, the prognosis can be established earlier than with traumatic brain injury. In traumatic coma, there is a 95% death rate in individuals whose pupillary reflexes or reflective eye movements are absent 6 hours after onset of coma and a 91% death rate if pupils are nonreactive at 24 hours.[11] In nontraumatic coma, absence of any two of the following is an unfavorable sign in the first hours after admission: pupil reflexes, corneal reflexes, or oculovestibular responses. Absence of eye opening and muscle tone in 24 hours predicts death or severe disability.[11]

Recovery of consciousness within 2 weeks is associated with favorable outcomes. Recovery of consciousness after 6 months is correlated with severe disability on the Glasgow Outcome Scale.[11] No recovery without severe disability has ever been documented after 1 year in coma.[11] No emergence from a VS can be expected after 3 months in a VS from hypoxic-ischemic injury and after 1 year from TBI.

Emergence from MCS is confirmed when there is reliable and consistent demonstration of either (1) interactive communication, that is, the ability to answer basic "yes/no" or "single word answered" personal or environmental questions, and (2) functional use of objects, that is, the ability to appropriately discriminate among objects.[11] Failure to emerge from MCS within 12 months predicts the likelihood of remaining in an MCS.[11]

Seizures

A **seizure** is caused by abnormal excessive hypersynchronous discharges of CNS neurons[16] and is characterized by a sudden, transient alteration in brain function. Depending on the distribution of the discharges, this abnormal CNS activity can be various manifestations[16] involving motor, sensory, autonomic, or psychic clinical manifestations and an alteration in level of arousal. The alteration in level of arousal is temporary. The term **convulsion**, sometimes applied to seizures, refers to the tonic-clonic (jerky, contract-relax) movement associated with some seizures. A seizure produces a brief disruption in brain electrical function.[16]

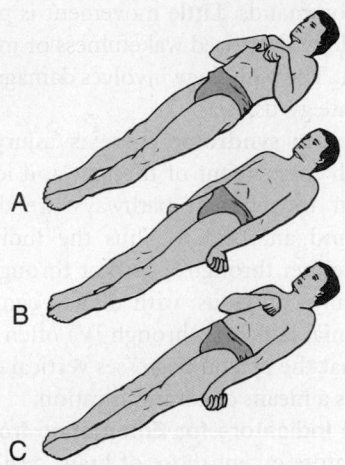

Figure 16-6 Decorticate and decerebrate responses. **A,** *Decorticate response.* Flexion of arms, wrists, and fingers with adduction in upper extremities. Extension, internal rotation, and plantar flexion in lower extremities. Both sides **B,** *Decerebrate response.* All four extremities in rigid extension, with hyperpronation of forearms and plantar extension of feet. **C,** *Decorticate response on right side of body and decerebrate response on left side of body.* (From Rudy EB: *Advanced neurological and neurosurgical nursing,* St Louis, 1984, Mosby.)

Types of Seizures

Seizures are classified in different ways—by clinical manifestations, site of origin, EEG correlates, or response to therapy.[17] A simplified version of the international classification of epileptic seizures is presented in Table 16-9. **Generalized seizures,** 30% of seizures, involve neurons bilaterally, often do not have a local (focal) onset, and usually originate from a subcortical or deeper brain focus. Generalized seizures result from cellular, biochemical, or structural abnormalities of a widespread nature.[16] With a generalized seizure, consciousness always is impaired or lost. **Partial seizures (focal seizures)** involve neurons only unilaterally, often have a local (focal) onset, and originate from discrete areas usually associated with structural abnormalities localized to the cortical brain tissue, thereby having a superficial focus. Consciousness may be maintained as long as the seizure activity is limited to one hemisphere in simple partial seizures, but partial seizures may become generalized to involve neurons of the other hemisphere and the deeper brain nuclei. This process is called **secondary generalization.** Consciousness is lost at the point of generalization. In complex partial seizures, consciousness is impaired; that is, the person is unable to respond normally to exogenous stimuli. Sixty percent of seizures are either complex partial seizures or seizures with secondary generalization.

Status epilepticus in adults is a state of continuous seizures lasting more than 5 minutes or rapidly recurring seizures before the person has fully regained consciousness from the preceding seizure or a single seizure lasting more than 30 minutes.[18] The person is still in a **postictal state** (state that follows a seizure) when the next seizure begins. Status epilepticus most often results from abrupt discontinuation of antiseizure medications but also may occur in untreated or inadequately treated persons with seizure disorders. The situation is a medical emergency because of the resulting cerebral hypoxia. Mental retardation, dementia, other brain damage,

Table 16-8	Comparative Clinical Features of Coma, Vegetative State, and Minimally Conscious State		
Diagnosis	**Arousal**	**Awareness**	**Communication**
Minimally conscious state	Eyes open spontaneously; normal to abnormal sleep-wake cycle; arousal level ranges from obtunded to normal	Inconsistent evidence of perception, communication ability, or purposeful motor activity; visual tracking often intact	Inconsistent verbalization, and gesturing
Locked-in syndrome	Full arousal; sleep wake cycle present; quadriplegic	Perceptions and emotions intact	Cannot speak or move muscles except vertical eye movement and blinking
Akinetic mutism	Eyes open spontaneously; normal sleep-wake cycle; arousal level is normal	Visual tracking present; little or no following of commands	Little or no volitional speech or movement
Coma	Eyes do not open spontaneously or in response to stimulation	No evidence of perception, communication ability, only reflexes and postural responses	None
Persistent vegetative state	Eyes open spontaneously; no visual tracking; sleep-wake cycle resumes or state of chronic wakefulness; arousal often sluggish	No evidence of cognitive function or purposeful motor activity	None

Data from Giacino JT et al: *Neurology* 58(3):349-353, 2002; Owen AM: *Ann N Y Acad Sci* 1125:225-238, 2008.

Table 16-9	International Classification of Epileptic Seizures
Traditional Terminology	**New Nomenclature**

Focal motor; jacksonian seizures (occasionally become secondarily generalized)	I. Partial seizures (seizures beginning locally)
	  A. Simple (without impairment of consciousness)
	    1. With motor signs
	    2. With special sensory or somatosensory symptoms
	    3. With autonomic symptoms or signs
	    4. With psychic symptoms

Temporal lobe or psychomotor seizures	B. Complex (with impairment of consciousness)
	    1. Simple partial onset followed by impaired consciousness
	    2. Impaired consciousness at onset—with or without automatisms
	  C. Secondarily generalized (partial onset evolving to generalized tonic-clonic seizures)
	II. Generalized seizures (bilaterally symmetric and without local onset)

Petit mal	A. Absence
	    1. Typical
	    2. Atypical
	  B. Myoclonic
	  C. Clonic
	  D. Tonic

Grand mal	E. Tonic-clonic

Drop attack	F. Atonic (astatic, akinetic)
	III. Unclassified epileptic seizures
	  A. Neonatal seizures
	  B. Infantile spasms

Table 16-10	Terminology Used to Describe a Seizure
Term	**Definition**
Aura	A partial seizure experienced as a peculiar sensation preceding the onset of a generalized seizure or complex partial seizure that may take the form of gustatory, visual, or auditory experience; a feeling of dizziness or numbness; or just "a funny feeling"
Prodroma	Early clinical manifestations, such as malaise, headache, or a sense of depression, that may occur hours to a few days before the onset of a seizure
Tonic phase	A state of muscle contraction in which there is excessive muscle tone
Clonic phase	A state of alternating contraction and relaxation of muscles
Postictal state	The period immediately following the cessation of seizure activity

and even death are serious threats. Aspiration also is a great risk. (Terminology associated with seizure activity is defined in Table 16-10.)

Diseases and Conditions Associated with Seizure Disorders

Any condition that changes the neuronal environment may produce seizure activity, so in theory, anyone can have a seizure. *Diseases* or other processes that involve the nervous system may cause a seizure disorder. The onset of seizures may point to the presence of an ongoing primary neurologic disease. Etiologic factors in seizures include (1) cerebral lesions, (2) biochemical disorders, (3) cerebral trauma, and (4) epilepsy. *Conditions* that may produce a seizure are metabolic defects, congenital malformations, genetic predisposition, perinatal injury, postnatal trauma, myoclonic syndromes, infection, brain tumor, vascular disease, fever, and drug or alcohol abuse or both.

Seizures also may be precipitated by hypoglycemia, fatigue or lack of sleep, emotional or physical stress, febrile illness, large amount of water ingestion, constipation, use of stimulant drugs, withdrawal from depressant drugs (including alcohol), hyperventilation (respiratory alkalosis), and some environmental stimuli, such as blinking lights, a poorly adjusted television screen, loud noises, certain odors, or merely being startled. Women immediately before or during menses may have increased seizure activity.

PATHOPHYSIOLOGY

Basic Pathologic Mechanisms

Seizures occur when there is disruption in the balance of excitation and inhibition.[19] The primary abnormality may be a membrane defect leading to instability in resting potential, abnormalities of potassium conductance or calcium channels, defects of the gamma-aminobutyric acid (GABA) inhibitory system, or an abnormality in excitatory transmission enhancement, particularly of the *N*-methyl-D-aspartate type.

In animal models, a defect in the GABA inhibitory system is the mechanism causing generalized seizures. Three groups of physiologic mechanisms are involved in seizures and epilepsies: (1) mechanisms of seizure initiation and propagation (excitation and inhibition), (2) mechanisms of epileptogenesis, and (3) genetics.[19]

Seizure initiation is characterized by two simultaneous events in a group of neurons: (1) high-frequency bursts of action potentials and (2) hypersynchronization. The burst activity is produced by a relatively long-lasting depolarization of the neuron caused by an influx of extracellular calcium that opens the voltage-dependent sodium channel. The influx of sodium generates repetitive action potentials.[16] The firing of involved neurons becomes increasingly greater in frequency and amplitude. With sufficient neuronal activation, recruitment of surrounding neurons occurs through a variety of mechanisms. The discharge spreads or propagates to adjacent normal neurons through corticocortical synapses. If uninhibited at this point, the cortical excitation spreads through interhemispheric tracts to the contralateral cortex and through projection pathways to the subcortical areas of the basal ganglia, thalamus, and brainstem. The excitation spread to the subcortical, thalamic, and brainstem areas corresponds to the **tonic phase** (phase of muscle contraction with increased muscle tone) and is associated with *loss of consciousness*. Autonomic clinical manifestations also may emerge at this point, and *apnea* may be present for a few seconds. The excitation is further projected downward to the spinal cord neurons through the corticospinal and reticulospinal pathways.

The **clonic phase** (phase of alternating contraction and relaxation of muscles) begins as inhibitory neurons in the cortex, anterior thalamus, and basal ganglia begin to inhibit the cortical excitation. This inhibition causes an interruption in the seizure discharge, producing an intermittent contract-relax pattern of muscle contractions. The intermittent clonic bursts gradually become more and more infrequent until they finally cease. At this point the epileptogenic neurons are exhausted and the neuronal membranes probably are hyperpolarized.

The maintenance of seizure activity demands a 250% increase in adenosine triphosphate (ATP). Cerebral oxygen consumption is increased by 60%. Although cerebral blood flow also increases approximately 250% during seizure activity, available glucose and oxygen are readily depleted. With a severe seizure the brain tissue may require more ATP than can be produced by the tissues from the available oxygen and glucose. A deficiency of ATP, phosphocreatine, and glucose then occurs, and lactate accumulates in the brain tissues. Severe seizures thus may produce secondary hypoxia, acidosis, and lactate accumulation, all of which are imbalances that may result in progressive brain tissue injury and destruction. Cellular exhaustion and destruction are consequences of these events.

Epileptogenesis refers to the transformation of a normal neuronal network into one that is chronically hyperexcitable (**epileptogenic focus**).[20] A delay of months to years often occurs between the initiating injury and the first seizure. Some

---

Box 16-1 International Classification of the Epilepsies

1. Localization related (focal, partial)
   A. Idiopathic
      1. Benign childhood epilepsy with centrotemporal spikes
      2. Childhood epilepsy with occipital paroxysms
      3. Primary reading epilepsy
   B. Symptomatic
      1. Temporal lobe epilepsy
      2. Frontal lobe epilepsy
      3. Parietal lobe epilepsy
      4. Occipital lobe epilepsy
      5. Chronic progressive epilepsia partialis continua of childhood
   C. Cryptogenic defined by:
      1. Seizure type
      2. Clinical features
      3. Etiology
      4. Anatomic localization
2. Generalized
   A. Idiopathic
      1. Benign neonatal familial convulsions
      2. Benign neonatal convulsions
      3. Benign myoclonic epilepsy in infancy
      4. Childhood absence epilepsy
      5. Juvenile absence epilepsy
      6. Juvenile myoclonic epilepsy
      7. Epilepsies with grand mal seizures on awakening
      8. Other generalized idiopathic epilepsies
   B. Cryptogenic or symptomatic
      1. West syndrome
      2. Lennox-Gastaut syndrome
      3. Epilepsy with myoclonic-astatic seizures
      4. Epilepsy with myoclonic absences
      5. Other symptomatic generalized epilepsies
   C. Symptomatic
      1. Nonspecific etiology
      2. Early myoclonic encephalopathy
      3. Early infantile epileptic encephalopathy with suppression bursts
3. Undetermined epilepsies
   A. Generalized and focal features
      1. Neonatal seizures
      2. Severe myoclonic epilepsy in infancy
      3. Epilepsy with continuous spike wave during slow-wave sleep
      4. Acquired epileptic aphasia
4. Special syndromes
   A. Situation-related seizures
      1. Febrile convulsions
      2. Isolated seizures or isolated status epilepticus
      3. Seizures occurring only when there is an acute or toxic event due to factors such as alcohol, drugs, eclampsia, nonketotic hyperglycemia

Commission on classification and terminology of the International League Against Epilepsy: proposal for the classification of epilepsy and epileptic syndromes, *Epilepsia* 30:389-399, 1989. Used with permission of International League Against Epilepsy.

forms of epileptogenesis involve structural changes in the neuronal network. Reorganization or "sprouting" of surviving neurons also has been found to affect the excitability of the network.

If a seizure focus is active for a prolonged period, a secondary focus, called a **mirror focus**, may develop in normal tissue. This process apparently is caused by the interhemispheric communication, inasmuch as the mirror focus is located in the contralateral cortical area. Seizure threshold in some individuals is genetically lower. Research is in progress to identify alterations in gene transcription that affect seizure threshold.[21]

Types of Seizure Syndromes

Seizure disorders, the second most common neurologic disorder, represent a syndrome, not a specific disease entity. The term **epilepsy**, meaning "to be seized by a force from without," generally is applied to conditions in which no underlying correctable cause for the seizures is found so that the seizure activity recurs without treatment because of a primary underlying brain abnormality. Epilepsy therefore is a general term for the primary condition that causes the seizures.

Epileptic syndromes are epileptic disorders characterized by specific clusters of signs and symptoms.[22] The three categories are based on clinical history, EEG manifestations, and etiology: (1) localization related, (2) generalized, and (3) undetermined. Localization-related epilepsies and syndromes are typified by seizures that originate from a localized cortical region and are characterized by seizures that have a focal or partial onset. Generalized and undetermined epilepsies and epilepsy syndromes are characterized by seizures with initial activation of neurons within both cerebral hemispheres.

Epilepsy syndromes are further subdivided into idiopathic, symptomatic, or cryptogenic. **Idiopathic epilepsy** refers to syndromes that arise spontaneously without a known cause, presumably having a genetic basis. The genetic basis may be through a specific inherited trait in which the seizures are the principal expression of the genetic defect (e.g., childhood absence epilepsy). In two thirds of cases, the etiology of the epilepsy is not identified. **Symptomatic epilepsy** denotes epilepsies with an identified cause. One third of seizures can be classified as symptomatic (provoked or secondary). Some symptomatic epilepsies also have a genetic basis in which the

Table 16-11	Causes of Recurrent Seizures in Different Age Groups
Age at Onset	**Probable Cause**
Neonates (<1 month)	Acute CNS infection (sepsis, meningitis, encephalitis)
	Cortical malformation
	Drug withdrawal or toxicity
	Genetic disorders
	Intracranial hemorrhage and trauma
	Kernicterus
	Metabolic disturbances (hypoglycemia, hypocalcemia, hypomagnesemia, pyridoxine deficiency)
	Perinatal hypoxic and ischemic encephalopathy
Infants and children (1 month to 12 yr)	Degenerative disorders (i.e., tuberous sclerosis, neurofibromatosis, Tay-Sachs disease)
	Febrile seizures
	Genetic disorders (metabolic, degenerative, primary epilepsy syndromes)
	Idiopathic
	Infantile spasms
	Trauma
Adolescents (12 to 18 yr)	Acute CNS infection (sepsis, meningitis, encephalitis)
	Brain tumor
	Genetic disorders
	Idiopathic
	Illicit drug use (i.e., cocaine, amphetamines)
	Trauma
Young adults (18 to 35 yr)	Alcohol or drug withdrawal (i.e., barbiturates, benzodiazepines)
	Brain tumor
	Idiopathic
	Illicit drug use (i.e., cocaine, amphetamines)
	Trauma
Older adults (>35 yr)	Alcohol or drug withdrawal (i.e., barbiturates, benzodiazepines)
	Brain tumor
	Cerebrovascular disease (i.e., stroke, aneurysm, arteriovenous malformations)
	CNS degenerative diseases (i.e., Alzheimer disease, multiple sclerosis)
	Idiopathic
	Metabolic disorders (i.e., uremia, hepatic failure, electrolyte abnormalities, hypoglycemia)

Data from Goetz CG, editor: *Textbook of clinical neurology,* ed 3, Philadelphia, 2007, Saunders; Nabbout R, Dulac O: *Curr Opin Neurol* 21(2):16106, 2008; Waterhouse E, Towne A: *Cleve Clin J Med* 72(Suppl 3):S26-S37, 2005.

CNS, Central nervous system

Table 16-12   Clinical Manifestations Related to Seizure Types

Type	Clinical Manifestations	Site
I. Partial seizures		
A. Simple		
1. With motor symptoms		
a. Without jacksonian march (focal motor seizure—the motor movements do not extend into adjacent areas)	Motor activity is usually clonic. Motor movement elicited by the seizure activity depends on the anatomic-physiologic portion of the irritated cortex, but motor seizures most often begin in the face and hands. Focal seizures begin with slow, repetitive jerking of the body part, which increases in strength and rate over 5 to 15 seconds. The seizure can cease spontaneously, with a gradual decrease in clonic movement.	Primary motor area
b. With jacksonian march (jacksonian seizure—the seizure activity spreads in an orderly fashion to adjacent areas)	Seizure activity spreads to adjacent areas after the initial clonic movement increases; motor movements, for example, begin in the fingers of one side and spread to the hand, wrist, forearm, arm, face, and finally the lower extremity on the same side of the body. After spreading, the jerking movements in all areas spontaneously stop.	Primary motor area
c. Adversive seizure	Turning movement of hand and eyes to the side opposite the irritative focus occurs. Often it is associated with contractions of the trunk and extremities. It may remain local or develop into a generalized seizure.	Frontal lobe anterior to the primary motor area
2. With special sensory or somatosensory symptoms (focal sensory seizure); less common than focal motor seizures; any age may be affected	Sensory experience is subjective and confined to the primary sensory modalities (somesthetic, visual, auditory-vestibular, or olfactory). If sensory seizure begins on the hand area of the sensory cortex, the person experiences numbness, tingling, or "pins and needles" phenomena. Other sensory experiences include burning, a crawling sensation, or a feeling of movement of the body part. Areas most often affected include lips, fingers, and toes. May remain local or develop into a generalized seizure.	Sensory cortex Postcentral gyrus (parietal lobe) with involvement of the primary sensory area
B. Complex (temporal lobe or psychomotor seizure)		
1. Simple partial onset followed by impairment of consciousness—common seizures found in children and adults but in most persons occurs before 20 years of age	The person is able to interact with the environment with purposeful, although inappropriate, movements; although the body muscles stiffen, the person does not fall and may even continue the complex activity in which he or she was involved, such as driving (perseverative automatisms); the person may appear "wide eyed." A wide variety of sensory experiences precede the automatism and include illusions; formed hallucinations; primitive visceral, olfactory, and gustatory sensations; and affective and cognitive symptoms. Most characteristic event of a temporal lobe seizure is the automatism; common examples of automatisms are lip smacking, chewing, facial grimacing, swallowing movements, and patting, picking, or rubbing oneself or one's clothing. Temporal lobe seizures generally last 11 seconds to 8 minutes (average 2 minutes) and are followed by several minutes of postictal confusion.	Temporal lobe and its connections Frontal lobes Other areas
2. Impaired consciousness at onset—with or without automatisms	See B1 above	
C. Secondarily generalized	Unconsciousness appears. General symptoms are produced.	

Table 16-12	Clinical Manifestations Related to Seizure Types—cont'd	
Type	**Clinical Manifestations**	**Site**
II. Generalized seizures		
A. Absence (petit mal seizures)		Multifocal
1. Typical	Characterized by lapses in consciousness that rarely last longer than 10 seconds. Often associated with additional subtle signs and symptoms such as clonic movements, changes in postural tone, automatisms, and autonomic changes.	
	The child immediately returns to normal consciousness without a postictal period.	
2. Atypical	Hyperventilation will induce a typical absence seizure.	
	Lapses in consciousness occur almost always accompanied by motor signs, especially changes in tone and lasts from 10 to 25 seconds.	
	Often occurs on awakening and with drowsiness.	
	A postictal period of confusion may follow.	
	Hyperventilation does *not* induce an atypical absence seizure.	
B. Myoclonus and myoclonic seizures	Characterized by sudden uncontrollable jerking movements of one or more extremities or the entire body.	Multifocal
	Seizures usually occur in the morning.	
	Consciousness is thought to be preserved.	
	Person often is flung violently to the ground; injury is a real possibility.	
	Myoclonic seizures can occur in clusters.	
C. Clonic	Characterized by repetitive clonic jerks of constant amplitude and diminishing frequency.	
D. Tonic (affects infants and children)	Loss of postural tone without evidence of clonicity, with flexion of the upper limbs and extension of the lower limbs.	
E. Tonic-clonic (grand mal seizure) (affects children and adults)	Child assumes an abnormal posture for seconds or minutes without losing consciousness.	Multifocal
	A prodromal period of irritability and tension may precede a tonic-clonic seizure by several hours or days; however, usually seizures begin without warning.	
	Characteristically tonic-clonic seizures begin with a sudden loss of consciousness and brief flexion; the person falls to the ground and the body stiffens in an opisthotonos position with legs and, usually, arms extended; the jaw snaps shut; a shrill cry may be heard as a result of forceful exhalation of air through the closed vocal cords as the thoracic muscles initially contract; the bladder and, less often, the bowel may evacuate; during the tonic phase, the person is apneic with subsequent cyanosis; pupils are dilated and unresponsive to light.	
	The tonic phase lasts less than 1 minute (average 10-15 seconds).	
	The clonic phase is characterized by flexion spasm of whole body interrupted by muscular relaxation; muscular contractions are accompanied by strenuous hyperventilation; the face is contorted; the eyes roll, and there is excessive salivation with frothing from the mouth; profuse sweating and a rapid pulse are evident. The tongue is often bitten.	
	The clonic jerking subsides in frequency and amplitude over a period of about 30 seconds.	
	The tonic-clonic seizure lasts 2-5 minutes.	
	After the clonic phase, the person is in a stupor or coma for about 5 minutes; the extremities are limp; breathing is quiet; and the pupils begin to respond to light.	
	When the person awakens, he or she may be confused and disoriented with complaints of headache, muscle aching, and fatigue.	
	There is no recollection of the attack.	
	Tonic-clonic seizures may occur at any time of day or night, whether the person is awake or asleep.	
	The frequency of recurrence may vary from hours to weeks, months, or years.	
F. Atonic (drop attack)	Characterized by sudden loss of postural muscle tone; the tone loss may be mild, resulting in a head nod, or more dramatic, including falls.	Multifocal

inherited trait is expressed in a neurologic or systemic disorder that is associated with seizures (e.g., neurofibromatosis). The term **cryogenic epilepsy** describes syndromes that are presumed to be symptomatic but have no known etiology, and occur in persons with or without abnormalities on neurologic examination. Box 16-1 presents the international classification of epilepsies, and Table 16-11 groups the etiology of recurrent seizures by age group.

Epilepsy is estimated to affect 5 to 10 people per 1000 in the United States.[16,23] Forty to 50 new cases per 100,000 persons develop yearly. Three percent of people are diagnosed with epilepsy.[23] Incidence is highest in early childhood and declines to plateau in adulthood. However, incidence rises again in older people to early childhood levels.

CLINICAL MANIFESTATIONS The clinical manifestations associated with seizure depend on the type of seizure (Table 16-12). Two types of symptoms often signal an impending generalized tonic-clonic seizure: an **aura**, a partial seizure that immediately precedes the onset of a generalized tonic-clonic seizure, and a **prodroma**, an early manifestation that may occur hours to days before a seizure (see Table 16-10). Both manifestations may become familiar to the person experiencing recurrent generalized seizures and so may help in preventing injuries during the seizure.

EVALUATION AND TREATMENT Health history is the most critical aspect in diagnosing a seizure disorder and establishing the cause. The health history is supplemented by the physical examination and laboratory tests of blood and urine (blood glucose, serum calcium, blood urea nitrogen, urine sodium, and creatinine clearance) to identify any systemic diseases known to have seizures as a clinical manifestation. Skull x-ray films, computed tomography (CT) scan, magnetic resonance imaging (MRI), and cerebrospinal fluid (CSF) examination are useful for identifying any neurologic diseases associated with seizures. The EEG is useful in assessing the type of seizure and may help determine its focus (Figure 16-7).

Treatment for a seizure disorder is first to correct or control its cause, if possible. If this is not possible, the major means of management is the judicious administration of antiseizure medications. The therapeutic goal is complete suppression of seizure activity without intolerable side effects of the drug or drug resistance. Temporal lobectomy, amygdalohippocampectomy, or vagus nerve stimulation can improve seizure control and quality of life in people with drug-resistant temporal lobe epilepsy.[24] Vagus nerve stimulation can reduce seizure frequency in persons with drug-resistant partial seizures.[25] Educational programs may reduce seizure frequency and improve psychologic functioning but it is not known if behavioral and psychologic treatments are beneficial.[26]

Alterations in Awareness

Selective attention (orienting), or a second attentional network, refers to the ability to select from available, competing environmental and internal stimuli-specific information to be consciously processed (orienting to specific information of interest).[27] Certain structures have been demonstrated to contribute to selective attention. The disengagement mechanism is mediated by the right parietal lobe. The move component is mediated by the superior colliculi for visual orienting. The engage component is mediated by the pulvinar nucleus of the thalamus (Figure 16-8). A weak orienting network results in a neglect syndrome.

Sensory inattentiveness is a form of neglect and may be visual, auditory, or tactile. The person with sensory inattentiveness is able to recognize individual sensory input from the dysfunctional side when called on to do so but ignores (i.e., neglects, extinguishes) the sensory input from the dysfunctional side when stimulated from both sides. This phenomenon is called **extinction**. The entire complex of denial of dysfunction, loss of recognition of one's own body parts, and extinction is sometimes referred to as the **neglect syndrome**.

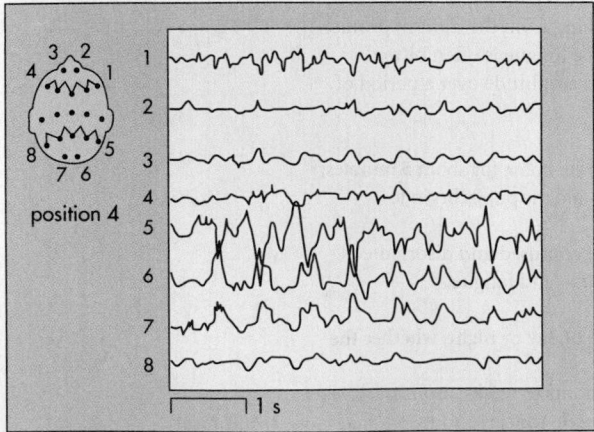

Figure 16-7 Electroencephalogram showing right posterior temporal sharp activity in individual with a microglioma. (From Perkin GD: *Mosby's color atlas and text of neurology*, London, 1998, Mosby-Wolfe.)

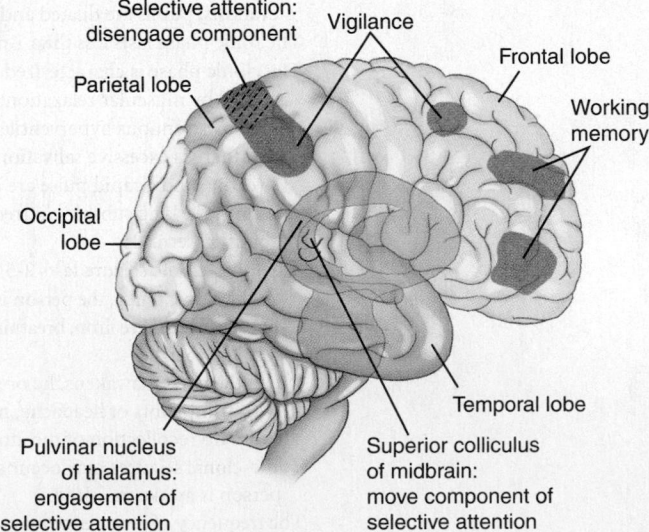

Figure 16-8 Right cortical, subcortical, and brainstem areas of the brain mediating cognitive functions. (From Boss BJ, Wilkerson R: Communication: language and pragmatics. In Hoeman SP, editor: *Rehabilitation nursing: prevention, intervention, & outcomes*, ed 4, p 508, St Louis, 2008, Mosby.)

An isolated (pure) **selective attention deficit (orientation)**, which manifests as a neglect syndrome, rarely, if ever, occurs clinically because typically other deficits also are present. A neglect syndrome may appear temporarily as a result of seizure activity or a postictal state. Temporary or permanent deficits may occur with contusions or subdural hematomas, encephalitis, and ischemic stroke. Progressive neglect deficits may be found with gliomas or metastatic tumor and in Alzheimer and Pick diseases.

Memory is the recording, retention, and retrieval of knowledge. Two types of memory exist: declarative and nondeclarative. **Declarative memory** involves the learning and remembrance of episodic memories (personal history, events, and experiences) and semantic memories (facts and information). Declarative memory is mediated by domain-specific cortical areas of the association areas of the temporal, parietal, and occipital lobes (Figure 16-9) where long-term memories are thought to be stored and by domain-independent areas of the medial temporal lobe, the diencephalon, and the basal forebrain (Figure 16-10) where it is thought distinct domain-specific features of an experience are related or bound.[28]

Nondeclarative memory (nonconscious), also called *reflexive, procedural,* or *implicit memory,* is the memory for actions, behaviors (habits), skills, and outcomes.[29] It is not a language memory but a motor memory. Nondeclarative memory involves the laying down of the motor pattern for the motor performance so that the action, behavior, or skill becomes more and more automatic. The striatum of the basal ganglia supports this learning across trials (stimulus-response learning), as well as probabilistic classification learning, which supports outcome prediction.[30] All skills and habits are stored in this memory network. *Cerebellar memory* was originally thought to be related to only motor learning but it is now believed to involve nonmotor functions.[31] *Emotional memory*

is mediated by the amygdala (see Figure 16-10). The amygdala attaches positive or negative dispositions to stimuli in the absence of conscious recollection of the circumstances of the emotional experience. Additionally, the amygdala modulates the event memory during and after the event (memory-enhancing effect).[32]

Dysmnesia is a disorder of the domain-independent declarative memory network defined as the loss of past memories (retrograde amnesia) coupled with an inability to form new memories (anterograde amnesia) despite intact attentional networks.[28] *Isolated (pure) domain-independent dysmnesia* is caused by only a limited number of conditions, such as transient global dysmnesia (episodic global dysmnesia), amnestic stroke, and Korsakoff psychosis (amnestic or dysmnestic syndrome), as well as after temporal lobectomy. Many disorders may temporarily or permanently produce domain-independent dysmnesia that accompanies other deficits of the cognitive systems. A *temporary domain-independent dysmnesia* is found during complex partial seizures that persist for a time in the postictal state, in postconcussive states, and in mild posttraumatic brain injury states. A *permanent domain-independent dysmnesia* may be seen after subarachnoid hemorrhage or moderate or severe posttraumatic brain injury states; in carbon dioxide poisoning and other hypoxic or anoxic states; in Wernicke encephalopathy, viral encephalitis, and granulomatous meningitides; in tumors; and in Alzheimer and Pick diseases.

A pure *auditory* or *visual domain–specific declarative memory deficit* manifests as an isolated agnosia (see Table 16-14). An isolated (pure) domain-specific declarative memory deficit of tactile sensations rarely occurs clinically because selective attention would likely be affected as well. A temporary auditory, visual, or tactile pattern recognition (remote memory) deficit may appear as a result of seizure activity or a postictal

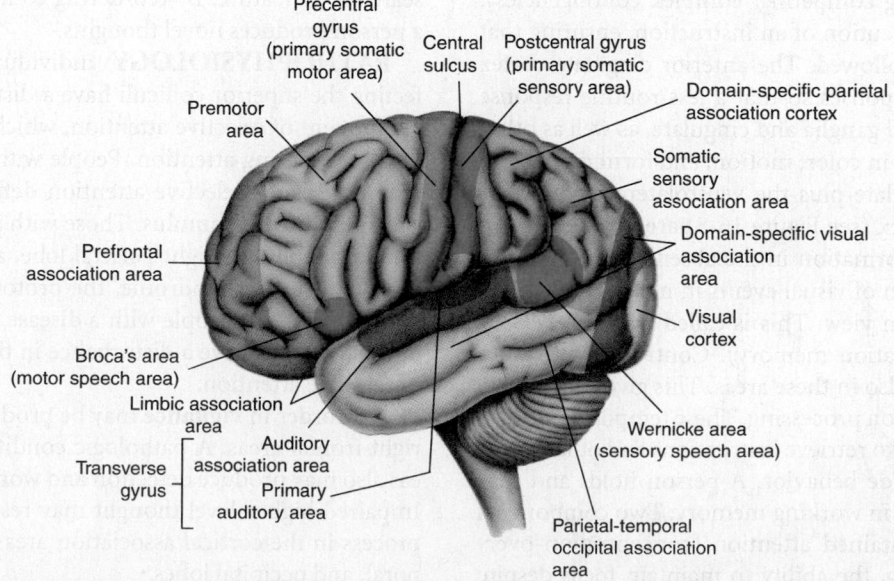

Figure 16-9 Cortical areas of the left (dominant) hemisphere. (From Patton KT, Thibodeau GA: *Anatomy & physiology,* ed 7, St Louis, 2010, Mosby.)

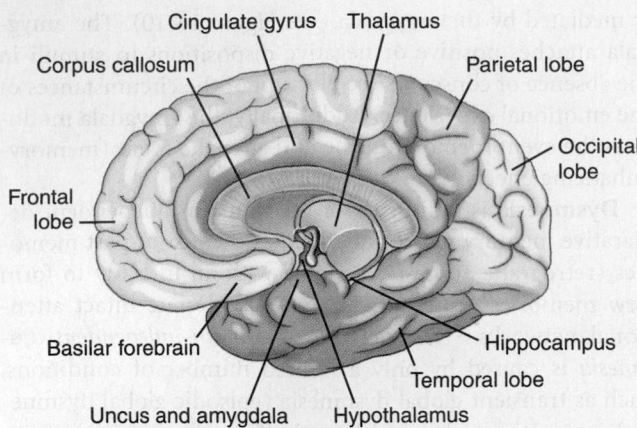

Figure 16-10 Midline cortical and deep areas of the cerebral hemisphere.

Labels: Cingulate gyrus · Thalamus · Corpus callosum · Parietal lobe · Occipital lobe · Frontal lobe · Basilar forebrain · Uncus and amygdala · Hypothalamus · Temporal lobe · Hippocampus

state. A temporary or permanent deficit can occur with temporal, occipital, or parietal lobe contusion; with subdural hematoma or ischemic stroke; and in encephalitis. A *progressive domain-specific declarative memory deficit* may occur in temporal, occipital, or parietal gliomas; in metastatic tumors; and in Alzheimer and Pick diseases.

The prefrontal areas mediate several cognitive functions, called *executive attention functions*. The *vigilance system* provides the person with the ability to maintain a sustained state of alertness for searching and scanning activities and involves the right frontal areas and the locus coeruleus (LC) located in the rostral pons (see Figure 16-8). Through the neurotransmitter norepinephrine from the LC, the speed of the orienting (selective attention) network is increased and the detection function of the anterior cingulate gyrus (see Figure 16-10) is decreased.

Detection is the recognition of the object's identity and the realization that the object fulfills a sought-after goal (i.e., target selection among competing, complex contingencies). There is conscious execution of an instruction, ensuring that the instructions are followed. The anterior cingulate cortex inhibits automatic responses so that a less routine response can be given. The basal ganglia and cingulate, as well as other frontal areas, function in color, motion, and form detection.

The anterior cingulate plus the ventrolateral and dorsolateral prefrontal cortex (see Figure 16-8) are involved in the representations of information in the absence of a stimulus, such as spatial position of visual events in memory when the event is removed from view. This is called *working memory* (short-term representation memory). Control of activation of these memories is also in these areas. This gives the person control over information processing. These temporary storage areas permit the brain to retrieve instructions and other information needed to guide behavior. A person holds and manipulates information in working memory. Two components are described: (1) sustained attention (concentration-over-time) and (2) tracking, the ability to maintain focus despite the presence of competing stimuli or the need to engage in alternating tasks.

Isolated (pure) vigilance, detection, and **working memory deficits** have been discussed in the literature, but their individual occurrence is uncommon because these deficits generally are present simultaneously. Akinetic mutism exemplifies a detection deficit. The person orients to external stimuli and can follow with his or her eyes but does not initiate other voluntary activity. There are no goals generated and no plans for carrying out the goals. The combination of vigilance, detection, and working memory deficits, accompanied by other deficits of the cognitive systems, is much more common. Whether the deficits are temporary or permanent depends on the cause and severity of injury. Deficits caused by CNS-depressant drugs, by seizure activity, and it is hoped, by neurosurgical procedures involving retraction of the frontal lobes are temporary. Deficits in postconcussive and mild traumatic brain injury states may prove to be temporary and resolve over time. Permanent deficits are more likely to be found with frontal lobe contusions, moderate or severe post-traumatic brain injury states, ischemic frontal lobe stroke, and neurosurgery that requires frontal lobe resection. Progressive deficits in vigilance, detection, and working memory functions are caused by frontal lobe gliomas, frontal lobe infarcts associated with hypertensive vascular disease, and late Alzheimer and Pick diseases. People with schizophrenia have difficulty in clearing working memory of information that is irrelevant to the task. Additionally, recently encountered visual material that is no longer in plain view cannot be preserved in working memory.

Higher-level thought involves the same neural areas used for sensory-specific computations, but when used voluntarily in thought, these areas are activated from the detection and work memory networks (top-down processing from the prefrontal cortex) rather than from bottom-up automatic processing (from the medial temporal lobe) beginning in sensory areas with a specific sensory stimulus. There is a voluntary search for a feature. By reordering component computation, a person produces novel thoughts.

PATHOPHYSIOLOGY Individuals with a disease affecting the superior colliculi have a disturbance in the move component of selective attention, which manifests as a slowness in orienting attention. People with parietal lobe disease may experience selective attention deficits related to disengagement from a stimulus. Those with parietal lobe dysfunction, especially the right parietal lobe, also may experience a unilateral neglect syndrome, the prototype of a selective attention disorder. People with a disease affecting the pulvinar of the thalamus have a disturbance in the engage component of selective attention.

A disorder in **vigilance** may be produced by disease in the right frontal areas. A pathologic condition in the frontal areas also may produce detection and working memory deficits. Impaired higher-level thought may result from a pathologic process in the cortical association areas of the parietal, temporal, and occipital lobes.

The exact pathophysiology of the various disorders of cognitive systems is not fully known. Researchers are studying the defects in the elementary operations (components) of each cognitive system. In the past, pathophysiology related to the memory systems was the most studied. Dysmnesia, also known as *amnesia*, originates from pathologic conditions in the hippocampus and related temporal lobe structures. Orienting and the executive attention network are receiving intense study.[33,34]

As a highly general statement, the primary pathophysiologic mechanisms that operate in cognitive systems disorders are (1) direct destruction because of direct ischemia and hypoxia or indirect destruction as a result of compression and (2) the effects of toxins and chemicals. Disinhibition resulting in overactivity, such as seen in some drug withdrawal states, is a pathologic mechanism that can produce detection deficits or a hypervigilant state. The pathophysiologic processes are summarized in Figure 16-11.

CLINICAL MANIFESTATIONS Clinical manifestations of selective attention deficits; domain-independent and domain-specific declarative deficits; and vigilance, detection, and working memory deficits are presented in Table 16-13.

EVALUATION AND TREATMENT Immediate medical management is directed at diagnosing the cause and treating reversible factors. Rehabilitative measures for cognitive system deficits generally are either compensatory or restorative in nature and have been greatly facilitated by computer technology and other electronic-assisted devices. Approaches based on behavioral techniques tend to be compensatory, whereas process-oriented approaches, it is hoped, are restorative.

Selective attention and executive attention deficits masquerade as other cognitive deficits. Differential diagnosis of other cognitive deficits is blocked, and learning potential is largely

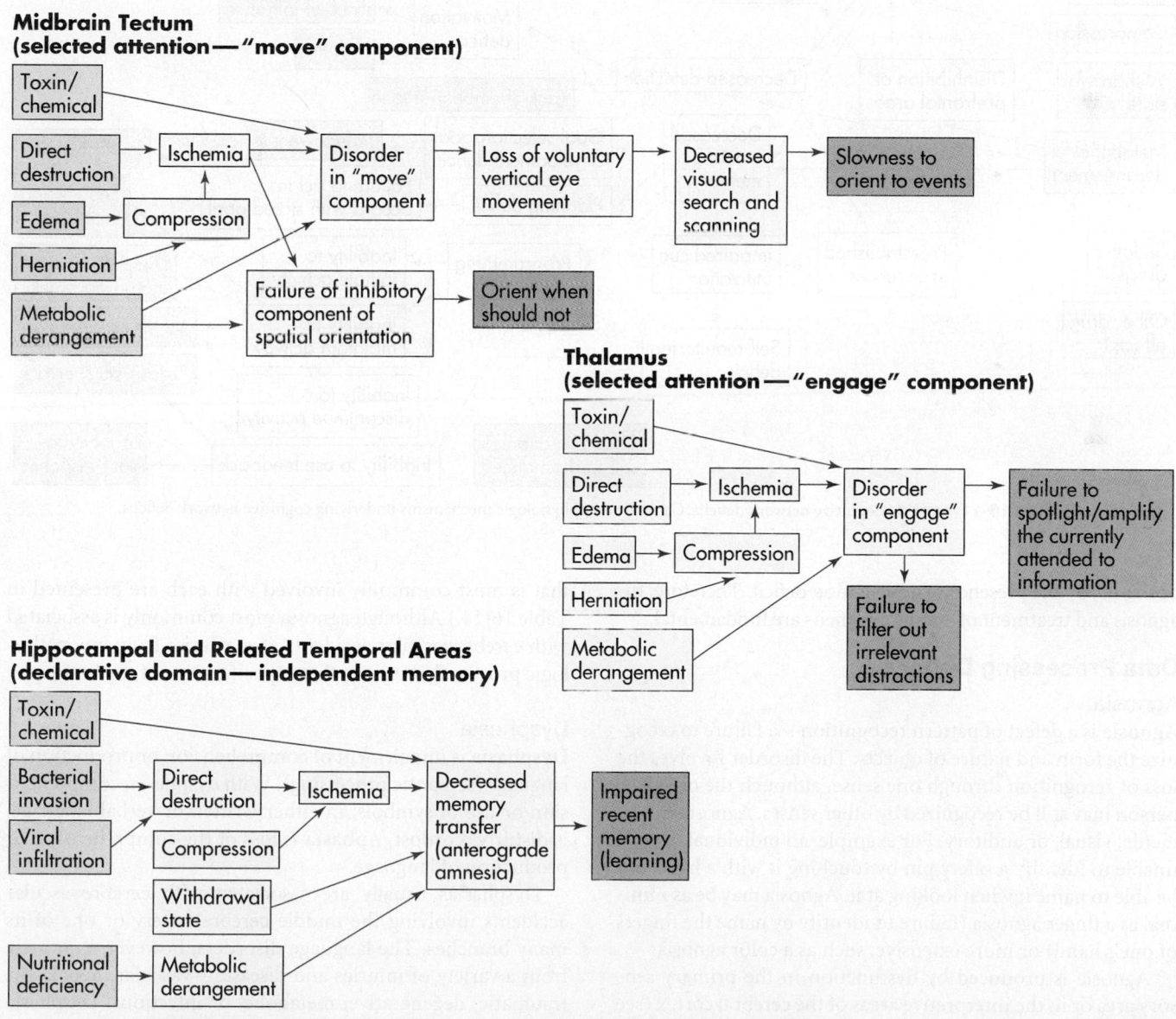

Figure 16-11 Cognitive network deficits. General pathophysiologic mechanisms underlying cognitive network deficits.

Continued

**Cortical Association Areas
(selective attention, disengage components, declarative domain—specific memory)
(image formation)**

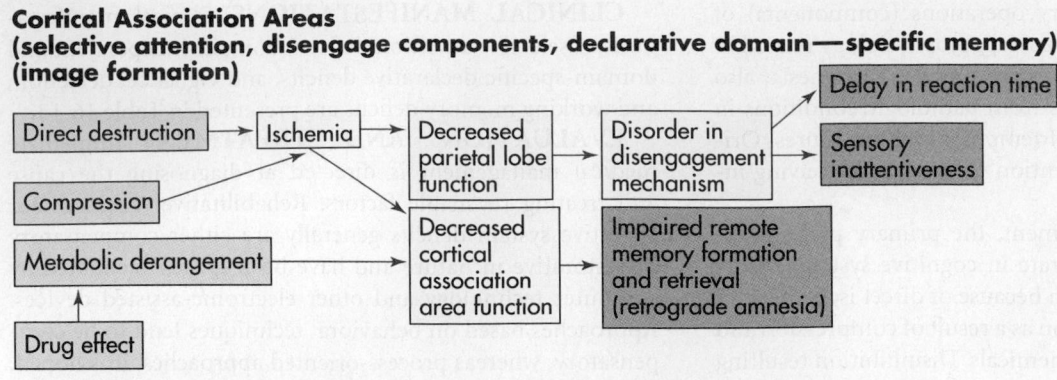

**Frontal Areas
(vigilance, detection, working memory)**

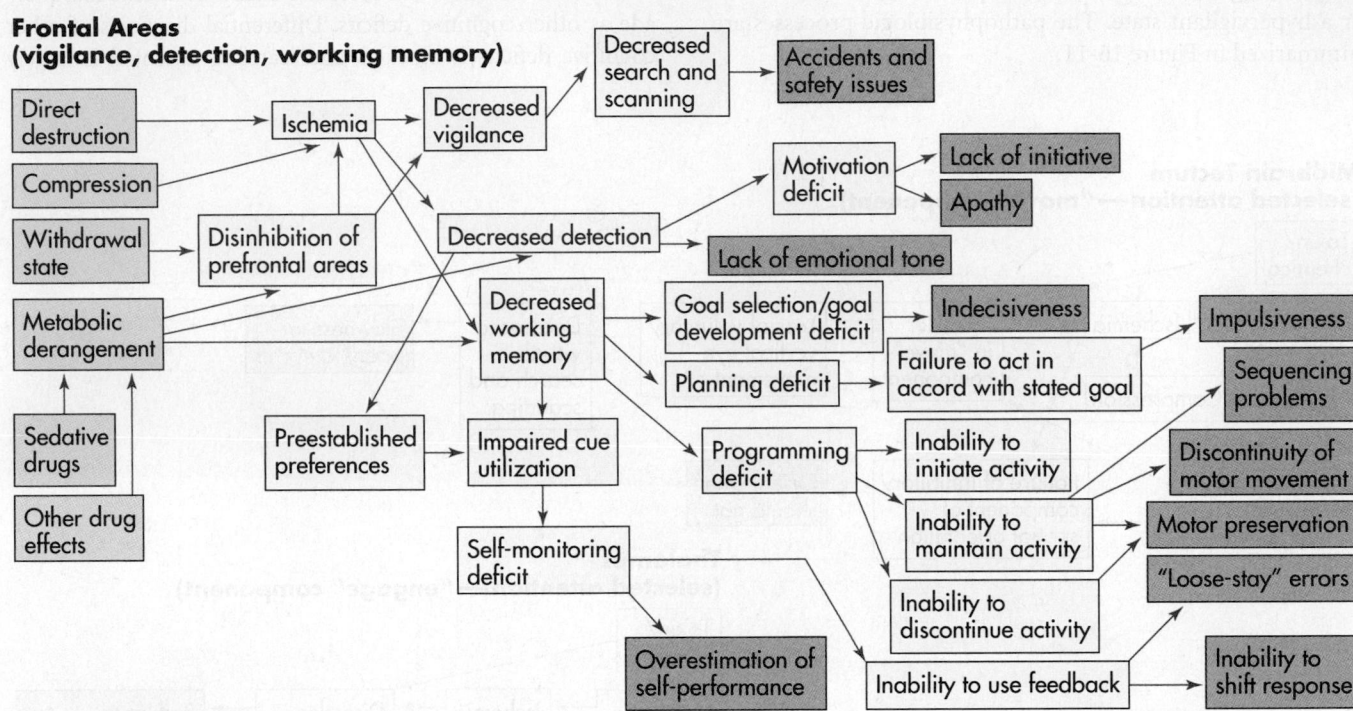

Figure 16-11 cont'd Cognitive network deficits. General pathophysiologic mechanisms underlying cognitive network deficits.

obscured, by the presence of an attention deficit. Therefore, diagnosis and treatment of attention deficits are fundamental.

Data Processing Deficits

Agnosia

Agnosia is a defect of pattern recognition—a failure to recognize the form and nature of objects. The disorder involves the loss of recognition through one sense, although the object or person may still be recognized by other senses. Agnosia can be tactile, visual, or auditory. For example, an individual may be unable to identify a safety pin by touching it with a hand but be able to name it when looking at it. Agnosia may be as minimal as a finger agnosia (failure to identify by name the fingers of one's hand) or more extensive, such as a color agnosia.

Agnosia is produced by dysfunction in the primary sensory area or in the interpretive areas of the cerebral cortex (see Figure 16-9). (The types of agnosia and the associated area

that is most commonly involved with each are presented in Table 16-14.) Although agnosia most commonly is associated with cerebrovascular accidents, it may arise from any pathologic process that injures these specific areas of the brain.

Dysphasia

Dysphasia is impairment of comprehension or production of language (semantic processing). With dysphasia, comprehension or use of symbols, in either written or verbal language, is disturbed or lost. **Aphasia** is loss of the comprehension or production of language.

Dysphasias usually are associated with cerebrovascular accidents involving the middle cerebral artery or one of its many branches. The language disorders, however, may arise from a variety of injuries and diseases—vascular, neoplastic, traumatic, degenerative, metabolic, or infectious. Dysphasia results from dysfunction in the left cerebral hemisphere, most

Table 16-13	Clinical Manifestations of Cognitive Network Deficits	
Deficit	**Clinical Signs**	**Symptoms**
Attention		
Selective attention (orienting)	Inability to focus attention; decreased eye, head, and body movements associated with focusing on the stimuli; decreased search and scanning; faulty orientation to stimuli causing safety problems	Person reports inability to focus attention, failure to perceive objects and other stimuli (history of injuries, falls, and safety problems)
Memory		
Domain-independent declarative	*Left hemisphere:* disorientation to time, situation, place, name, person (verbal identification); impaired language memory (e.g., names of objects); impaired semantic memory *Right hemisphere:* disorientation to self, person (visual), place (visual); impaired episodic memory (personal history); impaired emotional memory Either or both hemispheres: confusion; behavioral change	Person reports disorientation, confusion, "not listening," "not remembering"; reports by others of person being disoriented, not able to remember, not able to learn new information
Domain-specific declarative	*Left hemisphere:* inability to retrieve personal history, past medical history; unaware of recent current events *Right hemisphere:* inability to recognize persons, places, objects, music, etc., from the past	Person reports remote memory problems; others report that person cannot recall formerly known information
Image processing (semantic processing)	Inability to categorize (identify similarities and differences), sort; inability to form concepts; inability to analyze relationships; misinterpretation; inability to interpret proverbs	Reports by others of frequent misinterpretation of data; failure to conceptualize or generalize information
	Inability to perform deductive reasoning (convergent reasoning); inability to perform inductive reasoning (divergent reasoning); inability to abstract; concrete reasoning demonstrated; delusions	Reports by others of predominantly concrete thinking; lack of understanding of everyday situations, healthcare regimens, delusional thinking
Executive Attentional Network		
Vigilance	Failure to search and scan environment	Person reports accidents, safety issues
Detection	Lack of initiative (anergy); lack of ambition; lack of motivation; flat affect; no awareness of feelings; appears depressed, apathetic, and emotionless; fails to appreciate deficit; disinterested in appearance; lacks concern about childish or crude behavior	Reports by others of laziness or apathy, flat affect or lack of emotional expression, failing to exhibit or be aware of feelings
Mild	Responds to immediate environment but no new ideas; grooming and social graces are lacking	Reports by others of lack of ambition, motivation, or initiative, failure to carry out adult tasks, lack of social graces and new ideas
Severe	Motionless, lack of responding to even internal cues, does not respond to physical needs, does not interact with surroundings	Reports by others of failure to groom or toilet self, unawareness of surroundings and own physical needs
	Inability to use feedback regarding behavior; failure to recognize omissions and errors in self-care, speech, writing, and arithmetic; impaired cue utilization; overestimation of performance	Reports by others of not changing behavior when requested; unawareness of limitations; does not recognize and correct errors in dressing, grooming, toileting, eating; fails to recognize speech and arithmetic errors; careless speech
	Failure to shift response set; failure to change behavior when conditions change; cue utilization may be impaired	Reports by others of failure to use feedback; inability to incorporate feedback (does not correct when feedback is given)
Working memory	Inability to set goals or form goals; indecisiveness	Reports by others of failure to set goals, indecisiveness
	Failure to make plans; inability to produce a complete line of reasoning; inability to make up a story; appears impulsive	Reports by others of failure to plan, impulsiveness, "does not think things through"
	Failure to initiate behavior; failure to maintain behavior; failure to discontinue behavior; slowness to alternate response for the next step; motor perseveration	Reports by others of not knowing where to begin, inability to carry out sequential acts (maintain a behavior), inability to cease a behavior

Table 16-14   Types of Agnosia (Concept Disorders)

Type of Agnosia	Definition	Location of Injury
Tactile agnosia (astereognosis)	Inability to recognize objects by touch	Parietal lobe
Spatial agnosia	Incapacity to find one's way around familiar places; disturbance of perception of space (disorders of [1] topographic [extrapersonal] orientation or [2] topographic and geographic memory [construction])	Parietal lobe
Gerstmann syndrome	Loss of spatial orientation of fingers, body, sides, and numbers	Left angular gyrus (parietal lobe)
Finger agnosia (digital agnosia)	Inability to identify the names of one's fingers	
Right-left confusion	Inability to distinguish right from left	
Agraphia	Inability to write	
Acalculia	Inability to perform mathematic calculations	
Visual agnosia		
Object agnosia	Inability to recognize objects and pictures	Temporo-occipital area
Prosopagnosia	Inability to recognize faces	Temporo-occipital ventromesial region
Color agnosia	Inability to understand colors as qualities of objects; faulty color concepts and inability to evoke color images in the absence of color blindness; specific types: (1) "hue" problem, (2) color anomia (cannot name color)	Inferior occipital cortex in left hemisphere
Body image agnosias (may be spatial)		
Anosognosia	Ignorance or denial of existence of the disease	Right parietal lobe
Autotopagnosia	Loss of ability to identify the body, in whole or in part, or to recognize relationships among various parts	Right parietal lobe
Word blindness (alexia/dyslexia)	Inability to recognize written symbols	Left parietotemporal region
Auditory agnosia (pure word deafness)	Inability to recognize speech sounds	Superior temporal area
Amusia (music deafness)	Loss of capacity to recognize tones and melodies	Right superior temporal area

commonly in the frontotemporal region, particularly around the insula (see Figures 14-7 and 14-9). Genes located on several chromosomes have been linked to language development and disorders.[35,36] Most language disorders are caused by acute processes that either resolve or cause a chronic residual deficit. Some language disorders are caused by degenerative disorders that make the dysfunction progressive.

Dysphasias have been classified anatomically and functionally. Other classifications are linguistic and describe fluency, volume, or quantity of speech. Pure forms of any language dysfunction, however, are rare. Expressive dysphasias are characterized primarily by expressive deficits, but a verbal comprehension (auditory-receptive element) deficit may be present. Receptive dysphasias may have expressive deficits. (Table 16-15 compares types of dysphasias; Table 16-16 illustrates some of the language disturbances.)

Dysphasias, referred to as **transcortical dysphasias (transcortical sensory dysphasia, mixed transcortical dysphasia, isolated speech center)**, involve the ability to repeat (called **echolalia**) and recite. Speech is fluent but with striking paraphrases. The individual cannot read and write, and comprehension is impaired.

Transcortical dysphasias are caused by hypoxia from prolonged hypotension, carbon monoxide poisoning, or other mechanisms that destroy the border zone (watershed area) of the anterior, middle, and posterior cerebral arteries (see Figure 14-19). Blood supply is marginal in this region. Hypoxia

in this area occasionally may isolate the posterior speech areas or all the speech areas from the remainder of the cortex, although both areas remain intact. The sensory and motor speech areas therefore are functional, but connections with other sensory or motor areas are impaired. Information from the remaining areas of the cortex cannot be transmitted to the Wernicke area to be transformed into language.

Acute Confusional States

Acute confusional states (acute cerebral failure or **acute brain failure)** is an acquired mental disorder characterized by deficits in attention and coherence of thoughts and actions often associated with an altered level of arousal, global cognitive dysfunction, perceptual disturbances, sleep-wake cycle disruption, affective disturbance, and emotional liability.[37] Acute confusional states result from dysfunction secondary to such causes as drug intoxication, metabolic disorders, or nervous system disease. A common cause of an acute confusional state is withdrawal from alcohol, barbiturate, or other sedative drug ingestion. Acute confusional states of toxic origin may have either sudden or gradual onset, depending on the amount of exposure to the toxin. These states often occur with febrile illnesses, with systemic diseases such as heart failure, after head injury or anesthesia, postnatally, or with certain focal cerebral lesions.[38]

PATHOPHYSIOLOGY Acute confusional states arise from disruption of a widely distributed neural network

Table 16-15	Major Types of Dysphasia							
Type	Expression	Verbal Comprehension	Repetition	Name	Reading Comprehension	Writing	Location of Lesion	Cause of Lesion
Expressive (Broca Dysphasia, Motor)								
	Nonfluent; impairment of ability to find words, difficulty in writing	Relatively intact	Impaired	Impaired	Variable	Impaired	Left posteroinferior frontal lobe (Broca area)	Occlusion of one or several branches of middle cerebral artery MCA, trauma, tumor, infection, abscess
Receptive								
Wernicke dysphasia, sensory	Fluent; able to produce verbal language but language is meaningless; words are often inappropriate; words with similar sounds or words with similar meaning are substituted for the correct words; words that are not part of the language may be present; these neologisms may be so extensive as to make the speech entirely incomprehensible; because the person has no means to monitor the language for correctness, errors are not recognized; intonation, accent, cadence, rhythm, and articulation are normal	Impaired (disturbance in understanding all language)	Impaired	Impaired	Impaired	Impaired	Left posterosuperior temporal lobe (Wernicke area)	Occlusion of inferior or division of left middle cerebral artery, temporal abscess
Global (sensorimotor receptive-expressive)	Nonfluent; produces little speech; at best speaks a few words or phrases	Impaired or completely lost; person understands only the simplest things said	Impaired; not able to repeat	Impaired	Reading out loud—impaired or completely lost Reading silently intact	Impaired; produces little written language	Frontotemporal lobe (left sylvian region); anterior and posterior speech areas extensively impaired	Occlusion of the left middle cerebral artery of left internal carotid artery; trauma, infection, tumors, other mass lesions, and hemorrhage may be the cause

Continued

Table 16-15   Major Types of Dysphasia—cont'd

Type	Expression	Verbal Comprehension	Repetition	Name	Reading Comprehension	Writing	Location of Lesion	Cause of Lesion
Conduction	Fluent but with paraphrasia in self-initiated speech and writing or reading aloud	Relatively intact	Impaired; unable to repeat	Impaired	Variable	Impaired	Arcuate fasciculus, deep in supramarginal gyrus, disruption of the large bundle of fibers that arise from the temporal lobe and pass posteriorly around the sylvian fissure and then project anteriorly to the premotor area	Typical cause is embolic occlusion of the ascending parietal or posterior temporal branch of the middle cerebral artery, angular branch of middle cerebral artery
Anomic, nominal, amnesic (anomia)	Fluent but impaired ability to name objects, persons, qualities, or characteristics; knows what he or she wants to say but cannot find words; may even use desired word in another context but still cannot isolate word when needed	Relatively intact; able to recognize word when it is given	Intact	Impaired	Variable	Variable	Angular gyrus—posterosuperior temporal lobe	Residual of other aphasias, degenerative disorders
Transcortical motor	Nonfluent	Relatively intact	Intact	Impaired	Variable	Impaired	Left dorsolateral frontal cortex (anterior presylvian fissure)	Occlusion of left anterior cerebral artery or anterior border zone vascular infarct
Transcortical sensory	Fluent	Impaired	Intact	Impaired	Impaired	Impaired	Left temporoparietooccipital junction (posterior presylvian fissure)	Occlusion of left internal carotid with posterior border zone infarct, tumor, trauma, intracerebral hemorrhage, and degenerative disease

Table 16-16		Examples of Language Disturbances
Disorder		**Example**
Verbal paraphrasia	Question:	What did the car do?
	Response:	The car would spit sweetly down the road. (The car sped swiftly down the road.)
Literal paraphrasia	Request:	Say "persistence is essential to success."
	Response:	Mesastence is instans to success.
Neologism	Question:	What do you call this? (Pointing to a plant.)
	Response:	It's a logper.
Circumlocution	Question:	What do you call this? (Pointing to a plant.)
	Response:	Something that grows.
Anomia	Question:	What do you call this? (Pointing to a plant.)
	Response:	It's…
		or
	Question:	What did you do this morning?
	Response:	Reading.
	Question:	Were you reading a book or a newspaper?
	Response:	One of those.
Telegraphic style	Question:	Where is your daughter?
	Response:	New Orleans…home…Monday.

From Boss BJ: *J Neurosurg Nurs* 16(3):151, 1984.

involving the reticular activating system of the upper brainstem and its projections to the thalamus, basal ganglion, and specific association areas of the cortex and limbic areas. Delirium (hyperkinetic confusional states) is associated with right middle temporal gyrus or left temporo-occipital junction disruption.[37] These areas receive extensive input from the limbic areas and modulate motivational and affective aspects of attention. Hypokinetic confusional states are more likely associated with right-sided frontal-basal ganglion disruption.[37] These areas modulate motor exploratory aspects of attention.

Most metabolic disturbances that produce a confusional state interfere with neuronal metabolism or synaptic transmission. Many drugs and toxins also interfere with neurotransmission function at the synapse. Cholinergic pathways critical for attention and arousal are often disrupted.

CLINICAL MANIFESTATIONS The predominant features of an acute confusional state are impaired or lost detection. Because of dysfunction of the anterior cingulate gyrus (see Figures 16-10 and 14-7), the ability to focus, sustain, or shift attentional focus is seriously impaired or completely lost. The person is highly distractible and unable to concentrate on incoming sensory information or on any particular mental or motor task. Besides impaired attention, the person loses coherence of thought and actions. The person may persist in thoughts or actions that are no longer appropriate (perseveration) and be unable to monitor the environment for events of importance (impaired vigilance). The person demonstrates irrelevant or inappropriate responses.

The onset of an acute confusional state usually is abrupt rather than insidious. The first clinical manifestations are difficulty in concentration, restlessness, irritability, tremulousness, insomnia, and poor appetite. Later there are top-down processing problems, including misperception, illusion, hallucination, and delirium. Obsessions, compulsive behavior, and rituals may be evident.

In hypokinetic acute confusional states, the individual exhibits decreases in mental function. Alertness is decreased, as are attention span, accurate perception, and interpretation of the environment. Forgetfulness is prominent. Reactions to the environment are slowed and indecisive. The individual dozes frequently.

Delirium, an acute hyperkinetic confusional state, typically develops over 2 to 3 days. Early clinical manifestations include difficulty in concentrating, restlessness, irritability, insomnia, tremulousness, and poor appetite. Some persons experience seizures. Unpleasant, even terrifying, dreams may occur.

In a fully developed delirium state, the individual is completely inattentive and perceptions are grossly altered. Misperception and misinterpretation are predominant. Hallucinations may be present. The person appears distressed and often very perplexed. Conversation is incoherent. Frank tremor is evident, and a great deal of restless movement is common. Violent behavior may be present. The individual cannot sleep, is flushed, and has dilated pupils, a rapid pulse (tachycardia), temperature elevation, and perfuse sweating (diaphoresis). Delirium typically abates suddenly or gradually in 2 to 3 days, although occasional delirium states persist for several weeks.

EVALUATION AND TREATMENT An acute confusional state is an acute medical problem. The initial goal is to establish that the individual is confused, and the cause must be distinguished as organic or functional (Table 16-17). Next the goal is to determine whether the confusion is delirium, an acute hypokinetic confusional state, or an underlying dementia. The precise cause of an acute confusional state is established through the complete history and physical examination. Laboratory tests include an electrocardiogram and blood, urine, CSF, and radiologic studies.

Once the cause is established, treatment is directed at controlling the primary disorder. In an acute confusional state,

Table 16-17   Differences between Organic and Functional Confusion

Factor	Organic Confusion	Functional Confusion
Memory impairment	Recent, more impaired than remote	No consistent difference between recent and remote
Disorientation		
Time	Within own lifetime or reasonably near future	May not be related to individual's lifetime
Place	Familiar place or one where person might easily be	Bizarre or unfamiliar places
Person	Sense of identity usually preserved	Sense of identity diminished
	Misidentification of others as familiar	Misidentification of others based on delusion system
Hallucinations	Visual, vivid	Auditory more frequent
	Animals and insects common	Bizarre and symbolic
Illusions	Common	Not prominent
Delusions	Concern everyday occurrences and people	Bizarre and symbolic
Confusion	Spotty confusion	More consistent
	Clear intervals mixed with confused episodes	No tendency to become worse at night
	Worse at night	

From Morris M, Rhodes M: *Am J Nurs* 72(9):1632, 1972.

Box 16-2   World Health Organization Definition of Dementia

Dementia is a syndrome of disease of the brain, usually of a chronic or progressive nature, in which there is disturbance of multiple cortical functions, calculation, learning capacity, language, and judgment. Consciousness is not clouded. Impairments of cognitive function are commonly accompanied and occasionally preceded by deterioration in emotional control, social behavior, and motivation.

---

all drugs that may be contributing to or causing the condition are discontinued unless the problem is the result of drug withdrawal. Supportive measures are designed to enhance coping skills and to minimize the individual's need for altered cortical functions. Supportive and protective management also involves maintaining the person's intact cortical functions by promoting use of these functions. Agitated behavior is managed with neuroleptic medication.

Dementing Processes

Dementia is a syndrome that may be caused by a number of different illnesses. Dementia is the progressive failure (an acquired deterioration) of many cerebral functions that is not caused by an impaired level of consciousness.[39,40] Memory is the most common cognitive ability lost[41] but the dementias are all characterized by reduction in cognitive functions (intellectual function). Mental abilities are impaired, with a decrease in orienting, recent memory, remote memory, language, executive attentional functions, and alterations in behavior (Box 16-2). The greatest risk factor is age.[41]

Dementias can be classified according to etiologic factors (e.g., trauma, tumors, vascular disorders, infections) and to associated clinical and laboratory signs. Dementing processes have been grouped as cortical, subcortical, or both. Box 16-3 lists the most and least common causes of dementia. Alzheimer disease (AD) is the most common cause followed by vascular disease, then dementia associated with Parkinson disease.[41] In people younger than 60 years, frontotemporal dementia (FTD) rivals AD in terms of frequency.[41] Disruption in cerebral neural circuits is present. The culmination of

---

Box 16-3   Causes of Dementia

Potentially Reversible Causes of Dementia
Chronic Infection
  Neurosyphilis
  Meningitis
  Encephalitis
Normal Pressure Hydrocephalus
Chronic Subdural Hematoma
Nutritional Deficiencies
  Vitamin B$_1$ (thiamine) deficiency
  Vitamin B$_{12}$ (cobalamin) deficiency
  Nicotinic acid (pellagra)
Chronic Drug Intoxication
  Alcohol*
  Sedatives
Metabolic Disorders
  Thyroid abnormalities
  Chronic hepatic encephalopathy
  Cerebral vasculitis
  Sarcoidosis
Some Types of Tumors
  Frontal and temporal lobe
  Pseudodementia of depression
Medical Side Effects
  Anticholinergics
  Antihypertensives
  Antihistamines
Irreversible Causes of Dementia
Neurodegenerative Disorders
  Alzheimer disease*
  Dementia with Lewy bodies
  Frontotemporal dementia
  Pick disease
  Huntington disease
  Parkinson disease
Vascular Disease
  Binswanger disease* (diffuse white matter disease)
  Amyloid angiopathy
  Vascular dementia*
  Multi-infarct
  Strategic single infarct
Infection
  Creutzfeldt-Jakob disease (CJD)
  Postencephalitic dementia
  Dementia associated with HIV

*Most common; *HIV*, human immunodeficiency virus.

Table 16-18   The Molecular Basis for Degenerative Dementia

Dementia	Molecular Mechanism	Causal Genes and (Chromosome)	Susceptibility Genes and Chromosomes	Pathology
Alzheimer disease (familial)	Amyloid-beta protein (AB)	<2% carry these mutations APP (21), PSEN-1 (14), PSEN-2 (1) (most mutations are in PSEN-1)	apoE4 (19)	Amyloid plaques, neurofibrillary tangles
Creutzfeldt-Jakob disease	PrP^{SC} proteins type 1 and 2	Prion (20) (up to 15% of cases carry these dominant mutations)	PRNP codon 129 homozygosity for methionine or valine	Tau inclusions, spongiform changes, gliosis
Dementia with Lewy bodies	Alpha-synuclein	Very rare alpha-synuclein (4) (dominant)	Unknown	Alpha-synuclein inclusions (Lewy bodies)
Frontotemporal dementia	Microtubule-associated protein tau (MAPT) Progranulin (PGRN)	Tau exon and intron mutation (17) (about 10% of familial cases) PGRN (17) (10% of familial cases)	Tau haplotypes (H1 and H2)	Tau inclusions, Pick bodies, neurofibrillary tangles
Huntington disease (autosomal dominant)	Huntingtin protein (polyglutamine)	HD-IT15 (4) (trinucleotide repeat expansion)	None known	Neuronal degeneration, astrogliosis
Parkinson disease	Autosomal dominant alpha-synuclein Leucine-rich repeat kinase 2 Autosomal recessive parkin (juvenile onset) DJ-1 protein PTEN-induced putative kinase 1	SNCA(PARK1) (4) LRRK2- PARK8 (12) PARK2 (4) oncogene DJ-1 (PARK7) PINK1 (PARK6)	GBA (glucosidase beta acid) SNCAIP (alpha-synuclein interacting protein) NR4A2 (orphan nuclear receptor) UCH-L1 (PARK5) ubiquitin C-terminal hydrolase	Neuronal degeneration alpha-synuclein inclusions (Lewy bodies) gliosis

From Belin AC, Westerlund M: *FEBS J* 275(7):1377-1383, 2008; Borroni B et al: *Acta Neurol Scand* 117(5):359-366, 2008; Goldman JS et al: *Am J Alzheimers Dis Other Demen* 22(6):507-515, 2008; Graff-Radford NR, Woodruff BK: *Semin Neurol* 27(1):48-57, 2007; Waring SC, Rosenberg RN: *Arch Neurol* 65(3):329-334, 2007.

apoE, amyloid precursor protein (APP), apolipoprotein E; *PRNP*, prion protein; *PrP^{SC}*, prion protein; *PSEN*, presenilin.

a progressive dementing process is nerve cell degeneration and brain atrophy involving the cerebral cortex, diencephalon, and basal ganglia.

PATHOPHYSIOLOGY Mechanisms in dementing processes include (1) degeneration possibly caused by genetics, inflammation, or biochemical alterations; (2) atherosclerosis, multiple foci of infarction throughout the thalami, basal ganglia, cerebral projection pathways, and associated areas; (3) trauma, lesions in the cerebral convolutions, mainly frontal and temporal, corpus callosum, and mesencephalon; and (4) compression, increased intracranial pressure, and chronic hydrocephalus.

The major degenerative dementias are AD, FTD, dementia with Lewy bodies (DLB), Huntington disease (HD), and prion disorders including Creutzfeldt-Jakob disease (CJD). The molecular basis for these dementias is contrasted in Table 16-18. In some instances a familial history of dementia increases by four times the likelihood that dementia will develop. Environmental influences also may play a role in the pathogenesis of dementia. The exact nature of the influence of environmental factors, such as aluminum, is not clearly understood as yet.

CLINICAL MANIFESTATIONS A summary of the clinical manifestations of the degenerative dementias is presented in Table 16-19.

EVALUATION AND TREATMENT Establishing the cause for a dementing process may be complicated, but anyone evidencing the clinical manifestations of dementia should be evaluated with laboratory and neuropsychologic testing to identify underlying conditions that may be treatable.

If a specific treatable cause is identified, the appropriate treatment is initiated. For example, an infectious process requires the appropriate antibiotic, and a potentially resectable mass may require neurosurgery. Nutritional deficiencies are corrected. If the cause is metabolic, the imbalance is corrected or the metabolic disorder is treated, or both.

Unfortunately no specific treatment or cure exists for most progressive dementias. In such instances, therapy is directed at maintaining and maximizing the remaining capacities, restoring functions if possible, accommodating to lost abilities, and controlling behavioral changes. Delusions, paranoia, and hallucinations often respond to neuroleptic medications. If coexisting depression is suspected, a trial of antidepressants is appropriate. Assisting the family to understand the dementing process and to learn ways to assist the demented individual is an essential component of supportive management.

Alzheimer Disease

Alzheimer disease (dementia of Alzheimer type [DAT], senile disease complex) is a common neurologic disorder. Formerly believed to occur mostly in people younger than 65 years (familial, early onset dementia), AD has been

Table 16-19	Clinical Differentiation of the Major Degenerative Dementias

Disease	First Symptom	Mental Status	Neurobehavior	Neurologic Examination	Imaging
Alzheimer disease	Memory loss; impaired learning	Episodic memory loss	Initially normal, progressive cognitive impairment	Initially normal	Entorhinal cortex and hippocampal atrophy
Creutzfeldt-Jakob disease	Dementia, mood, anxiety, movement disorders	Variable, frontal/executive, focal cortical, memory	Depression, anxiety	Myoclonus, rigidity, parkinsonism	Cortical ribboning and basal ganglia or thalamus hyperintensity on diffusion/flare MRI
Dementia with Lewy body	Visual hallucinations, REM sleep disorder, delirium; Capgras syndrome, parkinsonism	Drawing and frontal/executive; spares memory; delirium prone	Visual hallucinations, depression, sleep disorder, delusions	Parkinsonism	Posterior parietal atrophy; hippocampi larger than in AD
Frontotemporal dementia	Apathy; poor judgment/reasoning, speech/language; hyperorality	Frontal/executive, language; spares drawing	Apathy, decline in personal or social conduct, hyperorality, euphoria, depression	Due to PSP/CBD overlap; vertical gaze palsy, axial rigidity, dystonia, alien hand	Frontal and/or temporal atrophy; spares posterior parietal lobe
Vascular dementia	Often but not always sudden, usually within 3 months of a stroke; variable; apathy, falls, focal weakness	Frontal/executive, cognitive slowing; memory can be intact	Apathy, delusions, anxiety	Usually motor slowing, spasticity; can be normal	Cortical and/or subcortical infarctions, confluent white matter disease

Adapted from Bird TD, Miller BL: Dementia. In Fauci AS et al, editors: *Harrison's principles of internal medicine*, ed 15, p 2538, New York, 2008, McGraw-Hill.
AD, Alzheimer disease; *CBD*, cortical basal degeneration; *MRI*, magnetic resonance imaging; *PSP*, progressive supranuclear palsy; *REM*, rapid eye movement.

demonstrated to be one of the most common causes of severe cognitive dysfunction in older adults. Its more prevalent forms are late-onset familial Alzheimer dementia (FAD) and nonhereditary, or sporadic, late-onset AD (70% of cases). FAD and sporadic, late-onset AD are known as senile dementia of the Alzheimer type (SDAT). AD is also associated with Down syndrome. It is estimated that 5 million Americans have AD.[42]

Early-onset FAD includes at least three gene defects: amyloid precursor protein (*APP*) gene on chromosome 21, presenilin 1 (*PSEN1*) on chromosome 14, and *PSEN2* on chromosome 1.[43,44] Late-onset FAD is linked to a defect in the apolipoprotein E (*apoE4*) gene on chromosome 19.[45] Presence of the *apoE4* allele is a marker of increased susceptibility rather than a genetic determinant.[40] The 3% of those who are homozygous for *apoE4* have an 85% risk, whereas the 25% who are heterozygous have a 45% to 50% risk.[40] The greatest risk factors are age and familial disposition (family history).[40,41,46]

Other risk factors include atherosclerosis, low education level, head injury, cardiovascular diseases, elevated serum homocysteine and cholesterol levels, and female gender estrogen deficit (Figure 16-12).[47] Protective factors include lifelong activity, *apoE2*, antioxidant substances, estrogen replacement, low caloric diet, nonsteroidal anti-inflammatory agents, and statins.[47]

PATHOPHYSIOLOGY The exact cause of AD is unknown. Several possible theories being investigated include

loss of neurotransmitter stimulation by choline acetyltransferase; mutation for encoding amyloid precursor protein; alteration in apoE, which binds amyloid-beta[48]; and pathologic activation of *N*-methyl-D-aspartate (NMDA) receptors resulting in an influx of excess calcium.

The pathogenesis of AD is linked to *amyloid-beta (AB)* peptide. AB peptide is derived from proteolysis of APP and released as AB 30 to AB 46, with AB 40 and AB 42 the most abundant isoforms produced.[47] These peptides have a strong tendency to form clusters of fibrils, especially AB 42.[47] A balance between production and catabolism (involving microglia, macrophages, and bulk flow across the blood-brain-barrier) is required.[47] Altered production and failure of clearance of amyloid from the brain occur in AD initiating accumulation (Figure 16-13). Fine diffuse plaques (**senile plaques**) are the initial accumulation of AB 42. This accumulation is followed by other AB depositions along with tau protein, activated glia, and, eventually, neurofibrillary tangles.[47] The abnormal AB is neurotoxic.

Microscopically the *tau protein* that normally stabilizes the microtubular transport system in the neurons detaches from the microtubule and forms insoluble helical filaments[40] called **neurofibrillary tangles** (see Figure 16-13). Tangles are flame shaped. Cortical nerve cell processes become twisted and dilated because of accumulation of the same filaments that form tangles. Amyloid also is deposited in cerebral arteries, causing an amyloid angiopathy. Senile plaques and neurofibrillary

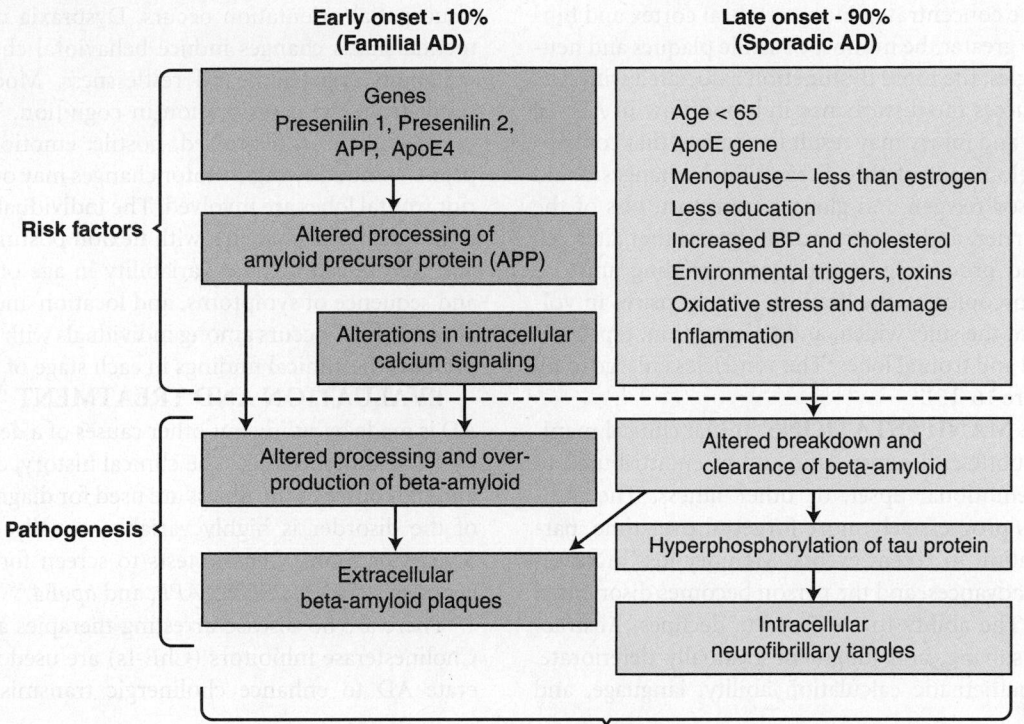

Early onset - 10%
(Familial AD)

Late onset - 90%
(Sporadic AD)

Risk factors

Genes
Presenilin 1, Presenilin 2,
APP, ApoE4

Age < 65
ApoE gene
Menopause— less than estrogen
Less education
Increased BP and cholesterol
Environmental triggers, toxins
Oxidative stress and damage
Inflammation

Altered processing of
amyloid precursor protein (APP)

Alterations in intracellular
calcium signaling

Pathogenesis

Altered processing and overproduction of beta-amyloid

Altered breakdown and
clearance of beta-amyloid

Extracellular
beta-amyloid plaques

Hyperphosphorylation of tau protein

Intracellular
neurofibrillary tangles

Loss of synaptic plasticity and neural transmission
Cholinergic dysfunction
Loss of neuronal repair and remodeling
Neurodegeneration
Dementia
Death

Figure 16-12 Proposed risk factors and pathogenesis of Alzheimer disease. *apoE*, apolipoprotein E; *APP*, amyloid precursor protein; *BP*, blood pressure. (Data from Bojarski L, Herms J, Kuznicki J: *Neurochem Inst* 52[4-5]:621-633, 2008; Ding Q, Dimayuga E, Keller JN: *Curr Alzheimer Res* 4[1]:73-79, 2007; Shah RS et al: *Biomed Pharmacother* 6[4]:199-207, 2008; Waring SC, Rosenberg RN: *Arch Neurol* 65[3]:329-334, 2008.)

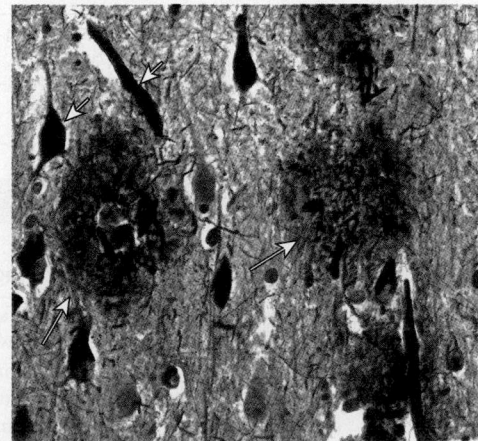

Figure 16-13 Major histopathologic changes in Alzheimer disease. Beta-amyloid protein deposits (plaques) in the neurophil *(long arrow)* and neurofibrillary tangles *(short arrow)*. (From Kumar V, Cotran RS, Robbins SL: *Robbins basic pathology,* ed 8, p 893, Philadelphia, 2007, Saunders.)

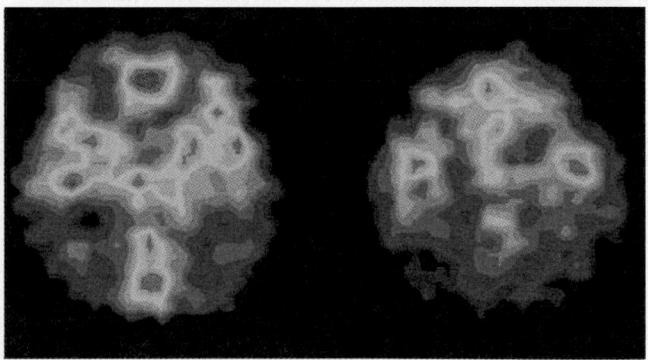

Figure 16-14 Altered cerebral blood flow in Alzheimer disease. Single photon emission computerized tomography scan showing reduction of temporoparietal blood flow *(right)* compared with normal blood flow *(left).* (From Perkin GD: *Mosby's color atlas and text of neurology,* London, 1998, Mosby-Wolfe.)

tangles are more concentrated in the cerebral cortex and hippocampus. The greater the number of senile plaques and neurofibrillary tangles, the more dysfunction associated with AD. Figure 16-14 shows the disturbance in blood flow in AD. In addition, aging and injury may result in changes that contribute to the development of this disease. Such changes could include decreased oxygen and glucose transport, loss of the blood-brain barrier, and mitochondrial defects that alter cell metabolism and processing of proteins, including amyloid (apoE4). Macroscopically, the brain in AD decreases in volume and weight, the sulci widen, and the gyri thin, especially in the temporal and frontal lobes. The ventricles enlarge to fill the space (Figure 16-15).

CLINICAL MANIFESTATIONS Initial clinical manifestations are subtle and nonspecific and often attributed to forgetfulness, emotional upset, or other illness. The individual becomes progressively more forgetful over time, particularly in relation to recent events. Memory loss increases as the disorder advances, and the person becomes disoriented and confused. The ability to concentrate declines. Abstraction, problem solving, and judgment gradually deteriorate. A failure in mathematic calculation ability, language, and visuospatial orientation occurs. Dyspraxia may appear. The mental status changes induce behavioral changes, including irritability, agitation, and restlessness. Mood changes also result from the deterioration in cognition. The person may become anxious, depressed, hostile, emotionally labile, and prone to mood swings. Motor changes may occur if the posterior frontal lobes are involved. The individual exhibits rigidity (paratonia, gegenhalten), with flexion posturing, propulsion, and retropulsion. Great variability in age of onset, intensity and sequence of symptoms, and location and extent of brain abnormalities occurs among individuals with AD. Table 16-20 presents the clinical findings in each stage of AD.

EVALUATION AND TREATMENT The diagnosis of AD is made by ruling out other causes of a dementing process by CT and blood tests. The clinical history, cognitive testing, and the course of the illness are used for diagnosis. The course of the disorder is highly variable, usually developing over 5 years or more. Genetic tests to screen for early onset AD genes are *PSEN1*, *PSEN2*, *APP*, and *apoE4*.[49,50]

There are no disease-arresting therapies available for AD. Cholinesterase inhibitors (ChE-Is) are used in mild to moderate AD to enhance cholinergic transmission. Drugs for

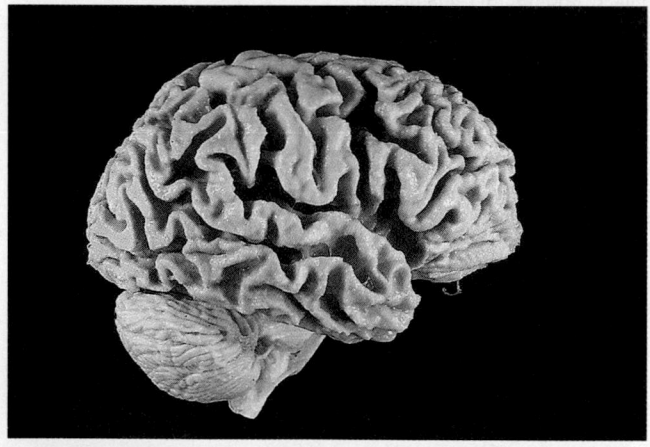

Figure 16-15 Alzheimer disease. The brain decreases in volume and weight, the sulci widen, and the gyri thin, especially in the temporal and frontal lobes. The ventricles enlarge to fill the space. (From Kumar V, Cotran RS, Robbins SL: *Robbins basic pathology*, ed 7 p 843, Philadelphia, 2007, Saunders.)

NUTRITION & DISEASE

Diet and Alzheimer Disease

Weight loss is a major concern for older adults with Alzheimer disease and it may precede onset of the classic motor symptoms. Weight loss may be a result of (1) increased incidence of infection, (2) increased energy output because of constant pacing, (3) olfactory and taste changes making food less appealing, (4) inadequate food intake, and (5) decreased independence and difficulty in self-feeding. Dementia may lead to memory loss, social isolation, depression, and poor food intake with resultant weight loss. Individuals may forget or refuse to eat, not communicate the need to eat, throw or hide food, eat spoiled food or nonfood substances, eat favorite foods to the exclusion of other foods, take a long time to eat, have difficulty in preparing foods, and be unable to feed themselves.

Data from Smith KL, Greenwood CE: *J Nutr Elder* 27(3-4):381-403, 2008: Shatenstein B et al: *J Nutr Health Aging* 12(7):461-469, 2008; Tamura BK, Masaki KH, Blanchette P: *J Nutr Elder* 26(3-4):21-38, 2007.

Table 16-20   Progression of Alzheimer Disease

Stage	Mild Cognitive Impairment	Early Stage	Middle Stage	Late Stage	End Stage
Cognitive	Mild memory loss	Measurable short-term memory loss; other cognition problems	Moderate to severe cognitive problems	Little cognitive ability; Language not clear	No significant cognitive function
Functional	Possibly depression (vs. apathy); mild anxiety	Mild IADL problems	IADL-dependent; some ADL problems	ADL dependent; incontinent	Nonambulatory/bedbound; unable to eat

Adapted from National Conference of Gerontological Nurse Practitioners and the National Gerontological Nursing Association, *Counseling Points* 1(1):6, 2008.
ADL, Activities of daily living; *IADL*, instrumental activities of daily living.

moderate to severe AD block the activity of glutamate and work as an uncompetitive NMDA receptor antagonist.[51,52]

Treatment of AD also is directed at decreasing the need for the impaired cognitive function by a compensation technique, such as memory aids, maintaining those cognitive functions that are not impaired, and maintaining or improving the general state of hygiene, nutrition, and health. Environmental management, counseling, education, pharmacotherapy, and health promotion measures provide the foundation on which a comprehensive treatment program is built.[51]

ALTERATIONS IN CEREBRAL HEMODYNAMICS

An injured brain reacts with structural, chemical, and pathophysiologic changes. Critical variables related to cerebral oxygenation include intracranial pressure, blood flow, and oxygen delivery. The pressure and oxygen delivery are critical management issues.

Cerebral Hemodynamics

Increased intracranial pressure (ICP) was the central management issue for many years. It is now recognized that cerebral oxygenation is the critical issue. Several relevant features of cerebral hemodynamics—cerebral blood volume (CBV), cerebral blood flow (CBF), and cerebral perfusion pressure (CPP)—relate to cerebral oxygenation (Box 16-4).

To guide therapeutic management, three critical categories related to cerebral hemodynamics are possible in the injured brain: (1) cerebral oligemia (also called *jugular fibrillation*), (2) CPP in the normal range (60 to 100 mmHg) but with an elevated ICP, and (3) cerebral hyperemia. In the treatment algorithms, oxygen saturation measured in the internal jugular vein (Sjo_2) is categorized as less than 55%, greater than 55% but less than 70%, or greater than 75%. After Sjo_2 is categorized, the ICP must be added to the equation as less than 20 mmHg or greater than 20 mmHg. Treatment algorithms are implemented depending on the Sjo_2 and ICP that address not only ICP but also CPP. The therapeutic goal is to balance ICP and Sjo_2. Target values for relevant clinical parameters are presented in Table 16-21.

Increased Intracranial Pressure

Intracranial pressure normally is 5 to 15 mmHg, or 60 to 180 cm H_2O. **Increased intracranial pressure** may result from an increase in intracranial content (as occurs with tumor growth), edema, excess CSF, or hemorrhage. A rise in intracranial pressure necessitates an equal reduction in volume of the other contents. The most readily displaced content of the cranial vault is CSF. If intracranial pressure remains high after CSF displacement out of the cranial vault, cerebral blood volume is altered, which causes stage 1 intracranial hypertension. Vasoconstriction and external compression of the venous system occur in an attempt to further decrease the intracranial pressure. Thus during the first stage of intracranial hypertension, intracranial pressure may not change because

---

Box 16-4 — Cerebral Hemodynamics

Cerebral blood volume (CBV) is the amount of blood in the intracranial vault at a given time (normally about 10%). Most of this CBV is in the low-pressure venous system. CBV is determined by autoregulatory mechanisms that control cerebral blood flow (CBF) with sensitivity to concentrations of carbon dioxide, hydrogen ion, and oxygen. CBF decreases 3% for every 1-mmHg decrease in CO_2 due to vasoconstriction. CBF increases at a Pao_2 of less than 50 mmHg; CBF is stable (maintained) at a Pao_2 of greater than 80 mmHg.

CBF to the brain is maintained at a rate that matches local metabolic needs of the brain, about 750 to 900 ml/minute (15% to 20% of the cardiac output). Blood flow to neuronal cell bodies of gray matter is about three to four times greater than white matter because of the increased metabolic activity. CBF is calculated as follows: CBF + CPP (cerebral perfusion pressure)/CVR (cardiovascular resistance). CPP is the net pressure gradient required to perfuse the cells of the brain. CPP is calculated as follows: CPP = MAP − ICP. Normal CPP is 60 to 100 mm Hg. The CPP determines CBF. As CPP decreases to 70 to 80 mmHg in the injured brain, vasodilation occurs, which increases CBV, also increasing ICP. An increased ICP will decrease CPP.

Oxygen saturation measured in the internal jugular vein (Sjo_2) at the jugular bulb reflects the amount of oxygen still bound as the blood leaves the cranial vault. Cerebral extraction of oxygen (CEO_2) is calculated using the formula $Sao_2 − Sjo_2/Sao_2 \times 100$. Normal CEO_2 is 20% to 24%; normal Sjo_2 is 55% to 70%. When oxygen demand exceeds oxygen supply, extraction increases, increasing the Sjo_2. A CEO_2 less than 24% or an Sjo_2 greater than 75% indicates cerebral hyperemia. Acid-base balance and temperature influence oxyhemoglobin dissociation (see Chapter 32).

Data from Steiner LA, Andrews PJ: *Br J Anaesth* 97(1):26-38, 2006; Verweij BH, Amelink GJ, Muizelaar JP: *Prog Brain Res* 161:111-124, 2007; Wright WL: *J Neurol Sci* 261(1-2):10-15, 2007.
ICP, Intracranial pressure; *MAP*, mean arterial pressure; *Sao₂*, oxygen saturation in arterial blood; *Sjo2*, oxygen saturation in the jugular vein.

Table 16-21 — Therapeutic Management Goals for Individuals with Altered Cerebral Hemodynamics

Clinical Parameter	Target Value
Central perfusion pressure	>70 mmHg
Intracranial pressure	<20 mmHg
Arterial CO_2 pressure ($Paco_2$)	35 mmHg
Mean arterial pressure	90 mmHg
Temperature	34°-36° C (93.2-96.8 F)
Pulmonary capillary wedge pressure	10-15 mmHg

---

of the effective compensatory mechanisms. CSF is reduced through increased reabsorption. Blood volume is reduced by compression of intracranial veins. Small increases in volume, however, cause an increase in pressure, and the pressure may take longer to return to baseline. Clinical manifestations at this stage usually are subtle and often transient and include episodes of confusion, drowsiness, and slight pupillary and breathing changes.

If ICP is still high, a state of intracranial hypertension occurs. With continued expansion of the intracranial content, the resulting increase in ICP may exceed the brain's compensatory capacity to adjust to the increasing pressure. In this state, the pressure begins to compromise neuronal oxygenation, and systemic arterial vasoconstriction occurs in an attempt to elevate the systemic blood pressure sufficiently to overcome the increased intracranial pressure. This is stage 2 of intracranial hypertension.

As intracranial pressure begins to approach arterial pressure, the brain tissues begin to experience hypoxia and hypercapnia and the individual's condition rapidly deteriorates. Clinical manifestations include decreasing levels of arousal, Cheyne-Stokes respiration or central neurogenic hyperventilation, pupils that become sluggish and dilated, widened pulse pressure, and bradycardia.

Dramatic sustained rises in intracranial pressure are not seen until all the compensatory mechanisms have been exhausted. Once decompensation begins, dramatic rises in ICP occur over a very short period. **Autoregulation**, the compensatory alteration in the diameter of the intracranial blood vessels designed to maintain a constant blood flow during changes in cerebral perfusion pressure, is lost with progressively increased intracranial pressure. Accumulating carbon dioxide may still cause vasodilation

at the local tissue level, but now, without autoregulation, this vasodilation causes the hydrostatic (blood) pressure in the vessels to drop and blood volume to increase. The brain volume is thus further enhanced, and ICP continues to rise. This is stage 3 of intracranial hypertension. Small increases in volume cause dramatic increases in ICP, and the pressure takes much longer to return to baseline. As the ICP begins to approach systemic blood pressure, cerebral perfusion pressure falls and cerebral perfusion slows dramatically. The brain tissues experience severe hypoxia and acidosis.

Increased ICP in one compartment of the cranial vault is not evenly distributed throughout the other vault compartments. In stage 4, the last stage of intracranial hypertension, brain tissue shifts (herniates) from the compartment of greater pressure to a compartment of lesser pressure (Figure 16-16). With this shift in brain tissue, the herniating brain tissue's blood supply is compromised, causing further ischemia and hypoxia in the herniating tissues. The herniated brain tissues increase the volume of content within the lower-pressure compartment, exerting pressure on the brain tissue that normally occupies that compartment, thus impairing that tissue's blood supply. Small hemorrhages frequently develop in the involved brain tissue. Obstructive hydrocephalus may develop. The herniation process markedly and rapidly

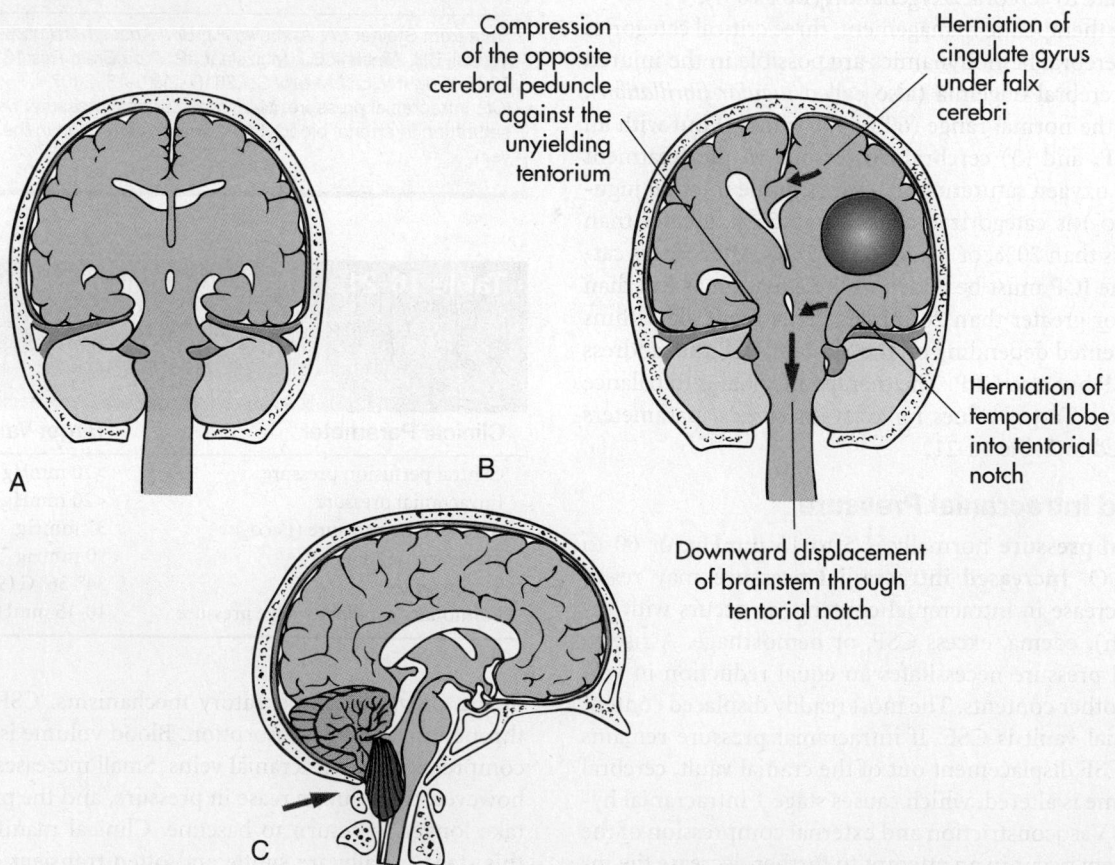

Compression of the opposite cerebral peduncle against the unyielding tentorium

Herniation of cingulate gyrus under falx cerebri

Herniation of temporal lobe into tentorial notch

Downward displacement of brainstem through tentorial notch

Figure 16-16 Herniation resulting from increased intracranial pressure. **A,** Normal relationship of intracranial structures. **B,** Shift of intracranial structures. **C,** Downward herniation of the cerebellar tonsils into the foramen magnum *(red arrow).*

increases ICP. Mean systolic arterial pressure soon equals ICP, and cerebral blood flow ceases at this point.

Herniation Syndromes

Supratentorial Herniation

The three types of supratentorial herniation syndromes are (1) uncal (temporal lobe, lateral transtentorial) herniation, (2) central (transtentorial) herniation, and (3) cingulate gyrus herniation. **Uncal herniation (hippocampal herniation, lateral mass herniation)** occurs when the uncus or hippocampal gyrus (or both) shifts from the middle fossa through the tentorial notch into the posterior fossa, compressing the ipsilateral third cranial nerve impairing parasympathetic function carried in periphery of the nerve, then the contralateral third cranial nerve, and finally the mesencephalon-inducing coma. Uncal herniation generally is caused by an expanding mass in the lateral region of the middle fossa. The earliest signs of uncal herniation are poor concentration, drowsiness, and the bilateral corticospinal tract signs of increased tone and a positive Babinski sign caused by pressure on the opposite cerebral peduncle in some cases.[2,6] The classic manifestations of uncal herniation are a decreasing level of consciousness, pupils that become sluggish before fixing and dilating (first the ipsilateral, then the contralateral pupil), Cheyne-Stokes respirations (which later shift to central neurogenic hyperventilation), the appearance of decorticate, then later decerebrate, posturing, and ipsilateral hemiplegia because of contralateral corticospinal tract compression.[6]

Central transtentorial herniation is the straight downward shift of the diencephalons (thalamic medial structures) through the tentorial notch. Causes of central herniation are injuries or masses located around the outer perimeter of the frontal, parietal, or occipital lobes; extracerebral injuries around the central apex (top) of the cranium; bilaterally positioned injuries or masses; and unilateral cingulate gyrus herniation. The heralding signs are miotic pupils and drowsiness.[2] The individual experiencing transtentorial herniation rapidly passes from a conscious to an unconscious state; from Cheyne-Stokes respirations to apnea; from small, reactive pupils to dilated and fixed pupils; and from decortication to decerebration.

Cingulate gyrus herniation (subfalcine or transfalcial herniation) occurs when the cingulate gyrus shifts under the falx cerebri. Little is known about the clinical manifestations of this type of herniation except that there are signs of a mass causing increased intracranial pressure.[6]

Infratentorial (Foraminal) Herniation

Two types of infratentorial (foraminal) herniation syndromes may occur. In the most common infratentorial herniation syndrome, a cerebellar tonsil shifts through the foramen magnum because of increased pressure within the posterior fossa. The clinical manifestations of this downward infratentorial herniation are an arched, stiff neck; paresthesias in the shoulder area; decreased consciousness; respiratory abnormalities

and arrest; and pulse rate variations. Occasionally the pressure force is such that an upward transtentorial herniation of a cerebellar tonsil or the lower brainstem results. No specific set of clinical manifestations is associated with this infratentorial herniation syndrome.

Cerebral Edema

Cerebral edema is an increase in the fluid content of brain tissue, a net accumulation of water within the brain (Figures 16-17 and 16-18). Cerebral edema causes an increase in extracellular or intracellular tissue volume after brain insult from trauma, infection, hemorrhage, tumor, ischemia, infarct, or hypoxia. The harmful effects of cerebral edema are caused by the distortion of blood vessels, the displacement of brain tissues, and the eventual herniation of brain tissue from one brain compartment to another.

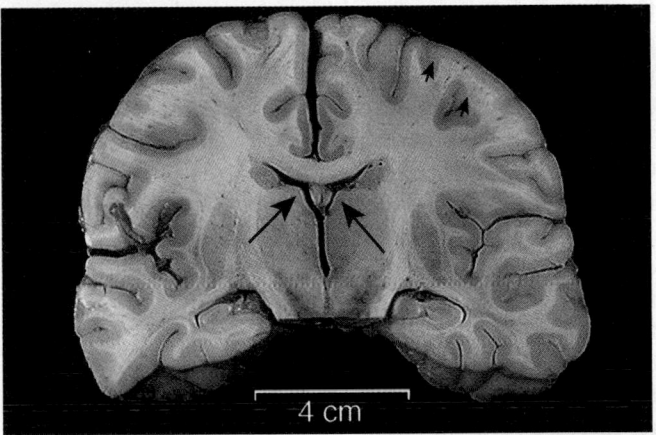

Figure 16-17 Cerebral edema. This coronal section of cerebrum demonstrates marked compression in the lateral ventricles *(long arrows)* and flattening of gyri *(short arrows)* from extensive bilateral cerebral edema. Edema increases intracranial pressure, leading to herniation. (From Klatt EC: *Robbins and Cotran atlas of pathology*, p 449, Philadelphia, 2006, Saunders.)

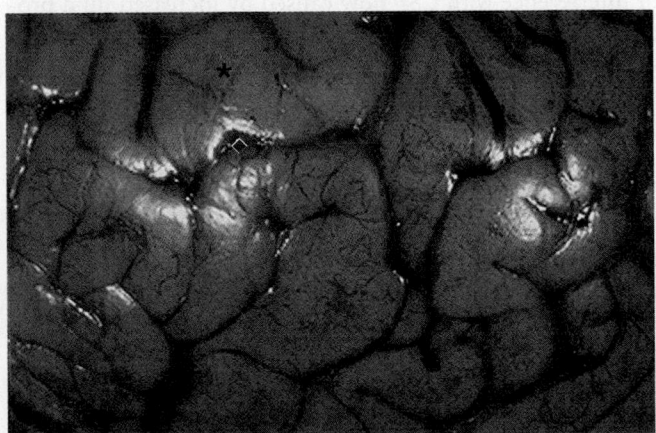

Figure 16-18 Cerebral edema, gross. The surface of the meninges of the brain with cerebral edema shows widened, flattened gyri (*) with narrowed sulci (♦). (From Klatt EC: *Robbins and Cotran atlas of pathology*, Philadelphia, 2006, Saunders, p 449.)

Three types of cerebral edema are (1) vasogenic edema, (2) cytotoxic (metabolic) edema, and (3) interstitial edema.[53] **Vasogenic edema** is clinically the most important type. It is caused by the increased permeability of the capillary endothelium of the brain after injury to the vascular structure. The result is a disruption in the blood-brain barrier. Plasma proteins leak into the extracellular spaces, drawing water to them, and the water content of the brain parenchyma increases. Vasogenic edema starts in the area of injury and spreads with preferential accumulation in the white matter of the ipsilateral side because the parallel myelinated fibers separate more easily. Edema then promotes more edema because of ischemia from increasing pressure.

Clinical manifestations of vasogenic edema include focal neurologic deficits, disturbances of consciousness, and a severe increase in intracranial pressure. Vasogenic edema resolves by slow diffusion.

In **cytotoxic (metabolic) edema**, toxic factors directly affect the cellular elements of the brain parenchyma (neuronal, glial, and endothelial cells), causing failure of the active transport systems. The blood-brain barrier is not disrupted. The cells lose their potassium and gain larger amounts of sodium. Water follows by osmosis into the cell so that the cells swell. Cytotoxic edema occurs principally in the gray matter and may increase vasogenic edema.

Interstitial edema is seen most often with noncommunicating hydrocephalus (see below and Chapter 19). The edema is caused by transependymal movement of CSF from the ventricles into the extracellular spaces of the brain tissues. The brain fluid volume thus is increased predominantly around the ventricles. The hydrostatic pressure within the white matter increases, and the size of the white matter is reduced because of the rapid disappearance of myelin lipids.

Hydrocephalus

The term **hydrocephalus** refers to a variety of conditions characterized by an excess of fluid within the cranial vault, subarachnoid space, or both. Hydrocephalus occurs because of interference with CSF flow caused by increased fluid production, obstruction within the ventricular system, or defective reabsorption of the fluid. A papilloma (i.e., epithelial tumor) may, in rare instances, cause overproduction of CSF (Figure 16-19).

Types of Hydrocephalus

Obstruction within the ventricular system, called **noncommunicating hydrocephalus** or *internal (intraventricular) hydrocephalus,* may result from congenital abnormalities in the ventricular system or mass lesions such as a tumor that compresses one of the structures of the ventricular system (see Chapter 19 for additional discussion). Impaired absorption of CSF from the subarachnoid space occurs when an obstructive process disrupts the flow of CSF through the subarachnoid space. The fluid is prevented from reaching the convex portion of the cerebrum, where the arachnoid granulations are located.

Hydrocephalus from impaired absorption may be caused by adhesions from inflammation, as with a meningitis or subarachnoid hemorrhage; compression of the subarachnoid space by a mass, such as a tumor; congenital abnormalities of the subarachnoid space; or high venous pressure within the sagittal sinus. This type of hydrocephalus is termed **communicating (extraventricular) hydrocephalus.** The most common causes of communicating hydrocephalus are subarachnoid hemorrhage, developmental malformation, head injury, and neoplasm.

One form of communicating hydrocephalus is **hydrocephalus ex vacuo**, which arises from cerebral atrophy. CSF fills the unoccupied space. The amount of CSF is increased, but the fluid is not under pressure. Another form of communicating hydrocephalus is **normal-pressure hydrocephalus (low-pressure, adult,** or **occult hydrocephalus)**, which occurs mostly in late middle age. The cause is thought to be arachnoid adhesions and thickening of the arachnoid that obstructs the subarachnoid space. This form of hydrocephalus is most often seen as a complication of head injury and subarachnoid hemorrhage.

Course of the Disease

Hydrocephalus may develop from infancy through adulthood. Congenital hydrocephalus (i.e., ventricular enlargement before birth) is rare. Noncommunicating hydrocephalus is more commonly seen in children. The more common type of hydrocephalus in adults is the communicating type. (Hydrocephalus in children is discussed in Chapter 19.)

Most cases of hydrocephalus develop gradually and insidiously over time. **Acute hydrocephalus,** however, may develop in several hours in persons who have sustained head injuries. Acute hydrocephalus contributes significantly to increased ICP.

PATHOPHYSIOLOGY The obstruction of CSF flow associated with hydrocephalus produces dilation of the ventricles proximal to the obstruction. Obstructed CSF is under pressure, causing atrophy of the cerebral cortex and degeneration of the white matter tracts. There is selective preservation of gray matter. When excess CSF fills a defect caused by atrophy, a degenerative disorder, or a surgical excision, this fluid is not under pressure; therefore, atrophy and degenerative changes are not induced.

CLINICAL MANIFESTATIONS The presentation of acute hydrocephalus is one of rapidly developing increased intracranial pressure. The person deteriorates rapidly into a deep coma if not promptly treated. Normal-pressure hydrocephalus has a long-term presentation and develops slowly over time. The individual or family of the individual complains of declining memory and cognitive function. An unsteady, broad-based gait with a history of falling is common. Additional clinical manifestations are apathy; inattentiveness; and indifference to self, family, and the environment. Urinary incontinence is present.[54]

EVALUATION AND TREATMENT The diagnosis is made on the basis of physical examination, CT scan, and

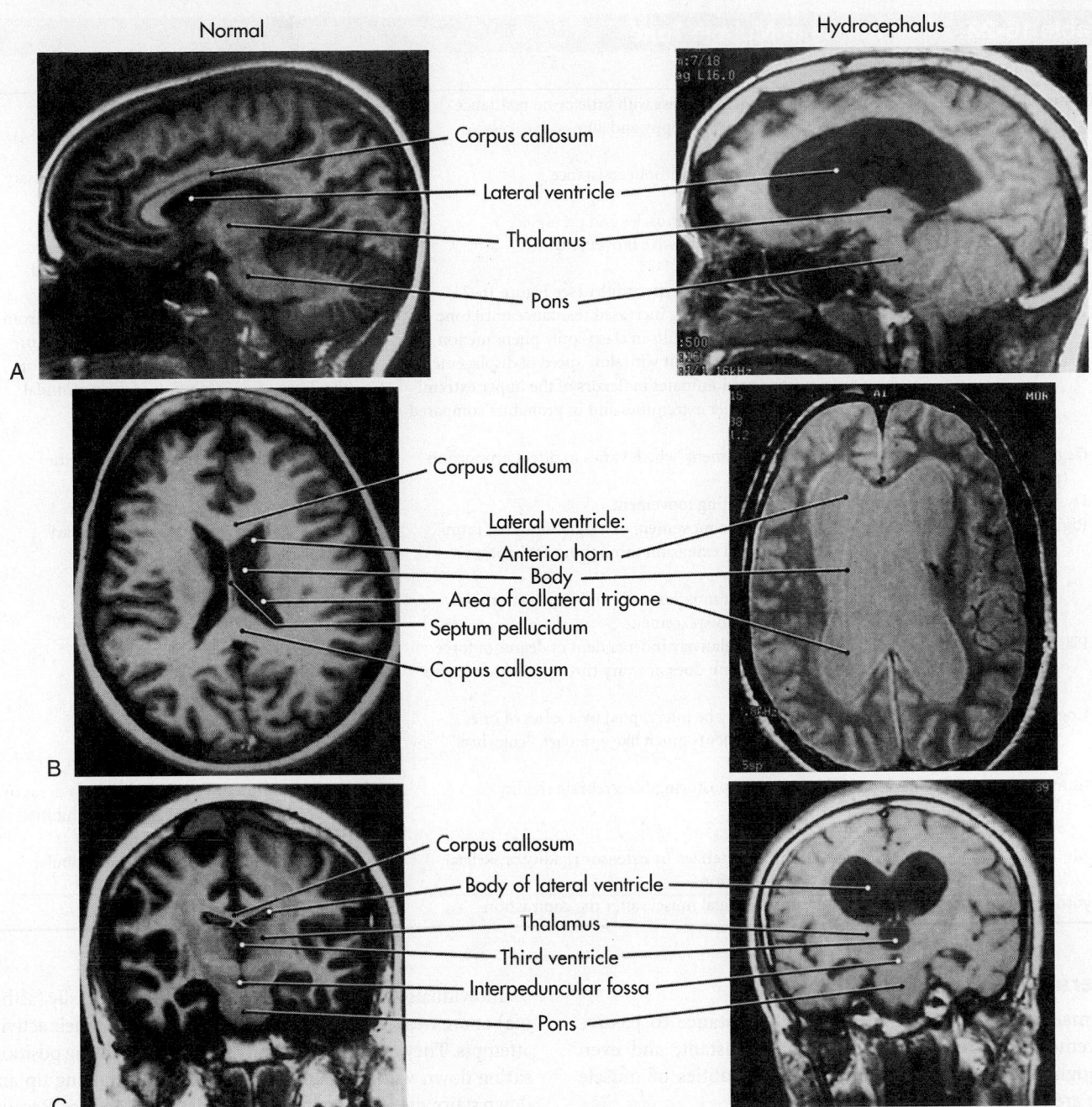

Figure 16-19 Comparison of normal and hydrocephalic brains. A, Sagittal; B, axial; and C, coronal planes as seen in magnetic resonance imaging (MRI). (From Haines DE, editor: *Fundamental neuroscience*, Philadelphia, 1997, Churchill Livingstone.)

MRI. A radioisotopic cisternogram may be performed to aid in diagnosing normal-pressure hydrocephalus. Hydrocephalus can be treated by surgery to resect cysts, neoplasms, or hematomas or by ventricular bypass into the normal intracranial channel or into an extracranial compartment using a shunt. Excision or coagulation of the choroid plexus is needed occasionally when a papilloma is present. In normal-pressure hydrocephalus, reduction in CSF through a diuresis regimen often is used.

ALTERATIONS IN MOTOR FUNCTION

Movements are complex patterns of activity controlled by the CNS. Movements are influenced by the cerebral cortex, the pyramidal system, the extrapyramidal system, and the motor units. Dysfunction in any of these areas can cause motor dysfunction. General motor dysfunctions may produce changes in muscle tone, movement, and complex motor performance.

Table 16-22 Alterations in Muscle Tone

Alterations	Characteristics	Cause
Hypotonia	Passive movement of a muscle mass with little or no resistance Difficult to detect; extremity is floppy and allows an excessive movement when displaced Muscles may be rapidly moved without resistance	Thought to be caused by decreased muscle spindle activity as a result of decreased excitability of neurons Occurs typically when nerve impulses necessary for muscle tone are lost
Flaccidity	Associated with limp, atrophied muscles and paralysis	
Hypertonia	Increased muscle resistance to passive movement May be associated with paralysis May be accompanied by muscle hypertrophy (see Figure 16-23)	Results when the lower motor unit reflex arc continues to function but is not mediated or regulated by higher centers
Spasticity	A gradual increase in tone causing increased resistance until tone suddenly is reduced, which results in clasp-knife phenomenon Velocity dependent (may be absent with slow speed of displacement) Selective distribution (predominates in flexors of the upper extremities and extensors of lower extremities and in pronators compared with supinators)	Exact mechanism unclear; appears to arise from an increased excitability of the alpha motor neurons to any input because of absence of the descending inhibition of the pyramidal systems
Gegenhalten (paratonia)	Resistance to passive movement, which varies in direct proportion to force applied	Exact mechanism unclear: associated with frontal lobe injury
Dystonia	Sustained involuntary twisting movement	Produced by slow muscular contraction
Rigidity	Muscle resistance to passive movement of a rigid limb that is uniform in both flexion and extension throughout the motion Not velocity dependent Activated by contraction of muscles in contralateral extremities Uniform through range in displacement	Occurs as a result of constant, involuntary contraction of muscle
Plastic, or lead-pipe	Increased muscular tone relatively independent of degree of force used in passive movement; does not vary throughout the passive movement	Associated with basal ganglion damage
Cogwheel	The uniform resistance may be interrupted by a series of brief jerks resulting in movements much like a ratchet, "cogwheel" phenomenon	Associated with basal ganglion damage
Gamma	Characterized by extensor posturing (decerebrate rigidity)	Loss of excitation of extensor inhibitory areas by the cerebral cortex decreasing the inhibition of alpha and gamma motor neurons
Alpha	Impaired relaxation characterized by extensor rigidity of skeletal muscle after the contraction	Loss of cerebellum input to lateral vestibular nuclei
Myotonia	Impaired relaxation of skeletal muscle after the contraction	

Alterations in Muscle Tone

Normal muscle tone involves a slight resistance to passive movement. The resistance is smooth, constant, and even throughout the range of motion. Abnormalities of muscle tone are presented in Table 16-22.

Hypotonia

In **hypotonia (decreased muscle tone)**, passive movement of a muscle occurs with little or no resistance. Hypotonia is thought to be caused by decreased muscle spindle activity secondary to decreased excitability of neurons. Hypotonia is caused by pure pyramidal tract damage (a rare occurrence) and cerebellar damage. A pure pyramidal tract injury produces hypotonia and weakness. The hypotonia contributes to the ataxia and intention tremor in cerebellar damage and manifests with minimal weakness, with normal or slightly exaggerated reflexes. Hypotonia, often described as flaccidity (a state in which the muscle may be moved rapidly without resistance), occurs when nerve impulses necessary for muscle tone are lost, such as in spinal cord injury or cerebrovascular accident.

Individuals with hypotonia report that they tire easily (asthenia) or are weak, signs that can be observed during their activity attempts. They may have difficulty rising from a sitting position, sitting down without using arm support, and walking up and down stairs, as well as an inability to stand on their toes. Because of their weakness, accident proneness during locomotion and self-care activities is common. Inasmuch as the joints become hyperflexible in hypotonic states, people with hypotonia may be able to assume positions that require extreme joint mobility. The joints may appear loose, and the knee jerks are pendulous.

The muscle mass atrophies because of decreased input entering the motor unit. Muscle cells gradually are replaced by connective tissue and fat. The muscles are flabby on palpation and are flat in appearance. Fasciculations may be present in some cases.

Hypertonia

In **hypertonia (increased muscle tone)**, passive movement of a muscle occurs with resistance. Four types of hypertonia are described: spasticity, gegenhalten (paratonia), dystonia, and rigidity.

Spasticity results from hyperexcitability of the stretch reflexes (overactivation of the alpha motor neurons) and is associated with damage to the motor, premotor, and supplementary motor areas, as well as lateral corticospinal tract damage (Figure 16-20). Spasticity is accompanied by increased deep tendon reflexes (hyperreflexia) and the spread of reflexes (clonus).

Gegenhalten (paratonia) manifests as resistance to passive movement that varies in direct proportion to the force applied and is associated with frontal lobe injury. Paratonia is not truly an increase in tone but an increase in resistance by the person. Dystonia manifests as sustained, involuntary twisting movements caused by slow muscle contraction and may be caused by a failure in appropriate reciprocal inhibition of the muscles (Figures 16-21 and 16-22). Injury to the putamen or its outflow tracts also is associated with hemidystonia.

Rigidity produced by tonic reflex activity mediated by gamma motor neurons may be continuous or intermittent. The involved muscles are firm and tense; the increase in muscle movement is even and uniform throughout the range of passive movement. Four types of rigidity are described: plastic, or lead-pipe; cogwheel; gamma; and alpha (Table 16-23).

Individuals with hypertonia may tire easily (asthenia) or be weak. Passive and active movement is equally affected, except in paratonia, in which more active than passive movement is possible. As a result of hypertonia and weakness, accident proneness during locomotion and self-care activities is common.

The muscles may atrophy because of decreased use of the muscles. However, hypertrophy occasionally may occur in some diseases. Hypertrophy results from overstimulation of muscle fibers. Overstimulation occurs when the motor unit reflex arc remains intact and functioning but is not inhibited by higher centers. The loss of inhibition and the constant state of excitation cause continual muscle contraction, resulting in

Table 16-23	UK Medical Research Council Classification of Muscle Power
Grade	**Definition**
0	Total paralysis
1	Flicker of contraction
2	Movement with gravity eliminated
3	Movement against gravity
4	Movement against resistance but incomplete
5	Normal power

UK, United Kingdom.

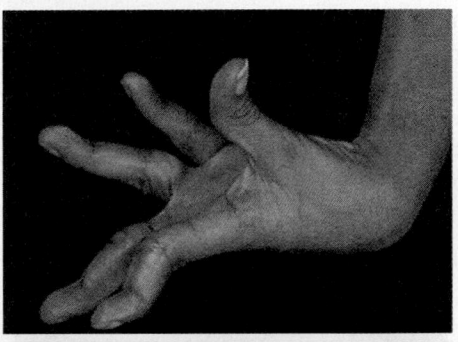
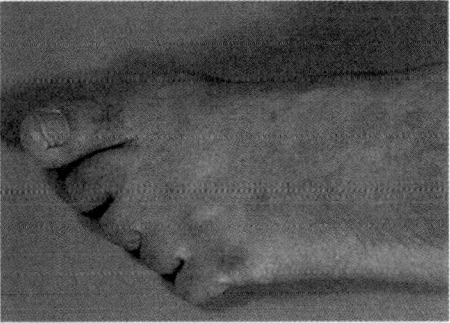

Figure 16-21 Dystonic posturing of the hand and foot. (From Perkin GD: *Mosby's color atlas and text of neurology,* London, 1998, Mosby-Wolfe.)

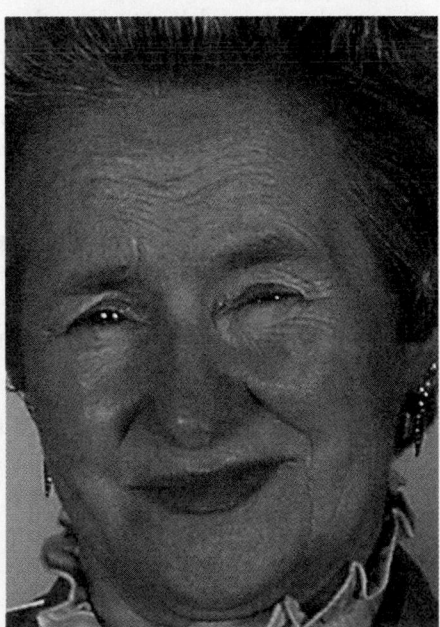

Figure 16-20 Left-sided hemifacial spasm. (From Perkin GD: *Mosby's color atlas and text of neurology,* London, 1998, Mosby-Wolfe.)

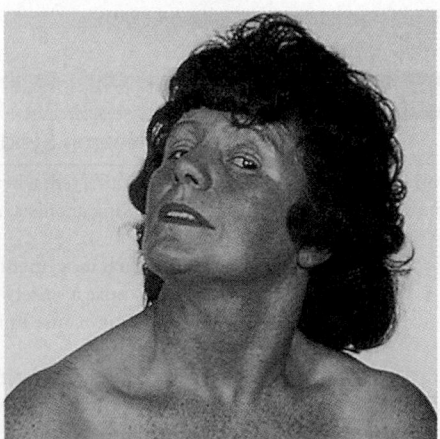

Figure 16-22 Spasmodic torticollis. A characteristic head posture. (From Perkin GD: *Mosby's color atlas and text of neurology,* London, 1998, Mosby-Wolfe.)

enlargement of the muscle mass (Figure 16-23). The muscles are firm on palpation.

Alterations in Movement

Movement requires a change in the contractile state of muscles. Abnormal movements may occur when a variety of CNS dysfunctions alter muscular innervation. Movement disorders are not well understood. Current knowledge has come predominantly from the areas of neuropharmacology and experimental therapeutics. The neurotransmitter *dopamine* has an apparent role in motor function. Some movement disorders (e.g., the akinesias) result from too little dopaminergic activity, whereas others (e.g., chorea, ballism, tardive dyskinesia) result from too much dopaminergic activity. Still others are not related primarily to dopamine function. Movement disorders are not associated necessarily with mass, strength, or tone but are neurologic dysfunctions with either a decreased amount of movement or an excess of movement. Muscle strength is quantitatively evaluated on a scale of 0 to 4+ or 0 to 5, in which 4+ or 5 is normal and 0 indicates an inability to move against gravity (see Table 16-23).

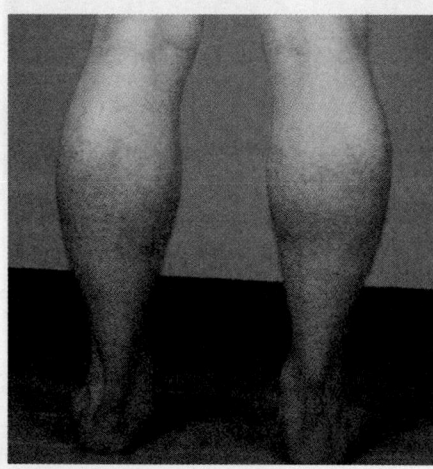

Figure 16-23 Pseudohypertrophy of the calf muscles. (From Perkin GD: *Mosby's color atlas and text of neurology,* London, 1998, Mosby-Wolfe.)

Paresis and Paralysis

Paresis (weakness) is impairment of motor function, that is, partial paralysis with incomplete loss of muscle power. **Paralysis** is loss of motor function, that is, inability of a muscle group to overcome gravity. Two subtypes of paresis and paralysis are described: upper motor neuron paresis and paralysis and lower motor neuron paresis and paralysis (Table 16-24).

Upper Motor Neuron Syndromes

Upper motor neuron paresis and paralysis is known also as spastic paresis and paralysis, and many different terms are used to describe a specific paresis or paralysis. **Hemiparesis** or **hemiplegia** is paresis or paralysis, respectively, of the upper and lower extremities on one side. **Diplegia** is the paralysis of both upper or lower extremities as a result of cerebral hemisphere injuries. **Paraparesis** or **paraplegia** refers to weakness or paralysis, respectively, of the lower extremities. **Quadriparesis** or **quadriplegia** refers to paresis or paralysis of all four extremities. Paraparesis or paraplegia and quadriparesis or quadriplegia may be caused by dysfunction of the spinal cord. Upper cord damage results in quadriparesis or quadriplegia, and lower cord damage preserves upper extremity function and causes paraparesis or paraplegia (spinal cord injury is discussed in Chapter 17).

Upper motor neuron paresis or paralysis is associated with a pyramidal motor syndrome. The **pyramidal motor syndrome** is a series of motor dysfunctions that result from interruption of the pyramidal system (Figures 16-24 and 16-25). The injury may be in the cerebral cortex, the subcortical white matter, the internal capsule, the brainstem, or the spinal cord. The clinical manifestations of a pure pyramidal injury without other damage are not known, but bilateral interruption of the pyramidal system in monkeys causes hypotonic paralysis, although much control of movement eventually returns. In humans, however, injury generally involves more than merely the interruption of the pyramidal system, so that an upper motor neuron paralysis occurs, which indicates involvement of several motor pathways.

The distribution of clinical manifestations varies, depending on the location of the lesion, although certain features are

Table 16-24	Upper and Lower Motor Neuron Syndromes	
Factor	Upper Motor Neuron Syndromes*	Lower Motor Neuron Syndromes†
Distribution of affected muscles	Muscle groups are affected; when movement is possible, the proper relationship among agonists, antagonists, synergists, and fixators is preserved	Individual muscles may be affected
	Synkinesias (residual movements) are present; attempts to move paralyzed part cause a variety of associated movements; movements of normal limb may cause imitative or mirror movements in the paralyzed limb	Individual muscles may be affected
Muscle tone	Hypertonia, specifically spasticity	Hypotonia, flaccidity
Tendon reflexes	Hyperreflexia with extensor plantar reflex present	Hyporeflexia, no abnormal reflexes present
Atrophy	Slight, caused by disuse	Pronounced atrophy
Fasciculations	Absent	May be present

*Pyramidal motor syndromes.
†All are motor unit syndromes.

constant. Excessive movements such as clonus and spasms occur regularly, and much variation exists, depending on the suddenness of onset and the age of the individual.

When the pyramidal system is destroyed below the level of the pons, spinal shock occurs. **Spinal shock** is the complete cessation of spinal cord functions below the lesion. It is characterized by complete flaccid paralysis, absence of reflexes, and marked disturbances of bowel and bladder function. The reasons for spinal shock are not fully understood, but a major factor is the sudden destruction of the efferent pathways. If destruction occurs more slowly, spinal shock may not develop (see Chapter 17).

If the pyramidal system is interrupted above the level of the pons, the hand and arm muscles are greatly affected. Paralysis rarely involves all the muscles on one side of the body, however, even when the hemiplegia results from complete damage to the internal capsule. Bilateral movements, such as those of the eye, jaw, and larynx, are affected only slightly, if at all. Predominantly the limbs are affected. Because of their bilateral control, trunk muscles are much less influenced.

Paralysis associated with a pyramidal motor syndrome rarely remains flaccid for a prolonged time. After a few days or weeks, a gradual return of spinal reflexes marks the end of spinal shock. Reflexes then become hyperactive, and muscle tone is increased significantly, particularly in antigravity muscles. Spasticity is common, although rigidity occasionally occurs. Most often, passive range of motion causes the "clasp-knife" phenomenon, probably because of the activation of the two varieties of stretch receptors: (1) the muscle spindles and (2) the Golgi tendon organ. (Muscle function is discussed in Chapter 41.) With pyramidal motor syndrome, predominantly the flexors of the arms and extensors of the legs are affected.

Lower Motor Neuron Syndromes

Lower (primary, alpha) motor neurons are the large motor neurons in the anterior (ventral) horn of the spinal cord and the motor nuclei of the brainstem. The axons from these nerve cell bodies bring nerve impulses from upper motor neurons to the skeletal muscles via the anterior spinal roots or cranial nerves. (Figure 16-26). Dysfunction in this motor

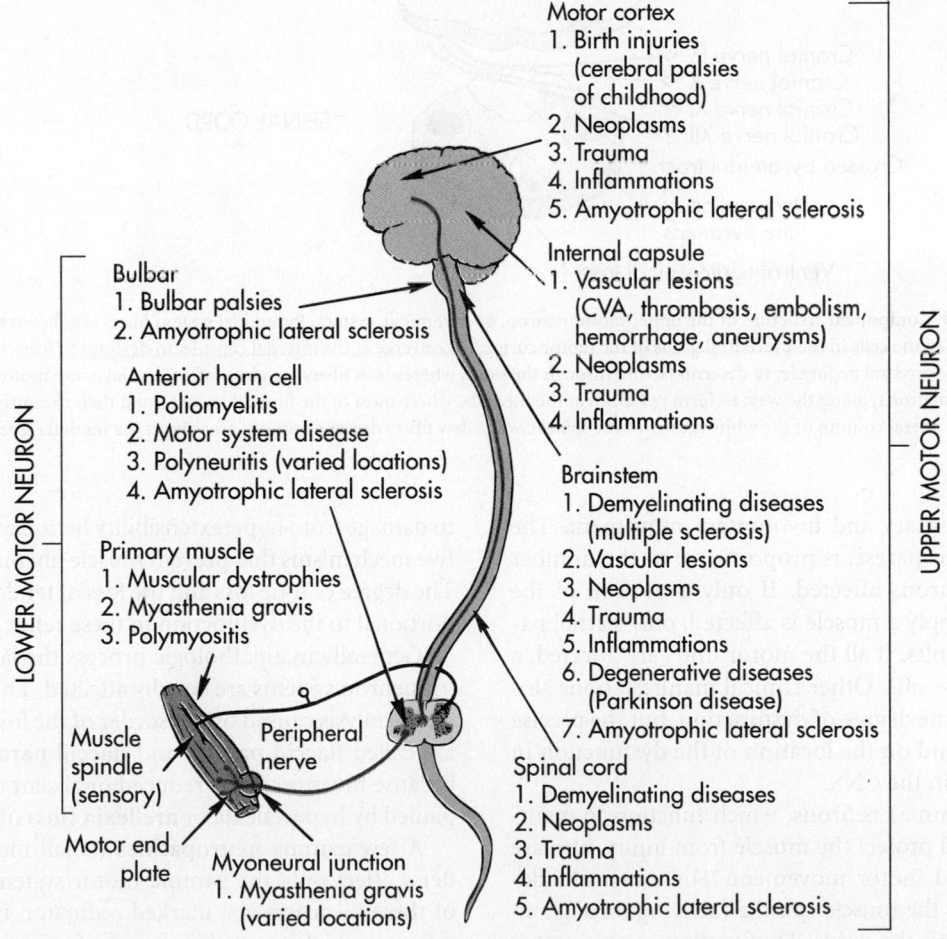

Figure 16-24 Disturbances in motor function. Disturbances in motor function are classified pathologically along upper and lower motor neuron structures. It should be noted that neoplasms occur at more than one site in an upper motor neuron *(above right)*. A few pathologic conditions, such as amyotrophic lateral sclerosis, involve upper and lower motor neuron structures. Other lesion sites include myoneural junction and primary muscle, making it possible to classify conditions as neuromuscular and muscular, respectively. *CVA,* Cerebrovascular accident.

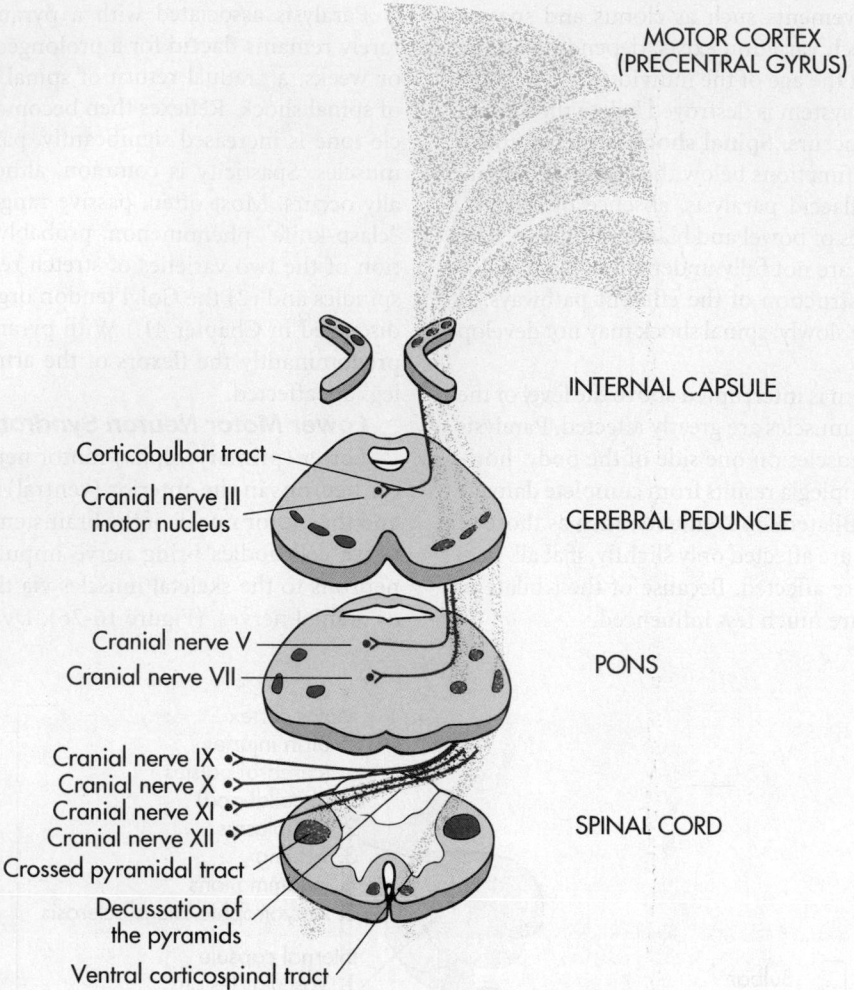

MOTOR CORTEX
(PRECENTRAL GYRUS)

INTERNAL CAPSULE

Corticobulbar tract

Cranial nerve III
motor nucleus

CEREBRAL PEDUNCLE

Cranial nerve V

Cranial nerve VII

PONS

Cranial nerve IX
Cranial nerve X
Cranial nerve XI
Cranial nerve XII

SPINAL CORD

Crossed pyramidal tract

Decussation of
the pyramids

Ventral corticospinal tract

Figure 16-25 Component structure of the upper motor neuron, or pyramidal, system. Pyramidal system fibers are shown to originate primarily in the cells in the precentral gyrus of the motor cortex; to converge at the internal capsule; to descend to form the central third of the cerebral peduncle; to descend farther through the pons, where small fibers are given off to cranial nerve motor nuclei (lower motor neurons) along the way; to form pyramids at the medulla, where most of the fibers decussate; and then to continue to descend in the lateral column of the white matter of the spinal cord. A few fibers descend without crossing at the medulla level.

system impairs voluntary and involuntary movement. The degree of paralysis or paresis is proportional to the number of lower motor neurons affected. If only a portion of the motor units that supply a muscle is affected, only partial paralysis or paresis results. If all the motor units are affected, a complete paralysis results. Other clinical manifestations also are proportional to the degree of dysfunction, but the precise manifestations depend on the location of the dysfunction in the motor unit and in the CNS.

Small motor (gamma) neurons, which function to maintain muscle tone and protect the muscle from injury, also are necessary for normal motor movement. These neurons depend on input from the muscle spindle (arriving through an afferent limb rising to the cord). Dysfunction in this motor system impairs tone and reduces the tendon reflexes, causing hyporeflexia. The muscle is lax and soft, with a decrease in normal tone, or hypotonia, which impairs voluntary and involuntary motor movements. The muscles become susceptible

to damage from hyperextensibility because the normal protective mechanisms that prevent muscle fiber injury are impaired. The degree of tone loss and the loss of tendon reflexes are proportional to the dysfunction in these reflex motor units.

Generally in a pathologic process the large and small motor neuron systems are equally affected. Therefore, the paresis and paralysis caused by a disorder of the lower motor neurons are called **flaccid paresis** and **flaccid paralysis**, respectively, because the muscle has reduced or absent tone and is accompanied by hyporeflexia or **areflexia** (loss of tendon reflexes).

A few **gamma neuropathies** (small motor neuron disorders) affect only the gamma motor system. A manifestation of these disorders is a marked reduction in the deep tendon reflexes, which are strikingly out of proportion to the degree of muscle weakness present.

Denervated muscles (i.e., muscles that have lost their nervous system input) undergo atrophy over weeks to months, mostly from disuse. Denervated muscles also demonstrate

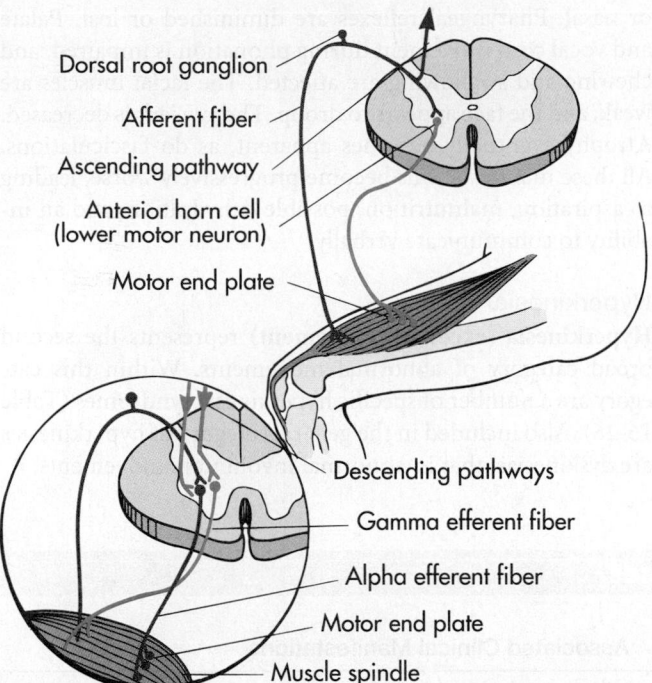

- Dorsal root ganglion
- Afferent fiber
- Ascending pathway
- Anterior horn cell (lower motor neuron)
- Motor end plate

- Descending pathways
- Gamma efferent fiber
- Alpha efferent fiber
- Motor end plate
- Muscle spindle

Figure 16-26 Component structure of a lower motor neuron, including motor (efferent) and sensory (afferent) elements. *Top,* Anterior horn cell (in anterior gray column of spinal cord and its axon), terminating in motor end plate as it innervates extrafusal muscle fibers in the quadriceps muscle. *Detailed enlargement,* Sensory and motor elements of the gamma loop system. The gamma efferent fiber is shown innervating the polar, or end, region of the muscle spindle (sensory receptor of skeletal muscle). Contraction of muscle spindle fibers stretches the central portion of the spindle and causes the afferent spindle fiber to transmit the impulse centrally to the cord. Muscle spindle afferent fibers in turn synapse on the anterior horn cell and are transmitted by way of gamma-efferent fibers to skeletal (extrafusal) muscle, causing it to contract. Muscle spindle discharge is interrupted by active contraction of extrafusal muscle fibers.

fasciculations, which are seen as muscle rippling or quivering under the skin. Occasionally denervated muscles cramp. Fibrillation (isolated contraction of a single muscle fiber) also may occur, although this manifestation is not visible clinically.

Amyotrophies

Lower motor neuron syndromes originating in the anterior horn cells or the motor nuclei of the cranial nerves are called **amyotrophies**. Paralytic poliomyelitis is the prototype of these disorders. It involves a severe inflammatory reaction in motor neurons, some of which do not survive, leaving a permanent lower motor neuron syndrome.

Several pathologic processes may give rise to an amyotrophy. A virally induced or postinfectious or postvaccination inflammatory process may injure or destroy anterior horn cells or cranial nerve cell bodies. Most of these inflammatory processes are mild and are followed by rapid cellular recovery (see What's New? Bell Palsy).

In the amyotrophies, muscle strength, muscle tone, and muscle bulk are affected in the muscles innervated by the involved motor neurons. The paresis and paralysis associated with anterior horn cell injury are segmental, but because each

WHAT'S NEW? Bell Palsy

There is increasing evidence that in addition to other etiologies, Bell palsy may be caused by reactivation of herpesviruses in cranial nerve VII (facial) ganglia. Herpes simplex-1 has been detected in up to 78% of cases and herpes zoster in 30% of cases. Severe pain with facial palsy and a vesicular rash in the ear or mouth suggest herpes zoster infection. Ramsay Hunt syndrome (herpes zoster oticus) is rare but complete recovery is less than 50%. Recovery from Bell palsy is usually complete. Both disorders are treated with antivirals, steroids, or both.

Data from Kawaguchi K et al: *Laryngoscope* 117(1):147-156, 2007; Khine H et al: *Pediatr Infect Dis J* 27(5):468-469, 2008; Tiemstra JD, Khatkhate N: *Am Fam Physician* 76(7):997-1002, 2007.

muscle is supplied by two or more roots, the segmental character of the weakness may be difficult to recognize. When cranial nerve motor nuclei are affected (these lack nerve roots and have only small rootlets near the point of exit from the brainstem), the distribution of the motor weakness follows that of the peripheral nerve. The weakness may involve distal muscles, proximal muscles, and the muscles of midline structures. Hypotonia and hyporeflexia or areflexia are present.

The atrophy associated with amyotrophy is segmental when the anterior horn cells of the spinal cord are involved and follows the distribution of the peripheral nerve when the motor nuclei of the cranial nerves are affected. The atrophy may be in distal, proximal, or midline muscles. Fasciculations are particularly associated with primary motor neuron injury, and muscle cramps are common. Mild fatigue is a common complaint. If the pathologic process is limited to the primary motor neuron, no sensory changes are evident.

Because degenerative disorders cause loss of nerve cells in the anterior horn or motor nuclei, the surviving cells are small, shrunken, and filled with lipofuscin. Lost neurons are replaced by astrocytes. The roots or rootlets are thin, and the muscles show denervation and atrophy.

Several brainstem syndromes involve damage to one or more of the cranial nerve nuclei. These are called **nuclear palsies** (Table 16-25) and may be caused by vascular occlusion, tumor, aneurysm, tuberculosis, or hemorrhage.

The anterior horn cells and the motor nuclei of the cranial nerves may be affected secondarily in many severe pathologic processes that primarily involve the peripheral nerves. The condition may extend proximally to affect the nerve roots or rootlets and the motor neurons themselves, a process commonly seen, for example, in Guillain-Barré syndrome. If sufficient numbers of motor neurons are destroyed, permanent loss of motor function results because regeneration of the damaged axons requires a living neuronal cell body.

A group of degenerative disorders principally cause progressive motor cell atrophy. One of these is **progressive spinal muscular atrophy**, in which the anterior horn cells of the spinal cord are the affected motor neurons. This disorder occurs in adults and closely resembles the familial progressive muscular atrophies that occur in infants and children and are considered inherited metabolic disorders (see Chapter 43). If the motor nuclei of the cranial nerves are affected instead of the anterior horn cells, the disorder is labeled **progressive bulbar palsy,** so named because the myelencephalon originally was called the *bulb* and a degenerative process causes a progressively more serious condition. When any lower motor neuron syndrome involves the cranial nerves that arise from the bulb (i.e., cranial nerves IX, X, and XII), the dysfunction is called a **bulbar palsy.**

The clinical manifestations of bulbar palsy include paresis or paralysis of the jaw, face, pharynx, and tongue musculature. Articulation is affected, especially articulation of the lingual *(r, n, l)*, labial *(b, m, p, f)*, dental *(d, t)*, and palatal *(k, g)* consonants. Modulation is impaired, making the voice rasping or nasal. Pharyngeal reflexes are diminished or lost. Palate and vocal cord movement during phonation is impaired, and chewing and swallowing are affected. The facial muscles are weak, and the face appears to droop. The jaw jerk is decreased. Atrophy eventually becomes apparent, as do fasciculations. All these manifestations become progressively worse, leading to aspiration, malnutrition, possible dehydration, and an inability to communicate verbally.

Hyperkinesia

Hyperkinesia (excessive movement) represents the second broad category of abnormal movements. Within this category are a number of specific hyperkinesia syndromes (Table 16-26). Also included in the general category of hyperkinesias are dyskinesias, that is, abnormal involuntary movements.

Table 16-25	Examples of Nuclear Palsy Syndromes	
Type of Nuclear Palsy	**Causes**	**Associated Clinical Manifestations**
Ocular	Upper brainstem tumor	Other cranial nerve signs
	Cerebrovascular disease in the vertebrobasilar system	Contralateral spastic hemiparesis/hemiplegia
	Aneurysm	Contralateral hyperreflexia
	Intramedullary bleeding	Contralateral extensor plantar reflex
Facial	Pontine tumor	Paresis/paralysis of both the upper and lower facial muscles for
	Cerebrovascular disease in the vertebrobasilar system	both voluntary movement and emotionally induced movement
Vagal	Intramedullary tumor	Ipsilateral loss of pain and temperature sensations of the face
	Cerebrovascular disease in the vertebrobasilar system	Contralateral spastic arm and leg paresis/hemiplegia
		Ipsilateral cerebellar signs
Hypoglossal	Intramedullary tumor	Contralateral loss of position sense and vibration in the arm and leg
	Cerebrovascular disease in the vertebrobasilar system	Contralateral spastic hemiparesis/hemiplegia

Table 16-26	Types of Hyperkinesia Syndromes	
Type	**Characteristics**	**Causes**
Chorea*	Nonrepetitive muscular contractions, usually of the extremities of the face; random pattern of irregular, involuntary rapid contractions of groups of muscles; disappears with sleep, decreases with resting; increases with emotional stress and attempted voluntary movement	Associated with excess concentration of or a supersensitivity to dopamine within basal ganglia
Athetosis*	Disorder of distal-muscle postural fixation; slow, sinuous, irregular movements most obvious in the distal extremities, more rhythmic than choreiform movements and always much slower; movements accompany characteristic hand posture; slowly fluctuating grimaces	Occurs most commonly as a result of injury to the putamen of the basal ganglion; exact pathophysiologic mechanism is not known
Ballism	Disorder of proximal-muscle postural fixation with wild flinging movement of the limbs; movement is severe and stereotyped, usually lateral; does not lessen with sleep; ballism is most common on one side of the body, a condition termed *hemiballism*	Results from injury to subthalamus nucleus (one of the nuclei that comprise the basal ganglia); thought to be caused by reduced inhibitory influence in the nucleus, a release phenomenon; hemiballism results from injury to the contralateral subthalamic nucleus
Hyperactivity	State of prolonged, generalized, increased activity that is largely involuntary but may be subject to some voluntary control; not highly stereotyped but rather manifests as continual changes in total body posture or in excessive performance of some simple activity, such as pacing under inappropriate circumstances	May be caused by frontal and reticular activating system injury

Table 16-26	Types of Hyperkinesia Syndromes—cont'd	
Type	**Characteristics**	**Causes**
Wandering	Tendency to wander without regard for environment	"Release" phenomenon; associated with bilateral injury to globus pallidus or putamen
Akathisia	Special type of hyperactivity; mild compulsion to move (usually more localized to legs); severe frenzied motion possible; movements are partly voluntary and may be transiently suppressed; carrying out the movement brings a sense of relief; a frequent complication of antipsychotic drugs	Dopaminergic transmission may be involved
Tremor at Rest	Rhythmic, oscillating movement affecting one or more body parts	Caused by regular contraction of opposing groups of muscles
Parkinsonian tremor	Regular, rhythmic, slow flexion-extension contraction; involves principally the metacarpophalangeal and wrist joints; alternating movements between thumb and index finger described as "pill rolling"; disappears during voluntary movement	Loss of inhibitory influence of dopamine in the basal ganglia, causing instability of basal ganglial feedback circuit within the cerebral cortex
Postural Tremor		
Asterixis (tremor of hepatic encephalopathy)	Irregular flapping movement of the hands accentuated by outstretching arms	Due to transient inhibition of muscles that maintain posture; thought to be related to accumulation of products normally detoxified by the liver
Metabolic	Rapid, rhythmic tremor affecting fingers, lips, and tongue; accentuated by extending the body part; enhanced physiologic tremor	Occurs in conditions associated with disturbed metabolism or toxicity, as in thyrotoxicosis (hyperthyroidism), alcoholism, and chronic use of barbiturates, amphetamines, lithium, amitriptyline (Elavil); exact mechanism responsible unknown
Essential (familial)	Tremor of fingers, hands, and feet; absent at rest but accentuated by extension of body part, prolonged muscular activity, and stress	Not associated with any other neurologic abnormalities; cause unknown
Intentional Tremor		
Cerebellar	Tremor initiated by movement, maximal toward end of movement	Occurs in disease of the dentate nucleus (one of the deep cerebellar nuclei responsible for efferent output) and the superior cerebellar peduncle (a stalk-like structure connected to the pons); caused by errors in feedback from the periphery and errors in preprogramming goal-directed movement
Rubral	Rhythmic tremor of limbs that originates proximally by movement	Results from lesions involving the dentatorubrothalamic tract (a spinothalamic tract connecting the red nucleus in the reticular formation and the dentate nucleus in the cerebellum)
Myoclonus	Series of shocklike, nonpatterned contractions of a portion of a muscle, entire muscle, or group of muscles that cause throwing movements of a limb; usually appear at random but frequently triggered by sudden startle; do not disappear during sleep	Associated with an irritable nervous system and spontaneous discharge of neurons; structures associated with myoclonus include the cerebral cortex, cerebellum, reticular formation, and spinal cord

*Choreoathetosis involves chorea and athetosis; precise pathophysiology unknown.

Paroxysmal dyskinesias are abnormal, involuntary movements that occur as spasms. The type of dyskinesia varies depending on the specific disorder.

Tardive dyskinesia is the involuntary movement of the face, trunk, and extremities. Although the condition occurs occasionally in individuals with Parkinson disease, it usually occurs as a side effect of prolonged first- or second-generation antipsychotic drugs.[55] The antipsychotic drugs cause denervation hypersensitivity so that it mimics the effect of too much dopamine. The most common symptom of tardive dyskinesia is rapid, repetitive, stereotypic movements. Most characteristic is continual chewing with intermittent protrusions of the tongue, lip smacking, and facial grimacing. Stereotypic movements are believed to be a form of excessive dopaminergic activity.

Other movement disorders under this category are (1) complex repetitive movements, including automatism, stereotype, complex tics, compulsions, perseverations, and mannerisms; (2) positivism (excessive reactions to certain stimuli); and (3) paroxysmal excessive activity, including cataplexy and excessive startle reaction.

Huntington Disease

Huntington disease (HD), also known as *chorea,* is a relatively rare, hereditary-degenerative disorder diffusely involving the basal ganglia and cerebral cortex. The onset of HD is usually between 25 and 45 years of age, when the trait may already have been passed to the victim's children. The disorder has a prevalence rate of approximately 2 to 8 per 100,000 persons and occurs in all races.[56]

PATHOPHYSIOLOGY HD is inherited as an autosomal dominant trait with high penetrance. The genetic defect is on the short arm of chromosome 4. There is an abnormally long polyglutamine tract in the huntingtin protein that is toxic to neurons caused by a cytosine-adenine-guanine (CAG) trinucleotide repeat expansion (40 to 70 repeats instead of 9 to 34).[57] Age of onset of symptoms is related to the length of the repeat sequences and mechanisms of toxicity. Increased length leads to progressively earlier presentations.

The principal pathologic feature of HD is severe degeneration of the basal ganglia, particularly the caudate and putamen nuclei, and the frontal cerebral cortex (Figures 16-27 and 16-28). Tangles of protein collect in brain cells and chains of glutamine on the abnormal molecules stick to each other.[58] Early in the disease, selective loss of the striatal GABA/enkephalin pathway to the lateral aspect of the pallidum occurs. The basal ganglia normally contain a preponderance of GABAergic (GABA-secreting) neurons, including the pathway between the basal ganglia and substantia nigra (pallidonigral pathway). Basal ganglia and nigral depletion of GABA, an inhibitory neurotransmitter, is the principal biochemical alteration in HD. Degeneration of the GABAergic pallidonigral pathway causes GABA depletion in the substantia nigra with decreased inhibitory GABA activity on dopaminergic neurons in the substantia nigra and a relative excess of dopaminergic activity in the basal ganglial feedback circuit within the cerebral cortex. A relative excess of dopaminergic activity in this circuit, as in HD, is manifested by hypotonia and hyperkinesia (involuntary, fragmentary movements such as chorea). Loss of excitatory glutamate may liberate the pathway from the thalamus to the premotor cortex, impairing modulation of movement later in the course of the disease. Within the neurons, producing the fuel for brain activity is difficult, with a resultant buildup of lactic acid.

CLINICAL MANIFESTATIONS The classic manifestations of HD are abnormal movement and progressive dysfunction of intellectual processes (dementia) and thought processes. Any one of these features may mark the onset of the disease. Chorea is the most common type of abnormal movement affecting individuals with HD. Choreiform movements begin in the face and arms, eventually affecting the

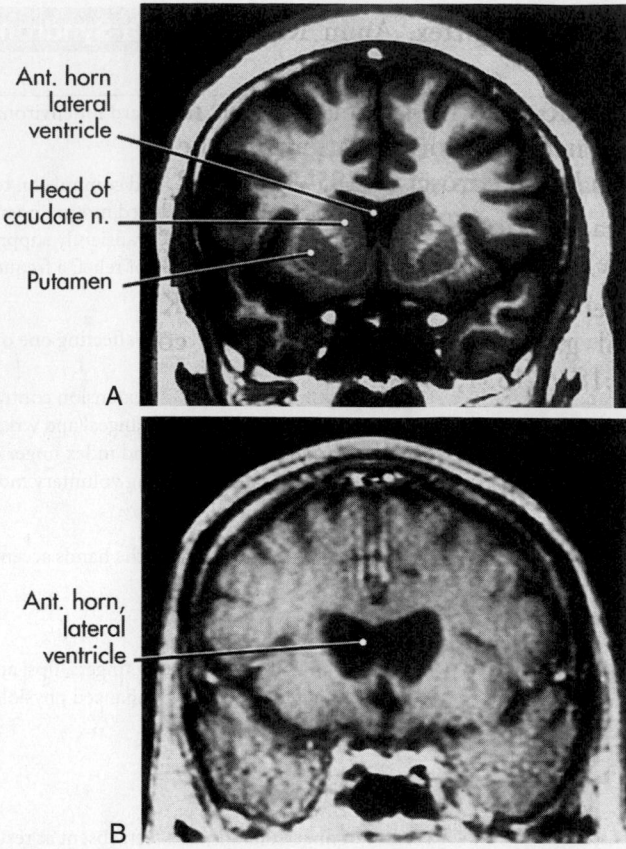

Figure 16-27 Coronal MRI through frontal lobe and head of the caudate nucleus. The head of the caudate normally forms a prominent bulge into the anterior horn of the lateral ventricle (**A,** inversion recovery image). Profound cell loss in the neostriatum of an individual with Huntington disease greatly diminishes the size of the caudate and renders the lateral wall of the ventricle flat (**B,** T1-weighted image). The slightly wavy appearance of the magnetic resonance imaging (MRI) in **B** is the result of movement (tremor) while the scan was being done. (From Haines DE, editor: *Fundamental neuroscience,* Philadelphia, 1997, Churchill Livingstone.)

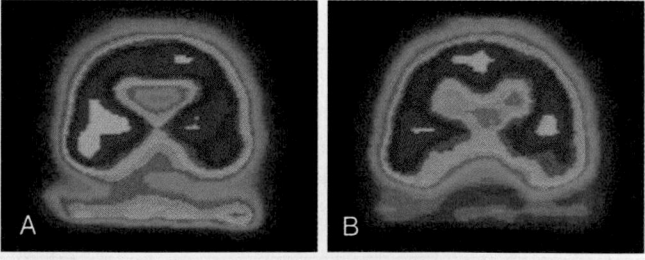

Figure 16-28 Caudate blood flow in Huntington disease. Single photon emission computed tomography scan showing reduced caudate blood flow (**A**) in Huntington disease compared with normal blood flow (**B**). (From Perkin DG: *Mosby's color atlas and text of neurology,* London, 1998, Mosby-Wolfe.)

entire body. Symptoms of frontal lobe dysfunction include executive attention deficits, short-term memory loss (working memory); reduced capacity to plan, organize, and sequence, as well as bradyphrenia (slow thinking); and apathy. Restlessness, disinhibition, and irritability are common. Affectively, euphoria or depression or both may be present.

EVALUATION AND TREATMENT The diagnosis of HD is based on family history, clinical presentation of the disorder, and genetic testing. No known treatment is effective in halting the degeneration or progression of symptoms. The discovery in 1983 of the HD marker, called *G8*, on chromosome 4 paves the way for presymptomatic diagnosis of the disorder and isolation of the HD gene. Recombinant genetic techniques and neuroprotective drug strategies may someday prevent or control the disorder.[59]

Hypokinesia

Hypokinesia (decreased movement) is loss of voluntary movement despite preserved consciousness and normal peripheral nerve and muscle function. Types of hypokinesia include akinesia, bradykinesia, and loss of associated movement.

Akinesia

Akinesia is an absence, poverty, or lack of control of associated and voluntary muscle movements. There is a disturbance in the time it takes to perform a movement. Akinesia is related to dysfunction of the extrapyramidal system, as in parkinsonism. Pathogenesis is related to either a deficiency of dopamine or a defect of the postsynaptic dopamine receptors, which occurs in parkinsonism (see Parkinson disease, page 572).

Bradykinesia

Bradykinesia is slowness of voluntary movements. There is a disturbance in the time it takes to perform a movement. In bradykinesia all voluntary movements become slow, labored, and deliberate. Bradykinesia consists of (1) difficulty in initiating movements, (2) difficulty in continuing movements smoothly, and (3) difficulty in performing synchronous (at the same time) and consecutive tasks. Difficulty in initiating movements ranges from slight hesitancy to severe **freezing** (transient, helpless immobility). Each intended movement requires effort. Difficulty in continuing motions smoothly causes jerky, irregular, rapid movements, which then decrease in rate and amplitude until they stop. The individual is scarcely aware of the cessation. Difficulty in performing synchronous and consecutive tasks means that each motor act is performed separately. The individual is unable to integrate

---

Box 16-5	Primary and Secondary Causes of Parkinsonism

Primary Parkinsonism
Sporadic (idiopathoic); most common form
Genetic: autosomal dominant; autosomal recessive
Phenotype may be influenced by gene-environment interactions

Secondary Parkinsonism
Neurodegenerative disorders (sporadic or genetic)
  Disorders associated with alpha-synuclein pathology
    Multiple system atrophies (glial and neuronal inclusions)
      Striatonigral degeneration
      Olivopontocerebellar atrophy
      Shy-Drager syndrome
      Motor neuron disease with PD features
    Dementia with Lewy bodies (cortical and brainstem neuronal inclusions)
  Disorders associated with primary tau pathology ("tauopathies")
    Progressive supranuclear palsy
    Corticobasal degeneration
    Frontotemporal dementia
  Disorders associated with primary amyloid pathology ("amyloidopathies")
    Alzheimer disease with parkinsonism
Genetically mediated disorders with occasional parkinsonian features
  Wilson disease
  Hallervorden-Spatz disease
  Chédiak-Higashi syndrome
  SCA-3 spinocerebellar ataxia
  X-linked dystonia-parkinsonism (*DYT3*)
  Fragile X permutation associated with ataxia-tremor-parkinsonism syndrome
  Huntington disease (Westphal variant)
  Prion disease

Miscellaneous acquired conditions
  Vascular parkinsonism: atherosclerosis, amyloid angiopathy
  Normal pressure hydrocephalus
  Catatonia
  Cerebral palsy
Repeated head trauma ("dementia pugilistica" with parkinsonian features)
Infectious and postinfectious diseases
  Postencephalitic PD
  Creutzfeldt-Jakob disease
  Neurosyphilis
Metabolic conditions
  Hypoparathyroidism or pseudohypoparathyroidism with basal ganglia calcifications
  Non-wilsonian hepatolenticular degeneration
Multiple sclerosis
Neoplastic disease
Drugs
  Neuroleptics (typical antipsychotics)
  Selected atypical antipsychotics
  Antiemetics (e.g., compazine, metoclopramide)
  Dopamine-depleting agents (reserpine, tetrabenazine)
  α-methyldopa
  Lithium carbonate
  Valproic acid
  Fluoxetine
Toxins
  1-Methyl-1,2,4,6 tetrahydropyridine (MPTP)
  Manganese
  Cyanide
  Methanol
  Carbon monoxide
  Carbon disulfide
  Hexane

Data from Delong MR, Juncos IL: Parkinson's disease and other extrapyramidal movement disorders. In Fauci AS et al, editors: *Harrison's principles of internal medicine*, ed 17, p 2553, New York, 2008, McGraw-Hill; Lang, A: Parkinsonism. In Goldman L, Ausiello D, editors: *Cecil medicine*, ed 23, p 2726, Philadelphia, 2008, Saunders.

two acts or to change from one motor pattern to the next with a single smooth motion.

Loss of Associated Movement

In hypokinesia the normal, habitually associated movements that provide skill, grace, and balance to voluntary movements are lost. Decreased associated movements accompanying emotional expression cause an expressionless face, a statue-like posture, absence of speech inflection, and absence of spontaneous gestures. Decreased associated movements accompanying locomotion cause reduction in arm and shoulder movements, in hip swinging, and in rotary motion of the cervical spine.

Parkinson Disease

Parkinson disease (PD) is a commonly occurring degenerative disorder of the basal ganglia (corpus striatum, globus pallidus, subthalamic nucleus, and substantia nigra) involving the dopaminergic (dopamine-secreting) nigrostriatal pathway. Nigrostriatal disorders produce a syndrome of abnormal movement called **parkinsonism (Parkinson syndrome, parkinsonian syndrome)**.

Etiologic classification of parkinsonism includes primary parkinsonism and secondary parkinsonism (Box 16-5). The onset of PD occurs after 40 years of age, with mean onset of 60 years of age.[60] Equal incidence occurs in both sexes.[23] PD is one of the most prevalent of the primary CNS disorders and a leading cause of neurologic disability in individuals older than 60 years. Approximately 1% to 2% of the U.S. population older than the age of 60 is affected—an estimated 1.5 million individuals. The familial form represents about 10% of PD; however, the majority of cases are sporadic or idiopathic. Several PD genes have been identified, the most significant of which are identified in Table 16-18.

PATHOPHYSIOLOGY The hallmark pathologic features of PD are loss of dopaminergic pigmented neurons in the substantia nigra (SN) pars compacta with dopaminergic deficiency in the putamen portion of the striatum (the striatum includes the putamen and caudate nucleus) (Figure 16-29). Dopamine loss in other brain areas including the brainstem, thalamus, and cortex also occurs.[61] Degeneration of the dopaminergic nigrostriatal pathway to the basal ganglia results in underactivity of the direct motor pathway (normally facilitates movement) (Figure 16-30) and overactivity of the indirect motor loop (normally inhibits movement). This results in inhibition of the motor cortex manifested with *bradykinesia and rigidity.* The subthalamic nucleus (STN) overactivity also influences the limbic system[60] accounting for emotional signs and symptoms. Neuronal loss within the cerebral cortex is found in one half of individuals with PD.

Lewy bodies, fibrillar intracellular eosinophilic inclusions, and high concentrations of alpha-synuclein, ubiquitin, tau protein, tuberculin, and other proteins, are found in the SN, LC, and other areas of the brain and are a marker for neuronal degeneration.[62] Degeneration of the LC, which contains noradrenergic neurons, also occurs in PD. Norepinephrine is thought to be neuroprotective and loss of LC neurons may be associated

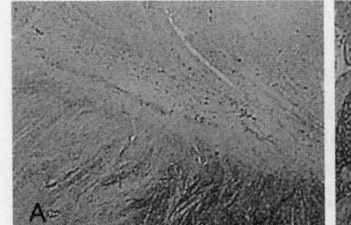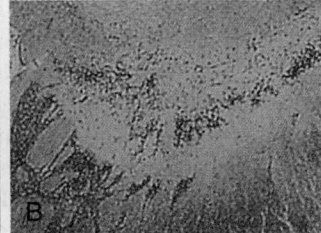

Figure 16-29 Atrophic substantia nigra (A) compared with normal control (B). (From Perkin DG: *Mosby's color atlas and text of neurology,* London, 1998, Mosby-Wolfe.)

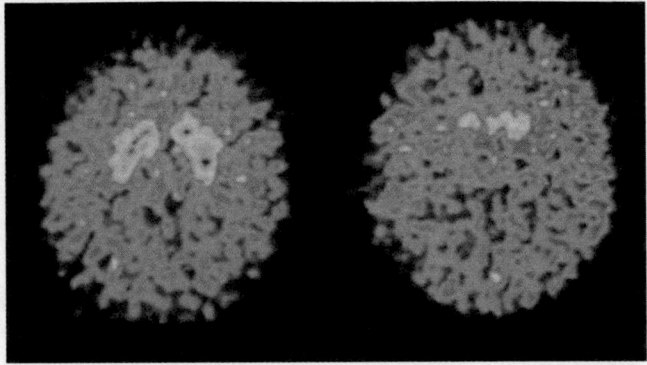

Figure 16-30 Reduced fluorodopa in Parkinson disease. Positron-emission tomography scan showing reduced fluorodopa uptake in the basal ganglia *(right)* compared with a normal control *(left).* (From Perkin DG: *Mosby's color atlas and text of neurology,* London, 1998, Mosby-Wolfe.)

with a worsening of disease progression and the behavioral symptoms of PD.[63] Molecular events thought to be associated with the neurodegeneration of PD include mitochondrial dysfunction, oxidative stress, abnormal folding and accumulation of alpha-synuclein, abnormal phosphorylation, and dysfunction of the ubiquitin proteosome system[64,65] (Figure 16-31).

CLINICAL MANIFESTATIONS Onset of symptoms is insidious and symptoms appear after a 70% to 80% loss of pigmented nigral neurons and a loss of 60% to 90% of striatal dopamine.[66] The classic motor manifestations of PD are bradykinesia, tremor at rest (resting tremor), rigidity (muscle stiffness), hypoakinesia (poverty of movement), and postural abnormalities. These manifestations may develop alone or in combination, but as the disease progresses, all four are usually present to at least some degree. There is no true paralysis. A modified Hoehn and Yahr scale[67] can be used to assess progression of symptoms:

0. No visible disease
1. Unilateral involvement, may have tremor of one limb
2. Bilateral involvement, balance intact
3. Bilateral involvement, slowing of body movement, mild to moderate postural instability, and gait difficulty
4. Bilateral involvement with severe postural instability, rigidity, and bradykinesia present
5. Bilateral involvement with inability to walk, confinement to wheelchair, cachexia present

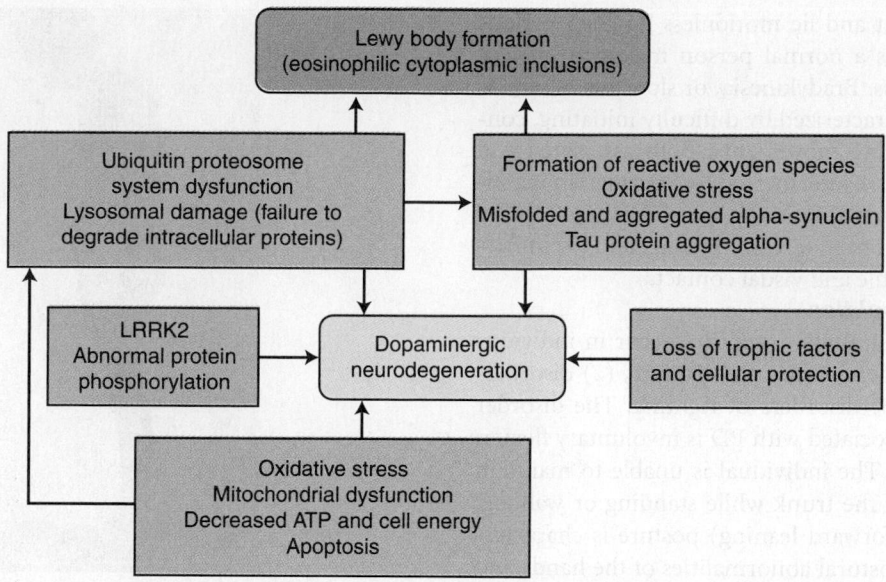

Figure 16-31 Proposed pathogenesis of dopaminergic neurodegeneration in Parkinson disease. *ATP,* Adenosine triphosphate; *LRRK2,* leucine-rich repeat kinase -2. (Data from Engelender S: *Autophagy* 4[3]:372-374, 2008; Lim KL, Tan JM: *BMC Biochem* 22:[8 Suppl 1]:S13, 2007; Mizuno Y et al: *Philos Trans R Soc Lond B Biol Sci* 363[1500]:2215-2227, 2008.)

In early stages of the disease, reflex, sensory, and mental status are usually normal. Nonmotor symptoms associated with PD include hyponosmia, fatigue, pain, autonomic dysfunction, sleep fragmentation, depression, and dementia with or without psychosis.[68]

Parkinsonian tremor, the most conspicuous and most variable symptom, is usually the first motor symptom to appear. It is an asymmetric, regular, rhythmic, low-amplitude tremor (4 to 6 cycles/second, with slowly alternating flexion-extension contraction).[69] Later the tremor becomes symmetric at 7 to 12 cycles per second. It is a tremor at rest, disappearing briefly during the course of a voluntary movement and reappearing when the limb is held in a stationary position. Intensity and amplitude of the tremor vary. The arm is more affected than the leg. The head is rarely involved. Seventy percent of individuals with PD have this tremor, and 20% have a postural (kinesic) tremor or both tremor types. All tremors are increased by stress and anxiety.

Parkinsonian tremor appears to result from instability of feedback from the basal ganglia to the cerebral cortex caused by loss of the inhibitory influence of dopamine in the basal ganglia. Increased oscillation in the normal feedback cycles of the motor outflow feedback circuit when the muscles are at rest produces the tremor. When the individual performs voluntary movements, the tremor becomes temporarily blocked, presumably because other motor control signals arriving in the thalamus override the abnormal basal ganglial signals. As the disorder worsens, tremor may lessen as rigidity supervenes. The postural tremor is associated with damage to the cerebellofugal pathway to the red nucleus, a pathway that subserves communication from muscle spindles to the thalamus and motor cortex.

Parkinsonian rigidity is an increased resistance to the passive movement of a joint that impedes active and passive movement. The first symptoms of rigidity may be painful muscle cramps in the toes or hands. More commonly the limb feels stiff, heavy, tired, or aching. **Plastic rigidity** is constant throughout the entire range of motion and is felt as lead-pipe resistance during passive movement. **Cogwheel rigidity,** brief palpable jerks, is accompanied by tremor. The mechanism underlying rigidity is unclear, but there is increased resting muscle activity of antagonistic muscle groups with enhancement of the long-latency component of the stretch reflex.[60]

Parkinsonian bradykinesia is poverty of associated and voluntary movements. It is the most prevalent and crippling symptom and often is overlooked in the early stages. The pathophysiology underlying the bradykinesia is an overactive subthalamic nucleus (STN) that inhibits the motor thalamus and motor cortex.[60] It is associated with dopamine deficiency and failure of the mechanism programming movement patterns manifested as a defect in the voluntary production of smooth motions at different speeds.[70]

All striated muscles—extremity, trunk, ocular, facial—are affected eventually, including muscles of mastication (chewing), deglutition (swallowing), and articulation. Micrographia is present. Extreme underactivity in the individual with PD makes the person appear stiff, even when resistance to passive movement cannot be felt. Bradykinesia is a separate phenomenon from rigidity and may be severe even in the presence of rigidity. Individuals state that they feel "wooden" (as though moving against resistance) and complain of rapid, severe fatigue.

Hypokinesia, or decreased frequency or absence of associated movements, is one of the earliest akinetic symptoms.

Individuals with PD sit and lie motionless for long periods without the little shifts a normal person makes to prevent discomfort and stiffness. Bradykinesia, or slowness of voluntary movements, is characterized by difficulty initiating, continuing, or synchronizing movements. Both associated and voluntary movements are interspersed by freezing (an inability to continue movement). Freezing may be precipitated by (1) increasing the effort to move, (2) turning, and (3) initiating certain types of tactile and visual contact.

Postural Abnormalities

Three types of postural abnormalities occur in individuals with PD: (1) disorders of postural fixation, (2) disorders of equilibrium, and (3) disorders of righting. The disorder of postural fixation associated with PD is involuntary flexion of the head and neck. The individual is unable to maintain an upright position of the trunk while standing or walking. The stooped (flexed, forward leaning) posture is characteristic (Figure 16-32). Postural abnormalities of the hands and feet also occur. Postural abnormalities are caused by a loss of normal postural reflexes.

Disorders of equilibrium result from loss of postural stability. The person with PD is unable to make the appropriate postural adjustment to tilting or falling and falls like a post when starting to tilt. The festinating gait (short, accelerating steps) of the person with PD is an attempt to maintain an upright position while walking (see Figure 16-32). Individuals also are unable to right themselves when changing from a reclining or crouching position to a standing position and when rolling over from a supine to a lateral or prone position.

Autonomic and Neuroendocrine Symptoms

Autonomic and neuroendocrine dysfunctions in PD produce nonmotor symptoms that are distressing but not incapacitating. The basal ganglia influences hypothalamic function (autonomic and neuroendocrine) through pathways connecting the hypothalamus with the basal ganglia and cerebral cortex. Common autonomic symptoms in PD include inappropriate diaphoresis, gastric retention, constipation, and urinary retention. Cardiac sympathetic denervation is common and causes neurogenic orthostatic hypotension.[71] A symptom attributed to neuroendocrine dysfunction is seborrhea. Hypothalamic hypersecretion of hormone-releasing factors acting on the anterior pituitary causes hypersecretion of androgenotropic hormones producing sebum hypersecretion by sebaceous glands. The resulting seborrhea is characterized by oily skin with seborrheic dermatitis along the hairline and in chin-nasal creases.

Cognitive-Affective Symptoms

Fifty percent of people with PD have a depression that is now believed to be an inherent part of the pathologic state of the disease (an endogenous depression), not a response to the situation. Thirty percent of individuals treated on an outpatient basis for PD have a dementia, and 80% of those with PD requiring institutional care have dementia as well. Dementia is more common in individuals older than 70 years. Pathologically, in those with dementia, findings include loss of cholinergic cells in the basal nucleus of Meynert; neuronal loss, senile plaques,

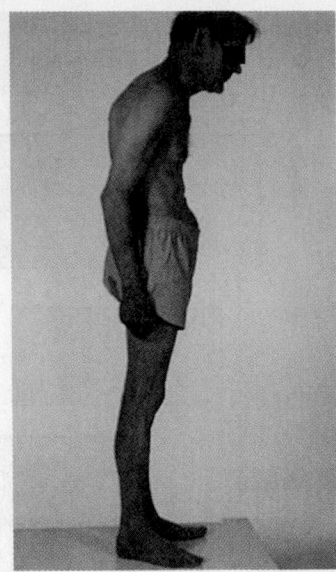

Figure 16-32 Stooped posture of Parkinson disease. (From Perkin DG: *Mosby's color atlas and text of neurology,* London, 1998, Mosby-Wolfe.)

and neurofibrillary tangles in the neocortex; and amyloid changes in small blood vessels. Lewy bodies are distributed diffusely in many neocortical neurons, making this a Lewy body dementia. The individual evidences disorientation; confusion; memory loss; distractibility; and difficulty with concept formation, abstraction, calculations, thinking, and judgment. Although the symptoms fluctuate, they progressively worsen. Anxiety disorders; impulse-control disorders; and punding, a disorder of stereotypical motor behavior in which there is intense fascination with repetitive handling and examining of mechanical objects, are recognized features of PD. A cognitive disorder unassociated with either a dementia or depression, called *bradyphrenia,* also is present. This disorder may appear early in the course of the disease and may progress to dementia. Bradyphrenia is caused by disruption of the caudal basal ganglion connections and outflows. The clinical manifestations are slowness of thinking, poverty of thought (diminished imagination and insight), and difficulty formulating thoughts (decreased ability to conceptualize, plan, decide, or improvise).

Nonmotor symptoms are common in PD including sensory dysfunction with anosmia, ageusia, pain, paresthesias, and disturbances in the sleep-wake cycle. Excessive daytime sleepiness is experienced in more than 50% of persons.[72,73]

Influence of Symptoms

Early in the disease, people often experience a sleep benefit; that is, symptoms decrease with sleep. Also symptoms fluctuate in an on-off pattern. Stress influences symptoms adversely, but the underlying mechanism is unclear. The person's mental status may be further compromised by the side effects of the medication taken to control symptoms.

The combination of all the parkinsonian symptoms gives the individual a characteristic appearance: a wide-eyed, unblinking, staring expression with the facial muscles smoothed out and almost immobile. Saliva frequently drools from the corners of the slightly open mouth. The skin of the face is frequently greasy. The gait is pathognomonic: the individual walks with slow, short, shuffling steps; the arms are flexed, abducted, and held stiffly at the side; and the trunk is bent slightly forward. The person may break into a run spontaneously or when pushed forward or backward. Because of the disorder of postural fixation, the tendency is to fall to the side. Postural instability, sleep disorders, and difficulty concentrating are some of the most depressing symptoms for people with PD.[74]

EVALUATION AND TREATMENT The diagnosis of PD is made on the basis of two of the four cardinal symptoms: (1) resting tremor, (2) bradykinesia, (3) cogwheel rigidity, and (4) postural instability. One of the two symptoms must be resting tremor or bradykinesia (criteria from Core Assessment Program for Intracerebral Transplantation [CAPIT]).[75] A combination of imaging techniques, clinical evaluations, biochemical markers, and genetic tests support the diagnosis of PD.[76] Median time between diagnosis and death is 9 years.[23]

The aim of drug therapy is to restore striatal dopamine using oral drugs such as levodopa (L-dopa), a precursor of dopamine (dopamine does not cross the blood-brain barrier), dopamine agonists that directly stimulate dopamine receptors, anticholinergic drugs, antihistamines, and amantadine. L-dopa is effective in reducing symptoms in early PD but can cause motor fluctuations, "off" periods, and dyskinesia in the long term. Monoamine oxidase B inhibitors, which inhibit the breakdown of endogenous dopamine, may improve symptoms, reduce motor fluctuations, and delay the need for L-dopa but can cause adverse effects. Adding catechol-O-methyltransferase (COMT) inhibitor prolongs the half-life of dopamine (COMT metabolizes dopamine in the synapse). Dopamine agonists to L-dopa or a dopamine agonist alone may reduce "off" time or improve symptoms but can also increase disability.[77] Surgery may be considered in later stages of PD. Thalamotomy and pallidotomy are being replaced with deep brain stimulation as an approach to controlling medically resistant motor symptoms and L-dopa–related peak dose dyskinesia.[78,79] Implants of stem cells, fetal cells, and gene therapy hold promise for future treatment.[80]

Dysphagia and general immobility are special problems of the individual with PD requiring preventive, symptomatic, supportive, and rehabilitative management, such as physiotherapy and speech therapy. Nursing interventions, occupational therapy (OT), physical therapy (PT), speech, language, and swallowing therapy are considered effective and safe for improving functional status.[81,82]

Alterations in Complex Motor Performance

The alterations in complex motor performance include disorders of posture (stance), disorders of gait, and disorders of expression.

Disorders of Posture (Stance)

An inequality of tone in muscle groups because of a loss of normal postural reflexes results in a posturing of limbs. Many reflex systems govern tone and posture, but the most important factor in posture control is the stretch reflex, in which stretching of extensor (antigravity) muscles causes increased extensor tone and inhibited flexor tone. Four types of disorders of posture are described: (1) dystonic posture, (2) decerebrate posture, (3) basal ganglion posture, and (4) senile posture. Equilibrium and balance are disrupted when postural disorders are present.

Dystonia is the maintenance of an abnormal posture through muscular contractions. When muscular contractions are sustained for several seconds, they are called **dystonic movements**, such as in choreoathetoid movements associated with high levels of L-dopa; when contractions last for longer periods, they are called **dystonic postures**, such as in torticollis. Dystonic postures may last for weeks, causing permanent fixed contractures. Dystonia has been associated with basal ganglia abnormality, but the exact pathophysiologic mechanisms are unknown (Box 16-6). One particularly relevant dystonic posture already discussed in this chapter is decorticate (striatal posture or upper motor neuron dysfunction posture), which may be unilateral or bilateral in occurrence. **Decorticate posture** (also referred to as **antigravity posture** or **hemiplegic posture**) is characterized by upper extremities flexed at the elbows and held close to the body and by lower extremities that are externally rotated and extended. Decorticate posture is believed to occur when the brainstem, which facilitates the antigravity position, is not inhibited by the motor function of the cerebral cortex. Upper motor neuron posture is more commonly described as the arm flexed at the elbow, with a wristdrop; the leg inadequately bent at the knee, with the hip excessively circumabducted; and the presence of a footdrop.

Decerebrate posture refers to increased tone in extensor muscles and trunk muscles, with active tonic neck reflexes. When the head is in a neutral position, all four limbs are rigidly extended. The decerebrate posture is caused by severe injury to the brain and brainstem, resulting in overstimulation of the postural righting and vestibular reflexes.

Box 16-6	Botulinum Toxin Therapeutic Effectiveness in Dystonia

Botulinum toxin, both A and B, is effective in relieving cervical dystonia (spasmodic torticollis) symptoms in adults and is the mainstay of modern treatment for focal dystonia. The effectiveness of other drugs (benodiazepines, gamma-aminobutyric acid [GABA] inhibitors, atypical anticonvulsants, dopaminergic agonists and antagonists) as well as the effect of surgical interventions or physical therapies is not empirically known.

Data from Benecke R, Dressler D: *Disabil Rehabil* 29(23):1769-1777, 2007; Ferreira JJ et al: *Expert Opin Pharmacother* 8(2):129-140, 2007; Pappert EJ et al: *Mov Disord* 23(4):510-517, 2008.

Basal ganglion posture refers to a stooped, hyperflexed posture with a narrow-based, short-stepped gait. This posture abnormality results from the loss of normal postural reflexes and not from defects in proprioceptive, labyrinthine, or visual function. Dysfunctional equilibrium results from the loss of postural stability, and thus the individual is unable to make the appropriate postural adjustment to tilting or loss of balance and falls instead. Dysfunctional righting is the inability to right oneself when changing from a lying or crouching to a standing position or when rolling from the supine to the lateral or prone position. Dysfunctional postural fixation is the involuntary flexion of the head and neck, causing the person difficulty in maintaining an upright trunk position while standing or walking. Basal ganglion dysfunction accounts for this posture.

Senile posture is characterized by an increasingly flexed posture similar to that caused by basal ganglion dysfunction. The posture is associated with frontal lobe dysfunction, but the primary pathophysiology is not well described.

Disorders of Gait

Four predominant types of gait disorder are (1) upper motor neuron dysfunction gait, (2) cerebellar (ataxic) gait, (3) basal ganglion gait, and (4) senile (frontal lobe, pseudoparkinsonian) gait. As with posture, equilibrium and balance are affected with gait disturbances.

Several upper motor neuron gaits exist. In the presence of mild upper motor neuron dysfunction, a footdrop may appear only with fatigue. The individual may complain of hip and leg pain. A **spastic gait**, which is associated with unilateral injury, is manifested by a shuffling gait with the leg extended and held stiff, causing a scraping over the floor surface. An impaired leg swing around the body rather than an appropriate lifting and placing of the leg is noted. The foot may drag on the ground, and the person tends to fall to the affected side. A **scissors gait** is associated with bilateral injury and spasticity. The legs are abducted, causing them to touch each other. As the person walks, the legs are still swung around the body but then cross in front of each other because of adduction. Injury to the pyramidal system accounts for these gaits.

A **cerebellar gait** manifests as a wide-based gait with the feet apart and often turned outward or inward for greater stability. The pelvis is held stiff, and it seems to be independent of the trunk. The individual staggers when walking. Cerebellar dysfunction accounts for this particular gait.

A **basal ganglion gait** and a **senile gait** are both broad-based gaits. The person walks with small steps and a decreased arm swing. The head and body are flexed and the arms are semiflexed and abducted, whereas the legs are flexed and rigid in more advanced states. Basal ganglion and frontal lobe dysfunction, respectively, account for these two gaits.

Disorders of Expression

Disorders of expression involve the motor aspects of communication and include (1) hypermimesis, (2) hypomimesis, and (3) dyspraxias and apraxias. Hypermimesis is a disinhibition phenomenon that most commonly manifests as pathologic laughter or crying. Pathologic laughter is associated with right hemisphere injury, and pathologic crying is associated with left hemisphere injury. The exact pathophysiology is not known. Hypomimesis manifests as aprosody, or the loss of voice modulation (pitch, speed, emphasis, emotion). Receptive aprosody involves an inability to *understand* emotion in speech and

Table 16-27	Dyspraxias and Apraxias	
Types	**Description**	**Location**
Ideomotor apraxia	Impairment in selecting, sequencing, and spatial orientation of movements involved in gestures (spatial and temporal production errors)	Left parietal cortex (angular gyrus) or supramarginal gyrus
Posterior form	Difficulty performing in response to command and imitation; cannot discriminate well between poorly performed and well-performed acts	Left parietal cortex (angular gyrus or supramarginal gyrus) lesion
Anterior form	Performs poorly to command and imitation but comprehends and discriminates pantomime	Lesions anterior to the supramarginal gyrus, which disconnects visual kinesthetic motor engrams from premotor and motor areas
Conduction apraxia	Greater impairment in performance when imitating movements than when pantomiming to command; comprehends pantomime and gesture but cannot perform the movements	Location unknown at this time
Disassociation apraxia	Inability to gesture normally to command and required verbal mediation has good performance with imitation and actual tools and objects	Callosal abnormalities but not all locations known
Ideational apraxia	Inability to carry out an ideational plan or a series of acts in the proper sequence	Location unclear at this time
Conceptual apraxia	Cannot recall type of action associated with specific tools, utensils, or objects (content and tool selection errors; may be unable to recall which tool is associated with a specific object or may have impaired mechanical knowledge)	Bilateral frontal and parietal dysfunction

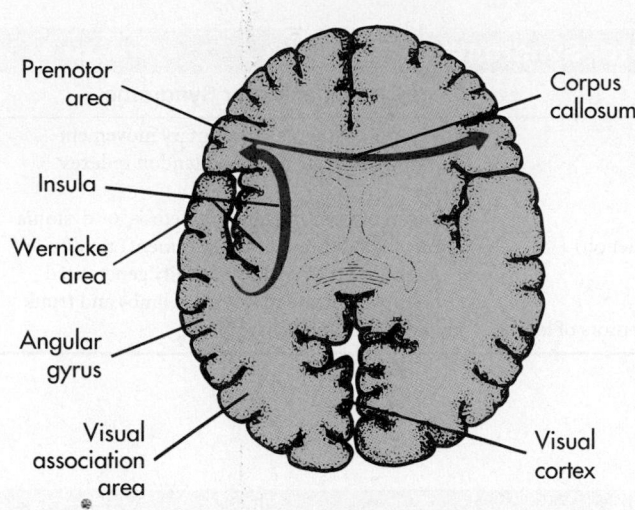

Figure 16-33 Pathways disrupted in dyspraxias. Formulation of the idea of the motor act is believed to originate in the region of the supramarginal gyrus in the inferior left parietal lobe. This area is connected via associational pathways to the left premotor cortex. The left premotor cortex is connected through the corpus callosum to the right premotor and motor areas. An injury that interrupts the pathways between the left supramarginal gyrus and the premotor region produces a dyspraxia that involves the entire body. An injury that disrupts the callosal pathways produces a dyspraxia of the left side of the body only.

facial expression, whereas expressive aprosody involves the inability to *express* emotion in speech and facial expression. Aprosody is associated with right hemisphere damage.

Dyspraxia is the partial inability and **apraxia** is the complete inability to perform purposeful or skilled motor acts in the absence of paralysis, sensory loss, abnormal posture and tone, abnormal involuntary movement, incoordination, or inattentiveness. These are disorders of learned skilled movements.[83] Dyspraxia and apraxia are associated with vascular disorders, trauma, tumor, degenerative disorders, infections, and metabolic disorders. The medial premotor cortex, including the supplementary motor area (SMA), appears to play a role in skilled movements as does the convexity premotor areas[83] (Table 16-27).

True dyspraxias occur when the connecting pathways between the left and right cortical areas are interrupted causing language-motor and motor representation disconnections between the hemispheres (Figure 16-33). Dyspraxias may result from any pathologic process that disrupts the cortical areas necessary for the conceptualization and execution of a complex motor act or the communication pathways within the left hemisphere or between the hemispheres.

Extrapyramidal Motor Syndromes

Because the extrapyramidal system encompasses all the motor pathways except the pyramidal system, two types of motor dysfunction make up the **extrapyramidal motor syndromes:** (1) the basal ganglia motor syndromes and (2) the cerebellar motor syndromes. Unlike pyramidal motor syndromes, both extrapyramidal motor syndromes result in movement or posture disturbance without significant paralysis, along with other distinctive symptoms (Table 16-28).

Basal Ganglia Motor Syndromes

Basal ganglia motor syndromes are movement disorders that involve either a paucity or an excess of movements. Stress and nervous tension typically worsen the symptoms, whereas relaxation improves motor performance. Akinesia may occur despite normal strength. Involuntary movements, such as tremor, chorea, ballism, athetosis, and dystonia, also may occur and probably are caused by the loss of the normal modulating effects of the corpus striatum and other parts of the basal ganglia.

Basal ganglia motor syndromes also are characterized by alterations in muscle tone and posture. Rigidity, together with the cogwheel phenomenon, is present in all muscle groups but is most prominent in those that maintain flexed position. Postural abnormalities result from the loss of normal postural reflexes. Dysfunctional equilibrium results from the loss of postural stability.

Cerebellar Motor Syndromes

Cerebellar motor syndromes involve the cerebellum and may result in (1) acute loss of muscle tone; (2) difficulty with coordination of voluntary movements (ataxia); (3) minor degrees of muscle weakness, tendency toward fatigue, and impairment of associated movements; and (4) disorders of equilibrium, posture, and gait. Cerebellar effects are chiefly ipsilateral (primarily affecting the same side of the body), so damage to the right cerebellum generally causes symptoms on the right side of the body. Predominant symptoms depend on the area of damage within the cerebellum. The three cerebellar syndromes are the rostral vermis, caudal vermis, and lateral syndromes[84] (Table 16-29).

Diagnosis of a cerebellar motor syndrome is based on the symptoms, but these may vary because of the individual's attempts at compensation. Further, the nervous system often can operate well despite destruction of parts of the cerebellum, although the mechanisms responsible for this retained function are not fully understood.

Table 16-28   Pyramidal versus Extrapyramidal Motor Syndromes

Manifestations	Pyramidal Motor Syndrome	Extrapyramidal Motor Syndrome
Unilateral movement	Paralysis of voluntary movement	Little or no paralysis of voluntary movement
Tendon reflexes	Increased tendon reflexes	Normal or slightly increased tendon reflexes
Babinski sign	Present	Absent
Involuntary movements	Absence of involuntary movements	Presence of tremor, chorea, athetosis, or dystonia
Muscle tone	Spasticity in muscles (e.g., clasp-knife phenomenon)	Plastic (equal throughout movement) rigidity or intermittent (cogwheel) rigidity generalized but predominate in flexors of limbs and trunk
	Hypertonia present in flexors of arms and extensors of legs	Hypotonia in cerebellar disease

Table 16-29   Cerebellar Motor Syndromes

Anatomic Location of Dysfunction	Characteristics
Rostral vermis (so-called *anterior lobe*)	Ataxia of stance and gait with varying degrees of instability of the trunk and ataxia of legs; anteroposterior body sway; presence of Romberg sign
Caudal vermis (including flocculonodular lobe)	Truncal, postural, and gait ataxia; omnidirectional body sway; Romberg negative; tendency to fall; saccadic slow pursuit, nystagmus; inability to suppress vestibulo-ocular reflex (doll's eyes)
Cerebellar hemisphere (neocerebellar syndrome)	Severe disturbance in ipsilateral limb movements; hypotonia in acute situation; dysmetria (extremity overshooting its target); decomposition of movement; kinetic tremor, past-pointing; deviation of gait; dysarthria
Pancerebellum	Ataxia of trunk and bilateral limbs; ataxia of gait and stance; dysarthria; oculomotor disturbance

Data from Timmann D, Diener HC: Coordination and ataxia. In Goetz GC, editor, *Textbook of clinical neurology,* St Louis, 2007, Saunders.

SUMMARY REVIEW

Alterations in Cognitive Systems

1. Full consciousness is an awareness of oneself and the environment and includes an ability to respond to external stimuli with a wide variety of responses.
2. Consciousness has two components: arousal and content of thought.
3. Decreased level of arousal can occur because of diffuse bilateral cortical dysfunction, bilateral subcortical (reticular formation, brainstem) dysfunction, or localized hemispheric dysfunction.
4. An alteration in breathing pattern and level of coma reflects the level of brain dysfunction.
5. Pupillary changes reflect changes in level of brainstem function, drug action, and response to hypoxia and ischemia.
6. Abnormal eye movements, including nystagmus and divergent gaze, reflect alterations in brainstem function.
7. Level of brain function manifests by changes in generalized motor responses or no responses.
8. Loss of cortical inhibition associated with decreased consciousness includes abnormal flexor and extensor movements.
9. Cerebral death or irreversible coma represents permanent brain damage; cardiac, respiratory, and other vital functions maintained.
10. Brain death or irreversible brain damage that includes an inability to maintain cardiac, respiratory, and other vital functions.
11. Arousal returns in the VS and MCS, but content of thought is absent or markedly reduced, respectively.
12. Seizures represent abnormal, excessive hypersynchronous discharges of cerebral neurons with transient alterations in brain function. Seizures may be generalized or focal. There are three categories of epileptic syndrome: location-related, generalized, and undetermined.
13. With a deficit in selective attention, mediated by the brainstem, parietal lobe structures, and the pulvinar nucleus of the thalamus, the individual cannot focus on selective stimuli and thus neglects those stimuli.
14. In dysmnesia and amnesia, some memories are not retrieved and new memories cannot be stored.
15. Frontal areas mediate vigilance, detection, and working memory. With a vigilance deficit, the person cannot maintain search and scanning activities. With a detection deficit, the person is unmotivated and unable to use feedback.
16. Some specific disorders of content of thought (cognition) are agnosias, dysphasias, acute confusional states, and dementias, including AD.
17. Agnosias are a defect of recognition and may be tactile, visual, or auditory. They are caused by dysfunction in the primary sensory area or the interpretive areas of the cerebral cortex.
18. Dysphasia is an impairment of comprehension or production of language. Dysphasia may be expressive or sensory.
19. Aphasia is loss of language comprehension or production.
20. Wernicke dysphasia is a disturbance in understanding all language—verbal and reading comprehension.

21. Conductive dysphasias result from disruption of temporal lobe fibers, with a failure to repeat words but an ability to initiate speech, writing, and reading aloud.
22. Anomic dysphasia is an inability to name objects, people, or qualities.
23. Transcortical dysphasias involve an ability to repeat and recite.
24. Broca aphasia is an expressive dysphasia of speech and writing but with retention of comprehension.
25. Global aphasia involves anterior and posterior speech areas, with expressive and receptive aphasia.
26. Acute confusional states are characterized chiefly by defects in attention and coherence of thoughts and actions and, in the case of delirium, an intense autonomic nervous system hyperactivity.
27. AD is a chronic, irreversible dementia.

Alterations in Cerebral Hemodynamics

1. Cerebral oxygenation is a critical management issue.
2. Cerebral perfusion pressure determines cerebral blood flow.
3. An injured brain may experience cerebral oligemia, normal cerebral blood flow but with increased intracranial pressure, or cerebral hyperemia.
4. Increased intracranial pressure may result from edema, excess CSF, hemorrhage, or tumor growth. When intracranial pressure approaches arterial pressure, hypoxia and hypercapnia produce brain damage.
5. Cerebral edema is an increase in the fluid content of the brain resulting from infection, hemorrhage, tumor, ischemia, infarct, or hypoxia.
6. The shifting or herniation of brain tissue from one compartment to another disrupts the blood flow of both compartments and damages brain tissue.
7. Supratentorial herniation involves temporal lobe and hippocampal gyrus shifting from the middle fossa to the posterior fossa; transtentorial herniation with a downward shift of the diencephalon through the tentorial notch; and shifting of the cingulate gyrus herniation under the falx.
8. The most common infratentorial herniation is a shift of the cerebellar tonsils through the foramen magnum.
9. Hydrocephalus comprises a variety of disorders characterized by an excess of fluid within the cranial vault, subarachnoid space, or both. Hydrocephalus occurs because of interference with CSF flow caused by increased fluid production or obstruction within the ventricular system or by defective reabsorption of the fluid.
10. Hydrocephalus can be treated by reducing CSF in the ventricles through the use of shunts and diuretic therapy if resection of the cause is not possible.

Alterations in Motor Function

1. Motor dysfunction may be characterized as alterations of motor tone, movement, and complex motor performance.
2. Hypotonia and hypertonia are the main categories of altered tone.
3. Four types of hypertonia exist: spasticity, gegenhalten, dystonia, and rigidity.
4. Paresis, paraplegia, hyperkinesia, and hypokinesia are the main categories of altered movement.
5. Two subtypes of paresis and paralysis are described: upper motor neuron and lower motor neuron.

6. An upper motor neuron syndrome is characterized by paresis or paralysis, hypertonia, and hyperreflexia.
7. Interruption of the pyramidal tract below the pons results in spinal shock.
8. Lower motor neuron syndromes manifest with impaired voluntary and involuntary movements.
9. Partial paralysis occurs with only partial loss of alpha motor neurons, and total paralysis is complete loss of alpha motor neurons. Loss of gamma motor neurons impairs muscle tone and decreases tendon reflexes.
10. Amyotrophy (e.g., poliomyelitis) is a lower motor neuron syndrome involving the anterior horn cells, with loss of muscle tone and strength resulting in segmental paresis and hyporeflexia.
11. Nuclear palsies involve damage to the cranial nerve nuclei.
12. Bulbar palsies involve cranial nerves IX, X, and XII.
13. Included in the category of hyperkinesia are chorea, athetosis, ballism, akathisia, tremor, and myoclonus.
14. HD (chorea) is a rare hereditary disease involving the basal ganglia and cerebral cortex. It is inherited as an autosomal dominant trait and commonly manifests between 25 and 45 years of age.
15. The major pathologic feature of HD is severe degeneration of the basal ganglia and the frontal cerebral cortex. The basal ganglia and the substantia nigra exhibit a depletion of neurons that secrete GABA (an inhibitory neurotransmitter). This depletion leads to an excess of dopaminergic activity that causes involuntary, fragmentary movements.
16. No known treatment is effective in halting the degenerative process in HD.
17. Types of hypokinesia include akinesia, bradykinesia, and loss of associated movements.
18. PD is a common degenerative disorder of the basal ganglia (corpus striatum) involving degeneration of the dopamine-secreting nigrostriatal pathway.
19. Degeneration of the dopaminergic nigrostriatal pathway allows overactivity by the STN to excessively inhibit motor thalamus and motor cortex causing rigidity and bradykinesia. Progressive dementia may be associated with an advanced stage of the disease.
20. Treatment of PD is symptomatic, involving levodopa (L-dopa), a precursor of dopamine.
21. Alterations in complex motor performance include disorders of posture (stance), disorders of gait, and disorders of expression.
22. Disorders of posture include dystonic posture, decerebrate posture, basal ganglion posture, and senile posture.
23. Disorders of gait include upper motor neuron gaits, cerebellar gait, basal ganglion gait, and senile gait.
24. Disorders of expression include hypermimesis, hypomimesis, and dyspraxia or apraxia.
25. Dyspraxia is an impairment of the conceptualization or execution of a complex motor act.
26. Extrapyramidal motor syndromes include basal ganglia and cerebellar motor syndromes.
27. Basal ganglia disorders manifest with alterations in muscle tone and posture, including rigidity, involuntary movements, and loss of postural reflexes.
28. Cerebellar motor syndromes result in loss of muscle tone, difficulty with coordination, and disorders of equilibrium and gait.

KEY TERMS

Acute confusional state (acute cerebral failure, acute brain failure), 548
Acute hydrocephalus, 560
Agnosia, 546
Akinesia, 571
Akinetic mutism (AM), 535
Alzheimer disease (dementia of Alzheimer type [DAT], senile disease complex), 553
Amyotrophy, 567
Aphasia, 546
Apraxia, 577
Areflexia, 566
Aura, 542
Autoregulation, 558
Basal ganglia motor syndrome, 577
Basal ganglion gait, 576
Basal ganglion posture, 576
Bradykinesia, 571
Brain death (brainstem death), 534
Bulbar palsy, 568
Central (transtentorial) herniation, 559
Cerebellar gait, 576
Cerebellar motor syndrome, 577
Cerebral death (irreversible coma), 534
Cerebral edema, 559
Cheyne-Stokes respiration, 531
Cingulate gyrus herniation (subfalcine herniation, transfalcial herniation), 559
Clonic phase, 538
Cogwheel rigidity, 573
Coma, 528
Communicating (extraventricular) hydrocephalus, 560
Content of thought, 528
Convulsion, 536
Cryogenic epilepsy, 542
Cytotoxic (metabolic) edema, 560
Decerebrate posture, 575
Declarative memory, 543
Decorticate posture (antigravity posture, hemiplegic posture), 575
Dementia, 543
Diplegia, 564
Dysmnesia, 543
Dysphasia, 546
Dyspraxia, 577

Dystonia, 575
Dystonic movement, 575
Dystonic posture, 575
Echolalia, 548
Epilepsy, 539
Epileptogenesis, 538
Epileptogenic focus, 538
Extinction, 542
Extrapyramidal motor syndrome, 577
Flaccid paralysis, 566
Flaccid paresis, 566
Freezing, 571
Gamma neuropathy, 566
Gegenhalten (paratonia), 563
Generalized seizure, 536
Hemiparesis, 564
Hemiplegia, 564
Huntington disease (HD), 570
Hydrocephalus, 560
Hydrocephalus ex vacuo, 560
Hyperkinesia, (excessive movement), 568
Hypertonia (increased muscle tone), 562
Hypokinesia (decreased movement), 571
Hypotonia (decreased muscle tone), 562
Idiopathic epilepsy, 539
Increased intracranial pressure, 557
Interstitial edema, 560
Intracranial pressure, 557
Isolated (pure) vigilance defect, 544
Locked-in syndrome, 535
Memory, 543
Minimally conscious state (MCS), 535
Mirror focus, 539
Neglect syndrome, 542
Neurofibrillary tangle, 554
Noncommunicating hydrocephalus, 560
Nondeclarative memory (nonconscious), 543
Normal-pressure hydrocephalus (low, adult, occult hydrocephalus), 560
Nuclear palsy, 567
Paralysis, 564
Paraparesis, 564
Paraplegia, 564
Paresis (weakness), 564
Parkinson disease (PD), 572

Parkinsonian bradykinesia, 573
Parkinsonian rigidity, 523
Parkinsonian tremor, 573
Parkinsonism (Parkinson syndrome, parkinsonian syndrome), 572
Paroxysmal dyskinesia, 569
Partial seizure (focal seizure), 536
Plastic rigidity, 573
Posthyperventilation apnea (PHVA), 531
Postictal state, 536
Prodroma, 542
Prognosis in coma, 535
Progressive bulbar palsy, 568
Progressive spinal muscular atrophy, 567
Pyramidal motor syndrome, 564
Quadriparesis, 564
Quadriplegia, 564
Rigidity, 563
Scissors gait, 576
Secondary generalization, 536
Seizure, 536
Seizure initiation, 538
Selective attention deficit (orientation), 543
Senile gait, 576
Senile plaque, 554
Senile posture, 576
Sensory inattentiveness, 542
Spastic gait, 576
Spasticity, 563
Spinal shock, 565
Status epilepticus, 536
Symptomatic epilepsy, 539
Tardive dyskinesia, 569
Tonic phase, 538
Transcortical dysphasia (transcortical sensory dysphasia, mixed transcortical dysphasia, isolated speech center), 548
Uncal herniation (hippocampal herniation, lateral mass herniation), 559
Vasogenic edema, 560
Vegetative state (VS), 535
Vigilance, 544
Working memory deficit, 544

REFERENCES

1. Stevens RD, Nyquist PA: Types of brain dysfunction in critical illness, *Neurol Clin* 26(2):469-486, 2008.
2. Ropper AH: Coma. In Fauci AS, et al, editors: *Harrison's principles of internal medicine*, ed 15 , New York, 2008, McGraw-Hill.
3. Posner JB et al: *Plum and Posner's diagnosis of stupor and coma*, ed 4, New York, 2007, Oxford University Press.
4. McNett M: A review of the predictive ability of Glasgow Coma Scale scores in head-injured patients, *J Neurosci Nurs* 39(2):68-75, 2007.
5. Saatman KE et al: Classification of traumatic brain injury for targeted therapies, *J Neurotrauma* 25(7):719-738, 2008.
6. Bleck TP: Levels of consciousness and attention. In Gottez CG, editor: *Textbook of clinical neurology,* Philadelphia, 2003, Saunders.
7. Drazkowski J: Determining brain death: back to the basics, *Semin Neurol* 27(4):393-399, 2007.
8. Greer DM et al: Variability of brain death determination guidelines in leading US neurologic institutions, *Neurology* 70(4):284-289, 2008.
9. Task Force for the Determination of Brain Death in Children: guidelines for the determination of brain death in children, *Arch Neurol* 44(6):587-588, 1987.
10. Young GB et al: Brief review: the role of ancillary test in the neurological determination of death, *Can J Anaesth* 53(6):62-67, 2006.
11. Boss BJ, Fletcher A: Severe brain injury rehabilitation: what's going to happen after critical care? *Crit Care Nurs Clin* 13(3):421-431, 2001.
12. Owen AM et al: Detecting awareness in the vegetative state, *Science* 313(5792):1402, 2006.

13. Owen AM: Disorders of consciousness, *Ann N Y Acad Sci* 1124:225-238, 2008.

14. Widjdicks EF, Cranford RE: clinical diagnosis of prolonged states of impaired consciousness in adults, *Mayo Clin Proc* 80(8):1037-1046, 2005.

15. Smith E, Delargy M: Locked-in syndrome, *BMJ* 330(7488):406-409, 2005.

16 Lowenstein DH: Seizures and epilepsy. In Fauci AS, et al, editors: *Harrison's principles of internal medicine*, ed 15, New York, 2008, McGraw-Hill.

17. Tuxhorn I, Kotagal P: Classification, *Semin Neurol* 28(3):277-288, 2008.

18. Feen ES, Bershad EM, Suarez JI: Status epilepticus, *South Med J* 101(4):400-406, 2008.

19. Scharfman HE: The neurobiology of epilepsy, *Curr Neurol Neurosci Rep* 7(4):348-354, 2007.

20. Pitkanen A et al: Epileptogenesis in experimental models, *Epilepsia* 48(Suppl 2):13-20, 2007.

21. Crino PB: Gene expression, genetics, and genomics in epilepsy: some answers, more questions, *Epilepsia* 48(Suppl 2):42-50, 2007.

22. Berg AT, Blackstone NW: Concepts in classification and their relevance to epilepsy, *Epilepsy Res* 70(Suppl 1):S11-S19, 2006.

23. *BMJ clinical evidence handbook*, London, 2007, BMJ Publishing Company.

24. Bate H et al: The seizure outcome after amygdalohippocampectomy and temporal lobectomy, *Eur J Neurol* 14(1):90-94, 2007.

25. Ramani R: Vagus nerve stimulation therapy for seizures, *J Neurosurg Anesthesiol* 20(1):29-35, 2008.

26. Elliott J, Shneker B: Patient, caregiver, and health care practitioner knowledge of, beliefs about, and attitudes toward epilepsy, *Epilepsy Behav* 12(4):547-556, 2008.

27. Boss BJ, Wilkerson R: Communication: language and pragmatics. In Hoeman SP, editor: *Rehabilitation nursing: prevention, intervention, & outcomes*, ed 4, St Louis, 2008, Mosby.

28. Gabrieli JDE et al: Memory. In Goetz CG, editor: *Textbook of clinical neurology*, Philadelphia, 2003, Saunders.

29. LaVoie DJ, Cobia DJ: Recollecting, recognizing and other act of remembering: an overview of human memory, *J Neurol Phys Ther* 31(3):135-144, 2007.

30. Manns JR, Eichenbaum H: Learning and memory: brain systems. In Squire LR et al, editors: *Fundamental neuroscience*, ed 3, Burlington, MA, 2008, Academic Press.

31. Timmann D, Daum I: Cerebellar contributions to cognitive functions: a progress report after two decades of research, *Cerebellum* 6(3):159-161, 2007.

32. Buchanan TW: Retrieval of emotional memories, *Psychol Bull* 133(5):761-779, 2007.

33. Carbeza R: Role of the parietal regions in episodic memory retrieval: the dual attentional processes hypothesis, *Neurophsychologia* 46(7):1813-1827, 2008.

34. Osada T et al: Towards understanding of the cortical network underlying associative memory, *Philos Trans R Soc Lond B Biol Sci* 363(1500):2187-2199, 2008.

35. Fisher S: On genes, speech and language, *N Engl J Med* 353(16):1655-1657, 2005.

36. Haines J, Camarata S: Examination of candidate genes in language disorder: a model of genetic association for treatment studies, *Ment Retard Develop Res Rev* 10(3):208-217, 2004.

37. Josephson SA, Miller BL: Confusion and delirium. In Fauci AS et al, editors: *Harrison's principles of internal medicine*, ed 15, New York, 2008, McGraw-Hill.

38. Guntehr ML, Morandi A, Ely EW: Pathophysiology of delirium in the intensive care unit, *Crit Care Clin* 24(1):45-65, 2008.

39. Drachman DA: Aging of the brain, entropy, and Alzheimer disease, *Neurology* 67(8):1340-1352, 2006.

40. Caselli RJ, Boeve BF: The degenerative dementias. In Goetz CG, editor: *Textbook of clinical neurology*, Philadelphia, 2003, Saunders.

41. Bird TD, Miller BL: Dementia. In Fauci AS, et al, editors: *Harrison's principles of internal medicine*, ed 15, New York, 2008, McGraw-Hill.

42. Alzheimer's Association: *2006 national public policy program to conquer Alzheimer's disease*. Available at www.alz.org. Accessed November 30, 2007.

43. Bertram L, Tanzi RE: Thirty years of Alzheimer's disease genetics: the implications of systemic meta-analyses, *Nat Rev Neurosci* 9(10):768-778, 2008.

44. Bird TD: Genetic aspects of Alzheimer disease, *Genet Med* 10(4):231-239, 2008.

45. Ertekin-Taner N: Genetics of Alzheimer's disease: a centennial review, *Neurol Clin* 25(3):611-667, 2007.

46. Auerhalm C: Recognition of risk factors and screening tools: optimizing care for patients with Alzheimer's disease: emerging treatment strategies, *J Acad Nurs Pract* (Suppl) 16(1):4-5, 2004.

47. Jellinger KA: Alzheimer's disease. In Gilman S, editor: *Neurobiology of disease*, ed 1, Burlington, MA, 2007, Academic Press.

48. Mele D: Cognitive, functional and behavioral decline in Alzheimer's disease: optimizing care for patients with Alzheimer's disease: emerging treatment strategies, *J Acad Nurs Pract* (Suppl) 16(1):6-7, 2004.

49. Feldman HH et al: Diagnosis and treatment of dementia: 2 Diagnosis, *CMAJ* 178(7):825-836, 2008.

50. Wang XP, Ding HL: Alzheimer's disease: epidemiology, genetics and beyond, *Neurosci Bull* 24(2):105-109, 2008.

51. Hogan DB et al: Diagnosis and treatment of dementia: Approach to management of mild to moderate dementia, *CMAJ* 179(8):787-793, 2008.

52. van Marum RJ: Current and future therapy in Alzheimer's disease, *Fund Clin Pharmacol* 22(3):265-274, 2008.

53. Marmarou A: A review of progress in understanding the pathophysiology and treatment of brain edema, *Neurosurg Focus* 22(5):E1, 2007.

54. Factora R, Luciano M: When to consider normal pressure hydrocephalus in the patient with gait disturbance, *Geriatrics* 63(2): 332-337, 2008.

55. Correll CU, Schenk EM: Tardive dyskinesia and new antipsychotics, *Curr Opin Psychiatry* 21(2):151-156, 2008.

56. Olanow CW: Hyperkinetic movement disorders. In Fauci AS et al, editors: *Harrison's principles of internal medicine*, ed 15, New York, 2008, McGraw-Hill.

57. Imarisio S et al: Huntington's disease: from pathology and genetics to potential therapies, *Biochem J* 412(2):191-209, 2008.

58. Jankovic J: Movement disorders. In Goetz CG, editor: *Textbook of clinical neurology*, Philadelphia, 2003, Saunders.

59. Hersch SM, Rosas HD: Neuroprotection for Huntington's disease, *Neurotherapeutics* 5(2):226-236, 2008.

60. Galvcz-Jimincz H: Parkinson's disease. In Gilman S, editor: *Neurobiology of disease*, ed 1, Burlington, MA, 2007, Academic Press.

61. Galvan A, Wichmann T: Pathophysiology of parkinsonism, *Clin Neurophysiol* 119(7):1459-1474, 2008.

62. Wakabayashi K et al: The Lewy body in Parkinson's disease: molecules implicated in the formation and degradation of alpha-synuclein aggregates, *Neuropathology* 27(5):494-506, 2007.

63. Rommelfanger KS, Weinshenker D: Norepinephrine: the redheaded stepchild of Parkinson's disease, *Biochem Pharmacol* 74(2): 177-190, 2007.

64. Fasano M, Lopiano L: Alpha-synuclein and Parkinson's disease: a protcomic view, *Exp Rev Proteomics* 5(2):239-248, 2008.

65. Thomas B, Beal MF: Parkinson's disease, *Hum Mol Genet* 16(Spec No 2):R183-R194, 2007.

66. Probst A, Block A, Tolnay M: New insights into the pathology of Parkinson's disease: does the peripheral autonomic nervous system become central? *Eur J Neurol* 15(Suppl 1):1-4, 2008.

67. Hoehn M, Yahr M: Parkinsonism: onset, progression and mortality, *Neurology* 17(5):427-442, 1967.

68. Wolters E: Variablility in the clinical expression of Parkinson's disease: *J Neurol Sci* 266(1-2):197-203, 2008.

69. Rivlin-Etzion M et al: Basal ganglia oscillations and pathophysiology of movement disorders, *Curr Opin Neurobiol* 16(6):629-637, 2006.

70. Jankovic J: Parkinson's disease: clinical features and diagnosis, *J Neurol Neurosurg Psychiatry* 79(4):368-376, 2008.

71. Goldstein DS: Cardiac denervation in patients with Parkinson disease, *Cleve Clin J Med* 74(Suppl 1):S91-S94, 2007.

72. Dhawan V et al: Sleep-related problems of Parkinson's disease, *Age Ageing* 35(3):220-228, 2006.

73. Troung DD, Bhidayasiri R, Wikters E: Management of non-motor symptoms in advanced Parkinson disease, *J Neurol Sci* 266(1-2):216-228, 2008.

74. Baker JH: The symptom experience of patients with Parkinson disease, *J Neurosci Nurs* 38(1):51-57, 2006.

75. Defer GL et al: Core assessment program for surgical interventional therapies in Parkinson's disease (CAPSIT-PD), *Mov Disord* 14(4):572-584, 1999.

76. Geriach M et al: Early detection of Parkinson's disease: unmet needs, *Neurodegener Dis* 5(3-4):137-139, 2008.

77. Jankovic J, Stacy M: Medical management of levodopa-associated motor complications in patients with Parkinson's disease, *CNS Drugs* 21(8):677-692, 2007.

78. Guridi J et al: L-Dopa-induced dyskinesia and stereotactic surgery for Parkinson's disease, *Neurosurgery* 62(2):311-323, 2008.

79. Yu H, Neimat JS: The treatment of movement disorders by deep brain stimulation, *Neurotherapeutics* 5(1):26-36, 2008.

80. Goya RL, Kuah WL, Barker RA: The future of cell therapies in the treatment of Parkinson's disease, *Expert Opin Biol Ther* 7(10):1487-1498, 2007.

81. Chan DK, Cordato DJ, O'Rourke F: Management for motor and non-motor complications in late Parkinson's disease, *Geriatrics* 63(5):22-27, 2008.

82. Sapir S, Ramig L, Fox C: Speech and swallowing disorders in Parkinson disease, *Curr Opin Otolaryngol Head Neck Surg* 16(3):205-210, 2008.

83. Heilman KM, Watson RT, Gonzalez-Rothi LJ: Praxis. In Goetz CG, editor: *Textbook of clinical neurology*, Philadelphia, 2003, Saunders.

84. Timmann D, Diener HC: Coordination and ataxia. In Goetz GC, editor: *Textbook of clinical neurology*, Philadelphia, 2003, Saunders.

DISORDERS OF THE CENTRAL AND PERIPHERAL NERVOUS SYSTEMS AND THE NEUROMUSCULAR JUNCTION

BARBARA J. BOSS

MEDIA RESOURCES

 Evolve Website (http://evolve.elsevier.com/McCance/)
- Review Questions and Answers
- Animations
- Glossary (with audio pronunciation for selected terms)
- WebLinks

Online Course
- Module 10

CHAPTER OUTLINE

CENTRAL NERVOUS SYSTEM DISORDERS
Trauma
Degenerative Disorders of the Spine
Cerebrovascular Disorders
Headache
Tumors of the Central Nervous System
Infection and Inflammation of the Central Nervous
    System

Demyelinating Disorders
Neurodegenerative Disorders
**PERIPHERAL NERVOUS SYSTEM
AND NEUROMUSCULAR JUNCTION DISORDERS**
Peripheral Nervous System Disorders
Neuromuscular Junction Disorders

Alterations in central nervous system (CNS) function are caused by traumatic injury, vascular disorders, tumor growth, infectious and inflammatory processes, metabolic derangements (including those arising from nutritional deficiencies and drugs/chemicals), and degenerative processes. Alterations in peripheral nervous system function involve the nerve roots (radiculopathies), a nerve plexus, or the nerves themselves (neuropathies). Disorders of the neuromuscular junction also occur.

CENTRAL NERVOUS SYSTEM DISORDERS

Trauma

Brain Trauma

Traumatic brain injury (TBI) is defined by the Brain Injury Association of America as a traumatic insult to the brain capable of producing physical, intellectual, emotional, social, and vocational changes. Of the 1.4 million traumatic brain injuries in the United States each year, 1.1 million are treated and released from emergency departments and 235,000 require hospitalization[1]: 80% have mild TBIs, 10% moderate

TBIs, and 10% severe TBIs.[2] The Glasgow Coma Scale (GCS) is used to describe injury severity by the international and United States National Traumatic Coma Data Banks. The hallmark of a severe TBI is loss of consciousness for 6 hours or more. TBI classifications using the GCS are (1) mild TBI with GCS of 13 to 15, associated with mild concussion; (2) moderate TBI with GCS of 9 to 12, associated with structural injury such as hemorrhage or contusion; and (3) severe TBI with GCS of 3 to 8, associated with cognitive and/or physical disability or death. Age and admission GCS are important diagnostic factors in TBI.[2]

At highest risk for TBI are young persons 15 to 35 years of age, infants 6 months to 2 years, young school-age children, and adults older than 70 years of age. Males are 1.5 times as likely to sustain a TBI.[1] TBI is highest among blacks in lower-median income families. Persons living in high-crime areas are at greater risk and blacks have the highest mortality rates.[1]

TBI is broadly categorized into **blunt (closed, nonmissile) trauma** and **open (penetrating, missile) trauma.** Blunt trauma, the more common injury, involves the head striking a hard surface or a rapidly moving object striking the head. The dura mater remains intact, and brain tissues are not exposed to the environment. Blunt trauma may result in both focal brain injuries and diffuse axonal injuries (Table 17-1). When a break in (penetration of) the dura mater results in exposure of the cranial contents to the environment, open trauma has occurred, which results in focal brain injuries.

The most common types of brain injury are mild concussion and classic cerebral concussion (see page 590). Of all head injuries, 75% to 90% are not severe. Focal brain injury and diffuse axonal injury (DAI) each account for half of all injuries. Focal brain injury accounts for more than two thirds of head injury deaths; DAI, for less than one third. However, DAI accounts for the greatest number of severely disabled survivors, including persons who persist in an unresponsive state or reduced level of consciousness.

In recent years the surviving TBI population has changed, mostly because of focus on reducing severity of injury (e.g., passive seat restraints, air bags), reduced transport time, and improved on-the-scene medical management. Management of secondary and tertiary injury has improved; acute care professionals are focusing more on morbidity than mortality. As a result, individuals with more severe TBIs are admitted to rehabilitation programs.

Causes of Brain Trauma

Most TBIs are caused by falls (28%), motor vehicle crashes (20%), being struck by moving objects or moving against stationary objects (19%), and assaults (11%).[1] Sports-related events also account for a portion of TBIs. Blasts are the leading cause of TBIs for active duty personnel.[3]

Compound fractures are caused by objects striking the head with great force or by the head striking an object forcefully. The comments regarding contusion (see page 585) hold true for compound fractures. Temporal blows, related to basilar skull fractures, may produce a fracture involving the middle fossa. An occipital blow may result in a basilar fracture down the occipital bone and across the petrous pyramid. The cervical vertebrae upwardly impacting the base of the skull can produce a posterior fossa **basilar skull fracture.**

Causes of **penetrating injuries** are missiles (most commonly bullets fired from rifles and handguns) and sharp projectiles (e.g., knives, ice picks, axes, screwdrivers). Most through-and-through (enter the head on one side and exit on the other) injuries are from high-velocity bullets.

Brain damage originates from primary and secondary brain injury. *Primary injury* is caused by the direct impact and involves the initial tear, neural injury and hemorrhage. In primary glial injury, oligodendroglia are affected by axon injury and by direct mechanical disruption caused by debris and leakage. *Secondary injury* includes intracranial and extracranial causes of brain damage. Intracranial brain damage is complex and occurs as a result of impairment of cerebral blood flow autoregulation, alterations in the blood-brain barrier, cerebral edema, increased intracranial pressure (ICP),

Table 17-1   Severity of Trauma Related to Injury, Onset, and Persistence

| Severity of Trauma | Trauma State Induced | | Onset of Clinical Manifestations | Persistence of DAI Clinical Manifestations |
	Focal Injury	DAI		
Mild blunt trauma		Mild concussion	Immediate	Hours to days
Moderate blunt trauma		Classic cerebral concussion	Immediate	Up to 6 months or longer
	Paraplegia (associated with injury to top of head)		Immediate	
	Blindness (associated with occipital injury)		Immediate	
	Delayed development of unresponsiveness (vasomotor or vasovagal syncopal episode)		Delayed	
Severe blunt trauma		Mild DAI	Immediate	Permanent residual
		Moderate DAI	Immediate	
		Severe DAI	Immediate	
	Acute epidural hemorrhage		Immediate to delayed (2-3 hours)	
	Acute contusional swelling		Delayed onset (few hours after injury)	
	Acute subdural hematoma		Delayed onset (few hours to 1 week after injury)	
	Subacute subdural hematoma*		Delayed onset (1 to few weeks)	
	Subdural hygroma		Delayed onset	
	Traumatic cerebral hemorrhage*		Delayed onset (as late as 1 week after injury)	

*May be seen after moderate head injury, especially in older adults.
DAI, Diffuse axonal injury.

brain herniation, a decrease in cerebral perfusion pressure and inflammation. Significant to secondary injury is tissue hypoxia arising from cerebral ischemia (inadequate perfusion and tissue hypoxia). Consequences of ischemia are as follows: (1) ischemic neurons release substances that produce glial permeability to sodium (cytotoxic edema); (2) with energy failure, influxes of calcium through incompetent channels produce axonal injury, mitochondrial swelling, and cell death; and (3) lactic acidosis. Tertiary causes of brain injury occur from compromised systemic circulation with hypotension and shock or inadequate pulmonary ventilation, or both. Traumatic brain injury can be focal or diffuse. Focal injury occurs in a specific area of the brain and includes contusions and hematomas. Diffuse injury involves more than one area and includes diffuse axonal injury and concussion.

Focal Brain Injury. **Focal brain injury** is specific and involves grossly observable brain lesions. The force of impact (translational acceleration) typically produces brain contusions (bruises from blood seeping from microhemorrhages into brain tissue) and intracranial bleeding that displaces brain tissue (i.e., extradural, subdural, and intracerebral hematomas). Contusion and bleeding occur because of small tears in blood vessels resulting from these forces. The focal injury may be **coup** (directly below the point of impact) or **contrecoup** (on the pole opposite the site of impact) (Figure 17-1). Objects (e.g., baseball bat, weapon) striking the front of the head usually produce only coup injuries (contusions and fractures) because the inner skull in the occipital area is smooth. Objects striking the back of the head usually result in both coup and contrecoup injuries because of the irregularity of the inner surface of the frontal bones (see Figure 17-1). Objects striking the side of the head may produce coup or contrecoup injuries. The same is true when the head strikes an immovable object with little velocity (e.g., a short fall). Brain edema forms around and in damaged neural tissues, contributing to the increasing ICP. Within the contused areas are infarction and necrosis, multiple hemorrhages, and edema. The tissue has a pulpy quality. The maximum effects of injury related to contusion, bleeding, and edema peak 18 to 36 hours after severe head injury.

Contusions (Figure 17-2) are found most commonly in the frontal lobes, particularly at the poles and along the inferior orbital surfaces; in the temporal lobes, especially in the anterior poles and along the inferior surface; and at the frontotemporal junction. The severity of contusion is associated with the amount of energy transmitted by the skull to underlying brain tissue. In addition, the smaller the area of impact, the greater the severity of injury because the force is concentrated into a smaller area. Contusions result in changes in attention, memory, executive attentional function (motivation, goal selection or formation, planning, self-monitoring, and use of feedback), affect, emotion, and behavior. Less commonly, contusions occur in the parietal and occipital lobes. Focal cerebral contusions are superficial, involving just the gyri. Hemorrhagic contusions may coalesce into a large, confluent intracranial hematoma.

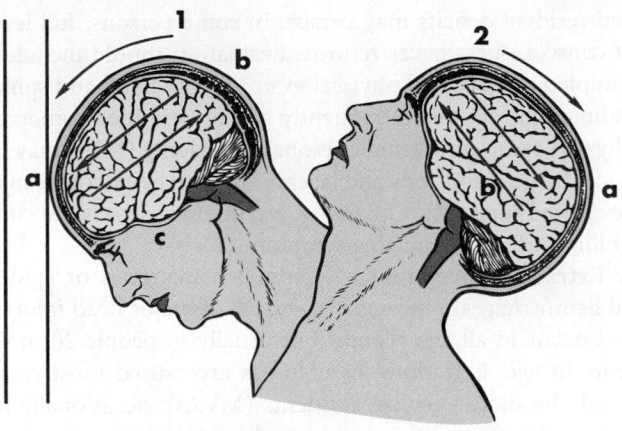

Figure 17-1 Coup and contrecoup brain injury following blunt trauma. 1, Coup injury: impact against object; *a*, site of impact and direct trauma to brain; *b*, shearing of subdural veins; *c*, trauma to base of brain. 2, Contrecoup injury: impact within skull, *a*, site of impact from brain hitting opposite side of skull; *b*, shearing forces through brain. These injuries occur in one continuous motion—the head strikes the wall (coup) and then rebounds (contrecoup). (Modified from Rudy EB: *Advanced neurological and neurosurgical nursing*, St Louis, 1984, Mosby.)

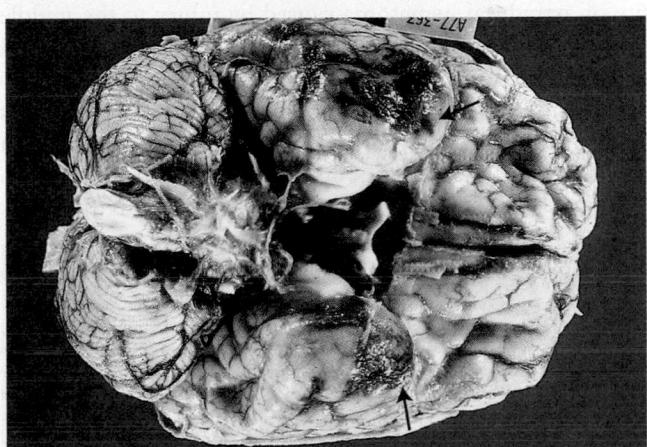

Figure 17-2 Cerebral contusions. The temporal poles are discolored by areas of hemorrhage *(arrows)*. Such lesions represent "bruises" on the surface of the brain caused by violent contact between the delicate brain parenchyma and the hard inner surface of the skull. (From Kumar V, Cotran RS, Robbins SL: *Robbins basic pathology*, ed 7, Philadelphia, 2003, Saunders.)

The clinical manifestations of a *contusion* may include immediate loss of consciousness (generally accepted to last no longer than 5 minutes); loss of reflexes, which results in the individual falling to the ground; transient cessation of respiration; brief period of bradycardia; and decrease in blood pressure (lasting 30 seconds to a few minutes). A momentary increase in cerebrospinal fluid (CSF) pressure and changes on electrocardiogram (ECG) and electroencephalogram (EEG) have been demonstrated to occur on impact. Vital signs may stabilize to normal values in a few seconds. Reflexes return next and the person begins to regain consciousness. Returning to being fully awake and alert can vary from minutes to days. Regaining a full level of consciousness may be extremely slow and residual deficits may persist. In some persons, full level of consciousness never returns. Evaluation should include a complete history and physical examination. Skull and spinal radiographs are taken frequently and a computed tomography (CT) scan or magnetic resonance imaging (MRI) may be done. Large contusions and lacerations with hemorrhage may be excised surgically. Otherwise, treatment is directed at controlling ICP and managing symptoms.

Extradural hematomas (epidural hematomas or epidural hemorrhages) represent 1% to 2% of major head injuries and occur in all age groups, but usually in people 20 to 40 years of age. Extradural hematomas are caused most commonly by motor vehicle accidents (MVAs), occasionally by minor falls and sporting accidents. A temporal fracture causes 90% of temporal lobe extradural hematomas. Direct frontal lobe trauma is associated with frontal extradural hematomas. Posterior extradural hematomas are associated with a fracture across the transverse sinus from an occipital blow.

An artery is the source of bleeding in 85% of extradural hematomas (Figure 17-3); 15% result from injury to the meningeal vein or dural sinus. Ninety percent of individuals also have a skull fracture. The temporal fossa is the most common site of extradural hematoma caused by injury to the middle meningeal artery or vein. The resulting shift of the temporal lobe medially precipitates uncal and hippocampal gyrus herniation through the tentorial notch. Extradural hemorrhages are found occasionally in the subfrontal area (especially in the young and older adult populations), caused by injury to

the anterior meningeal artery or a venous sinus, and in the occipital-suboccipital area, which results in herniation of the posterior fossa contents through the foramen magnum. CT and MRI show a lens-shaped mass over the surface of the cortex.

Individuals with classic *temporal extradural hematomas* (i.e., over the temporal lobe) experience loss of consciousness at the time of injury, followed by a lucid period that lasts from a few hours to a few days in one third of individuals (if bleeding from a vein). As the hematoma accumulates, a headache of increasing severity, vomiting, drowsiness, confusion, seizure, and hemiparesis may develop. Level of consciousness may dwindle rapidly as temporal lobe herniation begins. Clinical manifestations of temporal lobe herniation also include ipsilateral pupillary dilation and contralateral hemiparesis.

The diagnosis of an extradural hematoma is usually made by CT or MRI. In some instances, diagnosis is made by history and clinical findings, because time for a CT or MRI is not available. The prognosis is usually good if intervention is initiated before bilateral dilation of the pupils. Surgical therapy is evacuation of the hematoma through burr holes, followed by ligation of the bleeding vessel or vessels. Extradural hematomas are almost always medical emergencies.

Subdural hematomas arise in 10% to 20% of TBIs. MVAs are the most common cause of subdural hematomas; 50% of subdural hematomas are associated with skull fractures. Falls, especially in older adults or in those with long-term alcohol abuse, are associated with chronic subdural hematomas.

Acute subdural hematomas rapidly develop (within 48 hours) and usually are located at the top of the skull (the cerebral convexities). On CT they appear as a high-density mass. Bilateral hematomas occur in 15% to 20% of persons. Subacute subdural hematomas develop more slowly, often over 48 hours to 2 weeks. On CT they appear as a mixed-density mass. Chronic subdural hematomas (commonly found in older adults and those who abuse alcohol who have some degree of brain atrophy with a subsequent increase in the extradural space) develop over weeks to months. Tearing of the bridging veins is the major cause of rapidly developing and subacutely developing subdural hematomas, although torn cortical veins or venous sinuses and contused tissue may be the source. These subdural hematomas act as expanding masses, giving rise to increased ICP that eventually compresses the bleeding vessels (Figures 17-4 and 17-5). The displacement of brain tissue can result in a herniation syndrome.

In *acute, rapidly developing subdural hematomas* the expanding clots directly compress the brain, giving rise to the clinical manifestations. As the ICP rises the bleeding veins are compressed and thus bleeding is self-limiting, although cerebral compression and displacement of brain tissue can cause temporal lobe herniation.

An *acute subdural hematoma* classically begins with headache, drowsiness, restlessness or agitation, slowed cognition, and confusion. These symptoms worsen over time and progress to loss of consciousness, respiratory pattern changes, and pupillary dilation (the symptoms of temporal lobe herniation). These manifestations are more pronounced than focal

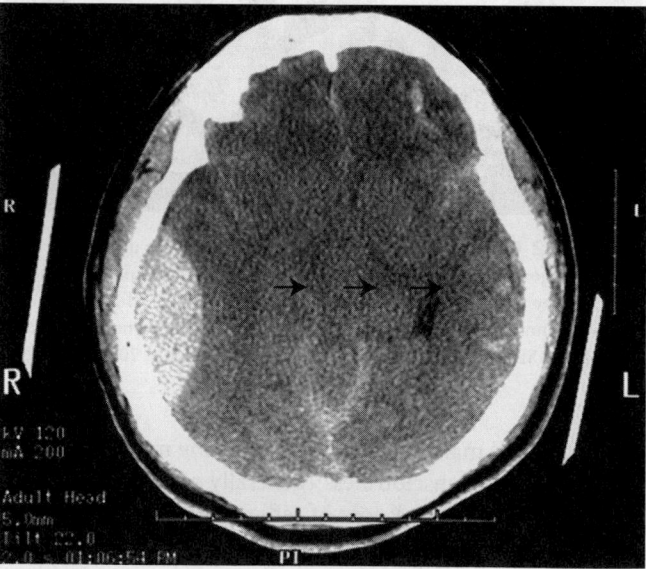

Figure 17-3 Epidural hematoma, CT image. Note the large right epidural hematoma with a lens-shaped outline as the smooth dura becomes indented against the underlying cortex on the right lateral aspect of the cerebrum. The epidural hematoma is confined within an area bounded by cranial sutures where the dura is firmly adherent to the skull. Note the mass effect with effacement of the lateral ventricles and the shift of midline to the left (*arrows*). In this case the individual fell from a height and struck the right side of his head, severing the middle meningeal artery. This epidural hematoma collected within hours. *CT,* Computed tomography. (From Klatt EC: *Robbins and Cotran atlas of pathology,* Philadelphia, 2006, Saunders.)

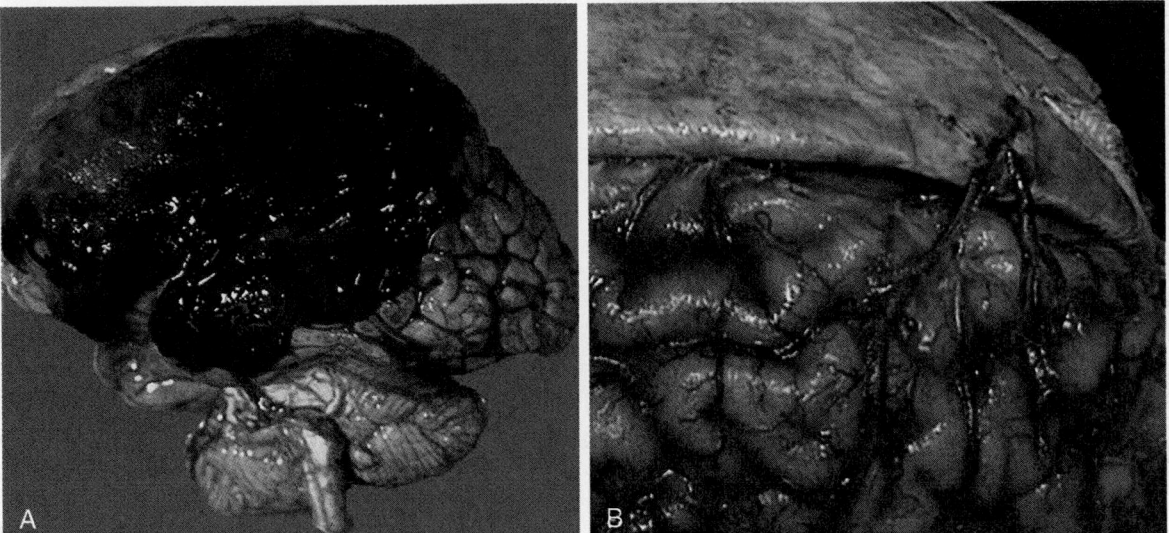

Figure 17-4 Subdural hematoma, gross, and bridging veins, gross. A large subdural hematoma (A) is seen in the frontoparietal region. A subdural hematoma forms after head trauma that severs the bridging veins from dura to brain, shown in the right panel (B) where the dura has been reflected to reveal the normal appearance of the bridging veins that extend across to the superior aspect of the cerebral hemispheres. Older adultss and the very young are at greater risk because their cerebral veins are more vulnerable to injury. Because the bleeding is venous, blood collects over hours to weeks, with variable onset of symptoms. Because the blood collects beneath the dura, a subdural hematoma can be seen to cross the region of cranial sutures. (From Klatt EC: *Robbins and Cotran atlas of pathology*, Philadelphia, 2006, Saunders.)

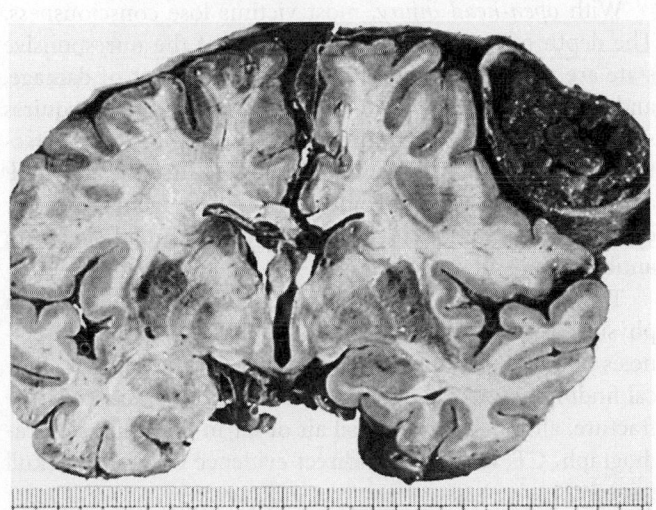

Figure 17-5 Chronic subdural hematoma. Compression of underlying brain and lateral ventricle. Note bone formation in falx and uncal herniation on the side of hematoma. (From Kissane JM, editor: *Anderson's pathology*, ed 9, St Louis, 1993, Mosby.)

manifestations such as dysphasia, dyspraxia, or hemiparesis. Other clinical manifestations may include homonymous hemianopia (defective vision in either the right or the left field), disconjugate gaze, and gaze palsies.

The pathogenesis of a *chronic subdural hematoma* is different. The existing subdural space gradually fills with blood. A vascular membrane forms around the hematoma in approximately 2 weeks. Further enlargement takes place in some persons, but the mechanism of this enlargement is unclear.

Presenting manifestations of *chronic subdural hematomas* vary. Of those affected, 80% have chronic headaches and tenderness over the hematoma on percussion. Most appear to have a progressive dementia accompanied by generalized rigidity (paratonia).

Whereas most acute and subacute subdural hematomas are treated with clot evacuation through a burr hole, chronic subdural hematomas (and some that are subacute) require a craniotomy to evacuate the gelatinous blood. The membrane around a chronic subdural hematoma is then dissected away from the dura mater and arachnoid membranes. A technique for percutaneous drainage for chronic subdural hematomas has proved successful.

Intracerebral hematomas (intraparenchymal hemorrhages)[4] occur in 2% to 3% of head injuries usually associated with MVAs and falls from some distance. Intracerebral hematomas may be single or multiple, and they are associated with contusions. Although most commonly located in the frontal and temporal lobes, intracerebral hematomas may occur in the hemispheric deep white matter. Small blood vessels are traumatized by penetrating injury or shearing forces. The intracerebral hematoma then acts as an expanding mass, resulting in increased ICP and compression of brain tissues with resultant edema (Figure 17-6). Delayed intracerebral hematomas may appear 3 to 10 days after the head injury.

A decreasing level of consciousness is associated with an *intracerebral hematoma*. Coma or a confusional state from other injuries, however, can make the cause of this increasing unresponsiveness difficult to detect. Contralateral hemiplegia also may occur. As the ICP rises, clinical manifestations of temporal lobe herniation may appear. In delayed intracerebral

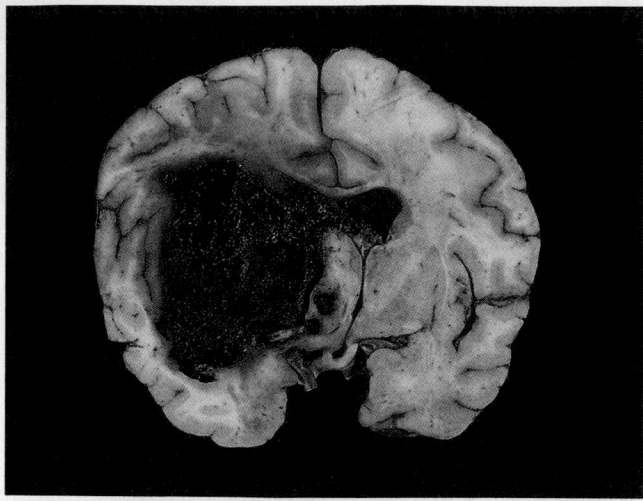

Figure 17-6 Acute intracerebral hemorrhage. A fresh hematoma has disrupted and expanded the left cerebral hemisphere, causing the midline structures to shift to the right. Uncontrolled hypertension is an important cause of this catastrophic lesion. (From Kumar V, Cotran RS, Robbins SL: *Robbins basic pathology*, ed 7, Philadelphia, 2003, Saunders.)

hematoma, the presentation is similar to that of hypertensive brain hemorrhage: sudden, rapidly progressive decreased level of consciousness with pupillary dilation; breathing pattern changes; hemiplegia; and bilateral positive Babinski reflexes.

Evacuation of a singular intracerebral hematoma has only occasionally been helpful, mostly for subcortical white matter hematomas. Otherwise, treatment is directed at reducing the ICP and allowing the hematoma to reabsorb slowly.

Open trauma produces discrete (focal) injuries and includes compound fractures and missile injuries. A compound fracture opens a communication between the cranial contents and the environment and should be investigated whenever there are lacerations of the scalp, tympanic membrane, a sinus, an eye, or mucous membranes. Such fractures may involve the cranial vault or the base of the skull (basilar skull fracture). The injury incurred from bone fragments is mainly a tangential injury (injury caused by direct contact) and occasionally a penetrating injury. Bone fragments may lacerate or contuse brain tissues or blood vessels. In addition, cranial nerves may be damaged with a basilar skull fracture.

Missiles include bullets, rocks, shell fragments, knives, and blunt instruments. The mechanisms of injury are crush injury and stretch injury. Crush injury is the laceration and crushing of whatever tissue the missile touches, with the amount of crush related to the degree of fragmentation, deformity, size, and shape. A tangential injury is injury to the coverings of the brain (scalp lacerations), skull fractures, laceration of the meninges, and cerebral lacerations. Projectiles and debris from scalp and skull injury, when driven into the brain substance, produce a penetrating brain injury. Occasionally projectiles are so forceful that they exit the cranial vault in addition to entering it, producing a through-and-through injury. Primary damage is localized along the path of the penetrating object, and direct tissue disruption along the projectile tract

results. A high-velocity bullet produces contusions at the site of entry, caused by bone striking the brain tissue on impact. Bone fragments are driven inward.

Stretch injury involves blood vessels and nerves that are damaged without direct contact due to the amount of tissue stretched secondary to shape, deformation, and striking velocity. Air compressed in front of a bullet exerts an explosive effect on entry, producing extreme distant tissue damage and an immediate primary increase in ICP; a cavity many times greater than the size of the bullet is produced because the brain tissue is propelled away from the tract. The cavity and pressure produce contrecoup injuries. The intracranial volume is increased directly by the projectile and the debris. The temporary cavity collapses back onto itself, leaving a smaller, permanent cavity. Intracranial bleeding occurs into the permanent cavity and may cause the cavity to expand. Edema in and around the injured brain tissue rapidly develops; edema and bleeding contribute markedly to ICP. This second rise in ICP to 60 to 100 mmHg may last 2 to 5 minutes. Because of acute ischemic damage to the tract, necrosis of tissue begins. Within hours after bullet-induced injury, tissue within 1 cm adjacent to the tract disintegrates. Demyelination of white matter affected by hemorrhage and edema occurs by the second day. Unconsciousness, flaccidity, or decerebrate posture (see Chapter 16) are associated with a 94% mortality.

With *open-head injury*, most victims lose consciousness. The depth of the coma and the length of the unresponsive state are related to the location of injury, extent of damage, and amount of bleeding. Open-head injury often requires surgery to débride the traumatized tissues to prevent infection and to remove blood clots to help reduce the ICP. ICP also is managed with steroids, dehydrating agents, osmotic diuretics, or a combination of these drugs. Broad-spectrum antibiotics are administered.

The diagnosis of a compound fracture is made through physical examination, skull radiographs, or both. The diagnosis of a basilar skull fracture is made on the basis of clinical findings. Skull radiographs often do not demonstrate the fracture, although intracranial air or air in the sinuses on radiograph, CT, or MRI is indirect evidence of a basilar skull fracture.

A compound linear fracture is débrided nonsurgically in cooperative adults and surgically in children and uncooperative adults. Cranioplasty with insertion of bone or an artificial graft may be necessary but often is delayed until antibiotics have been given. Antibiotics are administered after surgery.

Bed rest and close observation for meningitis and other complications are prescribed for a basilar skull fracture. Use of prophylactic antibiotics is controversial because studies have failed to demonstrate that they reduce the rate of infection.

Diffuse Brain Injury. Diffuse brain injury (**diffuse axonal injury [DAI]**) results from a shaking effect (inertial effects of mechanical input to the head associated with high levels of acceleration and deceleration, effects of head motion). Rotational acceleration (twisting movement) is the primary mechanism of injury, producing strains and distortions within the brain (see Figure 17-1). The brain tissues experience shearing stresses set up by the rotational forces that operate when a freely moving head is struck because of the skull's motion from its attachment to the neck. Shearing, tearing, or stretching of nerve fibers with subsequent axonal damage results. Forces applied axially as a result of centrifugal acceleration of the head establish a gradient of injury severity from the hemispheres to the brain stem. The most severe axonal injuries are located more peripheral to the brainstem, thus accounting for the tremendous cognitive and affective impairments seen in survivors of traumatic brain injury from MVAs. The frontal and temporal axonal tracts are particularly vulnerable. Damage reduces the speed of informational processing and responding and disrupts attention.

The common pathologic substrate in diffuse brain injury is axonal damage (disruption). Pathophysiologically, at the time of injury, the damage can be seen only with an electron microscope and involves either numerous axons alone or axonal injury in conjunction with actual tissue tears (Figure 17-7). Areas where axons and small blood vessels are torn appear as small hemorrhages, located particularly in the corpus

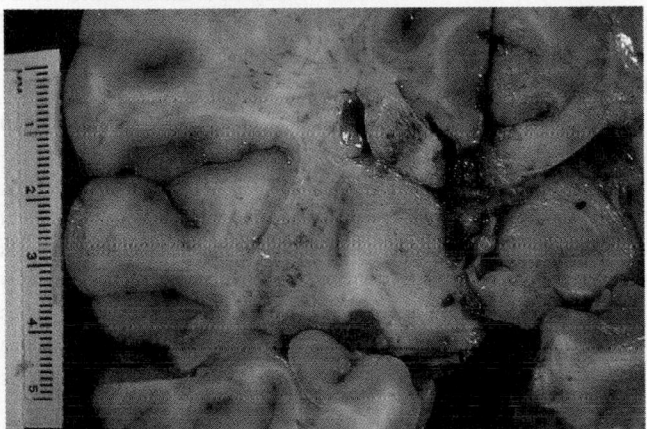

Figure 17-7 Diffuse axonal injury. Gross photograph demonstrating characteristic hemorrhage lesions within the corpus callosum. Courtesy of Walter Kemp, MD, Department of Pathology, University of Texas Southwestern Medical School, Dallas.) (From Kumar V, Cotran RS, Robbins SL: *Robbins basic pathology,* ed 7, Philadelphia, 2003, Saunders.)

callosum and dorsolateral quadrant of the rostral brain stem at the superior cerebellar peduncle.

Oxygen-free radicals contribute to secondary injury. Free radicals damage proteins and the phospholipid components of cells and organelle membranes. Membrane depolarization caused by the trauma permits nonselective opening of voltage-sensitive calcium channels, resulting in abnormal calcium accumulation in neurons and glial cells. These calcium shifts are associated with activation of lipolytic and proteolytic enzymes, protein kinases, protein phosphatases, dissolution of microtubules, and altered gene expression. Abnormal calcium influx occurs through activation of excitatory amino acid receptors. Widespread *exotoxicity* occurs after trauma, resulting in cell swelling, vacuolization, and death.[4]

Progressively increasing numbers of damaged axons are visible 12 hours to several days after the injury. Chromatolysis of the neurons involving eccentric relocation of the nucleus, swelling of the axon hillock, and redistribution of the rough endoplasmic reticulum in the cell body is evident. During this time the torn axons, which resemble dilated sausage links, also regress into round balls called *retraction balls*. These retraction balls are visible with light microscopy.

The number of retraction balls increases during the first week or two but begins to diminish in 2 to 3 weeks. Clusters of microglia appear in their place. Lastly, astrocytosis (gliosis, equivalent to scarring) occurs at the sites of axonal damage. Demyelination is seen particularly in the long axon tracts of the upper brainstem.

Severity of the diffuse injury correlates with the direction and velocity of rotation, that is, how much shearing force was applied to the brainstem. Figure 17-8 illustrates the spectrum of the diffuse injury as the magnitude increases. DAI is not associated with intracranial hypertension soon after injury, but acute brain swelling (increased intravascular blood within the brain, vasodilation, and increased cerebral blood volume) is seen often.

Several categories of diffuse brain injury exist: mild concussion, classic concussion, mild DAI, moderate DAI, and severe DAI. An organic component is present within each category, in contrast to the previous conceptualization that concussion had no structural injury component.

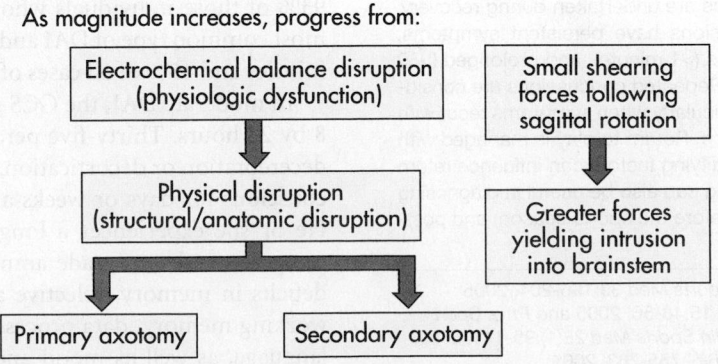

Figure 17-8 Spectrum of diffuse brain injury.

Mild concussion involves temporary axonal disturbances. Cerebrocortical dysfunction related to attentional and memory systems results, but consciousness is not lost. Three forms have been described:

Grade I: Confusion and disorientation accompanied by amnesia (momentary)

Grade II: Momentary confusion and retrograde amnesia that develops after 5 to 10 minutes (memory loss involves only events occurring several minutes before injury)

Grade III: Confusion and retrograde amnesia present from impact (also anterograde amnesia) (persists for several minutes)

Recommended guidelines for return to play after sports-related concussive injuries are contained in What's New? Sports-Related Concussion.

Mild concussion is characterized by an immediate onset of clinical manifestations at the time of injury and the transitory nature of clinical manifestations. A momentary rise in CSF pressure and changes in ECG and EEG have been demonstrated to occur on impact in the laboratory. No loss of consciousness is experienced. The initial confusional state exists for a moment to several minutes. Amnesia for events preceding the trauma (retrograde amnesia) may be experienced. Anterograde amnesia may exist transiently. Persons may experience head pain and complain of nervousness and "not being oneself" for up to a few days.

Classic cerebral concussion (*grade IV*) involves diffuse cerebral disconnection from the brainstem reticular activating system and is a phenomenon of physiologic, neurologic dysfunction without substantial anatomic disruption. Evidence of this disconnection is the immediate loss of consciousness, which lasts less than 6 hours. Retrograde and anterograde (posttraumatic) amnesia is present. This type of diffuse injury frequently is associated with focal pathologic findings, especially cerebral contusions that yield focal signs, not loss

of consciousness. There are two forms of classic cerebral contusion: uncomplicated classic cerebral concussion (without focal injury) and complicated classic cerebral concussion (accompanied by focal injury).

In classic cerebral concussion loss of consciousness lasts as long as 6 hours and reflexes are lost, causing falls. Reflexes are regained as responsiveness returns. Transient cessation of respiration, brief periods of bradycardia, and a decrease in blood pressure lasting 30 seconds or less occur. Vital signs stabilize within a few seconds to within normal limits. Retrograde and anterograde amnesia exist. A confusional state persists for hours to days. The individual experiences head pain, nausea, and fatigue. Attentional and memory system impairments may persist for weeks to months and may include inability to concentrate and forgetfulness. Mood and affect changes may persist for weeks to months and may include nervousness, anxiety reactions, depression, irritability, fatigability, and insomnia.

Some of the effects of a concussion may persist for weeks or months, depending on the severity of the injury. Fifty percent of persons have a **postconcussive syndrome** that includes headache, cognitive impairments, psychologic and somatic complaints, and cranial nerve signs and symptoms.[4] Treatment entails reassurance and symptomatic relief. Close observation for 24 hours by a reliable individual is indicated so that immediate intervention can be obtained if delayed effects become severe.

DAI produces prolonged traumatic coma lasting more than 6 hours because of axonal disruption. Three forms of DAI exist: mild, moderate, and severe. In **mild diffuse axonal injury,** posttraumatic coma lasts 6 to 24 hours. Death is uncommon but residual cognitive, psychologic, and sensorimotor deficits may persist. Mild DAI is a relatively uncommon lesion, occurring in 8% of all severe head injuries and 19% of all cases of DAI. In mild DAI 30% of persons display decerebrate or decorticate posturing; they may experience prolonged periods of stupor or restlessness (see Figure 16-5).

In **moderate diffuse axonal injury,** widespread physiologic impairment exists throughout the cerebral cortex and diencephalon. Actual tearing of some axons in both hemispheres occurs. Basal skull fracture, a focal injury, is commonly associated with moderate DAI. Prolonged coma lasting more than 24 hours is present but prominent brainstem signs do not exist with moderate DAI. Recovery often is incomplete in 93% of those individuals who survive. Moderate DAI is the most common type of DAI and is found in 20% of severe head injuries and 45% of all cases of DAI.

In moderate DAI, the GCS score is 4 to 8 initially and 6 to 8 by 24 hours. Thirty-five percent of victims have transitory decerebration or decortication. The person often remains unconscious for days or weeks and on awakening is confused. He or she experiences a long period of posttraumatic anterograde and retrograde amnesia and often has permanent deficits in memory, selective attention, vigilance, detection, working memory, data processing, vision or perception, and language, as well as mood and affect changes ranging from mild to severe.

WHAT'S NEW?   Sports-Related Concussion

The 2004 Prague Consensus statement distinguished simple versus complex concussions and the 2008 International Conference on Concussion in Sports updated the concensus statment. Simple concussion progressively resolves without complications over 7 to 10 days. Activities are limited while the athlete is still symptomatic but no further interventions are undertaken during recovery. Athletes with complex concussions have persistent symptoms, prolonged loss of consciousness (>1 minute), and prolonged (>30 minutes) cognitive impairment. Repeated concussions are considered complex concussions, particularly when symptoms recur with impacts of lesser and lesser force. Return to play is managed with rest and graduated activity. Modifying factors can influence return to play. Neuropsychologic testing can also be useful in diagnosing the concussion with baseline (before the sports season) and postconcussion assessment.

Data from McCrory P et al: *Br J Sports Med* 39:196-204, 2005 (co-published in *Clin J Sport Med* 15:48-56, 2005 and *Phys Sport Med* 33:29-44, 2005); Lovell M: *Clin Sports Med* 28(1):95-111, 2009; McCrory P et al: *J Clin Neurosci* 16(6):755-763, 2009.

Severe diffuse axonal injury, formerly called *primary brainstem injury* or *brainstem contusion,* involves severe mechanical disruption of many axons in both cerebral hemispheres and those extending to the diencephalon and brainstem. Severe DAI represents 16% of all severe head injuries and 36% of all cases of DAI. With an initial GCS score of 3, the mortality rate is 78%[2]; with an initial score between 3 and 8, the mortality rate is 36%; and 16% of persons have either a moderate or severe disability and 5% survive in a coma (unresponsive) state.[2]

Severe DAI is associated with brainstem signs that disappear in a few weeks. The person experiences immediate autonomic dysfunction that resolves in a few weeks. Increased ICP appears 4 to 6 days after injury. Pulmonary complications occur frequently, with profound sensorimotor and cognitive system deficits. Severely compromised coordinated movements and verbal and written communication, inability to learn and reason, and inability to modulate behavior also are found.

CT scan and MRI are the diagnostic tests of choice for TBI.[2,5] There is no strong research evidence that any treatment reduces the complications of moderate to severe TBI, although various treatment protocols are instituted. Specifically, the evidence is inconclusive about the effectiveness of hyperventilation, mild hypothermia, and use of mannitol.[2] Barbiturates have not been shown to be effective in reducing intracranial pressure or preventing adverse outcomes after TBI.[2] The Corticosteroid Randomisation After Significant Head Injury (CRASH) trial showed corticosteroids increase mortality with acute TBI, so these drugs are no longer used. Carbamazepine and phenytoin may reduce the occurrence of early seizures but have not been shown to reduce the onset of late seizures, neurologic disability, or death.[2] Prophylactic antibiotics also have not been shown to reduce the risk of meningitis or death with a skull fracture.[2] Extensive research is under way to discover effective therapeutic interventions. The role of fluid and nutrition management has emerged as critically important in the care of individuals with severe brain injuries.[6]

Genetics of Head Injury

Certain genes are up-regulated and others are down-regulated after head trauma. Researchers' attention has been focused predominantly on the *apolipoprotein E (apoE)* gene and its various alleles. Certain alleles have been correlated with increased susceptibility to and severity of head injury. Other alleles have been associated with improved or diminished recovery after head injury. The clinical significance of these findings is not clearly known.[4,7]

Spinal Cord Trauma

The number of spinal cord injuries (SCIs) in the United States is approximately 235,000, with 11,000 annually; of these, 77.8% are men, mostly young adults.[8] The average age is 38 years; however, the percent of SCI in individuals older than 60 years of age has increased to 11.5%, up 4.7% since 2000.[8] At discharge, since 2000, the extent of injury has been 34.1% incomplete quadriplegia, 18.3% complete quadriplegia, 18.5% incomplete paraplegia, and 23.0% complete paraplegia.[8] MVAs have accounted for 46.9% of reported SCI cases since 2000. Falls are now the next most common cause followed by acts of violence, primarily gunshot wounds, then recreational sporting activities.[8] Older adults, because of preexisting degenerative vertebral disorders, are particularly at risk for minor trauma resulting in serious spinal cord injury, especially from falls.

PATHOPHYSIOLOGY Spinal cord injuries most commonly occur because of vertebral injuries, as a result of acceleration, deceleration, or deformation forces most frequently applied at a distance. These forces injure the vertebral or neural tissues by compressing the tissues, pulling or exerting a traction (tension) on the tissues, or shearing tissues so that they slide into one another. These forces may be exerted on the vertebral and neural tissues by hyperextension, hyperflexion, vertical compression, or rotation of the spine (Figures 17-9 to 17-12). The bones, ligaments, and joints of the vertebral column may be damaged. The vertebral column may incur fracture and often compression of one or more elements, dislocation of its elements, or both fracture and dislocation (see Figure 14-16 for the structure of the vertebral column). Vertebral injuries can be classified as (1) simple fracture, a single break usually affecting transverse or spinous processes; (2) compressed (wedged) vertebral fracture, in which a vertebral body is compressed anteriorly; (3) comminuted (burst) fracture, in which a vertebral body is shattered into several fragments; and (4) dislocation.

Vertebrae fracture readily with direct and indirect trauma. When the supporting ligaments are torn, the vertebrae move out of alignment, and dislocations occur. A horizontal force moves the vertebrae straight forward; if the individual is in a flexed position at the time of injury, the vertebrae are then in an angulated position. Flexion and extension injuries may result in dislocations. (Mechanisms of vertebral injury are presented in Table 17-2.) Vertebral injuries occur mostly at vertebrae C1-C2 (cervical), C4-C7, and T1-L2 (thoracic-lumbar) (see Figure 14-10). These are the most mobile portions of the vertebral column. The cord occupies most of the vertebral canal in the cervical and lumbar regions. The size makes the cord in these areas more easily injured. The *primary spinal cord injuries* are summarized in Table 17-3. Noncontiguous vertebral injuries are not uncommon. Further, primary injury

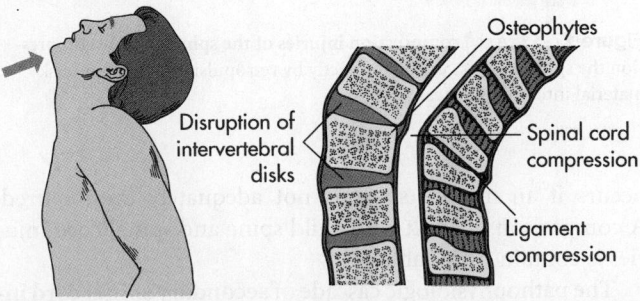

Figure 17-9 Hyperextension injuries of the spine. Hyperextension can result in fracture or nonfracture injuries with spinal cord damage.

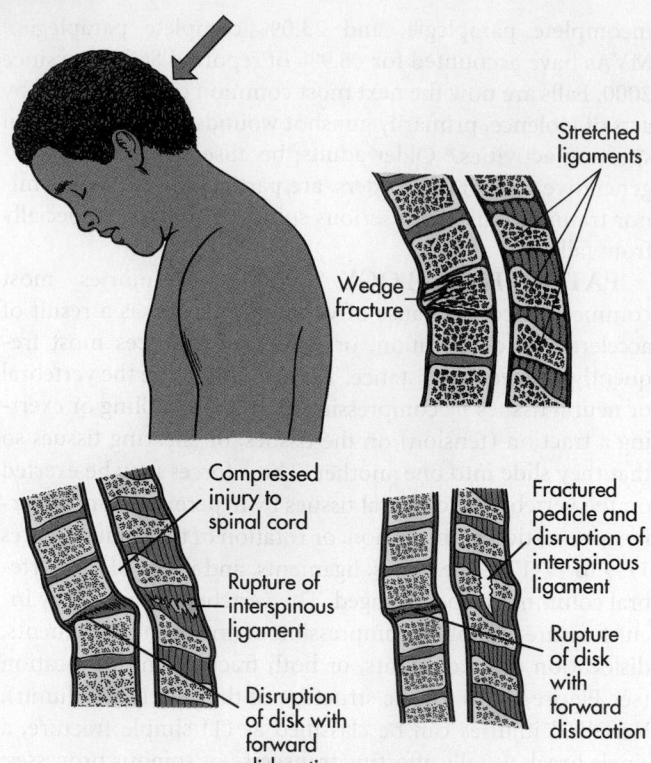

Figure 17-10 **Hyperflexion injury of the spine.** Hyperflexion produces translation (subluxation) of vertebrae, which compromises the central canal and compresses spinal cord parenchyma or vascular structures.

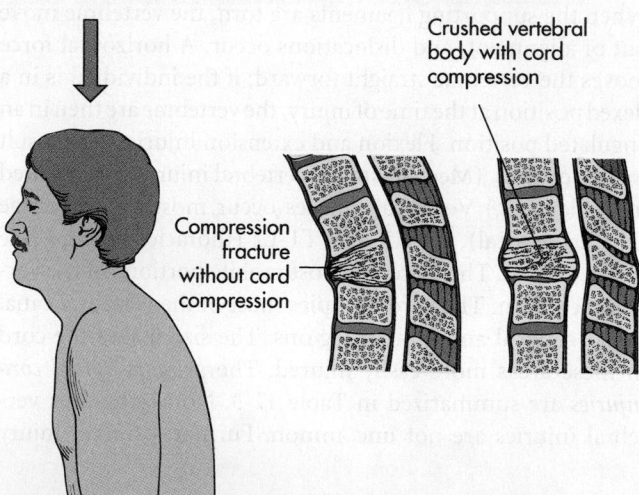

Figure 17-11 **Axial compression injuries of the spine.** In axial compression the spinal cord is contused directly by retropulsion of bone or disk material into the spinal canal.

occurs if an injured spine is not adequately immobilized. A comparison of adult with child spine and spinal cord injuries is contained in Table 17-4.

The pathophysiologic cascade of **secondary spinal cord injury** begins within a few minutes after injury. *Microscopic hemorrhages* appear in the central gray matter and pia arachnoid

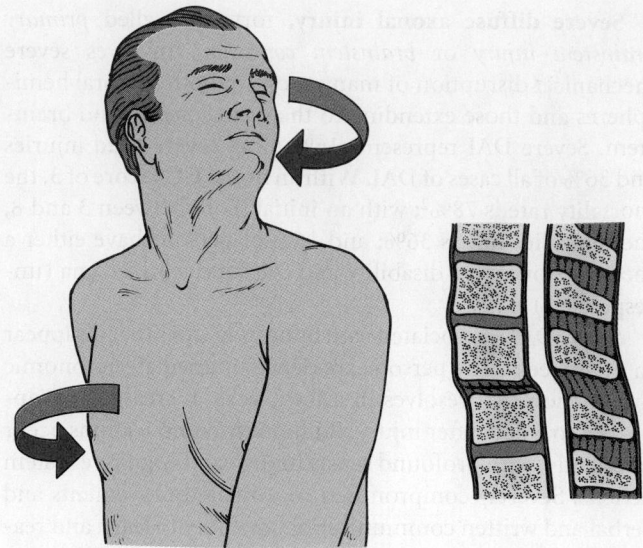

Figure 17-12 Flexion-rotation injuries of the spine.

that increase in size within 2 hours. *Edema* in the white matter occurs, impairing the microcirculation of the cord. Within 4 hours, numerous swollen axis cylinders develop. Localized hemorrhaging and edema therefore are followed by loss of autoregulation, vasospasm, impaired venous drainage, and reduced vascular perfusion with *development of ischemic areas.* Oxygen tension in the tissue at the injury site is decreased. The microscopic hemorrhages and edema are maximal at the level of injury and for two cord segments above and below it.

Cellular and subcellular alterations and *tissue necrosis* occur. By 5 minutes after injury, venules of the gray matter are congested and distended by erythrocytes. In 15 to 30 minutes, small hemorrhages occur with extravasation of erythrocytes into perivascular spaces of postcapillary and muscular venules. Within 4 hours, disruption of myelin, axonal degeneration, and ischemic endothelial injury occur.

Chemical and metabolic changes in spinal cord tissues include release of toxic excitatory amino acids, accumulation of endogenous opiates, lipid hydrolysis with production of active metabolites, and local free radical release. These changes may produce further ischemia, vascular damage, and necrosis of tissues (autodestruction). Necrosis consumes 40% of cross-sectional cord within 4 hours of trauma and 70% within 24 hours. Cord swelling increases an individual's degree of dysfunction so that distinguishing the functions to be lost permanently from those that are impaired just temporarily becomes difficult. In the cervical region, cord swelling may be life threatening because of the possibility of resulting impairment of the diaphragm function (phrenic nerves exit C3-C5) and vegetative functions mediated by the medulla oblongata. Within the first few days of injury, progressive axonal changes occur and necrotic zones develop. Progressive cavitation and coagulation necrosis at the site of injury are termed *posttraumatic infarction.*

Circulation in the white matter tracts of the spinal cord returns to normal in about 24 hours, but gray matter circulation

Table 17-2	Mechanisms of Vertebral Injury		
Mechanisms of Injury	Vertebral Injury	Forces of Injury	Location of Injury
Hyperextension	Fracture and dislocation of posterior elements such as spinous processes, transverse processes, laminae, pedicles, or posterior ligaments	Results from forces of acceleration-deceleration and the sudden reduction in the anteroposterior diameter of the spinal cord	Cervical area
Hyperflexion	Fracture or dislocation of the vertebral bodies, disks, or ligaments	Results from sudden and excessive force that propels the neck forward or causes an exaggerated lateral movement of the neck to one side	Cervical area
Vertical compression (axonal loading)	Shattering fractures	Results from a force applied along an axis from the top of the cranium through the vertebral bodies	T12-L2
Rotational forces (flexion-rotation)	Ruptures support ligaments in addition to producing fractures	Adds shearing force to acceleration–acceleration forces	Cervical area

Table 17-3	Spinal Cord Injuries	
Injury	Description	
Cord concussion	Results in a temporary disruption of cord-mediated functions	
Cord contusion	Bruising of the neural tissue causing swelling and temporary loss of cord-mediated functions	
Cord compression	Pressure on the cord causing ischemia to tissues; must be relieved (decompressed) to prevent permanent damage to the spinal cord	
Laceration	Tearing of the neural tissues of the spinal cord; may be reversible if only slight damage is sustained by the neural tissues; may result in permanent loss of cord-mediated functions if spinal tracts are disrupted	
Transection	Severing of the spinal cord, causing permanent loss of function	
Complete	All tracts in the spinal cord completely disrupted; all cord-mediated functions below the transection are completely and permanently lost	
Incomplete	Some tracts in the spinal cord remain intact, together with functions mediated by these tracts; has the potential for recovery although function is temporarily lost	
Preserved sensation only	Some demonstrable sensation below the level of injury	
Preserved motor nonfunctional	Preserved motor function without useful purpose; sensory function may or may not be preserved	
Preserved motor functional	Preserved voluntary motor function that is functionally useful	
Hemorrhage	Bleeding into the neural tissue because of blood vessel damage; usually no major loss of function	
Damage or obstruction of spinal blood supply	Causes local ischemia	

remains altered. Phagocytes appear 36 to 48 hours after injury. There is proliferation of microglia and changes in astrocytes. Red cells then begin to disintegrate, and resorption of hemorrhages begins. Degenerating axons are engulfed by macrophages in the first 10 days after injury. A cyst with fluid forms. The traumatized cord is replaced by acellular collagenous tissue (a scar), usually in 3 to 4 weeks. Meninges thicken as part of the scarring process.

CLINICAL MANIFESTATIONS Normal activity of the spinal cord cells at and below the level of injury ceases because of loss of the continuous tonic discharge from the brain or brainstem and inhibition of suprasegmental impulses immediately after cord injury, thus causing spinal shock. **Spinal shock** is characterized by a complete loss of reflex function in all segments below the level of the lesion. This condition involves all skeletal muscles, bladder, bowel, sexual function, and autonomic control. Severe impairment below the level of the lesion is obvious; it includes paralysis and flaccidity

in muscles, absence of sensation, loss of bladder and rectal control, transient drop in blood pressure, and poor venous circulation. The condition also results in disturbed thermal control because the sympathetic nervous system is damaged. This damage causes faulty control of sweating and radiation through capillary dilation. The hypothalamus cannot regulate body heat through vasoconstriction and increased metabolism; therefore, the individual assumes the temperature of the air.

Spinal shock may last for 7 to 20 days after onset; it may persist for as short a time as a few days or as long as 3 months. Indications that spinal shock is terminating include the reappearance of reflex activity, hyperreflexia, spasticity, and reflex emptying of the bladder. With cervical or upper thoracic cord injury, a form of distributive shock, called **neurogenic shock,** may be seen in addition to spinal shock, as a result of the loss of sympathetic outflow, causing vasodilation, hypotension, bradycardia, and hypothermia.

Table 17-4	Comparison of Spine and Spinal Cord Injuries in Adults and Children	
Characteristics	Adult	Pediatric
Most common mechanism of injury	Motor vehicle accidents	Falls
Level of Injury		
C1-C3	1% to 2%	60%
C3-C7	85%	30% to 40%
Thoracolumbar	10% to 15%	5%
Type of Injury		
Fracture-dislocation	>70%	25%
Subluxation	<20%	50%
SCIWORA	Rare	Up to 50%
Delayed neurological deficits	Rare	Up to 50%

From Evans RW, Wilberger JE: Traumatic disorders. In Goetz CG, editor, *Textbook of neurology,* Philadelphia, 2003, Saunders.
SCIWORA, Spinal cord injury without radiologic abnormalities.

Loss of motor and sensory function depends on the level of injury. All motor, sensory, reflex, and autonomic functions cease below any transected area and may cease below concussive, contused, compressed, or ischemic areas (Table 17-5). Paralysis of the lower half of the body with both legs involved is termed *paraplegia*. Paralysis involving all four extremities is termed *quadriplegia* (tetraplegia). In complete quadriplegia the level of injury is above C6, and all upper extremity function is lost. In incomplete quadriplegia, function at or above C6 is preserved, leaving the shoulder, upper arm, and some forearm muscle control intact. With acceleration injuries the greatest stress point is C4-C5. With a deceleration force the greatest stress point is at C5-C6.

Return of spinal neuron excitability occurs slowly. Depending on the degree of damage, either of the following can occur: (1) motor, sensory, reflex, and autonomic functions return to normal; or (2) autonomic neural activity in the isolated segment develops. The sequence of hyperactivity phases, which vary in length, may include (1) minimal reflex activity, (2) flexor spasms, (3) alternation between flexor and extensor spasms, and (4) predominant extensor spasms.

Table 17-5	Clinical Manifestations of Spinal Cord Injury
Stage	Manifestations
Spinal Shock Stage	
Complete spinal cord transection	Loss of motor function
	1. Quadriplegia with injuries of cervical spinal cord
	2. Paraplegia with injuries of thoracic spinal cord
	Muscle flaccidity
	Loss of all reflexes below level of injury
	Loss of pain, temperature, touch, pressure, and proprioception below level of injury
	Pain at site of injury caused by a zone of hyperesthesia above the injury
	Atonic bladder and bowel
	Paralytic ileus with distention
	Loss of vasomotor tone in lower body parts; low and unstable blood pressure
	Loss of perspiration below level of injury
	Loss or extreme depression of genital reflexes such as penile erection and bulbocavernous reflex
	Dry and pale skin, possible ulceration over bony prominences
	Respiratory impairment
Partial spinal cord transection	Asymmetric flaccid motor paralysis below level of injury
	Asymmetric reflex loss
	Preservation of some sensation below level of injury
	Vasomotor instability less severe than with complete cord transection
	Bowel and bladder impairment less severe than that seen with complete cord transection
	Preservation of ability to perspire in some portions of the body below level of injury
	Brown-Séquard syndrome (associated with penetrating injuries, hyperextension and flexion, locked facets, and compression fractures)
	1. Ipsilateral paralysis or paresis below level of injury
	2. Ipsilateral loss of touch, pressure, vibration, and position sense below level of injury
	3. Contralateral loss of pain and temperature sensations below level of injury
	Central cervical cord syndrome (acute cord compression between bony bars or spurs anteriorly and thickened ligamentum flavum posteriorly associated with hyperextension)
	1. Motor deficits in upper extremities, especially hands, more dense than in lower extremities
	2. Varying degrees of bladder dysfunction
	Burning hand syndrome (variant of central cord syndrome, half of cases have an underlying spine fracture/dislocation present)
	1. Severe burning parethesias and dysesthesias in the hands and/or feet

Table 17-5	Clinical Manifestations of Spinal Cord Injury—cont'd
Stage	**Manifestations**
	Anterior cord syndrome (compromise of anterior spinal artery by occlusion or pressure effect of disk)
	1. Loss of motor function below level of injury
	2. Loss of pain and temperature sensations below level of injury
	3. Touch, pressure, position, and vibration senses intact
	Posterior cord syndrome (associated with hyperextension injuries with fractures of vertebral arch)
	1. Impaired light touch and proprioception
	Conus medullaris syndrome (compression injury at T12 from disk herniation or burst fracture of body of T12)
	1. Flaccid paralysis of legs
	2. Flaccid paralysis of anal sphincter
	3. Variable sensory deficits
	Cauda equina syndrome (compression of nerve roots below L1 caused by fracture and dislocation of spine or large posterocentral intervertebral disk herniation)
	1. Lower extremity motor deficits
	2. Variable sensorimotor dysfunction
	3. Variable reflex dysfunction
	4. Variable bladder, bowel, and sexual dysfunction
	Syndrome of neuropraxia (seen postathletic injury, associated with congenital spinal stenosis)
	1. Dramatic but transient neurologic deficits including quadriplegia
	Horner syndrome (injury to preganglionic sympathetic trunk or postganglionic sympathetic neurons of superior cervical ganglion)
	1. Ipsilateral pupil smaller than contralateral pupil
	2. Sunken ipsilateral eyeball
	3. Ptosis of affected eyeball
	4. Lack of perspiration on ipsilateral side of face
Heightened Reflex Activity Stage	
	Emergence of Babinski reflexes, possibly progressing to a triple reflex; possible development of still later flexor spasms
	Reappearance of ankle and knee reflexes, which become hyperactive
	Contraction of reflex detrusor muscle, leading to urinary incontinence
	Appearance of reflex defecation
	Mass reflex with flexion spasms, profuse sweating, piloerection, and bladder and occasional bowel emptying may be evoked by an automonic stimulation of skin or from a full bladder
	Episodes of hypertension
	Defective heat-induced sweating
	Eventual development of extensor reflexes, first in muscles of hip and thigh, later in leg
	Possible paresthesias below level of transaction: dull, burning pain in lower back, abdomen, buttocks, and perineum

The initial clinical manifestations associated with acute spinal cord injury are rapid loss of (1) voluntary movement in body parts below the level of injury, (2) sensations in the lower extremities and possibly lower trunk (depending on the level of injury), and (3) spinal and autonomic reflexes below the level of injury. The duration of this areflexic state is highly variable. In most persons, reflex activity returns in 1 to 2 weeks.

Gradually reflexes return and become increasingly easier to elicit. A pattern of flexion reflexes emerges, first involving the toes and later the feet and legs. Reflex voiding and bowel elimination appear. Flexor spasms accompanied by profuse sweating, piloerection, and automatic bladder emptying (together called a **mass reflex**) may develop. The ability to sweat when overheated may be disrupted, and extensor spasms may develop, usually after full development of flexor spasms. Sometimes after several months, episodes of autonomic hyperreflexia are elicited.

Autonomic hyperreflexia (dysreflexia) is a syndrome of a sudden and dangerous increase in blood pressure that may occur at any time after spinal shock resolves. The syndrome is associated with a massive, uncompensated cardiovascular response to stimulation of the sympathetic nervous system (Figure 17-13). The condition is life threatening and requires immediate treatment. Individuals most likely to be affected have lesions at the T6 level or above. Autonomic hyperreflexia is characterized by paroxysmal hypertension (up to 300 mmHg systolic), a pounding headache, blurred vision, sweating above the level of the lesion with flushing of the skin, nasal congestion, nausea, piloerection caused by pilomotor spasm, and bradycardia (30 to 40 beats/minute).[9] The symptoms may develop singly or in combination (syndrome) and often are associated with a distended bladder or rectum.

Pathophysiology of hyperreflexia involves the stimulation of sensory receptors below the level of the cord lesion. The intact

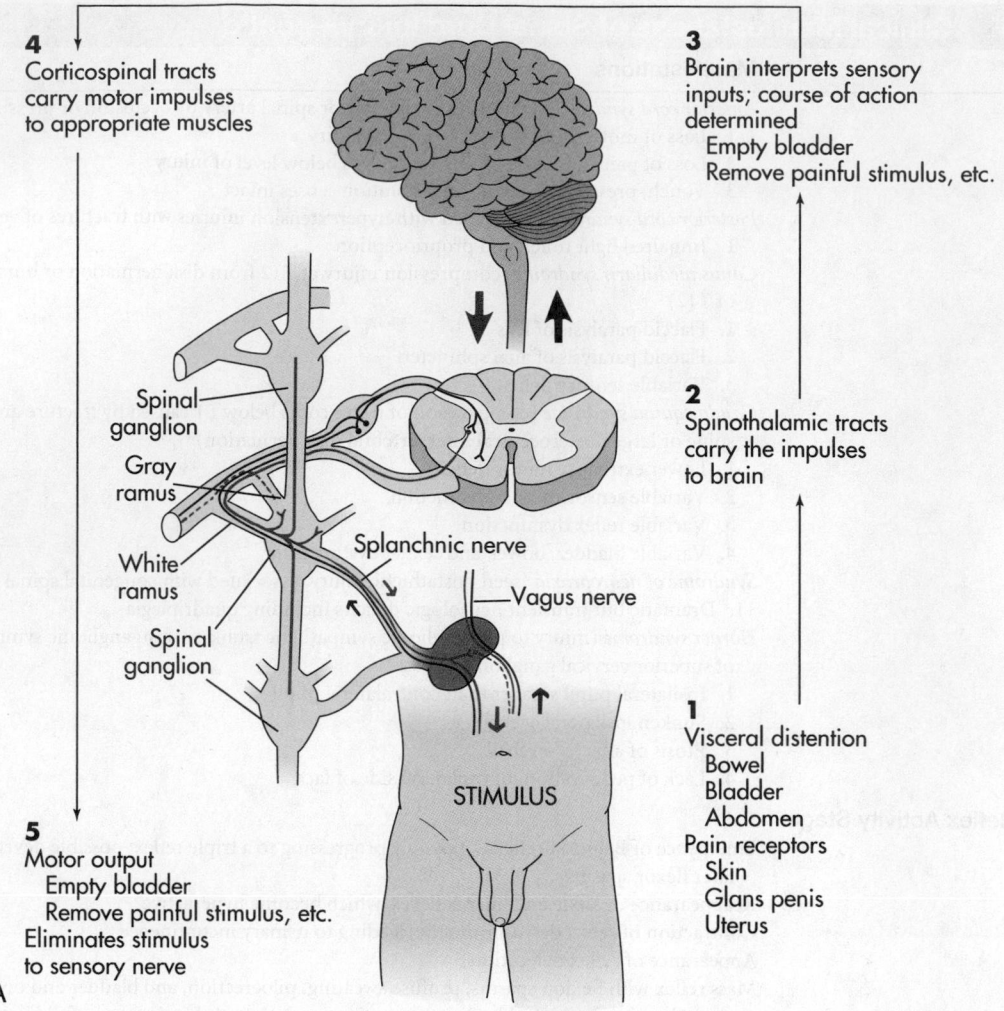

4
Corticospinal tracts
carry motor impulses
to appropriate muscles

3
Brain interprets sensory
inputs; course of action
determined
   Empty bladder
   Remove painful stimulus, etc.

Spinal
ganglion
Gray
ramus

White
ramus
Spinal
ganglion

Splanchnic nerve

Vagus nerve

2
Spinothalamic tracts
carry the impulses
to brain

STIMULUS

5
Motor output
   Empty bladder
   Remove painful stimulus, etc.
Eliminates stimulus
to sensory nerve

1
Visceral distention
   Bowel
   Bladder
   Abdomen
Pain receptors
   Skin
   Glans penis
   Uterus

A

Figure 17-13 Autonomic hyperreflexia. **A,** Normal response pathway. (Modified from Rudy EB: *Advanced neurological and neurosurgical nursing,* St Louis, 1984, Mosby.)

autonomic nervous system reflexively responds with an arteriolar spasm that increases blood pressure. Baroreceptors in the cerebral vessels, the carotid sinus, and the aorta sense the hypertension and stimulate the parasympathetic system. The heart rate decreases, but the visceral and peripheral vessels do not dilate because efferent impulses cannot pass through the cord.

The most common precipitating cause is a distended bladder or rectum, but any sensory stimulation can elicit autonomic hyperreflexia. Stimulation of the skin or stimulation of the pain receptors may cause autonomic hyperreflexia. Emptying of the bladder or bowel usually relieves the syndrome, and this may be facilitated by drugs, such as phenoxybenzamine.

EVALUATION AND TREATMENT Diagnosis of spinal cord injury is made on the basis of physical, radiologic, and myelographic examination; CT scan; and MRI. For a suspected or confirmed vertebral fracture or dislocation, regardless of the presence or absence of spinal cord injury, the immediate intervention is immobilization of the spine to prevent further injury. Decompression and surgical fixation may be necessary. Corticosteroids are given at the time of injury

to decrease secondary cord injury and continued for 24 to 48 hours, depending on time of initiation following injury. The only other agent continuing to show promise is GM-1 ganglioside.[4] Nutrition, lung function, skin integrity, and bladder and bowel management must be addressed. Plans for rehabilitation require early consideration.[10]

In cases of autonomic hyperreflexia, intervention must be prompt because cerebrovascular accident (CVA) is possible. The head of the bed should be elevated, and the stimulus should be found and removed. Medications may be used if these measures do not effectively reduce blood pressure.

Degenerative Disorders of the Spine

Degenerative Disk Disease

Degenerative changes occur in the vertebral disks. **Degenerative disk disease (DDD)** is a common finding in individuals 30 years of age and older. Only a small percentage of those persons have any functional incapacity because of pain. The causes of DDD include biochemical and biomechanical alterations of the tissue of the intervertebral disk. Fibrocartilage replaces

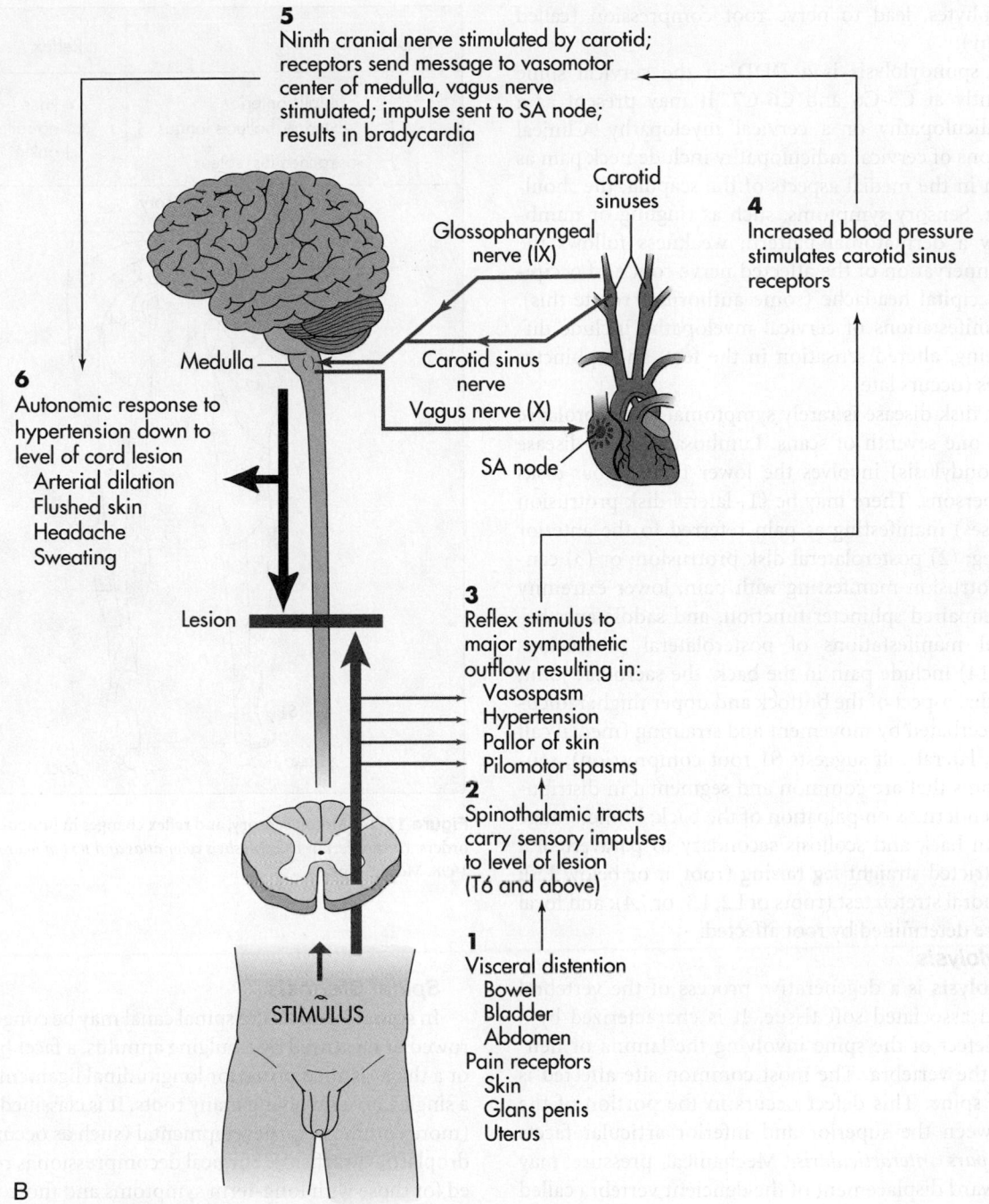

5
Ninth cranial nerve stimulated by carotid; receptors send message to vasomotor center of medulla, vagus nerve stimulated; impulse sent to SA node; results in bradycardia

Carotid sinuses

Glossopharyngeal nerve (IX)

4
Increased blood pressure stimulates carotid sinus receptors

Medulla

Carotid sinus nerve
Vagus nerve (X)

SA node

6
Autonomic response to hypertension down to level of cord lesion
Arterial dilation
Flushed skin
Headache
Sweating

Lesion

3
Reflex stimulus to major sympathetic outflow resulting in:
Vasospasm
Hypertension
Pallor of skin
Pilomotor spasms

2
Spinothalamic tracts carry sensory impulses to level of lesion (T6 and above)

1
Visceral distention
Bowel
Bladder
Abdomen
Pain receptors
Skin
Glans penis
Uterus

STIMULUS

B

Figure 17-13, cont'd Autonomic hyperreflexia. B, Autonomic dysreflexia pathway. *SA,* Sinoatrial. (Modified from Rudy EB: *Advanced neurological and neurosurgical nursing*, St Louis, 1984, Mosby.)

the gelatinous mucoid material of the nucleus pulposus as the disk changes with age. There may be splits in the annulus fibrosis, permitting herniation of elements of nucleus pulposus. There may be shrinkage of the nucleus pulposus that produces prolapse or folding of the annulus with secondary osteophyte formation at the margins of the adjacent vertebral body. The pathologic findings in DDD include disk protrusion, spondylolysis, and/or subluxation and degeneration of vertebrae (spondylolisthesis) and spinal stenosis.[11]

Symptoms result from either (1) disk or annulus protrusion or (2) narrowing of the spinal canal or intervertebral foramen by osteophytes. A congenital narrow canal or congenitally short pedicles may be present.

Posterior disk protrusion in the cervical and thoracic regions lead to cord compression, and cauda equina compression results in the lumbar area. Both situations are called *myelopathy*. Posterolateral disk protrusions, with or without a contribution from the vertebral body or apophyseal joint osteophytes, lead to nerve root compression (called *radiculopathy*).

Cervical spondylolysis is a DDD in the cervical spine predominantly at C5-C6 and C6-C7. It may present as a cervical radiculopathy or a cervical myelopathy. Clinical manifestations of cervical radiculopathy include neck pain as well as pain in the medial aspects of the scapula, the shoulder, or arm. Sensory symptoms, such as tingling or numbness, follow a dermatomal pattern; weakness follows the pattern of innervation of the affected nerve root and occipital or suboccipital headache (some authorities refute this). Clinical manifestations of cervical myelopathy include difficulty walking, altered sensation in the feet, and sphincter disturbances (occurs late).

Thoracic disk disease is rarely symptomatic, but prolapse is found in one seventh of scans. Lumbosacral disk disease (lumbar spondylosis) involves the lower two lumbar disks in 90% of persons. There may be (1) lateral disk protrusion (10% of cases) manifesting as pain referred to the anterior thigh and leg; (2) posterolateral disk protrusion; or (3) central disk protrusion manifesting with pain, lower extremity weakness, impaired sphincter function, and saddle anesthesia. Clinical manifestations of posterolateral protrusions (Figure 17-14) include pain in the back, the sacroiliac joint, and the medial aspect of the buttock and upper thigh; radicular pain exacerbated by movement and straining (medial calf suggests L5, lateral calf suggests S1 root compression); sensory symptoms that are common and segmental in distribution; focal tenderness on palpation of the back; limited range of motion in back and scoliosis secondary to paravertebral spasms; restricted straight-leg raising (root at or below L5); positive femoral stretch test (roots of L2, L3, or L4); and focal signs that are determined by root affected.

Spondylolysis

Spondylolysis is a degenerative process of the vertebral column and associated soft tissue. It is characterized by a structural defect of the spine involving the lamina or neural arch of the vertebra. The most common site affected is the lumbar spine. This defect occurs in the portion of the lamina between the superior and inferior articular facets called the *pars interarticularis*. Mechanical pressure may cause a forward displacement of the deficient vertebra called *spondylolisthesis*.

Heredity plays a significant role, and spondylolysis is associated with an increased incidence of other congenital spinal defects. As a result of torsional and rotational stress, "microfractures" occur at the affected site and eventually cause dissolution of the pars interarticularis.

Spondylolisthesis

Spondylolisthesis is a stress factor allowing a vertebra to slide forward in relation to the vertebra below, commonly occurring at L5-S1. Spondylolisthesis is graded from 1 to 4 on the basis of the percentage of slip that has occurred. Individuals with grade 3 or 4 are considered for operative decompression or stabilization or both. Grades 1 and 2 usually are managed symptomatically and with nonsurgical methods.

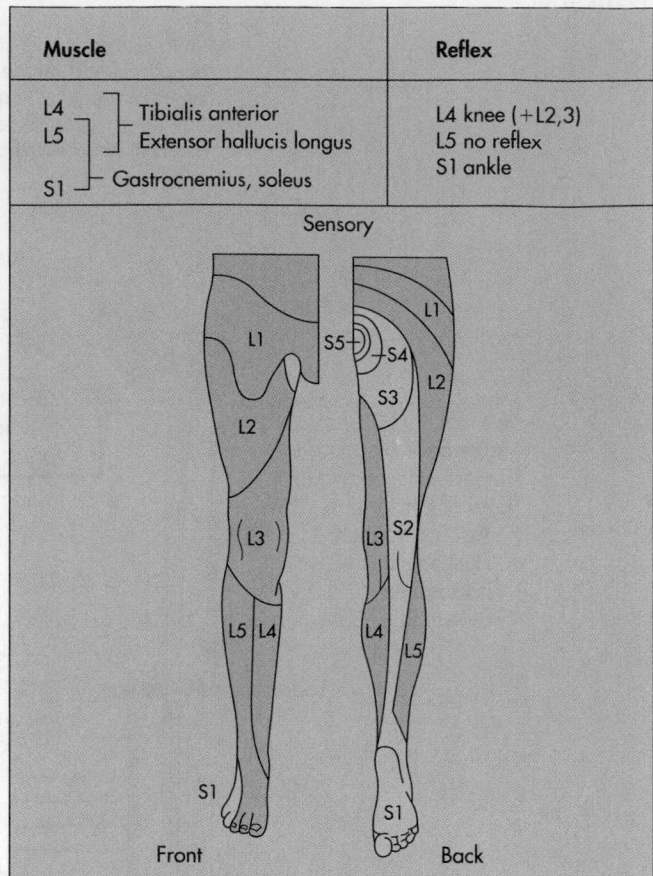

Figure 17-14 Motor, sensory, and reflex changes in lumbosacral root disorders. (From Perkin DG: *Mosby's color atlas and text of neurology*, London, 1998, Mosby-Wolfe.)

Spinal Stenosis

In **spinal stenosis** the spinal canal may be congenitally narrowed or narrowed by a bulging annulus, a facet hypertrophy, or a thick/ossified posterior longitudinal ligament entrapping a single nerve involving many roots. It is classified as acquired (more common) or developmental (such as occurs in achondroplastic dwarfism). Surgical decompression is recommended for those with long-term symptoms and those who remain unresponsive to medical management.

Low Back Pain

Low back pain affects the area between the lower rib cage and gluteal muscles and often radiates into the thighs. About 1% of individuals with acute low back pain have sciatica or pain in the distribution of the sciatic nerve or lumbar and sacral nerve roots. Sciatica often is accompanied by neurosensory and motor deficits, such as weakness.

The incidence of, or percentage of population affected with, low back pain at some point in life is 60% to 80%, and the annual incidence is 5%. Men and women are affected equally; however, women report low back symptoms more often after the age of 60 years.

PATHOGENESIS Most cases of low back pain are idiopathic, and clinicians are unable to provide a precise diagnosis for most individuals with this disorder. The local processes involved in low back pain range from tension caused by tumors or disk prolapse, bursitis, synovitis, rising venous and tissue pressure (found in degenerative joint disease), abnormal bone pressures, problems with spinal mobility, inflammation caused by infection (as in osteomyelitis), bony fractures, or ligamentous sprains to pain referred from viscera or the posterior peritoneum. General processes resulting in low back pain include bone diseases, such as osteoporosis or osteomalacia, and hyperparathyroidism.

Several risk factors have been identified in the pathogenesis of low back pain. They include involvement caused by occupations that require repetitive lifting in the forward bent-and-twisted position, exposure to vibrations caused by vehicles or industrial machinery, and perhaps cigarette smoking. Osteoporosis increases the risk of spinal compression fractures and may be the reason older adult women report more symptoms than men. Genetic predispositions for low back pain include isthmic spondylolisthesis (vertebra slides forward or slips in relation to a vertebra below), spinal osteochondrosis, and spinal stenosis associated with achondroplasia. Variations in posture, such as lordosis and scoliosis of less than 60 degrees, do not appear to increase the risk of low back pain or sciatica. Differences in weight, height, and leg length are controversial as risk factors.

Anatomically, low back pain must come from innervated structures, but deep pain is widely referred and varies from person to person. The nucleus pulposus has no intrinsic innervation; however, when extruded or herniated through a prolapsed disk, it irritates the dural membranes and is responsible for pain referred to the segmental area (see Figure 17-14). The interspinous bursae can be a source of low back pain between L3, L4, L5, and S1, but also may affect L1, L2, and L3 spinous processes, depending on the closeness of the adjacent pair of spines. The anterior and posterior longitudinal ligaments of the spine and the interspinous and supraspinous ligaments are abundantly supplied with pain receptors, as is the ligamentum flavum. All of these ligaments are vulnerable to traumatic tears (sprains) and fracture. The role of muscle injury in the production of low back pain remains uncertain, even though sprains and strains are the most common diagnoses. The muscle spasms that often are produced during sieges of low back pain are thought to be produced by as yet unknown sensory or motor-reflex pathways. The most commonly encountered causes of low back pain include lumbar disk herniation, degenerative disk disease, spondylolysis, spondylolisthesis, and spinal stenosis. (For a discussion of disk herniation and rupture, see following text.)

EVALUATION AND TREATMENT Diagnosis of low back injury is made by physical examination, electromyography (EMG), epidurography, diskography, and MRI; CT with or without myelography; and nerve conduction studies. Most individuals with acute low back pain benefit from a nonspecific short-term treatment regimen including bed rest, analgesic medications, exercises, physical therapy, and education. Surgical treatments may be indicated if individuals do not respond to medical management. Surgical treatments include diskectomy and spinal fusions. Individuals with chronic low back pain can be treated with anti-inflammatory and muscle relaxant medications, exercise programs, massage, topical heat, spinal manipulation, cognitive-behavioral therapy, and interdisciplinary care.[12]

Herniated Intervertebral Disk

Herniation of an intervertebral disk is a displacement of the disk material (nucleus pulposus or the annulus fibrosis) beyond the intervertebral disk space[2] (Figure 17-15). Men are more affected than women with a 2:1 ratio. The highest incidence is among those 30 to 50 years of age.[2] Between ages 25 and 55, 95% of herniated disks are in the lower lumbar spine (L4-L5); over age 55, herniation level is higher. Disk herniation occasionally occurs in the cervical area, usually at C5-C6 and C6-C7. Herniations at the thoracic level are extremely rare. Risk factors for herniation include smoking, weightbearing sports like weightlifting, and certain work activities such as repeated lifting.[2] Rupture of an intervertebral disk usually is caused by trauma or degenerative disk disease or both. Lifting with the trunk flexed and sudden straining when the back is in an unstable position are the most common causes. The injury may have an immediate onset or an onset within a few hours, or the manifestations of injury may take months to years to develop.

PATHOPHYSIOLOGY In a herniated disk the ligament and posterior capsule of the disk usually are torn, allowing the gelatinous material (the nucleus pulposus) to extrude. This extrusion compresses the nerve root. Occasionally the injury tears the entire disk loose, and it protrudes onto the nerve root or compresses the spinal cord. One or more nerve roots may be compressed. This multiple nerve root compression is found especially at the L5-S1 level, where the cauda equina may be compressed. Large amounts of extruded nucleus pulposus or complete disk herniation (i.e., of both the capsule and the nucleus pulposus) may compress the spinal cord.

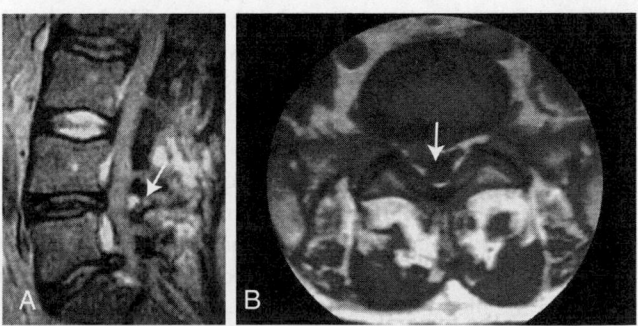

Figure 17-15 Posterolateral disk protrusion. Magnetic resonance imaging (MRI) scan, (**A**) sagittal (see arrow) and (**B**) axial (see arrow) sections. (From Perkin DG: *Mosby's color atlas and text of neurology*, London, 1998, Mosby-Wolfe.)

CLINICAL MANIFESTATIONS The location and size of the herniation into the spinal canal, together with the amount of space that exists inside the spinal canal, determine the clinical manifestations associated with the injury (see Figure 17-15). A herniated disk in the lumbosacral area is associated with pain that radiates along the sciatic nerve course over the buttock and into the calf or ankle. The pain occurs with straining, including coughing and sneezing, and usually on straight-leg raising. Other clinical manifestations include limited range of motion of the lumbar spine; tenderness on palpation in the sciatic notch and along the sciatic nerve; impaired pain, temperature, and touch sensation in the L5-S1 or L4-L5 dermatomes of the leg and foot; decreased or absent ankle jerk; and mild weakness of the foot.

With the herniation of a lower cervical disk, paresthesias and pain are present in the upper arm, forearm, and hand in the affected nerve root distribution. Neck and nerve root pain may be increased by neck motion and straining, including coughing and sneezing. Neck range of motion is diminished. Slight weakness and atrophy of biceps or triceps may occur; the biceps or triceps reflex may decrease. Occasionally signs of corticospinal and sensory tract impairments appear. These include motor weakness of the lower extremities, sensory disturbances in the lower extremities, and presence of a Babinski reflex.

EVALUATION AND TREATMENT Diagnosis of a herniated intervertebral disk is made on the basis of the history and physical examination, EMG, CT, MRI, myelography, and diskography; spinal radiography; and nerve conduction studies. Radiologic evidence of disk herniation does not reliably correlate with symptoms or predict low back pain. Many individuals with disk herniation on imaging have no symptoms.[13] Clinical improvement occurs in most people. Only about 10% have sufficient pain after 6 weeks to consider surgery. The herniated disk portion on serial imaging tends to regress over time.[2] There is little evidence to support drug treatments including the use of analgesics, antidepressants, or muscle relaxants.[14] Nonsteroidal anti-inflammatory drugs (NSAIDs), bed rest, or traction did not improve sciatica caused by herniation. Insufficient evidence exists to judge the effectiveness of epidural injections of nonsteroidals, activity, acupuncture, massage, exercise, heat, or ice.[2] However, standard diskectomy and microdiskectomy had self-reported improvement. A surgical approach is indicated if there is evidence of severe compression (weakness, decreased deep tendon reflexes and bladder/bowel reflexes).

Cerebrovascular Disorders

Cerebrovascular disease is the most frequently occurring neurologic disorder. More than 50% of persons admitted to general hospitals with neurologic problems have cerebrovascular disease. Any abnormality of the brain caused by a pathologic process in the blood vessels is referred to as a *cerebrovascular disease.* Included in this category are lesions of the vessel wall; occlusion of the vessel lumen by thrombus or embolus; rupture of the vessel; and alteration in vessel permeability, such as increased blood viscosity.

The brain abnormalities induced by cerebrovascular disease are of two types: (1) ischemia with or without infarction (death of brain tissues) accounting for 80% of CVAs and (2) hemorrhage. The common clinical manifestation of cerebrovascular disease is a **cerebrovascular accident (CVA, stroke),** which is a sudden, nonconvulsive focal neurologic deficit. Box 17-1 highlights the differences for strokes in children.

Cerebrovascular Accidents (Stroke Syndromes)
The incidence of new and recurrent stroke is 795,000 approximately 185,000 of these were recurrent.[15] CVAs are the third leading cause of death in the United States, resulting in 143,600 deaths (2005) or about one in seventeen deaths per year in the US.[15] Globally, 4.5 million people die from CVAs per year.[2] About 10% of persons with acute ischemic CVAs die within 30 days of onset. CVAs are the leading cause of disability in the United States—50% of individuals experience some level of disability after 6 months.[2] Five percent to 14% of stroke survivors have a second stroke within 1 year of the first CVA. By 5 years, 24% of females and 42% of males have a second stroke.

Fifty percent of CVAs occur in persons over 70 years of age.[2] Strokes, however, do occur in a 3:10 ratio (28%) in individuals younger than 65 years of age. Stroke tends to run in families. The incidence of stroke is 2.5 times higher in blacks than whites. Stroke prevalence in 2005 for black men was 2.3 million compared to 3.4 million in black women.[16] The risk of first ever stroke in blacks is almost twice that of whites.[16] Death rates in blacks was 74.9 in males and 65.5 in females compared to an overall death rate of 50 in whites. Mexican Americans have an increased incidence of stroke compared with non-Hispanic whites.[16] Blacks suffer greater physical impairments and are nearly twice as likely to die from their strokes. Intracranial atherosclerosis is more common in black and Asian populations, whereas extracranial disease is more common in the white population.

The mildest outcome of a CVA is so minimal as to be almost unnoticed. The most severe outcomes are hemiplegia, coma,

---

Box 17-1   Stroke in Children

- Risk factors different than adult (i.e., hypertension, atherosclerosis, diabetes, smoking, obesity)
- Important causes include congenital cardiac disease, sickle cell disease, arterial dissection, prothrombotic disorders, moyamoya disease, and head and neck trauma
- Vascular occlusion occurs more often in intracranial vessels, including internal carotid, middle cerebral and basilar arteries; infarcts more often limited to deep regions of the cerebral hemispheres, mostly basal ganglion and internal capsule areas
- Intracerebral hemorrhage and subaracnoid hemorrhage account for a much higher percentage of strokes in children

Data from Bernard TJ, Goldenberg NA: *Pediatr Clin North Am* 55(2):323-338,viii, 2008; Seidman C, Kirkham F, Pavlakis S: *Curr Opin Pediatr* 19(6):657-662, 2007.

and death. CVAs (stroke syndromes) are classified according to pathophysiology and thus are ischemic (thrombotic or embolic), global hypoperfusion (as in shock), or hemorrhagic. Risk factors for stroke include the following:

1. Arterial hypertension as well as elevated systolic and diastolic blood pressures are independent risk factors.
2. Smoking doubles the risk of stroke.
3. Diabetes is an independent risk factor and increases the risk of ischemic stroke between 2.5 and 3.5 times.[17]
4. Insulin resistance is an independent risk factor for ischemic stroke.
5. Polycythemia and thrombocythemia increase the risk for ischemic stroke.
6. Presence of elevated lipoprotein-a is an independent risk factor for ischemic stroke.
7. Impaired cardiac function increases the risk for ischemic stroke.
8. Hyperhomocysteinemia is a strong and independent risk factor for ischemic stroke.
9. Nonrheumatic atrial fibrillation is associated with a fivefold increase in the incidence of ischemic stroke.[18]
10. *Chlamydia pneumoniae* can increase the risk of stroke by infecting and injuring the endothelium.

Thrombotic Stroke. Thrombotic strokes (**cerebral thrombosis**) arise from arterial occlusions caused by thrombi formed in the arteries supplying the brain or in the intracranial vessels. The development of a cerebral thrombosis most frequently is attributed to atherosclerosis and inflammatory disease processes (arteritis) that damage arterial walls. Increased coagulation can lead to thrombus formation. Conditions causing inadequate cerebral perfusion (e.g., dehydration, hypotension, prolonged vasoconstriction from malignant hypertension) increase the risk of thrombosis. Over 20 to 30 years atheromatous plaques (stenotic lesions) tend to form at branchings and curves in the cerebral circulation. The smooth stenotic area can degenerate, forming an ulcerated area of vessel wall. Platelets and fibrin adhere to the damaged wall, and clots form, gradually occluding the artery. The thrombus may enlarge both distally and proximally in the vessel. Portions of the clot break off and travel up the vessel to distant sites where occlusion occurs, producing a stroke syndrome.

The distinction between transient ischemic attacks and thrombotic stroke is losing importance. With increasing use of brain imaging, many persons with symptoms lasting less than 24 hours are found to have had a brain infarction. The new definition for **transient ischemic attack (TIA)** is a brief episode of neurologic dysfunction caused by a focal disturbance of brain or retinal ischemia with clinical symptoms typically lasting less than 1 hour and without evidence of infarction.[17] TIAs probably represent thrombotic particles causing an intermittent blockage of circulation or spasm. Recurrence of symptoms is 10.7% at 90 days, 60% at 6 months, and 80% at 1 year without definitive treatment.[17]

Embolic Stroke. Cardioembolism accounts for 30% of all CVAs, 25% to 30% of strokes in persons less than 45 years of age.[19] An **embolic stroke** involves fragments that break from a thrombus formed outside the brain or in the heart, aorta, common carotid, or thorax. Emboli infrequently arise from the ascending aorta or common carotid artery. The embolus usually involves small vessels and obstructs at a bifurcation or other point of narrowing, thus causing ischemia. An embolus may plug the lumen entirely and remain in place or break into fragments and move up the vessel. High-risk sources for the onset of embolic stroke are atrial fibrillation (15% to 25% of strokes), left ventricular aneurysm or thrombus, left atrial thrombus, recent myocardial infarction, rheumatic valvular disease, mechanical prosthetic valve, nonbacterial thrombotic endocarditis, bacterial endocarditis, patent foramen ovale, and primary intracardiac tumors.[19,20] In persons who experience an embolic stroke, a second stroke usually follows at some point because the source of emboli continues to exist. The 7-day recurrence risk is 6.5%, in-hospital mortality is 27.3%, and 5-year prognosis is as high as 80%.[19] Embolization is usually in the distribution of the middle cerebral artery.

Hemorrhagic Stroke. Hemorrhagic stroke (**intracranial hemorrhage [ICH]**) is the third most common cause of CVA (10% of strokes) and accounts for 10% to 15% of CVAs in whites but 30% in blacks and Asians.[18] There are 40,000 ICHs in the United States per year.[21] The most common causes of spontaneous primary hemorrhagic strokes are hypertension (56% to 81%), ruptured aneurysms, arteriovenous malformation and fistula, amyloid angiopathy, and cavernous angioma.[21] ICH can occur secondary to TBI, bleeding into the ischemic brain infarction or tumor, or a bleeding disorder or anticoagulation. Risk factors for hemorrhagic stroke include hypertension, previous cerebral infarct, coronary artery disease, and diabetes mellitus.

A hypertensive hemorrhage is associated with a significant increase in systolic and diastolic pressure over several years and usually occurs within the brain tissue. A mass of blood is formed, and its volume increases. Adjacent brain tissue is displaced and compressed and rupture or seepage into the ventricular system occurs in many cases. Hemorrhages are described as massive, small, slit, or petechial. A massive hemorrhage is several centimeters in diameter; a small hemorrhage is 1 to 2 cm in diameter; a slit hemorrhage lies in the subcortical area; and a petechial hemorrhage is the size of a pinhead bleed. The most common sites for hypertensive hemorrhages are in the putamen of the basal ganglia (a portion of the lentiform nucleus) (40%), the thalamus (15%), the cortex and subcortex (22%), the pons (8%) (Figure 17-16), caudate (7%), and cerebellar hemispheres (8%).

Lacunar Stroke. A lacunar stroke (**lacunar infarct**) is a microinfarct smaller than 1 cm in diameter and involves the small perforating arteries, predominantly in the basal ganglia, internal capsules, and pons. Lacunar infarcts are caused by lipohyalinosis, subintimal lipid-loading foam cells, and fibrinoid materials that thicken the arterial walls and are associated with smoking,[18] hypertension, and diabetes mellitus. Because of the subcortical location and small area of infarction, these strokes may have pure motor and sensory deficits.

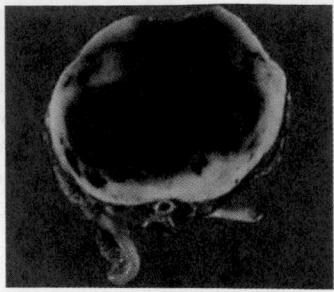

Figure 17-16 Hypertensive hemorrhage. Cross section of the pons showing a hypertensive hemorrhage. (From Perkin DG: *Mosby's color atlas and text of neurology*, London, 1998, Mosby-Wolfe.)

PATHOPHYSIOLOGY

Cerebral Infarction. Cerebral infarction results when an area of the brain loses blood supply because of vascular occlusion. The pathologic manifestation is either (1) a global process that affects neurons most susceptible to ischemia (pyramidal and striatal neurons), Purkinje cells of the cerebral hemispheres, and the border zones at the very end of the arteries' circulation; or (2) a focal process with a central zone of cell loss surrounded by a zone of injured cells, the ischemic penumbra, that if perfused in 1 hour will survive. Proposed pathogenesis may include (1) abrupt vascular occlusion (e.g., embolus), (2) gradual vessel occlusion (e.g., atheroma), and (3) vessels that are stenosed but not completely occluded. Cerebral thrombi and cerebral emboli are the most common causes of occlusion, but atherosclerosis and hypotension are the dominant underlying processes.

Cerebral infarctions are ischemic or hemorrhagic. In ischemic infarcts (pale infarcts, "white stroke"), cytotoxic ischemic events and interaction between blood elements and blood vessels combine to produce brain injury. The affected area becomes slightly discolored and softens about 6 to 12 hours after the occlusion. Necrosis, swelling around the insult, and mushy disintegration have appeared by 48 to 72 hours after infarction. At a microscopic level, neuronal cell bodies change, myelin sheaths and axis cylinders are interrupted and disintegrate, and there is loss of oligodendrites and astrocytes.

Cellular and biochemical events involve the loss of glucose and oxygen delivery resulting in depletion of high-energy phosphate compounds (failure of mitochondrial energy production) allowing cell membrane depolarization. With membrane depolarization, neurotransmitters, including glutamate, are released and cannot be reuptaken. Glutamate promotes excess entry of extracellular calcium. Unregulated, elevated calcium concentrations activate degrading enzymes.[22] Production and accumulation of lactic acid also result in an associated focal vasodilation. Infarcted areas may lose autoregulation of blood flow.

A syndrome of luxury perfusion in areas adjacent to the infarct develops first from the loss of autoregulation. The vascular bed in this area dilates. Later, capillary sprouting (neovascularization) supports this luxury perfusion syndrome.

In hemorrhagic infarcts ("red strokes"), bleeding occurs into the infarcted area as a result of restoration of blood flow. Reperfusion occurs when the embolus fragments, or lysis or compressive forces lessen, allowing blood flow to be reestablished into the infarcted area. Most hemorrhagic infarcts are located in the cerebral cortex. Unfortunately, reperfusion has been shown to compromise recovery by accelerating the sequence of metabolically damaging events including oxidative stress (reperfusion injury).

Cerebral Hemorrhage. The primary cause of cerebral hemorrhage is hypertension. (Aneurysms and arteriovenous malformations are discussed on pp. 606-608.) The pathogenesis of hypertensive cerebral hemorrhage is not fully understood. Hypertension involves primarily smaller arteries and arterioles, resulting in thickening of the vessel walls, and increased cellularity of the vessels and hyalinization. Necrosis may be present. Microaneurysms in these smaller vessels or arteriolar necrosis precipitates the bleeding.

A mass of blood is formed as bleeding continues into the brain tissue. In massive ICH (volume greater than 150 ml), cerebral perfusion falls to zero and cerebral blood flow stops, resulting in death.[21] Adjacent brain tissue is deformed, compressed, and displaced. Necrosis around the hematoma is present within 6 hours. Edema forms and the blood-brain barrier is disrupted. An inflammatory reaction in surrounding brain tissue appears rapidly and peaks in several days.[21] Figure 17-17 illustrates additional detail. Rupture or seepage of blood into the ventricular system occurs in many cases.

The cerebral hemorrhage resolves through reabsorption. Macrophages and astrocytes appear to clear away the blood. A cavity forms, surrounded by a dense gliosis after removal of the blood.

CLINICAL MANIFESTATIONS Because neurons surrounding the ischemic or infarcted areas undergo changes that disrupt plasma membranes, cellular edema results, causing further compression of capillaries. Most persons survive an initial hemispheric ischemic stroke unless massive cerebral edema develops. However, massive brain stem infarcts, caused by basilar thrombosis or embolism, are almost always fatal.

Clinical manifestations of thrombotic stroke vary, depending on the artery obstructed. Different sites of obstruction create different occlusion syndromes (Table 17-6).

With hemorrhagic stroke, clinical manifestations vary according to the location and size of the bleed. Focal neurologic deficits are found in 80% of individuals experiencing hemorrhagic strokes; altered consciousness occurs in 50%. Once a deep unresponsive state occurs the immediate prognosis is grave, and the individual rarely survives. If the person survives, however, recovery of function frequently is possible.

Individuals experiencing intracranial hemorrhage from a ruptured or leaking aneurysm have one of three sets of symptoms: (1) onset of an excruciating generalized headache with an almost immediate lapse into an unresponsive state; (2) headache, but with consciousness maintained; and (3) sudden lapse into unconsciousness. If the hemorrhage is confined to the subarachnoid space, there may be no local

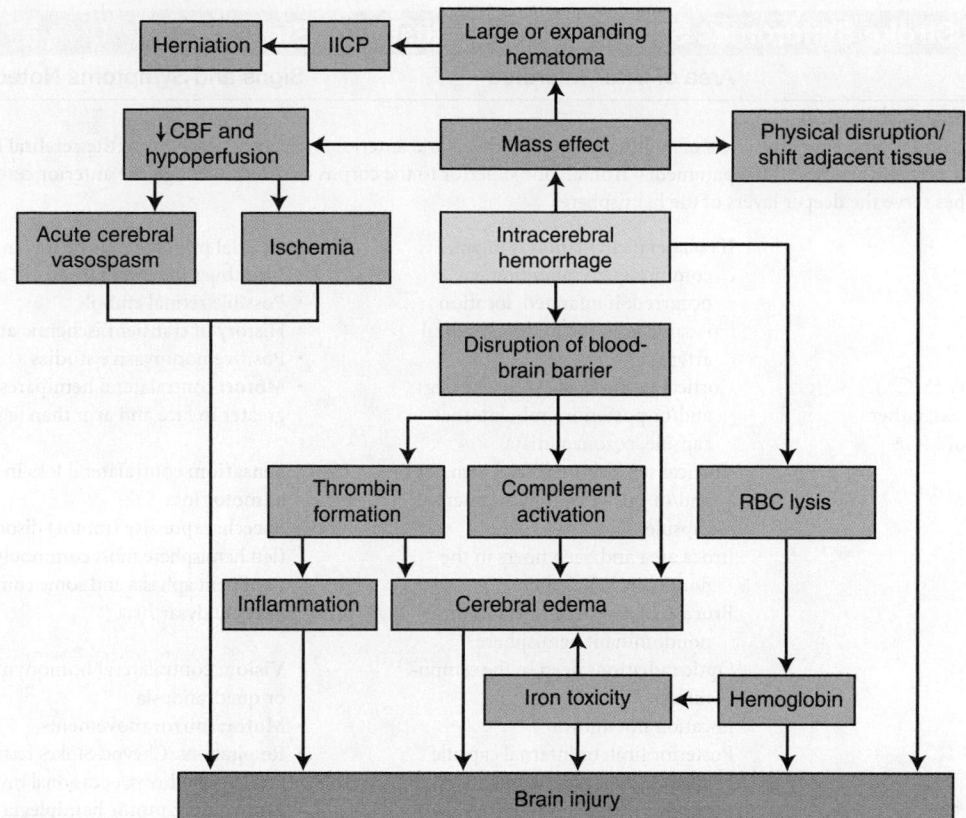

Figure 17-17 Injury mechanisms promoted by intracerebral hemorrhage. Hemorrhages can induce neuronal injury through mass effect, particularly in large hematomas that can *cause* increased intracranial pressure and herniation. Hemorrhages may also cause tissue damage through cerebral edema and "neurotoxic" mechanisms caused by activation of the coagulation cascade and inflammation. Not all potential interactions are shown (e.g., thrombin may potentiate iron-induced injury; the complement and inflammatory systems overlap and several factors contribute to cerebral edema). *CBF,* cerebral blood flow; *IICP,* increased intracranial pressure; *RBC,* red blood cell. (Data from Mocco J et al: *Neurosurg Focus* 15:22[5]:E7, 2007; Schubert GA, Thome C: *Front Biosci* 13:1594-603, 2008; Xi G, Keep RF, Hoff JT: *Lancet Neurol* 5[1]:53-63, 2006.)

signs. If bleeding spreads into the brain tissue, hemiparesis/paralysis, dysphasia, or homonymous hemianopia may be present. Warning signs of an impending aneurysm rupture may include headache, transient unilateral weakness, transient numbness and tingling, and transient speech disturbance. Warning signs, however, often are not present.

EVALUATION AND TREATMENT No identifiable cause can be established by conventional diagnostic tests in up to 40% of CVAs and are classified as having "undetermined" or "cryptogenic" mechanisms.[20] The principle of acute stroke treatment is "time is brain." Time to treatment is often too great considering the time limits for reversibility of brain ischemia. Treatment needs to be initiated within 6 hours of symptom onset. Research evidence related to acute stroke management is as follows:

1. Specialized stroke rehabilitation appears to be more effective than conventional care at reducing death and dependency and length of hospital stay.[23]
2. Aspirin has been shown to effectively reduce death and dependency at 6 months when given within 48 hours of ischemic stroke as are systemic anticoagulants (unfractionated heparin, low-molecular-weight heparin,

heparinoids, oral anticoagulants, or specific thrombin inhibitors) but with a lower risk of intracranial and extracranial hemorrhage.[2,24]

3. Thrombolysis (i.e., tissue plaminogen activator [tPA]) given within 3 hours of onset of symptoms reduces dependency at 6 months when the diagnosis of ischemic stroke has been confirmed. Streptokinase has been found to increase the risk of intracranial hemorrhage and is not used to treat acute ischemic stroke.[25]
4. Acute blood pressure lowering in acute ischemic stroke may actually lead to increased cerebral ischemia.
5. Disappointingly, neuroprotective agents (calcium channel antagonists, citicoline, gamma-aminobutyric acid (GABA) agonists, glycine antagonists, magnesium, N-methyl-D-aspartate antagonists, tirilazid) have not been shown to significantly reduce the risk of poor outcome including death or improve outcomes with ischemic stroke.[26]
6. Surgical evacuation does not appear to be an effective treatment for supratentorial ICHs but may be indicated in a few specific situations.[27]

Table 17-6 Stroke Syndromes Secondary to Occlusion or Stenosis

Location/Vessel	Area of Brain Infarcted	Signs and Symptoms Noted
Anterior and Central Circulation		
Note: The internal carotid artery enters the circle of Willis and supplies the lateral anterior and central portions of the cerebral hemispheres through the middle cerebral artery and the paramedial frontal lobe superior to the corpus callosum through the anterior cerebral artery; penetrating branches serve the deeper layers of the hemispheres		
Internal carotid	If collateral circulation is intact, commonly no infarction has occurred; if infarcted, location is same as in the middle cerebral artery	• Arterial pressure may be low in the retina • Bruit over the internal carotid artery • Possible retinal emboli • History of transient ischemic attacks (TIAs) • Positive noninvasive studies
Middle cerebral artery (MCA) (most common area); either stem or branches of MCA	Cortical motor area (face, arm, leg) and/or posterior limb, internal capsule, corona radiata	• **Motor:** contralateral hemiparesis or hemiplegia, greater in face and arm than leg
	Cortical sensory area (face, arm, leg) and/or posterior limb of internal capsule	• **Sensation:** contralateral loss in same distribution as motor loss
	Broca area and deep fibers in the dominant hemisphere	• **Speech:** expressive (motor) disorder with anomia (left hemisphere most commonly affected) with nonfluent aphasia and some comprehension defects
	Broca area and deep fibers in the nondominant hemisphere	• **Speech:** dysarthria
	Optic radiations deep in the temporal lobe	• **Vision:** contralateral homonymous hemianopsia or quadranopsia
	Location not known	• **Motor:** mirror movements
	Posterior limb or internal capsule and adjacent corona radiata	• Respirations: Cheyne-Stokes respirations, contralateral hyperhidrosis, occasional mydriasis • **Motor:** pure motor hemiplegia
	Penetrating branches of MCA (lenticulostriate branches) into the basal nuclei	• **Motor:** varying degrees of contralateral weakness of face, arm, or leg • **Sensory:** little or no loss; if present, contralateral following the motor distribution • **Speech:** transcortical sensory aphasia (communicating pathways are interrupted) • **Perception:** transient visual and sensory neglect on the left if a right lesion
Anterior cerebral artery (ACA) (least common)	Proximal segment: corona radiata (rarely)	• **Motor:** when present, a mild contralateral hemiparesis, greater in leg; with bilateral occlusion of ACA, cerebral paraplegia in both legs can occur
	Main stem (complete occlusion is uncommon, thus areas affected differ and collateral circulation may alleviate signs or symptoms); medial aspect of frontal lobes, caudate nucleus, and corpus callosum are supplied by the ACA	• **Motor:** contralateral paralysis or paresis (greater in foot and thigh); mild upper extremity weakness • **Sensory:** mild contralateral lower extremity deficiency with loss of vibratory and/or position sense, loss of two-point discrimination • **Speech:** may have transcortical motor and sensory aphasia if left hemisphere • Frontal lobe releasing signs • Apraxia
Posterior Circulation		
NOTE: The posterior circulation includes the posterior cerebral artery, the vertebral arteries, and the basilar artery; the anatomic territory covered includes the posterior aspects of the hemispheres, the central areas of the thalamus and midbrain, and the brainstem; occlusion of the vessels is most commonly by emboli; effects of infarct in these vessels and their penetrating vessels can be specific or devastatingly global; many complex syndromes have been identified		
Vertebral arteries	Medulla and spinal cord tracts, anterior spinal artery and penetrating branches (medial medullary syndrome)	• Motor: contralateral hemiparesis (face spared) and/or impaired contralateral proprioception; flaccid weakness or paralysis of the tongue and/or dysarthria

Table 17-6   Stroke Syndromes Secondary to Occlusion or Stenosis—cont'd

Location/Vessel	Area of Brain Infarcted	Signs and Symptoms Noted
Posterior Circulation—cont'd		
Basilar artery (three sets of branches)	Midline structures of pons (paramedian branches); three general areas of infarction are common: (1) medial inferior pontine syndrome, (2) medial midpontine syndrome, and (3) medial superior pontine syndrome Corticospinal and corticobulbar tracts in pons, sensory tracts of medial and lateral lemnisci, vestibular nuclei, inferior and middle cerebellar peduncles, cranial nerve nuclei and/or fibers, cerebellar connections in tectum, descending sympathetic pathways, central brainstem, pontine tegmentum (vertebrobasilar syndrome)	• **Motor:** contralateral hemiparesis or hemiplegia, ipsilateral lower motor neuron facial palsy, "locked-in syndrome" • **Sensory:** contralateral loss of vibratory sense, sense of position with dysmetria, loss of two-point discrimination, impaired rapid alternating movements • **Visual:** inferior pontine: diplopia; impaired abduction of ipsilateral eye: internuclear ophthalmoplegia; medial superior; diplopia, internuclear ophthalmoplegia, skewed deviation • **Motor:** upper motor neuron type of weakness: paralysis in combinations involving face, tongue, throat, and extremities; dysphagia, facial weakness, dysmetria, ataxia (either trunk or extremities), weak mastication muscles • **Sensation:** combinations of impaired sensation (vibratory, two-point, position sense, pain, temperature), facial hypesthesia, anesthesia of cranial nerve V
Posterior cerebral artery (PCA)	Central territory (thalamic area, dentothalamic tract, cerebral peduncle, red nucleus, subthalamic nucleus, and cranial nerve III)	• **Motor:** contralateral hemiplegia with possible dysmetria, dyskinesia, hemiballism or choreoathetosis, dystaxia, cerebellar ataxia, and tremor; contralateral upper motor neuron palsy; several syndromes are associated: (1) Weber: cranial nerve III palsy and contralateral hemiplegia; (2) thalamoperforate syndrome: superior, crossed cerebellar ataxia or inferior crossed cerebellar ataxia with cranial nerve III palsy (Claude syndrome); (3) decerebrate attacks • **Sensory:** contralateral sensory loss of all modalities without agraphia • **Function:** prosopagnosia (inability to recognize familiar faces), topographic disorientation, memory deficits, alexia, inability to read, color anomia • **Level of consciousness:** in bilateral PCA syndromes, coma with absent doll's eyes or loss of alertness may occur; if tegmentum of midbrain near hypothalamus and third ventricle is damaged, akinetic mutism may occur

Small Vessel Disease

NOTE: Small penetrating vessels in brain parenchyma that supply areas near the basal ganglia are most vulnerable to infarction although any small vessels can occlude deep in the brain and cause injury, producing neurologic signs or symptoms; such infarcts are commonly called *lacunes* (small pit or hollow), a term that is changing in meaning; they can be caused by emboli but are most commonly associated with microatheromas; although they can be found in otherwise healthy people, those with concurrent athersclerosis, arterial hypertension, and/or diabetes have a higher incidence of this type of infarct

	Internal capsule, most commonly	• **Motor:** contralateral hemiparesis on a single side, with equal deficit in face, arm, and leg; often unaccompanied by detectable signs of sensory, visual, and speech loss, depending on location; old term is "pure motor stroke" although evidence suggests that other neurologic signs are present but overlooked because of low intensity
	Thalamus, most commonly	• **Sensory:** complete or partial loss in face, arm, trunk, and leg that appears exactly midline; may be accompanied by pain, hyperesthesias, and uncomfortable sensations (hemisensory stroke)
	Pons	• Dysarthria, clumsy hand
	Pons, midbrain, capsule or parietal white matter	• Hemiparesis, ataxia on same side

Research evidence preventing a recurrence is as follows:

1. Antiplatelet therapy effectively reduces the risk of recurrence. No evidence shows that alternate antiplatelet regimens to low-dose aspirin are any more or less effective than aspirin alone.[2]

2. Lowering blood pressure reduces the risk of serious vascular events regardless of stroke etiology.[2]

3. Anticoagulation does not appear to be of benefit in preventing recurrence in persons with a normal sinus rhythm and the risk for intracranial and extracranial hemorrhage is increased. Oral anticoagulants reduce the risk of initial or recurrent stroke in atrial fibrillation.[28] Only 11% of persons with cardioembolic stroke had been receiving anticoagulation therapy[29] as reported in one study, and women are less likely to have anticoagulation therapy for atrial fibrillation.[30]

4. Carotid endarterectomy effectively reduces the risk of recurrence in cases with greater than 50% carotid stenosis, is not effective with 30% to 49% carotid stenosis, and increases the risk of stroke with less than 30% stenosis. No benefit was found for persons with near occlusion.[2]

5. Cholesterol reduction using statins appears to reduce primary or recurrence risk regardless of baseline cholesterol level or coronary artery disease status. Other methods of cholesterol reduction do not lower recurrence risk.[31]

6. Sufficient evidence to judge the efficacy of carotid and vertebral percutaneous transluminal angioplasty to prevent recurrence is not yet available.

Rehabilitation is indicated in thrombotic and embolic stroke. Treatment of an intracranial bleed, regardless of cause, is focused on stopping or reducing the bleeding, controlling the increased ICP, preventing a rebleed, and preventing vasospasm. Occasionally an attempt is made to evacuate or aspirate the blood.

Intracranial Aneurysm

Intracranial aneurysms may result from arteriosclerosis, congenital abnormality, trauma, inflammation, or infection. Cocaine use has been linked to aneurysm formation. The size of the aneurysm may vary from 2 mm to 3 cm. Most aneurysms are located at bifurcations in or near the circle of Willis, in the vertebrobasilar arteries, or within the carotid system (see Figure 14-19)—85% to 95% are in the anterior portion of the circle of Willis. Aneurysms may be single, but in 20% to 25% of cases, more than one is present. In these instances the aneurysms may be unilateral or bilateral. The incidence of rupture is 11 in 100,000 per year. Peak incidence of rupture is from 50 to 60 years of age. Women have a slightly greater incidence of aneurysms.

PATHOPHYSIOLOGY No single pathologic mechanism exists. A combination of genetic, congenital, and acquired factors is present.[32,33] Abnormalities in multiple layers of the blood vessel are found. The endothelial layer is thin, the internal elastic lamina is not present or fragmented, and the muscularis layer of the media ends at the aneurysm. Atherosclerotic changes are found. Aneurysm development is attributed to hemodynamic stress and is believed to be exacerbated by hypertension and certain connective tissue disorders in which there are abnormalities in the extracellular matrix.[33] The aneurysm wall is composed of fibrous tissue. Aneurysms may be classified on the basis of shape and form (Figure 17-18).

Saccular aneurysms (berry aneurysms) occur frequently (in approximately 2% of the population) and are the result of a combination of a congenital abnormality in the media of the arterial wall and degenerative changes.[18] The sac grows over time. A saccular aneurysm may be (1) round with a narrow stalk connecting it to the parent artery (Figure 17-19), (2) broad based without a stalk, or (3) cylindric. Saccular aneurysms are rare in childhood; their highest incidence of rupturing or bleeding is among people 20 to 50 years of age.

Fusiform aneurysms (giant aneurysms), by definition greater than 25 mm in diameter, make up 5% of all intracranial

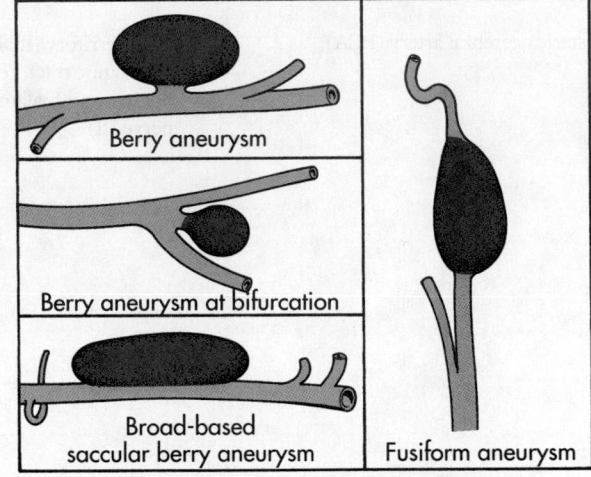

Figure 17-18 Types of aneurysms.

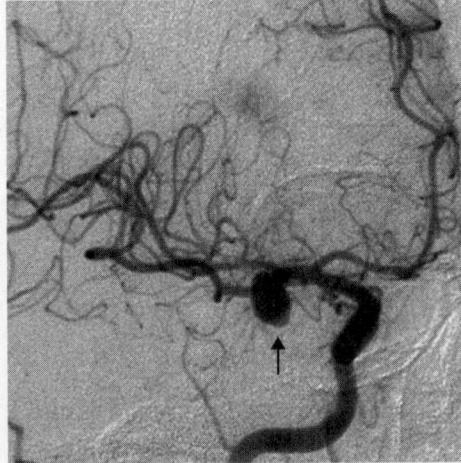

Figure 17-19 Berry aneurysm, angiogram. In this lateral view with contrast filling a portion of the cerebral arterial circulation can be seen a berry aneurysm *(arrow)* involving the middle cerebral artery of the circle of Willis at the base of the brain. (From Klatt EC: *Robbins and Cotran atlas of pathology,* Philadelphia, 2006, Saunders.)

aneurysms. They occur as a result of diffuse arteriosclerotic changes and are found most commonly in the basilar arteries or terminal portions of the internal carotid arteries. They act as space-occupying lesions. **Mycotic aneurysms** result from arteritis caused by bacterial emboli; these aneurysms are uncommon. **Traumatic (dissecting) aneurysms** are caused by a weakening of the arterial wall by a fracture line, by a penetrating missile, or after neurosurgical or imaging (e.g., angiographic) procedures.

What causes an aneurysm to rupture is not known[33] but rupture causes hemorrhage into the subarachnoid space with rapid spread, producing localized changes in the cerebral cortex and focal irritation of nerves and arteries (see Laplace law, Chapter 29). Because of compression, bleeding ceases with the formation of a fibrin-platelet plug at the point of rupture. Blood undergoes reabsorption through arachnoid villi within 3 weeks.

CLINICAL MANIFESTATIONS Aneurysms are frequently asymptomatic. In routine autopsy, 5% of persons are found to have one or more intracranial aneurysms. Clinical manifestations may arise from cranial nerve compression, but the signs vary, depending on the location and size of the aneurysm. Most often, cranial nerves III, IV, V, and VI are affected (see Table 14-6). Unfortunately the most common first indication of an aneurysm is an acute subarachnoid hemorrhage, intracerebral hemorrhage, or combined subarachnoid-intracerebral hemorrhage (see pages 601 and 607).

EVALUATION AND TREATMENT Diagnosis before a bleeding episode is made using arteriographic examination. After a subarachnoid or an intracerebral hemorrhage, a tentative diagnosis of an aneurysm that has bled is based on clinical manifestations, history, CT, and MRI. The treatment of choice for an aneurysm is surgical management. The location and size of the aneurysm and the person's clinical status determine whether invasive therapy is feasible.[34]

Vascular Malformations

Vascular formations are one tenth as common as aneurysms.[18] Four types of vascular malformation exist: arteriovenous malformation, cavernous angioma, capillary telangiectasis, and venous angioma. Most are sporadic, although multiple lesions are observed in families.[35] **Cavernous angiomas (malformations)** are sinusoidal collections of blood vessels without interspersed normal brain tissue. They rarely hemorrhage and comprise 8% to 15% of all vascular lesions. A **capillary telangiectasis** is dilated capillaries with interspersed normal brain tissue found deep in the brain, particularly in the brainstem; hemorrhage is rare. These vascular malformations are associated with Rendu-Osler-Weber disease. **Venous angioma,** the most common vascular malformation found at autopsy (3% of cases), is considered a subset of developmental venous anomalies that occur secondary to arrested development. The result is primitive embryologic veins in a radial pattern feeding a central vein. These rarely hemorrhage.[36]

In an **arteriovenous malformation (AVM)**, arteries feed directly into veins through a vascular tangle of malformed vessels (Figure 17-20). AVMs hemorrhage at a rate of 40% a year, occur in any part of the brain, and are usually cone shaped. Their size is highly variable, from malformations of a few millimeters to large ones that extend from the cortex to the ventricle. The large AVMs also may involve the dura mater, including the falx cerebri and the tentorium cerebelli. AVMs occur as frequently in males as in females, and occasionally are found in families. Although usually present at birth, AVMs exhibit a delayed age of onset and symptoms most commonly occur before 30 years of age. They usually rupture in the second and third decades of life.

PATHOPHYSIOLOGY AVMs, which are developmental abnormalities that represent persistence of embryonic patterns of blood vessels, do not have a normal blood vessel structure and are abnormally thin. The involved vessels are

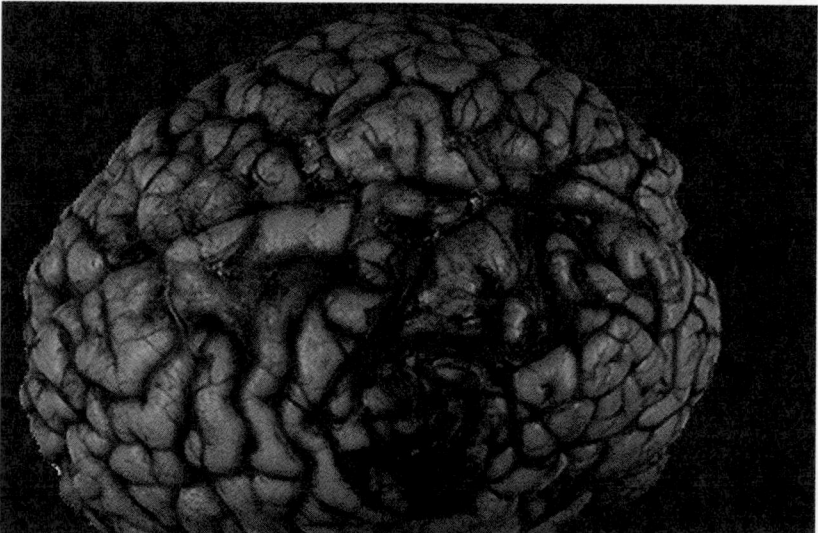

Figure 17-20 Vascular malformation, gross. A vascular malformation represented by a mass of irregular tortuous vessels over the left posterior parietal region of the brain. (From Klatt EC: *Robbins and Cotran atlas of pathology*, Philadelphia, 2006, Saunders.)

thought by some to enlarge over time. The AVM may be fed by one or several arteries. These feeder vessels become tortuous over time and often are dilated. With moderate to large AVMs, sufficient blood is shunted into the malformation to deprive surrounding tissue of adequate blood perfusion.

CLINICAL MANIFESTATIONS Clinical manifestations vary: 20% of persons with an AVM have a characteristic chronic nondescript headache, although some experience migraine; 50% experience seizure disorders caused by compression. Initially, the seizures tend to be focal or jacksonian; generalization often occurs over time. (Seizures are discussed in Chapter 16.) The other 50% suffer an intracerebral, a subarachnoid, or a subdural hemorrhage. Bleeding from an AVM into the subarachnoid space causes clinical manifestations identical to those associated with a ruptured aneurysm. If bleeding is into the brain tissue, focal signs that develop resemble a stroke-in-evolution. Ten percent of persons experience hemiparesis or other focal signs. Hemiparesis usually is caused by compression or rupture. At times, noncommunicating hydrocephalus (see Chapter 16) develops with a large AVM that extends into the ventricle lining. AVMs account for up to 1% of all sudden deaths.[37]

EVALUATION AND TREATMENT A systolic bruit over the carotid in the neck, the mastoid process, or (in a young person) the eyeball is almost diagnostic of an AVM. CT, magnetic resonance angiography (MRA), transcranial Doppler (TCD), and MRI are used in initial diagnosis, followed by an arteriogram to identify feeding vessels. Treatment options are direct surgical approach, embolization, or radiotherapy. The risk of bleeding is 6% in the first year and 2% to 4% each year thereafter with no intervention.

Subarachnoid Hemorrhage

With a **subarachnoid hemorrhage (SAH),** blood escapes from a defective or injured vasculature into the subarachnoid space (Figure 17-21). First-degree relatives of persons with SAH have seven times the risk of developing an SAH.[33] Heavy alcohol use, hypertension, smoking, anticoagulation, and oral contraceptive use are associated with SAH. Individuals at risk for a SAH are those with a saccular intracranial aneurysm (80% of cases), intracranial AVM, or hypertension and those who have sustained head injuries. There is a 50% overall mortality rate, and one third of survivors are dependent. SAHs often recur, especially from a ruptured intracranial aneurysm.

PATHOPHYSIOLOGY When a vessel is leaking, blood oozes into the subarachnoid space. When a vessel tears, blood under pressure is pumped into the subarachnoid space. The blood is extremely irritating to the meningeal and other neural tissues and so produces an inflammatory reaction in these tissues. Additionally, the blood coats nerve roots, clogs arachnoid granulations (impairing CSF reabsorption), and clogs foramina within the ventricular system (impairing CSF circulation). ICP immediately increases to almost diastolic levels. ICP returns to near baseline in about 10 minutes. Cerebral blood flow and cerebral perfusion pressure (CPP) decrease. The expanding hematoma acts like a space-occupying lesion, compressing and displacing brain tissue. Granulation tissue is formed, and scarring of the meninges with resulting impairment of CSF reabsorption and secondary hydrocephalus often results.

Subarachnoid hemorrhage has a unique pathophysiologic cascade triggered by the sudden appearance of blood in the subarachnoid space. Eighty percent of persons with SAH have infarction on MRI, which is the major cause of death and disability and 33% of persons have asymptomatic vasospasm in the first 2 weeks following an SAH.[33] The cause for **cerebral vasospasm (CVS)** and **delayed cerebral ischemia (DCI)** is unclear. DCI is related to but not explained by the CVS.

Development of CVS requires the presence of blood and its breakdown products as a consequence of the SAH. It also appears that oxyhemoglobin is a powerful precipitator of CVS.

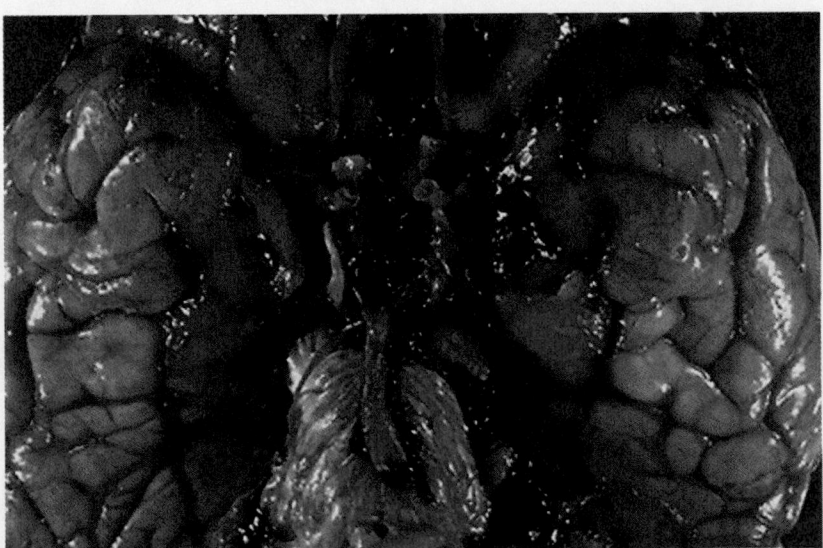

Figure 17-21 Subarachnoid hemorrhage, gross. Subarachnoid hemorrhage resulting from rupture of a berry aneurysm. (From Klatt EC: *Robbins and Cotran atlas of pathology,* Philadelphia, 2006, Saunders.)

It scavenges nitric oxide (a vasodilator), and its breakdown triggers a free radical cascade that disrupts multiple blood vessel layers and initiates release of inflammatory factors.[38] It appears that both CVS and disruption of cerebral autoregulation are necessary for DCI to occur. Autoregulation may be impaired in SAH and the combination of narrowed blood vessels, because of spasm and disrupted autoregulation, impairs perfusion, resulting in ischemia.[33]

CLINICAL MANIFESTATIONS Early manifestations associated with leaking vessels are episodic headache, transient changes in mental status or level of consciousness, nausea or vomiting, focal neurologic defects including visual or speech disturbances, cranial nerve palsies, or stiff neck. A ruptured vessel often is accompanied by a sudden throbbing, "explosive" headache that is associated with nausea and vomiting, visual disturbances, motor deficits, and loss of consciousness. These signs can be related to a dramatic rise in ICP. Meningeal irritation and inflammation often occur, causing neck stiffness (nuchal rigidity), photophobia, blurred vision, irritability, restlessness, and low-grade fever. A positive **Kernig sign** (in which straightening the knee with the hip and knee in a flexed position produces pain in the back and neck regions) and **Brudzinski sign** (in which passive flexion of the neck produces neck pain and increased rigidity) may appear. No localizing signs are present if the bleed is confined completely to the subarachnoid space.

The Hunt and Hess SAH grading system is based on description of the clinical manifestations (Table 17-7). Rebleeding is a significant risk with a high mortality (up to 70%). The period of greatest risk is the first month, with the peak incidence of rebleeding during the first 2 weeks after the initial bleed. Rebleeding is manifested by a sudden increase in blood pressure and ICP, along with a deteriorating neurologic status.

The peak time of CVS onset is 3 to 5 days, with maximal narrowing at 5 to 14 days after the initial bleed, but vasospasm may persist for 2 to 4 weeks. Seizures occur in 25% of SAHs.

Table 17-7	Subarachnoid Hemorrhage Classification Scale
Category	Description
Grade I	Neurologic status intact; mild headache, slight nuchal rigidity
Grade II	Neurologic deficit evidenced by cranial nerve involvement; moderate to severe headache with more pronounced meningeal signs (e.g., photophobia, nuchal rigidity)
Grade III	Drowsiness and confusion with or without focal neurologic deficits; pronounced meningeal signs
Grade IV	Stuporous with pronounced neurologic deficits (e.g., hemiparesis, dysphasia); nuchal rigidity
Grade V	Deep coma state with decerebrate posturing and other brainstem dysfunction

From Cook HA: Aneurysmal subarachnoid hemorrhage: neurosurgical frontiers and nursing challenges. In Winkleman C, editor: *AACN clinical issues in critical care nursing*, Philadelphia, 1991, Lippincott.

The incidence of hydrocephalus after a bleed is 20%. Hypothalamic dysfunction, manifested by salt wasting, hyponatremia, and ECG changes, is common.

EVALUATION AND TREATMENT The diagnosis of a subarachnoid hemorrhage is based on the clinical presentation, a noncontrast CT scan, and a lumbar puncture.[39] Arteriographic examination is the definitive diagnostic measure for defining and localizing an aneurysm or AVM. Treatment is directed at control of intracranial pressure, prevention of ischemia and hypoxia of neural tissues, and prevention of rebleeding episodes. Antifibrinolytic drugs may be used to stop rebleeding in selected cases. Blood pressure is allowed to remain in the high normal range or is elevated to that level. Platinum coils and balloon embolization to occlude the aneurysm are used, but microsurgical repair remains the treatment of choice. Calcium channel blockers, such as nimodipine, are used to prevent or reverse vasospasm. Volume expansion or hemodilution through continuous or bolus administration of hetastarch and plasma protein factors to maintain a hematocrit of 33% is used to expand blood volume and augment cerebral perfusion. Cerebral angioplasty can be tried for vasospasm. The primary problem must be diagnosed and corrected as well.

Headache

Headache is a common neurologic disorder and is usually a benign symptom. However, it can be associated with serious disease, such as brain tumor, meningitis, and giant cell arteritis. The headache syndromes discussed here are the chronic, recurring type not associated with structural abnormalities or systemic disease and include migraine, cluster, paroxysmal hemicrania, and tension headaches. Characteristics of the major types of headache syndromes are summarized in Table 17-8.

Migraine

Migraine is now viewed as a familial, episodic disorder whose marker is headache[40] and is defined as repeated, episodic headache lasting 4 to 72 hours. It is diagnosed when any two of the following features occur: unilateral head pain, worsening with movement, accompanied by photophobia or phonophobia; *and* presence of any one of the following: throbbing quality, moderate to severe nausea, or vomiting.[41] At least 12% of the general population experience an average of 18 migraine attacks per year,[41] two thirds of whom are female. Migraine is more common in those 25 to 55 years of age, and can occur in young children. The prevalence in women is highest at 20 to 40 years of age but remains higher than in men into older age. Onset after 50 years of age is rare. Hormonal factors account for most of the gender differences. A positive family history is common as is a genetic predisposition. Migraine is a multifactorial disorder caused by a combination of multiple genetic and environmental factors. Migraine sufferers have an increased risk for epilepsy, depression, anxiety disorders, and stroke.[40] Triggers believed to precipitate migraine attacks include altered sleep patterns (becoming tired or too much

Table 17-8   Characteristics of Common Headaches

| | Migraine | | Cluster Headache/ | Tension Type |
	Without Aura	With Aura	Proximal Hemicrania	of Headache
Age of onset	Childhood, adolescence, or young adulthood	Childhood, adolescence, or young adulthood	Young adulthood, middle age	Young adulthood, middle age
Gender	Female	Female	Male	Not gender specific
Family history of headaches	Yes	Yes	No	Yes
Onset and evolution	Slow to rapid	Slow to rapid	Rapid	Slow to rapid
Time course	Episodic	Episodic	Clusters in time	Episodic, may become constant
Quality	Usually throbbing	Usually throbbing	Steady	Steady
Location	Variable, often unilateral	Variable, often unilateral	Orbit, temple, cheek	Variable
Associated features	Prodrome, vomiting	Prodrome, vomiting	Lacrimation, rhinorrhea, Horner syndrome	None

sleep), skipping meals, overexertion, weather change, stress or relaxation from stress, hormonal changes (such as menstrual periods), excess afferent stimulation (bright lights, strong smells), and chemicals (alcohol or nitrates).[41]

The International Headache Society has broadly classified migraine with aura (previously called classic migraine) and migraine without aura (previously called common migraine).[41] In migraine with aura, at least some of the attacks are temporarily associated with distinct aura symptoms suggestive of focal brain dysfunction (flashing lights, visual loss). There are no associated focal neurologic symptoms in migraine without aura. Two thirds of those with migraines have migraine without aura.

The pathophysiologic basis for migraine is complex and includes neurologic, vascular, hormonal, and neurotransmitter components. The end point is hypothesized to be a disturbance of subcortical sensory modulation systems. The clinical phase of a migraine attack and associated pathophysiology follow:

1. *Premonitory phase*: up to one third have premonitory symptoms at least some of the time for several hours before aura or headache onset; the pathogenesis is unknown but evidence points to dopaminergic/hypothalamic involvement[42]

2. *Migraine aura*: up to one third have aura symptoms at least some of the time that may last 1 hour or sometimes much longer; migraine aura is defined as a spreading, focal, neurologic disturbance manifested as visual, sensory, or motor symptoms; pathophysiology appears to be a cortical spreading depression (CSD), reduction in electrical activity, and decrease in blood flow that slowly spreads across the cerebral cortex from the occipital region[43]

3. *Headache phase*: includes associated symptoms and may last from 4 to 72 hours (usually about a day); most research-supported pain mechanism is compensatory overactivity in the trigeminovascular system of the brain; activation of trigeminal sensory nerves produces release of vasoactive peptides that cause a sterile, inflammatory response around vessels in the meninges are present[44]

Migraine without aura is often located on one side. The pain is throbbing, of moderate to severe intensity, and aggravated by physical activity. In migraine with aura, the most common prodromal symptoms are visual (scotomas with luminous angles and scintillating edges, and hemianopsia). Sensory deficits and aphasia also may be present. The aura develops within 5 to 20 minutes and remits within 60 minutes, followed by headache and other symptoms, including nausea, vomiting, photophobia, scalp tenderness; 10% experience diarrhea.

In susceptible women, migraine occurs most frequently before and during menstruation and is decreased during pregnancy and menopause. The cyclic withdrawal of estrogens may trigger attacks of migraine.[45] Cyclic changes in estrogen are absent in pregnancy and after menopause, which could explain the less frequent attacks in some women. Estrogens may act directly on vascular smooth muscle, modulate activity of vasoactive substances at the neurovascular junction, and activate vasoregulatory responses in the hypothalamus. However, no direct evidence has been found to link circulating female sex hormones with the frequency and severity of migraine.

The diagnosis of migraine is made from medical history and physical examination. Clinicians must be skilled in their understanding of different types of headaches, risk factors, family history, and clinical features. Differential diagnosis is confirmed with CT, MRI, and EEG. A significant number of individuals with migraine have depression as a comorbidity.

The management of migraine includes education that migraine is a chronic physiologic, not psychosomatic, disorder. Avoidance of triggers, adequate sleep, regular eating habits, and daily relaxation and meditation can create a headache-protective environment. With the onset of acute migraine, a dark room, ice, and sleep can provide relief. The pharmacologic management of migraine varies with each individual and is related to the severity of the attack. Drug considerations should include antiemetics, NSAIDs, ergotamine and dihydroergotamine, and serotonin receptor agonists (e.g., sumatriptan).

Triptans, transcutaneous estrogen, and magnesium administration may help some women with menstrual migraine. Gastric absorption may be decreased during an attack, and routes of administration other than oral (e.g., nasal sprays, intravenous, and rectal) may be used.

The prophylaxis of migraine is considered when attacks cannot be treated effectively. Several drugs may be considered and should *not* be used in combination. Examples include beta-blockers, a calcium antagonist (flunarizine), serotonin antagonists (lisuride, methysergide), NSAIDs, dihydroergotamine (DHE), valproic acid, and amitriptyline.

Cluster Headache

Cluster headaches are one of a group of disorders referred to as trigeminal autonomic cephalagia[44] and occur primarily in men between 20 and 50 years of age. Cluster headache has been known also as *histamine cephalalgia, Horton syndrome,* and *erythromelalgia.* These headaches are known as cluster headaches because several attacks can occur during the day for a period of days followed by a long period of spontaneous remission. Cluster headache has an episodic and a chronic form.

The headache attack usually begins without warning and is characterized by severe, unilateral tearing, burning, periorbital, and retrobulbar or temporal pain lasting 30 minutes to 2 hours. One or several attacks may occur in a day, usually at the same time of day or night. The same side is affected in subsequent episodes, and the attack activates the trigeminal-autonomic reflex. Associated symptoms include lacrimation, reddening of the eye, nasal stuffiness, eyelid ptosis, and nausea. Pain often is referred to the midface and teeth. If the cluster of attacks occurs more frequently without sustained spontaneous remission, they are classified as *chronic cluster headaches* (20% of cases). Alcohol can stimulate an attack during a cluster headache in about 50% to 70% of cases, but it is not a triggering factor during remission.

The cause of trigeminal activation is unclear. The pathogenic mechanism for pain like migraine is probably release of vasoactive peptides and the formation of neurogenic inflammation. Autonomic dysfunction is characterized by sympathetic underactivity and parasympathetic activation.[44] The rhythmicity of attacks is associated with changes in the inferior posterior hypothalamus. There may be altered serotonergic nerve transmission but at different loci than in migraine headache.

Prophylactic drugs are used to treat cluster headache. The most effective are prednisone, lithium, methysergide, calcium channel antagonists, and valproate. Acute attacks are managed with oxygen inhalation, sumatriptan, and inhaled ergotamine.

Chronic Paroxysmal Hemicrania

Chronic paroxysmal hemicrania (CPH) is a cluster-type headache that occurs with more daily frequency (4 to 12 times per day) but with shorter duration (20 to 120 minutes). The remission phases are often shorter. The attacks are more common in women, usually after pregnancy. The symptoms are similar to cluster headache. As with cluster headache, there is an episodic and a chronic form. The pathophysiology involves a disorder of sympathetic hyperactivity, but the mechanism is different from cluster headache because there is effective relief of symptoms with indomethacin.

Tension-Type Headache

Tension-type headache is the most common type of headache, occurring in 69% of men and 88% of women. The average age of onset is during the second decade of life. Female/male ratio is 1:1. It is a mild to moderate bilateral headache with a sensation of a tight band or pressure around the head. The onset of pain is usually gradual. The headache occurs in episodes and may last for several hours or several days. It is not aggravated by physical activity. Chronic tension-type headache (CTTH) evolves from episodic tension-type headache and represents headache that occurs at least 15 days per month for at least 3 months.[41] Many individuals have both tension-type and migraine headaches.

Both a central mechanism and a peripheral mechanism operate in causing tension headache. The central mechanism probably involves hypersensitivity of pain fibers from the trigeminal nerve. The peripheral mechanism is probably related to contraction of jaw and neck muscles, but the exact mechanisms are unknown. Headache sufferers have more localized pain and tenderness of pericranial muscles.

Mild headaches are treated with ice, and more severe forms are treated with aspirin or NSAIDs. Chronic tension-type headaches are best managed with a tricyclic antidepressant, such as amitriptyline. Amitriptyline and mirtazapine are similarly effective for CTTH in decreasing the duration and frequency of the headache, however, amitriptyline has been found to have fewer adverse effects.[2] Cognitive behavioral therapy reduces symptoms of CTTH.[2] Naproxen is a second drug of choice. Long-term use of analgesics or other drugs, such as muscle relaxants, antihistamines, tranquilizers, caffeine, and ergot alkaloids, should be avoided.

Tumors of the Central Nervous System

The incidence of primary brain tumor has risen approximately 25% in the past two decades—a rise that may be attributable to better detection.[46] No proven causative agents have been established for tumors of the central nervous system (CNS). Carcinogenesis is discussed in Chapter 11.

Cranial Tumors

Tumors within the cranium can be either primary or metastatic. *Primary tumors* are classified as primary intracerebral tumors or primary extracerebral tumors. Primary intracerebral tumors originate from brain substance, neuroglia, neurons, cells of the blood vessels, and connective tissue (Table 17-9). Primary extracerebral tumors originate outside the substance of the brain and include meningiomas, acoustic nerve tumors, and tumors of the pituitary and pineal glands. *Metastatic tumors,* or *secondary tumors,* can be found inside or outside the brain substance. Sites of intracranial tumors are illustrated in Figure 17-22.

Table 17-9 Brain and Spinal Cord Tumors

Neoplasm	Location	Characteristics	Cell of Origin
Gliomas			
Pilocytic astrocytoma	Anywhere in brain or spinal cord	Slow growing, well circumscribed	Astrocytes
Diffuse astrocytoma	Anywhere in the brain	Slow-growing; marked cellular differentiation; infiltrative; undergoing malignant progression over time	Astrocytes
Oligodendroglioma	Most commonly in frontal lobes deep in white matter; may arise in brainstem, cerebellum, and spinal cord	Well differentiated; diffusely infiltrative; well-demarcated borders	Oligodendrocytes
Oligoastrocytoma	Same as with diffuse astrocytoma and oligodendroglioma	Most common mixed glioma	At least two distinct populations of neoplastic cell types—astrocytes and oligodendrocytes
Anaplastic astrocytoma	Anywhere in brain or spinal cord, but predominantly in cerebral hemispheres	Anaplastic features demonstrated	Astrocytes
Anaplastic oligoastrocytma	Same as with anaplastic astrocytoma	Same as anaplastic astrocytoma or anaplastic oligodendroglioma	Astrocytes and oligodendrocytes
Glioblastoma multiforme	Predominantly in cerebral hemispheres	Poorly differentiated neoplastic cells; extensive cellular heterogeneity; well-developed microvascular proliferation; necrosis	Astrocytes
Ependymoma	Intramedullary: wall of the ventricles, may arise in caudal tail of spinal cord	More common in children, variable growth rates; more malignant, invasive form is called *ependymoblastoma*; may extend into ventricle or invade brain tissue	Ependymal cells
Neuronal Cell			
Medulloblastoma	Posterior cerebellar vermis, roof of fourth ventricle	Well demarcated, rapid growing, fills fourth ventricle	Embryonic cells
Mesodermal Tissue			
Meningioma	Intradural, extramedullary: sylvian fissure region, superior parasagittal surface of frontal and parietal lobes, olfactory groove, wing of sphenoid bone, superior surface of cerebellum, cerebellopontine angle, spinal cord	Slow growing, circumscribed, encapsulated, sharply demarcated from normal tissues, compressive in nature	Arachnoid cells, may be from fibroblast
Choroid Plexus			
Papillomas	Choroid plexus of ventricular system, lateral ventricle in children, fourth ventricle in adults	Usually benign, slow expansion inducing hemorrhage and hydrocephalus; malignant tumor is rare	Epithelial cells
Cranial Nerves and Spinal Nerve Roots			
Neurilemmoma	Cranial nerves (most commonly vestibular division of cranial nerve VIII)	Slow growing	Schwann cells
Neurofibroma	Extramedullary—spinal cord	Slow growing	Neurilemma, Schwann cells
Pituitary Tumors			
	Pituitary gland; may extend to or invade floor of the third ventricle	Age linked, several types, slow growing, macroadenomas and microadenomas	Pituitary cells, pituitary chromophobes, basophils, eosinophils
Germ Cell Tumors			
	Neurohypophysis, hypothalamus, pineal region	Rare, 0.5% of all primary brain tumors; primarily in adolescents; male more common than female; variable prognosis	Several types: germinoma, embryonal carcinoma, yolk sac tumor, choriocarcinoma, teratoma, mixed germ cell tumor, with different cell origins
Blood Vessel Tumors			
Angioma	Predominantly in posterior cerebral hemispheres	Slow growing	Arising from congenitally malformed arteriovenous connections
Hemangioblastomas	Predominantly in cerebellum	Slow growing	Embryonic vascular tissue

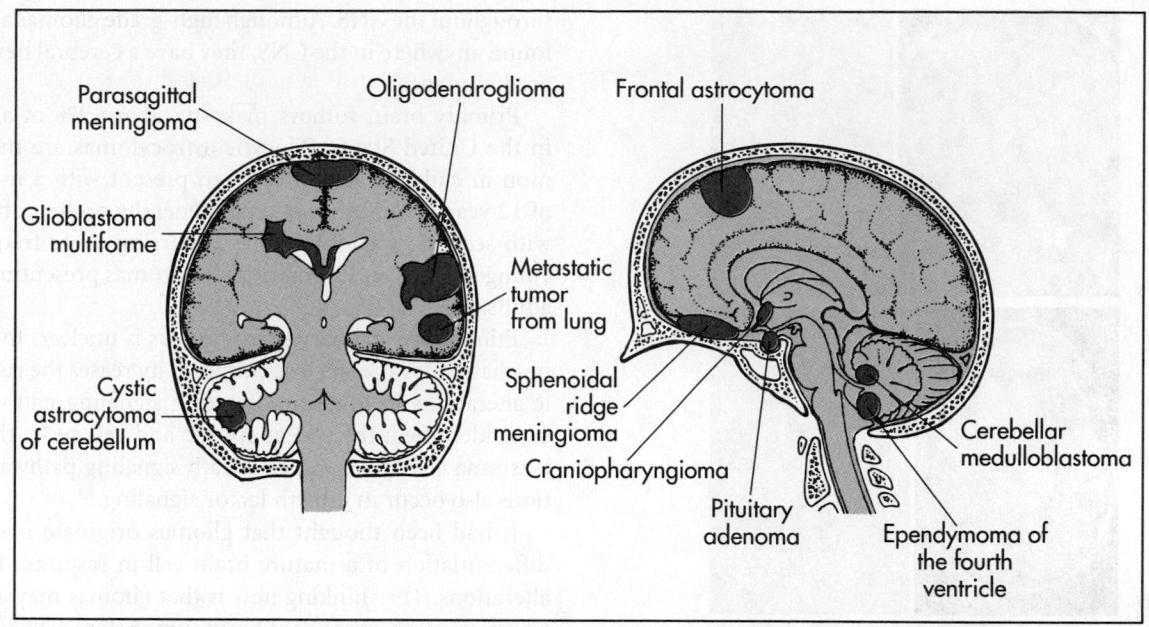

Figure 17-22 Common sites of intracranial tumors.

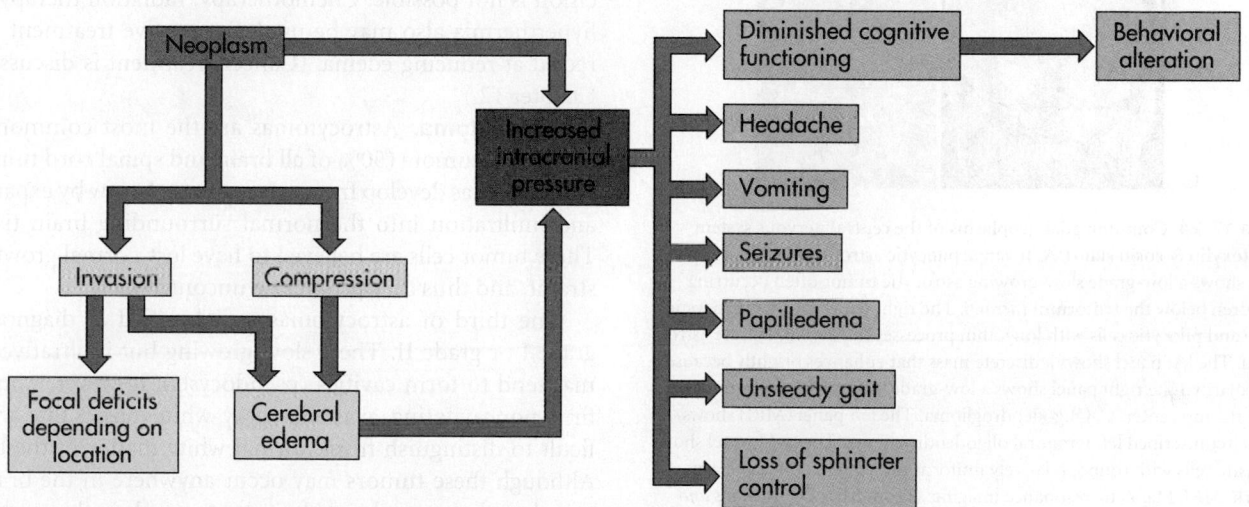

Figure 17-23 Origin of clinical manifestations associated with an intracranial neoplasm.

CNS tumors include brain and spinal cord tumors. The incidence is 10 per 100,000, which seems to increase up to 70 years of age and then decreases. These tumors represent the second most common group of tumors in children. Approximately 70% of all intracranial tumors in children are located infratentorially, and in adults 70% to 75% are located supratentorially. Peripheral nerve tumors are rare in children and common in adults.

Cranial tumors cause local and generalized clinical manifestations. The local effects are caused by the destructive action of the tumor itself on a particular site in the brain and compression causing decreased cerebral blood flow. The effects are varied and include seizures, visual disturbances, unstable gait, and cranial nerve dysfunction. The generalized effects result from increased ICP (Figure 17-23). Increased ICP may occur because of obstruction of the ventricular system, hemorrhages occurring in and around the tumor, or cerebral edema caused by tumors.

Intracranial brain tumors do not metastasize as readily as tumors in other organs because there are no lymphatic channels within the brain substance. If metastasis does occur, it is usually through seeding of cerebral blood, through CSF, during cranial surgery, or through artificial shunts.

Primary Brain (Intracerebral) Tumors

Primary brain (intracerebral) tumors, also called **gliomas,** comprise 50% to 60% of all adult brain tumors and include astrocytomas, oligodendrogliomas, mixed oligoastrocytomas, and ependymomas based on histologic and immunohistologic

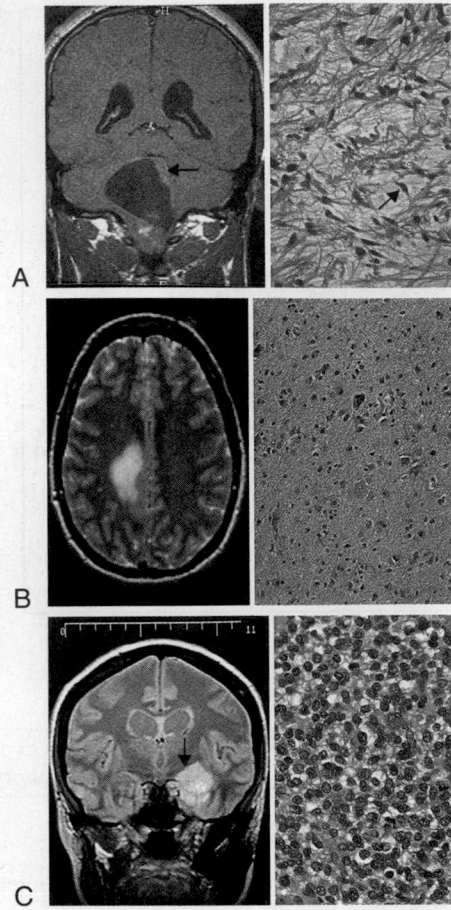

Figure 17-24 Common glial neoplasms of the central nervous system (hematoxylin & eosin stain). **A,** Juvenile pilocytic astrocytoma. The left panel (MRI) shows a low-grade slow-growing astrocytic tumor often occurring in children below the tentorium *(arrow)*. The right panel shows microcystic change and pilocytic cells with long, thin processes *(arrow)*. **B,** Diffuse astrocytoma. The left panel shows a discrete mass that enhances brightly because of vascularity. The right panel shows a low-grade tumor with pleomorphic cells at the top center. **C,** Oligodendroglioma. The left panel (MRI) shows a well-circumscribed left temporal oligodendroglioma. The right panel shows neoplastic cells with round, relatively uniform nuclei and a fine capillary network. *MRI,* Magnetic resonance imaging. (From Klatt EC: *Robbins and Cotran atlas of pathology,* Philadelphia, 2006, Saunders.)

characteristics (Figure 17-24).[47] The World Health Organization (WHO) divides gliomas into four grades based on histopathologic features of anaplasia-nuclear atypia, mitotic activity, microvascular proliferation, and/or necrosis.[47] Pilocytic astrocytomas (WHO grade I), diffuse astrocytomas (WHO grade II), and oligodendrogliomas (WHO grade II) are classified as low-grade gliomas. Anaplastic astrocytomas (WHO grade III), anaplastic oligodendrogliomas (WHO grade III), and anaplastic oligoastrocytomas (WHO grade III), along with glioblastoma multiforme (WHO grade IV), are classified as high-grade gliomas.[47] Glioblastomas are further subdivided into primary glioblastomas that start their development as grade IV gliomas, and secondary glioblastomas that arise from a low-grade precursor glioma through a sequence of genetic changes.[47] Low-grade gliomas are found

throughout the CNS. Although high-grade gliomas also can be found anywhere in the CNS, they have a cerebral hemispheric predominance.

Primary brain tumors make up about 2% of all cancers in the United States. Pilocytic astrocytomas are more common in children and most often present with a median age of 12 years.[48] All other gliomas generally present after age 30 with secondary glioblastomas occurring more frequently in younger adults and primary glioblastomas presenting in older adults.[47]

Etiology for primary brain tumors is unclear. Intracranial irradiation for therapeutic purposes increases the risk. Genetic alterations in three proliferation signaling pathways have been identified: the p53 apoptotic and cell cycle, the retinoblastoma cell cycle, and cell death signaling pathway. Alterations also occur in growth factor signaling.[49]

It had been thought that gliomas originate from loss of differentiation of a mature brain cell in response to genetic alterations. The thinking now is that gliomas may arise from transformation of resident brain tumor stem cells.[47,50]

The principal treatment for cerebral tumors is surgical or radiosurgical excision or surgical decompression if total excision is not possible. Chemotherapy, radiation therapy, and hyperthermia also may be used. Supportive treatment is directed at reducing edema. (Cancer treatment is discussed in Chapter 12.)

Astrocytoma. Astrocytomas are the most common primary CNS tumors (50% of all brain and spinal cord tumors). Astrocytomas develop from astrocytes and grow by expansion and infiltration into the normal surrounding brain tissues. These tumor cells are believed to have lost normal growth restraint, and thus they proliferate uncontrollably.

One third of astrocytomas are classified at diagnosis as grade I or grade II. These slow-growing but infiltrative gliomas tend to form cavities (pseudocysts); however, some are firm, noncavitating, avascular, gray-white masses that are difficult to distinguish from normal white matter of the brain. Although these tumors may occur anywhere in the brain or spinal cord, they are located most commonly in the cerebrum, hypothalamus, or pons. Low-grade astrocytomas in adults tend to have a lateral or supratentorial location, and they tend to be midline or near midline in position in children, often in the posterior fossa.

Headache and subtle neurobehavioral changes may be an early symptom. Approximately half of persons with low-grade astrocytomas experience a focal or generalized seizure. Onset of a focal seizure disorder between the second and sixth decades of life is suggestive of an astrocytoma. Other general or focal neurologic manifestations develop gradually. Increased ICP is usually a late clinical manifestation.

Grade I astrocytomas are treated with surgery and follow-up CT scans. Grade II astrocytomas are treated surgically if they are accessible or by conventional external radiation, local radiation, or stereotactic radiosurgery. Following surgery alone, the 5-year survival rate is 25%; with surgery followed by radiotherapy, the 5-year survival rate is 50%.

Grades III and IV astrocytomas are found predominantly in the frontal lobes and cerebral hemispheres (Figures 17-25 and 17-26). These tumors also may be located in the brainstem (Figure 17-27), cerebellum, and spinal cord. They are found twice as frequently in men as in women. Grades III and IV astrocytomas are the third most common cancer in the 15- to 34-year-old age group and the fourth most common in the 35- to 54-year-old age group.[46] Grades III and IV astrocytomas are often large and well circumscribed with a variegated pattern. The peripheral rim is pinkish gray and solid with a soft, yellow necrotic center and points of hemorrhage. Microscopically, there is increased cellularity, vascular

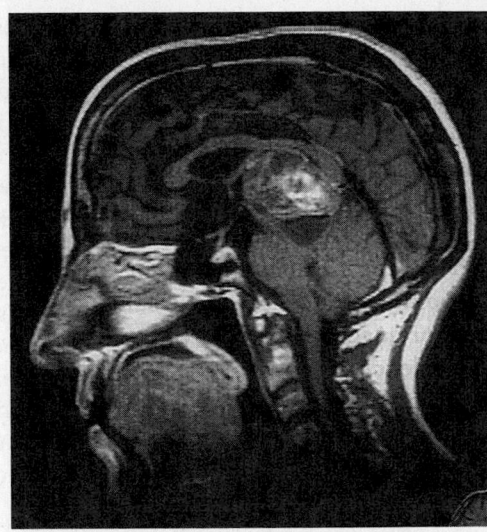

Figure 17-27 Magnetic resonance imaging (MRI) with gadolinium showing a high brainstem glioma. (From Perkin DG: *Mosby's color atlas and text of neurology,* London, 1998, Mosby-Wolfe.)

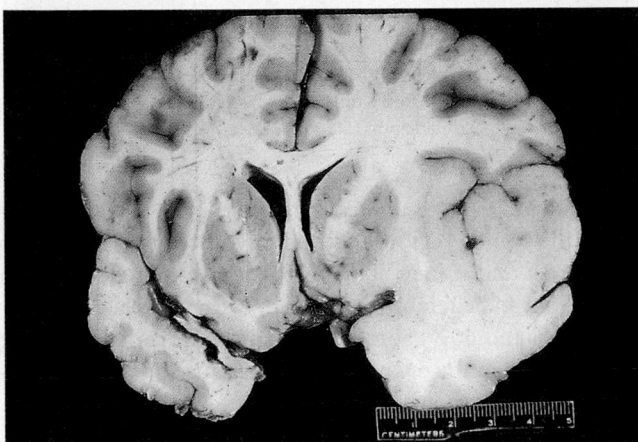

Figure 17-25 Well-differentiated infiltrating astrocytoma. The right temporal lobe contains an infiltrative, homogeneous lesion that has expanded the lobe and obscured the normal boundaries between gray and white matter (compare to left temporal lobe). Because of the ill-defined borders, surgical resection seldomly removes all of the tumor in such cases. (From Kumar V, Cotran RS, Robbins SL: *Robbins basic pathology,* ed 7, Philadelphia, 2003, Saunders.

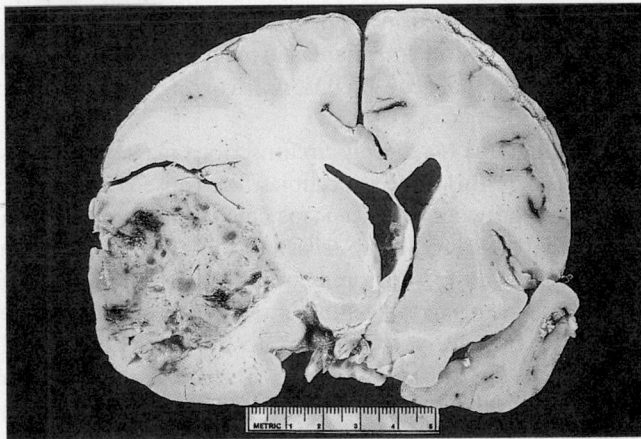

Figure 17-26 Glioblastoma multiforme. In contrast to the well-differentiated infiltrating astrocytoma in Figure 17-25, this glioblastoma contains irregular areas of discoloration and cystic change, reflecting the presence of necrosis and hemorrhage. These lesions are widely infiltrative and associated with considerable mass effect. Note the shift of midline structures to the right. (From Kumar V, Cotran RS, Robbins SL: *Robbins basic pathology,* ed 7, Philadelphia, 2003, Saunders.)

proliferation, cellular pleomorphism, and necrosis. Necrosis is the main histologic difference between an anaplastic grade III tumor and a grade IV glioblastoma multiforme.

Grade IV glioblastoma multiformes are highly vascular and extensively infiltrative. They may become large enough to extend from the meningeal surface through the ventricular wall. Fifty percent of glioblastomas are bilateral or at least occupy more than one lobe at the time of death. There are reports of grade IV astrocytomas found outside the central nervous system.[51]

The typical clinical presentation for a glioblastoma multiforme is that of diffuse, nonspecific clinical manifestations, such as headache, irritability, and personality changes, that progress to more clear-cut manifestations of increased ICP, such as headache on position change; papilledema; or vomiting. Of those affected, 30% to 40% experience seizure activity. Symptoms may progress to definite focal signs, such as hemiparesis, dysphasia, dyspraxia, cranial nerve palsies, and visual field deficits, in addition to the generalized signs from increased ICP.

Diagnosis of high-grade astrocytomas most commonly takes 3 to 6 months from onset of the first clinical manifestations because the person does not recognize the need to consult a healthcare provider.

Grade III astrocytomas are treated with surgery if they are accessible; radiotherapy; and chemotherapy possibly before, during, and after other therapies. Chemotherapy is given in cycles. With treatment, 1-year survival for grade III astrocytomas is 55% to 60%, 30% to 35% survive 2 years, and 10% survive longer than 5 years. Grade IV gliomas are also treated with surgery if accessible, radiotherapy and chemotherapy, or placement of wafers. The median survival rate is 3 years.[46]

Oligodendroglioma. A far less commonly occurring glioma is **oligodendroglioma,** comprising 2% of all brain tumors and 10% to 15% of all gliomas. Oligodendrogliomas are typically slow-growing well-differentiated tumors, often with cysts and calcification present. Most are macroscopically indistinguishable from other gliomas. They occur most often from 30 to 50 years of age and are more common in males than females. Their etiology is unknown. Most oligodendrogliomas are in the frontal and temporal lobes, often in deep white matter; 20% are in both hemispheres. They may be found also in other parts of the cerebrum, third ventricle, brainstem, cerebellum, and spinal cord. A high incidence of this tumor occurs in young adults with a history of temporal lobe epilepsy. Approximately half of these tumors generally classified as oligodendrogliomas (a grade II tumor) are actually oligoastrocytomas (a grade III tumor).[52] Malignant degeneration occurs in approximately one third of persons with oligodendrogliomas. If there is extension to the pia mater or ependymal wall (see Figure 14-15), oligodendrogliomas may metastasize to distant CNS sites through the ventriculoarachnoid spaces.

More than 50% of individuals experience a focal or generalized seizure as the first clinical manifestation; approximately half have experienced increased ICP at the time of diagnosis and surgery, and only one third develop any focal manifestations. The time from first clinical manifestation to surgical intervention often ranges from 2 to 6 years. Treatment options are surgery; radiotherapy (conventional external beam or stereotactic gamma knife and converged beam); and chemotherapy before, during, and after radiation. Median survival, when surgery and radiotherapy are both used, is 5 to 10 years.[46]

Ependymoma. **Ependymomas** are gliomas that arise from ependymal cells that form the walls of the ventricles and grow either into the ventricle or into adjacent brain tissue; they are not encapsulated (Figure 17-28 and see Table 17-9). They comprise 6% of all primary brain tumors in adults and 10% in children and adolescents. Among children and adolescents, 50% of those affected are younger than 5 years of age. Seventy percent of ependymomas occur in the fourth ventricle (i.e., in the posterior fossa) and manifest as difficulty with balance, unsteady gait, uncoordinated muscle movement, and difficulty with fine motor skills. Other common sites for ependymomas are the third ventricle, lateral ventricles, and caudal portion of the spinal cord. The clinical presentation of a lateral and third ventricle ependymoma that involves the cerebral hemispheres is seizures, visual changes, and contralateral weakness of a body part on one side of the body. Approximately 40% of infratentorial ependymomas occur in children younger than 10 years. Occurrence of cerebral (supratentorial) ependymomas is distributed among all ages but more common in adults. Etiology for these tumors is unknown.

Blockage of the CSF pathway by the tumor clinically results in the presence of headache, nausea, and vomiting related to the hydrocephalus produced. Brainstem or upper spinal cord ependymomas may cause neck pain as well.

Clinical manifestations and progression of dysfunction associated with ependymomas may follow a short or long course. The interval between first manifestations and surgery may be as short as 4 weeks with some ependymoblastomas to as long as 7 to 8 years with others.

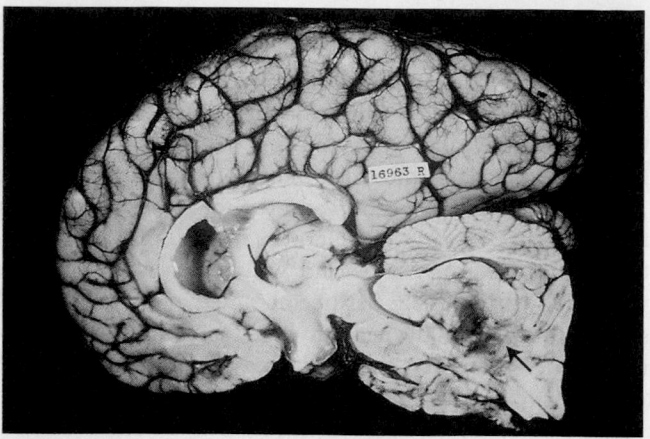

Figure 17-28 **Ependymoma.** These tumors may arise in both the intracranial compartment and the spine. Intracranial tumors typically originate from a ventricular surface, as in the case of this large lesion arising in the fourth ventricle *(arrow).* (From Kumar V, Cotran RS, Robbins SL: *Robbins basic pathology,* ed 7, Philadelphia, 2003, Saunders)

Ependymomas are treated surgically and with radiotherapy of the tumor region and operative site (possibly of the entire brain and spine); stereotactic radiosurgery focused on eradication; and chemotherapy. The 5-year survival rate is between 20% and 50%. Some persons benefit from a shunting procedure when the ependymoma has caused a noncommunicating hydrocephalus (see Chapter 16).

Primary Extracerebral Tumors

Meningioma. **Meningioma** constitutes about 20% of all intracranial tumors. The annual incidence is 6 cases per 100,000, with a peak incidence in the sixth and seventh decades, and is more common in women.[53] Predisposing factors to developing a meningioma are having neurofibromatosis (NF) type 2 (NF2, see p. 616) and ionizing radiation after a several-decade latency period.[54] Genetically, formation of benign meningiomas has been linked to *NF2* gene mutation and chromosome 22q loss along with *DAL-1* loss on chromosome 18. Atypical and anaplastic meningiomas have been linked to additional gene alterations involving multiple other chromosomes.[55]

A meningioma is a sharply circumscribed mass that derives its shape from the space it occupies; the cause is unknown. These slow-growing, often encapsulated tumors arise from arachnoidal (meningeal) cap cells in the dural coverings of the brain.[56] Rarely do meningiomas arise from arachnoid cells of the choroid plexus of the ventricles. Most are attached to the dura mater and arise within the intracranial cavity, the spinal cavity, or, rarely, the orbit (Figure 17-29).[56] A meningioma may extend to the dural surface and erode the cranial bones or produce an osteoblastic reaction. Small meningiomas (less than 2 cm in diameter) are often found on postmortem examination in middle-aged and older adults who had experienced no clinical manifestations and died of totally unrelated causes. A few meningiomas exhibit malignant, invasive qualities.

Only when meningiomas reach a certain size—at which time they begin to indent the brain parenchyma—do they

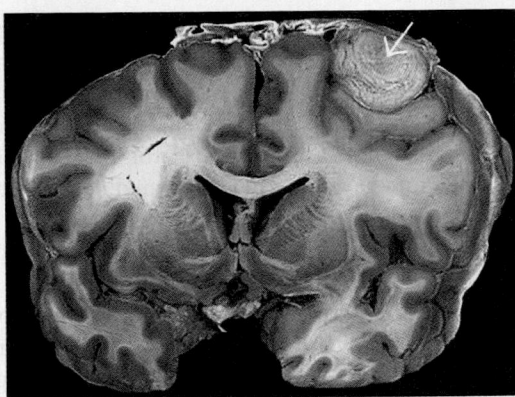

Figure 17-29 Meningioma, gross. Meningioma beneath the dura with compression of underlying cerebral hemisphere. (From Klatt EC: *Robbins and Cotran atlas of pathology*, Philadelphia, 2006, Saunders.)

begin to produce clinical manifestations. Focal seizures are frequently the first manifestation. Other clinical manifestations depend on the tumor's location. Clinical features based on site of origin are as follows:

1. *Sphenoidal wing:* ophthalmoplegia, mild proptosis, and involvement of the ophthalmic division of the trigeminal nerve
2. *Olfactory groove:* anosomia, personality change, and visual failure
3. *Parasagittal:* focal seizures of a focal motor or sensory deficit
4. *Parasellar:* evidence of chiasmatic compression; urinary incontinence; dementia; gradual paraparesis, hormonal failure; optic atrophy; bitemporal hemianopia
5. *Lateral convexity:* variable depending on structures compressed, including slow hemiparesis, speech abnormalities[46]

Because of the extremely slow-growing nature of most meningiomas, increased ICP is less common than with gliomas.

The most common symptom is seizures (40%). Diagnosis is made using contrast-enhanced CT, MRI, or both. The primary treatment is surgical resection. Sterotactic radiotherapy is used with incomplete resection or recurrence (20% rate). Conventional radiotherapy also is used. Hydroxyurea has been used in recurrence.[57]

Nerve Sheath Tumors. Nerve sheath tumors are either neurofibroma or schwannoma (neuroma, neurolemma). NF is an inherited autosomal dominant disorder accounting for 5% of all neuromas and are divided into two types: NF1 and NF2, which are clinically and genetically distinct disorders. The gene products are neurofibromin and merlin (schwannomin), both of which are thought to be tumor suppressors.[58] Alterations in chromosomes 17 (17q11.2 for NF1) and 22 (NF2) are associated with both neurofibromas and schwannomas.[59] NF1 is associated with cutaneous manifestations, iris hamartomas, and tumors primarily involving the peripheral nervous system and, occasionally, the CNS.[60] NF2 is associated with cataracts, hearing loss and tumors primarily in the CNS, most commonly vestibular schwannoma.[60] Criteria for the diagnosis

---

Box 17-2   Criteria for Diagnosis of Neurofibromatosis Types 1 and 2

Criteria for the Diagnosis of NF-1
Two of the following eight criteria:
- Six café-au-lait spots more than 15 mm in diameter (adults)
- Multiple axillary or inguinal freckles
- One plexiform neurofibroma or two or more neurofibromas of other types
- Optic nerve or chiasmatic glioma
- Lisch iris nodules (two or more)
- Thinning of the cortex of long bones
- Sphenoid dysplasia
- A first-degree relative with NF-1

Criteria for the Diagnosis of NF-2
Any one of the three following criteria:
- Bilateral eighth nerve tumors (as determined by CT or MRI)
- Unilateral eighth nerve tumor and first-degree relative with NF-2
- Any two of the following plus first-degree relative with NF-2
  a. Plexiform neurofibroma
  b. Neurofibroma of another type
  c. Meningioma
  d. Glioma
  e. Schwannoma
  f. Presenile posterior cataract

From Perkin GD: *Mosby's color atlas and text of neurology,* 1998, London, Mosby-Wolfe.
CT, Computed tomography; *MRI,* magnetic resonance imaging; *NF,* neurofibromatosis.

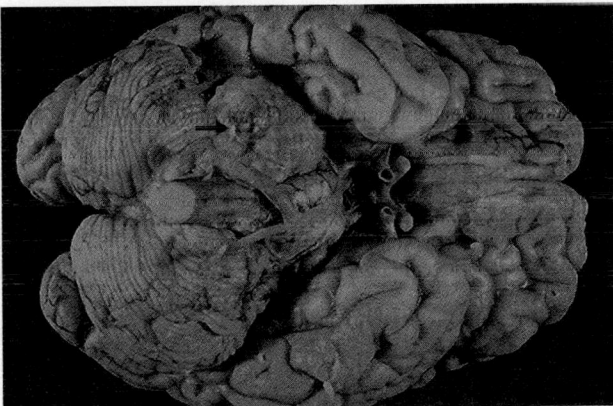

Figure 17-30 Acoustic neuroma (schwannoma), gross. A mass lesion arising in the right vestibular branch of the eighth cranial nerve at the cerebellopontine angle *(arrow).* (From Klatt EC: *Robbins and Cotran atlas of pathology,* Philadelphia, 2006, Saunders.)

of neurofibromatosis types 1 and 2 are presented in Box 17-2. The remainder of neuromas is benign tumors that arise from the sheath of Schwann cells surrounding the axons of the cranial nerves. The tumors most commonly affect people older than 50 years, women more often than men. The vestibular division of cranial nerve VIII is most commonly affected, although neuroma of the acoustic division of cranial nerves VIII, V, VII, and IX are found (Figure 17-30).

The tumor originates most commonly just distal to the junction between the nerve root and the brainstem. As the tumor grows, it extends into the posterior fossa to occupy the cerebropontine angle and compress adjacent nerves. Eventually the brainstem is displaced, and the CSF flow is obstructed.

Initial clinical manifestations may include headache, tinnitus, hearing loss, impaired balance, unsteady gait, facial pain, and loss of facial sensations. Later, vertigo with nausea and vomiting, a sense of pressure in the ear, and moderate to severe unsteadiness with rapid position changes may appear. CT or MRI can establish the diagnosis. Posterior fossa dye studies may be required. Treatment is by surgical excision and radiotherapy of the neuroma. Pituitary tumors are discussed in Chapter 21, and cerebral tumors in children are discussed in Chapter 19.

Brain Metastases. Brain metastases are approximately 10 times more common than primary brain tumors. The incidence may be as high as 200,000 cases per year. At autopsy, 20% to 40% of persons with metastases have brain metastases. Lung and breast are the most common tumors to have brain metastases within 1 to 3 years, but renal cell carcinoma, and malignant melanomas have an even higher brain metastasis incidence.[61] Carcinoma of the gallbladder, liver, thyroid, testes, uterus, ovary, and pancreas also may metastasize to the brain. Other tumors, besides carcinomas, that metastasize only occasionally are rhabdomyosarcomas, Ewing tumors, chorioepithelioma, and lymphoma.

Metastasis of a cancer to the brain parenchyma or the meninges is a late occurrence in the disease process. Metastasis to the brain parenchymna is believed to be hematogenous in origin.[62] Two thirds of metastatic tumors are located within the brain and one third are located in extradural spaces. The cerebral hemispheres are the site of 75% of metastases, most predominantly in the frontal lobes followed by the parietal, occipital, and temporal lobes in order of frequency of location. Tumors of the pelvis or retroperitoneal space have a predilection to metastasize to the cerebellum, pons, or their coverings.[63] In more than three fourths of persons with metastasis, the metastases are multiple and found in both the cerebrum and cerebellum in a scattered distribution. The metastatic tumors often are located in the meninges and near the brain surface in the gray matter and subcortical white matter. These tumors produce little glial cell reaction in the brain tissue but do cause vasogenic, peritumoral edema in the surrounding brain tissue due to blood-brain barrier incompetence.[62]

The brain metastatic process requires a series of sequential events, called the "metastatic cascade," as follows:
1. Invasion of primary tumor border
2. Extravasation of the circulatory system
3. Survival and persistence/quiescence in the circulation
4. Extravasation at the distant CNS site
5. Formation of micrometastasis
6. Progressive colonization and growth[61]

Hematogenesis metastasis to the CNS is an inherently inefficient process depending on an interaction between tumor cells with host defenses and the microenvironment. To produce brain metastasis, tumor cells must reach the brain vasculature by attaching themselves to the endothelial cells of the brain microvessels in the blood-brain barrier, extravasate

into the brain parenchyma, induce blood vessel development (angiogenesis), and proliferate in response to growth factors. Local brain invasion, in itself, is a process requiring mechanisms for cell motility, cell adhesion, and enzymatic remodeling of the extracellular components. Cytokines, chemokines, and growth factors have been demonstrated to participate in the process.[64]

The clinical manifestations of parenchymal brain metastasis are headache or alteration in cognition, mental status, and behavior,[62] although several unusual syndromes do exist. Carcinomatous encephalopathy causes headache, nervousness, depressed mood, trembling, confusion, and forgetfulness. In carcinomatosis of the cerebellum, headache, dizziness, and ataxia are found. Carcinomatosis of the craniospinal meninges (carcinomatous meningitis) manifests with headache, confusion, and manifestations of cranial or spinal nerve root dysfunction.

Contrasted enhancing imaging is the most sensitive imaging procedure for metastatic brain tumors. Prognosis is poor. If one to three tumors are found, surgical excision is indicated. Radiotherapy is commonly used to treat solitary as well as multiple tumors. Whole brain radiation prior to stereotactic radiosurgery improves regional control.[65] Chemotherapy is increasingly becoming part of the treatment plan.[65]

Spinal Cord Tumors

Spinal cord tumors are relatively rare. The most common primary spine tumors are listed in Box 17-3 and shown in Figure 17-31. Spinal cord tumors are named to reflect their cell type, growth rate, and structure of origin. They are classified as **intramedullary tumors** (originating within the neural tissues) or **extramedullary tumors** (originating from tissues outside the spinal cord). Extramedullary tumors arise from the meninges or roots (forming **intradural tumors**) or from epidural tissue or vertebral structure (forming **extradural tumors**). About 5% of spinal cord tumors seen in general hospital settings are intramedullary, 40% are intradural-extramedullary, and 55% are extradural.

The axial skeleton is the third most common site for metastasis behind lung and liver metastasis. Metastatic spinal cord tumors are three to four times more common than primary spinal cord tumors. They are usually carcinomas from

Box 17-3	Most Common Primary Spine Tumors

Benign Tumors
Osteoid osteoma/osteoblastoma
Giant cell tumors
Hemangiomas
Aneurysmal bone cyst

Malignant Tumors
Chondrosarcoma
Chordoma
Ewing sarcoma
Osteoarcoma

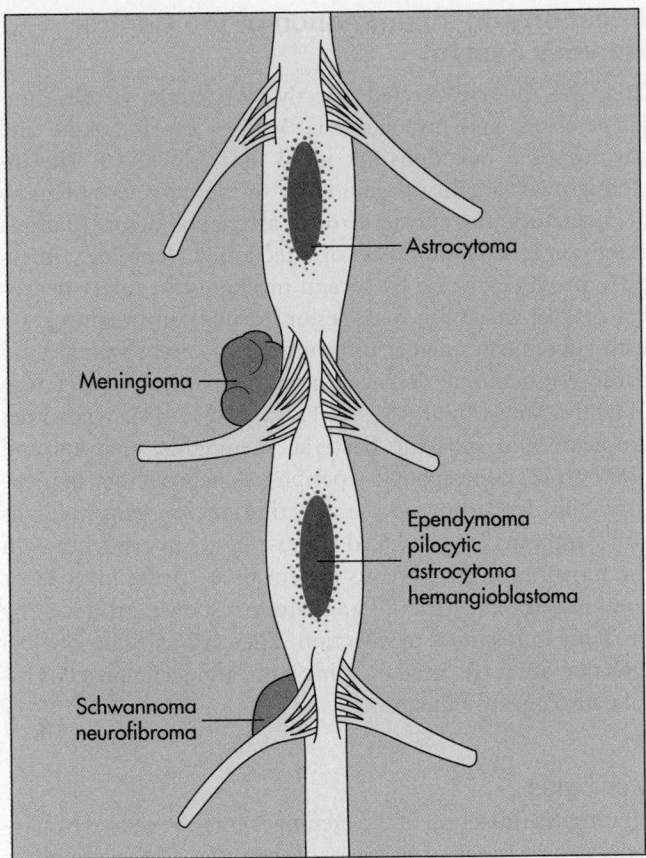

Figure 17-31 Distribution of some spinal tumors. (From Perkin DG: *Mosby's color atlas and text of neurology*, London, 1998, Mosby-Wolfe.)

breast, lung, and prostate; lymphomas; or myelomas; 25% to 70% involve the vertebral body and are asymptomatic. Metastatic spinal cord tumors are extradural in location. Of extradural tumors, 50% are metastatic and have spread to the spine through direct extension from tumors of the vertebral structures or from extraspinal sources extending through the interventricular foramen or through the bloodstream.

The most common primary extramedullary spinal cord tumors are neurofibromas and meningiomas. These tumors are intradural more often than extradural. Neurofibromas are found most commonly in the thoracic and lumbar regions. Meningiomas are more evenly distributed throughout the spine. Other extramedullary tumors in order of frequency of occurrence are sarcomas, vascular tumors, chordomas, and epidermoid and similar tumors. Of intradural-extramedullary tumors, 70% are meningiomas, neurofibromas, or sarcomas.

Intramedullary tumors have the same cellular origins as brain tumors. Ependymomas account for 40% of intramedullary spinal cord tumors. Astrocytomas, glioblastomas, oligodendrogliomas, ganglioneuromas, medulloblastomas, hemangiomas, and hemangioblastomas are more or less equally distributed in frequency of occurrence.

PATHOPHYSIOLOGY Extramedullary spinal cord tumors produce dysfunction by compression of adjacent tissue, not by direct invasion. The spinal cord is compressed by the tumor from without, and destruction of the white matter tracts occurs. The spinal canal around the cord becomes filled by tumor.

Intramedullary spinal cord tumors produce dysfunction by invasion and compression. The cord enlarges as a result of the tumor that is enlarging inside the cord. In addition, distortion of adjacent white matter tracts occurs. Metastases from spinal cord tumors occur from seeding through the CSF; medulloblastomas and ependymomas establish distant implants in this manner.

CLINICAL MANIFESTATIONS The acute onset of clinical manifestations suggests a vascular insult caused by thrombosis of vessels supplying the spinal cord. Clinical manifestations that are gradual and progressive suggest compression. The clinical manifestations associated with spinal cord tumors fall into three major categories: (1) a compressive syndrome (sensorimotor syndrome), (2) an irritative syndrome (radicular syndrome), and rarely (3) a syringomyelic syndrome.

The **compressive syndrome (sensorimotor syndrome)** is associated with compression and is caused less frequently by invasion and destruction of the spinal cord tracts. Symptoms are usually gradual and progressive, and initial manifestations may be asymmetric. With tumors located in the cervical area, the motor dysfunction usually has the following pattern: ipsilateral arm involvement, followed by ipsilateral and contralateral leg involvement, and finally involvement of the opposite arm. With thoracic tumors the pattern of motor involvement is paresis and spasticity of one leg, followed by involvement of the opposite leg. The sensory clinical manifestations of tingling paresthesias have a pattern similar to that of the motor signs. Pain and temperature dysfunctions are found more commonly than touch, vibration, and proprioceptive changes, although posterior column signs also are found frequently. Pain is less well localized than with an irritative syndrome caused by root involvement. Initially the pain and temperature changes are contralateral to the motor deficit (Brown-Séquard syndrome, see Table 17-5). Bladder and bowel deficits usually appear when paresis develops in the legs.

The **irritative syndrome (radicular syndrome)** combines the clinical manifestations of a cord compression with radicular pain, which is pain in the sensory root distribution and indicates root irritation. The segmental manifestations associated with root irritation include segmental sensory changes that include paresthesias and impaired pain and touch perception; motor disturbances, including cramps, atrophy, fasciculations, and decreased or absent deep tendon reflexes; and ache in the spine. Tenderness of the spinous processes over the tumor is present in about half of extramedullary tumors. The segmental changes may appear months and sometimes years before the clinical manifestations of compression in benign tumors. The compressive clinical manifestations include an asymmetric spastic paresis of the lower extremities with tumors in the thoracic or lumbar region, paresis of the arms and legs with tumors in the cervical area, decreased or absent pain and temperature perception below the tumor site, posterior column signs, and spastic bladder.

Because they involve the central gray matter of the cord, intramedullary spinal cord tumors (notably ependymomas) may produce a **syringomyelic syndrome,** or inflammation of the spinal cord. Inflammation results in the development of tubular (syrinx) cavities in the spinal cord. Occasionally an extramedullary tumor may produce the same effect, although the mechanisms are unknown.

EVALUATION AND TREATMENT The diagnosis of a spinal cord tumor is made through bone scan, needle biopsy guided by CT and positron-emission tomography (PET), or open biopsy. Benign or malignant spinal tumor staging may be done (Box 17-4). Involvement of specific cord segments is established.

Treatment varies, depending on the nature of the tumor and the person's clinical status. Indications for surgery include establishing a tissue diagnosis, neurologic palliation, spinal stabilization, pain relief, and cancer therapy. Surgical resection may involve curettage (piecemeal removal of the tumor) or may be performed en bloc (removal of tumor in one piece). Surgical approaches to the spine include posterior approach (decompression laminectomy), lateral approach, anterior approach (most favored), and combined approaches. Posterior and anterior reconstructive surgery may be necessary. Oncologic surgical procedures are classified as intralesional, marginal, wide excision, or radical excision. Indications for external radiation versus surgery are a radiosensitive tumor (e.g., lymphoma), soft tissue compression without instability, a person who is a poor surgical candidate, paraplegia or advanced paraparesis of greater than 24 hours' duration, and an expected survival of less than 3 to 4 months. Chemotherapy, hormonal therapy, and pain management protocols may be appropriate.

Box 17-4	Spinal Tumor Staging

Benign Spine Tumor Staging

S1	Latent, inactive, asymptomatic are bordered by a true capsule, often confined to vertebra
S2	Active, slowly growing, mildly asymptomatic; has thin capsule and layer of reactive tissue
S3	Aggressive, rapidly growing; often symptomatic; capsule very thin, incomplete, or absent; often invades neighboring compartments

Malignant Tumor Staging

Low-grade malignant: both 1A and 1B have no true capsule, but a thick pseudocapsule of reactive tissue with islands of tumor

Stage 1A	Tumor remains inside vertebra (intracompartmental)
Stage 1B	Tumor outside vertebra

High-grade malignant: rapid growth with continuous seeding nodules

Stage IIA	Inside vertebra with skip nodules present
Stage IIB	Outside vertebra
Stages IIIA and IIIB	Metastatic high grade intra- and extracompartmental

Infection and Inflammation of the Central Nervous System

The CNS may be affected directly by bacteria, viruses, fungi, parasites, and mycobacteria. Viruses causing acute and chronic CNS infections are listed in Table 17-10. The infecting microorganisms gain entry to the nervous system by (1) hematogenous spread through arterial blood or (2) direct extension from another site of infection.[66] Neurologic infections produce disease by several mechanisms: direct neuronal or glial infection; mass lesion formation; inflammation with subsequent edema; interruption of cerebrospinal fluid pathways; neuronal damage, or vasculopathy; and secretion of neurotoxins (Figures 17-32, 17-33, and 17-34). Syndromes are acute and subacute bacterial meningitis, epidural and brain abscess, encephalitis, peripheral neuropathy, or neurosyphilis depending on the infecting microorganism. Signs and symptoms are produced because of (1) interference with the function of the nervous system tissue being invaded or compressed or (2) the inflammatory response produced by the body in response to infection. The cardinal signs of CNS infection are fever, head or spine pain, and generalized or focal neurologic dysfunction.[67]

Meningitis

Meningitis (infection of the meninges) may be caused by bacteria, viruses, fungi, parasites, or other toxins. (The pathophysiology of infection is discussed in Chapter 9.) The infections are classified as acute, subacute, or chronic processes, and the pathophysiology, clinical manifestations, and treatment differ for each type of microorganism.

Bacterial meningitis is primarily an infection of the pia mater and arachnoid, the subarachnoid space, the ventricular system, and the CSF. A systemic or bloodstream infection or a direct extension from an infected area is the access route to the subarachnoid space. The bacterial infection originates in another part of the body. The incidence of bacterial meningitis is 2.5 to 3.5 cases per 100,000. The incidence is 20 per 100,000 annually for neonates, and 2 to 9 per 100,000 annually for those older than 60 years. The mortality is 25% in adults. Meningococcus (*Neisseria meningitidis*) and pneumococcus (*Streptococcus pneumoniae*) are the common causes of bacterial meningitis after the neonatal period. Pneumococcus and gram-negative enteric bacilli are the most common neonatal agents.

Meningococcus has been identified worldwide. Meningococcal meningitis occurs predominantly in men and boys and during the fall, winter, and spring. Epidemics of meningococcal meningitis occur in approximately 10-year cycles. Children and adolescents are affected predominantly; with pneumococcal meningitis, young persons and those older than 40 years are mostly affected.

Aseptic meningitis (viral meningitis, nonpurulent meningitis, lymphocytic meningitis) is an inflammation believed to be limited to the meninges. The most at-risk populations and the time of year when occurrences are

Table 17-10 Viruses Causing Acute and Chronic CNS Diseases

Virus	Family	Nucleic Acid	CNS Disease	Cell Tropism	Nonhuman Host	Route of Entry to CNS	Treatment
Viruses Causing Acute CNS Diseases							
Herpes simplex viruses-1 and -2	Herpesviridae	DNA	Meningoencephalitis	Neuron	ND	Intraneuronal	Acyclovir
Rabies virus	Rhabdoviridae	RNA	Encephalomyelitis	Neuron	Carnivores	Intraneuronal	Postexposure prophylaxis; RIG and vaccine
West Nile virus	Flaviviridae	RNA	Meningoencephalomyelitis	Neuron	Birds, horses	Hematogenous	IVIG, interferon-alpha
Nipah virus	Paramyxoviridae	RNA	Encephalitis	Neuron, endothelia	Pigs, fruit bats	Hematogenous	Ribavirin
Equine encephalitis viruses	Togaviridae	RNA	Meningitis, encephalitis	Neuron, astrocytes	Horses	Hematogenous	Supportive care
Mumps virus	Paramyxoviridae	RNA	Meningitis, encephalitis, myelitis	Neuron, ependymal cell	ND	Hematogenous	IVIG
Rubella virus	Togaviridae	RNA	Meningitis, encephalitis	Not specified	ND	Hematogenous	Plasmapheresis
Coxsackievirus, echovirus	Picornaviridae	RNA	Meningitis, meningoencephalitis, myelitis	Neuron	ND	Hematogenous	Pleconaril
Poliovirus	Picornaviridae	RNA	Meningitis, myelitis	Neuron	ND	Hematogenous	Pleconaril
California encephalitis virus	Bunyaviridae	RNA	Meningitis, encephalitis	Neuron	Small mammals	Hematogenous	Ribavirin
Viruses Causing Chronic CNS Disease							
Human immunodeficiency virus	Retroviridae	RNA	Encephalitis, meningitis, myelitis	Microglia, macrophage, astrocytes	ND	Hematogenous	HAART and neuroprotective agents
Human T-cell leukemia viruses-1 and 2	Retroviridae	RNA	Myelitis	Astrocyte, leukocyte	ND	Hematogenous	Zidovudine, lamivudine, glucocorticoids
JC virus	Polyomaviridae	DNA	Progressive multifocal leukoencephalopathy	Oligodendrocyte, astrocyte	ND	Hematogenous	Interferon-alpha, cidofovir
Varicella-zoster virus	Herpesviridae	DNA	Leukoencephalitis, cerebellitis, meningitis, myelitis	Neurons, satellite cell	ND	Hematogenous	Acyclovir
Measles virus	Paramyxoviridae	RNA	Encephalitis; SSPE	Neuron	ND	Hematogenous	Ribavirin, interferon-alpha, isoprinosine
Cytomegalovirus	Herpesviridae	DNA	Encephalitis	Neuron, ependymal cell, oligodendrocyte, monocytoid cell, endothelia	ND	Hematogenous	Foscarnet, ganciclovir
Epstein-Barr virus	Herpesviridae	DNA	Encephalitis, meningitis, myelitis	Infiltrating mononuclear cells	ND	Hematogenous	Acyclovir, ganciclovir (?)

From Lindquist L, Vapalahti O: *Lancet* 371(9627):1861-1871, 2008; Power C, Noorbakhsh F: Central nervous system viral infections: clinical aspects and pathogenic mechanism. In Gilman S, editor, *Neurobiology of disease*, pp 487-488, Burlington, MA, 2007, Elsevier.

CNS, Central nervous system; *DNA*, deoxyribonucleic acid; *HAART*, highly active retroviral therapy; *IVIG*, intravenous immunoglobulin; *JC*, John Cunningham; *ND*, not determined; *RIG*, rabies immune globulin; *RNA*, ribonucleic acid; *SSPE*, subacute sclerosing panencephalitis.

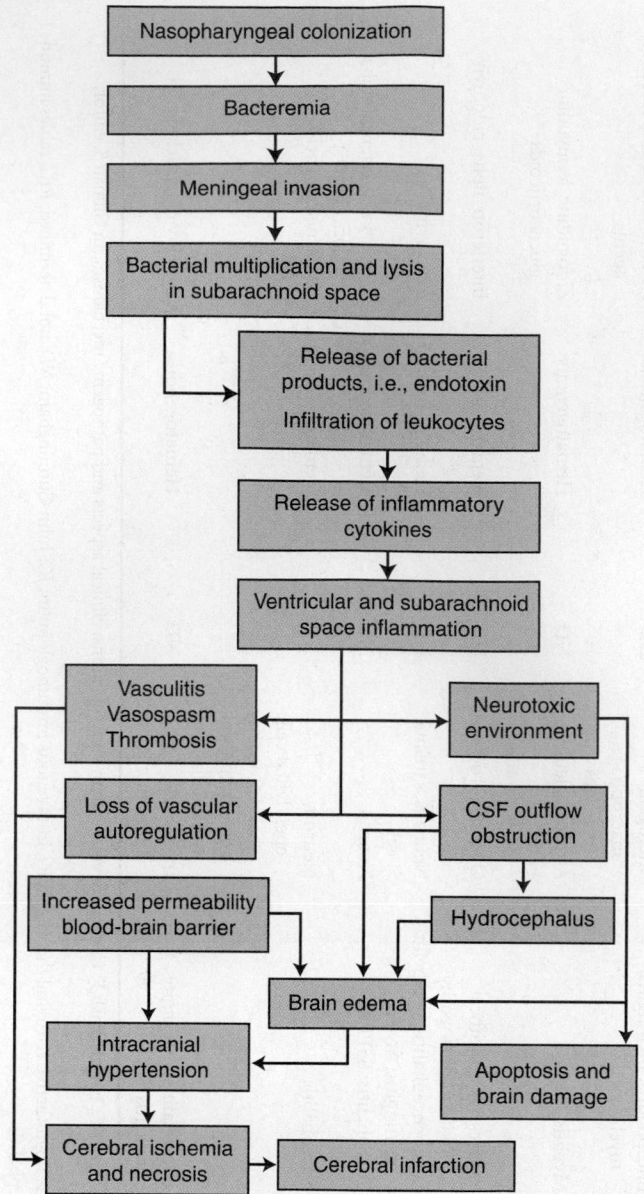

Figure 17-32 Pathogenesis of meningitis. (Adapted from Cohen J, Powderly WG: *Infectious diseases*, ed 2, Mosby, 2004, Edinburgh.)

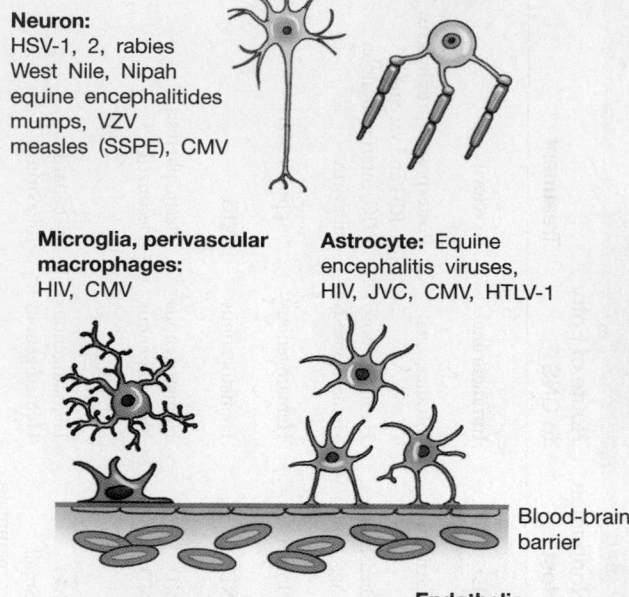

Oligodendrocyte: JCV, CMV

Neuron: HSV-1, 2, rabies West Nile, Nipah equine encephalitides mumps, VZV measles (SSPE), CMV

Microglia, perivascular macrophages: HIV, CMV

Astrocyte: Equine encephalitis viruses, HIV, JVC, CMV, HTLV-1

Blood-brain barrier

Endothelia: Nipah virus, CMV

Figure 17-33 Viral infection in the central nervous system (CNS). Viruses infect specific cell types within the CNS depending on the specific properties of the virus together with individual cell membrane proteins expressed on permissive cell types. Normally the brain is protected from circulating pathogens and toxins by the blood-brain barrier. *HIV,* Human immunodeficiency virus; *CMV,* cytomegalovirus; *HSV,* herpes simplex virus; *HTLV-1,* human T-cell lymphotropic virus (causes T-cell leukemia); *JCV,* John Cunningham virus (a polyomavirus causing progressive multifocal leukoencephalopathy); *SSPE,* subacute sclerosing panencephalitis; *VZV,* varicella zoster virus. (Adapted from Power C, Noorbakhsh G: Central nervous system viral infections: clinical aspects and pathogenic mechanisms. In Gilman S, editor, *Neurobiology of disease,* p 488, Burlington, MA, 2007, Elsevier.)

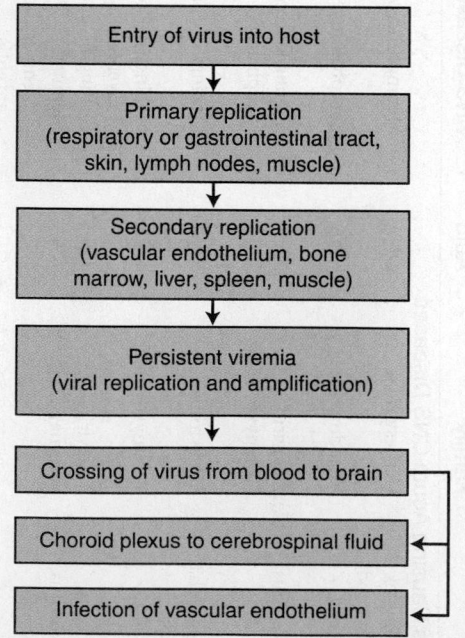

Figure 17-34 Hematogenous spread of viral pathogens to the central nervous system. (Adapted from Cohen J, Powderly WG: *Infectious diseases,* Mosby, 2007, Edinburgh.)

seen depend on the virus. Aseptic meningitis produces a variety of symptoms and is caused by a variety of infectious agents, most of which are viruses. They include enteroviral viruses (the most common) (echovirus, coxsackievirus, and nonparalytic poliomyelitis), mumps, herpes simplex types 1 and 2, St. Louis encephalitis virus, West Nile virus, California encephalitis virus, Venezuelan equine encephalitis, Colorado tick fever, lymphocytic choriomeningitis virus, Epstein-Barr virus, and influenzavirus types A and B.[68] Bacterial infections not adequately treated are another cause of aseptic meningitis.

Fungal meningitis is a chronic, much less common condition than bacterial or viral meningitis. The most common fungal infections of the nervous system are histoplasmosis, cryptococcosis, coccidioidomycosis, mucormycosis, candidiasis, and aspergillosis. Fungal meningitis most frequently occurs in persons with impaired immune responses or alterations in normal body flora. Fungal meningitis develops insidiously, usually over days or weeks. Syphilis, tuberculosis, and Lyme disease also are associated with chronic meningitis.

Tubercular meningitis, the most common and serious form of CNS tuberculosis, is again on the rise in the United States, especially in persons with acquired immunodeficiency syndrome (AIDS). Miliary tubercles form in the brain and meninges. At some point the tuberculomas erode the pia mater, and the mycobacteria enter the CSF, producing a hypersensitivity reaction that results in a purulent exudate involving the basal meninges, cerebrum, and spinal nerves. Cerebral ischemia and infarction occur from vasculitis. Symptoms include headache, low-grade fever, nausea and vomiting, irritability, difficulty sleeping, and fatigue. These signs and symptoms increase to confusion, stiff neck, significant behavioral changes, and seizures. Hydrocephalus and cranial nerve palsies or cerebral infarcts may occur. Recovery rate is 90% with early diagnosis and treatment with appropriate antituberculosis therapy.

PATHOPHYSIOLOGY The bacteria that commonly cause bacterial meningitis are common inhabitants of the nasopharynx, but a predisposing factor such as a prior upper respiratory infection must be present before the bacteria become blood-borne. Bacterial meningitis also may develop as a consequence of ear, dental, or paraspinal infections; impairment in the anatomic barrier from trauma or neurosurgery; and, rarely, when a brain abscess ruptures into the ventricular system or subarachnoid space.[67] The method of CNS entry is through the choroid plexuses or areas of altered blood-brain barrier or by hematogenous spread. Bacteria multiply in the subarachnoid space. The bacteria or their toxins function as irritants and induce an inflammatory reaction by the meninges (pia mater and arachnoid), the CSF, and the ventricles. The meningeal vessels undergo change, becoming hyperemic and increasingly permeable. Blood cells (neutrophils) migrate into the subarachnoid space, producing an exudate that thickens the CSF and interferes with normal CSF flow around the brain and spinal cord (Figure 17-35). The exudate has the potential to obstruct arachnoid villi and produce hydrocephalus and interstitial edema. The amount of purulent exudate increases rapidly (especially around the base of the brain), causing further inflammation. The exudate extends into the sheaths of the cranial and spinal nerves and into the perivascular spaces of the cortex. Meningeal cells become edematous. The exudate and vasogenic edema increase ICP. The small and medium-sized subarachnoid arteries, veins, and choroid plexuses undergo inflammatory changes and become engorged, disrupting blood flow and potentially producing thrombosis. Secondary infection of the brain may occur. The cortical neurons also show some changes, including an increase in the number of microglia and astrocytes.

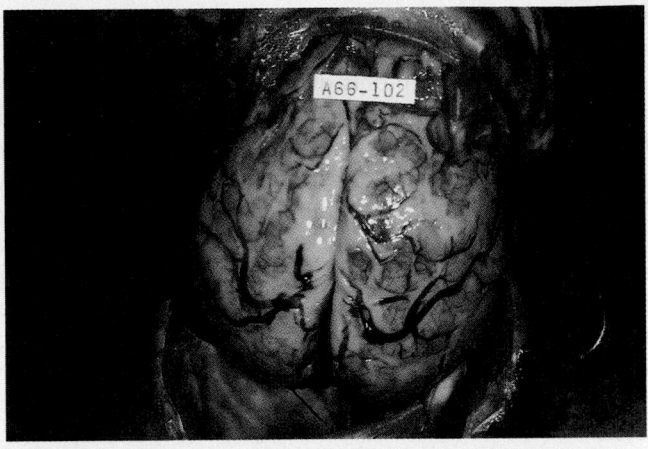

Figure 17-35 Acute leptomeningitis. The leptomeninges contain abundant creamy, purulent exudate, most prominently over the superior surface of the cerebrum. The underlying brain is swollen, and the vessels are congested. (From Kumar V, Cotran RS, Robbins SL: *Robbins basic pathology,* ed 7, Philadelphia, 2003, Saunders.)

Fungi in the nervous system usually produce a granulomatous reaction with formations of granulomas or gelatinous masses. These usually develop in the meninges at the base of the brain. Fungi also may extend along the perivascular sites in the subarachnoid space and into the brain tissue, producing arteritis with thrombosis, infarction, and communicating hydrocephalus. Meningeal fibrosis develops later in the inflammatory process. Cranial nerve dysfunction, caused by compression, often results from the granulomas and fibrosis.

CLINICAL MANIFESTATIONS The clinical manifestations of a bacterial meningitis can be grouped as (1) inflammation and irritation—generalized meningeal signs, throbbing headache that becomes more severe, photophobia that becomes more severe, nuchal rigidity, Kernig sign, and Brudzinski sign; (2) local tissue dysfunction—cranial nerve palsies, focal neurologic deficits (such as hemiparesis/hemiplegia, ataxia), and seizures; (3) mass effect—decreased level of consciousness, nausea, vomiting, and increased intracranial pressure; and (4) vascular compromise. The irritation and damage to the cranial nerves produced by the inflamed sheaths manifest as follows:

Cranial nerve II: papilledema, blindness

Cranial nerves III, IV, and VI: ptosis, visual field deficits, diplopia

Cranial nerve V: photophobia

Cranial nerve VII: facial paresis

Cranial nerve VIII: deafness, tinnitus, vertigo

Neck stiffness and pain, and possibly head retraction, reflect the irritability of spinal accessory and cervical spinal nerves. Often the vomiting center is irritated, causing projectile vomiting. Confusion and decreasing responsiveness are evidence of cortical involvement. In meningococcal meningitis, petechial or purpuric rash involving the skin and mucous membranes occurs. As ICP increases, papilledema may develop and delirium may progress to the point that the individual becomes unconscious.

The signs and symptoms of bacterial meningitis in neonates are subtle and nonspecific. Low-grade fever and mild behavioral changes with few meningeal signs may be the first signs. High fever, lethargy, irritability, hypothermia, seizures, bulging fontanels, poor feeding, vomiting, and respiratory distress may be present. Children may present with either a subacute infection that worsens over several days following an ear infection or upper respiratory infection, or as an acute fulminant illness that has developed rapidly over a few hours. Older adults often develop low-grade fever with confusion or other mild behavioral changes. Stupor or coma may appear later.

The clinical manifestations of aseptic meningitis are mild compared with those associated with bacterial meningitis. Mild generalized throbbing headache, mild photophobia, mild neck pain, stiffness, fever, and malaise are manifestations of aseptic meningitis.

Fungal meningitis develops slowly and insidiously. The first manifestations are often those of dementia or communicating hydrocephalus (see Chapter 16). The individual is characteristically afebrile.

EVALUATION AND TREATMENT Diagnosis of bacterial meningitis is based on physical examination, including skin rash, nasopharyngeal smear, and antigen tests. CSF is the gold standard for diagnosis. Bacterial meningitis and fungal meningitis are treated with appropriate antibiotic therapy, but resistant strains are an increasing problem. Other supportive measures may be needed. Aseptic meningitis is managed pharmacologically with antiviral drugs and steroids. Conjugate vaccines exist for meningococcal, pneumococcal, and hemophilic meningitis.[69] Chemoprophylaxis for exposure to meningococcal meningitis is rifampin, ciprofloxacin, or ceftriaxone.[70]

Suppurative Cerebral Masses

Localized pus-filled masses can develop with the CNS. The mass may be an abscess within the brain or spinal cord, a subdural empyema with the infection between the dura and the subarachnoid space, or an epidural abscess with the infection between the dura and skull or vertebrae. The latter two occur less commonly but have similar predisposing conditions, infectious agents, and clinical manifestations. Treatments are also similar. Subdural empyemas and epidural abscess generally spread locally from infections in an adjoining structure.

Abscess

Abscesses are localized collections of pus within the parenchyma of the brain and spinal cord. The incidence of abscesses is about 1 per 100,000 hospital admissions. Men experience abscesses more frequently than women, with a 2:1 ratio. The median age for abscess formation is 30 to 40 years of age. Abscesses occur (1) after open trauma and during neurosurgery; (2) in association with a contiguous focus of infection, such as the middle ear, mastoid cells, nasal

cavity, and nasal sinuses; (3) through metastatic or hematogenous spread from distant foci, such as the heart, lungs, pelvic organs, skin, tonsils, abscessed teeth, osteomyelitis in other than cranial bones, and dirty needles (especially in compromised hosts); and (4) cryptogenically, arising without other associated areas of infections. Streptococci, staphylococci, and bacteroids, often in combination with anaerobes, are the most common bacteria that cause abscesses; however, yeast and fungi also have been found in CNS abscesses. *Toxoplasma gondii* is producing an ever-increasing number of CNS abscesses in individuals with AIDS: 80% are located in the cerebrum and 20% are cerebellar. The frontal and temporal lobes are the most common sites (Figure 17-36). The abscesses are in more than one site in 5% to 20% of cases. The immunosuppressed are particularly at risk for abscesses.

Spinal cord abscesses are classified as epidural or intramedullary. Debilitated individuals with sepsis more frequently develop **intramedullary spinal cord abscesses** (those within the spinal cord).

PATHOPHYSIOLOGY Microorganisms gain entrance to the CNS from adjacent sites by direct extension from osteomyelitis or spread along the wall of a vein. Infective emboli carry the microorganisms from distant sites. Brain abscess evolves through four stages regardless of infecting microorganism except in the immunosuppressed host, where the process may be incomplete. The stages are as follows:

1. *Early cerebritis* (days 1 to 3): localized inflammatory process in which perivascular infiltration or inflammatory cells, composed of neutrophils, plasma cells, and mononuclear cells, surround a central core of coagulative necrosis; marked cerebral edema surrounds the area
2. *Late cerebritis* (days 4 to 9): necrotic center is surrounded by inflammatory infiltrate of macrophages and fibroblasts; rapid new blood vessel formation occurs around the abscess; a thin capsule of fibroblasts and reticular fibers gradually develops; the area is still surrounded by cerebral edema
3. *Early capsule formation* (days 10 to 13): necrotic center decreases in size; inflammatory infiltrate changes in character and contains an increasing number of fibroblasts and macrophages; mature collagen evolves forming a capsule
4. *Late capsule formation* (days 14 and longer): well-formed necrotic center surrounded by a dense collagenous capsule[67]

A free (nonencapsulated) abscess is associated with a higher mortality. A mature abscess has three layers: (1) a center of polymorphonuclear leukocytes, (2) a collagenous capsule, and (3) peripheral gliosis. Existing abscesses also tend to spread and form daughter abscesses.

Abscesses arising from the ear frequently are located in the middle or inferior temporal lobe or in the anterolateral cerebellar hemispheres. Abscesses originating from the oral and nasal area most commonly are located in the frontal and

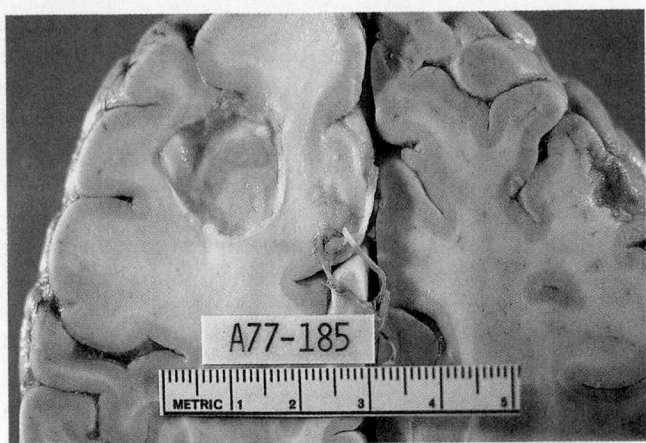

Figure 17-36 Brain abscess. The abcess is sharply demarcated, indicating that it has been present for some time. Purulent exudate is visible in the center of the abscess. Because antibiotics penetrate very poorly into abscesses, surgical drainage is often necessary to treat such lesions. (From Kumar V, Cotran RS, Robbins SL: *Robbins basic pathology*, ed 7, Philadelphia, 2003, Saunders.)

temporal lobes. Abscesses from distant foci often occur in multiple numbers in the distal portion of the middle cerebral arteries. In extradural abscesses, pus and granulation tissue accumulate in the extradural space.

CLINICAL MANIFESTATIONS Clinical manifestations of brain abscesses are associated with (1) intracranial infection, such as fever and increased sedimentation rate; or (2) an expanding intracranial mass, such as headache, nausea, vomiting, decreasing cognitive abilities, paresis, and seizures. Early clinical manifestations of brain abscesses are low-grade fever, headache, neck pain and stiffness with mild nuchal rigidity, confusion, drowsiness, sensory deficits, and communication deficits. Headache is the most common early symptom. Later clinical manifestations may include inattentiveness (distractibility), memory deficits, decreased visual acuity and

narrowed visual fields, papilledema, ocular palsy, ataxia, and dementia. Symptoms depend on the location of the abscess. The development of symptoms may be very insidious, often making an abscess difficult to diagnose. **Extradural brain abscesses** are associated with localized pain, purulent drainage from the nasal passages or auditory canal, fever, localized tenderness, and neck stiffness; occasionally the individual experiences a focal seizure. Clinical manifestations of spinal cord abscesses have four stages: (1) spinal aching; (2) root pain, which is usually severe, accompanied by spasms of the back muscles and limited vertebral movement because of pain and spasm; (3) weakness caused by progressive cord compression; and (4) paralysis.

EVALUATION AND TREATMENT The diagnosis is suggested on the basis of clinical features and confirmed by CT. MRI is helpful when the CT scan does not show an abscess even though it is suggested by clinical features. Surgery is indicated if the diagnosis is in doubt or there are space-occupying problems. Aspiration through a burr hole or excision through craniotomy with antibiotic therapy may be used. Multiple or surgically inaccessible abscesses are treated with antibiotics, often in conjunction with steroid therapy to treat the cerebral edema. In addition, ICP may have to be managed. Because decompression is necessary, spinal cord abscesses are treated with surgical excision or aspiration. Antibiotic and support therapy also is instituted.

Encephalitis

Encephalitis is an acute febrile illness, usually of viral origin, with nervous system involvement. The most common encephalitides are caused by arthropod-borne (mosquito-borne) viruses and herpes simplex, almost exclusively herpes simplex type 1 in adults (Figure 17-37). Etiologic agents for viral encephalitis are presented in Table 17-10. Referred to as *infectious viral encephalitides*, encephalitis also may occur as a complication of systemic viral diseases such as

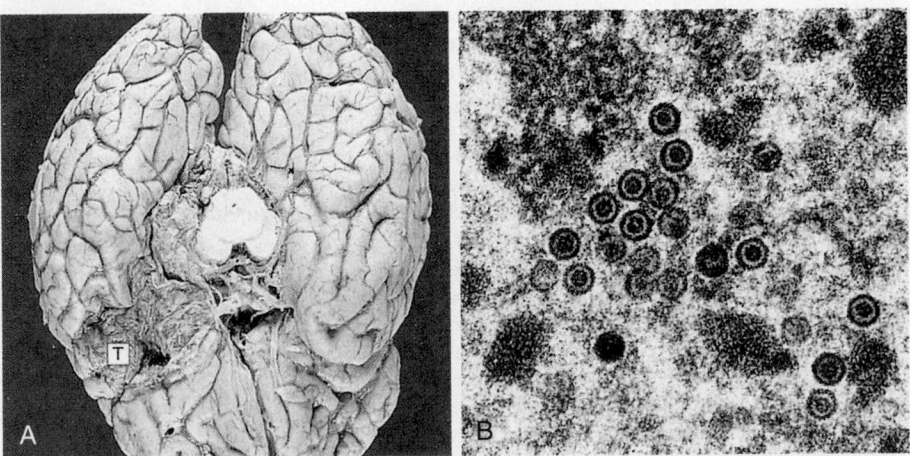

Figure 17-37 Herpes simplex encephalitis. In herpes simplex encephalitis (A) necrosis of the temporal lobes (T) is a typical development. Brain biopsy is useful in diagnosis when the virus can be seen by electron microscopy (B) as rounded particles with a dense core. Virus also can be identified by immunostaining or culture. In early cases, polymerase chain reaction (PCR) can be used to identify viral deoxyribonucleic acid (DNA) in cerebrospinal fluid samples. (From Stevens A, Lowe J: *Pathology*, ed 2, London, 2000, Mosby.)

poliomyelitis, rabies, or mononucleosis, or it may arise after recovery from some viral infection such as rubella or rubeola. Encephalitis also may follow vaccination with a live attenuated virus vaccine if the vaccine has an encephalitis component. Such vaccines include measles, mumps, and rubella. Typhus, trichinosis, malaria, and schistosomiasis also are associated with encephalitis. Toxoplasmosis may acutely reactivate in immunosuppressed hosts when the once-dormant parasite in cyst form disseminates in brain tissues (see p. 629).

With the exception of the California viral encephalitis, which is endemic, the arthropod-borne encephalitides occur in epidemics, varying in geographic and seasonal incidence (Table 17-11). Eastern equine encephalitis is the most serious but least common of the encephalitides.[67] West Nile virus is presented in Box 17-5.

PATHOPHYSIOLOGY Viruses gain access to the CNS through the bloodstream or through an intraneuronal route from peripheral nerves.[71] Evidence of meningeal involvement appears in all encephalitides. The arthropod-borne viral encephalitides cause widespread nerve cell degeneration. Edema and areas of necrosis with or without hemorrhage develop. Increased ICP develops and may progress to herniation. Large degenerative injuries are found in eastern equine encephalitis, whereas the other arthropod-borne viral encephalitides have microscopic areas of injury and degeneration.

Infectious encephalitis may result from a postinfectious autoimmune response to the virus or from direct invasion of the CNS by the virus. Herpes simplex type 1 has a tendency to infect the inferomedial surfaces of the temporal and frontal lobes and causes hemorrhagic necrosis.

CLINICAL MANIFESTATIONS Encephalitis may range from a mild infectious disease to a life-threatening disorder. The dramatic clinical manifestations of encephalitis are fever, delirium or confusion progressing to unconsciousness, seizure activity, cranial nerve palsies, paresis and paralysis, involuntary movement, and abnormal reflexes. Signs of marked ICP may be present.

EVALUATION AND TREATMENT Diagnosis is based on medical history and clinical presentation aided by CSF examination and culture, serologic examination, white blood cell (WBC) count, CT scan, or MRI. (Treatment available for the viral encephalitides is listed in Table 17-10.) Supportive therapy is initiated, and measures to control ICP are paramount.

Neurologic Complications of Acquired Immunodeficiency Syndrome

Approximately 40% to 60% of all persons with AIDS have neurologic complications (see Chapter 8 for the pathophysiology of AIDS). On postmortem examination, 75% have nervous system pathologic findings. The CNS pathologic findings result from (1) the primary human immunodeficiency virus

Table 17-11	Classification and Characteristics of Arthropod Viruses Causing Encephalitis					
Viruses	**Incubation Period (Days)**	**Virus**	**Location**	**Vector**	**Season**	**Affected Population**
Eastern equine encephalitis	5-15	Togaviridae Alphavirus (formerly group A arbovirus)	Atlantic, Gulf Coast, and Great Lake regions	Mosquito	Midsummer to early fall	Infants, children, and adults >50 years
Western equine encephalitis	5-10	Same as above	All parts of United States, especially western two thirds of country	Mosquito	Summer to early fall	Infants and young children
Venezuelan equine encephalitis	2-5	Same as above	Texas, Florida, Mexico; Central and South America	Mosquito	Year round	Infants and young children
St. Louis encephalitis	4-21	Flaviviridae Flavivirus group B (formerly group B arbovirus)	United States and Canada, especially Mississippi River, Pacific Coast, Texas, and Florida	Mosquito	Summer and fall	Adults >40 years; older adults more often affected than younger ages
California encephalitis including LaCrosse	5-15	Bunyaviridae Bunyavirus (California virus serogroup)	Midwestern United States, eastern seaboard, and Canada	Woodland mosquito	Late summer and early fall	Children <15 years
West Nile encephalitis	3-14	Same as above	Lower 48 states of the United States	Mosquito	Summer and fall	Older adults most seriously

Box 17-5   Emergence of West Nile Virus

West Nile (WN) virus, a flavivirus transmitted predominantly by the *Culex* mosquito, emerged in New York State in 1999. By the end of 2004, human cases had been found in the 48 contiguous states. Humans and horses, as well as other mammals, are incidental hosts. Birds and mosquitoes are life cycle hosts. Summer and fall are peak times of infection incidence. Besides mosquito transmission, WN virus can be transmitted through blood transfusions and organ transplants. Health experts believe transmission from mother to unborn child and through breast milk is possible.

Three clinical forms of West Nile have emerged: WN fever; WN encephalitis; and WN meningitis, although some individuals have other clinical manifestations. Some persons develop WN fever. The febrile illness of acute onset may be clinically unrecognizable as WN. About 20% of those infected have mild symptoms that last for 4 to 6 days that generally include fever and may include weakness, nausea, vomiting, headache, mental status changes, diarrhea, rash, and lymphadenopathy. WN encephalitis is marked by disorientation, stupor, coma, seizures, and movement disorders including tremor, ataxia, extrapyramidal signs, and paralysis. WN meningitis is characterized by meningeal signs of severe headache, high fever, and nuchal rigidity. Myelitis and polyradiculitis also may be present. Myocarditis, pancreatitis, and fulminant hepatitis are rare. Abnormalities in the thalamus, basal ganglia, and cerebellum are often seen on MRI in people with severe infection—about 1 in 150 develop nervous system involvement. Identifiable risk factors for this are advanced age and immunocompromise.

A preliminary diagnosis is made if IgM for the virus is found in serum or CSF. A rapid test became available in 2007. Plaque reduction neutralization assay (PRNA) is the confirmatory test. Interferon-alpha is used during treatment along with supportive care for those with severe infection. A new vaccine is being tested.

Data from National Institute on Allergy and Infectious Disease, Department of Health and Human Services, National Institutes of Health: *NIAID research on West Nile Virus, January 2008*, available at www.niaid.nih.gov.
CSF, cerebrospinal fluid; *IgM*, Immunoglobulin M; *MRI*, magnetic resonance imaging.

(HIV) infection; (2) the immune dysregulation of early HIV infection and progressive immunosuppression in late HIV infections resulting in opportunistic infections, neoplasms, and systemic illness; and (3) complications of therapy.[72]

A variety of CNS complications of HIV exist (Box 17-6). Multiple CNS pathologic conditions may be experienced by one person. The most common neurologic disorder is HIV-associated dementia; others are peripheral neuropathies, vacuolar (spongy softening) myelopathy, opportunistic infections of the CNS, and neoplasms.

HIV-infected macrophages/monocytes in blood are attracted to the brain by up-regulation of proinflammatory mediators such as monocyte chemoattractant protein-1 (MCP-1), tumor necrosis factor-alpha (TNF-α), and adhesion molecules on endothelial cells. Up-regulation enables transendothelial migration of activated macrophages/monocytes.

Human Immunodeficiency Virus–Associated Dementia

HIV-associated dementia (HAD) (HIV-associated cognitive dysfunction, HIV encephalopathy, subacute encephalitis, HIV-associated dementia complex, HIV cognitive motor complex, AIDS encephalopathy, AIDS dementia complex, or AIDS-related dementia) may affect adults and children and is characterized by progressive cognitive dysfunction in conjunction with motor and behavioral alterations[72] (Table 17-12). The syndrome typically develops later in the disease but may be an early or a singular manifestation. The syndrome is more prevalent in drug users with HIV.[73]

At the time of primary HIV infection, circulating HIV-infected leukocytes (activated leukocytes), including macrophages and lymphocytes, adhere to the endothelial lining of blood vessels within the nervous system. These cells subsequently enter the brain parenchyma. HIV infects the

Box 17-6   Nervous System Complications of HIV-1 Infections

CNS Complications of HIV-1 Infection
Diffuse cerebral disorders
  Minor cognitive and motor deficits (MCMDs)
  HIV-associated dementia
Meningitis
  Atypical aseptic meningitis
    Acute: typical meningitis signs
    Chronic: headache syndrome
  Nonviral infection
    Cryptococcus neoformans
  Other fungal infections
    Mycobacterial infections
Myelopathy
  Spinal vacuolar myelopathy
Focal brain disorders
  Opportunistic viral infections
    Progressive multifocal leukoencephalopathy
    Herpesviruses
  Nonviral infections
    Toxoplasma gondii
  Bacterial infections
Neoplasms
  Primary CNS neoplasms
  Metastatic neoplasms
Cerebrovascular complications
Complications resulting from systemic HIV therapy

Peripheral Nervous System Complications of HIV-1 Infections
Distal symmetric peripheral neuropathy (polyneuropathy)
Inflammatory demyelinating polyradiculoneuropathy
Mononeuropathy multiplex
Progressive polyradiculopathy
Other causes of peripheral nervous system dysfunction
Herpes zoster radiculitis
Cranial neuropathies

CNS, Central nervous system; *HIV*, human immunodeficiency virus.

Table 17-12	Classification of HIV-Associated Cognitive Dysfunction
Category	**Dysfunction**
1 (HIV-associated, minor)	0.5 SD below normal on standardized neuropsychologic tests
	Decline in work or other activities of daily living (ADLs)
	Symptoms for 1 month
	Criteria for HIV-1–associated dementia or delirium is absent
	No other etiology
2 (HIV-associated dementia)	Marked impairment in at least two ability domains
	Significant impairment in work and other ADLs
	Symptoms for 1 month
	No other etiology
	Free of delirium for a period sufficient to establish the presence of dementia
3 (HIV-associated delirium)	Clouding of consciousness
	Marked, rapid worsening of cognitive function in ≥2 domains

From Belman AL, Mirjana-Savatic M: Human immunodeficiency virus and acquired immunodeficiency syndrome. In Goetz CG, editor: *Textbook of clinical neurology*, ed 2, Philadelphia, 2003, Saunders. *HIV*, Human immunodeficiency virus; *SD*, standard deviation.

perivascular macrophages, the microglial cells in the area, and, to a lesser degree, the astrocytes in the area.[74] HIV preferentially affects the basal ganglia and deep white matter.[74] Affected macrophages, macrophage-derived multinucleated cells, and microglia cause an immune-mediated demyelination process in white matter. Some viral replication occurs in some of the glial cells and occasionally within neurons. Multiple small nodules containing inflammatory cells are scattered throughout the white matter and in subcortical gray matter, such as the basal ganglia and thalami. Perivascular inflammation is present. Focal and diffuse demyelination of white matter and spongy changes of the spinal cord are present. Factors other than direct cell damage are involved, such as released toxins, lymphokines, or other substances. Elevation in CSF levels of quinolinic acid, a neurotoxic metabolite of tryptophan, is correlated with the degree of dementia. A decreased concentration of adenosine triphosphate (ATP) and inorganic phosphates in the CNS produces a decrease in metabolism.

HIV-associated dementia is insidious in onset and unpredictable in its course. Most individuals experience a steady progression of mental slowing characterized by abrupt accelerations of signs over several months to more than 1 year, although some experience an abrupt onset or an accelerated course. The triad of clinical manifestations are neurocognitive impairment, behavioral disturbance, and motor abnormalities.

Early clinical manifestations of HIV-associated dementia may be vague. Impaired concentration and short-term memory and retrieval deficits commonly occur. Apathy and lack of motivation, social withdrawal, irritability, and emotional lability may appear. Later, difficulties with language, spatial or temporal disorientation, and visual construction appear. Some individuals manifest an organic psychosis with agitation, inappropriate behavior, and hallucinosis.

Generalized cognitive system deficits occur later in the course of HIV-associated dementia, often accompanied by psychomotor slowing and decreased speech spontaneity and fluency. Progressive loss of balance, ataxia, spastic paraparesis or paralysis, and generalized hyperreflexia are common motor signs. Decreased writing ability, tremor, myoclonus, and seizure are less commonly seen.

Diagnosis is difficult, especially in early stages. The individuals medical history along with physical examination findings and supporting CSF, CT, and MRI data help establish the diagnosis. Specific screening tools have been developed to assist in diagnosis. Antiretroviral, protease inhibitors, reverse transcriptase inhibitors, and adjunctive agents may be effective along with supportive treatment. However, highly active antiretroviral therapy (HAART) protocols have shown little efficacy in reversing HAD because it does not target the cause.[75]

HIV Myelopathy

HIV myelopathy involving diffuse degeneration of the spinal cord may occur with HIV. **Vacuolar myelopathy** is believed to be a direct consequence of HIV. The lateral and posterior columns of the lumbar spinal cord are affected. A progressive spastic paraparesis with ataxia is the predominant clinical manifestation. Leg weakness, upper motor neuron signs, incontinence, and posterior column sensory loss may be present. Diagnosis is made on the basis of history, physical findings, and supporting data from diagnostic procedures. Vacuolar myelopathy is treated supportively and does not respond to antiretrovirals.

HIV Neuropathy

Some HIV-related peripheral neuropathies occur early, may coincide with seroconversion, are immune-mediated, and respond to standard immunotherapies. Other peripheral neuropathies primarily develop with advanced HIV infection and immunocompromised states and are facilitated by HIV replication, neurotoxicity from antiretroviral therapies, and coinfection with opportunistic pathogens.[76]

HIV neuropathy may have one or a combination of several presentations: a predominantly sensory neuropathy, an autonomic neuropathy, a mononeuritis multiplex, a Guillain-Barré–like syndrome, and a myopathy. The peripheral nervous system may sustain injury in HIV, manifesting as a peripheral neuropathy or radiculopathy. A progressive radiculopathy of predominantly the dorsal roots of the lumbar and sacral nerves may occur, involving severe myelin and axonal loss. HIV-associated distal symmetric polyneuropathy, a sensory neuropathy occurring late in the disease, is the most commonly occurring neuropathy with slowly progressive numbness and paresthesias and burning sensations in the feet.[77]

HIV has been isolated from peripheral nerves, so it is believed that the virus may directly infect nerves. Individuals experience painful, burning dysesthesias and paresthesias, typically in the extremities. Weakness and decreased or absent distal reflexes may be present. Diagnosis is established through history, physical findings, laboratory data, nerve conduction studies, EMG, and possibly biopsy. The most common myopathy is polymyositis; it may be present initially or develop later. The muscle fiber is infiltrated, initiating inflammation that leads to cellular degeneration and necrosis. The individual experiences muscle weakness of extremities with myalgia and fatigue. Steroids are used therapeutically in polymyositis.

Aseptic Viral Meningitis

Some people develop an acute aseptic meningitis at approximately the time of seroconversion. This may well represent the initial infection of the nervous system by the HIV. Symptoms include headache, fever, and meningismus. Cranial nerve involvement, especially of nerves V and VII, may appear, but the disease is self-limiting and requires only symptomatic treatment. Aseptic meningitis might occur at any point in the disease.

Opportunistic Infections

Opportunistic infections may be bacterial, fungal, protozoal, or viral in origin and produce nervous system disease. Typically bacterial infections are caused by unusual microorganisms. Cryptococcal infection is the most common fungal disorder and the third leading cause of neurologic disease with HIV. In *Cryptococcus neoformans*, small granulomas and cysts are found in the cerebral cortex and later may be present in deep cerebral tissues. The symptoms are vague, such as fever, headache, malaise, and meningismus. Herpes encephalitis and herpes varicella-zoster radiculitis may develop. Papovavirus (especially JC virus) in the immunocompromised person with HIV may produce a demyelinating disorder called *progressive multifocal leukoencephalopathy (PML)*. This virus is found in 90% of healthy persons but is dormant. The virus reactivates to cause PML in 15% of HIV victims. Sensory and motor deficits, aphasia, and apraxia are common clinical manifestations. The condition is progressive.

Cytomegalovirus Infection. Cytomegalovirus encephalitis is common with AIDS but often not diagnosed while a person is alive. The encephalitis may be present as an acute illness with encephalitis features accompanied by nystagmus and cranial nerve signs. Retinitis is found in 50% of those affected.

Parasitic Infection. Toxoplasmosis is the most common opportunistic infection and occurs in one third of AIDS cases. CNS toxoplasmosis typically manifests as focal encephalitis. *Toxoplasma gondii*, a protozoan, is thought to reactivate from latent lesions to produce a well-demarcated necrotizing process. Inflammatory infiltrates, thrombotic lesions, and fibrinoid vascular walls are present at the necrotic edge. Marked edema is present adjacent to necrotic areas.

Lesions may be multiple and exist throughout the cerebral hemispheres.

Clinical manifestations of CNS toxoplasmosis are focal but highly variable and include clumsiness to hemiplegia, aphasia, seizures, ataxia, cognitive changes, and constitutional symptoms. Fever and headache are common. Toxoplasmosis is difficult to diagnose but is treated effectively with pyrimethamine and sulfadiazine. Allergic response to sulfadiazine can be a problem, and other drugs can be substituted. Individuals with HIV may develop meningitis, encephalitis, or fungal, mycobacterial, and bacterial brain abscesses.

Central Nervous System Neoplasms

CNS neoplasms associated with HIV include primary CNS lymphoma, systemic non-Hodgkin lymphoma, and metastatic Kaposi sarcoma. The precise mechanism of lymphoproliferation is not known. Primary CNS lymphoma is a large-cell lymphoma that presents as rapidly developing and expanding multicentric intracranial mass lesions. The meninges are invaded and, possibly, the cranial nerves and spinal cord are invaded as well in systemic non-Hodgkin lymphoma. Metastasis of a Kaposi sarcoma to the CNS is uncommon.

Other Central Nervous System Complications

Individuals with HIV may develop multifocal ischemic infarctions, hemorrhagic infarctions, hemorrhage into tumors, subdural hematomas, and epidural hemorrhage. The precise mechanism of these cardiovascular complications is not yet known. Reported neurologic symptoms produced by HIV therapeutics include extrapyramidal movements, myoclonus, dysphasia, delirium, and acute myelopathy.

Lyme Disease

Lyme disease, a tick-borne spirochette bacterial infection, is a common arthropod-borne infection in the United States. It affects all age groups and involves the peripheral and central nervous systems. Lyme disease is caused by *Borrelia burgdorferi* introduced by tick bite, requiring about 36 hours of attachment.[76] Transmission is most likely in the late summer or early fall. Infected ticks are endemic in the Midwest, western wooded and coastal areas, and the mid- to northeast Atlantic. The microorganism incubates for 3 to 32 days and then migrates to the skin, lymph nodes, and other body systems. The pathologic process progresses through three stages:

Stage I (acute localized): Within 1 month after the bite, the disease is characterized by a bull's-eye–like (5 cm in diameter) burning centrifugally expanding erythema migrans rash followed by acute disseminated disease with general malaise, flulike symptoms (fever, muscle pain), stiff neck, and headache.

Stage II: With acute widespread dissemination of antibodies and immune complexes, cardiac and neurologic involvement predominates. About 10% of cases show cardiac signs and symptoms (palpitations, dizziness, shortness of breath, dysrhythmias, and first-degree heart block). Neurologic signs occur in 10% to 15% and include headache, chronic aseptic (lymphocytic) meningitis, Bell palsy, encephalitis, and radiculitis. Pathologically there is meningeal inflammation, perivascular inflammatory cell formation, and focal demyelination.

Stage III (chronic stage): The third stage may occur up to 2 years after the bite and involves arthritis and involvement of brain parenchyma with encephalitis, chronic neuropathy, and encephalopathy.

Treatment of choice is antibiotic therapy. Minor recurring symptoms are common in 50% of individuals.

Demyelinating Disorders

Demyelinating disorders are the result of damage to the myelin nerve sheath. They can occur in either the central (i.e., multiple sclerosis) or peripheral (i.e., Guillain-Barré syndrome) nervous system. Causes of the disorders include genetics, infections, autoimmune reactions, environmental toxins, and unknown factors.

Multiple Sclerosis

Multiple sclerosis (MS) is an autoimmune disorder diffusely involving degeneration of CNS myelin and loss of axons. The peripheral nervous system is not involved. MS and its variants are primary demyelinating disorders. In secondary disorders, CNS demyelination is caused by disorders other than multiple sclerosis.

MS is a diffuse and progressive CNS disease that affects white and gray matter.[78] About 0.1% of the population is affected (400,000 persons in the United States and 2.5 million worldwide).[79] Prevalence rates vary with geographic location (higher in temperate regions far above the equator) and racial groups (highest in whites, although it occurs in all races).

The onset of MS is usually between 20 and 40 years of age with a peak of age 30. Male:female ratio is about 1:2. MS is the most prevalent CNS demyelinating disorder and a leading cause of neurologic disability in early adulthood. Life expectancy is not greatly altered by MS and the disease course often extends over 30 years.[80] Genetic and environmental factors and interactions are implicated in disease onset.[81] Although the disorder does not exhibit a defined inheritance pattern, 15% of those with MS have an affected relative. Multiple genes affect risk of development of MS. A genetic link exists in the human leukocyte antigen (HLA) complex, a large cluster of genes responsible for many immune functions. Two genes, the interleukin [IL]-2 receptor gene (*IL2RA*) and *IL7RA*, have been identified.[82] The first demyelinating event or "clinically isolated syndrome" (CIS), is a single episode of neurologic dysfunction lasting greater than 24 hours that can be a prelude to MS. Characteristic episodes include optic neuritis, solitary brainstem lesions, and transverse myelitis. MRI is used to assist diagnosis and assess prognosis although there are limitations to detecting the full extent of the lesions.[83]

PATHOPHYSIOLOGY MS is described as occurring when a previous viral insult to the nervous system has occurred in a genetically susceptible individual with a subsequent abnormal immune response in the CNS. The innate and adaptive immune systems are activated in the pathology of MS.[84] Various mechanisms cause the irreversible tissue damage (inflammation, oligodendrocyte injury, demyelination, and axonal degeneration) that characterizes MS. These degenerative processes begin early in the course of the disease and continue to progress throughout a person's life.[80] Early inflammation and demyelination lead to irreversible axonal degeneration and scarring or sclerosis. Demyelinated axons are more fragile and susceptible to further damage, and when degeneration exceeds self-repair ability (remyelination), permanent disability results.[85]

Myelin destruction and axonal damage begin prior to symptom onset (early inflammatory demyelination). As the disease progresses, inflammatory changes in the CNS increase, and loss of brain volume progresses more rapidly.[86] Box 17-7 describes the clinical courses of MS in relation to disease progression.

The immunopathology of MS involves:
1. CD8+ T-cell activation (autoreactive), cells cross the blood-brain barrier and enter CNS and attack myelin
2. IL-12 and IL-23 (proinflammatory cytokines)
3. Lack of IL-10 (an anti-inflammatory cytokine)
4. IL-17 (proinflammatory cytokine) production by T cells
5. Integrins expressed to facilitate adherence and passage of immune cells into the CNS
6. Chemokines promote the migration of immune cells and are up-regulated in MS
7. B lymphocytes and plasma cells contribute to the inflammatory response and directly damage myelin and axons; B cells are more active in chronic or progressive forms of MS (B cells produce autoantibodies, secrete inflammatory cytokines, and activate T cells by presenting antigen)[87]

Box 17-7   Clinical Course of Multiple Sclerosis (MS)

Relapsing-Remitting (RR) MS
Clear relapses (called *acute attacks* or *excerbations*) with either full recovery, or with partial recovery and lasting disability. Between attacks there is no progression (or worsening) of disease. RR is the most common course of MS (90% of cases).

Primary Progressive (PP) MS
Steady progression (or worsening) from onset, with only occasional plateaus or minor recovery. This is a fairly uncommon disease course and one that may involve different brain and spinal cord damage than do other forms of MS.

Secondary Progressive (SP) MS
Begins with a pattern of clear-cut relapses and recovery but becomes steadily progressive over time with continued worsening between acute attacks (develops in two thirds of individuals eventually).

Progressive-Relapsing (PR) MS
A rare type that is steadily progressive from onset but also has clear acute attacks.

8. Complement activation (promotes inflammation) during the acute phase; may be neuroprotective during relapse[88]

In addition, eosinophils, neutrophils, and macrophages are present. The demyelination disrupts sodium, calcium, and potassium ion channels and calcium influx is proinflammatory and neurotoxic in itself. Activated microglia and macrophages release nitric oxide and oxygen-free radicals. Activated immune cells also produce glutamate, a neurotoxin.[89]

MS is characterized not only by focal inflammatory changes but also diffuse injury throughout the CNS (MS lesions) (Figures 17-38 and 17-39). Four MS lesion pathologic patterns have been described (Box 17-8). MS lesions may occur anywhere in white or gray matter. In addition, other neurodegenerative processes that involve the entire CNS are taking place, including (1) changes in gray matter in the cortex, basal ganglia, brainstem, and spinal cord with substantial loss over time; (2) brain atrophy that begins early in the disease and is highly correlated with disability and progressive MS; and (3) direct dysfunction of or damage to oligodendrocytes that manufacture myelin.[80,90] Normal-appearing white matter also is highly abnormal microscopically with the presence of wallerian degeneration, diffuse inflammation, extensive microglial activation, neurotoxic substances, and gene activation that disrupt cellular processes.[80] In established disease the multifocal, multistaged feature of MS lesions gives rise to the aphorism that the lesions are "scattered in space and time." Symptoms therefore are multiple and variable.

CLINICAL MANIFESTATIONS A variety of events (e.g., infection, trauma, or pregnancy) occurring immediately before the onset or exacerbation of symptoms are regarded as precipitating factors related to MS. Most of the pregnancy-related exacerbations occur 3 months postpartum, suggesting a relation to the stresses of labor and the increased fatigue during the postpartum period rather than to the pregnancy itself.

The major classifications of MS are relapsing-remitting, primary progressive, secondary progressive, and progressive-relapsing (see Box 17-7). Initially 90% of persons present with a relapsing, remitting course; 10% present with a primary progressive course; and 90% develop a progressive course in 10 to 20 years after onset of the disease. However, once walking problems develop, disease progression occurs quickly regardless of disease type. Usually persons with late MS have one of the established syndromes—mixed, spinal, or cerebellar (Box 17-9). The initial syndrome depends on the portion of the CNS that is most involved. After years, 50% of individuals appear to have established syndromes of mixed involvement.

Mixed (General) Type

Twenty-five percent of persons initially experience retrobulbar or optic neuritis, the manifestations of optic nerve axonal loss.[91] The condition usually evolves rapidly over hours to days and is highly suggestive of MS. Involvement may be unilateral or bilateral. Subjective symptoms are impaired central vision (blurring, fogginess, haziness) and impaired color perception. Signs are decreased central visual acuity; central or paracentral scotoma (area of diminished vision); acquired color vision deficit, especially to red and green; and defective pupillary reaction to light. A variety of field defects may occur. In the acute phase these symptoms may reflect optic papillitis (inflammation and swelling of the optic disc) or retrobulbar neuritis with a normal disc. One third of persons recover completely, and most others improve significantly.

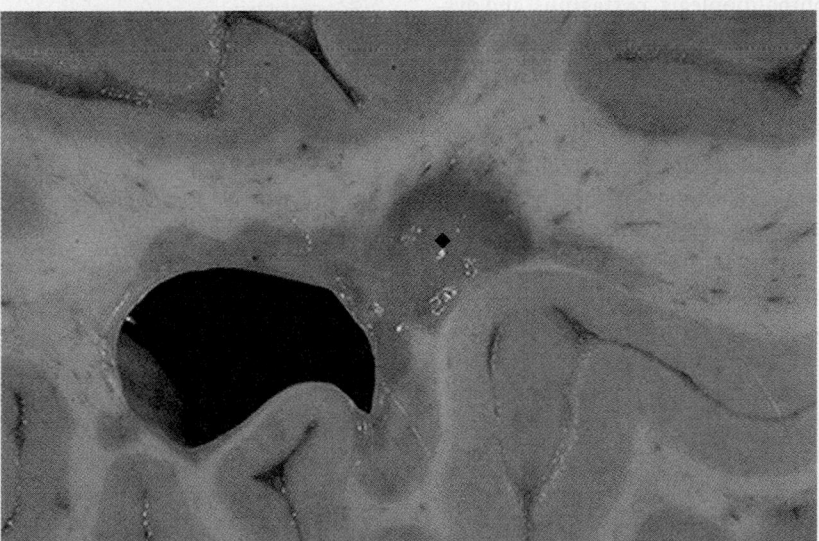

Figure 17-38 Multiple sclerosis, gross. Seen here in periventricular white matter is a large "plaque" (♦) of demyelination that has a sharp border with adjacent normal white matter. Such plaques have a gray-tan appearance and are typically associated with the clinical appearance of transient or progressive loss of neurologic function in multiple sclerosis (MS). Because MS is often multifocal, and the lesions appear in various white matter locations in the central nervous sytem over time, the clinical course and findings can be quite varied. (From Klatt EC: *Robbins and Cotran atlas of pathology*, Philadelphia, 2006, Saunders.)

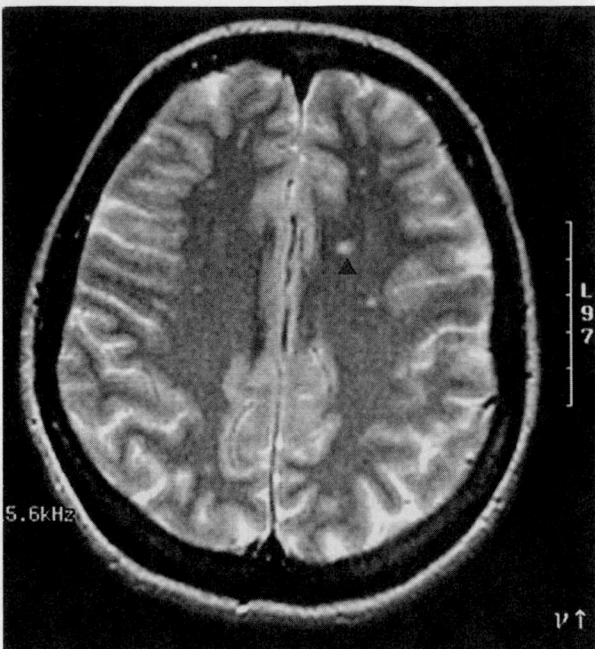

Figure 17-39 Multiple sclerosis (MS), MRI. This T2-weighted magnetic resonance image in axial view shows multiple bilateral small bright foci (▲) that represents areas of demyelinating plaque formation in an individual with an exacerbation of MS. White matter anywhere within the brain and spinal cord can be involved. (From Klatt EC: *Robbins and Cotran atlas of pathology*, Philadelphia, 2006, Saunders.)

Box 17-8   Multiple Sclerosis: Pathologic Patterns*

Pattern I
    Cell-mediated
    Macrophages, T cells
    Remyelination occurs
Pattern II
    Cell mediated
    IgG and complement in areas of active myelin damage
    Remyelination occurs
Pattern III
    Cellular infiltrate
    Macrophages, T cells, activated microglia
    No IgG or complement
    Oligodendrocyte apoptosis
    No remyelination
Pattern IV
    Cellular infiltrates
    No IgG
    Primary injury to oligodendrocytes?
    No remyelination

From Lucchinetti C et al: *Ann Neurol* 47(6):707-717, 2000.
*51 biopsies and 32 autopsy samples.
IgG, Immunoglobulin G.

Box 17-9   Established Syndromes of Multiple Sclerosis

Mixed or Generalized Type (50% of Persons)
Optic signs—optic neuritis
    Brainstem signs—internuclear ophthalmoplegia, diplopia, vertigo (vomiting), nystagmus, dysarthria
    Cerebellar signs—see page 633

Spinal Type (30% to 40% of Persons)
Spastic ataxia
    Deep sensory changes in the extremities
    Bladder and bowel symptoms

Cerebellar or Pontobulbar-Cerebral Type (5% of Persons)
Motor ataxia
    Hypotonia
    Asthenia

Amaurotic Form (5% of Persons)
Blindness

Later, pallor of the temporal half of the disc occurs from demyelination of a portion of the optic nerve. (Normal visual function is discussed in Chapter 15.)

The brainstem lesions involve cranial nerves III through XII at the root, nuclear, or corticobulbar (upper motor neuron) level. Internuclear ophthalmoplegia, nystagmus, and dysarthria are the most common brainstem symptoms, followed by deafness, vertigo and vomiting, tinnitus, facial weakness, and facial sensory deficit. Internuclear ophthalmoplegia is lateral gaze paralysis caused by involvement of the medial longitudinal fasciculus, the brainstem pathway that coordinates eye movement. Diplopia and eyeball pain are common complaints. Bilateral internuclear ophthalmoplegia in a young adult is virtually diagnostic of MS.

Cognitive dysfunction has been demonstrated to occur early in the disease course. The person experiences decreased short-term memory, recent memory impairment, decreased concentration, word-finding problems, and planning difficulties. Mood alterations are common in MS. Depression is far more common than euphoria.

Spinal Type
The spinal type of MS is the second most common type, chiefly involving the spinal tracts and dorsal column. Weakness, numbness, or both in one or more limbs are initial symptoms in 50% of cases of MS. Subjective corticospinal (upper motor neuron) symptoms (stiffness, slowness, weakness) are often unilateral and are a component of fatigability. Spinal signs are usually bilateral (symmetric), with lower limbs more often and more severely affected than upper limbs; spastic paraparesis is probably the most common single neurologic finding in MS.

Bladder and bowel symptoms occur with major spinal cord involvement. Urgency and hesitancy generally precede incontinence. Bladder dysfunction most often involves a small, spastic bladder, although occasionally a large, flaccid bladder may result with retention problems. Neurogenic impotence often occurs when sphincter symptoms are present. Bowel incontinence is rare, but constipation is common with severe disease. Subjective dorsal column symptoms are symmetric paresthesias (tingling and numbness) in an unpredictable pattern but with a predilection for lower extremities over upper extremities. Dorsal column signs are vibration, position, and two-point discrimination deficits. Sensory complaints often are not substantiated by objective physical findings but by further diagnostic tests.

Cerebellar Type

A nystagmus and ataxia presentation initially is not uncommon and reflects cerebellar and corticospinal involvement. Cerebellar deficits are usually symmetric, with all four limbs involved. With combined corticospinal and cerebellar involvement, the individual has a spastic ataxic gait and ataxia of the arms. Pure cerebellar symptoms are those of motor ataxia, hypotonia, and asthenia (weakness). Manifestations of motor ataxia are decomposition of movement, inability to perform rapid alternating movements (dysdiadochokinesia), and dysmetria. Charcot triad describes a combination of dysarthria, intention tremor, and nystagmus. Hypotonia is manifested by decreased resistance to passive movement, hypoactive deep tendon reflexes, and pendular knee jerk.

Short-lived attacks of neurologic deficits are the temporary appearance or worsening of symptoms. The mechanism of these attacks is complete reversible conduction block in partially demyelinated axons. Conditions that cause short-lived attacks include (1) minor increases in body temperature or serum Ca^{++} concentration and (2) functional demands exceeding conduction capacity. An increase in body temperature or serum Ca^{++} level increases current leakage through demyelinated neurons. Individuals with MS may become dramatically worse when body temperature is raised. Hypercalcemia induced by decreased serum pH may aggravate symptoms of MS. Physical and emotional stress imposes functional demands that may exceed conduction capacity of affected neurons.

Paroxysmal attacks are sensory or motor symptoms of abrupt onset and short duration (a few seconds or minutes). These symptoms include paresthesias, dysarthria and ataxia, and tonic head turning. The mechanism of paroxysmal attacks is nonsynaptic transmission in which nerve impulses are directly transmitted between adjacent demyelinated axons. These impulses arise focally and spuriously in the cervical portion of the spinal cord or in the brainstem. A common paroxysmal symptom, called *Lhermitte sign,* is the momentary paresthesia (shocklike or tingling sensation) that shoots down the trunk or limbs during active or passive flexion of the neck. Bending the neck evokes nonsynaptic impulses in demyelinated axons of the dorsal column in the spinal cord. A person with MS may have many paroxysmal attacks each day. Inciting events include sensory stimulation, voluntary movement, hyperventilation, and emotional stress. Paroxysmal attacks tend to persist for weeks or months and may be followed by progressive symptoms of MS.

EVALUATION AND TREATMENT The diagnostic criteria for MS were revised in 2001 and are known as the McDonald criteria. Clinical examination in combination with

Table 17-13	Diagnostic Tests for Multiple Sclerosis
Test	**Findings in Multiple Sclerosis**
Magnetic resonance imaging	
T2 weighted	Demyelinated plaques, both active and inactive
Gadolinium enhanced	Active demyelinating plaques
Cerebrospinal fluid analysis	Oligoclonal bands of immunoglobulin G
	Elevated immunoglobulin G index
Evoked potentials	Slowed nerve impulse conduction

From Chisholm-Burns MA, et al: *Pharmacotherapy principles and practices,* p 434, New York, 2008, McGraw-Hill.

MRI, to demonstrate MS lesions in time and space, and CSF findings are used to make the diagnosis earlier (Table 17-13) so that treatment may begin sooner. Persistently elevated CSF immunoglobulin G (IgG) index is found in about two thirds of individuals with MS, and oligoclonal bands of IgG on electrophoresis are found in more than 90% of persons. Evoked response (ER) studies aid diagnosis by detecting decreased conduction velocity in visual, auditory, and somatosensory pathways.

The treatment goal in MS is prevention of permanent neurologic damage. Acute relapses are treated with corticosteroids to speed recovery.[92] Evidence supports that corticosteroids may improve symptoms in acute relapse situations.[93] Disease-modifying drugs are used to decrease the number of relapses, prevent permanent CNS damage, and prevent disability.[94] Evidence supports that in relapsing-remitting multiple sclerosis (RRMS) glatiramer acetate, intravenous (IV) immunoglobulins, and azathioprine or other drug combinations may reduce relapses.[95] Interferon-beta and mitoxantrone may reduce relapses and disease progression but have serious adverse effects.[2] Treatments are in development to prevent demyelination, promote remyelination and repair, and suppress selective B-cell and T-cell function.[96,97]

Symptom management for fatigue, weakness, vertigo, ataxia, tremor, heat intolerance, spasticity, bladder dysfunction, bowel dysfunction, sexual dysfunction, sensory sensations, pain, cognitive difficulties, depression, and psychosocial issues is essential but many treatments are only partially effective, particularly for fatigue and spasticity.[2] Supportive and rehabilitative management is directed toward preventing the complications of immobility, especially pressure sores and infections of the pulmonary and genitourinary systems. Interdisciplinary inpatient rehabilitation may improve function in the short term.[98]

Neurodegenerative Disorders

Amyotrophic Lateral Sclerosis

Amyotrophic lateral sclerosis (ALS) (sporadic motor system disease, sporadic motor neuron disease, motor neuron disease) is a worldwide degenerative disorder diffusely involving lower and upper motor neurons resulting in progressive muscle weakness leading to respiratory failure and death, usually 2 to 5 years from symptom onset.[99,100] There are no racial, ethnic, or socioeconomic boundaries. The prevalence rate is about 1 to 3 cases per 100,000,[101] with 2 deaths per 100,000, and 5000 newly diagnosed cases per year in the United States. The term *amyotrophic* (without muscle nutrition or progressive muscle wasting) refers to the predominant lower motor neuron component of the syndrome. Lateral sclerosis, or scarring of the corticospinal tract in the lateral column of the spinal cord, refers to the upper motor neuron component of the syndrome. ALS differs from other motor neuron disorders in that upper and lower motor neurons are involved.

Classic ALS (Lou Gehrig disease) may begin at any time from the fourth decade of life; its peak occurrence is in the early 50s. Male/female ratio is 1:4 to 2:5,[100] equalizing after menopause. In familial ALS, mutations have been found in the superoxide dismutase *(SOD1)* gene on chromosome 21.[102] The defective *SOD1* gene leads to an autosomal dominant pattern with age-dependent penetrance and accounts for 15% to 20% of the cases of familial ALS. The *ALS2* gene is mapped to chromosome 2q33 and leads to a rare, recessively inherited ALS associated with deficiency of the gene product alsin and a juvenile form of ALS. The *ALS4* gene (senataxin) is linked to locus 9q34 and produces a rare juvenile form of familial ALS inherited in an autosomal dominant pattern. Several genes also alter the risk of developing sporadic ALS.[103]

ALS presentations include crural ALS, proximal or shoulder girdle ALS, and hemiplegic (Mills) ALS. Of persons with ALS, 20% have a benign form of the disease.

PATHOPHYSIOLOGY The pathogenesis of ALS is not clear. The molecular dysfunction caused by the *SOD1* is under study. Apoptotic factors, abnormal synthesis of filament units, defects in axonal transport, excitotoxicity and glutamate transports, oxidative stress, growth factors, mitochondrial dysfunction, and neuroinflammation are likewise under study for a possible contribution to the pathogenesis.

The principal pathologic feature of ALS is lower and upper motor neuron degeneration. The number of large motor neurons in the spinal cord, brainstem, and cerebral cortex (premotor and motor areas) is reduced, with ongoing degeneration in the remaining motor neurons. The nuclei of cranial nerves III, IV, and VI are not involved. Death of the motor neuron results in axonal degeneration and secondary demyelination with glial proliferation and sclerosis (scarring) along the corticospinal tract. Inclusion bodies containing the protein *ubiquitin* are found in surviving neurons. However, there also is widespread neural degeneration of nonmotor neurons in the spinal cord and motor cortices, as well as in the premotor, sensory, and temporal cortices.[100] Altered astrocytes and microglial functions are suspected to exist.

Lower motor neuron degeneration denervates motor units. Adjacent, still-viable lower motor neurons attempt to compensate by a process of distal intramuscular sprouting, reinnervation, and enlargement of motor units. The initial symptoms of the disease may be related to lower or upper motor neuron dysfunction or both. Fifty percent of persons with ALS present with hand weakness or incoordination, dysarthria, or leg weakness or incoordination.[104]

CLINICAL MANIFESTATIONS Weakness may begin in any or all muscles of the body. Muscle weakness in ALS exhibits the following characteristics:

1. Paresis usually begins in a single muscle group.
2. Corresponding muscle groups are asymmetrically affected in a mottled distribution.
3. Gradual involvement occurs in all striated muscles except extraocular muscles and heart and progresses to paralysis with no remissions.
4. Flaccid and spastic paresis may coexist in a single muscle group; flaccid paresis may mask spasticity, which is usually mild.
5. Urethral and anal sphincter weakness is uncommon.

The lower motor neuron syndrome of flaccid paresis consists of weakness of individual muscles, progressing to paralysis, associated with hypotonia and primary muscle atrophy (i.e., atrophy caused by denervation). Hypotonia is manifested by (1) decreased resistance to passive movement, (2) hypoactive or absent deep tendon reflexes, (3) absent abdominal and cremasteric reflexes, and (4) absent Babinski sign. Primary atrophy is manifested by (1) severe, irreversible muscular wasting; (2) fasciculations; (3) metabolically related changes in the skin and appendages; and (4) specific EMG findings. Fasciculations, along with fibrillations, are prominent features of ALS. Metabolic changes include (1) thinning of the skin, (2) thickening of the nails, (3) loss of body hair, and (4) decreased perspiration.

The upper motor neuron syndrome of spastic paresis consists of weakness of movement patterns, progressing to paralysis, associated with spasticity and, in some cases, atrophy secondary to disuse. Spasticity is manifested by (1) clasp-knife phenomenon, evident with passive movement; (2) hyperactive deep tendon reflexes and clonus with severe spasticity; (3) absent abdominal and cremasteric reflexes; and (4) presence of Babinski sign. The coexistence of a dementia has been demonstrated to be higher than previously thought.

EVALUATION AND TREATMENT The diagnosis of the syndrome is based predominantly on medical history and physical examination.[105] EMG and muscle biopsy verify lower motor neuron degeneration and denervation. Muscle biopsy usually is not needed to confirm the diagnosis. Riluzole (Rilutek), an antiglutamate, is the standard treatment for ALS, decreasing the risk of death by 35%.[100] Treatment is also directed at symptom relief, prevention of complications, maintenance of maximal function, and maintenance of optimal quality of life.[104] Special problems requiring preventive and symptomatic management are communication difficulty caused by dysmasesis and dysphonia, salivation problems with either thick saliva or excessively thin saliva (sialorrhea), and dyspnea caused by diaphragmatic and intercostal weakness. Ventilatory issues become prominent. Supportive and rehabilitation management is directed toward preventing complications of immobility. Psychologic support of the affected individual and the family is extremely important in this disorder.

PERIPHERAL NERVOUS SYSTEM AND NEUROMUSCULAR JUNCTION DISORDERS

Peripheral Nervous System Disorders

Neuropathies

The axons traveling to and from the brainstem and spinal cord neuronal cell bodies may be injured by a multitude of disease processes. Distinct anatomic areas of the axon may be injured or the spinal nerves may be affected at the spinal roots, at the plexus before peripheral nerve formation, or at the peripheral nerves themselves. Cranial nerves do not have roots or plexuses so are affected only within the nerves themselves. Autonomic nerve fibers may be injured as they travel within certain cranial nerves or emerge through the ventral root and plexuses to travel in the peripheral nerves of the body.

Neuropathies can be classified as (1) generalized symmetric polyneuropathies, (2) generalized neuropathies, and (3) focal or multifocal neuropathies. **Generalized symmetric polyneuropathies** are characterized by symmetric involvement of sensory, motor, or autonomic fibers although, with clinical signs, one type of fiber may predominate. Generalized symmetric polyneuropathies further subdivide into **distal axonal polyneuropathy** and **demyelinating polyneuropathy**. Distal axonal polyneuropathy affects peripheral axons and is the generalized peripheral neuropathy commonly seen. The clinical feature of distal axonal polyneuropathy is involvement of the longest nerve of the body, those going to the feet, first. Sensory impairment is greater than motor impairment. Symptoms are burning pain, tingling, and numbness of the feet. Small nerve fiber damage produces decreased pain and temperature sensation, as well as burning, numbness, and tingling. Large nerve fiber injury causes decreased light touch, vibration, and position sense. The two most common causes are diabetes mellitus and alcohol abuse; occasionally, neurotoxic therapeutic agents also are the cause. Within the classification of distal axonal neuropathies is another group of neuropathies called *autonomic neuropathy*.[106] This neuropathy can involve virtually any sympathetic or parasympthetic nerve fiber with impairment of cardiovascular, gastrointestinal, urogenital, thermoregulatory, sudomotor, and pupillomotor autonomic function.[107] Autonomic neuropathies have a progressive course and are usually reversible. The myelin or Schwann cells are affected in demyelinating polyneuropathy, which occurs far less frequently. Weakness is the predominant sign with far less sensory impairment. Acute and chronic inflammatory demyelinating neuropathies comprise this group, of which Guillain-Barré syndrome is the most widely recognized disorder (see p. 636).

Generalized neuropathies affect the cell body of only one type of peripheral neuron. The dorsal root ganglion cell is affected in sensory neuropathies, producing numbness that may begin in a focal or asymmetric distribution or in a distal symmetric pattern. **Sensory neuropathies** are seen in leprosy, some industrial solvent poisonings, some hereditary disorders, and chloramphenicol toxicity. The anterior horn in motor neuropathy is affected, causing weakness that may be symmetric or asymmetric. Motor neuropathies are caused by anterior horn cell disease, such as ALS or paralytic poliomyelitis.

Focal neuropathy or **multifocal neuropathies** affect sensory and motor fibers in one or more nerves as is seen in common compression neuropathies such as carpal tunnel syndrome (median nerve compression), ulnar nerve compression (at the elbow), peroneal nerve compression, or sciatic nerve compression. Focal neuropathies can involve one or more cranial nerves. Plexus injuries and radiculopathies also fall into this category.

PATHOPHYSIOLOGY Although distinct pathophysiologic processes are recognized in a neuropathy, these are not disease specific and may exist simultaneously in any one neuropathy. Wallerian degeneration, in which the axon and myelin distal to the site of axonal interruption degenerate, may be present (see Chapter 14). This type of degeneration is characteristic of a traumatic nerve injury in which the nerve is severed. In demyelinating neuropathies the axon may be spared and only the myelin degenerates. In **axonal degeneration** distal degeneration of the axon occurs first and is followed by degeneration of the myelin and the axis cylinder. Many pathologic processes may give rise to neuropathy, and one or more nerves may be involved.

CLINICAL MANIFESTATIONS When the axons are affected, muscle strength, muscle tone, and muscle bulk also are affected. Whole muscles or groups of muscles are paretic or paralyzed, and the muscles of the feet and legs often are affected first and more severely. These long, large axons are thought to (1) be more vulnerable to injury because of their size and length, (2) have more Schwann cells available to be injured, and (3) exhibit a "dying back" phenomenon caused by difficulty of the nerve cell body in maintaining the terminal portion of the axon. If unchecked, the pathologic process tends to involve the hands and arms because these have the next longest and largest axons.

Tone and the deep tendon reflexes in the affected muscles generally are decreased in a neuropathy. Atrophy is distributed according to the peripheral nerves involved. The degree and distribution of the atrophy probably depend on the extent of the injury. Fasciculation may be present, especially with associated ventral root or motor neuron changes or both, as in Guillain-Barré syndrome, diabetic neuropathy, and porphyric neuropathy. Mild fatigue may be experienced. A few disorders, notably Guillain-Barré syndrome, produce a pattern of paresis and paralysis that involves all limbs, the trunk, and the neck. Peripheral bifacial and other cranial nerve palsies may be seen with a variety of disorders. Tenderness of the nerve trunks and associated sensory alterations help to distinguish neuropathy from amyotrophy. These include paresthesias and dysesthesias as well as decreased or absent primary sensations (e.g., of temperature, touch, light pain, position, or vibration). Ataxia of gait or limb may arise from the loss of position and vibratory sensations (i.e., proprioceptive sensory loss) and may be enhanced by motor weakness.

Reflexes may be altered. Reflex-mediated autonomic nervous system functions, such as sweating and pupillary size, may be affected. Neuropathies associated with autonomic disturbances include diabetes mellitus, alcoholism and related nutritional neuropathies, amyloidosis, porphyria, Guillain-Barré syndrome, Riley-Day syndrome, and familial sensory neuropathy. In many chronic polyneuropathies the feet, hands, and spine become deformed. Metabolic changes may arise secondary to nerve dysfunction.

EVALUATION AND TREATMENT The diagnostic workup to determine the cause of a neuropathy is often extensive. Early diagnosis and treatment before irreversible neuronal cell damage ensues are of paramount importance. Although axonal regrowth and recovery of function may take months, many neuropathies can be reversed. The therapeutic management is directed first at elimination of the cause, if possible. At least the primary disorder, such as diabetes mellitus, should be controlled. Further damage to the axon must be prevented by avoiding (1) trauma from too-early demand for reuse of the nerve, (2) accidents that cause tissue damage, and (3) hypoxia and ischemia or other deprivation of essential substrates.

Guillain-Barré Syndrome

Guillain-Barré syndrome (GBS) (Landry-Guillain-Barré syndrome, idiopathic polyneuritis, acute inflammatory demyelinating polyradiculopathy, acute autoimmune neuropathy) is an acquired acute inflammatory demyelinating or axonal polyneuropathy with four subtypes. The subtypes and their clinical features are presented in Table 17-14. These subtypes occur throughout the world, affect children and adults of both genders and all age groups equally, and occur in all seasons of the year.

The annual incidence rate is 1 to 2 per 100,000 with a 4% to 6% mortality rate, and a 5% to 10% morbidity rate (permanent disabling weakness, imbalance, or sensory loss).

PATHOPHYSIOLOGY GBS is considered to be an autoimmune disease triggered by a preceding bacterial or viral infection. It has been recognized that glycolipids, particularly gangliosides, are immune targets in the subtypes of GBS. Different gangliosides predominate in different locations in peripheral nerves and in different nerve fiber types. Table 17-14 presents the pathology and pathogenesis of the four axonal subtypes of GBS.[108] The muscle innervated by the damaged peripheral nerves undergoes denervation and atrophy. If the cell body survives, regeneration of the peripheral nerve takes place and recovery of function is likely.

If the cell body dies from intense root involvement in the inflammatory-degenerative process, no regeneration is possible. Collateral reinnervation from surviving axons and regenerating axons may take place. In this case, motor recovery is less complete and residual deficits persist.

CLINICAL MANIFESTATIONS Clinical manifestations may vary depending on subtype. Typical first manifestations are numbness, pain, paraesthesias, or weakness in the limbs. Motor signs manifest as an acute or subacute progressive paralysis. Proximal muscles may be involved earlier and more significantly than distal muscles. The paresis/paralysis may be present in an ascending pattern involving limbs, respiratory muscles, and bulbar muscles. Only bulbar muscles may be involved, resulting in dysphagia and dysarthria. Weakness usually plateaus or improves by the fourth week in 90% of cases. After weakness plateaus, strength improves over a period of days to months, with the majority of individuals reaching activity levels similar to their predisease state. If sensory symptoms are present in the subtype they may include paresthesias/dysthesias (tingling, burning, shocklike sensations, particularly in the limbs), pain (throbbing, aching, particularly in the lower back, buttocks and legs), and numbness. Position and vibratory sensations are more affected than superficial sensation. Respiratory muscle weakness leads to the need for ventilatory support in 10% to 30% of individuals. Cranial nerve weakness manifests as facial weakness and bulbar weakness involving chewing, swallowing, and cough. Autonomic dysfunction may manifest as tachycardia or, less frequently, bradycardia; hypotension or hypertension; and loss of or significant increase in sweating in those more severely affected. Persons may undergo a respiratory arrest or cardiovascular collapse.[109] Hyponatremia caused by the syndrome of inappropriate antidiuretic hormone (SIADH) is common, especially in ventilated individuals.

EVALUATION AND TREATMENT Clinical history helps diagnose GBS and its subtypes. The major diagnostic tests are the examination of the CSF, nerve conduction studies, and EMG. The CSF findings include an unusually high protein level (500 mg/dl) without cellular abnormality. Nerve conduction studies help identify the subtype. Ventilatory support and management of the autonomic nervous system dysfunction are two dominant aspects of the therapeutic management. Plasmapheresis or plasma exchanges within the first 2 weeks of onset of clinical manifestations may be indicated. Intravenous immunoglobulin is used as well as combination therapy. After the disorder begins to remit, aggressive rehabilitation should be instituted.[110]

Radiculopathies

As the spinal roots emerge from or enter the vertebral canal, they may be injured or damaged by compression, infection, inflammation, ischemia, or direct trauma whereby the roots are stretched or torn. **Radiculopathies** are disorders of roots of spinal nerves. **Radiculitis (radiculoneuritis)** refers to an inflammatory disorder of the spinal nerve roots. One or more roots may be affected.

Table 17-14   Expanded Classification of Guillain-Barré Syndrome (GBS)

Subtypes	Clinical Features	Pathology	Pathogenesis
Acute inflammatory demyelinating polyneuropathy (AIDP accounts for most cases of GBS)	Ascending paralysis with typically distant start Early sensory symptoms Loss of DTRs	Macrophages invade myelin sheaths and denude axons Lymphocytic inflammation Demyelination Endoneurial edema Some degree of axon loss (all findings most prominent in the spinal roots and nerve terminals) CD4 and CD8 lymphocytes and macrophages are present Complement is deposited on the outermost Schwann cell plasmalemma	T-cell mediated Lymphocytic infiltration into nerves is common Antibody-mediated pathogenesis not yet demonstrated
Acute motor axonal neuropathy (AMAN)	Acute progressive weakness with no sensory impairment	Macrophages invade nodes of Ranvier, leaving the myelin sheath intact (absence of demyelination) Axonal degeneration in ventral root in severe cases Lymphocyte infiltration sparse	Selective antibody-mediated attack on axon (presence of IgG and complement deposits on axolemma along with macrophage recruitment) Likely GM1 antibodies play a direct pathogenic role
Acute motor and sensory axonal neuropathy (AMSAN)	Ascending paralysis Early sensory symptoms	Similar to AMAN Absence of demyelination Evidence of axonal loss in dorsal and ventral roots Lymphocytic infiltration sparse Extensive sensory nerve fiber degeneration	Undetermined
Fisher syndrome (FS) (5% of cases of GBS)	In purist form have ophthalmoparesis, areflexia, and ataxia In atypical FS also have features of AIDP Infections are common triggers for FS (*Campylobacter jejuni* enteritis)	Pathologic features similar to those in AIDP, but are atypical FS Deposition of antiganglioside antibodies Initially cause reversible conduction block followed by axonal degeneration.	Antigodies to ganglioside GQ1b measured in serum in 90% of cases Anti-GQ1b antibodies cross react with other gangliosides (typically GT1a, but in many cases with GD3, GD1b, and GT1b)

Data from: Hughes RA, Cornblath DR: *Lancet* 366(947):1653-1666, 2005; Kuwabara S: *Curr Neurol Neurosci Rep* 7(1):57-62, 2008; Overell JR et al: *Cochrane Database Syst Rev* (1):CD004761, 2007; Yuki N, Koga N: *Curr Opin Neurol* 19(5):451-457, 2007.
DTR, deep tendon reflex; *GM*, ganglioside GM 1; *IgG*, immunoglobulin.

PATHOPHYSIOLOGY Many different pathologic conditions may cause compression, inflammation, or tearing of nerve roots.[111] Roots may be traumatized by a forceful tearing of a nerve, termed *avulsion*, often associated with injuries to the head and shoulders. An acute intervertebral disk prolapse (herniated disk), degenerative spondyloarthropathies, or a benign tumor may compress nerve roots.

Metastatic tumors of the lung, breast, and gastrointestinal tract may produce a carcinomatous meningitis, causing compression and inflammatory changes in nerve roots. Other causes of inflammatory changes in nerve roots are chronic meningitis, neurosyphilis, sarcoidosis, and **inflammatory arachnoiditis** produced by myelography and lumbar punctures.

CLINICAL MANIFESTATIONS The strength, tone, and bulk of the muscles innervated by the involved roots are affected. The pattern and distribution of weakness and atrophy are similar to those of the amyotrophies. Tone and deep tendon reflexes are decreased, but rarely absent, because the involved muscles are usually innervated by two or more spinal roots. Fasciculations often are present, and mild fatigue may be experienced. Because pathologic processes usually affect the ventral as well as the dorsal roots, sensory alterations are common.

Diseases that involve spinal roots typically produce local pain; pain on local percussion; pain and paresthesias in the sensory root distribution (called **radicular pain** and **radicular paresthesia**); increased pain with movement, stretching of the root, and maneuvers that transiently increase CSF pressure; sensory loss in a radicular pattern; and spasms of the muscles surrounding the vertebral column (i.e., paravertebral muscle spasms).

EVALUATION AND TREATMENT Diagnostic measures may include spinal films, nerve conduction studies, EMG, lumbar puncture with CSF examination, myelography, and biopsy of tumor masses. Treatment is directed at the cause of the injury and may take the form of surgery, antibiotics, removal of the injurious agent, steroids, and radiation therapy and chemotherapy. Supportive management may include control of the discomfort, protection from further injury, prevention of complications, and rehabilitation when appropriate.

Plexus Injuries

Plexus injuries involve the nerve plexus distal to the spinal roots but proximal to the formation of the peripheral nerves. Such injuries may be caused by trauma, compression, or infiltration, or they may be iatrogenic, caused by positioning during surgery or by an intramuscular injection. Clinical manifestations include motor weakness, muscle atrophy, and sensory loss in affected areas. Paralysis can occur with complete plexus lesions.

The diagnosis is made on the basis of history and clinical manifestations. Therapeutic treatment is directed at removal of the cause, repair and approximation of nervous tissue, prevention of further injury, control of discomfort, prevention of complications, and rehabilitation when appropriate.

Neuromuscular Junction Disorders

Transmission of the nerve impulse at the neuromuscular junction requires the release of adequate amounts of neurotransmitter from the presynaptic terminals of the axon and effective binding of the released transmitter to the receptors on the membranes of muscle cells (see Figure 14-14). Four neuromuscular junction disorders (NMJD), whose pathogenesis is thought to be autoantibodies, are described: myasthenia gravis, muscle-specific kinase (MuSK) protein antibody-associated myasthenia gravis, Lambert-Eaton myasthenic syndrome, and acquired neuromyotonia. In addition, there are rare **inherited (congenital) myasthenic syndromes** that result from mutations in different key proteins for the acetylcholine receptor, ion channels, and motor end plates at the neuromuscular junction.[112,113] Nutritional deficits, certain drugs (e.g., reserpine or methyldopa [Aldomet]), certain toxins (e.g., botulism); some snake, scorpion, or spider venoms; certain plant extracts; and some insecticides also affect the neuromuscular junction. The most common autoimmune NMJD is myasthenia gravis caused by the binding of autoantibodies to the acetylcholine receptor on the postsynaptic membrane. MuSK antibody-associated myasthenia gravis is also postsynaptic and is a severe form of the disease.[114] Presynaptic autoimmune diseases include **neurotonia** with autoantibodies to the potassium channels and **Lambert-Eaton myasthenic syndrome** with autoantibodies to calcium channels (Figure 17-40 and Table 17-15).

Marked weakness results from interference with neuromuscular transmission. The distribution of affected muscles is mainly in the bulbar, respiratory, and proximal muscle groups. Botulism toxin has a predilection for the cranial nerves. Lambert-Eaton syndrome affects limb musculature, whereas myasthenia gravis predominantly involves ocular, bulbar, and proximal upper extremity muscles. There is marked fatigability. Muscle tone may be slightly reduced, as may deep tendon reflexes, but the muscle cells are not denervated. Atrophy, if present, is only mild, probably because the small motor system is intact so that tone is maintained to a large degree. Fasciculations or sensory alterations are not present.

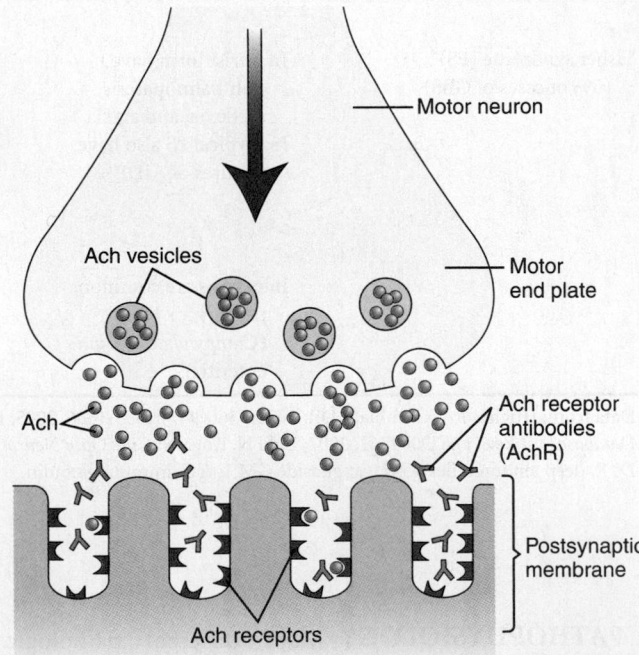

Figure 17-40 Antibodies and myasthenia gravis. Acetylcholine receptor antibodies block the acetylcholine receptor and inhibit the stimulating effect of acetylcholine on the postsynaptic membrane. *AChR,* Acetylcholine receptor. (Data from Juel VC, Massey JM: *Orphanet J Rare Dis* 2:44, 2007; Mahadeva B, Phillips LH 2nd, Juel VC: *Semin Neurol* 28[2]:212-227, 2008; Shigemoto K: *Acta Myol* 26[3]:185-191, 2007.)

Table 17-15   Antibodies and Mechanisms of Action at Neuromuscular Junction

Features	Myasthenia Gravis (MG)	Muscle-Specific Kinase MG	Lambert-Eaton Myasthenic Syndrome	Neuromyotonia
Target	AChR	MuSK	α1A VGCC	VGKC
Principal subclass of antibody	IgG1, IgG3 (autoantibodies against AChR)	IgG4 (autoantibody against MuSK)	Auto-antibodies not known (possibly IgG4)	IgG4 (autoantibody against K+ channels)
Principal mechanisms of action at NMJ	Complement-mediated destruction of folds (includes loss of AChR and sodium channels), increased turnover, direct block of function	Not clear yet May involve mutations in end-plate protein Dok-7	Increased turnover	Increased turnover
Compensatory mechanisms identified	Increased presynaptic ACh release, increased postsynaptic AChR synthesis	Not clear yet	Involvement of other VGCCs in release process	Probable up-regulation of other VGKCs

Data from Beeson D et al: *Ann N Y Acad Sci* 1132:99-103, 2008; Goodman BE: *Adv Physiol Edu* 32(2):127-135, 2008; Juel VC, Massey JM: *Orphanet J Rare Dis* 2:44, 2007; Vincent A: Myasthenia gravis and myasthenia syndromes. In Gilman S, editor: *Neurobiology of disease*, p 943, Burlington, MA, 2007, Elsevier.
AChR, Acetylcholine receptor; *Ig*, immunoglobulin; *MuSK*, muscle-specific kinase; *NMJ*, neuromuscular junction; *VGCC*, voltage-gated calcium channel; *VGKC*, voltage-gated potassium channel.

Myasthenia Gravis

Myasthenia gravis is a chronic autoimmune disease mediated by acetylcholine receptor (AChR) antibodies that act at the neuromuscular junction; it affects 20,000 to 70,000 people in the United States. The disease is characterized by exertional fatigue and weakness that worsens with activity, improves with rest, and recurs with resumption of activity. Myasthenia gravis is associated with an increased incidence of other autoimmune diseases, including systemic lupus erythematosus, rheumatoid arthritis, polymyositis, and thyrotoxicosis. (Autoimmune mechanisms are discussed in Chapter 8.) Transitory signs of myasthenia gravis are present in 10% to 15% of infants born to mothers with myasthenia gravis. The etiology of myasthenia gravis is unknown. Some persons have genetic susceptibility related to variants in AChR genes, as well as the major histocompatibility genes.

The subtypes of autoimmune myasthenia gravis are generalized AChR, ocular, and neonatal. Generalized AChR myasthenia gravis is further subdivided based on age and thymic pathology into:

1. Young persons, mostly female, with thymic hyperplasia
2. Older adults, both sexes, with normal or involuted thymus glands
3. Persons of both sexes with thymomas

In **neonatal myasthenia,** signs appear in 1 to 3 days after birth and persist for a few days to a few weeks. Myasthenia immunoglobulin is transferred from the mother to the neonate through the placenta. **Ocular myasthenia,** which is more common in males, involves weakness of the eye muscles and eyelids and may include swallowing difficulties and slurred speech as well. **Generalized AChR myasthenia** involves the proximal musculature throughout the body and has several courses: (1) a course with periodic remissions, (2) a slowly

progressive course, (3) a rapidly progressive course, or (4) a fulminating course. Classification by disease severity is:

Grade I: ocular disease
Grade II: generalized mild weakness
Grade IIa: mild weakness
Grade IIb: moderate weakness
Grade III: severe generalized weakness
Grade IV: myasthenic "crisis" with respiratory failure[115]

About 10% to 15% of those with signs and symptoms of myasthenia gravis, often involving severe swallowing and breathing (bulbar) problems, do not have AChR antibodies on testing. Some of these have MuSK antibodies (an IgG4). This is now subtyped as MuSK antibody-associated myasthenia gravis.

PATHOPHYSIOLOGY Myasthenia gravis results from a defect in nerve impulse transmission at the neuromuscular junction. The main defect is the formation of autoantibodies (an IgG antibody) against receptors at the ACh binding site on the postsynaptic membrane. The autoantibodies block the AChR or cause complement-mediated loss of AChRs from the neuromuscular junction (see Figure 17-40).[116] The cause of this autosensitization is not known. Eventually the destruction of receptor sites occurs, and the number of receptors on the plasma membrane is reduced. The destruction of receptor sites causes diminished transmission of nerve impulses across the neuromuscular junction. Muscle depolarization is incomplete or not achieved.

CLINICAL MANIFESTATIONS Myasthenia gravis typically has an insidious onset. Clinical manifestations may first appear during pregnancy, during the postpartum period, or in conjunction with the administration of certain anesthetic agents. The foremost complaint is muscular fatigue and progressive weakness. The individual often complains of fatigue after exercise and has a recent history of recurring upper respiratory tract infections. The muscles of the eyes, face, mouth, throat, and neck usually are affected first. The extraocular (eye) muscles and the levator muscles are most affected. Manifestations include diplopia, ptosis, and ocular palsies.

The muscles of facial expression, mastication, swallowing, and speech are the next most involved. The results are facial droop and an expressionless face; difficulty chewing and swallowing associated with dietary changes and weight loss; drooling; episodes of choking and aspiration; and a nasal, low-volume but high-pitched monotonous speech pattern.

The muscles of the neck, shoulder girdle, and hip flexors are affected less frequently. When these muscles do become involved, however, the person experiences fatigue requiring periods of rest, weakness of the arms and legs that improves with rest, and difficulty in maintaining head position. The respiratory muscles of the diaphragm and chest wall become weak, and ventilation is impaired. Impairment in deep breathing and coughing predisposes the individual to atelectasis and congestion. In the advanced stage of the disease, all the muscles are weak.

Myasthenic crisis occurs when severe muscle weakness causes extreme quadriparesis or quadriplegia, respiratory insufficiency with shortness of breath and a markedly decreased tidal volume and vital capacity, and extreme difficulty in swallowing. The individual in myasthenic crisis is in danger of respiratory arrest. Myasthenic crisis usually occurs 3 to 4 hours after the person takes medication.

Cholinergic crisis may arise secondary to drug overdose (anticholinesterase drug toxicity). The clinical picture resembles that of myasthenic crisis but the weakness occurs 30 to 60 minutes after taking anticholinergic medication. Other symptoms are also present. Intestinal motility increases and is associated with episodes of diarrhea and complaints of cramping; fasciculation, bradycardia, pupillary constriction, increased salivation, and increased sweating are present. These clinical manifestations are caused by the smooth muscle hyperactivity secondary to excessive accumulation of acetylcholine at the neuromuscular junctions and excessive parasympathetic-like activity. As in myasthenic crisis, the individual is in danger of respiratory arrest.

EVALUATION AND TREATMENT The diagnosis of myasthenia gravis is made on the basis of a response to edrophonium chloride (Tensilon), repetitive single-fiber EMG, and detection of AChR and MuSK antibodies. The antibodies are found in 80% of generalized autoimmune myasthenia and 70% of individuals with occular myasthenia. With intravenous administration of Tensilon, immediate improvement in muscle strength usually persists for 5 to 10 minutes The EMG is diagnostic in that the muscle fiber weakens readily. Mediastinal CT and MRI are used to determine whether a thymoma is present. The progression of myasthenia gravis is highly variable. In some individuals it is mild and spontaneously remits. There is usually a series of relapses, with symptom-free intervals ranging from weeks to months. Over time the disease can progress, leading to death. Ocular myasthenia has a very good prognosis.

Treatment of myasthenia gravis is individualized. Anticholinesterase drugs, steroids, immunosuppressant drugs, azathioprine, and cyclosporine are used to treat myasthenia gravis and myasthenic crisis.[115] Plasmapheresis may be lifesaving during myasthenic crisis, before and after thymectomy, and at the start of immunosuppressant therapy. For individuals with cholinergic crisis, treatment is to withhold anticholinergic drugs until blood levels fall out of the toxic range while providing ventilatory support and preventing respiratory complications. Thymectomy is the treatment of choice for a thymoma.[117]

SUMMARY REVIEW

Central Nervous System Disorders

1. MVAs are the major cause of traumatic CNS injury. Traumatic injuries are classified as closed-head trauma (blunt) or open-head trauma (penetrating). Closed-head trauma is the more common type of trauma.

2. Different types of focal brain injury include contusion (bruising of the brain), laceration (tearing of brain tissue), extradural hematoma (accumulation of blood above the dura mater), subdural hematoma (blood between the dura mater and arachnoid membrane), intracerebral hematoma (bleeding into the brain), and open-head trauma.

3. Open-head trauma involves a skull fracture with exposure of the cranial vault to the environment. The types of open-head trauma (compound fracture, perforated fracture) are linear, comminuted, compound, and basilar skull fracture (in the cranial vault or at the base of the skull).

4. DAI results from the effects of head rotation. The brain experiences shearing stresses resulting in axonal damage ranging from concussion to a severe DAI state.

5. Spinal cord injuries occur most often in young men who sustain various kinds of injuries (recreational or travel related) and older adults because of preexisting degenerative vertebral disorders.

6. Spinal cord injury involves damage to vertebral or neural tissues by compressing tissue, pulling or exerting tension on tissue, or shearing tissues so that they slide into one another.

7. Spinal cord injury often causes spinal shock with cessation of all motor, sensory, reflex, and autonomic functions below any transected area. Loss of motor and sensory function depends on the level of injury.

8. Paralysis of the lower half of the body with both legs involved is called paraplegia. Paralysis involving all four extremities is called quadriplegia.

9. Return of spinal neuron excitability occurs slowly. Reflex activity can return in 1 to 2 weeks in most people with acute spinal cord injury. A pattern of flexion reflexes emerges, involving first the toes and then the feet and legs. Eventually reflex voiding and bowel elimination appear, and mass reflex (flexor spasms accompanied by profuse sweating, piloerection, and automatic bladder emptying) may develop.

10. Immobilization of the spine is the immediate intervention for a suggested or confirmed vertebral fracture.

11. The pathologic findings in DDD include disk protrusion, spondylosis, and/or subluxation and degeneration of the vertebrae (spondylolisthesis) and spinal stenosis.

12. Low back pain is pain between the lower rib cage and gluteal muscles and often radiates into the thigh.

13. Low back pain has a high prevalence, affecting 75% to 90% of the population at some time. Sciatica affects about 1% of those with low back pain.

14. Most causes of low back pain are unknown; however, some secondary causes are disk prolapse, tumor, bursitis, synovitis, DDD, osteoporosis, fracture, inflammation, and sprain.

15. Diagnosis of injury to the lower back is made on the basis of physical examination, EMG, myelography, CT, and MRI.

16. Treatment for low back pain includes bed rest, use of analgesics and NSAIDs, exercise, PT, education, and surgery.

17. Herniation of an intervertebral disk is a protrusion of part of the nucleus pulposus. Herniation most commonly affects the lumbosacral disks (L5-S1 and L4-L5). The extruded pulposus compresses the nerve root, causing pain that radiates along the sciatic nerve.

18. Clinical improvement occurs in most cases; only 10% have sufficient pain after 6 weeks to consider surgery. There is little evidence that drug treatments are effective.

19. Cerebrovascular disease is the most frequently occurring neurologic disorder. Any abnormality of the blood vessels of the brain is referred to as a cerebrovascular disease.

20. Cerebrovascular disease is associated with two types of brain abnormalities: (a) ischemia with or without infarction and (b) hemorrhage.

21. The most common clinical manifestation of cerebrovascular disease is a CVA (stroke syndrome).

22. CVAs are classified according to pathophysiology and include global hypoperfusion and thrombotic (arterial occlusions caused by thrombi), embolic (fragments that break from a thrombus outside the brain), hemorrhagic (intracranial hemorrhage), and lacunar strokes.

23. Aspirin, systemic anticoagulation, and thrombolysis improve outcomes with ischemic stroke. Antiplatelet therapy and statins decrease recurrence. Endarterectomy is effective if carotid stenosis is greater than 50%.

24. Intracranial aneurysms result from defects in the vascular wall and are classified on the basis of form and shape. They are commonly asymptomatic, but the signs vary according to the location and size of the aneurysm.

25. In cerebral aneurysms, surgical intervention is the treatment of choice before rupture.

26. An AVM is a tangled mass of dilated blood vessels. Although sometimes present at birth, AVM exhibits a delayed age of onset.

27. Clinical manifestations of AVM range from headache and dementia to seizures and ICH or SAH.

28. A SAH occurs when blood escapes from defective or injured vasculature into the subarachnoid space. When a vessel tears, blood under pressure is pumped into the subarachnoid space. The blood produces an inflammatory reaction in these tissues.

29. Clinical manifestations of a SAH include headache, changes in mental status, transient motor weakness, and numbness and tingling. Vasospasm and delayed cerebral ischemia are serious complications. Treatment of vasospasm includes use of calcium channel blockers to prevent or reverse vasospasm and augmenting cerebral perfusion by volume expansion and hemodilution.

30. Migraine is now viewed as a familial episodic disorder whose marker is headache. Migraine is classified as a headache with and without aura and is precipitated by a triggering event.

31. The clinical phases of a migraine attack are the premonitory phase, the migraine aura, the headache phase, and the recovery phase.

32. Cortical spreading depression is thought to be followed by a compensatory overactivity of the trigeminovascular system of the brain.

33. Cluster headaches occur in episodes several times during a day for a period of days at different times of the year. The pain is unilateral, intense, tearing, and burning. Associated symptoms include ptosis, lacrimation, reddening of the eye, and nausea. The cause of trigeminal activation is unknown. There is sympathetic nervous system underactivity and parasympathetic overactivity. The two forms are acute and chronic.

34. Chronic paroxysmal hemicrania is a cluster headache with more frequent daily attacks; it occurs primarily in women. It responds to treatment with indomethacin.

35. Tension-type headache is the most common type of headache. Both a central mechanism and a peripheral mechanism are associated with the etiology. The headache is bilateral, with the sensation of a tight band around the head. The pain may last for hours or days. There are acute and chronic forms.

Continued

36. Two main types of tumors occur within the cranium: primary and metastatic. Primary tumors are classified as intracerebral or extracerebral. Metastatic tumors can be found inside or outside the brain substance.

37. CNS tumors cause local and generalized manifestations. The effects are varied; local manifestations include seizures, visual disturbances, loss of equilibrium, and cranial nerve dysfunction.

38. The principal treatment for brain tumors is surgical or radiosurgical excision or decompression if total excision is not possible. Chemotherapy and radiation therapy also are used.

39. Spinal cord tumors are classified as intramedullary (within the neural tissues) or extramedullary (outside the spinal cord). Metastatic spinal cord tumors are usually carcinomas, lymphomas, or myelomas.

40. Extramedullary spinal cord tumors produce dysfunction by compression of adjacent tissue, not by direct invasion. Intramedullary spinal cord tumors produce dysfunction by invasion and compression.

41. The onset of clinical manifestations of spinal cord tumors is gradual and progressive, suggesting compression. Specific manifestations depend on the location of the tumor; for example, there may be paresis and spasticity of one leg with thoracic tumors, followed by involvement of the opposite leg.

42. Spinal cord tumors are treated by surgery, radiation therapy, chemotherapy, and hormonal therapy.

43. Infection and inflammation of the CNS can occur by bacteria, viruses, fungi, parasites, and mycobacteria. The resulting infection by bacteria is pus producing, or pyogenic.

44. Meningitis (infection of the meninges) is classified as bacterial, aseptic (nonpurulent), or fungal. Bacterial meningitis is primarily an infection of the pia mater and arachnoid and of the fluid of the subarachnoid space. Aseptic meningitis is believed to be limited to the meninges. Fungal meningitis is a chronic less common type of meningitis.

45. The meningeal vessels become hyperemic, and neutrophils migrate into the subarachnoid space with bacterial meningitis. An inflammatory reaction occurs, and exudation ensues and increases rapidly.

46. The variety of clinical manifestations depends on the type of meningitis and ranges from throbbing headache to neck stiffness and rigidity and decreasing responsiveness. Specific cranial nerve dysfunction is a common occurrence.

47. Bacterial meningitis and fungal meningitis are treated with appropriate antibiotic therapy; aseptic meningitis is treated with antibiotics, antiviral drugs, and steroids.

48. Brain abscesses often originate from infections outside the CNS. Microorganisms gain access to the CNS from adjacent sites or spread along the wall of a vein. A localized inflammatory process develops with exudate formation, thrombosis of vessels, and degenerating leukocytes. After a few days the infection becomes delimited, with a center of pus and a wall of granular tissue.

49. Clinical manifestations of brain abscesses include headache, nuchal rigidity, confusion, drowsiness, and sensory and communication deficits. Treatment includes antibiotic therapy and surgical excision or aspiration.

50. Encephalitis is an acute febrile illness of viral origin with nervous system involvement. The most common encephalitides are caused by arthropod-borne viruses and herpes simplex virus. Meningeal involvement appears in all encephalitides.

51. Clinical manifestations of encephalitis include fever, delirium, confusion, seizures, abnormal and involuntary movement, and increased intracranial pressure.

52. Most encephalitides are treated with an antiviral agent or an immune globulin.

53. The common neurologic complications of AIDS are HIV neuropathy, HIV myelopathy, opportunistic infections, cytomegalovirus infection, parasitic infection, and neoplasms. Pathologically, there may be diffuse CNS involvement, focal pathologic findings, and obstructive hydrocephalus.

54. MS is a relatively common degenerative disorder involving CNS myelin. Immune system dysfunction produces the pathology but there are four different patterns. The demyelination is thought to result from an immunogenetic-viral cause. A previous viral insult to the nervous system in a genetically susceptible individual yields a subsequent abnormal immune response in the CNS.

55. The clinical manifestations of MS involve different types: mixed or generalized, spinal, and cerebellar.

56. There is no cure for MS. Steroid and immune therapy is used to acutely manage relapses or reduce frequency of relapses.

57. ALS is a degenerative disorder diffusely involving lower and upper motor neurons. The pathogenesis of ALS is not fully known; however, lower and upper motor neuron degeneration occurs as well as degeneration of the nonmotor neurons in the cortices and spinal cord.

58. Clinical manifestations of ALS may include weakness in all muscles. Flaccid paresis progressing to paralysis is characteristic of the lower motor neuron syndrome. One treatment is available to alter the time course of the ALS syndrome.

Peripheral Nervous System and Neuromuscular Junction Disorders

1. Neuropathies are the syndromes that result when the peripheral nerves are affected. Axon and myelin degeneration may be present. Neuropathies are classified as generalized symmetric polyneuropathies, generalized neuropathy, and focal or multifocal neuropathies.

2. Therapy for the neuropathies is directed at the primary cause, such as diabetes mellitus. Axonal regrowth and recovery of function may take months, but many neuropathies can be reversed.

3. Guillain-Barré syndrome is an acquired, acute inflammatory demyelinating or axonal disorder caused by a humoral or cell-mediated immunologic response, or both, directed at peripheral nerves. Four subtypes have been identified and clinical manifestations depend on the subtype.

4. Radiculopathies are disorders of the roots of spinal cord nerves. The roots may be compressed, inflamed, or torn. Clinical manifestations include local pain or paresthesias in the sensory root distribution. Treatment may involve surgery, antibiotics, steroids, radiation therapy, and chemotherapy.

5. Autoimmune myasthenia gravis is a disorder of voluntary muscles characterized by muscle weakness and fatigability, and has three subtypes.

6. Myasthenia gravis results from a defect in nerve impulse transmission at the neuromuscular junction. Autoantibodies complement deposits, and membrane attack complex destroys the receptor sites causing decreased transmission of the nerve impulse across the neuromuscular junction.

7. Clinical manifestations of myasthenia gravis include weakness of the muscles of the face and throat and may involve muscles of the diaphragm and chest wall.

8. Treatment of myasthenia gravis involves symptom relief and immunotherapy. The progression of the disease is highly variable; in some individuals it is mild and spontaneously remits.

KEY TERMS

Amyotrophic lateral sclerosis (ALS) (sporadic motor system disease, sporadic motor neuron disease, motor neuron disease), 633
Arteriovenous malformation (AVM), 607
Aseptic meningitis (viral meningitis, nonpurulent meningitis, lymphocytic meningitis), 620
Autonomic hyperreflexia (dysreflexia), 695
Axonal degeneration, 635
Bacterial meningitis, 620
Basilar skull fracture, 584
Blunt (closed, nonmissile) trauma, 583
Brudzinski sign, 609
Capillary telangiectasis, 607
Cavernous angioma (malformation), 607
Cerebral vasospasm (CVS), 608
Cerebrovascular accident (CVA, stroke), 600
Cholinergic crisis, 640
Chronic paroxysmal hemicrania (CPH), 611
Classic ALS (Lou Gehrig disease), 634
Classic cerebral concussion, 590
Cluster headache, 611
Compound fracture, 584
Compressive syndrome (sensorimotor syndrome), 619
Contrecoup injury, 585
Contusion, 585
Coup injury, 585
Degenerative disk disease (DDD), 596
Delayed cerebral ischemia (DCI), 608
Demyelinating polyneuropathy, 635
Diffuse axonal injury (DAI), 588
Diffuse brain injury, 588
Distal axonal polyneuropathy, 635
Embolic stroke, 601
Encephalitis, 625
Ependymoma, 616
Extradural brain abscess, 625
Extradural hematoma, 586
Extradural tumor, 618
Extramedullary tumor, 618
Focal brain injury, 585

Focal neuropathy, 635
Fungal meningitis, 622
Fusiform aneurysm (giant aneurysm), 606
Generalized AChR myasthenia, 639
Generalized neuropathy, 635
Generalized symmetric polyneuropathy, 635
Glioma, 613
Guillain-Barré syndrome (GBS) (Landry-Guillain-Barré syndrome, idiopathic polyneuritis, acute inflammatory polyradiculopathy, acute autoimmune neuropathy), 636
Hemorrhagic stroke (intracranial hemorrhage [ICH]), 601
HIV-associated dementia (HAD) (HIV-associated cognitive dysfunction, HIV encephalopathy, subacute encephalitis, HIV-associated dementia complex, HIV cognitive motor complex, AIDS encephalopathy, AIDS dementia complex, or AIDS-related dementia), 627
HIV myelopathy, 628
HIV neuropathy, 628
Inflammatory arachnoiditis, 637
Inherited (congenital) myasthenic syndrome, 638
Intracerebral hematoma (intraparenchymal hemorrhage), 587
Intradural tumor, 618
Intramedullary spinal cord abscess, 624
Intramedullary tumor, 618
Irritative syndrome (radicular syndrome), 619
Kernig sign, 609
Lacunar stroke (lacunar infarct), 601
Lambert-Eaton myasthenic syndrome, 638
Lyme disease, 629
Mass reflex, 595
Meningioma, 616
Meningitis, 620
Migraine, 609
Mild concussion, 590
Mild diffuse axonal injury, 590

Moderate diffuse axonal injury, 590
Multifocal neuropathy, 635
Multiple sclerosis (MS), 630
Myasthenia gravis, 639
Myasthenic crisis, 640
Mycotic aneurysm, 607
Neonatal myasthenia, 639
Neurogenic shock, 593
Neurotonia, 638
Ocular myasthenia, 639
Oligodendroglioma, 615
Open (penetrating, missile) trauma, 583
Penetrating injury, 584
Plexus injury, 638
Postconcussive syndrome, 590
Radicular pain, 638
Radicular paresthesia, 638
Radiculitis (radiculoneuritis), 636
Radiculopathy, 636
Saccular aneurysm (berry aneurysm), 606
Secondary spinal cord injury, 592
Sensory neuropathy, 635
Severe diffuse axonal injury (DAI), 591
Spinal cord abscess, 624
Spinal shock, 593
Spinal stenosis, 598
Spondylolisthesis, 598
Spondylolysis, 598
Subarachnoid hemorrhage (SAH), 608
Subdural hematoma, 586
Syringomyelic syndrome, 620
Tension-type headache, 611
Thrombotic stroke (cerebral thrombosis), 601
Toxoplasmosis, 629
Transient ischemic attack (TIA), 601
Traumatic (dissecting) aneurysm, 607
Traumatic brain injury (TBI), 583
Tubercular meningitis, 628
Vacuolar myelopathy, 628
Venous angioma, 607

REFERENCES

1. Langlois JT, Rutland W, Thomas KE: Traumatic brain injury in the United States: emergency department visits, hospitalizations, and deaths, Atlanta, 2006, Centers for Injury Prevention and Control.
2. BJM clinical evidence handbook, London, 2007, BJM Publishing Group Ltd.
3. Ivins BJ et al: Traumatic brain injury in U.S. army paratroopers: prevalence and character, J Trauma 55(4):617-621, 2003.
4. Evans RW, Wilberger JE: Traumatic disorders, In Goetz CG, editor: Textbook of clinical neurology, ed 2, Philadelphia, 2003, Saunders, pp 1129-1153.
5. Gallagher CN, Hutchinson PJ, Pickard JD: Neuroimaging in trauma, Curr Opin Neurol 20(4):402-409, 2007.
6. Hartl R et al: Effect of early nutrition on deaths due to severe traumatic brain injury, J Neurosurg 109(1):50-56, 2008.
7. Jordan BD: Genetic influences on outcome following traumatic brain injury, Neurochem Res 32(4-5):905-915, 2007.
8. Spinal Cord Injury Information Network: Facts and figures at a glance, June 2006. Available at www.spinalcord.uab.edu/show.asp?durki=21446. Accessed March 29, 2008.
9. Khastgir J, Drake MJ, Abrams P: Recognition and effective management of autonomic dysreflexia in spinal cord injuries, Expert Opin Pharmacother 8(7):945-956, 2007.
10. Branco F, Cardenas DD, Svircev JN: Spinal cord injury: a comprehensive review, Phys Med Rehabil Clin North Am 18(4):651-679, 2007.
11. Raj PP: Intervertebral disc: anatomy-physiology-pathophysiology-treatment, Pain Pract 8(1):18-44, 2008.
12. Chou R, Huffman LH: Nonpharmacologic therapies for acute and chronic low back pain: a review of the evidence from an American Pain Society/American College of Physicians clinical practice guideline, Ann Intern Med 147(7):492-504, 2007.
13. Modic MT, Ross JS: Lumbar degenerative disk disease, Radiology 245(1):43-61, 2007.

14. Legrand E et al: Sciatica from disk herniation: Medical treatment or surgery? *Joint Bone Spine* 74(6):530-535, 2007.

15. American Heart Association: *Heart disease and stroke statistics: 2009 update*, Dallas, 2009, American Heart Association.

16. American Heart Association: *Heart disease and stroke statistics: 2008 update.*, Dallas, 2008, American Heart Association.

17. Sacco RL et al: Guidelines for prevention of stroke in patients with ischemic stroke or transient ischemic attack, *Stroke* 37:577-617, 2006.

18. Chung CS, Caplan LR: Neurovascular disorders, In Goetz CG, editor: *Textbook of clinical neurology*, ed 2 , Philadelphia, 2003, Saunders.

19. Furie K: Cardioembolism. In Gilman S, editor: *Neurobiology of disease*, Burlington, MA, 2007, Elsevier.

20. Guercini F et al: Cryptogenic stroke: time to determine etiology, *J Thromb Haemost* 6(4):549-554, 2008.

21. Keep RF, Xi G, Hoff JT: Intracerebral hemorrhage and intraventricular hemorrhage-induced brain injury. In Gilman S, editor: *Neurobiology of disease*, Burlington, MA, 2007, Elsevier.

22. Wagner KR: Cerebral ischemic: molecular mechanism and protective therapies, In Gilman S, editor, *Neurobiology of disease*, Burlington, MA, 2007, Elsevier.

23. Foley N, Salter K, Teasell R: Specialized stroke services: a meta-analysis comparing three models of care, *Cerebrovasc Dis* 23(2-3):194-202, 2007.

24. Ovbiagele B: Antiplatelet therapy in management of transient ischemic attack: overview and evidence-based rationale, *J Emerg Med* 34(4):389-396, 2008.

25. Blakeley JO, Llinas RH: Thrombolytic therapy for acute ischemic stroke, *J Neurol Sci* 261(1-2):55-62, 2007.

26. Chcon MR et al: Neuroprotection in cerebral ischemia: emphasis on the SAINT trial, *Curr Cardiol Rep* 10(1):37-42, 2008.

27. Pantaz G et al: Early surgical treatment vs. conservative management for spontaneous supratentorial intracerebral hematomas: a prospective randomized study, *Surg Neurol* 66(5):492-501, 2006.

28. Sudlow C: Preventing further vascular events after a stroke or transient ischaemic attack: an update on medical management, *Pract Neurol* 8(3):141-157, 2008.

29. Roquer J, Campello AR, Gomis M: Sex differences in first-ever acute stroke, *Stroke* 34(7):1581-1585, 2003,

30. Glader EL et al: Sex differences in management and outcome after stroke, a Swedish national perspective, *Stroke* 34(8):1970-1975, 2003.

31. Athyros VG et al: Statins for the prevention of first or recurrent stroke, *Curr Vasc Pharmacol* 6(2):124-133, 2008.

32. Baumann F, Khan N, Yonekawa Y: Patient and aneurysm characteristics in multiple intracranial aneurysms, *Acta Neurochir Suppl* 103:19-28, 2008.

33. Palestrant D, Connolly S Jr: Subarachnoid hemorrhage. In Gilman S, editor: *Neurobiology of disease*, Burlington, MA, 2007, Elsevier.

34. Komotar RJ, Mocco J, Solomon RA: Guidelines for the surgical treatment of unruptured intracranial aneurysms: the first annual J. Lawrence Pool memorial research symposium—controversies in the management of cerebral aneurysms, *Neurosurgery* 62(1):183-193, 2008.

35. Brouillard P, Vikkula M: Genetic causes of vascular malformations, *Hum Mol Genet* 16(Spec No 2):R140-R149, 2007.

36. Topper R et al: Clinical significance of intracranial developmental venous anomalies, *J Neurol Neurosurg Psychiatry* 67(2):234-238, 1999.

37. Matschke J, Lockemann U, Schulz F: Intracranial arteriovenous malformations presenting as sudden unexpected death: a report of 3 cases and review of literature, *Am J Forensic Med Pathol* 28(2):173-176, 2007.

38. Rothoeri RD, Ringel F: Molecular mechanisms of cerebral vasospasm following aneurismal SAH, *Neurol Res* 29(7):636-642, 2007.

39. Edlow JA, Malek AM, Ogilvy CS: Aneurysmal subarachnoid hemorrhage: update for emergency physicians, *J Emerg Med* 34(3):237-251, 2008.

40. Ferrari MD, Goadsby PJ: Migraine as a cerebral ionopathy with abnormal central sensory processing. In Gilman S, editor: *Neurobiology of disease*, Burlington, MA, 2007, Elsevier.

41. Headache Classification Committee of the International Headache Society: The international classification of headache disorders, ed 2, *Cephalagia* 24(1):1-160, 2004.

42. Akerman S, Goadsby PJ: Dopamine and migraine: biology and clinical implications, *Cephalagia* 27(11):1208-1214, 2007.

43. Cutrer FM, Huerter K: Migraine aura, *Neurologist* 13(3):118-125, 2007.

44. O'Neilck: Pain management. In Chisholm-Burns MS, et al, editor: *Pharmacotherapy principles and practices*, New York, 2008, McGraw-Hill.

45. MacGregor EA: Menstural migraine, *Curr Opin Neurol* 21(3):309-315, 2008.

46. Janus TJ, Yung KA: Primary neurological tumors. In Goetz CG, editor: *Textbook of clinical neurology*, ed 2 , Philadelphia, 2003, Saunders.

47. Persson AI et al: Glioma. In Gilman S, editor: *Neurobiology of disease*, Burlington, MA, 2007, Elsevier.

48. Fisher JL et al: Epidemiology of brain tumors, *Neurol Clin* 25(4):867-890, vii, 2007.

49. Sauvageot CM, Kesari S, Stiles CD: Molecular pathogenesis of adult brain tumors and the role of stem cells, *Neurol Clin* 25(4):891-925, 2007.

50. Sanchez-Martin M: Brain tumour stem cells: implications for cancer therapy and regenerative medicine, *Curr Stem Cell Res Ther* 3(3):197-207, 2008.

51. Piccirilli M et al: Extra central nervous system metastases from cerebral glioblastoma multiforme in elderly patients, Clinico-pathological remarks on our series of seven cases and critical review of the literature, *Tumori* 94(1):40-51, 2008.

52. Belda-Iniesta C et al: Molecular biology of malignant gliomas, *Clin Transl Oncol* 8(9):635-641, 2006.

53. Marosi C et al: Meningioma, *Crit Rev Oncol Hematol* 67(2):153-171, 2008.

54. Lamszus K, Hagel C, Westphal M: Meningioma. In Gilman S, editor: *Neurobiology of disease*, Burlington, MA, 2007, Elsevier.

55. Simon M, Bostrom JP, Hartmann C: Molecular genetics of meningiomas: from basic research to potential clinical applications, *Neurosurgery* 60(5):787-798, 2007.

56. Whittle IR et al: Meningiomas, *Lancet* 363(9429):1535-1543, 2004.

57. Rockhill J, Mrugala M, Chamberlain MC: Intracranial meningiomas: an overview of diagnosis and management, *Neurosurg Focus* 23(4):E1, 2007.

58. Ferner RE, O'Doherty MJ: Neurofibroma and schwannoma, *Curr Opin Neurol* 15(6):679-684, 2002.

59. Farrell CJ, Plotkin SR: Genetic causes of brain tumors: neurofibromatosis, tuberous sclerosis, von Hippel-Lindau, and other syndromes, *Neurol Clin* 25(4):924-946, 2007.

60. Piersall MS, Gutmann DH: Neurofibromatosis 1. In Gilman S, editor: *Neurobiology of disease*, Burlington, MA, 2007, Elsevier.

61. Nathoo N et al: Pathobiology of brain metastases, *J Clin Pathol* 58(3):237-242, 2005.

62. Well JR: Central nervous system metastasis, In Gilman S, editor: *Neurobiology of disease*, Burlington, MA, 2007, Elsevier.

63. Benjamin RK, Das A, Hochberg FH: Metastatic neoplasms and paraneoplastic syndrome. In Goetz CG, editor: *Textbook of clinical neurology*, ed2, Philadelphia, 2003, Saunders,

64. Mareel M, Madani I: Tumour-associated host cells participating at invasions and metastasis: targets for therapy? *Acta Chir Belg* 106(6):635-640, 2006,

65. Winson BM, Friedman WA: Linear accelerator sterotactic radiosurgery for metastatic brain tumors: 17 years of experience at the University of Florida, *Neurosurgery* 62(5):1018-1031, 2008.

66. Bleck TP: Bacterial and fungal infections of the nervous system. In Gilman S, editor: *Neurobiology of disease*, Burlington, MA, 2007, Elsevier.

67. Roos KL: Nonviral infections. In Goetz CG, editor: *Textbook of clinical neurology*, ed 2 , Philadelphia, 2003, Saunders.

68. Lee BE, Davies HD: Aseptic meningitis, *Curr Opin Infect Dis* 20(3):272-277, 2007.

69. Bilukha O, Messonnier N, Fischer M: Use of meningococcal vaccines in the United States, *Pediatr Infect Dis J* 26(5):371-376, 2007.

70. Prasad K, Karlupia N: Prevention of bacterial meningitis: an overview of Cochrane systematic reviews, *Respir Med* 101(10):2037-2043, 2007.

71. Roos KL: Viral infections. In Goetz CG, editor: *Textbook of clinical neurology*, ed 2 , Philadelphia, 2003, Saunders.

72. Belman AL, Maleti-Savatic M: Human immunodeficiency virus and acquired immunodeficiency syndrome. In Goetz CG, editor: *Textbook of clinical neurology*, ed 2 , Philadelphia, 2003, Saunders.

73. Anthony IC, Bell JE: The neuropathology of HIV/AIDS, *Int Rev Psychiatry* 20(1):15-24, 2008.

74. Power C, Noorbakhsh F: Central nervous system viral infections: clinical aspect and pathogenic mechanisms. In Gilman S, editor: *Neurobiology of disease*, Burlington, MA, 2007, Elsevier.

75. Hult B et al: Neurobiology of HIV, *Int Rev Psychiatry* 20(1):3-14, 2008.

76. Twydell P, Herrmann DN: Neuropathies associated with infections. In Gilman S, editor: *Neurobiology of disease*, Burlington, MA, 2007, Elsevier.

77. Gonzalez-Duarte A, Cikurel K, Simpson DM: Managing HIV peripheral neuropathy, *Curr HIV/AIDS Rep* 4(3):114-148, 2007.

78. Stadelmann C et al: Cortical pathology in multiple sclerosis, *Curr Opin Neurol* 21(3):229-234, 2008.

79. Calabresi PA: Diagosis and management of multiple sclerosis, *Am Fam Physician* 70(10):1934-1944, 2004.

80. Costello K: *New insights into MS immunotherapy: implications for treatment and long-term outcomes*, New York, 2008, Bioscience Communications.

81. Ebers GC: Environmental factors and multiple sclerosis, *Lancet Neurol* 7(3):268-277, 2008.

82. International Multiple Sclerosis Genetics Consortium et al: Risk alleles for multiple sclerosis identified by a genomewide study, *N Engl J Med* 357(9):851-862, 2007.

83. Zivadinov R, Cox JL: Neuroimaging in multiple sclerosis, *Int Rev Neurobiol* 79:449-474, 2007.

84. Dhib-Jalbut S: Pathogenesis of myelin/oliogodendrocyte damage in multiple sclerosis, *Neurology* 68(22 Suppl 3):S13-S21, 2007.

85. Stadelmann C, Bruck W: Interplay between mechanisms of damage and repair in multiple sclerosis, *J Neurol* 255(Suppl 1):12-18, 2008.

86. Vollmer T: The natural history of relapses in multiple sclerosis, *J Neurol Sci* 256(Suppl 1):S5-S13, 2007.

87. Oh S et al: B-cells and humoral immunity in multiple sclerosis: implications for therapy, *Immunol Res* 40(3):224-234, 2008.

88. Rus H et al: Complement activation in autoimmune demyelination: dual role in neuroinflammation and neuroprotection, *J Neuroimmunol* 180(1-2):9-16, 2006.

89. Prat A, Antel J: Pathogenesis of multiple sclerosis, *Curr Opin Neurol* 18(3):225-230, 2005.

90. Zeis T, Schaeren-Wiemers N: Lame ducks or fierce creatures? The role of oligodendrocytes in multiple sclerosis, *J Mol Neurosci* 35(1):91-100, 2008.

91. Plant GT: Optic neuritis and multiple sclerosis, *Curr Opin Neurol* 21(1):16-21, 2008.

92. Ryan M: Multiple sclerosis. In Chisholm-Burns MA, et al: *Pharmacotherapy principles and practice*, New York, 2008, McGraw-Hill.

93. Froman EM et al: Corticosteroids for multiple sclerosis: I, Application for treating exacerbations, *Neurotherapeutics* 4(4):618-626, 2007.

94. Gold R: Combination therapies in multiple sclerosis, *J Neurol* 255(Suppl 1):51-60, 2008.

95. Stuart WH: Combination therapy for the treatment of multiple sclerosis: challenges and opportunities, *Curr Med Res Opin* 23(6):1199-1208, 2007.

96. DeAngelis T, Lublin F: Multiple sclerosis: new treatment trials and emerging therapeutic targets, *Curr Opin Neurol* 21(3):261-271, 2008.

97. Racke MK: The role of B cells in multiple sclerosis: rationale for B-cell targeted therapies, *Curr Opin Neurol* 21(Suppl 1):S9-S18, 2008.

98. Boissy AR, Cohen JA: Multiple sclerosis symptom management, *Exper Rev Neurother* 7(9):1213-1222, 2007.

99. Pirko I, Noseworthy JH: Demyelinating disorders of the central nervous system. In Goetz CG, editor: *Textbook of clinical neurology*, ed 2, Philadelphia, 2003, Saunders.

100. Maragakis NJ, Rothstein JD: Amyotrophic lateral sclerosis: idiopathic and inherited. In Gilman S, editor: *Neurobiology of disease*, Burlington, MA, 2007, Elsevier.

101. Logroscino G et al: Descriptive epidemiology of amyotrophic lateral sclerosis: new evidence and unsolved issues, *J Neurol Neurosurg Psychiatry* 79(1):6-11, 2008.

102. Valdmanis PN, Rouleau GA: Genetics of familial amyotrophic lateral sclerosis, *Neurology* 70(2):144-152, 2008.

103. Mitchell JD, Borasio GD: Amyotrophic lateral sclerosis, *Lancet* 369(9578):2031-2041, 2007,

104. Siddique N, Sufit R, Siddique T: Degenerative motor, sensory and autonomic disorders. In Goetz CG, editor: *Textbook of clinical neurology*, ed 2 , Philadelphia, 2003, Saunders.

105. Ferguson TA, Elman LB: Clinical presentation and diagnosis of amyotrophic lateral sclerosis, *NeuroRehabil* 22(6):409-416, 2007.

106. Reges T: Gastroparesis, an autonomic neuropathy: recognition, diagnosis and treatment, *AACN News* 21(2):14, 2004.

107. Freeman R: Autonomic peripheral neuropathy, *Neurol Clin* 25(1):277-301, 2007.

108. Teener JW, Albers JW: Acquired inflammatory demyelinating and axonal neuropathies. In Gilman S, editor: *Neurobiology of disease*, Burlington, MA, 2007, Elsevier.

109. Hughes RA, Cornblath DR: Guillain-Barre syndrome, *Lancet* 366(947):1653-1666, 2005.

110. Burns TM: Guillain-Barre syndrome, *Semin Neurol* 28(2):152-167, 2008.

111. Tsao B: The electrodiagnosis of cervical and lumbosacral radiculopathy, *Neurol Clin* 25(2):473-494, 2007.

112. Beeson D et al: Congenital myasthenic syndromes and the formation of the neuromuscular junction, *Ann N Y Acad Sci* 1132:99-103, 2008.

113. Newsome-Davis J: The emerging diversity of neuromuscular junction disorders, *Acta Myol* 26(1):5-10, 2007.

114. Wolfe GI, Oh SJ: Clinical phenotype of muscle-specific tyrosine kinase-antibody-positive myasthenia gravis, *Ann N Y Acad Sci* 1132:71-75, 2008.

115. Bartt R, Shannon KM: Autoimmune and inflammatory disorders. In Goetz CG, editor: *Textbook of clinical neurology*, ed 2, Philadelphia, 2003, Saunders.

116. Vincent A: Myasthenia gravis and myasthenic syndromes. In Gilman S, editor: *Neurobiology of disease*, Burlington, MA, 2007, Elsevier.

117. Juel VC, Massey JM: Myasthenia gravis, *Orphanet J Rare Dis* 2:44, 2007.

NEUROBIOLOGY OF SCHIZOPHRENIA, MOOD DISORDERS, AND ANXIETY DISORDERS

LOREY K. TAKAHASHI

MEDIA RESOURCES

evolve **Evolve Website** (http://evolve.elsevier.com/McCance/)
- Review Questions and Answers
- Animations
- Glossary (with audio pronunciation for selected terms)
- WebLinks

CHAPTER OUTLINE

SCHIZOPHRENIA
Etiology and Pathophysiology
Clinical Manifestations
Treatment
MOOD DISORDERS: DEPRESSION AND BIPOLAR DISORDER
Etiology and Pathophysiology
Clinical Manifestations
Treatment

ANXIETY DISORDERS
Panic Disorder
Generalized Anxiety Disorder
Posttraumatic Stress Disorder
Obsessive-Compulsive Disorder

Mental illnesses are common and have a long history of afflicting humanity. They appear in different cultures and across the socioeconomic spectrum. When mental disorders are left untreated, the consequences can be devastating. This chapter provides an introduction to the neurobiology of schizophrenia, mood disorders, and some anxiety disorders. The etiology and pathophysiology of these major mental illnesses are diverse and complex. Diagnostic criteria are constantly being updated to more precisely diagnose and effectively treat the disorders. Every mental disorder manifests a range of symptoms that vary in intensity for each individual. Symptom variations likely reflect individual differences in neural pathologic brain structures or functions, or both, which affect the options for treatment. To further complicate diagnosis and treatment, comorbid disorders such as depression and anxiety are often present.

Insight into the pathophysiologic basis of mental disorders has been greatly aided by the development of structural and functional neuroimaging techniques that provide a visual and quantitative evaluation of diseased brain

regions. In schizophrenia, neuroanatomic, functional, and neurochemical alterations associated with this debilitating disorder have been uncovered along with a host of candidate genes that confer risk. Similarly, in mood and anxiety disorders, brain scans provide new information on structural and functional abnormalities. Use and overuse, however, of brain scans is a continuing focus of concern and study. Many of the altered brain regions found in those with schizophrenia, mood, and anxiety disorders involve structures implicated in normal cognitive and emotional processes, suggesting that their exaggerated or diminished functions underlie the illness.

Knowledge of the pathophysiology associated with a specific mental illness has guided the development of pharmacologic medications. Although more effective second- and third-generation drugs with fewer side effects are available, many individuals continue to suffer. Future identification and characterization of diseased genes and how they contribute to psychopathology may eventually lead to medications that produce effective relief of symptoms and stop or reverse the neural alterations that produce the disorder.

SCHIZOPHRENIA

Schizophrenia is a serious psychiatric illness that strikes 1% of the world's population. The illness is equally prevalent in males and females and emerges in young adults during the late teens and early 20s, with a slightly earlier onset in males than in females. **Schizophrenia** is the term coined originally by Eugene Bleuler in 1911 to describe a collection of illnesses characterized by thought disorders. According to Bleuler, **thought disorders** reflected a break in reality or splitting of the cognitive from the emotional side of one's personality. A schizophrenic individual may exhibit a feeling of happiness when recollecting a terrible event or emotional indifference when describing a joyful occasion. Today, disorganized thought in schizophrenia is characterized by symptoms including hallucinations, delusions, and cognitive deficits. The impairment of cognitive functions, such as attention, planning, and social skills results in devastating effects on the individual and families. Although treatment of schizophrenia has been improving, the illness remains difficult to treat because of heterogeneity of the schizophrenia phenotype and the inability to identify the specific underlying neuropathology. However, advances in genetics, neurobiology, and neuroimaging provide unprecedented insights that hold promise for the effective treatment of schizophrenia.

Etiology and Pathophysiology

Genetic Predisposition

Genetic epidemiologic studies demonstrate that schizophrenia is a heritable disorder. In monozygotic twins, the concordance rate varies from 30% to 50%. This variability may stem from different diagnostic criteria and methodologic or sampling differences across studies. In dizygotic twins and siblings the concordance rate decreases to 12%, which is still considerably higher than the 1% figure found in the general population.

Nonetheless, schizophrenia is not a simple genetic disorder in which inherited disease alleles generally lead to illness. Schizophrenia likely involves several genes located on different chromosomes and differs from mendelian disorders, in which genes are fully penetrant. That is, in mendelian disorders, individuals with genes for a disease (e.g., Huntington disease) will usually develop the disorder. In contrast, as indicated by the 50% concordance rate in monozygotic twins, the genes for schizophrenia show reduced penetrance, resulting in individuals who may carry the disease genes without manifesting the illness. Further complicating the search for the genes that confer risk of schizophrenia is the variability in biologic and phenotypic traits among individuals who manifest the illness (see What's New? Novel Deletions and Duplications of Genes Controlling Neural Development Contribute to Schizophrenia).

Prenatal and Perinatal Factors

A leading hypothesis for the etiology of schizophrenia suggests that the illness results from neurodevelopmental defects that occur in fetal life. According to this hypothesis, environmental factors interfere with genetically programmed

WHAT'S NEW? Novel Deletions and Duplications of Genes Controlling Neural Development Contribute to Schizophrenia

Schizophrenia is a complex neurodevelopmental disorder that likely involves multiple genes and environmental factors. Researchers have found that genes disrupted by rare structural mutations are more than three times likely to occur in schizophrenic than unaffected individuals. Importantly, the structural mutations that disrupted genes (as opposed to deleting or duplicating entire genes) were found to compromise signaling pathways critical for brain development, including neuronal cell growth, migration, proliferation, differentiation, apoptosis, and synapse formation. Although a structural mutation may be rare, varying collections of rare mutations that alter the genetic regulation of brain development increase the risk of schizophrenia. Detecting rare structural mutations in a gene associated with schizophrenia is an important step in developing appropriate methods to address the alterations in the brain.

Data from Walsh T et al: Rare structural variants disrupt multiple genes in neurodevelopmental pathways in schizophrenia, *Science* 320(5875):539-543, 2008.

neural development, leading to alterations in brain structure and function.[1] An early brain defect may remain silent and not affect the individual until subsequent development requires extensive use of that brain structure.[2] Several early environmental factors have been suggested to increase the risk of developing schizophrenia including viral infection during pregnancy, prenatal nutritional deficiencies, and perinatal complications, such as birth defects and neonatal hypoxia.

Neuroanatomic and Functional Abnormalities

Neuroanatomic Alterations

The use of advanced neuroimaging techniques has provided strong evidence for structural brain abnormalities of individuals with schzophrenia.[3,4] A consistent finding is the enlargement of the lateral and third ventricles and widening of frontocortical fissures and sulci (Figure 18-1). Schizophrenic individuals with cerebral ventricular enlargement often exhibit cognitive impairments and negative symptoms, and respond poorly to treatment. Other imaging studies reveal reductions in the thalamus and temporal lobe (which includes the amygdala, hippocampus, and parahippocampal gyrus) brain areas important in emotional regulation and memory functions.[5] A reduction in thalamus size may disrupt communication between broad regions of the cortex and primary sensory and motor areas. Temporal lobe alterations may be responsible for the production of positive schizophrenic symptoms, such as hallucinations, delusions, thought disorder, and bizarre behavior.

Brain imaging work further reveals progressive loss of cortical gray matter in adolescent individuals with early onset schizophrenia (Figure 18-2). Loss of gray matter was found in temporal lobes, somatosensory and motor cortices, and the dorsolateral prefrontal cortex. Of particular concern is the

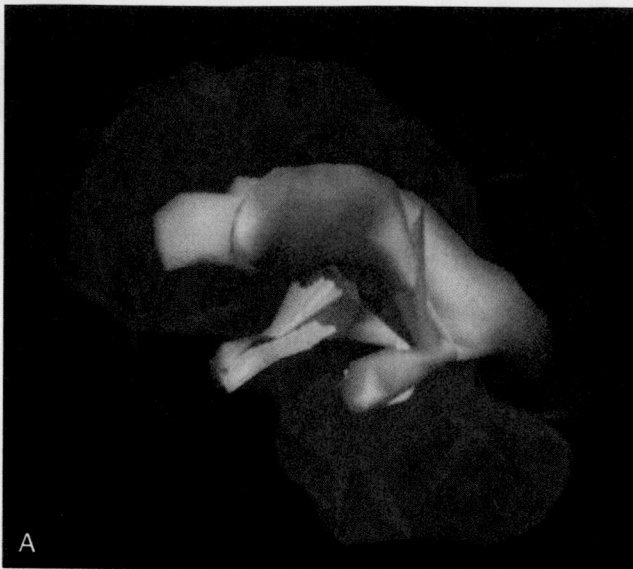

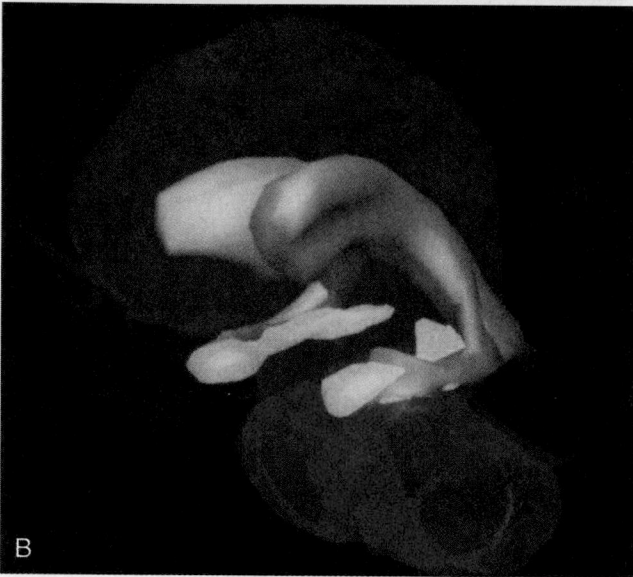

Figure 18-1 Magnetic resonance imaging (MRI) comparison of normal brain and brain with schizophrenia. Three-dimensional MRI reconstructions showing **A**, the cerebroventricles *(gray regions)* and hippocampus *(yellow regions)* of a schizophrenic patient, and **B**, a normal individual. Note enlarged cerebroventricles and reduced hippocampal volume of the brain of the schizophrenic individual. (From Gershon ES, Rieder RO: *Sci Am* 267:128, 1992. Original illustrations by Nancy C. Andreason, University of Iowa.)

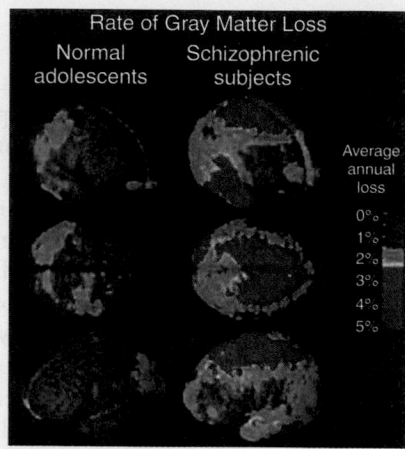

Rate of Gray Matter Loss

Figure 18-2 Accelerated gray matter loss in brains of early onset schizophrenic adolescents. Annual gray matter loss ranging from 2% to 5% was found in 13- to 18-year-old schizophrenics—compared with age-matched healthy—adolescents. (From Thompson PM et al: *Proc Natl Acad Sci U S A* 98:11650, 2001.)

The abnormalities documented in schizophrenic brains are believed to originate during the prenatal period of cell proliferation and migration. Reelin, an extracellular matrix protein involved in neuronal migration during development and synaptic function in the adult, is reduced in the prefrontal cortex and hippocampus of schizophrenic individuals.[7,8] Reelin is concentrated in interneurons that contain **gamma-aminobutyric acid (GABA),** the most widespread inhibitory neurotransmitter in the brain. Furthermore, in the dorsal prefrontal cortex of schizophrenic brains, glutamic acid decarboxylase, the major enzyme in GABA biosynthesis, is diminished, which likely impairs synaptic performance and cognitive and behavioral functions associated with this brain region.

Data suggest that the pathophysiologic processes in the dorsal prefrontal cortex are responsible for the negative symptoms of schizophrenia (Figure 18-3). In particular, the **dorsolateral prefrontal cortex (DLPFC)** is intricately involved in the initiation and maintenance of goal-directed activities and is actively involved in solving cognitive problems related to working memory. **Working memory** involves the brief storage and use of information that may be important in simple number calculations as well as complex tasks such as winning a chess match. Working memory is also essential in verbal comprehension and reasoning. During cognitive problem solving, blood flow and metabolism normally increase in the DLPFC. However, individuals with schizophrenia often perform poorly on these tests and fail to show an increase in cortical blood flow and metabolism. These studies suggest that the dorsal prefrontal cortex is hypoactive in schizophrenia.

Neurotransmitter Alterations

A long-standing neurotransmitter hypothesis of schizophrenia involves dopamine. The **dopamine hypothesis** initially suggested that abnormal elevation in dopaminergic transmission contributes to the onset of schizophrenia. This hypothesis was based on pharmacologic studies showing that

loss of cortical tissue, which is evident by the time the individual seeks treatment and progressively worsens throughout the course of the illness despite the use of antipsychotic medication.[6] In particular, the frontal lobe undergoes a progressive loss in volume that is accompanied by increased severity of negative symptoms and reduced cognitive functioning. These results highlight the progressive nature of the structural brain abnormalities and the ineffectiveness of current treatments in attenuating or reversing the frontal brain alterations present in schizophrenia.

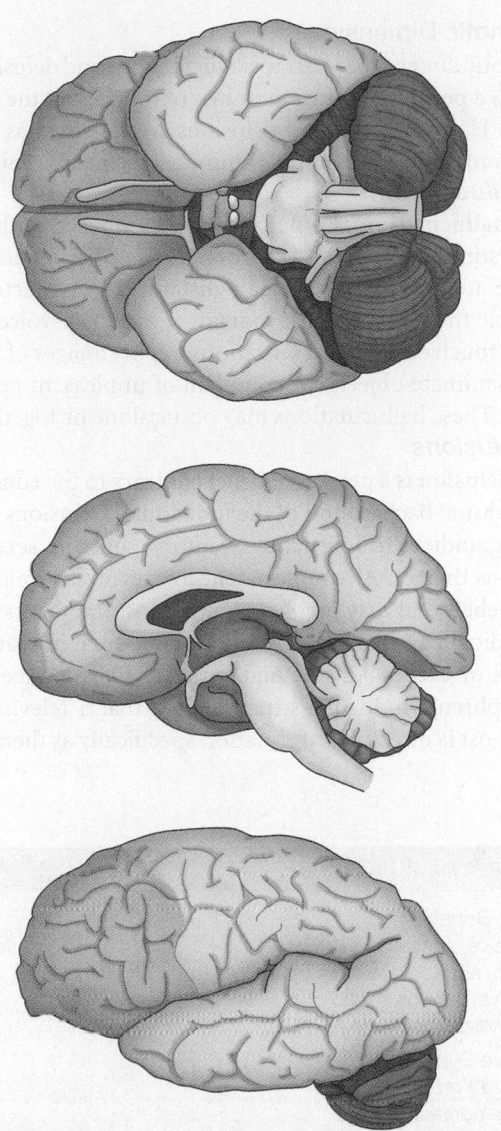

Figure 18-3 The prefrontal cortex. The prefrontal cortex consists of a dorsolateral (*blue*) and an orbitofrontal (*green*) region.

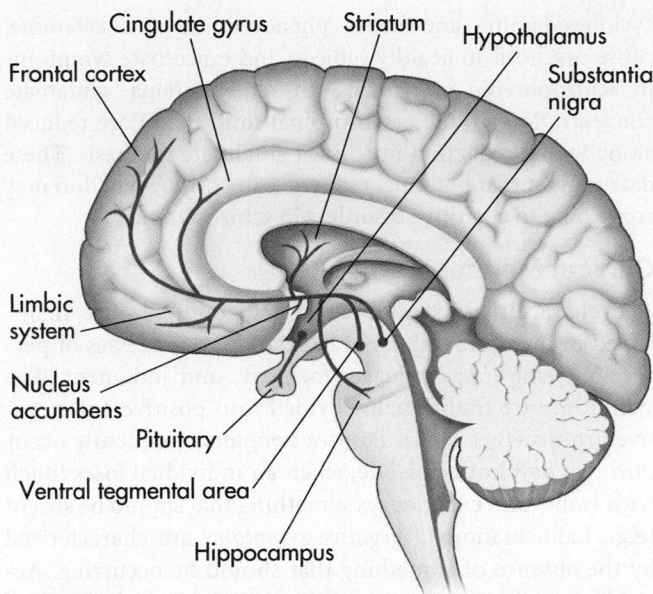

Figure 18-4 The dopamine system. Dopamine cell bodies are located in the substantia nigra, where they project to the stratum (nigrostriatal pathway); and in the ventral tegmental area where they project to the frontal and cingulate cortex (mesocortical pathway), the striatum, the hippocampus, and other limbic structures (mesolimbic pathway). Dopamine nuclei are also located in the hypothalamus and project to the pituitary.

antipsychotic drugs are potent blockers of brain dopamine receptors. A strong positive correlation is found between the clinical potencies of traditional antipsychotic drugs (e.g., chlorpromazine, fluphenazine, and haloperidol) and their affinity for the dopamine D_2 receptor. In addition, drugs that increase dopaminergic transmission—such as levodopa (L-dopa), cocaine, and amphetamine—produce schizophrenic-like psychosis at high doses. Dopamine blockers reverse these drug-induced psychotic states.

A more current view of the dopamine hypothesis of schizophrenia is that brain dopamine pathways are altered in different ways (Figure 18-4). For example, the mesocortical dopamine pathway plays an essential role in dorsal prefrontal cortical functions. Depletion of prefrontal cortical dopamine in monkeys produces deficits in cognition and affect. Some investigators suggest that negative symptoms of schizophrenia result from decreased dopaminergic neurotransmission

in frontocortical regions.[9] This hypodopaminergic transmission in the dorsal prefrontal cortex contrasts with the hypothesized hyperdopaminergic secretion in mesolimbic pathways. The mesolimbic dopamine pathway innervates temporal lobe structures including the hippocampal formation and amygdala, as well as the nucleus accumbens and anterior cingulate cortex. Hypersecretion of mesolimbic dopamine may contribute to the manifestation of positive symptoms.

Of additional relevance to brain dopamine systems and schizophrenia is the potential involvement of a genetic loci at chromosome 22q11.[10] Microdeletion of 22q11 causes velocardiofacial syndrome characterized by cardiac defects, learning impairments, and deformities of the palate and face. In addition, 25% to 30% of individuals with velocardiofacial syndrome exhibit psychotic symptoms. Deletion of 22q11 is also found in 2% of schizophrenic patients, a rate much higher than the 0.025% estimate occurring in the general population. Interestingly, 22q11 contains a gene encoding catechol-O-methyltransferase (COMT), an enzyme that catabolizes dopamine. COMT is normally active in dorsal prefrontal brain regions linked to schizophrenia. Thus deletion of a gene encoding an enzyme involved in dopamine regulation increases the risk of schizophrenia.

Another neurotransmitter system that may be involved in schizophrenia is the excitatory neurotransmitter glutamate and its actions on the N-methyl-D-aspartate (NMDA) receptor subtype.[11] This receptor is implicated in learning and memory, and NMDA antagonists, such as the cyclohexylamine anesthetics phencyclidine and ketamine, cause psychosis in healthy subjects and exacerbate symptoms in schizophrenic individuals. In schizophrenia, glutamate concentrations in the cerebrospinal fluid (CSF) are reduced along with a reduction in cortical glutamate synthesis. These data suggest that potential reduction in NMDA function may contribute to cognitive disorders in schizophrenia.

Clinical Manifestations

The characteristic symptoms of schizophrenia are manifested in the dysfunctions of basic human processes of perception, emotion, language, memory, and judgment. The symptoms are traditionally divided into positive and negative groups (Box 18-1). *Positive symptoms* frequently occur during a **psychotic episode**, when an individual loses touch with reality and experiences something that should be absent (e.g., hallucinations). *Negative symptoms* are characterized by the absence of something that should be occurring. According to the *Diagnostic and Statistical Manual of Mental Disorders (DSM-IV-TR)*,[11] schizophrenia is diagnosed when an individual exhibits delusions, hallucinations, negative symptoms, or social/occupational dysfunctions for at least 6 months.

Psychotic Dimension

Psychotic dimension refers to hallucinations and delusions and reflects a person's confusion or loss of touch with the external world. Hallucinations and delusions are classified as positive symptoms and are the most common in schizophrenia.

Hallucinations

A **hallucination** is a perception experienced without external stimulation of the sense organs. Sensory hallucinations can be auditory, tactile, visual, gustatory, and olfactory. For example the schizophrenic individual may hear voices, experience touch or electrical sensations, report images of animate and inanimate objects, or complain of unpleasant tastes and odors. These hallucinations may occur alone or together.

Delusions

A **delusion** is a persistent belief contrary to the educational and cultural background of the individual. Delusions may involve grandiose, nihilistic, persecutory, somatic, sexual, and religious themes. A common delusion revolves around paranoid beliefs that may involve spying, conspiracy, persecution, and ridicule. Delusions also may be referential in that certain stimuli or events become highly personalized. For example, schizophrenic individuals may believe that a television talk show host is directing information specifically at them.

Box 18-1 Major Symptoms of Schizophrenia

Positive Symptoms
Hallucinations
Auditory
Olfactory
Somatic-tactile
Visual
Voices commenting
Voices conversing

Delusions
Delusions of being controlled
Delusions of mind reading
Delusions of reference
Guilt
Grandiosity
Persecutory
Religious
Somatic
Thought broadcasting
Thought insertion
Thought withdrawal

Positive Formal Thought Disorder
Circumstantiality
Derailment
Distractible speech
Illogicality
Incoherence
Pressure of speech
Tangentiality

Bizarre Behavior
Aggressive, agitated
Clothing, appearance
Repetitive, stereotyped
Social, sexual behavior

Negative Symptoms
Affective Flattening
Affective nonresponsivity
Decreased spontaneous movements
Inappropriate affect
Lack of vocal inflections
Paucity of expressive gestures
Poor eye contact
Unchanging facial expression

Alogia
Blocking
Increase in response latency
Poverty of speech
Poverty of speech content

Anhedonia-Asociality
Few recreational interests
Few social relationships
Impaired intimacy
Little sexual interest

Attention
Social inattentiveness
Inattentiveness during testing

Avolition-Apathy
Impaired personal hygiene
Lack of persistence
Physical anergia

Disorganized Behavior

Disorganized behavior includes disorganized speech and disorganized or bizarre behavior. Incongruity of affect is another dimension of disorganized behavior.

Disorganized Speech

A common form of disorganized speech is **formal thought disorder,** which involves fluent speech that is difficult to comprehend. The speech is often incoherent as the individual moves from one topic to another unexpectedly (loose associations). Answers to questions are illogical or unrelated, and the person becomes easily distracted when talking.

Another form of disorganized speech is called **poverty of content.** In this case, the use of vocabularies to convey information is severely retarded despite a fair amount of spoken words. For instance, the same phrases are used repeatedly throughout a conversation.

Disorganized Behavior

Disorganized (or bizarre) behavior is the conceptual equivalent of disorganized speech. The individual has difficulty engaging in goal-directed activities. Behavior may be repetitive (e.g., stereotyped rocking) or aimless, and personal hygiene is poorly maintained. Another aspect is the incongruity of affect or the manifestation of inappropriate situational affect as exemplified by hostility without provocation or childlike silliness in sober situations.

Negative Dimensions

Negative dimensions reflect a deficit in normal functioning. These symptoms are disabling and include affective flattening, anhedonia, alogia (poverty of speech), and avolition. **Affective flattening** is the near absence of emotional or facial expression. A fixed expression is maintained throughout a conversation or in different situations. In **anhedonia,** individuals are unable to experience emotions such as pleasure or pain and report a sense of detachment from the environment. **Alogia** is the absence of spontaneous speech production for the purpose of answering questions or expressing oneself. **Avolition** is a deficit in spontaneous or goal-directed behavior in which an individual may sit for prolonged periods and must be prodded into completing simple daily tasks.

Treatment

Prior to the early 1950s, there was a steady increase in the number of schizophrenic patients requiring extensive hospitalization in mental institutions. The use of chlorpromazine dramatically changed the treatment of schizophrenia. The drug was especially effective in reducing positive symptoms such as hallucinations and delusions as well as thought disorders and hyperactivity. The widespread use of chlorpromazine and similar drugs such as haloperidol led to a marked reduction in the number of patients requiring hospitalization. These antipsychotic drugs are also known as **neuroleptics** from the Greek term "to clasp the neuron." The beneficial effects of these first-generation neuroleptics on positive symptoms were due to their ability to block the dopamine D_2-receptor subtype, especially in limbic and prefrontal brain regions associated with emotionality. The mesolimbic dopamine pathways are hypothesized to be overly active in schizophrenia, which contributes to the expression of positive symptoms. However, blockade of the D_2 receptor in brain regions such as the striatum also produced a notable neurologic side effect resembling Parkinson disease, a disorder associated with degeneration of dopamine cell bodies in the substantia nigra that projects to the striatum. Other side effects may include sedation, hypotension, akathisia (motor restlessness), constipation, weight gain, amenorrhea, and less frequently, hepatotoxicity and electrocardiographic changes. Although the pharmacologic blockade of D_2 receptors occurs rapidly, clinical efficacy does not appear until after 1 or 2 weeks of treatment. Thus the antipsychotic effects are not related directly to D_2-receptor blockade or acute suppression of dopamine hypersecretion.

Although the majority of schizophrenic individuals obtained some positive symptom relief from the first-generation or conventional antipsychotic drugs, approximately 20% failed to respond to D_2-blocking drugs (Box 18-2). Some of these treatment-resistant individuals responded to a second generation of drugs that became known as atypical antipsychotic drugs.[12] Some studies suggest that atypical antipsychotic drugs have superior efficacy in reducing not only the positive but also the negative symptoms in comparison with conventional neuroleptics. For example, clozapine may improve some cognitive functions, such as verbal fluency, verbal learning, and memory, and physical functions, such as psychomotor speed. In addition, the notable neurologic side effects that accompany the use of the conventional neuroleptics were diminished.

Although the mechanism of action of these drugs is not known, atypical medications clearly differ from conventional antipsychotic drugs in blocking a range of neurotransmitter receptors. For example, clozapine blocks a variety of receptors that include D_2 receptors, as well as D_1, D_3, D_4, and D_5 receptors and serotonin (5-hydroxytryptamine, i.e., HT_2, 5-HT_6,

---

Box 18-2   Medications Used in the Treatment of Schizophrenia

Conventional Antipsychotics
Chlorpromazine
Fluphenazine
Haloperidol
Perphenazine
Thioridazine
Thiothixene
Trifluoperazine

Second-Generation Atypical Antipsychotics
Aripiprazole
Clozapine
Olanzapine
Quetiapine
Risperidone
Ziprasidone

5-HT$_7$); norepinephrine; cholinergic, and histamine receptors. Risperidone and ziprasidone have higher affinity for blocking 5-HT$_2$ than D$_2$ receptors. The higher 5-HT$_2$:D$_2$-receptor–binding ratio of atypical antipsychotics in comparison with conventional neuroleptics may reflect a normalization of serotonin-dopamine interactions leading to clinical efficacy not observed with D$_2$-receptor blockade alone.

Atypical antipsychotics are not without adverse effects, most notably metabolic abnormalities including glucose regulation, lipids, and weight gain. Weight gain is a risk factor for diabetes and cardiovascular disease in schizophrenics who are maintained particularly on long-term clozapine or olanzapine treatment.

In conjunction with antipsychotic medication, psychosocial therapy can facilitate the management of schizophrenia. Psychosocial relationships may assist the individual in developing coping strategies and in identifying stressors and relapse symptoms. The addition of cognitive-behavioral therapy (CBT) may alleviate some of the schizophrenic symptoms resistant to medication.[13] An important benefit of psychosocial and family support is the encouragement of compliance with antipsychotic medication that requires a period before the emergence of clinical efficacy.

MOOD DISORDERS: DEPRESSION AND BIPOLAR DISORDER

Mood refers to a sustained emotional state as opposed to brief emotional feelings, which are termed *affective states.* Healthy individuals are normally capable of experiencing a variety of affective states including euphoria, joy, surprise, fear, sadness, anxiety, and depression. When emotional states, such as sadness, become predominant and uncontrollable, individuals may be diagnosed with a mood disorder called *depression.* The two major classifications of mood disorder are (1) unipolar or major depressive disorder, also known as *major depression* or *clinical depression,* which consists of episodes of depression; and (2) **bipolar disorder**, also known as *manic-depressive illness,* which is further classified into bipolar I and bipolar II disorders. Bipolar I disorder features manic episodes and at least one major depressive episode and bipolar II disorder is characterized by recurrent major depressive episodes with one or more hypomanic (milder than manic) episodes. Box 18-3 presents the major criteria of depression and bipolar disorder according to the American Psychiatric Association's *DSM-IV-TR.*[11]

Major (unipolar) depression is the most common mood disorder and the leading cause of disability in the United States and throughout the world. Unipolar depression appears in all age groups including young children. In the United States, the lifetime prevalence rate of depression is 16.2% of the population with a twofold greater risk in women than men after adolescence. In children and adolescents, 2% to 6% suffer from depression. The prevalence of bipolar disorder ranges from 3% to 5% in the general population. Bipolar I disorder occurs equally in men and women in comparison with bipolar

II disorder, which afflicts more women than men. When left untreated, a number of depressed and bipolar individuals are at risk of developing a host of medical illnesses, including cardiovascular disease, obesity, diabetes, and thyroid disease.

Etiology and Pathophysiology

Genetic Predisposition and Environmental Influences
Results from family and twin studies indicate a strong basis for mood disorders. A study using the Danish twin registry for bipolar disorder yielded concordance rates of 79% and 24% for monozygotic and dizygotic twins, respectively. For unipolar disorder, concordance rates of 54% and 19% have been reported in monozygotic and dizygotic twins, respectively. Even among adoptees with a biologic family history of mood disorders, the incidence of developing major depression or manic-depressive illness is higher than among control adoptees. The strong tendency for mood disorders to run in families has encouraged a search for the abnormal gene or genes. Interestingly, loci on chromosomes 18 and 22 have been linked to both bipolar disorder and schizophrenia. Bipolar individuals, who may exhibit psychotic behavior, have deficits in reelin expression linked to genetic loci, located on chromosome 22, which confers susceptibility to schizophrenia (see section on schizophrenia). However, the large variation in clinical symptoms suggests that developmental and environmental factors are as important as genetic factors in contributing to the etiology of mood disorders.

Box 18-3	Major Symptoms of Depression and Mania

Symptoms of Depression*
Depressed or irritable mood
Loss of interests and pleasure
Significant (>5%) weight gain or loss in a month
Insomnia or hypersomnia
Psychomotor agitation or retardation
Fatigue or loss of energy
Feelings of worthlessness or excessive guilt
Poor concentration or indecisiveness
Recent thoughts of death or suicide

Symptoms of Manic Episode†
Elevated mood
Irritable mood
Inflated self-esteem
Decreased need for sleep
Excessive talking
Racing/crowded thoughts
Distractibility
Increase in goal-directed activity
Excessive risky activities

---

*Five or more of symptoms are present in a 2-week period and at least one of the symptoms is either depressed mood or loss of interests or pleasure.
†Three or more symptoms (four if the mood is only irritable) during a distinct period of abnormally and persistently elevated, expansive, or irritable mood occurring for at least 1 week.

A current view of mood disorders is that the illness stems from a complex interplay between susceptible genes and environmental influences. For example, the interplay between life stressors and a potentially dysfunctional serotonin (5-HT) system appears to elevate the risk of depression.[14] In particular, researchers have identified a polymorphic variant of the serotonin transporter (5-HT-T) that exists either as a short *(s)* allele or long *(l)* allele. The serotonin transporter serves in the reuptake of serotonin at the synapse and may moderate the serotonergic response to stress. However, individuals with one or two copies of the *s* allele were more likely to develop major depression and have suicidal thoughts in response to stressful events than individuals homozygous for the *l* allele. In addition, among individuals who carry two s alleles, the risk of a major depressive episode increased twofold after experiencing four or more stressful events. This work[14] has implications for a gene-by-environment interaction underlying major depression by showing that adverse life events and a genetic alteration in 5-HT function increase the risk of a major depressive episode.

Neurochemical Dysregulation

Modern theories of the pathophysiology of mood disorders began with the important observation that imipramine reduced the reuptake of norepinephrine into presynaptic neurons, and the resultant increase in norepinephrine within the synapse was then responsible for antidepressant effects. This key finding, along with other studies work showing that drugs (e.g., reserpine) that deplete monoamines produce depression, led to the dominant **monoamine hypothesis of depression**. Accordingly, depression occurs following a deficit in brain norepinephrine, dopamine, and/or serotonin, whereas mania results from elevated concentrations of monoamines. The three major classes of antidepressant medications include monoamine oxidase inhibitors (MAOIs), tricyclic antidepressants (TCAs), and selective serotonin reuptake inhibitors (SSRIs). All available antidepressants share the common property, albeit through different mechanisms, that increasing monoamine neurotransmitter levels within the synapse is the basis for their antidepressant effects (Figure 18-5).

Further support for the monoamine hypothesis of depression came from examination of the major metabolites of norepinephrine (3-methoxy-4-hydroxyphenylglycol [MHPG]), dopamine (homovanillic acid [HVA]), and serotonin (5-hydroxyindoleacetic acid [5-HIAA]), in depressed individuals. The major metabolites of these monoamines were reduced in the CSF of depressed individuals. Other work demonstrated that dietary depletion of tryptophan, the precursor of serotonin synthesis, or alpha-methylparatyrosine (AMPT), a drug that inhibits dopamine and norepinephrine synthesis, produced a rapid return to depression in individuals who had been treated successfully with antidepressants.[15]

Although TCAs and SSRIs rapidly block synaptic reuptake of monoamines, resulting in elevations in synaptic monoamine concentrations, the onset of clinical efficacy requires several weeks or months of treatment. Antidepressant treatment appears to produce the delayed clinical effects through alterations in receptor-mediated functions. For example, the cyclic adenosine monophosphate (cAMP) signal transduction pathway is regulated by direct coupling of monoamine receptors to adenylyl cyclase or indirectly through other second messenger pathways. Antidepressants increase adenylyl cyclase leading to subsequent augmentation in cAMP signal transduction, phosphorylation of intracellular proteins and transcription factors, and genomic effects that may underlie the therapeutic actions of antidepressant drugs. Similarly, the mode of action of mood stabilizers for bipolar disorders appears to be mediated by altering postsynaptic signal transduction pathways. For example, the clinical effects of the mood stabilizer lithium result from an inhibition of the overactive phosphatidylinositol pathway (see Chapter 1).

Neuroendocrine Dysregulation
Hypothalamic-Pituitary-Adrenal System Dysregulation

The hypothalamic-pituitary-adrenal (HPA) system plays an essential role in an individual's ability to cope with stress (see Chapter 10). However, excessive activation of the HPA system resulting in elevated glucocorticoid secretion is found in a large percentage (30% to 70%) of people with major depression suggesting that mechanisms responsible for HPA hormone alterations contribute to the pathophysiology of depression.[16] Research has focused on inflammation, proinflammatory cytokines, and depression (see What's New? Does Inflammation Contribute to the Development of Depression?). Altered HPA function can be demonstrated in the dexamethasone suppression test.

WHAT'S NEW?   **Does Inflammation Contribute to the Development of Depression?**

Increasing evidence suggests that inflammation may be an important factor in the pathophysiology of depression. In medical illnesses, such as cardiovascular disease or cancer, markers of inflammation are often associated with symptoms of major depression. For example, inflammation is a significant contributor to coronary heart disease; the prevalence of comorbid depression in people with coronary heart disease is threefold higher than in the general population. Nonetheless, even among otherwise healthy individuals, exposure to pathogens or infections may increase the risk of developing depression.

Research shows that through systemic infection, activation of the immune system increases proinflammatory cytokines, such as interleukin (IL)-1α and IL-β, tumor necrosis factor-alpha (TNF-α), and IL-6. These cytokines produced in the periphery serve to regulate the inflammatory response to pathogens. However, proinflammatory cytokines will also enter the brain and modulate a widespread brain cytokine system consisting of neurons and glial cells with cytokine receptors involved in altering brain function. A major effect of cytokines on the brain is the induction of symptoms of sickness, such as loss of appetite, malaise, and avoidance of social interactions. Many of the symptoms of sickness overlap with key features of depression (e.g., fatigue, reduced appetite, altered mood and cognition). However, whereas sickness

Continued

behavior may be reversible by the efficacy of the immune system to clear the body of infectious pathogens, clinical depression can still develop in vulnerable individuals exposed to prolonged or intense inflammation (see Chapter 6).

The emerging recognition of a relationship between inflammation and depression is not limited to inflammation from peripheral infections. Uncontrolled stress is a well-known risk factor in depression, and research shows that psychosocial stress is capable of activating proinflammatory cytokines and their signaling pathways throughout the periphery and brain. In addition, activation of cytokines stimulates secretion of hypothalamic-pituitary-adrenal (HPA) hormones and nerve terminals of the sympathetic nervous system. One potential outcome of cytokine-induced activation is a dysregulation in feedback and feed-forward control mechanisms of the stress hormone–secreting system. The deleterious result of HPA dysregulation is persistent elevation in cortisol, as observed in depression, in conjunction with increased responsiveness to stress and production of proinflammatory cytokines, which in turn may compromise the body's immune systems to contain infectious diseases. Cytokine actions in the brain also are associated with alterations in monoamine metabolism of serotonin, norepinephrine, and dopamine, which may further contribute to the pathophysiology of depression.

The potential link between inflammation and depression offers novel insights into the mechanism of drug action in the treatment of depression. Studies report that available antidepressants effective in treating depressive symptoms also reduce activation of proinflammatory cytokines. In contrast, depressed individuals nonresponsive to antidepressant treatments continue to exhibit cytokine production such as IL-6. These observations raise exciting possibilities that cytokine antagonists or anti-inflammatory cytokines used in the treatment of inflammation may have the added benefit of ameliorating depressive symptoms. Some support for the use of anti-inflammatory drugs to treat depression is obtained using etanercept, the available TNF-α–blocking drug, administered to individuals with psoriasis. The development of drugs that target inflammation diminish stress-induced activation of the HPA system, or alter cytokine activation and signaling pathways through monoaminergic systems may yield a new class of therapeutic medications that inhibit inflammation and the development of depression.

Data from Dantzer R et al: *Nat Rev Neurosci* 9(1):46-56, review, 2008; Irwin MR, Miller AH: *Brain Behav Immun* 21(4):374-383, 2007.

Administration of dexamethasone, a potent synthetic glucocorticoid, normally suppresses adrenal cortisol secretion because of its negative-feedback effects on the HPA system. Individuals with depression, however, fail to suppress cortisol secretion after dexamethasone administration. In addition, whereas healthy individuals typically exhibit a diurnal rise in cortisol secretion at the onset of wakefulness followed by a trough 12 hours later, depressed people continue to exhibit elevated plasma cortisol levels throughout the evening and early morning hours. Notably, antidepressant drugs effective in normalizing the HPA system are associated with a good clinical response, whereas persistent HPA system dysregulation, as evidenced in the dexamethasone suppression test, is related to continued depression or relapse.

Hypothalamic-Pituitary-Thyroid System Dysregulation

Thyroid hormones are involved in the modulation of mood and behavior. Approximately 20% to 30% of persons with unipolar depression have an altered hypothalamic-pituitary-thyroid (HPT) system. These individuals exhibit increased CSF levels of thyrotropin-releasing hormone (TRH), blunted thyrotropin-stimulating hormone (TSH) response to TRH challenge, and decreased nocturnal rise in TSH that normally occurs between midnight and the early morning hours.[17] Persistent blunting of the TSH response to TRH is associated with an increased probability of relapse. Abnormalities in thyroid function, such as increased basal TSH concentrations with normal thyroxine levels, also are observed in bipolar disorder, especially among individuals with rapid cycling.

Neuroanatomic and Functional Abnormalities

The dorsal and median raphe nuclei, located in the central gray of the caudal mesencephalon and rostral pons, contain a large group of serotonin-synthesizing neurons that project extensively to all regions of the cortex, basal ganglia, limbic system, hypothalamus, cerebellum, and brainstem (Figure 18-6). Postmortem and/or brain imaging studies of depressed individuals revealed a widespread decrease in serotonin 5-HT$_{1A}$ receptor subtype binding in frontal, temporal, and limbic cortex as well as serotonin transporter binding in cerebral cortex and hippocampus. Mood disorders may reflect a dysfunctional raphe-serotonin system, which normally modulates homeostasis, emotionality, and tolerance to aversive experiences.

A group of norepinephrine-containing cells located in the locus ceruleus of the rostral pons project to vast areas of the forebrain, brainstem, and spinal cord (Figure 18-7). The locus ceruleus-norepinephrine system is implicated in global psychologic processes including attention, vigilance, and orientation to novel, aversive, or threatening stimuli. Activation of the locus ceruleus-norepinephrine system is also capable of inhibiting the raphe-serotonin system, suggesting an indirect role in modulating serotonin functions. Norepinephrine receptor alterations (e.g., α- and β-adrenergic receptor subtypes) are found in the frontal cortex of some suicide victims with major depression. Alterations in norepinephrine systems may be linked to attention or concentration difficulties as well as sleep and arousal disturbances in depression.

Postmortem and brain imaging studies further reveal structural and functional abnormalities associated with mood disorders, especially in frontal and limbic regions such as the amygdala.[18,19] Postmortem studies report a reduction in glial cell numbers in people with unipolar and bipolar disorders. There are also reports of reduced frontal lobe volume in depressed individuals and decreased or asymmetric temporal lobe volume in bipolar illness and depression. One study reported an increased volume of the amygdala in bipolar illness.

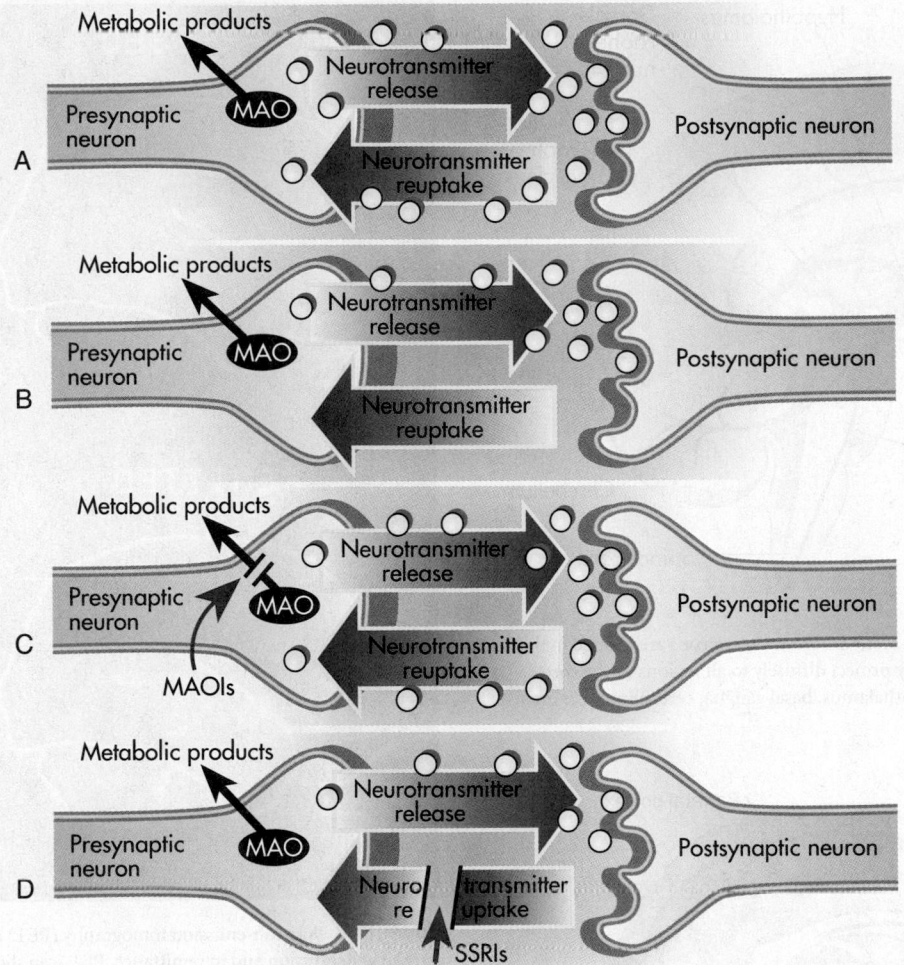

Figure 18-5 Schematic diagrams showing the sites of actions of antidepressants and their effects on neurotransmitter levels. **A,** In normal individuals an action potential generated in the presynaptic neuron results in neurotransmitter release into the synapse. Some neurotransmitters bind to receptors on the postsynaptic neuron that leads to activation of second messenger systems (not shown). Neurotransmitters are also removed from the synapse by reuptake into the presynaptic neuron and deaminated by monoamine oxidase (MAO). **B,** In depressed individuals, neurotransmitter levels are hypothesized to be reduced. The mechanisms responsible for this reduction are not understood. **C,** MAO inhibitors act by preventing the degradation of neurotransmitters, such as norepinephrine and serotonin. As a result, neurotransmitter levels are elevated. **D,** The tricyclic antidepressants (TCAs) and selective serotonin reuptake inhibitors (SSRIs) act by reducing the uptake of neurotransmitters from the synapse, leading to increased neurotransmitter levels. TCAs, such as nortriptyline and desipramine, tend to block norepinephrine reuptake, whereas amitriptyline and imipramine also have effects on serotonin reuptake. SSRIs are highly effective in blocking serotonin reuptake.

In some cases, specific brain abnormalities are associated with a subtype of depression. For instance, enlarged lateral ventricles are found more often in late onset or depressed older adults than in midlife depressed individuals, depressed older adults with an early age of illness, or bipolar individuals.

Functional neuroimaging studies indicate decreased cerebral blood flow and glucose metabolism in the dorsolateral and dorsomedial prefrontal cortex of major and bipolar individuals. Dorsolateral abnormalities in depression may be responsible for the retardation in cognitive processing and speech deficits similar to those found in schizophrenia. Dorsomedial frontal dysfunction may be associated with mnemonic and attentional impairments that accompany mood disorders. Other frontocortical regions, including the ventrolateral, ventromedial, and orbital areas, exhibit increased blood flow and

metabolism in unipolar depression (Figure 18-8). These frontal brain areas have extensive interconnections with the amygdala, and increased blood flow and metabolism, especially in the right amygdala, is positively related to negative affect in depressed individuals. These functional changes in brain activity begin to normalize with successful antidepressant treatments, suggesting they are state rather than trait related.

Clinical Manifestations

Depression

Major **depression** is characterized by unremitting feelings of sadness and despair (see Box 18-3). The **dysphoric mood** or intensely painful mood is accompanied frequently by insomnia, loss of appetite and body weight, and reduced interest in pleasurable activities and interpersonal relationships. Sleep

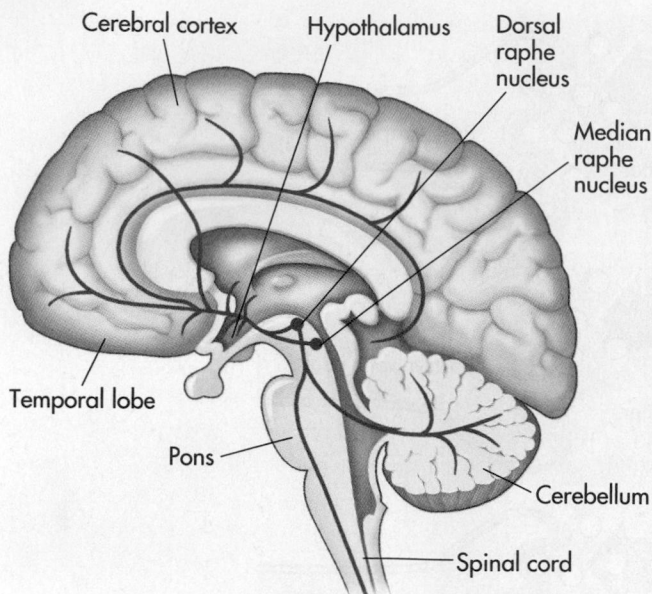

Figure 18-6 The serotonin system. Serotonin neurons are located in the brain stem raphe nuclei. They project diffusely to all regions of the cortex, temporolimbic regions, hypothalamus, basal ganglia, cerebellum, the brainstem, and spinal cord.

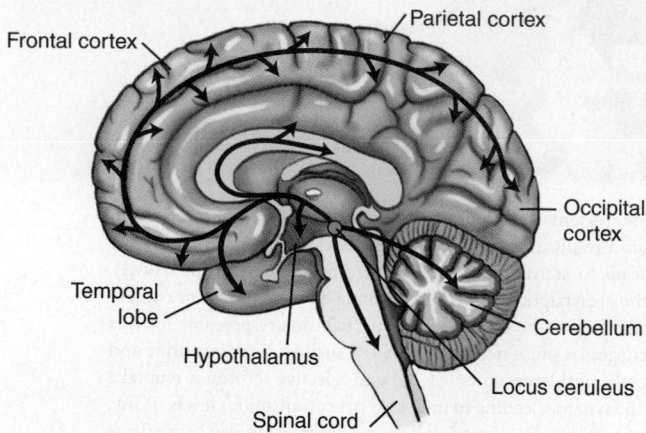

Figure 18-7 The norepinephrine system. The norepinephrine cell bodies originate in the locus ceruleus and project throughout the brain, including the hypothalamus, the temporal lobe, the entire cortex, the cerebellum, and spinal cord.

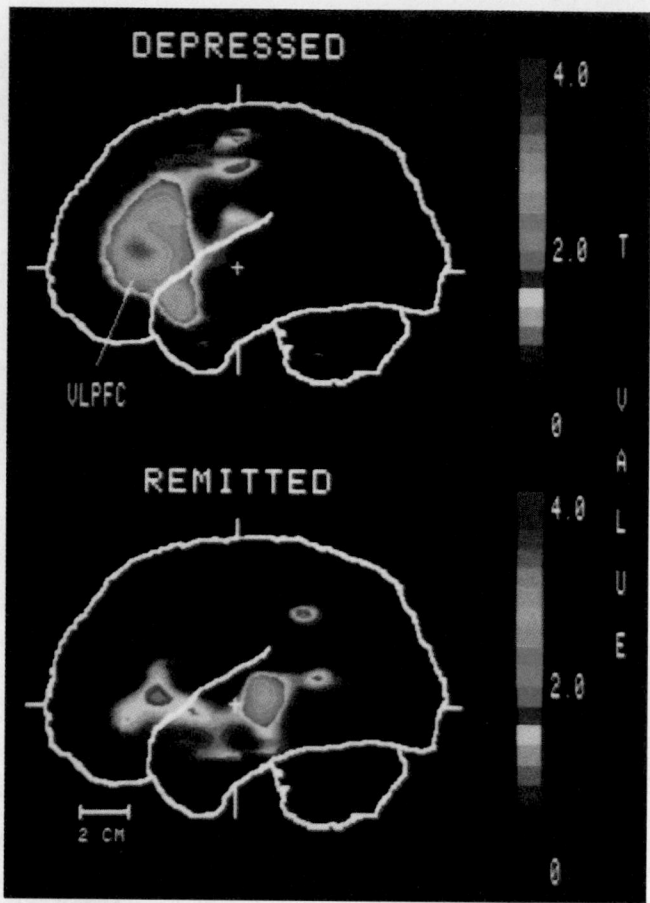

Figure 18-8 Positron-emission tomography (PET) comparison of brain activity in depression and in remittance. PET scan showing increased activity in the left prefrontal cortex in a depressed person but not in the remitted person. *VLPFC, Ventrolateral prefrontal cortex.* (From Drevets WC et al: *J Neurosci* 12:3628, 1992. Copyright ©1992 by the Society for Neuroscience.)

disturbances may include difficulty in initially falling asleep, awakening in the middle of the night and lying awake for several hours, and early morning wakefulness with an inability to subsequently fall asleep. Individuals may have reduced motor activity and suffer marked fatigue. Others complain of restlessness and agitation. Feelings of worthlessness and guilt are common, and pessimistic or negative outcomes are often perceived even in routine situations. The ability to function (e.g., work) and concentrate is greatly diminished. Suicidal risk increases in depression. Factors such as living alone or divorced, prior history of drug abuse or suicide attempt, or having depression at midlife or older ages than younger ages contribute to suicide in 10% to 15% of depressed individuals.

The symptoms of depression may occur suddenly or gradually for a period ranging from a few weeks to months or years. Depressive episodes recur in a substantial number of individuals and 20% may exhibit a chronic form of depression.

Bipolar Disorder: Mania

Manic individuals experience elevated levels of euphoria. Self-esteem and feelings of grandiosity are abnormally elevated and may result in psychoses such as delusions and hallucinations. Energy levels are greatly enhanced even after only a few hours of sleep each night. The increased energy, however, does not lead to organized plans and thoughts. The individual may show poor judgment in spending money, may become hypersexual, or may make poor business commitments. Other hallmarks of mania are excessive, rapid, loud, and pressured speech. The manic person frequently skips from one topic of conversation to another and is easily distracted both when speaking and when performing tasks. Approximately 50% of manic individuals develop psychotic symptoms, such as delusions or hallucinations, which require hospitalization. The onset and termination of manic symptoms (see Box 18-3) are usually abrupt and may last for a few days or months followed by depression. The risk of recurrence of bipolar disorder is high, especially without immediate treatment.

Treatment

Depression

Unipolar depression is one of the more treatable psychiatric disorders. Approximately 80% of depressed persons will respond to antidepressant drugs, psychotherapy, or a combination of both. MAOIs, TCAs, and SSRIs are used in the treatment of depression (Box 18-4). In addition, atypical antidepressants, such as nefazodone, trazodone, and mirtazapine, presumably produce their clinical effects by blocking specific receptors (e.g., 5-HT$_{2A}$). A new generation of antidepressants that selectively block serotonin and norepinephrine reuptake is available in the United States (i.e., venlafaxine) or Europe (i.e., milnacipran, reboxetine). Although SSRIs have become the standard first-line treatment for major depression, initial selection of an antidepressant often includes an assessment of the person's symptoms, age, side effects, safety, cost, and convenience. For example, medications that produce sedation may be helpful for the treatment of sleep disturbances. Approximately 50% of depressed individuals may not show a favorable response during initial treatment to an antidepressant drug, and 10% to 20% may continue to exhibit symptoms after 2 years. Individuals who are nonresponsive to a specific

antidepressant during a 2-month period may be given another antidepressant medication. At present, there are no criteria that indicate whether selection of the next antidepressant drug will be efficacious. Among children and adolescents, only fluoxetine, which is approved for use in children by the U.S. Food and Drug Administration (FDA), appears to have a favorable risk-benefit profile (see What's New? Advisory Warnings of SSRI Use in Pediatric Depression).[20]

In bipolar depression, antidepressant medications may lead to cycle acceleration or induction of mania. However, SSRIs and bupropion, which have effects on norepinephrine (NE) and dopaminergic function, may be less likely to induce these effects than MAOIs or TCAs.

A number of side effects are reported with MAOIs, TCAs, and SSRIs. Commonly reported side effects of MAOIs include sedation or agitation, insomnia, dry mouth, impotence, and weight gain. MAOIs also may induce acute and heightened elevations in blood pressure (e.g., hypertensive crisis) after intake of tyramine-rich foods, such as aged cheeses, sour cream, pods of broad beans, pickled herring, liver, canned figs, raisins, and avocados. In addition, MAOI interactions with TCAs,

---

Box 18-4	Medications Used in the Treatment of Depression and Anxiety Disorders

Monoamine Oxidase Inhibitors
Isocarboxazid
Phenelzine
Tranylcypromine

Tricyclics
Amitriptyline
Clomipramine
Desipramine
Doxepin
Imipramine
Nortriptyline

Selective Serotonin Reuptake Inhibitors
Citalopram
Escitalopram
Fluoxetine
Fluvoxamine
Paroxetine
Sertraline

Norepinephrine Reuptake Inhibitors
Reboxetine

Serotonin and Norepinephrine Reuptake Inhibitors
Venlafaxine

Atypical Antidepressants
Bupropion
Duloxetine
Mirtazapine
Nefazodone
Trazodone

WHAT'S NEW? Advisory Warnings of SSRI Use in Pediatric Depression

Approximately 60% of all suicides are committed by individuals suffering from mood disorders. Although antidepressant drugs are known to reduce the rate of suicide in depressed adults, concerns have been raised about the risks of antidepressant drugs, notably selective serotonin reuptake inhibitors (SSRIs), on increased suicide rates in children with depression. In 2003 the U.S. Food and Drug Administration and in 2004 the British and European regulatory agencies began to issue warnings about the risk of suicide associated with pediatric use of antidepressant medication. As a result, pediatric SSRI prescriptions declined throughout the United States and Europe. Two studies have evaluated the effects of the advisory warnings of SSRI prescriptions for pediatric depression. One study found that from 1999 to 2004, pediatric diagnosis of depression in the United States increased from 3 per 1000 to 5 per 1000 but decreased to 1999 levels after the advisory announcements. The reversal in diagnosis of pediatric depression was found in children treated by pediatric and nonpediatric primary care providers. In addition, there was no significant increase in the use of pharmacologic alternatives to antidepressants or psychotherapy. The authors concluded that the advisory warnings were associated with a significant reduction in diagnosis and treatment of pediatric depression. Another recent study further questioned whether the reduction in SSRI prescriptions produces safety benefits or increases the rate of suicide among children with depression. These authors reported that in the United States and the Netherlands, SSRI prescriptions for youths declined by approximately 22% but suicide rates jumped 14% in the United States between 2003 and 2004, and 49% in the Netherlands between 2003 and 2005. This study suggests that regulatory agencies' safety concerns of suicide risk with SSRI use in children with depression were associated with an increase in the rate of suicides when left untreated.

Data from Gibbons RD et al: *Am J Psychiatry* 164(9):1356-1363, 2007; Libby AM et al: *Am J Psychiatry* 164(6):884-891, 2007.

SSRIs, stimulants, and over-the-counter flu medications are dangerous and should be avoided. Because of these adverse side effect issues, MAOIs are used less often than other antidepressant medications.

TCAs may produce sedation, insomnia, orthostatic hypotension, seizures, and weight gain. Some TCAs have moderate anticholinergic side effects, including constipation, urinary hesitancy or retention, dry mouth, blurred vision, and memory impairment. These side effects may be an issue when considering TCA treatment of older adults, in which case, the TCAs desipramine and nortriptyline may be preferred because of their reduced anticholinergic, cardiovascular, and sedating effects.

Common side effects of SSRIs include sleep disturbances (e.g., insomnia) and nausea. However, agitation, allergic skin reactions, dry mouth, anxiety, altered appetite, and sexual dysfunction have been reported. Unlike MAOIs and TCAs, SSRIs do not have pronounced effects on the cardiovascular or cholinergic systems. SSRIs are potent inhibitors of cytochrome P-450 isoenzymes, which are involved in drug metabolism. Therefore, SSRIs may lead to dangerous elevations in blood concentrations of other psychiatric medications when taken together. SSRIs should not be taken with MAOIs or immediately after discontinuing MAOI treatment. A serotonin syndrome characterized by excitement or autonomic hyperactivity, abdominal pain, rigidity, and hyperthermia may develop, leading to coma or death.

Side effects of atypical antidepressants may include sedation, dry mouth, weight gain, and constipation. Nefazodone and trazodone have been associated with hepatic toxicity. Venlafaxine and reboxetine lack many of the serious side effects associated with TCAs; however, sweating, dry mouth, and some sedation may occur.

Electroconvulsive therapy (ECT) is used when individuals fail to respond to antidepressants or when they are severely depressed, pregnant, suicidal, or psychotic. ECT is effective in alleviating depressive symptoms in about 50% to 80% of people who may then begin to respond to antidepressant medications. Although the mechanism of action of ECT is not clear, the procedure is known to produce alterations in monoamine systems.

Bipolar Disorder

A number of FDA-approved treatments are available for bipolar disorders.[21] Individuals with bipolar I disorder are usually treated with lithium, the first choice of treatment that also reduces the risk of suicide. In some cases, lithium in combination with SSRIs is used to treat bipolar disorder. In addition to lithium, a number of medications for bipolar disorders, colloquially referred to as mood stabilizers, are available, including anticonvulsants (e.g., carbamazepine, divalproex, gabapentin, lamotrigine, topiramate) or atypical antipsychotics (e.g., clozapine, olanzapine). Some individuals also may benefit from thyroid augmentation (levothyroxine). As in depression, ECT is administered when manic individuals fail to respond to medication, are pregnant, or have cardiovascular disease.

Frequently reported side effects of lithium treatment include increased thirst, tremors, diarrhea, and weight gain, which diminish over time. A potentially serious side effect is lithium toxicity. Lithium is normally removed from the kidneys; however, when the body is sodium depleted, the kidneys will reabsorb sodium along with lithium. Individuals receiving lithium treatment are advised to avoid physically demanding activities that may dehydrate the body and to seek medical attention during fever or other conditions that may increase sweating. Anticonvulsant treatment may produce unsteadiness, dizziness, tremors, nausea, and blurry vision. Adverse effects of atypical antipsychotics may include movement problems (e.g., akathisia) and metabolic disturbances that lead to weight gain.

In addition to pharmacotherapy, psychotherapy can be beneficial for those who have difficulty with psychosocial stressors, such as self-esteem, legal problems, fear of recurrence, and interpersonal conflicts. Treatment involves a combination of making the individual aware of the bipolar disorder, coping with psychosocial stressors, facilitating drug compliance, and monitoring symptom recurrences.

Unlike the use of mood stabilizers to primarily treat the mania and rapid cycling in bipolar I disorder, a major focus in the treatment of bipolar II disorder is on the recurrent depressive symptoms. Although mood stabilizers are used, antidepressants alone (e.g., escitalopram, fluoxetine, venlafaxine) are reported to be effective in treating bipolar II disorder.

ANXIETY DISORDERS

Fear and anxiety are normal feelings expressed in threatening or harmful situations. The symptoms may include arousal, tenseness, and increased autonomic activity such as heart rate, blood pressure, and respiration. In addition, individuals often engage in protective behavioral responses such as flight or avoidance. These physiologic and behavioral responses reflect the individuals' evolutionary heritage. Their expression allowed humans to adapt and cope under a variety of situational challenges. However, when fear and anxiety become too intense and undermine the ability to function on a daily basis, the individual may develop an anxiety disorder. **Anxiety disorders** are the most prevalent psychiatric disorder, occurring in approximately 10% to 30% of the general population. Notably, many individuals with anxiety disorders develop major depression, and those with major depression often suffer from anxiety disorders. Comorbidity of anxiety disorders and depression suggest a common neural pathophysiologic basis linking these two mental illnesses.

Freud used the term *anxiety neurosis* to denote feelings of fearfulness, panic, terror, and doom. Anxiety neurosis is classified into a number of distinct anxiety disorders based on refined clinical observations. The *DMS-IV-TR* lists eight recognized anxiety disorders: panic disorder, agoraphobia, generalized anxiety disorder, social phobia, specific phobia, obsessive-compulsive disorder, posttraumatic stress disorder, and acute stress disorder. This section presents an overview of panic disorder, generalized anxiety disorder, posttraumatic stress disorder, and obsessive-compulsive disorder.

Panic Disorder

Panic disorder is a well-studied psychiatric condition that consists of multiple disabling panic attacks. Approximately 2% to 3% of women and 0.5% to 1.5% of men have panic disorder. Between panic attacks the individual spends an excessive amount of time worrying about future panic attacks. Panic attacks are characterized by intense autonomic arousal involving a wide variety of symptoms, including lightheadedness, a racing heart, difficulty breathing, chest discomfort, generalized sweating, general weakness, trembling, abdominal distress, and chills or hot flashes. In addition, the individual experiences the fear of losing control and dying. Symptoms originally occur spontaneously and vary in length from several minutes to an hour. If the symptoms are prolonged, they can be disabling.

A notable complication of panic disorder is the development of **agoraphobia** or phobic avoidance of places or situations where escape or help is not readily available. The agoraphobic individual will avoid being away from home, standing in line or in a crowd, or riding a train, plane, or automobile. Severe agoraphobia leads to individuals being housebound.

Etiology and Pathophysiology

Genetic factors appear to play a major role in panic disorder. The risk is nearly 20% among first-degree relatives of panic disorder individuals. The prevalence of panic disorder is about 1.5% in men and up to 3.0% in women with no family history of the illness. Some studies suggest that the cholecystokinin (CCK) receptor gene on chromosome 11p may be linked to panic disorder.[22]

Although the etiology of panic attacks is not known, some factors may be acting on vulnerable brainstem regions to provoke symptoms. For example, physiologic information from the peripheral cardiovascular and respiratory systems is regulated closely by cells in the brainstem, which may activate central autonomic pathways. Fearful perceptions and thoughts emanating from the cerebral cortex may further contribute by activating neural circuits in the temporal lobe and brainstem, which may then facilitate the production of panic symptoms.

Brain regions likely to be involved in panic attacks include the locus ceruleus–NE system and temporal lobe structures, including the amygdala and hippocampus[23] (see Figures 18-7 and 18-9). Both the hippocampus and locus ceruleus monitor internal and external signals and increase their activity when aroused. The locus ceruleus is sensitive to respiratory and cardiovascular changes in the periphery, such as hyperventilation. Abnormal firing of locus ceruleus neurons in response to peripheral autonomic signals may contribute to the onset of panic attacks.

Panic disorder also may involve the GABA-benzodiazepine (BZ) receptor system. BZ receptors and GABA$_A$ receptors are functionally coupled. BZ increases the GABA$_A$ ion channel response to GABA, thereby elevating chloride ion influx and

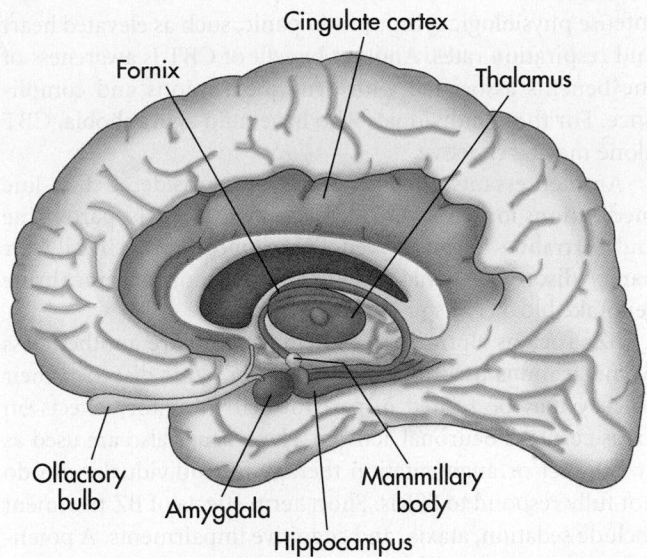

Figure 18-9 The limbic system. Structures of the limbic system play important roles in emotion, learning, and memory. Pathophysiology in limbic structures is frequently found in mental disorders.

producing a neuronal inhibitory effect. Brain imaging work reveals a reduction in BZ receptor binding in brain regions including the hippocampus, insular, and prefrontal cortex.[24] Thus an alteration in inhibitory neuromodulation may contribute to panic disorder.

Individuals with panic disorder respond to some pharmacologic challenges differently than do healthy controls. Physical symptoms of panic attacks are reproduced to a certain degree in panic-prone persons by inhalation of carbon dioxide, caffeine ingestion, sodium lactate, and NE receptor compounds. Many of these agents appear to directly or indirectly modulate the locus ceruleus–NE system, thereby contributing to the production of panic. For example, panic-prone individuals are sensitive to the anxiety-provoking effects of yohimbine, an α_2-adrenergic receptor antagonist, and exhibit elevated levels of plasma MHPG (a norepinephrine metabolite), cortisol, and cardiovascular responses. Clonidine, the α_2-adrenergic receptor agonist, produces less sedation and less plasma MHPG, but greater hypotension when given to individuals with panic disorder. Other drugs that block the benzodiazepine receptor or stimulate the cholecystokinin receptor are reported to increase panic attacks and feelings of anxiety in people with panic disorder. As indicated, these receptor systems may be involved in the pathophysiology of panic disorder.

Treatment

Panic disorder is highly treatable. Up to 80% of panic disorder individuals respond to CBT and antidepressant medication, either separately or in combination. In CBT, the individual learns that the physical symptoms are not fatal and attempts to exert control over the anxiety and panic. For example, breathing exercises to control hyperventilation serve to lessen the intense physiologic symptoms of panic, such as elevated heart and respiration rates. Another benefit of CBT is awareness of the benefits associated with drug medications and compliance. For those individuals who have mild agoraphobia, CBT alone may be effective.

Antidepressants such as SSRIs are considered first-line medications for panic disorder. Among the SSRIs, paroxetine and sertraline have received FDA approval specifically for panic disorder. Venlafaxine, a serotonin-norepinephrine reuptake blocker, also is effective.

BZs such as alprazolam and clonazepam are another class of medications used in the treatment of panic disorder; their efficacy may be related in part to their inhibitory effects on locus ceruleus neuronal activity. These drugs also are used as an adjunct or augmentation therapy for individuals who do not fully respond to SSRIs. Short-term effects of BZ treatment include sedation, ataxia, and cognitive impairments. A potential complication of long-term BZ treatment is physiologic and psychologic dependence. Abrupt BZ withdrawal may produce a withdrawal syndrome that includes a heightened reemergence or rebound of anxiety, insomnia, photophobia, and diarrhea. These symptoms may be lessened with gradual tapering off of BZ medication. Individuals taking BZs may benefit from CBT, which could reduce their reliance on these drugs.

Generalized Anxiety Disorder

Excessive and persistent worries are the hallmarks of **generalized anxiety disorder (GAD)**. The individual worries about life events such as marital relationships, job performance, health, money, or social status. The lifetime prevalence rates of GAD range from 4.1% to 6.6%, with somewhat higher rates in women than in men. GAD usually emerges in the early 20s, but can occur in childhood. Six major symptoms of GAD have been identified including restlessness, muscle tension, irritability, being easily fatigued, difficulty concentrating, and difficulty sleeping. The individual startles easily and frequently suffers from depression and panic attacks. The severity of symptoms fluctuates over time and may be linked to the changing nature of environmental stress. Although GAD tends to be a chronic disorder, the symptoms may become less severe with age. A frequent complication of GAD is the development of depression or substance abuse. The latter may occur as a result of self-medication with alcohol or drugs to relieve the symptoms.

Etiology and Pathophysiology

The etiology and pathophysiology of GAD are poorly understood. Female twin studies suggest a concordance rate of 30%, but disease genes linked to specific chromosomes have yet to be identified. Abnormalities in the norepinephrine and serotonin systems were reported in GAD.[25] For example, there is a reduction in α_2-adrenergic receptor binding, a decrease in serotonin levels in CSF, and reduced platelet binding of paroxetine, an SSRI.

A prominent alteration of GAD involves the GABA-BZ receptors. In GAD there is a reduction in peripheral BZ receptors, which increase after treatment with BZ drugs. Brain imaging work indicates GAD subjects have greater homogeneity of the cerebrum, BZ receptor distribution, and a significant reduction in the left temporal hemisphere.[26] The therapeutic effects of BZs may lie in part in their ability to normalize these BZ receptor alterations.

Treatment

GAD is diagnosed when an individual spends at least 6 months worrying excessively and exhibits at least three of the six symptoms.[11] 5-HT/NE reuptake inhibitors, such as venlafaxine or the SSRIs paroxetine and escitalopram, have become first-line therapeutics for managing GAD. These medications may produce relief of GAD symptoms within 1 week and are effective in treating comorbid symptoms of depression. Buspirone, which has affinity for serotonin receptors ($5\text{-}HT_{1A}$) is another treatment option, although the onset of clinical efficacy may take 2 weeks. The primary side effects of buspirone, which lessen over time, include dizziness, headaches, nausea, and mild nervousness. GAD nonresponders to 5-HT/NE reuptake inhibitors or buspirone may be placed on BZs. However, because GAD tends to be chronic, and comorbid with depression or other anxiety disorders,[27] BZs are usually limited to uncomplicated cases of GAD. SSRIs also have been used in the treatment of the young with GAD. In addition to drug therapy, treatment of GAD may involve behavioral therapy, during which the individual learns relaxation techniques to control anxiety.

Posttraumatic Stress Disorder

Exposure to a terrifying or life-threatening trauma may produce **posttraumatic stress disorder (PTSD)**.[28,29] Although the disorder was initially described in combat situations and called "shell shock," "war neurosis," or "traumatic neurosis," PTSD does not arise solely from exposure to the battlefield. Exposure to any major trauma, including serious accidents, natural disasters (such as earthquakes), child abuse, kidnapping, and violent attacks (such as rape or muggings), that involves intense fear, threat of death, or helplessness may induce PTSD. The disorder may develop within hours of the traumatic experience or after several months or years. In PTSD, the individual reexperiences the traumatic event as intrusive recollections or flashbacks during the day and during persistent nightmares. During a flashback, images, odors, sounds, and negative emotions are recalled and lead to marked distress. The duration of the flashback varies from seconds to hours or, in rare cases, several days. Nightmares replicate the traumatic experiences and often prevent further sleep. Exposure to cues associated with the life-threatening event also may trigger psychologic distress, intense autonomic arousal, and avoidance behavior. The individual shows emotional numbing or detachment from others and avoids activities that may lead to a recollection of thoughts, feelings, places, or people involved in the trauma. Persistent symptoms of PTSD include sleeping difficulties, irritability, lack of concentration, hypervigilance, and exaggerated startle response.

The lifetime prevalence rate of PTSD is 7% to 8%. In men, PTSD is usually found among combat veterans, whereas PTSD in women is often related to rape or assault. Abused children also may develop PTSD. Certain individuals appear to be vulnerable to PTSD. Those with a history of psychiatric illness (major depression, panic disorder) or those lacking strong social support are at increased risk and may be more sensitive to the effects of traumatic stress.

Etiology and Pathophysiology

The primary etiology of PTSD is exposure to a terrifying life-threatening event and may involve several neural structures and neurotransmitter systems. Structural brain imaging studies reported that combat-related PTSD victims have a smaller hippocampus, a brain structure susceptible to the damaging effects of the stress hormone cortisol and excitatory amino acids. Pediatric PTSD studies reveal a more generalized effect of trauma on reducing total brain volume. In functional imaging studies, PTSD individuals exposed to trauma-related stimuli generally exhibit increased activation in the amygdala and diminished activity in some prefrontal cortical areas. Reduced activation of the anterior cingulate cortex also has been reported in some but not all studies.[30]

As in panic disorder, BZ binding is altered in those with PTSD. Individuals with PTSD have reduced distribution of BZ receptor binding in the prefrontal cortex compared with healthy controls.[31] This reduction in BZ receptor distribution was not found in other brain regions.

These structural and functional data involving the hippocampus, amygdala, and prefrontal cortex are highly relevant to the pathophysiology of PTSD because these brain regions normally play important roles in how fearful memories are stored, retrieved, and forgotten. The pathogenesis of PTSD is hypothesized to stem from an altered fear-learning process that may involve, for example, amygdala hyperresponsiveness, lack of prefrontal cortical inhibition, hippocampal dysfunction, and/or susceptibility to the adverse effects of stress.[32] Support of this hypothesis is based on PTSD studies showing reduced hippocampal volume and increased metabolic activity in the amygdala. Continued dysfunction and deterioration of this fear-based memory system may underlie chronic PTSD.

Treatment

PTSD is diagnosed according to the duration and timing of symptoms (DSM-IV-TR). When the duration of symptoms is less than 3 months, PTSD is diagnosed as acute. PTSD is diagnosed as chronic when symptoms persist for 3 months or longer or when the delay of onset is longer than 6 months after the trauma. As in GAD, the severity of symptoms fluctuates over time. Chronic PTSD lasting for years may occur in 30% of diagnosed individuals. Treatment methods involve drug medications and CBT. The individual learns to control the anxiety symptoms and memories of the event during therapy. Among war veterans, group or family therapy is supported by the Veterans Administration.

Paroxetine and sertraline are considered first-line SSRI medications for chronic PTSD because of their tendency to lessen the recurrent nightmares and flashbacks. For chronic PTSD, long-term SSRI therapy is required for steady improvement of symptoms and quality of life. Other antidepressants such as the TCAs (amitriptyline and imipramine) have moderate effects and are second-line drugs. Some data suggest that nefazodone and bupropion may provide benefits. The tendency to use antidepressants is because of the high prevalence of comorbid depression and substance abuse. BZs may be used during the aftermath of a traumatic event to control hyperarousal symptoms such as irritability, insomnia, and muscle tension. However, there is no clear evidence that BZs have clinical efficacy or provide prophylaxis against the development of chronic PTSD—they should be carefully monitored among individuals with a history of drug abuse.

Obsessive-Compulsive Disorder

Repetitive, intrusive thoughts and/or compulsions are the hallmarks of **obsessive-compulsive disorder (OCD)**. These thoughts and acts are irrational, impair normal functioning, and may cause marked distress. Obsessions may involve a preoccupation with contamination, doubting, religious or sexual themes, or the belief that a negative outcome will occur if a specific act is not performed. Compulsions are physical and mental ritualized acts such as washing, cleaning, checking, counting, organizing, hoarding, and repeating specific thoughts or prayers. The lifetime prevalence rates of OCD range from 1.2% to 3.3% with an age of onset between 20 to 25 years. OCD occurs equally in adult men and women; however, many begin to experience symptoms during childhood or adolescence.

OCD individuals are often diagnosed when obsessions or compulsions cause severe distress, are time consuming, or interfere with normal daily activities.[11] In many cases the OCD individual may present with other psychiatric illnesses.[33] In adulthood, comorbidity with major depression, other anxiety disorders (especially panic disorders and GAD), and Tourette syndrome are common. Among children, tic disorders, attention deficit/hyperactivity disorder, and depression coexist with OCD.

Etiology and Pathophysiology

Family studies indicate a risk of about 10% to 12% among first-degree relatives. These first-degree relatives are also at increased risk (4.6%) of Tourette disorder and tics in comparison with control relatives (1%). Thus OCD and Tourette syndrome may share common genes and pathophysiology.

Abnormalities in the basal ganglia–frontocortical circuitry are found in OCD.[34] Some studies have shown increased orbitofrontal and thalamic volumes in OCD but not in the caudate nucleus of the basal ganglia (Figure 18-10). More consistent data are obtained from functional imaging studies, which report an increase in orbitofrontal and anterior cingulate cortical activity. Orbitofrontal and anterior cortical hyperactivity may be responsible for intrusive thoughts, obsessions,

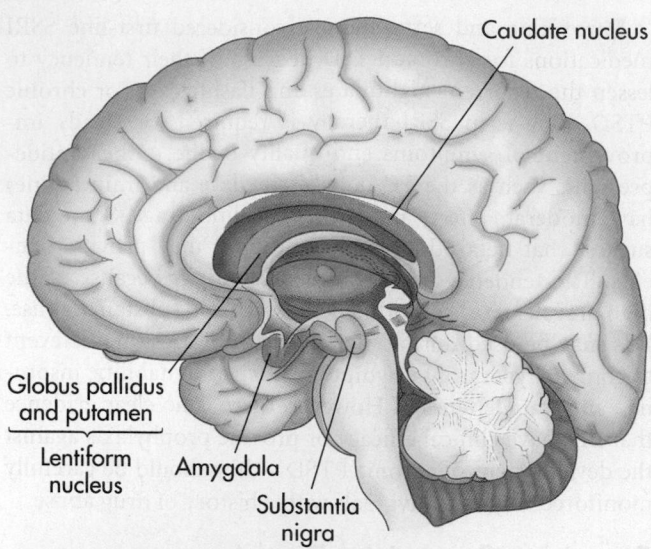

Figure 18-10 Basal ganglion. Structures of the basal ganglion, which include the caudate nucleus, putamen, globus pallidus, and substantia nigra, are important in movement.

and anxiety, which drives the basal ganglia to engage in compulsive ritualized acts as a means to alleviate the anxious obsessions. Studies further suggest that when provoked, OCD individuals consistently show increased activity in the orbito-frontal, anterior cingulate, and caudate nucleus areas of the brain. Of particular relevance to prognosis, OCD individuals with very high frontocortical activity are likely to respond more poorly to treatment than those with lower pretreatment activity in the orbitofrontal cortex.

Abnormalities in serotonin and dopamine functions may contribute to the pathophysiology of OCD. Serotonin agonists exacerbate the symptoms of OCD, and serotonin synthesis is decreased in the prefrontal cortex and caudate nucleus.

Stimulation of the dopamine system increases repetitive acts, which may be blocked by dopamine antagonists. However, the dopamine stimulant-induced compulsions are not accompanied by anxiety, which has led some investigators to suggest that lack of serotonin control over the dopamine system may be a primary defect in OCD.

Treatment

Because of the chronic nature of OCD, long-term treatment consisting of a combination of pharmacotherapy and CBT is often required. SSRIs, including citalopram, fluvoxamine, paroxetine, and sertraline, are the first drugs of choice for OCD.[35] Approximately 70% to 80% of OCD individuals will show a partial response that may be further improved by other medications. For example, clonazepam, a BZ, is found to improve the effects of fluoxetine and clomipramine therapy. Antipsychotic drugs, haloperidol and risperidone, in combination with SSRIs, are also effective especially in comorbid OCD and tic disorders. Normalization of dysfunctional serotonin and dopamine systems in OCD may be the basis for the therapeutic effects of SSRIs and dopamine receptor–related drugs.

CBT involves daily exposure to cues that elicit distress followed by preventing the individual from engaging in compulsive rituals for at least an hour or until the anxiety subsides. This exposure and response prevention therapy can produce long-term symptom remission and is effective in adults and children who are able to tolerate the exposure-induced anxiety component.

For individuals with severe treatment-resistant OCD, neurosurgery is performed to disconnect the basal ganglia from the frontal cortex.[36] This lesioning procedure results in significant relief of obsessions and compulsions in nearly 50% of individuals and provides further evidence of a pathophysiology in the basal ganglia–frontocortical circuitry in OCD.

SUMMARY REVIEW

Schizophrenia

1. Schizophrenia is a collection of symptoms characterized by thought disorders. Thought disorders reflect a break between the cognitive and the emotional sides of one's personality.
2. Schizophrenic symptoms are generally classified into positive and negative symptoms. Positive symptoms include hallucinations, delusions, formal thought disorder, and bizarre behavior. Negative symptoms include flattened affect, alogia, anhedonia, attention deficits, and apathy.
3. Schizophrenia has a strong genetic predisposition.
4. In early development, environmental factors (viral infection, nutritional deficiencies, or prenatal birth complications) may interfere with genetically programmed neural development leading to alterations in brain structure and function.
5. Structural brain abnormalities are present in schizophrenia. Brain imaging studies reveal an enlargement of the cerebroventricles and widening of the fissures and sulci in the frontal cortex. In addition, there is a reduction in the volume of the thalamus, which may disrupt communication among cortical

brain regions, and the temporal lobe, which may be responsible for the manifestations of positive symptoms.
6. In schizophrenia the frontal lobe shows a progressive loss in volume and a worsening of negative symptoms despite the use of antidepressant medications. Functional alterations in the dorsolateral prefrontal cortex, such as reduced blood flow and metabolism, compromise the ability to engage in goal-directed and cognitive problem-solving behavior.
7. Neurochemical abnormalities in dopamine and excitatory amino acid neurotransmission are found in schizophrenic brains.
8. The first generation of conventional antipsychotic drugs block the dopamine D_2 receptor. The second generation of effective treatment in schizophrenia is called atypical antipsychotic drugs, which block not only D_2 receptors but also a combination of dopamine, serotonin, and other neurotransmitter receptors. Antipsychotic drugs block the dopamine D_2 receptor or a combination of dopamine and serotonin receptors. Antipsychotic medications, however, are not always effective

SUMMARY REVIEW—cont'd

in treating individuals with severe negative symptoms. In addition to drug medications, psychosocial therapy is used to increase drug compliance and to encourage coping strategies.

Mood Disorders: Depression and Bipolar Disorder

1. Major depression and bipolar disorder are two common mood disorders. The former is characterized by an intense and sustained unpleasant state of sadness and hopelessness. Individuals with recurrent patterns of depression and mania, the latter characterized by extreme levels of energy and euphoria, have a bipolar illness.
2. Environmental triggers such as psychosocial stress appear to facilitate the onset of depression in individuals with a genetic vulnerability.
3. A reduction in brain monoamine neurotransmission is linked to depression, whereas an elevated monoamine level is associated with mania.
4. Individuals with major depression commonly have elevated levels of the stress hormone cortisol. Neuroendocrine abnormalities involving thyroid hormones also are found in depression.
5. Structural brain alterations that include reduced frontal lobe and limbic system volumes are found in depression and bipolar illness. Functional brain imaging studies show that depressed individuals have alterations in blood flow to prefrontal and limbic brain regions that include the amygdala, a structure implicated in emotional behavior.
6. Pharmacotherapy involving the use of MAOIs, TCAs, SSRIs, and atypical antidepressants is effective in the treatment of mood disorders. Manic and bipolar individuals are treatable with lithium or mood stabilizers. The clinical effects of drugs used in the treatment of mood disorders often take several weeks to develop. Severely depressed and manic people who do not respond to medication are administered ECT.

Anxiety Disorders

1. Fear and anxiety are normal emotional states that reflect individuals' evolutionary heritage. However, when these mental states persist and become uncontrollable, an individual may develop an anxiety disorder. Panic disorder, generalized anxiety disorder, PTSD, and OCD are examples of uncontrollable fear and anxiety states that require medical attention.

2. Panic disorder consists of panic attacks characterized by intense autonomic arousal that occurs spontaneously and may last for up to 1 hour. During a panic attack the individual experiences multiple symptoms including lightheadedness, a pounding heart, and difficulty breathing. In addition, the intense occurrence of autonomic responses is accompanied by heightened fear and anxiety that often continue between panic attacks.
3. Brain regions involved in the production of panic attacks are the locus ceruleus, hippocampus, and amygdala. A reduction in GABA$_A$-BZ receptor binding also may contribute to the pathophysiology of panic disorder.
4. Panic disorder is generally treatable with CBT and antidepressants such as TCAs and SSRIs. BZs are used as an adjunct or augmentation therapy for individuals who are nonresponsive to SSRIs or TCAs.
5. GAD is characterized by excessive and persistent worries about life events. Individuals exhibit varying levels of motor disturbances, irritability, and fatigue that may be linked to fluctuations in psychosocial stress. Many GAD individuals manifest symptoms of depression.
6. Pathophysiology in norepinephrine, serotonin, and GABA$_A$-BZ systems is found in those with GAD.
7. Treatment of GAD usually involves a combination of behavioral therapy and drug medications, especially serotonin/norepinephrine reuptake inhibitors.
8. PTSD develops after exposure to a life-threatening or traumatic experience. Individuals experience recurring thoughts and flashbacks and nightmares of the terrifying event.
9. In PTSD structural and/or functional alterations exist in the hippocampus, amygdala, and prefrontal cortex, which are neural components of a fear-based memory system.
10. Treatment of chronic PTSD is difficult. Methods involve psychotherapy and SSRI pharmacotherapy.
11. OCD is characterized by irrational thoughts and ritualized acts that impair normal functioning and cause severe distress.
12. Pathophysiology in the basal ganglia–frontocortical circuitry and serotonin and dopamine functions is linked to OCD.
13. OCD is a chronic illness that requires long-term treatment consisting of CBT and drug medication, such as SSRIs. Severe OCD may require neurosurgery to disconnect the basal ganglia from the frontal cortex.

KEY TERMS

Affective flattening, 651
Agoraphobia, 659
Alogia, 651
Anhedonia, 651
Anxiety disorder, 658
Avolition, 651
Bipolar disorder, 652
Delusion, 650
Depression, 655
Dopamine hypothesis, 648

Dorsolateral prefrontal cortex (DLPFC), 648
Dysphoric mood, 655
Formal thought disorder, 651
Gamma-aminobutyric acid (GABA), 648
Generalized anxiety disorder (GAD), 660
Hallucination, 650
Major (unipolar) depression, 652
Manic, 656
Monoamine hypothesis of depression, 653
Mood, 652

Neuroleptics, 651
Obsessive-compulsive disorder, 661
Panic disorder, 659
Posttraumatic stress disorder (PTSD), 660
Poverty of content, 651
Psychotic episode, 650
Schizophrenia, 647
Thought disorder, 647
Working memory, 648

REFERENCES

1. Lewis DA, Levitt P: Schizophrenia as a disorder of neurodevelopment, *Annu Rev Neurosci* 25:409-432, 2002.
2. Marenco S, Weinberger DR: The neurodevelopmental hypothesis of schizophrenia: following a trail of evidence from cradle to grave, *Dev Psychopathol* 12(3):501-527, 2000.
3. Berman KF, Meyer-Lindenberg A: Functional brain imaging studies in schizophrenia. In Charney DS, Nestler EJ, editors: *Neurobiology of mental illness*, ed 2, New York, 2004, Oxford.
4. Shenton LD et al: A review of MRI findings in schizophrenia, *Schizophr Res* 49(1-2):1-52, 2001.
5. Ross CA et al: Neurobiology of schizophrenia, *Neuron* 52(1):139-153, 2006.
6. Ho BC et al: Progressive structural brain abnormalities and their relationship to clinical outcome, *Arch Gen Psychiatry* 60:585-594, 2003.
7. Costa E et al: Dendritic spine hypoplasticity and downregulation of reelin and GABAergic tone in schizophrenia vulnerability, *Neurobiol Dis* 8(5):723-742, 2001.
8. Fatemi SH, Earle JA, McMenomy T: Reduction in reelin immunoreactivity in hippocampus of subjects with schizophrenia, bipolar disorder and major depression, *Mol Psychiatry* 5(6):654-663, 2000.
9. Duncan GE, Sheitman BB, Lieberman JA: An integrated view of pathophysiological models of schizophrenia, *Brain Res Brain Res Rev* 29(2-3):250-264, 1999.
10. Kennedy JL et al: The genetics of adult-onset neuropsychiatric disease: complexities and conundra? *Science* 302(5646):822-826, 2003.
11. American Psychiatric Association: *Diagnostic and statistical manual of mental disorders*, ed 4, Text Revision (DSM-IV-TR), Washington, DC, 2000, American Psychiatric Association.
12. Tamminga CA: Principles of the pharmacotherapy of schizophrenia. In Charney DS, Nestler EJ, editors: *Neurobiology of mental illness*, ed 2, New York, 2004, Oxford.
13. Rathod S et al: Cognitive-behavioral therapy for medication-resistant schizophrenia: a review, *J Psychiat Pract* 14(1):22-33, 2008.
14. Caspi A et al: Influence of life stress on depression: moderation by a polymorphism in the 5-HTT gene, *Science* 301(5631):386, 2003.
15. Heninger GR et al: The revised monoamine theory of depression: a modulatory role for monoamines, based on new findings from monoamine depletion experiments in humans, *Pharmacopsychiatry* 29(1):2-11, 1996.
16. Holsboer F: The corticosteroid receptor hypothesis of depression, *Neuropsychopharmacology* 23:477, 2000.
17. Bartalena L et al: Nocturnal serum thyrotropin (TSH) surge and the TSH response to TSH-releasing hormone: disassociative behavior in untreated depression, *J Clin Endocrinol Metab* 71(3):650-655, 1990.
18. Drevets WC: Prefrontal cortical-amygdalar metabolism in major depression, *Ann N Y Acad Sci* 877:614-637, 1999.
19. Rajkowska G: Depression: what we can learn from postmortem studies, *Neuroscientist*, 9(4):273-284, 2003.
20. Whittington CJ et al: Selective serotonin reuptake inhibitors in childhood depression: systematic review of published versus unpublished data, *Lancet* 363(9418):1341-1345, 2004.
21. Goldberg JF: What psychotherapists should know about pharmacotherapies for bipolar disorder, *J Clin Psychol* 63(5):475-490, 2007.
22. Kennedy JL et al: Investigation of cholecystokinin system genes in panic disorder, *Mol Psychiatry* 4(3):284, 1999.
23. Goddard AW, Charney DS: Toward an integrated neurobiology of panic disorder, *J Clin Psychiatry* 58(Suppl 2):4-11, 1997.
24. Malizia AL et al: Decreased brain GABA$_A$-benzodiazepine receptor binding in panic disorder, *Arch Gen Psychiatry* 55(8):715-720, 1998.
25. Jetty PV et al: Neurobiology of generalized anxiety disorder, *Psychiatr Clin North Am* 24(1):75, 2001.
26. Tiihonen J et al: Cerebral benzodiazepine receptor binding and distribution in generalized anxiety disorder, *Mol Psychiatry* 2(6):463-471, 1997.
27. Bruce SE: Infrequency of "pure" GAD: impact of psychiatric comorbidity on clinical course, *Depress Anxiety* 14(4):219-225, 2001.
28. Charney DS et al: Psychobiologic mechanisms of posttraumatic stress disorder, *Arch Gen Psychiatry* 50(4):294-305, 1993.
29. Southwick SM et al: Neurotransmitter alterations in PTSD: catecholamines and serotonin, *Semin Clin Neuropsychiatry* 4(4):242-248, 1999.
30. Pissota A et al: Neurofunctional correlates of posttraumatic stress disorder: a PET symptom provocation study, *Eur Arch Psychiatry Clin Neurosci* 252(2):68-75, 2002.
31. Bremner JD et al: Decreased benzodiazepine receptor binding in prefrontal cortex in combat-related posttraumatic stress disorder, *Am J Psychiatry* 157(7):1120-1126, 2000.
32. Bremner JD et al: Structural and functional plasticity of the human brain in posttraumatic stress disorder, *Prog Brain Res* 167:171-186, 2008.
33. Fireman B et al: The prevalence of clinically recognized obsessive-compulsive disorder in a large health maintenance organization, *Am J Psychiatry* 158(11):1904-1910, 2001.
34. Saxena S, Rauch SL: Functional neuroimaging and the neuroanatomy of obsessive-compulsive disorder, *Psychiatr Clin North Am* 23(3):563-586, 2000.
35. Swedo SE, Snider LA: The neurobiology and treatment of obsessive-compulsive disorder. In Charney DS, Nestler EJ, editors: *Neurobiology of mental illness*, ed 2, New York, 2004, Oxford.
36. Greenberg BD, Murphy DL, Rasmussen SA: Neuroanatomically based approaches to obsessive-compulsive disorder, *Psychiatr Clin North Am* 23(3):671-686, 2000.

ALTERATIONS OF NEUROLOGIC FUNCTION IN CHILDREN

BARBARA J. BOSS • SUE E. HUETHER

MEDIA RESOURCES

ⓔvolve **Evolve Website** (http://evolve.elsevier.com/McCance/)
- Review Questions and Answers
- Animations
- Glossary (with audio pronunciation for selected terms)
- WebLinks

CHAPTER OUTLINE

STRUCTURE AND FUNCTION OF THE NERVOUS SYSTEM IN CHILDREN
Myelin Sheath
Normal Growth and Development
STRUCTURAL MALFORMATIONS
Defects of Neural Tube Closure
ENCEPHALOPATHIES
Static Encephalopathies
Acute Encephalopathies
Human Immunodeficiency Virus Encephalopathy

CEREBROVASCULAR DISEASE IN CHILDREN
Occlusive Cerebrovascular Disease
Hemorrhagic Cerebrovascular Disease
CHILDHOOD TUMORS
Brain Tumors
Embryonal Tumors

Neurologic disorders in children can occur from infancy through adolescence and include congenital malformations, genetic defects in metabolism, brain injuries, infection, tumors, and other disorders that effect neurologic structure and function. The symptoms, diagnosis and management of neurologic disorders in children is often different than that of adults.

STRUCTURE AND FUNCTION OF THE NERVOUS SYSTEM IN CHILDREN

Embryology is a highly complex and often difficult science to understand fully. A basic knowledge of this science is essential because it is the process of embryonic development that explains many of the malformations that occur in children.

Environmental influences also play a significant role in nervous system development. Nutrition, hormones, oxygen levels, and external stimulation all affect normal growth. The proper proportions of essential nutrients are necessary for proliferation of the nervous system tissue (see Nutrition and Disease box). Maternal lifestyle, nutrition, and state of health also have a crucial effect on nervous system development at critical periods of fetal maturation.

The central nervous system (CNS) develops from a dorsal thickening of the ectoderm known as the **neural plate.** This plate appears around the middle of the third gestational week and unfolds to form a **neural groove** and **neural folds.** During the fourth gestational week the neural groove deepens, its folds develop laterally, and it closes dorsally to form the **neural tube,** epithelial tissue that ultimately becomes the CNS. The neural tube closes first in the cervical region and then "zippers" in two directions—cranially and caudally (Figure 19-1).

In the developmental process, some neuroectodermal cells separate from the neural tube but remain between the tube and the surface ectoderm, creating the **neural crest.** This cellular band develops into the cranial and spinal ganglia, more commonly referred to as the *peripheral nervous system.* Other

NUTRITION & DISEASE

Iron and Cognitive Function

Iron deficiency (ID) is the single most significant nutrient deficiency, affecting 15% of the world population and causing anemia in 40% to 50% of children. Iron is essential for neurologic activity, including synthesis of dopamine, serotonin, catecholamine, and, possibly, myelin formation. Children with ID have decreased attentiveness, short attention span, and perceptual restrictions. ID also may contribute to attention deficit/hyperactivity disorder. In some studies, cognitive deficits in iron can be reversed with iron supplements. Research is in progress to determine the effects of acute versus chronic ID and the relationships between severity of deficiency and cognitive functioning. Alterations in the hippocampus and the brain striatal dopaminergic-opiate system has been found in ID rate.

Data from Konofal E et al: *Arch Pediatr Adolesc Med* 158(12): 1113-1115, 2004; Lozoff B, Georgieff MK: *Semin Pediatr Neurol* 13(3):158-165, 2006; Manger MS et al: *Asia Pac J Clin Nutr* 13(Suppl):S46, 2004; McCann JC, Ames BN: *Am J Clin Nutr* 85(4):931-945, 2007; Youdin MB: *Neurotox Res* 14(1):45-56, 2008.

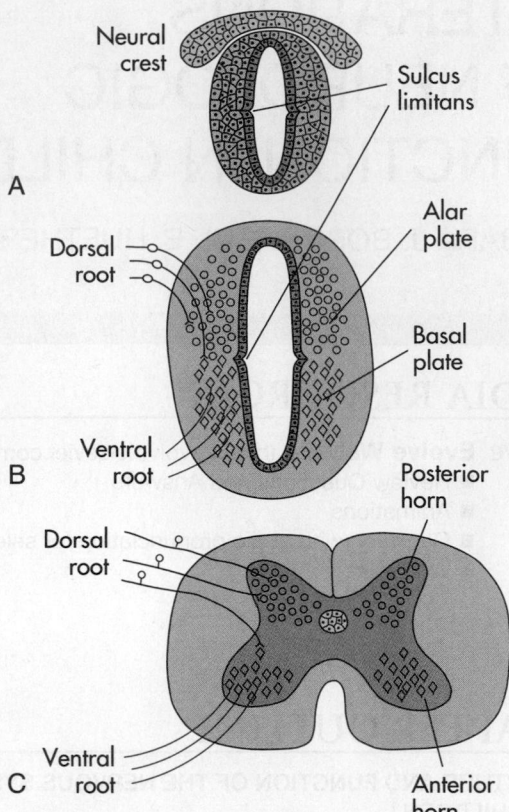

Figure 19-2 Sulcus limitans and alar and basal plates. **A,** Neural tube during the fourth week of gestation. **B,** Embryonic spinal cord during the sixth week of gestation; dorsal root ganglion cells, derived from the neural crest, send their central processes into the spinal cord to terminate mainly in alar plate cells; basal plate cells become motor neurons, whose axons exit in the ventral roots. **C,** Adult spinal cord.

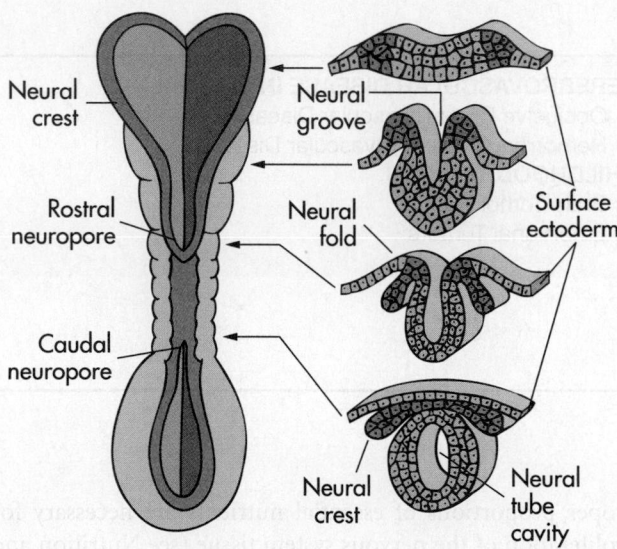

Figure 19-1 Neural tube at 3 weeks of gestation. Neural folds have begun to fuse at the cervical level of the future spinal cord. *Right,* Cross sections of the neural tube at four different levels; at any given level the embryonic central nervous system (CNS) goes through a series of stages resembling these four cross sections. Total length of neural tube at this time is about 2.5 mm.

structures associated with the nervous system arise from mesoderm (**somite**) and include blood vessels, microglial cells, dural and arachnoid layers of the meninges, the capsule of some peripheral sensory nerve endings, and peripheral nerve coverings.

The cranial end of the neural tube forms the brain, and the remainder develops into the spinal cord. The lumen of the neural tube becomes the ventricles of the brain and the central canal of the spinal cord (Figure 19-2). On either side of the neural tube's inner surface is a longitudinal groove (**sulcus limitans**). Anterior to this region (**basal plate**) the gray matter

differentiates into the nuclei of the lower motor neurons. The region posterior to the sulcus (**alar plate**) differentiates into the sensory nuclei of the spinal cord.

Embryonic development of the nervous system occurs in six stages: (1) dorsal (posterior) induction, (2) ventral (anterior) induction, (3) proliferation, (4) migration, (5) organization, and (6) myelination. (Figure 19-3 summarizes the embryonic development of the nervous system and identifies disorders associated with interference in any of these stages.) Many different events happen simultaneously, and critical periods must pass uninterrupted if the vulnerable fetus is to develop normally.

In the newborn the bones of the skull are separated, but definite **sutures** (bands of connective tissue) form shortly thereafter. The edges are several millimeters wide to allow for normal growth. At the junctions of the sutures are wider spaces of unossified membranous tissue called **fontanels.** Sutures and fontanels close as the skull and brain grow and develop.

On average the posterior fontanel closes within the first 3 months of life. By 6 months of age, a fibrous union of suture lines occurs and serrated edges interlock. By approximately 20 to 24 months, the anterior fontanel is closed (Figure 19-4). At approximately 8 years of age, ossification of the cranial bones

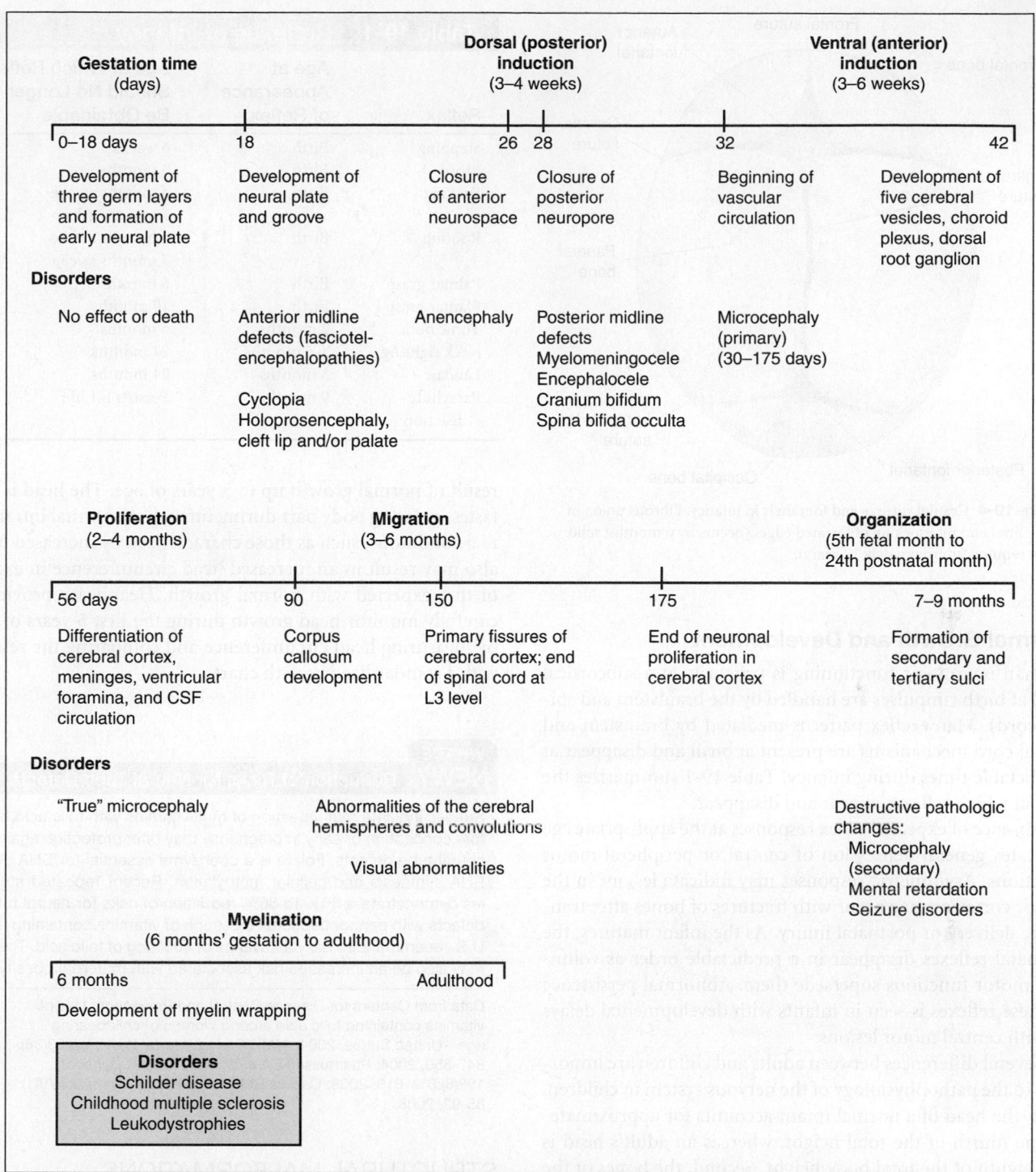

Gestation time (days)		Dorsal (posterior) induction (3–4 weeks)		Ventral (anterior) induction (3–6 weeks)	
0–18 days	18	26 28		32	42
Development of three germ layers and formation of early neural plate	Development of neural plate and groove	Closure of anterior neurospace	Closure of posterior neuropore	Beginning of vascular circulation	Development of five cerebral vesicles, choroid plexus, dorsal root ganglion
Disorders					
No effect or death	Anterior midline defects (fasciotel-encephalopathies) Cyclopia Holoprosencephaly, cleft lip and/or palate	Anencephaly	Posterior midline defects Myelomeningocele Encephalocele Cranium bifidum Spina bifida occulta	Microcephaly (primary) (30–175 days)	

Proliferation (2–4 months)		Migration (3–6 months)		Organization (5th fetal month to 24th postnatal month)	
56 days	90	150	175		7–9 months
Differentiation of cerebral cortex, meninges, ventricular foramina, and CSF circulation	Corpus callosum development	Primary fissures of cerebral cortex; end of spinal cord at L3 level	End of neuronal proliferation in cerebral cortex		Formation of secondary and tertiary sulci
Disorders					
"True" microcephaly		Abnormalities of the cerebral hemispheres and convolutions Visual abnormalities			Destructive pathologic changes: Microcephaly (secondary) Mental retardation Seizure disorders

Myelination (6 months' gestation to adulthood)	
6 months	Adulthood
Development of myelin wrapping	

Disorders
Schilder disease
Childhood multiple sclerosis
Leukodystrophies

Figure 19-3 Disorders associated with specific stages of embryonic development. *CSF*, Cerebrospinal fluid.

is complete; the sutures usually are completely fused and cannot be separated by 12 years of age, even in the presence of increased intracranial pressure (ICP).

Myelin Sheath

Axons are wrapped in concentric layers of myelin, a lipid-protein sheath (see Chapter 14). Specialized connective tissue cells, which in the peripheral nervous system are called Schwann cells, form membranes that wrap around the axon during embryonic development, laying down the lipoprotein lamellae of the myelin sheath. These axons are myelinated, whereas the axons that lack a sheath are thinner, unmyelinated fibers and conduct nerve impulses more slowly. During the first year of life, the presence or absence of various reflexes is indicative of the myelination that has occurred with growth of the infant.

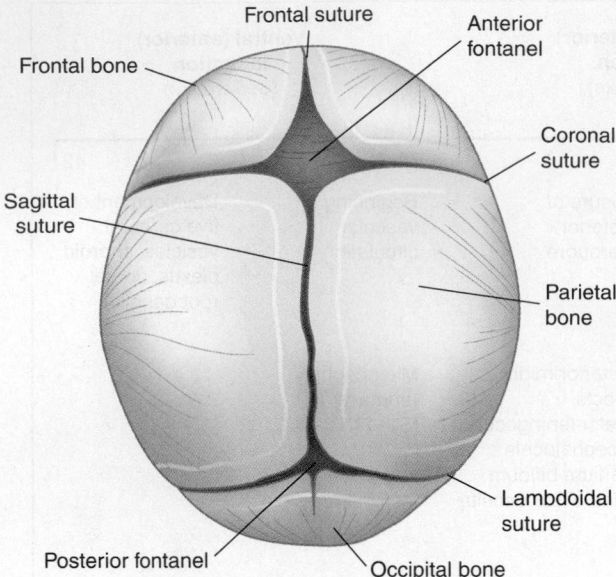

Figure 19-4 Cranial sutures and fontanels in infancy. Fibrous union of suture lines and interlocking of serrated edges (occurs by 6 months; solid union requires approximately 12 years).

Normal Growth and Development

Human neurologic functioning is primarily at a subcortical level at birth (impulses are handled by the brainstem and spinal cord). Many reflex patterns mediated by brainstem and spinal cord mechanisms are present at birth and disappear at predictable times during infancy. Table 19-1 summarizes the ages at which reflexes appear and disappear.

Absence of expected reflex responses at the appropriate age indicates general depression of central or peripheral motor functions. Asymmetric responses may indicate lesions in the motor cortex or may occur with fractures of bones after traumatic delivery or postnatal injury. As the infant matures, the neonatal reflexes disappear in a predictable order as voluntary motor functions supersede them. Abnormal persistence of these reflexes is seen in infants with developmental delays or with central motor lesions.

Several differences between adults and children are important to the pathophysiology of the nervous system in children. First, the head of a normal infant accounts for approximately one fourth of the total height, whereas an adult's head is one eighth of the total body height. Second, the bones of the infant's skull are separated at the suture lines, thus forming two fontanels or "soft spots": one diamond-shaped anterior fontanel and one triangular-shaped posterior fontanel. The posterior fontanel may be open until 2 to 3 months of age; the anterior fontanel normally closes by 18 months. Whereas the adult cranium is a closed cavity with sutures firmly holding the cranial bones together, the infant cranium has room for expansion through the fontanels. An adult's head size will not expand, regardless of intracranial events such as trauma or increased production of cerebrospinal fluid (CSF). The infant's head circumference, however, increases in size as a result of normal growth up to 5 years of age. The head is the fastest growing body part during infancy. Abnormal intracranial conditions, such as those characterized by increased ICP, also may result in an increased head circumference in excess of that expected with normal growth. Healthcare providers carefully monitor head growth during the first 5 years of life by measuring head circumference and comparing the results with a standardized growth chart.

Table 19-1	Reflexes of Infancy	
Reflex	Age at Appearance of Reflex	Age at Which Reflex Should No Longer Be Obtainable
Stepping	Birth	6 weeks
Moro	Birth	3 months
Sucking	Birth	4 months awake 7 months asleep
Rooting	Birth	4 months awake 7 months asleep
Palmar grasp	Birth	6 months
Plantar grasp	Birth	10 months
Tonic neck	2 months	5 months
Neck righting	4-6 months	24 months
Landau	3 months	24 months
Parachute reaction	9 months	Persists for life

WHAT'S NEW? Reduction of Risks for Neural Tube Defects

Studies indicate that ingestion of multivitamins with folic acid before conception or early in pregnancy may offer protection against neural tube defects. Folate is a coenzyme essential for DNA and RNA synthesis and cellular methylation. Recent repeated studies demonstrate a 60% to 86% reduction of risks for neural tube defects with periconceptional ingestion of vitamins containing the U.S. recommended daily allowance of 400 mcg of folic acid. There may also be an increased risk associated with maternal obesity.

Data from Centers for Disease Control and Prevention: Use of vitamins containing folic acid among women of childbearing age—United States, 2004, *MMWR Morb Mortal Wkly Rep* 53(36): 847-850, 2004; Rasmussen SA et al: *Am J Obstet Gynecol* 198(6):611-619, 2008; Cabera RM et al: *J Reprod Immunol* 79(1): 85-92, 2008.

STRUCTURAL MALFORMATIONS

Defects of Neural Tube Closure

Neural tube defects (NTDs) are caused by an arrest of the normal development of the brain and spinal cord and occur in about 3000 pregnancies in the United States each year.[1] There is a strong association of fetal death with NTDs, reducing their actual prevalence of neural defects at birth.[2] Maternal folate deficiency is associated with NTDs, but the specific mechanism that relates to how folate supplements prevent these anomalies is unknown.[3] Periconceptional supplementation with folic acid can reduce NTDs by up to 70%.[4]

Defects of neural tube closure are divided into two categories: posterior defects and anterior midline defects. Posterior defects are more common. These include anencephaly (*an,* "without"; *enkephalos,* "brain") and a group of disorders collectively referred to as the *myelodysplasias* (*dys,* "bad"; *plassein,* "to form"). Although **myelodysplasia** is defined as a defective formation of the spinal cord, the term is used to refer to anomalies of both the vertebral column and the spine (i.e., spina bifida and myelomeningocele).

Anterior midline defects are less common because the inductive processes occur in a relatively short period (2 to 3 days). These developmental defects may cause brain and skull abnormalities. The most extreme form is **cyclopia,** in which the child has a single midline orbit and eye with a protruding noselike appendage above the orbit.

Anencephaly

Anencephaly is an anomaly in which the soft, bony component of the skull and part of the brain are missing. This is a relatively common disorder, with an incidence rate of approximately 0.36 per 1000 total live births in the United States each year.[5] When development is arrested early in anterior closure of the neural tube, the cerebral hemispheres, diencephalon, mesencephalon, cerebellum, brainstem, or spinal cord may be affected. At birth the infant's head, viewed face-on, has a froglike appearance. These infants are stillborn or die within a few days after birth. Diagnosis is often made prenatally using ultrasound or evaluating maternal serum alpha fetoprotein (AFP).[6]

Encephalocele

Encephalocele refers to a herniation or protrusion of brain and meninges through a defect in the skull, resulting in a saclike structure. The incidence rate is approximately 1 in 5000 live births in the United States and Southeast Asia each year.[7,8]

PATHOPHYSIOLOGY Encephalocele occurs during the first weeks of pregnancy. When the defect contains only meninges, it is referred to as a **cranial meningocele.** Most encephaloceles occur in the occipital area, with the remainder found in the frontal, parietal, or nasopharyngeal regions.

CLINICAL MANIFESTATIONS Encephalocele usually is seen at birth as a midline skull defect through which a large mass protrudes (Figure 19-5). If the defect is located in the nasopharynx, no external anomaly is visible, but the child may experience nasal airway obstruction. On examination with a nasal speculum, a smooth, round mass will be visible in the nasal passages. A frontal encephalocele may extend into the orbit of the eye and produce proptosis on the affected side.

EVALUATION AND TREATMENT Diagnosis is based on clinical manifestations and examination of the meningeal sac. With cranial meningocele, surgical repair of the cranial defect affords a good prognosis for most affected infants whose intellectual and motor functioning is normal. An occipital encephalocele may be associated with other findings, such as blindness and cognitive impairment. The size,

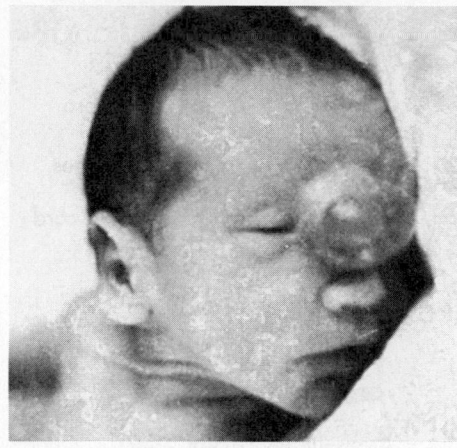

Figure 19-5 Newborn with frontal, nasal, interocular encephalocele. (Courtesy Dr. Charles Linder, Medical College of Georgia.)

location, and involvement of the encephalocele help determine a child's development and intellectual outcome.

Meningocele

Meningocele is a saclike cyst of meninges filled with spinal fluid. It develops during the first four weeks of pregnancy when the neural tube fails to close completely (Figure 19-6).

PATHOPHYSIOLOGY Meningocele is a sturctural anomaly of the posterior arch of the vertebra. The cystic dilation of meninges protrudes through the vertebral defect and around the malformed tube. The dura mater may be missing and the arachnoid layer of the meninges bulges beneath the skin. This defect does not involve the spinal cord. Meningoceles occur with equal frequency in the cervical thoracic and lumbar spine areas.

CLINICAL MANIFESTATIONS At birth the infant has a protruding sac on the back at the level of the defect. The sac may be covered by a thin layer of muscle and skin and usually appears as raw, fluid-filled tissue. Abnormal neurologic function sometimes is present. Talipes equinovarus (clubfoot), gait disturbance, bladder dysfunction, and upper extremity weakness also have been associated with meningocele. Hydrocephalus commonly is associated with this diagnosis.

EVALUATION AND TREATMENT The diagnosis is made on the basis of clinical manifestations and examination of the meningeal sac. In an effort to preserve neuronal function and minimize damage that may occur from infection and manipulation of the fragile sac, surgical closure is optimal during the first 72 hours of life. Functional implications depend on the level and severity of the defect (Table 19-2).

Myelomeningocele

Myelomeningocele (meningomyelocele; spina bifida cystica) is a hernial protrusion of a saclike cyst (containing meninges, spinal fluid, and a portion of the spinal cord with its nerves) through a defect in the posterior arch of a vertebra. Eighty percent of myelomeningoceles are located in the lumbar and lumbosacral regions, the last regions of the neural tube to

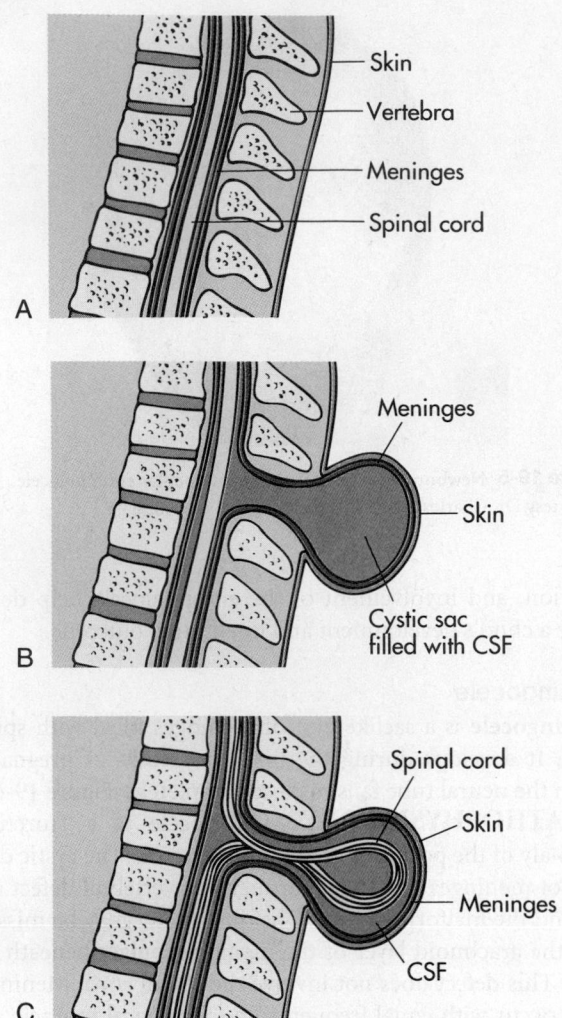

Figure 19-6 Comparison of normal spine and meningocele and myelomeningocele neural tube defects. Diagram depicts section through normal spine (A), spine with meningocele (B), and spine with myelomeningocele (C).

close. Myelomeningocele has an incidence rate ranging from 0.5 to 1 per 1000 pregnancies in the United States[9] and thus is one of the most common developmental anomalies of the nervous system.

PATHOPHYSIOLOGY A myelomeningocele is the failure of the neural tube to close, resulting in a cystic dilation of meninges and protuberance of the spinal cord through the vertebral defect. This defect occurs during the first 4 weeks of the gestational period; at the end of this time the neural tube is closed anteriorly and posteriorly.

CLINICAL MANIFESTATIONS A myelomeningocele is evident at birth as a pronounced skin defect on the infant's back (see Figure 19-6). The bony prominences of the unfused neural arches can be palpated at the lateral border of the defect. The defect usually is covered by a transparent membrane that may have neural tissue attached to its inner surface. This membrane may be intact at birth or may leak CSF, thereby increasing the risks of infection and neuronal damage. Until the defect is closed surgically, CSF may accumulate, resulting

Table 19-2	Functional Alterations in Myelodysplasia Related to Level of Lesion
Level of Lesion	**Functional Implications**
Thoracic	Flaccid paralysis of lower extremities; variable weakness in abdominal trunk musculature; high thoracic level may mean respiratory compromise; absence of bowel and bladder control
High lumbar	Voluntary hip flexion and adduction; flaccid paralysis of knees, ankles, and feet; may walk with extensive braces and crutches; absence of bowel and bladder control
Midlumbar	Strong hip flexion and adduction; fair knee extension; flaccid paralysis of ankles and feet; absence of bowel and bladder control
Low lumbar	Strong hip flexion, extension, and adduction and knee extension; weak ankle and toe mobility; may have limited bowel and bladder function
Sacral	Normal function of lower extremities; normal bowel and bladder function

Data from Farley JA, Dunleavy MJ: Myelodysplasia. In Allen PJ, Vessey JA, editors: *Primary care of the child with a chronic condition*, ed 4, St Louis, 2004, Mosby.

in further dilation and enlargement of the sac, which may risk more damage to the nervous system.

The actual involvement of the spinal cord has greater implications for the overall function of the infant throughout childhood (see Table 19-2). An absence of neurologic function may occur in some infants with myelomeningocele. Function may be attained if underlying fluid or pus accumulation is prevented from stretching and applying pressure to the neural tissue or if the biochemical alterations do not cause neural tissue to die. Residual neural tissue also may be lost temporarily or permanently at birth because of trauma to the tissue during delivery.

One serious, potentially life-threatening problem associated with myelomeningocele is the **Arnold-Chiari type II malformation.**[10] This deformity involves the downward displacement of the cerebellum, cerebellar tonsils, brainstem, and fourth ventricle (Figure 19-7). (Arnold-Chiari type I malformations also involve downward displacement but are not as great as those in type II; type I is seen more commonly in adults.) *Arnold-Chiari II* malformation compresses and essentially stretches the posterior region of the cerebellum and brainstem downward through the foramen magnum and into the cervical space. The brainstem houses 10 cranial nerves. Pressure on this region may result in altered function of these nerves or actual palsies.

Hydrocephalus occurs in 85% of these infants.[11] Seizures also occur in 30% of those with myelodysplasia.[12] Visual and perceptual problems, including ocular palsies, astigmatism,

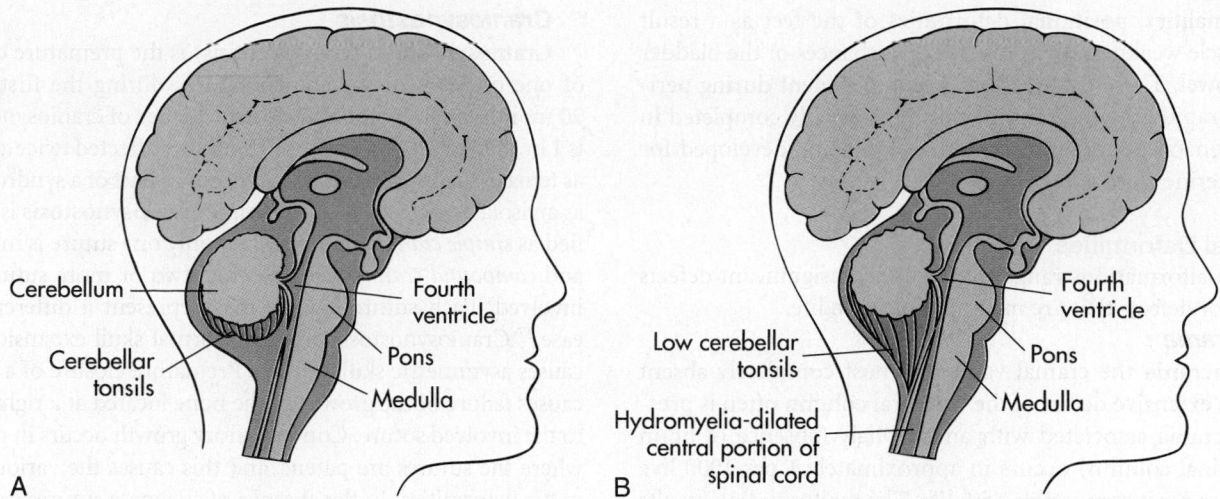

Figure 19-7 Comparison of normal brain and Arnold-Chiari type II malformation. Diagram depicts normal brain (**A**) and brain with Arnold-Chiari type II malformation (**B**).

and visuoperceptual deficits, are common, particularly with Arnold-Chiari type II malformation.[13] Motor and sensory functions below the level of the lesions are altered. This dysfunction may include degrees of weakness, paralysis, spasticity, and bowel and bladder dysfunction. Often these problems worsen as the child grows and the cord ascends within the vertebral canal, pulling primary scar tissue and tethering the cord.[14] Several musculoskeletal deformities are related to this diagnosis, including clubfoot, dislocation of hip or hips, and poor spinal alignment. Spinal deformities, such as scoliosis and kyphosis, are common.[15]

Tethered cord syndrome may develop in children with myelomeningocele, particularly after surgical correction.[16] The cord becomes abnormally attached or tethered as a result of scar tissue as it transcends the vertebral canal with growth and impairs oxidative metabolism.[17] Symptoms are related to excessive tension on the lumbosacral cord and can include scoliosis, altered gait pattern, changes in muscle strength at or below the lesion, disturbance in urinary and bowel patterns, and back pain.[18]

EVALUATION AND TREATMENT Diagnosis is based on clinical manifestations and examination of the meningeal sac. However, because the pathophysiology of myelodysplasia is determined early in gestation, prenatal diagnosis is possible through ultrasonography. In addition, the presence of a neural tube defect may result in an elevated amniotic fluid AFP level and subsequent maternal serum AFP levels. Prenatal diagnosis offers the parents the option to terminate the pregnancy or become a candidate for fetal intrauterine repair.[19,20] Cesarean delivery may be recommended to minimize trauma to the open myelomeningocele.[21]

Treatment for the infant with myelomeningocele is early surgical closure of the defect. Intrauterine surgery can be completed.[22] Because myelodysplasia affects several other body systems (e.g., renal, gastrointestinal, musculoskeletal), these infants require a lifetime, comprehensive, multidisciplinary approach to treatment. The prognosis depends on the extent of the involvement at birth and the success of prophylactic and acute treatment for potential and actual complications that affect the many body systems. Symptomatic Arnold-Chiari type II malformations require surgical decompression and/or placement of cerebrospinal fluid shunts.[11]

Spina Bifida and Spina Bifida Occulta

When defects of neural tube closure occur, such as meningocele and myelomeningocele, an accompanying vertebral defect allows the protrusion of the neural tube contents. Such a defect is called **spina bifida** (split spine). The cause of spina bifida is unknown. Periconceptual maternal folate deficiency and genetic alterations are commonly associated with the defect.[23] It also is possible for a defect to occur without any visible exposure of meninges or neural tissue. Because the defect is not apparent to the naked eye (i.e., it is "occult" or hidden), the term **spina bifida occulta** is used. In spina bifida occulta the posterior vertebral laminae have failed to fuse. This extremely common defect occurs to some degree in 10% to 25% of infants. Approximately 80% of these vertebral defects are located in the lumbosacral regions, most commonly in the fifth lumbar vertebra and the first sacral vertebra, and may be detected prenatally with ultrasonic scanning and AFP testing. About 3% of normal adults have spina bifida occulta of the atlas (cervical vertebra 1). The following cutaneous or subcutaneous abnormalities suggest underlying spina bifida:

- Abnormal growth of hair along the spine, which often is either very coarse or very silky
- A midline dimple with or without a sinus tract
- A cutaneous angioma, usually of the "port-wine" variety
- A subcutaneous mass, usually representing a lipoma or dermoid cyst

Spina bifida occulta usually causes no serious neurologic dysfunctions.[24] The spinal cord and spinal nerves generally are anatomically and functionally normal. When dysfunctions occur, the common lumbosacral defects cause gait abnormalities, positional deformities of the feet as a result of muscle weakness, or sphincter disturbances of the bladder and bowel. These dysfunctions become evident during periods of rapid growth. Surgical closure is usually completed in the neonatal period and techniques are being developed for intrauterine closure.[25]

Cranial Deformities

Skull malformations range from minor, insignificant defects to major defects that are incompatible with life.

Acrania

In **acrania** the cranial vault is almost completely absent and an extensive defect of the vertebral column often is present. Acrania associated with anencephaly (absence of brain and spinal column) occurs in approximately 1 per 1000 live births and is incompatible with life. The malformation results from a failure of the cranial end of the neural tube to close during the fourth gestational week. Subsequently, the cranial vault fails to form.

Craniosynostosis

Craniosynostosis (craniostenosis) is the premature closure of one or more of the cranial sutures during the first 18 to 20 months of an infant's life. The incidence of craniosynostosis is 1 in 1800 to 2200 live births.[26] Males are affected twice as often as females. Craniosynostosis can occur as part of a syndrome or as an isolated defect. **Nonsyndromic craniosynostosis** is classified as *simple craniosynostosis* when only one suture is involved and *compound craniosynostosis* when two or more sutures are involved. Each suture closure may represent a different disease.[27] Craniosynostosis prevents normal skull expansion and causes asymmetric skull growth. Premature closure of a suture causes failure of the growth of the bone located at a right angle to the involved suture. Compensatory growth occurs in regions where the sutures are patent, and this causes the various cosmetic deformities. In the absence of adequate sutures, cerebral growth may exceed the space present. Brain growth may be restricted, and compression may cause neurologic dysfunction from brain damage after 6 months of age (Figure 19-8).

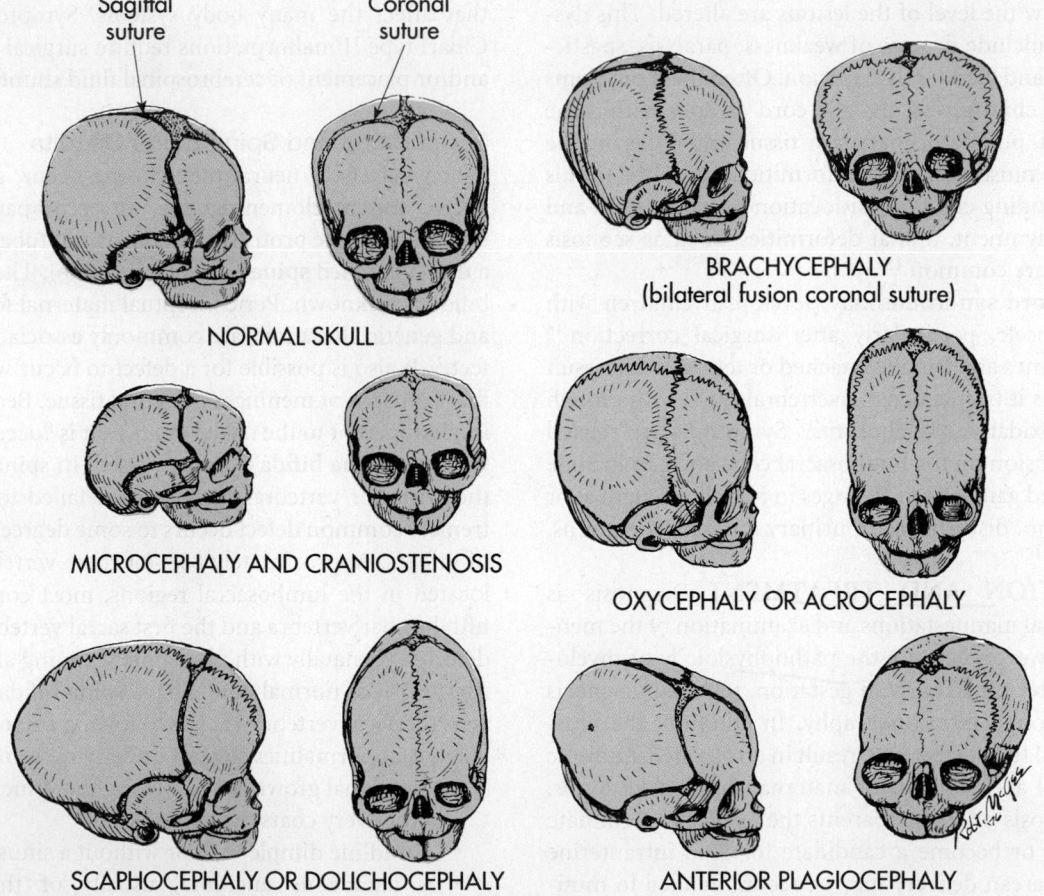

Figure 19-8 Craniosynostosis. Abnormal head configuration resulting from premature closing of cranial sutures. *Normal skull,* Bones separated by membranous seams until sutures gradually close. *Microcephaly and craniostenosis,* Microcephaly is head circumference more than 2 standard deviations below the mean for age, gender, race, and gestation and reflects a small brain; craniosynostosis is premature closure of sutures. *Scaphocephaly or dolichocephaly* (frequency 56%), Premature closure of sagittal suture, resulting in restricted lateral growth. *Brachycephaly,* Premature closure of coronal suture, resulting in excessive lateral growth. *Oxycephaly or acrocephaly* (frequency 5.8% to 12%), Premature closure of all coronal and sagittal sutures, resulting in accelerated upward growth and small head circumference. *Anterior plagiocephaly* (frequency 13%), Unilateral premature closure of coronal suture, resulting in asymmetric growth. (From Hockenberry JH et al: *Wong's nursing care of infants and children,* ed 7, St Louis, 2003, Mosby.)

PATHOPHYSIOLOGY The exact causes of craniosynostosis are unknown, but the condition represents more than a single disorder of embryonic development with mutations in multiple cytokine signaling pathyways.[28] **Syndromic craniosynostosis** involves mutations in several genes and accounts for about 30% of cases and chromosomal alterations account for another 10%.[29] More than 100 syndromes have been identified, with Apert and Crouzon syndromes as the most common, and involve fibroblast growth factor signaling pathways.[30] Most cases of craniosynostosis are nonsyndromic with no identifiable gene mutation.[31]

CLINICAL MANIFESTATIONS Craniosynostosis is classified according to head contour or suture involvement.[31] Final skull contour is determined by the sutures that close, the duration and order of closure, and the ability of other sutures to compensate by expansion. (The frequency and types of craniosynostosis are depicted in Figures 19-8 and 19-9.)

Premature closure of the sagittal suture, the most common form of craniosynostosis, causes elongation of the skull in the anteroposterior direction. Other anomalies are seen in 25% of these children. When the coronal suture fuses prematurely, the brain expands in a lateral direction. This type of craniosynostosis is associated with a 33% to 66% incidence of associated anomalies. Approximately half of these children are mentally retarded.

EVALUATION AND TREATMENT Craniosynostosis must be differentiated from the more benign skull deformity known as positional plagiocephaly (flattening of one side of the head).[31] Diagnosis is made on the basis of physical examination, head circumference measurements, and radiologic examination. Surgical treatment is indicated when closure of multiple sutures causes chronic increased intracranial pressure. Surgery then limits the extent of brain damage. In children with craniosynostosis of one suture, surgery often is performed for cosmetic purposes to limit the appearance of deformity.[32]

Microcephaly

Microcephaly is a rare defect in brain growth as a whole (see Figure 19-8). The word *microcephaly* is derived from the Greek (*mikro*, "small"; *kephale*, "head"). Cranial size is significantly below average for the infant's age, sex, race, and gestation. The small size of the skull reflects a small brain, except in infants with premature closure of the sutures. The condition is not treatable.

True (primary) microcephaly (present at birth) can be caused by genetic alterations, including autosomal dominant, autosomal recessive, or X-linked genes, or various chromosomal abnormalities. Environmental causes include toxin exposure during the period of induction and major cell migration (Box 19-1). Radiation, intrauterine infection, or chemical exposure may be the initiating factor. *Secondary microcephaly* (develops postnatally) is associated with a variety of causes including infection, trauma, metabolic disorders, maternal anorexia experienced during the third trimester of pregnancy, and the presence of other genetic syndromes.[33]

Microcephalic brain weight may be as low as 25% of normal, and the number and size of the cortical gyri may be diminished. Growth of the frontal lobes is severely stunted, and the cerebellum often is disproportionately large. In microcephaly caused by perinatal or postnatal disorders, neuronal loss and gliosis may be present in the cerebral cortex. The neurologic manifestations of microcephaly range from decerebrate posture, complete unresponsiveness, and autistic behavior to mild motor impairment, mental retardation, and hyperkinesis.

Congenital Hydrocephalus

Congenital hydrocephalus is characterized by an increased volume of CSF. This increase in volume may be caused by a blockage within the ventricular system in which the CSF flows, an imbalance in production of the CSF, or a reduced reabsorption of the CSF that results in ventricular enlargement and increased ICP. The pressure within the ventricular system

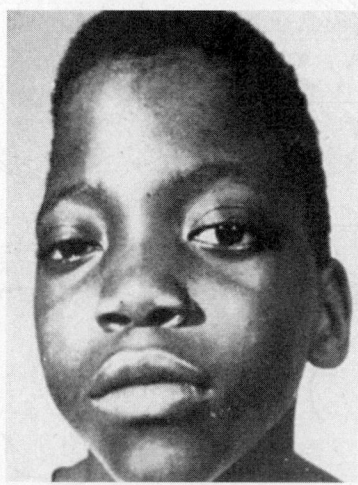

Figure 19-9 Dolichoscaphocephaly in 14-year-old boy. One of the less threatening types of craniosynostosis. (From Dyken PR, Miller MD: *Facial features of neurologic syndromes*, St Louis, 1980, Mosby.)

Box 19-1	Causes of Microencephaly

Defects in Brain Development
Hereditary (recessive) microcephaly
Down syndrome and other trisomy syndromes
Fetal ionizing radiation exposure
Maternal phenylketonuria
Seckel syndrome
Cornelia de Lange syndrome
Rubinstein-Taybi syndrome
Smith-Lemli-Opitz syndrome
Fetal alcohol syndrome

Intrauterine Infections
Congenital rubella
Cytomegalovirus infection
Congenital toxoplasmosis
Congenital syphilis

Perinatal and Postnatal Disorders
Intrauterine or neonatal anoxia
Severe malnutrition in early infancy
Neonatal herpesvirus infection

pushes and compresses the brain tissue against the skull cavity. When hydrocephalus develops before fusion of the cranial sutures, the skull has the capacity to increase its effort to accommodate this additional space-occupying volume and to preserve neuronal function. The overall incidence of hydrocephalus is approximately 3 per 1000 live births.[34] The incidence of hydrocephalus, excluding the hydrocephalus associated with myelomeningocele, is approximately 0.5 to 1 per 1000 live births, with aqueductal stenosis as the cause for approximately one third of these cases.[35] (Types of hydrocephalus are discussed in Chapter 16.)

PATHOPHYSIOLOGY Obstructive hydrocephalus is caused most commonly by congenital aqueduct stenosis. The cerebral aqueduct is narrowed or replaced by multiple channels, or "forks," that end blindly. In a small number of children the stenosis is transmitted as an X-linked recessive trait. The **Dandy-Walker malformation** is a congenital defect of midline cerebellar structures and fourth ventricle in which hydrocephalus is caused by atresia of the foramina of Luschka or Magendie, leading the ventricular flow of CSF into a "blind pouch." Other causes of obstructions within the ventricular system that can result in hydrocephalus include brain tumors, cysts, trauma, arteriovenous malformations, blood clots, and infections.

CSF travels throughout the ventricular system, surrounds the brain, and is reabsorbed into the venous system by the arachnoid villi. Blockage of the arachnoid villi may occur in conditions such as bacterial or viral meningitis, intraventricular hemorrhage, and subarachnoid hemorrhage, or may result from congenital malformations within this area. In this instance CSF flows or communicates effectively but is unable to be reabsorbed, resulting in hydrocephalus.

CLINICAL MANIFESTATIONS Congenital hydrocephalus may cause fetal death in utero, or the increased head circumference may require cesarean delivery of the infant. Symptoms of this condition depend directly on the cause and rate of hydrocephalus development. Infants may have no symptoms at birth. During the early weeks of life, the head begins to grow at an abnormal rate. Significant dilation of the ventricles may occur before an abnormal increase in head growth develops. The fontanels enlarge and become full and bulging (Figures 19-10 and 19-11). The separation of the cranial sutures leads to a resonant note when the skull is tapped, a manifestation termed **Macewen sign ("cracked-pot" sign).** The eyes may assume a staring expression, with sclera visible above the cornea, called *sunsetting.*

The infant may have difficulty holding the head upright. The scalp skin is thin and shiny, and scalp veins may become prominent. The large cranial vault and the face are disproportionate, and frontal bossing may be present. The infant's cry becomes high pitched as ICP rises; irritability, lethargy, vomiting, and other signs of increased ICP may develop. Dramatic head growth and enlargement, compression of the optic nerves, and optic chiasm occur in chronic, untreated hydrocephalus. However, because of early surgical intervention, these signs of hydrocephalus rarely are seen. When hydrocephalus develops late in childhood, the head may not have the capacity to enlarge, and evidence of increased ICP is present (see Chapter 16).

The relationship between hydrocephalus and mental retardation has been heavily debated. Correlation between the degree of hydrocephalus and impaired cognitive function often is a result of additional complications, such as severe congenital malformations, acute or chronic infections, or progressive brain tumors. Approximately two thirds of children with uncomplicated congenital hydrocephalus treated successfully with shunting may have normal to borderline intelligence.[36]

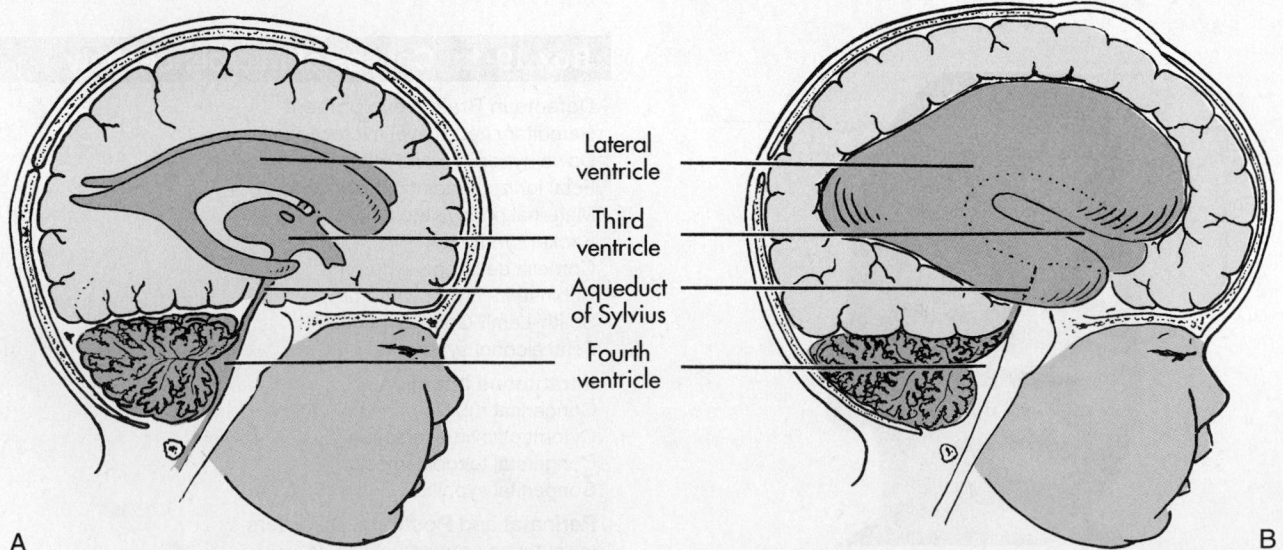

Lateral ventricle

Third ventricle

Aqueduct of Sylvius

Fourth ventricle

A   B

Figure 19-10 Hydrocephalus. A block in the flow of cerebrospinal fluid (CSF). **A,** Patent cerebrospinal fluid circulation. **B,** Enlarged lateral and third ventricles caused by obstruction of circulation—stenosis of aqueduct of Sylvius. (From Hockenberry MJ et al: *Wong's essentials of pediatric nursing,* ed 8, St Louis, 2009, Mosby.)

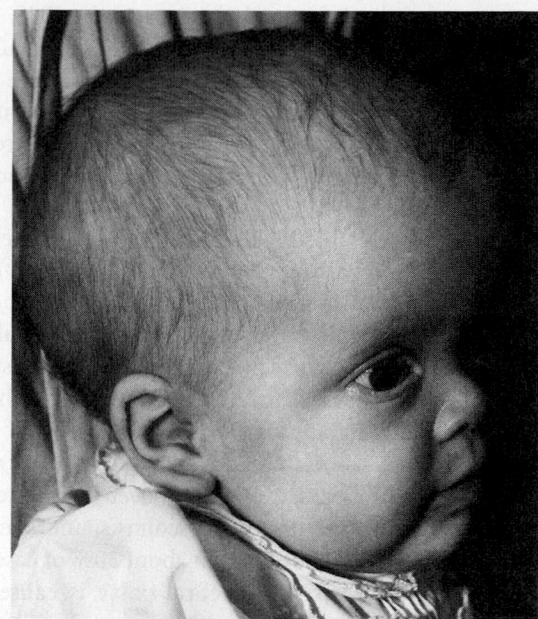

Figure 19-11 Child with enlarged head caused by hydrocephalus. (From McLaurin DC: *Pediatric neurosurgery,* ed 2, Philadelphia, 1989, Saunders.)

EVALUATION AND TREATMENT The definitive diagnostic tool for hydrocephalus is computed tomography (CT), and magnetic resonance imaging (MRI) may add information about the specific cause of the hydrocephalus. In infancy, head circumference measurements also are obtained and monitored. The treatment is surgical placement of a shunt to divert the excess CSF from the ventricular cavity to other areas of the body. Several types of shunts are available.[37] The main objective of any shunt system is to decrease ICP and preserve neuronal function. With neurosurgical intervention and follow-up, the 5-year survival usually is greater than 80%. Most deaths that occur within this category result from severe congenital malformations and/or progressive disorders such as brain tumors. Children with hydrocephalus depend on the internal shunt system to maintain safe ICPs and therefore are forever at risk for sudden failure of this system, which leads to acute increased ICP and death.

ENCEPHALOPATHIES

Encephalopathy, a pathology involving the brain, is a general category of syndromes and diseases that include infections, ischemia, and metabolic and toxic causes. Encephalopathies in children are associated with a great variety of known and suspected causes. These disorders may be acute or chronic and static or progressive.

Static Encephalopathies

Brain injury may occur during gestation or birth or at any time during childhood growth and development, causing a static, nonprogressive disorder. The clinical manifestations depend on the site and extent of the injury, as well as the age of the child and stage of development at the time of injury. Varying degrees of impairment may result from diffuse or localized injury to the cortex. For example, cerebral palsy results when the motor areas of the brain are injured. Injury to the occipital lobe of the cerebral cortex early in gestation can interfere with normal cerebral maturation and result in blindness. Cognitive impairment may follow diffuse cerebral injury. Seizures also may develop from cortical injury, particularly if scar tissue remains.

Prenatal factors that affect the developing nervous system may be endogenous or exogenous. The fetus may be affected by impaired embryo implantation, chromosomal abnormalities, infection, trauma, radiation, and toxic substances. Maternal toxemia, diabetes mellitus, and maternal nutritional deficiencies can produce neurologic damage in the fetus. The developing nervous system is most susceptible to injury occurring during the first trimester of pregnancy. Anoxia, trauma, and infections are the most common factors that cause injury to the nervous system in the perinatal period. Infections, metabolic disturbances (acute or a result of inborn errors), trauma, toxins, and vascular disease may injure the nervous system in the postnatal period.

Cerebral Palsy

Cerebral palsy (CP) is the term given to a diverse group of nonprogressive syndromes that affect the brain and cause motor dysfunction beginning in early infancy. Although cerebral palsy is by definition nonprogressive, its clinical manifestations change with growth and maturation of the child.

Cerebral palsy is one of the most common crippling disorders of childhood, affecting nearly 500,000 children in the United States alone. Although the exact incidence is unknown, studies suggest that the incidence is 1 to 2.3 cases of cerebral palsy per 1000 live births.[38,39] Causes of cerebral palsy are numerous, and genetic as well as environmental factors may be responsible. These factors can occur during the prenatal (most common), perinatal, or postnatal period (Table 19-3).

PATHOPHYSIOLOGY Several factors, alone or in combination, can produce brain damage that leads to cerebral palsy. Prenatal cerebral hypoxia, congenital malformations, and placental pathology can contribute to the systemic degeneration of immature areas of the brain white matter and interfere with cell maturation.[40] The severity of the damage depends on the gestational age at the time of the injury and the degree of injury sustained.

Low birth weight and birth asphyxia are commonly identified risk factors for cerebral palsy.[41,42] Hypoxia and asphyxia are known to cause edema in the brain. Lack of oxygen and the incorporation of amino acids during protein synthesis lead to acidosis. Carbon dioxide and lactic acid accumulate with acidosis, causing osmotic pressure changes. This condition contributes to generalized cerebral swelling and CNS damage. Magnesium sulfate in preterm newborns and head cooling during or after resuscitation at birth may reduce brain damage and risk of cerebral palsy.[43,44]

Table 19-3	Cerebral Palsy: Predisposing Factors and Known Causes	
Risk Factors	**Associated Causes**	
Prenatal		
Maternal	Metabolic diseases	
	Nutritional deficiencies (e.g., anemia)	
	Twin or multiple births	
	Bleeding	
	Toxemia	
	Blood incompatibilities	
	Exposure to radiation	
	Infection (e.g., rubella, toxoplasmosis, cytomegalic inclusion disease)	
	Premature labor	
Prematurity	Asphyxia leading to cerebral hemorrhage	
Genetic factors	Absence of corpus callosum, aqueductal stenosis, cerebellar hypoplasia	
Congenital anomalies of the brain	Unknown causes not evident on clinical examination	
Perinatal	Anesthesia or analgesia during labor and delivery	
	Mechanical trauma during delivery	
	Immaturity at birth	
	Metabolic disorders (e.g., hyperbilirubinemia, hypoglycemia, amino acid disorders, hyperosmolality)	
	Electrolyte disturbances (e.g., hypernatremia, hypoglycemia)	
Postnatal	Head trauma	
	Infections (e.g., meningitis, encephalitis)	
	Cerebrovascular accidents	
	Toxicosis	
	Environmental toxins (e.g., lead ingestion, methyl mercury ingestion from contaminated fish)	

Vascular abnormalities, arterial or venous stasis, and thrombosis can occur as a result of tissue hypoxia or as unrelated structural alterations. These anomalies may result in direct brain trauma that leads to infarction, intraventricular hemorrhage, and subarachnoid hemorrhage. Intraventricular hemorrhage is a common cause of death in newborn infants. Such injuries contribute to CNS damage.

Physical trauma to the central or peripheral nervous system can occur during the birthing process. Linear and depressed fractures are seen in newborns when head molding is extreme, with resultant hemorrhages and tears of the tentorium or falx cerebri. Tearing of the superficial cerebral veins is a relatively common occurrence and causes a thin layer of blood over the cerebral convexity. This blood may irritate the brain and result in CNS dysfunction. The infant's position during delivery may cause stretching and damage to nerves. Breech deliveries can cause traumatic injury to the brainstem or spinal cord, resulting in a more localized area of impairment. Malformations of the CNS play an important role in brain injury from perinatal trauma and predispose the infant

to a greater probability of sustained injury to the CNS. Both faulty maturation of the nervous system and a greater vulnerability to perinatal trauma and hypoxia are responsible for a high incidence of neurologic dysfunction in the preterm infant. Genetic, teratogenic, and early pregnancy influences on the development of cerebral palsy are multifactorial and not yet fully understood.[45]

CLINICAL MANIFESTATIONS The syndromes associated with cerebral palsy can be classified according to the areas of the brain that are damaged, pyramidal (spastic) and extrapyramidal (nonspastic). **Pyramidal/spastic cerebral palsy** results from damage or defects in the brain's corticospinal pathways (upper motor neuron) in either one or both hemispheres and accounts for approximately 70% to 80% of cerebral palsy cases. It is associated with increased muscle tone, prolonged primitive reflexes, exaggerated deep tendon reflexes, clonus, rigidity of the extremities, scoliosis, and contractures. Cognitive impairment occurs in about 30% of cases.[46]

Extrapyramidal/nonspastic cerebral palsy is caused by damage to cells in the basal ganglia, thalamus, or cerebellum and includes two subtypes: dyskinetic and ataxic. **Dyskinetic cerebral palsy** is associated with extreme difficulty in fine motor coordination and purposeful movements. Movements are jerky, uncontrolled, and abrupt, resulting from injury to the basal ganglia or thalamus. This form of cerebral palsy accounts for approximately 20% to 25% of cases. **Ataxic cerebral palsy** is associated damage to the cerebellum and manifests with gait disturbances and instability. The infant with this form of cerebral palsy may have hypotonia at birth, but stiffness of the trunk muscles develops by late infancy. This lack of flexibility exaggerates the infant's inability to balance body position without support. Persistence of this increased tone in truncal muscles affects the child's gait and ability to maintain equilibrium and depth perception. This form of cerebral palsy accounts for approximately 5% of cases. A child may have symptoms of each of these cerebral palsy types, which leads to a mixed-variety disorder that accounts for approximately 13% of cases.

Children with cerebral palsy often have associated neurologic disorders, such as seizures (35% to 50%), intellectual impairment ranging from mild to severe (50% to 75%), and visual impairment (50%). Because standardized intelligence tests do not allow for the physical handicaps of cerebral palsy, the incidence of associated cognitive impairment is uncertain. Other associated complications include but are not limited to hearing impairment, communication disorders, respiratory problems, bowel and bladder problems, and orthopedic disabilities.[46]

EVALUATION AND TREATMENT Diagnosis of cerebral palsy is made on the basis of neurologic examination and history. The management of children with cerebral palsy varies with age, type and severity of involvement, and associated disorders. Thus the scope of care required by the child and family includes ongoing medical, social and educational intervention, and a family-focused multidisciplinary team approach.[47]

Although the brain injury is static, the clinical picture of cerebral palsy may change with growth and development. The use of intrathecal baclofen pumps, botulinum toxin, and selective dorsal rhizotomy for spasticity has shown improvement in selected children with cerebral palsy.[48,49]

Inherited Metabolic Disorders of the Central Nervous System

A large number of inherited metabolic disorders have been identified. Because these disorders are inherited, their manifestations usually occur in infancy and childhood. Typically these metabolic disorders damage the entire CNS so extensively that these children do not survive to adulthood. The clinical syndromes of the inherited metabolic disorders depend on the nature of the biochemical defect and the stage of nervous system maturation. (Table 19-4 lists some of these inherited metabolic disorders.) Defects in amino acid and lipid metabolism are more common than rarely occurring defects in carbohydrate metabolism.

Defects in Amino Acid Metabolism

Biochemical defects in amino acid metabolism may be classified as (1) those in which the transport of amino acid is impaired, (2) those involving an enzyme or cofactor deficiency, and (3) those grouped around certain chemical components, such as sulfur-containing amino acids.[50] Most of the disorders in the literature described to date suggest that the absence of enzymatic activity most often is caused by the genetically determined absence of the enzyme protein.

Diseases caused by an enzymatic deficiency are associated with increased blood concentrations of the amino acid whose degradation pathway is impaired and with the presence of the amino acid in the urine. Because the normal pathway is blocked, small amounts of certain metabolites are found in the blood. Thus in certain diseases, an increase of compromised amino acids and unusual metabolites may appear in blood and urine concentrates.[51]

Phenylketonuria. Phenylketonuria (PKU) is an inborn error of metabolism characterized by the inability of the body to convert the essential amino acid phenylalanine to tyrosine (Figure 19-12). PKU is caused by phenylalanine hydroxylase deficiency and has a prevalence rate of 1 per 14,000 worldwide.[52] Because of its genetic component and distribution, this statistical prevalence varies widely on the basis of geographic and ethnic differences.[53] Most natural food proteins contain about 15% phenylalanine, an essential amino acid. Phenylalanine hydroxylase controls the conversion of this essential amino acid to tyrosine in the liver. The body uses tyrosine in the biosynthesis of protein, melanin, thyroxine, and the catecholamines in the brain and adrenal medulla. Phenylalanine hydroxylase deficiency causes an accumulation of phenylalanine in the serum and subsequently in the urinary excretion of abnormal metabolites called *phenyl acids*. One of these phenyl acids, phenylpyruvic acid, gives the urine a characteristic musty odor and is responsible for the name given to the disorder. Such high blood levels of phenylalanine prevent sufficient neutral amino acid entry into the brain,

Table 19-4	Inherited Metabolic Disorders of the Central Nervous System
Age of Onset	**Disorder**
Neonatal period	Pyridoxine dependency, galactosemia, maple syrup urine disease and its variant, phenylketonuria (PKU)
Early infancy	Tay-Sachs disease and its variants, infantile Gaucher disease, infantile Niemann-Pick disease, Krabbe disease (leukodystrophy), Farber lipogranulomatosis, Pelizaeus-Merzbacher disease and other sudanophilic leukodystrophies, spongy degeneration, Alexander disease, Alpers disease, Leigh disease (subacute necrotizing encephalomyelopathy), congenital lactic acidosis, Zellweger encephalopathy, Lowe disease (oculocerebrorenal disease)
Late infancy and early childhood	Disorders of amino acid metabolism, metachromatic leukodystrophy, late infantile GM1 gangliosidosis, late infantile Gaucher and Niemann-Pick diseases, neuroaxonal dystrophy, mucopolysaccharidosis, mucolipidosis, fucosidosis, mannosidosis, aspartylglycosaminuria, amaurotic idiocy (Jansky-Bielschowsky disease, Batten disease, Vogt-Spielmeyer disease, neuronal ceroid lipofuscinosis), Cockayne syndrome
Later childhood and adolescence	Progressive cerebellar ataxias of childhood and adolescence, hepatolenticular degeneration (Wilson disease), Hallervorden-Spatz disease, Lesch-Nyhan syndrome and other uremic states, familial calcification of vessels in basal ganglia and cerebellum, familial polymyoclonus, chronic familial leukodystrophy, homocystinuria, Fabry disease

which contributes to the neuropathologic process of PKU.[54] Abnormalities occur, such as anomalous development of the CNS, defective myelination, cystic degeneration of the gray and white matter, and disturbances in cortical layers. Unfortunately, brain damage occurs before the metabolites can be detected in the urine, and damage continues as long as phenylalanine levels remain high.

Clinical manifestations related to CNS damage range from mild to severe behavioral disturbances, self-abusive tendencies, and seizures. Because of the lack of tyrosine and its relationship to the biosynthesis of melanin, children with PKU have a characteristic phenotype that includes blond hair, blue eyes, and fair skin. Children with genetically darker complexions may be red haired or brunette.

Less severe variants of this disorder are caused by defects in the phenylalanine hydroxylase system rather than the phenylalanine hydroxylase itself. This related disorder, known as **hyperphenylalaninemia (HPA)**, occurs when plasma

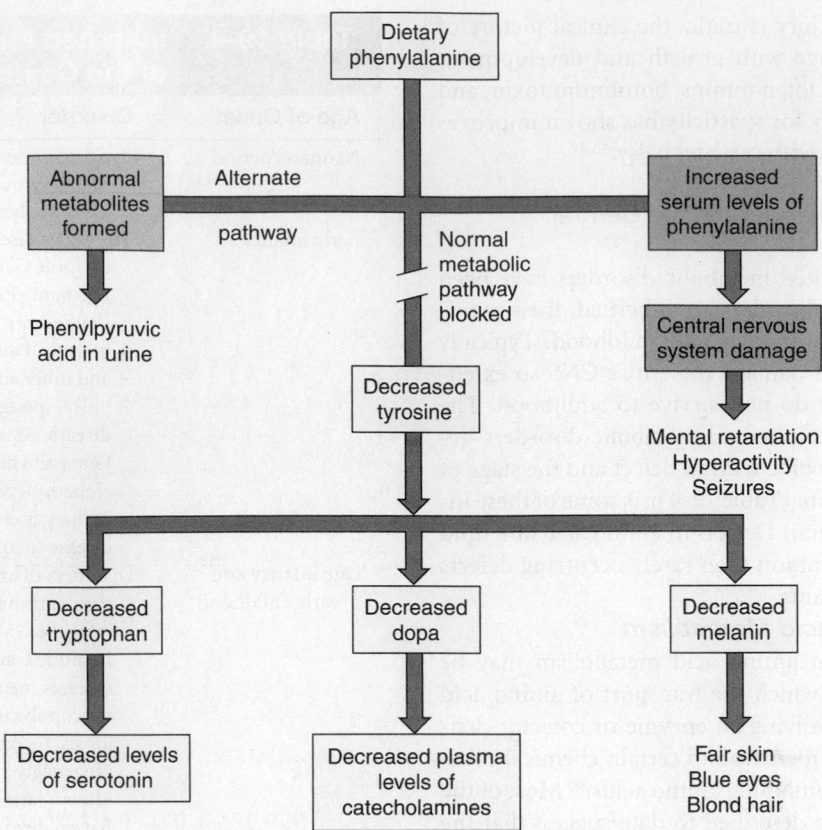

Figure 19-12 Metabolic errors and consequences in phenylketonuria. (Redrawn from Hockenberry MJ et al: *Wong's nursing care of infants and children*, ed 8, St Louis, 2007, Mosby.)

phenylalanine levels rise above normal but do not rise as high as in PKU.

Nonselective newborn screening is used to detect PKU and HPA in the United States and in more than 30 countries. Such programs are the greatest source of referrals and allow for accurate interpretation and follow-up of test results, including appropriate genetic and nutrition counseling.[53] Individuals with PKU also need to be screened for response to BH4 (6-R-L-erythro-5,6,7,8-tetrahydrobiopterin), which significantly decreases blood phenylalanine levels with oral supplements.[55]

Treatment for PKU involves restriction of phenylalanine in the diet to maintain a nontoxic level and supplement with phenylalanine free L-amino acids. The diet also must be supplemented with adequate sources of energy, protein, and nutrients to allow for optimum growth and brain development. Supplementation of tyrosine also may be required if plasma levels are low. Enzyme replacement and PKU gene therapy are under investigation.[56]

Defects in Lipid Metabolism

Disorders of lipid metabolism are termed **lysosomal storage diseases** because each disorder in this group can be traced to a missing lysosomal enzyme. (Lysosomes, the vesicles within the cell whose primary function is to degrade the breakdown products of cellular metabolism, are discussed in Chapter 1.) An estimated 25 to 30 enzymes within the lysosomes participate in the breakdown of lipids,

carbohydrates, proteins, and proteolipids A genetic defect results in a missing or defective enzyme and causes an excessive accumulation of a particular cell function. The enzyme defect may occur in the brain, liver, spleen, bone, or lung, thus involving several organ systems. Prenatal diagnosis is available. Therapy has been unsuccessful to date.

Tay-Sachs Disease. **Tay-Sachs disease** is a fatal autosomal recessive disorder (*HexA* gene on chromosome 15) caused by deficiency of the lysosomal enzyme hexosaminidase A (HexA), an enzyme that degrades GM2 gangliosides (fatty acids) within nerve cell lysosomes. Consequently there is accumulation of gangliosides (**gangliosidosis**) with toxicity to nerve cells.[57] Approximately 80% of individuals diagnosed are of Jewish ancestry, although sporadic cases appear in the non-Jewish population.[51] Prenatal screening is available.

In Tay-Sachs disease the pathologic changes predominate in the CNS, but neurons throughout the body contain characteristic changes in the cytoplasm. With time, neurons become distorted and balloon, and microglial cells, which also are swollen and filled with large granules, proliferate. Cystic degeneration of the cerebral white matter and atrophy of the cerebellar hemispheres often occur. The number of neurons is diminished. Changes in the spinal cord, particularly in the motor cells of the anterior horn of the cord, also are characteristic. Involvement of this region of the spinal cord results in hypotonia, hyporeflexia, and overall weakness.

Onset of this disease usually occurs when the infant is 3 to 6 months old. A loss of milestones is associated with an excessive startle response. Seizures, muscular rigidity, and blindness become prominent after the first year of life, and head size may increase. Death usually occurs by 2 to 5 years of age. No beneficial therapy has been developed. Genetic counseling programs are available, and some states require screening techniques for couples and those at risk who may be carriers.

Seizure Disorders in Children

Epilepsy

The incidence of epilepsy varies greatly with age. The incidence of epilepsy is estimated to be 0.5% to 1% of children with onset during infancy or childhood.[58] Infants are particularly susceptible during the first 12 months of life. The incidence decreases with age; 75% to 80% of epilepsy cases initially occur before 20 years of age, with 30% initially occurring within the first 4 years of life. Approximately 181,000 persons in the United States are newly affected each year.[58]

PATHOPHYSIOLOGY Seizures are the abnormal discharge of electrical activity within the brain. When a sufficient number of neurons become overexcited, they discharge abnormally, which sometimes results in clinical manifestations. If clinical manifestations develop, the specific physical activity that occurs may depend on the origin of the electrical activity and its extent within the brain. Repeated recurrence of seizure activity is known as **epilepsy.** Seizures may result from an underlying disorder of the CNS or a disorder that directly or indirectly affects normal CNS function (see Table 16-11). Certain types of seizures may have a genetic component or familial predisposition, or they can result from maternal diseases or congenital structural anomalies of the CNS. During the newborn period, asphyxia, intracranial hemorrhage, CNS infections, injury, electrolyte imbalances, and inborn errors of metabolism may cause seizures. Etiologic factors of seizures in older infants and children generally are the same as during the first month of life. Often the cause of seizures is unknown.

Seizures and seizure patterns may change as a child grows and develops. The differences between the immature and mature nervous systems may help explain the changing patterns of clinical seizures with age. The immature nervous system has a reduced capacity for sustaining well-organized seizures. Intracortical connections are poorly developed, and the sending of impulses throughout the cortex is limited. At the cellular level neurons are less capable of firing in repetitive high-frequency bursts. The excitatory output of a seizure focus is further diminished because the affected neurons do not act synchronously. In addition, changing neurotransmitters, immaturity of cells, and ongoing postnatal factors affect seizure expression in children.

CLINICAL MANIFESTATIONS The clinical manifestations at the time of diagnosis vary depending on the primary cause and the extent and involvement of abnormal electrical discharges within the neuronal tissue. Because of the diversities and complexities that seizure activity invariably displays, an international classification system was adopted (see Table 16-9).

This classification system groups seizures with similar clinical manifestations (see Table 16-10). Its general purpose is to assist the clinician with the assessment of the clinical course, the identification of the most appropriate treatment, and the evaluation of the individual's response to treatment.

The international classification system of epilepsy contains three major groupings: (1) partial seizures, (2) generalized seizures, and (3) unclassified epileptic seizures. Each major grouping is then divided into subsets on the basis of clinical manifestations and electroencephalogram (EEG) findings.

Partial seizures are characterized by seizure activity that begins in and usually is limited to one part of either the left or right hemisphere. A *simple partial seizure* refers to seizure activity that occurs without loss of consciousness. A *complex partial seizure* refers to seizure activity that occurs with impairment of consciousness. The clinical activity displayed by the individual is contingent on the particular part of the cortex from which the seizure is generated. For example, partial seizures may result in abnormal motor activity, such as twitching or loss of tone, or sensory changes, such as tingling or numbness.

Simple partial seizures generally are confined to one hemisphere, whereas a complex partial seizure involves both cerebral hemispheres. A simple or complex partial seizure may evolve into a generalized tonic-clonic, tonic, or clonic convulsion.

Generalized seizures are those in which the first clinical manifestations indicate that the seizure activity starts in or involves both cerebral hemispheres. Consciousness may be impaired in this grouping of seizures. The clinical manifestations may include convulsive activity (tonic-tonic, tonic, or clonic activity) or nonconvulsive activity (absence seizures). *Absence seizures* do not follow a mendelian pattern of inheritance that results from a single gene defect but rather have an autosomal dominant inheritance pattern.[59] Because both hemispheres are involved, the clinical manifestations almost always are bilateral.

Not all seizure disorders fit neatly into a classified grouping. These seizures are referred to as **unclassified epileptic seizures** and characteristically have a wide variety of abnormal clinical activity. Examples of this activity include rhythmic eye movements, chewing, and swimming movements. These activities are commonly seen in neonatal seizures.[60]

In addition to the seizures classified by the international system, there are several types of epileptic syndromes. These are seizure disorders that display a group of signs and symptoms that occur collectively and that characterize or indicate a particular condition. Several syndromes associated with epilepsy occur in infants and children. The three syndromes that occur most often are infantile spasms, Lennox-Gastaut syndrome, and juvenile myoclonic epilepsy.

Infantile spasms (also known as West syndrome) are a severe form of epilepsy characterized by a variety of clinical manifestations.[61] The infant may have episodes of sudden flexion or extension movements involving the neck, trunk, and extremities. Mutations in *ARX* and *CDKL5* genes and abnormal interneurons are involved in the pathogenesis of infantile spasms.[62] Clinical manifestations of the resulting spasms may range from subtle head nods to violent body contractions, commonly referred to as *jackknife seizures*. Onset of infantile spasms usually is between 4 and 8 months of age and may be idiopathic or may occur in response to a CNS insult.[63] An EEG will display the classic hypsarrhythmic chaotic pattern of epileptic spike and wave discharges on a slow, disorganized background. Infantile spasm manifests a typical clinical course. The "spasms" usually happen in clusters and occur 5 to 150 times per day. They usually are worse when the infant is waking up or falling asleep. Once begun, the seizure activity increases in intensity and severity over time. Invariably a loss of developmental milestones and disability is associated with this syndrome. Infantile spasms are also common (30%) in those with **tuberous sclerosis complex (TSC)**.[64] TSC develops from mutations in hamartin *(TSC1)* and tuberin *(TSC2)* genes. *Tubers* are cortical developmental malformations in the brain; they also form in other organs. Epilepsy associated with TSC is often difficult to treat and requires surgical intervention.[64]

Lennox-Gastaut syndrome is an epileptic syndrome characterized by an onset of seizures early in childhood, usually in males and around 1 to 5 years of age. This syndrome includes a variety of generalized seizures—predominantly tonic-clonic, atonic (drop attacks), akinetic, absence, and myoclonic activity. Mental retardation, delayed psychomotor development, personality disorders, and resistance to treatment are often associated with this syndrome.[65]

Juvenile myoclonic epilepsy is a primary generalized epilepsy that usually affects adolescents and young adults. Studies have indicated a possible locus on chromosomes 6p11, 15q14, 6q24, and 10q35 as a cause for this type of epilepsy.[66] It is a relatively benign form of epilepsy involving myoclonic jerks of the neck, shoulders, and arms. The seizures may occur singularly or repetitively. This form of epilepsy commonly is associated with a normal neurologic examination, normal intelligence, and a positive family history of seizures and is often underdiagnosed.[67]

EVALUATION AND TREATMENT Diagnosis of epilepsy and seizure classification are based on history, clinical presentation, physical and developmental examination, and the record of milestone achievements. Evaluation and testing include an EEG to isolate the focus or origin and involvement of seizure activity, MRI, or CT scan of the brain to investigate the presence of a lesion or abnormal tissue. A complete metabolic workup must be reviewed to explore the possibility of deficiency or malabsorption.[68]

Specific treatment for epilepsy is directed at the particular clinical manifestations or syndrome of seizure activity and its underlying causes. Treatment usually begins with the use of anticonvulsant medications. Often the epileptic pattern and clinical course require more than one drug to control the abnormal discharges.[69,70] A ketonic diet may be effective as a supplement treatment for epilepsy that is difficult to control with drugs[71,72] (see Nutrition & Disease: Ketogenic Diet in Children with Epilepsy).

NUTRITION & DISEASE

Ketogenic Diet in Children with Epilepsy

The goal of the ketogenic diet is to maintain a state of ketosis, which appears to facilitate reduced seizure frequency and severity for difficult-to-control seizures in children. The diet may be helpful to children who do not respond to conventional therapy or have intolerable side effects. Seizure reduction can occur within 5 to 14 days of initiating the diet. Two basic approaches to the ketogenic diet are (1) a traditional approach with four parts fat to one part carbohydrate/protein in the diet and (2) the medium-chain triglyceride (MCT) approach, in which MCTs make up about 50% to 70% of the diet. Either diet may be unpalatable and difficult to follow, particularly if the child has free access to food. Carbohydrates can be added by 5-g increments after 3 to 6 months if there has been no seizure activity, provided ketosis is maintained. Both dietary approaches include adequate protein for growth. A modified Atkins diet can also induce ketosis and does not restrict protein, fluid, or calories. The mechanisms are not clearly understood, but enhanced mitochondrial respiration, adenosine triphosphate (ATP) production, and decreasing kidney stones, reactive oxygen species may influence the dynamic of excitatory and inhibitory neurotransmitter systems in the brain and may be neuroprotective. Side effects can include acidosis, hypoglycemia, gastrointestinal distress, dehydration, lethargy, and poor growth.

Data from Zupec-Kania BA, Spellman E: *Nutr Clin Pract.* 23(6):589-596, 2009; Kossoff FH: *Epilepsia.* 49 Suppl 8:37-41, 2008; Vining EP: *Epilepsia.* 49 Suppl 8:27-29, 2008; Cross JH, Neal EG: *Epilepsia.* 49 Suppl 8:6-10, 2008; Kossoff EH et al: *Epilepsia.* 50(2):304-317, 2009; Neal EG et al: *Lancet Neurol* 7(6):500-506, 2008.

Surgery provides treatment for some forms of epilepsy that cannot be controlled with drugs. As with medical interventions, surgical therapy focuses on the particular clinical manifestations of seizure activity. Surgical interventions include resection of the epileptogenic zone of brain tissue (i.e., the temporal lobe for partial seizures or partial or complete severing of the corpus callosum for intractable generalized epilepsy). Children with intractable epilepsy have benefited somewhat from using the vagal nerve stimulator.[73]

Prognosis for epilepsy depends greatly on the type and severity of the disorder, the age of onset, coexisting factors, and the type and success of medical, surgical, and nutritional therapy. Several studies have estimated that approximately 40% to 50% of children diagnosed with epilepsy eventually will be seizure free.

Benign Febrile Seizures

Benign febrile seizures occur in 2% to 5% of children. These seizures usually are brief and self-limited and occur most often between the ages of 6 months and 5 years, with peak age at 14 to 18 months.[74,75]

PATHOPHYSIOLOGY The pathogenesis of benign febrile seizures is unknown. A familial incidence of benign febrile seizures indicates a genetic predisposition to the problem. Factors that contribute to susceptibility include age, degree and rate of temperature elevation, and nature of the particular fever-inducing illness. Any disorder producing a high fever may provoke benign febrile seizures in susceptible children.[76]

CLINICAL MANIFESTATIONS Characteristic features distinguish benign febrile seizures from seizures precipitated by fever:

1. Benign febrile seizures are rare before 9 months or after 5 years of age.
2. The convulsion occurs with a rise in temperature greater than 39° C (102.2 °F).
3. An acute respiratory or ear infection usually is present, with no evidence of CNS infection or inflammation.
4. Most seizures occur during the first 24 hours of the illness.
5. The convulsion is short (15 minutes or less), generalized, and predominantly tonic.
6. Interictal EEG is normal.
7. The seizure usually does not recur during the same infection.
8. No acute systemic metabolic disorder is present.

Complex febrile seizures have characteristic features similar to these except that (1) they have a longer duration than do benign febrile seizures, usually longer than 15 minutes; (2) they have focal characteristics; and (3) they usually occur more than once in a 24-hour period. Complex febrile seizures are considered a risk factor for the development of epilepsy and there may be a genetic predisposition.[77]

EVALUATION AND TREATMENT Reduction of elevated body temperature usually controls benign febrile seizures without anticonvulsant medication. In selected individuals, phenobarbital is the most effective medication for preventing recurrence of benign febrile seizures.

Status Epilepticus

Status epilepticus is defined as the state of continuing or recurring seizure activity in which the recovery from seizure activity is incomplete. Seizure activity is unrelenting and usually lasts for 30 minutes or more. Any one of the seizure activities discussed can evolve into status epilepticus. Status epilepticus is a medical emergency that requires immediate intervention.[78]

Acute Encephalopathies

Reye Syndrome

Reye syndrome is characterized by encephalopathy and fatty changes in a variety of organs, especially the liver. The incidence of Reye syndrome has declined sharply over the past 20 years, coinciding with increased public awareness of the association between ingestion of aspirin during illness and subsequent development of Reye syndrome.[79] Although Reye syndrome is becoming increasingly rare in the population, a brief overview of it is important for the following reasons:

1. It may be considered a prototype for acute hepatic encephalopathies.
2. The potential for recurrence is a factor.
3. The use of acetaminophen over aspirin should be considered important and discussed with the parents when obtaining a history.

PATHOPHYSIOLOGY Reye syndrome usually is associated with influenza B or varicella virus infections in children who have taken aspirin or aspirin-containing products. The exact cause of pathology is unknown, and inborn errors of metabolism can be a contributing factor.[80] A distinct clinical syndrome is apparent. The profound hypoglycemia, hypoketonemia, hyperammonemia, and increase in short-chain fatty acids in the serum after liver involvement are responsible for the cerebral manifestations. The liver shows diffuse deposits of lipids and absence of any inflammatory reaction or necrosis. Fatty degeneration of the kidneys leads to azotemia (excess urea in the blood). The brain is extremely edematous.[81,82]

The development of Reye syndrome has been linked to the administration of salicylates (aspirin). The American Association of Pediatrics has recommended not administering aspirin to children who have varicella or flulike symptoms. A direct relationship clearly exists between this recommendation and the overall decrease in incidence of Reye syndrome. A further reduction has occurred with administration of the varicella vaccine to children between 12 and 18 months of age.[83]

CLINICAL MANIFESTATIONS Typically Reye syndrome develops in a previously healthy child who is recovering from varicella, influenza B, upper respiratory infection, or gastroenteritis. The various clinical states are as follows:

Stage I—Vomiting, lethargy, drowsiness, nightmares

Stage II—Disorientation, delirium, aggressiveness and combativeness, central neurologic hyperventilation, shallow breathing, hyperactive reflexes, stupor

Stage III—Obtundation, coma, hyperventilation, decorticate rigidity

Stage IV—Deepening coma, decerebrate rigidity, loss of ocular reflexes, large fixed pupils, divergent eye movements

Stage V—Seizures, loss of deep tendon reflexes, flaccidity, respiratory arrest, extremely high blood ammonia levels, death

Death occurs in 30% to 40% of cases from brainstem dysfunction.[84]

EVALUATION AND TREATMENT According to the Centers for Disease Control and Prevention (CDC), the following conditions must be present for diagnosis of Reye syndrome:

1. Acute, noninflammatory encephalopathy documented by (a) alteration in level of consciousness and, if available, (b) a record of CSF containing leukocytes (8/mm³), and (c) a histologic specimen demonstrating cerebral edema without perivascular or meningeal irritation
2. Hepatomegaly documented by either a liver biopsy or autopsy
3. No more reasonable explanation for cerebral and hepatic abnormalities

The severity of the condition is inversely related to the age of the child at the onset of the illness.

The management of children with Reye syndrome ranges from simple monitoring to extremely complex neurointensive care. Treatment and outcome vary depending on the stage of involvement and the individual child's symptoms.

Intoxications of the Central Nervous System

Drug-induced encephalopathies always must be considered a possibility in the child with unexplained neurologic changes. Such encephalopathies may result from accidental ingestion, therapeutic overdose, intentional overdose, or ingestion of environmental toxins (the most commonly ingested poisons are listed in Box 19-2). About 2 million childhood poisonings that require medical attention occur each year, 1000 of which result in death.

High blood levels of lead occur in lead poisoning. If lead poisoning is not treated, lead encephalopathy will result and cause serious and irreversible neurologic damage[85,86] (Figure 19-13). Those at greatest risk are children 2 to 3 years of age and those prone to picas and living in lead-contaminated environments. **Pica** is the habitual, purposeful, and compulsive ingestion of nonfood substances such as clay, dirt, and paint chips. Lead intoxication also may occur from long-term exposure to smelters, sniffing of gasoline, lead-based paint, and ingestion of airborne lead.[87]

An estimated 275,000 to 810,000 U.S. children have excessive amounts of lead in their blood. Black children have a six times greater incidence of symptoms than white children. Most lead exposure is preventable.[87]

Meningitis

Meningitis is an inflammation of the meningeal coverings of the brain and spinal cord. The origin of such inflammation and acute encephalopathy can be caused by bacteria, viruses or other microorganisms. **Aseptic meninigitis** has no evidence of bacterial infection but may be associated with viral infection, systemic disease or drugs.

Bacterial Meningitis

Bacterial meningitis is one of the most serious infections to which infants and children are susceptible.[88] In the United States there are approximately 6000 cases per year of bacterial meningitis, of which half occur in children younger than 18 years of age. The microorganisms accountable for this illness are *Streptococcus pneumoniae* (1.1 per 100,000) and *Haemophilus influenza* type B (Hib) (0.2 per 100,000), especially in children beyond the neonatal period.

Before vaccines, *H. influenzae* type B was once the most common pathogen of bacterial meningitis in children younger than 5 years. The occurrence has dropped 95% with the advent of the Hib vaccine. Otitis media or sinusitis may be a precursor because the infections are almost always associated with a bacterium in the blood.

S. pneumoniae is the most common microorganism in children 1 to 23 months of age. Staphylococcal or streptococcal meningitis can occur in children of any age but shows a predilection for children who have had neurosurgery, skull fracture, or a complication of systemic bacterial infection. Infections that originate in the middle ear, sinuses, or mastoid cells also may lead to *S. pneumoniae* infection in children. In addition, this microorganism tends to occur in children with sickle cell disease or splenectomy. One in every 24 children with sickle cell disease develops pneumococcal meningitis by the age of 4 years. This incidence is 36 times greater than that found in the black population without sickle cell disease and 314 times greater than in white children. *Escherichia coli* and group B beta-hemolytic streptococci are the most common causes of meningitis in the newborn period.[89]

The second most common microorganism causing bacterial meningitis, particularly in children younger than 4 years, is *Neisseria meningitidis* (meningococcus) (groups A,B,C,Y and W135).[89] Approximately 2% to 5% of healthy children are carriers of *N. meningitidis*. The risk of meningitis in daycare center contacts of children with meningococcal disease is 1 per 1000.[90] During epidemics among military personnel, nasal and oral secretions from as many as 90% of those examined reveal *N. meningitidis*, suggesting a high rate of infectious transmission.

PATHOPHYSIOLOGY The cause of bacterial meningitis is related to the age of the child and to a number of factors that predispose the child to bacterial infection or that alter the child's response to an invading microorganism. Meningitis caused by *Staphylococcus aureus* or *Pseudomonas aeruginosa* may develop in the child with cystic fibrosis or severe burns. (For further discussion, see Chapter 17.) Infection with *N. meningitidis* is particularly virulent. Any microorganism may be pathogenic under the appropriate circumstances in a given individual.[91]

Pathogens enter the nervous system by direct extension from a contiguous (i.e., paranasal sinuses or mastoid cells) or, more commonly, by hematogenous spread (see Figure 17-32). Infection may spread through the blood to the meninges in children with infective endocarditis, pneumonia, thrombophlebitis, or after neurosurgical procedures. Many bacteria are very successful at evading normal defenses (see Chapter 9). Pathogens then cross the blood-brain barrier, enter the cerebrospinal fluid, and multiply. Bacterial toxins increase cerebrovascular permeability, causing alterations in blood flow and edema. Thrombosis and increased ICP can cause neurologic damage. Increased ICP may be increased further

---

Box 19-2	Common Poisons

Pharmacologic Agents	Heavy Metals	Miscellaneous Agents
Acetaminophen	Lead	Botulinum toxin
Amphetamines	Acute	Alcohols
Anticonvulsants	Chronic	Ethyl, isopropyl, methyl
Antidepressants	Mercury	Pesticides
Antihistamines	Thallium	Organophosphates
Atropine	Arsenic	Chlorinated
Barbiturates		hydrocarbons
Methadone		Mushrooms
Phencyclidine		Venoms
Salicylates		Snake bite
Tranquilizers		Tick paralysis
		Ethylene glycol

Data from Swaiman KF, Ashwal S: *Pediatric neurology: principles and practice,* vol 2, ed 3, St Louis, 1999, Mosby.

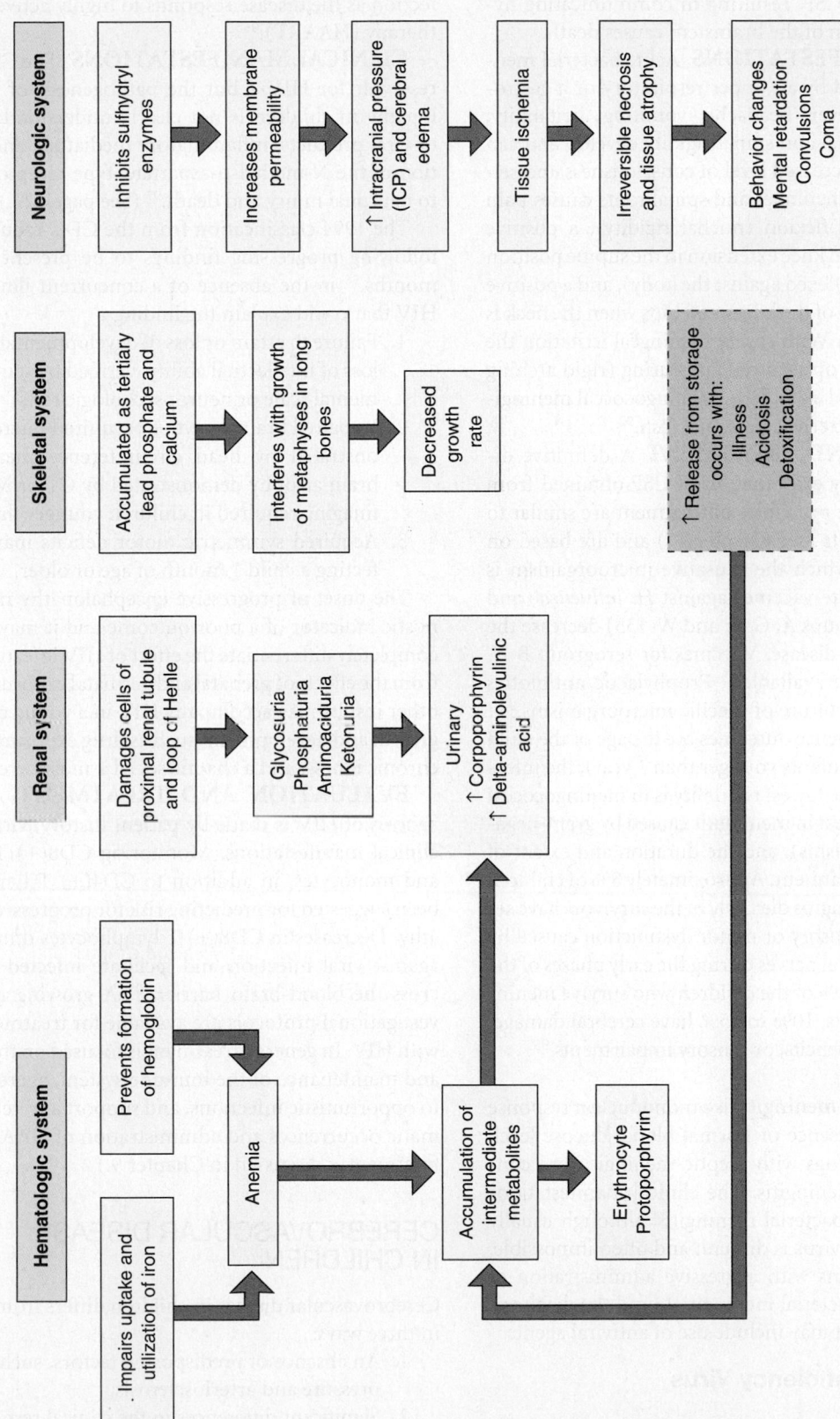

Figure 19-13 Systemic effects of increased lead absorption in children.

by obstruction to the CSF circulation. Thickened meninges and fibrous exudate in the subarachnoid space at the base of the brain obstruct the CSF, resulting in communicating hydrocephalus. Herniation of the brainstem causes death.

CLINICAL MANIFESTATIONS Acute bacterial meningitis often is preceded by an upper respiratory or a gastrointestinal infection. Fever, headache, vomiting, irritability, photophobia, and nuchal and spinal rigidity develop and can progress rapidly to a decreased level of consciousness and seizures. Irritation of the meninges and spinal roots causes pain and resistance to neck flexion (nuchal rigidity), a positive Kernig sign (resistance to knee extension in the supine position with the hips and knees flexed against the body), and a positive Brudzinski sign (flexion of the knees and hips when the neck is flexed forward rapidly). With severe meningeal irritation the child may demonstrate opisthotonic posturing (rigid arching of the back with the head extended). Meningococcal meningitis can produce a characteristic petechial rash.[92]

EVALUATION AND TREATMENT A definitive diagnosis is made only by examination of CSF obtained from a lumbar puncture. The principles of treatment are similar to those followed for adults (see Chapter 17) and are based on the culture results in which the causative microorganism is identified. The conjugate vaccines against *H. influenzae* and *N. meningitidis* (serogroups A, C, Y, and W-135) decrease the rate and spread of this disease. Vaccines for serogroup B *N. meningitidis* are not yet available.[93] Prophylactic antibiotics are effective guided by culture of specific microorganisms.[94]

The factors that influence outcomes are the age of the child (mortality is highest in infants younger than 1 year), the infective microorganisms (the lowest mortality is in meningococcal meningitis and the highest in meningitis caused by gram-negative enteric microorganisms), and the duration and extent of inflammation before treatment. Approximately 8% of children with *H. influenzae* meningitis die; 35% of the survivors have serious and permanent sensory or motor dysfunction caused by pressure on the peripheral nerves during the early phases of the illness. Approximately 5% of the children who survive meningitis have hearing deficits; 10% to 15% have cerebral damage, hydrocephalus, motor deficits, or sensory impairments.[95]

Viral Meningitis

The hallmark of **viral meningitis** is a mononuclear response in the CSF and the presence of normal blood glucose level. In some cases the findings with aseptic meningitis are consistent with bacterial meningitis. The clinical manifestations are similar to those in bacterial meningitis, although usually milder. Isolation of the virus is difficult and often impossible. Treatment usually begins with aggressive administration of antibiotics (potential bacterial meningitis) until the diagnosis is confirmed. Treatment may include use of antiviral agents.

Human Immunodeficiency Virus Encephalopathy

A particularly vulnerable site of human immunodeficiency virus (HIV) type-1 infection in infants and children is the CNS (see Chapter 9 for details of HIV infection).

PATHOPHYSIOLOGY Progressive HIV encephalopathy is an infrequent and reversible complication of HIV infection as the disease responds to highly active antiretroviral therapy (HAART).[96]

CLINICAL MANIFESTATIONS The CNS is a distinct reservoir for HIV-1 but the pathogenesis of HIV encephalopathy in children is not clearly understood. The presence of viral products, inflammatory mediators, and overstimulation of the *N*-methyl-D-aspartate–type receptor system leads to neuronal injury and death.[97] (See page 627.)

The 1994 classification from the CDC requires one of the following progressing findings to be present for at least 2 months,[98] in the absence of a concurrent illness other than HIV that could explain the findings:

1. Failure to attain or loss of developmental milestones, or loss of intellectual ability, verified by standard developmental scale or neuropsychologic tests
2. Impaired brain growth or acquired microcephaly demonstrated by head circumference measurements or brain atrophy demonstrated by CT or MRI with serial imaging required in children younger than 2 years
3. Acquired symmetric motor deficits manifested by affecting a child 1 month of age or older

The onset of progressive encephalopathy may be a prognostic indicator of a poor outcome and it may be difficult to completely differentiate the effect of HIV infection on the CNS from the effects of prenatal and perinatal exposure. In addition, other insults may accompany HIV in a young child and affect growth and development, such as drug exposure, prematurity, chronic illness, and a chaotic social atmosphere.[99,100]

EVALUATION AND TREATMENT A definite diagnosis of HIV is made by patient history, viral culture, and clinical manifestations. Monitoring CD8(+) T lymphocytes and monocytes, in addition to CD4(+) T lymphocytes, has been suggested for predicting risk for progressive encephalopathy. Decreases in CD8(+) T lymphocytes diminish defenses against viral infection and facilitate infected monocytes to cross the blood-brain barrier.[101] A growing number of investigational protocols are available for treatment of children with HIV. In general, treatment is focused on the preservation and maintenance of the immune system, aggressive response to opportunistic infections, and support and relief of symptomatic occurrences and administration of HAART.[97,102] (HIV treatment is discussed in Chapter 9.)

CEREBROVASCULAR DISEASE IN CHILDREN

Cerebrovascular disease in children differs from that in adults in three ways:

1. An absence of predisposing factors, such as high blood pressure and arteriosclerosis
2. Significant differences in the clinical response related to the developing nervous system and thus a greater capacity for the pediatric brain to recover from vascular insult
3. The anatomic site of the pathologic condition

Cerebrovascular disease can be divided into two categories: occlusive and hemorrhagic.

Occlusive Cerebrovascular Disease

Occlusive cerebrovascular disease is rare in children and may result from embolism, sinovenous thrombosis, or congenital or iatrogenic narrowing of vessels, which leads to a decreased flow of blood and oxygen to areas of the brain. Neonatal arterial ischemic stroke is estimated at 1 in 4000 live births and childhood stroke is about 2 to 8 in 100,000 in the United States. Sickle cell disease and cardiac anomalies are the most common disorders that lead to *arterial ischemic stroke*.[103]

Moyamoya disease is a rare, chronic, progressive vascular stenosis of the circle of Willis with obstruction of arterial flow to the brain. Moyamoya, a Japanese term, means "puff of smoke," which describes its appearance on CT examination. The vascularity may be a congenital anomaly, or it can develop as a result of cranial radiation therapy. Complications are developmental delay, mental retardation, and cerebral hemorrhage.[104,105] Treatment is surgical bypass of the occluded region.

Hemorrhagic Cerebrovascular Disease

PATHOPHYSIOLOGY Congenital cerebral arteriovenous malformations are the most common cause of intracranial bleeding and hemorrhagic stroke in children.[106] Hemorrhagic disease may result from vascular anomalies that lead to rupture, such as aneurysm, or from congenital arteriovenous malformation. The rupture and symptomatic development of a cerebral aneurysm is rare in children younger than 19 years. Intraventricular hemorrhage associated with premature birth is related to unstable blood pressure, and cerebral blood flow are contributing factors.[107]

CLINICAL MANIFESTATIONS The extent of the pathologic condition usually is less extensive in children than in adults. Symptoms may include degrees of hemiplegia (flaccid, spastic), weakness, seizures, headache, high fever, nuchal rigidity, hemianopia, sensory changes, facial palsy, and temporary aphasia.

EVALUATION AND TREATMENT Diagnosis of cerebrovascular disease is made through a series of tests, including CT, MRI, magnetic resonance angiography (MRA), angiogram, and echocardiogram.[108] History of evolving symptoms and past medical history are of vital importance in attaining an accurate diagnosis. Causative factors in the change in vascular flow often are not determined. Malformations vary in size, location, and symptoms, and these factors determine treatment. Options include surgery, radiation therapy, and embolic occlusion of the malformation[109] (see Chapter 17).

Excellent collateral circulation in the child's brain allows for more rapid recovery of motor function. The developing brain, however, may suffer more global, long-term effects, leading to mental retardation, behavior disorders, and seizures.

CHILDHOOD TUMORS

Brain Tumors

Brain tumors are the most common solid tumor and the second most common primary neoplasm in children, second only to leukemia. Approximately 50% of solid tumors in children are nonmalignant.[110] Overall, brain tumors account for nearly 20% of all childhood cancers, with an annual incidence of 2.4 to 4 per 100,000 in the United States; approximately 2000 cases are diagnosed each year.[111] Brain tumors remain the leading cause of death from disease in children ages 1 to 15 years.[112]

The cause of brain tumors is largely unknown, although genetic, environmental, and immune factors have been implicated in some tumor development. Other factors that have been investigated include familial tendencies, radiation, oncologic viruses, and chemical carcinogens.[113] An important area of study has been the relationship of parental occupation to subsequent brain tumors in offspring. Associations have been found with tumors and parental employment, for example, parental exposure to hydrocarbons and employment in the aircraft and paper/pulp industries. Alterations in embryologic development also may play a part in the development of childhood brain tumors. This theory suggests that tumors arise from cells that are "misplaced" during embryonic development, never maturing but later proliferating in this immature form. Chromosomal work has implicated the deletion of chromosomes 22 and 17 in some pediatric brain tumors. Further studies are being conducted that may affect the course of treatment for these children.[114] None of these factors, however, has proved significant.

PATHOPHYSIOLOGY Most childhood brain tumors arise from glial tissue, the supportive tissue of the brain. Tumors also may originate in other tissue such as nerve cells, cranial nerves, the pineal and pituitary glands, blood vessels, or neuroepithelium. Brain tumors are classified by the tissue and location from which they arise. Because a uniform pathologic nomenclature has yet to be established, inconsistencies occur when statistical data are compared.

Two thirds of all pediatric brain tumors are found in the posterior fossa region of the brain. This area also may be referred to as *infratentorial* because it is located below the tentorium. The tentorium is the layer of dura mater that separates the cerebellum from the hemispheres or cerebrum. Thus the area above the tentorium is referred to as the *supratentorial region*. Approximately one third of childhood brain tumors are located in the supratentorial space, whereas, in the adult population two thirds of brain tumors are located in the supratentorial region and only one third in the infratentorial region. The types and characteristics of childhood brain tumors are summarized in Table 19-5.

Brain tumors, by virtue of their location, have unique characteristics that distinguish them from tumors found elsewhere in the body. A number of brain tumors in children may be considered histologically benign yet clinically malignant and life threatening because of their location. For example, a tumor located in the brainstem region may appear benign under the microscope, but the clinical presentation threatens and all too often overrides the vital functions of the brainstem.

Table 19-5	Brain Tumors in Children
Type	**Characteristics**
Astrocytoma	Arises from astrocytes, often in the cerebellum or lateral hemisphere
	Slow growing, solid or cystic
	Often very large before diagnosed
	Varies in degree of malignancy
Optic nerve glioma	Arises from optic chiasm or optic nerve
	Slow-growing, low-grade astrocytoma
Medulloblastoma (infiltrating glioma)	Often located in cerebellum, extending into fourth ventricle and spinal fluid pathway
	Rapidly growing malignant tumor
	Can extend outside central nervous system
Brainstem glioma	Arises from pons or myeloencephalon
	Numerous cell types
	Compresses cranial nerves V through X
Ependymoma	Arises from ependymal cells lining ventricles
	Circumscribed, solid, nodular tumors
Craniopharyngioma	Arises near pituitary gland, optic chiasm, and hypothalamus
	Cystic and solid tumors that affect vision, pituitary, and hypothalamic functions

Types

Medulloblastoma, ependymoma, astrocytoma, brainstem glioma, craniopharyngioma, and optic nerve glioma make up approximately 75% to 80% of all pediatric brain tumors.[115] The location of brain tumors in children is illustrated in Figure 19-14; specific characteristics, treatment strategies, and prognoses are listed in Tables 19-5 and 19-6.

CLINICAL MANIFESTATIONS The actual location of the brain tumor dictates the presenting signs and symptoms (discussed in greater detail with each particular brain tumor type). In addition to tumor location and cell type, the rate of growth of the tumor also determines the presenting signs and symptoms. The ability of the brain and intracranial cavity to compensate for tumor growth is directly related to the rate of its growth. This compensatory mechanism allows the components of the intracranial space (blood, brain, and CSF) to adapt temporarily to slow changes in ICP. Therefore slow-growing tumors can grow to enormous size before signs and symptoms are apparent. Conversely, fast-growing tumors allow little time for compensation of the space-occupying lesion, and clinical symptoms occur quickly.

Signs and symptoms of brain tumors in children vary from generalized and vague to those that are localized and related specifically to the anatomic area. If the tumor is located in the posterior fossa region, the fourth ventricle may become blocked, which leads to hydrocephalus and signs of increased ICP. Increased ICP also may occur because of the additional mass volume within the fixed container of the skull vault. The symptoms of increased ICP include headache, vomiting, lethargy, and irritability. If a young child complains of a headache,

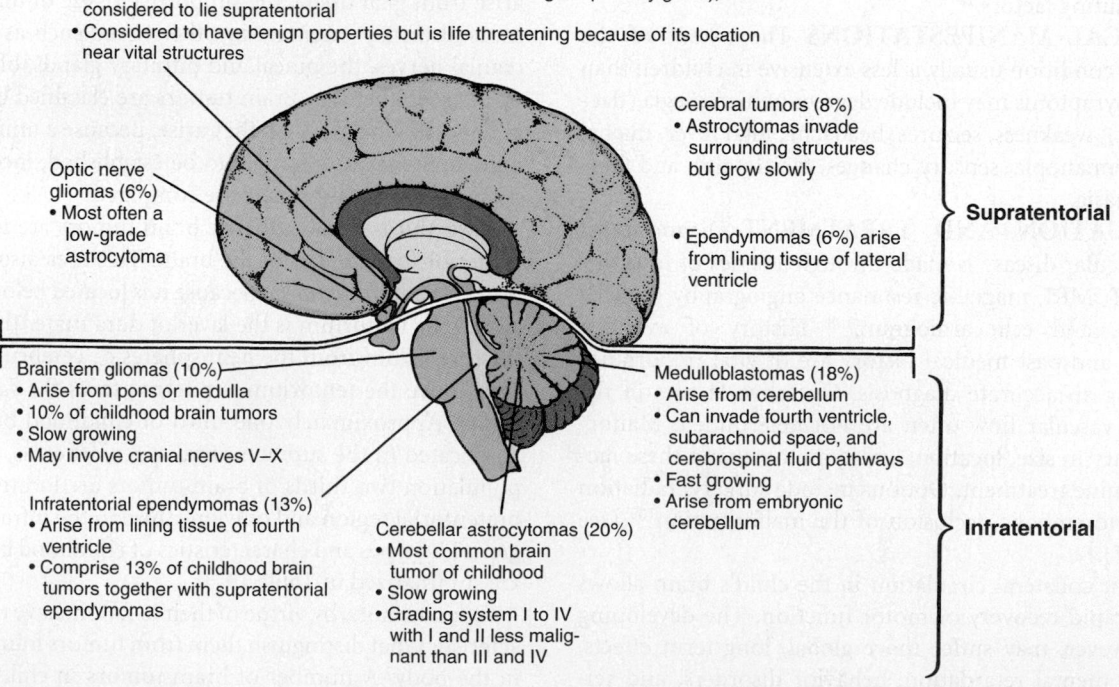

Figure 19-14 Location of brain tumors in children.

Table 19-6	Treatment Strategies for Childhood Brain Tumors
Tumor Type	**Treatment and Prognosis**
Cerebellar astrocytoma	Surgery; possibly curative
	Radiation and chemotherapy not proven successful but may delay recurrence
	Survival rate of more than 5 years in 50% to 75%; if tumor recurs, it does so very slowly
Medulloblastoma	Surgery, primarily as a partial resection to relieve increased intracranial pressure and "debulk" the tumor
	Type of treatment is age dependent
	Radiation is the primary treatment; may include spinal radiation
	Chemotherapy shows promise in conjunction with craniospinal radiation
	35% 5-year survival rate
Brainstem glioma	Surgery, resection occasionally possible
	Radiation, primarily palliative treatment
	Chemotherapy not yet proven beneficial, but new protocols being studied
	20% to 40% 5-year survival rate depending on total resection
Ependymoma	Tumor possibly indolent for many years
	Surgery rarely curative; risk of resecting an infratentorial tumor is too great
	Radiation for palliation (controversy regarding whether local or craniospinal radiation is better)
	Chemotherapy used for recurrent disease but with disappointing results
	20% to 80% 5-year survival rate depending on total resection
Craniopharyngioma	Surgery possibly successful when a complete resection is performed (partial resection usually requires further treatment)
	Radiation after partial surgical resection
	Chemotherapy not commonly used
	75% to 85% 5-year survival rate
Optic nerve glioma	Initial treatment controversial
	Surgery used for diagnosis or relief of hydrocephalus
	Radiation useful, particularly if the tumor is not treated by surgery
Cerebral astrocytoma	Surgery used if resection is possible
	Radiation useful for all grades of astrocytoma
	Chemotherapy beneficial in higher-grade tumors, but further study required

a thorough investigation should take place because headache is an uncommon complaint in young children. Headache caused by increased ICP usually is worse in the morning and gradually improves during the day when the child is upright and venous drainage is enhanced. Frequency of headache and other symptoms worsens as the tumor grows. A headache related to increased ICP generally occurs because of expansion of the lateral ventricle and cerebral hemisphere, which causes a stretching of the pain-sensitive dura mater. Irritability or possible apathy and increased somnolence also may result from increased ICP. Like headache, vomiting occurs more commonly in the morning. It frequently is not preceded by nausea and may become projectile, differing from a gastrointestinal disturbance in that the child may be ready to eat immediately after vomiting. Other signs and symptoms that can accompany increased ICP include increased head circumference with bulging fontanel in children younger than 2 years, cranial nerve palsies, and papilledema.

Localized findings relate to the degree of disturbance in physiologic functioning in the area where the tumor is located (see Table 17-9). Infratentorial tumors exhibit localized signs of impaired coordination and balance, including ataxia, gait difficulties, truncal ataxia, and loss of balance. A **medulloblastoma** is an embroynal tumor and the most common childhood malignant tumor. It occurs as an invasive tumor that develops in the vermis of the cerebellum and

may extend into the fourth ventricle.[116] Angiogenesis is the hallmark of progressive medulloblastomas. The **ependymoma** develops in the fourth ventricle and arises from the ependymal cells that line the ventricular system. The histology of the ependymoma varies, which makes the treatment course and prognosis difficult to establish. Because both tumors are located in the posterior fossa region along the midline, presenting signs and symptoms are similar. In addition to those already described, they may obstruct the fourth ventricle, resulting in hydrocephalus and generalized increased ICP, headache, nausea and vomiting, and nystagmus (involuntary eye movement).

In contrast, **cerebellar astrocytomas** are located on the surface of the right or left cerebellar hemisphere and cause unilateral symptoms (occurring on the same side of the tumor), such as head tilt, limb ataxia, and nystagmus when the eyes are turned toward the tumor.

Brainstem gliomas often cause a combination of cranial nerve involvement, cerebellar signs of ataxia, and corticospinal tract dysfunction. A common clinical pattern includes unilateral paralysis of cranial nerves with contralateral paralysis of the arm and leg, hyperreflexia, and extensor plantar responses. Increased ICP generally does not occur. Children with diffuse tumors usually die within 1 to 2 years.[117]

The area of the sella turcica, the structure containing the pituitary gland, is the site of several childhood brain tumors, including **craniopharyngioma** (the most common) and pituitary adenoma (see Chapter 21). These tumors may originate from the pituitary gland or the hypothalamus. They are usually slow growing and may be quite large by the time of diagnosis. Symptoms include headache, seizures, diabetes insipidus, early onset of puberty, and growth delay. Other tumors located in this region of the brain include **optic gliomas.** Tumors that involve the optic tract may cause complete unilateral blindness and hemianopia of the other eye. Optic atrophy is another common finding.

Supratentorial tumors of the cerebral hemispheres in children are not very common. Tumors located in the cortex may cause focal cerebral dysfunction, weakness, hemiparesis, seizures, and visual changes. Involvement of particular lobes may result in more specific localized symptoms. For example, a tumor located in the frontal lobe may cause changes in affect and behavior, and a tumor in the occipital lobe may cause cortical blindness or blindness in half of the visual field.

EVALUATION AND TREATMENT A child with signs and symptoms of a brain tumor requires a complete workup, including a neurologic, developmental, and ophthalmic examination. CT with contrast enhancement allows direct visualization of the tumor mass. MRI provides advanced, dramatic examination of the brain and neoplasms. Small low-grade tumors not seen on CT may be detected by MRI. Although less commonly used, MRA is very helpful in assessing vascularity of the tumor and its relationship to major blood vessels. Myelographic examination may be used to evaluate tumor dissemination along the spinal column. Lumbar puncture to examine CSF for tumor cells also is an option. Tumors more likely to spread throughout the neuraxis include medulloblastomas and ependymomas.

The most useful treatment for brain tumors is surgical resection.[118] Surgery to establish the diagnosis by biopsy or to excise the tumor is part of the initial treatment for most brain tumors. Some brain tumors may be cured with complete resection alone, such as low-grade cerebellar astrocytomas. Contraindications to such interventions are tumors in which surgical resection and biopsy carry a high risk of mortality or serious morbidity (brainstem gliomas). In these instances, diagnosis is made on radiologic evidence and clinical manifestations.

Most brain tumors require additional radiation and chemotherapy.[119] Although these treatments are essential for potential eradication of the brain tumor, radiation to the child's brain is associated with significant morbidity, including acute and long-term sequelae. Prognosis varies according to the type and location of the brain tumor. Historically, survival rates have been low; however, advances have been made with the combination of surgery, radiation therapy, and chemotherapy. Comprehensive care and management of these children and their families are vital. Multidisciplinary teams composed of neurosurgeons, neurologists, neuropathologists, radiation therapists, oncologists, nurses, social workers, physical therapists, and other providers are necessary to provide the continuity and consistency needed to care for these children.

Embryonal Tumors

Neuroblastoma

Neuroblastoma is an embryonal aggressive tumor that originates in neural crest cells that normally give rise to the sympathic nervous system (sympathetic ganglia and the adrenal medulla). The primitive neural crest cells (also called *sympathogonia*) are pluripotential (i.e., they give rise to several cell types). They mature into sympathetic ganglion cells, pheochromocytes (which are found in the sympathetic nervous system), or neurofibrous tissue. Thus tumors that develop from neural crest cells reflect the varying degrees of differentiation of the cells. **Ganglioneuroblastomas** are tumors of an intermediate level of cellular differentiation. The most differentiated tumor is a **ganglioneuroma,** which is considered benign and does not metastasize.

Because neuroblastoma involves a defect of embryonal tissue, it is diagnosed most commonly in young children and infants. Most tumors are diagnosed during the first 2 years of life, and 75% are found before the child is 5 years of age. Occasionally these tumors have been diagnosed at birth with metastasis apparent in the placenta. Neuroblastomas also are known to regress or mature into benign lesions.[120] Although it accounts for 8% to 10% of pediatric malignancies, neuroblastoma causes approximately 50% of all solid tumors in children in the first year, and 15% of cancer deaths in children of all ages.[121]

PATHOPHYSIOLOGY Neuroblastoma is the most primitive, or immature, form of the sympathetic nervous system tumors. Areas of necrosis and calcification often are present in the tumor.

The cause of neuroblastoma is elusive. The tumor has been associated with a number of conditions, including neurofibromatosis and Hirschsprung disease, but most children with neuroblastoma have neither of these conditions. Although familial tendency has been noted in individual cases, a nonfamilial or sporadic pattern occurs in most children with neuroblastoma. Familial cases of neuroblastoma are considered to have an autosomal dominant pattern of inheritance (mechanisms of inheritance are discussed in Chapter 4).

The most common genetic aberration is amplification of *N-myc* oncogene (myelocytomatosis viral-related oncogene, neuroblastoma derived) and loss of the short arm of chromosome 1, which is believed to represent the loss of a tumor response gene. The greater the number of copies of the *N-myc* oncogene, the more rapidly progressive and lethal the disease is.[122] The human multidrug-resistant gene (*MDR1* at chromosomes 3p and 11q1) has been identified and is associated with chemotherapy failure. The *MDR1* gene is amplified in some neuroblastoma cells after initial treatment with chemotherapy, and the increased presence of *MDR1* is associated with chemotherapy resistance. Chromosome 17q may be overexpressed.[123] Other molecular markers (i.e., neurotrophins) for neuroblastoma are being considered to support risk stratification and guidance of treatment.[124,125]

CLINICAL MANIFESTATIONS The clinical manifestations of neuroblastoma depend on the location of the tumor. Because neuroblastoma originates where there are elements of sympathetic nervous tissue, the tumor can arise in the sympathetic chain (column of sympathetic ganglia that parallels the spinal column), ganglia of effector organs, peripheral ganglia, adrenal medulla, bladder, and inner genitalia. The most common location is in the abdomen (65%) and most often in the adrenal medulla. The tumor is evident as an abdominal mass and may cause anorexia, bowel and bladder alteration, and sometimes spinal cord compression.[126]

The second most common location of neuroblastoma is the mediastinum (area separating the lungs) (15% of cases). There the tumor may cause dyspnea or infection related to airway obstruction. If the tumor is large, compression of the trachea, bronchi, lymphatic vessels, and mediastinal veins often results. Neck and facial edema may then be caused by superior vena cava syndrome. Less commonly, neuroblastoma may arise from the cervical sympathetic ganglion (3% to 4% of cases). Cervical neuroblastoma often causes Horner syndrome, which consists of miosis (pupil contraction), ptosis (drooping eyelid), enophthalmos (backward displacement of the eyeball), and anhidrosis (sweat deficiency).

The initial signs and symptoms of neuroblastoma often are related to metastatic disease. About half of children present with metastatic disease at the time of diagnosis. Common sites of metastasis include the skin, with characteristic blue or purple nodules; the liver, causing enlargement; bone, causing pain and pathologic fracture; and bone marrow infiltration, occurring in more than 50% of children. A unique but uncommon site of metastasis is the orbit of the eye, causing an ecchymotic discoloration of the upper and lower eyelids and a "raccoon" eye appearance. Opsoclonus-ataxia, also called "dancing eye syndrome," occurs in about 2% to 4% of cases, and these children have long-term neurologic complications.[127]

A number of systemic signs and symptoms are characteristic of neuroblastoma, including weight loss, irritability, fatigue, and fever. Intractable diarrhea occurs in 7% to 9% of children and is caused by tumor secretion of the hormone *vasoactive intestinal polypeptide (VIP).*

Neuroblastoma, more than any other cancer, has been associated with spontaneous remission, commonly in infants who have liver, bone marrow, or skin involvement in addition to the primary site. Remission has been estimated to occur in approximately 7% of cases but may occur much more often. Neuroblastoma in situ (i.e., noninvasive tumor) has been found during autopsies of infants who died of other causes.

More than 90% of children with neuroblastoma have increased amounts of catecholamines and associated metabolites in their urine. High levels of urinary catecholamines and serum ferritin are associated with a poorer prognosis.

EVALUATION AND TREATMENT Initial diagnostic studies are dictated by the location of the primary tumor. Diagnosis begins with a complete physical and neurologic examination. Visualizing examinations, including intravenous pyelogram, CT scan, or MRI of the primary site, provide further information. Investigation of metastatic disease includes skeletal survey, bone scan, liver scan, and bone marrow aspiration and examination. Newer nuclear medicine imaging studies for neuroblastoma, such as ^{123}I-metaiodobenzylguanidine (^{123}I-MIBG) and tumor-specific monoclonal antibody scan, may be helpful. Urinary catecholamine levels are measured by two metabolites: vanillylmandelic acid (VMA) and homovanillic acid (HVA). Other laboratory analyses are likely to include ferritin; serum neuron-specific enolase (NSE), an enzyme produced by neuronal tissues; and gangliosides, lipid molecules that may be shed from the surface of tumor cells.[128]

The diagnosis of neuroblastoma is confirmed by surgical biopsy and histopathology. A pathology classification system has been developed for neuroblastoma; for many years, however, there was no agreement on a risk staging system for neuroblastoma.[129] The International Neuroblastoma Risk Group is completing a consensus document for neuroblastoma risk stratification, which combined with the International Neuroblastoma Staging System, is used to guide treatment for low-, intermediate-, and high-risk patients.[129] A special stage (IV-S) is designated for infants who otherwise would be classified as having early stage disease but who also have metastatic disease involving the liver, skin, or bone.[128]

Treatment is based on the extent of the disease and prognostic markers, such as age, *N-myc* copy numbers, and high serum ferritin or NSE levels. Low-risk disease is treated surgically. Chemotherapy is used if there is recurrence. Intermediate-risk tumors are treated with surgery and chemotherapy. High-risk neuroblastomas are being treated with high-dose chemotherapy and radiotherapy followed by transplantation of purged autologous bone marrow. Additional treatment may include 13-*cis* retinoic acid. These combined treatments have increased survival rate in some to 3 years.

Stage IV-S disease requires very little treatment, primarily because of the high rate of spontaneous regression. Low-dose radiation treatment or single-course chemotherapy may be used to reduce large tumors. Approximately 60% of children with high-risk disease will die despite intensive therapy.[130]

Retinoblastoma

Retinoblastoma is a rare congenital eye tumor of young children that originates in the retina of one or both eyes (Figure 19-15). Retinoblastoma demonstrates both an inherited and

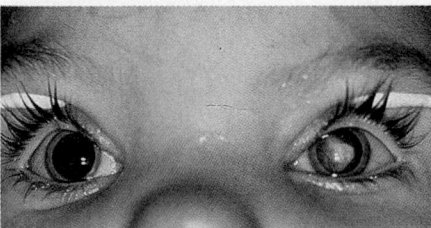

Figure 19-15 Retinoblastoma. The tumor occupies a large portion of the inside of the eye bulbus. (From Damjanov I: *Pathology for the health professions*, ed 3, St Louis, 2006, Saunders. Courtesy Dr. Walter Richardson and Dr. Jamsheed Khan, Kansas City, Kansas.)

an acquired form. Retinoblastoma rarely is diagnosed after the child is 5 years of age. The inherited form of the disease generally is diagnosed during the first year of life and often involves multiple tumors and sometimes both eyes (40%).[131] The acquired disease is commonly diagnosed in children 2 to 3 years of age and involves unilateral disease. Although retinoblastoma is the most common pediatric intraocular tumor, the prevalence rate is estimated between 1 in 15,000 and 20,000 live births.[131]

PATHOPHYSIOLOGY Approximately 40% of retinoblastomas are inherited as an autosomal dominant disorder caused by mutations in the *RB1* tumor-suppressor gene.[132] The remaining 60% are acquired. In the early 1970s Knudson[133] proposed the "two-hit" hypothesis to explain the occurrence of hereditary and acquired forms of the disease. This

hypothesis predicts that two separate transforming events or "hits" must occur in a normal retinoblast cell to cause the cancer. Further, it proposes that in the inherited form the first hit or mutation occurs in the germ cell (inherited from either parent), and the mutation is contained in every cell of the child's body. Only a second, random mutation in a retinoblast cell is necessary to transform that cell into cancer. Multiple tumors are observed in the inherited form because these second mutations are likely to occur in several of the approximately 1 to 2 million retinoblast cells. In contrast, the acquired form of retinoblastoma requires that two independent hits or mutations occur in the same somatic cell (after the egg is fertilized) for transformation to cancer. This is much less likely to happen. Figure 19-16 illustrates the two-mutation model for these two patterns of mutation.

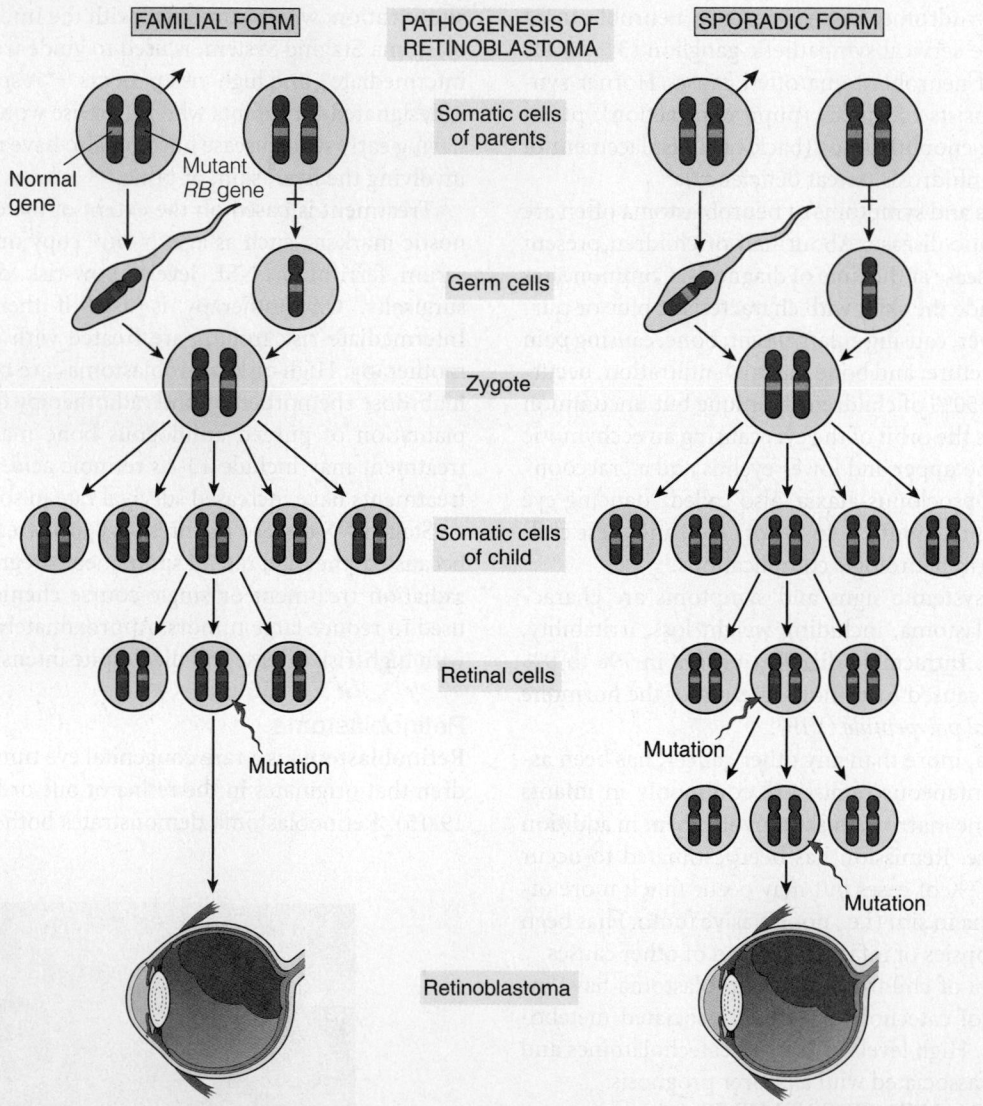

Figure 19-16 The two-mutation model of retinoblastoma development. In inherited (familial) retinoblastoma, mutations of the *RB* locus on chromosome 13q14 lead to neoplastic proliferation of retinal cells. The first mutation is transmitted through the germline of an affected parent. The second mutation occurs somatically in a retinal cell, leading to development of the tumor. In sporadic retinoblastoma, development of a tumor requires two somatic mutations. (From Kumar V, Cotran RS, Robbins SL: *Robbins basic pathology,* ed 7, p 184, Philadelphia, 2003, Saunders.)

The gene location in which the initial retinoblastoma mutation occurs is on the long arm of chromosome 13, band q14.[134] The gene responsible for retinoblastoma, a tumor suppressor gene, is called the *RB* gene. The first hit inactivates one allele of the *RB* gene, and the second hit inactivates the other allele of the gene. Without the normal functioning of the *RB* gene, production of protein growth regulators that control retinal cell growth is lacking. Because the gene is inactivated, lack of cell growth control results in unregulated proliferation and tumor development.[135]

The *RB* gene also has been implicated in other cancers, and survivors of hereditary retinoblastoma may be at increased risk for second cancers, particularly osteosarcoma but also cancer of the lung, breast, prostate, and bladder. Although retinoblastoma occurs in the very young child, second tumors can develop when survivors are in their 20s and 30s; such tumors generally are resistant to therapy.

Retinoblastoma grows as one or more tumors in the retina and extends into the vitreous humor. Free-floating, small tumors in the vitreous humor may attach to the surface of the retina in multiple areas and proliferate (Figure 19-17). The tumor also can invade the optic nerve by infiltrating the cribriform plate of the ethmoid bone or can spread through the sheath around the nerve. In either case the tumor can gain access to the subarachnoid space and the CNS. The tumor spreads into the choroid in 25% of children with retinoblastoma. Because the choroid is highly vascular, metastasis by means of hematogenous spread is possible. When hematogenous spread occurs, metastatic sites include the bone marrow, long bones, lymph nodes, and liver. If the tumor invades the orbit, lymphatic spread is possible. Spontaneous regression occurs, although infrequently, and may be caused by the tumor outgrowing its blood supply.

CLINICAL MANIFESTATIONS The two most frequent symptoms of retinoblastoma are leukokoria, a white pupillary reflex also called *cat's-eye reflex* caused by the mass behind the lens (see Figure 19-15), and strabismus. At that point the tumor is large enough that a light shone into the eye is reflected back by the tumor, making the pupil appear white. Other signs and symptoms include a red, painful eye and limited vision. Any of these signs and symptoms in a child younger than 4 years of age warrants careful ophthalmologic examination of both eyes. Similarly, any newborn with a known genetic risk for retinoblastoma should have routine ophthalmologic examinations.

EVALUATION AND TREATMENT Diagnostic evaluation for retinoblastoma includes documentation of family history; complete ophthalmologic examination; and metastatic studies that include bone marrow aspiration, lumbar puncture for spinal fluid examination, bone scan, and additional ultrasound, radiologic, and CT studies of the orbit and brain. Because of the potential hereditary risk to a child's siblings, all siblings younger than 4 years also should receive ophthalmologic evaluations.

Retinoblastoma is a treatable tumor, and dual priorities are saving the child's life and restoring useful vision. Early diagnosis and new chemotherapeutic agents have led to a more conservative approach to treatment. Chemoreduction of the tumor occurs with intravenous chemotherapy to reduce tumor volume. Focal treatments using hyperthermia, laser photocoagulation, or cryotherapy then destroy residual tumor. Large or multiple tumors, indicating more advanced disease, require external beam or plaque radiotherapy and in some cases enucleation (removal) of the eye. Every attempt is made to preserve vision in at least one eye without jeopardizing the child's survival.[136,137]

The prognosis for most children with retinoblastoma is excellent, with a greater than 90% long-term survival, although children with bilateral or metastatic disease at diagnosis have a poor prognosis.[138] Approximately 75% of children have useful vision in the treated eye.

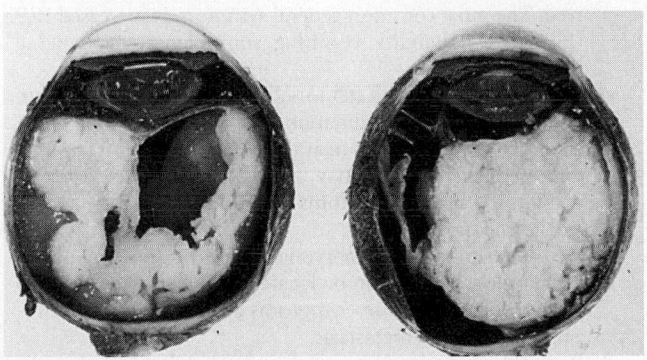

Figure 19-17 **Bilateral retinoblastoma.** Presence of white mass consisting of detached retina and neoplastic tissue immediately behind lens in each eye. (From Kissane JM, editor: *Anderson's pathology*, ed 8, St Louis, 1985, Mosby.)

SUMMARY REVIEW

Structure and Function of the Nervous System in Children

1. The central nervous system develops from the neural tube, which is ectodermal in origin. The cranial end of the tube forms the brain, and the spinal cord is formed from the remainder of the tube.
2. The cranial and spinal ganglia (peripheral nervous system) develop from the neural crest.
3. The nervous system develops in six stages, and disruption of any of the stages can lead to malfunction of the nervous system.
4. The bones of the skull are joined by sutures; the wide, membranous junctions of the sutures, known as *fontanels*, close by 20 months of age.
5. Myelin is a sheath that develops around axons to facilitate speed of nerve impulse conduction. Progressive development of reflexes corresponds to normal maturation of nerve tissue.
6. Neurologic functioning at birth is at the subcortical level with reflex patterns mediated by the brainstem and spinal cord. With maturation, neonatal reflexes disappear and voluntary motor functions develop.

(Continued)

SUMMARY REVIEW—cont'd

7. Head circumference is one fourth of the total height in infants compared with one eighth in adults. The fontanels allow for cranial expansion because the head is the fastest growing body part during infancy.

Structural Malformations

1. Defects of neural tube closure include anencephaly (absence of part of the brain and soft, bony part of skull), encephalocele (protrusion of brain and meninges through a skull defect), meningocele (cystlike defect with protrusion of spinal fluid–filled meninges through a vertebral defect), and myelomeningocele (a defect like meningocele only also containing the spinal cord).
2. Failure of the vertebrae to close with protrusion of neural tube contents is known as *spina bifida*.
3. Acrania is nearly complete absence of the cranial vault.
4. Premature closure of the cranial sutures causes craniosynostosis and prevents normal skull expansion and compression of growing brain tissue.
5. Microcephaly is lack of brain growth and retarded mental and motor development.
6. Congenital hydrocephalus results from an imbalance between the production and reabsorption of cerebrospinal fluid.

Encephalopathies

1. Static encephalopathies (i.e., cerebral palsy and epilepsy) are nonprogressive disorders of the brain that can occur during gestation, birth, or childhood and can be caused by endogenous or exogenous factors.
2. Cerebral palsy is a group of nonprogressive syndromes that can be caused by prenatal cerebral hypoxia or perinatal or postnatal trauma with symptoms of mental retardation, seizure disorders, or developmental disabilities.
3. Inherited metabolic disorders that damage the nervous system include defects in amino acid metabolism (phenylketonuria) and lipid metabolism (Tay-Sachs disease) and result in abnormal behavior, seizures, and deficient psychomotor development.
4. Seizures are the abnormal discharge of electrical activity within the brain. Seizure disorders are associated with numerous nervous system disorders and more often are a generalized rather than a partial type of seizure. Epilepsy is recurrence of seizure activity.
5. Generalized forms of seizures include tonic-clonic, myoclonic, atonic, akinetic, and infantile spasms.
6. Partial seizures suggest more localized brain dysfunction.
7. Febrile seizures usually are limited to the ages of 9 months to 3 years, with a pattern of one seizure per febrile illness.

8. Reye syndrome is an acute encephalopathy associated with influenza B and varicella viruses and symptoms of hypoglycemia, hyperammonemia, and increased serum short-chain fatty acids. Progressive manifestations include lethargy, stupor, rigidity, seizures, and respiratory arrest.
9. Accidental poisonings from a variety of toxins can cause serious neurologic damage.
10. Bacterial meningitis is commonly caused by *H. influenzae, N. meningitidis,* or *S. pneumoniae* and may result from respiratory or gastrointestinal infections with symptoms of fever, headache, photophobia, seizure, rigidity, and stupor.
11. Viral meningitis presents similar to bacterial meningitis, and the specific virus is often unknown.
12. HIV-1 encephalopathy is a CNS infection that can occur in infants and children.

Cerebrovascular Disease in Children

1. Occlusive cerebrovascular disease may result from embolism, sinovenous thrombosis, or congenital or iatrogenic vessel narrowing.
2. Congenital arteriovenous malformations are the most common cause of intracranial bleeding and hemorrhagic stroke in children.

Childhood Tumors

1. Brain tumors are the most common tumors of the nervous system and the second most common type of childhood cancer.
2. Tumors in children are most often located below the tentorial membrane.
3. Fast-growing tumors produce symptoms early in the disease, whereas slow-growing tumors may become very large before symptoms appear.
4. Symptoms of brain tumors may be generalized or localized. The most common general symptom is increased ICP (headache, irritability, vomiting, somnolence, and bulging of fontanels).
5. Localized signs of infratentorial tumors in the cerebellum include impaired coordination and balance. Cranial nerve signs occur with tumors near the brainstem.
6. Supratentorial tumors may be located near the cortex or deep in the brain. Symptoms depend on the specific location of the tumor.
7. Neuroblastoma is an embryonal tumor of the sympathetic nervous system and can be located anywhere there is sympathetic nervous tissue. Symptoms are related to tumor location and size of metastasis.
8. Retinoblastoma is a congenital eye tumor that has a hereditary and a nonhereditary form.

KEY TERMS

Acrania, 672
Alar plate, 666
Anencephaly, 669
Arnold-Chiari type II malformation, 670
Aseptic meningitis, 681
Ataxic cerebral palsy, 676
Bacterial meningitis, 681
Basal plate, 666
Benign febrile seizure, 680
Brainstem glioma, 687
Cerebellar astrocytoma, 687

Cerebral palsy (CP), 675
Congenital hydrocephalus, 673
Cranial meningocele, 669
Craniopharyngioma, 688
Craniosynostosis, 672
Cyclopia, 669
Dandy-Walker malformation, 674
Dyskinetic cerebral palsy, 676
Encephalocele, 669
Encephalopathy, 675
Ependymoma, 687

Epilepsy, 679
Extrapyramidal/nonspecific cerebral palsy, 676
Fontanel, 666
Ganglioneuroblastoma, 688
Ganglioneuroma, 688
Gangliosidosis, 678
Generalized seizure, 679
Hyperphenylalaninemia (HPA), 677
Infantile spasm, 679
Juvenile myoclonic epilepsy, 680

KEY TERMS—cont'd

Lennox-Gastaut syndrome, 680
Lysosomal storage disease, 678
Macewen sign ("cracked-pot" sign), 674
Medulloblastoma, 687
Meningitis, 681
Meningocele, 669
Microcephaly, 673
Moyamoya disease, 685
Myelodysplasia, 669
Neural crest, 665
Neural fold, 665
Neural groove, 665

Neural plate, 665
Neural tube, 665
Neuroblastoma, 688
Nonsyndromic craniosynostosis, 672
Optic glioma, 688
Partial seizure, 679
Phenylketonuria (PKU), 677
Pica, 681
Pyramidal/spastic cerebral palsy, 676
Retinoblastoma, 689
Reye syndrome, 681
Schwann cell, 667

Somite, 666
Spina bifida, 671
Spina bifida occulta, 671
Sulcus limitans, 666
Suture, 666
Syndromic craniosynostosis, 673
Tay-Sachs disease, 678
Tethered cord syndrome, 671
Tuberous sclerosis complex (TSC), 680
Unclassified epileptic seizure, 679
Viral meningitis, 684

REFERENCES

1. Centers for Disease Control and Prevention (CDC): Use of supplements containing folic acid among women of childbearing age—United States, 2007, *MMWR Morb Mortal Wkly Rep* 57(1):5-8, 2008.
2. Kaufman BA: Neural tube defects, *Pediatr Clin North Am* 51(2):389-419, 2004.
3. Anthony TE, Heintz N: The folate metabolic enzyme ALDH1L1 is restricted to the midline of the early CNS, suggesting a role in human neural tube defects, *J Comp Neurol* 500(2):368-383, 2007.
4. Beaudin AE, Stover PJ: Folate-mediated one-carbon metabolism and neural tube defects: balancing genome synthesis and gene expression, *Birth Defects Res C Embryo Today* 81(3):183-203, 2007.
5. Merserau P et al: Spina bifida and ancephaly before and after folic acid mandate—United States 1995-1996 and 1999-2000, *MMWR Morb Mortal Wkly Rep* 53(17):362-365, 2004.
6. Dashe JS et al: Alpha-fetoprotein detection of neural tube defects and the impact of standard ultrasound, *Am J Obstet Gynecol* 195(6):1623-1628, 2006.
7. Pollack IF: Management of encephaloceles and craniofacial problems in the neonatal period, *Neurosurg Clin N Am* 9(1):121-139, 1998.
8. Bhattacharjee A, Chakraborty A, Purkaystha P: Frontoethmoidal encephalomeningocoele with colpocephaly: case report and clinical review, *J Laryngol Otol* 122(3):321-323, 2008.
9. Shaer CM, Chescheir N, Schulkin J: Myelomeningocele: a review of the epidemiology, genetics, risk facotrs for conception, prenatal diagnosis, and prognosis for affected individuals, *Obstet Gynecol Surv* 62(7):471-479, 2007.
10. Stevenson KL: Chiari type II malformation: past, present and future, *Neurosurg Focus* 16(2):E5, 2004.
11. Chakraborty A et al: Toward reducing shunt placement rates in patients with myelomeningocele, *J Neurosurg Pediatr* 1(15):361-365, 2008.
12. Reigel DH: Infancy through the school years. In Rowley-Kelly F, Reigel DH, editors: *Teaching the student with spina bifida*, Baltimore, 1993, Brookes.
13. Salman MS et al: Smooth ocular pursuit in Chiari type II malformation, *Dev Med Child Neurol* 49(4):289-293, 2007.
14. Olsson I et al: Medical problems in adolescents with myelomeningocele (MMC): an inventory of the Swedish MMC population during 1986-1989, *Acta Paediatr* 96(3):446-449, 2007.
15. Ko AL et al: Retrospective review of multilevel spinal fusion combined with spinal cord transection for treatment of kyphoscoliosis in pediatric myelomeningocele patients, *Spine* 32(22):2493-2501, 2007.
16. Yamada S, Won DJ: What is the true tethered cord syndrome? *Childs Nerv Syst* 23(4):371-375, 2007.
17. Yamada S et al: Pathophysiology of tethered cord syndrome and similar complex disorders, *Neurosurg Focus* 23(2):1-10, 2007.
18. Hudgins RJ, Gilreath CL: Tethered spinal cord following repair of myelomeningocele, *Neurosurg Focus* 16(2):E7, 2004.
19. Bliton MJ: Ethics: "life before birth" and moral complexity in maternal-fetal surgery for spina bifida, *Clin Perinatol* 30(3):449-464, 2003.

20. Zambelli H et al: Assessment of neurosurgical outcome in children prenatally diagnosed with myelomeningocele and development of a protocol for fetal surgery to prevent hydrocephalus, *Childs Nerv Syst* 23(4):421-425, 2007.
21. Rintoul NE et al: A new look at myelomeningocele: functional level, vertebral level, and the implication for fetal intervention, *Pediatrics* 109(3):409-413, 2002.
22. Bruner JP: Intrauterine surgery in myelomeningocele, *Semin Fetal Neonatal Med* 12(6):471-476, 2007.
23. Pitkin RM: Folate and neural tube defects, *Am J Clin Nutr* 85(1):285S-288S, 2007.
24. Behrman RE, Kleigman RM, Jenson HB: *Nelson's textbook of pediatrics*, ed 17, Philadelphia, 2004, Saunders.
25. Bruner JP et al: Intrauterine repair of spina bifida: preoperative predictors of shunt-dependent hydrocephalus, *Am J Obstet Gynecol* 190(5):1305-1312, 2004.
26. Hukki J, Saarinen P, Kangasniemi M: Single suture craniosynostosis: diagnosis and imaging, *Front Oral Biol* 12:79-90, 2008.
27. Boyadjiev SA et al: Genetic analysis of non-syndromic craniosynostosis, *Orthod Craniofac Res* 10(3):129-137, 2007.
28. Wan DC et al: Current treatment of craniosynostosis and future theraperutic directions, *Front Oral Biol* 12:209-220, 2008.
29. Passos-Bueno MR et al: Genetics of craniosynostosis: genes, syndromes, mutations and genotype-phenotype correlations, *Front Oral Biol* 12:107-143, 2008.
30. Rice DP: Clinical features of syndromic craniosynostosis, *Front Oral Biol* 12:91-106, 2008.
31. Kimonis V et al: Genetics of craniosynostosis, *Semin Pediatr Neurol* 14(3):150-161, 2007.
32. Clayman MA et al: History of craniosynostosis surgery and the evolution of minimally invasive endoscopic techniques: the University of Florida experience, *Ann Plast Surg* 58(30):285-287, 2007.
33. Abuelo D: Microcephaly syndromes, *Semin Pediatr Neurol* 14(3):118-127, 2007.
34. Garton HJ, Platt JH Jr: Hydrocephalus, *Pediatr Clin North Am* 51(2):305-325, 2004.
35. Jackson PL: Hydrocephalus. In Jackson PL, Vessey JA, editors: *Primary care of the child with a chronic condition*, ed 4, St Louis, 2003, Mosby.
36. Kestle JR: Pediatric hydrocephalus—current management, *Neurol Clin* 21(4):883-895, 2003.
37. Beni-Adani L et al: The occurrence of obstructive vs absorptive hydrocephalus in newborns and infants: relevance to treatment choices, *Childs Nerv Syst* 22(12):1543-1563, 2006.
38. Jacobsson B, Hagberg G: Antenatal risk factors for cerebral palsy, *Best Pract Res Clin Obstet Gynaecol* 18(3):425-436, 2004.
39. Murphy N, Such-Neibar T: Cerebral palsy diagnosis and management: the state of the art, *Curr Probl Pediatr Adolesc Health Care* 33(5):146-169, 2003.
40. Nelson KB, Chang T: Is cerebral palsy preventable? *Curr Opin Neurol* 21(2):121-135, 2008.
41. Lawson RD, Badawi N: Etiology of cerebral palsy, *Hand Clin* 19(4):547-556, 2003.

42. Rennie JM, Hagmann CF, Robertson NJ: Outcome after intrapartum hypoxic ischemia at term, *Semin Fetal Neonatal Med* 12(5):398-407, 2007.

43. Gunn AJ, Gluckman PD: Head cooling for neonatal encephalopathy: the state of the art, *Clin Obstet Gynecol* 50(3):636-651, 2007.

44. Degos V et al: Neuroprotective strategies for the neonatal brain, *Anesth Analg* 106(6):1670-1680, 2008.

45. Keogh JM, Badawi N: The origins of cerebral palsy, *Curr Opin Neurol* 19(2):129-134, 2006.

46. Jones MW et al: Cerebral palsy: introduction and diagnosis (part I), *J Pediatr Health Care* 21(3):146-152, 2007.

47. Wood E: The child with cerebral palsy: diagnosis and beyond, *Semin Pediatr Neurol* 13(4):286-296, 2007.

48. Steinbok P: Selection of treatment modalities in children with spastic cerebral palsy, *Neurosurg Focus* 21(2):e4, 2006.

49. Simpson et al: Botulinum neurotoxin for the treatment of spasticity (an evidence-based review): report of the Therapeutics and Technology Assessment Subcommittee of the American Academy of Neurology, *Neurology* 70(19):1691-1698, 2008.

50. Menkes JH, Sarnat HB: *Child neurology*, ed 6 , Philadelphia, 2000, Lippincott Williams & Wilkins.

51. Swaiman KF, Ashwal S: *Pediatric neurology: principles and practice*, ed 3, St Louis, 1999, Mosby.

52. Fusetti F et al: Structure of tetrameric human phenylalanine hydroxylase and its implications for phenylketonuria, *J Biol Chem* 273(27):16962–16927, 1998.

53. Schmidt K: Phenylketonuria. In Jackson PL, Vessey JA, editors: *Primary care of the child with a chronic condition*, ed 4, St Louis, 2003, Mosby.

54. Kaufman S: An evaluation of the possible neurotoxicity of metabolites of phenylalanine, *J Pediatr* 114(5):895-900, 1989.

55. Michals-MatalonK et al: Response of phenylketonuria to tetrahydrobiopterin, *J Nutr* 137(6 Suppl 1):1564S-1567S, 2007.

56. Williams RA, Mamotte CD, Burnett JR: Phenylketonuria: an inborn error of phenylalanine metabolism, *Clin Biochem Rev* 29(1):31-41, 2008.

57. Guetta E, Peleg L: Rapid detection of fetal Mendelian disorder: Tay-Sachs disease, *Meth Mol Biol* 444:147-159, 2008.

58. Jarrar RG, Buchhalter JR: Therapeutics in pediatric epilepsy, Part 1: the new antiepileptic drugs and the ketogenic diet, *Mayo Clin Proc* 78(3):359-370, 2003.

59. Leppik E: The expanding role of genetics in epilepsy, *Am J Electroneurodiagnostic Tech* 43(2):105-107, 2003.

60. Siverstein FS, Jensen FE: Neonatal seizures, *Ann Neurol* 62(2):112-120, 2007.

61. Frost JD Jr, Hrachovy RA: Pathogenesis of infantile spasms: a model based on developmental desynchronization, *J Clin Neurophysiol* 22(1):25-36, 2005.

62. Kato M: A new paradigm for West syndrome based on molecular and cell biology, *Epilepsy Res* 70(Suppl 1):S87-S95, 2006.

63. Guggenheim MA, Frost JD Jr, Hrachovy RA: Time interval from a brain insult to the onset of infantile spasms, *Pediatr Neurol* 38(1):34-37, 2008.

64. Curatolo P et al: Management of epilepsy in tuberous sclerosis complex, *Expert Rev Neurother* 8(3):457-467, 2008.

65. MacAllister WS, Schaffer SG: Neuropsychological deficits in childhood epilepsy syndromes, *Neuropsychol Rev* 17(4):427-444, 2007.

66. Grill MF, Losey TE, Ng YT: The hitchhiker's guide to the child neurologist's genetic evaluation of epilepsy, *Semin Pediatr Neurol* 15(1):32-40, 2008.

67. Renganathan R, Delanty N: Juvenile myoclonic epilepsy: under-appreciated and under-diagnosed, *Postgrad Med J* 79(298):78-80, 2003.

68. Wiebe S, Tellez-Zenteno JF, Shapiro M: An evidence-based approach to the first seizure, *Epilepsia* 49(Suppl 1):50-57, 2008.

69. Hadjiloizou SM, Bourgeois BF: Antiepileptic drug treatment in children, *Expert Rev Neurother* 7(2):179-193, 2007.

70. Wheless JW et al: Treatment of pediatric epilepsy: European expert opinion, 2007, *Epileptic Disord* 9(4):353-412, 2007.

71. Freeman JM, Kossoff EH, Hartman AL: The ketogenic diet: one decade later, *Pediatrics* 119(3):535-543, 2007.

72. Hartman AL et al. The neuropharmacology of the ketogenic diet, *Pediatr Neurol* 36(5):281-292, 2007.

73. Buchhalter JR, Jarrar RG: Symposium on seizures. Therapeutics in pediatric epilepsy, Part 2: epilepsy surgery and vagus nerve stimulation, *Mayo Clin Proc* 78(3):371-378, 2003.

74. Champi G, Gaffney-Yocum PA: Managing febrile seizures in children, *Dimens Crit Care Nurs* 20(5):2-10, 2001.

75. Shinnar S, Glauser TA: Febrile seizures, *J Child Neurol* 17(Suppl 1):S44-S52, 2002.

76. Waruiru C, Appleton R: Febrile seizures: an update, *Arch Dis Child* 89(8):751-756, 2004.

77. Fetveit A: Assessment of febrile seizures in children, *Eur J Pediatr* 167(1):17-27, 2008.

78. Neville BG, Chin RF, Scott RC: Childhood convulsive status epilepticus: epidemiology, management and outcome, *Acta Neurol Scand,* Suppl 186:21-24, 2007.

79. Monto AS: The disappearance of Reye's syndrome—a public health triumph, *N Engl J Med* 340(18):1423-1424, 1999.

80. Gosalakkal JA, Komoji V: Reye syndrome and Reye-like syndrome, *Pediatr Neurol* 39(3):198-200, 2008.

81. Belay ED et al: Reye's syndrome in the United States from 1981 though 1997, *New Engl J Med* 340(18):1377, 1999.

82. Ward MJ: Reye's syndrome: an update. *Nurs Pract* 22(12):45, 1997.

83. Bhutta AT et al: Reye's syndrome: down but not out, *South Med J* 96(1):43-45, 2003.

84. Schror K: Aspirin and Reye syndrome: a review of the evidence, *Paediatr Drugs* 9(3):195-204, 2007.

85. Bernard SM: Should the Center for Disease Control and Prevention's childhood lead poisoning intervention level be lowered? *Am J Public Health* 94(1):8-9, 2004.

86. Meyer PA et al: Surveillance for elevated blood lead levels among children—United States, 1997-2001, *MMWR Morb Mortal Wkly Rep* 52(10):1-21, 2003.

87. Woolf AD, Goldman R, Bellinger DC: Update on the clinical management of childhood lead poisoning, *Pediatr Clin North Am* 54(2):271-294, 2007.

88. Chang CJ et al: Bacterial meningitis in infants: the epidemiology, clinical features and prognostic factors, *Brain Dev* 26(3):168-175, 2004.

89. Mace SE: Acute bacterial meningitis, *Emerg Med Clin North Am* 26(2):218-317, 2008.

90. Nigrovic LE, Kuppermann N, Malley R: Development and validation of a multivariable predictive model to distinguish bacterial from aseptic meningitis in children in post–*Haemophilus influenzae* era, *Pediatrics* 110(4):712-719, 2002.

91. Milonovich LM: Meningococcemia: epidemiology, pathophysiology, and management, *J Pediatr Health Care* 21(2):75-80, 2007.

92. Feigin RD et al: Bacterial meningitis beyond the neonatal period. In Feigin RD, et al: editors: *Textbook of pediatric infectious diseases*, ed 5 , Philadelphia, 2003, Saunders.

93. Broker M, Fantoni S: Meningococcal disease: a review on available vaccines and vaccines in development, *Minerva Med* 98(5):575-589, 2007.

94. Prasad K, Karlupia N: Prevention of bacterial meningitis: an overview of Cochrane systematic reviews, *Respir Med* 101(10):2037-2043, 2007.

95. Ahmed MN, Steele RW: Meningitis in a young infant, *Clin Pediatr* 43(5):495-497, 2004.

96. Chirlboga CA et al: Incidence and prevalence of HIV encephalopathy in children with HIV infection receiving highly active anti-retroviral therapy (HAART), *J Pediatr* 146(3):402-407, 2005.

97. Mitchell CD: HIV-1 encephalopathy among perinatally infected children: neuropathogenesis and response to highly active antiretroviral therapy, *Ment Retard Dev Disabil Res Rev* 12(3):216-222, 2006.

98. Centers for Disease Control and Prevention: 1994 revised classification system for human immunodeficiency virus infection in children less than 13 years of age, *MMWR Morb Mortal Wkly Rep* 43(12):1, 1994. Available at www.cdc.gov/mmwr/preview/mmwrhtml/00032890.htm.

99. Fahrner R: Pediatric HIV infections and AIDS. In Jackson PL, Vessey JA, editors: *Primary care of the child with a chronic condition*, ed 4 , St Louis, 2003, Mosby.

100. Tardieu M: HIV-1 and the developing central nervous system, *Dev Med Child Neurol* 40(12):843-846, 1998.

101. Petito CK et al: Brain CD8+ and cytotoxic T lymphocytes are associated with, and may be specific for, human immunodeficiency virus type 1 encephalitis in patients with acquired immunodeficiency syndrome, *J Neurovirol* 12(4):272-283, 2006.

102. McKinney RE Jr, Cunningham CK: New treatments for HIV in children, *Curr Opin Pediatr* 16(1):76-79, 2004.

103. Bernard TJ, Goldenberg NA: Pediatric arterial ischemic stroke, *Pediatr Clin North Am* 55(2):323-338, 2008:viii.

104. Horn P et al: Arterio-embolic ischemic stroke in children with moyamoya disease, *Childs Nerv Syst* 21(2):104-107, 2004.

105. Osanai T et al: Moyamoya disease presenting with subarachnoid hemorrhage localized over the frontal cortex: case report, *Surg Neurol* 69(2):197-200, 2008.

106. Jordan LC, Hillis AE: Hemorrhagic stroke in children, *Pediatr Neurol* 36(2):73-80, 2007.

107. Whitelaw A, Odd D: Postnatal phenobarbital for the prevention of intraventricular hemorrhage in preterm infants, *Cochrane Database Syst Rev* (4):CD001691, 2007.

108. Golomb MR et al: Neonatal arterial ischemic stroke and cerebral sinovenous thrombosis are more commonly diagnosed in boys, *J Child Neurol* 19(7):493-497, 2004.

109. Hartmann A et al: Treatment of arteriovenous malformations of the brain, *Curr Neurol Neurosci Rep* 7(1):28-34, 2007.

110. Rashidi M et al: Nonmalignant pediatric brain tumors, *Curr Neurol Neurosci Rep* 3(3):200-205, 2003.

111. Walter AW: Brain tumors in children, *Curr Oncol Rep* 6(6):438-444, 2004.

112. Kline ME: Solid tumors in children, *J Pediatr Nurs* 18(2):96-102, 2003.

113. Baldwin RT, Preston-Martin S: Epidemiology of brain tumors in childhood—a review, *Toxicol Appl Pharmacol* 199(2):118-131, 2003.

114. Biegel JA: Genetics of pediatric central nervous system tumors, *J Pediatr Hematol Oncol* 19(6):492-501, 1997.

115. Sklar CA: Childhood brain tumors, *J Pediatr Endocrinol Metab* 15(Suppl 2):669-673, 2002.

116. Gilbertson RJ: Medulloblastoma: signalling a change in treatment, *Lancet Oncol* 5(4):209-218, 2004.

117. Korones DN: Treatment of newly diagnosed diffuse brain stem gliomas in children: in search of the holy grail, *Expert Rev Anticancer Ther* 7(5):663-674, 2007.

118. Heuer GG et al: Surgical management of pediatric brain tumors, *Expert Rev Anticancer Ther* 7(12 Suppl):S61-S68, 2007.

119. Partap S, Fisher PG: Update on new treatments and developments in childhood brain tumors, *Curr Opin Pediatr* 19(6):670-674, 2007.

120. Friedman GK, Castleberry RP: Changing trends of research and treatment in infant neuroblastoma, *Pediatr Blood Cancer* 49(7 Suppl):1060-1065, 2007.

121. Castel V et al: Molecular biology of neuroblastoma, *Clin Transl Oncol* 9(8):478-483, 2007.

122. Weinstein JL, Katzenstein HM, Cohn SL: Advances in the diagnosis and treatment of neuroblastoma, *Oncologist* 8(3):278-292, 2003.

123. Goldstein LJ et al: Expression of the multidrug resistance, *MDR1*, gene in neuroblastomas, *J Clin Oncol* 8(1):128, 1990.

124. Henry MC, Tashjian DB, Breuer C: Neuroblastoma update, *Curr Opin Oncol* 17(1):19-23, 2005.

125. Tomioka N et al: Novel risk stratification of patients with neuroblastoma by genomic signature, which is independent of molecular signature, *Oncogene* 27(4):441-449, 2008.

126. Golden CG, Feusner JH: Malignant abdominal masses in children: quick guide to evaluation and diagnosis, *Pediatr Clin North Am* 49(6):1369-1392, 2002.

127. Mitchell WG et al: Opsoclonus-ataxia caused by childhood neuroblastoma: developmental and neurologic sequelae, *Pediatrics* 109(1):86-98, 2002.

128. Maris JM: Neuroblastoma, *Lancet* 369(9579):2106-2120, 2007.

129. Park JR, Eggert A, Caron H: Neuroblastoma: biology, prognosis and treatment, *Pediatr Clin North Am* 55(1):97-120, 2008:x, 2008.

130. Goldsby RE, Matthay KK: Neuroblastoma: evolving therapies for a disease with many faces, *Paediatr Drugs* 6(2):107-122, 2004.

131. Aerts I et al: Retinoblastoma, *Orphanet J Rare Dis* 1:31, 2006.

132. Leiderman YI, Kiss S, Mukai S: Molecular genetics of the *RB1-retinoblastoma* gene, *Semin Ophthalmol* 22(4):247-254, 2007.

133. Knudson AG: Mutation and cancer: a statistical study of retinoblastoma, *Proc Natl Acad Sci U S A* 68:620, 1971.

134. Kivela T et al: Retinoblastoma associated with chromosome 13q14 deletion mosaicism, *Ophthalmology* 110(10):1983-1988, 2003.

135. Rubnitz JE, Crist WM: Molecular genetics of childhood cancer: implications for pathogenesis, diagnosis, and treatment, *Pediatrics* 100(1):101, 1997.

136. Munier FL et al: New developments in external beam radiotherapy for retinoblastoma: from lens to normal tissue sparing, *Clin Experiment Ophthalmol* 36(1):78-89, 2008.

137. Shields CL et al: Continuing challenges in the management of retinoblastoma with chemotherapy, *Retina* 24(6):849-862, 2004.

138. American Cancer Society: What are the key statistics for retinoblastoma, *Cancer Ref Inform*, revised July 9, 2008. Available at www.cancer.org/docroot/CRI/content/CRI_2_4_1X_What_are_the_key_statistics_for_retinoblastoma_37.asp?rnav=cri.

MECHANISMS OF HORMONAL REGULATION

VALENTINA L. BRASHERS • ROBERT E. JONES

MEDIA RESOURCES

CHAPTER OUTLINE

MECHANISMS OF HORMONAL REGULATION
Regulation of Hormone Release
Hormone Transport
Cellular Mechanisms of Hormone Action
STRUCTURE AND FUNCTION OF THE ENDOCRINE GLANDS
Hypothalamic-Pituitary Axis
Thyroid and Parathyroid Glands

Endocrine Pancreas
Adrenal Glands
Neuroendocrine Response to Stressors
Tests of Endocrine Function
Aging and the Endocrine System

The endocrine system is composed of various glands located throughout the body (Figure 20-1). These glands are capable of synthesizing and releasing special chemical messengers called **hormones.** The endocrine system has five general functions:

1. Differentiation of the reproductive and central nervous systems in the developing fetus
2. Stimulation of sequential growth and development during childhood and adolescence
3. Coordination of the male and female reproductive systems, which makes sexual reproduction possible
4. Maintenance of an optimal internal environment throughout the life span
5. Initiation of corrective and adaptive responses when emergency demands occur

Hormones convey specific regulatory information among cells and organs and are integrated with the nervous system to maintain communication and control. The mechanisms of communication include autocrine (within cell), paracrine (between local cells), and endocrine (between remote cells).[1]

MECHANISMS OF HORMONAL REGULATION

The endocrine glands respond to specific signals by synthesizing and releasing hormones into the circulation. Although a wide variety of hormones function within the body, they share certain general characteristics:

1. Hormones have specific rates and rhythms of secretion. Three basic secretion patterns are (1) circadian or diurnal patterns, (2) pulsatile and cyclic patterns, and (3) patterns that depend on levels of circulating substrates (e.g., calcium, sodium, potassium, or the hormones themselves).
2. Hormones operate within feedback systems, either positive or negative, to maintain an optimal internal environment.
3. Hormones affect only cells with appropriate receptors and then act on those cells to initiate specific cell functions or activities.
4. Hormones are either excreted directly by the kidneys or metabolized by the liver, which inactivates them and renders the hormone more water soluble for renal excretion.

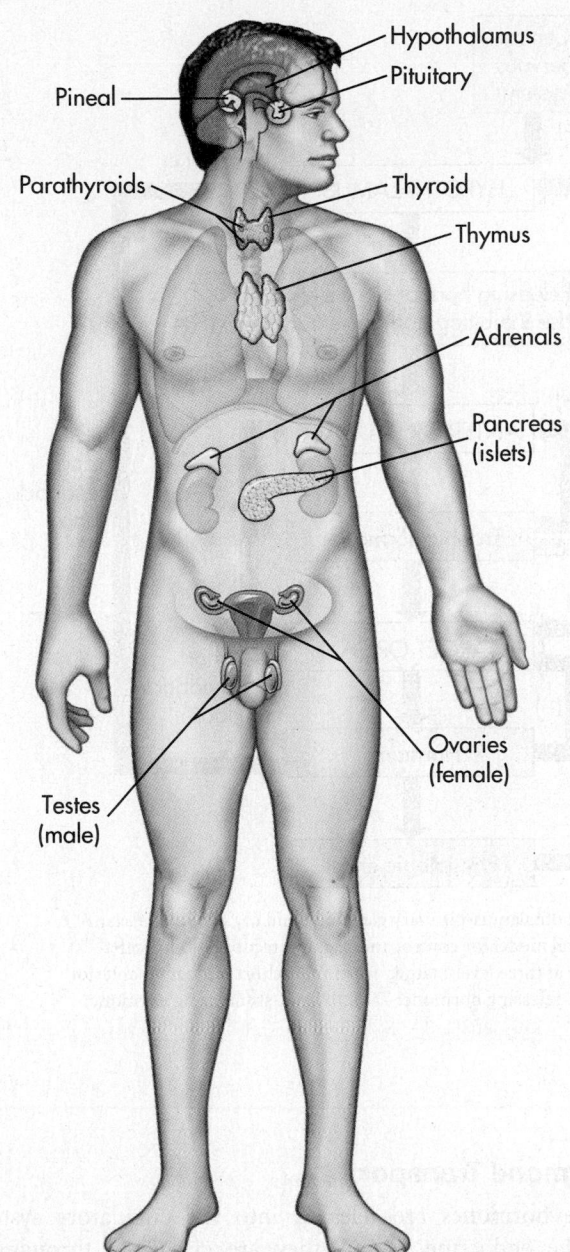

Figure 20-1 Principal endocrine glands. (From Patton KT, Thibodeau GA: *Anatomy & physiology,* ed 7, St Louis, 2010, Mosby.)

Table 20-1	Structural Categories of Hormones	
Structural Category	**Examples**	
Water Soluble		
Peptides	Growth hormone	
	Insulin	
	Leptin	
	Parathyroid hormone	
	Prolactin	
Glycoproteins	Follicle-stimulating hormone	
	Luteinizing hormone	
	Thyroid-stimulating hormone	
Polypeptides	Adrenocorticotropic hormone	
	Antidiuretic hormone	
	Calcitonin	
	Endorphins	
	Glucagon	
	Hypothalamic hormones	
	Lipotropins	
	Melanocyte-stimulating hormone	
	Oxytocin	
	Somatostatin	
	Thymosin	
	Thyrotropin-releasing hormone	
Amines	Epinephrine	
	Norepinephrine	
Lipid Soluble		
Thyroxine (an amine but lipid soluble)	Thyroxine (both thyroxine [T_4] and triiodothyronine [T_3])	
Steroids (cholesterol is a precursor for all steroids)	Estrogens	
	Glucocorticoids (cortisol)	
	Mineralocorticoids (aldosterone)	
	Progestins (progesterone)	
	Testosterone	
Derivatives of arachidonic acid (autocrine or paracrine action)	Leukotrienes	
	Prostacyclins	
	Prostaglandins	
	Thromboxanes	

Hormones may be classified according to their structure, gland of origin, effects, or chemical composition. (Table 20-1 categorizes hormones based on structure.) The secretion and mechanisms of action of hormones represent an extremely complex system of integrated responses. Although much has been learned about these complex systems, many of the specific mechanisms of action are not yet understood. The endocrine and nervous systems work together to regulate responses to the internal and external environments.

Regulation of Hormone Release

The release of hormones occurs either in response to an alteration in the cellular environment or in the process of maintaining a regulated level of certain hormones or certain substances.[2] Hormone release is regulated by one or more of the following mechanisms: (1) chemical factors (such as blood sugar or calcium levels); (2) endocrine factors (a hormone from one endocrine gland controlling another endocrine gland); and (3) neural control. Of these regulatory mechanisms, endocrine regulation by way of feedback circuits (systems) is perhaps the most important way in which hormonal secretion is maintained within a physiologic range.[1,2]

Negative feedback is the most common type of feedback system. In a negative-feedback system, plasma levels of one type of hormone influence the level of other types of hormones. An example of hormone negative feedback is shown in Figure 20-2, *A.* Increased anterior pituitary release of thyroid-stimulating hormone (TSH) stimulates the synthesis and secretion of thyroid hormones. TSH is inhibited by thyroxine (T_4) and to a lesser extent by triiodothyronine (T_3). TSH secretion is regulated by thyrotropin-releasing hormone

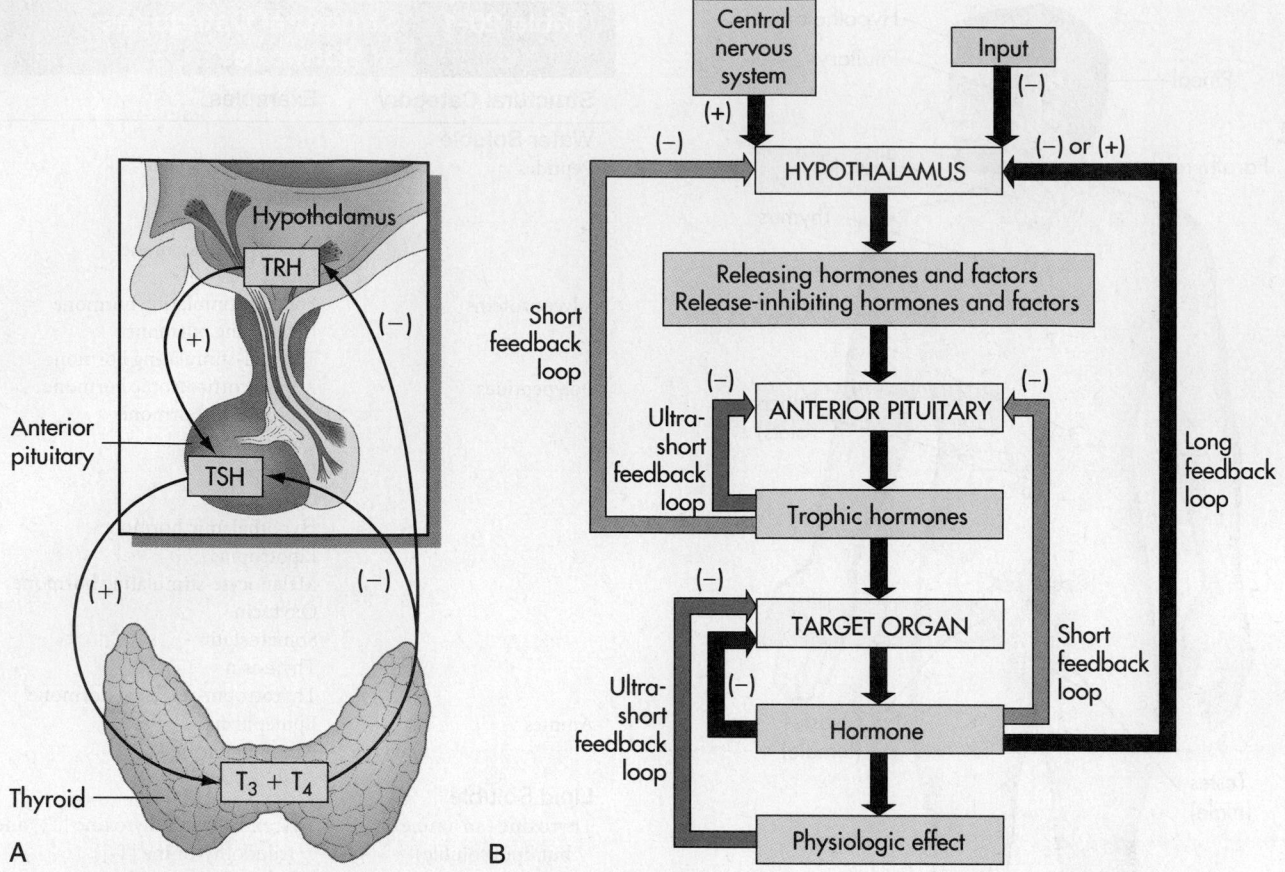

Figure 20-2 Feedback loops. **A,** Endocrine feedback loops involving the hypothalamus-pituitary gland and end organs; in this example, the feedback loops for the thyroid gland (endocrine regulation). **B,** General model for control and negative feedback to hypothalamic-pituitary target organ systems. Negative-feedback regulation is possible at three levels: target organ (ultrashort feedback), anterior pituitary (short feedback), and hypothalamus (long feedback). *TRH,* Thyroid-releasing hormone; *TSH,* thyroid-stimulating hormone; T_3, triiodothyronine; T_4, tetraiodothyronine-thyroxine.

primarily in the hypothalamus and by negative-feedback inhibition from thyroid hormones.

Negative-feedback systems are important in maintaining hormones within physiologic ranges. The lack of negative-feedback inhibition on hormonal release often results in pathologic conditions. As discussed in Chapter 21, various hormonal imbalances and related conditions are caused by excessive hormone production, which is the result of failure to "turn off" the system. These negative-feedback regulatory systems are diagrammed in Figure 20-2, *B.*

An example of neural regulation is the release of epinephrine from the adrenal medulla as a result of activation of the sympathetic division of the autonomic nervous system in response to stress. When the stress is removed, the nervous stimulation decreases and less epinephrine is released. Neural regulation is often integrated with temporal (e.g., circadian) and environmental stimuli. For example, the quantity and pattern of growth hormone secretion is a dynamic one affected by hypothalamic responses to stress, nutrients, adrenergic pathways, and other osmoreceptors.[2]

Hormone Transport

Once hormones are released into the circulatory system by the endocrine glands, they are circulated throughout the body. Peptide or protein hormones (insulin, pituitary, hypothalamic, parathyroid) are water soluble and circulate in free (unbound) forms. Water-soluble hormones generally have a short half-life because they are catabolized by circulating enzymes.[2] For example, insulin has a half-life of 3 to 5 minutes and is catabolized by insulinases. Lipid-soluble hormones, such as cortisol and adrenal androgens, are primarily circulated bound to a carrier or binding protein (Table 20-2). A small percentage of the lipid-soluble hormone circulates in a free or active form. For example, approximately 10% of the circulating cortisol is free, whereas 75% is bound to corticosteroid-binding globulin. Only free hormones can signal a target cell. A large change in the concentration of binding protein can affect the concentration of free hormones and therefore hormone effects (see Table 20-2). As is discussed later in this chapter, water-soluble hormones bind to one of four classes of cell surface receptors, whereas lipid-soluble hormones bind

Table 20-2	Binding Proteins, Their Hormones, and Variables That Affect Their Circulating Levels		
Binding Protein	Hormone	Factors That Increase Binding Protein Levels	Factors That Decrease Binding Protein Levels
Corticosteroid-binding globulin	Cortisol Progesterone	Estrogen	Liver disease
Sex hormone–binding globulin	Dihydrotestosterone Testosterone Estradiol	—	Androgens Hypothyroidism Liver disease
Thyroid-binding globulin	Thyroxine (T_4) Triiodothyronine (T_3)	Estrogen Hyperthyroidism	Testosterone Glucocorticoids Liver disease
Albumin	All lipid-soluble hormones	Estrogen	Liver disease Malnutrition Renal disease

to plasma membrane receptors or diffuse through the plasma membrane and bind to cytosolic or nuclear receptors.

Cellular Mechanisms of Hormone Action

When a hormone is released into the circulatory system, it is distributed throughout the body, but only those cells with appropriate receptors for that hormone are affected. The **target cell** hormone receptors have two main functions: (1) to recognize and bind with high affinity to their particular hormones and (2) to initiate a signal to appropriate intracellular effectors. See Chapter 1 for cell signaling pathways, particularly Figures 1-16 and 1-17 on pages 18-19. The binding of hormones with their receptors stimulates three general types of responses by:

1. Acting on preexisting channel-forming proteins to alter membrane channel permeability
2. Activating preexisting proteins through a second messenger system
3. Activating genes to cause protein synthesis

The sensitivity of the target cell to a particular hormone is related to the total number of receptors per cell. Low concentrations of hormone increase the number of receptors per cell; this is called **up-regulation** (Figure 20-3, A). High concentrations of hormone decrease the number of receptors; this is called **down-regulation** (Figure 20-3, B). Thus the cell can adjust its sensitivity to the concentration of the signaling hormone.

Hormones have two general types of effects on target cells: direct and permissive. **Direct effects** are the obvious changes in cell function that specifically result from stimulation by a particular hormone. **Permissive effects** are less obvious hormone-induced changes that facilitate the maximal response or functioning of a cell. For example, insulin has a direct effect on skeletal muscle cells with insulin receptors, causing increased glucose transport into these cells. Insulin also has a permissive effect on mammary cells, facilitating the response of these cells to the direct effects of prolactin.

Some hormones have biphasic pharmacologic effects that are dependent on the concentration of the hormone. For example, low or physiologic levels of antidiuretic hormone

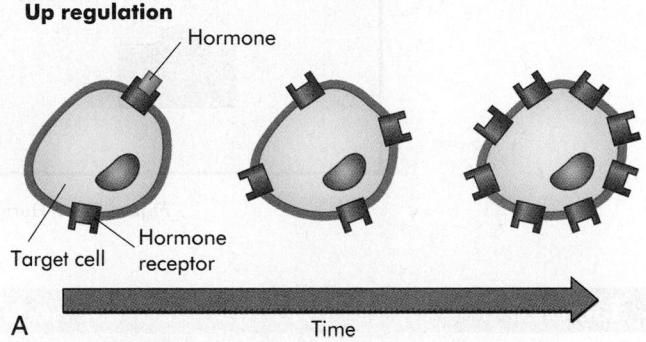

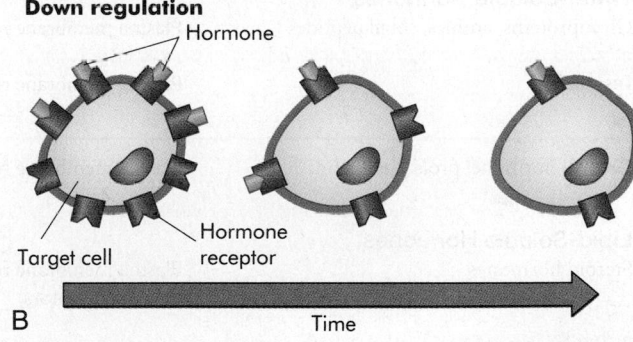

Figure 20-3 Regulation of target cell sensitivity. A, Low hormone level and up-regulation, or an increase in the number of receptors. B, High hormone level and down-regulation, or a decrease in the number of receptors. (From Thibodeau GA, Patton KT: *Anatomy & physiology*, ed 6, St Louis, 2007, Mosby.)

(ADH, or arginine vasopressin) stimulate renal tubular reabsorption of sodium and water. However, at supraphysiologic levels (i.e., those that can be achieved by exogenous administration), ADH acts as a vasoconstrictor.

Hormone Receptors

Hormone receptors may be located in or on the plasma membrane or in the intracellular compartment of the target cell (Figure 20-4). Water-soluble hormones (see Table 20-1)

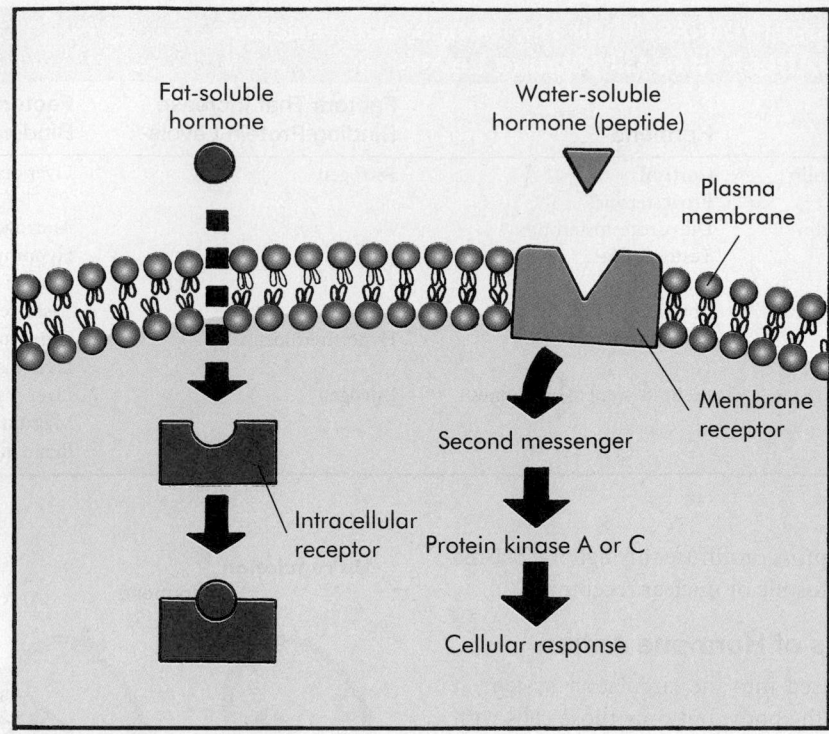

Figure 20-4　Hormone binding at target cell.

Table 20-3	Types of Hormones, Their Receptors, and Their Mechanisms of Action	
Hormone	**Type of Receptor**	**Mechanism of Action**
Water-Soluble Hormones		
Glycoproteins, amines, small peptides	Plasma membrane receptors	Second messengers; cAMP, cGMP, Ca^{++}, IP_3, DAG and proteins (except insulin)
Insulin	Plasma membrane receptors	Involves receptor autophosphorylation and activation of the receptor protein tyrosine kinase
Growth hormone, prolactin, leptin	Plasma membrane receptors	Involves intracellular JAK and activation of STAT pathway
Lipid-Soluble Hormones		
Steroid hormones	Plasma membrane receptors	Rapid nongenomic action
	Nuclear receptors	Nuclear translocation and altered genome transcription
Thyroid hormones (iodothyronines)	Nuclear receptor	Altered genome transcription
	Cytosolic receptors	Promote cytosolic signal transduction

cAMP, Cyclic adenosine monophosphate; *cGMP,* cyclic guanosine monophosphate; *DAG,* diacylglycerol; *IP₃,* inositol triphosphate; *JAK,* Janus family of tyrosine kinases; *STAT,* signal transducers and activators of transcription.

have a high molecular weight and cannot diffuse across the cell membrane. They interact or bind with receptors in or on the cell membrane.[3] Steroid hormones are lipid soluble. These hormones easily diffuse across the plasma membrane and bind to either cytosolic or nuclear receptors. The hormone-receptor complex binds to a specific region in the deoxyribonucleic acid (DNA) and alters the expression of a specific gene. The recent discovery of nongenomic rapid actions of thyroid and steroid hormones indicates plasma membrane receptors that activate second messenger systems

are also present.[4-6] (Types of hormones, their corresponding receptors, and the mechanisms by which they affect the cell are summarized in Table 20-3.)

Plasma Membrane Receptors and Signal Transduction

First Messenger

Receptors for most water-soluble hormones are located on the plasma membrane of a target cell. Sometimes a hormone or ligand that binds to a receptor is referred to as a **first**

messenger. This is because a hormone binding to its specific receptor represents the first signal within an elaborate signal transduction cascade. **Signal transduction** is the process by which extracellular signals (e.g., hormones) are communicated into a cell. In general, signal transduction involves a series of steps that includes receptor activation or binding of a hormone to its receptor, activation of a G protein (transducer) and membrane-associated enzyme (effector enzyme), and production of a second messenger (See Figure 1-20, page 22 and Figure 20-5). The final event is activation of an intracellular enzyme, such as protein kinase A or C, usually leading to alterations in gene transcription and the target cell response to the hormone.[7]

The signal transduction process begins at the receptor, which is a protein. Receptors on the plasma membrane are continuously synthesized and degraded, so the receptor number can vary from one cell type to another. Various physiochemical conditions can affect both the receptor number and the affinity at which the hormone binds to its receptor. Some of these physiochemical conditions are the fluidity and structure of the plasma membrane, pH, temperature,

ion concentration, diet, and the presence of other chemicals (e.g., drugs). Mutations in receptor structure also can affect target cell activation such that normal cellular responses are increased or decreased.[2]

Cell surface receptors usually are classified according to their function: (1) G protein–linked receptors, (2) ion-channel receptors, and (3) enzyme-linked receptors (including tyrosine-kinase, serine kinase, and the cytokine-receptor superfamily with intrinsic enzyme activity—such as the Janus family of tyrosine kinases [JAK] and signal tranducers and activators of transcription [STAT] molecules).[1,3,7,8] With the exception of insulin, growth hormone, and prolactin, most water-soluble hormones—such as adrenocorticotropic hormone (ACTH), glucagon, norepinephrine, and epinephrine—activate G protein–linked receptors.[3,8,9] Other hormones, such as angiotensin II, activate G protein–linked and ion-channel receptors. Insulin activates a tyrosine-kinase receptor. Growth hormones, prolactin, and cytokines—such as interleukins—activate the JAK/STAT receptors.[10]

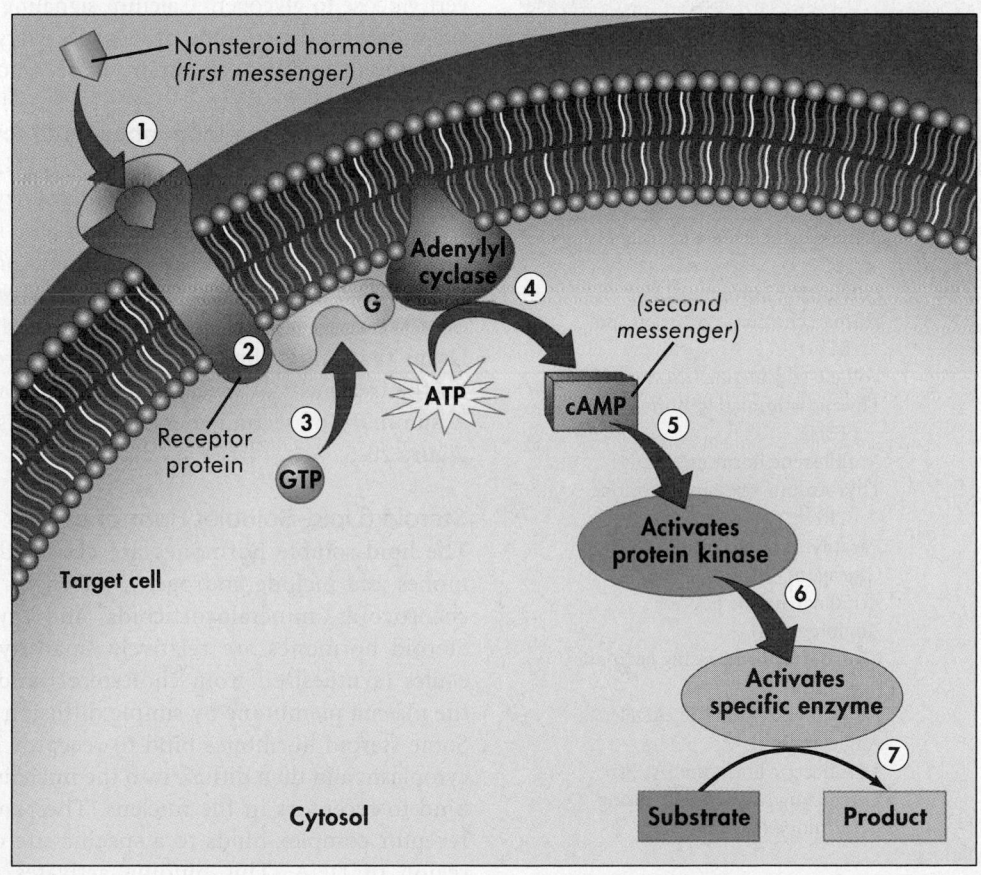

Figure 20-5 **Example of first- and second-messenger signaling.** A nonsteroid hormone (first messenger) binds to a fixed receptor of the target cell (1). The hormone-receptor complex activates the G protein (2). The activated G protein (G) reacts with guanosine triphosphate (GTP), which in turn activates the membrane-bound enzyme adenylyl cyclase (3). Adenylyl cyclase catalyzes the conversion of adenosine triphosphate (ATP) to cyclic adenosine monophosphate (cAMP; second messenger) (4). cAMP activates protein kinase (5). Protein kinases activate specific intracellular enzymes (6). These activated enzymes then influence specific cellular reactions and metabolic pathways, thus producing the target cell's response to the hormone (7). (From Thibodeau GA, Patton KT: *Anatomy & physiology,* ed 6, St Louis, 2007, Mosby).

Second-Messenger Molecules: cAMP, Ca⁺⁺, and cGMP

Cyclic Adenosine Monophosphate (cAMP). Second-messenger molecules are the initial link between the first signal (hormone) and the inside of the cell (Table 20-4). For example, binding of epinephrine to a β-adrenergic receptor subtype activates (through a stimulatory G protein [G_s]) the enzyme adenylyl cyclase. Adenylyl cyclase catalyzes the conversion of adenosine triphosphate (ATP) to the second messenger, 3′,5′-cAMP. Elevation of cAMP activates the enzyme cAMP-dependent *protein kinase A (PKA)*. Kinase enzymes, by adding a phosphate moiety to cellular proteins, either activate or deactivate intracellular proteins or enzymes. PKA phosphorylates and activates nuclear transcription factors (cAMP response element-binding [CREB] proteins) that influence numerous cellular functions.[11] Alterations in CREB activity have been implicated in many disease states including cancer and stroke.[12,13] In cardiac muscle, cAMP-dependent protein kinase phosphorylation of cellular membrane proteins associated with the L-type channel increase the influx of calcium into the cell. Increased intracellular calcium levels increase myocardial contractility. The actions of cAMP are terminated by the enzyme phosphodiesterase (PDE) III, which hydrolyzes cAMP into inactive adenosine monophosphate (AMP).

Calcium (Ca⁺⁺). In addition to being an important ion that participates in a multitude of cellular actions, Ca⁺⁺ is considered an important second messenger.[14,15] The binding of a hormone (such as norepinephrine or angiotensin II) to a surface receptor activates the enzyme *phospholipase C* through a G protein inside the plasma membrane. This enzyme breaks down membrane phospholipid phosphatidylinositol biphosphate (PIP_2) into second messengers **inositol triphosphate (IP₃)** and **diacylglycerol (DAG)** (See Figure 1-21, page 22). IP₃ mobilizes Ca⁺⁺ from intracellular stores (endoplasmic reticulum). In several cell types an increase in intracellular Ca⁺⁺ activates specific physiologic effects. For example, when Ca⁺⁺ binds with intracellular calmodulin, the Ca⁺⁺-calmodulin complex activates specific proteins.

DAG, together with Ca⁺⁺, activates *protein kinase C (PKC)*. Similar to other kinase enzymes, PKC either activates (by phosphorylation) or deactivates (dephosphorylates) other proteins or enzymes. PKC initiates a variety of cellular responses that are linked to cell metabolism and growth. For example, PKC activates glycogen synthase in liver cells to convert glucose to glycogen. Calcium signaling systems are crucial to healthy functioning of virtually every tissue system in the body including heart, brain, bone, smooth muscle, and many others.[14-18]

Cyclic Guanosine Monophosphate (cGMP). The production of the second messenger 3′,5′-cGMP is associated with the activation of the intracellular enzyme guanylyl cyclase. cGMP activates cGMP-dependent kinase, which in turn activates a number of physiologic processes. The effects of various ligands, such as atrial natriuretic factor and nitric oxide, are mediated by the second messenger cGMP. Drugs that target the actions of cGMP are being explored for the treatment of vascular and pulmonary disorders.[19,20] A summary of second messenger systems is presented in Figure 20-5.

Steroid (Lipid-Soluble) Hormones

The lipid-soluble hormones are classified as steroid hormones and include androgens, estrogens, progestins, glucocorticoids, mineralocorticoids, and thyroid hormones. Steroid hormones are relatively small hydrophobic molecules (synthesized from cholesterol) and therefore cross the plasma membrane by simple diffusion (see Chapter 1). Some steroid hormones bind to receptor molecules in the cytoplasm and then diffuse into the nucleus, whereas others bind to receptors in the nucleus. The resulting hormone-receptor complex binds to a specific site on the promoter region of DNA. This binding activates ribonucleic acid (RNA) polymerase, which stimulates DNA transcription and increased synthesis of specific proteins (increased gene expression) (Figure 20-6). Modulation of gene expression can take hours to days.

Recent studies indicate there are steroid hormone receptors in the plasma membrane associated with rapid response

Table 20-4	Second Messengers Identified for Specific Hormones	
Second Messenger	**Associated Hormones**
Cyclic AMP	Adrenocorticotropic hormone (ACTH)
	Luteinizing hormone (LH)
	Human chorionic gonadotropin (hCG)
	Follicle-stimulating hormone (FSH)
	Thyroid-stimulating hormone (TSH)
	Antidiuretic hormone (ADH)
	Thyrotropin-releasing hormone (TRH)
	Parathyroid hormone (PTH)
	Glucagon
Cyclic GMP	Atrial natriuretic peptide
Calcium	Angiotensin II
	Gonadotropin-releasing hormone (GnRH)
	Antidiuretic hormone (ADH)
IP₃ and DAG	Angiotensin II
	Antidiuretic hormone (ADH)
	Luteinizing hormone–releasing hormone (LHRH)
Tyrosine phosphorylation	
Tyrosine kinase	Insulin
JAK-STAT	Growth hormone
	Leptin
	Prolactin

AMP, Adenosine monophosphate; *DAG,* diacylglycerol; *GMP,* guanosine monophosphate; *IP₃,* inositol triphosphate; *JAK,* Janus family of tyrosine kinases; *STAT,* signal transducers and activators of transcription.

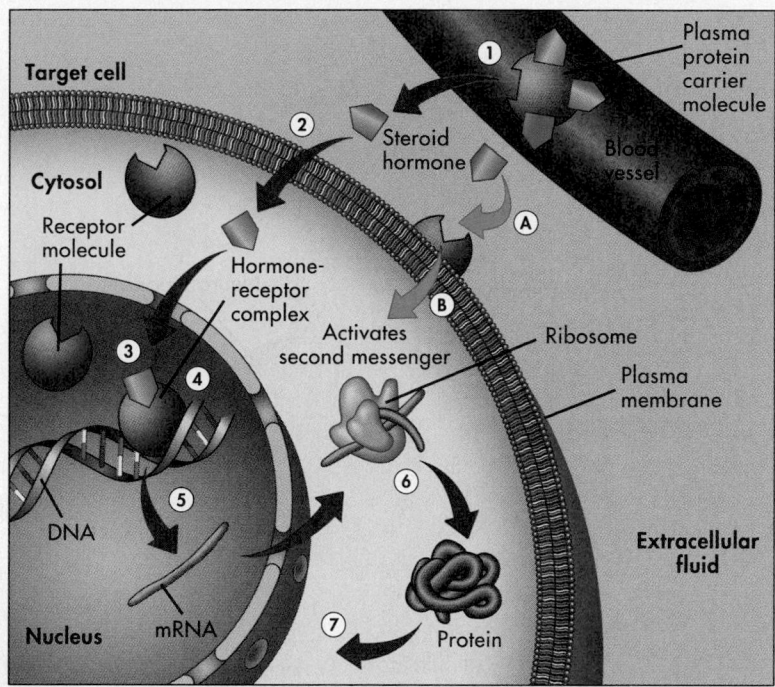

Figure 20-6 Steroid hormone mechanism. Lipid-soluble steroid hormone molecules detach from the carrier protein (1) and pass through the plasma membrane (2). Hormone molecules then diffuse into the nucleus, where they bind to a receptor to form a hormone-receptor complex (3). This complex then binds to a specific site on a DNA molecule (4), triggering transcription of the genetic information encoded there (5). The resulting messenger ribonucleic acid (mRNA) molecule moves to the cytosol, where it associates with a ribosome, initiating synthesis of a new protein (6). This new protein—usually an enzyme or channel protein—produces specific effects on the target cell (7). The classical genomic action is typically slow *(red arrows)*. Steroids also may exact rapid effects by binding to receptors on the plasma membrane (A) and activating an intercellular second messenger (B). (Modified from Patton KT, Thibodeau GA: *Anatomy & physiology,* ed 7, St Louis, 2010, Mosby.)

(seconds or minutes) that have nongenomic and genomic effects.[4,21-24] These receptors are still being explored, and it has been found that the nongenomic actions of steroid hormones involve many second messengers. Crosstalk between gene transcription and nongenomic responses modulates each other, allowing cells to adapt rapidly to environmental changes.[2] Thyroid hormone, a nonsteroid lipid-soluble hormone, also has been recently found to use a cell surface receptor for its nongenomic actions.[5,6] It first binds to an integrin receptor on the plasma membrane, then uses a specific transport mechanism to gain access to its nuclear receptors.[5]

STRUCTURE AND FUNCTION OF THE ENDOCRINE GLANDS

Hypothalamic-Pituitary Axis

The hypothalamic-pituitary axis (HPA) forms the structural and functional basis for central integration of the neurologic and endocrine systems, creating what is called the **neuroendocrine system**.[25] The HPA produces a number of releasing/inhibitory hormones and tropic hormones that affect a number of diverse body functions (Figure 20-7). For example, the functions of the thyroid gland, adrenal gland, and male and female reproductive glands, as well as somatic growth and lactation, are regulated by hormones originating from the HPA.

Hypothalamus

The hypothalamus is divided into several nuclei and nuclear areas and is located at the base of the brain (Figures 20-8 and 20-9). The pituitary gland is located at the sella turcica (a saddle-shaped depression on the superior surface of the sphenoid bone). The communication or anatomic connection (blood vessels and neural tract) between the hypothalamus and anterior and posterior pituitary is quite elaborate and well described. However, simply described, the hypothalamus is connected to the anterior pituitary by way of portal osmoreceptor blood vessels (Figure 20-10), whereas the hypothalamus is connected to the posterior pituitary by way of a nerve tract referred to as the *supraopticohypophsial tract* (see Figure 20-9). These connections are vital to the functioning of the hypothalamus-pituitary system.[25]

The special cells of the hypothalamus are like other neurons in that they have similar electrical properties, organelles, membranes, and synapses. Neurosecretory cells, however, can synthesize and secrete the hypothalamic-releasing hormones and synthesize the hormones of the posterior portion of the pituitary gland.[25] For example, **antidiuretic hormone (ADH) and oxytocin** are synthesized in hypothalamic neurons but are stored and secreted by the posterior pituitary. ADH and oxytocin travel to the posterior pituitary by way of the hypothalamohypophysial nerve tract. Releasing/inhibitory

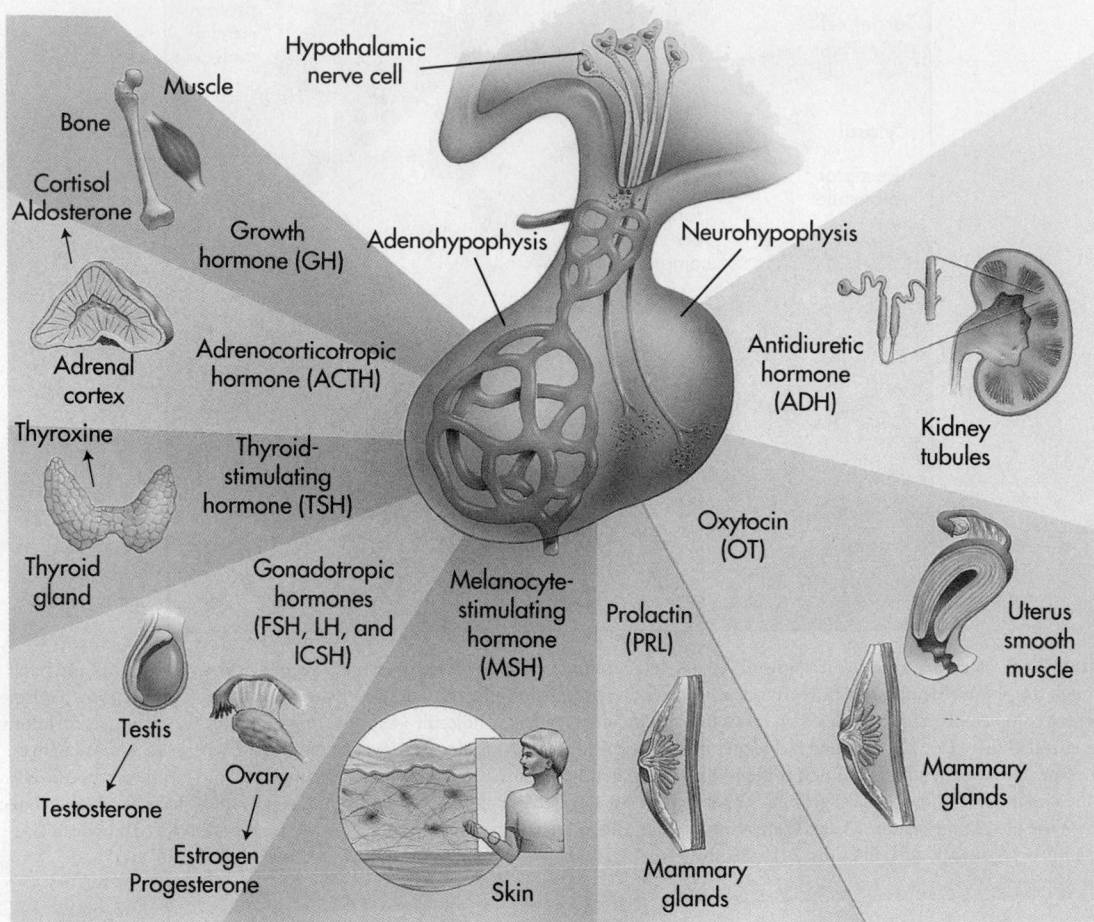

Figure 20-7 Pituitary hormones and their target organs. *FSH*, Follicle-stimulating hormone; *ICSH*, male analog of LH (interstitial cell–stimulating hormone) *LH*, luteinizing hormone. (Modified from Patton KT, Thibodeau GA: *Anatomy & physiology*, ed 7, St Louis, 2010, Mosby.)

hormones (see Figure 20-17, p. 716) are also synthesized in the hypothalamus and are secreted into the portal osmoreceptor blood vessels through which they travel to the anterior pituitary and control the release of tropic hormones. These releasing/inhibitory hormones from the hypothalamus include **prolactin-inhibiting factor** (PIF), **thyrotropin-releasing hormone** (TRH), **gonadotropin-releasing hormone** (GnRH), **somatostatin**, **growth hormone–releasing factor** (GRF), **corticotropin-releasing hormone** (CRH), and **substance P**. These hormones are summarized in Table 20-5.

Pineal Gland

The pineal gland is located within the brain itself (see Figure 20-1) and is composed of photoreceptive cells. It is innervated by noradrenergic sympathetic nerve terminals controlled by pathways within the hypothalamus.[25] The primary role of the pineal gland is to secrete the hormone melatonin. **Melatonin** release is stimulated by exposure to dark and inhibited by light exposure. It is synthesized from tryptophan. Tryptophan is first synthesized to serotonin and then to melatonin.

It regulates circadian rhythms and reproductive systems, including the secretion of GnRH and the onset of puberty.[25] It also plays an important role in immune regulation and is postulated to affect the aging process.[26,27] Further effects of melatonin include increasing nitric oxide release from blood vessels, removing toxic oxygen radicals, and decreasing insulin secretion.[28-30] Melatonin has been used therapeutically in humans to help with sleep disturbances, jet lag, and psychologic disorders, and its utility for numerous other disorders is being explored.[31]

Pituitary Gland

The **anterior pituitary** (adenohypophysis) accounts for 75% of the total weight of the pituitary gland. It is composed of three regions: (1) the pars distalis, (2) the pars tuberalis, and (3) the pars intermedia. The **pars distalis** is the major component of the anterior pituitary and the source of the anterior pituitary hormones. The **pars tuberalis** is a thin layer of cells on the anterior and lateral portions of the pituitary stalk. The **pars intermedia** lies between the two lobes of the pituitary

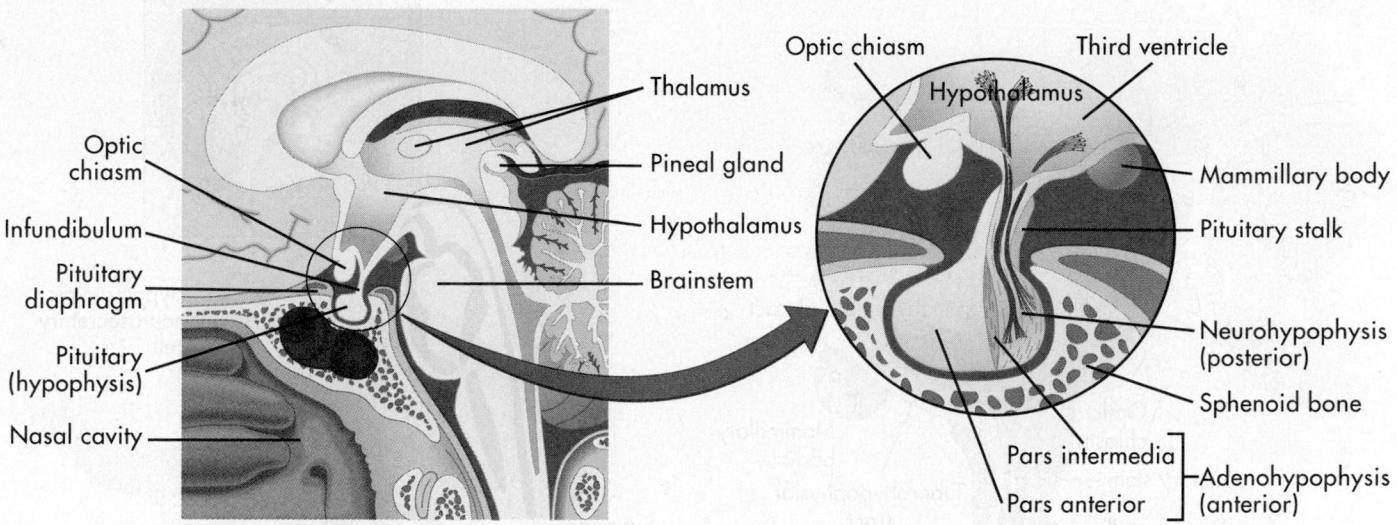

Figure 20-8 **Location and structure of the pituitary gland (hypophysis).** The pituitary gland is located within the sella turcica of the skull's sphenoid bone and is connected to the hypothalamus by a stalklike infundibulum. The infundibulum passes through a gap in the portion of the dura mater that covers the pituitary (the pituitary diaphragm). The inset shows that the pituitary is divided into an anterior portion, the adenohypophysis, and a posterior portion, the neurohypophysis. The adenohypophysis is further subdivided into the pars anterior and pars intermedia. The pars intermedia is almost absent in the adult pituitary. (Modified from Patton KT, Thibodeau GA: *Anatomy & physiology*, ed 7, St Louis, 2010, Mosby.)

gland. In the adult the distinct intermediate lobe disappears, and the individual cells are distributed diffusely throughout the pars distalis and **pars nervosa (neural lobe)**.

The **posterior pituitary** (neurohypophysis) arises embryologically from an outpouching of the floor of the third ventricle within the brain. The posterior pituitary consists of three parts: (1) the median eminence located at the base of the hypothalamus, (2) the pituitary stalk, and (3) the infundibular process, also known as the *pars nervosa* or *neural lobe*. The **median eminence** is composed largely of the nerve endings of axons that arise primarily in the ventral hypothalamus. The median eminence often is designated as part of the posterior pituitary but contains at least 10 biologically active hypothalamic-releasing hormones, as well as the neurotransmitters dopamine, norepinephrine, serotonin, acetylcholine, and histamine. The median eminence therefore might be more appropriately considered part of the hypothalamus. The **pituitary stalk** contains the axons of neurons that originate in the supraoptic and paraventricular nuclei of the hypothalamus. The pituitary stalk thus connects the pituitary gland to the brain. Axons originating in the hypothalamus terminate in the pars nervosa, which secretes the hormones of the posterior pituitary.

Because of the anatomic location and connection of the pituitary gland to the brain, several neurotransmitters as well as physical and emotional stressors influence the release of specific hypothalamic releasing–inhibitory hormones and their respective tropic hormones. For example, the neurotransmitter norepinephrine stimulates CRH, TRH, and GnRH secretion, whereas the neurotransmitter gamma-aminobutyric acid

(GABA) inhibits CRH, TRH, and GnRH secretion.[25] In terms of tropic hormone release from the anterior pituitary, norepinephrine stimulates the secretion of TSH, growth hormone (GH), luteinizing hormone (LH), and follicle-stimulating hormone (FSH), whereas the secretion of ACTH is inhibited. Physical (trauma) and emotional (pain) stress, starvation, and inflammation, as well as hypoglycemia, can influence the release of stimulating hormones, such as TRH and CRH, therefore ultimately affecting the amount of TSH and ACTH (the tropic hormones) released by the anterior pituitary.[25] This example emphasizes the integrated and coordinated function of the hypothalamic-pituitary axis.

Interestingly, hypothalamic hormones also are synthesized outside the HPA. For example, CRH is synthesized in cells of the immune system, female and male reproductive organs, and the placenta.[32] These peripherally synthesized neuropeptides are thought to play a role in the reproductive and immune responses to stress.[32,33]

Hormones of the Posterior Pituitary

The posterior pituitary secretes two polypeptide hormones: (1) ADH, also called *arginine vasopressin;* and (2) oxytocin. These peptide hormones are similar in structure, differing by only two amino acids. They are synthesized, along with their binding proteins, the neurophysins, in the supraoptic and paraventricular nuclei of the hypothalamus (see Figure 20-9). Once synthesized, these hormones and their carrier proteins are packaged in secretory vesicles. They are moved down the axons of the pituitary stalk to the pars nervosa for storage. The posterior pituitary thus can be seen as a storage

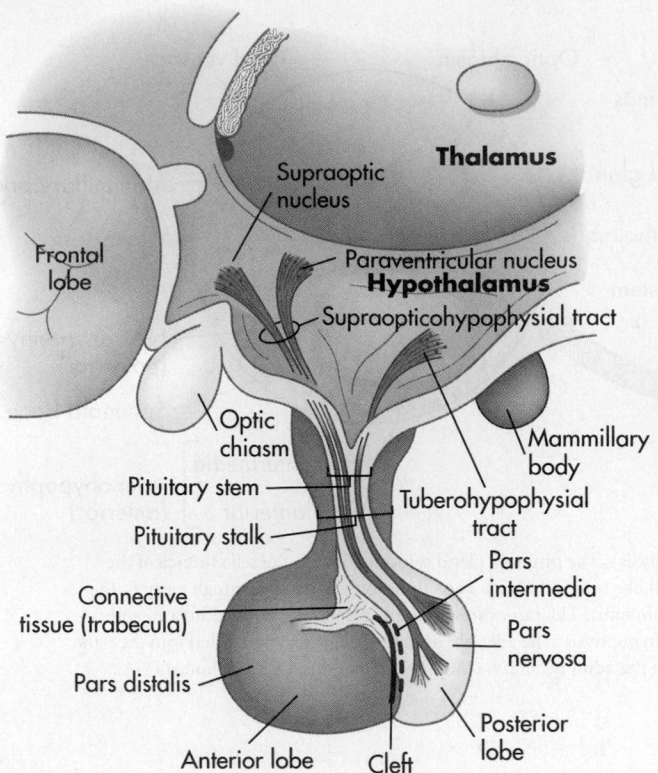

Figure 20-9 Nerve tracts from hypothalamus to posterior lobe of pituitary gland.

and releasing site for hormones synthesized in the hypothalamus.

Similar to the anterior pituitary hormones, the release of ADH and oxytocin is influenced by neurotransmitter release. The major stimulus to ADH and oxytocin release is glutamate, whereas the major inhibitory input is through GABA.[34]

Antidiuretic Hormone

The major homeostatic function of the posterior pituitary is the control of plasma osmolality, as regulated by ADH (see Chapter 3). At physiologic levels, ADH acts on the vasopressin 2 (V2) receptors of the renal tubular cells to increase their permeability (see Chapter 35). This increased permeability leads to an increase in water reabsorption into the blood and the production of more concentrated urine. These effects may be inhibited by hypercalcemia, prostaglandin E, and hypokalemia. ADH has no direct effect on electrolyte levels, but by increasing water reabsorption, serum electrolyte concentrations may decrease because of a dilutional effect.[34]

The secretion of ADH is regulated primarily by the osmoreceptors of the hypothalamus, located near or in the supraoptic nuclei (osmoreceptors are stimulated by increased osmolality). These osmoreceptors also control thirst. The plasma osmolality is maintained at the mean set point of approximately 280 mOsm/kg. As plasma osmolality increases, the rate of ADH secretion increases, more water is reabsorbed from the kidney, and the plasma is diluted back to its set-point osmolarity.

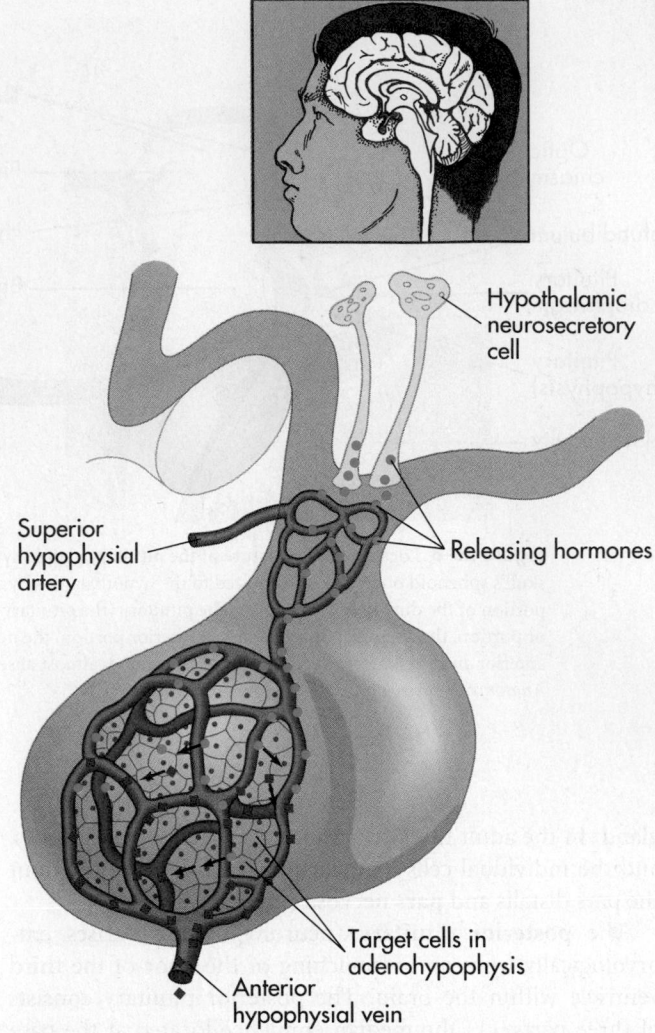

Figure 20-10 Hypophysial portal system. Neurons in the hypothalamus secrete releasing hormones into veins that carry the releasing hormones directly to the vessels of the adenohypophysis, thus bypassing the normal circulatory route. (From Patton KT, Thibodeau GA: *Anatomy & physiology,* ed 7, St Louis, 2010, Mosby.)

Other mechanisms also affect ADH secretion. ADH secretion is increased by changes in intravascular volume. Intravascular volume changes are monitored by mechanoreceptors in the left atrium and in the carotid and aortic arches. A volume loss of 7% to 25% acts through these receptors to stimulate ADH secretion. This mechanism for regulating ADH secretion is much less sensitive than that of the osmoreceptors. Stress, trauma, pain, exercise, nausea, nicotine, exposure to heat, and drugs such as chloroform and morphine also increase ADH secretion, apparently by activating cholinergic neurotransmitters in the hypothalamus. ADH secretion decreases with a decrease in plasma osmolality, an increase in intravascular volume, hypertension, estrogen, progesterone, angiotensin II, and alcohol ingestion.

ADH originally was named *vasopressin* because in extremely high doses it does cause vasoconstriction and a resulting increase in arterial blood pressure. This baroreceptor-mediated

Table 20-5   Hypothalamic Hormones (Hypophysiotropic Hormones)

Hormone	Target Tissue	Action
Thyrotropin-releasing hormone (TRH)	Anterior pituitary	Stimulates release of thyroid-stimulating hormone (TSH)
		Modulates prolactin secretion
Gonadotropin-releasing hormone (GnRH)	Anterior pituitary	Stimulates release of follicle-stimulating hormone (FSH) and luteinizing hormone (LH)
Somatostatin	Anterior pituitary	Inhibits release of growth hormone (GH) and TSH
Growth hormone–releasing hormone (GHRH)	Anterior pituitary	Stimulates release of GH
Corticotropin-releasing hormone (CRH)	Anterior pituitary	Stimulates release of adrenocorticotropic hormone (ACTH) and β-endorphin
Substance P	Anterior pituitary	Inhibits synthesis and release of ACTH
		Stimulates secretion of GH, FSH, LH, and prolactin
Dopamine	Anterior pituitary	Inhibits synthesis and secretion of prolactin
Prolactin-releasing factor (PRF)	Anterior pituitary	Stimulates secretion of prolactin

response is much less sensitive than the ADH response to changes in osmolarity. Therefore, physiologic levels of ADH do not significantly affect vessel tone. However, significant vasoconstriction may be achieved pharmacologically. For example, high doses of ADH (given as the drug vasopressin) may be administered to achieve hemostasis during hemorrhage and to raise blood pressure in shock states.[35,36]

Oxytocin

Oxytocin is primarily responsible for contraction of the uterus and milk ejection in lactating women and may have a role in sperm motility in men, although this effect has not yet been clearly elucidated. In both sexes, oxytocin has an antidiuretic effect similar to that of ADH. The mechanisms by which this effect is achieved appear to be similar to those of ADH, but the physiologic significance is not clear. (The function of this hormone is discussed in Chapter 22.)

The release of oxytocin has been studied more extensively in women than in men. In a woman, oxytocin is secreted in response to suckling and mechanical distention of the female reproductive tract.[34] Oxytocin is required for the milk "letdown" reflex. Stimulated by sucking, oxytocin binds to its receptors on myoepithelial cells in the mammary tissues and causes contraction of those cells. This results in increased intramammary pressure and milk expression.

Oxytocin also acts on the uterus to stimulate contractions. Its role in initiating labor has been debated because levels of oxytocin do not increase until near the end of labor. However, it is used clinically to induce uterine contraction. It is hypothesized that near the end of labor oxytocin functions to enhance effectiveness of contractions, to promote delivery of the placenta, and to stimulate postpartum contractions to prevent excessive bleeding.[37]

Oxytocin has been implicated in behavior responses, especially in women. It has been suggested that oxytocin reduces the brain's responsiveness to stressful stimuli, especially in the pregnant and postpartum states.[38,39] Its potential role in the treatment of a variety of anxiety disorders and autism is being explored.[38,40]

Hormones of the Anterior Pituitary

The anterior pituitary is composed of two main cell types: (1) the **chromophobes,** which appear to be nonsecretory, and (2) the **chromophils,** which are considered the secretory cells of the adenohypophysis. The chromophils are subdivided into six secretory cell types, each type secreting one or more specific hormones (Table 20-6). In general, the regulation of the anterior pituitary hormones is achieved by (1) feedback of hypothalamic releasing–inhibitory hormones and factors, (2) feedback from target gland hormones (i.e., cortisol, estrogen), and (3) direct effects of neurotransmitters.

The tropic hormones secreted by the anterior pituitary include ACTH, melanocyte-stimulating hormone (MSH), LH, GH, prolactin, FSH, and TSH. The actions of these anterior pituitary tropic hormones are summarized in Table 20-6. Even though six major stimulatory hormones are released by the anterior pituitary, they can be grouped into three categories: corticotropin-related hormones (ACTH, β-lipoprotein, MSH, and related endorphins), glycoproteins (LH, FSH, and TSH), and somatomammotropins (GH and prolactin). The corticotropin-related hormones are all derived from the precursor pro-opiomelanocortin (POMC). POMC is the precursor for ACTH and β-lipotropin; MSH exists within the ACTH amino acid sequence. β-endorphin and met-enkephalin are derived from β-lipotropin. (The role of ACTH is discussed later in this chapter. The glycoprotein gonadotropins FSH and LH control reproductive processes in men and women and are discussed in Chapter 22. TSH and its effects on the thyroid gland are discussed later in this chapter.) The somatomammotropins have diverse and important effects on body tissues.

Growth Hormone (GH)

GH secretion is controlled by two hormones from the hypothalamus: GnRH, which increases GH secretion, and somatostatin, which inhibits it.[41] GH is released from the pituitary in a pulsatile fashion, and overall secretion peaks during adolescence. This hormone is essential to normal tissue

Table 20-6 Tropic Hormones of the Anterior Pituitary and Their Functions

Hormone	Secretory Cell Type	Target Organs	Functions
Adrenocorticotropic hormone (ACTH)	Corticotropic	Adrenal gland (cortex)	Increased steroidogenesis (cortisol and androgenic hormones) Synthesis of adrenal proteins contributing to maintenance of the adrenal gland
Melanocyte-stimulating hormone (MSH)	Melanotropic	Anterior pituitary	Promotes secretion of melanin and lipotropin by anterior pituitary; makes skin darker
Somatotropic hormones Growth hormone (GH)	Somatotropic	Muscle, bone, liver	Regulates metabolic processes related to growth and adaptation to physical and emotional stressors, muscle growth, increased protein synthesis, increased liver glycogenolysis, increased fat mobilization
		Liver	Induces formation of somatomedins, or insulin-like growth factors (IGFs) that have actions similar to insulin
Prolactin	Lactotropic	Breast	Milk production
Glycoprotein hormones Thyroid-stimulating hormone (TSH)	Thyrotropic	Thyroid gland	Increased production and secretion of thyroid hormone Increased iodide uptake Promotes hypertrophy and hyperplasia of thymocytes
Luteinizing hormone (LH)	Gonadotropic	In women: granulosa cells	Ovulation, progesterone production
		In men: Leydig cells	Testicular growth, testosterone production
Follicle-stimulating hormone (FSH)	Gonadotropic	In women: granulosa cells	Follicle maturation, estrogen production
		In men: Sertoli cells	Spermatogenesis
β-Lipotropin	Corticotropic	Adipose cells	Fat breakdown and release of fatty acids
β-Endorphins	Corticotropic	Adipose cells Brain opioid receptors	Analgesia; may regulate body temperature, food and water intake

growth and maturation, and affects aging, sleep, nutritional status stress, and reproductive hormones.[42] In the bone, GH stimulates epiphyseal growth and increases osteoclast and osteoblast activity, resulting in increased bone mass.[41] GH also increases amino acid transport in muscles. Other functions of GH include lipolysis and enhancement of hepatic protein synthesis.

Many of the anabolic functions of GH are mediated, at least in part, by the insulin-like growth factors (IGFs), also known as the somatomedins.[41] There are two primary forms of IGF: IGF-1 and IGF-2, of which IGF-1 is the most biologically active. They both circulate bound to a group of binding proteins (IGFBP). IGF-1 binds to both insulin receptors, providing an insulin-like effect on skeletal muscle, and with the IGF-1 receptor, which mediates the anabolic effects of GH. The IGF-2 receptor causes a negative effect on tissue growth,

thus balancing the activity of the IGF-1 receptor.[43] IGF and IGFBPs have been linked to many forms of cancer because of their growth-stimulating effects.[43,44]

Prolactin

Prolactin primarily functions to induce milk production during pregnancy and lactation. It also has effects on ovulation and immune function. Its synthesis is stimulated by vasoactive intestinal polypeptide, serotonin, and growth factors. Its release is inhibited by dopamine. Hyperprolactinemia is a complication of tumors of the pituitary gland and some medications.[41]

Thyroid and Parathyroid Glands

The thyroid gland, located in the neck just below the larynx, produces hormones that control the rates of metabolic processes throughout the body. The four parathyroid glands are located near the posterior side of the thyroid and function to control serum calcium levels.

Thyroid Gland

The **thyroid gland** is composed of two lobes that lie on either side of the trachea, inferior to the thyroid cartilage (Figure 20-11). The lobes are joined by a small band of tissue, the **isthmus,** which crosses the anterior surface of the trachea and larynx at the cricoid cartilage. The normal thyroid gland is not visible on inspection, but it may be palpated on swallowing, which causes upward displacement of the gland.

The thyroid gland is composed of **follicles** (Figure 20-12). The follicles are composed of follicular cells that surround a viscous substance called *colloid.* The follicular cells synthesize and secrete some of the thyroid hormones. Neurons terminate on blood vessels within the thyroid gland and on the follicular cells themselves. Acetylcholine, catecholamines, and other peptides directly affect secretory activity of the follicular cells and thyroid blood flow.

Also found in the tissue of the thyroid are parafollicular cells, or **C cells** (see Figure 20-12). The C cells secrete various polypeptides, including calcitonin and somatostatin. **Calcitonin,** also called *thyrocalcitonin,* acts to lower serum calcium levels by inhibition of bone-resorbing osteoclasts. High levels of calcitonin are required for these effects, and deficiencies of calcitonin do not lead to hypocalcemia. (Bone resorption is explained in Chapter 41.) Consequently, the metabolic consequences of calcitonin deficiency or excess do not appear to be significant in humans (Table 20-7). However, calcitonin is used for treatment of osteoporosis, osteoarthritis, Paget bone disease, hypercalcemia, osteogenesis imperfecta, and metastatic cancer of the bone.[45-47] The precursor molecule to calcitonin, called procalcitonin, is a stress hormone that is elevated in significant infections and systemic inflammatory disorders.[48] Its measurement can aid in the diagnosis of these serious diseases.[48,49]

Regulation of Thyroid Hormone Secretion

Thyroid hormone (TH) is regulated through a negative-feedback loop involving the hypothalamus, the anterior pituitary, and the thyroid gland (see Figure 20-2). (Figure 20-12 illustrates the thyroid and parathyroid glands.) The initiating hormone is termed **thyrotropin-releasing hormone (TRH),** and it is synthesized and stored within the hypothalamus. TRH is released into the hypothalamic-pituitary portal system and circulates to the anterior pituitary, where it stimulates the release of TSH. TRH is increased with exposure to cold, stress, and decreased levels of thyroxine (T_4).

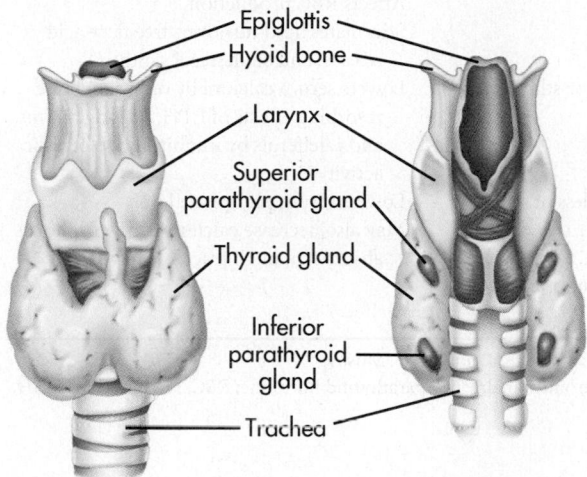

Figure 20-11 Thyroid and parathyroid glands. Note the relationship of the thyroid and parathyroid glands to each other, to the larynx (voice box), and to the trachea. (From Patton KT, Thibodeau GA: *Anatomy & physiology,* ed 7, St Louis, 2010, Mosby.)

Labels in figure: Epiglottis, Hyoid bone, Larynx, Superior parathyroid gland, Thyroid gland, Inferior parathyroid gland, Trachea

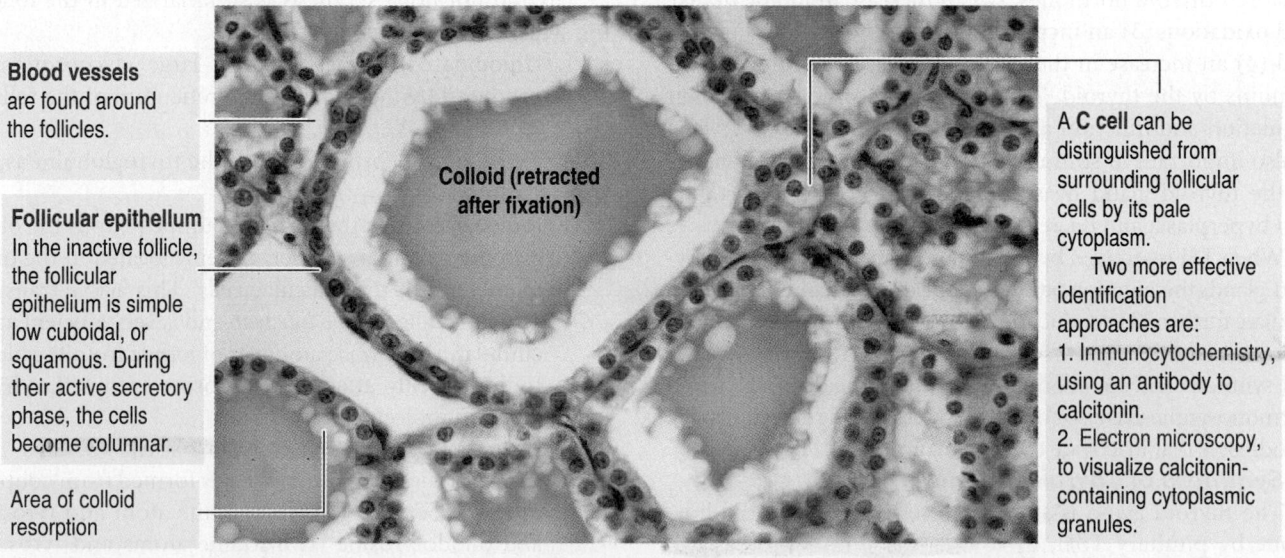

Blood vessels are found around the follicles.

Follicular epithelium In the inactive follicle, the follicular epithelium is simple low cuboidal, or squamous. During their active secretory phase, the cells become columnar.

Area of colloid resorption

Colloid (retracted after fixation)

A **C cell** can be distinguished from surrounding follicular cells by its pale cytoplasm.

Two more effective identification approaches are:
1. Immunocytochemistry, using an antibody to calcitonin.
2. Electron microscopy, to visualize calcitonin-containing cytoplasmic granules.

Figure 20-12 Thyroid follicle cells. (From Kierszenbaum A: *Histology and cell biology: an introduction to pathology,* ed 2, St Louis, 2007, Mosby.)

Table 20-7	Thyroid Gland Hormones and Their Regulation and Functions	
Hormone	Regulation	Functions

Thyroxine (T_4) and triiodothyronine (T_3)	T_4 and T_3 levels are controlled by TSH
	Released in response to metabolic demand
	Influences on amount secreted:
	    Gender
	    Pregnancy
	    Gonadal and adrenocortical-increased
	        steroids = ↑ levels
	    Exposure to extreme cold = ↑ levels
	    Nutritional state
	    Chemicals
	        GHIH = ↓ levels
	        Dopamine = ↓ levels
	        Catecholamines = ↑ levels
		Regulates protein, fat, and carbohydrate
		    catabolism in all cells
		Regulates metabolic rate of all cells
		Regulates body heat production
		Insulin antagonist
		Maintains growth hormone secretion, skeletal
		    maturation
		Affects CNS development
		Necessary for muscle tone and vigor
		Maintains cardiac rate, force, and output
		Maintains secretion of GI tract
		Affects respiratory rate and oxygen utilization
		Maintains calcium mobilization
		Affects RBC production
		Stimulates lipid turnover, free fatty acid
		    release, and cholesterol synthesis

Calcitonin	Elevated serum calcium—major stimulant for
	    calcitonin
	Other stimulants
	    Gastrin
	    Calcium-rich foods (regardless of serum
	        Ca^{++} levels)
	    Pregnancy
	Lowered serum calcium—suppresses
	    calcitonin release
		Lowers serum calcium by opposing bone-
		    resorbing effects of PTH, prostaglandins,
		    and calciferols by inhibiting osteoclastic
		    activity
		Lowers serum phosphate levels
		May also decrease calcium and phosphorus
		    absorption in GI tract

From Monahan FD, et al: *Phipps' medical-surgical nursing: health and illness perspective*, ed 8, St Louis, 2007, Mosby.
CNS, Central nervous system; *GHIH*, growth hormone–inhibiting hormone; *GI*, gastrointestinal; *PTH*, parathyroid hormone; *RBC*, red blood cell; *TSH*, thyroid-stimulating hormone.

Thyroid-stimulating hormone (TSH) is a glycoprotein hormone synthesized and stored within the anterior pituitary. Once TSH is secreted by the anterior pituitary, it circulates to bind with TSH receptor sites located on the outer side of the thyroid cell's plasma membrane. The effects of TSH on the thyroid include (1) an immediate increase in the release of stored thyroid hormones, (2) an increase in iodide uptake and oxidation, (3) an increase in thyroid hormone synthesis, and (4) an increase in the synthesis and secretion of prostaglandins by the thyroid. Thyroid gland hormones and their regulation and function are summarized in Table 20-7. TSH is also important in stimulating the growth and maintenance of the thyroid gland by stimulating thymocyte hypertophy and hyperplasia and decreasing apoptosis.[50]

When TH is secreted by the thyroid gland, it acts on the thyroid gland, the anterior pituitary, and the median eminence to regulate further TH production. Thyroid hormones have a negative-feedback effect and inhibit TRH and TSH, which decreases TH synthesis and secretion. Recent studies suggest that thyroid hormone synthesis is also controlled by circulating enzymes called deiodinases that inactivate the precursor molecule thyroxine.[51]

Synthesis of Thyroid Hormone

The thyroid gland is stimulated to produce thyroid hormone by pituitary TSH, by low serum iodide levels, or by drugs interfering with the thyroid gland's uptake of iodide from the blood. (Iodide is the inorganic or ionic form of iodine and is the form in which iodine enters the thyroid gland.) Iodide is oxidized to iodine in the presence of thyroidal peroxidase. The major naturally occurring source of iodine is seafood; in the United States iodine is added to salt and flour. Approximately 25% of ingested iodine is trapped by the thyroid gland.

Thyroid hormone synthesis is summarized in the following steps:

1. Uniodinated thyroglobulin (a large glycoprotein) is produced by the endoplasmic reticulum of the follicular cells.
2. Tyrosine is incorporated into the thyroglobulin as it is synthesized.
3. Iodide is actively transferred (pumped) from the blood into the colloid by carrier proteins located in the outer membrane of the follicular cells. This active transport system is called the *iodide trap* and is very efficient at accumulating the trace amounts of iodide from the blood.
4. Iodide quickly attaches to tyrosine within the thyroglobulin molecule.
5. Coupling of iodinated tyrosine forms thyroid hormones. Triiodothyronine (T_3) is formed from coupling of monoiodotyrosine (one iodine atom and tyrosine) and diiodotyrosine (two iodine atoms and tyrosine). Tetraiodothyronine (T_4), commonly known as thyroxine, is formed from coupling of two diiodotyrosines.

6. Thyroid hormones are stored attached to thyroglobulin within the colloid until it is released into the circulation. The thyroid gland normally produces 90% T$_4$ and 10% T$_3$. In the body tissues, however, T$_4$ is converted to T$_3$, and T$_3$ has the greatest metabolic effect. Once released into the circulation, T$_3$ and T$_4$ are primarily transported bound to one of three carrier proteins: thyroxine-binding globulin, thyroxine-binding prealbumin (transthyretin), or albumin. A small amount of thyroid hormone is also carried by lipoproteins.[52]

Thyroid hormones affect many body tissues, primarily by affecting growth and maturation of tissues. Similar to some steroid hormones, thyroid hormones bind to intracellular receptor complexes and then influence the genetic expression of specific proteins. Thyroid hormones also affect cell metabolism by altering protein, fat, and glucose metabolism and, as a result, heat production and oxygen consumption are increased. Thus these hormones are essential for maintaining healthy metabolic processes, and their use is being explored for the therapy of many metabolic disorders.[53]

It is important to note that thyroid hormones exert a number of permissive effects on many organs, which are rather modest at physiologic thyroid hormone levels. However, these effects can become very pronounced when there is either high or low levels of circulating thyroid hormones. For example, in the heart, T$_3$ stimulates the synthesis of specific contractile proteins (e.g., α-myosin heavy chain), sarcolemmal ion pumps (Na$^+$/K$^+$-ATPase pump, Ca^{++}-ATPase pump) and membrane receptors (β-adrenergic receptors). Therefore, in hyperthyroidism, which is associated with elevated levels of thyroid hormones, cardiac effects include increased heart rate and cardiac output, as well as the development of a cardiomyopathy. Thyroid hormones also affect the respiratory center, contributing to the normal hypoxic and hypercapnic drive. In severe hypothyroidism, ventilation can become very depressed. Thyroid hormone also stimulates bone resorption, and hyperthyroidism is associated with osteopenia, hypercalcemia, and hypercalciuria.[54] Thyroid hormone is essential for normal neurologic development in the fetus and infant and affects neurologic functioning in adults.[55] Other manifestations of thyroid hormone alteration are explained in Chapter 21.

Parathyroid Glands

Two pairs of parathyroid glands normally are present, but the number may range from two to six. They are small and located behind the upper pole of the thyroid gland and behind the lower pole (see Figure 20-11).

The parathyroid glands produce **parathyroid hormone (PTH),** a regulator of serum calcium. PTH is regulated primarily by the level of ionized plasma calcium, although how these regulatory mechanisms work is not precisely clear. Calcium also increases intraparathyroid destruction of PTH but apparently does not affect the rate of PTH synthesis.

Magnesium and phosphate levels also affect PTH secretion. Hypomagnesemia in persons with normal calcium levels acts as a mild stimulant to PTH secretion. In hypocalcemic individuals, hypomagnesemia decreases PTH secretion. Hyperphosphatemia leads to hypocalcemia because of calcium-phosphate precipitation in soft tissue and bone. Alterations in serum phosphate levels therefore may indirectly influence PTH secretion by affecting serum calcium levels (Figure 20-13). The overall effect of PTH is to increase serum calcium and to decrease serum phosphate concentration.

Once the parathyroid gland is stimulated, PTH is secreted. On release, PTH enters the circulation in unbound form. The hormone attaches to plasma membrane receptors in target tissues, where the biologic effects of PTH are mediated primarily by activation of the adenylyl cyclase system (see Chapter 1).

PTH is the single most important factor in the regulation of serum calcium levels (Figure 20-14). To achieve

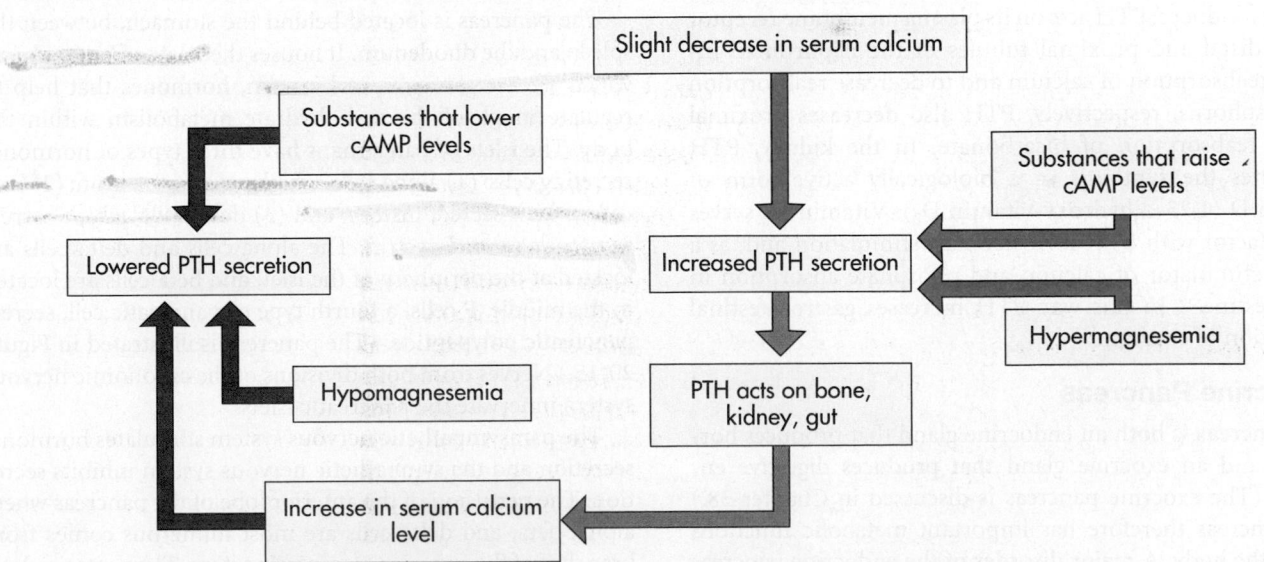

Figure 20-13 Variables affecting parathyroid hormone (PTH) secretion. *cAMP,* Cyclic adenosine monophosphate.

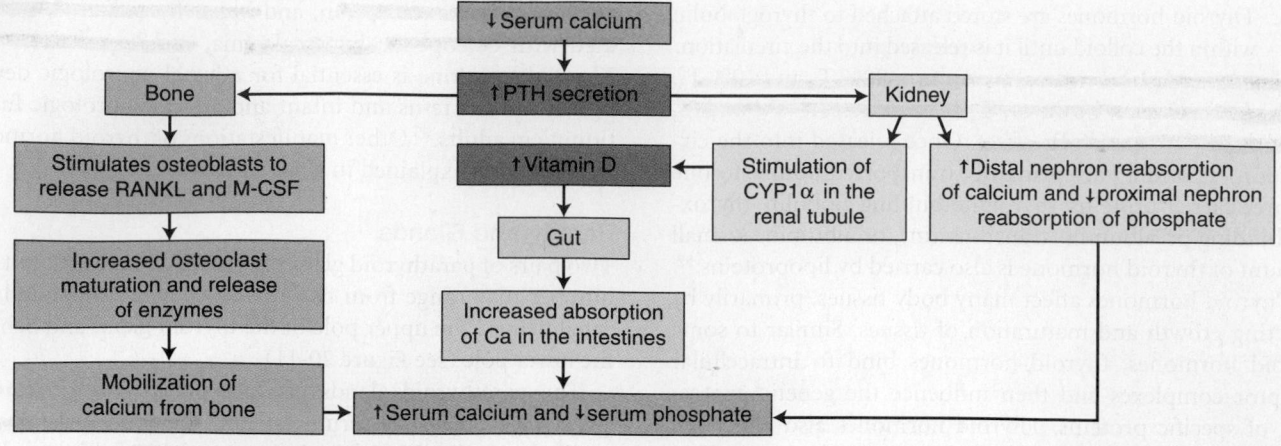

Figure 20-14 Normal calcium metabolism regulated by PTH and vitamin D. *CYP1*α-hydrolase, cytochrome P4501a-hydrolase; *M-CSF*, macrophage-colony stimulating factor; *PTH*, Parathyroid hormone; *RANKL*, Receptor activator of NF-ƙβ ligand.

regulation of serum calcium, PTH acts directly on bone and the kidneys. In bone, PTH has at least two effects. In acute hypocalcemia, PTH secretion stimulates osteoblasts to release receptor activator for nuclear factor-kappa beta (NF-ƙβ) ligand (RANKL) and macrophage-colony stimulating factor (M-CSF) which results in osteoclast proliferation, maturation, and release of acidic enzymes, such as cathepsin. These enzymes mobilize calcium from bone which increases the serum calcium. Chronic stimulation by PTH results in bone remodeling, a process in which bone is broken down and reformed. Chronic stimulation can occur because of parathyroid tumors (primary hyperparathyroidism) or because of chronic hypocalcemia like that seen in end-stage renal disease (secondary hyperparathyroidism). This process can weaken the bone, leading to an increased risk for fracture (e.g., renal osteodystrophy).[56] Paradoxically, intermittent therapeutic bursts of PTH can actually strengthen bone and are used in individuals with osteoporotic fractures.[57,58]

In the kidneys, PTH acts on its plasma membrane receptor in the distal and proximal tubules of the nephron to increase reabsorption of calcium and to decrease reabsorption of phosphorus, respectively. PTH also decreases proximal tubule reabsorption of bicarbonate. In the kidney, PTH stimulates the synthesis of a biologically active form of vitamin D (1,25-dihydroxy-vitamin D_3). Vitamin D_3 serves as a cofactor with PTH for osteoblast stimulation and, as a potent stimulator of calcium and phosphate absorption in the intestine.[59] In this way PTH increases gastrointestinal absorption of calcium.

Endocrine Pancreas

The **pancreas** is both an endocrine gland that produces hormones and an exocrine gland that produces digestive enzymes. (The exocrine pancreas is discussed in Chapter 38.) The pancreas therefore has important metabolic functions within the body. A major disorder of the endocrine pancreas is diabetes mellitus.

WHAT'S NEW?   Recombinant Parathyroid Hormone (rPTH)

Sustained PTH secretion leads to a reduction in bone density and increased bone fragility by stimulating osteoclasts to resorb bone and release calcium into the bloodstream. PTH stimulates bone resorption by first interacting with osteoblast receptors, resulting in osteoblast release of inflammatory stimulants for osteoclast activation. However, intermittent administration of rPTH (teriparatide) can be used therapeutically to strengthen bone, especially in individuals with osteoporotic fractures. Intermittent exposures to rPTH (once a day) increase bone turnover such that osteoblasts are stimulated more than osteoclasts and bone mineral density is increased. Furthermore, there is improvement in bone architecture as well as density (bone quality as well as quantity).

Data from Bergenstock MK, Partridge NC: *Ann N Y Acad Sci* 1116:354-359, 2007; Deal C: *Nat Clin Pract Rheumatol* 5(1):20-27, 2009; Khosla S, Westendorf JJ, Oursler MJ: *J Clin Invest* 118(2): 421-428, 2008.

The pancreas is located behind the stomach, between the spleen and the duodenum. It houses the islets of Langerhans, which secrete glucagon and insulin, hormones that help to regulate much of the carbohydrate metabolism within the body. The islets of Langerhans have three types of hormone-secreting cells: (1) alpha cells, which secrete glucagon; (2) beta cells, which secrete insulin; and (3) delta cells, which secrete somatostatin and gastrin. The alpha cells and delta cells are located at the periphery of the islet, and beta cells are located in the middle. F cells, a fourth type of pancreatic cell, secrete pancreatic polypeptide. (The pancreas is illustrated in Figure 20-15.) Nerves from both divisions of the autonomic nervous system innervate the pancreatic islets.

The parasympathetic nervous system stimulates hormonal secretion and the sympathetic nervous system inhibits secretion. The perfusion of the anterior lobe of the pancreas where alpha, beta, and delta cells are most numerous comes from branches of the superior mesenteric artery. The posterior lobe is perfused by branches of the celiac artery. The pancreatic

A

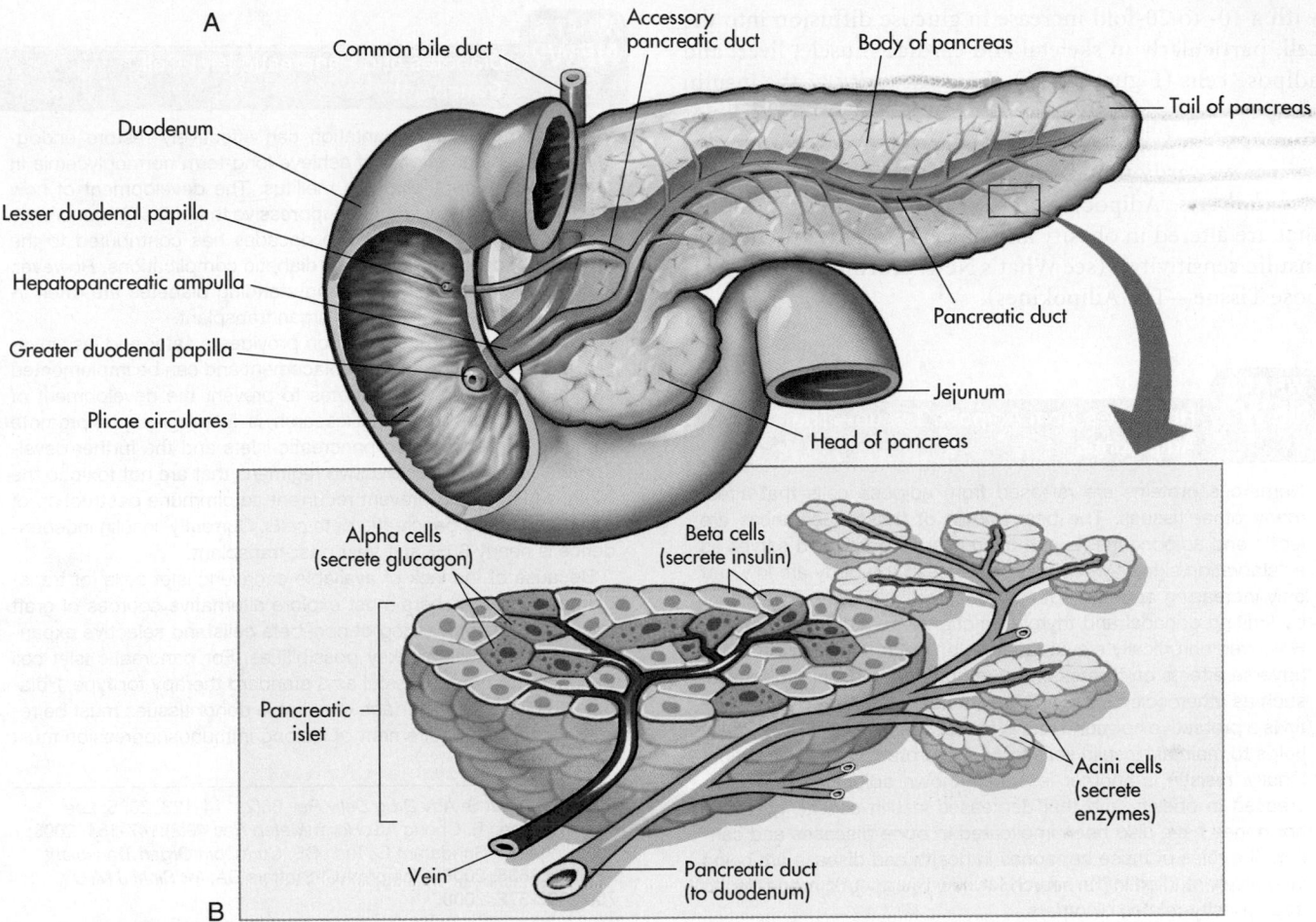

Common bile duct

Accessory pancreatic duct

Body of pancreas

Tail of pancreas

Duodenum

Lesser duodenal papilla

Hepatopancreatic ampulla

Greater duodenal papilla

Plicae circulares

Pancreatic duct

Jejunum

Head of pancreas

Alpha cells (secrete glucagon)

Beta cells (secrete insulin)

Pancreatic islet

Acini cells (secrete enzymes)

Vein

Pancreatic duct (to duodenum)

B

Figure 20-15 The pancreas. **A,** Pancreas dissected to show main and accessory ducts. The main duct may join the common bile duct, as shown here, to enter the duodenum by a single opening at the major duodenal papilla, or the two ducts may have separate openings. The accessory pancreatic duct is usually present and has a separate opening into the duodenum. **B,** Exocrine glandular cells (around small pancreatic ducts) and endocrine glandular cells of the pancreatic islets (adjacent to blood capillaries). Exocrine pancreatic cells secrete pancreatic juice, alpha endocrine cells secrete glucagon, and beta cells secrete insulin. (From Thibodeau GA, Patton KT: *Anatomy & physiology,* ed 5, St Louis, 2003, Mosby.)

islets receive 10% of the pancreatic blood flow but represent only 1% of pancreatic mass. This is necessary for oxygenation and delivery of islet hormones to target cells.

Insulin

The **beta cells** of the pancreas synthesize **insulin** from the precursor, proinsulin. Proinsulin is formed from a larger and earlier precursor molecule, preproinsulin. Proinsulin is composed of an A peptide and a B peptide connected by a C peptide and two disulfide bonds. C peptide is cleaved by proteolytic enzymes, leaving the A and B peptide chains connected by the disulfide bonds. The bonded A and B chains become insulin. Insulin circulates freely in the plasma and is not bound to a carrier. C peptide can be measured in the blood as an indirect measure of serum insulin synthesis. Recent studies have shown that C peptide has biologic activity and binds to cells through a G protein receptor resulting in increased intracellular calcium levels.[60] Its role in health and disease is being explored.[60-62]

Secretion of insulin is regulated by chemical, hormonal, and neural control. Insulin secretion is promoted by increased blood levels of glucose, amino acids (arginine and lysine), serum free fatty acids, and gastrointestinal hormones, and by parasympathetic stimulation of the beta cells. Insulin secretion diminishes in response to low blood levels of glucose (hypoglycemia), high levels of insulin (through negative feedback to the beta cells), and sympathetic stimulation of the alpha cells in the islets. Prostaglandin (PGE$_2$) also inhibits insulin secretion.

Insulin facilitates the rate of glucose uptake into many cells within the body. Binding of insulin to its tyrosine-kinase receptor subtype initiates a series of events that involves autophosphorylation of the insulin receptor substrate 1 (IRS-1) and the activation (phosphorylation) of other proteins, including GRB2, a PI-3 kinase, and a tyrosine phosphatase. The net effect is that glucose transporters (GLUT) migrate from the cytosol to the cell surface. Translocation of the GLUT4 transporter is associated with a 10- to 20-fold increase in glucose diffusion into the cell, particularly in skeletal and cardiac muscle, liver, and adipose cells (Figure 20-16). The sensitivity of the insulin receptor is a key component in maintaining normal cellular function, and insulin resistance has been implicated in numerous cardiovascular diseases, including hypertension and diabetes. Adipocytes release a number of hormones that are altered in obesity and have an important effect on insulin sensitivity[63] (see What's New? Hormones from Adipose Tissue—The Adipokines).

WHAT'S NEW? Hormones from Adipose Tissue—The Adipokines

Numerous proteins are released from adipose cells that affect many other tissues. The best known of these substances are leptin and adiponectin. Leptin decreases appetite and serves as a "starvation signal" when energy stores in the body are low, not only increasing appetite but also decreasing energy expenditure by limiting gonadal and thyroid function and increasing cortisol. However, chronically elevated levels of leptin can result in many adverse effects on tissues and contributes to vascular diseases, such as atherosclerosis and hypertension. In contrast, adiponectin is a protective hormone that is decreased in obesity. It normally helps to maintain insulin sensitivity and protect vascular function. Finally, resistin is another less well-known adipokine that is increased in obesity and that decreases insulin sensitivity. These hormones have also been implicated in bone diseases and cancer. The roles of these hormones in health and disease are being intensively studied in the search for new therapeutic modalities to treat obesity-related disorders.

Data from Antuna-Puente B et al: *Diabetes Metab* 34(1):2-11, 2008; Beltowski J, Jamroz-Wisniewska A, Widomska S: *Cardiovas Hematol Disord Drug Targets* 8(1):7-46, 2008; Guerre-Millo M: *Diabetes Metab* 34(1):12-18, 2008; Jarde T et al: *Oncol Rep* 19(4):905-911, 2008; Myers MG, Cowley MA, Munzberg H: *Ann Rev Physiol* 70:537-556, 2008; Smith SR, Ravussin E: Role of the adipocyte in metabolism and endocrine function. In DeGroot LJ, Jameson JL, editors: *Endocrinology*, ed 5, St Louis, 2006 Saunders.

Insulin is an anabolic hormone that promotes the synthesis of proteins, lipids, and nucleic acids. The major sites of insulin-promoted synthesis are the liver, muscle, and adipose tissue (Table 20-8). The net effect of insulin in these tissues is to stimulate cellular metabolism. Overall, however, the major consequence of insulin release is to decrease blood glucose. Insulin also facilitates the intracellular transport of potassium. The brain and red blood cells do not require insulin for glucose transport.

Insulin is metabolized in the liver and kidney by enzymes that split disulfide bonds. Very little insulin is excreted unchanged in the urine.

Amylin

Amylin is a peptide hormone co-secreted with insulin in response to nutrient stimuli. It regulates blood glucose by delaying nutrient uptake and suppressing glucagon secretion

---

WHAT'S NEW? Diabetes and Pancreatic Islet Cell Transplant

Whole pancreas transplantation can effectively restore endogenous insulin secretion and achieve long-term normoglycemia in people with type 1 diabetes mellitus. The development of new procedures and new immunosuppressive therapies for pancreatic transplant during the past two decades has contributed to the prevention, delay, or reversal of diabetic complications. However, secondary complications of long-standing diabetes are often irreversible at the time of whole organ transplant.

Pancreatic islet transplantation provides a safer and less invasive alternative for beta cell replacement and can be implemented earlier in the course of diabetes to prevent the development of secondary complications. Research is in progress to promote longevity of transplanted pancreatic islets and the further development of immunosuppressive regimens that are not toxic to the islets, which would prevent recurrent autoimmune destruction of the transplanted pancreatic beta cells. Currently, insulin independence is nearly 60% at 1 year post-transplant.

Because of the lack of available cadaveric islet cells for transplantation, researchers must explore alternative sources of graft material. Cell engineering of non–beta cells and selective expansion of stem cells are key possibilities. For pancreatic islet cell transplant to be successful as a standard therapy for type 1 diabetes mellitus, the shortage of suitable donor tissues must be resolved and the requirement of lifelong immunosuppression must be minimized.

Data from Efrat S: *Adv Drug Deliv Rev* 60(2):114-123, 2008; Lee DD, Grossman E, Chong AS: *Horm Metab Res* 40(2):147-154, 2008; Vaithilingam V, Sundaram G, Tuch BE: *Curr Opin Organ Transplant* 13(6):633-638, 2008; Claiborn KC, Stoffers DA: *Mt Sinai J Med* 75(4):362-372, 2008.

---

after meals. Amylin also has a satiety effect. Through these mechanisms, amylin has an antihyperglycemic effect.[64]

Glucagon

Glucagon is produced by the alpha cells of the pancreas and by a number of cells lining the gastrointestinal tract. High glucose levels cause glucagon release to be inhibited; low glucose levels and sympathetic stimulation promote glucagon release, particularly in the liver. Amino acids, such as alanine, glycine, and asparagine, also stimulate glucagon secretion. A protein-rich meal has the same effect.

Glucagon acts primarily in the liver and increases blood glucose by stimulating glycogenolysis and gluconeogenesis. Glucagon acts as an antagonist to insulin. Much controversy exists regarding the role of glucagon in carbohydrate regulation, both normally and in diabetes mellitus.[64] Glucagon also stimulates lipolysis, which has a ketogenic effect caused by the metabolism of free fatty acids in the liver.

Somatostatin

Pancreatic **somatostatin** is produced by delta cells of the pancreas and is a hormone essential in carbohydrate, fat, and protein metabolism (i.e., homeostasis of ingested nutrients). It differs from hypothalamic somatostatin, which inhibits release

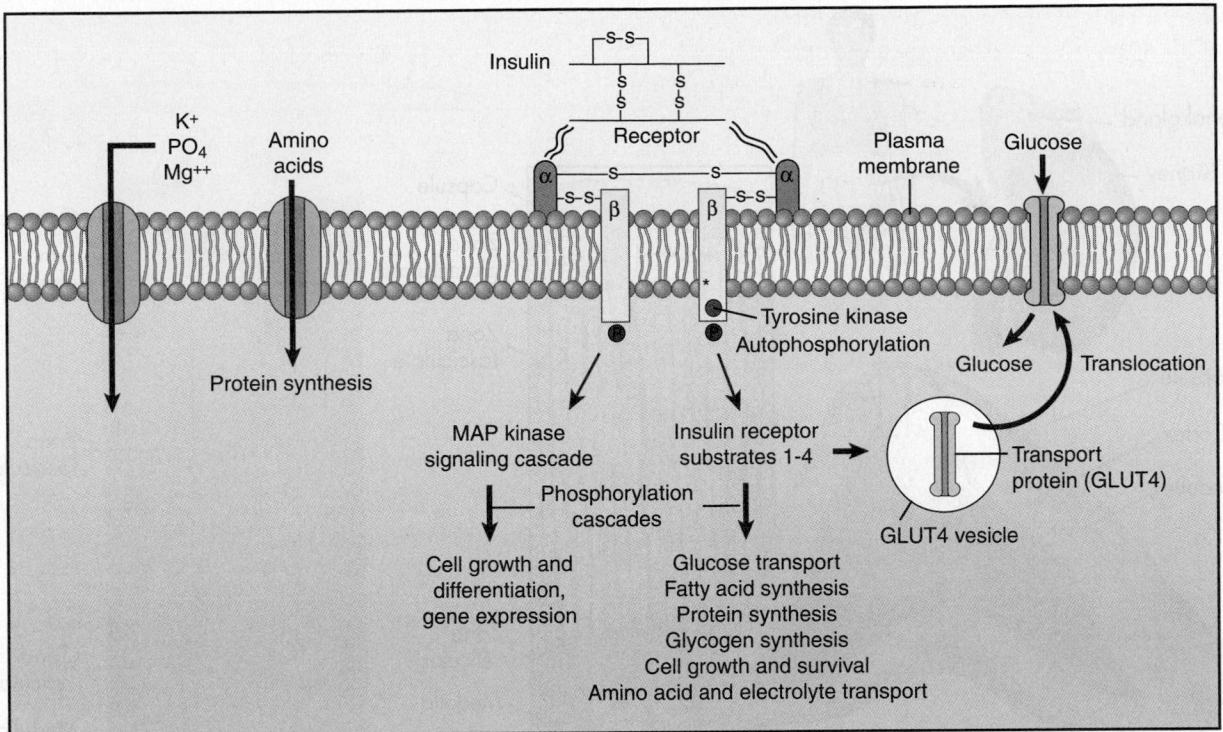

Figure 20-16 **Insulin action on cells.** Binding of insulin to its receptor causes autophosphorylation of the receptor, which then itself acts as a tyrosine kinase that phosphorylates insulin receptor substrate 1 (IRS-1). Numerous target enzymes, such as protein kinase B and MAP kinase are activated, and these enzymes have a multitude of effects on cell function. The glucose transporter, GLUT4, is recruited to the plasma membrane, where it facilitates glucose entry into the cell. The transport of amino acids, potassium, magnesium, and phosphate into the cell is also facilitated. The synthesis of various enzymes is induced or suppressed, and cell growth is regulated by signal molecules that modulate gene expression. *MAP,* mitogen-activated protein. (Redrawn from Berne RM, Levy MN: *Principles of physiology,* ed 3, St Louis, 2000, Mosby.)

Table 20-8	Insulin Actions		
	Sites of Insulin-Promoted Synthesis		
Actions	**Liver Cells**	**Muscle Cells**	**Adipose Cells**
Glucose uptake	Increased	Increased	Increased
Glucose use	—	—	Increased glycerol phosphate
Glycogenesis	Increased	Increased	—
Glycogenolysis	Decreased	Decreased	—
Glycolysis	Increased	Increased	Increased
Gluconeogenesis	Increased	—	—
Other	Increased fatty acid synthesis	Increased amino acid uptake	Increased fat esterification
	Decreased ketogenesis	Increased protein synthesis	Decreased lipolysis
	Decreased urea cycle activity	Decreased proteolysis	Increased fat storage

of growth hormone and TSH. Little is known about pancreatic somatostatin, but in animal studies it has been found to be involved in the regulation of alpha cell and beta cell function within the islets.[65] Presumably, somatostatin inhibits glucagon and insulin secretion, and it may prevent excess secretion of insulin.

Gastrin, Grehlin, and Pancreatic Polypeptide

The function of pancreatic **gastrin** has not been established; however, it likely controls the secretion of glucagon.[64] **Grehlin** stimulates GH secretion, controls appetite, and plays a role in the regulation of insulin sensitivity. **Pancreatic polypeptide**

is released by F cells in response to hypoglycemia and protein-rich meals and signals satiety.[66] It also inhibits gallbladder contraction and exocrine pancreas secretion and increases gastric acid secretion. It is frequently increased in pancreatic tumors and in diabetes.

Adrenal Glands

The **adrenal glands** are paired pyramid-shaped organs located behind the peritoneum and close to the upper pole of each kidney. Each gland is surrounded by a capsule embedded in fat and well supplied with blood from the phrenic and renal

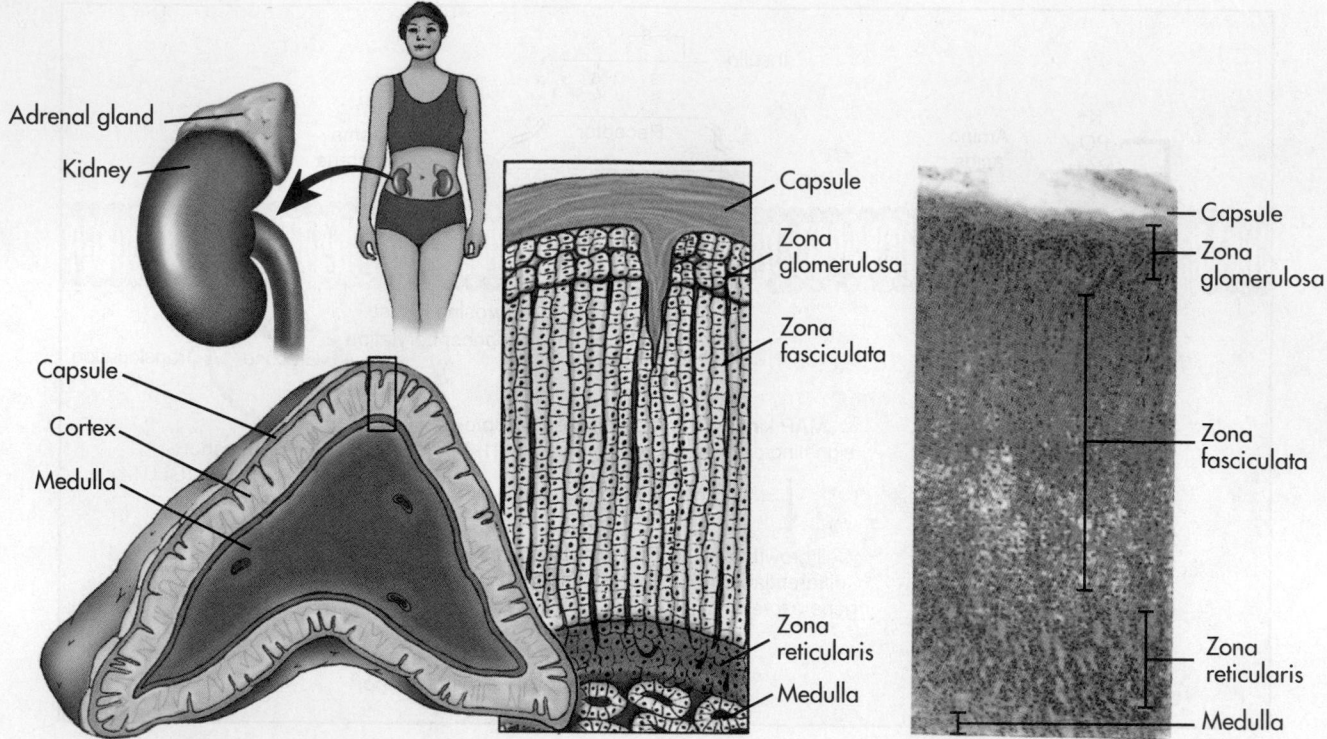

Figure 20-17 Structure of the adrenal gland showing cell layers (zones) of the cortex. Zona glomerulosa secretes aldosterone. Zona fasciculata secretes abundant amounts of glucocorticoids, chiefly cortisol. Zona reticularis secretes minute amounts of sex hormones and glucocorticoids. A portion of the medulla is visible at lower right in the photomicrograph ($\times$ 35) and at the bottom of the drawing. (From Patton KT, Thibodeau GA: *Anatomy & physiology*, ed 7, St Louis, 2010, Mosby.)

arteries and the aorta. Venous return on the left is to the renal vein and on the right is to the inferior vena cava.

Each adrenal gland consists of two separate portions: an inner medulla and an outer cortex. These two portions have different embryonic origins, different structures, and different hormonal functions. In effect, each adrenal gland functions like two separate glands, although there are interrelationships between functions of each portion (Figure 20-17).

The **adrenal cortex,** or outer region of the gland, accounts for 80% of the weight of the adult gland. The cortex is histologically subdivided into three zones. The outer layer, the **zona glomerulosa,** constitutes approximately 15% of the cortex and primarily produces the mineralocorticoid aldosterone. The middle layer, the **zona fasciculata** (78% of the cortex), and the inner layer, the **zona reticularis** (7% of the cortex), secrete other mineralocorticoids, the adrenal androgens and estrogens, and the glucocorticoids.[67] The **adrenal medulla,** accounting for 20% of the gland's total weight, secretes the catecholamines epinephrine (adrenaline), and norepinephrine (noradrenaline). Sympathetic and parasympathetic cholinergic fibers innervate the adrenal medulla; the adrenal cortex does not appear to be directly innervated.

Adrenal Cortex
The cells of the adrenal cortex are stimulated by the anterior pituitary hormone **adrenocorticotropic hormone (ACTH).** The adrenal cortex secretes several steroid hormones, including the glucocorticoids (mainly cortisol), the mineralocorticoids (mainly aldosterone), and the adrenal androgens and estrogens. These hormones are all synthesized from cholesterol. The best-known pathway of steroidogenesis involves the conversion of cholesterol to pregnenolone, which is then converted to the major corticosteroids.[67]

Glucocorticoids
The glucocorticoids have metabolic, neurologic, antiinflammatory, and growth-suppressing effects. They act through nuclear and nongenomic pathways in the cell.[21,68] The term **glucocorticoid** refers to those steroid hormones that have direct effects on carbohydrate metabolism. These hormones increase blood glucose concentration by promoting gluconeogenesis in the liver and by decreasing uptake of glucose into muscle cells, adipose cells, and lymphatic cells.[67] In extrahepatic tissues the glucocorticoids stimulate protein catabolism and inhibit amino acid uptake and protein synthesis. In hepatic tissue, however, glucocorticoids act primarily to stimulate glucose formation and synthesis of enzymes that mediate glucocorticoid effects. The ultimate effect on the body is protein breakdown (catabolism).

The glucocorticoids act at several sites to influence immune and inflammatory reactions (described in Chapters 6 and 10). They affect innate immunity through several pathways, including decreasing the activity of pattern receptors on the surface of macrophages (see Chapter 6).[69] Another major immune suppressant effect is a glucocorticoid-mediated decrease in the proliferation of T lymphocytes, primarily T-helper lymphocytes. There is a greater effect on T-helper 1 cytokine production (including antiviral interferons) than there is T-helper 2 cytokine production and therefore greater depression of cellular immunity than humoral immunity (see Chapter 7). Glucocorticoids also decrease immune and inflammatory responses by decreasing natural killer cell activity, promoting microphage phagocytosis of apoptotic granulocytes, and suppressing the synthesis, secretion, and actions of chemical mediators involved in inflammatory and immune responses. Glucocorticoids suppress the inflammatory response by blocking phospholipase A and the synthesis of prostaglandins, thromboxanes, and leukotrienes; and by inhibiting inflammatory gene expression.[67] In addition, glucocorticoids stimulate anti-inflammatory cytokines (e.g., IL-10 and transforming growth factor-beta). Lysosomal membranes are also stabilized, decreasing the release of proteolytic enzymes. This suppression of innate and adaptive immunity by glucocorticoids means that infection and poor wound healing are some of the most problematic complications of the use of glucocorticoids in the treatment of disease. Similarly, psychologic and physiologic stress increases glucocorticoid production, which provides a pathway for the well-described decrease in immunity seen in both acute and chronic stress conditions (see Chapter 10).

Pathologically high levels of glucocorticoids include increasing circulating erythrocytes, leading to polycythemia; increasing the appetite; promoting fat deposits in the face and cervical areas; increasing uric acid excretion; decreasing serum calcium levels, possibly by inhibiting gastrointestinal absorption of calcium; and suppressing GH secretion so that somatic growth is inhibited. The glucocorticoids also have important "permissive" effects, sensitizing arterioles to the vasoconstrictive effects of norepinephrine. Glucocorticoids appear to potentiate the effects of catecholamines, thyroid hormone, and GH on adipose tissue. It also has been speculated that a metabolite of cortisol may act like a barbiturate and depress nerve cell function in the brain. This may account for the noted effects on mood associated with steroid fluctuation in disease or stress.

The most potent of the naturally occurring glucocorticoids is **cortisol.** It is the main secretory product of the adrenal cortex and is necessary for the maintenance of life and for protection from stress (see Chapter 10, particularly Figure 10-2). Cortisol has a biologic half-life of approximately 90 minutes, with the liver primarily responsible for its deactivation.

The secretion of cortisol is regulated primarily by the hypothalamus and the anterior pituitary gland (Figure 20-18). In the hypothalamus, CRH is produced in several nuclei and stored in the median eminence. Once released, CRH travels through the portal vessels to stimulate the production of ACTH from POMC, β-lipotropin, γ-lipotropin, endorphins, and enkephalins by the anterior pituitary. ACTH is the main regulator of cortisol secretion and adrenocortical growth.

Three factors appear to be primarily involved in regulating the secretion of ACTH: (1) high circulating levels of cortisol and synthetic glucocorticoids suppress CRH and ACTH, whereas low cortisol levels stimulate their secretion; (2) diurnal rhythms affect ACTH and cortisol levels (in persons with regular sleep-wake patterns, ACTH peaks 3 to 5 hours after sleep begins and declines throughout the day; and cortisol levels follow a similar pattern, peaking right before awakening); and (3) stress has been shown to increase ACTH secretion, leading to increased cortisol levels. (Neuroendocrine mechanisms regulating sleep are discussed in Chapter 15.) ACTH secretion also is controlled by hypothalamic arginine vasopressin.[67] A form of ACTH (i.e., irACTH) also is produced by the cells of the immune system. It is detectable through laboratory techniques, and physiologically it appears to exert the usual feedback effects (see Chapter 10). This mechanism may account in part for integration of the immune and endocrine systems.

Once ACTH is secreted, it binds to specific plasma membrane receptors on the cells of the adrenal cortex and on other extra-adrenal tissues. Because both adrenal and extra-adrenal tissues have ACTH receptors, a number of effects result from stimulation by ACTH. (These are summarized in Box 20-1.) Both adrenal and extra-adrenal effects appear to be mediated through the activation of the adenylyl cyclase system. Melanocyte-stimulating hormone is also synthesized from the precursor POMC and increases skin pigmentation.

Once ACTH stimulates the cells of the adrenal cortex, cortisol synthesis and secretion immediately occur. In the normal person the secretory patterns of ACTH and cortisol are nearly identical. After secretion, most cortisol circulates in bound form: 15% to 30% is bound to albumin, and 55% to 75% is tightly but reversibly bound to a plasma glycoprotein called *transcortin,* or corticosteroid-binding globulin. The levels of transcortin play a role in the HPA feedback system controlling cortisol secretion.[70] Transcortin levels are significantly elevated by increased estrogen levels that occur with pregnancy and hormone therapy—10% to 15% of the cortisol secreted circulates unbound. The unbound portion is free to diffuse into cells, but only those cells with specific intracellular glucocorticoid receptors respond to cortisol stimulation. ACTH is rapidly inactivated in the circulation, and the liver and kidneys remove the deactivated hormone.

Mineralocorticoids: Aldosterone

Mineralocorticoid steroids directly affect ion transport by epithelial cells, causing sodium retention and potassium and hydrogen loss. **Aldosterone** is the most potent of the naturally occurring mineralocorticoids and acts to conserve sodium by increasing the activity of the sodium pump of the epithelial cells. (The sodium pump is described in Chapter 1.)

The initial stages of aldosterone synthesis occur in the zona fasciculata and zona reticularis. The final conversion of corticosterone to aldosterone, however, apparently is confined to the zona glomerulosa. Aldosterone synthesis and secretion are regulated primarily by the renin-angiotensin-aldosterone system (described in Chapter 3 and Chapter 35; see Figure 35-10), although other factors also may be involved. Sodium and potassium levels may directly affect aldosterone secretion;

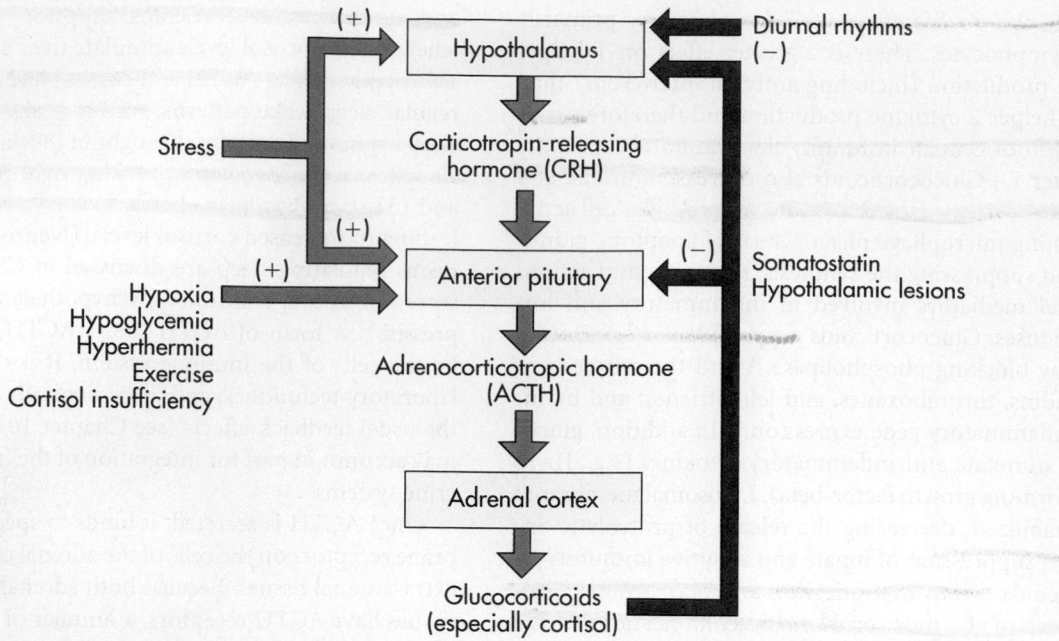

Figure 20-18 Feedback control of glucocorticoid synthesis and secretion.

however, the mechanisms involved are not understood. ACTH may transiently stimulate aldosterone synthesis but does not appear to be a major regulator of aldosterone secretion.

Aldosterone synthesis and secretion are stimulated by angiotensin II. The conversion of angiotensin I to angiotensin II is stimulated by the enzyme angiotensin I–converting enzyme (Figure 20-19). The conversion of angiotensinogen to angiotensin I is stimulated by renin. Renin secretion is stimulated primarily by decreased renal blood flow because of sodium and water depletion and a diminished effective blood volume. Renin secretion also is stimulated by increased serum potassium.

When sodium and potassium levels are within normal limits, normal serum levels of aldosterone are 5-30 mg/d; 50% to 75% of the secreted aldosterone bind to plasma proteins, including albumin, transcortin, and an α_1-acid glycoprotein (AAG). The relatively large proportion of unbound aldosterone contributes to its rapid metabolic turnover in the liver,

its low plasma concentration, and its short half-life of approximately 15 minutes. The main site of aldosterone degradation is the liver, with the metabolic end products being excreted by the kidney.

In the kidney aldosterone primarily acts on the epithelial cells of the nephron collecting duct to increase sodium ion reabsorption (thus promoting water reabsorption) and increase potassium and hydrogen ion excretion. High levels of aldosterone may result in alkalosis and hypokalemia (see Chapter 3). (Kidney function is discussed in Chapter 35.) This renal effect takes 1½ to 6 hours to occur after stimulation by aldosterone. Aldosterone also reduces sodium in sweat, saliva, and gastric juice.

Aldosterone affects many other tissues in the body, especially the cardiovascular system. Pathologically elevated levels of aldosterone have been implicated in hypertension, atherosclerosis, and heart failure.[71]

Adrenal Estrogens and Androgens

Estrogen secretion by the normal adrenal cortex is so minimal as to be considered physiologically unimportant. The adrenal cortex also secretes androgens. Adrenal androgen secretion is regulated by ACTH rather than the gonadotropins.[67] Some of the weak androgenic substances secreted by the cortex are then converted by peripheral tissues to stronger androgens, such as testosterone, thus accounting for some androgenic effect initiated by the adrenal cortex. An increased capacity for peripheral conversion of adrenal androgens to estrogens occurs in particular cases, however, including aging, obesity, liver disease, and hyperthyroidism. The biologic effects and metabolism of the adrenal sex steroids do not vary from those produced by the gonads (see Chapter 22).

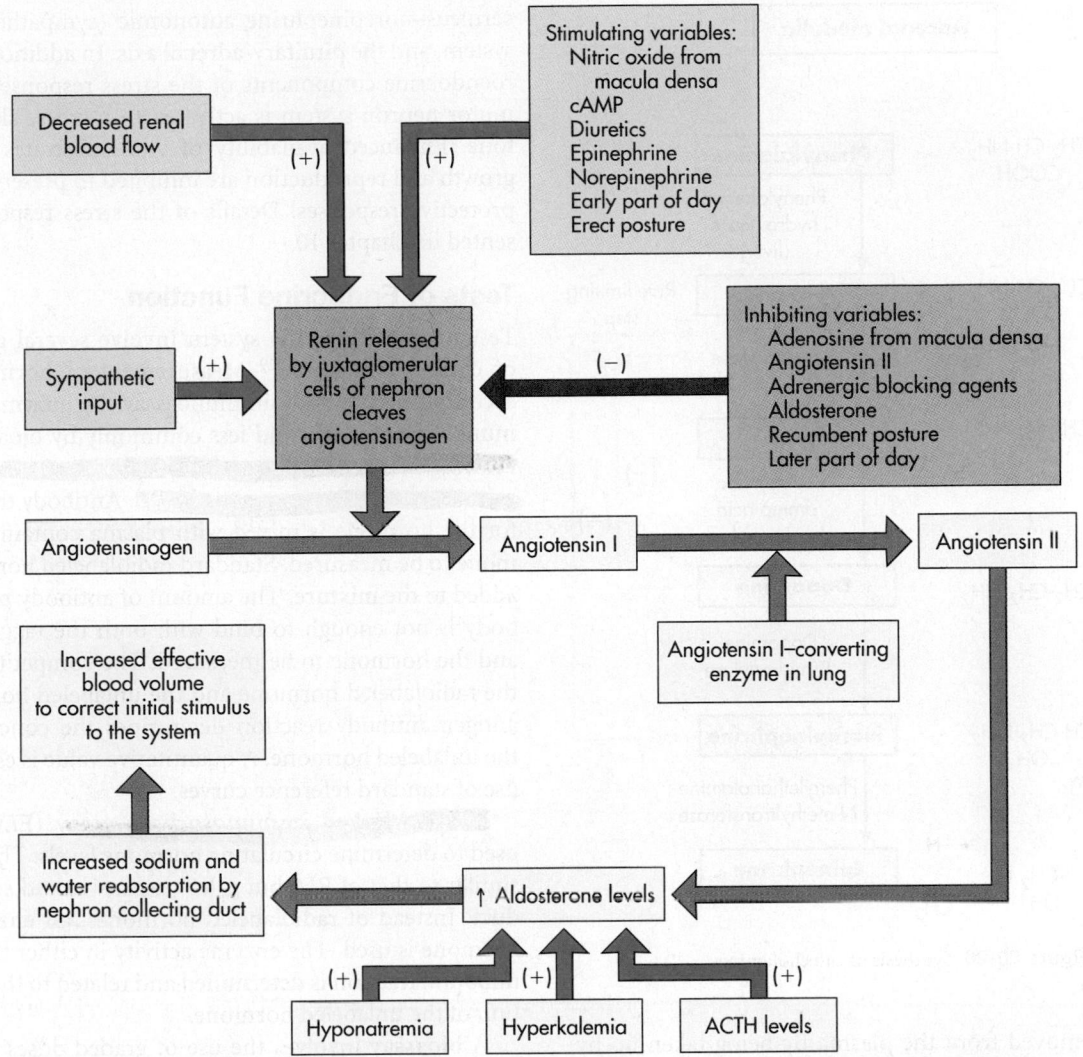

Figure 20-19 The feedback mechanisms regulating aldosterone secretion. *ACTH*, Adrenocorticotropic hormone; *cAMP*, cyclic adenosine monophosphate.

Adrenal Medulla

The adrenal medulla, together with the sympathetic divisions of the autonomic nervous system, is embryonically derived from neural crest cells. **Chromaffin cells (pheochromocytes) are the cells of the adrenal medulla.** The major products secreted by the chromaffin cells are the catecholamines epinephrine (adrenaline) and norepinephrine, although the medulla is only a minor source of norepinephrine. The adrenal medulla functions as a sympathetic ganglion without postganglionic processes. Sympathetic cholinergic preganglion fibers terminate on the chromaffin cells and secrete catecholamines directly into the bloodstream.[72] The catecholamines are therefore hormones and not neurotransmitters.

Only 30% of circulating epinephrine comes from the adrenal medulla. The other 70% is released from nerve terminals. Catecholamine production in the adrenal medulla consists of approximately 75% to 85% epinephrine and approximately 15% to 25% norepinephrine. Epinephrine is about 10 times more potent than norepinephrine in producing direct metabolic effects. The adrenal medulla synthesizes the catecholamines from the amino acid phenylalanine (Figure 20-20).

Adrenal catecholamines are stored in secretory granules within the chromaffin cells. Physiologic stress to the body (e.g., traumatic injury, hypoxia, hypoglycemia, and many others) triggers release of adrenal catecholamines through acetylcholine (from the preganglionic sympathetic fibers), which depolarizes the chromaffin cells.[72] Depolarization causes exocytosis of the storage granules from the chromaffin cells with release of epinephrine and norepinephrine into the bloodstream. The control of exocytosis probably involves calcium, although this mechanism is not fully understood.[72] Secretion of adrenal catecholamines is also increased by ACTH and the glucocorticoids.

Once released, the catecholamines remain in the plasma for only seconds to minutes. The catecholamines exert their biologic effects after binding to a plasma membrane receptors (α_1, α_2, β_1, β_2, β_3) in target cells (see Table 14-7). This binding activates the adenylyl cyclase system. Catecholamines

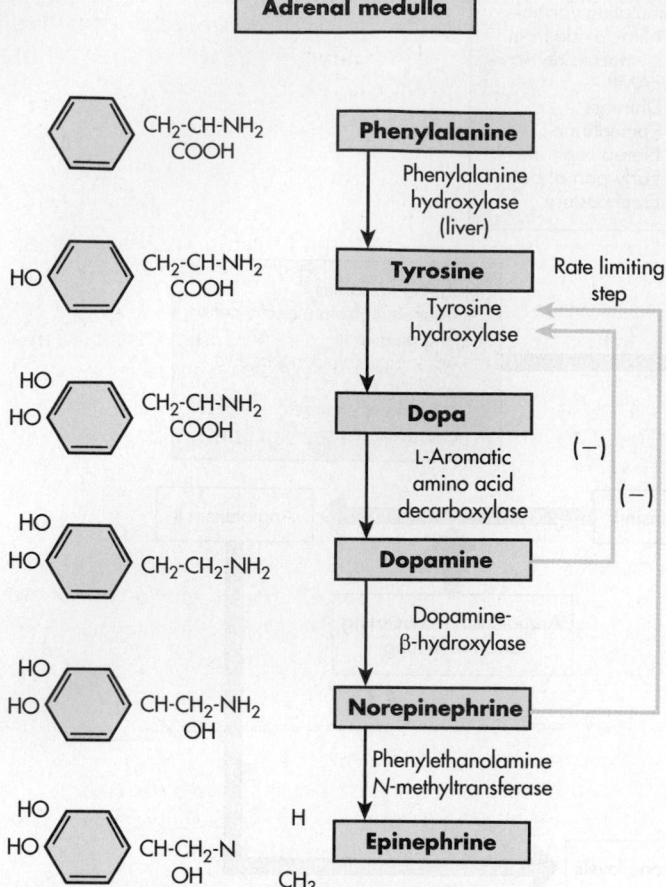

Figure 20-20 Synthesis of catecholamines.

are rapidly removed from the plasma by being taken up by neurons for storage in new cytoplasmic granules, or they may be metabolically inactivated and excreted in the urine.

Catecholamines have diverse effects on the entire body. Their release and the body's response have been characterized as the "fight or flight" response (see Chapter 10). In general, the metabolic effects of catecholamines promote hyperglycemia through a variety of mechanisms and through interfering with usual glucose regulatory feedback mechanisms.

Neuroendocrine Response to Stressors

The endocrine system acts together with the nervous system to respond to stressors. The integrated response to stressors also includes the immune system. Hormones of the neuroendocrine system affect components of the immune system, and mediators produced by immune components regulate the neuroendocrine response.

Perception that an event is stressful may be essential to the emotional arousal and initiation of the stress response (discussed in Chapter 10). Some events, such as bacterial invasion, can activate the stress response without emotional arousal. The hypothalamus receives input from a variety of areas within the brain and ultimately directs the neuroendocrine response to stress through the actions of CRH, the locus

ceruleus–norepinephrine autonomic (sympathetic) nervous system, and the pituitary-adrenal axis. In addition to the neuroendocrine components of the stress response, the gamma motor neuron system is activated to increase skeletal motor tone. Enhanced availability of vital substrates occurs, and growth and reproduction are inhibited to preserve energy for protective responses. Details of the stress response are presented in Chapter 10.

Tests of Endocrine Function

Tests of the endocrine system involve several general types of clinical evaluation.[29] Measurement of hormone level is accomplished by radioimmunoassay, by enzyme-linked immunosorbent assay, and less commonly by bioassay. **Radioimmunoassay (RIA)** is a technique for measuring the minute quantities of hormones in the blood. Antibody that is specific for the hormone is mixed with plasma containing the hormone to be measured. Standard radiolabeled hormone is also added to the mixture. The amount of antibody present in the body is not enough to bind with both the tagged hormone and the hormone to be measured. The competition between the radiolabeled hormone and the unlabeled hormone in an antigen-antibody reaction determines the concentration of the unlabeled hormone. A quantitative value is established by use of standard reference curves.

Enzyme-linked immunosorbent assay (ELISA) also is used to determine circulating hormone levels. This method is similar to that of RIA but is less expensive and easier to conduct. Instead of radiolabeled hormones, an enzyme-labeled hormone is used. The enzyme activity in either the bound or unbound fraction is determined and related to the concentration of the unlabeled hormone.

A **bioassay** involves the use of graded doses of hormone in a reference preparation and then comparison of the results with an unknown sample. Bioassays are used more commonly in investigative endocrinology than in clinical laboratories.

The concentration of hormones in serum can be measured to assess endocrine function in health and disease. If the serum level is greater or less than the reference values, more definitive tests are required to determine the source of the problem. Measurement of individual hormones does not always permit differentiation between normal and abnormal values when hormone levels are changing over time. For an accurate interpretation, the broad normal range of some hormones requires a knowledge of previous hormonal levels and timed sampling.

The major problems in evaluating the endocrine system include (1) the complexity of the clinical presentation because of multiple organ system involvement, (2) the nonspecific nature of complaints frequently associated with endocrine dysfunction, and (3) the inappropriate use of laboratory test interpretations.

Aging and the Endocrine System

The precise relationship between aging and the endocrine system is not clear. Perhaps most important, the question of whether changes in endocrine function are a consequence or a cause of aging has yet to be resolved. These relationships have been difficult to identify, in part because of a number of age-related variables that may coexist, such as acute and chronic nonendocrine disease; use of medications; alterations in diet, body composition, and weight; and changes in sleep-wake cycles. However, the endocrine system is so integral to health that changes in endocrine function have been used as "biomarkers" for unhealthy aging.[73]

Theories About the Effects of Aging

Investigation into the role of the endocrine glands and their interactions in the aging process has generated much data, although the evidence is contradictory. There are complex changes within the HPA, and altered biologic activity of hormones, altered circulating levels of hormones, altered secretory response of the endocrine glands, altered metabolism of hormones, and loss of circadian control of hormone secretion are among the findings. The most studied changes in hormone function with aging affect the levels of reproductive hormones and gonadotropins (menopause and andropause) (discussed in Chapter 22). Two of the most important endocrine changes associated with aging affect the pancreas and the thyroid gland.[74] Other important hormone changes associated with aging include a decline in serum levels of growth hormone, IGF-1, and dehydroepiandrosterone.[75]

Theories of cellular damage deal with adverse cellular conditions that produce the biologic effects associated with aging. (These theories are discussed in Chapter 2.) The endocrine system has not been specifically implicated in any of these theories, particularly as a causative variable. The cellular changes or consequences described by these theories, however, do affect specific endocrine glands and might contribute to endocrine gland dysfunction or alterations in responsiveness of target organs.

Theories of stress and adaptation suggest that body structures wear out from overuse or are no longer able to adapt to the cumulative effects of physiologic stress. One such endocrine function that may be affected is the sympathoadrenal axis. Exhaustion of this axis may be associated with an inability of the body to respond effectively to stressors.

Theories of programmed change are concerned with genetic control of cell function. Certain secretory cells may be programmed genetically to secrete hormones for a prescribed length of time. Changes seen with female reproductive function may represent the phenomenon of programmed change. Reduced signaling of insulin and insulin-like peptides is associated with increased life spans.

All changes in cellular activity—as a result of damage, programmed change, or wear and tear—may affect neuroendocrine regulation. Changes in secretion of hypothalamic regulatory factors and hormones or changes in hypothalamic feedback sensitivity may contribute to alterations in control of an optimal internal environment. The dynamic equilibrium of the endocrine system also may be affected by altered secretion of neurotransmitters within certain areas of the brain, affecting hypothalamic and pituitary function. Such alterations may include an excess or deficit in secretion of pituitary hormones and loss of appropriate secretory pattern of those hormones. Loss of endocrine steady states may be associated with or contribute to aging.

Effects of Aging on Specific Glands and Hormones

Thyroid Gland

Changes in thyroid structure and function occur with aging. Structurally, some glandular atrophy and fibrosis occur with nodularity and increasing inflammatory infiltrates. These infiltrative changes may reflect age-related autoimmune damage. Overall, it is estimated that there is some evidence of thyroid dysfunction in 5% to 10% of older adult women.[74] The presence of thyroid nodules increases after the age of 70 years.[76]

Changes relative to thyroid hormone and its function are more difficult to assess. One difficulty is finding older adults who are free of all systemic and thyroid-related illness, so that the resulting changes can be attributed to aging. Much of the available data are contradictory. Most evidence, however, supports the following age-related changes[74]:

1. Overall TSH secretion is diminished.
2. Responsiveness of plasma TSH concentration to TRH administration is reduced, especially in men.
   a. T_4 secretion and degradation are decreased.
   b. Plasma levels of T_3 decline, especially in men, but are generally in the normal range.
   c. Hypothyroidism is seen with increasing frequency as age advances.

In addition, the average dose for TH replacement appears to be lower in older adults because the peripheral metabolism of TH decreases with age. TH must be replaced slowly in elderly individuals with coronary artery disease to prevent angina and myocardial infarction. Clinical signs of thyroid disease are more difficult to detect in older adults.[76]

Pancreas

It is estimated that 40% to 50% of individuals older than age 65 have impaired glucose tolerance or diabetes.[74] With aging, the pancreatic cells are increasingly replaced with fat tissue. Dysfunction of the pancreas with decreased insulin secretion of the beta cells, insulin receptors, and cellular responses to insulin are all noted. These changes have significant implications for many target organs, particularly the cardiovascular system, which is increasingly at risk for both vascular (hypertension, atherosclerosis, glomerulosclerosis) and cardiac (infarction, failure) disorders. Exciting research is exploring the relationship between insulin and activation of genes for the "sirtuins," which are a group of proteins that have been linked with the aging process.[77]

Growth Hormone and Insulin-like Growth Factors

The amounts of GH and IGF decline with aging, a process that has been called the "somatopause." This decline in anabolic stimuli is linked to decreases in muscle size and function, fat and bone mass, and changes in reproductive and cognitive function.[42,74] Clinical findings related to somatotropic hormone changes with aging include increases in visceral fat, decreased lean body mass, and decreased bone density. Despite the initial enthusiasm for the use of therapeutic doses of GH as a way to slow the aging process, studies have not been consistently positive and the risk for GH- and IGF-mediated oncogenesis is being explored.[42]

Parathyroid Glands

An age-related alteration in PTH secretion has been proposed to explain alterations in calcium homeostasis that have been noted in older adults.[78] Such an alteration, however, has not been documented consistently. Calcium intake, especially in women, tends to decrease with aging and may contribute to osteoporosis (see Chapter 42). The average daily intake of 450 to 500 mg/day causes a negative calcium balance greater than 40 mg/day and may be related to the absolute bone loss of approximately 1.5% per year. Older adults show decreased intestinal adaptation to variations in calcium intake. Hyperparathyroidism may occur secondary to calcium malabsorption and hypocalcemia with increased bone remodeling that results in cortical bone thinning and porosity. Elevated levels of parathyroid hormone have been linked with an increase in mortality in older adults,[79] many of whom also have a mild, persistent hypercalciuria, which indicates a defective renal mechanism for responding to decreased calcium intake. Decreased circulating levels of vitamin D are common in older adults, especially those in long-term care institutions.[78] Vitamin D deficiency has been linked to not only osteoporosis but also cancer, autoimmune diseases, diabetes, cardiovascular disease, and mental health disorders.[80]

The decrease in calcium intake, an age-related decrease in circulating vitamin D, and a blunted response in older adults to PTH may explain these changes seen in aging. Additional investigation into mechanisms of altered calcium metabolism is required before the age-associated alterations can be explained.

Adrenal Glands

The adrenal cortex loses some weight and has more fibrous tissue after the age of 50 years. Age does not appear to affect the feedback mechanisms involved in maintaining glucocorticoid levels, but the decrease in the metabolic clearance rate of the glucocorticoids is age related.

The metabolic clearance of cortisol decreases with an age-related decline in liver and kidney function. Further, less cortisol appears to be used by the body when aging is accompanied by a loss of lean body mass. Decreased clearance and reduced use of cortisol contribute to higher circulating cortisol levels, but diurnal variation is maintained. Because feedback mechanisms are intact, the higher cortisol levels cause a decrease in cortisol secretion. Circadian patterns of ACTH and cortisol secretion may change with aging.

Plasma levels of the adrenal androgens, as well as urinary excretion of the metabolic end products, decrease gradually but dramatically with age, to as much as 50% to 70% of the young adult level. This change in adrenal function has been called the "adrenopause" and is correlated with decreased synthesis activity of dehydroepiandrosterone (DHEA).[74,75] This change appears to reflect a decline in the function of the zona reticularis. In postmenopausal women, this decline in adrenal androgen secretion is especially important because nearly all sex steroids after menopause come from adrenal and ovarian production of androgen precursors converted to estrogens in the periphery. In older adult men, adrenal androgen production accounts for more than half of circulating testosterone levels.

Antidiuretic Hormone

Although hyponatremia is a common finding in older adults, it appears related to changes in renal function rather than to ADH-related mechanisms. Morphologic studies have not shown significant age-related degenerative changes in the neuroendocrine pathways that regulate the synthesis and secretion of ADH. It appears that ADH secretion is augmented when stimulated by changes in osmotic concentration, whereas baroreceptor-mediated ADH secretion is reduced.

Mechanisms of Hormonal Regulation

1. The endocrine system has diverse functions, including sexual differentiation, growth and development, and continuous maintenance of the body's internal environment.
2. Hormones are chemical messengers synthesized by endocrine glands and released into the circulation.
3. Hormones have specific negative- and positive-feedback mechanisms. Most hormone levels are regulated by negative feedback, in which tropic hormone secretion raises the level of a specific hormone. The elevated level of the specific hormone then causes negative feedback decreasing secretion of the tropic hormone.
4. Endocrine feedback is described in terms of short, long, and ultrashort feedback loops.
5. Water-soluble hormones circulate throughout the body in unbound form, whereas lipid-soluble hormones (i.e., steroid and thyroid hormones) circulate throughout the body bound to carrier proteins.
6. Hormones serve as first messengers and affect only target cells with appropriate receptors and then act on those cells to initiate specific cell functions or activities.
7. Hormones have two general types of effects on cells: direct effects, or obvious changes in cell function, and permissive effects, or less obvious changes that facilitate cell function.
8. Receptors for hormones are proteins and may be located on or in the plasma membrane or in the cytosol or nucleus of the target cell. Receptors may be G protein–linked, ion channels, or enzyme linked.
9. Water-soluble hormones act as first messengers, binding to receptors on the cell's plasma membrane. The signals initiated by hormone-receptor binding are then transmitted into the cell by the action of second messengers.
10. Second messengers that have been identified include cAMP, cGMP, and calcium, which associates with IP_3, and DAG to produce physiologic effects.
11. For cells that have cAMP as their second messenger, a series of interactions within the plasma membrane must activate adenylyl cyclase.
12. For cells that have calcium as their second messenger, a rise in intracellular calcium causes calcium to bind with calmodulin, a regulatory protein. This step then initiates other intracellular processes.
13. Cells that have cGMP as their second messenger are activated by the enzyme guanylyl cyclase.
14. Lipid-soluble hormones (including steroid and thyroid hormones) may have rapid effects by binding to a plasma membrane or receptor or crossing the plasma membrane through diffusion. These hormones then either bind to cytoplasmic proteins or diffuse directly into the cell nucleus and bind to nuclear receptors.

Structure and Function of the Endocrine Glands

1. The pituitary gland, consisting of anterior and posterior portions, is connected to the central nervous system through the hypothalamus.
2. The hypothalamus regulates anterior pituitary function by secreting releasing hormones into the portal circulation.
3. Hypothalamic hormones include dopamine, which inhibits prolactin secretion; TRH, which affects release of thyroid hormones; GnRH, which facilitates release of ACTH and endorphins; and substance P, which inhibits ACTH release and stimulates release of a variety of other hormones.
4. The pineal gland produces melatonin, which affects sleep, immune function, and aging.

5. The posterior pituitary secretes ADH, also called arginine vasopressin, and oxytocin.
6. ADH controls serum osmolality, increases permeability of the renal tubules to water, and causes vasoconstriction when administered pharmacologically in high doses. ADH also may regulate some central nervous system functions.
7. Oxytocin causes uterine contraction and lactation in women and may have a role in sperm motility in men. In men and women, oxytocin has an antidiuretic effect similar to that of ADH.
8. Hormones of the anterior pituitary are regulated by (a) secretion of hypothalamic-releasing hormones or factors, (b) negative feedback from hormones secreted by target organs, and (c) mediating effects of neurotransmitters.
9. Hormones of the anterior pituitary include ACTH, MSH, somatotropic hormones (GH and prolactin), and glycoprotein hormones (FSH, LH, and TSH).
10. Growth hormone stimulates growth of bone, increased protein metabolism in muscles, and lipolysis. Its effects are mediated in part by IGFs.
11. Prolactin functions to produce milk during pregnancy and lactation.
12. The two-lobed thyroid gland contains follicles, which secrete some of the thyroid hormones, and C cells, which secrete calcitonin and somatostatin.
13. Regulation of TH levels is complex and involves the hypothalamus, anterior pituitary, thyroid gland, and numerous biochemical variables.
14. TH secretion is regulated by thyroid-releasing hormone through a negative-feedback loop that involves the anterior pituitary and hypothalamus.
15. TSH, which is synthesized and stored in the anterior pituitary, stimulates secretion of TH by activating intracellular processes, including uptake of iodine necessary for the synthesis of TH.
16. Synthesis of TH depends on the glycoprotein thyroglobulin, which contains a precursor of TH, tyrosine. Tyrosine then combines with iodide to form precursor molecules of the thyroid hormones T_4 and T_3.
17. When released into the circulation, T_3 and T_4 are bound by carrier proteins in the plasma that store these hormones and provide a buffer for rapid changes in hormone levels.
18. Thyroid hormones alter protein synthesis and have a wide range of metabolic effects on proteins, carbohydrates, lipids, and vitamins. TH also affects heat production and cardiac function.
19. The paired parathyroid glands normally are located behind the upper and lower poles of the thyroid. These glands secrete PTH, an important regulator of serum calcium levels.
20. PTH secretion is regulated by levels of ionized calcium in the plasma and by cAMP within the cell. Some other substances—hormones, neurotransmitters, and ions—affect PTH secretion by inhibiting cAMP or by changing calcium levels.
21. In bone, PTH causes bone breakdown and resorption. In the kidney PTH increases reabsorption of calcium, decreases reabsorption of phosphorus and bicarbonate, and stimulates synthesis of vitamin D.
22. The endocrine pancreas contains the islets of Langerhans, which secrete hormones responsible for much of the carbohydrate metabolism in the body.
23. The islets of Langerhans consist of alpha cells, beta cells, and delta cells. Delta cells secrete somatostatin, which inhibits glucagon and insulin secretion. Beta cells secrete preproinsulin, which is ultimately converted to insulin.

Continued

24. Insulin is a hormone that regulates blood glucose concentrations and overall body metabolism of fat, protein, and carbohydrates.

25. Alpha cells produce glucagon, which is secreted inversely to blood glucose concentrations.

26. The paired adrenal glands are situated on the kidneys. Each gland consists of an adrenal medulla, which secretes catecholamines, and an adrenal cortex, which secretes steroid hormones.

27. The steroid hormones secreted by the adrenal cortex are all synthesized from cholesterol. These hormones include glucocorticoids, mineralocorticoids, and adrenal androgens and estrogens.

28. Glucocorticoids directly affect carbohydrate metabolism by increasing blood glucose concentration through gluconeogenesis in the liver and by decreasing use of glucose. Glucocorticoids also inhibit immune and inflammatory responses.

29. Cortisol secretion is related to secretion of ACTH, which is stimulated by CRH. ACTH binds with receptors of the adrenal cortex, which activates intracellular mechanisms (specifically cAMP) and leads to cortisol release.

30. Mineralocorticoids, especially aldosterone, are steroid hormones that directly affect ion transport by epithelial cells, causing sodium retention and potassium and hydrogen loss.

31. Aldosterone secretion is controlled by the renin-angiotensin-aldosterone system and acts by binding to a site on the cell nucleus and altering protein production within the cell. Its principal site of action is the kidney, where it causes sodium reabsorption and potassium and hydrogen excretion.

32. Androgens and estrogens secreted by the adrenal cortex act in the same way as those secreted by the gonads.

33. The adrenal medulla secretes the catecholamines epinephrine and norepinephrine. Catecholamines are synthesized from the amino acid phenylalanine. Their release is stimulated by sympathetic nervous system stimulation, ACTH, and glucocorticoids.

34. Catecholamines bind with various target cells and are taken up by neurons or excreted in the urine. They cause a range of metabolic effects that generally are characterized as the "flight or fight" response.

35. The endocrine system acts together with the nervous and immune systems to respond to stressors, providing an integrated and protective response.

36. Several assay methods are used to measure levels of hormones in the plasma. RIA compares the proportion of radiolabeled and non-radiolabeled hormone against standard reference curves.

37. ELISA is a method similar to RIA, but uses a radiolabeled enzyme rather than a radiolabeled hormone.

38. Bioassays use graded doses of hormone in a reference preparation and then compare the results with an unknown sample to determine the hormone level.

Aging and the Endocrine System

1. Endocrine changes that may be associated with aging include altered biologic activity of hormones, altered circulating levels of hormones, altered secretory responses of endocrine glands, altered metabolism of hormones, and loss of circadian control of hormone release.

2. Cellular damage associated with aging, genetically programmed cell change, and chronic wear and tear may contribute to endocrine gland dysfunction or alterations in responsiveness of target organs.

3. Aging apparently causes atrophy of the thyroid gland and is associated with infiltrative glandular changes. Secretion of thyroid hormones may diminish with age.

4. Aging causes pancreatic fat deposition and is associated with a decrease in insulin secretion and insulin sensitivity.

5. Growth hormone levels decrease with aging leading to decreased bone and muscle mass.

6. Aging is associated with alterations in calcium steady states, which may be related to alterations in PTH secretion from the parathyroid glands.

7. Age-related changes in adrenal function include decreased clearance of glucocorticoids and a decrease in levels of adrenal androgens. The effects of these changes, however, are offset by feedback mechanisms that maintain glucocorticoid levels and by gonadal secretion of androgens.

KEY TERMS

Adrenal cortex, 716
Adrenal gland, 715
Adrenal medulla, 715
Adrenocorticotropic hormone (ACTH), 716
Aldosterone, 717
Amylin, 714
Anterior pituitary, 704
Antidiuretic hormone (ADH), 703
Beta cell, 713
Bioassay, 720
C cell, 709
Calcitonin, 709
Chromaffin cell (pheochromocyte), 719
Chromophil, 707
Chromophobe, 707
Corticotropin-releasing hormone (CRH), 704
Cortisol, 717
Diacylglycerol (DAG), 702
Direct effect, 699
Down-regulation, 699
Enzyme-linked immunosorbent assay (ELISA), 720

First messenger, 700
Follicle, 709
Gastrin, 715
Gonadotropin-releasing hormone (GnRH), 704
Grehlin, 715
Growth hormone–releasing factor (GRF), 704
Glucagon, 714
Glucocorticoid, 716
Hormone, 696
Hormone receptor, 699
Inositol triphosphate (IP$_3$), 702
Insulin, 713
Islets of Langerhans, 712
Isthmus, 709
Median eminence, 705
Melatonin, 704
Mineralocorticoid, 717
Neuroendocrine system, 703
Oxytocin, 703
Pancreas, 712
Pancreatic polypeptide, 715

Parathyroid hormone (PTH), 711
Pars distalis, 704
Pars intermedia, 704
Pars nervosa (neural lobe), 705
Pars tuberalis, 704
Permissive effect, 699
Pituitary stalk, 705
Posterior pituitary, 705
Prolactin-inhibiting factor (PIF), 704
Radioimmunoassay (RIA), 720
Signal transduction, 701
Somatostatin, 714
Substance P, 704
Target cell, 699
Thyroid gland, 709
Thyroid hormone (TH), 709
Thyroid-stimulating hormone (TSH), 710
Thyrotropin-releasing hormone (TRH), 704, 709
Up-regulation, 699
Zona fasciculata, 716
Zona glomerulosa, 716
Zona reticularis, 716

REFERENCES

1. Jameson LJ, Degroot LJ: Endocrinology: impact on science and medicine. In DeGroot LJ, Jamerson JL, editors: *Endocrinology*, ed 5, St Louis, 2006, Saunders.
2. Kronenberg HM et al: Principles of endocrinology. In Kronenberg HM et al, editors: *Williams textbook of endocrinology*, ed 11, Philadelphia, 2008, Saunders.
3. Spiegel A, Carter-Su C, Taylor SI: Mechanisms of action of hormones that act at the cell surface. In Kronenberg HM et al, editors: *Williams textbook of endocrinology*, ed 11, Philadelphia, 2008, Saunders.
4. Losel R, Wehling M: Nongenomic actions of steroid hormones, *Nat Rev Mol Cell Biol* 4(1):46-56, 2003.
5. Davis PJ, Leonard JL, Davis FB: Mechanisms of nongenomic actions of thyroid hormone, *Front Neuroendocrinol* 29(2):211-218, 2008.
6. Oetting A, Yen PM: New insights into thyroid hormone action, *Best Pract Res Clin Endocrinol Metab* 21(2):193-208, 2007.
7. Avruch J: Hormone signaling via tyrosine kinase receptors. In DeGroot LJ, Jamerson JL, editors: *Endocrinology*, ed 5, St Louis, 2006, Saunders.
8. Gonzales-Maeso J, Sealfon SC: Hormone signaling via G protein-coupled receptors. In DeGroot LJ, Jamerson JL, editors: *Endocrinology*, ed 5, St Louis, 2006, Saunders.
9. Lohse MJ et al: Kinetics of G-protein-coupled receptor signals in intact cells, *Br J Pharmacol* 153(Suppl 1):S125-S132, 2008.
10. Debrincat MA, Hilton DJ: Hormone signaling via cytokine receptors. In DeGroot LJ, Jamerson JL, editors: *Endocrinology*, ed 5, St Louis, 2006, Saunders.
11. Takemori H: Transcription factor cAMP response element-binding protein CREB, *FEBS J* 274(13):3201, 2007.
12. Kitagawa K: CREB and cAMP response element-mediated gene expression in the ischemic brain, *FEBS J* 274(13):3210-3217, 2007.
13. Siu YT, Jin DY: CREB—a real culprit in oncogenesis, *FEBS J* 274(13):3224-3232, 2007.
14. Bers DM: Calcium cycling and signaling in cardiac myocytes, *Annu Rev Physiol* 70:23-49, 2008.
15. Colomer J, Means AR: Physiological roles of the Ca2+/CaM-dependent protein kinase cascade in health and disease, *Subcell Biochem* 45:169-214, 2007.
16. Blair HC et al: Calcium signalling and calcium transport in bone disease, *Subcell Biochem* 45:539-562, 2007.
17. Friel DD, Chiel HJ: Calcium dynamics: analyzing the Ca2+ regulatory network in intact cells, *Trends Neurosci* 31(1):8-19, 2008.
18. Jude JA et al: Calcium signaling in airway smooth muscle, *Proc Am Thorac Soc* 5(1):15-22, 2008.
19. Omori K, Kotera J: Overview of PDEs and their regulation, *Circ Res* 100(3):309-327, 2007.
20. Sallustio F et al: Saving the ischemic penumbra: potential role for statins and phosphodiesterase inhibitors, *Curr Vasc Pharmacol* 5(4):259-265, 2007.
21. Haller J, Mikics E, Makara GB: The effects of non-genomic glucocorticoid mechanisms on bodily functions and the central neural system. A critical evaluation of findings, *Front Neuroendocrinol* 29(2):273-291, 2008.
22. Losel RM, Wehling M: Classic versus non-classic receptors for nongenomic mineralocorticoid responses: emerging evidence, *Front Neuroendocrinol* 29(2):258-267, 2008.
23. Michels G, Hoppe UC: Rapid actions of androgens, *Front Neuroendocrinol* 29(2):182-198, 2008.
24. Vasudevan N, Pfaff DW: Non-genomic actions of estrogens and their interaction with genomic actions in the brain, *Front Neuroendocrinol* 29(2):238-257, 2008.
25. Low MJ et al: Neuroendocrinology. In Kronenberg HM et al, editor: *Williams textbook of endocrinology*, ed 11, Philadelphia, 2008, Saunders.
26. Karasek M: Does melatonin play a role in aging processes? *J Physiol Pharmacol* 6 (58 Suppl):105-113, 2007.
27. Szczepanik M: Melatonin and its influence on the immune system, *J Physiol Pharmacol* 6 (58 Suppl):115-124, 2007.
28. Paulis L, Simko F: Blood pressure modulation and cardiovascular protection by melatonin: potential mechanisms behind, *Physiol Res* 56(6):671-684, 2007.
29. Peschke E: Melatonin, endocrine pancreas and diabetes, *J Pineal Res* 44(1):26-40, 2008.
30. Reiter RJ et al: Melatonin defeats neurally derived free radicals and reduces the associated neuromorphological and neurobehavioral damage, *J Physiol Pharmacol* 58(Suppl 6):5-22, 2007.
31. Maharaj DS, Glass BD, Daya S: Melatonin: new places in therapy, *Biosci Rep* 27(6):299-320, 2007.
32. Kalantaridou S et al: Peripheral corticotropin-releasing hormone is produced in the immune and reproductive systems: actions, potential roles and clinical implications, *Front Biosci* 12:572-580, 2007.
33. Smith EM: Neuropeptides as signal molecules in common with leukocytes and the hypothalamic-pituitary-adrenal axis, *Brain Behav Immun* 22(1):3-14, 2008.
34. Robinson AG, Verbalis J: Posterior pituitary. In Kronenberg HM et al, editors: *Williams textbook of endocrinology*, ed 11, Philadelphia, 2008, Saunders.
35. Dunser MW, Westphal M: Arginine vasopressin in vasodilatory shock: effects on metabolism and beyond, *Curr Opin Anaesthesiol* 21(2):122-127, 2008.

36. Franchini M: The use of desmopressin as a hemostatic agent: a concise review, *Am J Hematol* 82(8):731-735, 2007.

37. Su LL, Chong YS, Samuel M: Oxytocin agonists for preventing postpartum haemorrhage, *Cochrane Database Syst Rev* (3):CD005457, 2007.

38. Neumann ID: Stimuli and consequences of dendritic release of oxytocin within the brain, *Biochem Soc Trans* 35(Pt 5):1252-1257, 2007.

39. Slattery DA, Neumann ID: No stress please! Mechanisms of stress hyporesponsiveness of the maternal brain, *J Physiol* 586(2):377-385, 2008.

40. Carter CS: Sex differences in oxytocin and vasopressin: implications for autism spectrum disorders? *Behav Brain Res* 176(1):170-186, 2007.

41. Reiter EO, Rosenfield RG: Normal and aberrant growth. In Kronenberg HM et al, editor: *Williams textbook of endocrinology*, ed 11, Philadelphia, 2008, Saunders.

42. Sherlock M, Toogood AA: Aging and the growth hormone/insulin like growth factor-I axis. *Pituitary* 10(2):189-203, 2007.

43. Samani AA et al. The role of the IGF system in cancer growth and metastasis: overview and recent insights, *Endocr Rev* 28(1):20-47, 2007.

44. Ryan PD, Goss PE: The emerging role of the insulin-like growth factor pathway as a therapeutic target in cancer, *Oncologist* 13(1):16-24, 2008.

45. Karsdal MA et al: Calcitonin affects both bone and cartilage: a dual action treatment for osteoarthritis? *Ann N Y Acad Sci* 1117:181-195, 2007.

46. Mercadante S, Fulfaro F: Management of painful bone metastases, *Curr Opin Oncol* 19(4):308-314, 2007.

47. Simon LS: Osteoporosis, *Rheum Dis Clin North Am* 33(1):149-176, 2007.

48. Müller B: Endocrine aspects of critical illness, *Ann Endocrinol (Paris)* 68(4):290-298, 2007.

49. Becker KL, Snider R, Nylen ES: Procalcitonin assay in systemic inflammation, infection, and sepsis: clinical utility and limitations, *Crit Care Med* 36(3):941-952, 2008.

50. Szkudlinski MS, Kazlauskaite R, Weintraub BD: Thyroid stimulating hormone and regulation of the thyroid axis. In DeGroot LJ, Jamerson JL, editors: *Endocrinology*, ed 5, St Louis, 2006, Saunders.

51. Gereben B et al: Activation and inactivation of thyroid hormone by deiodinases: local action with general consequences, *Cell Moll Life Sci* 65(4):570-590, 2008.

52. Larsen PR et al: Thyroid physiology and diagnostic evaluation of patients with thyroid disorders. In Kronenberg HM, editor: *Williams textbook of endocrinology*, ed 11, Philadelphia, 2008, Saunders.

53. Grover GJ, Mellstrom K, Malm J: Therapeutic potential for thyroid hormone receptor-beta selective agonists for treating obesity, hyperlipidemia and diabetes, *Curr Vasc Pharmacol* 5(2):141-154, 2007.

54. Wexler JA, Sharretts J: Thyroid and bone, *Endocrinol Metab Clin North Am* 36(3):673-705, vi, 2007.

55. Rivas M, Naranjo JR: Thyroid hormones, learning and memory, *Genes Brain Behav* 6(Suppl 1):40-44, 2007.

56. Schumock GT, Sprague SM: Clinical and economic burden of fractures in patients with renal osteodystrophy, *Clin Nephrol* 67(4):201-208, 2007.

57. Bergenstock MK, Partridge NC: Parathyroid hormone stimulation of noncanonical Wnt signaling in bone, *Ann N Y Acad Sci* 1116:354-359, 2007.

58. Khosla S, Westendorf JJ, Oursler MJ: Building bone to reverse osteoporosis and repair fractures, *J Clin Invest* 118(2):421-428, 2008.

59. Heaney RP: Vitamin D endocrine physiology, *J Bone Miner Res* 22(Suppl 2):V25-V27, 2007.

60. Hills CE, Brunskill NJ: Intracellular signalling by C-peptide, *Exp Diabetes Res* 51(8):1534-1543, 2008.

61. Ekberg K, Johansson BL: Effect of C-peptide on diabetic neuropathy in patients with type 1 diabetes, *Exp Diabetes Res* 2008:457912, 2008.

62. Wilhelm B, Kann P, Pfutzner A: Influence of C-peptide on glucose utilization, *Exp Diabetes Res* 2008:769483, 2008.

63. Smith SR, Ravussin E: Role of the adipocyte in metabolism and endocrine function. In DeGroot LJ, Jamerson JL, editors: *Endocrinology*, ed 5, St Louis, 2006, Saunders.

64. Drucker DJ: The role of gut hormones in glucose homeostasis, *J Clin Invest* 117(1):24-32, 2007.

65. Ehrman MM et al: Regulation of pancreatic somatostatin gene expression by insulin and glucagon, *Mol Cell Endocrinol* 235(1-2):31-37, 2005.

66. Wren AM: Gut and hormones and obesity, *Front Horm Res* 36:165-181, 2008.

67. Stewart PM: The adrenal cortex. In Kronenberg HM et al, editor: *Williams textbook of endocrinology*, ed 11, Philadelphia, 2008, Saunders.

68. Heitzer MD et al: Glucocorticoid receptor physiology, *Rev Endocr Metab Disord* 8(4):321-330, 2007.

69. Chinenov Y, Rogatsky I: Glucocorticoids and the innate immune system: crosstalk with the toll-like receptor signaling network, *Mol Cell Endocrinol* 275(1-2):30-42, 2007.

70. Kumsta R et al: Cortisol and ACTH responses to psychosocial stress are modulated by corticosteroid binding globulin levels, *Psychoneuroendocrinol* 32(8-10):1153-1157, 2007.

71. Marney AM, Brown NJ: Aldosterone and end-organ damage, *Clin Sci* 113(6):267-278, 2007.

72. Young WF: Endocrine hypertension. In Kronenberg HM et al, editor: *Williams textbook of endocrinology*, ed 11, Philadelphia, 2008, Saunders.

73. Simm A et al: Potential biomarkers of ageing. *Biol Chem* 389(3): 257-265, 2008.

74. Lambers SW: Endocrinology and aging. In Kronenberg HM et al, editor: *Williams textbook of endocrinology*, ed 11, Philadelphia, 2008, Saunders.

75. Chahal HS, Drake WM: The endocrine system and ageing, *J Pathol* 211(2):173-180, 2007.

76. Peeters RP: Thyroid hormones and aging, *Hormones* 7(1):28-35, 2008.

77. Engel N, Mahlknecht U: Aging and anti-aging: unexpected side effects of everyday medication through sirtuin1 modulation, *Int J Mol Med* 21(2):223-232, 2008.

78. Adami S et al: Relationship between serum parathyroid hormone, vitamin D sufficiency, age, and calcium intake, *Bone* 42(2):267-270, 2008.

79. Bjorkman MP, Sorva AJ, Tilvis RS: Elevated serum parathyroid hormone predicts impaired survival prognosis in a general aged population, *Eur J Endocrinol* 158(5):749-753, 2008.

80. Holick MF: Vitamin D deficiency, *N Engl J Med* 357:266-281, 2007.

ALTERATIONS OF HORMONAL REGULATION

ROBERT E. JONES • VALENTINA L. BRASHERS • SUE E. HUETHER

CHAPTER OUTLINE

MECHANISMS OF HORMONAL ALTERATIONS
ALTERATIONS OF THE HYPOTHALAMIC-PITUITARY
SYSTEM
  Diseases of the Posterior Pituitary
  Diseases of the Anterior Pituitary
ALTERATIONS OF THYROID FUNCTION
  Hyperthyroidism
  Hypothyroidism
ALTERATIONS OF PARATHYROID FUNCTION
  Hyperparathyroidism
  Hypoparathyroidism

DYSFUNCTION OF THE ENDOCRINE PANCREAS:
  DIABETES MELLITUS
  Types of Diabetes Mellitus
  Acute Complications of Diabetes Mellitus
  Chronic Complications of Diabetes Mellitus
ALTERATIONS OF ADRENAL FUNCTION
  Disorders of the Adrenal Cortex
  Disorders of the Adrenal Medulla

Function of the endocrine system involves complex interrelationships and interactions that maintain dynamic steady-states, provide growth and reproductive capabilities, and allow for adoptive changes in times of stress. Dysfunction of the endocrine system initially was described in terms of excessive or insufficient function of the endocrine gland with alterations in hormone levels. Alterations in function were thought to be caused by either hypersecretion or hyposecretion of the various hormones, leading to abnormal hormone concentrations in the blood. Techniques for studying the various components of the endocrine system have improved, and evidence has shown that dysfunction may also result from abnormal receptor function or from altered intracellular response to the hormone-receptor complex.

MECHANISMS OF HORMONAL ALTERATIONS

Significantly elevated or depressed hormone levels may result from a variety of causes (Table 21-1). Dysfunction of an endocrine gland may involve the gland's failure to produce adequate amounts of biologically free or active hormone forms. This failure may occur when the secretory cells are unable to produce or obtain an adequate quantity of required hormone precursors or when they are unable to convert the precursors to the active hormone. A gland also may synthesize or release excessive amounts of hormone. In addition, feedback systems that recognize the need for a particular hormone may fail to function properly or may respond to

Table 21-1	Mechanisms of Hormone Alterations

Inappropriate Amounts of Hormone Delivered to Target Cell	Inappropriate Response by Target Cell
Inadequate hormone synthesis Inadequate quantity of hormone precursors Secretory cell unable to convert precursors to active hormone **Failure of feedback systems** Do not recognize positive feedback leading to inadequate hormone synthesis Do not recognize negative feedback leading to excessive hormone synthesis **Hormones inactive** Inadequate biologically free hormone Hormone degraded at an altered rate Circulating inhibitors **Dysfunctional delivery system** Inadequate blood supply Inadequate carrier proteins Ectopic production of hormones	**Cell surface receptor–associated disorders** Decrease in the number of receptors Impaired receptor function (altered affinity for hormones) Presence of antibodies against specific receptors Unusual expression of receptor function **Intracellular disorders** Acquired defects in postreceptor signaling cascades Inadequate synthesis of a second messenger Intracellular enzymes or proteins are altered Alterations in nuclear co-regulators Altered protein synthesis

inappropriate signals (see Chapter 20). Once hormones are released into the circulation, they may be degraded at an altered rate or they may be inactivated by antibodies before reaching the target cell. Ectopic sources of hormones (hormones produced by nonendocrine tissues) may result also in abnormally elevated hormone levels; i.e., bronchopulmonary tumors that release adrenocortictropic hormone (see page 765). This mechanism operates without benefit of the normal feedback system for hormone control. In these cases the ectopic hormone production is said to be *autonomous.*

Research has been directed toward understanding causes for the failure of the target cell to respond to its hormone (*hormone insensitivity*). The general types of abnormal target cell responses currently recognized are receptor-associated disorders and intracellular disorders. Receptor-associated disorders have been identified primarily in water-soluble hormones, such as insulin. These types of disorders usually involve one of the following: (1) a decrease in the number of receptors, leading to decreased or defective hormone-receptor binding; (2) impaired receptor function, resulting in insensitivity to the hormone; (3) presence of antibodies against specific receptors that either reduce available binding sites or mimic hormone action, exaggerating target cell response; or (4) unusual expression of receptor function, as occurs in some tumor cells with abnormal receptor activity.

Intracellular disorders may involve inadequate synthesis of the second messenger, such as cyclic adenosine monophosphate (cAMP), needed to transduce the hormonal signal into intracellular events. The target cell for water-soluble hormones may have a faulty response to hormone-receptor binding and thus fail to generate the required second messenger. The cell also may have an abnormal response to the second messenger if levels of intracellular enzymes or proteins are altered. (Second messengers for various hormones are listed in Table 20-4.) Both of these pathogenic mechanisms result in failure of the target cell to express the usual hormonal effect.

Pathogenic mechanisms affecting target cell response for lipid-soluble hormones, such as thyroid hormone or glucocorticoids, either occur less often or are recognized less often than those affecting the water-soluble hormones. These hormone-resistant states have been generally linked to mutations in the nuclear receptor for the hormone or, in some instances, to alterations in nuclear co-regulators.[1] The number of receptors may be decreased, or those receptors may have an altered affinity for hormones.[2] Both mechanisms would affect hormone-receptor binding. Alterations in generation of new messenger ribonucleic acid (mRNA) or absence of substrates for new protein synthesis also may occur, resulting in altered target cell response.[3,4]

ALTERATIONS OF THE HYPOTHALAMIC-PITUITARY SYSTEM

Documenting abnormal release of hypothalamic-releasing hormones has been difficult because of the relative inaccessibility of the hypothalamic-pituitary unit in the brain and the short half-life and small concentrations of the hypothalamic hormones. Perhaps the most common cause of apparent hypothalamic dysfunction is interruption of the pituitary stalk caused by destructive lesions, rupture after head injury, surgical transection, or tumor. In these cases, interruption of the physical connections between the hypothalamus and the pituitary gland causes apparent pituitary disease. For example, diabetes insipidus (antidiuretic hormone [ADH] insufficiency) may result, depending on the location at which the infundibular stem is interrupted. If the lesion is close to the hypothalamus, diabetes insipidus is likely; the farther away the lesion is from the hypothalamus, the less likely is the occurrence of diabetes insipidus.

The absence of hypothalamic releasing or inhibiting hormones (Figure 21-1) causes a variety of manifestations. For example, if there is an absence of gonadotropin-releasing hormone (GnRH) from the hypothalamus, then there is a lack of stimulation of gonadotropin follicle-stimulating hormone (FSH) and luteinizing hormone (LH) from the pituitary, thus the menses cease in women and spermatogenesis is impaired in men.

Diseases of the Posterior Pituitary

Diseases of the posterior pituitary that cause clinically significant alterations in hormone function usually are related to abnormal secretion of antidiuretic hormone (ADH, arginine vasopressin). An excess amount of this hormone results in water retention and a hypoosmolar state, whereas deficiency in the amount or response to ADH results in serum

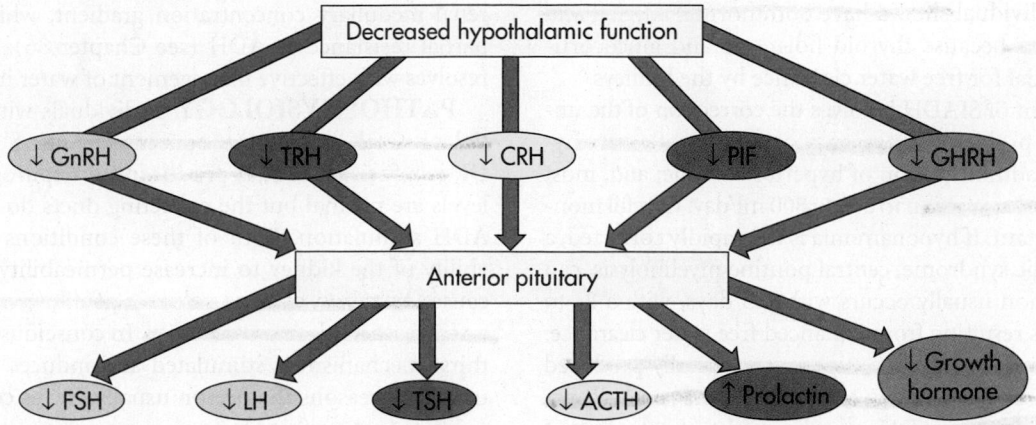

Figure 21-1 Loss of hypothalamic hormones. *ACTH,* Adrenocorticotropic hormone; *CRH,* corticotropin-releasing hormone; *FSH,* follicle-stimulating hormone; *GHRH,* growth hormone-releasing hormone; *GnRH,* gonadotropin-releasing hormone; *LH,* luteinizing hormone; *PIF,* prolactin-releasing inhibiting factor (likely dopamine); *TRH,* thyrotropin-releasing hormone; *TSH,* thyroid-stimulating hormone.

hyperosmolarity. These complex pathophysiologic states not only have significant clinical effects on the modulation of body fluids and electrolytes, but also affect cognitive and emotional responses to stress.[5]

Syndrome of Inappropriate Antidiuretic Hormone Secretion

Syndrome of inappropriate antidiuretic hormone (SIADH) secretion is characterized by high levels of ADH in the absence of normal physiologic stimuli for its release. SIADH can complicate malignancies, pulmonary disorders, central nervous system disorders, surgical procedures and the use of certain medications.

The most common cause of elevated levels of ADH is ectopically produced ADH. SIADH is associated with some forms of cancer, apparently because of the ectopic secretion of ADH by tumor cells. Tumors that have been reported in association with SIADH include small cell carcinoma of the lung, duodenum, stomach, and pancreas; cancers of the bladder, prostate, and endometrium; lymphomas; and sarcomas.[6] Pulmonary disorders associated with SIADH include pneumonia (e.g., tuberculosis), asthma, cystic fibrosis, and respiratory failure requiring mechanical ventilation. Central nervous system disorders that may cause SIADH include encephalitis, meningitis, intracranial hemorrhage, tumors, and trauma.[6]

Any surgery can result in postoperative fluid volume shifts that result in increased ADH secretion for as long as 5 to 7 days after surgery. The precise mechanism is uncertain but is likely related to fluid and volume changes following surgery, the amount and type of intravenous fluids given, and the use of narcotic analgesics. Transient SIADH is especially common after pituitary surgery because stored ADH is released in an unregulated fashion. Medications are an important cause of SIADH, especially in older adults. These include hypoglycemic medications (chlorpropamide), antidepressants, antipsychotics, narcotics, general anesthetics, chemotherapeutic agents, nonsteroidal anti-inflammatory drugs, and synthetic

ADH analogs.[6] These drugs serve either to simulate ADH release or enhance the physiologic effects of ADH or have a biologic action similar to ADH.

PATHOPHYSIOLOGY The cardinal features of SIADH are the result of enhanced renal water retention. Water retention results from the action of ADH on renal collecting ducts, where it increases their permeability to water thus increasing water reabsorption by the kidneys. (Renal function is discussed in Chapter 35.) This results in an expansion of extracellular fluid volume that leads to dilutional hyponatremia (low serum sodium), hypoosmolarity, and urine that is inappropriately concentrated with respect to serum osmolarity.[6,7]

CLINICAL MANIFESTATIONS The symptoms of SIADH are primarily the result of hypotonic (dilutional) hyponatremia. The severity and rapidity of onset of the hyponatremia determine the extent of the symptoms. Thirst, impaired taste, anorexia, dyspnea on exertion, fatigue, and dulled sensorium occur when the serum sodium decreases rapidly from 140 to 130 mEq/L. Peripheral edema is usually absent. Symptoms resolve with correction of hyponatremia. Severe gastrointestinal symptoms, including vomiting and abdominal cramps, occur with a drop in sodium from 130 to 120 mEq/L. With a serum sodium level below 115 mEq/L, confusion, lethargy, muscle twitching, and convulsions may occur. Even if hyponatremia develops slowly, serum sodium levels below 110 to 115 mEq/L are likely to cause severe and sometimes irreversible neurologic damage.

EVALUATION AND TREATMENT A diagnosis of SIADH requires the following signs: (1) serum hypoosmolality (<280 mOsm/kg) and hyponatremia (serum sodium <135 mEq/l); (2) urine hyperosmolarity (i.e., the osmolality of the urine is greater than expected for the concomitant serum osmolality); (3) urine sodium excretion that matches sodium intake; (4) normal renal, adrenal, and thyroid function; and (5) absence of conditions that can alter volume status (e.g., recent diuretic use, heart failure, hypervolemia from any cause, or renal insufficiency).[6,8] In order to make the diagnosis of

SIADH, the individual should have both normal adrenal and thyroid function because thyroid hormone and glucocorticoids are essential for free water clearance by the kidneys.[6]

The treatment of SIADH involves the correction of the underlying causal problems; emergency correction of severe hyponatremia by administration of hypertonic saline; and, most importantly, fluid restriction to 600 to 800 ml/day. Careful monitoring is important. If hyponatremia is too rapidly corrected, a severe neurologic syndrome, central pontine myelinolysis, can ensue.[6] Resolution usually occurs within 3 days, with a 2- to 3-kg weight loss resulting from enhanced free water clearance. No drug therapy is available to suppress ectopically produced ADH; however, demeclocycline, which causes the renal tubules to develop resistance to ADH, may be used to treat resistant or chronic SIADH. An ADH-receptor agonist, conivaptan, has been approved for the treatment of hospitalized individuals with hyponatremia caused by ADH excess.[6,9] Oral forms of ADH receptor antagonists are being developed.[9,10]

Diabetes Insipidus

Diabetes insipidus (DI) is an insufficiency of ADH, leading to polyuria (frequent urination) and polydipsia (frequent drinking).[11,12] There are two forms: neurogenic (central), and nephrogenic (renal). Neurogenic DI is the form encountered most often in clinical practice and is caused by insufficient amounts of ADH.[13] The nephrogenic form is caused by an inadequate renal response to ADH.[14]

Neurogenic DI occurs when any organic lesion of the hypothalamus, pituitary stalk, or posterior pituitary interferes with ADH synthesis, transport, or release.[12,13] Causative lesions include primary or secondary brain tumors, hypophysectomy, aneurysms, thrombosis, infections, and immunologic disorders. DI is a well-recognized complication of closed-head trauma.[15] Genetic mutations have been identified as a cause of central DI, including those that affect ADH genes directly and those that affect ADH copeptides.[12] Uncommonly, central DI can be a hereditary disorder (1% to 2% of cases) characterized by structural changes in the pituitary gland.

Nephrogenic DI is associated with an insensitivity of the renal collecting tubules to ADH. The nephrogenic form of DI can be genetic or acquired.[16] Several genetic abnormalities that affect the vasopressin receptor have been noted in DI.[12,14,17,18] One of the best described is a mutation in the gene that codes for aquaporin-2, which is one of the four water transport channels in the renal tubule.[18,19] Acquired nephrogenic DI is generally related to disorders and drugs that damage the renal tubules or inhibit the generation of cAMP in the tubules. These disorders include pyelonephritis, amyloidosis, destructive uropathies, polycystic disease, and intrinsic renal disease, all of which lead to irreversible DI. Drugs that may induce a reversible form of nephrogenic DI include lithium carbonate, colchicines, amphotericin B, loop diuretics, general anesthetics such as methoxyflurane, and demeclocycline.[12,14,16]

Psychogenic (primary) polydipsia may be confused with a partial deficiency of ADH. It is caused by the chronic ingestion of extremely large quantities of fluid that wash out the renal medullary concentration gradient, which results in a partial resistance to ADH (see Chapter 36). This condition resolves with effective management of water ingestion.

PATHOPHYSIOLOGY Individuals with DI have partial or total inability to concentrate urine. In neurogenic DI, insufficient ADH is produced. In nephrogenic DI, ADH levels are normal but the collecting ducts do not respond to ADH stimulation. Both of these conditions lead to an inability of the kidney to increase permeability to water. This causes excretion of large volumes of dilute urine, leading to an increase in plasma osmolality. In conscious individuals the thirst mechanism is stimulated and induces polydipsia. For unknown reasons the person usually craves cold drinks. The urine output is varied but can increase from the normal output of 1 to 2 L/day to as much as 8 to 12 L/day. The urine specific gravity is low, from 1.00 to 1.005, which is consistent with the failure to reabsorb water. Dehydration develops rapidly without ongoing fluid replacement. If the individual with DI cannot keep up with the urinary loss of water, serum hypernatremia and hyperosmolality occur. Other serum electrolytes generally are not affected.

CLINICAL MANIFESTATIONS The signs and symptoms of DI include polyuria, nocturia, continuous thirst, and polydipsia. Untreated individuals with long-standing DI may develop a large bladder capacity and hydronephrosis (see Chapter 36).

Idiopathic neurogenic DI usually has an abrupt onset, and many individuals can specifically recall the date of onset of their symptoms. Those with posttraumatic or postneurosurgical DI may develop a classic three-phase syndrome.[15,20] Initially, significant diuresis occurs, apparently as a result of acute damage to the hypothalamic centers involving ADH secretion.[13] The second phase is one of antidiuresis, which may represent necrosis of denervated tissue of the posterior pituitary with release of ADH into the circulation. The final phase is one of polyuria and polydipsia, reflecting a permanent loss of the ability to secrete adequate amounts of ADH, which does not have to be completely absent for polyuria and polydipsia to occur. Nephrogenic DI usually has a more gradual onset.

EVALUATION AND TREATMENT DI must be distinguished from other polyuric states, including diabetes mellitus, osmotically induced diuresis, and psychogenic polydipsia. The basic criteria for the diagnosis of DI includes polyuria, polydipsia, low urine specific gravity (<1.010), low urine osmolality (<200 mOsml/kg), hypernatremia, high serum osmolality (300 mOsm or more depending on adequate water intake), and continued diuresis despite a serum sodium of 145 mEq/L or greater.[11-13]

The diagnosis of DI is generally established through water deprivation testing and by correlating the clinical presentation with serum osmolarity and plasma ADH levels.[14] Water restriction is a useful test because people without DI respond with a rapid decrease in urine volume and an increase in urine osmolality. People with DI have no decrease in urine volume or increase in urine osmolarity, thus serum osmolality is always higher than urine osmolality in DI after 8 hours of water deprivation. In individuals with severe DI, water deprivation testing can be hazardous. If the individual loses more than 3% of the pretest body weight, circulatory collapse and shock can ensue. The diagnosis of psychogenic polydipsia can be extremely difficult, and differentiation from nephrogenic DI (caused by the washout of renal concentrating gradient) is based on plasma ADH levels.

Treatment for neurogenic DI is based on the extent of the ADH deficiency and on individual variables such as age, endocrine and cardiovascular status, and lifestyle. Individuals who have a urine output in excess of 9 L/day and a urine osmolality of less than 100 mOsm/kg after a dehydration or water restriction test generally require ADH replacement. Replacement therapy for symptomatic neurogenic DI includes administration of the synthetic vasopressin analog desmopressin acetate (DDAVP) given intranasally or orally. Drugs that potentiate the action of otherwise insufficient amounts of endogenous ADH, such as chlorpropamide, carbamazapine, and clofibrate, may be used in individuals with incomplete ADH deficiency.[12]

Treatment for nephrogenic DI requires treatment of any reversible underlying disorders, discontinuation of etiologic medications, and correction of associated electrolyte disorders. Although the use of thiazide diuretics has been implicated as a cause for DI, they improve salt and water absorption at the proximal tubule and may be helpful in moderate DI.[12,14,16]

Diseases of the Anterior Pituitary

Disorders of the anterior pituitary may involve either hypofunction or hyperfunction of the gland. Hypopituitarism can range in presentation from the absence of selective pituitary trophic hormones to complete failure of hormonal functions of the anterior pituitary. **Hypopituitarism** results from either an inadequate supply of hypothalamic-releasing hormones, damage to the pituitary stalk, or an inability of the gland to produce hormones.[21-23] Spontaneous mutations of the *prophet of pituitary transcription factor (PROP-1)* gene involved in early embryonic pituitary development leads to combined hormonal deficiencies.[24,25] The hormones include thyroid-stimulating hormone (TSH), growth hormone (GH), adrenocorticotropic hormone (ACTH), and prolactin and cause failure to thrive and short stature in children. Hyperfunction of the anterior pituitary usually results from an adenoma composed of secretory pituitary cells or may, rarely, result from the ectopic production of hypothalamic-releasing peptides.

Hypopituitarism

The most common causes of hypopituitarism lie within the pituitary gland itself. Anterior pituitary hypofunction may result from infarction of the gland, removal or destruction of the gland, or space-occupying lesions such as pituitary adenomas or aneurysms. Adenomas and aneurisms may compress otherwise normal secreting pituitary cells and lead to compromised hormonal output.[21,22]

One cause of hypopituitarism is pituitary infarction (death of tissue). Infarction may be seen in conjunction with Sheehan syndrome (ischemic pituitary necrosis) caused by severe postpartum hemorrhage. Pituitary infarction is also seen with shock, pituitary apoplexy, sickle cell disease, and during pregnancy in women with diabetes mellitus. Other more common causes of hypopituitarism are genetic abnormalities, head trauma, pituitary tumors, infections (e.g., meningitis, syphilis, tuberculosis), vascular malformations, subarachnoid hemorrhage, surgical ablation related to tumor removal, and granulomatous lesions.[22,26]

PATHOPHYSIOLOGY The pituitary gland is highly vascular and is therefore extremely vulnerable to ischemia and infarction. In addition, the pituitary relies heavily on portal blood flow from the hypothalamus. In traumatic brain injury, disruption of blood flow can cause infarction with subsequent necrosis and fibrosis of pituitary tissue.[21,26] After tissue necrosis, edema with swelling of the gland occurs. Expansion of the pituitary within the fixed compartment of the sella turcica further impedes blood supply to the pituitary. Over time the pituitary undergoes shrinkage, and symptoms of hypopituitarism develop.[27]

The likelihood of infarction is increased during pregnancy when there is increased size and vasculature of the gland and a rare condition known as **Sheehan syndrome** may develop. In 1961 Sheehan and Stanfield proposed that the primary pathologic mechanism in postpartum pituitary infarction is vasospasm of the artery supplying the anterior pituitary. A commonly identified cause is some event that leads to circulatory collapse (such as postpartum hemorrhage) and compensatory vasospasm. If vasospasm is sustained for more than several hours, tissue necrosis occurs. The pituitary gland may be particularly susceptible to necrosis because its blood supply, through the hypophyseal system, is already partially deoxygenated and, especially in the hyperplastic pituitary of pregnancy, oxygen demands are increased. A second mechanism that may be involved in pituitary infarction in the postpartum woman with Sheehan syndrome is an increased risk for intravascular coagulation. In such individuals, excessive fibrin is deposited in the pituitary vessels, predisposing the woman to decreased blood supply and infarction of the pituitary.

CLINICAL MANIFESTATIONS The signs and symptoms of hypofunction of the anterior pituitary are highly variable and depend on the affected hormones. If all hormones are absent (a condition termed **panhypopituitarism**), the individual experiences cortisol deficiency from lack of ACTH, thyroid deficiency from lack of TSH, and gonadal failure and loss of secondary sex characteristics from absence of FSH and LH. A decrease in GH and, consequently, insulin-like growth factor-1 results in delayed growth in children (Figure 21-2) and a vague, multisymptom syndrome in adults.[21,22] Children also have **dwarfism** with GH insensitivity (Laron syndrome), in which the GH receptor is altered.[28] Menses may cease from absence of FSH and LH. In addition, postpartum women are unable to lactate because of the absence of prolactin.

ACTH deficiency is a potentially life-threatening disorder because cortisol is required for many aspects of cellular

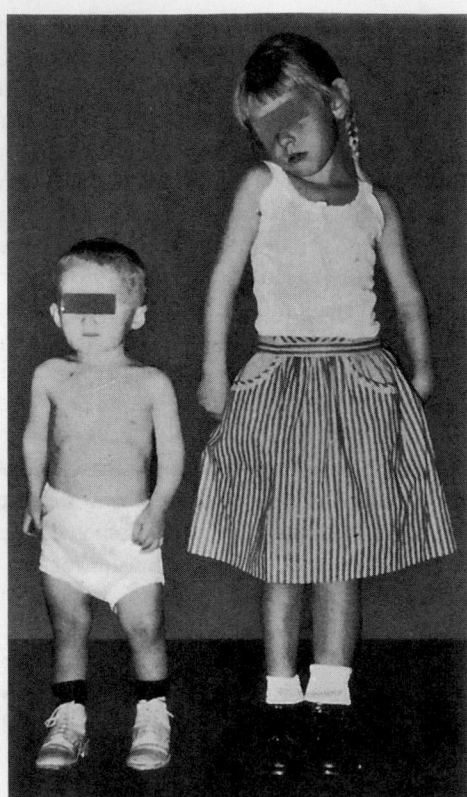

Figure 21-2 Hypopituitary dwarfism. A 4-year-old boy whose height is 25 inches. The girl is also 4 years old and has a normal height of 39 inches. Dwarf has a normal face, as well as head, trunk, and limbs of approximately normal proportions. (From Brashear HR, Raney RB: *Shand's handbook of orthopaedic surgery,* ed 10, St Louis, 1986, Mosby.)

metabolism. ACTH deficiency is usually encountered with generalized pituitary hypofunction and rarely occurs as an isolated event. Within 2 weeks of the complete absence of ACTH, symptoms of cortisol insufficiency develop, including nausea, vomiting, anorexia, fatigue, and weakness. Hypoglycemia is caused by increased insulin sensitivity, decreased glycogen reserves, and decreased gluconeogenesis associated with hypocortisolism. In women, loss of body hair and decreased libido may be caused by decreased adrenal androgen production. ACTH deficiency has a limited effect on aldosterone secretion.

TSH deficiency also is rarely seen in isolation but most often occurs in conjunction with other pituitary hormone deficiencies. The effects of decreased TSH levels may become apparent 4 to 8 weeks after the onset of hypothyrotropinemia. Cold intolerance, dryness of skin, mild myxedema, lethargy, and decreased metabolic rate occur as a result of hypothyroidism induced by decreased TSH levels. The symptoms are usually less severe than those associated with primary hypothyroidism, in which lack of thyroxine is related to disease in the thyroid gland (see p. 739).

The onset of **FSH and LH deficiencies** in women of reproductive age is associated with amenorrhea and atrophic vagina, uterus, and breasts. In postpubertal males, atrophy of the testes and decreased beard growth occur. Men as well as women experience a decrease in body hair and diminished libido. FSH and LH deficiencies often occur as a result of pressure on the gonadotropes from other sources, such as tumors. If there is enlargement caused by tumor, symptoms may include headache and visual disturbances with blurring and field defects from pressure on the optic chiasm.

GH deficiency occurs in children and adults. In children it may be genetic or it may be the result of tumors such as craniopharyngiomas.[28,29] Several genetic defects have been identified in the GH axis that account for impaired GH action.[30] The more common type is a recessive mutation in the *GHRH* gene resulting in a failure of GH secretion. A rare mutation, loss of the *GH* gene itself, has been observed. Mutations that cause GH insensitivity also have been reported. These mutations may involve the GH receptor, insulin-like growth factor 1 (IGF-1) biosynthesis, IGF-1 receptors, or defects in GH signal transduction.[30,31] Individuals with GH insensitivity do not respond normally to exogenously administered GH. Lastly, structural lesions of the pituitary or hypothalamus also may cause GH deficiency and may be associated with other anterior pituitary hormone deficiencies. In adults, GH deficiency is most often caused by structural or functional abnormalities of the pituitary. A decline in GH production is an inevitable consequence of aging and the significance of this phenomenon is poorly understood.[32]

GH deficiency in children is manifested by growth failure, but not all children with short stature have GH deficiency. Other causes of growth failure not related to GH deficiency include systemic illness, hypothyroidism, malnutrition, and emotional deprivation. Another feature of GH deficiency in children is fasting hypoglycemia, likely due to impaired substrate mobilization for gluconeogenesis and enhanced insulin sensitivity.

An *adult GH deficiency syndrome* has been described in those who have complete or even partial failure of the anterior pituitary. Symptoms of adult GH deficiency syndrome are vague and include social withdrawal, fatigue, loss of motivation, and a diminished feeling of well-being. Several studies also have documented increased mortality in adults who are GH deficient. Osteoporosis and alterations in body composition (i.e., reduced lean body mass) are common concomitants of adult GH deficiency.

GH replacement therapy has become relatively simple with the introduction of recombinant human growth hormone. In children, GH replacement therapy is monitored by measuring linear growth and IGF-1 levels.[28] GH replacement in adults is much more controversial and is generally reserved for those with symptomatic hypopituitarism.[21,33]

EVALUATION AND TREATMENT The diagnostic evaluation of suspected pituitary disease is often challenging and must be carefully interpreted together with the individual's signs and symptoms. Simultaneous measurements of the tropic hormones from the pituitary and target endocrine glands are crucial and, in some cases, dynamic testing of the various axes is indicated.[21,22] Radiographic assessment of the pituitary (magnetic resonance imaging [MRI] or computed tomography [CT] scans) may demonstrate enlargement of the pituitary, abnormal areas of enhancement suggestive of an adenoma, deviation of the pituitary stalk, or evidence of a locally aggressive tumor. However, some radiographic findings may be nonspecific and require clinical correlation to establish a diagnosis.

In general, treatment of hypopituitarism involves replacing target gland hormone(s) that are deficient because of lack of tropic anterior pituitary hormones.[21,22,34] In cases of circulatory collapse, immediate therapy with glucocorticoids and intravenous fluids is critical. Thyroid and cortisol replacement therapy must be maintained. Gender-specific sex steroid replacement therapy is also initiated to improve general well-being and to prevent osteoporosis.

Hyperpituitarism: Primary Adenoma

Pituitary adenomas are usually benign slow-growing tumors that arise from cells of the anterior pituitary, most commonly those that secrete GH and prolactin. The molecular pathogenesis of pituitary adenomas is not clearly understood. The incidence of pituitary adenomas may be as high as 22%, but most of these are microadenomas found incidentally on high-resolution MRI scanning and are asymptomatic.[35] The vast majority of pituitary microadenomas are hormonally silent and do not pose significant hazards to the individual.[36] More significant adenomas are associated with morbidity and mortality attributable to alterations in hormone secretion or to invasion or impingement of surrounding structures. Primary pituitary carcinomas are rare, representing about 0.2% of all pituitary tumors.[37]

PATHOPHYSIOLOGY Local expansion of pituitary adenomas may cause both neurologic and secretory defects. Neurologically, the tumor may impinge on the optic chiasm if it extends upward from the sella turcica. This causes a variety of visual disturbances, depending on the area of the optic chiasm that is compressed. If the tumor is locally aggressive, it may invade the cavernous sinus and cause cavernous sinus thrombosis with impairment of the function of the oculomotor, trigeminal, trochlear, and abducens cranial nerves, evoking symptoms relative to their function. Extension also may involve the hypothalamus, disturbing hypothalamic control of wakefulness, thirst, appetite, and temperature.

The adenomatous tissue secretes the hormone of the cell type from which it arose, without regard to physiologic needs and without benefit of regulatory feedback mechanisms. GH-, LH-, and FSH-secreting cells in the pituitary are most sensitive to pressure from expanding tumors within the rigid sella turcica, and as a consequence, hyposecretion of these hormones is most often seen in people with a large pituitary gland.

CLINICAL MANIFESTATIONS The clinical manifestations of pituitary adenomas are related to tumor growth and hormone hypersecretion or hyposecretion. Effects from an increase in tumor size include such nonspecific complaints as headache and fatigue. Visual changes produced by pressure on the optic chiasm include visual field impairments (occasionally beginning in one eye and progressing to the other)

and temporary blindness. If the tumor infiltrates other cranial nerves, neurologic function is affected.

Pituitary adenomas arise from hormone-producing cells of the pituitary, and most often are associated with increased secretion of GH and prolactin. Paradoxically, the pressure produced by a pituitary adenoma is also associated with decreased function of neighboring anterior pituitary cells, which results in hyposecretion of other anterior pituitary hormones. For example, gonadotropic hyposecretion often results in menstrual irregularity in women, decreased libido, and receding secondary sex characteristics in men and women. If the tumor exerts sufficient pressure, thyroid and adrenal hypofunction may occur because of lack of TSH and ACTH. These result in the symptoms of hypothyroidism and hypocortisolism.

EVALUATION AND TREATMENT Diagnosis of pituitary adenoma involves physical and laboratory evaluations, including pertinent hormone assays and radiographic examination of the skull. This may be accomplished by CT scanning or dynamic MRI used in conjunction with contrast material. Dynamic MRIs provide superior imaging and greater sensitivity for small lesions in comparison with CT scans.[38]

The goal of treatment is to protect the individual from the effects of tumor growth and to control hormone hypersecretion or hyposecretion while minimizing damage to appropriately secreting portions of the pituitary. Depending on the tumor size and type, individuals may be treated with specific medications to suppress tumor growth, transsphenoidal tumor resection, or radiation therapy.[39]

Hypersecretion of Growth Hormone: Acromegaly

Acromegaly occurs in adults who are exposed to continuously excessive levels of GH and concomitant elevation of IGF-1.[40] In children and adolescents whose epiphyseal plates have not yet closed, the effect of increased GH levels on long bone growth is termed **giantism** (Figure 21-3).

Acromegaly is a rare disease with an estimated prevalence of 70 persons per million.[40] Approximately 15% of all pituitary tumors release excessive GH. The most common cause of acromegaly is a primary autonomous GH-secreting pituitary adenoma.[40,41] Acromegaly occurs more often in women than men and is diagnosed most often in adults in their 40s and 50s, although the disease is usually present for years preceding the diagnosis.

Acromegaly is a slowly progressive disease that if untreated is associated with a decreased life expectancy. The increased number of deaths associated with acromegaly are caused by cardiac hypertrophy, hypertension, atherosclerosis, and type 2 diabetes mellitus that lead to coronary artery disease.[42] Malignancies, including colon, breast, and lung cancer, are also more common in individuals with acromegaly.[40,41]

PATHOPHYSIOLOGY With a GH-secreting adenoma, the usual GH baseline secretion pattern is lost, as are sleep-related GH peaks. A totally unpredictable secretory pattern ensues. With only slight elevations of GH, IGF-1 levels increase, stimulating growth. In the adult, epiphyseal closure has occurred and increased amounts of GH and IGF-1 cannot

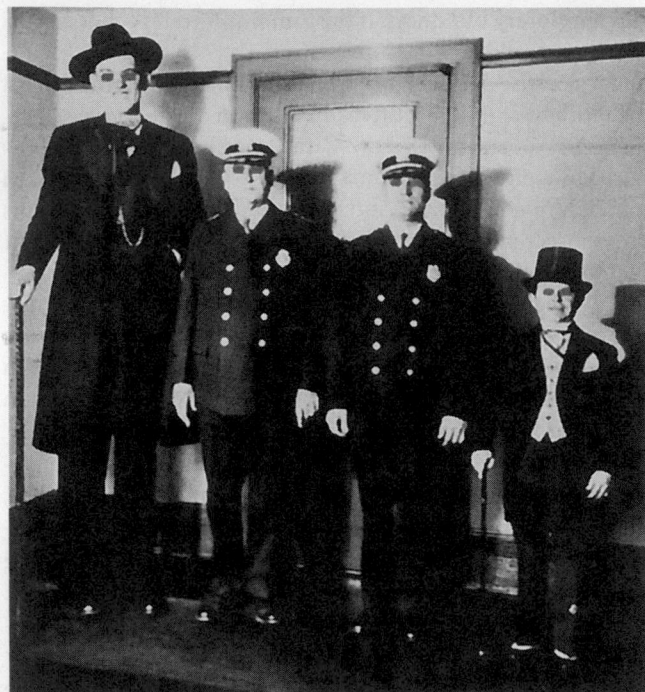

Figure 21-3 Giantism. A pituitary giant and dwarf contrasted with normal-size men. Excessive secretion of growth hormone by the anterior lobe of the pituitary gland during the early years of life produces giants of this type, whereas deficient secretion of this substance produces well-formed dwarfs. (From Patton K, Thibodeau GA: *Anatomy & physiology*, ed 7, St Louis, 2010, Mosby.)

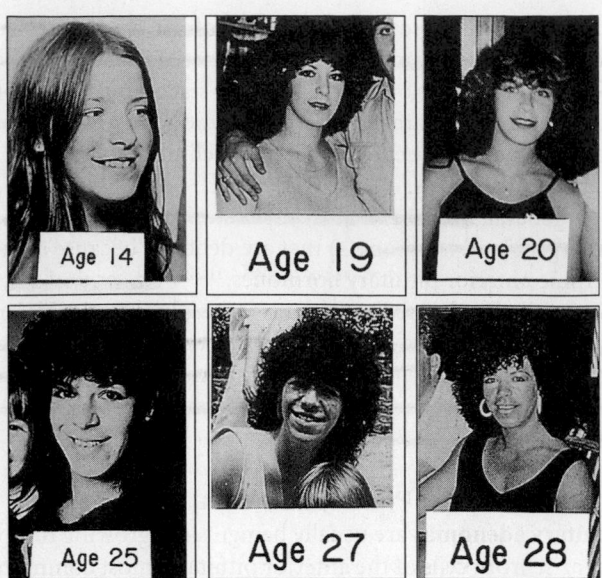

Figure 21-4 Acromegaly. Chronologic sequence of photographs showing slow development of acromegaly. (From Belchetz P, Hammond P: *Mosby's color atlas and text of diabetes and endocrinology*, Edinburgh, 2003, Mosby.)

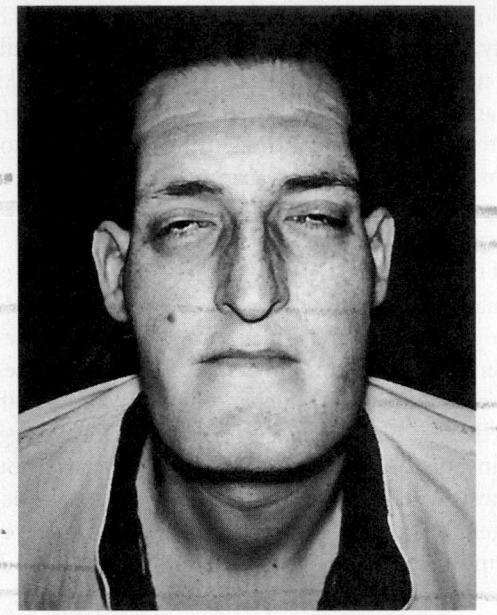

Figure 21-5 Acromegaly. Note large head, forward projection of jaw, and protrusion of frontal bone. (From Thibodeau GA: *Anatomy & physiology*, St Louis, 1987, Mosby.)

stimulate further long bone growth. Instead, these elevations cause connective tissue proliferation, an increase in the extracytoplasmic matrix, and bony proliferation. Thickening of the articular cartilage with fibrosis is followed by narrowing of the joint spaces and formation of osteophytes, leading to chronic arthritis. These changes affect large joints and the vertebrae, limiting mobility and causing pain.[40]

GH acts on the renal tubules to increase phosphate reabsorption, leading to mild hyperphosphatemia. The metabolic effects of GH hypersecretion include impaired carbohydrate tolerance and increased metabolic rate. Hyperglycemia may be seen as a result of GH's inhibition of peripheral glucose uptake and increased hepatic glucose production, followed by insulin resistance and, finally, compensatory hyperinsulinism. Not surprisingly, because of the aforementioned changes in glucose use, approximately one third of people with GH abnormalities have glucose intolerance and half of those individuals develop type 2 diabetes mellitus.[40] Type 2 diabetes mellitus occurs when the pancreas is unable to secrete enough insulin to offset the effects of GH.

CLINICAL MANIFESTATIONS As a result of connective tissue proliferation, individuals with acromegaly have enlarged tongues, interstitial edema, increase in the size and function of sebaceous and sweat glands (leading to increased body odor), and coarse skin and body hair. The coarse skin condition becomes very apparent when procedures such as inserting an intravenous needle are performed; the skin is

very thick and difficult to penetrate. Bony proliferation results in large joint arthropathy with swelling and decreased range of motion and periosteal vertebral growth, which causes kyphosis.[40] Enlargement of the facial bones and the bones of the hands and feet result in protrusion of the lower jaw and forehead and a need for increasingly larger sizes of shoes, hats, rings, and gloves (Figures 21-4 and 21-5).

Because IGF-1 stimulates cartilaginous growth, the increased IGF-1 levels cause elongation of ribs at the bone-cartilage junction, leading to a barrel-chest appearance and increased proliferation of cartilage in joints. This in turn causes backache, arthralgia, and arthritis. These are early manifestations of acromegaly. When shaking hands with an individual with acromegaly, one can palpate the large soft tissues. With bony and soft tissue overgrowth, entrapment of nerves may occur, leading to peripheral nerve damage as manifested by weakness, muscular atrophy, footdrop, and sensory changes in the hands.

Although the associated pathophysiology is not clearly understood at present, hypertension and left heart failure are seen in one third to one half of individuals with acromegaly. Cardiomyopathy associated with progressive and unrestrained myocardial growth is a significant factor.[40] Headache occurs in 50% to 87% of cases and does not appear related to GH levels, size of the tumor, or presence of hypertension. Because of a space-occupying lesion, central nervous system symptoms of headache, seizure activity, visual disturbances (e.g., bitemporal hemianopia from compression of the optic chiasm), papilledema, and compression hypopituitarism may occur.

If compression hypopituitarism does occur because of a large GH-secreting adenoma, the secretion of the gonadotropins may be affected. This causes amenorrhea in women and loss of libido and erectile dysfunction in men because of pituitary stalk compression. Dopamine delivery to the anterior pituitary is impaired in 30% to 40% of individuals with acromegaly resulting in hyperprolactinemia. In addition, co-secretion of GH and prolactin by the same neoplastic cell line has been documented.[40]

EVALUATION AND TREATMENT Diagnosis of acromegaly is accomplished by documenting GH suppression during oral glucose tolerance testing and elevated IGF-1 levels.[41] The goals of treatment are to normalize GH and IGF-1 serum levels, restoring normal pituitary function and relieving or preventing complications related to tumor expansion. The treatment of choice for acromegaly is transsphenoidal surgical removal of the GH-secreting adenoma.[43] Treatment by radiation therapy may be effective when rapid control of GH levels is not essential, when the individual is not a good surgical candidate, or when hyperfunction persists after subtotal resection. Octreotide, octreotide long acting and lanreotide are somatostatin analogs that have been shown to be effective in lowering elevated GH levels, reversing many of the clinical manifestations of the disease, and causing tumor shrinkage in nearly half of individuals.[40,43,44] Pegvisomant is an effective drug that induces tissue insensitivity to GH.[40,45]

Hypersecretion of Prolactin: Prolactinoma

Pituitary tumors that secrete prolactin are called **prolactinomas** and are the most common of the hormonally active pituitary tumors encountered in clinical medicine.[46,47] The physiologic actions of prolactin include breast development during pregnancy, postpartum milk production, and suppression of ovarian function in nursing women.

In addition to pituitary tumors, many conditions or medications can elevate prolactin in the absence of pituitary pathologic condition. For example, renal failure, polycystic ovarian disease (see Chapter 22), primary hypothyroidism, breast

stimulation, or even venipuncture can increase prolactin levels.[47,48] Prolactin is under tonic inhibitory hypothalamic control through the secretion of dopamine (prolactin inhibitor factor [PIF]).[46] Thus medications that block the effects of dopamine at the pituitary can increase prolactin and stimulate proliferation of prolactin-secreting cells (lactotrophies). These include antipsychotics (risperidone, chlorpromazine), metoclopramide, tricyclic antidepressants, methyldopa, and estrogens.[46] Any process that interferes with the delivery of dopamine from the hypothalamus to the lactotrophies (pituitary stalk tumor, pituitary stalk transection, or compressive pituitary tumor) also results in hyperprolactinemia. Because thyrotropin-releasing hormone (TRH) stimulates prolactin secretion in addition to enhancing TSH release, prolactin may be elevated in individuals with primary hypothyroidism.

PATHOPHYSIOLOGY The hallmark of a prolactinoma is sustained increases in serum prolactin. Indeed, tumor size roughly correlates with the degree of prolactin elevation. **Hyperprolactinemia** has several reproductive consequences. Prolactin suppresses GnRH pulses at the hypothalamus, impairs pulsatile pituitary gonadotropin release, and blunts the gonadal responsiveness to gonadotropins. In estrogen- and progesterone-primed breasts, milk production is stimulated.

CLINICAL MANIFESTATIONS Pathologic elevation of prolactin in women results in amenorrhea, nonpuerperal milk production (galactorrhea), hirsutism (excessive body hair in a masculine distribution pattern), and osteopenia caused by estrogen deficiency.[46,47] Menstrual abnormalities and galactorrhea are alarming symptoms in women, and, as a result, women generally present earlier in the course of the illness and are found to have microadenomas (less than 1 cm in size). Men, on the other hand, are more likely to have larger tumors at the time of diagnosis with associated compressive or impingement symptoms such as headache or visual impairment. Hyperprolactinemia in men causes hypogonadism, erectile dysfunction, impaired libido, oligospermia, and diminished ejaculate volume.[47]

EVALUATION AND TREATMENT The diagnostic evaluation of hyperprolactinemia starts with a careful history to exclude medications that may cause elevations in prolactin. Symptoms of hypothyroidism should be elicited, and screening with a serum TSH is mandatory. A careful search for a nonpituitary cause should be pursued if prolactin is less than 50 ng/ml. Prolactin levels more than 200 ng/ml are usually associated with a prolactinoma and are an indication for MRI scanning of the pituitary.[46,47]

Dopaminergic agonists (bromocriptine, cabergoline, and pergolide) are the treatment of choice for prolactinomas, and their use is often associated with both a rapid reduction in the size of the tumor and a reversal of the gonadal effects of hyperprolactinemia.[46,47] Restoration of fertility in previously anovulatory women is common. Although there is an association between valvular heart disease and cabergoline or pergolide used in the treatment of parkinsonism, those individuals receive much higher doses of these medications than those used for prolactinoma. Studies on the long-term safety of cabergoline in treatment of prolactinoma are underway.[49] Alternatives to dopaminergic agonists are being developed including somatostatin analogs and prolactin receptor antagonists.[47] In individuals resistant or intolerant to these medications, transsphenoidal surgery and radiotherapy are options.[47,48]

ALTERATIONS OF THYROID FUNCTION

Disorders of thyroid function develop as a result of primary dysfunction or disease of the thyroid gland or, secondarily, as a result of pituitary or hypothalamic alterations. Primary thyroid disorders result in alterations of thyroid hormone (TH) levels with secondary feedback effects on pituitary TSH. For example, when there are primary elevations in TH, TSH will secondarily decrease because of negative feedback. When TH is decreased because of a condition affecting the thyroid gland, TSH will be elevated. Secondary disorders of the thyroid gland are related to disorders of pituitary gland TSH production. When there is excessive TSH production, TH is elevated secondary to the primary elevation of TSH. The reverse is true with inadequate TSH production.

Hyperthyroidism

Thyrotoxicosis

PATHOPHYSIOLOGY Thyrotoxicosis is a condition that results from any cause of increased levels of circulating TH. The terms *thyrotoxicosis* and *hyperthyroidism* are often used interchangeably. The prevalence of hyperthyroidism is estimated to be 1.2% in the United States, of which 0.7% is subclinical.[50] Thyrotoxicosis has a variety of causes. Identifying the cause is important because the treatment and expected outcome vary accordingly. **Primary hyperthyroidism** is a form of thyrotoxicosis in which excess TH is synthesized and secreted by the thyroid gland. Specific diseases that can cause primary hyperthyroidism include Graves disease, toxic multinodular goiter, solitary hyperfunctioning nodules, and, very rarely, follicular thyroid carcinoma. Thyrotoxicosis also can occur transiently in subacute thyroiditis (viral, postpartum, painless, or de Quervain thyroiditis) because of the release of preformed TH; however, this is not considered a cause of true hyperthyroidism because an abnormal amount of TH synthesis does not occur, and therefore the thyrotoxicosis is not sustained.[50] Another cause of thyrotoxicosis is ingestion of excess TH medication, sometimes called thyrotoxicosis factitia (Figure 21-6). **Secondary hyperthyroidism** is very rare and is caused by TSH-secreting pituitary adenomas. Although each of these conditions is associated with specific pathophysiology and manifestations, all forms of thyrotoxicosis share some common characteristics.

CLINICAL MANIFESTATIONS The clinical features of thyrotoxicosis are attributable to the metabolic effects of increased circulating levels of TH (Figure 21-7). This usually results in an increased metabolic rate with heat intolerance and increased tissue sensitivity to stimulation by the sympathetic division of the autonomic nervous system. The major manifestations are summarized in Table 21-2. Enlargement of

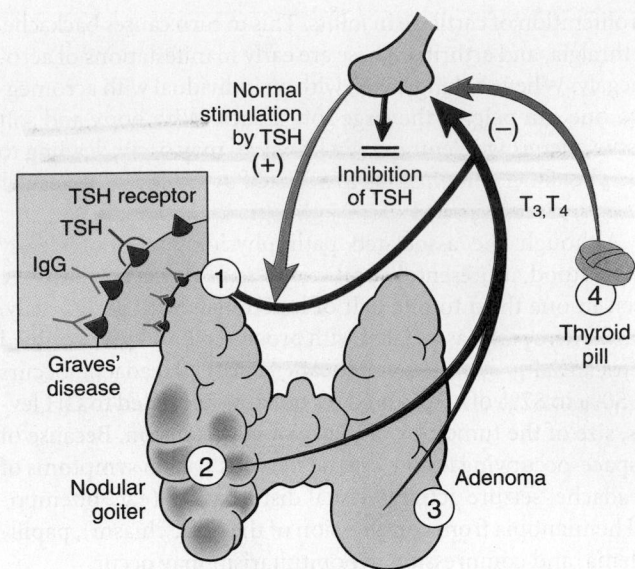

Figure 21-6 Hyperthyroidism may have several causes, among them: 1, Grave disease; 2, toxic multinodular goiter; 3, follicular adenoma; 4, thyroid medication. (From Damjanov I: *Pathology for the health professions*, St Louis, 2006, Saunders.)

the thyroid gland (goiter) is common in hyperthyroid conditions caused by stimulation of TSH receptors.

EVALUATION AND TREATMENT The diagnosis of thyrotoxicosis is based on symptoms of TH excess and documentation of increased circulating thyroid hormone levels. Elevated serum free thyroxine (T_4) and triiodothyronine (T_3) are found in all forms of thyrotoxicosis. In primary hyperthyroidism, TSH is decreased and in secondary hyperthyroidism it is increased. Radioactive iodine uptake (RAIU) can be used in evaluating the etiology of thyrotoxicosis[50] (Figure 21-8).

Treatment is directed at controlling excessive TH production, secretion, or action. The major types of therapy currently used to achieve these goals include antithyroid drug therapy (methimazole or propylthiouracil), radioactive iodine therapy, and surgery. One of the major complications of both radioactive iodine and surgical treatment of hyperthyroidism is excessive ablation of the gland, resulting in hypothyroidism.

Hyperthyroid Conditions

Graves Disease

Graves disease is an autoimmune disease that results in stimulation of the thyroid gland and resultant hyperthyroidism. It is the underlying cause of 50% to 80% of cases of hyperthyroidism and has a prevalence of approximately 0.5% in the U.S. population.[51] It occurs more commonly in women. This disease is characterized as a multisystem syndrome consisting of one or more of the following: (1) hyperthyroidism, (2) diffuse thyroid enlargement (goiter), (3) ophthalmopathy, and (4) dermopathy.

Genetic factors interacting with environmental triggers play an important role in the pathogenesis of autoimmune thyroid disease.[50-52] Variants in several major histocompatibility complex (MHC) genes have been associated with Graves

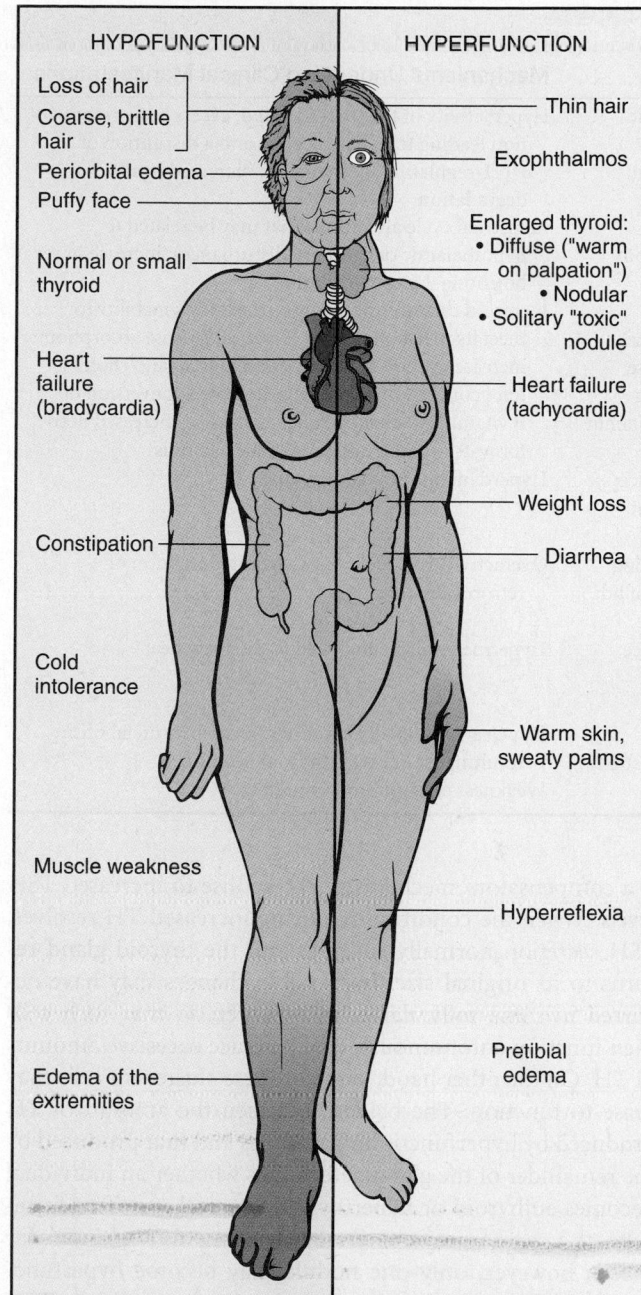

Figure 21-7 Clinical manifestations of hyperthyroidism and hypothyroidism. (From Damjanov I: *Pathology for the health professions,* St Louis, 2006, Saunders.)

disease, and it has a concordance rate of 35% for monozygotic twins.[51,52] Triggers for the onset of Graves symptoms include stressful life events, recent childbirth, and infection.[51]

The pathology of Graves disease indicates that normal regulatory mechanisms are overridden by abnormal immunologic mechanisms. T lymphocytes are sensitized to thyroid antigens and stimulate B cells to produce immunoglobulin G (IgG) antibodies that bind to TSH receptors in the thyroid gland and stimulate the synthesis and secretion of excess TH. These autoantibodies are called *thyroid-stimulating immunoglobulins (TSI)* (also called thyroid-stimulating antibodies [TSAb] or

thyroid receptor antibodies [TRAb]) and are found in more than 95% of people with Graves disease.[50] The hyperfunction of the thyroid gland leads to suppression of TSH and TRH because of the normal negative feedback from elevated levels of TH. The hyperfunction of the thyroid gland is reflected in a dramatically increased iodide uptake and increased rate of thyroid gland metabolism, which may in turn contribute to hypervascularity and enlargement of the gland (goiter). There is a disproportionate increase in T_3 production that reflects long-term hyperstimulation of the thyroid gland.

A small number of individuals with Graves disease and very high levels of TSI experience **pretibial myxedema (Graves dermopathy),** characterized by subcutaneous swelling on the anterior portions of the legs and by indurated and erythematous skin.[53] Thyroid-associated dermopathy is associated with thyrotropin receptor antigens on fibroblasts and recruited T lymphocytes. These manifestations occasionally appear on the hands giving the appearance of clubbing of the fingers (thyroid acropachy).[54]

Many individuals with Graves disease experience ocular manifestations (Figure 21-9). Two categories of ocular manifestations are associated with Graves disease: (1) functional abnormalities resulting from hyperactivity of the sympathetic division of the autonomic nervous system and (2) infiltrative changes involving the orbital contents with enlargement of the ocular muscles.[55] Functional abnormalities occur in most individuals with Graves disease. These abnormalities include a lag of the globe on upward gaze or a lag of the upper lid on downward gaze and are caused by overactivity of Müeller (eyelid) muscles. This manifestation does not affect ocular function and resolves with treatment for hyperthyroidism.[56]

Infiltrative ophthalmopathy occurs in 50% to 70% of individuals with Graves disease. It is characterized by orbital fat accumulation and inflammation with edema of the orbital contents resulting in protrusion of the globe (**exophthalmos**).[55] These changes result in extraocular muscle weakness leading to diplopia (double vision). The individual also may experience irritation, pain, lacrimation, photophobia, and blurred vision. Occasionally, decreased visual acuity, papilledema (edema of the optic nerve), visual field impairment, exposure keratopathy, and corneal ulceration may occur.

Therapy for Graves disease includes antithyroid drugs (propylthiouracil and methimazole), radioactive iodine, or surgery. Unfortunately, current treatment for Graves disease does not reverse the infiltrative ophthalmopathy or the pretibial myxedema. An experienced oculoplastic surgeon and glucocorticoids can help many individuals with progressive ophthalmopathy.[56] Skin lesions rarely require treatment, but if they are symptomatic they may respond to topical glucocorticoids.[53]

Hyperthyroidism Resulting from Nodular Thyroid Disease

The thyroid gland normally enlarges in response to an increased secretion of TSH that may occur in puberty, pregnancy, or iodine deficiency. The increased number of follicles

Table 21-2	Systemic Manifestations of Hyperthyroidism	
System	**Clinical Manifestations**	**Mechanisms Underlying Clinical Manifestations**
Endocrine	Enlarged thyroid gland (goiter) (97%-99% of cases); systolic or continuous bruit over thyroid; increased cortisol degradation; hypercalcemia and decreased PTH secretion; diminished sensitivity to exogenous insulin	Hyperactivity of the thyroid gland; excess bone resorption leading to hypercalcemia and a disruption of PTH-regulating mechanisms; increased insulin degradation
Reproductive	Oligomenorrhea or amenorrhea; erectile dysfunction and decreased libido; increased serum estradiol and estrone but lower than normal levels of free estradiol and estrone	Menstrual cycle alterations that may be related to hypothalamic or pituitary disturbances; increase in sex hormone–binding globulin
Gastrointestinal	Weight loss; increased peristalsis leading to less formed and more frequent stools; nausea, vomiting, anorexia, abdominal pain; increased use of hepatic glycogen stores and of adipose and protein stores; decrease in serum lipid levels (including triglycerides, phospholipids, and cholesterol); changes in vitamin metabolism leading to decrease in tissue stores of vitamins	Increased catabolism leading to the body's inability to meet its metabolic needs; increased glucose absorption; increase in cholesterol excretion in feces and cholesterol conversion to bile salts; impaired conversion of B vitamins to their coenzymes, causing increased need for water-soluble and fat-soluble vitamins
Integumentary	Excessive sweating, flushing, and warm skin; heat intolerance; hair fine, soft, and straight; temporary hair loss; nails that grow away from nail beds, palmar erythema	Hyperdynamic circulatory state
Sensory (eyes)	Ocular manifestations including elevated upper eyelid leading to decreased blinking and a staring quality; fine tremor of lid; infiltrative ocular changes associated with Graves disease	Overactivity of Mueller muscle; inflammation of retroorbital contents
Cardiovascular	Increased cardiac output and decreased peripheral resistance; tachycardia at rest; loud heart sounds; supraventricular dysrhythmias, left ventricular dilation and hypertrophy	Hypermetabolism and need to dissipate heat
Nervous	Restlessness; short attention span; compulsive movement; fatigue; tremor; insomnia; increased appetite; emotional lability	Not clearly defined; alterations in cerebral metabolism resulting from excess thyroid hormone
Pulmonary	Dyspnea; reduced vital capacity	Weakness of respiratory muscles

PTH, Parathyroid hormone.

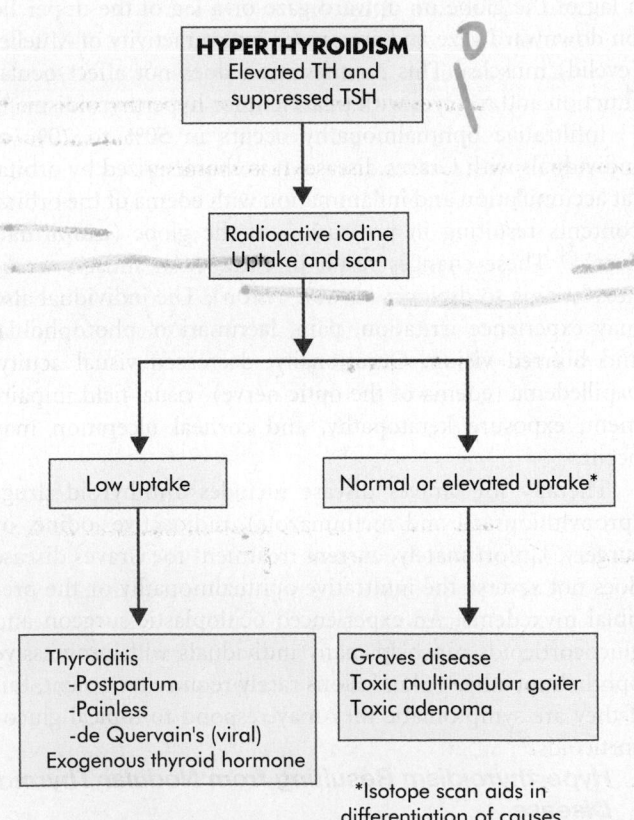

Figure 21-8 Evaluation of hyperthyroidism. Radioactive iodine is used in the differential diagnosis of hyperthyroidism. *TH*, Thyroid hormone; *TSH*, thyroid-stimulating hormone.

is a compensatory mechanism in response to increased TSH levels. When the condition requiring increased TH resolves, TSH secretion normally subsides and the thyroid gland returns to its original size. Irreversible changes may have occurred in some follicular cells, however, so that such cells then function autonomously and produce excessive amounts of TH. On the other hand, some of these clusters of cells may cease to function. The balance between the amount of TH produced by hyperfunctioning nodules and that produced by the remainder of the gland determines whether an individual becomes euthyroid or hyperthyroid. Once thyrotoxicosis results, the condition generally is termed **toxic multinodular goiter**; however, only one nodule may become hyperfunctioning and is termed **toxic adenoma**. Mutations of the TSH receptor have been found in most of the solitary, hyperfunctioning thyroid adenomas.[50]

Manifestations of hyperthyroidism resulting from toxic multinodular goiter or a toxic adenoma are similar to those of Graves disease, although infiltrative ophthalmopathy and myxedema do not occur. The symptoms usually develop slowly and appear over time. The incidence of malignancy in toxic nodular goiter is estimated to be as high as 9%, so most individuals should undergo MRI or fine-needle aspiration biopsy prior to treatment.[57,58] Treatment consists of a combination of antithyroid drugs, radioactive iodine, and surgery.[59]

Thyrotoxic Crisis

Thyrotoxic crisis (thyroid storm) is a rare but dangerous worsening of the thyrotoxic state, in which death can occur within 48 hours without treatment. The condition may

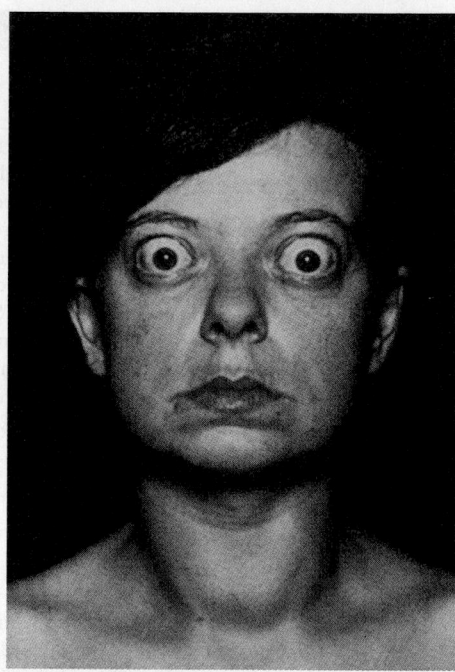

Figure 21-9 Thyrotoxicosis (Graves disease). Note large and protruding eyeballs in association with a large goiter. (From Seidel et al: *Mosby's guide to physical examination,* ed 4, St Louis, 1999, Mosby.)

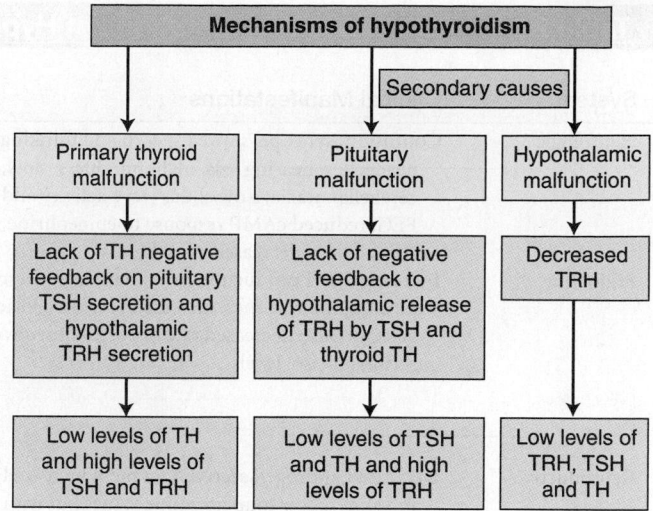

Figure 21-10 Mechanisms of primary and secondary hypothyroidism.

develop spontaneously, but it occurs most often in individuals who have undiagnosed or partially treated severe hyperthyroidism and who are subjected to excessive stress from other causes. These causes may include infection, pulmonary or cardiovascular disorders, trauma, burns, seizures, surgery (especially thyroid surgery), obstetrical complications, emotional distress, or dialysis.[60]

The systemic symptoms of thyrotoxic crisis include hyperthermia; tachycardia, especially atrial tachydysrhythmias; high-output heart failure; agitation or delirium; and nausea, vomiting, or diarrhea contributing to fluid volume depletion.[61-63] Treatment includes (1) the use of drugs that block TH synthesis (i.e., propylthiouracil), (2) the use of beta-blockers for control of cardiovascular symptoms, and (3) supportive care.[60,61]

Hypothyroidism

Hypothyroidism is the most common disorder of thyroid function and affects between 0.1% and 2% of individuals in the United States.[64] **Hypothyroidism** is caused by a deficient production of TH by the thyroid gland. Hypothyroidism may be primary or secondary. Primary hypothyroidism causes include (1) defective hormone synthesis resulting from autoimmune thyroiditis, endemic iodine deficiency, or iatrogenic loss of thyroid tissue after surgical or radioactive treatment for hyperthyroidism; and (2) congenital defects.[64] **Secondary (central) hypothyroidism**, which is much less common, includes conditions that cause either pituitary or hypothalamic failure with failure to stimulate normal thyroid function.[65]

PATHOPHYSIOLOGY In primary hypothyroidism the loss of functional thyroid tissue leads to a decreased production of TH (see Chapter 20). Without the negative feedback of TH on the pituitary, there is an increased secretion of TSH that may lead to goiter. On the other hand, the cellular infiltration that occurs in autoimmune thyroiditis also may cause thyroid enlargement independently of the trophic actions of TSH. Secondary hypothyroidism is caused most commonly by failure of the pituitary to synthesize adequate amounts of TSH, thus it is characterized by low TH levels in association with inappropriately low TSH or TRH levels (Figure 21-10). Pituitary adenomas that compress surrounding pituitary cells or as a result of their treatment are the most common causes of secondary hypothyroidism. Other causes include traumatic brain injury, subarachnoid hemorrhage, or Sheehan syndrome.[65]

CLINICAL MANIFESTATIONS Hypothyroidism generally affects all body systems, with the extent of the symptoms closely related to the degree of TH deficiency (see Figure 21-7). The onset is usually insidious over months or years. The lowered levels of TH result in decreased energy metabolism and heat production. The individual develops a low basal metabolic rate, cold intolerance, lethargy, tiredness, and slightly lowered basal body temperature. Many organ systems are affected (Table 21-3). The decrease in TH leads to increases in TSH production and may cause goiter.

The characteristic sign of severe or long-standing hypothyroidism is **myxedema,** which is histologically similar to the pretibial myxedema deposits that often occur with Graves disease. Myxedema is a result of an alteration in the composition of the dermis and other tissues. The connective fibers are separated by an increased amount of protein and mucopolysaccharides.

This protein-mucopolysaccharide complex binds water, producing nonpitting, boggy edema, especially around the eyes, hands, and feet and in the supraclavicular fossae (Figure 21-11). Myxedema is also responsible for thickening

Table 21-3 Systemic Manifestations of Hypothyroidism

System	Clinical Manifestations	Mechanisms Underlying Clinical Manifestations
Neurologic	Confusion, syncope, slowed speech and thinking, memory loss; lethargy, headaches, hearing loss, night blindness; slow, clumsy movements; cerebellar ataxia; slow alpha-wave activity and loss of amplitude in EEG; reduced cAMP response to epinephrine, glucagons, and PTH stimulation; decreased appetite	Decreased cerebral blood flow leading to cerebral hypoxia; reduced intracellular processes caused by decreased β-adrenergic activity that may be related to a decrease in the number of β-adrenergic receptor sites
Endocrine	Increased TSH production in primary hypothyroidism; enlarged pituitary thyrotropes, increase in serum prolactin levels with galactorrhea; decreased rate of cortisol turnover but with normal serum cortisol levels	Impaired TH synthesis or defects in iodide trapping leading to compensatory TSH production; chronic overstimulation of thyrotropes of TRH and by TSH synthesis; stimulation of lactotropes by TRH related to increased prolactin levels; decreased deactivation of cortisol
Reproductive	Decreased androgen secretion in men, increased estriol formation in women; low total hormone values but with increased amounts of unbound hormone; anovulation, decreased libido, and a high incidence of spontaneous abortion in women; erectile dysfunction, decreased libido, and oligospermia in men	Altered metabolism of estrogens and androgens; decreased levels of sex hormone–binding globulin
Hematologic	Decrease in red cell mass leading to normocytic, normochromic anemia; macrocytic anemia associated with vitamin B_{12} deficiency and inadequate folate or iron absorption in the gastrointestinal tract	Decreased basal metabolic rate and reduced oxygen requirements, decreased production of erythropoietin, possible relationship between TH and optimal hematologic response to vitamin B_{12}
Cardiovascular	Reduction in stroke volume and heart rate causing lowered cardiac output; increased peripheral vascular resistance to maintain systolic blood pressure; normal response to exercise but with alterations in circulatory system at rest (prolonged circulation time and decreased blood flow to tissues); cool skin and cold tolerance; enlarged heart; decreased intensity of heart sounds and variety of ECG changes (sinus bradycardia, prolonged PR interval, depressed P waves, flattened or inverted T waves, and low-amplitude QRS complexes); cardiac tamponade (although rare) (see Chapter 30)	Decreased metabolic demands and loss of regulatory and rate-setting effects of TH; protein-mucopolysaccharide-rich fluid in the pericardial sac associated with enlarged heart; pericardial effusions associated with heart sounds and ECG changes
Pulmonary	Dyspnea; myxedematous changes in respiratory muscles leading to hypoventilation and carbon dioxide retention, which contribute to myxedema coma	Pleural effusions associated with dyspnea, although effusions may be asymptomatic
Renal	Reduced renal blood flow and glomerular filtration rate leading to decreased renal excretion of water; increase in total body water and dilutional hyponatremia; reduced production of erythropoietin	Hemodynamic alterations associated with reduced blood flow and filtration; increased total body water related to decreased excretion and mucinous deposits in tissue
Gastrointestinal	Constipation, weight gain, and fluid retention; decreased absorption of most nutrients; decreased protein metabolism leading to retarded skeletal and soft-tissue growth and slightly positive nitrogen balance; edema; decreased glucose absorption and delayed glucose uptake; elevated serum lipid values	Reduced intake and reduced peristaltic activity that may progress to fecal impaction; water absorption related to prolonged transit time; fluid retention associated with myxedematous changes; edema associated with high concentrations of exchangeable albumin in the extravascular space caused by increased capillary permeability to proteins; depressed insulin degradation; depressed lipid synthesis and degradation
Musculoskeletal	Muscle aching and stiffness; slow movement and slow tendon jerk reflexes; decreased bone formation and resorption, increased bone density; aching and stiffness in joints	Decreased rate of muscle contraction and relaxation contributing to slow movement and reflexes
Integumentary	Dry, flaky skin; dry, brittle head and body hair; reduced growth of nails and hair, slow wound healing	Reduced sweat and sebaceous gland secretion
	Myxedema	Accumulation of hyaluronic acid, which binds water and causes a puffy appearance
	Cool skin	Decreased circulation to skin

cAMP, Cyclic adenosine monophosphate; ECG, electrocardiogram; EEG, electroencephalogram; PTH, parathyroid hormone; TH, thyroid hormone; TRH, thyrotropin-releasing hormone; TSH, thyroid-stimulating hormone.

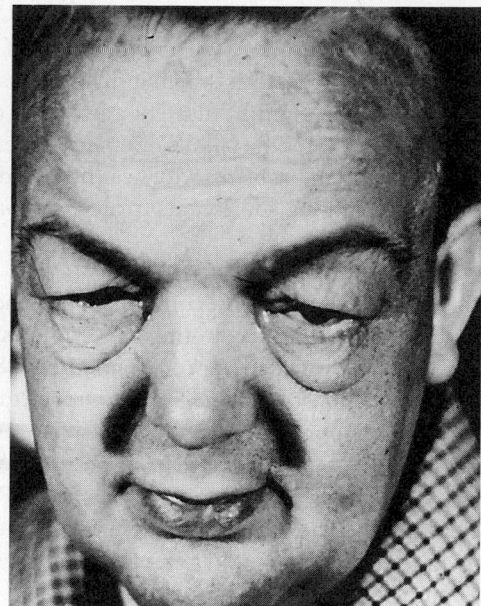

Figure 21-11 Myxedema. Note edema around eyes and facial puffiness. (From Thibodeau GA: *Anatomy & physiology*, St Louis, 1987, Mosby.)

of the tongue and the laryngeal and pharyngeal mucous membranes. This results in thick, slurred speech and hoarseness, both of which are common in hypothyroidism.

Myxedema coma, a medical emergency, is a diminished level of consciousness associated with severe hypothyroidism.[60,66] Signs and symptoms include hypothermia without shivering, hypoventilation, hypotension, hypoglycemia, and lactic acidosis. Older individuals with severe vascular disease and with moderate or untreated hypothyroidism are particularly at risk for developing myxedema coma. It also may occur after overuse of narcotics or sedatives or after an acute illness in hypothyroid individuals.

EVALUATION AND TREATMENT The diagnosis of primary hypothyroidism is made by documentation of the clinical symptoms of hypothyroidism, and measurement of increased levels of TSH and decreased TH (total T_3 and both total and free T_4). When hypothyroidism is caused by pituitary deficiencies, serum TSH levels are decreased or are inappropriately normal in the face of low levels of TH.[65] Hormone replacement therapy is the treatment of choice for hypothyroidism.[67] TH is available as a synthetic hormone (levothyroxine), which is preferred over the crude extract from animal thyroid glands (desiccated thyroid). Treatment of myxedema coma with TH combined with circulatory and ventilatory support is usually effective; however, mortality can be as high as 40% in severe cases.[66,68] **Subclinical hypothyroidism** is estimated to occur in 4% to 8% of U.S. adults and is defined as an elevation in TSH with normal levels of circulating TH.[64,69] Treatment of subclinical hypothyroidism remains controversial.[67,70]

The restoration of normal TH levels should be timed appropriately; a regimen of hormonal therapy depends on the individual's age, the duration and severity of the hypothyroidism, and the presence of other disorders, particularly cardiovascular disorders. The goal is maximal metabolic restoration consistent with the individual's overall well-being and normalization of TSH levels in individuals with primary hypothyroidism.[67]

Hypothyroid Conditions
Primary Hypothyroidism

There are several causes of **primary hypothyroidism**. Some are associated with spontaneous recovery and resultant euthyroidism, whereas others are linked to permanent hypothyroidism. **Iodine deficiency (endemic goiter)** is the most common cause of hypothyroidism worldwide, but is relatively rare in the United States. The most common cause of hypothyroidism in the United States is **autoimmune thyroiditis (Hashimoto disease, chronic lymphocytic thyroiditis)**, which results in gradual inflammatory destruction of thyroid tissue by infiltration of lymphocytes and circulating thyroid autoantibodies (antithyroid peroxidase and antithyroglobulin antibodies).[71] Variants in MHC antigens have been associated with autoimmune thyroiditis that are different from those found in Graves disease.[52,72] Hashimoto disease occurs in genetically predisposed individuals and is associated with high iodine intake, selenium deficiency, smoking, and chronic hepatitis C.[73] In addition to thyroid autoantibodies, autoreactive T lymphocytes, antibody activation of natural killer cells (antibody dependent cell mediated cytotoxicity), cytokines, and induction of apoptosis also are involved in the tissue destruction seen in Hashimoto thyroiditis.[71,74,75] Goiter formation is commonly observed.

Spontaneous recovery of thyroid function is seen in three conditions: subacute thyroiditis, painless thyroiditis, and postpartum thyroiditis. **Subacute thyroiditis** is a nonbacterial inflammation of the thyroid often preceded by a viral infection. It is accompanied by fever, tenderness, and enlargement of the thyroid.[76] The inflammatory process initially results in elevated levels of TH caused by release of stored thyroglobulin, then is associated with transient hypothyroidism before the gland recovers normal activity.[50] Symptoms may last for 2 to 4 months and nonsteroidal anti-inflammatory agents, beta-blockers, and, possibly, TH supplementation may be required during the course of the illness. **Painless thyroiditis** has a course similar to subacute thyroiditis but is pathologically identical to Hashimoto disease. **Iatrogenic hypothyroidism** results from radioiodine thyroid ablation, thyroidectomy, and medications (lithium and amiodarone). **Postpartum thyroiditis** generally occurs within 6 months of delivery, occurs in up to 7% of all women, and has a course similar to painless thyroiditis. Pathologic specimens suggest it is related to Hashimoto disease. Spontaneous recovery is seen in most women affected with this form of thyroiditis; however, persistent hypothyroidism does occur.[77]

Congenital Hypothyroidism

Congenital hypothyroidism, classified as a rare form of primary hypothyroidism, occurs in infants as a result of absent thyroid tissue (thyroid agenesis) and hereditary defects in

TH synthesis. Thyroid agenesis occurs more often in female infants, with permanent abnormalities in 1 of every 3000 to 4000 live births. There is evidence that the incidence of congenital hypothyroidism is increasing in the United States, although the cause of this increase is not known.[78]

TH is essential for embryonic growth, particularly of brain tissue. The infant will be mentally retarded if there is no T_4 during fetal life, but this can be significantly reversed with administration of T_4 immediately after birth.

Clinical manifestations of hypothyroidism may not be evident until after 4 months of age. Signs and symptoms include difficulty eating, hoarse cry, and protruding tongue caused by myxedema of oral tissues and vocal cords; hypotonic muscles of the abdomen with constipation, abdominal protrusion, and umbilical hernia; subnormal temperature; lethargy; excessive sleeping; slow pulse; and cold, mottled skin. Skeletal growth is stunted because of impaired protein synthesis, poor absorption of nutrients, and lack of bone mineralization. The individual will become dwarfed, with short limbs, if not treated (cretinism) (Figure 21-12). Dentition is often delayed. Mental retardation is a function of the severity of hypothyroidism and the delay before initiation of treatment.

Hypothyroidism is difficult to identify at birth, but high birth weight, hypothermia, delay in passing meconium, and neonatal jaundice are suggestive signs. Cord blood can

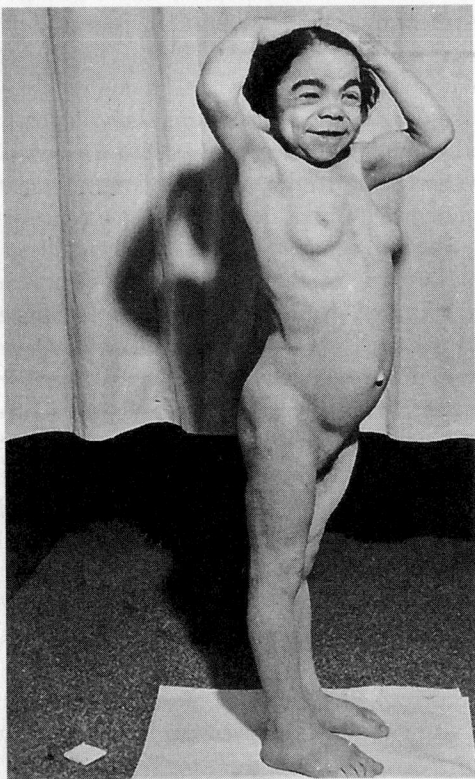

Figure 21-12 **Adult cretin.** Note characteristic facial features, dwarfism (44 inches), absent axillary and scant pubic hair, poorly developed breasts, potbelly, and small umbilical hernia. (From Schneeberg NG: *Essentials of clinical endocrinology,* St Louis, 1970, Mosby.)

be examined in the first days of life for T_4 and TSH levels.[79] Treatment is administration of T_4. The probability of normal growth and intellectual function is high if treatment is started before the child is 3 or 4 months old. The earlier TH replacement is initiated, the better the child's outcome. Recent studies suggest that persistent problems with health-related quality of life are common among adolescents treated for congenital hypothyroidism.[80,81]

Thyroid Carcinoma

Thyroid carcinoma is the most common endocrine malignancy but is relatively rare, accounting for 37,200 estimated new cases and 1630 estimated cancer deaths in 2008 in the United States.[82] The most consistent causal risk factor in the development of thyroid cancer appears to be exposure to ionizing radiation, especially exposure during childhood or puberty. Iodine deficiency also affects incidence.[83] Papillary and follicular thyroid carcinomas are the most frequent, and medullary and anaplastic thyroid carcinomas are less common. Most tumors are well differentiated.

Most individuals with thyroid carcinoma have normal T_3 and T_4 levels and are therefore euthyroid. Thyroid cancer typically is discovered as a small thyroid nodule or as a metastatic tumor most commonly occurring in the regional lymph nodes, lungs, brain, or bone. Changes in voice and swallowing and difficulty in breathing are related to tumor growth impinging on the trachea or esophagus. The diagnosis of thyroid carcinoma is generally made by fine-needle aspiration of a thyroid nodule.[83] Ultrasonography and radioisotope scanning may be helpful in assessing the malignant potential of a thyroid nodule; however, ultrasound-guided aspiration biopsy of small (less than 1 cm) thyroid nodules is very helpful in providing an earlier diagnosis and earlier institution of therapy.

Treatment for well-differentiated thyroid carcinoma remains somewhat controversial mainly because of its protracted nature and the relatively low mortality regardless of the method of treatment. Treatment of well-differentiated tumors includes a near-total or total thyroidectomy, postoperative radioactive iodine, and suppression of TSH with levothyroxine. Anaplastic thyroid carcinoma carries a grave prognosis, and palliation with surgical debulking, external beam radiotherapy, or chemotherapy may be offered.[83,84]

ALTERATIONS OF PARATHYROID FUNCTION

Hyperparathyroidism

Hyperparathyroidism is characterized by a greater than normal secretion of parathyroid hormone (PTH). The causes of hyperparathyroidism are classified as either primary or secondary, and their associated pathophysiologic mechanisms are somewhat different.

PATHOPHYSIOLOGY Primary **hyperparathyroidism** is characterized by inappropriate excess secretion of PTH by one or more of the parathyroid glands.[85-87] It is one of the most common endocrine disorders: 80% to 85% of cases are caused by parathyroid adenomas, another 10% to 15% result from parathyroid hyperplasia, and approximately 1% are caused by parathyroid carcinoma.[85] In primary hyperparathyroidism, normal feedback mechanisms, such as elevated serum levels of ionized calcium, fail to normally inhibit PTH secretion by the parathyroid gland.

The cause of primary hyperparathyroidism is unknown; however, recent data suggest that there are two mechanisms for the development of this condition. The first is a clonal proliferation of parathyroid cells with a higher threshold for calcium feedback, and the second is generalized growth of parathyroid tissue. The former is most likely the cause of adenomas, and the latter is probably the cause for hyperplasia. There is also a familial form of the disease that includes a wide range of inherited endocrine disorders such as multiple endocrine neoplasia type 1 (MEN-1).[85] Hypercalcemia and hypophosphatemia are the hallmarks of primary hyperparathyroidism. The effects of excessive PTH secretion and primary hyperparathyroidism on various organ systems are summarized in Table 21-4.

Secondary hyperparathyroidism is caused by an increase in PTH secondary to a chronic disease state, such as chronic renal failure or intestinal malabsorption, which causes a decrease in serum ionized calcium levels (hypocalcemia). Hypercalcemia does not occur in secondary hyperparathyroidism because the parathyroid tissue is not autonomous and is only responding to a physiologic stimulus (hypocalcemia).

The most common cause of secondary hyperparathyroidism is chronic renal failure (with failure of glomerular filtration), which results in hyperphosphatemia, reduced levels of activated vitamin D, and hypocalcemia, which stimulates PTH secretion. Disturbances in calcium and vitamin D metabolism that arise in chronic renal disease diminish activation of the parathyroid calcium-sensing receptor leading to increases in PTH secretion.[88] Because vitamin D metabolism is impaired in renal failure, eucalcemia cannot be restored unless vitamin D supplements are administered.

Other causes of secondary hyperparathyroidism include dietary deficiency in vitamin D or calcium; decreased intestinal absorption of vitamin D or calcium; and ingestion of drugs, such as phenytoin, phenobarbital, and laxatives, which either accelerates the metabolism of vitamin D or decreases intestinal absorption of calcium.

Two other conditions must be differentiated from primary and secondary hyperparathyroidism. **Pseudohypoparathyroidism** is an inherited condition that presents with increased PTH levels and hypocalcemia. These individuals are resistant to PTH and cannot produce cAMP in response to PTH. **Familial hypocalciuric hypercalcemia (FHH)** is a condition that can mimic hyperparathyroidism and is characterized by a high serum calcium, low serum phosphate, and low urine calcium excretion. It is caused by a mutation in the calcium-sensing receptor in the parathyroid gland. It can be differentiated from primary hyperparathyroidism by measurement of 24-hour urine calcium excretion.

CLINICAL MANIFESTATIONS Hypersecretion of PTH in primary and secondary hyperparathyroidism causes excessive osteoclastic activity, resulting in bone resorption. (Bone resorption is discussed in Chapter 41.) Pathologic bone changes include pathologic fractures, kyphosis (curvature) of

Table 21-4	Manifestations of Primary Hyperparathyroidism	
Symptoms	**Responsible Derangements**	**Mechanisms**
Renal colic, nephrolithiasis, recurrent urinary tract infections, renal failure	Hypercalciuria, hyperphosphaturia, proximal renal tubular bicarbonate leak, urine pH >6	Calcium phosphate salts precipitate in alkaline urine, renal pelvis, and collecting ducts; calcium oxalate stones also formed
Abdominal pain, peptic ulcer disease	Hypercalcemia-stimulated hypergastrinemia	Elevated hydrochloric acid secretion
Pancreatitis	Hypercalcemia	Etiology of relationship unknown
Bone disease, osteitis fibrosa and osteitis cystica, osteoporosis	PTH-stimulated bone resorption, metabolic acidosis	Osteoporosis now more commonly encountered, but other disorders are more specific for hyperparathyroidism
Muscle weakness, myalgia	PTH excess, possible direct effect on striated muscle and on nerves	Characteristic myopathic changes in muscle histology (neuropathy of type I and type II muscle fibers)
Neurologic and psychiatric problems (impaired memory, confusion, stupor, coma)	Hypercalcemia	Neuropathy; electroencephalographic changes present
Polyuria, polydipsia	Hypercalcemia	Direct effect on renal tubule to decrease responsiveness to antidiuretic hormone
Constipation	Hypercalcemia	Decreased peristalsis of gastrointestinal tract
Anorexia, nausea, and vomiting	Hypercalcemia	Central stimulation of vomiting center
Hypertension	Renal disease, direct effect of calcium on arterial smooth muscle, pheochromocytoma	Plasma rennin activity elevated or normal
Arthralgia and arthritis	Gout, pseudogout, periarticular classification	Hyperuricemia, chronic renal failure with high calcium × phosphate product

From Harden RH et al, editors: *William's textbook of endocrinology*, ed 10, Philadelphia, 2002, Saunders.

the dorsal spine, and compression fractures of the vertebral bodies.

In primary hyperparathyroidism, hypercalcemia affects proximal renal tubular function, causing hypercalciuria, metabolic acidosis, and production of an abnormally alkaline urine.[87] PTH also enhances the renal excretion of phosphate, which results in hypophosphatemia (low serum phosphate) and hyperphosphaturia (increased urine phosphate). The combination of these three variables—hypercalciuria, alkaline urine, and hyperphosphaturia—predisposes the individual to the formation of calcium stones.[87] Kidney stones are often formed in the renal pelvis or in the renal collecting ducts and may be associated with infections. Kidney stones and renal infection may lead to impaired renal function. Hypercalcemia also impairs the concentrating ability of the renal tubule by decreasing its response to ADH. Chronic hypercalcemia of hyperparathyroidism is associated with mild insulin resistance, necessitating increased insulin secretion to maintain normal glucose levels. Hypercalcemia also affects the muscular, nervous, and gastrointestinal systems.[87] (The clinical symptoms of primary hyperparathyroidism are summarized in Table 21-4.)

Secondary hyperparathyroidism caused by renal disease presents clinically not only with bone resorption but also the symptoms of hypocalcemia and hyperphosphatemia. Hypocalcemia can cause many significant clinical problems (see Chapter 3). Hyperphosphatemia can cause deleterious effects on the cardiovascular system.[89]

EVALUATION AND TREATMENT The diagnosis of hyperparathyroidism is relatively straightforward. The concurrent findings of increased ionized calcium in the face of elevated or inappropriately normal intact PTH (which documents an abnormal feedback mechanism) are suggestive of primary hyperparathyroidism. Sestamibi (a radioisotope) scanning, CT, or ultrasound is used to localize adenomas prior to surgery.[85,86] The definitive treatment of primary hyperparathyroidism is surgery. Surgery is generally reserved for individuals with documented complications of hyperparathyroidism (osteoporosis, nephrolithiasis, or gastrointestinal or neuropsychiatric complications), severely elevated serum calcium levels (more than 1 mg/dl above the upper limit or normal for the laboratory), marked hypercalciuria (more than 400 mg/24 hr), or individuals younger than 50 years of age. In those individuals who fail surgery, other treatments such as bisphosphonates, corticosteroids, and a new class of calcium-lowering drugs, called calcimimetics (e.g., cinacalcet), may be considered.[86,90]

If hypercalcemia is documented but PTH levels are low, the differential diagnosis shifts to hypercalcemia of malignancy, granulomatous diseases (sarcoidosis), excessive calcium ingestion, or to hypervitaminosis A or D. Treatment of these conditions depends on the underlying cause.

If serum calcium is low but PTH is elevated, secondary hyperparathyroidism is likely. Evaluation for renal function frequently documents chronic renal disease. Treatment for secondary hyperparathyroidism in chronic renal disease requires calcium replacement, dietary phosphate restriction and phosphate binders, and vitamin D replacement.[91] Treatment also

may include calcimimetics that work to increase the parathyroid calcium receptor sensitivity, thus lowering PTH levels.[92,93]

Hypoparathyroidism

Hypoparathyroidism (abnormally low PTH levels) most commonly is caused by damage to the parathyroid glands during thyroid surgery.[94] Postoperative hypoparathyroidism occurs in approximately 0.5% to 6.6% of all individuals undergoing thyroid surgery.[95] This is caused by the anatomic proximity of the parathyroid gland to the thyroid gland. Hypoparathyroidism also is associated with genetic syndromes, including familial hypoparathyroidism and DiGeorge syndrome (velocaridofacial syndrome).[94,96] Hypomagnesemia also can cause a decrease in PTH secretion and function.[94] An idiopathic or autoimmune form of hypoparathyroidism also is recognized.

PATHOPHYSIOLOGY In hypoparathyroidism a lack of circulating PTH causes a depressed serum calcium level and an increased serum phosphate level. In the absence of PTH the abilities to resorb calcium from bone and to regulate calcium reabsorption from the renal tubules are impaired. The phosphaturic effects of PTH are lost, resulting in hyperphosphatemia.

The effects of hypomagnesemia on the peripheral metabolism and clearance of PTH are not clearly understood. Once serum magnesium levels return to normal, however, PTH secretion returns to normal, as does peripheral tissues' responsiveness to PTH. Hypomagnesemia may be related to chronic alcoholism, malnutrition, malabsorption, increased renal clearance of magnesium caused by the use of aminoglycoside antibiotics or certain chemotherapeutic agents, or prolonged magnesium-deficient parenteral nutritional therapy.

CLINICAL MANIFESTATIONS Symptoms associated with hypoparathyroidism are related to hypocalcemia. Hypocalcemia causes a lowering of the threshold for nerve and muscle excitation so that a nerve impulse may be initiated by a slight stimulus anywhere along the length of a nerve or muscle fiber. This is manifested as muscle spasms, hyperreflexia, tonic-clonic convulsions, laryngeal spasms, and in severe cases, death from asphyxiation. Chvostek and Trousseau signs may be used to evaluate for neuromuscular irritability. Chvostek sign is elicited by tapping the cheek resulting in twitching of the upper lip. Trousseau sign is elicited by sustained inflation of a sphygmomanometer placed on the upper arm to a level above the systolic blood pressure with resultant painful carpal spasm.[94]

Other symptoms of hypocalcemia are caused by mechanisms that are not yet understood. These symptoms include dry skin, loss of body and scalp hair, hypoplasia of developing teeth, horizontal ridges on the nails, cataracts, basal ganglia calcifications (which may be associated with a parkinsonian syndrome), and bone deformities, including brachydactyly and bowing of the long bones.

Phosphate retention caused by increased renal reabsorption of phosphate is associated also with hypoparathyroidism. Hyperphosphatemia is associated with inhibition of the renal enzyme necessary for the conversion of vitamin D to its most active form. This enzyme, 25-OH vitamin D 1α hydroxylase also is required by PTH. This tends to depress serum calcium levels further by reducing gastrointestinal absorption of calcium.

EVALUATION AND TREATMENT A low serum calcium level and high phosphorus level in the absence of renal failure, intestinal disorders, or nutritional deficiencies suggest hypoparathyroidism. Intact PTH levels are low in hypoparathyroidism, and measurement of serum magnesium and urinary calcium excretion can help in diagnosis.[94] There is an inherited condition associated with hypocalcemia but with normal levels of PTH, called pseudohypoparathyroidism (see p. 743).

The treatment of hypoparathyroidism is directed toward the alleviation of hypocalcemia. In acute states this involves parenteral administration of calcium, which allows correction of serum calcium within minutes. Maintenance of serum calcium is achieved with pharmacologic doses of an active form of vitamin D and oral calcium. Injectable human PTH (teriparatide) has been explored in several recent studies, and results are encouraging.[94,97] As serum calcium levels return to normal, phosphaturia usually is stimulated. This leads to a return to normal serum phosphate levels. In some individuals, however, the absence of the phosphaturic effect of PTH causes a persistent hyperphosphatemia. Significant elevations of phosphorus should be treated with drugs that inhibit gastrointestinal absorption of phosphate (phosphate binders).[94]

DYSFUNCTION OF THE ENDOCRINE PANCREAS: DIABETES MELLITUS

Diabetes mellitus is not a single disease but a group of clinically heterogeneous disorders that have glucose intolerance in common. It encompasses many causally unrelated diseases and includes many different etiologies of disturbed glucose tolerance. The term *diabetes mellitus* is used to describe a syndrome characterized by chronic hyperglycemia and other disturbances of carbohydrate, fat, and protein metabolism. The American Diabetes Association classifies four categories of diabetes mellitus (Table 21-5):

1. Type 1 (absolute insulin deficiency)
2. Type 2 (insulin resistance with an insulin secretory deficit)
3. Other specific types
4. Gestational diabetes

Types 1 and 2 diabetes are the most common and are discussed in greatest detail in this text.

The criteria for the diagnosis of diabetes include symptoms, elevated fasting plasma glucose (FPG) concentration, and/or abnormal oral glucose tolerance test (OGTT)[98] (Box 21-1). Two conditions associated with a high risk for diabetes, impaired fasting glucose (IFG) and impaired glucose tolerance (IGT), are considered **prediabetes**.[98]

A normal fasting glucose is less than 100 mg/dl. IFG is defined as a fasting glucose greater than or equal to 100 mg/dl but less than 126 mg/dl. Glucose tolerance is normal if the 2-hour postload glucose level is less than 140 mg/dl. IGT is defined as a 2-hour postload glucose level greater than or equal to 140 but less than 200 mg/dl. IGT results from reduced suppression of hepatic glucose output and reduced pancreatic islet cell function.

Any abnormality of glucose tolerance has potentially serious consequences. Numerous epidemiologic studies have shown an increased risk of cardiovascular disease and premature death in individuals with glucose intolerance. In addition, individuals with abnormal glucose tolerance have a 3% to 7% yearly risk of developing overt diabetes. In comparison, a healthy individual's *lifetime* risk of acquiring diabetes is around 7% to 10%.

Types of Diabetes Mellitus

Type 1 Diabetes Mellitus

Diabetes mellitus is the most common pediatric chronic disease and affects 0.17% of U.S. children.[99] The common form of **type 1 diabetes mellitus** is the result of an autoimmune-mediated specific loss of beta cells in the pancreatic islets. The incidence of the condition is increasing in some areas, with other areas showing no change in incidence.[99] Table 21-6 summarizes the epidemiology of diabetes mellitus.

Type 1 diabetes mellitus is thought to be the result of a genetic-environmental interaction. Between 10% and 13% of individuals with newly diagnosed type 1 diabetes have a first-degree relative (parent or sibling) with type 1 diabetes. Diagnosis has a seasonal distribution, with more cases reported during autumn and winter in the northern hemisphere. Diagnosis is rare during the first 9 months of life and peaks at 12 years of age.

PATHOPHYSIOLOGY Two distinct types of type 1 diabetes have been identified: autoimmune and nonimmune. In autoimmune-mediated diabetes mellitus, environmental-genetic factors are thought to trigger cell-mediated destruction of pancreatic beta cells. Autoimmune type 1 diabetes is called *type 1A*. Nonimmune type 1 diabetes is far less common than immune. It occurs secondary to other diseases, such as pancreatitis, or to a more fulminant disorder termed *idiopathic (type 1B) diabetes*. Type 1B diabetes occurs mostly in people of Asian or African descent and affected individuals have varying degrees of insulin deficiency.[100]

Genetic Susceptibility

The exact nature of genetic susceptibility to type 1A diabetes is not clearly understood. The strongest association is with MHC (histocompatibility leukocyte antigen [HLA]) class II alleles HLA-DQ and HLA-DR).[100-102] The HLA-DR marker is associated with other autoimmune disorders, such as Graves, Hashimoto, and Addison diseases.[101] The risk of developing type 1 diabetes increases 5 to 8 times when one of those specific markers is present. When the individual is heterogeneous for HLA-DR3 and HLA-DR4, the risk is 20 to 40 times higher than that of the general population. Specific human antigens also are thought to decrease the risk of developing type 1 diabetes. For example, HLA-DR2 is associated with an

Table 21-5   Classification and Characteristics of Diabetes Mellitus

Name	Characteristics
Type 1 (beta cell destruction leading to absolute insulin deficiency)	Cellular-mediated autoimmune destruction of pancreatic B cells
	Individual prone to ketoacidosis
Immune-mediated diabetes is most common form (≈90%)	Little or no insulin secretion
	Insulin dependent
	75% of individuals develop before 30 years of age; can occur up to the tenth decade
	Usually not obese
Idiopathic (≈10%)	No defined etiologies; absolute requirement for insulin replacement therapy in affected individuals may come and go
Type 2 (may range from predominantly insulin resistant with relative insulin deficiency to a predominantly secretory defect with insulin resistance)	Usually not insulin dependent but may be insulin requiring
	Individual not ketosis prone (but may form ketones under stress)
	Obesity common in the abdominal region
	Generally occurs in those older than 40 years, but the frequency is rapidly increasing in children
	Strong genetic predisposition
	Often associated with hypertension and dyslipidemia
Other Specific Types	
Genetic defects of beta cell function	Genetic abnormalities that decrease the ability of the beta-cell to secrete insulin:
	1. Maturity-onset diabetes of youth (MODY) includes 6 specific autosomal dominant mutations including genes for hepatocyte nuclear factor-1α (HNF-1α; MODY 3), glucokinase (MODY 2), HNF-4α (MODY 1), insulin-promoter factor-1(IPF-1; MODY 4), HNF-1β (MODY 5) and NeuroD1 (MODY 6)
	2. Defects in mitochondrial deoxyribonucleic acid (DNA)
	3. Other (including an inability to convert proinsulin to insulin)
Genetic defects in insulin action	Mutations in the insulin receptor with hyperinsulinism or hyperglycemia or severe diabetes
Diseases of the exocrine pancreas	Any process that diffusely injures the pancreas including pancreatitis, neoplasia, and cystic fibrosis)
Endocrinopathies	Endocrine disorders including acromegaly, Cushing syndrome, glucagonoma, pheochromocytoma, hyperthyroidism, somatostatinoma, and aldosteronoma
Drug- or chemical-induced B cell dysfunction	Commonly associated drugs include glucocorticoids and thiazide diuretics, although many others may be implicated
Infections	B cell destruction by viruses including cytomegalovirus, congenital rubella
Uncommon forms of immune-mediated diabetes mellitus	Anti-insulin receptor antibodies
	Reported with "stiff man syndrome" and individuals receiving interferon-α
Other genetic syndromes sometimes associated with diabetes mellitus	Down, Klinefelter, Turner and Wolfram syndromes
Gestational Diabetes Mellitus (GDM)	
Any degree of glucose intolerance with onset or first recognition during pregnancy.	Insulin resistance combined with inadequate insulin secretion in relation to hyperglycemia
	Women who are obese, older than 25 years of age, have a family history of diabetes, have a history of previous GDM, or are of certain ethnic groups (Hispanic, Native Americans, Asian, or African-American) are at increased risk of developing GDM
	The metabolic stress of pregnancy may uncover a genetic tendency for type 2 diabetes mellitus

Data from American Diabetes Association (Committee Report): *Diabetic Care* 26(Suppl. 1):S5-S20, 2003; Agency for Healthcare Quality and Research, U.S. Preventive Services Task Force (USPSTF): *Screening for Gestational Diabetes Mellitus Recommendation Statement* May 2008. Available at http://www.ahqr.gov/clinic/uspstf08/gestdiab/gdrs.htm

unusually low risk. Current theories of causation hold that islet cell destruction occurs predominantly in genetically susceptible people.

Environmental Factors

Environmental factors are thought to have a significant contribution to the development of type 1 diabetes mellitus. Some types of viral infections have been implicated with autoimmune damage to beta cells, including congenital rubella, cytomegaloviruses, mumps, and Epstein-Barr virus.[102,103] Bovine serum albumin, a major constituent of cow's milk, may be involved in triggering beta cell autoantibodies.[102] Stress may advance development of type 1 diabetes mellitus by stimulating secretion of counterregulatory hormones and affecting immune responses (see Chapter 10). Specific environmental

factors linked to type 1 diabetes mellitus are presented in Box 21-2.

Immunologically Mediated Destruction of Beta Cells

Type 1 diabetes mellitus is a slowly progressive autoimmune T cell–mediated disease that occurs in genetically susceptible individuals (Figure 21-13 and see Chapter 8). Environmental mechanisms are thought to play a role in triggering an autoimmune response to beta cells. The destruction of beta cells progresses through the following stages:

1. *Lymphocyte and macrophage infiltration of the islets resulting in inflammation (insulinitis) and islet beta cell death.* Autoantigens are expressed on the surface of pancreatic islet cells and circulate in the bloodstream

Box 21-1   Criteria for the Diagnosis of Diabetes Mellitus

1. Symptoms of diabetes plus casual plasma glucose (CPG) concentration ≥200 mg/dl (11.1 mmol/L). Casual is defined as any time of day without regard to time since last meal. The classic symptoms of diabetes include polyuria, polydipsia, and unexplained weight loss.
2. FPG ≥126 mg/dl (7 mmol/L). Fasting is defined as no caloric intake for at least 8 hours.
3. Two-hour postload glucose ≥200 mg/dl (11.1 mmol/L) during an oral glucose tolerance test (OGTT).

In the absence of unequivocal hyperglycemia, these criteria should be confirmed by repeat testing on a different day. The third measure (OGTT) is not recommended for routine clinical use.

Data from American Diabetes Association: *Diabetes Care* 30(Suppl 1): S42-S47, 2007.

and lymphatics (see Figure 21-13). Circulating autoantigens are ingested by antigen-presenting cells that activate CD4+ T helper lymphocytes.[100,104] The activated T helper lymphocytes secrete interleukin 2 (IL-2) that activates beta cell autoantigen-specific T cytotoxic lymphocytes, causing them to proliferate and attack many more islet cells through secretion of toxic perforins and granzymes.[104,105] The T helper lymphocytes also secrete interferon that activates macrophages and stimulates the release of inflammatory cytokines (including IL-1 and tumor necrosis factor [TNF]), which cause further B-cell destruction and apoptosis.[100,104,106]

2. *Production of autoantibodies against islet cells, insulin, glutamic acid decarboxylase (GAD), and other cytoplasmic proteins.* T helper lymphocytes also produce IL-4, which stimulates B lymphocytes to proliferate and

Table 21-6   Epidemiology and Etiology of Diabetes Mellitus in the United States

	Type 1 Diabetes: Primary B Cell Defect or Failure	Type 2 Diabetes: Insulin Resistance with Inadequate Insulin Secretion
Incidence		
Frequency	One of the most common childhood diseases (5%-10% of all cases of diabetes mellitus) Prevalence rate is 0.17%	Accounts for most cases (≈90%-95%) Prevalence rate for ages 45 to 64 yr is 10.5%, for ages 65-74 yr is 18.4%
Change in incidences	No documented increase in incidence in the United States	Incidence in all age groups has doubled since 1980
Characteristics		
Age at onset	Peak onset at age 11 to 13 yr (slightly earlier for girls than for boys) Rare in children younger than 1 yr and adults older than 30 yr	Risk of developing diabetes increases after age 40 yr; in general, incidence increases with age into the 70s; among Pima Indians, incidence peaks between ages 40 and 50 yr, then falls
Gender	Similar in males and females	Similar in males and females overall, although black females have the highest incidence and prevalence of all groups
Racial distribution	Rates for whites 1.5-2 times higher than for nonwhites Higher rates for those of Scandinavian descent than for those of central or southern European descent	Risk is highest for blacks and Native Americans
Obesity	Generally normal or underweight	Frequent contributing factor to precipitate type 2 diabetes among those susceptible; a major factor in populations recently exposed to westernized environment Increased risk related to duration, degree, and distribution of obesity
Etiology		
Common theory	*Autoimmune:* genetic and environmental factors, resulting in gradual process of autoimmune destruction in genetically susceptible individuals *Nonautoimmune:* Unknown Strong association with *HLA-DQA* and *HLA-DQB* genes	Disease results from genetic susceptibility (polygenic) combined with environmental determinants and other risk factors; inherited defects in beta cell mass and function combined with peripheral tissue insulin resistance Associated with long-duration obesity
Heredity	Risk to sibling: 5%-10%; risk to offspring: 2%-5%	Risk to first-degree relative (child or sibling): 10%-15%
Presence of antibody	Islet cell autoantibodies (ICA) and/or autoantibodies to insulin, and autoantibodies to glutamic acid decarboxylase (GAD$_{65}$) and tyrosine phosphatases IA-2 and IA-2β are present in 85%-90% of individuals when fasting; hyperglycemia is initially detected	Islet cell antibodies not present
Insulin resistance	Insulin resistance at diagnosis is unusual, but insulin resistance may occur as the individual ages and gains weight	Insulin resistance is generally caused by altered cellular metabolism and an intracellular postreceptor defect
Insulin secretion	Severe insulin deficiency or no insulin secretion at all	Typically increased at time of diagnosis, but progressively declines over the course of the illness

Data from American Diabetes Association: *Diabetic Care* 30(Suppl 1):S42-S47, 2007.

produce antibodies (see Figure 21-13). Islet cell autoantibodies (ICAs) precede evidence of beta cell deficiency and can be found in the serum years before symptoms occur.[100,102,106,107] Antiglutamic acid decarboxylase (antiGAD$_{65}$) antibodies (an enzyme in beta cells that is involved in glucagon synthesis) are more persistent which makes them clinically useful in differentiating the etiology of diabetes in a given individual.[100] Autoantibodies against insulin (insulin autoantibodies [IAAs]) also have been noted. It is likely that IAAs may form during the process of active islet cell and beta cell destruction.

Another mechanism being explored in the pathogenesis of type 1 diabetes is a relative inactivity of T regulatory cells. These T lymphocytes normally serve to inhibit the immune response. Mutations affecting T regulatory cells have been found in a rare form of diabetes called *neonatal diabetes*, leading investigators to hypothesize about a role for T regulatory cell dysfunction in type 1A diabetes.[101,108]

Over time these immune mechanisms lead to a decrease in beta cell mass and insulin production. C-peptide, a component of proinsulin cleaved during insulin synthesis, declines. C-peptide may play a protective role in preventing beta cell destruction; therefore, decreasing amounts of this important peptide may accelerate the decline in beta cells.[109] C-peptide deficiency also has been implicated in the glomerular and neuronal complications of diabetes.[110-113] There may be further effects on beta cell decline as the individual ages. For example, the "accelerator hypothesis" suggests that increased body weight and associated proinflammatory state are contributors to worsening hyperglycemia in type 1 and type 2 diabetes.[114]

Hyperglycemia, Glucagon, and Hyperketonemia

Before hyperglycemia occurs, 80% to 90% of the function of the insulin-secreting beta cells in the islet of Langerhans must be lost. Beta cell abnormalities are present long before the acute clinical onset of type 1 diabetes.

A disequilibrium of hormones produced by the islets of Langerhans occurs in diabetes mellitus. Normally the paracrine action of insulin suppresses secretion of glucagon. Alpha and beta cell functions are abnormal, and a lack of insulin and a relative excess of glucagon (produced by alpha cells) exist in type 1 diabetes. The ratio of insulin to glucagon in the portal vein controls hepatic glucose and fat metabolism. Considerable data have documented that high levels of glucagon relative to insulin levels contribute to the generation of hyperglycemia and hyperketonemia. Relative hyperglucagonemia occurs in every form of diabetes mellitus. Thus the full metabolic syndrome seen in diabetes is caused by both hormones,

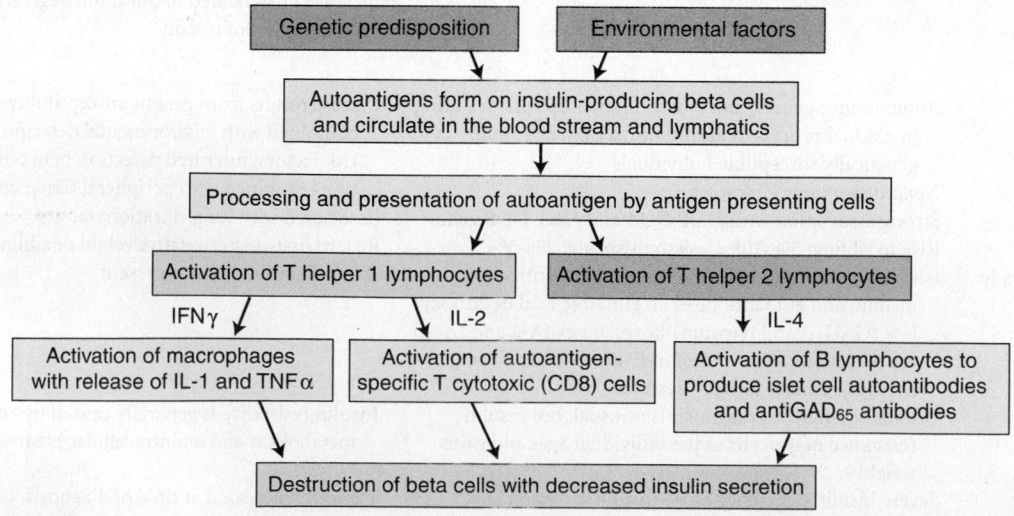

Figure 21-13 Pathophysiology of type 1 diabetes mellitus. *GAD$_{65}$*, glutamic acid decarboxylase; *INF-γ* Interferon-gamma; *IL*, interleukin; *TNF-α*, tumor necrosis factor-alpha.

a finding that ultimately may provide an entirely new therapeutic approach to its management.

Insulin normally stimulates lipogenesis and inhibits lipolysis, thus preventing fat catabolism. With insulin deficiency, lypolysis is enhanced and there is an increase in the amount of nonesterified fatty acids delivered to the liver. The consequence is increased glyconeogenesis contributing to hyperglycemia and production of ketone bodies (acetoacetate, hydroxybutyrate, and acetone) by the mitochondria of the liver at a rate that exceeds peripheral use. Accumulation of ketone bodies causes a drop in pH and triggers the buffering system associated with metabolic acidosis. Diabetic ketoacidosis (DKA), caused by increased levels of circulating ketones in the absence of the antilipolytic effect of insulin, may occur (p. 755).

CLINICAL MANIFESTATIONS Historically, type 1 diabetes mellitus has been thought to have an abrupt onset. More recently, however, prospective studies show a distinctive natural history involving a long preclinical period with gradual destruction of beta cells, eventually leading to insulin deficiency and hyperglycemia. Generally, this latent period is longer in older individuals and often results in misclassification of an older type 1 individual as having type 2 diabetes.

Type 1 diabetes mellitus affects the metabolism of fat, protein, and carbohydrates. Glucose accumulates in the blood and appears in the urine as the renal threshold for glucose is exceeded, producing an osmotic diuresis and symptoms of polyuria and thirst. Wide fluctuations in blood glucose levels occur. In addition, protein and fat breakdown occur because of the lack of insulin, resulting in weight loss (Table 21-7).

EVALUATION AND TREATMENT The diagnosis of diabetes is not difficult when the symptoms of polydipsia, polyuria, polyphagia, weight loss, and hyperglycemia are present in fasting and postprandial states. Nearly half of children ages 4 years and younger and nearly one quarter of those between the ages of 5 and 15 with type 1 diabetes are first diagnosed when they present with the signs and symptoms of DKA.[100] Acidosis causes a compensatory increase in the respiratory rate and depth known as Kussmaul respirations. Acetone (a ketone body) is blown off, giving the breath a sweet or fruity odor.

If the diagnosis is equivocal, based on FPG, then an OGTT may be needed. In nonpregnant women, an OGTT consists of the administration of a 75-g oral glucose load after a 10-hour fast followed by measurement of plasma glucose 2 hours later. Another mechanism that can be used to identify the plasma glucose concentration over time is the measurement of **glycosylated hemoglobin** or, more precisely, **hemoglobin A_{1c}** (HgbA$_{1c}$). In the normal 120-day life span of a red blood cell, glucose molecules join hemoglobin, forming glycosylated hemoglobin. In individuals with persistent hyperglycemia, increases in the quantities of three glycosylated hemoglobins (A_{1a}, A_{1b}, and A_{1c}) are noted. A buildup of glycosylated hemoglobin within the red cell reflects the average level of glucose to which the cell has been exposed during its life cycle (approximately 120 days). HgbA$_{1c}$ can be used for screening chronic hyperglycemia and to assess the effectiveness of therapy by monitoring long-term serum glucose regulation.

C-peptide, a component of proinsulin released during insulin production, can be measured in the serum as a surrogate for insulin levels and is indicative of residual beta cell mass and function. Other important aspects of evaluation include looking for evidence of the acute and chronic complications of type 1 diabetes, including DKA and renal, nervous system, cardiac, peripheral vascular, retinal, and bony tissue damage (see pp. 754 and 758).

Many different kinds of therapies are being tested to prevent the autoimmune destruction of beta cells that is characteristic of type 1 diabetes. These include immunosuppression with antirejection drugs (e.g., mycophenolate mofetil, rituximab, monoclonal antibodies to CD3, and cyclosporine), immunomodulation therapies (e.g., nicotinamide, bacille Calmette-Guérin, vitamin D, and DiaPep277), and oral or intranasal insulin.[101,107,115] Some of these studies are ongoing; however, the results so far have shown some potential for slowing disease progression but not in preventing diabetes. Many new clinical trials are planned.

Treatment regimens are designed to achieve optimal glucose control (as measured by the HgbA$_{1c}$) without causing episodes of significant hypoglycemia. The Diabetes Control and Complications Trial (DCCT) compared individuals whose blood sugars were tightly controlled (with blood glucose checks four times per day, three or more insulin injections daily or insulin pump, and meal planning) with

Table 21-7	Clinical Manifestations and Rationale for Type 1 Diabetes Mellitus
Manifestations	**Rationale**
Polydipsia	Because of elevated blood sugar levels, water is osmotically attracted from body cells, resulting in intracellular dehydration and hypothalamic stimulation of thirst
Polyuria	Hyperglycemia acts as an osmotic diuretic; the amount of glucose filtered by the glomeruli of the kidneys exceeds that which can be reabsorbed by the renal tubules; glycosuria results, accompanied by large amounts of water lost in the urine
Polyphagia	Depletion of cellular stores of carbohydrates, fats, and protein results in cellular starvation and a corresponding increase in hunger
Weight loss	Weight loss occurs because of fluid loss in osmotic diuresis and the loss of body tissue as fat and proteins are used for energy as a result of the effects of insulin deficiency
Fatigue	Metabolic changes result in poor use of food products, contributing to lethargy and fatigue; sleep loss from severe nocturia also contributes to fatigue

those who received standard treatment. Intensively treated individuals who achieve near-normal glucoses (HgbA₁c less than 7%) can expect a 50% to 75% reduction in the risk of developing or progression of retinopathy, neuropathy, and nephropathy after 8 to 9 years.[116] Although long-term complications were decreased in the tightly controlled group, achieving near-normal glucose levels was accompanied by risks, such as severe hypoglycemia and weight gain. However, the benefits of tight glucose control in the intensively treated group continued to be evident for more than 20 years.[100,117,118] Successful management requires individual planning according to type of disease, age, and activity level. All individuals with type 1 diabetes require some combination of insulin, meal planning, exercise, and self-monitoring of blood glucose.[100,118,119] Several different types of insulin preparations are available, as well as new technologies for more physiologic insulin delivery systems.[120] Blood glucose monitoring also is an essential part of management for which there are numerous types of monitoring devices. Finally, islet cell and whole pancreas transplantation has been successful in selected individuals (see What's New? Islet Transplant and Type 1 Diabetes Mellitus). Individuals should be screened at least yearly for complications of diabetes.

Type 2 Diabetes Mellitus

In the United States, **type 2 diabetes mellitus** affects 10.5% of those ages 45 to 64 years (up from 5.6% in 1985) and 18.4% of those ages 65 to 74 years (up from 10.2% in 1985).[99] The incidence of diabetes has doubled in all adult age groups in the past two decades. Prevalence varies by ethnic group and gender. Although the increase in overall prevalence of diabetes has increased the most in white men (116% increase since 1980), the condition remains most common in black women with an overall prevalence of 8.8% and a prevalence of 34% in those ages 65 to 74.[99] There also is an increased prevalence of type 2 diabetes in children, especially in Native American children ages 15 to 19[99] and in obese children[121-123] (see Table 21-6).

An environmental-genetic interaction appears to be responsible for type 2 diabetes. The most well-recognized risk factors are age, obesity, hypertension, physical inactivity, and family history. The metabolic syndrome is a constellation of disorders (central obesity, dyslipidemia, prehypertension, and a fasting blood glucose more than or equal to 100 mg/dl) that together confer a high risk of developing type 2 diabetes and associated cardiovascular complications (see What's New? Metabolic Syndrome and Diagnosis). Other novel risk factors being investigated include elevated C-reactive protein, decreased adiponectin, increased leptin, and increased IL-6.[124] A unique manifestation of insulin resistance in women of reproductive age is polycystic ovary syndrome (PCOS), which is associated with a risk of diabetes seven times the average risk for women without PCOS.

PATHOPHYSIOLOGY Many genes have been identified that are associated with type 2 diabetes, including those that code for beta cell mass, beta cell function (ability to sense

WHAT'S NEW? Islet Transplant and Type 1 Diabetes Mellitus

Type 1 diabetes mellitus is an irreversible, unpreventable disease. Transplantation of pancreatic islets is a treatment option that restores euglycemia, eliminates the occurrence of hypoglycemia associated with insulin therapy, and prevents the chronic complications of hyperglycemia. Islet transplant is relatively noninvasive although availability of donor islets is limited. The duration of effectiveness of islet transplant declines significantly with only 10% of recipients achieving sustained insulin independence over a period of 5 years. Transplant rejection and autoimmune attack of transplanted islets lead to ultimate loss of transplanted cells. An immediate blood-mediated inflammatory reaction that destroys islet cells is particularly problematic, requiring tissue from more than one donor to achieve insulin independence. However, even partial graft function improves glucose control and hypoglycemic events. Ongoing research is in progress to overcome recurrent autoimmunity, alloimmune rejection, and less toxic immunosuppression. Xenotransplantation (e.g., pig islets) or stem cell sources of islet cells also are being explored.

Data from: Hogan A, Pileggi A, Ricordi C: *Front Biosci* 13:1192-1202, 2008; Huang X et al: *Endocr Rev* 29(5):603-630, 2008; Leitao CB et al: *Curr Diabetes Rep* 8(4):324-331, 2008.

blood glucose levels, insulin synthesis, and insulin secretion), proinsulin and insulin molecular structure, insulin receptors, hepatic synthesis of glucose, glucagon synthesis, and cellular responsiveness to insulin stimulation.[125-128] These genetic abnormalities combined with environmental influences, such as obesity, result in the basic pathophysiologic mechanisms of type 2 diabetes: insulin resistance and decreased insulin secretion by beta cells (Figure 21-14). Both of these mechanisms are essential to the development of type 2 diabetes. Although many individuals with risk factors for type 2 diabetes (including obesity, metabolic syndrome, and hypertension) are insulin resistant, only those individuals who are genetically predisposed to beta cell dysfunction (and therefore a relative deficiency in insulin) will develop type 2 diabetes.[129-130]

Insulin resistance is defined as a suboptimal response of insulin-sensitive tissues (especially liver, muscle, and adipose tissue) to insulin. Several mechanisms are involved in abnormalities of the insulin signaling pathway and contribute to insulin resistance. These include an abnormality of the insulin molecule, high amounts of insulin antagonists, down-regulation of the insulin receptor, decreased or abnormal activation of postreceptor kinases, and alteration of glucose transporter (GLUT) proteins.[131] Obesity is present in 60% to 80% of those with type 2 diabetes and is a major contributor to insulin resistance through several important mechanisms:

1. Adipokines are hormones produced in adipose tissue. A nuclear receptor, called peroxisome proliferator-activated receptor gamma (PPARγ), is highly expressed in adipose cells and is responsible for modulating the changes in adipokines, including increased serum levels

of leptin (leptin resistance) and resistin and decreased levels of adiponectin.[128,130-133] These changes are associated with decreased insulin sensitivity. Although the specific mechanisms by which these adipokines alter insulin sensitivity are still being explored, a group of insulin-sensitizing drugs, called the thiazolidinediones

WHAT'S NEW? Metabolic Syndrome and Diagnosis

The **metabolic syndrome** also has been called the *insulin resistance syndrome* or *syndrome X*. It is a clustering of clinical traits occurring together that increase the risk for accelerated cardiovascular disease and type 2 diabetes mellitus. Metabolic syndrome was recently defined by the National Cholesterol Education Program's Adult Treatment Panel III as the identification of three of the following five traits:

- Increased waist circumference (>40 inches in men; >35 inches in women)
- Plasma triglycerides ≥150 mg/dl
- Plasma high-density lipoprotein (HDL) cholesterol <40 mg/dl (men) or <50 mg/dl (women)
- Blood pressure ≥130/85 mmHg
- Fasting plasma glucose ≥100 mg/dl

The syndrome is associated with insulin resistance and behaviorally modifiable risk factors, such as smoking, exercise, and diet. Approximately 55 million Americans meet the criteria for metabolic syndrome. These individuals should be screened on a regular basis for diabetes mellitus. Recent studies indicate that the syndrome develops during childhood and is highly prevalent among overweight children and adolescents. Early recognition and treatment, including vigorous lifestyle changes, are critical to reducing cardiovascular events and improving clinical outcomes. Treatment includes decreasing dietary calories, exercise, weight loss, treating dyslipidemias, and enhancing insulin sensitivity.

Data from Ford ES, Li C, Sattar N: *Diabetes Care* 31(9):1898-1904, 2008; Gallagher EJ, LeRoith D, Karnieli E: *Endocrinol Metab Clin North Am* 37(3):559-579, vii, 2008; Lusis AJ, Attie AD, Reue K: *Nat Rev Genet* 9(11):819-830, 2008.

that modulate PPARγ activity, have been used in the treatment of type 2 diabetes for many years.

2. Elevated serum free fatty acids (FFAs) and intracellular deposits of triglycerides and cholesterol are also found in obese individuals who have what has been termed "metabolic overload" (high caloric and lipid intake). These changes interfere with intracellular insulin signaling and thus decrease tissue responses to insulin. Increases in fatty acids also cause alterations in insulin secretion within the beta cell.[131,133-135]

3. Inflammatory cytokines (TNF-α, IL-6) are released from intra-abdominal adipocytes or adipocyte-associated mononuclear cells and induce insulin resistance through a postreceptor mechanism.[132,135-138]

4. Obesity is correlated with hyperinsulinemia and decreased insulin receptor density.

Compensatory hyperinsulinemia prevents the clinical appearance of diabetes for many years. Eventually, however, **beta cell dysfunction** develops and leads to a relative deficiency of insulin activity. The islet dysfunction may be caused by a decrease in beta cell mass, abnormal function of the beta cells, or some combination. A progressive decrease in the weight and number of beta cells occurs in type 2 diabetes, and several different mechanisms have been implicated. Beta cells are extremely sensitive to high levels of glucose and free fatty acids, and under these so-called glucolipotoxic conditions, beta cells undergo apoptotic cell death.[128,130,132,139] The adipokine leptin decreases insulin synthesis in the beta cell. A variety of inflammatory cytokines, including TNF-α and IL-1β, have also been shown to be toxic to beta cells.[128,130,132,140] Thus many of the obesity-related causes of insulin resistance (elevated free fatty acids [FFA] hyperglycemia, adipokines, and inflammatory cytokines) also promote programmed cell death in B cells. Beta cell "exhaustion" from increased demand for insulin biosynthesis, associated with intracellular oxidative stress and endoplasmic reticulum dysfunction, also has been implicated in beta cell apoptosis.[132,141]

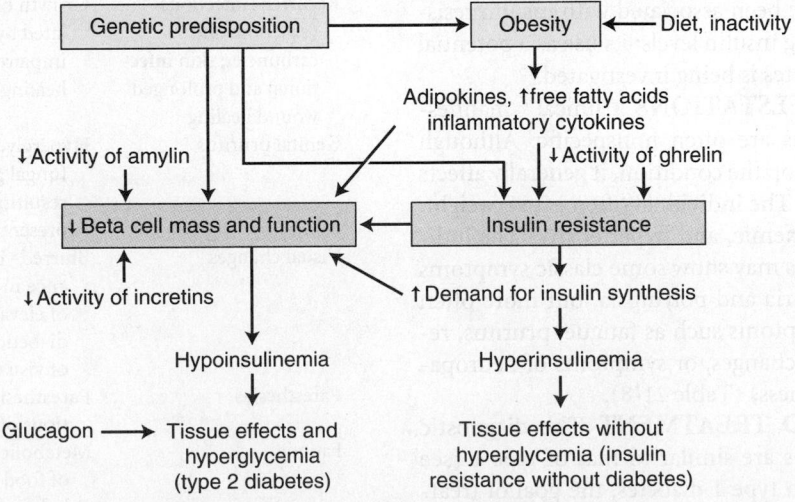

Figure 21-14 Pathophysiology of type 2 diabetes mellitus.

Glucagon is a hormone produced by the alpha cells of the pancreas and acts primarily in the liver to increase blood glucose by stimulating glycogenolysis and gluconeogenesis. Glucagon acts as an antagonist to insulin. In healthy individuals, high glucose levels cause glucagon release to be inhibited. In type 2 diabetes, pancreatic alpha cells are less responsive to glucose inhibition resulting in increased glucagon secretion.[142,143] These abnormally high levels of glucagon have long been known to play a role in the increased hepatic production of glucose and resultant hyperglycemia seen in type 2 diabetes.

Amylin is a hormone co-secreted with insulin by the beta cells. A deficiency of amylin in type 1 and type 2 diabetes parallels the reduction in insulin secretion. Amylin inhibits glucagon secretion, and problems with glycemic control may be related to altered glucagon control or assimilation of nutrients in relation to the deficit of amylin. Drugs aimed at improving amylin function are being studied.[144] Amyloid deposition in the pancreas resulting in islet cell destruction also may be related to changes in amylin function.[132,145,146] However, the role of amyloid accumulation in the pathogenesis of type 2 diabetes is unclear.

The **incretins** are a class of peptides released from the gastrointestinal tract in response to food intake that increase the sensitivity of beta cells to circulating glucose levels, thus improving insulin responsiveness to meals. **Glucagon-like peptide 1 (GLP-1)** is cleaved from proglucagon in the intestinal mucosa. Another incretin is **glucose-dependent insulinotropic polypeptide (GIP)**, which is synthesized in the duodenum and jejunum. These incretins bind to receptors on beta cells and increase the synthesis and secretion of insulin in response to glucose levels.[147] They are then inactivated by the enzyme **dipeptidyl peptidase IV (DPP-IV)**. Currently one GLP-1 agonist and one DPP-IV inhibitor are approved for use in the United States and others are being evaluated for the treatment of type 2 diabetes[147-150] (see What's New? Incretin Hormones for Diabetes Mellitus Therapy).

Ghrelin is a peptide produced in the stomach and pancreatic islets that stimulates GH receptors. Decreased levels of circulating ghrelin have been associated with insulin resistance and increased fasting insulin levels; its use as a potential treatment for type 2 diabetes is being investigated.[151]

CLINICAL MANIFESTATIONS Clinical manifestations of type 2 diabetes are often nonspecific. Although younger people may develop the condition, it generally affects those older than 30 years. The individual often is overweight, dyslipidemic, hyperinsulinemic, and hypertensive. The individual with type 2 diabetes may show some classic symptoms of diabetes, such as polyuria and polydipsia, but more often will have nonspecific symptoms such as fatigue, pruritus, recurrent infections, visual changes, or symptoms of neuropathy (paresthesias or weakness) (Table 21-8).

EVALUATION AND TREATMENT The diagnostic criteria for type 2 diabetes are similar to that of type 1 (see Box 21-1, p. 747). As with type 1 diabetes, the goal of treatment for individuals with type 2 diabetes is the restoration of

---

> **WHAT'S NEW?** Incretin Hormones for Diabetes Mellitus Therapy
>
> The incretin hormone system is being explored as a possible therapeutic target in diabetes. Incretin hormones are secreted by enteroendocrine cells of the large and small intestines. The major component of this system, glucagon-like peptide-1 (GLP-1), has many positive effects on glucose metabolism. GLP-1 augments glucose-dependent insulin secretion without causing hypoglycemia, stimulates insulin gene expression, inhibits glucagon secretion, delays gastric emptying, and induces a feeling of satiety through an effect on the central nervous system. GLP-1 also has been shown to induce new beta cell differentiation (neogenesis) from pancreatic ductal cells and to protect beta cells from apoptosis (programmed cell death). Considering the actions of GLP-1, it should be able to dramatically improve metabolic control in people with diabetes, assist individuals with weight loss, and augment endogenous insulin secretion. Because GLP-1 has an extremely short half-life (1 to 3 minutes), analogs with similar properties have been developed, and compounds, such as dipeptidyl peptidase-IV (DPP-IV) inhibitors, that inhibit the degradation of GLP-1 are being explored. Exenatide and liraglutide are GLP-1 receptor agonists that have been used in the management of type 2 diabetes. In addition to improving glucose control, many people are able to lose weight; however, dramatic improvements in B cell function are rarely seen. Sitagliptin and vildagliptin DPP-IV inhibitor, provide modest improvement in glucose control without weight loss.
>
> Data from Raman VS, Heptulla RA: *Pediatr Res* 65(4):370-374, 2009; Knop FK, Vilsbøll T, Holst JJ: *Curr Protein Pept Sci* 2009 Feb; 10(1):46-55, 2009; Holst JJ, Vilsbøll T, Deacon CF: *Mol Cell Endocrinol* 2009 Jan 15;297(1-2):127-136, 2009; Pratley RE: *Diabetes Educ* 35 (Suppl 1):4S-11S, 2009; McGill JB: *Postgrad Med* 121(1):46-58, 2009.

Table 21-8 | **Clinical Manifestations and Rationale for Type 2 Diabetes Mellitus**

Manifestation	Rationale
Recurrent infections (e.g., boils and carbuncles; skin infections) and prolonged wound healing	Growth of microorganisms is stimulated by increased glucose levels; impaired blood supply hinders healing
Genital pruritus	Hyperglycemia and glycosuria favor fungal growth; candidal infections, resulting in pruritus, are a common presenting symptom in women
Visual changes	Blurred vision occurs as water balance in the eye fluctuates because of elevated blood glucose levels; diabetic retinopathy is another cause of visual loss
Paresthesias	Paresthesias are common manifestations of diabetic neuropathies
Fatigue	Metabolic changes result in poor use of food products, contributing to lethargy and fatigue

near-euglycemia (a normal blood glucose level) and correction of related metabolic disorders.

Dietary measures, including restriction of the total caloric intake, are of primary importance in both the prevention and treatment of type 2 diabetes.[119,121,152] As the obese individual loses weight, the body's resistance to insulin often diminishes so that weight loss results in improved glucose tolerance. Nonobese individuals with type 2 diabetes should consume calories consistent with their ideal weight and pattern of activity. The emphasis of medical nutrition therapy (MNT) in type 2 diabetes mellitus should be focused on achieving glucose, lipid, and blood pressure goals (see Nutrition & Disease: Medical Nutrition Therapy [MNT] for Prevention and Treatment of Diabetes).

Exercise is an important aspect of prevention and treatment of type 2 diabetes.[119,121] Exercise reduces postprandial blood glucose levels, diminishes insulin requirements, lowers triglyceride and cholesterol levels, and increases the level of high-density lipoprotein (HDL) cholesterol. In addition, exercise is a valuable adjunct to weight loss for the overweight individual. Hypoglycemia may result, however, when the exercising individual receives sulfonylurea or insulin therapy.

In those individuals with morbid obesity unresponsive to diet and exercise interventions, bariatric surgery may be indicated. Recent studies suggest that gastric bypass surgery is associated with a decrease in the incidence of type 2 diabetes and marked improvements in glycemic control in those with established diabetes.[152-155]

Although the first approach to treatment of the individual with type 2 diabetes is appropriate meal planning and exercise, medications are usually needed for optimal management. Sulfonylurea, biguanide, thiazolidinediones, DPP-IV inhibitors, and α-glucosidase inhibitors are useful in treating some individuals with type 2 diabetes (Table 21-9). Use of oral hypoglycemic agents requires a pancreas capable of secreting insulin. Sulfonylureas acutely augment beta cell insulin secretion. Biguanides (metformin) inhibit hepatic glucose production and increase the sensitivity of peripheral tissue to insulin. α-Glucosidase inhibitors decrease postprandial hyperglycemia through delaying carbohydrate digestion and absorption. The thiazolidinedione class of insulin-sensitizing compounds activate a nuclear receptor termed the peroxisome proliferator-activated receptor (PPARγ), which in turn regulates cellular carbohydrate and lipid metabolism. As discussed previously, DPP-IV inhibitors increase GLP-1 levels that in turn help augment endogenous insulin secretion. Insulin therapy may be needed in the later stages of type 2 diabetes because of loss of beta cell function.[156] There is some evidence that exogenous insulin may help prevent further beta cell apoptosis.[157] Because the pathogenesis of type 2 diabetes involves a combination of insulin resistance and a relative insulin deficiency, it is common to combine therapeutic agents from different classes of oral agents in order to achieve acceptable glycemic control.

NUTRITION & DISEASE

Medical Nutrition Therapy (MNT) for Prevention and Treatment of Diabetes

Dietary intervention for the prevention and treatment of diabetes must be individualized. Structured programs are most helpful. Dietary strategies should include reduced intake of fats and carbohydrates. Carbohydrate monitoring can be achieved through carbohydrate counting, exchanges, or glycemic index. Saturated fat intake should be less than 7% of total calories and trans-fat intake should be minimized. Individuals also should consume foods that contain whole grains with a goal of dietary fiber intake of 14 g/100 kcal. Alcohol intake should be limited to one drink per day or less for adult women and two drinks per day or less for adult men. Routine supplementation with antioxidants or chromium cannot be recommended. These dietary interventions should be combined with exercise programs (150 minutes/week). The goal is to achieve moderate weight loss and a lowering of the hemoglobin A_{1C} to less than 7%.

Data from American Diabetes Association Executive Summary: *Diabetes Care* 31:S5-S11, 2008.

Table 21-9	Types of Oral Hypoglycemic Drugs
Drug Type	**Mechanism of Action**
α-Glycosidase inhibitor	Delays carbohydrate absorption in gut by inhibiting disaccharidases
Biguanide (metformin)	Decreases hepatic glucose production Increases insulin sensitivity and peripheral glucose uptake
Meglitinides (glinides)	Stimulate insulin release from pancreatic beta cells
Amino acid derivatives	Stimulates insulin release from pancreatic beta cells
Sulfonylureas	Stimulates insulin release from pancreatic beta cells
Thiazolidinediones	Increases insulin sensitivity, particularly in adipose tissue
DPP-IV inhibitors	Increases GLP-1 levels which promotes insulin secretion

DPP-IV, Dipeptidyl peptidase-IV; *GLP-1*, glucagon-like peptide 1.

Other Specific Types of Diabetes Mellitus and Gestational Diabetes Mellitus

As described in Table 21-5 (p. 746), the American Diabetes Association (ADA) classification of diabetes mellitus includes not only the most common forms of diabetes (type 1 and type 2) but also "other specific types of diabetes mellitus" and "gestational diabetes mellitus."[98] Other specific types of diabetes include genetic defects in beta cell function, genetic defects in insulin action, diseases of the exocrine pancreas, endocrinopathies, drug- or chemical-induced beta cell dysfunction, infections, and other uncommon autoimmune and inherited disorders that are associated with diabetes.

The most well-described of these other specific types of diabetes is termed **maturity-onset diabetes of youth (MODY)**.

Table 21-10	Causes of Hypoglycemia	
Cause	Predisposing Factor	Occurrence
Exogenous		
Insulin	Intentional or accidental overdose; may be combined with inadequate food intake, unusually increased exercise, decrease in insulin requirement, or potentiating medications	Most common cause of hypoglycemia
Sulfonylurea agents	Intentional or accidental overdose; may be combined with inadequate food intake, increased exercise, or potentiating medications	Frequent cause of hypoglycemia
Alcohol	Particularly likely in chronically malnourished or acutely food-deprived individuals	Occurs within 6-36 hr of ingesting moderate to large amounts of alcohol
Other agents	Salicylates, hypoglycines, pentamidine	Common in children younger than 2 yr
Exercise	Increased duration and intensity of exercise increase glucose uptake and normally decrease insulin secretion	Occurs with both insulin and sulfonylurea administration, and intense exercise but may be unpredictable in onset
Endogenous		
Organic hypoglycemia	Insulinoma	Uncommon neoplasm of B cells of islets of Langerhans
	Nesidioblastosis and B cell hyperplasia	Rare disease causing persistent hypoglycemia of infancy
Extrapancreatic neoplasms	May be mesenchymal tumors, hepatomas, adrenocortical carcinomas, gastrointestinal tumors, lymphomas, or leukemias	Rare; most common in adults 40-70 yr of age
Inborn errors of metabolism	Hereditary fructose intolerance	Rare autosomal recessively inherited inborn error of metabolism
	Fructose-1,6-disphosphatase deficiency	Rare autosomal recessive disease
	Galactosemia	Autosomal recessive disease; hypoglycemia less common than in fructose intolerance
	Phosphoenolpyruvate carboxykinase deficiency	Reported in a few infant cases
	Inborn errors in glycogen metabolism, leucine sensitivity	Reported in von Gierke disease, Hers disease, and type IXb glycogen storage disease

MODY includes six specific autosomal dominant mutations including genes for hepatocyte nuclear factor-1α (HNF-1α; MODY 3), glucokinase (MODY 2), HNF-4α (MODY 1), insulin promoter factor-1 (IPF-1; MODY 4), HNF-1β (MODY 5), and NeuroD1 (MODY 6).[158-160] Individuals with these genetic defects have a strong family history of diabetes mellitus, are of normal weight, and are usually diagnosed before age 25. MODY was previously classified as a form of type 2 diabetes because insulin levels are often in the normal range yet are inappropriately low for the degree of hyperglycemia. However, weight gain is not a prominent feature of MODY, whereas it is an important contributor to type 2 diabetes. Interestingly, the gene mutations found in MODY are not commonly found in type 2 diabetes.[159-161] Diagnosis and management are similar to type 2 diabetes.

Gestational diabetes mellitus (GDM) is defined as any degree of glucose intolerance with onset or first recognition during pregnancy.[98] GDM complicates approximately 4% of all pregnancies and represents approximately 90% of pregnancies complicated by diabetes.[98,162] The exact mechanism of GDM is unknown, but insulin resistance and inadequate insulin secretion are contributing factors. Diagnosis of GDM is based on the presence of risk factors (older age, family history, history of glucose intolerance, obesity, membership in certain ethnic or racial group, and history of poor obstetric outcomes, infant weighing greater than 9 pounds), plus the

measurement of an elevated fasting or casual FPG. OGTT can also be used to confirm the diagnosis. Often there are no symptoms and careful glucose control prenatally, during pregnancy, and after delivery are essential to both the short- and long-term health of mother and baby.[162-164] There is an increased risk for type-2 diabetes later in life in women who develop gestational diabetes.

Acute Complications of Diabetes Mellitus

Hypoglycemia

Hypoglycemia is a lowered plasma glucose level. Its causes may be exogenous, endogenous, or functional (Tables 21-10, 21-11, and 21-12 contain summaries of causes). In general, hypoglycemia occurs when blood glucose levels are less than 35 mg/dl in newborns for the first 48 hours of life and less than 45 to 60 mg/dl in children and adults. Some individuals may become symptomatic before glucose levels decrease to 60 mg/dl if the decrease is relatively rapid. Hypoglycemia occurs most often in individuals with diabetes mellitus treated with insulin (see Table 21-10 for a list of both endogenous and exogenous causes of hypoglycemia). It occurs in more than 90% of those with type 1 diabetes (especially in those on multiple daily injections of insulin) and limits the management of the disease.[100,165] Hypoglycemia in diabetes is sometimes called *insulin shock* or *insulin reaction*. Individuals with type 2 diabetes are at less risk for hypoglycemia than those with type 1 diabetes because they

Table 21-11   Functional Causes of Hypoglycemia

Dysfunction	Precipitating Factor	Occurrence
Alimentary hypoglycemia	Rapid dumping of carbohydrates into the upper small intestine	Postgastrectomy
Spontaneous reactive hypoglycemia	Syndrome of unknown cause with symptoms such as diaphoresis, tachycardia, tremulousness, headache, fatigue, drowsiness, and irritability	Rarely diagnosed throughout the world; widely diagnosed in United States, prompting American Diabetes Association and Endocrine Society to issue statement that entity is probably overdiagnosed; it is a benign condition
Alcohol-promoted reactive hypoglycemia	Drinking on an empty stomach	More common with drinks containing both alcohol and glucose or saccharin (e.g., beer, gin and tonic, rum and cola, whisky and ginger ale)
Posthyperalimentation hypoglycemia	Rapid discontinuation of total parenteral alimentation	Easily prevented by gradually reducing parenteral administration (alimentation)
Endocrine-deficiency states	Glucocorticoid deficiency	A danger for any person with adrenal insufficiency
	Growth hormone deficiency	Particularly during a prolonged fast in children
Severe liver deficiency	Insufficient glucose output by the liver	Fasting hypoglycemia
Lack of body stores for protein, fat, and carbohydrates	Profound malnutrition	Frequent; also found with relative frequency in kwashiorkor
Prolonged muscular exercise	Metabolism of energy-producing substances	Occurs if exercise is too prolonged or severe or if nutritional intake and carbohydrate stores are insufficient
Functional or transient hypoglycemia in infancy	Transient neonatal hypoglycemia	Occurs in 10% of live births, during first 3 days of life
	Maternal diabetes	Caused by beta cell hyperplasia and possibly relative hypoglucagonemia
	Erythroblastosis fetalis	Frequently associated with erythroblastosis fetalis
	Leucine-induced hypoglycemia	Generally in infants younger than 6 months of age; severe hypoglycemia attacks may occur postprandially or after short periods of fasting
	Ketotic or ketogenic hypoglycemia	One of the most common forms of hypoglycemia in childhood, occurs after food deprivation in children 1-8 yr old; generally, spontaneous recovery before 10 yr old

retain relatively intact glucose counterregulatory mechanisms.[166] However, hypoglycemia does occur in type 2 diabetes when treatment involves insulin secretagogues (e.g., sulfonylureas) or exogenous insulin.[156,166-168] Hypoglycemia also can occur as a result of many functional causes unrelated to diabetes (see Table 21-11).

Symptoms of hypoglycemia result from either activation of the sympathetic nervous system (adrenergic symptoms) or from an abrupt cessation of glucose delivery to the brain (neuroglycopenic symptoms) or both.[60] Symptoms commonly vary among individuals but tend to be consistent for each person. Adrenergic reactions occur when the decrease in blood glucose is rapid with tachycardia, palpitations, diaphoresis, tremors, pallor, and arousal anxiety.[169] The response is probably generated when the hypothalamus senses decreased glucose levels. Reduced substrate delivery to the brain (neuroglycopenia) causes changes in neuronal kinase activity and firing rates,[170] thus producing further symptoms including headache, dizziness, irritability, fatigue, poor judgment, confusion, visual changes, hunger, seizures, and coma. Hypoglycemia unawareness is a phenomenon that occurs in individuals without appropriate autonomic warning symptoms before development of neuroglycopenia. These individuals should be advised to raise their glycemic targets to avoid severe hypoglycemia.[119] If an individual is receiving a

beta-blocking medication, the autonomic symptoms may be blunted, and recovery from hypoglycemia may be delayed because of impaired glycogenolysis and hampered delivery of gluconeogenic substrates to the liver.

When hypoglycemic symptoms are nonspecific, the safest treatment is to provide some form of glucose because failure to provide glucose may precipitate convulsions, coma, and death. The ADA recommends that glucose (15 to 20 g) be given to a conscious patient with hypoglycemia, and that at-risk individuals and caregivers should be instructed in glucagon administration.[119] Prevention of hypoglycemia episodes through alternate therapeutic regimens, individualizing target blood glucose levels, frequent self-monitoring of blood glucose, and proper education should be the goal.[118,166-168,171]

Diabetic Ketoacidosis

Ketoacidosis, a serious complication of diabetes mellitus, is a common cause for hospital admissions. Although average mortality rates throughout the United States are less than 2%, the highest rates of mortality are observed in older adults and those with other severe underlying illnesses.[172] **Diabetic ketoacidosis (DKA)** develops when there is an absolute or relative deficiency of insulin. This is most common in individuals with type 1 diabetes but can occur in those with type

2 diabetes as well.[60,172-174] In addition, a syndrome called *ketosis-prone diabetes (KPD)* has been described in which affected individuals do not fit into the traditional ADA categories for diabetes and are more likely to be persons of African, African American, or Hispanic origin.[175] The most common precipitating factor for DKA is intercurrent illness, such as infection, trauma, surgery, or myocardial infarction. Interruption of insulin administration also may result in DKA. In 20% to 30% of cases, no precipitating factors are noted. Emotional factors and stress, particularly in children, are thought to contribute to the development of DKA. The frequency of DKA peaks in adolescence.

PATHOPHYSIOLOGY In a state of relative insulin deficiency there is an increase in insulin counterregulatory hormones including catecholamines, cortisol, glucagon, and GH. Catecholamines, cortisol, glucagon, and GH antagonize insulin by increasing glucose production. In addition, these hormones decrease use of glucose. Profound insulin deficiency results in decreased glucose uptake, increased fat mobilization with release of fatty acids, and accelerated gluconeogenesis and ketogenesis (Figure 21-15). Relatively increased glucagon levels also contribute to activation of the gluconeogenic (glucose-forming) and ketogenic (ketone-forming) pathways in the liver. Because of the insulin deficiency, hepatic overproduction of β-hydroxybutyrate and acetoacetic acids causes increased ketone concentrations.[173] Ordinarily ketones are used by tissues as an energy source to regenerate bicarbonate. This balances the loss of bicarbonate, which occurs when the ketone is formed. Hyperketonemia (increased blood ketone levels) may be a result of impairment in the use of ketones by peripheral tissue, which permits strong organic acids to circulate freely. Bicarbonate buffering then does not occur, and the individual develops a metabolic acidosis.

CLINICAL MANIFESTATIONS The signs and symptoms of DKA are fairly nonspecific. Polyuria and dehydration result from the osmotic diuresis associated with hyperglycemia. Here the plasma glucose level is higher than the individual's renal threshold, allowing much glucose to be lost in the urine. Sodium, phosphorus, and magnesium deficits are common. The most important electrolyte disturbance, however, is a marked deficiency in total body potassium. Although the serum potassium may appear normal or elevated because of volume contraction and a shift of potassium out of the cell and into the blood caused by metabolic acidosis, the total body deficiency of potassium may reach 3 to 5 mEq/kg. Symptoms of diabetic ketoacidosis include Kussmaul respirations (hyperventilation in an attempt to compensate for the acidosis), postural dizziness, central nervous system depression, ketonuria, anorexia, nausea, abdominal pain, thirst, and polyuria.

EVALUATION AND TREATMENT The diagnosis of ketoacidosis is suggested when individuals have symptoms of vomiting, abdominal pain, dehydration, an acetone odor on the breath, and change in sensorium. The ADA criteria for diagnosis of DKA include a serum glucose of more than 250 mg/dl, a serum bicarbonate of less than 18 mg/dl, a serum pH of less than 7.30, presence of an anion gap, and presence of urine and serum ketones.[176]

Treatment of DKA involves continual administration of low-dose insulin to decrease glucose levels.[60,172] Fluids are administered to replace lost fluid volume, and electrolytes—particularly sodium, potassium, and phosphorus—are administered as needed. Fluids and electrolytes should be

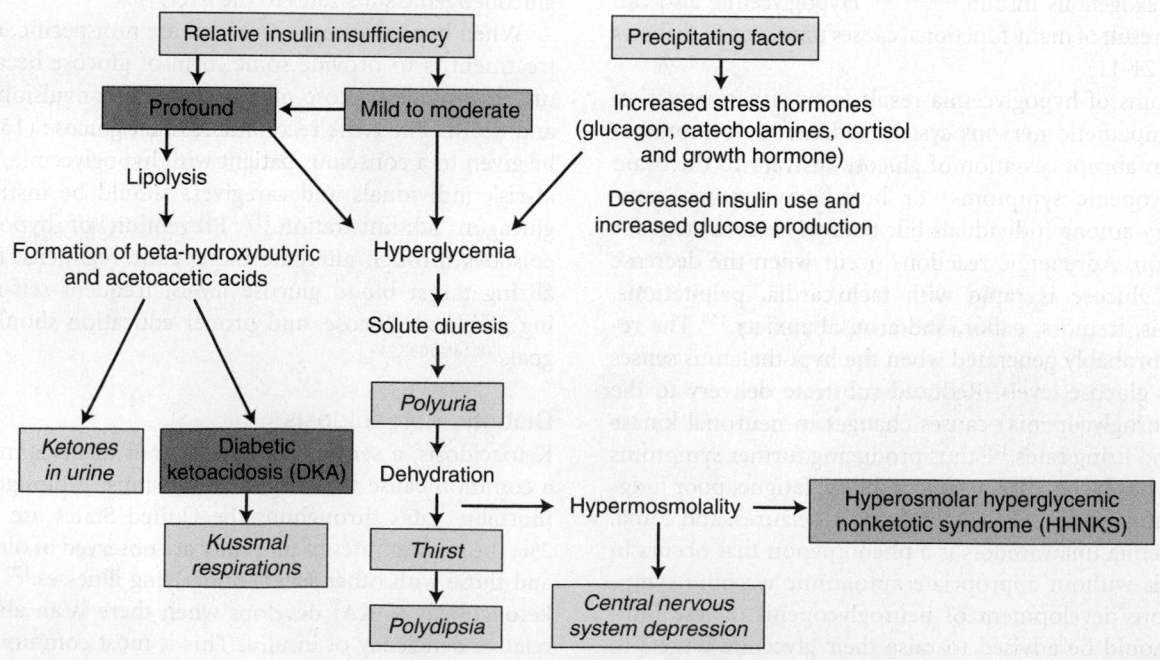

Figure 21-15 Pathophysiology of DKA and HHNKS in diabetes mellitus.

Table 21-12   Common Acute Complications of Diabetes Mellitus (DM)

Hypoglycemia in Persons with DM	Diabetic Ketoacidosis	Hyperglycemic Nonketotic Syndromes
Synonyms		
Insulin shock, insulin reaction	Diabetic coma syndrome	Hyperosmolar hyperglycemia nonketotic coma
Persons at Risk		
Individuals taking insulin	Individuals with type 1 diabetes	Older adults or very young individuals with
Individuals with rapidly fluctuating blood sugar	Individuals with nondiagnosed diabetes	type 2 diabetes, nondiabetic individuals with predisposing factors, such as pancreatitis;
Individuals with type 2 diabetes taking sulfonylurea agents		individuals with undiagnosed diabetes
Predisposing Factors		
Excessive insulin or sulfonylurea agent intake, lack of sufficient food intake, excessive physical exercise, abrupt decline in insulin needs (e.g., renal failure, immediately postpartum), simultaneous use of insulin-potentiating agents or beta-blocking agents that mask symptoms	Stressful situation such as infection, accident, trauma, emotional stress; omission of insulin; medications that antagonize insulin	Infection, medications that antagonize insulin, comorbid condition
Typical Onset		
Rapid	Slow	Slowest
Presenting Symptoms		
Adrenergic reaction: pallor, sweating, tachycardia, palpitations, hunger, restlessness, anxiety, tremors	Malaise, dry mouth, headache, polyuria, polydipsia, weight loss, nausea, vomiting, pruritus, abdominal pain, lethargy, shortness of breath, Kussmaul respirations, fruity or acetone odor to breath	Polyuria, polydipsia, hypovolemia, dehydration (parched lips, poor skin turgor), hypotension, tachycardia, hypoperfusion, weight loss, weakness, nausea, vomiting, abdominal pain, hypothermia, stupor, coma, seizures
Neurogenic reaction: fatigue, irritability, headache, loss of concentration, visual disturbances, dizziness, hunger, confusion, transient sensory or motor defects, convulsions, coma, death		
Laboratory Analysis		
Serum glucose <30 mg/dl in newborn (first 2-3 days) and <55-60 mg/dl in adults	Glucose levels >250 mg/dl, reduction in bicarbonate concentration, increased anion gap, increased plasma levels of β-hydroxybutyrate, acetoacetate, and acetone	Glucose levels >600 mg/dl, lack of ketosis, serum osmolarity >320 mOsm/L, elevated blood urea nitrogen and creatinine

monitored closely. Electrolyte deficits become apparent as fluid volume is replaced. After the administration of insulin, the concentration of β-hydroxybutyrate promptly begins to decrease and after a slight increase, acetoacetate also begins to decrease. A persistent ketonuria may be observed for several days after treatment. Continuous monitoring of the individual is essential to ensure an uncomplicated recovery from DKA. Cerebral edema is the most common cause of morbidity and mortality during the first day of treatment for DKA in children. The mechanisms are poorly understood.[177] Health teaching emphasizes predisposing factors and strategies for avoiding DKA.

Hyperosmolar Hyperglycemic Nonketotic Syndrome

Hyperosmolar hyperglycemic nonketotic syndrome (HHNKS) is a life-threatening emergency most often precipitated by infections, medications, nonadherence to diabetes treatment, or coexisting disease.[174,176] HHNKS is more commonly seen with type 2 diabetes. It can also occur in individuals with pancreatic destruction from other causes such as chronic pancreatitis.

PATHOPHYSIOLOGY HHNKS differs from DKA in the degree of insulin deficiency (which is more profound in DKA) and the degree of fluid deficiency (which is more marked in HHNKS) (see Figure 21-15).[176] Levels of free fatty acids in HHNKS are consistently lower than those found in DKA. HHNKS is characterized also by a lack of ketosis. Because the amount of insulin required to inhibit fat breakdown is less than that needed for effective glucose transport, insulin levels are sufficient to prevent excessive lipolysis but not to use glucose properly. Glucose levels are considerably higher in HHNKS than in DKA because of volume depletion.

CLINICAL MANIFESTATIONS The clinical features of HHNKS include a serum glucose of more than 600 mg/dl, a serum pH greater than 7.30, a serum bicarbonate greater than 15 mg/dl, a serum osmolarity greater than 320 mOsm/L, and either absent or small ketones in the urine and serum.[176] Glycosuria and polyuria in HHNKS result from the extreme serum glucose elevation. As much as 19 g of glucose per hour may be lost in diuresis, which also causes severe volume depletion, increased serum osmolarity, intracellular dehydration, and loss of electrolytes including potassium. Neurologic changes, such as stupor, correlate with the degree of hyperosmolarity and are more common in HHNKS than in DKA.[60]

EVALUATION AND TREATMENT The serum ketone concentration is normal or only mildly elevated and only minimal acidosis is seen in HHNKS, otherwise DKA and HHNKS show considerable overlap in symptoms and treatment. Insulin infusion should be combined with fluid repletion over 24 hours.[60,176] An important distinction, however, is that the dehydration in HHNKS is far more severe than that in DKA. Thus fluid replacement, with both crystalloids and colloids, is more rapid. Potassium deficits may be so extreme in HHNKS that more than 1 week of potassium repletion may be needed to correct the total body deficits. Phosphorus and sodium also may be needed. HHNKS is a significant risk factor for venous thrombosis and recent studies suggest that anticoagulant prophylaxis should be considered.[60,178] Mortality is also high in HHNKS, and is related to the age of the individual and comorbid conditions including the severity of the precipitating illness (see Table 21-12 for a comparison of the three acute complications described thus far).

Somogyi Effect

The **Somogyi effect** is a unique combination of hypoglycemia followed by rebound hyperglycemia. The problem is more common in individuals with type 1 diabetes mellitus, particularly in children, and should be investigated whenever fluctuations in blood sugar levels are serious.[179]

PATHOPHYSIOLOGY The Somogyi effect occurs when hypoglycemia stimulates glucose counterregulation, including epinephrine, GH, cortisol, and glucagon release.[180] These hormones serve to increase blood glucose by gluconeogenesis (formation of glucose from nonglucose sources) and glycogenolysis (breakdown of glycogen into glucose). They mobilize fatty acids and proteins while inhibiting peripheral glucose use. These hormones may cause insulin resistance for 12 to 48 hours. Commonly, excessive carbohydrate intake may be a major contributor to rebound hyperglycemia. Also hypoglycemia generally occurs during the peak of injected insulin; therefore, as counterregulatory hormones are activated and carbohydrate is consumed by the individual, insulin levels are on the decline, which contributes to the subsequent hyperglycemia.[180] The frequency of this phenomenon is debated, and recent studies suggest that it is much less common than previously reported.

CLINICAL MANIFESTATIONS In addition to fluctuating glucose levels, subtle symptoms of hypoglycemia occur. If an individual has nocturnal hypoglycemia, there may be complaints of nightmares and early morning headaches. Ketonuria may occur if the mobilization of energy sources overshoots the body's need for glucose and exogenous insulin is depleted.

EVALUATION AND TREATMENT If the individual has nocturnal hypoglycemia, diagnosis involves the measurement of plasma glucose during the night using monitors capable of continuous glucose sensing.[179] Treatment consists of decreasing insulin dosage or changing the time of administration.

Dawn Phenomenon

The **dawn phenomenon** is an early morning rise in blood glucose concentration with no hypoglycemia during the night. It appears to be related to nocturnal elevations of GH, a counterregulatory hormone that causes hyperglycemia by decreasing peripheral (other than liver) glucose uptake. Increased clearance of plasma insulin also may be involved. Altering the time and dose of insulin manages the problem.[181] Treating dawn phenomenon may result in the Somogyi effect and vice versa.

Chronic Complications of Diabetes Mellitus

A number of serious complications are associated with any type of diabetes mellitus and include microvascular (e.g., retinopathy, nephropathy, and neuropathies) and macrovascular disease (e.g., coronary artery disease, stroke, and peripheral vascular disease), and infection. Most complications are associated with metabolic alterations, primarily hyperglycemia. Strict control of blood glucose significantly reduces complications. Five metabolic events are associated with the tissue-damaging effects of chronic hyperglycemia and the pathogenesis of diabetic complications: shunting of glucose to the polyol pathway, activation of protein kinase C, induction of reactive oxygen species (oxidative stress), production of advanced glycation end products, and accumulation of hexosamines.[182-184]

Hyperglycemia and the Polyol Pathway

Tissues that do not require insulin for glucose transport, such as kidney, red blood cells (RBCs), blood vessels, eye lens, and nerves, use an alternate metabolic pathway for glucose metabolism known as the **polyol pathway.** With hyperglycemia, glucose is shunted to this pathway and is converted to sorbitol (a polyol) by the enzyme **aldose reductase.** Sorbitol is then slowly converted to fructose by sorbitol dehydrogenase.[185] The accumulation of sorbitol and fructose increases intracellular osmotic pressure and attracts water, leading to cell injury. This is particularly evident in the lens of the eye and leads to swelling with visual changes and cataracts. In nerves, sorbitol interferes with ion pumps, damages Schwann cells, and disrupts nerve conduction. RBCs become swollen and stiff and interfere with perfusion. Aldose reductase inhibitors may slow or prevent some diabetic complications, particularly neuropathies, although their effectiveness has been limited.[186]

Protein Kinase C

Protein kinase C (PKC) is an enzyme that is inappropriately activated in different tissues by hyperglycemia, particularly the diacylglycerol (DAG)-PKC pathway. Various consequences have been observed, including insulin resistance, production of extracellular matrix and cytokines, vascular cell proliferation, enhanced contractility, and increased permeability.[187] These effects may contribute to the macrovascular, microvascular, and neurologic complications of diabetes. Specific PKC inhibitors are under investigation and have shown some promise in stabilizing or preventing retinopathy, nephropathy, and neuropathy.[188]

Hyperglycemia and Nonenzymatic Glycosylation

Nonenzymatic glycosylation is the reversible attachment of glucose to proteins, lipids, and nucleic acids without the action of enzymes. With recurrent or persistent hyperglycemia, glucose becomes irreversibly bound to collagen and other proteins in red blood cells (e.g., glycated hemoglobin), blood vessel walls, and interstitial tissue. The products of this binding are known as **advanced glycosylation end product (AGE)** and their receptor (RAGE) have a number of properties that may cause tissue injury or pathologic conditions associated with diabetes[189-192]:

1. Cross-linking and trapping of proteins, including albumin, low-density lipoprotein (LDL), immunoglobulin, and complement, with thickening of the basement membrane or increased permeability in blood vessels and nerves
2. Binding to cell receptors, such as macrophages and glomerular mesangial cells, and inducing release of cytokines and growth factors that stimulate cellular proliferation in the glomeruli, smooth muscle of blood vessels, and collagen synthesis with fibrosis
3. Induction of lipid oxidation, oxidative stress, and inflammation
4. Inactivation of nitric oxide with loss of vasodilation and diminished endothelial function
5. Procoagulant changes on endothelial cells with promotion of platelet adhesion and reduced fibrinolysis

Pharmacologic agents that inhibit AGE formation or block their receptor (RAGE) are being evaluated.[189]

Hyperglycemia and Oxidative Stress

Chronic hyperglycemia increases the production of reactive oxygen species (ROS) and the detrimental effects of oxidative stress. AGEs, defects in the polyol pathway, uncoupling of nitric oxide synthase, xanthine oxidase, and nicotinamide adenine dinucleotide phosphate (NADPH) oxidase generate ROS, which damage large and small vessels and contribute to atherogenesis, cardiovascular disease, nephropathy, and neuropathy. Direct cellular injury, as well as the formation of gene products that cause cellular injury, contribute to these late complications of diabetes mellitus.[193,194]

Hyperglycemia and the Hexosamine Pathway

Chronic hyperglycemia causes shunting of excess intracellular glucose into the hexosamine pathway and leads to O-linked glycosylation of several enzymes and proteins with alteration in signal transduction pathways and oxidative stress. The O-linked attachment of N-acetylglucosamine (O-GlcNAc) on serine and threonine residues of nuclear and cytoplasmic proteins is associated with insulin resistance and cardiovascular complications of diabetes mellitus.[195,196]

Microvascular Disease

Diabetic microvascular complications are a leading cause of blindness, end-stage renal failure, and various neuropathies.[197] Thickening of the capillary basement membrane, endothelial cell hyperplasia, thrombosis, and pericyte degeneration are characteristic of diabetic microangiopathy and emerges over a period of 1 to 2 years. The thickening eventually results in decreased tissue perfusion. Hyperglycemia is a prerequisite for these microvascular changes and may be related to glycation of structural proteins, which results in the accumulation of AGEs. The frequency of the lesions appears to be proportional to the duration of the disease and blood glucose levels. In the DCCT study, individuals with tightly controlled blood glucose were half as likely to have renal and eye complications as those who received standard treatment.[198] Hypoxia and ischemia of various organs may result from microangiopathy. Three areas often affected are the retina, the kidney, and nerves.

Retinopathy

The retina is the most metabolically active structure per weight of tissue in the body. Thus the retina is a vulnerable target for microvascular disease in diabetes mellitus. **Diabetic retinopathy** appears to be a response to retinal ischemia resulting from blood vessel changes and red blood cell aggregation (Figure 21-16). Low-grade inflammation and poorly controlled hypertension is a risk factor for worsening of retinopathy. Vascular endothelial growth factors and GH appear to play a role in developing retinopathy, and therapeutic strategies have been developed to exploit this phenomenon.[199] The prevalence and severity of the retinopathy are strongly related to the age of the individual and duration of the diabetes and glycemic control. Retinopathy may be present in individuals at the time of diagnosis of type 2 diabetes as a result of the long preclinical latency of this form of diabetes. The vast majority of individuals with diabetes mellitus have some degree of retinopathy, and retinopathy is closely associated with systemic vascular complications including nephropathy, cardiovascular complications, and stroke.[200]

The three stages of retinopathy are described in Table 21-13. *Nonproliferative retinopathy* (stage I) is characterized by an increase in retinal capillary permeability, vein dilation, microaneurysm formation, superficial (flame-shaped) and deep (blot) hemorrhages, cotton wool spots from nerve damage, and macular edema. *Preproliferative retinopathy* (stage II) is a progression of retinal ischemia with areas of poor perfusion that culminate in infarcts. *Proliferative diabetic retinopathy* (stage III) is the result of neovascularization and fibrous tissue formation within the retina or optic disc. Traction of the new vessels on the vitreous humor may cause retinal detachment or hemorrhage into the vitreous humor.[201]

Maculopathy is a progressive process that may accompany the increased retinal capillary permeability, vessel occlusion, and ischemia. If formation of exudates, edema, or ischemia

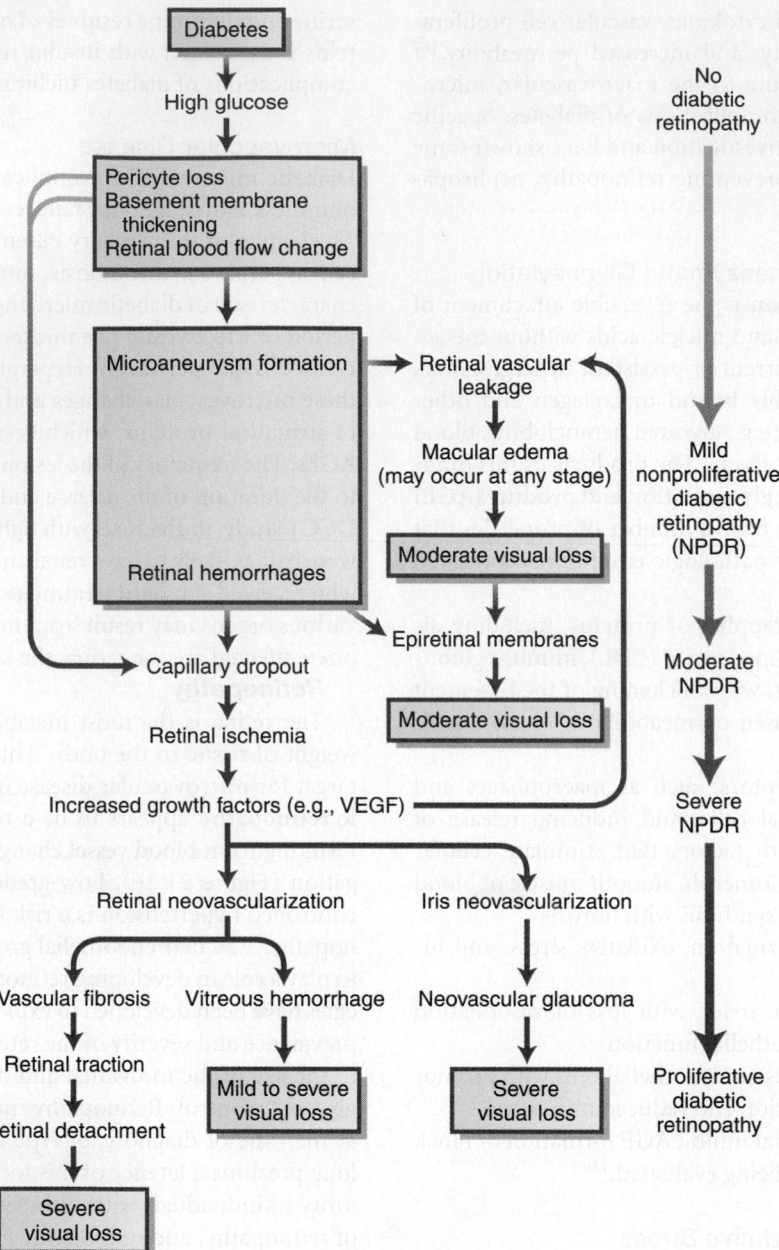

Figure 21-16 Diabetic retinopathy. *VEGF*, Vascular endothelial growth factor. (From Kronenberg et al: *Williams textbook of endocrinology,* ed 11, Philadelphia, 2008, Saunders.)

occurs near the fovea, serious loss of vision may result. Laser treatments are used to reduce the rate of vision loss from diabetic macular edema and neovascularization. Vitrectomy is a surgical procedure used to treat an intravitreal hemorrhage secondary to rupture of a neovascular capillary tuft. Cataracts, optic neuropathy and defects in eye muscle function are also associated with the chronic complications of hyperglycemia and diabetes mellitus.

Diabetic Nephropathy

Diabetes is the most common cause of end-stage renal disease in the Western world. Without appropriate management, approximately 30% of individuals with type 1 and 40% of those with type 2 diabetes develop nephropathy.[202] The

early phases of nephropathy are asymptomatic and begin to develop after 10 years in type 1 diabetes or 5 to 8 years in type 2 diabetes. There are some differences in renal lesions in type 1 and type 2 diabetes, with glomerular changes in type 1 being most prominent; however, hyperglycemia is the major initiating factor in both types.[203]

The exact process responsible for destruction of kidneys in diabetes is unknown. Multiple mechanisms contribute to nephropathy, including hyperglycemia, systemic hypertension, hyperperfusion, hyperfiltration, increased blood viscosity, increased glomerular pressure, albuminuria, protein kinase C, growth factors, advanced glycation end products, inflammatory cytokines, oxidative stress, the

Table 21-13 | Findings in Diabetic Retinopathy

Stages of Retinopathy	Pathologic Findings
Nonproliferative Retinopathy (Stage I)	
Venous abnormalities	Increased tortuosity, dilation with irregular constriction; frequency increases with increased severity of retinopathy
Microaneurysms	Mostly thin walled, 15-50 mcg in diameter, pathogenesis controversial
Interretinal hemorrhage	Circular and small; may take several months to resorb
Macular edema	Caused by serum leakage through incompetent vessel walls, may resorb in several weeks
Hard exudates	Characteristically "hard" exudates with pattern of exudation irregular in shape and sharply defined may appear and disappear over months to years; common with hypertension; "soft" exudates may appear and disappear more often; related to increased retinal capillary permeability
Preproliferative Diabetic Retinopathy (Stage II)	
Cotton-wool patches	Infarcts of the nerve fiber layer caused by retinal ischemia
Intraretinal microvascular shunts	Tortuous shunts between patent and occluded retinal vessels
Proliferative Diabetic Retinopathy (Stage III)	
Neovascularization	New vessels surrounded by connective tissue; five distinct groups representing different hazards to the eye
Glial proliferation	Often produced to reinforce neovascularization; may occur on optic disc and along vascular arcades
Vitreoretinal traction hemorrhage; retinal detachment	Traction occurring from the vitreous jelly; eventually causes small blood vessels to hemorrhage and retinal detachment to occur

renin-angiotensin-aldosterone system, and hypercholesterolemia.[204-206] Genetic factors may confer susceptibility or resistance to diabetic nephropathy in type 1 diabetes.[207] The glomeruli are injured by at least two mechanisms: protein denaturation by high glucose levels and adverse effects of intraglomerular microcirculatory hypertension. Renal glomerular changes can occur early in diabetes mellitus and occasionally may precede the overt manifestations of the disease (Figure 21-17). Glomerular enlargement and glomerular basement membrane (GBM) thickening, resulting in diffuse intercapillary glomerulosclerosis, develop during the first few years of diabetes. The Kimmelstiel-Wilson nodule, with thickening at the center of the glomerular lobules and thickening of the peripheral basement membrane, is distinctive in individuals with diabetes.[208] Increased mesangial matrix occurs contributing to resistance of glomerular capillary blood flow and decreased glomerular filtration rates. The tubular basement membrane also thickens in parallel with GBM thickening and mesangial expansion.

Microalbuminuria is the first manifestation of renal dysfunction (30 to 300 mg/day). Continuous untreated proteinuria generally heralds a life expectancy less than 10 years. Microalbuminuria is also an independent risk factor for cardiovascular disease.[209] The determinants of proteinuria in diabetic nephropathy are not completely understood. Glycated albumin generates ROS and directly damages glomerular membrane epithelial cells, vascular smooth muscle, and mesangial cells. Glomerular endothelial dysfunction also promotes albuminuria.[210,211] As renal failure progresses, extensive vascular and extravascular changes occur.

Before the development of clinical proteinuria (more than 300 mg/day), no clinical signs or symptoms of progressive glomerulosclerosis are likely to be evident. Later, hypoproteinemia, reduction in plasma oncotic pressure, fluid overload, anasarca (generalized body edema), and hypertension may occur.[212] Microalbuminuria and clinical proteinuria are risk factors for cardiovascular disease and progressive renal impairment.[213]

As renal function continues to deteriorate, individuals with type 1 diabetes may experience hypoglycemia, which necessitates a decrease in insulin therapy. The hypoglycemia occurs because the kidney's ability to metabolize insulin is lost along with other renal functions. As the glomerular filtration rate drops below 10 ml/minute, uremic signs such as nausea, lethargy, acidosis, anemia, and uncontrolled hypertension occur (see Chapter 36 for a discussion of renal failure). Impaired kidney function also accelerates retinopathy and cardiovascular disease.[214]

The development of more sensitive tests has permitted the detection of small amounts of urinary albumin, microalbuminuria. Earlier intervention with tight glucose control and angiotensin-converting enzyme (ACE) inhibitors or angiotensin II receptor blockers has reduced proteinuria and slowed the progression of nephropathy. Aggressive treatment of hypertension is another therapeutic intervention definitively shown to slow the progression of established renal disease.[215]

Diabetic Neuropathies

Diabetic neuropathy is the most common cause of neuropathy in the Western world and is probably the most common complication of diabetes. Nerves do not require insulin for glucose transport and are particularly vulnerable to the pathologic effects of hyperglycemia. The prevalence of neuropathy is similar for type 1 and type 2 diabetes.[216] Neuropathy in type 1 diabetes has more severe structural and functional changes and more rapid progression.[217] Neuropathy and other long-term complications are thought to result from the interaction of multiple metabolic, genetic, and environmental factors.

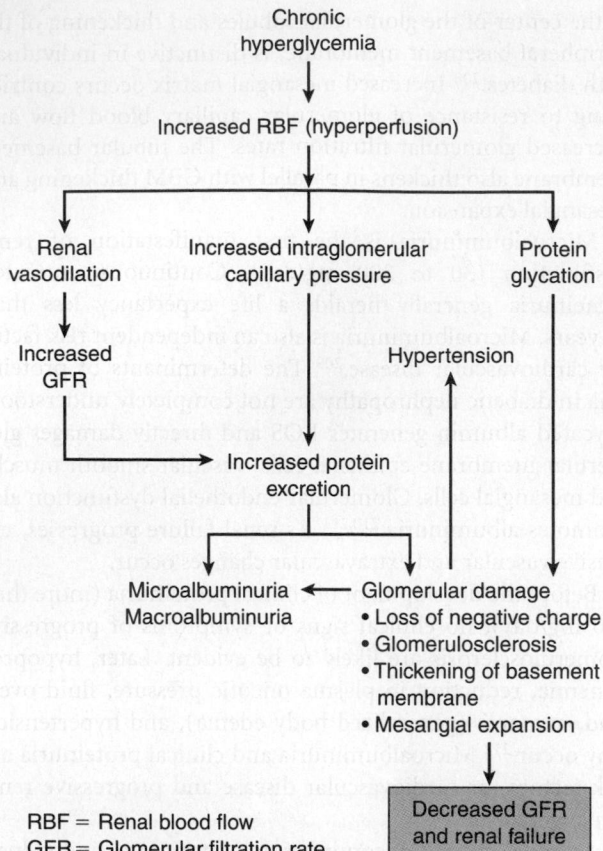

RBF = Renal blood flow
GFR = Glomerular filtration rate

Figure 21-17 Diabetic nephropathy.

The underlying pathophysiology is complex and related to chronic hyperglycemia. A combination of mechanisms is likely, including microangiopathy, oxidative stress, growth factor deficiency, abnormal signaling from AGE-RAGE interaction, polyol flux, and inflammation[218] (Figure 21-18). Neuropathy is classified into two stages: subclinical and clinical. In the subclinical stage, there is electromyographic (EMG) evidence of peripheral nerve dysfunctions, such as slowed motor and sensory nerve conduction, without clinical signs. In the clinical stage, symptoms or clinically detectable neurologic deficits are present.

Diabetic neuropathy is a form of "dying back" neuropathy, in which the distal portions of the neurons are initially and eventually more severely affected. The earliest morphologic change in both the peripheral nerves and central nervous system is axonal degeneration that preferentially involves sensory nerve fibers, particularly the smaller polymodal unmyelinated peripheral C fibers and the larger myelinated A-delta fibers. Metabolic activity of Schwann cells is disturbed, causing segmental loss of myelin and a characteristic pattern of demyelination and remyelination observed in long-term diabetic neuropathy. The location of the pathologic condition can include the spinal cord, the posterior root ganglia, or the peripheral nerves. These changes may occur alone or in combination. Nerve degeneration begins in

the periphery. Sensory nerve injury generally precedes motor nerve injury.[219]

Distal symmetric polyneuropathy (sensory, autonomic, and motor nerve involvement) is the most common neuropathy with involvement of both large and small nerve fibers. Loss of small nerve fiber function includes neuropathic pain, loss of sensation, and carries high risk for development of foot ulceration with subsequent gangrene and amputation. Large nerve fiber involvement results in sensory loss of proprioception and vibration with ataxia, loss of coordination, and risk for falls and fractures.[220]

Involvement of the autonomic nervous system can also occur early. Multiple alterations can develop affecting gastrointestinal enteric nerves (nausea, bloating, gastroparesis, diarrhea, or constipation), bladder and sexual function (loss of bladder sensation, urine retention, recurrent infection, erectile dysfunction), sweating, and body temperature regulation. Cardiovascular autonomic neuropathy may occur early particularly in type 1 diabetes with heart rate variability,

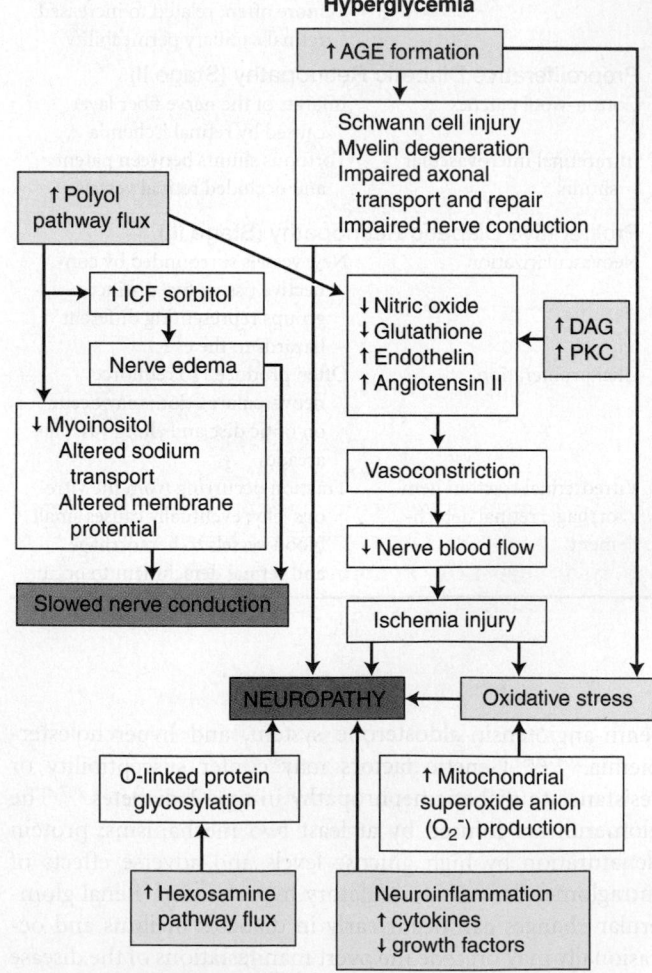

Figure 21-18 Multifactorial pathogenesis of diabetic neuropathy. The yellow boxes represent the consequences of chronic hyperglycemia in the development of neuropathy. *AGE,* Advanced glycosylation end product; *DAG,* diacylglycerol; *ICF,* intracellular fluid; *PKC,* protein kinase C.

changes in baroreceptor reflexes, postural hypotension, dysrhythmias, exercise intolerance, and painless myocardial infarction.[221,222]

Alterations in cognitive function and increased risk for dementia may accompany long-term complications in the brain particularly in type 2 diabetes. Cognitive alterations in type 1 diabetes are more controversial.[223,224]

Alterations in sensory perception and motor nerve conduction velocity and electromyography have shown abnormalities at the onset of diabetes and there are varying manifestations of diabetic neuropathies involving both the somatic and autonomic nerves (Table 21-14). Some of the neuropathic syndromes are progressive, but many—such as painful peripheral neuropathy, mononeuropathy (wristdrop, footdrop), diabetic amyotrophy, diabetic neuropathic cachexia, and visceral manifestations associated with autonomic neuropathy (e.g., diabetic diarrhea and orthostatic hypotension)—may spontaneously improve. *Charcot neuroarthropathy* (Charcot joint) is the progressive degeneration and structural disorganization of a joint, particularly in the foot of people with long-term diabetes. The pathogenesis is not clear but may be related to loss of sensation or neurally mediated alterations in osteoclastic bone resorption, or both.[225] The DCCT demonstrated a 60% reduction in results related to the appearance of clinical neuropathy and parameters of subclinical nerve dysfunction in the intensive insulin therapy cohort.[198] Similar results were seen in the Kumamoto trial[226] and the United Kingdom Prospective Diabetes Study.[227] Much investigation regarding the pathophysiology and progression of diabetic neuropathies remains to be done.

Macrovascular Disease

Macrovascular disease is a major cause of morbidity and mortality, particularly among individuals with type 2 diabetes mellitus. Children with poorly controlled type 2 diabetes have high risk for macrovascular disease within one or two decades.[228] The premature atherosclerosis of diabetes has many contributing factors, including hyperinsulinemia (insulin resistance), hyperglycemia, hypertriglyceridemia, low HDL, high LDL, lipoprotein oxidation, inflammation, vascular consequences of AGEs and their endothelial receptors (RAGEs), and altered endothelial function. The fibrous plaques of atherosclerosis are associated with the proliferation of subendothelial smooth muscle in the arterial wall. Other factors in the serum of individuals with diabetes also stimulate this proliferation (Figure 21-19).

In addition, deposition of lipids in vascular lesions may be facilitated in individuals with diabetes. Triglyceride elevations with low levels of the protective HDL cholesterol are common in individuals with type 2 diabetes mellitus in association with increased quantities of small, dense (very atherogenic) LDL cholesterol and endothelial cell and platelet abnormalities.[229] Increased levels of the atherogenic oxidized LDL also are seen in hyperglycemic individuals. Hypertension can increase capillary wall pressure, damage endothelium, increase capillary permeability, decrease nitric oxide

Table 21-14	Classification of Diabetic Neuropathies
Type of Neuropathy	**Characteristics**
Hyperglycemic neuropathy	Hyperesthesia, tingling and pain associated with hyperglycemia that resolves with glycemic control
Distal symmetric polyneuropathy (sensorimotor neuropathy)	Loss of large and small myelinated and unmyelinated nerve fibers
	Longest nerves affected first with numbness, tingling, and pain (sharp, burning, aching) in toes and feet then ascending to hands (stocking and glove pattern); loss of vibration and proprioception (large nerve fiber); loss of sensory light touch and temperature and pain (small nerve fiber)
	Motor nerves affected later with weakness, depressed reflexes and gait disturbances
Autonomic neuropathy	Cardiovascular: postural hypotension; exercise intolerance; silent myocardial infarction
	Gastrointestinal: decreased esophageal motility, gastroparesis and delayed gastric emptying, diabetic constipation or diarrhea
	Genitourinary tract: neurogenic bladder, urine retention, erectile dysfunction and retrograde ejaculation in men
	Sudomotor: anhydrosis, gustatory sweating
	Cranial nerve III: pain and ptosis and may spare the pupil
Mononeuropathies (focal neuropathies)	Compression and entrapment syndromes: carpel tunnel syndrome, radial nerve (wrist drop), peroneal nerve (foot drop), femoral nerve
	Cranial neuropathies: cranial nerve III, pain and ptosis and may spare the pupil
	Truncal mononeuropathy: abdominal or lower chest pain or hyperesthesia, abdominal muscle weakness
	Asymmetric lower limb neuropathy (diabetic amyotrophy; diabetic polyradiculopathy): involvement of lower thoracic and lumbar nerve roots (upper leg weakness, upper leg muscle atrophy, diminished knee and ankle tendon reflexes); may have paresthesia, hyperesthesia, pain

synthesis, and decrease autoregulation of blood flow.[230,231] Further work is needed to clarify the complexities of macrovascular complications.

Coronary Artery Disease

The risk of coronary artery disease (CAD) for those individuals with type 2 diabetes is higher than for the general population even when hypertension and hyperlipidemia are taken into account. CAD is the most common cause of death in individuals with type 2 diabetes and is common in those with type 1.[232] In general, the prevalence of CAD increases with the duration but not the severity of diabetes.

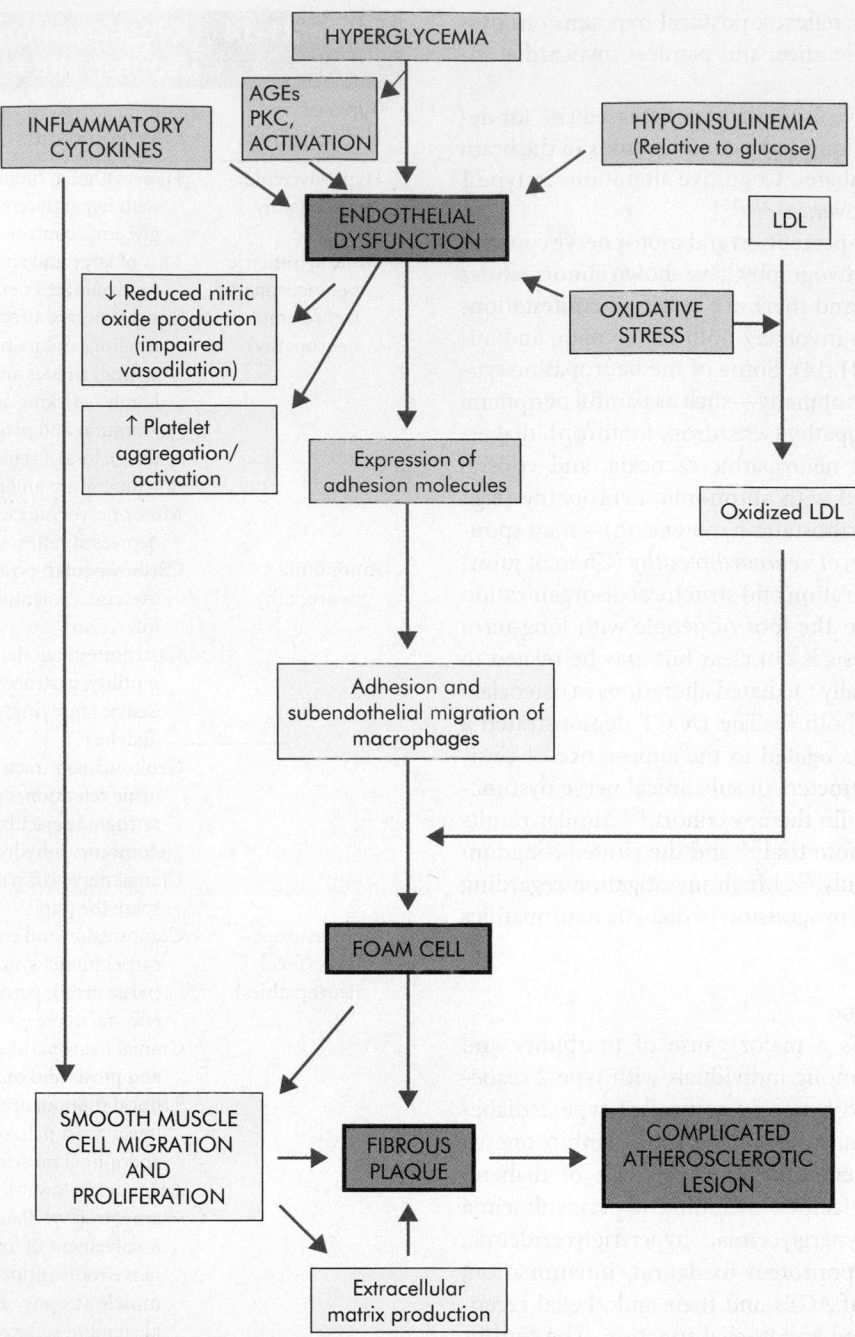

Figure 21-19 Diabetes mellitus and atherosclerosis. Diabetes with its associated hyperglycemia, relative hypoinsulinemia, oxidative stress, and proinflammatory state contributes to atherogenesis by causing arterial endothelial dysfuncton (impaired vasodilation, adhesion of inflammatory cells and alteration in permeability), dyslipidemia and smooth muscle proliferation resulting in atherosclerotic lesions. *AGEs*, Advanced glycosylation end products; *LDL*, low-density lipoprotein; *PKC*, protein kinase C.

Myocardial infarction (death of heart muscle as a result of coronary artery occlusion) is the cause of death in 20% of those with diabetes, and individuals with diabetes mellitus have a higher mortality during the acute phase of myocardial infarctions than do nondiabetic individuals. Increased platelet adhesion and decreased fibrinolysis promote thrombus formation and vascular occlusion.[233] In addition, the incidence of cardiomyopathy (myocardial dysfunction in the absence of coronary artery disease [CAD] and hypertension) is higher in

individuals with diabetes. The reason is unclear but may be related to the presence of increased amounts of collagen in the ventricular wall, which reduces the mechanical compliance of the heart during filling, inflammation, and changes in calcium handling. Diastolic dysfunction is the earliest symptom.[234]

Stroke

Stroke is twice as common in those with diabetes as in the nondiabetic population.[235] Ischemic stroke is more common than hemorrhagic stroke. The survival rate for an individual with diabetes after a massive stroke is typically shorter than for a person without diabetes. Hypertension, hyperglycemia, and dyslipidemia are definite risk factors (see Chapter 30), and aggressive management of blood pressure, hyperglycemia, and lipidemia in individuals with diabetes has been shown to reduce the incidence of stroke.[236]

Peripheral Arterial Disease

The increased incidence of peripheral arterial disease (PAD), neuropathy, gangrene, and amputation in diabetic persons has been documented in many studies, particularly in individuals with type 2 diabetes.[237,238] Many individuals with type 2 diabetes have evidence of peripheral vascular disease at the time of their initial diagnosis. The atherosclerotic process in diabetic persons is more common, appears at a younger age, advances more rapidly than vascular changes in nondiabetic persons, and increases the risk of cardiac death.[239] The prevalence of PAD is nearly equal in males and females with diabetes. Age, duration of diabetes, glycemic control, genetics, and additional risk factors influence the development of PAD.

Because of occlusions of the small arteries and arterioles, most of the gangrenous changes of the lower extremities occur in patchy areas of the feet and toes.[240] Smaller vessels often have more advanced disease than larger vessels in the same individuals. Figure 21-20 illustrates how foot lesions of diabetes can lead to amputation. Fifty percent of nontraumatic amputations in the United States are performed on individuals with diabetes. Hospital mortality for individuals with diabetes who undergo major amputation is between 10% and 23%. The survival rate after surgery is only about 40% at the end of 5 years.[237]

Infection

Increased morbidity and mortality from infectious agents have been documented in those with diabetes.[241] The individual with diabetes is at increased risk for infection throughout the body for several reasons:

1. Impaired vision caused by retinal changes and impaired touch caused by neuropathy diminish the prevention of breaks in the skin by decreasing the early warning systems. Once breaks in skin integrity occur, tissues may have increased susceptibility to infection because of hypoxia, a second reason for susceptibility to infection.
2. Microvascular and macrovascular complications cause decreased oxygen supply to tissues. In addition, the increased content of glycosylated hemoglobin in the red blood cell impedes the release of oxygen to tissues.
3. Pathogens are able to multiply rapidly once they have gained access to the tissues. Some pathogens proliferate rapidly because the increased glucose in body fluids provides an excellent source of energy.
4. Decreased blood supply resulting from vascular changes decreases the supply of white blood cells to the affected area.
5. Function of the white cells is impaired by ischemia and hyperglycemia. Chemotaxis is abnormal, and phagocytosis is defective.

6. Inflammatory responses to microbial invasion are diminished and clinical signs of infection may be absent.
7. Sensory neuropathy leads to loss of protective sensation with injury and repeated trauma that leads to open wounds and soft tissue or osseous infection.

The risk of infection is especially high for individuals undergoing surgery and for those taking immunosuppressant medications.[242,243]

ALTERATIONS OF ADRENAL FUNCTION

Disorders of the Adrenal Cortex

Disorders of the adrenal cortex are related to either hyperfunction or hypofunction. Hyperfunction that causes increased levels of circulating cortisol leads to Cushing disease, or Cushing syndrome; hyperfunction that causes increased secretion of adrenal androgens and estrogens leads to virilization or feminization; and hyperfunction that causes increased levels of aldosterone leads to hyperaldosteronism, which may be primary or secondary. Hypofunction of the adrenal cortex leads to Addison disease.

Adrenocortical Hyperfunction: Cushing Disease, Cushing Syndrome

Cushing disease is caused by excessive anterior pituitary secretion of ACTH. **Cushing syndrome** is an uncommon disorder and occurs whenever there is an excessive level of cortisol regardless of the cause. Cushing syndrome is the most common complication of Cushing disease. Cushing-like syndrome may develop as a result of the exogenous administration of glucocorticoids.[244] Endogenous Cushing syndrome is divided into two main forms: corticotropin dependent and corticotropin independent. *Corticotropin-dependent Cushing syndrome* is the most common (80% to 85% of cases), primarily because of ACTH-secreting pituitary tumors and is more common in women. The remaining cases are usually derived from ACTH-secreting carcinoid tumors or small-cell carcinoma of the lung. *Corticotropin-independent Cushing syndrome* is less common (15% to 20% of cases) and is usually caused by an adrenal tumor or, more rarely, corticotropin-independent macronodular adrenal hyperplasia, primary pigmented nodular adrenal disease.[245] Adrenal tumors, rather than pituitary tumors, are more common in children, especially girls.[246] In Cushing disease there is a loss of normal feedback inhibition by cortisol because there appears to be a higher set point for cortisol feedback on corticotropin-releasing hormone (CRH) and ACTH secretion.

PATHOPHYSIOLOGY Although the origin of Cushing disease remains incompletely understood, the vast majority of individuals with Cushing disease have a pituitary microadenoma, which secretes ACTH.[247] Ectopic ACTH-secreting tumors are nonpituitary tumors that synthesize and hypersecrete ACTH, leading to hypercortisolism. Some tumors may hypersecrete CRH, which results in oversecretion of ACTH from the pituitary. Tumors associated with episodic secretion of ACTH and hypercortisolism include small cell carcinomas of

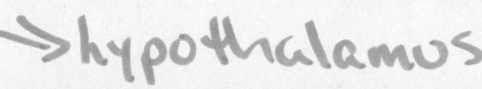
→ hypothalamus

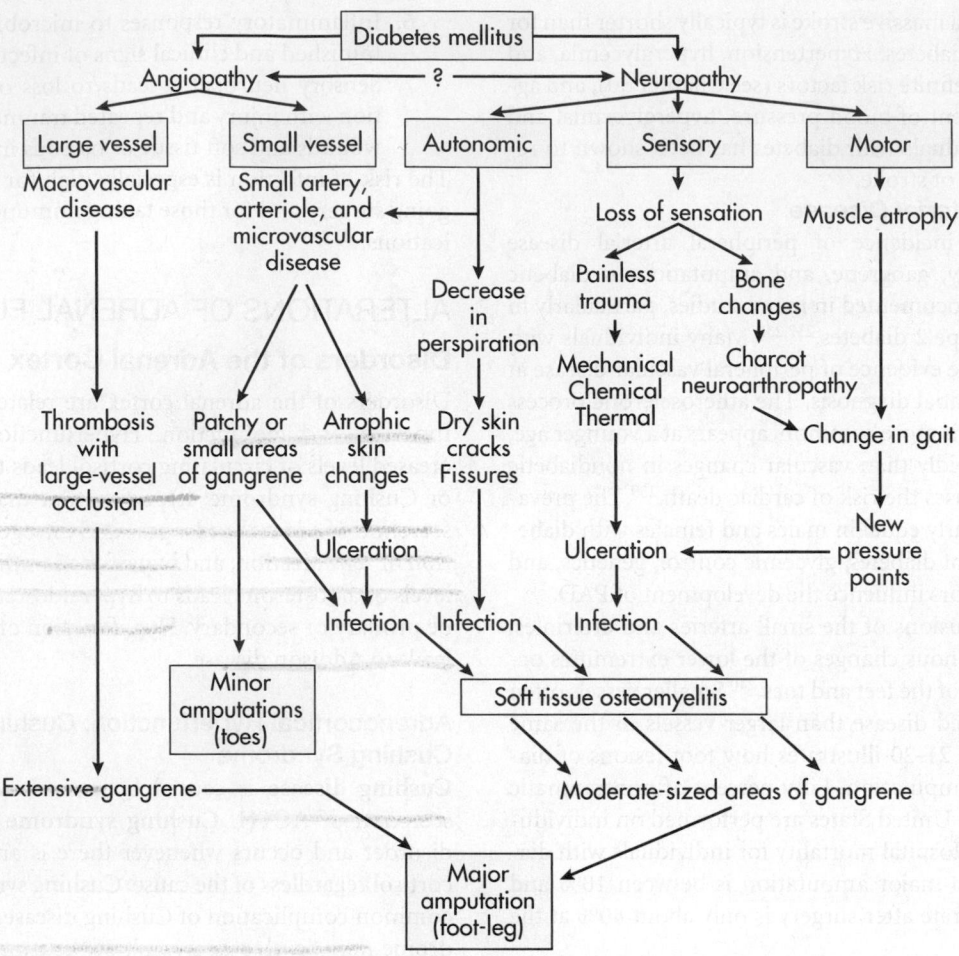

Figure 21-20 How foot lesions of diabetes can lead to amputation. (From Levin ME, O'Neal LW, Bowker JH: *The diabetic foot,* ed 5, St Louis, 1993, Mosby.)

the lung, thymoma, pancreatic cell tumors, carcinoid tumors, medullary carcinoma of the thyroid, and pheochromocytoma tumors. Even though the secretion of ectopic ACTH from the neoplasm is not under hypothalamic-pituitary control, the normal pituitary release of ACTH is inhibited by the elevated levels of cortisol. However, cortisol fails to inhibit the release of ACTH from the ectopic source. Autonomous secretion of cortisol can be the result of either an adrenal adenoma or, less commonly, adrenal cortical carcinoma.[248]

Elevated cortisol levels suppress CRH and ACTH release secretion from the hypothalamus and anterior pituitary, respectively, which leads to low levels of ACTH. Low levels of ACTH cause atrophy of the remaining normal portions of the adrenal cortex, which over time will alter the cortisol-secreting activity of normal cells. The normal diurnal variation in cortisol secretion is lost in individuals with hypercortisolism regardless of the underlying cause.

CLINICAL MANIFESTATIONS Most of the clinical signs and symptoms of Cushing syndrome are caused by hypercortisolism.[249] Weight gain is the most common feature and results from the accumulation of adipose tissue in the trunk, facial, and cervical areas. These characteristic patterns of fat

deposition have been described as "truncal [central] obesity," "moon face," and "buffalo hump" (Figures 21-21 and 21-22). Transient weight gain from sodium and water retention may be present because of the mineralocorticoid effects of cortisol, exhibited when cortisol is present in high levels.

Glucose intolerance occurs because of cortisol-induced insulin resistance and increased gluconeogenesis and glycogen storage by the liver. Overt diabetes mellitus develops in approximately 20% of individuals with hypercortisolism. Polyuria, which is sometimes seen in hypercortisolism, is a manifestation of hyperglycemia and resultant glycosuria.

Protein wasting is commonly observed in hypercortisolism and is caused by the catabolic effects of cortisol on peripheral tissues. Muscle wasting leads to muscle weakness and is especially obvious in the muscles of the extremities with thinning of the limbs. Hypercortisolism increases bone resorption, inhibits bone formation, decreases intestinal calcium absorption, and increases renal calcium excretion. This leads to osteoporosis, with pathologic fractures, vertebral compression fractures, bone and back pain, kyphosis, and reduced height. Hypercalciuria may result in renal stones, which are experienced by approximately 20% of individuals with this disease.

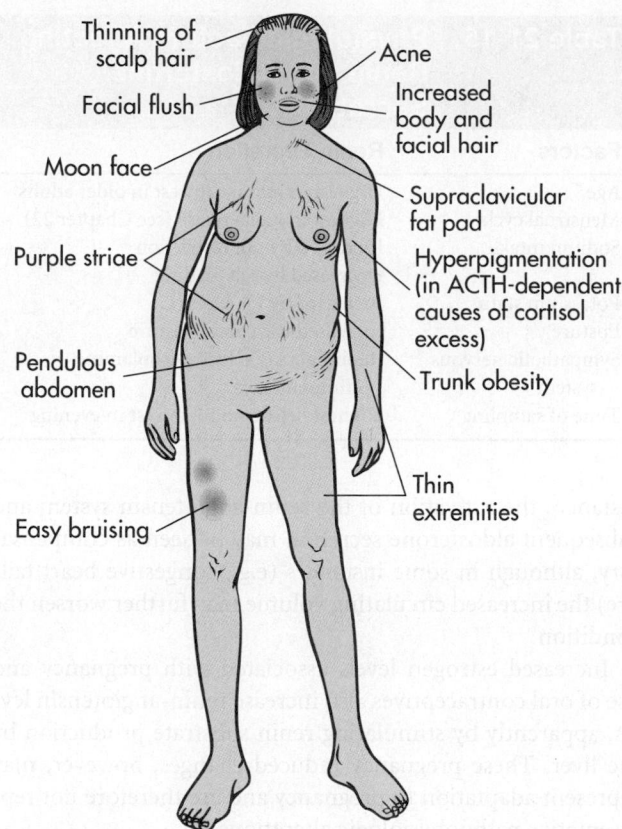

Figure 21-21 Symptoms of Cushing disease. *ACTH*, Adrenocorticotropic hormone.

Loss of collagen also leads to thin, weakened integumentary tissues through which capillaries are more visible; the tissues are easily stretched by adipose deposits. Together these changes account for the characteristic purple striae most often observed in the truncal area. Loss of collagenous support around small vessels makes them susceptible to rupture, leading to easy bruising, even with minor trauma. Thin, atrophied skin is also easily damaged, leading to skin breaks and ulcerations.

Hyperpigmentation in Cushing syndrome is associated with very high serum levels of ACTH, believed to be caused by increased melanocyte-stimulating hormones resulting from excess conversion of pro-opiomelanocortin when ACTH is elevated.[250] The pigmentation involves the mucous membranes, hair, and skin, all of which acquire a characteristic brownish or bronze color.

Cortisol has a permissive effect on the actions of the catecholamines. With elevated cortisol levels, vascular sensitivity to catecholamines is increased significantly, leading to vasoconstriction and hypertension. Metabolic syndrome with abdominal obesity, hypertension, glucose intolerance, and dyslipidemias is a common complication (see p. 751). Chronically elevated cortisol levels also cause suppression of the immune system and increased susceptibility to infections. Consequently, individuals with hypercortisolism experience poor wound healing and are particularly susceptible to superficial fungal infections.

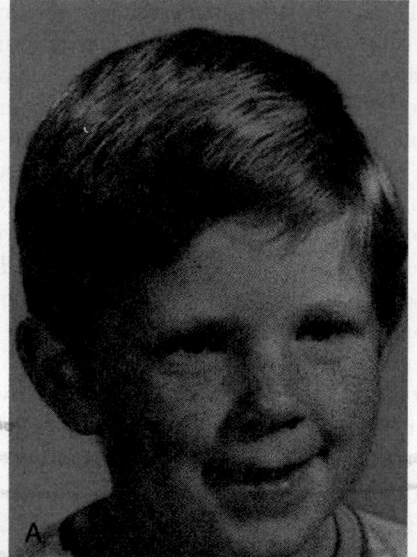

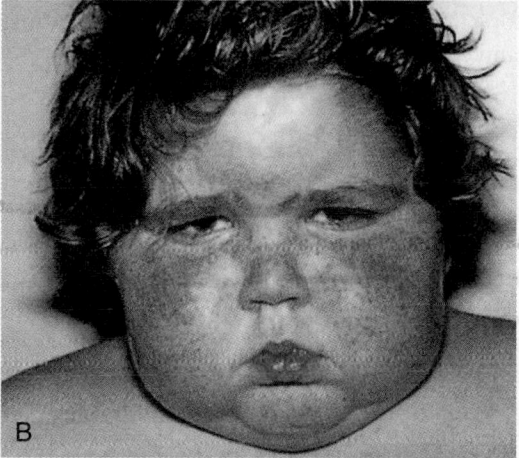

Figure 21-22 Cushing syndrome. **A,** Patient before onset of Cushing syndrome. **B,** Patient 4 months later. Moon facies is clearly demonstrated. (From Zitelli BJ, Davis HW: *Atlas of pediatric physical diagnosis*, ed 4, London, 2002, Gower.)

Approximately 50% of individuals with Cushing syndrome experience alterations in their mental status and include effects of cortisol on hippocampal neurons and the implications for learning and memory and other neurologic functions when cortisol is elevated. These may range from irritability and depression to severe psychiatric disturbances such as schizophrenia.[251,252] The effects of glucocorticoids on mood are complex.

Females may experience symptoms of increased adrenal androgen levels, increased hair growth (especially facial hair), acne, and oligomenorrhea. Androgen levels rarely become high enough to cause changes of the voice, recession of the hairline, and clitoral hypertrophy unless an adrenal carcinoma is involved. Infertility is common in men and women.[253] Routine laboratory examinations may reveal hyperglycemia, glycosuria, hypokalemia, and metabolic alkalosis.

EVALUATION AND TREATMENT A variety of laboratory tests must be used to diagnose hypercortisolism and to determine the underlying disorder.[254] These include urinary free cortisol higher than 50 mcg per 24 hours, abnormal dexamethasone suppressibility of either urinary or serum cortisol, and simultaneous measurement of ACTH and cortisol. Late evening salivary cortisol levels are used as a screening test and to document alterations in the diurnal variation of cortisol. Visualizing procedures, including pituitary MRI or abdominal scanning, are essential in the evaluation. Selective catheterization of the veins draining the pituitary (inferior petrosal sinus sampling) is very helpful in determining the cause of hypercortisolism and in localizing pituitary tumors.[249] The diagnosis and evaluation of hypercortisolism is one of the most challenging problems in endocrinology.[255]

Without treatment, approximately 50% of individuals with Cushing syndrome die within 5 years of onset. Major causes of death are overwhelming infection, suicide, complications from generalized arteriosclerosis, and hypertensive disease. Treatment is specific for the cause of hypercorticoadrenalism and includes medication, radiation therapy, and surgery.[256,257] Therefore, it is essential to differentiate between pituitary, adrenal, and ectopic causes of the hypercortisolism.

Hyperaldosteronism

Hyperaldosteronism is characterized by excessive aldosterone secretion by the adrenal cortex. The excessive secretion can result from a primary adrenal disorder, such as an aldosterone-secreting adenoma, or from excessive stimulation of the normal adrenal cortex by substances such as angiotensin II, ACTH, or elevated potassium. Both primary and secondary forms of hyperaldosteronism can occur in individuals. **Primary aldosteronism (primary hyperaldosteronism)** refers to an excessive secretion of aldosterone caused by an abnormality of the adrenal cortex. Several different subtypes have been identified.[258] **Secondary aldosteronism (secondary hyperaldosteronism)** involves excessive aldosterone secretion from an extra-adrenal stimulus, most often angiotensin II through a renin-dependent mechanism.

Primary aldosteronism (Conn disease, primary hyperaldosteronism) presents a clinical picture of hypertension, hypokalemia, renal potassium wasting, and neuromuscular manifestations. The most common cause of primary aldosteronism are a benign, single aldosterone-producing adrenal adenoma (30% to 40% of cases) and idiopathic bilateral adrenal hyperplasia (60%). Other rare tumors account for the remainder of cases.[259] The incidence of primary hyperaldosteronism is not known, but 5% to 13% of individuals with hypertension have primary aldosteronism.[260]

Secondary aldosteronism can be expected to result from sustained elevated renin release and activation of angiotensin II because aldosterone secretion is normally stimulated by the renin-angiotensin system. (Factors that affect renin and aldosterone secretion are summarized in Table 21-15.) Increased renin-angiotensin secretion occurs in a variety of situations. In general, these include decreased circulating blood volume (e.g., in dehydration, shock, or hypoalbuminemia) and decreased delivery of blood to the kidneys (e.g., renal artery stenosis, heart failure, or hepatic cirrhosis). In many of these

Table 21-15   Physiologic Factors Affecting Renin and Aldosterone Secretion

Factors	Renin Secretion
Age	Highest in infants; lowest in older adults
Menstrual cycle	Highest in luteal phase (see Chapter 22)
Sodium intake	Increased by salt restriction
	Decreased by salt loading
Potassium status	Increased by K^+ excess
Posture	Increased with erect posture
Sympathetic nervous system	Renin increased by catecholamine stimulation
Time of sampling	Highest before noon; lowest in evening

instances the activation of the renin-angiotensin system and subsequent aldosterone secretion may be seen as compensatory, although in some instances (e.g., congestive heart failure) the increased circulating volume may further worsen the condition.

Increased estrogen levels associated with pregnancy and use of oral contraceptives also increase renin-angiotensin levels, apparently by stimulating renin substrate production by the liver. These pregnancy-induced changes, however, may represent adaptation to pregnancy and are therefore not representative pathophysiologic alterations.

Other causes of secondary hyperaldosteronism include Bartter syndrome, which is a heterogeneous autosomal recessive disorder associated with reduced or absent salt transport by the thick ascending limb of the loop of Henle. Symptoms include salt wasting and low blood pressure, hypokalemia, metabolic acidosis, and hypercalciuria.[261] Renin-secreting tumors of the kidney also cause secondary hyperaldosteronism. Diuretic use is perhaps the most common cause of secondary hyperaldosteronism. (Renal disorders are discussed in Chapter 36.) Apparent mineralocorticoid excess can be seen in individuals who consume excess licorice (glycyrrhizic acid) or chewing tobacco.

PATHOPHYSIOLOGY In *primary hyperaldosteronism*, pathophysiologic alterations are caused by excessive aldosterone secretion and the fluid and electrolyte imbalances that ensue. Hyperaldosteronism promotes increased sodium reabsorption with corresponding hypervolemia (see Chapter 3). The extracellular fluid volume overload and suppression of normal feedback mechanisms of renin secretion are characteristic of primary disorders.

Edema usually does not occur with primary aldosteronism, possibly because of the renal tubular "escape" phenomenon that is activated in chronic hyperaldosteronism. The escape phenomenon changes or resets the rate of sodium excretion and prevents more severe sodium retention. The escape phenomenon operates in the proximal tubules and causes additional sodium to pass to the distal tubules, where the sodium is, to some extent, reabsorbed in exchange for potassium. This mechanism, while protecting from excessive sodium reabsorption and edema, increases urinary losses of potassium

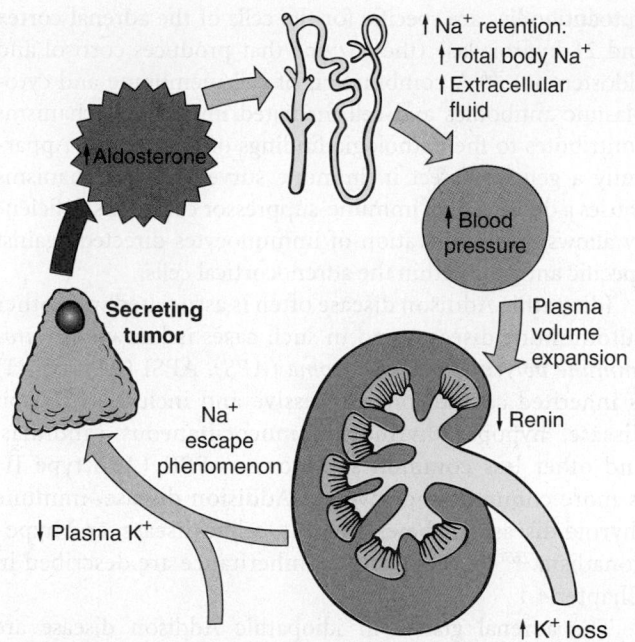

Figure 21-23 Primary hyperaldosteronism. Pathophysiology of mineralocorticoid excess syndromes in primary hyperaldosteronism.

and causes hypokalemia (Figure 21-23). Metabolic syndrome (hypertension, obesity, dyslipidemia, and hyperglycemia) also is associated with primary aldosteronism and may be related to insulin resistance that is related to aldosterone action on insulin receptor function.[262]

In *secondary hyperaldosteronism* the effect of increased extracellular volume on renin secretion may vary. If renin secretion is being stimulated by variables other than pressure-initiated cellular changes at the juxtaglomerular apparatus (see Chapter 35), increased circulating blood volume may not decrease renin secretion through feedback mechanisms. This physiologic process is normal in pregnancy and related to increased plasma estrogen.

In **Bartter syndrome** a state of hypokalemia develops because of defective renal tubular reabsorptive mechanisms. The hypokalemic state may induce the formation of prostaglandins (especially PGE_2) by the renal cells, which stimulates renin and hence aldosterone secretion. The stimulatory effect on aldosterone secretion is offset somewhat by the aldosterone-suppressing effects of hypokalemia.

Potassium secretion also is promoted by aldosterone, so that with excessive circulating levels of aldosterone, hypokalemia occurs (see Chapter 3). In hyperaldosteronism, hypokalemic alkalosis, changes in myocardial conduction, and skeletal muscle alterations may be seen, particularly with severe potassium depletion (i.e., the renal tubules may become insensitive to ADH, thus promoting excessive loss of free water). Rarely, this may result in mild hypernatremia because water is not able to follow the sodium that is reabsorbed.

CLINICAL MANIFESTATIONS Hypertension, and less commonly hypokalemia, and metabolic alkalosis are the hallmarks of hyperaldosteronism.[263] Hypertension may result from increased intravascular volume or from a state of aldosterone-mediated vasoconstriction, although the latter mechanism requires very high levels of aldosterone. If hypertension is sustained, the long-term effects of elevated arterial pressure become evident, which include the development of left ventricular dilation and hypertrophy. Because of the increased arterial pressure, renin secretion is typically suppressed, although it is elevated in secondary hyperaldosteronism, which provides a means to clearly differentiate between these conditions.

Aldosterone-stimulated potassium loss can be variable. Serum potassium levels below 3.0 mEq/L result in the typical manifestations of hypokalemia. Hypokalemic alkalosis is caused by the movement of potassium from the intercellular to extracellular space in exchange for hydrogen ions as well as renal loss of hydrogen ions to facilitate sodium reabsorption (see Chapter 3).

EVALUATION AND TREATMENT A variety of clinical and laboratory measurements are useful in the assessment of hyper aldosteronism.[264] These include blood pressure, serum and urinary electrolyte levels, serum and urinary levels of aldosterone and renin, plasma aldosterone concentration to plasma renin activity ratio, and aldosterone suppression testing. Blood pressure is elevated, serum sodium may be normal or elevated, serum potassium may be normal or depressed, and urinary potassium is elevated (i.e., more than 30 mmol/day). Serum aldosterone, as measured by radioimmunoassay, usually is greater than 15 ng/dl. Plasma renin activity is generally less than 1 ng/ml/hr for individuals with primary aldosteronism. A plasma aldosterone (in nanograms/dl)-to-renin (in nanograms/ml/hr) activity ratio of ≥ 20ng/dl is very suspicious for primary hyperaldosteronism. Serum aldosterone and plasma renin activity both must be measured under controlled situations and after careful dietary regulation of sodium and potassium intake (see Table 21-15). Aldosterone suppression testing commonly is accomplished with fludrocortisone acetate (Florinef) or salt loading. Imaging techniques, such as CT and nuclear magnetic resonance (NMR), may be used to localize an aldosterone-secreting adenoma. Selective venous catheterization of both adrenal veins is also useful.

Treatment includes management of hypertension and hypokalemia, as well as correction of any underlying causal abnormalities. If an aldosterone-secreting adenoma is present, it is generally approached surgically; however, medical management with spironolactone or eplerenone, a new drug without the side effects of spironolactone, is a viable option in complicated cases.[265]

Adrenocortical Hypofunction

Hypocortisolism (low levels of cortisol secretion) develops because of either inadequate stimulation of the adrenal glands by ACTH or a primary inability of the adrenals to produce and secrete the adrenocortical hormones. In some syndromes, however, there is partial dysfunction of the adrenal cortex so that only synthesis of cortisol and aldosterone or the adrenal androgens is affected. Hypofunction of the adrenal cortex may affect glucocorticoid or mineralocorticoid secretion or a combination of both.

Primary adrenal insufficiency is termed **Addison disease.** Addison disease is relatively rare, occurring most often in adults 30 to 60 years of age, although it may appear at any time throughout the life span. Addison disease, caused by autoimmune mechanisms, is more common in women.

The most common cause of Addison disease in the United States is autoimmune destruction of the adrenal cortex. Other causes include infections (tuberculosis, fungal, human immunodeficiency virus [HIV]), infiltrative diseases (amyloidosis, metastatic carcinoma), or bilateral adrenal hemorrhage. Adrenoleukodystrophy and adrenomyeloneuropathy are two rare types of X-linked adrenal deficiency that lead to symptoms of hypocortisolism and progressive neurologic symptoms.

PATHOPHYSIOLOGY Addison disease is characterized by elevated serum ACTH levels with inadequate corticosteroid synthesis and output. Before clinical manifestations of hypocortisolism are evident, more than 90% of total adrenocortical tissue must be destroyed.

Idiopathic Addison Disease

Idiopathic Addison disease (organ-specific autoimmune adrenalitis), which causes adrenal atrophy and hypofunction, generally is recognized as an organ-specific autoimmune disease. (Autoimmunity is discussed in Chapter 8.) It may occur in childhood (type 1) or adulthood (type 2). Autoantibodies are present in 50% to 70% of individuals with idiopathic Addison disease, and this percentage increases in younger persons and in those with other autoimmune diseases. The autoantibodies are specific for the cells of the adrenal cortex and 21-hydroxylase (the enzyme that produces cortisol and aldosterone).[266] A combination of cell membrane and cytoplasmic antibodies and cell-mediated immune mechanisms contributes to the pathologic findings of the disease. Apparently a genetic defect in immune surveillance mechanisms causes a deficiency of immune-suppressor cells. This deficiency allows the proliferation of immunocytes directed against specific antigens within the adrenocortical cells.

Idiopathic Addison disease often is associated with other autoimmune diseases and in such cases is known as *autoimmune polyendocrine syndrome (APS).* APSI (APS type I) is inherited as autosomal recessive and includes Addison disease, hypoparathyroidism, mucocutaneous candidias, and other less common symptoms. APSII (APS type II) is more common and involves Addision disease, immune thyroid disease, diabetes mellitus, celiac disease, and hypogonadism.[267] (Mechanisms of inheritance are described in Chapter 4.)

The adrenal glands in idiopathic Addison disease are smaller than normal and may be misshapen. Microscopically, gland atrophy is evident throughout the cortex, although the medulla appears intact. Extensive diffuse cortical lymphocytic infiltrate supports the immune component of the disease process.

Secondary Hypocortisolism

Secondary hypocortisolism is characterized by low to absent ACTH levels, which cause inadequate adrenal stimulation, adrenal atrophy, and ultimately decreased corticosteroidogenesis. The exogenous administration of glucocorticoids for nonendocrine disease results in this form of hypocortisolism. Successful surgical removal of cortisol-secreting tumors also results in postoperative hypocortisolism. In these cases, increased glucocorticoid levels suppress ACTH production through normal feedback mechanisms. With decreased ACTH levels, corticosteroid synthesis by remaining adrenal tissue is suppressed. Pituitary hypofunction (as occurs in postpartum pituitary infarction [Sheehan syndrome] and panhypopituitarism, hypophysectomy, or isolated ACTH deficiency) causes inadequate ACTH production and secretion and absence of pituitary responsiveness to normal stimulatory mechanisms. In all instances of low ACTH levels, adrenal atrophy occurs, and endogenous adrenal steroidogenesis is depressed.

Clinical manifestations of secondary hypocortisolism are similar to those of Addison disease. One difference is that with the typically low levels of ACTH seen in secondary hypocortisolism, hyperpigmentation does not occur. Second, the renin-angiotensin system is usually normal in these individuals; therefore, aldosterone and potassium levels also tend to be normal.

CLINICAL MANIFESTATIONS The symptoms of Addison disease are primarily a result of hypocortisolism and hypoaldosteronism and include weakness and fatigue, anorexia, weight loss, nausea, diarrhea, and orthostatic hypotension. Hyperpigmentation is associated with elevated ACTH levels.

Decreased adrenal androgen secretion is usually not clinically obvious in men because the adrenals are not a major source of male androgens. Women may experience a loss of some secondary sex characteristics, such as pubic and axillary hair, normally maintained by the adrenal androgens.[268] Disturbances in mood and motivation are common.[269] The symptoms of Addison disease are summarized in Table 21-16.

EVALUATION AND TREATMENT Serum and urine levels of cortisol are depressed with hypocortisolism. In primary adrenal insufficiency (Addison disease), ACTH levels are clearly elevated, and ACTH levels are low in secondary adrenal insufficiency. ACTH levels can be interpreted only in the face of a simultaneous measurement of cortisol. Individuals may develop azotemia caused by dehydration, and hyponatremia is common. Hyperkalemia is seen only in Addison disease, but hypoglycemia may be seen in hypocortisolism from any cause. Anemia, eosinophilia, and lymphocytosis are also common with symptoms of fatigue. The ACTH stimulation test may be used to evaluate adrenocortical function. This is achieved by administering ACTH and monitoring the serum cortisol levels.

The treatment of Addison disease involves glucocorticoid and possibly mineralocorticoid replacement therapy, together with dietary modifications. All individuals with hypocortisolism require lifetime daily glucocorticoid replacement therapy. In the event of acute stressors, additional cortisol must be administered to approximate the amount of cortisol that might be expected to be secreted if normal adrenal function were present (approximately 100 to 300 mg/day). Fludrocortisone is used for mineralocorticoid replacement therapy.[270]

The individual's diet should include at least 150 mEq of sodium per day, with sodium intake increased in the event of excessive sweating or diarrhea. Treatment also must include correction of any underlying disorders.

Hypersecretion of Adrenal Androgens and Estrogens

Hypersecretion of adrenal androgens and estrogens may be caused by adrenal tumors, either adenomas or carcinomas, Cushing syndrome, or defects in steroid synthesis. The clinical syndrome that results depends on the hormone secreted, the gender of the individual, and the ages at which the hypersecretion was initiated. Hypersecretion of estrogens causes **feminization,** the development of female sex characteristics. Hypersecretion of androgens causes **virilization,** the development of male sex characteristics (Figure 21-24).

Table 21-16	Clinical Manifestations and Pathophysiologic Mechanisms of Addison Disease

Clinical Manifestations	Pathophysiologic Mechanism
Weakness and easy fatigability that worsens as the day progresses, seen especially after exposure to stressors	Not known, may be related to hypoglycemia, hypotension, decreased metabolism of proteins
Gastrointestinal disturbances: anorexia, nausea, vomiting, diarrhea, abdominal pain, weight loss	May be associated with celiac disease or electrolyte abnormalities
Hypoglycemia, manifested by fatigue, mental confusion, apathy, psychosis	Absence of cortisol leads to decreased gluconeogenesis, decreased glycogen storage by liver, decreased metabolism of proteins, increased insulin sensitivity
Hyperpigmentation	Elevations of ACTH that lead to stimulation of melanocytes
Vitiligo (white patchy areas of depigmented skin)	Autoimmune destruction of melanocytes
Addisonian crisis: severe hypotension and vascular collapse	Combined effects of hypocortisolism, hypoaldosteronism, extracellular volume depletion, and some precipitating stressor (e.g., infection, vomiting, diarrhea); decreased vasomotor tone caused by cortisol deficiency

ACTH, Adrenocorticotropic hormone.

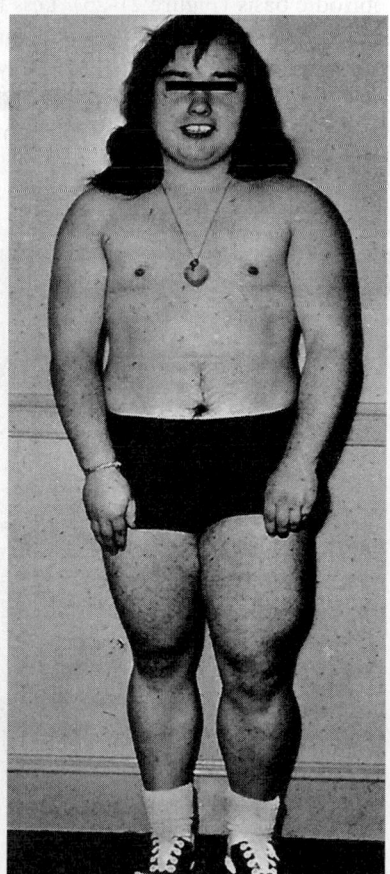

Figure 21-24 Virilization. Virilization of a young girl by an androgen-secreting tumor of the adrenal cortex. Masculine features include lack of breast development, increased muscle bulk, and hirsutism. (From Thibodeau GA: *Anatomy & physiology,* St Louis, 1987, Mosby.)

The effects of an estrogen-secreting tumor are most evident in men and result in gynecomastia (breast enlargement) (98% of cases), testicular atrophy, and decreased libido. In female children such tumors may lead to early development of secondary sex characteristics. An androgen-secreting tumor indicates changes more easily observed in women, including hirsutism, clitoral enlargement, deepening of the voice, amenorrhea, acne, and breast atrophy. In children, virilizing tumors promote precocious sexual development and bone aging. Treatment of androgen-secreting tumors usually involves surgical excision.

Disorders of the Adrenal Medulla

Adrenal Medulla Hypofunction

No known physiologic alterations are associated with hypofunction of the adrenal medulla. Bilateral adrenalectomy, for example, is followed by a rapid decrease in urinary excretion of epinephrine, but excretion of norepinephrine remains relatively stable. Pathophysiologic alterations are instead associated with hyperfunctioning of the adrenal medulla.

Adrenal Medulla Hyperfunction

Adrenomedullary hyperfunction is caused by tumors derived from the chromaffin cells of the adrenal medulla. These tumors, known as **pheochromocytomas,** secrete catecholamines on a continual or episodic basis (Figure 21-25). Less than 10% of these tumors are malignant; those that are malignant may metastasize to the lungs, liver, bones, or paraaortic lymph nodes. Most pheochromocytomas produce norepinephrine, although large tumors secrete epinephrine and norepinephrine.

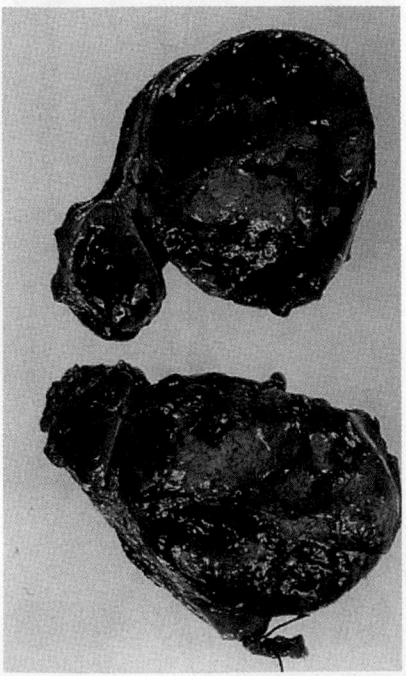

Figure 21-25 Pheochromocytoma. Gross appearance of adrenal pheochromocytoma. (From Rosai J: *Akerman's surgical pathology,* ed 8, St Louis, 1996, Mosby.)

The true incidence of pheochromocytoma in the general population is not known. About one tenth of one percent of the adult hypertensive population has a pheochromocytoma.[271] The tumors are most common in people 40 to 60 years of age, with men and women equally affected. Familial forms of the disease are associated with mutations in the *RET* protooncogene, the Von Hippel-Lindau *(VHL)* gene, a tumor-suppressor gene that encodes succinate dehydrogenase.[272]

PATHOPHYSIOLOGY Pheochromocytomas cause excessive production of catecholamines attributable to autonomous functioning of the tumor. Approximately 5% of people with pheochromocytomas have no symptoms because the tumor appears to be nonfunctioning; however, these tumors can release catecholamines in response to stressors, such as abdominal surgery.

CLINICAL MANIFESTATIONS The clinical manifestations of a pheochromocytoma are related to the chronic effects of catecholamine secretion and include persistent hypertension associated with diaphoresis, tachycardia, palpitations, and severe headache.[273] Hypertension is a result of increased peripheral vascular resistance and may be sustained or paroxysmal. Headaches appear because of sudden changes in catecholamine levels in the blood, affecting cerebral blood flow. Hypermetabolism is related to chronic activation of sympathetic receptors in adipocytes, hepatocytes, and other tissues. Glucose intolerance may occur because of catecholamine-induced inhibition of insulin release by the pancreas. Complaints of warmth, heat intolerance, weight loss, and constipation are common despite a normal or an increased appetite.

An acute episode of hypertension related to hypersecretion of catecholamines may follow specific events. Exercise, excessive ingestion of tyrosine-containing foods (aged cheese, red wine, beer, yogurt), ingestion of caffeine-containing foods, external pressure on the tumor, and induction of anesthesia all can increase secretion of catecholamines by the tumor.

These tumors tend to be extremely vascular and can rupture. Such an event can cause massive and potentially fatal hemorrhage. Rupture of a pheochromocytoma is characterized by a sudden, unexplained decrease in blood pressure; sudden, severe abdominal pain; and a rigid abdomen.

EVALUATION AND TREATMENT A diagnosis of pheochromocytoma is made when increased catecholamine production is demonstrated in the blood or urine. Individuals with this disorder can have total urine catecholamine levels greater than 250 mg/day. After elevation of urinary or plasma catecholamines is documented, the site of the tumor is determined using MRI; because of the possibility of metastasis, whole-body scanning may be done.

The usual treatment of pheochromocytoma is laparoscopic surgical excision of the tumor with adjunctive radiopharmaceuticals or chemotherapy. Medical therapy is used to stabilize blood pressure before surgery. Drugs used include α-adrenergic blocking agents and, possibly later, β-adrenergic blocking agents. Open resection is completed for large tumors or when metastasis is suspected.[274]

Mechanisms of Hormonal Alterations

1. Abnormalities in endocrine function may be caused by hypersecretion or hyposecretion of hormones, causing alterations in normal hormone levels.
2. Endocrine abnormalities also may be caused by alterations in receptor function through a variety of mechanisms: (a) a decrease in number of receptors, (b) receptor insensitivity to the hormone, (c) antibodies against specific receptors, and (d) defects in second messenger generation or postreceptor defects.
3. Abnormally high levels of circulating hormones sometimes are caused by hormone release from tissues outside the endocrine system (ectopic foci) that may not respond to normal feedback mechanisms, in which case they are said to function autonomously.

Alterations of the Hypothalamic-Pituitary System

1. Dysfunction in the release of hypothalamic hormones probably is related to interruption of the connection between the hypothalamus and pituitary—namely, the pituitary stalk.
2. Disorders of the posterior pituitary include SIADH secretion and DI. SIADH secretion is characterized by abnormally high ADH secretion; DI is characterized by abnormally low ADH secretion.
3. In SIADH, high ADH levels interfere with renal free water clearance, leading to hyponatremia and hypoosmolality. SIADH secretion is associated with certain forms of cancer, apparently because of ectopic secretion of ADH by tumor cells.
4. DI may be neurogenic, caused by insufficient amounts of ADH, or nephrogenic, caused by an inadequate response to ADH. Its principal clinical features are failure to concentrate urine with polyuria and polydipsia.
5. Hypopituitarism is dysfunction of the anterior pituitary that causes failure of hormonal functions. Symptoms may be mild to severe.
6. The most common cause of hypopituitarism is a tumor of the pituitary or subsequent treatment of the tumor (surgical or radiation therapy). Symptoms are variable depending on which hormones are deficient (i.e., TSH, ACTH, GH, etc.).
7. Hyperpituitarism is caused by pituitary adenomas. These are usually benign slow-growing tumors that arise from cells of the anterior pituitary.
8. Expansion of a pituitary adenoma causes neurologic and secretory effects. Pressure from the expanding tumor causes hyposecretion of cells, dysfunction of the optic chiasm (leading to visual disturbances), and dysfunction of the hypothalamus and some cranial nerves.
9. Hypersecretion of GH causes acromegaly, in which GH secretion becomes high and unpredictable. Pituitary adenoma is the most common cause of acromegaly.
10. Prolonged, abnormally high levels of GH lead to proliferation of body and connective tissues. Renal, thyroid, and reproductive dysfunction develop slowly, together with a change in bony proportions.
11. GH deficiency in children results in growth failure and fasting hypoglycemia. Adult GH deficiency results in fatigue, osteoporosis, and increased mortality.
12. Pituitary prolactinomas, renal failure, and medications can result in increased prolactin and affects reproductive organs and function in both men and women.

Alterations of Thyroid Function

1. Thyrotoxicosis is a general condition in which TH levels are elevated and produce an exaggerated physiologic response in tissues. The condition can be caused by a variety of specific diseases, each of which has its own pathophysiology and course of treatment.
2. In general, hyperthyroidism has a range of endocrine, reproductive, gastrointestinal, integumentary, and ocular manifestations. These are caused by increased circulating levels of TH and by stimulation of the sympathetic division of the autonomic nervous system.
3. Graves disease, the most common form of hyperthyroidism, is caused by an autoimmune mechanism that overrides normal mechanisms for control of TH secretion.
4. Manifestations of Graves disease can include symptoms of hyperthyroidism, diffuse thyroid enlargement, disorders of the skin, and enlargement of extraocular muscles.
5. The cutaneous manifestation of Graves disease is pretibial myxedema, a condition characterized by subcutaneous swelling of the legs and, occasionally, the hands.
6. Ocular manifestations of Graves disease are caused by hyperactivity of the sympathetic division of the autonomic nervous system and by immune-induced infiltration of extraocular muscles.
7. Toxic nodular goiter and toxic multinodular goiter occur when hyperplastic regions of the thyroid become autonomous.
8. Toxic nodular goiters are follicular-cell adenomas that produce symptoms similar to those of Graves disease.
9. Toxic multinodular goiters result from multiple functioning adenomas.
10. Thyrotoxic crisis is a severe form of hyperthyroidism that often is associated with physiologic stress. Without treatment, death occurs quickly.
11. Hypothyroidism is caused by deficient production of TH by the thyroid gland. The condition may be primary or secondary.
12. Primary hypothyroidism transiently occurs in either subacute or painless thyroiditis and spontaneous resolution of hypothyroidism is nearly universal. Chronic lymphocytic thyroiditis, an autoimmune disease, is associated with permanent hypothyroidism.
13. Subacute thyroiditis, a form of hypothyroidism, is a self-limited nonbacterial inflammation of the thyroid gland. The inflammatory process damages follicular cells, causing leakage of triiodothyronine (T_3) and thyroxine (T_4). Hyperthyroidism then is followed by transient hypothyroidism, which is corrected by cellular repair and a return to normal levels in the thyroid.
14. Autoimmune thyroiditis is associated with infiltration or fibrosis of the thyroid, circulating thyroid antibodies, and gradual loss of thyroid function. Autoimmune thyroiditis occurs in those individuals with a genetic susceptibility to an autoimmune mechanism that causes thyroid damage and eventual hypothyroidism.
15. Hypothyroidism also can be caused by hypothalamic-pituitary dysfunction in which TRH and TSH are not produced in sufficient amounts.
16. Thyroid carcinoma is a relatively rare cancer. The most consistent causal risk factor associated with thyroid carcinoma is exposure to ionizing radiation, especially in childhood.

Continued

17. Hypothyroidism affects all body systems. Symptoms depend on the degree of TH deficiency. Common manifestations include decreased energy metabolism and heat production.

18. Myxedema is the characteristic sign of hypothyroidism. Myxedema is caused by alterations in connective tissue with water-binding proteins. The excess water leads to edema and thickened mucous membranes.

19. Myxedema coma is a severe form of hypothyroidism, which may be life threatening without emergency medical treatment.

20. Congenital hypothyroidism occurs with thyroid agenesis and results in hypothyroidism, growth failure, and mental retardation from absence of thyroxine.

21. Thyroid carcinoma is probably caused by exposure to ionizing radiation, particularly during childhood, with the development of nodules and normal thyroxine levels.

Alterations of Parathyroid Function

1. Hyperparathyroidism may be primary or secondary and is characterized by greater than normal secretion of PTH.

2. Primary hyperparathyroidism is caused by an interruption of the normal mechanisms that regulate calcium and PTH levels, usually a parathyroid adenoma. Manifestations include chronic hypercalcemia, increased bone resorption, and hypercalciuria.

3. Secondary hyperparathyroidism is a compensatory response to hypocalcemia and often occurs with chronic renal failure.

4. Pseudohypoparathyroidism and familial hypocalciuric hypercalcemia are inherited conditions. In pseudohypoparathyroidism there is resistance to PTH action and familial hypocalciuric hypercalcemia mimics hyperparathyroidism with failure of calcium sensing by the parathyroid gland.

5. Hypoparathyroidism, defined by abnormally low PTH levels, is caused by thyroid surgery, autoimmunity, or genetic mechanisms.

6. The lack of circulating PTH in hypoparathyroidism causes depressed serum calcium levels, increased serum phosphate levels, decreased bone resorption, and eventual hypocalciuria.

Dysfunction of the Endocrine Pancreas: Diabetes Mellitus

1. Diabetes mellitus is a complex syndrome associated with glucose intolerance and hyperglycemia in genetically susceptible individuals that causes a number of metabolic and vascular changes. The two most common types of diabetes mellitus are type 1 and type 2.

2. Type 1 diabetes mellitus includes an autoimmune (most common) and a nonimmune type. The immune type is associated with autoantibody, T cell, and macrophage destruction of pancreatic beta cells with loss of insulin production and a relative excess of glucagon. Antibodies also can be formed against glutamic acid decarboxylase and insulin.

3. In type 1 diabetes mellitus, lack of insulin and excess glucagon cause hyperglycemia and subsequent loss of glucose in the urine. Polyuria and polydipsia result from osmotic diuresis. Weight loss is a classic symptom of type 1 diabetes.

4. Ketoacidosis is caused by abnormally low levels of insulin and increased levels of glucagon resulting in increased lypolysis, increased gluconeogenesis, and production of ketone bodies leading to ketoacidosis.

5. A diagnosis of diabetes mellitus is based on elevated plasma glucose concentrations and classic signs and symptoms.

6. Type 2 diabetes mellitus is caused by genetic susceptibility that is triggered by environmental factors. The most compelling environmental risk factor is obesity. Insulin production continues but the weight and number of beta cells decrease.

7. Several mechanisms of insulin resistance (hyperinsulinemia) cause reduced glucose uptake and metabolism in type 2 diabetes. These mechanisms include alteration in production of adipokines by adipose tissue (i.e., leptin resistance), elevated serum free fatty acids and intracellular lipid deposits, release of inflammatory cytokines from adipose tissue, and obesity-associated insulin resistance.

8. In type 2 diabetes myelin deficiency results in increased glucagon secretion and hyperglycemia. Deposition of amyloid in the pancrease contributes to beta cell loss.

9. Decreased gherlin levels have been associated with insulin resistance in type 2 diabetes.

10. Other specific types of diabetes mellitus include MODY associated with autosomal dominant gene mutations, and gestational diabetes with onset of glucose intolerance during pregnancy.

11. Acute complications of diabetes mellitus include hypoglycemia, DKA, HHNKS, the Somogyi effect, and the dawn phenomenon.

12. Hypoglycemia is a lowered blood glucose level that may be related to exogenous (i.e., insulin shock or insulin reaction), endogenous, or functional causes.

13. Symptoms of hypoglycemia are divided into adrenergic, caused by activation of the sympathetic nervous system; and neuroglycopenic, reflecting defective central nervous system metabolism resulting from impaired energy generation.

14. DKA develops when there is an absolute or relative deficiency of insulin and an increase in the insulin counterregulatory hormones of catecholamines, cortisol, glucagon, GH, and FFAs with accelerated gluconeogenesis and ketogenesis.

15. HHNKS is pathophysiologically similar to DKA, although levels of FFAs are lower in HHNKS and lack of ketosis indicates that some level of insulin is present. The hyperosmolar state can cause osmotic diuresis and profound dehydration.

16. The Somogyi effect is a combination of hypoglycemia with rebound hyperglycemia caused by effects of counterregulatory hormones. It is most common in persons with type 1 diabetes mellitus and in children.

17. The dawn phenomenon is an early morning rise in glucose levels caused by nocturnal elevations of GH.

18. Chronic complications of diabetes mellitus include diabetic neuropathies, microvascular disease (e.g., retinopathy, nephropathy and neuropathy), macrovascular disease (e.g., CAD, stroke, peripheral vascular disease), and infection. Metabolic changes contributing to complications include shunting of glucose to the polyol pathway, activation of protein kinase C, induction of ROS (oxidative stress), formation of AGEs, and accumulation of hexosamines.

19. Microvascular complications are associated with vascular alterations in endothelium, the basement membrane, and thrombosis.

20. Diabetic retinopathy is caused by several mechanisms including microvascular changes and thrombosis that lead to microvascular occlusion, increased vascular permeability, retinal ischemia and hemorrhages.

SUMMARY REVIEW—cont'd

21. Diabetic nephropathy is related to hyperglycemia, hyperperfusion, oxidative stress, and inflammation with glomerular enlargement and glomerular basement membrane thickening, diffuse intercapillary glomerulosclerosis, expansion of the mesangial matrix, and progressive renal failure.

22. Diabetic neuropathies may be caused by vascular and metabolic mechanisms, or a combination of both, with axonal and Schwann cell degeneration and abnormalities in sensory and motor nerve conduction velocity, including involvement of the autonomic nervous system.

23. Macrovascular disease associated with diabetes mellitus is associated with hyperglycemia, hyperlipidemia, inflammation, and altered endothelial function.

24. Incidence of coronary heart disease, peripheral vascular disease, and stroke is greater in persons with diabetes than in nondiabetic individuals.

25. CAD and stroke in diabetes are a consequence of accelerated atherosclerosis, hypertension, and increased risk for thrombus formation.

26. Peripheral vascular disease is a consequence of occlusion of large and small arteries with an increased risk of ischemia, necrosis, and amputation.

27. Individuals with diabetes are at risk for a variety of infections related to sensory impairment, vascular complications, impaired white blood cells and suppressed immunity, rapid proliferation of pathogens, and delayed wound healing.

Alterations of Adrenal Function

1. Disorders of the adrenal cortex are related to hyperfunction or hypofunction. No known disorders are associated with hypofunction of the adrenal medulla, but medullary hyperfunction causes clinically defined syndromes.

2. Hypercortisolism is divided into ACTH-dependent (Cushing disease or ectopic ACTH syndrome) and ACTH-independent (adrenal adenoma or adenocarcinoma) mechanisms.

3. Cushing disease is excessive anterior pituitary ACTH production most commonly by an ACTH-secreting pituitary microadenoma.

4. Cushing syndrome occurs whenever there is an excessive level of cortisol regardless of cause. Exogenous forms result from exogenous administration of glucocorticoids. Endogenous forms are either corticotropin dependent (most common and caused by an ACTH-secreting pituitary tumor) or corticotropin independent, usually caused by an adrenal cortical tumor.

5. Individuals with Cushing disease lose diurnal and circadian patterns of ACTH and cortisol secretion, and they lack the ability to increase secretion of these hormones in response to a stressor. Individuals experience weight gain, glucose intolerance, protein wasting, bone disease, hyperpigmentation, and immunosuppression.

6. Primary hyperaldosteronism is a disorder of the adrenal cortex usually caused by an adrenal adenoma or bilateral nodular hyperplasia. The condition is characterized by hypertension, hypokalemia, renal potassium wasting, and neuromuscular manifestations.

7. Secondary hyperaldosterone secretion is related to a variety of conditions associated with elevated renin release and activation of angiotensin II. These include decreased circulating blood volume, decreased renal blood supply, elevated estrogen levels, Bartter syndrome, and renin-secreting tumors.

8. Hyperaldosteronism promotes increased sodium reabsorption, corresponding hypervolemia, increased extracellular volume (which is variable), hypertension, and hypokalemia.

9. Adrenal tumors, either adenomas or carcinomas, can autonomously secrete androgens or estrogens.

10. Hypofunction of the adrenal cortex can affect glucocorticoid or mineralocorticoid secretion or both. Hypofunction can be caused by a deficiency of ACTH or by a primary deficiency in the gland itself.

11. Hypocortisolism (low levels of cortisol) is caused by inadequate adrenal stimulation by ACTH or by primary cortisol hyposecretion. Primary adrenal insufficiency is termed Addison disease.

12. Addison disease is characterized by elevated ACTH levels with inadequate corticosteroid synthesis and output. Causes include idiopathic autoimmune disease, tuberculosis of the adrenal gland, familial adrenal insufficiency, amyloidosis, metastatic destruction of the adrenal glands, and adrenal hemorrhage.

13. Secondary hypercortisolism is characterized by low to absent ACTH levels, leading to inadequate adrenal stimulation, adrenal atrophy, and decreased corticosteroidogenesis. The most common cause is withdrawal of exogenous administration of glucocorticoids.

14. Manifestations of Addison disease are related to hypocortisolism and hypoaldosteronism. Symptoms include weakness, fatigability, hypoglycemia and related metabolic problems, lowered response to stressors, vitiligo, hyperpigmentation, and manifestations of hypovolemia and hyperkalemia.

15. Hyperfunction of the adrenal medulla is caused by a pheochromocytoma, which is a catecholamine-producing tumor. Symptoms of catecholamine excess are related to their sympathetic nervous system effects and include hypertension, palpitations, tachycardia, glucose intolerance, excessive sweating, and constipation.

KEY TERMS

Acromegaly, 733
ACTH deficiency, 731
Addison disease (primary adrenal insufficiency), 770
Advanced glycosylation end product (AGE), 759
Aldose reductase, 758
Amylin, 752

Autoimmune thyroiditis (Hashimoto disease, chronic lymphocyte thyroiditis), 741
Bartter syndrome, 769
Beta cell dysfunction, 751
Congenital hypothyroidism, 741
Cushing disease, 765
Cushing syndrome, 765

Dawn phenomenon, 758
Diabetes insipidus (DI), 730
Diabetes mellitus, 745
Diabetic ketoacidosis (DKA), 755
Diabetic neuropathy, 762
Diabetic retinopathy, 759
Dipeptidyl peptidase VI (DPP-IV), 752
Distal symmetric polyneuropathy, 762

Continued

KEY TERMS—cont'd

Dwarfism, 731
Exopthalmos, 737
Familial hypocalciuric hypercalcemia (FHH), 743
Feminization, 771
FSH deficiency, 732
Gestational diabetes mellitus (GDM), 754
GH deficiency, 732
Ghrelin, 752
Giantism, 733
Glucagon, 752
Glucagon-like peptide (GLP-1), 752
Glucose-dependent insulinotropic polypeptide (GIP), 752
Glycosylated hemoglobin, 749
Graves disease, 736
Hemoglobin A_{1c}, 749
Hyperaldosteronism, 768
Hyperosmolar hyperglycemic nonketotic syndrome (HHNKS), 757
Hyperparathyroidism, 742
Hyperprolactinemia, 735
Hypocortisolism, 770
Hypoglycemia, 754
Hypoparathyroidism, 744
Hypopituitarism, 731
Hypothyroidism, 739
Iatrogenic hypothyroidism, 741

Idiopathic Addison disease (organ-specific autoimmune adrenalitis), 770
Incretin, 752
Insulin resistance, 750
Iodine deficiency (endemic goiter), 741
LH deficiency, 732
Maculopathy, 759
Maturity-onset diabetes of youth (MODY), 753
Metabolic syndrome, 751
Myxedema, 739
Myxedema coma, 741
Nephrogenic diabetes insipidus, 730
Neurogenic diabetes insipidus, 730
Nonenzymatic glycosylation, 759
Painless thyroiditis, 741
Panhypopituitarism, 731
Pheochromocytoma, 772
Pituitary adenoma, 733
Polyol pathway, 758
Postpartum thyroiditis, 741
Prediabetes, 745
Pretibial myxedema (Graves dermopathy), 737
Primary adrenal insufficiency (Addison disease), 770
Primary aldosteronism (primary hyperaldosteronism), 768

Primary hyperparathyroidism, 742
Primary hyperthyroidism, 736
Primary hypothyroidism, 741
Prolactinoma, 735
Protein kinase C (PKC), 758
Pseudohyperparathyroidism, 743
Secondary aldosteronism (secondary hyperaldosteronism), 768
Secondary hyperparathyroidism, 743
Secondary hyperthyroidism, 736
Secondary hypocortisolism, 770
Secondary (central) hypothyroidism, 739
Sheehan syndrome, 731
Somogyi effect, 758
Subacute thyroiditis, 741
Subclinical hypothyroidism, 741
Syndrome of inappropriate antidiuretic hormone (SIADH) secretion, 729
Thyroid carcinoma, 742
Thyrotoxic crisis (thyroid storm), 738
Thyrotoxicosis, 736
Toxic adenoma, 738
Toxic multinodular goiter, 738
TSH deficiency, 732
Type 1 diabetes mellitus, 745
Type 2 diabetes mellitus, 750
Virilization, 771

REFERENCES

1. Kim TJ, Travers S: Case report: thyroid hormone resistance and its therapeutic challenges, *Curr Opin Pediatr* 20(4):490-493, 2008.
2. Tonacchera M et al: Identification of TSH receptor mutations in three families with resistance to TSH, *Clin Endocrinol* 67(5):712-718, 2007.
3. Chen H, Hewison M, Adams JS: Control of estradiol-directed gene transactivation by an intracellular estrogen-binding protein and an estrogen response element-binding protein, *Mol Endocrinol* 22(3):559-569, 2008.
4. Visser WE et al: Thyroid hormone transport in and out of cells, *Trends Endocrinol Metab* 19(2):50-56, 2008.
5. Frank E, Landgraf R: The vasopressin system—from antidiuresis to psychopathology, *Eur J Pharmacol* 583(2-3):226-242, 2008.
6. Ellison DH, Berl T: Clinical practice. The syndrome of inappropriate antidiuresis, *N Engl J Med* 356(20):2064-2072, 2007.
7. Multz AS: Vasopressin dysregulation and hyponatremia in hospitalized patients, *J Intensive Care Med* 22(4):216-223, 2007.
8. Decaux G, Musch W: Clinical laboratory evaluation of the syndrome of inappropriate secretion of antidiuretic hormone, *Clin J Am Soc Nephrol* 3(4):1175-1184, 2008.
9. Ali F et al: Therapeutic potential of vasopressin receptor antagonists, *Drugs* 67(6):847-858, 2007.
10. Soupart A et al: Successful long-term treatment of hyponatremia in syndrome of inappropriate antidiuretic hormone secretion with satavaptan (SR121463B), an orally active nonpeptide vasopressin V2-receptor antagonist, *Clin J Am Soc Nephrol* 1(6):1154-1160, 2006.
11. Ball SG: Vasopressin and disorders of water balance: the physiology and pathophysiology of vasopressin, *Ann Clin Biochem* 44(Pt 5):417-431, 2007.
12. Makaryus AN, McFarlane SI: Diabetes insipidus: diagnosis and treatment of a complex disease, *Cleve Clin J Med* 73(1):65-71, 2006.
13. Loh JA, Verbalis JG: Disorders of water and salt metabolism associated with pituitary disease, *Endocrin Metab Clin North Am* 37(1):213-234, x, 2008.
14. Sands JM et al: Nephrogenic diabetes insipidus, *Ann Intern Med* 144(3):186-194, 2006.

15. Einaudi S, Bondone C: The effects of head trauma on hypothalamic-pituitary function in children and adolescents, *Curr Opin Pediatr* 19(4):465-470, 2007.
16. Khanna A: Acquired nephrogenic diabetes insipidus, *Semin Nephrol* 26(3):244-248, 2006.
17. Robben JH, Knoers NV, Deen PM: Cell biological aspects of the vasopressin type-2 receptor and aquaporin 2 water channel in nephrogenic diabetes insipidus, *Am J Physiol Renal Physiol* 291(2):F257-F270, 2006.
18. Spanakis E, Milord E, Gragnoli C: AVPR2 variants and mutations in nephrogenic diabetes insipidus: review and missense mutation significance, *J Cell Physiol* 217(3):605-617, 2008.
19. Schrier RW: Aquaporin-related disorders of water homeostasis, *Drug News Perspect* 20(7):447-453, 2007.
20. Agha A, Phillips J, Thompson CJ: Hypopituitarism following traumatic brain injury (TBI), *Br J Neurosurg* 21(2):210-216, 2007.
21. Schneider HJ et al: Hypopituitarism [see comment], *Lancet* 369(9571):1461-1470, 2007.
22. Toogood AA, Stewart PM: Hypopituitarism: clinical features, diagnosis, and management, *Endocrinol Metab Clin North Am* 37(1):235-261, x, 2008.
23. Rupp D, Molitch M: Pituitary stalk lesions, *Curr Opin Endocrinol Diabetes Obes* 15(4):339-345, 2008.
24. Mullis PE: Genetics of growth hormone deficiency, *Endocrinol Metab Clin North Am* 36(1):17-36, 2007.
25. Aikawa S et al: High level expression of Prop-1 gene in gonadotropic cell lines, *J Repro Develop* 52(2):195-201, 2006.
26. Behan LA, Agha A: Endocrine consequences of adult traumatic brain injury, *Hormone Res* 68(Suppl 5):18-21, 2007.
27. Kaplun J et al: Sequential pituitary MR imaging in Sheehan syndrome: report of 2 cases, *AJNR Am J Neuroradiol* 29(5):941-943, 2008.
28. Richmond EJ, Rogol AD: Growth hormone deficiency in children, *Pituitary* 11(2):115-120, 2008.
29. Buzi F et al: Growth hormone receptor polymorphisms, *Endocr Dev* 11:28-35, 2007.
30. Mullis PE: Genetics of growth hormone deficiency, *Endocrinol Metab Clin North Am* 36(1):17-36, 2007.

31. Clemmons DR: Value of insulin-like growth factor system markers in the assessment of growth hormone status, *Endocrinol Metab Clin North Am* 36(1):109-129, 2007.

32. Thorner MO, Nass R: Human studies of growth hormone and aging, *Pediatr Endocrinol Rev* 4(3):233-234, 2007.

33. Johannsson G: Management of adult growth hormone deficiency, *Endocrinol Metab Clin North Am* 36(1):203-220, 2007.

34. Auernhammer CJ, Vlotides G: Anterior pituitary hormone replacement therapy—a clinical review, *Pituitary* 10(1):1-15, 2007.

35. Ezzat S et al: The prevalence of pituitary adenomas: a systemic review, *Cancer* 101(3):613-619, 2004.

36. Zhang HW et al: Diagnosis and treatment of pituitary microadenoma: report of 80 cases, *Neurol Res* 30(6):587-593, 2008.

37. Li-Ng M, Sharma M: Invasive pituitary adenoma, *J Clin Endocrinol Metab* 93(9):3284-3285, 2008.

38. Kanou Y et al: Clinical implications of dynamic MRI for pituitary adenomas: clinical and histologic analysis, *J Clin Neurosci* 9(6): 659-663, 2002.

39. Zhang Y et al: Endoscopic transsphenoidal treatment of pituitary adenomas, *Neurol Res* 30(6):581-586, 2008.

40. Ben-Shlomo A, Melmed S: Acromegaly, *Endocrinol Metab Clin North Am* 37(1):101-122, viii, 2008.

41. Cordero RA, Barkan AL: Current diagnosis of acromegaly, *Rev Endocr Metab Disord* 9(1):13-19, 2008.

42. Ayuk J, Sheppard MC: Does acromegaly enhance mortality? *Rev Endocr Metab Disord* 9(1):33-39, 2008.

43. Katznelson L: An update on treatment strategies for acromegaly, *Exp Opin Pharmacother* 9(13):2273-2280, 2008.

44. Vallette S, Serri O: Octreotide LAR for the treatment of acromegaly, *Exp Opin Drug Metab Toxicol* 4(6):783-793, 2008.

45. Roelfsema F et al: The role of pegvisomant in the treatment of acromegaly, *Exp Opin Biol Ther* 8(5):691-704, 2008.

46. Prabhakar VK, Davis JR: Hyperprolactinaemia, *Best Pract Res Clin Obstet Gynaecol* 22(2):341-353, 2008.

47. Mancini T, Casanueva FF, Giustina A: Hyperprolactinemia and prolactinomas, *Endocrinol Metab Clin North Am* 37(1):67-99, viii, 2008.

48. Chahal J, Schlechte J: Hyperprolactinemia, *Pituitary* 11(2):141-146, 2008.

49. Kars M et al: Cabergoline and cardiac valve disease in prolactinoma patients: additional studies during long term treatment are required, *Eur J Endocrinol* 159(4):363-367, 2008.

50. Nayak B, Hodak SP: Hyperthyroidism. *Endocrinol Metab Clin North Am* 36(3):617-656, v, 2007.

51. Brent GA: Clinical practice. Graves' disease, *N Engl J Med* 358(24):2594-2605, 2008.

52. Caturegli P et al: Autoimmune thyroid diseases, *Curr Opin Rheumatol* 19(1):44-48, 2007.

53. Fatourechi V: Pretibial myxedema: pathophysiology and treatment options, *Am J Clin Dermatol* 6(5):295-309, 2005.

54. Mota A, Borrione P, Santiago M: Thyroid acropachy, *J Clin Rheumatol* 13(6):360, 2007.

55. Khoo TK, Bahn RS: Pathogenesis of Graves' ophthalmopathy: the role of autoantibodies, *Thyroid* 17(10):1013-1018, 2007.

56. Wiersinga WM: Management of Graves' ophthalmopathy, *Nat Clin Pract Endocrinol Metab* 3(5):396-404, 2007.

57. Cerci C et al: Thyroid cancer in toxic and non-toxic multinodular goiter, *J Postgrad Med* 53(3):157-160, 2007.

58. Tunca F et al: The preoperative exclusion of thyroid carcinoma in multinodular goiter: dynamic contrast-enhanced magnetic resonance imaging versus ultrasonography-guided fine-needle aspiration biopsy, *Surgery* 142(6):992-1002, 2007.

59. Porterfield JR Jr et al: Evidence-based management of toxic multinodular goiter (Plummer's disease), *World J Surg* 32(7):1278-1284, 2008.

60. Kearney T, Dang C: Diabetic and endocrine emergencies, *Postgrad Med J* 83(976):79-86, 2007.

61. Ngo SY, Chew HC: When the storm passes unnoticed—a case series of thyroid storm, *Resuscitation* 73(3):485-490, 2007.

62. Dahl P, Danzi S, Klein I: Thyrotoxic cardiac disease, *Curr Heart Fail Rep* 5(3):170-176, 2008.

63. Kung AW: Neuromuscular complications of thyrotoxicosis, *Clin Endocrinol* 67(5):645-650, 2007.

64. Devdhar M, Ousman YH, Burman KD: Hypothyroidism, *Endocrinol Metab Clin North Am* 36(3):595-615, v, 2007.

65. Yamada M, Masatomo M: Mechanisms related to the pathophysiology and management of central hypothyroidism, *Nat Clin Pract Endocrinol Metab* 4(12):683-694, 2008.

66. Kwaku MP, Burman KD: Myxedema coma, *J Intensive Care Med* 22(4):224-231, 2007.

67. Vaidya B, Pearce SH: Management of hypothyroidism in adults, *BMJ* 337:a801, 2008.

68. Beynon J, Akhtar S, Kearney T: Predictors of outcome in myxoedema coma, *Crit Care (Lond)* 12(1):111, 2008.

69. Herrick B: Subclinical hypothyroidism, *Am Family Phys* 77(7):953-955, 2008.

70. Villar HC et al: Thyroid hormone replacement for subclinical hypothyroidism, *Cochrane Database Syst Rev* (3):CD003419.

71. Takami HE, Miyabe R, Kameyama K: Hashimoto's thyroiditis, *World J Surg* 32(5):688-692, 2008.

72. Zeitlin AA et al: Analysis of HLA class II genes in Hashimoto's thyroiditis reveals differences compared to Graves' disease, *Genes Immun* 9(4):358-363, 2008.

73. Duntas LH: Environmental factors and autoimmune thyroiditis, *Nat Clin Pract Endocrinol Metab* 4(8):454-460, 2008.

74. Kimura H, Caturegli P: Chemokine orchestration of autoimmune thyroiditis, *Thyroid* 17(10):1005-1011, 2007.

75. Wang SH, Baker JR: The role of apoptosis in thyroid autoimmunity, *Thyroid* 17(10):975-979, 2007.

76. Nishihara E et al: Clinical characteristics of 852 patients with subacute thyroiditis before treatment, *Intern Med* 47(8):725-729, 2008.

77. Lucas A et al: Postpartum thyroiditis: long-term follow-up, *Thyroid* 15(10):1177-1181, 2005.

78. Harris KB, Pass KA: Increase in congenital hypothyroidism in New York state and in the United States, *Mol Genet Metab* 91(3):268-277, 2007.

79. Gruters A, Krude H: Update on the management of congenital hypothyroidism, *Hormone Res* 68(Suppl 5):107-111, 2007.

80. Arenz S et al: Intellectual outcome, motor skills and BMI of children with congenital hypothyroidism: a population-based study, *Acta Paediatr* 97(4):447-450, 2008.

81. van der Sluijs Veer L et al: Quality of life, developmental milestones, and self-esteem of young adults with congenital hypothyroidism diagnosed by neonatal screening, *J Clin Endocrinol Metab* 93(7):2654-2661, 2008.

82. American Cancer Society, Inc., Surveillance and Health Policy Research: Estimated New Cancer Cases and Deaths by Sex, U.S. 2009 available at: http://www.cancer.org/downloads/stt/CFF2009_EstCD_3.pdf.

83. Fitzgibbons SC, Brams DM, Wei JP: The treatment of thyroid cancer, *Am Surgeon* 74(5):389-399, 2008.

84. Brown RL: Standard and emerging therapeutic approaches for thyroid malignancies, *Semin Oncol* 35(3):298-308, 2008.

85. DeLellis RA, Mazzaglia P, Mangray S: Primary hyperparathyroidism: a current perspective, *Arc Pathol Lab Med* 132(8):1251-1262, 2008.

86. Rodgers SE, Lew JI, Solorzano CC: Primary hyperparathyroidism, *Curr Opin Oncol* 20(1):52-58, 2008.

87. Sitges-Serra A, Bergenfelz A: Clinical update: sporadic primary hyperparathyroidism, *Lancet* 370(9586):468-470, 2007.

88. Goodman WG, Quarles LD: Development and progression of secondary hyperparathyroidism in chronic kidney disease: lessons from molecular genetics, *Kidney Int* 74(3):276-288, 2008.

89. Hruska KA et al: Hyperphosphatemia of chronic kidney disease, *Kidney Int* 74(2):148-157, 2008.

90. de Francisco AL: New strategies for the treatment of hyperparathyroidism incorporating calcimimetics, *Exp Opin Pharmacother* 9(5):795-811, 2008.

91. Komaba H, Tanaka M, Fukagawa M: Treatment of chronic kidney disease-mineral and bone disorder (CKD-MBD), *Intern Med* 47(11):989-994, 2008.

92. Evenepoel P: Calcimimetics in chronic kidney disease: evidence, opportunities and challenges, *Kidney Int* 74(3):265-275, 2008.

93. Schlieper G, Floege J: Calcimimetics in CKD-results from recent clinical studies, *Pediatr Nephrol* 23(10):1721-1728, 2008.

94. Shoback D: Clinical practice, Hypoparathyroidism, *N Engl J Med* 359(4):391-403, 2008.

95. Asari R et al: Hypoparathyroidism after total thyroidectomy: a prospective study, *Arch Surg* 143:132-137, 2008.

96. Kobrynski LJ, Sullivan KE: Velocardiofacial syndrome, DiGeorge syndrome: the chromosome 22q11.2 deletion syndromes, *Lancet* 370(9596):1443-1452, 2007.

97. Angelopoulos NG, Goula A, Tolis G: Sporadic hypoparathyroidism treated with teriparatide: a case report and literature review, *Exp Clin Endocrinol Diabetes* 115(1):50-54, 2007.

98. American Diabetes Association: Diagnosis and classification of diabetes mellitus, *Diabetes Care* 30(Suppl 1):S42-S47, 2007.

99. Center for Disease Control and Prevention: *Diabetes data and trends.* Available at http://apps.nccd.cdc.gov/DDTSTRS/default.aspx.

100. Daneman D: Type 1 diabetes, *Lancet* 367:847-858, 2006.

101. Eisenbarth GS: Update in type 1 diabetes, *J Clin Endocrinol Metab* 92(7):2403-2407, 2007.

102. Jahromi MM, Eisenbarth GS: Cellular and molecular pathogenesis of type 1A diabetes, *Cell Mol Life Sci* 64(7-8):865-872, 2007.

103. Richer MJ, Horwitz MS: Viral infections in the pathogenesis of autoimmune diseases: focus on type 1 diabetes, *Front Biosci* 13:4241-4257, 2008.

104. Kaminitz A et al: The vicious cycle of apoptotic beta-cell death in type 1 diabetes, *Immunol Cell Biol* 85(8):582-589, 2007.

105. Chistiakov DA, Voronova NV, Chistiakov PA: The crucial role of IL-2/IL-2RA-mediated immune regulation in the pathogenesis of type 1 diabetes, an evidence coming from genetic and animal model studies, *Immunol Lett* 118(1):1-5, 2008.

106. Meier JJ: Beta cell mass in diabetes: a realistic therapeutic target? *Diabetologia* 51(5):703-713, 2008.

107. Sherr J et al: Prevention of type 1 diabetes: the time has come, *Nat Clin Pract Endocrinol Metab* 4(6):334-343, 2008.

108. Aguilar-Bryan L, Bryan J: Neonatal diabetes mellitus, *Endocr Rev* 29(3):265-291, 2008.

109. Hills CE, Brunskill NJ: Intracellular signalling by C-peptide, *Exp Diabetes Res* 2008:635158, 2008.

110. Ekberg K, Johansson BL: Effect of C-peptide on diabetic neuropathy in patients with type 1 diabetes, *Exp Diabetes Res* 2008:457912, 2008.

111. Forst T et al: Role of C-Peptide in the regulation of microvascular blood flow, *Exp Diabetes Res* 2008:176245, 2008.

112. Rebsomen L et al: C-Peptide effects on renal physiology and diabetes, *Exp Diabetes Res* 2008:281536, 2008.

113. Sima AA, Kamiya H: Is C-peptide replacement the missing link for successful treatment of neurological complications in type 1 diabetes? *Curr Drug Targets* 9(1):37-46, 2008.

114. Wilkin TJ: Diabetes: 1 and 2, or one and the same? Progress with the accelerator hypothesis, *Pediatr Diabetes* 9(3 Pt 2):23-32, 2008.

115. Pozilli P: Immuno-intervention and preservation of beta-cell function in type 1 diabetes, *Diabetes Metab Res Rev* 23:255-256, 2007.

116. Diabetes Control and Complications Trial Research Group: The effect of intensive treatment of diabetes on the development and progression of long-term complications in insulin-dependent diabetes mellitus, *N Engl J Med* 329(14):977-986, 1993.

117. Danne T, Lange K, Kordonouri O: New developments in the treatment of type 1 diabetes in children, *Arch Dis Child* 92(11):1015-1019, 2007.

118. Unger J: Management of type 1 diabetes, *Prim Care* 34(4):791-808, vi-vii, 2007.

119. American Diabetes AssociationExecutive Summary: Standards of medical care in diabetes—2008, *Diabetes Care* 31:S5-S11, 2008.

120. Shalitin S, Phillip M: The role of new technologies in treating children and adolescents with type 1 diabetes mellitus, *Pediatr Diabetes* 8 (Suppl 6):72-79, 2007.

121. Cali AM, Caprio S: Prediabetes and type 2 diabetes in youth: an emerging epidemic disease? *Curr Opin Endocrinol Diabetes Obes* 15(2):123-127, 2008.

122. Peterson K et al: Management of type 2 diabetes in youth: an update, *Am Fam Physician* 76(5):634-637, 2007.

123. Shaw J: Epidemiology of childhood type 2 diabetes and obesity, *Pediatr Diabetes* 8(Suppl 9):8-15, 2007.

124. Sattar N, Wannamethee SG, Forouhi NG: Novel biochemical risk factors for type 2 diabetes: pathogenic insights or prediction possibilities? *Diabetologia* 51(6):926-940, 2008.

125. Jafar-Mohammadi B, McCarthy MI: Genetics of type 2 diabetes mellitus and obesity—a review, *Ann Med* 40(1):2-10, 2008.

126. Lindgren CM, McCarthy MI: Mechanisms of disease: genetic insights into the etiology of type 2 diabetes and obesity, *Nat Clin Pract Endocrinol Metab* 4(3):156-163, 2008.

127. Moore AF, Florez JC: Genetic susceptibility to type 2 diabetes and implications for antidiabetic therapy, *Annu Rev Med* 59:95-111, 2008.

128. Romao I, Roth J: Genetic and environmental interactions in obesity and type 2 diabetes, *J Am Diet Assoc* 108(4 Suppl 1):S24-S28, 2008.

129. Florez JC: Newly identified loci highlight beta cell dysfunction as a key cause of type 2 diabetes: where are the insulin resistance genes? *Diabetologia* 51(7):1100-1110, 2008.

130. Maedler K: Beta cells in type 2 diabetes—a crucial contribution to pathogenesis, *Diabetes Obes Metab* 10(5):408-420, 2008.

131. Muoio DM, Newgard CB: Mechanisms of disease: molecular and metabolic mechanisms of insulin resistance and beta-cell failure in type 2 diabetes, *Nat Rev Mol Cell Biol* 9(3):193-205, 2008.

132. Meier JJ: Beta cell mass in diabetes: a realistic therapeutic target? *Diabetologia* 51(5):703-713, 2008.

133. Guilherme A et al: Adipocyte dysfunctions linking obesity to insulin resistance and type 2 diabetes, *Nat Rev Mol Cell Biol* 9(5):367-377, 2008.

134. Hojlund K et al: Mitochondrial dysfunction in type 2 diabetes and obesity, *Endocrinol Metab Clin North Am* 37(3):713-731, x,2008.

135. Schenk S, Saberi M, Olefsky JM: Insulin sensitivity: modulation by nutrients and inflammation, *J Clin Invest* 118(9):2992-3002, 2008.

136. Glund S, Krook A: Role of interleukin-6 signalling in glucose and lipid metabolism, *Acta Physiologica* 192(1):37-48, 2008.

137. Guest CB et al: The implication of proinflammatory cytokines in type 2 diabetes, *Front Biosci* 13:5187-5194, 2008.

138. Heilbronn LK, Campbell LV: Adipose tissue macrophages, low grade inflammation and insulin resistance in human obesity, *Curr Pharm Des* 14(12):1225-1230, 2008.

139. Poitout V, Robertson RP: Glucolipotoxicity: fuel excess and beta-cell dysfunction, *Endocr Rev* 29(3):351-366, 2008.

140. Donath MY et al: Cytokines and beta-cell biology: from concept to clinical translation, *Endocr Rev* 29(3):334-350, 2008.

141. Scheuner D, Kaufman RJ: The unfolded protein response: a pathway that links insulin demand with β-cell failure and diabetes, *Endocr Rev* 29(3):317-333, 2008.

142. Burcelin R, Knauf C, Cani PD: Pancreatic alpha-cell dysfunction in diabetes, *Diabetes Metab* 34(Suppl 2):S49-S55, 2008.

143. Göke B: Islet cell function: alpha and beta cells—partners towards normoglycaemia, *Int J Clin Pract Suppl* (159):2-7, 2008.

144. Lebovitz HE: New treatments of diabetes: the beta-amylin agonists, *Annales d Endocrinologie* 69(2):147-150, 2008.

145. Haataja L et al: Islet amyloid in type 2 diabetes, and the toxic oligomer hypothesis, *Endocr Rev* 29(3):303-316, 2008.

146. Khemtemourian L et al: Recent insights in islet amyloid polypeptide-induced membrane disruption and its role in beta-cell death in type 2 diabetes mellitus, *Exp Diabetes Res* 2008:421287, 2008.

147. Salehi M, Aulinger BA, D'Allesio DA: Targeting β-cell mass in type 2 diabetes: promise and limitations of new drugs based on incretins, *Endocr Rev* 29(3):367-379, 2008.

148. Madsbad S et al: Glucagon-like peptide receptor agonists and dipeptidyl peptidase-4 inhibitors in the treatment of diabetes: a review of clinical trials, *Curr Opin Clin Nutr Metab Care* 11(4):491-499, 2008.

149. McIntosh CH: Dipeptidyl peptidase IV inhibitors and diabetes therapy, *Front Biosci* 13:1753-1773, 2008.

150. Richter B et al: Dipeptidyl peptidase-4 (DPP-4) inhibitors for type 2 diabetes mellitus, *Cochrane Database Syst Rev* (2):CD006739, 2008.

151. Dezaki K, Sone H, Yada T: Ghrelin is a physiological regulator of insulin release in pancreatic islets and glucose homeostasis, *Pharmacol Ther* 118(2):239-249, 2008.

152. Crandall JP et al: The prevention of type 2 diabetes, *Nat Clin Pract Endocrinol Metab* 4(7):382-393, 2008.

153. Cummings S, Apovian CM, Khaodhiar L: Obesity surgery: evidence for diabetes prevention/management, *J Am Diet Assoc* 108(4 Suppl 1): S40-S44, 2008.

154. Moo TA, Rubino F: Gastrointestinal surgery as treatment for type 2 diabetes, *Curr Opin Endocrinol Diabetes Obes* 15(2):153-158, 2008.

155. Schernthaner G, Morton JM: Bariatric surgery in patients with morbid obesity and type 2 diabetes, *Diabetes Care* 31(Suppl 2):S297-S302, 2008.

156. Tibaldi J: Initiating and intensifying insulin therapy in type 2 diabetes mellitus, *Am J Med* 121(6 Suppl):S20-S29, 2008.

157. Leibiger IB, Berggren PO: Insulin signaling in the pancreatic beta-cell, *Annu Rev Nutr* 28:233-251, 2008.

158. Fajans SS, Bell GI, Polonsky KS: Molecular mechanisms and clinical pathophysiology of maturity-onset diabetes of the young, *N Engl J Med* 345:971-980, 2001.

159. Holmkvist J et al: Common variants in maturity-onset diabetes of the young genes and future risk of type 2 diabetes, *Diabetes* 57(6):1738-1744, 2008.

160. Vaxillaire M, Froguel P: Monogenic diabetes in the young, pharmacogenetics and relevance to multifactorial forms of type 2 diabetes, *Endocr Rev* 29(3):254-264, 2008.

161. Winckler W et al: Evaluation of common variants in the six known maturity-onset diabetes of the young (MODY) genes for association with type 2 diabetes, *Diabetes* 56(3):685-693, 2007.

162. Bentley-Lewis R et al: Gestational diabetes mellitus: postpartum opportunities for the diagnosis and prevention of type 2 diabetes mellitus, *Nat Clin Pract Endocrinol Metab* 4(10):552-558, 2008.

163. Galtier F et al: Optimizing the outcome of pregnancy in obese women: from pregestational to long-term management, *Diabetes Metab* 34(1):19-25, 2008.

164. Khandelwal M: GDM: postpartum management to reduce long-term risks, *Curr Diabetes Rep* 8(4):287-293, 2008.

165. Pickup JC, Sutton AJ: Severe hypoglycaemia and glycaemic control in type 1 diabetes: meta-analysis of multiple daily insulin injections compared with continuous subcutaneous insulin infusion, *Diabetic Med* 25(7):765-774, 2008.

166. Boyle PJ, Zrebiec J: Impact of therapeutic advances on hypoglycaemia in type 2 diabetes, *Diabetes Metab Res Rev* 24(4):257-285, 2008.

167. Amiel SA et al: Hypoglycaemia in type 2 diabetes, *Diabetic Med* 25(3):245-254, 2008.

168. Qayyum R et al: Systematic review: comparative effectiveness and safety of premixed insulin analogues in type 2 diabetes, *Ann Intern Med* 149(8):549-559, 2008.

169. Hoffman RP: Sympathetic mechanisms of hypoglycemic counterregulation, *Curr Diabetes Rev* 3(3):185-193, 2007.

170. McCrimmon R: The mechanisms that underlie glucose sensing during hypoglycaemia in diabetes, *Res Diabetic Med* 25(5):513-522, 2008.

171. Rossetti P et al: Prevention of hypoglycemia while achieving good glycemic control in type 1 diabetes: the role of insulin analogs, *Diabetes Care* 31(Suppl 2):S113-S120, 2008.

172. Kitabchi AE et al: Thirty years of personal experience in hyperglycemic crises: diabetic ketoacidosis and hyperglycemic hyperosmolar state, *J Clin Endocrinol Metab* 93(5):1541-1552, 2008.

173. Davis SN, Umpierrez GE: Diabetic ketoacidosis in type 2 diabetes mellitus—pathophysiology and clinical presentation, *Nat Clin Pract Endocrinol Metab* 3(11):730-731, 2007.

174. Pinhas-Hamiel O, Zeitler P: Acute and chronic complications of type 2 diabetes mellitus in children and adolescents, *Lancet* 369(9575): 1823-1831, 2007.

175. Balasubramanyam A et al: Syndromes of ketosis-prone diabetes mellitus, *Endocrin Rev* 29:292-302, 2008.

176. Kitabchi AE, Nyenwe EA: Hyperglycemic crises in diabetes mellitus: diabetic ketoacidosis and hyperglycemic hyperosmolar state, *Endocrinol Metab Clin North Am* 35(4):725-751, 2006:viii.

177. Levin DL: Cerebral edema in diabetic ketoacidosis, *Pediatr Crit Care Med* 9(3):320-329, 2008.

178. Keenan CR, Murin S, White RH: High risk for venous thromboembolism in diabetics with hyperosmolar state: comparison with other acute medical illnesses, *J Thromb Haemostasis* 5(6):1185-1190, 2007.

179. Guillod L et al: Nocturnal hypoglycaemias in type 1 diabetic patients: what can we learn with continuous glucose monitoring? *Diabetes Metab* 33(5):360-365, 2007.

180. Hoi-Hansen T, Pedersen-Bjergaard U, Thorsteinsson B: The Somogyi phenomenon revisited using continuous glucose monitoring in daily life, *Diabetologia* 48(11):2437-2438, 2005.

181. Carroll MF, Schade DS: The dawn phenomenon revisited: implications for diabetes therapy, *Endocr Pract* 11(1):55-64, 2005.

182. Aronson D: Hyperglycemia and the pathobiology of diabetic complications, *Adv Cardiol* 45:1-16, 2008.

183. Graves DT, Kayal RA: Diabetic complications and dysregulated innate immunity, *Front Biosci* 13:1227-1239, 2008.

184. Kakehi T, Yabe-Nishimura C: NOX enzymes and diabetic complications, *Semin Immunopathol* 30(3):301-314, 2008.

185. Lorenzi M: The polyol pathway as a mechanism for diabetic retinopathy: attractive, elusive, and resilient, *Exp Diabetes Res* 2007 61038, 2007.

186. Oates PJ: Aldose reductase, still a compelling target for diabetic neuropathy, *Curr Drug Targets* 9(1):14-36, 2008.

187. Noh H, King GL: The role of protein kinase C activation in diabetic nephropathy, *Kidney Int Suppl (106)* :S49-S53, 2007.

188. Das Evcimen N, King GL: The role of protein kinase C activation and the vascular complications of diabetes, *Pharmacol Res* 55(6):498-510, 2007.

189. Jandeleit-Dahm K, Cooper ME: The role of AGEs in cardiovascular disease, *Curr Pharm Des* 14(10):979-986, 2008.

190. Meerwaldt R et al: The clinical relevance of assessing advanced glycation endproducts accumulation in diabetes, *Cardiovasc Diabetol* 7:29, 2008.

191. Yamagishi S et al: Advanced glycation end products (AGEs) and cardiovascular disease (CVD) in diabetes, *Cardiovasc Hematol Agents Med Chem* 5(3):236-240, 2007.

192. Yan SF, Ramasamy R, Schmidt AM: Mechanisms of disease: advanced glycation end-products and their receptor in inflammation and diabetes complications, *Nat Clin Pract Endocrinol Metab* 4(5):285-293, 2008.

193. Forbes JM, Coughlan MT, Cooper ME: Oxidative stress as a major culprit in kidney disease in diabetes. *Diabetes* 57(6):1446-1454, 2008.

194. Son SM: Role of vascular reactive oxygen species in development of vascular abnormalities in diabetes, *Diabetes Res Clin Pract* 77(Suppl 1):S65-S70, 2007.

195. Copeland RJ, Bullen JW, Hart GW: Cross-talk GlcNAcylation and phosphorylation: roles in insulin resistance and glucose toxicity, *Am J Physiol Endocrinol Metab* 295(1):E17-E28, 2008.

196. Fulop N, Marchase RB, Chatham JC: Role of protein O-linked N-acetyl-glucosamine in mediating cell function and survival in the cardiovascular system, *Cardiovasc Res* 73(2):288-297, 2008.

197. Krentz AJ, Clough G, Byrne CD: Interactions between microvascular and macrovascular disease in diabetes: pathophysiology and therapeutic implications, *Diabetes Obes Metab* 9(6):781-791, 2007.

198. Diabetes Control and Complications Trial Research Group: The effect of intensive treatment of diabetes on the development and progression of long-term complications in insulin-dependent diabetes mellitus, *N Engl J Med* 329(14):977-986, 1993.

199. Lang GE: Pharmacological treatment of diabetic retinopathy, *Ophthalmologica* 221(2):112-117, 2008.

200. Cheung N, Wong TY: Diabetic retinopathy and systemic vascular complications, *Prog Retin Eye Res* 27(2):161-176, 2008.

201. Gunduz K, Bakri SJ: Management of proliferative diabetic retinopathy, *Compr Ophthalmol Update* 8(5):245-256, 2007.

202. Dronavalli S, Duka I, Bakris GL: The pathogenesis of diabetic nephropathy, *Nat Clin Pract Endocrinol Metab* 4(8):444-452, 2008.

203. Fioretto P, Mauer M: Histopathology of diabetic nephropathy, *Semin Nephrol* 27(2):195-207, 2007.

204. Forbes JM, Fukami K, Cooper ME: Diabetic nephropathy: where hemodynamics meet metabolism, *Exp Clin Endocrinol Diabetes* 115(2):69-84, 2007.

205. Navarro-Gonzalez JF, Mora-Fernandez C: The role of inflammatory cytokines in diabetic nephropathy, *J Am Soc Nephrol* 19(3):433-442, 2008.

206. Yamagishi S et al: Molecular mechanisms of diabetic nephropathy and its therapeutic intervention, *Curr Drug Targets* 8(8):952-959, 2007.

207. Rogus JJ et al: High-density single nucleotide polymorphism genome-wide linkage scan for susceptibility genes for diabetic nephropathy in type 1 diabetes: discordant sibpair approach, *Diabetes* 57(9):2519-2526, 2008.

208. Harris RD et al: Global glomerular sclerosis and glomerular arteriolar hyalinosis in insulin dependent diabetes, *Kidney Int* 40(1):107-114, 1991.

209. Battisti WP, Palmisano J, Keane WE: Dyslipidemia in patients with type 2 diabetes. Relationships between lipids, kidney disease and cardiovascular disease, *Clin Chem Lab Med* 41(9):1174-1181, 2003.

210. Khosla N, Sarafidis PA, Bakris GL: Microalbuminuria, *Clin Labor Med* 26(3):635-653, 2006.

211. Stachell SC, Tooke JE: What is the mechanism of microalbuminuria in diabetes: a role for the glomerular endothelium? *Diabetologia* 51(5):714-725, 2008.

212. Steffes MW, Mauer SM: Diabetic nephropathy: a disease causing and complicated by hypertension, *Clin Chem* 37(10 Pt 2):1838-1842, 1991.

213. Basi S, Lewis JB: Microalbuminuria as a target to improve cardiovascular and renal outcomes in diabetic patients, *Curr Diab Rep* 7(6):439-442, 2007.

214. Aso Y: Cardiovascular disease in patients with diabetic nephropathy, *Curr Mol Med* 8(6):533-543, 2008.

215. Sonkodi S, Mogyorosi A: Treatment of diabetic nephropathy with angiotensin II blockers, *Nephrol Dial Transplant* 18(Suppl 5):v21-23, 2003.

216. Vinik AI, Mehrabyan A: Diabetic neuropathies, *Med Clin North Am* 88(4):947-999, xi:2004.

217. Sima AA: The heterogeneity of diabetic neuropathy, *Front Biosci* 13:4809-4816, 2008.

218. Zochodne DW: Diabetes mellitus and the peripheral nervous system: manifestations and mechanisms, *Muscle Nerve* 36(2):144-166, 2007.

219. Zochodne DW, Ramji N, Toth C: Neuronal targeting in diabetes mellitus: a story of sensory neurons and motor neurons, *Neuroscientist* 14(4):311-318, 2008.

220. Casellini CM, Vinik AI: Clinical manifestations and current treatment options for diabaetic neuropathies, *Endocr Pract* 13(5):550-566, 2007.

221. Chandrasekharan B, Srinivasan S: Diabetes and the enteric nervous system, *Neurogastroenterol Motil* 19(12):951-960, 2007.

222. Vinik AI et al: Diabetic autonomic neuropathy, *Diabetes Care* 26(5):1553-1579, 2003.

223. Biessels GJ et al: Cognitive dysfunction and diabaetes: implications for primary care, *Prim Care Diabetes* 1(4):187-193, 2007.

224. Diabetes Control and Complications Trial/Epidemiology of Diabetes Interventions and Complications Study Research Group et al: Long-term effect of diabetes and its treatment on cognitive function, *N Engl J Med* 356(18):1842-1852, 2007.

225. La Fonaine J et al: Levels of endothelial nitric oxide synthase and calcitonin gene-related peptide in the Charcot foot: a pilot study, *J Foot Ankle Surg* 47(5):424-429, 2008.

226. Ohkabo Y et al: Intensive insulin therapy prevents the progression of diabetes microvascular complications in Japanese patients with non-insulin–dependent diabetes mellitus: a randomized, prospective 6-year study, *Diabetes Res Clin Pract* 28(2):103-117, 1995.

227. UK Prospective Diabetes Study (UKPDS) Group: Intensive blood-glucose control with sulphonylureas or insulin compared with conventional treatment and risk of complications in patients with type 2 diabetes (UKPDS 33), *Lancet* 352(9131):837-853, 1998.

228. Chiarelli F, Mohn A: Angiopathy in children with diabetes, *Minerva Pediatr* 54(3):187-201, 2002.

229. Coccheri S: Approaches to prevention of cardiovascular complications and events in diabetes mellitus, *Drugs* 67(7):997-1026, 2007.

230. Sowers JR: Insulin resistance and hypertension, *Am J Physiol Heart Circ Physiol* 286(5):H1597-H1602, 2004.

231. Orasanu G, Plutzky J: The pathologic continuum of diabetic vascular disease, *J Am Coll Cardiol* 53(5 Suppl):S35-42, 2009.

232. Retnakaran R, Zinman B: Type 1 diabetes, hyperglycaemia, and the heart, *Lancet* 371(9626):1790-1799, 2008.

233. Natarajan A, Zaman AG, Marshall SM: Platelet hyperactivity in type 2 diabetes: role of antiplatelet agents, *Diab Vasc Dis Res* 5(2):138-144, 2008.

234. Guha A, Harmancey R, Taegtmeyer H: Nonischemic heart failure in diabetes mellitus, *Curr Opin Cardiol* 23(3):241-248, 2008.

235. Bell DS: Stroke in the diabetic patient, *Diabetes Care* 17(3):213-219, 1994.

236. Furie K, Inzucchi SE: Diabetes mellitus, insulin resistance, hyperglycemia, and stroke, *Curr Neurol Neurosci Rep* 8(1):12-19, 2008.

237. Gazis A et al: Mortality in patients with diabetic neuropathic osteoarthropathy (Charcot foot), *Diabetes Med* 21(11):1243-1246, 2004.

238. Al-Delaimy WK et al: Effect of type 2 diabetes and its duration on the risk of peripheral arterial disease among men, *Am J Med* 116(4): 236-240, 2004.

239. Mohler ER 3rd: Therapy insight: peripheral arterial disease and diabetes-from pathogenesis to treatment guidelines, *Nat Clin Pract Cardiovasc Med* 4(3):151-162, 2007.

240. Bowering CK: Diabetic foot ulcers: pathophysiology, assessment, and therapy, *Can Fam Physician* 47:1107-1116, 2001.

241. Jude EB, Unsworth PF: Optimal treatment of infected diabetic foot ulcers, *Drugs Aging* 21(13):833-850, 2004.

242. Gardner SE, Grantz RA: Wound bioburden and infection-related complications in diabetic foot ulcers, *Biol Res Nurs* 10(1):44-53, 2008.

243. Peleg AY et al: Common infections in diabetes: pathogenesis, management and relationship to glycaemic control, *Diabetes Metab Res Rev* 23(1):3-13, 2007.

244. Bolland MJ et al: Cushing's syndrome due to interaction between inhaled corticosteroids and itraconazole, *Ann Pharmacother* 38(1): 46-49, 2004.

245. Newell-Price J et al: Cushing's syndrome. *Lancet* 367:1605-1617, 2006.

246. Stratakis CA: Cushing syndrome caused by adrenocortical tumors and hyperplasias (corticotropin-independent Cushing syndrome), *Endocr Dev* 13:117-132, 2008.

247. Aghi MK: Management of recurrent and refractory Cushing disease, *Nat Clin Pract Endocrinol Metab* 4(10):560-568, 2008.

248. Pivonello R et al: Cushing's syndrome, *Endocrinol Metab Clin North Am* 37(1):135-149, ix:2008.

249. Schuff KG: Issues in the diagnosis of Cushing's syndrome for the primary care physician, *Prim Care* 30(4):791-799, 2003.

250. Newell-Price J: Proopiomelanocortin gene expression and DNA methylation: implications for Cushing's syndrome and beyond, *Endocrinology* 177(3):365-372, 2003.

251. Findling JW, Raff H: Diagnosis and differential diagnosis of Cushing's syndrome, *Endocrinol Metab Clin North Am* 30(3):729-747, 2001.

252. Sonimo N, Fava GA: Psychiatric disorders associated with Cushing's syndrome. Epidemiology, pathophysiology, and treatment, *CNS Drugs* 15(5):361-373, 2001.

253. Pecori Giraldi F, Moro M, Cavagnini F: Gender-related differences in the presentation and course of Cushing's disease, *J Clin Endocrinol Metab* 88:1554-1558, 2003.

254. Reimondo G et al: Laboratory differentiation of Cushing's syndrome, *Clin Chim Acta* 388(1-2):5-14, 2008.

255. Davies JS et al: Diagnostic dilemmas in Cushing's syndrome, *Ann Clin Biochem* 37(Pt1):85-89, 2000.

256. Biller BM et al: Treatment of adrencorticotropin-dependent Cushing's syndrome: a concensus statement, *J Clin Endocrinol Metab* 93(7):2454-2462, 2008.

257. Shalet S, Mukherjee A: Pharmacological treatment of hypercortisolism, *Curr Opin Endocrinol Diabetes Obes* 15(3):234-238, 2008.

258. Young WF: Primary aldosteronism: renaissance of a syndrome, *Clin Endocrinol Oxf* 66(5):607-618, 2007.

259. Karagiannis A et al: Medical treatment as an alternative to adrenalectomy in patients with aldosterone-producing adenoma, *Endocr Relat Cancer* 15(3):693-700, 2008.

260. Young WF Jr: Minireview: primary aldosteronism—changing concepts in diagnosis and treatment, *Endocrinology* 144(6):2208-2213, 2003.

261. Herbert SC: Bartter syndrome, *Curr Opin Nephrol Hypertens* 12(4): 527-532, 2003.

262. Fallo F et al: The metabolic syndrome in primary aldosteronism, *Curr Diab Rep* 8(1):43-47, 2008.

263. Mattsson C, Young WF Jr: Primary aldosteronism: diagnostic and treatment strategies, *Nat Clin Pract Nephrol* 2(4):198-208, 2006.

264. Boscaro M et al: Diagnosis and management of primary aldosteronism, *Curr Opin Endocrinol Diabetes Obes* 15(4):332-338, 2008.

265. Rossi GP, Pessina AC, Heagerty AM: Primary aldosteronism: an update on screening, diagnosis and treatment, *J Hypertens* 26(4):613-621, 2008.

266. Falorni A et al: Italian Addison network study: update of diagnostic criteria for the etiological classification of primary adrenal insufficiency, *J Clin Endocrinol Metab* 89(4):1598-1604, 2004.

267. Larsen RP et al: *Williams textbook of endocrinology*, ed 10, Philadelphia, 2003, Saunders.

268. Nieman LK: Chanco Turner ML: Addison's disease, *Clin Dermatol* 24(4):276-280, 2006.

269. Anglin RE, Rosebush PI, Mazurek MF: The neuropsychiatric profile of Addison's disease, revisiting a forgotten phenomenon, *J Neuropsychiatry Clin Neurosci* 18(4):450-459, 2006.

270. Lovas K, Husebye ES: Replacement therapy for Addison's disease: recent developments, *Expert Opin Invest Drugs* 17(4):497-509, 2008.

271. Opocher G et al: Clinical and genetic aspects of phaeochromocytoma, *Horm Res* 59(Suppl 1):59-61, 2003.

272. Mittendorf EA et al: Pheochromocytoma: advances in genetics, diagnosis, localization, and treatment, *Hematol Oncol Clin North Am* 21(3):509-525, 2007.

273. Bravo EKL, Pheochromocytoma: *Cardiol Rev* 10(1):44-50, 2002.

274. Chrisoulidou A et al: The diagnosis and management of malignant phaeochromocytoma and paraganglioma, *Endocr Relat Cancer* 14(3):569-585, 2007.

STRUCTURE AND FUNCTION OF THE REPRODUCTIVE SYSTEMS

ANGELA DENERIS • SUE E. HUETHER

CHAPTER

22

MEDIA RESOURCES

evolve Evolve Website (http://evolve.elsevier.com/McCance/)
- Review Questions and Answers
- Animations
- Glossary (with audio pronunciation for selected terms)
- WebLinks

CHAPTER OUTLINE

DEVELOPMENT OF THE REPRODUCTIVE SYSTEMS
    Sexual Differentiation and Hormone Production In Utero
    Puberty
THE FEMALE REPRODUCTIVE SYSTEM
    External Genitalia
    Internal Genitalia
    Female Sex Hormones
    The Menstrual Cycle
THE MALE REPRODUCTIVE SYSTEM
    External Genitalia
    Internal Genitalia
    Spermatogenesis
    Male Sex Hormones

STRUCTURE AND FUNCTION OF THE BREAST
    The Female Breast
    The Male Breast
TESTS OF REPRODUCTIVE FUNCTION
    Infection and Cancer Tests
    Fertility Tests
        Aging and Reproductive Function
    Aging and the Female Reproductive System
    Aging and the Male Reproductive System

The male and female reproductive systems have several anatomic and physiologic features in common. Most obvious is their major function, reproduction, through which a 23-chromosome female gamete, the **ovum,** and a 23-chromosome male gamete, the **spermatozoon (sperm cell),** unite to form a 46-chromosome zygote that is capable of developing into a new individual. The male reproductive system produces sperm and delivers them to the female reproductive tract. The female reproductive system produces the ovum and, if it is fertilized, can nurture and protect it (at that point called the **embryo** and **developing fetus**) and expel it at birth. These functions are determined not only by anatomic structures but also by complex hormonal, neurologic, and psychogenic factors.[1]

DEVELOPMENT OF THE REPRODUCTIVE SYSTEMS

The structure and function of male and female reproductive systems depend on steroid hormones called **sex hormones.** Hormonal effects on the reproductive systems begin well before birth and continue for life.

Sexual Differentiation and Hormone Production in Utero

During embryonic development, the initial reproductive structures of male and female embryos are homologous (the same) and consist of one pair of primary sex organs, or **gonads,** and two pairs of ducts, the mesonephric ducts

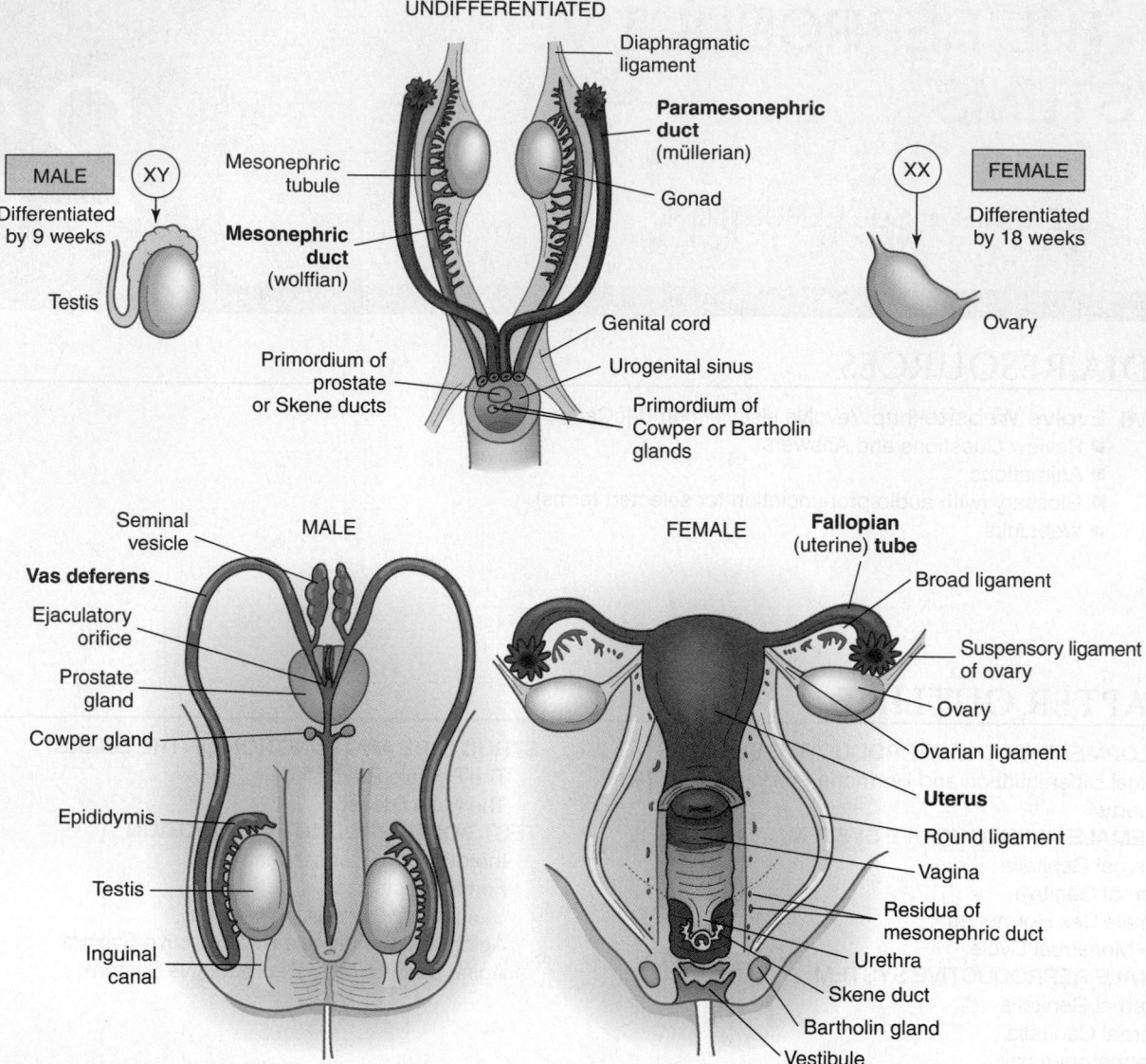

Figure 22-1 Internal genitalia development. Embryonic and fetal development of the internal genitalia.

(wolffian ducts) and the paramesonephric ducts (müllerian ducts) (Figure 22-1). Both pairs of ducts empty into an opening called the *urogenital sinus.*

Between 6 and 7 weeks' gestation, the male embryo will differentiate under the influence of testes-determining factor (TDF). The TDF is from a gene in the sex-determining region on the Y chromosome (SRY). This gene stimulates the gondal development of testes, which in turn produces antimüllerian hormone (AMH) and testosterone. AMH inhibits the formation of müllerian ducts. As the testes begin to differentiate, Sertoli cells appear and aggregate to form testicular cords. Mature Sertoli cells will produce inhibin and androgen-binding protein (ABP), which is important for spermatogenesis. Leydig cells differentiate at the beginning of the eighth week and the secretion of testosterone begins.[1,2] Under the influence of testosterone, the male gonads develop into two testes that produce sperm after puberty. The paramesonephric

ducts degenerate and the mesonephric ducts develop (wolffian system) into the vas deferens—the two tubes that carry sperm from the testes to the urethra (see Figure 22-1). By 9 months' gestation the male gonads (testes) have descended into the scrotum.

In female embryos the gonads produce the primary female sex hormone, estrogen. In the absence of testosterone there is a loss of the Wolffian system and the two gonads develop into ovaries at 6 to 8 weeks' gestation. There is rapid mitotic multiplication of germ cells and by 16 to 20 weeks there is a peak of 6 to 7 million oogonia. Oogonia are transformed into oocytes throughout the remainder of the pregnancy, when they enter the first meiotic division. This will remain stable until puberty. Just before ovulation a single ovum will be formed from two meiotic divisions of the oocytes. By birth only 1 to 2 million oocytes remain.[1] In females the mesonephric ducts deteriorate and the lower ends of the paramesonephric ducts

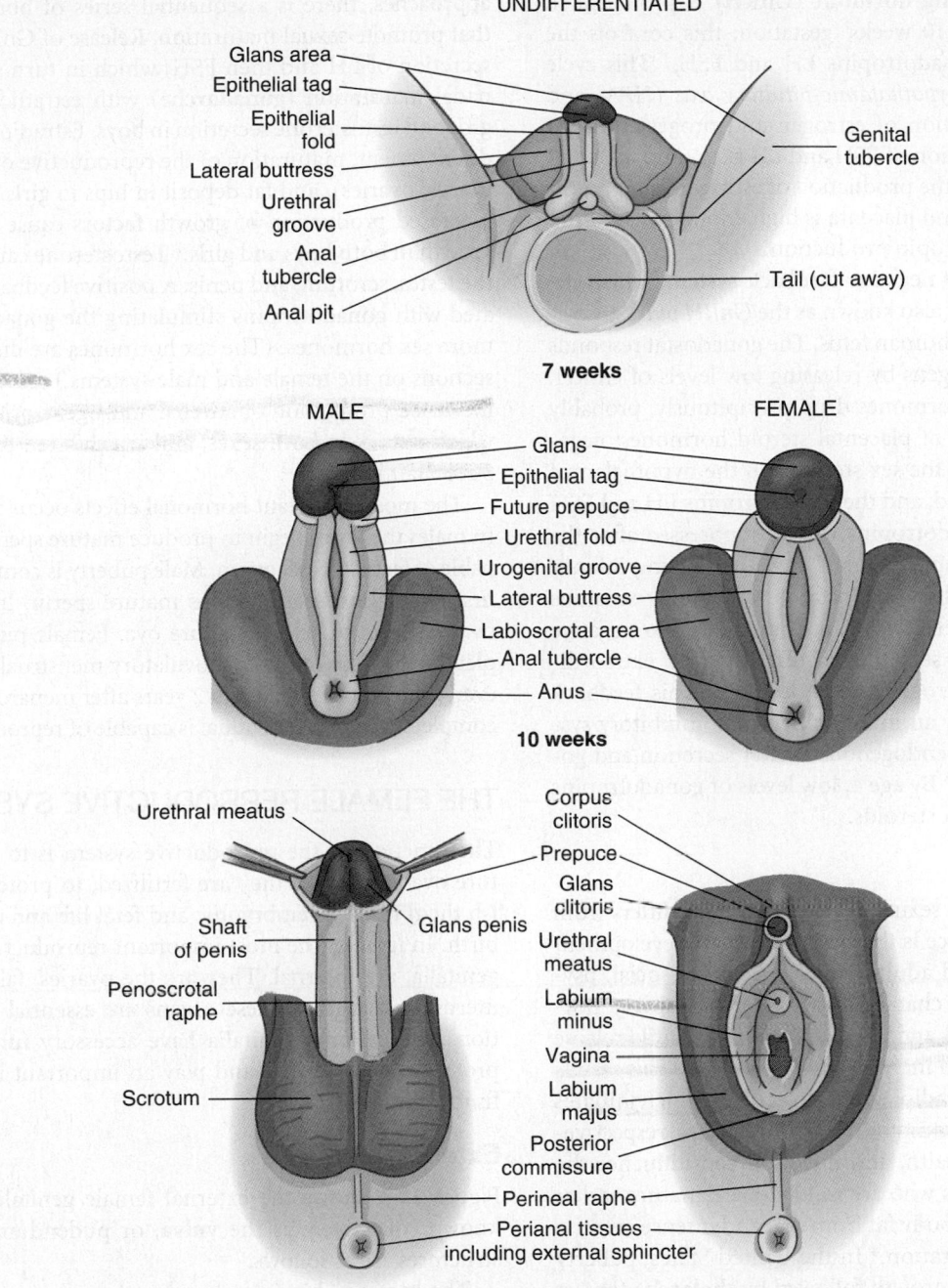

UNDIFFERENTIATED

Glans area
Epithelial tag
Epithelial fold
Lateral buttress
Urethral groove
Anal tubercle
Anal pit

Genital tubercle

Tail (cut away)

7 weeks

MALE | FEMALE

Glans
Epithelial tag
Future prepuce
Urethral fold
Urogenital groove
Lateral buttress
Labioscrotal area
Anal tubercle
Anus

10 weeks

Urethral meatus
Shaft of penis
Glans penis
Penoscrotal raphe
Scrotum

Corpus clitoris
Prepuce
Glans clitoris
Urethral meatus
Labium minus
Vagina
Labium majus
Posterior commissure
Perineal raphe
Perianal tissues including external sphincter

Near 40 weeks

Figure 22-2 External genitalia development. Embryonic and fetal development of the external genitalia.

join to become the uterus, fallopian tubes, cervix, and upper two thirds of the vagina. The upper portions of the paramesonephric ducts develop into the fallopian (uterine) tubes (Figure 22-2). These two ducts carry ova from the ovaries to the uterus.

Like the internal reproductive structures, the external structures develop from homologous embryonic tissues. During the first 7 to 8 weeks of gestation, both male and female embryos develop an elevated structure called the *genital tubercle*. Figure 22-2 shows how the undifferentiated genital tubercle develops

into the external reproductive organs. Under hormonal influence, male genitalia develop when testosterone is present. Female genitalia will develop if testosterone or testosterone receptors are absent even in the absence of ovaries.

Anterior pituitary development starts between the fourth and fifth weeks of fetal life and the vascular connection between the hypothalamus and the pituitary is established by the twelfth week. In the female fetus, high levels of two gonadotropins, **follicle-stimulating hormone** (FSH) and **luteinizing hormone** (LH) are excreted by the anterior pituitary.

Gonadotropin-releasing hormone (GnRH) is produced in the hypothalamus by 10 weeks' gestation; this controls the production of the gonadotropins LH and FSH.[1] This cycle is referred to as the *hypothalamic-pituitary axis (HPA)* and stimulates the production of estrogen and progesterone by the ovary. The production of FSH and LH rises until about 28 weeks' gestation, until the production of estrogen and progesterone by the ovaries and placenta is high enough to result in the decline of gonadotropin production.

At term, a sensitive negative-feedback system, which includes the **gonadostat** (also known as the *GnRH pulse generator*), is operative in the human fetus. The gonadostat responds to high placental estrogens by releasing low levels of GnRH. Soon after birth, sex hormones drop precipitously, probably because of withdrawal of placental steroid hormones; negative feedback action of the sex steroids on the hypothalamus and pituitary is removed; and the gonadotropins LH and FSH are released. The gonadotropins will be suppressed after the first year of life until approximately age 10. During infancy and early childhood, the gonadostat is remarkably sensitive (6 to 15 times more sensitive than in the adult) to negative feedback,[1] and GnRH secretion is restrained by extraordinarily low levels of estrogen or testosterone. This feedback mechanism is probably an intrinsic neuronal inhibitory system, which suppresses endogenous GnRH secretion and gonadotropin synthesis.[1,3] By age 4, low levels of gonadotropins parallel low levels of sex steroids.

Puberty

Puberty is the onset of sexual development and differs from adolescence. Adolescence is the stage of human development between childhood and adulthood and includes social, psychologic, and biologic changes. The onset of puberty normally begins between 8 and 14 years with a pulsatile release of GnRH followed by an increase in LH and FSH. This results in episodic peaks of estradiol and testosterone, which initiates the secondary sexual maturation in girls and boys, respectively. Genetics, general health, and nutrition can influence the timing of puberty. Girls who are mildly obese mature earlier and girls who have low body fat from diet and intense exercise will have delayed maturation.[4] In the United States, puberty begins with accelerated growth followed by **thelarche** (breast development) at about 9 years of age in white girls and 8 years of age in black girls. Early puberty in girls has been linked to obesity and more recently to increased levels of **leptin,** a hormone secreted from adipose tissue, which acts on central nervous system (CNS) neurons that regulate appetite.[3,5,6] Leptin levels increase through childhood until the onset of puberty and then decrease as puberty advances. Leptin probably contributes to increased adipose tissue, thereby allowing maturation to occur.[1]

Puberty is a process that involves a complex series of interrelated physiologic changes leading to reproductive maturation.[3] Reproductive maturation involves the hypothalamic-pituitary-gonadal (H-P-G) axis, the central nervous system, and the endocrine system (Figure 22-3). As puberty approaches, there is a sequential series of hormonal events that promote sexual maturation. Release of GnRH stimulates secretion of LH and then FSH, which in turn stimulates gonadal maturation (**gonadarche**) with estradiol secretion in girls and testosterone secretion in boys. Estradiol causes breast development, maturation of the reproductive organs (vagina, uterus, ovaries), and fat deposit in hips in girls. Estrogen and increased production of growth factors cause rapid skeletal growth in both boys and girls.[7] Testosterone causes growth of the testes, scrotum, and penis. A positive feedback loop is created with gonadotropins stimulating the gonads to produce more sex hormones. (The sex hormones are discussed in the sections on the female and male systems.) **Adrenarche** is the increased production of adrenal androgens prior to puberty, which occurs in both sexes, and is exhibited by axillary and pubic hair growth.[1,3]

The most important hormonal effects occur in the gonads. In males the testes begin to produce mature sperm that are capable of fertilizing an ovum. Male puberty is complete with the first ejaculation that contains mature sperm. In females, the ovaries begin to release mature ova. Female puberty is complete at the time of the first ovulatory menstrual period; however, this can take up to 1 to 2 years after menarche. Puberty is complete when an individual is capable of reproduction.

THE FEMALE REPRODUCTIVE SYSTEM

The function of the reproductive system is to produce mature ova and, when they are fertilized, to protect and nourish them through embryonic and fetal life and expel them at birth. In females the most important reproductive organs, or genitalia, are internal. They are the ovaries, fallopian tubes, uterus, and vagina. These organs are essential to reproduction. The external genitalia have accessory functions. They protect body openings and play an important role in sexual functioning.[1,8,9]

External Genitalia

Figure 22-4 shows the external female genitalia, which are known collectively as the **vulva,** or pudendum. The major structures are as follows.

The **mons pubis** (also known as *mons veneris*) is a fatty layer of tissue over the pubic symphysis (joint of the pubic bones). During puberty the mons pubis becomes covered with pubic hair, and its sebaceous and sweat glands become more active. Estrogen causes fat to be deposited under the skin, giving the mons pubis a moundlike shape. This cushion of tissue protects the pubic symphysis during sexual intercourse.

The **labia majora** (*singular,* **labium majus**) are two folds of skin that arise at the mons pubis and extend back to the fourchette, forming a cleft. Like the mons pubis, the labia majora undergo changes at puberty: the amount of fatty tissue increases, pubic hair grows on the lateral surfaces, and sebaceous glands on the hairless medial surfaces begin to secrete lubricants. Because of an extensive network of nerve endings, the labia majora are highly sensitive to temperature, touch,

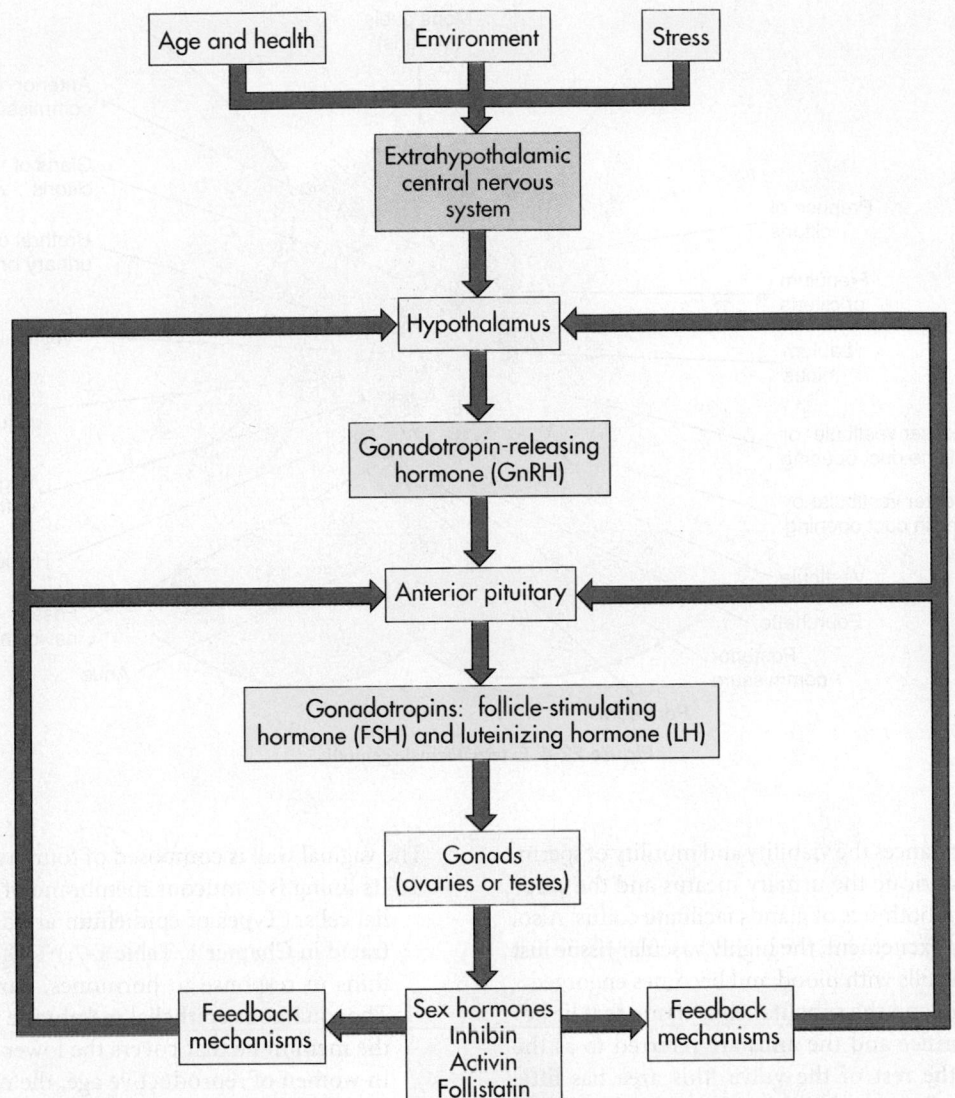

Figure 22-3 Hormonal stimulation of the gonads. The hypothalamic-pituitary-gonadal axis.

pressure, and pain and are homologous to the male scrotum (see Figure 22-2 and Figure 22-13). The principal function of the labia majora is to protect the inner structures of the vulva.

The **labia minora** (*singular,* **labium minus**), two smaller, thinner folds of skin, lie within the labia majora. Anteriorly they form the clitoral hood, or prepuce, and frenulum, then split to enclose the vestibule, and converge near the anus, forming the fourchette. The labia minora are hairless, pink, and moist and are well supplied with nerves, blood vessels, and sebaceous glands. These glands secrete a bactericidal fluid that has a distinctive odor and that lubricates and waterproofs the vulvar skin. During sexual arousal the labia minora become swollen with blood.

The **clitoris** is a richly innervated, erectile organ that lies anterior, between the labia minora. It is a small, cylindrical structure having a glans that is visible and a shaft that lies beneath the skin (see Figure 22-4). The clitoris is homologous

to the male penis. Like the penis, the clitoris is a major site of sexual stimulation and orgasm. With sexual arousal, erectile tissues in the clitoris fill with blood, causing it to enlarge somewhat. Similar to other vulvar glands, the clitoris secretes a fluid, called *smegma,* which has a unique odor and may be erotically stimulating to the male.

The **vestibule** is the area protected by the labia minora and contains the external opening of the vagina, which is called the **introitus,** or vaginal orifice. A thin, perforated membrane called the **hymen** may cover the introitus. The vestibule also contains the opening of the urethra, or **urinary meatus** (orifice). These structures are lubricated by two pairs of glands: Skene glands and Bartholin glands. The ducts of **Skene glands** (also called the **lesser vestibular** or **paraurethral glands**) open on both sides of the urinary meatus. The ducts of **Bartholin glands** (**greater vestibular** or **vulvovaginal glands**) open on either side of the introitus. In response to sexual stimulation, Bartholin glands secrete mucus that lubricates the inner labial

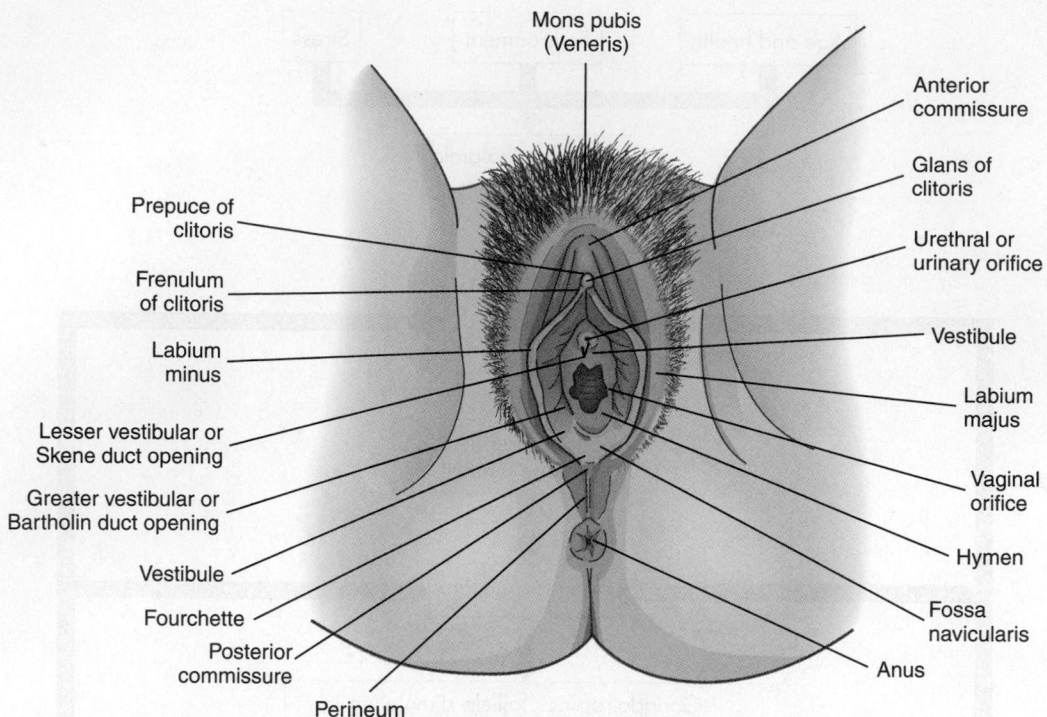

Figure 22-4 External female genitalia.

surfaces, as well as enhances the viability and motility of sperm. Skene glands help lubricate the urinary meatus and the vestibule. Secretions from both sets of glands facilitate coitus. Also, in response to sexual excitement, the highly vascular tissue just beneath the vestibule fills with blood and becomes engorged.

The less hairy skin and the subcutaneous tissue that lie between the vaginal orifice and the anus are referred to as the **perineum.** Unlike the rest of the vulva, this area has little subcutaneous fat so that the skin is close to the underlying muscles. The perineum covers the muscular **perineal body,** a fibrous structure that comprises elastic fiber, connective tissue, and the common attachment of the bulbocavernosus, the external anal sphincter, and the levator ani muscles (see Figure 22-4). The perineum varies in length from 2 to 5 cm or more and stretches remarkably. The length of the perineum and the elasticity of the perineal body influence tissue resistance and injury during childbirth.

Internal Genitalia

Vagina

The **vagina** is an elastic fibromuscular canal, 9 to 10 cm long in a reproductive-aged female, which extends up and back from the introitus to the lower portion of the uterus. As Figure 22-5 shows, it lies between the urethra (and part of the bladder) and the rectum. Mucosal secretions from the upper genital organs, menstrual fluids, and products of conception leave the body through the vagina, which also receives the penis during coitus. During sexual excitement the vagina lengthens and widens and the anterior third becomes congested with blood.

The vaginal wall is composed of four layers:

1. Its lining is a mucous membrane of squamous epithelial cells. (Types of epithelium are described and illustrated in Chapter 1, Table 1-7.) This layer thickens and thins in response to hormones, particularly estrogen. The squamous epithelial membrane is continuous with the membrane that covers the lower part of the uterus. In women of reproductive age, the mucosal layer is arranged in transverse wrinkles, or folds, called **rugae** (*singular,* **ruga**) that permit stretching during coitus and childbirth.
2. Fibrous connective tissue containing numerous blood and lymphatic vessels.
3. Smooth muscle.
4. Connective tissue and a rich network of blood vessels.

The upper part of the vagina surrounds the cervix, the lower end of the uterus (see Figure 22-5). The recessed space around the cervix is called the **fornix** of the vagina. The posterior fornix is "deeper" than the anterior fornix because of the angle at which the cervix meets the vaginal canal. In most women this angle is about 90 degrees. A pouch called the **cul-de-sac** separates the posterior fornix and the rectum.

Its elasticity and relatively sparse nerve supply enhance the vagina's function as the birth canal. During sexual arousal the vaginal wall becomes engorged with blood, like the labia minora and clitoris. Engorgement pushes some fluid to the surface of the mucosa, enhancing lubrication. The vaginal wall does not contain mucus-secreting glands; rather, secretions drain into the vagina from the endocervical glands or enter from the vestibule, from the Bartholin and Skene glands.

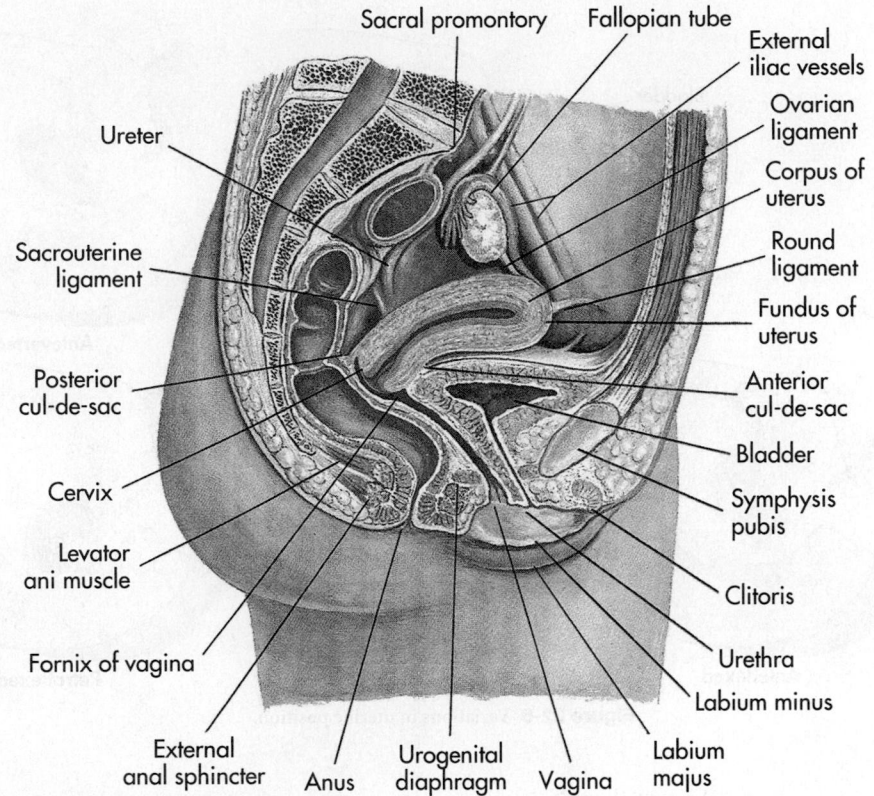

Figure 22-5 Internal female genitalia and other pelvic organs. Midsagittal view. (Modified from Seidel HM et al: *Mosby's guide to physical examination,* ed 6, St Louis, 2006, Mosby.)

Two factors help maintain the self-cleansing action of the vagina and defend it from infection, particularly during the reproductive years: (1) an acid-base balance that discourages the proliferation of most pathogenic bacteria and (2) the thickness of the vaginal epithelium. Before puberty, vaginal pH is about 7 (neutral) and the vaginal epithelium is thin. At puberty, the pH becomes more acidic (4 to 5) and the squamous epithelial lining thickens. These changes are maintained until menopause (cessation of menstruation), at which time the pH rises again to more alkaline levels and the epithelium thins out. Therefore, protection from infection is greatest during the years when a woman is most likely to be sexually active. Between puberty and menopause, vulnerability to infection varies somewhat with cyclic changes in pH and epithelial thickness. Both defenses are greatest when estrogen levels are high and the vagina contains a normal population of *Lactobacillus acidophilus,* a harmless resident bacterium that helps maintain pH at acidic levels. Any condition that causes vaginal pH to rise, such as douching or use of vaginal sprays or deodorants, low estrogen levels, or destruction of *L. acidophilus* by antibiotics, lowers vaginal defenses against infection.

Uterus

The **uterus** is a hollow pear-shaped organ whose lower end opens into the vagina. The functions of the uterus are to anchor and protect a fertilized ovum, provide an optimal environment while it develops, and push the fetus out at birth.

In addition, the uterus plays an important role in sexual response and conception. During sexual excitement the opening of the uterus (the cervix) dilates slightly. At the same time, the uterus increases in size and moves upward and backward, creating a tenting effect in the midvagina that results in the cervix "sitting" in a pool of semen. During orgasm, rhythmic contractions facilitate movement of sperm through the cervical os while also enhancing physical pleasure.

At puberty the uterus attains its adult size and proportions and descends from the abdomen to the lower pelvis, between the bladder and the rectum (see Figure 22-5). The uterus of a mature, nonpregnant female is approximately 7 to 9 cm long and 6.5 cm wide, with muscular walls 3.5 cm thick. It is held loosely in position by ligaments, peritoneal tissue folds, and pressure of adjacent organs, especially the urinary bladder, sigmoid colon, and rectum. In most women the uterus is anteverted; that is, it is tipped forward so that it rests on the urinary bladder. However, it may be retroverted, or tipped backward. Various degrees of flexion are normal (Figure 22-6).

Figure 22-7 shows a cross section of the uterus. The uterus has two major parts: the body, or **corpus,** and the cervix. The top of the corpus, above the insertion of the fallopian tubes, is called the **fundus.** The diameter of the uterine cavity is widest at the fundus and narrowest at the **isthmus,** which is the narrowed part of the corpus just above the cervix. The **cervix,** or "neck of the uterus," extends from the isthmus to the vagina. The passageway between the cervix's upper opening (the

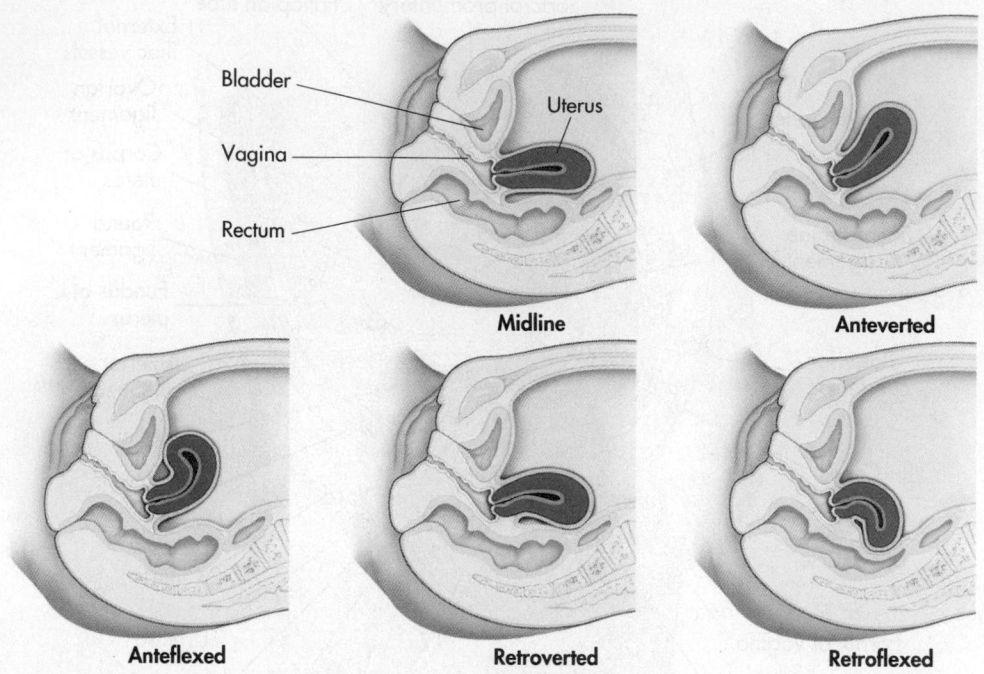

Bladder

Uterus

Vagina

Rectum

Midline

Anteverted

Anteflexed

Retroverted

Retroflexed

Figure 22-6 Variations in uterine position.

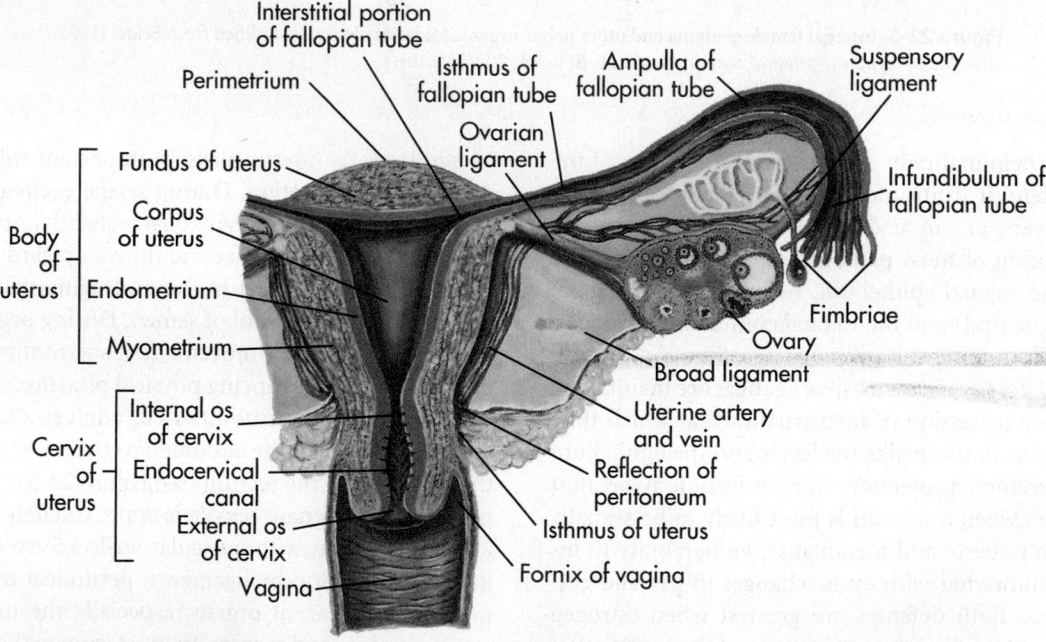

Interstitial portion
of fallopian tube

Isthmus of
fallopian tube

Ampulla of
fallopian tube

Suspensory
ligament

Perimetrium

Ovarian
ligament

Fundus of uterus

Infundibulum of
fallopian tube

Corpus
of uterus

Body
of
uterus

Endometrium

Myometrium

Fimbriae

Ovary

Broad ligament

Internal os
of cervix

Uterine artery
and vein

Cervix
of
uterus

Endocervical
canal

Reflection of
peritoneum

External os
of cervix

Isthmus of uterus

Fornix of vagina

Vagina

Figure 22-7 Cross section of uterus, fallopian tube, and ovary. (From Seidel HM et al: *Mosby's guide to physical examination,* ed 6, St Louis, 2006, Mosby.)

internal os) and its lower opening (the external os) is called the **endocervical canal.** The entire uterus, like the upper vagina, is innervated exclusively by motor and sensory fibers of the autonomic nervous system.

The uterine wall is composed of three layers: the perimetrium, the myometrium, and the endometrium (see Figure 22-7). The **perimetrium (parietal peritoneum)** is the outer

serous membrane that covers the uterus. The **myometrium** is the thick muscular middle layer. The myometrium is thickest at the fundus, apparently to facilitate birth. The **endometrium,** or uterine lining, is composed of a functional layer (superficial compact layer and spongy middle layer) and a basal layer. The functional layer of the endometrium is responsive to sex hormones. Between puberty and menopause this layer proliferates and sloughs off monthly. The basal layer, which is attached to the myometrium, regenerates the functional layer after it sloughs (menstruation).

The endocervical canal does not have an endometrial layer. Rather, it is lined with columnar epithelial cells (see Table 1-7). The endocervical lining is continuous with that of the outer cervix and vagina, but it is not made up of the same type of epithelial cells. The point at which the columnar epithelium of the cervix meets the squamous epithelium of the vagina is called the *transformation zone,* or the **squamous-columnar junction.** The transformation zone is especially susceptible to the oncogenic human papillomavirus (HPV), which leads to cervical dysplasia and, ultimately, cervical cancer; these are the cells sampled during a Papanicolaou test (Pap test).[10]

The cervix acts as a mechanical barrier to infectious microorganisms that may be present in the vagina. The external cervical os is a very small opening that contains thick, sticky mucus (the *mucous plug*) during the luteal phase of the menstrual cycle and all of pregnancy. During ovulation, the mucus changes under the influence of estrogen and forms watery strands, or spinnbarkeit mucus, to facilitate the transport of sperm into the uterus. In addition, the downward flow of cervical secretions moves microorganisms away from the cervix and uterus. In women of reproductive age, the pH of these secretions is inhospitable to most bacteria. Further, mucosal secretions contain enzymes and antibodies (mostly immunoglobulin A) of the secretory immune system. (The secretory immune system is discussed in Chapter 7.) These defenses do not always prevent infection, even if they are intact. Besides infection, uterine pathophysiology includes displacement of the uterus within the pelvis, benign growths (fibroids) of the uterine wall, hyperplasia of the endometrium, endometriosis, and cancer.

Fallopian Tubes

The two **fallopian tubes (oviducts, uterine tubes)** enter the uterus bilaterally just beneath the fundus (see Figure 22-7). Their function is to conduct the ova from the spaces around the ovaries to the uterus. From the uterus the fallopian tubes curve up and over the two ovaries. Each tube is 8 to 12 cm long and about 1 cm in diameter, except at its ovarian end, which flares out like the bell of a trumpet. This widened end, called the **infundibulum,** is fringed or fimbriated. The **fimbriae** (*singular,* fimbria) (fringes) move, creating a current that draws the ovum into the infundibulum. Once the ovum has entered the fallopian tube, cilia and peristalsis (muscle contractions) keep it moving toward the uterus.

The ampulla, or distal third, of the fallopian tube is the usual site of fertilization (see Figure 22-7). Sperm released into the vagina travel upward through the endocervical canal and uterine cavity and enter the fallopian tubes. If an ovum is present in either tube, fertilization can occur. Whether or not the ovum encounters sperm, it continues to travel through the fallopian tube to the uterus. If fertilized, the ovum (then called a *blastocyst*) implants itself in the endometrial layer of the uterine wall. If not fertilized, the ovum breaks down within 12 to 24 hours.

Disorders that affect the fallopian tubes can block the path of sperm and ovum and cause infertility or ectopic (tubal) pregnancy. Such disorders include congenital malformations, infection, and inflammation.

Ovaries

The **ovaries,** or the female gonads, are the primary female reproductive organs. They have two main functions: secretion of female sex hormones and development and release of female gametes, or ova.

The almond-shaped ovaries are located on both sides of the uterus and are suspended and supported by the mesovarian portions of the broad ligament, ovarian ligaments, and suspensory ligaments (see Figure 22-7). The ovaries are smaller than their male homologs, the testes. In women of reproductive age, each ovary is 3 to 5 cm long, 2.5 cm wide, and 2 cm thick and weighs 4 to 8 g. Size and weight vary somewhat from phase to phase of the menstrual cycle (see p. 792).

Figure 22-8 shows a cross section of an ovary. The central part, or medulla, is composed of connective tissue and contains many small arteries, veins, and lymphatics that enter at the hilum. Surrounding the medulla is the cortex. At birth the cortex of each ovary contains approximately 2 million ova within immature **ovarian follicles.** Follicles grow and undergo atresia continuously and irrevocably during a woman's life. By puberty the number ranges between 300,000 and 500,000 ova. During puberty some of the follicles and the ova within them begin to mature. Between puberty and menopause the ovarian cortex always contains follicles and ova in various stages of development. Once every menstrual cycle (about every 28 days), usually only one of the follicles reaches maturation and discharges its ovum through the ovary's outer covering, the germinal epithelium. During the reproductive years, 400 to 500 ovarian follicles mature completely and release an ovum, an event termed **ovulation.** The rest either fail to develop at all or degenerate without maturing completely.[1]

Having ejected a mature ovum, the follicle develops into another structure, the **corpus luteum** (see Figure 22-8). The immediate fate of the corpus luteum depends on whether the ejected ovum is fertilized. If fertilization occurs, the corpus luteum enlarges and begins to secrete hormones that maintain and support pregnancy. If fertilization does not occur, the corpus luteum secretes these hormones for approximately 14 days and then degenerates, which triggers the maturation of another follicle. The **ovarian cycle**—the process of follicular maturation, ovulation, corpus luteum development, and corpus luteum degeneration—is continuous from puberty to menopause, except during pregnancy or hormonal contraceptive use. At menopause, this process ceases and the ovaries atrophy to the point that they cannot be felt during pelvic examination.

Four types of cells within the ovarian cortex secrete sex hormones: cells of the stroma, or tissue matrix; two types of cells in the ovarian follicle, **granulosa cells** and **theca cells,** and cells of the corpus luteum (Figure 22-9). These cells all contain receptors for the gonadotropins (LH and FSH) or for the sex hormones, which are discussed in the next section.

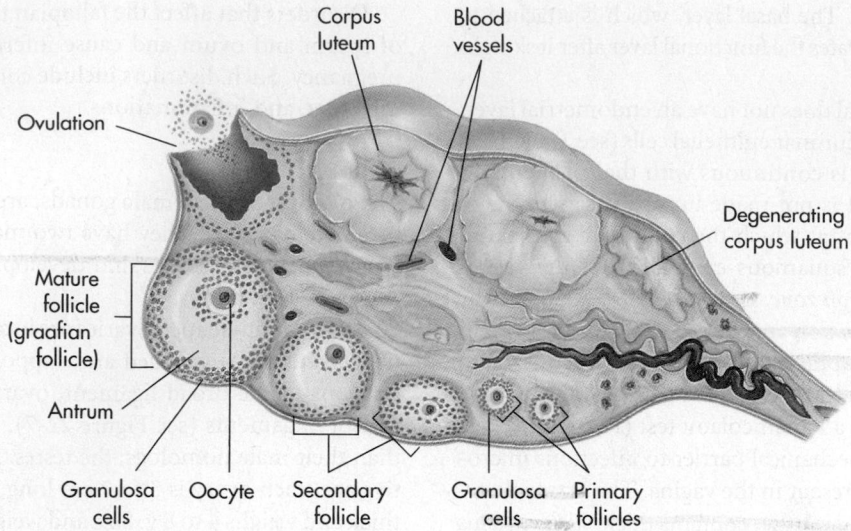

Figure 22-8 Cross section of ovary during reproductive years. (From Patton KT, Thibodeau GA: *Anatomy & physiology,* ed 7, St Louis, 2010, Mosby.)

Because gonadotropins and hormones regulate ovarian function, any disorder that disrupts this process, such as abnormal pituitary or thyroid function, or reception by target cells can cause ovarian dysfunction and infertility. Benign or malignant growths, cysts, infection, or inflammation also can cause ovarian pathologic conditions.[1]

Female Sex Hormones

The sex hormones are all steroid hormones, that is, they are synthesized from cholesterol (see Chapter 20 and Chapter 22). Male and female sex hormones are present in all adults. However, the female body contains low levels of testosterone and other androgens, and the male body contains low levels of estrogen. Individual effects of sex hormones depend on their amount and concentration in the blood.

The dominant female sex hormones, estrogen and progesterone, are produced primarily by the ovaries. During fetal development, infancy, and childhood, sex hormone production is low. At puberty hormone production surges, triggering sexual maturation and development of secondary sex characteristics. From puberty to menopause, the sex hormones control the menstrual cycle and are produced cyclically, that is, production surges and diminishes monthly, creating the ovarian and uterine changes associated with the menstrual cycle. These hormones are also produced in higher levels during pregnancy by the placenta and inhibit ovulation. Androgens are produced in small amounts by the ovaries and the adrenals and have important functions in women.

Estrogens

Estrogen is a generic term for three similar hormones: estradiol, estrone, and estriol. **Estradiol (E2)** is the most potent and plentiful of the three and is principally produced by the ovaries (ovarian follicle and corpus luteum). The ovary secretes about 95% of circulating estradiol, with limited amounts

secreted by the adrenal cortex. Androgens are converted to estrone in ovarian and peripheral adipose tissue, and estriol is the peripheral metabolite of estrone and estradiol.

Estrogen has numerous biologic effects, many of which involve interactions with other hormones. Estrogen is needed for maturation of reproductive organs, development of secondary sex characteristics, closure of long bones after the pubertal growth spurt, regulation of the menstrual cycle, and endometrial regeneration after menstruation. Estrogen also has metabolic effects on the bones, liver, blood vessels, brain and central nervous system, kidneys, and skin. After menopause, ovarian production of estradiol and estrone is markedly diminished. For this reason, postmenopausal women are susceptible to osteoporosis, a condition in which bone density is reduced. At this time, the majority of estrogen is derived from extraovarian and extraglandular production of estrones.[1] (Hormone levels during perimenopause are discussed in the section on menopause, p. 807.)

Like other steroid hormones, estrogens are derived from cholesterol in a complex, enzyme-mediated series of reactions. (Mechanisms of hormone synthesis and action are described in Chapter 20.) The hypothalamus secretes GnRH in a pulsating manner that stimulates gonadotropin (LH and FSH) release from the anterior pituitary. Gonadotropins trigger ovarian production of estrogen. The primary function of LH is to stimulate theca cells of the ovarian follicle to produce androgens, mainly androstenedione. (Androgens are discussed further on p. 800 and in the section on male reproductive function.) Some of these androgens are converted to estrogen by the theca cells themselves, and others diffuse into the granulosa cells. Within the granulosa layer, FSH induces conversion (aromatization) of androgens to estrogens. Estrogens are then released into the bloodstream. Estrogen and FSH together increase FSH receptors in the follicle, stimulating additional granulosa cells until a dominant follicle is determined.

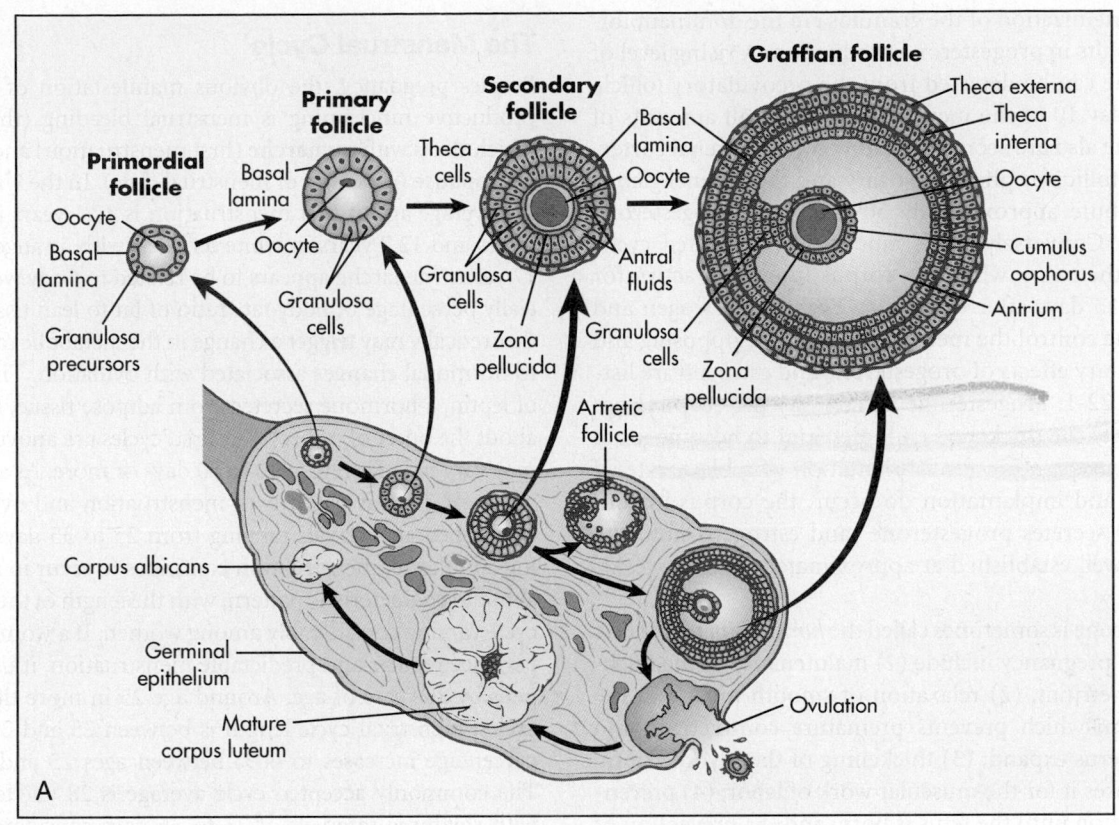

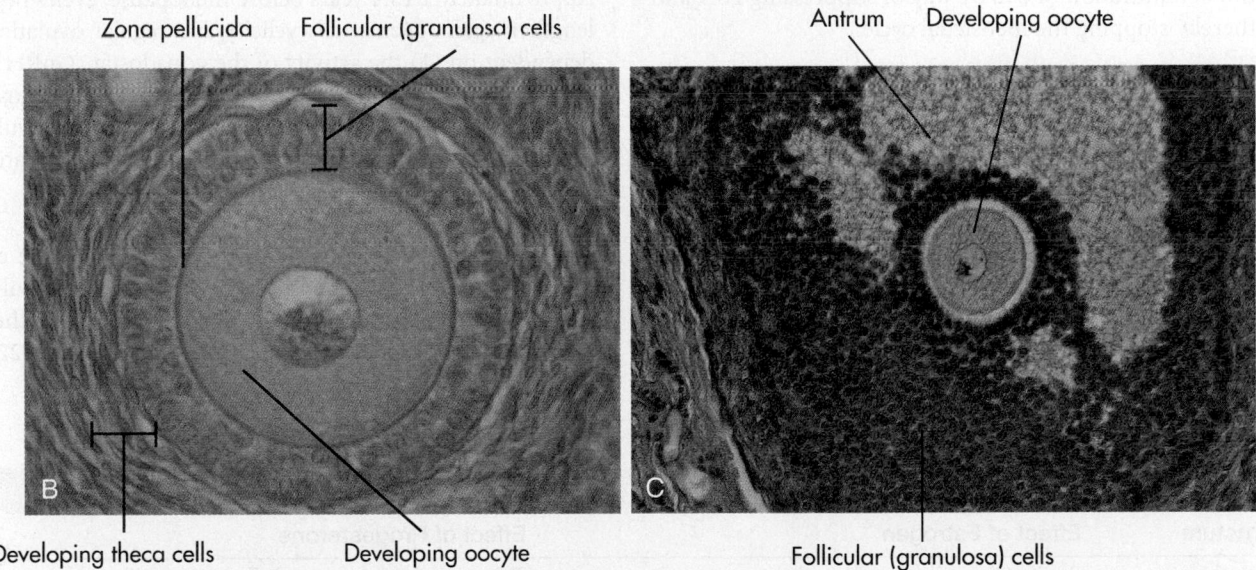

Figure 22-9 Development of an ovarian follicle. **A,** Schematic representation (not to scale) of the structure of the ovary, showing the various stages in the development of the follicle and its successor structure, the corpus luteum. **B,** A developing oocyte surrounded by hormone-secreting follicular (granulosa) cells. **C,** A more mature ovarian follicle has a fluid-filled cavity called the *antrum*. (**A** from Berne RM, Levy MN, editors: *Physiology,* ed 5, St Louis, 2003, Mosby. **B** and **C** from Patton KT, Thibodeau GA: *Anatomy & physiology,* ed 7, St Louis, 2010, Mosby.)

Disturbances of estrogen production can be caused by abnormalities that affect (1) secretion of GnRH by the hypothalamus, (2) secretion of LH or FSH by the anterior pituitary, (3) hormonal feedback mechanisms, or (4) structural integrity of the ovaries. Estrogen's role in the menstrual cycle is described on p. 794.

Progesterone

Luteinizing hormone (LH) stimulates the ovary to release the ova and secrete **progesterone,** the second major female sex hormone. LH surge occurs when there is a peak level of estrogen, about 24 to 36 hours before ovulation. LH promotes luteinization of the granulosa in the dominant follicle and results in progesterone production. A rising level of progesterone can be detected from the preovulatory follicle as early as day 10 of the menstrual cycle. Small amounts of progesterone also are secreted steadily by the adrenal cortex. During the follicular phase the ovary and the adrenal glands each contribute approximately 50% of total progesterone production. Conversely, large amounts are secreted cyclically from the ovary while the corpus luteum is active for about 9 to 13 days after ovulation. Together, estrogen and progesterone control the menstrual cycle. The opposing and complementary effects of progesterone and estrogen are listed in Table 22-1. Progesterone secreted by the corpus luteum stimulates the thickened endometrium to become more complex in preparation for implantation of a blastocyte. If conception and implantation do occur, the corpus luteum persists and secretes progesterone (and estrogen) until the placenta is well established at approximately 8 to 10 weeks' gestation.

Progesterone is sometimes called the *hormone of pregnancy*. Its effects in pregnancy include (1) maintenance of the thickened endometrium; (2) relaxation of smooth muscle in the myometrium, which prevents premature contractions and helps the uterus expand; (3) thickening of the myometrium, which prepares it for the muscular work of labor; (4) prevention of lactation until the fetus is born; and (5) prevention of additional maturation of ova by way of suppressing FSH and LH, thereby stopping the menstrual cycle.

Androgens

Although **androgens** are primarily male sex hormones, small amounts are produced in the ovary and adrenal cortex in women. Some androgens are precursors of female sex hormones, notably androstenedione. At puberty, androgens contribute to the skeletal growth spurt and cause growth of pubic and axillary hair. The androgens also activate sebaceous glands, accounting for some cases of acne during puberty, and play a role in libido.

The Menstrual Cycle

Besides pregnancy, the obvious manifestation of female reproductive functioning is menstrual bleeding (the menses), which starts with **menarche** (first menstruation) and ends with **menopause** (cessation of menstrual flow). In the United States the average age of first menstruation is 12.1 years in black females and 12.7 years in white females, with a range from 9 to 17 years. Menarche appears to be related to body weight, especially percentage of body fat (ratio of fat to lean tissue), which theoretically may trigger a change in the metabolic rate and lead to hormonal changes associated with ovulation. The presence of leptin, a hormone secreted from adipose tissue, helps bring about the onset of pubery.[3] At first, cycles are anovulatory and may vary in length from 10 to 60 days or more. As adolescence proceeds, regular patterns of menstruation and ovulation are established at intervals ranging from 25 to 35 days.[11-13] During adulthood, menstruation continues to recur in a recognizable and characteristic pattern, with the length of the menstrual cycle varying considerably among women. If a woman is to experience regular and predictable menstruation, it usually happens by 20 years of age. Around age 25 in more than 40% of cycles, menstrual cycle length is between 25 and 28 days; the percentage increases to 60% between ages 25 and 35 years.[1] The commonly accepted cycle average is 28 (27 to 30) days, with rhythmic intervals of 21 to 35 days considered normal. Approximately 2 to 4 years before menopause, cycles begin to lengthen again. Menstrual cyclicity and regular ovulation are dependent on (1) the activity of the gonadostat (GnRH pulse generator); (2) the pituitary secretion of gonadotropins; and (3) estrogen (estradiol) positive feedback for the preovulatory LH surge, oocyte maturation, and corpus luteum formation.[3]

Phases

The menstrual cycle consists of three phases of one event, ovulation. The three phases are the follicular/proliferative phase; the luteal/secretory phase; and the ischemic/menstrual phase, known as *menstruation* (Figure 22-10).

Table 22-1	Complementary and Opposing Effects of Estrogen and Progesterone	
Structure	**Effect of Estrogen**	**Effect of Progesterone**
Vaginal mucosa	Proliferation of squamous epithelium; increase in glycogen content of cells; layering (cornification) of cells	Thinning of squamous epithelium; decornification
Cervical mucosa	Production of abundant fluid secretions that favor survival and enhance motility of sperm	Production of thick, sticky secretions that tend to "plug" the cervical os
Fallopian tube	Increase of motility and ciliary action	Decrease of motility and ciliary action
Uterine muscle	Increase of blood flow; increase of contractile proteins and uterine muscle and myometrial excitability and action potential; increase of sensitization to oxytocin	Relaxation of myometrium; decrease of sensitization to oxytocin
Endometrium	Stimulation of growth; increase in number of progesterone receptors	Activation of glands and blood vessels; accumulation of glycogen and enzymes; decrease in number of estrogen receptors
Breasts	Growth of ducts; promotion of prolactin effects	Growth of lobules and alveoli; inhibition of prolactin effects

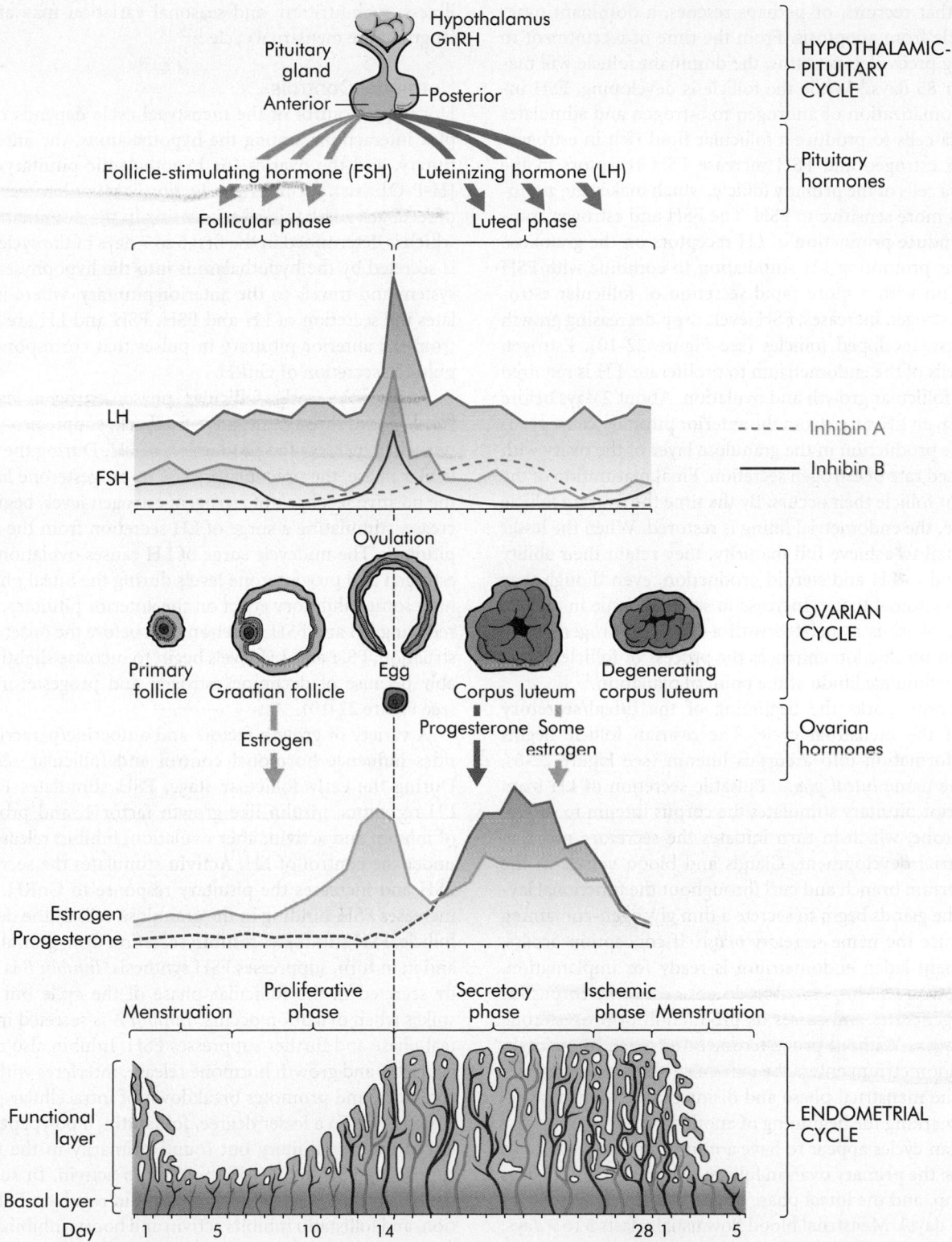

Figure 22-10 The menstrual cycle. (From Lowdermilk DL, Perry SE, Bobak IM: *Maternity and women's health care,* ed 8, St Louis, 2004, Mosby.)

During ovulation an ovum from a mature ovarian follicle is released.

During **menstruation (menses),** the functional layer of the endometrium disintegrates and is discharged through the vagina. Menstruation is followed by the **follicular/proliferative**

phase (FP). This phase is named for two simultaneous processes: maturation of an ovarian follicle and proliferation of the endometrium (see Figure 22-10). During the follicular/proliferative phase, a number of follicles are stimulated to mature. The anterior pituitary gland has a pulsatile secretion of FSH that recruits, or perhaps rescues, a dominant ovarian follicle from apoptosis. From the time of recruitment to achieving preovulatory status, the dominant follicle will mature over 85 days.[1] While the follicle is developing, FSH induces aromatization of androgen to estrogen and stimulates granulosa cells to produce a follicular fluid rich in estrogen. Together estrogen and FSH increase FSH receptors in the granulosa cells of the primary follicle, which makes the granulosa cells more sensitive to FSH. The FSH and estrogen combine to induce production of LH receptors on the granulosa cells, thus promoting LH stimulation to combine with FSH stimulation with a more rapid secretion of follicular estrogen. As estrogen increases, FSH levels drop decreasing growth of the less-developed follicles (see Figure 22-10). Estrogen causes cells of the endometrium to proliferate. LH is required for final follicular growth and ovulation. About 2 days before ovulation, an LH surge from the anterior pituitary causes progesterone production in the granulosa layer of the ovary with a decreased rate of estrogen secretion. Final maturation of the dominant follicle then occurs. By the time the ovarian follicle is mature, the endometrial lining is restored. When the lesser follicles fail to achieve full maturity, they retain their ability to respond to LH and steroid production, even though they return to stromal tissue. Increase in stromal tissue in the late follicular phase is associated with a rise in androgen levels. Androgen production enhances the process of follicle atresia and may stimulate libido at the point of ovulation.[1]

Ovulation marks the beginning of the **luteal/secretory phase** of the menstrual cycle. The ovarian follicle begins its transformation into a corpus luteum (see Figure 22-8), hence the name *luteal phase.* Pulsatile secretion of LH from the anterior pituitary stimulates the corpus luteum to secrete progesterone, which in turn initiates the secretory phase of endometrial development. Glands and blood vessels in the endometrium branch and curl throughout the functional layer, and the glands begin to secrete a thin glycogen-containing fluid, hence the name *secretory phase.* If conception occurs, the nutrient-laden endometrium is ready for implantation. If conception and implantation do not occur, the corpus luteum degenerates and ceases its production of progesterone and estrogen. Without progesterone or estrogen to maintain it, the endometrium enters the ischemic (blood-starved) portion of the menstrual phase and disintegrates. Menstruation occurs, marking the beginning of another cycle.

Ovarian cycles appear to have a minimum length of 24 to 26.5 days: the primary ovarian follicle requires 10 to 12.5 days to develop, and the luteal phase appears relatively fixed at 14 days (±3 days). Menstrual blood flow usually lasts 3 to 7 days, but it may last as long as 8 days or stop after 1 to 2 days and still be considered within normal limits. Bleeding is consistently scant to heavy and varies from 30 to 80 ml, with most blood loss occurring during the first 3 days of menses. Menstrual discharge consists of blood, mucus, and desquamated endometrial tissue and does not clot under normal circumstances. It is usually dark and produces a characteristic musty odor on oxidation. Factors such as severe emotional stress,

illness, malnutrition, and seasonal variation may affect the length of the menstrual cycle.[1,12-14]

Hormonal Controls

Hormonal control of the menstrual cycle depends on complex interactions among the hypothalamus, the anterior pituitary, and the ovaries (or hypothalamic-pituitary-ovarian [H-P-O] axis).[14] GnRH production is stimulated as a result of feedback mechanisms originating in the dominant follicle, which is determined in the first 5 to 7 days of the cycle. GnRH is secreted by the hypothalamus into the hypophyseal portal system and travels to the anterior pituitary, where it stimulates the secretion of LH and FSH. FSH and LH are released from the anterior pituitary in pulses that correspond to the pulsatile secretion of GnRH.

During the early follicular phase, estrogen levels rise steadily and, through negative feedback, suppresses FSH and positively increase the production of LH. During the late follicular phase, the preovulatory rise in progesterone facilitates the positive feedback of estrogen; estrogen levels begin to increase, stimulating a surge of LH secretion from the anterior pituitary. The midcycle surge of LH causes ovulation. Rising estrogen and progesterone levels during the luteal phase may have some inhibitory effect on the anterior pituitary, thereby reducing LH and FSH secretion. Just before the onset of menstruation, FSH and LH levels begin to increase slightly, probably because of declining estrogen and progesterone levels (see Figure 22-10).

A variety of growth factors and autocrine/paracrine peptides influence hormonal control and follicular response.[1] During the early follicular stage, FSH stimulates FSH and LH receptors, insulin-like growth factor 1, and production of inhibin and activin; after ovulation, inhibin release comes under the control of LH. **Activin** stimulates the secretion of FSH and increases the pituitary response to GnRH. Activin increases FSH-binding in the granulosa cells in the dominant follicle. FSH stimulates **inhibin** secretion from granulosa cells and it, in turn, suppresses FSH synthesis. *Inhibin B* is primarily secreted in the follicular phase of the cycle but sharply spikes when ovulation occurs. *Inhibin A* is secreted in the luteal phase and further suppresses FSH. Inhibin also restrains prolactin and growth hormone release, interferes with GnRH receptors, and promotes breakdown of intracellular gonadotropins.[15,16] To a lesser degree, **follistatin,** a polypeptide produced by the pituitary but found primarily in the follicles, suppresses FSH activity by binding to activin. In summary, the balance between activin and inhibin regulates FSH secretion, and follistatin inhibits activin and boosts inhibin activity. Inhibin and activin also regulate LH stimulation of androgen synthesis in theca cells. Figure 22-10 summarizes fluctuating estrogen, progesterone, gonadotropin, and inhibin levels during the menstrual cycle.[1]

Interestingly, inhibins, activins, and follistatins are structurally similar, belonging to the same family of nonsteroidal polypeptides, and are synthesized by granulosa cells in response to FSH. Inhibin is synthesized and secreted from both granulosa and luteal ovarian cells, activin from granulosa cells only, and follistatin from pituitary cells. These peptides are secreted into the follicular fluid and ovarian venous effluent. The expression of these peptides is not limited to the ovary; they are present in many tissues throughout the body and serve as regulators.[3] Understanding of the function and structural complexity of these polypeptides and their interaction with GnRH, gonadotropins, and sex hormones has increased monumentally over the past decade. New information is gained through research and published on a regular basis.

Ovarian Cycle

By stimulating follicles, gonadotropins initiate their growth and maturation. The most important hormonal event is a rise in FSH. The decline in the late luteal phase of estrogen, progesterone, and inhibin secretion allows FSH to rise; concurrently there is a slight increase in LH levels (see Figure 22-10). More specifically, FSH stimulates granulosa cell growth and initiates estrogen production in these cells in the next cycle. At this time a group of ovarian follicles is recruited and begins to mature; the exact number depends on the remaining pool of inactive follicles. As the follicles mature, granulosa cells multiply, increasing estradiol secretion. Within a few days of the cycle, one follicle becomes dominant and the others atrophy. The mechanism for follicular recruitment or dominance is unknown. Once dominance is acquired, it is not transferable but may be related to FSH receptors, blood supply, or the ability to convert androgens to estradiol. The dominant follicle begins to secrete progressively larger amounts of estradiol, which exerts a positive-feedback effect causing the LH surge. (The dynamic process of follicular growth is outlined in Box 22-1.) Ovulation generally occurs 1 to 2 hours before the final progesterone surge, or about 12 to 36 hours after the onset of the LH surge; specific timing may reflect seasonal variations.

Box 22-1   Dynamic Process of Follicular Growth

Follicles grow and undergo atresia under all physiologic circumstances. Growth and atresia continue during pregnancy, ovulation, or periods of anovulation and occur at all ages from fetal development to menopause. A maximum number of oocytes (follicles) is found in the fetus at approximately 16 to 20 weeks of gestation. By birth, the number has diminished from 6 to 7 million to 1 to 2 million. By puberty, only about 300,000 oocytes remain. During a woman's reproductive years, fewer than 500 oocytes will mature and be released during ovulation. The number of follicles that begin developing during each cycle depends on the residual pool. Follicular atresia will occur at a steady state regardless of how many anovulatory cycles there are in a woman's life (because of pregnancy or hormonal contraception). As a woman ages, fewer numbers of follicles are recruited. Follicular loss accelerates about 10 to 15 years before menopause.

Data from Speroff L, Fritz MA: *Clinical gynecology, endocrinology, and infertility*, ed 7, Baltimore, 2005, Williams & Wilkins.

Progesterone, proteolytic enzymes, and prostaglandins (E and F series) trigger mechanisms controlling follicular rupture and release of the ovum.[1] Possible mechanisms include thinning, stretching, degradation, and digestion of the follicular wall and contraction of smooth muscle cells of the follicle. The role of prostaglandins is essential to ovulation, and infertility patients should be advised to avoid the use of drugs that inhibit prostaglandin synthesis.[17]

The LH surge also transforms the granulosa cells of the ovulatory follicle into the corpus luteum. The corpus luteum secretes estrogen and progesterone in amounts that depend in part on adequate development of the follicle before ovulation. Progesterone acts centrally and locally within the ovary to suppress new follicular growth during the early and midluteal phases. If pregnancy does not occur, the corpus luteum persists for 11 to 14 days and then regresses and eventually disappears. An increase in pulse frequency of GnRH from a low level reactivates hormonal control of the menstrual cycle.

Uterine Phases

Uterine phases of the menstrual cycle—proliferative, secretory, and ischemic/menstrual phases—involve cyclic endometrial changes controlled by estrogen and progesterone. Hormonal effects are influenced by the presence of receptors and numerous growth factors, peptides, and enzymes that act as intermediaries between the sex steroids and the endometrium.[3] During the midfollicular phase, increasing levels of estrogen contribute to endometrial repair and proliferation, thus increasing endometrial thickness. Once ovulation occurs and serum progesterone levels increase, the endometrial tissue develops secretory characteristics. If implantation of a fertilized ovum does not take place, endometrial tissue begins to break down approximately 11 days after ovulation. The period of breakdown is sometimes called the *ischemic phase* (see Figure 22-10). Sloughing of tissue (menstrual bleeding) begins about 14 days after ovulation.

Cervical mucus also undergoes cyclic changes. During the proliferative phase the cervical mucus is thin and watery. Peak estrogen levels occur just before ovulation and maximally stimulate the cervical glands to produce mucus. Cervical mucus becomes abundant and more elastic (spinnbarkeit). In the presence of estrogen, tiny channels develop in the mucus, which allows sperm access to the interior of the uterus. Changes in the consistency of cervical mucus can be used to identify fertile intervals.

Vaginal Response

Vaginal endothelium also responds to cyclic hormonal changes. Under the influence of estrogen, epithelial cells of the vagina grow maximally during the follicular/proliferative phase. After ovulation, layers of keratinized cells overgrow the basal epithelium, a process known as **cornification.** Near the end of the luteal phase, leukocytes invade vaginal epithelium, removing the outer layers in a process termed **decornification.**

Body Temperature

Basal body temperature (BBT) undergoes characteristic biphasic changes during menstrual cycles in which ovulation occurs. During the follicular phase the BBT fluctuates around 37° C (98° F). During the luteal phase, the average temperature increases by 0.2° to 0.5° C (0.4° to 1.0° F). At the end of the luteal phase, 1 to 3 days before the onset of menstruation, BBT declines to follicular-phase levels. The shift in temperature is related to ovulation, corpus luteum formation, and increased serum progesterone levels. Progesterone probably acts on the thermoregulatory center of the hypothalamus to increase body temperature. Changes in BBT are used to document ovulatory cycles but are not useful to predict the exact timing of ovulation.

THE MALE REPRODUCTIVE SYSTEM

In men the external genitalia perform the major functions of reproduction, which are to produce sperm and deliver them to the female reproductive tract. Sperm are produced in the male gonads, the testes, and delivered to the female vagina by the penis. The internal male genitalia have a more accessory function. They consist of conducting tubes and fluid-producing glands, all of which aid in the transport of sperm from the testes to the urethral opening of the penis. The male reproductive and urinary structures are shown in Figure 22-11.

External Genitalia

Testes

In men the **testes** (*singular,* testis) are the essential organs of reproduction. Like the ovaries, the testes have two functions: (1) production of gametes (in this case, sperm) and (2) production of sex hormones (in this case, androgens and testosterone). The testes are suspended outside the pelvic cavity because sperm production requires an environment that is 1° or 2° C (34° or 36° F) cooler than body temperature.

During embryonic and fetal life, the testes develop within the abdomen (see Figure 22-1). Then, about 3 months before birth, the testes start to descend toward the developing scrotum. About 1 month before birth, they enter twin passageways called **inguinal canals.** The inguinal canals are vaginal processes created by outpouchings of the peritoneum (lining of the abdominal cavity). The descent of a testis is shown in Figure 22-12. Each testis moves down outside the peritoneum until it is suspended in the scrotal sac by its supply lines: the ducts, blood vessels, lymphatic vessels, and nerves of the **spermatic cord.** When descent is complete, the abdominal end of each vaginal process closes up and the inguinal canal disappears. If peritoneal closure at the site of the inguinal canal is incomplete or weak, an inguinal hernia may occur later in life. The scrotal end of each vaginal process becomes the outer covering of the testis, the **tunica vaginalis.**

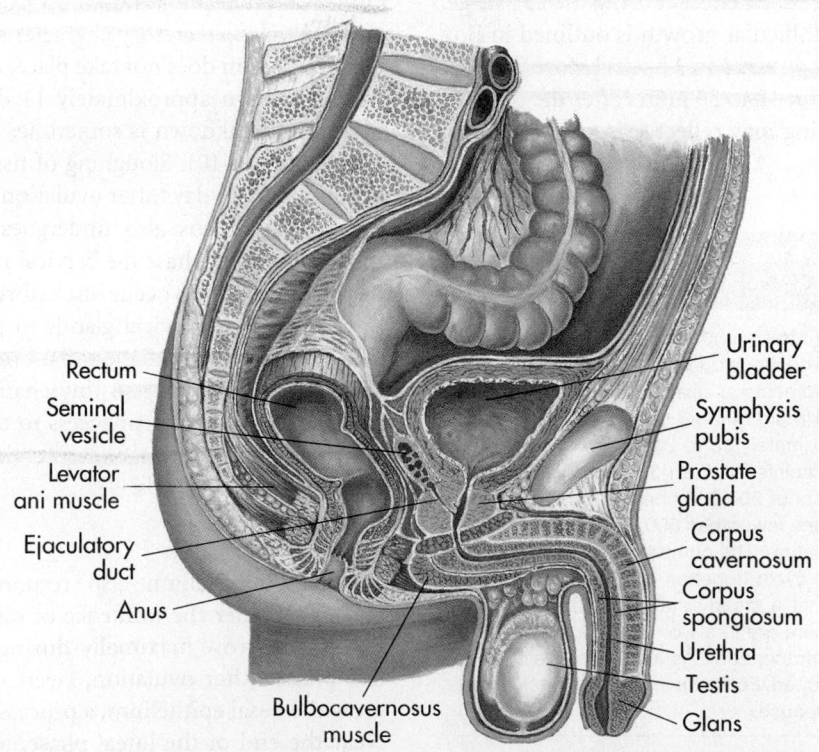

Rectum
Seminal vesicle
Levator ani muscle
Ejaculatory duct
Anus
Bulbocavernosus muscle

Urinary bladder
Symphysis pubis
Prostate gland
Corpus cavernosum
Corpus spongiosum
Urethra
Testis
Glans

Figure 22-11 Structure of the male reproductive organs. (From Seidel HM et al: *Mosby's guide to physical examination,* ed 6, St Louis, 2006, Mosby.)

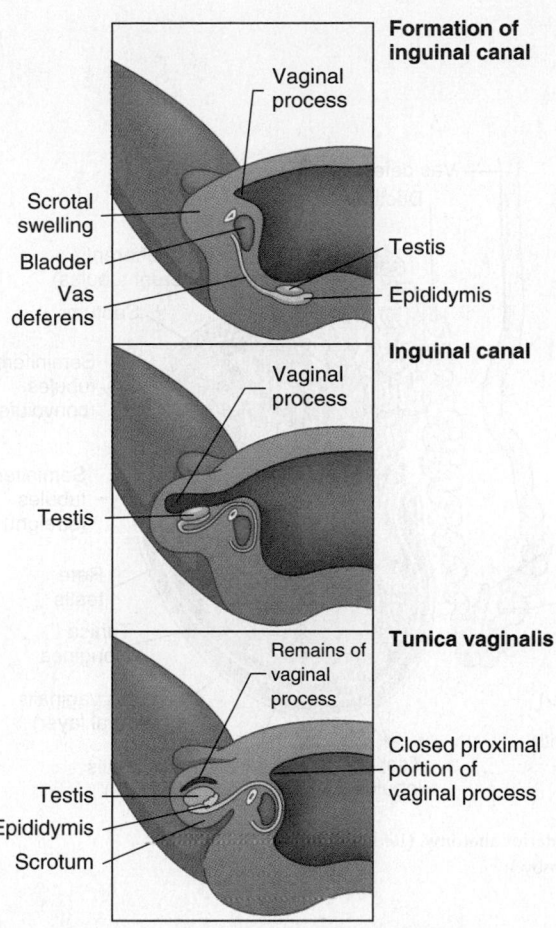

Formation of inguinal canal
- Vaginal process
- Scrotal swelling
- Bladder
- Vas deferens
- Testis
- Epididymis

Inguinal canal
- Vaginal process
- Testis

Tunica vaginalis
- Remains of vaginal process
- Closed proximal portion of vaginal process
- Testis
- Epididymis
- Scrotum

Figure 22-12 Descent of a testis. The testes descend from the abdominal cavity to the scrotum during the last 3 months of fetal development.

Figure 22-13 shows a sagittal section of a mature testis. The adult testis is ovoid and varies considerably in length (3 to 6 cm), width (2 to 3.5 cm), depth (3 to 4 cm), and weight (10 to 40 g). The testis is almost entirely surrounded by an outer covering, the tunica vaginalis, which separates the testis from the scrotal wall, and an inner covering, the **tunica albuginea.** Inward extensions of the tunica albuginea form septa that separate the testis into about 250 compartments, or lobules, each of which contains several tortuously coiled ducts called **seminiferous tubules.** The seminiferous tubules constitute the bulk (80%) of testicular volume and are the site of sperm production. (Sperm production, termed **spermatogenesis,** is described on p. 800.) Tissue surrounding these ducts contains blood and lymphatic vessels, fibroblastic support cells, macrophages, mast cells, and Leydig cells. **Leydig cells,** which occur in clusters and account for about 1% to 5% of testicular volume, produce androgens, chiefly testosterone.

The two ends of each seminiferous tubule join and leave the lobule through a short, straight section called the **tubulus rectus.** Sperm travel from the seminiferous tubules into these straight sections, which lead to the central portion of the testis, the **rete testis.** From the rete testis, sperm move through the **efferent tubules,** or vasa efferentia, to the epididymis, where they mature.

The testes are innervated by adrenergic fibers, whose sole function apparently is to regulate blood flow to the Leydig cells. The testes receive arterial blood from the internal spermatic and differential arteries. Arterial blood flows over the surface of the testes before entering the parenchyma (functional tissues). Surface flow cools the blood to temperatures that promote spermatogenesis, approximately 1° to 2°C (34° to 36° F) below body core temperature.[18]

Epididymis

The **epididymis** (plural, epididymides) is a comma-shaped structure that curves over the posterior portion of each testis (see Figure 22-13). It consists of a single highly packed and markedly coiled (60 to 70 cm when uncoiled) duct measuring 5 cm long, whose structural function is to conduct sperm from the efferent tubules to the vas deferens. The duct can become inflamed from infection by microorganisms that ascend the urethra or from the prostate, causing epididymitis. The epididymis has physiologic functions as well. When sperm enter the head of the epididymis, they are not fully mature or motile, nor are they capable of fertilizing an ovum. During the 12 days (or more) sperm take to travel the length of the epididymis, they receive nutrients and testosterone from the epididymal epithelium, and some biochemical or physiologic mechanism enhances their capacity for fertilization.[19]

The tail of the epididymis is continuous with the **vas deferens (ductus deferens),** a duct with muscular layers capable of powerful peristalsis that transports sperm toward the urethra. After traveling the length of the epididymis, sperm are stored in the epididymal tail and vas deferens. The vas deferens enters the pelvic cavity through the spermatic cord.

Scrotum

The testes, epididymides, and spermatic cord are enclosed and protected by the scrotum. The **scrotum** is a skin-covered fibromuscular sac that is homologous to the female labia majora (see Figure 22-2). The skin of the scrotum is thin and has rugae (wrinkles or folds), which enable it to enlarge or relax away from the body. At puberty the scrotal skin darkens, develops active sebaceous glands, and becomes sparsely covered with hair. Just under the skin lies a layer of connective tissue (fascia) and smooth muscle, the tunica dartos (see Figure 22-13). The **tunica dartos** also forms a septum that separates the two testes. Exposure to cold temperatures causes the tunica dartos to contract, pulling the testes close to the warm body. In warm temperatures the tunica dartos relaxes, suspending the testes away from body heat. These mechanisms promote optimal temperatures for spermatogenesis. In addition, scrotal sensitivity to touch, pressure, temperature, and pain protects the testes against potential harm. During sexual excitement, the scrotal skin and tunica thicken, the scrotum tightens and lifts, and the spermatic cords shorten, partially elevating the testes toward the body. As excitement plateaus, the engorged testes increase 50% in size, rotate anteriorly, and flatten against the body, signaling impending ejaculation.

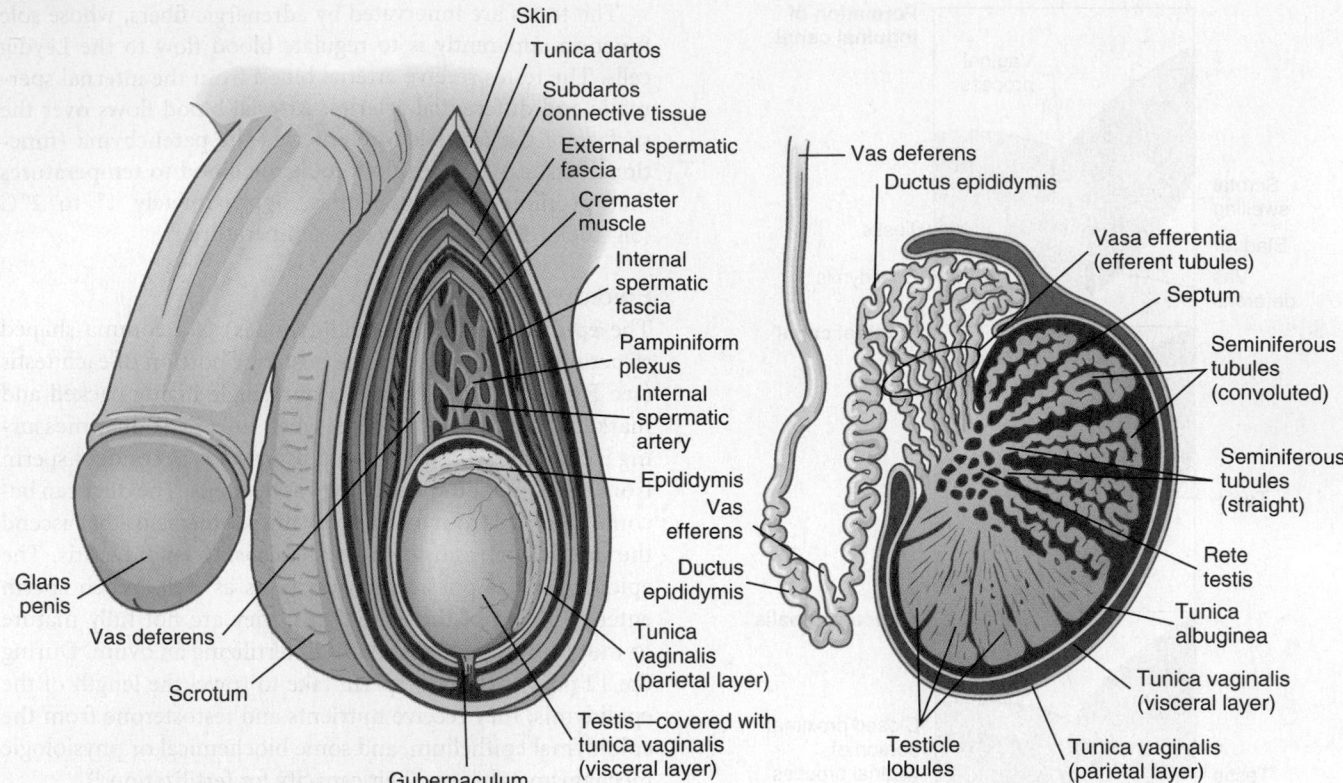

Figure 22-13 The testes. External and sagittal views showing interior anatomy. (Redrawn from Seidel HM et al: *Mosby's guide to physical examination*, ed 6, St Louis, 2006, Mosby.)

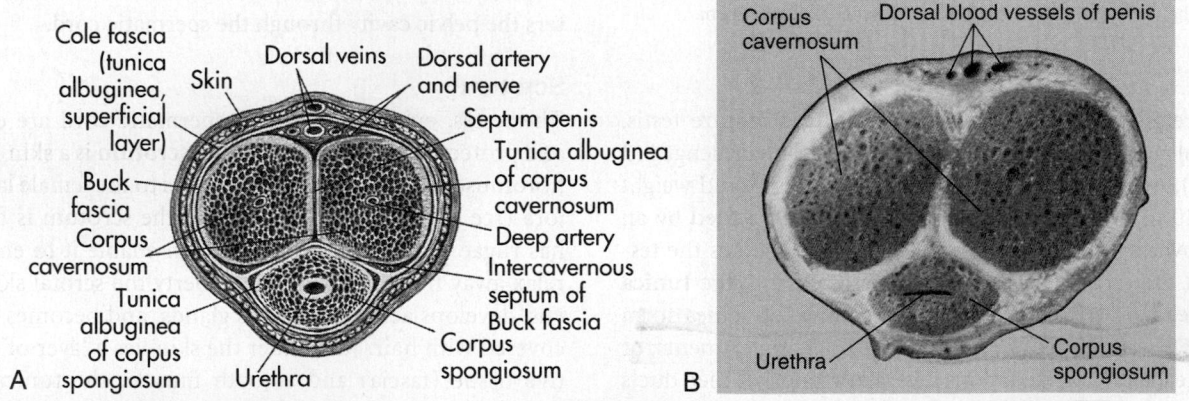

Figure 22-14 The penis. **A,** Cross section of the penis. **B,** Cross section of the shaft of the penis showing three columns of erectile, or cavernous, tissue. (**A** from Thompson JM et al: *Mosby's clinical nursing*, ed 5, St Louis, 2002, Mosby. **B** from Patton KT, Thibodeau GA: *Anatomy & physiology*, ed 7, St Louis, 2010, Mosby.)

Penis

The **penis** has two main functions: delivery of sperm to the female vagina and elimination of urine. (Urine formation and excretion are the subjects of Chapter 35.) Embryonically, the penis is homologous to the female clitoris (see Figure 22-2).

Figure 22-11 shows a sagittal section of the adult penis and its anatomic relation to other urogenital structures. Externally the penis consists of a shaft with a tip, the **glans,** which contains the opening of the urethra. For protection, the skin of the glans folds over the tip of the penis, forming the prepuce, or **foreskin.** At birth, the foreskin is adhered to the glans. Penile erections, which commonly occur, cause the adhesions to break so that by age 3 years the foreskin becomes completely retractable. The skin of the penis is continuous with that of the groin, scrotum, and inner thighs. It is hairless, movable, and darker than surrounding skin.

Internally, the penis consists of the urethra and three compartments: two **corpora cavernosa** and the **corpus** spongiosum (Figure 22-14). The three compartments are separated by Buck fascia and, like the testes, are enclosed by a tunica albuginea. The **urethra** passes through the corpus spongiosum and ends at a sagittal slit in the glans. If the urethra is not completely surrounded by the corpus spongiosum, the meatus may open on the ventral surface of the penile shaft (hypospadias) or on the dorsal surface (epispadias).

Penetration of the female vagina is made possible by the **erectile reflex,** a process in which erectile tissues within the corpora cavernosa and corpus spongiosum become engorged with blood, generally 20 to 50 ml. The erectile tissues consist of vascular spaces, or chambers, which are supplied with blood by arterioles (small arteries). Most of the time the arterioles are constricted through tonic noradrenaline release from sympathetic nerves so that not much blood flows through the erectile tissues. Sexual stimulation, however, causes the arterioles to dilate through release of nitric oxide and fill with blood.[20] Their rapid expansion fills the erectile tissues, causing an erection. Erection apparently is maintained by compression or constriction of veins that drain the corpora cavernosa and corpus spongiosum. When sexual stimulation ceases or orgasm and ejaculation occur, these veins open up, blood flows out of the arterioles, and the penis becomes flaccid (soft and pendulous).

Erection is under the control of the autonomic nervous system but can be stimulated or inhibited by central nervous system input. Stimulation of mechanoreceptors of the penis, particularly of the glans, causes parasympathetic nerves of the autonomic nervous system to relax smooth muscle in the walls of penile arterioles. At the same time the effects of sympathetic nerves, which normally cause arteriolar smooth muscle to constrict, are inhibited.

Erections begin in utero and continue throughout life, but ejaculation does not occur until sperm production begins at puberty. Growth of the penis and scrotal contents continues well past puberty, however, and may not be complete until the late teens or early 20s. Penis size, when flaccid, varies considerably; with an erection, differences in penis size diminish. Sexual excitement causes the corpora cavernosa to increase in length and width and become rigid; the penis becomes erect. Stimulation of the glans, which is endowed with copious sensitive nerve endings, provides maximum erotic sensation. With sexual arousal, skin color deepens, the glans doubles in size, and the urethral meatus dilates. Ejaculation occurs with frequent, strong contractions of the vas deferens, epididymis, seminal vesicles, prostate, urethra, and penis.[21]

Internal Genitalia

Figure 22-13 shows the anatomy of the internal genitalia and their relation to other pelvic organs. The internal genitalia consist of ducts and glands. The ducts—the two vasa deferentia, the ejaculatory duct, and the urethra—conduct sperm and glandular secretions from the testes to the urethral opening of the penis. The glands—the prostate gland, two seminal vesicles, and two Cowper (or bulbourethral) glands—secrete fluids that serve as a vehicle for sperm transport and create an alkaline, nutritious medium that promotes sperm motility and survival. Together the sperm and the glandular fluids comprise **semen.**

Sperm leave the epididymides and travel rapidly through the internal ducts in a process called **emission.** Emission occurs just seconds before ejaculation, at the moment when sexual arousal peaks. Emission always leads to ejaculation.

Emission occurs as smooth muscle in the walls of the epididymides and vasa deferentia begins to contract rhythmically, pushing sperm and epididymal secretions through the vasa deferentia. Each vas deferens is a firm, elastic fibromuscular tube that begins at the tail of the epididymis, enters the pelvic cavity within the spermatic cord, loops up and over the bladder, and ends in the prostate gland (Figure 22-15; see also Figure 22-11). Sperm are moved along by peristaltic contractions of smooth muscle in the walls of the vas deferens.

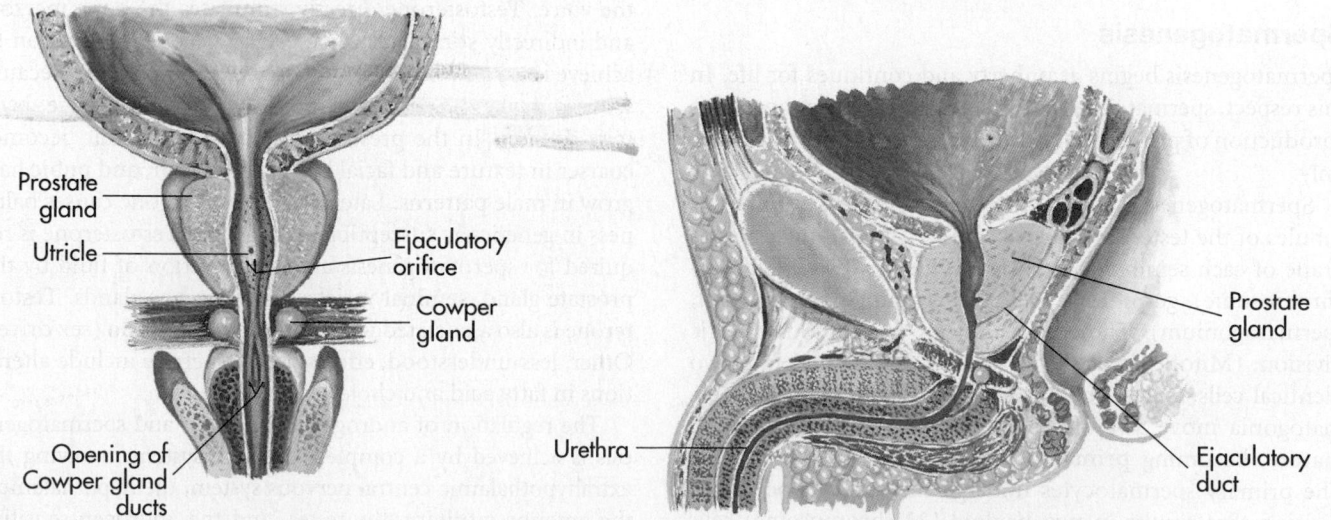

Figure 22-15 Anatomy of the prostate gland and seminal vesicles. (From Seidel HM et al: *Mosby's guide to physical examination*, ed 6, St Louis, 2006, Mosby.)

As sperm leave the ampulla (wide portion) of the vas deferens, the seminal vesicles secrete a nutritive glucose-rich fluid into the ejaculate (semen). The **seminal vesicles** are a pair of glands, each about 4 to 6 cm long, that lie behind the urinary bladder and in front of the rectum. The seminal vesicles provide fructose as a source of energy for ejaculated sperm, and secrete prostaglandins that promote smooth muscle contraction assisting with sperm transport. The ducts of the seminal vesicles join the ampulla of the vas deferens to become the **ejaculatory duct,** which contracts rhythmically during emission and ejaculation. As can be seen in Figures 22-11 and 22-15, the ejaculatory duct joins the urethra, where both pass through the prostate gland. During emission and ejaculation a sphincter (muscle surrounding a duct) closes, preventing urine from entering the prostatic urethra.[21]

The **prostate gland** is composed of alveoli and ducts embedded in fibromuscular tissue. It measures 4 cm in diameter and weighs approximately 20 g. While semen moves through the prostatic portion of the urethra, the prostate gland contracts rhythmically and secretes prostatic fluid into the mixture. Prostatic fluid is a thin, milky substance with an alkaline pH that helps sperm survive in the acid environment of the female reproductive tract. In addition, clotting enzymes and fibrinolysin in prostatic fluids help mobilize sperm after ejaculation.

Cowper glands (bulbourethral glands), whose ducts secrete mucus into the urethra near the base of the penis, are the last pair of glands to add fluid to the ejaculate. Ejaculation occurs as semen reaches the base of the penis and muscles there begin the rhythmic contractions that push semen out. Normally a man ejaculates between 2 and 6 ml of semen, containing 75 million to 400 million sperm. About 98% of the ejaculate consists of glandular fluids; 60% to 70% of volume comes from the seminal vesicles and 20% from the prostate. Therefore, the ejaculate of a man who has undergone vasectomy (a surgical procedure that prevents sperm from entering the vas deferens) is not reduced by much: about 2%.

Spermatogenesis

Spermatogenesis begins at puberty and continues for life. In this respect, spermatogenesis differs markedly from oogenesis (production of primordial ova), which occurs during fetal life only.

Spermatogenesis takes place within the seminiferous tubules of the testes (see Figure 22-13). The basement membrane of each seminiferous tubule is lined with diploid (46-chromosome) germ cells called **spermatogonia** (*singular, spermatogonium*). These cells undergo continuous mitotic division. (Mitotic division, in which a cell divides into two identical cells, is described in Chapter 1.) Some of the spermatogonia move away from the basement membrane and mature, becoming **primary spermatocytes** (Figure 22-16). The primary spermatocytes undergo meiosis, a type of cell division that results in two haploid (23-chromosome) cells called **secondary spermatocytes.** (Meiosis is described and illustrated in Chapter 4.) The two secondary spermatocytes

then undergo meiosis, resulting in four **spermatids.** It is the spermatids that differentiate into spermatozoa, or sperm, each of which contains 23 chromosomes (Figure 22-17).

The development of spermatids into sperm depends on the presence of **Sertoli cells (nondividing support cells)** within the seminiferous tubules. The spermatids attach themselves to Sertoli cells, from which they receive the nutrients and the hormonal signals they need to develop into sperm.[22]

The process of spermatogenesis, from mitotic division of a spermatogonium to maturation of the spermatids, takes about 70 to 80 days. Mature sperm migrate from the seminiferous tubules to the epididymis, where their capacity for fertilization continues to develop. Although they are completely mature by the time they are ejaculated, the sperm do not become motile (capable of movement) until they are activated by biochemicals in semen and in the female reproductive tract.

Male Sex Hormones

The male sex hormones are androgens. **Testosterone,** the primary male sex hormone, is an androgen. Mainly Leydig cells of the testes and, to a lesser degree, the adrenal glands produce testosterone and other androgens. In men, sex hormone production is relatively constant with some diurnal variation.

The androgens have a number of physiologic actions related to growth and development of male tissues and organs. They are responsible for fetal differentiation and development of the male urogenital system and have some effects on the fetal brain. After birth, the Leydig cells become quiescent until activated by the gonadotropins during puberty. At puberty, androgens cause the sex organs to grow and secondary sex characteristics to develop.

Testosterone affects nervous and skeletal tissues, bone marrow, skin and hair, and sex organs. It has an anabolic effect on skeletal muscle tissue, thereby contributing to the difference in body weight and composition between men and women. Testosterone also stimulates growth of the musculature and cartilage of the larynx, causing a permanent deepening of the voice. Testosterone directly stimulates the bone marrow and indirectly stimulates renal erythropoietin production to achieve increased hemoglobin and hematocrit levels. Because sebaceous gland activity is stimulated by testosterone, acne may develop. In the presence of testosterone, hair becomes coarser in texture and facial hair, axillary hair, and pubic hair grow in male patterns. Later in life, testosterone causes baldness in genetically susceptible individuals. Testosterone is required for spermatogenesis and for secretion of fluid by the prostate gland, seminal vesicles, and Cowper glands. Testosterone is also associated with an increase in **libido** (sex drive). Other, less-understood, effects of testosterone include alterations in fatty acid and cholesterol metabolism.

The regulation of androgen production and spermatogenesis is achieved by a complex feedback system involving the extrahypothalamic central nervous system, the hypothalamus, the anterior pituitary, the testes, and the androgen-sensitive end organs. These relationships, which are essentially the same in women, are summarized in Figure 22-3. Extrahypothalamic

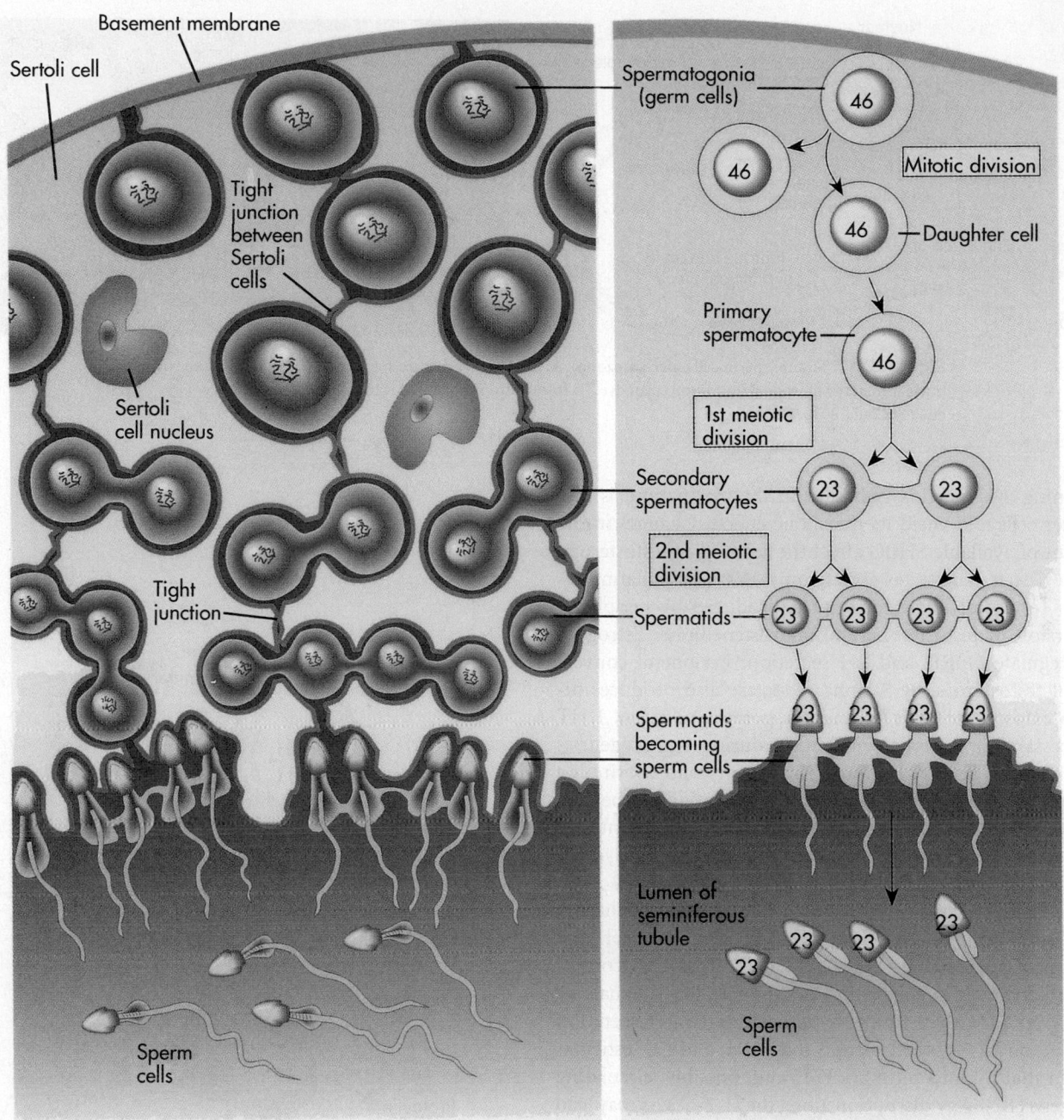

Figure 22-16 Seminiferous tubule. Section shows process of meiosis and sperm cell formation. (From Patton KT, Thibodeau GA: *Anatomy & physiology*, ed 7, St Louis, 2010, Mosby.)

influences include such variables as physiologic and psychologic stress, which may inhibit or augment hypothalamic activity. In the hypothalamus, neurotransmitters regulate GnRH synthesis and pulsatile release (about every 3 hours) into the hypophyseal portal veins. Norepinephrine stimulates GnRH secretion, and serotonin and dopamine inhibit GnRH secretion. GnRH is transported by portal flow to the median eminence of the pituitary gland, where it binds to receptors and stimulates the synthesis and secretion of gonadotropins, LH, and FSH. LH and FSH, which are named for their effects in the female reproductive system, have important effects on the male system as well.

LH acts on the Leydig cells to regulate testosterone secretion. FSH acts on the seminiferous tubule Sertoli cells to promote spermatogenesis. FSH secretion is inhibited by inhibin secreted by the Sertoli cells. Similar to their action in the female gonad, inhibin functions as an autocrine/paracrine regulator in the male gonad. Inhibin inhibits proliferation of spermatogonia by regulating pituitary FSH levels. In addition, inhibin facilitates LH stimulation of androgen biosynthesis in Leydig cells.

Ninety-eight percent of testosterone, the major steroid hormone produced by the testis, binds to either **sex hormone–binding globulin (SHBG)** (40%) or albumin (48%). The

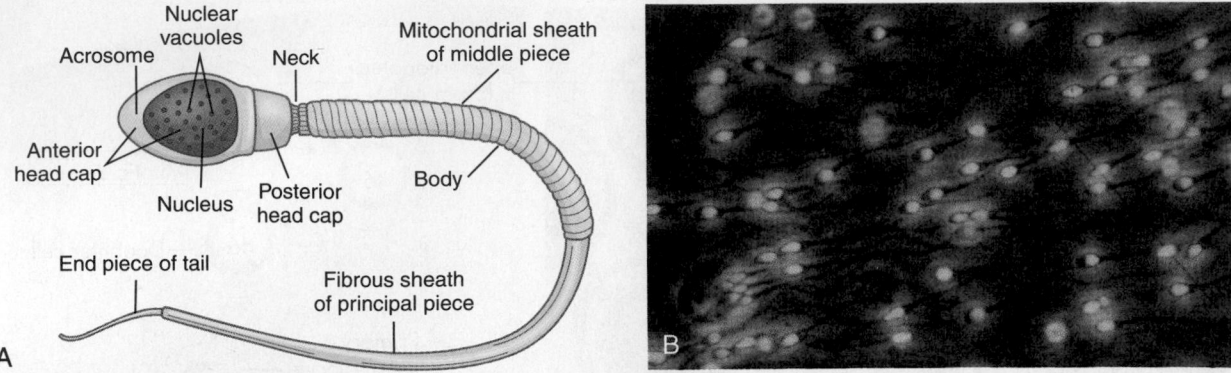

Figure 22-17 Mature sperm cell (spermatozoon). **A,** Anatomy of mature sperm cell. **B,** Human sperm with nuclear material glowing with a fluorescent dye. (B from Patton KT, Thibodeau GA: *Anatomy & physiology,* ed 7, St Louis, 2010, Mosby.)

remaining 2% remains unbound in the plasma and is free to enter cells and wield its metabolic effects. Changes in the amount of available SHBG affect the amount of testosterone within tissues. The testes secrete only 25% of circulating estrogen (estradiol). The majority is produced by peripheral conversion of testosterone and androstenedione. Estrogens help regulate GnRH and LH secretion. Peripheral conversion of testosterone by 5-alpha-reductase also produces **dihydrotestosterone (DHT),** another potent androgen. DHT is necessary for external virilization during embryogenesis and androgen activity beginning at puberty and continuing throughout adulthood. **Prolactin,** a polypeptide synthesized and secreted from the pituitary, helps maintain biosynthesis of testosterone. However, elevated prolactin levels may suppress biosynthesis.[23]

In summary, hormones secreted at each level of the hypothalamic-pituitary-testicular (H-P-T) axis control and coordinate testicular function (Figure 22-18). This control is exerted through positive and negative feedback signals by (1) sex steroids that inhibit hypothalamic GnRH secretion and pituitary LH responsiveness to GnRH; and (2) testicular inhibin that inhibits pituitary FSH and, possibly, circulating estrogens (E2). Any disruption along the H-P-T axis may lead to hypogonadism or infertility.

STRUCTURE AND FUNCTION OF THE BREAST

The **breasts** are modified sebaceous glands that lie on the ventral surface of the thorax, within the superficial fascia of the chest wall. They extend vertically from the second rib to the sixth or seventh intercostal space and laterally from the side of the sternum to the midaxillary line. Breast tissue also may extend into the axilla; this tissue is known as the *tail of Spence.*

The Female Breast

The female breast is composed of 15 to 20 pyramid-shaped lobes that are separated and supported by Cooper ligaments (Figure 22-19). Each lobe contains 20 to 40 lobules that are

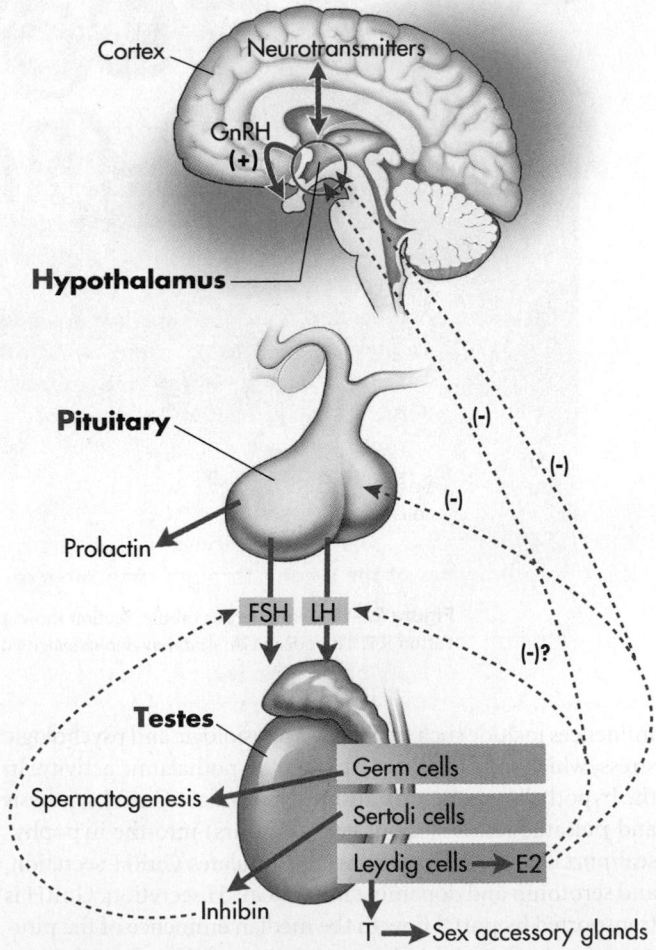

Figure 22-18 Schematic representation of activity along the hypothalamus-pituitary-testicular (H-P-T) axis. *E2,* Estrogen; *FSH,* follicle-stimulating hormone; *GnRH,* gonadotropin-releasing hormone; *LH,* luteinizing hormone; *T,* testosterone.

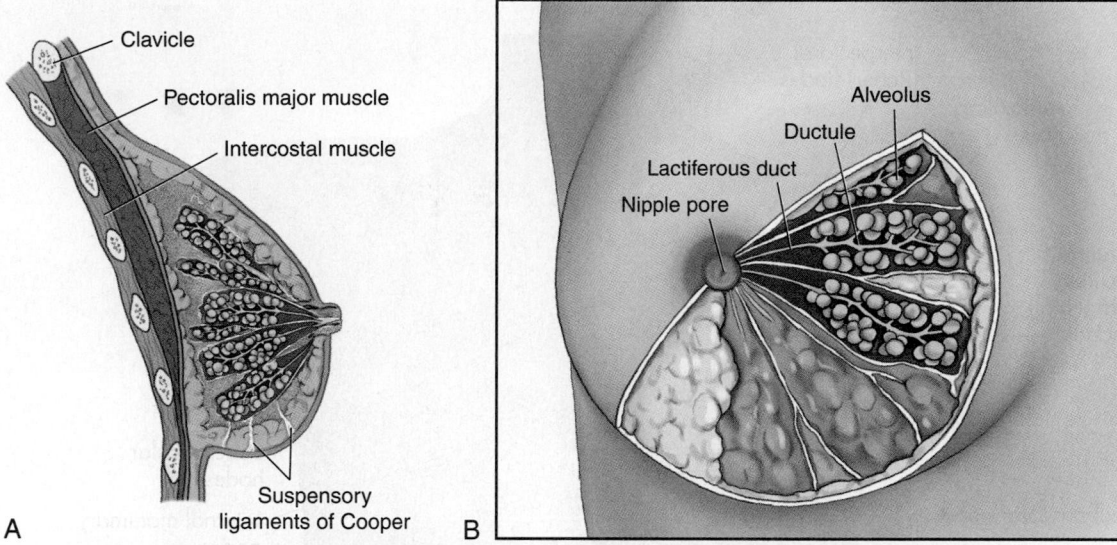

Figure 22-19 Schematic diagram of breast. (From Riordan J: *Breastfeeding and human lactation*, ed 3, Sudbury, MA, 2005, Jones and Bartlett.)

subdivided into glandular alveoli. The alveoli are composed of secretory acini that synthesize milk (lactation) after pregnancy (see Figure 22-19). Milk is continuously secreted into the alveolar lumen and is stored there until the myoepithelial cells are stimulated by oxytocin, which triggers the let-down reflex.[24] The alveoli empty into a network of lactiferous ducts. These ducts reach the skin through 9 or 10 openings (pores) in the nipple. The lobes and lobules are surrounded and separated by muscle strands and fatty connective tissue. The amount of fatty connective tissue varies from individual to individual, depending on weight and genetic and endocrine factors, and contributes to the diversity of breast size and shape.

An extensive capillary network surrounds the alveoli and is supplied by perforating branches of the internal mammary artery, the thoracoacromial artery, the internal and lateral thoracic arteries, and the intercostal arteries. Venous return follows arterial supply, with relatively rapid emptying into the superior vena cava. The breasts receive sensory innervation from branches of the second through sixth intercostal nerves and the cervical plexus. This accounts for the fact that breast pain may be referred to the chest, back, scapula, medial arm, and neck. Lymphatic drainage of the breast occurs largely through axillary nodes, but approximately 25% occurs through transpectoral and other draining nodes (Figure 22-20).[2,25]

The **nipple** is a pigmented, cylindrical structure that is usually located at the fourth or fifth intercostal space. It measures 0.5 to 1.3 cm in diameter and is approximately 10 to 12 mm in height when erect. On its surface lie multiple openings, one from each lobe. The **areola** is the pigmented circular area around the nipple. It may be 15 to 60 mm in diameter. A number of sebaceous glands, the **glands of Montgomery,** are located within the areola and aid in lubrication of the nipple during lactation. The nipple and areola contain smooth

muscles that receive motor innervation from the sympathetic nervous system. Breast-feeding, sexual stimulation, and exposure to cold cause the nipple to become erect.

The fetal and early postnatal development of breast tissue does not depend on hormones, although fetal breast tissue does become progressively responsive to hormonal stimulation. During childhood, breast growth is latent and growth of the nipple and areola keeps pace with body surface growth. (Male breast development normally does not progress any further.) At the onset of puberty in the female, estrogen secretion stimulates mammary growth. Breast development, or **thelarche,** is usually the first sign of puberty in the female. Full differentiation and maturation of breast tissue occur over approximately 4 years and are mediated by a variety of hormones, including estrogen, progesterone, prolactin, growth hormone, thyroxine, insulin, and cortisol. Estrogen promotes the increase in size of the breast by the formation of a mass of tissue under the areola, increases the size and pigmentation of the areola, and development of the lobular ducts. During pregnancy increased levels of estrogen promote further development of the lobular ducts. Progesterone stimulates development of cells lining the alveoli to produce milk. Lactation (milk production) occurs after childbirth in response to increased levels of prolactin. Prolactin secretion, in turn, increases by continued breast-feeding. Oxytocin, another hormone released during and after delivery, controls milk ejection from alveolar cells. Variations in breast development are listed in Box 22-2.

During the reproductive years, the breast undergoes cyclic changes in response to changes in the levels of estrogen and progesterone associated with the menstrual cycle. During the follicular/proliferative phase of the menstrual cycle, high estradiol levels increase the vascularity of breast tissue and stimulate proliferation of ductal and alveolar tissue.

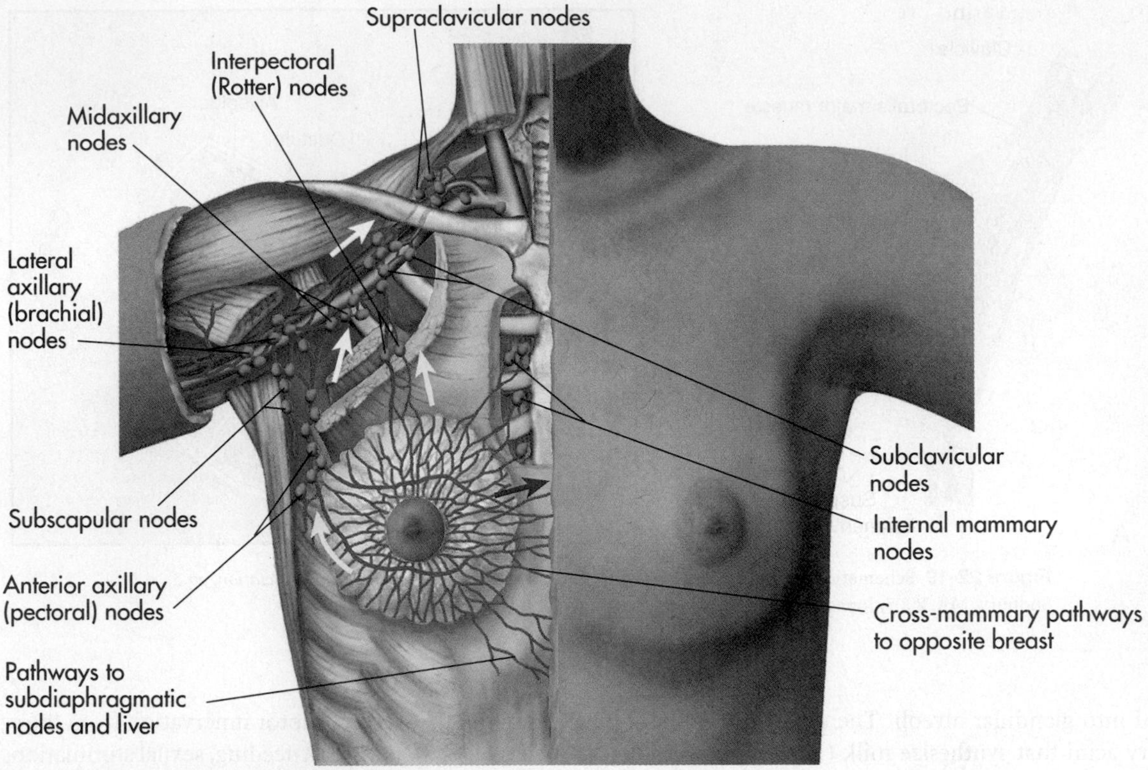
Supraclavicular nodes
Interpectoral (Rotter) nodes
Midaxillary nodes
Lateral axillary (brachial) nodes
Subscapular nodes
Anterior axillary (pectoral) nodes
Pathways to subdiaphragmatic nodes and liver
Subclavicular nodes
Internal mammary nodes
Cross-mammary pathways to opposite breast

Figure 22-20 **Lymphatic drainage of the female breast.** (From Seidel HM et al: *Mosby's guide to physical examination,* ed 6, St Louis, 2006, Mosby.)

Box 22-2 Variations in Breast Development

- Ectopic breast development may occur in males and females with tissue in the axilla, abdomen, labia in females, or back and buttocks (less common). The breast tissue develops from the milk line, an embryonic mammary ridge of ectoderm.
- Accessory nipples (polythelia) or mammary glands (polymastia) are caused by cellular migration along the milk line; polythelia occurs in approximately 1% of the population and is slightly more common in men.
- Inverted nipples usually revert to normal during the first month; persistence into adulthood may cause concerns with lactation.
- Failed development of the nipple (athelia) or entire mammary gland (amastia) is rare and may include a complete lack of development, unilateral failure, or extreme asymmetry. This is caused by complete involution of the mammary ridge.
- Symmetric or asymmetric hyperplasia occurs in approximately 1% to 4% of all females.

Data from Greydanus DE, Matytsina L, Gains M: *Prim Care* 33(2): 455-502, 2006; Jenkins RR: The breast. In Kliegman RM et al editors: *Nelson textbook of pediatrics*, ed 18, p 834, Philadelphia, 2007, Saunders.

This effect is sustained into the luteal/secretory phase of the cycle. During this phase, progesterone levels influence the growth of the alveoli and increase and contribute to the breast changes induced by estradiol. Specific effects of estrogen and progesterone include dilation of the ducts and conversion of the alveolar cells into secretory cells; and fluid secretion, mitotic activity, and deoxyribonucleic acid (DNA) production of nonglandular tissue and glandular epithelium.[1] Most women experience some degree of premenstrual breast fullness, tenderness, and increased nodularity. Breast volume may increase as much as 10 to 30 ml. Because the length of the menstrual cycle does not allow for complete regression of new cell growth, breast growth continues at a slow rate until approximately 35 years of age. Because of the cyclic changes that occur in breast tissue, clinical breast examination is recommended at the conclusion of or a few days after menses, when hormonal effects are minimal and breasts are at their smallest and least tender.

The function of the female breast is primarily to provide a source of nourishment for the newborn. Physiologically, breast milk is the most appropriate nourishment for newborns. Not only does its composition change over time to meet the changing digestive capabilities and nutritional requirements of the infant but it also contains immune cells, specific immunoglobulins, especially immunoglobulin A (IgA), and nonspecific antimicrobial factors, such as lysozymes and lactoferrin, that protect the infant against infection and allergies and asthma. Evidence suggests breast-feeding decreases future incidence in the infant of adult obesity, lowers atherosclerotic disease, and lowers the incidence of types 1 and 2 diabetes.[26] During lactation, high prolactin levels interfere with hypothalamic-pituitary hormones that stimulate ovulation. Lactation usually suppresses the menstrual cycle (lactational amenorrhea) and prevents ovulation for the first 6 months postpartum.[27] In many parts of the world lactational amenorrhea is a means of contraception. Breasts are also a source of pleasurable sexual sensation and in Western cultures have become a sexual symbol.

The Male Breast

Until puberty, development of the male breast is similar to that of the female breast. In the absence of sufficiently high levels of estrogen and progesterone, the male breast does not develop any further. The normal male breast consists of a small, underdeveloped nipple; some fatty and fibrous tissue; and a few ductlike structures in the subareolar area. The male breast may appear enlarged in obese men because of accumulation of fatty tissue. During puberty some males experience gynecomastia, a condition in which the breasts enlarge temporarily as a result of hormonal fluctuations. Thirty percent to 60% of men may have palpable breast tissue related to circulating or local production of estrogen from elevated aromatase activity, particularly in adipose tissue.[28]

TESTS OF REPRODUCTIVE FUNCTION

Diagnostic tests of the male and female reproductive systems are performed to determine the cause of infertility, to detect the presence of cancerous lesions, or to identify the presence of sexually transmitted infections. (Alterations of the reproductive systems are discussed in Chapter 23; sexually transmitted infections are discussed in Chapter 24.) Procedures include laboratory tests, such as cultures, tests, stains, biopsies, serologic testing, and hormonal assays. Radiographic procedures are performed to identify abnormal growths or structures. Direct observation of reproductive organs is completed by laparoscopy or colposcopy.

Infection and Cancer Tests

Tests, stains, cultures, and serologic testing commonly are used to detect infectious diseases. Tests are prepared by spreading a layer of specimen material on a glass slide. The specimen may be evaluated microscopically as a wet mount or dried and stained with different dyes. Gram staining is a technique that allows the differential identification of two categories of bacteria according to the tendency of the microorganism to selectively absorb different components of the stain. Fluorescent antibody testing and DNA probe testing (nucleic acid hybridization detection method) are fairly quick, inexpensive, and accurate methods that can be used to detect some bacterial and viral infections.

A **culture** is the growth of microorganisms in a nutrient medium selectively prepared to support the growth of particular microorganisms that are obtained from body secretions or tissues. Bacteria as well as viruses, such as cytomegalovirus, can be cultured.

Serologic testing identifies whether an antigen-antibody reaction has occurred in response to an infectious microorganism. Several different techniques can be used to identify the formation of antigen-antibody complexes. With immunofluorescent testing, fluorescein-labeled antibodies react with specific antigen, such as the spirochetes of syphilis. The fluorescent pattern of the reaction can be microscopically observed under ultraviolet light. The flocculation (agglutination) test is the precipitation of clumped cells caused by the reaction of antigen with homologous antiserum. The Venereal Disease Research Laboratory (VDRL) test for syphilis is a type of flocculation test. Certain viral diseases can be diagnosed using specific serologic antibody markers, for example, the diagnosis of hepatitis A and hepatitis B viruses. Radioimmunoassay (RIA) and enzyme-linked immunosorbent assay (ELISA) are more specific tests used to document viral infections. Tests used for the diagnosis of sexually transmitted infections are presented in Table 22-2.

Tissue biopsy is the surgical resection of a tissue specimen from a suspected site. The biopsy provides cells and tissues to be used to identify infectious processes and to differentiate benign from malignant conditions and primary from metastatic lesions. In the reproductive tract, tissue may be obtained from the vagina, cervix (by cone or brush biopsy), endometrium of the uterus (by curettage), ovary, testis, prostate, or penis.

Needle biopsy is a technique of aspirating small amounts of tissue by positioning a needle in the tissue and applying negative pressure by pulling back on the plunger of the attached syringe as the needle is moved back and forth at the biopsy site. There is relatively less discomfort with this procedure than with a tissue biopsy that requires opening the surface of

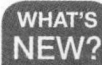

WHAT'S NEW? Human Papillomavirus (HPV) Vaccine and Cervical Cancer Prevention

A quadravalent HPV vaccine has been approved by the U.S. Food and Drug Administration to prevent genital infection from four types of HPV (6, 11, 16, and 18). These types of HPV are oncogenic and can cause cervical dysplasia and cervical cancer. HPV is responsible for 99.7% of cervical cancer cases and is estimated to cause 5% of all cancers worldwide. HPV can also cause cancer of the vulva, vagina, anus, penis, and oropharynx and genital warts. Symptoms of infection are often silent, and approximately 50% of women are estimated to be infected, usually during adolescence. The vaccine is administered by intramuscular injection and the recommended schedule is a three-dose series with the second and third doses administered 2 and 6 months after the first dose. The recommended age for vaccination of females is 11 to 12 years. The vaccine can be administered as young as age 9 years. Catch-up vaccination is recommended for females ages 13 to 26 years who have not been previously vaccinated. The vaccine is not disease treatment and disease may develop related to non-vaccine related HPV infection. Pap smear screening for cervical cancer should be continued. Efforts are in progress to make the vaccine affordable in less-developed countries with the hope of eradicating cervical cancer.

Data from Markowitz LE et al: *MMWR Recom Rep* 56(RR-2):1-24, 2007; Smith JS et al: *J Adolesc Health* 43(4 Suppl):S5-25.e1-41, 2008; Castellsaque X: *Gynecol Oncol* 110(3 Suppl 2):S4-S7, 2008; Beller U, Abu-Rustum NR: *Ostet Gynecol* 113(2 pt 2):550-552, 2009.

Table 22-2   Diagnosis of Sexually Transmitted Infections

Test	Description	Normal Value
Serologic Test for Syphilis	Detection of antibodies to *Treponema pallidum*	Negative or nonreactive
VDRL	Venereal Disease Research Laboratory (nonspecific)	
RPR	Rapid plasma reagin (more specific)	
FTA	Fluorescent treponemal antibody absorption test (more specific; confirmatory test)	
Other Test for Syphilis		
Darkfield examination	Direct smear of serous exudate from moist lesions to detect *T. pallidum* with corkscrew appearance	Negative
Tests for Gonorrhea		
Target amplified nucleic acid probe	Results reported in 1 to 2 days May collect from urine, endocervical or vaginal swabs, or male urethral swabs	
DNA probe (1-2 days)	Direct detection of DNA (inexpensive and quick) Female endocervical or male urethral swab—gross blood may interfere with test	Negative
Culture (1-3 days)	Isolation and detection of *Neisseria gonorrhoeae* in urethral, cervical, anal, or pharyngeal secretions	No growth
Tests for *Chlamydia*		
Target amplified nucleic acid probe	Results reported in 1 to 2 days May collect from urine, endocervical or vaginal swabs, or male urethral swabs	
Antigen detection of DNA probe	Direct immunofluorescent staining of cervical or urethral specimens to detect monoclonal antibodies or genetic probe to detect DNA sequence—gross blood may interfere with test results Not recommended for pediatric patient	Negative
Culture (1-3 days)	Isolation and detection of *Chlamydia trachomatis* from epithelial cells of rectum, eye, endocervix and urethra, or nasopharyngeal aspirate of the newborn	No growth
Tests for HIV Infections		
ELISA (enzyme-linked immunosorbent assay)	Detects the presence of antibodies to human immunodeficiency virus (HIV)	Nonreactive
IFA (indirect fluorescent antibody)	A more specific test for HIV	Nonreactive
WB (Western blot)	A more specific test for HIV	Nonreactive
Tests for Viral Infections		
TORCH test	Detects elevations of IgA or IgM caused by *Toxoplasma*, rubella, cytomegalovirus, syphilis and other infections, and herpes simplex in mother and newborn infant; herpes requires more specific testing when result is positive	No elevation in antibodies
Cytomegalovirus (herpesvirus 5) (liquid base, Pap smear)	Can be grown in cell culture with samples from urine, cervix, semen, saliva, blood	No growth
HPV testing	Detects human papillomavirus, a primary cause of cervical cancer	Negative
Herpes simplex virus by PCR (polymerase chain reaction)	Reported 1-3 days from ocular, amniotic, or vesicle fluid or from serum	

DNA, Deoxyribonucleic acid; *HPV,* human papillomavirus; *IgA,* immunoglobulin A; *IgM,* immunoglobulin M; *TORCH,* toxoplasmosis, rubella, syphilis and other infections (hepatitis B, coxsackie virus, Epstein-Barr virus, varicella-zoster virus, and human parvovirus), cytomegalovirus, herpes simplex.

the skin to localize the tissue site. Normal findings indicate no abnormal cells or tissues on histologic examination.

The **Papanicolaou (Pap) test** is a procedure commonly used for the **cytologic examination** of the female reproductive tract. Cells from body tissues and fluids (from the vagina or endocervix) are stained and examined for the number and types of cells and abnormalities in their morphology. Specimens also may be obtained from the mouth; nipple discharge; or amniotic, pleural, or spinal fluid aspirations. The Pap test

is particularly useful for diagnosis of premalignant (dysplastic), malignant, atypical, and inflammatory cells usually as a result of HPV infection. Because of the increased prevalence of Pap test screening, the rate of invasive cervical cancer has declined steadily over the past 30 years from 55% to 16%. Pap test screening is no longer necessary annually if the woman is older than 30, has had three negative Pap tests, and is in a mutually monogamous relationship. She may consider Pap tests every 2 to 3 years.[2] Liquid-based methods can test for

HPV. If the high-risk type is detected, further evaluation with colposcopy (magnification of rapid growing cells) with biopsy may be required.[25]

Evaluations of the breast are commonly performed to detect tumors or to differentiate solid masses from cysts and benign from malignant tumors. Screening or diagnostic **mammography,** surgical or **fine-needle biopsy (aspiration),** and **ultrasonography** are specific examination techniques. Less common tests include thermography, which is used for screening; chest x-rays, which are used to detect pulmonary metastases; and computed tomography (CT) scanning, which is used when liver or brain metastases are suspected. Mammography is a low-dose radiographic examination used to identify nonpalpable (less than 1 cm) or unrecognized lesions. Breast cancer can be detected by radiography 2 to 3 years before its clinical presentation, providing an excellent prognosis for cure. The American Cancer Society recommends clinical breast examinations yearly and annual mammograms starting at age 40. Earlier mammograms are recommended if a woman has a first-degree relative with early onset breast cancer, or is positive for the *BRCA* gene.[25]

Ultrasonography is performed chiefly to differentiate cystic from solid lesions; it is not diagnostic of malignancy. Fine-needle aspiration, an inexpensive and relatively simple procedure, is used to aspirate cysts or to obtain a specimen for cytologic examination. The main problem with any needle biopsy, or aspiration, is sampling error caused by improper positioning of the needle, which creates false-negative test results. The rate of false-positive results with fine needle aspiration is 1% to 2%; the rate of false-negative results is 10%.[9]

Fertility Tests

Tests of reproductive function are performed most commonly when infertility exists. Both partners are examined, and several diagnostic evaluations may be completed. The types of tests and their normal values are summarized in Tables 22-3 and 22-4. The man is evaluated for number, amount, structure, and motility of sperm and obstruction along the reproductive tract. Tests for women determine whether (1) the reproductive tract (cervix, uterus, fallopian tubes) is adequately patent to allow for passage of ovum and sperm, (2) ovulation occurs normally, (3) the endometrium is responding normally to hormones, and (4) reproductive tissues are free of tumors or infections. Hormonal assays evaluate the adequacy of pituitary function and target organ response. The position and size of organs or the presence of tumors can be detected by direct observation procedures using a laparoscope or by radiographic studies, such as plain films, computerized scans, or tomography.[16]

Aging and Reproductive Function

Aging and the Female Reproductive System

Menopause is a normal developmental event that is experienced universally by midlife women. In the United States, women reach menopause between ages 48 and 55 years, at a median age of 51.4 years. The mean age for smokers is 2 years sooner than nonsmokers (50 versus 52 years).[16] Age of menopause tends to be genetically predetermined and does not appear to be affected by age at menarche, childbearing or lactation, use of oral contraceptives, socioeconomic class, or race. If a woman stops menstruating before 40 years of age it is called **premature ovarian failure,** and occurs in about 1% of the population. Besides smoking, younger age at menopause has been associated with abnormalities of the X chromosome causing gonadal dysgenesis and undernourishment. Thinner women experience menopause at a slightly younger age, probably related to body fat. Irregular menses in women in their early 40s also may be a predictor of an earlier menopause. Alcohol consumption has been associated with later menopause, perhaps because of higher blood and urinary levels of estrogen.[16]

Perimenopause is the transitional period between reproductive and nonreproductive years, a transition lasting 2 to 8 years.[1,16] Five to 10 years before menopause, approximately 90% of women note mild to extreme variability in frequency and quality of menstrual flow. Perimenopause symptoms depend on the sensitivity of the target tissue receptors. Symptoms usually begin with a lengthening of the menstrual cycle, which correlates with anovulatory cycles. Unpredictable or irregular ovulation uniformly precedes menopause.[1] The perimenopause experience varies among women and from cycle to cycle in the same woman. How individual women experience symptoms is unpredictable. Estradiol levels remain in the normal to slightly elevated range until about 1 year before menopause.[1]

Around 37 to 38 years of age, 10 to 15 years before menstruation ceases, women experience accelerated follicular loss that begins when the total number of follicles reaches about 25,000 and ends when the supply of follicles is depleted (see discussion under Hormonal Controls, earlier in this chapter). This loss correlates with a subtle but definite increase in FSH and a decrease in inhibin. Increased FSH stimulation seems to accelerate follicular loss, and declining inhibin production disturbs the negative feedback influence over pituitary secretion of FSH. Perimenopausal cycles are marked by elevated FSH, decreased inhibin, normal LH, and slightly elevated estradiol levels[1] (Figure 22-21). A hallmark characteristic of impending menopause is the initial "monotropic" FP increase in FSH without corresponding changes in LH levels. Lower inhibin B and increased activin A (a potent stimulator of FSH) levels contribute to this phenomenon.[1]

Increased FSH levels and reduced ovarian secretion of inhibin reflect quality and capability of aging follicles. In a study of pregnancy rates during in vitro fertilization (IVF), women older than 40 years of age had as many oocytes recovered during laparoscopy, equal estrogen and progesterone levels, and similar pregnancy rates when compared with younger women. Yet, despite similar estradiol (E2) levels, inhibin response to exogenous hyperstimulation was significantly lower in the older women. Further, inhibin levels were significantly related to progesterone levels. In this study, 60% of women more

Table 22-3 Tests and Normal Values of Reproductive Function/Fertility

Test	Description	Normal Value
Basic Assessment		
Semen analysis (two samples at least 2 weeks apart)	Determines number, motility, and structure of sperm cells	Volume = 2-6 ml Number = >20 million/ml Motility = >50% with forward progression Morphology = >50% normal shape
White blood cells	Determines presence of bacteria/leukocytes	Immunobead test = <20% with adherent particles
Immunological tests	Detects antibody to sperm	Sperm MAR test (mixed antiglobulin reaction) = <10% with adherent particles <10^6 WBC/ml No sperm agglutinins present
Intermediate Assessment		
Basal body temperature	Determines whether ovulation has occurred	Decrease in basal body temperature before ovulation followed by a rise in temperature at the time of ovulation
FSH level	Day 3 of cycle	Lab specific results
Estradiol	Days 2-4 of cycle	TSH thyroid-stimulating prolactin level Luteal phase progesterone level Lab-specific results
Cervical mucus	Evaluates presence of ovulation from estrogenic effects at ovulation; mucus also may be examined for pH, glucose, or proteins or cultured for presence of infection	Fern pattern appears when cervical mucus dries on a clean slide; mucus is clear, watery, and elastic (spinnbarkeit ≥8-10 cm) with no inflammatory cells
Postcoital cervical mucus (Sims-Huhner test)	Tests ability of sperm to penetrate and maintain motility in cervical mucus 2-4 hours after coitus approximately 1 day before ovulation	≥10 motile sperm in each high-power field; motility in one direction; previous sperm analysis normal
Zona binding test or Hamster penetration test	Nonliving oocytes are surgically removed and bisected; sperm added to the hemi-oocyte to test fertilizing capability	Bonding <30% predicted failed fertilization 70% of the time Bonding >30% predicted successful fertilization 85% of the time Results may vary with lab
Ultrasound vaginal scanning	Provides superior quality resolution of the uterine, fallopian, and ovarian structures; also can be used to study folliculogenesis, ovulation, and luteogenesis to detect abnormalities	Normal structures visualized
More Specialized Tests		
Endometrial biopsy	Determines whether ovulation has occurred by obtaining endometrial tissue on day 26 of 28-day menstrual cycle (or postovulatory day 12)	Finding is "secretory-type" endometrium if ovulation has occurred; read in conjunction with day of cycle and serum progesterone levels
Hysterosalpingogram	Assessment of uterus and fallopian tubes for obstructions using transuterine injection of contrast material and radiography; performed 1-2 days after cessation of menses	No obstruction evident
Laparoscopy (pelvic endoscopy)	Visualization of reproductive organs using a laparoscope inserted within the pelvic cavity through the abdomen to assess structure or determine presence of adhesions, endometriosis tumors, or infection	Normal structure and position of organs
Hysteroscopy	Visualization of uterine cavity using modified cystoscope inserted through cervical os; best done during first 14 days of cycle	Absence of intrauterine lesions

FSH, Follicle-stimulating hormone; *TSH,* thyroid-stimulating hormone; *WBC,* white blood cells.

Table 22-4	Serum Hormone Values
Hormone	**Value**
Serum progesterone	Normal = >10 ng/dl, presumptive evidence of ovulation; draw level between days 20-25 of 28-day cycle or 6-10 days postovulation <10 ng/ml = inadequate luteal function <3 ng/ml suggests anovulation
Serum testosterone	Normal = 300-1200 ng/dl; must be interpreted with serum LH and FSH levels
Resulting from diurnal and pulsatile pattern, need serial blood draws	Low values in male hypogonadism
Serum FSH and LH Resulting from diurnal and pulsatile pattern, need serial blood draws	FSH = <22 international units/L LH = 4-24 international units/L High levels in males indicate primary testicular disease; low levels in males indicate hypogonadism caused by hypothalamic-pituitary dysfunction

FSH, Follicle-stimulation hormone; *LH,* luteinizing hormone.

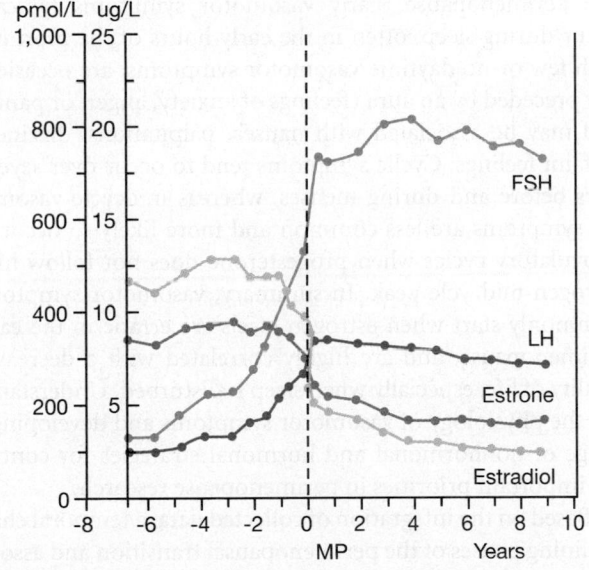

Figure 22-21 The perimenopausal hormone transition. Mean circulating hormone levels. *FSH,* Follicle-stimulating hormone; *LH,* luteinizing hormone.

than 40 years of age who became pregnant through IVF spontaneously aborted, compared with 30% of younger women.[29]

In summary, hormonal findings during the years surrounding menopause indicate that the process of folliculogenesis changes (Box 22-3). Initially, FSH levels are significantly elevated, whereas pulsatile secretion by the pituitary is maintained. Later, LH levels rise. In younger women, FSH stimulates inhibin, which in turn suppresses FSH. However, through an undetermined mechanism, perimenopausal women produce high levels of FSH in early FP and lower FP

Box 22-3	Changes in Ovarian Folliculogenesis During the Perimenopause Leading to Endogenous Overstimulation

- ↑ FSH → ovarian hyperstimulation → ↑ number of follicles recruited (net effect of follicular depletion) → ↑ estrogen (E2)
- ↓ Follicular reserve → ↓ inhibin and ↑ activin in FP and LP → ↑ FSH → ↑ number of follicles recruited, partial development, infrequent ovulation → ↑ estrogen (E2) and ↓ progesterone

FP, Follicular phase; *FSH,* follicle-stimulating hormone; *LP,* luteal phase.

Table 22-5	Endocrine Events Associated with Perimenopause
Hormone Changes	**Effects**
Estradiol (E2) levels Mean FP level 1 greater than mean FP level in younger women	Erratic and intermittent increase First in FP (inverse relationship between length of FP and estradiol level)
FP level may be greater than midcycle peak level in fertile women	Later during premenstrual phase
Ovulatory cycles	Short or insufficient LP (decreased fertility)
Progesterone levels	Decreased in ovulatory cycle; minimal during anovulatory cycles
Anovulatory cycles	Increased to about 50%; perhaps more in later perimenopause
FSH levels	Variable, then increased
LH levels	Normal initially, then increased
Inhibin levels	Correlate with progesterone levels

FP, Follicular phase; *FSH,* follicle-stimulating hormone; *LH,* luteinizing hormone; *LP,* luteal phase.

inhibin levels. The ovary, in response to high FSH, recruits increasing numbers of follicles; these follicles only partially develop, with a net effect of irregular ovulation, lower progesterone levels, and depleted follicle reserve. The increase in developing follicles leads to increased E2 levels. It is believed that lower levels of inhibin and higher levels of activin counteract the usual effect of the negative feedback loop found in younger women.[1] Table 22-5 summarizes endocrine events occurring during the perimenopause.

The majority of health concerns and public health issues focus on menstrual cycle changes, **vasomotor symptoms,** or hot flashes/flushes, potential for bone loss (osteoporosis is discussed in Chapter 42), and the emotional symptoms that may accompany the perimenopausal transition.[1,30] Heavy menstrual bleeding, menorrhagia (flooding), is one of the most distressing complaints and affects approximately 50% of women. It is also the complaint that in the past put women at high risk for hysterectomy. Increased endometrial bleeding is correlated with a change from ovulatory to anovulatory

Table 22-6	Impact of High Estrogen Levels on Menstrual Cycle and Symptomatology
Associated Physiologic Change	**Signs/Symptoms**
Short follicular phase (FP)	Short cycles
Long FP	Long cycles
Thickened endometrium*	Heavy, long, or unpredictable flow (including clotting and flooding)*
Increase in glandular cells without stromal support produced by progesterone → unstable endometrium	Midcycle spotting
	Menorrhagia
Possible increased production of prostaglandins within endometrial tissue	Metrorrhagia
	Dysmenorrhea
	Breast tenderness, modularity, enlargement
	Water retention
	Emotional stress; new or unpredictable mood swings
	Weight gain
	Vasomotor symptoms
	New onset of migraine headaches; exacerbation of headaches
	Increased premenstrual symptoms

*Symptoms aggravated by anovulatory cycles; leads to dysfunctional uterine bleeding (see Chapter 23).

cycles and is associated with unopposed high E2 levels the week before menses. Estrogen causes endometrial tissue to thicken. Because women with anovulatory cycles have longer exposure to periods of unopposed estrogen, the mean thickness of their endometrium, as measured by ultrasound, can be greater than that of ovulatory women.[29,30] Thicker endometrium without corresponding stromal support from progesterone production leads to heavier periods, menorrhagia, or midcycle bleeding, metrorrhagia[9] (Table 22-6).

In the United States, most women and clinicians link hot flashes/flushes, or **vasomotor flush,** with menopause and low estrogen levels. However, a rapid change in estrogen levels (withdrawal or increase), rather than low estrogen levels, induces hot flushes. Vasomotor symptoms are characterized by a rise in skin temperature, dilation of peripheral blood vessels, increased blood flow to the hands, increased skin conductance, and transient increase in heart rate (average of 9 beats per minute and up to 20), followed by a temperature drop and profuse perspiration over the area of flush distribution. Vasomotor flush usually occurs in the face and neck and may radiate into the chest and other parts of the body. Dizziness, nausea, headaches, or palpitations may accompany the flush. Vasomotor symptoms vary in frequency, intensity, and duration, lasting 1 to 5 minutes (mean 2.7 minutes). Anywhere from 11% to 85% of menopausal women experience vasomotor flushes.[29,30] Most (about 60% to 65%) have symptoms for 1 to 5 years, 25% for 6 to 10 years, and 10% to 15% for 10 to 15 years or longer.

Women with higher cyclic E2 levels, that is, premenopausal women with premenstrual vasomotor symptoms and women who report breast, fluid, and premenstrual mood symptoms during the early stages of the perimenopause, are predisposed to withdrawal vasomotor symptoms later in the perimenopausal transition. Anecdotal reports from participants in various research studies suggest that vasomotor symptoms occur just before flow and may be used to predict

menstruation.[30] Cyclic vasomotor symptoms, which typically begin early in the perimenopausal transition, differ from noncyclic vasomotor symptoms, which are experienced in late perimenopause. Early vasomotor symptoms typically occur during sleep, often in the early hours of the morning, with few or no daytime vasomotor symptoms; are occasionally preceded by an aura (feelings of anxiety, anger, or panic); and may be associated with nausea, palpitations, dizziness, or faint feelings. Cyclic symptoms tend to occur over several days before and during menses, whereas midcycle vasomotor symptoms are less common and more likely to occur in anovulatory cycles when progesterone does not follow high estrogen midcycle peak. In summary, vasomotor symptoms commonly start when estrogen levels are erratic in the early perimenopause, and are highly correlated with a decreased quality of life, especially when sleep is disturbed. Understanding the physiology of vasomotor symptoms and developing a range of nonhormonal and hormonal strategies for control are important priorities in perimenopause research.

Based on the integration of collected data, a temporal chart outlining phases of the perimenopausal transition and associated endocrine changes and symptoms has been developed.[29] Although the transition is divided into five phases, the vast variability in timing and degree of symptoms experienced by individual women may make clear predictions impossible. The information outlined in Table 22-7 provides a template to visualize the complex physiology of the perimenopause and the dynamic changes that occur during this time.

Several other physiologic changes are associated with the postmenopausal period. These changes affect breast tissue, urogenital structures, bone density or risk for osteoporosis, risk for heart disease and possible memory loss or Alzheimer disease. Only changes in the breast and urogenital structures are addressed here (other topics are addressed in appropriate chapters).

As ovarian function changes, breast tissue involutes. Two phases of involution have been described: the premenopausal

Table 22-7	Postulated Perimenopausal Transition Timeline		
Phase	Menstrual Physiology	Hormonal Changes	Symptomatology
A	Regular, ovulatory cycles Short cycles, short FP	Intermittent ↑ E2 FSH usually normal Intermittent ↑ FP FSH Low inhibin	Increased breast tenderness, mood swings, fluid retention, premenstrual symptoms Early morning night sweats (vasomotor symptoms) Weight gain, migraine headaches, heavy flow
B	Regular cycles with disturbances in ovulation Short LP Insufficient LP Anovulatory cycles	Intermittent ↑ FP FSH E2 often ↑ Inhibin inappropriately low	Heavy flow ↑ Premenstrual symptoms ↑ Dysmenorrhea Predictable or ↑ vasomotor symptoms before flow
C	Onset of perimenopause Alternating short, long, or skipped cycles	E2 often quite ↑ E2 normal or low ↑ FSH (slight) ↑ LH Low inhibin	Vasomotor symptoms during waking hours Vasomotor symptoms more persistent, remain cyclic before flow
D	Onset of oligomenorrhea 50% of cycles anovulatory Heavy flow may predict onset of oligomenorrhea	↑ Progesterone with ovulation Persistent ↓ FSH ↑ LH ↑ E2 Low inhibin	↑ Vasomotor symptoms ↑ Signs/symptoms of high estrogen after long periods without flow Flow light but unpredictable
E	Final menstrual period plus 1 year	↑ FSH and LH ↓ or normal E2 Consistent low inhibin ↓ Progesterone	↑ Intensity and frequency of vasomotor symptoms (although vasomotor symptoms may disappear) ↓ Cramps and premenstrual-type symptoms without subsequent flow ↓ Breast, mood, and fluid symptoms

E2, Estradiol; *FP*, follicular phase; *FSH*, follicle-stimulating hormone; *LP*, luteal phase.

phase and the postmenopausal phase. The premenopausal phase occurs between 35 and 45 years of age. During this phase there is a moderate decrease in mammary tissue. During the postmenopausal phase, glandular breast tissue is significantly reduced and there is some increase of fat deposits and connective tissue. These changes contribute to the reduction in size and firmness of breast tissue.

The urogenital tract undergoes a number of changes. The ovaries begin to decrease in size around age 30 years, and shrinkage accelerates after age 60 years. Gradually, over the years, the uterus atrophies and decreases in size. The vagina shortens, narrows, and loses some of its elasticity. Vaginal walls lose their ability to lubricate quickly. Intercourse before adequate lubrication may be painful. The vaginal pH, usually maintained at 4 to 6 before menopause, increases to between 6.5 and 8 and contributes to a higher incidence of vaginitis. The cervix atrophies and the cervical os decreases in size. The vaginal epithelium also atrophies; this atrophy can cause vaginal irritation, burning, itching (pruritus), white discharge (leukorrhea), painful intercourse (dyspareunia), and vaginal bleeding. The labia majora and minora become less prominent, and some pubic hair is lost. Urethral tone declines, as does muscle tone throughout the pelvic area. Urinary frequency, urgency, and incontinence are associated with estrogen deficiency.

Sexually active women have less vaginal atrophy; presumably, sexual activity and stimulation maintains vaginal vasculature and circulation.[1] Regular intercourse (once or twice per week) and masturbation are associated with vaginal pliability, vaginal function, and continued lubrication with arousal.

Aging and the Male Reproductive System

Men maintain reproductive capacity longer than women. There is no known discrete event, comparable to menopause, that characterizes aging of the male reproductive system, although the term *andropause* is sometimes used to describe the hypogonadism associated with male aging.[31] Gradual changes do occur, and aging in the male reproductive system is characterized by hypogonadism, testosterone deficiency, erectile dysfunction, and proliferative disorders of the prostate gland (see Chapter 23).[32] Aging changes are also influenced by chronic diseases and use of medications.

Components of male sexual behavior include both sexual drive and erectile and ejaculatory capacity. Libido, or sexual drive, is a complex phenomenon that requires a baseline hormonal milieu but is influenced significantly by health status and environmental, social, and psychologic factors. Aging causes specific physical changes that influence erectile and ejaculatory capabilities. Alterations in sexual response include the need for longer stimulation to achieve full erection; slower and less forceful ejaculation, with less pelvic muscle involvement; decreased vasocongestive response; and longer refractory period (time during which erection and ejaculation are not possible), up to 24 hours in some men.

The testes undergo several age-related structural changes, including decreased weight, atrophy, and softening. Degenerative changes in the seminiferous tubules may include thickening of the basement membrane; increase in lumen size; germ cell (spermatogonium) arrest and a decrease in spermatogenic activity; and collapse of tubules, followed by complete obstruction caused by sclerosis and fibrosis. Areas of mild to severe degenerative change may be interspersed with areas having intact tubules. These morphologic changes may result from atherosclerosis (arterial clogging) in the testicular vascular bed.[33] Alterations of the seminiferous tubules do not appear to diminish sperm counts, but they do reduce fertility because a greater percentage of the sperm lack motility or have structural abnormalities.

Aging probably causes changes in the production of male sex hormones, levels of SHBG, and responsiveness of target tissues. Hormone synthesis by the testes and testicular responsiveness to the gonadotropins (FSH and LH) are diminished, and pituitary secretion of these gonadotropins are elevated.[32,34] The reduced levels of testosterone may be related to alterations in the Leydig cells, the testosterone producers of the testes. The number of Leydig cells decreases as age increases, perhaps because of atherosclerotic changes in arteries that supply blood to the testes.[35] Even if testosterone levels are not decreased, older men may have less unbound testosterone in their blood, decreasing the amount of unbound hormone available to stimulate target tissues. Decreased testosterone levels have several effects, including functional deterioration of the accessory sex organs (the prostate gland, seminal vesicles, epididymis, and ductus deferens); loss of muscle mass, strength, and endurance; increased visceral fat, osteopenia, and cognitive decline; and, in many men, decrease in libido. This last effect also may be caused by alterations in other variables that affect libido.[36,37] Modifiable risk factors for low testosterone and symptoms of androgen deficiency include health status and waist circumference.[38]

SUMMARY REVIEW

Development of the Reproductive Systems

1. Differentiation of female and male genitalia begins around weeks 7 to 8 of embryonic development, when the gonads of genetically male embryos begin to secrete male sex hormones, primarily testosterone. Until that time the primitive reproductive organs of males and females are homologous (the same).

2. The structure and function of male and female reproductive systems are controlled by the H-P-G axis, a set of complex neurologic and hormonal interactions that accelerate at puberty and lead to sexual maturation and reproductive capability.

3. Extrahypothalamic factors cause the hypothalamus to secrete GnRH, which stimulates the anterior pituitary to secrete gonadotropins—FSH and LH—that stimulate the gonads (ovaries or testes) to secrete female or male sex hormones. Paracrine hormones (inhibin, activin, and follistatin) influence the positive and negative feedback loops that occur along the H-P-G axis.

4. Production of primitive female gametes (ova) occurs solely during fetal life. From puberty to menopause, one female gamete matures per menstrual cycle. Production of the male gametes (sperm) begins at puberty; after that, millions are produced daily, usually for life.

The Female Reproductive System

1. The function of the reproductive system is to produce mature ova and, when fertilized, to protect and nourish them through embryonic and fetal life, and expel them at birth.

2. The external female genitalia are the mons pubis, labia majora, labia minora, clitoris, vestibule (urinary and vaginal openings), Bartholin glands, and Skene glands.

3. The internal female genitalia are the vagina, uterus, fallopian tubes, and ovaries.

4. The vagina is a fibromuscular canal that receives the penis during sexual intercourse and is the exit route for menstrual fluids and products of conception. The vagina leads from the introitus (its external opening) to the cervical portion of the uterus.

5. The uterus is the hollow, muscular organ in which a fertilized ovum develops. The uterine walls have three layers: the endometrium (lining), myometrium (muscular layer), and perimetrium (outer covering, which is continuous with the pelvic peritoneum). The endometrium proliferates (thickens) and sloughs off in response to cyclic hormonal changes. The cervix is the narrow, lower portion of the uterus that opens into the vagina.

6. The two fallopian tubes extend from the uterus to the ovaries. Their function is to conduct ova from the spaces around the ovaries to the uterus. Fertilization normally occurs in the distal third of the fallopian tubes.

7. From puberty to menopause, the ovaries are the site of (1) ovum maturation and release and (2) production of female sex (estrogen and progesterone) and male (androgens) hormones. Female sex hormones predominate and are involved in sexual differentiation and development, the menstrual cycle, pregnancy, and lactation. Androgens in women contribute to prepubertal growth spurt, pubic and axillary hair growth, and activation of sebaceous glands.

8. Developing ovarian follicles (structures that enclose the ovum) produce estrogen (primarily estradiol). The corpus luteum, the structure that develops from the ruptured ovarian follicle after ovulation or ovum release, produces progesterone. Androgens are produced within the ovarian follicle, adrenal glands, and adipose tissue.

9. The average menstrual cycle lasts 27 to 30 days and consists of three phases, which are named for ovarian and endometrial changes: the follicular/proliferative phase, the luteal/secretory phase, and menstruation.

10. Ovarian events of the menstrual cycle are controlled by gonadotropins. High FSH levels stimulate follicle and ovum maturation (follicular phase); then a surge of LH causes ovulation, which is followed by development of the corpus luteum (luteal phase).

11. Ovarian hormones control the uterine (endometrial) events of the menstrual cycle. During the follicular phase of the ovarian cycle, estrogen produced by the follicle causes the endometrium to proliferate (proliferative phase) and induces the LH surge and progesterone production in the granulosa layer. During the luteal phase, estrogen maintains the thickened endometrium and progesterone causes it to develop blood vessels and secretory glands (secretory phase). As the corpus luteum degenerates, production of both hormones drops sharply, and the "starved" endometrium degenerates and sloughs off, causing menstruation.

12. Cyclic changes in hormone levels also cause thinning and thickening of the vaginal epithelium, thinning and thickening of cervical secretions, and changes in basal body temperature.

The Male Reproductive System

1. The function of the male reproductive system is to produce male gametes (sperm) and deliver them to the female reproductive tract.

2. The external male genitalia are the testes, epididymides, scrotum, and penis. The internal genitalia are the vas deferens, ejaculatory duct, prostatic and membranous sections of the urethra, seminal vesicles, prostate gland, and Cowper glands.

3. The testes (male gonads) are paired glands suspended within the scrotum. The testes have two functions: spermatogenesis (sperm production) and production of male sex hormones (androgens, chiefly testosterone).

4. The epididymis is a long, coiled tube arranged in a comma-shaped compartment that curves over the top and rear of the testis. The epididymis receives sperm from the testis and stores them while they develop further. Sperm travel the length of the epididymis and then are ejaculated into the vas deferens.

5. The scrotum is a skin-covered fibromuscular sac that encloses the testes and epididymides, which are suspended within the scrotum by the spermatic cord. The scrotum keeps these organs at optimal temperatures for sperm survival (about 1° to 2° C lower than body temperature) by contracting in cold environments and relaxing in warm environments.

6. The penis is a cylindrical organ consisting of three longitudinal compartments (two corpora cavernosa and one corpus spongiosum) and the urethra. The urethra runs through the corpus spongiosum. The corpora cavernosa and corpus spongiosum consist of erectile tissue. Externally the penis consists of a shaft and a tip, which is called the *glans*. The glans contains sebaceous glands and the opening of the urethra and is covered by a flap of skin (the foreskin).

7. The penis has two functions: delivery of sperm to the female vagina and elimination of urine. These two fluids are never in the urethra at the same time.

8. Sexual intercourse is made possible by the erectile reflex, in which tactile or psychogenic stimulation of the parasympathetic nerves causes arterioles in the corpora cavernosa and corpus spongiosum to dilate and fill with blood, causing the penis to enlarge and become firm.

9. Emission, which occurs at the peak of sexual arousal, is the movement of semen from the epididymides to the penis. Ejaculation, which is a continuation of emission, is the pulsatile ejection of semen from the penis. Both emission and ejaculation involve rhythmic contractions of smooth muscle within the internal glands and ducts.

10. Spermatogenesis is a continuous process because spermatogonia, the primitive male gametes, undergo continuous mitosis within the seminiferous tubules of the testes. Some of the spermatogonia develop into primary spermatocytes, which divide meiotically into secondary spermatocytes and then spermatids. The spermatids develop into sperm with the help of nutrients and hormonal signals from Sertoli cells.

11. Production of the male sex hormones is controlled (like production of the female sex hormones) by the H-P-G axis and by complex feedback mechanisms. The male hormones are produced steadily, with diurnal variations.

Structure and Function of the Breast

1. Until puberty the female and male breasts are similar, consisting of a small underdeveloped nipple, some fatty and fibrous tissue, and a few ductlike structures under the areola. At puberty, however, a variety of hormones (estrogen, progesterone, prolactin, growth hormone, insulin, cortisol) cause the female breast to develop into a system of glands and ducts that is capable of producing and ejecting milk.

2. The basic functional unit of the female breast is the lobe, a system of ducts that branches from the nipple to milk-producing units called *lobules*. The lobules contain alveolar cells, which are convoluted spaces lined with epithelial cells that secrete milk and subepithelial cells that contract, moving the milk into the system of ducts that leads to the nipple.

3. Each breast contains 15 to 20 lobes, which are separated and supported by Cooper ligaments.

4. Milk production occurs in response to prolactin, a hormone that is secreted in larger amounts after childbirth. Milk ejection is under the control of oxytocin, another hormone of pregnancy and parturition.

5. During the reproductive years, breast tissue undergoes cyclic changes in response to hormonal changes of the menstrual cycle.

Tests of Reproductive Function

1. Diagnostic tests are performed to evaluate fertility or presence of tumors, infection, or sexually transmitted infections.

2. Tests, stains, cultures, and serologic tests are used to diagnose infections. These tests specifically identify microorganisms or types of infections.

3. Tissue biopsy can be performed by resection or needle aspiration. Specimen analysis permits identification of abnormal cells.

4. The Pap test is a cytologic examination of cells taken from body fluids and tissues. Although cells can be obtained from many sites, the test is most commonly used (with endocervical cells) for diagnosis of cervical carcinoma.

5. Mammography is a low-dose radiographic examination of the breast for cancer detection.

6. Evaluation of fertility includes reproductive hormone assays and assessment of structural alteration or infections and the determination of normal ovulation or adequate sperm motility and count.

Aging and Reproductive Function

1. In women the transition from fertility to menopause (perimenopause) starts about 2 to 8 years before the last menstrual period and ends the following year. During this transition period, the ovaries produce erratic and high levels of estrogen that contribute to such symptoms as hot flashes, breast tenderness and nodularity, and migraine headaches. Menstrual cycles shorten and then become irregular as anovulation occurs. Menstruation ceases, and women move into menopause.

Continued

SUMMARY REVIEW—cont'd

2. Menopause is defined as 1 year after the cessation of menstruation and occurs at the average age of 51.4 years. Levels of sex hormones decrease with the last menstrual cycle.

3. In response to reduced levels of female sex hormones, the reproductive organs atrophy, the vaginal epithelium thins, and glandular secretions diminish and become more alkaline. Continued sexual activity and orgasm reduce vaginal changes.

4. Nonreproductive effects of reduced estrogen levels may include increased risk of osteoporosis and coronary artery disease.

5. Male reproductive function diminishes with age, but it does not cease in healthy men.

6. The testes atrophy and produce less testosterone, and some seminiferous tubules may degenerate and become fibrotic. These changes affect sex drive (libido) and sperm morphology. Although sperm count remains normal, the semen tends to contain more defective and nonmotile sperm.

7. The erectile reflex is somewhat diminished and occurs more slowly as age advances.

8. Reduced testosterone levels cause some loss of function in the internal genitalia and enlargement (hypertrophy) of the prostate gland.

KEY TERMS

Activin, 794
Adrenarche, 784
Androgens, 792
Areola, 803
Bartholin gland (greater vestibular or vulvovaginal gland), 785
Breast, 802
Cervix (neck of the uterus), 787
Clitoris, 785
Cornification, 795
Corpus cavernosum (pl., corpora cavernosa), 798
Corpus luteum, 789
Corpus spongiosum, 798
Corpus of uterus (body of uterus), 787
Cowper gland (bulbourethral gland), 800
Cul-de-sac, 786
Culture, 805
Cytologic examination, 806
Decornification, 795
Developing fetus, 781
Dihydrotestosterone (DHT), 802
Efferent tubule, 797
Ejaculatory duct, 800
Embryo, 781
Emission, 799
Endocervical canal, 788
Endometrium, 788
Epididymis, 797
Erectile reflex, 799
Estradiol (E2), 790
Estrogen, 790
Fallopian tube (oviduct, uterine tube), 789
Fimbria (pl., fimbriae), 789
Fine-needle biopsy (aspiration), 807
Follicle-stimulating hormone (FSH), 783
Follicular/proliferative phase, 793
Follistatin, 794
Foreskin (prepuce), 798
Fornix, 786
Fundus of uterus, 787
Glands of Montgomery, 803

Glans, 798
Gonad, 781
Gonadarche, 784
Gonadostat, 784
Gonadotropin-releasing hormone (GnRH), 784
Granulosa cell, 789
Hymen, 785
Infundibulum, 789
Inguinal canal, 796
Inhibin, 794
Introitus, 785
Isthmus of the uterus, 787
Labium majus (pl., labia majora), 784
Labium minus (pl., labia minora), 785
Leptin, 784
Leydig cell, 797
Libido, 800
Luteal/secretory phase, 794
Luteinizing hormone (LH), 783, 791
Mammography, 807
Menarche, 792
Menopause, 792
Menstruation (menses), 793
Mons pubis, 784
Myometrium, 788
Needle biopsy, 805
Nipple, 803
Ovarian cycle, 789
Ovarian follicle, 789
Ovaries, 789
Ovulation, 789
Ovum, 781
Papanicolaou (Pap) test, 806
Penis, 798
Perimenopause, 807
Perimetrium (parietal peritoneum), 788
Perineal body, 786
Perineum, 786
Premature ovarian failure, 807
Primary spermatocyte, 800
Progesterone, 791

Prolactin, 802
Prostate gland, 800
Puberty, 784
Rete testis, 797
Ruga (pl., rugae; pertains to vagina and testes), 786
Scrotum, 797
Secondary spermatocyte, 800
Semen, 799
Seminal vesicle, 800
Seminiferous tubule, 797
Serologic testing, 805
Sertoli cell (nondividing support cell), 800
Sex hormone, 781
Sex hormone–binding globulin (SHBG), 801
Skene gland (lesser vestibular or paraurethral gland), 785
Spermatic cord, 796
Spermatids, 800
Spermatogenesis, 797
Spermatogonium (pl., spermatogonia), 800
Spermatozoon (sperm cell), 781
Testis (pl., testes), 786
Testosterone, 800
Theca cell, 789
Thelarche, 784, 803
Tissue biopsy, 805
Tubulus rectus, 797
Tunica albuginea, 797
Tunica dartos, 797
Tunica vaginalis, 796
Ultrasonography, 807
Urethra, 799
Urinary meatus, 785
Uterus, 787
Vagina, 786
Vas deferens (ductus deferens), 797
Vasomotor flush, 810
Vasomotor symptom, 809
Vestibule, 785
Vulva, 784

REFERENCES

1. Speroff L, Fritz MA: *Clinical gynecology, endocrinology, and infertility*, ed 7, Baltimore, 2005, Williams & Wilkins.
2. Coad J, Dunstall M: *Anatomy and physiology for midwives*, ed 2, London, 2006, Churchill Livingstone.
3. Gordon K, Oehninger S: Reproductive physiology. In Copeland LJ, Farrell JF, editors: *Textbook of gynecology*, ed 2 , Philadelphia, 2000, Saunders.
4. Di Vall SA, Radovick S: Pubertal development and menarche, *Ann N Y Acad Sci* 1135:19-28, 2008.
5. Kaplowitz PB: Link between body fat and the timing of puberty, *Pediatrics* 121(Suppl 3):S208-S217, 2008.
6. Klein KO et al: Effect of obesity on estradiol level, and its relationship to leptin, bone maturation, and bone mineral density in children, *J Clin Endocrinol Metab* 83(10):3469, 1998.
7. Chagin AS, Savendahl L: Estrogens and growth: review, *Pediatr Endocrinol Rev* 4(4):329-334, 2007.
8. Berne RM, Levy MN, editors: *Physiology*, ed 5, St Louis, 2003, Mosby.
9. Lowdermilk DL, Perry SE: *Maternity and women's health care*, ed 8, St Louis, 2004, Mosby.
10. Schiffman M et al: Human papillomavirus and cervical cancer, *Lancet* 370(9590):890-907, 2007.
11. Rics FJ et al: A cross-cultural study of menstrual cycle characteristics of women practicing the sympto-thermal method of natural family planning. In Komenich P et al, editors: *The menstrual cycle*, vol 2, New York, 1981, Springer.
12. Trealor AE et al: Variation of the human menstrual cycle through reproductive life. *Int J Fertil* 12:77-126, 1970.
13. Adams Hillard PJ: Menstruation in young girls: a clinical perspective, *Obstet Gynecol* 99(4):655-662, 2002.
14. Golub S: *Periods: from menarche to menopause*, Newbury Park, NJ, 1992, Sage.
15. deKretser DM et al: Inhibins, activans and follistatin in reproduction, *Hum Reprod Update* 8(6):529-541, 2002.
16. Stenchevor MA et al: *Comprehensive gynecology*, ed 4 , St Louis, 2001, Mosby.
17. Sirois J et al: Cyclooxygenase-2 and its role in ovulation: a 2004 account, *Hum Reprod Update* 19(5):373-385, 2004.
18. Jung A, Schuppe HC: Influence of genital heat stress on semen quality in humans, *Andrologia* 39(6):203-215, 2007.
19. Cooper TG: Sperm maturation in the epididymis: a new look at an old problem, *Asian J Androl* 9(4):533-539, 2007.
20. Prieto D: Physiological regulation of penile arteries and veins, *Int J Impot Res* 2(1):17-29, 2007.
21. Ohi DA et al: Anejaculation and retrograde ejaculation. *Urol Clin North Am* 35(2):211-220, viii, 2008.
22. Sofikitis N et al: Hormonal regulation of spermatogenesis and spermiogenesis, *J Steroid Biochem Mol Biol* 109(3-5):323-330, 2008.
23. Buvat J: Hyperprolactinemia and sexual function in men: a short review, *Int J Impot Res* 15(5):373-377, 2003.
24. Riordan J: *Breastfeeding and human lactation,* ed 3 , Sudbury, MA, 2005, Jones and Bartlett.
25. Shuiling KD, Likis FE: *Women's gynecologic health*, Sudbury, MA, 2006, Jones and Bartlett.
26. Hosea Blewett HJ et al: The immunological components of human milk, *Adv Food Nutr Res* 54:45-80, 2008.
27. King J: Contraception and lactation, *J Midwifery Womens Health* 52(6):614-620, 2007.
28. Narula HS, Carlson HE: Gynecomastia, *Endocrinol Metab Clin North Am* 36(2):497-519, 2007.
29. Prior JC: Perimenopause: the complex endocrinology of the menopause transition, *Endocr Rev* 19(4):397, 1998.
30. Dagwood MY: Menopause. In Copeland LJ, Farrell JE, editors: *Textbook of gynecology*, ed 2 , Philadelphia, 2000, Saunders.
31. Kevorkian R: Andropause, *Mo Med* 104(1):68-71, 2007.
32. Sampson N et al: The ageing male reproductive tract, *J Pathol* 211(2):206-218, 2007.
33. Hafez ESE, Hafez B, Hafez SD: *An atlas of reproductive physiology in men*, London, 2003, Taylor & Francis Group.
34. Shulman C, Lunenfeld B: The ageing male. *World J Urol* 20(1):4-10, 2002.
35. Haider SG: Cell biology of Leydig cells in the testis, *Int Rev Cytol* 233:181-241, 2004.
36. Raynor MC et al: Androgen deficiency in the aging male: a guide to diagnosis and testosterone replacement therapy, *Can J Urol* 14 (Suppl 1):63-68, 2007.
37. Valenti G, Ceresini G, Maggio M: Androgen deficiency in older men, *Minerva Ginecol* 59(1):43-49, 2007.
38. Hall SA et al: Correlates of low testosterone and symptomatic androgen deficiency in a population-based sample, *J Clin Endocrinol Metab* 93(10):3870-3877, 2008.

ALTERATIONS OF THE REPRODUCTIVE SYSTEMS

GWEN A. LATENDRESSE • KATHRYN L. McCANCE •
KATHERINE MORGAN

MEDIA RESOURCES

CHAPTER OUTLINE

ALTERATIONS OF SEXUAL MATURATION
Delayed Puberty
Precocious Puberty
DISORDERS OF THE FEMALE REPRODUCTIVE SYSTEM
Hormonal and Menstrual Alterations
Infection and Inflammation
Pelvic Organ Prolapse (POP)
Benign Growths and Proliferative Conditions
Cancer
Sexual Dysfunction
Impaired Fertility

DISORDERS OF THE MALE REPRODUCTIVE SYSTEM
Disorders of the Urethra
Disorders of the Penis
Disorders of the Scrotum, Testis, and Epididymis
Disorders of the Prostate Gland
Sexual Dysfunction
Impairment of Sperm Production and Quality
DISORDERS OF THE BREAST
Disorders of the Female Breast
Disorders of the Male Breast

Alterations of the reproductive system span a wide range of concerns, from delayed sexual development and suboptimal sexual performance to structural and functional abnormalities. Many common reproductive disorders carry potentially serious physiologic or psychologic consequences. Sexual or reproductive dysfunction, such as impotence or infertility, can dramatically affect self-concept, relationships, and overall quality of life. Conversely, organic and psychosocial problems, such as alcoholism, depression, situational stressors, chronic illness, and medications, can affect ovulation and menstruation, sexual performance, and fertility and may be risk factors for the development of some types of reproductive tract cancers.[1] Prostate cancer is the second leading cause of cancer death in men, breast cancer is the second leading cause of cancer death in women. Diagnosis and treatment of reproductive system disorders are complicated because of the stigma and symbolism associated with the reproductive organs and the emotion-laden beliefs and behaviors related to reproductive health. Treatment and diagnosis for related problems may be delayed because of embarrassment, guilt, fear, or denial.

ALTERATIONS OF SEXUAL MATURATION

The process of sexual maturation, or puberty, is marked by the development of secondary sexual characteristics, rapid growth, and, ultimately, the ability to reproduce. A variety of congenital and endocrine disorders can disrupt the timing of puberty, or sexual maturation. These disorders may cause puberty to occur too late (delayed puberty) or too early (precocious puberty). Both types involve a disrupted onset of sex hormone production by the gonads.

Although there are conflicting and inconsistent reports, the age of pubertal onset appears to be decreasing for girls.[2]

This earlier onset appears primarily in breast development not age of menarche. There is little change in the age of puberty for boys. On average breast development begins at age 10.4 for white girls and 9.5 years for black girls. The average age for menarche is 12.6 years for white girls and 12.2 black girls.[3-5]

Delayed Puberty

About 3% of children in North America experience delayed development of secondary sex characteristics.[6] The first sign of puberty in girls is usually thelarche, or breast development. Thelarche should begin by the time a girl is 13 years old. Normally boys tend to mature later than girls, around 14 to 14.5 years of age. In boys the first sign is enlargement of the testes and thinning of the scrotal skin. Puberty is considered delayed if there are no clinical signs of puberty by age 13 in girls or age 14 in boys (2 standard deviation [SD] above the mean age of pubertal onset). Clinical diagnosis also can be made in the absence of menarche by age 15 or 16. Boys especially tend to be embarrassed by sexual immaturity[7]; therefore, early diagnosis and treatment are recommended, as well as reassurance for boys as well as girls.

In 95% of cases, delayed puberty is a physiologic delay, that is, hormonal levels are normal and the hypothalamic-pituitary-gonadal (HPG) axis is intact, but maturation is happening slowly.[8] This constitutional delay tends to be familial and is much more common in boys than in girls. Physiologic delay is difficult to distinguish from isolated gonadotropin deficiency and is usually diagnosed retrospectively once pubertal progression is complete.

Delayed puberty also may be related to consequences of any chronic condition that delays bone aging (i.e., lung disease, renal failure, cystic fibrosis) (Box 23-1).[6] Many clinicians recommend intervention (i.e., exogenous sex steroid administration) in physiologic cases of delayed puberty to reduce the psychologic effects (e.g., self-esteem issues, embarrassment) often associated with delayed puberty.[8,9]

The other 5% of cases are caused by a disruption of the hypothalamic-pituitary-gonadal axis of various etiologies (see Box 23-1).[10] Human gonadal function is partially controlled by luteinizing hormone (LH) and follicle-stimulating hormone (FSH), the release of which is regulated by the pulsatile secretion of hypothalamic gonadotropin-releasing hormone (GnRH).[8,10] Most recently, the G-protein–coupled receptor 54 (GPR54) has been identified as the gatekeeper gene for activation of the GnRH axis based on loss of function studies in mice and humans. GPR54 is required for the normal function of this axis, and data suggest that the ligand kisspeptin-1 may act as a neurohormonal regulator of the GnRH axis.[11] The mechanisms of childhood inhibition of GnRH release and activation are poorly understood but appear to involve feedback inhibition by sex steroids and presumably other central nervous system (CNS) pathways.[12] Given the myriad etiologies contributing to the occurrence of delayed puberty, a thorough evaluation should be conducted that includes physical examination and medical and family history. Such evaluation should specifically target known contributors to delayed puberty.[6,8] Laboratory workup generally consists of x-ray studies for bone age, measurement of thyroid function, serum levels of prolactin and adrenal and gonadal steroids, radioimmunoassay of plasma gonadotropins, and screening for systemic disorders. Adolescents with high gonadotropin levels require a karyotype, to rule out genetic causes, and those with low levels need skull imaging (lateral skull film, computed tomography [CT], or magnetic resonance imaging [MRI]) to rule out pituitary or other CNS infiltrate or tumor.[6] Treatment of delayed puberty depends on the cause; the goal of treatment is the development of secondary sex characteristics and fertility, when possible. Insufficient sex hormone secretion can be corrected by hormone replacement therapy, such as estrogen for girls and testosterone for boys.[13] Idiopathic hypogonadotropic hypogonadism is treated with synthetic GnRH or sex hormone administration, or both, and may be lifelong.[6,8,13]

Box 23-1	Causes of Delayed Absent Puberty

Constitutional (Physiologic) Delay (Most Common)
Chronic or Systemic Conditions
Chronic renal disease
Cystic fibrosis
Diabetes mellitus
Excessive exercise
Hematologic diseases
Hypothyroidism
Irritable bowel diseases
Poor nutrition (eating disorders, GI diseases, poverty)
Gonadal dysgenesis
   Klinefelter syndrome (genetic karyotype 47, XXY)—males
   Turner syndrome (genetic karyotype 45, XO)—females
Bilateral gonadal failure
   Autoimmune
   Congenital anorchia
   Postsurgical, postirradiation, post-chemotherapy
   Traumatic or infectious

Hypogonadotropic Hypogonadism (Deficient FSH/LH)
Central nervous system defects (GnRH deficiency)
   Craniopharyngioma
   GPR54 mutations
   Hemochromatosis
   Hypopituitarism
   Kallmann syndrome, Bardet-Biedl syndrome, Prader-Willi syndrome
   Marijuana use
   Pituitary adenoma/tumor
   Prolactinomas

Disordered Puberty

Data from Burchett MLR, Hanna CE, Steiner RD: Endocrine and metabolic diseases. In Burns CF, Brady MA, Dunn AM, editors: *Pediatric primary care*, ed 4, St Louis 2009, Saunders; Jospe N: Disorders of pubertal development. In Osborn LM et al, editors: *Pediatrics*, Philadelphia, 2005, Mosby; Karagiannis A, Harsoulis F: *Eur J Endocrinol* 152(4):501-513, 2005.
FSH, Follicle-stimulating hormone; *GI*, gastrointestinal; *GnRH*, gonadotropin-releasing hormone; *LH*, luteinizing hormone.

Precocious Puberty

Precocious puberty is a rare event, affecting about 1 in 10,000 girls and less than 1 in 50,000 boys. Recently, precocious puberty has been redefined as sexual maturation before age 6 in black girls or age 7 in white girls, and before age 9 in boys.[3] This reflects a trend toward earlier puberty, primarily for breast development in girls (see What's New? Precocious Puberty). All cases of precocious puberty require thorough evaluation.

Precocious puberty may be partial, complete, or mixed (heterosexual) types (Box 23-2) and can be further categorized into central (GnRH-dependent) and peripheral (GnRH-independent) (Box 23-3). **Central precocious puberty** is GnRH-dependent and occurs when the hypothalamic-pituitary-gonadal axis is working normally but prematurely. Besides the premature development of secondary sex characteristics, precocity causes premature closure of the epiphysis of long bones, which results in shorter stature. Central precocious puberty results from failure of central inhibition of the GnRH pulse generator (the gonadostat). The diagnosis of central precocious puberty is one of exclusion. Because a CNS lesion may be missed, children with presumed central precocious puberty require long-term surveillance. Peripheral puberty is GnRH-independent and develops when sex hormones are produced by some mechanism other than stimulation by the gonadotropins. Sex steroid–producing tumors (i.e., gonadal tumors), testotoxicosis, and exposure to exogenous sex steroids (i.e., hormonal contraceptives and environmental endocrine disruptors) are some of the causes (see Box 23-3).

Complete precocious puberty refers to the onset and progression of all pubertal features (i.e., thelarche, pubarche, and menarche).

Partial precocious puberty is the partial development of appropriate secondary sex characteristics alone or in combination. A girl with incomplete precocious puberty might undergo thelarche or pubarche and, rarely, premature menarche. Premature thelarche is seen in girls between 6 months and 2 years of age. Premature pubarche tends to occur

---

WHAT'S NEW?　Precocious Puberty

Studies implicate obesity, leptin, ghrelin, and environmental endocrine disruptor chemicals (EDCs) as possible contributors to precocious puberty in girls. Obesity may affect the production and secretion of leptin and ghrelin, powerful communicators of satiety, hunger, metabolic rate, and in timing of puberty. EDCs may mimic, block, or alter the normal signaling systems involved in sex hormone secretion, uptake, and use. EDCs include agrochemicals, widespread industrial compounds, and persistent pollutants.

Data from Bluher S, Mantzoros CS: *Curr Opin Endocrinol Diabetes Obes* 14(6):458-464, 2007; Buck Louis GM et al: *Pediatrics* 121 (Suppl 3):S192-S207, 2008; Caserta DL et al: *Hum Reprod Update* 14(1):59-72, 2008; Euling SY et al: *Pediatrics* 121(Suppl 3):S167-S171, 2008; Kaplowitz PB: *Pediatrics* 121(Suppl 3):S208-S217, 2008; Rasier G et al: *Mol Cell Endocrinol* 254-255:187-201, 2006; Tena-Sempere M: *Vitam Horm* 77:285-300, 2008.

Box 23-2　Primary Forms of Precocious Puberty

Complete Precocious Puberty
Premature development of appropriate characteristics for the child's sex
Hypothalamic-pituitary-ovarian axis working normally but prematurely
In about 10% of cases, lethal central nervous system tumor may be the cause

Partial Precocious Puberty
Partial development of appropriate secondary sex characteristics
Premature thelarche (breast budding) seen in girls between 6 months and 2 years of age
Does not progress to complete puberty (ovulation and menstruation)
Premature adrenarche (growth of axillary and pubic hair) tends to occur between 5 and 8 years of age
Can progress to complete precocious puberty; may be caused by estrogen-secreting neoplasms or may be a variant of normal pubertal development

Mixed Precocious Puberty
Causes the child to develop some secondary sex characteristics of the opposite sex
Common causes: adrenal hyperplasia or androgen-secreting tumors

Data from Burchett MLR et al: Endocrine and metabolic diseases. In Burns CE et al, editors: *Pediatric primary care*, St Louis, 2009, Saunders; Jospe N: Disorders of pubertal development. In Osborn LM et al, editors: *Pediatrics*, Philadelphia, 2005, Mosby.

Box 23-3　Causes of Precocious Puberty

Central (Gonadotropin-Releasing Hormone [GnRH] Dependent)
Idiopathic
Central nervous system (CNS) disorders
　Congenital anomalies (hydrocephalus)
　Hypothalamic hamartoma
　Postinflammatory/infectious condition
　Trauma
　Tumors (hypothalamic, pineal, other)
Hypothyroidism (severe)

Peripheral Puberty (GnRH Independent)
Adrenal hyperplasia or tumor
Environmental endocrine disruptors
Exogenous sex steroid exposure
Exogenous anabolic steroids
Familial Leydig cell hyperplasia
Gonadal tumors or cysts
Human chorionic gonadotropin (hCG)–secreting tumors (hepatoblastomas, intracranial lesions)
McCune-Albright syndrome
Testotoxicosis

From Bhagavath B, Layman LC: *Semin Reprod Med* 25(4): 272-286, 2007; Burchett MLR et al: Endocrine and metabolic diseases. In Burns CE et al, editors: *Pediatric primary care*, St Louis, 2009, Saunders; Caserta DL et al: *Hum Reprod Update* 14(1):59-72, 2008; Cesario SK, Hughes LA: *J Obstet Gynecol Neonatal Nurs* 36(3): 263-274, 2007; Jospe N: Disorders of pubertal development. In Osborn LM et al, editors: *Pediatrics*, Philadelphia, 2005, Mosby.

between ages 5 and 8 years. Premature pubarche is usually the consequence of an early increase in the adrenal androgens that leads to early growth of pubic hair and possibly a transient acceleration in growth and bone maturation that has no significant effect on timing of puberty or final height. Sparse hair growth on the genitalia, in the absence of thelarche or menarche, does not represent precocious puberty.

The diagnosis and cause of premature development are often obvious. A thorough history and physical examination are done to determine the velocity of the process and to rule out life-threatening CNS, ovarian, or adrenal neoplasms. Family occurrence helps exclude tumors. Children with precocious puberty also have a tendency toward obesity.[14-16]

Treatment for all forms of precocious puberty includes identifying and removing the underlying cause or administering appropriate hormones (see Boxes 23-2 and 23-3). In many cases, precocious puberty can be reversed. Management goals include diagnosing and treating intracranial disease; arresting maturation until early teen years; maximizing eventual adult height; reducing emotional problems; and providing contraception, if necessary. The most common form, central precocious puberty, is usually treated with potent GnRH agonist analogs, which induce reversible, selective suppression of the hypothalamic-pituitary-gonadal axis. Treatment does not seem to affect body composition or increase obesity in children with central precocious puberty. Because many of these children are obese and childhood obesity is predictive of morbidity in adolescence and adulthood, it is important for clinicians to include assessment and management of obesity as part of the treatment for central precocious puberty.

Mixed precocious puberty (virilization of a girl or feminization of a boy) causes the child to develop some secondary sex characteristics of the opposite sex. This condition is usually evident at birth and is rare in older children (Box 23-4).

Box 23-4	**Causes of Mixed Precocious Puberty**

Female (Virilization)
Congenital adrenal hyperplasia
Androgen-secreting tumors
   Adrenal
   Ovarian
   Teratoma
   Exogenous androgens

Male (Feminization)
Estrogen-producing tumors
   Adrenal
   Teratoma
   Hepatoma
   Testicular
Exogenous estrogens
Increased peripheral conversion of androgens to estrogens

From Jospe N: Disorders of pubertal development. In Osborn LM et al, editors: *Pediatrics,* Philadelphia, 2005, Mosby.

DISORDERS OF THE FEMALE REPRODUCTIVE SYSTEM

Hormonal and Menstrual Alterations

Primary Dysmenorrhea

Primary dysmenorrhea is painful menstruation associated with the release of prostaglandins in ovulatory cycles, but not with pelvic disease. The severity of dysmenorrhea is directly related to the duration and amount of menstrual flow. Between 50% and 90% of women ages 15 to 25 years are affected, some (10% to 15%) severely enough to miss work or school. Primary dysmenorrhea usually begins with the onset of ovulatory cycles, around age 15 or 16 years. The incidence peaks in women during the late teens and early 20s, and decreases slowly thereafter.[17] **Secondary dysmenorrhea** is related to pelvic pathology, manifests in later reproductive years, and may occur any time in the menstrual cycle.[18]

PATHOPHYSIOLOGY Dysmenorrhea is primarily the result of the effects of excessive endometrial prostaglandin production, enhanced by progesterone. Women with painful periods produce 10 times as much prostaglandin F ($PGF_2\alpha$), a potent myometrial stimulant and vasoconstrictor, as asymptomatic women. Elevated levels of prostaglandins (especially $PGF_2\alpha$ and $PGE_2\alpha$) are found in endometrial fluid of dysmenorrheic women and correlate positively with pain. Compared with proliferative endometrium, secretory endometrium produces three times the amount of prostaglandins, and the discharged endometrium produces even more.[19] In addition, leukotrienes heighten sensitivity of pain fibers in the uterus and vasopressin contributes to myometrial hypersensitivity, constriction of endometrial blood vessels, and resultant ischemia, endometrial bleeding, and pain caused by prostaglandins. Prostaglandins are primarily released during the first 48 hours of menstruation, when symptoms are the most intense. Women who are anovulatory because they use oral contraceptives do not have primary dysmenorrhea. Secondary dysmenorrhea results from disorders such as endometriosis, pelvic adhesions, inflammation, cervical stenosis, uterine fibroids, polyps, tumors, cysts, intrauterine devices (IUDs), or imperforate hymen. Dysmenorrhea may be more severe in women who are obese, who smoke, are nulliparous, have delayed childbearing, and are sexually inactive.[20]

CLINICAL MANIFESTATIONS The chief symptom of dysmenorrhea is pelvic pain associated with the onset of menses. The pain often radiates into the groin and may be accompanied by backache, anorexia, vomiting, diarrhea, syncope, and headache. The latter symptoms are caused by entry of prostaglandins and prostaglandin metabolites into the systemic circulation. Usually, the discomfort associated with primary dysmenorrhea begins shortly before the onset of menstruation and rarely persists beyond the second day.

EVALUATION AND TREATMENT Primary dysmenorrhea can be differentiated from secondary dysmenorrhea by a thorough history and pelvic examination. In women who desire contraception, dysmenorrhea may be relieved with hormonal contraceptives. Hormonal contraception stops ovulation and creates an atrophic endometrium, thereby decreasing prostaglandin synthesis and myometrial contractility. Nonsteroidal anti-inflammatory medication (e.g., ibuprofen) is the treatment of choice. Prostaglandin inhibitors work in the majority of women with primary dysmenorrhea and are most effective if started at the first sign of bleeding or cramping.[21] Regular exercise and stress reduction are thought to prevent or reduce symptoms.[22] Other comfort measures include local application of heat, massage, relaxation techniques, vitamin B, and magnesium supplementation, and high-frequency transcutaneous electrical nerve stimulation (TENS).[23,24] Orgasm may relieve or worsen symptoms.

Amenorrhea

Amenorrhea means lack of menstruation, the most common cause of which is pregnancy. **Primary amenorrhea** is the failure of menarche and the absence of menstruation by age 14 years without the development of secondary sex characteristics or by age 16 years regardless of the presence of secondary sex characteristics (see p. 817 for discussion of delayed puberty). Primary amenorrhea differs from delayed puberty in that most cases of delayed puberty require only reassurance, but when the diagnosis of primary amenorrhea is reached, a thorough evaluation must be undertaken. **Secondary amenorrhea** is the absence of menstruation for a time equivalent to three or more cycles or 6 months in women who have previously menstruated.

PATHOPHYSIOLOGY   There are numerous classifications of the etiologies of primary amenorrhea. One approach to understanding the pathophysiology is through compartmentalization. *Compartment IV disorders* include CNS disorders, in particular hypothalamic disorders. In some of the congenital syndromes that cause primary amenorrhea, the hypothalamic-pituitary-ovarian (HPO) axis is dysfunctional. The hypothalamus is unable to synthesize GnRH, so the pituitary fails to secrete LH and FSH. Therefore, the ovary does not receive the hormonal signals that normally initiate the ovarian and endometrial changes of the menstrual cycle, and ovulation and menstruation do not occur. Because the ovarian hormones are absent, estrogen-dependent sex characteristics do not develop.

Compartment III disorders are disorders of the anterior pituitary, including tumors. Some anatomic defects of the CNS, whether congenital or acquired, impinge on the hypothalamic-pituitary unit so as to interfere with or interrupt the secretion of GnRH or FSH and LH. Examples of such defects include hydrocephalus, craniopharyngiomas, and other space-occupying lesions of the CNS (see Box 23-1). Again the target organ, the ovary, does not receive the necessary signals, and ovulation and menstruation do not occur. In some cases these lesions develop between the onset and conclusion of puberty. Therefore, skeletal growth may occur and secondary sex characteristics may develop, but sexual maturation is interrupted before menarche, which normally concludes puberty.

Compartment II disorders involve the ovary. Several genetic disorders are associated with primary amenorrhea. These include gonadal dysgenesis (Turner syndrome), androgen insensitivity syndrome (AIS), formerly known as *testicular feminizing syndrome* or *male pseudohermaphroditism*. Among all the chromosomal abnormalities of Turner syndrome (45,X/46,XX; structural X or Y abnormalities; mosaicism),[25] the ovaries lack gametes and ovarian failure is complete. Without primitive gametes and follicles, follicular development and estrogen secretion cannot occur. Lack of estrogen accounts for failure of secondary sex characteristic development and amenorrhea, although there are high levels of circulating FSH and LH. In AIS, the individual is male genetically but female morphologically. The individual does not develop male genitalia because androgen receptors are absent in undifferentiated target organs. The gonads are found either in the abdomen or in the inguinal canal, and they produce both androgens and estrogens. Because target tissues lack androgen receptors but have estrogen receptors, most individuals with AIS have female external genitalia and female secondary sex characteristics. With the exception of a small vagina, internal female genitalia are absent, accounting for amenorrhea and infertility.

Compartment I disorders are anatomic defects of the outflow tract associated with primary amenorrhea. They include congenital absence of the vagina and uterus and congenital uterine hypoplasia (infantile uterus). Females without a uterus or vagina usually have normal ovarian function. Therefore, skeletal growth occurs and secondary sex characteristics develop in the proper sequence, but menstruation does not occur. In cases of uterine hypoplasia the uterus does not respond to hormonal stimulation during puberty.

CLINICAL MANIFESTATIONS   The major clinical manifestation of primary amenorrhea is the absence of the menses. The cause of the amenorrhea determines whether secondary sex characteristics and height are affected.

EVALUATION AND TREATMENT   Diagnosis of primary amenorrhea is based on history and physical examination. If ovarian steroid hormone levels are low, the individual has the appearance of an immature female. Physical examination may show structural or physiologic alterations. Laboratory studies may be required to document karyotype, abnormal levels of gonadotropins, and ovarian hormones. Diagnostic imaging is used to document structural abnormalities (Figure 23-1).

Treatment involves correction of any underlying disorders and hormone replacement therapy to induce the development of secondary sex characteristics as necessary (see p. 817 for a discussion of delayed puberty). Although surgical alteration of the genitalia may be undertaken to correct structural abnormalities, surgery should be delayed until the affected individual can make a truly informed decision. Hormonal manipulation or embryo transplantation may make pregnancy possible for women with primary amenorrhea who have a uterus.

Secondary Amenorrhea

A wide variety of disorders and physiologic conditions are associated with secondary amenorrhea. Besides disease, secondary amenorrhea can be triggered by dramatic

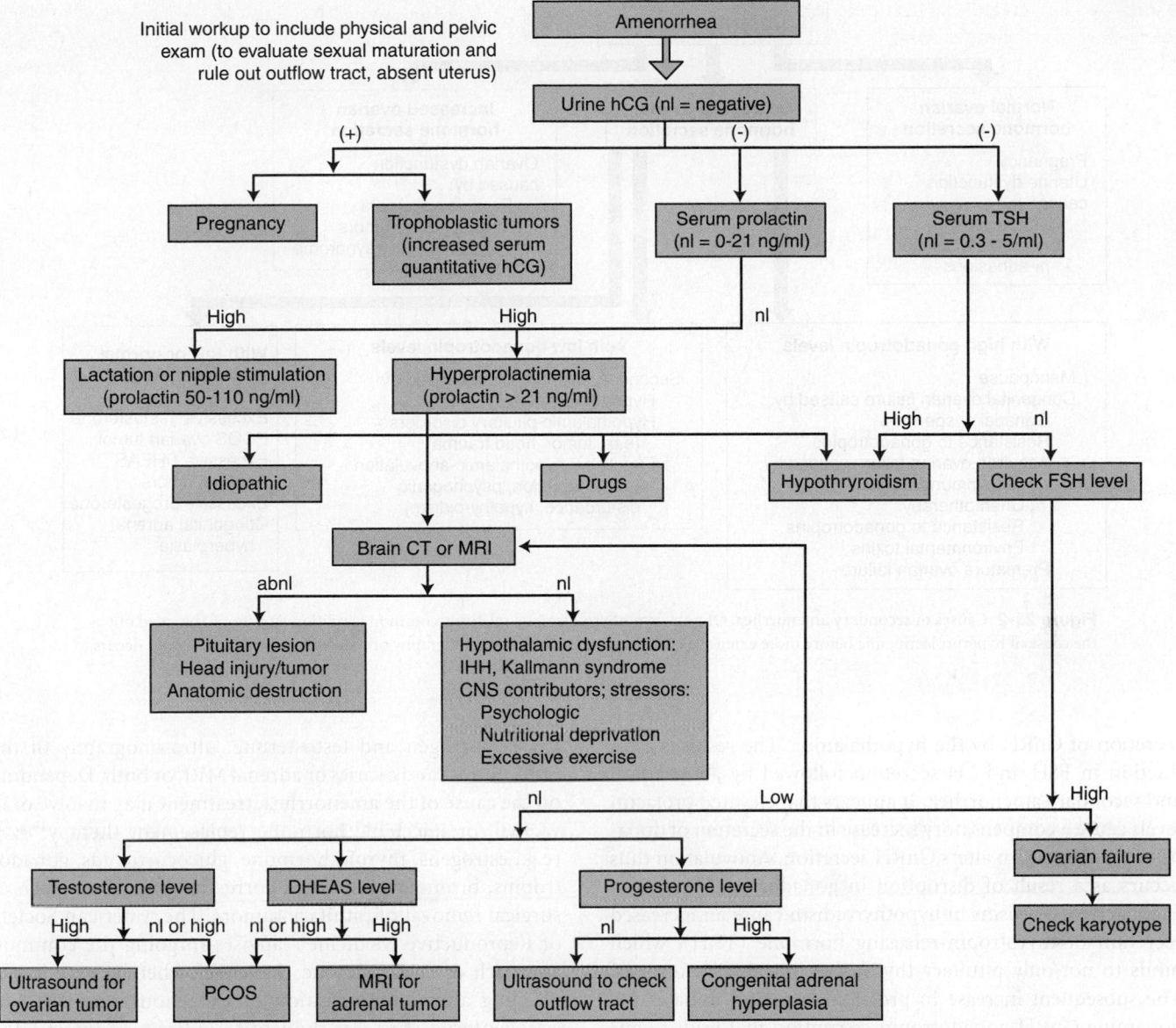

Initial workup to include physical and pelvic exam (to evaluate sexual maturation and rule out outflow tract, absent uterus)

Figure 23-1 Diagnosis of amenorrhea. Pregnancy is the most common cause of amenorrhea. *abnl,* Abnormal; *CNS,* central nervous system; *CT,* computed tomography; *DHEAS,* dehydroepiandrosterone sulfate; *FSH,* follicle-stimulating hormone; *hCG,* human chorionic gonadotropin; *IHH,* idiopathic hypogonadotropic hypogonadism; *MRI,* magnetic resonance imaging; *nl,* normal; *PCOS,* polycystic ovary syndrome; *TSH,* thyroid stimulating hormone. (Adapted from Schorge JO et al, editors: *Williams gynecology,* New York, 2008, McGraw-Hill.)

weight loss, whether the loss results from malnutrition or excessive exercise. Secondary amenorrhea is common during early adolescence and the perimenopausal period, pregnancy, and lactation. The most common causes (after pregnancy) are thyroid disorders (e.g., hypothyroidism), hyperprolactinemia, HPO interruption secondary to excessive exercise, stress, weight loss, and polycystic ovary syndrome (PCOS).

PATHOPHYSIOLOGY The causes of secondary amenorrhea are summarized in Figure 23-2. In women with normal ovarian steroid hormone levels, secondary amenorrhea may be caused by structural abnormalities (müllerian anomalies), Asherman syndrome (removal of the endometrial decidua basalis), or removal of the uterus. In women with

elevated ovarian steroid hormone levels, inhibited ovulation leads to amenorrhea. An excess of ovarian hormones disrupts feedback relationships within the HPO axis, preventing ovulation. Depressed ovarian hormone levels, which are associated with a variety of clinical disorders, also cause amenorrhea by preventing ovulation. Lack of ovulation, termed **anovulation,** may result from increased levels of prolactin, decreased levels of gonadotropins, irregular secretion of gonadotropins, or abnormally low levels of CNS neurotransmitters (i.e., dopamine and GnRH). Any of these variables alters the feedback effects that the ovarian hormones have on the hypothalamus and pituitary.

Hyperprolactinemia (overproduction of prolactin by the pituitary) may have indirect effects that lead to decreased

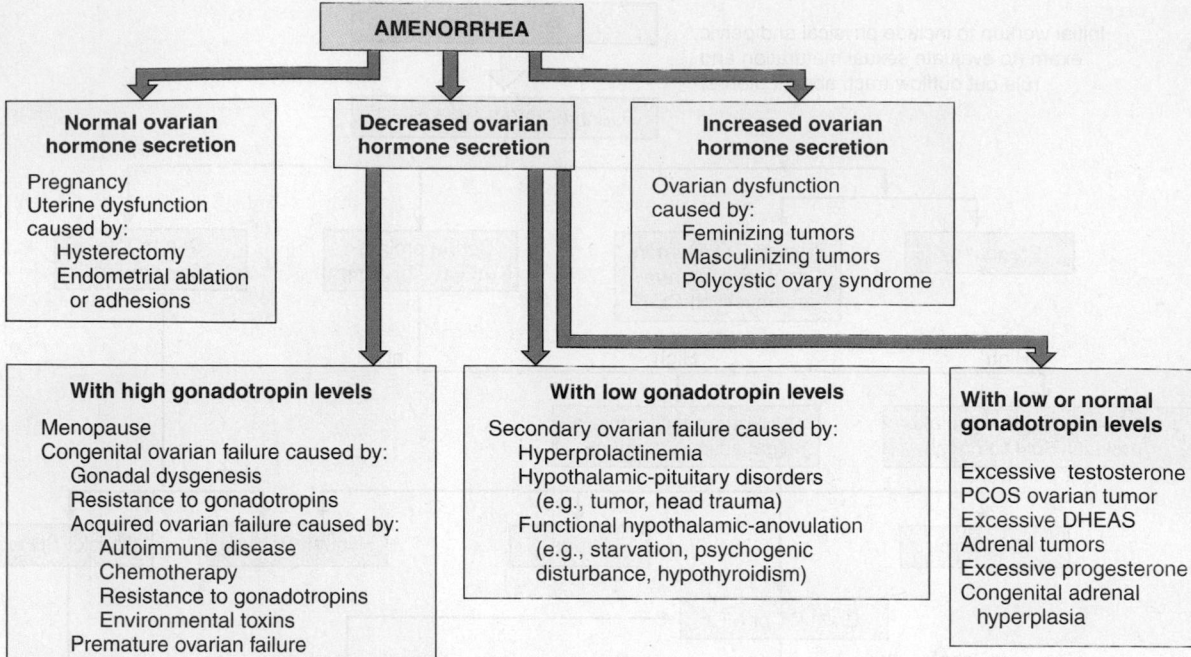

Figure 23-2 Causes of secondary amenorrhea. Of note, hypothyroidism is a relatively common condition and should be ruled out as the cause of hyperprolactinemia before more extensive evaluation (i.e., computed tomography or magnetic resonance imaging) occurs.

secretion of GnRH by the hypothalamus. The result is a reduction in FSH and LH secretion followed by anovulation and secondary amenorrhea. It appears that elevated prolactin levels cause a compensatory increase in the secretion of dopamine, which in turn alters GnRH secretion. Anovulation thus occurs as a result of disruption in gonadotropin secretion. Feedback mechanisms in hypothyroidism cause an increased secretion of thyrotropin-releasing hormone (TRH), which binds to not only pituitary thyrotopes but also lactotropes. The subsequent increase in prolactin secretion initiates the dopamine-GnRH-gonadotropin disruption that leads to anovulation and amenorrhea.[26]

CLINICAL MANIFESTATIONS The major manifestation of secondary amenorrhea is the absence of menses. Infertility, vasomotor flushes, vaginal atrophy, acne, osteopenia, and **hirsutism** (abnormal hairiness) also may be present, depending on the underlying cause of the amenorrhea.

EVALUATION AND TREATMENT Pregnancy is the most common cause of amenorrhea and must be ruled out prior to other evaluations. Diagnosis of secondary amenorrhea involves the identification of underlying hormonal or anatomic alterations. A woman with secondary amenorrhea and normal secondary sex characteristics should have a complete history and physical examination. After ruling out pregnancy, initial evaluation includes measurement of thyroid-stimulating hormone (TSH) and prolactin levels (see Figure 23-1). Elevated prolactin levels warrant brain CT or MRI if TSH levels are normal. Hypothyroidism is treated with thyroid replacement. If the initial tests are normal, further testing would include measurement of gonadotropins

(FSH), estrogen and testosterone, ultrasonography of the outflow tract and ovaries or adrenal MRI, or both. Depending on the cause of the amenorrhea, treatment may involve oral, vaginal, or injectable hormone replacement therapy[19,27-29] (e.g., estrogens, thyroid hormone, glucocorticoids, gonadotropins, bromocriptine) or a corrective procedure, such as surgical removal of pituitary tumors. The American Society of Reproductive Medicine[30] advises forgoing the common approach of "progesterone challenge" whereby withdrawal bleeding after administration of exogenous progestins or estrogen/progestins was thought to indicate an intact HPO axis, intact endometrium, and patent outflow tract. A diagnosis of PCOS might be treated with an insulin-sensitizing agent, such as metformin, as well as ovulation-inducing drugs if fertility is desired (a discussion of PCOS is contained on p. 824).

Abnormal Uterine Bleeding

Menstrual irregularity or abnormal bleeding patterns (Table 23-1) account for approximately 33% of all gynecologic visits. Anovulatory cycles (failure to ovulate) because of various etiologies (age, stress, endocrinopathy) are the most common cause of cycle irregularity. Other causes include uterine tumors, polyps, ovarian cysts, pregnancy and its complications, and bleeding disorders (e.g., von Willebrand disease). Common causes of abnormal uterine bleeding based on age group and frequency are listed in Table 23-2. Pathophysiology and treatment options vary and are based on etiology.[31]

Dysfunctional uterine bleeding (DUB) is heavy or irregular bleeding in the absence of organic disease, such as

Table 23-1	Abnormal Menstrual Bleeding
Term	**Definition**
Polymenorrhea	Cycles shorter than 3 wk; may indicate disturbance in endocrine control of ovulation
Oligomenorrhea	Cycles longer than 6-7 wk; may indicate disturbance in endocrine control of ovulation
Metrorrhagia	Intermenstrual bleeding or bleeding of light character occurring irregularly between cycles; may be a sign of organic disease
Hypermenorrhea	Excessive flow; may be a sign of organic disease
Menorrhea	Prolonged duration of flow
Menorrhagia	Increased amount and duration of flow
Menometrorrhagia	Prolonged flow associated with irregular and intermittent spotting between bleeding episodes

Table 23-2	Common Causes of Abnormal (Vaginal/Genital) Bleeding in Descending Order of Frequency
Age Group	**Cause**
Prepubescence	Sexual assault
	Trauma
	Foreign bodies
	Precocious puberty
Adolescence	Anovulation (immature hypothalamic pituitary-ovarian axis)
	Trauma and sexual abuse
Reproductive years	Pregnancy
	Pelvic inflammatory disease
	Coagulation disorder
	Hormonal contraceptives
	Endometriosis
	Anovulation
	IUDs
	Ovarian cysts
	Uterine polyps/tumors
	PCOS
	Bleeding disorders (e.g., von Willebrand)
	Trauma/rape
Perimenopause	Anovulation
	Malignancy
	Pregnancy
	Endometriosis
	Benign neoplasms (myomas, adenomyosis)
Postmenopause	Malignancy
Other: Non–age specific	Chronic conditions
	Adrenal conditions
	Thyroid disorders
	Liver disease
	Diabetes mellitus
	Obesity
	Hypertension

IUD, Intrauterine device; *PCOS,* polycystic ovary syndrome.

submucous fibroids, endometrial polyps, blood dyscrasias, pregnancy, infection, or systemic disease. The diagnosis of DUB is made once these other causes have been excluded. DUB affects 15% to 20% of all women at some time during their menstrual life and accounts for 70% of all hysterectomies and almost all endometrial ablation procedures.[32] Perimenopausal women are by far the most affected by DUB.

PATHOPHYSIOLOGY More than 80% of DUB is associated with anovulatory cycles, and the remaining 20% is due to corpus luteum defects or atrophic endometrium.[33] Although DUB may occur at any time during the reproductive years, 20% of cases occur in adolescents, and more than 50% of cases occur in perimenopausal women ages 40 to 50 years. Symptoms of hypomenorrhea, followed by missed periods or prolonged intervals between menses, could mark the onset of physiologic perimenopause or may be an early sign of pathologically premature ovulatory failure and secondary amenorrhea. Other conditions associated with chronic anovulation include PCOS, immaturity of the HPO axis, obesity, hyperthyroidism and hypothyroidism, and estrogen-secreting ovarian neoplasms.

DUB secondary to ovarian dysfunction is a result of either progesterone deficiency or relative estrogen excess. In perimenopausal women in their 40s and 50s, inhibin B and progesterone secretion is absent or low, yet estrogen (estradiol [E_2]) continues to be secreted by the granulosa–theca cell complex, and levels are often erratic and high.[34-36] (See Chapter 22 for a description of the many hormonal changes associated with the time before and just after menopause.) In the absence of growth-limiting progesterone and periodic desquamation, the endometrium attains an abnormal height with increasing hypervascularity and back-to-back glandularity, but without an intervening stromal support matrix. Menstrual flow may become irregular (metrorrhagia) and excessive (menorrhagia) or both (menometrorrhagia), resulting from the large quantity of tissue available for bleeding and the random breakdown of tissue that results in exposure of vascular channels. In the absence of adequate progesterone levels, usual endometrial control mechanisms are missing, such as vasoconstrictive rhythmicity, tight coiling of spiral vessels, and orderly collapse, and stasis does not occur. Unopposed estrogen induces a progression of endometrial responses beginning with proliferation, hyperplasia, and adenomatous hyperplasia; over a course of many years, unopposed estrogen may end with atypia and carcinoma. *endometrial hyperplasia*

DUB in ovulatory cycles is not common, and mechanisms underlying the bleeding are associated with organic lesions or corpus luteum defects.[33] Excessive fibrinolytic activity and changes in prostaglandin production may be implicated.

CLINICAL MANIFESTATIONS Anovulatory DUB is characterized by unpredictable and variable bleeding in terms of amount and duration. Especially during perimenopause, dysfunctional bleeding also may involve flooding and the passage of large clots, which often indicate excessive blood loss. Excessive bleeding can lead to iron deficiency anemia and associated symptoms (fatigue, shortness of breath). Iron supplementation may be required.

EVALUATION AND TREATMENT Treatment goals include preventing or controlling abnormal bleeding, identifying underlying disease, and inducing regular menstrual cycles. Although no gold standard approach has been identified, usual therapy is hormonal and may consist of progestin-estrogen combination therapy (i.e., low-dose oral contraceptives), estrogen-only therapy (for acute episodes only), or progesterone-only therapy.[31,37] For the woman with idiopathic menorrhagia not associated with anovulatory cycles, prostaglandin synthetase inhibitors may be effective in decreasing blood loss. Desmopressin, a synthetic analog of arginine vasopressin, is used to treat abnormal uterine bleeding in women with coagulation disorders (von Willebrand disease, which affects about 1% of the population).[33] Recalcitrant bleeding may be controlled by suppression of the endometrium followed by surgical ablation. Total or partial ablation of the endometrium has replaced dilation and curettage (D&C) or hysterectomy as the surgical technique of choice for treatment of menorrhagia. Various techniques have been developed, including cryoablation, thermal balloon, circulated hot fluid, and electro- or microwave energy ablation.[38] The best results are obtained if the endometrium is suppressed for 4 to 6 weeks with either high-dose progestin, GnRH agonist, or danazol. Endometrial ablation is successful in approximately 90% of women; only 50% become amenorrheic. The major indication for a D&C is diagnostic or as a curative procedure in the removal of products of conception, polyps, or focal endometrial hyperplasia.

More recently, the levonorgestrel-intrauterine system (LNG-IUS), a contraceptive hormonal IUD, is being used with success as effective as hysterectomy or ablation, or both, and is much less expensive. The LNG-IUS decreases blood loss by 86% to 97% by decreasing endometrial proliferation.

Polycystic Ovary Syndrome

Polycystic ovary syndrome (PCOS) has at least two of the following conditions: oligo-ovulation or anovulation, elevated levels of androgens, or clinical signs of hyperandrogenism and polycystic ovaries. Polycystic ovaries do not have to be present to diagnose PCOS, and conversely their presence alone does not establish the diagnosis. PCOS remains one of the most common endocrine disturbances affecting women, especially young women, and is a leading cause of infertility in the United States, where prevalence rates are estimated at between 4% and 12%, afflicting between 3.2 and 5.4 million young women.[39] PCOS appears to be familial, and various features of the syndrome may be differentially inherited.[40,41] Confusing the issue is the frequency, expression, and timing of PCOS (polycystic ovaries can be detected in prepubescent children). From 22% to 30% of women have polycystic ovaries on ultrasound, with 80% having one or more symptoms of the syndrome; 80% of women with normal ovaries also experience one or more PCOS symptoms. Signs and symptoms of women with PCOS may change over time, with metabolic syndrome becoming more prominent with age. In addition,

polycystic ovaries may be associated with Cushing syndrome, acromegaly, premature ovarian failure, simple obesity, congenital adrenal hyperplasia, thyroid disease, androgen-producing adrenal tumors or ovarian tumors (Figure 23-3), and syndromes with hyperprolactinemia. Thus several factors contribute to difficulties in the diagnosis.

PATHOPHYSIOLOGY Although the underlying cause of PCOS is unknown, a genetic basis is suspected. Initial identification of genes involved in steroid biosynthesis, androgen biosynthesis, and insulin receptors within the ovary indicate genetic involvement. No single factor fully accounts for the abnormalities of PCOS.[41-44] A hyperandrogenic state is a cardinal feature in the pathogenesis of PCOS. However, glucose intolerance/insulin resistance (IR) and hyperinsulinemia often run parallel and markedly aggravate the hyperandrogenic state, thus contributing to the severity of signs and symptoms of PCOS.[41,45] Obesity adds to and worsens IR. Although 50% of normal weight women with PCOS have IR, all obese women

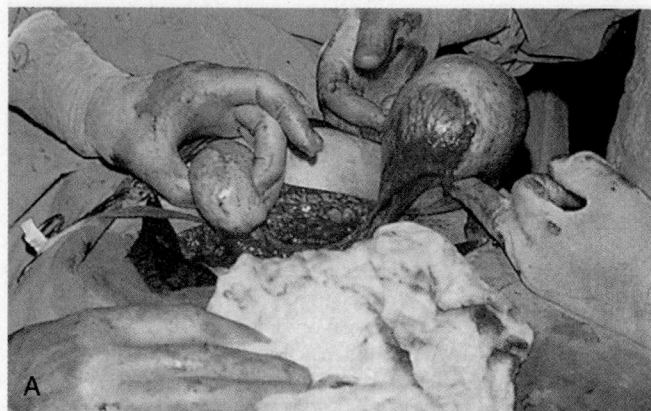

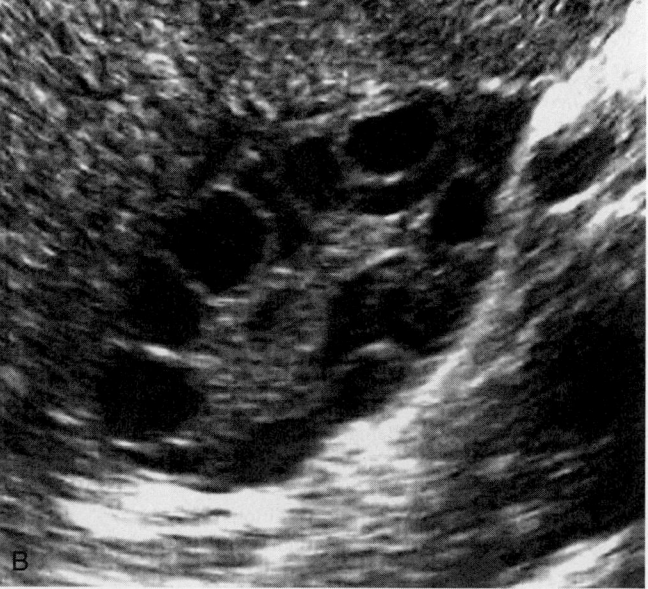

Figure 23-3 Polycystic ovary. **A,** Surgical view of polycystic ovaries. **B,** Ultrasound of polycystic ovary. (**A** from Symonds EM, Macpherson MBA: *Diagnosis in color: obstetrics and gynecology,* London, 1997, Mosby-Wolfe; **B** from King J: Polycystic ovary syndrome: *J Midwifery Womens Health* 51[6]:415-422, 2006. Reprinted with permission.)

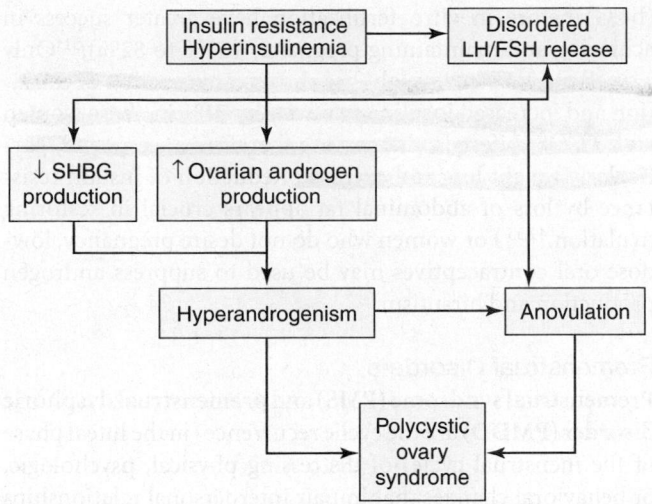

Figure 23-4 Insulin resistance and hyperinsulinemia in polycystic ovary syndrome (PCOS). See text. *FSH,* Follicle-stimulating hormone; *LH,* luteinizing hormone; *SHBG,* sex hormone–binding globulin.

with PCOS do. Insulin stimulates androgen secretion by the ovarian stroma and reduces serum sex hormone–binding globulin (SHBG) directly and independently. The net effect is an increase in free testosterone levels. Excessive androgens affect follicular growth, and insulin affects follicular decline by suppressing apoptosis and enabling follicles, which would normally disintegrate, to survive[46] (Figure 23-4). Further, there appears to be a genetic ovarian defect in PCOS, which makes the ovary either more susceptible to or sensitive to insulin's stimulation of androgen production. Recent research suggests that decreased intraovarian receptors for estrogen receptor-α or insulin-like growth factor 1 (IGF-1), increased leptin levels, or direct insulin resistance within selective ovarian cells (fibroblasts) may contribute to this phenomenon.[46] Intrauterine and early childhood environments may also contribute to the development of PCOS (see What's New? Early Programming for PCOS?).

Weight gain tends to aggravate symptoms, whereas weight loss may ameliorate some of the endocrine and metabolic events and thus decrease symptoms. Women with PCOS tend to have increased leptin levels (leptin levels are increased in thin as well as overweight women with PCOS).[47] Leptin influences the hypothalamic pulsatility of GnRH and consequent interaction along the entire HPO axis. Feedback from the polycystic ovary is disturbed because of changes in ovarian steroid and nonsteroidal (inhibins and related proteins) hormones.

In PCOS there is dysfunction in follicle development.[46] Inappropriate gonadotropin secretion triggers the beginning of a vicious cycle that perpetuates anovulation. Typically, levels of FSH are low or below normal and LH levels and LH bioactivity are elevated. An increased frequency of GnRH pulses appears to cause increased frequency of LH pulses.[33,48] Persistent LH elevation causes an increase in androgens (dehydroepiandrosterone sulfate [DHEAS] from the adrenal glands and testosterone, androstenedione, and DHEA from the ovary). Androgens are converted to estrogen in peripheral tissues,

and increased testosterone levels cause a significant reduction (approximately 50%) in SHBG, which in turn causes increased levels of free estradiol. Elevated estrogen levels trigger a positive-feedback response in LH and a negative-feedback response in FSH. Because FSH levels are not totally depressed, new follicular growth is continuously stimulated, but not to full maturation and ovulation. The accumulation of follicular tissue in various stages of development allows an increased and relatively constant production of steroids in response to gonadotropin stimulation. Thus PCOS is characterized by excessive production of both androgen and estrogen.

Increased androgen secretion by the ovaries contributes to premature follicular failure (atresia) and persistent anovulation. In turn, persistent anovulation causes enlarged polycystic ovaries characterized by a smooth, pearly white capsule. This characteristic appearance is caused by an increase of surface area and increased volume of up to 2.8 times, doubling of growing and atretic follicles, thickening of the tunica (outermost area) by 50%, increasing cortical stromal thickening by one third and a fivefold increase in subcortical stroma, and escalating hyperplasia. With advancing age, menstrual irregularities may improve while metabolic syndrome and type 2 diabetes mellitus increases.

CLINICAL MANIFESTATIONS Clinical manifestations of PCOS usually appear within 2 years of puberty but may appear after a variable period of normal menstrual function and, possibly, pregnancy. The symptoms are related to anovulation and hyperandrogenism and include dysfunctional bleeding or amenorrhea, hirsutism, acne, and infertility. Approximately 41% of women with PCOS are obese.[42] Box 23-5 contains a list of signs and symptoms, summary of hormonal disturbances, and complications of PCOS.

EVALUATION AND TREATMENT Diagnosis of PCOS is based on evidence of androgen excess, chronic anovulation, and inappropriate gonadotropin secretion. Tests for impaired glucose tolerance are recommended. As stated, polycystic ovaries do not have to be present and, conversely, their presence alone does not establish the diagnosis. Goals of treatment include reversing signs and symptoms of androgen excess, instituting cyclic menstruation, restoring fertility, and ameliorating any associated metabolic or endocrine, or both,

Box 23-5	Clinical Manifestations of Polycystic Ovary Syndrome

Presenting Signs and Symptoms (% of Women Affected)
Obesity (41%)
Menstrual disturbance (70% [i.e., dysfunctional uterine bleeding])
Oligomenorrhea (47%)
Amenorrhea (19%)
Regular menstruation (48%)
Hyperandrogenism (69% to 74%)
Infertility (73% of anovulatory infertility)
Asymptomatic (20% of those with polycystic ovary syndrome)

Hormonal Disturbances
Increased insulin (independent of obesity)
Decreased SHBG
Increased androgens (testosterone, androstenedione)
Increased DHEA (occurs in 50% of women)
Increased LH (genetic variant LH-β subunit)
Increased prolactin
Increased leptin, especially in obesity (independent of insulin)
Suggested decreased insulin-like growth factor (IGF-1) receptors on theca cells
Possible decreased estrogen receptors (intraovarian and along hypothalamic-pituitary axis)

Possible Late Sequelae
Dyslipidemia: increased low-density lipoproteins, decreased high-density lipoproteins, increased triglycerides
Diabetes mellitus (30% of women with or without obesity will develop type 2 diabetes mellitus by age 30)
Cardiovascular disease; hypertension
Endometrial hyperplasia and carcinoma (anovulatory women are hyperestrogenic)

Other
Women with PCOS are at increased risk of gestational diabetes mellitus, pregnancy-induced hypertension, preterm birth, and perinatal mortality

Adapted from Azziz R et al: *Fertil Steril*, October 22, 2008 [Epub ahead of print]; Boomsma CM et al: *Semin Reprod Med* 26(1):72-84, 2008; Diamanti-Kandarakis E: *Expert Rev Mol Med* 10(2):e3, 2008; Simoni M et al: *Hum Reprod Update* 14(5):459-484, 2008.
DHEA, Dehydroepiandrosterone; *LH,* luteinizing hormone; *PCOS,* polycystic ovary syndrome; *SHBG,* sex hormone–binding globulin.

disturbances.[49,50] Traditionally, treatment of PCOS focused on correcting anovulation and the effects of hyperandrogenism with combined oral contraceptives (COCs), antiandrogens, and fertility agents. With a greater understanding of the role that insulin resistance and hyperinsulinemia play in this disease, insulin sensitizers, such as metformin,[50,51] may be used to decrease insulin, prevent diabetes and heart disease (by reducing microvascular events), and restore fertility. Progesterone therapy is recommended to oppose estrogen's effects on the endometrium and as a means to initiate monthly withdrawal bleeding (at the expense of continued hirsutism). For infertile women, clomiphene citrate, an antiestrogen, can be used to facilitate ovulation, although better effects are achieved (75% ovulation rates and 30% to 40% pregnancy rates) if therapy is combined with an insulin sensitizer.[52-54] Women who are primed with human chorionic gonadotropin

(hCG) before in vitro fertilization have greater success in achieving and maintaining pregnancy (58% to 82%).[51] Only a small reduction of weight has shown a restoration of ovulation and increased insulin sensitivity by 71% in obese women with PCOS. Lifestyle changes are therefore encouraged, particularly weight loss and exercise. Reduction of insulin resistance by loss of abdominal fat appears crucial in restoring ovulation.[49,55] For women who do not desire pregnancy, low-dose oral contraceptives may be used to suppress androgen production and hirsutism.

Premenstrual Disorders

Premenstrual syndrome (PMS) and **premenstrual dysphoric disorder (PMDD)** are the cyclic recurrence (in the luteal phase of the menstrual cycle) of distressing physical, psychologic, or behavioral changes that impair interpersonal relationships or interfere with usual activities.[33] PMDD is listed as a mood disorder in the American Psychiatric Association's *Diagnostic and Statistical Manual of Mental Disorders (DSM-IV)* (Box 23-6). The prevalence of PMS and PMDD is difficult to determine. It has been estimated that 5% to 10% of menstruating women have severe to disabling premenstrual symptoms, 3% to 8% have cyclic dysphoria warranting treatment, and 20% or more have mild to moderately distressing symptoms.[56] To confuse matters, it seems that (1) symptoms are experienced to some degree by most adolescent and adult women and can occur throughout all menstrual phases, (2) the presence and severity of symptoms in any one woman may be inconsistent from month to month, (3) menstrual phase for peak symptom severity may differ depending on the population studied, and (4) inconsistent and overlapping use of terminology and criteria are used to describe these syndromes. PMDD is the term often used to refer to the premenstrual disorder with a predominant psychosocial or functional impairment similar to dysthymia and minor depression.[33,57]

It is thought that PMS/PMDD is the result of abnormal tissue response to the normal changes of the menstrual cycle. This biologic response may be triggered by fluctuating estrogen and progesterone levels. Given that premenstrual disorders occur almost exclusively in ovulatory cycles, it has been theorized that symptoms are triggered by the preovulatory estrogen peak or postovulatory increase in progesterone, or both.[58] However, the mechanisms involved are not known. Furthermore, the neurotransmitters serotonin, gamma-aminobutyric acid (GABA), and noradrenaline may have mediating or moderating roles on symptom manifestation. These neurotransmitters have demonstrated interactions with estrogen and progesterone and *all* of these are neuroactive with known mood and behavior effects, including negative mood, irritability, aggression, and impulse control.[33] Sex steroids also interact with the renin-angiotensin-aldosterone system (RAAS), which could explain some PMS/PMDD signs and symptoms (e.g., water retention, bloating, weight gain). A predisposition to PMS runs in families, perhaps because of genetics or shared environment. A woman's menstrual experience tends to be similar to her mother's or her sister's

Box 23-6	DSM-IV 2000 Diagnostic Criteria for Premenstrual Dysphoric Disorder

A. In most menstrual cycles during the past year, five (or more) of the following symptoms were present for most of the time during the last week of the luteal phase, began to remit within a few days after the onset of the follicular phase, and were absent in the week postmenses, with at least one of the symptoms being either (1), (2), (3), or (4):

   (1) Markedly depressed mood, feelings of hopelessness, or self-deprecating thoughts

   (2) Marked anxiety, tension, feelings of being "keyed up," or "on edge"

   (3) Marked affective lability (e.g., feeling suddenly sad or tearful or increased sensitivity to rejection)

   (4) Persistent and marked anger or irritability or increased interpersonal conflicts

   (5) Decreased interest in usual activities (e.g., work, school, friends, hobbies)

   (6) Subjective sense of difficulty in concentrating

   (7) Lethargy, easy fatigability, or marked lack of energy

   (8) Marked change in appetite, overeating, or specific food cravings

   (9) Hypersomnia or insomnia

  (10) A subjective sense of being overwhelmed or out of control

  (11) Other physical symptoms, such as breast tenderness or swelling, headaches, joint or muscle pain, a sensation of "bloating," weight gain

NOTE: In menstruating females, the luteal phase corresponds to the period between ovulation and the onset of menses, and the follicular phase begins with menses. In nonmenstruating females (e.g., those who have had a hysterectomy), the timing of luteal and follicular phases may require measurement of circulating reproductive hormones.

B. The disturbance markedly interferes with work or school or with usual social activities and relationships with others (e.g., avoidance of social activities, decreased productivity and efficiency at work or school).

C. The disturbance is not merely an exacerbation of the symptoms of another disorder, such as major depressive disorder, panic disorder, dysthymic disorder, or a personality disorder (although it may be superimposed on any of these disorders).

D. Criteria A, B, and C must be confirmed by prospective daily ratings during at least two consecutive symptomatic cycles. (The diagnosis may be made provisionally prior to this confirmation.)

Data from American Psychiatric Association: *DSM-IV-TR diagnostic and statistical manual of mental disorders,* ed 4, Washington, DC, 2000, American Psychiatric Association.

Box 23-7	American College of Obstetricians and Gynecologists (ACOG) Criteria

A problem with premenstrual dysphoric disorder (PMDD) diagnosis is that many women with clinically relevant premenstrual syndrome/premenstrual dysphoric disorder (PMS/PMDD) symptoms do not meet the full criteria of the *Diagnostic and Statistical Manual of Mental Disorders-IV* (DSM-IV). The ACOG attempts to rectify this problem by using the following definitions: "Presence of at least one psychological or physical symptom that causes significant impairment and is confirmed by means of prospective ratings (i.e., 2 cycles of a symptom diary)."

Data from American College of Obstetricians and Gynecologists: *ACOG Pract Bull* 15, 2000; Yonkers KA et al: *Lancet* 371(9619): 1200-1210, 2008.

symptoms have been attributed to PMS/PMDD. Emotional symptoms, particularly depression, anger, irritability, and fatigue, have been reported as the most prominent and the most distressing, whereas physical symptoms seem to be the least prevalent and problematic. Approximately 6% of women have classic PMS, as defined earlier, and 7% report premenstrual magnification of symptoms that occur during the entire cycle. Underlying physical or psychologic disease may be aggravated premenstrually and must be diagnosed and treated independently from PMS/PMDD.

EVALUATION AND TREATMENT Diagnosis of PMS/PMDD is based on prospective health history and symptoms. Diagnostic criteria for PMDD are presented in Box 23-7. Because the cause of PMS is not known and cannot be reduced to a single biologic explanation, and because the occurrence and severity of PMS are mediated by lifestyle and social and psychologic factors, treatment for PMS is symptomatic. Nonpharmacologic therapies, with or without medication, tend to be more effective in controlling symptoms than medication alone.

Initial treatment focuses on validation of the premenstrual experience, education on PMS and self-help techniques, and elimination of contributing factors or treatment of coexisting or underlying disorders. Individual, marriage, or family counseling; anger management and conflict resolution; and stress-reduction techniques, including biofeedback, relaxation and imagery, regular exercise, adequate rest, and time management, are recommended. Dietary changes, such as eating six small meals each day; increasing intake of complex carbohydrates, fiber, and water; and decreasing caffeine, alcohol, sugar, and animal fat can be beneficial (see Nutrition & Disease: Premenstrual Syndrome).

After a trial of nonpharmacologic therapies or if criteria for PMDD are met, medications may be added to the treatment regimen. Drugs often prescribed include vitamin and mineral supplements, selective serotonin reuptake inhibitors (SSRIs; some have been U.S. Food and Drug Administration (FDA) approved for use in PMDD), antiprostaglandins, and alprazolam. SSRIs relieve symptoms in about 60% to 90% of women and may be given continually or only during the

experience. Although research is limited, further evidence supports a relationship between the severity and frequency of premenstrual symptoms and reports of low general well-being, history of major affective disorder, and personality characteristics, such as perfectionism, increased stress, poor nutrition, lack of exercise, low self-esteem, history of sexual abuse, and family conflict. In turn, when premenstrual symptoms are perceived as distressing, the quality of interpersonal relationships and self-image are negatively affected.

CLINICAL MANIFESTATIONS The pattern of symptom frequency and severity is more important than specific complaints. Nearly 300 physical, emotional, and behavioral premenstrual period. Long-acting SSRIs, such as fluoxetine, should be tapered to prevent withdrawal symptoms. The rapid action of SSRIs suggests that it is indeed the serotonin effects as opposed to the antidepressant effects of these drugs that obtain the positive results observed with their use in PMS/PMDD treatment.[56] Progesterone is often used, but has failed to show efficacy for severe PMS/PMDD in large randomized placebo controlled trials.[59] However, progesterone's muscle relaxant and sedative properties may be beneficial. Because the edema associated with PMS is a result of local fluid shifts rather than fluid retention, diuretics are not recommended.

In severe cases, menses can be abolished, which eliminates cyclic ovarian hormones and thus the biologic trigger for PMS. Elimination of menses can be accomplished with the use of oral contraceptives, medroxyprogesterone acetate, or GnRH agonists; emotional symptoms may not be relieved with the latter. In addition, if GnRH analogs are used, then continuous estrogen replacement therapy is needed because of the "medical menopause" that results.[60] Of interest is that women with PMS may experience similar symptoms with synthetic hormones.[61] Continuous administration of low-dose oral contraceptives for extended periods with fewer hormone-free days (3 to 4 days every 3 months) may reduce the frequency and severity of PMS/PMDD symptoms.[62]

Infection and Inflammation

Infections of the genital tract may result from exogenous or endogenous microorganisms. Exogenous pathogens are most often sexually transmitted (see Chapter 24). Endogenous causes of infection include microorganisms that are normally present in the vagina, bowel, or vulva. Infection occurs if these microorganisms migrate to a new location or overproliferate or if the immune system and other defense mechanisms are impaired.

A number of skin disorders can affect the vulva. They include reactive dermatitis, contact dermatitis, psoriasis, and impetigo. (For a discussion of skin disorders, see Chapter 44.) Most infectious disorders that affect the vulva and vagina are sexually transmitted, however. These disorders are described in Chapter 24.

Pelvic Inflammatory Disease

Pelvic inflammatory disease (PID) is an acute inflammatory process caused by infection (Figure 23-5). PID may involve any organ, or combination of organs, of the upper genital tract—the uterus, fallopian tubes, or ovaries—and, in its most severe form, the entire peritoneal cavity. (Inflammation of the fallopian tubes is termed **salpingitis** [Figure 23-6]; inflammation of the ovaries is called **oophoritis.**) Sexually transmitted microorganisms, such as chlamydia and gonorrhea, that migrate from the vagina to the uterus, fallopian tubes, and ovaries cause most cases of PID.

PATHOPHYSIOLOGY The development of upper genital tract infections is mediated by the failure of a number of defense mechanisms that usually are effective in preventing PID. Virulence of the organism, size of the inoculum, and defense status of the individual determine whether an infectious process results.

PID usually is considered a polymicrobial infection.[63,64] Although initiated by gonorrhea or chlamydia, the majority of cases (up to 84%) are caused by mixed nongonococcal/nonchlamydial bacteria, including anaerobes (*Bacteroides* species and peptostreptococci), facultative organisms (*Gardnerella vaginalis, Haemophilus influenzae,* and streptococci), and genital tract mycoplasmas (*Mycoplasma hominis, Mycoplasma genitalis* and *Ureaplasma urealyticum*). *M. hominis* and *U. urealyticum* have been isolated from the endocervix but not the fallopian tubes. *Escherichia coli* has been overemphasized as a causal agent but may contribute to pelvic infections in older women. Recovery of *Neisseria gonorrhoeae* (37% to 44%), *Chlamydia trachomatis* (10% to 45%), or both (9% to 12%) is variable; however, facultative or anaerobic bacteria have been isolated in about 50% of women with acute PID. About 25% to 50% of the time, only facultative or anaerobic microorganisms are recovered.[65]

PID develops when pathogenic microbes ascend from an infected cervix along the endometrial tissue to infect the uterus and adnexae. Gonorrhea or chlamydia may induce changes in the columnar epithelium that lines the upper reproductive tract, causing damage and facilitating invasion by other microorganisms. This observation is supported from the recovery of cytokines, such as interleukin 6 (IL-6), from the cervix and endometrium of women with acute PID,[66] and the presence of antibodies to a chlamydial protein (CHSP60) in animal studies of chronic PID.[67] The resultant inflammatory response leads to tubonecrosis with repeated infections and may predispose a woman to PID.[63] Other mechanisms that

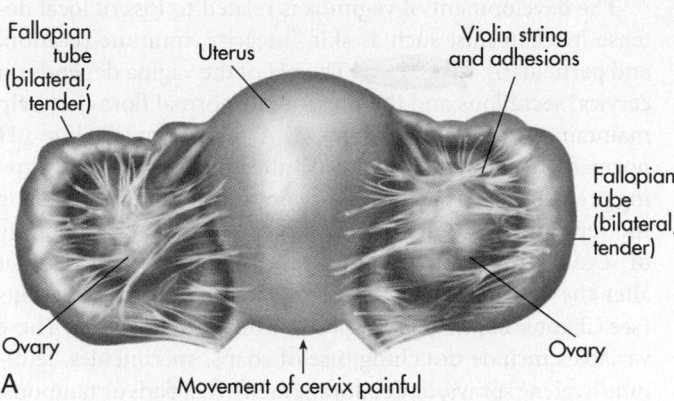

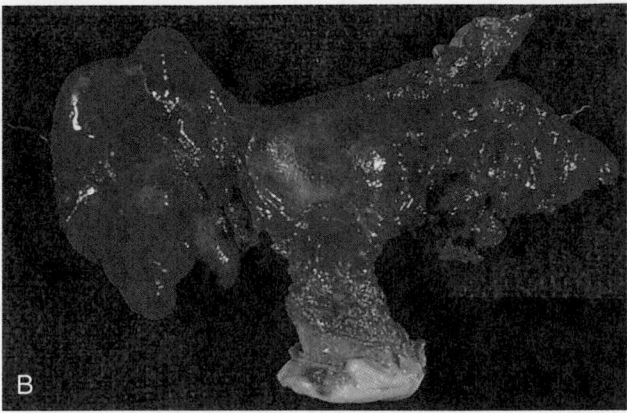

Figure 23-5 Pelvic inflammatory disease. **A,** Involvement of both ovaries and fallopian tubes. **B,** Total abdominal hysterectomy and bilateral salpingo-oophorectomy specimen showing unilateral pyosalpinx. (A from Seidel H et al: *Mosby's guide to physical examination,* ed 4, St Louis, 1999, Mosby. B from Morse SA, et al: *Atlas of sexually transmitted diseases and AIDS,* ed 3, London, 2003, Mosby.)

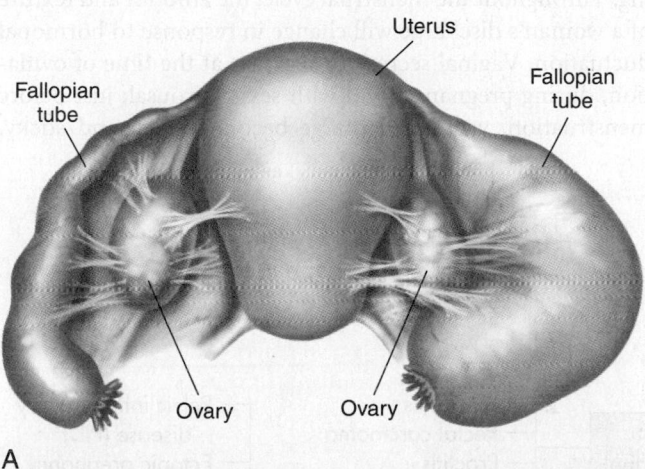

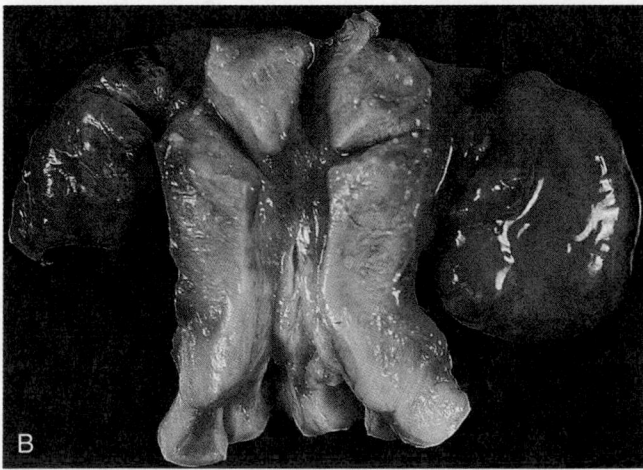

Figure 23-6 Salpingitis. **A,** Advanced pyosalpinx. Note the swollen fallopian tubes. **B,** Bilateral, retort-shaped, swollen, sealed tubes and adhesions of ovaries are typical of salpingitis. (A from Seidel H et al: *Mosby's guide to physical examination,* ed 4, St Louis, 1999, Mosby. B from Damjanov I, Linder J, editors: *Anderson's pathology,* ed 10, St Louis, 1996, Mosby.)

may contribute to PID include lymphatic drainage with parametrial spread of the infection or the adherence of sexually transmitted bacteria to sperm that travel through the genital tract. Several investigators report that bacterial vaginosis (BV), a bacterial overgrowth of the vagina, and mycoplasma genitalis has been linked to clinical findings of PID and histologic endometritis. Women with BV are nine times more likely to develop PID[63,68] and *M. genitalis* is found in 14% of nongonococcal and non-chlamydial PID.[69] (See Chapter 24 for further discussion of BV.) After one episode of pelvic infection, 15% to 25% of women develop long-term sequelae, such as infertility, ectopic pregnancy, chronic pelvic pain, dyspareunia, pelvic adhesions, perihepatitis, and tubo-ovarian abscess. The incidence of complications increases markedly with repeated infections. Tubal infertility occurs in 8% to 11% of women after one episode, 20% to 30% after two episodes, and 40% to 50% after three episodes.[70,71] The mortality rate associated with PID is 0.29 deaths per 100,000 women ages 14 to 44.[33] Most deaths resulting from PID are caused by septic shock (see Chapter 46).

CLINICAL MANIFESTATIONS The clinical manifestations of PID vary from sudden, severe abdominal pain with fever to no symptoms at all. An asymptomatic cervicitis may be present for some time before PID develops. Of women with salpingitis, 67% to 75% may have a subclinical infection. The first sign of the ascending infection may be the onset of low bilateral abdominal pain, most often characterized as dull and steady with a gradual onset. Symptoms are more likely to develop during or immediately after menstruation. The pain of PID may worsen with walking, jumping, or intercourse. Other manifestations of PID include dysuria (difficult or painful urination) and irregular bleeding.

EVALUATION AND TREATMENT The diagnosis of PID is based on history, abdominal tenderness with or without rebound, presence of uterine and cervical movement tenderness on bimanual pelvic examination, mucopurulent discharge at the cervical os, white blood cells on Gram stain or wet mount of cervical discharge, leukocytosis, and increased erythrocyte sedimentation rate. To support the diagnosis, chlamydia and gonorrhea testing is done; sonography, laparoscopy, and culdocentesis are indicated when a woman has recurrent symptoms or symptoms unresponsive to outpatient treatment regimen, fever greater than 38.3° C (100.9 ° F), or an adnexal mass. Other conditions that cause pelvic pain must be excluded, including ectopic pregnancy, threatened abortion, ovarian torsion, or appendicitis (Figure 23-7).

Because of the significance of the complications of PID, aggressive treatment is recommended. Treatment involves bed rest, avoidance of intercourse, and combined antibiotic therapy (Box 23-8). From 25% to 40% of women require hospitalization for intravenous administration of antibiotics and treatment of peritonitis or a tubo-ovarian abscess. To prevent recurrence, sexual partners also are treated with antibiotic combinations.[72] Fluoroquinolone-resistant gonorrhea has become widespread in the United States, prompting changes in Centers for Disease Control and Prevention (CDC) recommendations for antibiotic regimens in PID treatment.[73]

Vaginitis

Vaginitis is infection of the vagina. The major causes of vaginitis are sexually transmitted pathogens (see Chapter 24) and *Candida albicans*. The incidence of sexually transmitted vaginitis remains highest in young women 15 to 24 years of age.[72]

The development of vaginitis is related to loss of local defense mechanisms, such as skin integrity, immune reaction, and particularly vaginal pH. The pH of the vagina depends on cervical secretions and the presence of normal flora that help maintain an acidic environment. A neutral or alkaline pH normally occurs before puberty, after menopause, and during pregnancy. The acidic nature of vaginal secretions during the reproductive years provides protection against a variety of sexually transmitted pathogens. Therefore, variables that alter the vaginal pH or the bactericidal nature of secretions (see Chapter 22) may predispose a woman to infection. These variables include douching; use of soaps, spermicides, feminine hygiene sprays, or deodorant menstrual pads or tampons; and conditions associated with increased glycogen content of vaginal secretions, such as pregnancy or diabetes. Antibiotics often destroy normal vaginal flora, facilitating overgrowth of *C. albicans,* causing a yeast vaginitis.

Normally, vaginal discharge is a clear, milky, or cloudy secretion with a slippery or clumpy texture. It is nonirritating, has a mild inoffensive odor, and turns yellow after drying. Throughout the menstrual cycle, the amount and texture of a woman's discharge will change in response to hormonal fluctuation. Vaginal secretions increase at the time of ovulation, during pregnancy, and with sexual arousal; just before menstruation, vaginal discharge becomes thick and sticky.

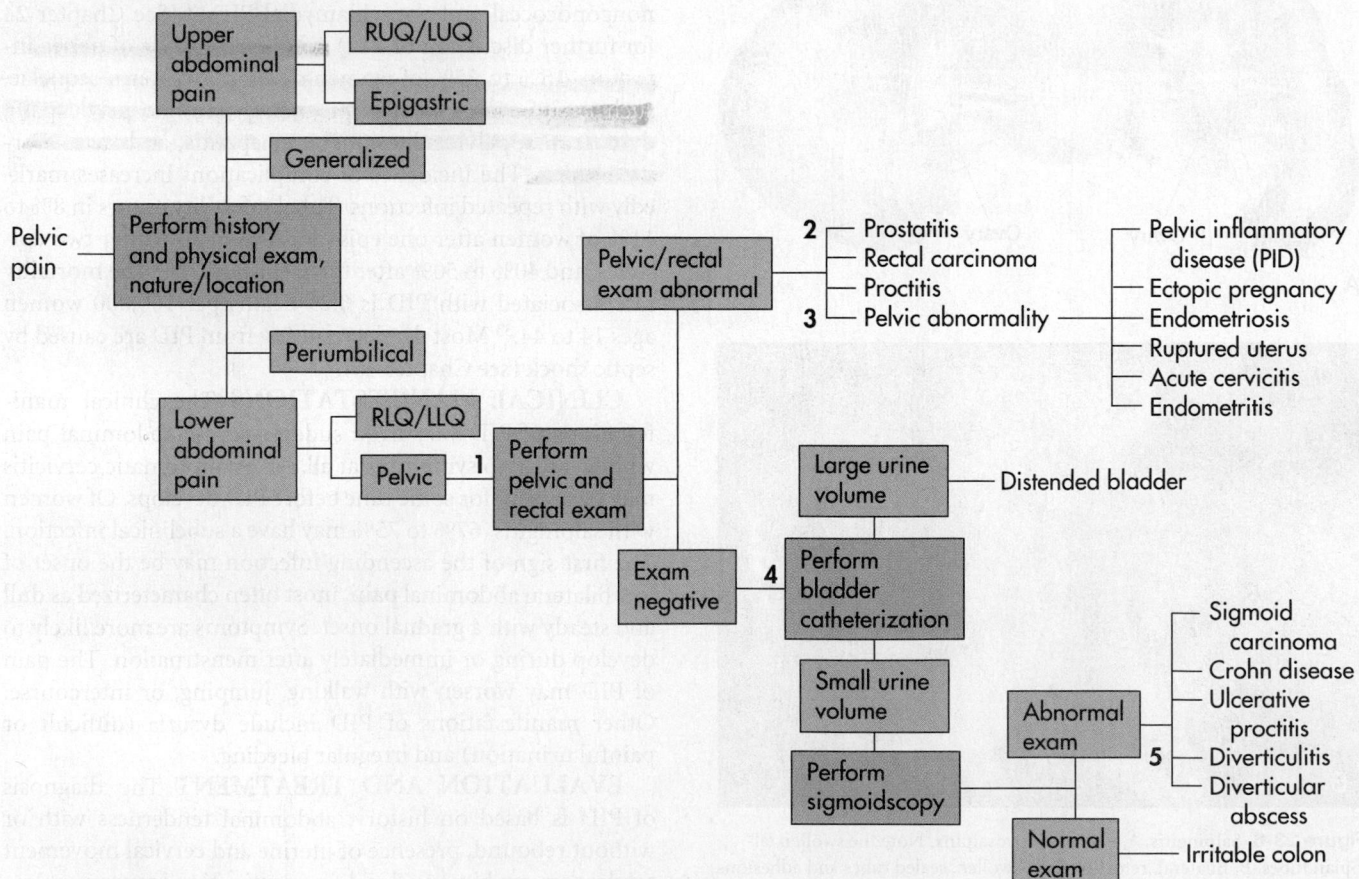

Figure 23-7 Diagnostic algorithm for pelvic pain. *LLQ,* Left lower quadrant; *LUQ,* left upper quadrant; *RLQ,* right lower quadrant; *RUQ,* right upper quadrant.

Box 23-8   CDC Recommended Treatment for Acute Pelvic Inflammatory Disease (2006)

Parenteral

Regimen A

Cefotetan, 2 g IV every 12 hours

or

Cefoxitin, 2 g IV every 6 hours

plus

Doxycycline, 100 mg orally or IV every 12 hours

NOTE: Because of pain associated with infusion, doxycycline should be administered orally when possible, even when the individual is hospitalized. Both oral and IV administration of doxycycline provides similar bioavailability.

Parenteral therapy may be discontinued 24 hours after an individual improves clinically, and oral therapy with doxycycline (100 mg twice a day) should continue to complete 14 days of therapy. When tubo-ovarian abscess is present, many healthcare providers use clindamycin or metronidazole with doxycycline for continued therapy rather than doxycycline alone because it provides more effective anaerobic coverage.

Clinical data are limited regarding the use of other second- or third-generation cephalosporins (e.g., ceftizoxime, cefotaxime, and ceftriaxone), which also may be effective therapy for PID and may replace cefotetan or cefoxitin. However, these cephalosporins are less active than cefotetan or cefoxitin against anaerobic bacteria.

Regimen B

Clindamycin, 900 mg IV every 8 hours

plus

Gentamicin, loading dose IV or IM (2 mg/kg of body weight) followed by a maintenance dose (1.5 mg/kg) every 8 hours; single daily dosing may be substituted

Although use of a single daily dose of gentamicin has not been evaluated for the treatment of PID, it is efficacious in other analogous situations. Parenteral therapy can be discontinued 24 hours after a woman improves clinically; continuing oral therapy should consist of doxycycline 100 mg orally twice a day or clindamycin 450 mg orally four times a day to complete a total of 14 days of therapy. When tubo-ovarian abscess is present, many healthcare providers use clindamycin for continued therapy rather than doxycycline because clindamycin provides more effective anaerobic coverage.

Alternative Parenteral Regimens

Limited data support the use of other parenteral regimens, but the following three regimens have been investigated in at least one clinical trial, and they have broad-spectrum coverage.

Ampicillin/sulbactam, 3 g IV every 6 hours

plus

Doxycycline, 100 mg orally or IV every 12 hours

with or without

Metronidazole, 500 mg IV every 8 hours

Intravenous ofloxacin has been investigated as a single agent; however because of concerns regarding its spectrum, metronidazole may be included in the regimen. Ampicillin/sulbactam plus doxycycline has good coverage against *C. trachomatis, N. gonorrhoeae,* and anaerobes and is effective for women who have tubo-ovarian abscess.

Oral Treatment

Oral treatment can be considered for women with mild to moderately severe PID, as the clinical outcomes among women treated with oral antibiotics are similar to those treated with parenteral antibiotics. Women who do not respond to oral therapy within 72 hours should be reevaluated to confirm the diagnosis and should be administered parenteral therapy on either an outpatient or inpatient basis.

Regimen C

Ceftriaxone, 250 mg IM in a single dose

or

Cefoxitin, 2 g IM in a single dose and **Probenecid,** 1 g orally administered concurrently in a single dose

or

Other parenteral third-generation **cephalosporin** (e.g., **ceftizoxime** or **cefotaxime**)

plus

Doxycycline, 100 mg orally twice a day for 14 days

with or without

Metronidazole, 500 mg orally twice a day for 14 days

The optimal choice of a cephalosporin is unclear; although cefoxitin has better anaerobic coverage, ceftriaxone has better coverage against *N. gonorrhoeae.* Clinical trials have demonstrated that a single dose of cefoxitin is effective in obtaining short-term clinical response in women who have PID; however, the theoretic limitations in its coverage of anaerobes may require the addition of metronidazole to the treatment regimen. The metronidazole also will effectively treat BV, which is frequently associated with PID. No data have been published regarding the use of oral cephalosporins for the treatment of PID. Limited data suggest that the combination of oral metronidazole plus doxycycline after primary parenteral therapy is safe and effective.

Alternative Oral Regimens

If parenteral cephalosporin treatment is not feasible, use of fluoroquinolones (levofloxacin 500 mg daily dose or ofloxacin 400 mg twice daily for 14 days) with or without metronidazole may be considered if community prevalence and individual risk of gonorrhea are low. Testing for gonorrhea must be performed prior to instituting treatment; if the test is positive, the individual is managed as follows:

1. If NAAT test is positive, parenteral cephalosporin is recommended.

2. If culture for gonorrhea is positive, treatment should be based on the results of antimicrobial susceptibility. If isolate is quinolone-resistant *N. gonorrhoeae,* or the antimicrobial susceptibility cannot be assessed, parenteral cephalosporin is recommended.

Although information regarding other outpatient regimens is limited, amoxicillin/clavulanic acid and doxycycline (or azithromycin) with metronidazole have demonstrated short-term clinical cure. No data have been published regarding use of oral cephalosporins for the treatment of PID. In one randomized study, azithromycin was demonstrated to be an effective regimen for acute PID.

Follow-Up

Women should demonstrate substantial clinical improvement (e.g., defervescence; reduction in direct or rebound abdominal tenderness; and reduction in uterine, adnexal, and cervical motion tenderness) within 3 days after initiation of therapy. Those who do not improve within this period usually require hospitalization, additional diagnostic tests, and surgical intervention.

If the healthcare provider prescribes outpatient oral or parenteral therapy, a follow-up examination should be performed within 72 hours using the criteria for clinical improvement described previously. If the individual has not improved, hospitalization for parenteral therapy and further evaluation are recommended. Some specialists also recommend rescreening for *C. trachomatis* and *N. gonorrhoeae* 4 to 6 weeks after therapy is completed in women with documented infection with these pathogens. All women diagnosed with PID should be offered HIV testing.

Continued

| Box 23-8 | CDC Recommended Treatment for Acute Pelvic Inflammatory Disease (2006)—cont'd |

NOTE: Ongoing data from the CDC's Gonorrhea Isolate Surveillance Project demonstrated that fluoroquinolone-resistant gonorrhea is continuing to spread and is now widespread in the United States; as a consequence, this class of antibiotics is no longer recommended for the treatment of gonorrhea. Treatment recommendations have been updated from 2006 to 2007.

Modified from Centers for Disease Control and Prevention (CDC): *2006 Sexually transmitted diseases: treatment guidelines*, Washington DC, 2006, U.S. Department of Health and Human Services; Centers for Disease Control and Prevention (CDC): *MMWR Morb Mort Wkly Rep* 56(14):332-336, 2007.
BV, Bacterial vaginosis; *HIV,* human immunodeficiency virus; *IM,* intramuscular; *IV,* intravenous; *NAAT,* nucleic acid amplification test *PID,* pelvic inflammatory disease.

Although the amount of vaginal discharge alone is not an indication of infection, any other change in discharge may indicate a problem. Infection is suggested with a marked change in color or if the discharge becomes copious, malodorous, or irritating.

Diagnosis is based on history, physical examination, and examination of the discharge by wet mount. Treatment involves developing and maintaining an acidic environment, relieving symptoms (usually pruritus), and administering antimicrobial or antifungal medications to eradicate the infectious organism. If the infection can be sexually transmitted, a woman's partner also will be treated.

Cervicitis

Cervicitis is a nonspecific term used to describe inflammation of the cervix prior to the identification of pathogens. **Mucopurulent cervicitis (MPC)** usually is caused by one or more sexually transmitted pathogens, such as *Trichomonas,* gonorrhea, *Chlamydia, Mycoplasma,* or *Ureaplasma.* Infection causes the cervix to become red and edematous. A mucopurulent (mucus- and pus-containing) exudate drains from the external cervical os, and the individual may report vague pelvic pain, bleeding, or dysuria. The cervix often becomes friable, bleeding easily during sexual intercourse or with pelvic examinations and Papanicolaou (Pap) smears. The infectious microorganisms are cultured or identified by immunoassay. Definitive diagnosis is followed by oral antibiotic therapy to prevent reinfection; sexual partners are treated as well.[72]

Vulvovestibulitis

Vulvovestibulitis (VV) (also referred to as vulvitis, vestibulitis, or vulvodynia) is inflammation of the vulva or vestibule of the genitalia, or both. In many cases, it may represent several disorders without an identifiable cause.[74] VV is fairly common, affecting approximately 10% of women at some point in life. While the inflammation of VV may be caused by contact dermatitis (i.e., exposure to soaps, detergents, lotions, sprays, shaving, menstrual pads/tampons, perfumed toilet paper, tight-fitting clothes), the condition may be more complex and represent abnormalities in three interdependent systems: vestibular mucosa, pelvic floor musculature, and central nervous system pain regulatory pathways.[75,76] The condition may also represent an autoimmune reaction, similar to fibromyalgia. The mechanisms are poorly understood, thus VV is often a difficult condition to evaluate and treat and many women suffer through years of misdiagnosis as a result.[77] After ruling out and treating conditions that may contribute to or cause vulvar inflammation (e.g., *Candida,* sexually transmitted infection, seborrhea, psoriasis, lichen sclerosus, and contact dermatitis) there are few treatment options. Studies are limited but suggest that women may benefit from behavioral treatment (35% to 83% of women benefit) or vestibulectomy (61% to 94% success rate), a procedure that is understandably unacceptable to many women because of the invasiveness of the procedure.[78] Other approaches with little or no research to support them include use of hydrocortisone cream, applying a water barrier (such as thick skin cream or solid vegetable shortening) during a period of healing, and overnight lidocaine applications.[79] Women are advised to avoid potential irritants and to wear loose, cotton clothing. VV may increase susceptibility to vaginal infection; likewise, VV may be caused by vaginal infections (e.g., candidiasis, trichomoniasis) that spread to the labia, where they cause inflammation and edema. Other skin diseases, such as tinea cruris, psoriasis, lichen sclerosus, and inflammation of the apocrine (sweat) glands, can involve the vulva (see Chapter 44).

Bartholinitis

Bartholinitis, or **Bartholin cyst,** is an inflammation of one or both of the ducts that lead from the introitus (vaginal opening) to the Bartholin glands (Figure 23-8). The usual causes of bartholinitis are microorganisms that infect the lower female reproductive tract, such as streptococci, staphylococci, and sexually transmitted pathogens. Acute bartholinitis may be preceded by an infection, such as cervicitis, vaginitis, or urethritis.

Infection or trauma causes inflammatory changes that narrow the distal portion of the duct, leading to obstruction and stasis of glandular secretions. The obstruction, or cyst, varies from 1 to 8 cm in diameter and is located in the posterolateral portion of the vulva. The cyst is usually reddened and painful, and pus may be visible at the opening of the duct; this exudate should be cultured. The individual may have symptoms of the initiating infection, fever, and malaise.

Most Bartholin cysts are asymptomatic and require no treatment. Chronic bartholinitis is characterized by the presence of a small cyst that is slightly tender but otherwise is

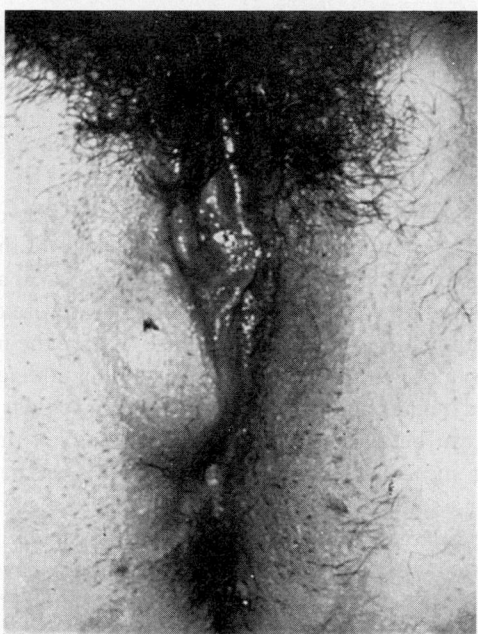

Figure 23-8 Inflammation of Bartholin gland. (From Gardner HL, Kaufman RH: *Benign diseases of the vulva and vagina*, St Louis, 1969, Mosby.)

asymptomatic. Symptoms occur if an exacerbation of infection causes an abscess to form in the gland itself.

Diagnosis of bartholinitis is based on the clinical manifestations and the identification of infectious microorganisms. Antibiotics are given to treat infection, and pain is relieved with analgesics and warm sitz baths. If an abscess forms, it is surgically drained.

Pelvic Organ Prolapse (POP)

The bladder, urethra, and rectum are supported by the endopelvic fascia and the perineal muscles, particularly the levator ani group. This muscular and fascial tissue loses tone and strength with aging and may fail to maintain the pelvic organs in the proper position. Progressive descent of the pelvic support structures may cause pelvic floor disorders, such as urinary and fecal incontinence and pelvic organ prolapse. Nearly 24% of women experience at least one pelvic floor disorder.[80] Pelvic organ prolapse is thought to be caused by direct trauma, such as childbirth or pelvic surgery or damage to pelvic innervation, particularly the pudendal nerve. Pelvic organ descent is progressive and is related to the inherent strength or weakness of the woman's musculofascial tissue. Prolapse of the bladder, urethra, rectum, or uterus may occur many years after an initial injury to the supporting structure. A strong familial tendency and possibly a multifactorial genetic component place some women at risk for the development of prolapse. Black and Asian women have the lowest risk of POP, and Hispanic women appear to have the highest risk.[81] Risk factors in nulliparous women, which mimic the effects of childbirth, tend to be occupational activities that require heavy lifting or chronic medical conditions, such as chronic lung disease or refractory constipation. Some women at risk for pelvic organ prolapse have neural abnormalities that interfere with the innervation of the levator ani. A list of risk factors is contained in Box 23-9. (Chapter 22 contains a discussion of pelvic support structures.) Pelvic organ prolapse is the third most common indicator for hysterectomy in the United States. At least 30% of women will have repeat surgical procedures.[82]

The trend is to use terminology that describes physical examination findings, thus avoiding assumptions about structural involvement (Box 23-10). The terms *cystocele* and *rectocele* may be used when the structures involved (bladder, rectum) have been definitively identified (i.e., an anterior vaginal wall prolapse may or may not be a cystocele involving the urinary bladder) (see Figure 23-10, p. 835). Having a woman stand and strain maximally provides the best information about the degree of pelvic organ relaxation. Physical examination may be augmented with imaging by ultrasound, fluoroscope, or magnetic resonance. There are several systems used to describe prolapse. One in widespread clinical use is based on physical examination findings (see Box 23-10) and uses a grading system to describe the extent of the prolapse observed (Box 23-11). Subjective reports regarding the symptoms and effects of POP can be assessed through direct questioning or commonly used questionnaires, such as the Pelvic Floor Impact Questionnaire or the Pelvic Floor Distress Inventory.

Uterine prolapse is descent of the cervix or entire uterus into the vaginal canal (Figure 23-9). In severe cases the uterus falls completely through the vagina and protrudes from the introitus. Grade 1 uterine prolapse is not treated unless it causes discomfort. Grades 2 through 4 prolapse cause feelings of fullness, heaviness, and collapse through the vagina. Symptoms of other pelvic floor disorders also may be present. Treatment in these cases is the insertion of a **pessary,** which is a removable mechanical device that holds the uterus in position. The pelvic fascia may be strengthened through Kegel exercises (repetitive isometric tightening and relaxing of the pubococcygeal muscles) or by a course of estrogen therapy in menopausal women. Maintaining a healthy body mass index, preventing constipation, and treating chronic cough may help prevent prolapse. Surgical repair with or without hysterectomy is the treatment of last resort.

Figure 23-10 shows vaginal prolapse caused by cystocele and rectocele. **Cystocele** is descent of a portion of the posterior bladder wall and trigone into the vaginal canal and usually is caused by the trauma of childbirth. In severe cases the bladder and anterior vaginal wall bulge outside the introitus. Usually symptoms are insignificant in mild to moderate cases. Increased bulging and descent of the anterior vaginal wall and urethra can be aggravated by vigorous activity, prolonged standing, sneezing, coughing, or straining and can be relieved by rest or assumption of a recumbent or prone position. If the prolapse is large, women may complain of vaginal pressure or the feeling of "sitting on a ball." A prolapse caused by a cystocele may be interpreted as incomplete bladder emptying, which can be controlled by a second voiding a few minutes after the first void or by manually reducing the anterior vaginal wall prolapse during voiding. Occasionally a cystocele causes significant residual urine and bladder infection.

Although commonly associated with urinary stress incontinence, cystocele does not cause it. Stress incontinence is

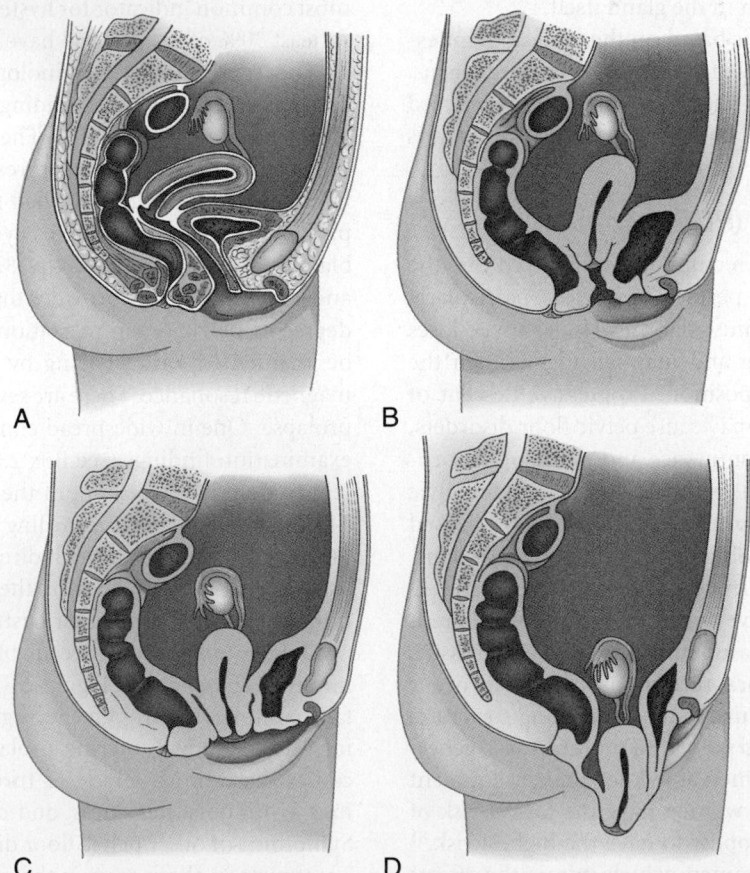

Figure 23-9 Degrees of uterine prolapse. **A**, Normal uterus (grade 0). **B**, Grade 1 prolapse: descent within the vagina. **C**, Grade 2 prolapse: descent to the hymen. **D**, Grade 4 prolapse: maximal possible descent of the uterus. Grade 3 prolapse not shown.

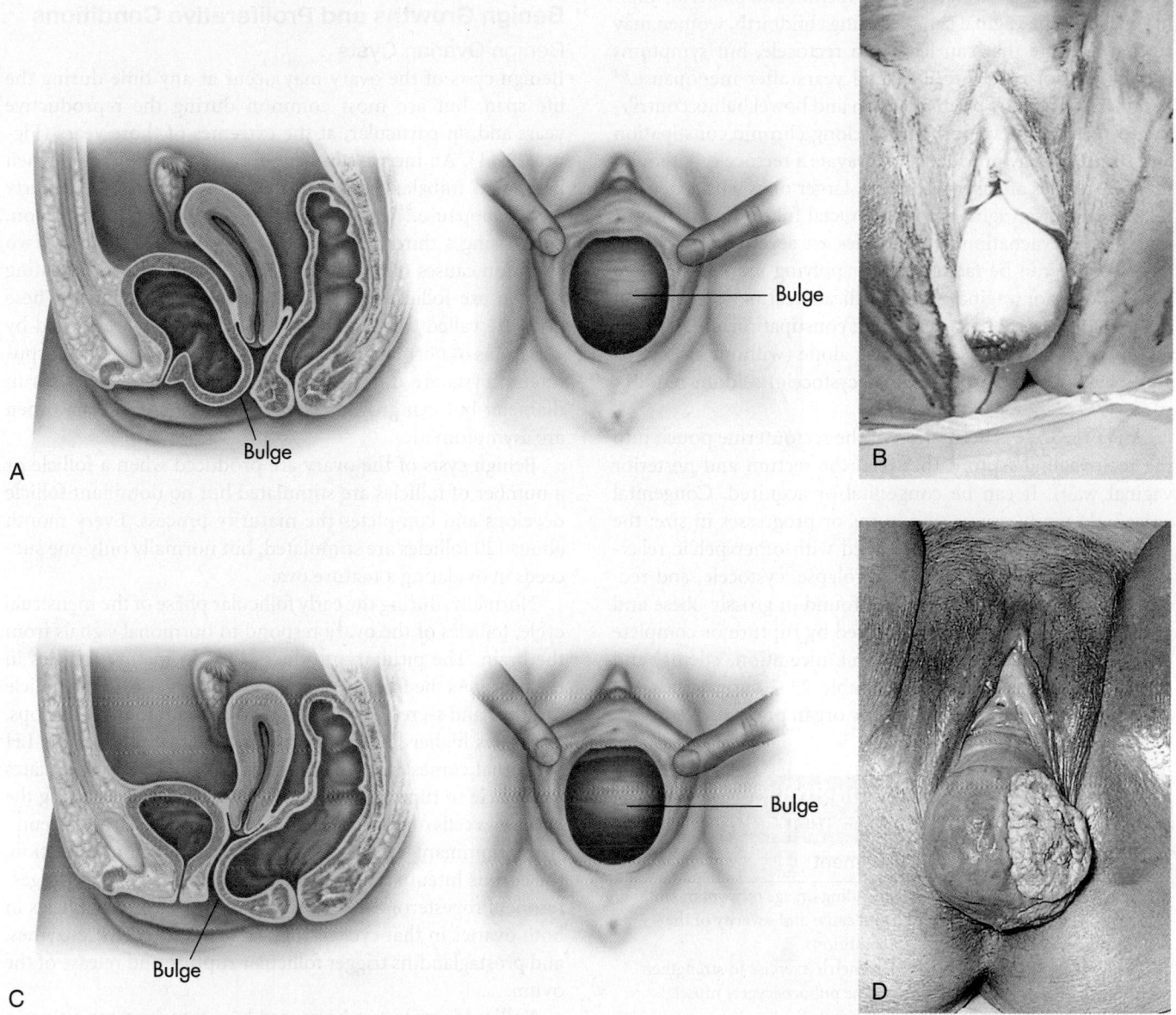

Figure 23-10 Cystocele and rectocele. **A,** Grade 2: anterior vaginal wall prolapse. **B,** Grade 4: prolapse. **C,** Grade 2: posterior wall prolapse. **D,** Grade 4: associated with ulceration of vaginal wall. Grades 1 and 3 not shown. (A and C from Seidel H et al: *Mosby's guide to physical examination,* ed 4, St Louis, 1999, Mosby. B and D from Symonds EM, Macpherson MBA: *Color atlas of obstetrics and gynecology,* London, 1994, Mosby-Wolfe.)

likely the result of relaxation of the musculofascial supporting tissues of the urethra that also contribute to the cystocele. Operative correction of a large cystocele may actually cause rather than correct stress incontinence.[83]

Medical management includes vaginal pessary; Kegel exercises (prophylactic use produces best outcome); estrogen therapy for postmenopausal women; and, most important, reassurance that pressure symptoms are not the result of a serious condition. Surgical correction is used for severe anatomic injury unresponsive to medical treatment, and its success depends on treatment of generalized urogenital musculofascial supporting tissue relaxation, correction of underlying paravaginal defects, and elimination or prevention

of contributing factors that increase intra-abdominal pressure, such as pregnancy, constipation, obesity, large pelvic tumors, bronchitis, and heavy manual labor.[84]

Urethrocele, or sagging of the urethra, is commonly associated with cystocele, especially in women with urinary stress incontinence. Like cystocele, urethrocele does not cause urinary incontinence. Urethrocele may be caused by the shearing effect of the fetal head on the urethra during childbirth. However, **cystourethrocele** may occur in nulliparous women and is most likely caused by congenital weakness and relaxation of the musculature of the pelvic floor or the endopelvic connective tissues or fascia. Treatment may be necessary after menopause.

A **rectocele** is the bulging of the rectum and posterior vaginal wall into the vaginal canal. During childbirth, women may sustain damage that can lead to a rectocele, but symptoms usually do not occur until several years after menopause.[84] Familial and genetic predisposition and bowel habits contribute to rectocele development. Lifelong chronic constipation and straining may produce or aggravate a rectocele. Although most rectoceles are asymptomatic, larger ones with extensive relaxation cause vaginal pressure, rectal fullness, and incomplete bowel evacuation. If rectoceles are severe, defecation is difficult and can be facilitated by applying manual pressure to the posterior vaginal wall. Medical treatment focuses on the management and prevention of constipation and, if needed, the use of a pessary. Rectocele alone (without associated enterocele, uterine prolapse, and cystocele) seldom requires surgery.

An **enterocele** is herniation of the rectouterine pouch into the rectovaginal septum (between the rectum and posterior vaginal wall). It can be congenital or acquired. Congenital enterocele rarely causes symptoms or progresses in size; the acquired form usually is associated with other pelvic relaxation disorders such as uterine prolapse, cystocele, and rectocele. Most large enteroceles are found in grossly obese and older adults and can be complicated by rupture or complete eversion of the vagina with trophic ulceration, edema, and fibrosis. Treatment is surgical. Table 23-3 summarizes the symptoms and treatments of pelvic organ prolapse.

Table 23-3	Pelvic Organ Prolapse: Symptoms and Treatments
Symptoms	**Treatment**
Urinary Sensation of incomplete emptying of bladder Urinary incontinence Urinary frequency/urgency Bladder "splinting" to accomplish voiding **Bowel** Constipation or feeling of rectal fullness or blockage Difficult defecation Stool or flatus incontinence **Urgency** Manual "splinting" of posterior vaginal wall to accomplish defecation **Pain and Bulging** Vaginal, bladder, rectum Pelvic pressure, bulging, pain Lower back pain **Sexual** Dyspareunia Decreased sensation, lubrication, arousal	Depending on age of woman and cause and severity of the condition: Isometric exercise to strengthen the pubococcygeal muscle (Kegels) Estrogen to improve tone and vascularity of fascial support (postmenopausal) Pessary (a removable device) to hold pelvic organs in place **Surgical:** Reconstructive: autologus grafts; synthetic mesh/sling Obliterative (most extreme) Weight loss Avoidance of constipation Treatment of cough/lung conditions

Benign Growths and Proliferative Conditions

Benign Ovarian Cysts

Benign cysts of the ovary may occur at any time during the life span, but are most common during the reproductive years and, in particular, at the extremes of those years (Figure 23-11). An increase in benign ovarian cysts occurs when hormonal imbalances are more common, around puberty and menopause.[85] Benign ovarian cysts are quite common, comprising a third of gynecologic hospital admissions. Two common causes of benign ovarian enlargement in ovulating women are follicular cysts and corpus luteum cysts. These cysts are called **functional cysts** because they are caused by variations of normal physiologic events. Follicular and corpus luteum cysts are unilateral. They are typically 5 to 6 cm in diameter but can grow as large as 8 to 10 cm. Most women are asymptomatic.

Benign cysts of the ovary are produced when a follicle or a number of follicles are stimulated but no dominant follicle develops and completes the maturity process. Every month about 120 follicles are stimulated, but normally only one succeeds in ovulating a mature ova.

Normally, during the early follicular phase of the menstrual cycle, follicles of the ovary respond to hormonal signals from the brain. The pituitary produces FSH to mature follicles in the ovary. As the follicles enlarge, granulosa cells in the follicle multiply and secrete estradiol. As a dominant follicle develops, it secretes higher levels of estradiol, which stimulates the LH surge that comes from the pituitary. The LH surge stimulates the follicle to rupture, releasing the ova and transforming the granulosa cells of the dominant follicle into the corpus luteum. If the dominant follicle develops properly before ovulation, the corpus luteum becomes vascularized and secretes progesterone. Progesterone arrests development of other follicles in both ovaries in that cycle. Progesterone, proteolytic enzymes, and prostaglandins trigger follicular rupture and release of the ovum.

Follicular cysts can be caused by a transient condition in which the dominant follicle fails to rupture or one or more of the nondominant follicles fail to regress. This disturbance is not well understood. It may be that the hypothalamus does

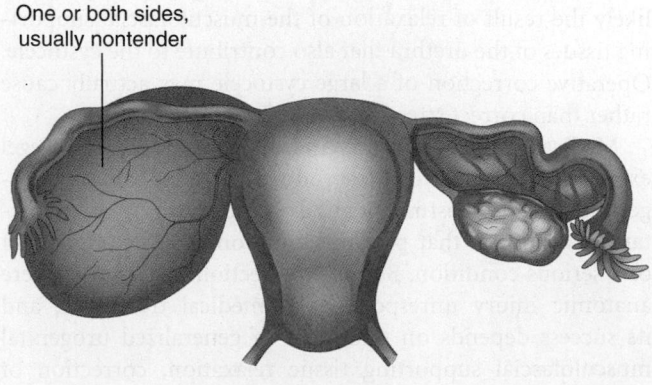

One or both sides, usually nontender

Figure 23-11 Ovarian cyst.

not receive or send a message strong enough to increase FSH levels needed to develop or mature a dominant follicle. The hypothalamus monitors blood levels of estradiol and progesterone; when FSH is low, estradiol does not increase enough to stimulate LH. Recent evidence indicates that when progesterone is not being produced, the hypothalamus releases GnRH to increase the FSH level.[86] FSH continues to stimulate follicles to mature, and the granulosa cells grow and, presumably, estradiol increases. This abnormal cycle continues to stimulate follicular size and causes follicular cysts to develop. Clinical symptoms of follicular cysts or even a single cyst is bloating, swollen and tender breasts, and heavy or irregular menses. After several subsequent cycles in which hormone levels once again follow a regular cycle and progesterone levels are restored, cysts usually are absorbed or regress.

Follicular cysts can vary in size and symptoms from one episode to the next and often can recur. Most are fluid filled; the more solid an ovarian cyst, the greater the chance of malignancy.

A **corpus luteum cyst** may develop because of a hormonal imbalance in low LH and progesterone levels causing an inadequate development of the corpus luteum. There is an intracystic hemorrhage that occurs in the vascularization stage, and the affected cyst then consists of blood. In normal cysts the blood is replaced by a clear fluid that accumulates in the cavity of the corpus luteum.

Corpus luteum cysts are less common than follicular cysts, but luteal cysts typically cause more symptoms, particularly if they rupture. Manifestations include dull pelvic pain and amenorrhea or delayed menstruation, followed by irregular or heavier than usual bleeding. Rupture occasionally occurs and can cause massive bleeding with excruciating pain; immediate surgery may be required. Corpus luteum cysts usually regress spontaneously in nonpregnant women. Oral contraceptives may be used to prevent future cysts from forming.

Dermoid cysts are ovarian teratomas that contain elements of all three germ layers; they are common ovarian neoplasms. These growths may contain mature tissue including skin, hair, sebaceous and sweat glands, muscle fibers, cartilage, and bone. Dermoid cysts are usually asymptomatic and are found incidentally on pelvic examination. Dermoid cysts have malignant potential and should be removed.

Torsion of the ovary may occur as a complication of ovarian cysts or tumors or enlargement of the ovary associated with infertility treatments. Ovarian torsion is rare but is a gynecologic emergency when present. Individuals present with acute, severe unilateral abdominal or pelvic pain related to a change of position.

Endometrial Polyps

An **endometrial polyp** is a benign mass of endometrial tissue, covered by a surface epithelium, and contains a variable amount of glands, stoma, and blood vessels. Endometrial polyps are usually solitary and originate at the fundus but also may be multiple (20% of the cases) or originate from the lower uterine segment or upper endocervix and contain

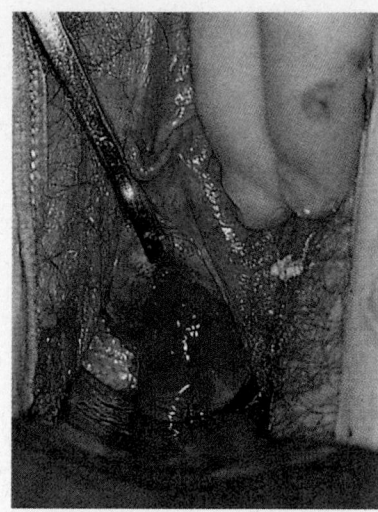

Figure 23-12 **Endometrial polyp.** It is protruding through the cervical os. (From Symonds EM, Macpherson MBA: *Color atlas of obstetrics and gynecology,* London, 1994, Mosby-Wolfe.)

mixed epithelium. Polyps are morphologically diverse and usually classified as hyperplastic, atrophic (or inactive), or functional. In the last case, the surface epithelium may be "out of phase" with other endometrial tissue. Hyperplastic polyps are often pedunculated and may be mistaken for endometrial hyperplasia or, if large, adenosarcoma (Figure 23-12). Although polyps most often develop in women between ages 40 and 50, they can occur at all ages. These are often related to estrogen stimulation. As many as 35% of women with abnormal uterine bleeding are found to have polyps.[87]

Endometrial polyps are a common cause of intermenstrual or excessive menstrual bleeding. Diagnosis is made by transvaginal sonography or hysteroscopy. Risk factors include obesity, tamoxifen use, hypertension, and estrogenic states (i.e., anovulatory cycles and unopposed estrogen). Malignancy is extremely rare (1% to 2%), and coexistence of a separate endometrial atypical hyperplasia or adenocarcinoma is common. Women with polyps less than 1.5 cm can be observed. Uterine polyps have a high rate of spontaneous resolution. Polypectomy can be performed through hysteroscopy for symptomatic women or those with risk factors for malignancy.[88]

Leiomyomas

Leiomyomas, commonly called **myomas** or **uterine fibroids,** are benign smooth muscle tumors in the myometrium (Figure 23-13). Leiomyomas are the most common benign tumors of the uterus, affecting as many as 70% to 80% of all women, and most remain small, asymptomatic, and clinically insignificant.[89] Prevalence increases in women ages 30 to 50 but decreases with menopause. The incidence of leiomyomas in black and Asian women is two to five times higher than that in white women.[90]

The cause of uterine leiomyomas is unknown, although their size appears to be related to estrogen, progesterone, growth factors, angiogenesis, and apoptosis. Leiomyomas are estrogen-and

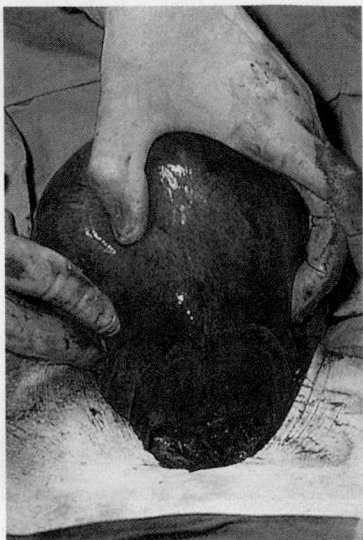

Figure 23-13 Uterine fibroid. The uterus is irregular because it contains multiple fibroids. (From Symonds EM, Macpherson MBA: *Color atlas of obstetrics and gynecology,* London, 1994, Mosby-Wolfe.)

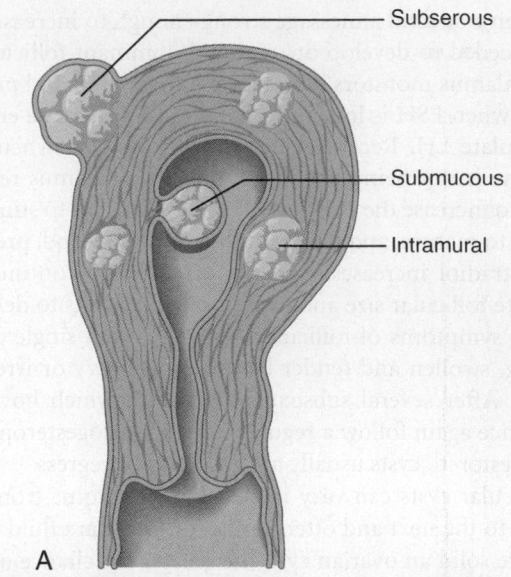

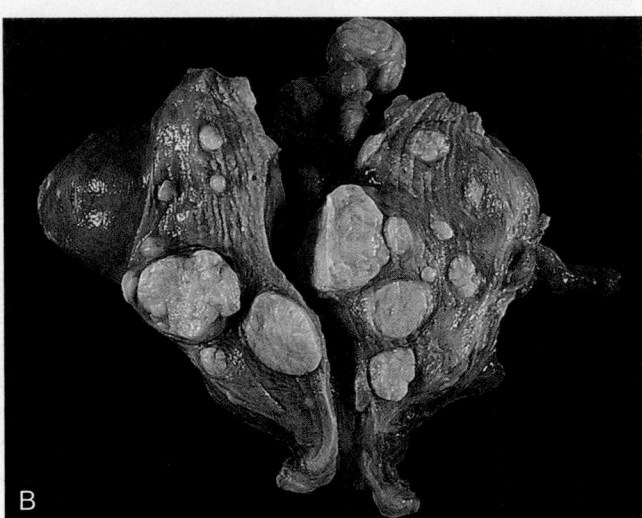

Figure 23-14 Leiomyomas. **A,** Uterine section showing whorl-like appearance and locations of leiomyomas, which are also called *uterine fibroids.* **B,** Multiple leiomyomas in sagittal section. Typical, well-circumscribed, solid, light gray nodules distort uterus. (**B** from Damjanov I, Linder J: *Pathology: a color atlas,* St Louis, 2000, Mosby.)

progesterone-sensitive and are found to have increased numbers of estrogen receptors.[89] Uterine leiomyomas are not seen before menarche, and those that develop during the reproductive years generally decrease in size after menopause. Occurrence is thought to be related to increased estrogen exposure. Tumors in pregnant women enlarge rapidly but often decrease in size after termination of the pregnancy. Risk factors include heredity, nulliparity, obesity, PCOS, diabetes mellitus, and hypertension.

PATHOPHYSIOLOGY Most leiomyomas occur in multiples in the fundus of the uterus, although they may occur singly and throughout the uterus. Leiomyomas are classified as subserous, submucous, or intramural according to their location within the various layers of the uterine wall (Figure 23-14). Uterine leiomyomas are usually firm and surrounded by a connective tissue layer. Degeneration and necrosis may occur when the leiomyoma outgrows its blood supply and therefore are more common in larger tumors and may be accompanied by pain.

CLINICAL MANIFESTATIONS The major clinical manifestations of leiomyomas are abnormal uterine bleeding, pain, and symptoms related to pressure on nearby structures. They also may contribute to infertility and subfertility. The leiomyoma tends to make the uterine cavity larger, thereby increasing the endometrial surface area. This increase may account for the increased menstrual bleeding that is associated with leiomyomas. Pain is not an early symptom but tends to occur with the devascularization of larger leiomyomas. It is also associated with blood vessel compression that limits blood supply to adjacent structures. Symptoms of abdominal pressure are slow to develop, apparently because the tumor is relatively slow growing, enabling adjacent structures to adapt to pressure. Pressure on the bladder may contribute to urinary frequency, urgency, and dysuria. Pressure on the ureter may cause it to become distended "upstream" from

the pressure point; rectosigmoid pressure may lead to constipation. A sensation of abdominal or genital heaviness may be felt with larger tumors.

EVALUATION AND TREATMENT Uterine leiomyomas are suspected when the bimanual examination discloses uterine enlargement and irregular, nontender nodularity of the uterus. Pelvic sonography confirms diagnosis.[90] Treatment depends on the symptoms, tumor size, age, reproductive status, and overall health of the individual. Most myomas are asymptomatic and can be managed by observation only. Medical treatment for symptomatic or subfertile women is aimed at shrinking the myoma. Some leiomyomas shrink in response to oral contraceptives, however, oral contraceptive pills (OCPs) may enhance growth so should be monitored carefully. GnRH agonists are usually a temporary management for those close to menopause or as a presurgical treatment. GnRH side effects related to decreased estrogen, including hot flashes and osteoporosis, limit its usefulness. Various selective estrogen receptor modulators have been studied in conjunction with GnRH agonists and appear safe and effective.[91] Antidepressants, such as mifepristone (RU486) have also shown some effectiveness in shrinking leiomyomas. Myomectomy may be undertaken and remains the standard of cure for women wishing to preserve their fertility. Hysterectomy is also an option. Newer experimental treatments that show promise include uterine artery embolization, laser ablation treatment with mifepristone, and the levonorgestrel intrauterine system. With each of these new therapies, benefits and risks should be carefully explored.[92]

Adenomyosis

Adenomyosis is the presence of islands of endometrial glands surrounded by benign endometrial stroma within the uterine myometrium. Endometrial cells migrate into the myometrial layer because of an unknown mechanism. Estrogen and progesterone likely play a role and, perhaps, metaplasia of müllerian tissue. Unlike endometriosis, this tissue does not respond to cyclic hormone changes. It commonly develops during the late reproductive years, with the highest incidence among women in their 40s and women on tamoxifen. Adenomyosis has been found in 18% of hysterectomy specimens and 53% of specimens from women taking tamoxifen. Ninety percent of all adenomyosis is found in parous women. Adenomyosis may be asymptomatic or may be associated with abnormal menstrual bleeding, dysmenorrhea, uterine enlargement, and uterine tenderness during menstruation. Secondary dysmenorrhea becomes increasingly severe as disease progresses. On bimanual examination the uterus is diffusely enlarged, globular, and most tender just before or after menstruation. Diagnosis is confirmed with ultrasonography or MRI. Treatment is symptomatic, similar to dysmenorrhea (i.e., nonsteroidal anti-inflammatory drugs [NSAIDs], COCs, and perhaps levonorgestrel-containing IUDs). Surgical treatment includes resection of localized areas of adenomyosis or, if severe, hysterectomy. GnRH and danazol are experimental.[90]

Endometriosis

Endometriosis is the presence of functioning endometrial tissue or implants outside the uterus. Like normal endometrial tissue, the ectopic (out of place) endometrium responds to the hormonal fluctuations of the menstrual cycle.

The incidence of endometriosis is difficult to determine, particularly in asymptomatic adolescent and fertile women. It is estimated that 2% to 22% of reproductive-age women and 2% to 4% of menopausal women have endometriosis. In addition, as many as 50% of women evaluated for pelvic pain, infertility, or a pelvic mass are diagnosed as having endometriosis, and 4% to 8% of fertile women have endometriosis. Moreover, the frequency and severity of symptoms do not correlate well with the extent or site of lesions.[93]

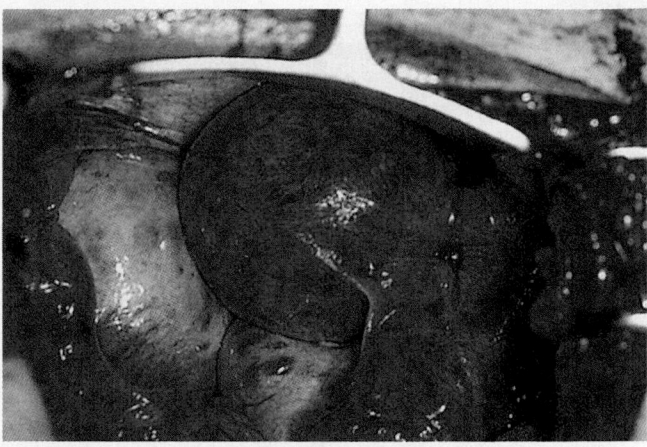

Figure 23-15 Endometriosis. The uterus is distended, and retrograde spill of menstrual loss has led to the development of endometriosis (*dark purple patches*). (From Symonds EM, Macpherson MBA: *Color atlas of obstetrics and gynecology*, London, 1994, Mosby-Wolfe.)

A large study has found that women with endometriosis are at greater risk for cancers (ovarian and non-Hodgkin lymphoma, endocrine, and brain), in particular for those with long-standing disease or early diagnosis, or both.[94]

The cause of endometriosis is not known, but several theories have been proposed. In 1927 Sampson[95] proposed that endometriosis is caused by the implantation of endometrial cells during **retrograde menstruation,** in which menstrual fluids move through the fallopian tubes and empty into the pelvic cavity (Figure 23-15). It is now known that retrograde menstruation occurs in almost all women; however, not all women develop endometriosis.

Another theory is that women with endometriosis have impaired cellular and humoral immunity. Alterations in cytokine and growth factor signaling have been identified. Cytotoxic T cell and natural killer (NK) cell activity has been found to be depressed. At the same time, increased numbers of macrophages appear to be stimulating endometrial cell proliferation outside the uterus. An autoimmune response is also suspected.[93] Such alterations may cause the body to tolerate ectopic implantation of endometrial cells. Researchers also have proposed that endometrial cells spread through the lymphatic or vascular systems or that multipotential cells in the epithelial coverings of reproductive organs are somehow stimulated to develop into endometrial and metaplastic cells. A genetic predisposition to endometriosis has been documented. Studies show that incidence and severity of disease are greatest among women with female relatives who also have endometriosis.[93] Some genetic polymorphisms have been identified. Environmental toxins have also been implicated (see What's New? Do Environmental Toxins Contribute to Endometriosis?).

PATHOPHYSIOLOGY Endometrial implants can occur throughout the body but generally occur in the pelvic and abdominal cavities. The most common sites of implantation are the ovaries, uterine ligaments, rectovaginal septum, and pelvic peritoneum (Figure 23-16). Other sites of implantation are the sigmoid colon, small intestine, rectum, appendix,

WHAT'S NEW? Do Environmental Toxins Contribute to Endometriosis

Dioxin and dioxin-like compounds—byproducts of industrial processing—are associated with an increased prevalence of endometriosis and with infertility in women with endometriosis. These compounds may increase interleukin levels, activate cytochrome P-450 enzymes, and create tissue remodeling. Together with estrogen, they stimulate endometriosis formation and blocking of normal progesterone-induced regression of endometrial tissue.

Data from Caserta D et al: *Hum Reprod Update* 14(1):59-72, 2008.

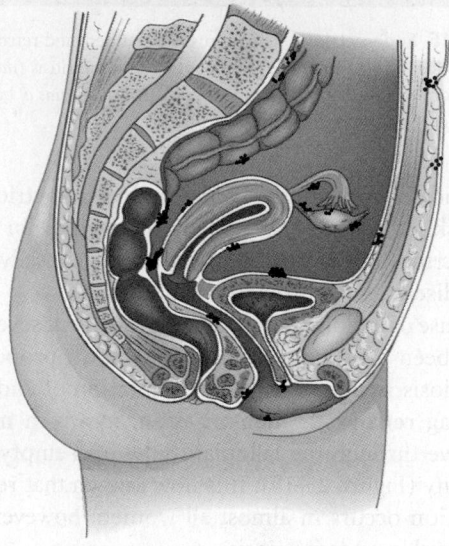

Figure 23-16 Pelvic sites of endometrial implantation. Endometrial cells may enter the pelvic cavity during retrograde menstruation.

bladder, uterus, vulva, vagina, cervix, lymph nodes, extremities, pleural cavity, lungs, laparotomy scars, and hernial sacs.

Cyclic changes depend on the blood supply of the implants and the presence of glandular and stromal cells. Given that blood supply is sufficient, the ectopic endometrium proliferates, breaks down, and bleeds in conjunction with the normal menstrual cycle. The bleeding causes inflammation, triggering a cascade of cellular inflammatory mediators, including cytokines, chemokines, growth factors, and protective factors such as secretory leukocyte protease inhibitor and superoxide dismutase.[93] Pain occurs in surrounding tissues. The inflammation may lead to fibrosis, scarring, and adhesions.

CLINICAL MANIFESTATIONS   The clinical manifestations of endometriosis can mimic other disease processes (i.e., pelvic inflammatory disease, irritable bowel syndrome, ovarian cysts, dysmenorrhea) and are variable in frequency and severity. These include primarily infertility and pain,[93] dysmenorrhea, dyschezia (pain on defecation), dyspareunia (pain on intercourse), and less commonly, constipation, abnormal vaginal bleeding, and if implants are located within the pelvis, an asymptomatic pelvic mass having irregular, movable nodules and a fixed, retroverted uterus. Most symptoms of endometriosis can be explained by the proliferation, breakdown, and bleeding of the ectopic endometrial tissue with subsequent formation of adhesions. In most instances, however, the degree of endometriosis is not related to the frequency or severity of symptoms. Dysmenorrhea, for example, does not appear to be related to the degree of endometriosis. With involvement of the rectovaginal septum or the uterosacral ligaments, dyspareunia develops. Dyschezia, a hallmark symptom of endometriosis, occurs with bleeding of ectopic endometrium in the rectosigmoid musculature and subsequent fibrosis.

Twenty-five percent to 40% of women with infertility have endometriosis. The link between endometriosis and infertility is strong, yet the degree of disease and infertility is not as closely associated. That is, women with untreated minimal to mild disease may have high pregnancy rates or may experience infertility. The exact mechanism for infertility in women with endometriosis is unknown. Infertility may result from mechanical interference with ovulation or ovum transport through the fallopian tube because of adhesions and the effects of inflammation and cytokine activity. There are conflicting reports regarding the effect of endometriosis on sperm activity. An increased phagocytosis of spermatozoa by macrophages has been observed. Some researchers suggest impairment in follicle development as well as embryo development.[96] Implantation defects also are postulated to be present (e.g., decreased uterine receptivity).[93] Oxidative stress is thought to contribute to decreased ovarian and tubal function and further decreases uterine receptivity.[97]

EVALUATION AND TREATMENT   A presumptive diagnosis can be made based on clinical manifestations but laparoscopy is required for definitive diagnosis of endometriosis. A uniform classification system that includes both extent and severity has been developed (Table 23-4) but still does not correlate well with a woman's symptoms. Treatment is aimed at preventing or decreasing progression and spread, alleviating pain, and restoring fertility. Current therapies include suppression of ovulation with noncyclic estrogen-progestin COCs, depot medroxyprogesterone acetate (DMPA), danazol (which diminishes midcycle LH surge), GnRH agonists/analogs (to create a medical oophorectomy), gestrinone (a 19-nortestosterone derivative and antiprogestational steroid), mifepristone (RU486) (an antiprogestational and antiglucocorticoid agent that can inhibit ovulation and disrupt endometrial integrity), and atrophy of endometrium with progestins, including DMPA, oral progestins, or a levonorgestrel-containing IUD.[98,99] A newer therapy is an injectable GnRH antagonist, which produces immediate inhibition of gonadotropin release. GnRH antagonists are shorter acting than GnRH but release histamine at the site of injection. Conservative surgical treatment includes laparoscopic removal of endometrial implants with conventional or laser techniques and presacral neurectomy for severe dysmenorrhea. Effectiveness may be increased when medical regimens are combined with surgical techniques. All treatments have risks or side effects, and recurrent symptoms develop in as many as 74% of women within a few years.[99]

Table 23-4	Classification System for Endometriosis (Requires Laparoscopic Visualization)
Stage	Degree of Invasiveness
I	Minimal
II	Mild
III	Moderate

Classification system also documents the location of lesions and presence of adhesions.

Data from: Practice Committee of the American Society for Reproductive Medicine: *Fertil Steril* 67(5):817-821, 1997.

Cancer

Malignant tumors of the female reproductive system are common. Endometrial carcinoma accounts for approximately 5.8% of all cancers in women, ovarian tumors account for 3.1% of all cancers, and cervical cancers account for 1.6%.[1] Malignant neoplasms of the female reproductive tract account for about 1 in 8 (13.3%) diagnosed cancers and 1 in 9 (11.3%) cancer deaths in women in the United States.[1]

Cervical Cancer

Cancer of the cervix is the most common cancer in women worldwide; however, in the United States, it is the 14th most common type of cancer in women.[1] In the United States, the rates of invasive cancer have steadily decreased (a 75% reduction since the 1960s) and mortality rates caused by cervical cancer have declined (more than 45% since the early 1970s) largely because of the increased prevalence and frequency of cervical cancer screening with the Pap smear. The incidence rate in black women (11.4 per 100,000) exceeds the rate in white women (8.5 per 100,000); the mortality rate is more than double (4.9 per 100,000) for black women compared to the mortality rate for white women (2.3 per 100,000). In 2009, the American Cancer Society estimated 11,270 new cases of cervical invasive cancer and 4070 cervical cancer deaths.[1]

It is now widely know that cervical cancer is almost exclusively caused by cervical human papillomavirus (HPV) infection. Infection with "high-risk" (oncogenic) types of HPV (predominantly 16 and 18) is a necessary precursor to development of the precancerous dysplasia of the cervix that leads to invasive cancer (also see Chapter 11). Precancerous dysplasia, also called *cervical intraepithelial carcinoma (CIN)* or *cervical carcinoma in situ (CIS)*, occurs more often in younger women. Fifty percent of adolescents and young women acquire HPV (predominantly high-risk types) within 3 years of initiation of sexual intercourse; half of these are within 3 months (also see Chapter 24).[100] However, most of these infections are spontaneously cleared by the immune system; the vast majority of these cases do not go on to develop into CIS or invasive cervical cancer.[101] Smoking, immunosuppression, and poor nutrition are considered cofactors, perhaps explaining why some HPV infections do progress to cervical cancer. Infection with *C. trachomatis* also may be a cofactor in

Table 23-5	Cervical Epithelial Cell Abnormalities (Precancerous Cervical Neoplasias)
Cytology Report	Type of Intraepithelial Lesion
Atypical Squamous Cells	
Of undetermined significance (ASC-US)	Suggestive of but do not meet criteria for LSIL (mild dysplasia)
Cannot exclude HSIL (ASC-H)	Do not meet criteria for HSIL but does not preclude HSIL (potentially CIN I/II; moderate to severe dysplasia)
LSIL	CIN I (mild dysplasia)
HSIL	CIN II and III (moderate to severe dysplasia and CIS

ASC-H, Atypical squamous cells, cannot exclude high-grade squamous intraepithelial lesion; *ASC-US*, atypical squamous cells of undetermined significance; *CIN*, cervical intraepithelial neoplasia; *CIS*, carcinoma in situ; *HSIL*, high-grade squamous intraepithelial lesion; *LSIL*, low-grade squamous intraepithelial lesion.

the development of one type of cervical cancer; squamous cell invasive cervical cancer.[102] Human immunodeficiency virus (HIV)–positive women also are at greater risk for developing cervical cancer.[101,103] Specific guidelines for screening and follow-up of abnormal cytology or positive HPV testing for HIV-positive women are available.[103]

PATHOGENESIS   Cervical cancer is a slowly progressive disease that is staged according to histology (Tables 23-5 and 23-6). Testing for high-risk HPV is often positive for many years (10 or more) before dysplasia progresses to a high-grade squamous intraepithelial lesion (HSIL) prior to invasive cervical cancer. Other than HPV infection, the genetics of cervical cancer remains poorly understood. Several chromosome regions with recurrent loss of heterozygosity (LOH) have been identified (also see Chapter 11). However, the problematic tumor suppressor genes located on these chromosomal locations are yet to be identified. Recurrent amplifications have been mapped to the short arm of chromosome 3 in invasive cancer. Like other cancers, cervical cancer requires the accumulation of genetic alterations for carcinogenesis to occur.

The progressive changes of cervical cells are classified on a continuum from cervical intraepithelial neoplasia (dysplasia), to cervical carcinoma in situ (full epithelial thickness of the cervix is involved), to invasive carcinoma (see Tables 23-5 and 23-6). Cervical dysplasia is replacement of some epithelial cells by atypical, neoplastic cells, and is "staged" depending on the depth of epithelial involvement (Figure 23-17). In cervical CIN III or HSIL, all or most of the cervical epithelium shows cellular features of carcinoma, but underlying tissue is not affected. Risk of progression to invasive carcinoma rises steadily with the severity of dysplasia. Women with CIN I (low grade intraepithelial lesion [LSIL] or mild dysplasia) have an 11% chance of progression to CIS and a 1% chance of progression to cervical invasion. Women with CIN II have a 22% chance of progression to CIS and a 5% chance of invasive lesions. At least 12% of women with CIN III (CIS) progress to cervical invasion. More than half (57%) of women with CIN I, 43% of women with CIN II, and 32% of women with CIN III will have a natural "regression" of lesions. At least a third or more of all cervical intraepithelial lesions will simply persist without progression or regression.

Carcinoma in situ is most likely to develop in the squamous-columnar junction—the so-called transformation zone—where the columnar epithelium of the cervical lining meets the squamous epithelium of the outer cervix and vagina (Figure 23-18). In this zone, columnar epithelium is constantly being replaced by squamous epithelium in a process known as *metaplasia*. Metaplasia is thought to be affected by hormonal levels; change in cervical epithelium is not understood as well as endometrial tissue change in response to fluctuating hormones. Because metaplastic cells are at increased risk of incorporating foreign or abnormal genetic material, neoplastic changes are most common in the transformation zone.

Carcinoma in situ is generally a precursor of invasive carcinoma of the cervix. A number of factors, including tumor type, contribute to the rate at which carcinoma in situ becomes invasive. **Invasive carcinoma of the cervix** consists of direct invasion into adjacent tissues and metastasis through the lymphatics. Adjacent tissues most often involved are the ureters and structures of the lateral pelvic wall, the vaginal stroma and epithelium, and the lower uterine segment and myometrium. The internal, external, and common iliac lymph nodes and the obturator nodes are common sites of lymphatic involvement. A staging system for carcinoma of the cervix is shown in Table 23-6.

CLINICAL MANIFESTATIONS Because cervical neoplasms are asymptomatic, regular Pap test or HPV screening is necessary. About 90% of cervical cancer cases can be detected early through the use of regular screening tests (see What's New? Is the Pap Smear for Cervical Cancer Screening Obsolete?). If symptoms exist, they may include vaginal bleeding or abnormal discharge. Bleeding is variable

Table 23-6	Clinical Staging for Cancer of the Cervix
Stage	**Characteristics**
0	Cancer in situ, intraepithelial carcinoma; earliest stage of cancer; cancer confined to its original site
I	Carcinoma confined to cervix (extension to corpus disregarded)
IA	Earliest form of stage I; there is very small amount of cancer, which is visible only under a microscope
IA1	Area of invasion is <3 mm (about 1/8 inch) deep and <7 mm (about 1/3 inch) wide
IA2	Area of invasion is between 3 mm and 5 mm (about 1/5 inch) deep, and <7 mm (about 1/3 inch) wide
IB	Includes cancers that can be seen without a microscope; also includes cancers seen only with a microscope that have spread deeper than 5 mm (about 1/5 inch) into connective tissue of the cervix or are wider than 7 mm
IB1	A IB cancer that is no larger than 4 cm (about 1 3/5 inches)
IB2	A IB cancer that is >4 cm
II	Cancer has spread beyond the cervix to the upper part of the vagina; cancer does not involve the lower third of the vagina
IIA	Cancer has spread beyond the cervix to the upper part of the vagina; cancer does not involve the lower third of the vagina
IIB	Cancer has spread to the tissue next to the cervix, called the *parametrial tissue*
III	Cancer has spread to the lower part of the vagina or the pelvic wall; cancer may be blocking the ureters (tubes that carry urine from the kidneys to the bladder)
IIIA	Cancer has spread to the lower third of the vagina but not to the pelvic wall
IIIB	Cancer extends to the pelvic wall, blocks urine flow to the bladder, or both
IV	Most advanced stage of cervical cancer; cancer has spread to other parts of the body
IVA	Cancer has spread to the bladder or rectum, which are organs close to the cervix
IVB	Cancer has spread to distant organs beyond the pelvic area, such as the lungs

Reprinted from the American Cancer Society's Cancer Information Database with permission.

WHAT'S NEW?

Is the Pap Smear for Cervical Cancer Screening Obsolete?

The problem with the use of the conventional Papanicolaou (Pap) smear in screening for cervical cancer is the low sensitivity of the test, which ranges between 44% and 77%. This means that a large number of cervical abnormalities (23% to 56%) can be missed with a single test! Thus the success of Pap smear screening in reducing cervical cancer in the United States lies in the frequency of screenings (annually for most women) and the fact that cervical cancer is almost always a slowly progressive condition. However, a high frequency of Pap smear screenings is often not feasible, either economically, socially, culturally, or logistically, in many countries and in some regions and populations in the United States leading to much higher rates of invasive cervical cancer for women in such populations or locales. Multiple, large, well-conducted studies have demonstrated that human papillomavirus (HPV) testing is considerably more sensitive (between 97% and 98%) than either conventional or liquid-based Pap testing. HPV infection is known to be the required precursor to cervical cancer. With sensitive HPV tests now widely available, requiring less frequent screening (every 3 years), and with rapid return of results, the future of cervical cancer screening may rely almost exclusively on this newer technology, not on conventional cervical cytology testing. For those women with a positive HPV screening test, management decisions may still require at least a "reflexive" cytology (Pap) test that can be conducted on the same cervical sample collected for the HPV screening or colposcopy or both.

Data from Koliopoulos G et al: *HPV testing versus cervical cytology for screening for cancer of the uterine cervix (protocol)*, The Cochrane Collaboration, 2008; Widdice LE, Moscicki AB: *J Adolesc Health* 43(4 Suppl):S41-S51, 2008; Wright TC Jr: *Clin Obstet Gynecol* 50(2):313-323, 2007.

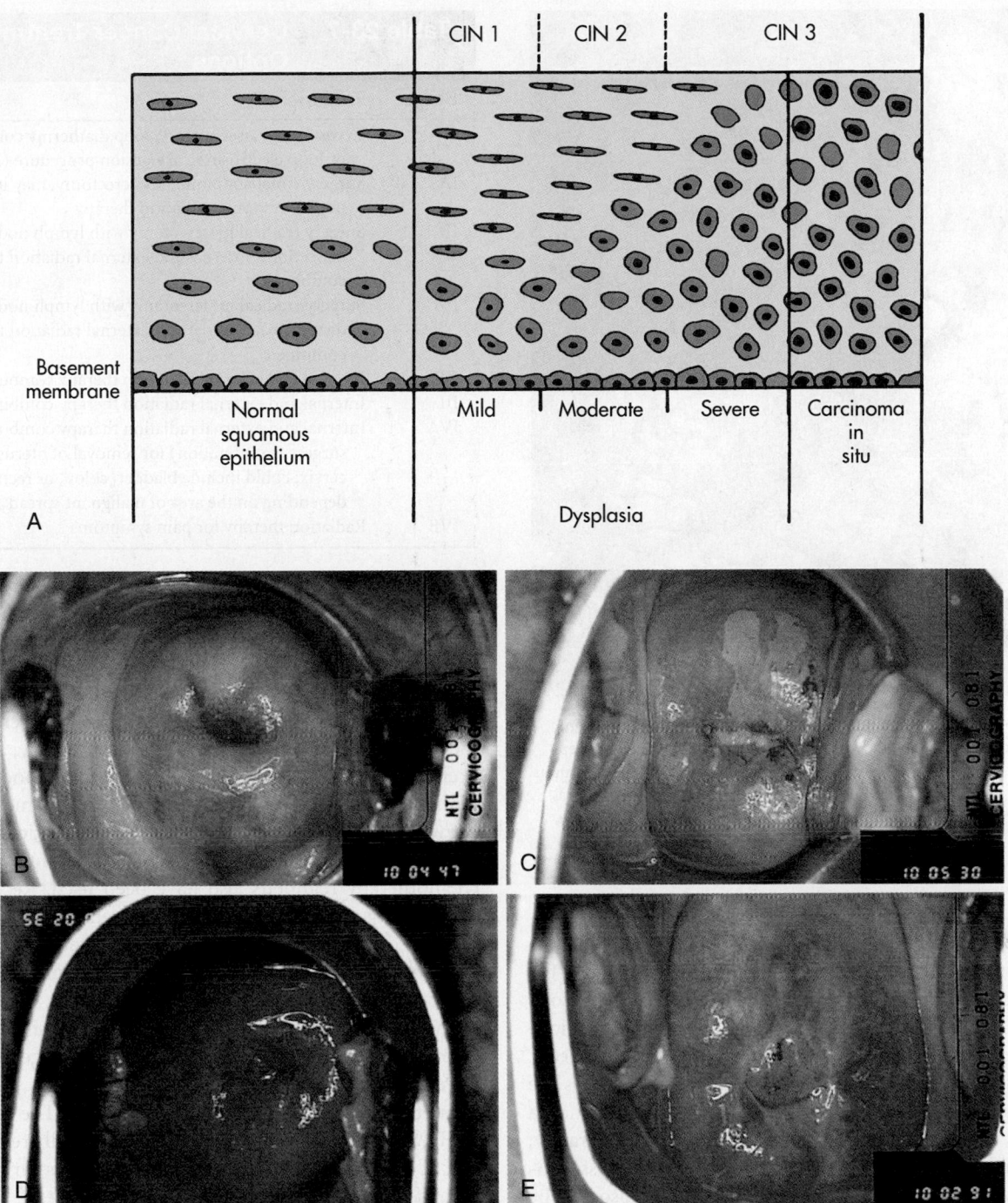

Figure 23-17 Cervical intraepithelial neoplasia (CIN). A, Diagram of cervical endothelium showing progressive degrees of CIN. B, Normal multiparous cervix. C, CIN stage 1. Note the white appearance of part of the anterior lip of the cervix associated with neoplastic changes. D, CIN stage 2. Lesions reflected in distant capillaries. E, CIN stage 3. Lesion predominantly around the external os. (A from Herbst AL et al: *Comprehensive gynecology*, ed 2, St Louis, 1992, Mosby. B-E, from Symonds EM, Macpherson MBA: *Color atlas of obstetrics and gynecology*, London, 1994, Mosby-Wolfe.)

and may occur after intercourse or between menstrual periods. At times, women will complain of abnormal menses or postmenopausal bleeding. Vaginal discharge is a less common presenting symptom and may be serosanguineous or yellowish. A new or foul odor also may be present. Bleeding and discharge are subtle and are likely to be disregarded by premenopausal women, who mistake these signs for variations of normal processes. Postmenopausal women are more likely to seek medical attention if these signs appear. With severe bleeding, symptoms of anemia may occur. Pelvic or epigastric pain is experienced only with large lesions. Advanced disease may cause urinary or rectal symptoms and pelvic or back pain.

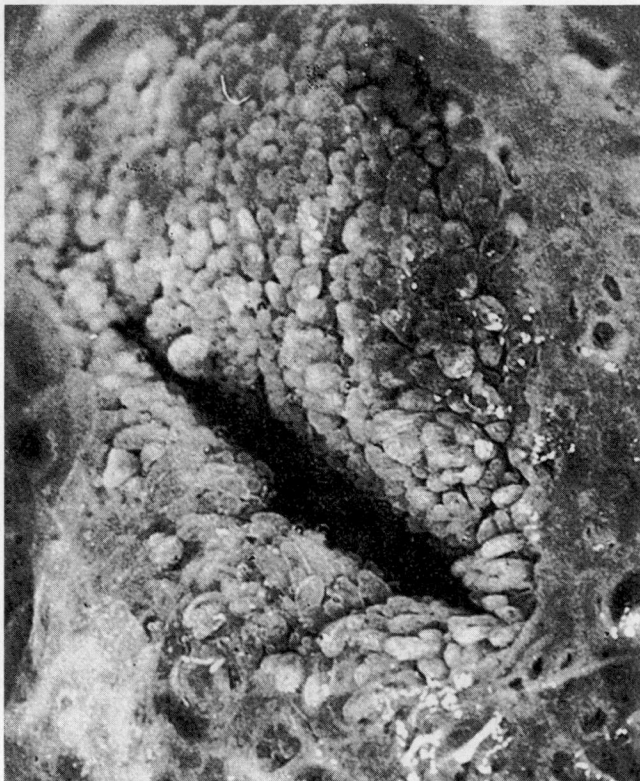

Figure 23-18 Cervical carcinoma in situ. Typical transformation zone, where the columnar (grapelike) epithelium is replaced by metaplastic epithelium. At its outer edge, the metaplastic epithelium adjoins the squamous epithelium, which extends into the vagina. (From Coppleson M, Pixley E, Reid B: *Colposcopy: a scientific approach to the cervix in health and disease,* Springfield, IL, 1971, Charles C Thomas.)

Table 23-7	Cervical Cancer Treatment Options
Stage	**Treatment**
0	Cryosurgery, laser surgery, loop diathermy conization, or loop electrosurgical excision procedure (LEEP)
IA	Surgery (total abdominal hysterectomy, may include oophorectomy), radiation therapy
IB	Surgery (radical hysterectomy with lymph node dissection), internal and external radiation therapy combined
IIA	Surgery (radical hysterectomy with lymph node dissection), internal and external radiation therapy combined
IIB	Internal and external radiation therapy combined
III	Internal and external radiation therapy combined
IVA	Internal and external radiation therapy combined; surgery (exenteration) for removal of uterus, vagina, cervix; could include bladder, colon, or rectum depending on the area of malignant spread
IVB	Radiation therapy for pain symptoms

EVALUATION AND TREATMENT Cervical cytology is most accurate if cells are obtained from both the endo- and ectocervix. When dysplasia is detected, colposcopy is usually indicated to identify lesions and for obtaining biopsies of the ectocervix and curettage biopsy of the endocervix. The transformation zone moves higher into the cervix as age increases, making biopsy more difficult. If invasive carcinoma is found, lymphangiography, CT scan, ultrasonography, or radioimmunodetection methods are used to assess lymphatic involvement. Cystoscopy and proctoscopy also may be performed.

The treatment depends on the degree of neoplastic change, the size and location of the lesion, and the extent of metastatic spread. For premalignant change or CIS (stage 0), cryosurgery or carbon dioxide laser therapy is commonly used; laser treatment may produce better results in the multiparous cervix. Loop diathermy conization and the loop electrosurgical excision procedure (LEEP) are alternative treatments. In LEEP, a small, looped wire with electric current generates heat and burns off cancer cells. Conization is removal of a cone-shaped section of tissue that includes the cancer; high-frequency current is used with cold-knife conization. The amount of tissue removed depends on the location of the lesion. None of these measures affects fertility or childbearing.

For invasive cervical carcinoma, treatment depends on the stage of the tumor (Table 23-7). Surgical intervention may include a hysterectomy, pelvic lymphadenectomy, and pelvic exenteration (radical removal of contents of body cavity). Radiation therapy is used most often in cases of small cell cancer with lymphatic involvement. External radiation usually is combined with one or two intracavitary implants. Multidrug chemotherapy regimens also have been used. Recent phase 3 trials suggest significant improvement in survival with combined chemotherapy and radiation therapy.[104] Smokers tend to have a higher stage of disease at diagnosis, and their cancer is more resistant to radiation treatment.

With early detection and treatment, prognosis is excellent. Overall, the 5-year survival rate is 95% for stage IA or lower (e.g., early detection). A cure rate of 100% is possible for women with dysplasia or carcinoma in situ.[1] The prevention of HPV infection may be the key to substantially reducing the risk of cervical cancer. FDA-approved vaccines for two of the high-risk types of HPV show excellent promise.[105,106]

Vaginal Cancer

Cancer of the vagina is the rarest of the female genital cancers and accounts for less than 2% of gynecologic cancers.[107] About 90% are squamous cell-type cancers; the remaining 10% of tumors are adenocarcinomas, sarcomas (rare), and melanomas (rare). Women with either an in situ or an invasive cervical or vulvar squamous cell cancer are at increased risk for squamous cell abnormality of the vagina, and may have a similar etiology.[108] The mean age of women with invasive cancer of the vagina is 55 years; carcinoma in situ occurs about 10 years earlier. However, vaginal neoplasia is increasingly seen in younger women, likely because of an increase in HPV infection at younger ages. Vaginal sarcomas develop in children younger than 5 years and in women in the fifth to sixth decades. Clear-cell carcinomas, the most common form of adenocarcinomas, occur in conjunction with vaginal adenosis in young women with a history of in utero diethylstilbestrol (DES) exposure. Metastatic adenocarcinomas arise from the urethra, Bartholin gland, rectum, bladder, endometrium, endocervix, ovary, or a distant organ.[108]

Vaginal and cervical cancers are thought to have similar epidemiology. Both start as intraepithelial lesions, occur in sexually active women, and are associated with HPV infection.[108,109] As mentioned, prior carcinoma of the cervix places a woman at higher risk for developing vaginal cancer. In utero exposure to nonsteroidal estrogens also has been considered a risk factor. It has been estimated that 100,000 to 160,000 women were exposed in utero to such nonsteroidal estrogens as DES, dienestrol, or hexestrol from 1960 to 1970. Apparently, exposure to such hormones during the first 3 months of gestation inhibits the normal replacement of columnar epithelium by squamous epithelium in the vagina of the fetus. The columnar epithelium, which is not normally found in the vagina, then may undergo malignant transformation. Not all women exposed to DES in utero develop neoplastic changes in the vagina, however. Between 0.14 and 1.4 cases of vaginal cancer develop per 1000 women at risk. Nineteen years is the average age at which clear-cell carcinoma develops as a result of DES exposure.

Like cervical neoplasms, vaginal cancers are classified as intraepithelial neoplasia (dysplasia), carcinoma in situ, or invasive carcinoma and are staged based on extension into local tissues and metastasis to distant organs. Vaginal cancer is generally asymptomatic, discovered by vaginal cytologic examination, and confirmed by colposcopy and biopsy. The major symptom of invasive cancer, independent of type, is vaginal bleeding (bloody discharge). Advanced disease causes vaginal discharge, vulvar pruritus, rectal or bladder symptoms, and pain or leg edema.

Biopsy techniques confirm the tumor type and determine its size, location, and extent. Treatment depends on these findings and the age of the individual. Vaginal dysplasia or carcinoma in situ is excised with upper vaginectomy, laser ablation or loop electrosurgical excision, cryotherapy, or laser surgery.[108] Topical 5-fluorouracil (5-FU) also may be used. If the lesion is invasive, surgery may include hysterectomy and pelvic bilateral inguinal lymphadenectomy. Radiation and chemotherapy may follow surgery. Approximately 40% of individuals with invasive vaginal cancer develop recurrent cancer, which usually is confined to the pelvic area. The 5-year survival rate is 70% to 75% for early disease, 30% to 40% for stage III, and rare for stage IV.

Vulvar Cancer

Cancer of the vulva is responsible for about 3% to 5% of all gynecologic cancers[107]; an incidence of 3580 new cases was estimated for 2009.[1] The majority (90%) are squamous cell carcinomas, although melanoma (5%), Bartholin gland

carcinoma (2%), sarcoma (2%), and adenosquamous carcinoma (1%) may occur.[110] A history of HPV infection is a risk factor but less so than with cervical or vaginal lesions. Squamous dysplasia of the vagina or cervix is a major risk factor,[109] as are smoking and coffee use.[110] Although it usually affects postmenopausal women (median age of presentation is women in their 60s), vulvar cancer has been diagnosed in women between ages 30 and 90. Although leukoplakia and lichen sclerosus were believed to be precursors, no prospective studies have been able to confirm such a relationship. Usually, women have a long history of vulvar irritation and pruritus (70%); urinary symptoms and discharge are less common. In addition, women may have a hard ulcerated area of the vulva, large cauliflower lesions, or lesions similar to those of chronic dermatitis. Biopsy confirms the diagnosis. Treatment options include primarily ablative or excisional surgery, and sometimes radiation with or without chemotherapy.[110] Topical treatments under investigation include imiquimod cream, cidofovir emulsion, and 5-FU cream. Prognosis depends on lesion size and location, histology, and lymph involvement; risk of metastasis increases with tumor size. The 5-year survival rate is 85% to 90% for stage I and decreases to 20% for stage IV cancer.[110]

Endometrial Cancer and Uterine Sarcoma

Endometrial carcinomas arise within the glandular epithelium of the uterine lining. Cancer of the endometrium is the most common cancer of the pelvic region in women and accounts for 5.8% of all cancers in women. Estimates include 40,100 new cases in 2008, with approximately 3470 deaths.[1,107] Although incidence rates are higher in white than in black women, mortality rates in black women are nearly twice as high. Most cases occur in postmenopausal women (Figure 23-19), with peak incidence occurring in the late 50s to early 60s.[111] One in 30 American women will develop endometrial cancer. The primary risk factor is unopposed estrogen exposure with resultant hyperplasia.[111] The World Health Organization has divided endometrial hyperplasia into two major categories according to whether cytologic atypia is present;

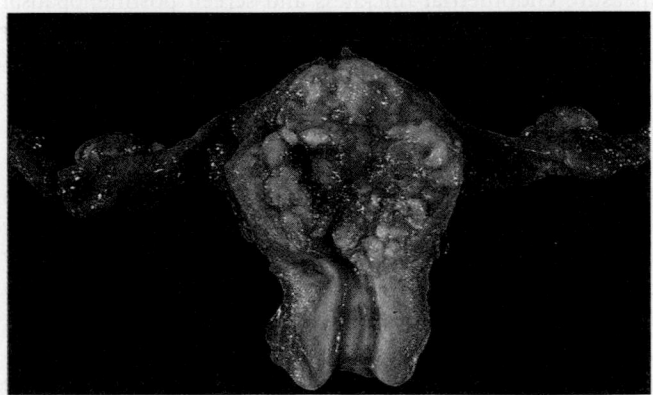

Figure 23-19 Endometrial cancer. Tumor fills the endometrial cavity. Obvious myometrial invasion is seen. (From Damjanov I, Linder J, editors: *Anderson's pathology*, ed 10, St Louis, 2000, Mosby.)

only atypical hyperplasia has a significant risk of progressing to well-differentiated endometrial carcinoma. Estrogen-related exposures include unopposed (without an accompanying progestin) estrogen replacement therapy, tamoxifen, early menarche, late menopause, never having children, and a failure to ovulate (i.e., PCOS and anovulatory cycles typical of the late reproductive years). Obesity also is a known source of endogenous estrogen and is a risk factor for endometrial cancer. Other coexisting factors include diabetes, gallbladder disease, and hypertension likely related to obesity effects. A family history of colon, endometrial, or ovarian cancer could signal hereditary nonpolyposis colorectal cancer (HNPCC) and indicates further genetic testing.[112]

Pregnancy and the use of combined hormonal contraceptives (i.e., COCs) containing synthetic estrogen and progestin have a protective effect as do progestin-containing IUDs.[113] After 12 months of COC use, the risk of endometrial cancer is half that among women who have never used COCs; this effect seems to persist for at least 10 to 20 years after birth control pills are discontinued.[111] Controlling obesity, hypertension, and diabetes may reduce an individual's risk of endometrial cancer. A review of modifiable risk factors and prevention for endometrial hyperplasia and cancer indicates that obesity, inactivity, and dietary habits are considerable risk factors.[114] The review authors advise that endometrial cancer prevention should also target these modifiable risk factors to include exercise, weight reduction, and increased fiber.[115]

About 75% of endometrial cancers are adenocarcinomas. Abnormal vaginal bleeding is the most common clinical manifestation of endometrial cancer. The bleeding is caused by disruption of the endometrial surface by neoplastic processes. Pain and weight loss are symptoms of late disease.

Screening methods for early detection of endometrial cancer are as effective as those for cervical cancer. Pap tests, which are highly effective in detecting cervical dysplasia, are ineffective in detecting early endometrial cancer.[111] Endometrial biopsies, which allow for direct cytologic sampling of the endometrium, are required for diagnosis and are recommended to screen high-risk women at menopause and periodically. Transvaginal ultrasound (TVUS) may be used to measure endometrial thickness and screen postmenopausal and high-risk premenopausal women. An endometrial depth of less than 5 mm is suggestive of atrophic endometrium.[111] Although cancer antigen (CA-125) is not a useful screen for endometrial cancer, it may predict the presence of extrauterine diseases that contribute to an undesired estrogenic environment (i.e., ovarian granulosa cell tumors increase estrogen levels and have an associated 30% risk of endometrial cancer).[111] Once cancer is confirmed by biopsy, a laparoscopy may be performed to determine stage of disease. Evaluation for metastasis includes routine blood work, metabolic studies, chest x-rays, intravenous pyelography (IVP), barium enema, ultrasonography, lymphangiography, CT, MRI, and bone scans.

Treatment is based on the extent of the disease. For women with nonatypical hyperplasia, progestin therapy (orally or through levonorgestrel-containing IUD) may often suffice. However, treatment for atypical hyperplasia usually includes surgical intervention, such as curettage for carcinoma in situ, total abdominal hysterectomy with bilateral salpingo-oophorectomy, and lymphadenectomy. Chemotherapy, radiation, or hormone therapy with progestins also may be used in combination. The 1-year relative survival rate for endometrial cancer is 93%; the 5-year relative survival rate is 95% with early diagnosis and 64% if diagnosis occurred in the late stage. Relative survival rates for white women exceed those for black women by at least 18% at every stage.

Uterine sarcomas are rare neoplasms that arise from myometrial smooth muscle, endometrial stroma, or more rarely ubiquitous connective tissue elements. Uterine sarcomas constitute 2% to 8% of all uterine malignancies. The average age at diagnosis is the early 50s. The very low occurrence of these tumors explains the lack of epidemiologic data. Thus relatively few risk factors have been identified. However, chronic excess estrogen exposure, tamoxifen, and black race have been cited as risks. Symptoms include abnormal uterine bleeding, awareness of a mass, and pelvic pressure or pain. Vaginal discharge may be profuse and foul. Gastrointestinal and genitourinary complaints are common. The uterus often enlarges rapidly. Most commonly, serendipitous diagnosis occurs at the time of surgery for leiomyomas. Treatment consists of total hysterectomy with bilateral salpingo-oophorectomy and selective lymphadenectomy followed by radiation therapy. Five-year survival rates range from 50% in early disease to 5% in advanced disease. Like most cancers, stage is the most important determinant of prognosis. The survival rate at 5 years for stage I disease is 50%. Few women survive advanced-stage disease.[116]

Ovarian Cancer

The incidence of ovarian cancer is estimated as 21,550 women in the United States in 2009.[1] In 2009 ovarian cancer accounted for 3% of all cancers among women and caused more deaths (14,600) than any other female reproductive cancer.[1] From 2001 to 2005, the incidence declined at a rate of 3% per year. Ovarian cancer in women older than 40 years is associated with early menarche, late menopause, nulliparity, and the use of fertility drugs. Race and prior pelvic radiation also appear to increase risk. Factors that suppress ovulation decrease the risk of ovarian cancer and include multiple pregnancies, prolonged lactation, and the use of oral contraceptives. Oral contraceptives inhibit ovulation, and progestins likely have a direct biologic effect on ovarian tissue.[117]

PATHOGENESIS   The cause of ovarian cancer is unknown at present. The great majority (approximately 90%) of ovarian cancers are sporadic and not associated with a known pattern of inheritance.[118] Of the 5% to 10% that are familial, the majority are associated with the breast cancer susceptibility gene 1 (*BRCA1*) and a smaller number with mutations of *BRCA2* or mismatched repair genes (HNPCC syndrome). Various pathways have been proposed, including the aberrant cellular proliferation that occurs with repetitive ovulatory tissue repair in the ovary. Spontaneous *TP53* (a tumor-suppressor gene) mutations accompany this proliferation and likely play a major role in carcinogenesis activity.[119] In sporadic ovarian cancer, *BRCA1* and *BRCA2* are rarely mutated.

The two major types of ovarian cancer are epithelial ovarian neoplasms and germ-cell neoplasms. Most ovarian malignancies are epithelial ovarian neoplasms that usually develop from the surface epithelium of the ovary or that which line cysts immediately beneath the ovarian surface. Most epithelial cancers arise from a single cell (i.e., clonal), involve loss of tumor suppressor genes, and activate oncogenes (see Chapter 11). Therefore, a number of abnormalities, including LOH, and amplification of several chromosomes are observed. Epithelial ovarian tumors may be serous, mucinous, endometrioid, or undifferentiated. These tumors are classified as (1) benign, (2) borderline malignant, or (3) frankly malignant (Figure 23-20). The malignant forms are collectively classed as ovarian adenocarcinomas and account for 90% of all ovarian malignancies. Of the ovarian adenocarcinomas, 40% to 50% are serous epithelial malignancies, which usually involve both ovaries and tend to be bulky. Serous tumors generally affect women from 50 to 55 years of age and are extremely rare in prepubertal girls. The 5-year survival rate is 90% if treated in stage I; however, only 25% of ovarian cancers are diagnosed this early. Five-year survival rates decline with stage of disease: 40% to 60% of women with stage II disease survive 5 years, 15% to 20% with stage III disease survive 5 years, and less than 5% with stage IV disease survive 5 years.[120]

Germ-cell tumors are derived from the primitive germ cells (gametes) of the embryonic gonad and may be malignant or benign. The benign cystic teratoma accounts for approximately 10% of all ovarian tumors. If the germ-cell tumor is malignant, it tends to be a highly aggressive and rapidly growing tumor with a poor prognosis. Germ-cell tumors almost always occur in children or adolescents.

CLINICAL MANIFESTATIONS   Given the location of the ovaries, assessing abnormalities on routine gynecologic examination poses difficulty. Furthermore, early disease is commonly asymptomatic. Thus the disease is frequently diagnosed after metastasis has occurred. Consequently, ovarian cancer is often termed the *silent killer*. The intrapelvic location of the ovaries and the range of tumor activity (from slow to rapid and relentless growth) cause diverse signs and symptoms. The most obvious symptoms are pain and abdominal swelling that arise from the primary ovarian mass or ascites and abdominal distention (Figure 23-21). Gastrointestinal manifestations may include dyspepsia, vomiting, and alterations in bowel habits caused by mechanical obstruction. Abnormal vaginal bleeding may occur if the postmenopausal endometrium is stimulated by a hormone-secreting tumor. The tumor also may cause ulcerations through the vaginal wall that result in bleeding. There also can be a feeling of pressure in the pelvis and leg pain.

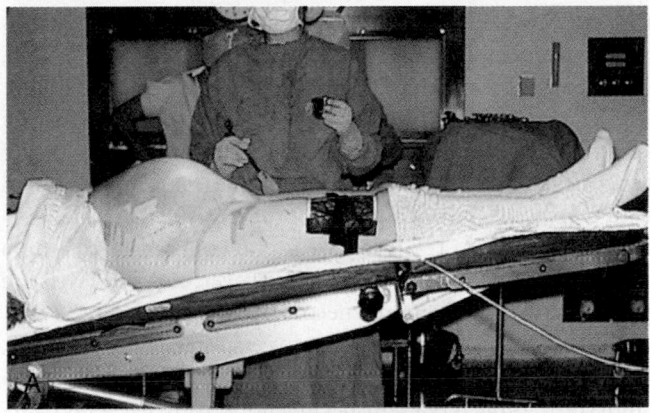

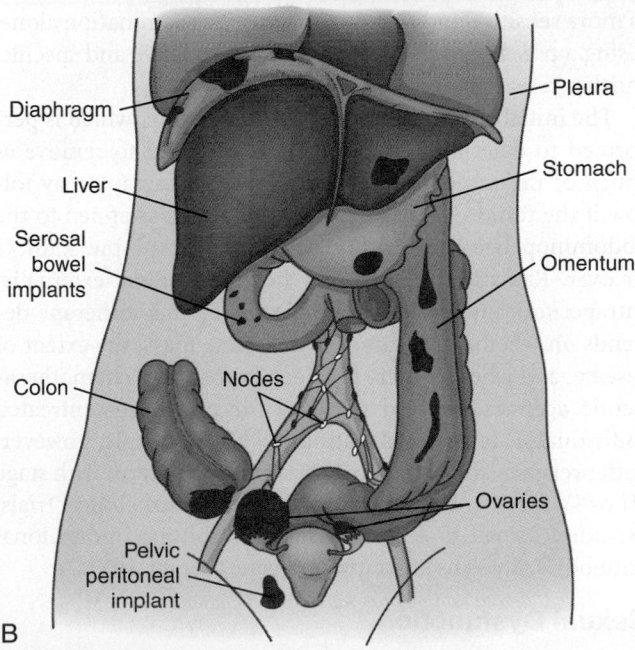

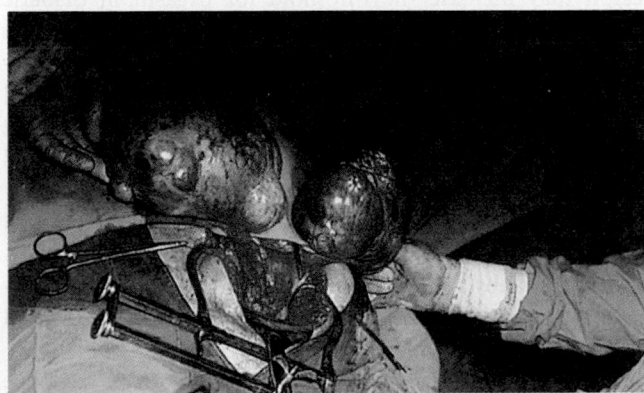

Figure 23-20 Ovarian tumors. Bilateral multicystic ovarian tumors. (From Symonds EM, Macpherson MBA: *Color atlas of obstetrics and gynecology,* London, 1994, Mosby-Wolfe.)

Figure 23-21 Large malignant ovarian tumor and metastasis of ovarian cancer. A, Tumor has caused massive abdominal distention. B, Pattern of spread for epithelial cancer of the ovary. (A from Symonds EM, Macpherson MBA: *Color atlas of obstetrics and gynecology,* London, 1994, Mosby-Wolfe.)

Systemic manifestations of nonmetastatic malignant disease include connective tissue inflammation (dermatomyositis), abnormal pigmentation (acanthosis nigricans), and subacute cerebellar degeneration. Tumor obstruction of vascular channels can cause venous and, occasionally, arterial thrombosis. Alterations in coagulability also occur, contributing to clot formation. Metastasis often causes pleural effusion.

EVALUATION AND TREATMENT Because ovarian cancer has no early symptoms and no effective screening techniques can detect it, disease usually is advanced by the time treatment is sought. Diagnosis is confirmed by biopsy, and extent of the disease is determined by ultrasound, CT, MRI, or other imaging techniques. Women undergoing surgery for early-stage ovarian cancer need thorough checking for spread to the abdomen and lymph nodes. Staging of disease requires exploratory surgery. The International Federation of Gynecologists and Obstetricians (FIGO) staging system is described in Table 23-8. Other preoperative studies may be used to determine the extent of metastasis. These include an upper gastrointestinal series, barium enema, IVP, mammography, and lymphography.

The search for a tumor marker that could be used as a screening tool for ovarian cancer is ongoing. Some types of germ cells and, rarely, adenocarcinoma may be associated with increased levels of alpha fetoprotein (AFP), hCG, or CA-125. Increased CA-125 levels are found in about 78% to 80% of nonmucinous ovarian cancers; however, elevated levels are produced in 29% of nongynecologic tumors and in a variety of noncancerous conditions, for example, endometriosis, PID, benign ovarian cysts, myomas, and pregnancy. Carcinoembryonic antigen is a nonspecific, nonsensitive test for ovarian cancer; when combined with transvaginal ultrasound, it is more sensitive and accurate than pelvic examination alone. Using a panel of markers may be more sensitive and specific. Further research is needed.[121]

The initial approach to treatment is surgery, which is performed to determine the stage of disease and to remove as much of the tumor as possible. Radiation therapy may follow if the tumor is smaller than 2 cm and is confined to the abdominopelvic area without involvement of the kidneys or liver. Radiation therapy may be administered externally, intraperitoneally, or both. The success of chemotherapy depends on whether the tumor is a discrete mass, the extent of disease, and whether there has been exposure to chemotherapeutic agents. The gold standard for previously untreated individuals is taxane and platinum.[122] Most people, however, suffer relapses and less than 20% survive long term with stage III or IV disease. New therapies have extended clinical trials, including small-molecular-weight inhibitors, monoclonal antibodies, antisense therapy, and gene therapy.[122]

Sexual Dysfunction

Increased awareness of female sexual dysfunction is relatively new, and most of what is known comes from clinical observations and anecdotal reports from women. Adequate research is still needed. Both organic and psychosocial disorders

Stage	Characteristics
I	Growth limited to the ovaries
IA	Growth limited to one ovary; no ascites
IA1	No tumor on the external surface; capsule intact (90% 5-year survival with treatment)
IA2	Tumor present on the external surface, or capsule(s) ruptured, or both
IB	Growth limited to both ovaries; no ascites
IB1	No tumor on the external surface; capsule intact
IB2	Tumor present on the external surface, or capsule(s) ruptured, or both
IC	Tumor either stage IA or stage IB, with ascites present or with positive peritoneal washings
II	Growth involving one or both ovaries with pelvic extension
IIA	Extension and/or metastases to the uterus and/or tubes
IIB	Extension to other pelvic tissues
IIC	Tumor either stage IIA or stage IIB but with ascites present or with positive peritoneal washings
III	Growth involving one or both ovaries with intraperitoneal metastases outside the pelvis, or positive retroperitoneal nodes, or both; tumor limited to the true pelvis with histologically proven malignant extension to small bowel or omentum
IV	Growth involving one or both ovaries with distant metastases; if pleural effusion is present, there must be positive cytology to allot a case to stage IV; parenchymal liver metastases indicate stage IV
Special category	Unexplored cases that are thought to be ovarian carcinoma

FIGO, International Federation of Gynecologists and Obstetricians.

can be implicated in sexual dysfunction. Organic problems may be the underlying cause in 10% to 20% of cases and can contribute to another 15%. The exact cause may not always be identified.

As in men, chronic illness can affect sexual functioning and response in women. For example, neuropathy in the pelvic region may increase the threshold for orgasm in diabetic women. Diminished intensity and gradual decline in orgasm may be analogous to the development of impotence in diabetic men. For women with heart disease, problems in sexual functioning more often are related to drug therapy than the disease itself. Table 23-9 outlines possible effects of specified chronic diseases on female sexual functioning.

Disorders of desire (inhibited sexual desire, decreased libido) may be a biologic manifestation of depression, alcohol or other substance abuse, prolactin-secreting pituitary tumors, or testosterone deficiency. β-Adrenergic blockers used for heart disease also may inhibit sexual desire.

Vaginismus is an involuntary muscle spasm in response to attempted penetration. Common causes include prior sexual trauma or fear of sex; organic causes are less common and are similar to those that cause dyspareunia, including

Table 23-9	Possible Effects of Chronic Disease on Sexual Functioning in Women
Disease	**Sexual Function**
Cerebral palsy	Intact genital sensations, decreased lubrication; difficulty with sexual activity/positioning because of muscle spasticity, rigidity, and/or weakness; pain with positioning caused by contracture of knees and hips or because of increased spasms with arousal
Cerebrovascular accident (CVA)	Difficulties in sexual positioning and sensitivity because of impaired motor strength, coordination or paralysis; decreased sex drive with stroke on the dominant side of the brain
Diabetes	Diminished intensity of orgasm and gradual decline in ability to achieve orgasm; decreased lubrication and/or recurrent vaginal infections with resultant dyspareunia
Chronic renal failure	Decreased arousal; increasingly rare and less intense orgasms; decreased lubrication
Rheumatoid arthritis (RA)	Painful sexual activity/positions because of swollen, painful joints, muscular atrophy and joint contracture; decreased sex drive because of pain, fatigue, and/or medication; genital sensations remain intact
Systemic lupus erythematosus (SLE)	Similar to RA; decreased lubrication and vaginal lesions result in painful penetration
Myocardial infarction (MI)	Most literature male oriented; problems related to medications
Multiple sclerosis (MS)	Diminished genital sensitivity; decreased lubrication; declining orgasmic ability; difficulty with sexual activity because of muscle weakness, pain, or incontinence
Spinal cord injury	Reflex sexual response with injury above sacral area; disrupted response with lesion at or below sacrum; loss of sensation, decreased lubrication; spasticity, incontinence, or pain with arousal; continued orgasmic sensations or sensations diffused in general or to specific body parts, such as breast or lips

vulvovestibulitis. Even after the underlying organic problem is detected and successfully treated, vaginismus may persist.

Anorgasmia or **orgasmic dysfunction** is the inability of the woman to reach or achieve orgasm. Dysfunction follows a continuum from difficulty in arousal to lack of orgasm. Any chronic illness may affect arousal. Orgasmic dysfunction is linked to organic causes in less than 5% of cases. Diabetes, alcoholism, neurologic disturbances, hormonal deficiencies, and pelvic disorders, such as infections, trauma, and surgical scarring, are specific disorders that may block orgasm.

Narcotics, tranquilizers, antidepressants, and antihypertensive medications also can inhibit orgasm.

Rapid orgasm is a relatively new diagnosis and seems to be rare. In this instance, once orgasm occurs there is little interest in further sexual activity. Rapid orgasm has no known organic cause.

Dyspareunia (painful intercourse) is common. Women may experience pain during arousal, at the time of orgasm, at the initiation of intercourse, midway during intercourse, or after intercourse. The pain may have a burning, sharp, searing, or cramping quality and may be described as external, vaginal, deep abdominal, or pelvic. A variety of psychosocial and organic causes have been identified. Inadequate lubrication may make penetration or intercourse difficult or painful. Drugs with a drying effect, such as antihistamines, certain tranquilizers, and marijuana, and disorders such as diabetes, vaginal infections, and estrogen deficiency can decrease lubrication. Other causes of dyspareunia include skin problems around the introitus or affecting the vulva; irritation or infection of the clitoris; disorders of the vaginal opening, such as scarring from episiotomy, intact hymen, or chronically infected hymenal remnants; bartholinitis; disorders of the urethra or anus; disorders of the vagina, such as infections, thinning of the walls caused by aging or decreased estrogen, or irritation caused by spermicides or douches; and pelvic disorders, such as infection, tumors, cervical or uterine abnormalities, and torn uterine ligaments.

Sexual dysfunction may develop as a coping mechanism. Women with a history of sexual trauma—rape, incest, or molestation—often have problems of desire, arousal, or orgasm or experience pain with sexual activity. In extreme cases total sexual aversion may develop. At other times, sexual dysfunction may be a symptom of marital or relationship problems. Unresolved anger may manifest as inhibited desire or diminished arousal. A population study indicated that relationship factors are more important in decreasing libido than age or menopause, whereas physiologic and psychologic factors are more prominent in genital arousal with decreased organic functioning.[123]

Impaired Fertility

Infertility affects approximately 15% of all couples and is defined as the inability to conceive after 1 year of unprotected intercourse with the same partner. Fertility can be impaired by factors in the man or the woman or both partners. Male factors include diminished quality and production of sperm and female factors are associated with malfunctions of the fallopian tubes, ovaries, or reproductive hormones. Adhesions from pelvic infection may cause blockage of one or both fallopian tubes, preventing access of the sperm to the ovum. Hormonal or local factors may disrupt ovulation or prevent a fertilized egg from implantation. Hyperthyroidism in males may affect production of sperm and motility.[124] Hypothyroidism in females is also related to infertility as previously discussed. A number of diagnostic procedures are required in the routine investigation of the infertile couple (see Table 22-3). In many instances no cause may be identified.

Treatment of infertility is aimed toward correcting problems identified during the diagnostic workup. The best treatment for infertility is prevention, specifically of sexually transmitted infection that can result in scarring and adhesion formation in the reproductive tract of a man or woman.

Fertility Tests

Tests of reproductive function are performed most commonly when infertility exists. Both partners are examined, and several diagnostic evaluations may be completed. The types of tests and their normal values are summarized in Table 21-4. The man is evaluated for number, amount, structure, and motility of sperm and obstruction along the reproductive tract. Tests for women determine whether (1) the reproductive tract (cervix, uterus, fallopian tubes) is adequately patent to allow for passage of ovum and sperm, (2) ovulation occurs normally, (3) the endometrium is responding normally to hormones, and (4) reproductive tissues are free of tumors or infections. Hormonal assays evaluate the adequacy of pituitary function and target organ response. The position and size of organs or the presence of tumors can be detected by direct observation procedures using a laparoscope or by radiographic studies, such as plain films, or CT. Before testing and treatment, assessing knowledge of fertility with timing of sexual intercourse is essential. A mature ovum remains viable for 12 to 24 hours, and sperm retain their fertility for up to 5 days. A prospective study showed that almost all pregnancies resulted from sexual intercourse during a 6-day period ending on the day of ovulation.[125]

DISORDERS OF THE MALE REPRODUCTIVE SYSTEM

Disorders of the Urethra

Urethritis and urethral strictures are common disorders of the male urethra. Urethral carcinoma occurs in men older than 60 years, but it is an extremely rare form of cancer.

Urethritis

Urethritis is an inflammatory process of the urethra without concurrent bladder infection that is usually, but not always, caused by a sexually transmitted microorganism. Biologic agents associated with infectious urethritis in males include *N. gonorrhoeae* and *C. trachomatis, U. urealyticum,* and other, less common, mycobacteria; parasites (e.g., *Trichomonas vaginalis*); and viruses (herpes simplex virus [HSV]).[126,127] Infectious urethritis caused by *N. gonorrhoeae* often is called *gonococcal urethritis (GU);* infection caused by other microorganisms is called *nongonococcal urethritis (NGU).*[128] (Sexually transmitted urethritis is described in Chapter 24.) Nonsexual origins of urethritis include inflammation or infection as a result of urologic procedures, insertion of foreign bodies into the urethra, anatomic abnormalities, or trauma.

Noninfectious urethritis is rare and is associated with the ingestion of wood alcohol, ethyl alcohol, or turpentine. It is seen also with Reiter syndrome, which involves a number of mucocutaneous lesions.

Symptoms of urethritis include urethral tingling, itching, or burning sensation on urination (dysuria), frequency, and urgency. The individual may note a purulent or clear mucus-like discharge from the urethra. Nucleic acid detection amplification tests allow easy detection of *N. gonorrhoeae* and *C. trachomatis* in first-void urine.[128] Treatment consists of appropriate antibiotic therapy for infectious urethritis and avoidance of future chemical or mechanical irritation.

Urethral Stricture

A **urethral stricture** is a fibrotic narrowing of the urethra caused by scarring. The scars may be congenital but are more likely to result from trauma or untreated or severe urethral infections, most often from long-term use of indwelling urinary catheters. Large catheters and instruments cause internal trauma and ischemia, whereas external trauma, such as pelvic fracture, can partially or completely sever the urethra and cause severe and complex strictures.[129] In addition, a report has concluded that stricture may occur decades after initial hypospadias surgery.[130] Urethral carcinoma is a less common cause of urethral stricture. Prostatitis and infection secondary to urinary stasis are common complications. Severe and prolonged obstruction can result in hydronephrosis and renal failure. In addition, chronic, severe strictures may lead to urethral fistulas and periurethral abscesses.[129]

The clinical manifestations of urethral stricture are caused by bladder outlet obstruction. The primary symptom is diminished force and caliber of the urinary stream; other symptoms include urinary frequency and hesitancy, mild dysuria, double urine stream or spraying, and postvoiding dribbling. Symptoms of acute urinary retention may occur in the presence of infection or urinary obstruction. Induration at the stricture site may be palpable. Tender, enlarged masses along the urethra usually indicate periurethral abscesses.

Urethral stricture is diagnosed on the basis of history, physical examination, urinary flow rates, voiding cystourethrogram, and urethroscopy; biopsy confirms carcinoma. Treatment is usually surgical and may involve urethral dilation, urethrotomy, or a variety of open surgical techniques. The choice of surgical intervention depends on the age of the individual and the severity of the problem. Strictures may recur up to 1 year after treatment. Follow-up is necessary during this time; urinary flow measurements and urethrogram help determine extent of residual obstruction.

Disorders of the Penis

Phimosis and Paraphimosis

Phimosis and paraphimosis are disorders in which the foreskin (prepuce) is "too tight" to be moved easily over the glans penis. **Phimosis** is a condition in which the foreskin cannot be retracted back over the glans, whereas **paraphimosis** is the opposite: the foreskin is retracted and cannot be moved forward (reduced) to cover the glans (Figure 23-22). Both conditions can cause penile pathologic conditions.

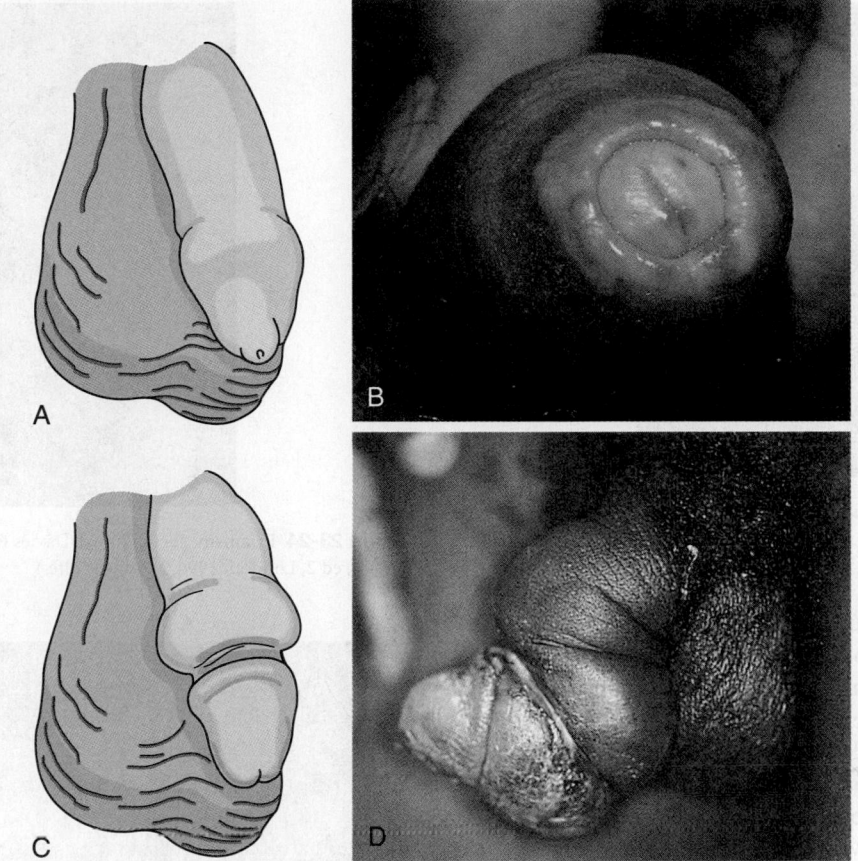

Figure 23-22 Phimosis and paraphimosis. **A,** Phimosis: the foreskin has a narrow opening that is not large enough to permit retraction over the glans. **B,** Lesions on the prepuce secondary to infection cause swelling, and retraction of foreskin may be impossible. **C,** Paraphimosis: the foreskin is retracted over the glans but cannot be reduced to its normal position. Here it has formed a constricting band around the penis. **D,** Ulcer on the retracted prepuce with edema. (**A, C** from Phipps WP, Sand JK, Marek JF: *Medical-surgical nursing: concepts and clinical practice,* ed 6, St Louis, 1999, Mosby; **B** from Taylor PK: *Diagnostic picture tests in sexually transmitted diseases,* London, 1995, Mosby-Wolfe, **D** from Morse SA, Moreland AA, Holmes KK: *Atlas of sexually transmitted diseases and AIDS,* ed 2, London, 1996, Mosby-Wolfe.)

The inability to retract the foreskin is normal in infancy and is caused by congenital adhesions. During the first 3 years of life, these adhesions separate naturally with penile erections and are not an indication for circumcision. Although most cases occur in uncircumcised males, stenosis and resultant phimosis can occur in males with excessive skin remaining after circumcision.[129] Phimosis can occur at any age and is caused most commonly by poor hygiene and chronic infection. Chronic balanoposthitis (inflammation of the glans and prepuce) predisposes older diabetic men to phimosis. It rarely occurs with normal foreskin.

Edema, erythema, and tenderness of the prepuce and purulent discharge are usually the reasons for seeking treatment; inability to retract the foreskin is a less common complaint. Circumcision, if needed, is performed after infection has been eradicated. Complications of phimosis include inflammation of the glans (balanitis) or prepuce (posthitis) and paraphimosis. There is a higher incidence of penile carcinoma in uncircumcised males, but chronic infection, most likely with HPV, is usually the underlying factor in such cases.[131,132]

Paraphimosis, in which the foreskin is retracted, can constrict the penis, causing edema of the glans. If edema is such that the foreskin cannot be reduced manually, surgery must be performed to prevent necrosis of the glans caused by constricted blood vessels. Severe paraphimosis is a surgical emergency and phimosis may require immediate release if there is urinary obstruction.

Peyronie Disease

Peyronie disease (bent nail syndrome) is a fibrotic condition of the tunica albuginea of the penis resulting in varying degrees of curvature and sexual dysfunction[133] (Figure 23-23). Peyronie disease develops slowly and is characterized by tough, fibrous thickening of the fascia in the erectile tissue of the corpora cavernosa. A dense fibrous plaque is usually palpable on the dorsum of the penile shaft. The problem usually affects middle-age men and is associated with painful erection, painful intercourse (for both partners), and poor erection distal to the involved area. In some cases, impotence or unsatisfactory penetration occurs. There is no pain when the penis is flaccid.

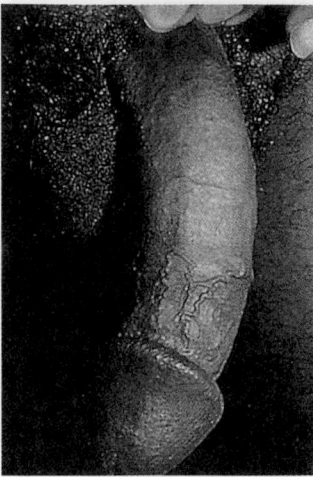

Figure 23-23 Peyronie disease. (From Taylor PK: *Diagnostic picture tests in sexually transmitted diseases,* London, 1995, Mosby-Wolfe.)

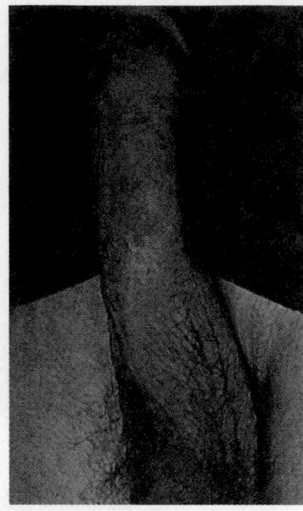

Figure 23-24 Priapism. (From Lloyd-Davies RW et al: *Color atlas of urology,* ed 2, London, 1994, Mosby-Wolfe.)

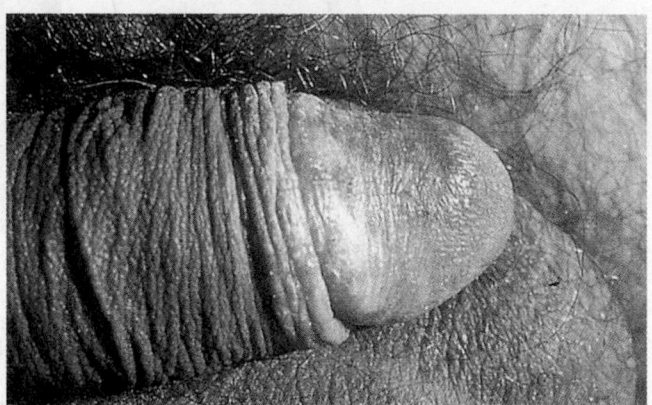

Figure 23-25 Balanitis. Itchy, red rash on glans of penis secondary to *Candida albicans.* (From Taylor PK: *Diagnostic picture tests in sexually transmitted diseases,* London, 1995, Mosby-Wolfe.)

Although the exact cause is unknown, a local vasculitis-like inflammatory reaction occurs and decreased tissue oxygenation results in fibrosis and calcification. Peyronie disease is associated with Dupuytren contracture (a flexion deformity of the fingers or toes caused by shortening or fibrosis of the palmar or plantar fascia), diabetes, tendency to develop keloids, and in rare cases, use of beta-blocker medications.

There is no definitive treatment for Peyronie disease. Spontaneous remissions occur in as many as 50% of cases. Treatment with pharmacologic therapies include colchicine, aminobenzoate potassium (Potaba), L-carnitine, and liposomal superoxide dismutase.[133] Placation, as well as surgical resection of the fibrous plaque followed by grafting, has been successful.[129]

Priapism

Priapism is an uncommon condition of prolonged penile erection. It is usually painful and is not associated with sexual arousal (Figure 23-24). Priapism is idiopathic in 60% of cases; the remaining 40% of cases are associated with spinal cord trauma, sickle cell disease, leukemia, pelvic tumors or infections, or penile trauma. Priapism also has been associated with cocaine use.[134] Intracavernous injection therapy for impotence seems to be the most common cause. Prolonged sexual stimulation often is associated with initial development of the idiopathic type.[129] The two corpora cavernosa within the erect penis are filled with blood and are tender to palpation; neither the corpus spongiosum nor the glans is engorged. The vascular congestion is thought to be associated with venous obstruction. If the erection remains over a period of days, edema and fibrosis develop, leading to erectile dysfunction (impotence).

Priapism is a urologic emergency. Treatment within hours is effective and prevents impotence. Conservative approaches include iced saline enemas, ketamine administration, and spinal anesthesia. Needle aspiration of blood from the corpus through the dorsal glans is often effective and is followed by catheterization and pressure dressings to maintain decompression. More aggressive surgical treatments include the creation of vascular shunts to maintain blood flow. Erectile dysfunction results in up to 50% of prolonged cases.

Balanitis

Balanitis is an inflammation of the glans penis (Figure 23-25) and usually occurs in conjunction with posthitis, an inflammation of the prepuce. It is associated with poor hygiene and phimosis. The accumulation under the foreskin of glandular secretions (smegma), sloughed epithelial cells, and *Mycobacterium smegmatis* can irritate the glans directly or lead to infection. Skin disorders (e.g., psoriasis, lichen planus, eczema) and candidiasis must be differentiated from inflammation resulting from poor hygienic practices. Balanitis is seen most commonly in men with poorly controlled diabetes mellitus and candidiasis. Antimicrobials are used to treat infection. Circumcision can prevent recurrences and can be considered after the inflammation has subsided.

Penile Cancer

In the United States, carcinoma of the penis is rare and affects about 1 in 100,000 men. Approximately 1290 cases and 290 deaths were estimated in the year 2009.[1] Although rare in North America and Europe, where it accounts for about 0.2% of cancers and 0.1% of cancer deaths in men, penile cancer may account for up to 10% of cancers in African and South American men.

In the United States it is twice as common in black men than in white men[131] and in men older than age 50.[135] Major risk factors include infection with HPV (mainly serotypes 16, 18, 33, 35, and 45), smoking, and psoriasis treated with a combination involving the drug psoralen and ultraviolet (UV) light. Men circumcised at birth have less than half the chance of getting penile cancer than those who were not.[131] Penile cancer is more common in men with phimosis and those with AIDS.[131] About two thirds of men with penile cancer are diagnosed at more than 65 years of age. [1]

Before the development of penile cancer, signs of premalignant cancer or epidermal cancer in situ are present.[136] These include thick white plaque (leukoplakia) that typically involves the meatus; red, inflamed areas of Paget disease; red, velvety, ulcerative lesions of erythroplasia of Queyrat that usually involve the glans; large, invasive, scaly growths of Buschke-Löwenstein tumor; red plaque with encrustations of Bowen disease; and in situ carcinoma that generally affects the penile shaft. Men with leukoplakia or erythroplasia of Queyrat may have concurrent invasive penile carcinoma.[131,137] Pain and bleeding are late signs of penile cancer. Condylomata (genital warts) caused by HPV may be involved in the development of precancerous lesions (see Chapter 24 for a discussion of HPV). At times the penis might be the site of metastatic spread of solid tumors from the bladder, prostate, rectum, or kidney. Early squamous cell carcinoma and premalignant epidermal lesions are easily treated but are often ignored. Delays in seeking treatment are attributed to denial, embarrassment, failure to detect lesions under a phimotic foreskin, fear, guilt, and ignorance.

Penile cancer is mostly squamous cell carcinoma, which usually begins as a small, fat, ulcerative or papillary lesion on the glans or foreskin that grows to involve the entire penile shaft (Figure 23-26). Extensive lesions are associated with metastases and a poor prognosis. These lesions are not as painful as the amount of tissue involvement would seem to indicate. The regional femoral and iliac nodes are common metastatic sites. Rarely the urethra and bladder are involved. Weight loss, fatigue, and malaise accompany chronic suppurative lesions. Untreated, progressive disease causes death within 2 years.

The specific diagnosis is made by biopsy after examination to document the location, size, and fixation of the lesion. After a positive biopsy, the extent of cancer spread is determined by imaging tests such as ultrasound, CT, or MRI. Fine-needle aspiration of lymph tissue confirms absence or presence of regional adenopathy.[131] About 30% of penile cancers spread to lymph nodes before diagnosis.[135] Distant metastases occur in less than 10% of cases and may involve lung, liver, bone,

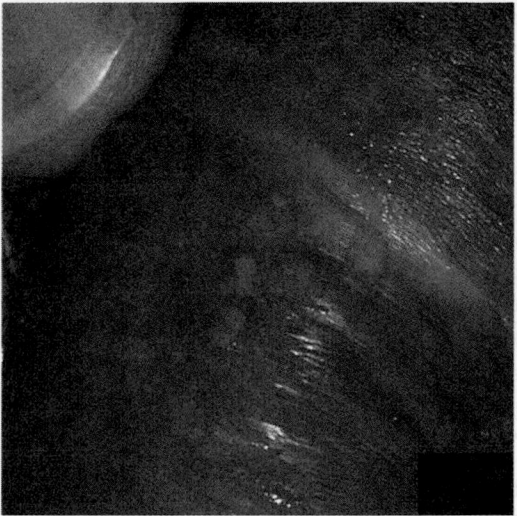

Figure 23-26 Carcinoma in situ of penis. Flat papules turn white after diagnostic treatment with acetic acid. (From Morse SA, et al: *Atlas of sexually transmitted diseases* and *AIDS*, ed 3, London, 2003, Mosby.)

Box 23-12	Tumor, Node, Metastasis (TNM) Staging for Penile Cancer

Stage 0	Stage III
T_{is}, N_0, M_0	T_1, N_2, M_0
T_a, N_0, M_0	I_2, N_2, M_0
Stage I	T_3, N_0, M_0
T_1, N_0, M_0	T_3, N_1, M_0
Stage II	T_3, N_2, M_0
T_1, N_1, M_0	T_2, N_1, M_0
T_2, N_0, M_0	**Stage IV**
T_2, N_1, M_0	T_4, any N, M_0
	Any T, N_3, M_0
	Any T, any N, M_1

Recurrent

Any local or distant penile cancer that returns after treatment.

*See Figure 11-25, p. 386 for TNM definitions.

or brain.[137] Staging of penile cancer uses a system created by the American Joint Committee on Cancer (AJCC) and the International Union Against Cancer (IUCC). The AJCC/IUCC staging system is also known as the tumor, node, metastasis (TNM) system.[1] Although this system initially seems cumbersome, it is a simple and easy method of communicating degree of cancer (Box 23-12).

For invasive penile carcinoma, complete excision leaving adequate tumor-free margins is the goal. A simple circumcision may be sufficient for localized lesions of the prepuce. If the primary site is glans and distal shaft, removal of the penis may be necessary. Although conventional radical surgery continues to be an effective approach, the emasculating nature of the treatment has serious psychologic and sexual consequences. Recent studies have challenged the conventional belief that a 2-cm margin was required for adequate cancer control.[138] Newer innovative surgical techniques can now preserve as much penile tissue and functional integrity as possible without compromising cancer control. Inguinal lymph nodes also are removed if metastasis to these structures is known or suspected. Palliative treatment with radiation or chemotherapy may be used when the disease is inoperable and bulky inguinal metastases have occurred. Options for individuals with carcinoma in situ include local excision, radiation, laser surgery, cryosurgery, chemosurgery, or chemotherapy with topical (5%) 5-FU. Differentiation, tumor stage, and age influence prognosis.[139] The 5-year survival rate for stage I disease is greater than 80%[1,135]; average 5-year survival rate for all stages is 50%.[1,131]

Disorders of the Scrotum, Testis, and Epididymis

Disorders of the Scrotum

Men may seek treatment for painful or painless scrotal masses. Masses may be serious (cancer or torsion) or benign (hydrocele or cyst); they may require immediate surgical

intervention or allow for careful observation. A flow diagram for diagnosing scrotal masses[140] is provided in Figure 23-27.

Varicocele, hydrocele, and spermatocele are common intrascrotal disorders.[141-143] A **varicocele** is an abnormal dilation of a vein within the spermatic cord and is classically described as a "bag of worms" (Figure 23-28). Most (95%) occur on the left side and may be painful or tender. Varicocele occurs in 10% of males and is seen most often after puberty. Sudden development of a varicocele in an older man is a late sign of renal tumor.[142] Unilateral right-sided varicoceles are rare and result from compression or obstruction of the inferior vena cava by a tumor or thrombus. Color Doppler ultrasonography is used to confirm the diagnosis.[140]

The cause of varicocele is incompetent or congenitally absent valves in the spermatic veins. The valves that normally prevent backflow are absent or do not close adequately, permitting blood to pool in the veins rather than flow into the venous system. Varicocele decreases blood flow through the testis. This interferes with spermatogenesis and is a cause of infertility.[141,142] If infertility is a problem, treatment consists of ligation of the spermatic vein or occlusion of the vein by

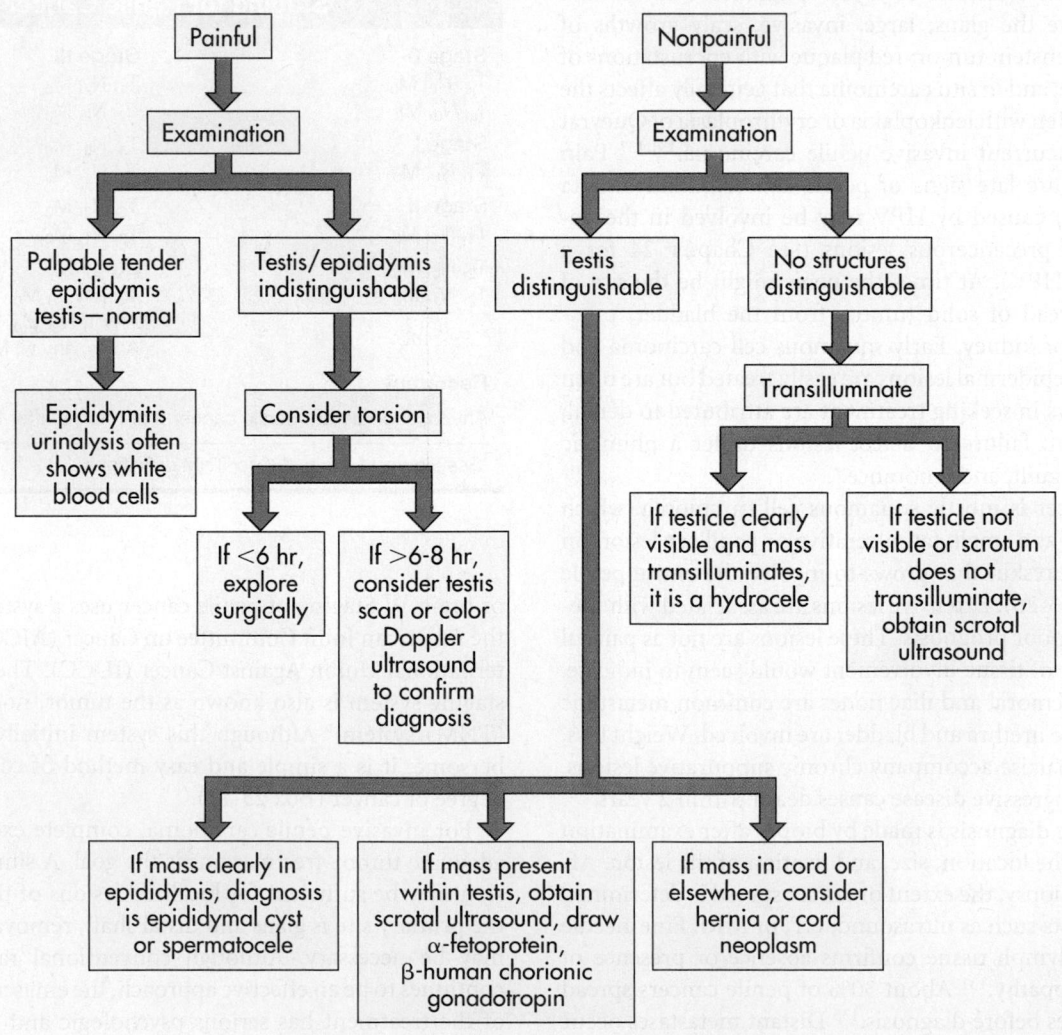

Figure 23-27 Diagnostic algorithm of a scrotal mass.

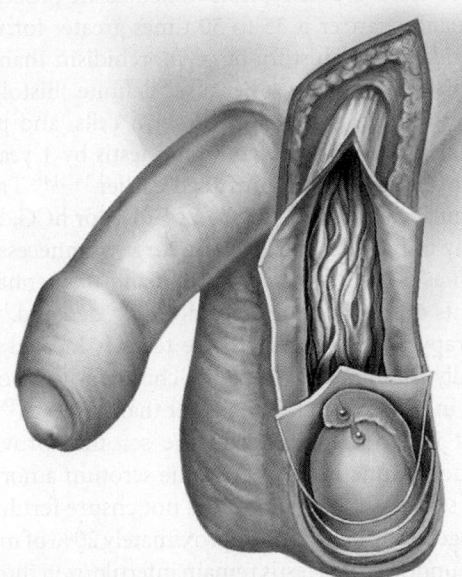

Figure 23-28 Varicocele. Dilation of veins within the spermatic cord. (From Seidel H et al: *Mosby's guide to physical examination*, ed 4, St Louis, 1999, Mosby.)

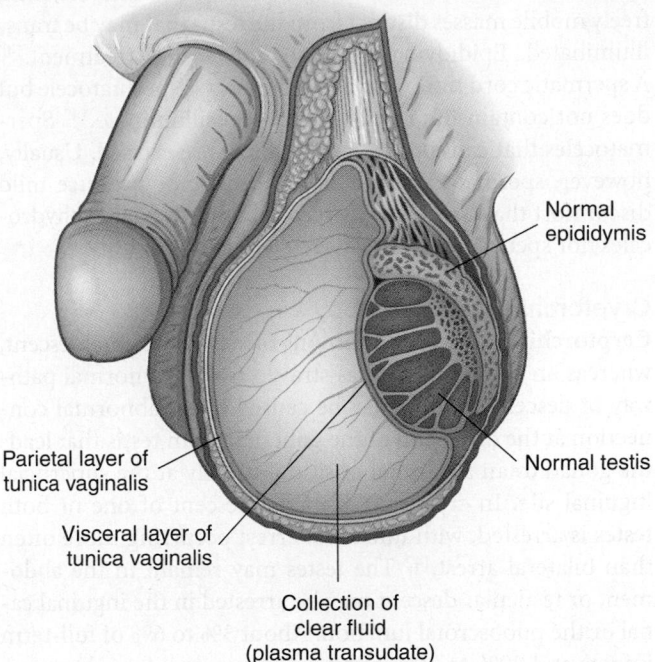

Figure 23-29 Hydrocele. Accumulation of clear fluid between the visceral and parietal layers of the tunica vaginalis.

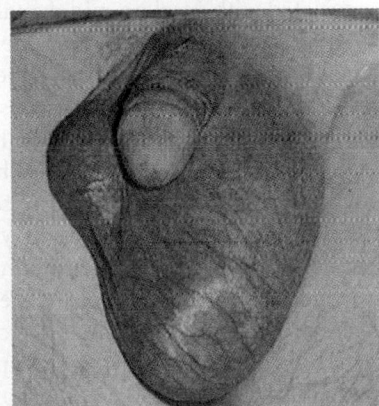

Figure 23-30 Spermatocele. Retention cyst of the head of the epididymis or of an aberrant tubule or tubules of the rete testis. The spermatocele lies outside the tunica vaginalis; therefore, on palpation it can be readily distinguished and separated from the testis. (From Lloyd-Davies RW, Gow JG, Davies DR: *Color atlas of urology*, ed 2, London, 1994, Mosby-Wolfe.)

percutaneous methods, such as balloon catheter and sclerosing fluids.[142,144] If varicocele is mild and fertility is not an issue, a scrotal support usually is sufficient to relieve symptoms of scrotal heaviness or "dragging."

A **hydrocele** is a collection of fluid within the tunica vaginalis[140-142] (Figure 23-29). It is the most common cause of scrotal swelling. Hydroceles occur in 6% of male newborns and are congenital malformations (patent processus vaginalis) that often resolve spontaneously in the first year of life. Surgical ligation is recommended if hydrocele persists after age 1 year.[143] Hydroceles in adults may be caused by an imbalance between the secreting and absorptive capacities of scrotal tissues. Hydroceles range in size from slightly larger than the testes to the size of a grapefruit or larger and may be flaccid or tense. Compression of testicular blood supply may lead to atrophy.

The exact mechanism of idiopathic hydrocele is unknown. Secondary hydrocele may result from trauma or infection of the testis or epididymis or from a testicular tumor. Rapid accumulation of fluid occurs after local injury, radiotherapy, or infection (epididymitis or orchitis), or it may accompany testicular neoplasm. Chronic hydroceles are more common and occur in men older than 40 because of an imbalance between fluid secretion and reabsorption in the tunica vaginalis. A painless, extratesticular mass that easily transilluminates is found on physical examination. Ultrasonography of a large hydrocele, which may conceal a testicular tumor, is recommended. Treatment is usually not required unless a large, bulky hydrocele causes considerable physical discomfort or undesirable cosmetic appearance.[141] Treatment for uncomplicated hydrocele is aspiration of the fluid and injection of a sclerosing agent into the scrotal sac.[140,145] The goal of

treatment is to remove the hydrocele and prevent recurrence by sclerosing or excising the tunica vaginalis.

A **spermatocele** is a painless diverticulum of the epididymis located between the head of the epididymis and the testis. In other words, efferent ducts of the epididymis have potential for cystic dilation to form a spermatocele[140,142] (Figure 23-30). Spermatoceles are filled with milky fluid that contains sperm. Spermatocele is differentiated from a hydrocele in that aspiration of the hydrocele recovers a clear, yellow fluid, and unlike a hydrocele, a spermatocele does not cover the entire anterior surface of the testis. An epididymal cyst is similar to a spermatocele but does not communicate with the epididymis.

Spermatoceles and epididymal cysts manifest as discrete, firm, freely mobile masses distinct from the testis that may be transilluminated. Epididymal cysts do not require treatment.[140] A spermatic cord tumor may feel like a tense spermatocele but does not contain fluid and will not transilluminate.[142] Spermatoceles that cause pain or discomfort are excised. Usually, however, spermatoceles are asymptomatic or produce mild discomfort that is relieved by scrotal support. Neither hydroceles nor spermatoceles are associated with infertility.

Cryptorchidism and Ectopy

Cryptorchidism is a condition of testicular maldescent, whereas an **ectopic testis** has strayed from the normal pathway of descent. Ectopy may be caused by an abnormal connection at the distal end of the gubernaculum testis that leads the gonad to an abnormal position, usually at the superficial inguinal site. In cryptorchidism the descent of one or both testes is arrested, with unilateral arrest occurring more often than bilateral arrest.[142] The testes may remain in the abdomen, or testicular descent may be arrested in the inguinal canal or the puboscrotal junction. About 3% to 6% of full-term infants and 20% to 30% of premature male infants have undescended testes at birth[143]; half of such testes descend in the first month of life and a few more at puberty. The incidence of cryptorchidism in adults is 0.7% to 0.8%.[142] Cryptorchidism is commonly associated with vasal or epididymal abnormalities. These congenital anomalies affect about one third to two thirds of newborns with cryptorchidism. Other structural anomalies include posterior urethral valves (less than 5%), upper tract abnormalities (less than 5%), and hypospadias. The presence of hypospadias as well as cryptorchidism raises the suspicion of mixed gonadal dysgenesis (intersex infant). It has been hypothesized that cryptorchidism may result from an absence or abnormality of the gubernaculum, a cordlike structure that extends from the lower pole of the testis to the scrotum; a congenital gonadal or dysgenetic defect that makes the testis insensitive to gonadotropins (a likely explanation for unilateral cryptorchidism); or lack of maternal gonadotropins (a likely explanation for bilateral cryptorchidism of prematurity).[142] Mechanical possibilities include a short spermatic cord, fibrous bands or adhesions in the normal path of the testes, or a narrowed inguinal canal. Chromosomal studies do not support a genetic component. Physiologic cryptorchidism, also called *retractile* or *migratory testis,* is an involuntary retraction of the testes out of the scrotum that occurs with excitement, physical activity, or exposure to cold and is caused by the small mass of prepubertal testis and the strength of the cremaster muscle. This is a common phenomenon that is self-limiting (descent occurs at puberty).

Physical examination discloses the absence of one or both testes in the scrotum and an atrophic scrotum on the affected side. If the undescended testis is in a vulnerable position, for example, over the pubic bone, an individual may complain of severe pain secondary to trauma. The adult male with bilateral cryptorchidism may be infertile. Ultrasonography, CT, or MRI can be used to locate an intra-abdominal or nonpalpable testis.

Undescended testes are susceptible to neoplastic processes: the risk of testicular cancer is 35 to 50 times greater for men with cryptorchidism or a history of cryptorchidism than for the general male population. Because definite histologic change (decreased Leydig cells, loss of germ cells, and peritubular fibrosis) occurs in the cryptorchid testis by 1 year of age, surgical correction is recommended earlier.[142,146] Treatment often begins with administration of GnRH or hCG, hormones that may initiate descent, making surgery unnecessary. GnRH is given as a nasal spray in Europe and may enhance germ-cell counts even when the testis does not descend.[146] If hormonal therapy is not successful, the testis is located and moved surgically (orchiopexy) in young children or removed (orchiectomy) in adults and children older than 10 years.[142,146] The testis that is properly placed in the scrotum provides adequate hormonal function and gives the scrotum a normal appearance. A successful operation does not ensure fertility if the testis is congenitally defective. Approximately 20% of males with unilateral undescended testis remain infertile even though orchiopexy is performed by age 1 year; most individuals with treated or untreated bilateral testicular maldescent have poor fertility. In addition, placement of the cryptorchid testis into the scrotal sac does not decrease the potential for malignancy; it does facilitate examination and tumor detection.

Torsion of the Testis

Torsion of the testis is rotation of a testis, which twists blood vessels in the spermatic cord. It causes an acute scrotum, which is testicular pain and swelling (Figure 23-31). Differentiation between testicular torsion and two other common

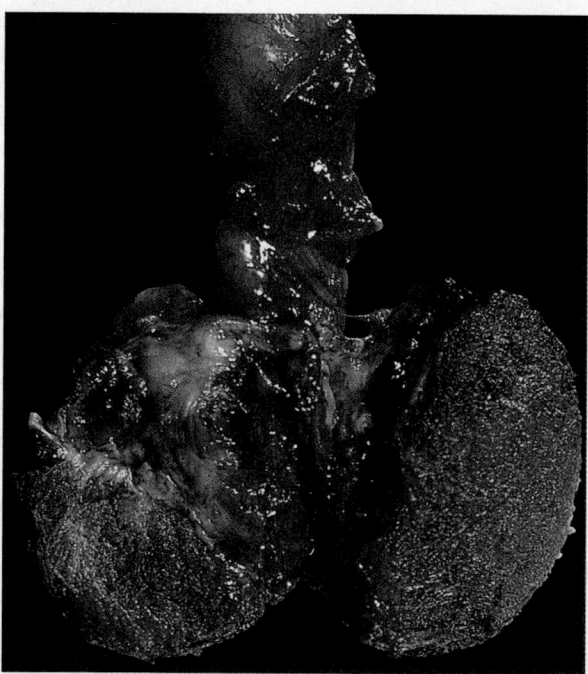

Figure 23-31 Torsion of the testes. The testes appear dark red and partially necrotic owing to hemorrhagic infarction. (From Damjanov I, Linder J, editors: *Anderson's pathology,* ed 10, St Louis, 1996, Mosby.)

Table 23-10	Diagnosis of Selected Conditions Responsible for the Acute Scrotum					
Condition	Onset of Symptoms	Age	Tenderness	Urinalysis	Cremasteric Reflex	Treatment
Testicular torsion	Acute	Early puberty	Diffuse	Negative	Negative	Surgical exploration
Appendiceal torsion	Subacute	Prepubertal	Localized to upper pole	Negative	Positive	Bed rest and scrotal elevation
Epididymis	Insidious	Adolescence	Epididymal	Positive or negative	Positive	Antibiotics

causes of an acute scrotum is based on physical examination and history[140,143] (Table 23-10). This event is most common among neonates and pubertal adolescents, but it can occur in males at any age.[140,143] Onset may be spontaneous or follow physical exertion or trauma. Torsion twists the arteries and veins in the spermatic cord, reducing or stopping circulation to the testis. Vascular engorgement and ischemia develop, causing scrotal swelling and pain. These manifestations are not relieved by scrotal elevation (Prehn sign), rest, or scrotal support. On physical examination, men have a tender, high-riding testis, a thickened spermatic cord, and an absent cremasteric reflex. Unlike epididymitis, the epididymis cannot be differentiated from the testis.[143] Diagnostic testing includes urinalysis (to rule out infection) and color Doppler ultrasonography.[125,142,143] Torsion of the testis is a surgical emergency. If the torsion cannot be reduced manually, surgery must be performed within 6 hours after the onset of symptoms to preserve normal testicular function. Surgery includes untwisting the spermatic cord and anchoring both testes in correct position within the scrotum to prevent recurrences. With successful manual detorsion, surgical fixation should be done within a few days.

Orchitis

Orchitis is an acute inflammation of the testes (Figure 23-32) and is uncommon except as a complication of systemic infection or as an extension of an associated epididymitis[127] (see p. 859). Infectious microorganisms may reach the testes through the blood or the lymphatics or, most commonly, by ascent through the urethra, vas deferens, and epididymis. Most cases of orchitis are actually cases of epididymo-orchitis. Occasionally, in middle-age men, a nonspecific, apparently noninfectious, inflammatory process (called *granulomatis orchitis*) can occur. It seems to be an autoimmune disease that triggers a granulomatous response to spermatozoa.

Mumps is the most common infectious cause of orchitis and usually affects postpubertal males. The onset is sudden, occurring 3 to 4 days after the onset of parotitis. Signs and symptoms include high fever, reaching 40° C (104° F), marked prostration, bilateral or unilateral erythema, edema and tenderness of the scrotum, and leukocytosis. An acute hydrocele may develop. Urinary signs and symptoms, which accompany epididymitis, are absent. Atrophy with irreversible damage to spermatogenesis may result in 30% of affected testes. Bilateral orchitis does not affect androgenic function but may cause permanent sterility.

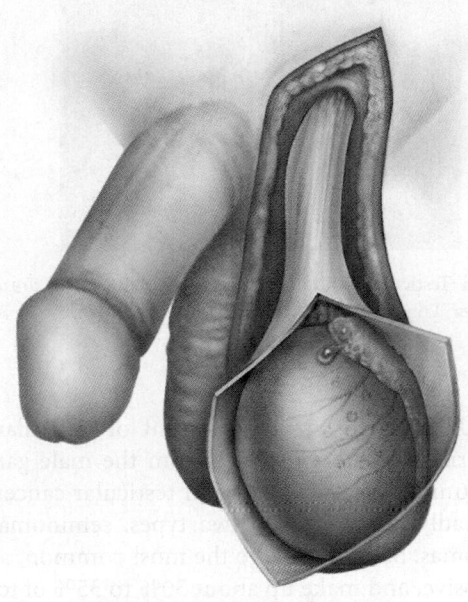

Figure 23-32 Orchitis. (From Seidel H et al: *Mosby's guide to physical examination*, ed 4, St Louis, 1999, Mosby.)

Treatment is supportive and includes bed rest, scrotal support, elevation of the scrotum, hot or cold compresses, and analgesic agents for relief of pain. If an acute hydrocele develops, it is aspirated. Testicular abscess usually requires orchiectomy (removal of the testis). Appropriate antimicrobial drugs should be used for bacterial orchitis, and corticosteroids are indicated in proved cases of nonspecific granulomatous orchitis.

Cancer of the Testis

Testicular cancer is among the most curable of cancers; for nearly all common types, cure rates are more than 95%. Overall, testicular cancers are rare, accounting for only 1% of cancers and 0.24% of cancer deaths[1] in men, yet they are the most common form of cancer in young men between ages 15 and 35. Approximately 8400 cases and 380 deaths were estimated for 2009.[1] In the United States, the lifetime probability of developing testicular cancer is 0.2% for white men, an incidence that is four times higher than for blacks. Testicular tumors are slightly more common on the right side than on the left, a pattern that parallels the occurrence of cryptorchidism; about 1% to 2% of primary testicular cancers are bilateral (Figure 23-33), and 50% of these tumors arise from treated or untreated cryptorchid testes.

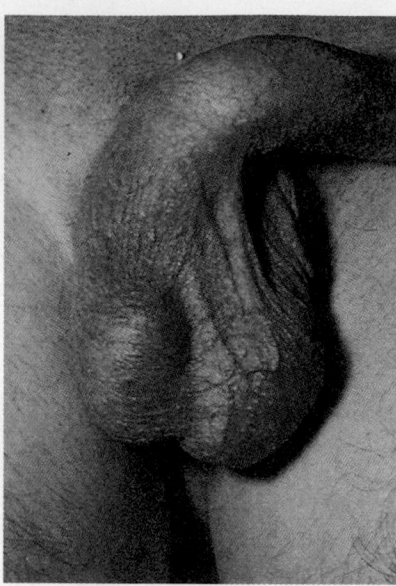

Figure 23-33 Testicular tumor. (From *400 Self-assessment picture tests in clinical medicine*, London, 1984, Wolfe Medical.)

PATHOGENESIS Ninety percent of testicular cancers are germ-cell tumors arising from the male gametes. Germ-cell tumors constitute 90% of testicular cancers and can be broadly classified into two types: seminomas and nonseminomas. Seminomas are the most common, are the least aggressive, and make up about 30% to 35% of testicular cancers. Nonseminomas include embryonal carcinomas, teratomas, and choriocarcinomas, the most aggressive but rare (less than 1%) form of testicular cancer. Testicular cancers can include a mix of types.[147] In addition, testicular tumors can arise from specialized cells of the gonadal stroma. These tumors, which are named for their cellular origins, are Leydig cell, Sertoli cell, granulosa cell, and theca cell tumors and constitute less than 10% of all testicular cancers.[148]

The cause of testicular neoplasms is unknown. A genetic predisposition is suggested by the fact that the incidence is higher among brothers, identical twins, and other close male relatives. Genetic predisposition is supported further by statistics showing that the disease is relatively rare among black Africans, black Americans, Asians, and native New Zealanders. Risk factors include history of cryptorchidism, abnormal testicular development, HIV and AIDS, Klinefelter syndrome, and history of testicular cancer.[147]

CLINICAL MANIFESTATIONS Painless testicular enlargement commonly is the first sign of testicular cancer. Enlargement is usually gradual and may be accompanied by a sensation of testicular heaviness or dull ache in the lower abdomen.[147,148] Occasionally, acute pain occurs because of rapid growth, resulting in hemorrhage and necrosis. Ten percent of affected men have epididymitis, 10% have hydroceles,[148] and 5% have gynecomastia or hydrocele. Incidence of gynecomastia increases considerably (30% to 45%)

in men with Sertoli or Leydig tumors. Approximately 10% of individuals already have symptoms related to metastases at the time of initial diagnosis, which correlates with the typical delay of 3 to 6 months from initial recognition to definitive treatment. Lumbar pain may be present and usually is caused by retroperitoneal node metastasis. Signs of metastasis to the lungs include cough, dyspnea, and bloody sputum (hemoptysis). Supraclavicular node involvement may cause difficulty swallowing (dysphagia) and neck swelling. Alterations in vision or mental status, papilledema, and seizures may be experienced with metastasis to the CNS. Approximately 10% of affected individuals are asymptomatic; the tumor may be detected by the man's sexual partner or incidentally following trauma.

EVALUATION AND TREATMENT An incorrect diagnosis at the initial examination occurs in as many as 25% of men with testicular cancer. Epididymitis and epididymoorchitis are the most common misdiagnoses; others include hydrocele and spermatocele. Evaluation begins with careful physical examination, including palpation of the scrotal contents with the individual in the erect and supine positions. The abdomen and lymph nodes are palpated to rule out metastases. Signs of testicular cancer include abnormal consistency, induration, nodularity, or irregularity of the testis. A firm, nontender testicular mass or diffuse enlargement is found in the majority of cases. Primary testicular cancer can be assessed rapidly and accurately by scrotal ultrasonography. Tumor markers are higher than normal in the presence of a tumor and may help detect a tumor that is too small to be palpated during physical examination or seen on imaging.[147] Tumor type is identified after inguinal biopsy or orchiectomy. Scrotal incisions may cause dissemination of the tumor and increase the risk of local recurrence and therefore are avoided. Chest x-ray, lymphangiogram, IVP, abdominal ultrasound, and CT are used in clinical staging of disease. Treatment is based on type of tumor, stage of disease, general health, and age. Besides surgery, treatment involves radiation and chemotherapy singly or in combination. A number of factors influence the prognosis (Table 23-11). They include histology of the tumor, stage of the disease, and selection of appropriate treatment. Serum markers, such as AFP, β-hCG, and lactate dehydrogenase, are useful for detecting metastases and assessing responses to therapy. Most individuals treated for cancer of the testis can expect a normal life span, although some have persistent paresthesias, Raynaud phenomenon, or infertility. Almost 90% of disease-related deaths occur in the first 2 years after cessation of therapy; disease-free survival of 3 years is considered a cure. Approximately 10% of men treated for testicular cancer will experience a relapse; if the relapse is discovered early and treated, 99% can be cured. Orchiectomy does not affect sexual function, but infertility can result from chemotherapy or surgical removal of affected abdominal lymph nodes if nerves necessary for ejaculation are severed. After orchiectomy, testicular silicone implants may be used to restore "normal" scrotal appearance.

Table 23-11　Testicular Tumors of Germ-Cell Origin

Cell Types	Occurrence	Metastatic Pattern	Prognosis/Remission Rate
A. Seminoma (germinoma)	30%-35% of all testicular tumors	Rarely to retroperitoneal lymph nodes	Excellent; tumor usually remains localized and is responsive to radiation; cure rate stages I and II >95%; stages III and IV >80%
B. Nonseminomatous tumors 1. Single cell	60% of all testicular tumors		
a. Embryonal carcinoma	20%-25% of all testicular tumors; most common testicular tumor in infants and children	Earlier to regional lymphatics, also lung, liver, bone	Good; complete remission rate stages I and II >95%; stages III and IV >70%-80%
b. Teratoma	5%-10% of all testicular tumors (occurs in children and adults)	Through lymphatics and bloodstream; affects same organ systems as embryonal type	Fair
c. Choriocarcinoma	<1% of all testicular tumors	Earliest and widest, initially through bloodstream	Poor; early metastasis
2. Mixed tumors	30%-40% of all testicular tumors		
a. Teratocarcinoma	20%-25% of all testicular tumors	Mixed pattern; depends on cell types	Variable; prognosis becomes that of the most malignant element
b. Other i. Teratocarcinoma with seminoma ii. Embryonal cancer with seminoma iii. Teratoma with seminoma iv. Any combination with choriocarcinoma	10%-15% of all testicular tumors	Mixed pattern; depends on cell types	Variable; prognosis becomes that of the most malignant element
3. Non–germ-cell tumors (Leydig cell, Sertoli cell, granulosa cell, and thecal cell tumors)	<10%		

Data from American Cancer Society. In *Cancer response system document #10029*, New York, 1995, The Society; Cancer Net: *Cancer facts: questions and answers about testicular cancer*, National Cancer Institute, 2000. Available at www.cancernet.nci.nih.gov.

Epididymitis

Epididymitis, or inflammation of the epididymis, generally occurs in sexually active young males (younger than 35 years) and is rare before puberty (Figure 23-34). In young men the usual cause is a sexually transmitted microorganism, such as *N. gonorrhoeae* or *C. trachomatis*. Men who practice unprotected anal intercourse may acquire sexually transmitted epididymitis because of *E. coli, H. influenzae,* tuberculosis (especially in regions where incidence of pulmonary tuberculosis is high), *Cryptococcus,* or *Brucella*.[149] In men older than 35 years, Enterobacter (intestinal bacteria) and *Pseudomonas aeruginosa* associated with urinary tract infections and prostatitis also may cause epididymitis. Besides an infectious etiology, epididymitis may result from a chemical inflammation caused by the reflux of sterile urine into the ejaculatory ducts.[149,150] It is associated with urethral strictures, congenital posterior valves, and excessive physical straining in which increased abdominal pressure is transmitted to the bladder. Chemical epididymitis is usually self-limiting and does not require evaluation or intervention unless it persists.

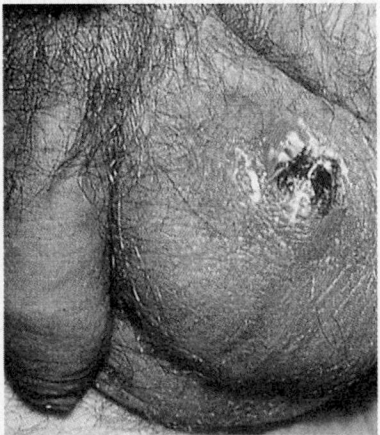

Figure 23-34 Epididymitis secondary to gonorrhea or nongonococcal urethritis. Secondary to gonorrhea or nongonococcal urethritis, this infection spread to the testes, and rupture through the scrotal wall is threatened. (From Taylor PK: *Diagnostic picture tests in sexually transmitted diseases,* London, 1995, Mosby-Wolfe.)

PATHOPHYSIOLOGY The pathogenic microorganism usually reaches the epididymis by ascending the vasa deferentia from an already infected urethra or bladder. The presence of bacteria initiates the inflammatory response, causing symptoms of bacterial epididymitis. Epididymitis caused by heavy lifting or straining results from reflux of urine from the bladder into the vas deferens and epididymis. Urine is extremely irritating to the epididymis and initiates an inflammatory response called *chemical epididymitis.*

CLINICAL MANIFESTATIONS Pain is the main symptom of epididymitis. Scrotal or inguinal pain is caused by inflammation of the epididymis and surrounding tissues. The pain is usually acute and severe. Flank pain may occur if, as the urethra passes over the spermatic cord, edematous swelling of the cord obstructs the urethra. The individual may have pyuria and bacteriuria and a history of urinary symptoms, including urethral discharge. The scrotum on the involved side is red and edematous as a result of inflammatory changes. The tail of the epididymis near the lower pole of the testis usually swells first; then swelling ascends to the head of the epididymis. The spermatic cord also may be swollen and tender.

Complications of epididymitis include abscess formation, infarction of the testis, recurrent infection, and infertility. Infarction probably is caused by thrombosis (obstruction by blood clots) of the prostatic vessels secondary to severe inflammation. Recurrent epididymitis may result from inadequate initial treatment or failure to identify or treat predisposing factors. Chronic epididymitis can cause scarring of the epididymal endothelium. Once scarring has occurred, treatment with antibiotics is ineffective because adequate antibiotic levels cannot be achieved within the epididymis.[149,150]

EVALUATION AND TREATMENT A history of recent urinary tract infection or urethral discharge suggests the diagnosis of epididymitis. The relief of pain when the inflamed testis and epididymis are elevated (Prehn sign) is also diagnostic. Definitive diagnosis is based on culture or Gram stain of a urethral swab. Epididymal aspiration may be necessary to obtain a specimen, especially if the individual has been taking antibiotics and has sterile urine.

Treatment includes antibiotic therapy for the infection itself (see Chapter 24) and various measures to provide symptomatic relief. Bed rest and scrotal elevation are recommended until the scrotum is no longer tender. Scrotal elevation facilitates maximal lymphatic and venous drainage. Abscess formation is rare with antibiotic therapy. If an abscess occurs and persists, it is drained surgically and an orchiectomy may be indicated. Complete resolution of swelling and pain may take several weeks to months. The individual's sexual partner should be treated with antibiotics if the causative microorganism is a sexually transmitted pathogen.

Disorders of the Prostate Gland

Benign Prostatic Hyperplasia

Benign prostatic hyperplasia (BPH), also called **benign prostatic hypertrophy,** is the enlargement of the prostate gland (Figure 23-35). (Because the major prostatic changes

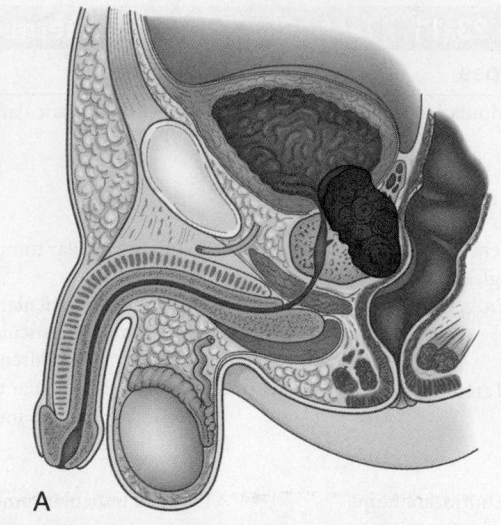

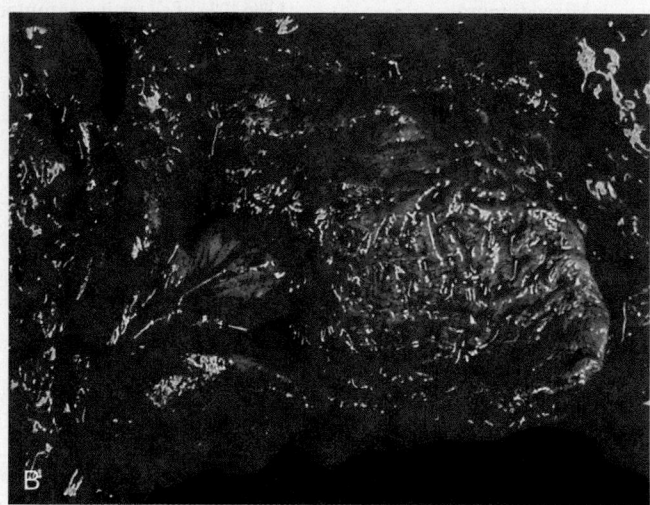

Figure 23-35 Benign prostatic hyperplasia (BPH). **A,** Condition becomes a problem as prostatic tissue compresses the urethra. **B,** Gross appearance of BPH showing transition zone resulting from bulging nodules of varying size. (B from Damjanov I, Linder J, editors: *Anderson's pathology,* ed 10, St Louis, 1996, Mosby.)

are caused by hyperplasia, not hypertrophy, benign prostatic hyperplasia is the preferred term.) This condition becomes problematic as prostatic tissue compresses the urethra, where it passes through the prostate. The prevalence among U.S. men 60 years and older is about 50% and among men 70 years or older 90%.[151] BPH is common and involves a complex pathophysiology with several endocrine and local factors and remodeled microenvironment. Its relationship to aging is well documented. At birth the prostate is pea sized, and growth of the gland is gradual until puberty. A period of rapid development continues until the third decade of life, when the prostate reaches adult size. Around 40 to 45 years of age, benign hyperplasia begins and continues slowly until death. Although dihydrotestosterone (DHT) is necessary for normal prostatic development, its role in BPH remains unclear. Among all androgen-metabolizing enzymes within the human prostate, 5α-reductase is the most powerful. This reductase corresponds to an age-dependent DHT level. Therefore, although 5α-reductase and DHT decrease with age in the epithelium, they remain relatively constant in the stroma of the prostate gland.

PATHOGENESIS   Current causative theories of BPH focus on levels and ratios of endocrine factors such as androgens, estrogens, gonadotropins, and prolactin and changes in the balance between autocrine/paracrine growth-stimulatory and growth-inhibitory factors. These factors include insulin-like growth factors (IGFs), epidermal growth factor, nerve growth factor, fibroblast factors, IGF binding proteins, and transforming growth factor-beta (TGF-β).[152]

Aging and circulating androgens are associated with BPH and enlargement. These factors are predisposed as disrupting the *balance* of growth factor signaling pathways and stromal/epithelial interactions creating a growth-promoting and tissue remodeling microenvironment.[153] All together these interactions lead to an increase in prostate volume. The remodeled stroma promotes local inflammation with altered cytokine, reactive oxygen/nitrogen species, and chemoattractants.[153] The resultant increased oxygen demands of proliferating cells causes a local hypoxia that induces angiogenesis and changes to fibroblasts. Functional and phenotypic changes (transdifferentiation) of fibroblasts to the myofibroblasts is a hallmark of the remodeled microenviroment.[153]

BPH begins in the periurethral glands, which are the inner glands or layers of the prostate. The prostate enlarges as nodules form and grow (nodular hyperplasia) and glandular cells enlarge (hypertrophy). The development of BPH occurs over a prolonged period, and changes within the urinary tract are slow and insidious.

CLINICAL MANIFESTATIONS   Clinical manifestations are a result of complex interactions involving prostatic urethral resistance to the mechanical and spastic effects of BPH, intravesical pressure during voiding, detrusor muscle strength, neurologic functioning, and general physical health.

During the early stages of urethral obstruction, the detrusor muscle hypertrophies to help the bladder force urine out against increasing resistance. Symptoms are considered obstructive (weak urinary stream, prolonged voiding, abdominal straining, hesitancy, intermittency, incomplete bladder emptying, postmicturitional dribble) or irritative (frequency and repeated urination, nocturia, urgency, incontinence, and bladder pain and dysuria)[154] and may wax and wane.[155] As obstruction progresses, often over a period of several years, the detrusor muscle decompensates and the bladder is unable to empty all of the urine. Increasing volumes of urine are retained until urine retention is chronic. The volume of urine retained may be great enough to produce uncontrolled "overflow incontinence" with any increase in intra-abdominal pressure. At this stage the force of the urinary stream is reduced significantly and much more time is required to initiate and complete voiding.

Progressive bladder distention causes sacculations or diverticular outpouchings of the bladder wall, and some neural degeneration of smooth muscle cells occurs. The ureters may be obstructed where they pass through the hypertrophied detrusor muscle. Hematuria, bladder or kidney infection, bladder calculi, acute urinary retention hydroureter, hydronephrosis, and renal insufficiency are common complications.[154] Some men initially have signs of uremia and renal failure. On digital rectal examination (DRE) the hyperplastic prostate is a soft or firm enlargement with smooth mucosal surface and no discernible distinction between lobes; asymmetry is common. The palpated prostate does not always reflect the degree of BPH because a substantial portion of the enlargement is intravesicular.[156] Thirty percent of men with mild to moderate symptoms improve with watchful waiting.

There is no way to reverse progressive BPH, but the hyperplasia is not always progressive. For these reasons, timing of intervention is variable and depends on severity of symptoms and the presence of complications. Annual DREs are used to screen men older than 40 years for BPH. If marked enlargement, moderate to severe symptoms, or complications are present, transrectal ultrasound (TRUS) is used to determine bladder and prostate volume and residual urine. Urinalysis, serum creatinine and blood urea nitrogen, uroflowmetry, postvoid residual (PVR) urine, pressure-flow study, cystometry, and cystourethroscopy are used to determine kidney and bladder function.[154] Physical examination with DRE and prostate-specific antigen (PSA) is conducted to determine hyperplasia.[157] PSA density (PSAD) is helpful in differentiating BPH from prostatic cancer. PSAD is calculated by dividing PSA serum levels by the volume of prostate tissue, which is determined by TRUS. When necessary, the hyperplastic tissue may be removed surgically to prevent the serious consequences of urethral obstruction. Glands less than 60 g are treated by transurethral resection, laser therapy, or microwave thermotherapy,[158] whereas larger glands are removed surgically (prostatectomy). A permanent indwelling catheter is inserted if the individual cannot tolerate surgery. BPH has been treated successfully with drugs. α₁-Adrenergic blockers (prazosin and tamsulosin) are used to relax the smooth muscle of the bladder and prostate. Antiandrogen agents, such as finasteride (Proscar), selectively block androgens at the prostate cellular level and cause the prostate gland to shrink.[159] These drugs offer an alternative to surgery for as many as 75% of men with mild prostate enlargement.[159] Neither α₁-adrenergic blockers nor finasteride seems to affect sexual desire or potency; finasteride may cause bone loss and lower levels of PSA. PSA is used as a screen for prostate cancer.

Prostatitis

Prostatitis is an inflammation of the prostate. Some degree of prostatic inflammation is present in 4% to 36% of the male population. This percentage increases to 50% in older men. Inflammation is usually limited to a few of the gland's excretory ducts (Figure 23-36).

Prostatitis is characterized as (1) acute bacterial prostatitis, (2) chronic bacterial prostatitis, or (3) nonbacterial prostatitis. **Prostatodynia** (pain in the prostate) is sometimes

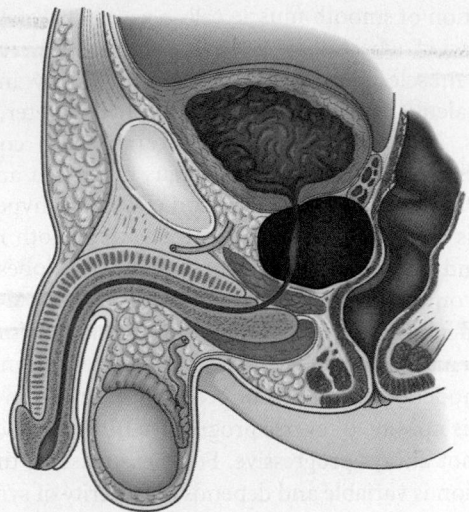

Figure 23-36 Prostatitis.

considered a form of nonbacterial prostatitis. Men with prostatodynia have the same clinical manifestations as those with nonbacterial prostatitis, but physical and laboratory examinations do not show prostatic pathology. Prostatodynia may not be caused by a pathologic condition of the prostate but rather by spasms in the genitourinary tract or tension in the muscles of the pelvic floor.

A number of defense mechanisms normally protect the lower urogenital tract from infection. Mechanical defenses include urethral length, micturition (urination), and ejaculation. Structural malformations and instrumentation of the genitourinary tract may weaken these defense mechanisms. Chemical defenses include antimicrobial substances in the prostatic fluid. The most important of these is a zinc-containing polypeptide known as *prostatic antibacterial factor.* Coliform bacteria, particularly *Enterobacter, E. coli, Enterococcus, Klebsiella,* and *Pseudomonas,* are common pathogens of bacterial prostatitis. *Ureaplasma* and *C. trachomatis* also may be causative agents of infectious prostatitis.[150]

Bacterial Prostatitis

Acute bacterial prostatitis is an ascending infection of the urinary tract that tends to occur in men between ages 30 and 50 years but is also associated with BPH in older men. Infection stimulates an inflammatory response in which the prostate becomes enlarged, tender, and firm or boggy. The onset of prostatitis may be acute and unrelated to previous illnesses, or it may follow catheterization or cystoscopy.

Clinical manifestations of acute bacterial prostatitis are those of acute cystitis or pyelonephritis. Sudden onset of malaise, low back and perineal pain, high fever (up to 40° C [104° F]), and chills is common, as are dysuria, inability to empty the bladder, nocturia, and urinary retention. Myalgia and arthralgia also may occur. The individual also may have symptoms of lower urinary tract obstruction, such as a slow, small, narrowed urinary stream, which may be a medical emergency. Men are acutely ill and may look toxic. Prostatic

pain may occur, especially when the individual is in an upright position, because the pelvic floor muscles tighten with standing and compression of the prostate gland occurs. Some individuals experience low back pain, painful ejaculation, and rectal or perineal pain. Palpation discloses an extremely tender, swollen prostate with normal to "boggy" consistency that may be warm to the touch.

Because acute bacterial prostatitis usually is associated with a bladder infection caused by the same microorganism, urine cultures disclose its identity. Prostatic massage may express enough secretions from the urethra for direct bacterial examination, but massage may be painful and increases the risk that the infection will ascend to adjacent structures or enter the bloodstream and cause septicemia. For these reasons, prostatic massage generally is contraindicated; transurethral instrumentation also is contraindicated.

Long-term, broad-spectrum antibiotic therapy with fluoroquinolone agents or trimethoprim-sulfamethoxazole for at least 30 to 42 days is recommended to resolve the infection and control its spread. In severe cases the individual is hospitalized and treated with combination intravenous antibiotics, usually an aminoglycoside (gentamicin sulfate, kanamycin sulfate, or tobramycin) and ampicillin for 1 week followed by 4 to 6 weeks of oral antibiotics. Pain relievers, antipyretics, bed rest, and adequate hydration also are therapeutic. Complications include urinary retention that resolves with antibiotic therapy; prostatic abscess that may rupture into the urethra, rectum, or perineum; epididymitis; bacteremia; and septic shock. Urinary retention requiring drainage is best managed with a suprapubic catheter; Foley catheterization is contraindicated during acute infection.

Chronic bacterial prostatitis is characterized by recurrent urinary symptoms and persistence of pathogenic bacteria (usually gram negative) in urine or prostatic fluid.[150] This form of prostatitis is the most common recurrent urinary tract infection in men. Symptoms are variable and may be similar to those of an acute bladder infection: frequency, urgency, dysuria, perineal discomfort, low back pain, and sexual dysfunction. The prostate may be only slightly enlarged or boggy, but fibrosis caused by repeated infections can cause it to be firm and irregular in shape.

When the initial urine sample is bacteria free, prostatic massage is used to express secretions. Subsequently, the first 10 ml of voided urine is collected and examined microscopically. Prostatic secretions showing more than 10 white blood cells per high-power field and macrophages containing fat indicate bacterial infection; diagnosis is confirmed by culture. Prostatic calculi may be seen on pelvic x-ray or TRUS.

Treatment of chronic bacterial prostatitis is difficult because it is often caused by prostatic calculi. Calculi are silent and are found in up to 50% of men with prostatitis, and infected calculi can serve as a source of bacterial persistence and relapsing urinary tract infections.[150] Calculi harbor pathogens within the stone, and consequently pathogens cannot be eradicated from the urinary tract. Permanent cure is achieved by surgical removal of the stones through transurethral prostatectomy, which may not be a viable option for young men. More common symptoms are tempered with chronic suppressive therapy. Quinolones, because of their bioavailability and penetration into prostatic tissue, are the treatment of choice; drug therapy lasts for a minimum of 3 to 4 weeks. If symptoms do not subside, other infectious microorganisms are considered and treated accordingly.[150] Comfort measures include nonsteroidal anti-inflammatory drug therapy and liberal use of sitz baths.

Nonbacterial Prostatitis

Nonbacterial prostatitis is the most common prostatitis syndrome and consists of prostatic inflammation without evidence of bacterial infection. Symptoms tend to be milder but are persistent and annoying. Presumably, noninfectious prostatitis or prostatodynia is caused by reflux of sterile urine into the ejaculatory ducts as a result of high-pressure voiding.[150] Reflux may be triggered by spasms of the external or internal sphincters. Some men may actually have interstitial cystitis and should be treated accordingly.

Men with nonbacterial prostatitis may complain of pain or a dull ache that is continuous or spasmodic in the suprapubic, intrapubic, scrotal, penile, or inguinal area. Other symptoms are pain on ejaculation and urinary symptoms, such as frequency of urination. The prostate gland generally feels normal on palpation.

Digital examination of the prostate, bacterial cultures of the urogenital tract, microscopic examination of expressed prostatic fluid, urethroscopy, and urodynamic studies are used to verify the diagnosis of nonbacterial prostatitis. Nonbacterial prostatitis is a diagnosis by exclusion.

Therapy is individualized and aimed at decreasing symptoms. α_1-Adrenergic blockers (e.g., terazosin, doxazosin, and tamsulosin) may be helpful in decreasing spasms of the prostate muscle. Other treatments include skeletal muscle relaxants, pelvic floor relaxation using biofeedback, and prostatic thermotherapy.[150] Additional treatments may include hot sitz baths, bed rest, anticholinergics, and anti-inflammatory drugs.

Cancer of the Prostate

Prostate cancer is among the most common male cancers but the incidence varies greatly worldwide (Figure 23-37). It is the most common cancer in American males but the third most common cancer worldwide. In the United States it accounts for more than 14% of all cancer deaths; only lung cancer accounts for more deaths. Among countries with reliable cancer statistics, prostate cancer rates are highest in westernized countries, such as the United States and Western Europe and lowest in Asian countries. It also is rare in Africa, Central America, and South America. Screening with PSA can amplify the incidence

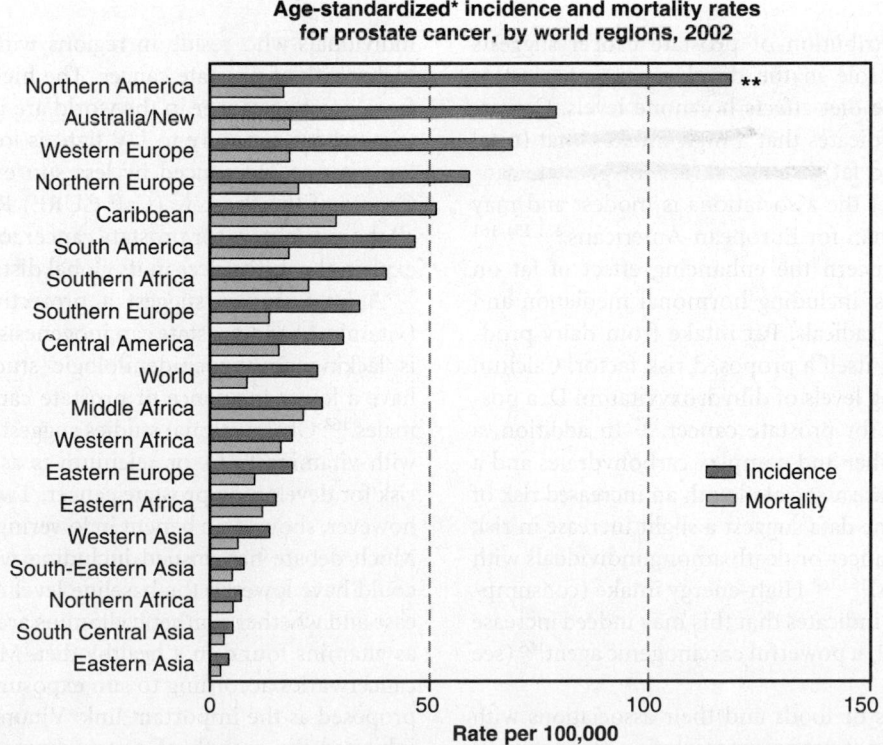

Age-standardized* incidence and mortality rates for prostate cancer, by world regions, 2002

Northern America, Australia/New, Western Europe, Northern Europe, Caribbean, South America, Southern Africa, Southern Europe, Central America, World, Middle Africa, Western Africa, Eastern Europe, Eastern Africa, Western Asia, South-Eastern Asia, Northern Africa, South Central Asia, Eastern Asia

Rate per 100,000 — 0, 50, 100, 150

Incidence / Mortality

* to the World Standard population
**One reason for the large incidence in the USA is the frequent use of PSA testing.

Figure 23-37 Age-standardized* incidence and mortality rates for prostate cancer by world regions, 2002. (Data from Cancer Research, UK Cancer Incidence Statistics updated November 2008, News & Resources.)

of prostate cancer by allowing detection of prostate lesions that although meeting the pathologic criteria for malignancy, many believe to have low potential for growth and metastasis; however, this is controversial. Thus screening can amplify the incidence of prostate cancer by including the detection of these localized lesions. Therefore, the incidence rates in some countries, such as the United States, reflect clinical as well as latent (preclinical) disease compared with other countries that report only clinical disease. Comparing data in the pre-PSA era does reflect less extreme incidence rates, but the United States still has the highest rates. Data from the Surveillance, Epidemiology, and End Results (SEER) program show that incidence rates in the United States for white men increased 80% from 1983 to 1987 and 1988 to 1992 (possibly because of increased screening in asymptomatic men).[160]

A small decline in the death rate has been noted during the past few years in the United States and other developing countries. The overall mortality rates are mostly in men older than 65; within younger groups, mortality has been stable across decades. Incidence increases with advancing age; more than 75% of all prostate cancer is diagnosed in men older than 65.[1] By age 85, about one in six American men will develop prostate cancer in their lifetime and about 3% will die from it. With aging, most of the androgen-metabolizing enzymes undergo significant alteration. The incidence is low in black African men worldwide; however, black African-American men have the highest rate of prostate cancer in the world and in the United States.

Dietary Factors

The worldwide distribution of prostate cancer suggests that diet may play a role in the development of prostate cancer, especially if the diet affects hormone levels. Consistency across studies indicates that a high intake of fat (total and especially saturated fat) is a risk factor for prostate cancer, but the strength of the associations is modest and may be greater for blacks than for European-Americans.[151,154-161] Several hypotheses concern the enhancing effect of fat on prostate carcinogenesis, including hormonal mediation and the generation of free radicals. Fat intake from dairy products increases calcium, itself a proposed risk factor. Calcium can suppress circulating levels of dihydroxyvitamin D, a possible protective factor for prostate cancer.[162] In addition, a low intake of dietary fiber and complex carbohydrates and a high intake of protein are associated with an increased risk of prostate cancer.[161] Some data suggest a slight increase in risk of advanced prostate cancer or death among individuals with a high body mass index.[163,164] High-energy intake (consumption of excess calories) indicates that this may indeed increase insulin levels and IGF-1, a powerful carcinogenic agent[165] (see Pathogenesis p. 865).

Individual nutrients or foods and their associations with prostate cancer risk are not strong, yet migration of individuals from low-risk geographic areas of the world, such as Japan, to high-risk countries, such as the United States, increases risk considerably.[166] These changes in risk probably reflect differences in lifestyle and dietary habits. Geographically,

individuals who reside in regions with less sunlight have a higher risk of prostate cancer. The highest rates of mortality from prostate cancer in the world are in Scandinavian countries, where exposure to UV light is low; the possible link is less vitamin D induced by less sun exposure. The Cure of Cancer of the Prostate (CaP CURE) Report[167] states that of all the risk factors for prostate cancer, only nutrition seems to explain the differences in its global distribution.

Animal studies suggest a protective effect of retinoids (vitamin A) and prostate carcinogenesis; however, consistency is lacking among epidemiologic studies. Vegetarian men have a lower incidence of prostate cancer than omnivorous males.[168] Observational studies suggest that supplementation with vitamins E, C, or selenium is associated with a lower risk for developing prostate cancer. Two recent clinical trials, however, showed no benefit in lowering prostate cancer.[169,170] Much debate has ensued including whether PSA screening could have lowered the baseline level of more advanced disease and whether synthetic vitamins are possibly not the same as vitamins found in a healthy diet. Mortality from prostate cancer varies according to sun exposure; vitamin D has been proposed as the important link. Vitamin D (1,25-[OH]2D3) inhibited the growth of certain human prostate cancer cell lines by an androgen-dependent mechanism.[171] Higher selenium levels of vitamin D were significantly related to a better prognosis in individuals with prostate cancer.[172] Lycopene, a carotenoid found in large amounts in tomatoes that gives

---

NUTRITION & DISEASE

Nutrition and Risk Reduction for Prostate Cancer

- Avoid saturated fat and red meat.
- Avoid specific polyunsaturated fats, including omega-6 fat, linoleic acid (found in safflower and soybean oil), and omega-3 fat α-linolenic acid (found in red meat, mayonnaise, soybean oil, rapeseed oil, and margarine)
- Avoid foods with hydrogenated or partially hydrogenated oil.
- Substitute oils with olive oils (use sparingly).
- Decrease total energy intake from calories; avoid refined sugars.*
- Increase vegetables (cruciferous), fruits, garlic, green tea.
- Increase lycopene (reddest tomatoes available, tomato juice, soup, salads).
- Increase soy (genistein).
- Increase sunshine exposure for daily requirement of vitamin D or vitamin D_3 supplementation.
- Maintain calcium intake at 1000 mg (19 to 50 years old), 1200 mg (51 and older); switch from cow's milk† to soy milk.
- Increase fiber (whole grains, beans, cereals).
- Folic acid (high dose) is not supported for prevention.‡

For documented studies see Arnot R: *The prostate cancer protection plan: the foods, supplements and drugs that could save your life,* Boston, 2000, Little, Brown.
*Emerging as very important for decreasing insulin-like growth factor (IGF-1).
†Cow's milk with inceased levels of IGF-1.
‡Data from Figueiredo JC: *J Natl Cancer Inst* 101:432, 2009.

them their color, has been associated with a lower risk of prostate cancer.[173,174]

Hormones

Prostate cancer develops in an androgen-dependent epithelium and is usually androgen sensitive. In addition, a few case reports exist of prostate cancer in men who used androgenic steroids as anabolic agents or for medical purposes, suggestive of a causal relationship.[166,175-177] Population studies have not, however, provided clear and convincing patterns about associations between circulating hormone concentrations and prostate cancer risk.[166] Only a few associations with prostate cancer risk have been observed consistently (in at least three studies), and their associations are weak: (1) slightly higher circulating testosterone and estrogen levels and lower DHEA (sulfate) levels in high-risk black men as compared with lower-risk European-American men; and (2) a cytosine-adenine-guanine (CAG) repeat-length polymorphism in the androgen-receptor gene associated with increased risk and increased receptor activity (androgen receptor). Evidence for involvement of activity of the enzyme 5α-reductase, which is critical in androgen activity in the prostate, is contradictory and inconsistent.[166] In men younger than 50 years, circulating levels of androgens and estrogens appear to be higher in men of African descent than in European-American men.

Androgens promote prostatic epithelial growth during fetal and prepubertal periods. In adults androgens act through reciprocal homeostatic stromal (microenvironment; see Chapter 11) epithelial interactions to maintain normal differentiation and halt growth[178] (see Pathogenesis).

Investigations directed at understanding the hormonal basis of prostate (as well as breast) carcinogenesis have numerous problems. The complexities of interacting hormones and separating out the effects of a single hormone are profound. In addition, only single *blood* samples are generally available, *tissue* hormone samples important for paracrine signaling are not consistently measured, and within-subject variations over time and differences in circadian rhythms cannot be adequately measured. The results of several animal studies do support elevation of bioavailable and bioactive androgens in the circulation and in target tissue as an important risk factor. Animal studies also indicate that increased biologic activity of the androgen receptor may be associated with prostate cancer. See the Pathogenesis section for a more thorough discussion of the role of hormones in the pathogenesis of prostate cancer.

Vasectomy

Vasectomy has been identified as a possible risk factor for prostate cancer in case-controlled and cohort studies.[170,179,180] Three mechanisms by which vasectomy could increase risk are (1) elevation of circulating androgens; (2) immunologic mechanisms involving antisperm antibodies; and (3) reduction of seminal fluid levels of 5α-dihydrotestosterone, the active metabolite of testosterone in the prostate, in vasectomized men. Other investigators reported a decrease in SHBG and an increase in the ratio of testosterone to SHBG.[181] These results suggest an elevation of circulating free testosterone following

vasectomy.[166] However, with these combined mechanisms it is unlikely that vasectomy plays a causal role.[162]

Genetic and Epigenetic Factors

Other possible causes are genetic predisposition (familial and hereditary forms). Genetic studies suggest that strong familial predisposition may be responsible for 5% to 10% of prostate cancers.[1] Compared with men with no family history, those with one first-degree relative with prostate cancer have twice the risk and those with two first-degree relatives have five times the risk.[182] Men with *BRCA2* (suppressor tumor) germline mutations have a 20-fold increase in risk. A common type of somatic mutation that gives rise to chromosomal rearrangements is the *ETS* gene. The most common epigenetic alteration in prostate cancer is hypermethylation of the glutathione S-transferase (*GST P1*) gene. This gene is located on chromosome 11 and is part of the pathway that helps protect against carcinogen damage.[183] A number of other epigenetic modifications found on tumor suppressor genes include *PTEN, RB, p16/INK4a, MLH1, MSH21,* and *APC*.[182] The hereditary form constitutes about 9% of all prostate cancers and approximately 43% of cancers in men less than 55 years of age.[156] There is no clear evidence of a causal link between BPH and prostate cancer even though they may often occur together. Variations in several other genes related to inflammatory pathways might affect the probability of developing prostate cancer.[184]

PATHOGENESIS   More than 95% of prostatic neoplasms are adenocarcinomas,[185] and most occur in the periphery of the prostate. Most hyperplasias, however, arise in the transitional zone (Figure 23-38). Several histologic grading systems have been developed on the basis of the glandular pattern, the degree of differentiation (anaplasia) of the cancer cells, or both. The biologic aggressiveness of the neoplasm appears to be related to the degree of differentiation rather than the size of the tumor (see Box 23-13 on p. 869).

Hormonal

Just as the testicles are the male equivalent of the female ovaries, the prostate is the male equivalent of the female uterus; in both situations they originate from the same embryonic cells. This may be important in understanding the role of the associated hormones testosterone, dihydrotestosterone, and estradiol in prostate carcinogenesis. Testosterone and DHT are the most important androgens in the adult male. Testosterone is the major *circulating* androgen, whereas DHT predominates in prostate tissue and binds to the androgen receptor (AR) with greater affinity than does testosterone.[186]

Testosterone is the major androgen from the interstitial cells of the testis (Leydig cells). Its production in men is almost 5 mg/day. The adrenal cortex contributes the far less potent androstenedione as its major androgen, at about 3 mg/day. In the target tissues and, to a lesser extent, in the testes themselves, testosterone is converted to DHT by the enzyme type 2 5α-reductase (Figure 23-39). Type 2 5α-reductase is located mostly in stromal cells. Thus DHT is the most potent intraprostatic androgen. About half of circulating testosterone is bound to SHBG, about half binds to albumin, and about

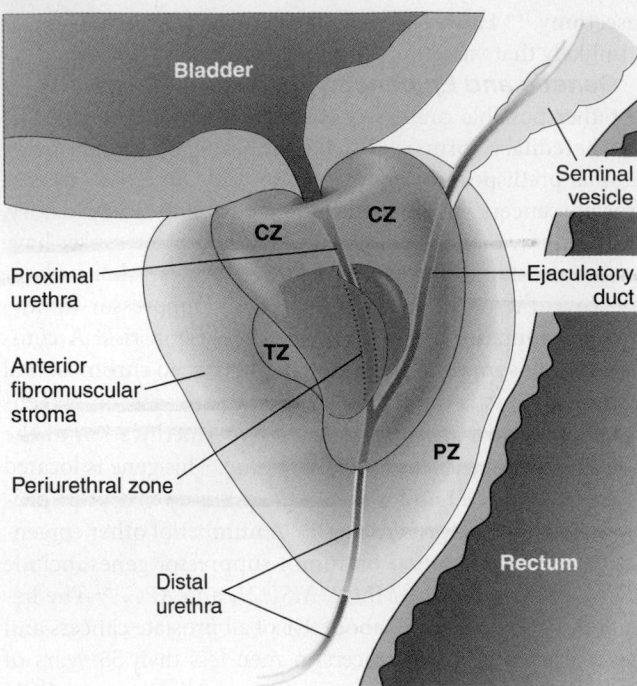

Figure 23-38 Adult prostate. The normal prostate contains several distinct regions, including a central zone (CZ), a peripheral zone (PZ), a transitional zone (TZ), and a periurethral zone. Most carcinomas arise from the peripheral glands of the organ and may be palpable during digital examination of the rectum. Nodular hyperplasia, in contrast, arises from more centrally situated glands and is more likely to produce urinary obstruction early than is carcinoma. (From Epstein JI: The lower urinary tract and male genital system. In Kumar V, Abbas AK, Fausto N, editors: *Robbins and Cotran pathologic basis of disease,* ed 8, Philadelphia, 2009, Saunders.)

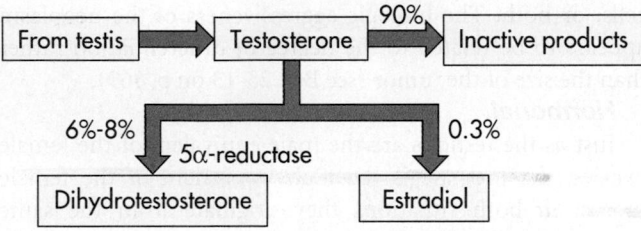

Figure 23-39 Testosterone and conversion to dihydrotestosterone (DHT).

1% to 2% exists in a free state. Free testosterone, including testosterone disassociated from albumin and possibly SHBG, enters the prostate cell, where it is converted to DHT.[186] DHT is a paracrine hormone because it affects the local environment or stroma. Several intraprostatic enzymes encoded by genes, *HSD3A* and *HDS3B*, are activated by DHT and are important components of intraprostatic androgen regulation. The conjugated byproduct, 3α-androstenediol glucuronide (AAG), a terminal metabolite of DHT, can be measured in the circulation and used as an indicator of DHT levels. The drug finasteride, an inhibitor of intraprostatic 5α-reductase type II enzyme, decreases AAG levels. Thus AAG is a marker of intraprostatic 5α-reductase activity and androgen levels.

Normally a small amount of estrogen is produced per day—65 mcg of estrone and 45 mcg of estradiol—by the aromatization of androstenedione and testosterone, respectively. This reaction is catalyzed by the enzyme system aromatase. A very small quantity of estradiol is released by the testes (see Figure 23-39); the rest of the estrogens in males are produced by adipose tissue, liver, skin, brain, and other nonendocrine tissue. Thus testosterone is a precursor of the two hormones, DHT and estradiol.

Most of the androgen-metabolizing enzymes undergo a significant age-dependent alteration. In epithelium, both the 5α-reductase activity and the DHT level decrease with age; whereas in stroma not only is 5α-reductase activity rather constant over the whole age range but also the DHT level is constant. In contrast to the relatively unaltered DHT level, the estrogen content follows an age-dependent increase. Thus the age-dependent decrease of the DHT accumulation in epithelium and the concomitant increase of the estrogen accumulation in stroma lead to a tremendous increase with age of the estrogen/androgen ratio in the human prostate. In animal studies, chronic exposure to testosterone plus estradiol is strongly carcinogenic, whereas testosterone alone is weakly carcinogenic.[166] The mechanism is not clearly understood but appears to involve estrogen-generated oxidative stress and DNA toxicity, and it requires androgen and estrogen receptor–mediated processes, such as changes in sex steroid metabolism and receptor status.[166] In addition, there are changes in the balance between autocrine/paracrine growth-stimulatory and growth-inhibitory factors, such as IGFs, epidermal growth factor (EGF), nerve growth factor (NGF), IGF-binding proteins, and TGF-β.

Stromal Environment

A precursor lesion, *prostatic intraepithelial neoplasia (PIN)* has been described. PIN may be more concentrated in prostates containing cancer and are noted in proximity to cancer.[182] The final fate of PIN is, however, unknown including the possibilities of latency invasion and even regression (Figure 23-40). The microenvironment (stroma) surrounding the prostatic tumor actively fuels the progression of prostate cancer from localized growth, to invasion, to development of distant metastases.[187] Several types of stromal cells in the surrounding microenvironment are recruited to tumors, enhancing cancer growth and metastases.[187] Important are the microenvironment balances of proliferation and apoptosis to suppress malignancy, but perturbations in the stroma, for example by chronic inflammation, override the protective mechanisms and shift the tissue microenvironment to a growth-promoting malignant state.[187]

Androgens drive prostatic epithelial growth during fetal and prepubertal periods and in adulthood androgens participate through reciprocal homeostatic stromal-epithelial interactions to maintain differentiation but *arrest* growth.[178] Intercellular communication between prostate tumor cells and organ-specific stroma involve diffusible molecules from stromal cell types (e.g., endothelial cells, pericytes, fibroblasts) and bone marrow-derived cells (BMDCs, macrophages,

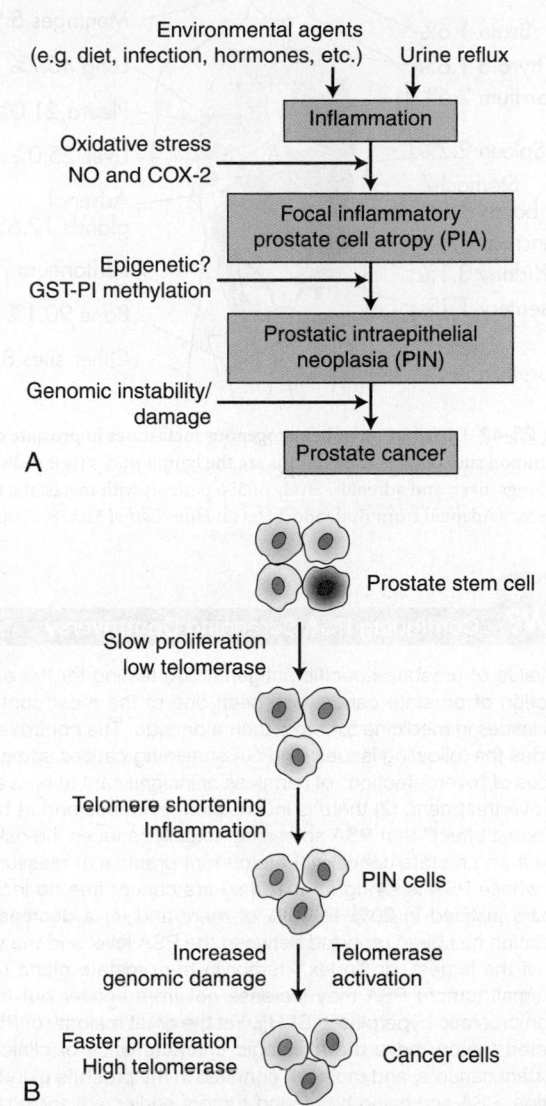

Environmental agents
(e.g. diet, infection, hormones, etc.)   Urine reflux

Inflammation

Oxidative stress
NO and COX-2

Focal inflammatory
prostate cell atropy (PIA)

Epigenetic?
GST-PI methylation

Prostatic intraepithelial
neoplasia (PIN)

Genomic instability/
damage

Prostate cancer

A

Prostate stem cell

Slow proliferation
low telomerase

Telomere shortening
Inflammation

PIN cells

Increased
genomic damage   Telomerase
activation

Faster proliferation
High telomerase   Cancer cells

B

Figure 23-40 Hypothetical models of prostate carcinogenesis: inflammation and telomerase. A, Inflammation may happen early from repeated injuries or infection, or both, or from refluxed urine into the prostate. Manifestations of inflammation include oxidative stress damage with the generation of ROS. Thus, the microenvironment is inflammatory and products like nitric oxide (NO) and cyclooxygenase (COX-2) can cause genetic and epigenetic alterations. Inflammatory infiltrates can produce "focal" atrophy. In this model, proliferative inflammatory atrophy (PIA) may be considered the precursor lesion to prostatic intraepithelial neoplasia (PIN). If the oxidant damage is not detoxified by the glutathione enzyme (GST P1) the cells continue to produce PIN. Interesting is that estrogen, through ER-B, influences the protective mechanism of glutathione transferase and can cause epigenetic alterations that increase inflammation. Elevation of estrogens in the presence of testosterone results in prostate-specific inflammation. With the loss of GST P1 continued inflammation causes the transition of PIN to increased prostate cancer. **B,** Telomerase is an enzyme in the normal stem cell population thought to regulate telomere length and homeostasis during cell renewal (see Chapter 11). Although unknown, prostate stem cells are thought to have low levels of telomerase activity. Studies reveal that telomere length of high grade PIN were shorter than normal cells and that a subset of PIN cells activate telomerase causing cells to become immortal and progress to prostate cancer. (Data from Marian CO, Shay JW: *Biochimica Biophysics Acta* 2009 Mar 2 [Epub ahead of print]; Sciarra A et al: *Eur Urol* 52[4]:964-972, 2007.)

neutrophils, mast cells). All together these released mediators result in malignant progression (also see Chapter 11, p. 377). In addition, the periepithelial stroma undergoes progressive loss in smooth muscle with the appearance of **carcinoma-associated fibroblasts (CAFs).** Thus the stromal microenvironment is a necessary determinant of benign versus malignant growth.[178,187]

From all of these observations, the following multifactorial general hypothesis of prostate carcinogenesis emerges: (1) androgens act as tumor promoters through androgen receptor–mediated mechanisms to (2) enhance the carcinogenic activity of strong endogenous DNA toxic carcinogens, including reactive estrogen metabolites and estrogen—and prostatic-generated reactive oxygen species—(3) alterations in autocrine/paracrine growth-stimulating and growth-inhibiting factors between the prostate tumor cells and microenvironment, and (4) possibly unknown environmental-lifestyle carcinogens. All of these factors are modulated by diet and genetic determinants, such as hereditary susceptibility genes and polymorphic genes (especially steroid 5α-reductase type II *[SRD5A2]*), that encode receptors and enzymes involved in the metabolism and action of steroid hormones.[166,186]

The most common sites of distant metastasis are the lymph nodes, bones, lungs, liver, and adrenals. The pelvis, lumbar spine, femur, thoracic spine, and ribs are the most common sites of bone metastasis. Local extension is usually posterior, although late in the disease the tumor may invade the rectum or encroach on the prostatic urethra and cause bladder outlet obstruction (Figure 23-41; see Clinical Manifestations). The spread through blood vessels is illustrated in Figure 23-42.

CLINICAL MANIFESTATIONS Prostatic cancer often causes no symptoms until it is far advanced. The first manifestations of disease are those of bladder outlet obstruction: slow urinary stream, hesitancy, incomplete emptying, frequency, nocturia, and dysuria. Unlike the symptoms of obstruction caused by BPH, the symptoms of obstruction caused by prostatic cancer are progressive and do not remit. Local extension of prostatic cancer can obstruct the upper urinary tract ureters as well. If rectal obstruction occurs, a man may experience a large bowel obstruction or difficulty in defecation. Symptoms of late disease include bone pain at sites of bone metastasis, edema of the lower extremities, enlargement of lymph nodes, liver enlargement, pathologic bone fractures, and mental confusion associated with brain metastases.

EVALUATION AND TREATMENT The most significant test used in the diagnosis and management of prostate cancer is **prostate-specific antigen (PSA).** DRE may detect early prostatic carcinomas but is has low sensitivity and specificity.[182] A transrectal biopsy is required to confirm the diagnosis. The cut-off point between normal and abnormal PSA is a serum level of 4 ng/mL. Yet this simplified approach to serum PSA tests has led to the delay in diagnosis of prostate cancer and has caused considerable controversy (see What's New? Continuing PSA Screening Controversy). In addition,

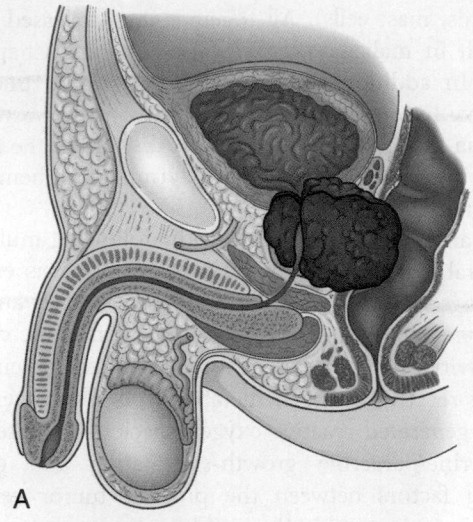

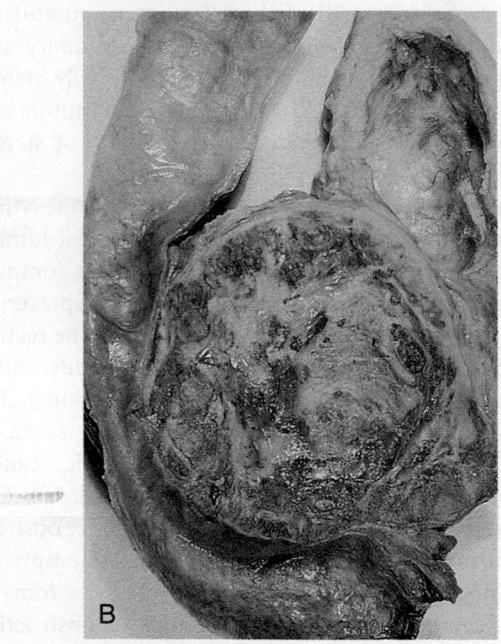

Figure 23-41 Carcinoma of prostate. A, Schematic of prostate tumor. **B,** Carcinoma of the prostate extending into the rectum and urinary bladder. (B from Damjanov I, Linder J, editors: *Pathology: a color atlas,* St Louis, 2000, Mosby.)

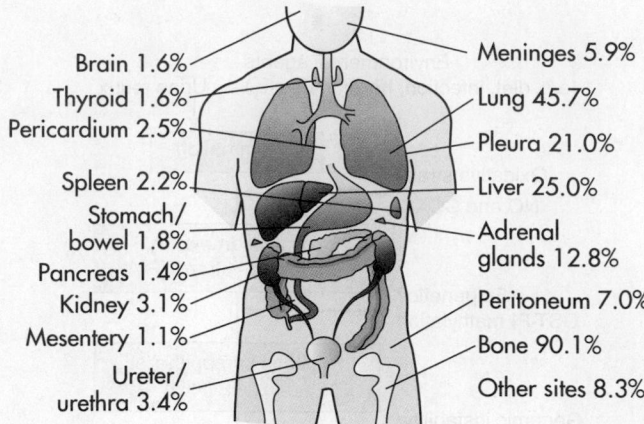

Brain 1.6%	Meninges 5.9%
Thyroid 1.6%	Lung 45.7%
Pericardium 2.5%	Pleura 21.0%
Spleen 2.2%	Liver 25.0%
Stomach/bowel 1.8%	Adrenal glands 12.8%
Pancreas 1.4%	Peritoneum 7.0%
Kidney 3.1%	
Mesentery 1.1%	Bone 90.1%
Ureter/urethra 3.4%	Other sites 8.3%

Figure 23-42 Distribution of hematogenous metastases in prostate cancer. Common sites of distant metastasis are the lymph nodes (not shown), bones, lungs, liver, and adrenals. Study of 556 patients with metastatic prostate cancer. (Adapted from Budendorf L et al: *Hum Pathol* 31:578, 2000.)

WHAT'S NEW? Continuing PSA Screening Controversy

The value of prostate-specific antigen (PSA) testing for the early detection of prostate cancer has been one of the most contentious issues in medicine for more than a decade. The controversy includes the following issues: (1) PSA screening causes some instances of "overdetection" of harmless or insignificant tumors and thus overtreatment; (2) there is inconsistent evidence and at best a "modest effect" that PSA screening actually reduces the risk of death from prostate cancer; (3) the current practice of reassuring men whose PSA is ≤4 ng/ml that they are cancer free no longer appears justified in 20% to 40% of men; and (4) a decreasing correlation has been reported between the PSA level and the volume of the largest, or "index," tumor in the prostate gland (i.e., with small tumors PSA may increase not from cancer but from benign prostatic hyperplasia [BPH]). Yet the great majority of PSA-detected tumors have the histologic characteristics of clinically important cancers, and most are confined in the prostate gland. In addition, PSA screening has found tumors earlier, advancing the date of diagnosis by 5 to 13 years, and prostate cancer–specific mortality rates in the United States have decreased by about 4% per year since 1992, 5 years after the beginning of PSA screening. Adding fuel to the controversy is the most recent finding that as many as 15% of men with a "normal" PSA level had prostate cancer emphasizes the need to consider changes in the approach to diagnosing prostate cancer. The dilemma of overtreating the clinically unimportant disease that will be detected if the PSA threshold for biopsy is lowered or undertreating potentially clinically important disease will go undetected if biopsy is not performed in men with a PSA level of 4 ng/ml or less needs resolution.

Data from Andriole GL et al: *N Engl J Med* 360:1310-1319, 2009; Ries LAG et al: National Cancer Institute, Bethesda, MD, 2008, available at http://seer.cancer.gov/csr/1975_2005; Schröder FH et al: *N Engl J Med* 360:1320-1328.

because PSA is organ specific and not cancer specific, it can increase and overlap with BPH, prostatitis, infarct, manipulation from instrumentation, and ejaculation.[182] Several progressions of PSA values have been proposed. These include (1) *PSA density* or the ratio between the serum PSA value and volume of prostate gland, (2) *PSA velocity* or the rate of change in PSA value with time, (3) age-specific PSA reference ranges, and (4) total PSA or the ratio of free and bound PSA in the serum. Serial measures of PSA have great utility in determining the response to treatment.

Screening earlier than 50 years of age with the PSA test is recommended for men at high risk for prostate cancer, such as blacks or relatives of men who have had prostate cancer.[156,188] It is important to note that PSA levels tend to be higher in blacks at baseline and all stages of cancer.[189] When TRUS is added to the annual DRE and PSA testing, the ability to predict cancer rises significantly, from 41% to greater than 78%. Lymph node biopsy, bone scans, MRI, and

| Box 23-13 | Determining the Grade of Prostate Cancer with the Gleason Score |

Grade 1: The cancer cells closely resemble normal cells. They are small, uniformly shaped, evenly spaced, and well differentiated (i.e., they remain separate from one another).

Grade 2: The cancer cells are still well differentiated, but they are arranged more loosely and are irregular in shape and size. Some of the cancer cells have invaded the neighboring prostate tissue.

Grade 3: This is the most common grade. The cells are less well differentiated (some have fused into clumps) and are more variable in shape.

Grade 4: The cells are poorly differentiated and highly irregular in shape. Invasion of the neighboring prostate tissue has progressed further.

Grade 5: The cells are undifferentiated. They have merged into large masses that no longer resemble normal prostate cells. Invasion of the surrounding tissue is extensive.

CT may be used to determine metastasis to lymph, bone, or other adjacent tissue.

The 5-year survival rate of men with localized cancer is 100% with or without treatment. However, before screening most men with prostate cancer had advanced disease and died within a few years of diagnosis. Therefore, it is unclear which men will benefit from early screening and which will not. The most important observation for pathologists to make to facilitate cure of any individual of prostate cancer is that of accurately measuring the size of the index (longest) tumor and Gleason score (degree of differentiation) (Box 23-13).[190] Molecular diagnostic tests include glutathione-5-transferase P1 (GST P1) gene promoter hypermethylation, TPRSS2:EFG fusion transcripts, and prostate cancer-specific gene 3, formerly called DDS. The annual rate by which PSA rises (i.e., PSA velocity) is one way to improve the prognostic accuracy of PSA screening.[191]

Treatment of prostatic cancer depends on the stage of the neoplasm (see Box 23-13); the anticipated effects of treatment; and the age, general health, and life expectancy of the individual. The TNM method of staging has been used to determine extent of disease (see Chapter 11, p. 386. Options include no treatment; surgical treatments such as total prostatectomy, transurethral resection of the prostate (TURP), or cryotherapy; nonsurgical treatments such as radiation therapy, hormone therapy, or chemotherapy; watchful waiting; and any combination of these. In addition, new approaches are using immunotherapy.[192] Palliative treatment is aimed at relieving urinary, bladder outlet, or colon obstruction; spinal cord compression; and pain. Treatments at an early stage can cure the disease in most, if not all, men, and treatment for advanced stage cancer can extend life and reduce tumor size, thus preventing or relieving pain. Prognosis and survival rates have improved steadily over the past 50 years. Currently, 85% of all prostate cancers are discovered in the local and regional stages; in

these stages the 5-year survival rate is 100%; survival rates decline at 10 years (84%) and 15 years (56%).[1]

Treatment for prostate cancer may lead to loss of urinary control, which may return to normal after several weeks or months. Stress incontinence can occur after surgery and mild urge incontinence can occur after radiation therapy. Prostate cancer and its treatment can affect sexual functioning. Sensation of orgasm is not usually affected, but smaller amounts of ejaculate will be produced or men may experience a "dry" ejaculate because of retrograde ejaculation.

Sexual Dysfunction

In men the normal sexual response involves three processes: erection, emission, and ejaculation. **Sexual dysfunction** is the impairment of any or all of these processes. Impairment can be caused by a number of physiologic and psychologic factors.

Until the late 1970s, most cases of male sexual dysfunction were thought to be psychogenic. Studies of this problem indicate that in men older than 40 years, organic factors are involved in more than 50% of cases. The causes of organic sexual dysfunction include (1) vascular, endocrine, and neurologic disorders; (2) chronic disease, including renal failure and diabetes mellitus; (3) penile diseases and penile trauma; and (4) iatrogenic factors, such as surgery and pharmacologic therapies. Most of these disorders cause erectile dysfunction.

PATHOPHYSIOLOGY Vascular disorders can prevent erection. Some arterial diseases diminish or interrupt circulation to the penis. This prevents engorgement of erectile tissues in the corpora cavernosa and corpus spongiosum. Rarely, excessive venous drainage of the corpora cavernosa prevents erection.

Endocrine disorders that reduce testosterone production affect sexual function and libido. The reduction may be caused by inadequate secretion of the gonadotropins caused by pituitary dysfunction or hyperprolactinemia. Feminizing tumors and estrogen therapy reduce relative levels of testosterone. Testicular atrophy from any cause also decreases testosterone levels and contributes to sexual dysfunction.

Neurologic disorders can interfere with the important sympathetic, parasympathetic, and CNS mechanisms required for erection, emission, and ejaculation. They include spinal cord injury or tumor, multiple sclerosis, and disorders that cause peripheral neuropathies, such as diabetes mellitus and chronic renal failure. Spinal cord injuries or tumors can alter one or more components of the sexual response, depending on the location of the lesion. For example, in most men with upper motor neuron lesions, reflexogenic erection is possible but emission and ejaculation (i.e., orgasm) are not possible. Lesions affecting the lower motor neurons usually prevent erection. In approximately 40% of such cases, emission and ejaculation are prevented.

Many chronic diseases are associated with sexual dysfunction. In some conditions the sexual dysfunction has a specific physiologic cause. Diabetes mellitus, for example, causes peripheral vascular and neurologic pathology that can lead to erectile dysfunction. Impotence occurs in about 50% of men undergoing dialysis due to decreased testosterone levels, autonomic neuropathy, accelerated vascular disease, multiple medications, worsening of primary disease, and psychologic stress. Potency may be restored by successful renal transplantation, except in bilateral transplantation if arterial flow is diminished or interrupted. Cirrhosis of the liver, scleroderma, chronic debilitation, and cachexia also are known to cause impotence. Emotional and psychologic response to chronic illness, such as anxiety, depression, and loss of self-esteem, can affect sexual functioning. In other chronic conditions, sexual dysfunction is associated with low energy levels and loss of libido. The pathophysiologic mechanisms responsible for such changes are not known.

Priapism causes fibrosis of trabeculae (erectile tissues) within the corpora cavernosa, making erection difficult. The penile curvature caused by Peyronie disease does not make erection impossible but may make it extremely painful and intercourse impossible. Penile trauma can damage the erectile tissue, disrupt the posterior urethra, and disrupt the pudendal arteries or nerves.

Iatrogenic factors, including drugs and surgery, have a significant effect on erectile function. The following surgical procedures carry the risk of erectile dysfunction: radical pelvic surgery; radical prostatectomy; transurethral, suprapubic, or simple retropubic prostatectomy; and aortoiliac surgery. Erectile dysfunction is caused by the severing of small nerve branches that are essential for erection. Aortoiliac surgery, retroperitoneal lymphadenectomy, and sympathectomy cause the loss of ejaculation capacity in some individuals.

A few pharmacologic agents enhance the sexual response, but most have the opposite effect. Men who are taking antihypertensives, antidepressants, antihistamines, antispasmodics, sedatives or tranquilizers, barbiturates, diuretics, sex hormone preparations, narcotics, or psychoactive drugs may experience some degree of sexual dysfunction. Drug-induced sexual dysfunction consists of decreased desire, decreased erectile ability, or decreased ejaculatory ability. Ethyl alcohol may induce alcoholic neuropathy or increased estrogens because of hepatic dysfunction; marijuana depresses testosterone levels; and cigarette smoking contributes to vasoconstriction and venous leakage. A number of pharmacologic agents also diminish the quality or quantity of sperm. A few may cause priapism. Drugs can assist in maintaining an erection.

EVALUATION AND TREATMENT Evaluation of sexual dysfunction includes a physical examination, with particular attention to the genitalia, prostate, and nervous system, and basic laboratory tests to identify the presence of endocrinopathies or other underlying disorders that can cause the dysfunction. If no physiologic cause is found and the condition does not improve with psychotherapy, the man is referred for further investigation of organic causes. Psychologic evaluation is indicated for younger men with a sudden onset of sexual dysfunction or men of any age who are able to achieve but not maintain an erection.

Sophisticated diagnostic techniques can be used to assess penile blood flow, erectile tissue anatomy, nervous system function, and occurrence of erection or emission during sleep (nocturnal emission). Penile blood flow is measured by Doppler techniques and penile arteriography. Corpus cavernosography, in which contrast material is injected into the corpora cavernosa, provides anatomic information about the erectile tissue of the penis. Neuropathic causes of sexual dysfunction are evaluated by measuring the speed of the bulbocavernous reflex. Nocturnal penile tumescence monitoring measures the frequency of nocturnal erections. Depending on the equipment used, this information may be correlated to rapid eye movement (REM) or non-REM sleep.

Treatments for organic sexual dysfunction include medical and surgical interventions. Nonsurgical interventions include correction of underlying disorders, particularly drug-induced dysfunction and endocrinopathy-related (e.g., reduced testosterone associated with chronic renal failure) dysfunction. Vasodilators and cessation of smoking can benefit individuals with vasculogenic erectile dysfunction. Surgical interventions include penile implants, penile revascularization, and correction of other anatomic defects contributing to sexual dysfunction.

Impairment of Sperm Production and Quality

Spermatogenesis requires adequate secretion of FSH and LH by the pituitary; sufficient secretion of testosterone by the Leydig cells; sufficient function of the Sertoli cells, including secretion of androgen-binding protein, growth factors, inhibin B, and a number of other important (but poorly understood) peptides; and adequate spermatogonia.[193,194] The Leydig cells are located in the testicular interstitium *between* the tubules, and the Sertoli cells and spermatogonia are located *within* the seminiferous tubules. The Sertoli cells extend from the basement membrane to the lumen, display tight junctions between adjacent cells, and form the blood-testis barrier. Inadequate secretion of gonadotropins may be caused by hypothyroidism, hyperadrenocortisolism, hyperprolactinemia, or hypogonadotropic hypogonadism. In these situations, gonadotropin levels are low because of feedback inhibition or idiopathic hyposecretion. In the absence of adequate gonadotropin levels, the Leydig cells are not stimulated to secrete testosterone and sperm maturation is not promoted in the Sertoli cells. Spermatogenesis depends not only on appropriate stimulation by the gonadotropins but also on an appropriate response by the testes. Defects in testicular response to the gonadotropins result in decreased secretion of testosterone and inhibin B and, as a result of normal feedback mechanisms, high levels of circulating gonadotropins. In the absence of adequate testosterone levels, spermatogenesis is impaired. Newer research demonstrates the significance of inhibin B as an important marker of the competence of Sertoli cells and spermatogenesis. Inhibin B is strongly correlated with severity of spermatogenic effects. A positive correlation exists between serum inhibin B levels and sperm concentration and testicular volume, and lower levels have been associated with azoospermia, testicular disorders, and infertility.[194]

Impaired spermatogenesis also can be caused by genetic disorders (such as Klinefelter syndrome), myotonic dystrophy, or testicular trauma. Other conditions associated with impaired spermatogenesis include systemic illness, such as renal failure, hepatic disease, or sickle cell disease; exposure to gonadotoxins, such as chemotherapy or radiation; varicocele; and cryptorchidism.

Fertility is adversely affected if spermatogenesis is normal but the sperm are chromosomally or morphologically abnormal or are produced in insufficient quantities. Chromosomal abnormalities are caused by genetic factors and by external variables, such as exposure to radiation or toxic substances. Ongoing research using small ribonucleic acids (RNAs) is elucidating the molecular mechanisms regulating spermatogenesis.[195] A sperm count of 20 million sperm per milliliter of semen has been suggested as the minimum concentration required for fertility. Average fertile men have 50 to 100 million sperm per milliliter.[144,193]

Sperm motility is another important variable affecting fertility. Motility appears to be affected by the sperm's chemical environment, that is, the characteristics of semen. Prostatic dysfunction, excessive semen viscosity, presence of drugs or toxins in the semen, and presence of antisperm antibodies are associated with impaired sperm motility. Approximately 3% to 7% of infertile males have antisperm antibodies in their semen. Antisperm antibodies may develop as a result of epididymitis or other inflammation of the genitourinary tract, testicular injury or torsion, a previous vasectomy or biopsy, and cryptorchidism. Antisperm antibodies may be (1) cytotoxic antibodies, which attack sperm and reduce their number in the semen; or (2) sperm-immobilizing antibodies, which impair sperm motility and reduce their ability to traverse the endocervical canal. Intrinsic, biologic factors leading to the production of antisperm antibodies seem to play a greater role than extrinsic factors. The exact mechanism remains unclear.[193]

A male factor contributes to the cause of up to 50% of cases of infertility. As understanding of the male factor in infertility increases, evaluation becomes more complex and essential to appropriate treatment (Box 23-14). Treatment for impaired spermatogenesis involves correction of any underlying disorders and avoidance of radiation or toxins. Androgens, human gonadotropins, and antiestrogens (e.g., clomiphene citrate, tamoxifen citrate) may enhance spermatogenesis. Semen can be modified to improve sperm motility. If conception is desired, the semen is obtained by masturbation (or mechanical device),[193] after which it can be diluted, concentrated, or washed to remove antisperm antibodies. These alterations are followed by artificial insemination.

DISORDERS OF THE BREAST

Disorders of the Female Breast

Galactorrhea

Galactorrhea (inappropriate lactation) is the persistent and sometimes excessive secretion of a milky fluid from the breasts of a woman who is not pregnant or nursing an infant. It can occur in men, may involve one or both breasts and is not associated with breast cancer.

Box 23-14	**Evaluation of Male Partner of Infertile Couples**

Thorough history and physical, including imaging for varicocele
Two semen analyses and quantification of serum FSH, LH, testosterone levels, and prolactin if indicated
Semen and urethral cultures
Serum assays or monoclonal antibody testing for white blood cells
Immunobead monoclonal antibody test
Postcoital testing of semen activity and function
Sperm penetration assay
Inhibin B assays or testicular biopsy
Vasogram, TRUS, or other imaging studies

FSH, Follicle-stimulating hormone; *LH,* luteinizing hormone; *TRUS,* transrectal ultrasonography.

Incidence is difficult to estimate because of differences among definitions of the condition, examination techniques, and populations of women who have been studied. Prevalence has been documented as 0.1% to 32% of all women.

PATHOPHYSIOLOGY Galactorrhea is a manifestation of pathophysiologic processes in the body, rather than a breast disorder. These processes are chiefly hormone imbalances caused by hypothalamic-pituitary disturbances, pituitary tumors, or neurologic damage. Exogenous causes include drugs, estrogen, and manipulation of the nipples. When caused by hyperprolactinemia it is manifested by the spontaneous appearance of a milky secretion from multiple duct openings, usually from both breasts. Galactorrhea caused by oral contraceptives (OCs) is more likely to occur with high-dose use; is characterized by clear, serous, or milky discharge from multiple ducts; and is noticeable during the drug-free interval between OC packets. In premenopausal women, unilateral or bilateral spontaneous multiple duct discharge that increases before menstruation often is caused by fibrocystic change. Unilateral, spontaneous, serous, or serosanguineous discharge from a single duct usually is caused by an intraductal papilloma; bloody discharge suggests cancer; bilateral, sticky, multicolored discharge from multiple ducts is often caused by duct ectasia; and purulent discharge indicates a subareolar abscess.[196]

The most common cause of galactorrhea is **nonpuerperal hyperprolactinemia,** or excessive amounts of prolactin (the pituitary hormone that stimulates milk production) in the blood not related to pregnancy or childbirth. Nonpuerperal hyperprolactinemia can be caused by any factor that (1) stimulates or overstimulates the prolactin-secreting units of the pituitary gland; (2) interferes with production of **prolactin-inhibiting factor (PIF),** a neurotransmitter (probably dopamine) that inhibits prolactin secretion; or (3) interferes with pituitary receptors for PIF. A variety of exogenous agents (such as drugs) and disorders can trigger one of these three mechanisms, thereby causing hyperprolactinemia (Box 23-15).

Hypothyroidism causes increased secretion of hypothalamic TRH that stimulates prolactin release from the pituitary.

Hypothyroidism also is associated with reduced metabolic clearance of prolactin, which prolongs its effects.

Many types of pituitary tumors cause hyperprolactinemia. Prolactinomas cause hyperprolactinemia by secreting prolactin, decreasing production of PIF, or putting pressure on the pituitary stalk such that delivery of PIF to the anterior pituitary is prevented. Growth hormone–secreting pituitary tumors may cause galactorrhea through the intrinsic lactogenic effect that growth hormone appears to have on mammary tissue. Prolactin-secreting lung and kidney tumors also cause hyperprolactinemia.

Chronic stress may cause hyperprolactinemia by inhibiting PIF release. Cervical spinal injuries, head trauma, encephalitis, meningitis, herpes zoster, or thoracotomy scars may stimulate the afferent portion of the suckling reflex arc, which is carried in the second to sixth thoracic nerves. The suckling reflex increases prolactin secretion.

Persistent and repeated sucking or squeezing of the nipples can induce galactorrhea, and has been documented in women who manipulate their breasts and nipples daily.[197] Monthly examination of the breasts for nipple discharge usually is not associated with the development of galactorrhea.

CLINICAL MANIFESTATIONS A small amount of breast milk expressed from the nipple of parous women usually is not a concern, and normal breast milk color can be other than white. Inappropriate lactation is manifested by the appearance of a milky breast secretion in nonpregnant, nonlactating women from one or both breasts. Most women with galactorrhea experience menstrual abnormality. If a pituitary process is involved, the woman usually experiences hirsutism and infertility; if a hypothalamic lesion is present, she may report such CNS symptoms as intractable headache, visual field disturbances, sleep disturbances, and abnormal temperature, thirst, or appetite.[198]

EVALUATION AND TREATMENT Galactorrhea requires evaluation when it (1) occurs in nulliparous women or in parous women who have not been pregnant or have not breastfed for 12 months or (2) is associated with amenorrhea, headache, visual field abnormalities, or other symptoms implying systemic illness. Evaluation includes a variety of diagnostic tests. When amenorrhea accompanies galactorrhea, the assessment is the same as for amenorrhea. Breast secretions are examined for fat globules and neoplastic cells to verify their source. Serum prolactin levels are measured. Because such variables as eating, sleeping, stress, and breast examinations increase prolactin levels, at least two positive results are needed for a diagnosis of hyperprolactinemia. Prolactin levels greater than 25 to 30 ng/ml (by radioimmunoassay) are elevated. Those in the range of 75 to 100 ng/ml are considered to be caused by a pituitary tumor until proved otherwise. Serum thyroxine and TSH levels are measured to rule out hypothyroidism, and LH and FSH levels are obtained if the individual is amenorrheic. CT, MRI, and carotid angiography may assist in the localization of adenomas.

Treatment is specific to the underlying cause and occurs after identification of the cause. Medical and surgical therapies may be involved. A pituitary microadenoma may be surgically removed, or treated medically with bromocriptine (Parlodel), which controls the tumor but does not cure it. A pituitary macroadenoma usually is treated medically because surgical and radiologic therapies seldom succeed.

Benign Breast Disease and Conditions

Benign breast disease (BBD) is a condition of noncancerous changes in the breast. Numerous benign alterations in ducts and lobules occur in the breast, including irregular lumps, cysts, sensitive nipples, and itching. The most common symptoms reported by women are pain, palpable mass, or nipple discharge; the majority of these prove to have a benign cause. However, histologic features, age at biopsy, and degree of family history have been found as major determinants of the risk of breast cancer after a diagnosis of BBD.[199] This risk varies according to the histologic category of BBD (moderate in women with proliferative lesions without atypia and substantial in women with atypical (atypia) hyperphasia [AH])[200] (see p. 875). Among premenopausal women, the risk appears to be greater for those with atypical lobular hyperplasia (ALH) than with atypical ductal hyperplasia (ADH) (see p. 875). For postmenopausal women the risk of breast cancer was similar between those with ALH or ADH.[200] Family history is reported as an independent risk factor for breast cancer. Women with atypia and a family history had a breast cancer risk four times the expected risk.[199] Risk was lower among those with atypia and no family history.

The College of American Pathologists has classified biopsy tissue according to breast cancer risk. These classifications are listed in Box 23-16. Benign epithelial lesions can be broadly classified according to their future risk of developing breast cancer as (1) nonproliferative breast lesions, (2) proliferative breast disease, and (3) atypical (atypia) hyperplasia.

Box 23-16   Classification of Breast Biopsy Tissue According to Risk for Breast Cancer

No Increased Risk
Adenosis (sclerosing or florid)
  Apocrine metaplasia
  Macrocysts or microcysts
  Fibroadenoma
  Fibrosis
Mild hyperplasia
  Mastitis or periductal mastitis
  Squamous metaplasia

Slightly Increased Risk (1.5 to 2 Times)
Moderate or florid hyperplasia
  Papilloma

Moderately Increased Risk (4 to 5 Times)
Atypical hyperplasia (ductal or lobular)

Nonproliferative Breast Lesions

The term *nonproliferative* has been used to discriminate from the *proliferative* changes commonly associated with increased risk for development of breast cancer. This group includes **fibrocystic changes** (FCCs)—the most widely accepted term—for physiologic nodularity and breast tenderness that wax and wane with the menstrual cycle. On palpation, breasts are lumpy or bumpy and, in radiologic studies, breast tissue appears dense with cysts. These lesions cause women to seek medical attention because the lesions mimic carcinoma and produce palpable lumps or nipple discharge. **Cysts** (fluid-filled sacs) are a specific type of lump that commonly occurs in women in their 30s, 40s, and early 50s. Cysts feel "squishy" when they occur close to the surface of the breast but when deeply embedded they can feel hard (Figure 23-43). It has become increasingly clear that FCC is a heterogeneous group of lesions that should be diagnosed separately. An estimated 50% to 80% of women normally experience some of these changes. The prevalence of fibrocystic lesions is probably related to hormonal changes, which in turn are affected by genetic background, age, parity, history of lactation, caffeine consumption, and use of exogenous hormones.[201] Based on experimental animal studies, it is assumed that breast cysts are the result of ovarian alterations, but the exact mechanism is unknown. Calcifications, found in cysts and adenosis or an increase in the number of acini per lobule, can form mammographically suspicious alterations.[202] Cysts also can be associated with unilateral nipple discharge. A variety of substances are secreted into cyst fluid, including polypeptide

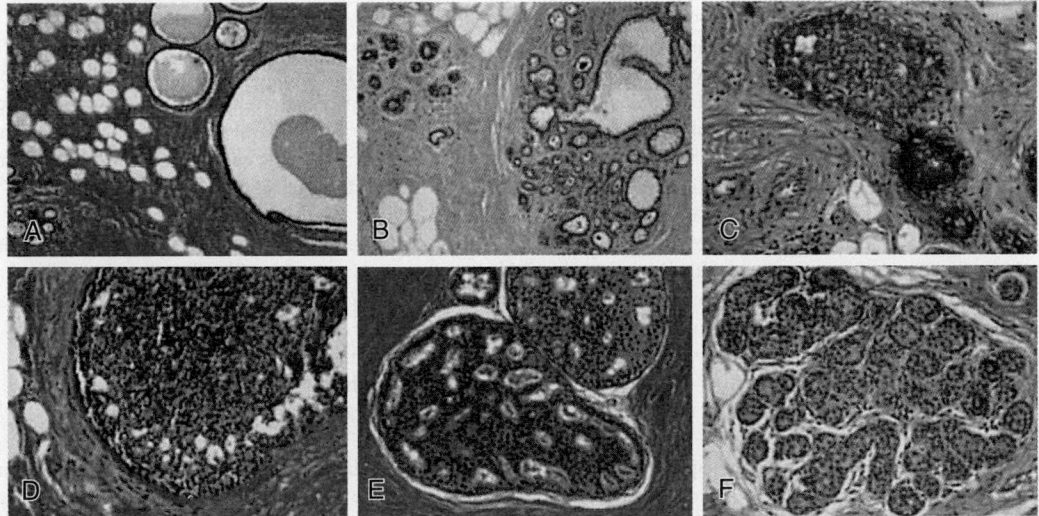

Figure 23-43 Benign breast disease. **A,** Nonproliferative fibrocystic changes. The architecture of the terminal-duct lobular unit is distorted by the formation of microcysts, associated with interlobular fibrosis. **B,** Proliferative hyperplasia without atypia. This is adenosis, a distinctive form of hyperplasia characterized by the proliferation of lobular acini, forming crowded glandlike structures. For comparison, a normal lobule is on the left side. **C,** Proliferative hyperplasia without atypia. There is moderate ductal hyperplasia, which is characterized by a duct that is partially distended by hyperplastic epithelium within the lumen. **D,** Proliferative hyperplasia without atypia, which is florid ductal hyperplasia. The involved duct is greatly expanded by a crowded, jumbled-appearing epithelial proliferation. **E,** Atypical ductal hyperplasia. These proliferations are complex and partially formed secondary lumens and mild nuclear hyperchromasia in the epithelial-cell population. The peripheral spaces are irregular and slitlike. **F,** Atypical lobular hyperplasia. Monomorphic, small, rounded, loosely cohesive cells fill the lumens of partially distended acini in this terminal-duct lobular unit. (Hematoxylin and eosin.) (From Elmore JG, Gigerenzer G: *N Engl J Med* 353[3]:231, 2005.)

hormones and male and female sex steroid hormones. Cysts often rupture with release of secretory material into the adjacent tissue. The resulting chronic inflammation and scarring fibrosis contribute to the palpable firmness of the breast.[202] Fibrous tissue increases progressively until menopause and regresses thereafter.

In addition to FCC, many women experience benign breast tumors (Table 23-12 and Figure 23-44). In general, the frequency of chromosome abnormalities is lower in benign lesions than in breast cancer. Genetic aberrations are more common in proliferative than in nonproliferative lesions.[202] The *multiplicity* of benign breast lesions, sometimes called *heterogeneous benign breast disease (HBBD)* in a biopsy appears to be a risk factor for progression to breast cancer.[203]

Proliferative Breast Lesions without Atypia

These disorders are characterized by proliferation of ductal epithelium and/or stroma without cellular signs of malignancy and in addition to fibroadenoma with complex features including the following structurally diverse lesions[202]:

1. **Epithelial hyperplasia** is defined by the presence of *more* than two cell layers above the basement membrane. In the normal breast, only myoepithelial cells and a single layer of luminal cells are present above the basement membrane.[202] Moderate to **florid hyperplasia** is more than four cell layers above the basement membrane. The proliferating epithelium fills and distends the ducts and lobules by both luminal and myoepithelial cells.

2. **Sclerosing adenosis** is present when the number of acini per terminal duct is greater than twice the number found in uninvolved lobules. Calcification is commonly present within the lumens; however, the normal lobular arrangement is maintained. The acini are structurally altered and myoepithelial cells are prominent. Occasionally, stromal fibrosis may mimic the appearance of invasive carcinoma.[202]

3. **Complex sclerosing lesion ([radial scar] radial sclerosing lesions, sclerosing papillary proliferation)** refers to an irregular, radial proliferation of ductlike small tubules entrapped in a dense central fibrosis. The term *scar* refers to the structural appearance only because these lesions are not associated with prior injury or surgery. Radial scars (RSs) have been implicated as an independent risk factor for invasive breast cancer. However, a retrospective study of 9556 women found that although RSs mildly elevate the risk of invasive breast cancer, the risk was largely attributed to the coexistent presence of

Table 23-12   Benign Breast Tumors

Benign Breast Tumor	Risk Factors	Pathophysiology	Clinical Manifestations	Treatment
Fibroadenoma	Puberty, early adulthood; occurs earlier and more frequently in young black women	Slow-growing lesion composed of variable proportions of epithelial and connective tissue; thought to be under influence of estrogen	Painless, firm, elastic, solitary, well-circumscribed mass ≈1-5 cm in diameter	Excision with person under local anesthesia; or careful observation
Phyllodes tumor	Middle age	Fibroepithelial tumor characterized by marked proliferation of connective tissue stroma and great size; initially slow growing; 10%-25% may be malignant	Spheric, firm, usually well-circumscribed multinodular tumor with a diameter of 2-20 cm; trophic cutaneous ulceration is a late manifestation	Local excision of benign or small tumor; simple mastectomy if voluminous or malignant tumor
Intraductal papilloma	Ages 30-50 yr; relatively uncommon	Subareolar tumor consists of epithelial vegetation with central connective tissue axis; found in lactiferous duct	Spontaneous or induced watery, serous, or bloody nipple discharge; small soft, friable, yellow or red, ≈5 mm, papillomatous growth attached to duct wall by short, thin stalk; rare nipple retraction	Excision of involved duct
Mammary duct ectasia	After menopause or during pregnancy and lactation	Principal lactiferous ducts become dilated and filled with cellular debris; secondary inflammatory reaction; possible rupture of ducts	Subareolar induration or nipple retraction; spontaneous, bloody, sticky, thick, multiple duct discharge; burning pain and swelling of areolar area; palpable mass after rupture	Antibiotic and anti-inflammatory therapy
Fat necrosis	Ages 14-80 yr; average age 50 yr; increased in women with fatty, voluminous breasts; trauma	50% are posttraumatic; necrosis secondary to inflammation is more rare	Poorly circumscribed indurated area with yellow or gray necrotic foci	Leave alone or local excision

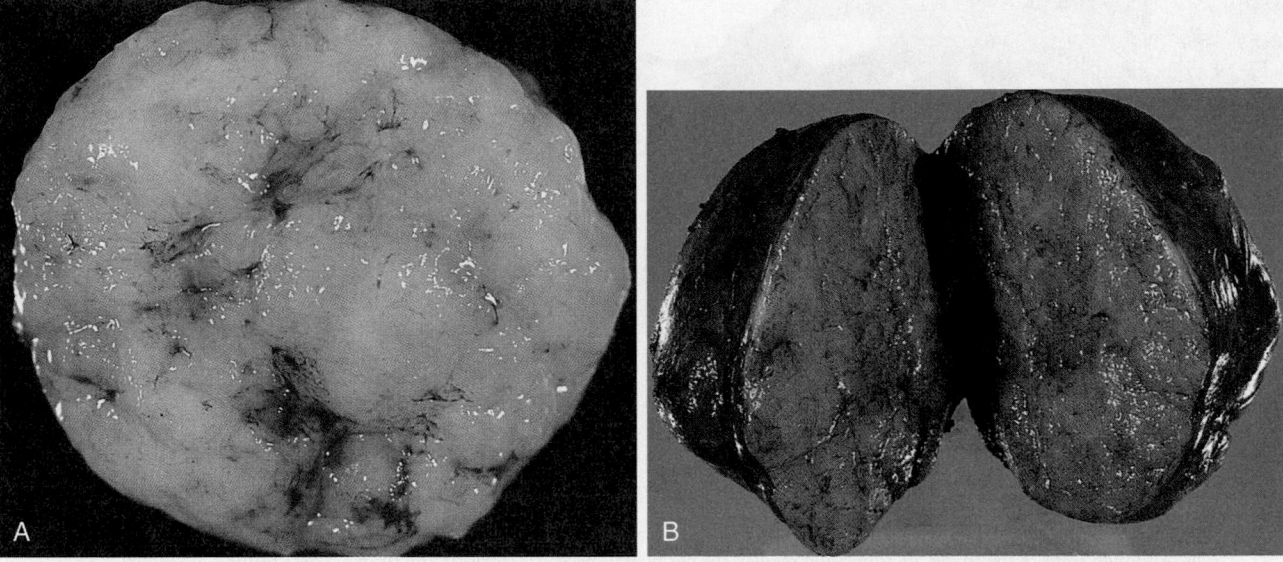

Figure 23-44 Fibroadenoma. **A,** Myxoid type of fibroadenoma, showing pale, lobulated, translucent tissue. **B,** Juvenile fibroadenoma showing well-circumscribed mass of tan, fleshy, lobulated tissue. (From Damjanov I, Linder J, editors: *Anderson's pathology,* ed 10, St Louis, 1996, Mosby.)

proliferative disease.[204] Invasive breast cancer risk was further increased in women with AH.[204,205] The appearance in mammograms of RSs, as well as the gross and microscopic appearance, can cause it to be confused with infiltrating ductal carcinoma.[206]

4. **Papillomas** consist of multiple finger-like projections or branching axes lined by myoepithelial cells and luminal cells. They constitute an important subset of mammary fibrocystic changes with about 5% of those with proliferative changes. Hyperplasia and metaplasia are often present within the ducts. Atypical hyperplasia may be present within or adjacent to papilloma, making the distinction from ductal carcinoma in situ (DCIS) difficult (see p. 898). The presence of atypia (ductal or lobular) coexisting with a single papilloma (atypical papilloma) does not appreciably modify the breast cancer risk attributable to just atypia.[207] A single papilloma without atypia conveys a risk similar to proliferative fibrocystic lesions, whereas multiple papillomas, even without identified atypia, increase breast cancer risk significantly.[207] Small-duct papillomas increase the risk of subsequent carcinoma; it is unknown whether large duct papillomas do as well.

Proliferative Breast Lesions with Atypia

Proliferative breast lesions with some abnormal structure or *atypia* include ADH and ALH.[202] **Atypical hyperplasia (AH)** is an increase in the number of cells with some variation in cellular structure. Studies continue to indicate that women with AH have an increased risk (about fourfold) of breast cancer compared with women who have nonproliferative lesions.[200] From the Nurses' Health Study, time of benign breast biopsy appeared to influence the degree of later breast cancer risk among women with AH.[200] Among premenopausal women at the time of their benign biopsy, the risk of breast cancer was substantially increased among women with AH (OR, 7.3) than among women with ADH (OR, 2.72). The risks for women who were postmenopausal at the time of benign biopsy were similar for women with ALH and those with ADH.[200]

Ductal hyperplasia is an increased number of cells mostly within the lumen of the terminal ducts (Figure 23-45, *A*). It includes a continuum of changes—cell structure and placement—ranging from an increase in cellularity to features of ductal carcinoma in situ (DCIS; see p. 898). In ADH, the cells fail to completely fill ductal spaces as compared with DCIS. Although still controversial, isoflavone exposure has been associated with a decreased risk of proliferative benign fibrocystic changes, nonproliferative changes, and breast cancer.[208]

Lobular hyperplasia refers to proliferation of small, uniform cells in the lumen of lobular units. The abnormal cells of **atypical lobular hyperplasia (ALH)** and lobular carcinoma in situ (LCIS) are identical, but the cells in ALH do not distend more than 50% of the acini within a lobule[202] (see Figure 23-45, *B*). ALH can extend into ducts, and this is associated with an increased risk of invasive carcinomas.[202] Other benign conditions are summarized in Table 23-13.

EVALUATION AND TREATMENT   Breast problems should be diagnosed from a multimodal approach that combines physical examination, mammogram when applicable, sonogram, possibly MRI, aspiration of lumps, and surgical or needle biopsy if warranted. Breast biopsy is used to make a definitive diagnosis and assess an individual's risk for the development of breast cancer. The principal mammographic signs of breast carcinoma are densities and calcifications. However, the dense breast tissue often seen in young women can make interpretation extremely difficult (see also What's New? Screening Mammograms: Far from Perfect in

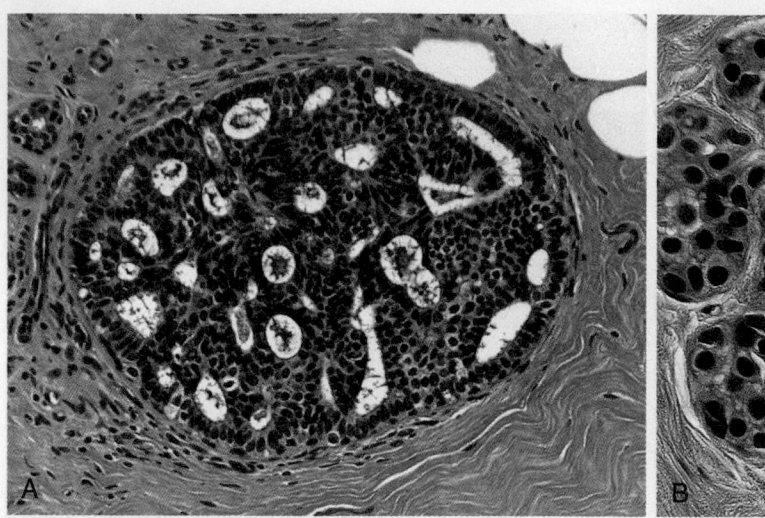
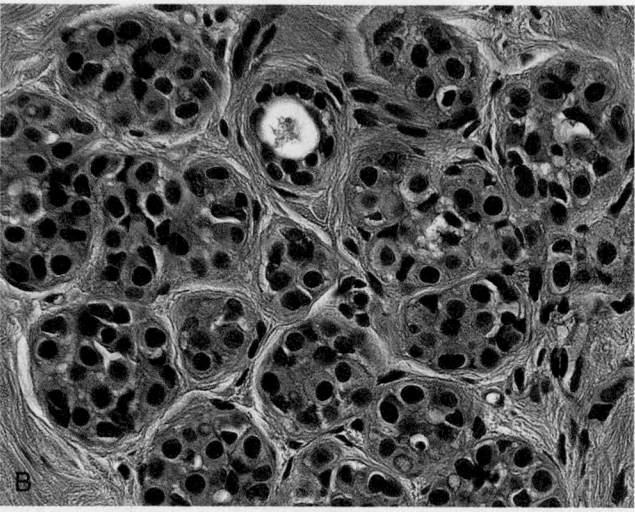

Figure 23-45 Atypical ductal and lobular hyperplasias. **A,** Atypical ductal hyperplasia. A duct is filled with a mixed population of cells. Although some of the spaces are round and regular, the peripheral spaces are irregular and slitlike. These features are highly atypical but fall short of a diagnosis of ductal carcinoma in situ (DCIS). **B,** Atypical lobular hyperplasia. A population of monomorphic small, rounded, loosely cohesive cells partially fill a lobule. (From Kumar V: *Robbins and Cotran pathologic basis of disease*, ed 8, Philadelphia, 2008, Saunders.)

Table 23-13	Other Benign Breast Conditions
Type	**Comment**
Developmental	
Milk-line remnants	Increase in number of nipples or breasts results from persistent epidermal thickening along the milk line
Accessory axillary breast tissue	Ductal system may extend into subcutaneous tissue of the chest wall and axillary region; this tissue can undergo lactational changes and give rise to tumors
Congenital nipple inversion	Is common and may be unilateral; can spontaneously correct during pregnancy; can be confused with retraction of nipple, which is sometimes part of invasive cancer or inflammation
Macromastia	Juvenile hypertrophy may be caused by unusual tissue response to hormonal stimulus
Iatrogenic	
Reconstruction or augmentation	Breast tissue can be replaced or augmented by skin and muscle flaps for synthetic prostheses; silicone implants, the most common, are rubbery silicone filled with either silicone gel or saline; a common complication of implants is formation of a thick fibrous capsule (i.e., chronic inflammatory responses) that can cause cosmetic deformity; the capsule can limit the spread of a ruptured implant but if the capsule ruptures silicone gel can escape; long-term consequences of rupture are unknown
Inflammation	
Acute mastitis	Inflammatory diseases of the breast are rare; acute mastitis is confined to the lactating period of nursing; the nipples can become dry, cracked, and fissured, increasing risk of bacterial infection; infection may lead to abscess formation
Periductal mastitis	Women or men present with a painful subareolar mass thought to be infectious; not associated with lactation; 90% of individuals are smokers; vitamin A deficiency associated with smoking may alter the differentiation of the ductal epithelium; keratin is trapped within the ductal system causing dilation and rupture; antibiotic therapy and surgery are usually indicated
Mammary duct ectasia	Affects 50- and 60-year-olds, usually multiparous women, not associated with smoking; dilation of ducts with chronic granulomatous inflammatory reaction; fibrosis may eventually lead to skin and nipple retraction, thus mistaken for cancer; may have white nipple secretions
Fat necrosis	Painless, palpable mass, skin thickening or retraction; mammographic density or calcification; may have hemorrhage; most women will give a history of prior surgery or trauma; can be confused with breast carcinoma
Lymphocytic mastopathy	Single or multiple hard, palpable masses; can be so hard that interferes with biopsy; lesion includes collagenized stroma surrounding atrophic ducts and lobules; the breast membrane is frequently thickened; a prominent lymphocytic infiltrate surrounds epithelium and blood vessels; most common in women with type 1 diabetes or autoimmune thyroid disease

Data from Lester SC: The breast. In Kumar V, Abbas AK, Fausto N, editors: *Robbins and Cotran pathologic basis of disease*, ed 7, Philadelphia, 2005, Saunders.

Chapter 11, p. 386). Ultrasonography (ultrasound) is used to differentiate a solid mass from a cystic (fluid-filled) mass, which is generally benign.

Treatment consists largely of relieving symptoms. Breast pain may be minimized by wearing a brassiere that provides good support. Reduction of caffeinated beverages, cola, root beer, and chocolate, which can cause overstimulation of breast tissue for some women, may reduce pain and nodularity. Given time the cysts may disappear without treatment.

Iodine deficiency may increase fibrocystic breast change, thus may be useful for relieving pain (see Nutrition & Disease: Diet and Breast Cancer Risk Updates, p. 892).[209] Although unknown, increasing omega-3 fatty acids may decrease associated pain caused by inflammation as well as the application of castor oil packs to the breasts. The use of aspirin for decreasing breast alterations is being investigated (see below and What's New? Inflammation, Breast Carcinogenesis, Aspirin, and NSAIDs). Drugs used to treat severe breast pain are listed in Table 23-14.

WHAT'S NEW? Inflammation, Breast Carcinogenesis, Aspirin, and NSAIDs

The role of inflammation in breast disorders and cancer is a hot topic (see Figures *A* & *B* below). Specifically the role of the inflammatory enzymes cyclooxygenase (COX)-1 and COX-2 and drugs that inhibit COX-2 (see Chapters 6 and 11). COX-2 has been found to be associated with some cancers, including breast cancer. Inactivating COX-2 may interrupt carcinogenesis by several pathways: inhibition of angiogenesis, promotion of apoptosis, alteration of insulin, signaling pathways that result in insulin resistance, and suppression of estrogen synthesis through decreased aromatase activity (see Figure *B* on p. 878). Interleukin-6 (IL-6) is a cytokine reported to be involved in inflammation, insulin, and estrogen pathways, and IL-6 may be associated with breast cancer through several pathways (see Figure A). Several epidemiologic studies have examined the association between nonsteroidal antiinflammatory drugs (NSAIDs) and breast cancer with inconclusive and inconsistent results. Most case-control studies, but not all, have found relative risk reductions from 20% to 40%.[227, 228] Eight prospective studies found no association, six studies found a reduced risk, and one study found a U-shaped curved association.[229] Alternate-day use of low-dose aspirin for a mean of 10 years in a randomized Women's Health Study did not reduce the incidence of breast cancer.[230] The American Association of Retired Persons (AARP) Diet and Health Study found breast cancer risk was not significantly associated with NSAID use, but daily aspirin (unknown dose) was correlated with a modest reduction in ER+ breast cancer.[229] In 2004, investigators reported that aspirin use in women is associated with a significant reduction in the risk of breast cancer, especially for hormone receptor–positive tumors.[231] This was the first report to examine whether the protective effects of aspirin varied with estrogen receptor (ER) or progesterone receptor (PR) status. Aspirin has been associated with a reduction in mortality from cardiovascular disease and colorectal cancer.[232, 233] In mice, Chang and colleagues[234] defined the molecular mechanisms by which COX-2 derived prostaglandin E$_2$ (PGE$_2$; proinflammatory) induced tumor-associated angiogenesis and initiation or progression of mammary cancer. These investigations reported that PGE$_2$ induced angiogenesis at the earliest stage of tumor development, even before PGE$_2$-induced *mammary gland hyperplasia!* From the Mayo Clinic Benign Breast Cohort (n = 9343), 40 of the 247 women with atypia have developed breast cancer. Of those atypia samples, investigators found significantly higher COX-2 staining intensity.[235] Terry and colleagues[231] found the inverse association between aspirin use and breast cancer was evident for every patient subgroup except those with negative hormone receptor status (ER–, PR–). The association was strongest among frequent aspirin users, unfortunately the dose was not identified. Acetaminophen was not associated with protection in any group. Aspirin showed more effects than ibuprofen (NSAID). These findings suggest possible mechanistic connections between aspirin and estrogen. In 1996, investigators suggested genetic activation of COX-2 in transformed mammary epithelial cells.[236] The COX-2

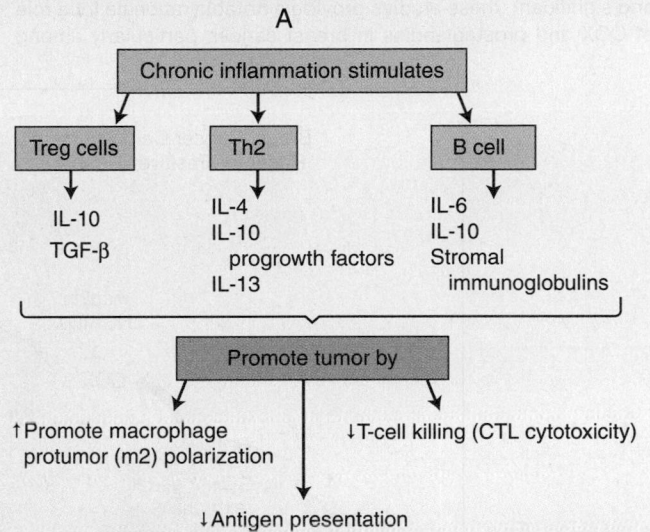

A, Chronic activated lymphocytes increase inflammation. Chronic activation of immune response when tissue injury/damage is not resolved results in accumulation of regulatory T cells (Treg), T-helper (Th2) cells, and activated B lymphocytes. These cells in turn cause the secretion of progrowth factors (i.e., interleukin 4 [IL-4], IL-6, IL-10, IL-13), transforming growth factor-beta (TGF-β), and immunoglobulins. Stromal infiltrating immunoglobulins may activate innate or inflammatory responses promoting disease progression. Retrospective studies reveal that the presence or maturation of immunoglobulin G (IgG) correlates with increases in disease stage (stage 1 versus stage 11) and in total tumor burden. Immunoglobulins found in the stroma are predominant lymphocyte populations (e.g., more than early ductal carcinoma in situ [DCIS]). These observations have been found in other types of solid tumors. Although immunoglobulins play a role in carcinogenesis, the specific mechanisms are unclear. A 2002 meta-analysis found tissue macrophage density was associated with a poor prognosis. Polarized macrophages (M1 and M2) are like Th1 and Th2 designations; that is, different macrophage phenotypes and functions. M2 cells participate in polarized Th2 reactions; promote killing of parasites; are present in tumors; and promote progression, tissue repair (thus paradoxical function), and remodeling. M2 increases production of inflammatory cytokines. Macrophages enhance angiogenesis by promoting angiogenic factors, including vascular endothelial growth factor (VEGF) and remodel the extracellular matrix, especially collagen fibrils (fibrillogenesis). Thus tumor invasion is enhanced because mobile and invasive tumor cells track along collagen fibers that are anchored to blood vessels—all potentiated by macrophages (M2). Activation of Th2 cells increases IL-4, IL-5, IL-6, IL-10, and IL-13, which induce immune unresponsiveness or T-cell anergy and *loss* of T-cell–mediated cytotoxicity (CTL). (Data from Bingle L, Brown NJ, Lewis CE: *J Pathol* 196:254-265, 2002; DeNardo NG, Coussens LM: *Breast Cancer Res* 9:212, 2007; Pollard JW: *J Leuk Biol* 84(3):623-630, 2008.)

continued

gene is normally inactive (quiescent) but becomes active in response to infection, inflammation (e.g., from arthritis), and growth factors. COX-2 has been found in precancerous breast disease (hyperplasia, hyperplasia with atypia) and noninvasive and invasive breast cancer. In the same year, Zhao and colleagues[237] demonstrated that PGE_2 can induce the enzyme aromatase leading to increased estrogen production in mammary adipose stromal cells. In 1999, investigators found that COX-2 is up-regulated in the *normal adjacent* epithelium to ductal carcinoma in situ and that COX-2 overexpression correlates with local areas of p16(INKA) hypermethylation (see Chapter 11) in vivo that might represent *early* neoplastic changes leading to breast cancer.[238,239] All together and significant, these studies provide a notable rationale for a role of COX and prostaglandins in breast cancer, particularly among postmenopausal women. In vitro and animal studies have shown that NSAIDs inhibit COX-1 and COX-2, which oxygenate arachidonic acid and, ultimately, produce prostaglandins. Inhibiting COX-1 reduces platelet aggregation and gastrointestinal mucosa protection. Blocking or inactivating COX-2 may interrupt breast carcinogenesis and other tumors through multiple pathways (e.g., angiogenesis, apoptosis, aromatase, and estrogen synthesis).[229] Emerging is inconsistent evidence of aspirin use in ER+ and PR+ breast cancers. Questions about the dosage; timing and duration of treatments; and management of side effects, such as gastric irritation and bleeding, and aspirin allergies and how to manage this risk need to be evaluated. Studies are ongoing to determine whether COX-2 selective inhibitors, either alone or in combination with other drugs, help prevent breast cancer.

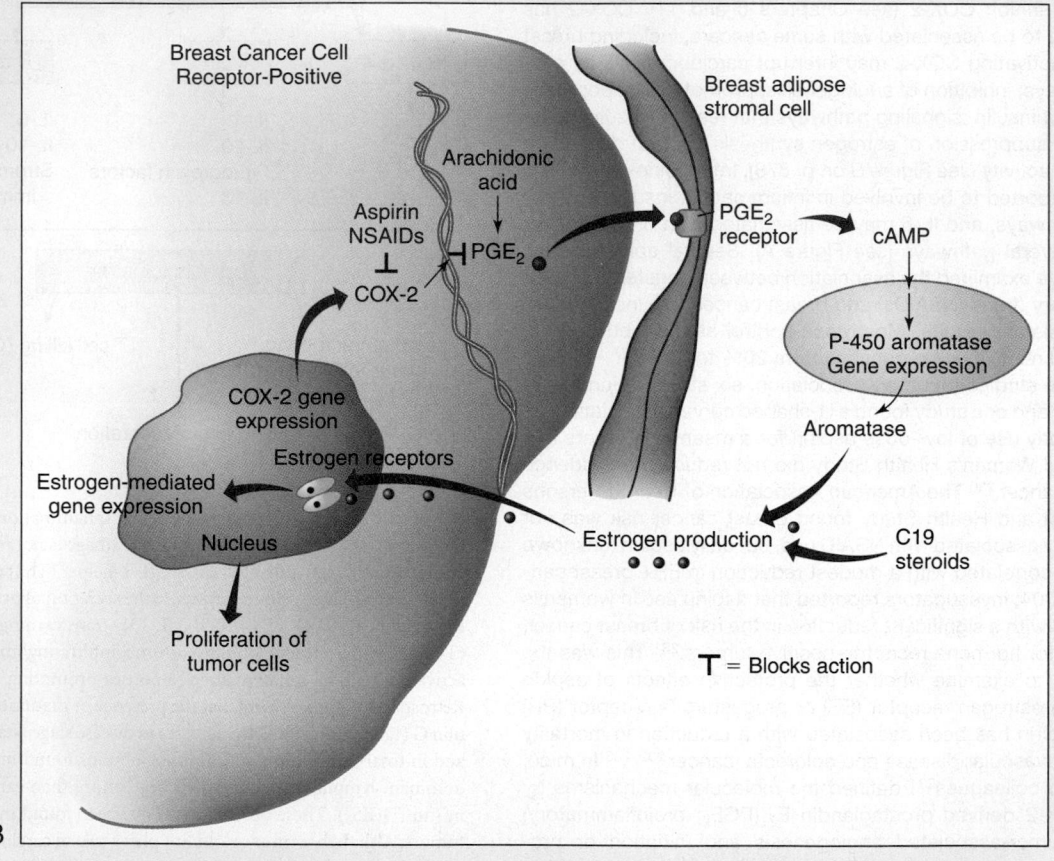

B, Proinflammatory PGE_2 produced by breast cancer cells stimulates aromatase in breast stromal cells. Increased COX-2 can occur in precancerous breast disease (hyperplasia, hyperplasia with atypia) and noninvasive and invasive breast cancer. Here COX-2 in breast cancer cells leads to changes in tumor biology from increased PGE_2 levels (i.e., can affect apoptosis, cell invasion, immune function, and angiogenesis). PGE_2 can induce expression of local tissue levels of aromatase through increased cyclic adenosine monophosphate (cAMP) production in breast stromal cells. Thus estrogen synthesis is enhanced, which can increase proliferation of tumor cells. This paracrine loop (which is not associated with blood levels of estrogen) could explain why inhibition of COX-2 activity could decrease estrogen and decrease proliferation of hormone receptor-positive breast cancers. (Adapted from DuBois RN: *JAMA* 291:2488-2489, 2004.)

NUTRITION & DISEASE

Revisiting Iodine and Breast Alterations

The last national nutritional survey revealed that 15% of the U.S. adult female population are iodine deficient by the World Health Organization (WHO) standard, that is, less than 0.05 mg/L urine.[210] Recommendations by the WHO, United Nations International Children's Emergency Fund, and the International Council for the Control of Iodine Deficiency Disorders set 10 mcg/dl as the minimum urinary iodine concentration for iodine sufficiency.[211] This amount corresponds to a daily intake of 150 mcg iodine. Large segments of Europe continue to have iodine deficiency. Significant deficiency is present in 45 countries in Africa, 15 in the Americas, 24 in Europe and Central Asia, 11 in Southeast Asia, 10 in the Middle East, and 9 in the Far East. Iodine deficiency is a common endocrine problem, presumably easy to correct, and the most preventable cause of mental retardation in many underdeveloped countries. Iodine is found in abundance in marine plants and animals in deposits of organic origin, in certain natural mineral waters, in phosphate rock, and in association with mineral deposits. A small fraction is from drinking water. Important factors in the depletion of iodine have been glaciation, which removes old soil and scrapes virgin rocks, the substitution of bromine for iodine in bread manufacturing, and decreases in iodinated salt intake.

Although several extrathyroidal organs and tissues can concentrate and organify iodine, compelling evidence for iodine is its effects on the mammary gland. Intriguing is the concept that iodine deficiency causes fibrocystic changes in rodents and that iodine, and to a lesser extent iodide, induced relief of breast pain in two large uncontrolled trials and in one placebo-controlled trial.[212, 213] In estradiol-treated rats, iodine deficiency has been shown to lead to pathologic changes similar to those noted in benign breast disease—cystic changes, periductal fibrosis, and lobular hyperplasia.[214]

Most studies on iodine function in humans and animals have focused on thyroid function. Little attention has been devoted to extrathyroidal tissues in which an important function of iodine is as an antioxidant in humans, including the eye, thyroid, and breast. The antioxidant properties of dietary iodide depend on redox reactions from iodination of tyrosine to the formation of thyroid hormones.[215]

Although thyroid-stimulating hormone has no role in promoting iodide intake into mammary cells, these cells have been shown to possess the sodium iodide symporter (transporter).[216, 217] Uptake of iodide into mammary cells can be promoted by prolactin and other hormones (oxytocin, estrogens). Iodoproteins have been detected in breast tissue but it is not known how their facilitation occurs. Free radicals have been associated with carcinogenesis, including breast cancer. Although no direct evidence exists that iodide acts as an antioxidant in the breast, increased rates of breast cancer have been reported in iodine-deficient populations.[218] Iodine deficiency also has been linked to increased fibrosis and adenosis of the mammary gland and administration of iodine has been used in the treatment of breast pain.[212,219] It has been suggested that a combination of deficiency of iodine and selenium may facilitate the development of breast cancer.[215,220] Funahashi and colleagues[221,222] found that administration of Lugol's iodine or iodine-rich wakame seaweed to rats treated with dimethylbenz(a)-anthracene (DMBA, a carcinogen) suppressed the development of mammary tumors. In addition, the same researchers documented that seaweed-induced apoptosis in human breast cancer cells had a stronger effect than fluorouracil (a strong chemotherapeutic agent) used to treat breast cancer. This finding led these authors and others to hypothesize that "seaweed may be applicable for prevention of breast cancer."[223] This hypothesis is intriguing because of the relatively low incidence of breast cancer in Japan in men and women who consume a diet rich in seaweed and with increasing breast cancer rates in Japanese women who emigrate to the West or consume a Western diet.[224-226] The antioxidant potential of iodide may require its oxidation to iodine. Eskin and colleagues[214] have postulated that normal physiologic function of mammary tissue requires iodine. Careful consideration of iodine deficiency is warranted because iodine replacement can promote problems with thyroid and extrathyroidal tissue function.

Table 23-14	Drugs Used to Treat Severe Breast Pain (Mastalgia)
Agents	**Comments**
Definitely Effective	
Danazol	Causes a decrease in cyclic pain and nodularity believed to reduce estrogen; also used for endometriosis; some side effects include changes in menstrual cycle regularity, weight gain, acne, and flushing
Bromocriptine	Decreases cyclic pain, nodularity, and tenderness; decreases prolactin levels and may alter dopamine receptors; is also used to suppress lactation after childbirth; can cause nausea, vomiting, hypotension, and dizziness
Tamoxifen	As an antiestrogen it can decrease cyclic pain; increase clot formation (phlebitis, emboli, strokes); cause hot flashes, amenorrhea, weight gain, and increased risk of uterine cancers
Evening primrose oil (linoleic acid)	Can decrease cyclic pain, nodularity, and tenderness; women with mastalgia believed to have low levels of breast linoleic acid; reduces PGE_2 prostaglandins and inflammation; too much oil, however, has been associated with increasing inflammation (>1000 mg/day)
Possibly Effective	
Iodine	Can decrease cyclic pain and nodularity (see Nutrition & Disease above)
Vaginal progesterone	Decrease in cyclic pain and tenderness; not as effective for decreasing tenderness; antagonist to estrogen; can cause weight gain
Insufficiently Studied	
Progestins	May decrease estrogenic effects, however, related to endothelial vasospasms, weight gain, and increased risk of breast cancer

Cancer

Breast cancer, the most common cancer in American women, is the leading cause of death in women ages 40 to 44 years and the second most common killer after lung cancer of women of all ages. The incidence of breast cancer has risen steadily since 1950 and is leveling off at about 126 cases per 100,000 women per year. The highest absolute lifetime (calculated to age 85) risk of breast cancer is 1 in 8 for non-Hispanic white women, 1 in 14 for black women, 1 in 21 for New Mexican Hispanics, and 1 in 40 for New Mexican American Indians[240] (Table 23-15). In women younger than 50 years of age, blacks experience higher incidence of early onset breast cancer and higher breast cancer mortality.[241] Black women in all age groups experience the highest mortality rates for breast cancer although the reason for this disparity is not clearly understood.[242] More than two thirds of breast cancer cases occur in women older than 55 years. The median age for breast cancer diagnosis is

Table 23-15	Chance of Being Diagnosed with Breast Cancer
By Age (years)	**By Ratio**
30-39	1 in 238
40-49	1 in 69
50-59	1 in 38
60-69	1 in 27
Ever*	1 in 8
Never	7 in 8

NOTE: These calculations are averages. An individual's risk may be higher or lower depending on several factors (e.g., family history, reproductive history, race ethnicity, and others).
*Absolute lifetime risk.
Data from Reis LAG et al: *Cancer statistics review, 1975-2005*, Bethesda, MD, 2008, National Cancer Institute. Available at http://seer.cancer.gov/csr/1975_2005. Based on November 2007 SEER data, posted SEER website, 2008.

Table 23-16	Factors Associated with Increased Risk of Breast Cancer*	
Category	**Risk Factor**	**Relative Risk†**
Race	Blacks have higher incidence up to age 40 yr; whites have higher incidence after age 40 yr	1.1-1.9
Family history	Breast cancer in first-degree relative before age 60 yr	2-3
	Premenopausal or bilateral breast cancer	>4
	Postmenopausal in first-degree relative	≤2
	Breast cancer in two first-degree relatives	4-6
	BRCA1 or *BRCA2*	≤4
	TP53 (Li-Fraumeni syndrome)	≤4
Previous medical history	Moderate or florid mammary hyperplasia	1.5-2
	Mammary papilloma	1.5-2
	Atypical mammary hyperplasia	4-5
	DCIS, LCIS‡	8-10
Estrogen exposure	Early menarche (before age 12 yr)	1.1-1.9
	Late menopause (after age 55 yr)	1.1-1.9
	Postmenopausal hormone therapy	1.4
	Oral contraceptive use	1.5
Pregnancy	Nulliparous or late first pregnancy (after age 35 yr)	1.1-1.9
Radiation	Atomic bomb	3
	Repeated fluoroscopy	1.5-2§
Obesity and stature	Postmenopausal	1.2
	Tallness	≤2
Dietary/alcohol	High alcohol consumption	1.4-2
	High energy intake	≤2
	Advanced age	2-4
	Xenobiotics	≤2
Social	Smoking	2-4
	Higher socioeconomic status	≤2
	Low physical activity	≤2
Environmental	Excess radiation to breasts	??‡
	Chemical carcinogens	≤2-??
	Infectious agents	≤2-??

*Normal lifetime risk in white non-Hispanic women: 1 in 8.
†Relative risk is defined and discussed in Chapter 5.
‡Data from Lester SC: The breast. In Kumar V, Abbas AK, Fausto N, editors: *Robbins and Cotran pathologic basis of disease*, ed 7, Philadelphia, 2005, Saunders.
§Currently being debated.
DCIS, Ductal carcinoma in situ; *LCIS,* lobular carcinoma in situ.

61 years of age. The median age at death for breast cancer is 69 years of age.[242] Because DCIS is almost exclusively detected by mammography, the large increase in incidence over the past 20 years can be attributed to screening.

Risk factors and possible causes of breast cancer can be classified as reproductive, hormonal, environmental and lifestyle, and familial (Table 23-16). However, two factors emerging as important are postpartum involution of the mammary gland and breast density, which are not as easily classified.

Reproductive Factors: Pregnancy

A clearer understanding of mammary gland structure (morphology) and function from fetal development, to puberty, pregnancy, and aging will help elucidate fundamental changes to breast development and disease. A key element is "branching morphogenesis," in which the mammary gland produces and delivers copious amounts of milk by forming a rootlike network of branched ducts from a rudimentary epithelial bud.[243] Branching morphogenesis begins in fetal development, pauses after birth, starts again in response to estrogens at puberty, and is modified by cyclic ovarian hormonal action. This systemic hormonal action elicits local paracrine interactions between the developing epithelial ducts and their adjacent mesenchyme (embryonic) or postnatal stroma. Then the local cellular crosstalk directs the tissue remodeling, ultimately producing a mature ductal tree.[243] The gland is unique as it undergoes most of its branching during adolescence and not fetal development. This allows experimental manipulation of the gland not possible with any other organ.[244]

A woman's age when her first child is born affects her risk for developing breast cancer—the younger she is, the lower the risk. A complete pregnancy before age 20 reduces the risk of breast cancer by 20% to 50%.[245-247] The protective factor is especially observed in the years of peak incidence, the postmenopausal years.[248] Paradoxically, however, a transient *increase* in breast cancer risk lasting 3 to 5 years after pregnancy is reported in women 25 years of age or older during pregnancy.[245,249,250] In addition, pregnancy induces a *lifelong*, not *transient increase*, in breast cancer risk in women who are more than 30 at the time of first pregnancy.[251] Why age affects this transient increase in breast cancer risk is unknown. A hypothesis for risk at any age is that gland *involution* after pregnancy and lactation uses some of the same tissue remodeling pathways activated during wound healing (i.e., proinflammatory pathways). The proinflammatory environment, although physiologically normal, promotes tumor progression. The presence of macrophages in the involuting mammary gland may contribute to carcinogenesis.[252] (Involution is an important topic discussed on p. 882.)

The main mechanisms for the *protective* effect of pregnancy are controversial including (1) induction of breast differentiation with lasting protective phenotypic (morphologic) changes; (2) altered cell fate with removal or modification of vulnerable cells; (3) enhancement of the ability for DNA repair or apoptosis, or both; (4) altered systemic hormonal regulation and possible persistent changes in intracellular pathways regulating proliferation; (5) decreased proliferation in the parous involuted

| Box 23-17 | Well-Established Evidence Concerning Pregnancy and Breast Cancer |

Epidemiologic

Early age at first-term pregnancy is related to lifetime decrease in breast cancer risk.

Increasing parity is associated with long-term risk reduction, even when controlling for age at first birth.

The additional long-term protective effect of young age at subsequent term pregnancies is not as strong as for first pregnancy.

A nulliparous woman has about the same risk as a woman with a first term birth around age 30.

Breast cancer risk is transiently *increased* after a term pregnancy (before it has a lasting *reduced* risk).

Induced abortion is not associated with an increase in breast cancer risk.

Known spontaneous abortion is not associated with an increase in breast cancer risk.

Long duration of lactation provides a small additional reduction in breast cancer risk after consideration of age at and number of term pregnancies.

Animal Models

Pregnancy protects against subsequent chemical carcinogen-induced breast cancer in rats and mice.

Estrogen and progesterone combinations and hCG protect against carcinogen-induced cancer in rodents by mimicking pregnancy.

Short-term estrogen exposure at levels of estrogen mimicking pregnancy is protective for carcinogen-induced cancer in rats.

From National Cancer Institute. National Cancer Institute Board of Scientific Advisors (BSA) and Board of Scientific Counselors: NCI summary report: early reproductive events and breast cancer, 2003. Available at www.cancerblog/cancerinfo/ere-workshop-report. *hCG*, Human chorionic gonadotropin.

gland; and (6) early-life hormonal and dietary exposures.[248] Although contradictory evidence exists the majority of data suggest that lasting changes and decreased proliferation are not closely related to hormone-induced protection. In animal models, hormone levels mimicking pregnancy, including estrogen and progesterone combinations and human chorionic gonadotropin, protect against carcinogen-induced cancer[253] (Box 23-17). The mechanism whereby protection is caused by an increase in apoptosis has been implicated in the *post-pregnancy treatment* experimental animal model. Studies of in utero and prepubertal exposures and subsequent breast cancer risk have yielded inconclusive results.

Thus the two prevailing hypotheses, not mutually exclusive, of protective mechanisms induced by pregnancy are (1) the induction of an altered *systemic hormonal pattern* and (2) an altered cell fate or persistent changes in intracellular regulatory circuits (loops).[248] The first hypothesis involves systemic levels of hormones, including growth hormone and prolactin, and their cascading downstream effectors as modifying the chemical-carcinogen–initiated mammary cells (see p. 883). The second hypothesis emphasizes that hormones induce a molecular switch in stem cells that result in cells with long-lasting changes in regulatory circuits regulating proliferation and response to DNA damage.[248] Still controversial, stem cells are proposed to be the origin for breast cancer.[254-256] Although further research is needed data indicate that reduced stem cells may help explain why early pregnancy reduces the risk of breast cancer. In addition, cancers may result from *errant* stem or progenitor cells misguided by their microenvironment (stroma) or from mutated somatic cells that interact with stem cells causing dysfunctional signaling that leads to carcinogenesis.[257] Much research is devoted to the concept that stem cells are controlled by their microenvironment, systemic hormones, and local growth factors.[258] A series of experiments demonstrated that estrogen facilitates epithelial proliferation and morphogenesis by a paracrine mechanism.[259] **Amphiregulin (AREG)** was found to be a major paracrine-mediator of ductal morphogenesis and plays an important role in mammary stem cell self-renewal and differentiation.[258] These studies are important because they help elucidate factors in mammary stem differentiation and breast cancer initiation, progression, and protection. Thus hierarchical models are emerging of hormones, growth factors, and transcription factors in which all types of epithelial cells in the mammary gland possibly originate from a single common multipotent stem cell.[258] As part of the second hypothesis, investigators are focusing on the *TP53* tumor-suppressor gene, which has been demonstrated to be important in pregnancy-related hormone-induced protection. The function of *TP53* is required for hormone-mediated protection against the carcinogens dimethylbenz(a)anthracene (DMBA)-induced carcinogenesis in mice.[244] Russo and colleagues[260] have found that the post-pregnancy involuted mammary gland exhibits elevated expression of genes involved in DNA repair and apoptosis.

Lobular Involution and Age

Part of the uniqueness of the mammary gland is its profound physiologic changes throughout the phases of a woman's life: puberty, pregnancy, lactation, postlactational involution, and aging. The human breast is organized to 15 to 20 major lobes, each with lobules containing milk-forming acini (see Figure 22-19). With aging, breast lobules regress or involute with a decrease in the number and size of acini per lobule and replacement of the intralobular stroma with the more dense collagen of connective tissue.[261] Over time the glandular elements and collagen are replaced with fatty tissue. This process is called **lobular involution** whereby, over many years, the parenchymal elements progressively atrophy and disappear. A first study of its kind found lobular involution was associated with reduced risk of breast cancer.[261-263] Breast cancer risk decreased with increasing extent of involution in both high- and low-risk subgroups defined by family history of breast cancer, epithelial atypia, reproductive history, and age.[261] Based on pathologic and epidemiologic factors, these investigators propose that delayed involution (persistent glandular epithelium) is a major risk factor for breast cancer.[261-263] Widely appreciated is that as women age, their risk of breast cancer increases. But the *rate* of increase of breast cancer *slows* at about 50 years of age.[264,265] This slowing has been attributed to a reduction in ovarian hormone production. Milanese and colleagues[261] observed a definite increase in the process of involution at about 50 years of age with complete involution present in 5.8% of women ages 40 to

49 years and 21.6% of women ages 50 to 59 years. Investigators propose that involution may contribute to this slowing in the rate of increase of breast cancer among women older than 50 years.[263] Importantly, investigators found an inverse association between lobular involution and parity.[261] Other investigators have reported that the more children a woman has, the more likely she is to have persistent lobular tissue,[266,267] which Milanese and colleagues[261] found was associated with increased risk of breast cancer. However, multiparity also has been found to reduce risk of breast cancer.[268,269] This apparent contradiction may be explained by studies documenting that full-term pregnancies after 35 years of age are correlated with an increased risk of breast cancer.[270] In the Milanese study, age of the mother at each child's birth was unknown.

Henson and colleagues[271] propose that late pregnancy with its concomitant increase in the proliferation of the ductal-alveolar epithelium is likely to interrupt the process of involution, which typically begins between 30 and 40 years of age. The activated stromal environment in the process of involution is similar to that in invasive breast cancer. The long-term protective effects of pregnancy with hormones released during pregnancy affect remodeling of the stromal microenvironment by causing apoptosis and involution. However, a short-term increase in breast cancer risk following pregnancy may be caused by the process of mammary gland involution which returns the tissue back to its prepregnant state and is co-opted by processes of wound healing resulting in a proinflammatory environment that although physiologically normal can promote carcinogenesis.[252]

Interestingly, oophorectomy, which is associated with a decrease in risk of breast cancer, leads to atrophy of breast parenchyma in young women as is noted in older women. Thus the risk reduction of oophorectomy may be caused by an accelerated involution.[271]

Risk data are needed on the age of a woman at pregnancy and at breast biopsy to evaluate the relationship of parity, involution, and breast cancer risk. In addition, the Milanese and colleagues[261] study had a large number ($n = 5197$) of women with partial involution only; they propose better quantitative measures of degree of involution are needed. However, they hypothesize that given the inverse association of complete involution and multiparity, the breast cancer risk modification associated with parity is independent of involution. An important finding in their study is that the extent of involution was independent of all known breast cancer risk factors.[261]

The biologic mechanisms suggested by which involution or lack thereof alters breast cancer risk include that (1) complete involution causes a decrease in epithelial cell number so fewer cells undergo carcinogenesis; (2) aberrant involution or prolonged involution activates tissue remodeling pathways during wound healing, resulting in proinflammatory pathways that although physiologically normal, promote carcinogenesis (see Pregnancy and Breast Cancer, p. 881)[252]; and (3) failure to involute allows prolonged exposure to intrinsic or extrinsic factors, and genetic, epigenetic, or oxidative stressors. Elucidation on the mechanisms of lobular involution is very important for understanding breast carcinogenesis and factors that reduce breast cancer risk.

Hormonal Factors

The link between breast cancer and hormones is based on six factors that affect risk: (1) the protective effect of an early (i.e., in the 20s) first pregnancy; (2) the protective effect of removal of the ovaries and pituitary gland; (3) the increased risk associated with early menarche, late menopause, and nulliparity; (4) the relationship between types of fat, free estrogen levels, and oxidative changes in estrogen metabolism; (5) the hormone-dependent development and differentiation of mammary gland structures; and (6) the efficacy of antihormone therapies for treatment and prevention of breast cancer. Throughout its existence, the mammary gland epithelium proceeds through critical "exposure periods" of rapid growth or cycles of proliferation, including neonatal growth, pubertal development, pregnancy lactation, and involution (after pregnancy and postmenopause; see p. 882).[242,252]

Our understanding of the role of systemic hormones as powerful regulators of mammary gland development is shifting. Evidence is pointing to the wide-ranging effects of systemic hormones as possibly not due to their *direct* hormone action but rather their *induced* actions from multiple secondary paracrine effectors—thus the term *hierarchical*.[243] Unraveling is a complex model of hormone, paracrine, and adhesion molecule-signaling pathways affecting epithelial and stromal cell fate in development and cancer (Figure 23-46). Despite differences between the organized process of development and the less, even chaotic, environment of invasive cancer, both processes share many identical mechanisms and signaling pathways. Key is *tissue remodeling* that applies to pubertal growth, immediately after pregnancy and during involution (see previous section).[252,272-273]

A vast majority of breast cancers are *initially* hormone-dependent (estrogen-receptor positive [ER+] and/or progesterone-receptor positive [PR+]), with estrogens playing a crucial role in their development.[274] Estrogens control processes critical for cellular functions by regulating activities and expression of key signaling molecules. These processes include regulation of receptor activity, its interaction with other intracellular proteins, and DNA.[274] Estrogens thus play prominent roles in cellular proliferation, differentiation, and apoptosis.[274-276] It is now appreciated that estrogen has both nuclear (genomic) and non-nuclear (nongenomic) actions (Figure 23-47, *A*). Studies reveal 58 target genes of estradiol (E_2), some of which may be relevant to *onset* and proliferation of breast cancer (see Figure 23-47, *B*).[275-277] It is well documented that in addition to direct regulation of gene expression (genomic), steroid hormones (e.g., estrogen) regulate cytoplasmic cell-signaling cascades or rapid nongenomic effects.[275] In hormone-dependent breast cancers, estrogens, especially the potent 17β-E_2 contribute greatly to the development of carcinoma cells, and some carcinomas require estrogen for continued growth.[278]

Most of our understanding of carcinogenicity of estrogens is based on animal studies. Two main mechanisms of

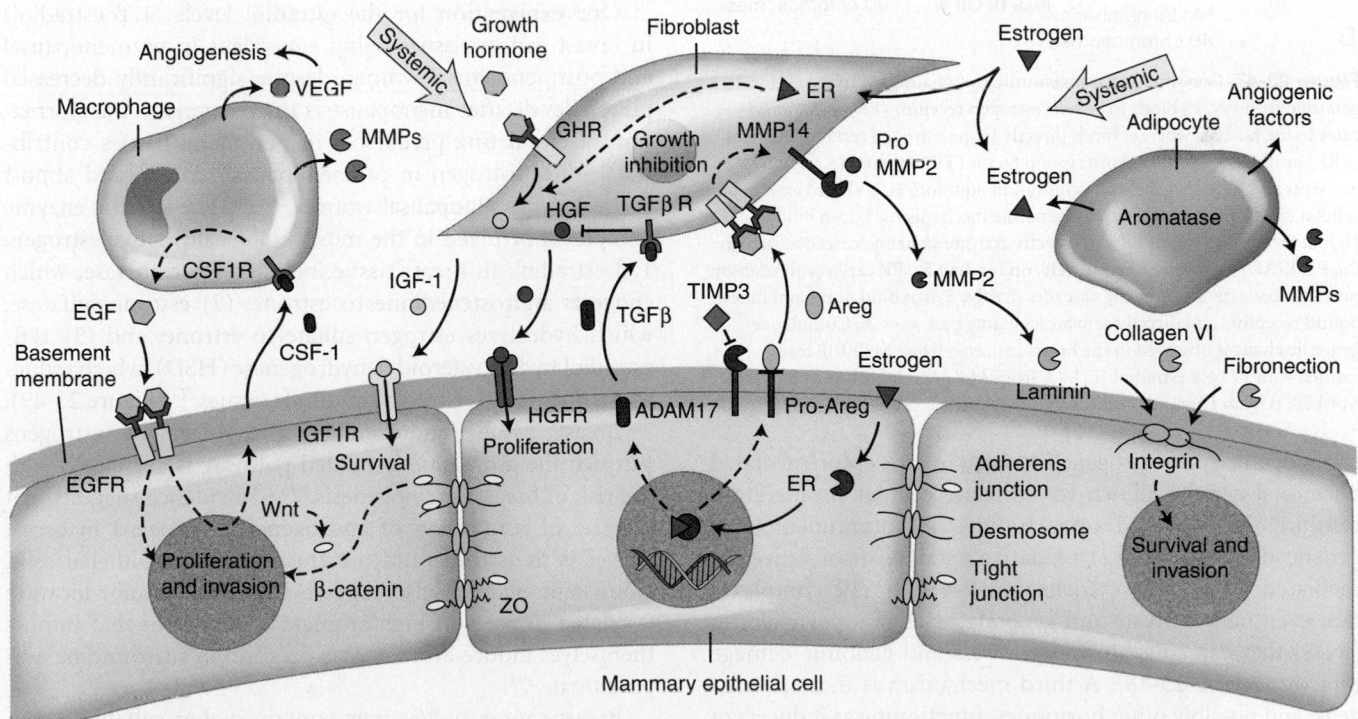

Figure 23-46 Figure of the current hypothesis of mammary gland during development and cancer. A tissue model of interacting endocrine, paracrine, and adhesion signaling pathways that modulate epithelial and stromal cell behavior. Some of the pathways depicted are not exclusive to one type of stromal cell. *Dotted arrows* indicate indirect interactions. (From Lanigan F et al: *Cell Mol Life Sci* 64:3165, 2007.)

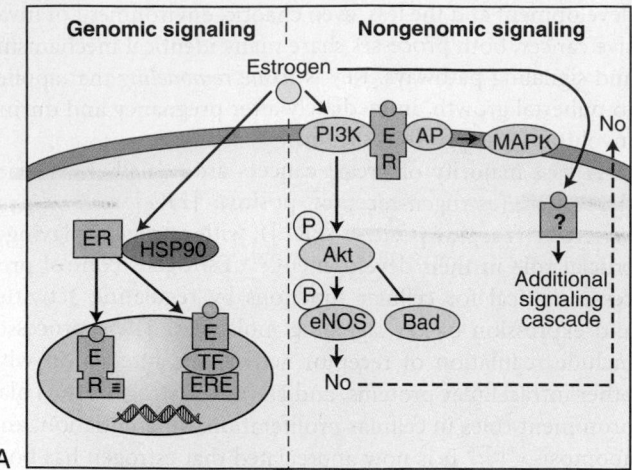

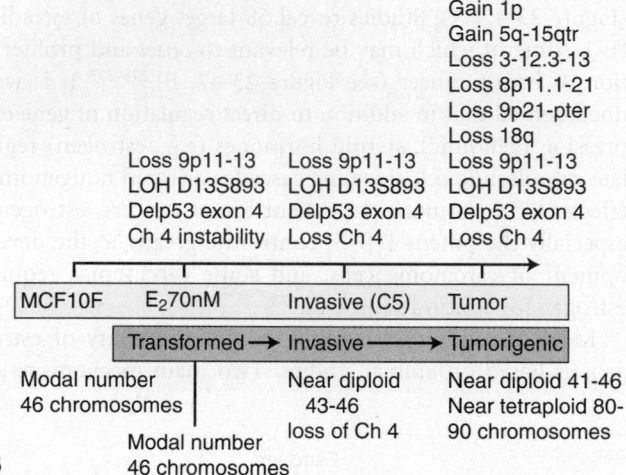

Figure 23-47 Genomic and nongenomic E_2 signaling. **A,** In the classical genomic pathway, E_2 binds to *cystolic* estrogen receptor (ER) and translocates to the nucleus where it binds directly to the estrogen receptor element (ERE) or binds to another transcription factor (TF) tethered to response elements and induces gene transcription. In addition, E_2 is able to exert *rapid* cellular effects through several nongenomic mechanisms. E_2 can bind to *plasma membrane-bound* ER and directly activate signaling cascades, such as the PI3K/AKT pathway. Alternatively, on binding E_2, ER can recruit adaptor proteins that activate signaling cascades. Lastly, E_2 can bind nonmembrane-bound receptors and directly activate signaling pathways. **B,** Cumulative genomic changes observed in the breast cancer cell line MCF10F transformed with 17 beta estradiol (E_1). (**A** from *Mol Med* published online 2008 April 20. **B** from *J Steroid Biochem Mol Biol* 102[1-5]:89-96, 2006.)

carcinogenicity of estrogens involve (1) a receptor-mediated hormonal activity shown to stimulate cellular proliferation resulting in increased opportunities for accumulation of genetic damage, and (2) oxidative catabolism of estrogens mediated by various cytochrome P-450 (CYP) complexes that eventually activate and generate reactive oxygen species (ROS) that can cause oxidative stress and genomic damage directly (Figure 23-48). A third mechanism is that of estrogens, and possibly other hormones, functioning as inducers of aneuploidy (gain or loss of chromosomes). LOH, and aneuploidy are crucial events during carcinogenesis. However, it is not clear whether aneuploidy is a result of neoplastic development or a cause.

Estrogens affect microtubules that are essential for establishing cell shape and cell polarity, processes necessary for epithelial gland organization.[274] In addition, the centrosomes, which are necessary for segregating chromosomes into daughter cells, are affected by estrogen. Centrosomes facilitate the coordination of intracellular activities, including cell cycle progression and cell cycle checkpoints (see Chapter 1). Although the mechanisms that promote the formation of abnormal centrosomes are unclear, several possibilities have been proposed in regard to the development of cancer,[274] including centrosome amplification in breast tumors and hyperplastic gland development prior to tumor formation,[279] progestins may facilitate aneuploidy,[280] and bisphenol-A (BPA, found in plastics) induces the same pattern of aneuploidy found by estrogens.[281] Women taking hormone replacement therapy (HRT) (estrogen plus progestin) have increased mammographic breast density and increased breast cancer risk compared with women taking only estrogen[282-284] (see discussion following).

Evidence is emerging on the roles of estrogen and other hormones as initiators. An experimental system has demonstrated that the natural estrogen 17β-E_2, by itself, or its metabolites 2-hydroxy, 4-hydroxy, and 16-a-hydroxy-estradiol induced carcinogenesis of human breast epithelial cells (HBECs).[285]

Other studies suggest that *local* (in situ; paracrine) formation of estrogens in breast tumors may be more important than circulating estrogens in *plasma* for the growth and survival of estrogen-dependent breast cancer in postmenopausal women.[274,286,287]

One explanation for the estradiol levels (17β-estradiol) in breast cancer tissues being equivalent in premenopausal and postmenopausal women despite significantly decreased plasma levels after menopause is that enzymatic transformation of circulating precursors in peripheral tissues contribute 75% of estrogen in premenopausal women and almost 100% in postmenopausal women.[288,289] The specific enzyme complexes involved in the most biologically active estrogen, 17β-estradiol, in breast tissue include (1) aromatase, which converts androstenedione to estrone; (2) estrone sulfatase, which hydrolyzes estrogen sulfate to estrone; and (3) 17β-estradiol hydroxysteroid dehydrogenase (HSD), which reduces estrone to 17β-estradiol in tumor tissues[274] (Figure 23-49).

Breast tissue (endogenous) metabolism of estrogens through the aromatase-mediated pathway is correlated with the risk of breast carcinogenesis.[290,291] Evidence suggests that the site of conversion of androgens to estrogens in breast cancer is the stroma and not the malignant epithelial cells. Consistent evidence also suggests that either tumor location is related to areas of high aromatase activity or that tumors themselves induce aromatase expression in surrounding adipose tissue.[292]

Breast cancer tissues may contain higher sulfatase activity than aromatase activity and produce estrone through the hydrolysis of estrone sulfate[274,293-295] (see Figure 23-49). In addition, estrone sulfate has a longer half-life than estrone.[295] Thus quantitatively estrone sulfate may be the most

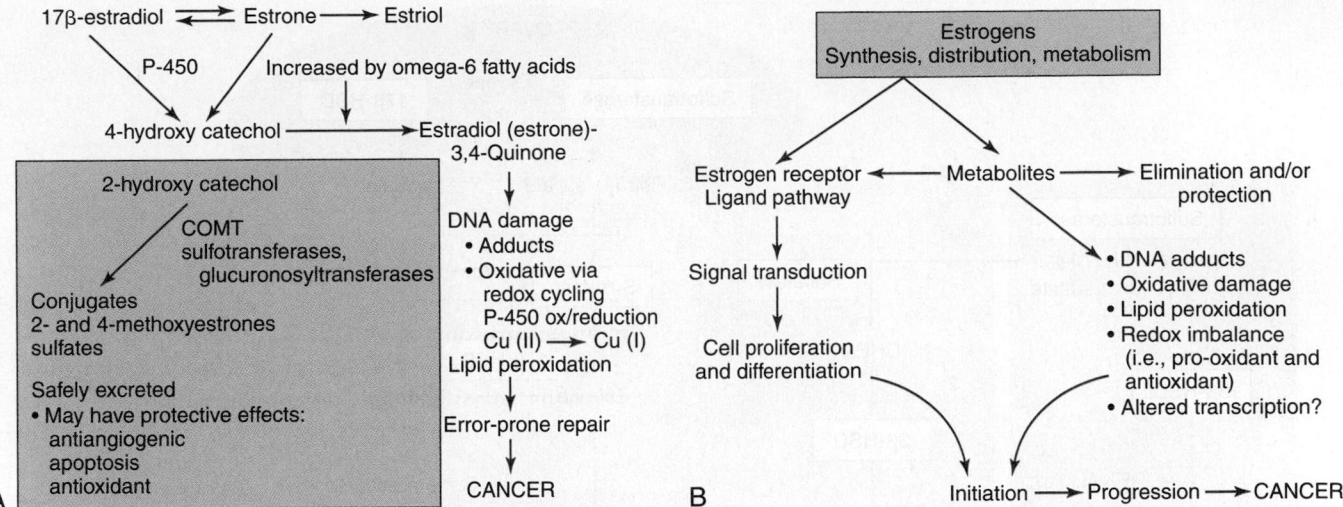

Figure 23-48 Metabolites of estrogen and their associated carcinogenic effects. **A,** Metabolites of estrogen and carcinogenic pathway. Genotoxicity can be produced by the 4-hydroxy catechol metabolite. A redox cycle catalyzed by microsomal P-450 and cytochrome P-450-reductase can locally generate superoxide ($O_2\cdot$) and hydroxyl radicals to produce additional DNA damage. Catechol estrogens also have been shown to interact with breast tissue nitric oxide, a potent oxidant that induces DNA strand breakage. Unstable polyunsaturated fats (omega-6) can increase the production of quinones. Unstable omega-6 fatty acids can be transformed by the effects of oxygen and heat into carriers of free radicals. 2-Hydroxy catechol, when methylated, may have protective effects against tumor development. Several enzymes are involved with the metabolism of estrogen, including specific cytochrome P-450 isoforms, sulfotransferases, and catechol-O-methyltransferase (COMT). These enzymes may be influenced by environmental factors, including fats, alcohol, and xenobiotic exposures. These enzymes also are polymorphic and their distributions may differ among different ethnic populations. **B,** Estrogen receptor and estrogen metabolites on cancer initiation and progression. (**B** adapted from Yager JD: *J Natl Cancer Inst Monogr* 27:67, 2000; additional data from Russo J, Russo I: *Molecular basis of breast cancer: prevention and treatment,* Germany, 2004, Springer; Cavalieri EL, Rogan EG: *Ann N Y Acad Sci* 1028:247-257, 2004.)

important circulating estrogen in women; it increases the reservoir for the production of estrone and, ultimately, estradiol. Furthermore, sulfatase levels have independently predicted breast cancer relapse-free survival.[295,296] The association between sulfatase and poor prognosis was significant only in individuals with ER+ tumors. Miyoshi and colleagues found high sulfatase expression was associated with a poorer prognosis in premenopausal *and* postmenopausal women with ER+ tumors. These results suggest a possibility that, even in premenopausal women, the intratumoral estrogen biosynthesis plays an important role in the growth stimulation of breast tumors.[296] Unknown are the relative contributions of estradiol to the intratumoral synthesized estradiol from the ovary versus the total intratumoral quantities. Aromatase inhibitors (anastrozole, letrozole, and exemestane) are extremely effective and very selective (targeted) for this enzyme. Estrogen formation from estrone sulfatase cannot be blocked by aromatase inhibitors.

The first sulfatase inhibitor, 667 COUMATE, was used in a phase 1 clinical trial in postmenopausal women with hormone-dependent breast cancer. Although a small number (five of eight) of women showed evidence of stable disease with 667 COUMATE, all had been unresponsive (refractory) to aromatase inhibition.[297]

Recent studies in mice illustrate the complex and paradoxical roles of hormones in mammary tissue. On the one hand, *short* duration of exposure to estrogen and progesterone, or estrogen alone, imparts a *protective* effect on breast

carcinogenesis.[298] On the other hand, *continuing* the same dose of hormones for a prolonged period strongly *stimulates* the development of tumors in the same mouse models. Different mechanisms have been suggested for the short-term protective effect, including (1) a different cellular developmental fate or (2) a systemic effect involving down-regulation of pituitary hormones (e.g., growth or prolactin hormones, or both). A short duration of hormones or blocking the same hormone pathway (i.e., tamoxifen) produces a similar result or decrease in tumor development. Overwhelming data, however, show that prolonged exposure to estradiol and progesterone (progestins) increase the risk of breast cancer.[298]

IGFs regulate cellular functions involving cell proliferation, differentiation, and apoptosis. Emerging evidence indicates that members of the IGF family play important roles in the development and progression of cancer. The IGF-1 receptor (IGF-1R), overexpressed in cancer cells, mediates the effects of IGFs and plays a role in cell transformation.[299] IGFs are potent mitogens for ER+ breast cell lines. Interruption of IGF action can inhibit estrogenic stimulation of breast cancer cells, evidence of cellular crosstalk between the insulin growth factors and estrogen receptors.[300] IGF-binding protein 3 (IGFBP-3) regulates the mitogenic and metabolic effects of IGFs; *TP53* may regulate apoptosis in tumor cells through IGFBP-3.[274] The protective effects of IGFBP-3 may be modulated by hCG that facilitates differentiation of the mammary gland. Increased levels of IGFBP-3 in the more differentiated Lob 3 compared with Lob 1 is a finding that requires further study.[274]

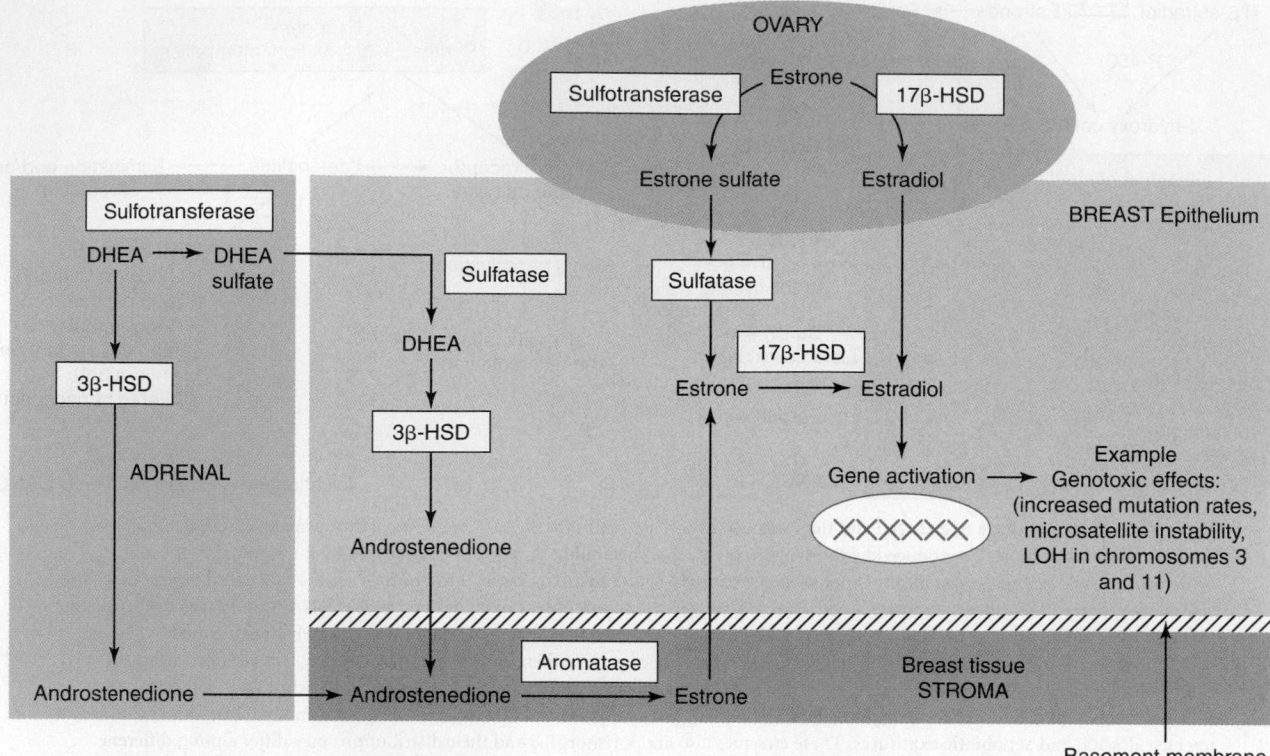

Figure 23-49 Local biosynthesis of estrogens. Three main enzyme complexes (yellow) involved in estrogen formation in breast tissue, including aromatase, sulfatase, and 17β-estradiol hydroxysteroid dehydrogenase (HSD). Thus despite low levels of circulating estrogens in postmenopausal women with breast cancer, the tissue levels are several-fold higher than these in plasma, suggesting tumor accumulation of these estrogens. Data suggest that most abundant is sulfatase in premenopausal and postmenopausal women with breast cancer. Numerous agents can block the aromatase action, exploration of progesterone, and various progestins to inhibit sulfatase and 17β-HSD or stimulate sulfotransferase (i.e., breast cancer cells cannot inactivate estrogens because they lack sulfotransferase) to provide new possibilities for treatment. (Adapted from Russo J, Russo I: *Molecular basis of breast cancer: prevention and treatment,* Germany, 2004, Springer.)

During the first trimester of pregnancy hCG increases, then rapidly declines to a slow steady state maintained throughout the rest of pregnancy. The action of hCG is mediated by a G-protein–coupled receptor, which also binds LH. Low levels of these receptors are present in breast tissue. This coupled with the epidemiologic findings of a decreased breast cancer risk in women who complete full-term pregnancy at a young age and a protective effect of hCG against carcinogen-induced mammary tumor development in rats, suggests that hCG may be protective against breast cancer.[274,301] Treatment of human breast cancer cells (MCF-7) with hCG resulted in a modest dose-dependent decrease in cell proliferation but a dramatic decrease in cell invasion.[301] Experiments showed not only inhibition of genes involved in cell proliferation and invasion but also activation of genes involved in cell differentiation, apoptosis, and DNA repair.[302] hCG down-regulates ER levels through an epigenetic mechanism (CpG island methylation, see p. 374) leading to a protective effect.[303] Treatment with hCG, however, can stimulate breast cancer growth in animals with overexpressed *HER-2/neu* oncogene.[304] Nonetheless, the antiproliferative and anti-invasive effect may be useful in developing new therapies.

Investigators also have proposed that persistent alteration in the hypothalamic-hypophyseal axis (e.g., occurring during pregnancy) results in reduced circulating levels of mammary hormones, including growth hormone and prolactin that have been identified as important promoters of breast carcinogenesis.[298]

Hormonal Therapy: Estrogen Only

Data based on an overview of all epidemiologic studies on the effect of menopausal estrogen therapy (ET) show that ET causes a 2% mean increase in breast cancer risk per year of use,[305,306] or a 10% increase in risk after 5 years of use.[306] Analysis of hormonal therapy risks, however, seems to differ according to body mass index (BMI). The effects of obesity reveal that increases in non–SHBG bound E_2 exceeding about 10.2 pg/ml have no *further* effect on breast cancer risk.[306] The increased risk of ET (0.6251 mg/day) is more evident in slender women, estimated at 30% increase in risk in a woman with a BMI of 20 kg/m² decreasing to an 8% increase in risk in a woman with a BMI of 30 kg/m².[305-308] The equivalent figures for estrogen-progestin therapy (EPT) are 50% in slender women (BMI 20 kg/m²) and 26% in heavier women (i.e., 30 kg/m²). Interestingly, according to these risk estimates, reducing the dose of estrogen in ET and EPT by as much as half has little or no effect on risk.[306] These data differ from the randomized Women's Health Initiative (WHI) with women who had hysterectomy that found a decrease in risk with use of ET.[309] These findings are confusing because of other inconsistent data: (1) increased *serum* levels of estrogen are associated with increased risk[310-313]; (2) increasing postmenopausal weight increases breast cancer risk, an association between weight and increased serum levels of estrogen[311-313]; and (3) treating the original breast cancer with aromatase inhibitors sharply reduces risk of contralateral breast cancer. Thus ET increases breast cancer risk; the effect is greatest in slender women and difficult to discern in women with a BMI greater than 30 kg/m^2.

Estrogen-Progestin Therapy. To compare risks among several studies Lee and colleagues[314] standardized measures to enable data from the WHI randomized trial, cohort studies, and case-control studies to be expressed in the same relative risk terms. The summary of all studies showed a weighted average relative risk at the end of 5 years of use of EPT to be 1.44. The relative risk for the studies from the United States was 1.29 and 1.53 for the Scandinavian studies, a statistically significant difference. The continuous-combined (estrogen-progestin) therapy from the United States studies was associated with a slightly lower risk than the sequential therapy, that is, a 20% increased risk after 5 years. In comparison, there is a 32% increase in risk with sequential therapy. The opposite findings were found for the Scandinavian studies in which the continuous-combined regimens were associated with an 8.8% increase risk compared with a 40% increase with sequential.[306] These differences are explained by different continuous-combined progestin doses in the United States and Scandinavia; additionally U.S. women have a greater BMI.[306] Importantly, the greater risk in the Scandinavian studies compared to the United States studies is explained by a *greater* relative effect of EPT on breast cancer risk in leaner women.[306,307]

In conclusion, ET use is associated with a statistically significant increased risk of breast cancer, especially in slender women.[306] An explanation for this risk may be related to the so-called ceiling (effect) to the carcinogenic risk of estrogen on the breast. Slender women may be more vulnerable to the additional exogenous estrogen because endogenously they may have lower serum levels of estrogen than obese women. Thus additional estrogen has no further effect (i.e., ceiling effect) on breast cancer risk in heavier women.[306] Heavier women on EPT could likely reduce their breast cancer risk by reducing the progestin dose. In terms of ceiling effect, progestins appear to act independently on estrogen without the estrogen ceiling decreasing the progestin effect.[306] A French study showed no increase in breast cancer risk with micronized progesterone instead of progestin (i.e., in EPT therapy),[315] and an experimental study in macaques showed no effect of micronized progesterone on breast cell proliferation.[316] Micronized progesterone, however, increased mammographic density in a randomized trial.[317] An Italian retrospective study found long-term use with EPT using either micronized progesterone or transdermal progesterone were both associated with breast cancer risk; however, transdermal use was associated with a lower risk (RR 1.27 versus 2.14).[318]

Depending on the tissue, progesterone is classified as either a proliferative or differentiative hormone. Its effects also vary depending on whether it is used in combination with estrogen or alone. The conclusion from studies[319,320] is that progesterone is neither inherently proliferative nor antiproliferative but it is capable of stimulating or inhibiting cell growth depending on whether treatment is transient or continuous. Continuous treatment may decrease sensitivity of the cells to the proliferative effects of epidermal growth factor. Investigators reported that different signal transduction pathways are used by natural versus synthetic progestins for the induction of vascular endothelial growth factor (VEGF), which promotes angiogenesis. This distinction may represent the different pathologies reported in progesterone versus synthetic progestin medroxyprogesterone acetate (MPA)–induced breast tumors in mice or the different potencies exhibited by natural and synthetic progestins for inducing proliferation of breast cancer cells in vitro.[321] The safe use of progesterone-progestins, in terms of breast cancer, however, is not yet established.

Some studies have shown that OC use increases a young woman's risk of breast cancer, especially current use.[322,323] Other studies have found that the most important variable is the total months of use, with an increase of 38% (relative risk) for 10 years of use.[324] A study of women between 35 and 64 years of age that included current and former OC users showed no significant association with increased breast cancer risk.[325] A small study ($n = 25$) showed that baby boomers who took OCs for 10 years and then took hormone therapy for 3 or more years (the first group to do this) had a relative risk of 3.2—more than triple the risk of women who never used either.[326] Controversy remains about the relationship between OC use and breast cancer risk; however, the efficacy of OCs in protecting against ovarian cancer and endometrial cancer is well established.

Mammographic Breast Density

Mammographic density (MD) is the radiologic appearance of the breast reflecting variations in breast tissue composition (Figure 23-50). Mammographic density in more than 60% to 75% of the breast is associated with a four- to sixfold greater risk for breast cancer.[327] Thus extensive breast density is one of the strongest risk factors for developing breast cancer and second only to age and carrying a *BRCA1* or *BRCA2* mutation.[328] Increased MD is common among 26% to 32% of women in the general population having densities of 50% or greater. Estimates of attributable risk reveal that densities of more than 50% of the breast may account for 16% to 21% of breast cancers, and possibly greater among premenopausal women.[329] The strongest correlations of MD with other breast cancer risk factors is with BMI and age. Importantly, MD appears to be an *independent* risk factor for breast cancer because of its robust association with breast cancer after adjusting for other breast cancer risk factors.[330,331]

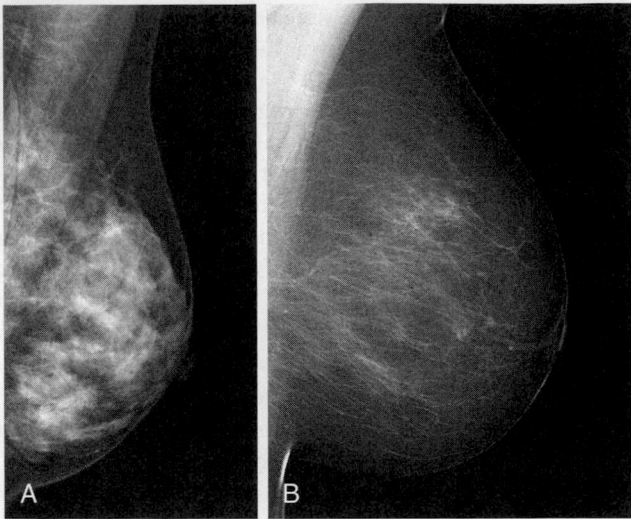

Figure 23-50 Breast density varies among women. The sensitivity of mammography for detecting malignancy is significantly reduced if the breast consists of a high proportion of fibroglandular (dense) breast tissue (**A**) compared to a breast that is fatty (**B**). (From O'Malley FP, Pinder SE, editors: *Breast pathology*, New York, 2006, Churchill Livingstone.)

The Minnesota Breast Cancer Family Study[332] demonstrated that the factors of baseline percent density (PD), postmenopausal hormone use, and BMI (inverse relationship) predict changes in MD trends during adult life. Height has been shown to be positively associated with percent of mammographic density and with increased risk of breast cancer. However, these factors all together account for only 20% to 30% of the variation in the population. Investigators detected increased risks of breast cancer in women with MD that persisted for at least 8 years after entry into the study and were greater in younger than in older women. Their data also showed that more extensive mammographic density was strongly associated with greater risk of breast cancer detected by screening and an increased risk of detection of breast cancer between screens. Consistent with other studies, risk of breast cancer was positively correlated with the area of dense tissue but unlike other studies, less so than overall percent density. Because definitive diagnosis by mammography of breast cancer is more difficult in women with dense breasts, the optimal approach for detection remains to be determined.[333]

Histologic studies of breast biopsy sections and from mastectomy specimens have shown that epithelial and stromal proliferation were associated with mammographic density.[333] These data suggest that genetic and environmental factors affecting risk of breast cancer affect the proliferative activity and quantity of epithelial and stromal tissue in the breast, and that these effects are possibly related to differences in mammographic density among women of the same age (see Figure 23-50). It has been shown that the dense area noted by mammogram is related to risk of breast cancer but percent density may be a stronger risk factor. Mammographic density appears to play a large role in explaining variance in the mammographic areas of dense and nondense tissue and, because

MD is a continuous trait, is likely to be influenced by multiple genes. Finding the genes involved in MD may help explain why it is a strong risk factor. Evaluation of younger women to understand the pathogenesis of MD holds a promise for improved risk prediction; however, the controversy surrounding mammograms (see Chapter 11 and p. 386) and radiation in younger women speaks for alternative imaging modalities to provide an MD estimate for risk models in these women.[329] How MD is related to involution is unknown.

Environmental Factors and Lifestyle

The environmental causes of breast cancer possibly affect the breast the most during critical phases or "windows" of development including early differential stages—that is, undifferentiated cells to alveolar buds and then lobules, puberty, pregnancy and lactation, involution, and menopause. During early phases, mitotic activity and cell division are greater than later in life.

Radiation. Ionizing radiation is a known risk factor for breast cancer. To date, only accidentally or medically induced radiation has been demonstrated to exert a carcinogenic effect on the breast. There are many sources of ionizing radiation, including x-rays, CT scans, fluoroscopy, and other medical radiologic procedures. According to the National Cancer Institute (NCI), CT scans "comprise about 10% of diagnostic radiologic procedures in large U.S. hospitals"; however, they contribute an estimated 65% of the effective radiation dose to the public from all medical x-ray examinations.[334] Scientists and clinicians have expressed concern about the increasing number of CT scans performed, particularly for children, because of the high dose radiation exposure and subsequent cancer risk, which has the potential to become a public health issue in the future.[335]

Between 1950 and 1991 the incidence of breast cancer in the United States increased dramatically as did screening, leading some to suggest that increased exposure may have been a contributing factor.[336] However, since the 1980s, screening has resulted in increased detection of small invasive carcinomas and in situ carcinomas. The duration of increased risk from radiation is unknown, but increased risk appears to have lasted at least 35 years in women treated for mastitis, those treated with fluoroscopy, and Atom-bomb survivors.

The type of cancer that can result from radiation exposure depends on the area exposed and the age of the individual at time of exposure. Radiologic exposure of the upper spine, heart, ribs, lungs, shoulders, and esophagus also can expose breast tissue to radiation. X-rays and fluoroscopy of infants may constitute whole body irradiation. The younger the age, the higher the risk. Evidence indicates that childhood exposure to radiation creates the greatest cancer risk whereas exposure after age 40 confers the lowest.[334] Breast cancer rates in atomic bomb survivors in Japan were highest among women younger than 20 years of age at time of exposure. An important finding among the Atom-bomb survivors is that those who had early full-term pregnancies were at significantly lower risk than those who had not.[337] Therefore, interacting factors can modulate the risks from radiation.

Radiobiologists have long been struggling to estimate the health risks for low doses of radiation (less than 10 cGy). Cancer induction and exposure to low doses of radiation are controversial and the topic of much debate and research. Biologic understanding related to low doses of radiation is presented in Chapters 2 and 12 and a few of these points are relevant here. Data among Japanese A-bomb survivors suggest that for solid tumors the dose response relationship is a *linear* function of doses between 10 and 250 cGy.[338] Estimates of cancer risks at low doses—except for those from direct epidemiologic observations—are obtained by a mathematical model of linear extrapolation from these higher doses. Qualitative and quantitative differences in responses to doses of irradiation are important for understanding whether the biologic effects of low- and high-dose ionizing radiation are linearly distributed. Because cellular responses from low doses may be different than from high doses linear extrapolation may not be accurate.[339] Specifically, the concerns of cellular responses from low doses including bystander effects, adaptive response, and potential radiation hypersensitivity responses in certain population subgroups (e.g., hypersensitive to low doses).[340] The first study to use global gene expression changes for investigating the effects of extremely low radiation doses and high radiation doses on the cell yielded intriguing results.[341] The percentage of total genes responding to the low dose at all experimental times was lower than that for genes responding to high doses. However, the groups of genes responding were *different* for low- than high-dose exposures. The cellular responses to high doses were apoptosis and cell proliferation. The most dominant response to low-dose irradiation were cell-cell signaling, DNA damage responses, and signal transduction.[341] Several types of cellular responses to ionizing radiation, such as the bystander effect or the adaptive response, may distinguish it from the effects from high doses. Further, low-dose-induced alterations are predictive of subsequent genomic damage.[342]

Considerable attention is being addressed to the low dose (less than 10 cGy) radiation. Glandular doses from screening mammography are low, typically around 2.5 to 4.5 mGy (two-view; 1.76 mGy digital mammography) of about 26 to 30 kVp low energy x-rays.[343] Renewed debate has emerged concerning the benefits and harms of routine screening mammography.[344-348] The goal of screening is to decrease the death rate from the disease. Thus the debate has centered on whether screening mammography actually saves lives (see Box 11-2). Most study trials covered the age range from 45 to 64 years.[345] The U.S. Preventive Services Task Force, however, (ages 40 to 49) and Cochrane Review (ages 45 to 64) both found a 15% relative reduction in the death rate and 0.05% absolute reduction in the death rate in risk from screening for women,[345,346] but the Armstrong study estimated that 30 to 200 per 100,000 women ages 40 to 49 will die after annual screening mammography as a result of radiation-induced breast cancer.[344] Results of recent studies have led to questioning whether benefits outweigh the harms because risk reduction is *low* and the potential for overdiagnosis and overtreatment results in risk increase.

It is questionable whether further research on the benefits of screening will enable better estimation of the ratio of benefit to harm in the 40- to 49-year-old group. However, much more research on the harms is needed because they remain too uncertain in this ratio. Toward that end, the rest of this discussion summarizes the experimental biologic data on low-level radiation and breast tissue.

The underlying mechanisms of radiation-induced carcinogenesis are not completely understood. The historical viewpoint has been that the biologic effects of ionizing radiation occur in irradiated cells as a result of DNA damage. This viewpoint implies that (1) these alterations only occur in directly irradiated cells, (2) radiation movement through the cell nucleus is necessary to producing a biologic response, and (3) the target in the cell is DNA.[349] Emerging evidence points to radiation-induced non-DNA targeted effects including mutations, chromosomal aberrations, and changes in gene expression (phenotype) in the cells not directly irradiated (non-hit). These phenomena include radiation-induced genomic instability (RIGI) in which the biologic effects include increased frequency of mutations and chromosomal aberrations that occur in *descendants* of irradiated cells (see Chapter 12 for a discussion of RIGI). Another phenomenon is the "bystander effect," the so-called innocent cells that did not receive radiation directly but still experience biologic effects. These effects include damaged cell-to-cell signaling, presumably through gap junction channels, and may be the result of oxidative stress[350,351] (see Chapters 2 and 12, and Figure 12-11). Together these effects are often called nontargeted effects. A major paradigm shift in radiation biology has occurred because of work involving the bystander effect.[351] Clearly, radiation-induced signaling contributes to nontargeted effects.[352] Investigators[351,353] have shown in vitro and in vivo that radiation activates the inflammatory response and induces activation of multiple signaling pathways. Thus evidence is emerging of a multicellular program of tissue response to damage that also includes surveillance and selective apoptosis of abnormal cells.[354-356] Yet normal signaling can be altered by radiation, compromising surveillance and apoptosis of abnormal cells, and causing genomically unstable cells to accumulate and proliferate. Data provide evidence that centrosome deregulation is a mechanism involved in the generation of RIGI[352] (Figure 23-51, *A*; see also Chapter 12).

Maxwell and colleagues[352] also showed that the cytokine TGF-β has a surveillance role in RIGI. In their experiments using human mammary epithelial cells (HMEC) TGF-β signaling in irradiated tissues could either promote carcinogenesis—causing stromal remodeling from activation of inflammatory responses leading to epithelial tissue transitioning to mesenchymal tissue (EMT)—or reestablish homeostasis by eliminating RIGI cells by activating a *TP53*-dependent apoptosis, thus inhibiting carcinogenesis. However, with continued chronic exposure to radiation, TGF-β induces the remaining population of stromal cells to undergo tissue transformation or EMT facilitating a neoplastic process (see Figure 23-51, *B*). Thus, TGF-β, a regulatory cytokine, can exert tumor-suppressor effects or paradoxically can cause tissue changes that facilitate cell invasion and immune regulation, transforming the microenvironment into a malignant environment (see Figure 23-51).[357]

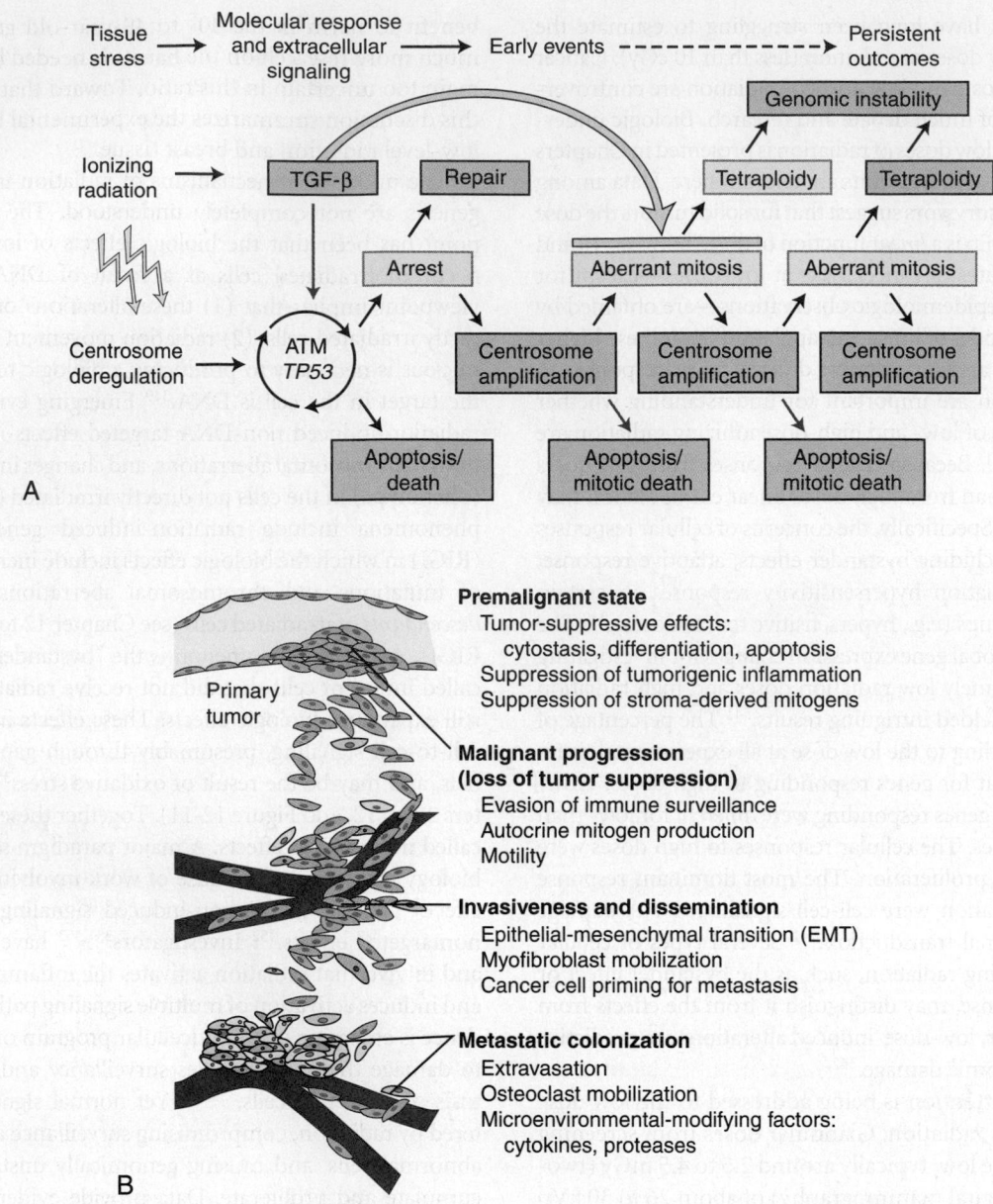

Figure 23-51 Roles of transforming growth factor-beta (TGF-β). **A,** Roles of TGF-β in response to IR. **B,** Roles of TGF-β in cancer.

Other investigators studied low-dose ionizing radiation of the breast stromal microenvironment.[358] These studies showed that human mammary stromal fibroblasts respond to protracted (repeated overtime) low-dose ionizing radiation by displaying a "senescence-like phenotype," thus an epigenetic mechanism. Senescent cells persist overtime, are irreversible, and accumulate in aging tissues.[359,360] One hypothesis is that accumulation of senescent cells in the stroma may serve as a means of stromal activation, subsequent inflammation, and stromal remodeling. Fibroblasts respond to a variety of chronic stressors including oxidative stress, UV light, inflammatory cytokines, and numerous genotoxic agents. The combination of these effects may represent a long-term outcome of cellular stress, including genotypic and phenotypic (epigenetic) changes. So in addition to replicative senescence, accumulating

evidence indicates that chronic stress to tissue may cause the accumulation of senescent cells in the stroma.[358]

Ionizing radiation may be only one type of environmental stress creating perturbed mammary stromal changes. Tsai and colleagues[358] found that with radiation-induced senescence-like fibroblasts, other disruptions included cytoskeletal alterations, increased extracellular matrix degradation, mammary ductal alterations (e.g., enlarged cystic structures), disorganized cell masses, and changes in cellular death (i.e., apoptosis) pathways. Breast cancer cells growing in this type of stromal environment lead to dysregulated cell-cell and cell-matrix interactions, thereby enabling malignancy.[358] Overall, these investigators suggest that protracted, low-dose ionizing radiation exposure fostered an oncogenic environment.

Normal stroma suppresses tumor growth by releasing growth-inhibiting biochemical signals whereas oncogenic stroma promotes tumor growth.[358] The tumor effects of stromal fibroblasts have been attributed to their production of matrix metalloproteinases (MMPs; see Chapter 11). MMP-3 has recently been shown to regulate the branching developments of mammary epithelial cells in response to senescent fibroblasts.[361] MMPs have been linked in vivo to breast cancer invasion and metastasis.[362]

Because some human cancers arise from the accumulation of multiple genetic abnormalities, the age at which mammography begins and the total number of mammograms received may be important factors in the development of radiation-induced breast cancer. Women at high risk for developing breast cancer—those with mutations of the *BRCA1* or *BRCA2* genes or have a first degree relative (parent, sibling, or child) with such a mutation and women who received radiation to the chest for Hodgkin disease—are recommended to start mammography screening with MRI at age 30. However, low-dose ionizing radiation has been shown to increase the risk of breast cancer significantly among *BRCA1* and *BRCA2* mutation carriers.[363] A retrospective cohort study of 1601 female *BRCA1* and *BRCA2* mutation carriers found an association with reported chest x-ray exposure and significantly increased risk of breast cancer (hazard ratio 1.54). Also a review showed a strong association (odds ratio 3.21) between CHEK2*1100delC carrier status, history of chest x-rays and breast cancer risk.[364] Continuing research will help to determine if high-risk women should be screened with MRI. It is true that MRI can find lesions that mammograms miss, and women are not exposed to ionizing radiation. However, MRIs can increase the detection of cancers that would not be clinically relevant (i.e., not become invasive) and lead to unnecessary treatment, including mastectomies. Thus the role of MRIs is still being investigated and more study is needed to fully understand all its benefits and harms.

In conclusion, the risk of radiation-induced breast cancer depends strongly on when radiation exposure occurs. Exposure before the age of 20 years carries the greatest risk. Biologic mechanisms of low-dose and subsequent cellular effects are emerging. Other factors that also may influence risk include age at first-term pregnancy, parity, possibly a history of benign breast disease and injury, exposure while pregnant, endogenous hormone levels and ratios, and genetic factors.[365] Overall, mammography screening, which is convenient and efficient, has a modest effect on breast cancer mortality, in absolute terms. The death rate after 10 years of screening is reduced by 0.05% (i.e., 1 death prevented of 2000 women screened).[245] However, the harms include overdiagnosis and overtreatment of healthy women (i.e., 30% more surgery, 20% more mastectomies, and more use of radiotherapy). Unclear from screening and/or overtreatment with radiotherapy are the exact numbers of women that develop radiation-induced breast cancer, heart disease, and lung disturbances. Newer understandings of the biology of breast cancer challenge the widely held view that breast cancer is a uniformly progressive disease

not cured unless caught early. It is now understood that breast cancer is a heterogenous disease that may be metastatic from the very start of it and may never metasasize. Women need information on both benefits and harms to make a rational decision about screening (see What's New: Screening Mammograms: Far from Perfect, p. 386, in Chapter 11).

Diet. Prospective epidemiologic studies on diet and breast cancer risk fail to show an association that is consistent, strong, and statistically significant except for alcohol intake, being overweight, and weight gain after menopause (see discussion following).[366] Dietary fat and breast cancer risk is the subject of much study, controversy, and debate. Potential biologic mechanisms between fat intake and breast cancer risk include (1) that fat may stimulate endogenous steroid hormone production (also affect weight gain, age of menarche), (2) they interfere with immune or inflammatory function, and (3) they influence gene expression. Evidence from large, prospective cohort studies has been mostly unsupportive and clinical trials have not supported a strong association with total fat intake.[367] Cohort studies, however, suggest a modest positive association between fat intake and the risk of breast cancer,[368] but so far more than 70 studies of dietary fat during midlife on risk of breast cancer show the relationship is likely to be small.

Another area of study is how consumption of red meat could increase breast cancer risk. The hypotheses range from available iron content, growth-promoting hormones used in the cattle industry, and carcinogenic heterocyclic amines released from cooking the fatty acid content. Case-control and cohort studies have shown a modest association of red meat intake with breast cancer incidence but no association in a pooled analysis of prospective studies.[369] Research has reported an increased risk with red meat consumption.[370-372] For other updates on diet and breast cancer risk see Nutrition & Disease: Diet and Breast Cancer Risk Updates.

Studies in animal models and recent observations in humans have provided some evidence that a high intake of omega-6-polyunsaturated fatty acids (omega-6 PUFAs) stimulates several stages in the development of mammary and colon cancer and possibly prostate cancer—from an increase in oxidative DNA damage that affects cell proliferation and increased free estrogen levels that affect hormonal catabolic products.[373-376] The prospective Malmo diet and cancer cohort ($n = 11,699$) found after a 10-year follow-up that omega-6 PUFAs may promote breast cancer.[377] Conversely, fish oil–derived omega-3 fatty acids may help to prevent cancer by influencing the activity of enzymes and proteins related to intracellular signaling, inflammation, and eventually cell proliferation.[378,379] Studies that show protective effects of fish oil and decreased cancer risk have been confined to countries with high fish intake.

Investigators have identified potential carcinogens in breast fluid in normal women, especially cholesterol derivatives.[380] Breast fluid represents secretions from the cells lining the breast ducts, which is where the majority of breast cancers develop.[381] These breast secretions have been related to the fat content of the diet. Estrogen levels are also substantially higher in breast secretions than in blood. Thus fat tissue in the breast may be a

NUTRITION & DISEASE

Diet and Breast Cancer Risk Updates

Total fat intake and reductions in fat uptake—Do not support a strong relationship (see p. 891).

Red meat intake—Some consistent evidence of raising breast cancer risk slightly (see p. 891).

Fruits and vegetables (see isothiocyanates below)—From eight prospective cohort studies (large European prospective study) lack of association of intake for lowering breast cancer risk (Women's Health Eating and Living Trial); women with early-stage breast cancer randomized to a diet high in fruits and vegetables, fiber, and low in fat showed no reduction in breast cancer recurrence or mortality.

Micronutrients

Folic acid—Two recent meta-analyses found a positive protective effect for women who drink alcohol; this meta-analysis found folate increments of 200 µg/day was not associated with breast cancer risk in prospective studies and for total folate was significantly associated with a protective effect in case-control studies.

Vitamin D—Vitamin D has been inversely (i.e., protective) related to breast cancer in the Nurses' Health Study and meta-analyses; high serum levels of vitamin D were inversely related to risk of breast cancer in a dose-dependent manner.

Carotenoids, retinols, tocopherols—The roles of carotenoids, retinol, and tocopherols in breast cancer risk have been inconclusive; although some studies have shown significant protective effects of high serum carotenoid levels; studies of dietary intake are inconclusive.

Caffeine—Was not linked to breast cancer risk in a large prospective Swedish study.

Soy and phytoestrogens—Two meta-analyses of published studies on soy intake noted a decreasing (highest doses about 30%) breast cancer risk with increasing doses of soy; possible protective effects are strongest during puberty (rats) or adolescence (girls); Japanese researchers, however, reported genistein and diadzein causes oxidative deoxyribonucleic acid (DNA) damage and other data on soy-based phytoestrogens may have opposing effects on tamoxifen.

Alcohol—From animal and epidemiologic studies, alcohol consistently predicts higher incidence of breast cancer; a meta-analysis of cohort studies showed a 10% increase in risk for every 10 g of alcohol/day and similar in two pooled analyses; all together 53 studies included alcohol increased relative risk by 7.1% for each daily serving; even one drink a day is related to modest elevation in risk; adequate folic acid intake (from vitamins), however, may reduce or eliminate the excess risk of alcohol.

Early life exposures—Carcinogenic exposure in the "sensitive window" (after menarche and before first pregnancy) may increase sensitivity and susceptibility to breast cancer; nutrition can affect height and age at menarche; studies on dairy products and breast cancer risk are inconsistent; total carbohydrate was not linked to either premenopausal or postmenopausal breast cancer (12 prospective cohort studies)

Fiber—Was not linked to either premenopausal or postmenopausal breast cancer

Dairy—Case-control studies of diet in adolescence reported a decreased risk for cancer with diets high in fat from dairy; however, other epidemiologic studies have indicated a relationship between dairy consumption and risk in premenopausal women; cow's milk can increase IGF-1 levels and premenopausal women with higher IGF-1 levels have an increased risk of breast cancer; in addition the recombinant bovine growth hormone (rBGH) can be found in U.S. dairy products

Isothiocyanates (sulforaphone [SFN])—Found in vegetables (broccoli, Brussels sprouts [highest amounts], cabbage, cruciferous vegetables); cancer cell line research and animal studies reveal their role to promote apoptosis of breast cancer cells, disruptors of ER alpha, inhibit proliferation of cultured human breast cells by stabilizing microtubules similar to the drugs Paclitaxel and vincristine.

Data from Azarenko O et al: *Carcinogenesis* 29(12):2360-2368, 2008; Bertone-Johnson ER et al: *Cancer Epidemiol Biomarkers Prev* 14:1991-1997, 2005; Hankinson SE et al: *J Natl Cancer Inst* 87:1297-1302, 1995; Kang L, Ding L, Wang ZY: *Oncol Rep* 21(1):185-192, 2009; Knight JA et al: *Epidemiol Biomarkers Prev* 16:422-429, 2007; Larsson SC, Giovannucci E, Wolk A: *J Natl Cancer Inst* 99:64-76, 2007; Hamajima N et al: *Br J Cancer* 87:1234-1245, 2002; Lowe LC et al: *Eur J Cancer* 41:1164-1169, 2005; Michels JB et al: *Ann Epidemiol* 12:21-26, 2002; Nakamura Y, Miyoshi N: *Biofactors* 26(2):123-134, 2006; Pierce JP et al: *JAMA* 298:289-298, 2007; Pryor M et al: *Cancer Res* 49:2161-2167, 1989; Shin MH et al: *J Natl Cancer Inst* 94:1301-1311, 2002; Smith-Warner SA et al: *JAMA* 279:535-540, 1998; Tamini RM et al: *Am J Epidemiol* 161:153-160, 2005; Trock BJ, Hilakivi-Clarke L, Clarke R: *J Natl Cancer Inst* 18:459-471, 2006; Wu AJ et al: *Carcinogenesis* 23:1491-1496, 2002; Zang S et al: *JAMA* 281:163201637, 1999; Zang SM et al: *J Natl Cancer Inst* 95:373-380, 2003; Zang SM et al: *Am J Epidemiol* 165:667-676, 2007.

source of high concentrations of fat-soluble chemicals (including estrogens), some of which may be carcinogens.[381]

Further studies are needed to evaluate the benefits of substantially lowering fat intake (20% or less of total calories) and the roles of micronutrient imbalances and childhood nutrition in the development of breast cancer. The role of obesity in breast cancer is complex and seems to be related to fat distribution, type of fatty acids consumed, and sex hormone levels.[382]

Obesity has been associated with a *reduced* risk of *premenopausal* breast cancer. One mechanism suggested is the direct relationship between irregular menstrual cycling, especially obesity and anovulatory cycling, which would result in a decrease in estrogens and progesterone and thus decrease the risk of breast cancer. It is possible that in obese women with hyperinsulinemia the higher insulin levels increase the enzymatic conversion of testosterone to dihydrotestosterone, rather than estradiol, lowering their estrogen levels.[381]

Obesity, however, is related to *increased* risk of breast cancer in *postmenopausal* women. Despite strong links with endogenous estrogen levels, body fat has been consistently but *weakly* related to increased postmenopausal risk.[383] This observation has been surprising because obese postmenopausal women have endogenous estrogen levels (estrone and estradiol) nearly double those of lean women.[383,384] This weak association is possibly related to two factors. First, the premenopausal reduction in breast cancer risk related to being overweight possibly persists, opposing the adverse effect of elevated estrogens after menopause. Thus *weight gain* should be more strongly related to postmenopausal breast cancer risk than attained weight. In two case-control studies and prospective studies, this was indeed true.[385-388] A pooled analysis of prospective cohort studies showed women with a BMI of 28 kg/m^2 or higher were 26% more likely to develop postmenopausal breast cancer compared with leaner women.[389]

Premenopausal and postmenopausal weight gain is also associated with higher estradiol and estrone levels and lower SHBG as a transporter protein; low levels cause higher bioavailable estrogen.[390] This increase in estrogens, particularly estradiol, is from aromatization in the adipose tissue. Second, use of exogenous hormones postmenopausally obscures the variation in endogenous estrogens caused by adiposity and elevates breast cancer risk regardless of body weight.[383] Excess body fat and weight gain are stronger risk factors for women who do not use hormone therapy. A recent prospective study found weight gained at multiple time points throughout adulthood of 20 to 29 kg was associated with a 56% higher risk of breast cancer, and weight gain of 40 to 49 kg doubled the risk of breast cancer among hormone users.[391]

Weight loss after menopause reduces circulating estrogens and increases SHBG, making weight loss a potentially important prevention strategy especially for those women not on hormone therapy. Weight loss and postmenopausal cancer risk have been examined in prospective studies. In one of the largest studies, women who lost 10 kg or more after menopause and maintained this weight loss halved their risk for breast cancer. This relationship was clearer in nonhormone users.[392]

Obesity is associated with poor survival among women with breast cancer, and the association of obesity with mortality from breast cancer appears to be stronger than its association with incidence.[383,387] Thus the increase in breast cancer risk with increasing BMI among postmenopausal women largely results from increased estrogen, especially estradiol.[383]

Soy products are a hot topic because of their consumption in Asian countries that have low rates of cancer (see Nutrition & Disease: Diet and Breast Cancer Risks Update, p. 892). These isoflavone compounds, including diadzen and genistein, can bind estrogen receptors but are far less potent than estradiol. Soy may act like other antiestrogens, such as tamoxifen, by blocking the action of endogenous estrogens to reduce breast cancer risk. Thus depending on the estradiol concentration and the timing of administration, soy exhibits weak estrogenic or antiestrogenic activity. Isoflavones can influence transcription and cell proliferation. They modulate enzyme activities, as well as signal transduction, and have antioxidant properties.[393] Results of clinical studies on the effects of soy products or isolated isoflavones on vasomotor symptoms are contradictory. Epidemiologic studies, however, have shown a decrease in the prevalence of hot flashes in women from countries with high isoflavone intake, such as Japan, more so than in Western countries. Evidence from epidemiologic, animal, in vitro data, and human clinical trials show isoflavones are promising agents for breast cancer prevention.[208,394-399] However, there are concerns that soy or isoflavones may increase proliferating cells. A study of nipple aspirate fluid from women who had ingested high-soy diets and were either premenopausal or took estrogen replacement therapy showed an increase in proliferating cells.[400] Controversy has ensued on whether breast cell proliferation can equal breast cancer growth. Soy may cause breast cells to grow; however, in vitro properties of soy for blocking invasion and antiangiogenesis may be more important in preventing breast cancer. In vitro

and animal studies show that soy inhibits breast cancer growth, and additional work showed this effect on cancer cells that are both ER+ and ER−.[399] In addition, soy may optimize extrarenal $1,25(OH)2$ cholecalciferol or vitamin D_3 (a prodifferentiating vitamin D metabolite), which could result in growth control and, conceivably, inhibition of tumor progression.[394]

Environmental Chemicals. Evidence for linking chemicals to the cause of breast cancer is difficult. It is challenging because it is a life history of exposure that is important—not just a single chemical but also complex mixtures of chemicals and their interaction with endogenous hormones and with radiation. The highest rates of breast cancer are found in superindustrialized countries—North America and Europe—and the lowest rates in central Africa and Asia. With industrial development, breast cancer rates increase. An estimated 85,000 synthetic chemicals are registered for use today in the United States, another 1000 or more are added each year, and toxicologic screening for these chemicals is minimal—only about 7%.[401] Chemicals persist in the environment, accumulate in adipose tissue, interact with local adipose tissue physiology in an endocrine-paracrine manner, and remain in breast tissue for decades. Some of these chemicals are known human carcinogens and many have been linked to mammary tumors in animals. Women who emigrate to the United States from Asian countries experience an enormous percent increase in risk within one generation. A generation later their daughters' risk approaches that of women born in the United States. This change in risk suggests that in utero exposures affect subsequent disease risk. However, it is difficult to know whether these changes in risk come from nutritional content, pollutants, cosmetics, food additives, or other factors.

Xenoestrogens are synthetic chemicals that mimic the actions of estrogens and are found in many pesticides, fuels, plastics, detergents, and drugs.[206] Because many factors correlated with breast cancer (early menarche, delayed pregnancy and breast-feeding, late menopause, etc.) are associated with lifetime exposure to estrogens, investigators reasoned that environmental chemicals affect estrogen metabolism and contribute to breast cancer. The most significant chemicals may be polychlorinated biphenyls (PCBs), pesticides, BPA (pervasive in polycarbonate plastics), tobacco smoke (active and passive), dioxins, alkyphenols, metals, phthalates, parabens, food additives, HRT, and others (see Table 23-17). Many chemicals are fat soluble with estrogenic effects. Because the amount of these environmental estrogens is presumably minute, their effect may be secondary to an abnormal (e.g., mutagenic) response of the estrogen receptor and DNA or catabolized products of estrogen. (Human studies related to HRT are exhaustive and discussed on p. 883.) Human studies of women exposed to DDT during childhood and early adolescence was associated with a fivefold increase in risk of developing breast cancer.[402] Other human studies include heptachlor,[403,404] environmental tobacco smoke,[405] benzene among enlisted women in the U.S. Army,[406] and benzene among women in different professions in Israel related to increased rates of breast cancer.[407] Further, a long-term follow-up (30 years) of women who were exposed to DES shows

Table 23-17   Selected Chemicals and Risk of Breast Cancer

Chemical	Comments
Bisphenol-A (BPA)	Studies have shown altered reproductive systems and breast tissue when exposed to BPA in utero[408]
	BPA is commonly found in plastics[410]
Polyvinyl chloride (PVC)	Used in food packaging, medical products, appliances, cars, toys, credit cards, rain wear[409]
	Has been found in the air near waste sites, landfills, and tobacco smoke
	Has been linked to increased mortality from breast and liver cancer among manufacturing workers[411, 412]
Pesticides: aldrin and dieldrin (organochlorines)	Used in crops like corn and cotton from 1950s to 1970s
	Banned by the EPA in 1975 except for termite control; completely banned in 1987
	In vitro assays showed estrogenic activity and dieldrin found in 78% of women diagnosed with breast cancer[413]
	High incidence of breast cancer in Massachusetts study found associations with higher income and regular use of lawn services, termite treatments, and home pesticides[414]
Household products: methylene chloride	Spray paints and paint removers may contain methylene chloride, documented breast cancer in lab animals[415]
Diethylstilbestrol (DES)	Prescribed for women to avert miscarriages between 1941 and 1971
	Exposed daughters known to have higher rates of vaginal cancer, and in the mothers slight increased risk of breast cancer[416, 417]
	Daughters now known to have slight increased risk of breast cancer[418]
Solvents (e.g., benzene, toluene, trichloroethylene, chlorinated organic solvents)	Used in manufacture of computers, also some in cosmetics
	In 2003 a Taiwanese study documented increased risk of breast cancer among electronic workers exposed to chlorinated organic solvents[419]
	A Danish study of women 22 to 55 years of age employed in industries (fabricated metal, lumber, furniture, printing, textiles) using solvents doubled the risk of breast cancer[420]
Styrene, carbon tetrachloride, formaldehyde	A 1995 study suggested increased risk with occupational exposure—validation in Finland, Sweden, and Italy[421-424]
Ethylene glycol methyl ether (EGME)	A Duke University study found it acts as hormone sensitizer in vivo and in vitro[425,426]
	Compounds are found in semiconductor industry, varnishes, paints, dyes, and fuel additives
Valproic acid (anticonvulsant medication)	Found to be hormone sensitizing and prescribed for migraines and bipolar disorder[425,426]
1,3-butadiene	Air pollutant and synthetic rubber product and some fungicides and tobacco smoke
	Causes mammary and ovarian tumors in female mice and rats[427,428]
Aromatic amines (heterocyclic, polycyclic, moncyclic)	Found in plastics, tobacco smoke, grilled meats and fish, combustion of wood chips and rubber
	Exposure in adolescence before full-term pregnancy may increase risk[429]
Dichlorodiphenyltrichloroethane (DDT) and polychlorinated biphenyls (PCBs)	PCB used in manufacture of electrical equipment[430]
	PCB and DDT are banned in the United States since 1970s but are still found in body fat, as well as breast milk[431]
	DDT was used as pesticide for insects on farms and swamps
	PCB deteriorates slowly in soil
	PCB is difficult to study because it is a diverse class of compounds
	A 1999 in vitro study showed PCBs proliferate in breast cancer cells[432]
	Conflicting results; several large studies failed to show relationship with PCBs
Polycystic aromatic hydrocarbons (PAH, including tobacco)	Found in soot and fumes from fuels
	Increased DNA damage (DNA adducts) implicated from the Long Island Breast Cancer Study Project[433]
	Tobacco smoke also contains PAHs
	Smokers who began smoking as adolescents have an increased risk of breast cancer[434-436]
	In 2004 the California EPA concluded that environmental tobacco smoke (ETS) increases the risk of breast cancer, and the association appears stronger for premenopausal women[437]
	Tobacco smoke also contains the carcinogens polonium-210, vinyl chloride, benzene, and 1-3 butadiene[438]
Dioxin	Products containing PVC, PCBs, or other chlorinated compounds release dioxin from incineration
	Declared a known carcinogen by the EPA in 2000
	It may be the most prevalent of all toxic chemicals
	Occurs in meat, poultry, dairy products, and human breast milk
	A United Kingdom study linked dioxin to the development of mammary tumors in mice[439]
	A study in Seveso, Italy, connected dioxin with breast cancer[440]
Ethylene oxide	Used to sterilize surgical instruments and in some cosmetics
	Linked to breast cancer in women exposed to ethylene oxide in commercial sterilization facilities[441]

a small increased risk of breast cancer (relative risk 1.35) and no increasing risk over time.[381] Table 23-17 contains information on selected studies, chemicals, and risk of breast cancer.

Physical Activity. Regular physical activity may reduce overall risk of breast cancer, especially in premenopausal or young postmenopausal women.[440-442] Yet selection bias in studies related to recreational physical activity during adulthood and random error in the measurements of activity remain concerns.[443] A large prospective study found walking for 1 hour per day and additional weekly exercise seemed to be protective against breast cancer regardless of menopausal status.[444] Mechanisms for this protective effect are not known but include alterations in endogenous free radical formation and oxidative damage, effects on DNA repair capacity, alteration in carcinogen-metabolizing enzymes, increased intestinal transit times (i.e., reduced exposures to carcinogens), weight loss, and changes in endogenous sex hormone levels.[441,442]

Familial Factors and Tumor-Related Genes

Genetically, breast cancer can be divided into three main groups: (1) sporadic, the majority or 40% of women with breast cancer have no known family history; (2) inherited dominant cancer gene syndromes, in which the gene is passed to future generations by an autosomal dominant mechanism; and (3) probable polygenic, in which there is family history but it is not passed on to future generations as a dominant gene. Yet to be determined are the number of genes in the polygenic model that could be involved, the nature of the interactions among these genes, and their interaction with environmental factors. The major risk factors for sporadic cancer are related to hormone exposure including age at menarche and menopause, reproductive history, breast-feeding history, and endogenous and exogenous estrogens (see p. 886). Radiation exposure is known to increase risk. Chemical exposures during critical windows of development may also be important (see p. 893). The majority of these cancers occur in postmenopausal women with increased ER expression.

A history of breast cancer in first-degree relatives (mother or sister) increases a woman's risk two to three times. Risk increases even more if two first-degree relatives are involved, especially if the disease occurred before menopause and was bilateral. In some families, breast cancer occurs at an earlier age and the frequency of bilateral tumors is greater. Women with inherited breast or ovarian cancer have tumors characterized by alterations in particular genes, mainly *BRCA1* and *BRCA2* breast cancer susceptibility genes, but also *CHEK2* (Li-Fraumeni syndrome), ataxia telangiectasia *(AT)*, and *STK11* (Peutz-Jeghers syndrome). An obvious hereditary predisposition and strongly penetrant mutations in genes such as *BRCA1* and *BRCA2* are responsible for 5% to 10% of all breast cancer, or 18,000 individuals per year.[445] The probability that a mutation will be present in family kindred increases if the family history includes disease at early ages, clustering of both breast and ovarian cancers *(BRCA1)*, male breast cancer *(BRCA2)*, and other rare cancers, such as sarcomas.[445] Even in families with more than four individuals with breast cancer, a germline mutation in *BRCA1* or *BRCA2* was found in only

65% of people.[446] Unexplained familial breast cancer possibly includes other more common lower-penetrant genes.

Investigators estimate that 45% of families with apparent autosomal dominant transmission of breast cancer susceptibility and about 90% of families with dominant inheritance of both breast and ovarian cancer have *BRCA1* germline mutations[447] (Figure 23-52). The *BRCA1* and *BRCA2* genes include several "founder" mutations identified in various populations. Most common in the United States are three mutations of the Eastern European population: two in *BRCA1* (185delAg and 5382insC) and the 6174delT mutation in *BRCA2*.[445] The penetrance, or lifetime risk, of developing breast cancer and ovarian cancer from *BRCA* mutations is the subject of intense research. Breast cancer risk associated with mutations in *BRCA1* have been estimated in the range of 50% to 80% and in 40% to 70% for *BRCA2*.[446,448] The ovarian cancer risk among *BRCA1* carriers is about 40% lifetime, exceeding the risk of 20% for *BRCA2* carriers. The risk for ovarian cancer is not the same for all *BRCA2* mutations, which depend on the location of the gene mutation.[449] In premenopausal women, a modifier of risk for breast cancer has been prophylactic oophorectomy, reducing lifetime risk by 50%.[450,451] Thus the risk associated with an inherited predisposition can be reduced significantly by modifying endogenous, and possibly exogenous, hormonal exposures. The risk for other cancers, such as pancreatic, prostate, melanoma, and others, is increased in *BRCA2* carriers.[445]

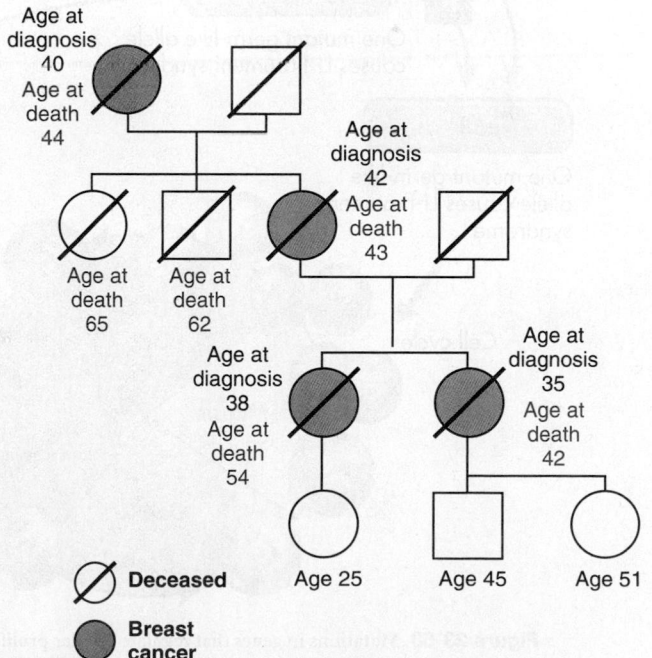

Figure 23-52 Example of family pedigree for breast cancer. Family pedigree showing cases of breast cancer associated with typical dominant transmission of breast cancer. Other possible genetic alterations related to risk of breast cancer include changes in *TP53* and alterations in the estrogen receptor. Numerous somatic mutations in the expression of oncogenes in breast cancer cells have been reported.

Genes important to the development of cancer regulate diverse cellular pathways, including the progression of cells through the cell cycle, resistance to apoptosis, and the response to signals that direct cellular differentiation.[452] The inactivation of genes (e.g., tumor-suppressor genes) that contribute to the stability of the genome itself can favor errors in other genes that regulate proliferation. The importance of this latter pathway is exemplified by two studies linking the function of the *BRCA1* gene with that of the gene for ataxia-telangiectasia mutation (ATM) (Figure 23-53).

Other tumor-related genes or proteins include *p53, Bcl-2, HER-2/neu,* and *c-myc.* About 40% of breast carcinomas reveal high levels of stabilized, often mutant *p53* protein in their cells; *p53*-related defects in tumor cells correlate with a poor prognosis.

Production of the proto-oncogene *Bcl-2* decreases or inhibits apoptosis and thereby promotes breast and other cancers. However, the College of American Pathologists has classified it as belonging to category III, meaning there is insufficient evidence to support it as a prognostic factor.[453]

HER-2/neu, another oncogene, is overexpressed in 25% to 30% of breast cancer cells. It transmits a growth signal to the nucleus. The drug trastuzumab (Herceptin) blocks the signal in about 35% of those affected, thereby decreasing the growth of the tumor.

C-myc is a proto-oncogene expressed in cells and is one of the immediate, early growth response genes that are rapidly induced when quiet cells receive a signal to divide. Mutation of *c-myc* is amplified in breast, colon, lung, and many other cancers.

PATHOGENESIS   Breast cancer is as varied as the breast itself. Table 23-18 lists the different types of breast carcinomas and summarizes their major characteristics. Most breast cancers arise from the ductal epithelium (Figure 23-54). Tumors of the infiltrating ductal type do not become large, but they metastasize early. This type accounts for the majority of breast cancers.

Breast cancer is a heterogeneous disease with diverse molecular, phenotypic, and pathologic changes. Despite heroic efforts, this diversity has greatly challenged the understanding

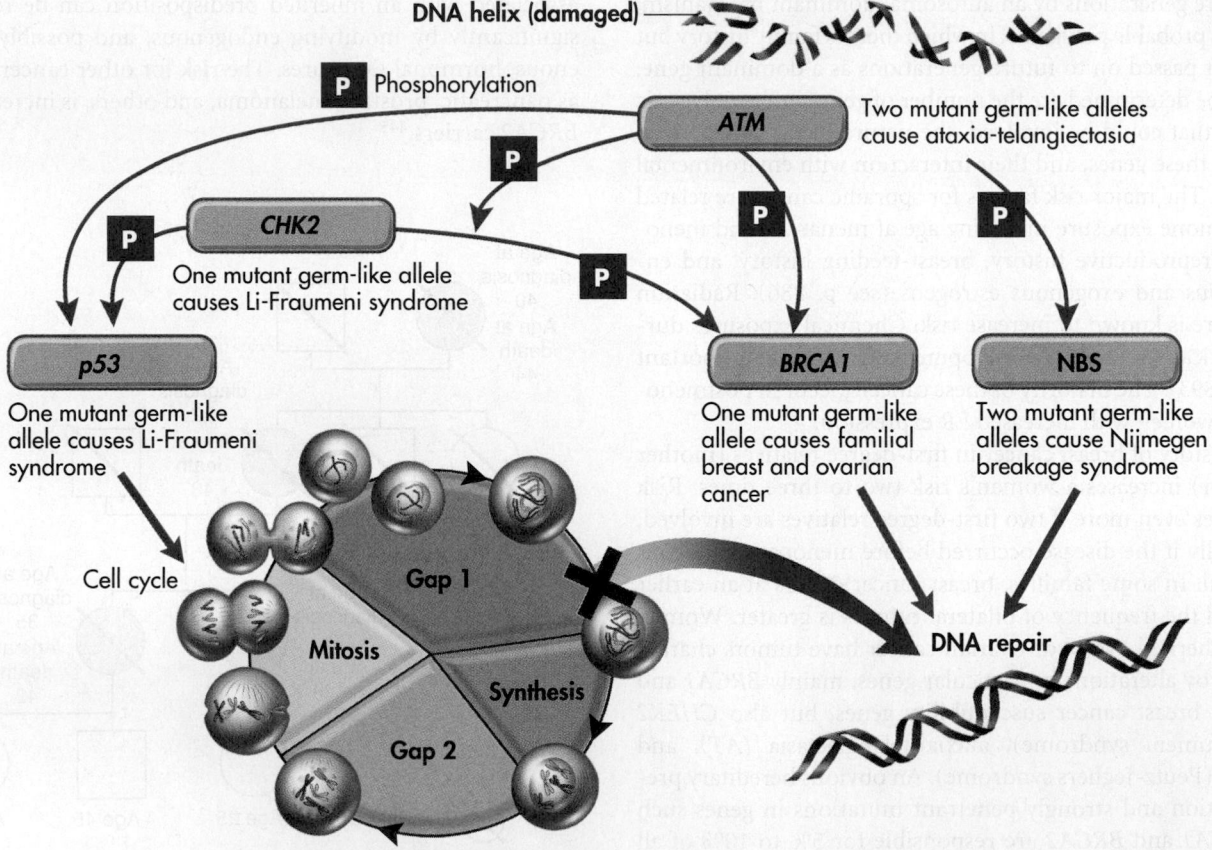

Figure 23-53 Mutations in genes that regulate cellular proliferation and repair of deoxyribonucleic acid (DNA) and lead to breast carcinogenesis. The ataxia-telangiectasia mutated *(ATM)* gene encodes a protein kinase that activates (through phosphorylation) the tumor-suppressor *p53* protein either directly or indirectly by activating *CHK2* (a gene that encodes a protein kinase that activates *p53* by adding a phosphate group to it) in response to damage to DNA. The *p53* protein then triggers the arrest of the cell cycle, increasing time for DNA to be repaired. More simply, the *ATM* gene is necessary to accomplish DNA repair. The *BRCA1* and Nijmegen breakage syndrome (NBS) proteins are also activated by the *ATM* gene and are thought to be directly involved in the repair of damaged DNA. The inactivating mutations in the genes that encode these proteins increase the risk of breast cancer. (Redrawn from Haber D: *N Engl J Med* 343[21]:1566, 2000.)

Table 23-18	Types of Breast Carcinomas and Major Distinguishing Features
Histologic Type	**Distinguishing Features**
Carcinoma of Mammary Ducts	
Papillary	Well-delineated cystic masses in multiple areas; hemorrhage often present; majority appear in 40- to 60-year age group; often involves skin
Intraductal (comedo)	Often accompanied with evidence of inflammation; well-circumscribed tumors within the duct; well-differentiated tumor cells; rarely ulcerates the skin
Infiltrating Carcinoma	
Ductal (no specific type [NST])	Fibrous, firm, glistening, gray-tan mass with chalky streaks, mixture of patterns; may cause discharge from the nipple; represents about 79% of all breast cancer
Mucinous	Usually large (>3 cm in diameter), circumscribed, and encapsulated, glistening appearance, varies in color; two types: pure and mixed; pure tumor is surrounded by mucin; infrequent; found in the lateral half of the breast; tends to occur in women after age 70 years
Medullary	Encapsulated and grows to be very large (7-8 cm in diameter); commonly surrounded by lymphocytic inflammatory infiltrate; occurs after age 50 years
Tubular	Well differentiated with orderly tubules in center (stroma) of mass; can be associated with noninfiltrating ductal carcinoma; occurs in women about 50 years of age; nodal metastasis infrequent; occurrence rare
Adenoid cystic	Very rare; well-circumscribed, painless mass arising from the nipple and areola
Metaplastic	Involves cartilage or bone; mixed tumors or osteogenic sarcomas
Squamous cell	Frequent in blacks; originates in ductal epithelium
Carcinoma of Mammary Lobules	
Lobular carcinoma in situ	Found in individuals with fibrocystic disease; localized to upper breast quadrants; risk of 15%-35% becoming invasive; occurs frequently in mid-40s; infiltrating variety occurs in early 50s
Infiltrating lobular	Infiltrates from duct; firm mass with chalky streaks
Paget disease	Eczema of the nipple that extends to the areola; cancer usually found underneath the nipple; poorly circumscribed; large Paget cells arise from the duct and directly invade nipple; history of scaly, red rash spreading from the nipple; lesion palpable beneath the nipple, often bilateral; occurs in middle age
Inflammatory carcinoma	Not a histologic type; fairly diffuse within the breast tissue, diffuse edema of the overlying skin; extremely undifferentiated, very rare, most metastasize to axilla
Sarcoma of the Breast	
Cytosarcoma phyllodes	Usually large (>17 cm in diameter); mostly localized but can rupture through the skin; rarely metastasizes to lymph nodes; history of painless nodule present for years before it forms a large mass; ulceration and bleeding of skin often present; occurs in wide age range (ages 13-77 years)
Fibrosarcoma	Well circumscribed, firm, and usually does not involve the skin or nipple; well differentiated to extremely undifferentiated; arises from connective tissue; extremely rare (e.g., liposarcoma, angiosarcoma)

of breast cancer evolution. Recent research suggests that breast cancer may be heterogeneous from its initial preinvasive stages.[454] The historic multistep model of breast carcinogenesis proposing tissue transition through a single pathway of sequential molecular alterations from normal epithelium to invasive carcinoma (e.g., nontypical, atypical hyperplasia, in situ carcinoma) is an important model for understanding colon carcinogenesis (Figure 23-55, *A*). However, emerging evidence indicates that for breast cancer this model may be oversimplified or flawed, and that other alternative models are possible and have been proposed[454,455] (see Figure 23-55). All together three models are proposed for breast carcinogenesis including (1) the multistep (hits and stepwise) sequential acquisition model, (2) the telomere crisis model, and, (3) the imprinted stem cell model. Models are necessary because in humans, carcinogenesis or progression from one lesion to the

next cannot be experimentally tested. Nevertheless, several biologic associations are known. DCIS (see p. 898) is associated with invasive cancer at the site of clinical diagnosis.[454] This characteristic implies a direct "clonal" progression from DCIS to invasive carcinoma and is the basis for current DCIS treatment.[456] Hyperplasia and atypical hyperplasia, however, are not known to have invasive cancer at the *site* of the lesion (see p. 872). Instead, they are deemed markers of risk throughout the *entire* breast.[454] In addition, from the multistep model where the programmed malignant potential depends on sequential acquisition of genetic alterations with specific "hits" responsible for the transition from DCIS to invasive cancer remain unknown—despite tremendous study (see Figure 23-55, *A*). Instead, several lines of evidence suggest there may be multiple molecular genetic pathways of complex crosstalking networks that progress toward malignancy.

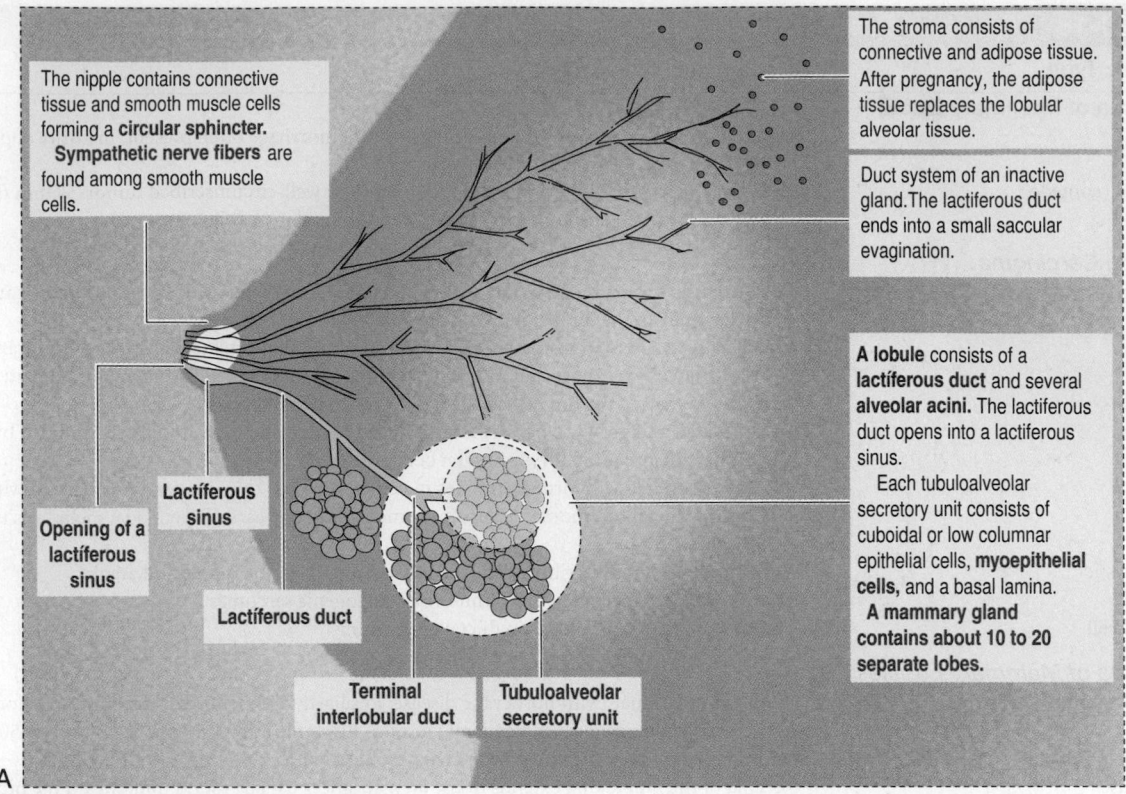

The nipple contains connective tissue and smooth muscle cells forming a **circular sphincter.**
Sympathetic nerve fibers are found among smooth muscle cells.

The stroma consists of connective and adipose tissue. After pregnancy, the adipose tissue replaces the lobular alveolar tissue.

Duct system of an inactive gland. The lactiferous duct ends into a small saccular evagination.

A lobule consists of a **lactiferous duct** and several **alveolar acini.** The lactiferous duct opens into a lactiferous sinus.
Each tubuloalveolar secretory unit consists of cuboidal or low columnar epithelial cells, **myoepithelial cells,** and a basal lamina.
A mammary gland contains about 10 to 20 separate lobes.

Opening of a lactiferous sinus

Lactiferous sinus

Lactiferous duct

Terminal interlobular duct

Tubuloalveolar secretory unit

A

Figure 23-54 Normal breast and breast cancer. **A,** Normal breast. (From Kierszenbaum AL: *Histology and cell biology: an introduction to pathology,* ed 2, Philadelphia, 2007, Mosby.)

The telomere crisis model of breast carcinogenesis[457] involves the initiation of cancer occurring through telomere shortening and genetic instability (see Figure 23-55, *B* and Chapter 11). Hyperplasia results in shortening telomeres and increasing genetic instability (telomere crisis). Certain genetic changes may eventually become stabilized with reactivation of the enzyme telomerase, stabilizing the aberrant genomic composition, and immortalizing (cancerizing) the cell. Overall these genetic changes might be considered the origin or "birth" of the cancer-initiating cell or cancer stem cell. This model—imprinted stem cell model—suggests that this "birth" occurs as the tissue becomes DCIS or the cancer stem cell is "born" at the precancer stage. From other experiments, Damonte and colleagues[454] modified this model slightly by showing that genetic instability is not required. Instead, these investigators show that overexpression of a single gene is sufficient and that the modifications in the precancer stem cell might be epigenetic as well as genetic. The continuing "low level" genetic changes and epigenetic changes may contribute to heterogeneity and are not required for neoplastic progression (see Figure 23-55, *C*). Thus this model suggests that the precancer stem cell is programmed from the beginning and is not dependent on multihits as the origin of invasive cancer. The risk for advancing to invasive breast cancer from human DCIS will therefore be predictable at the precancer stage possibly requiring the understanding of the interactions between the DCIS epithelium and stroma.[454]

Ductal Carcinoma In Situ

Ductal carcinoma in situ (DCIS) refers to a heterogeneous group of proliferations limited to ducts and lobules (Figure 23-56, *B*). DCIS occurs predominantly in women but can occur in men. The cells sometimes extend to the overlying skin without crossing the basement membrane and mistakenly appear as Paget disease[202] (see Table 23-18). Since 1980, with the increased use of mammography, the incidence and presentation have changed dramatically.[458] Today DCIS represents at least 15% to 30% of all newly screen-detected breast carcinomas.[459] DCIS presents as microcalcifications (low grade) or rod-shaped branching (high grade) on a mammogram (see Figure 23-56, *A*).

Molecular genetics has helped define the complexities of DCIS. From genome—wide molecular techniques—the DCIS lesions demonstrate differences in number and type of unbalanced or aberrant chromosome changes as well as intermediate, and poorly differentiated types. These changes seem to mirror the aberrant chromosomal changes observed in invasive breast carcinomas. Still controversial, DCIS does not appear to progress from sequential steps of low grade or risk types to higher grades or risk types en route to cancer or recurrence. This property therefore suggests a stable population. Emerging evidence suggests that DCIS may have programmed potential for phenotype, including progression to invasion, metastasis, hormone receptor expression, and treatment resistance.[454] The main issue and challenge revolve

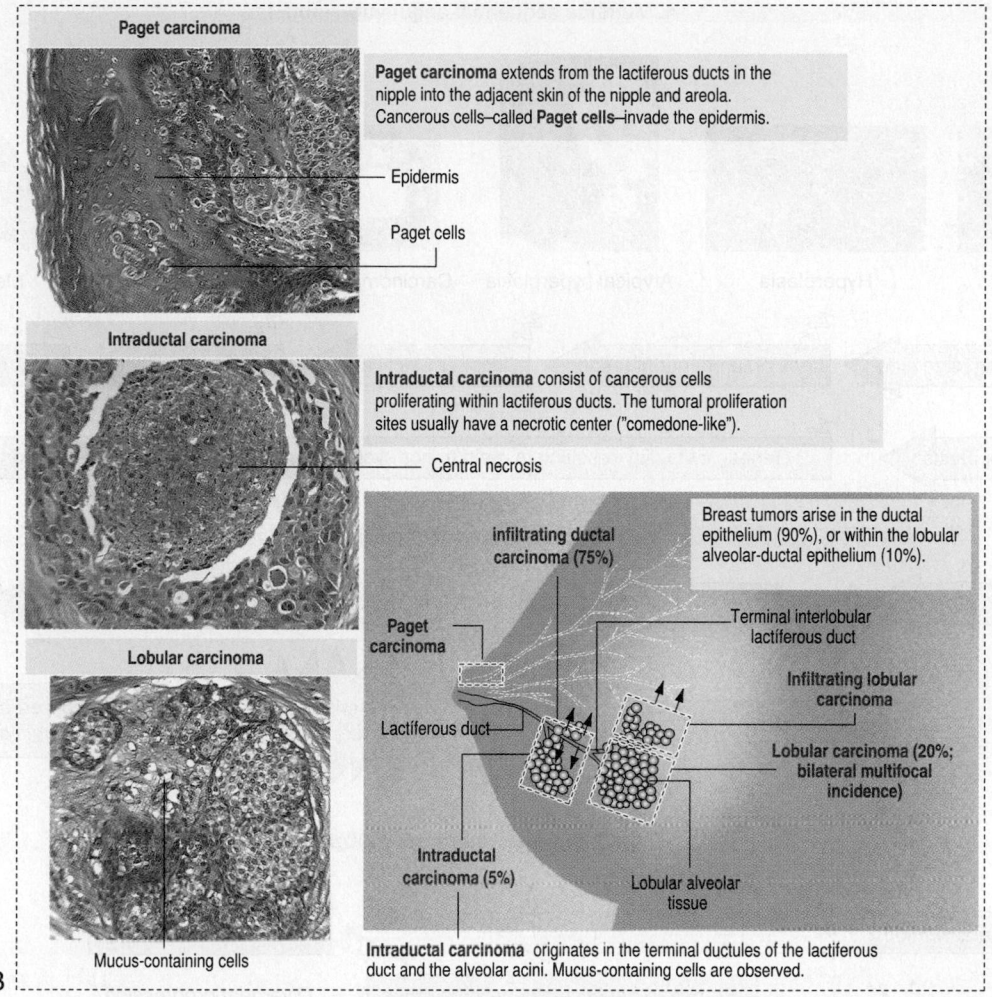

Paget carcinoma

Paget carcinoma extends from the lactiferous ducts in the nipple into the adjacent skin of the nipple and areola. Cancerous cells–called **Paget cells**–invade the epidermis.

— Epidermis

— Paget cells

Intraductal carcinoma

Intraductal carcinoma consist of cancerous cells proliferating within lactiferous ducts. The tumoral proliferation sites usually have a necrotic center ("comedone-like").

— Central necrosis

Breast tumors arise in the ductal epithelium (90%), or within the lobular alveolar-ductal epithelium (10%).

infiltrating ductal carcinoma (75%)

Terminal interlobular lactiferous duct

Paget carcinoma

Infiltrating lobular carcinoma

Lactiferous duct

Lobular carcinoma (20%; bilateral multifocal incidence)

Lobular carcinoma

Intraductal carcinoma (5%)

Lobular alveolar tissue

Mucus-containing cells

Intraductal carcinoma originates in the terminal ductules of the lactiferous duct and the alveolar acini. Mucus-containing cells are observed.

B

Figure 23-54, cont'd B, Breast cancer.

around which lesions of the category DCIS become invasive and how soon that happens.[458] In a study of 110 autopsies of young and middle-aged women (20 to 54 years), 14% were found to have DCIS,[460] suggesting that the preclinical prevalence (subtle histologic distortion and/or nonpalpable mass) is significantly higher than the clinical expression. Other autopsy series show that not all DCIS lesions progress to invasion or become clinically significant.[161,167,460,461] DCIS is detected more often in younger women than in older women.

Although there is no universally accepted histopathologic classification, historically most pathologists divided DCIS into five subtypes (papillary, micropapillary, cribriform, solid, and comedo) and often compare the first four types, noncomedo, with comedo. In a single biopsy, however, several types may be mixed and some noncomedo types may express characteristics of the comedo type. Although the term *comedo type* is widely used it does not specify a grade or an architecture, so newer categories most often use nuclear grade

(high, intermediate, or low) and record the architectural pattern separately.[459]

Lobular Carcinoma in situ

Lobular carcinoma in situ (LCIS) originates from the terminal duct–lobular unit (see Figure 23-54, *B*). Unlike DCIS, LCIS has a uniform appearance in which the cells occur in noncohesive (discohesive) clusters primarily in lobules. Research, however, suggests that some lobular and ductal carcinomas are closely related.[462] LCIS is not associated with calcifications or a stromal involvement that would form a density (lump). Thus it is usually an incidental finding from biopsy for something else. LCIS is fairly uncommon (up to 3.8% of all specimens).[463] LCIS is bilateral in 20% to 40% of women, and the majority (80% to 90%) occur before menopause. Although the cells of LCIS and invasive lobular carcinoma are identical,[202] whether LCIS is a true neoplasm or a marker of breast cancer risk remains controversial. Evidence to support LCIS as a precursor lesion of invasive carcinoma comes from molecular genetic data highlighting chromosomal alterations

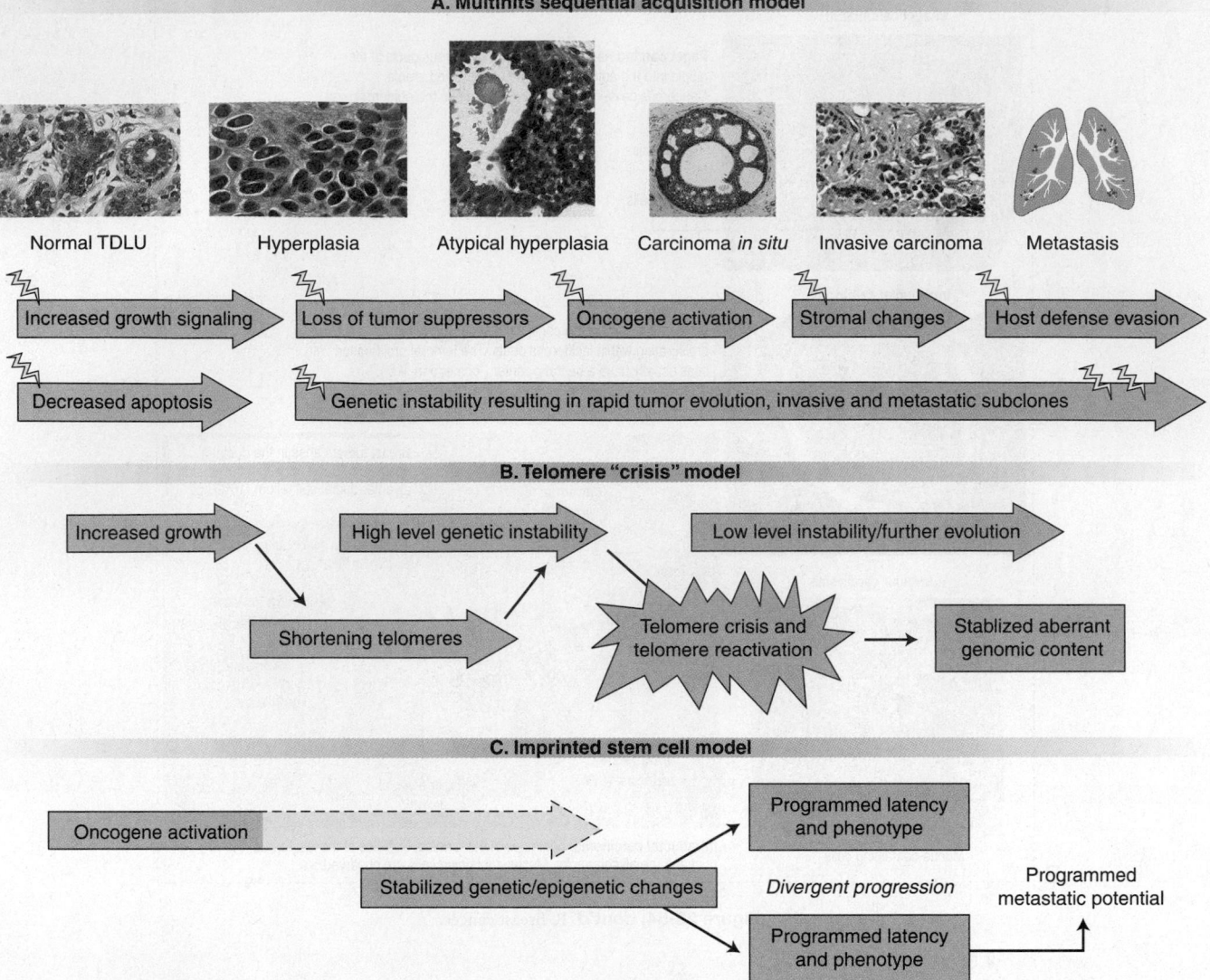

Figure 23-55 Conceptual models of breast carcinogenesis. A, Multihits sequential acquisition model (schematic as lightning bolts) corresponds to structural changes with cancer progression (also see Chapter 11). **B,** Hyperplasia increases the shortening of telomeres, swiftly increasing genetic instability known as "telomere crisis," with eventual stability after the enzyme telomerase reactivation, those individual cells reactivating telomerase with this genetic profile give rise to ductal carcinoma in situ (DCIS) and later invasive carcinoma. **C,** Genetically stable precancer stem cells are turned on through activation of oncogenes with divergent programmed behavior through epigenetic encoding and possible genetic, although not required, content changes. With progression, intermediate structural and molecular events are not required. These cells initiate DCIS and have innate built-in latency to invade with a built-in (innate) metastatic potential. (From Damonte P et al: *Breast Cancer Res* 10[3]:R50, 2008.)

and that LOH on chromosome 16q is present in LCIS and invasive carcinoma.[43,464] Invasive carcinoma develops in 25% to 35% of women with LCIS, and the contralateral (opposite) breast also is at risk.[465]

Inflammatory Stroma in Breast Cancer

Dominating the cancer field is the idea that epithelial function depends on the *entire* tissue, including the stroma or microenvironment. There is compelling evidence that cancer is a tissue-based disease with a possible abnormal aberrant wound healing and **inflammatory stromal (reactive stroma) component** (see Chapter 11). Early alterations in the stroma that occur with wound healing and inflammation

include activation of (1) mesenchymal cells (embryonic) fibroblasts; (2) endothelial cells; and (3) immune cells, including macrophages. Evidence of this type of activation is noted adjacent to tumors and is pathologically known as *desmoplastic stroma.*

Similar to mesenchymal cells, tumor cells appear to be stimulated, if not initiated, by such proinflammatory microenvironments.[466] Inflammation has been correlated with increased cancer incidence and a worse prognosis, or both, for cancers of the prostate, stomach, intestine, liver, and lung. In addition to these clinical data, laboratory data demonstrate how a wound can promote carcinogenesis.[467,468]

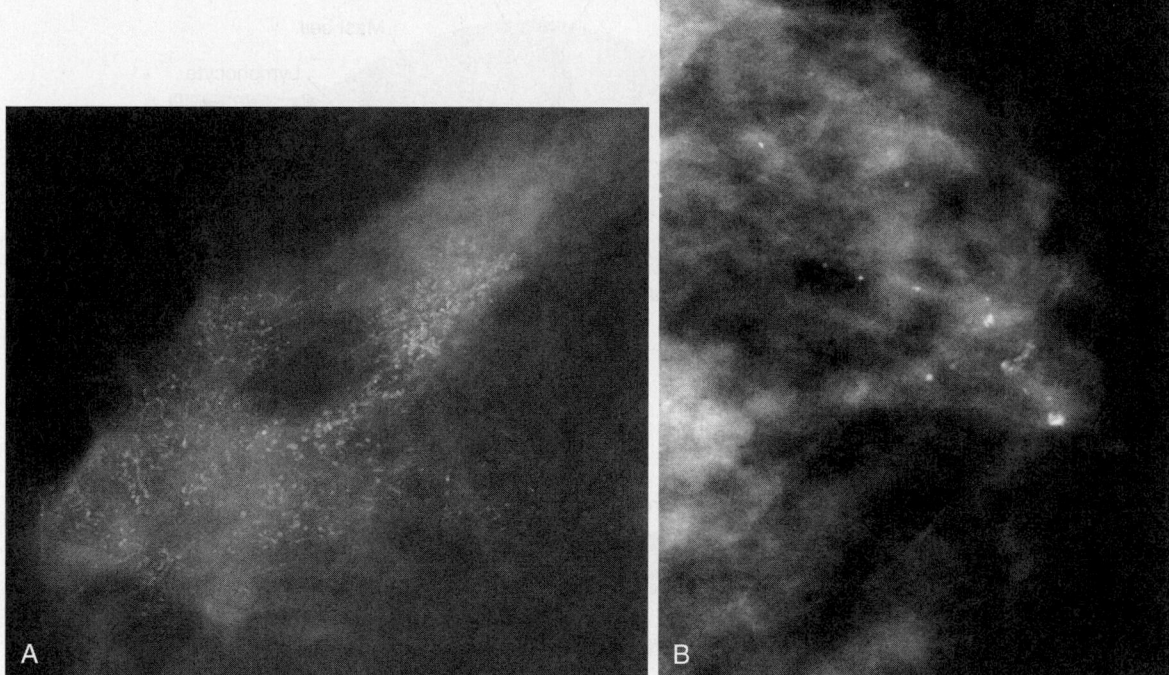

Figure 23-56 Ductal carcinoma in situ (DCIS). **A,** Malignant microcalcifications. Extensive area of pleomorphic microcalcifications; granular, rod-shaped, and branching microcalcifications can be identified. The appearances are typical of high-grade DCIS. **B,** Cranio-caudal mammography reveals fine and course granular calcifications. Histopathology revealed low-grade DCIS. (A from O'Malley FP, Pinder SE, editors: *Breast pathology,* New York, 2006, Churchill Livingstone/Elsevier. B from Donegan WL, Spratt JS: *Cancer of the breast,* ed 5, Philadelphia, 2002, Saunders.)

Evidence of the link between wound healing and carcinogenesis is based on the fact that these two distinct pathologies share a common "footprint" or "signature," a common molecular gene expression signature.[466] Furthermore, the genetic expression profile from a wound-healing model of fibroblasts actually predicted metastasis and death in several epithelial cancers. The "activated fibroblast gene signature" also was shown to be an independent marker for local recurrence of breast cancer.[469,470]

The wound response is based on the theory that "tumors are wounds that do not heal,"[471] and that cells involved in angiogenesis and the wound-healing response, including endothelial cells, immune cells, and fibroblasts have a prominent role in carcinogenesis and metastasis.[471] Fibroblasts are associated with cancer cells at all stages (Figure 23-58), and their structural and functional roles are emerging. Reactive tumor stroma is associated with an increased number of fibroblasts, increased capillary density, type-I collagen, and fibrin deposition. Thus reactive stroma provides oncogenic signals to promote carcinogenesis (see Figure 23-58).[471] Emerging evidence suggests that the development of this wound-reactive pattern and change in tumor tissue architecture create a distinctive phenotype change called **epithelial-mesenchymal transition (EMT)** (see p. 904).[472] EMT is normally activated during early embryogenesis and following injury of some epithelial tissues.[473] Therefore, it is possible that cancer cells "reactivate" a latent molecular program usually confined to embryonic

development and tissue repair but exaggerated and uncontrolled in cancer.[474] The EMT phenotype encourages the "migration step" for tumor invasion, enabling metastasis.[475] Interestingly, the tumor cells that undergo EMT have been shown to acquire the characteristics of cancer stem cells.[476] Once the metastasizing cancer cells settle in another tissue, they might reestablish the EMT epithelial phenotype.[473]

Another cell that is gaining importance for cancer invasion is the macrophage.[477] In one meta-analysis, investigators found that an abundance of macrophages in tumor stroma correlates with a poor prognosis.[478] Experimental evidence of the relationship between macrophages and poor prognosis comes from mouse models of breast cancer. In established tumors, tumor-derived cytokines induce the differentiation of the M2 macrophage phenotype. M1 macrophage phenotype is produced mainly in inflamed noncancerous tissue.[473] The M2 phenotype stimulates angiogenesis and ECM breakdown from the production of angiogenic growth factors and MMPs, thus promoting carcinogenesis.[479] Macrophages may provide a notable "whammy" at the tumor invasive front not only by promoting tumor cell migration, invasion, and intravasation but also by increasing the number of blood vessels as targets for intravasation.[477]

Invasive Breast Carcinoma

Invasive breast carcinoma is a malignant invasive epithelial lesion derived from the terminal duct lobular unit (Figure 23-54, *B,* p. 899). It can arise from anywhere in the

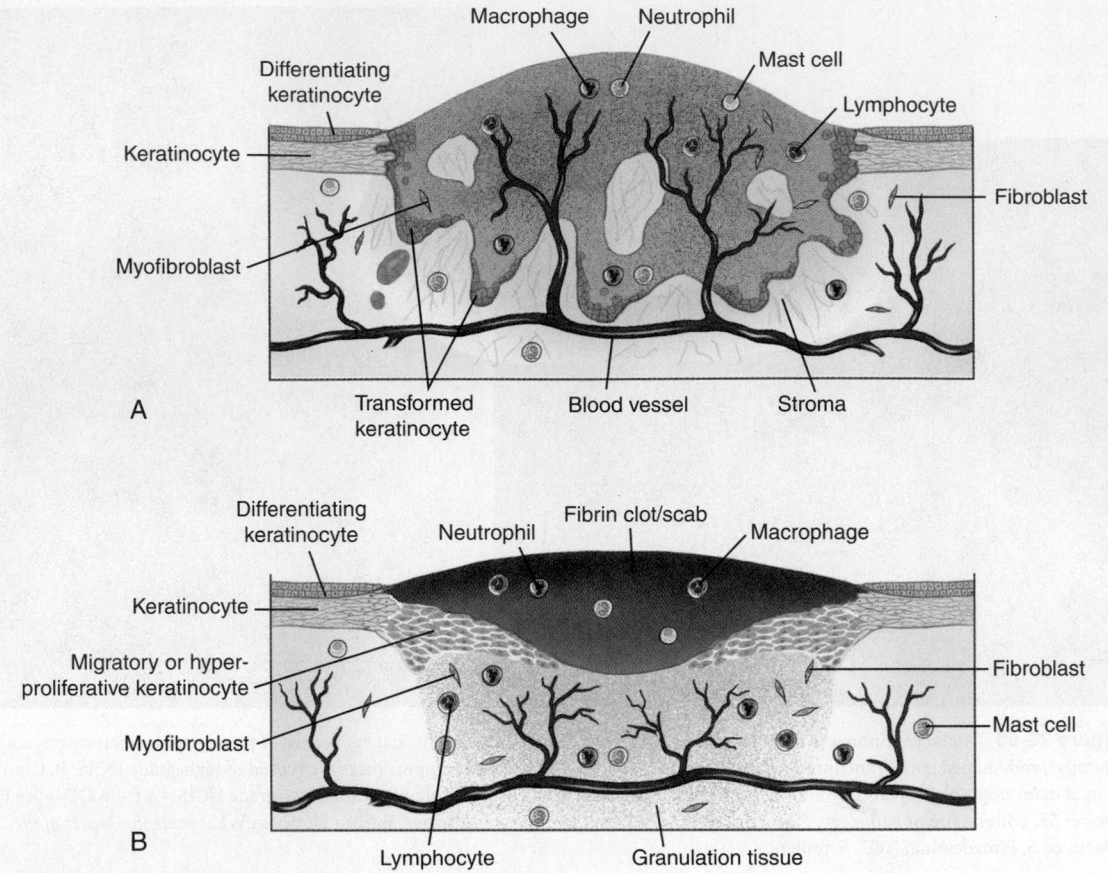

Figure 23-57 Schematic figure comparing a wound and invasive tumor. Invasive epithelial tumor (**A**) and a skin wound (**B**) in the phase of new tissue formation 3 to 10 days after wounding. Both types of tissue are characterized by the presence of a fibrin clot, inflammatory cells (neutrophils, macrophages, mast cells, and lymphocytes), newly formed vessels, and a large number of fibroblasts and myofibroblasts. These are components of the wound granulation tissue, which strongly resembles the tumor stroma. In addition, migrating and proliferating keratinocytes are present in the wound and in the cancer tissue. The main difference between tumors and wounds is the invasive growth of the transformed keratinocytes (which fill the tumor). (From Schäfer M, Werner S: *Nat Rev Mol Cell Biol* 9, 628-638, 2008.)

breast parenchyma or accessory breast tissue but it appears to be more common in the upper outer quadrant. The exact molecular events leading to invasion are complex and not completely understood. Unlike the colon cancer multistep model, in which some carcinomas arise sequentially from the preexisting adenoma, breast carcinomas are a group of different disease entities showing parallel progression pathways probably involving crosstalk of multiple signaling pathways.[480] From newer data using the stem cell model of breast carcinogenesis, the origin of invasion is hypothesized as the precancer stem cell. Accordingly, the precancer stem cell has an intrinsic programmed latency to invasion and metastases. This newer model suggests that the risk for advancing to invasive breast cancer from human DCIS is predictable at the precancer stage and may depend on the interactions between the DCIS epithelium and the surrounding stroma. It also suggests that these events may involve epigenetic interactions and that genomic alterations may play a role in the programming but their role

in neoplastic progression to malignancy and metastasis is unknown.[454]

Studies of human mammary epithelial cells (HMECs) from *healthy* individuals are providing insights into how epigenetic and genomic factors fuel cancer progression.[481] Hypermethylation of a key cell cycle regulator **p16 INK4A,** an epigenetic change, creates a previously unknown premalignant lesion (preclonal phase) in healthy disease-free women. These so-called **variant HMECs (vHMECs)** are thus characterized by lack of p16 INK4A activity and proliferate for an extended period of time with disappearing telomere sequences. These cells exhibit telomere dysfunction and generate chromosomal abnormalities noted in the earliest lesions of breast cancer.[482] The existence of this subpopulation of vHMECs with the accompanying telomeric and centrosomal dysfunction may be important early events in breast carcinogenesis.[481] Bean and colleagues[483] tested this hypothesis in high-risk women and found the frequency of INK4A/ARF promotes hypermethylation and

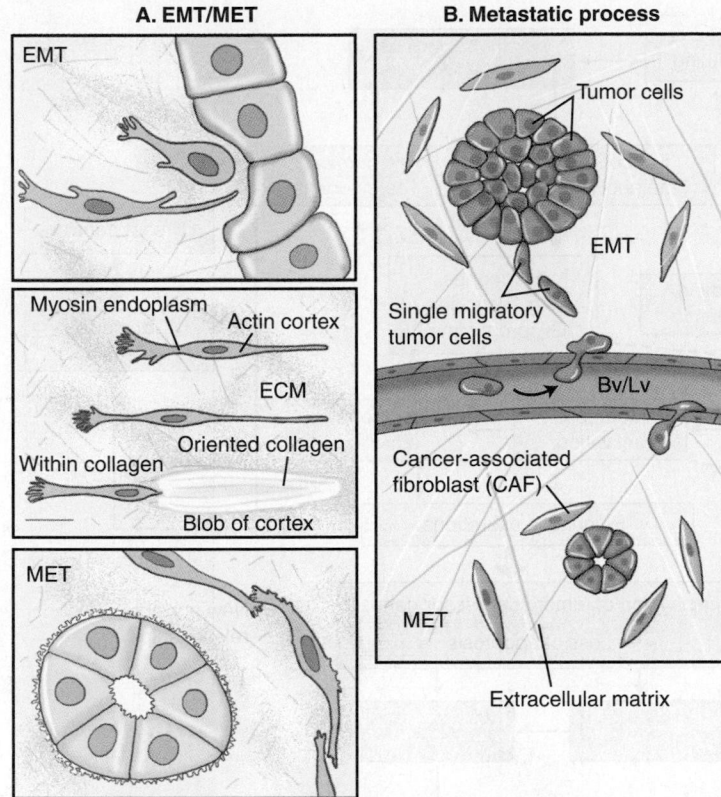

A. EMT/MET

EMT

Myosin endoplasm
Actin cortex
ECM
Within collagen
Oriented collagen
Blob of cortex

MET

B. Metastatic process

Tumor cells

EMT

Single migratory tumor cells

Bv/Lv

Cancer-associated fibroblast (CAF)

MET

Extracellular matrix

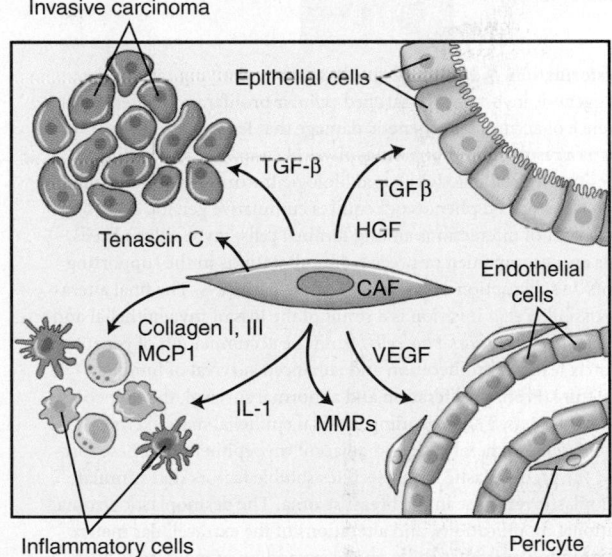

C. Cancer-associated fibroblasts communication

Invasive carcinoma

Epithelial cells

TGF-β

TGFβ

Tenascin C

HGF

Endothelial cells

CAF

Collagen I, III
MCP1

VEGF

IL-1

MMPs

Inflammatory cells

Pericyte

Figure 23-58 The epithelial-mesenchymal transition in cancer (past, present, and future) and functions of activated fibroblasts in the tumor stroma. **A,** Betty Hey, well known professor of cell biology and embryology, coined the term epithelial-to-mesenchymal (EMT) transformation some 40 years ago and left us beautiful drawings that show not only the transformation to mesenchyme but also the transient nature of the process and the reversion to the epithelial character. This is why the preferred term is now epithelial-to-mesenchymal transition. **B,** The EMT, as an initial step in the metastatic cascade, has until recently remained a matter of debate; however, powerful imaging tools have convincingly shown that individual cells delaminate (also see Figure 23-59, *B*) from primary tumors (possibly from decreased cell adhesion) because of dismantling of E cadherin. **C,** Fibroblasts communicate with cancer cells, resident epithelial cells, endothelial cells, pericytes, and inflammatory cells through the secretion of growth factors and chemokines. Through the increased deposition of collagen types I and III and de novo expression of tenascin C, fibroblasts induce an altered extracellular-matrix microenvironment that potentially provides additional oncogenic signals. Fibroblasts mediate the inflammatory response by secreting chemokines such as monocyte chemotactic protein 1 (MCP1) and interleukins such as IL-1. Fibroblasts interact with the microvasculature by secreting matrix metalloproteinases (MMPs) and vascular endothelial growth factor (VEGF). Fibroblasts also provide potentially oncogenic signals such as transforming growth factor-β (TGF-β) and hepatocyte growth factor (HGF) to resident epithelia, and directly stimulate cancer-cell proliferation and invasion by secreting growth factors such as TGF-β and stromal-cell–derived factor 1 (SDF1). *Bv,* Blood vessels; *ECM,* extracellular matrix; *Lv,* lymphatic vessels. (A and B from Acloque H, Thiery JP, Nieto MA: *EMBO Rep* 9[4]:322-326, 2008. C from Kalluri R, Zeisburg M: *Nat Rev Cancer* 6:392-401, 2006.)

was associated with the combined frequency of other epigenetic hypermethylation changes of the retinoic acid receptor-beta 2 (RARβ), estrogen receptor gene (ESR-1), and *BRCA1* genes. In another study (small sample), Bean and colleagues[484] found *BRCA1* promoter hypermethylation was associated with age and the combined frequency of promoter hypermethylation of the *RARβ* gene, *ESR-1* gene, and *p16 (INK4A)* gene. Lui and colleagues[485] found *p16 INKA* methylation and γ-tubulin gene amplification had a synergistic effect on promoting tumor progression.

Both of these effects were found to increase in atypical ductal hyperplasia and in situ carcinomas. Hypermethylated p16 promoter sequences, and others, could continue to proliferate, thereby generating chromosomal abnormalities that may increase carcinogenesis (Figure 23-59). The continued alterations in the *variant* cells could occur from microenvironment stromal contributions. Other investigators observed that *p16* modulates *TP53* in HMEC but not in fibroblasts (see next section).[486] How this interaction between signaling pathways is regulated—stroma or intrinsic

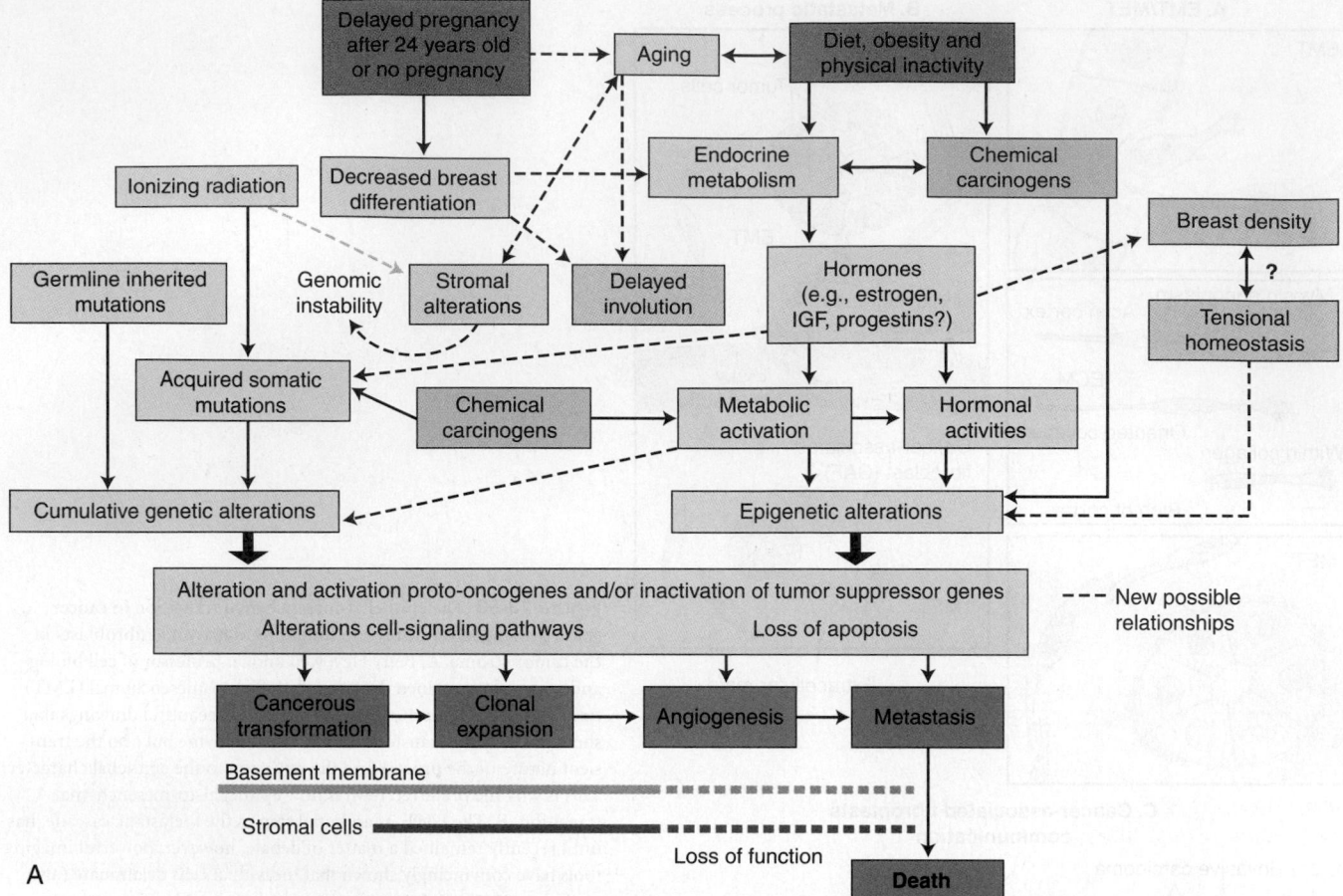

A

Figure 23-59 Model of breast carcinogenesis and breast tissue transformation. A, Molecular mechanisms underlying each of the risk factors for breast cancer are not completely defined. Breast carcinogenesis involves uncontrolled cellular proliferation, alterations in cell signaling pathways, aberrance or loss of apoptosis as a consequence of accumulated genetic damage that lead to activation, and alteration of germline mutation or acquired as somatic mutations as a result of environmental physical *(peach)* (e.g., ionizing radiation), chemical *(blue)*, lifestyle *(purple)* (e.g., pregnancy, diet, obesity, physical inactivity), and biologic factors *(green)* (e.g., aging, endocrine/hormonal milieu); unclassified *(pink)*. The expression of the transformed phenotype requires cumulative genetic alterations and epigenetic alterations. The normal breast is maintained by a complex set of interactions among luminal cells, myoepithelial cells, the basement membrane, and stromal cells. Changes in malignant cells are accompanied or preceded by alterations in the supporting myoepithelial and stromal cells because of genetic and epigenetic events and disruption of normal signaling pathways. The final alteration, invasion of the stroma, is the least understood. Emerging is the possibility that invasion is a result of the loss of myoepithelial and stromal cells to maintain the basement membrane. **B,** Breast tissue transformation *(dark blue cells)* from the accumulation of genetic and epigenetic alterations in the epithelium and an altered stromal matrix leads to proliferation and enhanced survival of luminal epithelial cells within the ductal tree compromising normal ductal structure. From proliferation and abnormal survival, the preneoplastic luminal mammary epithelial cells eventually expand to fill the breast ducts. The expanding luminal epithelial mass exerts outward projecting compression forces of increasing magnitude on the basement membrane and adjacent myoepithelium. These forces are countered by an inward projecting resistance force. Importantly, the preneoplastic lesion secretes soluble factors that stimulate immune cell infiltration and activation of fibroblasts to induce a desmoplastic response in the breast stroma. The desmoplastic stroma stiffens over time because of changes in the composition, post-translational modifications, and alterations of the extracellular matrix (ECM). This rigid parenchyma exerts a progressively greater inward projecting resistance force on the expanding preneoplastic duct. Eventually, the number of myoepithelial cells surrounding the preneoplastic mass decreases and the basement membrane thins, probably owing to increased matrix metalloproteinase (MMP) activity, decreased protein deposition, and compromised assembly. A buildup of interstitial fluid pressure continues, contributed by a leaky vasculature and lymphatic drainage. Responding to their genetic modifications and the altered materials properties of the matrix, the preneoplastic luminal epithelial cells exhibit altered tensional homeostasis and respond to the combination of forces and stromal cues to invade the breast parenchyma. Some fibroblasts transdifferentiate into myofibroblasts and increase tumor migration and invasion by promoting the assembly of collagen fibrils surrounding the distended preneoplastic epithelial ducts. (**B** from Butcher DT, Alliston T, Weaver VM: *Nat Rev Cancer* 9:108-122, 2009.)

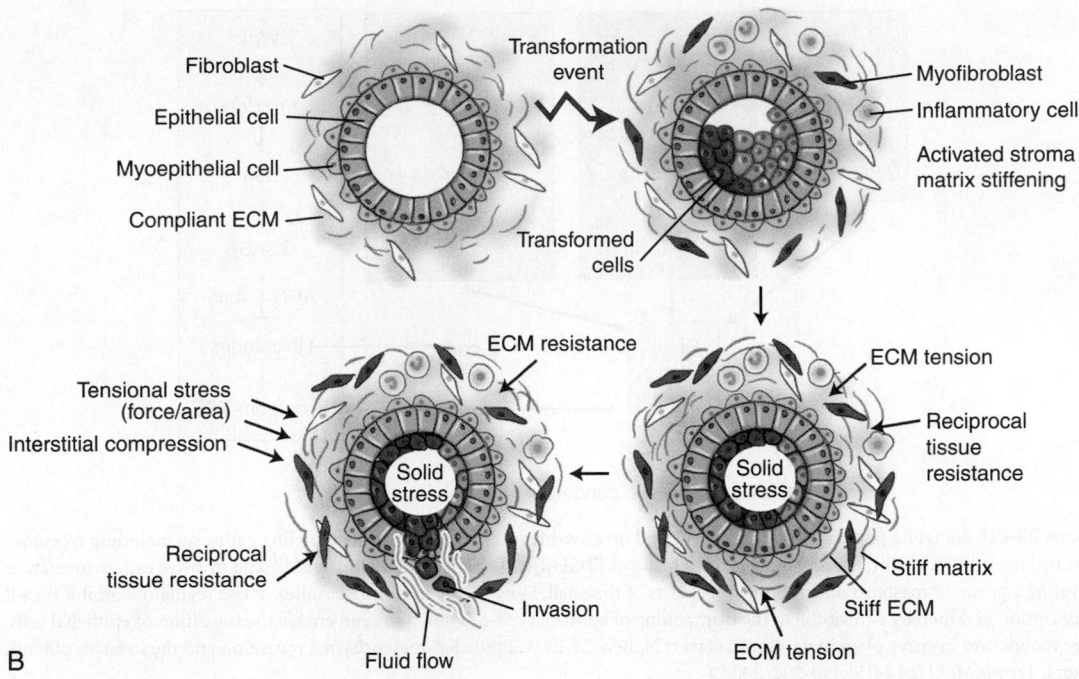

Figure 23-59, cont'd. Model of breast carcinogenis and breast tissue transformation. **B,** Breast tissue transformation.

cell factors—is unknown and potentially important for understanding carcinogenesis. This model differs from the classic view in that it identifies a potentially *vulnerable* stage of cancer cells.[484]

While all of these changes are occurring, parallel changes also occur because of mutation, epigenetic alterations (see Chapters 11 and 12), or abnormal signaling pathways resulting in altered cellular interactions and tissue structure. Loss of these normal functions also occurs with aging, which may contribute to breast cancer in older women.

The last step in carcinogenesis, the transition of carcinoma in situ to invasive carcinoma, is the subject of emerging evidence. Research shows that tumor-associated stroma undergoes extensive gene expression changes as does the malignant epithelium. Up-regulated genes in the stroma include those of the extracellular matrix, matrix metalloproteinases, and cell cycle-related genes (also see Chapter 11). Important is restoration of normal microenvironment signaling has been shown to revert features of the malignant phenotype despite the mutations in tumor cells.[487] Cells of importance in the microenvironment include inflammatory cells, endothelial cells, and stromal fibroblasts. Fibroblasts may play a dominant role in modulating epithelial cell function, promoting tumor progression, and even initiating epithelial cell carcinogenesis.[488] Tumor-derived fibroblasts exhibit higher levels of invasion-promoting capacity (IPC) than normal fibroblasts, and this role is enhanced by releasing the matrix metalloproteinases (MMPs) (Figures 23-58 and 23-59).[488] Various stimuli within the tumor microenvironment promote EMT of carcinoma cells. Most of the exogenous EMT stimuli are potentially exhibited by cancer-associated fibroblasts.[489] The development of this "reactive stromal change" in tumor

tissue architecture creates a phenotype normally seen in early embryogenesis that in cancer is reactivated, exaggerated, uncontrolled, and just might acquire the characteristics of cancer stem cells (see Inflammatory Stroma section, p. 900). Numerous signaling pathways (RGKs, Wnt, TGF-β, NF-$_κ$β) can induce both EMT and invasive cancer by activating master families of transcriptional regulators (Snail, Slug, Twist, ZeB1). These activated regulators inhibit E-cadherin (cell adhesion molecule) causing the dismantling of epithelial cell-cell junctions, which enables the transition of epithelial cells to become motile and invade surrounding tissue (Figure 23-60).[490]

Newer techniques, such as microarray technologies (gene chips) that survey many changes in DNA, RNA, and proteins of carcinomas, provide molecular patterns of the overall biologic diversity of invasive breast carcinomas. The four main molecular classes are discussed below.

CLINICAL MANIFESTATIONS Invasive carcinoma of the breast generally presents as a nontender palpable mass or thickened area.[202] Lumps caused by breast tumors do not have any classic characteristics. If the local lymphatics are blocked, the subsequent lymphedema and thickening of the skin causes a change called *peau d'orange* (orange peel skin). Tethering of the skin by Cooper ligaments to the breast mimics the look of an orange peel (Figure 23-61). If the central portion of the breast is involved, retraction of the nipple can occur. Other signs include nipple discharge, palpable nodes in the axilla, or bone pain caused by metastasis to the vertebrae or other skeletal area. Table 23-19 summarizes the clinical manifestations of breast cancers. Manifestations vary according to the type of tumor and stage of disease.

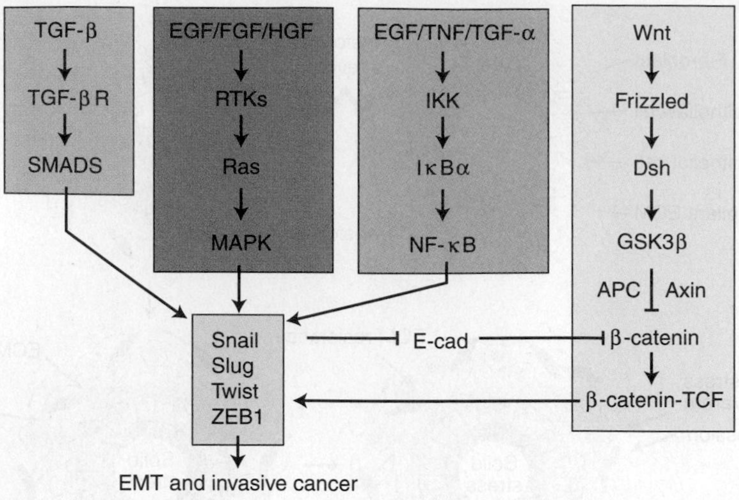

```
┌──────────┐  ┌──────────────┐  ┌──────────────┐  ┌──────────────┐
│  TGF-β   │  │ EGF/FGF/HGF  │  │ EGF/TNF/TGF-α │  │     Wnt      │
│    ↓     │  │      ↓       │  │      ↓        │  │      ↓       │
│  TGF-β R │  │    RTKs      │  │     IKK       │  │  Frizzled    │
│    ↓     │  │      ↓       │  │      ↓        │  │      ↓       │
│  SMADS   │  │    Ras       │  │    IκBα       │  │     Dsh      │
│          │  │      ↓       │  │      ↓        │  │      ↓       │
│          │  │    MAPK      │  │    NF-κB      │  │   GSK3β      │
│          │  │              │  │               │  │  APC │ Axin  │
└──────────┘  └──────────────┘  └──────────────┘  └──────────────┘
```

Snail
Slug   ── ┤ E-cad ├── β-catenin
Twist   ↓
ZEB1 ←──────────────────── β-catenin-TCF
  ↓
EMT and invasive cancer

Figure 23-60 **Signaling pathways to induce EMT and invasive breast cancer.** Numerous signaling pathways including receptor tyrosine kinase (RTKs, Wnt, transforming growth factor-β [TGF-β], NF-kappa$_{K}$β can induce EMT and invasive cancer formation by activating a group of master transcriptional regulators of the Snail, Slug, Twist, and ZEB1 families. These regulators inhibit E-cadherin transcription and thereby contribute to the dismantling of epithelial cell-cell junctions and enable the transition of epithelial cells to a more mobile and invasive phenotype. (From Gavert N, Ben-Zé-Ev A: Epithelial-mesenchymal transition and the invasive potential of tumors, *Trends Mol Med* 14[5]:199-208, 2008.)

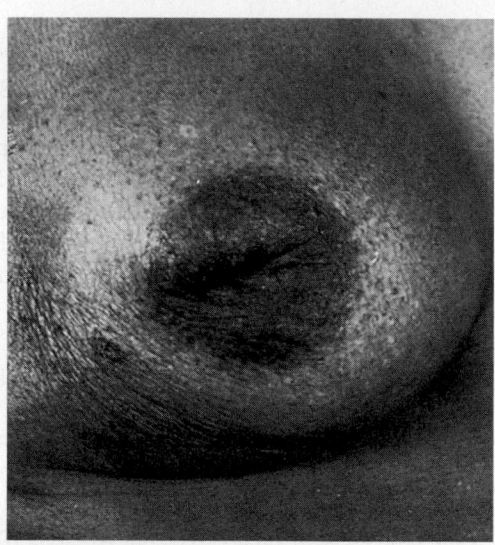

Figure 23-61 Retraction of nipple caused by carcinoma. (From del Regato JA, Spjut HJ, Cox JD: *Ackerman and del Regato's cancer: diagnosis, treatment, and prognosis,* ed 6, St Louis, 1985, Mosby.)

The most common histologic types of breast carcinomas are listed in Table 23-18 (p. 897). Invasive carcinomas of no special type (NST) constitute the majority (70% to 80%) of tumors, however, they cannot be specifically classified. Carcinomas of NST have varying amounts of DCIS. In the future, gene expression profiling may specifically identify subtypes and enable understanding of the clinical relevance (e.g., etiology, presentation, prognosis, or treatment).

EVALUATION AND TREATMENT Approximately 50% of carcinomas of the breast occur in the upper outer quadrant because most of the glandular tissue of the breast is

there. Most lymphatic vessels in the breast connect to axillary lymph nodes. Other important lymph nodes are the internal mammary nodes and those close to the collar bone—the infraclavicular and supraclavicular nodes. The lymphatic spread of cancer to the opposite breast, to lymph nodes in the base of the neck, and to the abdominal cavity is caused by obstruction of the normal lymphatic pathways or destruction of lymphatic vessels by surgery or radiation. The less common inner-quadrant tumors may spread to mediastinal nodes or Rotter nodes, which are located between the pectoral muscles. Internal mammary chain nodes are common sites of metastasis. Metastases from the vertebral veins can involve the vertebrae, pelvic bones, ribs, and skull. The brain, lungs, liver, spinal cord, kidneys, adrenal glands, ovaries, and pituitary gland also are sites of metastasis.

Mammography, digital mammography, MRI, ultrasonography, percutaneous needle aspiration, biopsy or minimally invasive biopsy called *mammotome,* palpation, hormone receptor assays, and gene expression profiling are used to evaluate an individual's breast cancer, plan treatment, and predict outcome.[491] Gene expression profiling results support the hypothesis that estrogen-receptor (ER)–negative (–) and ER-positive (+) cancers originate from distinct cell types and has uncovered biologic processes that govern metastatic progression.[492] Four main molecular classes of breast cancer have been identified by profiling, including (1) basal-like (ER–, PR–, HER-2 negative, thus called "triple negative" tumors), (2) luminal-A cancers (mostly ER+ [low grade]), (3) luminal B cancers (mostly ER+ low levels of hormone receptors and often high grade) and (4) HER-2 positive with amplification of the *ERBB2* gene and several others of the *ERBB2* family. According to Sotiriou and Pusztai[492] these subgroups correspond reasonably well

Table 23-19 Clinical Manifestations of Breast Cancer

Clinical Manifestation	Pathophysiology
Chest pain	Metastasis to the lung
Dilated blood vessels	Obstruction of venous return by a fast-growing tumor; obstruction dilates superficial veins
Dimpling of the skin	Can occur with invasion of the dermal lymphatics because of retraction of Cooper ligament or involvement of the pectoralis fascia
Edema	Local inflammation or lymphatic obstruction
Edema of the arm	Obstruction of lymphatic drainage in the axilla
Hemorrhage	Erosion of blood vessels
Local pain	Local obstruction caused by the tumor
Nipple/areolar eczema	Paget disease
Nipple discharge in a nonlactating woman	Spontaneous and intermittent discharge caused by tumor obstruction
Nipple retraction	Shortening of the mammary ducts
Pitting of the skin (similar to the surface of an orange [peau d'orange])	Obstruction of the subcutaneous lymphatics, resulting in the accumulation of fluid
Reddened skin, local tenderness, and warmth	Inflammation
Skin retraction	Involvement of the suspensory ligaments
Ulceration	Tumor necrosis

Data from Griffiths MJ, Murray KH, Russo PC: *Oncology nursing: pathophysiology, assessment, and intervention*, New York, 1984, Macmillan.

Box 23-18 Staging of Breast Cancer—TNM Method

T—Primary Tumor Size	N—Regional Lymph Nodes	Stage Grouping			
T_x Primary tumor cannot be assessed	N_x Regional lymph nodes cannot be assessed (e.g., previously removed)	Stage 0	Tis	N0	M0
T_0 No evidence of primary tumor		Stage I	T_1	N0	M0
		Stage IIa	T_0	N0	M0
T_{is} Carcinoma in situ: intraductal carcinoma, lobular carcinoma in situ, or Paget disease of the nipple with node	N_0 No regional lymph node metastasis		T_1	N_1	M0
	N_1 Metastasis to movable ipsilateral axillary lymph node or nodes		T_2	N0	M0
T_1 Tumor 2 cm or less in greatest dimension	N_2 Metastasis to ipsilateral axillary lymph node(s) fixed to one another or to other structures	Stage IIB	T_2	N_1	M0
T_2 Tumor more than 2 cm but not more than 5 cm in greatest dimension	N_3 Metastasis to ipsilateral internal mammary lymph node or nodes		T_3	N0	M0
T_3 Tumor more than 5 cm in greatest dimension	M—Distant Metastasis	Stage IIIA	T_0	N_2	M0
			T_1	N_2	M0
			T_2	N_2	M0
			T_3	N_1	M0
			T_3	N_2	M0
T_4 Tumor of any size with direct extension to chest wall or skin	M_x Presence of distant metastasis cannot be assessed	Stage IIIB	T_4	Any N	M0
			Any T	N_3	M0
NOTE: Paget disease associated with a tumor is classified according to the size of the tumor	M_0 No distant metastasis M_1 Distant metastasis (includes metastasis to ipsilateral supraclavicular lymph node or nodes)	Stage IV	Any T	Any N	M_1

Data from Beahrs OH, Hutter RV, Kennedy BJ, editors: *Breast manual for staging of cancer*, ed 45, Philadelphia, 1992, Lippincott.

to clinical features on the basis of ER and HER2 status. Responding to the need for earlier, more accurate, safer, and cost-effective methods for cancer detection, investigators are studying other methods, including traveling wave and MRI, ultrasound, infrared (thermography), elastography, optical imaging, and others.[493,494] Surgical biopsy is the definitive diagnostic test.

Treatment is based on the extent or stage of the cancer (Box 23-18). The extent of the tumor at the primary site, the presence and extent of lymph node metastasis, and the presence of any distant metastases are all evaluated to determine the stage of disease.

Ovarian ablation in some women younger than 50 years of age with early breast cancer significantly improves long-term survival.[495] Radiation therapy is used to prevent metastasis of a small tumor (0.2 cm) or if the cancer is near bone or the edge of the breast that has been surgically excised. Not all women with breast cancer need radiation. The long-term effect of radiotherapy on mortality from breast cancer and other causes remains uncertain. It is especially important to protect the heart and lungs from radiation exposure. Chemotherapy and hormone therapy are most successful as an adjunct to surgery in premenopausal women with hormone-dependent tumors, and are used in individuals with advanced disease. Trastuzumab, the antibody to the *HER-2* oncogene, is available and blocks the growth-promoting signal produced by *HER-2/neu*. Other biologic therapies under investigation are based on discovered relationships between COX-2 and VEGF. Hypoxia upregulates COX-2, which increases proinflammatory prostaglandins (PGE_2). Therefore, COX-2 or VEGF inhibitors (e.g., bevacizumab) may be an additional therapeutic choice. Endocrine therapy may be used to prolong survival time and is thought to be most effective in women with ER+ and PR+ tumors. Long-term antiestrogen therapy, such as tamoxifen, has proven efficacy (improves 10-year survival) in individuals with ER+ tumors, and in those with unknown ER status.[496] Use of tamoxifen for many years, however, can increase tumor resistance as well as the risk of adverse effects such as blood clots and endometrial cancer. Thus tamoxifen use should not exceed 5 years, and some data support switching to anastrozole or other aromatase inhibitors.[497,498] According to a Cochrane Review,[436] adjuvant tamoxifen needs further study for women with ER-tumors. Currently, tamoxifen is not recommended as an agent for prevention of breast cancer in those without breast cancer. In early postmenopausal breast cancer, aromatase inhibitors, such as anastrozole, have increased disease-free survival rates more than has tamoxifen[499,500] (see p. 883).

Strategies are being studied that have high affinity for breast estrogen receptors but weak affinity for receptors in the uterus, such as the drug raloxifene. Results from the Multiple Outcomes of Raloxifene Evaluation (MORE), a randomized study, found that among postmenopausal women with osteoporosis, raloxifene decreased the risk of invasive breast cancer by 76% (13 cases in 5129 women versus 27 cases in the 2579 placebo group).[501] Results from the STAR (study of tamoxifen and raloxifene) trial showed raloxifene to be as effective as tamoxifen in reducing the risk of invasive breast cancer. Raloxifene also has a lower risk of thromboembolic events and cataracts but a nonsignificant higher risk of noninvasive breast cancer. The risk of other cancers, fractures, ischemic heart disease, and stroke were similar for both drugs.[501] Coumate 667 (STX 64), a steroid sulfatase inhibitor, has completed a phase 1 trial in postmenopausal women with breast cancer (see Hormones, p. 885). STC 64 is a potent, apparently well-tolerated steroid sulfatase inhibitor, which showed decreases in serum concentrations of steroids with estrogenic properties.[502] The effectiveness of sulfatase inhibitors needs further study.

Disorders of the Male Breast

Gynecomastia

Gynecomastia is the overdevelopment of breast tissue in a male. Gynecomastia accounts for approximately 85% of all masses that develop in the male breast and affects 32% to 40% of the male population. If only one breast is involved, it is typically the left. Incidence is greatest among adolescents and men older than 50 years.

Gynecomastia results from hormonal alterations, which may be idiopathic or caused by systemic disorders, drugs, or neoplasms. It usually involves an imbalance of the estrogen/testosterone ratio, which can be altered in one of two ways. First, estrogen levels may be excessively high, although testosterone levels are normal, as in drug-induced and tumor-induced cases of hyperestrogenism. Second, testosterone levels may be extremely low although estrogen levels are normal, as is the case in hypergonadism. Gynecomastia also can be caused by alterations in breast-tissue responsiveness to hormonal stimulation. Breast tissue may have increased responsiveness to estrogen or decreased responsiveness to androgen. Alterations of responsiveness may cause many cases of idiopathic gynecomastia.

Besides puberty and aging, estrogen-testosterone imbalances are associated with hypogonadism, Klinefelter syndrome, and testicular neoplasms. Hormone-induced gynecomastia is usually bilateral. Pubertal gynecomastia is a self-limiting phenomenon that usually disappears within 4 to 6 months. Senescent gynecomastia usually regresses spontaneously within 6 to 12 months.

Systemic disorders associated with gynecomastia include obesity, cirrhosis of the liver, infectious hepatitis, chronic renal failure, chronic obstructive lung disease, hyperthyroidism, tuberculosis, and chronic malnutrition. It may be that these disorders ultimately alter the estrogen/testosterone ratio, initiating the gynecomastia.

Gynecomastia is often seen in men receiving estrogen therapy, either in preparation for a sex-change operation or for prostatic carcinoma. Other drugs that can cause gynecomastia include digitalis, cimetidine, spironolactone, reserpine, thiazide, isoniazid, ergotamine, tricyclic antidepressants, amphetamines, vincristine, and busulfan. Gynecomastia is usually unilateral in these instances.

Malignancies of the testes, adrenals, or liver can cause gynecomastia if they alter the estrogen/testosterone ratio. Pituitary adenomas and lung cancer also are associated with gynecomastia.

PATHOPHYSIOLOGY The breast enlargement consists of hyperplastic stroma and ductal tissue. Hyperplasia results in a firm, palpable mass, at least 2 cm in diameter located beneath the areola.

EVALUATION AND TREATMENT The diagnosis of gynecomastia is based on physical examination. Identification and treatment of the cause are likely to be followed by resolution of the gynecomastia. The man should be taught to perform breast self-examination and is examined at 6- and

12-month intervals if the gynecomastia persists. All unilateral breast enlargement in men warrants an evaluation for malignancy; workup includes fine-needle aspiration, cytology, mammography, ultrasound, and biopsy.

Cancer

Male breast cancer (MBC) accounts for 1% of all male cancers and less than 1% of all breast cancers. Breast cancer in men has increased 25% over the past 25 years.[503] It occurs most commonly after age 60, with the peak incidence between 60 and 69 years. It has, however, been reported in males as young as 6 years and in adolescents. Possible risk factors include gynecomastia, radiation of the chest wall, family history of breast cancer, Klinefelter syndrome, and especially with germline mutation in BRCA1 or BRCA2. Other genetic factors include CYP17 polymorphism, Cowden syndrome, CHEK2, and AR gene mutations.[444] Obesity increases the risk of MBC. Testicular disorders, including cryptorchidism, mumps, orchitis, and orchiectomy are related to risk.[504] The relationship between these factors and risk of disease is not clearly defined.

Male breast tumors often resemble carcinoma of the breast in women (see p. 880). The majority of MBCs express estrogen and progesterone receptors.[505] The malignant male breast lesion is usually a unilateral solid mass located near the nipple. Because the nipple is commonly involved, crusting and nipple discharge are typical clinical manifestations. Other findings include skin retraction, ulceration of the skin over the tumor, and axillary node involvement. Patterns of metastasis are similar to those in females.

The diagnosis of cancer is confirmed by biopsy. Because of delays in seeking treatment, male breast cancer tends to be advanced at the time of diagnosis and therefore tends to have a poor prognosis. Treatment protocols are similar to those for female breast cancer, but endocrine therapy is used more often for males because a higher percentage of male tumors are hormone dependent. The mainstay of treatment is modified mastectomy with axillary node dissection to assess stage and prognosis.[506] Orchiectomy is performed to treat metastatic disease.

SUMMARY REVIEW

Alterations of Sexual Maturation

1. Sexual maturation, or puberty, should begin in girls between ages 8 and 13 years and in boys between ages 9 and 14 years. Delayed puberty is the onset of sexual maturation after these ages; precocious puberty is onset before these ages. The average age of puberty has been occurring earlier than previously defined for girls.
2. Alterations of sexual maturation can be idiopathic or caused by a disease or congenital anomaly. In most cases of delayed puberty, the hypothalamic-pituitary-gonadal axis is intact but the surge of activity that stimulates puberty is delayed. This situation is common in boys. Precocious puberty, more common in girls, also can be caused by mistiming of the stimulatory surge in a child whose HPG system is otherwise normal.
3. Precocious puberty can be complete (sex appropriate), mixed (not sex appropriate), or partial (development of one secondary sex characteristic only). Causes of delayed or incomplete puberty can be divided into categories based on gonadotropic secretion: hypergonadotropism (increased levels of FSH and LH), and hypogonadotropism (decreased LH and FSH levels).

Disorders of the Female Reproductive System

1. The female reproductive system can be altered by hormonal imbalances, infectious microorganisms, inflammation, structural abnormalities, and benign or malignant proliferative conditions.
2. Menstrual disorders usually involve some disruption of the HPG axis and subsequent alteration of hormone production, reception by target organs, or feedback mechanisms.
3. Primary dysmenorrhea is painful menstruation not associated with pelvic disease. It results from excessive synthesis of prostaglandins, which cause the myometrium to contract and constrict blood vessels, resulting in ischemic pain.

4. Primary amenorrhea is the continued absence of menarche and menstrual function by 14 years of age without the development of secondary sex characteristics or by age 16 years if these changes have occurred.
5. Secondary amenorrhea is the absence of menstruation for a time equivalent to more than three cycles or 6 months in women who have previously menstruated. Secondary amenorrhea is usually associated with anovulation.
6. Categorization of amenorrhea as primary or secondary has no clinical significance. Instead, amenorrhea is divided into compartments that reflect the underlying disorder: compartment I, disorders of the outflow tract or uterine target organ; compartment II, disorders of the ovary; compartment III, disorders of the anterior pituitary; and compartment IV, disorders of the CNS or hypothalamic factors.
7. DUB is heavy or irregular bleeding caused by a disturbance of the menstrual cycle.
8. PCOS is a difficult syndrome to diagnose because several factors are involved. It is a syndrome when at least two of the following are present: oligo-ovulation or anovulation, elevated levels of androgens, or clinical signs of hyperandrogenism and polycystic ovaries. Prolonged anovulation leads to infertility, menstrual bleeding disorders, hirsutism, acne, endometrial hyperplasia, cardiovascular disease, and diabetes mellitus in women with hyperinsulinemia.
9. PMS is the cyclic recurrence of physical, psychologic, or behavioral changes distressing enough to disrupt normal activities or interpersonal relationships. More than 200 emotional, physical, and behavioral symptoms have been attributed to PMS. Emotional symptoms, particularly depression, anger, irritability, and fatigue, are reported as the most distressing; physical symptoms tend to be less problematic. Treatment is symptomatic and includes self-help techniques, lifestyle changes, counseling, and SSRIs.

Continued

10. Infection and inflammation of the female genitalia can result from microorganisms from the environment or over-proliferation of microorganisms that normally populate the genital tract.

11. PID is an acute ascending polymicrobial infection of the upper genital tract and is sexually transmitted.

12. Vaginitis, or vaginal infection, is usually caused by sexually transmitted pathogens or *C. albicans,* which causes candidiasis. Development is related to the overall health of a woman and local defense mechanisms, particularly vaginal pH. Variables such as antibiotics, douching, soaps, feminine hygiene sprays, and pregnancy alter vaginal pH or the bactericidal nature of secretions and predispose a woman to infection.

13. Cervicitis, which is inflammation of the cervix, can be acute (mucopurulent cervicitis) or chronic. Its most common cause is a sexually transmitted pathogen.

14. Vulvovestibulitis is an inflammation of the skin of the vulva. It can be caused by chemical and mechanical irritants, allergens, skin disorders, or vaginal infections, such as candidiasis.

15. Bartholinitis, also called Bartholin cyst, is an inflammation of the ducts that lead from the *Bartholin glands* to the surface of the vulva. Inflammation blocks the glands, preventing the outflow of glandular secretions, and is caused by trauma or infection.

16. Pelvic organ prolase—uterine prolapse, cystocele, rectocele, and urethrocele—are caused by loss of support provided by the pelvic muscles and fascia. Age and pelvic trauma are associated. Women with a familial or genetic predisposition have a higher risk.

17. Benign growths and proliferative conditions of the female reproductive tract tend to affect the ovaries (benign ovarian cysts) or uterine tissues (endometrial polyps, leiomyomas, and endometriosis).

18. Benign ovarian cysts develop from mature ovarian follicles that do not release their ova (follicular cysts) or from a corpus luteum that persists abnormally instead of degenerating (corpus luteum cyst). Cysts usually regress spontaneously.

19. Endometrial polyps are overgrowths of endometrial tissue and often cause abnormal bleeding in the premenopausal woman.

20. Leiomyomas, also called *uterine fibroids,* are tumors arising from the muscle layer of the uterus, the myometrium. Incidence increases in women between ages 30 and 50; most myomas remain small and asymptomatic. Adenomyosis is the presence of endometrial glands and stroma within the uterine myometrium.

21. Endometriosis is the presence of functional endometrial tissue (i.e., tissue that responds to hormonal stimulation) at sites outside the uterus. Endometriosis causes an inflammatory reaction at the site of implantation and is a cause of infertility.

22. Most cancers of the female genitalia involve the uterus (particularly the cervix) and the ovaries. Cancer of the vagina is rare.

23. Infection with high-risk HPV is a necessary precursor to developing CIN and cervical cancer. Smoking, immuno-suppression, and poor nutrition are cofactors. HPV vaccination can substantially reduce the risk of cervical cancer.

24. Cervical cancer arises from the cervical epithelium and is considered a sexually transmitted disease. The progressively serious neoplastic alterations are (1) cervical intraepithelial neoplasia (cervical dysplasia), (2) cervical carcinoma in situ, and (3) invasive cervical carcinoma.

25. Risk factors for vaginal cancer are in utero DES exposure and prior or concurrent cervical cancer. Like cervical cancers, vaginal cancers arise from the epithelium and are identified as intraepithelial neoplasia (dysplasia), carcinoma in situ, or invasive carcinoma. Most are secondary in nature. Mean age is 55 years for invasive cancer, 45 years for precursor lesions.

26. The major risk for vulvar cancer is a history of HPV infection or squamous dysplasia of the vagina or cervix. Symptoms include chronic vulvar irritation, pruritus, bloody discharge, and a hard, ulcerated area of the vulva or large cauliflower lesions. Peak incidence is in postmenopausal women, but women age 40 years or younger can be affected.

27. Endometrial cancer is the most common cancer of the pelvic region. Risk factors for endometrial cancer include unopposed estrogen exposure, obesity, infertility, failure to ovulate, early menarche or late menopause, and tamoxifen. Oral contraceptive use protects against endometrial and ovarian cancers. Peak incidence occurs at 58 to 60 years of age, approximately 10 years later than peak incidence of precursor lesions.

28. Risk factors for ovarian cancer include early menarche, late menopause, nulliparity, use of fertility drugs, and associations with breast cancer–susceptibility genes. Ovarian cancer causes more deaths than any other genital cancer in women.

29. Awareness of sexual dysfunction is relatively new. Chronic illness, medications, infection, sexual trauma, and a variety of psychosocial concerns have been implicated as causes.

30. Infertility, or the inability to conceive after 1 year of unprotected intercourse, affects approximately 15% of all couples. Fertility can be impaired by factors in the male, female, or both partners.

Disorders of the Male Reproductive System

1. Disorders of the urethra include urethritis (inflammation of the urethra) and urethral strictures (narrowing or obstruction of the urethral lumen caused by scarring).

2. Although noninfectious urethritis can occur, most cases of urethritis result from sexually transmitted pathogens. Symptoms of urethritis include dysuria, frequency, urgency, urethral tingling or itching, and clear or purulent discharge. Treatment consists of appropriate antibiotic therapy and avoidance of future chemical or mechanical irritation.

3. Acquired or congenital scarring that causes urethral stricture can be caused by trauma or by severe or untreated urethral infection. The primary symptom is diminished force and caliber of the urinary stream; other symptoms include urinary frequency and hesitancy, mild dysuria, double urine stream or spraying, and postvoiding dribbling. Treatment is usually surgical.

4. Phimosis and paraphimosis are penile disorders involving the foreskin (prepuce). In phimosis the foreskin cannot be retracted over the glans. In paraphimosis the foreskin is retracted and cannot be returned to its normal anatomic position over the glans. Phimosis is caused by poor hygiene and chronic infection and can lead to paraphimosis. Paraphimosis can constrict the penile blood vessels, preventing circulation to the glans.

5. Peyronie disease consists of fibrosis, affecting the corpora cavernosa, which causes penile curvature during erection. Fibrosis prevents engorgement on the affected side, causing a lateral curvature that can prevent intercourse.

6. Priapism, a prolonged painful erection not stimulated by sexual arousal, is a urologic emergency. The corpora cavernosa (but not the corpus spongiosum) fills with blood that does not drain out, probably because of venous obstruction. Priapism is associated with spinal cord trauma, sickle cell disease, leukemia, and pelvic tumors. It can also be idiopathic.

7. Balanitis is an inflammation of the glans penis and usually occurs in conjunction with posthitis. It is associated with phimosis, inadequate cleansing under the foreskin, skin disorders, and infections.

8. Cancer of the penis is rare; major risk factors include HPV, smoking, and consequences of treatment for psoriasis. Penile carcinoma in situ tends to involve the glans; invasive carcinoma of the penis involves the shaft as well.

9. A varicocele is an abnormal dilation of the veins within the spermatic cord caused by either congenital absence of valves in the internal spermatic vein or acquired valvular incompetence.

10. A hydrocele is a collection of fluid between the testicular and scrotal layers of the tunica vaginalis. Hydroceles can be idiopathic or caused by trauma or infection of the testes.

11. A spermatocele is a cyst located between the testis and epididymis that is filled with fluid and sperm.

12. Cryptorchidism is a congenital condition in which one or both testes fail to descend into the scrotum. Treated or untreated cryptorchidism is associated with infertility and a significantly increased risk of testicular cancer.

13. Testicular torsion is the rotation of a testis, which twists blood vessels in the spermatic cord. This interrupts blood supply to the testis, resulting in edema and, if not corrected within 4 to 6 hours, necrosis and atrophy of testicular tissues.

14. Orchitis is an acute inflammation of the testes. Pathogenic organisms may reach the testes through the blood or the lymphatics; most commonly, they reach the testes by ascending through the vas deferens and epididymis. Complications of orchitis include hydrocele and atrophy. Granulomatis orchitis, an autoimmune disease, is a nonspecific, noninfectious, inflammatory process that occurs in middle-aged men.

15. Testicular cancer is the most common malignancy in males ages 15 to 35 years. Although its cause is unknown, high androgen levels, genetic predisposition, and a history of cryptorchidism, trauma, or infection may contribute to tumorigenesis. Most testicular neoplasms are germ-cell tumors.

16. Epididymitis, an inflammation of the epididymis, is usually caused by a sexually transmitted pathogen that ascends through the vasa deferentia from an already infected urethra or bladder.

17. BPH is enlargement of the prostate gland. Symptoms are obstructive or irritative in nature and include urge to urinate often, delay in starting urination, and decreased force of stream. BPH can be treated surgically, with laser therapy, microwave thermotherapy, or medications.

18. Prostatitis can be bacterial or nonbacterial and chronic or acute. Bacterial prostatitis is an infection of the prostate. Acute bacterial prostatitis causes an inflammatory response in which the prostate becomes enlarged, tender, and firm. Chronic bacterial prostatitis is recurrent prostatic infection that eventually causes fibrosis. Nonbacterial prostatitis is prostatic inflammation without evidence of bacterial infection.

19. Prostate cancer is the most common cancer in American men, and the incidence varies greatly worldwide. Possible causes involve dietary and hormonal factors, obesity, and age. Only nutrition seems to explain the differences in global incidence. Incidence is greatest among northwestern European and North American men (particularly blacks) older than 65 years.

20. Most cancers of the prostate are adenocarcinomas that develop at the periphery of the gland. Because there are no early symptoms, disease is often advanced at the time of diagnosis.

21. A multifactorial model of prostate carcinogenesis includes (1) androgens act as tumor promoters through receptor mechanisms; (2) to enhance endogenous DNA toxic carcinogens, including ROS and reactive estrogen metabolites and estrogen; and (3) unknown environmental carcinogens. In addition, there are changes in the balance between autocrine/paracrine growth promoting and inhibiting factors, such as IGFs.

22. The microenvironment fuels the metastatic growth of prostate cancer.

23. Sexual dysfunction in males can be caused by any physical or psychologic factor that impairs erection, emission, or ejaculation. Impairment can be caused by a number of physiologic, psychologic, and emotional factors.

24. Spermatogenesis (sperm production by the testes) can be impaired by disruptions of the hypothalamic-pituitary-gonadal axis that reduce testosterone secretion and by testicular trauma or atrophy from any cause. Sperm production is also impaired by neoplastic disease, cryptorchidism, or any factor that causes testicular temperature to rise.

25. Sperm quality is impaired by chromosomal abnormalities resulting from genetic factors, irradiation, or toxins. Sperm motility can be impaired by unfavorable constituents or characteristics of semen.

Disorders of the Breast

1. Most disorders of the breast are disorders of the mammary gland, that is, the female breast.

2. Galactorrhea, or inappropriate lactation, is the persistent secretion of a milky substance by one or both breasts in nonpregnant, nonlactating women. Its most common cause is nonpuerperal hyperprolactinemia, a rise in serum prolactin levels that is not associated with pregnancy and childbirth. Hyperprolactinemia can be caused by medications, pituitary tumors, hypothyroidism, chronic stress, or persistent and repeated suckling.

3. Numerous benign conditions occur in ducts and lobules in the breast. Benign lesions are broadly classified as (1) nonproliferating breast lesions, (2) proliferative breast disease, and (3) atypical (atypia) hyperplasia.

4. The term *nonproliferative lesions* is used to discriminate such lesions from the "proliferative" changes associated with increased risk of breast cancer.

5. FCC is the most widely accepted term for physiologic nodularity and breast tenderness that waxes and wanes with the menstrual cycle. These changes are nonproliferative. Symptoms affect women ages 30 to 50 and include cyclic bilateral breast tenderness and transient breast lumps.

6. Proliferative breast lesions without atypia are characterized by proliferation of ductal epithelium and/or stroma without cellular signs suggestive of malignancy. These diverse lesions include (1) epithelial hyperplasia, (2) sclerosing adenosis, (3) complex sclerosing lesion (radial scar), (4) and papillomas.

7. Proliferative breast lesions with atypia include ADH and ALH. ADH is an increased number of cells mostly within the lumen of the terminal ducts. It includes a continuum of changes—cell structure and placement—ranging from an

continued

SUMMARY REVIEW—cont'd

increase in cellularity to features of DCIS. The cells in ALH do not distend more than 50% of the acini within a lobule.

8. Breast cancer is the most common form of cancer in American women and second only to lung cancer as the most frequent cause of cancer death. Most breast cancer occurs in women older than 50 years. The major risk factors for breast cancer are reproductive, such as nulliparity; familial, such as inherited gene syndromes; and environmental and lifestyle, such as radiation exposure. Important factors not easily classified are involution of the mammary gland and breast density.

9. Most breast cancers arise from the ductal epithelium and then may metastasize to the lymphatics, opposite breast, abdominal cavity, lungs, bones, kidneys, liver, adrenal glands, ovaries, and pituitary glands.

10. Breast cancer is a heterogeneous disease with diverse molecular, phenotypic, and pathologic changes. It may be heterogeneous from its initial preinvasive stages. Altogether three models are proposed for breast carcinogenesis including (1) the multistep sequential acquisition model, (2) the telomere crisis model, and (3) the imprinted stem cell model. Several lines of evidence suggest multiple genetic pathways of complex crosstalking networks that progress toward malignancy.

11. DCIS refers to a malignant heterogeneous group of lesions limited to ducts and lobules. Because not all DCIS lesions progress to invasion or become clinically significant, the main concern is which DCIS lesions become invasive. LCIS originates from the duct-lobular unit and appears not to be associated with stromal involvement.

12. Dominating the cancer field is the idea that epithelial function depends on the *entire* tissue including the stroma or microenvironment. Breast cancer and other types of cancer are getting known as tissue-based diseases with a possible abnormal aberrant wound healing and inflammatory stromal (reactive stroma) component. Early alterations in the stroma include (1) mesenchymal cells (embryonic) fibroblasts; (2) endothelial cells; and (3) immune cells, including macrophages.

13. Epithelial-mesenchymal transition (EMT) is the distinctive phenotype created from the change in tumor tissue architecture (remodeled tissue) resulting from the wound-heal-ing response. Pathologically, this tissue change is known as desmoplastic stroma.

14. The exact molecular events leading to breast cancer invasion are complex and not completely understood. These events involve genetic and epigenetic alterations with telomere dysfunction and chromosomal alterations. Numerous signaling pathways induce both EMT and invasive cancer by activating master families of transcriptional regulators (Snail, Slug, Twist, ZeB1). These regulators inhibit cell adhesion molecules (e.g., E-cadherin) causing the dismantling of epithelial cell-cell junctions enabling the epithelial cells to become motile and invade surrounding tissue.

15. The first clinical manifestation of breast cancer is usually a small, painless lump in the breast. Other manifestations include palpable lymph nodes in the axilla, dimpling of the skin, nipple and skin retraction, nipple discharge, ulcerations, reddened skin, and bone pain associated with bony metastases.

16. Treatment is based on the extent or stage of the cancer and includes surgery, radiation, chemotherapy, hormone therapy, and biologic therapy.

17. Gynecomastia is the overdevelopment (hyperplasia) of breast tissue in a male. It is first seen as a firm, palpable mass at least 2 cm in diameter located in the subareolar area. Gynecomastia affects 32% to 40% of the male population. Incidence is greatest among adolescents and men older than 50 years.

18. Gynecomastia is caused by hormonal or breast tissue alterations that cause estrogen to dominate. These alterations can result from systemic disorders, drugs, neoplasms, or idiopathic causes.

19. Although breast cancer is relatively uncommon in men, it has a poor prognosis because men tend to delay seeking treatment. Most breast cancers in men are ER+. Incidence is greatest in men in their 60s and incidence has been increasing.

20. Possible risk factors for male breast cancer include gynecomastia, radiation of the chest wall, germline mutations in BRCA1 or BRCA2, family history of breast cancer, Klinefelter syndrome, testicular disorders, obesity, and other genetic factors.

KEY TERMS

Acute bacterial prostatitis, 862
Adenomyosis, 839
Amenorrhea, 820
Amphiregulin (AREG), 882
Anorgasmia (orgasmic dysfunction), 849
Anovulation, 821
Atypical lobular hyperplasia (ALH), 875
Atypical hyperplasia (AH), 875
Balanitis, 852
Bartholinitis (Bartholin cyst), 832
Benign breast disease (BBD), 872
Benign prostatic hyperplasia (BPH) (benign prostatic hypertrophy), 860
Carcinoma-associated fibroblast (CAF), 867
Central precocious puberty, 818
Cervical dysplasia, 841

Cervicitis, 832
Chronic bacterial prostatitis, 862
Complete precocious puberty, 818
Complex sclerosing lesion (radial scar), 874
Corpus luteum cyst, 837
Cryptorchidism, 856
Cyst, 873
Cystocele, 834
Cystourethrocele, 835
Dermoid cyst, 837
Disorders of desire (inhibited sexual desire, decreased libido), 848
Ductal carcinoma in situ (DCIS), 898
Ductal hyperplasia, 875
Dysfunctional uterine bleeding (DUB), 822
Dyspareunia (painful intercourse), 849

Ectopic testis, 856
Endometrial polyp, 837
Endometriosis, 839
Enterocele, 836
Epididymitis, 859
Epithelial-mesenchymal transition (EMT), 901
Epithelial hyperplasia, 874
Fibrocystic change (FCC), 873
Florid hyperplasia, 874
Follicular cyst, 836
Functional cyst, 836
Galactorrhea (inappropriate lactation), 871
Gynecomastia, 909
Hirsutism, 822
Hydrocele, 855

KEY TERMS—cont'd

Hyperprolactinemia, 821
Infertility, 849
Inflammatory stromal (reactive stroma) component, 900
Invasive breast carcinoma, 901
Invasive carcinoma of the cervix, 842
Leiomyoma (myoma, uterine fibroid), 837
Lobular carcinoma in situ (LCIS), 899
Lobular hyperplasia, 875
Lobular involution, 882
Mammographic density (MD), 887
Mixed precocious puberty, 819
Mucopurulent cervicitis (MPC), 832
Nonbacterial prostatitis, 863
Nonpuerperal hyperprolactinemia, 871
Oophoritis, 828
Orchitis, 857
p16 (INK4A), 902
Papilloma, 875
Paraphimosis, 850

Partial precocious puberty, 818
Pelvic inflammatory disease (PID), 828
Pessary, 833
Peyronie disease (bent nail syndrome), 851
Phimosis, 850
Polycystic ovary syndrome (PCOS), 824
Precocious puberty, 818
Premenstrual dysphoric disorder (PMDD), 826
Premenstrual syndrome (PMS), 826
Priapism, 852
Primary amenorrhea, 820
Primary dysmenorrhea, 819
Prolactin-inhibiting factor (PIF), 871
Prostate-specific antigen (PSA), 867
Prostatitis, 861
Prostatodynia, 861
Radial sclerosing lesions, 874
Rapid orgasm, 849
Rectocele, 836

Retrograde menstruation, 839
Salpingitis, 828
Sclerosing adenosis, 874
Sclerosing papillary proliferation, 874
Secondary amenorrhea, 820
Secondary dysmenorrhea, 819
Sexual dysfunction, 869
Spermatocele, 855
Torsion of the testis, 856
Urethral stricture, 850
Urethritis, 850
Urethrocele, 835
Uterine prolapse, 833
Uterine sarcoma, 846
Vaginismus, 848
Vaginitis, 830
Variant HMEC (vHMEC), 902
Varicocele, 854
Vulvovestibulitis (VV), 832
Xenoestrogen, 893

REFERENCES

1. American Cancer Society: *Cancer facts & figures—2009*, Atlanta, 2009, American Cancer Society.
2. Slyper AH: The pubertal timing controversy in the USA and a review of possible causative factors for the advance in timing of onset of puberty, *Clin Endocrinol* 65(1):1-8, 2006.
3. Euling SY et al: Examination of US puberty-timing data from 1940 to 1994 for secular trends: panel findings, *Pediatrics* 121(Suppl 3):S172-S191, 2008.
4. Kaplowitz P: Pubertal development in girls: secular trends, *Curr Opin Obstet Gynecol* 18(5):487-491, 2006.
5. McDowell MA et al: Has age at menarche changed? Results from the National Health and Nutrition Examination Survey (NHANES) 1999-2004, *J Adolesc Health* 40(3):227-231, 2007.
6. Jospe N: Disorders of pubertal development. In Osborn LM et al, editors: *Pediatrics*, Philadelphia, 2005, Mosby.
7. Healtheon/WebMD: Hypothalamic disorders. In *Scientific American Medicine*, 1999. Available at www.samed.com/sam/forms/index.htm.
8. Burchett MLR et al: Endocrine and metabolic diseases. In Burns CE et al, editors: *Pediatric primary care*, St Louis, 2009, Saunders.
9. DiVasta AD, Gordon CM: Hormone replacement therapy for the adolescent patient, *Ann N Y Acad Sci* 1135:204-211, 2008.
10. Foster DL et al: Programming of GnRH feedback controls timing puberty and adult reproductive activity, *Mol Cell Endocrinol* 254-255:109-119, 2006.
11. Kauffman AS et al: Emerging ideas about kissepeptin-GPR54 signaling in the neuroendocrine regulation of reproduction, *Trends Neurosci* 30(10):504-511, 2007.
12. Parent AS et al: The timing of normal puberty and the age limits of sexual precocity: variations around the world, secular trends, and changes after migration, *Endocr Rev* 24(5):668-693, 2003.
13. Fenichel P: Delayed puberty, *Endocr Dev* 7:106-128, 2004.
14. Carel JC, Leger J: Clinical practice. Precocious puberty, *N Engl J Med* 358(22):2366-2377, 2008.
15. Muir A: Precocious puberty, *Pediatr Rev* 27(10):373-381, 2006.
16. Papathanasiou A, Hadjiathanasiou C: Precocious puberty, *Pediatr Endocrinol Rev* 3(Suppl 1):182-187, 2006.
17. Dawood MY: Primary dysmenorrhea: advances in pathogenesis and management, *Obstet Gynecol* 108(2):428-441, 2006.
18. Marjoribanks J, Proctor ML, Farquhar C: Nonsteroidal anti-inflammatory drugs for primary dysmenorrhea, *Cochrane Database Syst Rev* (4):CD001751, 2003.
19. Speroff L, Fritz MA: *Clinical gynecologic endocrinology and infertility*, ed 7, Philadelphia, 2005, Lippincott Williams & Wilkins.
20. Latthe PL et al: Factors predisposing women to chronic pelvic pain: systematic review, *Br J Med* (7544):749-755, 2006.
21. French L: Dysmenorrhea in adolescents: diagnosis and treatment, *Paediatr Drugs* 10(1):1-7, 2008.
22. Daley AJ: Exercise and primary dysmenorrhoea: a comprehensive and critical review of the literature, *Sports Med* 38(8):659-670, 2008.
23. Harel Z: Dysmenorrhea in adolescents and young adults: from pathophysiology to pharmacological treatments and management strategies, *Exp Opin Pharmacother* 9(15):2661-2672, 2008.
24. Proctor ML et al: Transcutaneous electrical nerve stimulation and acupuncture for primary dysmenorrhea, *Cochrane Database Syst Rev* (1):CD002123, 2002.
25. Saenger P: Growth-promoting strategies in Turner's syndrome, *J Clin Endocrinol Metab* 84(12):4345, 1999.
26. Halvorson LM: Amenorrhea. In Schorge JO et al, editors: *Williams gynecology*, pp 512-531, New York, 2008, McGraw-Hill.
27. Reid RL: Amenorrhea. In Copeland LJ, Farrell JF, editors: *Textbook of gynecology*, ed 2, Philadelphia, 2000, Saunders.
28. Wetzel W: Micronized progesterone: a new option for women's health care, *Nurse Pract* 24(5):62, 1999.
29. Warren MP, Biller MK, Shangold MD: A new clinical option for hormone replacement therapy in women with secondary amenorrhea: effects of cyclic administration of progesterone from the sustained-release vaginal gel Crinone (45 and 8%) on endometrial morphologic features and withdrawal bleeding, *Am J Obstet Gynecol* 180(1):42, 1999.
30. Practice Committee of the American Society for Reproductive Medicine: Practice guideline: current evaluation of amenorrhea, *Fertil Steril* 86(5 Suppl):S148-S155, 2006.
31. Ely JW et al: Abnormal uterine bleeding: a management algorithm, *J Am Board Fam Med* 19(6):590-602, 2006.
32. Pitkin J: Dysfunctional uterine bleeding, *Br J Med* 334(7603):1110-1111, 2007.
33. Schorge JO et al, editors: *Williams gynecology*, New York, 2008, McGraw-Hill.
34. Prior JC: Perimenopause: the complex endocrinology of the menopausal transition, *Endocr Rev* 19(4):397, 1998.
35. Burger HG et al: Cycle and hormone changes during perimenopause: the key role of ovarian function, *Menopause* 15(4 Pt 1):603-612, 2008.
36. Dasgupta A, Rehman HU: Neuroendocrinology of menopause, *Minerva Ginecol* 58(1):25-33, 2006.

37. Hickey MJ et al: Progestogens versus oestrogens and progestogens for irregular uterine bleeding associated with anovulation, *Cochrane Database Syst Rev* (4):CD001895, 2007.

38. Sharp HT: Assessment of new technology in the treatment of idiopathic menorrhagia and uterine leiomyomata, *Obstet Gynecol* 108:990-1003, 2006.

39. Azziz R et al: The Androgen Excess and PCOS Society criteria for the polycystic ovary syndrome: the complete task force report, *Fertil Steril*, October 22, 2008, [Epub ahead of print].

40. Ehrmann DA: Genetic contributions to glucose intolerance in polycystic ovary syndrome, *Reprod Biomed Online* 9(1):28-34, 2004.

41. Franks S et al: Development of polycystic ovary syndrome: involvement of genetic and environmental factors, *Int J Androl* 29(1):278-285, 2006.

42. Ehrmann DA: Polycystic ovary syndrome, *N Engl J Med* 352(12): 1223-1236, 2005.

43. Milsom I: The levonorgestrel-releasing intrauterine system as an alternative to hysterectomy in peri-menopausal women, *Contraception* 75(6 Suppl):S152-S154, 2007.

44. Simoni M et al: Functional genetic polymorphisms and female reproductive disorders: part I: polycystic ovary syndrome and ovarian response, *Hum Reprod Update* 14(5):459-484, 2008.

45. Diamanti-Kandarakis E: Insulin resistance in PCOS, *Endocrine* 30(1):13-17, 2006.

46. Norman RJ et al: Polycystic ovary syndrome, *Lancet* 370(9588): 685-697, 2007.

47. Mendonca HC et al: Positive correlation of serum leptin with estradiol levels in patients with polycystic ovary syndrome, *Braz J Med Biol Res* 37(5):729-736, 2004.

48. Diamanti-Kandarakis E: Polycystic ovarian syndrome: pathophysiology, molecular aspects and clinical implications, *Expert Rev Mol Med* 10(2):e3, 2008.

49. King J: Polycystic ovary syndrome, *J Midwifery Womens Health* 51(6):415-422, 2006.

50. Teede HJ et al: Insulin resistance, the metabolic syndrome, diabetes, and cardiovascular disease risk in women with PCOS, *Endocrine* 30(1):45-53, 2006.

51. Palomba S et al: Outlook: metformin use in infertile patients with polycystic ovary syndrome: an evidence-based overview, *Reprod Biomed Online* 16(3):327-335, 2008.

52. Palomba S et al: Role of metformin in patients with polycystic ovary syndrome: the state of the art, *Minerva Ginecol* 60(1):77-82, 2008.

53. Nader S: Ovulation induction in polycystic ovary syndrome, *Minerva Ginecol* 60(1):53-61, 2008.

54. Sinawat S et al: Long versus short course treatment with metformin and clomiphene citrate for ovulation induction in women with PCOS, *Cochrane Database Syst Rev* (1):CD006226, 2008.

55. Moran LJ et al: Dietary therapy in polycystic ovary syndrome, *Semin Reprod Med* 26(1):85-92, 2008.

56. Yonkers KA et al: Premenstrual syndrome, *Lancet* 371(9619): 1200-1210, 2008.

57. Halbreich U: The etiology, biology, and evolving pathology of premenstrual syndromes, *Psychoneuroendocrinology* 28(3): 55-99, 2003.

58. Halbreich U, Monacelli E: Some clues to the etiology of premenstrual syndrome/premenstrual dysphoric disorder, *Prim Psychiatry* 11:33-40, 2004.

59. Freeman EW: Luteal phase administration for agents for the treatment of premenstrual dysphoric disorder, *DNS Drugs* 18(7):435-468, 2004.

60. Wyatt KM et al: The effectiveness of GnRHa with and without 'add-back' therapy in treating premenstrual syndrome: a meta analysis, *BJOG* 111(6):585-593, 2004.

61. Rapkin AJ: Premenstrual symptoms: current concepts in diagnosis and treatment, *J Reprod Med* 51(4):337-338, 2006.

62. Yonkers KA et al: Efficacy of a new low-dose oral contraceptive with drospirenone in premenstrual dysphoric disorder, *Obstet Gynecol* 106(3):492-501, 2005.

63. Banikarim C, Chacko MR: Pelvic inflammatory disease in adolescents, *Semin Pediatr Infect Dis* 16(3):175-180, 2005.

64. Centers for Disease Control and Prevention (CDC): Sexually transmitted diseases treatment guidelines, *MMWR Mortal Morb Wkly Rep* :1-94, 2006.

65. Saini S et al: Role of anaerobes in acute pelvic inflammatory disease, *Indian J Med Microbiol* 21(3):189-192, 2003.

66. Richter HE et al: The association of interleukin-6 with clinical and laboratory parameters of acute pelvic inflammatory disease, *Am J Obstet Gynecol* 181(4):940, 1999.

67. Peeling RW et al: Antibody response to the chlamydial heat-shock protein 60 in an experimental model of chronic pelvic inflammatory disease in monkeys, *J Infect Dis* 180(3):774-779, 1999.

68. Ness RB et al: A cluster analysis of bacterial vaginosis-associated microflora and pelvic inflammatory disease, *Am J Epidemiol* 162(6):585-590, 2005.

69. Haggerty CL et al: *Mycoplasma genitalium* among women with nongonococcal, nonchlamydial pelvic inflammatory disease, *Infect Dis Obstet Gynecol* 2006:30184, 2006.

70. Haggerty CL, Ness RB: Diagnosis and treatment of pelvic inflammatory disease, *Womens Health (Lond Engl)* 4(4):383-397, 2008.

71. Pellati D et al: Genital tract infections and infertility, *Eur J Obstet Gynecol Reprod Biol* 140(1):3-11, 2008.

72. Centers for Disease Control and Prevention (CDC): *Sexually transmitted disease surveillance, 2006*, Atlanta, 2007, US Department of Health and Human Services.

73. Centers for Disease Control and Prevention (CDC): Update to CDC's sexually transmitted diseases treatment guidelines, 2006: Fluoroquinolones no longer recommended for treatment of gonococcal infections, *MMWR* 332-336, 2007.

74. Goldstein AT, Burrows L: Vulvodynia, *J Sex Med* 5(1):5-14, quiz 15, 2008.

75. Farage MA et al: Determining the cause of vulvovaginal symptoms, *Obstet Gynecol Surv* 63(7):445-464, 2008.

76. Zolnoun DK et al: A conceptual model for the pathophysiology of vulvar vestibulitis syndrome, *Obstet Gynecol Surv* 61(6):395-401, quiz 423, 2006.

77. Gunter J: Vulvodynia: new thoughts on a devastating condition, *Obstet Gynecol Surv* 62(12):812-819, 2007.

78. Landry TS et al: The treatment of provoked vestibulodynia: a critical review, *Clin J Pain* 24(2):155-171, 2008.

79. Zolnoun DA et al: Overnight 5% lidocaine ointment for treatment of vulvar vestibulitis, *Obstet Gynecol* 102(1):84-87, 2003.

80. Nygaard I et al: Prevalence of symptomatic pelvic floor disorders in US women, *JAMA* 300(11):1311-1316, 2008.

81. Kim S et al: A review of the epidemiology and pathophysiology of pelvic floor dysfunction: do racial differences matter? *J Obstet Gynaecol Can* 27(3):251-259, 2005.

82. Jelovsek JE et al: Pelvic organ prolapse, *Lancet* 369(9566):1027-1038, 2007.

83. Wai CY: Urinary incontinence. In Schorge JO et al, editors: *Williams gynecology*, pp 512-531, New York, 2008, McGraw-Hill.

84. Hughes D: Pelvic organ prolapse. In Schorge JO et al, editors: *Williams gynecology*, pp 532-555, New York, 2008, McGraw-Hill.

85. Hoffman BL: Pelvic mass. In Schorge JO et al, editors: *Williams gynecology*, pp 187-224, New York, 2008, McGraw-Hill.

86. McCartney CR et al: Hypothalamic regulation of cyclic ovulation: evidence that the increase in gonadotropin-releasing hormone pulse frequency during the follicular phase reflects the gradual loss of the restraining effects of progesterone, *J Clin Endocrin Metab* 87(5):2194-2200, 2002.

87. Silberstein T et al: Endometrial polyps in reproductive-age fertile and infertile women, *Isr Med Assoc J* 8(3):192-195, 2006.

88. Machtinger R et al: Transvaginal ultrasound and diagnostic hysteroscopy as a predictor of endometrial polyps: risk factors for premalignancy and malignancy, *Int J Gynecol Cancer* 15(2):325-328, 2005.

89. Okolo S: Incidence, aetiology and epidemiology of uterine fibroids, *Best Pract Res Clin Obstet Gynaecol* 22(4):571-588, 2008.

90. Hoffman BL: Pelvic mass. In Schorge JO et al, editors: *Williams gynecology*, pp 197-224, New York, 2008, McGraw-Hill.

91. Palomba S et al: Long-term effectiveness and safety of GnRH agonist plus raloxifene administration in women with uterine leiomyomas, *Hum Reprod* 19(6):1308-1314, 2004.

92. Olive DL, Lindeheim SR, Pritts EA: Non-surgical management of leiomyoma: impact on fertility, *Curr Opin Obstet Gynecol* 16(3): 239-243, 2004.

93. Carr BR: Endometriosis. In Schorge JO et al, editors: *Williams gynecology*, pp 225-243, New York, 2008, McGraw-Hill.

94. Melin AP et al: Endometriosis and the risk of cancer with special emphasis on ovarian cancer, *Hum Reprod* 21(5):1237-1242, 2006.

95. Sampson JA: Peritoneal endometriosis due to the menstrual dissemination of endometrial tissue into the peritoneal cavity, *Am J Obstet Gynecol* 14:422, 1927.

96. Suzuki T et al: Impact of ovarian endometrioma on oocytes and pregnancy outcome in in vitro fertilization, *Fertil Steril* 83(4):908-913, 2005.

97. Gupta S et al: Pathogenic mechanisms in endometriosis-associated infertility, *Fertil Steril* 90(2):247-257, 2008.

98. Chwalisz K et al: Selective progesterone receptor modulator development and use in the treatment of leiomyomata and endometriosis, *Endocr Rev* 26(3):423-438, 2005.

99. Ozkan S et al: Endometriosis and infertility: epidemiology and evidence-based treatments, *Ann N Y Acad Sci* 1127:92-100, 2008.

100. Widdice LE, Moscicki AB: Updated guidelines for Papanicolaou tests, colposcopy, and human papillomavirus testing in adolescents, *J Adolesc Health* 43(4 Suppl):S41-S51, 2008.

101. Griffith WF: Preinvasive lesions of the lower genital tract. In Scorge JO et al, editors: *Williams gynecology*, pp 617-645, New York, 2008, McGraw-Hill Medical.

102. Smith JS et al: *Chlamydia trachomatis* and invasive cervical cancer: a pooled analysis of the IARC multicentric case-control study, *Int J Cancer* 111(3):431-439, 2004.

103. Danso DF et al: Cervical screening and management of cervical intraepithelial neoplasia in HIV-positive women, *Int J STD AIDS* 17(9):579-584; quiz 585-587, 2006.

104. Research report: Combination therapy for cervical cancer, *Womens Health Prim Care* 2(60):479, 1999.

105. Conner MR, Collins MM: Human papillomavirus infection and the HPV vaccine: what are the facts? *JAAPA* 21(10):32-34, 2008:37, 2008.

106. Dunne EF et al: A review of prophylactic human papillomavirus vaccines: recommendations and monitoring in the US, *Cancer* 113 (10 Suppl):2995-3003, 2008.

107. National Cancer Institute: *Cancer statistic fact sheet 2008*, Bethesda, MD, 2008, National Institutes of Health.

108. Nishida KJ: Vaginal cancer. In Schorge JO et al, editors: *Williams gynecology*, pp 677-686, New York, 2008, McGraw-Hill.

109. Centers for Disease Control and Prevention: *HPV fact sheet*, Atlanta, 2007, Department of Health and Human Services.

110. Lea JS: Invasive cancer of the vulva. In Schorge JO et al, editors: *Williams gynecology*, pp 665-676, New York, 2008, McGraw-Hill.

111. Miller DS: Endometrial cancer. In Schorge JO et al, editors: *Williams gynecology*, pp 687-705, New York, 2008, McGraw-Hill.

112. Lu HK, Broaddus RR: Gynecologic cancers in Lynch syndrome/HNPCC, *Fam Cancer* 4(3):249-254, 2005.

113. Tao MH et al: Oral contraceptive and IUD use and endometrial cancer: a population-based case-control study in Shanghai, China, *Int J Cancer* 119(9):2142-2147, 2006.

114. Bandera EV et al: Association between dietary fiber and endometrial cancer: a dose-response meta-analysis, *Am J Clin Nutr* 86(6):1730-1737, 2007.

115. Linkov F et al: Endometrial hyperplasia, endometrial cancer and prevention: gaps in existing research of modifiable risk factors, *Eur J Cancer* 44(12):1632-1644, 2008.

116. Schorge JO: Uterine sarcoma. In Schorge JO et al, editors: *Williams gynecology*, pp 706-715, New York, 2008, McGraw-Hill.

117. Schildkraut JM et al: Impact of progestin and estrogen potency in oral contraceptives on ovarian cancer risk, *J Natl Cancer Inst* 94(1):32-38, 2002.

118. Blast RC, Mills GB: Molecular pathogenesis of ovarian cancer. In Mendelsohn J et al, editors: *The molecular basis of cancer*, ed 2, Philadelphia, 2001, Saunders.

119. Corney DC et al: (2008). Role of p53 and Rb in ovarian cancer, *Adv Exp Med Biol* 622:99-117, 2008:2008, 2008.

120. Schorge JO: Epithelial ovarian cancer. In Schorge JO et al, editors: *Williams gynecology*, pp 716-737, New York, 2008, McGraw-Hill.

121. Schorge JO: Ovarian germ cell and sex cord-stromal tumors. In Schorge JO et al, editors: *Williams gynecology*, pp 738-754, New York, 2008, McGraw-Hill.

122. See HT, Kavanagh JJ: Novel agents in epithelial ovarian cancer, *Cancer Invest* 22(Suppl 2):29-44, 2004.

123. Hayes RD et al: Risk factors for female sexual dysfunction in the general population: exploring factors associated with low sexual function and sexual distress, *J Sex Med* 5(7):1681-1693, 2008.

124. Krassas GE, Pontikides N: Male reproductive function in relation with thyroid alterations, *Best Pract Res Clin Endocrinol Metab* 18(2):183-195, 2004.

125. Wilcox AJ, Weinberg CR, Baird DD: Timing of sexual intercourse in relation to ovulation, *N Engl J Med* 33(23):1517, 1995.

126. Cunningham KA, Beagley KW: Male: genital tract chlamydial infection: implications for pathology and infertility, *Bio Reprod* 79(2):180-189, 2008.

127. LaRock DR, Sant GR: Lower urinary tract infections in men. In Nseyo UO, Weinman E, Lamm DL, editors: *Urology for primary care physicians*, Philadelphia, 1999, Saunders.

128. Taylor-Robinson D: Nongonoccal urethritis and antibiotic-resistant *Mycoplasma genitalium* infection, *Clinical Infectious Diseases* 47:1554-1555, 2008.

129. McAninch JW: Disorders of the penis and male urethra. In Tanagho EA, McAninch JW, editors: *Smith's general urology*, ed 17, Norwalk, CT, 2008, McGraw Hill Lange.

130. Tang SH et al: Adult urethral stricture disease after childhood hypospadias repair, *Adv Urol* 150315:2008, [Epub 2008 Nov 4].

131. American Cancer Society: *Penile cancer resource center*, 2008. Available at www.cancer.org

132. Madsen BS et al: Risk factors for squamous cell carcinoma of the penis—population-based case-control study in Denmark, *Biomarkers Prev* 17(10):2683-2691, 2008.

133. Smith JF, Walsh TJ, Lue TF: Peyronie's disease: a critical appraisal of current diagnosis and treatment, *Int J Impot Res* 20(5):445-459, 2008.

134. Altman AL et al: Cocaine associated priapism, *J Urol* 161(6):1817-1818, 1999.

135. American Cancer Society: *Penile cancer*. In *Cancer response system document #10005*, New York, 1995, The Society.

136. Nasca MR, Innocenzi D, Micali G: Penile cancer among patients with genital lichen sclerosus, *J Am Acad Dermatol* 41(6):911-914, 1999.

137. Presti JC, Herr HW: Genital tumors. In Tanagho EA, McAninch JW, editors: *Smith's general urology*, ed 14, Norwalk, CT, 1995, Appleton & Lange.

138. Hegarty PK: Penile preserving surgery and surgical strategies to maximize penile form and function in penile cancer: recommendations from the United Kingdom experience, *World J Urol* 2008 Jul 18. [Epub ahead of print].

139. Lindegarrds JC et al: A retrospective analysis of 82 cases of cancer of the penis, *Br J Urol* 77(6):883, 1996.

140. Kolon TF, Albertsen PC: Diagnosis and treatment of scrotal abnormalities, *Clin Advisor* 47(47-48):53-56, 2000.

141. Benoff S, Marmar JL, Hurley IR: Molecular and other predictors for infertility in patients with varicoceles, *Front Biosci* 14:3641-3672, 2009.

142. McAninch JW: Disorders of the testis, scrotum, and spermatic cord. In Tanagho EA, McAninch JW, editors: *Smith's general urology*, ed 14, Norwalk, CT, 1995, Appleton & Lange.

143. Galejs LE, Usaf M: Diagnosis and treatment of the acute scrotum, *Am Fam Physician* 59(4):817, 1999.

144. Del Pizzo JJ, Jarow JP: Management of male infertility. In Nseyo UO, Weinman E, Lamm DL, editors: *Urology for primary care physicians*, Philadelphia, 1999, Saunders.

145. Rosenthal MS: *The fertility sourcebook*, Los Angeles, 1998, Lowell House.

146. Walsh TJ et al: Prepubertal orchiopexy for crytorchidism may be associated with lower risk of testicular cancer, *J Urol* 178(4 Pt 1):1440-1446, 2007.

147. CancerNet: *Cancer facts: questions and answers about testicular cancer*, National Cancer Institute, 2000, Available at www.cancernet.nci.nih.gov.

148. Lanum DL: Carcinoma of the genitourinary system. In Nseyo UO, Weinman E, Lamm DL, editors: *Urology for primary care physicians*, Philadelphia, 1999, Saunders.

149. Gebrosky NP, Nseyo UO: Sexually transmitted diseases. In Nseyo UO, Weinman E, Lamm DL, editors: *Urology for primary care physicians*, Philadelphia, 1999, Saunders.

150. LaRock DR, Sant GR: Lower urinary tract infections. In Nseyo UO, Weinman E, Lamm DL, editors: *Urology for primary care physicians*, Philadelphia, 1999, Saunders.

151. Benign Prostatic hyperplasia (BPH)/Enlarged Prostate www.urology channel.com 2009

152. Lucia MS, Lambert JR: Growth factors in benign prostatic hyperplasia: basic science implications, *Curr Urol Rep* 9(4):272-278, 2008.

153. Sampson N, Madersbacher S, Berger P: [Pathophysiology and therapy of benign prostatic hyperplasia], *Wien Klin Wochenschr* 120(13-14):390-401, 2008.

154. Jepson JV, Bruskewitz RC: Clinical manifestations and indications for treatment. In Lepor H, editor: *Prostatic diseases*, Philadelphia, 2000, Saunders.

155. Barry MJ, Meigs JB: Benign prostatic hyperplasia. In Lepor H, editor: *Prostatic diseases*, Philadelphia, 2000, Saunders.

156. Narayan P: Neoplasms of the prostate gland. In Tanagho EA, McAninch JW, editors: *Smith's general urology*, ed 14, Norwalk, CT, 1995, Appleton & Lange.

157. Roehrborn CG: The role of guidelines in the diagnosis and treatment of benign prostatic hyperplasia. In Lepor H, editor: *Prostatic diseases*, Philadelphia, 2000, Saunders.

158. d'Ancona FC: Nonablative minimally invasive thermal therapies in the treatment of symptomatic benign prostatic hyperplasia, *Curr Opin Urol* 18(1):21-27, 2008.

159. Chiu KY, Yong CR: Effects of finasteride on prostate volume and prostate specific antigen, *J Chin Med Assoc* 67(11):571-574, 2004.

160. Shibata A, Ma J, Whittemore AS: Prostate cancer incidence and mortality in the United States and the United Kingdom, *J Natl Cancer Inst* 90(16):1230-1231, 1998.

161. Ma RW, Chapman K: A systematic review of the effect of diet on prostate cancer prevention and treatment, *J Hum Nutr Diet* April 1, 2009[Epub ahead of print].

162. Signorello LB, Adami H: Prostate cancer. In Adami H, Hunter D, Trichopoulos D, editors: *Textbook of cancer epidemiology*, New York, 2002, Oxford Press.

163. Calle EE et al: Overweight, obesity, and mortality from cancer in a prospectively studied cohort of U.S. adults, *N Engl J Med* 348(17):1625-1638, 2003.

164. Rodriquez C et al: Body mass index, height, and prostate cancer mortality in two large cohorts of adult men in the United States, *Cancer Epidemiol Biomarkers Prev* 10(4):345-353, 2001.

165. Platz EA: Energy imbalance and prostate cancer, *J Nutr* 132(11 Suppl):3471S-3481S, 2002.

166. Bosland MC: The role of steroid hormones in prostate carcinogenesis, *J Natl Cancer Inst Monogr* 27:39-66, 2000.

167. Heber D, Fair WR, Ornish D: Nutrition and prostate cancer: a monograph from the CaP CURE Nutrition Project, ed 2, Santa Monica, CA, 1998, CaP CURE.

168. Denis L et al: Diet and its preventive role in prostatic disease, *Eur Urol* 35(5-6):377, 1999.

169. Gaziano JM et al: Vitamins E and C in the prevention of prostate cancer and total cancer in men: the Physicians' Health Study II randomized controlled trial, *J Am Med Assoc* 301:52-62, 2009.

170. Lippman SM et al: Effect of selenium and vitamin E on risk of prostate cancer and other cancers: the Selenium and Vitamin E Cancer Prevention Trial (SELECT), *J Am Med Assoc* 301:39-51, 2009.

171. Zhao XY et al: 1-Alpha,25-dihydroxyvitamin D3 inhibits prostate cancer cell growth by androgen-dependent and androgen-independent mechanisms, *Endocrinology* 141(7):2548, 2000.

172. Tretli S et al: Association between serum 25(OH)D and death from prostate cancer, *Br J Cancer* 100(3):450-454, 2009.

173. Arnot R: *The prostate cancer protection plan: the powerful foods, supplements, and drugs that could save your life*, Boston, 2000, Little, Brown.

174. Giovannucci E et al: Intake of carotenoids and retinol in relation to risk of prostate cancer, *J Natl Cancer Inst* 87(23):1767, 1995.

175. Ebling DW et al: Development of prostate cancer after pituitary dysfunction: a report of 8 patients, *Urology* 49(4):564, 1998.

176. Oosthuizen JM et al: Melatonin and steroid-dependent carcinomas, *Andrologia* 21(5):429, 1989.

177. Roberts JT, Essehigh DM: Adenocarcinoma of prostate in 40-year-old body builders, *Lancet* 2(8509):742, 1986.

178. Cunha GR et al: Role of the stromal microenvironment in carcinogenesis of the prostate, *Int J Cancer* 107(1):1-10, 2003.

179. Giovannucci E et al: A prospective cohort study of vasectomy and prostate cancer in US men, *JAMA* 269(7):873, 1993.

180. Peterson RE et al: Vasectomy and the risk of prostate cancer, *Am J Epidemiol* 135(3):324, 1992.

181. Honda GD et al: Vasectomy, cigarette smoking, and age at first sexual intercourse as risk factors for prostate cancer in middle-aged men, *Br J Cancer* 57(3):326, 1988.

182. Epstein JI: The lower urinary tract and male genital system. In Kumar V, Abbas AK, Fausto N, editors: *Robbins and Cotran pathologic basis of disease*, ed 8, Philadelphia, 2009, Saunders.

183. Carmen J et al: Quantitation of GSTP1 methylation in non-neoplastic prostatic tissue and organ-confined prostate adenocarcinoma, *J Natl Cancer Inst* 93:1671, 2001.

184. Sciarra A et al: Inflammation and chronic prostatic diseases: evidence for a link? *Eur Urol* 52(4):964-972, 2007.

185. Brown SL, Resnick MI: Transrectal ultrasound and the prostate biopsy: clinical and pathologic issues. In Lepor H, editor: *Prostatic diseases*, Philadelphia, 2000, Saunders.

186. Parnes HL, Thompson IM, Ford LG: Review article: prevention of hormone-related cancers: prostate cancer, *J Clin Oncol* 23(2):368-377, 2005.

187. Joyce JA, Pollard JU: Microenvironment regulation of metastasis, *Nat Rev Cancer* 9:239-252, 2009.

188. Tanejo SS: The rationale for early detection of prostate cancer. In Lepor H, editor: *Prostatic diseases*, Philadelphia, 2000, Saunders.

189. Moule JW et al: Prostate-specific antigen values at the time of prostate cancer diagnosis in African-American men, *JAMA* 274(16):1277, 1995.

190. Boorjian SA et al: The impact of discordance between biopsy and pathological Gleason scores on survival after radical prostatectomy, *J Urol* 181(1):95-104, 2009.

191. Schwenk TL: PSA screening lacks value, *N Engl J Med* 25(10):7-8, 2005.

192. Salgaller ML: Prostate cancer immunotherapy at the dawn of the new millennium, *Expert Opin Investig Drugs* 9(6):1217, 2000.

193. Kim ED, Lipshultz ED: Male infertility. In Copeland LJ, Farrell JF, editors: *Textbook of gynecology*, ed 2, Philadelphia, 2000, Saunders.

194. Pierik FH et al: Serum inhibin B as a marker of spermatogenesis, *J Clin Endocrinol Metab* 83(9):3110, 1998.

195. He Z et al: Small RNA molecules in the regulation of spermatogenesis, *Reproduction* 2009 Mar 24 [Epub ahead of print].

196. Harney KA, Smith LF: The breast. In DeCherney AH, Pernoll ML, editors: *Current obstetric and gynecologic diagnosis and treatment*, ed 8, Norwalk, CT, 1994, Appleton & Lange.

197. Haagensen CD: *Diseases of the breast*, Philadelphia, 1986, Saunders.

198. Kase N, Weingold AB, Gershenon DM, editors: *Principles and practice of clinical gynecology*, ed 2, New York, 1990, Churchill Livingstone.

199. Hartmann LC et al: Benign breast disease and the risk of breast cancer, *N Engl J Med* 353(3):229-237, 2005.

200. Collins LC et al: Magnitude and laterality of breast cancer risk according to histologic type of atypical hyperplasia: results from the Nurses' Health Study, *Cancer* 109(2):180-187, 2006.

201. Friedenreich C et al: Risk factors for benign proliferative breast disease, *Int J Epidemiol* 29(4):634, 2000.

202. Lester SC: The breast. In Kumar V, Abbas AK, Fausto N, editors: *Robbins and Cotran pathologic basis of disease*, ed 7, Philadelphia, 2005, Saunders.

203. Warsham MJ et al: Multiplicity of benign lesions is a risk factor for progression to breast cancer, *Clin Cancer Res* 13(18 Part 1):5474-5479, 2007.

204. Sanders ME et al: Interdependence of radial scar and proliferative disease with respect to invasive breast carcinoma risk to patients with benign breast biopsies, *Cancer* 106(7):1453-1461, 2006.

205. Berg JC et al: Breast cancer risk in women with radial scars in benign breast biopsies, *Breast Cancer Res Treat* 108(2):167-174, 2008.

206. Sharkey FE, Allred DC, Valente PT: Breast. In Damjanov I, Linder J, editors: *Anderson's pathology*, ed 10, St Louis, 1996, Mosby.

207. Lewis JT et al: An analysis of breast cancer risk in women with single, multiple, and atypical papilloma, *Am J Surg Pathol* 30(6):665-672, 2006.

208. Lampe JW et al: Plasma isoflavones and fibrocystic breast conditions and breast cancer among women in Shanghai, China, *Cancer Epidemiol Biomarkers Prev* 16(12):2579-2586, 2007.

209. Rohan TE et al: A randomized controlled trial of calcium plus vitamin D supplementation and risk of benign proliferative breast disease, *Breast Cancer Res Treat*, 2008 Oct 14 [Epub ahead of print.]

210. Hollowell JG et al: Iodine nutrition in the United States. Trends and public health implications: iodine excretion data from National Health and Nutrition Examination Surveys I and II (1971-1974 and 1988-1994), *J Clin Endocrinol Metab* 83(10):3401-3408, 1998.

211. World Health Organization, United Nations International Children's Emergency Fund, International Council for the Control of Iodine Deficiency Disorders: *Indicators for assessing iodine deficiency disorders and their control through salt iodination*, Geneva, 1994, World Health Organization.

212. Ghent WR et al: Iodine replacement in fibrocystic disease, *Can J Surg* 36(5):453-460, 1993.

213. Medeiros-Neto G: Iodine deficiency disorders. In DeGroot LJ, Jameson JL, editors: *Endocrinology*, ed, 4, Philadelphia, 2001, Saunders.

214. Eskin BA et al: Different tissue responses for iodine and iodide in rat thyroid and mammary glands, *Biol Trace Elem Res* 49(1):9-19, 1995.

215. Smyth PP: Role of iodine in antioxidant defense in thyroid and breast disease, *Biofactors* 19(3-4):121-130, 2003.

216. Tazebay UH et al: The mammary gland iodide transporter is expressed during lactation and in breast cancer, *Nat Med* 6(8):871-878, 2000.

217. Wapnir IL et al: Immunohistochemical profile of the sodium/iodide symporter in thyroid, breast, and other carcinomas using high density tissue microarrays and conventional sections, *J Clin Endocrinol Metab* 88(4):1880-1888, 2003.

218. Bogardus GM, Finley JW: Breast cancer and thyroid disease, *Surgery* 49:461-468, 1961.

219. Eskin BA et al: Iodine metabolism and breast cancer, *Trans N Y Acad Sci* 11:911-947, 1970.

220. Cann SA, van Netten JP, van Netten C: Hypothesis: iodine, selenium, and the development of breast cancer, *Cancer Causes Control* 11(2):121-127, 2000.

221. Funahashi H et al: Suppressive effect of iodine on DMBA-induced breast tumor growth in the rat, *J Surg Oncol* 61(3):209-213, 1996.

222. Funahashi H et al: Wakame seaweed suppresses the proliferation of 7,12-dimethylbenz(a)-anthracene-induced mammary tumors in rats, *Jpn J Cancer Res* 90(9):922-927, 1999.

223. Funahashi H et al: Seaweed prevents breast cancer? *Jpn J Cancer Res* 92(5):483-487, 2001.

224. LeMarchand K, Kolonel LN, Nomura AM: Breast cancer survival among Hawaii Japanese and Caucasian women: ten-year rates and survival by place of birth, *Am J Epidemiol* 122(4):571-578, 1985.

225. Minami Y et al: Trends in the incidence of female breast and cervical cancer in Miyagi prefecture, Japan 1959-1987, *Jpn J Cancer Res* 87(1):10-17, 1996.

226. Tajima N, Tsukuma H, Oskima A: Descriptive epidemiology of male breast cancer in Osaka, Japan, *J Epidemiol* 11(1):1-7, 2001.

227. Bosetti C, Gallus S, LaVecchia C: Aspirin and cancer risk: an updated quantitative review to 2005, *Cancer Causes Control* 17:871-888, 2006.

228. Mangiapane S, Blettner M, Schlattmann P: Aspirin use and breast cancer risk: a meta-analysis and meta-regression of observational studies from 2001 to 2005, *Pharmocoepidemiol Drug Saf* 17:115-124, 2008.

229. Gierach GL et al: Nonsteroidal anti-inflammatory drugs and breast cancer risk in the National Institutes of Health AARP diet and health study, *Breast Cancer Res* 10(2):R38, 2008.

230. Cook NR et al: Low-dose aspirin in the primary prevention of cancer: the Women's Health Study: a randomized control trial, *JAMA* 294:47-55, 2005.

231. Terry MB et al: Association of frequency and duration of aspirin use and hormone receptor status with breast cancer risk, *JAMA* 291(20):2433-2440, 2004.

232. Mueller RL, Scheidt S: History of drugs for thrombotic disease: discovery, development, and directions for the future, *Circulation* 89(1):432-449, 1994.

233. Smalley WE, DuBois RN: Colorectal cancer and nonsteroidal anti-inflammatory drugs, *Adv Pharmacol* 39:1-20, 1997.

234. Chang SH et al: Role of prostaglandin E2-dependent angiogenic switch in cyclooxygenase-2-induced breast cancer progression, *Proc Natl Acad Sci U S A* 101(2):591-596, 2004.

235. Hartmann LC et al: *COX-2 expression in atypia: correlation with breast cancer risk.* Presented at the 97th American Association for Cancer Research Annual Meeting, April 1-5, 2006, Washington, DC.

236. Subbaramaiah K et al: Transcription of cyclooxygenase-2 is enhanced in transformed mammary epithelial cells, *Cancer Res* 56(19): 4424-4429, 1996.

237. Zhao Y et al: Estrogen biosynthesis proximal to a breast tumor is stimulated by PGE$_2$ via cyclic AMP, leading to activation of promoter II of the CYP19 (aromatase) gene, *Endocrinology* 137(12):5739-5742, 1996.

238. Crawford YG et al: Histologically normal human mammary epithelia with silenced p16(INK4a) overexpress COX-2, promoting a premalignant program, *Cancer Cell* 5(3):263-273, 2004.

239. Shim V et al: Cyclooxygenase-2 expression is related to nuclear grade in ductal carcinoma in situ and is increased in its normal adjacent epithelium, *Cancer Res* 63(10):2347-2350, 2003.

240. Berg JW: Clinical implications of risk factors for breast cancer, *Cancer* 53(3 Suppl):589-591, 1984.

241. Axelrod D et al: Breast cancer in young women, *J Am Coll Surg* 206(3):1193-1203, 2008.

242. Reis LAG et al: *Cancer statistics review, 1975-2005*, Bethesda, MD, 2008, National Cancer Institute. Available at http://seer.cancer.gov/csr/1975_2005/

243. Sternlicht MD et al: Hormonal and local control of mammary branching morphogenesis, *Differentiation* 74:365-381, 2006.

244. Medina D: Mammary developmental fate and breast cancer risk, *Endocr Relat Cancer* 12:483-495, 2005.

245. Clarke LH et al: Differentiation of mammary gland as a mechanism to reduce breast cancer risk, *J Nutr* 136:2697S-2699S, 2006.

246. Trichopoulos D et al: Age at any birth and breast cancer risk, *J Int Cancer* 321:701-704, 1983.

247. White E: Projected changes in breast cancer incidence due to the trend toward delayed childbearing, *Am J Public Health* 77:495-497, 1987.

248. Medina D: Breast cancer: the protective effect of pregnancy, *Clin Cancer Res* 10(1 Pt 2):380S-384S, 2004.

249. Hsieh C et al: Dual effect of parity on breast cancer risk, *Eur J Cancer* 30A:969-973, 1994.

250. Williams EM et al: Short term increase in risk of breast cancer associated with full pregnancy, *BMJ* 300:578-579, 1990.

251. MacMahon B et al: Age at first birth and breast cancer, *Bull World Health Organ* 43:209-221, 1970.

252. Schedin P et al: Microenvironment of the involuting mammary gland mediates mammary cancer progression, *J Mammary Gland Biol Neoplasia* 12:71-82, 2007.

253. National Cancer Institute: National Cancer Institute Board of Scientific Advisors (BSA) and Board of Scientific Counselors: NCI summary report: early reproductive events and breast cancer, 2003. Available at http://www.cancerblog/cancerinfo/ere-workshop-report

254. Li Z et al: ETV6-NTRK3 fusion oncogenes initiate breast cancer from committed progenitors via activation of AP1 complex, *Cancer Cell* 12:542-558, 2007.

255. Shackleton M et al: Generation of a functional mammary gland from a single stem cell, *Nature* 439:84-88, 2006.

256. Siwko SK et al: Evidence that an early pregnancy causes a persistent decrease in the number of functional mammary epithelial stem cells—implications for pregnancy-induced protection against breast cancer, *Stem Cells*, September 11, 2008 [Epub ahead of print].

257. LaBarge MA, Petersen OW, Bissell MJ: Microenvironments and mammary stem cells, *Stem Cell Rev* 3:137-146, 2007.

258. LaMarca HL, Rosen JM: Hormones and mammary cell fate—what will I become when I grow up? *Endocrinol* 149(9):4317-4321, 2008.

259. Ciarloni L, Mallepell S, Brisken C: Amphiregulin is an essential mediator of estrogen receptor alpha function in mammary gland development, *Proc Natl Acad Sci U S A* 104:5455-5460, 2007.

260. Russo J et al: The protective role of pregnancy in breast cancer, *Breast Cancer Res* 8(3):131-142, 2005.

261. Milanese TR et al: Age-related lobular involution and risk of breast cancer, *J Natl Cancer Inst* 98(2):1600-1607, 2006.

262. Henson DE, Tarone RE: On the possible role of involution in the natural history of breast cancer, *Cancer* 71(6 Suppl):2154-2156, 1993.

263. Henson DE, Tarone RE: Involution and the etiology of breast cancer, *Cancer* 74(1 Suppl):424-429, 1994.

264. Clemmesen J: The Danish cancer registry: problems and results, *Acta Pathol Microbiol Scand* 25:26-30, 1948.

265. Cutler SY, Young JL: Third National Cancer Survey: incidence data, *Natl Cancer Inst Monog* 41, 1975.

266. Vorrherr H, editor: *The breast: morphology, physiology, and lactation*, New York, 1974, Academic Press.

267. Geschickter CD: *Diseases of the breast*, ed 2, Philadelphia, 1945, Lippincott.

268. Kelsey JL, Gammon MD, John EM: Reproductive factors and breast cancer, *Epidemiol Rev* 15:36-47, 1993.

269. Ursin G et al: Reproductive factors and subtypes of breast cancer defined by hormone receptor and histology, *Br J Cancer* 93:364-371, 2005.

270. Trichopoulos D et al: Age at any birth and breast cancer risk, *Int J Cancer* 31:701-704, 1983.

271. Henson DE, Tarone RE, Nsouli H: Lobular involution: the physiologic prevention of breast cancer, *J Natl Cancer Inst* 98(22):1589-1590, 2006.

272. Fenton SE: Endocrine-disrupting compounds and mammary gland development: early exposure and later life consequences, *Endocrinology* 147(6 Suppl):S18-S24, 2006.

273. Lanigan F et al: Molecular links between mammary gland development and breast cancer, *Cell Mol Life Sci* 64:3161-3184, 2007.

274. Russo J, Russo I: *Molecular basis of breast cancer: prevention and treatment,* Germany, 2004, Springer.

275. Cheskis BJ et al: Signaling by estrogens: mini review, *J Cell Physiol* 213(3):610-617, 2007.

276. Cheskis BJ et al: MNAR plays an important role in ERa activation of Src/MAPK and P13K/Akt signaling pathways, *Steroids* 73(9-10): 901-905, 2008.

277. Kininis M et al: Genomic analyses of transcription factor binding, histone acetylation, and gene expression reveal mechanistically distinct classes of estrogen-regulated promoters, *Mol Cell Biol* 27(14): 5090-5014, 2007.

278. Sasano H et al: New development in intracrinology of breast carcinoma: review, *Breast Cancer* 13(2):129-136, 2006.

279. Milliken EL: Ovarian hyperstimulation induces chromosome amplification and aneuploid mammary tumors independently of alterations in p53 in a transgenic mouse model of breast cancer, *Oncogene* 27(12):1759-1766, 2008.

280. Goepfert TM et al: Progesterone facilitates chromosome instability (aneuploidy) in *p53* null normal mammary epithelial cells, *FASEB J* 14(14):2221-2229, 2000.

281. Quick EL, Parry EM, Parry JM: Do oestrogens induce chromosome specific aneuploidy in vitro similar to the pattern of aneuploidy seen in breast cancer? *Mutat Res* 651(1-2):46-55, 2008.

282. Greendale GA et al: Effects of estrogen and estrogen-progestin on mammographic parenchymal density, *Ann Int Med* 130(4 Part 1): 262-269, 1999.

283. Ross RK et al: Effect of hormone replacement therapy on breast cancer risk: estrogen versus estrogen plus progestin, *J Natl Cancer Inst* 92(4):328-332, 2000.

284. Schairer C et al: Menopausal estrogen and estrogen-progestin replacement therapy and breast cancer risk, *JAMA* 283(4):485-491, 2000.

285. Russo J et al: 17 beta estradiol induces transformation and tumorigenesis in human breast epithelial cells, *FASEB J* 20:1-13, 2006.

286. Chetrite GS et al: Comparison of estrogen concentrations, estrone sulfatase and aromatase activities in normal and in cancerous, human breast tissues, *J Steroid Biochem Mol Biol* 72(1-2):23-27, 2000.

287. Pasqualine JR et al: Concentrations of estrone, estradiol, and estrone sulfate and evaluation of sulfatase and aromatase activities in pre- and postmenopausal breast cancer patients, *J Clin Endocrinol Metab* 81(4):1460-1464, 1996.

288. Labrie F: Intracrinology, *Mol Cell Endocrinol* 78:C113-C118, 1991.

289. Labrie F et al: Structure, regulation and role of 3 beta-hydroxysteroid dehydrogenase, 17 beta-hydroxysteroid dehydrogenase and aromatase enzymes in the formation of sex steroids in classical and peripheral intracrine tissues, *Bailliere's Clin Endocrinol Metab* 8(2):451-474, 1994.

290. Dowsett M: Future uses for aromatase inhibitors in breast cancer, *J Steroid Biochem Mol Biol* 61(3-6):261-266, 1997.

291. Miller WR, O'Neill J: The importance of local synthesis of estrogen within the breast, *Steroids* 50(4-6):537-548, 1987.

292. Foster PA: Steroid metabolism in breast cancer, *Minerva Endocrinology* 33:27-37, 2008.

293. Falany JL, Falany CN: Regulation of estrogen activity by sulfation in human MCF-7 breast cancer cells, *Oncol Res* 9(11-12):589-596, 1997.

294. Martel C et al: Distribution of 17 beta-hydroxysteroid dehydrogenase gene expression and activity in rat and human tissues, *J Steroid Biochem Mol Biol* 41(3-8):597-603, 1992.

295. Utsumi T et al: Steroid sulfatase expression is an independent predictor of recurrence in human breast cancer, *Cancer Res* 59(2): 377-381, 1999.

296. Miyoshi Y et al: High expression of steroid sulfatase in mRNA predicts poor prognosis in patients with estrogen receptor-positive breast cancer, *Clin Cancer Res* 9(6):2288-2293, 2003.

297. Stanway SJ et al: Phase 1 study of STX 64 (667 COUMATE) in breast cancer patients: the first study of a steroid sulfatase inhibitor, *Clin Cancer Res* 12:1585-1592, 2006.

298. Rajkumar L et al: Short-term exposure to pregnancy levels of estrogen prevents mammary carcinogenesis, *Proc Natl Acad Sci USA* 98(20): 11755-11759, 2001.

299. Yu H, Berkel H: Insulin-like growth factors and cancer, *J La State Med Assoc* 151(4):218, 1999.

300. Yee D, Lee AV: Crosstalk between the insulin-like growth factors and estrogens in breast cancer, *J Mammary Gland Biol Neoplasia* 5(1):107, 2000.

301. Rao ChV et al: Human chorionic gonadotropin decreases proliferation and invasion of breast cancer MCF-7 cells by inhibiting NF-κB and AP-1 activation, *J Biol Chem* 279(24):25503-25510, 2004.

302. Janssens JP et al: Human chorionic gonadotropin (hCG) and prevention of breast cancer, *Mol Cell Endocrinol* 269(1-2):93-98, 2007.

303. Russo IH, Russo J: Primary prevention of breast cancer by hormone-induced differentiation, *Recent Results Cancer Res* 174:111-130, 2007.

304. Tanaka Y et al: Gonadotropins stimulate growth of MCF-7 human breast cancer cells by promoting intercellular conversion of adrenal androgens to estrogens, *Oncol* 59(Suppl 11):19-23, 2000.

305. Collaborative Group on Hormonal Factors in Breast Cancer: Breast cancer and hormone replacement therapy: collaborative reanalysis of data from 51 epidemiological studies of 52,705 women with breast cancer and 108,411 women without breast cancer, *Lancet* 350: 1047-1059, 1997.

306. Pike MC et al: Estrogens, progestins, and risk of breast cancer, *Ernst Schering Found Symp Proc* (1):127-150, 2007.

307. Beral V, Reeves G, Banks E: Current evidence about the effect of hormone replacement therapy in the incidence of major conditions in postmenopausal women, *Br J Obstet Gynaecol* 112:692-695, 2005.

308. Million Women Study Collaborators: Breast cancer hormone-replacement therapy in the Million Women Study, *Lancet* 362: 419-427, 2003.

309. Women's Health Initiative: Effects of conjugated equine estrogen in postmenopausal women with hysterectomy, *JAMA* 291:1701-1712, 2004.

310. Adyl L et al: Serum concentrations of estrogens, sex hormone-binding globulin, and androgens and risk of breast cancer in postmenopausal women, *Int J Cancer* 119(10):2402-2407, 2006.

311. Endogenous Hormones and Breast Cancer Collaborative Group: Body mass index, serum sex hormones, and breast cancer risk in postmenopausal women, *J Natl Cancer Inst* 95:1218-1226, 2003.

312. Endogenous Hormones and Breast Cancer Collaborative Group: Free estradiol and breast cancer risk in postmenopausal women: comparison of measured and calculated values, *Cancer Epidemiol Biomarkers Prev* 12:1457-1461, 2003.

313. Miyoshi Y et al: Association of serum estrone levels with estrogen receptor-positive breast cancer risk in postmenopausal Japanese women, *Clin Cancer Res* 9(6):2229-2233, 2003.

314. Lee SA, Ross RK, Pike MC: An overview of menopausal oestrogen-progestin hormone therapy and breast cancer risk, *Br J Cancer* 92(11):2049-2058, 2005.

315. Fournier A et al: Brest cancer risk in relation to different types of hormone replacement therapy in the E3N-EPIC cohort, *Int J Cancer* 114:448-454, 2005.

316. Wood CE et al: Effects of estradiol with micronized progesterone or medroxyprogesterone acetate on risk markers for breast cancer in postmenopausal monkeys, *Breast Cancer Res Treat* 101:125-134, 2007.

317. Greendale GA et al: Postmenopausal hormone therapy and change in mammographic density, *J Natl Cancer Inst* 95:30-37, 2003.

318. Corrao G et al: Menopause hormone replacement therapy and cancer risk: an Italian record linkage investigation, *Ann Oncol* 19(1):150-155, 2008.

319. Groshong SD et al: Biphasic regulation of breast cancer cell growth by progesterone: role of the cyclin-dependent kinase inhibitors, p21 and p27 (Kip1), *Mol Endocrinol* 11(11):1593-1607, 1997.

320. Lange CA, Richer JK, Horwitz KB: Hypothesis: progesterone primes breast cancer cells for cross-talk with proliferative or antiproliferative signals, *Mol Endocrinol* 13(6):829-836, 1999.

321. Wu J, Brandt S, Hyder SM: Ligand- and cell-specific effects of signal transduction pathway inhibitors on progestin-induced vascular endothelial growth factor levels in human breast cancer cells, *Mol Endocrinol* 19(2):312-326, 2005.

322. Collaborative Group on Hormonal Factors in Breast Cancer (CGHFBC): Breast cancer and hormonal contraceptives: collaborative reanalysis of individual data on 53,297 women with breast cancer and 100,239 women without breast cancer from 54 epidemiological studies, *Lancet* 347(9017):1713-1727, 1996.

323. Ursin G et al: Use of oral contraceptives and risk of breast cancer in young women, *Breast Cancer Res Treat* 50(2):175-184, 1998.

324. Bernstein L, Ross R, Henderson B: Relationship of hormone use to cancer risk, *Monogr Natl Cancer Inst* 12:137, 1992.

325. Marchbanks PA et al: The NICHD Women's Contraceptive and Reproductive Experiences Study: methods and operational results, *Ann Epidemiol* 12(4):213-221, 2002.

326. Brinton LA et al: Breast cancer risk among women under 55 years of age by joint effects of usage of oral contraceptives and hormone replacement therapy, *Menopause* 5(3):145-151, 1998.

327. McCormack VA, dos Santos Silva I: Breast density and parenchymal patterns as markers of breast cancer risk: a meta-analysis, *Cancer Epidemiol Biomarkers Prev* 15:1159-1169, 2006.

328. Ginsburg ON et al: Mammographic density, lobular involution, and risk of breast cancer, *Br J Cancer* 4(99):1369-1374, 2008.

329. Vachon CM et al: Strong evidence of a genetic determinant for mammographic density, a major risk factor for breast cancer, *Cancer Res* 67:8412-8418, 2007.

330. Boyd NF et al: Mammographic breast density as an intermediate phenotype for breast cancer, *Lancet Oncol* 6:798-808, 2005.

331. Bryne C et al: Mammographic features and breast cancer risk: effects with time, age, and menopause status, *J Natl Cancer Inst* 87:1622-1629, 1995.

332. Kelemen LE et al: Can genes from mammographic density inform cancer etiology? *Nat Rev Cancer* 8(10):812-813, 2008.

333. Boyd WF et al: Mammographic density: a heritable risk factor for breast cancer, *Methods Mol Biol* 472:343-360, 2009.

334. National Cancer Institute: Radiation risks and pediatric computed tomography (CT): a guide for health care providers, 2002. Available at www.cancer.gov.

335. Brenner DJ, Hall EJ: Computed tomography-an increasing source of radiation exposure, *N Engl J Med* 357(22):2277-2284, 2007.

336. National Cancer Institute: *SEER cancer statistics review 1975-2001,* 2001. Available at http://seer.cancer.gov/csr1975_2001/results_merged/topic_inc_mor_trends.pdf.

337. Land CD: Radiation and breast cancer risk, *Prog Clin Biol Res* 396:115-124, 1997.

338. Pierce DA, Preston DL: Radiation-related risks at low doses among atomic bomb survivors, *Radiat Res* 154:178, 2000.

339. Morgan WF: Will radiation-induced bystander effects or adaptive responses impact on the shape of the dose response relationship at low doses of ionizing radiation? *Dose Response* 4(4):257-262, 2006.

340. Wang HP et al: Identification of differentially transcribed genes in human lymphoblastoid cells irradiated with 0.5 Gy of gamma-ray and the involvement of low dose radiation inducible *CHD6* gene in cell proliferation and radiosensitivity, *Int J Radiat Biol* 82(3):181-190, 2006.

341. Ding LH et al: Gene expression profiles of normal human fibroblasts after exposure to ionizing radiation: a comparative study of low and high doses, *Radiat Res* 164(1):17-26, 2005.

342. Coleman MA et al: Low-dose irradiation alters the transcript profiles of human lymphoblastoid cells including genes associated with cytogenetic radioactive response, *Radiat Res* 164(4 pt 1):369-382, 2005.

343. Young KC, Burch A: Radiation doses received in the UK Breast Screening Programme in 1997 and 1978, *Br J Radiol* 73(867):278-287, 2000.

344. Armstrong K et al: Screening mammography in women 40-49 years of age: a systematic review for the American College of Physicians, *Ann Intern Med* 146(7):516-526, 2007.

345. Gøtzsche PC, Nielsen M: Screening for breast cancer with mammography, *Cochran Database Syst Rev* 18(4):CD001877, 2006.

346. Humphrey L et al: Breast cancer screening: a summary of the evidence for the U.S. Preventive Services Task Force, *Ann Intern Med* 137:344-346, 2002.

347. Miettinen OS et al: Mammographic screening: no reliable supporting evidence? *Lancet* 359(9304):404-405, 2002.

348. Olsen O, Gøtzsche PC: Cochrane review of screening for breast cancer with mammography, *Lancet* 358(9290):1340-1342, 2001.

349. Little JB, Lauriston S: Taylor lecture: nontargeted effects of radiation: implications for low dose exposures, *Health Phys* 91(5):416-426, 2006.

350. Azzam EI, de Toledo SM, Little JB: Expression of CONNEXINS43 is highly sensitive to ionizing radiation and other environmental stresses, *Cancer Res* 63(21):7128-7135, 2003.

351. Zhou H et al: Mitochondrial function and nuclear factor-kappa B-mediated signaling in radiation-induced bystander effects, *Cancer Res* 68(7):2233-2240, 2005.

352. Maxwell CA et al: Targeted and nontargeted effects of ionizing radiation that impact genomic instability, *Cancer Res* 68:8304-8311, 2008.

353. Wright EG, Coates PJ: Untargeted effects of ionizing radiation: implications for radiation pathology, *Mutat Res* 597(1-2):119-132, 2006.

354. Zhou H et al: Mechanism of radiation-induced bystander effect: role of the cyclooxygenase-2 signaling pathway, *Proc Natl Acad Sci U S A* 102(41):1461-1466, 2005.

355. Bauer G: Low dose radiation and intercellular induction of apoptosis: potential implications for the control of oncogenesis, *Int J Radiat Biol* 83(11-12):873-888, 2007.

356. Chaudhry, MA: Bystander effect: biological endpoints and microarray analysis 597(1-2):98-112, 2006.

357. Massagué J: TGFbeta in cancer, *Cell* 134(2):215-230, 2008.

358. Tsai KK et al: Cellular mechanisms for low-dose ionizing radiation-induced perturbation of the breast tissue microenvironment, *Cancer Res* 65(15):6734-6744, 2005.

359. Krtolica AS, Campisi J: Cancer and aging: a model for the cancer promoting effects of the aging stroma, *Int J Biochem Cell Biol* 34:1301-1313, 2002.

360. Krtolica A, Campisi J: Integrating epithelial cancer, aging stroma and cellular senescence, *Adv Gerontol* 11:109-116, 2003.

361. Parrinello S et al: Stomal-epithelial interactions in aging and cancer: senescent fibroblasts after epithelial cell differentiation, *J Cell Sci* 118(pt 3):485-496, 2005.

362. Duffy MJ et al: Metalloproteinases: a role in breast carcinogenesis, invasion and metastasis, *Breast Cancer Res* 2(4):252-257, 2000.

363. Andrieu N et al: Effect of chest x-rays on the risk of breast cancer among *BRCA1/2* mutation carriers in the international *BRCA 1/2* carrier cohort study: a report from the EMBRACE, GENEPSO, GEO_HEBON, and IBCCS Collaborators' Group, *J Clin Oncol* 24:3361-3366, 2006.

364. Bernstein JL et al: The CHEK2*1100delC allelic variant and risk of breast cancer: screening results from the Breast Cancer Family Registry, *Cancer Epidemiol Biomarkers Prev* 15:348-352, 2006.

365. Ronckers CM, Erdmann CA, Land CE: Radiation and breast cancer: a review of current evidence, *Breast Cancer Res* 7(1):21-32, 2005.

366. Michels KB et al: Diet and breast cancer: a review of the prospective observational studies, *Cancer* 109(12 Suppl):2712-2749, 2007.

367. Mahoney MC et al: Opportunities and strategies for breast cancer prevention through risk reduction, *CA Cancer J Clin* 58(6):347-371, 2008.

368. Smith-Warner SA, Stampfer MJ: Fat intake and breast cancer revisited, *J Natl Cancer Inst* 99(6):418-419, 2007.

369. Missner SA et al: Meat and dairy food consumption and breast cancer: a pooled analysis of cohort studies, *Int J Epidemiol* 31:78-85, 2002.

370. Cho E et al: Red meat intake and risk of breast cancer among premenopausal women, *Arch Intern Med* 166:2258-2259, 2006.

371. Taylor EF et al: Meat consumption and risk of breast cancer in the UK Women's Cohort Study, *Br J Cancer* 96:1139-1146, 2007.

372. Egeberg R et al: Meat consumption, N-acetyl transferase 1 and 2 polymorphism and risk of breast cancer in Danish postmenopausal women, *Eur J Cancer Prev* 17:39-47, 2008.

373. Bartsch H et al: Dietary polyunsaturated fatty acids and cancer of the breast and colorectum: emerging evidence for their role as risk modifiers, *Carcinogenesis* 20(12):2209, 1999.

374. Cognault S et al: Effect of an alpha-linolenic acid–rich diet on rat mammary tumor growth depends on the dietary oxidative status, *Nutr Cancer* 36(1):33, 2000.

375. Nakagawa H et al: Effects of genstein and synergistic action in combination with eicosapentaenoic acid on the growth of breast cancer cell lines, *J Cancer Res Clin Oncol* 126(8):448, 2000.

376. Thoennes SR et al: Differential transcriptional activation of peroxisome proliferator-activated receptor gamma by omega-3 and omega-6 fatty acids in MCF-7 cells, *Mol Cell Endocrinol* 160(1-2):67, 2000.

377. Sonestedt E et al: Do both heterocyclic amines and omega-6 polyunsaturated fatty acids contribute to the incidence of breast cancer in postmenopausal women of the Malmo diet and cancer cohort? *Int J Cancer* 123(7):1637-1643, 2008.

378. Straume T: High-energy gamma rays in Hiroshima and Nagasaki: implications for risk and war, *Health Phys* 69(6):954-956, 1995.

379. Simopoulos AP: The importance of the ratio of omega-6/omega-3 essential fatty acids, *Biomed Pharmacother* 56(8):365-379, 2002.

380. Petrakis NL: Nipple aspirate fluid in epidemiologic studies of breast disease, *Epidemiol Rev* 15(1):188-195, 1993.

381. Kuller LH: The etiology of breast cancer—from epidemiology to prevention, *Public Health Rev* 23(2):157-213, 1995.

382. Deslypere JP: Obesity and cancer, *Metabolism* 44(suppl 9):14, 1995.

383. Holmes MD, Willett WC: Does diet affect breast cancer risk? *Breast Cancer Res* 6(4):170-178, 2004.

384. Hankinson SE et al: Alcohol, height, and adiposity in relation to estrogen and prolactin levels in post-menopausal women, *J Natl Cancer Inst* 87(17):1297-1302, 1995.

385. Wenten M et al: Associations of weight, weight change, and body mass with breast cancer risk in Hispanic and non-Hispanic white women, *Ann Epidemiol* 12(6):435-444, 2002.

386. Trentham-Diaz A et al: Weight change and risk of postmenopausal breast cancer (United States), *Cancer Causes Control* 11(6):533-542, 2000.

387. Le Marchand L et al: Body size at different periods of life and breast cancer risk, *Am J Epidemiol* 128(1):137-152, 1988.

388. Morimoto LM et al: Obesity, body size, and risk of postmenopausal breast cancer: the Women's Health Initiative (United States), *Cancer Causes Control* 13(8):741-751, 2002.

389. van den Brandt PA et al: Pooled analysis of prospective cohort studies on height, weight, and breast cancer risk, *Am J Epidemiol* 152:514-527, 2000.

390. Endogenous Hormones Breast Cancer Collaborative Group: Body mass index, serum sex hormones, and breast cancer risk in postmenopausal women, *J Natl Cancer Inst* 95(6):1218-1226, 2003.

391. Ahn J et al: Adiposity, adult weight gain, and postmenopausal breast cancer risk, *Arch Intern Med* 167:2091-2102, 2007.

392. Harvie M et al: Association of gain and loss of weight before and after menopause with risk of postmenopausal breast cancer in the Iowa Women's Health Study, *Cancer Epidemiol Biomarkers Prev* 14:656-661, 2005.

393. Wolters M, Hahn A: Soy isoflavones—a therapy for menopausal symptoms, *Wein Med Wochenschr*, 2004.

394. Cross HS et al: Phytoestrogens and vitamin D metabolism: a new concept for the prevention and therapy of colorectal, prostate, and mammary carcinomas, *J Nutr* 134(5):1207S-1212S, 2004.

395. Ito T, Warnken SP, May WS: Protein synthesis inhibition of flavinoids: roles of eukaryotic initiation factor 2 alpha kinase, *Biochem Biophys Res Com* 265(2):3890–3894, 1999.

396. Kumar N et al: Isofavones in breast cancer chemoprevention: where do we go from here? *Front Biosci* 9:2927-2934, 2004.

397. Lu LJ et al: Effects of soy consumption for one month on steroid hormones in premenopausal women: implications for breast cancer risk reduction, *Cancer Epidemiol Biomarkers Prev* 5:63-70, 1996.

398. McMichael-Phillips DF et al: Effects of soy-protein supplementation on epithelial proliferation in the histologically normal human breast, *Am J Clin Nutr* 68(Suppl):1431S-1435S, 1998.

399. Shao Z-M et al: Genistein exerts multiple suppressive effects on human breast carcinoma cells, *Cancer Res* 58(21):4851-4857, 1998.

400. Petrakis NL et al: Stimulatory influence of soy protein isolate on breast secretion in pre- and postmenopausal women, *Cancer Epidemiol Biomarkers Prev* 5(10):785-794, 1996.

401. Bennett LM, Davis BJ: Identification of mammary carcinogens in rodent bioassays, *Environ Mol Mutagen* 39(2-3):150-157, 2002.

402. Cohn BA et al: DDT and breast cancer in young women: new data on the significance of age at exposure, *Environ Health Perspect* 115:1406-1414, 2007.

403. Cassidy RA et al: The link between the insecticide heptachlor epoxide, estradiol, and breast cancer, *Breast Cancer Res Treat* 90:55-64, 2005.

404. Khanjani N et al: An ecological study of organochlorine pesticides and breast cancer in rural Victoria, Australia, *Arch Environ Contam Toxicol* 50:454-461, 2006.

405. Lee PN, Hamling J: Environmental tobacco smoke exposure and risk of breast cancer in nonsmoking women: a review with meta-analyses, *Inhalation Toxicol* 18:1053-1070, 2006.

406. Rennix CP et al: Risk of breast cancer among enlisted army women occupationally exposed to volatile organic compounds, *Am J Ind Med* 48:157-167, 2005.

407. Shaham J et al: The risk of breast cancer in relation to health habits and occupational exposures, *Am J Ind Med* 49:1021-1030, 2006.

408. Markey CM et al: In utero exposure to bisphenol A alters the development and tissue of organization of the mouse mammary gland, *Biol Reprod* 65(4):1215-1223, 2001.

409. Chiazze L Jr, Ference LD: Mortality among PVC fabricating employees, *Env Health Perspect* 41:137-143, 1981.

410. Infante PF, Pesak J: A historical perspective of some occupationally related diseases of women, *J Occup Med* 36(8):826-831, 1994.

411. Hoyer AP et al: Organochlorine exposure and risk of breast cancer, *Lancet* 352(9143):1816-1820, 1998.

412. Maxwell NI et al: *Newton Breast Cancer Study*, Newton, MA, 1999, Silent Spring Institute.

413. National Toxicology Program (NTP): *Chemicals associated with site-specific tumor induction in mammary glands*, 2003. Available at http://ntp-server.niehs.nih.gov/htdocs/sites/MAMM.html.

414. Colton T et al: Breast cancer in mothers prescribed diethylstilbestrol in pregnancy. Further follow-up, *JAMA* 269(16):2096-2100, 1993.

415. Herbst AL, Scully RE: Adenocarcinoma of the vagina in adolescence: a report of 7 cases including 6 clear cell carcinomas (so-called mesonephromas), *Cancer* 25(4):745-757, 1970.

416. Palmer JR et al: Risk of breast cancer in women exposed to diethylstilbestrol in utero: preliminary studies (United States), *Cancer Causes Control* 13(8):753-758, 2002.

417. Chang YM et al: A proportionate cancer morbidity ratio study of workers exposed to chlorinated organic solvents in Taiwan, *Indust Health* 41(2):77-87, 2003.

418. Hansen J: Breast cancer risk among relatively young women employed in solvent-using industries, *Am J Ind Med* 36(1):43-47, 1999.

419. Belli S et al: Mortality study of workers employed by the Italian National Institute of Health, 1960-1989, *Scand J Work Environ Health* 18(1):64-67, 1992.

420. Walrath J et al: Causes of death among female chemists, *Am J Public Health* 75(8):883-885, 1985.

421. Weiderpass E et al: Breast cancer and occupational exposures in women in Finland, *Am J Ind Med* 36(1):48-53, 1999.

422. Wennborg H et al: Mortality and cancer incidence in biomedical laboratory personnel in Sweden, *Am J Ind Med* 35(4):382-389, 1999.

423. Almekinder JL et al: Toxicity of methoxyacetic acid in cultured human luteal cells, *Fund Appl Toxicol* 38(2):191-194, 1997.

424. Jansen MS et al: Short-chain fatty acids enhance nuclear receptor activity through mitogen-activated protein kinase activation and histone deacetylase inhibition, *Proc Natl Acad Sci USA* 101(18):7199-7204, 2004.

425. Melnick RL et al: Multiple organ carcinogenicity of inhaled chloroprene (2-chloro-1,3-butadiene) in F334/N rats and B6C3F1 mice and comparison of dose-response in 1,3-butadiene in mice, *Carcinogenesis* 20(5):867-878, 1999.

426. National Toxicology Program (NTP), US Department of Health and Human Services: Toxicology and carcinogenesis studies of 1,3-butadiene (CAS No 106-99-0) in B6C3F1 mice (inhalation studies), NTP TR 434, NIH Pub No 93-3165, Research Triangle Park, NC, 1993, National Institute of Health.

427. DeBruin LS, Josephy PD: Perspectives on the chemical etiology of breast cancer, *Environ Health Perspect* 110(S1):119-128, 2002.

428. Evans N: *State of the evidence: what is the connection between the environment and breast cancer?*, ed 3, San Francisco, Calif, 2004, Breast Cancer Fund.

429. Zheng T et al: DDE and DDT in breast adipose tissue and risk of female breast cancer, *Am J Epidemiol* 150(5):453-458, 1999.

430. Hatakeyama M, Matsumura F: Correlation between the activation of Neu tyrosine kinase and promotion of foci formation induced by selected organochlorine compounds in the MCF-7 model system, *J Biochem Molec Toxicol* 13(6):296-302, 1999.

431. Gammon MD et al: Environmental toxins and breast cancer on Long Island. I. Polycyclic aromatic hydrocarbon DNA adducts, *Cancer Epidemiol Biomark Prev* 11(8):677-685, 2002.

432. Band PR et al: Carcinogenic and endocrine disrupting effects of cigarette smoke and risk of breast cancer, *Lancet* 360(9339):1044-1049, 2002.

433. Calle EE et al: Cigarette smoking and risk of fatal breast cancer, *Am J Epidemiol* 139(10):1001-1007, 1994.

434. Johnson KC, Hu J, Mao Y: Passive and active smoking and breast cancer risk in Canada, 1994-1997, The Canadian Cancer Registries Epidemiology Research Group, *Cancer Causes Control* 11(3):211-221, 2000.

435. California Environmental Protection Agency: Air Resources Board: Proposed identification of environmental tobacco smoke as a toxic air contaminant, *Draft Report Part B, chap 7* :147, 2004.

436. Kilthau GF: Cancer risk in relation to radioactivity in tobacco, *Radiol Tech* 67(3):217-222, 1996.

437. Brown NM et al: Prenatal TCDD and predisposition to mammary cancer in rats, *Carcinogenesis* 19(9):1623-1629, 1998.

438. Warner MB et al: Serum dioxin concentrations and breast cancer risk in the Seveso Women's Health Study, *Environ Health Perspect* 110(7):625-628, 2002.

439. Steenland K et al: Ethylene oxide and breast cancer incidence in a cohort study of 7576 women, *Cancer Causes Control* 14(6):531-539, 2003.

440. Dorn J et al: Lifetime physical activity and breast cancer risk in pre- and postmenopausal women, *Med Sci Sports Exercise* 35(2):278-285, 2003.

441. Friedenreich CM, Orenstein MR: Physical activity and cancer prevention: etiologic evidence and biological mechanisms, *J Nutr* 132(11 Suppl):3464S-3465S, 2002.

442. Kaaks R, Lukanova A: Effects of weight control and physical activity in cancer prevention: role of endogenous hormone metabolism, *Ann N Y Acad Sci* 963:268-281, 2002.

443. Maruti SS et al: Physical activity and premenopausal breast cancer: an examination of recall and selection bias, *Cancer Causes Control*, 2008 Nov 15 [Epub ahead of print].

444. Suzuki S et al: Effect of physical activity on beast cancer risk: findings of the Japan Collaborative Cohort Study, *Cancer Epidemiol Biomarkers Prev* 17(12):3396-3401, 2008.

445. Garber JE, Offit K: Hereditary cancer predisposition syndromes, *J Clin Oncology* 23(2):276-292, 2005.

446. Ford D et al: Genetic heterogeneity and penetrance analysis of the *BRCA1* and *BRCA2* genes in breast cancer families. The Breast Cancer Linkage Consortium, *Am J Hum Genet* 62(3):676-689, 1998.

447. Weber B: Genetic testing for breast cancer, *Sci Am Sci Med* 3(1):12, 1996.

448. Antoniou A et al: Average risks of breast and ovarian cancer associated with *BRCA1* and *BRCA2* mutations detected in case series unselected for family history: a combined analysis of 22 studies, *Am J Hum Genet* 72(2):1117-1130, 2003.

449. Thompson D, Easton D, Breast Cancer Linkage Consortium: Variation in cancer risks by mutation position in *BRCA2* mutation carriers, *Am J Hum Genet* 68(2):410-419, 2001.

450. Kauff ND et al: Risk reducing salpingo oophorectomy in women with *BRCA1* or *BRCA2* mutation, *N Engl J Med* 346(21):1609-1615, 2002.

451. Rebbeck TR et al: Prophylactic oophorectomy in carriers of *BRCA1* or *BRCA2* mutations, *N Engl J Med* 346(21):1616-1622, 2002.

452. Haber D: Roads leading to breast cancer, *N Engl J Med* 343(21):1566, 2000.

453. Waxman J: A new understanding of the hormonal regulation of endocrine dependent cancer, *Br Med Bull* 47(1):197, 1991.

454. Damonte P et al: Mammary carcinoma behavior is programmed in the precancer stem cell, *Breast Cancer Res* 10(3):R50, 2008.

455. Namba R et al: Heterogeneity of mammary lesions represent molecular differences, *BMC Cancer* 6:275, 2006.

456. Burnstein HJ et al: Ductal carcinoma *in situ* of the breast, *N Engl J Med* 350:1420-1444, 2004.

457. Chin K et al: In situ analyses of genome instability in breast cancer, *Nat Genet* 36:984-988, 2004.

458. Silverstein MJ, Baril NB: In situ carcinoma of the breast. In Donegan WL, Spratt JS, editors: *Cancer of the breast*, Philadelphia, 2002, Saunders.

459. Pinder SE, O'Malley FP: Morphology of ductal carcinoma in situ. In O'Malley FP, Pinder SE, editors: *Breast pathology*, Edinburgh, 2006, Churchill Livingstone.

460. Nielsen M et al: Breast cancer and atypia among young and middle-aged women: a study of 110 medicolegal autopsies, *Br J Cancer* 56(6):814-819, 1987.

461. Alpers CE, Wellings SR: The prevalence of carcinoma in situ in normal and cancer-associated breasts, *Hum Pathol* 16(8):796-807, 1985.

462. Hanby AM, Hughes TA: In situ and invasive neoplasia of the breast, *Histopathology* 52(1):58-66, 2008.

463. Reis-Filho JS, Lakhani SR: Molecular genetics of ADH/DCIS and ALH/LCIS. In O'Malley FP, Pinder SE, editors: *Breast pathology*, New York, 2006, Churchill Livingstone/Elsevier.

464. Lakhani SR: Molecular genetics of solid tumors: translating research into clinical practice. What we could do now: breast cancer, *Mol Pathol* 54(5):281-284, 2001.

465. Page DL et al: Atypical lobular hyperplasia as a unilateral predictor of breast cancer risk: a retrospective cohort study, *Lancet* 361(9352):125-129, 2003.

466. Schedin P et al: Microenvironment of the involuting mammary gland mediates mammary cancer progression, *J Mammary Gland Biol Neoplasia* 12(1):71-82, 2007.

467. Barcellos-Hoff MH, Ravani SA: Irradiated mammary gland stroma promotes the expression of tumorigenic potential by unirradiated epithelial cells, *Cancer Res* 60(5):1254-1260, 2000.

468. Martins-Green M, Boudreau N, Bissell MJ: Inflammation is responsible for the development of wound-induced tumors in chickens infected with Rous sarcoma virus, *Cancer Res* 54(16):4334-4341, 1994.

469. Chang HY et al: Robustness, scalability, and integration of a wound-response gene expression signature in predicting breast cancer survival, *Proc Natl Acad Sci U S A* 102(10):3738-3743, 2004.

470. Nuyten DS et al: Predicting a local recurrence after breast-conserving therapy by gene expression profiling, *Breast Cancer Res* 8(5):R62, 2006.

471. Kalluri R, Zeisberg M: Fibroblasts in cancer, *Nat Rev Cancer* 6:392-401, 2006.

472. Acloque H, Thiery JP, Nieto MA: The physiology and pathology of the EMT, *EMBO Rep* 9(4):322-326, 2008.

473. Schäfer M, Werner S: Cancer as an overhealing wound: an old hypothesis revisted, *Nat Rev Mol Biol* 9(8):628-638, 2008.

474. Tse JC, Kalluri R: Mechanisms of metastasis: epithelial-to-mesenchymal transition and contribution of tumor microenvironment, *J Cell Biochem* 101:816-829, 2007.

475. Guarino M, Rubino B, Ballabio G: The role of epithelial-mesenchymal transition in cancer pathology, *Pathology* 39(3):305-318, 2007.

476. Mani SA et al: The epithelial-mesenchymal transition generates cells with properties of stem cells, *Cell* 133:704-715, 2008.

477. Pollard J: Macrophages define the invasive microenvironment in breast cancer, *J Leuk Biol* 84(3):623-630, 2008.

478. Bingle L, Brown NJ, Lewis CE: The role of tumor-associated macrophages in tumor progression: implications for new anticancer therapies, *J Pathol* 196:254-265, 2002.

479. Allavena P et al: The yin-yang of tumor-associated macrophages in neoplastic progression and immune surveillance, *Immunol Rev* 222:155-161, 2008.

480. Harris G, Pinder SE, O'Malley FP: Invasive carcinoma—special types. In O'Malley FP, Pinder SE, editors: *Breast pathology*, New York, 2006, Churchill Livingstone.

481. Berman H et al: Genetic and epigenetic changes in mammary epithelial cells identify a subpopulation of cells involved in early carcinogenesis, *Cold Spring Harb Symp Quant Biol* 70:317-327, 2005.

482. Romanov SR et al: Normal human mammary epithelial cells spontaneously escape senescence and acquire genomic changes, *Nature* 409(6820):633-637, 2001.

483. Bean GR et al: Morphologically normal-appearing mammary epithelial cells obtained from high-risk women exhibit methylation silencing of INK4a/ARF, *Clin Cancer Res* 13(22Part 1):6834-6841, 2007.

484. Bean GR et al: Hypermethylation of the breast cancer-associated gene 1 promoter does not predict cytologic atypia or correlate with surrogate end points of breast cancer risk, *Cancer Epidemiol Biomarkers Prev* 16(1):50-56, 2007.

485. Liu T et al: Increased γ-tubulin expression and p16 INK4a promoter methylation occur together in preinvasive lesions and carcinomas of the breast, *Ann Oncol*, 2009 Jan 8 [Epub ahead of print.]

486. Zhang J et al: p16 INK4a modulates p53 in primary human mammary epithelial cells, *Cancer Res* 66(21):10325-10331, 2006.

487. Bissell MJ, Radisky D: Putting tumors in context, *Nat Rev Cancer* 1:46-54, 2001.

488. Holliday DL et al: Intrinsic genetic characteristics determine tumor-modifying capacity of fibroblasts: matrix metalloproteinase-3 5A/5A genotype enhances breast cancer cell invasion, *Breast Cancer Res* 9(5):R67, 2007.

489. Kalluri R, Zeisburg M: Fibroblasts in cancer, *Nat Rev Cancer* 6(5):392-401, 2006.

490. Gavert N, Ben-Zé-Ev A: Epithelial-mesenchymal transition and the invasive potential of tumors, *Trends Mol Med* 14(5):199-208, 2008.

491. Nuyten DSA et al: Combining biological gene expression signatures in predicting outcome in breast cancer: an alternative to supervised classification, *Eur J Cancer* 44:2319-2329, 2008.

492. Sotiriou C, Pusztai L: Gene-expression signatures in breast cancer, *N Engl J Med* 360(8):790-800, 2009.

493. Brenner RG, Parisky Y: Alternative breast-imaging approaches, *Radiol Clin North Am* 45:907-923, 2007.

494. Conant EF, Maidment ADA: Breast cancer imaging, *Sci Am Sci Med* 3(1):22, 1996.

495. Clarke MJ: Ovarian ablation for early breast cancer, *Cochrane Database Syst Rev* (4):CD000485, 2008.

496. Clarke MJ: Tamoxifen for early breast cancer, *Cochrane Database Syst Rev* (4):CD000486, 2008.

497. ATAC Group: Effect of anastrozole and tamoxifen as adjuvant treatment for early-stage breast cancer: 100-month analysis of the ATAC trial, *Lancet Oncol* 9(1):45-53, 2008.

498. Jakesz R et al: Switching of postmenopausal women with endocrine-responsive early breast cancer to anastrozole after 2 years' adjuvant tamoxifen: combined results of ABCSG trial 8 and ARNO 95 trial, *Lancet* 366(9484):455-462, 2005.

499. Aydiner A, Tas F: Meta-analysis of trials comparing anastrozole and tamoxifen for adjuvant treatment of postmenopausal women with early breast cancer, *Trials* 9:47, 2008.

500. Baum M: Anastrozole alone or in combination with tamoxifen versus tamoxifen alone for adjuvant treatment of postmenopausal women with early breast cancer: first results of the ATAC randomized trial, *Lancet* 359(9324):2129–2131, 2002.

501. Vogel VG et al: Effects of tamoxifen vs raloxifene on the risk of developing invasive breast cancer and other disease outcomes, *JAMA* 295(23):2727-2741, 2006.

502. Stanway SJ et al: Phase 2 study of STX 64 (667 Coumate) in breast cancer patients: the first study of a steroid sulfatase inhibitor, *Clin Cancer Res* 12(5):1585-1592, 2006.

503. Giordano SH et al: Breast carcinoma in men: a population based study, *Cancer* 101(1):51-57, 2004.

504. Weiss JR, Moysich KB, Swede H: Epidemiology of male breast cancer, *Cancer Epidemiol Biomarkers Prev* 14(1):20-26, 2005.

505. Clark JL et al: Prognostic variables in male breast cancer, *Am Surg* 66(5):501, 2000.

506. Jepson AS, Fentiman IS: Male breast cancer, *Int J Clin Pract* 52(8):571, 1998.

SEXUALLY TRANSMITTED INFECTIONS

LISA KALOCZI • GWEN A. LATENDRESSE •
KATHERINE MORGAN

MEDIA RESOURCES

CHAPTER OUTLINE

SEXUALLY TRANSMITTED UROGENITAL INFECTIONS
  Bacterial Infections
  Chlamydial Infections
  Viral infections
  Parasitic Infections

SEXUALLY TRANSMITTED INFECTIONS OF OTHER BODY SYSTEMS
  Gastrointestinal Infections
  Systemic Diseases

Throughout recorded history, infectious diseases have threatened humans. Even into the twentieth century, epidemics of diphtheria, typhoid, tuberculosis, cholera, and other catastrophic infections have decimated entire communities almost overnight (see Chapter 9). Despite medical advances, improved living standards, and better nutrition, epidemics still arise as major public health problems, and some pose lethal threats to individuals and communities. Some of these epidemics are caused by sexually transmitted infections (STIs). At this time, many people consider the number of individuals with acquired immunodeficiency syndrome (AIDS), human immunodeficiency virus (HIV), and human papillomavirus (HPV) infections to be at epidemic levels.

Sexually contracted infections affect more than 19 million Americans per year, and half of those are younger than 25 years,[1] and account for about one third of the reproductive mortality in the United States. Complications of STIs include pelvic inflammatory disease, infertility, ectopic pregnancy, chronic pelvic pain, neonatal morbidity and mortality, and genital cancers. Long-term sequelae of untreated or undertreated STIs may be disastrous and can affect a person's physical, emotional, and financial well-being.

In the past an infection transmitted through sexual intercourse was called a *venereal disease*. Because of its limited scope, the term venereal disease has been replaced with *sexually transmitted infection (STI)*. STIs are contracted by intimate, as well as sexual, contact and include systemic infections, such as tuberculosis and hepatitis, that can be spread to a sexual partner. Etiology of an STI may be bacterial, viral, protozoal, parasitic, or fungal (Table 24-1). Although the majority of STIs can be treated, virally induced STIs are considered incurable. The current increase in severity and incidence of STIs can be attributed to earlier onset of sexual activity and a greater number of lifetime sexual partners. Many infected individuals do not seek treatment because symptoms are absent, minor, or transient or because health services are inaccessible. Increased numbers of single individuals, bisexuality, and premarital or extramarital sexual affairs contribute to rising numbers of lifetime sexual partners and exposure to STIs. Indulgence in high-risk sexual behaviors and poor health habits, such as failure to use a condom in nonmonogamous or new relationships, and drug use, increases an individual's risk of exposure or the severity of infection if exposed. Perhaps partly because of risk-taking behavior (unprotected intercourse or selection of high-risk partners), adolescents have the greatest risk for STI exposure and infection. In addition, adolescent women may have a physiologically increased susceptibility to infection because of increased cervical immaturity and lack of immunity. Rates of gonorrhea, chlamydia, vaginitis, cervical condyloma, genital warts, and pelvic inflammatory disease (PID) are highest in adolescents and young women and decline exponentially

Table 24-1	Currently Recognized Sexually Transmitted Infections
Causal Microorganism	**Infection**
Bacteria	
Campylobacter	Campylobacter enteritis
Calymmatobacterium granulomatis	Granuloma inguinale
Chlamydia trachomatis	Urogenital infections; lymphogranuloma venereum
Polymicrobial	
Gardnerella vaginalis interaction with anaerobes (*Bacteroides* and *Mobiluncus spp.*) and genital mycoplasmas	Bacterial vaginosis
Haemophilus ducreyi	Chancroid
Mycoplasma	Mycoplasmosis
Neisseria gonorrhoeae	Gonorrhea
Shigella	Shigellosis
Treponema pallidum	Syphilis
Viruses	
Cytomegalovirus	Cytomegalic inclusion disease
Hepatitis B virus (HBV)	Hepatitis
Hepatitis C virus (HCV)	Hepatitis
Herpes simplex virus (HSV)	Genital herpes
Human immunodeficiency virus (HIV)	Acquired immunodeficiency syndrome (AIDS)
Human papillomavirus (HPV)	Condylomata acuminata, cervical dysplasia, and cervical cancer
Molluscum contagiosum virus	Molluscum contagiosum
Protozoa	
Entamoeba histolytica	Amebiasis; amebic dysentery
Giardia lamblia	Giardiasis
Trichomonas vaginalis	Trichomoniasis
Ectoparasites	
Phthirus pubis	Pediculosis pubis
Sarcoptes scabiei	Scabies
Fungus	
Candida albicans	Candidiasis

with increasing age. Women and infants bear the greatest burden from STIs.

STIs are stereotyped as occurring only among urban poor and minority populations. Because the Centers for Disease Control and Prevention (CDC) do not require that all STIs be reported, private physicians may not report them. Thus reported STIs often come from public health clinics, giving the impression that a greater number of the urban poor and minority populations are infected with STIs. In fact, STIs are prevalent in all socioeconomic groups.

SEXUALLY TRANSMITTED UROGENITAL INFECTIONS

Bacterial Infections

Gonorrhea

Gonorrhea is caused by **gonococci** (singular, *gonococcus*), which are microorganisms of the species *Neisseria gonorrhoeae*. Neisser first identified gonococci in stained smears of vaginal, urethral, and conjunctival exudate in 1879. Until 1994 gonorrhea was the most commonly reported communicable

infection in the United States. After declining 74% between 1974 and 1997, the rates for gonorrhea have remained relatively stable in the United States. The number of reported cases in 2007 was 355,991,[2] but the actual number of cases is estimated to be twice as high.

Infection rates are highest in the southern region of the country, but appear to be stable.[3] The number of reported cases decreased in all racial and ethnic groups between 2006 and 2007, except for blacks. The gonorrhea rate is now about 19 times greater for blacks than for non-Hispanic whites, down from 23 times higher in 1999.[2] Other demographic and lifestyle risk factors may include transient or urban residence, early onset of sexual activity, multiple serial or consecutive sex partners, drug use, prostitution, and previous gonorrheal or concurrent STI.[2] The risk of developing gonorrhea from intercourse with an infected male partner is 50% to 80% for women, and with an infected female partner, it is 20% to 30% for men. The risk increases threefold to fourfold for men after four exposures to an infected partner.

Transmission of gonococcal infection generally requires contact of epithelial (mucosal) surfaces, such as occurs during sexual, oral, or anal intercourse. A pregnant woman also can

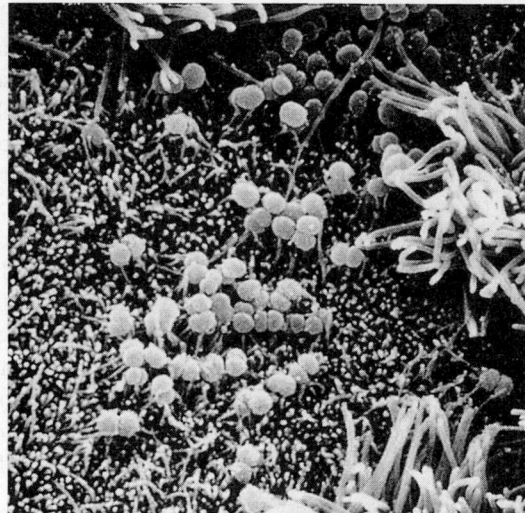

Figure 24-1 Gonococci. Scanning electron microscopy showing gonococci attaching to the nonciliated cells of human fallopian tube mucosa. (From Morse SA et al, editors: *Atlas of sexually transmitted diseases and AIDS*, ed 3, London, 2003, Mosby.)

transmit gonorrhea to her fetus. The infection passes from mother to child across the amniotic membranes, by direct inoculation with a fetal scalp electrode during labor monitoring, or during passage through the birth canal. **Fomites** (contaminated objects) are rarely involved in the transmission of *N. gonorrhoeae*, primarily because the gonococcus requires a rich medium (e.g., body fluids) and an environment high in carbon dioxide (5% to 10%) for growth.

PATHOPHYSIOLOGY Humans are the only natural hosts for *N. gonorrhoeae*, which is an aerobic, non–spore-forming, oxidase-positive gram-negative coccal (round) microorganism that usually appears in pairs (diplococci), with the adjacent sides slightly flattened. Hairlike filaments, called *pili*, appear to help the microorganisms attach themselves to host cells: the epithelial cells of mucous membranes (Figure 24-1). Columnar, transitional, and stratified squamous epithelial cells are infected most often. First the microorganisms become attached to the plasma membranes (cell walls) of these cells, and then they invade the cells and begin to damage the mucosa. Generally a quick leukocytic (inflammatory) response and exudation at the site of infection occur.

In women the endocervical canal (inner portion of the cervix) is the usual site of original gonococcal infection, although urethral colonization and infection of Skene or Bartholin glands also are common. Several factors can facilitate ascent of gonococci into the uterus and the fallopian tubes, where they cause pelvic inflammatory disease (PID). Among these factors are (1) disintegration of the cervical mucous plug and

a rise in vaginal pH above 4.5 during menstruation, (2) uterine contraction that may cause retrograde menstruation into the fallopian tubes, and (3) various microbes that possess virulent potentiating factors for chlamydia or gonococcal PID. Bacteria (*N. gonorrhoeae*, *Chlamydia trachomatis*) also may adhere to sperm and be transported to the fallopian tubes. In the fallopian tubes, progressive mucosal and submucosal invasion and sloughing of normal, ciliated tubal epithelium are accompanied by marked inflammatory response, causing the fallopian tubes to fill with exudate (see Chapter 23 for more on PID). In men the gonococci typically infect the urethra. Untreated urethral infection causes epididymitis in 1% to 2% of men and, rarely, urethral stricture and sterility. Commonly, concurrent oropharyngeal and anorectal infection can be found in infected men and women.[4-6] Virulence is determined by variations in the bacterial properties and host response.

CLINICAL MANIFESTATIONS The clinical manifestations of gonorrhea can be categorized as local or systemic and uncomplicated or complicated. Uncomplicated local infections are seen as urethral infections in men and urogenital infections in women. In men the incubation period for urethritis is 3 to 10 days with a range of 12 hours to 3 months.[7] Without treatment, urethritis persists for 3 to 7 weeks, with 95% of men becoming asymptomatic after 3 months. Approximately 60% of men infected suddenly experience marked dysuria (painful or difficult urination) and spontaneous, profuse, mucopurulent discharge from the urethra. However, some individuals have little discharge or urethral itching only, and 5% to 10% never have signs or symptoms. Most cases of untreated gonococcal urethritis resolve spontaneously after several weeks, and more than 95% of individuals are asymptomatic by 6 months after infection. Some men develop urethritis even after being appropriately treated.

In women the incubation period varies, but those who typically develop symptoms do so within 10 days of exposure or within 1 to 2 days after the next menstrual period. The clinical manifestations of uncomplicated gonorrhea in women may be absent (50% of women have asymptomatic infection) or severe; they can include dysuria, increased vaginal discharge, abnormal menses (increased flow or dysmenorrhea), or dyspareunia. Physical examination may disclose cervical friability and erythema (redness) and purulent or mucopurulent discharge from the cervical os (Figure 24-2). There may be a discharge from the Skene or Bartholin glands if these sites are involved.

Anal and rectal gonococcal infection is found in 30% to 50% of women diagnosed with urogenital gonorrhea. In women, anorectal infection is usually asymptomatic and not necessarily related to anal intercourse. Anorectal gonorrhea most commonly occurs in homosexual men with a history of receptive anorectal intercourse. About 50% of these infected men have symptoms.[7]

Symptoms of anorectal gonorrhea range from mild anal pruritus (itching), mucopurulent rectal discharge, and slight rectal bleeding to severe rectal pain, tenesmus (painful and ineffectual straining at stool), and constipation. Physical examination may disclose anal erythema and discharge and evidence of mucosal damage to the anus and rectum, such as friability, edema, and purulent exudate.

Gonococcal pharyngitis occurs primarily in homosexual or bisexual men or heterosexual women after fellatio (oral sexual contact) with an infected partner. Symptomatic pharyngitis is indistinguishable from any other bacterial pharyngitis and can include fever, lymphadenopathy, and tonsillitis. Approximately 60% of these infections are asymptomatic.

Other sites of uncomplicated local infections include the eye, leading to conjunctivitis; however, this is rare in adults. Primary cutaneous infection also has been reported

and is usually manifested as a localized ulcer of the genitalia, perineum, proximal lower extremities, or fingers. It is important to determine whether such infections are the result of *N. gonorrhoeae* or secondary colonization by a preexisting lesion.

Localized gonococcal infections can be complicated by prostatitis, epididymitis, lymphangitis, and urethral stricture in men and salpingitis, PID, and bartholinitis in women. Chronic salpingitis or perididymitis can cause scarring and tubal adhesions that lead to sterility. Anyone who is infected and remains untreated is at risk for disseminated gonococcal infection.[4-6]

Before the advent of antimicrobial therapy, approximately 20% of infected men developed acute epididymitis. Men with this condition report unilateral testicular pain and swelling and commonly have overt urethritis at the same time. Penile lymphangitis is a rare complication with an unclear pathogenesis.[4] Before modern antibiotics, individuals with this condition were at risk for developing urethral strictures; however, this complication is now uncommon if treatment is sought and therapy instituted properly.

Acute salpingitis, or PID, is the most common local complication in women. Approximately 10%[2] of women with untreated cervical gonorrhea develop this condition. Salpingitis is significant in its development because of the potential long-term sequelae associated with it, namely, infertility and ectopic pregnancy.

The onset of symptoms may be rapid and usually occurs during menses. Women may experience chills, fever, nausea, vomiting, and lower abdominal pain that worsen with coughing, sneezing, or intercourse. Abdominal palpation often discloses bilateral lower quadrant tenderness and rebound tenderness resulting from peritoneal irritation caused by tubal exudate. Marked tenderness of the internal genitalia is often noted during pelvic examination. Enlargement or masses also may be palpable in the upper genital tract. Abscess of Skene and Bartholin glands is also a local complication associated with gonococcal infection in women. Tubal infertility is found in 8% of women after one episode of PID. If a woman has three or more episodes of PID, she has a 40% risk of tubal infertility.[8] Apart from PID, abscess formation of Bartholin glands is the most common complication of gonorrhea in women.

Disseminated gonococcal infection (DGI) is a rare systemic complication brought about by the spread of infection through the bloodstream. Less than 1% of individuals with untreated gonococcal infection develop this complication.[9] Men are affected more than women. Symptoms include fever, rash, and joint swelling or pain.

Spread of *N. gonorrhoeae* to the liver causes a condition known as **perihepatitis** or Fitz-Hugh–Curtis syndrome. *C. trachomatis* also has been identified as a causative agent. Inflammation of the capsule of the liver is the primary pathologic manifestation and produces sudden and intense right upper quadrant pain.[10] This complication usually develops after acute salpingitis and is very rare in men.

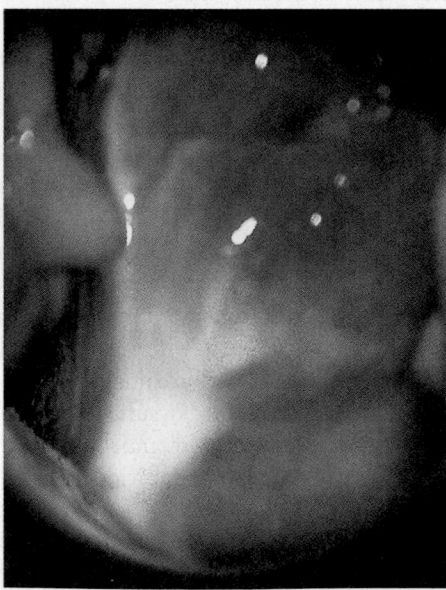

Figure 24-2 Gonococcal cervicitis. The cervix is involved in 85% to 90% of cases in women, but the resultant discharge is profuse enough to be recognized in only 10%. (From McMillan A, Scott GR: *Sexually transmitted infections,* ed 2, London, 2000, Churchill Livingstone.)

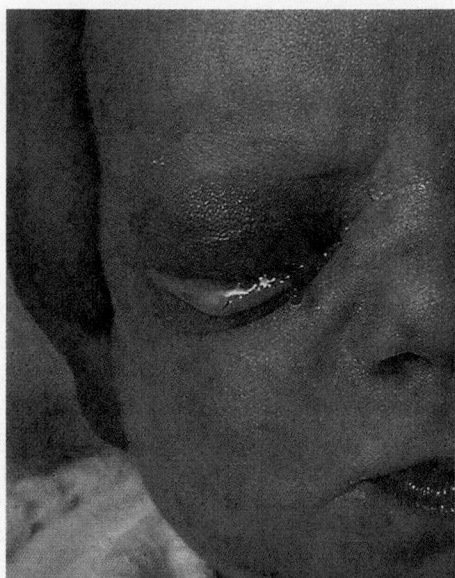

Figure 24-3 Gonococcal ophthalmia neonatorum. (Examiner would be gloved.) (From McMillan A, Scott GR: *Sexually transmitted infections*, ed 2, London, 2000, Churchill Livingstone.)

Newborns are at risk most commonly for gonococcal eye infection (**ophthalmia neonatorum**) (Figure 24-3) but also may acquire rhinitis, anorectal infection, or an abscess at the site of electrode placement for fetal monitoring. Onset of symptoms generally occurs 1 to 12 days after birth, with a mean of 4 to 6 days. Affected newborns usually are born to mothers who have had prolonged ruptured membranes. In these cases, immediate treatment with a topical antibiotic is not effective because the infection is already established. Established infection causes bilateral corneal ulceration, with a profuse yellow or gray purulent exudate and is followed by necrosis, scarring, and compromised vision. Signs of systemic disease are seldom apparent.

EVALUATION AND TREATMENT Clinical signs and symptoms are not sufficient for the differential diagnosis of gonococcal infections. Microscopic evaluation of Gram-stained slides of clinical specimens is deemed positive for *N. gonorrhoeae* if gram-negative diplococci with typical "kidney bean" morphology are seen inside polymorphonuclear leukocytes. Such a finding is considered adequate for the diagnosis of gonococcal urethritis in a symptomatic man. For women the Gram-stain technique is less accurate and reliable and is replaced with a single culture of endocervical secretions. Most clinic settings now use ligase chain reaction (LCR), polymerase chain reaction (PCR) testing, or deoxyribonucleic (DNA) testing because these samples do not require an anaerobic incubation, are highly sensitive, and can be easily transported to a laboratory for testing. Because of the large percentage of infected women without symptoms, routine screening for at-risk women is recommended. Tests should be obtained from any site that may be exposed.[11]

The many different strains of *N. gonorrhoeae* vary with respect to pathogenicity, virulence, and susceptibility to antibiotics. Several types of drug-resistant strains have been identified, including penicillinase-producing *N. gonorrhoeae* (PPNG), which is resistant to penicillin; tetracycline-resistant *N. gonorrhoeae* (TRNG), which is resistant to tetracycline; chromosomal control of mechanisms of resistance of *N. gonorrhoeae* (CMRNG), which is resistant to penicillin and tetracycline; and increasingly a fluoroquinolone-resistant *N. gonorrhoeae* (QRNG).[12,13] Of all the isolates collected in 2006 by the Gonococcal Isolate Surveillance Project (GISP), 25.6%[2] were resistant to penicillin, tetracycline, ciprofloxacin, or some combination of these antibiotics.[2] In the United States the overall percentage of PPNG isolates has declined every year since 1991.[12] However, QRNG has been increasing in Asia, the Pacific Islands, Hawaii, and has now become widespread in the United States. The CDC no longer recommends fluoroquinolone treatment for the treatment of gonococcal infections and associated conditions, such as pelvic inflammatory disease, and issued an important treatment update in 2007. Until 2007, fluoroquinolones were the first line treatment recommended by the CDC. The only class of drugs still recommended for treatment of gonorrhea are the cephalosporins.[14]

Another major concern is the coexistence of chlamydial infection with gonorrhea.[15] (Chlamydial infections are discussed on p. 935.) Approximately 20% to 30% of men and a higher proportion of women have coexistent chlamydia infections. In the absence of gonorrhea, chlamydia may go undetected until complications such as PID or urethritis manifest themselves.

Treatment for gonorrhea is influenced by three factors: (1) the spread of infection caused by drug-resistant strains, (2) the high frequency of chlamydia infection accompanying gonorrhea, and (3) recognition of the serious complications of chlamydia and gonorrheal infections. CDC treatment guidelines are updated regularly, and the most recent edition should be used. Current CDC treatment guidelines for uncomplicated gonorrheal infections are listed in Box 24-1; complicated infections require intravenous antibiotic therapy and possibly hospitalization.

Sexual partners also are assessed and treated according to these protocols, and sexual contact is avoided until treatment is completed. Condoms are strongly recommended to prevent future infection.

Syphilis

Syphilis, a disease with local and systemic manifestations, has been well known throughout history. Many famous figures from the ancient world and from the royal families of Europe were thought or known to have had syphilis.[16] In the early half of the 1900s, an estimated 1 in 4 to 1 in 20 Americans were infected.[17] With the advent of antibiotics and intensive public health efforts during and after World War II, the prevalence of syphilis declined sharply to 3 in 100,000 Americans in 2002. Rates of syphilis declined in the 1990s and reached an all-time low in 2000 (2.2 cases per 100,000). However, between 2000 and 2007, the syphilis rate in the

Box 24-1	Outpatient Treatment for Uncomplicated Gonorrhea Infection[3]

- One of the following:
    Ceftriaxone, 125 mg IM in a single dose
    or
    Cefixime, 400 mg oral tablet or 400mg by suspension (200mg/5 ml) in a single dose
    or
    Spectinomycin, 2 g IM (if allergic to penicillin)
- Followed by one of these regimens for presumptive coexistent chlamydia:
    Azithromycin, 1 g PO in a single dose
    or
    Doxycycline, 100 mg PO bid × 7 days
    or Alternatives treatments
    Erythromycin, 500 mg PO qid × 7 days
    or
    Erythromycin E, 800 mg PO qid X 7 days
    or
    Ofloxacin 300mg PO bid X 7 days
    or
    Levofloxacin 500 mg PO once daily X 7 days

United States increased. Between 2006 and 2007, the national primary and secondary rate increased 15.2%, from 3.3 to 3.8 cases per 100,000 population, with the number of cases increasing from 9756 to 11,466 between 2006 and 2007.[4] The rate of primary and secondary syphilis has risen 54% among men in the past 5 years. Data suggest this increase is driven by increased transmission of primary and secondary syphilis among men who have sex with men (MSM), and accounts for 65% of these cases. The rate of primary and secondary syphilis is now nearly six times greater in men than women, whereas rates were almost equivalent a decade ago. Syphilis remains a problem in certain geographic regions, particularly in the South. Syphilis facilitates the transmission of HIV infection and seems to contribute to HIV transmission in those parts of the United States where rates of both infections are high. The rates of syphilis increased for all groups except for blacks between 2000 and 2003. Since 2003 the rates have increased for all groups; in 2007 the reported rate among non-Hispanic whites was 2.0 per 100,000, among Hispanics the rate was 4.3 per 100,000, among Asian/Pacific Islanders the rate was 1.2 per 100,000, among Native American/Alaskan Natives the rate was 3.8, and among Blacks the rate was 14 per 100,000. Rates in women have also increased; 10% between 2006 and 2007.[18] Subsequently, the yearly 14% percent decrease in congenital syphilis since 1996 ended in 2005 with increases of 11% and 15.4% for 2006 and 2007. The subsequent result is a reported 10.5 cases of congenital syphilis per 100,000 (it had been reported at 0.8 per 100,000 in 2003). During pregnancy, untreated early syphilis results in perinatal death in as many as 40% of cases and, if acquired in the previous 4 years, may lead to fetal infection in more than 70% of cases.[19]

Race, ethnicity, and gender alone do not alter STI risk but rather act as risk markers that correlate with other more fundamental determinants of health status, such as poverty, access to quality care, and health-seeking behavior. Higher infection rates have been associated with urban areas, with the exchange of sex for drugs, especially crack cocaine, and with prison populations.[3,20] A growing concern is the incidence of coinfection with HIV among MSM.[3,18]

PATHOPHYSIOLOGY *Treponema pallidum*, the cause of syphilis, is an anaerobic bacterium that cannot be cultured in vitro. The treponema (individual microorganism) looks like a corkscrew, with regular, tight spirals and a rotary motion; it can infect any body organ or tissue. Because the bacterium is present in exudate from moist mucosal or cutaneous lesions, the spirochete is transmitted during the first few years of infection. Transmission generally occurs through minor abrasions during sexual intercourse but can occur extragenitally as well. Approximately 30% to 50% of partners who have sexual intercourse with an individual in early stage syphilis develop the disease.[16]

Syphilis becomes a systemic disease shortly after infection and can be transmitted from a pregnant woman to her fetus as early as the ninth week of gestation. The risk of transmission to the fetus gradually declines with each subsequent pregnancy; therefore, a mother who has had several children with severe congenital syphilis may go on to bear a healthy child. After about 8 years, even without treatment, the mother's infection is not transmitted to her fetus.[17]

The course of untreated syphilis consists of four stages: primary, secondary, latent, and tertiary (Box 24-2).

Primary syphilis begins at the site of bacterial invasion (Figure 24-4). There *T. pallidum* multiplies in the epithelium, producing a granulomatous tissue reaction called a **chancre.** Some microorganisms drain with lymph into adjacent lymph nodes. Within the nodes and at the site of the chancre, the cell-mediated and humoral immune responses are stimulated.

Secondary syphilis is systemic. During this stage, blood-borne bacteria spread to all major organ systems. The secondary stage is followed by a period during which the immune system is able to suppress the infection. Even without treatment, spontaneous resolution of the skin lesions occurs and the individual enters the latent stage of infection.

Box 24-2	Progression of Untreated Syphilis

Stage I, primary syphilis—local invasion: *Treponema pallidum* multiplies in epithelium, producing granulomatous tissue reaction (chancre); lymph-containing microorganisms drain into adjacent lymph nodes and stimulate immune responses
Stage II, secondary syphilis—systemic disease: blood-borne bacteria spread to all major organ systems; immune system suppresses infection and symptoms regress spontaneously
Stage III, latent syphilis—silent infection: transmission of infection possible even though there are no clinical signs of infection
Stage IV, tertiary syphilis—noninfectious disease: significant morbidity and mortality occur; destructive skin, bone, and soft tissue lesions, or gummas, result from severe hypersensitivity; cardiovascular complications (aneurysms, heart valve insufficiency, heart failure) and neurosyphilis develop

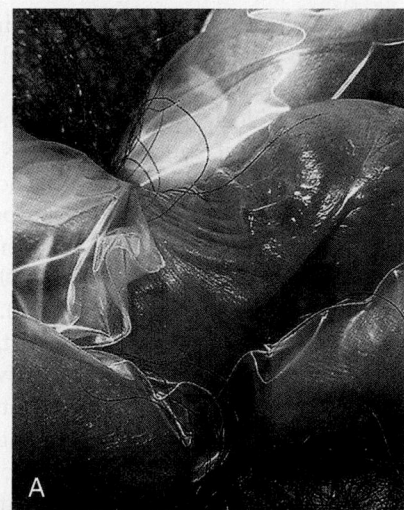

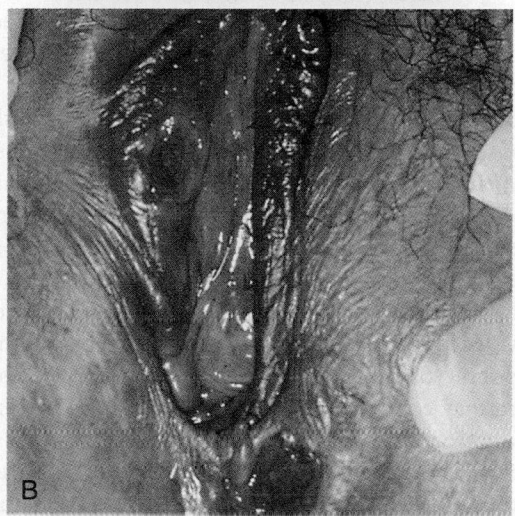

Figure 24-4 Primary syphilis. **A,** Penile chancre. **B,** Vulval chancres; the the labia and perineum show induration and edema of chancres. (**A** from McMillan A, Scott GR: Sexually transmitted infections, ed 2, London, 2000, Churchill Livingstone; **B** from Morse SA et al, editors: *Atlas of sexually transmitted diseases and AIDS,* ed 3, London, 2003, Mosby.)

Latent syphilis may be subdivided into early and late stages; however, no specific criteria delineate one from the other.[20] Medical history and serologic studies show that syphilis is present, but the individual has no clinical manifestations. Transmission is possible during the late and early latent stages.

Tertiary syphilis is the most severe stage, involving significant morbidity and mortality. The pathogenesis of syphilitic manifestations at this stage remains unclear. The destructive skin, bone, and soft tissue lesions (called **gummas**) of tertiary syphilis probably are caused by a severe hypersensitivity reaction to the microorganism. Within the cardiovascular system, infection with *T. pallidum* may cause aneurysms, heart valve insufficiencies, and heart failure. Within the central nervous system (CNS), the presence of *T. pallidum* in cerebrospinal fluid may cause the manifestations of **neurosyphilis.**[17]

The risk of acquiring congenital syphilis (CS) is estimated at 50% in primary and secondary syphilis, 40% in early latent

syphilis, and 10% in late latent syphilis.[21] Intrauterine infection causes fetal or perinatal death in 40% of affected infants.[19,22]

CLINICAL MANIFESTATIONS

Primary Stage. In adults the incubation period of syphilis ranges from 12 days to 12 weeks after exposure and averages 3 weeks. At the site of treponemal entry a sore, or *hard chancre,* develops. Typically the chancre is an eroded, painless, firm, and indurated (hard) ulcer that may be a few millimeters to 2 cm in diameter. Firm, enlarged, and nontender regional lymph nodes accompany chancres. Figure 24-4 shows typical chancres of the penis and vulva. Syphilitic chancres are not always typical, however, and syphilis should be considered in the presence of any open lesion. Secondary infection can cause chancres to become necrotic and painful, and lesions on the fingers may be dry, scaly, and papular or moist and vegetative. If left untreated, the chancre of primary syphilis heals in 2 to 8 weeks and then spontaneously disappears, usually without leaving a scar.

Secondary Stage. Clinical manifestations of secondary syphilis usually develop 6 weeks after the first appearance of the chancre but may overlap with those of the primary stage. Typically this stage presents with variable systemic symptoms, including low-grade fever, malaise, sore throat, hoarseness, anorexia, generalized adenopathy, headache, joint pain, and skin or mucous membrane lesions or rashes. Cutaneous (skin) rashes are generally papulosquamous (raised and scaly), but any variation or combination of macular (flat), papular (raised), and pustular (pus-filled) lesions may be seen. Often lesions are widespread and bilateral and appear on the palms and soles (Figure 24-5). Some lesions become hypertrophied, flat, moist, and wartlike or vegetative (e.g., cauliflower-like). These lesions, called **condylomata lata,** are highly contagious and develop on the perineum, vulva, and groin of women (Figure 24-6) and around the inner thigh and the anal area in men and women. Besides skin sores, oral mucous membrane lesions (known as mucous patches), lymphadenopathy, pruritus, and alopecia are common. Some individuals develop anemia, leukocytosis, increased sedimentation rate, hepatitis, transitory proteinuria, arthritis, electrocardiographic abnormalities, and CNS symptoms. Regardless of whether treatment is given, the cutaneous lesions generally heal in 2 to 10 weeks, but relapses may occur for several years.[21]

Latent and Tertiary Stages. The asymptomatic, latent stage of syphilis may be as short as 1 year or as long as a lifetime. After the latent stage, tertiary syphilis may present with gummas, cardiovascular lesions, and neurosyphilis. These manifestations of tertiary syphilis are quite rare because antibiotics can cure syphilis.

Congenital Syphilis. Congenital syphilis is characterized by vasculitis, necrosis, fibrosis, and distribution of *T. pallidum* throughout the tissues; it is divided into early and late stages. Signs and symptoms of early CS manifest in the first 2 years of life, and clinical manifestations of the late stage often occur near puberty. Affected newborns often are premature and show evidence of intrauterine growth restriction,

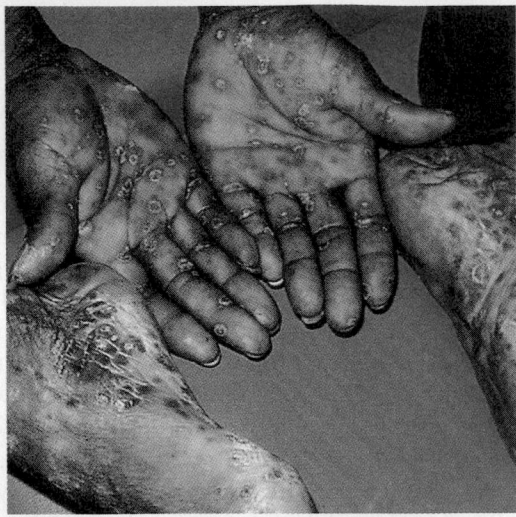

Figure 24-5 **Secondary syphilis.** Secondary syphilis to the palms and plantar surfaces. (From Morse S et al, editors: *Atlas of sexually transmitted diseases and AIDS*, ed 3, London, 2003, Mosby.)

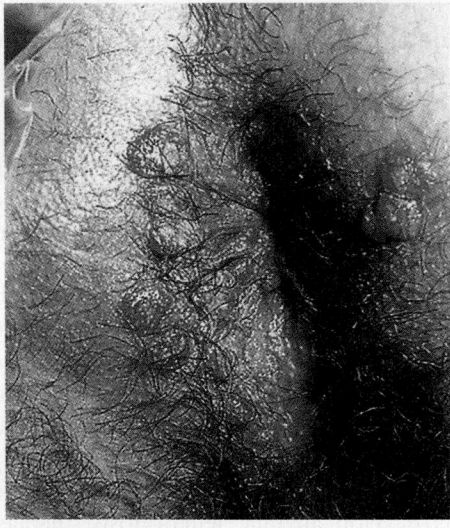

Figure 24-6 **Condylomata lata.** Broad-based, moist, darkfield-positive condylomata lata of the perineum. (From McMillan A, Scott GR: *Sexually transmitted infections*, ed 2, London, 2000, Churchill Livingstone.)

hepatosplenomegaly, bone marrow depression, destructive bone and skin lesions (see Figure 24-5), retinal inflammation, glaucoma, blood dyscrasia, nephrotic syndrome, and varying degrees of CNS involvement.[17] Late manifestations of classic congenital syphilis correspond to those of tertiary syphilis in the adult and are rare.

EVALUATION AND TREATMENT Because *T. pallidum* cannot be cultured in vitro, early definitive diagnosis of primary or secondary syphilis depends on darkfield microscopy of a specimen taken from a chancre, regional lymph node, or other lesion. If the initial result is negative, the darkfield examination is repeated on 2 successive days. When suspicion of syphilis—based on history and physical

examination—persists, serologic testing is required. An algorithmic approach to the diagnosis of genital ulcers is presented in Figure 24-7.

Two categories of serologic testing exist: nontreponemal antigen tests and treponemal antibody tests.[23] Nontreponemal antigen tests, which demonstrate the presence of *reagin* (a group of antibodies present in syphilis) in serum, provide indirect evidence of infection. Examples of nontreponemal analysis are the Venereal Disease Research Laboratory (VDRL) antigen and the rapid plasma reagin (RPR) tests (Box 24-3). These tests yield a positive result (presence of reagin) in more than 50% of individuals with primary syphilis and 100% of individuals with secondary disease. When the serologic test is negative and another stage of syphilis is suspected, the test is repeated. If latent or tertiary syphilis is suspected, a treponemal serologic test is done. Treponemal tests are serologic-specific tests that are used to assess antibody response to *T. pallidum* and include the fluorescent treponemal antibody absorption (FTA-ABS) test and the microhemagglutination (MHA-TP) test.

Numerous dermatologic disorders can mimic the skin lesions of secondary syphilis, making differential diagnosis difficult. Again, laboratory confirmation is important; darkfield microscopy of scrapings from the condylomata lata or other skin lesions discloses the treponemata. Serologic tests are almost always strongly positive in this stage.

During the latent stage, individuals continue to have serologic evidence of untreated disease, but confirmation through darkfield microscopy is difficult. Examination of cerebrospinal fluid may confirm that the treponemata are present and the insidious onset of neurosyphilis has begun.

Preferred treatment for all stages of syphilis is parenteral injection of benzathine penicillin G. If the individual has had signs of the disease for less than 1 year, a single dose is appropriate. If signs have been present for more than 1 year, the treatment is three weekly injections. This therapy is also appropriate for pregnant women. There is no evidence to date that *T. pallidum* has developed resistance to penicillin. In fact, it is highly sensitive but because of the slow replication time serum levels must be maintained for 7 to 14 days. Duration of therapy depends on estimated length of infection. Treatment for 14 days is recommended if the individual has been infected less than 1 year; treatment is for 28 days if the individual has been infected for longer than 1 year. Individuals who are allergic to penicillin may receive oral doxycycline, 100 mg twice daily for 14 days. Pregnant women with a penicillin allergy should be desensitized and then treated with benzathine penicillin G as recommended by the CDC.[14] Because treatment failures do occur, all individuals should have follow-up evaluation. Sexual partners also are examined and treated, and the use of condoms is recommended.

Definitive diagnosis of CS is made by microscopic identification of *T. pallidum* in material from skin lesions or nasal discharge. Probable diagnosis is assumed on the basis of a rising or persistently reactive FTA-ABS value and clinical manifestations. In all cases of maternal syphilis, the goal

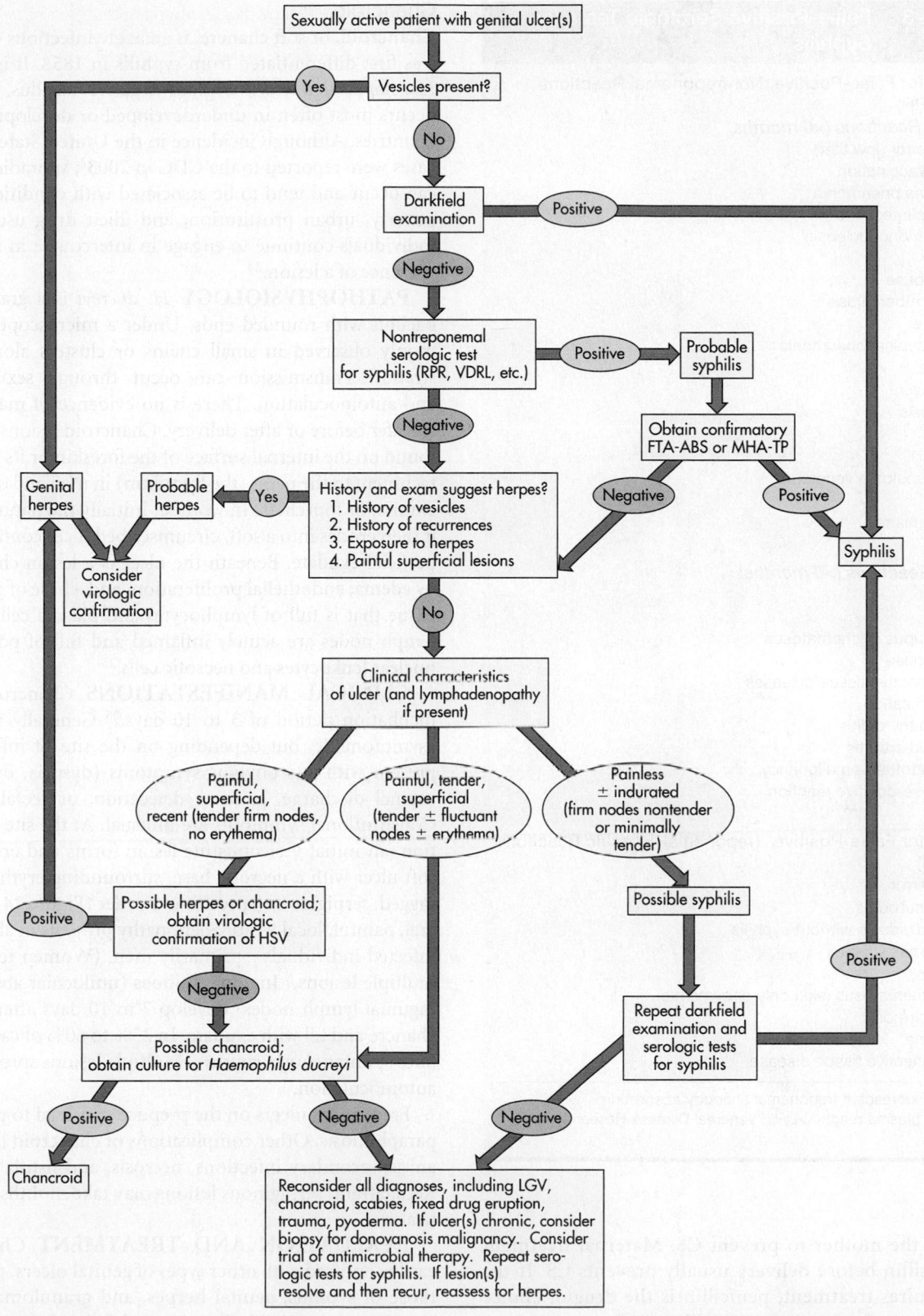

Figure 24-7 **Genital ulceration.** Algorithm outlining an approach to the diagnosis of an individual who presents with a genital ulceration. *FTA-ABS,* Fluorescent treponemal antibody absorption; *HSV,* herpes simplex virus; *LGV,* lymphogranuloma venereum; *MHA-TP,* microhemagglutination assay–*Treponema pallidum; RPR,* rapid plasma reagin; *VDRL,* Venereal Disease Research Laboratory. (Redrawn from Pitot P, Plummer FA. In Holmes KK et al, editors: *Sexually transmitted diseases,* ed 2, New York, 1990, McGraw-Hill.)

Box 24-3	False-Positive Serologic Tests for Syphilis

Reasons for False-Positive, Nontreponemal Reactions (VDRL, RPR)

Transient Reactions (<6 months)
Technical error (low titer)
Smallpox vaccination
Mycoplasma pneumonia
Enterovirus infections
Infectious mononucleosis
Pregnancy
Narcotic abuse
Advanced tuberculosis
Scarlet fever
Viral and atypical pneumonia
Brucellosis
Rat-bite fever
Leptospirosis
Measles
Mumps
Lymphogranuloma venereum
Malaria
Trypanosomiasis
Varicella

Chronic Reactions (>6 months)
Malaria
Leprosy
Systemic lupus erythematosus
Narcotic abuse
Other connective tissue diseases
Elderly population
Hashimoto thyroiditis
Rheumatoid arthritis
Reticuloendothelial malignancy
Familial false-positive reaction
Idiopathic

Reasons for False-Positive, Treponemal-Specific Reactions (FTA-ABS)
Technical error
Inefficient sorbents
Healthy individuals without syphilis
Genital herpes simplex
Pregnancy
Lupus erythematosus (skin only or systemic)
Alcoholic cirrhosis
Scleroderma
Mixed connective tissue disease

FTA-ABS, Fluorescent treponemal antibody absorption; *RPR,* rapid plasma reagin; *VDRL,* Venereal Disease Research Laboratory.

is to treat the mother to prevent CS. Maternal treatment with penicillin before delivery usually prevents CS. If the infant requires treatment, penicillin is the drug of choice because allergy does not pose a problem in the neonatal period. Such infants are then given serologic tests for syphilis every 2 to 3 months until the test becomes nonreactive or the titer has decreased fourfold. Nearly all tests become nonreactive (negative) by the time the infant is 6 months of age.[19]

Chancroid

Chancroid, or soft chancre, is an acute infectious disease that was first differentiated from syphilis in 1852. It is caused by *Haemophilus ducreyi,* a gram-negative bacillus. Chancroid occurs most often in underdeveloped or developing tropical countries. Although incidence in the United States is low, 54 cases were reported to the CDC in 2003[2]; sporadic outbreaks can occur and tend to be associated with conditions such as poverty, urban prostitution, and illicit drug use, in which individuals continue to engage in intercourse in spite of the presence of a lesion.[24]

PATHOPHYSIOLOGY *H. ducreyi* is a gram-negative bacillus with rounded ends. Under a microscope it is commonly observed in small chains or clusters along mucous strands. Transmission can occur through sexual contact and autoinoculation. There is no evidence of maternal-fetal transfer before or after delivery. Chancroid lesions usually are found on the internal surface of the foreskin or its point of attachment to the penis (the frenulum) in men and on the labia, clitoris, or fourchette in women. Initially the papule enlarges; it then erodes into a soft, circumscribed ulcer containing a superficial exudate. Beneath the ulcer is a lesion characterized by edema, endothelial proliferation, and a base of granulation tissue that is full of lymphocytes and plasma cells. Adjacent lymph nodes are acutely inflamed and full of polymorphonuclear leukocytes and necrotic cells.[25]

CLINICAL MANIFESTATIONS Chancroid has an incubation period of 3 to 10 days.[26] Generally women are asymptomatic, but depending on the site of infection, can present with less obvious symptoms (dysuria, dyspareunia, vaginal discharge, pain on defecation, or rectal bleeding). Constitutional symptoms are unusual. At the site of inoculation, an initial vesicopustule lesion forms and erodes into a soft ulcer with a necrotic base, surrounding erythema, and a ragged, serpiginous (spreading) border (Figure 24-8). Unilateral, painful, local lymphadenopathy presents in about half of infected individuals—primarily men. (Women tend to have multiple lesions.) Inguinal **buboes** (unilocular abscess of the inguinal lymph nodes) develop 7 to 10 days after the initial chancre and fill with exudate. In 25% to 60% of cases, the buboes spontaneously rupture. Multiple lesions spread through autoinoculation.

Frequently, ulcers on the prepuce may lead to phimosis or paraphimosis. Other complications of chancroid include balanitis, secondary infections, necrosis, and fistula formation. Recalcitrant, serpiginous lesions may take months or years to heal.

EVALUATION AND TREATMENT Chancroid is easily confused with other types of genital ulcers, particularly those of syphilis, genital herpes, and granuloma inguinale (see Figure 24-8). Unlike the syphilitic ulcer, chancroidal ulcer is painful, tender, and nonindurated. Microscopic analysis of a gram-stained smear from the chancroid helps to identify the microorganism. Definitive diagnosis depends on recovery of *H. ducreyi* from cultured specimens. Fluorescent monoclonal antibody stains and PCR provide more specific

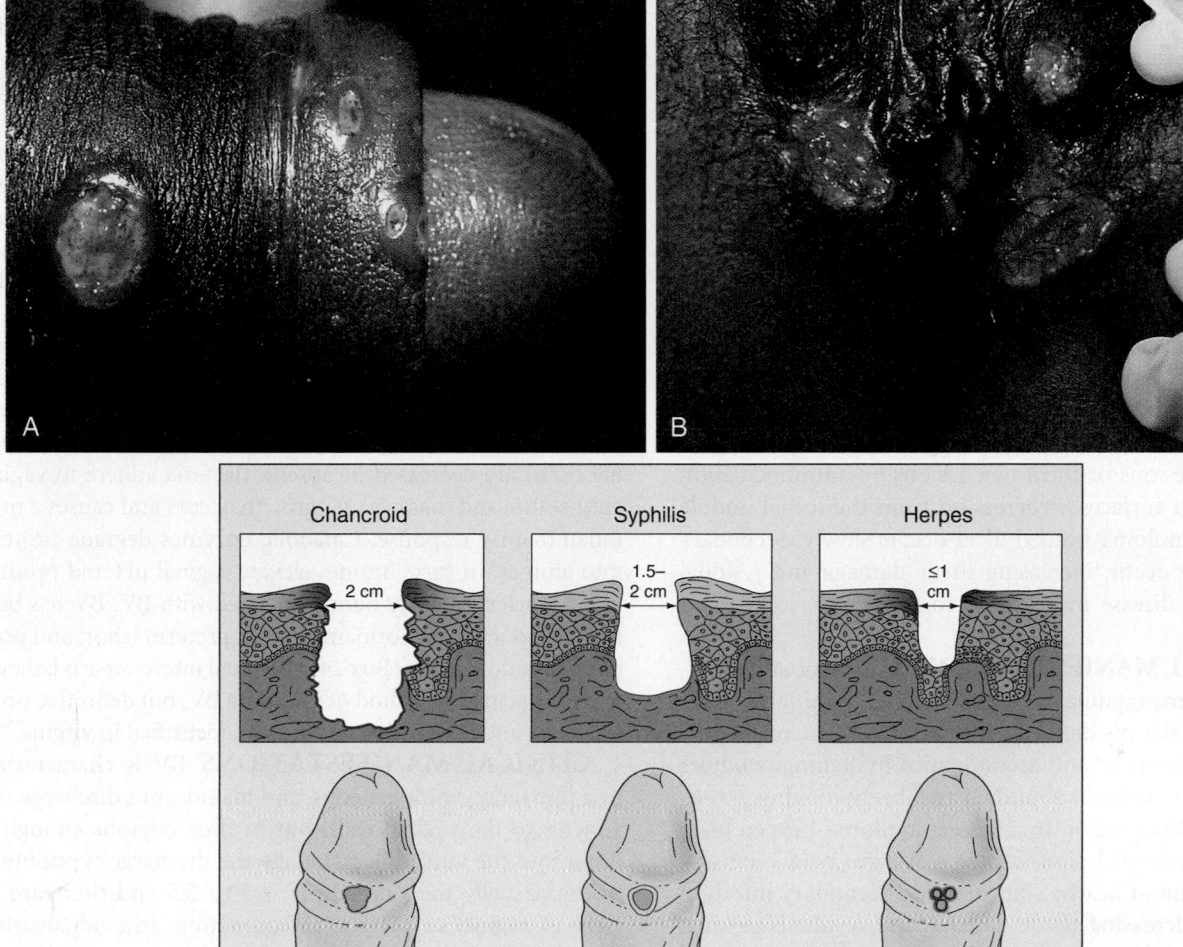

Figure 24-8 Chancroid. A, Ulcers on the penile shaft. B, Multiple vulvar lesions. C, Differences in clinical appearance among chancroid, syphilis, and genital herpes. (From Morse SA et al, editors: *Atlas of sexually transmitted diseases and AIDS*, ed 3, London, 2003, Mosby.)

diagnosis but are not routinely available. Because 10% of infected individuals are coinfected with syphilis or herpes simplex virus (HSV), testing includes serologic examination for syphilis and viral culture for HSV. In addition, HIV testing is recommended: chancroid is a cofactor for transmission of HIV.

Resistance to recommended antibiotics has emerged in isolated instances worldwide. Recent treatment recommendations include a single intramuscular injection of ceftriaxone (250 mg) or a single dose of oral azithromycin (1 g). Effective oral multiple-dose regimens include ciprofloxacin, 500 mg orally twice daily for 3 days; or erythromycin, 500 mg three times daily for 7 days. Persons infected with HIV have higher rates of treatment failure with single-dose therapy and may require a longer treatment regimen. As a palliative measure, buboes can be aspirated through adjacent, healthy skin. In approximately 5% of cases, relapses at the site of original ulcer have occurred.[26,27] Simultaneous treatment of sexual partners and condom use are recommended to prevent reinfection.

Granuloma Inguinale

Granuloma inguinale (donovanosis) is a chronic, progressively destructive bacterial infection caused by *Calymmatobacterium granulomatis,* recently reclassified as *Klebsiella granulomatis.*[24] Although sexually transmissible, granuloma inguinale is only mildly contagious and repeated exposure is necessary to cause disease. Often, individuals are coinfected with syphilis.[28]

Indigenous granuloma inguinale no longer occurs in the United States (cases that occur are imported).[26] Yet in some parts of the world (India, New Guinea, Africa, central Australia, and to a lesser extent the Caribbean and Brazil), granuloma inguinale is among the most prevalent of the present STIs. Incidence of infection is found in tropical and subtropical environments with sustained high temperature and high relative humidity. Infection is usually acquired through sexual intercourse with an individual who has active disease or asymptomatic rectal infection. As with all genital ulcerative diseases, granuloma inguinale plays a role in HIV transmission.[24]

PATHOPHYSIOLOGY *C. granulomatis* is a gram-negative, nonsporing, nonmotile, encapsulated rod that is not easily isolated in the laboratory. After exposure the bacteria survive and multiply within vacuoles of large histiocytic cells or polymorphonuclear leukocytes. The bacteria reproduce within these cells until a vacuole may contain 20 to 30 microorganisms. These bacteria-filled vacuoles were identified by Donovan in 1905 and are termed **Donovan bodies.** The presence of Donovan bodies in tissue smears of material from the lesions is considered the gold standard for diagnosis of lymphogranuloma inguinale.[28,29]

The initial lesion is an indurated subcutaneous nodule that is often preceded and accompanied by itching. The primary sites for development of the lesions are the distal penis in men and the introitus in women. Single lesions often coalesce with nearby lesions or form new lesions by autoinoculation of nearby skin surfaces. Progression from the initial nodule to a large, granuloma-heaped ulcer occurs slowly. Secondary infection may occur, increasing tissue damage and residual scarring. The disease may spread to the bones, joints, and liver.

CLINICAL MANIFESTATIONS The incubation period of granuloma inguinale is 8 to 80 days. The initial lesion is an indurated, sharply defined, painless, subcutaneous nodule that is often preceded and accompanied by itching. Nodules bleed easily and contain abundant red, beefy-looking granulation tissue. Progression to a large granuloma-heaped ulcer occurs slowly; single lesions coalesce or form new lesions by autoinoculation of nearby skin surfaces. Secondary infection may occur, increasing tissue damage and residual scarring. Although systemic symptoms are rare, the disease may spread to the bones, joints, and liver. In some cases, infection spreads to the inguinale area and produces **pseudobuboes.** In these instances, the affected lymph nodes are not directly affected, but the surrounding area may be infected and abscessed.

EVALUATION AND TREATMENT Although the clinical manifestations of this disease are important for diagnosis, confirmation involves microscopic examination in which Donovan bodies are found in a smear or biopsy specimen. No FDA-cleared PCR tests for the detection of *K. granulomatis* DNA exists, but such an assay would be helpful.[14]

Many antibiotics have been used successfully against *K. granulomatis.* Because other STIs frequently coexist, individuals should be tested for chlamydia, gonorrhea, syphilis, hepatitis B, and HIV. Because of the indolent nature of the disease, duration of therapy tends to be relatively long. With effective antibiotic treatment, lesions begin to heal in 7 days, but treatment is continued for at least 3 weeks and until all lesions are completely healed. Oral therapy includes doxycycline (100 mg) twice a day, azithromycin (1 g) once a week, ciprofloxacin (750 mg) twice a day, erythromycin base (500 mg) four times a day, or trimethoprim-sulfamethoxazole (160 mg/800 mg, double-strength tablet) twice a day. Relapses can occur 6 to 18 months later despite effective initial therapy, so prolonged follow-up is necessary, as is treatment of sexual partners.

Bacterial Vaginosis

Bacterial vaginosis (BV)—previously called nonspecific vaginitis; nonspecific vaginosis; or *Haemophilus, Corynebacterium,* or *Gardnerella* vaginitis—is a sexually associated condition, but is not necessarily considered an STI. Bacterial vaginosis occurs almost exclusively in sexually active women of reproductive age and is uncommon in sexually inexperienced women. Prevalence rates vary from 17% among women in family planning clinics to 37% among some groups of pregnant women.[1] Fifty percent of women with signs of BV are asymptomatic.

PATHOPHYSIOLOGY The exact etiology of BV is unknown. *Gardnerella vaginalis* and various anaerobes, including *Mycoplasma hominis, Bacteroides,* and *Mobiluncus,* interact and proliferate when lactobacilli (the normal predominant vaginal flora) are decreased or absent. Bacteria adhere to vaginal epithelium, and massive overgrowth occurs and causes a noninflammatory response. Catabolic enzymes degrade proteins into amines. In turn, amines elevate vaginal pH and produce the characteristic fishy odor associated with BV. BV has been implicated in PID, chorioamnionitis, preterm labor, and postpartum endometritis (Box 24-4). Sexual intercourse is believed to be the primary method of initiating BV, but definitive proof is lacking and the syndrome has been identified in virgins.[28,30]

CLINICAL MANIFESTATIONS BV is characterized by a thin, gray, homogeneous, and malodorous discharge that adheres to the vaginal walls but is often copious enough to drain into the vulva. Occasionally the discharge is bubbly or frothy. Usually the vaginal pH is 5 to 5.5 and there are no signs of vaginal or cervical inflammation. Individuals often complain of a strong, foul, fishy vaginal odor, particularly after intercourse and during menses. Odor is caused by contact with alkaline secretions, including semen and menstrual discharge. Male partners of infected women may harbor the microorganisms that are responsible for BV but have no signs or symptoms of active disease.

EVALUATION AND TREATMENT Diagnosis of BV can be made based on three of four of the following criteria: (1) presence of adherent gray vaginal discharge, (2) pH

Box 24-4 | **Is Bacterial Vaginosis a Risk Factor for Preterm Delivery?**

Eighteen studies with 20,232 subjects were reviewed as a meta-analysis to evaluate bacterial vaginosis as a risk factor for preterm delivery. It was found that bacterial vaginosis increased the risk of preterm delivery twofold. Higher risks were calculated for subgroups of studies that screened for bacterial vaginosis at <16 weeks of gestation or at <20 weeks of gestation. Bacterial vaginosis also significantly increased the risk of spontaneous abortion and maternal infection. No significant results, however, were calculated for the outcome of neonatal infection or perinatal death. In conclusion, it was determined that bacterial vaginosis, early in pregnancy, is a strong risk factor for preterm delivery and spontaneous abortion.

Data from Leitich H et al: *Am J Obstet Gynecol* 289(1):139-247, 2003.

greater than 4.5, (3) positive amine odor, and (4) presence of clue cells on wet mount.[32] Clue cells are considered pathognomonic for BV. The saline wet mount also may show absence of lactobacilli and few or no leukocytes. Clue cells are vaginal epithelial cells that are covered with bacteria and look as if pepper has been sprinkled on them. When a drop of potassium hydroxide (KOH) solution is added to the slide, a characteristic amine odor is released immediately. Cultures are neither useful nor recommended; however, individuals should be screened for gonorrhea and chlamydia.

The most commonly used treatment for *Gardnerella*-associated BV is a course of oral metronidazole (Flagyl), 500 mg twice daily for 7 days, or 0.75% vaginal gel once daily for 5 days. Alternative regimens include oral clindamycin (300 mg) twice daily for 7 days or 2% vaginal cream once daily for 7 days. Clindamycin vaginal suppositories have been newly approved for use as a 3-day treatment regimen in nonpregnant women. Clindamycin cream is oil based, and for up to 72 hours after completing therapy, it may weaken latex condoms. BV treatment in women infected with HIV is the same for HIV-negative patients. It is especially important in women who are pregnant, because BV and chorioamnionitis may increase the risk of perinatal transmission of HIV.[27] No evidence indicates that treatment of sexual partners reduces recurrence and is not recommended.[31]

Chlamydial Infections

Urogenital Infections

Chlamydia is the common name for infections caused by *Chlamydia trachomatis* (CT). *C. trachomatis* is responsible for a variety of syndromes, including acute urethral syndrome, nongonococcal urethritis (NGU), mucopurulent cervicitis, and PID. Chlamydia, the most common bacterial STI in the United States, affects about 3 million individuals annually[5] and is the leading cause of preventable infertility and ectopic pregnancy. In 2007, 1,108,374 cases of chlamydial infections were reported. This is more than three times the number of reported gonorrhea infections. The rate of chlamydia in 2007 was 544 cases per 100,000 population, and has increased for all race/ethnic groups except among Native Americans/Alaskan Natives. This increase probably reflects the continued expansion of screening efforts and increased use of more sensitive diagnostic tests as well as a frank increase in incidence.[32] Approximately 75% of women with CT infection are asymptomatic. In addition, *C. trachomatis* can be recovered from the urethra in 25% to 60% of men with NGU, in 4% to 35% of men with gonorrhea, in 28% of asymptomatic men whose partners have chlamydial cervicitis, and in 0% to 7% of men without urethritis who are seen in STI clinics.

Chlamydia is most common among young (less than 20 years old) heterosexuals who have new or multiple partners, are economically disadvantaged, are entering juvenile detention centers, and have been diagnosed with gonorrhea.[5] The incidence of CT infection in pregnancy has been estimated at between 2% and 30%. Age younger than 25 years (with highest rates in women younger than 20 years), a new sexual partner and first pregnancy were strongly and independently associated with infection in a study of more than 7000 pregnant women who were screened for CT at their first prenatal visit. Like gonorrhea, *Chlamydia* infection is transmitted from mother to infant through the infected birth canal. Estimated rate of transmission ranges from 60% to 70%.[33]

PATHOPHYSIOLOGY *C. trachomatis* is an obligate, gram-negative intracellular bacterium that lacks the ability to reproduce independently. Like viruses, *Chlamydia* can reproduce only within host cells. It is differentiated from other bacteria by its unique two-part growth cycle. The first part consists of an elementary body that is small, resilient, metabolically inert, and able to survive extracellularly. Once this elementary body attaches itself to a receptor host cell, it is able to enter by endocytosis. Once inside the cell, the second part of the cycle begins and the microorganism becomes a metabolically active parasite, reproducing within the cell until the cell is destroyed and ruptures, disseminating up to 1000 new elementary bodies. Rarely does this cause a secondary infection. Infection with *C. trachomatis* produces a mononuclear inflammatory reaction rather than a polymorphonuclear inflammatory reaction. The former reaction produces permanent scarring of tissues.[34]

Chlamydia microorganisms are always pathogens; they are not part of the normal flora of the urogenital tract, despite the fact that infection is often asymptomatic. Numerous serotypes, or strains, of *C. trachomatis* have been identified. Some cause urogenital infection; some, ocular trachoma; and others, lymphogranuloma venereum, which is discussed in the next section.

The strains of *C. trachomatis* that cause urogenital infection apparently require squamous-columnar and columnar-epithelial cells as hosts. *C. trachomatis* infects and disrupts epithelial tissues but does not seem to invade or destroy deeper tissues or organs. Urogenital chlamydial infections may have a fairly self-limited acute course followed by a chronic, low-grade, persistent infection that lasts for years.[34]

In newborns, several sites may be inoculated with *Chlamydia* during passage through the infected maternal cervix. These include the eye, nasopharynx, rectum, and vagina. The infant also may aspirate infected secretions with its first breaths, resulting in chlamydial pneumonitis and substantial newborn morbidity.

CLINICAL MANIFESTATIONS Asymptomatic chlamydial infection is common. Urogenital infections caused by *Chlamydia* closely parallel those caused by gonorrhea. Both microorganisms infect superficial genital tract tissues, such as mucosa of the urethra and cervix, and both can invade the epididymides, fallopian tubes, and hepatic capsule. Table 24-2 lists the pathophysiologic similarities of chlamydial and gonococcal infections.

Chlamydial infection accounts for 50% to 60% of cases of NGU in men. Clinically, urethritis caused by gonorrhea and chlamydia cannot be differentiated: both have a 7- to 21-day incubation period and cause dysuria. Although urethral

Table 24-2	Similarity of Clinical Syndromes Caused by *Chlamydia trachomatis* and *Neisseria gonorrhoeae*	
	Clinical Syndrome	
Site of Infection	N. gonorrhoeae	C. trachomatis
Men		
Urethra	Urethritis	Nongonococcal urethritis; postgonococcal urethritis
Epididymis	Epididymitis	Epididymitis
Rectum	Proctitis	Proctitis
Conjunctiva	Conjunctivitis	Conjunctivitis
Systemic	Disseminated gonococcal infection	Reiter syndrome
Women		
Urethra	Acute urethral syndrome	Acute urethral syndrome
Bartholin gland	Bartholinitis	Bartholinitis
Cervix	Cervicitis	Cervicitis; cervical atypia
Fallopian tube	Salpingitis	Salpingitis
Conjunctiva	Conjunctivitis	Conjunctivitis
Liver capsule	Perihepatitis	Perihepatitis
Systemic	Disseminated gonococcal infection	Arthritis-dermatitis syndrome

Data from Stamm WE, Holmes KK: Chlamydia trachomatis infections in the adult. In Holmes KK et al, editors: *Sexually transmitted diseases,* ed 2, New York, 1990, McGraw-Hill.

discharge in men may be similar in the two infections, chlamydial discharge tends to be more clear and gonococcal discharge more purulent. Men might note a clear, mucous discharge on rising in the morning; dry, clear discharge on their underwear; or mild burning with urination. Chlamydial urethritis is generally milder than gonorrheal urethritis and more likely to be asymptomatic. Symptoms may be intermittent or unnoticeable. Gram-stained smears of the urethral discharge show numerous polymorphonuclear leukocytes, which indicates ongoing inflammation. Screening men without symptoms is not cost effective at this time.

Chlamydial epididymitis can accompany chlamydial urethritis and is characterized by fever and a unilaterally painful, swollen scrotum. Chlamydial infection also causes proctitis (rectal inflammation) in homosexual men and occasionally in heterosexual women and is linked to the practice of receptive anal intercourse. Chlamydial proctitis is generally mild, although it may, like gonorrheal proctitis, cause rectal bleeding, mucous discharge, and diarrhea. Reiter syndrome (urethritis, conjunctivitis, arthritis, and characteristic mucocutaneous lesions) is also associated with untreated chlamydial infections of the urogenital tract.

Chlamydia infection is the leading cause of tubal infertility in women. Risk factors for infertility include numbers of chlamydial infections and duration and severity of infection. Even women with asymptomatic salpingitis have a risk of subsequent infertility. This may reflect an antigen-antibody response rather than inflammatory damage.[35]

In young sexually active women, *C. trachomatis* is a cause of **acute urethral syndrome** (dysuria, urinary frequency, and presence of sterile pus in the urine). *C. trachomatis* also causes asymptomatic urethral infection in women. Chlamydial infection of Bartholin glands can cause purulent discharge and formation of a Bartholin cyst. Women with chlamydial cervicitis may be asymptomatic or may have a yellow mucopurulent

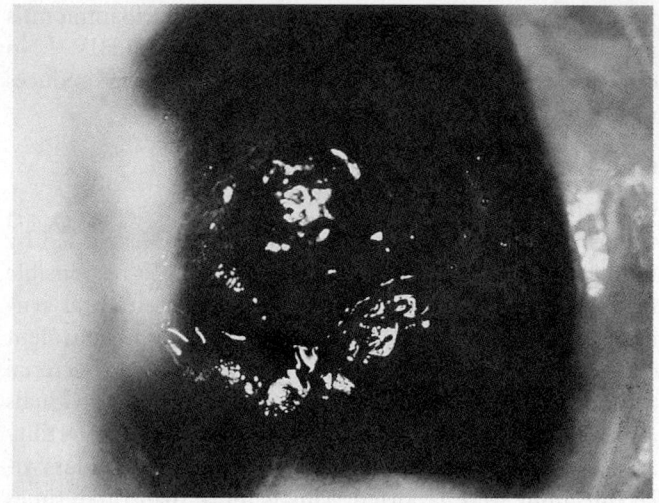

Figure 24-9 Chlamydial cervicitis. Beefy red mucosa of columnar epithelium of cervix. (From Morse SA et al, editors: *Atlas of sexually transmitted diseases and AIDS,* ed 3, London, 2003, Mosby.)

discharge from the cervical os and a hypertrophic, edematous, and friable area of cervical ectopy. The woman also may report intermenstrual or postcoital spotting. Although ectopy alone does not indicate a pathologic condition, a raised, erythematous, raw, and friable ectopy is abnormal and strongly suggestive of chlamydial cervicitis (Figure 24-9).

The most common clinical manifestations of chlamydial infections in the newborn are conjunctivitis and pneumonia. Like gonococcal infection, prophylactic treatment with antibiotic eye ointment at birth does not provide complete protection against neonatal conjunctivitis and does not protect against neonatal pneumonia. Chlamydial conjunctivitis begins between 5 and 14 days after delivery, when the infant's eyes begin to water. This discharge may become purulent, and both eyes may become red and swollen (Figure 24-10).

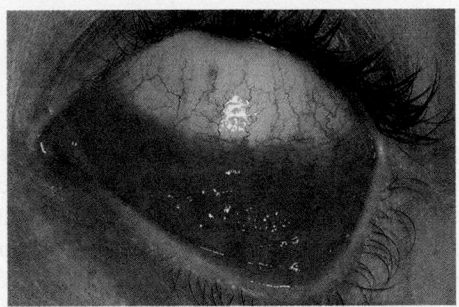

Figure 24-10 Chlamydial ophthalmia. (From McMillan A, Scott GR: *Sexually transmitted infections,* ed 2, London, 2000, Churchill Livingstone.)

Scarring of the conjunctivae may result, but this infection does not cause blindness, as does the ophthalmia neonatorum caused by *N. gonorrhoeae.* The pneumonia is mild or severe and may accompany the conjunctivitis. Infants with chlamydial pneumonia are seen at 3 to 11 weeks of age with staccato coughing spells, nasal congestion, dyspnea, and minimal fever. Other signs include otitis media, tachypnea, wheezing, bronchospasm, crepitant inspiratory rales, and apneic spells.

EVALUATION AND TREATMENT Methods for diagnosing chlamydial infections include tissue culture techniques, direct chlamydia enzyme immunoassay, fluorescein-labeled monoclonal antibody tests, and DNA probe testing. Currently, tests using chlamydia-specific nucleic acid sequences (LCR, PCR, and DNA) are the most sensitive and cost-effective tests available.[33] Concurrent DNA testing for gonorrhea can be done using the same swab.

C. trachomatis is susceptible to inexpensive, readily accessible antibiotics. Treatment includes antibiotic therapy for infected individuals and all sexual contacts; abstinence or use of condoms during treatment is recommended. Azithromycin is given 1 g orally, as a single dose or a 7-day course of oral doxycycline, 100 mg twice daily. Alternative regimens include a 7-day course of oral erythromycin, 500 mg four times a day, or erythromycin E 800 mg four times daily for 7 days. Ofloxacin 300 mg, twice daily or levofloxacin 500 mg once daily for 7 days are also effective alternatives.[5] Azithromycin is the drug of choice in pregnancy. Because of the asymptomatic nature of *Chlamydia* and the potential sequelae of untreated infection, extensive widespread screening is warranted.

Lymphogranuloma Venereum
C. trachomatis (invasive serovars of strains L1, L2, or L3) can cause a chronic STI known as **lymphogranuloma venereum (LGV),** which may be confused with syphilis, herpes, or chancroid. Although LGV is rare in the United States, it has been endemic in Asia and Africa. The infection is acquired during sexual intercourse or through contact with contaminated exudate from active lesions. Inapparent infections and latent disease are rare.[36]

PATHOPHYSIOLOGY The strain of *C. trachomatis* that causes LGV probably penetrates skin and mucous membranes through tiny abrasions. LGV begins as a skin lesion and spreads to genital and rectal lymphatic tissue, where it causes marked inflammation, necrosis, buboes, abscesses of inguinal lymph nodes, and infection of surrounding tissues. Healing occurs by fibrosis after several weeks or months and results in scarring, which damages the lymph nodes and disrupts nodal function. Affected nodes become chronically swollen, hardened, and enlarged. *C. trachomatis* also spreads systematically through the bloodstream and can enter the CNS.[37]

CLINICAL MANIFESTATIONS The primary lesion of LGV appears after an incubation period of 5 to 21 days. The lesion is most commonly a herpetiform (multivesicular) ulcer, but it can take various forms. The ulcer generally is asymptomatic and inconspicuous and heals rapidly, leaving no scar. In men the lesion is found most commonly on the penis or scrotum; in women it is found on the vaginal wall, cervix, or labia. Other signs of primary LGV include a large, tender lymphatic nodule or bubo, urethritis, and cervicitis.

The secondary stage of untreated LGV in men is characterized by inflammation and swelling of the lymph nodes. At first the inguinal bubo is a firm, somewhat painful mass. As the bubo gradually enlarges, it becomes very painful, thereby restricting mobility, and deep blue. This color change signals impending rupture of the bubo through the skin. Thick yellow pus may drain from the site for weeks or months. Healing is slow and results in scar formation. Systemic manifestations of secondary LGV include meningitis, pneumonitis, and other major infections. In some cases the bubo does not rupture but rather involutes and becomes firm. Bubo formation is most common in men. In women the inguinal lymph nodes are involved in less than one third of cases.

Anorectal LGV may be caused by direct inoculation during anal intercourse, or it may be a chronic or late manifestation of lymphatic spread from the inguinal area. Most individuals with anorectal LGV are women or homosexual men. Clinical symptoms include multiple ulcerations of the rectal mucosa, chronic inflammation, mucopurulent rectal discharge, and rectovaginal fistulas in women. Individuals may have fever, rectal pain, and tenesmus. Rectal strictures, perirectal abscesses, and anal fissures may develop and are the cause of most of the severe morbidity associated with LGV.

EVALUATION AND TREATMENT Clinical manifestations and laboratory tests are used to diagnose LGV. Tests include the LGV complement-fixation test, isolation of the microorganism in tissue culture, and monoclonal antibody tests. The diagnosis usually is made serologically and by excluding other causes of genital ulcers or inguinal lymphadenopathy. LGV is treated with oral doxycycline, 100 mg twice daily for 21 days. A 21-day course of erythromycin is also effective. Sex partners also should be treated.

Nongonococcal or Nonspecific Urethritis
Nongonococcal urethritis (NGU), also known as *nonspecific urethritis,* is a nonreportable STI. In student health centers and STI clinics, more than 50% of individuals with urethritis have NGU. The morbidity is equal to or greater than that associated with gonorrhea. Approximately 2 million men are

affected each year. Most commonly it affects heterosexual men and men of higher socioeconomic status. NGU may be complicated by epididymitis in heterosexual men younger than 35 years, proctitis in homosexual men, and Reiter syndrome.

PATHOPHYSIOLOGY Nongonococcal urethritis is a syndrome caused by a variety of microbes, including *C. trachomatis* and *Ureaplasma urealyticum*. Postgonococcal urethritis occurs in 15% to 35% of men diagnosed with gonorrhea. These men usually have coexistent gonorrheal and chlamydial infection and develop biphasic illness because of the longer incubation period of CT. Chlamydial infections are discussed earlier in this chapter (see p. 935).

C. trachomatis is the most common cause of NGU (15% to 55%). *Trichomonas vaginalis* and HSV sometimes cause NGU. However, *Ureaplasma, U. urealyticum,* and possibly *Mycoplasma* are implicated in as many as one third of the cases of NGU.[2] Genital colonization with *U. urealyticum* occurs with an increasing number of sexual partners. That is, urethral cultures of men with a history of three to five lifetime sexual partners yield *U. urealyticum* whether those men have urethritis or not. The difference in symptomatology may be the result of infection by different serotypes. Some of the 14 different serotypes of *U. urealyticum* may be more pathogenic than others—20% to 30% of men with acute urethritis are negative for *N. gonorrhoeae, C. trachomatis,* and *U. urealyticum*. Some of these men respond to antibiotic treatment; others experience persistent and recurrent infection. No clear association has been found between NGU and infection caused by herpes simplex virus, trichomonads, cytomegalovirus, and other microorganisms.

CLINICAL MANIFESTATIONS Clinically, NGU infection caused by CT cannot be differentiated from NGU caused by another microbe. In both cases, men present after a 7- to 21-day incubation period with complaints of dysuria and mild to moderate white or clear urethral discharge. Discharge may be absent, and urethral itching may be the only symptom. Asymptomatic infection is common.

EVALUATION AND TREATMENT NGU is a diagnosis of exclusion. Urethral exudate is Gram stained, and an endourethral swab is taken for testing or culture. Urine sediment also may be examined. All individuals who have urethritis should be evaluated for the presence of gonococcal and chlamydial infection. A treatment of a single 1-g oral dose of azithromycin should be initiated as soon as possible after diagnosis. Doxycycline, 100 mg orally twice a day for 7 days, is also effective. Single-dose regimens have the advantage of improved compliance and of directly observed therapy.[2]

Viral Infections

Genital Herpes

Genital herpes, which causes blisters (cold sores), is the most common infectious genital ulceration in the United States. In fact, genital infection with HSV is an epidemic in the United States. Genital herpes can be caused by either of the two serotypes of HSV: HSV-1 or HSV-2. Although infections caused by the serotypes are clinically indistinguishable, serologic studies show that more than 80% of initial and 98% of recurrent genital HSV infections are caused by HSV-2.

Herpes simplex virus is not a reportable disease, and any reporting that is done is nonstandardized, so national statistics are not available. However, primary HSV infections are estimated to affect 1 million individuals each year. Recurrent infections are mostly asymptomatic (50% to 70%) and affect an estimated 50 million Americans annually.[1] The seroprevalence of HSV-2 is estimated to range from 16% to 20% of the total adult population to 35% to 60% for subgroups, for example, STI clinic patients and black women. The incidence of HSV infection tends to be highest in the teen to young adult age group (12 to 29 years) and in non-white lower socioeconomic groups.[2] Infection with HSV is not commonly associated with other STIs, for example, gonorrhea.[19]

Herpes simplex virus infection is transmitted through intimate contact with a person who is shedding the virus in a secretion or from a peripheral lesion or mucosal surface. Persons without symptoms probably transmit most infections. Transmission rates are not well identified; however, it is estimated that a woman has an 80% to 90% risk of developing genital herpes after being exposed to an infected man. In 1992 Mertz and colleagues[38] studied monogamous heterosexual couples in which one partner had HSV-2 infection. The noninfected partner seroconverted in 10% of couples over a 1-year period. As many as 70% of such infections seem to be acquired during periods of asymptomatic shedding. Uninfected female partners were at greater risk than men, especially if they were seronegative for HSV-1 antibodies as well. The likelihood of nonsexual transmission of genital herpes, through aerosolized secretions of other fomites, is quite rare and unlikely.[5,34]

Neonatal infections can occur in utero or, more commonly, during the intrapartum or postpartum period. The risk of transmission of HSV to the neonate varies from <1% among women with recurrence of known herpes at term who acquired HSV during the pregnancy and up to 30% to 50% in women who are exposed and acquire HSV near term.[14] Perinatal transmission can cause extensive morbidity and mortality.

Intrauterine transmission can occur through transplacental or ascending infection and can cause spontaneous abortion or premature delivery.[19] Most infections are transmitted intrapartally. Infants are at greatest risk if the mother has a primary infection acquired near the time of delivery rather than a recurrent infection or an infection acquired during the first half of pregnancy. Ruptured membranes have a role in the development of HSV. Membranes that have been ruptured for more than 4 hours increase the risk for contracting HSV. Internal fetal monitoring devices also increase the risk of the infant contracting HSV.[39]

PATHOPHYSIOLOGY After initial exposure and entry of the virus at mucocutaneous sites or abraded skin, the virus undergoes replication locally in the dermis and epidermis. This leads to cell destruction, transudation, and vesicle formation. The virus spreads to contiguous cells and eventually into sensory nerves. Eventually the virus is transported intra-axonally to the dorsal root, where it remains in a latent stage until it becomes reactivated. During the latent period the genome for the virus is maintained in the host cell nucleus without causing the death of the cell. After oral infection the latent virus resides in the trigeminal ganglion; after genital infection it resides in the dorsal sacral nerve roots.

Latent infections can become reactivated and cause a recurrent infection with similar manifestations. Reactivation of the HSV-2 infection is twice as common as HSV-1 infections, and the likelihood of HSV-2 recurrent infections is 8 to 10 times. Reactivation of HSV is not well understood but may be attributable to physical, hormonal, and immunologic stimuli. Other triggering events may be menstruation, stress, and sun exposure.[33] During reactivation the viral genomes are transported through the peripheral sensory nerves back to the dermal surface.

CLINICAL MANIFESTATIONS Three distinct syndromes associated with HSV infection are first-episode primary genital infection, first-episode nonprimary HSV, and recurrent infections. The manifestations of each one depend on the individual's previous immune state. First-episode primary genital infection occurs when an individual has no antibodies to HSV-1 or HSV-2. Up to 60% of primary infections with HSV-2 and one third of primary infections with HSV-1 are asymptomatic.[40] If symptoms occur, the individual may have small (1 to 2 mm), multiple, vesicular lesions that are generally located on the labia minora, fourchette, or penis (Figure 24-11). They also may appear on the cervix, buttocks, and thighs and are often painful and pruritic. These lesions usually last about 10 to 20 days. The lesions of HSV-1 and HSV-2 are indistinguishable to the naked eye. These wet lesions actively shed virus for about 10 to 14 days, after which they heal by reepithelialization. Small lesions may coalesce into larger ulcers and become secondarily infected.

Systemic manifestations often accompany primary HSV infection, and an individual may experience fever, malaise, myalgias, lymphadenopathy, and urinary retention. Pharyngitis, aseptic meningitis, and hepatitis also may accompany primary HSV infection. Figure 24-12 illustrates the clinical course of primary genital HSV.

First-episode nonprimary HSV occurs in individuals who have preexisting antibodies. In some individuals the primary infection may not have had any clinical manifestations. The HSV becomes latent within the nerve root and is reactivated at a later date. Compared with primary infection, the first episode of nonprimary HSV is often milder with fewer lesions that are less painful and heal faster. Fewer systemic manifestations occur and viral shedding is of shorter duration.

Recurrent infections produce mild local symptoms. The number of lesions is greatly reduced, and the lesions are less painful. Lesions are often unilateral, with crusting within 4 to 5 days. Recovery and healing are usually complete within 10 days.[41] Asymptomatic viral shedding can occur with both HSV-1 and HSV-2.

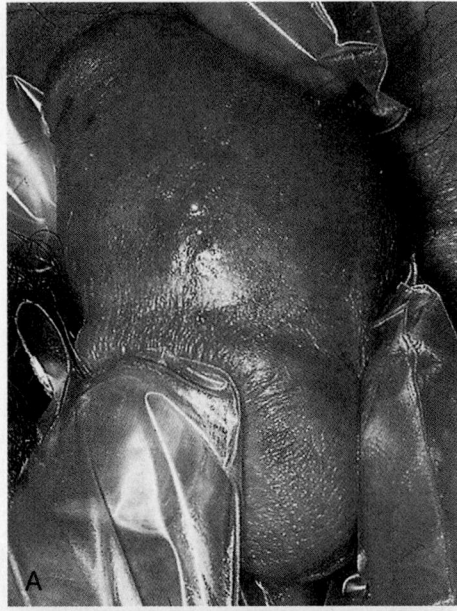
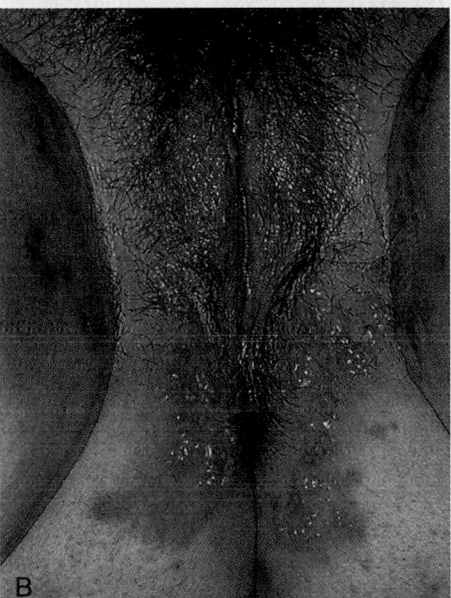

Figure 24-11 Herpes lesions. **A,** Herpetic vesicles on the penis. **B,** Herpetic ulceration of the vulva. (From McMillan A, Scott GR: *Sexually transmitted infections,* ed 2, London, 2000, Churchill Livingstone.)

Individuals affected with HSV-2 are more likely to experience recurrent infections. Recurrent infections occur an average of five to eight times per year but may be as frequent as every month or as rare as every few to many years. Individuals may experience prodromal symptoms (e.g., pruritus, tingling, dysesthesias) a few hours to 2 days before the eruption of lesions. Women may experience a vaginal discharge and dysuria, and 44% of men have dysuria. Symptomatic HSV infection of the newborn may occur any time in the first month of life. Manifestations range from a local infection of the eyes, skin, or mucous membranes to a severe disseminated infection with CNS involvement. About 70% of affected infants present with skin lesions. CNS involvement includes seizures

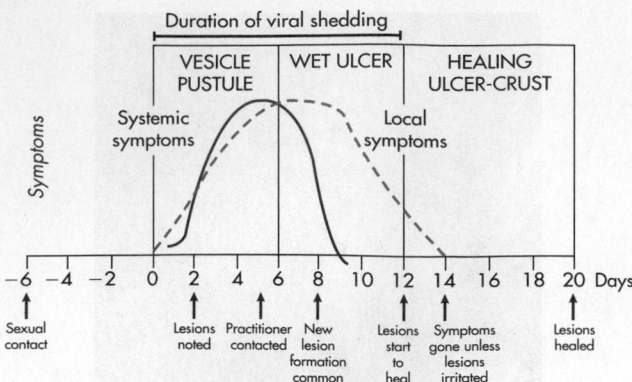

Figure 24-12 Clinical course of primary genital herpes. (From Corey L: Genital herpes. In Holmes KK et al, editors: *Sexually transmitted diseases,* ed 2, New York, 1990, McGraw-Hill.)

and is associated with a mortality of more than 50% and extensive neurologic sequelae in survivors.

EVALUATION AND TREATMENT Genital HSV infection is suggested if typical genital lesions are present. A presumptive diagnosis of HSV-associated infection is supported by the identification in a Papanicolaou (Pap) test of multinucleated giant cells with intranuclear inclusions. Definitive diagnosis is made after viral tissue culture. HSV-1 and HSV-2 are distinguished by fluorescent antibody, neutralization, or serologic tests. Serologic testing may be useful in identifying symptomatic carriers of HSV, for use in discordant couples and to screen pregnant women.

No curative treatment for HSV infection is known. A vaccine is in development but is only effective in women who have not been infected with HSV-1; however, it is not yet available.[42] Oral acyclovir, valacyclovir, penciclovir, and famciclovir are used for primary and periodic outbreaks and to prevent recurrences. Neither valacyclovir nor famciclovir is approved by the U.S. Food and Drug Administration for use in children younger than 12 years.[4] Intravenous acyclovir is reserved for severely immunocompromised individuals.[43] Acyclovir-resistant strains of HSV have been identified periodically; no specific definitive resistant strains are known to exist. Suppressive treatment is recommended for individuals with more than six recurrences per year. Suppressive treatment also may reduce asymptomatic viral shedding. Although condoms offer some protection, individuals with HSV should refrain from all genital contact when symptomatic and understand that an undetermined risk of transmission exists even during asymptomatic periods.

Human Papillomavirus Infection

Human papillomavirus (HPV) infection is the most common symptomatic viral STI in the United States. Although more than 5.5 million cases are diagnosed yearly, prevalence is considered underestimated because HPV infection is often subclinical. More sensitive measures of HPV indicate that 57% to 60% of all sexually active young women are infected with the virus. Currently the incidence of HPV is at epidemic

proportions; an estimated 75% of the reproductive-age population has been infected with HPV.[1]

More than 120 different types of HPV have been identified. More than 30 serotypes are unique to the stratified squamous epitheliums of the genital area. These are divided into serotypes that have a high risk of causing cervical cancer and low-risk serotypes, which are associated with benign lesions: *condylomata acuminata* of the vulva, vagina, penis, and perianal areas. High-risk types 16 and 18 are the most common, found in more than half of cases of cervical dysplasia.[44] High-risk type 18 is associated with adenocarcinoma of the cervix.[44] Serotypes associated with genital warts include types 6 and 11, among others. These lesions can coexist with the high-risk types but do not cause cancer. Although rare, these types also may cause oral lesions. It is now known that infection with persistent, high-risk serotypes of HPV are necessary for the development of cervical cancer (see also Chapters 11 and 23). Fortunately, most cases of HPV are transient and resolve by 2 years.[44] Persistence of the virus, immune response, and the presence of cofactors, including smoking and hormonal contraceptive exposure, may play a role in the development of cervical dysplasia and cancer following HPV exposure.[45] HPV infection is closely associated with multiple sexual partners and early onset of sexual activity and is most common in teens and young adults, 16 to 25 years of age.

Genital warts are quite contagious, with transmission rates among individuals estimated to be between 38% and 95%. Such a wide range is attributable to the subclinical nature of some infections and various influencing factors that include number of exposures, HPV type, location of lesions, and cellular immunity response. Infants and children also have been identified as being infected with HPV. Infants can be infected in utero and by passage through an infected birth canal. HPV infection in children has been traced to child sexual abuse; however, reports vary in making this connection.[4,46]

PATHOPHYSIOLOGY HPV is a nonenveloped, circular, double-stranded DNA virus, one of the papovaviruses, that belongs to the Papovaviridae family.[47] Information about HPV was not readily available until the late 1970s, when it became possible to clone the viral genomes directly from infected tissues by recombinant DNA technology.[48]

Transmission of the virus is believed to occur through sexual contact; however, the exact transmissibility of the virus into the cell is unknown. The initial infection follows trauma to the epithelium that allows the virus to reach and infect the basal cells of the epithelium, which appear to be supportive of viral propagation. Such minor trauma may occur during sexual intercourse. Epithelial cells that are infected with HPV undergo transformation, proliferate, and form a warty growth. HPV manifestations appear in about 2 to 3 months.

CLINICAL MANIFESTATIONS **Condylomata acuminata** are soft, skin-colored, whitish pink to reddish brown discrete growths. They may occur singly or in clusters and may be broad based or pedunculated and feathery or smooth (Figure 24-13). Sometimes the warts enlarge to form cauliflower-like masses on the male frenulum, glans, foreskin, urinary meatus,

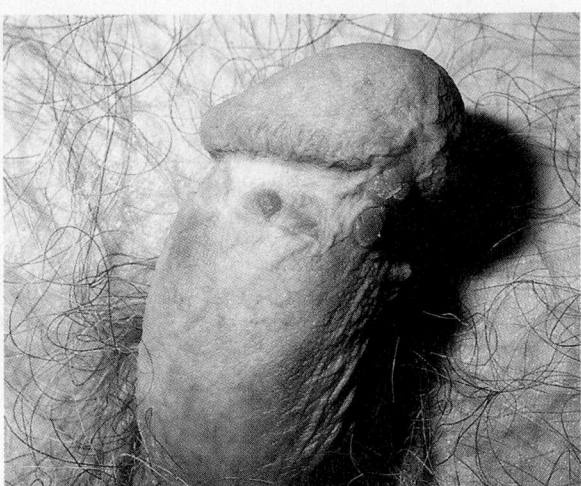

Figure 24-13 Condylomata acuminata—penile. Asymptomatic, flesh-colored papules are present on the shaft of the penis. (From Morse SA et al, editors: *Atlas of sexually transmitted diseases and AIDS*, ed 3, London, 2003, Mosby.)

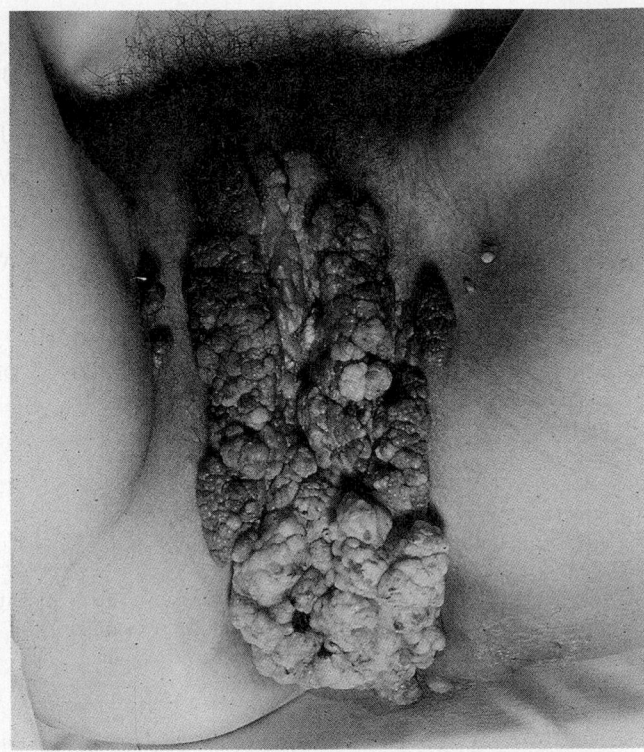

Figure 24-14 Condylomata acuminata—vulva and perineum. The clinical diagnosis was giant condylomata of Buschke and Löwenstein. Such large and confluent lesions should be carefully examined and multiple biopsies obtained to rule out underlying malignancy. (From Morse SA et al, editors: *Atlas of sexually transmitted diseases and AIDS*, ed 3, London, 2003, Mosby.)

shaft, scrotum, or anus and on the female labia, clitoris, perineum, vagina, or anus (Figure 24-14). Although the lesions are usually not painful, they may cause dyspareunia (painful intercourse) and may be friable and bleed easily. Some individuals complain of pruritus. Cervical lesions are generally flattened and may not be seen easily without colposcopy.[16] Urethral condylomata may occur in men, are always preceded by skin lesions, and can become cancerous.[49] Ninety percent of lesions are found in the distal urethra.

Laryngeal papillomas can occur in infants whose mothers had genital warts at the time of delivery. Clinical manifestations of laryngeal warts include stridor, hoarseness, abnormal cry, cough, and respiratory distress.[50] Many women with HPV may develop cytologic changes detected by Pap testing. These cell changes may be transient or may progress to dysplasia and, ultimately, cancer.

EVALUATION AND TREATMENT Generally, diagnosis of condylomata acuminata is made on the basis of clinical manifestations. Verrucose, fleshy pink lesions caused by HPV must be differentiated from condylomata lata (the whitish gray, flat lesions) of secondary syphilis. Because HPV infection often accompanies other STIs, gonorrhea culture, chlamydia culture, serologic test for syphilis, and wet mount for other vaginal microorganisms also should be performed.

HPV infection is associated with the development of squamous cell carcinoma; therefore, all atypical or persistent lesions should have a biopsy examination. HPV testing can be useful in the triage of abnormal Pap tests or can be used in conjunction with Pap testing to identify women at risk for the development of cervical dysplasia.

Treatments for external genital warts are considered cosmetic—not curative—and include patient-applied therapies (podofilox and imiquimod) and provider-administered therapies (cryotherapy, podophyllin resin, trichloroacetic acid [TCA], bichloroacetic acid [BCA], interferon, and surgery). Cervical and extensive vaginal lesions may be treated with 5-fluorouracil cream or surgical excision with CO_2 laser surgery, cryosurgery, or electrosurgery. Interferons that have general antiviral, antiproliferative, and immunomodulating effects have been used successfully in treating stubborn genital warts. Success of treatment depends on response of the immune system. Approximately one third of individuals experience a cure, and another one third experience a decrease in wart size.[19] Surgical excision is the treatment for laryngeal warts in infants. A vaccine against HPV serotypes 16 and 18 is available and has shown to be effective in prevention of primary cervical infection with those strains, which are associated with cervical cancer[51] (Table 24-3 and see What's New? HPV Vaccine; also see Chapter 23 What's New? Pap Test for Cervical Screening Obsolete?).

Molluscum Contagiosum

Molluscum contagiosum is a benign viral infection of the skin in children and adults. Primarily the face, hands, lower abdomen, and genitalia are affected; papules found on other parts of the skin or widely distributed are not uncommon. Individuals with AIDS may develop extensive lesions over the face, neck, and genital region.

Molluscum contagiosum occurs throughout the world and has been a common childhood disease in Papua New

Table 24-3 Recent Recommendations for Cervical Cancer Screening

Parameter	American Cancer Society (ACS) Guidelines (November 2002)	U.S. Preventive Services Task Force (USPSTF) (January 2003)	American College of Obstetricians and Gynecologists (ACOG) Practice Bulletin (August 2003)
Age to start screening	3 years after onset of sexual activity but no later than 21 years of age	Within 3 years of onset of sexual activity or age 21, whichever comes first	3 years after onset of sexual activity but no later than 21 years of age
Age to stop screening	At 70 years—if three consecutive normal Pap tests and no history of CIN in last 10 years and no history of DES exposure or immunosuppression	Women >65 years with negative tests, who are not otherwise at high risk for cervical cancer	It is difficult to set an upper age limit—determine on an individual basis as regards medical history and risk factors for CIN
Screening post-hysterectomy for benign disease	Not indicated if documented that hysterectomy was for benign disease	Discontinue testing if hysterectomy for benign reasons	Not indicated if documented that hysterectomy was for benign disease
Cytologic screening—interval up until age 30 years	Annually with conventional Pap or every 2 years with liquid-based cytology	At least every 3 years	Annual screening
Cytologic screening—interval after age 30 years	After three consecutive negative Pap tests on screen, every 2-3 years unless history of CIN, DES exposure, or immunosuppression	At least every 3 years	After three consecutive negative Pap tests on screen, every 2-3 years; women with HIV, immunosuppression, or DES exposure may require more frequent screening
Use of HPV DNA testing and Pap after age 30 years	HPV DNA testing and cervical cytology is an acceptable screening approach	Insufficient evidence	Acknowledges the FDA approval for using a combination of HPV DNA testing and cervical cytology
HPV DNA testing and Pap after age 30—screening	No more frequently than every 3 years	Insufficient evidence	If negative on both tests—repeat no more frequently than every 3 years

Data from American College of Obstetricians and Gynecologists (ACOG): *Int J Gynaecol Obstet* 83(2):237-247, 2003; Saslow D et al: *CA Cancer J Clin* 52:342-362, 2002 (available at: http://caonline.amcancersoc.org/cgi/content/full/52/6/342); US Preventive Services Task Force (USPSTF): *Screening for cervical cancer,* January 2003 (available at: htp//www/ahcpr.gov/clinic/uspstf/uspscerv.htm; also see http://www.acog.org/from_home/publications/press_releases/nr07-31-03.cfm.
CIN, Cervical intraepithelial neoplasia; *DES,* diethylstilbestrol; *DNA,* deoxyribonucleic acid; *FDA,* Food and Drug Administration; *HPV,* human papillomavirus; *Pap,* Papanicolaou.

Guinea and Fiji. It is much less common in the United States, where incidence is highest among young adults. The childhood disease is transmitted by skin-to-skin contact and fomites (swimming pools, towels, gymnasium equipment) and affects the face, trunk, and limbs. Adult disease is more commonly sexually transmitted and affects the lower abdomen, genitalia, and perianal area.[52] Molluscum contagiosum is most common in men 20 to 29 years of age and in those with multiple sexual partners. The molluscum contagiosum virus is taken into epithelial cells by phagocytosis and replicates within the cytoplasm, where it produces cytoplasmic inclusions (**molluscous bodies**) and cellular hyperplasia. The underlying skin usually is not affected.[53]

After an incubation period of 2 to 7 weeks, white or flesh-colored, round or oval dome-shaped papules appear. The lesions are relatively small (3 to 5 mm) but occasionally may coalesce to form larger lesions up to 15 mm. The surface has a characteristic central umbilication, from which a thick, creamy core material can be expressed (Figure 24-15). Generally the lesions are not painful or pruritic unless secondarily infected. The papules may last several months or several years and spread by autoinoculation.

The appearance of the lesions is generally all that is needed to make the diagnosis, although direct microscopic examination of stained material from the core of the papule discloses molluscous bodies within the swollen and rounded epithelial cells. The lesions often heal spontaneously after several months. Other effective means of removing the lesions include curettage and application of liquid nitrogen (cryotherapy) or silver nitrate. Topical acids have been used also but cause scarring. Individuals tend to have lifetime immunity once lesions are healed completely.

Parasitic Infections

Trichomoniasis

Originally discovered in 1836, *T. vaginalis* was at first thought to be a harmless commensal microorganism. *T. vaginalis* is now known to be a common cause of sexually transmitted lower genital tract infection and urethritis.

Every year in the United States:

- About 12,000 women are diagnosed with cervical cancer
- Almost 4000 women die from this disease

Gardasil is available in the United States to vaccinate against high-risk human papillomavirus (HPV) types 16 and 18

- Recommended for women as early as age 9 or 10 years and up to age 26 years; effectiveness in men has not yet been established and administration of the vaccine to men is not recommended
- Given in a series of three shots over 6 months; administration of all thee doses recommended as efficacy, not established if series not completed
- Highly effective in preventing high-risk HPV types associated with cervical cancer; proven safe and effective by the Centers for Disease Control and Prevention (CDC), ongoing safety monitoring
- Not recommended for pregnant women because safety is not yet established
- A Papanicolaou (Pap) smear is not necessary prior to initiation of the HPV vaccine; however, women still need cervical cancer screening at regular intervals because the vaccine will not protect against all HPV types
- The vaccine costs approximately $125 per shot or $375, is covered by most insurance plans, Medicaid, and the Vaccines for Children (VFC) program if individuals meet eligibility requirements, including age and financial need

For more information, contact the Centers for Disease Control and Prevention's STD hotline at 1-800-277-8922 or visit the website at www.cdc.gov/std

Data from Centers for Disease Control and Prevention: *HPV vaccine information, 2008*, Atlanta, 2008, U.S. Department of Health and Human Services. Available at www.cdc.gov/std/Hpv/STDFact-HPV-vaccine.htm.

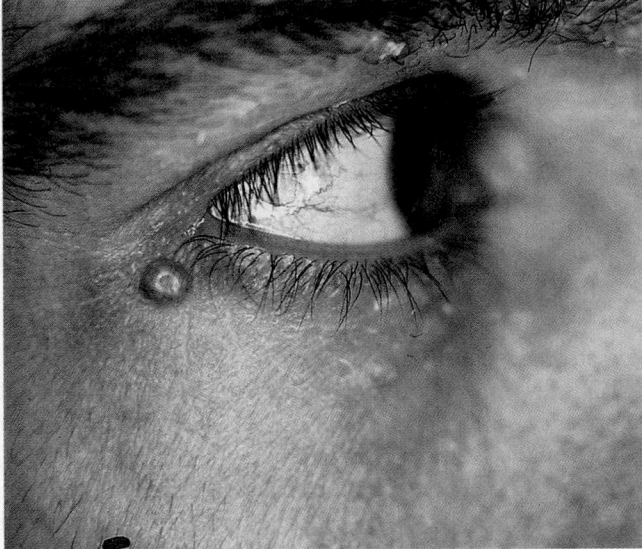

Figure 24-15 Molluscum contagiosum. Flesh-colored papules of molluscum may be distinguished by their umbilicated centers. The papules contain a white cheesy substance that may be stained for the presence of viral inclusion bodies. (From Morse SA et al, editors: *Atlas of sexually transmitted diseases and AIDS,* ed 3, London, 2003, Mosby.)

Because **trichomoniasis** (infection by *T. vaginalis*) is not a reportable disease, its prevalence can only be estimated. The latest estimates suggest that as many as 5 million cases of trichomoniasis occur each year in the United States,[1] and that *T. vaginalis* accounts for one of four cases of infectious vaginitis. Trichomoniasis is usually found in both sexual partners and often coexists with gonorrhea. Although sexual transmission is clearly the most common means of disease spread, transmission through fomites is theoretically possible. To cause infection, the fomite would have to introduce an inoculum of about 10,000 microorganisms directly into the vagina.[54]

PATHOPHYSIOLOGY *T. vaginalis* is an anaerobic, unicellular, flagellated, parasitic protozoan that adheres to and damages squamous epithelial cells. Because this protozoan selectively affects squamous epithelia, vaginal and urethral tissue is often infected, as are Skene and Bartholin glands. The endocervical canal is not affected because it is lined with columnar epithelium. In men the urethra is the most common site of infection, although the protozoa, called **trichomonads,** also can infect the epididymis and (rarely) the prostate. Zinc, which has potent antibacterial

properties, is found in high concentrations in the prostate. Hence many trichomonads are cleared from the male urethra during ejaculation. This action makes urethral trichomoniasis a fairly self-limiting infection in men. Most infections of the male urethra clear up within 2 weeks.

Trichomoniasis is most common in men and women of reproductive age, and it is primarily an infection of the vagina. *T. vaginalis* can induce a marked inflammatory response in the vagina, causing a copious discharge that contains large numbers of polymorphonuclear neutrophils. Trichomonads adhere to but do not invade the squamous epithelial cells.

CLINICAL MANIFESTATIONS Manifestations of vaginal trichomoniasis range from none to severe, with some women reporting an increase in distressing symptoms immediately after menses. Vaginal discharge and internal pruritus are the most common complaints. Dyspareunia and dysuria are also fairly common. Secretions are usually copious, frothy, malodorous, and yellow-green to a gray-green. The vaginal walls may appear erythematous and sore. Rarely, small, punctate red marks, sometimes called *strawberry spots,* are visible. Vaginal pH is usually more than 4.2.

Most men with trichomoniasis remain asymptomatic. Possible clinical manifestations include scant intermittent discharge, slight pruritus, and mild dysuria.

EVALUATION AND TREATMENT History and symptoms are inadequate for diagnosis of trichomoniasis. Fresh secretions have a pH higher than 4.7 and a positive amine odor when mixed with 10% KOH (positive "whiff test").

Microscopic confirmation of the presence of the trichomonads in vaginal secretions or urine provides a definitive diagnosis. In a fresh wet mount preparation that has been warmed slightly, the epithelial cells have relatively clean and sharp edges, the ratio of polymorphonuclear leukocytes to epithelial cells exceeds 1:1, and the trichomonads are visible. The ovoid microorganism is slightly larger than a polymorphonuclear leukocyte and has one rounded, flagellated end and one slightly pointed, flagellated end. The flagella give the trichomonads their characteristic twisting motility. In an acidic environment, such as urine, the trichomonads assume a "balled-up" or spherical shape and become less motile.

The treatment of choice for trichomoniasis is a single dose of metronidazole (Flagyl). The single-dose therapy is effective, has few side effects, and obviates the need for individual compliance with longer regimens. Sexual partners, even if asymptomatic, also are treated and examined for coexisting STIs. The 2-g single dose of metronidazole can be used to treat pregnant women. However, lactating women should suspend breast-feeding for 24 hours after single-dose therapy.[55]

Scabies

Scabies is a rather benign, common parasitic infection that can be spread by skin-to-skin and sexual contact. Discovered by Bonomo in 1687, it is considered to be the first human disease with a known cause.[56]

Scabies has a worldwide distribution, but actual prevalence is unknown.[24] Traditionally the disease was attributed to conditions of poverty, overcrowding, uncleanliness, and sexual promiscuity. Today it is recognized that scabies occurs in individuals with good personal hygiene and is not limited to any social class. Outbreaks of scabies occur every 30 years or so and last about 15 years. The most recent outbreak in the United States began in 1971 and subsided in the 1980s.

Transmission of scabies requires prolonged close skin-to-skin contact, which typically occurs within families or between sexual partners. Nonsexual transmission from patient to nurse has been reported in hospitals during sponge baths and lotion application, and mites have been transferred through infested bedding, clothes, and other fomites.[5]

PATHOPHYSIOLOGY The adult female itch mite, *Sarcoptes scabiei*, is 0.3 to 0.4 mm long and has a life span of about 30 days. Once deposited on human skin, it burrows through the horny layer of the stratum granulosum. Within hours of burrowing, the female begins laying two or three large eggs per day, each of which progresses through larval and nymphal stages to become an adult itch mite in about 10 days. The most common places for scabies to burrow are on the hands (between the fingers) and on the flexor surfaces of the wrists and the extensor surfaces of the elbows. Characteristic lesions may occur on the nipples of women and as pruritic papules on the penile shaft and glans and on the scrotum.[52,57] Pruritic papules may be seen on the buttocks also.[57] Figure 24-16 shows the typical sites of scabies burrows.

CLINICAL MANIFESTATIONS The classic symptom of scabies is intense pruritus, which may be pronounced at night. The typical burrow of the *S. scabiei* is a short, linear,

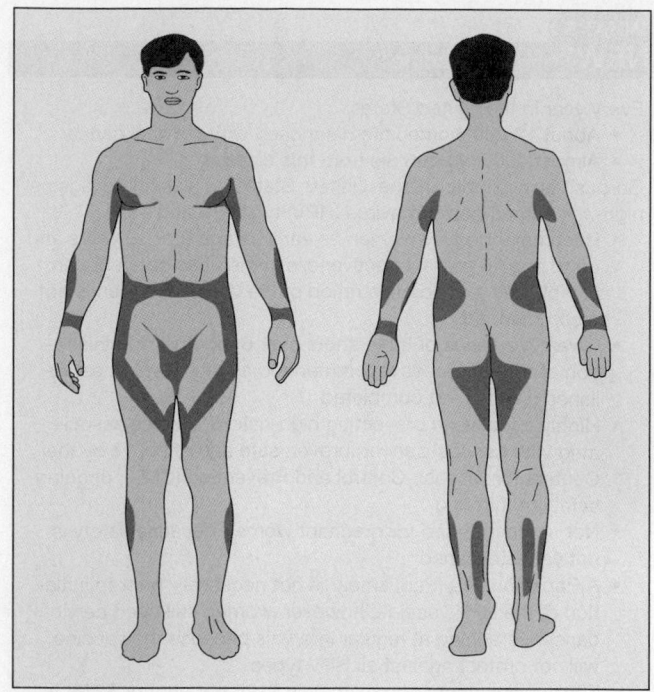

Figure 24-16 Distribution of skin lesions of *Sarcoptes scabiei* infestation. Unshaded areas are rarely affected in healthy adults. (From Morse SA et al, editors: *Atlas of sexually transmitted diseases and AIDS,* ed 3, London, 2003, Mosby.)

curved, or S-shaped line (Figure 24-17). There may be small, erythematous, excoriated larval papules near the burrows. Secondary infections are common and are caused by scratching. In some individuals a hypersensitivity reaction occurs a month or more after the infestation and causes multiple, reddish brown, pruritic nodules to develop on the covered portions of the body—most commonly, the upper thighs, buttocks, male genitalia, and axillary regions. These nodules may persist for more than 1 year despite treatment with a scabicide.

EVALUATION AND TREATMENT Although the diagnosis is often made on clinical grounds, microscopic identification of the mite or its eggs, larvae, or feces is recommended because the symptoms of scabies can imitate those of many other dermatologic conditions. Superficial scrapings from a recently developed unexcoriated papule or burrow can be observed easily under the microscope; the addition of KOH allows easier visualization of the mite.

Preferred treatment is topical application of 5% permethrin massaged and left for 8 to 14 hours. Also effective is Lindane (1%) lotion or cream applied thinly to all areas of the body below the neck and washed thoroughly at 8 hours and 10% crotamiton applied to the body below the neck nightly for 2 nights and washed thoroughly 24 hours after the second application.[55,57] Close household and sexual contacts should be treated also. Permethrin has been used safely in infants as young as 2 months and is the treatment of choice for children. Pregnant women should be treated with permethrin only if infestation with scabies can be documented.[55,57]

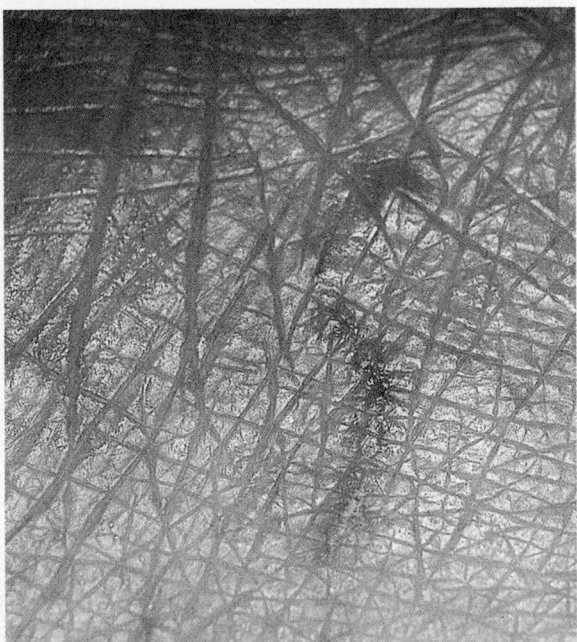

Figure 24-17 **Scabies burrow.** An S-shaped burrow with a tiny vesicle at one end. (From Habif TP et al: *Skin disease: diagnosis and treatment,* St Louis, 2001, Mosby.)

To prevent reinfestation, clothing and bed linens should be machine washed and dried at high temperatures, or dry-cleaned.

Pediculosis Pubis

Phthirus pubis, the crab louse, is one of three species of lice that infest humans. *P. pubis* is commonly transmitted sexually and causes **pediculosis pubis,** or "crabs." Adolescents and young children are most commonly infected.

P. pubis is transmitted primarily by intimate sexual contact or contact with infected bed linens or clothing. It is highly contagious; there is a 95% chance of contracting the disease during a single sexual encounter. The transfer of lice from pubic hair is probably mechanical, assisted by animated scratching; fingernails; towels; and other similar means rather than by self-propulsion. Pubic lice usually infect the perineal and axillary hair and occasionally the hair of the trunk, beard, scalp, and eyelashes.

PATHOPHYSIOLOGY The crab louse has a 25- to 30-day life cycle from egg to egg that consists of five stages: an egg (or nit) stage, three nymphal stages, and an adult stage, all of which occur in the host. The nits of crab lice are found "glued" to hairs; they are oval, 0.8 by 0.3 mm, and whitish, and they hatch in 5 to 10 days (Figure 24-18). In the adult stage, pubic lice are grayish, are approximately 1 mm in length, and have a segmented body and claws particularly designed for clinging to pubic hairs. Because lice depend on blood for nutrition, they bite into the skin to obtain food.

CLINICAL MANIFESTATIONS Symptoms range from mild pruritus to severe, intolerable itching, depending on the individual's sensitivity to louse bites. Allergic

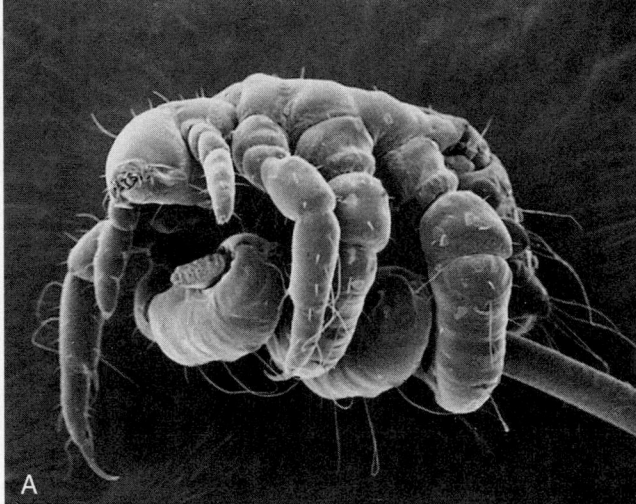

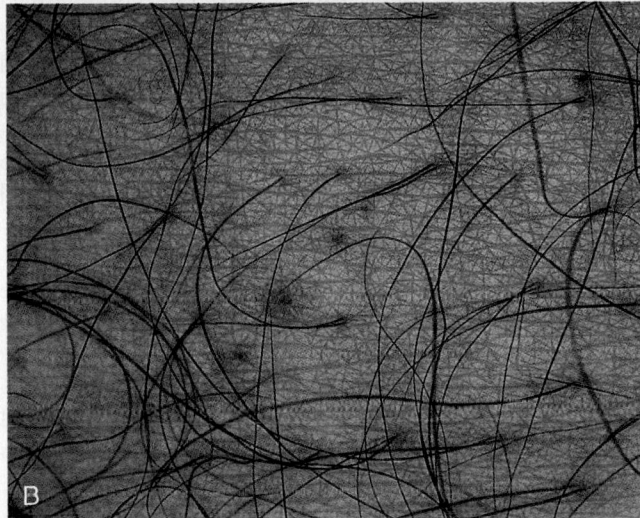

Figure 24-18 **Pubic louse and crab louse. A,** Pubic louse *(Phthirus pubis)* encircling a pubic hair; the clawlike legs produce a firm grip. **B,** Crab louse bites *(P. pubis).* (From Morse SA et al, editors: *Atlas of sexually transmitted diseases and AIDS,* ed 3, London, 2003, Mosby.)

sensitization occurs in about 5 days, when itching, erythema, and inflammation may worsen. Excessive scratching may lead to secondary infection.

EVALUATION AND TREATMENT The individual's history usually discloses a recent exposure and the typical symptoms of infestation. Because the lice and nits are visible to the naked eye, a thorough clinical examination permits definitive diagnosis. Pediculosis pubis is treated with 1% permethrin cream rinse or 1% lindane lotion, cream, or shampoo or with over-the-counter pyrethrin or piperonyl butoxide. The pediculicide is applied to infested and adjacent hairy areas and removed after a specified length of time by thorough washing. Remaining nits can be removed with a fine-toothed comb. Permethrin is recommended for young children and pregnant women and has less potential toxicity with inappropriate use. On the other hand, lindane is the least expensive and nontoxic if used correctly. Lindane should not be used after a bath, or by persons with extensive dermatitis, by pregnant or lactating women, or by children less than 2 years of age.[55] Sexual contacts and any other intimate household contacts also should be examined and treated, and clothing and bed linens should be dry-cleaned or machine washed and dried at high temperatures. Treatment can be repeated in 7 days to eradicate any newly hatched lice.

SEXUALLY TRANSMITTED INFECTIONS OF OTHER BODY SYSTEMS

Gastrointestinal Infections

Shigellosis and *Campylobacter* Enteritis

A variety of enteric bacterial pathogens are now recognized as being sexually transmitted, particularly among homosexual men. The bacteria most commonly involved include species of *Shigella* and *Campylobacter*. *Shigella* infection, termed **shigellosis,** is transmitted by contact with infected feces. Few microorganisms are needed to cause infection. Anal-oral spread occurs easily through household contact and anal-oral sexual practices. *Campylobacter jejuni,* which causes **Campylobacter enteritis,** is primarily an animal pathogen but also may be transmitted among humans through anal-oral sexual practices. Again, few microorganisms are necessary for inoculation and infection.

PATHOPHYSIOLOGY *Shigella* microorganisms are nonmotile gram-negative rods that are related to *Escherichia coli.* They invade and kill intestinal epithelial cells, thereby inducing a marked inflammatory response and diarrhea. *Campylobacter* microorganisms are highly motile, curved gram-negative rods that also invade and kill intestinal cells and cause bloody, inflammatory exudate and diarrhea.

CLINICAL MANIFESTATIONS Either microorganism may cause a mild self-limited gastroenteritis or severe dysentery. After a 24- to 48-hour incubation period, shigellosis begins with fever, abdominal distress, and diarrhea. It may resolve completely or progress to dysentery with severe cramping, abdominal pain, tenesmus, and bloody mucoid discharge from the rectum. *Campylobacter* enteritis typically begins, after a 1- to 7-day incubation period, with sudden fever and abdominal pain followed by diarrhea. Malaise, anorexia, headache, arthralgia, and myalgia are common.

EVALUATION AND TREATMENT Clinical manifestations and cultures of fresh stool samples are used to diagnose shigellosis. Culturing *Campylobacter* is expensive; therefore, microscopic analysis of a Gram-stained smear of rectal exudate may be used as a diagnostic aid.

Treatment for mild illness includes correction of fluid and electrolyte imbalance. Antidiarrheals are avoided because they may delay clearance of the microorganism. Because *Shigella* and *Campylobacter* are highly contagious, antibiotic treatment may be advisable even for mild cases. The preferred treatment for shigellosis is oral ciprofloxacin, 500 mg, twice daily for 3 days. However, susceptibility testing of a stool culture should be performed because of an increasing number of antibiotic-resistant strains of *Shigella.* Oral ciprofloxacin, 500 mg twice daily for 3 to 5 days, or erythromycin, 500 mg four times daily for 5 days, is effective against *Campylobacter* enteritis.[55] Sexual partners are examined and treated, and individuals are instructed to avoid anal-oral contact until the infection is cured.

Giardiasis and Amebiasis

Two enteric protozoa that are sexually transmitted, primarily among homosexual men, are *Giardia lamblia,* the cause of **giardiasis,** and *Entamoeba histolytica,* the cause of **amebiasis.** The incidence of these infections in the male homosexual population has decreased over the past years, presumably because of safer sex practices.[58] Although the principal route of transmission is contaminated drinking water, giardiasis and amebiasis are transmitted also by anal-oral or genital-anal contact.

PATHOPHYSIOLOGY *G. lamblia* and *E. histolytica* are parasites having two forms, cysts and **trophozoites** (uncysted protozoa). The cysts are the infective form because they can survive in moist environments outside the host. Giardiasis commonly begins with ingestion of a small number of *G. lamblia* cysts. Once in the upper small bowel, each cyst becomes a trophozoite, which multiplies and attaches to the bowel mucosa. Enzyme deficiencies, inflammation, and immunologic damage then apparently occur, resulting in intestinal malabsorption. Amebiasis begins similarly: the ingested cysts pass to the small or large bowel, where each returns to the trophozoite state, multiplies quickly, and begins to invade the mucosa through cytotoxic activity. Mucosal invasion results in the development of ulcers and an inflammatory response. Individuals infected with *E. histolytica* may excrete up to 45 million cysts per day.

CLINICAL MANIFESTATIONS Giardiasis begins with sudden, explosive diarrhea, distention, and flatulence. Upper gastrointestinal symptoms are also prominent and may include epigastric pain; vomiting; foul, sulfuric burping; and nausea. After the acute illness, which usually lasts several days, milder symptoms may persist for months, with evidence of malabsorption and weight loss. Amebiasis is often asymptomatic. Symptoms that do occur range from mild diarrhea to severe dysentery. Amebiasis may spread from the intestine to other organs, such as the liver.

EVALUATION AND TREATMENT Diagnosis of both entities usually is made by history and microscopic examination of fresh stool specimens for either trophozoites or cysts. Small bowel biopsy may aid in the diagnosis of giardiasis; rectal biopsy may aid in the diagnosis of amebiasis. Serologic testing is useful in the differential diagnosis of symptomatic individuals with amebiasis. Metronidazole is the treatment of choice in the United States, usually 250 mg three times daily for 5 to 7 days.[59] Other nitroimidazoles as well as other agents including quinacrine are also effective. The dosage of metronidazole for amebiasis depends on the severity of the infection.[55]

Hepatitis B

Hepatitis is a liver infection that can be caused by six types of viruses: hepatitis A, hepatitis B, hepatitis C, hepatitis D, hepatitis E, and hepatitis G. Each virus causes a syndrome of acute, icteric (jaundice-producing) liver inflammation. Of the three types, the **hepatitis B virus (HBV)** is known to be sexually transmitted. (Hepatitis A, like most other predominantly enteric infections, may be considered an STI because of anal-oral transmission.) Although hepatitis C (HCV) is not recognized as an STI, the CDC has listed sexual exposure as an HCV risk factor (Figure 24-19). Data indicate sexual transmission of HCV appears to occur, but the virus is inefficiently spread through this manner.[14] Additional information about hepatitis is found in Chapter 39.

The prevalence of HBV infection varies dramatically worldwide. In Southeast Asia and Africa, 60% to 80% of the population may harbor serologic evidence of past or current infection. In the United States, approximately 5% to 20% of the general population has evidence of HBV infection. Seropositivity generally increases with age. Serologic tests of STI clinic patients show evidence of past infection in 28% of individuals ages 25 years and older and 7% in those younger than 25 years.[55] At risk for HBV infection are those with low socioeconomic status, blacks, Indochinese refugees, healthcare workers, and male homosexuals. In groups of male homosexuals, the seropositivity rates may be as high as 80%. Other groups at risk are intravenous drug users, institutionalized mentally retarded persons, hemodialysis patients, and heterosexual partners of HBV carriers.[60]

Transmission of HBV can occur through needle puncture, blood transfusion, cuts or abrasions in the skin, and absorption by mucosal surfaces. Direct contact with infected body fluids, such as tears, cerebrospinal fluid, synovial fluid, gastric juices, pleural fluid, semen, and urine, may pass the infection. Fomites also can transmit hepatitis: HBV can survive on inanimate objects for up to 1 week.[61]

Perinatal transmission of HBV is relatively common. Neonates whose mothers are infectious have a 90% chance of becoming infected with HBV during labor or delivery; almost all become chronic carriers.[62,63] HBV can be found in maternal vaginal secretions, blood, amniotic fluid, saliva, and breast milk.[61]

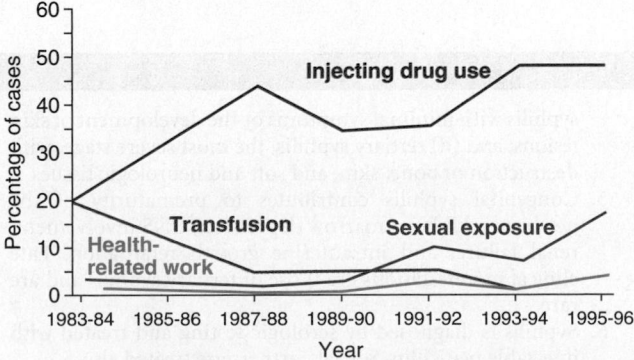

Figure 24-19 Risk for hepatitis C exposure. Comparison of injecting drug use *(blue)*, transfusions *(purple)*, health-related work *(green)*, and sexual exposure *(red)*. Note the rise in sexually transmitted incidences. (From Centers for Disease Control and Prevention: *Hepatitis C: what clinicians and other health professionals need to know*, 2000. Available at www.cdc.gov/ncidod/diseases/hepatitis/c_training/edu/intro.)

Hepatitis delta agent is a defective virus that is similar to HBV antigen but cannot cause hepatitis B by itself, requiring the presence of HBV to cause hepatitis. Hepatitis delta infection is rare in the United States, but cases have been documented in intravenous drug users and their sexual contacts and in recipients of contaminated blood. It commonly is found in homosexuals, persons requiring kidney dialysis, and healthcare workers.

PATHOPHYSIOLOGY After exposure, HBV passes through the bloodstream to the liver, where it infects liver cells and multiplies. The infection is usually self-limiting, with most patients mounting an effective immune response. Approximately 6% to 10% of infected individuals cannot eradicate the virus and become chronic carriers of HBV.

CLINICAL MANIFESTATIONS Most HBV infections are clinically unapparent and result in solid and permanent immunity. Symptoms of hepatitis usually develop only after a certain HBV antigen has been circulating in the blood for 3 to 6 weeks. Approximately 15% to 20% of individuals develop a prodromal syndrome that is similar to serum sickness. This syndrome is characterized by an erythematous rash, urticaria, polyarthralgias, and arthritis. Symptoms of infection also may include lassitude, anorexia, nausea, vomiting, headache, fever, dark urine, jaundice, and moderate liver enlargement with tenderness. Long-term sequelae include chronic persistent and chronic active hepatitis, cirrhosis, hepatocellular carcinoma, hepatic failure, and death. In neonates who contract HBV, the disease may be manifested in many ways, from mild illness to a severe, fulminant infection with a mortality of 75%.

EVALUATION AND TREATMENT HBV infection is clinically indistinguishable from other types of hepatitis. Diagnosis can be made only through serologic testing.

No specific therapy exists for HBV infection in adults. Treatment consists of supportive care and relief of symptoms. Vaccinations of only high-risk groups has proven to be ineffective. Thus a comprehensive strategy to eliminate HBV and its sequelae has been implemented by the CDC. This involves testing of all pregnant women and vaccinations of susceptible infants, children, and high-risk adults.[64]

The infant who is born to a mother with infectious HBV is given HBV immunoglobulin and HBV vaccine within 12 hours of birth. The HBV vaccine is administered again at 1 and 6 months if serologic tests show that a chronic carrier state has not developed.

Systemic Diseases

Epstein-Barr Virus

Recent investigations have indicated that the **Epstein-Barr virus (EBV),** which is transmitted orally, is also capable of being harbored within the male and female genital tracts and transmitted sexually. Further research is needed to specifically identify the role that EBV plays in STIs; however, the significance of EBV infection of the genital tract relates to its ability to transform cells and potentially contribute to the development of cancers in the genital tract.[65]

Acquired Immunodeficiency Syndrome

Epidemiology, modes of transmission, pathophysiology, clinical manifestations, and evaluation and treatment of AIDS are discussed in detail in Chapter 9.

Cytomegalovirus Infection

Cytomegalovirus (CMV) is a sexually transmissible herpesvirus. It is associated with a number of clinical syndromes in newborns, otherwise healthy adults, and immunosuppressed individuals.

CMV infection causes no specific genital disease, but its incidence is high in individuals being treated for other STIs. CMV infection is prevalent worldwide, especially in developing countries and lower socioeconomic groups. The virus is found in semen, cervical secretions, urine, blood, saliva, breast milk, and stool, and transmission is associated with close (although not always genital) interpersonal contact or direct transfer of cells or body fluids. It is more common in homosexual men and in young women with multiple sexual partners. Intrauterine CMV infection is the most common congenital infection and occurs in 0.5% to 3% of all live births. Like HSV, primary maternal infection carries the greatest risk of transmission and severe consequences. Infected infants can be asymptomatic or may experience varying degrees of sensorineural hearing loss or severe cognitive and psychomotor developmental deficits.[2,67] Perinatal transmission of CMV may occur across the placenta, by contamination with infected secretions during passage through the birth canal, or during breast-feeding.

PATHOPHYSIOLOGY After CMV infects a human cell, it may replicate and destroy the infected cell or become incorporated into the host cell's DNA. Local CMV infections can persist despite the presence of large quantities of systemic antibody to CMV. Cell-mediated immunity seems to have a particular role in protecting against CMV infections. Depression of CMV-specific cell-mediated immunity has been noted in otherwise normal hosts with CMV infection. This may be caused by injury of T cells or macrophages by the cytomegalovirus.[67]

CLINICAL MANIFESTATIONS In healthy individuals, CMV infection can cause a number of mild subclinical or nonspecific illnesses, including mononucleosis, pneumonitis, hemolytic anemia, and thrombocytopenia purpura. In contrast, a CMV infection in an immunocompromised individual, such as a transplant recipient or an individual with AIDS, can cause a devastating, life-threatening illness.

Congenital CMV infection is the most common serious viral infection among infants. Approximately 1% of all infants (40,000) are born with congenital CMV. Of these, 10% (4000) demonstrate typical manifestations of the infection, such as hepatosplenomegaly, intracranial calcifications, microcephaly, smallness for gestational age, and hearing impairments. An additional 10% to 15% of these are asymptomatic at birth; however, they begin to develop manifestations of the infection within the first few months of life. Recent evidence suggests that symptomatic infection of infants is caused by a primary infection of the mother during her pregnancy and not necessarily by reinfection or reactivation of a prior infection.

EVALUATION AND TREATMENT The most definitive diagnostic test for CMV is isolation of the virus, usually through growth in human fibroblast cell culture. Several methods for measuring antibodies to CMV are available, including complement-fixation (CF) tests and indirect immunofluorescent antibody (IFA) tests. These methods commonly are used in clinical situations.

With the increased incidence of CMV infection among immunocompromised individuals (persons with AIDS or transplants), various treatment modalities have been investigated. Ganciclovir is similar to acyclovir and inhibits viral DNA polymerase (see Chapter 4). Relapses of CMV infection are frequent after therapy ceases; thus lifelong therapy is particularly indicated in individuals with AIDS.[48] Acyclovir has been used, but optimum therapeutic benefits have not been established. Future therapies still under investigation include ganciclovir plus CMV immunoglobulin and vaccine.

Experimental antiviral drugs may prove helpful in the treatment of severe CMV infection, and preliminary studies to develop a vaccine appear promising. No treatment is indicated, however, in most cases of CMV infection.

SUMMARY REVIEW

Sexually Transmitted Urogenital Infections

1. Gonorrhea is a sexually transmitted communicable disease that can be local or systemic. Complications include PID; sterility; and disseminated infection, which is spread through the bloodstream to the skin, joints, and heart.
2. Gonorrhea passed to the fetus from the mother typically manifests as an eye infection and develops 1 to 12 days after birth. Usually ophthalmic antibiotic prophylaxis is not sufficient to prevent infection.
3. Antibiotic coverage for penicillin-resistant strains and chlamydial coinfection is recommended for all individuals diagnosed with gonorrhea and their partners.
4. Syphilis is an STI that becomes systemic shortly after infection. The four stages of the disease are (a) primary syphilis with a chancre at the site of infection; (b) secondary syphilis with systemic spread to all body systems; (c) latent syphilis with minimal symptoms or the development of skin lesions; and (d) tertiary syphilis, the most severe stage, with destruction of bone, skin, and soft and neurologic tissues.
5. Congenital syphilis contributes to prematurity of the newborn with bone marrow depression, CNS involvement, renal failure, and intrauterine growth retardation. Late clinical manifestations are those of tertiary syphilis and are rare.
6. Syphilis is diagnosed by serologic testing and treated with injectable penicillin. Sexual partners are treated also.
7. With chancroid infection, women are generally asymptomatic and men may develop inflamed, painful genital ulcers and inguinal buboes. Incubation period is 1 to 14 days. Single-dose therapy with injectable ceftriaxone or oral azithromycin for both partners is recommended. Persons with HIV may require a longer treatment regimen.

8. Granuloma inguinale (donovanosis) is rare in the United States. The bacteria are gram negative and survive within macrophages. Localized nodules coalesce to form granulomas and ulcers on the penis in men and labia in women. Antibiotics provide effective treatment. Although rare and mildly infectious, granuloma inguinale is a chronic, progressively destructive bacterial infection. Often individuals diagnosed with granuloma inguinale are coinfected with syphilis.

9. BV is a sexually associated condition caused by an overgrowth of anaerobic bacteria that produce aromatic amines and raise the pH of the vagina, promoting further bacterial growth (without an inflammatory response) and a fishy odor. "Clue cells" are found on the wet mount. Metronidazole (Flagyl) provides effective treatment. BV has been associated with PID, chorioamnionitis, preterm labor, and postpartum endometritis. Treatment of male sexual partners is not recommended.

10. Chlamydia is the most common bacterial STI in the United States and the leading preventable cause of infertility and ectopic pregnancy. The causative organism, *C. trachomatis*, localizes to epithelial tissue and can spread throughout the urogenital tract or pass from infected mother to the eyes and respiratory tract of newborn infants during birth. As with gonorrhea, prophylactic eye antibiotic treatment is insufficient to prevent infection. *C. trachomatis* is susceptible to inexpensive, readily accessible antibiotics. Single-dose azithromycin is the drug of choice. Antibiotic therapy for infected individuals and all sexual contacts is recommended. Because of the asymptomatic nature of chlamydia and the potential sequelae of untreated infection, extensive and widespread screening is warranted.

11. Lymphogranuloma venereum is a chronic STI that is uncommon in the United States. The lesion begins as a skin infection and spreads to the lymph tissue, causing inflammation, necrosis, buboes, and abscesses of the inguinal lymph nodes. Primary lesions appear on the penis and scrotum in men and on the cervix, vaginal wall, and labia in women. Secondary lesions involve inflammation and swelling of the lymph nodes with formation of large blue buboes that rupture and form draining ulcerative lesions. A 21-day course of oral doxycycline or erythromycin is effective. Treatment of sexual partners is recommended.

12. Genital herpes is the most common genital ulceration in the United States and is caused by either HSV-1 or HSV-2. Lesions initially appear as groups of vesicles that progress to ulceration with pain, lymphadenopathy, and fever. Herpes simplex virus passes from mother to fetus and can cause spontaneous abortion or prematurity. Acyclovir reduces symptoms but does not cure the disease.

13. Three distinct syndromes are associated with HSV infection: (a) first-episode primary infections, (b) first-episode nonprimary infections, and (c) recurrent infections. Recurrent infections are most often attributable to HSV-2 and are generally milder and of shorter duration.

14. HPV is associated with the development of cervical dysplasia and cancer as well as condylomata acuminata. The high-risk strains of HPV (HR-HPV) that are precursors to the development of cervical cancer do not cause genital warts. Testing is available to detect HR-HPV, as well as a vaccine for HPV types 16 and 18, which have the highest risk for cervical cancer.

15. Condylomata acuminata (genital warts) are associated with multiple sexual partners and are highly contagious. The velvety cauliflower-like lesions occur in the genital and anal areas, vagina, and cervix and are painless. They can be transmitted to the infant at birth.

16. Molluscum contagiosum is a benign viral infection of the skin. It is transmitted by skin-to-skin contact in children and adults. In adults it tends to occur on the genitalia and to be transmitted by sexual contact.

17. Trichomoniasis (*T. vaginalis*) causes vaginitis in women, and urethritis in men. Both partners usually are infected. Women usually have a copious, malodorous, gray-green discharge with pruritus. Men usually are asymptomatic. Metronidazole is the treatment for both partners.

18. Scabies is a common parasitic infection that can be spread by skin-to-skin contact and sexual contact. The scabies mite burrows through the skin, depositing two or three large eggs per day. Intense pruritus, especially at night, is the most pronounced clinical manifestation. Treatment consists of topical application of a pediculicide.

19. Pediculosis pubis (crabs) is commonly transmitted sexually and is caused by the crab louse, *P. pubis*. The lice bite into the skin for nutrition. Symptoms include mild and severe pruritus. Topical application of prescription or over-the-counter pediculicides is effective treatment.

Sexually Transmitted Infections of Other Body Systems

1. Various enteric bacterial pathogens are now recognized as being sexually transmitted, particularly among homosexual men. The infections include shigellosis, *Campylobacter* enteritis, giardiasis, amebiasis, and hepatitis A.

2. Shigellosis is transmitted by contact with infected feces. *Campylobacter* enteritis can be transmitted through anal-oral sexual practices.

3. Giardiasis and amebiasis are transmitted primarily through contaminated drinking water, but they can be transmitted by anal-oral and genital-anal contact.

4. Transmission of HBV can occur through needle puncture, blood transfusion, cuts in the skin, and contact with infected body fluids.

5. Hepatitis B infection poses significant health risks including chronic liver disease and hepatocellular cancer. Immunization against hepatitis B is the most effective means of preventing transmission. Universal vaccination of infants and children is recommended, as well as vaccination of high-risk adults.

6. Perinatal transmission of HBV is relatively common.

7. Hepatitis C is generally transmitted percutaneously but sexual transmission appears possible.

8. Systemic diseases known to be sexually transmitted include AIDS (see Chapter 8), cytomegalovirus infection, and Epstein-Barr virus.

9. Epstein-Barr virus may be harbored in the genital tract and passed on through sexual encounters.

10. CMV is a sexually transmissible herpesvirus. The infection causes no specific genital disease, but its incidence is high in individuals being treated for other STIs. The virus is found in semen, cervical secretions, urine, blood, saliva, breast milk, and stool.

11. CMV infection is more common in homosexual men and in young women with multiple sexual partners. It is the most common congenital infection.

12. CMV infection can cause mononucleosis, pneumonitis, hemolytic anemia, and thrombocytopenia purpura. A CMV infection in an immunosuppressed individual can cause a life-threatening illness. No treatment is indicated in most cases of CMV infection.

KEY TERMS

Acute urethral syndrome, 936
Amebiasis, 946
Bacterial vaginosis (BV), 934
Buboes, 932
Campylobacter enteritis, 946
Chancre, 928
Chancroid, 932
Chlamydia, 935
Condylomata acuminata, 940
Condylomata lata, 929
Congenital syphilis (CS), 929
Cytomegalovirus (CMV), 948
Disseminated gonococcal infection (DGI), 926
Donovan body, 934

Epstein-Barr virus (EBV), 947
Fomite, 925
Genital herpes, 938
Giardiasis, 946
Gonococcus, 924
Gonorrhea, 924
Granuloma inguinale (donovanosis), 933
Gummas, 929
Hepatitis B virus (HBV), 947
Hepatitis delta agent, 947
Human papillomavirus (HPV), 940
Latent syphilis, 929
Lymphogranuloma venereum (LGV), 937
Molluscous body, 942
Molluscum contagiosum, 941

Neurosyphilis, 929
Nongonococcal urethritis (NGU), 937
Ophthalmia neonatorum, 927
Pediculosis pubis, 945
Perihepatitis, 926
Primary syphilis, 928
Pseudobuboes, 934
Scabies, 944
Secondary syphilis, 928
Shigellosis, 946
Syphilis, 927
Tertiary syphilis, 929
Trichomonad, 943
Trichomoniasis, 943
Trophozoite, 946

REFERENCES

1. National Center for HIV/AIDS, Viral Hepatitis, STD, and TB Prevention. Annual Report 2008. U.S. Department Health and Human Services CDC and Prevention Available. www.cdc.gov/std/stats
2. Centers for Disease Control and Prevention. *Sexually Transmitted Disease Surveillance, 2007*. Atlanta, GA: U.S. Department of Health and Human Services; December 2008. www.cdc.gov/std/stats
3. Centers for Disease Control and Prevention. *Sexually Transmitted Disease Surveillance 2007 Supplement, Gonococcal Isolate Surveillance Project (GISP) Annual Report 2007*. Atlanta, GA: U.S. Department of Health and Human Services, Centers for Disease Control and Prevention, March 2009. www.cdc.gov/std/stats.
4. Centers for Disease Control and Prevention. *Sexually Transmitted Disease Surveillance 2007 Supplement, Syphilis Surveillance Report*. Atlanta, GA: U.S. Department of Health and Human Services, Centers for Disease Control and Prevention, March 2009. www.cdc.gov/std/stats.
5. Centers for Disease Control and Prevention. *Sexually Transmitted Disease Surveillance 2007 Supplement, Chlamydia Prevalence Monitoring Project Annual Report 2007*. Atlanta, GA: U.S. Department of Health and Human Services, Centers for Disease Control and Prevention; January 2009. www.cdc.gov/std/stats.
6. Centers for Disease Control and Prevention: Trends in reportable sexually transmitted diseases in the United States, 2007: National data on chlamydia, gonorrhea and syphilis. In *STD surveillance 2007*. Available at www.cdc.gov/std/stats/trends2007.htm.
7. Hook EW III, Handsfield HH: Gonococcal infections in the adult. In Holmes KK, et al: *Sexually transmitted diseases*, ed 4, New York, 2008, McGraw-Hill.
8. Pelouze PS: *Gonorrhea in the male and female*, Philadelphia, 1941, Saunders.
9. Whittington W et al: Gonorrhea. In Morse SA, Moreland AA, Holmes KK, editors: *Atlas of sexually transmitted diseases and AIDS*, ed 3, London, 2003, Mosby-Wolfe.
10. Krieger JN: Sexually transmitted diseases in men. In Tanagho EA, McAninch JW, editors: *Smith's general urology*, ed 17, New York, 2007, McGraw-Hill.
11. Westrom L et al. Pelvic inflammatory disease and fertility: a cohort study of 1,844 women with laparoscopically verified disease and 657 control women with normal laparoscopic results, *Sex Trans Dis* 19(4):184-1982, 1992.
12. Zenilman JM: Gonorrhea: clinical and public health issues, *Hosp Pract* 28(2a):29, 1993.
13. Sperling RS: Infection protocols: perihepatitis, *Contemp OB/GYN* 37(6):51, 1992.
14. Emmert DH, Kirchner JT: Sexually transmitted diseases in women: gonorrhea and syphilis, *Postgrad Med* 107(2):181-184, 189-190, 193-197, 2000.

15. Centers for Disease Control and Prevention: *Sexually transmitted disease surveillance 2006 supplement, gonococcal isolate surveillance project (GISP) annual report*, Atlanta, 2008, U.S. Department of Health and Human Services.
16. Centers for Disease Control and Prevention: *Sexually transmitted disease surveillance 2006 supplement, syphilis surveillance project*, Atlanta, 2007, U.S. Department of Health and Human Services.
17. Centers for Disease Control and Prevention: Sexually transmitted diseases treatment guidelines 2002, *MMWR* 51(RR-11):1-94, 2006.
18. Leu RH: Complications of coexisting chlamydial and gonococcal infections, *Postgrad Med* 89(7):56-60, 1991.
19. Brandt AM: *No magic bullet: a social history of venereal disease in the United States since 1880, expanded edition*, New York, 1987, Oxford University Press.
20. Sparling PF: Clinical manifestations of syphilis. In Holmes KK, et al, editors: *Sexually transmitted diseases*, ed 4, New York, 2008, McGraw-Hill.
21. Schultz KF et al: Congenital syphilis. In Holmes KK et al, editors: *Sexually transmitted diseases*, ed 4, New York, 2008, McGraw-Hill.
22. Hook EW, Marra CM: Medical progress: acquired syphilis in adults, *N Engl J Med* 326(16):1060, 1992.
23. Thin RN: Early syphilis in the adult. In Holmes KK, et al, editors: *Sexually transmitted diseases*, ed 4, New York, 2008, McGraw-Hill.
24. Wooldridge WE: Syphilis: a new visit from an old enemy, *Postgrad Med* 89(1):193-196, 199-202 , 1991.
25. Tillman J: Syphilis an old disease, a contemporary problem, *J Obstet Gynecol Neonat Nurs* 21(3):209, 1992.
26. Jacobs RA: Infectious diseases: spirochetal. In McTierney LM, McPhee SJ, Papadakis MS, editors: *Current medical diagnosis & treatment*, ed 47, Norwalk, CT, 2008, Appleton & Lange.
27. O'Farrell N: Tropical medicine series: donovanosis, *Sex Transm Infect* 78(6):452-457, 2002.
28. Para MF, Baird IM: Genital ulcer syndromes. In Spagna VA, Prior RB, editors: *Sexually transmitted diseases: a clinical syndrome approach*, New York, 1985, Marcel Dekker.
29. Committee on Infectious Disease: *Red Book 2000*, Elk Grove Village, IL, 2000, American Academy of Pediatrics.
30. Ronald AR, Albritton W: Chancroid and *Haemophilus ducreyi*. In Holmes KK, et al, editors: *Sexually transmitted diseases*, ed 2, New York, 1990, McGraw-Hill.
31. Richens J: The diagnosis of treatment of donovanosis (granuloma inguinale), *Genitourin Med* 67(6):441-452, 1991.
32. Hart G, Donovanosis: In Holmes KK, et al, editors: *Sexually transmitted diseases*, ed 4, New York, 2008, McGraw-Hill.
33. Hillier SL et al: Association between bacterial vaginosis and preterm delivery of a low-birth-weight infant, *N Engl J Med* 333(26):1737-1742, 1995.
34. Amsel R et al: Nonspecific vaginitis. Diagnostic criteria ad microbial and epidemiologic associations, *Am J Med* 74(1):14-22, 1983.

35. Kellogg ND et al: Comparison of nucleic acid amplification tests and culture techniques in the detection of *Neisseria gonorrhoeae* and *Chlamydia trachomatis* in victims of suspected child sexual abuse, *J Pediatr Adolesc Gynecol* 17(5):331-339, 2004.

36. Sargent SJ: The "other" sexually transmitted diseases: chlamydial, herpes simplex virus, and human papillomavirus infections, *Postgrad Med* 91(4):359-362, 371-374, 377, 1992.

37. Schachter J, Barnes R: Infections caused by *Chlamydia trachomatis*. In Morse SA, Moreland AA, Holmes KK, editors: *Atlas of sexually transmitted diseases and AIDS*, ed 2, London, 1996, Mosby-Wolfe.

38. Westrom LV: Chlamydia and its effect on reproduction, *J Br Fer Soc* 1(1):23-30, 1996.

39. Chambers HF: Infectious diseases: bacterial and chlamydial. In McTierney LM, McPhee SJ, Papadakis MA, editors: *Current medical diagnosis and treatment*, ed 35, Norwalk, CT, 1996, Appleton & Lange.

40. Perine PI, Osoba AO: Lymphogranuloma venereum. In Holmes KK, et al, editors: *Sexually transmitted diseases*, ed 2, New York, 1990, McGraw-Hill.

41. Mertz GJ et al: Risk factors for the sexual transmission of genital herpes, *Ann Intern Med* 116(3):197, 1992.

42. Stagno S, Whitley RJ: Herpesvirus infection in the neonate and children. In Holmes KK, et al, editors: *Sexually transmitted diseases*, ed 2, New York, 1990, McGraw-Hill.

43. Landenberg AG et al: A prospective study of new infections with herpes simplex virus type 1 and type 2. Chiron HSV Vaccine Study Group, *N Engl J Med* 341(19):1432-1438, 1999.

44. Koelle DM, Wald A: Herpes simplex virus: the importance of asymptomatic shedding, *J Antimicrob Chemother* 45(Suppl T3):1-8, 2000.

45. Stephenson J: Genital herpes vaccine shows limited promise, *JAMA* 284(15):1913-1914.

46. Rose FB, Camp CJ: Genital herpes: how to relieve patients' physical and psychological symptoms, *Postgrad Med* 84(3):81-86, 1988.

47. Wright TC et al: Interim guidance for the use of human papillomavirus DNA testing as an adjunct to cervical cytology for screening, *Obstet Gynecol* 103(2):304-309, 2004.

48. Woodman CB et al: Natural history of cervical human papillomavirus infection in young women: a longitudinal cohort study, *Lancet* 357(9271):1831-1836, 2001.

49. Derksen DJ: Children with condylomata acuminata, *J Fam Pract* 34(4):419-423, 1992.

50. Alary M et al: Strategy for screening pregnant women for chlamydial infection in a low-prevalence area, *Obstet Gynecol* 82(3):399, 1993.

51. Shah KV: Biology of genital tract human papillomaviruses, *Urol Clin North Am* 19(1):63-69, 1992.

52. McAninch JW: Disorders of the penis and male urethra. In Tanagho EA, McAninch JW, editors: *Smith's general urology*, Norwalk, CT, 1995, Appleton & Lange.

53. Camisa C: Condyloma acuminatum and other human papillomavirus-induced diseases. In Spagna VA, Prior RB, editors: *Sexually transmitted disease: a clinical syndrome approach*, New York, 1985, Marcel Dekker.

54. Harper DM et al: Efficacy of a bivalent L1 virus-like particle vaccine in prevention of infection with human papillomavirus types 16 and 18 in young women: a randomised controlled trial, *Lancet* 364(9447): 1757-1765, 2004.

55. Berger TG: Skin diseases of the external genitalia. In Tanagho EA, McAninch JW, editors: *Smith's general urology*, Norwalk, CT, 1995, Appleton & Lange.

56. Lambert DR, Yoder FW: Ectoparasites and molluscum contagiosum. In Spagna VA, Prior RB, editors: *Sexually transmitted diseases: a clinical syndrome approach*, New York, 1985, Marcel Dekker.

57. Rein MR, Holmes KK: Nonspecific vaginitis, vulvovaginal candidiasis, and trichomoniasis: clinical features, diagnosis, and management. In Remington J, Schwartz MN, editors: *Current clinical topics in infectious diseases*, New York, 1983, McGraw-Hill.

58. Bartlett JG: *Pocket book of infectious disease therapy*, Baltimore, 1995, Williams & Wilkins.

59. Orkin M, Maibach HI: Scabies. In Holmes KK, et al, editors: *Sexually transmitted diseases*, ed 2, New York, 1990, McGraw-Hill.

60. Hammerschlag MR, Laraque D: Inappropriate use of nonculture tests for the detection of chlamydia trachomatis in suspected victims of child sexual abuse: a continuing problem, *Pediatrics* 104(5):1137, 1999.

61. Quinn TC, Stamm WE: Proctocolitis, enteritis, and esophagitis in homosexual men. In Holmes KK, et al, editors: *Sexually transmitted diseases*, ed 2, New York, 1990, McGraw-Hill.

62. Gardner TB, Hill DR: Treatment of giardiasis, *Clin Microbiol Rev* 14(1):114-128, 2001. Available at http://cmr.asm.org/cgi/content/full/14/1/114?view=long&pmid=11148005.

63. Lemon SM, Newbold JE: Viral hepatitis. In Holmes KK, et al, editors: *Sexually transmitted diseases*, ed 4, New York, 2008, McGraw-Hill.

64. Klein MB: Hepatitis B virus: perinatal management, *J Perinat Neonat Nurs* 1(4):12, 1988.

65. Beasley RP et al: The e antigen and vertical transmission of hepatitis B surface antigen, *Am J Epidemiol* 105(2):94-98, 1977.

66. Stevens CE et al: HBeAg and anti-HBe detection by radioimmunoassay: correlation with vertical transmission of hepatitis B virus in Taiwan, *J Med Virol* 3(3):237-241, 1979.

67. Immunization Practices Advisory Committee: Hepatitis B virus: a comprehensive strategy for eliminating transmission in the United States through universal childhood vaccination: recommendations of the Immunization Practice Advisory Committee (ACIP), *MMWR* 40(RR-13):1-19, 1991.

STRUCTURE AND FUNCTION OF THE HEMATOLOGIC SYSTEM

NEAL S. ROTE • KATHRYN L. McCANCE

MEDIA RESOURCES

CHAPTER OUTLINE

COMPONENTS OF THE HEMATOLOGIC SYSTEM
Composition of the Blood
Lymphoid Organs
DEVELOPMENT OF BLOOD CELLS
Hematopoiesis
Development of Erythrocytes
Development of Leukocytes
Development of Platelets
MECHANISMS OF HEMOSTASIS
Function of Blood Vessels
Function of Platelets

Function of Clotting Factors
Control of Hemostatic Mechanisms
Lysis of Blood Clots
CLINICAL EVALUATION OF THE HEMATOLOGIC SYSTEM
Tests of Bone Marrow Function
Blood Tests
Pediatrics and the Hematologic System
Aging and the Hematologic System

All the body's tissues and organs require oxygen and nutrients to survive. These essential needs are provided by the blood that flows through miles of vessels throughout the human body. The red blood cells provide the oxygen and remove carbon dioxide, and the fluid portion of the blood carries the nutrients and ions for proper acid-base balance. The blood also cleans discarded waste from the tissues, transports hormones, conveys cells (white blood cells), platelets, and other ingredients that are necessary for protecting the entire body from injury and infection and initiating healing, and provides thermal regulation to maintain organs and tissues within an acceptable range of temperatures.

COMPONENTS OF THE HEMATOLOGIC SYSTEM

Composition of the Blood

Blood consists of various cells that circulate in the cardiovascular system suspended in a solution of protein and inorganic materials (plasma), which is approximately 90% water

and 10% dissolved substances (solutes). The blood volume amounts to about 6 quarts (5.5 L) in adults. The continuous movement of blood guarantees that critical components are available to all parts of the body to carry out their chief functions: (1) delivery of substances needed for cellular metabolism in the tissues, (2) removal of the wastes of cellular metabolism, (3) defense against invading microorganisms and injury, and (4) maintenance of acid-base balance.

Plasma and Plasma Proteins

In adults, plasma accounts for 50% to 55% of blood volume. **Plasma** is a complex aqueous liquid containing a variety of organic and inorganic elements (Table 25-1). The concentration of these elements varies depending on diet, metabolic demand, hormones, and vitamins. Plasma differs from serum in that **serum** is plasma that has been allowed to clot in the laboratory in order to remove fibrinogen and other clotting factors that may interfere with some diagnostic tests.

The plasma contains a large number of proteins (**plasma proteins**) that constitute about 7% of the total plasma weight. These vary in structure and function and can be classified into two major groups, albumin and globulins. Most plasma proteins are produced by the liver. The major exception is antibodies (immunoglobulins), which are produced by plasma cells in the lymph nodes and other lymphoid tissues (see Chapter 7).

Albumin (about 60% of total plasma protein at a concentration of about 4 g/dl) serves as a carrier molecule for normal components of blood as well as drugs that have low solubility in water (e.g., free fatty acids, lipid-soluble hormones, thyroid hormones, bile salts). Its most essential role is regulation of the passage of water and solutes through the capillaries. Albumin molecules are large and do not diffuse freely through the vascular endothelium, and thus they maintain the critical colloidal osmotic pressure (or oncotic pressure) that regulates the passage of water and solutes into the surrounding tissues (see Chapters 1 and 3). Water and solute particles tend to diffuse out of the arterial portions of the capillaries because the blood pressure is greater in arterial than in venous blood

vessels (see Chapter 3). Water and solutes move from tissue cells into the venous portions of the capillaries where the pressures are reversed, oncotic pressure being greater than intravascular pressure or hydrostatic pressure. In the case of decreased production (e.g., cirrhosis, other diffuse liver diseases, protein malnutrition) or excessive loss of albumin (e.g., certain kidney diseases, extensive burns), the reduced oncotic pressure leads to excessive movement of fluid and solutes into the tissue and decreased blood volume.[1]

The remaining plasma proteins, or **globulins,** are often classified by their properties in an electric field (serum electrophoresis). Under the normal conditions used to perform serum electrophoresis, albumin is the most rapidly moving protein. The globulins are classified by their movement relative to albumin: alpha (α) globulins (those moving most closely to albumin), beta (β) globulins, and gamma (γ) globulins (those with the least movement). Depending on the electrophoretic procedure the alpha and beta globulins may be subdivided

Table 25-1	Organic and Inorganic Components of Arterial Plasma	
Constituent	**Amount/Concentration**	**Major Functions**
Water	93% of plasma weight	Medium for carrying all other constituents
Electrolytes	Total <1% of plasma weight	Maintain H_2O in extracellular compartment; act as buffers; function in membrane excitability
Na^+	142 mEq/L (142 mM)	
K^+	4 mEq/L (4 mM)	
Ca^{2+}	5 mEq/L (2.5 mM)	
Mg^{2+}	3 mEq/L (1.5 mM)	
Cl	103 mEq/L (103 mM)	
HCO_3^-	27 mEq/L (27 mM)	
Phosphate (mostly HPO_4^-)	2 mEq/L (1 mM)	
SO_4^{2-}	1 mEq/L (0.5 mM)	
Proteins	7.3 g/dl (2.5 mM)	Provide colloid osmotic pressure of plasma; act as buffers; bind other plasma constituents (lipids, hormones, vitamins, minerals, etc.); clotting factors; enzymes; enzyme precursors; antibodies (immune globulins); hormones; transporters
Albumin	4.5 g/dl	
Globulins	2.5 g/dl	
Fibrinogen	0.3 g/dl	
Transferrin	250 mg/dl	
Ferritin	15-300 mcg/L	
Gases		
CO_2 content	22-32 mmol/L plasma	Byproduct of oxygenation, most CO_2 content is from HCO_3 and acts as a buffer
O_2	Pao_2 80 torr or greater (arterial); Pvo_2 30-40 torr (venous)	Oxygenation
N_2	0.9 ml/dl	By-product of protein catabolism
Nutrients		Provide nutrition and substances for tissue repair
Glucose and other carbohydrates	100 mg/dl (5.6 mM)	
Total amino acids	40 mg/dl (2 mM)	
Total lipids	500 mg/dl (7.5 mM)	
Cholesterol	150-250 mg/dl (4-7 mM)	
Individual vitamins	0.0001-2.5 mg/dl	
Individual trace elements	0.001-0.3 mg/dl	
Iron	50-150 mcg/dl	
Waste products		
Urea (blood urea nitrogen [BUN])	7-18 mg/dl (5.7 mM)	End product of protein catabolism
Creatinine (from creatine)	1 mg/dl (0.09 mM)	End product from energy metabolism
Uric acid (from nucleic acids)	5 mg/dl (0.3 mM)	End product from protein metabolism
Bilirubin (from heme)	0.2-1.2 mg/dl (0.003-0.018 mM)	End product of red blood cell destruction
Individual hormones	0.000001-0.05 mg/dl	Functions specific to target tissue

Data from Vander AJ, Sherman JH, Luciano DS: *Human physiology: the mechanisms of body function*, ed 8, New York, 2001, McGraw-Hill.

into subregions (α_1, α_2, β_1, or β_2-globulins). Fibrinogen is a major plasma protein (about 4% of total plasma protein) that would move between the beta and gamma regions but is removed during the formation of serum. The gamma globulin region consists primarily of immunoglobulin G (IgG) (see Chapter 7).

Plasma proteins can also be classified into groups by function: clotting, defense, transport, or regulation. The **clotting factors** promote coagulation and stop bleeding from damaged blood vessels. Fibrinogen is the most plentiful of the clotting factors and is the precursor of the fibrin clot. Proteins involved in defense, or protection, against infection include antibodies and complement proteins (see Chapters 6 and 7). Transport proteins specifically bind and carry a variety of inorganic and organic molecules, including iron (transferrin), copper (ceruloplasmin), steroid hormones, and vitamins (e.g., retinol-binding protein). The plasma lipids, triglycerides, phospholipids, cholesterol, and fatty acids are carried through the blood as complexes with plasma proteins; they are known as *lipoproteins* (see Chapters 1 and 30). Regulatory proteins include a variety of enzymatic inhibitors (e.g., α_1-antitrypsin) that protect the tissues from damage, precursor molecules (e.g., kininogen) that are converted into active

biologic molecules when needed, and protein hormones (e.g., cytokines) that communicate between cells.

Plasma also contains several charged inorganic ions (electrolytes) that regulate cell function, osmotic pressure, and blood pH. (Electrolytes are described in Chapters 1 and 3.)

Cellular Components of the Blood

The cellular elements of the blood are broadly classified as red blood cells (RBCs) (i.e., erythrocytes), white blood cells (WBCs) (i.e., leukocytes), and platelets (thrombocytes). The components of the blood are listed in Table 25-2.

Erythrocytes

In 1628 Robert Burton described blood as a "hot, temperate red humor whose office is to nourish the whole body, to give it strength and color being dispersed by the veins through every part of it."[2] A few years later, with the invention of the microscope, researchers learned that erythrocytes give blood its red color.

Erythrocytes (red blood cells [RBCs]) are the most abundant cells of the blood, occupying approximately 48% of the blood volume in men and about 42% in women. Erythrocytes are primarily responsible for tissue oxygenation. The erythrocyte contains hemoglobin, which

Table 25-2	Cellular Components of the Blood			
Cell	Structural Characteristics*	Normal Amounts of Circulating Blood	Function	Life Span
Erythrocyte (red blood cell)	Non-nucleated cytoplasmic disk containing hemoglobin	4.2-6.2 million/mm³	Gas transport to and from tissue cells and lungs	80-120 days
Leukocyte (white blood cell)	Nucleated cell	5000-10,000/mm³	Body defense mechanisms	See below
Lymphocyte	Mononuclear immunocyte	25%-33% of leukocyte count (leukocyte differential)	Humoral and cell-mediated immunity (see Chapter 6)	Days or years depending on type
Monocyte and macrophage	Large kidney-shaped mononuclear phagocyte	3%-7% of leukocyte differential	Phagocytosis; mononuclear phagocyte system	Months or years
Eosinophil	Segmented polymorphonuclear granulocyte with granules stainable by eosin dyes	1%-4% of leukocyte differential	Phagocytosis, response to parasites, control of allergic reactions	8-12 days
Neutrophil	Segmented polymorphonuclear granulocyte with granules stainable by neutral staining	57%-67% of leukocyte differential	Phagocytosis, particularly during early phase of inflammation, bacterial killing	4 days
Basophil	Lobate nuclear granulocyte with granules stainable by basic dyes	0%-0.75% of leukocyte differential	Similar to mast cell, secretes inflammatory mediators (e.g., histamine, chemotactic factors for eosinophils and neutrophils), involved with allergic reactions	Few hours to days
Platelet	Irregularly shaped cytoplasmic fragment (not a cell)	140,000-340,000/mm³	Hemostasis following vascular injury; normal coagulation and clot formation/retraction	8-11 days

*See bottom row of Figure 25-9 for illustrations of cells.

carries the gases, and electrolytes, which regulate diffusion through a cell's plasma membrane. The mature erythrocyte lacks a nucleus and cytoplasmic organelles (e.g., mitochondria), so it cannot synthesize protein or carry out oxidative reactions. Because it cannot undergo mitotic division, the erythrocyte has a limited life span (approximately 120 days), ages, and is removed from the circulation to be replaced by new erythrocytes.

The erythrocyte's size and shape are ideally suited to its function as a gas carrier. An RBC is a small disk with two unique properties: (1) a *biconcave* shape and (2) the capacity to be *reversibly deformed* (Figure 25-1).[3] The flattened, biconcave shape provides a surface area/volume ratio that is optimal for gas diffusion into and out of the cell. During its life span, the erythrocyte, which is 6 to 8 μm in diameter, repeatedly circulates through sinusoids of the spleen and capillaries that are only 2 μm in diameter. Reversible deformity enables the erythrocyte to assume a more compact torpedo-like shape, squeeze through the microcirculation, and return to normal.

Leukocytes

Leukocytes (white blood cells [WBCs]) defend the body against microorganisms that cause infection and remove debris, including dead or injured cells of all kinds (Figure 25-2). The leukocytes act primarily in the tissues but are transported in the circulation. The average adult has approximately 5000 to 10,000 leukocytes/mm³ of blood.

Leukocytes are classified according to structure as either **granulocytes** or **agranulocytes** and according to function as either **phagocytes** or **immunocytes.** The granulocytes, which include neutrophils, basophils, and eosinophils, are all phagocytes. (Phagocytic action is described in Chapter 6.) Of the agranulocytes, the monocytes and macrophages are phagocytes, whereas the lymphocytes are immunocytes (cells that create immunity; see Chapter 7).

Granulocytes. Granulocytes have many membrane-bound granules in their cytoplasm. These granules contain enzymes capable of killing microorganisms and catabolizing debris ingested during phagocytosis. The granules also contain powerful biochemical mediators with inflammatory and immune functions. These mediators, along with the digestive enzymes, are released from granulocytes in response to specific stimuli. The biochemical mediators have vascular and intercellular effects and the enzymes participate in the breakdown of debris from sites of infection or injury. Granulocytes are capable of amoeboid movement, by which they migrate through vessel walls (diapedesis) and then to sites where their action is needed (see Chapter 6).

The **neutrophil (polymorphonuclear neutrophil [PMN])** is the most numerous and best understood of the granulocytes (Figure 25-3, *A*). Neutrophils constitute about 55% of the total leukocyte count in adults. The cytoplasm of neutrophils contains small lysosomal granules and a central nucleus with two to five distinct lobes. Immature neutrophils are called *bands* or *stabs*. Mature neutrophils are called *segmented neutrophils* because of the characteristic appearance of their nucleus.

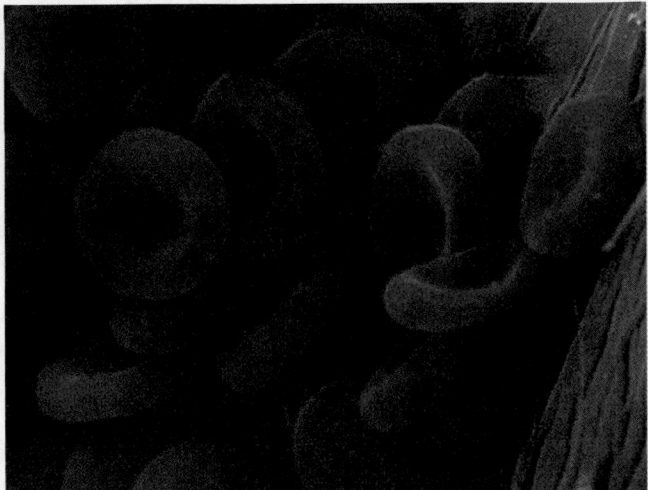

Figure 25-1 Mature erythrocytes. Scanning electron micrograph of mature erythrocytes on cell wall. (Copyright Dennis Kunkel Microscopy, Inc.)

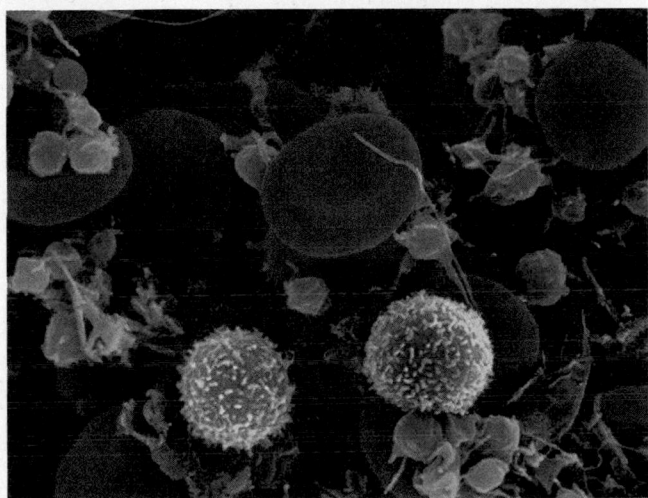

Figure 25-2 Blood cells. Leukocytes are spherical and have irregular surfaces with numerous extending pili (appear as yellow). Erythrocytes are flattened spheres with a depressed center. Activated platelets are green. (Copyright Dennis Kunkel Microscopy, Inc.)

Neutrophils reach a fully mature state in the bone marrow, and these mature neutrophils are called the *marrow neutrophil reserve.* Normally it takes about 14 days for neutrophils to develop from early precursors, but this process is accelerated by infection and treatment with colony-stimulating factors.

Neutrophils are the chief phagocytes of early inflammation. Soon after bacterial invasion or tissue injury, neutrophils migrate out of the capillaries and into the inflamed site, where they ingest and destroy microorganisms and debris and then die in 1 or 2 days. The dissolution of dead neutrophils releases digestive enzymes from their cytoplasmic granules. These enzymes dissolve cellular debris and prepare the site for healing. (This final function, called *débridement,* is described in Chapter 6).

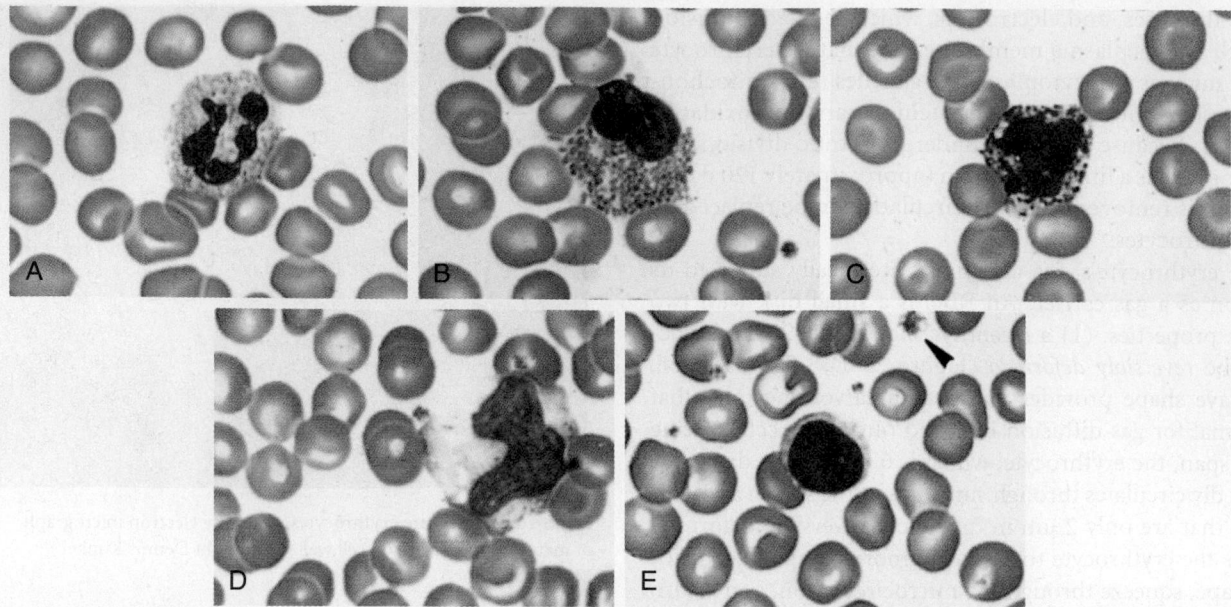

Figure 25-3 Leukocytes. An example of leukocytes in a human blood smear. A, Neutrophil. B, Eosinophil. C, Basophil. D, Monocyte. E, Lymphocyte. (From Erlandsen S, Magney J: *Color atlas of histology*, St Louis, 1992, Mosby.)

Eosinophils. **Eosinophils,** which have large, coarse granules, constitute only 1% to 4% of the normal leukocyte count in adults (see Figure 25-3, *B*). Like neutrophils, eosinophils are capable of amoeboid movement and phagocytosis.[4] Unlike neutrophils, which ingest cellular debris, eosinophils ingest antigen-antibody complexes, and viruses and are induced by mast cell chemotactic factors to attack parasites. Eosinophil granules contain chemicals (e.g., major basic protein, eosinophil cationic protein, eosinophil peroxidase, eosinophil-derived neurotoxin) that are highly destructive to parasites and viruses. The eosinophil granules contain a variety of enzymes (e.g., histaminase) that help to control inflammatory processes. (Their function in inflammation and defense against parasites is described in Chapters 6 and 7.) Type I hypersensitivity allergic reactions and asthma are characterized by high numbers of circulating eosinophils, which may be involved in a dual role of regulation of inflammation and may contribute to the destructive inflammatory processes observed in the lungs of asthmatics (see Chapter 8).

Basophils, which make up less than 1% (0.01% to 0.3%) of the leukocytes, contain cytoplasmic granules that contain an abundant mixture of biochemical mediators, including histamine, chemotactic factors, proteolytic enzymes, and an anticoagulant (heparin) (see Figure 25-3, *C*). Stimulation of basophils also induces synthesis of vasoactive lipid molecules (e.g., leukotrienes) and cytokines.[5] Basophils are a particularly rich source of the cytokine interleukin-4 (IL-4), which preferentially guides B-cell differentiation toward plasma cells that secrete IgE (see Chapter 7).

The precise function of basophils is poorly understood, but numbers of basophils are often increased at sites of allergic inflammatory reactions and parasitic infection, particularly

exoparasites (e.g., ticks). IgE receptors on the basophil would induce degranulation at sites of IgE-mediated hypersensitivity reactions and contribute to the local inflammatory response.

Mast cells are highly similar to basophils, but are generated from a different set of precursor cells in the bone marrow, from which they migrate in an immature form into tissues.[5] They reside in vascularized connective tissues just beneath body epithelial surfaces, including the submucosal tissues of the gastrointestinal and respiratory tracts and the dermal layer that lies just below the surface of the skin. Mast cells play a central role in inflammation, and their activation and degranulation affects a great number of cells, including those involved in inflammation (e.g., vascular endothelial cells, smooth muscle cells, circulating platelets and leukocytes, nerves) and healing (e.g., fibroblasts), as well as glandular cells and cells of the immune system. Their activation contributes greatly to increased permeability of blood vessels and smooth muscle contraction (see Figure 6-8).

Agranulocytes. The **agranulocytes**—monocytes, macrophages, and lymphocytes—differ from the granulocytes in that they contain relatively fewer granules in their cytoplasm. The lymphocytes do not contain any enzyme-filled digestive vacuoles, and the digestive vacuoles of the monocytes and macrophages are larger and fewer than those of the granulocytes.

Lymphocytes constitute approximately 36% of the total leukocyte count and are the primary cells of the immune response (see Figure 25-3, *E* and Chapter 7). Most lymphocytes transiently circulate in the blood and eventually reside in secondary lymphoid tissues as mature T cells, B cells, or plasma cells. The life span of the lymphocyte can be days, months, or years, depending on its type and subtype. (Lymphocyte function and dysfunction are described in detail in Unit III.)

Natural killer (NK) cells, which resemble large granular lymphocytes, kill some types of tumor cells (in vitro) and some virus-infected cells without being induced by previous exposure to these antigens (see Chapters 6 and 7). Hence they are named *natural killer cells* to differentiate them from T cytotoxic cells, which are induced by antigen. NK cells also have the capacity to activate T cells and phagocytes and produce a variety of cytokines that can regulate immune responses. The predominant form of NK cells develops in the bone marrow and circulates in the blood, where it accounts for 5% to 10% of the circulating lymphoid pool, and is found mainly in the peripheral blood and spleen. NK cells develop independent of a thymus, although some NK precursors are found in the thymus and may develop into NKT cells that have markers of NK and T cells.

The monocytes and macrophages make up the **mononuclear phagocyte system (MPS),** formerly called the *reticuloendothelial system (RES).*[6] Monocytes and macrophages are active phagocytes that participate in the immune and inflammatory responses. They also ingest dead or defective host cells, particularly blood cells.

Monocytes are the largest normal blood cell and have a horseshoe-shaped nucleus (see Figure 25-3, *D*). They are formed and released by the bone marrow into the bloodstream. Monocytes migrate into a variety of tissues and fully mature into tissue **macrophages** and myeloid **dendritic cells** (Table 25-3). Other monocytes may mature into macrophages in the circulation and migrate out of the vessels in response to infection or inflammation. Macrophages are generally larger and are more active as phagocytes than monocytes. Dendritic cells frequently extend projections *(dendrites)* into the tissue and take on a "neuron-like" appearance. The origin and turnover of many of the tissue macrophages are not precisely known. It seems clear that once monocytes leave the circulation, they do not return. They can survive many months or even years.

The normal role of macrophages is to remove old and damaged cells and large-molecular substances from the blood. Cellular targets of macrophage phagocytosis include circulating senescent or damaged erythrocytes and platelets (removed primarily in spleen), dead neutrophils (in the circulation and at sites of inflammation), and cells undergoing apoptosis. Noncellular targets include antigen-antibody complexes, cellular debris, products of coagulation, and macromolecules (such as lipids and carbohydrates synthesized by the body as the result of faulty metabolism, as in storage diseases). Macrophages remove and kill contaminating microorganisms in the blood (mostly in the liver and spleen) and at sites of infection. Macrophages and, particularly, dendritic cells are the major "antigen-processing" and "antigen-presenting" cells that initiate immune responses (see Chapter 7). Macrophages initiate wound healing and tissue remodeling and if activated by cytokines from T cells secrete a large array of biologically active chemicals that if uncontrolled result in chronic inflammation and tissue injury (see Chapter 6). Osteoclasts are multinucleated cells specialized for the function of lacunar bone resorptions and remodeling in addition to phagocytosis.

Table 25-3	Mononuclear Phagocyte System*
Name of Cell	**Location**
Committed Stem Cells[†]	Bone marrow
Monoblasts	Bone marrow
Promonoblasts	Bone marrow
Monocytes	Bone marrow and peripheral blood
Macrophages	Tissue
Kupffer cells	Liver macrophages
Alveolar macrophages	Lung
Histiocytes	Connective tissue
Macrophages	Bone marrow
Fixed and free macrophages	Spleen and lymph nodes
Pleural and peritoneal macrophages	Serous cavities
Adipose macrophages	Adipose (fat) tissue
Microglial cells	Nervous system
Mesangial cells	Kidney
Osteoclasts	Bone
Langerhans cells	Skin
Dendritic cells	Lymphoid tissue, lining of respiratory and gastrointestinal tracts

Modified from Kumar V et al: *Robbins and Cotran pathologic basis of disease,* ed 7, Philadelphia, 2005, Saunders.
*Formerly called the reticuloendothelial system.
†Development of blood cells from stem cells in the marrow is described on this page and illustrated in Figure 25-9.

Platelets

Platelets (thrombocytes) are not true cells but disk-shaped cytoplasmic fragments that are essential for blood coagulation and control of bleeding. They are formed by fragmentation of very large (40 to 100 μm in diameter) cells known as **megakaryocytes** (Figure 25-4). They lack a nucleus, have no deoxyribonucleic acid (DNA), and are incapable of mitotic division. They do, however, contain cytoplasmic granules (i.e., dense granules, alpha granules) capable of releasing biochemical mediators (e.g., adenosine diphosphate [ADP], adenosine triphosphate [ATP], calcium, serotonin from dense granules; coagulation factors, platelet-derived growth factor [PDGF], platelet factor 4 from alpha granules) when stimulated by injury to a blood vessel. Activation also stimulates synthesis of arachidonic acid pathway products (e.g., thromboxane-A_2) (see Chapter 6).

There are approximately 140,000 to 340,000 platelets/mm³ of circulating blood. An additional one third of the body's available platelets are in a reserve pool in the spleen. A platelet circulates for approximately 10 days, ages, and is removed by macrophages of the MPS, mostly in the spleen.

Lymphoid Organs

The lymphoid system is closely integrated with the circulatory system. The lymphoid organs, some of which are merely aggregations of lymphoid tissue, are classified as primary or

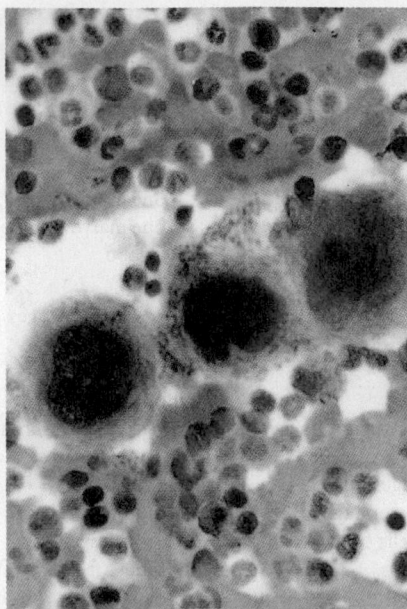

Figure 25-4 Megakaryocyte and platelets. Note the large number of platelets (purple) surrounding the large megakaryocytes in the center. (From Miale JB, *Laboratory medicine: hematology*, ed 6, St Louis, 1982, Mosby.)

secondary. The primary lymphoid organs are the thymus and the bone marrow. The secondary lymphoid organs consist of the spleen, lymph nodes, tonsils, and Peyer patches of the small intestine (see Figure 7-3). All of the lymphoid organs link the hematologic and immune systems in that they are sites of residence, proliferation, differentiation, or function of lymphocytes and mononuclear phagocytes (monocytes and macrophages). (The liver, which also has hematologic functions, is primarily a digestive organ and is described in Chapter 38.)

Spleen

The spleen is the largest of the secondary lymphoid organs. It is a site of fetal hematopoiesis; its mononuclear phagocytes filter and cleanse the blood; its lymphocytes mount an immune response to blood-borne microorganisms; and it serves as a blood reservoir (see Chapter 27).

The spleen is a concave, encapsulated organ that weighs about 150 g and is about the size of a fist. It is located in the left upper abdominal cavity, curved around a portion of the stomach (see Figure 7-3). Strands of connective tissue (trabeculae) extend from the capsule, dividing the spleen into compartments (Figure 25-5). The compartments contain masses of lymphoid tissue called *splenic pulp*. The spleen is interlaced with many blood vessels, some of which are capable of distending to store blood. Blood that circulates through the spleen comes from the splenic artery, which branches from the descending aorta and reenters the circulatory system through the splenic vein and into the portal vein.

The portion of arterial blood that enters the spleen first encounters the white splenic pulp, which consists of masses of lymphoid tissue containing macrophages and lymphocytes, primarily T lymphocytes in proximity to the arterioles (see Figure 25-5, *B* and *E*). Cellular clumps (lymphoid follicles) are formed in the white pulp around the splenic arterioles. The lymphoid follicles consist primarily of B lymphocytes. These are the chief sites of immune function within the spleen. Here blood-borne antigens encounter lymphocytes, initiating the immune response and the conversion of lymphoid follicles into germinal centers (see Chapter 7).[7]

Some of the blood that enters the terminal capillaries continues through the microcirculation and enters highly distensible storage areas called venous sinuses in the red pulp of the spleen. The venous sinuses are capable of storing more than 300 ml of blood. Passive dilation of the venous sinuses enables the spleen to increase its storage capacity as needed by the body. Sudden reductions in blood pressure cause the sympathetic nervous system to stimulate constriction of the sinuses, resulting in expulsion of as much as 200 ml of blood into the venous circulation, which helps restore blood volume and increases the hematocrit by as much as 4%.

The endothelial lining of the venous sinuses is discontinuous (having gaps between endothelial cells) and therefore extremely permeable so that blood cells are allowed to exit the circulation (Figure 25-6). The red pulp contains a system of loosely interconnected resident macrophages that provide the principal site of splenic filtration. Because of the slow circulation in the sinuses, the macrophages easily phagocytose old, damaged, or dead blood cells of all kinds (but chiefly erythrocytes), microorganisms, macromolecules, and particles of debris. Hemoglobin from phagocytosed erythrocytes is catabolized, and heme (iron) is stored in the cytoplasm of the macrophages or released back into the blood (see Figure 25-16). The macrophages also can remove particulate inclusions containing denatured hemoglobin (Heinz bodies) from erythrocytes without harming the cells themselves. Blood that filters through the red pulp also finds its way into the venous sinuses and hence into the portal circulation.

The spleen is not absolutely necessary for life or for adequate hematologic function. However, splenic absence from any cause (atrophy, traumatic injury, or removal because of disease) has several secondary effects on the body. For example, leukocytosis (high levels of circulating leukocytes) often occurs after splenectomy, suggesting that the spleen exerts some control over the rate of proliferation of leukocyte stem cells in the bone marrow or their release into the bloodstream. Circulating levels of iron may also decrease, reflecting the spleen's role in the iron cycle. The immune response to encapsulated bacteria (e.g., *Streptococcus pneumoniae* [pneumococcus], *Neisseria meningitidis* [meningococcus], *Haemophilus influenzae*), which is primarily an IgM response, may be severely diminished resulting in increased susceptibility to disseminated infections. Loss of the spleen results in an increase in morphologically defective blood cells in the circulation, confirming the spleen's role in removing old or damaged cells.

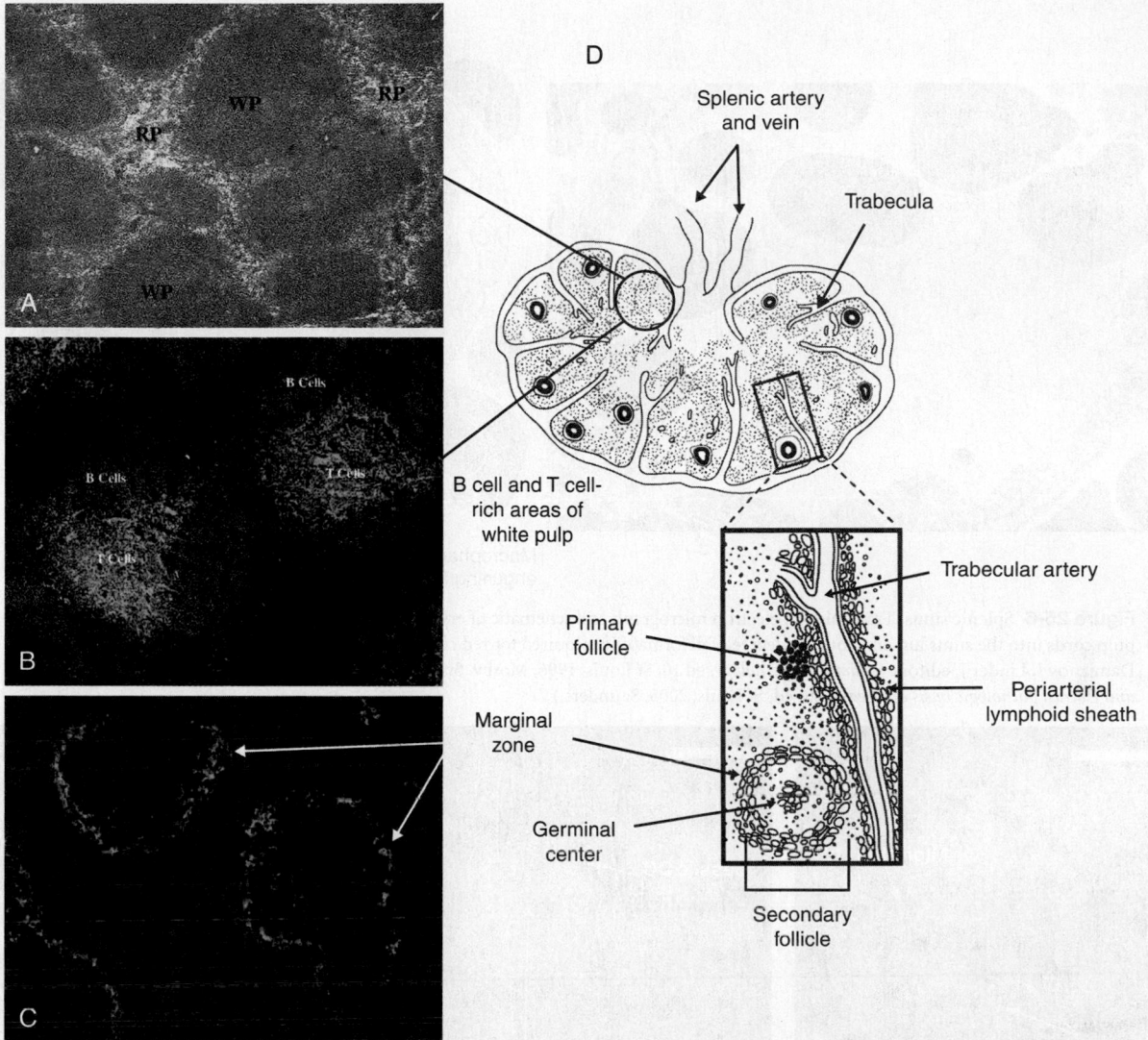

Figure 25-5 Spleen architecture. **A,** Spleen section stained with hematoxylin and eosin shows areas of densely packed cells, referred to as the *white pulp* (WP), separated by areas with more dispersed cell populations, referred to as the *red pulp* (RP). **B,** Spleen section that has been stained with fluorescently labeled antibodies specific for B cells *(orange)* and T cells *(green)* shows the distinct localization of B cells and T cells within the white pulp. **C,** Staining for macrophages *(orange)* and the splenic marginal zone *(green)* shows the density of macrophages and phagocytic cells in the red pulp and marginal zone. **D,** The spleen is enclosed in a capsule with the interior pulp divided into compartments by strands of connective tissue (trabeculae). The splenic pulp contains regions that are rich in lymphocytes (white pulp) and those containing erythrocytes (red pulp). Arteries residing near the trabeculae (tubercular arteries) are frequently surrounded by a periarterial lymphoid sheath, primarily containing T cells and macrophages, with adjacent lymphoid follicles. (A, B, and C from Mandell G, Bennett J, Dolin R: *Principles and practice of infectious diseases,* ed 6, Philadelphia, 2005, Churchill Livingstone; D from Hoffman R et al: *Hematology: basic principles and practice,* ed 4, Philadelphia, 2005, Churchill Livingstone.)

Lymph Nodes

Structurally, lymph nodes are part of the lymphatic system. Lymphatic vessels collect interstitial fluid from the tissues and transport it, as lymph, through vessels of increasing size to the thoracic duct, which drains into the superior vena cava returning the lymph to the circulation. Lymph nodes are distributed throughout the body and provide filtration of the lymph during its journey through the lymphatics. Each lymph node is enclosed in a fibrous capsule, branches of which (trabeculae) extend inward to partition the node into several compartments (Figure 25-7). Reticular fibers of connective tissue divide the compartments into a meshwork throughout the lymph node. The node consists of outer (cortex) and inner (paracortex) cortical areas and an inner medulla. Lymph enters through multiple small afferent lymphatic vessels into the subcapsular sinus, just beneath the capsule, drains into the cortical sinuses to the medullary sinuses, from which the lymph is collected and leaves the node by way of the efferent lymphatic vessel. Blood flows into the lymph nodes through the lymphatic artery, which ends in groups of postcapillary venules disturbed throughout the outer cortex. The blood is drained through the lymphatic vein.

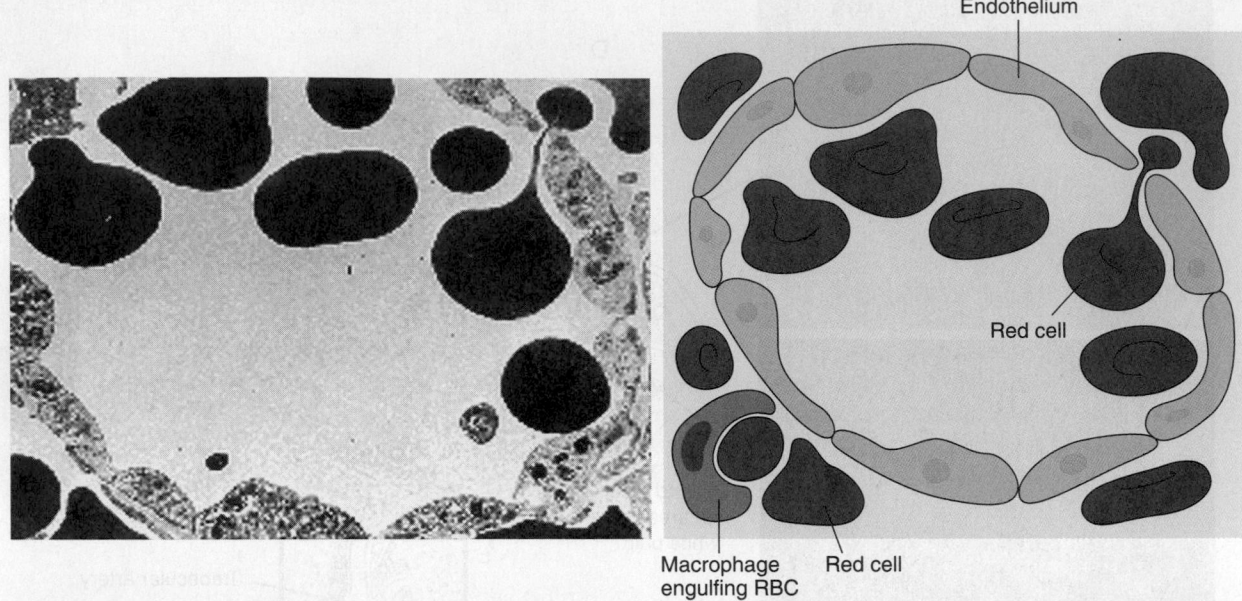

Figure 25-6 Splenic sinus. Transmission electron micrograph and schematic of erythrocytes in the process of squeezing from the red pulp cords into the sinus lumen. Note the degree of deformability required for red cells to pass through the wall of the sinus. (From Damjanov I, Linder J, editors: *Anderson's pathology,* ed 10, St Louis, 1996, Mosby. Schematic from Kumar V, Fausto N, Abbas A: *Robbins and Cotran pathologic basis of disease,* 7th ed, St Louis, 2005, Saunders.)

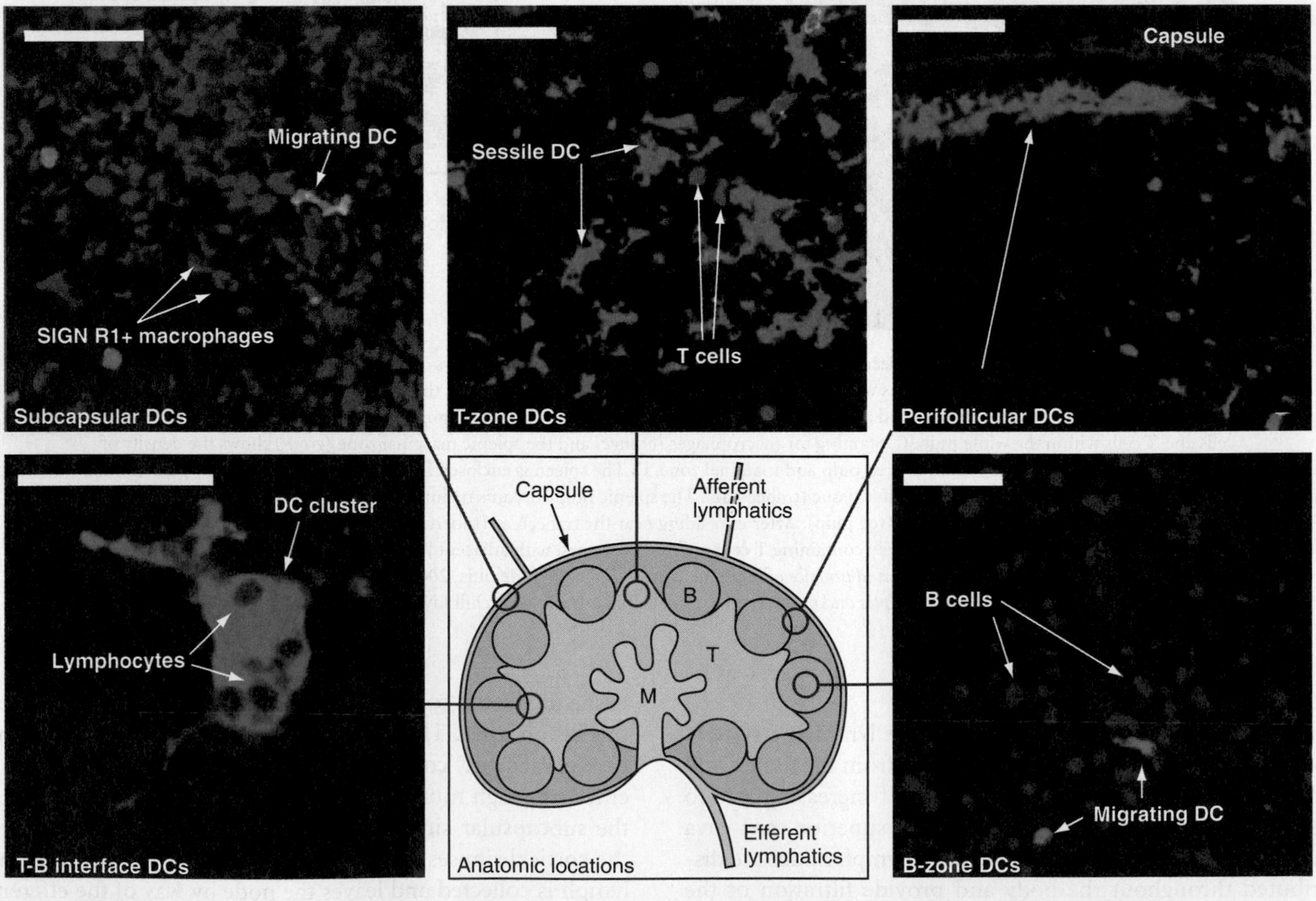

Figure 25-7 Lymph node architecture. *Drawing in lower center:* Lymph enters via the afferent lymphatics and exits via the efferent lymphatics. T cells enter the lymph nodes via the high endothelial venules and exit via medulla to the efferent lymphatics. *B,* B-cell follicles; *M,* medullary cords; *T,* T-cell zone. Other structures are labeled. Stained microscopic images: all images are linked to the drawing of the lymph node. *DC,* Dendritic cell. (All scale bars 50 µm.) (From Lindquist RL et al: *Nat Immunol* 5:1243-1250, 2004 by permission from Macmillan Publishers Ltd.)

Functionally, however, lymph nodes are part of the hematologic and immune systems and are the primary site for the first encounter between antigen and lymphocytes. Lymphocytes enter the lymph node from the blood through the postcapillary venules by means of diapedesis across the endothelial lining. B lymphocytes tend to migrate preferentially to nodes in the cortex and medulla, whereas T lymphocytes predominantly migrate to the paracortex (see Figure 25-7). Macrophages reside in the lymph node, help filter the lymph of debris, foreign substances, and microorganisms, and provide antigen-processing functions. The dendritic cells encounter and process antigens and microorganisms in other tissues, enter the lymph node through the afferent lymph vessels, and migrate throughout the nodes. The reticular network provides adhesive surfaces for trapping large numbers of phagocytes and lymphocytes and facilitating their organization into follicles or primary nodules.[8] The presence of antigen, either removed from the lymph by macrophages or presented on the surface of dendritic cells, results in the production of secondary nodules containing germinal centers. In the germinal centers lymphocytes, particularly B cells, respond to antigenic stimulation by undergoing proliferation and further differentiation, including class-switch, into memory cells and plasma cells (see Chapter 7). Plasma cells migrate to the medullary cords. The B lymphocyte proliferation in response to a great deal of antigen (e.g., during infection) may result in lymph node enlargement and tenderness (reactive lymph node).

DEVELOPMENT OF BLOOD CELLS

Hematopoiesis

The typical human requires about 100 billion new blood cells per day. Blood cell production, termed **hematopoiesis**, is constantly ongoing, occurring in the liver and spleen of the fetus and only in bone marrow (*medullary hematopoiesis*) after birth (see Chapter 28). This process involves the biochemical stimulation of populations of relatively undifferentiated cells to undergo mitotic division (i.e., proliferation) and maturation (i.e., differentiation) into mature hematologic cells (Table 25-4). Although proliferation and differentiation are usually sequential, certain blood cells proliferate and differentiate simultaneously. Erythrocytes and granulocytes generally differentiate fully before entering the blood, but monocytes and lymphocytes continue to mature in the blood and in secondary lymphatic organs.

Hematopoiesis continues throughout life, increasing in response to a need to replenish destroyed circulating cells (e.g., during hemorrhage, hemolytic anemia [peripheral destruction of erythrocytes], consumptive thrombocytopenia) or in response to infection. In general, long-term stimuli, such as chronic diseases, cause a greater increase in hematopoiesis than acute conditions, such as hemorrhage.

Table 25-4	Human Hematopoietic Growth Factors (cytokines, colony-stimulating factors)	
Factor	**Cell Origin**	**Primary Cell Stimulated**
M-CSF	Macrophage, lymphocyte, fibroblast, endothelial cell, osteoblast	Monocyte progenitor to monocyte
GM-CSF	Macrophage, T cell, endothelial cell, fibroblast, mast cell	Common myeloid progenitor to granulocyte progenitor and monocyte progenitor
G-CSF	Macrophage, fibroblast, endothelial cell	Granulocyte progenitor to neutrophil
IL-2	Th cell	T-cell progenitor to T cell
IL-3	T cell, monocyte/macrophage, stromal cell	Common myeloid progenitor to progenitors for megakaryocyte, erythroid, granulocyte, and monocyte series
IL-4	Th cell	B-cell progenitor to B cell
IL-5	Th cell, mast cell	Common myeloid progenitor to eosinophil
IL-7	Stromal cell, intestinal epithelium	Hematopoietic stem cell to common lymphoid progenitor
		Common lymphoid progenitor to pro B cell, pro NK cell, and pro T cell
		Pro T cell to T cell and pro B cell to B cell
IL-11	Stromal cell	Megakaryocyte progenitor to megakaryocyte
IL-15	Monocyte/macrophage	NK progenitor to NK cell
Erythropoietin	Peritubular kidney cell and Kupffer cell	Common myeloid progenitor to erythrocyte progenitor; Erythrocyte progenitor to erythrocyte
Thrombopoietin	Liver, kidney, skeletal muscle	All cells in megakaryocyte lineage from common myeloid progenitor to platelet
Stem cell factor (steel factor)	Stromal cell in bone marrow and many other cells	Hematopoietic progenitor to common myeloid progenitor
		Common myeloid progenitor to progenitors for megakaryocyte, erythroid, granulocyte, and monocyte series

G-CSF, Granulocyte colony-stimulating factor; *GM-CSF,* granulocyte-macrophage colony-stimulating factor; *IL,* interleukin; *M-CSF,* macrophage colony-stimulating factor; *NK,* natural killer; *Th,* T helper.

Various abnormalities in medullary hematopoiesis have been identified and is discussed in Chapter 26. Extramedullary hematopoiesis—blood cell production in tissues other than bone marrow—of apparently normal blood cells has been reported in the spleen, liver, and, less frequently, lymph nodes, adrenal glands, cartilage, adipose tissue, intrathoracic areas, and kidneys. In adults, however, extramedullary hematopoiesis is usually a sign of disease, occurring in pernicious anemia, sickle cell anemia, thalassemia, hemolytic disease of the newborn (erythroblastosis fetalis), hereditary spherocytosis, and certain leukemias.

Bone Marrow

Bone marrow is confined to the cavities of bone and is the primary site of residence of hematopoietic stem cells (Figure 25-8). Adults have two kinds of bone marrow: red, or active

(hematopoietic), marrow (also called **myeloid tissue**) and yellow, or inactive, marrow. The large quantity of fat in inactive marrow gives its characteristic yellow color. Not all bones contain active marrow. In adults, active marrow is found primarily in the flat bones of the pelvis (34%), vertebrae (28%), cranium and mandible (13%), sternum and ribs (10%), and in the extreme proximal portions of the humerus and femur (4% to 8%). Inactive marrow predominates in cavities of other bones. (Bones are discussed further in Chapter 41.)

Hematopoietic marrow is vascularized by the primary arteries of the bones, which terminate in a capillary network forming large venous sinuses. Hematopoietic marrow and fat fill the spaces surrounding the network of venous sinuses. Newly produced blood cells traverse narrow openings between endothelial cells in the venous sinus walls and thus

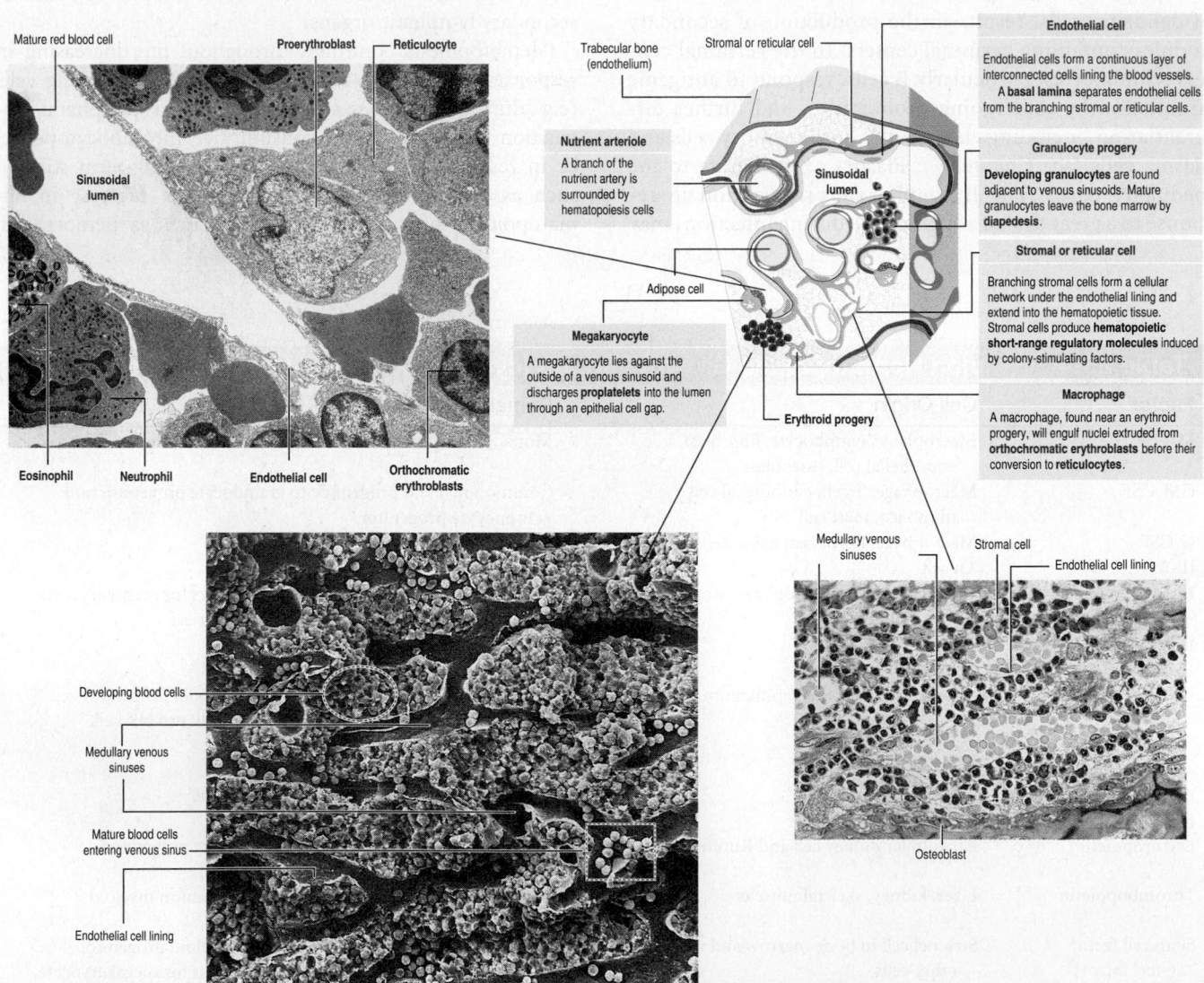

Figure 25-8 Bone marrow: structure and vascularization. (From Kierszenbaum A: *Histology and cell biology: an introduction to pathology*, 2nd ed, Philadelphia, 2006, Mosby. Scanning electron micrograph from Kessel RG, Kardon RH: *Tissues and organs*, New York, WH Freeman, 1979.)

enter the circulation. Normally, immature cells have not developed the appropriate surface receptors to interact with the endothelium and enter the circulation.

The stromal compartment of the bone marrow contains a variety of cell types, including **mesenchymal stem cells**, macrophages/osteoclasts, and endothelial-like cells.[9] The mesenchymal stem cells can differentiate into fibroblasts, osteoblasts, or adipocytes. Bone marrow fibroblasts secrete a large variety of cytokines (e.g., macrophage colony-stimulating factor [M-CSF], granulocyte-macrophage colony-stimulating factor [GM-CSF], IL-6) that are necessary for hematopoiesis (see Table 25-4). Osteoblasts are responsible for the formation of new bone.[10] Additionally, osteoclasts secrete cytokines that drive hematopoietic cell differentiation. Adipocytes are fat cells containing large depositions of lipid. Adipocytes secrete several growth factors, as well as leptin. Leptin preferentially stimulates mesenchymal stem cells to differentiate into osteoblasts.

Macrophages and osteoclasts have common monocytic precursors. Bone marrow macrophages secrete cytokines and chemokines that regulate proliferation of hematopoietic progenitor cells. Other monocytic cells differentiate under the direction of stromal cells and osteoblasts and undergo intercellular fusion into large multinucleate osteoclasts. Osteoclasts remodel bone by resorption and can produce cytokines that affect proliferation of hematopoietic cells.

The hematologic compartment of the bone marrow consists of a variety of cellular niches that favor differentiation of various hematopoietic progenitor cells.[11] The niches are distinguished by a variety of locally produced cytokines and growth factors, so that one niche may be more likely to support differentiation of erythroid precursors into erythrocytes, whereas granulocytes may differentiate in a different site.

Cell Differentiation

Each type of blood cell originates from common **hematopoietic stem cells** that proliferate and differentiate under control of a variety of cytokines and growth factors (Figure 25-9 and see Table 25-4). During this process some hematopoietic stem cells undergo different paths of differentiation into more differentiated stem cells that are committed to a particular line of blood cells.

All humans originate from a single cell (the fertilized egg) that has the capacity to proliferate and eventually differentiate into the huge diversity of cells of the human body. After fertilization, the egg divides over a 5-day period to form a hollow ball (blastocyst) that implants on the uterus. Until about 3 days after fertilization, each cell (blastomere) is undifferentiated and retains the capacity to differentiate into any cell type. In the 5-day blastocyst, the outer layer cells have undergone differentiation and commitment to become the placenta. Cells of the inner cell mass (*embryonic stem cells*), however, continue to have unlimited differentiation potential (currently referred to as being *pluripotent*) and can grow into different kinds of tissue—blood, nerves, heart, bone, and so forth. After implantation, cells of the inner cell mass begin

differentiation into other cell types. Differentiation is a multistep process and results in intermediate groups of stem cells (*multipotent stem cells*) with more limited, but still impressive, abilities to differentiate into many different types of cells (see Figure 25-9).[12]

The hematopoietic organs contain a population of hematopoietic stem cells that have partially differentiated.[13] They have the capacity to differentiate easily into any of the hematologic cell populations but are very difficult to differentiate into other cell types, like nerve or muscle cells.[12] The challenge of getting any partially committed multipotent stem cells to differentiate reliably involves coaxing them with identical chemical signals that the body uses naturally for differentiation. This is a daunting task with potentially astonishing clinical implications. For example, bone marrow might become the reservoir from which stem cells are harvested and then stimulated to produce nerve cells to help with the treatments of spinal cord injuries.

As with all stem cells, the hematopoietic stem cells are self-renewing (they have the ability to proliferate without further differentiation) so that a relatively constant population of stem cells is available.[12] Some hematopoietic stem cells will continue differentiation into hematopoietic progenitor cells. Progenitor cells retain proliferative capacity but are committed to possible further differentiation into particular types of hematologic cells: lymphoid (lymphocytes, NK cells), granulocyte-monocyte (granulocytes, monocytes, macrophages), and megakaryocyte-erythroid (platelets, erythrocytes) progenitor cells (see Figure 25-9).

As with all other forms of cellular differentiation, successful hematopoiesis requires that progenitor cells interact with neighboring cells (e.g., **stromal cells** of the bone marrow) through a variety of adhesion molecules and are exposed to particular signaling molecules (e.g., cytokines) (see Table 25-4).[14] Stromal cells apparently express **steel factor**, a stem cell factor, which activates stem cells to develop. Several cytokines participate in hematopoiesis, particularly **colony-stimulating factors** (**CSFs** or **hematopoietic growth factors**), which stimulate the proliferation of progenitor cells and their progeny and initiate the maturation events necessary to produce fully mature cells (see Figure 25-9).[15] Multiple cell types in the hematopoietic organs, including endothelial cells, fibroblasts, and lymphocytes, produce CSFs.

Hematopoiesis in the bone marrow occurs in two separate pools, the stem cell pool and the bone marrow pool (Figure 25-10). The stem cell pool is responsible for maintaining the number of pluripotent stem cells and partially committed progenitor cells. The bone marrow pool contains cells that are proliferating and maturing in preparation for release into the circulation and mature cells that are stored for later release into the peripheral blood. The peripheral blood also contains two pools of cells; those in the circulation and those stored around the walls of the blood vessels (often called the **marginating storage pool**). The marginating storage pool primarily consists of neutrophils

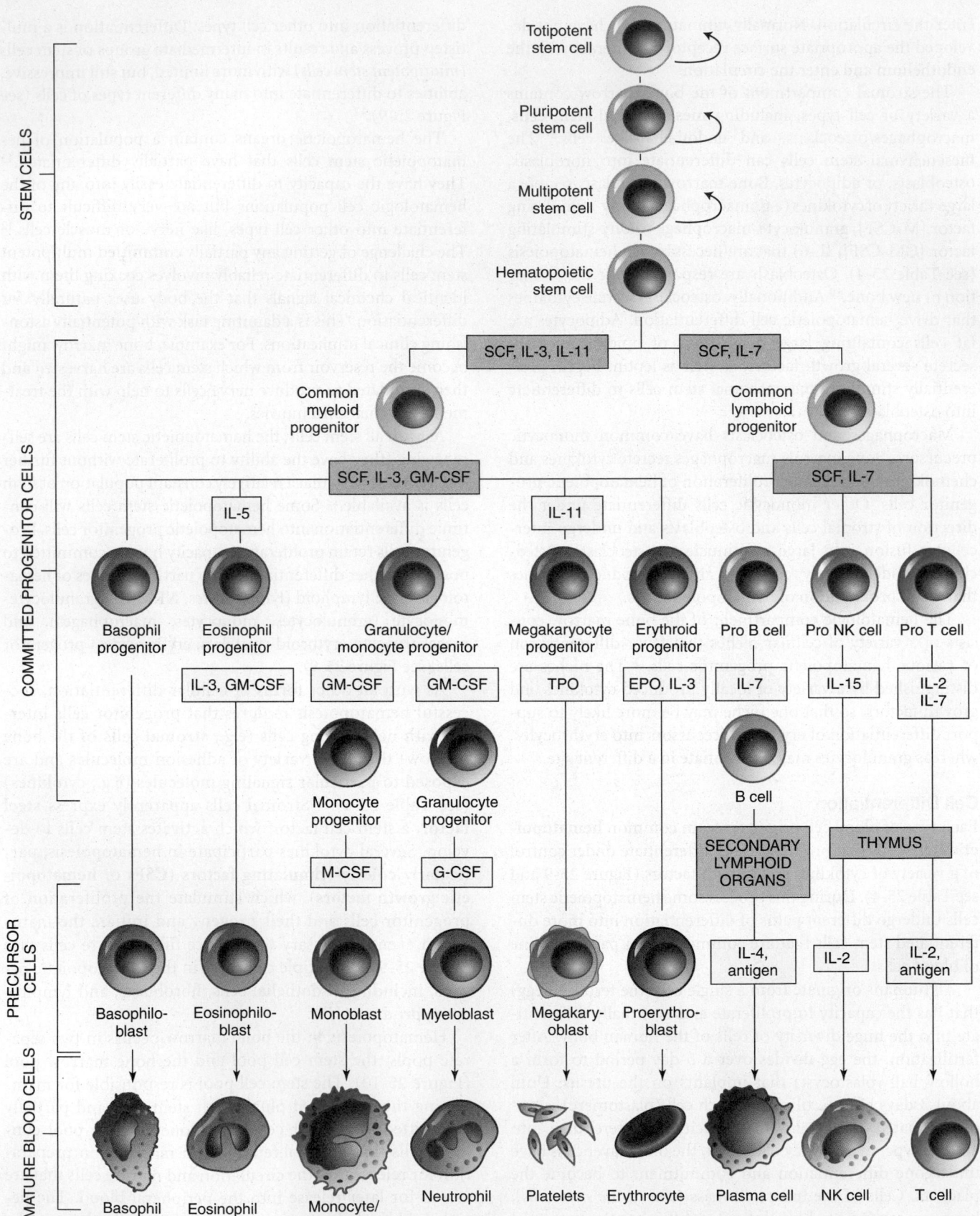

Figure 25-9 **Differentiation of hematopoietic cells.** Curved arrows indicate proliferation and expansion of pre-hematopoietic stem cell populations. *EPO,* erythropoietin; *G-CSF,* granulocyte colony-stimulating factor; *GM-CSF,* granulocyte-macrophage colony-stimulating factor; *IL,* interleukin; *M-CSF,* macrophage colony-stimulating factor; *NK,* natural killer; *SCF,* stem cell factor; *TPO,* thrombopoietin.

that adhere to the endothelium in vessels where the blood flow is relatively slow. These cells can rapidly move into tissues and mucous membranes when needed in an inflammatory response. The infiltrating cells are replenished from the circulating pool.

Under certain conditions of rapid depletion of the circulating pool, the circulating hematologic cells need to be rapidly replenished. Medullary hematopoiesis can be accelerated by any or all of three mechanisms: (1) conversion of yellow bone marrow, which does not produce blood cells, to hematopoietic red marrow by the actions of **erythropoietin** (a hormone that stimulates erythrocyte production); (2) faster differentiation of progenitor cells; and (3) faster proliferation of stem cells into progenitor cells (see Table 25-4).

Clinical Uses of Colony-Stimulating Factors

Neutrophils are normally present in the blood in the range of 4000 to 6000 cells/μL, and in response to a bacterial infection, numbers usually increase to 10,000 to 20,000 cells/μL. Susceptibility to infection develops when normal levels drop below 1000 cells/μL, such as during congenital neutropenia or as a consequence of cytotoxic therapy for cancer. Similarly normal levels of other hematologic cells may be suppressed, e.g., congenital or acquired immune deficiencies and anemia (see Chapters 8 and 9).

The numbers of circulating hematologic cells are under the control of CSFs (see Table 25-4). Administration of CSFs can raise white cell numbers to extremely high levels in healthy individuals. These excessive levels of white blood

cells may result in production of toxic products and tissue damage. Therapy with CSFs has been tested in individuals with subnormal levels of circulating blood cells, such as acquired immunodeficiency syndrome (AIDS), aplastic anemia, or congenital neutropenia or as a consequence of cytotoxic therapy lymphoma or leukemia (Figure 25-11). CSF therapy can stimulate increases in circulating granulocyte-monocyte populations, but the degree of response depends on the available numbers of stem and progenitor cells that have survived chemotherapy or the effects of disease. CSF treatment has corrected some cases of congenital neutropenia and resulted in reconstitution of hematopoiesis after bone marrow transplantation.[16] CSF treatment can result in shorter periods of intensive nursing and hospitalization. Recombinant CSFs (e.g., granulocyte colony-stimulating factor [G-CSF], GM-CSF, erythropoietin) are being mass-produced for therapeutic use.

Development of Erythrocytes

For almost 100 years it was believed that erythrocytes developed from lymphocytes that were transformed in the spleen. It was not until the 1850s that the bone marrow was identified as the site of **erythropoiesis,** or development of red blood cells.

Erythropoiesis

In the confines of the bone marrow erythroid progenitor cells proliferate and differentiate into large, nucleated **proerythroblasts,** which are committed into producing cells of the

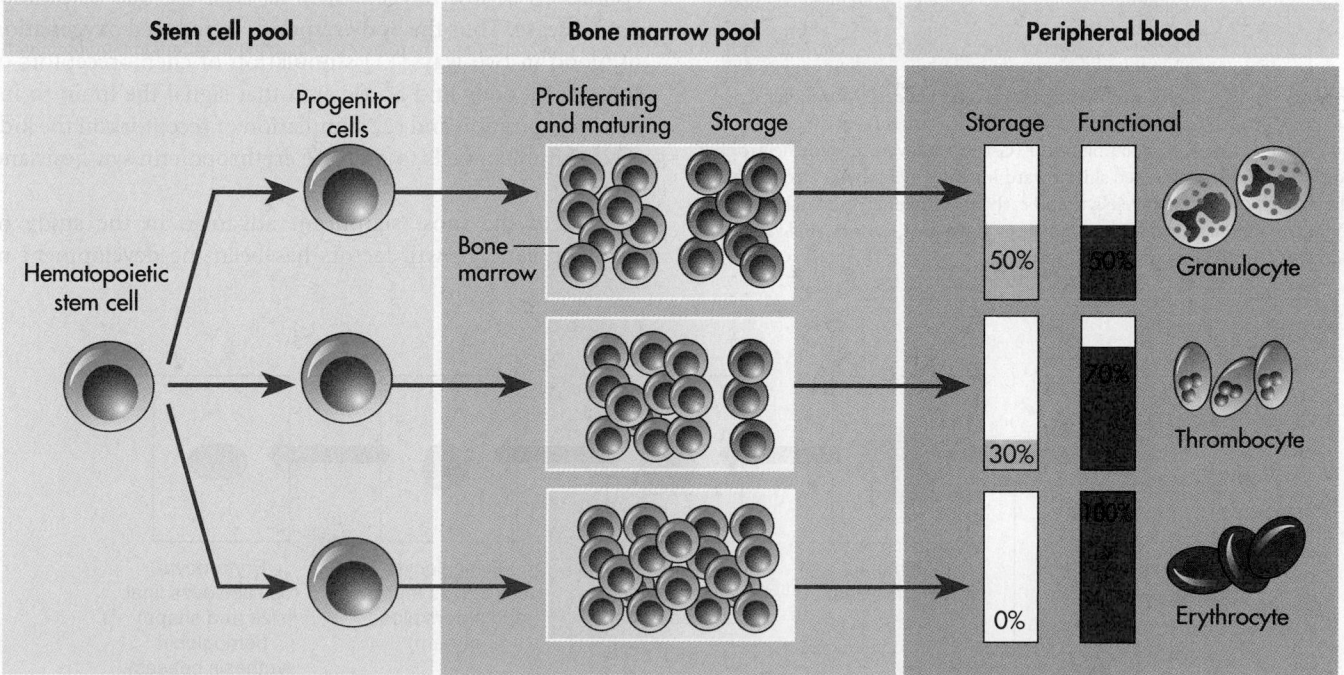

Figure 25-10 Hematopoiesis. Hematopoiesis from the stem cell pool; activity mainly in the bone marrow and in the peripheral blood. (Modified from Harmening DM, editor: *Clinical hematology and fundamentals of hemostasis,* ed 3, Philadelphia, 1997, FA Davis.)

erythroid series (Figure 25-12). Erythroid development from the proerythroblast onward is contained in a compartment referred to as the *erythron*.[17] The proerythroblast, which has ribosomes and can produce protein, differentiates through several intermediate forms of **erythroblast** while synthesizing hemoglobin and progressively eliminating most intracellular structures, including the nucleus. Thus the maturing erythroblast becomes more compact and progressively assumes the shape and characteristics of an erythrocyte. Hemoglobin is readily apparent and increases in quantity as nuclear size shrinks throughout the basophilic and polychromatophilic stages. The orthochromatic erythroblast (**normoblast**) is the smallest of the nucleated erythrocyte precursors.

The last immature form of erythroblast is the **reticulocyte**, which is anucleate and contains a meshlike (reticular) network of ribosomal ribonucleic acid (RNA) that is visible microscopically after staining with certain dyes. The

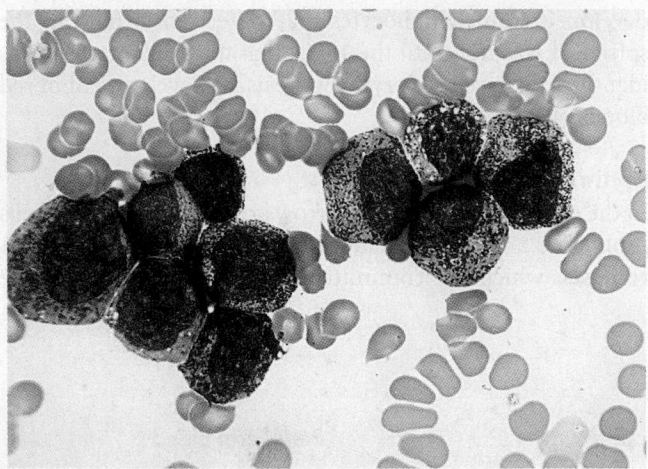

Figure 25-11 Colony-stimulating factor (CSF) effects. Morphologic effects of growth factor. Marrow aspirate from a patient receiving granulocyte colony-stimulating factor (G-CSF) showing an early neutrophil response. There is a marked shift toward immaturity in the neutrophils with the majority at the promyelocyte and early myelocyte stages of maturation (Wright-Giemsa stain). (From Damjanov I, Linder J, editors: *Anderson's pathology,* ed 10, St Louis, 1996, Mosby.)

reticulocyte contains polyribosomes (for globin synthesis) and mitochondria (for oxidative metabolism and heme synthesis). The reticulocyte matures into an erythrocyte within 24 to 48 hours. During this period, mitochondria and ribosomes disappear and the cell becomes smaller and more disk like. With these final changes, the erythrocyte loses its capacity for hemoglobin synthesis and oxidative metabolism. Reticulocytes remain in the marrow approximately 1 day and are released into the venous sinuses. They continue to mature in the bloodstream and may travel to the spleen for several days of additional maturation. The normal reticulocyte count is 1% of the total red blood cell count. Approximately 1% of the body's circulating erythrocyte mass normally is generated every 24 hours. Therefore, the reticulocyte count is a useful clinical index of erythropoietic activity and indicates whether new red cells are being produced.

Regulation of Erythropoiesis

In healthy individuals, the total volume of circulating erythrocytes remains surprisingly constant. Most steps of erythropoiesis are primarily under the control of a feedback loop involving the glycoprotein erythropoietin (see Table 25-4). In conditions of tissue hypoxia, erythropoietin is secreted by the liver and, primarily, by the peritubular cells of the kidney (Figure 25-13). Rising levels of circulating erythropoietin cause a compensatory increase in proliferation and differentiation of proerythroblasts in the bone marrow. The density of cellular erythropoietin receptor decreases progressively during erythroid maturation to almost undetectable levels on reticulocytes. The normal steady-state rate of production of approximately 2.5 million erythrocytes per second can increase to 17 million per second during anemia or under conditions of low oxygen, such as high-altitude or pulmonary disease. Thus the body responds to reduced oxygenation of blood in two ways: (1) stimulation of chemoreceptors of the carotid body and aortic arch that signal the brain to increase respiration and (2) stimulation of receptors on the kidney peritubular cells to increase erythropoietin synthesis and release.

One of the most significant advances in the study of hematopoietic growth factors has been the development of

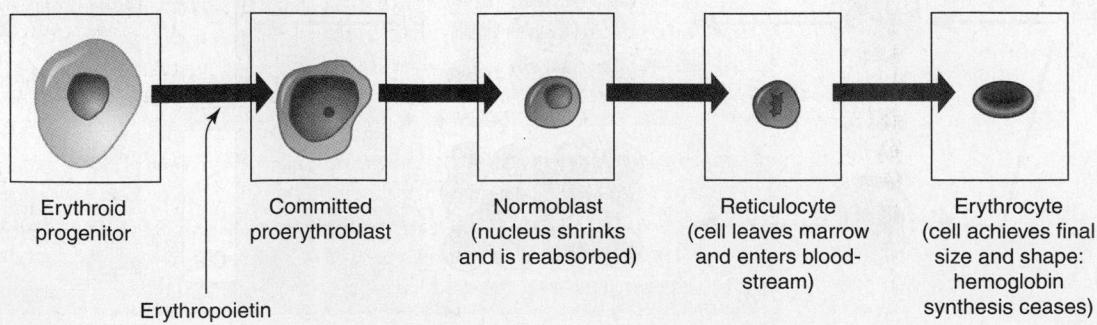

Figure 25-12 Erythrocyte differentiation. Erythrocyte differentiation from large nucleated progenitor cells to small nonnucleated erythrocytes.

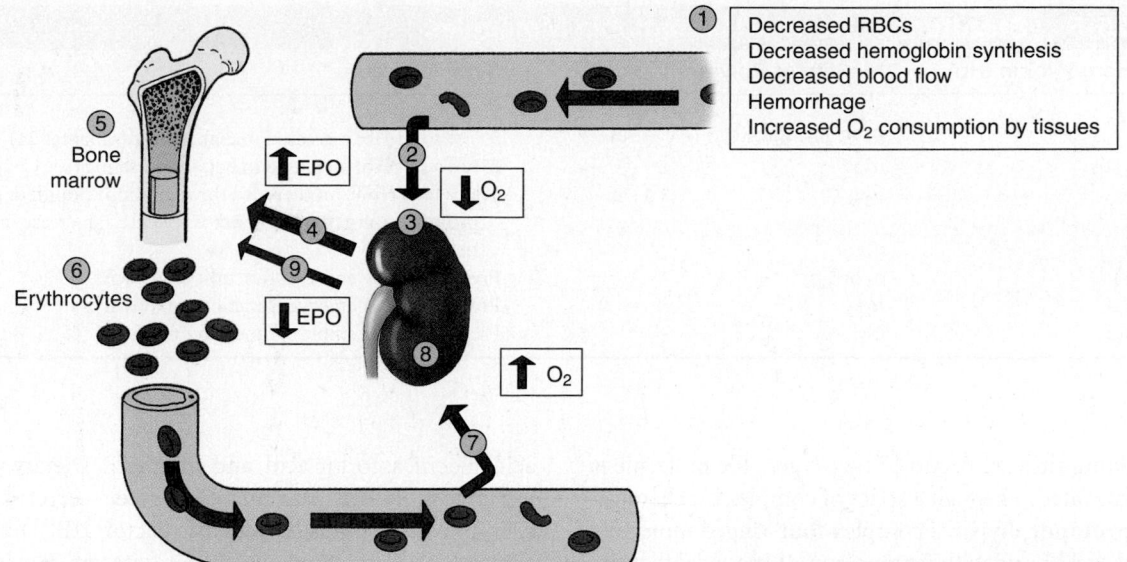

Figure 25-13 Role of erythropoietin in regulation of erythropoiesis. (1) Decreased arterial oxygen levels result in (2) decreased tissue oxygen (hypoxia) that (3) stimulates the kidney to increase (4) production of erythropoietin. Erythropoietin is carried to the bone marrow (5) and binds to erythropoietin receptors on proerythroblasts, resulting in increased red cell production and maturation and expansion of the erythron (6). The increased release of red cells into the circulation frequently corrects the hypoxia in the tissues (7). (8) Perception of normal oxygen levels by the kidney causes (9) diminished production of erythropoietin (negative feedback) and return to normal levels of erythrocyte production. *EPO,* Erythropoietin; O_2, oxygen in the blood and tissue; *RBCs,* red blood cells.

erythropoietin for use in individuals with chronic renal failure. In 1986 large amounts of recombinant human erythropoietin (r-HuEPO) became widely available for clinical research. Erythropoietin is administered intravenously or subcutaneously for the treatment of anemia caused by decreased production of erythropoietin. An immediate effect of increased endogenous or exogenous erythropoietin is an increase in the blood reticulocyte count, followed by increasing levels of erythrocytes. The most significant side effect associated with r-HuEPO is increased blood pressure.

Hemoglobin Synthesis

Hemoglobin (Hb), the oxygen-carrying protein of the erythrocyte, constitutes approximately 90% of the cell's dry weight. Hemoglobin-packed blood cells take up oxygen in the lungs and exchange it for carbon dioxide in the tissues. A single erythrocyte can contain as many as 300 hemoglobin molecules. Hemoglobin increases the oxygen carrying capacity of blood by 100-fold. Each hemoglobin molecule is composed of two pairs of polypeptide chains (the **globins**) and four colorful complexes of iron plus protoporphyrin (the hemes) (Figure 25-14).[18] Hemoglobin is responsible for blood's ruby-red color.

Several variants of hemoglobin exist, but they differ only slightly in primary structure based on the use of different polypeptide chains; alpha, beta, gamma, delta, epsilon, or zeta (α, β, γ, δ, ε, or ζ) (Table 25-5). Each polypeptide chain contains approximately 150 amino acids and is arranged in the knotted-sausage configuration shown in Figure 25-14. The chains assemble to form a tetrahedron containing two pairs of identical chains. Hemoglobin A, the most common type in

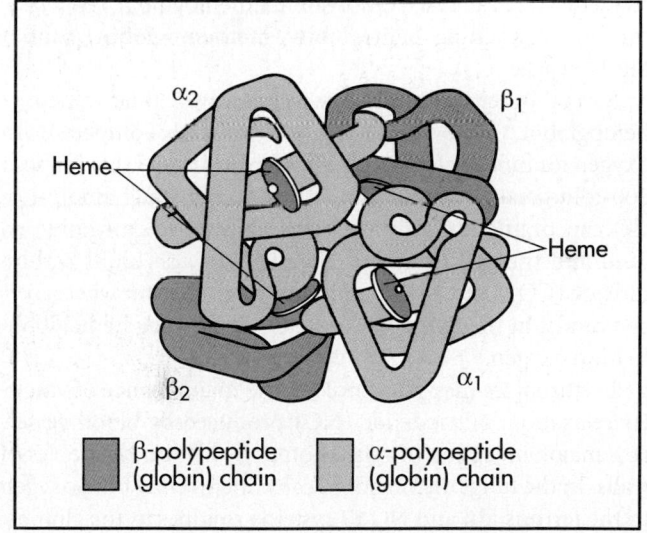

Figure 25-14 Molecular structure of hemoglobin. Molecule is a spherical tetramer weighing approximately 64,500 daltons. It contains a pair of α-polypeptide and a pair of β-polypeptide chains and several heme groups.

adults, is composed of two α- and two β-polypeptide chains ($\alpha 2\beta 2$). A normal variant, fetal hemoglobin (hemoglobin F) is a complex of two α- and two γ-polypeptide chains ($\alpha 2\gamma 2$) that binds oxygen with a much greater affinity than adult hemoglobin.

Heme is a large, flat, iron-protoporphyrin disk that is synthesized in the mitochondria and can carry one molecule of oxygen (O_2). Thus an individual hemoglobin molecule with its four hemes can carry four oxygen molecules. If all four

Table 25-5	Structure of Normal Hemoglobin Molecules	
Type of Hemoglobin (Hb)	Identity of Polypeptide Chain	Significance
HbA	$\alpha_2\beta_2$	92% of adult Hb
HbA$_{1c}$	α_2 (β-NH-glucose)	5% of adult Hb; increased in diabetes (see Chapter 21)
HbA$_2$	$\alpha_2\delta_2$	2% of adult Hb; increased in beta-thalassemia (see Chapter 28)
HbF	$\alpha_2\gamma_2$	Major fetal Hb from the third through ninth month of gestation; promotes oxygen transfer across platelets; increase in beta-thalassemia
Hb Gower I	ε_4 or $\zeta_2\varepsilon_2$	Present in early embryo; function unknown
Hb Gower II	$\alpha_2\varepsilon_2$	Present in early embryo; function unknown
Hb Portland	$\zeta_2\gamma_2$	Present in early embryo; function unknown

NH, amine.

oxygen-binding sites are occupied by oxygen, the molecule is said to be saturated. Through a series of complex biochemical reactions, **protoporphyrin,** a complex four-ringed molecule, is produced and bound with ferrous iron. It is crucial that the iron be correctly charged; reduced ferrous iron (Fe^{2+}) can bind oxygen in the lungs and release it in the tissues, where oxygen concentration is less, whereas ferric iron (Fe^{3+}) cannot. Binding of oxygen to ferrous iron (**oxyhemoglobin**) temporally oxidizes Fe^{2+} to Fe^{3+}, but after the release of oxygen the body reduces the iron to Fe^{2+} (**deoxyhemoglobin** [reduced hemoglobin]) and reactivates the hemoglobin's capacity to bind oxygen. Without reactivation by methemoglobin reductase, the Fe^{3+}-containing hemoglobin (**methemoglobin**) cannot bind oxygen.

Several other molecules can competitively bind to deoxyhemoglobin. Carbon monoxide (CO) directly competes with oxygen for binding to ferrous ion with an affinity that is about 200-fold greater than oxygen. Thus even a small amount of CO can dramatically decrease the ability of hemoglobin to bind and transport oxygen. Hemoglobin also binds carbon dioxide (CO_2), but at a binding site separate from where oxygen binds. In the lungs, CO_2 is released allowing hemoglobin to bind oxygen.

Erythrocytes may play a role in the maintenance of vascular relaxation. Nitric oxide (NO) produced by blood vessels is a major mediator of relaxation and dilation of the vessel walls. In the lungs, hemoglobin can concurrently bind oxygen to the ferrous ion and NO to cysteine residues in the globins. As hemoglobin transfers its oxygen to tissue, it may also shed small amounts of nitric oxide, contributing to dilation of the blood vessels and helping get the oxygen into tissues.

Nutritional Requirements for Erythropoiesis

Normal development of erythrocytes and synthesis of hemoglobin depends on an optimal biochemical milieu and adequate supplies of the necessary building blocks, including protein, vitamins, and minerals (Table 25-6). If these components are lacking for a prolonged time, erythrocyte production slows and anemia (insufficient numbers of functional erythrocytes) may result (see Chapter 26).

Erythropoiesis cannot proceed in the absence of vitamins, especially B$_{12}$, folate (folic acid), B$_6$, riboflavin, pantothenic

acid, niacin, ascorbic acid, and vitamin E. Dietary vitamin B$_{12}$ is a large molecule that requires a protein secreted by parietal cells into the stomach (intrinsic factor [IF]) for transport across the ileum. Once absorbed, vitamin B$_{12}$ is stored in the liver and used as needed in erythropoiesis. Defects in IF production lead to decreased B$_{12}$ absorption and pernicious anemia.

Folate is the second most important vitamin for erythrocyte production and maturation. Folate is necessary for DNA synthesis, being a component of three of the four DNA bases (thymine, adenine, and guanine), and RNA synthesis. Folate absorption occurs principally in the upper small intestine and is stored in the liver. Folate deficiency is more common than vitamin B$_{12}$ deficiency and occurs more rapidly. Folate stores can be depleted within a few months, whereas vitamin B$_{12}$ depletion can take years. Folate supplements are prescribed for pregnant women because pregnancy increases the demand for folate and may cause anemia.

Normal Destruction of Senescent Erythrocytes

After about 100 to 120 days in the circulation, old erythrocytes are removed by tissue macrophages, primarily in the spleen. Although mature erythrocytes lack nuclei, mitochondria, and endoplasmic reticulum, they do have cytoplasmic enzymes capable of glycolysis (anaerobic glucose metabolism) and production of small quantities of ATP, which provides the energy needed to maintain cell function and membrane pliability. Metabolic processes diminish as the erythrocyte ages, so less ATP is available to maintain plasma membrane function. The senescent red cell becomes increasingly fragile and loses its reversible deformability, becoming susceptible to rupture while passing through narrowed regions of the microcirculation.

Additionally, the plasma membrane of senescent red cells undergoes phospholipid rearrangement that is recognized by receptors on macrophages (primarily in the spleen) that selectively remove and sequester the red cells. If the spleen is dysfunctional or absent, macrophages in the liver (Kupffer cells) take over.

The erythrocytes are digested by proteolytic and lipolytic enzymes in the phagolysosomes (digestive vacuoles) of the macrophage. The heme and globin of methemoglobin

Table 25-6	Nutritional Requirements for Erythropoiesis	
Nutrient	**Role in Erythropoiesis**	**Consequence of Deficiency**
Protein (amino acids)	Structural component of plasma membrane	Decreased strength, elasticity, and flexibility of membrane; hemolytic anemia
	Synthesis of hemoglobin	Decreased erythropoiesis and life span of erythrocytes
Cobalamin (vitamin B_{12})	Synthesis of DNA, maturation of erythrocytes, facilitator of folate metabolism	Macrocytic (megaloblastic) anemia
Folate (folic acid)	Synthesis of DNA and RNA, maturation of erythrocytes	Macrocytic (megaloblastic) anemia
Vitamin B_6 (pyridoxine)	Heme synthesis	Microcytic-hypochromic anemia
Vitamin B_2 (riboflavin)	Oxidative reactions	Normocytic-normochromic anemia
Vitamin C (ascorbic acid)	Iron metabolism, acts as a reducing agent to maintain iron in its ferrous (Fe^{2+}) form	Normocytic-normochromic anemia
Pantothenic acid	Heme synthesis	Unknown in humans[*]
Niacin	None, but needed for respiration in mature erythrocytes	Unknown in humans
Vitamin E	Heme synthesis (?); protection against oxidative damage in mature erythrocytes	Hemolytic anemia with increased cell membrane fragility; shortens life span of erythrocytes in individuals with cystic fibrosis
Iron	Hemoglobin synthesis	Iron deficiency anemia
Copper	Required for optimal mobilization of iron from tissues to plasma	Microcytic-hypochromic anemia

Data from Strine-Martin EA, Lotspeich-Steininger CA, Koepke JA: *Clinical hematology: principles, procedures, correlations,* ed 2, Philadelphia, 1998, Lippincott.
[*]Although pantothenic acid is important for optimal synthesis of heme, experimentally induced deficiency *failed* to produce anemia or other hematopoietic disturbances.
DNA, Deoxyribonucleic acid; *RNA,* ribonucleic acid.

dissociate easily, and the globin is broken down into its component amino acids. The iron in hemoglobin is oxidized, forming Fe^{+3} (methemoglobin), and recycled (see following section).

Porphyrin is reduced to bilirubin, which is transported to the liver, conjugated, and finally excreted in the bile as glucuronide (Figure 25-15). Approximately 6 g of hemoglobin is catabolized daily, producing 200 mg of bilirubin. Bacteria in the intestinal lumen transform conjugated bilirubin into urobilinogen. Although a small portion is reabsorbed to be either metabolized further by the liver or excreted by the kidney into the urine, most urobilinogen is excreted in feces. Conditions causing accelerated erythrocyte destruction increase the load of bilirubin for hepatic clearance, leading to increased serum levels of unconjugated bilirubin and increased urinary excretion of urobilinogen. Gallstones (cholelithiasis) can result from a chronically elevated rate of bilirubin excretion.

Iron Cycle

Approximately 67% of total body iron is bound to heme in erythrocytes (hemoglobin) and muscle cells (**myoglobin**), and approximately 30% is stored in mononuclear phagocytes (i.e., macrophages) and hepatic parenchymal cells as either ferritin or hemosiderin. The remaining 3% (less than 1 mg) is lost daily in urine, sweat, bile, and epithelial cells in the gut.

Iron is continually recycled.[19] The methemoglobin released from the breakdown of senescent or damaged erythrocytes (see preceding section) is dissociated by the enzyme

heme oxygenase, and the iron released into the bloodstream, where it is free to bind again to transferrin, or stored in the macrophage's cytoplasm as ferritin or hemosiderin (Figure 25-16). A minute amount of iron is stored in muscle cells by the heme-containing protein myoglobin. Unavailable stores of iron are present in cytochromes, catalases, and peroxidase enzymes.

The protein ferritin is the major intracellular iron storage protein. **Apoferritin,** which is ferritin without attached iron, can store thousands of atoms of iron. Several (24) apoferritin complexes combine to form the micelle ferritin. Large aggregates of micelles (if a large amount of iron is present) produce numerous ferritin micelles, known as **hemosiderin.** Hemosiderin is visible as an iron-based pigment under a light microscope as cell inclusions. The iron within deposits of hemosiderin is poorly available to supply iron when needed. Conditions leading to large amounts of iron include hemolysis, severe congestion, unusual increases in dietary iron consumption, increased absorption, or decreased loss. The most common cause of hemosiderin deposition is simple bruising. Hemosiderin in small amounts within iron-rich tissues (i.e., spleen, liver, bone marrow) is considered normal. Large aggregates or its presence in tissue such as the lungs or subcutaneous tissue suggest a pathologic condition.

Iron balance is maintained through controlled absorption rather than excretion. Dietary iron (primarily as Fe^{2+}) is transported by a divalent metal ion transporter directly across the membranes of epithelial cells in the duodenum and proximal jejunum.[20] (Transport mechanisms are described

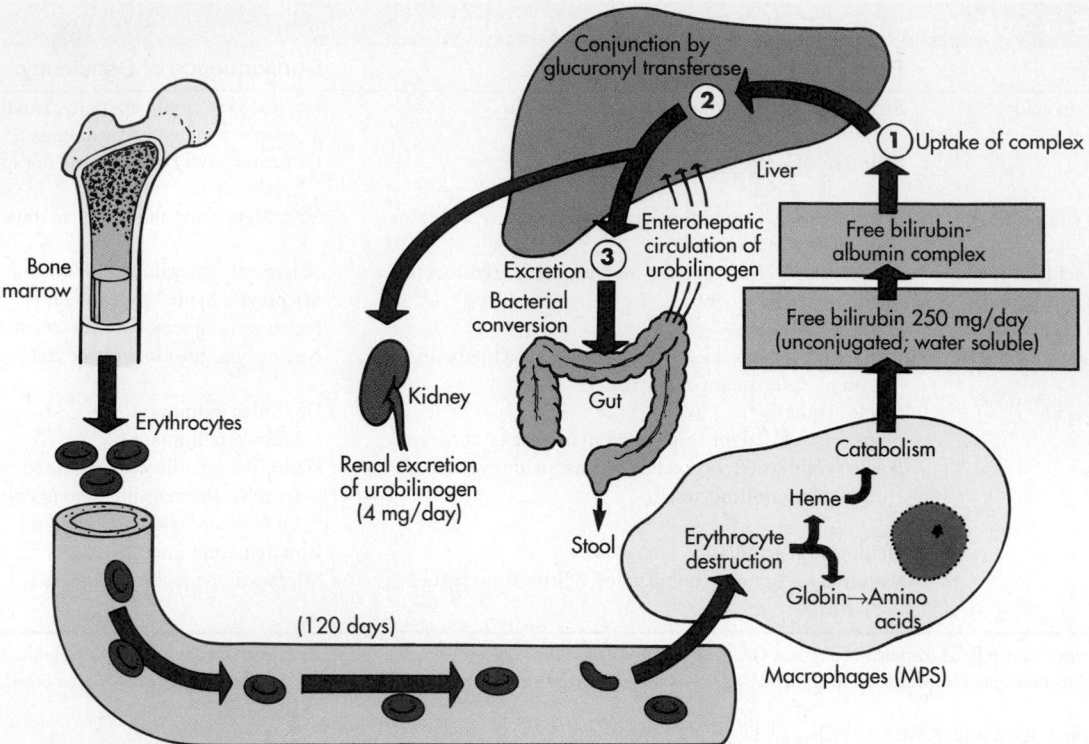

Figure 25-15 Metabolism of bilirubin released by heme breakdown.

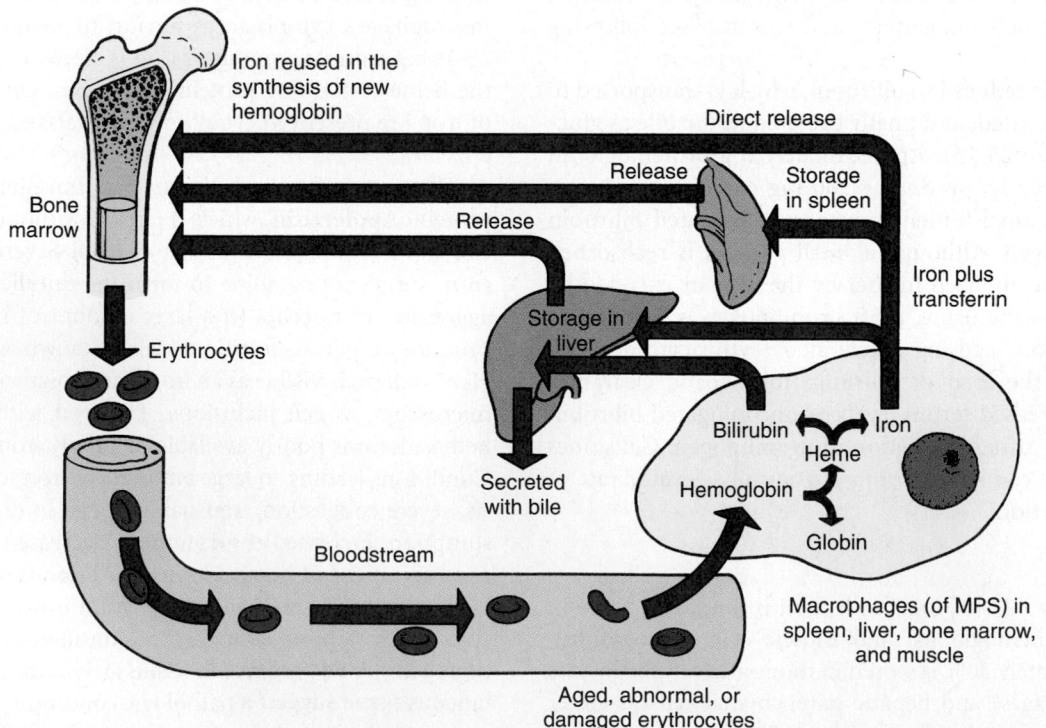

Figure 25-16 Iron cycle. Iron (Fe) released from gastrointestinal epithelial cells circulates in the bloodstream associated with its plasma carrier, transferrin. It is delivered to erythroblasts in bone marrow, where most of it is incorporated into hemoglobin. Mature erythrocytes circulate for approximately 100 to 120 days, after which they become senescent and are removed by the mononuclear phagocyte system (MPS). Tissue macrophages (mostly in spleen) break down ingested erythrocytes and return iron to the bloodstream directly or after storing it as a ferritin or hemosiderin.

in Chapter 1.) Regulation of iron transport across the plasma membrane of gastrointestinal epithelial cells is related to the cells' iron content and the overall rate of erythropoiesis. If the body's iron stores are low or the demand for erythropoiesis increases, iron is transported rapidly through the epithelial cell and into the plasma. If body stores are high and erythropoiesis is not increased, iron transport is shut down, although iron can cross the epithelial cells' plasma membrane passively and is stored as ferritin. Excretion of iron occurs when the epithelial cells of the intestinal mucosa slough off.

Iron from either dietary sources or erythrocyte catabolism is transported in the blood bound to **apotransferrin**, which is then called **transferrin;** under normal conditions, only one third of the iron-binding sites on transferrin molecules are occupied. Apotransferrin is a glycoprotein synthesized primarily by hepatocytes in the liver but also produced in small quantities by tissue macrophages, submaxillary and mammary glands, and ovaries or testes. Iron for hemoglobin production is carried by transferrin to the bone marrow, where it binds to transferrin receptors on erythroblasts. Transferrin receptors are on the plasma membrane of all nucleated cells, although at particularly high levels on erythroid precursors and rapidly proliferating cells (e.g., lymphocytes), and are thought to be the only route of cellular entry for transferrin-attached iron. Transferrin is recycled (transferrin cycle) in the following manner:

1. The transferrin-iron complex binds to a transferrin receptor on the erythroblast's plasma membrane.
2. The complex moves into the cell by receptor-mediated endocytosis.
3. Iron is released (dissociated) from transferrin.
4. The dissociated transferrin is returned to the bloodstream for reuse.

The iron is transported to the erythroblast's mitochondria (the site of hemoglobin production), where the enzyme heme synthetase inserts ferrous iron into protoporphyrin to form heme. Heme then is bound to globin to form hemoglobin. Iron not used in erythropoiesis is stored temporarily as ferritin or hemosiderin and later excreted.

Development of Leukocytes

Leukocytes consist of lymphocytes, granulocytes, and monocytes. Most of the leukocytes arise from stem cells in the bone marrow (their pathways of differentiation are shown in Figure 25-9). Hematopoietic stem cells differentiate into two populations of progenitor cells: common lymphoid progenitors and common myeloid progenitors. Lymphoid progenitors that remain in the bone marrow undergo differentiation into the B-cell lineage, after which they are released into the circulation and undergo further maturation in the secondary lymphoid organs (described in Chapter 7 [see Figure 7-12]). The common myeloid progenitors futher differentiate into progenitors for basophils, mast cells, eosinophils, and megakaryocytes, and granulocyte/monocyte progenitors. The granulocyte/monocyte progenitors further differentiate into monocyte progenitors and granulocyte progenitors, which develop into monocytes/macrophages and neutrophils, respectively. Development from hematopoietic stem cell to common granulocyte-monocyte progenitors primarily is under the control of stem cell factor, IL-3, and GM-CSF, whereas further differentiation into granulocytic and monocytic progenitors is controlled by G-CSF and M-CSF, respectively (see Table 25-4).

Monocytic progenitors undergo development into monocytes within 24 hours and are released into the circulation. Monocytes mature into various forms of macrophages, which is usually complete within 1 or 2 days after release (see Table 25-3).[21]

Progenitor cells for granulocytes normally fully mature in the bone marrow into neutrophils, eosinophils, and basophils. The ultimate phenotype is determined by relative local bone marrow concentrations of early and late-acting cytokines, including GM-CSF, G-CSF, IL-3, IL-5, stem cell factor, and others (see Table 25-4). Granulocytes are released into the blood within 14 days of development. The bone marrow selectively retains immature granulocytes as a reserve pool that can be rapidly mobilized in response to the body's needs.

Most leukocytes exist in the body from days to years, depending on type. Maintenance of optimal levels of granulocytes and monocytes in the blood depends on the availability of pluripotent stem cells in the marrow, induction of these into committed stem cells, timely release of new cells from the marrow, and mobilization of the granulocyte reserve pool. Leukocyte production increases in response to infection, to the presence of steroids, and to reduction or depletion of reserves in the marrow. It is also associated with strenuous exercise, convulsive seizures, heat, intense radiation, paroxysmal tachycardias, pain, nausea and vomiting, and anxiety.

Development of Platelets

Platelets (thrombocytes) are derived from stem cells and progenitor cells that differentiate into megakaryocytes.[22] During thrombopoiesis, the megakaryocyte progenitor is programmed to undergo an endomitotic cell cycle (**endomitosis**) during which DNA replication occurs, but anaphase and cytokinesis are blocked (see Chapter 1). Thus the megakaryocyte nucleus enlarges and become extremely polyploidy (up to 100-fold or more of the normal amount of DNA) without cellular division. Concurrently, the numbers of cytoplasmic organelles (e.g., internal membranes, granules) increase, and the cell develops cell surface elongations and branches that progressively fragment into platelets. A single megakaryocyte may produce thousands of platelets. Like erythrocytes, platelets released from the bone marrow lack nuclei.

About two thirds of platelets enter the circulation, and the remainder reside in the splenic pool. Platelets circulate in the bloodstream for about 10 days before losing their ability to carry out thrombogenic activity. Senescent platelets are sequestered and destroyed in the spleen by mononuclear cell phagocytosis.

An adequate level of committed platelet precursors (megakaryoblasts) in the bone marrow and differentiation into circulating platelets are controlled by specific interactions between megakaryocyte progenitors and stromal cells in the bone marrow as well as thrombopoietin (TPO), a hormonal growth factor primarily produced by the liver, and various cytokines and colony-stimulating factors and interleukins (see Table 25-4). Platelets express high affinity receptors for TPO, and when circulating platelet levels are normal, TPO is adsorbed onto the platelet surface and prevented from accessing the bone marrow and initiating further platelet production.[23] TPO stimulates committed cells at further stages of differentiation to differentiate faster so that rates of megakaryocyte development, endomitosis, and platelet release are increased. During inflammation IL-6 induces increased production of TPO, which increases production of newly formed platelets, which are more thrombogenic.

MECHANISMS OF HEMOSTASIS

Hemostasis is defined as arrest of bleeding (Figure 25-17). As a result of hemostasis, damaged blood vessels maintain a relatively steady state of blood volume, pressure, and flow. The importance of hemostasis clearly varies with vessel size. Damage to large vessels cannot easily be controlled by hemostasis but requires vascular contraction and dramatically decreased blood flow into the damaged vessels.

Three equally important components of hemostasis are the vasculature (endothelial cells and subendothelial matrix), platelets, and blood proteins (clotting factors). The general sequence of events in hemostasis are (1) vascular injury leads to a transient arteriolar vasoconstriction to limit blood flow to the affected site; (2) damage to the endothelial cell lining of the vessel exposes prothrombogenic subendothelial connective tissue matrix leading to platelet adherence and activation and formation of a *hemostatic plug* to prevent further bleeding (primary hemostasis); (3) tissue factor, produced by the endothelium, collaborates with secreted platelet factors and activated platelets to activate the clotting (coagulation) system to form fibrin clots and further prevent bleeding (secondary hemostasis); and (4) the fibrin/platelet clot contracts to form a more permanent plug, and regulatory pathways are activated (fibrinolysis) to limit the size of the plug and begin the healing process.

Function of Blood Vessels

The vessel walls consist of a layer of endothelial cells that adhere to an underlying matrix of connective tissue. The matrix contains a variety of proteins, including collagen, fibronectin, and laminins. Endothelial cells adhere to the matrix and to each other through receptors (e.g., vascular endothelial cell-specific cadherin [VE-cadherin], platelet-endothelial cell adhesion molecule-1 [PECAM-1], integrins [especially $\alpha2\beta1$ and $\alpha5\beta1$]) that are expressed only on the intercellular and basal surfaces.

Under normal conditions the endothelium actively regulates blood flow and prevents spontaneous activation of platelets and the clotting system (see Figure 25-17). Endothelial cells produce **nitric oxide (NO)** from L-arginine and **prostacyclin (PGI$_2$)** from arachidonic acid. Both NO, via cGMP, and PGI$_2$ are vasodilators that work in concert with endothelin (a vasoconstrictor) to maintain blood flow and pressure.[24] NO and PGI$_2$ also inhibit platelet adhesion and aggregation. Synergism between PGI$_2$ and NO is significant. PGI$_2$ production varies a great deal in response to stimuli, whereas NO is released continually to regulate vascular tone. NO has other biologic functions including cell signaling, free radical production, and possibly others. Endothelium also produces adenosine diphosphatase, which degrades ADP (a potent activator of platelets).

The endothelial cell surface contains antithrombotic molecules, such as glycosaminoglycans (e.g., heparan sulfate), thrombomodulin, and plasminogen activators. These limit platelet activation and fibrin deposition. Although thrombomodulin and plasminogen activators help control hemostasis in normal vessels, their effects are magnified during vascular damage and clot formation; therefore, further information is provided on these molecules in the following section on control of hemostatic mechanisms.

As a result of damage to the vessels, the endothelial cell barrier is frequently compromised, remaining endothelial cells activated by product of tissue damage, and the underlying matrix exposed. Endothelial cells contain intracellular structures (Weibel-Palade bodies) that contain von Willebrand factor (vWF) that is released during damage. The matrix, in addition to collagen and other connective tissue, contains vWF and can bind additional vWF released by the endothelium.[25] The matrix itself and vWF are potent activators of platelets.

Function of Platelets

Platelets normally circulate freely, suspended in plasma, in an unactivated state. The role of platelets is to (1) contribute to regulation of blood flow into a damaged site by induction of vasoconstriction (vasospasm), (2) initiate platelet-to-platelet interactions resulting in formation of a platelet plug to stop further bleeding, (3) activate the coagulation (or clotting) cascade to stabilize the platelet plug, and (4) initiate repair processes including clot retraction and clot dissolution (**fibrinolysis**). The normal platelet count ranges from 140,000 to 340,000/mm^3. If platelet counts drop below 100,000/mm^3 an individual is usually considered thrombocytopenic (abnormally low numbers of platelets) and may experience prolongation of normal clotting but is usually not at risk for spontaneous major bleeding episodes unless the platelet count falls below 20,000/mm^3. If platelet numbers are elevated (thrombocytosis) the risk for spontaneous blood clots (thrombosis), stroke, or heart attack is increased.

The state of platelet activation is primarily under the control of endothelial cells lining the vessels. Damage to the vessel initiates a process of platelet activation; (1) increased platelet adhesion to the damaged vascular wall; (2) activation leading to secretion of chemicals from platelet granules, which stimulate changes in platelet shape and biochemistry; and

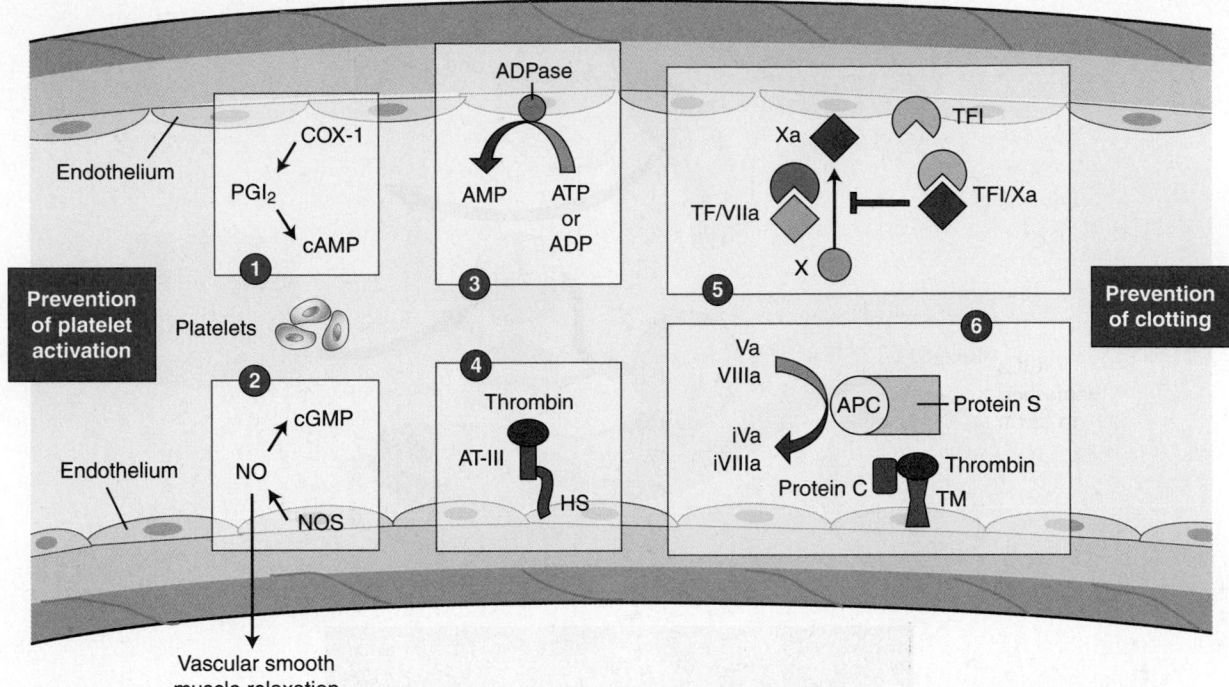

Figure 25-17 Hemostasis. Endothelium controls hemostasis by preventing platelet activation (1-3) and preventing activation of the clotting system (4-6). **(1) Prostacyclin production.** Injury activates inflammation (COX-1 arachidonic acid). Enzymes convert arachidonic acid into prostacylin I_2 (PGI_2) in endothelial cells. PGI_2 eventually increases intracellular cyclic adenosine monophosphate (cAMP); cAMP inhibits platelet aggregation and induces vasodilation. Nitric oxide (NO) formation is induced by NO synthases (NOS) and NO causes increased cyclic guanosine monophosphate (cGMP). **(2) Nitric oxide system.** Endothelial cell NOS produces nitric oxide, which controls platelet activation through cGMP-mediated signaling. **(3) ADPase.** Endothelial cells express a surface bound ADPase (CD39) that converts circulating ADP and ATP to AMP. **(4) Antithrombin III–heparan sulfate system.** Antithrombin III (AT-III) inhibits thrombin slowly when heparan sulfate (HS) is absent. When HS is present, it quickly activates thrombin because it binds to a specific site on AT-III that causes an instant conformational change in AT-III, allowing it to quickly activate thrombin. **(5) Tissue factor inhibitor (TFI) system.** Expression of TFI on the endothelial cells and secreted into the circulation complexes with factor IXa to form a competitive inhibitor of the tissue factor/factor VIIa complex (TF/VIIa) and prevent further activation of factor X to Xa. **(6) Protein C/protein S pathway (thrombomodulin).** Thrombin in the circulation binds to thrombomodulin on the endothelial cell creating a complex that can bind and activate protein C to activated protein C (APC) that complexes in the blood or on the surface of active platelets with protein S. This complex degrades circulating clotting factors Va and VIIIa to inactive forms (iVa, iVIIIa) to prevent further activation of clotting.

(3) aggregation as platelet-vascular wall and platelet-platelet adherence increases.[26] This process leads to activation of the clotting system and development of an immobilizing meshwork of platelets and fibrin (Figure 25-18).

Adhesion

Normally, platelets are generally observed "rolling" along the margins of vessels. At sites of vessel injury, however, platelets become adherent to the site of endothelial damage where the subendothelial matrix is exposed and endothelial cells have released vWF and decreased their antithrombotic activities (Figure 25-19).[25] **Platelet adhesion** is mostly mediated by the binding of platelet surface receptor glycoprotein-Ib (GPIb) (in a complex with clotting factors IX and V) to **von Willebrand factor (vWF)** (Figure 25-20).[27] The vWF protein is found in the subendothelial matrix and is released by endothelial cells and platelets. Deficiencies in GPIb (Bernard-Soulier syndrome) or of vWF (von Willebrand disease) lead to highly defective hemostasis and congenital bleeding

disorders. Platelet adhesion narrows the diameter of the blood vessel resulting in increasing shear forces that could strip platelets off the vessel surface. However, those same forces induce conformational changes in the vWF molecule that result in increased affinity with GPIb, thus stabilizing the adherent platelet.[28]

Platelet adhesion is also facilitated by other interactions between platelet receptors and exposed molecules of the subendothelial matrix. For instance, adhesion is increased through binding of the platelet collagen receptor GPVI to exposed collagen in the matrix.

Activation

As a result of interactions with the endothelium or the subendothelial matrix, as well as exposure to inflammatory mediators produced by the endothelium and other cells, the platelets are activated. Activation results in dynamic changes in platelet shape from smooth spheres to those with spiny projections and degranulation (also called the **platelet-release reaction**)

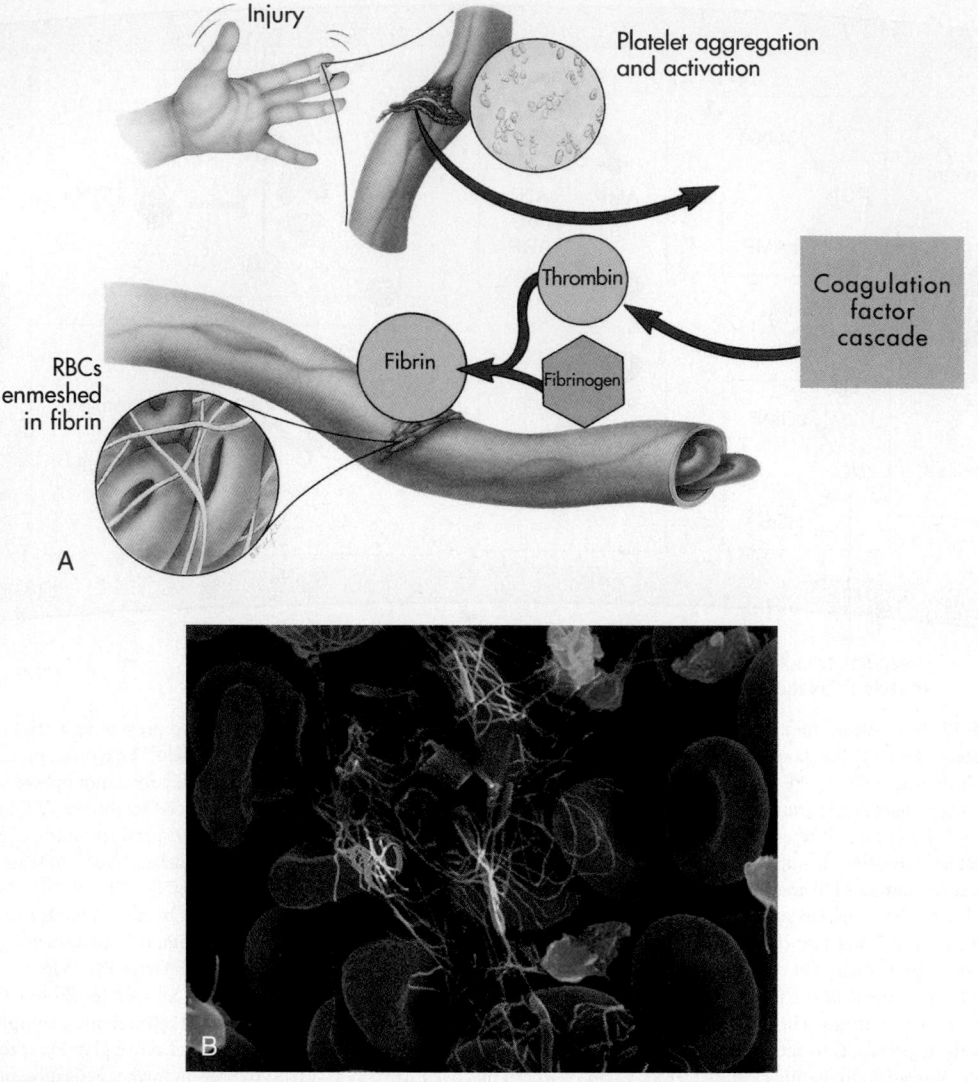

Figure 25-18 Blood clotting mechanism. A, The clotting mechanism involves release of platelet factors at the injury site, formation of thrombin and trapping of red blood cells (RBCs) in fibrin to form a clot. **B,** An electron micrograph showing entrapped RBCs in a fibrin clot. (**A** from Thibodeau GA, Patton KT: *Anatomy & physiology,* ed 5, St Louis, 2003, Mosby; **B** copyright Dennis Kunkel Microscopy, Inc.)

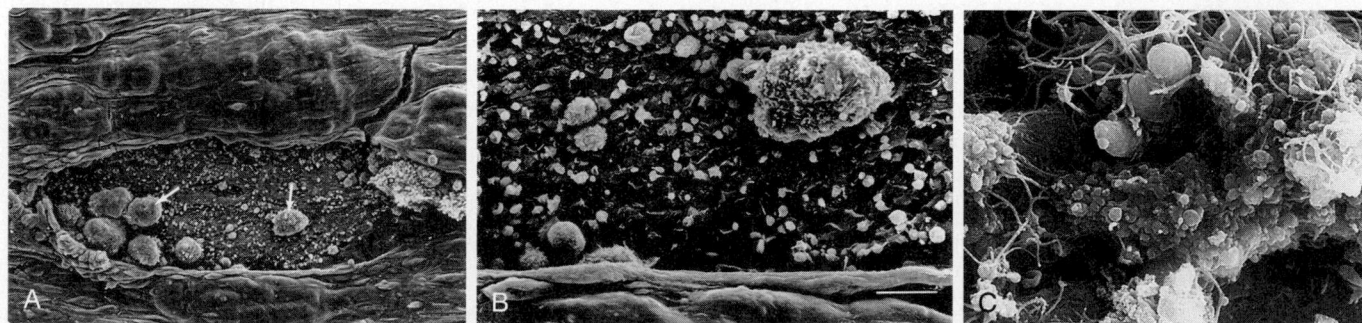

Figure 25-19 Platelet activation. A, After endothelial denudation, platelets and leukocytes adhere to the subendothelium in a monolayer fashion. **B,** Higher-power view showing leukocytes and platelets adherent to the subendothelium. **C,** High magnification of a thrombus showing a mixture of red cells and platelets incorporated into the fibrin meshwork. (**A** and **B** from Libby P, et al: *Braunwald's heart disease: a textbook of cardiovascular medicine,* ed 8, Philadelphia, 2007, Saunders, as reproduced from Faggiotto A, Ross R: Studies of hypercholesterolemia in the nonhuman primate. II. Fatty streak conversion to fibrous plaque. *Arteriosclerosis* 341-356, 1984; **C** from Damjanov I, Linder J, editors: *Anderson's pathology,* ed 10, St Louis, 1996, Mosby.)

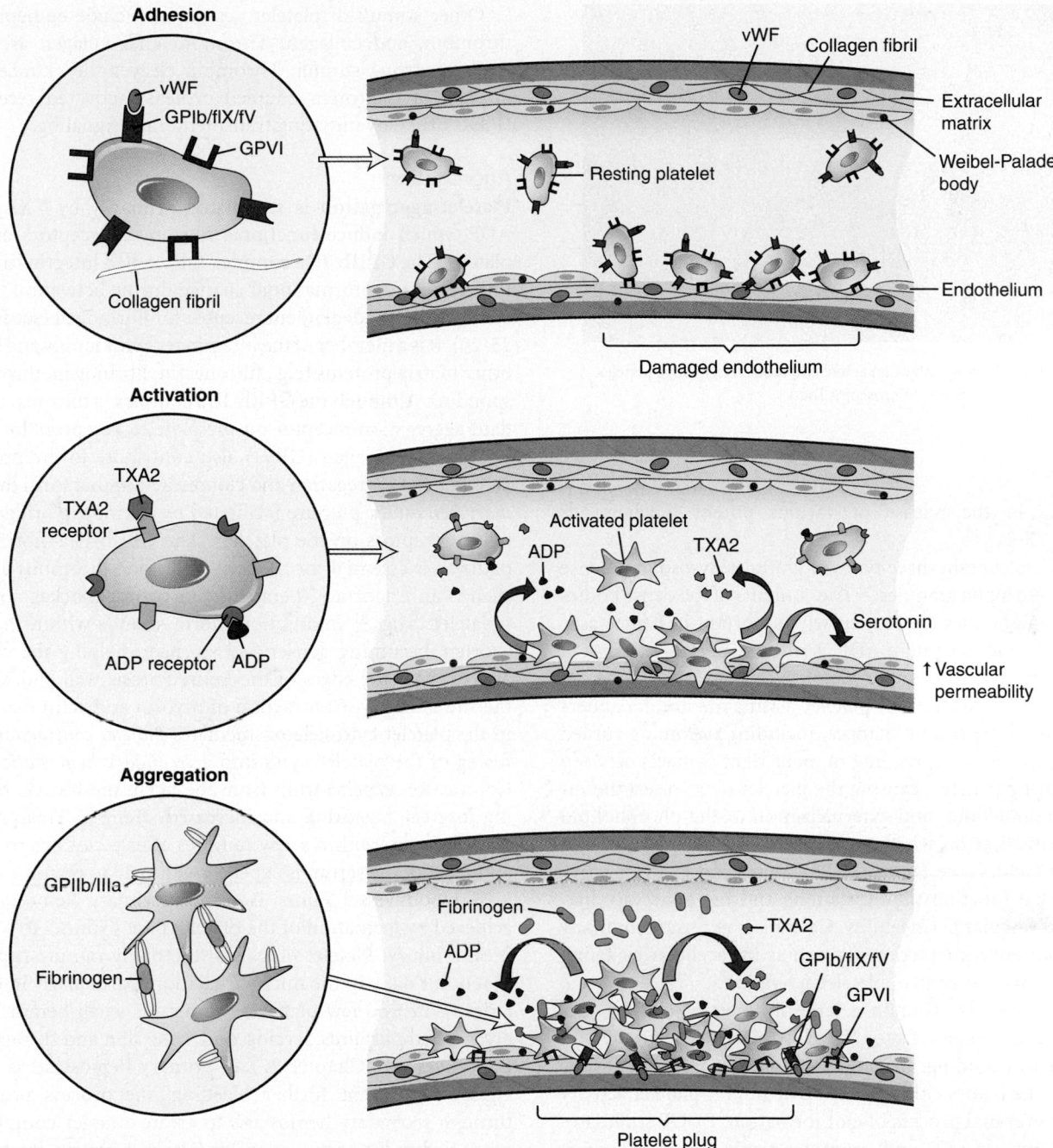

Figure 25-20 Platelet adhesion, activation, aggregation. *Adhesion.* Damage to a vessel may result in the removal of endothelial cells covering the extracellular matrix. The matrix contains collagen and von Willebrand factor (vWF) that was stored in the Weibel-Palade bodies of endothelial cells and secreted. Resting platelets express receptors for collagen (GPVI) and for vWF (GPIb in a complex with factor IX and factor V, GPIb/fIX/fV) that mediate adherence to the exposed matrix. *Activation.* Adhesion leads to activation of the platelets with a change in morphology and release of mediators contained in alpha and dense granules; adenosine diphosphate (ADP) and thromboxane (TXA$_2$) acting through specific receptors are primarily responsible for recruitment and activation of more platelets to the clot, as well as platelet spreading and complete coverage of the exposed matrix. Mediators such as serotonin enhance the inflammatory response by binding to neighboring endothelial cells and inducing further vascular permeability. *Aggregation.* The platelet plug is consolidated by further production of ADP and TXA$_2$, which induce expression of platelet receptors (GPIIb-IIIa) for fibrinogen. The binding of fibrinogen to the fibrinogen receptors on adjacent facilitates platelet aggregation by triggering further platelet spreading and clot retraction. Aggregation is further facilitated by continuing interactions between platelet receptors and collagen and vWF in the matrix.

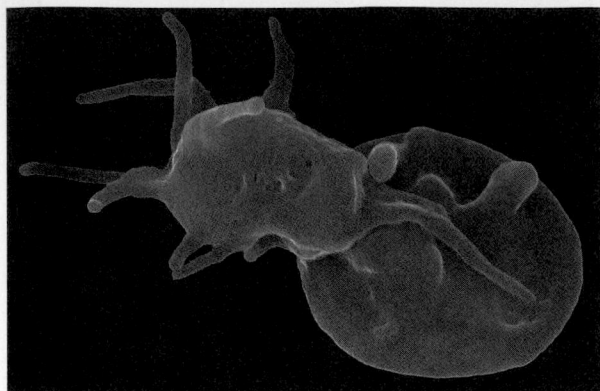

Figure 25-21 Micrograph of an active and moderately active platelet. (Copyright Dennis Kunkel Microscopy, Inc.)

resulting in the release of various potent biochemicals (Figure 25-21).[29]

Platelets contain three types of granules: lysosomes, dense bodies, and alpha granules.[30] The contents of the dense bodies and alpha granules are particularly important in hemostasis. The dense bodies contain ADP, serotonin, and calcium. ADP recruits and activates other platelets through specific receptors. During activation the platelet plasma membrane undergoes several important changes, including becoming ruffled and sticky, cellular spreading to make tight contacts between neighboring platelets causing the platelet plug to seal the injured endothelium, and externalization of the phospholipid phosphatidylserine, which provides a matrix for activation of clotting factors (see Figure 25-20). Serotonin is a vasoactive amine that functions like histamine and increases vasodilation and vascular permeability. Calcium is necessary for many of the adhesive interactions as well as intracellular signaling mechanisms that control platelet activation.

Alpha granules contain a large number of clotting factors (e.g., fibrinogen, factor V), growth factors (e.g., PDGF), and heparin-binding proteins (e.g., platelet factor 4). Many of these mediators either promote or inhibit platelet activity and the eventual process of clot formation. PDGF stimulates smooth muscle cells and promotes tissue repair. Heparin-binding proteins enhance clot formation at the site of injury.

Platelets also initiate production of the prostaglandin derivative **thromboxane-A_2 (TXA$_2$)**, which counters the effects of PGI$_2$ that is produced by endothelial cells (see Figure 25-20). TXA$_2$ promotes the degranulation of platelets, increases expression of platelet fibrinogen receptors, and stimulates platelet aggregation. The balance between TXA$_2$ and PGI$_2$ affects platelet aggregation, which is favored by TXA$_2$ excess and inhibited by PGI$_2$ excess. An isoform of **cyclooxygenase (COX-1)** converts arachidonic acid to TXA$_2$ in platelets. Aspirin at low doses specifically and irreversibly inactivates COX-1, decreasing production of TXA$_2$ and decreasing platelet activation.[31] A few days of low doses of aspirin lead to more than 95% inhibition of TXA$_2$.

Other stimuli of platelet activation include epinephrine, thrombin, and collagen. Thrombin and collagen are particularly strong stimuli. Thrombin cleaves the extracellular domain of G-protein–coupled protease-activated receptors (PARs), thereby initiating transmembrane signaling.

Aggregation

Platelet aggregation is stimulated primarily by TXA$_2$ and ADP, which induce functional fibrinogen receptors on the platelet. The **GPIIb-IIIa complex** (also called integrin αIIbβ3) undergoes a conformational change during activation to become a calcium-dependent receptor for fibrinogen (see Figure 25-20). It is a member of the integrin receptor family and binds other matrix proteins (e.g., fibronectin, fibrinogen, thrombospondin). Although the GPIIb-IIIa complex is the most abundant aggregation receptor on the platelet, receptors for vWF (GPIb) and collagen (GPVI) also contribute to the process. Interplatelet aggregation and clot retraction that form the *primary hemostatic plug* are facilitated by fibrinogen bridges between receptors on the platelets. The GPIIb-IIIa–fibrinogen pathway is essential for the formation of a thrombus and as such is an important therapeutic target for blockage by antiplatelet drugs.[31] In addition, fibrin strands within the clot shorten, becoming denser and stronger, helping the clot to approximate the edges of the injured vessel wall and sealing the site of injury. Contraction of myosin and actin filaments in the platelet cytoskeleton mediates *platelet contraction* and fusing of the platelet mass into a *secondary hemostatic plug*. Contraction expels serum from the fibrin meshwork, resulting in greater packing and increased strength. This process usually begins within a few minutes after a clot has formed, and most of the serum is expelled within 20 to 60 minutes.[32]

If blood vessel injury is minor, primary hemostasis is achieved by formation of the platelet plug within 3 to 5 minutes of injury. Platelet plugs seal the many minute ruptures that occur daily in the microcirculation, particularly in capillaries. With too few platelets, numerous small hemorrhagic areas called *purpuras* develop under the skin and throughout the tissues (see Chapter 27). If primary hemostasis is inadequate to prevent further bleeding, the process proceeds through secondary hemostasis to create a larger complex of more tightly interactive platelets within a matrix created by activation of the clotting system.

Function of Clotting Factors

A **blood clot** is a meshwork of protein strands that stabilizes the platelet plug and traps other cells, such as erythrocytes, phagocytes, and microorganisms. The strands are made of fibrin, which is produced by the **clotting (coagulation) system**. The clotting system was described in Chapter 6 and consists of a family of proteins that circulate in the blood in inactive forms (proenzymes). Initiation of the system results in sequential enzymatic activation (cascade) of multiple members of the system until a fibrin clot is created (Table 25-7).

The clotting system is usually presented as two pathways of initiation (intrinsic and extrinsic pathways) that join in a

Table 25-7	Coagulation Factors and Synonyms	
Factor	**Synonym**	**Primary Function**
I	Fibrinogen	Source of fibrin to form clot
II	Prothrombin	Source of thrombin that activates fibrinogen, V, VII, VIII, XI, XIII, protein C, platelets
Tissue factor	Previously called factor III	Cofactor for factor VIIa
Calcium	Previously called factor IV	Cofactor for clotting factor binding to phosphatidylserine
V	Labile factor	Va is cofactor in the prothrombinase complex
VII	Stable factor, proconvertin	VIIa forms a complex with tissue factor and activates factors IX and X
VIII	Antihemophilic factor	VIIIa is a component of tenase complex
IX	Christmas factor	IXa is a component of tenase complex, activates factor X
X	Stuart-Prower factor	Xa is component of prothrombinase complex, activates prothrombin
XI	Plasma thromboplastin antecedent	XIa activates factor IX
XII	Hageman (contact) factor	XIIa activates factor XI
XIII	Fibrin-stabilizing factor	XIIIa cross-links fibrin

common pathway (Figure 25-22).[26] The intrinsic pathway is activated when Hageman factor (factor XII) in plasma contacts negatively charged subendothelial substances exposed by vascular injury. The extrinsic pathway is activated when membrane-bound or soluble **tissue factor (TF)** (also called **tissue thromboplastin**), a substance released by damaged endothelial cells, reacts with a high affinity with activated factor VII (TF/VIIa).[33] The resultant complexes of both pathways are enzymatically active with factor X as the substrate.[34]

Activated platelets are important participants in clotting. The phosphatidylserine-rich surface produced during activation provides a matrix on which several important complexes of clotting factors are formed. These include the intrinsic pathway's *tenase complex* (factor X and activated factors VIII and IX) that activates factor X and the *prothrombinase complex* (prothrombin and activated factors X and V) that activates prothrombin into thrombin (see Figure 25-22). Thrombin then converts fibrinogen into fibrin, which polymerizes into a fibrin clot. Thrombin has broad reactivity in the inflammatory response.[35] In addition to producing fibrin, thrombin is an activator of other coagulation proteins (e.g., factors V, VIII, XI, XIII), platelets (e.g., aggregation, degranulation), endothelial cells (e.g., up-regulation of adhesion molecules for leukocytes, increased NO, PGI_2, PDGF), and monocytes (e.g., cytokine secretion, increased receptors for endothelial cells).

The extrinsic pathway is clearly predominant; individuals with deficiencies in intrinsic pathway components (i.e., factor XI, factor XII) do not have prolonged bleeding.[36] As with the complement cascade, the clotting system is complex with a large number of alternative activators and inhibitors, and the relative importance of particular factors may differ between in vivo hemostasis and in vitro testing of clotting or may depend on the particular mechanism by which the pathway is activated.[37] Also there is interaction between components of the intrinsic and extrinsic pathways so that an activated member of one pathway may activate a member of the other pathway (e.g., factor VIIa of the extrinsic pathway can directly activate factor IX of the intrinsic pathway).

Another similarity with the complement system is that some complexes may have biologic activities outside the predominantly described pathway. For instance, in vitro studies have showed that TF/VIIa complex activates protease-activated receptors (PARs); thus TF may contribute to other biologic processes by facilitating signaling in vascular cells (Figure 25-23). Abnormal TF expression in the vessel wall and/or low circulating cells initiates life-threatening thrombosis in various diseases. TF also contributes to inflammation, tumor angiogenesis and metastasis, and cell migration (Figure 25-24).

Control of Hemostatic Mechanisms

The endothelium is the major site of hemostasis. Despite the continual presence of clotting factors and platelets in the circulation, blood normally remains fluid. Thus the major regulatory factors that control hemostasis reside where the greatest probability of clotting would occur: on the endothelial cell surface (see Figure 25-17). The primary anticoagulant mechanisms include thrombin inhibitors (e.g., antithrombin III), tissue factor inhibitors (e.g., tissue factor pathway inhibitor), and mechanisms for degrading activated clotting factors (e.g., protein C).[38] Antithrombotic mechanisms are listed in Table 25-8.

Table 25-8	Antithrombotic Mechanisms of Endothelial Cells
Function Regulated	**Substances Involved**
Clotting cascade	Tissue factor pathway inhibitor Antithrombin III Heparan sulfate Thrombomodulin/protein C/protein S
Vessel and platelet activity	Cover prothrombotic intercellular matrix molecules Prostacyclin (PGI_2) Nitric oxide (NO) Adenosine diphosphate
Eliminate fibrin clot	Plasminogen activators

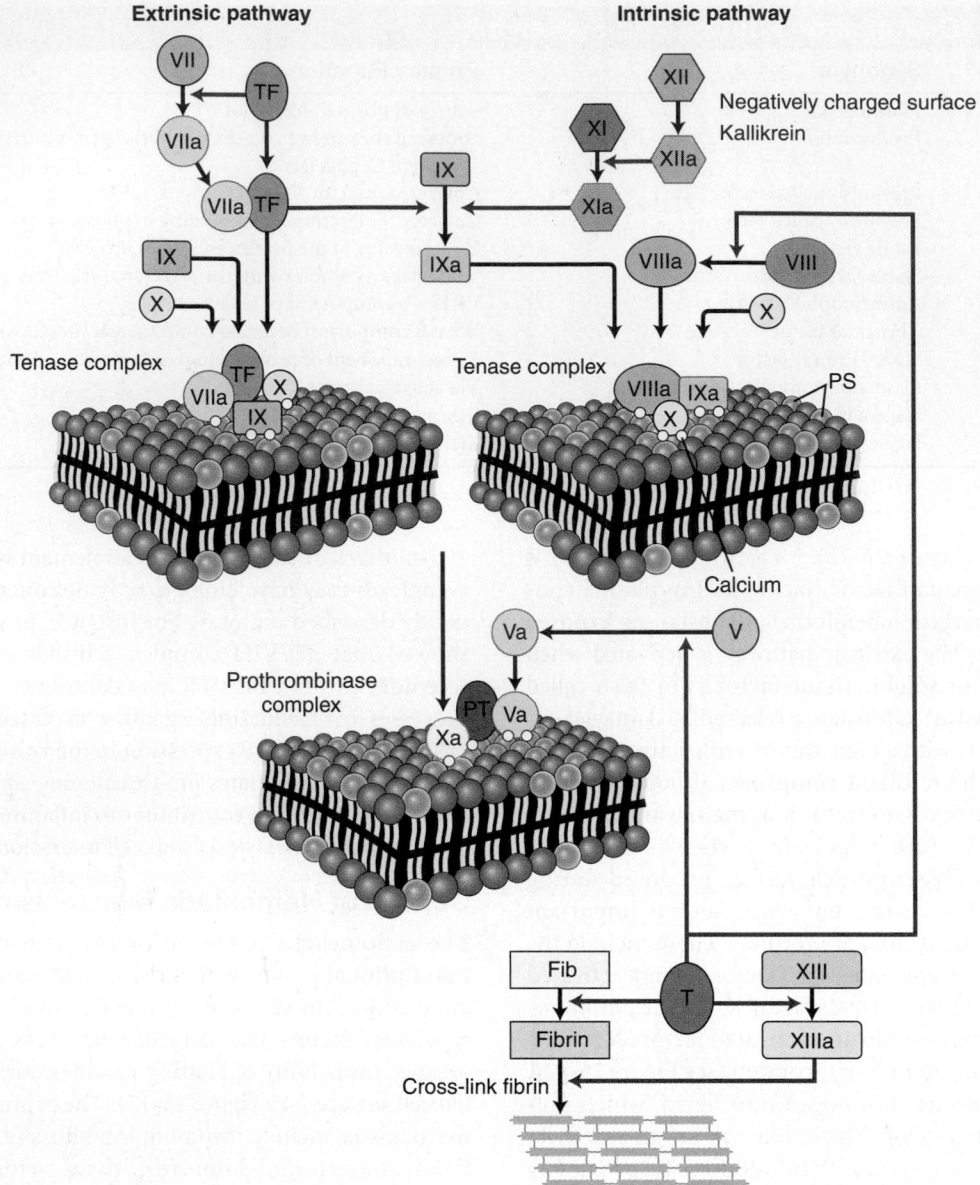

Figure 25-22 The clotting system. The clotting system is frequently presented with two routes of initiation: the intrinsic and extrinsic pathways. The intrinsic pathway is initiated by activation of factor XII to XIIa by negatively charged molecules or surfaces or by the action of kallikrein, a member of the kinin system. Factor XIIa induces enzymatic activation of factor XI to XIa, which activates IX to IXa. A complex of factors IXa/VIIIa/X and calcium aggregate on the surface of activated platelets that have externalized the plasma membrane phospholipid phosphatidylserine (PS). The IXa/VIIIa complex is an active enzyme ("tenase") that can activate factor X to Xa. The extrinsic pathway is the primary physiologic route of activation and is activated by exposure of tissue factor (TF) on endothelial cells or in the circulation. TF activates factor VII in the blood to factor VIIa. The TF/VIIa complex associates with circulating factors IX and X and calcium on the PS-rich surface of activated platelets. The TF/VIIa/IX complex is a tenase that produces Xa. The VIIa/TF complex also can activate factor IX to IXa and facilitate the formation of the VIIIa/IXa tenase. Factor Xa associates with activated factor V (Va) and prothrombin (PT) in a PS and calcium-dependent complex that is a "prothrombinase," which converts PT to thrombin (T). Thrombin is an active enzyme that converts fibrinogen (Fib) to fibrin. Thrombin also activates factor XIII to XIIIa, which cross-links fibrin into a matrix that seals clots. Thrombin amplifies the clotting process by activating factor VIII to VIIIa and facilitating formation of the VIIIa/IXa tenase and by activating factor V to Va to create further prothrombinase complexes.

Antithrombin III (AT-III) is a circulating plasma serine protease inhibitor produced by the liver. Specifically, it inhibits thrombin and several activated clotting factors (e.g., VIIa, IXa, Xa, XIa, XIIa). Clinically administered heparin or heparan sulfate (on the surface of endothelial cells) binds to AT-III and induces a conformational change that greatly enhances its activity. Under normal conditions the presence of endothelial cell heparan sulfate and available AT-III in the circulation cooperate to protect the vessels from the effects of spontaneously activated thrombin (see Figure 25-17).

Acquired AT-III deficiencies can result from infection with bacteria that produce AT-III inhibitors, sepsis, liver disease, and nephrotic syndrome and lead to venous thrombosis and pulmonary embolism.

Tissue factor pathway inhibitor (TFPI) is produced by endothelial cells and complexes to, and reversibly inhibits, factor Xa. The resultant TFPI/Xa complex inhibits TF/VIIa, which mediates feedback inhibition of tissue factor as well as factor VIIa (see Figure 25-17). Although the majority of TFPI remains associated with endothelial surfaces, about

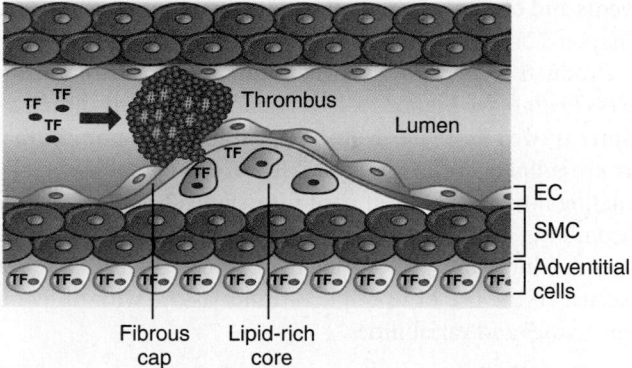

Figure 25-23 Tissue factor (TF) in thrombus formation after rupture of an atherosclerotic plaque. In atherosclerosis TF is expressed by macrophage-derived foam cells and within atherosclerotic plaque. High levels of TF exposed on rupture trigger thrombosis and myocardial infarction. In addition, blood-borne TF may contribute to thrombus propagation. TF is also expressed by adventitial cells *(blue). EC,* Endothelial cells; *SMC,* smooth muscle cells. (Modified from Mackman N: *Arterioscler Thromb Vasc Biol* 24[6]:1015-1022, 2004.)

20% circulates in plasma with lipoproteins. Heparin increases plasma levels of TFPI, which may contribute to heparin's antithrombotic effects.

Thrombomodulin is a membrane thrombin-binding protein on the surface of endothelial cells. **Protein C** in the circulation binds to thrombomodulin in a thrombin-dependent manner and is converted to activated protein C (see Figure 25-17). Activated protein C, in association with a cofactor **(protein S),** degrades factors Va and VIIIa. Deficiencies of AT-III, protein C, or protein S are important causes of hypercoagulation (increased clotting).[39] Expression of thrombomodulin and the endothelial cell protein C receptor is down-regulated by cytokines and other products of inflammation (e.g., IL-1α, tumor necrosis factor-alpha [TNF-α], endotoxin). Decreased expression prevents protein C activation, thereby enhancing clot formation. Activated protein C inhibits the adhesion of neutrophils to the endothelium, but during inflammation the neutrophil enzyme elastase enzymatically removes thrombomodulin from the endothelial cell surface.[40]

Lysis of Blood Clots

Concurrent with activation of coagulation is the activation of pathways that limit the size of the clot and remove the clot after bleeding has ceased and repair has begun. The primary mechanism for lysis (breakdown) of blood clots is the **fibrinolytic system (plasminogen-plasmin system)** that produces plasmin. **Plasmin** (also called *fibrinase* or *fibrinolysin*) is a serine protease that degrades fibrin polymers in clots.[41]

The inactive precursor of plasmin is **plasminogen**, which is produced in the liver (Figure 25-25). Plasminogen activation may occur by several means, although the most physiologically

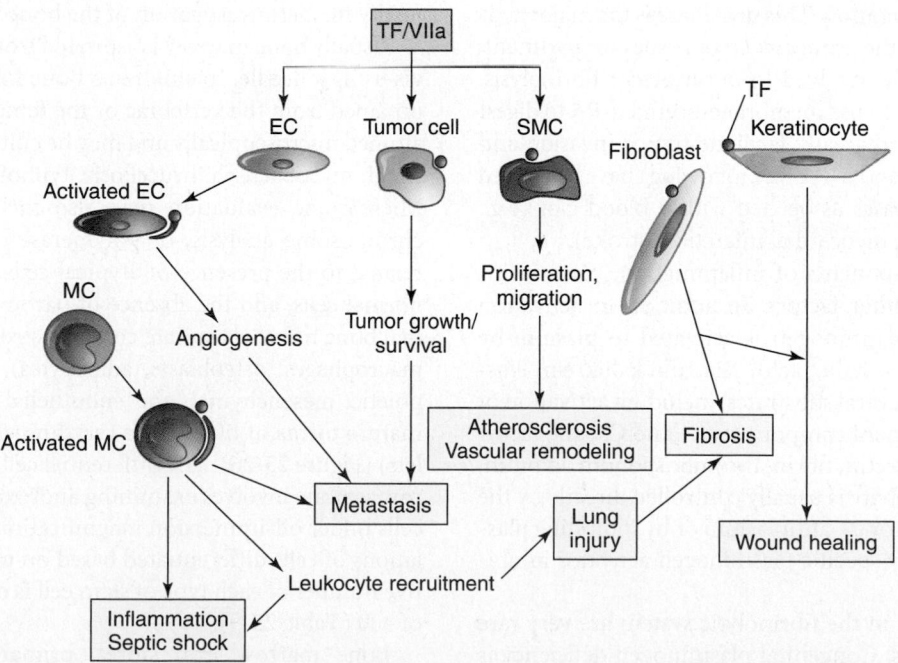

Figure 25-24 Factor VIIa signaling through tissue factor (TF) expressed on the surface of cells mediates changes in disease-related cellular activities, *EC,* Endothelial cell; *MC,* monocyte/macrophage; *SMC,* smooth muscle cell. (Modified from Rao LV, Pendurthi UR: *Arterioscler Thromb Vasc Biol* 25[1]:47-56, 2005.)

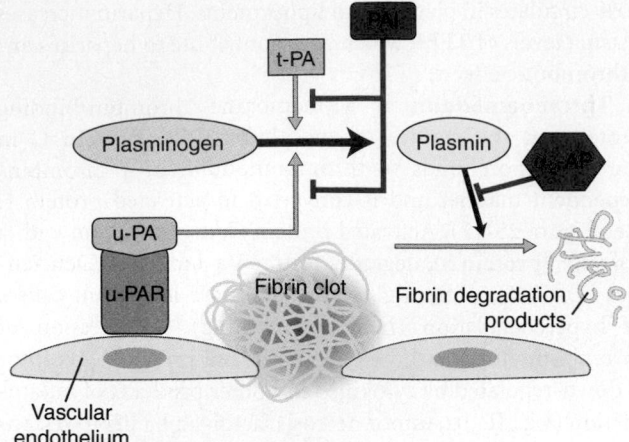

Figure 25-25 The fibrinolytic system. Fibrinolysis is initiated by the binding of plasminogen to fibrin. Although tissue plasminogen activator (t-PA) initiates intravascular fibrinolysis, urokinase plasminogen activator (u-PA) is the major activator of fibrinolysis in tissue (extravascular). Inhibitors *(indicated by red lines)* of fibrinolysis include α_2-antiplasmin (α_2-AP) that inhibits plasmin and plasminogen activator inhibitor-1 (PAI-1) that inhibits t-PA. Plasmin digests the fibrin into smaller soluble pieces (fibrin degradation products). *u-PAR,* urokinase-like plasminogen activator receptor.

important is by the action of **tissue plasminogen activator (t-PA)**.[42] Endothelial cells at a site of vascular injury express t-PA, which is also a serine protease that reaches maximum enzymatic activity after binding to fibrin and proteolytically activates plasminogen to plasmin. Another activator of plasminogen is **urokinase-like plasminogen activator (u-PA)**. The u-PA is a serine protease that can bind to a specific cellular u-PA receptor (u-PAR) causing activation of plasminogen resulting in plasmin generation. This urokinase is the major activator of fibrinolysis in the *extravascular* or tissue compartment, whereas t-PA is largely involved in *intravascular* fibrinolysis. Several cancers appear to use membrane-bound u-PA to digest intercellular matrix and greatly facilitate tumor invasion and metastasis. Both t-PA and u-PA (see following) have been used clinically to treat diseases associated with a blood clot (e.g., pulmonary embolism, myocardial infarction, stroke).

As with most components of inflammation, plasmin interacts greatly with other factors. In addition to activation by t-PA and u-PA, plasminogen is activated to plasmin by thrombin, fibrin, factor XIIa, factor XIa, and kallikrein. Plasmin is proteolytic to several substrates, including activation of collagenases, complement components C1 and C3, and factor XII and cleaves fibronectin, fibrin, thrombospondin, laminin, and vWF. Plasmin activity is usually controlled directly by the serine protease inhibitor α_2-antiplasmin or by inhibiting plasminogen activation by specific plasminogen activator inhibitors (PAIs).

Congenital defects in the fibrinolytic system are very rare and variable in effects. Congenital plasminogen deficiency is associated with venous thrombosis if the plasminogen level is decreased by more than 50%. Apparent defects in plasminogen may result from dysfunctional plasminogen or an absence of fibrinogen. Congenital deficiencies of plasminogen activator or abnormal increases in plasminogen activator inhibitor also may increase the chance for spontaneous thrombosis. Alternative routes of fibrin degradation may mitigate the severity of symptoms in these deficiencies. Other enzymes released during inflammation (e.g., leukocyte elastase, cathepsin G, metalloproteinases [MMPs]) are fibrinolytic.

Cross-linked fibrin is deposited in tissues around wounds, inflammatory sites, and tumors. Fibrin removal is an important biologic process, for intravascular and extravascular spaces, with various controlling mechanisms that can lead to abnormalities of fibrin accumulation, and thrombotic events and can be a structural barrier to tumor invasion (see Chapter 12).

Products of fibrinolysis include **fibrin degradation products (FDPs)** (see Figure 25-25). A major FDP is D-dimer. **D-dimer** is two D domains from adjacent fibrin monomers that are cross-linked by factor XIIIa. Measurement of levels of circulating D-dimer has been used for diagnosis of deep venous thrombosis (DVT) or pulmonary embolism (PE).[43] Despite extensive literature, the diagnostic role of D-dimer is unclear because of the use of multiple D-dimer assays with different sensitivities and variabilities.

CLINICAL EVALUATION OF THE HEMATOLOGIC SYSTEM

Tests of Bone Marrow Function

The bone marrow is the soft spongy tissue found within bones, especially the sternum, pelvis, and femur. Several abnormal conditions in the numbers or morphology of circulating blood cells or suspected infection of the marrow may justify further investigation of the bone marrow.

Usually bone marrow is aspirated from the sternum or pelvis using a needle. In children a bone marrow aspirate can be obtained from the vertebrae or the femur. The aspirate is examined microscopically and may be cultured if infection (e.g., fungi, mycobacteria, brucellosis, typhoid fever) is suspected. Microscopic evaluation may also include flow cytometry, chromosome analysis, or polymerase chain reaction (PCR) related to the presence of atypical cells, atypical numbers of normal cells, and the absence of particular cell types. A normal bone marrow aspirate contains stromal cells (fibroblasts, macrophages, osteoblasts, adipocytes), stem cells (hematopoietic, mesenchymal, and endothelial), and immature and mature forms of blood cells (erythrocytes, leukocytes, platelets) (Figure 25-26). The differential cell count of a bone marrow aspirate involves examining approximately 400 nucleated cells under oil-immersion magnification and counting populations of cells differentiated based on morphology. The relative number of each type of stem cell is expressed as a fraction of 400 (Table 25-9).

Bone marrow iron stores, primarily in macrophages, can be examined using special stains (e.g., Prussian blue) for iron-containing granules. A direct measure of iron stores also can be obtained only from liver biopsy specimens, although

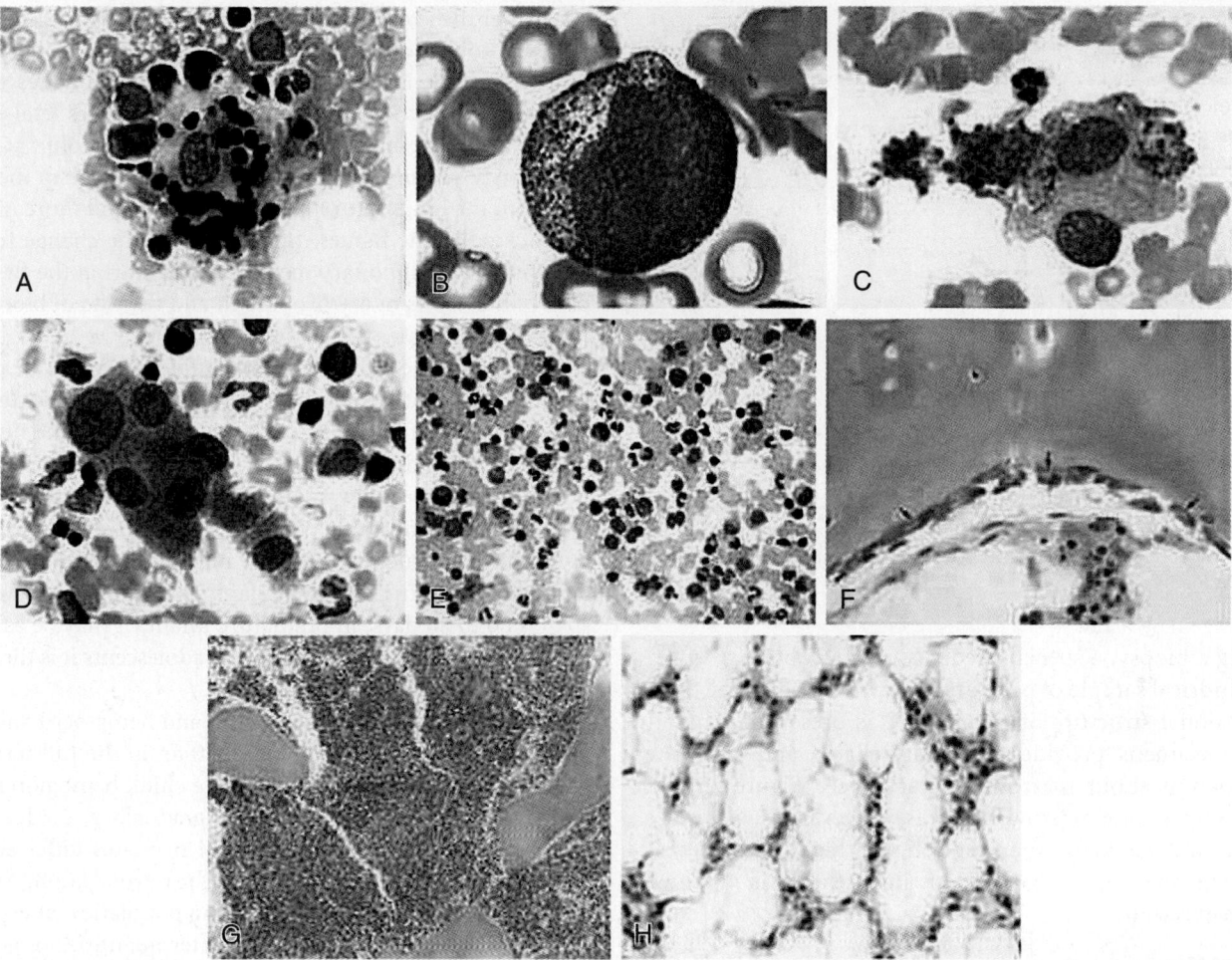

Figure 25-26 **Bone marrow samples.** Images A through D contain bone marrow aspirates; images E through H contain bone marrow biopsy specimens; images A through F are examples of normal bone marrow. **A,** An erythroblastic island in which several erythroid precursors cluster around a central "nursing" histiocyte. **B,** An early promyelocyte within which primary granules are prominent and a centrosome is present. **C,** A megakaryocyte with clusters or chains of platelets (small, darkly staining objects) being shed. **D,** Osteoclasts containing multiple nuclei that are separated by cytoplasm. These cells may be confused with megakaryocytes. **E,** Low-power scan of a normal bone marrow with a heterogeneous population of cells. **F,** Bone marrow biopsy illustrating the linear distribution of the osteoblasts along the bony trabecula. **G,** Bone marrow biopsy of a 63-year-old male who was being evaluated for anemia. A discrete germinal center is present (left-center of image) in this otherwise normal marrow biopsy. **H,** High-power view of a bone marrow biopsy from an individual with aplastic anemia showing markedly hypocellular marrow containing mainly fat cells. (Sources for photographs: **A,** American Society of Hematology Image Bank (ASHIB); 2004:101123; **B,** ASHIB; 2005:101355; **C,** ASHIB; 2005:101324; **D,** ASHIB; 2005:101358; **E,** ASHIB; 2005:101401; **F,** ASHIB; 2002:100504; **G,** ASHIB; 2004:101190; **H** from Kumar V et al: *Robbins and Cotran pathologic basis of disease,* ed 7, Philadelphia, 2005, Saunders.)

bone marrow is preferred as a safer procedure and because the bone marrow is the immediate source of iron destined for erythrocyte production.

Bone marrow aspiration is an important diagnostic test for severe central defects in hematopoiesis (e.g., aplastic anemia, metabolic anemias arising from insufficient iron or inadequate erythropoietin, thrombocytopenia, neutropenia; see Chapters 26 and 27). Examination of the bone marrow is also useful to diagnosis B lymphocyte immune deficiencies (see Chapter 8), nonmalignant myeloproliferative disorders (e.g., polycythemia vera), lymphoid/monocytic malignancies (e.g., leukemias, myelomas, lymphomas; see Chapters 27 and 28). This test can also be used to monitor the effects of chemotherapy on malignancies that have invaded the bone marrow (see Figure 25-26). A marrow aspirate that is richly cellular implies normal or increased hematopoiesis but does not indicate whether marrow activity is effective.

Results from bone marrow aspiration are sometimes limited because this technique disturbs the architecture of the marrow and only provides an analysis of the general cellularity (numbers of constituent cells) of the marrow. On occasion, analysis of an aspirate may only suggest the presence of a malignancy or a central defect in hematopoiesis without being clearly confirmatory, or the sample may be inadequate for diagnosis of bone marrow fibrosis. In these cases the need for a bone marrow biopsy may be indicated.

Table 25-9	Differential Cell Counts in Bone Marrow with Age				
Developing Cells in Marrow	Birth	1 mo-1 yr	1-4 yr	4-12 yr	Adult
Erythrocytic series	14	8	19	21	20
Lymphocytic series	14	47	22	18	17
Eosinophilic series	3	3	6	3	3
Neutrophilic series	60	33	50	52	57
Myeloid/ erythroid ratio	4:3	4:0	1:3	2:5	1:3

NOTE: Values are percentages of cell types counted during examination of a marrow specimen containing approximately 400 nucleated cells.

During a biopsy, a special needle is used to obtain a "core" or cylindrical sample of bone and marrow in which the three dimensional structure of the marrow is preserved. The biopsy specimens provide the most reliable and complete information about marrow cellularity (see Figure 25-26). Obtaining a bone marrow biopsy is, however, usually more painful and expensive than aspiration. Therefore, biopsy is not performed unless insufficient information is obtained from aspiration.

Blood Tests

Blood tests provide information about the absolute and relative numbers of blood cells in a specimen of blood, as well as various structural and functional characteristics of the cells, and usually provide the initial justification for performing a bone marrow aspiration. Deviations from the normal differential distribution and the presence of abnormal or immature cells can reflect disease, physiologic states (e.g., pregnancy, infancy, old age), injury, or dysfunction in almost any part of the body. Blood tests that reflect chiefly hematologic disorders are listed in Table 25-10.

Pediatrics and the Hematologic System

Blood cell counts tend to rise above adult levels at birth and then decline gradually throughout childhood. Table 25-11 lists normal ranges during infancy and childhood. The immediate rise in values is the result of accelerated hematopoiesis during fetal life, increased numbers of cells that result from the trauma of birth, and cutting of the umbilical cord.

Average blood volume in the full-term neonate is 85 ml per kilogram of body weight. The premature infant has a slightly larger blood volume of 90 ml per kilogram of body weight, with the mean increasing to 150 mg/kg during the first few days after birth. In both full-term and premature infants, blood volume decreases during the first few months.

Thereafter the average blood volume is 75 to 77 ml/kg, which is similar to that of older children and adults.

The hypoxic intrauterine environment stimulates erythropoietin production in the fetus and accelerates fetal erythropoiesis, producing polycythemia (excessive proliferation of erythrocyte precursors) of the newborn. After birth the oxygen from the lungs saturates arterial blood, and more oxygen is delivered to the tissues. In response to the change from a placental to a pulmonary oxygen supply during the first few days of life, levels of erythropoietin and the rate of blood cell formation decrease.

The very active rate of fetal erythropoiesis results in a large number of immature erythrocytes (reticulocytes) in the peripheral blood of full-term neonates. After birth the number of reticulocytes decreases about 50% every 12 hours so that it is rare to find an elevated reticulocyte count after the first week of life. During this period of rapid growth, the rate of erythrocyte destruction is greater than that in later childhood and adulthood. In full-term infants, normal erythrocyte life span is 60 to 80 days; in premature infants it may be as short as 20 to 30 days; and in children and adolescents it is the same as that in adults—120 days.

The postnatal fall in hemoglobin and hematocrit values is more marked in premature infants than in the full-term infant. In the preschool and school-age child, hemoglobin, hematocrit, and red blood cell counts gradually rise. Metabolic processes within the erythrocytes of neonates differ significantly from those of erythrocytes in the normal adult. Among other differences, the relatively young population of erythrocytes in the newborn consumes greater quantities of glucose than do erythrocytes in adults.

At birth, the lymphocyte count is high and continues to rise during the first year of life, and then steadily declines until lower adult values are reached. The lymphocytes of children also tend to have more cytoplasm and less compact nuclear chromatin than do the lymphocytes of adults. A possible explanation is that children tend to have more frequent viral infections, some of which are subclinical, and are receiving vaccinations, both of which are associated with atypical lymphocytes.

The neutrophil count, like the lymphocyte count, is high at birth and rises during the first days of life. After 2 weeks the neutrophil count falls to within or below the normal adult range. By approximately 4 years of age, the neutrophil count is the same as that of an adult. The eosinophil count is high in the first year of life and higher in children than in teenagers or adults. Monocyte counts also are high in the first year of life but then decrease to adult levels. Platelet counts in full-term neonates are comparable with platelet counts in adults and remain so throughout infancy and childhood.

Aging and the Hematologic System

Blood composition changes little with age. Erythrocyte life span in older adults is normal, although erythrocytes are replenished more slowly after bleeding, probably because of

Table 25-10   Blood Tests for Hematologic Disorders

Cell Type and Test	Properly Evaluated by Test	Possible Hematologic Cause of Abnormal Findings
Erythrocyte		
Red cell count	Number (in millions) of erythrocytes/μL of blood	Altered erythropoiesis, anemias, hemorrhage, Hodgkin disease, leukemia
Mean corpuscular volume	Size of erythrocytes	Anemias, thalassemias
Mean corpuscular hemoglobin (MCH)	Amount of hemoglobin in each erythrocyte (by weight)	Anemias, hemoglobinopathy
Mean corpuscular hemoglobin concentration (MCHC)	Concentration of hemoglobin in each erythrocyte (percentage of erythrocyte occupied by hemoglobin)	Anemias, hereditary spherocytosis
Hemoglobin determination	Amount of hemoglobin (by weight)/dl of blood	Anemias
Hematocrit determination	Percentage of a given volume of blood that is occupied by erythrocytes	Hemorrhage, polycythemia, erythrocytosis, anemias, leukemia
Reticulocyte count	Number of reticulocytes/μL of blood (also expressed as percentage of reticulocytes in total red cell count)	Hyperactive or hypoactive bone marrow function
Erythrocyte osmotic fragility test	Cellular shape (biconcavity), structure of plasma membrane	Anemias, hemolytic disease caused by ABO or Rh incompatibility, Hodgkin disease, polycythemia vera, thalassemia major
Hemoglobin electrophoresis	Relative percentage of different types of hemoglobin in erythrocytes	Sickle cell disease, sickle cell trait, hemoglobin C disease, hemoglobin C trait, thalassemias
Sickle cell test	Presence of hemoglobin S in erythrocytes	Sickle cell trait, sickle cell anemia
Glucose-6-phosphate dehydrogenase (G6PD) deficiency test	Deficiency of G6PD in erythrocytes	Hemolytic anemia
Hemoglobin Metabolism		
Serum ferritin determination	Depletion of body iron (potential deficiency of heme synthesis)	Iron deficiency anemias
Total iron-binding capacity (TIBC)	Amount of iron in serum plus amount of transferring available in serum (mcg/dl)	Hemorrhage, iron deficiency anemia, hemochromatosis, hemosiderosis, iron overload, anemias, thalassemia
Transferrin saturation	Percentage of transferrin that is saturated with iron	Acute hemorrhage, hemochromatosis, hemosiderosis, sideroblastic anemia, iron deficiency anemia, iron overload, thalassemia
Porphyrin analysis (protoporphyrin analysis)	Concentration of protoporphyrin in erythrocytes (mcg/dl); an indicator of iron-deficient erythropoiesis	Megaloblastic anemia, congenital erythropoietic porphyria
Direct antiglobulin test (DAT)	Antibody binding to erythrocytes	Hemolytic disease of the newborn, autoimmune hemolytic anemia, drug-induced hemolytic anemia, transfusion reaction
Antibody screen (indirect Coombs test)	Detection of antibodies to erythrocyte antigens (other than the ABO antigens)	Same as for DAT
Leukocytes		
Differential white cell count (absolute number of a type of leukocyte/μL of blood)	See below	See below
Neutrophil count	Neutrophils/μL	Myeloproliferative disorders, hematopoietic disorders, hemolysis, infection, immune deficiency
Lymphocyte count	Lymphocytes/μL	Infectious lymphocytosis, infectious mononucleosis, hematopoietic disorders, anemias, leukemia, lymphosarcoma, Hodgkin disease, primary immune deficiency
Plasma cell count	Plasma cells/μL	Infectious mononucleosis, lymphocytosis, plasma cell leukemia, primary immune deficiency
Monocyte count	Monocytes/μL	Hodgkin disease, infectious mononucleosis, monocytic leukemia, non-Hodgkin lymphoma, polycythemia vera, primary immune deficiency

Data from Byrne CJ et al: *Laboratory tests: implications for nursing care*, Menlo Park, CA, 1986, Addison-Wesley; Bick RL et al: *Hematology: clinical and laboratory practice*, St Louis, 1993, Mosby.
NOTE: See Figure 25-23 and Table 25-7 for information about clotting factors and their sequence of activation in the coagulation cascade.

Continued

Table 25-10   Blood Tests for Hematologic Disorders—cont'd

Cell Type and Test	Properly Evaluated by Test	Possible Hematologic Cause of Abnormal Findings
Eosinophil count	Eosinophils/µL	Hematopoietic disorders
Basophil count	Basophils/µL	Chronic myelogenous leukemia, hemolytic anemias, Hodgkin disease, polycythemia vera
Platelets and Clotting Factors		
Platelet count	Number of circulating platelets (in thousands)/µL of blood	Anemias, multiple myeloma, myelofibrosis, polycythemia vera, leukemia, disseminated intravascular coagulation (DIC), hemolytic disease of the newborn, idiopathic thrombocytopenic purpura, transfusion reaction, lymphoproliferative disorders
Bleeding time	Duration of bleeding following a standardized superficial puncture wound of the skin, integrity of the platelet plug, measured in minutes following puncture	Leukemia, anemias, DIC, fibrinolytic activity, purpuras, hemorrhagic disease of the newborn, infectious mononucleosis, multiple myeloma, clotting factor deficiencies, thrombasthenia, thrombocytopenia, von Willebrand disease
Clot retraction test	Platelet number and function, fibrinogen quantity and use, measured in hours required for expression of serum from a clot incubated in a test tube	Acute leukemia, aplastic anemia, factor XIII deficiency, increased fibrinolytic activity, Hodgkin disease, hyperfibrinogenemia or hypofibrinogenemia, idiopathic thrombocytopenic purpura, multiple myeloma, polycythemia vera, secondary thrombocytopenia, thrombasthenia
Platelet adhesion studies	Ability of platelets to adhere to foreign surfaces	Anemia, macroglobulinemia, Bernard-Soulier syndrome, multiple myeloma, myeloid metaplasia, plasma cell dyscrasias, thrombasthenia, thrombocytopathy, von Willebrand disease
Platelet aggregation tests	Ability of platelets to adhere to one another	Afibrinogenemia, Bernard-Soulier syndrome, thrombasthenia, hemorrhagic thrombocythemia, myeloid metaplasia, plasma cell dyscrasias, platelet release defects, polycythemia vera, preleukemia, sideroblastic anemia, von Willebrand disease, Waldenström macroglobulinemia, hypercoagulability
Whole blood clotting time (Lee-White coagulation time)	Overall ability of blood to clot, as measured in minutes in a test tube	Afibrinogenemia, clotting factor deficiencies, excessive fibrinolysis, hemorrhagic disease of the newborn, hypofibrinogenemia, hypoprothrombinemia, leukemia
Circulating anticoagulants (immunoglobulin G [IgG] or M [IgM] antibodies that inhibit coagulation)	Presence of antibodies that neutralize clotting factors and inhibit coagulation, as indicated by prolonged clotting time, prothrombin time, or partial thromboplastin time	Afibrinogenemia, presence of fibrin-fibrinogen degradation products, macroglobulinemia, multiple myeloma, DIC, plasma cell dyscrasias
Partial thromboplastin time (PTT)	Effectiveness of clotting factors (except factors VII and VIII), effectiveness of intrinsic pathway of coagulation cascade, as measured by a test tube (in seconds)	Presence of circulating anticoagulants, DIC, clotting factor deficiencies, excessive fibrinolysis, hemorrhagic disease of the newborn, hypofibrinogenemia and afibrinogenemia, prothrombin deficiency, von Willebrand disease, acute hemorrhage
Prothrombin time	Effectiveness of activity of prothrombin, fibrinogen, and factors V, VII, and X; effectiveness of vitamin K–dependent coagulation factors of the extrinsic and common pathways of the coagulation cascade as measured in a test tube (in seconds)	Hypofibrinogenemia, dysfibrinogenemia, and afibrinogenemia; presence of circulating anticoagulants; DIC; deficiency of factors V, VII, or X; presence of fibrin degradation products, increased fibrinolytic activity, hemolytic jaundice, hemorrhagic disease of the newborn; acute leukemia, polycythemia vera, prothrombin deficiency, multiple myeloma
Thrombin time	Quantity and activity of fibrinogen as measured in a test tube (in seconds)	Hypofibrinogenemia, dysfibrinogenemia, and afibrinogenemia; presence of circulating anticoagulants; hemorrhagic disease of the newborn, polycythemia vera; increase in fibrin-fibrinogen degradation products; increased fibrinolytic activity

Table 25-10	Blood Tests for Hematologic Disorders—cont'd	

Cell Type and Test	Properly Evaluated by Test	Possible Hematologic Cause of Abnormal Findings
Fibrinogen assay	Amount of fibrinogen available for fibrin formation	Acute leukemia, congenital hypofibrinogenemia or afibrinogenemia, DIC, increased fibrinolytic activity, severe hemorrhage
Fibrin-fibrinogen degradation products (fibrin-fibrinogen split products)	Fibrinogenic activity as measured by levels of fibrin-fibrinogen degradation products (in mcg/ml of blood)	Transfusion reactions, DIC, internal hemorrhage in the newborn, deep vein thrombosis, pulmonary embolism

Table 25-11	Hematologic Values During Infancy and Childhood								
				Differential Counts					
Age	Hemoglobin (g/dl):Mean	Hematocrit (%):Mean	Reticulocytes (%):Mean	Leukocytes (WBC/mm³):Mean	Neutrophils (%):Mean	Lymphocytes (%):Mean	Eosinophils (%):Mean	Monocytes (%):Mean	Platelets (10^3/mm³)
Cord blood	16.8	55	5.0	18,000	61	31	2	6	290
2 wk	16.5	50	1.0	12,000	40	48	3	9	252
3 mo	12.0	36	1.0	12,000	30	63	2	5	140-340
6 mo-6 yr	12.0	37	1.0	10,000	45	48	2	5	140-340
7-12 yr	13.0	38	1.0	8,000	55	38	2	5	140-340
Adult	13.0	40	1.0	8,000	55	35	2	5	140-340
Female	14	41	0.8-4.1	7,400	54-62	25-33	1-4	3-7	140-340
Male	16	47	0.8-2.5	7,400	54-62	25-33	1-4	3-7	140-340

WBC, White blood cell.

iron depletion. Total serum iron, total iron-binding capacity, and intestinal iron absorption are all decreased in older adults. Iron deficiency is often responsible for the low hemoglobin levels noted in older adults. The plasma membranes of erythrocytes become increasingly fragile, presumably because of physical trauma inflicted during circulation.

Lymphocyte function decreases with age (see Chapters 7 and 8), causing changes in cellular immunity with some decline in T cell function. The humoral immune system is less able to respond to antigenic challenge. No changes in platelet numbers or structure have been observed in elderly persons, yet platelet adhesiveness probably increases. Although fibrinogen levels and factors V, VII, and IX tend to be increased in older adults, evidence concerning hypercoagulability is inconclusive.

SUMMARY REVIEW

Components of the Hematologic System

1. Blood consists of cells suspended in a solution of about 90% water and 10% solutes. In adults the total blood volume is approximately 5.5 L.
2. Plasma, the liquid portion of the blood, contains two major groups of proteins: albumins and globulins.
3. The cellular elements of blood are the erythrocytes (red blood cells), leukocytes (white blood cells), and platelets (thrombocytes).
4. Erythrocytes are the most abundant cells of the blood, occupying approximately 48% of the blood volume in men and approximately 42% in women. Erythrocytes are responsible for tissue oxygenation.
5. Leukocytes are fewer in number than erythrocytes and constitute approximately 5000 to 10,000 cells/mm^3 of blood. Leukocytes defend the body against infection and remove dead or injured host cells.
6. Leukocytes are classified as either granulocytes (neutrophils, basophils, eosinophils) or agranulocytes (monocytes, macrophages, lymphocytes).
7. The neutrophil is the most abundant leukocyte (approximately 55% of the leukocytes) and is the primary granulocyte that defends against infections.
8. Lymphocytes are the primary cells of the immune response.
9. Platelets are not cells—they are disk-shaped cytoplasmic fragments. Platelets are essential for blood coagulation and control of bleeding.
10. The lymphoid organs are classified as primary (thymus and bone marrow) or secondary (spleen, lymph nodes, tonsils, and Peyer patches of the small intestine).
11. The lymphoid organs are sites of residence, proliferation, differentiation, and function of lymphocytes and mononuclear phagocytes.
12. The spleen is the largest of the secondary lymphoid organs and functions as the site of hematopoiesis in the fetus, filters and cleanses the blood, and is a reservoir for lymphocytes and other blood cells.
13. The lymph nodes are the site of development or activity of large numbers of lymphocytes, monocytes, and macrophages.
14. The MPS is composed of macrophages in tissue and lymphoid organs.
15. The MPS is the main line of defense against bacteria in the bloodstream and cleanses the blood by removing old, injured, or dead blood cells; antigen-antibody complexes; and macromolecules.

Development of Blood Cells

1. Hematopoiesis, or blood cell production, occurs in the liver and spleen of the fetus and in the bone marrow after birth.
2. Hematopoiesis involves two stages: (1) proliferation and (2) maturation.
3. Hematopoiesis continues throughout life to replace blood cells that grow old and die, are killed by disease, or are lost through bleeding.
4. Bone marrow consists of red (hematopoietic) marrow (blood vessels, mononuclear phagocytes, stem cells, blood cells in various stages of differentiation, stromal cells) and yellow marrow (fatty tissue).
5. The bone marrow contains multiple populations of *stem cells*; mesenchymal stem cells develop into fibroblasts, osteoclasts, and adipocytes; and hematopoietic stem cells develop into blood cells.

6. Regulation of hematopoiesis possibly occurs two ways: (1) by stromal cells involved in cell contact processes and (2) by cytokines or regulatory molecules.
7. Specific hematopoietic growth factors (e.g., colony-stimulating factors) are necessary for the adequate production of myeloid, erythroid, lymphoid, and megakaryocytic lineages.
8. Erythropoiesis (production of erythrocytes) is regulated by erythropoietin. Erythropoietin is secreted by the kidneys in response to tissue hypoxia and causes a compensatory increase in erythrocyte production if the oxygen content of the blood decreases because of anemia, high altitude, or pulmonary disease.
9. Hemoglobin, the oxygen-carrying protein of the erythrocyte, enables the blood to transport 100 times more oxygen than could be transported dissolved in plasma alone.
10. The iron cycle reutilizes iron released from old or damaged erythrocytes. Iron binds to transferrin in the blood, is transported to macrophages of the MPS, and is stored in the cytoplasm as ferritin.
11. Granulocytes and monocytes in the blood develop from common myeloid progenitor cells in the bone marrow under the direction of several growth factors, including stem cell factor, IL-3, and GM-CSF.
12. Platelets develop from megakaryocytes by a process called *endomitosis*, which is controlled by thrombopoietin. During endomitosis the megakaryocytes undergo mitosis but not cell division and the cytoplasm and plasma membrane fragment into platelets.

Mechanisms of Hemostasis

1. Hemostasis, or arrest of bleeding in damaged vessels, involves (1) vasoconstriction, (2) damage to the endothelium and exposure of connective tissue resulting in formation of a platelet plug, (3) activation of the clotting cascade, (4) formation of a blood clot, and (5) activation of fibrinolysis for clot retraction and clot dissolution.
2. Platelet activation involves three linked processes: (1) adhesion, (2) activation, and (3) aggregation.
3. A blood clot is a meshwork of protein strands that stabilizes the platelet plug. The strands are made of fibrin. Fibrin is the end product of the coagulation cascade.
4. The coagulation cascade is composed of intrinsic and extrinsic pathways, with the extrinsic pathway being dominant. The intrinsic pathway is initiated by TF that forms a complex with TF/VIIa complex.
5. The endothelium prevents the formation of spontaneous clots in normal vessels by several anticoagulant mechanisms, including production of NO and PGI$_2$, thrombin inhibitors (antithrombin III), tissue factor inhibitors (tissue factor pathway inhibitors), and degrading activated clotting factors (thrombomodulin-protein C).
6. Fibrinolysis (breakdown of blood clots) is the function of the plasminogen-plasmin system. Plasmin is a degrading enzyme of fibrin clots. It is produced from plasminogen by activated by plasminogen activators (t-PA, u-PA), thrombin, fibrin, factor XIIa, factor XIa, and kallikrein.
7. Products of fibrinolysis include fibrin degradation products, such as D-dimer.

Clinical Evaluation of the Hematologic System

1. Tests of bone marrow function include bone marrow aspiration and bone marrow biopsy.
2. Cells contained in the marrow specimen are assessed with respect to (1) relative numbers of stem cells and their developing daughter cells and (2) morphologic structure.

SUMMARY REVIEW—cont'd

Pediatrics and the Hematologic System

1. Blood cell counts rise above adult levels at birth and then gradually decline throughout childhood.
2. The average blood volume of an infant is 75 to 77 ml/kg, which is similar to that of older children and adults.
3. In response to the change from a placental to a pulmonary oxygen supply during the first few days of life, levels of erythropoietin and the rate of blood cell formation decrease.
4. The normal erythrocyte life span is 60 to 80 days in full-term infants, 20 to 30 days in premature infants, and 120 days in children, adolescents, and adults.
5. The lymphocyte count is high at birth, rises further during the first year of life, and steadily declines until lower adult volumes are reached.
6. The neutrophil count is very high at birth, falls to adult ranges after 2 weeks, and is the same as for adults by 4 years of age.
7. The eosinophil count is high in the first year of life and is higher in children than in adolescents and adults. Monocyte counts are high in the first year of life and decrease to adult levels.
8. Platelet counts in full-term infants are comparable with those in adults and remain so throughout childhood.

Aging and the Hematologic System

1. Blood composition changes little with age. A delay in erythrocyte replenishment may occur after bleeding, presumably because of iron deficiency.
2. Lymphocyte function appears to decrease with age. Particularly affected is a decrease in cellular immunity.
3. Platelet adhesiveness probably increases with age.

KEY TERMS

Agranulocyte, 955, 956
Albumin, 953
Antithrombin III (AT-III), 978
Apoferritin, 969
Apotransferrin, 971
Basophil, 956
Blood clot, 976
Bone marrow, 962
Clotting (coagulation) system, 976
Clotting factor, 954
Colony-stimulating factor (CSF, hematopoietic growth factor), 963
Cyclooxygenase (COX-1), 976
D-dimer, 980
Dendritic cell, 957
Deoxyhemoglobin, 968
Endomitosis, 971
Eosinophil, 956
Erythroblast, 966
Erythrocyte (red blood cell [RBC]), 954
Erythropoiesis, 965
Erythropoietin, 965
Fibrin degradation product (FDP), 980
Fibrinolysis, 972
Fibrinolytic system (plasminogen-plasmin system), 979
Globin, 967
Globulin, 953

GPIIb-IIIa complex, 976
Granulocyte, 955
Hematopoiesis, 961
Hematopoietic stem cell, 962
Heme, 967
Hemoglobin (Hb), 967
Hemosiderin, 969
Hemostasis, 972
Immunocyte, 955
Leukocyte (white blood cell [WBC]), 955
Lymphocyte, 956
Macrophage, 957
Marginating storage pool, 963
Mast cell, 956
Megakaryocyte, 957
Mesenchymal stem cell, 961
Methemoglobin, 968
Monocyte, 957
Mononuclear phagocyte system (MPS), 957
Myeloid tissue, 962
Myoglobin, 969
Natural killer (NK) cell, 957
Neutrophil (polymorphonuclear neutrophil [PMN]), 955
Nitric oxide (NO), 972
Normoblast, 966
Oxyhemoglobin, 968
Phagocyte, 955

Plasma, 952
Plasma protein, 952
Plasmin, 979
Plasminogen, 979
Platelet (thrombocyte), 957
Platelet adhesion, 973
Platelet aggregation, 976
Platelet-release reaction, 973
Proerythroblast, 965
Prostacyclin (PGI), 972
Protein C, 979
Protein S, 979
Protoporphyrin, 968
Reticulocyte, 966
Serum, 952
Steel factor, 963
Stromal cell, 963
Thrombomodulin, 979
Thromboxane A_2 (TXA$_2$), 976
Tissue factor (TF, tissue thromboplastin), 977
Tissue factor pathway inhibitor (TFPI), 979
Tissue plasminogen activator (t-PA), 980
Transferrin, 971
Urokinase-like plasminogen activator (u-PA), 980
von Willebrand factor (vWF), 973

REFERENCES

1. Chuang VT, Otagiri M: Recombinant human serum albumin, *Drugs Today* 43(8):547-561, 2007.
2. Babior BM, Stossel TP: *Hematology: a pathophysiological approach*, New York, 1984, Churchill Livingstone.
3. Mohandas N, Gallagher PG: Red cell membrane: past, present, and future, *Blood* 112(10):3939-3948, 2008.
4. Karikyawasam HH, Robinson DS: The eosinophil: the cell and its weapons, the cytokines, its locations, *Semin Respir Crit Care Med* 27(2):117-127, 2006.
5. Prussin C, Metcalfe DD: IgE, mast cells, basophils, and eosinophils, *J Allergy Clin Immunol* 117(2 Suppl):S450-S456, 2006.
6. Hume DA: The mononuclear phagocyte system, *Curr Opin Immunol* 18(1):49-53, 2005.
7. Junt T, Scandella E, Ludewig B: Form follows function: lymphoid tissue microarchitecture in antimicrobial immune defense, *Nat Rev Immunol* 8(10):764-775, 2008.
8. Mueller SN, Ahmed R: Lymphoid stroma in the initiation and control of immune responses, *Immunol Rev* 224(1):284-294, 2008.
9. Ross FP, Christiano AM: Nothing but skin and bones, *J Clin Invest* 116(5):1140-1149, 2006.
10. Bar-Shavit Z: The osteoclast: a multinucleated, hematopoietic-origin, bone-resorbing osteoimmune cell, *J Cell Biochem* 102(5):1130-1139, 2007.

11. Yin T, Li L: The stem cell niches in bone, *J Clin Invest* 116(5): 1195-1201, 2006.
12. *Stem cell information*, Bethesda MD, 2009. National Institutes of Health, U.S. Department of Health and Human Services [cited, January 17, 2009]. Available at http://stemcells.nih.gov/info.
13. Ratajczak MZ: Phenotypic and functional characterization of hematopoietic stem cells, *Curr Opin Hematol* 15(4):293-300, 2008.
14. Valtieri M, Sorrentino A: The mesenchymal stromal cell contribution to homeostasis, *J Cell Physiol* 217(2):296-300, 2008.
15. Möhle R, Kanz L: Hematopoietic growth factors for hematopoietic stem cell mobilization and expansion, *Semin Hematol* 44(3):193-202, 2007.
16. Pusic I, DiPersio JF: The use of growth factors in hematopoietic stem cell transplantation, *Curr Pharm Des* 14(20):1950-1961, 2008.
17. Chasis JA, Mohandas N: Erythroblastic islands: niches for erythropoiesis, *Blood* 112(3):470-478, 2008.
18. Schechter AN: Hemoglobin research and the origins of molecular medicine, *Blood* 112(10):3927-3938, 2008.
19. Edison ES, Bajel A, Chandy M: Iron homeostasis: new players, newer insights, *Eur J Haematol* 81(6):411-424, 2008.
20. West AR, Oates PS: Mechanisms of heme iron absorption: current questions and controversies, *World J Gastroenterol* 14(26):4101-4110, 2008.
21. Naito M: Macrophage differentiation and function in health and disease, *Path Int* 58(3):143-155, 2008.
22. Kaushansky K: Historical review: megakaryopoiesis and thrombopoiesis, *Blood* 111(3):981-986, 2008.
23. Marcucci R, Romano M: Thrombopoietin and its splicing variants: structure and functions in thrombopoiesis and beyond, *Biochim Biophys Acta* 1782(7-8):427-432, 2008.
24. Freestone B, Lip GY: The endothelium and atrial fibrillation. The prothrombotic state revisited, *Hamostaseologie* 28(4):207-212, 2008.
25. Reininger AJ: Function of von Willebrand factor in haemostasis and thrombosis, *Haemophilia* 14(Suppl 5):11-26, 2008.
26. Furie B, Furie BC: Mechanisms of thrombus formation, *N Engl J Med* 359(9):938-949, 2008.
27. Reininger AJ: VWF attributes—impact on thrombus formation, *Thromb Res* 122(Suppl 4):S9-S13, 2008.
28. Andrews RK, Berndt MC: Platelet adhesion: a game of catch and release, *J Clin Invest* 118(9):3009-3011, 2008.
29. Ren Q, Ye S, Whiteheart SW: The platelet release reaction: just when you thought platelet secretion was simple, *Curr Opin Hematol* 15(5):537-541, 2008.
30. Gleissner CA, von Hundelshausen P, Ley K: Platelet chemokines in vascular disease, *Arterioscler Thromb Vasc Biol* 28(11):1920-1927, 2008.
31. Krötz F, Sohn H-Y, Klauss V: Antiplatelet drugs in cardiological practice: established strategies and new developments, *Vasc Health Risk Manag* 4(3):637-645, 2008.
32. De Gaetano G, Crescente M, Cerletti C: Current concepts about inhibition of platelet aggregation, *Platelets* 19(8):565-570, 2008.
33. Hoffman M: Some things I thought I knew about tissue factor that turn out to be wrong, *Thromb Res* 122(Suppl 1):S73-S77, 2008.
34. Pendurthi UR, Rao LV: Factor VIIa interaction with tissue factor and endothelial cell protein C receptor on cell surfaces, *Semin Hematol* 45(2 Suppl 1):S21-S24, 2008.
35. Di Cera E, Thrombin, *Mol Aspects Med* 29(4):203-254, 2008.
36. Müller F, Renné T: Novel roles for factor XII-driven plasma contact activation system, *Curr Opin Hematol* 15(5):516-521, 2008.
37. Henry BL, Desai UR: Recent research developments in the direct inhibition of coagulation proteinases—inhibitors of the initiation phase, *Cardiovasc Hematol Agents Med Chem* 6(4):323-336, 2008.
38. Wang L, Bastarache JA, Ware LB: The coagulation cascade in sepsis, *Curr Pharm Des* 14(19):1860-1869, 2008.
39. Castoldi E, Hackeng TM: Regulation of coagulation by protein S, *Curr Opin Hematol* 15(5):529-536, 2008.
40. Jackson CJ, Xue M: Activated protein C—an anticoagulant that does more than stop clots, *Int J Biochem Cell Biol* 40(12):2692-2697, 2008.
41. Weisel JW, Litvinov RI: The biochemical and physical process of fibrinolysis and effects of clot structure and stability on the lysis rate, *Cardiovasc Hematol Agents Med Chem* 6(3):161-180, 2008.
42. Zorio E et al: Fibrinolysis: the key to new pathogenetic mechanisms, *Curr Med Chem* 15(9):923-929, 2008.
43. Righini M et al. D-dimer for venous thromboembolism diagnosis: 20 years later, *J Thromb Haemost* 6(7):1059-1071, 2008.

ALTERATIONS OF ERYTHROCYTE FUNCTION

NEAL S. ROTE • KATHRYN L. McCANCE

MEDIA RESOURCES

 Evolve Website (http://evolve.elsevier.com/McCance/)
- Review Questions and Answers
- Animations
- Glossary (with audio pronunciation for selected terms)
- WebLinks

Online Course
- Module 13

CHAPTER OUTLINE

ANEMIA
  Classification
  Macrocytic-Normochromic Anemias
  Microcytic-Hypochromic Anemias
  Normocytic-Normochromic Anemias

MYELOPROLIFERATIVE RED BLOOD CELL DISORDERS (POLYCYTHEMIA)

Alterations of erythrocyte function involve either insufficient or excessive numbers of erythrocytes in the circulation or normal numbers of cells with abnormal components. Anemias are conditions in which there are too few erythrocytes or an insufficient volume of erythrocytes in the blood. Polycythemias are conditions in which erythrocyte numbers or volume is excessive. Each of these conditions has many causes and is a pathophysiologic manifestation of a variety of disease states.

ANEMIA

Strictly speaking, **anemia** is a reduction in the total number of erythrocytes in the circulating blood or a decrease in the quality or quantity of hemoglobin. Anemias commonly result from (1) impaired erythrocyte production, (2) blood loss (acute or chronic), (3) increased erythrocyte destruction, or (4) a combination of these three.

Classification

Anemias are classified by their causes or to changes in their morphology (size, shape, or hemoglobin content) (Box 26-1). The most common classification is based on changes that affect the size or hemoglobin content of the erythrocyte (Table 26-1). The terminology reflects these characteristics; terms that end in "-cytic" refer to cell size, whereas "-chromic" refers to hemoglobin content (Table 26-2). Additional descriptors of erythrocytes associated with some anemias include **anisocytosis** (assuming various sizes) or **poikilocytosis** (assuming various shapes) (Figure 26-1).

CLINICAL MANIFESTATIONS The fundamental physiologic manifestation of anemia is a reduced oxygen-carrying capacity of the blood resulting in tissue hypoxia. Symptoms of anemia vary, depending on the body's ability to compensate for hypoxia (Figure 26-2). Anemia that is mild and develops gradually, so-called *asymptomatic anemia*, is usually easier to compensate for and may cause problems for the individual only during physical exertion. As the reduction in red blood cells (RBCs) continues, symptoms become more pronounced and alterations of specific organs and compensatory effects become more apparent. Compensation generally involves the cardiovascular, respiratory, and hematologic systems. (Hematologic findings associated with various anemias are listed in Table 26-3 and progression and manifestations of anemias are shown in Figure 26-2.)

The initial manifestations of anemia are apparent in the cardiovascular system. With hemorrhage, a reduction in the number of RBCs results in reduced blood volume. Compensation for a reduced blood volume causes fluids to move from the interstitium into the intravascular space (osmotic gradient), expanding plasma volume. This compensatory

Box 26-1   Etiologic (Pathophysiologic) Classification of Anemias

Decreased or Defective Production of Erythrocytes
Altered hemoglobin synthesis
  Iron deficiency
  Thalassemia
  Anemia of chronic inflammation
Altered deoxyribonucleic acid (DNA) synthesis resulting from deficient nutrients
Pernicious anemia (decreased B_{12}, folate)
Stem cell dysfunction
  Aplastic anemia
  Myeloproliferative leukemia
Bone marrow infiltration
  Carcinoma
  Lymphoma
Pure red cell aplasia

Increased Erythrocyte Destruction
Blood loss
  Acute—hemorrhage, trauma
  Chronic—gastrointestinal bleeding, menorrhagia
Hemolysis (intracorpuscular defect)
  Membrane—hereditary spherocytosis
  Hemoglobin—sickle cell trait or disease
  Glycolysis—pyruvate kinase
  Oxidation—glucose-6-phosphate dehydrogenase (G6PD) deficiency
Hemolysis (extracorpuscular defect)
  Immune mechanisms—warm antibody/cold antibody
  Infection—clostridial, malarial
  Trauma to erythrocyte—hemolytic uremic syndrome
  Splenic sequestration—hypersplenism

mechanism maintains adequate blood volume, increasing venous return, preload, and stroke volume, but the viscosity (thickness) decreases causing the blood to become diluted. The diluted blood flows faster and more turbulently than normal blood.

Hypoxemia, reduced oxygen levels in the blood, further contributes to cardiovascular dysfunction by causing systemic arterial dilation leading to decreased vascular resistance, which effectively reduces afterload (the pressure necessary to eject blood from the left ventricle into the aorta). Additionally, anemia activates the sympathetic nervous system, causing the heart rate to increase.

These hemodynamic alterations—increased preload, heart rate, and stroke volume, and a reduced afterload—all contribute to increased cardiac output in an effort to maintain adequate oxygen delivery. Without timely interventions, cardiac compensatory mechanisms fail and precipitate the development of congestive heart failure. (Mechanisms of congestive heart failure are described in Chapter 30.)

Tissue hypoxia creates additional demands and compensatory actions on the pulmonary and hematologic systems. The rate and depth of breathing increase in an attempt to increase the availability of oxygen. These demands are accompanied by an increase in the release of oxygen from hemoglobin because of an increase in 2,3-diphosphoglycerate (DPG) in the erythrocytes. (Mechanisms of oxygen transport and release by hemoglobin are described in Chapter 32.) When compensatory mechanisms fail, individuals may experience shortness of breath (dyspnea), a rapid, pounding heartbeat (palpitations), dizziness, and fatigue even at rest. In mild, chronic conditions, these symptoms might be experienced only when demand for oxygen is increased (i.e., during physical exertion), but in severe conditions they may be experienced at rest. Decreased blood supply to skeletal and cardiac muscle also may contribute to the development of muscle pain (claudication) and cardiac angina.

Manifestations of anemia may be observed in other parts of the body. The skin, mucous membranes, lips, nail beds, and conjunctivae become pale as a result of reduced hemoglobin concentration. If anemia is caused by RBC destruction (hemolysis), the skin may become yellowish because of accumulation of the products of hemolysis. Tissue hypoxia also affects the skin causing impaired healing and loss of elasticity, as well as thinning and early graying of the hair.

Affects on the nervous system can occur if the anemia is caused by a vitamin B_{12} deficiency. Myelin degeneration may occur with the resultant loss of fibers in the spinal cord, producing paresthesias (numbness), gait disturbances, extreme weakness, spasticity, and reflex abnormalities. Decreased oxygen supply to the gastrointestinal (GI) tract often produces abdominal pain, nausea, vomiting, and anorexia. A low-grade fever of less than 38.5° C (less than about 101° F) occurs in some anemic individuals and may be the result of leukocyte pyrogens released from ischemic tissues.

When the anemia is severe or rapid in onset (i.e., hemorrhage), peripheral blood vessels constrict, diverting blood flow to vital organs. Decreased blood flow detected by the kidneys activates the renal renin-angiotensin response. This lifesaving maneuver causes vasoconstriction and increases salt and water retention to increase blood volume and improve kidney perfusion. These situations are emergencies and require immediate intervention to stop the acute loss of blood; consequently, long-term compensatory mechanisms do not develop.

Interventions for slowly developing anemic conditions require treatment of the underlying disorder and palliation of associated symptoms. Therapeutic interventions include control of bleeding, transfusions, dietary correction, and administration of supplemental vitamins or iron.

Macrocytic-Normochromic Anemias

The **macrocytic (megaloblastic) anemias** are characterized by unusually large stem cells (megaloblasts) in the marrow that mature into erythrocytes that are unusually large in size (macrocytes), thickness, and volume.[1] The hemoglobin content is normal (normochromic). These anemias are the result of defective erythrocyte precursor DNA synthesis commonly caused by deficiencies of vitamin B_{12} (cobalamin) or folate, coenzymes that are required for nuclear maturation and the DNA synthesis pathway. More than half the residents in nursing homes are anemic, and about a third of those cases are caused by deficiencies in vitamin B_{12}, folate, or iron.[2,3] Vitamin

Table 26-1	Morphologic Classification of Anemias	
Morphology of Remaining Erythrocytes	**Name and Mechanism of Anemia**	**Primary Cause**
Macrocytic-normochromic anemia: large, abnormally shaped erythrocytes but normal hemoglobin concentrations	Pernicious anemia: lack of vitamin B_{12} (cobalamin) for erythropoiesis; abnormal deoxyribonucleic acid (DNA) and ribonucleic acid (RNA) synthesis in the erythroblast; premature cell death	Congenital or acquired deficiency of intrinsic factor (IF); genetic disorder of DNA synthesis
	Folate deficiency anemia: lack of folate for erythropoiesis; premature cell death	Dietary folate deficiency
Microcytic-hypochromic anemia: small, abnormally shaped erythrocytes and reduced hemoglobin concentration	Iron deficiency anemia: lack of iron for hemoglobin production; insufficient hemoglobin	Chronic blood loss; dietary iron deficiency, disruption of iron metabolism or iron cycle (see Chapter 25)
	Sideroblastic anemia: dysfunctional iron uptake by erythroblasts and defective porphyrin and heme synthesis	Congenital dysfunction of iron metabolism in erythroblasts, acquired dysfunction of iron metabolism as a result of drugs or toxins
	Thalassemia: impaired synthesis of α- or β-chain of hemoglobin A; phagocytosis of abnormal erythroblasts in the marrow	Congenital genetic defect of globin synthesis
Normocytic-normochromic anemia: normal size, normal hemoglobin concentration	Aplastic anemia: insufficient erythropoiesis	Depressed stem cell proliferation resulting in bone marrow aplasia
	Posthemorrhagic anemia: blood loss	Acute or chronic hemorrhage that stimulates increased erythropoiesis, which eventually depletes body iron
	Hemolytic anemia: premature destruction (lysis) of mature erythrocytes in the circulation	Increased fragility of erythrocytes
	Sickle cell anemia: abnormal hemoglobin synthesis, abnormal cell shape with susceptibility to damage, lysis, and phagocytosis	Congenital dysfunction of hemoglobin synthesis
	Anemia of chronic disease: abnormally increased demand for new erythrocytes	Chronic infection or inflammation; malignancy

Table 26-2	Terms Used in Assessment of Erythrocytes	
	Erythrocyte Volume	**Hemoglobin Content**
Normal	Normocytic	Normochromic
Increased	Macrocytic (higher mean corpuscular volume [MCV])	Hyperchromic (higher mean corpuscular hemoglobin concentration [MCHC])
Decreased	Microcytic (lower MCV)	Hypochromic (lower MCHC)

B_{12} deficiency in older adults often goes unrecognized because of the subtle nature of manifestations that are potentially serious, particularly hematologically and neurologically.

In spite of defective DNA synthesis in megaloblasts, ribonucleic acid (RNA)–controlled processes (RNA replication and hemoglobin synthesis) occur at a normal rate, resulting in the unequal growth and development of the cytoplasm and nucleus. Asynchronous development leads to a larger than normal normoblast with a disproportionally small nucleus. With each cell division the disproportion between RNA and DNA becomes more obvious. The chromatin in the nucleus fails to clump normally, resulting in finely distributed chromatin throughout the nucleus. The altered pattern of chromatin deposition allows for microscopic differentiation of normoblasts from megaloblasts. Hemoglobin increases in proportion to the size of the cell; thus the mean corpuscular hemoglobin concentration (MCHC) remains normal and the megaloblastic anemias, in the absence of complications, are normochromic.

Immature precursors of the megaloblastic RBCs have a greater chance of dying during maturation than do normoblastic precursors. Phagocytosis of these cells occurs within the bone marrow, resulting in a reduction of reticulocytes and erythrocytes in the circulation. Additionally there is an increase in lactic dehydrogenase, reflecting cellular destruction, and indirect bilirubin, from the breakdown of heme. Both of these substances may be measured in the blood, providing biochemical evidence of ineffective erythropoiesis.

Defective DNA synthesis also may result in significant enlargement of neutrophil precursors creating giant metamyelocytes with a tendency to have more nuclear lobes than normal. Other cells throughout the body also may demonstrate enlargement and nuclear abnormalities. Cells lining epithelium and those with high turnover rates are most affected.

Pernicious Anemia

Pernicious anemia (PA), the most common type of megaloblastic anemia, is caused by vitamin B_{12} deficiency, which is often associated with the end stage of type A chronic atrophic

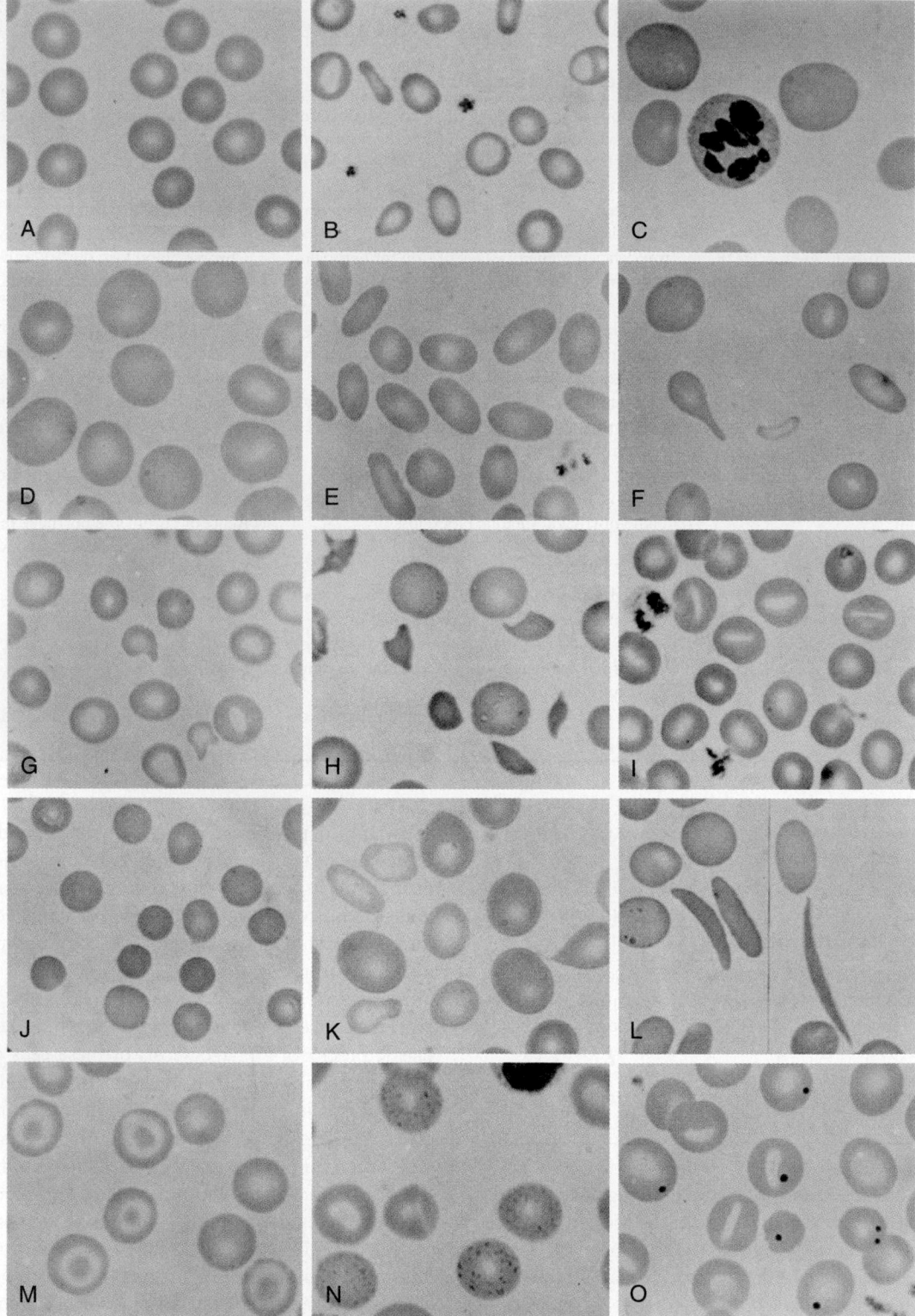

Figure 26-1 Appearance of red blood cells in various disorders. **A,** Normal blood smear. **B,** Microcytic-hypochromic anemia (iron deficiency). **C,** Macrocytic anemia (pernicious anemia). **D,** Macrocytic anemia in pregnancy. **E,** Hereditary elliptocytosis. **F,** Myelofibrosis (teardrop). **G,** Hemolytic anemia associated with prosthetic heart valve. **H,** Microangiopathic anemia. **I,** Stomatocytes. **J,** Spherocytes (hereditary spherocytosis). **K,** Sideroblastic anemia; note the double population of red blood cells. **L,** Sickle cell anemia. **M,** Target cells (after splenectomy). **N,** Basophil stippling in case of unexplained anemia. **O,** Howell-Jolly bodies (after splenectomy). (From Wintrobe MM et al: *Clinical hematology,* ed 8, Philadelphia, 1981, Lea & Febiger.)

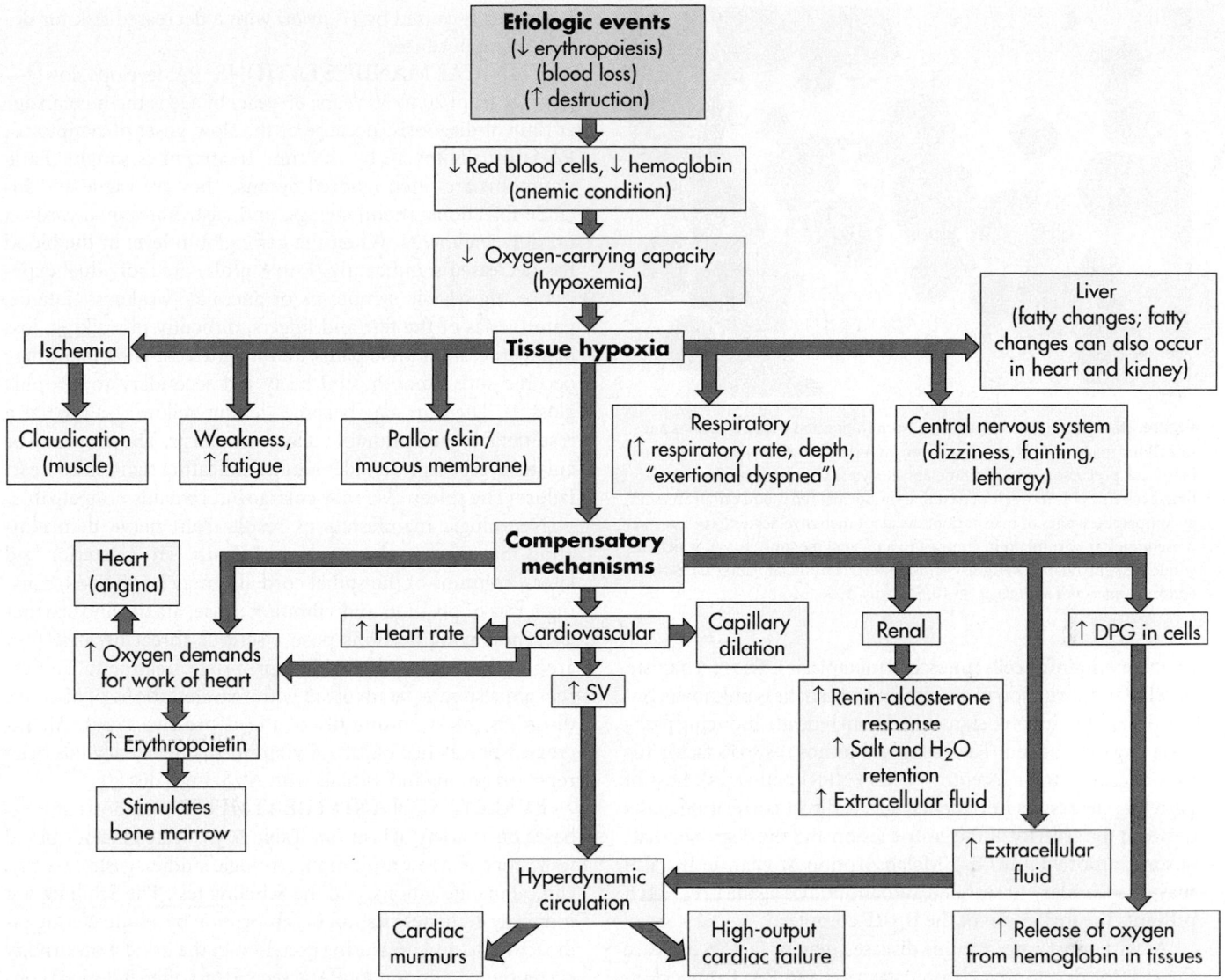

Figure 26-2 Progression and manifestations of anemia. *DPG*, Diphosphoglycerate; *SV*, stroke volume.

(congenital or autoimmune) gastritis (see Figure 26-1, *C*; Figure 26-3). *Pernicious* means highly injurious or destructive and reflects the fact that this condition was once fatal. It most commonly affects individuals older than the age of 50 who are of Northern European descent, as well as blacks and Hispanics. Females are more prone to develop PA, with black females having an earlier onset.

PATHOPHYSIOLOGY The principal disorder in PA is an absence of **intrinsic factor (IF),** a transporter required for absorption of dietary vitamin B_{12}. Vitamin B_{12} catalyzes the action of methionine synthase and R-methylmalonyl-coenzyme A (CoA) mutase, which acts to promote nuclear maturation and DNA synthesis in erythrocytes. IF, along with hydrochloric acid, is secreted by gastric parietal cells and complexes with dietary vitamin B_{12} in the small intestine. The B_{12}-IF complex binds to cell surface receptors in the ileum and is transported across the intestinal mucosa. Deficiency in IF secretion may be congenital or result from adult onset

gastric mucosal atrophy and destruction of parietal cells. In older adults, virtually all the vitamin B_{12}-deficiency anemia is caused by a failure of IF-related absorption.[4] Congenital IF deficiency is a genetic disorder that demonstrates an autosomal recessive inheritance pattern. Gastric atrophy commonly occurs in the presence of type A chronic gastritis and may be autoimmune. Autoantibodies against gastric parietal cells are frequently observed.[5] The autoantibodies are directed against H^+, K^+-ATPase, an enzyme responsible for secretion of hydrogen ions by parietal cells in exchange for potassium ions. Other characteristics associated with chronic gastric atrophy include achlorhydria, low serum levels of pepsinogen I, hypergastrinemia, and gastric carcinoids.

Early in the disease process the gastric submucosa becomes infiltrated with inflammatory cells, eventually extending into the lamina propria and causing degeneration of the parietal and zymogenic cells. Late in the course of the disease, the parietal and zymogenic cells are destroyed and replaced by

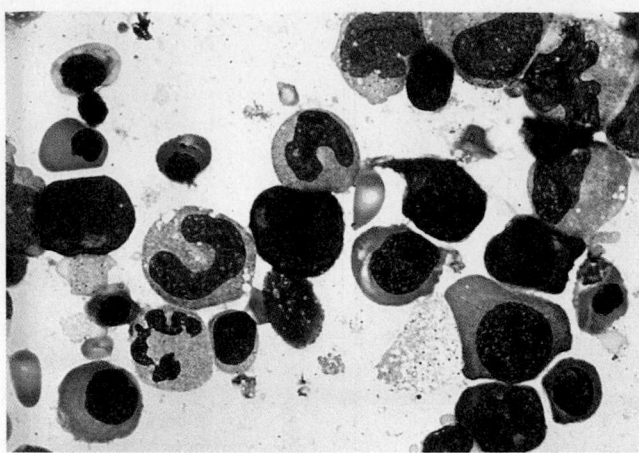

Figure 26-3 Bone marrow aspirate from individual with pernicious anemia. Bone marrow aspirate smear from an individual with megaloblastic red blood cell precursors and giant metamyelocytes. The chromatin in the red blood cell nuclei is more dispersed than in normal red blood cell precursors at comparable stages of maturation; the giant metamyelocytes have dispersed nuclear chromatin in contrast to a normal metamyelocyte, which has condensed chromatin (Wright-Giemsa stain). (From Damjanov I, Linder J, editors: *Anderson's pathology*, ed 10, St Louis, 1996, Mosby.)

mucus-containing cells (intestinal metaplasia). The mechanism of cellular destruction in autoimmune gastritis is unknown, but it is thought to involve signaling through death-inducing pathways (e.g., Fas ligand [Fas/FasL] and tumor necrosis factor/tumor necrosis factor receptor [TNF/TNFR] pathways). Loss of parietal cells results in IF deficiency. A direct correlation exists between the severity of the gastric lesion and the degree of malabsorption of vitamin B_{12}. Malabsorption of vitamin B_{12} also may be secondary to secreted autoantibodies against IF, which prevents the formation of the B_{12}-IF complex.[5]

As with most autoimmune diseases, genetic factors increase the risk for developing chronic gastritis and PA. Family clusters have been identified; 20% to 30% of individuals related to persons with PA also have PA. These relatives, particularly first-degree female relatives, also demonstrate a higher frequency of the presence of gastric autoantibodies.

PA also is associated with other autoimmune conditions, particularly those affecting the endocrine system, including chronic autoimmune thyroiditis (Hashimoto thyroiditis), type 1 diabetes mellitus, Addison disease, primary hypoparathyroidism, Graves disease, and myasthenia gravis.

Environmental conditions also may lead to chronic gastritis. These include excessive alcohol ingestion, hot tea, and smoking. Complete or partial gastrectomy causes IF deficiency. *Helicobacter pylori* has been identified as a causative agent in the development of vitamin B_{12} deficiency.[6] Drugs known as proton pump inhibitors (PPIs) are used to decrease gastric acidity, but also may decrease cobalamin absorption, although it is not thought that they actually cause PA. Individuals with type A chronic gastritis PA are at risk for developing gastric adenocarcinoma of the noncardia stomach from intestinal metaplasia and esophageal squamous cell carcinoma. The incidence of carcinoma in these individuals is 2% to 3%. Type

B gastritis is caused by *H. pylori* with a decreased risk for development of cancer.

CLINICAL MANIFESTATIONS PA develops slowly—possibly from 20 to 30 years; 60 years of age is the median age at time of diagnosis. Because of the slow onset of symptoms, PA is usually severe by the time treatment is sought. Early symptoms are often ignored because they are vague and include infections, mood swings, and gastrointestinal, cardiac, or kidney ailments. When the hemoglobin level in the blood has decreased significantly (7 to 8 g/dl), the individual experiences the classic symptoms of anemia—weakness, fatigue, paresthesias of the feet and fingers, difficulty in walking, loss of appetite, abdominal pains, and weight loss. The tongue may become sore, smooth, and beefy red secondary to atrophic glossitis. The skin may become "lemon yellow" (sallow) as a result of a combination of pallor and icterus. The liver may be enlarged, especially in older adults, indicating right-sided heart failure. The spleen also may enlarge but remains nonpalpable.

Neurologic manifestations result from nerve demyelination that may produce neuronal death. The posterior and lateral columns of the spinal cord also may be affected, causing a loss of position and vibration sense, ataxia, and spasticity. These complications pose a serious threat because they are not reversible, even with appropriate treatment. The cerebrum also may be involved with manifestations of affective disorders, most commonly of the depressive types. An increased prevalence of serum vitamin B_{12} deficiency has been reported among individuals with Alzheimer disease.

EVALUATION AND TREATMENT Diagnosis of PA is based on a variety of tests (see Table 26-3), which include blood tests, bone marrow aspiration, serologic studies, gastric biopsy, clinical manifestations, and the Schilling test. The Schilling test indirectly evaluates vitamin B_{12} absorption by administering radioactive B_{12} and measuring excretion in the urine. Low urinary excretion is significant for PA. A second test often is done to confirm the diagnosis. In the second test, IF may be administered to see whether urinary excretion increases. If urinary excretion does not increase, other causes of PA must be considered.

Serologic studies, however, have replaced the Schilling test for diagnosing PA. Measuring methylmalonic acid and homocysteine levels, which are elevated early in PA, is more sensitive. The presence of circulating antibodies against parietal cells and intrinsic factor is also useful in diagnosis.[5] Gastric biopsy reveals total achlorhydria (absence of hydrochloric acid), which is diagnostic for PA because it occurs only in the presence of this gastric lesion.

Replacement of vitamin B_{12} (cobalamin) is the treatment of choice. Cyanocobalamin or hydroxocobalamin (1000 mcg) is administered parenterally on a monthly schedule. Initial injections are administered weekly until the deficiency is corrected. Conventional wisdom and practice assumed that oral preparations were ineffective because there was no IF to facilitate absorption. Recent experience, however, has determined that vitamin B_{12} will be absorbed across the small bowel so that oral administration is beneficial in dosages higher than parenteral dosages.

The effectiveness of cobalamin replacement therapy is determined by a rising reticulocyte count. Within 5 to 6 weeks, blood counts return to normal. PA cannot be cured, so maintenance therapy is lifelong. Blood transfusions are given if the individual shows signs of circulatory collapse, heart failure, or severe angina pectoris.

Untreated PA is fatal, usually because of heart failure. Death occurs after a course of remissions and exacerbations lasting from 1 to 3 years. Since 1926, when replacement therapy began, mortality has been reduced significantly. Today, death from PA is rare, and any relapses that occur are usually the result of noncompliance with therapy.

Folate Deficiency Anemia

Folate (folic acid) is an essential vitamin for erythrocyte production and maturation. Humans totally depend on dietary intake of folate, requiring 50 to 200 mcg/day, with pregnant and lactating females requiring increased amounts. Folate synthesis takes place in the human intestine, although not in quantities sufficient to make any significant contribution.

Absorption of folate occurs primarily in the upper small intestine and does not depend on the presence of any other facilitating factor. From the small intestine it is circulated to and through the liver where it is stored. Folate deficiency is more common than cobalamin deficiency, particularly in alcoholics and individuals with chronic malnourishment. Alcohol interferes with folate metabolism in the liver, causing a profound depletion of folate stores. Fad diets and diets low in vegetables also may cause folate deficiency because of the absence of plant sources of folate. At least 10% of North Americans have a folate deficiency, although the incidence has been on the decrease in the United States since the fortification of food with folate and the increased use of folate supplements.

Folates are coenzymes required for the synthesis of thymine and purines (adenine and guanine) and the conversion of homocysteine to methionine. Deficient production of thymine, in particular, affects cells undergoing rapid division (e.g., bone marrow cells undergoing erythropoiesis). The clinical manifestations of folate deficiency become apparent when the synthesis of thymidylate is critically impaired and progresses to the development of megaloblastic anemia.

PATHOPHYSIOLOGY Impaired DNA synthesis secondary to a folate deficiency results in megaloblastic cells with clumped nuclear chromatin. Anemia may result from apoptosis of erythroblasts in the late stages of erythropoiesis. In addition to anemia, folate deficiency in pregnant women is associated with neural tube defects of the fetus. Folate is necessary for the reduction of circulating levels of homocysteine, a risk factor for the development of atherosclerosis (see Chapter 30), thus a folate deficiency increases the risk for developing coronary artery disease. A deficiency of folate also is implicated in the development of cancers, specifically colorectal cancers.

CLINICAL MANIFESTATIONS Clinical manifestations of folate deficiency anemia are similar to the cachectic, malnourished appearance of individuals with PA. Specific symptoms include severe cheilosis (scales and fissures of the lips and corners of the mouth), stomatitis (inflammation of the mouth), and painful ulcerations of the buccal mucosa and tongue. Gastrointestinal symptoms may be present and include dysphagia (difficulty swallowing), flatulence, and watery diarrhea, as well as histologic and roentgenographic changes of the GI tract suggestive of the chronic malabsorption syndrome, sprue. Neurologic manifestations, such as those that occur in PA, are generally not seen in folate deficiency anemia. Any neurologic symptoms are usually caused by a thiamine deficiency, which often accompanies folate deficiency.

EVALUATION AND TREATMENT Determination of a folate deficiency is based on measurement of serum folate levels and symptoms. Successful treatment requires daily oral administration of folate preparations until adequate blood levels are obtained and clinical symptoms are reduced or eliminated. One milligram per day is sufficient for most individuals, although persons with alcoholism may require 5 mg. Prophylactic dosages of 0.1 to 0.4 mg/day are sometimes given during pregnancy. Parenteral administration of folic acid (citrovorum factor or leucovorin) generally is not used except in situations in which an individual has been using drugs that inhibit dihydrofolate reductase. After administration of folate, the manifestations of anemia disappear within 1 to 2 weeks.

After the folate deficiency has been corrected, long-term treatment with folate is not necessary if the appropriate dietary adjustments are made to maintain adequate intake. An intake of folate (400 mcg/day) is recommended as a measure to prevent heart disease.

Microcytic-Hypochromic Anemias

The **microcytic-hypochromic anemias** are characterized by erythrocytes that are abnormally small and contain abnormally reduced amounts of hemoglobin (see Figure 26-1, *B*). Hypochromia occurs even in cells of normal size.

Microcytic-hypochromic anemia results from a wide variety of conditions that are related to (1) disorders of iron metabolism, (2) disorders of porphyrin and heme synthesis, or (3) disorders of globin synthesis. Specific disorders include iron deficiency anemia, sideroblastic anemia, and thalassemia (thalassemia is discussed in Chapter 28).

Iron Deficiency Anemia

Iron deficiency anemia (IDA) is the most common type of anemia worldwide, occurring in both developing and developed countries and affecting as many as one fifth of the world population. Those at greatest risk for developing hypoferremia and IDA are the chronic poor, women of childbearing age, and children. Iron deficiency in children is associated with numerous adverse health-related manifestations, especially cognitive impairment, which may be irreversible. Teens who had iron deficiency as infants are likely to score lower on cognitive and motor tests, even if the iron deficiency was identified and treated in infancy.

Children in developing countries often are affected by chronic parasite infestations that result in intestinal blood and iron loss that outpaces dietary intake.[7] Treatment of helminth infections results in an improvement in the anemia as well as in appetite and growth. Iron deficiency also occurs in individuals with lead poisoning. Treatment of the iron deficiency is associated with a decrease in lead levels.

In the United States, 720,000 children (9%) ages 1 to 2 years are estimated to be iron deficient, of whom 240,000 (3%) are anemic, which may be a result of increased iron requirements with growth. Females demonstrate a higher incidence of hypoferremia (13.9%) than do males (8.3%), as well as IDA; 4% to 6% in females and 4% in males. The incidence peaks in females during their reproductive years and decreases after menopause. In females, menorrhagia (excessive bleeding during menstruation) is a common cause of primary IDA. Those at highest risk are black females living in urban poverty.[8] Males demonstrate a higher incidence during childhood and adolescence, a decrease occurring during young adulthood, and an upswing during late adulthood. An increased prevalence of iron deficiency has been demonstrated in overweight children. The most common cause of IDA in well-developed countries is pregnancy and chronic blood loss.[4] Blood loss of 2 to 4 ml/day (1 to 2 mg of iron) is sufficient to cause iron deficiency and may result from erosive esophagitis, gastric and duodenal ulcers, colon adenomas, and cancers. *H. pylori* infections also have been found to cause IDA of unknown origin, although *H. pylori* impairs iron uptake.

Other causes of IDA are (1) medications that cause gastrointestinal bleeding (aspirin, nonsteroidal anti-inflammatory drugs [NSAIDs]); (2) surgical procedures that decrease stomach acidity, intestinal transit time, and absorption; (3) insufficient dietary intake of iron; and (4) eating disorders, such as pica, which is the craving and eating of nonnutritional substances.

Iron is the essential for several biologic processes. As a component of hemoglobin, iron is in constant demand for use in normal erythropoiesis. Iron is recyclable; therefore, the body maintains a balance between iron that is contained in hemoglobin and iron that is in storage and available for future hemoglobin synthesis. Iron metabolism for erythropoiesis is complex and not well understood. Sources of iron include a small portion absorbed from the duodenum and, to a lesser extent, from the stomach, ileum, and colon. A much larger portion is available through recycling of iron from senescent RBCs (see Chapter 25).

Iron also contributes to immune function by regulating immune effector mechanisms (i.e., cytokine activities [interferon-gamma (INF-γ)], nitric oxide formation, and T-cell proliferation).

Acquired hypoferremia may be part of the body's response to infection. Anemia can be part of the nonspecific acute phase response to any type of inflammation of sufficient degree. Many pathogens require iron for survival; thus hypoferremia would hamper their growth. However, the precise benefits or detriments of iron deficiency and immunity are still controversial.

PATHOPHYSIOLOGY IDA can be classified as arising from one of two different etiologies or a combination of both. Nutritional iron deficiency results from inadequate dietary intake or excessive blood loss. In both instances there is no intrinsic dysfunction in iron metabolism; however, both deplete iron stores and result in IDA caused by reduced hemoglobin synthesis. A second category is a metabolic or functional iron deficiency in which various metabolic disorders lead to either insufficient iron delivery to bone marrow or impaired iron use within the marrow. Paradoxically, iron stores may be sufficient but delivery is inadequate to maintain heme synthesis, thus producing a functional or relative iron deficiency.

IDA occurs when the demand for iron exceeds the supply and develops slowly through three overlapping stages. In stage I, the body's iron stores are depleted. Erythropoiesis proceeds normally, with the hemoglobin content of RBCs remaining normal. In stage II, iron transportation to bone marrow is diminished, resulting in iron deficiency erythropoiesis. Stage III begins when the small hemoglobin-deficient cells enter the circulation in sufficient numbers to replace the normal mature erythrocytes that have been removed from the circulation. Manifestations of IDA appear in stage III when iron stores are depleted and there is diminished hemoglobin production.

CLINICAL MANIFESTATIONS Symptoms of IDA begin gradually, and the symptoms are usually not severe enough for individuals to seek medical attention until hemoglobin levels have decreased to about 7 to 8 g/dl. Early symptoms include fatigue, weakness, and shortness of breath. Pale earlobes, palms, and conjunctivae (Figure 26-4) are also common signs.

Progressive IDA causes more severe alterations, with structural and functional changes apparent in epithelial tissue (see Figure 26-4). The nails become brittle, thin, coarsely ridged, and spoon-shaped or concave (koilonychia) as a result of impaired capillary circulation (Figure 26-5). The tongue becomes red, sore, and painful, which is caused by atrophy of the papillae (glossitis) (Figure 26-6). The degree of pain experienced is directly associated with the amount of iron deficiency. Individuals also experience dryness and soreness in the epithelium at the corners of the mouth, known as *angular stomatitis*. Difficulty in swallowing is associated with an esophageal "web," a thin, concentric, smooth extension of

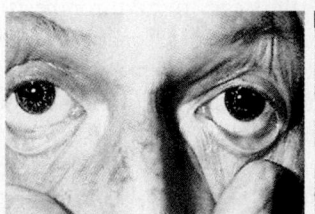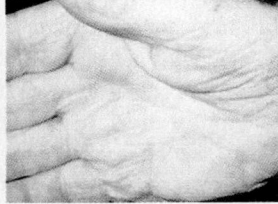

Figure 26-4 Pallor and iron deficiency. Pallor of the skin, mucous membranes, and palmar creases in an individual with hemoglobin of 9 g/dl. Palmar creases become as pale as the surrounding skin when the hemoglobin level approaches 7 g/dl. (Courtesy Hoffbrand AV, Pettit JE, editors: *Sandoz atlas of clinical hematology,* London, 1988, Gower Medical.)

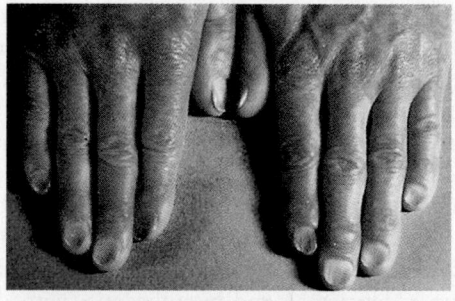

Figure 26-5 Koilonychia. The nails are concave, ridged, and brittle. (Courtesy Hoffbrand AV, Pettit JE, editors: *Sandoz atlas of clinical hematology,* London, 1988, Gower Medical.)

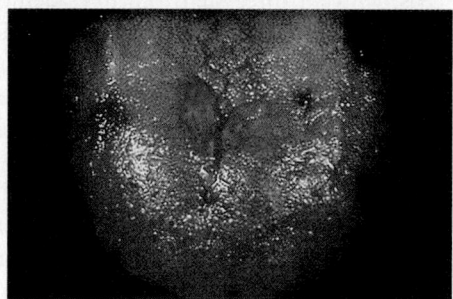

Figure 26-6 Glossitis. Tongue of individual with iron deficiency anemia has bald, fissured appearance caused by loss of papillae and flattening. (Courtesy Hoffbrand AV, Pettit JE, editors: *Sandoz atlas of clinical hematology,* London, 1988, Gower Medical.)

normal esophageal tissue consisting of mucosa and submucosa at the juncture between the hypopharynx and esophagus. The duration of iron deficiency required for web formation is uncertain. Dysphagia also is exacerbated by hyposalivation. The pathophysiology associated with these epithelial lesions is not well understood, but the lesions have the potential to become cancerous.

Nonheme iron is a component of many enzymes in the body (e.g., cytochromes, myoglobin, catalases, peroxidases), particularly those involved in the metabolism of amine neurotransmitters, reduction of nucleotides, and biosynthesis of methionine. Abnormalities and deficiencies of iron-dependent enzymes may account for many of the clinical manifestations of IDA. Individuals with IDA also exhibit gastritis, neuromuscular alterations, irritability, headache, numbness, tingling, and vasomotor disturbances. The pathogenesis of neurologic symptoms is unknown but may be caused by hypoxia in already compromised cerebral vessels. Gait disturbances are rare. Mental confusion, memory loss, and disorientation often are associated with anemia in older adults and may be wrongly perceived as "normal" events related to aging.

EVALUATION AND TREATMENT Initial evaluation is based on the presence of a decreased hemoglobin and hematocrit. Additional measurements, however, are needed to determine the cause of the anemia (see Table 26-3). Iron stores may be measured directly by bone marrow biopsy and iron staining or indirectly by laboratory tests for serum ferritin, transferrin saturation, or total iron-binding capacity.

Serum ferritin is a widely accepted and available measurement of iron status that has been used for the past 25 years; 1 mcg/L serum ferritin corresponds to 8 to 10 mg or 120 mcg of storage iron/kg body weight.[8] Serum ferritin level has demonstrated its superiority over other measures (i.e., mean corpuscular volume [MCV], transferrin saturation). One limit to the serum ferritin is the elevation of values independent of iron status that accompanies acute or chronic inflammation, malignancy, liver disease, or alcoholism.

An indicator of iron levels is the level of serum transferrin receptor (sTfR). Transferrin receptors are membrane glycoproteins that bind circulating transferrin for transport into cells. Soluble forms of the receptor are found in serum. The ratio of serum levels of transferrin receptor to ferritin (R/F) reliably and accurately estimate body iron stores and differentiate primary IDA from anemia secondary to chronic disease. A major drawback, however, is the lack of proper standardization for the sTfR assay.

The first step in treatment of IDA is to identify and eliminate sources of blood loss.[9] With ongoing bleeding, any pharmacologic therapy is likely to be ineffective. Iron replacement therapy is very effective in the treatment of nutritional deficient anemia. In fact, the most conclusive evidence for the diagnosis of IDA is an increase in hemoglobin of 1 to 2 g/dl after iron therapy is initiated. Iron is available in ferrous or ferric forms; however, ferrous is preferable because it is more readily absorbed. The ferrous form is available as sulfate, gluconate, or fumarate. Ferrous sulfate is the cheapest and most commonly used.

Initial iron replacement therapy is 150 to 200 mg/day; however, recent studies have found that dosages as low as 60 mg/day are effective in certain individuals. Once therapy has begun, individuals demonstrate a rapid decrease in fatigue, lethargy, and other associated symptoms. Hematocrit levels should improve within 1 to 2 months of therapy; however, the serum ferritin level is a more precise measurement of improvement and total body stores of iron. Once the serum ferritin level reaches 50 mcg/L, adequate replacement of iron has occurred. Replacement therapy is usually continued for 3 to 6 months after bleeding has been contained; however, therapy may continue for as long as 24 months. Daily therapy (60–120 mg/day) for menstruating females may be required until menopause.

Parenteral iron replacement is used in instances of uncontrolled blood loss, intolerance to oral iron, intestinal malabsorption, and poor adherence to oral therapy. Iron dextran has been the only parenteral agent available in the United States. Intramuscular injection is the recommended method; however, intravenous administration is generally preferred because of the ability to administer larger doses. A significant concern in the use of IV dextran is the potential for severe anaphylactic reaction. Delayed allergic reactions are also major concerns.

Newer medications that have recently been approved for parenteral therapy in treating IDA are sodium ferric gluconate complex in sucrose (Ferrlecit) and iron sucrose injection

(Venofer). Iron dextran is recommended as the first choice in spite of its higher rate of adverse reactions. For individuals who are intolerant of iron dextran, the two newer agents are safe and effective alternatives. Drawbacks to their use include higher cost and the need for multiple infusions.

Sideroblastic Anemia

Sideroblastic anemias (SAs) are a heterogeneous group of disorders characterized by anemia of varying severity caused by a deviation in mitochondrial metabolism leading to ineffective iron uptake and dysfunctional heme synthesis.[10] Ringed sideroblasts within the bone marrow are diagnostic of SA. **Ringed sideroblasts** are erythroblasts that contain iron granules that have not been synthesized into hemoglobin, but instead are arranged in a perinuclear collar around one third or more of the nucleus (see Figure 26-1, *K*). Individuals with SA also have increased levels of iron in their tissue. The blood contains hypochromic erythrocytes, either microcytic or macrocytic depending on the form of the disease.

PATHOPHYSIOLOGY SAs have multiple etiologies but all share the commonality of altered mitochondrial heme synthesis in the erythroid cells in bone marrow. Mitochondrial aminolevulinic acid (ALA) synthase uses glycine to convert succinyl CoA into ALA.[11] ALA undergoes further enzymatic modification in the cytoplasm to the porphyrin structure becoming coproporphyrinogen III, which reenters the mitochondria. Within the mitochondria the molecule is progressively converted to protophorphyrin IX, which has ferrous iron (Fe^{2+}) inserted by the enzyme ferrochelatase. Disruptions to this pathway lead to the accumulation of iron in the mitochondria and the characteristic sideroblasts.

SAs are either hereditary or acquired. Hereditary SAs are rare and occur almost exclusively in males, suggesting a predominant recessive X-linked transmission. An occasional autosomal recessive transmission occurs with mitochondrial mutations and deficiencies of ferrochelatase.[12] The anemia of hereditary SA is usually present in infancy or childhood, but may remain undetected until midlife. In some instances, other symptoms (e.g., diabetes or cardiac failure resulting from tissue iron overload) may be the first manifestation of SA. Differentiation of SA from idiopathic hemachromatosis needs to be confirmed because both are characterized by tissue iron deposition.

The severity of the anemia is quite variable, and qualitative alterations of the erythrocytes (e.g., decreased MCV and increased RBC volume distribution width) may be evident even when anemia is not present. **Dimorphism,** in which normocytic and normochromic cells are seen concomitantly with microcytic-hypochromic cells, may be present and is seen more commonly in individuals with mild anemia, female carriers, or those receiving treatment with pyridoxine. Anisocytosis and poikilocytosis also are seen on examination of the blood smear.

Hereditary SA (X-linked sideroblastic anemia [XLSA]) has been linked to missense mutations in the erythroid-specific ALAS-E gene *Xp11.21*.[12] More than 25 missense mutations

have been identified. ALAS is the first and rate-limiting enzyme in the heme biosynthesis pathway, and mutations lead to reduced synthesis of protoporphyrin IX and the characteristic accumulation of iron in the erythrocyte.

Acquired sideroblastic anemias (ASAs) are the most common SAs. The causes of primary forms of ASA are unknown (idiopathic) or associated with other myeloproliferative or myeloplastic disorders. Another form, reversible SAs, is secondary to various conditions, such as alcoholism, drug reactions, copper deficiency, and hypothermia, with drugs and toxins being the leading cause.

The leading known cause of primary ASA, **myelodysplastic syndrome (MDS)**, is a group of disorders of hematopoietic stem cells, with all three stem cell lines demonstrating dysplastic characteristics.[13] Initially, all ASAs associated with myelodysplastic syndrome were considered to be one and the same and identified as refractory anemia with ringed sideroblasts. This classification proved unsatisfactory because different outcomes were observed in individuals who had the same apparent disease. Further investigations discovered morphologic and chromosomal characteristics that predicted different clinical courses. Two subsets of myelodysplastic ringed sideroblasts were identified based on which cell lines were affected. In one subset dysplastic features were limited to the erythroid line and was classified as pure SA. Individuals with pure SA require transfusions, which may produce iron overload.[14] With adequate chelation therapy, they are able to survive and thrive for many years. A significant outcome of this condition is the rare occurrence of conversion to leukemia.

The second subset was characterized by abnormalities of multiple cell lineages. In addition to SA, major alterations of neutrophil and platelet were observed. Infections, frequently fatal, are common secondary to neutropenia and neutrophil dysfunction. Bleeding from thrombocytopenia and platelet dysfunction also are prevalent. Of those who survive, 40% develop acute (myeloblastic) leukemia.

Reversible SA, the most prevalent form of ASA, is a result of several factors (predominantly drugs or toxins [e.g., lead, zinc]) that affect heme biosynthesis, and anemia related to these causes is reversible with reduced exposure to the toxin or drug. The most frequent cause of reversible SA is alcohol abuse. Excessive alcohol inhibits pyridoxal phosphate, which is a cofactor for ALA-synthase in mitochondria. Alcohol abuse may also secondarily result in nutritional deficiencies that may affect heme biosynthesis, such as pyridoxine and copper. Copper is a cofactor for mitochondrial ferrochelatase, which controls the insertion of iron into protoporphyrin IX to form heme. Other drugs that are copper chelators (e.g., penicillamine) have similar effects leading to SA.

Other drugs that cause ASA include antituberculous agents (isoniazid [INH], pyrazinamide, and cycloserine) and chloramphenicol. Antituberculous agents interfere with vitamin B_6 metabolism, which reduces ALA synthesis, thus decreasing heme generation. Chloramphenicol causes direct mitochondrial injury by inhibiting mitochondrial membrane proteins and thus mitochondrial respiration. Additionally, therapeutic drug levels are known to inhibit erythroid colony growth but not granulocyte colony growth.

CLINICAL MANIFESTATIONS The anemias of SA are generally moderate to severe, with hemoglobin levels varying from 4 to 10 g/dl. In addition to the cardiovascular and respiratory manifestations common to all anemias, individuals with SA demonstrate signs of iron overload known as **erythropoietic hemochromatosis.** Mild to moderate enlargement of the spleen (splenomegaly) and liver (hepatomegaly) occurs; however, liver function remains normal or only slightly impaired. Occasionally abnormal skin pigmentation (bronze colored) is seen. Neurologic and epithelial alterations commonly associated with other anemias are nonexistent. Heart rhythm disturbances, along with congestive heart failure, are major life-threatening complications related to cardiac iron overload. These manifestations are fortunately rare and occur late in the progression of the disease. Young children and infants who are severely affected may demonstrate growth and developmental impairment.

EVALUATION AND TREATMENT Initially, SA may be mistaken for deficiency of stem cells in the marrow (**hypoplastic anemia**) or IDA (laboratory findings are listed in Table 26-3). Bone marrow examination establishes the diagnosis. The marrow is packed with erythrocyte stem cells, and mononuclear phagocytes in the marrow are loaded with iron in the form of hemosiderin. Platelet and leukocyte values are generally normal; however, they may be reduced if splenomegaly is evident. The presence of sideroblasts confirms the diagnosis of SA.

Initial treatment of SA is directed toward identification of a causative agent (i.e., drugs or toxins).[15] Treatment is supportive, with transfusions being the primary intervention. Following removal of the agent, oral pyridoxine (100 mg/day) may be administered on a trial basis. Acquired SA related to alcohol abuse and pyridoxine antagonists often demonstrates a complete response to pyridoxine. SA caused by other etiologies does not demonstrate the same improvement.

Individuals with hereditary XLSA also are initially treated with pyridoxine therapy in doses of 50 to 200 mg/day. Approximately one third of individuals with hereditary SA respond to this therapy. An optimal response is related to reticulocytosis with blood hemoglobin levels returning to normal within 1 to 2 months and low free erythrocyte protoporphyrin levels also returning to normal. Morphologic abnormalities of cells (microcytosis), however, do not disappear, even in the presence of normal ALA synthase activity and hemoglobin. Hemoglobin levels also may increase in response to therapy but stabilize at less than normal levels. When a response to pyridoxine therapy is observed, lifelong maintenance therapy at a lowered dosage is instituted. Discontinuing therapy initiates a relapse. Individuals not responding to pyridoxine require blood transfusions to relieve symptoms and permit growth and development.

Individuals who demonstrate evidence of iron overload require iron depletion therapy to prevent or minimize organ damage. Phlebotomies are generally well tolerated and preferable for individuals who have a mild to moderate anemia without other complications, such as heart disease. Once all

Test	Pernicious Anemia	Folate Deficiency Anemia	Iron Deficiency Anemia	Sideroblastic Anemia	Aplastic Anemia	Posthemorrhagic Anemia	Hemolytic Anemia	Anemia of Chronic Disease
Hemoglobin	Low	Low	Low	Low	Low or normal	Normal or low	Low	Low
Hematocrit	Low	Low	Low	Low	Low or normal	Normal or low	Low	Low
Reticulocyte count	Low	Low	Normal or slightly high or low	Normal or slightly high	Low	Increased	High	Normal
Mean corpuscular volume	High	High	Low	Low	Normal or slightly high	Slightly low	Normal or high	Normal or low
Plasma iron	High	High	Low	High	High	Normal	Normal or high	Low
Total iron-binding capacity	Normal	Normal	High	Normal	Normal	Normal	Normal	Low
Ferritin	High	High	Low	High	Normal	Normal	Normal	Normal
Serum B₁₂	Low	Normal	Normal	Normal	Normal	Normal	Normal	Normal
Folate	Normal	Low	Normal	Normal	Normal	Normal	Normal	Normal
Bilirubin	Slightly high	Slightly high	Normal	High	Normal	Normal	Slightly high	Normal
Free erythrocyte protoporphyrin	Normal	Normal	High	Increased or normal	High	Normal	Normal	Normal or slightly high
Transferrin	Slightly high	Slightly high	Low	High	Normal	Normal	Normal	Slightly low

Table 26-3   Laboratory Findings for Various Anemias

the stored iron is removed, maintenance phlebotomies are performed on a continuing basis. Individuals who have severe anemia and/or depend on transfusions become extremely overloaded with iron. When this occurs, iron chelation therapy with desferrioxamine is necessary to eliminate excess iron.

As stated, individuals with acquired SA infrequently respond to pyridoxine. Fortunately, these individuals are rarely incapacitated by SA. In the absence of abnormalities of other blood cells and without iron overload, progression takes place over many years. Transfusion and chelation therapy are the same as for hereditary SA when indicated.

Recent advances in treatment for SAs include prolonged administration of erythropoietin and stem cell transplant. Treatment with recombinant human erythropoietin improves anemia in 30% of those with myelodysplastic syndrome.[16] Those with the subset of MDS identified as refractory anemia have the overall best response rate. Stem cell transplant has been found to successfully treat congenital SA; however, this treatment is in the early stages of use, and long-term efficacy has not yet been established. Death from SA is relatively rare and often secondary to complications, such as infection, bone marrow failure, liver failure, or cardiac failure or arrhythmias, or both.

Normocytic-Normochromic Anemias

Normocytic-normochromic anemias are characterized by erythrocytes that are relatively normal in size and hemoglobin content but insufficient in number. These anemias have no common etiology, pathologic mechanisms, or morphologic characteristics. They are less frequent than macrocytic-normochromic and microcytic-hypochromic anemias. NNAs include five distinct groups: aplastic, posthemorrhagic (acute blood loss), hemolytic, sickle cell, and anemia of chronic inflammation. (Sickle cell anemia is discussed in Chapter 28).

Aplastic Anemia

Aplastic anemia (AA) is a critical condition characterized by **pancytopenia,** a reduction or absence of all three blood cell types, resulting from failure or suppression of bone marrow to produce adequate amounts of blood cells (Figure 26-7). The rate or decline in the quantity of blood cells is related to their respective life span; thus RBCs (life span about 120 days) are last to demonstrate a reduction in numbers.

The incidence of AA is relatively rare (annual rate of 2 to 5 new cases per million per year). The incidence in developing countries is somewhat higher and is thought to be caused by unregulated use of and exposure to certain chemicals known to cause AA. The incidence is bimodal, with one peak occurring between 15 and 25 years of age and a second peak occurring in individuals older than age 60. AA is equally distributed between genders.

AAs are the most common type, with idiopathic AA (primary acquired) accounting for approximately 75% of all confirmed cases. Secondary AA, which accounts for approximately 15% of cases, is caused by a variety of known chemical agents and ionizing radiation. Chemical agents include benzene, arsenic, and multiple drugs, including chloramphenicol

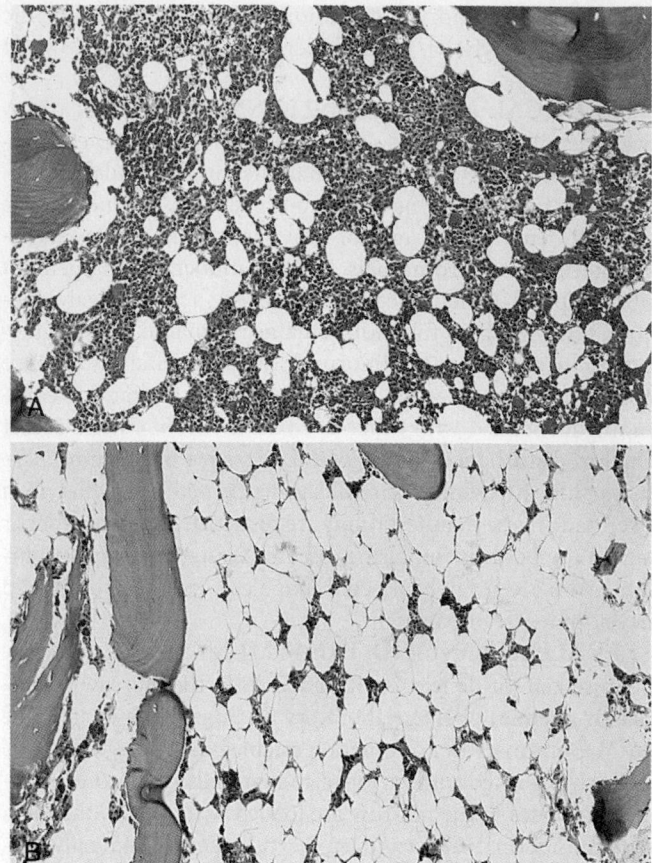

Figure 26-7 Aplastic anemia. **A,** Normal bone marrow of an adult. Hematopoietic cells account for approximately 40% of marrow's cellularity. **B,** There is a marked reduction in hematopoietic cells with expansion of fat cells. (From Damjanov I, Linder J: *Pathology: a color atlas,* St Louis, 2000, Mosby.)

and alkylating and antimetabolite chemotherapeutic drugs (6-mercaptopurine, vincristine, and busulfan).[17] Other drugs known to cause AA are identified in Table 26-4. The development of AA with use of these agents is generally dose related, and the effect can be controlled with diminished dosages. In other instances, AA might develop after the use of small amounts of these drugs (idiosyncratic), with the anemia following a severe, rapid, irreversible progression. Liver disease is also recognized as a cause of AA.

AA is constitutional or familial in origin or is associated with one or more somatic abnormalities in approximately 5% to 10% of affected individuals. A subset of these is found to have defective telomerase RNA resulting in shortened telomeres. This abnormality also is found in some individuals with idiopathic AA.

Total body irradiation also causes AA and in certain instances may be used therapeutically for this effect. Infections are also known to cause AA, with viruses being the most common agent. Viral infections identified as causing AA include the human immunodeficiency virus (HIV) infections, Epstein-Barr virus, and hepatitis (non-A, non-B, non-C, and non-G virus). Persistent parvovirus B19 infection also has

Table 26-4   Anemias Secondary to Drug Effects

Drug	Hemolytic	Megaloblastic	Sideroblastic	Aplastic
Antibiotics				
Amphotericin B				X
Trimethoprim-sulfamethoxazole (Bactrim)		X		
Chloramphenicol (Chloromycetin)			XX	XXXX
Erythromycin	X			X
Sulfisoxazole (Gantrisin)				X
Penicillin	XXX			X
Sulfanilamide/sulfonamides	XX			X, X*
Streptomycin	X			X
Anticonvulsants				
Phenytoin (Dilantin)		XXX		XXX, X*
Mephenytoin		XXX		XXX
Primidone (Mysoline)		XX		
Phenobarbital		XX		
Trimethadione (Tridione)				XXX
Anti-inflammatories				
ASA (aspirin)				X*
Colchicine		X?		
Gold compounds				XX
Ibuprofen (Motrin)	X			X
Indomethacin (Indocin)				X
Phenacetin	XXX			X
Phenylbutazone				XX, X*
Antihypertensive/Diuretics				
Methyldopa (Aldomet)	XXX			
Acetazolamide (Diamox)				X
Thiazides	X			
Tranquilizers				
Chloridazepoxide (Librium)				X
Chlorpromazine (Thorazine)	XX			X
Meprobamate				X
Oral Hypoglycemics				
Chlorpropamide (Diabinese)	X			
Tolbutamide (Orinase)				X, X*
Immunosuppressants				
Azathioprine (Imuran)			X	X*
Cyclosporine	X			
Miscellaneous Agents				
Benzene	XX			XX
Cimetidine (Tagamet)				X
Heparin				X*
INH (isoniazid)	XX			
PASA (para-aminosalicylic acid)	XX	X		
Pyridium (phenazopyridine HCl				XX
Potassium perchlorate				XX
Quinine/quinidine	XX			
Acetaminophen (Tylenol)	X			X

INH, PASA, Pyridium bracketed: Antituberculous agents

X, Rare number of reported cases; *XXXX*, substantial number of reported cases; *XX, XXX*, intermediate number of reported cases; *X**, "pure red cell" aplasia.

been identified as producing bone marrow failure resulting in AA. Parvovirus B19 has been identified as the cause of aplastic crisis in children who have sickle cell hemoglobinopathies and hereditary spherocytosis.

Another condition associated with AA is **pure red cell aplasia (PRCA),** in which only the RBCs are affected. PRCA is a rare disorder and has been associated with autoimmune, viral, and neoplastic (leukemias) disorders; infiltrative disorders of the bone marrow (myelofibrosis); renal failure; hepatitis; mononucleosis; and systemic lupus erythematosus.[17] It also is a well recognized but infrequent complication of allogeneic bone marrow transplantation, particularly when there is donor-recipient ABO mismatch. A thymoma often is found in association with PRCA and is also present in Diamond-Blackfan syndrome, a congenital disorder.

A very small percentage of AA cases is linked to genetic alterations or predisposition. **Fanconi anemia** is a rare genetic anemia characterized by pancytopenia resulting from defects in DNA repair. This anemia develops early in life and is accompanied by multiple congenital anomalies.

PATHOPHYSIOLOGY The characteristic lesion of AA is a hypocellular bone marrow that has been replaced with fat. Most cases of AA result from an autoimmune disease directed against hematopoietic stem cells.[18] The evidence supporting an autoimmune process includes the response of AA to immunosuppressive therapy including depletion of T-cells by antithymocyte antibodies. Cytotoxic T cells (Tc cells) appear to be the main culprits, although the causative antigen has yet to be identified. Th1 cytokines (involved in the differentiation of Tc cells), such as INF-γ and TNF-α, as well as cellular contact with Tc cells through FasL, induce apoptosis of CD34+ target cells, which includes most of the hematopoietic progenitors.

CLINICAL MANIFESTATIONS The onset of symptoms is insidious and related to the rapidity with which the bone marrow is destroyed and replaced.[17] Approximately 50% of AA cases progress rapidly, with a high risk of death from overwhelming infection or bleeding. In some cases the rate of decline is slow and the individual may adapt progressively to a new level of hematologic function. This condition is referred to as *hypoplastic anemia* rather than aplastic anemia.

Initial symptoms depend on which cell line is affected. Rapidly progressing disease is usually associated with hypoxemia, pallor (occasionally with a brownish pigmentation of the skin), and weakness along with fever and dyspnea with rapidly developing signs of hemorrhaging if platelets are affected (e.g., unexplained bruising, nosebleeds, bleeding gums, bleeding in the GI tract, prolonged bleeding at sites of minor injury). A slower onset over weeks or months is characterized by progressive weakness and fatigue with developing signs of hemorrhaging. Major hemorrhage may occur from any organ; however, it is generally observed in the late stages and is often secondary to other events. Menorrhagia and purpura also may be evident; however, purpura is not necessarily a classic indication of AA and may not be representative of the degree of thrombocytopenia. In both rapid and slow onset AA, diminished leukocyte production may result in a progressive frequency and prolongation of infections.

Late manifestations of the condition include ulcerations of the mouth and pharynx or a low-grade cellulitis in the neck. Splenomegaly is extremely rare, and if present, other conditions that may imitate AA should be ruled out. Neurologic changes are only evident when hemorrhages have occurred within the system; however, some individuals have complained of paresthesias.

EVALUATION AND TREATMENT Diagnosis is made by blood tests and bone marrow biopsy. AA is suspected if levels of circulating erythrocytes, leukocytes, and platelets are diminished; a granulocyte count less than 500/μL, a platelet count less than 20,000/μL, and an absolute reticulocyte count less than or equal to 40×10^9/L. The diagnosis is confirmed by a bone marrow biopsy. The bone marrow usually has reduced cellularity (i.e., less than 25% normal cellularity). The morphology of the few remaining hematopoietic cells is usually normal. Occasionally the RBCs are macrocytic, with anisocytosis and poikilocytosis, and may appear immature.

Marrow biopsied from individuals with typical AA contains yellowish white material consisting mainly of fat, fibrous tissue, and lymphocytes. Pancytopenia is usually characterized by decreased stem cell and progenitor cell populations to approximately 1% or less of normal.

Up until the past 20 years, treatment involved determining the cause, removal of exposure to the potential causative agent, transfusion, and prevention and treatment of infection and hemorrhage. Stimulation of blood cell production also was used, and in some instances splenectomy was recommended. The prognosis with these forms of treatment was extremely poor. In acute cases, 25% of individuals succumbed within 4 months, and approximately 70% died within 5 years; only about 10% experienced complete recovery. Newer forms of treatment, such as bone marrow transplant (BMT), immunosuppression, and identification of high-risk individuals, has decreased mortality significantly.[18]

Bone marrow and, most recently, peripheral blood stem cell transplantation from a histocompatible sibling often cures the underlying bone marrow failure.[19] Survival rates of 75% to 80% have been reported, and mortality rates within the first 100 days have decreased. Before transplantation the recipient usually received radiation or chemotherapy to deplete the bone marrow of disease-causing lymphocytes. Thus an unsuccessful transplantation may leave the recipient with a depleted immune system and an increased vulnerability to infection. Graft-versus-host (GVH) disease remains a risk and is a major contributor to premature death.[20] Children demonstrate higher survival than adults.

For those individuals unable to undergo bone marrow transplantation or who lack a suitable sibling donor, immunosuppression remains the treatment of choice.[20] Antithymocyte globulin (ATG) specifically suppresses lymphocytes, including those autoreactive lymphocytes destroying the bone marrow cells. Drugs like cyclosporine, which is often used in combination with ATG, broadly suppress the activity of immune cells. Response rates, that is, increased blood cell counts, of 40% to 50% may occur in individuals who receive ATG. The addition of cyclosporine has increased the response and survival rates to as much as 70% to 80%, with a 5-year survival rate between 80% and 90%. Cyclosporine as a single therapeutic agent is not as effective. Corticosteroids are often used concurrently with ATG and cyclosporine. Cyclophosphamide also has been used as an immunosuppressive agent and has produced the same effects as ATG; however, its use has been discontinued because of its toxicity. The addition of recombinant hematopoietic growth factors, such as granulocyte-macrophage colony-stimulating factor (GM-CSF), IL-6, and epoetin, to immunosuppressive therapy has produced significant additional benefit in both children and adults.

Immunosuppressive therapy is not without risk. Individuals receiving immunosuppressive therapy are at risk of experiencing treatment failure or late clonal/malignant conditions or both. Late clonal/malignant conditions include paroxysmal nocturnal hemoglobinuria (PNH), MDS, acute leukemia, or solid tumor. Although quite rare (less than 3%), administration of ATG may cause an anaphylactic reaction in some individuals.

Posthemorrhagic Anemia (Acute Blood Loss)

Posthemorrhagic anemia is a normocytic-normochromic anemia caused by acute blood loss. Initial manifestations of this event depend on the severity of blood loss. If blood loss is severe, the significant manifestations are related to loss of blood volume rather than loss of hemoglobin.

A normal, healthy young adult can tolerate a blood loss of 500 to 1000 ml (10% to 20% of volume) without experiencing any symptoms. Additional losses up to 1500 ml do not cause obvious symptoms if the individual is recumbent—symptoms appear only when assuming an upright position. When blood loss exceeds 1500 ml, symptoms are apparent even in a recumbent position (Table 26-5).

Volume loss reduces mean systemic filling pressure, resulting in decreased venous return. The initial manifestations (increased sympathetic nerve activation and a reduction in blood pressure, cardiac output, and central venous pressure) are caused by cardiovascular adaptations to blood volume depletion. If blood loss exceeds 2000 ml, severe shock, lactic acidosis, and death occur. (Shock is discussed in Chapter 46.)

If the acute blood loss is not severe (does not cause the preceding manifestations), complete recovery is possible. Within 24 hours of blood loss, lost plasma is replaced by mobilizing water and electrolytes from tissues and interstitial spaces into the vascular system. The hemodilution that results lowers the hematocrit; concurrently, there is often a rapid elevation of circulating neutrophils and platelets. Neutrophils can rise to levels between 10,000 and 30,000/μL within a few hours as a result of a shift of marginated leukocytes into the circulation and a release of leukocytes from the bone marrow. The platelet count can rise to levels of about 1million/μL. In severe blood loss, more immature cells—metamyelocytes, myelocytes, and nucleated red blood cells—may enter the circulation. Reduction in tissue oxygenation stimulates production of erythropoietin and increasing production of RBCs (reticulocytes) in the bone marrow. Iron recovery from destroyed RBCs may occur if the acute blood loss is internal; however, if blood is lost externally, iron stores may be depleted and erythropoiesis may be impeded. Hemorrhage that is chronic (occult [i.e., bleeding ulcer or neoplasm]) produces adaptations that are less prominent, but the individual may experience an IDA when iron reserves become depleted.

Initial treatment for acute blood loss is restoration of blood volume by intravenous administration of saline, dextran,

Table 26-5	Clinical Manifestations of Acute Blood Loss of Increasing Severity

Volume Lost		Clinical Manifestations
% TBV	ml	
10	500	None; rarely notice vasovagal syncope in blood donors
20	1000	When person is at rest, it is difficult, if not impossible, to detect volume loss; tachycardia is common with exercise and a slight drop in blood pressure with postural change
30	1500	Neck veins are flat in supine position; exercise tachycardia and postural hypotension are usually present; resting supine blood pressure and pulse can still be normal
40	2000	Central venous pressure, cardiac output, and arterial blood pressure are below normal even at rest and supine position; person commonly has air hunger; a rapid, thready pulse; and cold, clammy skin
50	2500	Severe shock, lactic acidosis, death

Adapted from Hillman RS: Acute blood loss anemia. In Beutler E et al, editors: *Williams hematology,* ed 5, New York, 1995, McGraw-Hill. Data based on a 70-kg person with a total blood volume of 5000 ml. *TBV,* Total blood volume.

albumin, or plasma. Large volume losses may require transfusion of fresh whole blood.

Successful therapy is first indicated by a return of erythrocytes to their normal size and shape. As the bone marrow begins to produce more erythrocytes, an increase in reticulocytes (10% to 15% after 7 days) is seen. Changes in the appearance of RBCs (polychromatophilia and macrocytosis) associated with reticulocytosis may give the impression that an underlying hemolytic process is occurring. A normal erythrocyte count is usually noted in 4 to 6 weeks, but hemoglobin restoration may take 6 to 8 weeks.

Hemolytic Anemia

The predominant event in **hemolytic anemias** is premature accelerated destruction of erythrocytes, either episodically or continuous. The consequences of the anemia are elevated levels of erythropoietin to induce accelerated production of erythrocytes and an increase in the products of hemoglobin catabolism.

Hemolytic anemias may be either congenital or acquired. Congenital hemolytic anemias result from intrinsic defects in erythrocytes, including the red cell membrane (e.g., hereditary spherocytosis, paroxysmal nocturnal hemoglobinuria), enzymatic pathways (e.g., glucose-6-phosphate dehydrogenase deficiency), and hemoglobin synthesis (e.g., the thalassemia syndromes, sickle cell anemia). (Glucose-6-phosphate dehydrogenase deficiency, thalassemia, and sickle cell disease are discussed in Chapter 28.) Acquired hemolytic anemias are usually immunologic (immune hemolytic anemias), such as RBC destruction caused by autoantibodies against erythrocyte antigens (e.g., autoimmune hemolytic anemia), isohemagglutinins (e.g., mismatched RBC transfusions), or allergic reactions against drug antigens adsorbed onto the erythrocyte surface (drug-induced hemolytic anemia). (Isohemagglutinins, erythrocyte antigens, autoantibodies, and allergic reactions are discussed in Chapter 8.) Acquired hemolytic anemia may also be secondary to erythrocyte damage caused by cardiac valve prostheses or by increased shear stresses in narrowed small vessels (e.g., during disseminated intravascular coagulation). Causes of acquired and hereditary hemolytic anemias are listed in Table 26-6.

PATHOPHYSIOLOGY Hemolytic anemias can be classified by a variety of parameters, although no system is entirely satisfactory. Dividing these anemias into inherited or acquired is the preferred and most useful method. Pathophysiologic mechanisms also can be discussed in the context of where hemolysis occurs. Hemolysis occurs within blood vessels (intravascular) or lymphoid tissues (extravascular) that filter blood—that is, spleen and liver. Intravascular hemolysis is the least common and typically caused by physical destruction of RBCs in the circulation, frequently by antibody and complement. Extravascular hemolysis results from removal of damaged or opsonized erythrocytes by cells of the mononuclear phagocyte system (MPS). Erythrocytes continuously circulate through the spleen, passing through the thin-walled splenic cords into the splenic sinusoids, a sponge-like labyrinth of macrophages with long dendritic processes. Normally, RBCs are able to alter their shape to allow passage through openings in the splenic cords. Macrophages will phagocytose RBCs with structure alterations of the membrane surface or that have become more rigid are incapable of maneuvering through this network. In some cases, IgG antibodies or complement component C3b can coat erythrocytes without causing hemolysis, but can function as opsonins that are recognized by macrophages.

Table 26-6   Causes of Hemolytic Anemias

Type of Hemolytic Disorder	Primary Cause or Associated Disorder	Mechanisms of Erythrocyte Destruction
Acquired Forms		
Immune system–mediated hemolysis	Transfusion reaction Hemolytic disease of the newborn (see Chapter 28) Autoimmune hemolytic anemia (see text)	Antibody-mediated: intravascular hemolysis by activation of complement system; extravascular hemolysis by phagocytosis of antibody-coated erythrocytes in spleen (see Chapter 8)
Traumatic hemolysis	Presence of prosthetic heart valves Structural abnormalities of the heart Hemolytic uremic syndrome Disseminated intravascular coagulation Hemodialysis	Physical destruction of erythrocytes by "mechanical" means (trauma)
Infectious hemolysis	Bacterial infection Viral infection Protozoal infection Helminthic infection	Bacterial hemolysins (e.g., *Escherichia coli* 0157:H7 shiga toxin; *Clostridium perfringens* toxin) Initiate autoimmune hemolysis (e.g., *Mycoplasma pneumoniae*: cold agglutinin) Affects erythrocytes (e.g., parvovirus B19: infects erythroid progenitors) Infects erythrocytes (e.g., malaria) Intestinal bleeding (e.g., hookworm)
Drug or toxic (chemical) hemolysis	Exposure to toxic chemical agents Hemodialysis or uremia Venoms	Chemical injury of erythrocytes (see Chapter 2)
Physical hemolysis	Burns Radiation	Heat or radiation injury (see Chapter 2)
Hypophosphatemic hemolysis	Hypophosphatemia (phosphate deficiency in plasma; see Chapter 3)	Diminished cellular production of substances required for erythrocyte life and function
Hereditary Forms		
Structural defects	Plasma membrane defects	Fragility of the erythrocyte
Plasma membrane protein mutation	Deficient complement regulatory proteins (i.e., paroxysmal nocturnal hemoglobulinuria)	Complement activation on erythrocyte surface, intravascular lysis
Enzyme deficiencies	Deficiency of glycolytic enzymes Deficiency of metabolic enzymes (i.e., glucose-6-phosphate dehydrogenase deficiency)	Diminished cellular function
Defects of globin synthesis or structure	Sickle cell anemia	Increased membrane fragility and deformation during sickle crises
	Thalassemia	Defective hemoglobin structure and function
	Miscellaneous hemoglobin defects	Defective hemoglobin structure and function

From Lee GR et al: *Wintrobe's clinical hematology*, ed 9, Philadelphia, 1993, Lea & Febiger.

Paroxysmal nocturnal hemoglobinuria may be congenital or acquired secondarily to acquired aplastic anemia. The disease results from a mutation in the X-linked gene for phosphatidylinositol glycan—class A (*PIG-A*), which results in a defect in expression of glycosylphosphatidylinositol (GPI) in hematologic stem cells.[21] GPI is a lipid anchor that is necessary for attachment of a large number of proteins to the plasma membrane. Several GPI-anchored proteins on erythrocytes are complement regulatory proteins, including CD55 and CD59. Normally low levels of complement are activated on cell surfaces through the alternative pathway (see Chapter 6). Erythrocytes are protected from complement-mediated damage by CD55, which accelerates the degradation of any C3 convertase that forms on the cell surface, and by CD59, which prevents C9 aggregation and pore formation by the the the membrane attack complex. Thus RBCs deficient in CD55 and CD59 undergo complement-mediated intravascular lysis and release of hemoglobin. In addition to anemia and hemoglobinuria, affected individuals also present with severe fatigue, abdominal pain, and thrombosis.[22] The cause of death is usually thrombosis of the abdominal or cerebral veins.[23] Thrombosis most likely results from a depletion of vascular nitric oxide (NO) by free hemoglobin, which has a high affinity for NO. The result is dysregulation of normal hemostasis and increased platelet vascular adherence and clot formation (see Chapter 25).

Autoimmune hemolytic anemias (AIHAs) are acquired disorders caused by autoantibodies against antigens normally on the surface of erythrocytes.[24] Three types of AIHAs have been described: (1) warm reactive antibody type, (2) cold agglutinin type, and (3) cold hemolysin type (paroxysmal cold hemoglobinuria). This classification is based on the optimal temperature at which the antibody binds to erythrocytes and the mechanism of RBC destruction.

Warm autoimmune hemolytic anemia is uncommon (incidence of about 1 per 80,000 population annually), although it is the most common form of AIHA (80 to 90% of cases), and generally occurs in individuals older than the age of 40.[25] Approximately half of the cases are secondary to other diseases, especially lymphomas but also chronic lymphocytic leukemia, other neoplastic disorders, or systemic lupus erythematosus (SLE). The anemia is caused by IgG that binds optimally to erythrocytes at normal body temperature (98.6° F, 37° C). Most cases are related to antibody against Rh-related antigens other than the D epitope (Rh antigens are discussed in Chapter 8). The spectrum of antibody specificities includes antibodies against the e, E, or c antigens of the Rh complex. Other cases are caused by IgG antibodies against erythrocyte antigens outside the Rh complex and include antibodies against Wr^b, En^a, the Kell blood group, and many others. The warm reactive IgG antibodies usually do not activate complement because of the rather sparse distribution of antigens on the RBC surface. (Activation of complement by antibody is discussed in Chapters 6, 7, and 8.) RBC destruction is caused by extravascular processes. The IgG-coated RBCs bind to the Fc receptors on monocytes and splenic macrophages and are removed by phagocytosis.

Cold agglutinin autoimmune hemolytic anemia is mediated by immunoglobulin M (IgM) antibodies and occurs less often than warm antibody hemolysis, affecting mostly the middle-aged and older adults.[26] Cold antibodies optimally bind to RBCs at colder temperatures (lower than 31° C [87.8° F])with maximal binding capacity at 4° C (39.2° F). Cold agglutinin autoantibodies may appear acutely during recovery of certain infectious disorders, particularly infectious mononucleosis and mycoplasma pneumonia. With these conditions, the individuals are usually younger than those with primary disease; the anemia may be severe but may be self-limiting. Chronic cold agglutinin AIHAs also can occur in association with lymphoid neoplasm and other unknown or idiopathic conditions.[27]

The IgM autoantibody is usually monoclonal and directed against erythrocyte carbohydrate antigens of the I system (i.e., i, I) or the P system (i.e., Pr).[26] In the colder areas of the body, particularly during cold weather (e.g., fingers, toes, nose, ears, exposed skin), the IgM autoantibodies bind to circulating erythrocytes. The IgM is rapidly released when the blood recirculates and warms. IgM is an extremely efficient activator of complement, resulting in the stable deposition of C3b on the cell surface. If an adequate amount of complement is deposited, the erythrocytes become vulnerable to recognition and rapid phagocytosis by mononuclear phagocytes in the liver and spleen (also see Chapter 8). The severity of hemolysis is variable and may result in a progressive chronic anemia. If the level of antibody is high or has particularly strong binding, hemagglutination may occur in the capillaries of exposed sites, such as fingers, toes, and ears, when temperatures are below 30° C (86° F). Obstruction of blood flow caused by RBC agglutination may lead to a bluish discoloration of the skin (acrocyanosis) that resolves as the skin is warmed. Prolonged exposure to the cold may lead to gangrene. **Cold hemolysin autoimmune hemolytic anemia (paroxysmal cold hemoglobinuria)** is a disorder in which exposure to cold initiates acute and severe intravascular hemolysis that unlike cold agglutinin anemia results in hemoglobulinuria.[26] The chronic form of this anemia is extremely rare, but an acute form of paroxysmal cold hemoglobinuria is frequently observed (30% to 40% of cases) in AIHA of childhood. The acute form occurs primarily in young children younger than the age of 10 and is usually preceded by an upper respiratory tract infection or flulike symptoms. Infections with measles, mumps, *Mycoplasma* (pneumonia), and *Varicella* have also been linked to an onset of paroxysmal cold hemoglobinuria. The anemia may be rapidly progressing and severe and associated with fever, reddish brown urine, hemoglobinuria, jaundice, abdominal pains, and pallor, with about 25% of individuals presenting with hepatomegaly and splenomegaly.

Paroxysmal cold hemoglobinuria is generally caused by IgG autoantibodies against the P blood group antigen.[26] Antibody binding occurs in the colder portions of the body. As the erythrocyte recirculates, enzymes of the complement cascade are activated, and cells are destroyed in the vasculature by complement-mediated lysis. The involved antibody, also called *Donath-Landsteiner antibody*, was first recognized in individuals with anemia secondary to chronic syphilis infection. A transfusion reaction is an example of alloimmune hemolytic anemia (also see Chapter 8). Transfused blood that is mismatched for ABO antigens is destroyed by preexisting isohemagglutinins in the recipient. Isohemagglutinins, which are generally IgM antibodies, activate complement, resulting in a rapid intravascular hemolysis. The individual may immediately experience fever, chills, dyspnea, and hypotension and may progress to shock. In some cases the hemolytic reaction may be delayed and develop 3 to 10 days after transfusion. The delayed reaction is caused by a low titer of preexisting antibodies to minor RBC antigens.

Drug-induced hemolytic anemia is a form of immune hemolytic anemia usually resulting from an allergic reaction against foreign antigens (e.g., antibiotics) (also see Chapter 8). Usually the drug is small molecular weight and functions as a hapten and binds to proteins on the surface of erythrocytes. This is sometimes called the *hapten model* and is based on anemia caused by penicillin, cephalosporins (more than 90% of cases), and, very recently, hydrocortisone (Figure 26-8).[28] IgG antibody against the drug or against the unique antigen formed by the interface of the drug and erythrocyte protein is formed and binds to the erythrocyte at normal body temperature. Hemolysis is usually extravascular because the opsonized RBCs are removed by phagocytes in the spleen and liver, although complement-dependent intravascular hemolysis may occur in some individuals. This form of drug-induced anemia usually follows a large intravenous infusion of an antibiotic and occurs 1 to 2 weeks after the initiation

of therapy. Cessation of administration of the drug results in rapid resolution of the anemia.

The erythrocyte plasma membrane contains receptors of components of the complement system, such as C3b, and can bind circulating immune complexes that have activated the complement cascade (see Chapter 8 for a discussion of immune complexes). This forms the basis for the *immune complex model* of drug-induced hemolytic anemia and was first described for anemia resulting from administration of the drug quinidine. The drug or a metabolite of the drug, both of which are haptens, initially binds to plasma proteins and becomes immunogenic (see Chapter 7). The circulating drug/protein complex reacts with the resultant antibody (usually IgM, although IgG complexes have also been described) and activate the complement system resulting in the deposition of C3b into the complex. Binding of the immune complexes to the erythrocyte surface results in further complement activation and intravascular hemolysis. This mechanism also may explain some of the anemia observed in other immune complex conditions, such as SLE.

In at least one instance, administration of the drug α-methyldopa induces an immune response against normal erythrocyte antigens and thus initiates a true AIHA *(autoantibody model)*. The autoantibody is usually against Rh blood group antigens. It is estimated that 20% of individuals taking α-methyldopa develop detectable antibodies, but only 1% actually develop clinically significant anemia. The mechanism by which α-methyldopa induces autoantibodies against the erythrocytes is unknown.

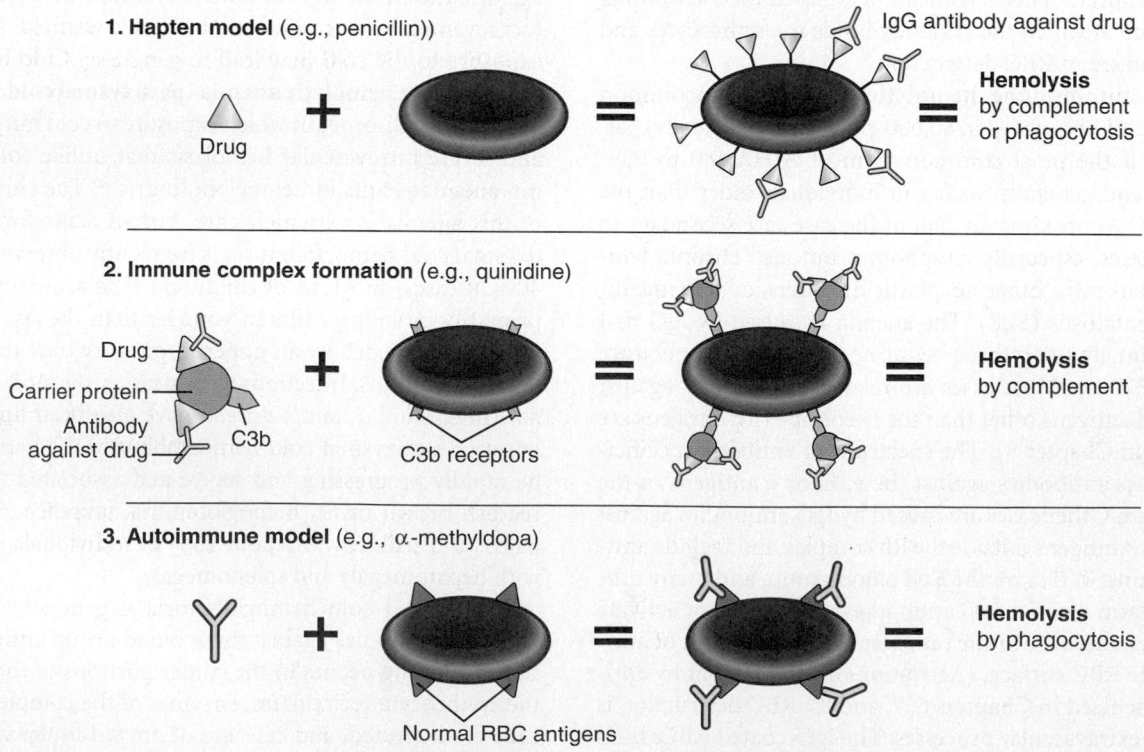

1. Hapten model (e.g., penicillin))

Drug

IgG antibody against drug

Hemolysis by complement or phagocytosis

2. Immune complex formation (e.g., quinidine)

Drug
Carrier protein
Antibody against drug
C3b

C3b receptors

Hemolysis by complement

3. Autoimmune model (e.g., α-methyldopa)

Normal RBC antigens

Hemolysis by phagocytosis

Figure 26-8 Models of drug-induced hemolytic anemia. (See discussion in text). *IgG,* Immunoglobulin G; *RBC,* red blood cell.

CLINICAL MANIFESTATIONS The presence and severity of signs and symptoms of hemolytic anemia depend on the degree of anemia and hemolysis and the success of compensatory erythropoiesis. Adaptation to red cell destruction is facilitated by increased red cell production. Bone marrow is capable of increasing red cell production up to eight times its normal rate. Accelerated RBC production that is incapable of keeping up with destruction develops into a true hemolytic anemia.

The severity of anemia varies widely from individual to individual, even in individuals who have the same illness. Severe disease is commonly diagnosed shortly after birth or within the first year of life. Mild to moderate anemia is more common because the shortened erythrocyte survival time is offset by increased erythropoiesis. Some individuals have no symptoms of anemia, and the underlying hemolytic process remains undetected unless some other complication develops during the course of the disease.

Jaundice (icterus) is present when heme destruction exceeds the liver's ability to conjugate and excrete bilirubin. Jaundice is first noticed in the neonatal period. Children and adults with congenital hemolytic anemia may not have icterus, or it may be mild enough that it goes unnoticed. In some individuals, faint scleral icterus may be the only indication of hemolytic disease.

Acute conditions that disrupt the delicate equilibrium of accelerated erythropoiesis and RBC destruction may precipitate a crisis. The most common type of crisis is aplastic and results from failure of bone marrow RBC production. The most common cause of aplastic crisis is human parvovirus B19 infection.

Commonly individuals with congenital hemolytic disorders demonstrate splenomegaly, which is often only mild in nature. In some cases the spleen may become quite enlarged and may cause discovery of the underlying hemolytic disorder. Another underlying condition that may be the cause of inadvertently determining the presence of the anemic disorder is the development of gallstones.

Children who have hemolytic anemia often demonstrate skeletal abnormalities caused by expansion of erythroid bone marrow during the active phase of growth and development. These alterations are more pronounced in the bony structures of the face and skull and may result in pathologic fractures (see Chapter 28). Cardiovascular and respiratory manifestations vary with the degree of anemia. In spite of the disorder being characterized as hemolytic in nature, thromboembolism may occur. Pulmonary embolism is a common finding during autopsies of individuals with immune hemolytic anemia.

EVALUATION AND TREATMENT Diagnosis is based on clinical manifestations, bone marrow studies, and blood tests (see Table 26-3). Abnormally increased numbers of erythrocyte stem cells are found in the marrow, a finding termed *erythroid hyperplasia*. Accelerated erythropoiesis causes large numbers of fragile and immature erythrocytes (stem cells and reticulocytes) to be released prematurely into the circulation. These cells are observed in blood smears. If the bone marrow is able to consistently maintain adequate compensation, the hemoglobin may remain stable. The mean corpuscular volume, however, may be decreased in the presence of reticulocytes. A blood smear is helpful in determining the presence of spherocytes or schistocytes, as well as examining white blood cells and platelets for coexisting hematologic or malignant conditions.

Acquired hemolytic anemias are treated by removing the cause or treating the underlying disorder. Acute fulminating hemolytic anemia (hemolytic crisis) is treated with fluid and electrolyte replacement to prevent shock and renal damage, which may be caused by RBC debris clogging the kidney tubules. Transfusions of blood products sometimes are given. Splenectomy is performed if the spleen is the major site of hemolysis and splenomegaly is significant.

Folate also is used in treating chronic hemolytic disease to prevent megaloblastic crisis because long-term erythrocyte turnover increases folate requirements. The use of monoclonal antibody therapy has proven beneficial. Rituximab is a monoclonal antibody directed against the CD20 antigen and specifically depletes or suppresses B cells throughout the body. CD20 is expressed on most cells in the B-cell lineage, except hematopoietic stem cells and plasma cells. Rituximab is used to treat a variety of leukemias and lymphomas and autoimmune diseases (e.g., rheumatoid arthritis, idiopathic thrombocytopenia, multiple sclerosis, type 1 diabetes mellitus, systemic lupus erythematosus). It is used successfully in several types of immune hemolytic anemias.[29] Eculizumab is a monoclonal antibody against complement protein C5, which blocks the enzymatic activation of C5 to C5a and C5b.[23] Thus treatment with eculizumab prevents the formation of the membrane attack complex and complement-mediated cell lysis (see Chapter 6). Eculizumab has been used in multiple trials to treat paroxysmal nocturnal hemoglobinuria.[30] Treatment has rapidly decreased serum markers for intravascular hemolysis, the need for transfusions, and the risk for thrombosis and diminished many other symptoms, including fatigue and abdominal pains.[30,31] Blockage of C5 activation mimics individuals who have congenital deficiencies in C5 (see Chapter 8). Lack of C5 increases the risk for disseminated infections with *Neisseria* sp., particularly *Neisseria meningitidis*. Thus immunization with the meningococcal vaccine is recommended before treatment with eculizumab.[31]

Anemia of Chronic Disease

Anemia of chronic disease (ACD) is a mild to moderate anemia resulting from decreased erythropoiesis in individuals with conditions of chronic systemic disease or inflammation (e.g., cancer, infections, autoimmune diseases).[11] These conditions include acquired immunodeficiency disease (AIDS), rheumatoid arthritis, SLE, malaria, acute and chronic hepatitis, and chronic renal failure. This form of anemia also is commonly noted in the presence of congestive heart failure (CHF). The anemia develops after 1 to 2 months of disease activity. The severity of anemia is related to that of the underlying disorder. Individuals may be asymptomatic, or the anemia may be a coincidental clinical finding. Morphologically, ACD is initially normocytic-normochromic, but as the condition progresses it becomes hypochromic and microcytic. ACD is characterized by normal iron stores with low circulating iron (less than 60 mcg/dl).

ACD is one of the most common conditions encountered in medicine and is probably only secondary to IDA in overall incidence. In individuals older than age 65 anemia is present in 10% of those who live in the community and more than 50% of those who reside in nursing homes[3]; two thirds of which is ACD or unexplained anemia. Older adults may be predisposed to ACD related to age-associate hematopoietic restriction. Additionally, older adults demonstrate increased concentrations of inflammatory cytokines, which play a significant role in the development of ACD. Older adult who present with characteristics of ACD without an underlying malignancy or inflammatory condition are described as having primary defective iron-utilization syndrome.

PATHOPHYSIOLOGY ACD results from a combination of (1) decreased erythrocyte life span, (2) suppressed production of erythropoietin, (3) ineffective bone marrow erythroid progenitor response to erythropoietin, and (4) altered iron metabolism and iron sequestration in macrophages.[32-35] During chronic inflammation a large variety of cytokines are released by lymphocytes and macrophages, including TNF-α, INF-γ, interleukin-1β (IL-1β), (IL-3, and IL-6) (also see Chapter 7).[32,35]

The precise mechanism by which RBC destruction is mediated remains unclear, but it is thought to result from activation of macrophages by TNF-α. Macrophages are responsible for removal of senescent or damaged erythrocytes. Increased erythrocyte sensitivity to phagocytosis may be a result of bacterial toxins or factors released from tumors. The erythropoietic defect in ACD is failure to increase erythropoiesis in response to decreased numbers of RBCs. In part, decreased erythropoiesis results from diminished production of erythropoietin by the kidneys. The kidney is frequently affected by chronic inflammatory processes through the production of circulating immune complexes and other factors that deposit in the kidney and activate secondary inflammatory mechanisms. In addition, the failure in erythropoiesis may reflect decreased responsiveness of erythroid progenitors to erythropoietin. Decreased availability of iron (discussed following) would diminish the rate of erythropoiesis. Proliferation of erythroid cells is also inhibited by proinflammatory cytokines, especially TNF-α, INF-γ, and IL-1β. TNF-α also directly induces apoptosis of erythroid progenitors, thus diminishing the number of responsive cells. In individuals who had anemia secondary to rheumatoid arthritis, the bone marrow contained elevated levels of IL-3, which correlated with diminished expression of integrins on the surface of cells of the erythroid series.[33] Loss of integrins may prevent adequate interaction with stromal cells and matrix proteins and inhibit erythropoiesis.

Impaired iron metabolism is partially the result of iron sequestration. IL-6 in particular affects hepatocytes and increases the release of the peptide hepcidin, which regulates the activity of ferroportin. Ferroportin is the primary transporter for the export of iron from macrophages to the plasma. Increased levels of hepcidin result in decreased ferroportin activity and suppression of iron release[11] (Figure 26-9). Additionally, normal iron transport by transferrin may be decreased as a result of competitive iron binding by inflammation-related increases in circulating lactoferrin and apoferritin. **Lactoferrin** is a member of the transferring family of nonheme iron-binding glycoproteins, and under normal conditions is present in the blood in only small amounts. During inflammation neutrophils release lactoferrin to bind iron and reduce its availability for bacteria. However, the affinity of iron for lactoferrin is 260 times greater than for transferrin. Lactoferrin-bound iron is removed by the mononuclear-phagocyte system and converted into ferritin, the storage form of iron. **Apoferritin** also has a higher affinity for iron and affects available iron in a similar manner.

CLINICAL MANIFESTATIONS ACD has fewer and milder manifestations than most other anemias. The anemia is usually in the mild to moderate range. If hemoglobin levels drop significantly, clinical manifestations of IDA appear.

EVALUATION AND TREATMENT The most significant finding of ACD is a very-high total body iron storage, although inadequate iron is available in the bone marrow for erythropoiesis. Very often the first indication of ACD is a failure to respond to conventional iron replacement therapy. Levels of erythropoietin are generally lower than expected for the degree of anemia. The affected individuals also frequently present with low or normal total iron binding capacity (TIBC), normal or high serum ferritin levels, and low concentrations of soluble transferrin receptor (blood test findings are listed in Table 26-3). Occasionally it may be difficult to differentiate ACD from IDA; however, measurement of sTfR may be useful. Levels of sTfR do not respond to iron supplementation in ACD but do so in IDA.

Use of erythropoietin in treatment of ACD associated with arthritis, malignancies, and AIDS has met with limited success. Transfusion of critically ill individuals may worsen the outcome and increase morbidity and mortality.[36] The principal treatment is alleviation of the underlying disorder. Individuals who have ACD but demonstrate no evidence of inflammatory or infectious conditions are screened for the presence of malignancies.

MYELOPROLIFERATIVE RED BLOOD CELL DISORDERS (POLYCYTHEMIA)

Hematologic dysfunction results from an overproduction of cells as well as a deficiency. One or more hematopoietic lines may be overproduced in the marrow in response to exogenous (e.g., radiation, drugs) or endogenous (physiologic compensatory responses, immune disorders) signals. Excessive RBC production is classified as **polycythemia**. Polycythemia exists in two forms: relative and absolute. **Relative polycythemia** results from hemoconcentration of the blood associated with dehydration that may be caused by decreased water intake,

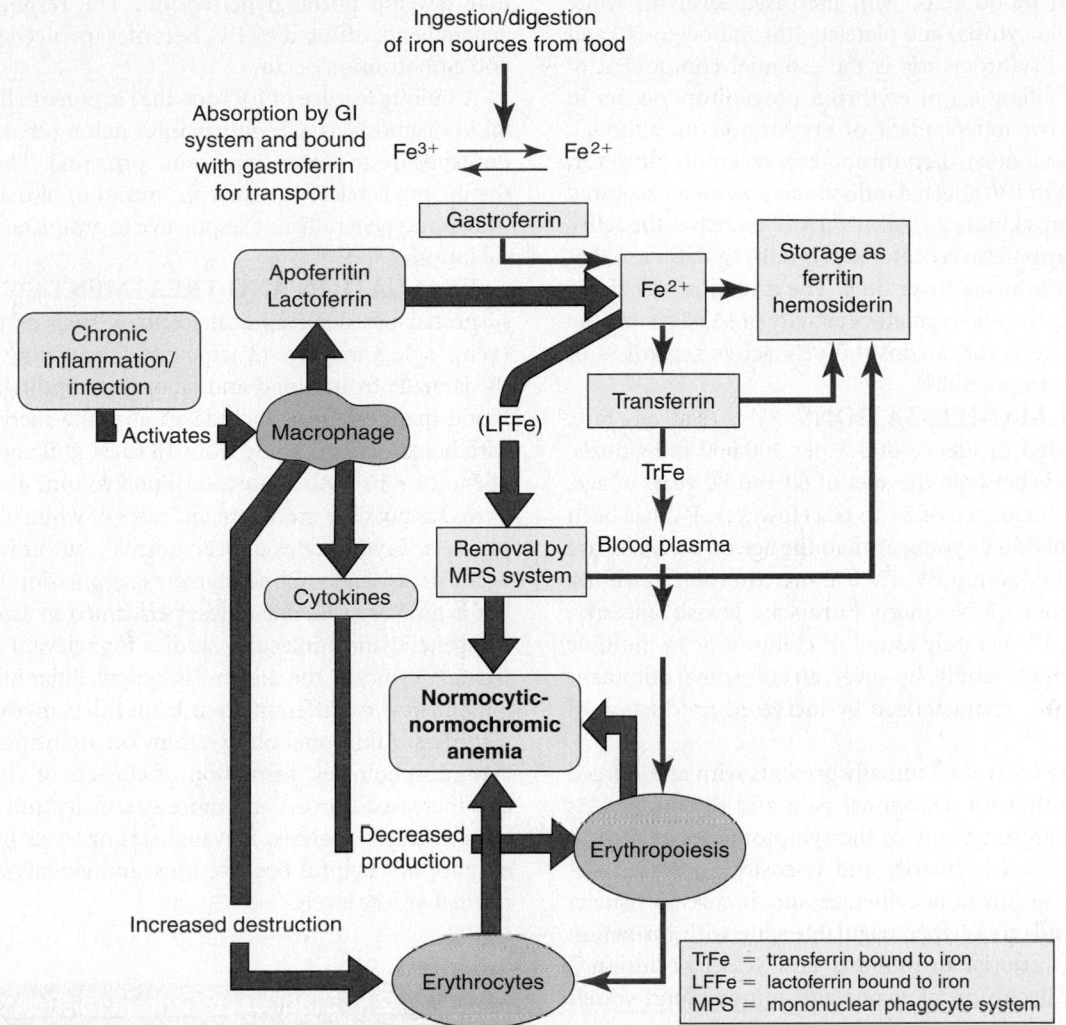

Figure 26-9 Pathophysiology of anemia of chronic disease. Normal iron metabolism is indicated by the narrow arrows. Abnormal mechanisms that are instrumental in the development of anemia of chronic inflammation are indicated by thick arrows. (See discussion in text.) *GI,* Gastrointestinal.

diarrhea, excessive vomiting, or increased use of diuretics. It is usually of minor consequence development and resolves with fluid administration or treatment of the underlying condition.

Absolute polycythemia consists of two forms: primary or secondary. *Secondary polycythemia,* the more common type, is caused by an increase in erythropoietin as a physiologic response to chronic hypoxia. This hypoxia is noted in individuals who live at higher altitudes (i.e., above 10,000 ft), smokers with increased levels of carbon monoxide (CO), and individuals with chronic obstructive pulmonary disease and congestive heart failure. Abnormal types of hemoglobin (e.g., Hb$_{San Diego}$ or Hb$_{Chesapeake}$), which have a greater affinity for oxygen, also cause secondary polycythemia, as does secretion of erythropoietin by certain tumors (e.g., renal cell carcinoma, hepatoma, cerebral hemiangioblastoma).

Primary polycythemia (known as *polycythemia vera*) is one of several disorders collectively known as *chronic myeloproliferative disorders* (CMPDs).[37] Others in this group include essential thrombocytosis, chronic idiopathic myelofibrosis, chronic myeloid leukemia, chronic neutrophilic leukemia, and chronic eosinophilic leukemia.[38] All of these disorders result from abnormal regulation of the multipotent hematopoietic stem cells. The major characteristics shared by these disorders are (1) involvement of a multipotent hematopoietic progenitor cell; (2) overproduction of one or more of the formed elements of the blood in the absence of a defined stimulus; (3) dominance of a transformed progenitor cell over the nontransformed progenitor cells; (4) marrow hypercellularity or fibrosis; (5) cytogenetic abnormalities; (6) predisposition to thrombus formation and hemorrhage; and (7) spontaneous transformation to acute leukemia. Determining a precise distinction between the CMPDs is difficult if not impossible because of overlapping clinical features and a lack of specific molecular markers. As a result, diagnosis is quite challenging.

PATHOPHYSIOLOGY Polycythemia vera (PV) is a neoplastic, nonmalignant condition characterized by an increase in red blood cells, with increased levels of white blood cells (leukocytosis) and platelets (thrombocytosis), and splenomegaly. Erythrocytosis is the essential component of PV. Clonal proliferation of erythroid progenitors occurs in the bone marrow independent of erythropoietin, although the cells express a normal erythropoietin receptor. However, more than 95% of PV-affected individuals possess an acquired mutation in Janus kinase 2 (JAK2).[39] JAK2 increases the activity of the erythropoietin receptor and is self-regulatory so that JAK2 activity diminishes over time. The mutation associated with PV negates the self-regulatory activity of JAK2 so that the erythropoietin receptor is constitutively active regardless of the level of erythropoietin.[40]

CLINICAL MANIFESTATIONS PV is relatively rare, with an estimated incidence of 2.3 per 100,000 individuals, peak incidence is between the ages of 60 and 80 years of age, with a median incidence of 55 to 60. However, PV has been observed in individuals younger than the age of 40. Males are twice as likely to develop PV. PV is more common in whites, particularly those of Northern European Jewish ancestry, than in blacks. PV is rarely found in children or in multiple members of a single family; however, an autosomal dominant form exists that is characterized by increased production of erythropoietin.

Almost every individual initially presents with an enlarged spleen, frequently with abdominal pain and discomfort. As the disease progresses many of the symptoms are related to the increased blood cellularity and viscosity. Increased viscosity, as well as thrombocythemia and increased platelet dysfunction, leads to a hypercoagulable state with formation of venous and arterial thrombosis and vessel occlusion.[41] Thrombi with occlusion of major and minor blood vessels lead to tissue and/or organ ischemia or infarction (tissue injury and/or death). Extreme thrombocythemia (greater than 1,5000,000/mm³ of blood) increases the risk for excessive bleeding, rather than thrombosis.

Increased blood viscosity results in a variety of circulatory alterations in PV, such as plethora (ruddy, red color of the face, hands, feet, ears, and mucous membranes) and engorgement of the retinal and cerebral vessels. Individuals also may experience headache, drowsiness, delirium, mania, psychotic depression, chorea, and visual disturbances. The risk for death from cerebral thrombosis is increased approximately fivefold in individuals with PV.

Cardiac workload and output remain essentially unchanged; however, increased blood volume may lead to elevated blood pressure. Coronary blood flow may be affected and lead to the onset of angina, although myocardial infarctions caused by PV are relatively rare. Other evidence of cardiovascular involvement is the development of Raynaud phenomenon and thromboangiitis obliterans.

Additionally, gastrointestinal gastric and duodenal thrombosis may occur with resultant hemorrhaging. The development of mesenteric thrombosis requires immediate medical intervention. Splenomegaly and hepatomegaly result from pooling of blood in these organs; consequently individuals may develop portal hypertension. The respiratory system, generally not affected by PV, becomes involved if thrombosis and embolization occur.

A unique feature of PV, one that is potentially instrumental in diagnosis, is extreme, painful itching that is intensified on exposure to water (aquagenic pruritus). The intensity of the itching is related to the concentration of mast cells in the skin, but is generally not responsive to antihistamines or topical lotions.

EVALUATION AND TREATMENT PV is frequently suspected based on clinical features, such as a thrombotic event, splenomegaly, or aquagenic pruritus. Diagnosis of PV is made from blood and laboratory findings (Box 26-2). Blood manifestations include an absolute increase in RBCs, with hematocrits ranging from 18 to 24 g/dl and RBC counts of 7 to 10×10^{12}. Absolute total blood volume also is increased as well as possible moderate increases of white blood cells and platelets. Erythrocytes appear normal, but anisocytosis may occur occasionally. Bone marrow examination may be done, but is not very valuable unless performed in association with cytogenetic and molecular studies for relevant mutations in JAK2.[42] Typically the marrow is hypercellular but not in such a manner as to differentiate it from other myeloproliferative disorders. Additional observations on abnormal megakaryocyte morphologies, formation of clusters of abnormal cells, and increased fibrosis add more specificity and usefulness to bone marrow analysis. Elevated serum levels of erythropoietin are not helpful because most individuals with PV have normal or low levels.

Box 26-2 Diagnostic Criteria for Polycythemia Vera

Major Criteria (A)
Increased total red blood cell (RBC) volume (RBC mass):
  > 25% above normal predicted value
  M ≥36 ml/kg (Hgb >18.5 g/dl)
  F ≥32 ml/kg (Hgb >16.5 g/dl)
O_2 saturation ≥92%
Splenectomy
Clonal genetic abnormality other than Philadelphia chromosome or *bcr/abl* fusion gene in marrow*
Endogenous erythroid formation in vitro*

Major Criteria (B)
Platelets ≥400,000 μL
WBC count ≥12,000 μL
LAP score >100
Serum B_{12} >900 pg/ml
$UB_{12}BC$ >2200 pg/ml
Panmyelosis (myeloid metaplasia with abnormal immature blood cells in spleen and/or liver) with prominent erythroid/megakaryocytic hyperplasia on marrow biopsy*
Decreased serum erythropoietin levels*

---

*World Health Organization (WHO) Criteria for Diagnosis: Elevated red cell mass (RCM) and any other major criteria or elevated RCM and any two minor criteria.
LAP, Leukocyte alkaline phosphatase; *UB₁₂BC*, unbound B₁₂-binding capacity; *WBC*, white blood cell.

Treatment of PV is challenging and directed toward minimizing the risk of thrombosis and preventing progression to myelofibrosis and acute leukemia. In low-risk individuals (e.g., those younger than age 60 or with no history of thrombosis and without risk factors for cardiovascular disease), the recommended therapy is phlebotomy and low-dose aspirin.[39] The guideline for phlebotomy (300 to 500 ml at a time to reduce erythrocytosis and blood volume) is maintenance of the hematocrit at less than 45%. The initial phlebotomies are performed two or three times a week until the hematocrit drops, and are repeated every 3 to 4 months to maintain a safe hematocrit. Aspirin is used for its antithrombotic (decrease in thromboxane) properties.

The recommended therapy for those at high risk includes use of hydroxyurea, an antimetabolite that blocks DNA synthesis and reduces vascular cellularity. Unlike other similar drugs, hydroxyurea reduces the risk of thrombotic complications, but does not increase the risk for developing leukemia.[39] INF-α has been used when other forms of treatment have failed. Interferon inhibits the growth of the abnormal progenitors and inhibits the actions of cytokines that may lead to the development of myelofibrosis. Therapy with INF-α is complicated by its proinflammatory activities, thus fever, flu-like symptoms, and more severe complications are common. INF-α is not consistently effective in high-risk adult cases, but is considered in individuals who are intolerant to hydroxyurea, younger individuals, and pregnancy.

Radioactive phosphorus (^{32}P) has been used to suppress erythropoiesis. It is generally effective for an extended time, and as many as 18 months may elapse between treatments. Side effects of ^{32}P treatment include suppression of hematopoiesis resulting in anemia, leukopenia, or thrombocytopenia. Development of acute leukemia is also a major side effect of ^{32}P, occurring after 7 or more years of treatment, making this therapy more useful in older adults.

Without proper treatment, 50% of individuals with PV die within 18 months of the onset of initial symptoms. The primary cause of death is thrombosis, which is more prevalent in older individuals and those with prior vascular complications. Hemorrhage is rare but more common in individuals with high platelet counts and those taking antiplatelet drugs. Conversion to acute myeloid leukemia (AML) occurs in 10% of individuals within 15 years, increasing to 50% within 20 years. This leukemia is generally refractory to conventional treatment and remains a significant potential adverse outcome of PV. Conversion to AML is more common in individuals who were treated with alkylating agents, whereas those treated only with INF or hydroxyurea had the same incidence of conversion as those who received no treatment. Although PV is a chronic disorder and remissions occur with appropriate therapy, the prevention of significant morbidity and mortality is possible, and survival for 10 to 15 years is common.

SUMMARY REVIEW

Anemia

1. Anemia is defined as a reduction in the number or volume of circulating RBCs or a decrease in hemoglobin. Polycythemias are excessive levels of RBCs or volume.
2. Anemias can be classified according to (1) erythrocyte size or concentration of hemoglobin or (2) their cause.
3. Clinical manifestations of anemia may be demonstrated in all organs and tissues (tissue hypoxia) throughout the body. Decreased oxygen delivery to tissues causes fatigue, dyspnea, syncope, angina, compensatory tachycardia, and organ dysfunction.
4. Macrocytic-normochromic, or megaloblastic-normochromic, anemias are characterized by larger than normal RBCs with normal levels of hemoglobin. They most commonly are caused by deficiency of vitamin B_{12} (PA) or folate.
5. PA results from inadequate vitamin B_{12} absorption because of autoantibodies against the B_{12} transporter IF. Folate deficiency anemia is caused by inadequate dietary intake of folate. Both anemias respond to replacement therapy.
6. Microcytic-hypochromic anemias are characterized by abnormally small RBCs with insufficient hemoglobin content. This disorder results from disorders of (1) iron metabolism (IDA), (2) porphyrin and heme synthesis (SAs), or globin synthesis (thalassemia).
7. IDA is the most common type of anemia worldwide. It usually develops slowly, with gradual insidious onset of symptoms. Fatigue, weakness, dyspnea, alteration of various epithelial tissues, and vague neuromuscular complaints result.

8. IDA is usually a result of blood loss or poor nutritional intake. Individuals at highest risk for developing IDA; older adults, women, infants, and those living in poverty. Anemia is also recognized as part of the nonspecific acute phase response to any type of inflammation. Once the source of blood loss is identified and corrected, oral iron replacement therapy can be initiated.
9. SA results from defects in mitochondrial metabolism leading to ineffective iron uptake and dysfunctional heme synthesis. The characteristic cell in the bone marrow, a ringed sideroblast, is an erythroblast containing iron granules arranged around the nucleus. SAs may be hereditary or acquired, and treatment varies depending on the cause.
10. Normocytic-normochromic anemias are characterized by insufficient numbers of normal erythrocytes. Included in this category are aplastic, posthemorrhagic, and hemolytic anemias and ACD.
11. AA is a critical condition characterized by a reduction or absence of all three blood cell types (pancytopenia). Unless the cause is determined, bone marrow aplasia results in death.
12. Acute blood loss from hemorrhage results in posthemorrhagic anemia with the severity depending on the amount of hemorrhage. Restoration of blood volume by plasma expanders or transfusions may diminish subjective symptoms of anemia. Hemoglobin restoration may take 6 to 8 weeks.
13. Hemolytic anemia is a result of excessive destruction of erythrocytes and may be acquired or hereditary. Of the acquired forms, autoimmune reaction (immunohemolytic) and drug-induced hemolysis are the most common.

Continued

14. AIHAs include (1) warm reactive antibody type, (2) cold agglutinin type, and (3) cold hemolysin type (paroxysmal cold hemoglobinuria).
15. ACD results from decreased erythropoiesis secondary to chronic diseases. The anemia is mild to moderate and one of the most common conditions encountered in medicine.
16. Mechanisms associated with ACD include (1) decreased erythrocyte life span, (2) reduced production of erythropoietin, (3) ineffective bone marrow response to erythropoietin, and (4) iron sequestration in macrophages. In particular, the proinflammataory cytokine IL-6 increases hepatocyte release of hepcidin, which suppresses ferroportin transport of iron out of macrophages.

Myeloproliferative RBC Disorders (Polycythemia)

1. Polycythemia vera is a myeloproliferative disorder characterized by excessive proliferation of erythrocyte precursors in the bone marrow. Signs and symptoms result directly from increased blood volume and viscosity and a predisposition to thrombosis.
2. Therapeutic phlebotomy to remove excessive blood volume and the use of hydroxyurea have been helpful in decreasing the excessive RBC population.

KEY TERMS

Absolute polycythemia, 1009
Anemia, 989
Anemia of chronic disease (ACD), 1007
Anisocytosis, 989
Aplastic anemia (AA), 1000
Apoferritin, 1008
Autoimmune hemolytic anemia (AIHA), 1005
Cold agglutinin autoimmune hemolytic anemia, 1005
Cold hemolysin autoimmune hemolytic anemia (paroxysmal cold hemoglobinuria), 1005
Dimorphism, 998

Drug-induced hemolytic anemia, 1006
Erythropoietic hemochromatosis, 999
Fanconi anemia, 1002
Folate (folic acid), 995
Hemolytic anemia, 1003
Hypoplastic anemia, 999
Hypoxemia, 990
Intrinsic factor (IF), 993
Iron deficiency anemia (IDA), 995
Lactoferrin, 1008
Macrocytic anemia (megaloblastic anemia), 990
Microcytic-hypochromic anemia, 995
Myelodysplastic syndrome (MDS), 998

Normocytic-normochromic anemia, 1000
Pancytopenia, 1000
Paroxysmal nocturnal hemoglobinuria, 1005
Pernicious anemia (PA), 991
Poikilocytosis, 989
Polycythemia, 1008
Polycythemia vera (PV), 1009
Posthemorrhagic anemia, 1003
Pure red cell aplasia (PRCA), 1001
Relative polycythemia, 1008
Ringed sideroblast, 998
Sideroblastic anemia (SA), 998
Warm autoimmune hemolytic anemia, 1005

REFERENCES

1. Aslinia F, Mazza JJ, Yale SH: Megaloblastic anemia and other causes of macrocytosis, *Clin Med Res* 4(3):236-241, 2006.
2. Gaskell H et al: Prevalence of anaemia in older persons: systemic review, *BMC Geriat* 8(January 14):1-8, 2008.
3. Patel KV: Epidemiology of anemia in older adults, *Semin Hematol* 45(4):210-217, 2008.
4. Carmel R: Nutritional anemias and the elderly, *Semin Hematol* 45(4):225-234, 2008.
5. Vojdani A: Antibodies as predictors of complex autoimmune diseases, *Int J Immunopathol Pharmacol* 21(2):267-278, 2008.
6. Desai HG, Gupte PA: *Helicobacter pylori* link to pernicious anaemia, *J Assoc Physicians India* 55(12):857-859, 2007.
7. West AR, Oates PS: Mechanisms of heme iron absorption: current questions and controversies, *World J Gastroenterol* 14(26):4101-4110, 2008.
8. Killip S, Bennett JM, Chambers MD: Iron deficiency anemia, *Am Fam Physician* 75(5):671-678, 2007.
9. Alleyne M, Horne MK, Miller JL: Individualized treatment for iron-deficiency anemia in adults, *Am J Med* 121(11):943-948, 2008.
10. Finsterer J: Hematological manifestations of primary mitochondrial disorders, *Acta Haematol* 118(2):88-98, 2007.
11. Edison ES, Bajel A, Chandy M: Iron homeostasis: new players, newer insights, *Eur J Haematol* 81(6):411-424, 2008.
12. Camaschella C: Recent advances in the understanding of inherited sideroblastic anaemia, *Brit J Haematol* 143(1):27-38, 2008.
13. Koppel A, Schiller G: Myelodysplastic syndrome: an update on diagnosis and therapy, *Curr Oncol Rep* 10(5):372-378, 2008.
14. Dreyfus F: The deleterious effects of iron overload in patients with myelodysplastic syndromes, *Blood Rev* 22(Suppl 2):S29-S34, 2008.
15. Malcovati L, Nimer SD: Myelodysplastic syndromes: diagnosis and staging, *Cancer Contr* 15(Supp):4-13, 2008.
16. Moyo V et al: Erythropoiesis-stimulating agents in the treatment of anemia in myeodysplastic syndromes: a meta-analysis, *Ann Hematol* 87(7):527-536, 2008.
17. Young NS, Calado RT, Scheinberg P: Current concepts in the pathophysiology and treatment of aplastic anemia, *Blood* 108(8): 2509-2519, 2006.
18. Bacigalupo A: Aplastic anemia: pathogenesis and treatment, *Hematol 2007* 2007:23-28, 2007.
19. Armand P, Antin JH: Allogeneic stem cell transplantation for aplastic anemia, *Biol Blood Marrow Transplant* 13(5):505-516, 2007.
20. Davies JK, Guinan EC: An update on the management of severe idiopathic aplastic anaemia in children, *Brit J Haematol* 136(4):549-564, 2007.
21. Brodsky RA: Narrative review: paroxysmal nocturnal hemoglobinuria: the physiology of complement-related hemolytic anemia, *Ann Intern Med* 148(8):587-595, 2008.
22. Ziakas PD, Poulou LS, Pomont A: Thrombosis in paroxysmal nocturnal hemoglobinuria at a glance: a clinical review, *Curr Vasc Pharmacol* 6(4):347-353, 2008.
23. Brodsky R: Advances in the diagnosis and therapy of paroxysmal nocturnal hemoglobinuria, *Blood Rev* 22(2):65-74, 2008.
24. Valent P, Lechner K: Diagnosis and treatment of autoimmune haemolytic anaemias in adults: a clinical review, *Wien Klin Wochenschr* 120(5–6), 2008.
25. Packman CH: Hemolytic anemia due to warm autoantibodies, *Blood Rev* 22(1):17-31, 2008.
26. Petz LD: Cold antibody autoimmune hemolytic anemias, *Blood Rev* 22(1):1-15, 2008.
27. Berentsen S, Belske K, Tjønnfjord GE: Primary chronic cold agglutinin disease: an update on pathogenesis, clinical features and therapy, *Hematology* 12(5):361-370, 2007.
28. Martinengo M et al: The first case of drug-induced immune hemolytic anemia due to hydrocortisone, *Transfusion* 48(9):1925-1929, 2008.

29. Garvey B: Rituximab in the treatment of autoimmune haematological disorders, *Brit J Haematol* 141(2):149-169, 2008.

30. Charneski L, Patel PN: Eculizumab in paroxysmal nocturnal haemoglobinuria, *Drugs* 68(10):1341-1346, 2008.

31. Hill A: Update on eculizumab for the treatment of paroxysmal nocturnal hemoglobinuria, *Clin Adv Hematol Oncol* 6(7):499-500, 2008.

32. Handelman GJ, Levin NW: Iron and anemia in human biology: a review of mechanisms, *Heart Fail Rev* 13(4):393-404, 2008.

33. Jaworski J et al: Decreased expression of integrins by hematopoietic cells in patients with rheumatoid arthritis and anemia: relationship with bone marrow cytokine levels, *J Investig Allerg Clin Immunol* 18(1):17-21.

34. Foley RN: Erythropoietin: physiology and molecular mechanisms, *Heart Fail Rev* 13(4):405-414, 2008.

35. Zarychanski R, Houston DS: Anemia of chronic disease: a harmful disorder or an adaptive, beneficial response? *Can Med Assoc J* 179(4):333-337, 2008.

36. Asare K: Anemia of critical illness, *Pharmacotherapy* 28(10):1267-1282, 2008.

37. Levine RL, Gilliland DG: Myeloproliferative disorders, *Blood* 112(6):2190-2198, 2008.

38. National Institutes of Health, U.S. Department of Health and Human Services. *Chronic myeloproliferative disorders treatment: health professional version*, Bethesda, MD, 2008, Available at http://cancer. gov/cancertopics/pdq/treatment/myeloproliferative/healthprofessoinal/. Accessed January 22, 2009.

39. Finazzi G, Barbui T: Evidence and expertise in the management of polycythemia vera and essential thrombocythemia, *Leukemia* 22(8):1494-1502, 2008.

40. Chen G, Prchal JT: Polycythemia vera and its molecular basis: an update, *Best Pract Res Clin Haemotol* 19(3):387-397, 2006.

41. Landolfi R, Cipriani MC, Novarese L: Thrombosis and bleeding in polycythemia vera and essential thrombocythemia: pathogenetic mechanisms and prevention, *Best Pract Res Clin Haematol* 19(3): 617-633, 2006.

42. Tefferi A: The diagnosis of polycythemia vera: new tests and old dictums, *Best Pract Res Clin Haematol* 19(3):455-469, 2006.

ALTERATIONS OF LEUKOCYTE, LYMPHOID, AND HEMOSTATIC FUNCTION

NEAL S. ROTE • KATHRYN L. McCANCE

MEDIA RESOURCES

 Evolve Website (http://evolve.elsevier.com/McCance/)
- Review Questions and Answers
- Animations
- Glossary (with audio pronunciation for selected terms)
- WebLinks

Online Course
- Module 14

CHAPTER OUTLINE

ALTERATIONS OF LEUKOCYTE FUNCTION
  Quantitative Alterations of Leukocytes
  Infectious Mononucleosis
  Leukemias
ALTERATIONS OF LYMPHOID FUNCTION
  Lymphadenopathy
  Malignant Lymphomas
  Plasma Cell Malignancies

ALTERATIONS OF SPLENIC FUNCTION
ALTERATIONS OF PLATELETS AND COAGULATION
  Disorders of Platelets
  Disorders of Coagulation

The many disorders involving leukocytes range from deficiencies in the quality and quantity of leukocytes (leukopenia) to increased numbers of leukocytes (leukocytosis) in response to infections to proliferative disorders, such as leukemia. Many hematologic disorders are malignancies, and many nonhematologic malignancies metastasize to bone marrow, affecting leukocyte production. Thus a large portion of this chapter is devoted to malignant disease.

The primary role of clotting (hemostasis) is to stop bleeding through an interaction among vascular endothelium, platelets, and the clotting system. Many disease states are associated with clinically significant aberrations in any of these three necessary components of clotting. This chapter discusses various components of clotting and their control systems.

ALTERATIONS OF LEUKOCYTE FUNCTION

Leukocyte function is affected if too many or too few white cells are present in the blood or if the cells that are present are structurally or functionally defective. **Quantitative leukocyte disorders** result from decreased production in the bone marrow or accelerated destruction of cells in the circulation. Other quantitative alterations, however, occur in response to infections.

Qualitative leukocyte disorders consist of disruptions of leukocyte function. Phagocytic cells (granulocytes, monocytes, macrophages) may lose their capacity to function as effective phagocytes. Lymphocytes may lose their capacity to respond to antigens. (Qualitative disruptions of inflammatory and immune processes caused by leukocyte disorders are described in Chapter 8.) Other leukocyte alterations include infectious mononucleosis and cancers of the blood—leukemia and multiple myeloma.

Quantitative Alterations of Leukocytes

Leukocytosis is a leukocyte count that is higher than normal; conversely, **leukopenia** is a count that is lower than normal. Leukocytosis or leukopenia may affect all cell types or only a specific type of leukocyte and may result from a variety of physiologic conditions and alterations.

Leukocytosis occurs as a normal protective response to physiologic stressors, such as infection, strenuous exercise, emotional changes, temperature changes, anesthesia, surgery, pregnancy, and some drugs, hormones, and toxins. It is also caused by pathologic conditions, such as malignancies and hematologic disorders. Unlike leukocytosis, leukopenia is never normal. When the leukocyte count decreases to less than 1000/mm^3, the individual is at increased risk for infection. With counts less than 500/mm^3, the possibility for life-threatening infections is high. Leukopenia can be caused by radiation, anaphylactic shock, autoimmune disease (e.g., systemic lupus erythematosus), immune deficiencies (see Chapter 8), and exposure to certain chemotherapeutic agents.

Granulocytes and Monocytes

Increased numbers of circulating granulocytes (neutrophils, eosinophils, basophils) and monocytes are primarily a response to infection. Increased numbers also occur as a result of myeloproliferative disorders (i.e., polycythemia vera, chronic myelogenous leukemia, chronic neutrophilic leukemia, chronic eosinophilic leukemia) that increase stem cell proliferation in bone marrow.

Decreased numbers occur when infectious processes exhaust the supply of circulating granulocytes and monocytes by drawing them out of the circulation and into infected tissues faster than they can be replaced. Decreases also can be caused by disorders that suppress marrow function.

Granulocytosis—an increase in granulocytes (neutrophils, eosinophils, basophils)—begins with the release of stored leukocytes from the venous sinuses of the marrow. **Neutrophilia** is another term that may be used to describe *granulocytosis* because neutrophils are the most numerous of the granulocytes (Table 27-1). Neutrophilia occurs in the early stages of infection or inflammation and is established when the absolute neutrophil count exceeds 7500/μL. Stored neutrophils are approximately 20 to 40 times greater in number than circulating neutrophils. When the neutrophil count increases greatly—more than 100,000/μL (usually seen only in those with myelocytic leukemia)—the blood viscosity may increase greatly so that thrombosis or occlusion of blood vessels occurs. Release and depletion of stored neutrophils from the venous sinuses stimulate granulopoiesis to replenish neutrophil reserves. Specific conditions associated with neutrophilia are identified in Table 27-1.

When the demand for circulating mature neutrophils exceeds the supply, the marrow begins to release immature neutrophils (and other leukocytes) into the blood. Premature release of the immature white cells is responsible for the phenomenon known as a **shift-to-the-left** or **leukemoid reaction.** This refers to the microscopic detection of disproportionate numbers of immature leukocytes in peripheral blood smears. Many diagrams present cellular differentiation and maturation progressing from left to right within the drawing, instead of vertically as shown in Figure 25-9. An early release of immature leukocytes would shift the distribution of cells in the blood toward those on the left side of the diagram. This phenomenon is also seen in the blood smear of individuals with leukemia, hence the term *leukemoid reaction*. As infection or inflammation diminishes and as granulopoiesis replenishes circulating granulocytes, a return to normal occurs.

Neutropenia is a condition associated with reduction in circulating neutrophils. Clinically, neutropenia exists when the neutrophil count is less than 2000/μL.[1] A reduction in neutrophils occurs in severe prolonged infections when production of granulocytes cannot keep up with demand. Neutropenia is considered mild with a neutrophil count between 1000 and 1500/μL. Moderate neutropenia is a neutrophil count between 500 and 1000/μL, and severe neutropenia is a count less than 500/μL. Neutrophil reduction results from severe or prolonged infections when granulocyte production does not keep up with demand.

Other causes of neutropenia, in the absence of infection, may be (1) decreased neutrophil production or ineffective granulopoiesis, (2) reduced neutrophil survival, and (3) abnormal neutrophil distribution and sequestration. Neutropenia also is categorized as primary or secondary; primary disorders are further identified as congenital or acquired.

Congenital defects in neutrophil production include cyclic neutropenia and neutropenia with congenital immunodeficiency diseases, as well as multiple syndromes (e.g., Kostmann, Shwachman-Diamond, Diamond-Blackfan, Griscelli, Chédiak-Higashi, and Barth syndromes). Primary acquired neutropenia is associated with multiple conditions, for example, hypoplastic anemia or aplastic anemia, leukemia (acute myelogenous leukemia [AML]/chronic lymphocytic leukemia [CLL]), lymphomas (Hodgkin, non-Hodgkin), and myelodysplastic syndrome (MDS). The megaloblastic anemias (vitamin B$_{12}$ and folate deficiency) as well as starvation and anorexia nervosa cause neutropenia because of an inadequate supply of vitamins and nutrients for protein production.

Reduced neutrophil survival and abnormal distribution and sequestration are usually secondary to other disorders. Neutropenia occurs in a variety of immunologic disorders, particularly systemic lupus erythematosus, rheumatoid arthritis, Felty and Sjögren syndromes, splenomegaly, and drug-related causes.

Severe **granulocytopenia** (less than 500/μL) or **agranulocytosis** (complete absence of granulocytes in blood) is usually secondary to arrested hematopoiesis in the bone marrow or massive cell destruction in the circulation. Chemotherapeutic agents used to treat hematologic and other malignancies cause generalized bone marrow suppression. Several other drugs and large doses of ionizing radiation cause agranulocytosis, which occurs rarely but carries a high mortality rate (10% to 50%). Clinical manifestations of agranulocytosis include recurrent and persistent life-threatening infection (particularly of the respiratory system) leading to septicemia, general malaise, fever, tachycardia, and ulcers in the mouth and colon. If untreated, sepsis caused by agranulocytosis results in death within 3 to 6 days.

Eosinophilia is an absolute increase (more than 450/μL) in the total numbers of circulating eosinophils. Allergic disorders (type I hypersensitivity) associated with asthma, hay fever, and drug reactions, as well as parasitic infections (particularly

Table 27-1 Other Conditions Associated with Neutrophils, Eosinophils, Basophils, Monocytes, and Lymphocytes

Condition	Cause	Example
Neutrophil		
Neutrophilia (granulocytosis)	Inflammation or tissue necrosis	Surgery, burns, MI, pneumonitis, rheumatic fever, rheumatoid arthritis
	Infection	Bacterial: gram-positive (staphylococci, streptococci, pneumococci), gram-negative (*Escherichia coli, Pseudomonas* species)
	Physiologic	Exercise, extreme heat or cold, third-trimester pregnancy, emotional distress
	Hematologic	Acute hemorrhage, hemolysis, myeloproliferative disorder, chronic granulocytic leukemia
	Drugs or chemicals	Epinephrine, steroids, heparin, histamine, endotoxin
	Metabolic	Diabetes (acidosis), eclampsia, gout, thyroid storm
	Neoplasm	Liver, GI tract, bone marrow
Neutropenia	Decreased marrow production	Radiation, chemotherapy, leukemia, aplastic anemia, abnormal granulopoiesis
	Increased destruction	Splenomegaly, hemodialysis, autoimmune disease
	Infection	Gram-negative (typhoid), viral (influenza, hepatitis B, measles, mumps, rubella), severe infections, protozoal infections (malaria)
Eosinophil		
Eosinophilia	Allergy	Asthma, hay fever, drug sensitivity
	Infection	Parasites (trichinosis, hookworm), chronic (fungal, leprosy, TB)
	Malignancy	CML, lung, stomach, ovary, Hodgkin disease
	Dermatosis	Pemphigus, exfoliative dermatitis (drug-induced)
	Drugs	Digitalis, heparin, streptomycin, tryptophan (eosinophilia-myalgia syndrome), penicillins, propranolol
Eosinopenia	Stress response	Trauma, shock, burns, surgery, mental distress
	Drugs	Steroids (Cushing syndrome)
Basophil		
Basophilia	Inflammation	Infection (measles, chickenpox), hypersensitivity reaction (immediate)
	Hematologic	Myeloproliferative disorders (CML, polycythemia vera, Hodgkin lymphoma, hemolytic anemia)
	Endocrine	Myxedema, antithyroid therapy
Basopenia	Physiologic	Pregnancy, ovulation, stress
	Endocrine	Graves disease
Monocyte		
Monocytosis	Infection	Bacterial (subacute bacterial endocarditis, TB), recovery phase of infection
	Hematologic	Myeloproliferative disorders, Hodgkin disease, agranulocytosis
	Physiologic	Normal newborn
Monocytopenia	Rare	
Lymphocyte		
Lymphocytosis	Physiologic	4 months to 4 years
	Acute infection	Infectious mononucleosis, CMV infection, pertussis, hepatitis, mycoplasma pneumonia, typhoid
	Chronic infection	Congenital syphilis, tertiary syphilis
	Endocrine	Thyrotoxicosis, adrenal insufficiency
	Malignancy	ALL, CLL, lymphosarcoma cell leukemia
Lymphocytopenia	Immunodeficiency syndrome	AIDS, agammaglobulinemia
	Lymphocyte destruction	Steroids (Cushing syndrome), radiation, chemotherapy, Hodgkin lymphoma, CHF, renal failure, TB, SLE, aplastic anemia

AIDS, Acquired immunodeficiency syndrome; *ALL*, acute lymphocytic leukemia; *CHF*, congestive (left) heart failure; *CLL*, chronic lymphocytic leukemia; *CML*, chronic myelogenous leukemia; *CMV*, cytomegalovirus; *GI*, gastrointestinal; *MI*, myocardial infarction, *SLE*, systemic lupus erythematosus; *TB*, tuberculosis.

with metazoal parasites) are often cited as causes. Hypersensitivity reactions and the normal defense against parasites trigger the release of eosinophil chemotactic factor of anaphylaxis (ECF-A) from mast cells, attracting eosinophils to the area. (These processes are described and illustrated in Chapters 7 and 8.) Tissues with abundant mast cells, such as the respiratory and gastrointestinal tracts, are particularly common sites for eosinophil invasion. Mast cells also release interleukin-5 (IL-5), which stimulates the bone marrow to produce and release more eosinophils into the blood. Eosinophilia may also be associated with dermatologic disorders, such as atopic dermatitis, eczema, and pemphigus. Various types of eosinophilic scleroderma-like diseases also have been reported to occur in association with hemato-oncogenic disorders (i.e., eosinophilic cellulitis [Wells syndrome] and eosinophilic fasciitis [Schulman syndrome]). Increased numbers of eosinophils have been observed in individuals with eosinophilia-myalgia syndrome (EMS), which is associated with ingestion of tryptophan, and a relationship between EMS and fibromyalgia syndrome (FMS) has been suggested.

Eosinopenia, a decrease in circulating numbers of eosinophils, generally is caused by migration of eosinophils into inflammatory sites. It also may be seen in Cushing syndrome and as a result of stress caused by surgery, shock, trauma, burns, or mental distress. Other conditions causing eosinopenia are detailed in Table 27-1.

Basophilia, an increase in circulating numbers of basophils, is rare and generally is a response to inflammation and immediate hypersensitivity reactions. Basophils contain histamine that is released during an allergic reaction. An increase in levels of basophils is seen also in myeloproliferative disorders, such as chronic myeloid leukemia and myeloid metaplasia. Other conditions associated with basophilia are listed in Table 27-1.

Basopenia (also known as *basophilic leukopenia*), a decrease in circulating numbers of basophils, is seen in hyperthyroidism, acute infection, and long-term therapy with steroids. A decrease in basophils may be seen during ovulation and pregnancy. Other conditions associated with basopenia are listed in Table 27-1.

Monocytosis is an increase (generally greater than 800/µL) in numbers of circulating monocytes. The condition is often transient and not related to a dysfunction of monocyte production. When present, it most commonly occurs with neutropenia associated with bacterial infections, particularly in the late stages or recovery stage, when monocytes are needed to phagocytize surviving microorganisms and debris. Monocytosis often is seen in chronic infections, usually with intracellular bacteria, such as tuberculosis (TB), brucellosis, and listeriosis, and subacute bacterial endocarditis (SBE). Peripheral monocytosis has been found to correlate with the extent of myocardial damage following myocardial infarction. Increased numbers of monocytes also may indicate marrow recovery from agranulocytosis. Other conditions associated with monocytosis are identified in Table 27-1.

Monocytopenia, a decrease in numbers of circulating monocytes, is rare, and not much is known about this condition because of the small numbers of monocytes generally present in the blood. Monocytopenia, however, has been identified with hairy cell leukemia and prednisone therapy.

Lymphocytes

Quantitative alteration of lymphocytes occurs when lymphocytes are activated by antigenic stimuli, usually microorganisms (see Chapter 7). A **lymphocytosis** is rare in acute bacterial infections and occurs most commonly in acute viral infections, particularly those caused by the Epstein-Barr virus (EBV), a causative agent in infectious mononucleosis. Other specific disorders associated with lymphocytosis are listed in Table 27-1.

Lymphocytopenia may be attributable to (1) abnormalities of lymphocyte production associated with neoplasias and immune deficiencies, and (2) destruction by drugs, viruses, or radiation. It also can occur in individuals for no apparent reason. Other conditions associated with lymphocytopenia are identified in Table 27-1. The lymphocytopenia associated with heart failure and other acute illnesses may be caused by elevated levels of cortisol. Lymphocytopenia is a major problem in acquired immunodeficiency syndrome (AIDS) in which the human immunodeficiency virus (HIV) is cytopathic for T helper lymphocytes. (For a more detailed discussion of AIDS, see Chapter 9.)

Infectious Mononucleosis

Infectious mononucleosis (IM) is an acute, self-limiting, neoplastic lymphoproliferative clinical syndrome characterized by acute viral infection of B lymphocytes (B cells). The most common etiologic agent is EBV, a ubiquitous, lymphotrophic, gamma-group herpesvirus, which was first recognized as the causative agent in IM in the late 1960s. EBV accounts for approximately 85% of all IM cases. Other etiologic agents that may cause symptoms resembling IM are viruses (cytomegalovirus [CMV], adenovirus, HIV, hepatitis A, influenza A and B, and rubella), as well as the bacteria *Toxoplasma gondii*, *Corynebacterium diphtheriae*, and *Coxiella burnetii*. IM caused by CMV is generally noted in older individuals, with fever and malaise the major complaints; the major manifestations of EBV-induced IM are the classic triad of symptoms of pharyngitis, lymphadenopathy, and fever.

Approximately 50% to 85% of children are infected with EBV by age 4, and more than 90% of adults have indications of subclinical EBV infections. These early infections are usually asymptomatic and provide immunity to EBV, thus early EBV infections rarely develop into IM. IM may arise when the initial infection occurs during adolescence or later, but still only results in IM in 35% to 50% of these individuals. Symptomatic IM usually affects young adults between ages 15 and 35 years, with the peak incidences occurring between 15 and 19 years; males have a later peak (18 to 23 years) than females. The overall incidence rate for this age group is 6 to 8 cases per 1000 persons per year. Children from low socioeconomic environments are particularly susceptible to infections with EBV. IM is uncommon in individuals over age 40 years, but if it does occur, it is more commonly caused by CMV.

Transmission of EBV is usually by saliva through personal contact (e.g., kissing, hence the term "kissing disease"). The virus also may be present in other mucosal secretions of the genital, rectal, and respiratory tract, as well as blood. No evidence of aerosol transmission through sneezing or coughing has been documented. The disease begins with widespread infection of B lymphocytes, all of which possess receptors for EBV. The virus initially infects the oropharynx, nasopharynx, and salivary epithelial cells with later spread to the lymphoid tissue and B cells. Infection of B cells permits the virus to enter the bloodstream, which spreads the infection systemically.

In the immunocompetent individual, unaffected B cells produce antibodies (IgG, IgM, IgA) against the virus. Concomitantly, there is a massive activation and proliferation of cytotoxic T cells (CD8) directed against EBV-infected cells; CD8 lymphocytes can account for greater than 50% of the total circulating lymphocytes. The immune response against EBV-infected cells (cellular infiltration, production of cytokines) is largely responsible for the cellular proliferation in the lymphoid tissues (lymph nodes, spleen, tonsils, occasionally liver). Sore throat and fever, two of the earliest manifestations, are caused by inflammation at the site of viral entry and initial infection (the mouth and throat).

CLINICAL MANIFESTATIONS The incubation period of IM is approximately 30 to 50 days (4 to 8 weeks). Flu-like symptoms such as headache, malaise, fatigue, arthralgia, fever, chills, and dysphagia, may appear within the first 3 to 5 days, although some individuals remain asymptomatic. These symptoms may vary in severity for the next 7 to 20 days. At the time of diagnosis the individual usually has the classic triad of symptoms: fever, pharyngitis, and lymphadenopathy of the cervical lymph nodes. The pharyngitis is usually diffuse and often accompanied by a whitish or grayish green, thick exudate. It also is quite painful and is the symptom that most often causes the individual to seek treatment. IM is usually self-limiting, and recovery occurs in a few weeks. Fatigue may last for 1 to 2 months after resolution of the infection.

Although severe clinical complications are rare, as the condition progresses, generalize lymph node enlargement may develop and enlargement of the spleen and liver also may occur. Splenomegaly is clinically evident 50% of the time and is demonstrated radiologically 100% of the time. Difficulty in detecting splenomegaly with physical examination contributes to the underestimation of actual enlargement. Splenic rupture is rare (only 0.1% to 0.15% of all cases) and can occur spontaneously as a result of mild trauma, occurring primarily in males between days 4 and 21 after the onset of symptoms. It is the most common cause of death related to IM. Other causes of fatalities are hepatic failure, extensive bacterial infection, or viral myocarditis.

Other organ systems are rarely involved, but such involvement may result in additional symptoms, such as meningitis, encephalitis, Guillain-Barré syndrome, Bell palsy, optic neuritis, mental impairment, transverse myelitis, cerebellar ataxia, and demyelinating diseases. Ocular manifestations may include eyelid and periorbital edema, dry eyes, keratitis, uveitis, conjunctivitis, retinitis, oculoglandular syndrome, choroiditis, papillitis, and ophthalmoplegia. In children, Reye syndrome also has been associated with EBV infection.

Pulmonary involvement is rare, but when present may include hilar and mediastinal lymphadenopathy, interstitial pneumonitis, and pleural effusion. Pneumonia and respiratory failure have been documented; however, they are more likely to develop in immunocompromised individuals. Approximately 3% to 10% of adults older than 40 years of age have never been infected with EBV and are susceptible to IM later in life. In these individuals the classic symptoms are not generally present, making diagnosis more difficult. If an older individual has an elevated temperature that cannot be explained and persists for more than 2 weeks, EBV infection should be suspected, particularly in the presence of abnormal liver function tests with hepatomegaly and jaundice. Other neurologic manifestations that may be present include peripheral neuropathy and Guillain-Barré syndrome.

EVALUATION AND TREATMENT The blood of affected individuals contains an increased number of atypical lymphocytes (Figure 27-1). Diagnosis of IM is commonly based on Hoagland's criteria of at least 50% lymphocytes and at least 10% atypical lymphocytes in the blood in the presence of fever, pharyngitis, and adenopathy confirmed by a positive serologic test. Serologic tests are used to determine a heterophile antibody response.[2] **Heterophile antibodies** are a heterogeneous group of immunoglobulin M (IgM) antibodies that are agglutinins against nonhuman red blood cells (e.g., sheep, horse) and are detected by qualitative (Monospot) or qualitative methods (heterophile antibody test).

The Monospot test is limited because other infections (e.g., CMV, adenovirus) and toxoplasmosis also produce heterophilic antibodies. Thus 5% to 15% of Monospot tests yield false-positive results. Levels of heterophilic antibodies in the blood increase as the condition progresses, although some individuals and children younger than age 4 years do not produce them. These individuals give a false-negative result. Specificity for diagnosis of EBV infection may be increased with viral-specific serology tests that identify EBV-specific antibodies (e.g., IgG or IgM against the viral capsid antigen [VCA], or IgG against the EBV nuclear antigen [EBNA]). These tests are more expensive and labor intensive so are reserved for instances in which the Monospot test is not appropriate.

Because IM is usually self-limiting, medical intervention is rarely required. Treatment of IM is supportive and includes rest and alleviation of symptoms with analgesics and antipyretics. Ibuprofen, *not aspirin,* is used with children and adolescents because of the reported incidence of Reye syndrome associated with EBV infection. Pharyngitis of streptococcal origin, which occurs in 20% to 30% of cases, is treated with penicillin or erythromycin. Ampicillin is contraindicated because it causes a rash in most individuals with IM.

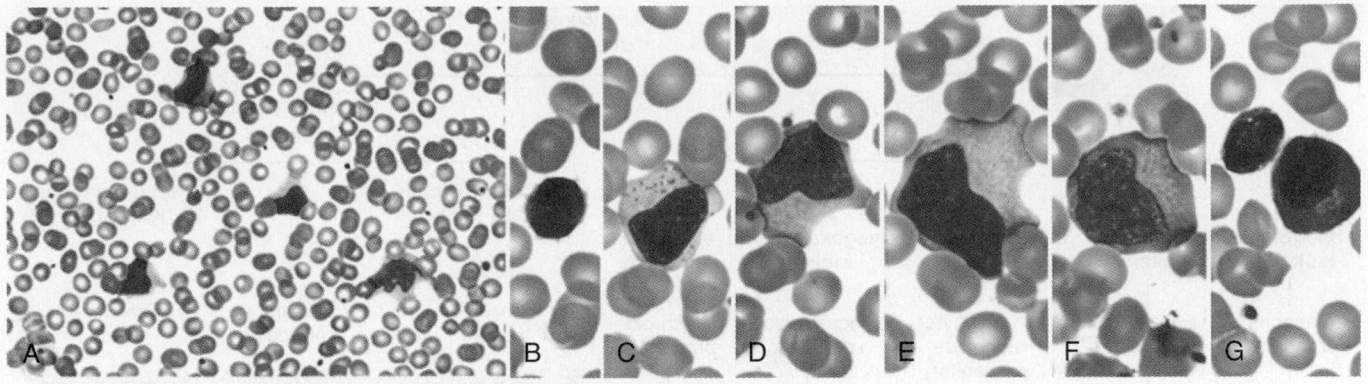

Figure 27-1 Peripheral blood smear in infectious mononucleosis. Low power (A) shows moderately high white blood cell count and high number of reactive, or "atypical" lymphocytes. Higher power (B-G) illustrates spectrum of lymphoid morphology, including small resting lymphocyte (B) for comparison, large granular lymphocyte (C), atypical forms (D-F), also referred to as "reactive" lymphs, and circulating plasma cell (G). (From Hoffman R, et al: *Hematology: basic principles and practice*, ed 5, Philadelphia, 2009, Churchill Livingstone.)

Bed rest and avoidance of strenuous activity should be included in the therapy. Steroids may be used, but only in the presence of severe complications (e.g., impending airway obstruction) or other organ system involvement (e.g., nervous system manifestations, thrombocytopenic purpura, myocarditis, pericarditis). Acyclovir has been used with immunosuppressed individuals; however, clinical improvement has been minimal and therefore it is not recommended for standard treatment.

In the rare event of splenic rupture, the treatment has been removal of the spleen and continues to be the choice in hemodynamically unstable individuals. More recent practice has been to repair the spleen to avoid overwhelming postoperative infection (OPSI). Children are at greater risk of OPSI than adults. Postsplenectomy vaccinations for *Streptococcus pneumoniae*, *Haemophilus influenzae*, and *Meningococcus* are essential because these microorganisms are responsible for 92% of fatal infections. Treatment may also be necessary for airway obstruction from massive edema of the Waldeyer ring or for autoimmune hemolytic anemia, which occurs in approximately 3% to 5% of cases.

Fatal IM also is expressed with the inherited X-linked lymphoproliferative (XLP) syndrome. The underlying cause leading to death is the absence of a functional SAP protein that allows for the unregulated proliferation of cytotoxic T cells and the concomitant production and release of cytokines.

Leukemias

Leukemia is a clonal malignant disorder of leukocytes in the blood and blood-forming organs. The common feature of all forms of leukemia is an uncontrolled proliferation of malignant leukocytes, causing an overcrowding of bone marrow and decreased production and function of normal hematopoietic cells. The first description of a "leukemic" individual was written by Velpeau in 1827.[3] Virchow, a pathologist, coined the term *white blood (Weissus blut)* and later originated the term *leukemia*. Since Virchow's initial discovery, the overall classification of leukemia has become increasingly complex and undergone several permutations. The current classification of leukemia is based on (1) the predominant cell of origin (either myeloid or lymphoid) and (2) the rate of progression, which usually reflects the degree at which cell differentiation was arrested when the cell became malignant (acute or chronic) (Figure 27-2). **Acute leukemia** is characterized by undifferentiated or immature cells, usually a blast cell, and the onset of disease is abrupt and rapid with a short survival time. In **chronic leukemia** the predominant cell is more differentiated but does not function normally, with a relatively slow progression. Thus there are four types of leukemia: acute lymphocytic (ALL), acute myelogenous (AML), chronic lymphocytic (CLL), and chronic myelogenous (CML). In 1976 the French-American-British Cooperative Group developed more extensive criteria for the classification of acute leukemias. This system is based on characteristics that may provide significant therapeutic prognostic information, such as structure, number of cells, genetics, identification of surface markers, and histochemical staining.

Leukemia occurs with varying frequencies at different ages and is more common in adults than children (Figure 27-3). It is estimated that more than 44,000 cases of leukemia were newly diagnosed in 2008, with males having a slightly higher incidence than females (Table 27-2).[4] In all types of leukemia males have a higher incidence rate (56%) as do Americans of European descent. White children have higher rates of leukemia than children of other groups. ALL is the least common type overall, but is the most common in children (approximately 61% of ALL cases are diagnosed before the age of 20). Leukemia accounts for about 30% of all childhood cancers, and ALL accounts for almost 78% of all new cases of leukemia in children. CLL and AML are the most common types in adults. CML is found mostly in adults.

Over the past two decades the rates of induced remission and survival in most forms of leukemia have increased. Current survival rates range from 25% for AML to 75% for CLL.

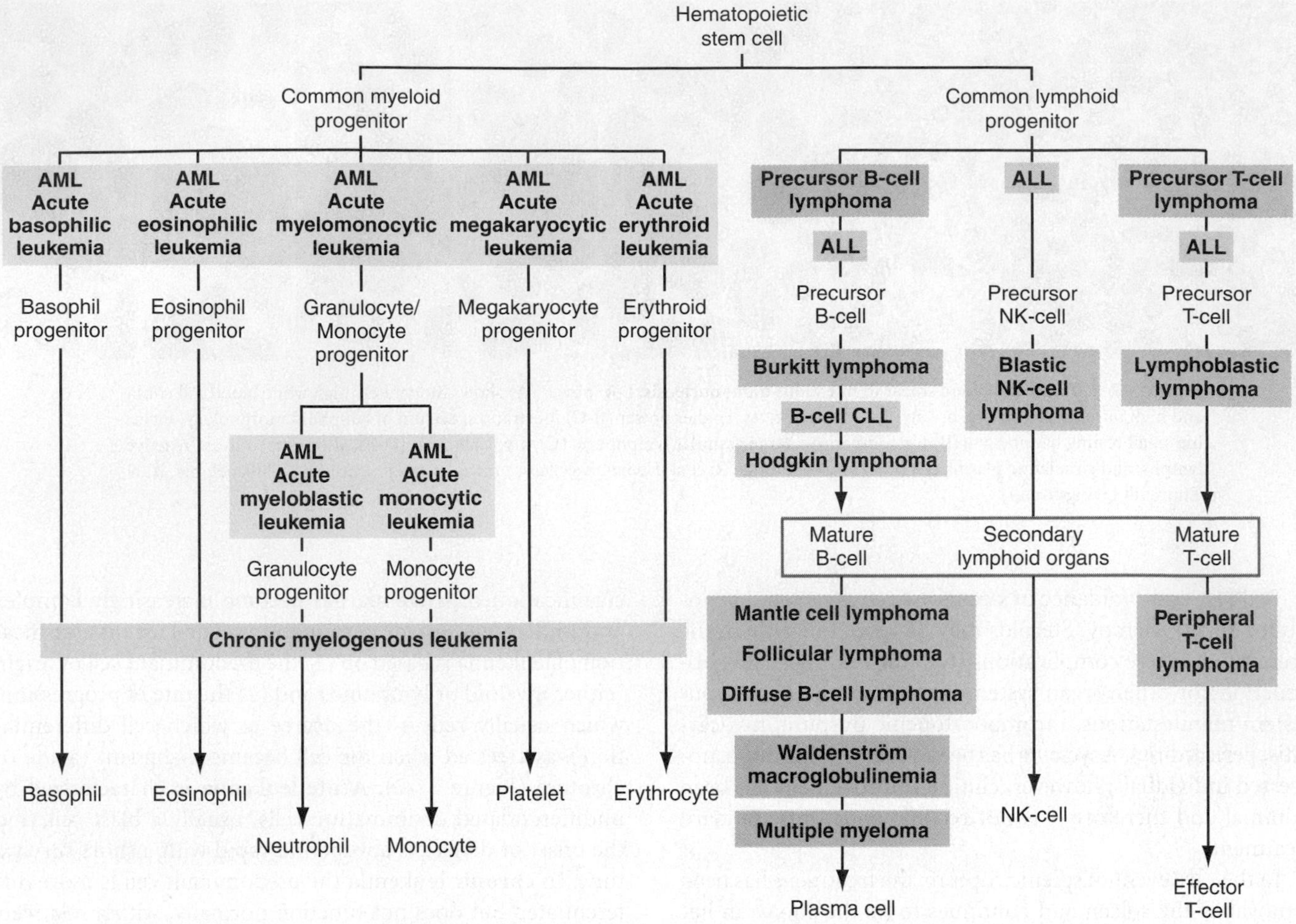

Hematopoietic stem cell
Common myeloid progenitor
Common lymphoid progenitor
AML Acute basophilic leukemia
AML Acute eosinophilic leukemia
AML Acute myelomonocytic leukemia
AML Acute megakaryocytic leukemia
AML Acute erythroid leukemia
Precursor B-cell lymphoma
ALL
Precursor T-cell lymphoma
ALL
ALL
Basophil progenitor
Eosinophil progenitor
Granulocyte/ Monocyte progenitor
Megakaryocyte progenitor
Erythroid progenitor
Precursor B-cell
Precursor NK-cell
Precursor T-cell
Burkitt lymphoma
Blastic NK-cell lymphoma
Lymphoblastic lymphoma
B-cell CLL
Hodgkin lymphoma
AML Acute myeloblastic leukemia
AML Acute monocytic leukemia
Mature B-cell
Secondary lymphoid organs
Mature T-cell
Granulocyte progenitor
Monocyte progenitor
Mantle cell lymphoma
Follicular lymphoma
Diffuse B-cell lymphoma
Peripheral T-cell lymphoma
Chronic myelogenous leukemia
Waldenström macroglobulinemia
Multiple myeloma
Basophil
Eosinophil
Platelet
Erythrocyte
NK-cell
Neutrophil
Monocyte
Effector T-cell
Plasma cell

Figure 27-2 **Origins of leukemias and lymphomas.** Differentiation pathways of blood-forming cells and reported sites from which specific leukemias and lymphomas originate. Tumors of similar types are given the same background coloring. *ALL*, acute lymphocytic leukemia; *AML*, acute myelogenous leukemia; *CLL*, chronic lymphocytic leukemia; *NK*, natural killer.

Incidence (per 100,000)
35
30
25
20
15
10
5
0
<1
1–4
5–9
10–14
15–19
20–24
25–29
30–34
35–39
40–44
45–49
50–54
55–59
60–64
65–69
70–74
75–79
80–84
85+
Age at diagnosis
ALL
AML
CLL
CML

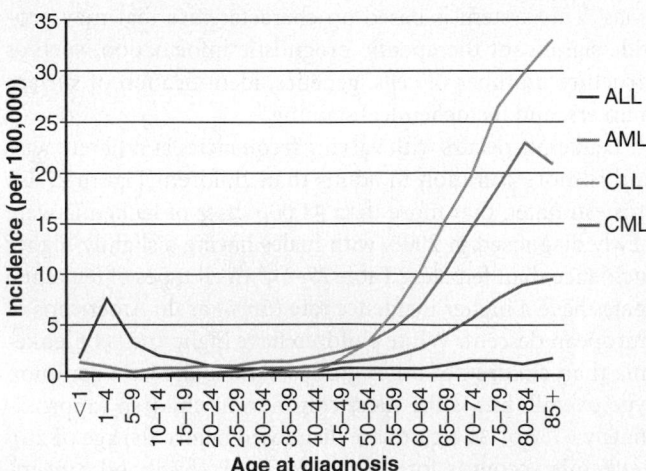

Figure 27-3 **Age-related incidence at diagnosis of leukemias.** The incidences of acute myelogenous leukemia (AML), chronic lymphocytic leukemia (CLL), and chronic myelogenous leukemia (CML) are relatively stable until middle age and then increase dramatically. The incidence of acute lymphocytic leukemia (ALL) peaks in childhood, then diminishes until middle age when the incidence begins rising slowly with age. Data obtained from http://seer.cancer.gov/csr/1975_2005/results_merged/sect_13_leukemia.pdf.

This progress is the result of more effective chemotherapeutic agents, improved blood product and antimicrobial support, and specialized nursing care. Chemotherapy and bone marrow transplants have significantly increased the survival time for individuals with acute leukemia.

PATHOPHYSIOLOGY All leukemias have certain pathophysiologic features in common. Although the exact cause of leukemia is unknown, several risk factors and related genetic aberrations are associated with the onset of malignancy. There is a statistically significant tendency for leukemia to reappear in families. There is also an increased incidence of leukemia in association with other hereditary abnormalities such as Down syndrome, Fanconi aplastic anemia, Bloom syndrome, trisomy 13, Patau syndrome, and some immune deficiencies (i.e., ataxia-telangiectasia, Wiskott-Aldrich syndrome, and congenital X-linked agammaglobulinemia; see Chapter 8).

Genetic translocations (mitotic errors) are observed in leukemic cells. The most common genetic abnormality is the reciprocal translocation between chromosomes 9 and 22 t(9;22)(q34;q11), the **Philadelphia chromosome.**[5] The

| Table 27-2 | Estimated New Cases and Deaths: Leukemia and Lymphoma in the United States in 2008 |

	Estimated Number and Proportion (%) of New Cases			Estimated Number of Deaths			5-Year Survival Rate (1996-2004)	
Type	Total	Male	Female	Total	Male	Female	Overall	<5 Years of Age
Leukemias	44,270	25,180	19,090	22,570	12,540	10,030		
Acute lymphocytic leukemia	5430 (12.3%)	3220	2210	1490	850	640	66.1%	91.2%
Chronic lymphocytic leukemia	15,110 (34.1%)	8750	6360	4600	2520	2080	76.2%	
Acute myelogenous leukemia	13,290 (30.0%)	7200	6090	9000	5040	3960	21.3%	55.2%
Chronic myelogenous leukemia	4830 (11.0%)	2800	2030	850	430	420	46.7%	
Other leukemias	5610 (12.7%)	3210	2400	6630	3700	2930		
Lymphomas	74,340	39,850	34,490	20,510	10,490	10,000		
Hodgkin lymphoma	8220 (11.1%)	4400	3820	1350	700	650	86%	
Non-Hodgkin lymphoma	66,120 (88.9%)	35,450	30,670	19,160	9700	9370	64%	
Multiple myeloma	19,920	11,190	8730	10,690	5640	5050	34%	

Data from *Cancer Facts and Figures 2008,* American Cancer Society.

Philadelphia chromosome was first observed in persons with CML, and is present in 95% of those with CML, 3% of individuals with AML, and 20% of those with ALL (primarily adults).[6] This translocation results in the novel fusion of the *BCR1* gene region from chromosome 22 and the proto-oncogene *ABL1* from chromosome 9 (Figure 27-4). The *BCR-ABL1* joining results in the expression of a unique fused oncoprotein BCR-ABL1.[5] The ABL1 protein is a tyrosine kinase in the signaling pathway that promotes cell proliferation. The BCR-ABL1 variant possessed greater tyrosine kinase activity and proved to be essential for transformation into leukemic cells. BCR-ABL1 appears to excessively activate intracellular pathways leading to increased proliferation, decreased sensitivity to apoptosis, and premature release of immature cells into the circulation. In most leukemias and lymphomas a single major genetic abnormality, such as the t(9;22) translocation, does not lead to an aggressive malignancy. The initial event is usually followed by a series of secondary genetic changes.[7] Thus the original tumor becomes genetically unstable and diverse.

Risk factors for the onset of leukemia include environmental factors as well as other diseases. Increased risk in adults has been linked to cigarette smoke, exposure to benzene, and ionizing radiation. Large doses of ionizing radiation particularly result in an increased incidence of myelogenous leukemia. Infections with HIV or hepatitis C virus increase the risk for leukemia, and it is now widely accepted that some types of leukemia are caused by infection with the human T-cell leukemia/lymphoma virus-1 (HTLV-1). Drugs that cause bone marrow depression (e.g., chloramphenicol, phenylbutazone, and certain alkylating agents, such as cytoxan) also can predispose an individual to leukemia. AML is the most frequently reported secondary cancer after high doses of chemotherapy for Hodgkin lymphoma, non-Hodgkin lymphoma, multiple myeloma, ovarian cancer, and breast cancer. Acute leukemia also may develop secondary to certain acquired disorders, including CML, CLL, polycythemia vera, myelofibrosis, Hodgkin lymphoma, multiple myeloma, ovarian cancer, and sideroblastic anemia.

Leukemias are considered clonal disorders in that a single progenitor cell undergoes malignant transformation. The leukemia blasts literally "crowd out" the marrow and cause cellular proliferation of the other cell lines to cease. Normal granulocytic-monocytic, lymphocytic, erythrocytic, and megakaryocytic progenitor cells cease to function, resulting in **pancytopenia** (a reduction in all cellular components of the blood). An interesting observation is that leukemic cells apparently divide more *slowly* and take longer to synthesize deoxyribonucleic acid (DNA) than other blood precursors. Leukemic cells accumulate relentlessly in the bone marrow causing overcrowding of the marrow, and they compete with cellular proliferation and function of normal hematopoietic cells. Thus leukemia has been termed an *accumulation* disorder, as well as a *proliferation* disorder. In the majority of cases, leukemic cells are ejected into the blood, where they accumulate. These cells also may infiltrate and accumulate in the liver, spleen, lymph nodes, and other organs throughout the body. The presentation of large numbers of leukemic cells in the blood may be one of the most dramatic indicators of leukemia; however, leukemia is still a primary disruption of the bone marrow.

Acute Leukemias

Acute leukemias consist of two types: **acute lymphocytic leukemia (ALL)** and **acute myelogenous leukemia (AML).** Acute leukemias are seen in both genders and in all ages, with the incidence increasing dramatically in individuals older

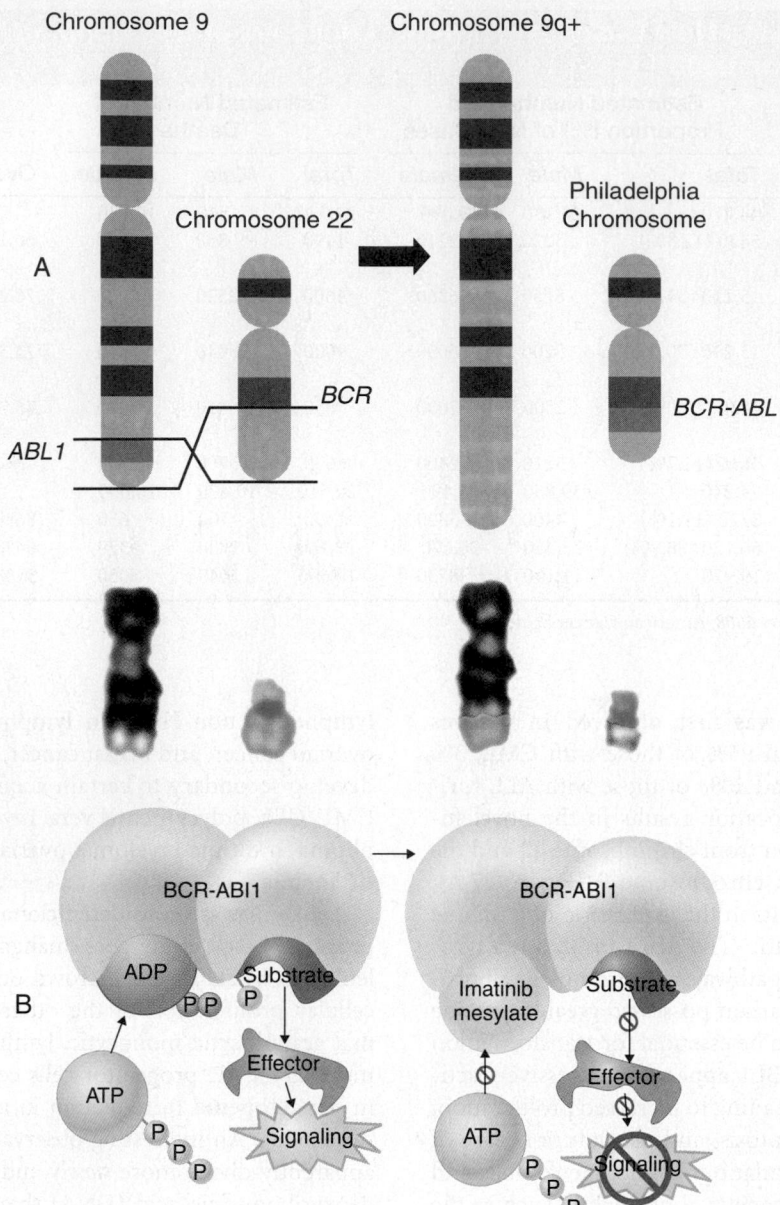

Figure 27-4 Philadelphia chromosome. The Philadelphia chromosome is an example of a reciprocal chromosomal translocation that results in an abnormal gene product responsible for a clinical disorder. **A,** An exchange occurs between the long arm of chromosome 9 (black chromosome) and the long arm of chromosome 22 (blue chromosome); t(9;22)(q34;q11). **B,** Mechanism of action of imatinib. By occupying the ATP-binding pocket of the ABL kinase domain, imatinib prevents substrate phosphorylation and downstream activation of signals, thus inhibiting the leukemogenic effects of BCR-ABL1 on cells in chronic myelogenous leukemia. *ADP,* adenosine diphosphate; *ATP,* adenosine triphosphate; *P,* phosphate group. (**A,** Top portion from Rakel R, Bope E: *Conn's current therapy 2008,* Philadelphia, 2008, Saunders. **A,** Lower portion from Yanoff M, Duker J: *Ophthalmology,* ed 3, Edinburgh, 2009, Mosby. **B** from Goldman L, Ausiello D: *Cecil medicine,* ed 23, Philadelphia, 2008, Saunders.)

than 50 years. Mortality for all acute leukemias in the United States is about 7 per 100,000. In children younger than 15 years, leukemia accounts for a third of all deaths from cancer. North American and Scandinavian countries have the highest mortality; Eastern European countries, Asia (except Japan), and Central America have the lowest mortality. Japan's higher mortality is the result of the atomic bombs dropped in World War II. Blacks have consistently shown a lower mortality than whites. More than 5400 new cases of ALL and 4800 cases of

AML occurred in 2008, with more than 1400 deaths attributed to ALL and 450 to AML.[4,8]

PATHOPHYSIOLOGY ALL is a progressive neoplasm defined by the presence of greater than 30% lymphoblasts in the bone marrow or blood. Most cases of ALL occur in children (80% of ALL), and it is the most common leukemia in children, most often occurring in the first decade. The median age of diagnosis of ALL is age 13. Although adults with ALL account for only 20% of all cases, their mortality rate is significantly higher (see Table 27-2). The significant difference between the incidence of ALL in adults and children is thought to be determined by differences in the biology of the disease.

Immunotyping of leukemic blast cells allows for the identification of subtypes of ALL. Approximately 75% of ALL in children originate from transformed precursor B cells, whereas adult ALL is a mixture of cancers of precursor B-cell or precursor T-cell origin. A small percentage of ALL cases have neither B- nor T-cell origination and are called *null cell* (Table 27-3). Precursor B-cell ALL can be subdivided into different phenotypes, depending on their progression through the B-cell maturation process before becoming malignant.[9,10] The general phenotype of precursor B-cell ALL expresses CD19, human leukocyte antigen DR (HLA-DR), and other B-cell–associated antigens in the cytoplasm. The most immature form (pro-B ALL) occurs in about 5% of precursor B-cell ALL and is characterized by lack of expression of CD10. CD10 (common acute lymphocytic leukemia antigen [CALLA]) is a cell surface metalloprotease. Lack of CD10 is frequently associated with translocation of the myeloid/lymphoid leukemia *(MLL)* gene and a poor prognosis. The common precursor B-cell ALL makes up approximately 80% of precursor B-cell ALL cases; these express surface CD10, but have not yet undergone rearrangement of the immunoglobulin genes. The remaining individuals have a more mature form of precursor B-cell ALL (pre–B-cell ALL) in which the cells express immunoglobulin molecules in the cytoplasm. Less common variations include cells that are intermediate between the common precursor and pre–B-cell phenotypes and express immunoglobulin heavy chain, but no light chain, and cells that are more mature than the pre–B-cell ALL and express surface immunoglobulin and the absence of staining for the enzyme—terminal deoxynucleotidyl transferase (TdT).

The T-cell lineage ALL (precursor T-cell ALL) is distinguished by T-cell–associated markers.[9,10] Cytoplasmic CD3 is the most common T-cell lineage specific marker, but CD7, CD2, and CD5 are frequently used. In addition to lymphoid markers, T-cell receptor (TCR) gene rearrangements are the most common genetic alteration in T-cell ALL. No specific cytogenetic abnormality, however, has been linked to the subtype of T-cell ALL. ALL blast cells also can express myeloid markers in 15% to 50% of adults and 5% to 35% of children.

Precursor B-cell ALL is strongly associated with aneuploidy of various types, ranging from hypodiploid to hyperdiploid with more than 50 chromosomes.[6,9,10] Individuals with hyperdiploid ALL usually have a better prognosis than those with fewer than 46 chromosomes. Precursor T-cell ALL generally have fewer cytogenetic abnormalities, and the majority involve deletions. Genetic translocations between the *MYC* locus on chromosome 8 and one of the loci for the Ig heavy or light-chain genes (14q32, 2p12, and 22q11) are characteristic (also see Chapters 7 and 11). Several other translocations are commonly observed in ALL, including the Philadelphia chromosome and translocations involving the *ETV6* (formerly *TEL*) and *MLL* genes (Figure 27-5).[6] Philadelphia chromosome–positive ALL carries the worst prognosis

of all types of ALL and is found in 25% to 30% of adult ALL cases but less than 5% of childhood ALL cases. A translocation between chromosomes 12 and 21 (t[12;21]) results in fusion of the *ETV6* oncogene from chromosome 12 with the *AML1* (acute myeloid leukemia 1) gene on chromosome 21 to produce a fusion protein, ETV6-AML1. AML1 is a transcription factor for several genes important in hematopoiesis (e.g., IL-3, granulocyte-macrophage colony-stimulating factor [GM-CSF], CSF1 receptor).[6] The t(12;21) translocation occurs in 25% to 30% of childhood pre–B-cell ALL cases but in only 2% of adult ALL cases. This translocation significantly affects the prognosis of childhood ALL; children younger than 10 years with pre–B-cell ALL and the *ETV6-AML1* translocation have a 5-year cure rate of 90%, compared with 60% to 65% in those without the translocation.

Translocations of the *MLL* gene on chromosome 11 occur in about 10% of individuals with ALL and in 70% of infants with AML or ALL.[6] Infants and adults with this translocation develop a very aggressive form of leukemia with a very poor prognosis and frequent treatment failure, although children with this abnormality have better outcomes. The most common translocations involving *MLL* are t(4;11) and t(11;19). The t(4;11) translocation results in a fusion of *MLL* with the *AFF1* (ALL1 fused gene from chromosome 4) gene, and the t(11;19) translocation fuses *MLL* with the *MLLT1* (formerly *ENL*) gene.

Specific causes of ALL are unknown, but multiple factors may contribute to its development.[9,10] Risk factors for childhood ALL include prenatal exposure to x-rays and postnatal exposure to high-dose radiation. Individuals with Down syndrome have an increased risk for developing ALL and AML. Increased risk for ALL is also seen in individuals with other genetic conditions, including neurofibromatosis, Shwachman syndrome, Bloom syndrome, and ataxia telangiectasis (see Chapter 8). A unique characteristic of ALL, unlike other forms, is that ALL develops at different rates in different locations. Individuals in developed countries and in higher socioeconomic categories have an increased incidence of ALL. Prevention is almost impossible because there are no known causes.

AML is the most common adult leukemia; the mean age of diagnosis is 67 years of age. It results from an abnormal proliferation of myeloid precursor cells, decreased rate of apoptosis, and an arrest in cellular differentiation.[11] Therefore, the bone marrow and peripheral blood are characterized by leukocytosis and a predominance of blast cells. As the immature blasts increase, they replace normal myelocytic cells, megakaryocytes, and erythrocytes. This displacement eventually leads to complications of bleeding, anemia, and infection. AML increases with age, peaking in the sixth decade of life. Certain risk factors have been identified as possible causes, including exposure to radiation, benzene, and chemotherapy. Hereditary conditions, such as Down syndrome, Fanconi aplastic anemia, Bloom syndrome, ataxia telangiectasis, trisomy 13 (Patau syndrome), Wiskott-Aldrich syndrome, and congenital X-linked agammaglobulinemia, are known to be associated with a higher risk for AML (see Table 27-2). AML subtypes are classified based on the stage of development

Table 27-3	Immunophenotype of Adult Acute Lymphocytic Leukemia						
Lineage	TdT	HLA–DR	CD34	CD19	CD22	CD79a
Precursor B-cell ALL						
Pro-B ALL	+	+	+	+	+	+
CALL	+	+	−	+	+	−
Pre-B ALL	+	+	−	+	+	−
Transitional precursor B-cell ALL	±	+	−	+	+	−
Mature B-cell ALL	−	+	−	+	±	−
T-lineage ALL						
Pro-T ALL	+	±	±			
Pre-T ALL	+	±	±			
Cortical T ALL	+	−	−			
Mature T ALL	+	−	−			

From Faderl S et al: *Cancer* 98:1337-1354, 2003.

*Usually no surface light chain (L) expression.

ALL, Acute lymphoblastic leukemia; *cALL*, common acute lymphoblastic leukemia; *cy*, cytoplasmic; *TdT*, terminal deoxynucleotidyl transferase.

myeloblasts have reached at the time of diagnosis. These subtypes are included in Box 27-1.

More than 150 structural chromosomal abnormalities and several duplications or deletions within genes have been identified in AML.[6] The most common abnormalities are balanced translocations or inversions that disrupt genes critical to hematopoiesis of myeloid cells. The most common translocation is between chromosomes 8 and 21 in which the *RUNX1T1* (formerly *ETO*) (encodes a transcription factor) gene on chromosome 8 is fused with the *AML1* gene on chromosome 21 resulting in an *AML1-RUNX1T1* fusion gene and a fusion gene product, AML1-RUNX1T1. Production of AML1-RUNX1T1 disrupts the normal hematopoiesis process for myeloid cells and directly leads to the AML malignant phenotype.

Many kinds of mutations have been found in AML; however, a mutation in the receptor tyrosine kinase FLT3 occurs in about one third of AML persons. FLT3 conveys a proliferation signal normally expressed early in the development of bone marrow stem cells, but mutated FLT3 remains active and promotes blast cell proliferation. Several FLT3 inhibitors are in various stages of clinical development. Another mutation in receptor tyrosine kinases is *KIT*, which also provides a proliferative and/or survival signal to progenitor cells. Together these mutations result in proliferation but not differentiation.

CLINICAL MANIFESTATIONS The clinical manifestations of all the varieties of acute leukemia are generally similar. (Mechanisms associated with common manifestations are summarized in Table 27-4.) Signs and symptoms related to bone marrow depression include fatigue caused by anemia, bleeding resulting from thrombocytopenia (reduced numbers of circulating platelets), and fever caused by infection. Sites of infection include the oral cavity, throat, respiratory tract, lower colon, urinary tract, and skin. Common organisms include the gram-negative bacilli *Escherichia coli*, *Pseudomonas aeruginosa*, and *Klebsiella pneumoniae*. Fever is an early sign, often accompanied by chills. Bleeding can occur

in skin, gums, mucous membranes, and gastrointestinal and genitourinary tracts. Visible signs of bleeding include petechiae and ecchymosis, as well as discoloration of the skin, gingival bleeding, hematuria, and midcycle or heavy menstrual bleeding.

Anorexia can occur in all varieties of acute leukemia and is associated with weight loss, diminished sensitivity to sour and sweet tastes, wasting away of muscle, and difficulty in swallowing. Liver, spleen, and lymph node enlargement is more common in ALL than in AML (Figure 27-6). Splenomegaly and hepatomegaly usually occur together. The leukemic individual often experiences abdominal pain and tenderness and breast tenderness. Pain in the bones and joints is thought to result from leukemia infiltration with secondary stretching of the periosteum.

Central nervous system (CNS) involvement is common and may be caused by either leukemic infiltration or cerebral bleeding. Headache, vomiting, papilledema, facial palsy, blurred vision, auditory disturbances, and meningeal irritation can occur if leukemic cells infiltrate the cerebral or spinal meninges. CNS involvement at the time of diagnosis is rare, and less than 5% of children and less than 10% of adults are affected. Without CNS prophylaxis, approximately one third of individuals will develop CNS complications. Interventions associated with CNS prophylaxis include cranial irradiation, chemotherapy, and high doses of systemic chemotherapy. Specific treatment modalities or combinations of treatment vary and are determined by age and risk status.

EVALUATION AND TREATMENT Leukemia is often confused with other conditions, making early detection difficult. Persistent symptoms need intensive medical investigation. The diagnosis is made through examination of blood cells and bone marrow. A stained peripheral blood smear will exhibit low red blood cell and platelet counts along with the presence of leukemic blast cells (Figure 27-7). Examination of bone marrow demonstrates hypercellularity with 60% to 100% blast cells, an occasional normal myeloid, and erythroid precursors and rare to no megakaryocytes.

CD10	Cyμ	cgκ/λ	sIgH/L	cyCD3	CD7	CD1a	CD2	CD5	sCD3	Frequency (%)
										5-10
−	−	−	−							40-50
+	−	−	−							10
±	+	−	−							1
−	−	−	+*							1
−	−	+	+							5
				+	+	−	−	−	−	5
				+	+	−	+	+	−	
				+	+	+	+	+	−	10-15
				+	+	−	+	+	+	5-10

Chemotherapy, used in varying combinations, is the treatment of choice for leukemia.[9,10,12] Supportive measures include blood transfusions, antibiotics, antifungals, and antivirals. Allopurinol is used for preventing production of uric acid (which is elevated from cellular death because of treatment). Stem cell transplantation is now considered standard therapy for selected individuals with leukemia.

Bone marrow transplantation as a treatment has been increasing during the past two decades. Two controversial treatments are immunotherapy agents that induce differentiation of immature granulocytes (i.e., *cis*-retinoic acid) and marrow transplants. Although there has not been a marked improvement in response or survival of AML, dramatic improvements in survival and response of people with ALL have occurred.

The 5-year survival rate for those with leukemia is 38%, largely because of poor survival rates of individuals with certain types of leukemia (e.g., acute myelogenous). Since the 1970s, 5-year survival rates for those with ALL have increased from 38% to 65% for adults and from 53% to 85% for children. Factors influencing increased survival rate include the use of combined and multimodality treatment methods, improved supportive services such as blood banking and nutritional support, and antimicrobial treatment. The presence of the Philadelphia chromosome (observed in about 5% of children with ALL, in 30% of adults with ALL, and occasionally in AML) is a poor prognostic indicator.

Stimulation of blood cell growth and development with hematopoietic drugs has increased neutrophil recovery during chemotherapy and bone marrow transplant. Blood granulocyte numbers (e.g., eosinophils, neutrophils, basophils or mast cells) are normally in the range of 4000 to 6000 cells/μL, and susceptibility to infection develops below 1000 cells/μL. During a natural response to a bacterial infection, granulocytes usually rise in number to 10,000 to 20,000 cells/μL. Leukemia itself as well as the chemotherapeutic agents used to treat the disease can result in dramatic decreases in circulating granulocytes. The administration of colony-stimulating factors (CSFs) can raise white cell numbers and afford protection from infections.

Chronic Leukemias

The two main types of chronic leukemia are (1) **chronic myelogenous leukemia (CML)** and (2) **chronic lymphocytic leukemia (CLL)** (see Table 27-2). Several forms of CML can occur, depending on the lineage of the malignant cells (e.g., chronic neutrophilic leukemia [CNL], chronic eosinophilic leukemia [CEL]). Unlike cells in acute leukemia, chronic leukemic cells are well differentiated and can be readily identified. Individuals with chronic leukemia have a longer life expectancy, usually extending several years from the time of diagnosis.

The chronic leukemias account for the majority of cases in adults, accounting for approximately 30% of leukemias in the Western world. It is estimated that in 2008 more than 15,000 cases of CLL and 4500 cases of CML will be newly diagnosed in the United States.[13,14] The incidences of CLL and CML increase significantly in individuals older than 40 years, with prevalence in the sixth through eighth decades. CML is a group of diseases called *myeloproliferative disorders,* which also include polycythemia vera, primary thrombocytosis, and idiopathic myelofibrosis (invasion of bone marrow by fibrous tissue).

PATHOPHYSIOLOGY CLL involves malignant transformation and progressive accumulation of monoclonal B lymphocytes; rarely (less than 5%) are CLL malignancies of T-cell origin. The characteristic immunophenotype is expression of CD5, CD19, and CD23 molecules and low amounts of surface membrane Ig and CD20 molecules.[15] CD5 is a signal transduction molecule linked to the B-cell receptor (BCR), CD19 is a low-affinity antigen receptor expressed on maturing B cells, but is lost in plasma cells, and CD23 is a low-affinity receptor for the Fc portion of IgE. Thus CLL is derived from transformation of a partially mature B cell that has not yet encountered antigen. The gene for the variable region of the antibody heavy chain (*IGHV*) is frequently mutated (30% to 40% of persons). (See Chapter 7 concerning immunoglobulin heavy-chain structure.)

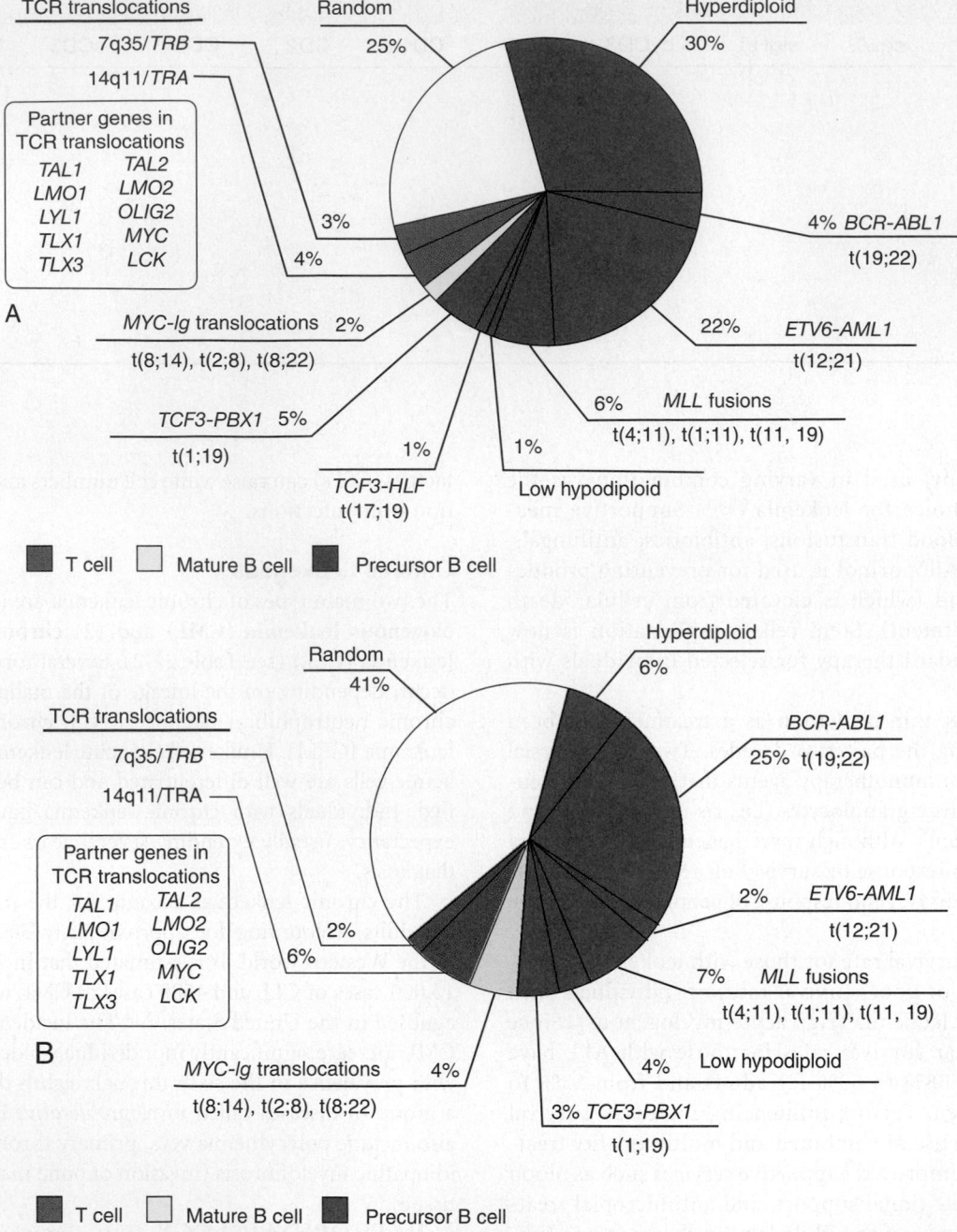

Figure 27-5 Frequency of the major chromosomal translocations in (A) pediatric and (B) adult acute lymphocytic leukemia (ALL). The genes affected by chromosomal translocation are shown in boldface type. TCR translocations in T-ALL can activate a number of different proto-oncogenes as shown in the insert, including *TAL1, LMO1/2, TLX1, TLX3,* and *MYC.* (Modified from Hoffman R, et al: *Hematology: basic principles and practice,* ed 5, Philadelphia, 2009, Churchill Livingstone.)

Clients with a mutated *IGHV* tend to have a more benign condition with a more slowly developing and less malignant disease.

The etiology of CLL is unknown. A familial tendency suggests a genetic linkage; first-degree relatives have a three times greater risk of developing the disease. It is rare in individuals less than 45 years of age, and when diagnosed, 95% of individuals are older than age 50. Genetic anomalies occur in approximately 90% of cases, frequently as deletions, although none has been linked to the etiology of CLL.

CLL cells that accumulate in the marrow do not interfere with normal blood cell production to the extent found in acute leukemias. This is a significant feature explaining the reduced severity in the beginning stage of disease. Accumulation of malignant B cells is the result of cell cycle arrest in the G_0/G_1 phase. CLL cells tend to express increased levels of proapoptotic proteins (e.g., BCL2) and suppress antiapoptotic proteins (e.g., BCL2L1), which reduces their sensitivity to apoptosis. Because the major pathophysiologic deficit in CLL is the failure of B cells to mature into plasma cells that

---

Box 27-1   Classification of Acute Myeloid Leukemias

Acute myeloblastic leukemia, minimally differentiated (AML-M0)
Acute myeloblastic leukemia without maturation (AML-M1)
Acute myeloblastic leukemia with maturation (AML-M2)
Acute promyelocytic leukemia (AML-M3)
   Hypergranular type
   Microgranular variant
Acute myelomonocytic leukemia (AML-M4)
   Increased marrow eosinophils (AML-M4-EO)
Acute monocytic leukemia (AML)
   Acute monoblastic leukemia (AML-M5A)
   Acute monocytic leukemia, differentiated (AML-M5B)
Erythroleukemia (AML-M6)
Acute megakaryoblastic leukemia (AML-M7)

From Damjanov I, Linder J: *Pathology: a color atlas,* St Louis, 2000, Mosby.

---

synthesize immunoglobulin, this often results in hypogammaglobulinemia (60% of clients).

CML is a member of the family of myeloproliferative disorder that also includes polycythemia vera (see Chapter 26), essential thrombocythemia, chronic idiopathic myelofibrosis (invasion of bone marrow by fibrous tissue), chronic neutrophilic leukemia, and chronic eosinophilic leukemia. CML is clonal and thought to arise from a hematopoietic stem cell. The cells observed in CML are heterogeneous in differentiation, depending on the stage of the disease.[16] During the chronic phase the predominant cell is a long-lasting hematopoietic stem cell. A leukemic granulocyte-monocyte progenitor cell is seen. The Philadelphia chromosome is present in more than 95% of CML, and the presence of the BCR-ABL1 protein is responsible for initiation of CML. In advanced disease, the accumulation of additional mutations leads to the more aggressive leukemic phenotype.

CLINICAL MANIFESTATIONS Chronic leukemia advances slowly and insidiously. Approximately 70% of individuals with CLL are asymptomatic at the time of diagnosis. When symptoms do appear, the most common finding is lymphadenopathy. The most significant effect of CLL is

---

Table 27-4   Clinical Manifestations and Related Pathophysiology in Leukemia

Clinical Manifestations	Laboratory Abnormalities	Cause	Comments
Anemia	Key is the relative *proportion* of erythroblasts to total count (decreased in anemia)	Decreased stem cell input or ineffective erythropoiesis or both	In acute leukemia, anemia is usually present from the beginning, often the first symptom noticed, and severe; mild form without symptoms is common in CML and CLL; hemorrhage common in acute forms, occasional in CML, but rare in CLL
Bleeding (purpura, petechiae, ecchymosis, hemorrhage)	Decreased and possibly abnormal platelets	Reduction in megakaryocytes leading to thrombocytopenia	Bleeding more common in acute than in chronic leukemia
Infection	Increased multisegmented neutrophils	Opportunistic organisms; decreased protection resulting from granulocytopenia or immune deficiency secondary to chemotherapy, corticosteroids, and the disease process	Major sites of infection: oral cavity, throat, lower colon, urinary tract, lungs, and skin; prevention of infection focuses on restoration of host defenses, decreasing invasive procedures, and reducing colonization of organisms
Weight loss	Decreased 24-hr urinary creatinine excretion; hypoalbuminemia	Condition can be attributed to pain, depression, chemotherapy, radiation therapy, loss of appetite, and alterations in taste	Severe weight loss may be related to excess production of TNF-α
Bone pain	Often no radiographic evidence of bone problems	Result of bone infiltration by leukemic cells or intramedullary infection	If combination drug regimens are ineffective, radiation therapy is used
Liver, spleen, and lymph node enlargement	Biopsy abnormal for liver and spleen	Leukemic cell infiltration; lymph nodes also undergo leukemia proliferation in CLL	
Elevated uric acid	Normal excretion of uric acid is 300-500 mg/day; the leukemic individual can excrete 50 times more	Increased catabolism of protein and nucleic acid; urate precipitation increased from dehydration caused by anorexia or fever and drug therapy	Hyperuricemia is present in both acute leukemia and CML; increasing urine pH or decreasing acid production with the drug allopurinol

CLL, Chronic lymphocytic leukemia; *CML,* chronic myelogenous leukemia; *TNF,* tumor necrosis factor.

of the terminal phase, which then resembles AML, blast cells or promyelocytes predominate, and the individual experiences a blast crisis.

The acute effects of CML resemble those of acute leukemia but with more prominent and painful splenomegaly. Liver function rarely is altered despite enlargement, and lymphadenopathy generally is found only in the acute phase of the disease. Hyperuricemia invariably is present and produces gouty arthritis. Infections, fever, and weight loss are common findings in clients with CML.

EVALUATION AND TREATMENT Diagnosis of chronic leukemia depends on laboratory analyses of peripheral blood and bone marrow. Diagnosis of CLL is based on detection of a monoclonal B-cell lymphocytosis in the blood. The cells must have the immunophenotype characteristic of CLL (CD5+, CD19+, CD20 [weak], CD23+), at levels in excess of 5000 cells/μL, over a sustained period of time (usually 4 weeks). Bone marrow may contain more than 30% lymphocytes and be normocellular or hypercellular.

Treatment is frequently based on prognostic indicators. Typically, individuals with CLL survive 10 years or more. However, those with certain risk markers have a more aggressive disease that shortens survival to less than 3 years. Markers of high risk include anemia, thrombocytopenia, and no mutations in the *IGHV* gene. Mutations in *IGHV* correlate very closely with levels of intracellular ZAP-70, detection of which may be substituted for tests of *IGHV* mutation. ZAP-70 is a tyrosine kinase that is linked to the T-cell receptor (see Chapter 7). It is not normally detected in CLL cells with mutated *IGHV*, but is easily detectable by immunohistology in cells with an unmutated *IGHV*.

Chlorambucil, administered with or without corticosteroids, on a daily or intermittent schedule is the most common treatment for individuals with the most aggressive disease. Relief of symptoms is often achieved, but there is no substantial effect on survival. Combination therapy (CHOP) that includes **C**yclophosphamide, **H**ydroxydaunomycin (Adriamycin), vincristine (**O**ncovin), and **P**rednisone has an improved response rate but still does not demonstrate improved survival. Fludarabine, a purine analog, has a higher response rate and disease-free intervals, although survival is not affected. Promising results also have been obtained with the use of monoclonal antibodies (rituximab and alemtuzumab). Stem cell (autogenic and allogeneic) transplant also is being investigated as treatment; however, the advanced age at which individuals contract CLL makes its use less desirable.

Present treatment modalities for CML do not cure the disease, prevent blastic transformation, or prolong the average survival time. Standard treatment consists of combined chemotherapy, biologic response modifiers, and allogeneic stem cell transplant. Although transplantation is potentially curative, its use is limited by donor availability and high toxicity in older adults thus limiting use to those older than 65 years. Allogeneic bone marrow transplantation had increased survival time significantly (20% to 30%) when used after high-dose radiation and chemotherapy and with

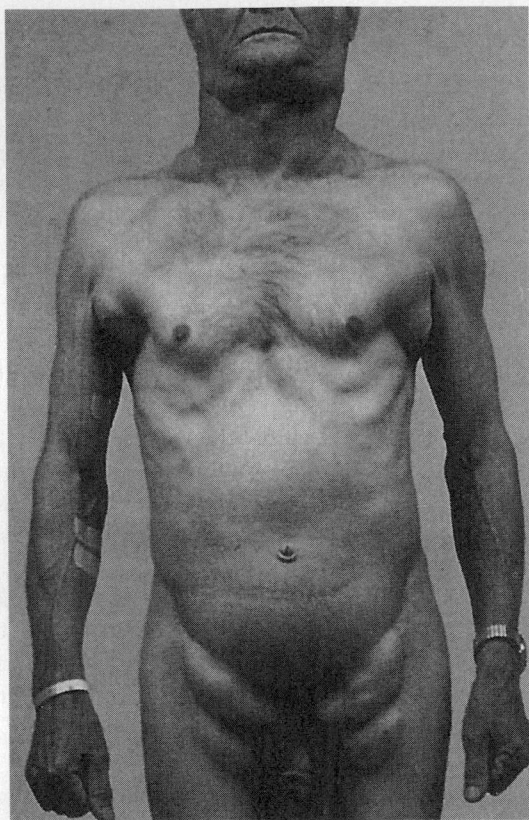

Figure 27-6 Lymphadenopathy. Individual with lymphocyte leukemia with extreme but symmetric lymphadenopathy. (Courtesy Dr. A.R. Kagan, Los Angeles. From del Regato JA, Spjut HJ, Cox JD: *Ackerman and del Regato's cancer*, ed 2, St Louis, 1985, Mosby.)

suppression of humoral immunity and increased infection with encapsulated bacteria. Frequently the level of neutrophils is depressed, which adds to the risk of infection. Invasion of most organ cells is uncommon but infiltration does occur in lymph nodes, liver, spleen, and salivary glands. CNS involvement is rare. Approximately 10% of individuals develop a more aggressive malignancy, usually a diffuse large B-cell lymphoma. In these individuals, extreme fatigue, weight loss, night sweats, low-grade fever, and elevated levels of the enzyme lactic dehydrogenase, hypercalcemia, anemia, and thrombocytopenia are common.

Individuals with CML may progress through three phases of the disease; a chronic phase lasting 2 to 5 years during which symptoms may not be apparent, an accelerated phase of 6 to 18 months during which the primary symptoms develop, and a terminal blast phase ("blast crisis") with a survival of only 3 to 6 months. The accelerated phase is characterized by excessive proliferation and accumulation of malignant cells. Splenomegaly is the most common finding, which is prominent and painful, but lymphadenopathy generally is not present. Liver enlargement also occurs, but liver function is rarely altered. Hyperuricemia is common and produces gouty arthritis. Infections, fever, and weight loss also are seen often. The terminal blast phase is characterized by rapid and progressive leukocytosis with an increase in basophils. In the later stages

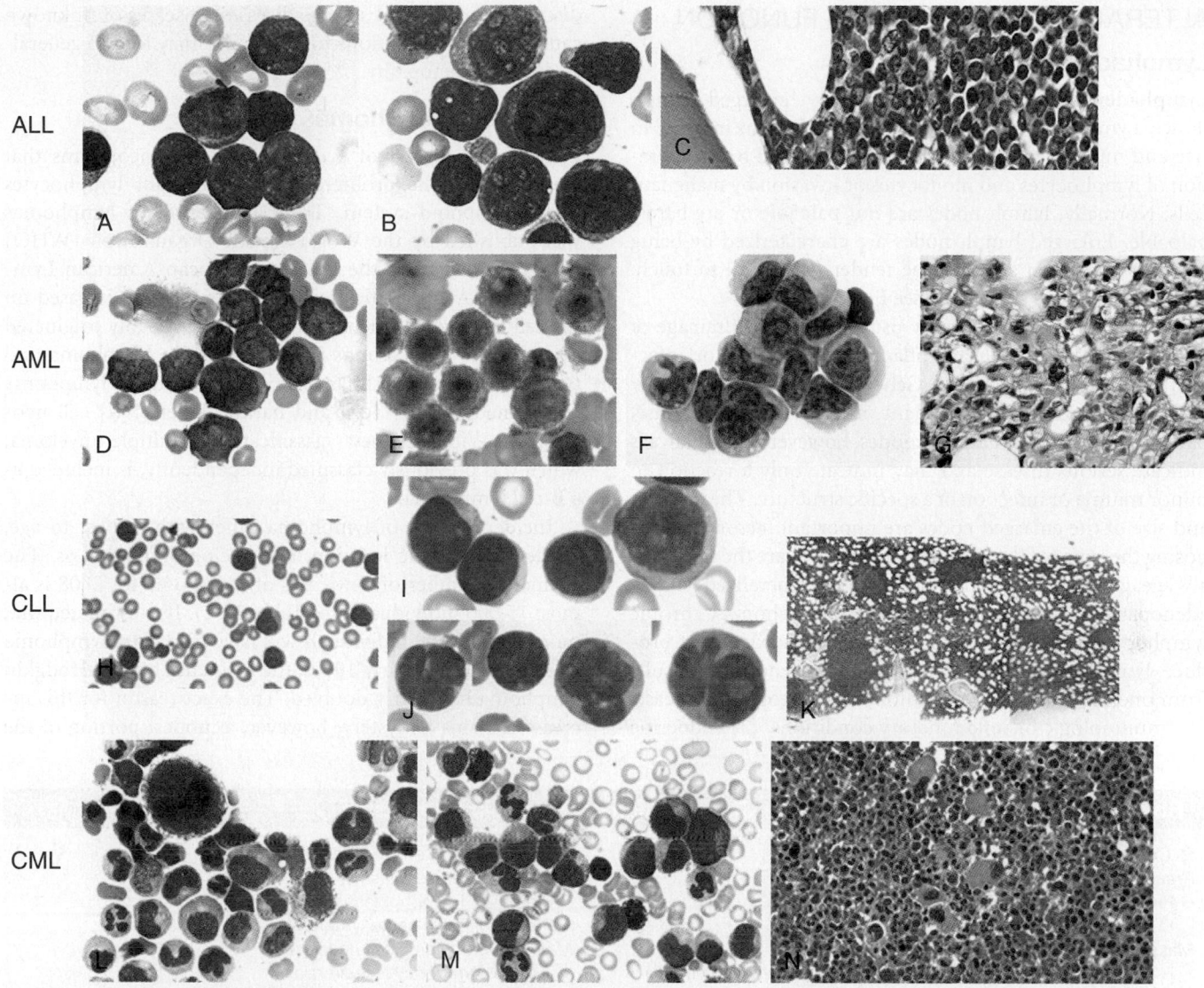

Figure 27-7 Morphologic aspects of leukemia cells. *Acute lymphoblastic leukemia* (ALL) (A-C). A, Typical uniform lymphoblasts with intermediate-sized nuclei, fine but "smudgy" chromatin, absence of nucleoli, and scant cytoplasm. B, Lymphoblasts with more cytologic variation, including variability in size, number of nucleoli, and amount of cytoplasm. C, Histologic features of ALL in bone core biopsy. *Acute myeloid leukemia (AML) (D-G).* D, Acute myeloblastic leukemia with minimal or no maturation. The cells are myeloblasts with dispersed chromatin and variable amounts of agranular cytoplasm. Some display medium-sized, poorly defined nucleoli. E, Acute monoblastic leukemia; characteristic monoblasts with round nuclei and delicate chromatin and prominent nucleoli. Cytoplasm is abundant. F, Acute monocytic leukemia with most of the cells in this field being promonocytes. Monoblasts and an abnormal monocyte also are present. G, Marrow biopsy of acute megakaryoblastic leukemia containing large and small blasts and atypical megakaryocytes. *Chronic lymphocytic leukemia (CLL) (H-K).* H, Peripheral blood smear typically shows lymphocytosis. Cytologic features of CLL cells differ. I, Classic cells have a small nucleus with a "soccer ball" chromatin pattern. J, Some cases have increased large cells, or prolymphocytes, with more open chromatin and prominent "punched-out" nucleoli (prolymphocyte, right side). K, The bone marrow can show nodular infiltrates of CLL cells. *Chronic myelogenous leukemia (CML) (L-N).* L, Peripheral smear shows marked leukocytosis due to a granulocytic proliferation of all stages with particularly increased myelocytes and absolute basophilia. M, Bone core biopsy illustrates markedly hypercellular marrow due to granulocytic proliferation and increased small hypolobated megakaryocytes. N, Bone marrow aspirate shows granulocytic proliferation and small, "dwarf" megakaryocyte. (A-C, H-N from Hoffman R, et al: *Hematology: basic principles and practice*, ed 5, Philadelphia, 2009, Churchill Livingstone. D-G from Abeloff M, et al: *Abeloff's clinical oncology*, ed 4, Philadelphia, 2008, Churchill Livingstone.)

concurrent treatment with interferon. Traditional chemotherapy agents used are hydroxyurea and busulfan. The development and introduction of the tyrosine kinase inhibitor imatinib mesylate (Gleevec) as a treatment modality have changed current management of CML. Imatinib mesylate is highly specific for CML and suppression of BCR-ABL kinase

activity. Suppression of hematologic symptoms occurs in 97% of treated individuals, and the use of imatinib mesylate has become the standard of care for CML. A small percentage of clients develop additional mutations in BCR-ABL that confer resistance to imatinib mesylate.[17] Several new tyrosine kinase inhibitors are under investigation as treatments for CML.

ALTERATIONS OF LYMPHOID FUNCTION

Lymphadenopathy

Lymphadenopathy is characterized by enlarged lymph nodes. Lymph node enlargement is caused by an increase in size and number of its germinal centers caused by proliferation of lymphocytes and monocytes or invasion by malignant cells. Normally, lymph nodes are not palpable or are barely palpable. Enlarged lymph nodes are characterized by being palpable and often also may be tender or painful to touch, although not in all situations (see Figure 27-6).

Localized lymphadenopathy usually indicates drainage of an area associated with an inflammatory process or infection (reactive lymph nodes). Generalized lymphadenopathy is generally a result of malignant or nonmalignant disease, particularly in adults. Palpable nodes, however, do not always indicate serious disease and may indicate only a reaction to minor trauma or infection of a specific structure. The location and size of the enlarged nodes are important factors in diagnosing the cause of the lymphadenopathy, as are the individual's age, gender, and geographic location. Generalized lymphadenopathy occurs with non-Hodgkin lymphomas, chronic lymphocytic leukemia, histiocytosis, and disorders that produce lymphocytosis. In general, lymphadenopathy results from one of four types of conditions: (1) neoplastic disease, (2) immunologic or inflammatory conditions, (3) endocrine disorders, or (4) lipid storage diseases. Diseases of unknown cause, including reactions to drugs, also may lead to generalized lymphadenopathy.

Malignant Lymphomas

Lymphomas consist of a diverse group of neoplasms that develop from the proliferation of malignant lymphocytes in the lymphoid system. The classification of lymphomas was published by the World Health Organization (WHO) and is derived from the Revised European-American Lymphoma (REAL) classification. This classification is based on the cell type from which the lymphoma probably originated (Box 27-2).[18] The groups include Hodgkin lymphoma and two that were previously classified as non-Hodgkin lymphoma (B-cell neoplasms, T-cell and natural killer [NK] cell neoplasms). With the new classification, multiple myeloma, which was previously classified independently, is included as a B-cell lymphoma.

Incidence rates of lymphoma differ with respect to age, gender, geographic location, and socioeconomic class. The estimated number of new cases of lymphoma for 2008 is almost 75,000 individuals (see Table 27-2). It is estimated that more than 20,000 individuals will have died from lymphoma in 2008. Since the early 1970s, the incidence of non-Hodgkin lymphoma has nearly doubled. The exact reason for this increase remains a mystery; however, a modest portion of the

---

Box 27-2	World Health Organization Classification of Lymphoid Neoplasms

B-Cell Neoplasms

Precursor B-cell neoplasms
  Precursor B-lymphoblastic leukemia/lymphoma
  Precursor B-cell acute lymphoblastic leukemia

Mature (peripheral) B-cell neoplasms
  B-cell chronic lymphocytic leukemia/small lymphocytic lymphoma
  B-cell prolymphocytic leukemia
  Lymphoplasmacytoid lymphoma
  Splenic marginal zone B-cell lymphoma (with/without villous lymphocytes)
  Hairy cell leukemia
  Plasma cell myeloma/plasmacytoma
  Extranodal marginal zone B-cell lymphoma of mucosa-associated lymphoid tissue (MAL type)
  Nodal marginal zone B-cell lymphoma (with/without monocytoid B cells)
  Follicular lymphoma
  Mantle-cell lymphoma
  Diffuse large B-cell lymphoma
    Mediastinal large B-cell lymphoma
    Primary effusion lymphoma
  Burkitt lymphoma/Burkitt cell leukemia

T-Cell and NK-Cell Neoplasms

Precursor T-cell neoplasms
  Precursor T-lymphoblastic lymphoma/leukemia
  Precursor T-cell acute lymphoblastic leukemia

Mature (peripheral) T-cell neoplasms
  T-cell prolymphocytic leukemia
  T-cell granular lymphocytic leukemia
  Aggressive NK-cell leukemia
  Adult T-cell lymphoma/leukemia (HTLV-1 positive)
  Extranodal NK/T-cell lymphoma, nasal type
  Enteropathy-type T-cell lymphoma
  Hepatosplenic gamma-delta T-cell lymphoma
  Subcutaneous panniculitis-like T-cell lymphoma
  Mycosis fungoides/Sézary syndrome
  Anaplastic large-cell lymphoma, T/null cell, primary cutaneous type
  Peripheral T-cell lymphoma, not otherwise characterized
  Angioimmunoblastic T-cell lymphoma
  Anaplastic large-cell lymphoma, T/null cell, primary systemic type

Hodgkin Lymphoma (Hodgkin Disease)
Nodular lymphocyte predominant Hodgkin lymphoma
Classical Hodgkin lymphoma
  Nodular sclerosis Hodgkin lymphoma (grades 1 and 2)
  Lymphocyte-rich classical Hodgkin lymphoma
  Mixed cellularity Hodgkin lymphoma
  Lymphocyte depletion Hodgkin lymphoma

From: National Institutes of Health, National Cancer Institute, Surveillance Epidemiology and End Results (SEER) Program, http://training.seer.cancer.gov/module_coding_primary/table_who_class_hemo_2.html.
NK, Natural killer; *HTLV,* Human T-cell leukemia virus.

increase had been attributed to lymphomas developing in association with immune deficiencies, including AIDS and organ transplants. Conversely, the incidence of Hodgkin lymphoma has declined over the same time period, especially among older adults.

In general, lymphomas are the result of genetic mutations or viral infection. Malignant transformation produces a cell with uncontrolled and excessive growth that accumulates in the lymph nodes and other sites, producing tumor masses. Lymphomas usually start in the lymph nodes or lymphoid tissues of the stomach or intestines.

Hodgkin Lymphoma

Hodgkin lymphoma (HL) is a malignant lymphoma first characterized by Thomas Hodgkin in 1832. It is estimated that more than 8000 individuals will be newly diagnosed with HL in 2008 (see Table 27-2). The incidence of HL is approximately 3.1 per 100,000 men and 2.5 per 100,000 women.[19] The median age of diagnosis is age 38. Incidence rates for HL have declined, especially among older adults. The decrease in incidence in older adults is attributed to improved diagnostic accuracy. The incidence is greater in whites than blacks. Denmark, the Netherlands, and the United States have the highest incidence of HL, and Japan and Australia have the lowest incidence. HL peaks at two different ages: early in life in the second and third decades and later in life during the sixth and seventh decades.

PATHOPHYSIOLOGY HL is characterized by its progression from one group of lymph nodes to another, the development of systemic symptoms, and the presence of **Reed-Sternberg (RS) cells** (Figure 27-8). It is widely accepted that the RS cell represents the malignant transformed lymphocyte. The RS cells are often large and binucleate, with occasional mononuclear variants. The RS cells are necessary for the diagnosis of HL; however, they are not specific to HL.

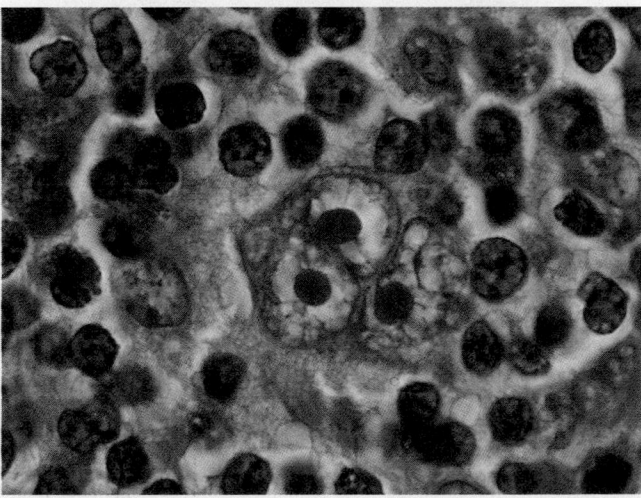

Figure 27-8 Reed-Sternberg cell. A large multinucleated or multilobed cell *(center of photograph)* with inclusion body–like nucleoli surrounded by a halo of clear nucleoplasm. (From Damjanov I, Linder J, editors: *Anderson's pathology*, ed 10, St Louis, 1996, Mosby.)

In rare instances, cells resembling them can be found in benign illnesses, as well as in other forms of cancer, including non-Hodgkin lymphomas and solid tissue cancers and in infectious mononucleosis.

The triggering mechanism for the malignant transformation of cells remains unknown. Classical HL appears to be derived from a B cell in the germinal center that has not undergone successful immunoglobulin gene rearrangement (see Chapter 7) and would normally be induced to undergo apoptosis. Survival of this cell may be linked to infection with EBV. Laboratory and epidemiologic studies have linked HL with EBV infections and EBV DNA. RNA, and proteins are frequently observed in HL cells. The RS cells secrete and release cytokines (e.g., IL-10, transforming growth factor-beta (TGF-β) that result in the accumulation of inflammatory cells that produces the local and systemic effects. HL is subcategorized into two main types: classical Hodgkin and nodular lymphocyte–predominant Hodgkin. Classical HL is subclassified into four types (Table 27-5) based on the morphology of RS cells, and the characteristics of the inflammatory cell infiltrate in the tumor.

The molecular events causing malignant transformation remain controversial; although RS cells are apparently from B-cell lineage, they express very few B-cell markers and express markers normally not found on B cells. For instance, RS cells do not express immunoglobulin, but do express CD15 (a carbohydrate adhesion molecule found on neutrophils), TARC (a Th2-cell specific chemokine), and T-cell–associated antigens (e.g., β-chain of the T-cell receptor).[18] The precise genetic defects leading to development of HL are unknown, although several have been suggested. These generally include defects in immunoglobulin variable region gene rearrangement or defects in other B-cell–specific differentiation genes.

CLINICAL MANIFESTATIONS Many of the characteristic clinical features (Box 27-3) of HL can be explained by the complex action of cytokines and other growth factors that are secreted by the malignant cells. These substances induce infiltration and proliferation of inflammatory cells, resulting in an enlarged, painless lymph node in the neck (often the first sign of HL) (Figure 27-9). The discovery of an asymptomatic mediastinal mass on routine chest x-ray is not uncommon and is often an initial sign of HL. The cervical, axillary, inguinal, and retroperitoneal lymph nodes are commonly affected in HL (Figure 27-10). Local symptoms caused by pressure and obstruction of the lymph nodes are the result of the lymphadenopathy.

About one third of individuals will have some degree of systemic symptoms.[20] Intermittent fever, without other symptoms of infection, drenching night sweats, itchy skin (pruritus), and fatigue are relatively common. These constitutional symptoms accompanied by weight loss are associated with a poor prognosis. The Cotswold staging classification system used for HL is able to establish a correlation between the anatomic extent of the disease and prognosis (Table 27-6). This classification system is based on the individual's medical history, examination (presence of symptoms and palpable

Table 27-5   Subtypes of Hodgkin Lymphoma

Subtype	Incidence	Presentation
Nodular sclerosis Hodgkin lymphoma (HL)	Most common subtype in developing countries Found in all ages but most common in adolescents and young adults (median age of onset is about 28 years) Incidence in females exceeds that in males	Large tumor nodules with RS cells surrounded by collagen and fibrous bands
Mixed cellularity HL	Second most common subtype Incidence in males exceeds that in females	RS cells with mixed inflammatory cell (lymphocytes, monocyte/macrophage, eosinophils, plasma cells) infiltrates
Lymphocyte-rich classical HL	Uncommon subtype Found in all ages but most common in adults Incidence in males exceeds that in females	Few RS cells and predominantly lymphocytic infiltration Usually localized at diagnosis Survival is long with or without treatment
Lymphocyte depletion HL	Uncommon subtype Most common type in older adults, HIV-positive individuals, and persons in nonindustrialized countries Incidence in males exceeds that in females	Large number of RS cells with less additional cellular infiltrate Usually widespread disease: abdominal lymphadenopathy; spleen, liver, and bone marrow involvement, without peripheral lymphadenopathy Stage is usually more advanced at diagnosis

HIV, Human immunodeficiency virus; *RS*, Reed-Sternberg.

Box 27-3   Clinical Manifestations of Hodgkin Lymphoma

Physical Findings
Adenopathy
Mediastinal mass
Splenomegaly
Abdominal mass

Symptoms
Fever, weight loss, night sweats
Pruritus

Laboratory Findings
Thrombocytosis
Leukocytosis
Eosinophilia
Elevated erythrocyte sedimentation rate (ESR)
Elevated alkaline phosphatase
Paraneoplastic syndromes

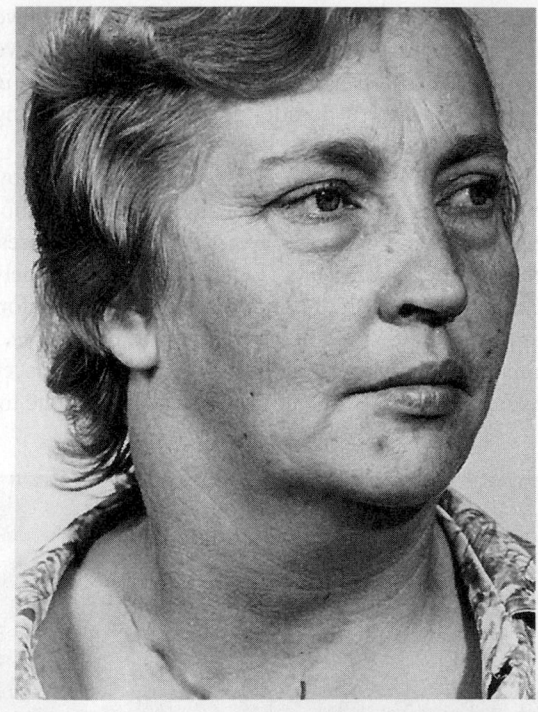

Figure 27-9 Hodgkin lymphoma and enlarged cervical lymph node. Typical enlarged cervical lymph node in the neck of a 35-year-old woman with Hodgkin lymphoma. (From del Regato JA, Spjut HJ, Cox JD: *Ackerman and del Regato's cancer*, ed 2, St Louis, 1985, Mosby.)

---

lymph nodes), and other radiologic and hematologic results. Prognostic indicators include clinical stage, histologic type, tumor cell concentration and tumor burden, constitutional symptoms, and age.

Although HL rarely arises in the lung, mediastinal and hilar node adenopathy can cause secondary involvement of the trachea, bronchi, pleura, or lungs. Retroperitoneal nodes can involve vertebral bodies and nerves, causing displacement of ureters. Spinal cord involvement is more common in the dorsal and lumbar regions than in the cervical region. Although uncommon, skin manifestations include psoriasis and eczematoid lesions, causing itching and scratching.

As a result of direct invasion from mediastinal lymph nodes, pericardial involvement can cause pericardial friction rub, pericardial effusion, and engorgement of the neck veins. The gastrointestinal (GI) tract and urinary tract rarely are involved. Anemia often is found in individuals with HL, accompanied by a low serum iron and iron-binding capacity. Other laboratory findings include elevated sedimentation rate, leukocytosis, and eosinophilia. Leukopenia occurs in advanced states of HL.

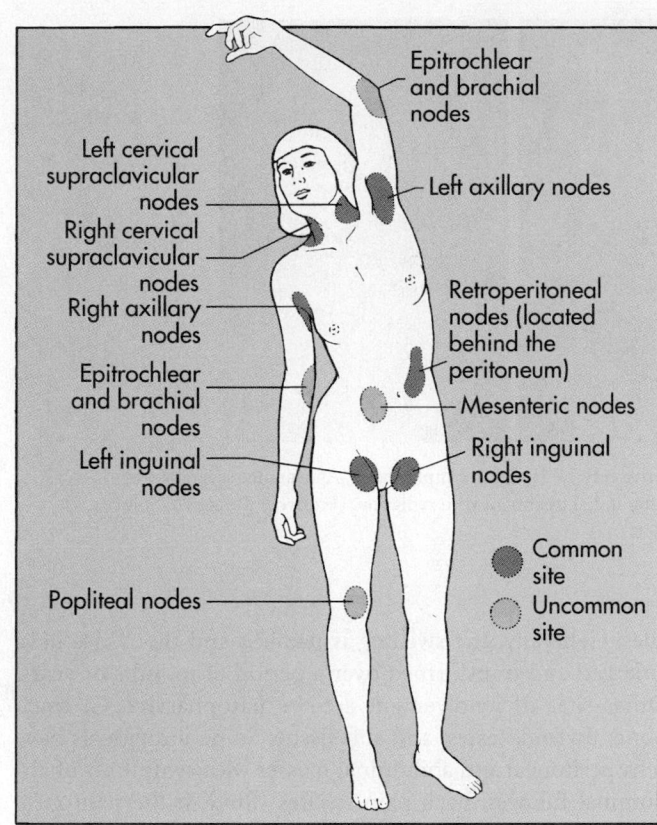

Figure 27-10 Common and uncommon involved lymph node sites for Hodgkin lymphoma.

Table 27-6	Cotswold Staging Classification System

Stage	Criteria
I	Involvement of a single lymph node region or single extranodal organ or site
II	Involvement of two or more lymph node regions on the same side of the diaphragm or a single extranodal organ or site and its regional lymph nodes
III	Involvement of lymph node regions or structures on both sides of the diaphragm
IV	Disseminated involvement of one or more extralymphatic organs or an isolated extralymphatic organ with distant nodal involvement
	Modifying characteristics for all four stages
	A: No B symptoms
	B: Unexplained fever of >38° C (100.4° F), drenching night sweats, unexplained loss of >10% of body weight in the 6 months preceding diagnosis
	E: Large mediastinal mass with direct extension into extranodal sites

Data from Lister TA, Crowther D: Staging for Hodgkin's disease, *Semin Oncol* 17:696, 1990.

Splenic involvement of HL depends on histopathologic type (see Table 27-5). The spleen is involved in 60% of cases of mixed cellularity and lymphocytic depletion types. With lymphocyte predominance and nodular sclerosis types, only 34% of cases reveal splenic involvement.

EVALUATION AND TREATMENT Because of the variability in symptoms, early definitive detection may be difficult. Asymptomatic lymphadenopathy can progress undetected for several years. Careful evaluation, including chest x-rays, lymphangiography, and biopsy, should be carried out for individuals with fever of unknown origin and peripheral lymphadenopathy.[20] A lymph node biopsy with scattered RS cells and a cellular infiltrate is highly indicative of HL. The effectiveness of treatment is related to the age of the individual and the extent of the disease. Approximately 75% of individuals diagnosed with HL are cured, largely because of successful treatment with irradiation and chemotherapy (Figure 27-11). More recent treatments include high-dose chemotherapy with bone marrow or stem cell transplant. Monoclonal antibodies also are being developed and nonmyeloablative allogeneic stem cell transplant has been found to help certain individuals even though this treatment is still under development.

The 5-year survival rate varies depending on which stage is identified at diagnosis.[20] The 5-year survival rate for stage I and II is 90% to 95%, 80% to 85% for stage III, and 75% for stage IV. Those with stage I or II disease are candidates for chemotherapy, radiation therapy, or a combination of these.

Individuals with stage III or IV disease, bulky disease (more than 10-cm mass or mediastinal disease with a transverse diameter exceeding 33% of the transthoracic diameter), or presence of B symptoms require combined chemotherapy with or without additional radiation treatment. Other factors, if present, have an influence on survival. Poorer survival is related to a high white blood cell count (greater than 15,000) or low hemoglobin (Hb) (less than 10.5); low lymphocyte count (less than 600); and being male. Cure for HL can be achieved in 70% of cases with current therapies.

Non-Hodgkin Lymphoma

The previously used generic classification of **non-Hodgkin lymphoma (NHL)** has been reclassified in the WHO/REAL scheme into **B-cell neoplasms,** which includes a variety of lymphomas including myelomas that originate from B cells at various stages of differentiation, and **T-cell** and **NK-cell neoplasms,** which includes lymphomas that originate from either T or NK cells. These cancers are differentiated from HL by lack of RS cells and other cellular changes not characteristic of HL.

More than 66,000 cases of NHL and 19,000 deaths are predicted for 2008 (see Table 27-2).[21] The median age of diagnosis is 67 years of age. The incidence of NHL has increased from 8 persons per 100,000 in 1973 to 23.5 per 100,000 in 2006. Lymphomas from HIV and EBV have accounted for some of the increase but an actual cause has yet to be determined. Conversely, the mortality rate has risen at a slower rate. It is thought that newer treatment modalities are improving survival rates.

PATHOPHYSIOLOGY NHL is best described as a progressive clonal expansion of B cells, T cells, or NK cells. The genetic lesions affecting proto-oncogenes or tumor-suppressor

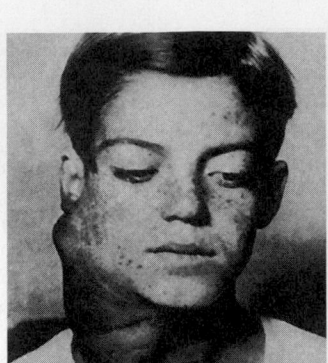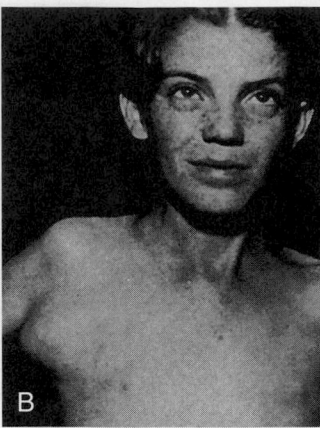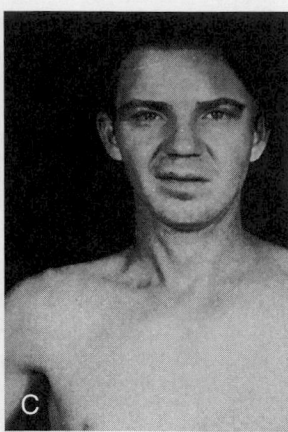

Figure 27-11 Cervical Hodgkin lymphoma. **A,** Young boy with extensive cervical Hodgkin lymphoma. **B,** Appearance several years later, when axillary manifestations developed. **C,** Appearance 23 years after initial treatment with radiation. (From del Regato JA, Spjut HJ, Cox JD: *Ackerman and del Regato's cancer,* ed 2, St Louis, 1985, Mosby.)

genes result in cell immortalization and the resultant increase in malignant cells. Oncogenes may be activated by chromosomal translocations or the tumor-suppressor loci may be inactivated by deletion or mutation of chromosomes. Oncogenic viruses also may alter the genome of certain subtypes. The various subtypes of NHL may be identified by specific diagnostic markers related to various cytogenic lesions.

Lymphomas most likely originate from mutations in cellular genes (many of which are environmentally induced) in a single cell that lead to loss of control of proliferation and other aspects of cell growth. The most common type of chromosomal alteration in NHL is translocation, which disrupts the genes encoded at the breakpoints. Risk factors include a family history, exposure to a variety of mutagenic chemicals, irradiation, infection with certain cancer-related viruses (e.g., EBV, human herpesvirus-8, HIV, HTLV-1, hepatitis C), and immune suppression related to organ transplantation. Gastric infection with *Helicobacter pylori* increases the risk for gastric lymphomas. NHL is a disease of middle age, usually found in individuals more than 50 years old.

B cells account for approximately 85% of NHLs, with T cells and NK cells accounting for the remaining 15%. A very small percent originates from macrophages. NHL tumors are categorized by the level of differentiation, cell of origin, and rate of cellular proliferation. Tumor aggressiveness of many B-cell NHLs may be predicted by the pattern of cell growth and size. Tumors with a characteristic nodular pattern, vaguely resembling lymphoid follicular structures, are generally less aggressive than lymphomas with a diffuse pattern of proliferation. Small lymphocyte lymphomas are less aggressive than large cell lymphomas, which are generally intermediate to high grade in aggressiveness. However, small cells are characteristic of some subtypes of high-grade lymphomas.

CLINICAL MANIFESTATIONS Clinical manifestations of NHL usually start out as localized or generalized lymphadenopathy, similar to HL. The cervical, axillary, inguinal, and femoral chains are the most commonly affected

sites. Generally, the swelling is painless and the nodes have enlarged and transformed over a period of months or years. Other sites of involvement are the nasopharynx, GI tract, bone, thyroid, testes, and soft tissue. Some individuals have retroperitoneal and abdominal masses with symptoms of abdominal fullness, back pain, ascites (fluid in the peritoneal cavity), and leg swelling.

Lymphomas are classified as low, intermediate, or high grade. A low-grade lymphoma, which also may be termed *indolent,* has a slow progression. Individuals with low-grade lymphoma commonly present with a painless, peripheral adenopathy. Spontaneous regression of these nodes may occur, mimicking the presence of an infection. Night sweats with an elevated temperature (more than 38° C [100.4° F]) and weight loss, as well as extranodular involvement, are not commonly present in the early stages but are common in advanced or end stage. Cytopenia, reflective of bone marrow involvement, is often observed. Hepatomegaly is common; however, splenomegaly is present in approximately 40% of individuals. Fatigue and weakness are more prevalent with advanced stages.

Immediate and high-grade lymphomas, which are more progressive, have a more varied clinical presentation. A high-grade lymphoma also may be termed *aggressive.* Adenopathy is common with more than one third of individuals having extranodal involvement. Common sites are the GI tract, skin, bone marrow, sinuses, genitourinary (GU) tract, thyroid, and CNS. Night sweats, with an increased temperature (more than 38° C [100.4° F]), as well as weight loss (more than 10% from baseline within 6 months) are present in approximately 30% to 40% of individuals. Some individuals have retroperitoneal and abdominal masses with symptoms of abdominal fullness, back pain, ascites (fluid in the peritoneal cavity), and leg swelling. Hepatomegaly and splenomegaly are often present. Differences in clinical features are noted in Table 27-7.

EVALUATION AND TREATMENT Biopsy is considered the primary means for diagnosis of NHL. Staging of NHL is necessary to identify treatment and make a prognosis.

Table 27-7	Clinical Differences Between Non-Hodgkin Lymphoma and Hodgkin Lymphoma	
Characteristic	Non-Hodgkin Lymphoma	Hodgkin Lymphoma
Nodal involvement	Multiple peripheral nodes	Localized to single axial group of nodes (i.e., cervical, mediastinal, para-aortic)
	Mesenteric nodes and Waldeyer ring commonly involved	Mesenteric nodes and Waldeyer ring rarely involved
Spread	Noncontiguous	Orderly spread by contiguity
B symptoms*	Uncommon	Common
Extranodal involvement	Common	Rare
Extent of disease	Rarely localized	Often localized

*Fever, weight loss, night sweats.

Table 27-8	Ann Arbor Staging for Hodgkin Lymphoma	
Stage	Criteria	
I	Involvement of single lymph node	
II	Involvement of two or more lymph node regions	
III	Involvement of lymph nodes on both sides of diaphragm	
IV	Diffuse involvement of one or more extra lymphatic organs with or without associated lymph node involvement	
Subclassifications		
E	Involvement of adjacent extra lymphatic site	
S	Involvement of spleen	
A	Asymptomatic	
B	Fever, night sweats, weight loss	

In addition to biopsy, computed tomography (CT) scans of the neck, chest, abdomen, and pelvis, as well as bilateral bone marrow aspirate, are performed. Data from all three procedures is necessary for appropriate staging. A common finding in NHL is noncontiguous lymph node involvement, which is not common in HL. The Ann Arbor staging system is most commonly used to stage NHL (Table 27-8). Treatment for NHL is quite diverse and depends on type (B cell or T cell) of tumor stage, histologic status (low, intermediate, or high grade), symptoms, age, and any comorbidities.

In general, treatment is initiated at the time of diagnosis; however, some low-grade lymphomas are widely disseminated at diagnosis, and because current therapy is not curative, observation without treatment may be the most appropriate choice. A partial remission may be achieved in some cases in which evidence of the disease remains but it does not progress.

Success of treatment is dependent on several parameters, including the type of lymphoma, stage of disease, cell type, involvement of organs outside the lymph nodes, age of the person, and the severity of the body's reaction to the disease (e.g., fever, night sweats, weight loss).[20,22] Treatment with chemotherapy alone may be adequate in many cases, although radiation therapy is frequently included. Low-dose chemotherapy has been followed by autologous stem cell transplantation in some NHLs or for recurrent disease. Treatment of B-cell lymphomas with rituximab has proven effective. Rituximab is a commercial monoclonal antibody against antigen CD20, which is expressed on the surface of all B cells, including those that are malignant. Administration of rituximab depletes most B cells and allows the replenishment of normal B cells from the lymphoid stem cell pool. It has also proven useful in a variety of autoimmune diseases, including immune thrombocytopenia purpura, autoimmune anemias, systemic lupus erythematosus, and rheumatoid arthritis.

Individuals with NHL can survive for extended periods.[20,22] Survival with nodular lymphoma ranges up to 15 years, but those with diffuse disease generally do not survive as long. Overall, the survival rates of NHL are less than for Hodgkin lymphoma. For NHL, the survival rates are 1 year, 77%; 5 years, 59%; and 10 years, 42%. Many investigators believe that more aggressive treatment increases the cure rate. High-grade NHL is seen with increasing frequency in persons with AIDS and has an extremely poor prognosis.

Burkitt Lymphoma

Burkitt lymphoma is a B-cell tumor with unique clinical and epidemiologic features that accounts for 30% of childhood lymphomas worldwide. It occurs in children from east-central Africa and New Guinea and is characterized by a rapidly growing tumor primarily in the jaw and facial bones (Figure 27-12). In the United States, Burkitt lymphoma is rare, usually involves the abdomen, and is characterized by extensive bone marrow invasion and replacement. EBV, found in nasopharyngeal secretions, is associated with Burkitt lymphoma in African children.

PATHOPHYSIOLOGY EBV is associated with almost all cases (more than 90%) of Burkitt lymphoma. It is suspected that suppression of the immune system by other illnesses (e.g., HIV infection, chronic malaria) increases the individual's susceptibility to EBV. B cells are particularly sensitive because of specific surface receptors for EBV. As a result, the B cell undergoes chromosomal translocations that result in overexpression of the *C-MYC* proto-oncogene and loss of control of cell growth (Figure 27-13). The most common translocation (75% of individuals) is between chromosomes 8 (containing the *C-MYC* gene) and 14 (containing the immunoglobulin heavy-chain genes). Other translocations have been reported between chromosome 8 and chromosomes 2 or 22, which contain genes for immunoglobulin light chains.

CLINICAL MANIFESTATIONS In non-African Burkitt lymphoma the most common presentation is abdominal swelling. More advanced disease may involve other organs—eye, ovaries, kidneys, glandular tissue (breast, thyroid, tonsil)—and presents with type B symptoms (night sweats, fever, weight loss).

EVALUATION AND TREATMENT The distribution of tumors and biopsies of enlarged lymph nodes or the bone marrow containing malignant B cells are usually indicative of Burkitt lymphoma. It is one of the most aggressive and quickly growing malignancies. However, the African variety in children has been successfully treated with radiotherapy and cyclophosphamide (60% survival overall; 90% survival with limited disease). The American type is more resistant to treatment.

Lymphoblastic lymphoma

Lymphoblastic lymphoma (LL) is a relatively rare variant of NHL (2% to 4%) but accounts for almost one third of cases of NHL in children and adolescents, with a male predominance. The vast majority of LL (more than 85%) is of T-cell origin, and the remainder arises from B cells. LL is similar to acute lymphoblastic leukemia and may be considered a variant of that disease.

PATHOPHYSIOLOGY The disease arises from a clone of relatively immature T cells that becomes malignant in the thymus. As with most lymphoid tumors, LL is frequently associated with translocations, primarily of the chromosomes that encode for the T-cell receptor (chromosomes 7 and 14). These aberrations result in increased expression of a variety of transcription factors and loss of growth control.

CLINICAL MANIFESTATIONS The first sign of LL is usually a painless lymphadenopathy in the neck. Peripheral

lymph nodes in the chest become involved in about 70% of individuals, mostly above the diaphragm. LL is a very aggressive tumor that presents as stage IV in most people. T-cell LL is associated with a unique mediastinal mass (up to 75%) because of the apparent origin of the tumor in the thymus.

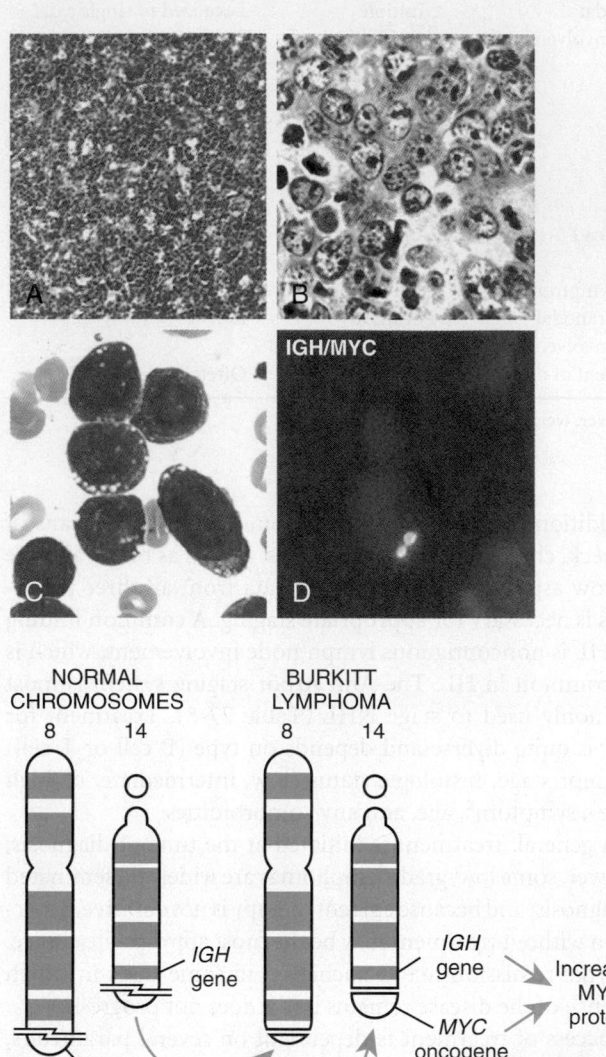

Figure 27-13 Burkitt lymphoma cells. **A,** A case of Burkitt lymphoma illustrated at low power showing the "starry sky" appearance. This is due to the dense proliferating cells producing the dark sky, and the scattered lighter-staining tingible body macrophages (stars) phagocytizing dying cells. **B,** Higher magnification illustrating the syncytia of intermediate-sized cells with coarse chromatin and multiple nucleoli. Note the tingible body macrophage with abundant light cytoplasm and ingested debris *(center bottom)*. **C,** Burkitt cells as seen on a Wright-stained bone marrow aspirate in a person with Burkitt leukemia. Notice deep blue cytoplasm with numerous vacuoles. **D,** Fluorescence in situ hybridization (FISH) with probes to *MYC* and *IGH* illustrate the IGH/MYC fusion. **E,** The 8, 14 chromosomal translocation and associated oncogenes in Burkitt lymphoma. (A-D, from Hoffman R, et al: *Hematology: basic principles and practice,* ed 5, Philadelphia, 2009, Churchill Livingstone. D, courtesy of Dr. Yanming Zhang, University of Chicago. E, from Kumar: *Robbins and Cotran pathologic basis of disease,* ed 7, Philadelphia, 2005, Saunders.)

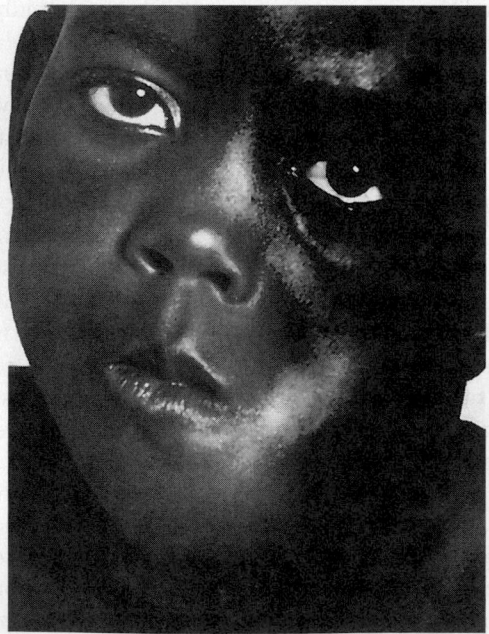

Figure 27-12 Burkitt lymphoma. Burkitt lymphoma involving the jaw in a young African boy. (Courtesy Dr. JNP Davies, Albany, NY. From del Regato JA, Spjut HJ, Cox JD: *Ackerman and del Regato's cancer,* ed 2, St Louis, 1985, Mosby.)

The mass results in chest pain and may cause compression of bronchi or superior vena cava. The tumor may infiltrate the bone marrow in about half of those affected, and suppression of bone marrow hematopoiesis leads to increased susceptibility to infections. Other organs, including the liver, kidney, spleen, and brain, may also be affected. Many individuals express type B symptoms: fever, night sweats, and significant weight loss.

EVALUATION AND TREATMENT The most common therapeutic approach is combined chemotherapy with multiple drugs. In early disease, the response rate is high with increased survival; the 5-year survival in children is 80% to 90%, and it is 45% to 55% in adults. Although LL is easily treated, there is a high relapse rate: 40% to 60% of adults.

Conditions That Mimic Lymphomas

Certain other clinical conditions mimic the malignant lymphomas. These conditions include TB, syphilis, systemic lupus erythematosus, lung cancer, and bone cancer. An important distinction between lymphomas and other conditions is that lymphomas usually involve localized lymphadenopathy. Infectious precursors of malignant lymphomas are characterized by more generalized lymphadenopathy with systemic signs and symptoms.

Plasma Cell Malignancies

The plasma cell is the end-stage cell of the humoral immune response (see Chapter 7). Immunocompetent B cells presented with antigen and stimulated with cytokines from T helper cells will undergo proliferation and differentiation into antibody-producing plasma cells. Antigen-reactive B cells have undergone rearrangement of immunoglobulin heavy-chain variable region genes *(V, D, J)* and express surface IgM or IgD, or both. After simulation with antigen, the B cells may not undergo any further genetic rearrangement and develop into plasma cells that secrete IgM or selectively rearrange the

immunoglobulin heavy-chain genes to irreversibly switch to secreting IgG, IgA, or IgE. During this process some cells may undergo malignant transformation, leading to one of several types of plasma cell malignancies (Figure 27-14). The most common and most aggressive plasma cell tumor is multiple myeloma. Other diseases in this classification include precursors to malignant myeloma (smoldering myeloma, monoclonal gammopathy of undetermined significance [MGUS]), solitary plasmacytoma of the bone, and Waldenström macroglobulinemia.[23] A common characteristic of these tumors is secretion of complete or partial immunoglobulin molecules.

Multiple Myeloma

Multiple myeloma (MM) is a clonal plasma cell cancer characterized by the slow proliferation of malignant cells as tumor cell masses in the bone marrow that usually results in destruction of the bone. Most MMs secrete large amounts of monoclonal proteins that resemble intact immunoglobulins. The reported incidence of myeloma has doubled in the past two decades, possibly as a result of more sensitive testing used for diagnosis. The annual incidence rate in the United States is 5.6 per 100,000, with almost 20,000 new cases and almost 11,000 deaths estimated for 2008.[24] Multiple myeloma occurs in all races, but the incidence in blacks is about twice that of whites. It rarely occurs before the age of 40 years—peak age of incidence is about 70 years. It is slightly more common in men than women. Neoplastic cells of multiple myeloma reside in the bone marrow and are usually not found in the peripheral blood. Occasionally it may spread to other tissues, especially in very advanced disease.

PATHOPHYSIOLOGY Many myelomas are aneuploidy, with chromosomal numbers ranging from 44 chromosomes to near tetraploid. Chromosomal translocations (break points) are responsible for development of myeloma in most individuals. The primary translocation involves the immunoglobulin heavy chain on chromosome 14 that

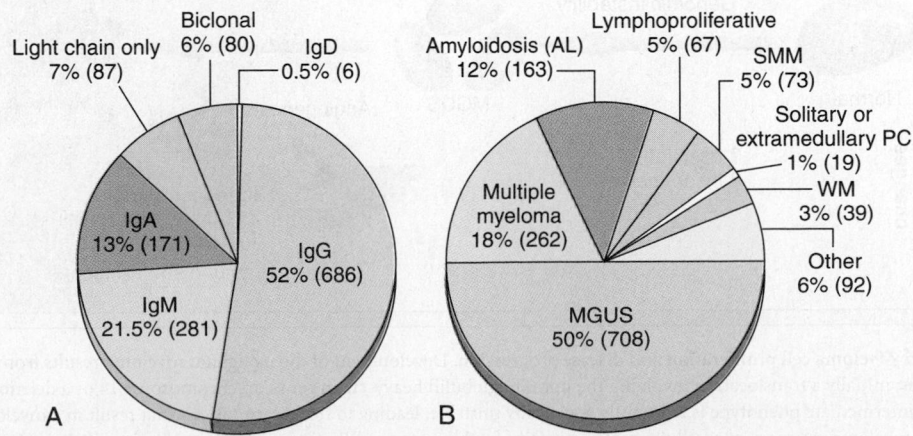

Figure 27-14 Distribution of monoclonal gammapathy types. **A,** Distribution of serum monoclonal proteins in 1311 clients seen at the Mayo Clinic during 2004. **B,** Diagnoses in 1423 cases of monoclonal gammopathy seen at the Mayo Clinic during 2004. *Ig,* Immunoglobulin; *MGUS,* monoclonal gammopathy of undetermined significance; *PC,* plasmacytoma; *SMM,* smoldering multiple myeloma; *WM,* Waldenström's macroglobulinemia. (From Goldman L, Ausiello D: *Cecil medicine,* ed 23, Philadelphia, 2008, Saunders.)

relocates to sites of containing genes that cell cycle (cyclins) on chromosomes 11(q13), 12(p13), and 6(p21); oncogenes on chromosomes 16(q23), 8(q24), and 20; and fibroblast growth factor receptor on chromosome 4(p16).[6] A progression of further secondary genetic alterations causes progression to an aggressive MM (Figure 27-15). The molecular pathogenesis of multiple myeloma also involves proto-oncogene mutations and, more rarely, inactivation of tumor-suppressor genes. The precise timing and reason for the genetic alteration and accumulation are unknown, but probably occur initially late in B-cell development after exposure to antigen.

Malignant plasma cells arise from one clone of B cells that produce abnormally large amounts of one class of immunoglobulin (usually IgG, occasionally IgA, and rarely IgD or IgE). The malignant transformation may begin early in B-cell development, possibly before encountering antigen in the secondary lymphoid organs. The myeloma cells return to either the bone marrow or other soft tissue sites. Their return is aided by cell adhesion molecules that help them target favorable sites that promote continued expansion and maturation.

Myeloma cells in the bone marrow directly secrete hepatocyte growth factor and parathyroid hormone–related peptide and adhere to stromal cells inducing their production of several cytokines (e.g., IL-6, IL-1, tumor necrosis factor-alpha (TNF-α), IL-11, macrophage inflammatory protein). (Lymphocytes and cytokines are described in Chapter 7.) All of these factors, IL-6 in particular, act as an osteoclast-activating factor and stimulate osteoclasts to reabsorb bone. This process results in bone lesions and hypercalcemia (high calcium levels in the blood) resulting from release of calcium from the breakdown of bone.

The antibody produced by the transformed plasma cell is usually defective, containing truncations, deletions, and other abnormalities, and is frequently referred to as a paraprotein (abnormal protein in the blood). Because of the large number of malignant plasma cells, the abnormal antibody, called the **M protein,** becomes the most prominent protein in the blood in 80% of myeloma clients (Figure 27-16). Suppression of normal plasma cells by the myeloma results in diminished or absent normal antibodies. The excessive amount of M protein may also contribute to many of the clinical manifestations of the disease. The myeloma may produce free immunoglobulin light chain (**Bence Jones protein**) that is present in the blood and urine in approximately 80% of clients and contributes to damage of renal tubular cells.

CLINICAL MANIFESTATIONS The common presentation of MM is characterized by elevated levels of calcium in the blood (hypercalcemia) (13% of persons), renal failure (19%), anemia (72% of persons), and bone lesions (80% of persons).[25] The hypercalcemia and bone lesions result from infiltration of the bone by malignant plasma cells and stimulation of osteoclasts to reabsorb bone. This process results in the release of calcium (hypercalcemia) and development

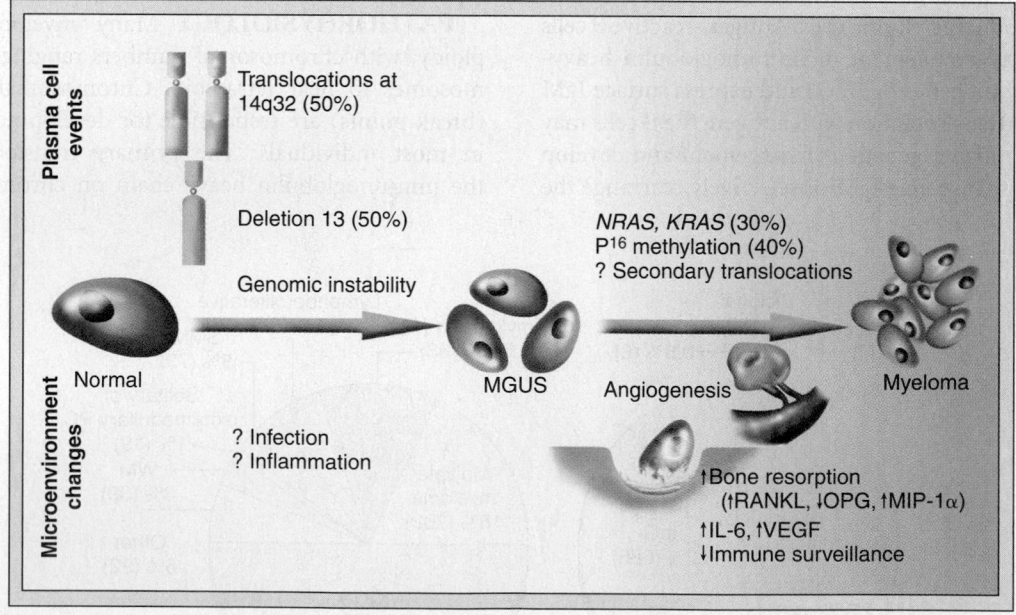

Figure 27-15 Myeloma cell proliferation and disease progression. Development of the malignant myeloma results from multiple genetic changes; initially a translocation involving the immunoglobulin heavy-chain genes on chromosome 14 or a deletion in chromosome 13. The intermediate phenotype is frequently genetically unstable, leading to further mutations that result in a myeloma. Interactions between myeloma cells and extracellular matrix proteins further increase adhesion molecule expression, antiapoptotic pathways, angiogenesis, bone resorption, and cytokine secretion. *IL-6,* Interleukin-6; *KRAS,* V-Ki-ras Z Kirsten rat sarcoma viral oncogene homolog; *MGUS,* monoclonal gammopathy of undetermined significance; *MIP-1α,* macrophage inflammatory protein-1α; *NRAS,* neuroblastoma RAS viral (v-ras) oncogene homolog; *OPG,* osteoprotegerin; *RANKL,* receptor activator of nuclear factor-κB ligand; *VEGF,* vascular endothelial growth factor. (From Abeloff M, et al: *Abeloff's clinical oncology,* ed 4, Philadelphia, 2008, Churchill Livingstone.)

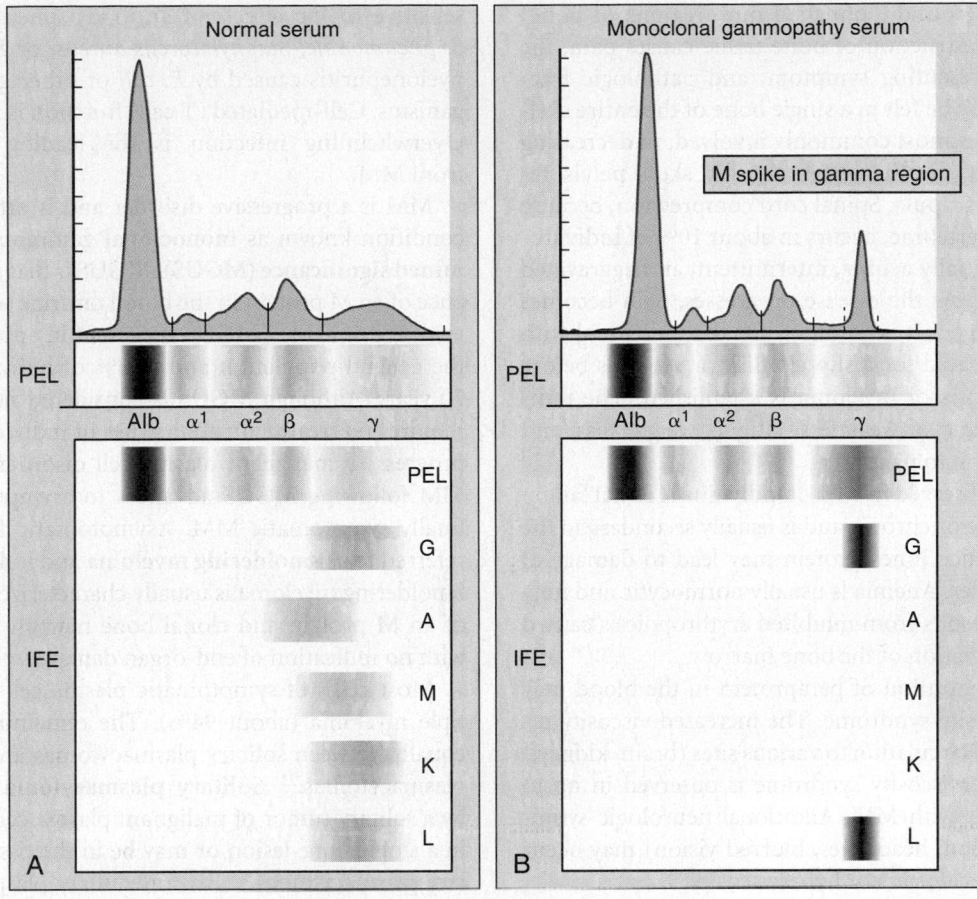

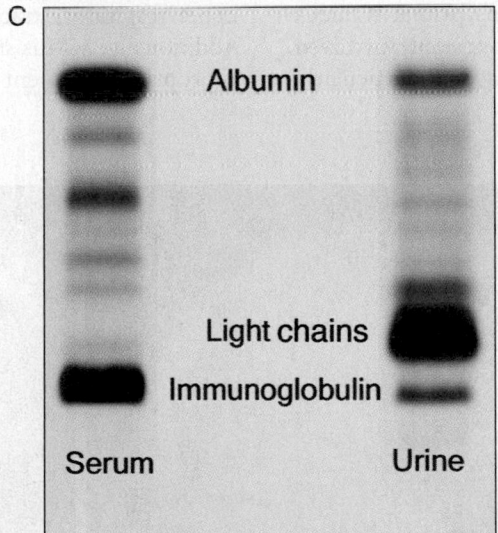

Figure 27-16 M protein. Serum protein electrophoresis (PEL) is used to screen for M proteins in multiple myeloma. **A,** In normal serum the proteins separate into several regions between albumin (Alb) and a broad band in the gamma (γ) region, where most antibodies (gamma globulins) are found. Immunofixation (IFE) can identify the location of IgG (G), IgA (A), IgM (M), and kappa (K) and lambda (L) light chains. **B,** Serum from an individual with multiple myeloma contains a sharp M protein (M spike). The M protein is monoclonal and contains only one heavy chain and one light chain. In this instance the IFE identifies the M protein as an IgG containing a lambda light chain. **C,** Serum and urine protein electrophoretic patterns in a client with multiple myeloma. Serum demonstrates an M protein (immunoglobulin) in the gamma region, and the urine has a large amount of the smaller-sized light chains with only a small amount of the intact immunoglobulin. (**A** and **B,** from Abeloff M, et al: *Abeloff's clinical oncology,* ed 4, Philadelphia, 2008, Churchill Livingstone. **C,** From McPherson R, Pincus M: *Henry's clinical diagnosis and management by laboratory methods,* ed 21, Edinburgh, 2006, Saunders.)

of "lytic lesions" (round, "punched out" regions of bone) (Figure 27-17). Destruction of bone tissue causes pain, the most common presenting symptom, and pathologic fractures. The pain may be felt in a single bone of the entire skeleton, and the bones most commonly involved, in decreasing order of frequency, are the vertebrae, ribs, skull, pelvis, femur, clavicle, and scapula. Spinal cord compression, because of the weakened vertebrae, occurs in about 10% of individuals. The pain is initially aching, intermittent, and aggravated by weight-bearing. As the disease progresses, pain becomes severe and prolonged. It is common for the individual with myeloma to be treated for a slipped disk or arthritis before the correct diagnosis of myeloma is established. The individual may complain of weakness, fatigue, weight loss, and anorexia in addition to pain.

Proteinuria is observed in 90% of individuals. Renal failure may be either acute or chronic and is usually secondary to the hypercalcemia. Bence Jones protein may lead to damage of the proximal tubules. Anemia is usually normocytic and normochromic and results from inhibited erythropoiesis caused by tumor cell infiltration of the bone marrow.

The high concentration of paraprotein in the blood may lead to hyperviscosity syndrome. The increased viscosity interferes with blood circulation to various sites (brain, kidneys, extremities). Hyperviscosity syndrome is observed in up to 20% of individuals with MM. Additional neurologic symptoms (e.g., confusion, headaches, blurred vision) may occur secondary to hypercalcemia or hyperviscosity.

Suppression of the humoral (antibody-mediated) immune response results in repeated infections, primarily pneumonias and pyelonephritis. The most commonly involved organisms are encapsulated bacteria that are particularly sensitive to the effects of antibody; pneumonia caused by *S. pneumoniae*, *Staphylococcus aureus*, or *K. pneumoniae* or pyelonephritis caused by *E. coli* or other gram-negative organisms. Cell-mediated (T cell) function is relatively normal. Overwhelming infection is the leading cause of death from MM.

MM is a progressive disorder and is often preceded by a condition known as **monoclonal gammopathy of undetermined significance (MGUS).** MGUS is diagnosed by the presence of an M protein in the blood or urine without additional evidence of MM.[25] MGUS is present in approximately 1% of the general population and in 3% of individuals older than 70 years. Although MGUS is considered nonpathologic and requires no treatment, about 16% of individuals with MGUS progress to malignant plasma cell disorders. Progression of MM following MGUS advances to asymptomatic MM and finally symptomatic MM. Asymptomatic MM also may be referred to as **smoldering myeloma** and indolent myeloma.[25] Smoldering myeloma is usually characterized by the presence of an M protein and clonal bone marrow plasma cells, but with no indication of end-organ damage.

Most cases of symptomatic plasma cell tumors are multiple myeloma (about 94%). The remaining 6% is divided equally between solitary plasmacytomas and extramedullary plasmacytomas.[23] **Solitary plasmacytoma** is characterized by a solitary tumor of malignant plasma cells that may result in a single bone lesion or may be in the tissues (extramedullary plasmacytoma).[25] Extramedullary plasmacytoma can be found in a variety of soft tissues, but commonly in those of the upper respiratory tract (e.g., tonsils, nasopharynx, sinuses). Additionally, MM is staged to help determine prognosis and appropriate treatment (Table 27-9).

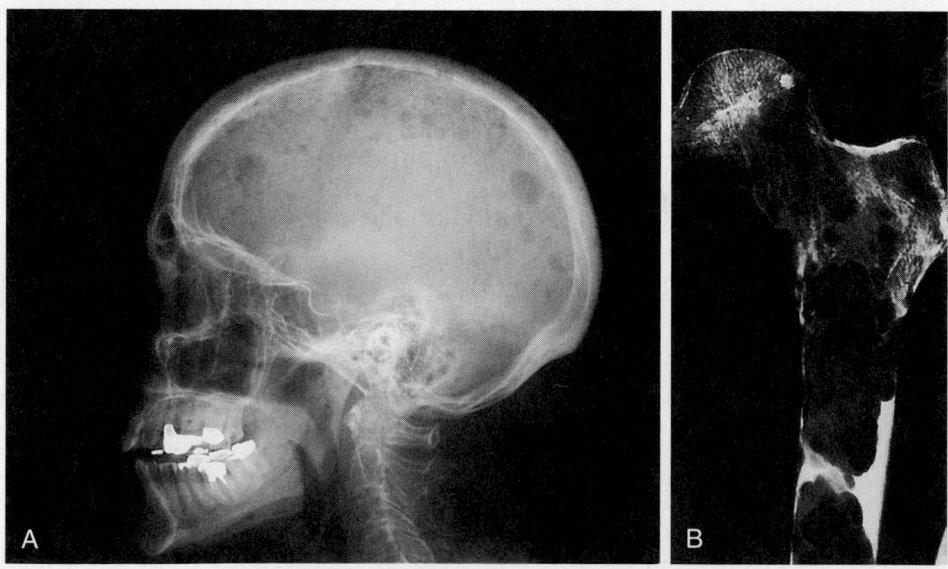

Figure 27-17 Osteolytic lesions in individuals with multiple myeloma. **A,** Lesions in the skull on radiograph in a client with myeloma. **B,** Roentgenogram of femur showing extensive bone destruction caused by tumor. Note absence of reactive bone formation. (**A** from Abeloff M, et al: *Abeloff's clinical oncology*, ed 4, Philadelphia, 2008, Churchill Livingstone. **B** from Kissane JM, editor: *Anderson's pathology*, ed 9, St Louis, 1990, Mosby.)

Table 27-9	International Staging System for Multiple Myeloma
Stage	**Criteria**
I	Serum β_2-microglobulin <3.5 mg/L
	Serum albumin ≥3.5 g/dl
II	Not stage I or III*
III	Serum β_2-microglobulin ≥5.5 mg/L

From Greipp PR et al: *J Clin Oncology* 23(15):3412-3420, 2005.
*There are two categories for stage II: serum β_2-microglobulin <3.5 mg/L but serum albumin <3.5 g/dl; or serum β_2-microglobulin 3.5 to <5.5 mg/L irrespective of the serum albumin level.

EVALUATION AND TREATMENT Diagnosis of MM is made by symptoms, radiographic and laboratory studies, and a bone marrow biopsy. Quantitative measurements of immunoglobulins (IgG, IgM, IgA) are usually performed. Typically, one class of immunoglobulin (the M protein produced by the myeloma cell) is greatly increased, whereas the others are suppressed. Serum electrophoretic analysis reveals increased levels of M protein. Because the M protein is monoclonal, each molecule has the same electric change and migrates at about the same site on electrophoresis, resulting in a highly concentrated protein (M spike). Bence Jones protein is observed in the urine or serum by immunoelectrophoresis or in the serum using enzyme-linked immunosorbent assay (ELISA) assays. Usually individuals with Bence Jones protein also have M protein in their blood. However, variants of MM include individuals in which free light chain only is produced and a rare variant that produces only free heavy chain, and approximately 1% are nonsecretory so that neither an M protein nor Bence Jones protein is produced. The amount of M protein in the blood may be used as a measure of the extent of the disease or as a measure of response to therapy. The serum level of another protein, free β_2-**microglobulin,** is a useful indicator of prognosis or effectiveness of therapy.

A bone marrow biopsy is performed to confirm the presence of myeloma cells in the marrow (Figure 27-18). Radiographic studies include x-ray, CT scans, and magnetic resonance imaging (MRI) to document the presence of bone lesions and areas of destruction. Diagnosis is based on findings and the degree of involvement. The individual must have all three major criteria (Box 27-4).

Combinations of chemotherapy, radiation therapy, and plasmapheresis (exchange), and marrow transplantation have been the standards of treatment.[23] Conventional combinations of chemotherapeutic agents have included melphalan and prednisone (MP); MP with vincristine, carmustine, and cyclophosphamide; vincristine, doxorubicin, and dexamethasone; and thalidomide and dexamethasone. The drug thalidomide disrupts the stromal marrow–MM cell interaction by modulating cell surface adhesion molecules and inhibiting angiogenesis. In addition, it increases apoptosis and G_1 growth arrest (i.e., the cell cycle gap 1; see Chapter 1) of MM cells.

Dose intensification improves the outcomes in younger clients; however, long-term remissions are obtained in a minority of clients. Thus intensive research measuring the effect of novel new therapies is the objective of ongoing trials. Gene expression profiling (GEP) helps improve the treatment of MM because it identifies prognostic subgroups and defines the molecular pathways associated with these subgroups. Newer agents (e.g., bortezomib, lenalidomide) have broadened the therapeutic regimens for end-stage myeloma.

High-dose chemotherapy followed by blood-forming stem cell transplantation (SCT) has become standard treatment for younger individuals (up to 70 years old in some trials).[23,26] Survival is increased with SCT compared with chemotherapy alone. SCT uses the client's own blood-forming stem cells (autologous) or a donor's cells (allogeneic). Survival may be prolonged by performing a second autologous transplant within 6 to 12 months from the first transplant.

Radiation with high-energy x-rays is used more for a localized effect rather than systemic. It is most often used to treat areas of the bone that have been damaged and are not responding to chemotherapy. In addition, it may be used to treat sites where tumor has led to collapse of vertebrae and spinal cord compression.

Additional interventions are used to prevent and treat complications arising from progression of the disease. Drugs that inhibit bone resorption—bisphosphonates—reduce the incidence of skeletal damage, which also reduces hypercalcemia and decreases bone pain. Hydration and diuretics may be used to maintain a high urine output, and antibiotics to treat recurring infections.

The prognosis for persons with MM remains poor. The median survival for all states of MM is 3 years. Individuals with

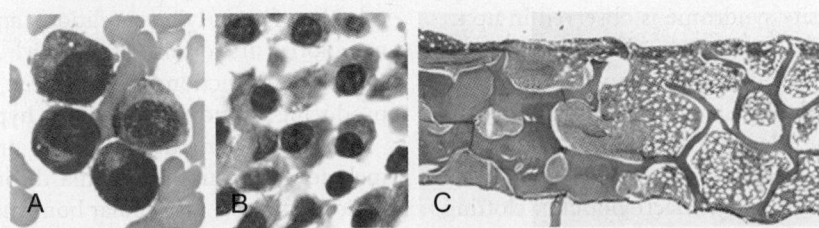

Figure 27-18 Myeloma cells. The typical myeloma type has fairly mature-appearing plasma cells with eccentric nuclei on bone marrow aspirate (**A**) and biopsy (**B**). **C,** Osteosclerotic myeloma in which the left side of the photograph shows bone sclerosis and the marrow cavity replaced by myeloma. (From Hoffman R, et al: *Hematology: basic principles and practice*, ed 5, Philadelphia, 2009, Churchill Livingstone.)

Box 27-4	Diagnostic Criteria for Multiple Myeloma

Major Criteria
Positive biopsy result
More than 30% plasma cells in bone marrow sample
Monoclonal antibody in blood/urine

Minor Criteria
10% to 30% plasma cells in bone marrow sample
Monoclonal antibody present but not enough to be a major criterion
Holes in bone from tumor seen on imaging studies
Normal antibody in blood abnormally low

multiple bone lesions, if untreated, rarely survive more than 6 to 12 months. Individuals with inactive (indolent) myeloma, however, can survive for many years. With chemotherapy and aggressive management of complications, median survival may increase to 24 to 30 months, with a 10-year survival rate of 3%.

Waldenström Macroglobulinemia

Waldenström macroglobulinemia (WM), also called **lymphoplasmacytic lymphoma,** is a rare type of slow-growing plasma cell tumor that secretes a monoclonal IgM molecule. Approximately 1500 new cases are diagnosed yearly in the United States; the median age of diagnosis is 63 years of age.[27] WM shares a great deal of similarity with multiple myeloma regarding its plasma cell origin, diagnosis, and treatment. However, the overproduction of the macromolecule IgM leads to certain unique clinical characteristics.

PATHOPHYSIOLOGY WM arises from plasma cells that have undergone genetic rearrangement of the variable region genes (V, D, J), but have not undergone class switch. Therefore, the principal secretory product of the tumor is IgM. Although no definitive genetic defect has been identified, WM may originate from aberrant B cell maturation and class switch.

Most of the pathology is associated with the production of large amounts of IgM, a large-molecular-weight protein (about 900,000 daltons). Excessive production leads to thickening of the blood and abnormally high blood viscosity (hyperviscosity syndrome). The increased viscosity interferes with circulation to various sites (e.g., eyes, brain, kidneys, extremities). IgM paraprotein may also result in cryoglobulins (proteins that precipitate from the blood at lower than body temperature). Hyperviscosity syndrome is observed in up to 20% of individuals with WM.

CLINICAL MANIFESTATIONS Many clients with WM are asymptomatic. The most common symptoms include weakness and fatigue, bleeding (from gums and nose), weight loss, and bruising. Bleeding may result secondary to formation of complexes among the macroglobulin, clotting factors, and platelets that diminish hemostatic capacity. If hyperviscosity syndrome occurs, the individual may develop neurologic problems (e.g., blurred vision, loss of vision, headaches, dizziness, vertigo), The macromolecules may also

precipitate in colder regions of the body (cryoglobulins) leading to Raynaud phenomenon.

Although the malignant plasma cells invade the bone marrow, erosion of the bone is not commonly observed; less than 5% of individuals have lytic bone lesions. The tumor often disseminates to other organs, including the spleen, lymph nodes, and liver. Anemia occurs in about 10% of clients, secondary to tumor infiltration of the bone marrow. Peripheral hemolysis can also result from production of cold agglutinins.

EVALUATION AND TREATMENT Diagnosis is made based on high levels of monoclonal IgM in the blood and the identification of malignant cells in bone marrow aspirates. Other hematologic abnormalities may be observed, especially anemia (80% of clients with symptomatic WM) but also thrombocytopenia and leukopenia. Bence Jones protein may be observed in almost half of individuals with WM.

Treatment is similar to that described for multiple myeloma.[28] First-line therapy includes combined chemotherapy with nucleoside analogs, alkylating agents, and monoclonal antibody (e.g., rituximab). Bone marrow stem cell transplantation has also proven effective in some individuals. The current recommendations include treatment with a combination of dexamethasone, rituximab, and cyclophosphamide, with the use of other drugs (e.g., doxorubicin, vincristine, and nucleoside analogs) in individuals with very high levels of M protein.

ALTERATIONS OF SPLENIC FUNCTION

The spleen has been an organ of mystery and perplexity in the study of medicine. Its relationship to other organs and disease processes, particularly the immune and hematologic systems, was not identified until the eighteenth century. The complexities of splenic function are not totally understood, and its mysteries are still being explored. The spleen is a useful organ, but its functions overlap those of other organs so that one is capable of living a normal, healthy life without the spleen. The relationship between asplenia and a higher risk for infection was not recognized until the early 1950s.

In the past, **splenomegaly** (enlargement of the spleen) was associated with various disease states. It is now recognized that splenomegaly is not necessarily pathologic; an enlarged spleen may be present in certain individuals without any evidence of disease. Splenomegaly may be, however, one of the first physical signs of underlying conditions, and its presence should not be ignored. In conditions in which splenomegaly is present, the normal functions of the spleen may become overactive, producing a condition known as **hypersplenism.**

Current criteria indicating the presence of hypersplenism include (1) anemia, leukopenia, thrombocytopenia, or combinations of these; (2) cellular bone marrow; (3) splenomegaly; and (4) improvement after splenectomy. Some individuals may seek treatment for problems even though they have not met all these clinical criteria; therefore, the relevance and significance of hypersplenism are still uncertain. Primary hypersplenism is recognized when no etiologic factor has been identified; secondary hypersplenism occurs in the presence of another condition.

PATHOPHYSIOLOGY Splenomegaly without a specific etiology is seen in 7% to 15% of individuals who are being evaluated for primary splenomegaly and is generally a diagnosis of exclusion. Specific conditions causing secondary splenomegaly and resulting hypersplenism are many and are related to all other categories of disease that affect individuals. Secondary splenomegaly may be classified according to the underlying cause. Specific conditions related to these various classifications of splenomegaly are detailed in Box 27-5. Different pathologic processes that produce splenomegaly are described briefly.

Acute inflammatory or infectious processes cause splenomegaly because of an increased demand for defensive activities. Acutely enlarged spleens secondary to infection may become so filled with erythrocytes that their natural rubbery resilience is lost and become fragile and vulnerable to blunt trauma. Splenic rupture is a complication associated with infectious mononucleosis; rupture occurs mostly in males between the fourth and twenty-first day of acute illness.

Congestive splenomegaly is accompanied by ascites, portal hypertension, and esophageal varices and is most commonly seen in those with hepatic cirrhosis. Splenic hyperplasia develops in disorders that increase splenic workload and is associated most commonly with various types of anemia (hemolytic) and chronic myeloproliferative disorders (i.e., polycythemia vera).

Infiltrative splenomegaly is caused by engorgement by the macrophages with indigestible materials associated with various "storage diseases." Tumors and cysts cause actual growth of the spleen. Metastatic tumors in the spleen are rare and may result from primary tumors of the skin, lung, breast, and cervix.

Box 27-5   Diseases Related to Classification of Splenomegaly

Inflammation or Infection
Acute: viral (hepatitis, infectious mononucleosis, cytomegalovirus), bacterial (*Salmonella,* gram negative), parasitic (typhoid)
Subacute or chronic: bacterial (subacute bacterial endocarditis, tuberculosis), parasitic (malaria), fungal (histoplasmosis), Felty syndrome, systemic lupus erythematosus, rheumatoid arthritis, thrombocytopenia

Congestive
Cirrhosis, heart failure, portal vein obstruction (portal hypertension), splenic vein obstruction

Infiltrative
Gaucher disease, amyloidosis, diabetic lipemia

Tumors or Cysts
Malignant: polycythemia vera, chronic or acute leukemias, Hodgkin lymphoma, metastatic solid tumors
Nonmalignant: hamartoma
Cysts: true cysts (lymphangiomas, hemangiomas, epithelial, endothelial); false cysts (hemorrhagic, serous, inflammatory)

CLINICAL MANIFESTATIONS Overactivity of the spleen results in hematologic alterations that affect all blood components. Sequestering of red blood cells, granulocytes, and platelets results in a reduction of all circulating blood cells. The spleen may sequester up to 50% of the red blood cell population, thereby upsetting the normal physiologic concentration of red blood cells in the circulation. The rate of splenic pooling is directly related to spleen size and the degree of increased blood flow through it. Sequestering exposes the red blood cells to splenic conditions that accelerate destruction, further contributing to the decreased red blood cell concentration. Anemia is the result of these combined activities. Anemia may be further potentiated by an increase in blood volume, which produces a dilutional effect on the already reduced concentration of red blood cells. The dilutional effect, as well as the removal and destruction of red blood cells, depends primarily on the degree of splenomegaly.

White blood cells and platelets also are affected by sequestering, although not to the same degree as the red blood cell. Again, the size of the spleen is the determining factor in the number of cells sequestered.

EVALUATION AND TREATMENT Treatment for hypersplenism is splenectomy; however, it is not always the treatment of choice. A splenectomy should be performed when its removal is considered necessary to alleviate the destructive effects on red blood cells. Clinical indicators should determine the need for splenectomy, not necessarily the specific condition. Splenectomy for splenic rupture no longer is considered mandatory in light of the possibility of overwhelming sepsis after removal. Repair and preservation of the ruptured spleen are now considered before the decision to remove the spleen. Splenectomy also may be performed as treatment for hairy cell leukemia, Felty syndrome, agnogenic myeloid metaplasia, thalassemia major, Gaucher disease, hemodialysis, splenomegaly, splenic venous thrombosis, and thrombotic thrombocytopenia purpura (TTP).

Individuals are able to lead normal lives after splenectomy, but hematologic abnormalities often exist after removal of the spleen. The red blood cells become thinner, broader, and wrinkled as a result of increases in surface area and membrane lipids. The white blood cell count increases dramatically 1 week after removal and then levels off to approximately 40% above normal. Platelets also rise immediately after surgery and then level off to above-normal levels for the duration of the individual's life. Increased platelet levels have been implicated in ischemic heart disease in males because of increased thrombocytosis and hypercoagulability.

A major postoperative complication following splenectomy is OPSI. Unless treated in time, OPSI may rapidly progress to septic shock and possibly disseminated intravascular coagulation (DIC). Initial statistics indicate a mortality rate of 50% to 70%, with most deaths occurring within the first 48 hours after hospitalization. Prompt medical attention can reduce the mortality rate to 10%.

ALTERATIONS OF PLATELETS AND COAGULATION

Hemostasis is dependent on adequate numbers of platelets and levels of coagulation factors. Diminished or excessive levels may lead to defective hemostasis or spontaneous and unnecessary activation of clotting. (Hemostasis is described in Chapter 25.) Diminished hemostasis results in either internal or external hemorrhage. Diffuse hemorrhage into skin tissues that is visible through the skin causes a red-purple discoloration identified as a **purpura.** Purpuric disorders occur when there are not enough normal platelets to plug damaged vessels or prevent leakage from the many minute tears that occur daily in normal capillaries. Disorders of the clotting system tend to result in more serious internal bleeding than platelet defects and usually are caused by a deficiency of one or several clotting factors. Disorders that result in spontaneous clotting can result from genetic disorders of clotting system components or from acquired diseases that activate clotting. These disorders are known collectively as **thromboembolic disease.**

Disorders of Platelets

Quantitative or qualitative abnormalities of platelets can interrupt normal blood coagulation and prevent hemostasis.[29] The quantitative abnormalities are thrombocytopenia, a decrease in the number of circulating platelets, and thrombocythemia, an increase in the number of platelets. Qualitative disorders affect the structure or function of individual platelets and can coexist with the quantitative disorders. Qualitative disorders usually prevent platelet adherence and aggregation, preventing formation of a platelet plug.

Thrombocytopenia

Thrombocytopenia is defined as a platelet count less than 150,000 platelets/mm³ of blood, although most health care providers do not consider the decrease of significance unless the count falls to less than 100,000 platelets/mm³ of blood.[30] Hemorrhage resulting from minor trauma does not usually occur until the count falls below 50,000/mm³. Spontaneous bleeding without apparent trauma can occur with counts between 10,000 and 15,000/mm³, resulting in petechiae, ecchymoses, larger purpuric spots, or frank bleeding from mucous membranes. Severe spontaneous bleeding may result if the count is less than 10,000/mm³ and can be fatal if it occurs in the gastrointestinal tract, respiratory system, or CNS.

Before the diagnosis of thrombocytopenia is made, **pseudothrombocytopenia** must be ruled out. This phenomenon occurs in approximately 1 in 1000 to 1 in 10,000 laboratory samples and is an in vitro artifact that may occur when a blood sample is analyzed by an automated cell counter. Platelets in the sample may become nonspecifically agglutinated by immunoglobulins in the presence of ethylenediaminetetraacetic acid (EDTA), a preservative in banked blood. The agglutinated platelets are not counted, thus giving an apparent, but false, thrombocytopenia. Thrombocytopenia also may be falsely diagnosed because of a dilutional effect observed after massive transfusion of platelet-poor packed cells to treat a hemorrhage. This occurs when more than 10 units of blood have been transfused within a 24-hour period. The hemorrhage that necessitated the transfusion also accelerates the loss of platelets, which further contributes to the pseudothrombocytopenic state. Splenic sequestering of platelets secondary to hypersplenism (congestive) induces an apparent thrombocytopenia, as does hypothermia (less than 25° C [77° F]), which is reversed when temperatures return to normal, suggesting an increased platelet sequestration in response to chilling.

PATHOPHYSIOLOGY Thrombocytopenia results from decreased platelet production, increased consumption, or both. The condition also may be congenital or acquired and primary or secondary to other acquired or congenital conditions. Thrombocytopenia secondary to congenital conditions occurs in a large number of different diseases, although each is relatively rare. These include thrombocytopenia with absence of radius (TAR) syndrome, Wiskott-Aldrich syndrome (see Chapter 8), various forms of *MYH9* gene mutation (e.g., May-Hegglin syndrome), X-linked thrombocytopenia, and many other examples.

Acquired thrombocytopenia is more common and may occur as a result of decreased platelet production secondary to viral infections (e.g., EBV, rubella, CMV, HIV), drugs (e.g., thiazides, estrogens, quinine-containing medications, chemotherapeutic agents, ethanol), nutritional deficiencies (vitamin B_{12} or folic acid in particular), chronic renal failure, bone marrow hypoplasia (e.g., aplastic anemia), radiation therapy, or bone marrow infiltration by cancer. Most common forms of thrombocytopenia are the result of increased platelet consumption. Examples include heparin-induced thrombocytopenia, idiopathic (immune) thrombocytopenic purpura, thrombotic thrombocytopenic purpura.

Heparin-Induced Thrombocytopenia

Heparin is a common cause of drug-induced thrombocytopenia. Approximately 4% of individuals treated with unfractionated heparin develop **heparin-induced thrombocytopenia (HIT).** The incidence is lower (about 0.1%) with the use of low-molecular-weight heparin. HIT is an immune-mediated, adverse drug reaction caused by IgG antibodies against the heparin-platelet factor 4 complex leading to platelet activation through platelet Fc γIIa receptors (Figure 27-19).[31] The release of additional platelet factor 4 from activated platelets and activation of thrombin lead to increased platelet consumption and a decrease in platelet counts beginning 5 to 10 days after administration of heparin.

CLINICAL MANIFESTATIONS The hallmark of HIT is thrombocytopenia. A decrease of approximately 50% in the platelet count is seen in more than 95% of individuals. However, 30% or more of those with thrombocytopenia are also at risk for venous or arterial thrombosis.[31] Venous thrombosis is most common and results in deep venous thrombosis and pulmonary emboli. Arterial thromboses affect the large

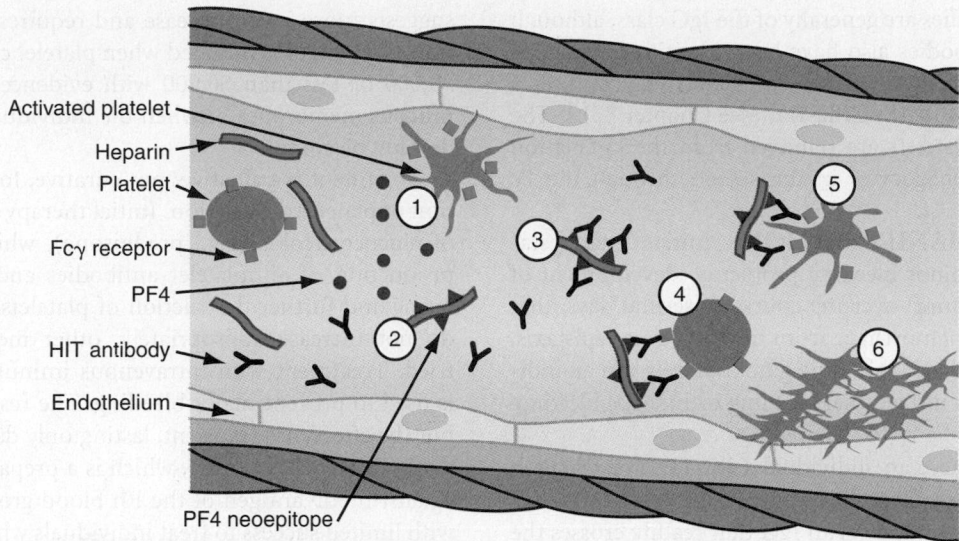

Figure 27-19 Pathogenesis of heparin-induced thrombocytopenia (HIT). (1) Activated platelets release procoagulant proteins from α-granules, including platelet factor 4 (PF4). Administered heparin binds PF4 (2), which undergoes a conformation change and expresses a new antigen (neoepitope). Individuals with HIT produce an immunoglobulin G (IgG) antibody that specifically reacts (3) with multiple identical neoepitopes on the heparin-PF4 complex. The reaction forms heparin-PF4-IgG immune complexes. Platelets express FcγRIIa receptors (Fcγ receptor) that react (4) with the Fc portion of IgG in immune complexes. Cross-linking of Fc receptors (5) results in FcγRIIa-dependent platelet activation. The activated platelets mediate a series of events that lead to further activation of the coagulation cascade, resulting in thrombin generation. Further release of PF4 from newly activated platelets leads to a cycle of continuing platelet activation and (6) formation of a primary clot. The reaction can be enhanced by the release of platelet-derived microparticles that are rich in surface phosphatidylserine and increase activation of coagulation and by the binding of heparin-PF4 complexes and HIT-IgG to the vascular endothelium (not shown).

arteries of the lower extremities, causing acute limb ischemia. Arterial thrombosis also may lead to cerebrovascular accidents and myocardial infarctions. Other major arteries (renal, mesenteric, upper limb) also may be affected. Bleeding is uncommon in HIT, even with low platelet counts.

EVALUATION AND TREATMENT Diagnosis is primarily based on clinical observations.[31] The individual presents with dropping platelet counts after 5 days or longer of heparin treatment. On average, platelet counts may reach 60,000/mm³. Because most clients are postsurgery, and the onset of symptoms, including thrombosis, may be delayed until after release from the hospital, other possible causes of thrombocytopenia (e.g., infection, other drug reactions) must be considered.

Tests are available to measure antibodies against heparin-platelet factor 4.[32] The test sensitivity is extremely high (more than 90%), but the specificity is less because of false-positive reactions (e.g., those on dialysis). HIT antibody titers may be measured, but the titers must be evaluated in the context of the clinical presentation. If HIT is not recognized and treated, intravascular aggregation of platelets causes rapid development of arterial and venous thrombosis. Although rare, heparin antibodies have caused anaphylactic shock.

Treatment is the withdrawal of heparin and use of alternative anticoagulants. A switch to low-molecular-weight heparin is not indicated, and warfarin should not be used until the symptoms of HIT have resolved because of an increased risk of initiating skin necrosis. The thrombocytopenia should progressively resolve. The chance of spontaneous blood clots

can be diminished using thrombin inhibitors (e.g., lepirudin, argatroban).[31]

Immune Thrombocytopenic Purpura

The most common cause of thrombocytopenia secondary to increased platelet destruction is **immune thrombocytopenic purpura (ITP).** The incidence of ITP is estimated to be 5.8 to 6.6 per 100,000 in the general population. ITP was formerly known as *idiopathic thrombocytopenic purpura;* however, it is widely recognized now as an immune process, hence the change from idiopathic to immune.[33] ITP may be acute or chronic. The acute form is frequently observed in children and typically lasts 1 to 2 months with a complete remission. In some instances it may last for up to 6 months, and some children (7% to 28%) may progress to the chronic condition. Acute ITP is usually secondary to infections (particularly viral) or other conditions that lead to large amounts of antigen in the blood, such as drug allergies or systemic lupus erythematosus (SLE) (see Chapter 8). Under these conditions the antigen usually forms immune complexes with circulating antibody, and it is thought that the immune complexes bind to Fc receptors on platelets, leading to their destruction in the spleen. The acute form of ITP usually resolves as the source of antigen is removed (e.g., the viral infection resolves).

Chronic ITP is associated with autoantibodies against platelet-specific antigens. This form is more commonly observed in adults, with highest prevalence in women between 20 and 40 years old, although it can develop at most any age. The chronic form tends to get progressively worse.

The autoantibodies are generally of the IgG class, although IgA and IgM antibodies also have been identified. They react against one or more of several platelet glycoproteins (e.g., GPIIb-IIIa, GPIb-IX, GPIa-IIa) (see Chapter 25).[34] The antibody-coated platelets are removed from the circulation by mononuclear phagocytes in the spleen through the Fc receptor.

CLINICAL MANIFESTATIONS Initial manifestations are usually minor bleeding problems (development of petechiae and purpura) over the course of several days, that progress to major hemorrhage from mucosal sites (epistaxis, hematuria, menorrhagia, bleeding gums). Rarely will an individual present with intracranial bleeding or internal bleeding at other sites.

During pregnancy, an individual with ITP may have a newborn that is also thrombocytopenic. In most individuals the antiplatelet antibody is an IgG that readily crosses the placenta (see Chapters 7 and 8). If the fetal platelets express the same antigen as the mother, the maternal antibody will coat the platelets potentially resulting in thrombocytopenia in utero. A variant of neonatal thrombocytopenia (neonatal alloimmune thrombocytopenia) occurs when the mother does not have ITP, but makes IgG antibodies against an antigen inherited from the father and found on fetal platelets but not on maternal platelets.[35] Alloimmune neonatal thrombocytopenia occurs in 1 of 2000 pregnancies. The most common antibody in this condition is against the human platelet antigen-a (HPA-a) antigen on the GPIIIa protein. Neonatal thrombocytopenia, either secondary to maternal autoimmune thrombocytopenia or as alloimmune thrombocytopenia, may occur to various degrees. The most severe form results in fetal platelet counts below 20,000/mm^3 with a high associated risk of intracranial hemorrhage.

EVALUATION AND TREATMENT Diagnosis of ITP is based on a history of bleeding and associated symptoms, such as weight loss, fever, and headache. Physical examination includes notations on the types of bleeding, location, and severity. Evidence of infections (bacterial, HIV and other viral), medication history, family history, and evidence of thrombosis are also assessed. Other diagnostic tests include complete blood count (CBC) and peripheral blood smear. Unlike some other forms of thrombocytopenia, splenectomy is rarely observed. Testing for antiplatelet antibodies is usually not helpful. Although most cases of ITP are associated with elevated levels of IgG on platelets, other forms of thrombocytopenia also have a high incidence of platelet-associated antibodies; thus the specificity is low (50% to 65%).[36] In addition, some cases of ITP will not present with elevated platelet-associated antibodies; the sensitivity is 75% to 94%, so that a negative test does not completely rule out ITP.

The acute form of ITP usually resolves without major clinical consequences. As with most autoimmune diseases, the course of the chronic form is variable, with multiple remissions and exacerbations. For many individuals the platelet count may remain adequate enough to avoid clinically serious bleeding. However, the presence of spontaneous bleeding suggests more severe disease and requires immediate attention. Treatment is initiated when platelet counts are less than 30,000 or less than 50,000 with evidence of bleeding from mucous membranes or when the individual is at high risk to develop bleeding.

Treatment is palliative, not curative, focusing on prevention of platelet destruction. Initial therapy for ITP is infusion of glucocorticoids (e.g., prednisone), which suppresses the production of antiplatelet antibodies and prevents sequestering and further destruction of platelets. If platelet counts do not increase appropriately, other medications may be tried. Treatment with intravenous immunoglobulin (IVIG) is used to prevent major bleeding. The response rate is 80%, but the effects are transient, lasting only days or a few weeks. Anti-(Rh$_o$)D (RhoGAM), which is a preparation of antibody against the D antigen of the Rh blood group, has been used with limited success to treat individuals who are Rh-positive.

If all other therapies are ineffective, splenectomy is considered to remove the primary site of platelet destruction.[37] The response rate (resolution of the thrombocytopenia) is 60% to 70%; however, the procedure is not without risk. Approximately 10% to 20% of individuals who undergo splenectomy suffer a relapse and require further treatment. It is thought that other reticuloendothelial organs, particularly the liver, can become major sites for platelet destruction. If splenectomy is unsuccessful and life-threatening thrombocytopenia persists, more aggressive immunosuppressive medications (e.g., azathioprine, cyclophosphamide) may be used. Because of potential major complications, these medications are reserved for individuals who are severely thrombocytopenic and refractory to other therapies.

Thrombotic Thrombocytopenic Purpura
Thrombotic thrombocytopenic purpura (TTP) is characterized by thrombotic microangiopathy in which platelets aggregate and cause occlusion of arterioles and capillaries within the microcirculation.[38] Aggregation may lead to increased platelet consumption and organ ischemia. TTP is relatively uncommon, occurring in about 5 per 1 million individuals per year. The incidence is increasing, which appears to be an actual increase in the number of affected individuals rather than a result of improved recognition. There are two forms of TTP: familial or acquired idiopathic. The familial form is the more rare and is usually chronic, relapsing, and seen in children. The child experiences predictable recurring episodes at approximately 3-week intervals and are responsive to treatment. Acquired TTP is more common, as well as more acute and severe. It occurs mostly in females in their 30s and is rarely observed in infants or older adults.

Platelet aggregation and microthrombi formation are found throughout the entire vascular system, causing damage to multiple organs. Organs most susceptible to damage are the kidney, brain, and heart. Other organs often affected are the pancreas, spleen, and adrenal glands. The thrombi are primarily composed of platelets with minimal fibrin and red cells, differentiating them from thrombi secondary to intravascular coagulation. Most cases of TTP are related to a dysfunction of the plasma metalloprotease ADAMTS13. This enzyme is responsible for digesting large precursor molecules of von Willebrand factor (vWF) produced by endothelial cells into smaller molecules. Defects in ADAMTS13 result in expression of large-molecular-weight vWF on the endothelial cell surface and the formation of large aggregates of platelets. The aggregates may break off and form occlusions in smaller vessels. Most individuals with TTP (about 80%) have less than 5% of normal plasma ADAMTS13 levels. TTP also is commonly associated with an IgG autoantibody against ADAMTS13 that is able to neutralize the enzyme's activity and accelerate its clearance from the plasma.

CLINICAL MANIFESTATIONS The rare familial **chronic relapsing TTP** observed in children is usually recognized and successfully treated. The acquired **acute idiopathic TTP** is much more common and more severe.[38] Early diagnosis and treatment is important because the disease may be fatal within 90 days of onset. TTP is clinically related to and must be distinguished from other thrombotic microangiopathic conditions, including hemolytic uremic syndrome, malignant hypertension, preeclampsia, or the pregnancy-induced HELLP (hemolysis, elevated liver enzymes, low platelet count) syndrome. Hemolytic uremic syndrome (HUS) shares many of the clinical characteristics of TTP; however, HUS often follows a hemorrhagic, diarrheal illness.

EVALUATION AND TREATMENT Acute idiopathic TTP is characterized by a "pathognomonic pentad" of symptoms. These include extreme thrombocytopenia (less than 20,000 platelets/mm³), intravascular hemolytic anemia, ischemic signs and symptoms most often involving the CNS (about 65% present with memory disturbances, behavioral irregularities, headaches, or coma), kidney failure (affecting about 65% of individuals), and fever (present in about 33%).[38] It is not mandatory that all five be present to begin treatment. A routine blood smear usually reveals fragmented red cells *(schizocytes)* produced by shear forces when red cells are in contact with the fibrin mesh in clots that form in the vessels. As a result of tissue injury, serum levels of lactate dehydrogenase (LDH) may be very high, and low-density lipoprotein (LDL) levels may be elevated. Tests for antibody on red cells are negative, excluding immune hemolytic anemia.

Untreated acute TTP has a mortality rate of 90%, which can be reduced to 12% to 20% with prompt treatment. Plasma exchange with fresh frozen plasma replenishes functional ADAMTS13 and is the treatment of choice achieving a response rate of 70% to 85%. Additionally, steroids (glucocorticoids) are administered. In the absence of major organ damage, this approach may lead to complete recovery with no long-term complications. Relapses do occur at a rate of 13% to 36%, and recurrences have been reported, some as far out as 9 years. Individuals who do not respond to conventional treatment may be candidates for splenectomy; however, postoperative hemorrhage remains a dangerous complication. Immunosuppressive (azathioprine) therapy has been successful in some individuals.

Thrombocythemia

Thrombocythemia (also called **thrombocytosis**) is defined as a platelet count greater than 400,000/mm³ of blood.[39] Thrombocythemia may be primary or secondary (reactive) and is usually asymptomatic until the count exceeds 1 million/mm³ of blood. Then intravascular clot formation (thrombosis), hemorrhage, or other abnormalities can occur.

PATHOPHYSIOLOGY Secondary thrombocythemia may occur after splenectomy because platelets that normally would be stored in the spleen remain in circulating blood. The increase in platelets may be gradual, with thrombocythemia not occurring for up to 3 weeks after splenectomy. Reactive thrombocythemia may occur during some inflammatory conditions, such as rheumatoid arthritis and cancers. In these conditions, excessive production of some cytokines (e.g., IL-6, IL-11) may induce increased production of thrombopoietin in the liver, resulting in increased megakaryocyte proliferation. Reactive thrombocythemia may also occur during a variety of physiologic conditions, such as after exercise. Because of the relatively self-resolving nature of secondary thrombocythemia, the remaining discussion will focus on the more severe primary form.

Essential (primary) thrombocythemia (ET) is a chronic myeloproliferative disorder characterized by excessive platelet production resulting from a defect in bone marrow megakaryocyte progenitor cells.[40] The overall incidence of ET is 0.8 per 100,000 in the United Kingdom, 2.53 in the United States, and 0.59 in Denmark. It is more common in middle-age individuals, with the majority of cases occurring between ages 50 and 60 years. There is no known gender preference. There also is a rare hereditary type of ET called *familial essential thrombocythemia (FET)* that is inherited in an autosomal dominant pattern.

The thrombocythemia is secondary to increased plasma thrombopoietin levels resulting from defects in the thrombopoietin receptor. The defective receptor cannot adequately bind and remove thrombopoietin from the blood, thus circulating levels remain high. Along with increased platelet levels, there may be a concomitant increase in red cells, indicating a myeloproliferative disorder; however, the increase in red cells is not to the extent seen in polycythemia vera (see Chapter 26). The bone marrow of affected individuals with ET is characterized by hyperplasia of megakaryocytes. The platelets of affected individuals appear to have a normal survival time, compatible with a defect in production rather than an increase in platelet life span.

RBCs in ET tend to aggregate and contribute to the blockage of flow in the microvasculature and altered interactions between platelets and the vascular endothelium.[41] Increased adherence of erythrocytes to the endothelium appears to result from a mutation in an erythrocyte Janus kinase 2 (JAK2) that is responsible for phosphorylation of the erythrocyte receptor for endothelial laminin.[42,43] The frequency of JAK2 mutations in ET is about 30%. Increased platelet aggregation arises from several mutations that result in altered platelet membrane glycoproteins, particularly resulting in increased expression of GPIV, and increased secretion of thromboxane.

CLINICAL MANIFESTATIONS Clinical manifestations vary significantly among individuals. Those with ET are at risk for large-vessel arterial or venous thrombosis, although the most common complication is **microvasculature thrombosis** leading to ischemia in the fingers, toes, or cerebrovascular regions.[41] The primary presenting symptoms of microvasculature thrombosis are erythromyalgia, headache, and paresthesias. **Erythromyalgia** is characterized by unilateral or bilateral warm, congested, red hands and feet with painful burning sensations, particularly in the forefoot sole and one or more toes. The lower extremities are affected more often, and only one side may be involved. The pain is initiated by standing, exercise, or warmth and relieved by elevation and cooling. In extreme situations, acrocyanosis and gangrene may result.

Arterial thrombosis is more common than venous thrombosis and may involve the coronary and renal arteries. The carotid, mesenteric, and subclavian arteries also may be affected. Myocardial ischemia and infarction have occurred without clear evidence of coronary artery disease. Deep venous thrombosis of the lower extremities and pulmonary embolism are the major sites for venous involvement. Intraabdominal venous thrombosis (portal and hepatic) also are common sites of venous thrombosis.

Microvascular thrombosis in the CNS is usually associated with headache and dizziness, with paresthesias, transient ischemic attacks, strokes, visual disturbances, and seizures also being reported. Major thrombotic events, not directly related to the platelet count, occur in about 20% to 30% of individuals with ET. Prior history of thrombotic events, advanced age, and duration of thrombocytosis are predictors of future thrombotic complications. Individuals older than age 60 are at greatest risk.

Although thrombosis is the most common symptom, hemorrhage can also occur. Sites for bleeding include the GI tract, skin, mucous membranes, urinary tract, gums, tooth sockets (after extraction), joints, eyes, and brain. GI bleeding may be mistaken for a duodenal ulcer. Hemorrhage is not severe, and generally occurs in the presence of very high platelet counts, and occasionally requires transfusion. Important is recognition that bleeding and clotting may exist simultaneously and individuals will not necessarily be "bleeders" or "clotters."

EVALUATION AND TREATMENT Initial diagnosis is not difficult; as many as two thirds of affected individuals are diagnosed from a routine CBC. Secondary thrombocytosis may present as a moderate rise in the platelet count that resolves with treatment or resolution of the underlying condition. ET is diagnosed by a platelet count greater than 600,000/mm^3 and remains elevated, with no other indicated cause, such as arthritis, iron deficiency anemia, cancer, or splenectomy. Many individuals present with a mild anemia and a slightly elevated white blood cell count.

After diagnosis, these individuals may recall events related to thrombosis or hemorrhage. Manifestations of ET may be mistaken for CML; therefore, differentiation of the two is important because treatment varies significantly. Identification of the Philadelphia chromosome is recommended in all cases of ET.

Treatment of ET is directed toward preventing thrombosis or hemorrhage.[44] Whether to reduce platelet count remains a significant treatment issue. Historically treatment of ET relied on the use of alkylating agents (busulfan) or radiophosphorus (^{32}P) to suppress platelet production. Hydroxyurea, a nonalkylating myelosuppressive agent, has been the drug of choice to suppress platelet production: however, long-term use may cause progression to other myelodysplastic disorders, particularly AML or myelofibrosis.[44] Conversion to myelofibrosis occurs approximately 8% of the time and conversion to AML occurs approximately 3.5% of the time when treated with Vhydroxyurea as a single cytotoxic agent, but increases to 14% when more than one cytotoxic agent is used.

Interferon (IFN) also may be used and has a response rate of 80%. IFN may not work for everyone because it has many side effects and 20% of individuals may be intolerant. Anagrelide is now considered to be the drug of choice. Anagrelide specifically interferes with platelet maturation rather than production, thus not affecting erythropoiesis or leukopoiesis.

Aspirin also is used in the treatment of ET; however, its action is not to reduce the platelet count but to prevent adherence of platelets to each other and prevent thrombus formation. Early studies with aspirin found hemorrhage to be a major contraindication for its use; however, in lower doses (80 to 160 mg/daily) it effectively alleviates erythromyalgia and transient neurologic manifestations.

Prognosis and survival of individuals with ET have been somewhat difficult to establish. ET is not necessarily considered life threatening, but in those older than age 60 and who have had previous incidences of thrombosis, complications are more common and have a higher risk of mortality.

Alterations of Platelet Function

Qualitative alterations in platelet function occur with an increased bleeding time in the presence of a normal platelet count. Associated clinical manifestations include spontaneous petechiae and purpura, bleeding from the GI tract, genitourinary tract, pulmonary mucosa, and gums. Congenital alterations in platelet function (thrombocytopathies) are quite rare and may be categorized into several types of disorders: (1) platelet-vessel wall adhesion, (2) platelet-platelet interactions, (3) platelet granules and secretion, (4) arachidonic acid pathways, and (5) membrane phospholipid regulation (coagulation protein-platelet interactions).[45]

Disorders of platelet-vascular wall adhesion result from aberrations of the platelet membrane glycoprotein GPIb-IX-V (Bernard-Soulier syndrome), the collagen receptor (GPVI) or deficiencies of vWF. The GPIb protein is the most commonly mutated in individuals with Bernard-Soulier syndrome. Lack of these proteins prevents platelets from adhering to collagen, resulting in impaired hemostasis and clinical hemorrhage.

Disorders of platelet-platelet interactions result in failure of platelets to aggregate in response to adenosine diphosphate

(ADP), collagen, epinephrine, or thrombin because of a deficiency in the glycoprotein (αIIbβ3) that acts as a receptor for fibrinogen, vWF, and fibronectin (Glanzmann thrombasthenia). Lack of this protein results in a failure to build "fibrinogen bridges" between platelets (see Figure 25-20). Defects also can occur in platelet receptors for platelet activators. These include mutations in the receptors for thromboxane or ADP.

Disorders of platelet granules and secretion and arachidonic pathways are characterized by initial normal platelet aggregation with collagen or ADP; however, there is failure of subsequent processes, specifically secretion of prostaglandins and release of granules. Defective α-granule numbers or release (gray platelet syndrome) results from mutations in several aspects of granule function, including biosynthesis or loading of proteins normally found in these granules. Defects in dense granules include Hermansky-Pudlak syndrome, Chédiak-Higashi syndrome, and delta-storage pool disease. These usually result from mutations in proteins involved in formation of dense granules or their movement to the plasma membrane. Defects in the thromboxane pathway prevent the release of this mediator.

Externalization of plasma membrane phosphatidylserine (PS) is necessary for effective platelet function. In Scott syndrome, the enzyme responsible for PS efflux is defective, thus platelets are unable to support the activation of factor X and prothrombin. The inreverse of Scott syndrome is Stormorken syndrome, in which platelets constitutively externalize PS.

Acquired disorders of platelet function are more common than the congenital disorders and may be categorized into three principal causes: (1) drug effects, (2) systemic inflammatory conditions, and (3) hematologic conditions.

Multiple drugs are known to affect platelet function in several ways: inhibition of platelet membrane receptors, inhibition of prostaglandin pathways, and inhibition of phosphodiesterase activity. Aspirin is the most commonly used drug that affects platelets and the only drug specifically used for its platelet effects. It irreversibly inhibits cyclooxygenase function for several days after administration. Nonsteroidal anti-inflammatory drugs also affect cyclooxygenase, although in a reversible fashion.

Systemic disorders that affect platelet function are chronic renal disease, liver disease, cardiopulmonary bypass surgery, severe deficiencies of iron or folate, and antiplatelet antibodies associated with autoimmune disorders. Hematologic disorders that cause platelet dysfunction are chronic myeloproliferative disorders, multiple myeloma, leukemias, myelodysplastic syndromes, and dysproteinemias.

Disorders of Coagulation

Disorders of coagulation usually are caused by defects or deficiencies of one or more of the clotting factors. (Normal function of the clotting factors is described in Chapter 25.) Qualitative or quantitative abnormalities of clotting factors interfere with or prevent the enzymatic reactions that transform circulating clotting proteins into a stable fibrin clot (see Figure 25-22).

Some clotting factor defects are inherited and usually involve a single factor, such as hemophilias and von Willebrand disease, caused by deficiencies of specific clotting factors (see Chapter 28). Other coagulation defects are acquired and tend to result from deficient synthesis of clotting factors by the liver. Causes include liver disease and dietary deficiency of vitamin K.

Other coagulation disorders are attributed to pathologic conditions that trigger coagulation inappropriately. For example, any cardiovascular abnormality that alters normal blood flow by speeding it up, slowing it down, or obstructing it can result in spontaneous coagulation within the vessels. Coagulation is also stimulated by the presence of tissue factor, which is released by damaged or dead tissues. **Vasculitis**, or inflammation of the blood vessels, as well as vessel damage, activates platelets, which in turn activates the coagulation cascade. In extensive or prolonged vasculitis, blood clot formation can suppress mechanisms that normally control clot formation and breakdown, leading to clogging of the vessels. In each of these acquired conditions, normal hemostatic function proves detrimental to the body by consuming coagulation factors excessively or by overwhelming the normal control of clot formation and breakdown (fibrinolysis).

Impaired Hemostasis

Impaired hemostasis, or the inability to promote coagulation and the development of a stable fibrin clot, is commonly associated with liver disorders, either resulting from the lack of vitamin K or specific diseases of the liver.

Vitamin K Deficiency

Vitamin K, a fat-soluble vitamin, is necessary for synthesis and regulation of prothrombin, procoagulant factors (VII, IX, X), and anticoagulant regulators (proteins C and S) within the liver.[46] Vitamin K is found in green leafy vegetables and is the primary dietary source. Vitamin K also is synthesized by intestinal flora, but its contribution to the overall supply of vitamin K is uncertain. The most common cause of vitamin K deficiency is parenteral nutrition in combination with broad-spectrum antibiotics that destroy normal gut flora. Rarely is a deficiency caused by lack of dietary intake; however, bulimia can suppress vitamin K–dependent activity. Clinical manifestations of vitamin K deficiency are caused by a reduction of vitamin K–dependent proteins. The severity of manifestations is related to the degree of deficiency and ranges from laboratory abnormalities to significant hemorrhage.

Parenteral administration of vitamin K is the treatment of choice and usually results in correction of the deficiency. Improvement of clotting tests is usually noted within 8 to 12 hours. Fresh frozen plasma may be administered but usually is reserved for individuals with life-threatening hemorrhages or who require emergency surgery.

Liver Disease

Individuals who have liver disease (e.g., acute or chronic hepatocellular diseases, cirrhosis, vitamin K deficiency) or major liver surgery present with a broad range of hemostasis derangements that may be characterized by defects in the clotting or fibrinolytic systems or platelet function.[46] The hepatic parenchymal cells produce most of the factors involved in hemostasis. Thus damage to the liver frequently results in diminished production of factors involved in clotting, usually in proportion to the degree of hepatic parenchymal cell damage. For instance, factor VII is most sensitive to liver damage because of its rapid turnover. Factor IX levels are less affected and do not decline until liver destruction is well advanced. The liver is also a major site for production of plasminogen and α_2-antiplasmin of the fibrinolytic system, as well as thrombopoietin and the metalloprotease ADAMTS13. Diminished thrombopoietin may lead to thrombocytopenia from decreased platelet production. Decreased production of ADAMTS13 results in increased levels of large precursor molecules of vWF, which leads to the formation of large aggregates of platelets.

In conditions of severe liver disease (e.g., cirrhosis) circulating levels of most clotting factors are significantly depressed. Concurrently production of clotting system regulators (e.g., antithrombin, protein C, protein S) and of fibrinogen is diminished. The fibrinolytic system is commonly active due to decreased levels of plasmin inhibitor and unaffected levels of fibrinolytic activators (e.g., tPA, uPA). The affected individuals also are thrombocytopenic because of diminished thrombopoietin and ADAMTS13, as well as increased platelet sequestration in the spleen, which is frequently enlarged in cirrhosis and is associated with portal hypertension. Thus the individuals with cirrhosis may appear to have a condition similar to DIC (see next section).

Treatment of hemostatic alterations in liver disease must be comprehensive to cover all aspects related to platelet, clotting, and fibrinolytic dysfunctions. Fresh frozen plasma administration is the treatment of choice, but not all individuals tolerate the volume needed to adequately replace all deficient factors. Alternative modalities include the addition of exchange transfusions and platelet concentration to plasma administration.

Consumptive Thrombohemorrhagic Disorders

Consumptive thrombohemorrhagic disorders are a heterogeneous group of conditions that demonstrate the entire range of hemorrhagic and thrombotic pathologic conditions. Symptoms range from subtle to devastating and generally are considered to be intermediary disease processes that complicate many primary disease states. These disorders also are characterized by confusion and controversy regarding diagnosis, treatment, and management. No one definition can cover all possible varieties of these disorders; however, disseminated intravascular coagulation is the most common term used in the clinical setting to describe a pathologic condition associated with hemorrhage and thrombosis.

Disseminated Intravascular Coagulation

Disseminated intravascular coagulation (DIC) is an acquired clinical syndrome characterized by widespread activation of coagulation resulting in formation of fibrin clots in medium and small vessels throughout the body. Disseminated

clotting may lead to blockage of blood flow to organs, resulting in multiple organ failure. The magnitude of clotting may result in consumption of platelets and clotting factors leading to severe bleeding. The Subcommittee on DIC of the International Society on Thrombosis and Hemostasis defined DIC as, "An acquired syndrome characterized by the intravascular activation of coagulation with loss of localization arising from different causes. It can originate from and cause damage to the microvasculature, which if sufficiently severe, can produce organ dysfunction."[47,48]

The clinical course of DIC largely is determined by the intensity of the stimulus, host response, and comorbidities and ranges from an acute, severe, life-threatening process that is characterized by massive hemorrhage and thrombosis to a chronic low-grade condition. The chronic condition is characterized by subacute hemorrhage and diffuse microcirculatory thrombosis. DIC may be localized to one specific organ or generalized, involving multiple organs.

Because of the complexity and wide variations in manifestations of DIC, diagnosis has been confusing and difficult. Minimally acceptable diagnostic criteria have been established and include a systemic thrombohemorrhagic disorder with laboratory evidence of (1) clotting activation, (2) fibrinolytic activation, (3) coagulation inhibitor consumption, and (4) biochemical evidence of end-organ damage or failure.

DIC is secondary to a wide variety of well-defined clinical conditions, specifically those capable of activating the clotting cascade (Box 27-6). These include (1) arterial hypotension, frequently accompanying shock; (2) hypoxemia; (3) acidemia; and (4) stasis of capillary blood flow.

Sepsis is the most common condition associated with DIC. Gram-negative microorganisms, as well as some gram-positive microorganisms, fungi, protozoa (malaria), and viruses (influenza, herpes) are capable of precipitating DIC by causing

---

Box 27-6   Major Etiologies Identified as Antecedents to the Initiation and Development of Disseminated Intravascular Coagulation (DIC)

- Malignancy: acute leukemias, metastatic solid malignancies
- Infections: bacterial (gram-negative endotoxin, gram-positive mucopolysaccharides), viral (hepatitis, varicella, cytomegalovirus), fungal, parasitic
- Pregnancy complications: eclampsia/preeclampsia, placental abruption, amniotic fluid embolism
- Severe trauma: head injury, burns, crush injuries, tissue necrosis
- Liver disease: obstructive jaundice, acute liver failure
- Intravascular hemolysis: transfusion reactions, drug-induced hemolysis
- Medical devices: aortic balloon, prosthetic devices
- Hypoxia and low blood flow states: arterial hypotension secondary to shock, cardiopulmonary arrest

Data from Bick, RL et al: *Hematology: clinical and laboratory practice*, St Louis, 1993, Mosby.

damage to vascular endothelium. Gram-negative endotoxins are the primary cause of endothelial damage; DIC may occur in up to 50% of individuals with gram-negative sepsis. DIC occurs in approximately 10% to 20% of individuals with metastatic cancer or acute leukemia. Direct tissue damage (ischemia and necrosis, surgical manipulation, crushing injury) also result in release of tissue factor (TF) by the endothelium. Severe trauma, especially to the brain, can induce DIC. DIC occurs in about two thirds of individuals with a systemic inflammatory response to trauma. Some complications of pregnancy also are associated with DIC; incidences range from 50% for women with placental abruptions to less than 10% for severe preeclampsia. Other causes of DIC have been identified, most notably blood transfusion. Transfused blood dilutes the clotting factors, as well as circulating naturally occurring antithrombins. In hemolytic transfusion reactions, the endothelium is damaged by complement-mediated reactions.

PATHOPHYSIOLOGY The coagulation system is designed to function at local areas of vascular damage, resulting in cessation of bleeding and activation of repair to the vessels. DIC results from abnormally widespread and ongoing activation of clotting (Figure 27-20). A variety of conditions are associated with DIC (see Box 27-6), primarily by activating the extrinsic clotting cascade. The common pathway for DIC appears to be excessive and widespread exposure of TF. This may occur by several mechanisms. Widespread damage to vascular endothelium results in exposure of subendothelial TF. Several types of cells, either after stimulation by cytokines or constitutively, express TF on their surfaces. Endothelial cells and monocytes do not normally express surface TF unless stimulated by inflammatory cytokines (particularly IL-6 and TNF-α).[49] Many tumors express surface TF or produce cytokines that stimulate TF expression by endothelium or monocytes or both.[50] These cytokines are abundantly produced during many of the conditions listed in Box 27-6. Endotoxin, in particular, triggers the release of multiple cytokines that play a significant role in the development and maintenance of DIC. Proinflammatory cytokines (TNF-α, interleukins [IL-1, IL-6, IL-8], and platelet activating factor [PAF]) are responsible for the clinical signs and symptoms associated with sepsis. They also contribute to the development of DIC by activating endothelial cells, causing release of TF and vWF, increasing plasminogen activator inhibitor-1 (PAI-1) synthesis and tissue factor activity, and decreasing thrombomodulin expression, thereby promoting development of thrombi. TF also may be released directly into the bloodstream from circulating white blood cells (monocyte/endotoxin interaction).

TF binds clotting factor VII, which leads to conversion of prothrombin to thrombin and formation of fibrin clots (see Figure 25-22). This pathway appears to be the primary route by which DIC is initiated; inhibition of TF or factor VIIa completely prevents the generation of thrombi by gram-negative bacterial endotoxin in animal models of DIC.

Not only is the clotting system extensively activated in DIC, but the predominant natural anticoagulants (tissue factor inhibitor, antithrombin III [AT III], protein C) are also greatly diminished (see Figure 25-17). During DIC the activation of clotting is prolonged by the increased rate of consumption because of persistent thrombin production, as well as decreased synthesis, of these inhibitors and protein S and by cytokine-mediated decreased expression of thrombomodulin on the endothelial cell surface. Hepatic dysfunction in sepsis results in decreased antithrombin synthesis and extravascular leakage of this protease inhibitor because of capillary leakage. Additionally, antithrombin is degraded by elastase released by activated neutrophils, and clotting is initiated concurrently with loss of regulation of the extent of thrombosis, thus the amount of thrombin produced during DIC exceeds the ability of the body's naturally occurring anticoagulants to regulate it.

The rate of fibrinolysis is also diminished in DIC. The primary component of the fibrinolysis is plasmin, which exists in the circulation as an inactive precursor, plasminogen (see Figure 25-25). Plasminogen is activated to plasmin that digests fibrin clots, thus controlling the extent of fibrin deposition in the vessels. During DIC the activity of plasmin is diminished by increased production of its natural inhibitor, PAI-1. Although some fibrinolytic activity remains, the level is inadequate to control the systemic deposition of fibrin. The slow breakdown of fibrin by plasmin produces FDPs that are released into the blood. These are potent anticoagulants that are normally removed from blood by fibronectin and macrophages. FDPs, along with thrombin, induce further cytokine release from monocytes, contributing to endothelial damage and TF release. During DIC the presence of fibrin degradation products is prolonged, probably because of diminished production of fibronectin. Fibronectin is a glycoprotein with adhesive properties that mediate removal of particulate matter (e.g., fibrin clumps). Low levels of fibronectin suggest a poor prognosis.

Although thrombosis is generalized and widespread, individuals with DIC are paradoxically at risk for hemorrhage. Hemorrhage is secondary to the abnormally high consumption of clotting factors and platelets, as well as the anticoagulant properties of FDPs, which interfere with polymerization of fibrin monomers. Both thrombin and FDPs have a high affinity for platelets and cause platelet activation and aggregation—an event that occurs early in the development of DIC—which facilitates microcirculatory coagulation and obstruction in the initial phase. However, platelet consumption exceeds production, resulting in a thrombocytopenia that increases bleeding. (Box 27-7).

Activation of clotting also leads to activation of other inflammatory pathways, including the kallikrein-kinin and complement systems (see Chapter 6). Factor XIIa, generated in DIC, converts prekallikrein to kallikrein, ultimately resulting in conversion to circulating kinins. Activation of these systems contributes to increased vascular permeability, hypotension, and shock. Activated complement components also induce platelet destruction, further contributing initially to the thrombosis and later to the thrombocytopenia.

The deposition of fibrin clots in the circulation interferes with blood flow, causing widespread organ hypoperfusion.

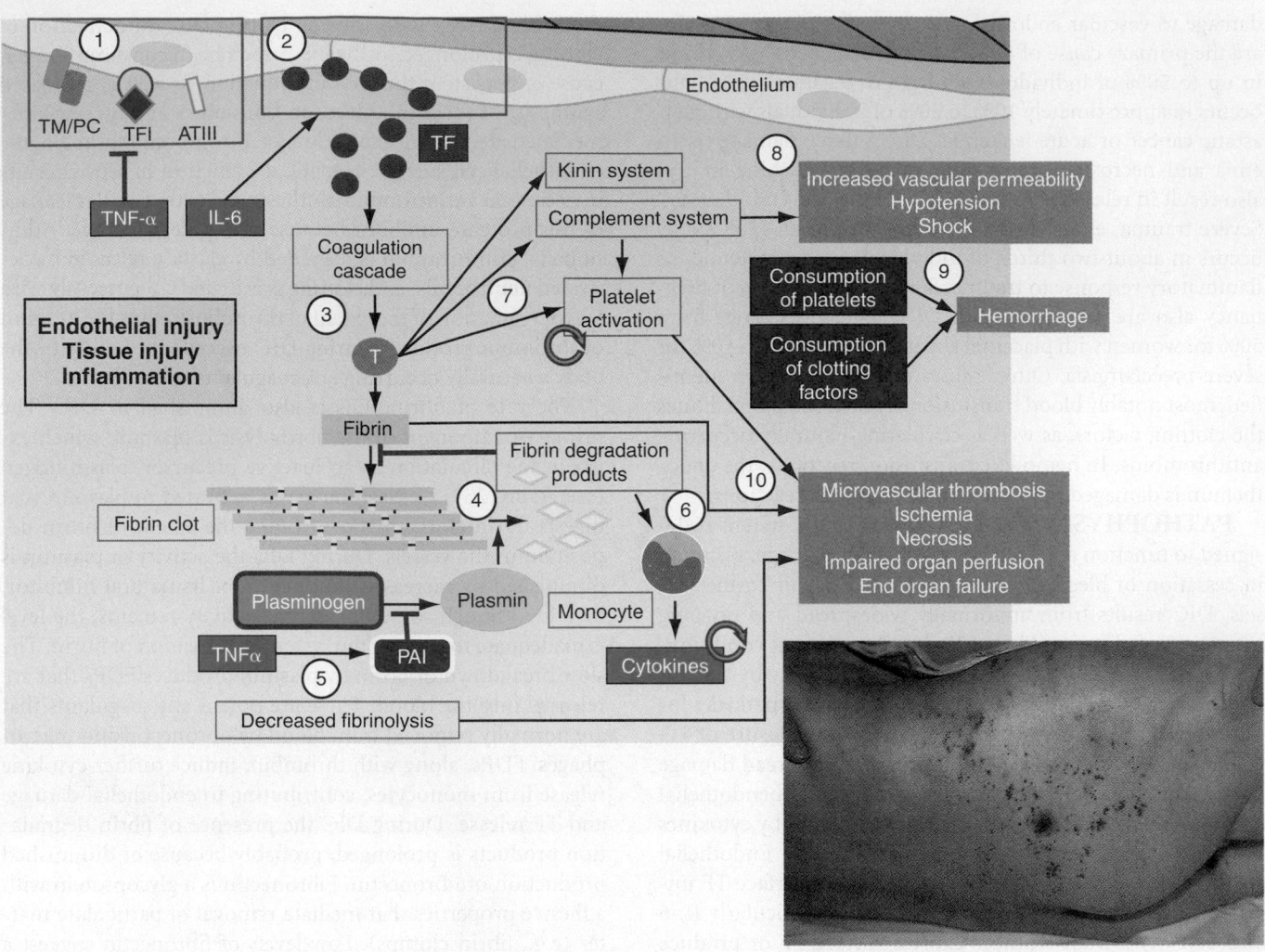

Figure 27-20 Pathophysiology of disseminated intravascular coagulation (DIC). DIC is initiated by a variety of factors (endothelial injury, tissue injury, inflammation, and others), most of which either directly or indirectly result in release of large amounts of tissue factor. Many cytokines create a procoagulant environment by concurrently (1) suppressing normal control of homeostasis and (2) inducing tissue factor release by endothelium or monocytes. Tissue factor initiates the coagulation cascade (3) leading to the activation of thrombin, production of fibrin, and polymerization into a fibrin clot. Fibrinolysis normally digests clots (4) through the activity of plasmin, resulting in the production of various fibrin degradation products. However, during DIC, factors, such as TNF-α, induce (5) inhibitors of plasmin generation, thus leading to diminished fibrinolysis. Fibrin split products possess several biological activities that affect DIC, including (6) the induction of further cytokine release by monocytes. Enzymatically active products of the coagulation cascade, including thrombin, activate (7) other inflammatory systems, including platelets and the kinin and complement systems. Activation of platelets and monocytes continue the procoagulant cycle (indicated by circular arrows) by inducing additional tissue factor and cytokines. Mediators produced from the kinin and complement system (8) affect vascular endothelium leading to increased vascular permeability that contributes to hypotension and potential shock. The uncontrolled consumption of platelets and clotting factors (9) compromises the normal hemostatic mechanisms resulting in potential systemic hemorrhages. Excess activation of the coagulation cascade and platelets, with decreased fibrinolysis, leads to systemic microvascular thrombosis (10) and blockage of the vessels with progressive ischemia. Uncontrolled DIC will eventually lead to multiple end-organ failure. For further details of these mechanisms see Chapters 6 and 25. *AT III,* Antithrombin III; *IL-6,* interleukin-6; *PAI,* plasminogen activator inhibitor; *T,* thrombin; *TF,* tissue factor; *TFI,* tissue factor inhibitor; *TM/PC,* thrombomodulin/protein C complex; *TNF-α,* tumor necrosis factor-alpha. Insert is an example of DIC resulting from staphylococcal septicemia. Note the characteristic skin hemorrhage ranging from small purpuric lesions to larger ecchymoses.

This condition may lead to ischemia, infarction, and necrosis, further potentiating and complicating the existing DIC process by causing further release of TF and eventually organ failure.

In addition to initiation of clotting by TF, DIC may be precipitated by direct proteolytic activation of factor X. This has been described as "thrombin mimicry" and is the result of activated factor X directly converting fibrinogen to fibrin. The proteases that activate factor X may come from snake venom, some tumor cells, or the pancreas and liver, where they are released during episodes of pancreatitis and various stages of liver disease. Direct proteolytic activity appears to be independent of any type of damage to the endothelium or tissue.

Box 27-7	Clinical Manifestation Associated with Disseminated Intravascular Coagulation (DIC)

Integumentary System
Widespread hemorrhage and vascular lesions
Oozing from puncture sites, incisions, mucous membranes
Acrocyanosis (irregularly-shaped cyanotic patches)
Gangrene

Central Nervous System
Subarachnoid hemorrhage
Altered state of consciousness (slight confusion to convulsions and coma)

Gastrointestinal System
Occult bleeding to massive gastrointestinal bleeding
Abdominal distention
Malaise
Weakness

Pulmonary System
Pulmonary infarctions
ARDS
Cyanosis
Tachypnea
Hypoxemia

Renal System
Hematuria
Oliguria
Renal failure

Modified from Bailes BK: Disseminated intravascular coagulation. Principles, treatment, nursing management, *AORN J* 55(2):517-529, 1992.
ARDS, Acute respiratory distress syndrome.

Vascular obstruction results from circulatory deposition of thrombin and clot formation that impedes blood flow, causing widespread organ hypoperfusion that can lead to tissue ischemia, infarction, and necrosis. The resulting tissue damage further potentiates and complicates the existing DIC process. Because organ perfusion is drastically impaired, manifestations of multisystem organ dysfunction and failure ultimately result. Multisystem organ dysfunction and failure are discussed in Chapter 46. Whatever initiates the process of DIC, the cycle of thrombosis and hemorrhage persists until the underlying cause of the DIC is removed or appropriate therapeutic interventions are used.

CLINICAL MANIFESTATIONS Clinical signs and symptoms of DIC present a wide spectrum of possibilities, depending on the underlying disease process that initiates DIC and whether the DIC is acute or chronic (see Box 27-7). Most symptoms are the result of either hemorrhage or thrombosis. Acute DIC presents with rapid development of hemorrhaging, such as oozing from venipuncture sites, arterial lines, and surgical wounds, or development of ecchymotic lesions (purpura, petechiae) and hematomas. Other sites of bleeding include the eyes (sclera and conjunctiva), the nose (epistaxis), and the gums. Most individuals with DIC demonstrate bleeding at three or more unrelated sites, and any combination may be observed. Shock of variable intensity, out of proportion to

the amount of apparent blood loss, also may be observed. Hemorrhaging into closed compartments of the body also can occur and may precede the development of shock.

DIC has been conceptualized as a systemic hemorrhagic disorder because bleeding, sometimes very extensive, is usually the initial observation. Symptoms of thrombosis are not always as evident, even though it is often the first pathologic alteration to occur and ultimately determines the degree of morbidity and risk for death. A large amount of microvascular and macrovascular occlusion may occur that is not clinically obvious. Several organ systems are susceptible to microvascular thrombosis that affects their function; these include the cardiovascular, pulmonary, central nervous, renal, and hepatic systems. Quick and accurate clinical diagnosis is critical to preventing further progression of DIC that may lead to multisystem organ dysfunction or failure. Indicators of multisystem failure include changes in level of consciousness, behavior, and mentation; confusion; seizure activity; oliguria; hematuria; hypoxia; hypotension; hemoptysis; chest pain; and tachycardia. Symmetric cyanosis of the fingers and toes ("blue finger/toe syndrome") and, in some instances, of the nose and breasts may be present. Symmetric parts are often affected and are indicative of microvascular thrombosis. This may progress to infarction and gangrene, requiring amputation. Jaundice also may be present and is believed to result from red blood cell destruction rather than hepatic dysfunction.

Individuals with chronic or low-grade DIC do not present with overt manifestations of hemorrhaging and thrombosis but instead have subacute bleeding and diffuse thrombosis and are described as having a **compensated DIC,** or non-overt DIC. The major characteristic of this state is an increased turnover and decreased survival time of the components of hemostasis: platelets and clotting factors. On occasion diffuse or localized thrombosis develops, but this is infrequent.

EVALUATION AND TREATMENT No single laboratory test can be used to effectively diagnosis DIC. Diagnosis is based primarily on clinical symptoms and confirmed by a combination of laboratory tests. The individual must present with a clinical condition that is known to be associated with DIC. The most commonly used combination of laboratory tests usually confirms thrombocytopenia or a rapidly decreasing platelet count on repeated testing, prolongation of clotting times, the presence of fibrin degradation products, and decreased levels of coagulation inhibitors. The relationships among these criteria are summarized in Box 27-8. Platelet counts less than $100,000/mm^3$ or a progressive decrease in platelet counts is very sensitive for DIC, although not greatly specific. These changes usually indicate consumption of platelets.

The standard coagulation tests (e.g., prothrombin time [PT], activated partial thromboplastin time [aPTT]) also have a high degree of sensitivity, but they are not highly specific for DIC. As a result of consumption of circulating clotting factors, these tests are usually abnormal, ranging from shortened to prolonged times. However, conditions other than DIC may prolong clotting times. Assays of specific clotting factors do not contribute meaningful diagnostic information.

Box 27-8	Laboratory Diagnostic Criteria for Disseminated Intravascular Coagulation (DIC)

Group I Tests (Indicators of Procoagulant Activation)
1. Elevated prothrombin fragment 1+2
2. Elevated fibrinopeptide A
3. Elevated fibrinopeptide B
4. Elevated thrombin-antithrombin (TAT) complex
5. Elevated D-dimer

Group II Tests (Indicators of Fibrinolytic Activity)
1. Elevated D-dimer
2. Elevated fibrin degradation products (FDPs)
3. Elevated plasmin
4. Elevated plasmin-antiplasmin (PAP) complex

Group III Tests (Indicators of Inhibitor Consumption)
1. Decreased antithrombin III
2. Decreased α_2-antiplasmin
3. Decreased heparin cofactor II
4. Decreased protein C or S
5. Elevated TAT complex
6. Elevated PAP complex

Group IV Tests (Indicators of End-Organ Damage/Failure)
1. Elevated lactic dehydrogenase (LDH)
2. Elevated creatinine
3. Decreased pH
4. Decreased Pao_2

Satisfactory criteria for laboratory diagnosis of DIC requires one abnormality in each of groups I through III and at least two abnormalities in group IV.

Data from Bick RL: *Semin Thromb Hemost* 24(1):3, 1998.

Detection of various fibrin degradation products is more specific for DIC; of these tests the detection of D-dimers is the most widely used, reliable and specific test.[51] A D-**dimer** is a molecule produced by plasmin degradation of crosslinked fibrin in clots. D-dimers in the blood can be quantified using enzyme-linked immunosorbent assay (ELISA) tests that include commercially available and highly specific monoclonal antibody against the D-dimer. Agglutination tests for other fibrin degradation products are available. Fibrin degradation products, in general, are elevated in the plasma in 95% to 100% of cases; however, they are less specific and only document the presence of plasmin and its action of fibrin, whereas detection of D-dimers measures a specific DIC-related product.

ELISAs for markers of thrombin activity are sometimes used. Normal conversion of prothrombin to thrombin produces an inactive prothrombin fragment 1.2 (PF1+2).[51] This fragment is released from the prothrombin molecule generating an intermediate factor, prethrombin 2. Once generated, prethrombin 2 can be split to produce thrombin that can then proteolyze fibrinogen, liberating fibrinopeptide A (FPA) or combine with its major antagonist, antithrombin, and form a stable inactive enzyme inhibitor complex, the thrombin-antithrombin (TAT) complex. Assays of these factors (PF1+2, FPA, TAT) are now generally available to quantify their blood levels, providing evidence of excessive factor Xa (PF1+2) and thrombin (FPA) generation.

Levels of coagulation inhibitors (e.g., AT III, protein C) can be measured by assays that rely on function or by ELISAs that quantify the amount of the specific inhibitor. AT III levels can provide key information for diagnosing and monitoring therapy of DIC. Initial levels of functional AT III are low in DIC because thrombin is irreversibly complexed with activated clotting factors and AT III.

Treatment of DIC is directed toward (1) eliminating the underlying pathology, (2) controlling ongoing thrombosis, and (3) maintaining organ function. Elimination of the underlying pathology is the initial intervention in the treatment phase in order to eliminate the trigger for activation of clotting. Once the stimulus is gone, production of coagulation factors in the liver leads to restoration of normal plasma levels within 24 to 48 hours.

Control of thrombosis is more difficult to attain. Heparin has been used for this; however, its use is controversial because its mechanism of action is binding to and activating AT III, which is deficient in many types of DIC. Currently heparin is indicated only in certain situations related to DIC. For instance, heparin seems to be effective in DIC caused by a retained dead fetus or associated with acute promyelocytic leukemia. Organ function is compromised by microthrombi, and there is a risk of losing an extremity because of vascular occlusion, thus heparin is also indicated in these conditions. Heparin's usefulness, however, for DIC that is precipitated by septic shock has not been established and so is contraindicated in that instance; heparin is also contraindicated when there is evidence of postoperative bleeding, peptic ulcer, or CNS bleeding.

Replacement therapy (interventions based on restoring the balance of coagulation factors, deficient coagulation factors, platelets, and other coagulation elements) is gaining recognition as an effective treatment modality. Components used in replacement therapy include platelets, fresh frozen plasma, and cryoprecipitate. Platelets are given for thrombocytopenia, plasma provides volume and replaces clotting factors, and cryoprecipitate replaces fibrinogen. Their use is not without controversy, however, because of the possible risk of adding components that will increase the rate of thrombosis. Clinical judgment is the key factor in determining whether replacement is to be used as a treatment modality.

Several clinical trials are evaluating replacement of anticoagulants (i.e., AT III, protein C). Replacement of AT III appears to be effective in DIC caused by sepsis. Low levels of AT III correlate with sepsis-initiated DIC, which makes a case for its use. AT III is an α_2-globulin that inactivates thrombin, factor Xa, factor IXa, and other activated components of the clotting system. Heparin augments AT III, but the increased benefit of a combination of heparin with AT III replacement has not been established. Antifibrinolytic drugs also are used in treatment but are limited to instances of life-threatening bleeding that have not been controlled by blood component replacement therapy.

Maintenance of organ function is achieved by fluid replacement to sustain adequate circulating blood volume and to maintain optimal tissue and organ perfusion. Fluids may be required to restore blood pressure, cardiac output, and urine output to normal parameters.

Thromboembolic Disease

Certain conditions within the blood vessels predispose an individual to develop clots spontaneously.[52] A stationary clot attached to the vessel wall is called a **thrombus** (Figure 27-21). A thrombus is composed of fibrin and blood cells and can develop in either the arterial or venous system. **Arterial thrombi** form under conditions of high blood flow and are composed mostly of platelet aggregates held together by fibrin strands. **Venous thrombi** form in conditions of low flow and are composed mostly of red cells with larger amounts of fibrin and few platelets.

A thrombus may eventually grow large enough to reduce or obstruct blood flow to tissues or organs, such as the heart, brain, or lungs, depriving them of essential nutrients critical to survival. A thrombus also has the potential of detaching from the vessel wall and circulating within the bloodstream (referred to as an **embolus**). The embolus may become lodged in smaller blood vessels, blocking blood flow into the local tissue or organ and leading to ischemia. Whether episodes of thromboembolism are life threatening depends on the site of vessel occlusion.

Therapy consists of removal or breakdown of the clot and supportive measures. Anticoagulant therapy is effective in treating or preventing venous thrombosis; it is not as useful in treating or preventing arterial thrombosis. Parenteral heparin

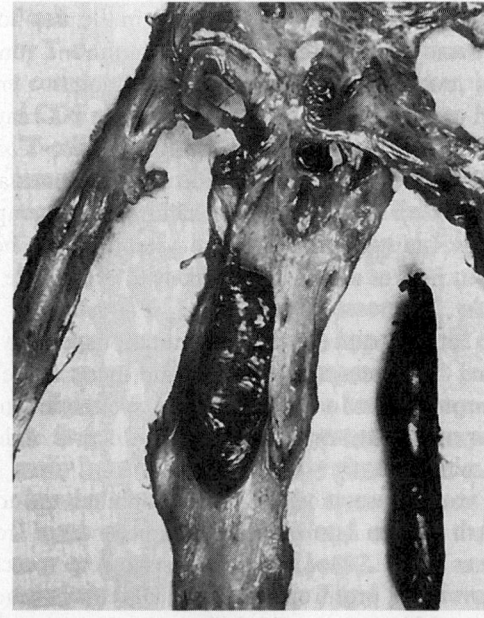

Figure 27-21 Thrombus. Thrombus arising in valve pocket at upper end of superficial femoral vein. Postmortem clot on the right is shown for comparison. (From McLachlin J, Paterson JC: *Surg Gynecol Obstet* 93:1, 1951.)

is the major anticoagulant used to treat thromboembolism. Oral coumarin drugs also are widely used, particularly for individuals not hospitalized. More aggressive therapy may be indicated for such conditions as pulmonary embolism, coronary thrombosis, or thrombophlebitis. Streptokinase and urokinase activate the fibrinolytic system and are administered to accelerate the lysis of known thrombi. Thrombolytic therapy has limited uses and is prescribed with a high degree of caution because it can cause hemorrhagic complications.

The risk for developing spontaneous thrombi is related to several factors, referred to as the **Virchow triad:** (1) injury to the blood vessel endothelium, (2) abnormalities of blood flow, and (3) hypercoagulability of the blood.

Vascular endothelial injury can result from atherosclerosis (plaque deposits on arterial walls). Atherosclerosis initiates platelet adhesion and aggregation, promoting the development of atherosclerotic plaques that enlarge, causing further damage and occlusion. Other causes of vessel endothelial injury may be related to hemodynamic alterations associated with hypertension and turbulent blood flow. Injury also is caused by radiation injury, exogenous chemical agents (toxins from cigarette smoke), endogenous agents (cholesterol), bacterial toxins or endotoxins, or immunologic mechanisms. Whatever the precipitating cause of endothelial injury, it is a potent thrombogenic agent.

Sites of turbulent blood flow in the arteries and stasis of blood flow in the veins are at risk for thrombus formation. In areas of turbulence, platelets and endothelial cells may be activated, leading to thrombosis. In sites of stasis, platelets may remain in contact with the endothelium for prolonged times, and clotting factors that would normally be diluted with fresh-flowing blood are not diluted and may become activated. The most common clinical conditions that predispose to venous stasis and subsequent thromboembolic phenomena are major surgery (e.g., orthopedic surgery), acute myocardial infarction, congestive heart failure, limb paralysis, spinal injury, malignancy, advanced age, the postpartum period, and bed rest longer than 1 week. Turbulence and stasis occur with ulcerated atherosclerotic plaques (myocardial infarction), hyperviscosity (polycythemia), and conditions with deformed red cells (sickle cell anemia).

Hypercoagulability, or **thrombophilia,** is the condition in which an individual is at risk for thrombosis. Hypercoagulability is differentiated according to whether it results from primary (hereditary) or secondary (acquired) causes. Primary causes include defects in proteins involved in hemostasis. Secondary causes include a variety of clinical disorders or conditions (Box 27-9). It is not well understood why there is not a greater incidence of thrombosis formation in hypercoagulable states associated with various disease states and conditions.

Hereditary Thrombophilias

A large number of inherited conditions have been identified that increase the risk of developing thrombosis (Box 27-10).[53] Most are autosomal dominant, thus individuals who

Box 27-9	Clinical Conditions Associated with High-Risk for Thrombosis or Thromboembolism

Arterial	Venous
Atherosclerosis	General surgery
Cigarette smoking	Orthopedic surgery
Hypertension	Arthroscopy
Diabetes mellitus	Trauma
LDL cholesterol	Malignancy
Hypertriglyceridemia	Immobility
Positive family history	Sepsis
Left ventricular failure	Congestive heart failure
Oral contraceptives	Nephrotic syndrome
Estrogens	Obesity
Lipoprotein A	Varicose veins
Polycythemia	Postphlebotic syndrome
Hyperviscosity syndrome	Oral contraceptives
Leukostasis syndrome	Estrogens
Thrombocythemia	Thrombocythemia

LDL, Low-density lipoprotein.

Box 27-10	Hereditary and Acquired Thrombophilic Disorders

Inherited Disorders (Primary)
Activated protein C resistance
    Factor V Leiden mutation
    Factor V Cambridge mutation
    Factor V Hong Kong
    Factor V HR2 mutation
    Prothrombin 20210A mutation
Factor XII deficiency (Hageman trait)
Dysfibrinogenemia
Hyperhomocysteinemia
Platelet defects
    Wein-Penzing defect
    Sticky-platelet syndrome

Inherited and Acquired Disorders
Antithrombin deficiency
Heparin cofactor II deficiency
Protein C deficiency
Protein S deficiency
Plasminogen deficiency
Other fibrinolytic system defects

Acquired Disorders (Secondary)
Antiphospholipid antibodies
    Anticardiolipin antibodies
    Lupus anticoagulant
    Subgroup phospholipid antibodies
Myeloproliferative syndromes
Trousseau syndrome

From Bick RL: *Hematol Oncol Clin North Am* 17(1):115-147, 2003.

are homozygous for the mutation are at greatest risk for thrombosis. These include mutations in coagulation proteins, fibrinolytic proteins, platelet receptors, and other factors. The particular mutations that have been most strongly linked as risk factors for venous thrombosis or for arterial thrombosis leading to coronary artery disease or stroke include those that affect fibrinogen, prothrombin (G20210A variant), factor V (factor V Leiden) of the coagulation system, PAI-1 of the fibrinolytic system, the platelet receptor GPIIIa, and methylenetetrahydrofolate reductase (MTHFR), as well as mutations that result in excessive levels of homocysteine (hyperhomocysteinemia). Other inherited thrombophilias are risk factors primarily for venous thrombosis.[54] These include deficiencies in protein C, protein S, and AT III.[55]

Factor V Leiden results from a single nucleotide mutation of guanine to adenine at nucleotide 1691 (G1691A). Activated factor V (Va) is usually inactivated by protein C, but this single mutation results in a change in amino acid 506 from arginine to glutamine. The change alters the site where protein C would cleave factor Va and confers partial resistance, resulting in prolonged high levels of Va and prolongation of clot formation.[56] Although this mutation increases the risk for thrombosis, most individuals with factor V Leiden do not have clinically relevant thrombotic events. It is the most common hereditary thrombophilia and is found in about 30% of individuals presenting with deep venous thrombosis (DVT) or pulmonary embolism. It is primarily observed in individuals of European ancestry and in about 5% of whites in the United States and Europe.

The second most common inherited thrombophilia is a mutation in the prothrombin gene, resulting in a replacement of guanine at nucleotide 20210 with an adenine (G20210A variant).[54] This mutation is observed in about 2% to 5% of individuals of European ancestry, but is found in 5% to 10% of individuals presenting with venous thrombosis. The G20210A variant leads to overproduction of prothrombin and prolongation of clot formation.

MTHFR mutation leads to alterations in the metabolism of the amino acid homocysteine into methionine and abnormally elevated levels of that amino acid in the blood (hyperhomocysteinemia).[57] Acquired hyperhomocysteinemia may result from deficiencies in vitamins B_6 or B_{12}, endocrine diseases (e.g., diabetes mellitus, hypothyroidism), pernicious anemia, inflammatory bowel disease, renal failure, and therapy with some drugs. Individuals with homocysteine levels above the 95th percentile are 2.5 times more likely to experience an episode of DVT.

More than 100 different known mutations lead to defects of proteins C, protein S, and AT III and increase the risk of venous thrombosis. Mutations may lead to either quantitative (low levels of protein) or qualitative (production of defective protein) changes.

Tests to diagnose inherited thrombophilias include prothrombin time, partial thromboplastin time, levels of protein C, protein S, and AT III. More elaborate tests to detect precise mutations in factor V, prothrombin, or MTHFR may be indicated.

Acquired Hypercoagulability

Deficiencies in protein S and C and AT III may be acquired and contribute to a hypercoagulable state.[56] Conditions associated with an acquired protein deficiency include DIC, liver disease, infection, DVT, acute respiratory distress syndrome, L-asparaginase therapy, HUS, and TTP. The postoperative state also predisposes an individual to protein C or S deficiency; however, its role in contributing to DVT remains unclear.

Acquired hypercoagulable states include the antiphospholipid syndrome (APS), an autoimmune syndrome characterized by autoantibodies against plasma membrane phospholipids and phospholipid-binding proteins. As with most autoimmune diseases, the predominantly affected individual is female and of reproductive age. Those with APS are at risk for arterial and venous thrombosis and a variety of obstetric complications, including pregnancy loss and preeclampsia or eclampsia (Figure 27-22).[58] In severe cases the patients may die from recurrent major thrombus formation.[59] The pathophysiology is related to autoantibodies directly reacting with platelets or endothelial cells (increasing the risk for thrombosis) or the placental surface (resulting in damage to the placenta). The predominant diagnostic tests measure prolongation of laboratory blood coagulation tests related to an antibody inhibitor (lupus anticoagulant) and specific ELISAs for antibodies against phospholipids (e.g., anticardiolipin antibody) or proteins that bind to phospholipids (e.g., β_2-glycoprotein I).[60] Highly effective therapy (i.e., unfractionated or low-molecular-weight heparin with low-dose aspirin) is available to prevent the obstetric complications.[61]

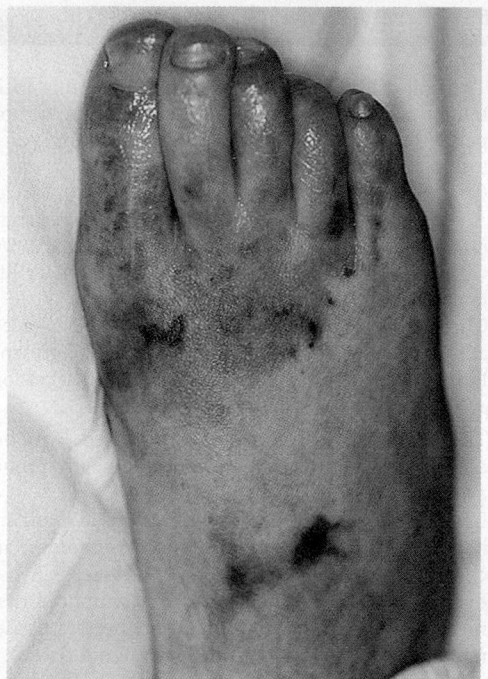

Figure 27-22 Arterial thrombosis associated with antiphospholipid antibodies. A 12-year-old girl with systemic lupus erythematosus and antiphospholipid antibodies with painful cutaneous vasculitis of the right foot. Arterial thrombosis documented by angiography resulted in cyanosis of the large toe. Symptoms resolved with treatment with heparin and corticosteroids. (From Kliegman R, et al: *Nelson textbook of pediatrics*, ed 18, Philadelphia, 2007, Saunders.)

SUMMARY REVIEW

Alterations of Leukocyte Function

1. Quantitative alterations of leukocytes (too many or too few) can be caused by bone marrow dysfunction or premature destruction of cells in the circulation. Many quantitative changes in leukocytes occur in response to invasion by microorganisms.
2. Leukocytosis is a condition in which the leukocyte count is higher than normal and is usually a response to stress and invasion of microorganisms.
3. Leukopenia is a condition in which the leukocyte count is lower than normal and is caused by pathologic conditions such as malignancies and hematologic disorders.
4. Granulocytosis (particularly as a result of an increase in neutrophils) occurs in response to infection. The marrow releases immature cells, causing a shift-to-the-left, when responding to an infection that has created a demand for neutrophils that exceeds the supply in the circulation.
5. Eosinophilia results most commonly from parasitic invasion and ingestion or inhalation of toxic foreign particles.
6. Basophilia is seen in hypersensitivity reactions because of the high content of histamine and subsequent release.
7. Monocytosis occurs during the late or recuperative phase of infection when macrophages (mature monocytes) phagocytose surviving microorganisms and debris.
8. Granulocytopenia, a significant decrease in neutrophils, can be a life-threatening condition if sepsis occurs; it is often caused by chemotherapeutic agents, severe infection, and radiation.

9. Infectious mononucleosis is an acute infection of B lymphocytes most commonly associated with EBV, a type of herpesvirus. Transmission of EBV is by personal contact, commonly through saliva, thus its nickname, the kissing disease.
10. Two of the earliest manifestations of mononucleosis are sore throat and fever caused by inflammation at the primary site of viral entry.
11. Most causes of EBV mononucleosis include fever lasting 7 to 10 days, sore throat, and enlargement and tenderness of the cervical lymph nodes. It is self-limiting, and treatment consists of rest and relief of symptoms.
12. The common pathologic feature of all forms of leukemia is an uncontrolled proliferation of leukocytes, overcrowding the bone marrow and resulting in decreased production and function of the other blood cell lines.
13. All leukemias are classified by the cell type involved, lymphocytic or myelogenous, and are differentiated by onset, acute or chronic. Thus there are four major types of leukemia: ALL, CLL, AML, and CML.
14. Although the exact cause of leukemia is unknown, it is considered a clonal disorder. A high incidence of acute leukemias and CLL is reported in certain families, suggesting a genetic predisposition.
15. The most common genetic abnormality in adult ALL is the Philadelphia chromosome. In about a third of clients with AML there is a mutation in the receptor tyrosine kinase FLT3.
16. In leukemia, blasts (precursor cells) "crowd out" the marrow and cause cellular proliferation of the other cell lines to cease.

Continued

17. The major clinical manifestation of leukemia includes fatigue caused by anemia, bleeding caused by thrombocytopenia, fever secondary to infection, anorexia, and weight loss.
18. Chemotherapy is the treatment of choice for leukemia. Acute leukemias are associated with an increasing survival rate of 80% to 90%, with long-term survival of 30% to 40%. Chronic leukemias are associated with a longer life expectancy than are acute leukemias.
19. Chronic leukemias progress differently than acute leukemias, advancing slowly and without warning. The presence of the Philadelphia chromosome is a diagnostic marker for CML.

Alterations of Lymphoid Function

1. The number of lymphocytes is decreased (lymphocytopenia) in most acute infections and in some immunodeficiency syndromes.
2. Lymphocytosis occurs in viral infections (IM and infectious hepatitis, in particular), leukemia, lymphomas, and some chronic infections.
3. Lymphomas are tumors of primary lymphoid tissue (thymus, bone marrow) or secondary lymphoid tissue (lymph nodes, spleen, tonsils, intestinal lymphoid tissue). The two major types of malignant lymphomas are Hodgkin lymphoma (HL) and non-Hodgkin lymphoma (NHL).
4. HL is associated with a highly distinctive cell, the Reed-Sternberg cell (RS), in the lymph nodes. The RS cell is derived from a malignant B cell that usually becomes binucleate.
5. A virus might be involved in the pathogenesis of HL. Some familial clustering suggests an unknown genetic mechanism.
6. An enlarged painless mass or swelling, most commonly in the neck, is an initial sign of HL. Local symptoms are produced by lymphadenopathy, usually caused by pressure or obstruction.
7. Treatment of HL includes radiation therapy and chemotherapy. A cure is possible regardless of the stage of HL; however, individuals treated with chemotherapy who relapse in less than 2 years have a poor prognosis.
8. The cause of lymph node enlargement and cancerous transformation in NHL is unknown. Immunosuppressed persons have a higher incidence of NHL, suggesting an immune mechanism.
9. Generally, with NHL, the swelling of lymph nodes is painless, and the nodes enlarge and transform over months or years.
10. Individuals with NHL can survive for long periods. Treatment is chemotherapy.
11. Burkitt lymphoma involves the jaw and facial bones and occurs in children from east-central Africa and New Guinea.
12. Multiple myeloma (MM) is a neoplasm of B cells (immature plasma cells) and mature plasma cells. It is characterized by multiple malignant tumor masses of plasma cells scattered throughout the skeletal system and sometimes found in soft tissue.
13. Myeloma cells usually secrete monoclonal protein (M protein) that is an abnormal antibody molecule. The myeloma cell may also secrete free antibody light chain that is excreted in the urine (Bence Jones protein).
14. The exact cause of MM is unknown, but genetic factors and chronic stimulation of the mononuclear phagocyte system by bacteria, viral agents, and chemicals have been suggested.

15. The major clinical manifestations for MM include recurrent infections caused by suppression of the humoral immune response and renal disease as a result of Bence Jones proteinuria.
16. Chemotherapy is the treatment of choice for MM. Survival is still only 2 to 3 years with chemotherapy, however. Treatment with thalidomide is showing promise as an effective therapeutic agent in producing long-term remissions.
17. Waldenström macroglobulinemia is a rare type of slow-growing plasma cell tumor that secretes a monoclonal IgM molecule.

Alterations of Splenic Function

1. Splenomegaly (enlargement of the spleen) may be considered normal in certain individuals, but its presence should not be ignored.
2. Splenomegaly results from (a) acute inflammatory or infectious processes, (b) congestive disorders, (c) infiltrative processes, and (d) tumors or cysts.
3. Hypersplenism (overactivity of the spleen) results from splenomegaly. Hypersplenism results in sequestering of the blood cells, causing increased destruction of red blood cells, which leads to the development of anemia.

Alterations of Platelets and Coagulation

1. Thrombocytopenia is characterized by a platelet count less than 100,000 platelets/mm^3 of blood; a count less than 50,000/mm^3 increases the potential for hemorrhage associated with minor trauma.
2. Thrombocytopenia exists in primary or secondary forms and is commonly associated with autoimmune diseases and viral infections; bacterial sepsis with DIC also results in thrombocytopenia.
3. Heparin-induced thrombocytopenia develops in approximately 4% of individuals receiving unfractionated heparin.
4. Immune thrombocytopenic purpura (ITP) is a major cause of platelet destruction, often affecting females, and results in hemorrhaging that ranges from minor development of petechiae to major bleeding from mucosal sites.
5. Thrombotic thrombycytopenic purpura (TTP) causes platelet aggregation leading to microcirculatory occlusion.
6. Thrombocythemia is characterized by a platelet count more than 400,000 platelets/mm^3 of blood and is symptomatic when the count exceeds 1 million/mm^3, at which time the risk for intravascular clotting (thrombosis) is high.
7. Thrombocythemia is caused by accelerated platelet production in the bone marrow.
8. Qualitative alterations in normal platelet adherence or aggregation prevent platelet plug formation and may result in prolonged bleeding times.
9. Prolonged bleeding can result from alterations in platelet function, including adhesion between platelets and the vessel wall, platelet-platelet adhesion, platelet granule secretion, arachidonic acid pathway activity, and membrane phospholipid regulation.
10. Disorders of coagulation are usually caused by defects or deficiencies of one or more clotting factors.
11. Coagulation is impaired when there is a deficiency of vitamin K because of insufficient production of prothrombin and synthesis of clotting factors II, VII, IX, and X, often associated with liver diseases.
12. DIC is a complex syndrome that results from a variety of clinical conditions that release tissue factor causing an increase in fibrin and thrombin activity in the blood and producing augmented clot formation and accelerated fibrinolysis. Sepsis is a condition that is often associated with DIC.

SUMMARY REVIEW—cont'd

13. DIC is characterized by a cycle of intravascular clotting followed by active bleeding caused by the initial consumption of coagulation factors and platelets and diffuse fibrinolysis.

14. Diagnosis of DIC is based on measurement in the blood of end products characteristic of dysfunctional coagulation activity. Treatment is complex and nonstandardized and focused on removing the primary cause, restoring hemostasis, and preventing further organ damage.

15. Thromboembolic disease results from a fixed (thrombus) or moving (embolus) clot that blocks flow within a vessel, denying nutrients to tissues distal to the occlusion; death can result when clots obstruct blood flow to the heart, brain, or lungs.

16. Hypercoagulability is the result of deficient anticoagulation proteins. Secondary causes are conditions that promote venous stasis.

17. The term *Virchow triad* refers to three factors that can cause thrombus formation: (1) injury to the vessel wall, (2) abnormalities of blood flow, and (3) alterations in the blood constituents leading to hypercoagulability.

18. Autoantibodies against phospholipids result in a state of acquired hypercoagulability, an increased risk for venous or arterial thrombosis, and a high incidence of pregnancy complications.

KEY TERMS

Acute idiopathic TTP, 1047
Acute leukemia, 1019
Acute lymphocytic leukemia (ALL), 1021
Acute myelogenous leukemia (AML), 1021
Agranulocytosis, 1015
Arterial thrombus(*pl.*, thrombi), 1055
Basopenia, 1017
Basophilia, 1017
B-cell neoplasms, 1033
Bence Jones protein, 1038
β_2-microglobulin, 1041
Burkitt lymphoma, 1035
Chronic leukemia, 1019
Chronic lymphocytic leukemia (CLL), 1025
Chronic myelogenous leukemia (CML), 1025
Chronic relapsing TTP, 1047
Compensated DIC, 1053
Congestive splenomegaly, 1043
Consumptive thrombohemorrhagic disorders, 1050
D-dimer, 1054
Disseminated intravascular coagulation (DIC), 1050
Embolus, 1055
Eosinopenia, 1017
Eosinophilia, 1015
Erythromyalgia, 1048
Essential (primary) thrombocythemia (ET), 1047

Granulocytopenia, 1015
Granulocytosis, 1015
Heparin-induced thrombocytopenia (HIT), 1044
Heterophile antibodies, 1018
Hodgkin lymphoma (HL), 1031
Hypercoagulability, 1055
Hypersplenism, 1042
Immune thrombocytopenic purpura (ITP), 1045
Impaired hemostasis, 1049
Infectious mononucleosis (IM), 1017
Infiltrative splenomegaly, 1043
Leukemia, 1019
Leukemoid reaction, 1015
Leukocytosis, 1014
Leukopenia, 1014
Lymphadenopathy, 1030
Lymphoblastic lymphoma (LL), 1036
Lymphocytopenia, 1017
Lymphocytosis, 1017
Lymphoplasmacytic lymphoma, 1042
Microvasculature thrombosis, 1048
Monoclonal gammopathy of undetermined significance (MGUS), 1040
Monocytopenia, 1017
Monocytosis, 1017
M protein, 1038
Multiple myeloma, (MM) 1037

Neutropenia, 1015
Neutrophilia, 1015
NK-cell neoplasms, 1033
Non-Hodgkin lymphoma (NHL), 1033
Pancytopenia, 1021
Philadelphia chromosome, 1020
Pseudothrombocytopenia, 1044
Purpura, 1044
Qualitative leukocyte disorder, 1014
Quantitative leukocyte disorder, 1014
Reed-Sternberg (RS) cell, 1031
Shift-to-the-left, 1015
Smoldering myeloma, 1040
Solitary plasmacytoma, 1040
Splenomegaly, 1042
T-cell neoplasms, 1033
Thrombocythemia, 1047
Thrombocytopenia, 1044
Thrombocytosis, 1047
Thromboembolic disease, 1044
Thrombophilia, 1055
Thrombotic thrombocytopenic purpura (TTP), 1046
Thrombus, 1055
Vasculitis, 1049
Venous thrombus, 1055
Virchow triad, 1055
Waldenström macroglobulinemia, 1042

REFERENCES

1. Marris JA: Care of patients with neutropenia, *Clin J Oncol Nurs* 10(2):164-166, 2006.
2. Bell AT, Fortune B, Sheeler R: Clinical inquiries: what test is the best for diagnosing infectious mononucleosis? *J Fam Pract* 55(9):799-802, 2006.
3. Gunz FW: The dreaded leukemias and the lymphomas: their nature and their prospects. In Wintrobe MM, editor: *Blood, pure and eloquent: a story of discovery, of people, and of ideas*, New York, 1980, McGraw-Hill.
4. *SEER stat fact sheets—acute lymphocytic leukemia*, Bethesda, MD, 2008, National Institutes of Health, U.S. Department of Health and Human Services. Available at http://seer.cancer.gov/statfacts/html/alyl.html. Accessed February 3, 2009.
5. Druker BJ: Translation of the Philadelphia chromosome into therapy for CML, *Blood* 112(13):4808-4817, 2008.
6. Keen-Kim D, Nooraie F, Rao PN: Cytogenetic biomarkers for human cancer, *Front Biosci* 13(May 1):5928-5949, 2008.
7. Dick JE: Stem cell concepts renew cancer research. *Blood* 112(13): 4793-4807, 2008.

8. *SEER stat fact sheets—acute myeloid leukemia*, Bethesda, MD, 2008, National Institutes of Health, U.S. Department of Health and Human Services. Available at http://seer.cancer.gov/statfacts/html/amyl.html. Accessed February 3, 2009.

9. *Childhood acute lymphoblastic leukemia treatment: health professional version*, Bethesda, MD, 2008, National Institutes of Health, U.S. Department of Health and Human Services. Available at www.cancer.gov/cancertopics/pdq/treatment/childALL/healthprofessional. Accessed February 3, 2009.

10. *Adult acute lymphoblastic leukemia treatment: health professional version*, Bethesda, MD, 2008, National Institutes of Health, U.S. Department of Health and Human Services. Available at www.cancer.gov/cancertopics/pdq/treatment/adultALL/healthprofessional. Accessed February 3, 2009.

11. Estey E, Dohner H: Acute myeloid leukemia, *Lancet* 368(9550): 1894-1907, 2006.

12. *Adult acute myeloid leukemia treatment: health professional version*, Bethesda, MD, 2008, National Institutes of Health, U.S. Department of Health and Human Services. Available at www.cancer.gov/cancertopics/pdq/treatment/adultAML/healthprofessional. Accessed February 3, 2009.

13. *SEER stat fact sheets—chronic lymphoblastic leukemia*, Bethesda, MD, 2008, National Institutes of Health, U.S. Department of Health and Human Services. Available at http://seer.cancer.gov/statfacts/html/clyl.html. Accessed February 3, 2009.

14. *SEER stat fact sheets—chronic myeloid leukemia*, Bethesda, MD, 2008, National Institutes of Health, U.S. Department of Health and Human Services. Available at http://seer.cancer.gov/statfacts/html/alyl.html. Accessed February 3, 2009.

15. Montserrat E, Moreno C: Chronic lymphocytic leukemia: a short overview, *Ann Oncol* 19(Suppl 7):vii320-vii325, 2008.

16. Savona M, Talpaz M: Getting to the stem of chronic myeloid leukemia, *Nat Rev Cancer* 8(5):341-350, 2008.

17. Kantarjian HM et al: New insights into the pathophysiology of chronic myeloid leukemia and imatinib resistance, *Ann Intern Med* 145(12):913-923, 2006.

18. Jaffe ES et al: Classification of lymphoid neoplasms: the microscope as a tool for disease discovery, *Blood* 112(12):4384-4399, 2008.

19. *SEER stat fact sheets—Hodgkin lymphoma*, Bethesda, MD, 2008, National Institutes of Health, U.S. Department of Health and Human Services. Available at http://seer.cancer.gov/statfacts/html/hodg.html. Accessed February 3, 2009.

20. *What you need to know about Hodgkin lymphoma*, Bethesda, MD, 2008, National Institutes of Health, U.S. Department of Health and Human Services. Available at http://cancer.gov/cancertopics/wyntk/hodgkin. Accessed February 12, 2009.

21. *SEER stat fact sheets—non-Hodgkin lymphoma*, Bethesda, MD, 2008, National Institutes of Health, U.S. Department of Health and Human Services. Available at http://seer.cancer.gov/statfacts/html/nhl.html. Accessed February 3, 2009.

22. *Adult non-Hodgkin lymphoma treatment: health professional version*, Bethesda, MD, 2008, National Institutes of Health, U.S. Department of Health and Human Services. Available at www.cancer.gov/cancertopics/pdq/treatment/myeloma/healthprofessional. Accessed February 3, 2009.

23. *Multiple myeloma and other plasma cell neoplasms treatment: health professional version*, Bethesda, MD, 2008, National Institutes of Health, U.S. Department of Health and Human Services. Available at www.cancer.gov/cancertopics/pdq/treatment/adult-non-hodgkins/healthprofessional. Accessed February 3, 2009.

24. *SEER stat fact sheets—myeloma*, Bethesda, MD, 2008, National Institutes of Health, U.S. Department of Health and Human Services. Available at http://seer.cancer.gov/statfacts/html/mulmy.html. Accessed February 3, 2009.

25. Kyle RA, Rajkumar SV: Criteria for diagnosis, staging, risk stratification and response assessment of multiple myeloma, *Leukemia* 23(1):3-9, 2009.

26. Yasui H et al: Recent advances in the treatment of multiple myeloma, *Curr Pharm Biotechnol* 7(5):381-393, 2006.

27. *Waldenström macroglobulinemia: questions and answers: fact sheet*, Bethesda MD, 2008, National Institutes of Health, U.S. Department of Health and Human Services. Available at http://cancer.gov/cancertopics/factsheet/Sites-Types/WM. Accessed February 12, 2009.

28. Dimopoulos MA et al: Update on treatment recommendations from the fourth international workshop on Waldenström's macroglobulinemia, *J Clin Oncol* 27(1):120-126, 2009.

29. Nachman RL, Rafii S: Platelets, petechiae, and preservation of the vascular wall, *N Eng J Med* 359(12):1261-1270, 2008.

30. *Thrombocytopenia*, Bethesda, MD, 2008, National Institutes of Health, U.S. Department of Health and Human Services. Available at www.nhlbi.nih.gov/health/dci/Diseases/thcp/thcp_all.html. Accessed February 3, 2009.

31. Selleng K, Selleng S, Greinacher A: Heparin-induced thrombocytopenia in intensive care patients, *Semin Thromb Hemost* 34(5):425-438, 2008.

32. Warkentin TE, Sheppard J- AI: Testing for heparin-induced thrombocytopenia antibodies, *Transfus Med Rev* 20(4):259-272, 2006.

33. *Idiopathic thrombocytopenic purpura*, Bethesda, MD, 2008, National Institutes of Health, U.S. Department of Health and Human Services. Available at www.nhlbi.nih.gov/health/dci/Diseases/Itp/ITP.all.html. Accessed February 3, 2009.

34. Curtis BR: Genotyping for human platelet alloantigen polymorphisms: applications in the diagnosis of alloimmune platelet disorders, *Semin Thromb Hemost* 34(6):539-548, 2008.

35. Arnold DM, Smith JW, Kelton JG: Diagnosis and management of neonatal alloimmune thrombocytopenia, *Transfus Med Rev* 22(4):255-267, 2008.

36. Bennett CM, de Jong JLO, Neufeld EJ: Targeted ITP strategies: do they elucidate the biology of ITP and related disorders? *Pediatr Blood Cancer* 47(5 Suppl):706-709, 2006.

37. Psaila B, Bussel JB: Refractory immune thrombocytopenic purpura: current strategies for investigation and management, *Brit J Haematol* 143(1):16-26, 2008.

38. *Thrombotic thrombocytopenic purpura*, Bethesda, MD, 2008, National Institutes of Health, U.S. Department of Health and Human Services. Available at www.nhlbi.nih.gov/health/dci/Diseases/Itp/ITP.all.html. Accessed February 16, 2009.

39. *Thrombocytopenia & thrombocytosis*, Bethesda, MD, 2008, National Institutes of Health, U.S. Department of Health and Human Services. Available at www.nhlbi.nih.gov/health/dci/Diseases/thrm/thrm_all.html. Accessed February 3, 2009.

40. Harrison CN, Green AR: Essential thrombocythaemia, *Best Pract Res Clin Haematol* 19(3):439-453, 2006.

41. Landolfi R, Di Gennaro L, Falanga A: Thrombosis in myeloproliferative disorders: pathogenetic facts and speculation, *Leukemia* 22(11):2020-2028, 2008.

42. Kota J, Caceres N, Constantinescu SN: Aberrant signal transduction pathways in myeloproliferative neoplasms, *Leukemia* 22(10):1828-1840, 2008.

43. Tefferi A, Elliott M: Thrombosis in myeloproliferative disorders: prevalence, prognostic factors, and the role of leukocytes and *JAK2V617F*, *Semin Thromb Hemost* 33(4):313-320, 2007.

44. Barbui T, Finazzi G: Therapy for polycythemia vera and essential thrombocythemia is driven by the cardiovascular risk, *Semin Thromb Hemost* 33(4):321-329, 2007.

45. Salles II et al: Inherited traits affecting platelet function, *Blood Rev* 22(3):155-172, 2008.

46. Wada H, Usui M, Sakuragawa N: Hemostatic abnormalities and liver disease, *Semin Thromb Hemost* 34(8):772-778, 2008.

47. Taylor FB Jr et al: Towards definition, clinical and laboratory criteria, and a scoring system for disseminated intravascular coagulation, *Thromb Hemost* 86(5):1327-1330, 2001.

48. Furlong MA, Furlong BR: Disseminated intravascular coagulation. Available at www.emedicine.com/emerg/topic150.htm. Accessed March 16, 2005.

49. Kwaan HC, Vicuna B: Incidence and pathogenesis of thrombosis in hematologic malignancies, *Semin Thromb Hemost* 33(4):303-312, 2007.

50. Palumbo JS: Mechanisms linking tumor cell-associated procoagulant function to tumor dissemination, *Semin Thromb Hemost* 34(2):154-160, 2008.

51. Wada H, Sakuragawa N: Are fibrin-related markers useful for the diagnosis of thrombosis, *Semin Thromb Hemost* 34(1):33-38, 2008.

52. *Excessive blood clotting*, Bethesda, MD, 2008, National Institutes of Health, U.S. Department of Health and Human Services. Available at www.nhlbi.nih.gov/health/dci/Diseases/ebc/ebc_all.html. Accessed February 3, 2009.

53. Chan MY, Andreotti F, Becker RC: Hypercoagulable states in cardiovascular disease, *Circulation* 118(22):2286-2297, 2008.

54. Lippi G, Franchini M: Pathogenesis of venous thromboembolism: when the cup runneth over, *Semin Thromb Hemost* 34(8):747-761, 2008.

55. Middeldorp S, Vlieg AH: Does thrombophilia testing help in the clinical management of patients? *Brit J Haematol* 143(3):321-335, 2008.
56. Boekholdt SM, Kramer MHH: Arterial thrombosis and the role of thrombophilia, *Semin Thromb Hemost* 33(6):588-596, 2007.
57. Cohn DM, Roshani S, Middeldorp S: Thrombophilia and venous thromboembolism: implications for testing, *Semin Thromb Hemost* 33(6):573-581, 2007.
58. Tincani A et al: Lupus and the antiphospholipid syndrome in pregnancy and obstetrics: clinical characteristics, diagnosis, pathogenesis, and treatment, *Semin Thromb Hemost* 34(3):267-273, 2008.
59. Merrill JT, Asherson RA: Catastrophic antiphosholipid syndrome, *Nat Clin Pract Rheumatol* 2(2):81-89, 2006.
60. Pierangeli SS, Harris EN: A quarter of a century in anticardiolipin antibody testing and attempted standarization has led us to here, which is? *Semin Thromb Hemost* 34(4):313-328, 2008.
61. Heilmann L et al: Pregnancy outcome in women with antiphospholipid antibodies: report on a retrospective study, *Semin Thromb Hemost* 34(8):794-802, 2008.

ALTERATIONS OF HEMATOLOGIC FUNCTION IN CHILDREN

NANCY E. KLINE

MEDIA RESOURCES

€volve **Evolve Website** (http://evolve.elsevier.com/McCance/)
- Review Questions and Answers
- Animations
- Glossary (with audio pronunciation for selected terms)
- WebLinks

CHAPTER OUTLINE

FETAL AND NEONATAL HEMATOPOIESIS
POSTNATAL CHANGES IN THE BLOOD
Erythrocytes
Leukocytes and Platelets
DISORDERS OF ERYTHROCYTES
Acquired Disorders
Inherited Disorders

DISORDERS OF COAGULATION AND PLATELETS
Inherited Hemorrhagic Disease
Antibody-Mediated Hemorrhagic Disease
LEUKEMIA AND LYMPHOMA
Leukemia
Lymphomas

This chapter briefly explains fetal and neonatal hematopoiesis and postnatal changes in blood as a foundation for understanding the pathophysiology of specific blood disorders in childhood. Among the diseases that affect erythrocytes are acquired disorders, such as iron deficiency anemia, hemolytic disease of the newborn, and anemia of infectious disease; and inherited disorders, such as glucose-6-phosphate dehydrogenase (G6PD) deficiency, hereditary spherocytosis, sickle cell disease, and the thalassemias. Disorders of coagulation and platelets include inherited hemorrhagic diseases, such as the hemophilias, and antibody-mediated hemorrhagic diseases, which include idiopathic thrombocytopenic purpura, autoimmune neonatal thrombocytopenias, and autoimmune vascular purpuras. Finally, leukocyte disorders, such as leukemia and the lymphomas (non-Hodgkin lymphoma as well as Hodgkin disease), are discussed.

FETAL AND NEONATAL HEMATOPOIESIS

As the developing embryo becomes too large for oxygenation of tissues by simple diffusion, the production of erythrocytes begins within the vessels of the yolk sac. Shortly after 2 weeks of gestation, circulating erythrocytes play a major role in delivering oxygen to the tissues. At approximately the eighth week of gestation, the site of erythrocyte production shifts from the vessels to the liver sinusoids and the production of leukocytes and platelets begins in the liver and spleen. Erythropoiesis in the liver and, to a lesser extent, in the spleen and lymph nodes, reaches a peak at approximately 4 months. Hepatic blood formation declines steadily thereafter but does not disappear entirely during the remainder of gestation. By the fifth month of gestation, hematopoiesis begins to occur in the bone marrow and increases rapidly until hematopoietic (red) marrow fills the entire bone marrow space. By the time of delivery, the marrow is the only significant site of hematopoiesis.

In neonates and young infants, hematopoietic marrow progressively fills the bony cavities of the entire axial skeleton (skull, vertebrae, ribs, sternum), the long bones of the limbs, and many intramembranous bones. (These structures are described in Chapter 43.) Fatty (yellow) marrow gradually replaces hematopoietic marrow in some bones. During childhood, hematopoietic tissue retreats centrally to the vertebrae, ribs, sternum, pelvis, scapulae, skull, and proximal ends of the femur and humerus.

In diseases characterized by hemolysis, erythrocyte production can increase as much as eight times the normal because erythropoietin causes hematopoietic marrow to increase in volume. Initially, hematopoietic marrow expands from the ends of the long bones toward the middle of the shafts, replacing fatty marrow. Next, blood cell production begins to occur outside the marrow cavities, especially in the liver and spleen. Extramedullary hematopoiesis is more likely to occur in children than in adults because the bony cavities of children already are filled with red marrow (Figure 28-1). This is why hemolytic disease causes especially pronounced enlargement of the spleen and liver in children.

The erythrocytes undergo striking changes during gestation, particularly during the first two trimesters, at which time they nearly double in numbers and in hemoglobin content. A proportionate increase in hematocrit also occurs. By the end of gestation the erythrocyte count has more than tripled but the size of each erythrocyte has decreased.

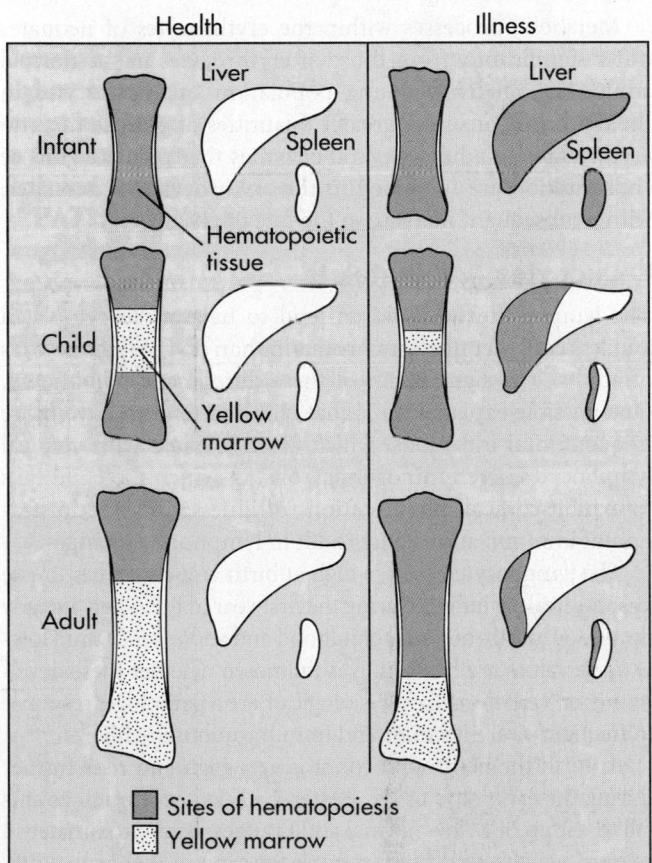

Figure 28-1 Sites of hematopoiesis in health and illness. With normal maturation, red marrow is partly replaced by yellow marrow in the shafts of the long bones. In adults, red marrow is largely restricted to the proximal ends of the femur and humerus. In response to hemolysis, red marrow replaces yellow marrow in the long bones. In infants, whose long bones already are filled with red marrow, additional hematopoiesis takes place in the liver and spleen. In children and adults, red marrow can replace yellow marrow in response to hemolysis, necessitating less hematopoiesis in the liver and spleen.

A biochemically distinct type of hemoglobin is synthesized during fetal life. The three **embryonic hemoglobins (Gower 1, Gower 2, and Portland)** and the **fetal hemoglobin (Hb F)** are composed of two α and two γ-chains of polypeptides, whereas the adult hemoglobins (Hb A and Hb A_2) are composed of two α-chains and two β-chains. (The structure of an adult hemoglobin molecule is illustrated in Figure 25-14, and types of hemoglobin are defined in Table 25-5.) Some unknown regulatory mechanism promotes γ-chain synthesis and inhibits β- and δ-chain synthesis in utero. This results in production of embryonic or fetal hemoglobin. After birth, γ-chain synthesis is inhibited, whereas β- and δ-chain synthesis is facilitated, resulting in production of adult hemoglobins.

Fetal hemoglobin has greater affinity for oxygen than does adult hemoglobin because it interacts less readily with an enzyme (2,3-diphosphoglycerate [DPG]) that inhibits hemoglobin-oxygen binding. The decreased inhibitory effects of 2,3-DPG enable fetal blood to transport oxygen despite the relative lack of oxygen in the uterine environment. The increased affinity for oxygen enables Hb F to bind with maternal oxygen in the placental circulation.

During the first trimester, nearly all of the hemoglobin in the fetus is embryonic, but some Hb A can be detected. Therefore, it is possible to identify as early as 16 to 20 weeks of gestation some disorders of adult hemoglobin, such as sickle cell anemia and thalassemia major. In the 6-month fetus, Hb F constitutes 90% of the total. This percentage then begins to decline. At birth, neonatal hemoglobin consists of 70% Hb F, 29% Hb A, and 1% Hb A_2. Between 6 and 12 months of age, normal adult hemoglobin percentages are established (see Chapter 25).

POSTNATAL CHANGES IN THE BLOOD

Blood cell counts tend to rise above adult levels at birth and then decline gradually throughout childhood. Table 28-1 lists normal ranges during infancy and childhood. The immediate rise in values is the result of accelerated hematopoiesis during fetal life, increased numbers of cells that result from the trauma of birth, and cutting of the umbilical cord. These events surrounding the birth also are accompanied by a "shift to the left," that is, the presence of large numbers of immature erythrocytes and leukocytes (particularly granulocytes) in peripheral blood (see Chapter 25). The shift to the left disappears as the infant develops, usually within the first 2 to 3 months of life. Other unique postnatal characteristics, particularly of lymphocytes, may be caused by exogenous factors, such as viral infections.

Average blood volume in the full-term neonate is 85 ml/kg of body weight. The premature infant has a slightly larger blood volume of 90 ml/kg of body weight, with the mean increasing to 150 mg/kg during the first few days after birth. In full-term and premature infants, blood volume decreases during the first few months. Thereafter the average blood volume is 75 to 77 ml/kg, which is similar to that of older children and adults.

Table 28-1   Hematologic Values During Infancy and Childhood

Age	Hemoglobin (g/dl)		Hematocrit (%)		Reticu-locytes (%)	MCV (fl)	Leukocytes (WBC/mm³)		Neutrophils (%)		Lympho-cytes (%)	Eosin-ophils (%)	Mono-cytes (%)
	Mean	Range	Mean	Range	Mean	Lowest	Mean	Range	Mean	Range	Mean*	Mean	Mean
Cord blood	16.8	13.7-20.1	55	45-65	5	110	18,000	(9000-30,000)	61	(40-80)	31	2	6
2 wk	16.5	13-20	50	42-66	1		12,000	(5000-21,000)	40		63	3	9
3 mo	12	9.5-14.5	36	31-41	1		12,000	(6000-18,000)	30		48	2	5
6 mo to 6 yr	12	10.5-14	37	33-42	1	70-74	10,000	(6000-15,000)	45		48	2	5
7-12 yr	13	11-16	38	34-40	1	76-80	8,000	(4500-13,500)	55		38	2	5
Adult													
Female	14	12-16	42	37-47	1.6	80	7,500	(5000-10,000)	55	(35-70)	35	3	7
Male	16	14-18	47	42-52		80							

fl, Femtoliters; *MCV*, mean corpuscular volume; *WBC*, white blood cells.
*Relatively wide range.
From Behrman R et al, editors: *Nelson textbook of pediatrics,* 17th ed, Philadelphia, 2004, Saunders.

Erythrocytes

The hypoxic intrauterine environment stimulates erythropoietin production in the fetus. This accelerates fetal erythropoiesis, producing polycythemia (excessive proliferation of erythrocyte precursors) of the newborn. After birth the oxygen from the lungs saturates arterial blood and the amount of oxygen delivered to the tissues increases. In response to the change from a placental to a pulmonary oxygen supply during the first few days of life, levels of erythropoietin and the rate of blood cell formation decrease. The very active rate of fetal erythropoiesis is reflected by the large numbers of immature erythrocytes (reticulocytes) in the peripheral blood of full-term neonates. After birth the number of reticulocytes decreases about 50% every 12 hours so it is rare to find an elevated reticulocyte count after the first week of life. A decrease in extramedullary hematopoiesis also occurs at this time. In the peripheral blood the erythrocyte count drops for 6 to 8 weeks after birth. During this period of rapid growth the rate of erythrocyte destruction is greater than that in later childhood and adulthood. In full-term infants, normal erythrocyte life span is 60 to 80 days; in premature infants it may be as short as 20 to 30 days; and in children and adolescents, it is the same as that in adults—120 days. (Mechanisms of hemolysis are described in Chapter 25.)

In the premature infant the postnatal fall in hemoglobin and hematocrit values is more marked than in the full-term infant. In the preschool and school-age child, there is a gradual rise in hemoglobin, hematocrit, and red blood cell (RBC) count. Values in males and females first begin to diverge in adolescence. In the female the gradual hemoglobin increase continues into early puberty, at which time it stabilizes. In the male the hemoglobin increase keeps pace with growth and maturation and eventually surpasses that of the female. This higher value in the mature male is related to androgen secretion.

Metabolic processes within the erythrocytes of neonates differ significantly from those of erythrocytes in the normal adult. The relatively young population of erythrocytes in the newborn consumes greater quantities of glucose than do erythrocytes in adults. Several enzymes that regulate glucose consumption are increased in the erythrocytes of neonates, with a subsequent increase in the rate of glycolysis.

Leukocytes and Platelets

The lymphocytes of children tend to have more cytoplasm and less compact nuclear chromatin than do the lymphocytes of adults. The significance of these differences is unknown. One possible explanation is that children tend to have more frequent viral infections, which are associated with atypical lymphocytes. Even minor infections, in which the child fails to exhibit clinical manifestations of illness, and administration of immunizations may result in lymphocyte changes.[1]

The lymphocyte count is high at birth and continues to rise in some healthy infants during the first year of life. Then a steady decline occurs throughout childhood and adolescence until lower adult values are reached. It is unknown whether these developmental variations are physiologic or are a pathologic response to frequent viral infections and immunizations in children.

At birth the neutrophil count is very high and rises further during the early days of life.[2] After 2 weeks, neutrophil counts fall to within or below normal adult ranges. By approximately 4 years of age, the neutrophil count is the same as that of an adult. White children have slightly higher counts than black children.[3]

Eosinophil count is high in the first year of life and is higher in children than in teenagers or adults.[4] Monocyte counts are high in the first year of life and then decrease to adult levels. No relationship between age and basophil count has been found. Platelet counts in full-term neonates are comparable to platelet counts in adults and remain so throughout infancy and childhood.[5]

DISORDERS OF ERYTHROCYTES

Anemia is the most common blood disorder in children. Like the anemias of adulthood, the anemias of childhood are caused by ineffective erythropoiesis or premature destruction of erythrocytes. The most common cause of insufficient erythropoiesis is iron deficiency, which may result from insufficient dietary intake or chronic loss of iron caused by bleeding. The hemolytic anemias of childhood may be divided into two large categories. The first category consists of disorders that result from premature destruction caused by intrinsic abnormalities of the erythrocytes, and the second category consists of disorders that result from damaging extraerythrocytic factors. The hemolytic anemias are inherited, congenital, or both.

The most dramatic form of acquired congenital hemolytic anemia is **hemolytic disease of the newborn (HDN),** also termed **erythroblastosis fetalis.** HDN is an alloimmune disease in which maternal blood and fetal blood are antigenically incompatible, causing the mother's immune system to produce antibodies against fetal erythrocytes. Fetal erythrocytes that have been attacked by (i.e., bound to) maternal antibodies are recognized as foreign or defective by the fetal mononuclear phagocyte system and are removed from the circulation by phagocytosis, usually in the fetal spleen. (For a complete discussion of HDN, see p. 1066.) Other acquired hemolytic anemias—some of which begin in utero—include those caused by infections or the presence of toxic chemicals.

The inherited forms of hemolytic anemia result from intrinsic defects of the child's erythrocytes, any of which can lead to erythrocyte removal by the mononuclear phagocyte system. Structural defects include abnormal cellular size and abnormalities of plasma membrane structure (spherocytosis). Intracellular defects include enzyme deficiencies, the most common of which is G6PD deficiency, and defects of hemoglobin synthesis, which manifest as sickle cell disease or thalassemia, depending on which component of hemoglobin is defective. These and other causes of childhood anemia, some more common than others, are listed in Table 28-2.

Acquired Disorders

Iron Deficiency Anemia

Iron deficiency anemia is the most common blood disorder of infancy and childhood, with the highest incidence occurring between 6 months and 2 years of age. Incidence is not related to gender or race, but socioeconomic factors are important because they affect nutrition, for example, the risk of iron deficiency anemia in children of single, homeless women.[6] However, greater use of iron-fortified products has decreased the prevalence of anemia in low-income infants.[7] Iron deficiency anemia is a common disorder in children because of their extremely high need for iron for normal growth to occur.

Between 4 years of age and the onset of puberty, dietary iron deficiency is uncommon. During adolescence, however, it is relatively common, especially in menstruating females. Rapid growth, together with the average teenager's dietary habits, causes iron depletion. (Mechanisms of iron depletion are described in Chapter 25.)

PATHOPHYSIOLOGY Although inadequate intake of iron is the most common cause of iron deficiency anemia during the first few years of life and during adolescence, blood loss is the most common cause in childhood. Chronic iron deficiency anemia from occult (hidden) blood loss may be caused by a gastrointestinal lesion, parasitic infestation, or hemorrhagic disease. As many as one third of infants with severe iron deficiency anemia have chronic intestinal blood loss induced by exposure to a heat-labile protein in cow's milk. Such exposure causes an inflammatory gastrointestinal reaction that damages the mucosa and results in diffuse hemorrhage.

The amount of iron available for hemoglobin synthesis in the infant depends on iron stores present at birth, rate of growth, the amount of dietary iron absorbed, and physiologic or pathologic loss of iron. During the period of inactive erythropoiesis immediately after birth, iron from erythrocytes that die at the end of their normal life span is stored, as hemosiderin, in bone marrow and liver tissue. This creates an iron reserve that can be used in lieu of dietary intake. The greatest stores are present 4 to 8 weeks after birth. Until erythropoiesis resumes, these iron stores are mobilized. In the premature infant, resumption of erythropoiesis depletes iron stores within 6 to 12 weeks; in the full-term infant, depletion takes longer—about 16 to 20 weeks. Once iron stores have been used, the infant depends on dietary iron.

The amount of dietary iron available for erythropoiesis depends on which foods are consumed. Iron-fortified cereals, green and yellow vegetables, fruits, and milk are common in the average 6-month-old infant's diet and provide iron in the amount of 0.9 to 1.5 mg/kg/day, amounts that satisfy the normal average daily requirement. Iron-fortified formulas are available commercially.

CLINICAL MANIFESTATIONS The symptoms of mild anemia—lethargy and lassitude—usually are not present or detectable in infants and young children, who are unable to describe these symptoms. Therefore, parents usually do not notice any change in the child's behavior or appearance until moderate anemia has developed. General irritability, decreased activity tolerance, weakness, and lack of interest in play are nonspecific indications of anemia. In mild to moderate iron deficiency anemia (hemoglobin of 6 to 10 g/dl), compensatory mechanisms of tissue oxygenation, such as increased amounts of 2,3-DPG within erythrocytes and a shift of the oxyhemoglobin dissociation curve, may be so effective that few clinical manifestations are apparent. When the hemoglobin falls below 5 g/dl, however, pallor, tachycardia, and systolic murmurs may occur.

Splenomegaly is evident in 10% to 15% of children with iron deficiency anemia, and if the condition is long-standing, the sutures of the skull may be widened. Chronic anemia also may result in decreased physical growth and developmental delays. Some children exhibit pica, a behavior in which nonfood

Table 28-2   Anemias of Childhood

Cause	Anemic Condition
Deficient Erythropoiesis or Hemoglobin Synthesis	
Decreased stem cell population in marrow (congenital or acquired pure red cell aplasia)	Normocytic-normochromic anemia
Decreased erythropoiesis despite normal stem cell population in marrow (infection, inflammation, cancer, chronic renal disease, congenital dyserythropoiesis)	Normocytic-normochromic anemia
Deficiency of a factor or nutrient needed for erythropoiesis	
Cobalamin (vitamin B$_{12}$), folate	Megaloblastic anemia
Iron	Microcytic-hypochromic anemia
Increased or Premature Hemolysis	
Alloimmune disease (maternal-fetal Rh, ABO, or minor blood group incompatibility)	Hemolytic disease of the newborn (HDN)
Autoimmune disease (idiopathic autoimmune hemolytic anemia, symptomatic systemic lupus erythematosus, lymphoma, drug-induced autoimmune processes)	Autoimmune hemolytic anemia
Inherited defects of plasma membrane structure (spherocytosis, elliptocytosis, stomatocytosis) or cellular size or both (pyknocytosis)	Hemolytic anemia
Infection (bacterial sepsis, congenital syphilis, malaria, cytomegalovirus infection, rubella, toxoplasmosis, disseminated herpes)	Hemolytic anemia
Intrinsic and inherited enzymatic defects (deficiencies of glucose-6-phosphate dehydrogenase [G6PD], pyruvate kinase, 5′-nucleotidase, glucose phosphate isomerase)	Hemolytic anemia
Inherited defects of hemoglobin synthesis	Sickle cell anemia Thalassemia
Disseminated intravascular coagulation (see Chapter 27)	Hemolytic anemia
Galactosemia	Hemolytic anemia
Prolonged or recurrent respiratory or metabolic acidosis	Hemolytic anemia
Blood vessel disorders (cavernous hemangioma, large vessel thrombus, renal artery stenosis, severe coarctation of the aorta) (see Chapter 31)	Hemolytic anemia

substances are eaten. Because children with iron deficiency anemia may be obese, underweight, or of normal weight, other manifestations of undernutrition must be identified.

Iron deficiency anemia may affect neurologic and intellectual function. Some research findings indicate that low iron in the blood affects attention span, alertness, and learning ability, even when anemia is not severe.

EVALUATION AND TREATMENT The most definitive test for differentiating iron deficiency from other microcytic states is the absence of iron stores in the bone marrow. However, measurement of serum ferritin iron concentration, transferrin saturation, iron-binding capacity, and, more recently, serum transferrin receptors may prevent proceeding to actual bone marrow evaluation. Evaluation and treatment of iron deficiency anemia in children are similar to evaluation and treatment in adults (see Chapter 26). Oral administration of simple ferrous salts usually is satisfactory, but additional vitamin C may be needed to promote absorption.[8] Administration of supplementary trace metals or other vitamins is not necessary. If malabsorption is the cause of the anemia (or if oral administration has not been successful), iron dextran (Imferon) is given intravenously. Iron therapy is continued for at least 2 months after erythrocyte indexes have returned to normal in order to replenish iron stores.[9]

Dietary modification is required to prevent recurrences of iron deficiency anemia. The child's intake of iron-rich foods is increased, and the intake of cow's milk may be restricted, with the exact amount depending on the child's age (from 16 to 32 ounces). Limiting milk intake makes the child hungrier for other iron-rich foods and prevents gastrointestinal blood loss in children whose anemia is aggravated or caused by inflammatory reactions to proteins in cow's milk.

Hemolytic Disease of the Newborn

HDN can occur only if antigens on fetal erythrocytes differ from antigens on maternal erythrocytes. The antigenic properties of erythrocytes are determined genetically: they may be type A, B, or O and may or may not include Rh antigen D. Erythrocytes that express Rh antigen D are Rh-positive; those that do not are Rh-negative. The frequency of Rh negativity is higher in whites (15%) than in blacks (5%), and is rare in Asians. Maternal-fetal incompatibility exists if mother and fetus differ in ABO blood type or if the fetus is Rh-positive and the mother is Rh-negative. (The antigenic properties of erythrocytes are described in Chapter 8.)

ABO incompatibility occurs in about 20% to 25% of all pregnancies, but only 1 in 10 cases of ABO incompatibility results in HDN. Rh incompatibility occurs in less than 10% of pregnancies and rarely causes HDN in the first incompatible fetus. Even after five or more pregnancies, only 5% of women have babies with hemolytic disease. Usually erythrocytes from the first incompatible fetus cause the mother's immune system to produce antibodies that affect the fetuses of subsequent incompatible pregnancies. Only one in three cases of HDN is caused by Rh incompatibility; most cases are caused by ABO incompatibility.

PATHOPHYSIOLOGY If the mother and fetus have antigenically incompatible erythrocytes, HDN will result (1) if the mother's blood contains preformed antibodies against fetal erythrocytes or produces them on exposure to fetal erythrocytes, (2) if sufficient amounts of antibody (usually immunoglobulin G [IgG]) cross the placenta and enter fetal blood, and (3) if IgG binds with sufficient numbers of fetal erythrocytes to cause widespread antibody-mediated hemolysis or splenic removal. (Antibody-mediated cellular destruction is discussed in Chapter 7.)

Individuals usually form IgM antibodies against the ABO antigen they do not express; against the A antigen if the mother is blood type O or B or against the B antigen if the mother is type O or A. These are produced early in life against gastrointestinal bacteria that make antigens similar to A and B. IgM antibodies do not cross the placenta or cause HDN. Occasionally, a blood type O individual may have also produced IgG against the A or B antigen. If the fetus is blood group A or B, the ABO incompatibility can cause HDN in the first pregnancy. The severity of HDN is usually not severe because A and B antigens are expressed on most cells, including the placenta, and much of the IgG against A or B will be absorbed before encountering fetal blood cells.

Anti-Rh antibodies, on the other hand, are formed *only* in response to the presence of incompatible (Rh-positive) erythrocytes in the blood of an Rh-negative mother. Sources of exposure include fetal blood that is mixed with the mother's blood at the time of delivery, transfused blood, and, rarely, previous sensitization of the mother by her own mother's incompatible blood.

The first Rh-incompatible pregnancy usually presents no difficulties because very few fetal erythrocytes cross the placental barrier during gestation. When the placenta detaches at birth, however, large numbers of fetal erythrocytes usually enter the mother's bloodstream. If the mother is Rh-negative and the fetus is Rh-positive, the mother produces anti-Rh antibodies. The capacity of the mother's immune system to produce anti-Rh antibodies depends on many factors, including her genetic capacity to make antibodies against the Rh antigen D, the amount of fetal-to-maternal bleeding, and the occurrence of any bleeding earlier in the pregnancy. Anti-Rh antibodies persist in the bloodstream for a very long time, and if the next offspring is Rh-positive, the mother's anti-Rh antibodies can enter the fetus's bloodstream and destroy the erythrocytes. Antibodies against Rh antigen D are of the IgG class and easily cross the placenta.

IgG-coated fetal erythrocytes are destroyed extravascularly, primarily by mononuclear phagocytes in the spleen. As hemolysis proceeds, the fetus becomes anemic. Erythropoiesis accelerates, particularly in the liver and spleen, and immature nucleated cells (erythroblasts) are released into the bloodstream (hence the name *erythroblastosis fetalis*) (Figure 28-2). The degree of anemia depends on the length of

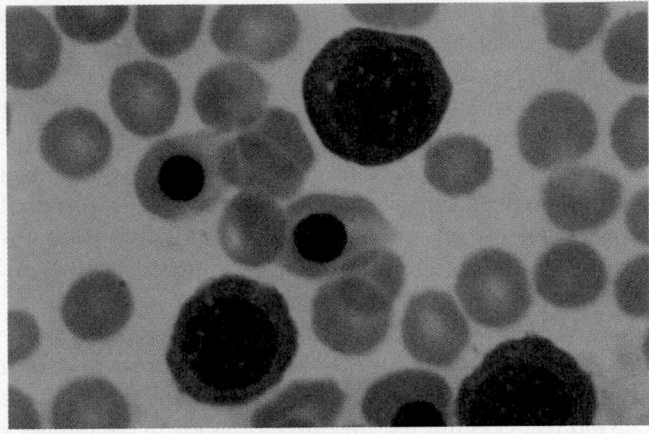

Figure 28-2 Rh incompatibility in hemolytic disease of the newborn. This micrograph shows immature red blood cells not normally found in blood. Large purple cells are erythroblasts; nucleated red blood cells are normoblasts. Normal red blood cells also are shown (× 500). (Copyright Ed Reschke.)

time the antibody has been in the fetal circulation, antibody concentration, and the ability of the fetus to compensate for increased hemolysis. Unconjugated (indirect) bilirubin, which is formed during breakdown of hemoglobin, is transported across the placental barrier into the maternal circulation and is excreted by the mother. **Hyperbilirubinemia** occurs in the neonate after birth because excretion of lipid-soluble unconjugated bilirubin through the placenta no longer is possible.

The pathophysiologic effects of HDN are more severe in Rh incompatibility than in ABO incompatibility. ABO incompatibility may resolve after birth without life-threatening complications. Maternal-fetal incompatibility in which a mother with type O blood has a child with type A or B blood usually is so mild that it does not require treatment.

Rh incompatibility is more likely than ABO incompatibility to cause severe or even life-threatening anemia, death in utero, or damage to the central nervous system (CNS). Severe anemia alone can cause death as a result of cardiovascular complications (see Chapter 26). Extensive hemolysis also results in increased levels of unconjugated bilirubin in the neonate's circulation. If bilirubin levels exceed the liver's ability to conjugate and excrete bilirubin, some of it is deposited in the brain, causing cellular damage and eventually, if the neonate does not receive exchange transfusions, death.

Fetuses that do not survive anemia in utero usually are stillborn, with gross edema in the entire body, a condition called **hydrops fetalis.** Death can occur as early as 17 weeks of gestation and results in spontaneous abortion.

CLINICAL MANIFESTATIONS Neonates with mild HDN may appear healthy or slightly pale, with slight enlargement of the liver and spleen. Pronounced pallor, splenomegaly, and hepatomegaly indicate severe anemia, which predisposes the neonate to cardiovascular failure and shock. Life-threatening Rh incompatibility is rare today, largely because of the routine use of Rh immune globulin.

Because the maternal antibodies remain in the neonate's circulatory system after birth, erythrocyte destruction can continue. This causes hyperbilirubinemia and **icterus neonatorum (neonatal jaundice)** shortly after birth. Without replacement transfusions, in which the child receives Rh-negative erythrocytes, the bilirubin is deposited in the brain, a condition termed **kernicterus.** Kernicterus produces cerebral damage and usually causes death (**icterus gravis neonatorum**). Infants who do not die may have mental retardation, cerebral palsy, or high-frequency deafness.

EVALUATION AND TREATMENT Routine evaluation of fetuses at risk for HDN (i.e., fetuses resulting from Rh- or ABO-incompatible matings) include the Coombs test. The indirect Coombs test measures antibody in the mother's circulation and indicates whether the fetus is at risk for HDN. The direct Coombs test measures antibody already bound to the surfaces of fetal erythrocytes and is used primarily to confirm the diagnosis of antibody-mediated HDN. Determining prior history of fetal hemolytic disease, as well as diagnostic tests, may help predict the severity of the disorder. Diagnostic measures include maternal antibody titers, fetal blood sampling, amniotic fluid spectrophotometry, and ultrasound fetal assessment.[10]

The key to treatment of HDN resulting from Rh incompatibility lies in prevention (immunoprophylaxis). One of the success stories of immunology has been the spectacular results obtained through the use of Rh immune globulin (RhoGAM), a preparation of antibody against Rh antigen D. If an Rh-negative woman is given Rh immune globulin within 72 hours of exposure to Rh-positive erythrocytes, she will not produce antibody against the D antigen and the next Rh-positive baby will be protected (Figure 28-3). The injected antibodies remain in the mother's bloodstream long enough to prevent her immune system from producing its own anti-Rh antibodies but not long enough to affect subsequent offspring. The mother must be given Rh immune globulin injections after the birth of each Rh-positive baby and after an miscarriage. Also the mother must be especially careful not to receive a transfusion containing Rh-positive blood, because this also would stimulate production of anti-Rh antibodies. In many hospitals, Rh immune globulin is given prophylactically at 28 weeks to all pregnant Rh-negative women with Rh-positive partners. Immunoprophylaxis with Rh immune globulin, unfortunately, appears to be underused in the United States. Failure to use immunoprophylaxis, such as in cases of unrecognized miscarriage, has led to a small increase in mothers who will require comprehensive treatment during subsequent pregnancies.[11]

If antigenic incompatibility of the mother's erythrocytes is not discovered in time to administer Rh immune globulin and a child is born with HDN, treatment consists of exchange transfusions in which the neonate's blood is replaced with new Rh-positive blood that is not contaminated with anti-Rh antibodies. This treatment is instituted during the first 24 hours of extrauterine life to prevent kernicterus. Phototherapy also is used to reduce the toxic effects of unconjugated bilirubin.

Jaundice and indirect hyperbilirubinemia are reduced when the infant is exposed to high-intensity light in the visible spectrum, the most effective being the blue range (from 420 to 470 nm). Bilirubin in the skin absorbs light energy, which, by photoisomerization, converts the toxic unconjugated bilirubin into conjugated isomers that are excreted in the bile. Phototherapy also causes autosensitization that results in oxidation reactions. Breakdown products from the oxidation reactions are excreted by the liver and kidney without need for conjugation. The therapeutic effect of phototherapy depends on the light energy emitted in the effective wavelengths, the distance between the infant and the light source, and the amount of skin exposed; the rate of hemolysis and the infant's ability to excrete bilirubin also are factors in determining the effectiveness of phototherapy in lowering serum bilirubin levels.

Anemia of Infectious Disease

Infections of the newborn, often initially acquired by the mother and transmitted to the fetus, may result in a hemolytic anemia with clinical manifestations similar to those of HDN. Congenital syphilis, toxoplasmosis, cytomegalic inclusion disease, rubella, coxsackievirus B infection, herpesvirus infection, and bacterial sepsis can cause hemolytic anemia in the neonate.

The exact mechanism of anemia caused by congenital infections is unclear. In some instances it is related to direct injury of erythrocyte membranes or erythrocyte precursors by the infectious microorganism. In other instances it results from traumatic destruction of erythrocytes during their passage through inflamed capillaries.

Inherited Disorders

A number of inherited and intrinsic erythrocyte defects are known to cause increased hemolysis (see Table 28-2). These defects may be associated with enzymatic abnormalities that disrupt metabolic processes and prevent normal biochemical balance within the cell, with alterations of hemoglobin structure or synthesis, or with plasma membrane defects accompanied by changes in erythrocyte size or shape.

Glucose-6-Phosphate Dehydrogenase Deficiency

Glucose-6-phosphate dehydrogenase (G6PD) deficiency is an inherited, X-linked recessive disorder, most fully expressed in homozygous males, although partial expression and a carrier state are possible in heterozygous females. (X-linked inheritance is discussed in Chapter 4.) The deficiency is present in 10% of blacks and tends to occur in Sephardic Jews, Greeks, Iranians, Chinese, Filipinos, and Indonesians, with a frequency ranging from 5% to 40%.

PATHOPHYSIOLOGY G6PD is an enzyme that normally enables erythrocytes to maintain metabolic processes despite injurious conditions, such as the presence of certain drugs (sulfonamides, antimalarial agents, salicylates, or naphthaquinolones); ingestion of fava beans (a dietary staple in some Mediterranean areas); hypoxemia; infection; fever; or

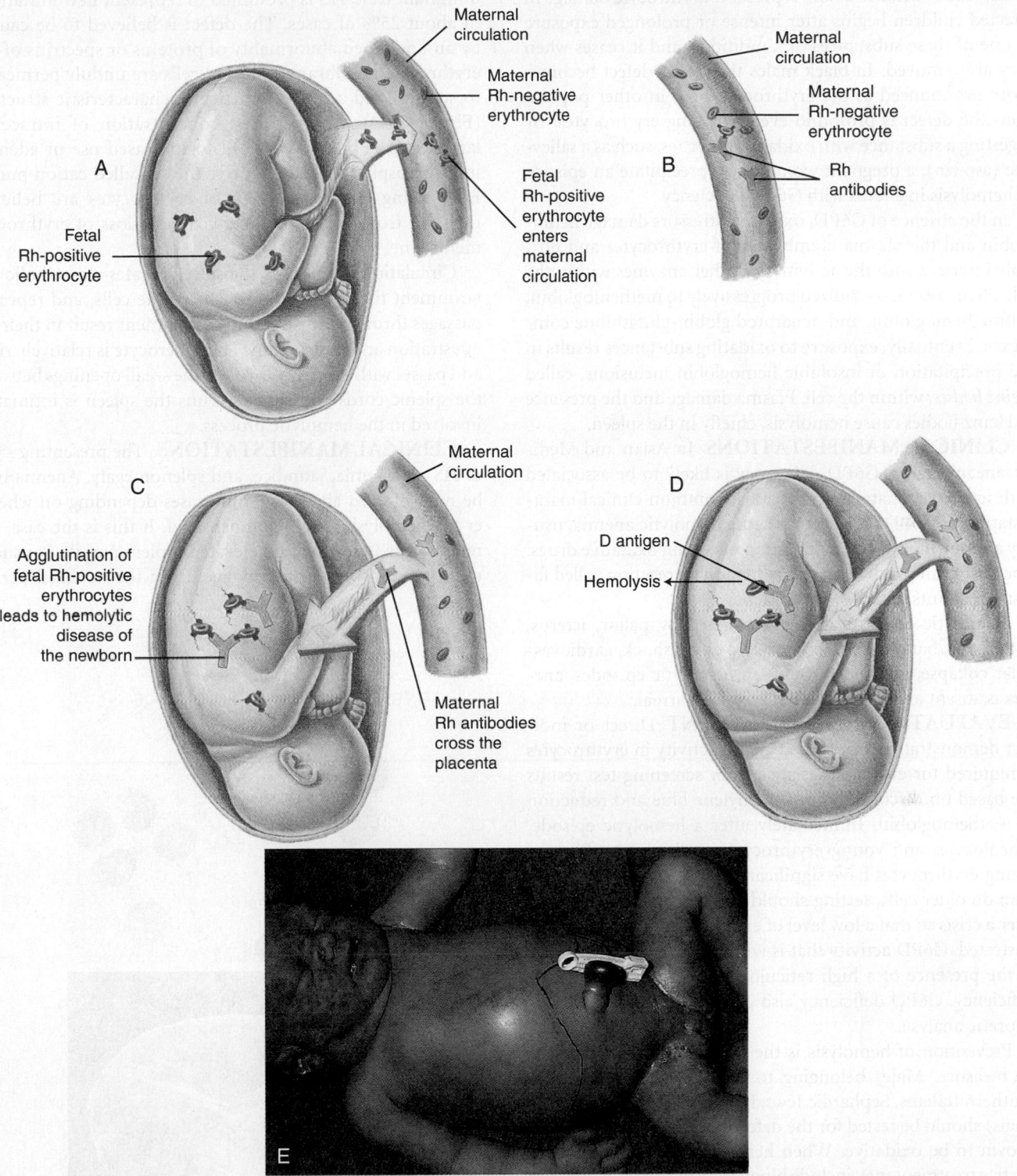

Figure 28-3 Hemolytic disease of the newborn (HDN). **A,** Before or during delivery, Rh-positive erythrocytes from the fetus enter the blood of an Rh-negative woman through a tear in the placenta. **B,** The mother is sensitized to the Rh antigen and produces Rh antibodies. Because this usually happens after delivery, there is no effect on the fetus in the first pregnancy. **C,** During a subsequent pregnancy with an Rh-positive fetus, Rh-positive erythrocytes cross the placenta, enter the maternal circulation, and **(D)** stimulate the mother to produce antibodies against the Rh antigen. The Rh antibodies from the mother cross the placenta, using agglutination and hemolysis of fetal erythrocytes, and HDN develops **(E).** (Modified from Seeley RR, Stephens TD, Tate P: *Anatomy and physiology,* ed 3, St Louis, 1995, Mosby.)

acidosis. Therefore, G6PD deficiency is usually asymptomatic unless one of these stressors is present. Erythrocyte damage in affected children begins after intense or prolonged exposure to one of these substances or conditions, and it ceases when they are removed. In black males the G6PD defect becomes more pronounced as the erythrocyte ages; in other populations the defect is profound even in young erythrocytes. By ingesting a substance with oxidant properties, such as a salicylate (aspirin), a pregnant woman may precipitate an episode of hemolysis in a fetus with G6PD deficiency.

In the absence of G6PD, oxidative stressors damage hemoglobin and the plasma membranes of erythrocytes and possibly interfere with the activities of other enzymes within the cell. Hemoglobin is oxidized progressively to methemoglobin, sulfmethemoglobin, and denatured globin-glutathione complexes. Eventually, exposure to oxidating substances results in the precipitation of insoluble hemoglobin inclusions, called *Heinz bodies*, within the cell. Plasma damage and the presence of Heinz bodies cause hemolysis, chiefly in the spleen.

CLINICAL MANIFESTATIONS In Asian and Mediterranean infants, G6PD deficiency is likely to be associated with icterus neonatorum. The most common clinical manifestation of G6PD deficiency is acute hemolytic anemia, usually after infections or the ingestion of certain oxidative drugs. The fava bean produces a severe hemolytic reaction called favism in infants with G6PD deficiency.[12]

Hemolytic episodes are characterized by pallor, icterus, dark urine, back pain, and, in severe cases, shock, cardiovascular collapse, and death. Between hemolytic episodes, anemia is absent and erythrocyte survival is normal.

EVALUATION AND TREATMENT Direct or indirect demonstration of reduced G6PD activity in erythrocytes is required for evaluation. Satisfactory screening test results are based on discoloration of methylene blue and reduction of methemoglobin. Immediately after a hemolytic episode, reticulocytes and young erythrocytes predominate. Because young erythrocytes have significantly higher enzyme activity than do older cells, testing should be performed a few weeks after a crisis so that a low level of enzyme activity can be demonstrated. G6PD activity that is within the low normal range in the presence of a high reticulocyte count suggests G6PD deficiency. G6PD deficiency also can be detected by electrophoretic analysis.

Prevention of hemolysis is the most important therapeutic measure. Males belonging to high-risk groups (Greeks, southern Italians, Sephardic Jews, Filipinos, Chinese, Africans, Thais) should be tested for the defect before being given drugs known to be oxidative. When hemolysis has occurred, supportive treatment may include blood transfusions and oral iron therapy. Spontaneous recovery generally follows treatment.

Hereditary Spherocytosis

Hereditary spherocytosis (HS), also known as *congenital hemolytic anemia* or *congenital acholuric jaundice*, is the most common of the hemolytic disorders in which there is no abnormality of hemoglobin.

PATHOPHYSIOLOGY Transmitted as an autosomal dominant trait, HS is presumed to represent new mutations in about 25% of cases. The defect is believed to be caused by an undefined abnormality of proteins or spectrins of the erythrocyte membrane. Affected cells are unduly permeable to sodium and acquire a particular characteristic structure (Figure 28-4). An increased concentration of intracellular sodium is believed to lead to increased use of adenosine triphosphate (ATP) to drive the so-called cation pump. Early aging and destruction of erythrocytes are believed to result from metabolic overwork and loss of erythrocyte membrane.[13]

Circulation of blood to the spleen creates a metabolic environment that is stressful to spherocyte cells, and repeated passages through this stressful environment result in their sequestration and destruction. The spherocyte is relatively rigid and passes with difficulty through the small openings between the splenic cords and sinuses. Thus the spleen is intimately involved in the hemolytic process.

CLINICAL MANIFESTATIONS The presenting signs of HS are anemia, jaundice, and splenomegaly. Anemia may be mild of even absent in some cases depending on whether the hemolysis is well compensated. If this is the case, the reticulocyte count will be elevated. Splenomegaly is usually mild. HS can present at any age, from the neonatal period

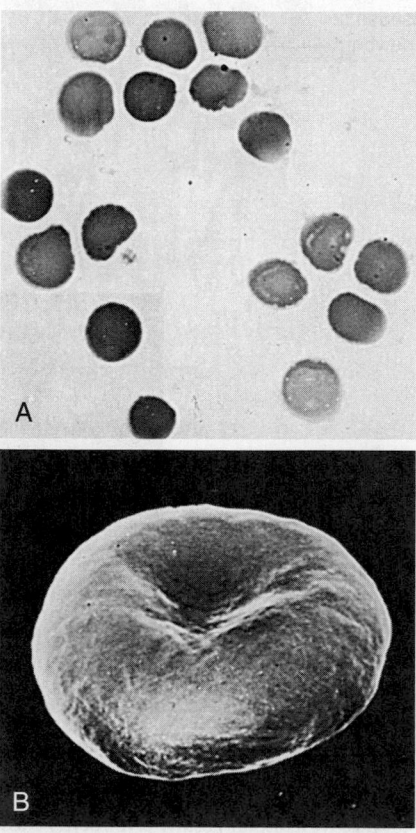

Figure 28-4 The microspherocyte. **A,** Blood smear from individual with hereditary spherocytosis (Wright stain). **B,** Scanning electron micrograph. (Courtesy Dr. M Bessis. From Miale JB: *Laboratory medicine: hematology,* ed 6, St Louis, 1982, Mosby.)

until older adulthood. More severe types of HS present with signs of hemolytic anemia and hyperbilirubinemia during the newborn period.[14] Children who suffer from HS may have values considerably lower than children who do not. These children therefore may have life-threatening anemia with clinical symptoms ranging from difficulty tolerating feeding, circumoral pallor, tachycardia, nasal flaring, diaphoretic episodes, and lethargy. These children also are at increased risk for gallstones because their bodies make extra bile pigment. Infection (specifically parvovirus), fever, and stress can stimulate the spleen to destroy more red blood cells than usual, leading to a worsening anemia in an already baseline anemic child.

EVALUATION AND TREATMENT It is important to ascertain family history of spherocytosis. Laboratory findings include spherocytes in the peripheral blood smear, elevated reticulocyte count with or without anemia, indirect hyperbilirubinemia, and a positive osmotic fragility test. An osmotic fragility test is performed by placing the individual's red blood cells in a saline solution for 24 hours. Spherocytes do not tolerate weak saline solutions, thus causing them to burst more readily than normal cells. Treatment of HS is based on disease severity. Although some children with severe HS will have severe anemia, blood transfusions are rarely required. Treatment before the age of 5 years consists of daily folic acid supplementation to help with production of healthy red blood cells. In the past, splenectomy was the first line of treatment. Currently, however, splenectomy is only recommended for those children older than 5 years of age with severe disease or those who develop symptomatic gallstones. Partial splenectomy, in which only a portion of the spleen is removed, is being performed on children with HS in an attempt to decrease the risk of postsplenectomy complications.[15]

Sickle Cell Disease

Sickle cell disease (SCD) is a group of disorders characterized by the presence of an abnormal form of hemoglobin—**hemoglobin S (Hb S)**—within the erythrocytes. Hb S is formed by a genetic mutation in which one amino acid (valine) replaces another (glutamic acid) (Figure 28-5, A). Hb S, the so-called sickle hemoglobin, reacts to deoxygenation and dehydration by solidifying and stretching the erythrocyte into an elongated sickle shape. This change has a variety of pathologic consequences, including hemolytic anemia.

SCD is an inherited autosomal recessive disorder that is expressed as sickle cell anemia, sickle cell–thalassemia disease, or sickle cell–Hb C disease, depending on mode of inheritance (Table 28-3). (See Chapter 4 for a discussion of genetic inheritance of disease.) **Sickle cell anemia,** a homozygous form, is the most severe. **Sickle cell–thalassemia disease** and **sickle cell–Hb C disease** are heterozygous forms in which the child simultaneously inherits another type of abnormal hemoglobin from one parent. **Sickle cell trait,** in which the child inherits Hb S from one parent and normal hemoglobin (Hb A) from the other, is a heterozygous carrier state that rarely has

clinical manifestations. All forms of SCD are lifelong conditions and have no known cure.

SCD tends to occur in people with origins in equatorial countries, particularly central Africa, the Near East, the Mediterranean area, and parts of India. In the United States, SCD is most common in blacks, with a reported incidence ranging from 1 in 400 to 1 in 500 live births. In the general population the risk of two black parents having a child with sickle cell anemia is 0.7%. Sickle cell–Hb C disease is less common (1 in 800 births), and sickle cell–thalassemia disease occurs in 1 in 1700 births.

Sickle cell trait occurs in 7% to 13% of blacks, whereas its incidence among East Africans may be as high as 45%. The sickle cell trait may provide protection against lethal forms of malaria, a genetic advantage to carriers who reside in endemic regions for malaria (Mediterranean and African zones) but no advantage to carriers living in the United States.

PATHOPHYSIOLOGY Deoxygenation is probably the most important variable in determining the occurrence of sickling.[16] The degree of deoxygenation required to produce sickling varies with the percentage of Hb S in the cells. Sickle trait cells will sickle at oxygen tensions of about 15 mm Hg, whereas those from an individual with SCD will begin to sickle at about 40 mmHg. Hb S that is not bound with oxygen forms aggregates of semisolid gel that become stacked within the erythrocyte, stretching it into an elongated crescent (Figures 28-5, C and 28-6). Sickled erythrocytes are stiff and cannot change shape as easily as normal cells when they pass through the microcirculation. (The reversible deformability of erythrocytes is described in Chapter 25.) As a result, sickled erythrocytes tend to plug the blood vessels, causing vascular occlusion, pain, and organ infarction. Sickled cells undergo hemolysis in the spleen or become sequestered there, causing blood pooling and infarction of splenic vessels. The anemia that follows triggers erythropoiesis in the marrow and, in extreme cases, in the liver.

Sickling usually is not permanent; most sickled erythrocytes regain a normal shape after reoxygenation and rehydration. Irreversible sickling is not caused by irreversible hemoglobin changes but rather by irreversible plasma membrane damage caused by sickling. The precise nature of the permanent membrane injury is not known, but it is known that while in the sickled state, the plasma membrane loses some of its capacity for active transport, permitting an influx of calcium ions. (Membrane transport and the effects of calcium influx are described in Chapters 1 and 2.) In people with sickle cell anemia, in which the erythrocytes contain a high percentage of Hb S (75% to 95%), up to 30% of the erythrocytes can become irreversibly sickled. Occasionally, irreversible sickling occurs in SCD but never in the carrier state (sickle cell trait).

Sickling is an occasional, intermittent phenomenon that can be triggered or sustained by one or more of the following stressors: decreased oxygen tension (Po_2) of the blood (i.e., hypoxemia), increased hydrogen ion concentration in the blood (decreased pH), increased plasma osmolality, decreased plasma volume, and low temperature (Figure 28-7).

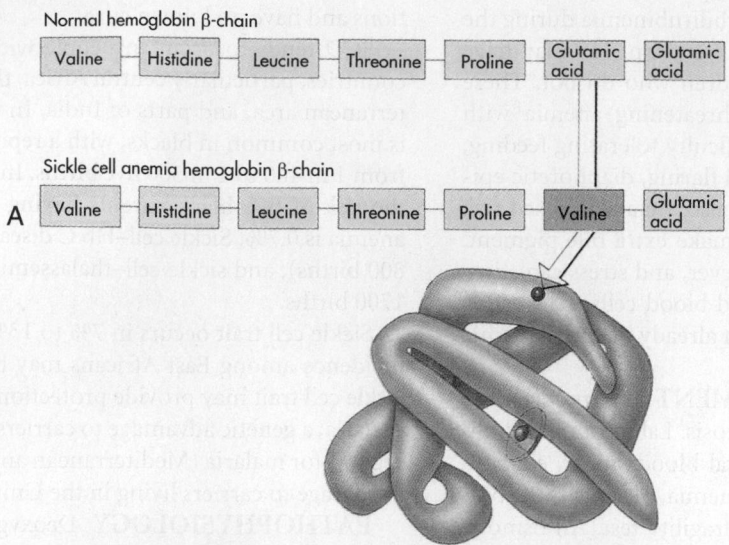

Normal hemoglobin β-chain

| Valine | Histidine | Leucine | Threonine | Proline | Glutamic acid | Glutamic acid |

Sickle cell anemia hemoglobin β-chain

A | Valine | Histidine | Leucine | Threonine | Proline | Valine | Glutamic acid |

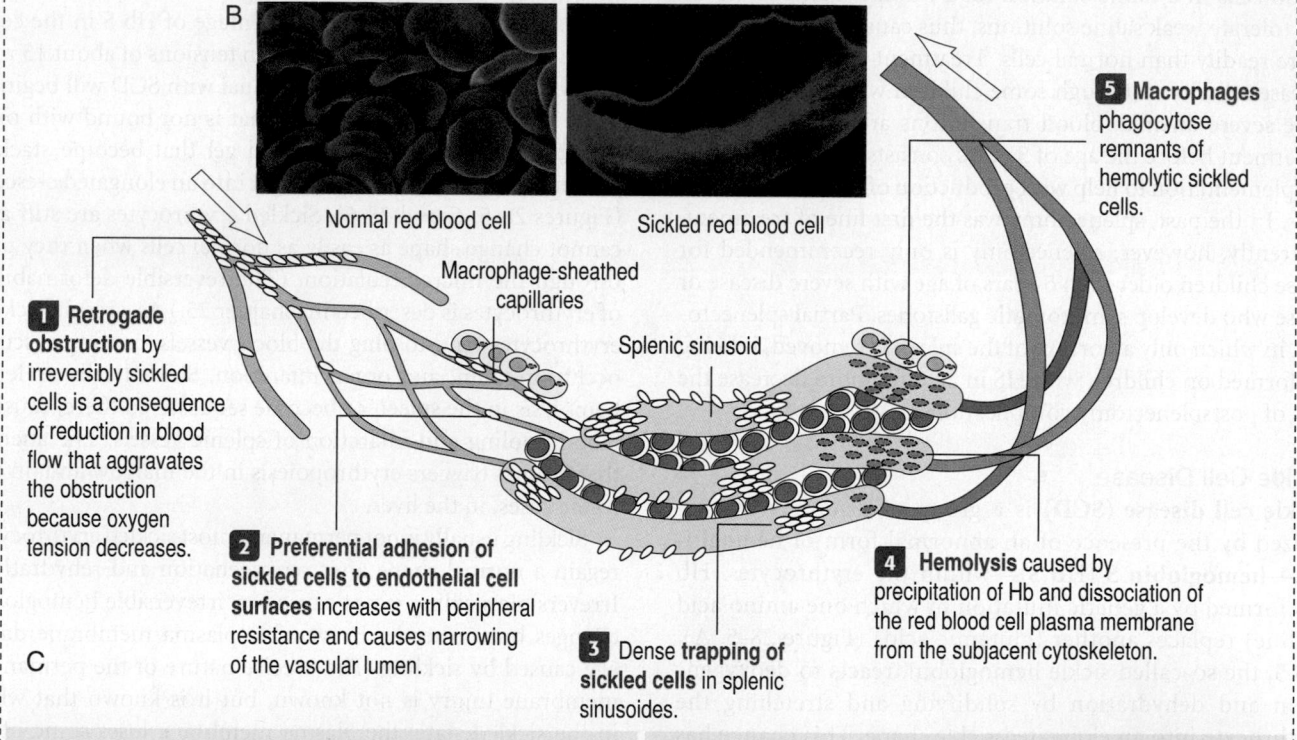

B

Normal red blood cell   Sickled red blood cell

Macrophage-sheathed capillaries

Splenic sinusoid

5 Macrophages phagocytose remnants of hemolytic sickled cells.

1 Retrogade obstruction by irreversibly sickled cells is a consequence of reduction in blood flow that aggravates the obstruction because oxygen tension decreases.

2 Preferential adhesion of sickled cells to endothelial cell surfaces increases with peripheral resistance and causes narrowing of the vascular lumen.

3 Dense trapping of sickled cells in splenic sinusoides.

4 Hemolysis caused by precipitation of Hb and dissociation of the red blood cell plasma membrane from the subjacent cytoskeleton.

C

Sickle cell anemia is determined by the substitution of normal hemoglobin (Hb A) by hemoglobin S (Hb S) caused by a point mutation (replacement of the nucleotide triplet CTC coding glutamic acid at the mRNA level [GAG] by the CAC triplet [GUG] coding for valine) that modifies the physicochemical properties of the β-globin chain of hemoglobin. All hemoglobin is abnormal in homozygous individuals for the mutant gene, and red blood cells

show a sickling deformity and hemolytic anemia in the presence or absence of normal oxygen tension. Heterozygous individuals contain a mixture of Hb A and Hb S, and sickling and anemia are observed when the tension of oxygen decreases.

Irreversibly sickled red blood cells are trapped within the splenic sinusoids and are destroyed by adjacent macrophages. Hemolysis may also occur in the macrophage-sheathed capillaries of the red pulp.

Figure 28-5 Sickle cell hemoglobin. **A,** Sickle cell hemoglobin is produced by a recessive allele of the gene encoding the β-chain of the protein hemoglobin. It represents a single amino acid change—from glutamic acid to valine at the sixth position on the chain. In this model of a hemoglobin molecule, the position of the mutation can be seen near the end of the upper arm. **B,** Color-enhanced electron micrograph shows normal erythrocytes. **C,** Illustration of the characteristic shape of a red blood cell containing the abnormal hemoglobin. (**A** from Raven PH, Johnson GB: *Biology,* ed 3, St Louis, 1992, Mosby. **B** copyright Dennis Kunkel Microscopy, Inc. **C** from Miale JB: *Laboratory medicine: hematology,* ed 6, St Louis, 1982, Mosby.)

Table 28-3	Inheritance of Sickle Cell Disease	
Hemoglobin (Hb) Inherited from First Parent	Hemoglobin Inherited from Second Parent	Form of Sickle Cell Disease in Child
Hb S (an abnormal Hb)	Hb S	Sickle cell anemia: homozygous inheritance in which the child's Hb is mostly Hb S, with the remainder fetal hemoglobin (Hb F)
Hb S	Defective or insufficient α- or β-chains of Hb A (alpha- or beta-thalassemia)	Sickle cell: thalassemia disease (heterozygous inheritance of Hb S and alpha- or beta-thalassemia)
Hb S	Hb C or D (both abnormal Hb)	Sickle cell: Hb C (or D) disease (heterozygous inheritance of Hb S and either Hb C or Hb D)
Hb S	Normal Hb (mostly Hb A)	Sickle cell trait, the carrier state (heterozygous inheritance of Hb S and normal Hb)

NOTE: See Chapter 25 for a description of normal fetal and adult hemoglobins.

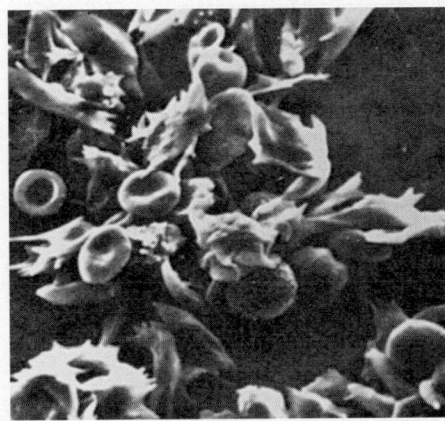

Figure 28-6 Normal and sickle-shaped blood cells. Scanning electron micrograph of normal and sickle-shaped red blood cells. The irregularly shaped cells are the sickle cells; the circular cells are the normal blood cells. (From Raven PH, Johnson GB: *Biology*, ed 3, St Louis, 1992, Mosby.)

The same decrease in Po_2 will cause the most sickling in persons with sickle cell anemia (high concentrations of Hb S), the second most in children with sickle cell thalassemia, the third most in those with sickle cell–Hb C disease, and the least or none in those with sickle cell trait. The duration of the Po_2 decrease also is important, because sickling tends to occur only after the inciting stimulus has been present for some time.

The level of Po_2 in the microcirculation also affects sickling because hemoglobin releases whatever oxygen it is carrying to tissues. The Po_2 normally is lower in the microcirculation. The added reduction in Po_2 caused by persistent hypoxemia—induced by stressors—eventually results in sickling in the microcirculation of all cells that contain Hb S in that site (not throughout the body). Sickling within the microcirculation decreases blood flow as sickled cells clog the vessels. Slow blood flow promotes hypoxemia and perpetuates sickling. Finally, decreased blood pH decreases hemoglobin's affinity for oxygen. As less oxygen is taken up by hemoglobin in the lungs, Po_2 drops, promoting sickling further.

Polymerization of sickle hemoglobin is central to the disorder. **Polymerization** stiffens the sickle erythrocyte, changing it from a flexible, nourishing cell to an inflexible obstacle that starves and damages tissues.

Increased osmolality of the plasma (increased concentration of solutes; see Chapters 1 and 3) draws water out of the erythrocytes. This promotes sickling by raising the relative Hb S content in erythrocytes. Decreased plasma volume, which occurs in states of dehydration, causes the blood to become viscous (thick and sticky). Increased viscosity of the blood is the final common pathway leading to many pathologic effects. Viscous blood flows slowly and promotes vascular obstruction by increasing opportunities for sickling while decreasing opportunities for reoxygenation in the lungs. This is an example of positive feedback in a vicious cycle of events. Low temperatures precipitate sickle crisis, presumably because of vasoconstriction.[16]

Once sickling begins, it tends to perpetuate itself until Po_2 returns to normal; then it ceases spontaneously. The extent, severity, and clinical manifestations of sickling depend to a great extent on the percentage of hemoglobin that is Hb S. That is why homozygous inheritance of Hb S produces the severest form of SCD—sickle cell anemia. Heterozygous inheritance of SCD results in less sickling because the individual's erythrocytes contain other forms of abnormal hemoglobin that although defective, do not participate in sickling to any great degree. Heterozygous inheritance (sickle cell trait), in which abnormal hemoglobin is inherited from one parent and normal hemoglobin from the other, rarely results in sickling because normal Hb F and Hb A do not participate in sickling at all. Anemia persists because Hb F does not live 120 days.

CLINICAL MANIFESTATIONS Clinical manifestations of SCD may first be seen at 6 to 12 months of age as fetal hemoglobin is replaced by Hb S. There are two characteristics of SCD that determine presentation. The first is its nature to be a chronic disease with acute exacerbations. The second is that it is a condition affecting red blood cells that supply oxygen to all cells of the body. Therefore, SCD can affect any part of the body. When sickling occurs, the general manifestations of hemolytic anemia—pallor, fatigue, jaundice, and irritability—sometimes are accompanied by acute manifestations called *crises*. Extensive sickling can precipitate four types of crises:

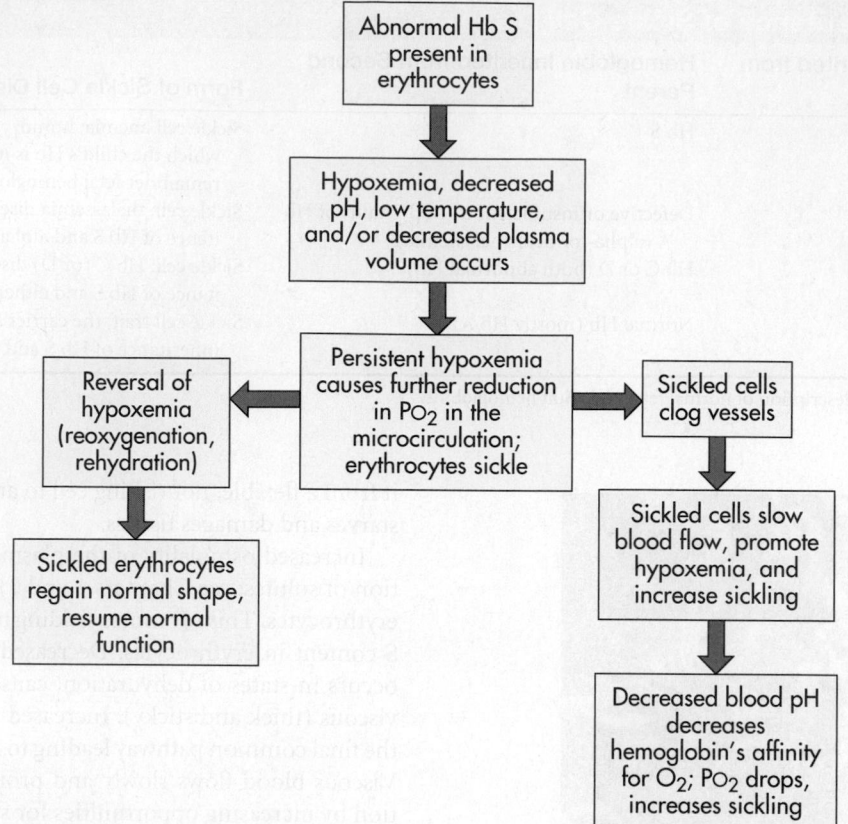

Figure 28-7 Sickling of erythrocytes.

(1) vasoocclusive (or thrombotic) crisis, (2) aplastic crisis, (3) sequestration crisis, or rarely (4) hyperhemolytic crisis. Sites of specific dysfunction are shown in Figure 28-8.

Vasoocclusive crisis (thrombotic crisis) begins with sickling in the microcirculation. As blood flow is obstructed by tangled masses of rigid, sickled cells, vasospasm occurs and a "logjam" effect brings all blood flow through the vessel to a halt. Unless the process is reversed, thrombosis and infarction (death caused by lack of oxygen) of local tissue follow. Vasoocclusive crisis is extremely painful and may last for days or even weeks, with an average duration of 4 to 6 days. The frequency of this type of crisis is variable and unpredictable.

Vasoocclusive crises may develop spontaneously or be precipitated by infection, exposure to cold, dehydration, low Po_2, acidosis (low pH), or localized hypoxemia. Symmetric, painful swelling of the hands and feet (hand-foot syndrome) caused by infarction in the small vessels of the extremities often is the initial manifestation of SCD in infancy. In older children and adults the large joints and surrounding tissue become painful and swollen. Priapism (persistent erection of the penis) may occur if penile veins become obstructed. Severe abdominal pains often are caused by infarction in abdominal structures. Strokes resulting from cerebral occlusion may leave the child with paralysis (usually hemiplegia) or other CNS deficits.

Aplastic crisis, a transient cessation in red blood cell production resulting in acute anemia, occurs as a result of a viral infection, almost always infection with parvovirus B19 which is the virus responsible for the common childhood infection known as fifth disease. The virus causes temporary shutdown of red blood cell production in the bone marrow, or reticulocytosis. However, hemolysis, a component of SCD, continues. The outcome is a severe drop in hemoglobin with an extremely low reticulocyte count.

In **sequestration crisis** large amounts of blood become acutely pooled in the liver and spleen. This type of crisis is seen only in a young child. Because the spleen can hold as much as one fifth of the body's blood supply at one time, mortality rates up to 50% have been reported, with death caused by cardiovascular collapse. If blood volume and pressure are maintained by hydration and blood transfusion, much of the sequestered blood eventually is remobilized. Removal of the spleen is the treatment for recurrent sequestration crises and may be performed after the child reaches 5 years of age.[17]

Hyperhemolytic crisis, an accelerated rate of red blood cell destruction, is unusual but may occur in association with certain drugs or infections. It is characterized by anemia, jaundice, and reticulocytosis. The concomitant presence of G6PD deficiency (see p. 1068) contributes to hyperhemolytic episodes, especially when combined with infections.

Acute chest syndrome is the presence of a new pulmonary infiltrate (involving at least one complete lung segment—not atelectasis) with chest pain, a temperature of more than 38.5° C (101.3° F) increased respiratory rate (tachypnea), wheezing,

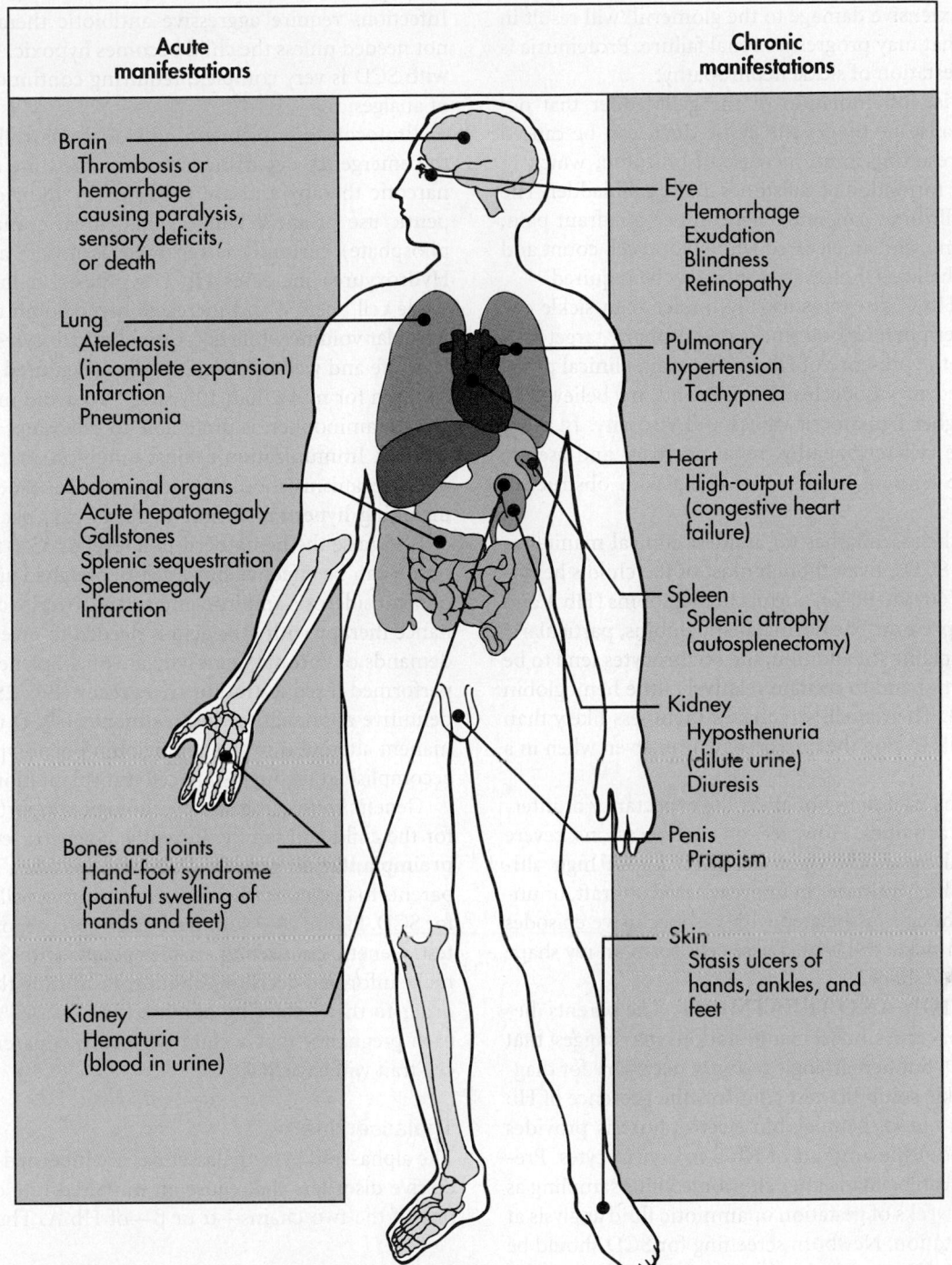

Figure 28-8 Clinical manifestations of sickle cell disease.

Acute manifestations

Brain
  Thrombosis or hemorrhage causing paralysis, sensory deficits, or death

Lung
  Atelectasis (incomplete expansion)
  Infarction
  Pneumonia

Abdominal organs
  Acute hepatomegaly
  Gallstones
  Splenic sequestration
  Splenomegaly
  Infarction

Bones and joints
  Hand-foot syndrome (painful swelling of hands and feet)

Kidney
  Hematuria (blood in urine)

Chronic manifestations

Eye
  Hemorrhage
  Exudation
  Blindness
  Retinopathy

Pulmonary hypertension
  Tachypnea

Heart
  High-output failure (congestive heart failure)

Spleen
  Splenic atrophy (autosplenectomy)

Kidney
  Hyposthenuria (dilute urine)
  Diuresis

Penis
  Priapism

Skin
  Stasis ulcers of hands, ankles, and feet

or cough in an individual with SCD. An injured, underventilated, and inflamed lung becomes "spleenlike" as sickled red cells attach to its endothelium, fails to be reoxygenated, and eventually undergoes more inflammation and lung infarction. The prognosis is poor, and infarction is a leading cause of morbidity. Acute chest syndrome is the cause of death in approximately 25% of all deaths in persons with SCD.[17]

Infection is the most common cause of death resulting from SCD. Sepsis and meningitis develop in as many as 10%

of children with sickle cell anemia during the first 5 years of life, with a mortality rate of 25%. Survival time is unpredictable, and many young adults die in their 20s.

Glomerular disease, characterized by damage to the glomeruli allowing protein and often red blood cells to leak into the urine, can be caused by sickling of red blood cells in the kidneys, which also can damage the glomeruli. The earliest manifestation of SCD in the kidney is hyposthenuria, or the ability to concentrate urine. In young children this often results in bed-wetting. Extensive damage to the glomeruli will result in nephropathy that may progress to renal failure. Proteinuria is an early manifestation of sickle nephropathy.

Cholecystitis, inflammation of the gallbladder that occurs when a gallstone blocks the cystic duct, can be caused by hemolysis resulting in an increase of bilirubin, which in turn causes the formation of gallstones in the gallbladder. The presence of gallstones can cause right upper quadrant pain, nausea, vomiting, and an elevated white blood cell count and alkaline phosphatase. Cholecystectomy may be required.

Sickle cell–Hb C disease is usually milder than sickle cell anemia. The peripheral blood smear reveals many target cells resulting from the presence of Hb C. The main clinical problems are related to vasoocclusive crises and are believed to result from higher hematocrit values and viscosity. In older children, sickle cell retinopathy, renal necrosis, and aseptic necrosis of the femoral heads occur along with obstructive crises.

Sickle cell–thalassemia has the mildest clinical manifestations of all the SCDs. Even though most of the child's hemoglobin is Hb S (60% to 90%), normal hemoglobins (Hb A and Hb F) also are present. The normal hemoglobins, particularly Hb F, inhibit sickling. In addition, the erythrocytes tend to be small (microcytic) and to contain relatively little hemoglobin (hypochromic). Their small size makes them less likely than normal-size cells to clog the microcirculation, even when in a sickled state.

The sickle cell trait does not affect life expectancy or interfere with daily activities. However, on rare occasions, severe hypoxia caused by shock, vigorous exercising at high altitudes, flying at high altitudes in unpressurized aircraft, or undergoing anesthesia is associated with vasoocclusive episodes in persons with sickle cell trait. These cells form an ivy shape instead of a sickle shape.

EVALUATION AND TREATMENT The parents' hematologic history and clinical manifestations may suggest that a child has SCD, but hematologic tests are necessary for diagnosis. If the sickle solubility test confirms the presence of Hb S in peripheral blood, hemoglobin electrophoresis provides information about the amount of Hb S in erythrocytes. Prenatal diagnosis can be made after chorionic villus sampling as early as 8 to 10 weeks of gestation or amniotic fluid analysis at 15 weeks of gestation. Newborn screening for SCD should be performed according to state law.

Treatment advances over the past 25 years have significantly decreased morbidity and mortality in children with SCD. Aggressive management of fever, early diagnosis of *acute chest syndrome* (hypoxia, decreased hemoglobin, progressive multilobar pneumonia, fat emboli), judicious use of transfusions, and proper treatment of pain can improve quality of life and prognosis for these children. Treatment of SCD consists of supportive care aimed at preventing consequences of anemia and avoiding crises. Crises can be prevented by avoiding fever, infection, acidosis, dehydration, constricting clothes, and exposure to cold. Immediate correction of acidosis and dehydration with appropriate intravenous fluids is imperative.

Infections require aggressive antibiotic therapy. Oxygen is not needed unless the child becomes hypoxic. Pain associated with SCD is very complex, requiring continuous adjustment of analgesics.

Protocols to implement individual-controlled analgesia in the emergency department shorten the time of initiation of narcotic therapy and are preferred by individuals.[18] Therapeutic use of antisickling agents (urea, cyanate, carbamoyl phosphate) currently is regarded as unsafe and ineffective. Hydroxyurea increases Hb F synthesis in individuals with sickle cell anemia and increases hemoglobin and mean corpuscular volume while decreasing reticulocytes and bilirubin. It is safe and well tolerated and has been used successfully in children for more than 10 years.[19] To avoid increased acidosis, acetaminophen is preferable to salicylates for antipyretic therapy. Immunization against influenza and pneumococcal microorganisms should be administered. Blood transfusion, including hypertransfusion therapy (e.g., packed red blood cells to raise the hematocrit to a level of 35% for a period of time), can be effective but must be weighed against the risks of hemosiderosis and iron and splenic overload. Oral maintenance therapy with folic acid is needed to meet the increased demands of chronic hemolytic anemia. Splenectomy may be performed if sequestration crises recur (Box 28-1). The most definitive approach to the treatment of SCD requires a permanent alteration in the hemoglobin phenotype. This can be accomplished through stem cell transplantation.

Genetic counseling and psychologic support are important for the child and family. Recently, a genetic technique called **preimplantation genetic diagnosis** has been performed on parents to diagnose whether their offspring will carry the gene for SCD. Figure 28-9 summarizes this prepregnancy sickle cell test. Genetic counseling enables people with SCD or trait to make informed decisions about transmitting this genetic disorder to their offspring because there is a 25% chance with each pregnancy that a child born to two parents with sickle cell trait will have SCD.

Thalassemias

The alpha- and beta-thalassemias are inherited autosomal recessive disorders that cause an impaired rate of synthesis of one of the two chains—α or β—of Hb A. The disorder was

---

Box 28-1   Laparoscopic Splenectomy

Laparoscopic splenectomy (LS) has been demonstrated to be safe and effective in children with hematologic disorders and is associated with minimal complications, zero mortality, and a short hospital stay. Between August 1995 and February 2001, 112 children underwent LS at a single pediatric facility. Three children required conversion to open splenectomy. Complications included ileus (4), acute chest syndrome (4), bleeding (2), pneumonia (1), and diaphragm perforation (1). None of the children died as a result of the procedure. Average length of stay was 1.51 days (range from 1 to 11 days).

Data from Rescorla FJ et al: *Am Surg* 68(3):297-301, 2002.

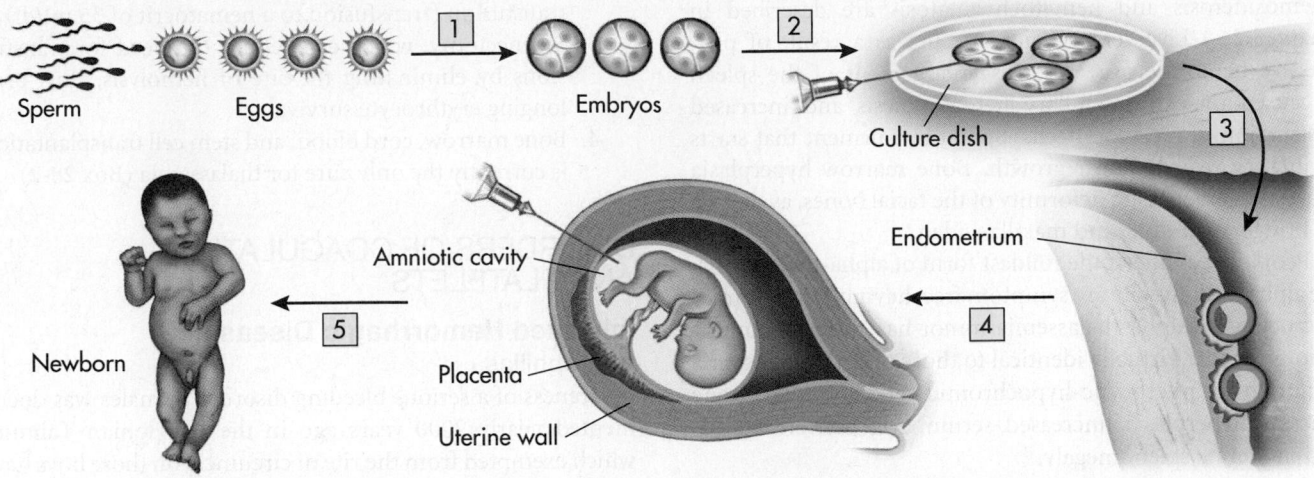

Figure 28-9 Prepregnancy sickle cell test. (This technique has potential for other inherited diseases.) 1, Fertilization produces several embryos. 2, The embryos are tested for the presence of the gene. 3, The embryo(s) without the gene are implanted. 4, Amniocentesis confirms whether the fetus (or fetuses) has the sickle cell gene. 5, Woman has a normal child.

named **thalassemia,** which is derived from the Greek word for *sea,* because it was defined initially in persons with origins near the Mediterranean Sea. Beta-thalassemia, in which synthesis of the β-globin chain is slowed or defective, is prevalent among Greeks, Italians, and some Arabs and Sephardic Jews. Alpha-thalassemia, in which the α-chain is affected, is most common among Chinese, Vietnamese, Cambodians, and Laotians. Both alpha- and beta-thalassemia are common among blacks.

Alpha- and beta-thalassemia can be major or minor, depending on how many of the genes that control α- or β-chain synthesis are defective and whether the defects are inherited homozygously (thalassemia major) or heterozygously (thalassemia minor). Pathophysiologic effects range from mild microcytosis to death in utero, depending on the number of defective genes and mode of inheritance. The anemic manifestation of thalassemia is microcytic-hypochromic hemolytic anemia.

PATHOPHYSIOLOGY Normally two genes control β-chain synthesis and four genes control α-chain synthesis. The number of genetic defects in the controlling genes determines the severity of the disorder. As in SCD the hemoglobin abnormality usually consists of the substitution of a single amino acid for another amino acid. Other molecular abnormalities that cause thalassemia are two amino acid substitutions, amino acid deletions or fusions, and synthesis of elongated chains.

The fundamental defect in beta-thalassemia is the uncoupling of α- and β-chain synthesis. β-Chain production is depressed—moderately in the heterozygous form, **beta-thalassemia minor,** and severely in the homozygous form, **beta-thalassemia major** (also called **Cooley anemia**). Depression of β-chain synthesis results in erythrocytes having a reduced amount of hemoglobin and accumulations of free α-chains. The free α-chains are unstable and easily precipitate

in the cell. Most erythroblasts that contain precipitates are destroyed by mononuclear phagocytes in the marrow, resulting in ineffective erythropoiesis and anemia. Some of the precipitate-carrying cells do mature and enter the bloodstream, but they are destroyed prematurely in the spleen, resulting in mild hemolytic anemia.

There are four forms of alpha-thalassemia:
1. **Alpha trait** (the carrier state), in which a single α-chain–forming gene is defective
2. **Alpha-thalassemia minor,** in which two genes are defective
3. **Hemoglobin H disease,** in which three genes are defective
4. **Alpha-thalassemia major,** a fatal condition in which all four alpha-forming genes are defective; death is inevitable because α-chains are absent and oxygen cannot be released to the tissues

Beta-thalassemia occurs more commonly than does alpha-thalassemia. Occasionally synthesis of γ- or δ-polypeptide chains is defective, resulting in gamma- or delta-thalassemia. (Hemoglobin chains are described in Chapter 25.)

CLINICAL MANIFESTATIONS Beta-thalassemia minor causes mild to moderate microcytic-hypochromic anemia, mild splenomegaly, bronze coloring of the skin, and hyperplasia of the bone marrow. The degree of reticulocytosis depends on the severity of the anemia, resulting in skeletal changes. Hemolysis of immature (and therefore fragile) erythrocytes may cause a slight elevation in serum iron and indirect bilirubin levels. Persons with beta-thalassemia minor usually are asymptomatic.

Persons with beta-thalassemia major may become quite ill. Anemia is severe and results in a significant cardiovascular burden, with high-output congestive heart failure. In the past, death resulted from cardiac failure. Today, blood transfusions can increase life span by one to two decades, and death usually is caused by hemochromatosis (from transfusions). (Hemosiderosis and hematochromatosis are described in Chapter 26.) Liver enlargement occurs as a result of progressive hemosiderosis, whereas enlargement of the spleen is caused by extramedullary hematopoiesis and increased destruction of red blood cells. Spinal impairment that starts in infancy retards linear growth. Bone marrow hyperplasia causes a characteristic deformity of the facial bones, as the nasal bridge, mandible, and maxilla widen.

People who inherit the mildest form of alpha-thalassemia, the alpha trait, usually are symptom free, having, at most, mild microcytosis. Alpha-thalassemia minor has clinical manifestations that are virtually identical to those of beta-thalassemia minor: mild microcytic-hypochromic reticulocytosis, bone marrow hyperplasia, increased serum iron concentrations, and moderate splenomegaly.

Signs and symptoms of alpha-thalassemia are similar to those of beta-thalassemia major but milder. Moderate microcytic-hypochromic anemia, enlargement of the liver and spleen, and bone marrow hyperplasia are evident.

Alpha-thalassemia major causes hydrops fetalis and fulminant intrauterine congestive heart failure. In addition to edema and massive ascites, the fetus has a grossly enlarged heart and liver. Diagnosis usually is made postmortem. Prenatal screening for this disorder can be performed by use of chorionic villus sampling. These cells can be analyzed, and a deoxyribonucleic acid (DNA) genetic map can be constructed and evaluated for the abnormalities characteristic of hydrops fetalis.

Alpha-thalassemia major and beta-thalassemia major are life threatening. Children with thalassemia major generally are weak, fail to thrive, show poor development, and experience cardiovascular compromise with high-output failure secondary to anemia. Untreated, they will die by 5 to 6 years of age.

EVALUATION AND TREATMENT Evaluation of thalassemia is based on familial disease history, clinical manifestations, and blood tests. Peripheral blood smears that show microcytosis and hemoglobin electrophoresis that demonstrates diminished amounts of α- or β-chains are used to make the diagnosis. Analysis of fetal DNA from withdrawn amniotic fluid is used as a screening test to detect hydrops fetalis (alpha-thalassemia major). Newborn screening for thalassemia should be done according to state law.

"Silent" carriers or those who have thalassemia minor generally have few if any symptoms and require no specific treatment. Therapies to support and prolong life are necessary, however, for thalassemia major. There is no cure for either condition. Prenatal diagnosis and genetic counseling may be the most important therapeutic measures offered.

At present, thalassemia major is treated with the following therapies:

1. Blood transfusions, which can return hemoglobin and hematocrit levels to normal thus alleviating the anemia-induced cardiac failure; iron overload and hemochromatosis are complications of transfusion therapy

2. Iron chelation therapy in combination with hypertransfusion (transfusion to a hematocrit of 35 ml/dl)

3. Splenectomy, which can reduce the need for transfusions by eliminating the site of hemolysis, thus prolonging erythrocyte survival

4. Bone marrow, cord blood, and stem cell transplantation is currently the only cure for thalassemia (Box 28-2)

DISORDERS OF COAGULATION AND PLATELETS

Inherited Hemorrhagic Disease

Hemophilias

Awareness of a serious bleeding disorder in males was documented nearly 2000 years ago in the Babylonian Talmud, which exempted from the rite of circumcision those boys having male relatives prone to excessive bleeding. In 1803 the first description of this disorder appeared in the medical literature, where it was noted to be X linked in nature and associated with joint bleeding and crippling.

Table 28-4 lists the coagulation factors. Until 1952 the term *hemophilia* was reserved for deficiency of factor VIII (antihemophilic factor). Since then two additional coagulation proteins, factor IX (plasma thromboplastin component [PTC]) and factor XI (plasma thromboplastin antecedent [PTA]), have been identified and their deficiency associated with similar clinical manifestations. Congenital deficiencies of these three plasma clotting factors—VIII, IX, XI—account for 90% to 95% of the hemorrhagic bleeding disorders collectively called *hemophilia*.

Types of Hemophilia

It is estimated that hemophilia occurs in 1 in 5000 male births. Eighty percent to 85% of those with hemophilia have hemophilia A and 10% to 15% have hemophilia B.[20]

Hemophilia A (classic hemophilia) is caused by factor VIII deficiency. It is the most common of the hemophilias. Hemophilia A is inherited as an X-linked recessive disorder that affects men and is transmitted by women.

Hemophilia B (Christmas disease), caused by factor IX deficiency, also is transmitted as an X-linked recessive trait

---

Box 28-2	Bone Marrow Transplantation for Beta-Thalassemia Major

Stem cell transplantation (SCT) remains the only cure for thalassemia major. Between 1991 and 2001, 55 children underwent SCT for thalassemia major in the United Kingdom. The median age at SCT was 6.4 years. Overall survival and thalassemia-free survival at 8 years following transplant were 94.5% and 81.8%, respectively. Transplant-related mortality was low (5.4%). The rejection rate was 4.6% of cases, acute graft-versus-host disease (GVHD) of grade II to IV occurred in 21%, and chronic GVHD occurred in 14.5%. These data suggest that allogeneic SCT is an important treatment option for children with beta-thalassemia major.

Data from Lawson SE et al: *Br J Haematol* 120(2):289-295, 2003.

Table 28-4	The Coagulation Factors	
Clotting Factors	**Synonym**	**Disorder**
I	Fibrinogen	Congenital deficiency (afibrinogenemia) and dysfunction (dysfibrinogenemia)
II	Prothrombin	Congenital deficiency or dysfunction
V	Labile factor, proaccelerin	Congenital deficiency (parahemophilia)
VII	Stable factor or proconvertin	Congenital deficiency
VIII	Antihemophilic factor (AHF)	Congenital deficiency is hemophilia A (classic hemophilia)
IX	Christmas factor	Congenital deficiency is hemophilia B
X	Stuart-Power factor	Congenital deficiency
XI	Plasma thromboplastin antecedent	Congenital deficiency, sometimes referred to as hemophilia C
XII	Hageman factor	Congenital deficiency is *not* associated with clinical symptoms
XIII	Fibrin-stabilizing factor	Congenital deficiency

and is clinically indistinguishable from factor VIII deficiency. Hemophilia A and hemophilia B occur with varying degrees of clinical severity, depending on concentrations of clotting factor VIII or IX in the blood. Severe hemophilia (concentration of clotting factors less than 1% of normal) is associated with spontaneous bleeding. In moderate hemophilia (1% to 5% of normal), bleeding usually occurs only after trauma; in the mild form (5% to 35% of normal), bleeding occurs only after severe trauma or surgery. The severity of hemophilia is similar in all affected members of a family.

Hemophilia C (factor XI deficiency) occurs as an autosomal recessive disease and occurs equally in men and women. Bleeding usually is less severe than in hemophilia A or B.

von Willebrand disease results from an inherited autosomal dominant trait with variable clinical manifestations and hematologic findings. The factor VIII deficiency differs from that of hemophilia A in mode of inheritance and response to treatment. In hemophilia A the deficiency is inherited as an X-linked recessive trait, whereas in von Willebrand disease, it is inherited as an autosomal dominant trait. The most important difference, however, is in responses to the infusion of plasma. In von Willebrand disease, infusion of plasma causes factor VIII activity to increase for several days because infusion of factor VIII temporarily induces endogenous synthesis of factor VIII.

PATHOPHYSIOLOGY Two types of defects dominate the hereditary defects of hemophilia to date: gene deletions and point mutations. Both types of genetic defects are associated with severe hemophilia A, in which no factor VIII circulates in the blood. Many different gene deletion mutations are associated with factor VIII and factor IX disease. The molecular defect that leads to the deletional mutation is identical among members of a given family.[21]

Point mutations, in which a single base in the DNA is mutated to another base, represent a second type of mutation that causes hemophilia. When a point mutation gives rise to a de novo stop codon (nonsense mutation), translation of the protein ceases and a shortened version of the protein is synthesized. Usually the protein is destroyed intracellularly and never reaches the plasma. This type of defect is associated with severe hemophilia, that is, with coagulant activity levels below 1%. Point mutations in which one amino acid is substituted for another can cause phenotypes of varying severity.

The mutation of an important amino acid can destroy protein function, activation, or folding; inhibit intracellular processing; or cause protein clearance.[22] Unlike deletional mutations, point mutations at the same site have been recorded in different families with hemophilia.

Table 28-4 summarizes the types of coagulation disorders. Not all the disorders are discussed in this chapter because some are extremely rare (congenital dysfibrinogenemias) and others have no clinical significance (e.g., Hageman factor deficiency, a condition in which profound laboratory deficiency of factor XII is associated with absolutely no clinical defects).

CLINICAL MANIFESTATIONS Children with severe hemophilia start to bleed at different ages. Although there is no transfer of maternal clotting factor to the fetus, many boys with hemophilia are circumcised without excessive bleeding. Normal hemostasis is achieved in these infants because clotting is activated through the extrinsic coagulation cascade, which does not involve factors VII, IX, or XI.

During the first year, spontaneous bleeding often is minimal, but hematoma formation may result from injections and from firm holding (e.g., under the arms). Many children present when reaching developmental milestones (i.e., crawling, pulling to stand) and become easily injured (i.e., increased bruising, swelling, redness at joints, mouth bleeding). By 3 to 4 years of age, 90% of children with hemophilia have had episodes of persistent bleeding from relatively minor traumatic lacerations (e.g., to the lip or tongue). This usually is the first clinical manifestation of hemophilia. Hemorrhage into the elbows, knees, and ankles cause pain, limit joint movement, and predisposes the child to degenerative joint changes. Spontaneous hematuria and epistaxis are troublesome but minor complications.

Recurrent bleeding—spontaneous and after minor trauma—is a lifelong problem. Many affected individuals experience phases or cycles of spontaneous bleeding episodes. Mechanisms that cause this phenomenon are unknown. Intracranial hemorrhage and bleeding into the neck or abdomen constitute life-threatening emergencies.

EVALUATION AND TREATMENT Although laboratory tests are of primary value in the evaluation of hemorrhagic disorders, the history and physical assessment also should be given careful consideration. The three phases of coagulation can be assessed individually by simple, reliable tests. In any hemorrhagic condition, the adequacy of phase III should be determined first. Unless adequate fibrinogen is present, the blood is incapable of coagulation; thus other laboratory tests that require formation of a visible clot will be invalid. Phase III can be evaluated by the **thrombin time,** the time required for plasma to clot after the addition of bovine thrombin. Fibrinogen can be measured by chemical or immunologic methods.

Phase II is assessed by the **prothrombin time (PT),** the time required for plasma to clot after the addition of thromboplastin and calcium. If phase III is intact, a prolonged prothrombin time indicates a deficiency involving factors II, V, VII, or X, alone or in combination. Specific assays for each of the factors are available.

Phase I, the most complex part of coagulation, can be evaluated by several tests. The **activated partial thromboplastin time (aPTT)** is the time required for clotting of plasma that has been activated by incubation with kaolin when calcium and platelets (or partial thromboplastin) are added. aPTT assesses the adequacy of factors XII, XI, IX, and VII. The **prothrombin consumption time** is a standard prothrombin test of serum instead of plasma. Because prothrombin is used up during coagulation, the serum normally contains little prothrombin and the serum prothrombin time is prolonged. Deficiencies of the phase I factors are associated with poor use of prothrombin. If the serum and plasma prothrombin times are similar, deficiency of a phase I factor is likely. The **thromboplastin generation test** is the most sensitive of all phase I tests. The test can precisely identify deficiencies of factors VIII and IX. If the aPTT, prothrombin consumption, or thromboplastin generation test results are abnormal, the way in which they can be corrected identifies the specific deficiency.

The treatment of hemophilia has advanced during the past 70 years. Plasma first was used in the 1920s, and by the 1940s it was used routinely to treat persons with hemophilia. The disadvantages of fresh frozen plasma (FFP), which is low in factor VIII per volume of plasma, led to the development of cryoprecipitate. In 1964 cryoprecipitate (quick-frozen precipitate), which is rich in factor VIII per volume, was used to treat persons with hemophilia. Although cryoprecipitate advanced the treatment of hemophilia A, it has several disadvantages. The most notable complication is the possibility of transmission of viral diseases. Factor VIII concentrates were first introduced in 1965. In addition to the predictable factor VIII content, other advantages of the early factor VIII concentrates included greater purity than cryoprecipitate and less contamination with other plasma proteins. The development of recombinant factor VIII resulted in new factor VIII products that minimize the risk of transmission of viral infection (e.g., HIV and hepatitis) and are potentially less expensive than plasma-derived factor VIII.

Recombinant antihemolytic factor plasma/albumin-free method (rAHF-PFM, Advate) is a product used for the prevention and control of bleeding episodes in individuals with hemophilia A, and in the perioperative management of those with hemophilia A. By excluding proteins or raw materials derived from human or animal sources in the final product, the risk of transmission of potentially infectious agents is removed.[23]

Primary prophylaxis consists of regular infusions of factor VIII or IX with the goal of preventing joint bleeding. It is usually given to children with severe hemophilia. A 5-year, multicenter trial found prophylaxis initiated in children between 6 and 30 months of age to be effective in the prevention of joint bleeding, structural joint damage, and frequency of bleeding in boys with factor VIII deficiency.[24]

Congenital Hypercoagulability and Thrombosis

Hereditary bleeding disorders, such as hemophilia, have been recognized and treated for centuries; however, the counterpart of these disorders, **thrombophilia,** has not been recognized until very recently. The inherited thrombophilic conditions generally are caused by defects in the clotting factors that inhibit clot formation; thus the balance between bleeding and clotting is directed toward the clotting aspects of hemostasis. Defects in specific proteins (C and S) and antithrombin (AT), as well as resistance to activated protein C (APC) and hyperhomocystinemia, are the major recognized causes of inherited thrombophilia.

Both proteins C and S are inhibitors of coagulation and depend on vitamin K for synthesis in the hepatocytes of the liver. Decreased levels of either of these proteins interfere with the normal homeostatic balance of procoagulant and anticoagulant activity at the endothelial level. Protein C and S deficiency states predispose affected individuals to thrombosis, especially venous thrombosis of the lower extremities.

Inheritance of **protein C deficiency** is autosomal dominant. Heterozygotes have protein C levels 50% to 60% of normal and may develop superficial thrombophlebitis, deep venous thrombosis, or pulmonary embolism in their late teens and early 20s. The majority of these thrombotic events (75%) occur spontaneously, whereas only 25% are the result of predisposing conditions.[25] Homozygotes have less than 1% of normal levels of protein C and tend to develop thrombosis of the cutaneous vessels with large areas of skin necrosis. It is rare for individuals with protein C deficiency to develop arterial thrombosis.

Protein C deficiency exists in two forms: types I and II. Type I, the more common form, involves a reduction in both biologic and immunologic activity of protein C. Type I is caused by deletion of the entire gene. In type II, the less common form, there is a normal level of protein C antigen but decreased functional levels of activity.

Neonatal purpura fulminans is a fatal syndrome found in infants who are homozygous or double heterozygous for types I and II protein deficiency. Manifestations of this syndrome are ecchymosis that becomes apparent on the first day of life and develops around the head, trunk, and extremities. These cutaneous manifestations often are accompanied by cerebral thrombosis and infarction. The lesions apparent on the skin often coalesce and demonstrate ulceration and necrosis. The condition is treated with fresh frozen plasma and heparinization, although the infant rarely survives.[25]

Treatment for protein C deficiency is heparin for acute episodes of thrombosis. Long-term therapy is required and consists of either oral warfarin sodium (Coumadin) or subcutaneous heparin (2500 to 5000 units) every 12 hours. Protein C concentrates have been developed; however, they have not yet been formally approved for treatment.

Protein S deficiency is similar to protein C deficiency, and the inheritance pattern (autosomal dominant) is also similar. Heterozygotes demonstrate a strong tendency for deep venous thrombosis, with the first incidence often occurring before age 25 years. Other manifestations include superficial thrombophlebitis and pulmonary emboli. There are predisposing conditions for thrombi development in some cases, with evidence of spontaneous thrombi development in most cases.

Protein S deficiency exists in two forms: type I and type II. Type I is identified as a quantitative deficiency and manifests as low levels of protein S antigen and activity, and type II is identified as a qualitative deficiency with low levels of free protein S and normal levels of free and total protein S antigen.[25]

Homozygotes demonstrate severe manifestations of the condition and may develop a form of purpura fulminans in the neonatal period. It also is possible that the homozygous state may lead to uterine death. Treatment with heparin and warfarin (Coumadin) is similar to that of protein C deficiency.

Antithrombin III (AT III) deficiency is inherited as an autosomal dominant condition, with the heterozygote state being the most common. AT III also exists in two forms, type I and type II, with type I being a quantitative deficiency of the AT III antigen. Type II is characterized as a dysfunctional form: normal levels of AT III are present but with reduced activity.

Individuals with AT III deficiency are at risk for early development of venous thrombosis and pulmonary embolism. These events often occur in the middle to late teens, and can occur as early as 10 years of age. The deep veins of the lower extremities most commonly are involved, with the iliofemoral vein being the most common site of involvement. Other sites include the mesenteric veins, vena cava, renal veins, and retinal veins. Cerebral thromboses also have been described. Arterial thrombotic events are rare. In some cases, thrombosis is precipitated by predisposing conditions, such as surgery, trauma, pregnancy, oral contraceptives, and infection.

The treatment of choice for AT III deficiency is heparin. Antiplatelet agents (e.g., aspirin, dipyridamole) may be used, as well as AT III concentrates.

Antibody-Mediated Hemorrhagic Disease

The antibody-mediated hemorrhagic diseases are a group of disorders caused by the immune response. Antibody-mediated destruction of platelets or antibody-mediated inflammatory reactions to allergens damage blood vessels and cause seepage into tissues. The thrombocytopenic purpuras may be intrinsic or idiopathic, or they may be transient phenomena transmitted from mother to fetus. The inflammatory, or "allergic," purpuras occur in response to allergens in the blood. All these disorders first appear during infancy or childhood.

Idiopathic Thrombocytopenic Purpura

Acute **idiopathic thrombocytopenic purpura (ITP) (auto-immune or primary thrombocytopenic purpura)** is the most common of the thrombocytopenic purpuras of childhood. It is a disorder of platelet consumption in which antiplatelet antibodies bind to the plasma membranes of platelets, causing platelet sequestration and destruction by mononuclear phagocytes in the spleen and other lymphoid tissues at a rate that exceeds the ability of the bone marrow to produce them.

PATHOPHYSIOLOGY Platelets have several tissue-specific antigens on their plasma markers that may be targets for antiplatelet antibody. In approximately 70% of cases of ITP, there is an antecedent viral disease (e.g., cytomegalovirus [CMV], Epstein-Barr virus [EBV], human immunodeficiency virus [HIV], parvovirus, or viral respiratory infection), thus suggesting that viral sensitization has occurred. The interval between infection and onset of purpura is 1 to 4 weeks. A comparison with purpura seen in adults has identified an immune mechanism as the basis for ITP. High levels of IgG have been found bound to platelets and may represent immune complexes on the platelet surface.[26]

CLINICAL MANIFESTATIONS One to 4 weeks after a viral infection, bruising and a generalized petechial rash often occur with acute onset. Asymmetric bleeding is typical and is found most often on the legs and trunk. Hemorrhagic bullae of the gums, lips, and other mucous membranes may be prominent. Epistaxis (nose bleeding) may be severe and difficult to control. Except for the signs of bleeding, the child appears well. The acute phase of the disease associated with spontaneous hemorrhages lasts 1 to 2 weeks, but thrombocytopenia often persists. Although its incidence is less than 1%, intracranial hemorrhage is the most serious complication of ITP. In some cases the onset is more gradual and clinical manifestations consist of moderate bruising and a few petechiae.

EVALUATION AND TREATMENT Laboratory examination reveals a reduced platelet count, and the few platelets observed on a peripheral blood smear are large in size, reflecting increased bone marrow production. The Ivy bleeding time is prolonged. Bone marrow aspiration reveals megakaryocytes in normal or increased numbers and normal erythrocytes and granulocytes.

Even without treatment, the prognosis for children with ITP is excellent—75% recover completely within 3 months. After the initial acute phase, spontaneous clinical manifestations subside. By 6 months after onset, 80% to 90% of affected children have regained normal platelet counts.[27]

Because of the short life span of platelets (10 days), fresh blood or platelets are of no value or of transient benefit; however, their use is indicated when life-threatening hemorrhage occurs. Corticosteroid therapy reduces the severity and shortens the duration of the initial phase by suppressing the immune attack on platelets. Recent evidence indicates that the use of high-dose methylprednisolone increases bone resorption and may cause osteonecrosis in children with ITP.[28] Intravenous IgG has been demonstrated to increase the platelet count in some children with ITP, but it is quite costly (see What's New? Monoclonal Antibody Therapy for Treatment of Idiopathic Thrombocytopenic Purpura [ITP]). A newer product, anti-D, is a gamma globulin fraction containing a high proportion of antibodies to the $Rh_O(D)$ antigen of the red blood cells. Intravenous anti-D is a safe and effective treatment for Rh-positive, nonsplenectomized individuals with ITP, although it is expensive. Intravenous anti-D is an effective treatment for Rh-positive nonsplenectomized children with ITP, although it is associated with side effects including chills, fever, headache, and a decrease in hemoglobin levels. Administration of steroids and antipyretics prior to the anti-D treatment may prevent side effects.[27]

Parents should be instructed to protect the child from falls or other trauma that might result in bleeding. Splenectomy should be reserved for chronic cases that fail to respond to nonsurgical intervention.

Autoimmune Neonatal Thrombocytopenias

Antibody-mediated thrombocytopenic purpura occurs in neonates in either autoimmune or alloimmune form. Both forms are characterized by the immunologic destruction of platelets by antibodies (IgG) against tissue-specific antigens expressed by the platelets (i.e., platelet-specific antigens).

Autoimmune neonatal thrombocytopenia was first noted in the early 1950s when it was observed that mothers with ITP often delivered infants who were transiently thrombocytopenic. Neonatal thrombocytopenia was observed in approximately 50% of infants at risk and lasted an average of 1 month. As platelet counts returned to normal, a concomitant drop in the level of maternal antiplatelet antibody on the child's platelets occurred. The antibody is directed against antigens common to maternal and neonatal platelets. The prognosis generally is favorable. The frequency of intracranial hemorrhage has been estimated to be 1% to 3% of cases. The principal aim of the management of affected infants is to prevent the deleterious consequences of severe thrombocytopenia by administering intravenous immunoglobulins.[29]

Neonatal alloimmune thrombocytopenic purpura (NATP) is less common, estimated to occur in 1 in 800 to 1000 live births. NATP is suspected in thrombocytopenic infants of mothers with normal platelet counts and no history of purpura. The disorder is caused by the production of a maternal antibody against a fetal platelet-specific antigen inherited from the father and not shared by the mother. More than 50% of NATP cases are associated with the presence of the P1^{A1} antigen on neonatal and paternal platelets but not on maternal platelets.

It is not known why NATP occurs in only half of the neonates genetically at risk for NATP. Because 98% of the population show P1^{A1} positivity, approximately 1 in 50 pregnancies would be expected to show maternal-fetal incompatibility, but the incidence of NATP is 100 times less. NATP does not develop in neonates born to some mothers with high antiplatelet antibody levels.

The diagnosis of NATP is confirmed by detection in the maternal serum of antibody that reacts with platelets from the infant and father but not with platelets from the mother. In approximately 75% to 85% of cases, NATP recurs in subsequent pregnancies. Purpura usually develops in the affected infant shortly after delivery, and intracranial, renal, and gastrointestinal hemorrhages are possible. The mortality rate from intracranial hemorrhage has been estimated at 10% to 15%. Following birth, maternal platelet transfusion (mother to infant) is the treatment of choice.[29]

Most of the life-threatening clinical manifestations of transient neonatal thrombocytopenia and NATP can be avoided through cesarean delivery. If the mother has antiplatelet disease, however, surgery can result in hemorrhage and serious maternal morbidity. Maternal morbidity resulting from NATP during pregnancy is low (less than 5%): the principal maternal risk is bleeding from surgical incisions during cesarean delivery. This poses a problem for the obstetrician. The incidence of transient thrombocytopenia in infants born to mothers with NATP is about 50%. If all deliveries were cesarean, half the mothers would undergo cesarean delivery unnecessarily. Conversely, if all deliveries were vaginal, half the infants—those with thrombocytopenia—would be at risk for intracranial bleeding.

A considerable amount of research has focused on methods of predicting whether the fetus is thrombocytopenic so that the route of delivery can be chosen to minimize the risks for both mother and child. No satisfactory method has been found, despite reports from many laboratories that fetal platelet counts correlate closely with levels of antiplatelet antibody on maternal platelets or in the maternal circulation. Equally unreliable are predictions of neonatal thrombocytopenia based on immunosuppression with corticosteroids. Research continues in areas such as the identification of specific subclasses of antiplatelet antibodies.

WHAT'S NEW? Monoclonal Antibody Therapy for Treatment of Idiopathic Thrombocytopenic Purpura (ITP)

Rituximab, a chimeric monoclonal antibody against the protein CD20, has been tested in children with ITP. Long-term follow-up at 39.5 months of 49 children with ITP who were treated with rituximab demonstrated an overall response rate of 69%: 21 children had platelet counts of greater than 50,000/mm³ at 20 months' post-treatment. Only mild and self-limited side effects were observed in 18%, and no major infections or long-term toxicities were reported.

Data from Parodi E et al: Br J Haematol 144(14):552-558, 2009.

Autoimmune Vascular Purpura

Autoimmune vascular purpura (allergic purpura) is caused by antibody-mediated injury of blood vessel walls, typically arterioles and capillaries. The inflammatory reaction is to foreign proteins or chemicals in the blood (microorganisms, drugs, or other chemicals).

Autoimmune vascular purpura usually is seen in children, with the incidence decreasing in adolescents and adults and occurring only rarely in older adults. The average age at onset is 5 years, with a slightly higher proportion of males affected. Purpura occurs as vessel integrity is disrupted by inflammatory processes, causing effusion of serosanguineous exudate to perivascular tissues.

Clinical manifestations vary and include headache, anorexia, fever, abdominal pain, arthralgias, and skin lesions (urticaria and erythema). The lesions usually are located symmetrically on the proximal portions of the extremities, particularly on the legs and buttocks, and may be accompanied by itching or paresthesias. Abdominal pain results from hemorrhage into the bowel, which may lead to colic, nausea, and vomiting. These symptoms may precede the appearance of skin lesions. The pain usually is midabdominal but may radiate to other parts of the abdomen. Constipation may occur.

Some forms of autoimmune vascular purpura may produce joint pain and tenderness. Periarticular swelling and edema of the hands and feet are common, but hemarthrosis does not occur. These symptoms may precede the onset of symptoms associated with abdominal pain and purpura. Subacute glomerulonephritis occurs in some cases but usually is reversible.

The characteristic skin lesions (purpura and cutaneous manifestations of allergy), accompanied by a history of joint and abdominal pain, are clues for diagnosis. Laboratory test results often reveal no major abnormalities. Attacks may last several weeks and may recur at odd intervals and with changing manifestations with each episode. Treatment, if necessary, consists of the alleviation of symptoms.

LEUKEMIA AND LYMPHOMA

Leukemia, the most common malignancy of childhood, represents approximately 40% of all childhood cancers. Childhood lymphoma is the third most common malignant neoplasm of children in the United States, representing approximately 11% of all childhood cancers. (See Chapter 27 for a discussion of leukemia in adults.)

Leukemia

Of the varieties of childhood leukemia, 80% to 85% of leukemias in children are acute lymphocytic leukemia (ALL) or acute undifferentiated leukemia (AUL). The remaining 15% to 20% are acute nonlymphocytic leukemias (ANLLs) (which include myeloblastic, promyelocytic, monocytic, and myelomonoblastic leukemias) and the very rare red blood cell leukemia, erythroleukemia. Because the vast majority of ANLLs involve the myeloblastic cell, many experts refer to the disease

as *acute myelogenous leukemia (AML)*. Leukemia accounts for 25% of cases of cancer in black children and 34% of cases of cancer in white children. Approximately 4900 new cases are diagnosed each year in the United States. Of those 4900 children, 75% to 80% are diagnosed with ALL.[30]

The peak incidence for childhood ALL is between 2 and 6 years of age. ALL affects more white and Hispanic than black children and more males than females. Male predominance is greater in T-cell disease. There also is a higher incidence of ALL in Western and industrialized nations.[30]

Types of Leukemia

A number of different classifications are used for the leukemias. First, acute leukemia is differentiated from chronic leukemia. Second, the cell line determines whether lymphoid cells or myeloid cells are involved. In acute leukemia this difference separates ALL from AML and vice versa. Within each of these categories, further subdivisions have been developed. (See Chapter 27 for a discussion of leukemias in adults.)

Cytogenic studies of leukemic cells are performed routinely at most major treatment centers during the diagnostic process. Abnormal morphologic characteristics, as well as abnormalities in the number of copies of chromosomes, are found in leukemic cells. Hyperdiploidy (increased number of chromosome copies) is associated with a good prognosis. Common translocations associated with ALL are TEL AML1, BCR ABL, and MLL. TEL-AML1 is the most common abnormality (in 20% to 30% of cases) and occurs when the *TEL* gene on chromosome 12p13 fuses with the *AML1* gene on chromosome 21q22. TEL-AML1 is associated with a favorable outcome. MLL arrangement, t(4;11), is located on chromosome 11q23. This translocation, the most common within this subtype, is found in infant ALL and is associated with a poor prognosis despite intensive therapy. Philadelphia chromosome positive (Ph+) leukemia expresses the BCR-ABL protein and is characterized by the presence of t(9;22)(q34;q11) translocation. Ph+ leukemia can be ALL or chronic myelocytic leukemia (CML), depending where the breakpoint on chromosome 22 occurs. In CML, the translocation can be detected in multiple cell lines. Ph+ ALL occurs in 2% to 3% of cases and responds poorly to conventional chemotherapy. In CML, 99% of cases are characterized by the presence of t(9;22).[31]

Classification of childhood leukemia has become a complex but essential process that determines treatment. Previous classification by the French-American-British Cooperative Group (FAB) was based primarily on the morphologic and biochemical system. A classification scheme developed by the World Health Organization (WHO) is based on a more comprehensive system that uses morphology, immunophenotyping, and cytogenic and clinical features. The three major classifications of childhood leukemia are ALL (75% to 80%), AML (15% to 20%), and CML (less than 5%).

Flow cytometric immunophenotyping has made distinguishing between lymphoblastic and nonlymphoblastic leukemia much easier than in the past, when the degree of immaturity of the cell sometimes made such distinction difficult.

Immunologic classification has been used on identification of various surface markers. Five categories of ALL have been identified on the basis of their presumed origin from thymic cells (T cells) and bursa-equivalent cells (B cells) of normal lymphocytes:

1. T-cell ALL—characterized by the presence of abnormal T lymphocytes and found more commonly in older boys whose diagnosis includes mediastinal masses, high white blood cell counts, and hepatosplenomegaly (20% of ALL)
2. B-cell ALL—characterized by the presence of abnormal B lymphoblasts and associated with a poor prognosis (5% of ALL)
3. Pre–B-cell ALL—characterized by the presence of pre-B lymphoblasts (20% of ALL)
4. Unclassified ALL—also known as *null cell* (meaning neither T nor B lymphoblasts), and now classified as early B-cell lineage (15% of ALL)
5. Common ALL—characterized by the presence of a specific antigen known as *common ALL antigen,* or common acute lymphocytic leukemia antigen (CALLA), recently designated cellular differentiation 10 or CD10, in which the actual cell usually is considered to be of the B lineage (39% of ALL)

PATHOGENESIS The exact cause of childhood leukemia is unclear. Investigations have focused on genetic susceptibility, environmental factors, and viral infections[32] (see Chapter 13). Observations of a familial tendency and links with a number of inherited disorders have implicated genetic factors in the origin of leukemia. Analysis of leukemia in twins has revealed a frequent prenatal origin and an early or initiating role for chromosome translocations. In addition, twin studies also suggest that there is a protracted latency and the need in ALL and AML for postnatal exposures or genetic events to produce clinical disease.[33] A positive family history of hematopoietic malignancies among first- or second-degree relatives has been associated with a slight increase for risk for childhood ALL, although it is modest (odds ratio 2.06).[34]

Inherited diseases that predispose a child to leukemia (ALL and AML) include Down syndrome, Fanconi anemia, Bloom syndrome, Diamond-Blackfan anemia, Klinefelter syndrome, Shwachman-Diamond syndrome, and ataxia-telangiectasia. Leukemia also has been associated with known genetic diseases, such as congenital agammaglobulinemia. AML in children sometimes is associated with loss or deletion of chromosome 7. AML can develop from preexisting myeloproliferative disorders that also are preleukemia syndromes (i.e., myelodysplastic syndrome).

Childhood exposure to ionizing radiation, drugs, or viruses has been associated with the risk of developing cancer. Retrospective research has shown a significant correlation between radiation-induced malignancies from radiotherapy (as cancer treatment) or from radiation exposure from diagnostic imaging. The relationship between childhood cancer and electromagnetic fields, small appliances, radon, and other sources has been the focus of many epidemiologic studies; however, no conclusive evidence has been observed.[32]

Although chemicals such as benzene have been associated with the development of AML in adults, no evidence suggests a similar chemical or drug association in childhood leukemia. Leukemia (primarily AML) has been reported as a secondary malignancy (development of a second cancer after the first) in children treated for Hodgkin disease and Wilms tumor, although such cases are rare. In most cases the children received chemotherapy (alkylating agents or dactinomycin) and radiation therapy for the primary cancer, perhaps accounting for the subsequent development of another cancer.

Leukemic "clusters" that represent a greater number of leukemia cases occurring in a particular geographic location have raised speculation about environmental factors or infectious patterns of transmission. Careful follow-up, however, has failed to document the abnormal clustering.[35]

The strongest association between viruses and the development of cancer in children has been EBV and Burkitt lymphoma, and nasopharyngeal carcinoma and Hodgkin disease. Children with AIDS have an increased risk of developing non-Hodgkin lymphoma and Kaposi sarcoma. However, with the use of highly active antiretroviral therapy in the developed world, the incidence of acquired immunodeficiency syndrome (AIDS)–related malignancies has declined dramatically.[36] Retroviruses have not been linked with childhood leukemia.

CLINICAL MANIFESTATIONS Few variations appear in the presenting symptoms of the various cell types of acute leukemias. The onset may be abrupt or insidious, but the most common symptoms reflect the consequence of bone marrow failure, which results in decreased red blood cells and platelets and changes in white blood cells. Pallor, fatigue, petechiae, purpura, bleeding, and fever generally are present. Approximately 45% of children have a hemoglobin level below 7 g/dl; in contrast to adults, children seem to demonstrate fewer symptoms. If acute blood loss occurs, however, characteristic symptoms of tachycardia, air hunger, restlessness, and thirst may be present. Epistaxis, excessive bruising, and hematuria often occur in children with severe thrombocytopenia. Three fourths of children with ALL have platelet counts less than 100,000/mm^3 at diagnosis, and 28% have platelet counts below 20,000/mm^3. Half of all children newly diagnosed with AML have platelet counts less than 50,000/mm^3. Disseminated intravascular coagulation occurs more commonly with AML, particularly with promyelocytic leukemia. The granules in the leukemic promyelocytes may then indicate thromboplastin activity.

Fever usually is present as a result of two causes: (1) infection associated with the decrease in functional neutrophils and (2) hypermetabolism associated with the ongoing rapid growth and destruction of leukemic cells. In most children with ALL, the total white blood count is less than 10,000/mm^3, and with AML most have white cell counts below 50,000/mm^3. In a few children, however, the peripheral white blood count can go well above 100,000/mm^3. White blood cell counts greater than 200,000/mm^3 can cause leukostasis, an intravascular clumping of cells that result in infarction and hemorrhage, usually in the brain and lung. The three most important favorable prognostic factors are age at diagnosis (2 to 10 years), initial leukocyte count (less than 50,000/mm³), and initial response to treatment.

Renal failure as a result of hyperuremia (high uric acid levels) can be associated with ALL, particularly at diagnosis. Cell breakdown results as a natural process in the presence of a high white blood cell count or as a result of cellular breakdown caused by chemotherapy. Uric acid levels rise as an end product of purine metabolism from cellular destruction. Because the major excretory pathway is through the kidney, urates can precipitate in renal tubules or ureters and can lead to oliguria and acute renal failure. Renal failure is preventable if uric acid levels are monitored and treatment is aimed at optimal hydration, alkalinization of urine to assist with the excretion of soluble urates, and blockage of further uric acid formation by administration of the drug allopurinol.

Extramedullary invasion with leukemic cells can occur in nearly all body tissue. Most children with ALL have some extramedullary involvement at diagnosis. Leukemic invasion of tissue other than bone marrow is believed to represent metastatic infiltration. Hepatosplenomegaly and lymphadenopathy, resulting from extramedullary hematopoiesis, occur in nearly one half of children with ALL, but they are less common in children with AML.

The CNS is a common site of infiltration of extramedullary leukemias, although less than 10% of children with ALL have CNS involvement at diagnosis. CNS infiltration manifests later in the course of the disease. Because successful chemotherapy prolongs the time of remission, the incidence of CNS involvement has increased. The most common symptoms of CNS involvement relate to increased intracranial pressure, causing early morning headaches, nausea, vomiting, irritability, and lethargy. Prophylactic CNS treatment therefore is necessary because systemic treatment with chemotherapy does not cross the blood-brain barrier.

Gonadal involvement, with testicular and ovarian infiltration, has been demonstrated in postmortem examination in 57% and 35% of children, respectively. Clinical detection of gonadal involvement is much less frequent. The incidence of testicular involvement, like CNS involvement, has increased with lengthened duration of remission. Prophylactic treatment has not been successful and currently is not recommended.

Leukemic infiltration into bones and joints is common in children. Reports of bone or joint pain actually lead to the diagnosis of leukemia in some children. In most children, bone pain is characterized as migratory, vague, and without areas of swelling or inflammation. If joint pain is the primary symptom and some swelling is associated with the pain, however, misdiagnoses of rheumatoid arthritis and rheumatic fever may occur.

Other organs reported to be sites of leukemic invasion include the kidneys, heart, lungs, thymus, eyes, skin, and gastrointestinal tract. Of these, the kidneys, lungs, and gastrointestinal tract are the most frequently reported sites. Skin involvement is more common in AML than in ALL.

EVALUATION AND TREATMENT Although blood test results can raise the clinician's suspicion of leukemia, a bone marrow aspiration is required to establish the diagnosis. The **blast cell** is the hallmark of acute leukemia (Figure 28-10). The blast cell is a relatively undifferentiated cell characterized by diffusely distributed nuclear chromatin, with one or more nucleoli and basophilic cytoplasm (Figure 28-11).

Healthy children have less than 5% blast cells in the bone marrow and none in the peripheral blood. The bone marrow is categorized on the basis of blast percentage. Normal bone marrow is called M1 marrow; M2 and M3 represent an increased percentage of blasts in the sample. This categorization

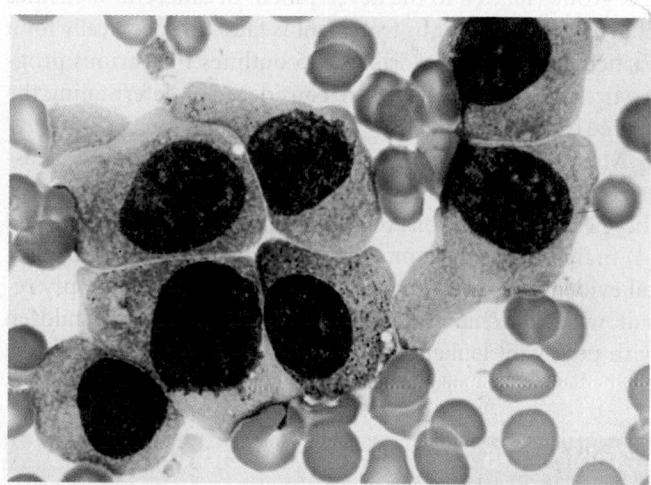

Figure 28-10 Monoblasts from acute monoblastic leukemia. Monoblasts in a marrow smear from an individual with acute monoblastic leukemia (M5A). The monoblasts are larger than myeloblasts and usually have abundant cytoplasm, often with delicate scattered azurophilic granules (an element that stains well with blue aniline dyes). (From Damjanov I, Linder J, editors: *Anderson's pathology*, ed 10, St Louis, 1996, Mosby.)

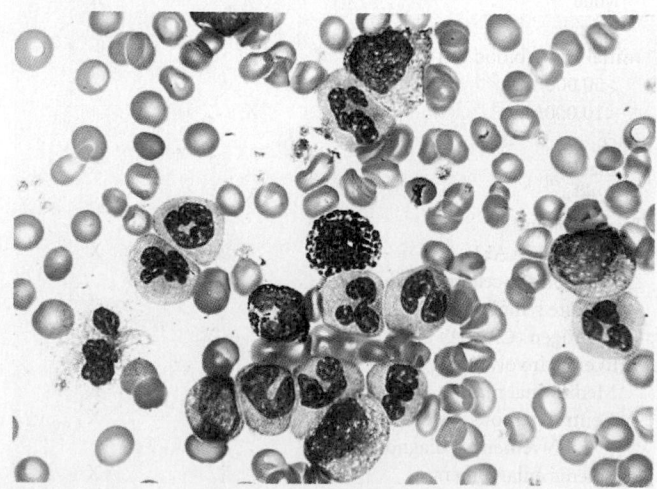

Figure 28-11 Leukocytosis and basophilia in chronic myeloid leukemia. Blood smear from a child with chronic myeloid leukemia (blasts) showing marked leukocytosis and basophilia. Karyotype analysis identified a Philadelphia chromosome (Wright-Giemsa stain). (From Damjanov I, Linder J, editors: *Anderson's pathology*, ed 10, St Louis, 1996, Mosby.)

system should not be confused with the similar terminology used to denote subtypes of AML. In ALL the bone marrow often is replaced by 80% to 100% blast cells, with a reduction in normally developing red blood cells and granulocytes. The marrow, which is considered hypercellular, is composed of a homogeneous population of cells. Occasionally, however, the marrow appears hypocellular, making the diagnosis difficult to differentiate from aplastic anemia. When this occurs, bone marrow biopsy or biopsy of extramedullary sites is necessary to confirm the diagnosis.

Combination chemotherapy, with or without radiation therapy to localized sites, such as the CNS, is the treatment of choice for acute leukemia. In ALL, identification of various risk groups has led to the development of different intensities of drug protocols. Thus treatment is tailored specifically for a particular risk group. (Table 28-5 outlines the various prognostic factors for ALL that are considered in determining the degree of risk.).

Most ALL treatment programs have four distinct phases: (1) induction of remission, (2) preventive therapy for the CNS, (3) intensification (also called *consolidation*), and (4) maintenance. In remission induction, the goal is no clinical evidence of disease and a normal bone marrow biopsy result, which is achieved in 95% of children with ALL. Children with persistent leukemia at the end of 1 month of induction

Table 28-5	Prognostic Factors in Acute Lymphoblastic Leukemia (ALL)		
Prognostic Factor		**Better Prognosis**	**Worse Prognosis**
Age*			
<2 yr or >10 yr			X
2-7 yr		X	
Gender*			
Male			X
Female		X	
Initial white blood cell count*			
>50,000/mm^3			X
<10,000/mm^3		X	
Race			
Black			X
White		X	
Immunology*			
T- or B-cell ALL			X
Early pre–B-cell or common acute lymphocytic leukemia antigen (CALLA)		X	
Leukemic involvement			
Mediastinal mass			X
Central nervous system involvement at diagnosis			X
Splenic enlargement			X

*The four most reliable prognostic factors. Initial prognostic factors become less effective predictors with increasing length of remission. Age and gender are not significant after 15 months of continuous remission, and white blood cell count is not significant after 24 months of continuous remission.

therapy have a dismal prognosis. Prophylactic CNS treatment historically included both chemotherapy and radiation, but therapy, although effective in preventing CNS leukemia, adversely affects neurologic and intellectual function. A marked incidence of learning disabilities has been identified in children previously treated to prevent CNS disease.[37] CNS radiation is no longer given and intrathecal regimens are less toxic. Once remission is achieved, an intensification phase of treatment begins. This treatment is necessary because leukemic cells will continue to be present despite successful remission. Thus the goal of the intensification phase is to further decrease and eliminate the remaining leukemic cells. Intensification therapy often overlaps prophylactic CNS treatment. The final phase of initial treatment is called *maintenance therapy*. The goal of this phase is to maintain disease control. The optimal duration of maintenance therapy is not well defined, but it usually continues for 2.5 to 3 years. During maintenance therapy, intermittent "pulses" of new drugs may be given. Periods of intensified therapy are believed to minimize development of drug-resistant leukemic cells.

ALL is a curable disease. This prognosis is a dramatic reversal of the outlook for a child diagnosed with this disease 40 years ago, when ALL was uniformly fatal and the average survival time was only 2 to 3 months. Today, with prompt and appropriate treatment, 75% to 85% of children with ALL are cured. Those children with the more favorable early pre–B-cell or CALLA-positive ALL have a survival rate of 90%.[30]

Prognostic factors in AML are not as well defined as they are for ALL because of the small number of affected children and their overall poor prognosis. The goal of treatment for AML is similar to that of ALL except that much more aggressive chemotherapy is administered. With intensive chemotherapy, significant bone marrow suppression is necessary but predisposes children to infection, bleeding, and anemia. The use of colony-stimulating factor (CSF), which stimulates the rapid proliferation of specific blood cell lines, is an advance that shortens this period of bone marrow aplasia (CSFs are discussed in Chapter 25). Although initial remission is achieved relatively easily in all cases of ALL, successful and lasting remission can be achieved in only 70% to 80% of children with AML.[30] If remission is achieved, further treatment, called *continuation therapy*, is required. The specific intensity, timing, and length of continuation therapy are controversial. The use of either a stem cell or bone marrow transplantation (BMT) is an important treatment consideration in AML. Because long-term remission and cure of AML are difficult to achieve with chemotherapy alone, transplant often is recommended after the first remission is achieved. Transplant is the treatment of choice after relapse of AML. The long-term survival rate for children with AML, whether treated with chemotherapy or chemotherapy and BMT, is approximately 45% to 50%.[30]

Lymphomas

Non-Hodgkin lymphoma (NHL) and Hodgkin disease make up approximately 15% of all childhood cancer. Approximately 800 cases of childhood lymphoma are diagnosed in the United

States annually.[30] Either group of diseases is rare before age 5 years, and the relative incidence increases throughout childhood. NHL is 1.5 times more common than Hodgkin disease in children. Boys are more likely to be diagnosed with a malignant lymphoma than are girls. There is an increased incidence of lymphoma in children with congenital immunodeficiency syndromes such as Wiskott-Aldrich syndrome, severe combined immunodeficiency (SCID), X-linked lymphoproliferative disease, and ataxia-telangiectasia, as well as those with AIDS. Increased incidence of NHL also is associated with immunosuppression after solid organ and stem cell transplants, particularly T-cell–depleted stem cell transplantation.

Non-Hodgkin Lymphoma

The classification of **non-Hodgkin lymphoma (NHL)** has been confusing because of the heterogeneity of this group of diseases. Generally most classification systems divide NHL into two categories—nodular or diffuse—on the basis of cellular pattern. Whereas one half of all adults with NHL have a nodular form of the disease, children rarely demonstrate this pattern. Nodular disease represents a less aggressive form of lymphoma. Almost without exception, childhood NHL becomes evident as a diffuse disease and can be further subdivided into three groups: (1) large cell (histiocytic), (2) lymphoblastic, and (3) small noncleaved cell (Burkitt or non-Burkitt lymphoma). Large cell NHL often involves chromosomal translocations. Disease sites commonly involve extranodal sites, such as brain, lung, bone, and skin. Lymphoblastic NHL also shows chromosomal translocations, particularly chromosomes 7 and 14. Disease sites commonly include the mediastinum and peripheral lymph nodes. Small noncleaved cell NHL involves chromosome translocations of 8 and 14. It is believed that this translocation triggers the *c-myc* oncogene. Children with small noncleaved cell NHL commonly have intra-abdominal disease at diagnosis.

An area of intensive study concerns the apparent biologic similarities of NHL and ALL in children. These two diseases are cytologically identical, and the histologic distinction between them is indicated by the degree of infiltration in the blood and bone marrow. The more bone marrow involvement and the less nodal and organ infiltration present, the more likely the disease is to be classified as ALL. Childhood NHL also is much more like ALL in its clinical manifestations and much less like Hodgkin disease or adult NHL.

As in ALL, immunophenotyping is an important part of the classification of childhood NHL. Almost 45% of the disease in children originates from T cells; an equal number originates from B cells. The remaining group, which represents 10% of childhood NHLs, is classified as non-T, non-B.

PATHOGENESIS The origin of NHL in childhood is still elusive. Although defective host immunity is implicated in most children in whom NHL develops, an immune deficit cannot be identified. Viral etiology is suggested, but the role in development of human lymphoma is still unclear. The strongest correlation exists between EBV and African Burkitt lymphoma. This form of NHL is associated with a breakpoint on chromosome 8 that is located near the *c-myc* oncogene.[38] The relationship between EBV infection and Burkitt lymphoma outside Africa is weak, however, even though the tumor is histopathologically and clinically indistinguishable. Chronic immunostimulation also has been suggested as a factor in the development of lymphomas because these diseases are seen more often when chronic persistent antigenic stimulation occurs from infection, such as malaria or intestinal parasites. Genetic susceptibility also may play a role in the process of malignant transformation.

CLINICAL MANIFESTATIONS In children, NHL has been found to arise from any lymphoid tissue. Signs and symptoms therefore are specific for the site involved. Some children have such widespread involvement that no original site can be determined. Because childhood NHL is a rapidly progressive disease, symptoms generally are present only a few weeks before diagnosis is made. Rapidly enlarging lymphoid tissue and painless lymphadenopathy are common in about one third of children with abdominal sites of involvement, usually representing a gastrointestinal origin for the disease. Symptoms often include abdominal pain and vomiting, but a palpable mass is not always present. Most children with abdominal symptoms have diffuse, small noncleaved cell NHL (Burkitt or non-Burkitt) of B-cell origin. If the tumor recurs, it appears again in the abdomen before distant spread.

The other common site of childhood NHL is the chest region. An anterior mediastinal mass, with or without pleural effusion, often is present. If the mass is large enough, respiratory compromise, tracheal compression, and superior vena cava syndrome may arise, which constitute a medical emergency. Children with anterior mediastinal involvement often are male adolescents and usually have diffuse lymphoblastic lymphoma of T-cell origin. This form of diffuse lymphoblastic lymphoma often evolves into extensive bone marrow involvement and is considered to be an overt leukemic phase (Figure 28-12); therefore, it is referred to as *leukemic transformation*. CNS involvement and testicular infiltration often then occur. CNS involvement occurs in about 30% of individuals with NHL, usually causing multiple deep-seated lesions within the brain parenchyma. In children with AIDS, NHL is the most common mass lesion found in the brain.

Bone marrow involvement is less common than other primary sites, whereas CNS involvement is common. Relatively few children (10% to 20%) with NHL have lymphoid tissue involvement of the head and neck (Waldeyer ring, nasopharynx, sinuses). Signs and symptoms include tonsillitis, sinusitis, and a painless nasopharyngeal mass. In African Burkitt lymphoma, involvement of facial bones, particularly the jaw, is common, although this occurs infrequently in non-African cases.

EVALUATION AND TREATMENT Diagnosis is made by biopsy of disease sites, usually the involved lymph nodes. Other sites of biopsy include the tonsils, bone marrow, spleen, liver, bowel, or skin. Advances in understanding the disease and progress in treatment strategies have meant that most children with NHL are cured of the disease. The

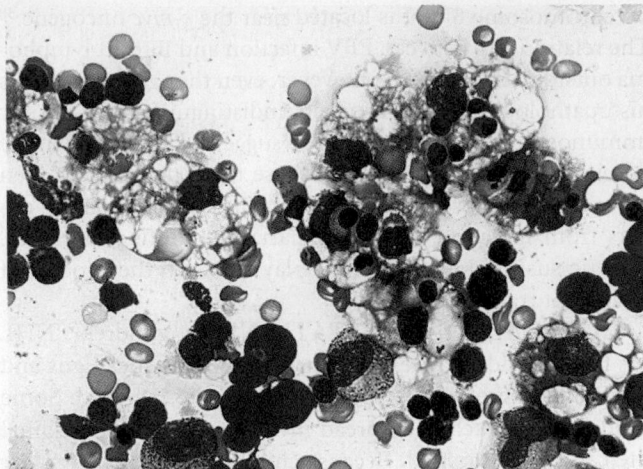

Figure 28-12 Bone marrow aspirate from a child with T-cell lymphoma in a lymph node biopsy. There is marked histiocytic hyperplasia. Two of the histiocytes contain phagocytosed red cells. The histiocytic hyperplasia regressed with disease remission and recurred with relapse of the lymphoma (Wright-Giemsa stain). (From Damjanov I, Linder J, editors: *Anderson's pathology*, ed 10, St Louis, 1996, Mosby.)

primary therapeutic modality for childhood NHL is chemotherapy, regardless of stage or site(s) of the disease. The tumor responds to many different agents. Many children with NHL receive intrathecal agents (methotrexate [Mexate] or cytarabine [cytosine arabinoside], or both) for CNS prophylaxis. Radiation is not routinely used to treat childhood NHL, with the exception of emergent situations when airway, intestinal, or spinal obstruction requires immediate reduction in tumor size. Cranial radiation therapy (XRT) may be used for children with T-cell lymphoblastic lymphoma.

Children with advanced small noncleaved cell lymphoma of the abdomen have the poorest prognosis. Although remission occurs in more than 90% of these children, most experience subsequent relapses. Even in the presence of advanced lymphoblastic lymphoma, however, 70% to 80% of children can be cured. Children with localized disease in more easily

treated sites are likely to be cured with prompt and appropriate treatment. Overall, children with localized diseases have a 90% survival rate and those with advanced disease have a 70% to 80% survival rate.[39]

Hodgkin Lymphoma

Hodgkin lymphoma accounts for 6% of all childhood cancers with a significant male-to-female dominance of 4:1 in young children. There is an increased incidence in children with immunologic disorders, whether caused by genetics, infection, or iatrogenic agents. EBV has been associated with Hodgkin lymphoma. Approximately 15% to 25% of adolescents and young adults have EBV-positive Hodgkin lymphoma.[40]

Clustering of cases within families may suggest a genetic predisposition to the disease or common exposure to a causative agent.[41]

Hodgkin lymphoma accounts for 6% of all childhood cancers. It occurs infrequently in children younger than 2 years, and few cases are observed before age 5 years. A gradual rise in incidence occurs through age 11 years, with a marked increase through adolescence that continues into the 30s.

Individuals typically have painless supraclavicular or cervical adenopathy. These nodes are firm and rubbery and may be sensitive to palpation if they have grown rapidly. At least two thirds of individuals have mediastinal involvement that may cause symptoms ranging from a nonproductive cough to tracheal or bronchial compression leading to airway obstruction. Systemic symptoms may include fatigue, anorexia, weight loss, fever, drenching night sweats, and pruritus.

The Ann Arbor staging system considers extent and location of disease, as well as substage classifications that consider systemic symptoms (presence of fever of 38° C [100.4° F] for three consecutive days, drenching night sweats, or unexplained loss of 10% or more of body weight in the 6 months preceding diagnosis). Combination chemotherapy used in conjunction with involved field low-dose radiation has been shown to be an effective treatment, with long-term cure rates reported from 90% to 95%.[40]

SUMMARY REVIEW

Fetal and Neonatal Hematopoiesis

1. After 2 weeks of gestation, circulating erythrocytes play a major role in delivering oxygen to the tissues.
2. Erythropoiesis in the liver and, to a lesser extent, in the spleen and lymph nodes reaches a peak at about 4 months.
3. By the fifth month of gestation, hematopoiesis begins to occur in the bone marrow, and by the time of delivery it is the only significant site of hematopoiesis.
4. A biochemically distinct type of hemoglobin is synthesized during fetal life, including Gower 1, Gower 2, and Portland.

Postnatal Changes in the Blood

1. Blood cell counts tend to rise above adult levels at birth and then decline gradually throughout childhood.
2. The immediate rise in blood cell counts is the result of increased hematopoiesis during fetal life, trauma of birth, and cutting of the umbilical cord.
3. The active rate of fetal erythropoiesis is observed in the large numbers of reticulocytes in the peripheral blood of the full-term neonate.
4. Erythrocyte values are age dependent, and values in males and females are apparent in adolescence.

SUMMARY REVIEW—cont'd

5. The lymphocyte count is high at birth, and continues to rise in some healthy infants during the first year of life.

6. Platelet counts in full-term neonates are comparable to platelet counts in children and adults.

Disorders of Erythrocytes

1. Iron deficiency anemia is the most common blood disorder of infancy and childhood; the highest incidence occurs between 6 months and 2 years of age.

2. HDN results from incompatibility between the maternal and the fetal blood, which may involve differences in Rh factors or blood type (ABO). Maternal antibodies enter the fetal circulation and cause hemolysis of fetal erythrocytes. Because the immature liver is unable to conjugate and excrete the excess bilirubin that results from the hemolysis, icterus neonatorum, or kernicterus or both can develop.

3. Kernicterus, which may result from other causes as well, results in increased breakdown of red blood cells or decreased liver output of enzymes.

4. Infections of the newborn, often acquired by the mother and transmitted to the infant, may result in hemolytic anemia.

5. G6PD deficiency is an inherited enzyme deficiency in erythrocytes that results in a disruption of a common pathway of glycolysis, shortening erythrocyte life span.

6. Hereditary spherocytosis is the most common of the hereditary hemolytic states in which there is no abnormality of hemoglobin. The basic defect is an undefined abnormality of the proteins or spectrins of the erythrocyte membrane in which affected cells are unduly permeable to sodium and acquire a characteristic structure.

7. SCD is a genetically determined defect of hemoglobin synthesis, inherited by an autosomal recessive transmission; it causes a change in the shape of a red blood cell that results in decreased oxygen or hydration. This disease is most common among Africans, blacks, and those of Mediterranean descent.

8. The thalassemias are a heterogeneous group of hereditary hypochromic anemias of varying severity. Basic genetic defects include abnormalities of messenger ribonucleic acid (mRNA) processing or deletion of genetic materials, resulting in a decrease in the chains for hemoglobin.

Disorders of Coagulation and Platelets

1. Hemophilia is a condition characterized by impairment of the coagulation of blood and subsequent tendency to bleed. The classic disease is hereditary and limited to males, being transmitted through the female to the second generation. Many similar conditions attributable to the absence of various clotting factors are recognized.

2. von Willebrand disease is a dominantly inherited disease characterized by a vascular abnormality that produces a prolongation of bleeding time and by decreased levels of clotting factor VIII. The platelets in von Willebrand disease have decreased adhesiveness because the plasma factor is absent.

3. Disorders of congenital hypercoagulability and thrombosis include protein C deficiency, protein S deficiency, neonatal purpura fulminans, and antithrombin III deficiency.

4. The acquired antibody-mediated hemorrhagic diseases include ITP, autoimmune neonatal thrombocytopenia, and autoimmune vascular purpura.

5. ITP, the most common of the childhood thrombocytopenic purpuras, is a disorder of platelet consumption in which antiplatelet antibodies bind to the plasma membranes of platelets. This results in platelet sequestration and destruction by mononuclear phagocytes at a rate that exceeds the ability of the bone marrow to produce them.

6. Autoimmune neonatal thrombocytopenia is an antibody-mediated disorder that occurs in either autoimmune or alloimmune form.

7. The autoimmune vascular purpuras (allergic purpuras) are caused by the body's responses to allergens in the blood.

Leukemia and Lymphoma

1. The most common types of childhood leukemia include, in order of their rate of incidence, ALL, and ANLL.

2. Although the cause of childhood leukemia is not known, it is probably the result of multiple interactions between hereditary or genetic predisposition and environmental influences.

3. Acute lymphoblastic leukemia is a potentially curable disease, with more than 75% to 80% of cases cured.

4. The lymphomas of childhood are non-Hodgkin lymphoma and Hodgkin lymphoma.

5. The origin of non-Hodgkin lymphoma is unknown. Factors that have been implicated include defective host immunity, a viral agent, chronic immunostimulation, and genetic predisposition.

6. Non-Hodgkin lymphoma has a favorable prognosis, with a 70% to 80% cure rate.

7. The risk of Hodgkin lymphoma is associated in part with infectious diseases, immune deficits, and genetic susceptibility.

8. Hodgkin lymphoma is a readily curable disease with long-term cure rates of 90% to 95%.

KEY TERMS

Activated partial thromboplastin time (aPTT), 1080
Acute chest syndrome, 1074
Alpha-thalassemia major, 1077
Alpha-thalassemia minor, 1077
Alpha trait, 1077
Antithrombin III (AT III) deficiency, 1081
Aplastic crisis, 1074
Autoimmune neonatal thrombocytopenia, 1082

Autoimmune vascular purpura (allergic purpura), 1083
Beta-thalassemia major (Cooley anemia), 1077
Beta-thalassemia minor, 1077
Blast cell, 1085
Cholecystitis, 1076
Embryonic hemoglobin (Gower 1, Gower 2, and Portland), 1063
Fetal hemoglobin (Hb F), 1063

Glomerular disease, 1075
Glucose-6-phosphate dehydrogenase (G6PD) deficiency, 1068
Hemoglobin H disease, 1077
Hemoglobin S (Hb S), 1071
Hemolytic disease of the newborn (HDN) (erythroblastosis fetalis), 1065
Hemophilia A (classic hemophilia), 1078
Hemophilia B (Christmas disease), 1078
Hemophilia C (factor XI deficiency), 1079

Continued

KEY TERMS—cont'd

Hereditary spherocytosis (HS), 1070
Hodgkin lymphoma, 1088
Hydrops fetalis, 1067
Hyperbilirubinemia, 1067
Hyperhemolytic crisis, 1074
Icterus gravis neonatorum, 1068
Icterus neonatorum (neonatal jaundice), 1068
Idiopathic thrombocytopenic purpura (ITP) (autoimmune or primary thrombocytopenic purpura), 1081
Kernicterus, 1068

Neonatal alloimmune thrombocytopenic purpura (NATP), 1082
Neonatal purpura fulminans, 1080
Non-Hodgkin lymphoma (NHL), 1087
Polymerization, 1073
Preimplantation genetic diagnosis, 1076
Protein C deficiency, 1080
Protein S deficiency, 1081
Prothrombin consumption time, 1080
Prothrombin time (PT), 1080
Sequestration crisis, 1074
Sickle cell anemia, 1071

Sickle cell disease (SCD), 1071
Sickle cell trait, 1071
Sickle cell–Hb C disease, 1071
Sickle cell–thalassemia disease, 1071
Thalassemia, 1077
Thrombin time, 1080
Thrombophilia, 1080
Thromboplastin generation test, 1080
Vasoocclusive crisis (thrombotic crisis), 1074
von Willebrand disease, 1079

REFERENCES

1. Graham BS: Pathogenesis of respiratory syncytial virus vaccine-augmented pathology, *Am J Resp Crit Care Med* 152:S63-S66, 1995.
2. Schelonka RL et al: Differentiation of segmented and band neutrophils during the newborn period, *J Pediatr* 127:298-300, 1995.
3. Bartlett JA et al: Immune function in healthy inner-city children, *Clin Diag Lab Immunol* 8:740-746, 2001.
4. Cunningham AS: Eosinophil counts—age and sex differences, *J Pediatr* 87:426-427, 1975.
5. Kühne T, Imbach P: Neonatal platelet physiology and pathophysiology, *Eur J Pediatr* 157:87-94, 1998.
6. Khan JL et al: Persistence and emergence of anemia in children during participation in the Special Supplemental Nutrition Program for Women, Infants, and Children, *Arch Pediatr Adolesc Med* 156(10):1028-1032, 2002.
7. Sherry B, Mei Z, Yip R: Continuation of the decline in prevalence of anemia in low-income infants and children in 5 states, *Pediatrics* 107:677-682, 2001.
8. Shah M et al: Effect of orange and apple juice on iron absorption in children, *Arch Pediatr Adolesc Med* 157:1232-1236, 2003.
9. Cook JD: Diagnosis and management of iron-deficiency anemia, *Bailliere's Best Pract Clin Hematol* 18:319-322, 2005.
10. Koelewijn JM et al: Effect of screening for red cell antibodies, other than anti-D, to detect hemolytic disease of the fetus and newborn: a population study in the Netherlands, *Transfusion* 48:941-952, 2008.
11. Chilcott J et al: The economics of routine antenatal anti-D prophylaxis for pregnant women who are rhesus negative, *Br J Obstet Gynecol* 111:903-907, 2004.
12. Luzzatto L: Glucose-6-phosphate dehydrogenase deficiency and hemolytic anemia. In Nathan DG et al, editors: *Hematology of infancy and childhood*, ed 6, pp 704-725, Philadelphia, 2003, Saunders.
13. Lanzkowsky P: Glucose-6-phosphate dehydrogenase deficiency. In Lanzkowsky P, editor: *Manual of pediatric hematology and oncology*, ed 4, pp 153-157, Burlington, Mass, 2005, Elsevier.
14. Delhommeau F et al: Natural history of hereditary spherocytosis during the first year of life, *Blood* 95:393-397, 2000.
15. Bolten-Maggs PH: Hereditary spherocytosis: new guidelines, *Arch Dis Childhood* 89:809-812, 2004.
16. Smith WR et al: Temperature changes, temperature extremes and their relationship to emergency department visits and hospitalizations for sickle cell disease, *Pain Manag Nurs* 4:106-111, 2003.
17. Driscoll CM: Sickle cell disease, *Pediatr Rev* 28:259-268, 2007.
18. Melzer-Lange MD et al: Patient-controlled analgesia for sickle-cell pain crisis in a pediatric emergency department, *Pediatr Emerg Care* 20:2-4, 2004.
19. Thornburg CD et al: A pilot study of hydroxyurea to prevent chronic organ damage in young children with sickle cell anemia,, *Pediatr Blood Cancer* : 2008 Dec 5, (Epub ahead of print).
20. Ross J, editor: *Perspectives of hemophilia carriers*, Montreal, Canada, 2004, World Federation of Hemophilia.
21. Peyvandi F et al: Genetic diagnosis of haemophilia and other inherited bleeding disorders, *Haemophilia* 12(Suppl 3):82-89, 2006.

22. Bowen DJ: Haemophilia A and haemophilia B: molecular insights, *Mol Pathol* 55(2):127-144, 2002.
23. Ananyeva N et al: Treating hemophilia A with recombinant blood factors: a comparison, *Exp Opin Pharmacother* 5:1061-1070, 2004.
24. Manco-Johnson MJ et al: Prophylaxis versus episodic treatment to prevent joint disease in boys with severe hemophilia, *N Engl J Med* 357:535-544, 2007.
25. Young G: Diagnosis and treatment of thrombosis in children: general principles, *Pediatr Blood Cancer* 46:540-546, 2006.
26. Kubota M et al: Serum immunoglobulin levels at onset: association with the prognosis of childhood idiopathic thrombocytopenic purpura, *Internat J Hematol* 77:304–304, 2003.
27. Gupta V, Tilak V, Bhatia BD: Immune thrombocytopenic purpura, *Indian J Pediatr* 75:723-728, 2008.
28. Yldrm ZK et al: Late side effects of high-dose steroid therapy on skeletal system in children with idiopathic thrombocytopenic purpura, *J Pediatr Hematol Oncol* 30:749-753, 2008.
29. Nugent DJ: Immune thrombocytopenic purpura of childhood, *Hematology Am Soc Hematol Educ Program* :97-103, 2006.
30. American Cancer Society: *Cancer facts and figures 2008*, Atlanta, 2008, American Cancer Society.
31. Plon SE, Malkin D: Childhood cancer and heredity. In Pizzo PA, Poplack DG, editors: *Principles and practice of pediatric oncology*, pp 14-37, Philadelphia, 2006, Lippincott Williams & Wilkins.
32. Buka I, Koranteng S, Osornio-Vargas AR: Trends in childhood cancer incidence: review of environmental linkages, *Pediatr Clin North Am* 54:177-203, 2007.
33. Greaves MF et al: Leukemia in twins: lessons in natural history, *Blood* 102:2321-2333, 2003.
34. Infante-Rivard C, Guiguet M: Family history of hematopoietic and other cancers in children with acute lymphoblastic leukemia, *Cancer Detect Prev* 28:83-87, 2004.
35. Laurier D et al: Epidemiological studies of leukaemia in children and young adults around nuclear facilities: a critical review, *Radiat Prot Dosimetry* : Oct 15, 2008, (Epub ahead of print).
36. Powles T et al: Head and neck cancer in patients with human immunodeficiency virus-1 infection: incidence, outcome and association with Epstein-Barr virus, *J Laryngol Otol* 118(3):207-212, 2004.
37. Koh S et al: Anterior lumbosacral radiculopathy after intrathecal methotrexate treatment, *Pediatr Neurol* 21:576-578, 1999.
38. Link MP, Weinstein HJ: Malignant non-Hodgkin lymphoma in children. In Pizzo PA, Poplack DG, editors: *Principles and practice of pediatric oncology*, pp 722-747, Philadelphia, 2006, Lippincott Williams & Wilkins.
39. Pinkerton R: Continuing challenges in childhood non-Hodgkin's lymphoma, *Br J Hematol* 130:480-488, 2005.
40. Hudson MM, Donaldson SS, Onciu M: Malignant non-Hodgkin lymphoma in children. In Pizzo PA, Poplack DG, editors: *Principles and practice of pediatric oncology*, pp 695-721, Philadelphia, 2006, Lippincott Williams & Wilkins.
41. Oliapuram Jose B et al: Pediatric Hodgkin's disease, *J Ky Med Assoc* 102(3):104-106, 2004.

STRUCTURE AND FUNCTION OF THE CARDIOVASCULAR AND LYMPHATIC SYSTEMS

VALENTINA L. BRASHERS • KATHRYN L. McCANCE

MEDIA RESOURCES

evolve **Evolve Website** (http://evolve.elsevier.com/McCance/)
- Review Questions and Answers
- Animations
- Glossary (with audio pronunciation for selected terms)
- WebLinks

CHAPTER OUTLINE

CIRCULATORY SYSTEM
THE HEART
   Structures That Direct Circulation Through the Heart
   Structures That Support Cardiac Metabolism: The
      Coronary Vessels
   Structures That Control Heart Action
   Factors Affecting Cardiac Output
SYSTEMIC CIRCULATION
   Structure of Blood Vessels
   Factors Affecting Blood Flow

   Regulation of Blood Pressure (Arterial Pressure)
   Regulation of Coronary Circulation
LYMPHATIC SYSTEM
TESTS OF CARDIOVASCULAR FUNCTION
   Cardiac and Coronary Artery Evaluation
   Systemic Vascular Evaluation
   Aging and the Cardiovascular System

The function of the circulatory system is to deliver oxygen, nutrients, and other substances to all the body's cells and to remove the waste products of cellular metabolism. Delivery and removal are achieved by a complex array of tubing—the blood vessels—connected to a pump—the heart. The heart pumps blood continuously through the blood vessels with cooperation from other systems, particularly the nervous and endocrine systems, which are intrinsic regulators of the heart and blood vessels. Nutrients and oxygen are supplied by the digestive and respiratory systems; gaseous wastes of cellular metabolism are blown off by the lungs; and other wastes are removed by the kidneys.

Of critical importance is the role of the vascular endothelium. It is a multifunctional organ whose health is essential to normal vascular physiology and whose dysfunction is an important factor in the pathogenesis of vascular disease.

CIRCULATORY SYSTEM

The heart pumps blood through two separate circulatory systems, one to the lungs and one to all other parts of the body. Structures on the right side of the heart, or **right heart,** pump blood through the lungs. (This system, termed the **pulmonary circulation,** is described in Chapter 32.) The left side of the heart, or **left heart,** sends blood throughout the **systemic circulation,** which supplies all of the body except the lungs (Figure 29-1). These two systems are serially connected, thus the output of one becomes the input of the other.

Arteries carry blood from the heart to all parts of the body, where they branch into even smaller vessels until they become a fine meshwork of capillaries. Capillaries allow the closest contact and exchange between the blood and the interstitial space, or interstitium—the environment in which the cells live. Veins channel blood from capillaries in all parts of the body back to the heart. The plasma passes through the walls

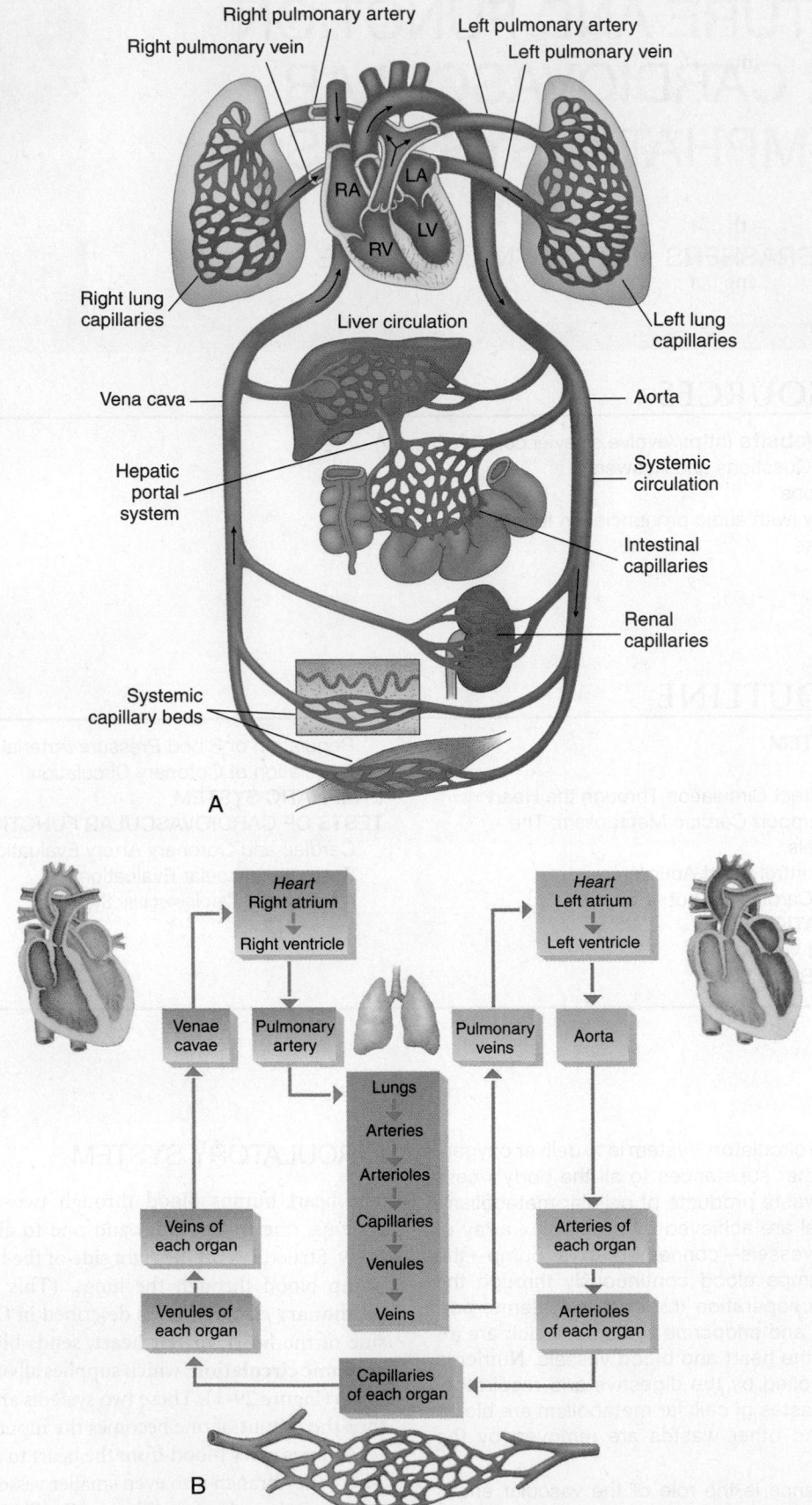

Figure 29-1 Diagram showing serially connected pulmonary and systemic circulatory systems and how to trace the flow of blood. **A,** Right heart chambers propel unoxygenated blood through the pulmonary circulation, and the left heart propels oxygenated blood through the systemic circulation. **B,** The direction of blood flow begins at the left ventricle of the heart, flows to the arteries, arterioles, capillaries of each body organ, venules, veins, right atrium, right ventricle, pulmonary artery, lung capillaries, pulmonary veins, left atrium, and then goes back to the left ventricle. *RA,* Right atrium; *RV,* right ventricle; *LA,* left atrium, *LV,* left ventricle. (B from Thibodeau GA, Patton KT: *Anatomy & physiology,* ed 5, St Louis, 2003, Mosby.)

of the capillaries into the interstitial space. This fluid eventually is returned to the cardiovascular system by vessels of the lymphatic system.

THE HEART

The adult heart weighs less than 1 pound and is about the size of a fist. It lies obliquely (diagonally) in the **mediastinum,** an area above the diaphragm and between the lungs. The heart of a normal woman is smaller and lighter than that of a normal man.

Heart structures can be categorized by function:

1. *Structural support of heart tissues and circulation of pulmonary and systemic blood through the heart.* This category includes the heart wall and fibrous skeleton, which enclose and support the heart and divide it into four chambers; the valves that direct flow through the chambers; and the great vessels that conduct blood to and from the heart.

2. *Maintenance of heart cells.* This category comprises vessels of the coronary circulation—the arteries and veins that serve the metabolic needs of all the heart cells—and the lymphatic vessels of the heart.

3. *Stimulation and control of heart action.* Among these structures are the nerves and specialized muscle cells that direct the rhythmic contraction and relaxation of the heart muscles, propelling blood throughout the pulmonary and systemic circulatory system.

Structures That Direct Circulation Through the Heart

Heart Wall

The heart wall has three layers—the pericardium, myocardium, and endocardium. The pericardium is a double-walled membranous sac that encloses the heart (Figure 29-2). The **pericardium** has several functions. It (1) prevents displacement of the heart during gravitational acceleration or deceleration, (2) is a physical barrier that protects the heart against infection and inflammation from the lungs and pleural space, and (3) contains pain receptors and mechanoreceptors that can elicit reflex changes in blood pressure and heart rate. The outer layer of the pericardium, the **parietal pericardium**, is composed of a surface layer of mesothelium over a thin layer of connective tissue. The **visceral pericardium,** or **epicardium,** is the inner layer of the pericardium. At one point the visceral pericardium folds back and becomes continuous with the parietal pericardium, allowing the large vessels to enter and leave the heart without breaching the pericardial layers.

The visceral and parietal pericardia are separated by a fluid-containing space called the **pericardial cavity.** The **pericardial fluid** (10 to 30 ml), which is secreted by cells of the mesothelium, lubricates the membranes that line the pericardial cavity, enabling them to slide over one another with a minimum of friction as the heart beats. The amount and character of the pericardial fluid are altered by inflammation of the pericardium (see Chapter 30).

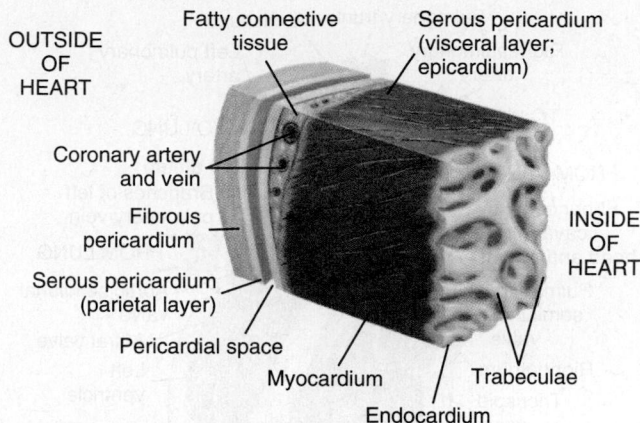

Figure 29-2 Wall of the heart. This section of the heart wall shows the fibrous pericardium, the parietal and visceral layers of the serous pericardium (with the pericardial space between them), the myocardium, and the endocardium. Note the fatty connective tissue between the visceral layer of the serous pericardium (epicardium) and the myocardium. Note also that the endocardium covers beamlike projections of myocardial muscle tissue, called *trabeculae.* (From Thibodeau GA, Patton KT: *Anatomy & physiology,* ed 5, St Louis, 2003, Mosby.)

The thickest layer of the heart wall, the **myocardium,** is composed of cardiac muscle and is anchored to the heart's fibrous skeleton. The thickness of the myocardium varies tremendously from one heart chamber to another. Thickness is related to the amount of resistance the muscle must overcome to pump blood from the different chambers. The internal lining of the myocardium is composed of connective tissue and a layer of squamous cells called the **endocardium** (see Figure 29-2). The endocardial lining of the heart is continuous with the endothelium that lines all the arteries, veins, and capillaries of the body, creating a continuous, closed circulatory system.

Chambers of the Heart

The heart has four chambers: the **right atrium, left atrium, right ventricle,** and **left ventricle.** (Blood flow through these chambers is illustrated in Figure 29-3.) The atria are smaller than the ventricles and have thinner walls. The wall of the right atrium is about 2 mm thick, and the wall of the left atrium is about 3 to 5 mm thick. The ventricles have a thicker myocardial layer and make up much of the bulk of the heart. The wall of the right ventricle is about 3 to 5 mm thick, and that of the left ventricle, the most muscular chamber, is about 13 to 15 mm. The ventricles are formed by a continuum of muscle fibers that take origin from the fibrous skeleton at the base of the heart (chiefly around the aortic orifice).

The myocardial thickness of each cardiac chamber depends on the amount of pressure or resistance it must overcome to eject blood. The two atria have the thinnest walls because they are low-pressure chambers that serve as storage units and conduits for blood that is emptied into the ventricles. Normally, there is little resistance to flow from the atria to the ventricles. The ventricles, on the other hand, must propel blood all the way through the pulmonary or systemic circulation. The ventricular myocardium also must be strong enough to pump

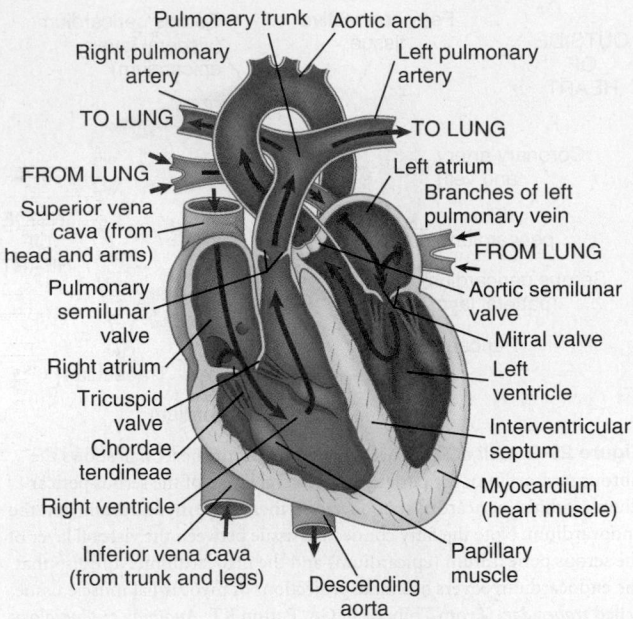

Figure 29-3 Structures that direct blood flow through the heart. Arrows indicate path of blood flow through chambers, valves, and major vessels.

against pressures in the pulmonary or systemic vessels. The mean pulmonary capillary pressure, which is the major force favoring movement of fluid out of the pulmonary capillaries into the interstitium, is only 15 mmHg. By comparison, the mean arterial pressure is about 92 mmHg. Pressure is greatest in the systemic circulation, driven by the left ventricle; the left ventricle's myocardium is several times thicker than that of the right ventricle.

The right ventricle is shaped like a crescent, or triangle, enabling it to function like a bellows and efficiently eject large volumes of blood through a very small valve into the low-pressure pulmonary system. The left ventricle is larger and bullet shaped, helping it to eject blood through a relatively large valve opening into the high-pressure systemic circulation.

The ventricles are structurally more complex than the atria. Each ventricle contains muscle fibers that divide it roughly into an **inflow tract,** which receives blood from the atrium, and an **outflow tract,** which sends blood to the circulation (see Figure 29-3).

Normally blood does not flow between the chambers of the right side of the heart and the chambers of the left side of the heart. The adult right and left sides of the heart are separated by an intact septal membrane. The atria are separated by the interatrial septum, and the ventricles by the interventricular septum. The interventricular septum is an extension of the fibrous skeleton of the heart. Indentations of the endocardium form valves that separate the atria from the ventricles and the ventricles from the aorta and pulmonary arteries.

Fibrous Skeleton of the Heart
Four rings of dense fibrous connective tissue provide a firm anchorage for the attachments of the atrial and ventricular musculature, as well as the valvular tissue. The fibrous rings

are adjacent and form a central, fibrous supporting structure collectively termed the anuli fibrosi cordis.

Valves of the Heart
One-way blood flow through the heart is ensured by the four heart valves. During ventricular relaxation the two **atrioventricular valves** open and blood flows from the higher-pressure atria to the relaxed ventricles. With increasing ventricular pressure these valves close and prevent backflow into the atria as the ventricles contract. The **semilunar valves** of the heart open when intraventricular pressure exceeds aortic and pulmonary pressures and blood flows out of the ventricles and into the pulmonary and systemic circulations. After ventricular contraction and ejection, intraventricular pressure falls and the **pulmonic** and **aortic semilunar valves** close, preventing backflow into the right and left ventricles (Figure 29-4; see also Figure 29-3).

The atrioventricular (AV) (tricuspid and mitral) valve openings are guarded by flaps of tissue called *leaflets or cusps* that are attached to the papillary muscles by the **chordae tendineae** (see Figure 29-3). The **papillary muscles** are extensions of the myocardium that pull the cusps together and downward at the onset of ventricular contraction, thus preventing their backward expulsion into the atria (see p. 1096 for a description of pressure changes and valvular function).

The right AV valve is called the **tricuspid valve** because it has three cusps. The tricuspid opening (orifice) has the largest diameter of all the heart valves. The left AV valve is a bicuspid (two cusps) valve called the **mitral valve.** The mitral valve resembles a cone-shaped funnel that extends into the cusps, which are connected by a fibrous tissue called the *commissure.* The anterior cusp of the mitral valve is continuous with supporting tissues of the aortic semilunar valve cusps and the left coronary valve cusps. (The coronary circulation is described on p. 1096.) Thus damage to this continuous tissue can alter function of the aortic as well as the mitral valves.

The tricuspid and mitral valves function as a unit because the atrium, fibrous rings, valvular tissue, chordae tendineae, papillary muscles, and ventricular walls are connected. Collectively, these six structures are known as the **mitral and tricuspid complex.** Damage to any one of the complex's six components can alter function significantly.

Blood leaves the right ventricle through the pulmonic semilunar valve, and it leaves the left ventricle through the aortic semilunar valve (see Figures 29-3 and 29-4). The pulmonic and aortic semilunar valves have three cup-shaped cusps that arise from the fibrous skeleton. The pulmonic cusps are slightly thinner than the aortic cusps. The lower edges of each cusp are suspended from the root of the pulmonary artery or aorta, with the upper valve edges freely projecting into the vessel lumen. When the ventricles contract, the cusps behave like one-way swinging doors. The force of the blood propels the cusps outward against the vessel wall. When the ventricles relax, blood fills the cusps and causes their free edges to meet in the middle of the vessel, closing the valve and preventing any backflow.

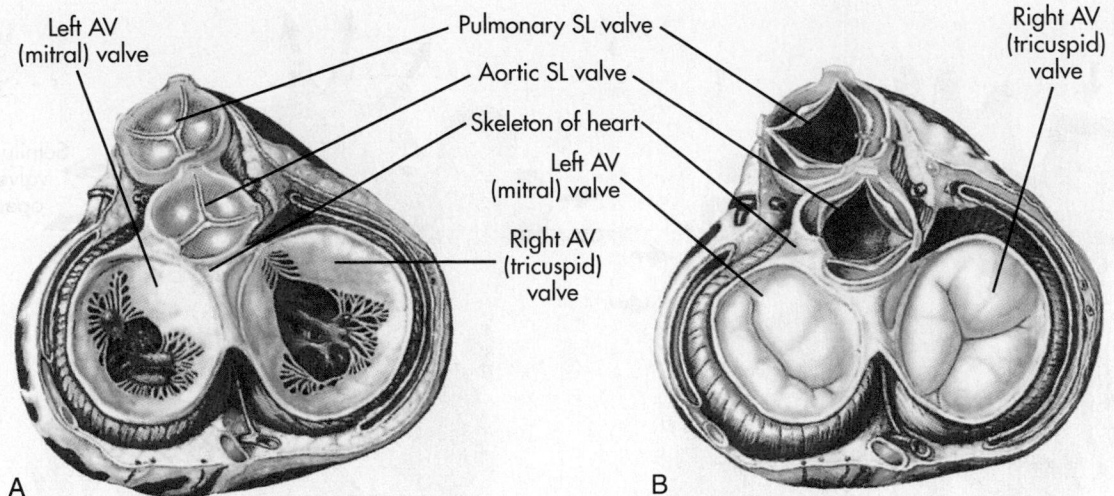

Figure 29-4 Structure of the heart valves. **A,** The heart valves in this drawing are depicted as viewed from above (looking down into the heart). Note that the semilunar (SL) valves are closed and the atrioventricular (AV) valves are open, as when the atria are contracting. **B,** Similar to A except that the semilunar valves are closed and the AV valves are open, as when the ventricles are contracting. (From Thibodeau GA, Patton KT: *Anatomy & physiology,* ed 5, St Louis, 2003, Mosby.)

Great Vessels

Blood moves in and out of the heart through several large vessels (see Figure 29-3). The right heart receives venous blood from the systemic circulation through the **superior vena cava** and the **inferior vena cava,** which enter the right atrium. Blood leaves the right ventricle and enters the pulmonary circulation through the pulmonary artery. The **pulmonary artery** divides into **right** and **left pulmonary arteries** to transport unoxygenated blood from the right heart to the right and left lungs. The pulmonary arteries branch further into the pulmonary capillary bed, where oxygen and carbon dioxide exchange occurs.

The four **pulmonary veins,** two from the right lung and two from the left lung, carry oxygenated blood from the lungs to the left side of the heart. The oxygenated blood moves through the left atrium and ventricle and out into the **aorta,** which delivers it to systemic vessels that supply the body.

Blood Flow During the Cardiac Cycle

The pumping action of the heart consists of contraction and relaxation of the myocardial layer of the heart wall. Each ventricular contraction and the relaxation that follows it constitute one **cardiac cycle.** (Blood flow through the heart during a single cardiac cycle is illustrated in Figure 29-5.) During relaxation, termed **diastole,** blood fills the ventricles. The contraction that follows, termed **systole,** propels the blood out of the ventricles and into the circulation. Contraction of the left ventricle is slightly earlier than contraction of the right ventricle.

During ventricular systole, blood from the veins of the systemic circulation enters the thin-walled right atrium from the superior vena cava and the inferior vena cava (see Figures 29-3 and 29-5). Venous blood from the coronary circulation enters the right atrium through the coronary sinus. The right atrium fills and distends, pushing open the right AV (tricuspid) valve. This permits blood to fill the right ventricle during ventricular diastole (sometimes called atrial systole). The same sequence

of events occurs a split second earlier in the left heart. The four pulmonary veins, two from the right lung and two from the left lung, carry blood from the pulmonary circulation to the left atrium. As the left atrium fills, it pushes the cusps of the mitral valve open and blood flows into the left ventricle. Left atrial contraction, "atrial kick," provides a significant increase of blood to the left ventricle. Filling of the right and left ventricles occurs during one period of diastole.

Five phases of the cardiac cycle can be identified (Figures 29-6 and 29-7):

Phase 1: Atrial systole (ventricular diastole) begins with opening of the mitral and tricuspid valves and ventricular filling from the atria occurs. The ventricles fill rapidly in early diastole and again in late diastole when the atria contract.

Phase 2: Ventricular systole begins with "isovolumic contraction," so-called because ventricular volume is constant; that is, the lengths of the muscle fibers remain relatively constant. Isovolumic contraction is the first detectable rise in ventricular pressure. Contraction pushes the AV valves shut. Their cusps bulge backward but are prevented from opening back into the atria by their anchors, the chordae tendineae (see Figure 29-3).

Phase 3: When ventricular pressure reaches that of the pulmonary artery and aorta, the semilunar valves open and ventricular ejection occurs. Intraventricular pressure and ventricular volume decrease rapidly.

Phase 4: With ventricular relaxation and decreased ventricular pressure, the aortic valve closes and "isovolumic relaxation" occurs.

Phase 5: When sufficient decreases exist in left ventricular pressure, the mitral valve opens and *passive ventricular filling occurs.*

As blood is pushed through the inflow and outflow tracts of the ventricles, it flows around the **crista supraventricularis—** the muscle that separates the inflow from the outflow

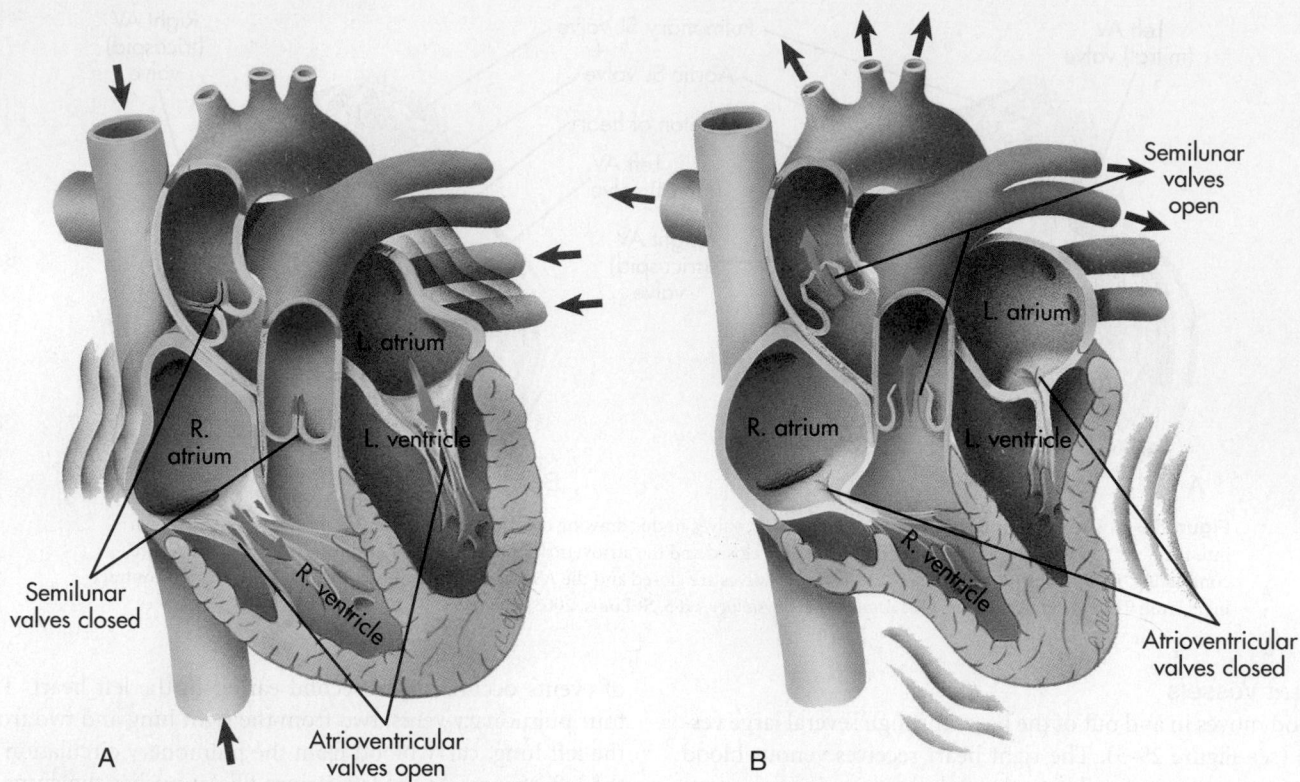

Figure 29-5 Chambers and valves of the heart. These illustrations depict the action of the heart chambers and valves when the atria contract (A), and when the ventricles contract (B). (From Thibodeau GA, Patton KT: *Anatomy & physiology*, ed 5, St Louis, 2003, Mosby.)

tracts—and is mixed by passing through the strands of the **trabeculae carneae.**

Normal Intracardiac Pressures

Normal intracardiac pressures are shown in Table 29-1 and Figures 29-6 and 29-8. Atrial pressure curves are composed of the **a wave,** which is generated by atrial contraction, and the **v wave,** which is an early diastolic peak caused by filling of the atrium from the peripheral veins. The **x descent** follows the a wave and is produced because of descent of the tricuspid valve ring and by the ejection of blood from both ventricles. The **y descent** follows the v wave and reflects the rapid flow of blood from the great veins and right atrium into the right ventricle. A small deflection, the **c wave,** occurs after the a wave in early systole and may represent bulging of the mitral valve into the left atrium during early systole. Ventricular pressures are illustrated by a peak systolic pressure and an end-diastolic pressure, which is the ventricular pressure immediately before the onset of systole. The minimal left ventricular pressure occurs in early diastole.

Structures That Support Cardiac Metabolism: The Coronary Vessels

The blood within the heart chambers does not supply oxygen and other nutrients to the cells of the heart. Like all other organs, including the lungs, heart structures are nourished by vessels of the systemic circulation. The branch of the systemic

circulation that supplies the heart is termed the *coronary circulation* and consists of coronary arteries, which receive blood through openings in the aorta, called the *coronary ostia.* The cardiac veins empty into the right atrium through another ostium, the opening of a large vein called the *coronary sinus* (Figure 29-9). (Regulation of the coronary circulation, which is similar to regulation of flow through systemic and pulmonary vessels, is described elsewhere.)

Coronary Arteries

The major coronary arteries are the **right coronary artery (RCA)** and the **left coronary artery (LCA)** (see Figure 29-9). These arteries traverse the epicardium and branch several times. The right coronary artery has greater flow than the left in 50% of individuals, the left greater than the right in 20%, and equal flow in each in 30%.[1] The pattern of branching through the visceral pericardium differs from heart to heart. The branches enter the myocardium and endocardium and branch further to become arterioles and then capillaries. Although the coronary arteries are smaller in women than men, this is attributable to differences in heart weight.

The left coronary artery arises from a single ostium (opening) behind the left cusp of the aortic semilunar valve. This artery ranges from a few millimeters to a few centimeters in length. It passes between the left atrial appendage and the pulmonary artery and generally divides into two branches—the left anterior descending artery and the circumflex artery.

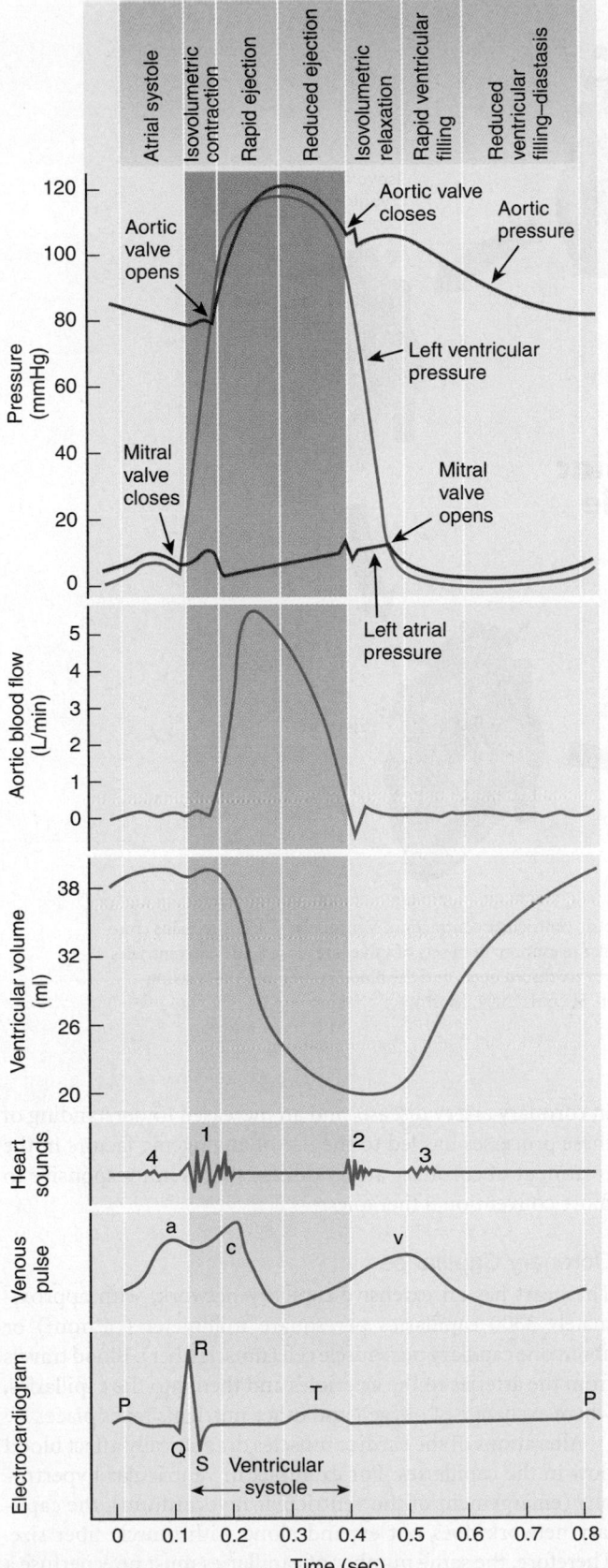

Figure 29-6 Composite chart of heart function. This chart is a composite of several diagrams of heart function (cardiac pumping cycle, blood pressure, blood flow, volume, heart sounds, venous pulse, and electrocardiogram [ECG]), all adjusted to the same time scale.

Other branches of the left main coronary artery are distributed diagonally across the free wall of the left ventricle.

The **left anterior descending artery (LAD),** also called the *anterior interventricular artery,* delivers blood to portions of the left and right ventricles and much of the interventricular septum. The left anterior descending artery travels down the anterior surface of the interventricular septum toward the apex of the heart.

The **circumflex artery** travels in a groove called the **coronary sulcus,** which separates the left atrium from the left ventricle, to the left border of the heart. It supplies blood to the left atrium and the lateral wall of the left ventricle. The circumflex artery often branches to the posterior surfaces of the left atrium and left ventricle (see Figure 29-9).

The right coronary artery originates from an ostium behind the right aortic cusp, travels behind the pulmonary artery, and extends around the right heart to the heart's posterior surface, where it branches to the atrium and the ventricle. The three major branches of the right coronary artery include the conus, which supplies blood to the upper right ventricle; the right marginal branch, which traverses the right ventricle to the apex; and the posterior descending branch, which lies in the posterior interventricular sulcus and supplies smaller branches to both ventricles.

Collateral Arteries

The **collateral arteries** are really connections, or anastomoses, between two branches of the same coronary artery or connections of branches of the right coronary artery with branches of the left. They are particularly common within the interventricular and interatrial septa, at the apex of the heart, over the anterior surface of the right ventricle, and around the sinus node. The epicardium contains more collateral vessels than the endocardium.

The functional importance of the collateral circulation is that it protects the heart from ischemia. The collateral circulation is responsible for supplying blood and oxygen to the myocardium that has been deprived of oxygen following narrowing of a major coronary artery (coronary artery disease). Gradual coronary occlusion results in the growth of coronary collaterals. New collateral vessels are formed through two processes, **arteriogenesis** (new artery growth from preexisting arteries) and **angiogenesis** (growth of new capillaries within a tissue).[2]

The stimulus to collateral arteriogenesis is the **shear stress** caused by increased blood flow velocity that occurs close to the site of occlusion. Shear stress activates the endothelium of the preexisting arterioles and stimulates the production of growth factors and cytokines, including monocyte chemoattractant protein-1 (MCP-1) and vascular endothelial growth factor (VEGF).[3] Monocytes/macrophages are called to the area of endothelial activation and release more growth factors and cytokines. Recent studies suggest that adequate monocyte numbers and function are critical to the growth of collaterals in individuals with coronary artery disease.[3] As the collaterals begin to accept coronary flow, flow stress and pressure changes cause them to be restructured and remodeled.

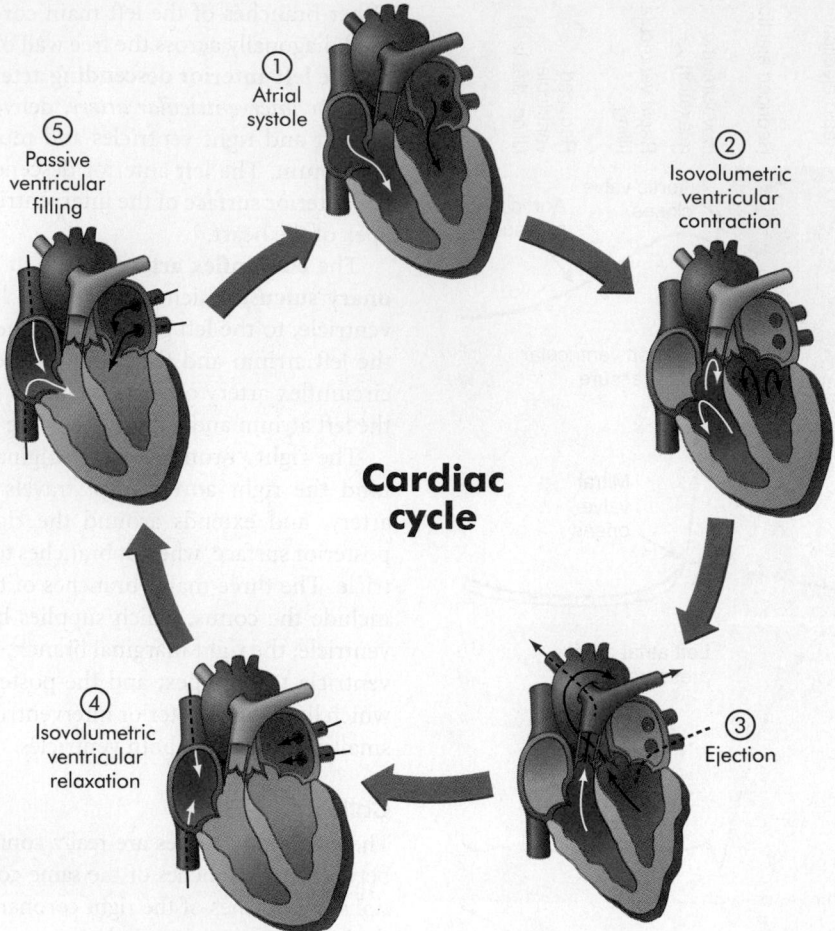

Cardiac cycle

① Atrial systole
② Isovolumetric ventricular contraction
③ Ejection
④ Isovolumetric ventricular relaxation
⑤ Passive ventricular filling

Figure 29-7 Phases of the cardiac cycle. **1,** Atrial systole. **2,** Isovolumetric ventricular contraction. Ventricular volume remains constant as pressure increases rapidly. **3,** Ejection. **4,** Isovolumetric ventricular relaxation. Both sets of valves are closed, and the ventricles are relaxing. **5,** Passive ventricular filling. The atrioventricular (AV) valves are forced open, and the blood rushes into the relaxing ventricles. (From Thibodeau GA, Patton KT: *Anatomy & physiology,* ed 6, St Louis, 2007, Mosby.)

Table 29-1	Normal Intracardiac Pressures	
	Mean (mmHg)	**Range (mmHg)**
Right atrium	4	0-8
Right ventricle		
Systolic	24	15-28
End-diastolic	4	0-8
Left atrium	7	4-12
Left ventricle		
Systolic	130	90-140
End-diastolic	7	4-12

Angiogenesis also is stimulated by numerous growth factors (VEGF, fibroblast growth factor [FGF]) and through the production of nitric oxide.[2,4] Unfortunately, diabetes, which predisposes to coronary artery disease, also impedes collateral formation because of increased production of antiangiogenic factors such as endostatin and angiostatin.[5] The presence of an effective collateral system has been shown to be protective in coronary artery disease, and an increased understanding of these processes has led to the use of angiogenic factors in the treatment of coronary artery disease that is not responsive to more conventional therapies.[6]

Coronary Capillaries

The heart has an extensive capillary network, with approximately 3300 capillaries per square millimeter (ca/mm²) or about one capillary per muscle cell (muscle fiber). Blood travels from the arteries to the arterioles and then into the capillaries, where exchange of oxygen and other nutrients takes place.

Alterations of the cardiac muscles dramatically affect blood flow in the capillaries. For example, in ventricular hypertrophy (enlargement of the ventricular myocardium), the capillary network does not expand along with muscle fiber size. Therefore, the same number of capillaries must now perfuse a larger area. This results in decreased exchange of oxygen and nutrients. At rest, the heart extracts 70% to 80% of the oxygen delivered to it and coronary blood flow is directly correlated with myocardial oxygen consumption.[1]

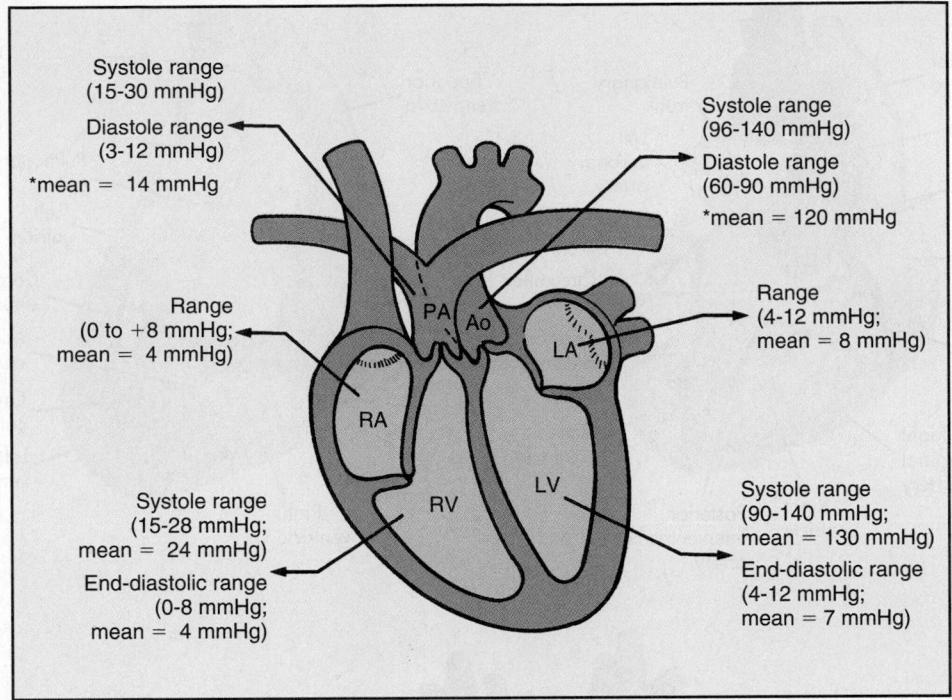

Figure 29-8 Normal intracardiac pressures. *Ao,* Aorta; *LA,* left atrium; *LV,* left ventricle; *PA,* pulmonary artery; *RA,* right atrium; *RV,* right ventricle. *Main mean pressure.

Coronary Veins and Lymphatic Vessels

After passing through the extensive capillary network, blood from the coronary arteries drains into the cardiac veins, which travel alongside the arteries. Most of the venous drainage of the heart occurs through veins in the visceral pericardium. The veins then feed into the great cardiac vein (see Figure 29-9) and coronary sinus on the posterior surface of the heart, between the atria and ventricles, in the coronary sulcus. Venous coronary blood empties into the right atrium from the coronary sinus. Blood from the left ventricular walls generally is drained through the coronary sinus and its tributaries, which together form the largest system of coronary veins. The **great cardiac vein** primarily drains the anterior surface of the heart. The **posterior vein of the left ventricle,** the largest on the posterior surface of the heart, branches from the coronary sinus and accompanies the circumflex artery.

The myocardium has an extensive system of lymphatic vessels. With cardiac contraction the lymphatic vessels drain fluid to lymph nodes in the anterior mediastinum that eventually empty into the superior vena cava. The lymphatics are important for protecting the myocardium against injury. (The lymphatic vessels are described on p. 1131.)

Structures That Control Heart Action

The continuous, rhythmic repetition of the cardiac cycle (systole and diastole) depends on the transmission of electrical impulses, termed **cardiac action potentials,** through the myocardium. (Action potentials are described in Chapters 1 and 3.) As an electrical impulse passes from cell to cell (fiber to fiber) in the myocardium, it stimulates the fibers to shorten. Shortening causes muscular contraction, or systole. After the action potential passes, the fibers relax and return to their resting length, causing diastole. The muscle fibers of the myocardium are uniquely joined so that action potentials pass from cell to cell very rapidly and efficiently. Therefore, an action potential generated in one part of the myocardium passes almost simultaneously through all its contiguous fibers, causing rapid contraction.

The myocardium differs from other muscle tissues in that it contains its own **conduction system**—specialized cells that enable it to generate and transmit action potentials without stimulation from the nervous system (Figure 29-10). These cells are concentrated at certain sites in the myocardium called **nodes.** Although the heart is innervated by the autonomic nervous system (sympathetic and parasympathetic fibers), neural impulses are not needed to maintain the cardiac cycle. Thus the heart will beat in the absence of any nervous connection. The cardiac cycle is stimulated by the nodes of specialized cells and "fine-tuned" as needed by the autonomic fibers. The sympathetic and parasympathetic nerves affect the speed of the cardiac cycle (**heart rate,** or beats per minute) and the diameter of the coronary vessels (Figure 29-11). The sympathetic nervous system increases heart rate and conduction through the nodes, the parasympathetic nervous system slows heart rate and prolongs intranodal conduction time, and both systems cause coronary vasodilation.[7]

Heart action is also influenced by substances delivered to the myocardium in coronary blood. Nutrients and oxygen are needed for cellular survival and normal function, and hormones and biochemicals affect the strength and duration of

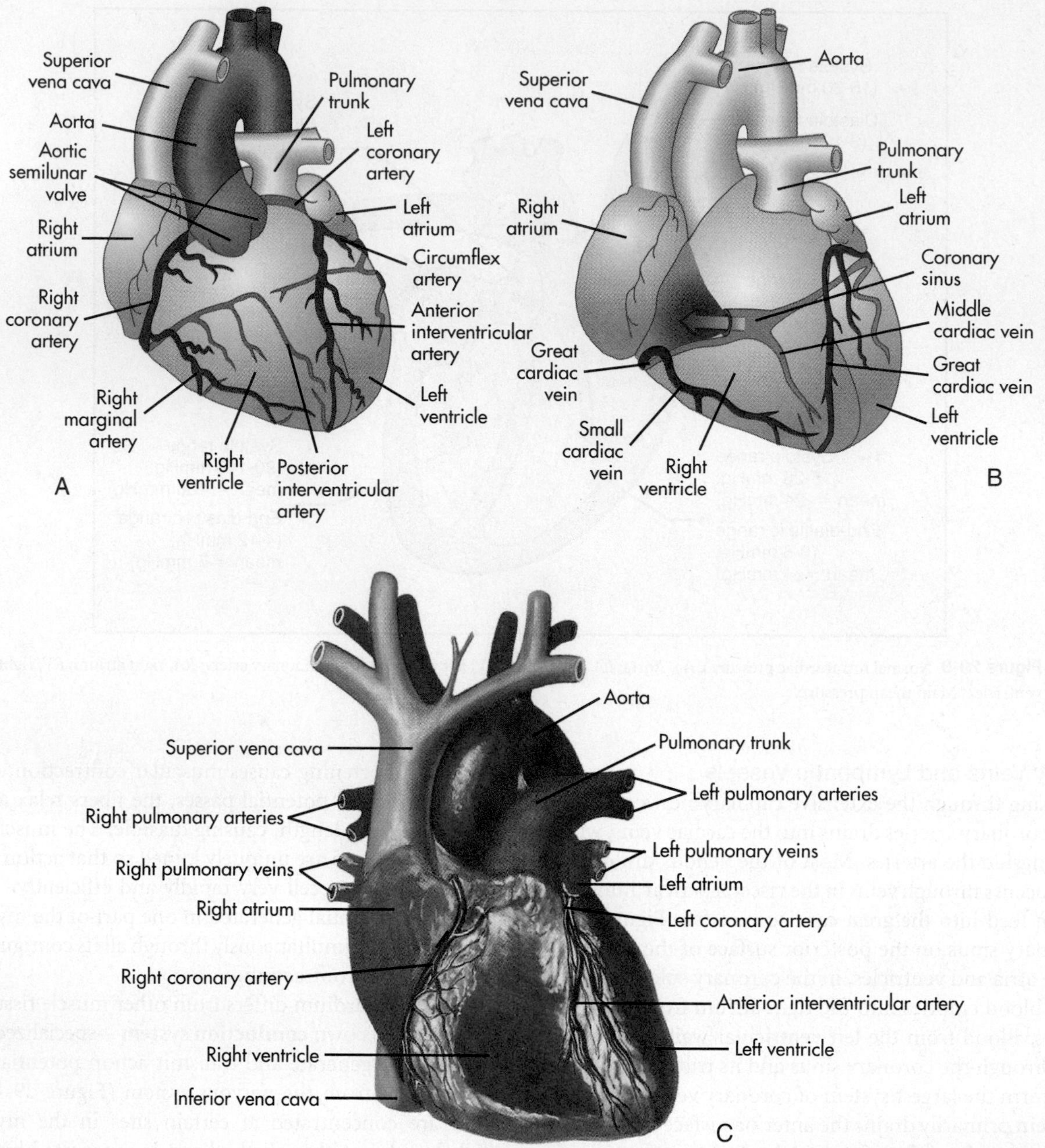

Figure 29-9 Coronary circulation. **A,** Arteries. **B,** Veins. Both **A** and **B** are anterior views of the heart. Vessels near the anterior surface are more darkly colored than vessels of the posterior surface seen through the heart. **C,** View of the anterior (sternocostal) surface. (**A** and **B,** modified from Thibodeau GA, Patton KT: *Anatomy & physiology,* ed 5, St Louis, 2003, Mosby. **C,** from Seeley RR, Stephens TD, Tate P: *Anatomy & physiology,* ed 3, St Louis, 1995, Mosby.)

myocardial contraction and the degree and duration of myocardial relaxation. Normal or appropriate function depends on the availability of these substances, which is why coronary artery disease can seriously disrupt heart function.

Conduction System

Normally electrical impulses arise in the **sinoatrial (SA) node (SA node, sinus node),** which is often called the *pacemaker of the heart.* The SA node is located at the junction of the right atrium and superior vena cava, just above the tricuspid valve (see Figure 29-10). The SA node lies only 1 mm or less beneath

the visceral pericardium, making it vulnerable to injury and disease, especially pericardial inflammation. The SA node is nourished by the sinus node artery, which passes through the center of the node. Numerous autonomic nerve endings are within the node. The SA node is heavily innervated by both sympathetic and parasympathetic nerve fibers.[7] The SA node's **P cells,** so-called because they are pale and primitive appearing, are assumed to be the site of impulse formation.

In the resting adult the SA node generates about 75 action potentials per minute. Each one travels rapidly from cell to cell and through special pathways in the atrial myocardium,

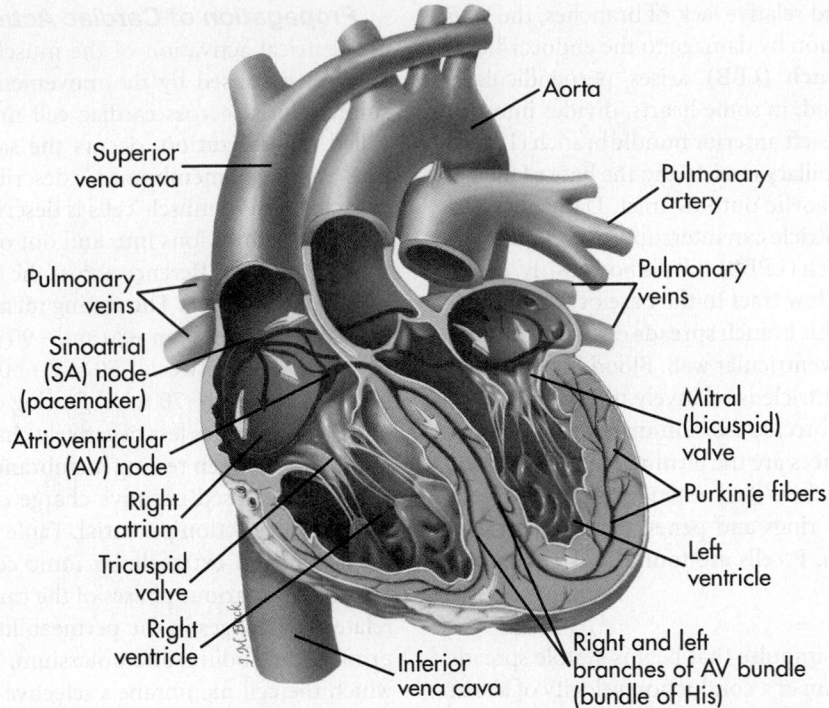

Figure 29-10 Conduction system of the heart. Specialized cardiac muscle cells in the wall of the heart rapidly conduct an electrical impulse throughout the myocardium. The signal is initiated by the SA node (pacemaker) and spreads to the rest of the atrial myocardium and to the AV node. The AV node then initiates a signal that is conducted through the ventricular myocardium by way of the AV bundle (of His) and Purkinje fibers. (Modified from Thibodeau GA, Patton KT: *Anatomy & physiology*, ed 5, St Louis, 2003, Mosby.)

causing both atria to contract, beginning systole. Ventricular contraction is delayed because the fibrous skeleton of the heart interrupts cell-to-cell transmission of the electrical impulses. The action potential is transmitted from the atrial to the ventricular myocardium through fibers of the conduction system, traveling first to the **atrioventricular (AV) node** then to the **bundle of His (atrioventricular bundle, common bundle),** and finally through the **bundle branches** of the interventricular septum to Purkinje fibers in the heart wall (see Figure 29-10).

The AV node is well situated for mediating conduction between the atria and ventricles. It is located in the right atrial wall above the tricuspid valve and anterior to the ostium of the coronary sinus. There is much variation from one heart to another in the size and length of the AV node fibers. Generally the AV node is thicker and shorter and has fewer P cells than the SA node. Behind the AV node are numerous autonomic parasympathetic ganglia. (The nervous systems are described in Chapter 14.) These ganglia may serve as receptors for the vagus nerve and cause slowing of impulse conduction through the AV node.[1]

Conducting fibers from the AV node converge to form the bundle of His. The bundle of His, which is triangular shaped, lies within the posterior border of the interventricular septum. The two lower ends of the triangle give rise to the right and left bundle branches. The **right bundle branch (RBB)** is thin and travels without much branching to the right ventricular apex.

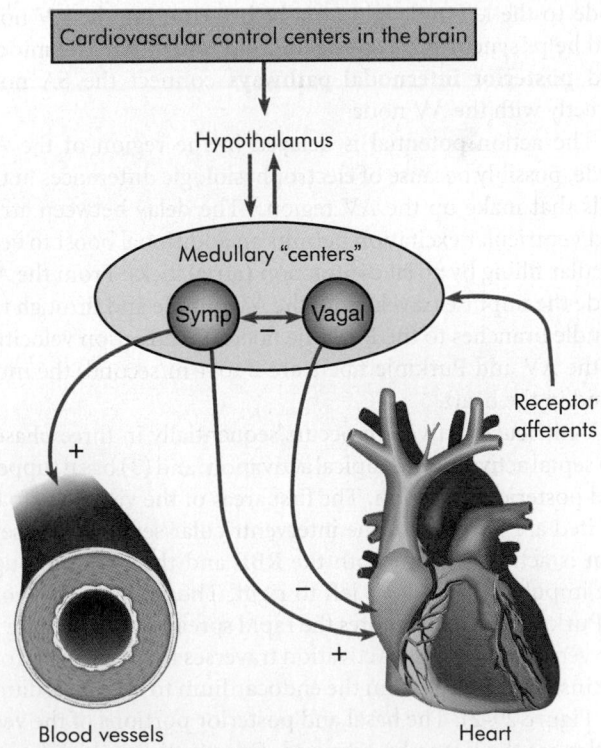

Figure 29-11 Autonomic innervation of cardiovascular system. +, Activation; −, inhibition; *symp*, sympathetic.

Because of its thinness and relative lack of branches, the RBB is susceptible to interruption by damage to the endocardium.

The **left bundle branch (LBB)** arises perpendicularly from the bundle of His and, in some hearts, divides into two branches, or fascicles. The left anterior bundle branch (LABB) passes the left anterior papillary muscle and the base of the left ventricle and crosses the aortic outflow tract. Damage to the aortic valve or the left ventricle can interrupt this branch. The left posterior bundle branch (LPBB) travels posteriorly, crossing the left ventricular inflow tract to the base of the left posterior papillary muscle. This branch spreads diffusely through the posterior inferior left ventricular wall. Blood flow through this portion of the left ventricle is relatively nonturbulent, so the LPBB is somewhat protected from injury caused by wear and tear. The **Purkinje fibers** are the terminal branches of the right and left bundle branches. They extend from the ventricular apices to the fibrous rings and penetrate the heart wall to the outer myocardium. P cells are found also among the Purkinje fibers.

Cardiac Excitation

From the SA node the impulse that begins systole spreads throughout the right atrium at a conduction velocity of about 1 m/second. Because impulses from the SA node arrive at the AV node very quickly, investigators have proposed that these nodes are connected by internodal pathways, called the anterior, middle, and posterior internodal pathways. These pathways consist of ordinary myocardial cells and specialized conducting fibers. The **anterior interatrial myocardial band** (or **Bachmann bundle**) conducts the impulse from the SA node to the left and right atria before entering the AV node and helps synchronize contractions of both atria. The **middle** and **posterior internodal pathways** connect the SA node directly with the AV node.

The action potential is delayed in the region of the AV node, possibly because of electrophysiologic differences in the cells that make up the AV region.[7] The delay between atrial and ventricular excitation permits an additional boost to ventricular filling by atrial contraction (atrial kick). From the AV node the impulse travels from the AV bundle and through the bundle branches to the Purkinje fibers. Conduction velocities in the AV and Purkinje fibers are 2 to 4 m/second, the most rapid in the heart.

Ventricular activation occurs sequentially in three phases: (1) septal activation, (2) apical activation, and (3) basal (upper) and posterior activation. The first areas of the ventricles to be excited are portions of the interventricular septum. The septum is activated from both the RBB and the LBB, although the impulse travels from left to right. The extensive network of Purkinje fibers promotes the rapid spread of the impulse to the ventricular apices. Activation traverses the heart wall from the inside outward (from the endocardium to the epicardium; see Figure 29-2). The basal and posterior portions of the ventricles are the last to be activated. Deactivation, which begins in diastole, occurs in the opposite direction, spreading from the outside inward (epicardium to endocardium). All areas of the ventricle recover at about the same time.

Propagation of Cardiac Action Potentials

Electrical activation of the muscle cells, termed **depolarization,** is caused by the movement of electrically charged solutes (ions) across cardiac cell membranes. Deactivation, called **repolarization,** occurs the same way. (Movement of ions across cell membranes is described in Chapter 1; electrical activation of muscle cells is described in Chapter 41.)

Movement of ions into and out of the cell creates an electrical (voltage) difference across the cell membrane called the *membrane potential.* The resting membrane potential of myocardial cells is between −80 and −90 millivolts (mV), whereas the SA node is between −50 and −60 mV and the AV node is between −60 and −70 mV.[7] During depolarization the inside of the cell becomes less negatively charged. In cardiac cells the difference between resting membrane potential (in millivolts) and the decreased negative charge caused by depolarization is the cardiac action potential. Table 29-2 summarizes the intracellular and extracellular ionic concentrations of cardiac muscle. The various phases of the cardiac action potential are related to changes in the permeability of the cell membrane, primarily to sodium and potassium. Threshold is the point at which the cell membrane's selective permeability to sodium and potassium is temporarily disrupted, leading to depolarization. If the resting membrane potential becomes more negative due to a decrease in extracellular potassium concentration (hypokalemia), it is termed *hyperpolarization.*

Normal myocardial cell depolarization and repolarization occur in five phases (Figure 29-12). Phase 0 consists of depolarization. This phase lasts 1 to 2 milliseconds (ms) and represents rapid sodium entry into the cell. Phase 1 is early repolarization, in which calcium slowly enters the cell. Phase 2, also called the *plateau,* is a continuation of repolarization, with slow entry of calcium and sodium into the cell. Potassium is moved out of the cell during phase 3, with a return to resting membrane potential in phase 4. The time between action potentials corresponds to diastole. If the resting membrane potential becomes more negative, for example, with a decrease in extracellular potassium concentration (hypokalemia), it is termed *hyperpolarization.*

The phases of depolarization and repolarization occur somewhat differently in the SA and AV node cells, a difference that enables these cells to generate cardiac action potentials independently. The cells of the Purkinje fibers, atria, and

Table 29-2	Intracellular and Extracellular Ion Concentrations in the Myocardium	
Ion	**Intracellular Concentration**	**Extracellular Concentration**
Sodium (Na+)	15 mM	145 mM
Potassium (K+)	150 mM	4 mM
Chloride (Cl−)	5 mM	120 mM
Calcium (Ca++)	10^{-7} M	2 mM

M, Moles; *mM,* millimoles per kilogram.

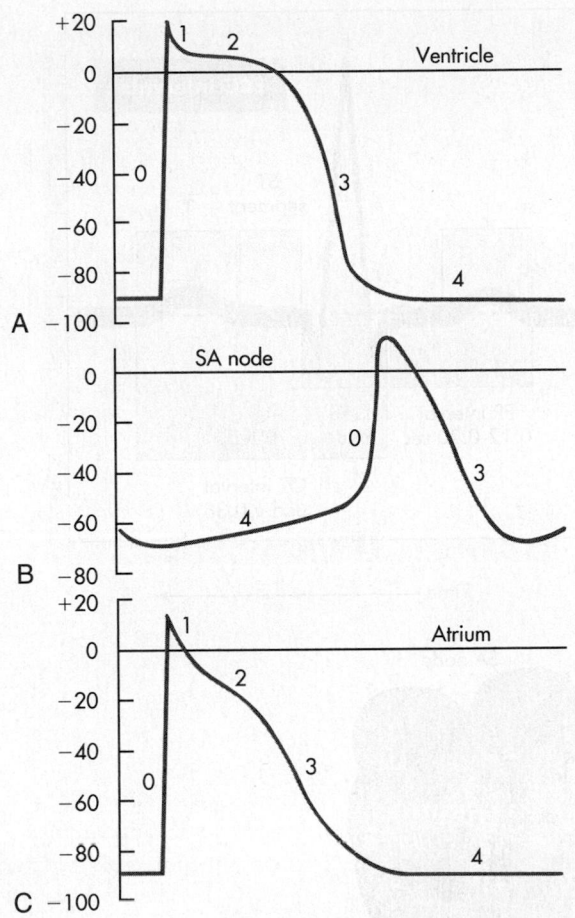

Figure 29-12 Cardiac action potentials. A, Ventricle. B, Sinoatrial (SA) node. C, Atrium. Sweep velocity in B is one half that in A or C. (Modified from Berne RM, Levy MN: *Cardiovascular physiology*, ed 8, St Louis, 2001, Mosby)

sodium and calcium influx (phase 0 through half of phase 3). A relative refractory period occurs near the end of repolarization, following the effective refractory period. During this time the membrane can be depolarized again but only by a greater than normal stimulus. Abnormal refractory periods as a result of disease can cause abnormal heart rhythms, or dysrhythmias, including ventricular fibrillation and cardiac arrest (see Chapter 30).

Normal Electrocardiogram. The genesis of the normal electrocardiogram is from electrical activity recorded by skin electrodes, that is, the sum of all cardiac action potentials (Figure 29-13). The **P wave** represents atrial depolarization. The **PR interval** is a measure of time from the onset of atrial activation to the onset of ventricular activation; it normally ranges from 0.12 to 0.20 second. The PR interval represents the time necessary to travel from the sinus node through the atrium, AV node, and His-Purkinje system to activate ventricular myocardial cells. The **QRS complex** represents the sum of all ventricular muscle cell depolarizations. The configuration and amplitude of the QRS complex vary considerably among individuals. The duration is normally between 0.06 and 0.10 second. During the **ST interval** the entire ventricular myocardium is depolarized. The **QT interval** is sometimes called the "electrical systole" of the ventricles. It lasts about 0.4 second, but it varies inversely with the heart rate.

Automaticity. **Automaticity,** or the property of generating spontaneous depolarization to threshold, enables the SA and AV nodes to generate cardiac action potentials without any stimulus. Cells capable of spontaneous depolarization are called **automatic cells.** The automatic cells of the cardiac conduction system can stimulate the heart to beat even when the heart is removed from the body. Spontaneous depolarization is possible in automatic cells because the membrane potential does not "rest" during phase 4. Instead, it slowly creeps toward threshold during the diastolic phase of the cardiac cycle. Because threshold is approached during diastole, phase 4 in automatic cells is called **diastolic depolarization.** The electrical impulse normally begins in the SA node because its cells depolarize more rapidly than other automatic cells.

Rhythmicity. **Rhythmicity** is the regular generation of an action potential by the heart's conduction system. The SA node sets the pace because normally it has the fastest rate, which is why it is called the *natural pacemaker of the heart.* The SA node depolarizes spontaneously 60 to 100 times per minute. If the SA node is damaged, the AV node will become the heart's pacemaker at a rate of about 40 to 60 spontaneous depolarizations per minute. Purkinje fibers are capable of spontaneous depolarization but at a rate of only 30 to 40 beats/minute.

Cardiac Innervation
Although the heart's nodes and conduction system generate cardiac action potentials independently, the autonomic nervous system influences the rate of impulse generation (firing), depolarization, and repolarization of the myocardium and the strength of atrial and ventricular contraction. Autonomic

ventricles begin with a negative resting membrane potential and proceed to a rapid upstroke, or depolarization (phase 0), a rapid early repolarization (phase 1), a plateau (phase 2), and a rapid later repolarization (phase 3) (see Figure 29-12, A, C). This fast inward current, mediated by sodium ions flowing through "fast channels" in the cell membrane, causes the rapid upstroke of the action potential in Purkinje fibers, atria, and ventricles. Cells of the SA and AV nodes begin with a less negative resting membrane potential, proceed to a slow upstroke (phase 0), and usually lack a plateau (phase 2) (see Figure 29-12, B). The slow inward current, mediated by calcium (transient and long-lasting channels) and sodium ions flowing through "slow channels" of the cell membrane, is responsible for the action potential of the SA node and the AV node. Hence, drugs that block calcium have profound effects on the slow inward current and can alter heart rate. Slow channel-blocking drugs, such as verapamil, are used to treat a variety of cardiovascular disorders.

A refractory period, during which no new cardiac action potential can be initiated by a stimulus, follows depolarization. This effective or absolute refractory period corresponds to the time needed for the reopening of channels that permit

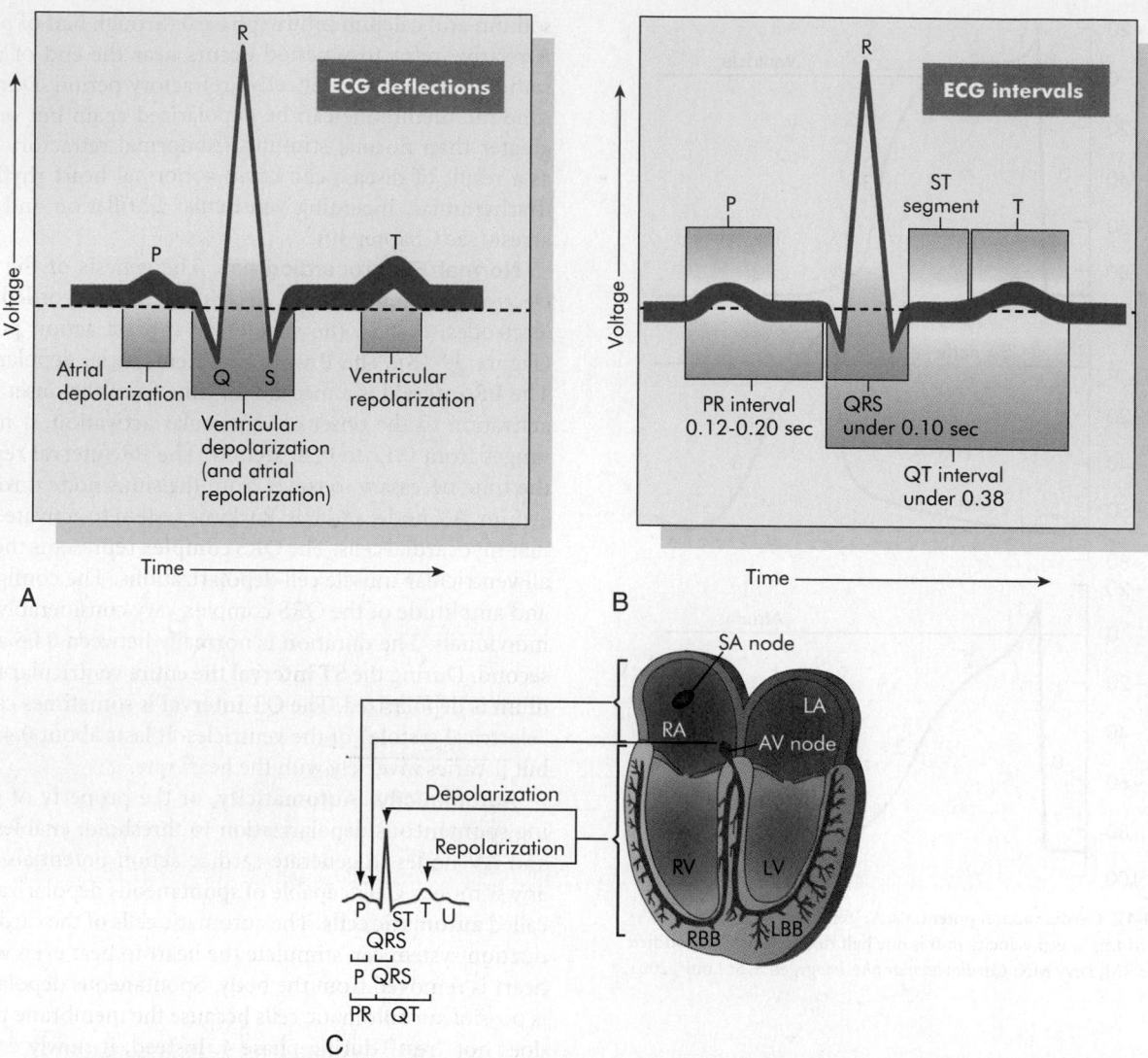

Figure 29-13 Electrocardiogram (ECG) and cardiac electrical activity. **A,** Normal ECG. Depolarization and repolarization. **B,** ECG intervals among P, QRS, and T waves. **C,** Schematic representation of ECG and its relationship to cardiac electrical activity. *RA,* right atrium; *LA,* left atrium; *AV,* atrioventricular; *RV,* right ventricle; *LV,* left ventricle; *LBB,* left bundle branch; *RBB,* right bundle branch. (A and B from Thibodeau GA, Patton KT: *Anatomy & physiology,* ed 5, St Louis, 2003, Mosby. C from Thibodeau GA: *Anatomy & physiology,* St Louis, 1987, Mosby.)

neural transmission produces changes in the heart and circulatory system faster than metabolic or humoral agents (see Figure 29-11). Speed is important, for example, in stimulating the heart to increase its pumping action during times of stress or fear, the so-called *fight-or-flight response.* Although increased delivery of oxygen, glucose, hormones, and other blood-borne factors sustains increased cardiac activity, the rapid initiation of increased activity depends on the sympathetic and parasympathetic fibers of the autonomic nervous system. (The autonomic nervous system is described and illustrated in Chapter 14.)

Sympathetic and Parasympathetic Nerves

Sympathetic and parasympathetic nerve fibers innervate all parts of the atria and ventricles and the SA and AV nodes. In general, sympathetic stimulation increases electrical conductivity and parasympathetic nerve activity, from vagal stimulation, slows conduction of action potentials through the heart.

Efferent sympathetic fibers originate in the thoracic spinal cord and branch into the superior middle and inferior cardiac nerves. They join at the **cardiac plexus,** a neural junction located at the root of the aorta in front of the trachea. Sympathetic nervous activity enhances myocardial performance. Catecholamines speed heart rate, shorten the conduction time through the AV node, and increase the rhythmicity of the AV pacemaker fibers. Neurally released norepinephrine or circulating catecholamines interact with β-adrenergic receptors on the cardiac cell membranes. The overall effect is an increased influx of Ca^{++} during the action potential plateau. The increased calcium increases the contractile strength of the heart.

The efferent parasympathetic fibers originate in the medulla oblongata and travel by way of the vagus nerves to join the sympathetic nerves in the cardiac plexus. Parasympathetic (vagal) activity causes the release of acetylcholine. Receptors for these neurotransmitters are found in the myocardium and coronary vessels of the heart. Acetylcholine decreases heart rate, slows conduction through the AV nodes, and can block cardiac action potentials transmitted from the atria.

Adrenergic Receptor Function

Sympathetic neural stimulation of the myocardium and coronary vessels depends on the presence of adrenergic receptors, which bind specifically with neurotransmitters of the sympathetic nervous system. (Receptor physiology is discussed in Chapter 1). The effects of sympathetic stimulation depend on whether (1) α- or β-adrenergic receptors are most plentiful on cells of the effector tissue and (2) the neurotransmitter is norepinephrine or epinephrine.

There are four types of adrenergic receptors: β_1, β_2, α_1, and α_2 (see Table 14-7). Overall, cardiovascular structures have more β than α receptors; therefore, effects mediated by the β receptors predominate. Epinephrine stimulates all four types of receptors strongly, whereas norepinephrine stimulates all four weakly or not at all.

The β_1 receptors are found mostly in the heart, specifically the conduction system (AV and SA nodes, Purkinje fibers) and the atrial and ventricular myocardium. Norepinephrine and epinephrine, binding with β_1 receptors, increase the rate of impulse generation (firing) and conduction and the strength of myocardial contraction during systole (positive inotropic effect). This enables the heart to pump more blood. Thus epinephrine and norepinephrine stimulate the heart.

The β_2 receptors are found mostly on coronary arterioles and cause coronary vasodilation when stimulated by epinephrine. This opposes the vasoconstrictor activity of α_1 receptor stimulation by norepinephrine (see following). When the sympathetic nervous system is activated, epinephrine-mediated β_2 receptor stimulation combines with the production of vasodilatory metabolites from actively metabolizing myocytes to override the effect of norepinephrine.[1] Thus sympathetic nervous system activation has the overall effect of increasing coronary blood flow. This activation supplies the hard-working myocardium with more oxygen and nutrients (see Table 14-7).

β_3 receptors are also found in the myocardium and coronary vessels. In the heart, stimulation of these receptors opposes the effects of β_1 receptor stimulation and decreases myocardial contractility (negative inotropic effect). Thus β_3 receptors may provide a "safety mechanism" to prevent overstimulation of the heart by the sympathetic nervous system.[8]

As noted, norepinephrine binding with α_1 receptors in the systemic and coronary arteries causes vasoconstriction. The α_2 receptors are located mostly on the sympathetic ganglia and nerve terminals. The effect of norepinephrine on the α_2 receptors is to inhibit release of more norepinephrine, which promotes vasodilation, thus providing another safety mechanism to prevent overactivity of the sympathetic nervous system. Dysfunction of adrenergic receptors can occur in many conditions (e.g., diabetes, hypertension) and has been implicated in the pathogenesis of many cardiac diseases, including heart failure, myocardial ischemia, and dysrhythmias.[9-11]

Myocardial Cells

The cells of cardiac muscle (the myocardium) and of skeletal muscle are nearly identical in structure, function, and microscopic appearance. (The properties of skeletal muscle are described in detail in Chapter 41.) Both types of muscle tissue are composed of long, narrow cells, called *fibers,* that contain basically the same structures: bundles of longitudinally arranged myofibrils; a nucleus (cardiac muscle) or many nuclei (skeletal muscle); mitochondria; an internal membrane system (the sarcoplasmic reticulum); cytoplasm (sarcoplasm); and a plasma membrane (the sarcolemma), which encloses the cell. Cardiac and skeletal muscle cells also have an "external" membrane system made up of transverse tubules (T tubules) formed by invaginations of the sarcolemma. The sarcoplasmic reticulum forms a network of channels that surround the muscle fiber.

The microscopic appearance of cardiac and skeletal muscle is somewhat similar as well (see Chapter 1, Table 1-8). Because the myofibrils in both types of fibers are made up of alternating light and dark bands of protein, the fibers appear striped, or striated. The dark and light bands of the myofibrils make up longitudinal repeating units called *sarcomeres.* The length of the sarcomeres, normally between 1.6 and 2.2 mm, is important because it determines the limits of myocardial stretch at the end of diastole and subsequently the force of contraction during systole.

Cardiac muscle differs from skeletal muscle in several respects that reflect heart function. Cardiac cells are arranged in branching networks throughout the myocardium, whereas skeletal muscle cells tend to be arranged in parallel throughout the length of the muscle. Cardiac fibers have only one nucleus, whereas skeletal muscle cells have many nuclei. Other differences enable cardiac fibers to (1) transmit action potentials quickly from cell to cell, (2) maintain high levels of energy synthesis, and (3) gain access to more ions, particularly sodium and potassium, in the extracellular environment.

Rapid transmission of electrical impulses from cardiac fiber to cardiac fiber is possible because the network of fibers is connected at specialized intercellular junctions called *intercalated disks.* **Intercalated disks** are thickened portions of the sarcolemma that enable electrical impulses to spread quickly in a continuous cell-to-cell (syncytial) fashion. The intercalated disks contain two junctions: desmosomes, which attach one cell to another; and gap junctions, which allow the electrical impulse to spread from cell to cell (see Chapter 1). Together these junctions provide a low-resistance pathway for impulse propagation.

Unlike skeletal muscle, the heart cannot rest and is in constant need of energy compounds, such as adenosine triphosphate (ATP). Therefore, the cytoplasm surrounding the bundles of myofibrils in each cardiac muscle cell contains a superabundance of mitochondria (25% of the cellular volume). Cardiac muscle cells have more mitochondria than

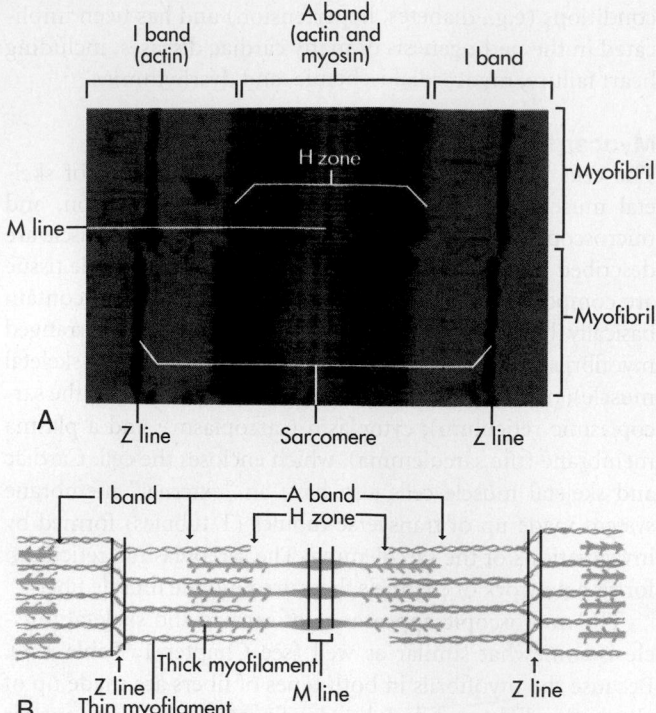

Figure 29-14 Sarcomere. A, Electron photomicrograph of sarcomere. B, Schematic of location and interaction of actin and myosin. (Modified from Thibodeau GA, Patton KT: *Anatomy & physiology*, ed 3, St Louis, 1996, Mosby.)

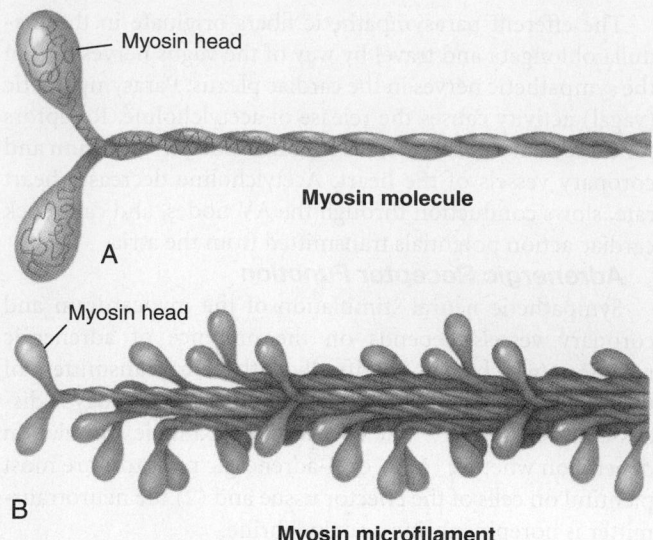

Figure 29-15 Structure of myosin. A, Each myosin molecule is a coil of two chains wrapped around one another. At the end of each chain is a globular region, much like a golf club, called the *head*. B, Myosin molecules usually are combined into filaments, which are stalks of myosin from which the heads protrude at regular intervals.

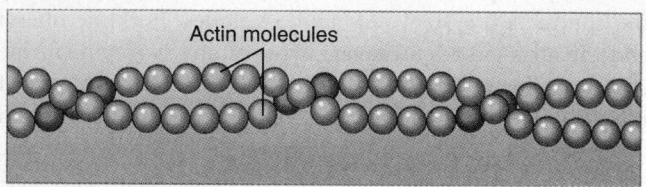

Figure 29-16 Actin microfilament. (From Raven RH, Johnson GB: *Understanding biology*, ed 3, Dubuque, IA, 1995, Brown.)

skeletal muscle cells. The large numbers of mitochondria provide the necessary respiratory enzymes for aerobic metabolism and supply quantities of ATP sufficient for the constant action of the myocardium.

The third major difference between cardiac and skeletal muscle cells has to do with the T tubule system. Cardiac fibers contain more T tubules than skeletal muscle fibers. This gives each myofibril in the myocardium ready access to molecules it needs for the continuous transmission of action potentials, a process that involves transport of sodium and potassium through the walls of the T tubules. (The mechanisms by which sodium and potassium transport causes transmission of cardiac action potentials are described in Chapters 1 and 41.) Because the T tubule system is continuous with the extracellular space and the interstitial fluid, it facilitates the rapid transmission of electrical impulses from the surface of the sarcolemma to the myofibrils inside the fiber. This activates all the myofibrils of one fiber simultaneously. The sarcoplasmic reticulum is located around the myofibrils. When an action potential is transmitted through the T tubules, it induces the sarcoplasmic reticulum to release its stored calcium, which activates the contractile proteins, actin and myosin.

Actin, Myosin, and the Troponin-Tropomyosin Complex

The thick filaments of **myosin** constitute the central dark band called the **anisotropic,** or **A, bands** (Figure 29-14). The myosin molecule resembles a golf club with two large bulbous

heads protruding from one end of a straight shaft (Figure 29-15). The bilobed heads contain an actin-binding site and a site of ATPase activity. A thick filament is composed of about 200 myosin molecules bundled together with the heads of the molecules (called *cross-bridges*) facing outward (see Figure 29-15). The actin molecules are part of the thin filaments (Figure 29-16). The light bands are called **isotropic,** or **I, bands** (see Figure 29-14). The thin filaments of actin appear light and extend from the **Z line,** a dense fibrous line that crosses the center of each I band. A sarcomere is the area from one dark Z line to an adjacent Z line with a length that varies from 1.6 to 2.2 mm. In the center of a sarcomere is the H zone, a somewhat less dense region. A thin, dark **M line** travels the center of the H zone. A single tropomyosin molecule (a relaxing protein) lies alongside seven actin molecules. **Troponin,** another relaxing protein, associates with the tropomyosin molecule, forming the **troponin-tropomyosin complex** (Figure 29-17). The troponin complex itself has three components. **Troponin T** aids in binding of the troponin complex to actin and tropomyosin; troponin I inhibits the ATPase of actomyosin; and **troponin C** contains binding sites for the calcium ions involved in contraction.

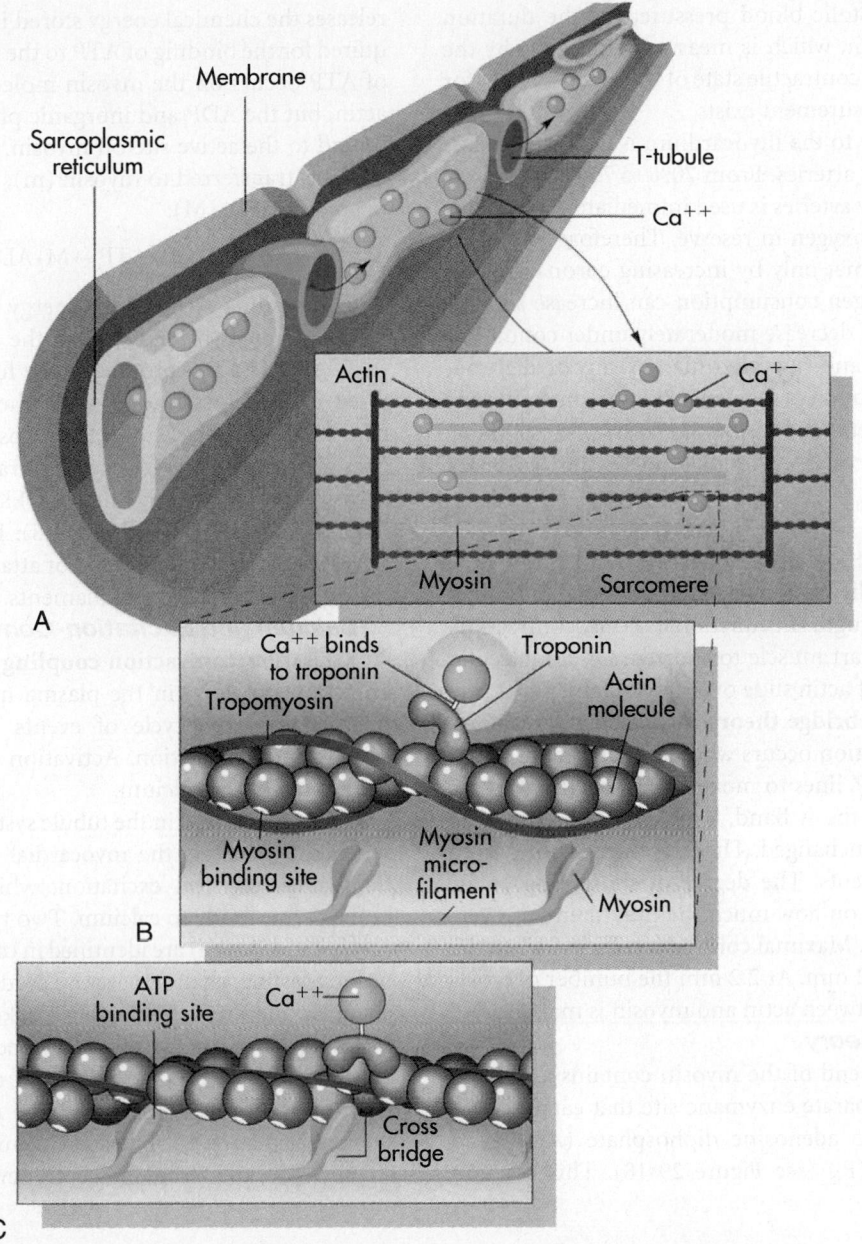

Figure 29-17 Myofilaments and mechanisms of muscle contraction. **A,** Thin and thick myofilaments. In resting muscle, calcium ions are stored in the sarcoplasmic reticulum. When an action potential reaches the muscle cell, the T tubules carry the action potential deep into the sarcoplasm. The action potential causes the sarcoplasmic reticulum to release the store of calcium ions. **B,** In resting muscle the myosin binding sites are covered by troponin and tropomyosin. The calcium ions released into the sarcoplasm as a result of action potential bind to the troponin. This binding causes the tropomyosin and troponin to move out of the way of the myosin binding sites, leaving the myosin heads free to bind to the actin microfilament. (From Raven PH, Johnson GB: *Understanding biology,* ed 3, Dubuque, IA, 1995, Brown.)

Myocardial Metabolism

Cardiac muscle, like other muscle tissue, depends on the constant production of ATP for energy. ATP is produced within the mitochondria mainly from glucose, fatty acids, and lactate. If the myocardium is inadequately perfused because of coronary artery disease, anaerobic metabolism becomes an essential source of energy (see Chapter 1). The energy produced by metabolic processes is used for muscle contraction and relaxation, electrical excitation, membrane transport,

and synthesis of large molecules. Normally, the amount of ATP produced supplies sufficient energy to pump blood systemically.

Cardiac work often is expressed in terms of **myocardial oxygen consumption ($M\dot{V}O_2$)**. Because oxidative metabolism is the main process of cardiac energy generation, the rate of $M\dot{V}O_2$ correlates closely with total cardiac energy requirements. $M\dot{V}O_2$ is determined by three major factors: (1) the amount of wall stress during systole, which can be estimated by measuring the systolic blood pressure; (2) the duration of systolic wall tension, which is measured indirectly by the heart rate; and (3) the contractile state of the myocardium, for which no clinical measurement exists.

The oxygen supply to the myocardium is delivered exclusively by the coronary arteries. From 70% to 75% of the oxygen from the coronary arteries is used immediately by cardiac muscle, leaving little oxygen in reserve. Therefore, increased energy needs can be met only by increasing coronary blood flow. Myocardial oxygen consumption can increase several-fold with exercise and decrease moderately under conditions such as hypotension and hypothermia. As myocardial metabolism and consumption of oxygen increases, the local concentration of local metabolic factors increases. One of these, adenosine, dilates coronary arterioles, increasing coronary blood flow.[1]

Myocardial Contraction and Relaxation

Myocardial contractility is a change in developed tension at a given resting fiber length. In functional terms, contractility is the ability of the heart muscle to shorten. On a molecular basis, thin filaments of actin slide over thick filaments of myosin, called the **cross-bridge theory of muscle contraction.** Anatomically, contraction occurs when the sarcomere shortens, causing adjacent Z lines to move closer together (Figure 29-18). The width of the A band, which contains the thick myosin filaments, is unchanged. The movement comes from the long sets of filaments. The degree of shortening of the muscle fibers depends on how much the thin filaments overlap the thick filaments. Maximal contraction occurs when the sarcomere length is 2.2 mm. At 2.2 mm the number of cross-bridge attachments between actin and myosin is maximal.

Cross-Bridge Theory

The globular head-end of the myosin contains a binding site for actin and a separate enzymatic site that catalyzes the breakdown of ATP to adenosine diphosphate (ADP) and inorganic phosphate (P_i) (see Figure 29-18). This reaction releases the chemical energy stored in ATP. Magnesium is required for the binding of ATP to the myosin site. The splitting of ATP occurs on the myosin molecule before it attaches to actin, but the ADP and inorganic phosphate released remain bound to the active site on myosin. The chemical energy released is transferred to myosin (m), producing a high-energy form of myosin (M):

$$M \cdot ATP \rightarrow M \cdot ADP + P_i$$

The binding of this high-energy form of myosin to actin through a cross-bridge releases the energy stored in myosin (e.g., ADP and P_i), producing the force necessary for movement of the cross-bridge. With the attachment of actin to myosin at the cross-bridge, the myosin head molecule undergoes a position change, exerting traction on the rest of the myosin bridge, causing the thin filaments to slide past the thick filaments (see Figure 29-18). During contraction each cross-bridge undergoes cycles of attachment, movement, and dissociation from the thin filaments.

Calcium and Excitation-Contraction Coupling

Excitation-contraction coupling is the process by which an action potential in the plasma membrane of the muscle fiber triggers the cycle of events leading to cross-bridge activity and contraction. Activation of this cycle depends on the availability of calcium.

Calcium is stored in the tubule system and the sarcoplasmic reticulum. It enters the myocardial cell from the interstitial fluid after electrical excitation, which increases the membrane permeability to calcium. Two types of calcium channels (L-type and T-type) are identified in cardiac tissues. The L-type, or long-lasting, channels are the predominant type of calcium channels and are the channels blocked by **calcium channel–blocking drugs** (verapamil, nifedipine, diltiazem). Their major effect is to decrease the strength of cardiac contraction. The T-type, or transient, channels are much less abundant in the heart and are not blocked by currently available calcium channel–blocking drugs, however, new types of T-type channel

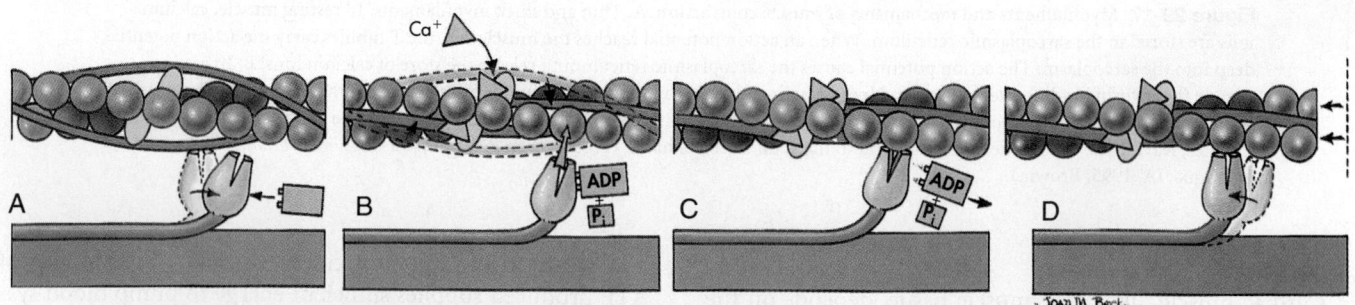

Figure 29-18 Cross-bridge theory of muscle contraction. **A,** Each myosin cross-bridge in the thick filament moves into a resting position after an adenosine triphosphate (ATP) molecule binds and transfers its energy. **B,** Calcium ions released from the sarcoplasmic reticulum bind to troponin in the thin filament, allowing tropomyosin to shift from its position blocking the active sites of actin molecules. **C,** Each myosin cross-bridge then binds to an active site on a thin filament, displacing the remnants of ATP hydrolysis— adenosine diphosphate (ADP) and inorganic phosphate (Pi). **D,** The release of stored energy from step **A** provides the force needed for each cross-bridge to move back to its original position, pulling actin along with it. Each cross-bridge will remain bound to actin until another ATP molecule binds to it and pulls it back into its resting position (**A**). (From Thibodeau GA, Patton KT: *Anatomy & physiology*, ed 4, St Louis, 1999, Mosby.)

blockers are being developed.[12] Calcium that enters the cell from the interstitial fluid triggers release of calcium from the storage sites. The storage sites most important for contraction are from the sarcoplasmic reticulum. Calcium from these sites diffuses toward the myofibrils, where it binds with troponin.

The calcium-troponin complex facilitates the contraction process. In the resting state, troponin I is bound to actin and the configuration of the tropomyosin molecule is such that it covers the sites where the myosin heads bind to actin. Thus interaction between actin and myosin is prevented. Calcium binding to troponin inhibits troponin C (which enhances troponin I–actin binding). This in turn causes tropomyosin to move away, thus uncovering the binding sites on the myosin heads. Myosin and actin can then form cross-bridges, and ATP can be dephosphorylated to ADP. Sliding of the thick and thin filaments can then occur, and the muscle contracts.

Myocardial Relaxation

Adequate relaxation is just as vital to optimal cardiac function as contraction, and calcium, troponin, and tropomyosin also facilitate relaxation. After contraction, free calcium ions are actively pumped out of the cell back into the interstitial fluid or reaccumulated in the sarcoplasmic reticulum and stored. Troponin releases its bound calcium. The tropomyosin complex blocks the active sites on the actin molecule, preventing cross-bridges with the myosin heads. Each tropomyosin molecule is held in this blocking position by a molecule of troponin. Troponin is bound to both tropomyosin and actin (see Figures 29-17, A, and 29-18).

Factors Affecting Cardiac Output

Cardiac output is the volume of blood flowing through either the systemic or the pulmonary circuit and is expressed in liters per minute. The cardiac output is determined by multiplying the heart rate (beats per minute) and the **stroke volume** (liters per beat). Normal cardiac output is about 5 L/minute for a resting adult. The ventricle does not eject all of the blood it contains; the amount ejected is called the **ejection fraction** or the stroke volume divided by the end-diastolic volume. The end-diastolic volume of the normal ventricle (VEDV) is about 70 to 80 ml/m² and the normal ejection fraction of the resting heart is about 60% to 75%.

Four factors affect cardiac output directly: preload, afterload, myocardial contractility, and heart rate (Figure 29-19). **Preload** (pressure generated at the end of diastole) and **afterload** (resistance to ejection during systole) depend on the heart as well as the vascular system. Contractility and heart rate are characteristics of the cardiac tissue per se and are influenced by neural and humoral mechanisms. To understand the role of these factors in cardiac performance, it is first necessary to understand two physical laws that explain the mechanisms of heart action: the Frank-Starling law of the heart and Laplace's law.

Frank-Starling Law of the Heart

Cardiac muscle, like other muscle, increases its strength of contraction when it is stretched. This relationship was described in 1914 by a British physiologist, Ernest Starling, who based his studies on the earlier work of a German physiologist, Otto Frank. In 1914 Starling wrote that "the output of any heart can be varied within wide limits by alterations of the venous inflow, and that within these limits it varies directly as the venous inflow. So long as the functional condition of the heart remains constant, the amount put out at each beat depends directly on the diastolic filling."[12a]

The **Frank-Starling law of the heart,** or the length-tension relationship of cardiac muscle, relates resting sarcomere

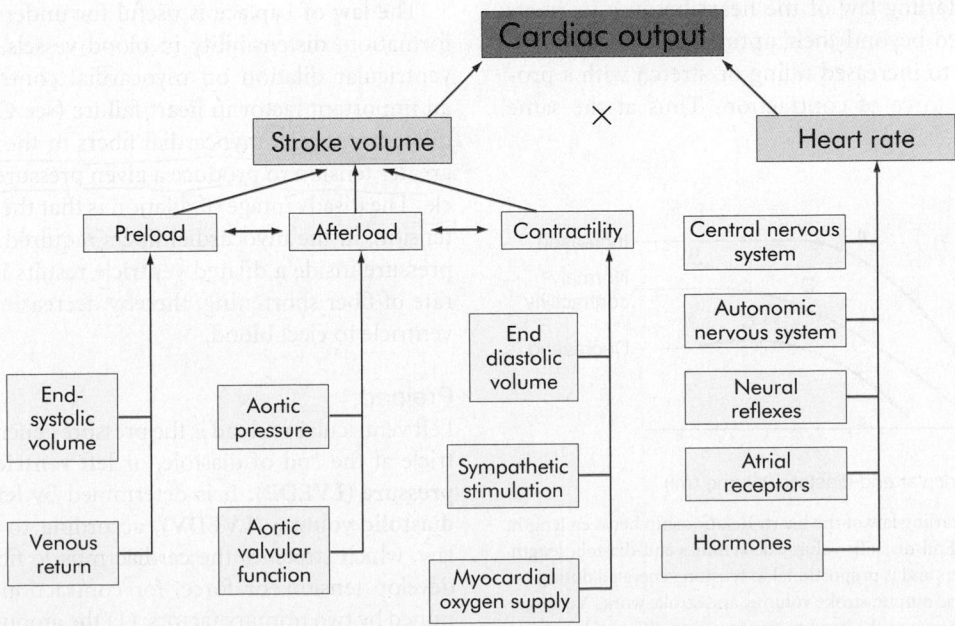

Figure 29-19 Factors affecting cardiac performance. Cardiac output, which is the amount of blood (in liters) ejected by the heart per minute, depends on heart rate (beats per minute) and stroke volume (milliliters of blood ejected during ventricular systole).

length, expressed as the volume of blood in the heart at the end of diastole, or **end-diastolic volume,** to tension generation, described as development of left ventricular pressure. Thus the volume of blood in the heart at the end of diastole (the length of its muscle fibers) is directly related to the force of contraction during the next systole. Although the change in pressure is related to volume of the ventricle and, consequently, to the length of the ventricular muscle fibers, it is common to use preload (i.e., filling pressure) as an index of ventricular volume. The length-tension mechanism is the major mechanism by which the normal right and left ventricles maintain equal minute outputs even though their stroke outputs may vary considerably during normal respiration. For example, changes in volume occur when an individual assumes a reclining position after being in a standing position; the volume of blood returning to the heart temporarily increases. The right ventricle stretches to accommodate this increase in volume and thereby increases its force of contraction. A larger stroke volume (i.e., the amount of blood ejected per beat) is pumped to the lungs, generating higher pressures. Pulmonary vascular pressure increases, causing a rise in the left ventricular filling pressure or preload. Left ventricular volume and pressure increase. The left ventricle pumps a larger stroke volume, and arterial vascular pressure rises.

The mechanical function of the heart is characterized by a number of length-tension curves (Figure 29-20). Factors that increase contractility (i.e., positive inotropic), such as sympathetic nerve stimulation, cause the heart to operate on a higher length-tension curve (curve *A* in Figure 29-20). A higher tension or increase in ventricular stroke volume is generated without a necessary change in left ventricular end-diastolic volume or fiber length. Heart failure (curve *C* in Figure 29-20) is characterized by a lower length-tension curve (see Chapter 30). The failing or dilated heart may not be able to use the Frank-Starling law of the heart because its fibers are already stretched beyond their optimal length. The failing heart responds to increased filling or stretch with a progressive decline in force of contraction. Thus at the same

left ventricular end-diastolic volume as curves *A* and *B* (see Figure 29-20), the force of contraction of stroke volume is decreased.

The cross-bridge theory partially accounts for the length-tension mechanism of cardiac muscle. According to the Frank-Starling law, the longer the initial resting length of the cardiac muscle fiber (optimal length is between 2.2 and 2.4 mm), the greater the strength of contraction. At 2.2 mm there is an optimal number of active cross-bridges between actin and myosin. If the fibers are stretched beyond 2.2 to 2.4 mm, the force of contraction decreases because actin and myosin become partially disengaged, disrupting many of the cross-bridges. Excessive stretching, to about 3.65 mm, causes actin and myosin to become completely disengaged and developed tension (force of contraction) to drop to zero. The relationship between stretch and contraction can be compared with that of a rubber band. To a certain point, the more the rubber band is stretched, the farther it will fly when one end is released; beyond that point, however, the rubber band will break.

Laplace's Law

In Laplace's law, wall tension is related directly to the product of intraventricular pressure and internal radius and inversely to the wall thickness. This relationship can be calculated by Laplace's equation:

$$T = (p \times r)/\mu m$$

where T = wall tension, p = intraventricular pressure, r = internal radius of the sphere, and μm = wall thickness. In other words, the amount of tension generated in the wall of the ventricle (or any chamber or vessel) to produce a given intraventricular pressure depends on the size (radius and wall thickness) of the ventricle.

The law of Laplace is useful for understanding aneurysm formation, distensibility in blood vessels, and the effects of ventricular dilation on myocardial contraction. Dilation is an important factor in heart failure (see Chapter 30). With a dilated ventricle, myocardial fibers in the wall must develop greater tension to produce a given pressure within the ventricle. The disadvantage of dilation is that the increased force, or tension, in the myocardial fibers required to develop a given pressure inside a dilated ventricle results in a decrease in the rate of fiber shortening, thereby decreasing the ability of the ventricle to eject blood.

Preload

Left ventricular preload is the pressure generated in the left ventricle at the end of diastole, or **left ventricular end-diastolic pressure (LVEDP).** It is determined by **left ventricular end-diastolic volume (LVEDV),** according to the Frank-Starling law, which stretches the cardiac muscle fibers, which in turn develop tension, or force, for contraction. Preload is determined by two primary factors: (1) the amount of venous return to the ventricle and (2) the blood left in the ventricle after systole (end-systolic volume). End-systolic volume is dependent

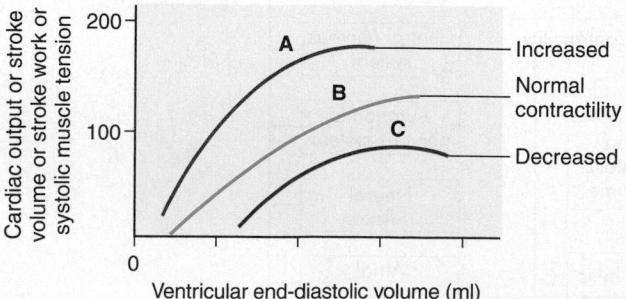

Figure 29-20 Frank-Starling law of the heart. Relationship between length and tension in the heart. End-diastolic volume determines end-diastolic length of ventricular muscle fibers and is proportional to tension generated during systole, as well as to cardiac output, stroke volume, and stroke work. A change in myocardial contractility causes the heart to perform on a different length-tension curve. A, Increased contractility; B, normal contractility; C, heart failure or decreased contractility. (See text.)

on the strength of ventricular contraction and the resistance to ventricular emptying. Within a physiologic range of muscle stretching (2.2 to 2.4 mm), increased preload increases cardiac output (volume of blood pumped per minute; see Figure 29-19). When preload exceeds the physiologic range, further muscle stretching causes a decline in cardiac output (see Frank-Starling law, p. 1109). In monitoring preload the clinician measures indexes of left ventricular end-diastolic pressure. Pressure changes are important because increased left ventricular filling pressures "back up" into the pulmonary circulation, where they force plasma out through vessel walls, causing fluid to accumulate in lung tissues (pulmonary edema; see Chapter 33). Treatment goals are to maintain an end-diastolic volume and pressure that will maintain or increase cardiac output.

Afterload

Left ventricular afterload is the resistance to ejection of blood from the left ventricle. Aortic systolic pressure is a good index of afterload. Low aortic pressures (decreased afterload) enable the heart to contract more rapidly, whereas high aortic pressures (increased afterload) slow contraction and cause higher workloads against which the heart must function so it can eject less blood. Pressure in the ventricle must exceed aortic pressure before blood can be pumped out during systole. Increased aortic pressure is usually the result of increased peripheral vascular resistance (PVR), also called total peripheral resistance (TPR). In individuals with hypertension, increased PVR means that afterload is chronically elevated resulting in increased ventricular workload and hypertrophy of the myocardium.

Myocardial Contractility

Stroke volume, or the volume of blood ejected during systole, depends on the force of contraction, which depends on myocardial contractility, or the degree of myocardial fiber shortening. Three major factors determine the force of contraction: (1) changes in the stretching of the ventricular myocardium caused by changes in ventricular volume (preload), (2) alterations in the sympathetic activation of the ventricles, and (3) adequacy of myocardial oxygen supply (see Figure 29-19). As discussed, increased blood flow from the veins into the heart distends the ventricle by increasing preload, which, within the physiologic range, increases the stroke volume and, subsequently, cardiac output.

Chemicals affecting contractility are called **inotropic agents.** The most important positive inotropic agents are epinephrine and norepinephrine released from the sympathetic nervous system. Other positive ionotropes include thyroid hormone and dopamine. The most important negative ionotropic agent is acetylcholine released from the vagus nerve. Many drugs have positive or negative ionotropic properties that can have profound effects on cardiac function.

Myocardial contractility also is affected by oxygen and carbon dioxide levels (tensions) in the coronary blood. With severe hypoxemia (arterial oxygen saturation less than 50%), contractility is decreased. With less severe hypoxemia (saturation more than 50%), contractility is stimulated. Moderate degrees of hypoxemia may increase contractility by enhancing the myocardial response to circulating catecholamines.[1]

Preload, afterload, and contractility all interact with one another to determine stroke volume and cardiac output. Changes in any one of these factors can result in deleterious effects on the others, resulting in heart failure (see Chapter 30).

Heart Rate

The average heart rate in healthy adults is about 70 beats/minute. The average heart rate is significantly greater in children. Heart rate diminishes by 10 to 20 beats/minute during sleep and can accelerate to more than 100 beats/minute during muscular activity or emotional excitement. In well-conditioned athletes at rest the heart rate is normally about 50 to 60 beats/minute. In highly trained or elite athletes the resting heart rate can be less than 50 beats/minute. The low resting heart rate is the result of increased vagal stimulation and lower sympathetic stimulation.

Highly trained athletes also have a greater stroke volume and lower peripheral resistance than they had before training. The lowered peripheral resistance is thought to be caused by an increase in the number of arterioles in skeletal muscle. The decrease in peripheral resistance increases the venous return. The slow heart rate (and therefore prolonged diastole) combined with the increased venous return results in a higher end-diastolic ventricular volume.[1,7] The increased end-diastolic fiber length increases stroke volume, which helps compensate for the decreased heart rate so that cardiac output is maintained.

Neural factors, including neural reflexes, and hormonal and chemical factors influence the heart rate. Neural control is exerted by the central and autonomic nervous systems. Hormonal factors include the catecholamines norepinephrine and epinephrine, thyroid hormones, growth hormones, and pancreatic hormones. (Hormonal function is described in Chapter 20. Stimulation by the sympathetic nervous system increases the rhythmicity of the cardiac pacemaker (SA node), whereas the parasympathetic stimulation has an inhibiting effect.

Cardiovascular Control Centers in the Brain

The major **cardiovascular control center** is in the brainstem in the medulla with secondary areas in the hypothalamus, the cerebral cortex, the thalamus, and complex networks of exciting or inhibiting interneurons (connecting neurons) throughout the brain. The hypothalamic centers regulate cardiovascular responses to changes in temperature; the cerebral cortex centers adjust cardiac reaction to a variety of emotional states; and the medullary control center regulates heart rate and blood pressure (see p. 1122 for blood pressure regulation). The medullary neurons often are classified as cardiac and vasomotor (vasoconstrictor or vasodilator) centers; however, because these centers are not discrete anatomic areas and actually constitute diffuse networks of interneurons, it is preferable to call the entire area the cardiovascular control center.

The nerve fibers from the cardiovascular control center synapse with the autonomic neurons (see Chapter 14 and Table 14-7). When the parasympathetic nerves to the heart are stimulated, the sympathetic nerves to the heart, arterioles, and veins usually are inhibited. The opposite also is true: when the sympathetic nerves are stimulated, the parasympathetic nerves usually are inhibited. Because parasympathetic excitation and simultaneous sympathetic inhibition generally depress cardiac function (e.g., decrease the heart rate), these interneurons often are referred to as the **cardioinhibitory center.** Excitation occurs with parasympathetic inhibition and sympathetic stimulation, and these interneurons are collectively called the **cardioexcitatory center.** Therefore, heart rate can be slowed by two simultaneous events that begin in the cardiovascular control center: (1) inhibition of sympathetic stimulation of the SA node and (2) activation of parasympathetic stimulation of the SA node. Conversely, heart rate can be increased by activation of sympathetic nerves and inhibition of parasympathetic nerves.

The resting heart rate in healthy individuals is primarily under the control of parasympathetic stimulation. While the individual is at rest, parasympathetic effects from the vagus nerves override sympathetic effects in the SA node. Interruption of the vagus nerves causes significant tachycardia (abnormally fast heart rate) because the inhibitory parasympathetic influence is lost.

Neural Reflexes

Two important neural reflexes that affect heart rate and rhythm are the Bainbridge reflex and the baroreceptor reflex. The **Bainbridge reflex** causes changes in the heart rate after intravenous infusions of blood or other fluid[13] (Figure 29-21). The changes in heart rate is thought to be caused by a reflex mediated by volume receptors in the atria that are innervated by the vagus nerves (volume receptors are thought to respond to increased plasma volume). The magnitude and direction of the change in heart rate depends on the initial heart rate. If the initial heart rate is slow, intravenous infusion usually accelerates it, but if the initial heart rate is rapid, infusions usually will slow it down.[13] Contractility usually is not affected by the Bainbridge reflex.

The **baroreceptor reflex** facilitates both blood pressure changes and heart rate changes. The baroreceptor reflex is mediated by tissue pressure receptors (pressoreceptors) in the aortic arch and carotid arteries. (Because the receptors respond to mechanical factors, they are also called *aortic and carotid mechanoreceptors.*) If blood pressure is decreased, the baroreceptor reflex accelerates heart rate and causes vessels to constrict. These responses raise blood pressure back toward normal. This reflex is critical to maintaining adequate tissue perfusion. Aging is associated with dysfunction of the baroreflex and can result in postural hypotension (orthostatic hypotension, see p. 1156).[14,15] Dysfunction of this reflex also plays a role in shock states.[16]

The baroreflex also serves to lower blood pressure when it gets too high. The pressoreceptors increase their rate of discharge when stretched by blood pressure elevations. Neural impulses are then transmitted over the glossopharyngeal nerve (ninth cranial nerve) from the carotid artery and through the vagus nerve from the aorta to the cardiovascular control centers in the medulla. These centers initiate an increase in parasympathetic activity and a decrease in sympathetic activity, causing blood vessels to dilate and heart rate to decrease. Responses to the baroreceptor reflex return the blood pressure to its previous level, which may or may not be normal. The higher the blood pressure, the greater the reflexive decrease in heart rate. This action of the baroreflex is being explored as a potential mechanism for the treatment of hypertension.[17]

Neural receptors in the lungs cause heart rate to increase during inspiration and decrease during expiration. The increase in heart rate during inspiration is caused by the stretching (activation) of vagal fibers in the lungs that cause heart rate to speed up by inhibiting the cardioinhibitory center of the medulla. Inhibition of this center allows unopposed sympathetic acceleration of heart rate.

Atrial Receptors

Receptors that influence heart rate exist in both atria. They are located in the right atrium at its junctions with the vena cava and in the left atrium at its junctions with the pulmonary veins.[13] Distension of these atrial receptors sends impulses via C-fiber afferents. Stimulation of these atrial

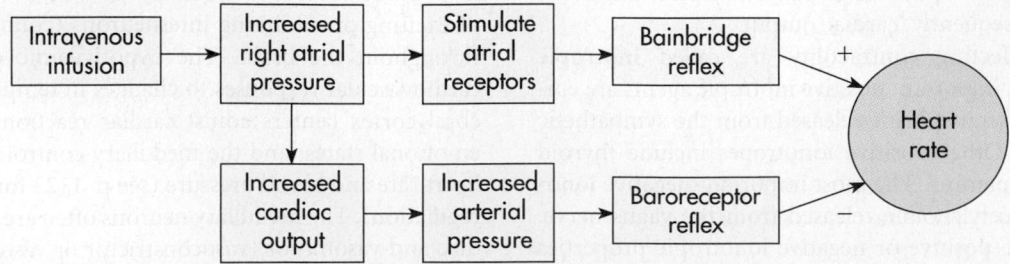

Figure 29-21 Heart rate and intravenous infusions. Intravenous infusions of blood or electrolyte solutions tend to increase heart rate through the Bainbridge reflex and to decrease heart rate through the baroreceptor reflex. The actual change in heart rate induced by such infusions is the result of these two opposing effects. (From Berne RM, Levy MN: *Cardiovascular physiology,* ed 8, St Louis, 2001, Mosby.)

receptors also increases urine volume because of a neurally mediated reduction in antidiuretic hormone and the release of natriuretic peptides.[1] Atrial natriuretic peptide (ANP) is released from atrial tissue in response to increased blood volume. ANP has powerful diuretic and natriuretic (salt excretion) properties, resulting in decreased blood volume and pressure.

Hormones and Biochemicals

Hormones and biochemicals affect the arteries, arterioles, venules, capillaries, and contractility of the myocardium. Norepinephrine increases heart rate, enhances myocardial contractility, and constricts blood vessels. Epinephrine dilates vessels of the liver and skeletal muscle and causes an increase in myocardial contractility. Some adrenocortical hormones, such as hydrocortisone, potentiate the effects of the catecholamines.

Thyroid hormones enhance sympathetic activity, promoting an increase in cardiac output. The exact mechanism by which this occurs is not known. A decrease in growth hormone, thyroid hormones, or adrenal hormones results in bradycardia (heart rate below 60 beats/minute), reduced cardiac output, and low blood pressure.

SYSTEMIC CIRCULATION

The arteries and veins of the systemic circulation are illustrated in Figure 29-22. Blood from the left side of the heart flows through the aorta and into the systemic arteries. The **arteries** branch into small **arterioles** that branch further into the smallest vessels, the **capillaries,** where nutrient exchange between the blood and tissues occurs. Blood from the capillaries then enters tiny **venules** that join to form the larger **veins,** which return venous blood to the right heart. **Peripheral vascular system** is an imprecise term used to describe the part of the systemic circulation that supplies the skin and the extremities, particularly the legs and feet.

Structure of Blood Vessels

Blood vessel walls are composed of three layers: the **tunica intima** (innermost or intimal layer), the tunica media (middle or medial layer), and the tunica externa or adventitia (outermost or external layer). These structures are illustrated in Figure 29-23 and 29-24. The tunica intima is composed of a layer of squamous epithelium or endothelium, a layer of connective tissue, and a basement membrane. (These cellular structures are described in Chapter 1.) The **tunica media** is composed of smooth muscle fibers mixed with elastic fibers. The **tunica externa,** or **adventitia,** has a thin layer of connective tissue containing elastic and collagenous fibers that run lengthwise in the vessel. Blood vessel walls vary in thickness depending on the thickness or absence of one or more of these three layers. Cells of the larger vessels are nourished by the **vasa vasorum,** small vessels located in the tunica externa. The vasa vasorum arise from the blood vessel itself or from other vessels nearby.

Arterial Vessels

Arterial walls are composed of elastic connective tissue, fibrous connective tissue, and smooth muscle. The two types of arteries are elastic and muscular. The **elastic arteries** have a very thick tunica media that contains more elastic fibers than smooth muscle fibers. Elastic arteries include the aorta and its major branches and the pulmonary trunk. Elasticity enables the vessel to stretch as blood is ejected from the heart during systole. During diastole, elasticity promotes recoil of the arteries, which is important for maintaining blood pressure within the vessels.

The **muscular arteries** are the medium-size and small arteries farther from the heart than the elastic arteries. They contain fewer elastic fibers and more muscle fibers than the elastic arteries because, being farther from the heart, they have less need of the properties of stretch and recoil. The function of the muscular arteries is to distribute blood to arterioles throughout the body. They also play a role in controlling blood flow because their smooth muscle can be stimulated to contract or relax. Contraction narrows the vessel **lumen** (the internal cavity of the vessel), which diminishes flow through the vessel. This condition is termed **vasoconstriction.** The smooth muscle layer also can be stimulated to relax, which permits more blood to flow through the vessel lumen. This state is called **vasodilation.**

An artery becomes an arteriole at the point where the diameter of its lumen narrows to less than 0.5 mm. The arterioles are composed almost exclusively of smooth muscle, with little elastic tissue. Arterioles regulate the flow of blood into the capillaries by vasoconstriction, which retards the flow of blood into the capillaries, and vasodilation, which permits blood to enter the capillaries freely (Figure 29-25, p. 1117). The thick, smooth muscle layer of the arterioles is a major determinant of the resistance blood encounters as it flows through the systemic circulation.

The capillary network is composed of connective channels, or thoroughfares, called **metarterioles,** and "true" capillaries (Figure 29-26, p. 1118). The capillaries branch from the metarterioles, meeting at a ring of smooth muscle called the **precapillary sphincters.** As the sphincters contract and relax, they regulate blood flow through the capillaries. Appropriately stimulated, the precapillary sphincters help maintain arterial pressure and regulate selective flow to vascular beds.

The capillary walls are very thin, making possible the rapid exchange of substrates, metabolites, and special products (e.g., hormones) between the blood and the interstitial fluid, from which they are taken up by the cells. The capillary wall consists of a single layer of endothelial cells surrounded by the thin basement membrane of the tunica intima. A single endothelial cell may form the entire vessel wall if the capillary has no tunica media or tunica externa. In some capillaries the endothelial cells contain oval windows or pores termed **fenestrations.** Fenestrations generally are covered by a thin diaphragm.

Substances pass between the capillary lumen and the interstitial fluid in several ways: (1) through junctions between endothelial cells, (2) through fenestrations in endothelial cells, (3) in vesicles moved by active transport across the endothelial cell membrane, or (4) by diffusion through the endothelial cell membrane. (Movement across cell membranes is described in Chapter 1.) A single capillary may be only 0.5 to 1 mm in length and 0.01 mm in diameter, but the capillaries are so numerous that their total surface area may be more than 600 m².

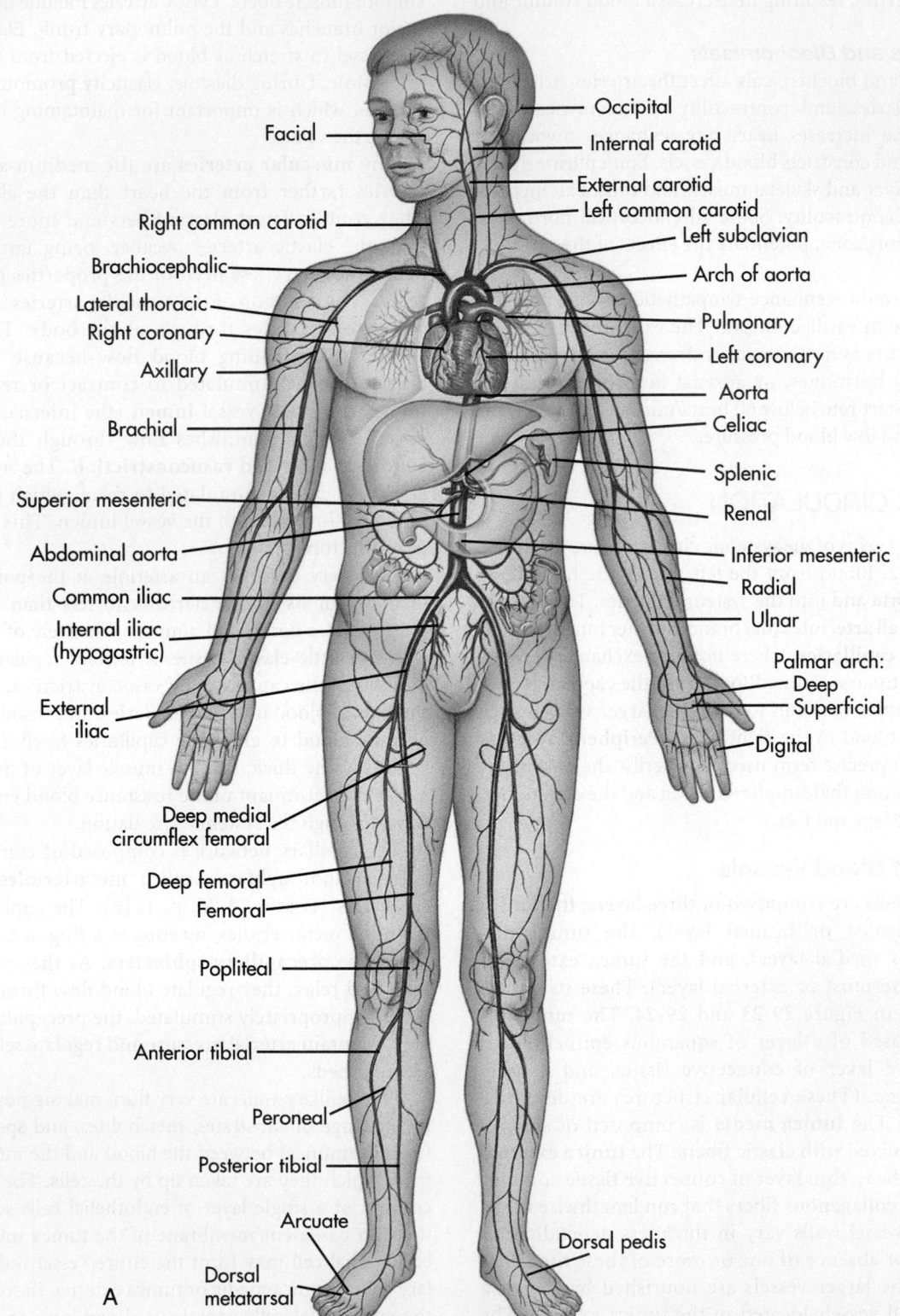

Figure 29-22 Circulatory system. A, Principal arteries of the body. (From Thibodeau GA, Patton KT: *Anatomy & physiology*, ed 5, St Louis, 2003, Mosby.)

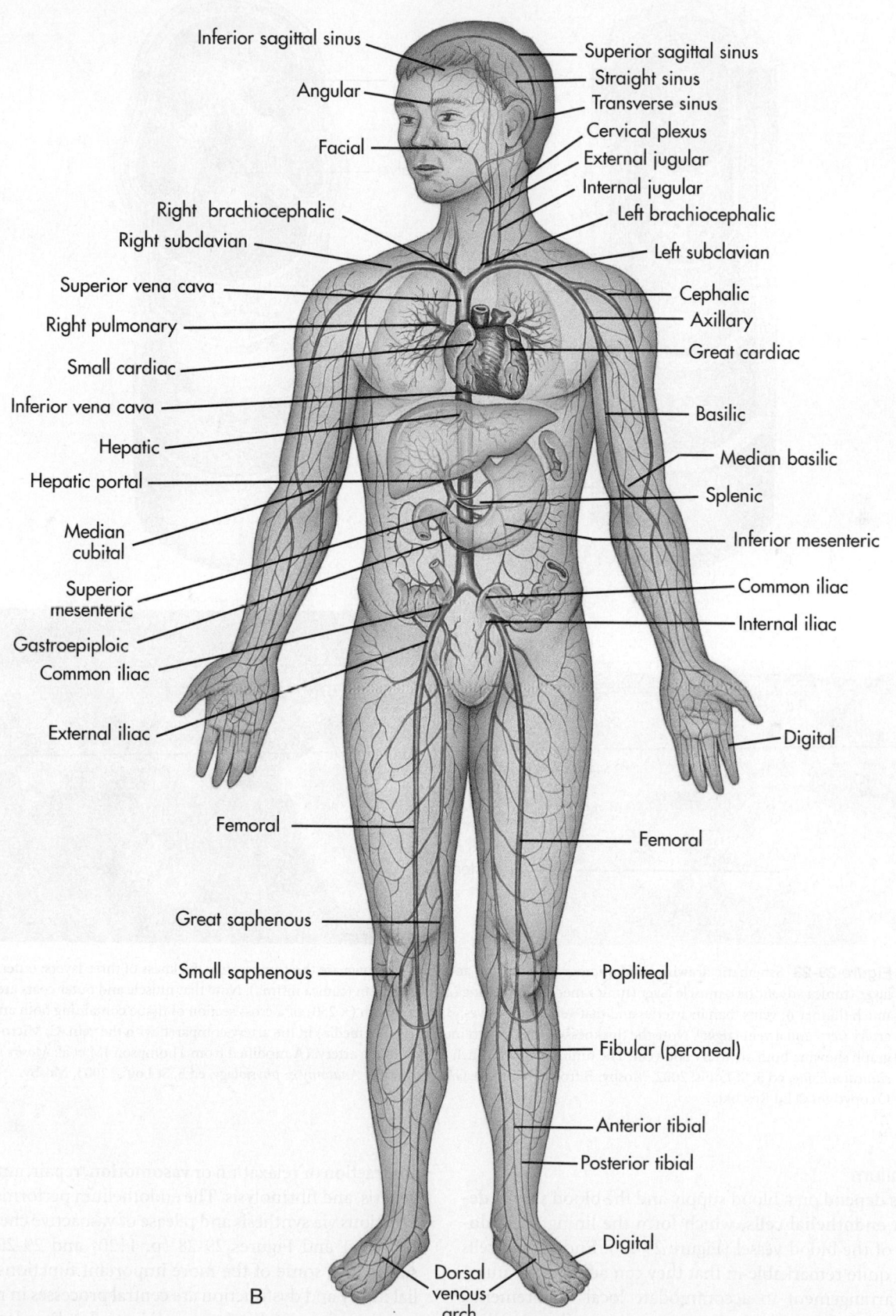

Inferior sagittal sinus
Angular
Facial
Right brachiocephalic
Right subclavian
Superior vena cava
Right pulmonary
Small cardiac
Inferior vena cava
Hepatic
Hepatic portal
Median cubital
Superior mesenteric
Gastroepiploic
Common iliac
External iliac
Femoral
Great saphenous
Small saphenous

Superior sagittal sinus
Straight sinus
Transverse sinus
Cervical plexus
External jugular
Internal jugular
Left brachiocephalic
Left subclavian
Cephalic
Axillary
Great cardiac
Basilic
Median basilic
Splenic
Inferior mesenteric
Common iliac
Internal iliac
Digital
Femoral
Popliteal
Fibular (peroneal)
Anterior tibial
Posterior tibial
Digital

Dorsal venous arch

B

Figure 29-22, cont'd B, Principal veins of the body.

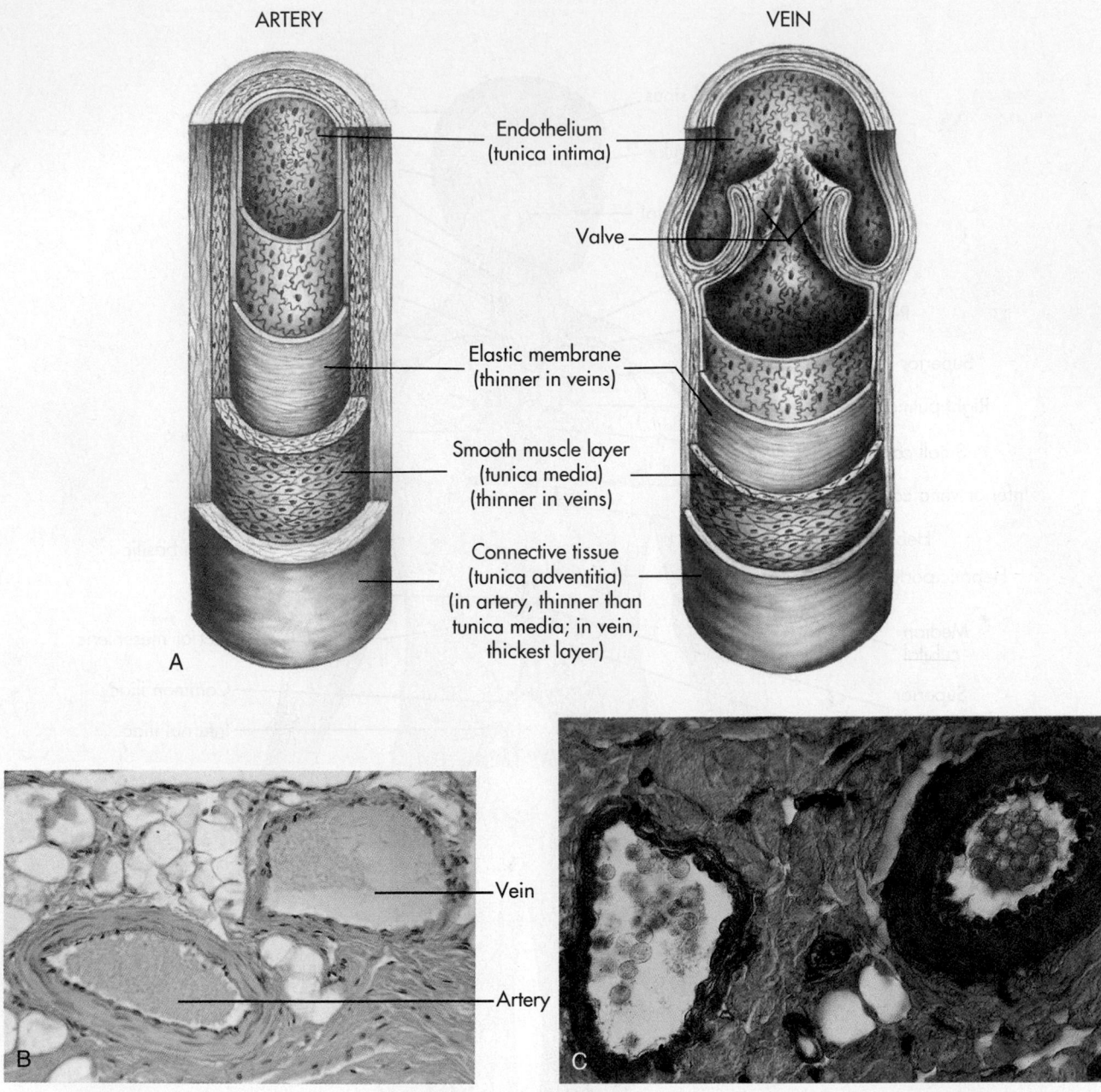

Figure 29-23 Schematic drawings and micrograph of artery and vein. **A,** Shown are the comparative thickness of three layers: outer layer (tunica adventitia), muscle layer (tunica media), and lining of endothelium (tunica intima). Note that muscle and outer coats are much thinner in veins than in arteries and that veins have valves. **B,** Micrograph (× 250) of a cross section of tissue containing both an artery *(left)* and a vein *(right)*. Note the thickness of the smooth muscle (tunica media) in the artery compared with the vein. **C,** Micrograph showing both an artery and vein. The tunica media is much thicker in the artery. (**A** modified from Thompson JM et al: *Mosby's clinical nursing,* ed 5, St Louis, 2002, Mosby. **B** from Thibodeau GA, Patton KT: *Anatomy & physiology,* ed 5, St Louis, 2003, Mosby. **C** copyright © Ed Reschke.)

Endothelium

All tissues depend on a blood supply and the blood supply depends on **endothelial cells,** which form the lining, or **endothelium,** of the blood vessel (Figure 29-27). Endothelial cells are really quite remarkable in that they can adjust their number and arrangement to accommodate local requirements. Thus they are a life-support tissue extending and remodeling the network of blood vessels to enable tissue growth, promote contraction or relaxation or **vasomotion,** repair, antithrombogenesis, and fibrinolysis. The endothelium performs these vital functions via synthesis and release of vasoactive chemicals.[18-20] Box 29-1 and Figures 29-28 (p. 1120) and 29-29 (p. 1121) summarize some of the more important functions. Endothelial injury and dysfunction are central processes in many of the most common and serious cardiovascular disorders including hypertension and atherosclerosis (see p. 1157).

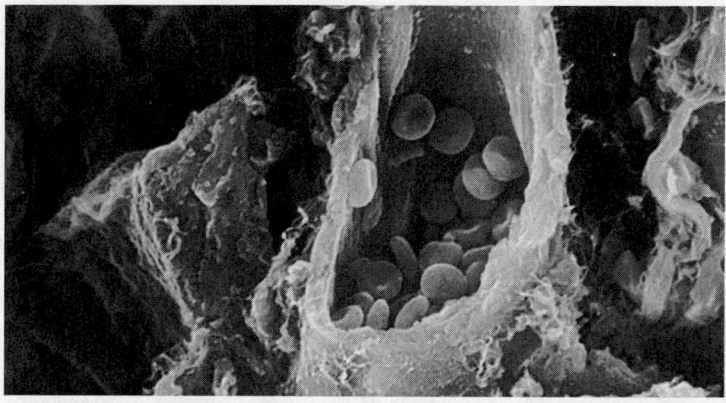

Figure 29-24 This ruptured tube is a blood vessel. It is full of red blood cells that move through blood vessels transporting oxygen and carbon dioxide from one place to another in the body. (From Raven RH, Johnson GB: *Biology*, ed 3, St Louis, 1992, Mosby)

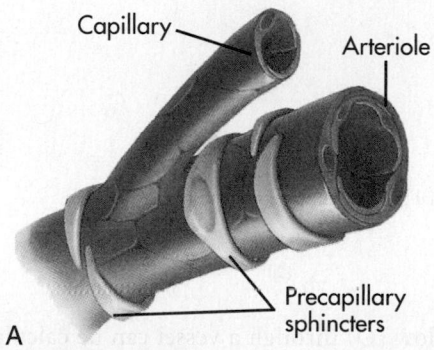

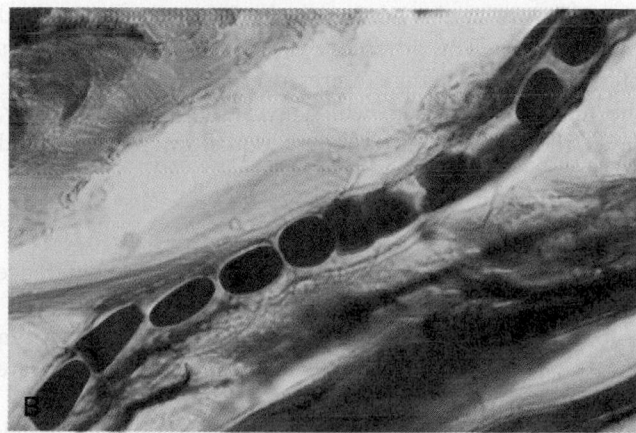

Figure 29-25 Capillary wall. A, Capillaries have a wall composed of only a single layer of flattened cells, whereas the walls of the larger vessels also have smooth muscle. B, Capillary with red blood cells in single file (× 500). (A from Thibodeau GA, Patton KT: *Anatomy & physiology*, ed 5, St Louis, 2003, Mosby; B copyright © Ed Reschke.)

Veins

The smallest venules closest to the capillaries have an inner lining composed of the endothelium of the tunica intima and surrounded by fibrous tissue. The largest venules, those farthest from the capillaries, are surrounded by a few smooth muscle fibers comprising a thin tunica media.

Compared with arteries, veins are thin walled and fibrous with a larger diameter (see Figure 29-23). A given vein is larger than the artery that lies within the same sheath. Veins are more numerous than arteries. In veins the tunica externa has less elastic tissue than in arteries, so veins do not recoil after distention as quickly as arteries. Like arteries, veins receive nourishment from the tiny vasa vasorum. Some veins, most commonly in the lower limbs, contain valves that regulate the one-way flow of blood toward the heart (Figure 29-30, p. 1121). These valves are folds of the tunica intima and resemble the semilunar valves of the heart. Backflow in veins of the legs is stopped as the flaps of the valves fill with blood and block the vessel. The position of the valves also facilitates blood flow in the proper direction during venous compression. When a person stands up, contraction of the skeletal muscles of the legs compresses the deep veins of the legs and assists the flow of blood toward the heart. This important mechanism of venous return is called the *muscle pump* (Figure 29-31, p. 1122).

Factors Affecting Blood Flow

Blood flow is the amount of fluid moved per unit of time and usually is expressed as liters or milliliters per minute (ml/min) or cubic centimeters per second (cm³/sec). Flow is regulated by the same physical properties that govern the movement of simple fluids in a closed, rigid system, that is, pressure, resistance, velocity, turbulent versus laminar flow, and compliance.

Pressure and Resistance

Blood flow is determined primarily by two factors: pressure and resistance. **Pressure** in a liquid system is the force exerted on the liquid per unit area and is expressed as dynes per square centimeter (dynes/cm²), millimeters of mercury (mmHg), or torr. Blood flow depends partly on the difference between pressures in the arterial and venous vessels supplying the organ. Fluid moves from the arterial "side" of the capillaries, a region of greater pressure, to the venous side, a region of lesser pressure.

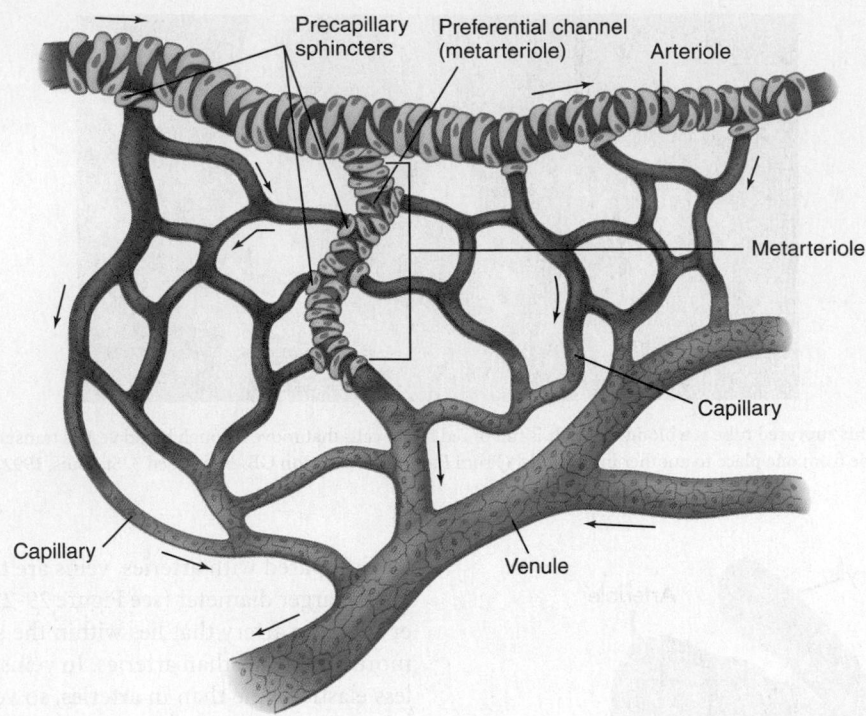

Figure 29-26 Capillary network. Blood enters the network as arterial blood and exits as venous blood.

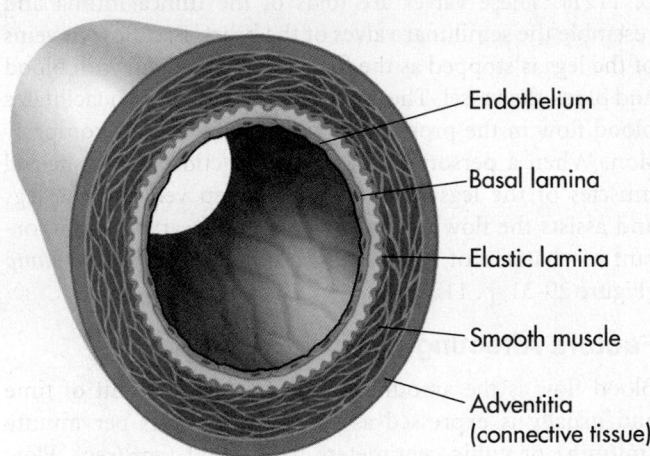

Figure 29-27 Endothelium. Practically imperceptible, the endothelial cells arrange themselves as a fine lining that has numerous life support functions.

Resistance is the opposition to force. In the cardiovascular system most opposition to blood flow is provided by the diameter and length of the blood vessels themselves. Therefore changes in blood flow through an organ result from changes in the vascular resistance within the organ. The major mechanisms causing changes in vascular resistance are an increase or a decrease in vessel diameter and the opening or closing of vascular channels. Resistance in a vessel is inversely related to blood flow; that is, increased resistance leads to decreased blood flow.

Blood flow *(Q)* through a vessel can be calculated from measurements of pressure at the inflow end of the vessel *(P₁)*, pressure at the outflow end of the vessel *(P₂)*, and resistance *(R)*. The difference between P_1 and P_2 often is referred to as the change in pressure and is expressed as δP. The following formula, which expresses Poiseuille's law, shows the relationship among blood flow, pressure, and resistance:

$$Q = \delta P / R$$

where Q = blood flow, δP = the pressure difference $(P_1 - P_2)$, and R = resistance.

Resistance to flow cannot be measured directly, but it can be calculated if the pressure difference and flow volumes are known.

Flow varies inversely with the viscosity of the fluid. Thick fluids move more slowly and cause greater resistance to flow than thin fluids. The viscosity of blood depends on its red cell content. The greater the percentage of red cells in the blood, the more viscous the blood. This relationship is expressed as the hematocrit—the ratio of the volume of red blood cells to the volume of whole blood (see Chapter 25). A high hematocrit reduces flow through the blood vessels, particularly the microcirculation (arterioles, capillaries, venules). Conditions in which the hematocrit is elevated, such as dehydration, cyanotic congenital heart disease (see Chapter 31), or polycythemia (see Chapter 26), can lead to increased cardiac work as a result of increased vascular resistance.

Box 29-1   Endothelium Functions and Vasoactive Substances

Dilators

Prostacyclin: A prostaglandin formed from arachidonic acid that can relax vascular smooth muscle through increases in cAMP. The primary function is to inhibit platelet adherence to the endothelium.

Nitric oxide (NO): Bradykinin prompts the endothelium to synthesize and release NO, a potent vasodilator. NO is anti-inflammatory and antithrombotic.

C-type natriuretic hormone: Made throughout the vasculature and works with NO and prostacyclin as a vasodilator.

Insulin: Insulin increases endothelial cell production of nitric oxide.

Estrogen: Triggers enzyme activation and release of NO.

Constrictors

Endothelin: A potent endothelium-derived constrictor.

Urotensin II: Another potent endothelium-derived constrictor

Angiotensin II (Ang II): A potent vasoconstrictor is produced both hormonally via the renin-angiotensin-aldosterone system and locally in vascular tissues. Ang II blocks the release of NO and prostacyclin. Ang II is also proinflammatory: it increases vascular permeability, recruits infiltrating monocytes, increases expression of adhesion molecules, and stimulates release of growth factors.

Thromboxane: Causes vasoconstriction and platelet adhesion.

Prostaglandins: Cause vasoconstriction especially during states of chronic inflammation.

Other Endothelial Functions

Platelet and monocyte adhesion: The endothelium helps regulate clotting and inflammation by modulating the number of platelets and inflammatory cells (monocytes and macrophages) that bind to the vessel wall. Endothelial-derived substances include von Willebrand factor, platelet-activating factor, heparan sulfate, t-PA, and others..

Filtration and permeability: The endothelium facilitates movement of large molecules through intercellular junctions and small molecules via vesicles and junctions.

Cell growth and inhibition: NO and prostacyclin inhibit cellular growth; Ang II stimulates growth.

Endothelial balance

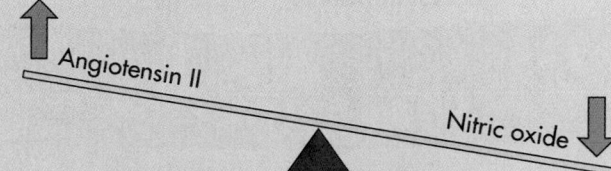

Endothelial dysfunction: levels of angiotensin II are increased and nitric oxide levels are decreased

Treatment: ACE inhibitors reestablishes balance

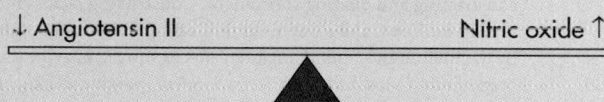

Figure adapted from Rocket JL: *Am J Nurs* 99(10):44, 1999. *ACE,* Angiotensin-converting enzyme; *cAMP,* cyclic adenosine monophosphate; *t-PA,* tissue-type plasminogen activator.

Data from Esper RJ et al: *Adv Cardiol* 45:17-43, 2008; Schafer A, Bauersachs J: *Curr Vasc Pharmacol* 6(1):52-60, 2008; Thijssen DH et al: *J Physiol* 586(2):319-324, 2008.

The viscosity of blood also increases if blood flow becomes very slow or stagnates (**anomalous viscosity**). Anomalous viscosity is generally not significant unless cardiac output is low. (Shock is described in Chapter 46.)

Poiseuille's formula for resistance to fluid flow through a tube takes into account the length of the tube, the viscosity of the fluid, and the radius of the tube's lumen. Resistance *(R)* is proportional to a constant 8/π, the viscosity of the blood (η), and the length of the vessel *(l)*, and it is inversely proportional to the fourth power of the lumen's radius (v⁴).[2] Thus

$$R = \frac{8\eta l}{\pi v 4}$$

Because this equation was derived using straight, rigid tubes with steady streamlined flow, it cannot be applied directly to the vascular system. Nevertheless, it is a useful model of vascular resistance.

The most important factor determining resistance in a single vessel is the caliber of the vessel's lumen, expressed in Poiseuille's formula as its radius and in Figure 29-32 as its diameter. Small changes in the lumen's radius lead to large changes in vascular resistance. Because vessel length is relatively constant, length is not as important as lumen size in determining flow through a single vessel.

Generally, resistance to flow is greater in longer tubes because resistance increases with length. That resistance increases with increased length is demonstrated by comparing flow of the same amount of blood under the same pressure through vessels arranged in different configurations. Blood flowing through the distributing arteries, beginning with branches off the aorta and ending at arterioles in the capillary bed, encounters more resistance than blood flowing through the capillary bed itself, where flow is distributed among many short, tiny branches arranged in parallel. This is because the distributing arteries comprise a long system of tubes connected in series (end-to-end), whereas the arterioles and capillaries comprise

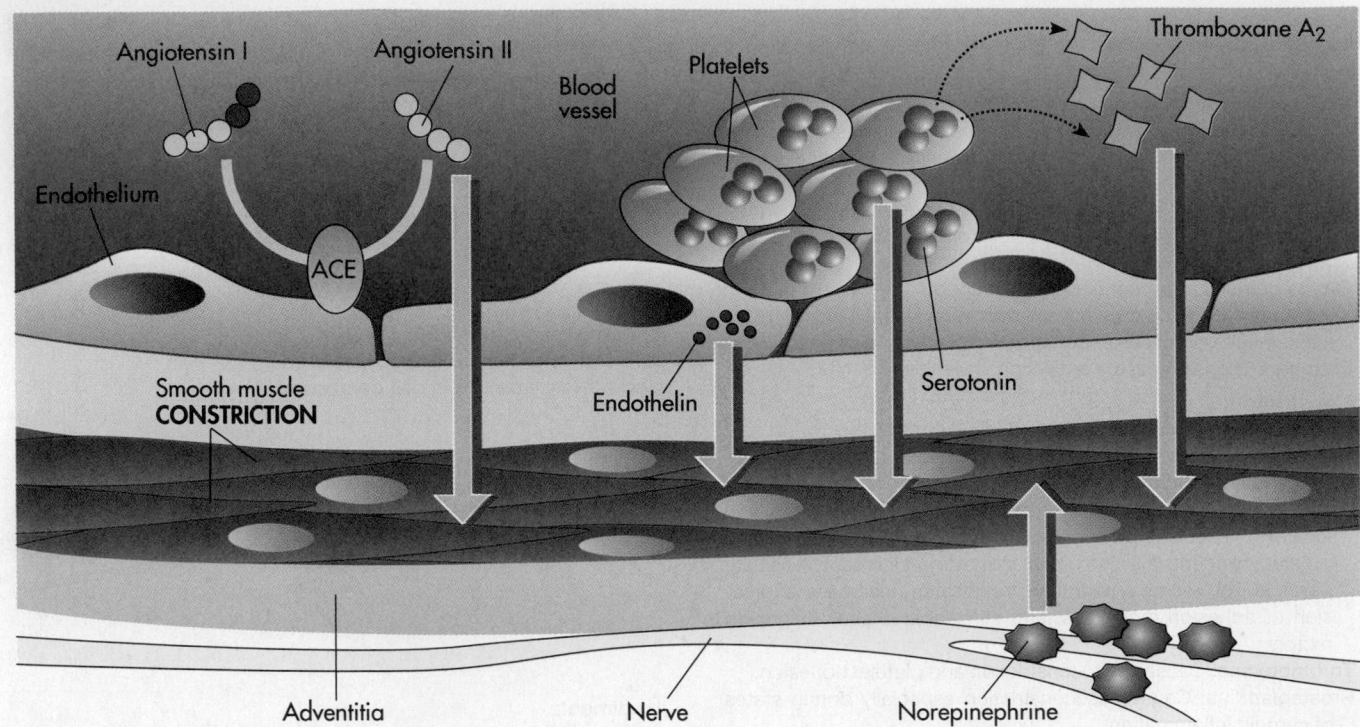

Figure 29-28 Endothelium regulation of vasomotion (constriction and dilation) and platelet aggregation by release of a variety of constricting and dilating substances. Constricting factors include arachidonic acid and metabolites, such as thromboxane A_2 (which aspirin inhibits), and a potent amino acid peptide called *endothelin*. The endothelium also converts angiotensin I into angiotensin II by the membrane-bound angiotensin-converting enzyme that also metabolizes the endogenous endothelium-dependent vasodilator, bradykinin. (Modified from Stern S: *Silent myocardial ischemia*, St Louis, 1998, Mosby.)

a short system of many vessels arranged in parallel (side by side) (Figure 29-33). Although the arterioles are arranged in series with the distributing arteries and the capillaries, they are arranged in parallel with other arterioles. Similarly, the capillaries are in series with the metarterioles, but they are in parallel with other capillaries.

Resistance to flow through a system of vessels, or **total resistance,** depends not only on characteristics of individual vessels but also on whether the vessels are arranged in series or in parallel (see Figure 29-30). For vessels arranged in series, total resistance equals the sum obtained by adding all the individual resistances calculated using Poiseuille's formula. For vessels arranged in parallel, total resistance equals the sum of the reciprocals *(I/R)* of the individual resistances.

Total resistance is related to the total cross-sectional area of a system of vessels in parallel and to the number of vessels in parallel that make up the total cross-sectional area. The larger the total cross-sectional area, as in the capillary system, the lower the resistance. However, if a cross-sectional area is made up of a very large number of parallel vessels, the overall resistance will be greater than it would be if the cross-sectional area were made up of only two or three parallel vessels. Therefore, resistance is greater in smaller vessels than in larger vessels. The total cross-sectional area of the arteriolar system is greater than that of the arterial system

(see Figure 29-32); the greater number of arterioles arranged in parallel, however, leads to greater resistance to flow in the arteriolar system. The pressure drop is greatest across the arterioles. Many capillaries arise from each arteriole so that the total cross-sectional area of the capillary bed is very large and resistance is low, despite the fact that the cross-sectional area of each capillary is less (which normally increases resistance) than that of each arteriole. As a result, blood flow becomes quite slow in the capillaries, analogous to water flow in a river. A narrow river whose bed widens flows more slowly through the wide section than through the narrow section. The slow velocity of flow in each vessel promotes optimal capillary-tissue exchange.

Velocity

Blood velocity is the distance blood travels in a unit of time, usually centimeters per second (cm/sec). Blood velocity is directly related to blood flow (amount of blood moved per unit of time) and inversely related to the cross-sectional area of the vessel in which the blood is flowing.

The relationship between velocity and flow can be understood by thinking of a river. The volume of water flowing in a river is the same whether the river is narrow or wide. Where the river narrows, the water flows quickly; where it widens, the water flows slowly. The volume of water moving between the riverbanks does not change. In the body,

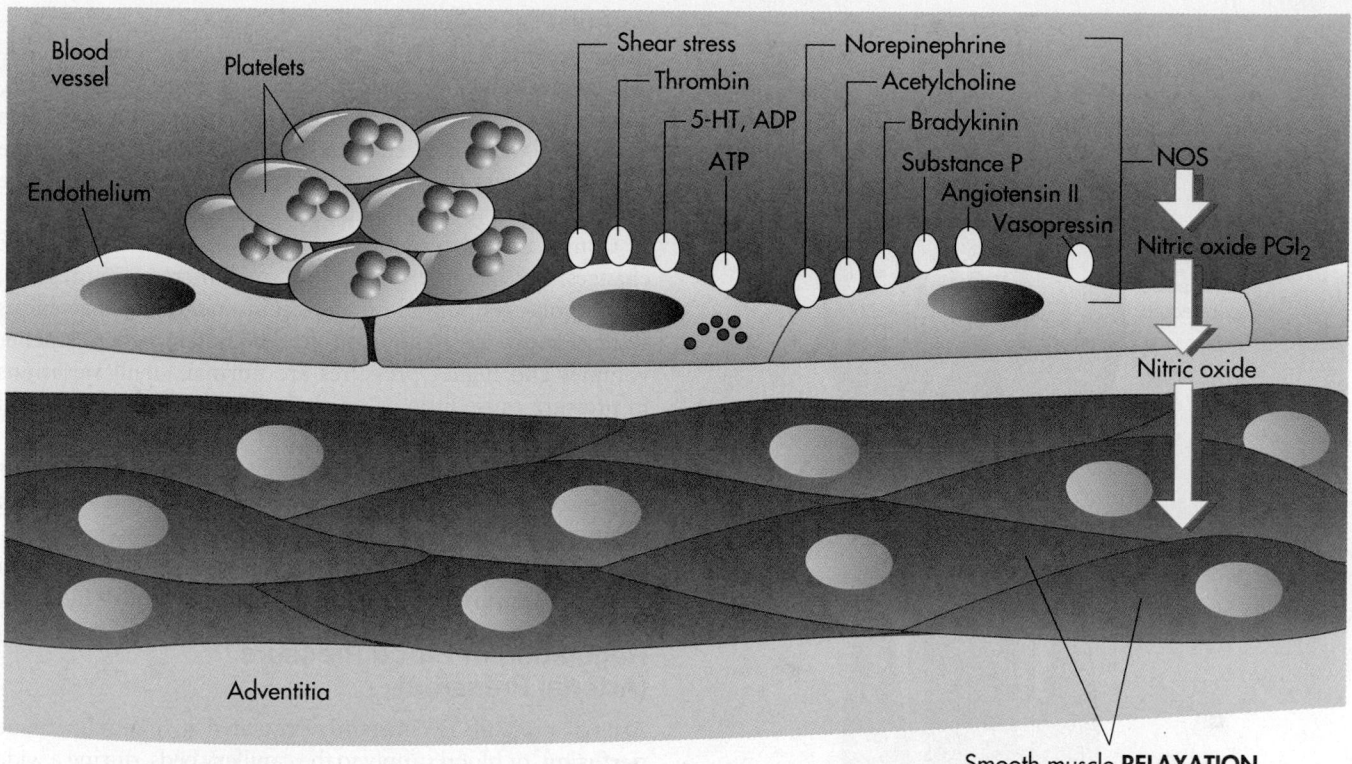

Figure 29-29 Factors causing endothelium-dependent vasodilation. A variety of exogenous pharmacologic substances, platelet-derived factors, and shear stress can promote release of nitric oxide by stimulating nitric oxide synthase (NOS). Prostacyclin (PGI₂) causes relaxation of vascular smooth muscle cells by cyclic adenosine monophosphate (cAMP)–dependent mechanism, and both nitric oxide and PGI₂ inhibit platelet aggregation. *5-HT,* Serotonin; *ADP,* adenosine diphosphate; *ATP,* adenosine triphosphate. (Modified from Stern S: *Silent myocardial ischemia,* St Louis, 1998, Mosby.)

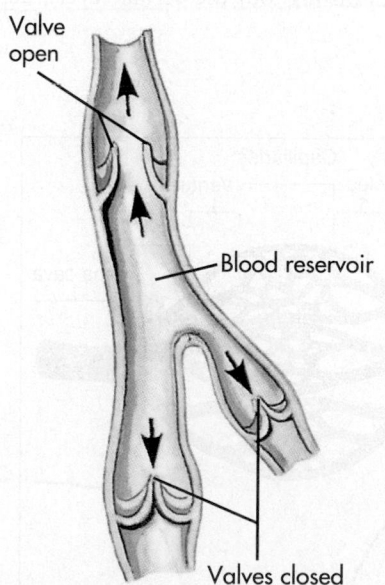

Figure 29-30 Valves of vein. Pooled blood is moved toward heart as valves are forced open by pressure from volume of blood downstream. (From Thibodeau GA, Patton KT: *Anatomy & physiology,* ed 5, St Louis, 2003, Mosby.)

as blood moves from the aorta to the capillaries, the total cross-sectional area of the vessels increases and velocity of flow decreases.

Laminar Versus Turbulent Flow

Flow through any tubular system is either laminar or turbulent. Normally, blood flow through the vessels is laminar. In **laminar flow,** concentric layers of molecules move "straight ahead." Each concentric layer flows at a different velocity (Figure 29-34). The cohesive attraction between the fluid and the vessel wall prevents the molecules of blood that are in contact with the wall from moving. The next thin layer of blood is able to slide slowly past the stationary layer and so on until, at the center, the blood velocity is greatest. The centermost concentric layer of fluid is not slowed by friction against the vessel wall. Large vessels have room for a large center layer; therefore, they have less resistance to flow and greater flow and velocity than smaller vessels.

Where flow is obstructed, the vessel turns, or blood flows over rough surfaces, it becomes **turbulent** with whorls or eddy currents that produce noise, causing a murmur to be heard on auscultation. Resistance increases with turbulence.

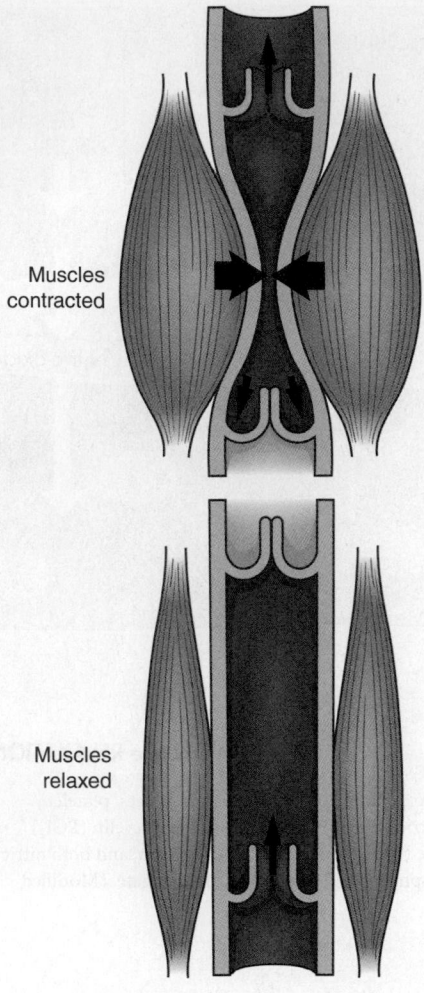

Figure 29-31 Muscle pump.

Vascular Compliance

Vascular compliance is the increase in volume a vessel is able to accommodate for a given increase in pressure (e.g., *C = VP*). Compliance depends on the ratio of elastic fibers to muscle fibers in the vessel wall. The elastic arteries are more compliant than the muscular arteries; the veins are more compliant than either type of artery and serve as storage areas for the circulatory system.

Compliance determines a vessel's response to pressure changes. For example, with a very small increase in pressure, a large volume of blood can be accommodated by the venous system. In the less compliant arterial system, where smaller volumes and higher pressures are normal, small variations in pressure cause little or no change in the volume of blood within the arterial vessels.

Stiffness is the opposite of compliance. Several conditions and disorders can cause stiffness, with the most common being arteriosclerosis (see Chapter 30). Arteriosclerosis increases the rigidity or stiffness of arterial walls, which in turn increases peak arterial pressure at a given volume of blood.

Regulation of Blood Pressure (Arterial Pressure)

Arterial pressure is constantly regulated to maintain tissue **perfusion,** or blood supply to the capillary beds, during a wide range of physiologic conditions, including changes in body position, muscular activity, and circulating blood volume. Arterial pressure is determined by the cardiac output (heart rate times stroke volume) and the peripheral resistance. Increases in one or both will raise arterial pressure, and decreases in one or both will lower the arterial pressure (see Table 29-3). The **mean arterial pressure (MAP),** which is the average pressure in the arteries throughout the cardiac cycle, depends on the

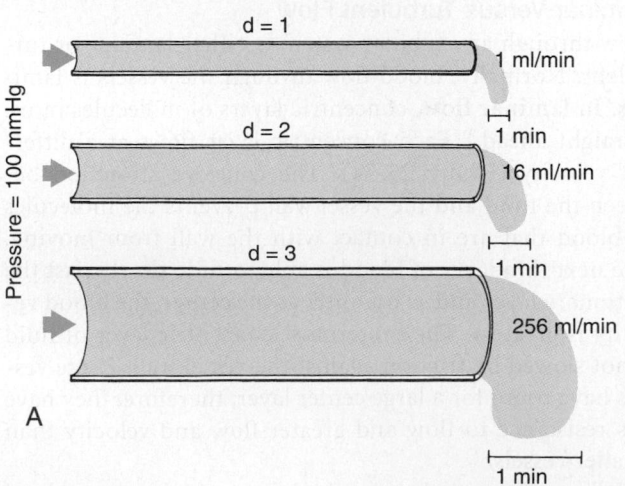

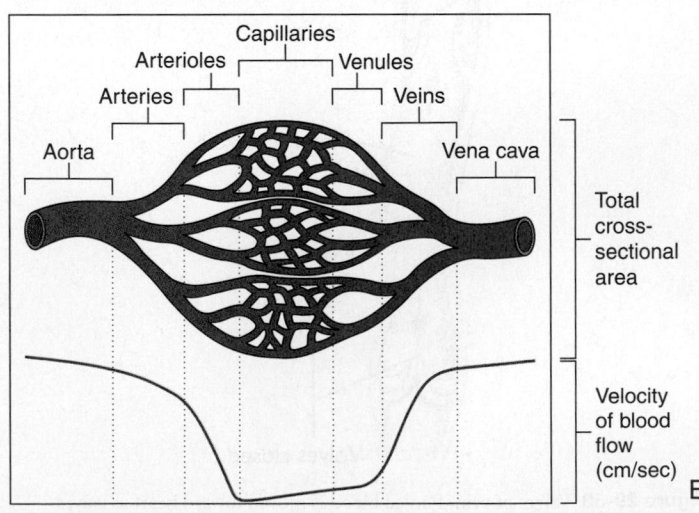

Figure 29-32 Lumen diameter, blood flow, and resistance. **A,** Effect of lumen diameter on flow through vessel. **B,** Blood flows with great speed in the large arteries. However, branching of arterial vessels increases the total cross-sectional area of the arterioles and capillaries, reducing the flow rate. When capillaries merge into venules and venules merge into veins, the total cross-sectional area decreases, causing the flow rate to increase. *d,* Diameter. (**B** from Thibodeau GA, Patton KT: *Anatomy & physiology,* ed 5, St Louis, 2003, Mosby.)

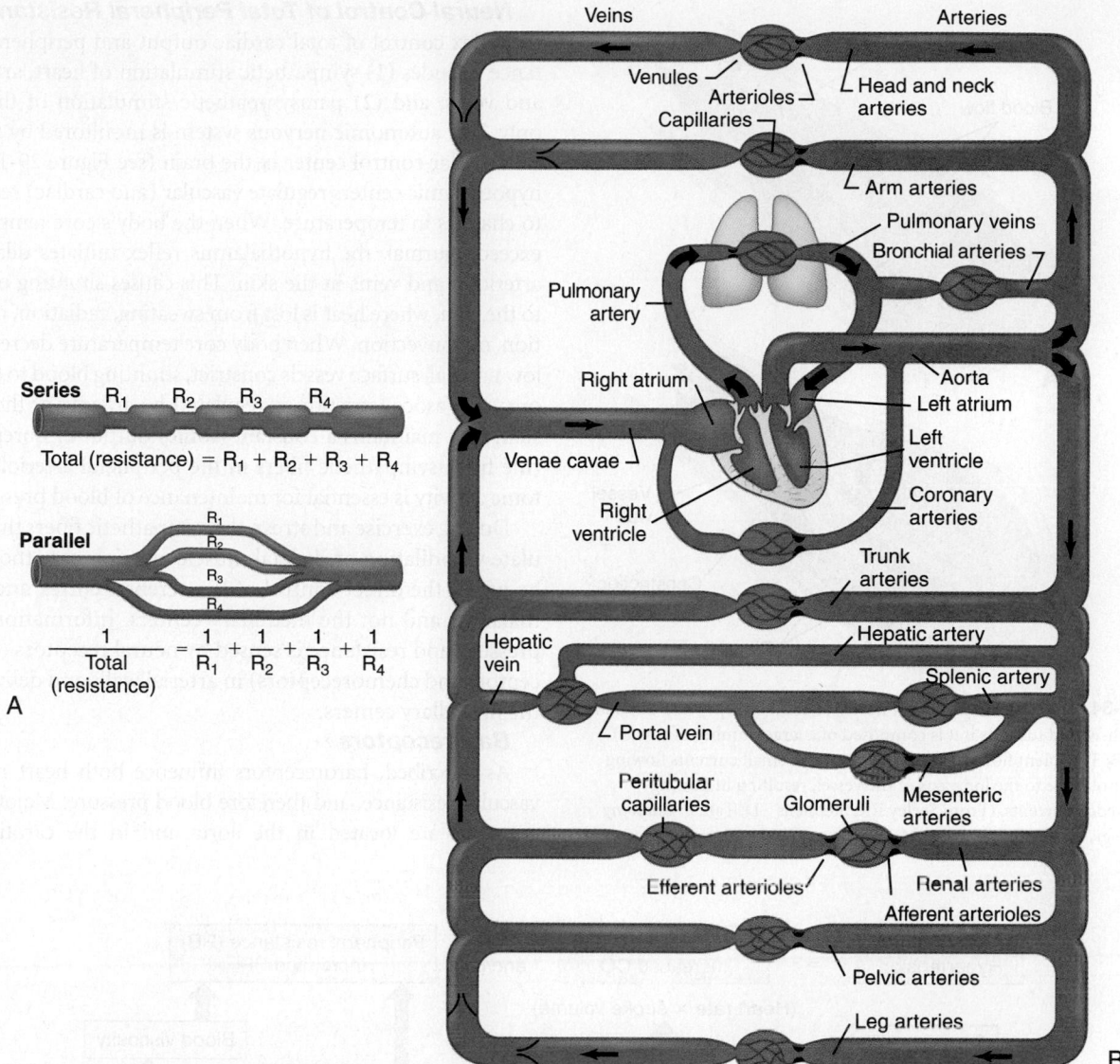

Figure 29-33 Schematic diagram of the parallel and series arrangement of the vessels composing the circulatory system. **A,** Resistance in blood vessels arranged in series or parallel. **B,** The capillary beds are represented by thin lines connecting the arterioles (on the right) and the veins (on the left). The crescent-shaped thickenings proximal to the capillary beds represent the arterioles (resistance vessels). *R,* Resistance in an individual vessel. (B modified from Berne RM, Levy MN: *Cardiovascular physiology,* ed 8, St Louis, 2001, Mosby.)

elastic properties of the arterial walls and the mean volume of blood in the arterial system. MAP can be approximated from the measured values of the systolic *(Ps)* and diastolic *(Pd)* pressures by means of the following formula:

$$MAP = Pd + \frac{1}{3}(ps - Pd, \text{ or pulse pressure})$$

The major factors and relationships that regulate arterial blood pressure are summarized in Figure 29-35.

Effects of Cardiac Output

The cardiac output (minute volume) of the heart can be changed by alterations in heart rate, stroke volume (volume of blood ejected during each ventricular contraction), or both.

An increase in cardiac output without a decrease in peripheral resistance will cause arterial volume and mean blood pressure to increase. The higher arterial pressure increases blood flow through the arterioles. On the other hand, a decrease in the cardiac output causes an immediate drop in mean arterial blood pressure and arteriolar flow (Table 29-3).

Effects of Total Peripheral Resistance and Blood Volume

Total resistance in the systemic circulation, sometimes called *total peripheral resistance,* is determined primarily by change in the diameter of the arterioles. Arteriolar constriction raises mean arterial pressure by preventing the free flow of blood into the capillaries. Dilation has the opposite effect.

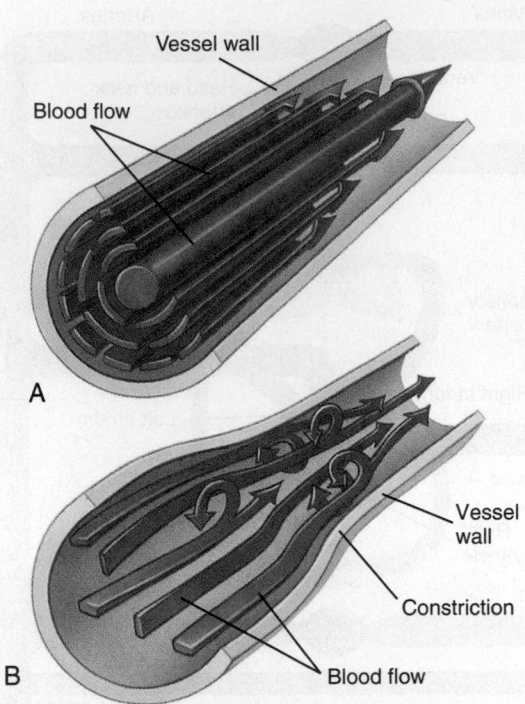

Vessel wall

Blood flow

A

Vessel wall

Constriction

Blood flow

B

Figure 29-34 **Laminar and turbulent flow. A,** Laminar flow. Fluid flows in long smooth-walled tubes as if it is composed of a large number of concentric layers. **B,** Turbulent flow is caused by numerous small currents flowing crosswise or oblique to the long axis of the vessel, resulting in flowing whorls and eddy currents. (From Seeley RR, Stephens TD, Tate P: *Anatomy and physiology,* ed 3, St Louis, 1995, Mosby.)

Neural Control of Total Peripheral Resistance

Reflex control of total cardiac output and peripheral resistance includes (1) sympathetic stimulation of heart, arterioles, and veins; and (2) parasympathetic stimulation of the heart only. The autonomic nervous system is monitored by the cardiovascular control center in the brain (see Figure 29-11). The hypothalamic centers regulate vascular (and cardiac) responses to changes in temperature. When the body's core temperature exceeds normal, the hypothalamus reflex initiates dilation of arterioles and veins in the skin. This causes shunting of blood to the skin, where heat is lost from sweating, radiation, conduction, or convection. When body core temperature decreases below normal, surface vessels constrict, shunting blood to the vital organs. Vasoconstriction is regulated by an area of the brainstem that maintains a constant (tonic) output of norepinephrine from sympathetic fibers in the peripheral arterioles. This tonic activity is essential for maintenance of blood pressure.

During exercise and stress, the sympathetic fibers that stimulate vasodilation of skeletal muscle arterioles are thought to be under the direct control of the cerebral cortex and hypothalamus and not the medullary centers. Information about pressure and resistance is sensed by neural receptors (baroreceptors and chemoreceptors) in arterial walls and delivered to the medullary centers.

Baroreceptors

As described, baroreceptors influence both heart rate and vascular resistance, and therefore blood pressure. Major stretch receptors are located in the aorta and in the carotid sinus

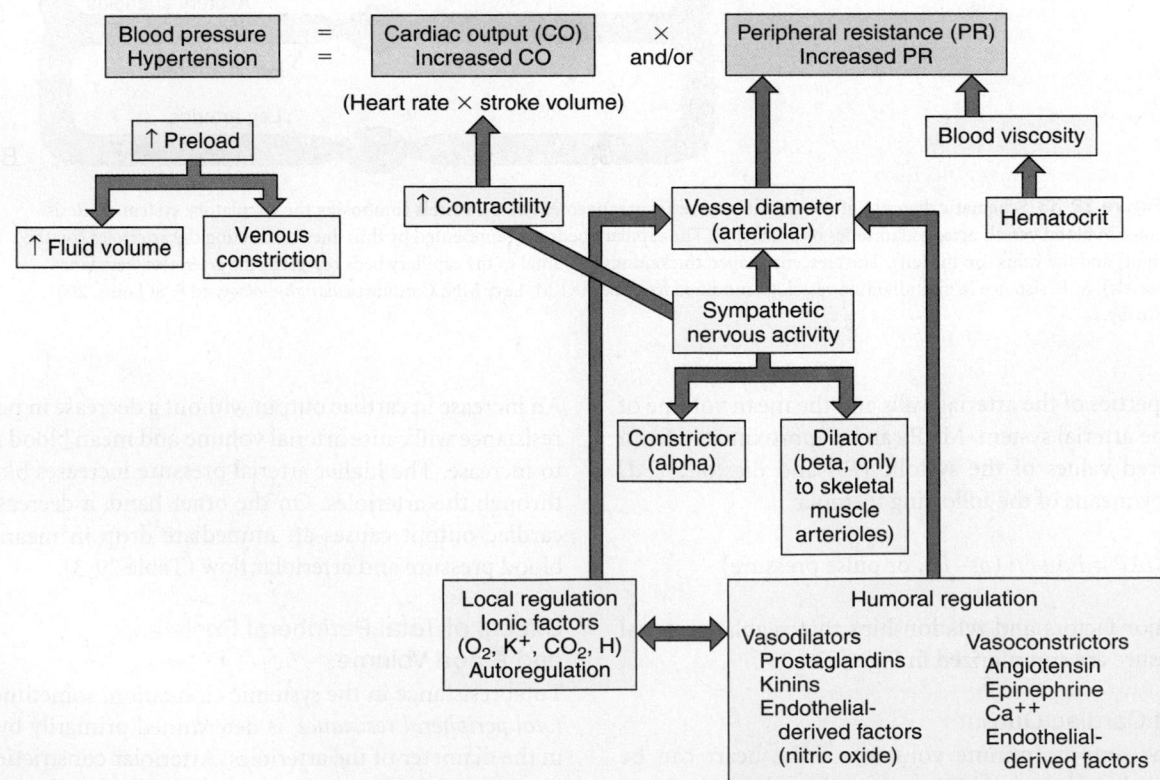

Figure 29-35 Factors regulating blood flow

Table 29-3	Factors That Affect Mean Arterial Pressure and Capillary Flow	
	Mean Arterial Pressure	Capillary Flow
Peripheral Resistance*		
Increased	Increased	Decreased
Decreased	Decreased	Increased
Heart Rate†		
Increased	Increased	Increased
Decreased	Decreased	Decreased
Stroke Volume‡		
Increased	Increased	Increased
Decreased	Decreased	Decreased

From Little RC: *Physiology of the heart and circulation,* ed 3, St Louis, 1985, Mosby.
*Cardiac output maintained constant.
†Peripheral resistance and stroke volume constant.
‡Peripheral resistance and heart rate constant.

(Figure 29-36). These baroreceptors respond to changes in smooth muscle fiber length by altering their rate of discharge and they supply sensory information to the cardiovascular center that regulates blood pressure.[14,15] (Technically they are mechanoreceptors but they usually are called *baroreceptors* or *pressoreceptors.*) The rate of firing of the baroreceptors increases and decreases with changes in blood pressure. An increase in arterial pressure increases the rate of firing of the carotid sinus and aortic arch baroreceptors. These impulses travel up the afferent nerves to the medulla (e.g., the cardiac control center) and (1) slow heart rate by decreasing sympathetic discharge and increasing parasympathetic discharge (vagus nerve), (2) decrease myocardial contractility by inhibiting sympathetic discharge, and (3) increase arteriolar and venous dilation by decreasing sympathetic discharge to smooth muscle. The net effect of this major blood pressure–regulating reflex is to reduce blood pressure to normal by decreasing cardiac output (heart rate and stroke volume) and peripheral resistance. Conversely, the baroreceptor response to decreased blood pressure results in an increase in heart rate, an increase in myocardial contractility, and peripheral vasoconstriction, thus raising the blood pressure. (Postural changes and the baroreceptor reflex are discussed in Chapter 30.)

Arterial Chemoreceptors

Specialized areas within the medulla oblongata and aortic and carotid arteries are sensitive to concentrations of oxygen, carbon dioxide, and hydrogen ions (pH) in the blood (see Figure 29-34, B). Although these receptors, called *chemoreceptors,* are more important for the control of respiration, they also transmit impulses to the medullary cardiovascular centers that regulate blood pressure. A decrease in arterial oxygen concentration or pH causes a reflexive increase in blood pressure, whereas an increase in carbon dioxide causes a decrease in blood pressure. Blood pressure changes are carried out by smooth muscle layers in the vessels. Vasoconstriction

raises blood pressure and vasodilation lowers it. The major chemoreceptive reflex is caused by alterations in arterial oxygen concentration. The effects of altered pH or carbon dioxide levels are minor.

Effect of Hyperemia

When metabolic activity is increased in the heart, skeletal muscle, and other muscular organs, it causes an increase in blood flow termed **hyperemia.** For example, the blood flow to exercising skeletal muscle increases in proportion to the activity of the muscle. This condition, known as *active (exercise) hyperemia,* is the result of arteriolar dilation and autoregulation of blood flow within the active organ. *Reactive hyperemia* refers to vasodilation in response to restoration of blood flow after a period of tissue ischemia and results from a buildup of vasodilatory metabolic byproducts in the ischemic tissue.

Effects of Hormones

Many hormones cause contraction or relaxation of arteriolar smooth muscle. By constricting or dilating arterioles in specific vascular beds, hormones can (1) increase the blood supply to vital organs requiring more flow in times of stress, (2) redistribute blood volume during hemorrhage or shock, and (3) regulate heat loss.

Epinephrine, the hormone released from the adrenal medulla, causes vasoconstriction in most vascular beds (exceptions are the coronary, liver, and skeletal muscle). However, the effects of **norepinephrine** (from the sympathetic nervous system and adrenal medulla) are quantitatively more vasoconstrictive than the effects of epinephrine.

Antidiuretic hormone (ADH) is released by the posterior pituitary and causes reabsorption of water by the kidney. With reabsorption the blood plasma volume will increase, increasing blood pressure. ADH, also known as arginine vasopressin, is a potent vasoconstrictor, thus it increases peripheral resistance (Figure 29-37, and see Chapters 3 and 35).

Renin is an enzyme synthesized and secreted by the juxtaglomerular cells of the kidney. It also has been found in the adrenal cortex, salivary gland, prolactin-producing and luteinizing hormone–producing cells of the pituitary, arterial smooth muscle cells in the vascular endothelium, brain, myocardium, and possibly other tissues.[21] The following factors control renin release:

1. A drop in blood pressure (detected by the juxtaglomerular cells as a decrease in blood flow to the kidney)
2. A decrease in the amount of sodium chloride delivered to the kidney
3. β-adrenergic stimuli (increase renin release) and β-adrenergic inhibitors (decrease renin release)
4. Angiotensin II (decreases renin release)
5. Low potassium concentrations in plasma (increases renin release)

Angiotensin II (Ang II) is created when renin splits off a polypeptide from angiotensinogen to generate **angiotensin I (Ang I).** Angiotensin I appears to be physiologically inactive. Angiotensin I, however, is converted by an enzyme, called angiotensin-converting enzyme (ACE), to Ang II. Ang II is a powerful vasoconstrictor and stimulates the secretion

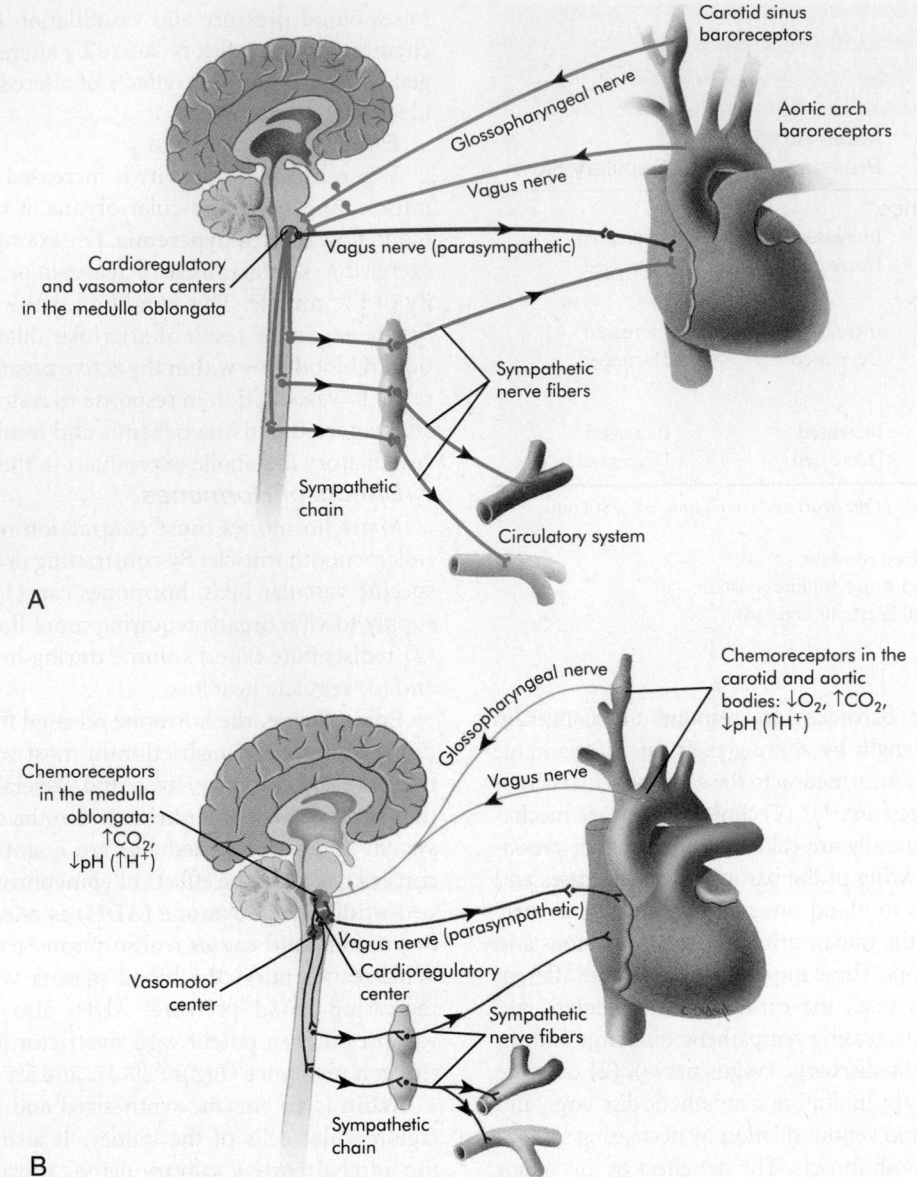

Figure 29-36 Baroreceptor and chemoreceptor reflex control of blood pressure. **A,** Baroreceptor reflexes. Baroreceptors located in the carotid sinuses and aortic arch detect changes in blood pressure. Action potentials are conducted to the cardioregulatory and vasomotor centers. The heart rate can be decreased by the parasympathetic system; the heart rate and stroke volume can be increased by the sympathetic system. The sympathetic system also can constrict or dilate blood vessels. **B,** Chemoreceptor reflexes. Chemoreceptors located in the medulla oblongata and in the carotid and aortic bodies detect changes in blood oxygen, carbon dioxide, or pH. Action potentials are conducted to the medulla oblongata. In response, the vasomotor center can cause vasoconstriction or dilation of blood vessels by the sympathetic system, and the cardioregulatory center can cause changes in the pumping activity of the heart through the parasympathetic and sympathetic systems. (From Seeley RR, Stephens TD, Tate P: *Anatomy & physiology*, ed 3, St Louis, 1995, Mosby.)

of aldosterone from the adrenal gland[22] (Figure 29-37; also see Figure 29-38). Ang II is also a growth promoter in cardiovascular tissues, resulting in myocyte and vascular hypertrophy and progression of hypertension.[21,22] Neural effects of Ang II include stimulation of thirst, release of antidiuretic hormone, and increases in sympathetic nervous system output (i.e., catecholamines). A second form of ACE, called ACE$_2$,

helps to degrade Ang II and therefore balance its effects on the vasculature[23] (see What's New? The Renin-Angiotensin-Aldosterone System Revisited, p. 1128).

This kidney-based **renin-angiotensin-aldosterone-system (RAAS)** serves as an important regulatory loop. For example, decreases in blood pressure or sodium delivery to the kidneys (macula densa), as might occur

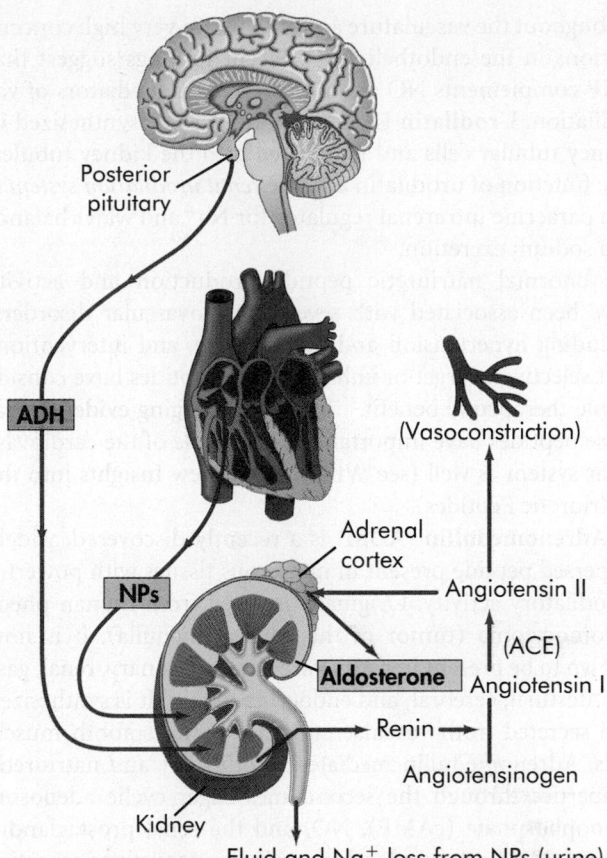

Figure 29-37 Three mechanisms that influence total plasma volume. The antidiuretic hormone (ADH) mechanism and renin-angiotensin and aldosterone mechanisms tend to increase water retention and thus increase total plasma volume. The natriuretic peptides antagonize these mechanisms by promoting water loss and sodium loss, thus promoting a decrease in total plasma volume. *NPs,* Natriuretic peptides; *ACE,* angiotensin-converting enzyme. (Modified from Thibodeau GA, Patton KT: *Anatomy & physiology,* ed 5, St Louis, 2003, Mosby.)

after hemorrhage or extracellular volume deficits (dehydration), stimulate secretion of renin, which forms Ang I, which is converted to Ang II and restores blood pressure. Sodium retention also results from increased secretion of aldosterone. Overall, the renin-angiotensin system is activated after volume depletion or hypotension or both, and it is suppressed after volume repletion and restoration of normal blood pressure. Basic knowledge of the renin-angiotensin system has advanced. Important is knowledge of a **tissue-based renin-angiotensin system** that can be regulated independently from the circulation. These new data are redefining our understanding of hypertension and other vascular disorders. The tissue renin-angiotensin system is activated in response to tissue injury. This system is involved in maladaptive alterations, such as ventricular and vascular remodeling, alterations in renal functions, and atherosclerosis[24,25] (see Chapter 30). Particularly significant is an increased recognition of the role of Ang II in these processes (see Figure 29-38).

Ang II has two primary subtypes of receptors, AT_1 and AT_2 (see Figure 29-38). Both subtypes are expressed in human hearts. $\mathbf{AT_1}$ is also found on vascular smooth muscle and endothelial cells, nerve endings, conduction tissues, adrenal cortex, liver, kidney and brain. $\mathbf{AT_2}$ receptors are found in fetal mesenchymal tissue, adrenal medulla, uterus and ovarian follicles, renal tubules, and vasculature. A third type of Ang II receptor, AT_4, has been described, although its effects are still being evaluated[26] (see What's New? The Renin-Angiotensin-Aldosterone System Revisited). The majority of Ang II actions are thought to occur through the AT_1 receptor, including growth promotion, vasoconstriction, antinatriuresis (save Na^+), aldosterone secretion, inhibition of renin synthesis and release, salt appetite, thirst, sympathetic outflow and stimulation of inflammation.[22,25-28] Treatments such as ACE inhibitors and angiotensin receptor antagonists that inhibit AT_1 receptor are a main target in preventive and reparative strategies in cardiovascular disease.

Although the majority of Ang II actions are mediated via the AT_1 receptor, evidence is emerging that AT_2 receptor opposes the AT_1 receptor, especially by inducing vasodilation instead of vasoconstriction.[29] AT_2 dilator action is mediated by nitric oxide (NO) in a bradykinin-dependent or independent manner (Figure 29-39). Vasodilation mediated by AT_2 receptors has been shown in microarteries of the coronary, mesenteric, and uterine circulation. In addition, continuous use of compounds that stimulate AT_2 receptor (agonists) cause sustained vasodilation and hypotension. Therapeutically, these data predict that AT_2 receptor stimulation would be a beneficial addition to AT_1 receptor blockage in the treatment of hypertension.

Ang II is now considered to be a growth promoter in cardiovascular tissues, and the resultant vascular hypertrophy is a significant factor in the pathogenesis of hypertension. Chronically elevated levels of Ang II in the heart, like that seen in hypertension, contribute to myocardial hypertrophy and heart failure (see Chapter 30). Ang II plays a role in the kidney, not only as a regulator of blood flow but also in the development of structural changes and proteinuria. Therefore treatments, such as ACE inhibitors and angiotensin receptor (ATR) antagonists that inhibit mostly AT_1 receptors are a main target in preventive and reparative strategies in cardiovascular diseases.

Aldosterone is released by the adrenal cortex in response to Ang II. It causes reabsorption of sodium and water in the kidneys. Aldosterone plays an important role in the pathogenesis of cardiovascular and renal disease. Aldosterone has a number of deleterious effects, including myocardial necrosis and fibrosis, vascular stiffening and injury, reduced fibrinolyses, endothelial dysfunction, catecholamine release, and promotion of dysrhythmias. These effects are caused by aldosterone, itself, and are independent of Ang II. Some mechanisms of aldosterone-induced cardiovascular dysfunction include activation of phospholipase C-mediated vasoconstriction, activation of the cyclooxygenase 2 pathway of inflammation, increased production of toxic oxygen radicals, and stimulation of smooth muscle cell proliferation.[30]

The natriuretic peptides include ANP, brain natriuretic peptide, C-type natriuretic peptide (CNP), and urodilatin.[31] These peptides help regulate urinary sodium excretion (natriuresis), diuresis, vasodilation, and antagonism of the renin-angiotensin system. All of these effects lead to the formation of a large volume of dilute urine that decreases blood volume and blood pressure. **Atrial natriuretic peptide (ANP) (or factor)** is a peptide secreted from cells (monocytes) in the right atrium when right atrial blood pressure increases. In addition, under pathologic conditions, the left ventricle may secrete ANP. ANP causes increased urine sodium excretion, leading to decreased blood volume and blood pressure.[32] **Brain natriuretic peptide (BNP)** was originally isolated from paracrine brain and named *brain natriuretic peptide*. The name is misleading, however, because BNP is mostly synthesized, stored, and secreted from cardiac cells (i.e., atria). BNP also contributes to urinary sodium excretion and is used both as a marker and as a treatment for acute heart failure.[33] **C-type natriuretic peptide (CNP)** is widely expressed throughout the vasculature and is found in very high concentrations in the endothelium.[34] Recent findings suggest that CNP complements NO and prostacyclin as mediators of vasodilation. **Urodilatin** is a natriuretic peptide synthesized in kidney tubular cells and is secreted into the kidney tubules. The function of urodilatin and the *renal urodilation system* is as a paracrine intrarenal regulator for Na^+ and water balance and sodium excretion.

Abnormal natriuretic peptide production and activity have been associated with several cardiovascular disorders, including hypertension and heart failure, and interventions that selectively target or enhance these peptides have considerable therapeutic benefit.[35] There is emerging evidence that these peptides have important roles outside of the cardiovascular system as well (see What's New? New Insights into the Natriuretic Peptides).

Adrenomedullin (ADM) is a recently discovered, widely dispersed peptide present in numerous tissues with powerful vasodilatory activity. Originally isolated from human pheochromocytoma (tumor of the adrenal medulla), it is now known to be present in cardiovascular, pulmonary, renal, gastrointestinal, cerebral, and endocrine tissues. It is synthesized and secreted from vascular endothelial and smooth muscle cells. Adrenomedullin mediates vasodilatory and natriuretic properties through the second messenger cyclic adenosine monophosphate (cAMP), NO, and the renal prostaglandin system. ADM acts as a local autocrine or paracrine vasoactive hormone and is increased in the plasma in various cardiorenal diseases such as hypertension, chronic renal failure, and congestive heart failure. Overall, ADM appears to play an important role in fluid and electrolyte balance and cardiorenal regulation. Recent studies in rats with myocardial infarction where ADM was administered revealed decreased left ventricle remodeling and heart failure.

ADM plays an important role in vascular protection by decreasing oxidative stress, limiting endothelial injury, causing vasodilation, and promoting angiogenesis.[36,37] Other

---

WHAT'S NEW? The Renin-Angiotensin-Aldosterone System Revisited

Exciting research is uncovering additional roles of the renin-angiotensin-aldosterone system (RAAS) in cardiovascular and systemic conditions:

1. A new type of angiotensin-converting enzyme (ACE_2) has been identified that decreases angiotensin II (Ang II) levels and may offer a whole new way of combating hypertension.
2. The RAAS has profound effects on glucose metabolism, endothelial cell function, and renal disease that has led to new uses for drugs that block angiotensin receptors, especially in individuals with diabetes and kidney disease.
3. Activation of angiotensin 1 receptor (AT_1) promotes systemic inflammation and mediates inflammatory myocyte hypertrophy, fibroblast proliferation, collagen synthesis, smooth muscle cell growth, endothelial adhesion molecule expression, and catecholamine synthesis. Thus there is likely an important role for the RAAS in many diseases including atherosclerosis, heart failure, and shock;
4. A new angiotensin receptor (AT_4) has been described that is concentrated in the brain and may be involved in cerebral processing, cerebroprotection, local blood flow, stress, anxiety, and depression.
5. Vaccines to Ang II and its receptors are being developed that might provide a more targeted and potent blockade of the RAAS.

Data from Lambert DW, Hooper NM, Turner AJ: *Biochem Pharmacol* 75(4):781-786, 2008; Perkins JM, Davis SN: *Curr Opin Endocrinol Diabetes Obes* 15(2):147-152, 2008; Skultetyova D et al: *Recent Patents Cardiovasc Drug Discov* 2(1):23-27, 2007; Widdop RE et al: *Clin Exp Pharmacol Physiol* 35(4):386-390, 2008; Wright JW, Yamamoto BJ, Harding JW: *Prog Neurobiol* 84(2):157-181, 2008; Zhu F, Zhou Z, Liao Y: *Curr Opin Invest Drugs* 9(3):286-2d94, 2008.

WHAT'S NEW? New Insights into the Natriuretic Peptides

Atrial natriuretic peptide (ANP), brain natriuretic peptide (BNP), C natriuretic peptide (CNP), and urodilantin have long been known to play a role in hypertension and heart failure through their ability to reduce blood volume. New and exciting roles for these unique peptides have been described, including effects on cartilage growth, immunity, asthma, myocardial hypertrophy, and vascular endothelial function. Although there is increasing appreciation for the complexity of these molecules and their receptors, much work is needed to better understand their potential in the therapy of many diseases.

Data from Chen H et al: *J Bio Chem* 283(7):4439-4447, 2008; Gardner DG et al: *Hypertension* 49(3):419-426, 2007; Pagel-Langenickel I et al: *J Mol Med* 85(8):797-810, 2007; Pejchalova K et al: *Mol Genet Metab* 92(3):210-215, 2007; Sandow SL, Tare M: *Trends Pharmacol Sci* 28(2):61-67, 2007.

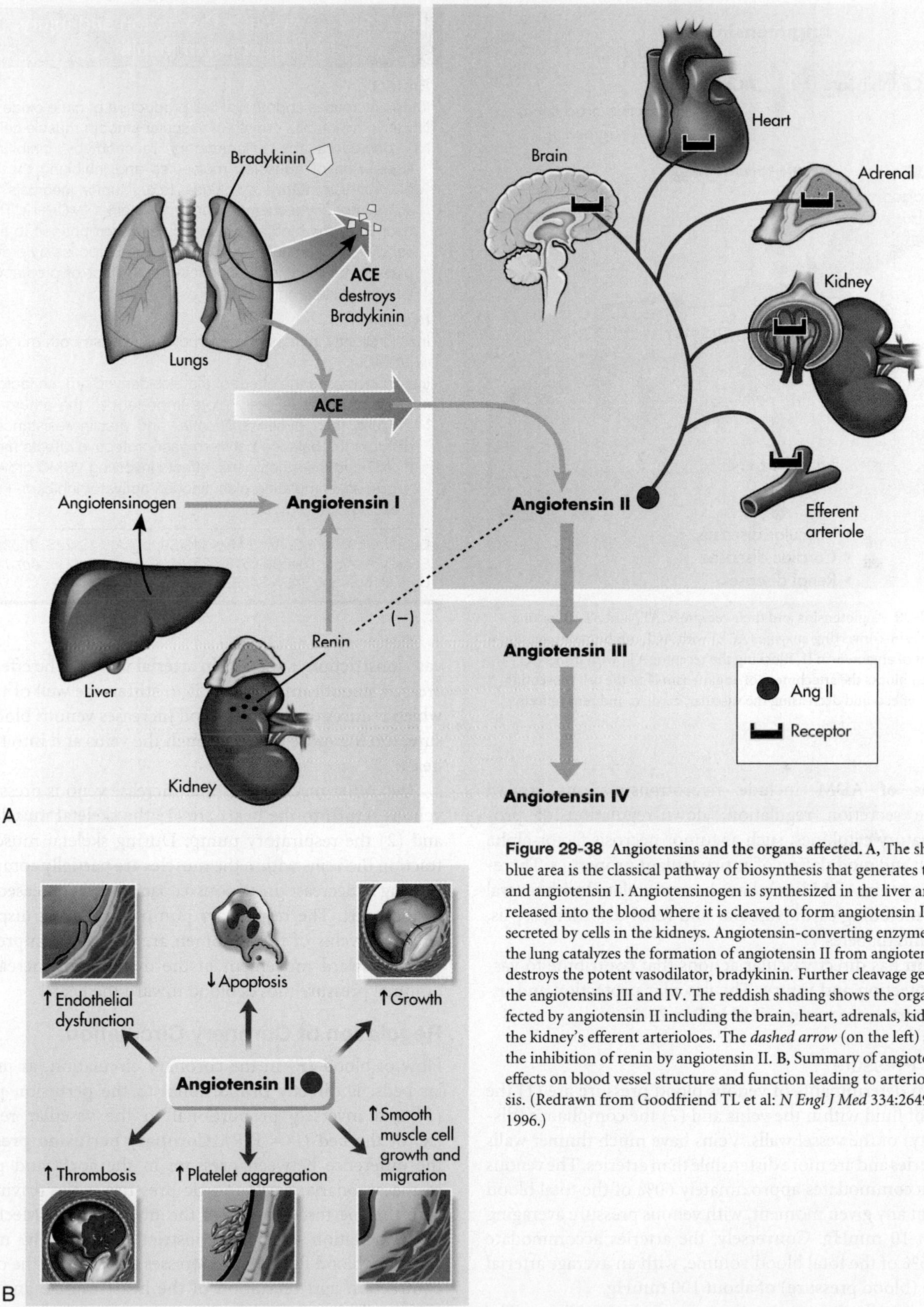

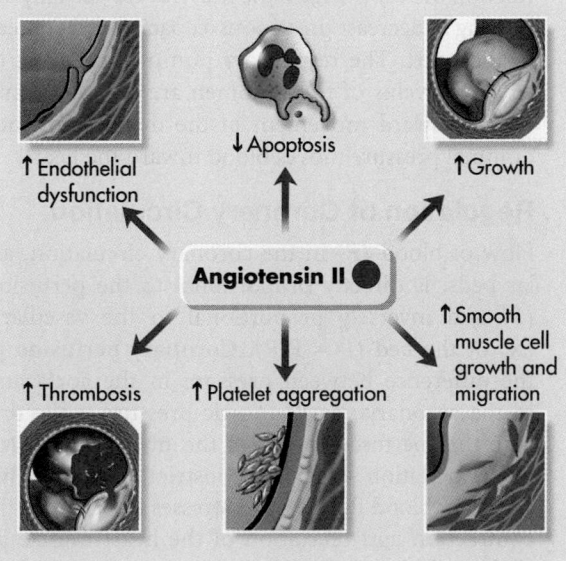

A

Bradykinin

ACE destroys Bradykinin

Lungs

ACE

Angiotensinogen → **Angiotensin I**

Liver

Renin

(−)

Kidney

Brain

Heart

Adrenal

Kidney

Angiotensin II ● ⊔ Efferent arteriole

● Ang II
⊔ Receptor

Angiotensin III

Angiotensin IV

B

↑ Endothelial dysfunction

↓ Apoptosis

↑ Growth

Angiotensin II ●

↑ Thrombosis

↑ Platelet aggregation

↑ Smooth muscle cell growth and migration

Figure 29-38 Angiotensins and the organs affected. **A,** The shaded blue area is the classical pathway of biosynthesis that generates the renin and angiotensin I. Angiotensinogen is synthesized in the liver and is released into the blood where it is cleaved to form angiotensin I by renin secreted by cells in the kidneys. Angiotensin-converting enzyme (ACE) in the lung catalyzes the formation of angiotensin II from angiotensin I, and destroys the potent vasodilator, bradykinin. Further cleavage generates the angiotensins III and IV. The reddish shading shows the organs affected by angiotensin II including the brain, heart, adrenals, kidney, and the kidney's efferent arterioloes. The *dashed arrow* (on the left) shows the inhibition of renin by angiotensin II. **B,** Summary of angiotensin II effects on blood vessel structure and function leading to arteriosclerosis. (Redrawn from Goodfriend TL et al: *N Engl J Med* 334:2649-2654, 1996.)

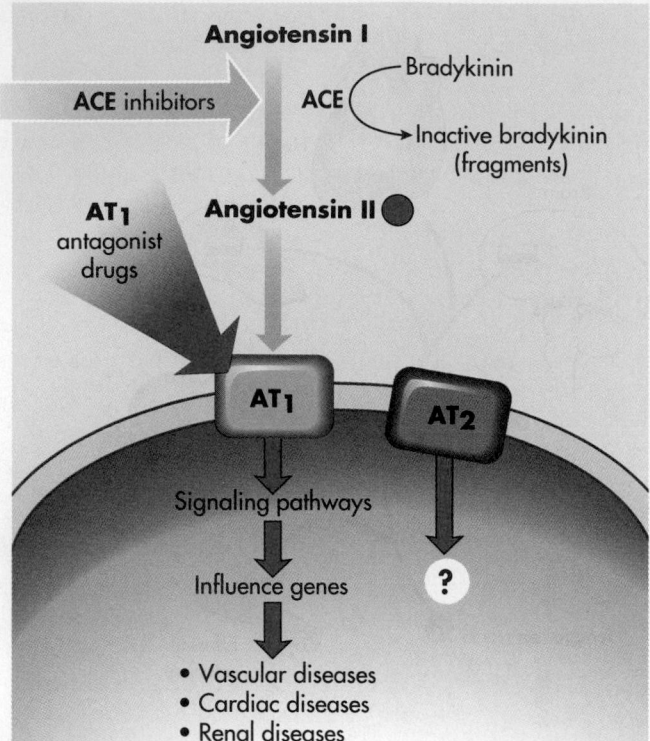

Figure 29-39 Angiotensins and their receptors, AT_1 and AT_2. Blocking the angiotensin-converting enzyme (ACE) with ACE inhibitors decreases the amount of angiotensin II. Blocking the receptor AT_1 with drugs (AT_1 antagonists) blocks the attachment of angiotensin II to the cell preventing the cellular effects and decreasing the vascular, cardiac, and renal effects.

<table>
<tr><td colspan="2">Box 29-2   Vascular Protection and Injury Properties of Insulin</td></tr>
</table>

Protection

Insulin increases endothelial cell production of nitric oxide (NO).

NO (in vitro) inhibits growth of vascular smooth muscle cells.

NO decreases the inflammatory reaction by inhibiting the expression of adhesion molecules and inhibiting the activity of proinflammatory cytokines (e.g., tumor necrosis factor-alpha, monocyte chemoattractant protein-1 [MCP-1]). Thus NO decreases the binding of monocytes/macrophages to the vessel wall. NO also inhibits the thrombotic process by preventing platelet adhesion and enhancing the effect of prostacyclin to inhibit platelet aggregation.

Injury

Insulin slightly increases growth of vascular smooth muscle cells (VSMCs).

Insulin increases the effect of platelet-derived growth factor.

Insulin resistance is likely more important to the atherogenesis process than *hyperinsulinemia,* and insulin resistance likely disrupts the balance between vasoprotective effects mediated by NO and the atherogenic effects involving VSMC growth and migration, stimulating plasminogen activator inhibitor-1 and increasing clot formation.

Data from Sobel BE: *Am J Med* 113(Suppl 6A):12S-22S, 2002; Sorisky A: *Am J Ther* 9(6):516-521, 2002; Tennyson GE: *Am J Manag Care* 8(16 Suppl):S450-S459, 2002.

---

functions of ADM include neurotransmission; growth hormone secretion regulation; down-regulation of proinflammatory cytokines, such as tumor necrosis factor-alpha (TNF-α); and modulation of anticoagulant properties. Therefore, changes in ADM levels have been correlated with several diseases including cardiovascular and renal disorders, sepsis, cancer, and diabetes.

Insulin has direct vascular actions that contribute to vascular protection and injury. The vascular protection and injury properties are summarized in Box 29-2.

Venous Pressure

The main determinants of venous blood pressure are (1) the volume of fluid within the veins and (2) the compliance (distensibility) of the vessel walls. Veins have much thinner walls than arteries and are more distensible than arteries. The venous system accommodates approximately 60% of the total blood volume at any given moment, with venous pressure averaging less than 10 mmHg. Conversely, the arteries accommodate about 15% of the total blood volume, with an average arterial pressure (blood pressure) of about 100 mmHg.

The sympathetic nervous system controls compliance. The walls of the veins are highly innervated by sympathetic fibers that when stimulated cause venous smooth muscle to contract. This increases smooth muscle tone rather than causing

vasoconstriction, as occurs in arterial vessels. The effect of increased smooth muscle tone is to stiffen the wall of the vein, which reduces distensibility and increases venous blood pressure, forcing more blood through the veins and into the right heart.

Two other mechanisms that increase venous pressure and venous return to the heart are (1) the skeletal muscle pump and (2) the respiratory pump. During skeletal muscle contraction the veins within the muscles are partially compressed, causing a decrease in venous capacity and increased return to the heart. The respiratory pump acts during inspiration, when the veins of the abdomen are partially compressed by the downward movement of the diaphragm. Increased abdominal pressure moves blood toward the heart.

Regulation of Coronary Circulation

Flow of blood *(F)* in the coronary circulation, as in vascular beds, is directly proportional to the perfusion pressure *(P)* and inversely proportional to the vascular resistance *(R)* of the bed *($F = P/R$)*. **Coronary perfusion pressure** is the difference between pressure in the aorta and pressure in the coronary vessels. Aortic pressure is the driving pressure that perfuses vessels of the myocardium. Mechanisms of vasodilation and vasoconstriction normally maintain coronary blood flow despite stresses imposed by the constant contraction and relaxation of the heart muscle and despite shifts (within a physiologic range) of coronary perfusion pressure.

Several anatomic factors influence coronary blood flow. Because of their location, the aortic valve cusps obstruct coronary blood flow by pushing against the openings of the coronary arteries during systole. Also during systole, the coronary arteries are compressed by ventricular contraction. These anatomic factors have a **systolic compressive effect,** which is particularly evident in the subendocardial layers of the left ventricular wall and can greatly increase resistance to coronary blood flow.[1] Therefore, most coronary blood flow in the left ventricle occurs during diastole. During the period of systolic compression, when flow is slowed or stopped, oxygen is supplied by **myoglobin,** a protein that is present in heart muscle that binds oxygen during diastole and then releases it when blood levels of oxygen fall during systole.

Autoregulation

Autoregulation (automatic self-regulation) enables individual vessels to regulate blood flow by altering their own arteriolar resistances. Autoregulation in the coronary circulation maintains constant blood flow at perfusion pressures (mean arterial pressure) between 60 and 180 mmHg when other influencing factors are held constant. Thus autoregulation ensures constant coronary blood flow despite shifts in the perfusion pressure within the stated range.

The mechanism of autoregulation is not known, but two explanations have been proposed: the myogenic hypothesis and the metabolic hypothesis. The myogenic hypothesis proposes that autoregulation originates in vascular smooth muscle, presumably of the arterioles, as a response to changes in arterial perfusion pressure. Increased coronary perfusion pressure increases the pressure against the vessel wall and the stretch increases the vessel's radius, resulting in an increase in wall tension. Initially, coronary blood flow increases with the abrupt distention of the blood vessels. The stretching eventually stimulates contraction of the smooth muscles, which increases vascular resistance. The return of more normal flow follows constriction of the arterioles. Because stretch of vascular smooth muscle increases intracellular Ca^{++}, it is proposed that an increase in transmural pressure activates membrane calcium channels.[1] This mechanism also works in the opposite direction; that is, vasodilation is stimulated by decreased arterial pressure.

The metabolic hypothesis of autoregulation, which is better documented, proposes that autoregulation of coronary vessels originates in the myocardium. The stimulus is a drop in coronary perfusion pressure or an increase in the metabolic needs of the myocardium (e.g., because of strenuous exercise). With an increased myocardial oxygen requirement, myocardial cells release substances that promote vasodilation. Substances implicated include CO_2, hydrogen ions (lactic acid), potassium ions, and adenosine. The best known of these substances is adenosine, a potent vasodilator released in response to a decrease in myocardial oxygenation.[1] An increased concentration of adenosine in the interstitial fluid decreases the resistance of the coronary arterioles and increases blood flow. Perfusion strongly correlates with the amount of adenosine released. When coronary perfusion pressure is increased, the increased flow washes out the vasodilatory substances.

As the dilators are washed out, vasoconstriction occurs and returns flow toward normal.

Autonomic Regulation

As described, stimulation of the sympathetic nerves to the heart causes a marked increase in coronary blood flow, even though it also causes vasoconstriction of the coronary vessels. The increased coronary flow is caused by the increase in myocardial metabolism created by the sympathetic stimulation of the heart rate and contractility. The release of vasodilatory metabolites, such as adenosine, from the increased myocardial activity tends to overwhelm the coronary vasoconstriction. Thus metabolic autoregulation overrides neurogenic influences, and the net effect of sympathetic stimulation is to increase coronary blood flow.[1]

LYMPHATIC SYSTEM

The **lymphatic system** is a special vascular system that picks up excess tissue fluid and returns it to the bloodstream. Normally, fluid is forced out of the blood at the arterial end of the capillary bed and is reabsorbed into the bloodstream at the venous end (Figure 29-40), yet capillary outflow exceeds venous reabsorption by about 3 L/day so some fluid lags behind in the interstitium. To maintain sufficient blood volume in the

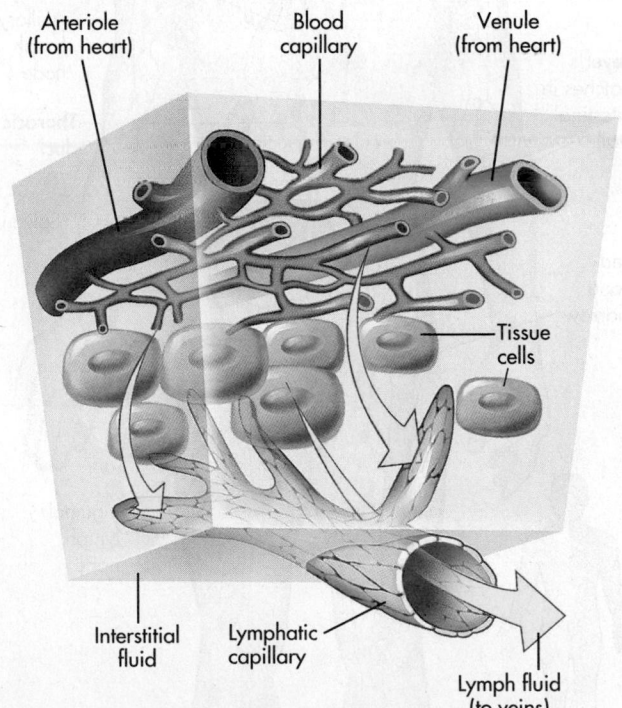

Figure 29-40 Role of the lymphatic system in fluid balance. Fluid from plasma flowing through the capillaries moves into interstitial spaces. Although much of this interstitial fluid is either absorbed by tissue cells or reabsorbed by capillaries, some of the fluid tends to accumulate in the interstitial spaces. As this fluid builds up, it tends to drain into lymphatic vessels that eventually return the fluid to the venous blood. (From Thibodeau GA, Patton KT: *Anatomy & physiology,* ed 5, St Louis, 2003, Mosby.)

cardiovascular system, this fluid must eventually rejoin the bloodstream, which is the function of the lymphatic system.

The lymphatic system consists of lymphatic vessels and the lymph nodes (Figure 29-41). (Lymph nodes and lymphoid tissues are described in Chapters 7 and 25.) In this pumpless system a series of valves ensures one-way flow of the excess interstitial fluid (then called *lymph*) toward the heart. The lymphatic capillaries are closed at the ends (Figure 29-42).

Lymph consists primarily of water and small amounts of dissolved proteins, mostly albumin, which are too large to be reabsorbed into the less permeable blood capillaries. Once within the lymphatic system, lymph travels successively through larger and larger vessels called **lymphatic venules** and **lymphatic veins.** The lymphatic vessels run in the same sheaths with the arteries and veins and eventually drain into one of two large ducts in the thorax—the right lymphatic duct and the thoracic duct. The **right lymphatic duct** drains lymph from the right arm and the right side of the head and thorax, whereas the larger thoracic duct receives lymph from the rest of the body (see Figure 29-41). The right lymphatic duct and the **thoracic duct** drain lymph into the right and left subclavian veins, respectively.

The lymphatic veins are thin walled, like the veins of the cardiovascular system. In the larger lymphatic veins, endothelial flaps form valves similar to those in the circulatory veins (see Figure 29-26). The valves permit lymph to flow in only one direction because lymphatic vessels are compressed intermittently by contraction of skeletal muscles, pulsatile expansion of an artery in the same sheath, and contraction of the smooth muscles in the walls of the lymphatic vessel.

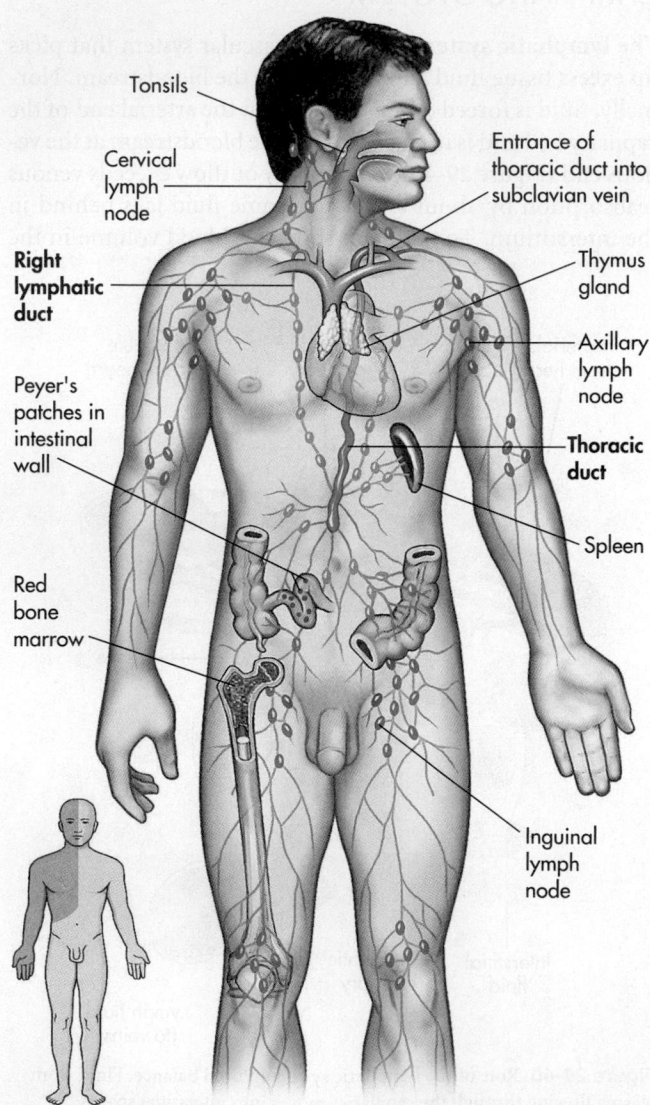

Figure 29-41 **Principal organs of the lymphatic system.** The inset shows the areas drained by the right lymphatic duct (green) and the thoracic duct (blue). (From Thibodeau GA, Patton KT: *Anatomy & physiology,* ed 5, St. Louis, 2003, Mosby.)

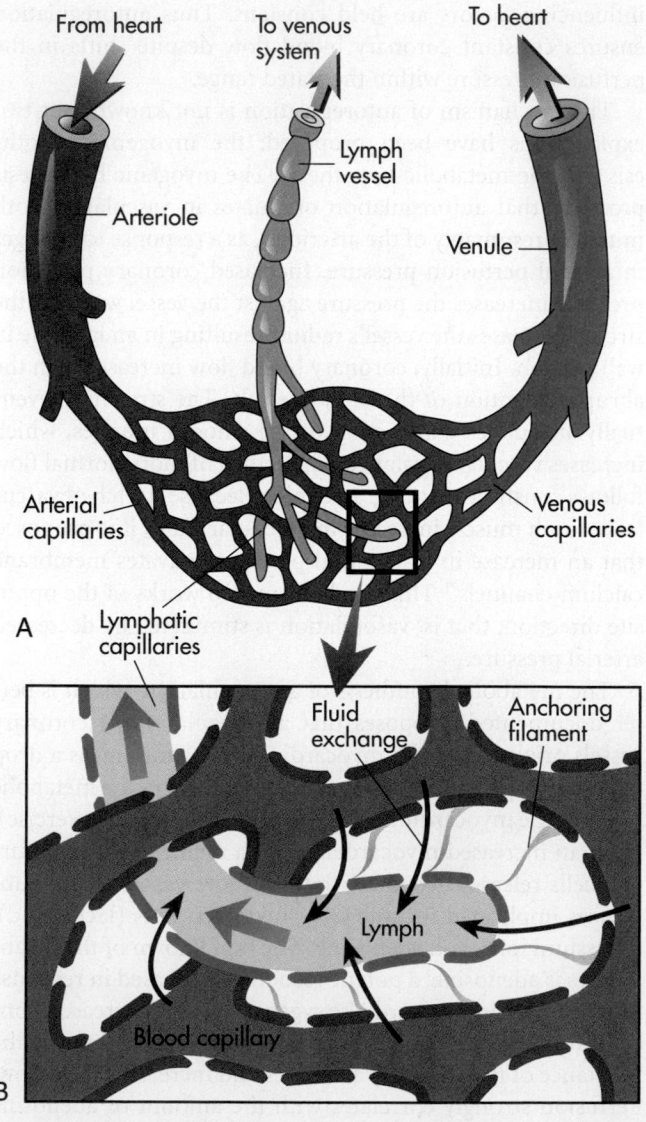

Figure 29-42 **Lymphatic capillaries. A,** Schematic representation of lymphatic capillaries. **B,** Anatomic components of microcirculation.

As lymph is transported toward the heart, it is filtered through thousands of bean-shaped lymph nodes clustered along the lymphatic vessels (see Figure 29-41). Lymph enters the node through several **afferent lymphatic vessels,** filters through the sinuses in the node, and leaves by way of **efferent lymphatic vessels.** Lymph flows slowly through the node, which facilitates the phagocytosis of foreign substances within the node and prevents them from reentering the bloodstream. (Phagocytosis is described in Chapter 6.)

TESTS OF CARDIOVASCULAR FUNCTION

The general approach to the individual with suspected cardiovascular disorders begins with a thorough history for risk factors and symptoms. This is followed by a careful physical examination looking for evidence of tissue ischemia, pulmonary congestion, and cardiac dysfunction. Nonspecific and specific serum laboratories are usually obtained. For many individuals, these basic steps will be complemented by the use of sophisticated methods to measure heart and vascular function. Cardiac function can be evaluated using indicators calculated from pressures and flow rates in the heart and vessels.

Table 29-4 defines the indicators most often used in the clinical setting.

Cardiac and Coronary Artery Evaluation

Many sophisticated tests can be obtained to evaluate individuals for cardiac or coronary artery disease, and new ones are being tested each year. Some of the more commonly used modalities include electrocardiography, chest x-ray, stress testing, echocardiography, computed tomography (CT) and magnetic resonance imaging (MRI), technetium scanning, electrophysiology, and catheterization with angiography.

Cardiography

Electrocardiography, typically the 12-lead electrocardiogram (ECG), gives information about heart rate and rhythm, the effects of electrolytes or drugs on the heart, and the electrical orientation of the cardiac muscle. An ECG gives no direct information about the contractile state or mechanical performance of the heart.

Serial 12-lead ECGs are of primary importance in establishing the presence of myocardial ischemia and infarction or conduction defects and dysrhythmias. This examination has become part of the routine hospital admission assessment,

Table 29-4	Indicators of Cardiac Function	
Indicator	**Definition***	**Common Cause of Abnormality**
Heart rate (HR)	Number of heartbeats (cardiac cycles) per min Normal adult value: 70 beats/min	Ischemia, electrolyte disturbances, drug toxicity
Cardiac output (CO)	Amount of blood (in liters) moved by the heart in 1 min Normal range: 4-8 L/min	Decrease indicates heart failure Increase indicates decreased systemic vascular resistance, common in sepsis
Cardiac index (CI)	Relationship between cardiac output and body surface area (BSA, in square meters) Normal range: 2.8-4.2 L/min/m²	Decrease indicates heart failure Increase indicates decreased systemic vascular resistance, common in sepsis
Stroke volume (SV)	Amount of blood (in milliliters) ejected by the left ventricle during systole (i.e., per beat) Normal range: 60-100 ml/beat	Decrease indicates heart failure Increase indicates deceased systemic vascular resistance, common in sepsis
Stroke volume index (SVI)	Relationship between stroke volume and body surface area Normal range: 33-47 ml/beat/m²	Decrease indicates heart failure Increase indicates deceased systemic vascular resistance, common in sepsis
Oxygen consumption index (V·O₂)	Amount of oxygen (in milliliters) consumed per minute in relation to BSA	Decrease: sedation, anesthesia, hypothermia Increase: elevated temperature, sepsis, seizures
Stroke work index (SWI)	Amount of work (expressed as done) by the left or right ventricle per systole per square meter of BSA Normal value: 35 g/m²	Decreases within specific ranges indicate cardiogenic or hypovolemic shock (see Chapter 46) Increase: elevated systemic vascular resistance
Systemic mean arterial pressure (MAP)	Mean blood pressure (in millimeters of mercury) in the systemic arteries Normal range: 70-100 mmHg	Elevated: epinephrine release, diseases of arteries, primary hypertension Decreased: cardiac failure, decreased vascular resistance of sepsis
Pulmonary vascular resistance (PVR)	Relationship among cardiac output, preload, and afterload, expressed as units of force of resistance per second per centimeter of water Normal value: less than 250 dynes/sec/cm⁻⁵	Increased: acute respiratory distress syndrome (ARDS), pneumonia, primary pulmonary hypertension, congestive heart failure Decreased: late shock
Systemic vascular resistance (SVR)	Same definition as for PVR Normal range: 770-1500 dynes/sec/cm⁻⁵	Increased: epinephrine release Decreased: inflammatory response

*Values given are for adults at rest.

even when the admitting diagnosis is not cardiac in nature, because it establishes baseline information about the electrical function of the heart. Also recent ECGs can be compared with ECGs obtained from the same individual in the past. Changes in the ECG over time assist in determining the cause, amount, or nature of changes in cardiac anatomy and physiology.

Chest Radiograph Examination

Chest x-rays allow for the examination of the size and contour of the heart and related structures. Evidence of chamber enlargement, pericardial disease, pulmonary edema, valvular calcification, and pathology of the great vessels may be visualized. Chest x-ray is also useful to look for appropriate placement of invasive cardiac devices and for any complications thereof (e.g., pneumothorax or hemothorax; see Chapter 33). A chest x-ray examination is a routine part of a cardiac examination. The most commonly obtained views are posteroanterior (PA) and lateral, with the individual standing upright and the lungs fully expanded. In those individuals confined to bed, an anteroposterior (AP) view may be obtained but is usually of lesser quality than the PA.

Stress Testing

Cardiac activity during exercise is examined during a stress test. Stress testing elicits signs and symptoms of heart disease and coronary artery disease that may not appear at rest. Continuous 12-lead ECG and blood pressure measurement are obtained before, during, and after the study. Cardiac stress from exercise is induced by having the individual walk on a treadmill. Other, less frequently used forms of exercise include static exercise (hand ergometry or chemical stress), stair climbing (the Stairmaster's double two-step), arm ergometry, and bicycle ergometry. The individual exercises until the maximal heart rate for gender and age is reached or until other subjective or objective indicators of cardiac dysfunction or distress appear. Subjective indicators include chest pain, extreme fatigue, extreme dyspnea, leg pain, or the individual's request to stop the test. Objective criteria are ST segment elevation or depression, SA node or atrial dysrhythmias, AV node dysrhythmias, ventricular dysrhythmias, elevated or decreased blood pressure, signs of cerebral hypoxia, and signs of circulatory insufficiency.

A stress test is useful also in determining the rate or progress of recovery from a myocardial infarction or cardiac surgery. Graded exercise in individuals with low- to moderate-risk chest pain evaluated in an emergency department can be used as a prognostic indicator of adverse cardiac events. When a differential diagnosis for chest pain has been difficult to determine, stress testing may help distinguish coronary artery insufficiency from other causes of pain. There is some risk associated with stress testing. The risk is greater when the test is performed soon after an acute ischemic event.

Stress testing with ECG monitoring may not be sensitive enough to detect and localize areas of the myocardium at risk for ischemia and infarction. Currently, most stress testing includes the injection of a radiotracer that is taken up by active heart cells. When the heart is scanned, during and after stress testing, areas where the radiotracer is not taken up by ischemic cells can be seen and therefore localizes areas of myocardial damage and risk.

Single-Photon Emission Computed Tomography

Single-photon emission computed tomography (SPECT) is the most commonly used tool for evaluating individuals for coronary artery disease and myocardial ischemia during stress testing. A radiotracer (usually thalium-201) is injected intravenously and is taken up by healthy myocytes and retained for some period of time.[38] Photons are emitted from the myocardium in proportion to perfusion of the tissue. A gamma camera visualizes the photons, and views are taken from 360 degrees by CT, which digitizes the information and provides a three-dimensional view. Data about where the myocardium take up the tracer normally, slowly, or not at all can be correlated with existing myocardial disease and can help quantify ischemic risk.

Echocardiography

Echocardiography is the most effective noninvasive modality for evaluating the structures of the heart. Ultrasound beams reflected by cardiovascular structures produce shapes that can be visualized and allow for recognition of altered cardiac anatomy.[38] It is used to evaluate for suspected heart failure, valvular disease, infective endocarditis, cardiomyopathies, pericardial disease, and congenital heart disease. Through the use of two-dimensional techniques with Doppler and color flow imaging, accurate assessments of cardiac output, ejection fraction, and valvular function can be obtained.

Computed Tomography and Magnetic Resonance Imaging

Initially, CT and MRI had limited roles in the evaluation of heart disease because they required structures to be still in order to provide clear images. New techniques, including ECG gating (timing of gathering the data to the cardiac cycle), have greatly expanded the use of these two modalities[38] that can evaluate cardiac anatomy and physiology. Improvements such as electron beam CT and spiral CT have improved the ability of tomography to visualize cardiac structures. The high resolution of CT can provide information about calcification of coronary vessels and cardiac valves. It is also an essential tool for evaluating large-vessel disease.

MRI is based on the principle that the frequency of energy (resonant frequency) given up by a nucleus is exactly proportional to the surrounding magnetic field[38] (see Chapter 14). Anatomy and physiology of the great blood vessels and myocardium are depicted in three dimensions with excellent resolution. Ventricular function can be evaluated using indices of ventricular function, such as ejection fraction. Rapidly moving sequences (MRI) can determine regional wall motion and myocardial deformation. Flow direction and velocity also can be quantitatively determined.

Technetium Scanning

Technetium pyrophosphate (^{99m}TcPYP) is injected intravenously into a resting individual during a "hot spot" imaging examination. Two hours after injection the distribution pattern of the radioactive solution is recorded by nuclear scan. During the 2-hour delay, the injected material will have been taken up by infarcted areas of the myocardium, particularly 1 to 3 days after the onset of symptoms. This study is not definitive during the first 12 hours after an infarct.

Technetium scanning is used when (1) there is a conflicting history for myocardial infarction, (2) there are equivocal ECG abnormalities, or (3) an individual's cardiac enzymes have been elevated because of surgery or trauma. Such small amounts of the injected material are used in this examination that the risks associated with radioactive substances are not an issue.

Electrophysiology Studies

In-depth evaluation of electrical conduction within the heart can provide important information about the nature and causes of dysrhythmias, such as atrial and ventricular tachycardias and heart block. There are many types of electrophysiology studies that are specific to certain conduction disorders but they have the common goal of documenting abnormal conduction pathways. Furthermore, the techniques used may also allow for ablation of unwanted pathways or the appropriate placement of stimulating devices (pacers).

One example of an electrophysiology study is AV bundle electrocardiography. Two electrode-tipped catheters are inserted percutaneously into the femoral vein, floated up the inferior vena cava, and positioned in or near the right atrium during AV bundle (His bundle) electrocardiography. AV bundle electrocardiography can detect secondary sites of impulse generation (ectopic foci), as well as accessory pathways of conduction. Other conduction defects and the effects of drugs on conduction also can be illuminated. Risks related to this procedure can be grave and include dysrhythmias, death, vessel or heart perforation, clot or plaque embolization, and kidney failure.

Cardiac Catheterization and Angiography

One or both sides of the heart can be examined using **cardiac catheterization.** This procedure requires the use of fluoroscopy and strict sterile techniques and takes place in a specially equipped catheterization laboratory. Local anesthesia is given, and a catheter is introduced percutaneously into the vasculature and passed caudally into the atrium and ventricle. For a right-heart catheterization, the catheter is placed in the jugular, subclavian, brachial, or femoral vein. The femoral artery is commonly used for a left-heart study. Once the catheter has been guided into the atrium, pressures are recorded, blood samples are obtained to examine oxygen content, and

a contrast medium is injected to visualize chamber function and valve patency. The catheter is then passed into the ventricles and the sequence is repeated.

Cardiac catheterization provides a means to visualize the chambers of the heart continuously, although for a short time. A great deal of information can be obtained about heart structure and function. Pressures in each chamber and across heart valves can be precisely measured, along with timing of events in the cardiac cycle. Of particular value is the ability to compare the oxygen content of blood in each heart chamber. Risks for this procedure have decreased over time. One of the most serious complications of cardiac catheterization is the development of dysrhythmias. Death usually is caused by cardiac arrest after ventricular fibrillation.

Fluoroscopic visualization of the coronary arteries and left-heart structures using contrast dye is called **coronary angiography** or arteriography. Like cardiac catheterization, this study takes place in a catheterization laboratory using local anesthesia and a sterile field. A catheter is threaded into the left ventricle through the femoral artery. A ventriculogram generally is performed first. Contrast dye is injected into the apex of the ventricle, and the next few cardiac cycles are visualized and filmed. Like cardiac catheterization, coronary angiography is used to gain information about the structure and function of the ventricles and related valves. After the ventriculogram, catheters are introduced individually into the ostia of the coronary arteries. When the catheter is in position, 5 to 10 ml of contrast dye is mechanically and rapidly injected into the artery and the results are visualized and filmed. Dye injection is repeated with the individual tilted at various angles to afford views of the artery other than the anteroposterior view. The catheter is then either moved to the next artery to be studied or withdrawn to conclude the study.

The risks of this procedure are similar to those of cardiac catheterization, with exceptions. Because the blood supply to the cardiac muscle is briefly interrupted when dye is introduced into the coronary arteries, angina (chest pain) caused by ischemia (lack of oxygen) is much more common. Coronary artery spasms also can occur. Interrupted flow also causes decreased heart rate (bradycardia), as well as some tachydysrhythmias, hypotension, and ST segment depression.

Systemic Vascular Evaluation

The systemic vascular system can be studied by a variety of techniques in order to evaluate for adequate flow rates, vascular obstruction, and structural defects. These techniques include pulse tracing, Doppler ultrasonography, CT and MRI, venography, and arteriography.

Pulse Tracing

Pulsation, described by the flow of blood through an artery during the cardiac cycle, can be drawn as a waveform plotting pressure against time (Figure 29-43). The waveform can be obtained noninvasively by placing a transducer on the skin over the carotid artery while the individual's head is turned slightly away from the transducer. The amplitude and shape

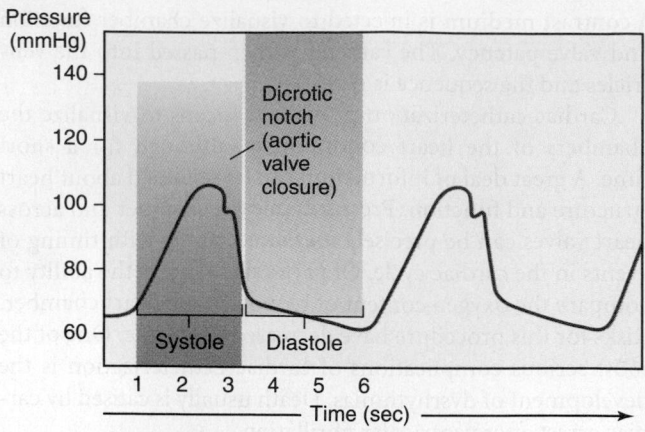

Figure 29-43 Arterial pulse waveforms.

of arterial waveforms can provide information about arterial stiffening and adequacy of perfusion.

Doppler Ultrasonography Studies

A Doppler study is made by using a handheld microphone placed on the skin over a lubricating gel. The microphone amplifies and can record sounds made by blood flowing in peripheral vessels. The Doppler microphone is placed over the vessel to be studied, and sounds related to obstructions to flow, vessel wall mobility, and heart murmurs are transmitted through the gel to the microphone. The microphone amplifies sound waves so that they are audible to the human ear. Ultrasound techniques can be used to digitize the audio findings into visual findings that can be analyzed for flow velocity and volume. These studies are useful in the evaluation for abnormalities of venous flow (e.g., deep venous thrombosis) and arterial flow (e.g., embolism).

Computed Tomography and Magnetic Resonance Imaging

CT and MRI, used to evaluate the systemic circulation, provide information about the structure of the great vessels. Either can be used to evaluate for aneurysms and dissections of the thoracic or abdominal aorta. CT also can be used to assess for vessel calcification and provide some insights into the risk for stroke and myocardial infarction through evaluation of the carotid and coronary vessels.

Venography and Arteriography

Radiopaque dye can be injected through intravenous or intra-arterial catheters to allow for visualization of the internal structure, diameter, and patency of veins and arteries. Venography is performed primarily in the lower extremity to assess for the presence of thrombi in the large veins of the leg. Arteriography (angiography) can be used in almost any vascular system, including the great vessels, pulmonary, coronary (see previously in this chapter), cerebral, mesenteric, renal, hepatic, and peripheral arteries. Risks include rupture, dissection,

thrombosis, embolization, or organ infarction involving the arterial system being studied.

Aging and the Cardiovascular System

Cardiovascular disease is the most common cause of hospitalization and death in older adults in Western society. The most common cardiovascular pathologic condition is hypertension followed by coronary atherosclerosis. It is difficult to describe normal physiologic changes in cardiac function with aging because many pathologic changes are usually present as well. Studies of the effect of age on cardiovascular function must be rigorous in their distinction between persons who are free of disease and those who have disease that may be evident only during stress testing. A consistent finding is the large variation in the older population for nearly every cardiovascular variable. These variations are in part the result of a sharp increase in the prevalence of hypertension and coronary disease with advancing age and in part the result of major age-associated changes in lifestyle (e.g., fitness status). The most relevant age-associated changes in cardiovascular performance are myocardial and blood vessel stiffening, changes in neurogenic control over vascular tone, and left ventricular hypertrophy and fibrosis.[39,40] These changes pose considerable consequences with increased demand for flow, changes in posture, or with disease.

Arterial stiffening occurs with aging even in the absence of clinical hypertension. It can, however, be an important contributor to systolic hypertension and its associated risks for cardiovascular events, dementia, and death. These changes result from alterations within the vascular media, including age-associated changes in cross-linking of collagen, an increase in the amount of collagen, and changes in the nature of elastin, and extracellular matrix, inflammatory molecules, endothelial cell function, and reactive oxygen species.[39] Other influences include glucose regulation, chronic renal disease, salt, and changes in neurohormonal (e.g., renin-angiotensin-aldosterone) regulation.[39] The increased arterial stiffness may not be related strictly to an age-associated change in vascular structure but may be caused by changes in baroreceptor activity. Baroreceptor activity may decrease with age, slowing physiologic adjustment to changes in blood pressure, and posture. The autonomic nervous system also is affected by the aging process, including changes in catecholamine receptor sensitivity.

Left ventricular hypertrophy and fibrosis also are more common in the aging population, even when controlled for hypertension. In the aging heart, disruption of growth factor function and an imbalance in collagen synthesis and degradation result in cardiac dysfunction and increased risk for heart failure.[40]

Stress testing is used to uncover changes in functional capacity that are not apparent at rest. In contrast to the subtle age effects on resting cardiac tests, more dramatic changes occur during exercise. Table 29-5 summarizes age-associated changes at rest and during exercise. Overall, long-term exercise conditioning in older individuals increases aerobic capacity and decreases arterial stiffness and left ventricular function. Cardiovascular diseases often can be prevented in older adults. A recent article indicates that although age plays a role in cardiovascular disease, much of the high prevalence of heart disease in older individuals is because of their lifelong exposure to traditional risk factors such as hypertension, diabetes, and dyslipidemia.[41] Although the risks and benefits of pharmacologic and invasive strategies must always be assessed carefully, many older adults can live longer and healthier lives if appropriate preventive and treatment regimens are offered, even quite late in life.

Table 29-5 Cardiovascular Function in Older Adults

Determinant	Resting Cardiac Performance	Exercise Cardiac Performance
Cardiac output	Unchanged or slightly decreased in women only	Declines because of a decrease in heart rate and stroke volume
Heart rate	Slight decrease	Increases less than in younger people, possibly because of decreased cardiovascular response to catecholamines; overall slight decrease
Stroke volume	Slight increase	Slight increase
Ejection fraction	Unchanged	Increases more from rest to exercise in younger people than in older people
Afterload	Increased	Uncertain
End-diastolic volume	Unchanged	Smaller for women
End-systolic volume	Unchanged	Lesser increase
Contraction	Increased because of prolonged relaxation	Decreases with vigorous exercise*
Cardiac dilation	No change	Increases at end-diastole and end-systole
$\dot{V}O_2$ max	Not applicable	Declines because of a decline in skeletal muscle mass

Data from Gerstenblith G, Lakatta EG: Aging and the cardiovascular system. In Willerson JT, Cohn JN, editors: *Cardiovascular medicine*, New York, 1995, Churchill Livingstone.

*As measured by end-systolic volume/systolic blood pressure (ESV/SBP), an index of contractility.

SUMMARY REVIEW

Circulatory System

1. The circulatory system is the body's transport system. It delivers oxygen, nutrients, metabolites, hormones, neurochemicals, proteins, and blood cells throughout the body and carries metabolic wastes to the kidneys and lungs for excretion.
2. The circulatory system consists of the heart and blood vessels and is made up of two separate, serially connected systems: the pulmonary circulation and the systemic circulation.
3. The pulmonary circulation is driven by the right side of the heart. The function of the pulmonary circulation is to deliver blood to the lungs for oxygenation.
4. The systemic circulation is driven by the left side of the heart, and its function is to move oxygenated blood throughout the body.
5. The lymphatic vessels collect fluids from the interstitium and return the fluids to the circulatory system.

The Heart

1. The heart consists of four chambers (two atria and two ventricles), four valves (two AV valves and two semilunar valves), a muscular wall, a fibrous skeleton, a conduction system, nerve fibers, systemic vessels (the coronary circulation), and openings where the great vessels enter the atria and ventricles.
2. The heart wall, which encloses the heart and divides it into chambers, is made up of three layers: the pericardium (outer layer), the myocardium (muscular layer), and the endocardium (inner lining).
3. The myocardial layer of the two atria, which receive blood entering the heart, is thinner than the myocardial layer of the ventricles, which must be stronger to squeeze blood out of the heart.
4. The right and left sides of the heart are separated by portions of the heart wall called the *interatrial septum* and the *interventricular septum*.
5. Unoxygenated (venous) blood from the systemic circulation enters the right atrium through the superior and inferior venae cavae. From the atrium the blood passes through the right AV (tricuspid) valve into the right ventricle. In the ventricle the blood flows from the inflow tract to the outflow tract and then through the pulmonic semilunar valve (pulmonary valve) into the pulmonary artery, which delivers it to the lungs for oxygenation.
6. Oxygenated blood from the lungs enters the left atrium through the four pulmonary veins (two from the left lung and two from the right lung). From the left atrium the blood passes through the left AV valve (mitral valve) into the left ventricle. In the ventricle the blood flows from the inflow tract to the outflow tract and then through the aortic semilunar valve (aortic valve) into the aorta, which delivers it to systemic arteries of the entire body.
7. The heart valves ensure the one-way flow of blood from atrium to ventricle and from ventricle to artery.
8. Oxygenated blood enters the coronary arteries through an opening in the aorta, and unoxygenated blood from the coronary veins enters the right atrium through the coronary sinus.
9. The pumping action of the heart consists of two phases: diastole, during which the myocardium relaxes and the chambers fill with blood; and systole, during which the myocardium contracts, forcing blood out of the ventricles. A cardiac cycle consists of one systolic contraction and the diastolic relaxation that follows it. Each cardiac cycle makes up one heartbeat.

Continued

10. The conduction system of the heart generates and transmits electrical impulses (cardiac action potentials) that stimulate systolic contractions. The autonomic nerves (sympathetic and parasympathetic fibers) can adjust heart rate and systolic force, but they do not stimulate the heart to beat.

11. The normal ECG is the sum of all action potentials. The P wave represents atrial depolarization; the QRS complex is the sum of all ventricular cell depolarizations. The ST interval occurs when the entire ventricular myocardium is depolarized.

12. Cardiac action potentials are generated by the SA node at the rate of about 75 impulses per minute. The impulses can travel through the conduction system of the heart, stimulating myocardial contraction as they go.

13. Cells of the cardiac conduction system possess the properties of automaticity and rhythmicity. Automatic cells return to threshold and depolarize rhythmically without outside stimulus. The cells of the SA node depolarize faster than other automatic cells, making it the natural pacemaker of the heart. If the SA node is disabled, the next fastest pacemaker, the AV node, takes over.

14. Each cardiac action potential travels from the SA node to the AV node to the bundle of His (AV bundle), through the bundle branches, and finally to the Purkinje fibers. There the impulse is stopped. It is prevented from reversing its path by the refractory period of cells that have just been polarized. The refractory period ensures that diastole (relaxation) will occur, thereby completing the cardiac cycle.

15. Adrenergic receptor number, type, and function govern autonomic (sympathetic) regulation of heart rate, contractile force, and dilation or constriction of coronary arteries. The presence of specific receptors (α_1, α_2, β_1, β_2) in the myocardium and coronary vessels determines the effects of the neurotransmitters norepinephrine and epinephrine.

16. Unique features that distinguish myocardial cells from skeletal cells enable myocardial cells to transmit action potentials faster (through intercalated disks), synthesize more ATP (because of a large number of mitochondria), and have readier access to ions in the interstitium (because of an abundance of transverse tubules). These combined differences enable the myocardium to work constantly, which skeletal muscle is not required to do.

17. Cross-bridges between actin and myosin enable contraction to occur. Calcium and its interaction with the troponin complex facilitate the contraction process. With troponin release of calcium, myocardial relaxation begins.

18. Cardiac performance is affected by preload, afterload, heart rate, and myocardial contractility.

19. Preload, or pressure generated in the ventricles at the end of diastole, depends on the amount of blood in the ventricle. Afterload is the resistance to ejection of the blood from the ventricle. Afterload depends on pressure in the aorta.

20. Heart rate is determined by the SA node and by components of the autonomic nervous system, including cardiovascular control centers in the brain, neuroreceptors in the atria and aorta, hormones, and catecholamines (epinephrine and norepinephrine).

21. Contractility is the potential for myocardial fiber shortening during systole. It is determined by the amount of stretch during diastole (i.e., preload) and by sympathetic stimulation of the ventricles.

22. The Frank-Starling law of the heart states that the myocardial stretch determines the force of myocardial contraction (the greater the stretch, the stronger the contraction).

23. Laplace's law states that the amount of contractile force generated within a chamber depends on the radius of the chamber and the thickness of its wall (the smaller the radius and the thicker the wall, the greater the force of contraction).

Systemic Circulation

1. Blood flows from the left ventricle into the aorta and from the aorta into arteries that eventually branch into arterioles and capillaries, the smallest of the arterial vessels. Oxygen, nutrients, and other substances needed for cellular metabolism pass from the capillaries into the interstitium, where they are available for uptake by the cells. Capillaries also absorb products of cellular metabolism from the interstitium.

2. Venules, the smallest veins, receive capillary blood. From the venules the venous blood flows into larger and larger veins until it reaches the venae cavae, through which it enters the right atrium.

3. Vessel walls consist of three layers: the tunica intima (inner layer), the tunica media (middle layer), and the tunica externa (outer layer).

4. Layers of the vessel wall differ in thickness and composition from vessel to vessel, depending on the vessel's size and location within the circulatory system. In general, the tunica media of arteries close to the heart contains a greater proportion of elastic fibers because these arteries must be able to distend during systole and recoil during diastole. Distributing arteries farther from the heart contain a greater proportion of smooth muscle fibers because these arteries must be able to constrict and dilate to control blood pressure and volume within specific capillary beds.

5. Blood flow into the capillary beds is controlled by the contraction and relaxation of smooth muscle bands (precapillary sphincters) at junctions between metarterioles and capillaries. The endothelium is probably a source of prostaglandins that control vasomotion.

6. Blood flow through the veins is assisted by the contraction of skeletal muscles (the muscle pump), and backflow in the lower body is prevented by one-way valves, particularly in the deep veins of the legs.

7. Blood flow is affected by blood pressure; resistance to flow within the vessels; blood consistency (which affects velocity); anatomic features that may cause turbulent or laminar flow; and compliance (distensibility) of the vessels.

8. Poiseuille's law describes the relationship of blood flow, pressure, and resistance as the difference between pressure at the inflow end of the vessel and pressure at the outflow end divided by resistance within the vessel.

9. According to Poiseuille's formula, resistance depends on the vessel's length and radius and on the viscosity of the blood. The greater the vessel's length and the blood's viscosity and the narrower the radius of the vessel's lumen, the greater the resistance within the vessel.

10. Total peripheral resistance, or the resistance to flow within the entire systemic circulatory system, depends on the combined lengths and radii of all the vessels within the system and on whether the vessels are arranged in series (greater resistance) or in parallel (lesser resistance).

11. Poiseuille's law and Poiseuille's formula are based on physical laws governing the behavior of fluids in a straight tube. In the body, blood flow is influenced also by neural stimulation (of vasoconstriction or vasodilation) and by anatomic features that cause turbulence within the vascular lumen (e.g., protrusions from the vessel wall, twists and turns, bifurcations).

12. Arterial blood pressure is influenced and regulated by factors that affect cardiac output (heart rate and stroke volume), total resistance within the system, and blood volume.

13. Many hormones alter vasomotion including epinephrine, norepinephrine, antidiuretic hormone, renin-angiotensin system, natriuretic peptides adrenomedullin and insulin.

14. Ang II has two subtypes of receptors, AT_1 and AT_2. The majority of Ang II actions are thought to be mediated by AT_1 receptor.

15. Venous blood pressure is influenced by blood volume within the venous system and compliance of the venous walls.

16. Blood flow through the coronary circulation is governed not only by the same principles as flow through other vascular beds but also by adaptations dictated by cardiac dynamics. First, blood flows into the coronary arteries during diastole rather than systole because during systole, the cusps of the aortic semilunar valve block the openings of the coronary arteries. Second, systolic contraction inhibits coronary artery flow by compressing the coronary arteries.

17. Autoregulation enables the coronary vessels to maintain optimal perfusion pressure despite systolic effects, and myoglobin in heart muscle stores oxygen for use during the systolic phase of the cardiac cycle.

Lymphatic System

1. The vessels of the lymphatic system run in the same sheaths in which the arteries and veins run.

2. Lymph (interstitial fluid) is absorbed by lymphatic venules in the capillary beds and travels through ever larger lymphatic veins until it is emptied through the right or left thoracic duct into the right or left subclavian vein.

3. As lymph travels toward the thoracic ducts, it is filtered by thousands of lymph nodes clustered around the lymphatic veins. The lymph nodes are sites of immune function.

Tests of Cardiovascular Function

1. The evaluation of an individual with known or suspected cardiovascular disease must include a careful history and physical examination including assessment of risk factors, symptoms, vital signs, level of consciousness, mucous membrane color, and cardiopulmonary functioning.

2. Important tests for cardiac disorders are ECG and Holter monitoring, which detect disturbances of impulse generation or conduction.

3. Stress tests elicit clinical manifestations of cardiovascular disease that might not be present at rest.

4. The sensitivity of stress testing is improved by the use of radiotracer imaging techniques such as SPECT.

5. Echocardiography detects structural and functional cardiac abnormalities over time.

6. Cardiac catheterization is used to measure the oxygen content and pressure of blood in the heart's chambers and to inject contrast media for x-ray examination of the size and shape of the chambers and valves. Injection of contrast medium into the coronary arteries (coronary angiography), on the other hand, permits visualization of the coronary circulation and every tissue perfused by the coronary arteries.

7. Evaluation of the systemic vascular system can include pulse tracings, Doppler ultrasonography, venography, and arteriography.

Aging and the Cardiovascular System

1. Much controversy exists regarding the effects of normal aging on the cardiovascular system. Separating the physiologic from the pathologic alterations is difficult because of the presence of arteriosclerosis in a majority of older adults.

2. Studies have documented no change in cardiac output, a slight decrease in heart rate, and a slight increase in stroke volume in healthy (lack of ischemic heart disease) older adults at rest. No changes were noted at rest in ejection fraction. A slight increase in afterload (e.g., as systolic blood pressure) and prolonged left ventricular relaxation was noted.

3. The most relevant age-associated changes in cardiovascular performance are myocardial and blood vessel stiffening, changes in neurogenic control over vascular tone, and left ventricular hypertrophy and fibrosis.

4. With active risk reduction and disease management, older adults can have markedly improved cardiovascular health.

a wave, 1096
Adrenomedullin (ADM), 1128
Afferent lymphatic vessel, 1133
Afterload, 1109
Aldosterone, 1127
Angiogenesis, 1097
Angiotensin I (Ang I), 1125
Angiotensin II (Ang II), 1125
Anisotropic band (A band), 1106
Anomalous viscosity, 1119
Anterior interatrial myocardial band (Bachmann bundle), 1102
Antidiuretic hormone (ADH), 1125
Aorta, 1095
Aortic semilunar valve, 1094
Arteriogenesis, 1097
Arteriole, 1113
Arteries, 1113

AT_1, 1127
AT_2, 1127
Atrial natriuretic peptide (ANP or factor), 1128
Atrioventricular (AV) node, 1101
Atrioventricular valve, 1094
Automatic cell, 1103
Automaticity, 1103
Bainbridge reflex, 1112
Baroreceptor reflex, 1112
Brain natriuretic peptide (BNP), 1128
Bundle branch, 1101
Bundle of His (atrioventricular bundle, common bundle), 1101
c-type natriuretic peptide (CNP), 1128
c wave, 1096
Calcium channel–blocking drug, 1108
Capillary, 1113

Cardiac action potential, 1099
Cardiac catheterization, 1135
Cardiac cycle, 1095
Cardiac output, 1109
Cardiac plexus, 1104
Cardioexcitatory center, 1112
Cardioinhibitory center, 1112
Cardiovascular control center, 1111
Chordae tendineae, 1094
Circumflex artery, 1097
Collateral artery, 1097
Conduction system, 1099
Coronary angiography, 1135
Coronary perfusion pressure, 1130
Coronary sulcus, 1097
Crista supraventricularis, 1095
Cross-bridge theory of muscle contraction, 1108

Continued

KEY TERMS–cont'd

Depolarization, 1102
Diastole, 1095
Diastolic depolarization, 1103
Efferent lymphatic vessel, 1133
Ejection fraction, 1109
Elastic artery, 1113
End-diastolic volume, 1110
Endocardium, 1093
Endothelial cells, 1116
Endothelium, 1116
Epinephrine, 1125
Excitation-contraction coupling, 1108
Fenestration, 1113
Frank-Starling law of the heart, 1109
Great cardiac vein, 1099
Heart rate, 1099
Hyperemia, 1125
Inferior vena cava, 1095
Inflow tract, 1094
Inotropic agent, 1111
Insulin, 1130
Intercalated disk, 1105
Isotropic band (I band), 1106
Laminar flow, 1121
Left anterior descending artery (LAD), 1097
Left atrium, 1093
Left bundle branch (LBB), 1102
Left coronary artery (LCA), 1096
Left heart, 1091
Left pulmonary artery, 1095
Left ventricle, 1093
Left ventricular end-diastolic pressure (LVEDP), 1110
Left ventricular end-diastolic volume (LVEDV), 1110
Lumen, 1113
Lymph, 1132
Lymphatic system, 1131
Lymphatic vein, 1132
Lymphatic venule, 1132
M line, 1106
Mean arterial pressure (MAP), 1122
Mediastinum, 1093

Metarterioles, 1113
Middle internodal pathway, 1102
Mitral and tricuspid complex, 1094
Mitral valve, 1094
Muscular artery, 1113
Myocardial contractility, 1108
Myocardial oxygen consumption ($M\dot{V}O_2$), 1107
Myocardium, 1093
Myoglobin, 1131
Myosin, 1106
Node, 1099
Norepinephrine, 1125
Outflow tract, 1094
P cell, 1100
P wave, 1103
Papillary muscle, 1094
Parietal pericardium, 1093
Perfusion, 1122
Pericardial cavity, 1093
Pericardial fluid, 1093
Pericardium, 1093
Peripheral vascular system, 1113
Poiseuille's formula, 1119
Posterior internodal pathway, 1102
Posterior vein of the left ventricle, 1099
Precapillary sphincter, 1113
Preload, 1109
Pressure, 1117
PR interval, 1103
Pulmonary artery, 1095
Pulmonary circulation, 1091
Pulmonary veins, 1095
Pulmonic semilunar valve, 1094
Purkinje fiber, 1102
QRS complex, 1103
QT interval, 1103
Renin, 1125
Renin-angiotensin aldosterone system (RAAS), 1126
Repolarization, 1102
Resistance, 1118
Rhythmicity, 1103

Right atrium, 1093
Right bundle branch (RBB), 1101
Right coronary artery (RCA), 1096
Right heart, 1091
Right lymphatic duct, 1132
Right pulmonary artery, 1095
Right ventricle, 1093
Semilunar valve, 1094
Shear stress, 1097
Sinoatrial node (SA node, sinus node), 1100
ST interval, 1103
Stroke volume, 1109
Superior vena cava, 1095
Systemic circulation, 1091
Systole, 1095
Systolic compressive effect, 1131
Thoracic duct, 1132
Tissue-based renin-angiotensin system, 1127
Total resistance, 1120
Trabeculae carneae, 1096
Tricuspid valve, 1094
Troponin, 1106
Troponin C, 1106
Troponin T, 1106
Troponin-tropomyosin complex, 1106
Tunica externa (adventitia), 1113
Tunica intima, 1113
Tunica media, 1113
Turbulent, 1121
Urodilatin, 1128
v wave, 1096
Vasa vasorum, 1113
Vascular compliance, 1122
Vasoconstriction, 1113
Vasodilation, 1113
Vasomotion, 1116
Vein, 1113
Venule, 1113
Visceral pericardium (epicardium), 1093
x descent, 1096
y descent, 1096
Z line, 1106

REFERENCES

1. Mohrman DE, Heller JA, editors: *Cardiovascular physiology*, ed 6, Philadelphia, 2006, McGraw-Hill.
2. Shireman PK: The chemokine system in arteriogenesis and hind limb ischemia, *J Vasc Surg* 45(Suppl A):A48-A56, 2007.
3. Kocaman SA et al: Increased circulating monocytes count is related to good collateral development in coronary artery disease, *Atherosclerosis* 197(2):753-756, 2008.
4. Maulik N, Thirunavukkarasu M: Growth factor/s and cell therapy in myocardial regeneration, *J Mol Cell Cardiol* 44(2):219-227, 2008.
5. Boodhwani M et al: Insulin treatment enhances the myocardial angiogenic response in diabetes, *J Thorac Cardiovasc Surg* 135(6): 1453-1460, 2007.
6. Molin D, Post MJ: Therapeutic angiogenesis in the heart: protect and serve, *Curr Opin Pharmacol* 7(2):158-163, 2007.
7. Zipes DP, Rubart M: Genesis of cardiac arrhythmias: electrophysiological considerations. In Peter L et al, editors: *Braunwald's heart disease: a textbook of cardiovascular medicine*, ed 8, Philadelphia, 2008, Saunders.

8. Gauthier C, Seze-Goismier C, Rozec B: Beta 3-adrenoceptors in the cardiovascular system, *Clin Hemorheol Microcirc* 37(1-2):193-204, 2007.
9. Feldman DS et al: Mechanisms of disease: detrimental adrenergic signaling in acute decompensated heart failure, *Nat Clin Pract Cardiovasc Med* 5(4):208-218, 2008.
10. Hassan M et al: Association of beta1-adrenergic receptor genetic polymorphism with mental stress-induced myocardial ischemia in patients with coronary artery disease, *Arch Intern Med* 168(7):763-770, 2008.
11. Schwartz PJ et al: Neural control of heart rate is an arrhythmia risk modifier in long QT syndrome, *J Am Coll Cardiol* 51(9):920-929, 2008.
12. Horiba M et al: T-type Ca2+ channel blockers prevent cardiac cell hypertrophy through an inhibition of calcineurin-NFAT3 activation as well as L-type Ca2+ channel blockers, *Life Sci* 82(11-12):554-560, 2008.
12a. Book Review: The Linacre lecture on the law of the heart given at Cambridge, 1915, *Nature* 101(2525):43, 1918.
13. Berne RM, Levy MN, editors: *Cardiovascular physiology*, ed 8, St Louis, 2001, Mosby.
14. Monahan KD: Effect of aging on baroreflex function in humans, *Am J Physiol Reg IntegrComp Physiol* 293(1):R3-R12, 2007.

15. Freeman R: Clinical practice, Neurogenic orthostatic hypotension, *N Engl J Med* 358(6):615-624, 2008.

16. Schmidt H et al: The alteration of autonomic function in multiple organ dysfunction syndrome,, *Crit Care Clin* 24(1):149-163, ix, 2008.

17. Filippone JD, Bisognano JD: Baroreflex stimulation in the treatment of hypertension, *Curr Opin Nephrol Hypertens* 16(5):403-408, 2007.

18. Esper RJ et al: Endothelial dysfunction in normal and abnormal glucose metabolism, *Adv Cardiol* 45:17-43, 2008.

19. Schafer A, Bauersachs J: Endothelial dysfunction, impaired endogenous platelet inhibition and platelet activation in diabetes and atherosclerosis, *Curr Vasc Pharmacol* 6(1):52-60, 2008.

20. Thijssen DH et al: Physical (in)activity and endothelium-derived constricting factors: overlooked adaptations, *J Physiol* 586(2): 319-324, 2008.

21. Gradman AH, Kad R: Renin inhibition in hypertension, *J Am Coll Cardiol* 51(5):519-528, 2008.

22. Coffman TM, Crowley SD: Kidney in hypertension: Guyton redux, *Hypertension* 51(4):811-816, 2008.

23. Lambert DW, Hooper NM, Turner AJ: Angiotensin-converting enzyme-2 and new insights into the renin-angiotensin system, *Biochem Pharmacol* 75(4):781-786, 2008.

24. Raizada V et al: Intracardiac and intrarenal renin-angiotensin systems: mechanisms of cardiovascular and renal effects, *J Invest Med* 55(7): 341-359, 2007.

25. Selektor Y, Weber KT: The salt-avid state of congestive heart failure revisited, *Am J Med Sci* 335(3):209-218, 2008.

26. Wright JW, Yamamoto BJ, Harding JW: Angiotensin receptor subtype mediated physiologies and behaviors: new discoveries and clinical targets, *Prog Neurobiol* 84(2):157-181, 2008.

27. Skultetyova D et al: The role of angiotensin type 1 receptor in inflammation and endothelial dysfunction, *Recent Patents Cardiovas Drug Discov* 2(1):23-27, 2007.

28. Perkins JM, Davis SN: The renin-angiotensin-aldosterone system: a pivotal role in insulin sensitivity and glycemic control, *Curr Opin Endocrinol Diabetes Obes* 15(2):147-152, 2008.

29. Widdop RE et al: Vascular angiotensin AT2 receptors in hypertension and ageing, *Clin Exp Pharmacol Physiol* 35(4):386-390, 2008.

30. Schiffrin EL: Effects of aldosterone on the vasculature, *Hypertension* 47(3):312-318, 2006.

31. Gardner DG et al: Molecular biology of the natriuretic peptide system: implications for physiology and hypertension, *Hypertension* 49(3): 419-426, 2007.

32. Chen H et al: Atrial natriuretic peptide-initiated cGMP pathways regulate vasodilator-stimulated phosphoprotein phosphorylation and angiogenesis in vascular endothelium, *J Bio Chem* 283(7):4439-4447, 2008.

33. Bettencourt P, Januzzi JL Jr: Amino-terminal pro-B-type natriuretic peptide testing for inpatient monitoring and treatment guidance of acute destabilized heart failure, *Am J Cardiol* 101(3A):67-71, 2008.

34. Sandow SL, Tare M: C-type natriuretic peptide: a new endothelium-derived hyperpolarizing factor? *Trends Pharmacol Sci* 28(2):61-67, 2007.

35. Lee CY, Burnett JC Jr: Natriuretic peptides and therapeutic applications, *Heart Fail Rev* 12(2):131-142, 2007.

36. Yanagawa B, Nagaya N: Adrenomedullin: molecular mechanisms and its role in cardiac disease, *Amino Acids* 32(1):157-164, 2007.

37. Temmesfeld-Wollbruck B et al: Adrenomedullin and endothelial barrier function, *Thromb Haemost* 98(5):944-951, 2007.

38. Fang JC, O'Gara PT: Evaluation of the patient. In Peter L et al, editors: *Braunwald's heart disease: a textbook of cardiovascular medicine*, ed 8, Philadelphia, 2008, Saunders.

39. Schwartz JB: Zipes DP: Cardiovascular disease in the elderly. In Peter L et al, editors: *Braunwald's heart disease: a textbook of cardiovascular medicine* ed 8, Philadelphia, 2008, Saunders.

40. Susic D, Frohlich ED: The aging hypertensive heart: a brief update, *Nat Clin Pract Cardiovasc Med* 5(2):104-110, 2008.

41. Sniderman AD, Furberg CD: Age as a modifiable risk factor for cardiovascular disease, *Lancet* 371(9623):1547-1549, 2008.

ALTERATIONS OF CARDIOVASCULAR FUNCTION

VALENTINA L. BRASHERS

MEDIA RESOURCES

 Evolve Website (http://evolve.elsevier.com/McCance/)
- Review Questions and Answers
- Animations
- Glossary (with audio pronunciation for selected terms)
- WebLinks

Online Course
- Module 15

CHAPTER OUTLINE

DISEASES OF THE VEINS
Varicose Veins and Chronic Venous Insufficiency
Thrombus Formation in Veins
Superior Vena Cava Syndrome
DISEASES OF THE ARTERIES
Aneurysm
Thrombus Formation
Embolism
Peripheral Arterial Diseases
Hypertension
Orthostatic (Postural) Hypotension
Atherosclerosis

Peripheral Artery Disease
Coronary Artery Disease, Myocardial Ischemia, and Acute Coronary Syndromes
DISORDERS OF THE HEART WALL
Disorders of the Pericardium
Disorders of the Myocardium: The Cardiomyopathies
Disorders of the Endocardium
Cardiac Complications in Acquired Immunodeficiency Syndrome
MANIFESTATIONS OF HEART DISEASE
Heart Failure
Dysrhythmias

Cardiovascular disease is the leading cause of death in the United States (Table 30-1) and in the world.[1] The pathophysiology of heart disease is now known to be much more complicated than just structural and hemodynamic changes. Today the focus is on the genetic, neurohumoral, and inflammatory mechanisms that underlie tissue and cellular processes, such as endothelial injury, remodeling, stunning, reperfusion injury, and autoimmune disease.

DISEASES OF THE VEINS

Varicose Veins and Chronic Venous Insufficiency

A **varicose vein** is a vein in which blood has pooled. Varicose veins typically involve the saphenous veins of the legs and are distended, tortuous, and palpable (Figure 30-1). Varicose veins are caused by (1) trauma to the saphenous veins that

damages one or more valves, or (2) gradual venous distention caused by the action of gravity on blood in the legs.

Veins are thin-walled, highly distensible vessels. Normally, the muscular pump in the legs moves venous blood up toward the heart and valves prevent backflow and pooling of blood (see Figures 29-30 and 29-31). If a valve is damaged, permitting backflow, a section of the vein is subjected to the pressure exerted by a larger volume of blood under the influence of gravity. The vein swells as it becomes engorged and surrounding tissue becomes edematous because increased hydrostatic pressure pushes plasma through the stretched vessel wall.

In individuals who habitually stand for long periods, wear constricting garments, or cross the legs at the knees, distention progresses until the pressure in the vein damages venous valves, rendering the valves incompetent. Damaged valves cannot maintain normal venous pressure, which causes hydrostatic pressure in the vein to increase. As the vein distends further, it becomes tortuous, and edema develops in the extremity.

Table 30-1	Death Rates and Percent of Total Deaths for the 15 Leading Causes of Death in the United States (Final Data Report 2006)		
Rank Order*	Cause of Death	Rate†	Percent of Total Deaths
1	Diseases of the heart	199.4	26.0
2	Malignant neoplasms	180.8	23.1
3	Cerebrovascular diseases	45.8	5.7
4	Chronic lower respiratory diseases	40.4	5.1
5	Accidents (unintentional injuries)	38.5	5.0
6	Diabetes mellitus	22.7	3.0
7	Alzheimer disease	23.3	3.0
8	Influenza and pneumonia	17.7	2.3
9	Nephritis, nephrotic syndrome, and nephrosis	14.3	1.9
10	Septicemia	10.9	1.4
11	Intentional self-harm (suicide)	10.6	1.4
12	Chronic liver disease and cirrhosis	8.7	1.1
13	Essential hypertension and hypertensive disease	7.6	1.0
14	Parkinson disease	6.3	0.8
15	Assault (homicide)	6	0.8

Data from National Center for Health Statistics: *National vital statistics report 57, No 14,* 2009, National Center for Health Statistics. Available at www.cdc.gov/nchs.
*Rank based on number of deaths.
†Rates per 100,000 population.

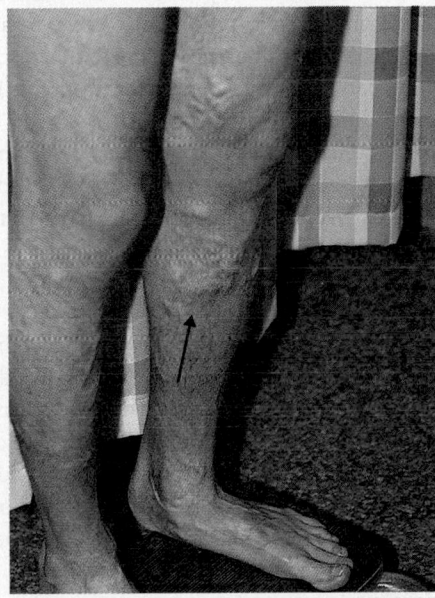

Figure 30-1 Varicose veins of the leg *(arrow).* (From Kumar V, et al: *Robbins basic pathology,* ed 8, Philadelphia, 2007, Saunders. Courtesy of Dr. Magruder C. Donaldson, Brigham and Women's Hospital, Boston.)

Varicose veins and valvular incompetence can progress to **chronic venous insufficiency (CVI).** CVI is inadequate venous return over a long period. Venous hypertension, circulatory stasis, and tissue hypoxia lead to an inflammatory reaction in vessels and tissue leading to fibrosclerotic remodeling of the skin and then to ulceration.[2] Symptoms include chronic pooling of blood in the veins of the lower extremities and hyperpigmentation of the skin of the feet and ankles. Edema in these areas may extend to the knees.

Circulation to the extremities can become so sluggish that the metabolic demands of the cells for oxygen, nutrients, and waste removal are barely met. Any trauma or pressure can therefore lower the oxygen supply and cause cell death and necrosis **(venous stasis ulcers).** Infection can occur because poor circulation impairs the delivery of the cells and biochemicals for the immune and inflammatory responses. This same sluggish circulation makes infection following reparative surgery a significant risk. Varicose veins and CVI may be associated with **deep venous thrombosis (in a deep vein, DVT)** in some individuals because of changes in collateral flow and shared risk factors; therefore, anyone with new onset varicose veins should be evaluated for the possibility of underlying DVT.

Treatment of varicose veins and CVI begins conservatively, and excellent wound healing results have followed noninvasive treatments, such as leg elevation, compression stockings, and physical exercise.[3] Invasive management includes endovascular ablation or surgical ligation and vein stripping.[4]

Thrombus Formation in Veins

A **thrombus** is a blood clot that remains attached to a vessel wall (Figure 30-2). A detached thrombus is a **thromboembolus.** Venous thrombi are more common than arterial thrombi because flow and pressure are lower in the veins than in the arteries. DVT occurs primarily in the lower extremity. Three factors (triad of Virchow) promote venous thrombosis: (1) venous stasis (e.g., immobility, obesity, prolonged leg dependency [e.g., air travel], age, congestive heart failure [CHF], (2) venous endothelial damage [e.g., trauma, medications], and (3) hypercoagulable states (e.g., inherited disorders, malignancy, pregnancy, oral contraceptives, hormone replacement, hyperhomocysteinemia, antiphospholipid syndrome).[5-9] All individuals who are hospitalized are at significant risk and orthopedic trauma or surgery, spinal cord injury, and obstetric/gynecologic conditions can be associated with up to a 100% likelihood of DVT. There are numerous genetic abnormalities

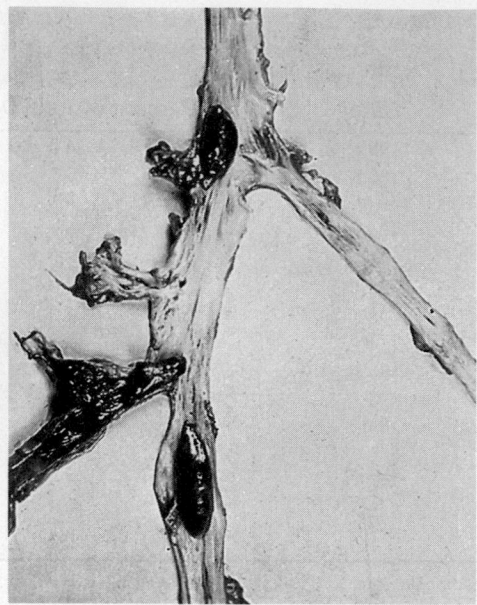

Figure 30-2 Multiple venous thrombi. (From Rosai J: *Ackerman's surgical pathology,* ed 8, vol 2, St Louis, 1996, Mosby.)

associated with an increased risk for venous thrombosis primarily related to states of hypercoagulability. These inherited abnormalities include factor V Leiden mutation; prothrombin mutations; and deficiencies of protein C, protein S, and antithrombin, and are commonly found in individuals who develop thrombi in the absence of the usual risk factors.[6,10,11]

Accumulation of clotting factors and platelets leads to thrombus formation in the vein, often near a venous valve. Inflammation around the thrombus promotes further platelet aggregation and the thrombus propagates or grows proximally.[12] This inflammation may cause local symptoms but because the vein is deep in the leg, it is usually not accompanied by clinical symptoms or signs. If the thrombus creates significant obstruction to venous blood flow, increased pressure in the vein behind the clot may lead to edema of the extremity.

Most thrombi will eventually dissolve without treatment, but untreated DVT is associated with a high risk of **thromboembolization** of a part of the clot from the leg to the lung (pulmonary embolism) (see Chapter 33).[13] Persistent venous outflow obstruction may lead to **post-thrombotic syndrome (PTS),** a frequent complication of DVT characterized by chronic, persistent pain, swelling, and ulceration of the affected limb.[14]

Because DVT is usually asymptomatic and difficult to detect clinically, prevention in at-risk individuals is crucial. If possible, individuals should be mobilized as soon as possible after illness, injury, or surgery. Prophylactic treatment can include low-molecular-weight heparin, antithrombin agents, warfarin, or pneumatic devices.[15-17] In individuals at high risk for pulmonary embolism but for whom anticoagulation is contraindicated, placement of an inferior vena caval filter may be necessary to prevent pulmonary embolism.[13]

Diagnosis is most often made by combining measurement of serum D-dimer concentration with lower extremity ultrasonography.[18,19] In selected individuals, computed tomography (CT) or magnetic resonance imaging (MRI) may be needed to make the diagnosis.[20,21] If noninvasive testing is nondiagnostic, a venogram may be indicated. DVT is treated with low-molecular-weight heparin, unfractionated intravenous heparin, antithrombin agents, or adjusted-dose subcutaneous heparin.[22,23] Fibrinolytic therapy may be used in selected individuals to dissolve the clot more quickly but is associated with a greater risk for bleeding than heparin.

Superior Vena Cava Syndrome

Superior vena cava syndrome (SVCS) is a progressive occlusion of the superior vena cava (SVC) that leads to venous distention in the upper extremities and head. The leading cause of SVCS is bronchogenic cancer (approximately 75% of cases), followed by lymphomas and metastasis of other cancers.[24] Benign causes of SVCS include thrombosis, histoplasmosis, tuberculosis, mediastinal fibrosis, cystic fibrosis, and benign tumors, such as retrosternal goiter.[25] Invasive therapies, including pacemaker wires, central venous catheters, and pulmonary artery catheters, can lead to acute and chronic SVCS.

The SVC is a relatively low-pressure vessel that lies in the closed thoracic compartment; therefore, tissue expansion can easily compress the SVC. The right mainstem bronchus abuts the SVC so that cancers occurring in this bronchus may press on the SVC. Additionally, the SVC is surrounded by lymph nodes and lymph chains that commonly become involved in thoracic cancers and compress the SVC during tumor growth. Because onset of SVCS is slow, collateral venous drainage to the azygos vein usually has time to develop.

Clinical manifestations of SVCS include edema and venous distention in the upper extremities and face, including the ocular beds. Individuals may complain of a feeling of fullness in the head, or tightness of shirt collars, necklaces, and rings. Cerebral and central nervous system edema may cause headache, visual disturbance, and impaired consciousness. The skin of the face and arms is purple and taut, and capillary refill time is prolonged. Respiratory distress may be present because of edema of bronchial structures or compression of the bronchus by a carcinoma.

Diagnosis is made by chest roentgenogram, Doppler studies, CT, MRI, and ultrasound. With slow onset and the development of collateral venous drainage, SVCS is generally not a vascular emergency but rather an oncologic emergency. Treatment includes radiation therapy, chemotherapy, and the administration of diuretics, steroids, and anticoagulants, as necessary.[24,25] Treatment also may include bypass surgery using various grafts; local and systemic thrombolysis; balloon angioplasty; and placement of intravascular stents.

DISEASES OF THE ARTERIES

Aneurysm

An **aneurysm** is a localized dilation or outpouching of a vessel wall or cardiac chamber. Laplace's law can provide an understanding of the hemodynamics of an aneurysm (Figure 30-3).

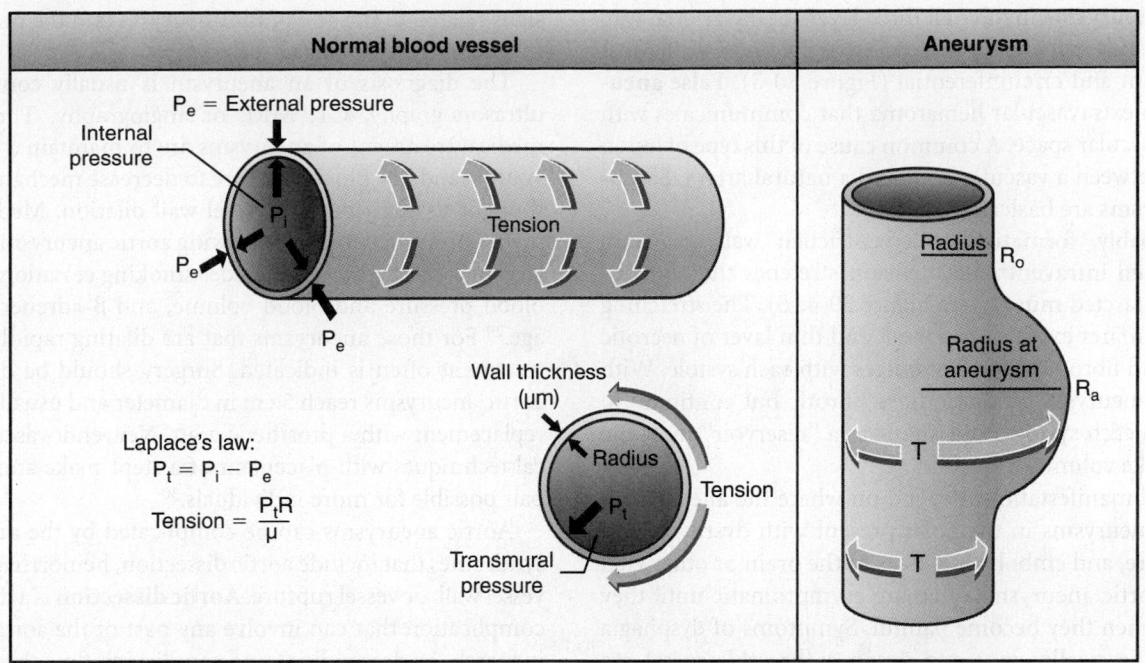

Figure 30-3 Pressure-tension and wall thickness relations in blood vessels or cardiac chambers (Laplace's law).

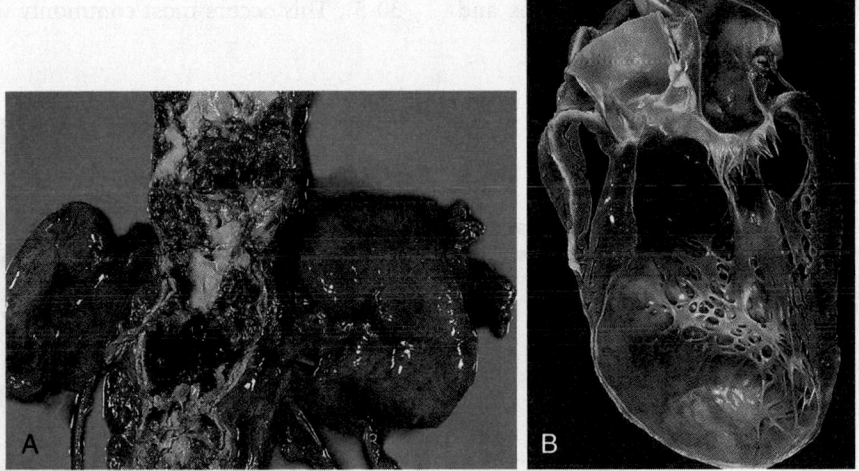

Figure 30-4 Aneurysms. A, Abdominal aortic atherosclerotic aneurysm. B, In a long-axis view of the left ventricle there is a large thin-walled apical aneurysm that does not contain thrombus. (From Damjanov I, Linder J, editors: *Anderson's pathology*, ed 10, St Louis, 1996, Mosby.)

(Laplace's law is discussed in detail in Chapter 29.) Aneurysms most commonly occur in the thoracic or abdominal aorta.

The aorta is particularly susceptible to aneurysm formation because of constant stress on the vessel wall and the absence of penetrating vasa vasorum in the media layer (Figure 30-4, *A*). It is estimated that up to 10% of older individuals have an aortic aneurysm, and about 15,000 persons in the United States die from aortic aneurysm rupture annually.[26] Arteriosclerosis and hypertension are found in more than half of all individuals with aneurysms. Chronic hypertension results in mechanical and shear forces that contribute to remodeling and weakening of the vessel wall. Atherosclerosis is a common cause of aneurysms because plaque formation erodes the vessel wall. Infections, such as syphilis, collagen disorders (such as Marfan syndrome), and traumatic injury to the chest or abdomen, also can cause aortic aneurysms. For those aortic aneurysms not clearly related to atherosclerosis, infection, Marfan syndrome or trauma, or numerous genetic susceptibilities have been identified including genes polymorphisms for the production of growth factors, myosin, and proteases.[26,27] Inflammation, with the production of toxic oxygen radicals, activates matrix degrading proteins and smooth muscle cell apoptosis resulting in loss of medial elastic lamellae and thinning of the tunica media. Autoimmunity and the production of metalloproteinases and elastases further contribute to the degradation of the vessel wall.[26,28]

True aneurysms involve all three layers of the arterial wall and are best described as a weakening of the vessel wall. Most are fusiform and circumferential (Figure 30-5). **False aneurysm** is an extravascular hematoma that communicates with the intravascular space. A common cause of this type of lesion is a leak between a vascular graft and a natural artery. **Saccular aneurysms** are basically spherical.

Presumably, formation of a ventricular wall aneurysm occurs when intraventricular tension stretches the noncontracting infarcted muscle (see Figure 30-4, *B*). The stretching produces infarct expansion, a weak and thin layer of necrotic muscle, and fibrous tissue that bulges with each systole. With time, the aneurysm becomes more fibrotic but continues to bulge with each systole, thus acting as a "reservoir" for some of the stroke volume.

Clinical manifestations depend on where the aneurysm is located. Aneurysms in the heart present with dysrhythmias, heart failure, and embolism of clots to the brain or other vital organs. Aortic aneurysms often are asymptomatic until they rupture, when they become painful. Symptoms of dysphagia (difficulty in swallowing) and dyspnea (breathlessness) are caused by the pressure of a thoracic aneurysm on surrounding organs. An abdominal aneurysm can impair flow to an extremity and cause symptoms of ischemia. Aneurysms that occur elsewhere in the body have variable symptoms and signs related to the size of the aneurysm and the potential for rupture and hemorrhage.

The diagnosis of an aneurysm is usually confirmed by ultrasonography, CT, MRI, or angiography. The goals of medical treatment of aneurysms are to maintain a low blood volume and low blood pressure to decrease mechanical forces thought to contribute to vessel wall dilation. Medical treatment is indicated for slow-growing aortic aneurysms, particularly in early stages, and includes smoking cessation, reducing blood pressure and blood volume, and β-adrenergic blockage.[29] For those aneurysms that are dilating rapidly, surgical treatment often is indicated. Surgery should be done when aortic aneurysms reach 5 cm in diameter and usually includes replacement with a prosthetic graft. New endovascular surgical techniques with placement of a stent make aneurysm repair possible for more individuals.[30]

Aortic aneurysms can be complicated by the acute aortic syndromes that include aortic dissection, hemorrhage into the vessel wall, or vessel rupture. **Aortic dissection** is a devastating complication that can involve any part of the aorta (ascending, arch, or descending) and can disrupt flow through arterial branches, thus creating a surgical emergency. Dissection of the layers of the arterial wall occurs when there is a tear in the intima and blood enters the wall of the artery (see Figure 30-5). This occurs most commonly when there is trauma to

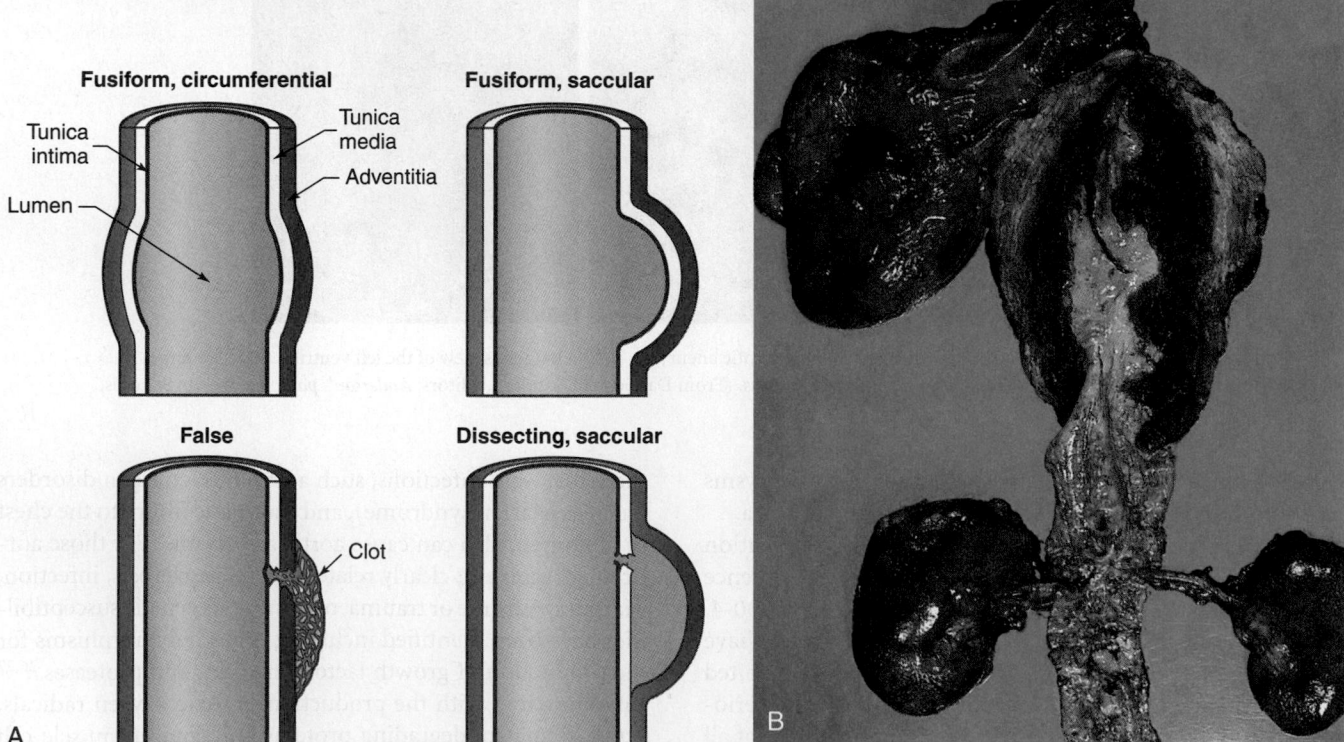

Figure 30-5 Longitudinal sections showing types of aneurysms. **A,** The fusiform circumferential and fusiform saccular aneurysms are true aneurysms, caused by weakening of the vessel wall. False and saccular aneurysms involve a break in the vessel wall, usually caused by trauma. **B,** Dissecting aneurysm of thoracic aorta. (**B** from Damjanov I, Linder J, editors: *Anderson's pathology,* ed 10, St Louis, 1996, Mosby.)

the aorta or when there is tissue ischemia and necrosis at the edge of an atherosclerotic plaque that weakens the intima. Persistent chronic hypertension and inflammation contribute to further degradation of the vessel wall with fibrotic obstruction of vessels that feed the arterial wall. Emergent evaluation and surgical intervention are indicated.[31]

Thrombus Formation

As in venous thrombosis, arterial thrombi tend to develop wherever intravascular conditions promote activation of the coagulation, or clotting, cascade. These conditions include intimal irritation and roughening, inflammation, traumatic injury, infection, and low blood pressures or obstructions that cause blood stasis and pooling within the vessels. (Mechanisms of coagulation are described in Chapter 25.) In the arteries, activation of the coagulation cascade usually is caused by roughening of the tunica intima by atherosclerosis. Invasion of the tunica intima by an infectious agent also roughens the normally smooth lining of the artery, causing platelets to adhere readily. Anatomic changes of an artery can stimulate thrombus formation, particularly if the change results in pooling of arterial blood. This can occur, for example, in blood that is pooled within an aneurysm. Thrombi form also on heart valves altered by calcification or bacterial vegetation. Valvular thrombi are associated most commonly with inflammation of the endocardium (endocarditis) and rheumatic heart disease.

Widespread arterial thrombus formation can occur in shock. Shock, particularly the type resulting from septicemia, can activate the intrinsic and extrinsic pathways of coagulation. The impaired cellular metabolism that occurs with all types of shock activates the extrinsic pathway of coagulation, whereas blood stasis caused by very low blood pressures activates the intrinsic pathway (see Chapter 25). Thrombus formation may be confined to one area or may progress to diffuse coagulopathy, such as disseminated intravascular coagulation (see Chapter 27).

Arterial thrombi pose two potential threats to the circulation. First, the thrombus may grow large enough to occlude the artery, causing ischemia in tissue supplied by the artery. Second, the thrombus may dislodge, becoming a thromboembolus that travels through the vascular system until it occludes flow into a distal systemic vascular bed.

Diagnosis of arterial thrombi is usually accomplished through the use of Doppler ultrasonography and angiography. Pharmacologic treatment involves the administration of heparin, warfarin derivatives, thrombin inhibitors, or thrombolytics. A balloon-tipped catheter also can be used to remove or compress an arterial thrombus. Various combinations of drug and catheter therapies are sometimes used concurrently.

Embolism

Embolism is the obstruction of a vessel by an **embolus**—a bolus of matter that is circulating in the bloodstream. The embolus may consist of a dislodged thrombus; an air bubble; an aggregate of amniotic fluid; an aggregate of fat, bacteria, or cancer cells; or a foreign substance. An embolus travels in the bloodstream until it reaches a vessel through which it cannot fit. No matter how tiny it is, an embolus eventually will lodge in a systemic or pulmonary vessel. The source of the embolus determines whether the embolus will lodge in a vessel of the pulmonary or systemic circulation. Pulmonary emboli originate in the venous circulation (mostly from the deep veins of the legs) or in the right heart (see p. 1143). Arterial emboli most commonly originate in the left heart and are associated with thrombi after myocardial infarction, valvular disease, left heart failure, endocarditis, and dysrhythmias.

Embolism causes ischemia or infarction in tissues distal to the obstruction. A limb that is ischemic because of arterial occlusion is characterized (1) by an almost waxy whiteness of the skin because the vasculature is devoid of erythrocytes, and (2) by numbness and pain resulting from neural ischemia.

Embolism of a central organ causes organic dysfunction and pain. For example, pulmonary artery embolism causes chest pain and dyspnea; renal artery embolism causes abdominal pain and oliguria; and mesenteric artery embolism causes abdominal pain and a paralytic, ischemic bowel. Infarction and subsequent necrosis of a central organ are life threatening, not only because of organ dysfunction but also because of sepsis. Necrotic tissue is a rich medium for the growth of bacteria from the lungs, bowel, and occasionally, bladder. Necrosis of the bladder, in particular, can quickly lead to peritonitis or septicemia.

Embolism of a coronary or cerebral artery is an immediate threat to life if the embolus severely obstructs a major vessel. Occlusion of a coronary artery will cause a myocardial infarction (see p. 1171), whereas occlusion of a cerebral artery causes a stroke (see Chapter 17).

Thromboembolism

Thromboembolism is a vascular obstruction resulting from a dislodged thrombus. The most common source of arterial thromboemboli to the systemic circulation is the heart. Mitral or aortic valvular disease, especially that associated with abnormal heart rhythms (atrial fibrillation and flutter), causes thrombus formation on roughened vascular surfaces and in atrial blood as a result of stasis. More than half of these thromboemboli lodge in the lower extremities (in the femoral and popliteal arteries). Others lodge in the coronary arteries and the cerebral vasculature. Heart failure also is associated with an increased risk of thrombotic complications, although the mechanism for this increased risk is unclear.

Air Embolism

Room air that enters the circulation through intravenous lines is probably the most common cause of air embolism. Room air is about 70% nitrogen. Although nitrogen dissolves quickly in blood, large amounts of air cannot be dissolved rapidly enough to prevent the displacement of blood in the arterioles and capillary beds. Ischemia and necrosis occur when air totally blocks a vessel.

Air also can be introduced into the bloodstream if trauma to the chest causes air from the lungs to enter the vascular space. For example, gunshot wounds and puncture wounds of the thorax sometimes introduce air emboli. Treatment for air embolism is supportive, including bed rest and supplemental oxygen, once the connection between the source of air and the vascular system is eliminated.

Amniotic Fluid Embolism

The great intra-abdominal pressures generated during labor and delivery may force amniotic fluid into the mother's bloodstream through the highly vascular uterine wall. Amniotic fluid not only displaces blood, reducing oxygen, nutrient, and waste exchange, but also introduces antigens, cells, and protein aggregates that trigger inflammation, coagulation, and the immune response within the bloodstream. Capillary beds usually are affected by amniotic fluid emboli, especially the capillary beds of the lungs and kidneys. Treatment is supportive and may include dialysis, particularly after a cesarean delivery or hysterectomy.

Bacterial Embolism

Isolated bacteria in the bloodstream do not cause embolism, but aggregates of bacteria may be large enough to do so. The most common cause of bacterial embolism is subacute bacterial endocarditis, during which clumps of vegetation are dislodged from infected cardiac valves and ejected into the pulmonary or systemic circulation. A less common cause is erosion of an artery or vein by bacteria at a source of infection, such as an abscess. Treatment for bacterial embolism includes bed rest, supplemental oxygen, and antibiotics to eradicate the source of infection.

Fat Embolism

Trauma to the long bones is associated with fat embolism, particularly in the lungs. Two mechanisms have been proposed to account for the generation of fat emboli after skeletal trauma. The first is that trauma to the bones initiates defective fat metabolism, causing globules of fat to form in the blood. Platelets adhere to these globules until the conglomerate is large enough to lodge in a capillary bed. The second possible explanation is that globules of fat are released from fatty bone marrow exposed by fracture. Again, platelets adhere to the fat globules and embolism occurs.

Treatment for fat embolism consists of prompt immobilization of fractures and supportive measures that include administration of supplemental oxygen, steroids, and glucose. Steroid administration may decrease the inflammation that occurs with vascular occlusion. Inflammation in the pulmonary bed is especially dangerous because it can cause acute respiratory distress syndrome (ARDS) (see Chapter 33).

Foreign Matter

Foreign matter can enter the bloodstream during trauma or through an intravenous or intra-arterial line. Small particles, such as drug precipitates, small glass shards, or fibers from linen, are sometimes introduced unintentionally into a vessel through intravenous injections or manipulation of monitoring lines. Once in the blood, these small particles initiate the coagulation cascade. The thromboemboli that form around the particles are large enough to occlude a vessel and result in ischemia. Treatment is aimed at preventing thrombus formation around the particle, dissolution of the particle, and supportive measures to alleviate ischemia. If the bolus of foreign matter is relatively large, it usually is removed surgically.

Peripheral Arterial Diseases

Thromboangiitis Obliterans (Buerger Disease)

Thromboangiitis obliterans (Buerger disease) is an inflammatory disease of the peripheral arteries. It is associated with smoking in approximately 95% of cases—the other 5% are related to frostbite, trauma, or the use of sympathomimetic drugs.[32] The incidence of Buerger disease has been steadily declining, presumably because of a decrease in cigarette smoking in men. The inflammatory lesions are accompanied by thrombi and sometimes by vasospasm of arterial segments.[32] Inflammation, thrombus formation, and vasospasm eventually can occlude and obliterate portions of small and medium-size arteries. Typically affected are the digital, tibial, and plantar arteries of the feet and the digital, palmar, and ulnar arteries of the hands. The pathogenesis of thromboangiitis obliterans is still being explored. There is evidence of significant T-cell activation and autoimmunity.[32]

The chief symptoms of thromboangiitis obliterans are pain and tenderness of the affected part. Clinical manifestations are caused by sluggish blood flow and include rubor (redness of the skin), which is caused by dilated capillaries under the skin, and cyanosis, which is caused by blood that remains in the capillaries after its oxygen has diffused into the interstitium. Chronic ischemia causes the skin to thin and become shiny and the nails to become thickened and malformed. In advanced disease, ischemia resulting from vessel obliteration can cause gangrene. Buerger disease has been associated with cerebrovascular disease and rheumatic symptoms (joint pain).

The most important part of treatment is cessation of cigarette smoking. All other measures are aimed at improving circulation to the foot or hand. Vasodilators are prescribed to alleviate vasospasm, and exercises are taught that use gravity to improve blood flow.[32,33] If vasospasm persists, sympathectomy may be performed.[33] Gangrene necessitates amputation.

Raynaud Phenomenon and Disease

Raynaud phenomenon and Raynaud disease are characterized by attacks of vasospasm in the small arteries and arterioles of the fingers and, less commonly, the toes. Although the clinical manifestations of the phenomenon and the disease are the same, their causes differ.

Raynaud phenomenon is secondary to systemic diseases, particularly collagen vascular disease (scleroderma), chemotherapy, cocaine use, hypothyroidism, pulmonary hypertension, thoracic outlet syndrome, serum sickness, vasculitis, malignancy, or long-term exposure to environmental conditions, such as cold or vibrating machinery in the workplace.[34] Raynaud phenomenon associated with malignancy can be especially severe and is an important clue to finding a previously undiagnosed cancer.

Raynaud disease is a primary vasospastic disorder of unknown origin. Raynaud disease tends to affect young women and to consist of vasospastic attacks triggered by brief exposure to cold or by emotional stress. It is estimated that the prevalence of Raynaud disease is 11% of women and 8% of men in the United States.[34] Blood vessels in these individuals demonstrate endothelial dysfunction with decreased nitric oxide production and increased endothelin-1 activity. Genetic predisposition may play a role in its development.

The clinical manifestations of the vasospastic attacks of either disorder are changes in skin color and sensation caused by ischemia. Vasospasm occurs with varying frequency and severity and causes pallor, numbness, and the sensation of cold in the digits. Attacks tend to be bilateral, and manifestations usually begin at the tips of the digits and progress to the proximal phalanges. Sluggish blood flow resulting in ischemia may cause the skin to appear cyanotic. Rubor follows as vasospasm ends and the capillaries become engorged with oxygenated blood. Rubor often is accompanied by throbbing and paresthesias. Skin color returns to normal after the attack, but frequent, prolonged attacks interfere with cellular metabolism, causing the skin of the fingertips to thicken and the nails to become brittle. In severe, chronic Raynaud phenomenon or disease, ischemia eventually can cause ulceration and gangrene. This outcome is rare, however.

The diagnostic criteria for Raynaud disease include not only the characteristic clinical manifestations described previously but also the absence of necrosis, no detectable underlying cause, normal capillaroscopy findings, normal laboratory tests for inflammation, and negative tests for antinuclear factors. Any condition causing Raynaud phenomenon will usually be detected if one of these evaluative tests is abnormal.

Treatment for Raynaud phenomenon consists of removing the stimulus or treating the primary disease process. When Raynaud phenomenon is associated with malignancy, surgical removal of the tumor may resolve the ischemia. For Raynaud phenomenon not associated with malignancy, treatment is limited to amelioration of symptoms with medications such as calcium channel blockers or other vasodilators. Attacks of vasospasm sometimes can be alleviated at their onset by an exercise in which the arms are swung forward and backward. This maneuver increases hydrostatic pressure (and perfusion pressure) in the arteries by means of centrifugal force.

Treatment of Raynaud disease is limited to prevention or alleviation of vasospasm itself, because no underlying disorder has been identified. Stimuli that trigger attacks (e.g., emotional stress, cold) are avoided, and cigarette smoking is stopped to eliminate the vasoconstricting effects of nicotine. Exercises that build centrifugal force in the extremities also are helpful in the early stages of vasospasm. If attacks of vasospasm become frequent or prolonged, pharmacologic management can include calcium channel blockers, nitric oxide agonists, alpha-blockers, prostaglandin analogs, and selective serotonin reuptake inhibitors.[34,35] Biofeedback may be helpful. Sympathectomy may be recommended in severe cases but is not always effective and has a high rate of recurrence. If ischemia leads to ulceration and gangrene, amputation is necessary.

Hypertension

Hypertension is consistent elevation of systemic arterial blood pressure. Hypertension is the most common primary diagnosis in the United States. Approximately 65% of Americans older than the age of 60 have hypertension and less than two thirds of those have adequately controlled hypertension.[36] Hypertension is defined by the Seventh Report of the Joint National Committee on Prevention, Detection, Evaluation, and Treatment of High Blood Pressure (JNC7)[37] as a sustained systolic blood pressure of 140 mmHg or greater or a diastolic pressure of 90 mmHg or greater (Table 30-2). Normal blood pressure is associated with the lowest cardiovascular risk, whereas those who fall into the prehypertension category are at risk for developing hypertension unless lifestyle modification is instituted (more than 90% will develop hypertension).[36,37] The prevalence of hypertension increases with age and is higher for blacks than for whites.[36]

Individuals with hypertensive disease may have combined systolic and diastolic hypertension or isolated systolic hypertension. **Isolated systolic hypertension** is elevated systolic blood pressure accompanied by normal diastolic blood pressure (less than 90 mmHg). Most cases of hypertension have no known cause and therefore are diagnosed as **primary hypertension.** Primary hypertension, also called **essential or idiopathic hypertension,** affects 90% to 95% of hypertensive individuals.[36,37] **Secondary hypertension** is caused by altered hemodynamics associated with a primary disease, such as renal disease. Although many diseases can cause secondary hypertension, this form of hypertension accounts for only 5% to 8% of cases. Hypertension is a complex disorder that affects the entire cardiovascular system, and all types and stages of hypertension are associated with increased risk for target organ disease events, such as myocardial infarction, kidney disease, and stroke.[36-38]

Table 30-2	Classification of Blood Pressure for Adults Age 18 Years or Older		
Category	Systolic (mmHg)		Diastolic (mmHg)
Normal	<120	AND	<80
Prehypertension	120-139	OR	80-89
Stage 1 hypertension	140-159	OR	90-99
Stage 2 hypertension	≥160	OR	≥100

Data from the JNC 7 Report, *JAMA* 289(19):2560-2572, 2003.

Factors Associated with Primary Hypertension

Hypertension is caused by increases in cardiac output or total peripheral resistance, or both. (The many factors affecting cardiac output and peripheral resistance are described in Chapter 29.) Cardiac output is increased by any condition that increases heart rate or stroke volume, whereas peripheral resistance is increased by any factor that increases blood viscosity or reduces vessel diameter, particularly arteriolar diameter.

A specific cause for primary hypertension has not been identified, and a combination of genetic and environmental factors is thought to be responsible for its development. Genetic predisposition to hypertension is thought to be polygenic. The inherited defects are associated with renal sodium excretion, insulin and insulin sensitivity, activity of the renin-angiotensin-aldosterone system (RAAS), cell membrane sodium or calcium transport, and sympathetic response to neurogenic hormones[39,40] (see What's New? Genes and the Risk of Hypertension). Risk factors associated with primary hypertension include (1) family history of hypertension; (2) advancing age; (3) gender (men younger than 55 and women older than 70 years); (4) black race; (5) high dietary sodium intake; (6) glucose intolerance (diabetes mellitus); (7) cigarette smoking; (8) obesity; (9) heavy alcohol consumption; and (10) low dietary intake of potassium, calcium, and magnesium.[36,37] Many of these factors are also risk factors for other cardiovascular disorders. In fact, hypertension, dyslipidemia, and glucose intolerance often are found together.

WHAT'S NEW?   Genes and the Risk of Hypertension

Heritability accounts for an estimated 30% to 40% of primary hypertension. Gene polymorphisms that have been implicated include angiotensin II receptor genes, angiotensinogen, and renin genes; endothelial nitric oxide synthetase genes; G protein receptor kinase gene; aldosterone genes, adrenergic receptor genes; calcium transport and sodium-hydrogen antiporter genes (affect salt sensitivity); and genes associated with insulin resistance, obesity, hyperlipidemia and hypertension as a cluster of traits.

Adducin is a membrane-skeleton protein that plays an important role in the determination of cellular morphology and motility and in the regulation of membrane ion transport. It interacts with Na^+, K^+-ATPase and thus regulates the sodium-potassium pump. Mutations (e.g., ADD1 Gly460Trp) of the gene that codes for adducin cause an increase in tubular renal reabsorption of sodium and are associated with an approximately 50% to 70% increase in risk for hypertension in whites. The presence of an adducin gene mutation indicates that the affected individual is more likely to be salt sensitive and to respond more effectively to diuretic treatment of hypertension. These discoveries have led to potential treatments for hypertension using gene therapy techniques.

Data from Kingwell B, Boutouyrie P: *Clin Exper Pharmacol Physiol* 34(7):652-657, 2007; Kohara K et al: *Hypertens Res Clin Exper* 31(2):203-212, 2008; Manunta P et al: *Pharmacogenomics* 8(5): 465-472, 2007; Perticone F et al: *J Hypertens* 25(11):2234-2239, 2007; Puddu P et al: *Acta Cardiol* 62(3):281-293, 2007; Weder AB: *J Clin Hypertens* 9(3):217-223, 2007.

Although populations with high dietary sodium intake have long been shown to have an increased incidence of hypertension, recent studies indicate that low dietary potassium, calcium, and magnesium intakes are also risk factors because without their intake sodium is retained.[41-43] The nicotine in cigarette smoke is a vasoconstrictor that can elevate systolic and diastolic blood pressure acutely. In habitual smokers an individual cigarette may not raise blood pressure, yet habitual smoking is associated with a high incidence of severe hypertension, myocardial hypertrophy, and death resulting from coronary artery disease (CAD). The incidence of hypertension is higher among heavy drinkers of alcohol (more than three drinks per day) than among abstainers, but moderate drinkers (two to four drinks per week) appear to have lower blood pressures, as well as lower cardiovascular mortality, than either abstainers or heavy drinkers. Obesity is recognized as an important risk factor for hypertension, even in children and adolescents.[44]

PATHOPHYSIOLOGY

Primary Hypertension. Primary hypertension is the result of a complicated interaction between genetics and the environment that increase vascular tone (increased peripheral resistance) and blood volume, thus causing sustained increases in blood pressure. Multiple pathophysiologic mechanisms mediate these effects including the sympathetic nervous system (SNS), the RAAS, and natriuretic peptides. Inflammation, endothelial dysfunction, obesity-related hormones, and insulin resistance also contribute to both increased peripheral resistance and increased blood volume. Increased vascular volume is related to a decrease in renal excretion of salt, often referred to as a shift in the pressure-natriuresis relationship. This means that for a given blood pressure, individuals with hypertension tend to secrete less salt in their urine. The pathophysiology of primary hypertension is summarized in Figure 30-6.

The SNS contributes to the pathogenesis of hypertension in many persons. In the healthy individual, the SNS contributes to the maintenance of adequate blood pressure and tissue perfusion by promoting cardiac contractility and heart rate (maintenance of adequate cardiac output) and by inducing arteriolar vasoconstriction (maintenance of adequate peripheral resistance). In individuals with hypertension, overactivity of the SNS can result from increased production of catecholamines (epinephrine and norepinephrine) or from increased receptor reactivity involving these neurotransmitters. Increased SNS activity causes increased heart rate and systemic vasoconstriction, thus raising the blood pressure. Additional mechanisms of SNS-induced hypertension include structural changes in blood vessels (vascular remodeling), renal sodium retention, insulin resistance, increased renin and angiotensin levels, and procoagulant effects.[36,45] The role of the SNS in the pathogenesis of cardiovascular disease is summarized in Figure 30-7.

In the healthy individual, the RAAS provides an important homeostatic mechanism for maintaining adequate blood pressure and therefore tissue perfusion (see Chapter 29). Dysfunction of this system in the hypertensive individual can lead to persistent increases in peripheral resistance and renal salt retention.[46]

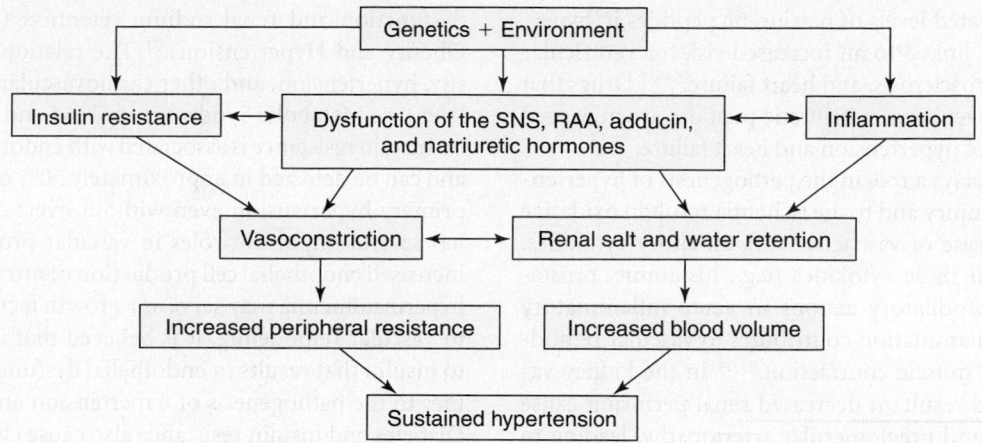

Figure 30-6 **Pathophysiology of hypertension.** Numerous genetic vulnerabilities have been linked to hypertension and these, in combination with environmental risks, cause neurohumoral dysfunction (sympathetic nervous system [SNS], renin-angiotensin-aldosterone system [RAAS], adducin, and natriuretic hormones) and promote inflammation and insulin resistance. Insulin resistance and neurohumoral dysfunction contribute to sustained systemic vasoconstriction and increased peripheral resistance. Inflammation contributes to renal dysfunction, which, in combination with the neurohumoral alterations, results in renal salt and water retention and increased blood volume. Increased peripheral resistance and increased blood volume are two primary causes of sustained hypertension.

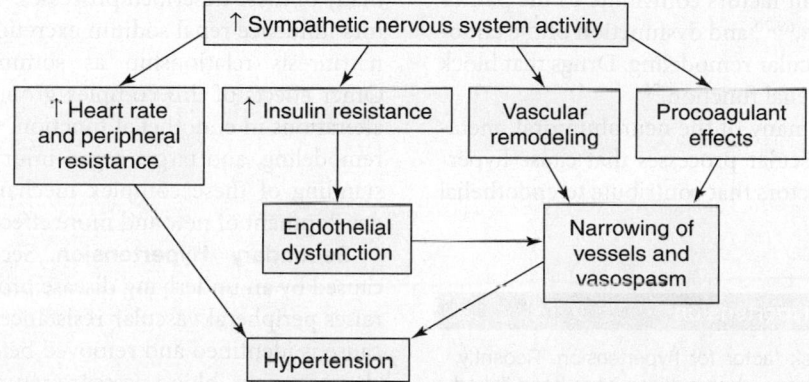

Figure 30-7 **Role of the sympathetic nervous system in the pathogenesis of hypertension.** Increased activity of the sympathetic nervous system (SNS) not only increases heart rate and peripheral resistance but also causes vascular remodeling with narrowing and vasospasm of arteries. The SNS contributes to insulin resistance, which is associated with endothelial dysfunction and decreased production of vasodilators, such as nitric oxide. The SNS also has procoagulant properties, making vascular spasm and thrombosis more likely. All of these factors contribute to sustained increases in blood pressure.

Angiotensin II also causes structural changes in blood vessels (remodeling) that contribute to permanent increases in peripheral resistance and make vessels more vulnerable to endothelial dysfunction and platelet aggregation.[36,46-49] Angiotensin II is also responsible for the hypertrophy of the myocardium and much of the renal damage associated with hypertension.[46,50,51] Aldosterone not only contributes to sodium retention by the kidney but also has further deleterious effects on the cardiovascular system.[52] An important effect of the RAAS is to contribute to insulin resistance.[53] Drugs that block renin, angiotensin-converting enzyme (ACE), or angiotensin and aldosterone receptors are used widely in the treatment of hypertension and have been shown to improve vascular, cardiac, and renal function and insulin sensitivity in select populations.[36,54-56]

Natriuretic peptides modulate renal sodium (Na^+) excretion and include atrial natriuretic peptide (ANP), brain natriuretic peptide (BNP), C-type natriuretic peptide (CNP), and urodilantin.[57,58] The function of these hormones can be affected by excessive sodium intake; inadequate dietary intake of potassium, magnesium, and calcium; and obesity.[41,57] Dysfunction of these hormones, along with alterations in the RAAS and the SNS, cause an increase in vascular tone and a shift in the pressure-natriuresis relationship.[42,47] Salt retention leads to water retention and increased blood volume, which contributes to increased blood pressure. Renal injury can result, with renal vasoconstriction and tissue ischemia. Tissue ischemia causes inflammation of the kidney and contributes to dysfunction of the glomeruli and tubules and promotes additional sodium retention.[43,47] Elevated levels of natriuretic peptides in hypertension have been linked to an increased risk for ventricular hypertrophy, atherosclerosis, and heart failure.[58-62] Drugs that increase the effectiveness of natriuretic peptides are now used for the treatment of hypertension and heart failure.

Inflammation plays a role in the pathogenesis of hypertension. Endothelial injury and tissue ischemia result in oxidative stress and the release of vasoactive inflammatory cytokines. Although many of these cytokines (e.g., histamine, prostaglandins) have vasodilatory actions in acute inflammatory injury, chronic inflammation contributes to vascular remodeling and smooth muscle contraction.[63,64] In the kidney vasoconstriction and resultant decreased renal perfusion cause tubular ischemia and preglomerular arteriopathy, leading to decreased sodium filtration and increased sodium retention, thus shifting the pressure-natriuresis curve and contributing to sustained hypertension.[42,43,47]

Endothelial dysfunction in primary hypertension is characterized by a decreased production of vasodilators, such as nitric oxide, and increased production of vasoconstrictors, such as endothelin (see Chapter 29, Box 29-1).[65-68] Increased expression of adhesion molecules and decreased endothelial production of anticoagulant factors contribute to the pathophysiology of hypertension,[69,70] and dysfunction of the endothelium contributes to vascular remodeling. Drugs that block the RAAS improve endothelial function.[56]

Obesity contributes to many of the neurohumoral, metabolic, renal, and cardiovascular processes that cause hypertension, especially those factors that contribute to endothelial

WHAT'S NEW? Obesity and Hypertension

Obesity is a well-known risk factor for hypertension. Recently, several obesity-related hormone abnormalities have been linked to the development of hypertension. Adipocytes (fat cells) secrete leptin and adiponectin. Leptin's primary function is to interact with the hypothalamus to control body weight and fat deposition through appetite inhibition and increased metabolic rate. However, chronically high levels of leptin associated with obesity result in resistance to these weight-reducing functions and have been found to increase sympathetic nervous system activity, decrease renal sodium excretion, promote inflammation, and stimulate myocyte hypertrophy. Adiponectin is a protein that is produced by adipose tissue but is reduced in obesity. Decreased adiponectin is associated with insulin resistance, decreased endothelial-derived nitric oxide (vasodilator) production, and activation of the sympathetic nervous and renin-angiotensin-aldosterone systems. Taken together, these obesity-related changes result in vasoconstriction, salt and water retention, and renal dysfunction that may contribute to the development of hypertension. Further studies aimed at achieving a better understanding of these mechanisms may lead to new treatments for obesity-related hypertension.

Data from Beltowski J: *J Hypertens* 24(5) 789-801, 2006; Boban M et al: *Am J Med Sci* 334(1)23-30, 2007; Biaggioni I: *Hypertension* 51(2):168-171, 2008; Campia B et al: *Am J Cardiol* 101(7):980-985, 2008; Karthikeyan VJ et al: *J Hum Hypertens* 21:8-11, 2007; Morris MJ: *Clin Exp Pharm Phys* 35:416-419, 2008; Patel JV et al: *J Hum Hypertens* 21(1):1-4, 2007; Wang ZV: *Hypertension* 5:8-14, 2008.

dysfunction and renal sodium retention (see What's New? Obesity and Hypertension).[71] The relationship among obesity, hypertension, and other cardiovascular risks is discussed later (see Metabolic Syndrome, p. 1164 and Chapter 21).

Insulin resistance is associated with endothelial dysfunction and can be detected in approximately 50% of individuals with primary hypertension even without overt diabetes.[53] Insulin has several important roles in vascular protection including increased endothelial cell production of nitric oxide. Although hyperinsulinemia may serve as a growth factor and contribute to vascular remodeling, it is believed that it is the resistance to insulin that results in endothelial dysfunction and contributes to the pathogenesis of hypertension and atherosclerosis. Diabetes and insulin resistance also cause changes in SNS and RAAS activity, cause renal glomerular dysfunction, and contribute to the target organ effects of hypertension.[53,72-74] It is interesting to note that blood pressure often declines in many diabetic individuals treated with drugs that increase insulin sensitivity, even in the absence of antihypertensive drugs, and insulin sensitivity improves in hypertensive individuals treated with drugs that inhibit the RAAS.[53,75]

Primary hypertension is the result of an interaction between many of these described processes. The majority of these factors influence renal sodium excretion and shift the pressure-natriuresis relationship as summarized in Figure 30-8. Other effects of this complex group of mechanisms include alterations in endothelial function, vasomotor tone, vascular remodeling, and target organ injury. Our increasing understanding of these complex mechanisms contributes to the development of new and more effective treatments.

Secondary Hypertension. Secondary hypertension is caused by an underlying disease process or a medication that raises peripheral vascular resistance or cardiac output. If the cause is identified and removed before permanent structural changes occur, blood pressure returns to normal. Table 30-3 summarizes the pathogenesis of major forms of secondary hypertension.

Complicated Hypertension. Chronic hypertension damages the walls of systemic blood vessels. Within the walls of arteries and arterioles, smooth muscle cells undergo hypertrophy and hyperplasia with associated fibrosis of the tunica intima and media in a process called vascular "remodeling" (Figure 30-9). Endothelial dysfunction, angiotensin II, catecholamines, insulin resistance, and inflammation contribute to this process. Once significant fibrosis has occurred, reduced blood flow and dysfunction of the organs perfused by these affected vessels is inevitable. Target organs for hypertension include the kidney, brain, heart, extremities, and eyes—these effects are summarized in Table 30-4.

Cardiovascular complications include left ventricular hypertrophy, angina pectoris, congestive heart failure (left heart failure), coronary artery disease, myocardial infarction, and sudden death. Myocardial hypertrophy in response to hypertension is mediated by several neurohormonal substances, including the SNS and angiotensin II. This results in changes in the myocyte proteins, apoptosis of myocytes, and deposition of collagen into

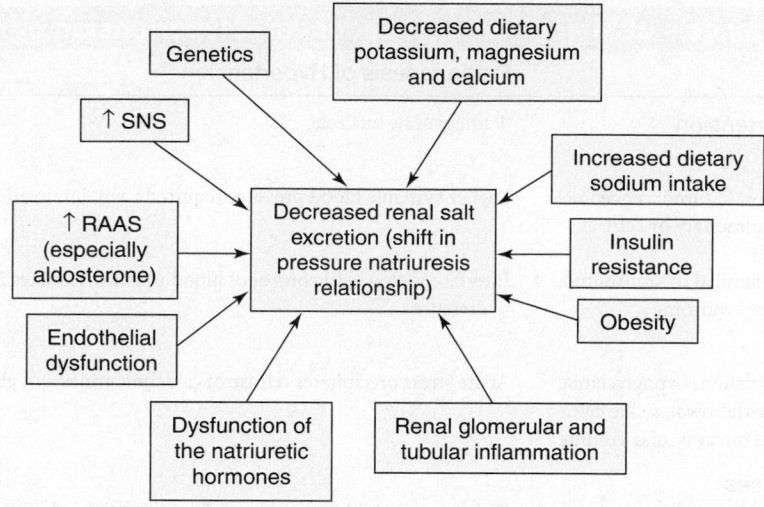

Figure 30-8 **Shift in the pressure-natriuresis relationship.** Numerous factors have been implicated in the pathogenesis of sodium retention in individuals with hypertension. These factors cause less renal excretion of salt than would normally occur with increased blood pressure. This is called a *shift in the pressure-natriuresis relationship* and is believed to be a central process in the pathogenesis of primary hypertension. *RAAS,* Renin-angiotensin-aldosterone system; *SNS,* sympathetic nervous system.

Table 30-3	Pathogenesis of Major Forms of Secondary Hypertension by Cause
Primary Disease	**Pathogenesis of Hypertension**
Renal Disorders	
Renal parenchymal disease	Disturbances in filtration and reabsorption of serum sodium, potassium, and calcium initiate the hemodynamics of early hypertension
Renovascular disease	Impaired blood flow and renal ischemia invoke the compensatory renin-angiotensin-aldosterone mechanism in an effort to raise the renal perfusion pressure
Renin-producing tumors	Elevated blood renin levels invoke elevations in angiotensin and aldosterone, which causes blood pressure to rise
Renal failure	Disturbances in filtration and reabsorption of serum sodium, potassium, and calcium initiate the hemodynamics of early hypertension
Primary sodium retention	Disturbance in filtration and/or reabsorption of serum sodium initiates the hemodynamics of early hypertension
Endocrine Disorders	
Acromegaly	Excess human growth hormone causes increased peripheral resistance
Hypothyroidism	Mucopolysaccharide deposits in vascular tissue increase resistance
Hypercalcemia	Calcium ion directly affects vascular tonicity; elevated serum calcium levels increase vascular tone and peripheral resistance
Hyperthyroidism	Increased inotropic effect on the heart elevates systolic pressure; diastolic pressure decreases as a result of decreased peripheral resistance
Adrenal disorders	Glucocorticoids facilitate sodium and water retention, initiating the hemodynamics of early hypertension
Cortical disturbances	
Cushing syndrome	
Primary aldosteronism	Excess aldosterone promotes sodium retention and initiation of the hemodynamics of early hypertension
Congenital adrenal hyperplasia	Excess production of adrenocortical hormones promotes sodium and water retention
Medullary disturbance: pheochromocytoma	Excess catecholamines raise vascular tone and increase peripheral resistance
Extra-adrenal chromaffin tumors	Excess catecholamines raise vascular tone and increase peripheral resistance
Vascular Disorders	
Coarctation of the aorta	Decreased blood flow in distal areas initiates maximum peripheral resistance as an autoregulatory effort to adjust perfusion pressure
Arteriosclerosis	Loss of elasticity in vessel walls results in increased peripheral resistance

Continued

Table 30-3   Pathogenesis of Major Forms of Secondary Hypertension by Cause—cont'd

Primary Disease	Pathogenesis of Hypertension
Pregnancy-Induced Hypertension	Pathogenesis unclear
Neurologic Disorders	
Elevated intracranial pressure (brain tumor, encephalitis, respiratory acidosis of pulmonary or central nervous system [CNS] origin)	Higher systemic blood pressure required to maintain adequate cerebral perfusion
Quadriplegia, acute porphyria, familial dysautonomia, lead poisoning, Guillain-Barré syndrome	Interface with neural control of blood pressure initiates increased systemic blood pressure
Acute Stress	
Surgery, psychogenic hyperventilation, hypoglycemia, burns, pancreatitis, alcohol withdrawal, sickle cell crisis, resuscitation, increased intravascular volume	Acute stress precipitates release of catecholamines and glucocorticoids
Drugs and Other Substances	
Oral contraceptives and estrogen	Unknown; possibly caused by sodium retention, plasma retention, weight gain, changes in levels and actions of renin, angiotensin, and aldosterone
Corticosteroids	Same as for Cushing disease
Sympathetic stimulants, appetite suppressants, antihistamines	Raises vascular tone and increases vascular resistance
Licorice	Contains glycerrhizic acid, a mineralocorticoid that causes salt and water retention
Monoamine oxidase inhibitors	Hypertension may develop in an individual who routinely takes a monoamine oxidase (MAO) inhibitor with ingestion of a food containing tyramine, such as aged cheese

From Kaplan NM: *Clinical hypertension*, ed 8, Baltimore, 2002, Lippincott Williams & Wilkins; Cheng J et al: Unclear is the role of viral infections, for example, recent data reveal CMV causes an increase in blood pressure, *PLoS Pathog* May 5(5), 2009. Epub ahead of print.

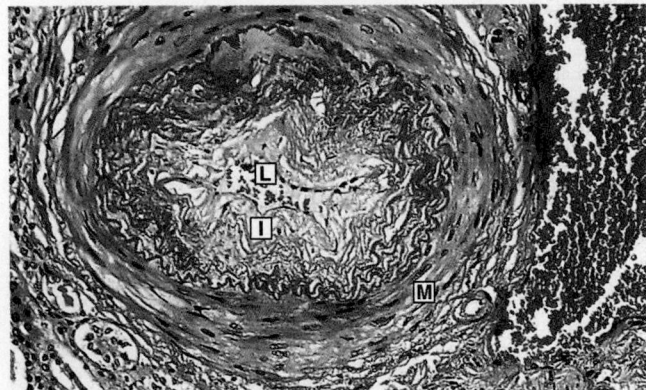

Figure 30-9 Dramatic hypertension change in small arterioles. Fibrous intimal proliferation *(I)* with reduction in lumen vessel caliber (radius) *(L)* and normal media *(M)*. (From Stevens A, Lowe J: *Pathology*, ed 2, St Louis, 2000, Mosby.)

the heart muscle. In addition, the increased size of the heart muscle increases demand for coronary perfusion, such that over time contractility of the heart is impaired and the individual is at increased risk for heart failure. Vascular complications include the formation, dissection, and rupture of aneurysms (outpouchings in vessel walls); intermittent claudication; and gangrene resulting from vessel occlusion. Renal complications are parenchymal damage, nephrosclerosis, renal arteriosclerosis, and renal insufficiency or failure.[51] Microalbuminuria (small amounts of protein in the urine) is an early sign of impending renal dysfunction and significantly increased risk for cardiovascular events.[51,76]

Changes in the vascular beds can be estimated by viewing the arterioles of the retina. Complications specific to the retina include retinal vascular sclerosis, exudation, and hemorrhage. Cerebrovascular complications are similar to those of other arterial beds and include transient ischemia, stroke, cerebral thrombosis, aneurysm, and hemorrhage. Chronic hypertension also has been linked to cognitive decline in older adults.[77]

Malignant hypertension (rapidly progressive hypertension in which diastolic pressure is usually above 140 mmHg) has been linked to dysfunction of renin and angiotensin genes and can cause encephalopathy, a profound cerebral edema that disrupts cerebral function and causes loss of consciousness.[78] Encephalopathy occurs because high arterial pressure renders the cerebral arterioles incapable of regulating blood flow to the cerebral capillary beds. Capillary permeability is increased by high hydrostatic pressures in the capillaries, and vascular fluid exudes into the interstitial space.[78] If blood pressure is not reduced, cerebral edema and cerebral dysfunction increase until death occurs. Organ damage resulting from malignant hypertension is life threatening. Besides encephalopathy, malignant hypertension can cause papilledema, cardiac failure, uremia, retinopathy, and cerebrovascular accident. This should be considered a hypertensive emergency and managed with rapid administration of parenteral vasodilators, such as nitrates or beta-blockers, with the goal of lowering the blood pressure by 10% to 25% within 2 hours.[79]

CLINICAL MANIFESTATIONS The early stages of hypertension have no clinical manifestations other than

Table 30-4	Pathologic Effects of Sustained, Complicated Primary Hypertension	
Site of Injury	**Mechanism of Injury**	**Potential Pathologic Effect**
Heart		
Myocardium	Increased workload combined with diminished blood flow through coronary arteries	Left ventricular hypertrophy, myocardial ischemia, left heart failure
Coronary arteries	Accelerated atherosclerosis (coronary artery disease)	Myocardial ischemia, myocardial infarction, sudden death
Aorta	Weakened vessel wall	Aneurysms, acute aortic syndromes (see p. 1144)
Kidneys	Renin and aldosterone secretion stimulated by reduced blood flow	Retention of sodium and water, leading to increased blood volume and perpetuation of hypertension
	Inflammation and ischemia	Tissue damage that compromises filtration
	High pressures in renal arterioles	Nephrosclerosis leading to renal failure
Brain	Reduced blood flow and oxygen supply; weakened vessel walls, accelerated atherosclerosis	Transient ischemic attacks, cerebral thrombosis, aneurysm, hemorrhage, acute brain infarction
Eyes (retinas)	Reduced blood flow	Retinal vascular sclerosis
	High arteriolar pressure	Exudation, hemorrhage
Arterial vessels of lower extremities	Reduced blood flow and high pressures in arterioles, accelerated atherosclerosis	Intermittent claudication, arterial thrombosis, gangrene

elevated blood pressure. Most important, no signs and symptoms cause the individual to seek healthcare; thus hypertension is called a **lanthanic (silent) disease.** Some hypertensive individuals never have signs, symptoms, or complications, whereas others become very ill, in which case hypertension can cause death. Still others have anatomic and physiologic damage caused by past hypertensive disease despite having current blood pressures within normal ranges.

The chance of developing primary hypertension increases with age, over and above the natural rise in blood pressure associated with aging. Although hypertension usually is thought to be an adult health problem, it is important to remember that hypertension does occur in children and is being diagnosed with increasing frequency. Usually, however, increased peripheral resistance and early hypertension develop in the second, third, and fourth decades of life. If elevated blood pressure is not detected and treated, it becomes established and may begin to accelerate its effect on tissues when the individual is 30 to 50 years of age. This sets the stage for the complications of hypertension that begin to appear during the fourth, fifth, and sixth decades of life.

The clinical manifestations of chronic hypertension tend to be specific for the organs or tissues affected. Evidence of heart disease, renal insufficiency, central nervous system dysfunction, impaired vision, impaired mobility, vascular occlusion, or edema can be caused by sustained hypertension. (See appropriate chapters for specific clinical manifestations of organ dysfunction.)

EVALUATION AND TREATMENT A single elevated blood pressure reading does not mean that a person has hypertension. Diagnosis requires the measurement of blood pressure on at least two separate occasions averaging two readings at least 2 minutes apart, with the individual seated, the arm supported at heart level, after 5 minutes rest, with no smoking or caffeine intake in the past 30 minutes.[36] The American Heart Association updated recommendations for the diagnosis of hypertension in 2005 to include 24-hour ambulatory blood pressure monitoring in selected individuals because of better correlation with end-organ damage and the ability to screen out "white coat hypertension (HTN)" (elevated blood pressure that occurs only in a clinic setting).[80,81] Ambulatory measurement also detects those who fail to have a nocturnal decrease in blood pressure and who may be at higher cardiovascular risk. It is especially recommended for individuals with drug resistance, hypotensive symptoms with medications, episodic HTN, and autonomic dysfunction.[81] Home blood pressure monitoring with approved devices can help manage hypertension.

Evaluation of the hypertensive individual should include a complete medical history and assessment of lifestyle and other risk factors for hypertension and cardiovascular disease, as well as evidence of possible secondary causes of hypertension. Physical examination should include examination of the optic fundi; calculation of body mass index; auscultation for carotid, abdominal, and femoral bruits; examination of the heart and lungs; palpation of the abdomen; assessment of lower extremity pulses and edema; and neurologic examination.[36] Further routine diagnostic tests for the evaluation of hypertension include hematocrit, urinalysis, biochemical blood profile (fasting glucose, sodium, potassium, calcium, creatinine, total cholesterol, high-density cholesterol, triglycerides), and an electrocardiogram (ECG). Optional tests include urinary albumin excretion or albumin/creatinine ratio.[36] Individuals who have elevated blood pressure are assumed to have primary hypertension unless their history, physical examination, or initial diagnostic screening indicates secondary hypertension.

Treatment of primary hypertension depends on its severity. Figure 30-10 illustrates an overview of the JNC7 recommendations.[37] Treatment begins with reducing or eliminating risk factors. Lifestyle modification can prevent hypertension from developing in those individuals who fall into the prehypertension category, may control the blood pressure in stage I hypertension, and can enhance the effects of drug treatment for those with more significant blood pressure elevation. The usual dietary recommendations are to restrict sodium intake to 2.4 g/day, to

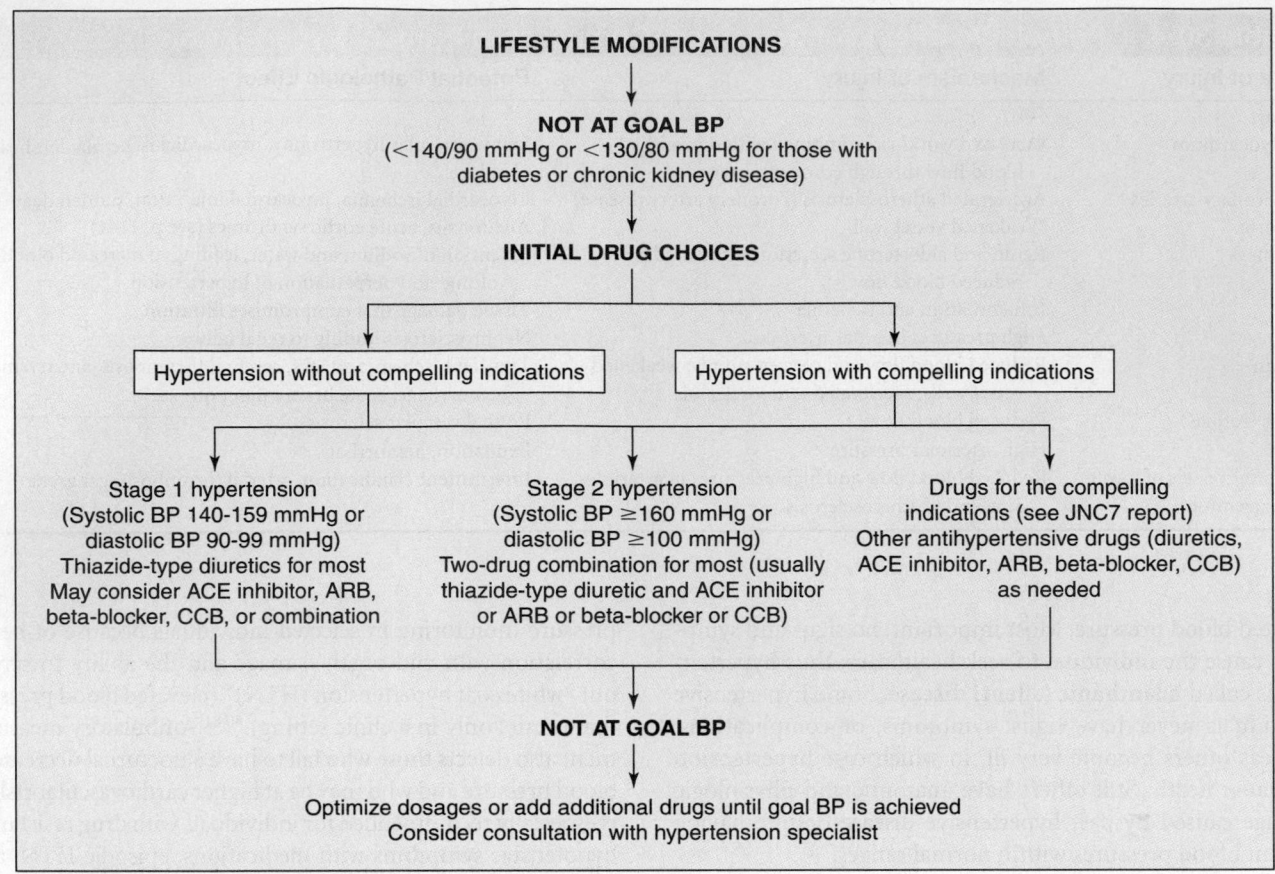

Figure 30-10 Summary of treatment for hypertension. *ACE,* Angiotensin-converting enzyme; *ARB,* angiotensin-receptor blocker; *BP,* blood pressure; *CCB,* calcium channel blocker. (Data from Chobanian AV et al: The Seventh Report of the Joint National Committee on Prevention, Detection, Evaluation, and Treatment of High Blood Pressure, *JAMA* 289:2560-2572, 2003.)

increase potassium intake, to restrict saturated fat intake, and to adjust calorie intake as required to maintain optimum weight. The Dietary Approaches to Stop Hypertension (DASH) diet is recommended. An exercise program that promotes endurance and relaxation usually is recommended. Physical training increases stroke volume, which has the effect of lowering heart rate and hence systolic blood pressure, and should consist of regular aerobic physical activity at least 30 minutes most days of the week.[37] Relaxation is expected to reduce levels of circulating catecholamines, which has the effect of reducing vascular tone and blood pressure. Individuals are counseled to stop smoking to eliminate vasoconstrictor effects of nicotine.

Pharmacologic treatment of hypertension reduces the risk of end-organ damage and prevents major diseases, such as myocardial ischemia and stroke. Thiazide diuretics have been shown to be the safest and most effective medications for lowering blood pressure and preventing the cardiovascular complications of hypertension.[37] Some individuals will have "compelling indications" for choosing a particular antihypertensive as a first-line medication. For example, individuals with heart failure, with chronic kidney disease, or who are post–myocardial infarction, or who have had recurrent stroke should begin antihypertensive treatment with an ACE inhibitor, angiotensin receptor blocker (ARB), or aldosterone

antagonist.[37,82] If the individual requires two drugs for blood pressure control, the recommendation is combinations of thiazide diuretics and other antihypertensives, such as beta blockers and ACE inhibitors.

Orthostatic (Postural) Hypotension

The term **orthostatic (postural) hypotension** means a decrease in systolic and diastolic arterial blood pressure on standing. The American Autonomic Society (AAS) and the American Academy of Neurology (AAN) define orthostatic hypertension as a systolic blood pressure decrease of at least 20 mmHg or a diastolic blood pressure decrease of at least 10 mmHg within 3 minutes of standing up.[83] It can be categorized as arteriolar, venular, or mixed.[84] When a normal individual stands up, the resultant gravitational changes on the circulation are compensated for by several mechanisms that include reflex arteriolar and venous constriction, increased heart rate, and mechanical factors, such as the closure of valves in the venous system, pumping of the leg muscles, and a decrease in intrathoracic pressure. The normally increased sympathetic activity during upright posture is mediated through stretch receptors (baroreceptors) in the carotid sinus and the aortic arch (see Chapter 29). Their reflex response to shifts in volume caused by postural changes leads to a prompt increase in heart rate and constriction of the systemic arterioles, which maintains a stable blood pressure. These compensatory mechanisms are not effective in maintaining a stable blood pressure in individuals with orthostatic hypotension.

Orthostatic hypotension may be acute and temporary or chronic. **Acute orthostatic hypotension,** or temporary type, is caused when the normal regulatory mechanisms are sluggish. This delay may be the result of (1) anatomic variation, (2) altered body chemistry, (3) drug action (e.g., antihypertensives or antidepressants), (4) prolonged immobility caused by illness, (5) starvation, (6) physical exhaustion, (7) any condition that produces volume depletion (e.g., massive diuresis, potassium or sodium depletion), and (8) venous pooling (e.g., pregnancy, extensive varicosities of the lower extremities). Older adults are susceptible to this type of orthostatic hypotension, in which postural reflexes are slowed as part of the aging process.

The two forms of **chronic orthostatic hypotension** are (1) secondary to a specific disease and (2) idiopathic or primary. The diseases that cause secondary orthostatic hypotension are endocrine disorders (e.g., adrenal insufficiency, diabetes mellitus), metabolic disorders (e.g., porphyria), or diseases of the central or peripheral nervous system (e.g., intracranial tumors, cerebral infarcts, Wernicke encephalopathy, peripheral neuropathies). Cardiovascular autonomic neuropathy is a common cause of orthostatic hypotension in diabetes and is a serious and often overlooked complication.

Idiopathic, or primary, orthostatic hypotension is the term for hypotension in which there is no known initial cause. It affects men more often than women and usually occurs between the ages of 40 and 70 years. Up to 18% of the older adult population may be affected by chronic orthostatic hypotension.[84] It is a significant risk factor for falls and associated injuries and has been associated with an increased risk for cardiovascular events. In addition to cardiovascular symptoms, impotence and bowel and bladder dysfunction often are found in this type. Orthostatic hypotension is also a feature of multiple system atrophy (MSA), in which there are multiple central nervous system degenerative changes.

Orthostatic hypotension often is accompanied by dizziness, blurring or loss of vision, and syncope or fainting. To assess hypotensive episode frequency, severity, and correlation with symptoms, 24-hour blood pressure monitoring is recommended.[85] No curative treatment is available for idiopathic orthostatic hypertension. In the secondary form, syncope ceases when the underlying disorder is corrected. Several treatments can help acute and chronic orthostatic hypotension, including liberalization of salt intake, raising the head of the bed, thigh-high stockings, volume expansion with mineralocorticoids, and vasoconstrictors such as midodrine.[84]

Atherosclerosis

Atherosclerosis is a form of arteriosclerosis in which thickening and hardening of the vessel are caused by the accumulation of lipid-laden macrophages within the arterial wall, which leads to the formation of a lesion called a **plaque.** Atherosclerosis is not a single disease but rather a pathologic process that can affect vascular systems throughout the body, resulting in ischemic syndromes that can vary widely in their severity and clinical manifestations. It is the leading contributor to coronary artery and cerebrovascular disease. (Atherosclerosis of the coronary arteries is described on p. 1160; atherosclerosis of the cerebral arteries is discussed in Chapter 17.)

PATHOPHYSIOLOGY Although there remains considerable controversy as to the pathophysiology of atherosclerosis and many questions remain to be answered, the most widely accepted theories of the mechanisms of atherosclerosis are based on the finding that atherosclerosis is an inflammatory disease.[86,87] Pathologically, the lesions progress from endothelial injury and dysfunction to fatty streak to fibrotic plaque to complicated lesion (Figures 30-11 and 30-12). Atherosclerosis begins with injury to the endothelial cells that line artery walls.[86-88] Possible causes of endothelial injury include the common risk factors for atherosclerosis, such as smoking, hypertension, diabetes, increased levels of low-density lipoprotein (LDL), decreased levels of high-density lipoprotein (HDL), and autoimmunity. Other causes of endothelial injury are called the nontraditional risk factors, such as elevated CRP, increased serum fibrinogen, insulin resistance, oxidative stress, infection, and periodontal disease. These risk factors are discussed in more detail in the following section on coronary artery disease (see p. 1160). Recent evidence indicates that individuals with a defect in the production of precursor endothelial cells in the bone marrow are at greater risk for atherosclerotic disease because these precursor cells are not available to repair injured endothelium.[89]

Once injury has occurred, endothelial dysfunction and inflammation lead to the following pathophysiologic events:

1. Injured endothelial cells become inflamed and cannot make normal amounts of antithrombotic and vasodilating cytokines[90-92] (see Figure 29-29).
2. Numerous inflammatory cytokines are released, including tumor necrosis factor-alpha (TNF-α), interferon-gamma (IFN-γ), interleukin-1 (IL-1), toxic oxygen radicals, and heat shock proteins.[86-88]
3. Macrophages adhere to injured endothelium by way of adhesion molecules, such as vascular cell adhesion molecule-1 (VCAM-1).[86-88]
4. These macrophages then release enzymes and toxic oxygen radicals that create oxidative stress, oxidize LDL, and further injure the vessel wall.[86-88,93]
5. Growth factors also are released, including angiotensin II, fibroblast growth factor, and platelet-derived growth factor, which stimulate smooth muscle cell proliferation in the affected vessel.[86-88,94]

The oxidation of LDL is an important step in atherogenesis. Inflammation with oxidative stress and activation of macrophages is the primary mechanism.[86,93] Diabetes, smoking, and hypertension (especially with increased levels of angiotensin II) are associated with increased LDL oxidation. Oxidized LDL is toxic to endothelial cells, causes smooth muscle proliferation, and activates further immune and inflammatory responses.[86-88,95] The oxidized LDL penetrates into the

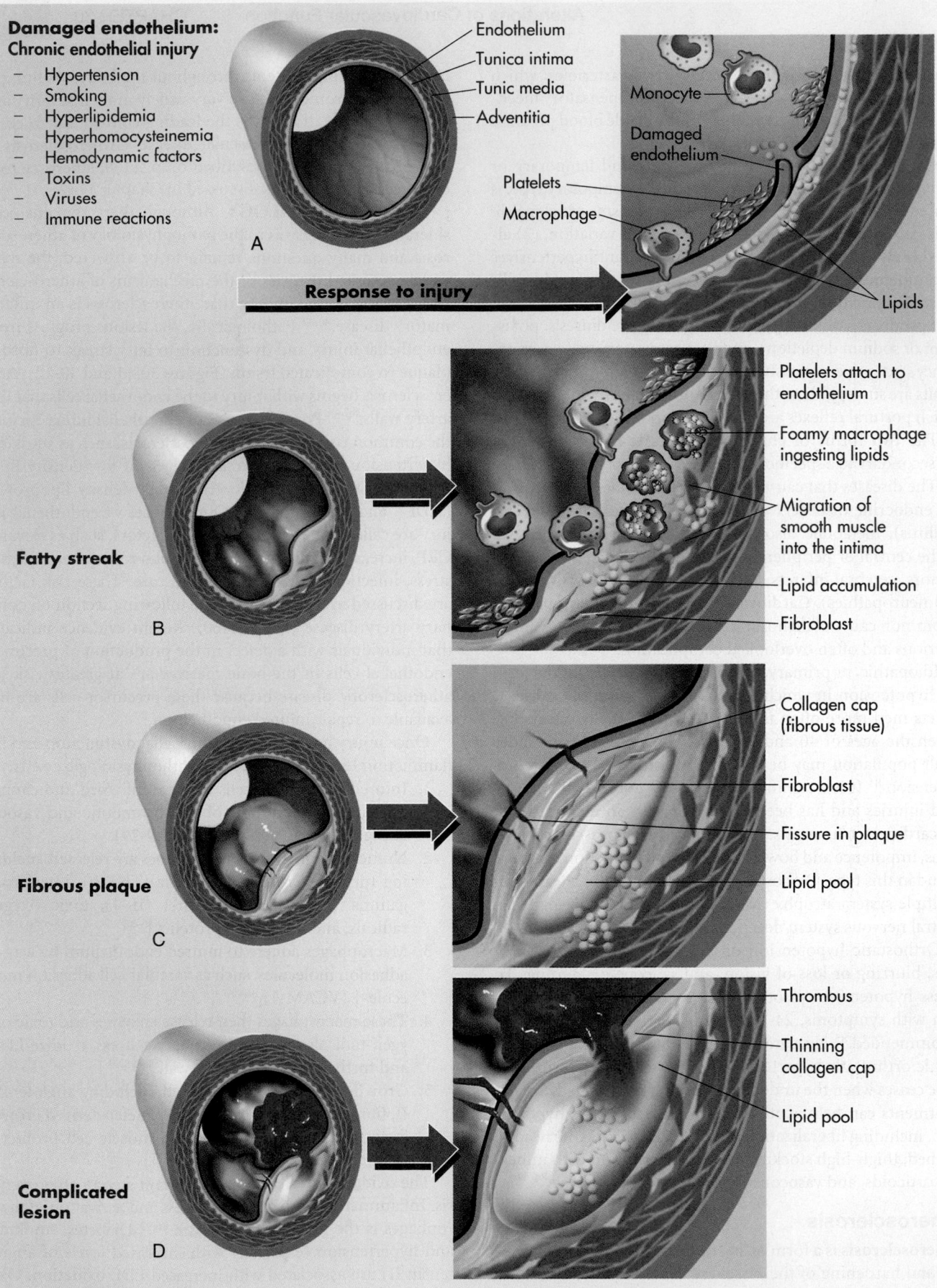

Figure 30-11 Progression of atherosclerosis. *A,* Damaged endothelium. *B,* Diagram of fatty streak and lipid core formation (see Figure 30-12 for a diagram of oxidized low-density lipoprotein [LDL]). *C,* Diagram of fibrous plaque. Raised plaques are visible: some are yellow; others are white. *D,* Diagram of complicated lesion; thrombus is red; collagen is blue. Plaque is complicated by red thrombus deposition.

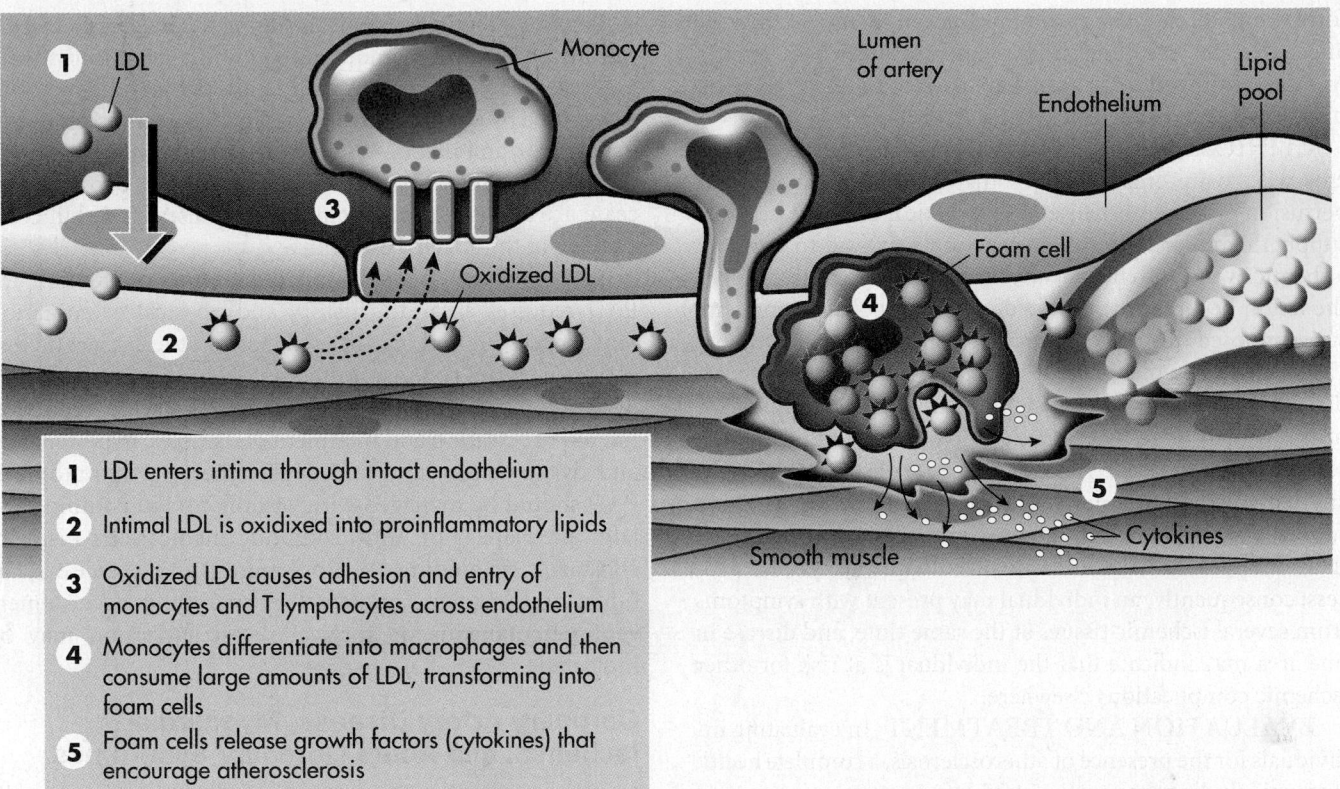

1 LDL enters intima through intact endothelium

2 Intimal LDL is oxidixed into proinflammatory lipids

3 Oxidized LDL causes adhesion and entry of
   monocytes and T lymphocytes across endothelium

4 Monocytes differentiate into macrophages and then
   consume large amounts of LDL, transforming into
   foam cells

5 Foam cells release growth factors (cytokines) that
   encourage atherosclerosis

Figure 30-12 Low-density lipoprotein oxidation. (1) Low-density lipoprotein (LDL) enters the arterial intima through an intact endothelium. In hypercholesterolemia, the influx of LDL exceeds the eliminating capacity and an extracellular pool of LDL is formed. This is enhanced by association of LDL with the extracellular matrix. (2) Intimal LDL is oxidized through the action of free oxygen radicals formed by enzymatic or nonenzymatic reactions. (3) This generates proinflammatory lipids that induce endothelial expression of the adhesion molecule; vascular cell adhesion molecule-1 activates complement and stimulates chemokine secretion. All of these factors cause adhesion and entry of mononuclear leukocytes, particularly monocytes and T lymphocytes. (4) Monocytes differentiate into macrophages. Macrophages up-regulate and internalize oxidized LDL and transform into foam cells. Macrophage update of oxidized LDL also leads to presentation of fragments of it to antigen-specific T cells. (5) This induces an autoimmune reaction that leads to production of proinflammatory cytokines. Such cytokines include interferon-γ, tumor necrosis factor-α, and interleukin-1, which act on endothelial cells to stimulate expression of adhesion molecules and procoagulant activity; on macrophages to activate proteases, endocytosis, nitric oxide (NO), and cytokines; and on smooth muscle cells *(SMCs)* to include NO production and inhibit growth, collagen, and actin expression. (Modified from Crawford MH, DiMarco JP, editors: *Cardiology,* London, 2001, Mosby-Wolfe.)

intima of the arterial wall and is engulfed by macrophages. Macrophages filled with oxidized LDL are called **foam cells** (see Figure 30-12).

Once these lipid-laden foam cells accumulate in significant amounts, they form a lesion called a **fatty streak** (see Figure 30-11). These lesions can be found in the walls of arteries of most people, even young children. Once formed, fatty streaks produce more toxic oxygen radicals and cause immunologic and inflammatory changes, resulting in progressive damage to the vessel wall. Decreasing levels of LDL can cause regression of atherosclerotic lesions and can improve endothelial function. Increasing attention is being given to the evaluation of children for dyslipidemia so that early dietary intervention to prevent atherosclerosis can be initiated.

At this point, smooth muscle cells proliferate, produce collagen, and migrate over the fatty streak forming a **fibrous**

plaque (see Figure 30-11). This process is mediated by many inflammatory cytokines, including growth factors (e.g., transforming growth factor-beta [TGF-β]).[96] The fibrous plaque may calcify, protrude into the vessel lumen, and obstruct blood flow to distal tissues, especially during exercise, which may cause symptoms (e.g., angina or intermittent claudication).

Many plaques, however, are "unstable," meaning they are prone to rupture even before they affect blood flow significantly, and are clinically silent until they rupture. Plaque rupture occurs because of the inflammatory activation of proteinases, such as the matrix metalloproteinases and the cathepsins, and can be accelerated by bleeding within the lesion (plaque hemorrhage).[97,98] Plaques that have ruptured are called **complicated plaques** (see Figure 30-11). Once rupture occurs, exposure of underlying tissue results in platelet adhesion, initiation of the clotting cascade, and rapid thrombus formation.[86,87,91,92] The thrombus may suddenly occlude the affected vessel, resulting in ischemia and infarction. Aspirin or other antithrombotic agents are used to prevent this complication of atherosclerotic disease.[99]

CLINICAL MANIFESTATIONS Atherosclerosis presents with symptoms and signs that result from inadequate perfusion of tissues because of obstruction of the vessels that supply them. Partial vessel obstruction may lead to transient ischemic events, often associated with exercise or stress. Once the lesion becomes complicated, increasing obstruction with superimposed thrombosis may result in tissue infarction. CAD caused by atherosclerosis is the major cause of myocardial ischemia and is one of the most important health issues in the United States. Atherosclerotic obstruction of the vessels supplying the brain is the major cause of stroke. Similarly, any part of the body may become ischemic when its blood supply is compromised by atherosclerotic lesions. Often more than one vessel will become involved with this disease process; consequently, an individual may present with symptoms from several ischemic tissues at the same time, and disease in one area may indicate that the individual is at risk for other ischemic complications elsewhere.

EVALUATION AND TREATMENT In evaluating individuals for the presence of atherosclerosis, a complete health history including the presence of risk factors and symptoms of cardiovascular disease is essential. Physical examination may detect arterial bruits and evidence of decreased blood flow to tissues. Serum should be tested for risk indicators, such as lipid profile and the highly sensitive C-reactive protein (hs-CRP). If coronary disease is suspected, evaluation of plaques in affected vessels can include roentgenography, electrocardiography, intravascular ultrasonography, CT, MRI, nuclear scanning, and angiography.[100-102]

Current management of atherosclerosis includes detection of "preclinical" lesion treatment with drugs aimed at stabilizing plaques before they rupture.[101,102] Once a lesion obstructs blood flow, the primary goal of management is to restore adequate flow to affected tissues. In situations in which the disease process does not require immediate intervention, management focuses on the reduction of risks to prevent continued endothelial injury and the prevention of plaque progression. Risk reduction includes smoking cessation, weight loss, and the control of hypertension, diabetes, and dyslipidemia through diet, exercise, and medication. Management of atherosclerotic risk factors is discussed further starting on p. 1161. If an individual presents with acute ischemia, such as myocardial infarction (MI) or stroke, interventions are specific to the diseased area (see Myocardial Infarction on p. 1191; see Stroke on p. 600).

Peripheral Artery Disease

Peripheral artery disease (PAD) refers to atherosclerotic disease of arteries that perfuse the limbs, especially the lower extremities. It is estimated that 12 million people in the United States have significant PAD.[36] The risk factors for PAD are the same as those for atherosclerotic disease, and it is especially prevalent in individuals with diabetes.

Lower-extremity ischemia, resulting from arterial obstruction in PAD, can be gradual or acute. In most individuals, gradually increasing obstruction to arterial blood flow to the legs caused by atherosclerosis in the iliofemoral vessels results in pain with ambulation called **intermittent claudication.** If a thrombus forms over the atherosclerotic lesion, perfusion can cease acutely with severe pain, loss of pulses, and skin color changes in the affected extremity.

PAD is often asymptomatic; therefore, evaluation for PAD requires a careful history and physical examination that focuses on looking for evidence of atherosclerotic disease (e.g., bruits) and noninvasive Doppler measurement of blood flow. Treatment includes risk factor reduction (smoking cessation and treatment of diabetes, hypertension, and dyslipidemia) and antiplatelet therapy. Symptomatic PAD should be managed with vasodilators in combination with antiplatelet or antithrombotic medications (aspirin, cilostazol, ticlopidine, or clopidogrel) and exercise rehabilitation.[103] If acute or refractory symptoms occur, emergent percutaneous or surgical revascularization may be indicated.

Coronary Artery Disease, Myocardial Ischemia, and Acute Coronary Syndromes

Coronary artery disease, myocardial ischemia, and myocardial infarction form a pathophysiologic continuum that impairs the pumping ability of the heart by depriving the heart muscle of blood-borne oxygen and nutrients. The earliest lesions of the continuum are those of **coronary artery disease (CAD)**—virtually any vascular disorder that narrows or occludes the coronary arteries. By far the most common cause of coronary artery obstruction is atherosclerosis (Figure 30-13). CAD can diminish the myocardial blood supply until deprivation impairs myocardial metabolism enough to cause **ischemia,** a local state in which the cells are temporarily deprived of blood supply. They remain alive but cannot function normally. Persistent ischemia or the complete occlusion of a coronary artery causes **acute coronary syndrome,** including infarction, or irreversible myocardial damage. **Infarction** constitutes the often-fatal event known as a *heart attack.*

Development of Coronary Artery Disease

More than 16 million people in the United States suffer from coronary artery disease—it is estimated that between 770,000 and 1 million people have a heart attack each year.[36] Despite a dramatic decline in mortality in the past decade, CAD causes one third of all deaths in the United States. More than half of men and nearly one third of women older than age 40 will develop CAD.[36] The primary cause of CAD is atherosclerosis of the coronary vessels; therefore, those factors that contribute to the development of atherosclerosis also are risk factors for CAD.

Risk factors for CAD can be categorized as conventional (major) versus nontraditional (novel) and modifiable versus nonmodifiable. Much new information has been obtained about the conventional risk factors that has markedly

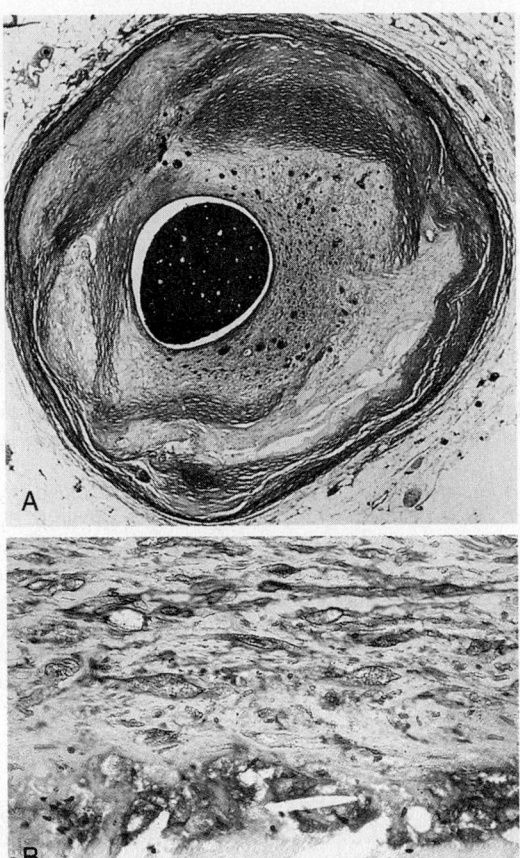

Figure 30-13 Atherosclerosis. **A,** Concentric coronary plaque. The lumen is central. Multiple new small blood vessels are shown within the plaque, the late result of disruption. **B,** Cell types in a fibrolipid plaque. The plaque cap (brownish) contains numerous elongated smooth muscle cells; some contain lipid. Macrophages are clustered on the edge of the core. (From Damjanov I, Linder J, editors: *Anderson's pathology,* ed 10, St Louis, 1996, Mosby.)

WHAT'S NEW? Women and Heart Disease

More women in the United States die from coronary artery disease (CAD) and stroke than from all cancers combined. Women have a higher rate of CAD-related mortality than men, in part because of underdiagnosis and treatment. Nearly two thirds of women who die from CAD had no warning symptoms. When women do have symptoms, they are often different from those classically seen in men. Common symptoms in women may include atypical chest pain, palpitations, sense of unease, weakness, mild discomfort in the back, and severe or sudden fatigue. In addition, they may not have any angina. One theory is that women have more microvascular coronary disease than men, which can cause fewer and less recognizable symptoms.

Women have a higher prevalence of avoidable risk factors than men, especially elevated cholesterol and physical inactivity, and women are less likely to receive counseling about nutrition, exercise, and weight control. CAD risk rises dramatically after menopause. Although many studies suggest that endogenous estrogen is protective of vascular function, several large prospective studies have determined that estrogen replacement regimens do not reduce the risk of CAD in postmenopausal women. In addition to lifestyle changes, the most effective interventions to reduce CAD risk in women have been found to be the 3-hydroxy-3-methylglutaryl-CoA (HMG-CoA) reductase drugs (statins) that lower cholesterol and exert anti-inflammatory and plaque-stabilizing effects. More studies, however, are needed on long-term effects of statins.

Data from Chambers TA et al: *Curr Opin Anaesthesiol* 20(1):75-82, 2007; Collins P: *Int J Cardiol* 124(3):275-282, 2008; D'Antono B et al: *Can J Cardiol* 24(4):285-291, 2008; Kuller LH: *Arterioscler Thromb Vasc Biol* 23(1):11-16, 2003; Morise AP: *Am J Cardiol* 97(3):367-371, 2006; Shaw LJ et al: *J Am Coll Cardiol* 47(Suppl)1s-71s, 2006.

improved prevention and management of CAD. In addition, nontraditional risk factors have been identified in recent years that have provided insight in to the pathogenesis of CAD and may lead to more effective interventions.

Conventional or major risk factors for CAD that are non-modifiable include (1) advanced age, (2) male gender or women after menopause, and (3) family history. Aging is associated with increased vulnerability to endothelial injury and decreased endothelial repair. The risk for CAD increases dramatically in women after menopause (see What's New? Women and Heart Disease). Family history may contribute to the risk for CAD through genetics and shared environmental exposures. Many gene polymorphisms have been identified that are related to the development of atherosclerosis and its many associated underlying risk factors.[104]

Major modifiable conventional risks include (1) dyslipidemia, (2) hypertension, (3) cigarette smoking, (4) diabetes and insulin resistance, (5) obesity, (6) sedentary lifestyle, and (7) an atherogenic diet (see Nutrition & Disease: The Basics on Fats). In individuals with known CAD, the vast majority have the risk factors of smoking, diabetes, dyslipidemia, or hypertension, and many have several of these risks. These traditional risk factors are often poorly controlled and are associated with the growing epidemic of obesity in the United States. If individuals receive appropriate preventive care, modification of these factors can dramatically reduce the risk for CAD.[101,105] Of great concern is a recent finding that exposure to particulate matter air pollution, which is a worsening global problem, can also cause a significant increase in cardiovascular risk.[106]

Dyslipidemia

The strong link between CAD and elevated plasma lipoprotein concentrations is well documented.[107] **Lipoprotein** refers to lipids, phospholipids, cholesterol, and triglycerides bound to carrier proteins. Lipids (cholesterol in particular) are required by most cells for the manufacture and repair of plasma membranes. Cholesterol is also a necessary component for the manufacture of such essential substances as bile acids and steroid hormones. Although cholesterol can easily be obtained from dietary fat intake, most body cells also can manufacture cholesterol.

The cycle of lipid metabolism is complex. Dietary fat is packaged into particles known as **chylomicrons** in the small intestine. Chylomicrons are required for absorption of fat; they function by transporting exogenous lipid from the intestine to the liver and peripheral cells. Chylomicrons are the least dense of the lipoproteins and primarily contain triglyceride.

NUTRITION & DISEASE

The Basics on Fats

Saturated fats are found in animal fats (butter, cheese, beef, pork, lamb, chicken) and some tropical oils (e.g., palm, kernel). Saturated fats consist of a long chain of atoms that take a longer time to burn than shorter-chained fats. The longer the fat takes to burn, the stickier it becomes. Those fats that become stickiest are more conducive to weight gain and heart disease. Healthy saturated fats for cooking include coconut and palm oils; look for extra virgin oils and not refined.

Unsaturated fats consist of two types: monounsaturated and polyunsaturated. Both contain essential fatty acids (EFAs), but polyunsaturated fats have more.

Monounsaturated fats are liquid at room temperature but more solid when refrigerated. They are found in especially high concentration in olive and canola oils that are high in the healthy oleic acid, a common monounsaturated fat. Monounsaturated fats are known to lower low-density lipoproteins (LDL) and raise high-density lipoprotein (HDL) levels. They are more stable in heat than other oils, thus they are often used for stir-frying and baking. Avocados are high in oleic oil. For healthy cooking avoid refined oils and chemically treated oils.

Polyunsaturated fats are liquid at any temperature and are found in vegetable oils, soy, fish, walnuts, pumpkin seeds, and flaxseed oil. They contain omega-6 and omega-3 EFAs in varying ratios. Today people are eating many more omega-6 EFAs than omega-3. Too much omega-6 can contribute to clot formation; omega-3 fats have the opposite effect, so to reduce the risk of heart disease one needs more omega-3 and less omega-6.

Omega-3 EFAs are found in fish oil, flaxseed (and flaxseed oil), canola oil, walnuts, pumpkins, and green leafy vegetables. Soy contains both omega-6 and omega-3. Populations that eat high amounts of omega-3 EFAs have a lower risk of heart disease

Omega-6 EFAs are found in vegetable oils such as corn, safflower, sunflower, cottonseed, peanut, sesame, grape seed, borage, primrose, and soy. Omega-6 EFAs have protective effects only when they are combined with omega-3 EFAs. Many advocate using only cold-pressed: high heat damages these fats.

Trans-fats are primarily found in artificially solidified (hydrogenated) oils (e.g., margarine and vegetable shortening). By becoming more solid they lose EFAs. They can raise LDL and lower HDL levels, and raise lipoprotein-a levels, which increases risk of heart disease. Trans-fats raise blood sugar levels and contribute to more weight gain than the same amount of other fats. "Partially hydrogenated" or "hydrogenated" on a food label means the food contains trans-fatty acids (e.g., cakes, cookies, crackers, processed cheese).

Table 30-5	Criteria for Dyslipidemia						
	Optimal	Near Optimal	Desirable	Low	Borderline	High	Very High
Total cholesterol			<200		200-239	≥240	
LDL	<100	100-129			130-159	160-189	≥190
Triglycerides			<150		150-199	200-499	≥500
HDL				<40		≥60	

Data from Expert Panel on Detection, Evaluation, and Treatment of High Blood Cholesterol in Adults, *JAMA* 285:2486-2497, 2001.

Some of the triglyceride may be removed and either stored by adipose tissue or used by muscle as an energy source. The chylomicron remnants, composed mainly of cholesterol, are taken up by the liver. A series of chemical reactions in the liver results in the production of several lipoproteins that vary in density and function. These include **very-low-density lipoproteins (VLDLs),** primarily triglyceride and protein; **low-density lipoproteins (LDLs),** mostly cholesterol and protein; and **high-density lipoproteins (HDLs),** mainly phospholipids and protein.

Dyslipidemia (or **dyslipoproteinemia**) refers to abnormal concentrations of serum lipoproteins as defined by the Third Report of the National Cholesterol Education Program[107] (Table 30-5). It is estimated that nearly half of the U.S. population has some form of dyslipidemia, especially among white and Asian populations.[36] These abnormalities are the result of a combination of genetic and dietary factors. Primary or familial dyslipoproteinemias result from genetic defects that cause abnormalities in lipid-metabolizing enzymes and abnormal cellular lipid receptors (Table 30-6). Secondary causes of dyslipidemia include several common systemic disorders, such as diabetes, hypothyroidism, pancreatitis, and renal nephrosis, as well as the use of certain medications such as certain diuretics, beta-blockers, glucocorticoids, interferons, and antiretrovirals.[108]

An increased serum concentration of LDL is a strong indicator of coronary risk.[36,108,109] LDL is responsible for the delivery of cholesterol to the tissues. Serum levels of LDL are normally controlled by hepatic receptors for LDL that bind LDL and limit liver synthesis of this lipoprotein. High dietary intake of cholesterol and fats, often in combination with a genetic predisposition to accumulations of LDL in the serum (e.g., dysfunction of the hepatic LDL receptor), results in high levels of LDL in the bloodstream.[108] The term LDL actually describes several types of LDL molecules; the "small dense" LDL particles are the most atherogenic. LDL oxidation, migration into the vessel wall, and phagocytosis by macrophages are key steps in the pathogenesis of atherosclerosis[86-88] (see p. 1157 and Figure 30-12). LDL also plays a role in endothelial injury, inflammation, and immune responses that have been identified as being important in atherogenesis. Aggressive reduction of LDL with diet and cholesterol-lowering drugs, such as the statins and ezetimibe, is associated with a dramatic decrease in risk for CAD.[108-112]

Table 30-6   Familial Dyslipoproteinemias

Name	Laboratory Findings	Clinical Features	Therapy
Type I: exogenous hyper-lipidemia; fat-induced hypertriglyceridemia	Cholesterol normal Triglycerides increased three times Chylomicrons increased	Abdominal pain Hepatosplenomegaly Skin and retinal lipid deposits Usual onset: childhood	Low-fat diet
Type IIa: hypercholesterolemia	Triglycerides normal LDL increased Cholesterol increased	Premature vascular disease Xanthomas of tendons and bony prominences Common Onset: all ages	Low-saturated-fat and low-cholesterol diet Cholestyramine[a] Colestipol[b] Lovastatin[c] Nicotinic acid[d] Neomycin[e] Intestinal bypass
Type IIb: combined hyperli-pidemia; carbohydrate-in-duced hypertriglyceridemia	LDL, VLDL increased Cholesterol increased Triglycerides increased	Same as IIa	Same as IIa; *plus* carbohydrate restriction Clofibrate[f] Gemfibrozil[g] Lovastatin
Type III: dysbetalipoproteine-mia	IDL or chylomicron remnants increased Cholesterol increased Triglycerides increased	Premature vascular disease Xanthomas of tendons and bony prominences Uncommon Onset: adulthood	Weight control Low-carbohydrate, low-saturated-fat, and low-cholesterol diet Alcohol restriction Clofibrate Gemfibrozil Lovastatin Nicotinic acid Estrogens[h] Intestinal bypass
Type IV: endogenous hyperli-pidemia; carbohydrate-in-duced hypertriglyceridemia	Glucose intolerance Hyperuricemia Cholesterol normal or increased VLDL increased Triglycerides increased	Premature vascular disease Skin lipid deposits Obesity Hepatomegaly Common onset: adulthood	Weight control Low-carbohydrate diet Alcohol restriction Clofibrate Nicotinic acid Intestinal bypass
Type V: mixed hyperlipidemia; carbohydrate and fat-in-duced hypertriglyceridemia	Glucose intolerance Hyperuricemia Chylomicrons increased VLDL increased LDL increased Cholesterol increased Triglycerides increased three times	Abdominal pain Hepatosplenomegaly Skin lipid deposits Retinal lipid deposits Onset: childhood	Weight control Low-carbohydrate and low-fat diet Clofibrate Lovastatin Nicotinic acid Progesterone[i] Intestinal bypass

IDL, Intermediate-density lipoprotein; *LDL,* low-density lipoprotein; *VLDL,* very-low-density lipoprotein.

[a]*Cholestyramine* (Questran), anion exchange resin; binds bile acids; enhances cholesterol excretion.

[b]*Colestipol* (Colestid), same as cholestyramine.

[c]*Lovastatin,* 3-hydroxy-3-methylglutaryl coenzyme A (HMG-CoA) reductase inhibitor; decreases cholesterol synthesis in the liver.

[d]*Nicotinic acid* (niacin), decreases release of free fatty acids from adipose tissue; increases lipogenesis in liver; decreases glucagon release; most effective for type V disorder.

[e]*Neomycin,* experimental medication; questionable mode of action; decreases LDLs.

[f]*Clofibrate* (Atromid-S), decreases release of free fatty acids from adipose tissue; decreases hepatic secretion of VLDL and increases catabolism of VLDL.

[g]*Gemfibrozil* (Lopid), similar to clofibrate but increases HDLs more.

[h]*Estrogens,* decrease IDL levels in type III disorders; experimental.

[i]*Progesterone,* decreases plasma triglycerides in type V disorders; experimental.

Low levels of HDL cholesterol also are a strong indicator of coronary risk, and high levels of HDL may be more protective for the development of atherosclerosis than low levels of LDL.[36,107,113,114] HDL is responsible for "reverse cholesterol transport," which returns excess cholesterol from the tissues to the liver, where it binds to hepatic receptors (including the LDL receptor) and is processed and eliminated as bile or converted to cholesterol-containing steroids.[113] HDL also participates in endothelial repair and decreases thrombosis.[113,114] It can be fractionated into several particle densities (HDL-2 and HDL-3) or sizes (large, medium, small) that have different effects on vascular function. HDL-2 is most effective at reverse cholesterol transport and its selective measurement is a better indicator of cardiovascular risk than total HDL levels.[113,114] It has been found that inflammation in early atherogenesis results in the production of toxic oxygen radicals that can reduce or eliminate the protective function of HDL.[115] Exercise, weight loss, fish oil consumption, and moderate alcohol use can result in modest increases in HDL. Niacin, fibrates, and statins are drugs that can cause modest increases in HDL. Newer drugs aimed specifically at increasing HDL include recombinant apolipoprotein A-I (ApoA-I) mimetics, thiazolidinediones (used to treat diabetes), and cholesteryl ester transfer protein inhibitors, although the safety of these medications is still being evaluated.[113,116]

Other lipoproteins associated with increased cardiovascular risk include elevated serum VLDL (triglycerides) and increased lipoprotein (a). Triglycerides are associated with an increased risk for CAD, especially in combination with other risk factors such as diabetes.[107] Because of this, the measurement of "non-HDL cholesterol" (LDL plus VLDL) is frequently used to assess cardiovascular risk rather than just LDL or HDL levels alone.[117] **Lipoprotein (a) (Lp[a])** is a genetically determined molecular complex between LDL and a serum glycoprotein called apoprotein (a) that has been shown to be an important risk factor for atherosclerosis, especially in women.[117]

Hypertension

Hypertension is responsible for a two- to threefold increased risk of atherosclerotic cardiovascular disease. It contributes to endothelial injury, a key step in atherogenesis (see p. 1157), and causes myocardial hypertrophy, which increases myocardial demand for coronary flow. The overactivity of the SNS and RAAS commonly found in hypertension also contributes to the genesis of coronary artery disease. Drugs that block the effects of the SNS and RAAS to treat hypertension have many positive effects on the vasculature.[118,119]

Cigarette Smoking

Direct and passive (environmental) smoking increase the risk of CAD. The mechanism by which smoking increases atherosclerosis is uncertain. Nicotine stimulates the release of catecholamines (epinephrine and norepinephrine), which increases heart rate and causes peripheral vascular constriction. As a result blood pressure increases, as do cardiac workload and oxygen demand. Cigarette smoking is associated with an increase in LDL and a decrease in HDL, and contributes to vessel inflammation and thrombosis. The risk of CAD increases with heavy smoking and decreases when smoking is stopped.

Diabetes Mellitus

Diabetes mellitus is an extremely important risk factor for CAD.[36] Diabetes and insulin resistance have multiple effects on the cardiovascular system. These effects can include endothelial damage, thickening of the vessel wall, increased inflammation and leukocyte adhesion, increased thrombosis, glycation of vascular proteins, and decreased production of endothelial-derived vasodilators such as nitric oxide.[120-122] Diabetes is also associated with dyslipidemia because of the resulting alteration of hepatic lipoprotein synthesis and increases in LDL oxidation.[122] Aggressive management of this additional risk factor can significantly improve CAD risk in individuals with diabetes.

Obesity and Sedentary Lifestyle

It is estimated that nearly two thirds of the adult population in the U.S. is overweight or obese resulting in a much increased risk for CAD and stroke.[36] An estimated 47 million residents have a combination of obesity, dyslipidemia, and hypertension (called the **metabolic syndrome**) (see Chapter 21), which is associated with an even higher risk for CAD events.[123] Obesity is caused by genetics, diet, and inadequate physical exercise. Abdominal obesity has the strongest link with increased CAD risk and is related to insulin resistance, decreased HDL, increased blood pressure, inflammation, and decreased levels of a recently described cardioprotective protein called *adiponectin*.[124-127] (see What's New? New Serum Markers of Cardiovascular Risk). A sedentary lifestyle not only increases the risk of obesity but also has an independent effect on increasing CAD risk. Physical activity and weight loss offer substantial reductions in risk factors for CAD.

Nontraditional Risk Factors

Nontraditional, or novel, risk factors for CAD include (1) increased serum markers for inflammation and thrombosis, (2) hyperhomocysteinemia, (3) adipokines, and (4) infection. The amount of risk conferred by these relatively newly identified factors is still being explored.

WHAT'S NEW? New Serum Markers of Cardiovascular Risk

A number of serum markers of inflammation have been found to be excellent predictors of cardiovascular risk, especially highly sensitive C-reactive protein (hs-CRP). Other inflammatory markers predictive of cardiovascular risk include fibrinogen, erythrocyte sedimentation rate, von Willebrand factor, interleukin-6, interleukin-1, tumor necrosis factor-α, uric acid, adhesion molecules (selectins, intercellular adhesion molecules [ICAMs]), and serum amyloid A. hs-CRP is made by the liver in response to inflammatory stimuli and has been demonstrated convincingly to be a good predictor of coronary artery disease. However, several problems remain in determining its use in clinical practice. hs-CRP must be measured by a high-sensitivity technique and it is a nonspecific marker of inflammation. It can therefore be elevated in many other inflammatory states and its use for the diagnosis of coronary artery disease (CAD) is limited to helping identify high-risk individuals and for following disease progression in individuals with known coronary disease. It should not be used to screen the general population. The 3-hydroxy-3-methyl-glutaryl-CoA (HMG-CoA) reductase drugs (statins) reduce hs-CRP levels. Another group of serum markers of cardiovascular risk are the adipokines, especially adiponectin. This hormone is secreted by fat cells and has anti-inflammatory and antiatherogenic properties. It is decreased in obesity, and low levels have been linked to CAD. Other adipokines being evaluated for their association with atherosclerotic disease include leptin, resitin, visfatin, apelin, vaspin, and hepcidin. Brain natriuretic peptide also is linked with increased cardiovascular risk, especially in those with known coronary artery disease. A better understanding of the role of these serum biomarkers in cardiovascular disease may lead to earlier detection and more effective therapies.

Data from Ferri C et al: *Curr Pharmaceut Des* 13(16):1631-1645, 2007; Menzaghi C et al: *Diabetes* 56(5):1198-1209, 2007; Palazzuoli A et al: *Minerva Cardioangiol* 55(4):491-496, 2007; Selcuk MT et al: *Coron Artery Dis* 19(2):79-84, 2008; Singh SK et al: *Ann Med* 40: 110-120, 2008; Steffens S et al: *Circulation Res* 102(2):140-142, 2008; Virani SS et al: *Curr Atheroscler Rep* 10(2):164-170, 2008.

Markers of Inflammation and Thrombosis. Of the numerous markers of inflammation that have been linked to an increase in CAD risk (hs-CRP, fibrinogen, protein C, plasminogen activator inhibitor), the relationship between serum levels of CRP and CAD has been explored in the greatest depth. **Highly sensitive C-reactive protein (hs-CRP)** is an acute phase reactant or protein mostly synthesized in the liver and is an indirect measure of atherosclerotic plaque-related inflammation.[128] Elevated levels of hs-CRP are associated with numerous other CAD risk factors including smoking, obesity, and diabetes. However, as a nonspecific serum marker for inflammation, its utility as a screening tool for cardiovascular risk continues to be debated.[101,129] Other markers of inflammation associated with CAD include erythrocyte sedimentation rate, von Willebrand factor concentration, uric acid, IL-6, IL-18, TNF-α, fibrinogen, and CD40 ligand.[129]

Hyperhomocysteinemia. Hyperhomocysteinemia occurs because of a genetic lack of the enzyme that breaks down homocysteine (an amino acid) or because of a nutritional deficiency of folate, cobalamin (vitamin B_{12}), or pyridoxine (vitamin B_6). It has been identified as a risk factor for CAD, although its significance in CAD and stroke continues to be explored.[130,131] Mechanisms by which it contributes to coronary disease include associated increases in LDL oxidation, decreases in endogenous vasodilators, increased smooth muscle proliferation, and an increased tendency for thrombosis.[131] Routine serum measurement of homocysteine is not currently recommended and prevention and management are focused on increasing the dietary intake of folate and B vitamins; however, the efficacy of vitamin supplementation in improving cardiovascular risk has not been proved.

Adipokines. Adipokines are a group of hormones released from adipose cells. The two that are most studied are adiponectin and leptin. Leptin is primarily implicated in hypertension (see p. 1149) but is also being explored as a factor in diabetes and degenerative joint disease.[132] Adiponectin is normally antiatherogenic and is decreased in obesity. It functions to protect the vascular endothelium and is anti-inflammatory. Decreased adiponectin in obese individuals has been linked to a significant increase in cardiovascular risk.[127,133,134] A more recently described adipokine is resistin, which has been linked to inflammation in vascular endothelial cells.[131] Weight loss, exercise, and treatment with statins improve adipokine levels and are correlated with improved cardiovascular risk.

Infection. Infection may play a role in atherogenesis and CAD risk, although cause and effect has not been proved. Several microorganisms, especially *Chlamydia pneumoniae*, *Helicobacter pylori*, and cytomegalovirus, are associated with atherosclerotic lesions and the presence of serum antibodies to microorganisms have been linked to an increased risk for CAD.[135,136] Periodontal disease also has been linked to an increased risk for CAD. One hypothesis is that systemic infection results in increased local inflammation of vessels and therefore contributes to vascular disease.[137] Unfortunately, the use of antibiotics for the prevention and treatment of CAD has not yielded consistently positive results.

Myocardial Ischemia

PATHOPHYSIOLOGY The coronary arteries normally supply blood flow sufficient to meet the demands of the myocardium as it labors under varying workloads. Oxygen extraction from these vessels occurs with maximal efficiency. If efficient exchange does not meet myocardial oxygen needs, healthy coronary arteries are able to dilate to increase the flow of oxygenated blood to the myocardium. A variety of pathologic mechanisms can interfere with blood flow through the coronary arteries, giving rise to myocardial ischemia. Narrowing of a major coronary artery by more than 50% impairs blood flow sufficiently to hamper cellular metabolism under conditions of increased myocardial demand (see Figure 30-13).

Myocardial ischemia develops if the supply of coronary blood cannot meet the demand of the myocardium for oxygen and nutrients. Imbalances between myocardial demand and coronary blood supply can result from a number of conditions. Common causes of increased myocardial demand for blood include tachycardia, exercise, hypertension (hypertrophy), and valvular disease. The most common cause of decreased coronary blood flow and resultant myocardial ischemia is the formation of atherosclerotic plaques in the coronary circulation. As the plaque increases in size, it may partially occlude the vessel lumina, thus limiting coronary flow and causing ischemia especially during exercise. Some plaques are "unstable," meaning they are prone to ulceration or rupture (see p. 1159 and Figure 30-20). When this occurs, underlying tissues of the vessel wall are exposed resulting in platelet adhesion and thrombus formation. This can suddenly cut off blood supply to the heart muscle, resulting in acute myocardial ischemia, and if the vessel obstruction cannot be reversed rapidly, ischemia will progress to infarction. Myocardial ischemia also can result from other causes of decreased blood and oxygen delivery to the myocardium, such as coronary spasm, hypotension, dysrhythmias, and decreased oxygen-carrying capacity of the blood (anemia, hypoxemia).

Myocardial cells become ischemic within 10 seconds of coronary occlusion. After several minutes the heart cells lose the ability to contract, and cardiac output decreases. Ischemia also causes conduction abnormalities that lead to changes in the electrocardiogram and may initiate dysrhythmias. Anaerobic processes take over, and lactic acid accumulates. Cardiac cells remain viable for approximately 20 minutes under ischemic conditions. If blood flow is restored, aerobic metabolism resumes, contractility is restored, and cellular repair begins. If the coronary artery occlusion persists beyond 20 minutes, myocardial infarction occurs (Figure 30-14).

CLINICAL MANIFESTATIONS Individuals with reversible myocardial ischemia present clinically in several ways. Chronic coronary obstruction usually results in recurrent predictable chest pain called **stable angina.** Abnormal vasospasm of coronary vessels results in unpredictable chest pain called **Prinzmetal angina.** Myocardial ischemia that does not cause detectable symptoms is called **silent ischemia.**

Stable Angina. Angina pectoris is chest pain caused by myocardial ischemia. The discomfort is usually transient,

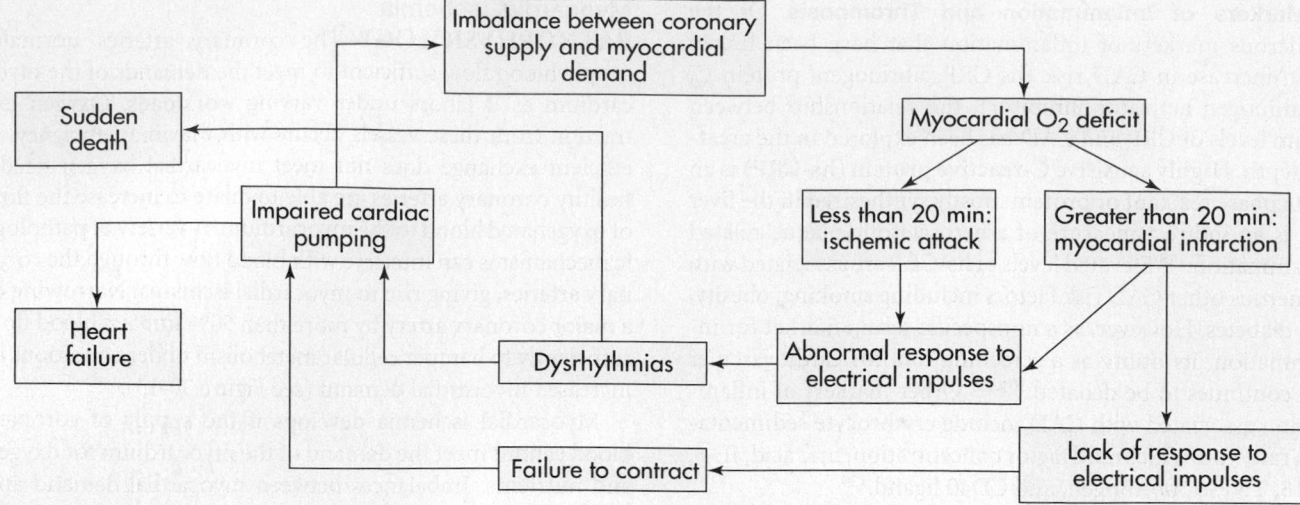

Figure 30-14 Cycle of ischemic events.

lasting approximately 3 to 5 minutes. If blood flow is restored, no permanent change or damage results. **Angina pectoris** is typically experienced as substernal chest discomfort, ranging from a sensation of heaviness or pressure to moderately severe pain. Individuals often describe the sensation by clenching a fist over the left sternal border. Discomfort may radiate to the neck, lower jaw, left arm, and left shoulder or, occasionally, to the back or down the right arm. Discomfort is commonly mistaken for indigestion. The pain is caused by the buildup of lactic acid or abnormal stretching of the ischemic myocardium that irritates myocardial nerve fibers. These afferent sympathetic fibers enter the spinal cord from levels C3 to T4, accounting for the variety of locations and radiation patterns of anginal pain.[138] Pallor, diaphoresis, and dyspnea may be associated with the pain. Stable angina is caused by gradual luminal narrowing and hardening of the arterial walls, so that affected vessels cannot dilate in response to increased myocardial demand associated with physical exertion or emotional stress. The pain is usually relieved by rest and nitrates; lack of relief indicates an individual may be developing infarction.

Myocardial ischemia in women may not present with typical anginal pain. Common symptoms in women include atypical chest pain, palpitations, sense of unease, and severe fatigue. Similarly, in individuals who have autonomic dysfunction, such as older adults or those with diabetes, angina may be mild, atypical, or even silent (see following).

Prinzmetal Angina. Prinzmetal angina (also called variant angina) is chest pain attributable to transient ischemia of the myocardium that occurs unpredictably and almost exclusively at rest. Pain is caused by vasospasm of one or more major coronary arteries with or without associated atherosclerosis. The pain often occurs at night during rapid eye movement sleep and may have a cyclic pattern of occurrence. The angina may result from hyperactivity of the SNS, increased calcium reflux in arterial smooth muscle, or impaired production or release of serotonin, histamine, endothelin, or thromboxane.[139] If the spasm persists long enough, infarction results. Angina is usually a benign condition, but can occasionally cause serious dysrhythmias.[140]

Silent Ischemia and Mental Stress (Induced Ischemia). Myocardial ischemia does not always cause angina and may be associated only with nonspecific symptoms such as fatigue, dyspnea, or feeling of unease[141] (see What's New? Women and Heart Disease, p. 1161). Ischemia can be totally asymptomatic and referred to as silent ischemia. Some individuals only have silent ischemia, and episodes of silent myocardial ischemia are common in individuals who also experience angina. One proposed mechanism for the absence of angina in silent myocardial ischemia is the presence of a global or regional abnormality in left ventricular sympathetic afferent innervation. Such an abnormality might occur as part of a metabolic dysfunction in diabetes mellitus, following surgical denervation during coronary artery bypass grafting (CABG) or cardiac transplantation, or following ischemic local nerve injury by myocardial infarction.

Another area that is receiving renewed interest is the lack of angina, even though an artery is occluded, in some individuals during mental stress (Figures 30-15, 30-16, and 30-17). Rozanski documented myocardial ischemia by radionuclide angiography (RNA) during mental stress; the majority of these cases (83%) were silent ischemias.[142] They also noted a smaller increase in heart rate during mental stress than during exercise, although the systolic blood response was comparable and the diastolic blood pressure response is even greater with mental stress. These observations suggest that increases in blood pressure and myocardial oxygen demand induced by mental stress play a role in the pathophysiology of myocardial ischemia. In addition, acute stress has been shown to increase markers of inflammation, such as CRP, and chronic stress has been linked to a hypercoagulable state that may contribute to acute ischemic events.[143,144] Although stress management has been associated with a reduction in CAD events in men, further research into the brain-heart pathways is under way to better elucidate appropriate interventions.[145]

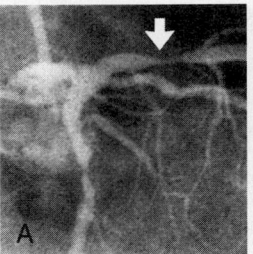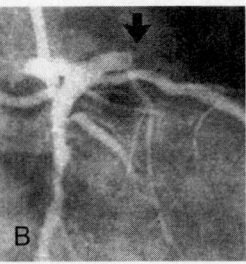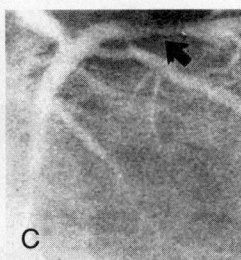

Figure 30-15 **Angiogram. A,** Baseline (*arrow* points to narrowing). **B,** Transient total occlusion of left anterior descending branch of the left coronary artery after mental stress *(arrow).* **C,** After administration of nitrates and nifedipine, artery reopened to same diameter as baseline *(arrow).* (From Stern S, editor: *Silent myocardial ischemia,* St Louis, 1998, Mosby.)

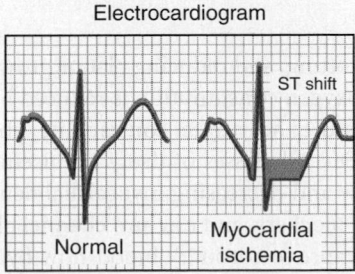

Mental stress

Ischemia usually painless

Coronary vasoconstriction

Myocardial ischemia

Electrocardiogram

ST shift

Normal

Myocardial ischemia

Figure 30-16 **The ischemic cost of aggravation.** Linkages among daily mental and emotional stimuli, brain activity, and coronary and myocardial physiology. (Modified from Papodemetrion V et al: *Am Heart J* 132:1299, 1996.)

Screening for silent ischemia is based on the presence of risk factors.[146] Silent ischemia is detected with greater sensitivity and specificity using stress radionucleotide imaging than by exercise electrocardiogram testing alone. Detection of silent ischemia is important because it is an indicator of increased risk for serious CVD events, and aggressive treatment may be indicated.[147]

EVALUATION AND TREATMENT Many individuals with reversible myocardial ischemia exhibit a normal physical examination between episodes. Physical examination of an individual experiencing myocardial ischemia may disclose tachycardia, extra heart sounds (gallops or murmurs), and pulmonary congestion indicating impaired left ventricular function. The presence of **xanthelasmas** (small fat deposits) around the eyelids or **arcus senilis** of the eyes (a yellow lipid ring around the cornea) suggests dyslipidemia and possible atherosclerosis. The presence of peripheral or carotid arterial bruits suggests probable atherosclerotic disease and increases the likelihood that CAD is present.

Electrocardiography is a critical tool for the diagnosis of myocardial ischemia. Because many individuals have normal ECGs in the absence of pain, diagnosis requires that electrocardiography be performed during an attack of angina. Transient ST segment depression and T wave inversion are characteristic signs of subendocardial ischemia frequently seen in angina. ST elevation, indicative of transmural ischemia, can be seen in individuals with variant angina but is more common in infarction (Figure 30-18). The ECG also can give some indication of which coronary artery is involved. Approximately 30% of individuals with angina have nondiagnostic ECG tracings and require other diagnostic studies.

Exercise stress testing is useful in differentiating angina from other types of chest pain, as well as detecting ischemic changes that occur in the absence of anginal pain (silent ischemia). Stress testing is made more sensitive when radioisotope imaging is added to the ECG as an indicator of myocardial ischemia. Currently, the modality of choice for the diagnosis of myocardial ischemia is single-photon emission computed tomography (SPECT), which is effective at identifying ischemia and estimating risk for coronary events. Radioisotope imaging with thallium-201 and stress echocardiography also are used.

Imaging the coronary arteries for the evaluation of atherosclerotic plaques involves the use of CT with and without

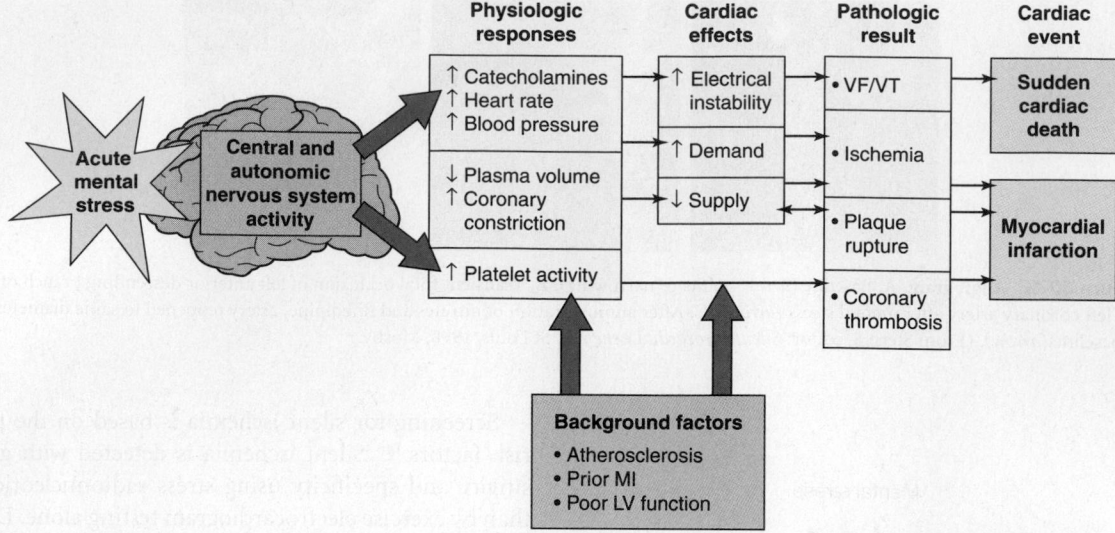

Figure 30-17 Pathophysiologic model of acute stress effects triggering cardiac clinical events. Acting via the central and autonomic nervous systems, stress can produce a cascade of physiologic responses that may lead to myocardial ischemia, potentially fatal dysrhythmia, plaque rupture, or coronary thrombosis. *LV,* Left ventricular; *MI,* myocardial infarction; *VF,* ventricular fibrillation; *VT,* ventricular tachycardia. (From Kranz DS et al: Mental stress as a trigger of myocardial ischemia and infarction. In Deedwania PC, Tofler GH, editors: *Triggers and timing of cardiac events,* ed 2, London, 1996, Saunders.)

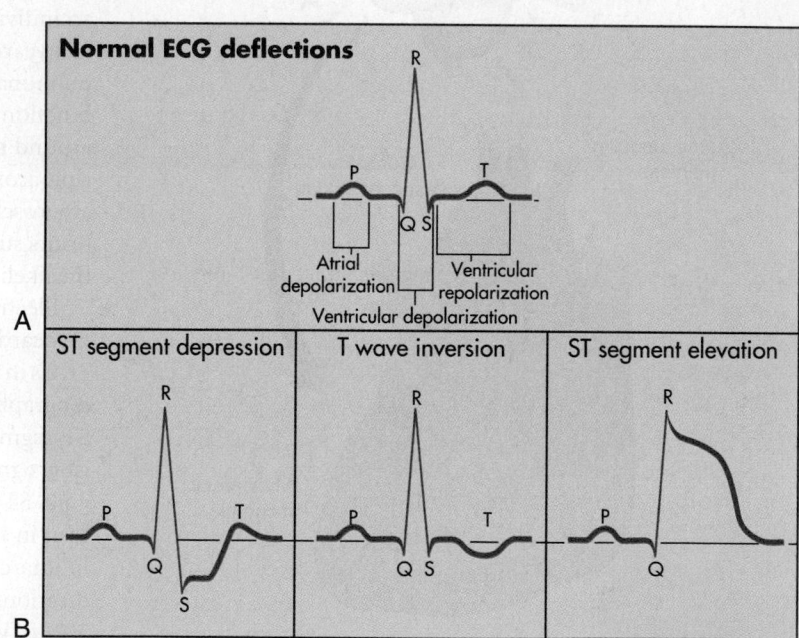

Figure 30-18 Electrocardiogram (ECG) and ischemia. **A,** Normal ECG. **B,** Electrocardiographic alterations associated with ischemia.

angiography, MRI, or intravascular ultrasound.[148] Coronary angiography is useful in determining the anatomic extent of CAD. The procedure is expensive and carries some risk; thus it is used primarily to evaluate for possible percutaneous coronary intervention (PCI) or CABG surgery for individuals whose noninvasive studies suggest severe disease.

The primary aim of therapy for myocardial ischemia and angina is to increase delivery of oxygen by improving coronary artery blood flow and to reduce myocardial oxygen consumption by favorably altering its various determinants. Coronary blood flow is improved by reversing vasoconstriction,

preventing clotting, and reducing plaque growth and rupture. Myocardial oxygen consumption is reduced by manipulation of blood pressure, heart rate, contractility, and left ventricular volume. Several classes of drugs are useful for increasing coronary flow and decreasing myocardial demand, especially nitrates, beta blockers, and calcium channel blockers.[149,150]

Nitrates improve coronary blood flow by reducing coronary artery spasm and thereby increase myocardial blood supply, but their actions are impaired in vessels with significant atherosclerosis. Nitrates also reduce myocardial demand by causing peripheral veins and, to a lesser extent, peripheral arteries to dilate. Dilation reduces peripheral vascular resistance and venous return to the heart (preload) and thereby reduces left ventricular filling pressure and decreases workload for the heart.

β-Adrenergic blockade also helps restore the balance between oxygen supply and myocardial demand. Beta blockers diminish catecholamine-induced elevations of heart rate, myocardial contractility, and blood pressure. Reduction in heart rate provides additional diastolic filling time for coronary perfusion, leading to enhanced oxygen delivery to the heart.

Calcium plays a key role in the electrical excitation of cardiac cells and in mechanical contraction of the myocardial and vascular smooth muscle cells (see Chapter 29). By blocking the influx of calcium into myocardial cells and vascular smooth muscle cells, the pacemaker activity of the sinoatrial (SA) node and conduction properties of the atrioventricular (AV) node can be modified so that myocardial oxygen demand is reduced. Thus calcium channel blockers can improve myocardial ischemia and reduce anginal symptoms; however, short-acting formulations should be used with caution because of potentially harmful effects on cardiac contractility and heart rate.[149]

Combinations of nitrates, beta-blockers, and calcium antagonists may provide dramatic relief from clinical manifestations of ischemic heart disease and make more invasive interventions unnecessary. However, they do not reverse the atherosclerotic process; thus the individual remains at risk for persistent or worsening CAD. Recommendations for appropriate diet, exercise, and risk reduction strategies have been widely distributed. Medications aimed at plaque stabilization, regression, and prevention of clotting also are indicated in the majority of individuals.[150] These include statins, ACE inhibitors or receptor blockers, and antithrombotics. Statins have been shown to significantly improve vascular function, help stabilize plaques, promote plaque regression, and reduce the risk of coronary events.[109-112,150,151] Angiotensin blockade lowers blood pressure, reduces myocardial hypertrophy, and improves vascular function.[149,150] Antithrombotics are important for reducing the risk of clot formation on vulnerable plaques and therefore reduce the risk for developing the acute coronary syndromes. Currently recommended antiplatelet agents include aspirin and clopidogrel, although some individuals may require warfarin.[150,152]

Percutaneous coronary intervention (PCI) is a procedure whereby stenotic (narrowed) coronary vessels are dilated with a catheter. Several different types of catheters can be used to open the blocked vessel. PCI is generally used to treat single-vessel disease, but it can be effective with multiple-vessel disease or restenosis of a CABG in selected individuals.[150,153] Restenosis of the artery is the major complication of the procedure; however, placement of a coronary stent can reduce this risk. Antithrombotic treatment with glycoprotein (GP) IIb-IIIa receptor antagonists after stenting also can greatly improve outcomes.[153]

Ischemic heart disease can be surgically treated by a **coronary artery bypass graft.** A saphenous vein from the lower leg is most commonly used to bypass the obstructed coronary artery. A technique using the left internal mammary artery (LIMA) rather than the saphenous vein has shown significant improvement in long-term graft patency. In selected individuals a procedure called **minimally invasive direct coronary artery bypass (MIDCAB)** can allow for effective bypass grafting of the heart, but with minimal disruption of the chest wall and without cardiopulmonary bypass or cardioplegia; thus recovery times are much shorter. One of the most common indications for bypass surgery is incapacitating angina in an individual who has good left ventricular function and technically operable coronary arteries but who has not responded to medical therapy and is not a candidate for PCI. When compared with PCI, CABG is more effective in relieving anginal symptoms but has more risks.[154] Although surgery has been shown to relieve angina, it does not halt the progression of atherosclerosis. Surgery also does not prolong life except when multiple coronary vessels are obstructed or when the left main coronary artery is blocked. A successful coronary artery bypass graft can, however, diminish the probability of lethal insult to the coronary tissues and can markedly improve quality of life.

Newer therapies for refractory angina include transmyocardial laser revascularization (TMR), gene therapy for myocardial angiogenesis, enhanced external balloon counterpulsation, spinal cord stimulation, laser revascularization, and percutaneous in situ coronary venous arterialization. Drugs being evaluated in the medical management of myocardial ischemic syndromes include ranolazine, trimetazidine, nicorandil, ivabradine, fasudil, and molsidomine.[149]

Acute Coronary Syndromes

The process of atherosclerotic plaque progression can be gradual. However, when there is sudden coronary obstruction caused by thrombus formation over a ruptured or ulcerated atherosclerotic plaque, acute coronary syndromes result (Figure 30-19). **Unstable angina** is the result of reversible myocardial ischemia and is a harbinger of impending infarction. **Myocardial infarction (MI)** results when there is prolonged ischemia causing irreversible damage to the heart muscle. MI can be further subdivided into **non–ST elevation MI (non-STEMI)** and **ST elevation MI (STEMI).** Sudden cardiac death can occur as a result of any of the acute coronary syndromes.

An atherosclerotic plaque that is prone to rupture is called unstable and has a core that is especially rich in deposited oxidized LDL and a thin fibrous cap (Figure 30-20.) Plaque disruption (ulceration or rupture) occurs because of shear forces, inflammation with release of multiple inflammatory mediators, secretion of macrophage-derived degradative enzymes, and apoptosis of cells at the edges of the lesions.[85-88,98,155,156] Exposure of the plaque substrate activates the clotting cascade.[91,92] In addition, platelet activation results in the release of coagulants and exposure of platelet GPIIb-IIIa surface receptors, resulting in further platelet aggregation and adherence.[91,92] The resulting thrombus can form very quickly. Vessel obstruction is further exacerbated by the release of vasoconstrictors such as thromboxane A_2 and endothelin. The thrombus may break up before permanent myocyte damage has occurred (unstable angina), or it may cause prolonged ischemia with infarction of the heart muscle

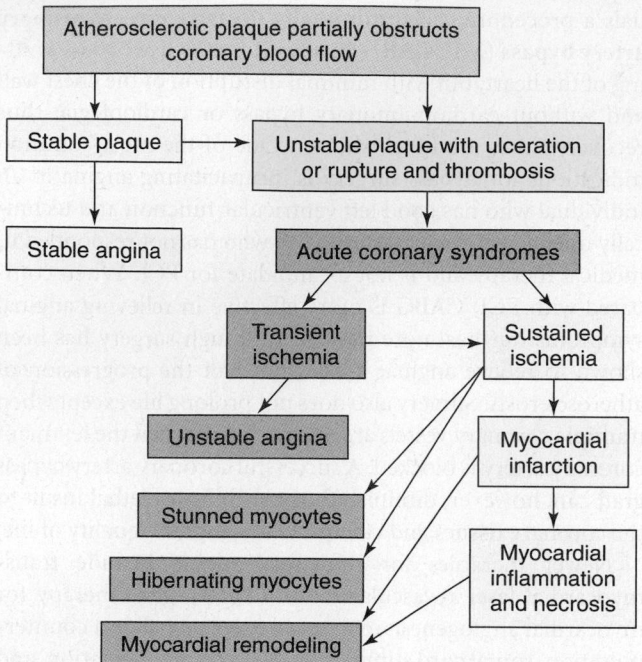

Figure 30-19 Pathophysiology of acute coronary syndromes. The atherosclerotic process can lead to stable plaque formation and stable angina or can result in unstable plaques that are prone to rupture and thrombosis. Thrombus formation on a ruptured plaque that disperses in less than 20 minutes leads to transient ischemia and unstable angina. If the vessel obstruction is sustained, myocardial infarction with inflammation and necrosis of the myocardium result. In addition, myocardial infarction is associated with other structural and functional changes, including myocyte stunning and hibernation and myocardial remodeling.

(myocardial infarction). Some individuals have sudden cardiac death without underlying histologic evidence of infarction most often caused by ischemia-initiated dysrhythmias.

Unstable Angina

Unstable angina is a form of acute coronary syndrome that results in reversible myocardial ischemia. Important, however, is that it signals that the atherosclerotic plaque has become complicated, and infarction may soon follow.

PATHOPHYSIOLOGY A fairly small fissuring or superficial erosion of the plaque leads to transient episodes of thrombotic vessel occlusion and vasoconstriction at the site of plaque damage.[156] This thrombus is labile and occludes the vessel for no more than 10 to 20 minutes, with return of perfusion before significant myocardial necrosis occurs.

CLINICAL MANIFESTATIONS Unstable angina presents as new-onset angina, angina that is occurring at rest, or angina that is increasing in severity or frequency (Box 30-1). Individuals may experience increased dyspnea, diaphoresis, and anxiety as the angina worsens. Those with unstable angina at rest have the greatest risk of subsequent infarction or death.

EVALUATION AND MANAGEMENT Physical examination may reveal evidence of ischemic myocardial dysfunction such as tachycardia, S_3 gallop, or pulmonary congestion. The ECG most commonly reveals ST segment depression and T wave inversion during pain that resolves as the pain is relieved. The ECG may be inconclusive in up to one third of individuals with unstable angina, for whom further evaluation is necessary. The cardiac biomarkers (troponins, creatine phosphokinase-myocardial bound [CPK-MB], and lactate dehydrogenase [LDH_1]) remain normal. Emergency echocardiography may reveal abnormal cardiac contraction. Approximately 20% of individuals with unstable angina progress to myocardial infarction or death within 30 days.[156] Management of unstable angina requires

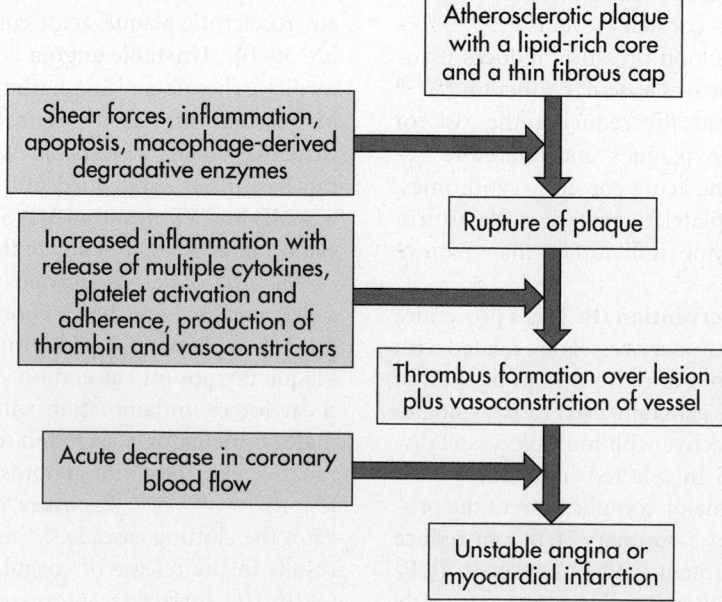

Figure 30-20 Pathogenesis of unstable plaques and thrombus formation.

immediate hospitalization with administration of oxygen, aspirin (if not contraindicated), nitrates, and morphine if pain is still present. Additional antithrombotic therapy with clopidogrel or GP IIb-IIIa platelet receptor antagonists may be indicated. Beta-blockers and ACE inhibitors, anticoagulants such as low-molecular-weight heparin, or direct thrombin inhibitors (e.g., fondaparinux) also can be given. Individuals with refractory angina and those with electrical or hemodynamic instability require immediate intervention with PCI or CABG.[156,157] Those who are stabilized with medications are then assessed for potential PCI or CABG. After discharge, individuals will continue on antithrombotics and also should be managed with risk factor reduction, including the use of statins.[156-159]

Myocardial Infarction

When coronary blood flow is interrupted for an extended period, myocyte necrosis occurs.[160] This results in MI. In the majority of cases of MI, the decrease in coronary flow is the result of atherosclerotic CAD; other causes include coronary spasm and coronary artery embolism.[161] Pathologically there

---

Box 30-1	Three Principal Presentations of Unstable Angina

Rest angina*—Angina occurring at rest and prolonged, usually >20 minutes
New-onset angina—New-onset angina of at least Canadian Cardiovascular Society (CCS) class III severity
Increasing angina—Previously diagnosed angina that has become distinctly more frequent, longer in duration, or lower in threshold (i.e., increased by ≥1 CCS class to at least CCS class III severity)

From Anderson J et al: *J Am Coll Cardiol* 50:e1-e157, 2007. Originally adapted from Braunwald E: *Circulation* 80:410-414, 1989.
*Individuals with non–ST elevation myocardial infarction (non-STEMI) usually present with angina at rest.

---

are two major types of myocardial infarction: subendocardial infarction and transmural infarction. Clinically, however, myocardial infarction is categorized as non-STEMI or STEMI.

PATHOPHYSIOLOGY Plaque progression, disruption, and subsequent clot formation is the same for myocardial infarction as it is for unstable angina (see Figures 30-19, 30-20, and 30-21). In this case, however, the thrombus is less labile and occludes the vessel for a prolonged period, such that myocardial ischemia progresses to myocyte necrosis and death. If the thrombus breaks up before complete distal tissue necrosis has occurred, the infarction will involve only the myocardium directly beneath the endocardium (subendocardial MI). This infarction usually presents with ST depression and T wave inversion without Q waves, so is termed non-STEMI. It is especially important to recognize this form of acute coronary syndrome because recurrent clot formation on the disrupted atherosclerotic plaque is likely unless some intervention is undertaken as soon as possible. If the thrombus lodges permanently in the vessel, the infarction will extend through the myocardium all the way from endocardium to epicardium (transmural MI), resulting in severe cardiac dysfunction. Clinically it is important to identify those individuals with transmural infarction who are at highest risk for serious complications and who should receive definitive intervention without delay. Those individuals usually have marked elevations in the ST segments on ECG and are categorized as having STEMI.

Cellular Injury. Cardiac cells can withstand ischemic conditions for about 20 minutes before cellular death takes place. After only 30 to 60 seconds of hypoxia, ECG changes are visible. Yet even if cells are metabolically altered and nonfunctional, they can remain viable if blood flow returns within 20 minutes. Reports suggest previous recurrent episodes of myocardial ischemia can result in myocyte adaptation to

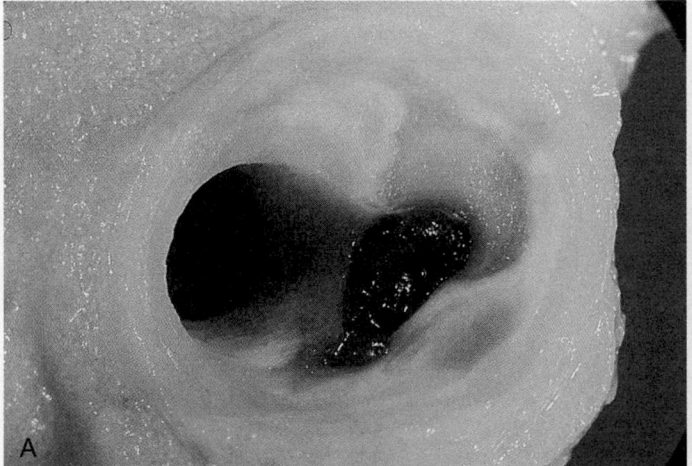
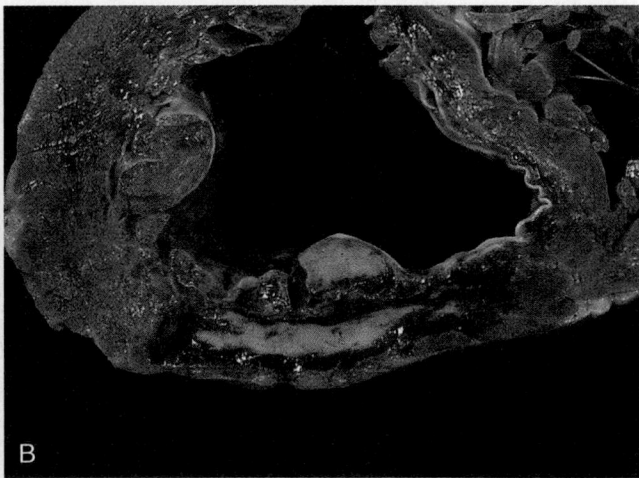

Figure 30-21 Plaque disruption and myocardial infarction. **A,** Plaque disruption. The cap of the lipid-rich plaque has become torn with the formation of a thrombus, mostly inside the plaque. **B,** Myocardial infarction. This infarct is 6 days old. The center is yellow and necrotic with a hemorrhagic red rim. The responsible coronary artery occlusion is probably in the right coronary artery. The infarct is on the posterior wall. (From Damjanov I, Linder J, editors: *Anderson's pathology*, ed 10, St Louis, 1996, Mosby.)

oxygen deprivation and preservation of myocardium. This process, termed **ischemic preconditioning,** is being studied to determine whether it has potential prophylactic or therapeutic uses. Although this phenomenon is now well described in other organs, such as the liver, its clinical utility in heart disease and surgery has yet to be determined.[161,162]

After 8 to 10 seconds of decreased blood flow, the affected myocardium becomes cyanotic and cooler. Myocardial oxygen reserves are used very quickly (within about 8 seconds) after complete cessation of coronary flow. Glycogen stores decrease as anaerobic metabolism begins. Unfortunately, glycolysis can supply only 65% to 70% of the total myocardial energy requirement and produces much less adenosine triphosphate (ATP) than aerobic processes. Hydrogen ions and lactic acid accumulate. Because myocardial tissues have poor buffering capabilities and myocardial cells are very sensitive to low cellular pH, accumulation of these products further compromises the myocardium.[161] Acidosis may make the myocardium more vulnerable to the damaging effects of lysosomal enzymes and may suppress impulse conduction and contractile function, thereby leading to heart failure.

Oxygen deprivation also is accompanied by electrolyte disturbances—specifically, loss of potassium, calcium, and magnesium from cells. Myocardial cells deprived of necessary oxygen and nutrients lose contractility, thereby diminishing the pumping ability of the heart. Ischemic myocardial cells release catecholamines (epinephrine and norepinephrine), predisposing the individual to serious imbalances of sympathetic and parasympathetic function, irregular heartbeats (dysrhythmia), and heart failure. Catecholamines mediate the release of glycogen, glucose, and stored fat from body cells. Therefore, plasma concentrations of free fatty acids and glycerol rise within 1 hour after onset of acute myocardial infarction. Excessive levels of free fatty acids can have a harmful detergent effect on cell membranes. Norepinephrine elevates blood sugar levels through stimulation of liver and skeletal muscle cells. It also suppresses pancreatic B-cell activity, which reduces insulin secretion and elevates blood glucose further. Not surprisingly, hyperglycemia is noted approximately 72 hours after an acute myocardial infarction.

Angiotensin II is released during myocardial ischemia and contributes to the pathogenesis of MI in several ways. First, it results in the systemic effects of peripheral vasoconstriction and fluid retention. These homeostatic responses are counterproductive in that they increase myocardial work and thus exacerbate the effects of the loss of myocyte contractility. Angiotensin II is also released locally, where it is a growth factor for vascular smooth muscle cells, myocytes, and cardiac fibroblasts; promotes catecholamine release; and causes coronary artery spasm.

Cellular Death. After about 20 minutes of myocardial ischemia, irreversible hypoxic injury causes cellular death and tissue necrosis.[161] (Types of necrosis are described in Chapter 2.) Necrosis of myocardial tissue results in the release of certain intracellular enzymes through the damaged cell membranes into the interstitial spaces. The lymphatics pick up the enzymes and transport them into the bloodstream, where they can be detected by serologic tests.

Structural and Functional Changes. Myocardial infarction results in structural and functional changes of cardiac tissues (Figure 30-22). Table 30-7 outlines the tissue changes that may follow myocardial infarction. Gross tissue changes in the area of infarction may not become apparent for several hours, despite almost immediate onset (within 30 to 60 seconds) of ECG changes. The infarcted myocardium is surrounded by a zone of hypoxic injury, which may progress to necrosis, undergo remodeling, or return to normal. Cardiac tissue surrounding the area of infarction also undergoes changes that can be categorized into (1) **myocardial stunning,** a temporary loss of contractile function that persists for hours to days after perfusion has been restored[161,163]; (2) **hibernating myocardium,** tissue that is persistently ischemic and undergoes metabolic adaptation to prolong myocyte survival until perfusion can be restored[161,163]; and (3) **myocardial remodeling,** a process

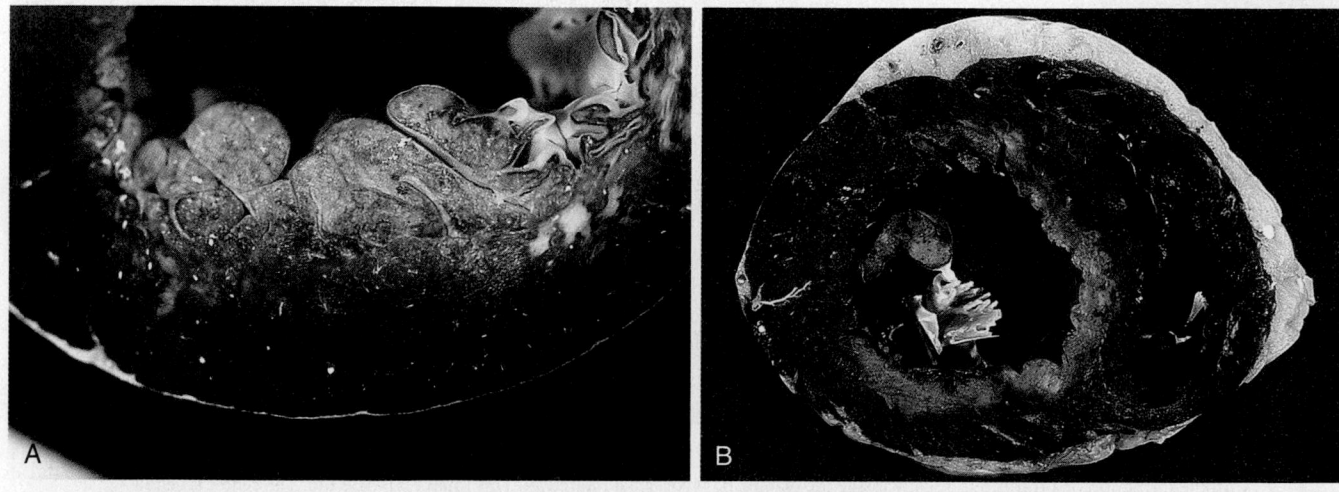

Figure 30-22 Myocardial infarction. **A,** Local infarct confined to one region. **B,** Massive large infarct caused by occlusion of three coronary arteries. (From Damjanov I, Linder J, editors: *Anderson's pathology,* ed 10, St Louis, 1996, Mosby.)

Table 30-7	Tissue Changes After Myocardial Infarction	
Time After Myocardial Infarction	**Tissue Changes**	**Stage of Healing Process**
6-12 hours	No gross changes; subcellular cyanosis with decreased temperature	Not begun
18-24 hours	Pale to gray-brown; slight pallor	Inflammatory response; intercellular enzyme release
2-4 days	Visible necrosis: yellow-brown in center and hyperemic around edges	Proteolytic enzymes remove debris; catecholamines, lipolysis, and glycogenolysis elevate plasma glucose and increase free fatty acids to assist depleted myocardium recovery from anaerobic state
4-10 days	Area soft, with fatty changes in center, regions of hemorrhage in infarcted area	Debris cleared; collagen matrix laid down
10-14 days	Weak, fibrotic scar tissue with beginning revascularization	Healing continues but area very mushy, vulnerable to stress
6 weeks	Scarring usually complete	Tough inelastic scar replaces necrotic myocardium

NOTE: Processes of tissue healing are described and illustrated in Chapter 6.

mediated by angiotensin II, aldosterone, catecholamines, adenosine, and inflammatory cytokines, which causes myocyte hypertrophy and loss of contractile function in the areas of the heart distant from the site of infarction.[161,164] All these changes can be limited through rapid restoration of coronary flow and the use of ACE inhibitors and beta-blockers after MI.[165]

The severity of functional impairment depends on the size and the site of infarction. Functional changes can include (1) decreased cardiac contractility with abnormal wall motion, (2) altered left ventricular compliance, (3) decreased stroke volume, (4) decreased ejection fraction, (5) increased left ventricular end-diastolic pressure, and (6) SA or AV node malfunction. Life-threatening dysrhythmias and heart failure often follow MI.

Repair. Myocardial infarction causes a severe inflammatory response that ends with wound repair (see Chapter 6). Repair consists of degradation of damaged cells, proliferation of fibroblasts, and synthesis of scar tissue. Many cell types, hormones, and nutrient substrates must be available for optimal healing to proceed. Within 24 hours, leukocytes infiltrate the necrotic area and proteolytic enzymes from scavenger neutrophils degrade necrotic tissue. A pseudodiabetic state often develops as catecholamines released from damaged cells stimulate release of glucose and free fatty acids. By the second week, insulin secretion increases to mobilize glucose from the repair processes. The collagen matrix that is deposited is initially weak, mushy, and vulnerable to reinjury. Unfortunately it is at this time in the recovery period (10 to 14 days after infarction) that individuals feel more capable of increasing activities and thus may stress the newly formed scar tissue. After 6 weeks the necrotic area is completely replaced by scar tissue, which is strong but unable to contract and relax like healthy myocardial tissue.

CLINICAL MANIFESTATIONS The first symptom of acute MI is usually sudden, severe chest pain. It is not possible to distinguish between angina and MI by symptoms alone, although the pain associated with MI tends to be more severe and prolonged. It may be described as heavy and crushing,

such as a "truck sitting on my chest." Radiation to the neck, jaw, back, shoulder, or left arm is common. Some individuals (especially older adults or those with diabetes) experience no pain, thereby having a "silent" infarction. Infarction often stimulates a sensation of unrelenting indigestion. Nausea and vomiting may occur because of reflex stimulation of vomiting centers by pain fibers. Vasovagal reflexes from the area of the infarcted myocardium also may affect the gastrointestinal tract. Catecholamine release results in sympathetic stimulation, producing diaphoresis and peripheral vasoconstriction that cause the skin to become cool and clammy.

EVALUATION AND TREATMENT The diagnosis of acute myocardial infarction is made on the basis of history, physical examination, ECG, and serial cardiac biomarker alterations (Box 30-2). A variety of cardiovascular changes may be found on physical examination. With an acute myocardial infarction, blood pressure may initially decrease. The drop in blood pressure reflexively activates the sympathetic nervous system to compensate and increase the heart rate in an effort to restore the blood pressure. Blood pressure may remain low (hypotension) or may become elevated depending on the severity of myocardial damage. Abnormal extra heart sounds (S_3, S_4) reflect left ventricular dysfunction. Inflammation can cause pericardial friction rub. Cardiac murmurs may indicate acute valvular insufficiency. The pulmonary examination may reveal inspiratory crackles consistent with pulmonary edema.

Cardiac troponins (troponin I and troponin T) are the most specific indicators of MI. A transient rise in these plasma biomarker levels can confirm the occurrence of MI and indicate its severity. Other biomarkers released by myocardial cells include CPK-MB and LDH. These isoenzymes exist in several different active molecular forms called *isoenzymes* and are present in different amounts within particular tissues. Blood is drawn for troponin and isoenzyme determinations as soon as possible after the onset of symptoms; serial serum levels of these biomarkers are assessed for several days. If serologic tests show abnormally high levels of troponin and isoenzymes, acute myocardial infarction probably has occurred.

Box 30-2	Universal Definition of Myocardial Infarction

The term *myocardial infarction* should be used when there is evidence of myocardial necrosis in a clinical setting with myocardial ischemia. Under these conditions any one of the following criteria meets the diagnosis for myocardial infarction:

- Detection of rise and/or fall of cardiac biomarkers (preferably troponin) with at least one value above the 99th percentile of the upper reference limit (URL) together with evidence of myocardial ischemia with at least one of the following:
  - Symptoms of ischemia
  - Electrocardiographic changes indicative of new ischemia (new ST-T changes or new left bundle branch block ([LBBB])
  - Development of pathologic Q waves in the electrocardiogram
  - Imaging evidence of new loss of viable myocardium or new regional wall motion abnormality
- Sudden, unexpected cardiac death, involving cardiac arrest, often with symptoms suggestive of myocardial ischemia, and accompanied by presumably new ST elevation, or new LBBB, and/or evidence of fresh thrombus by coronary angiography and/or at autopsy; but death occurring before blood samples could be obtained, or at a time before the appearance of cardiac biomarkers in the blood.
- For percutaneous coronary interventions (PCI) in patients with normal baseline troponin values, elevations of cardiac biomarkers above the 99th percentile URL are indicative of periprocedural myocardial necrosis. By convention, increases of biomarkers greater than 3 × 99th percentile URL have been designated as defining PCI-related myocardial infarction. A subtype related to a documented stent thrombosis is recognized.
- For coronary artery bypass grafting (CABG) in patients with normal baseline troponin values, elevations of cardiac biomarkers above the 99th percentile URL are indicative of periprocedural myocardial necrosis. By convention, increases of biomarkers greater than 5 × 99th percentile URL plus either new pathologic Q waves or new LBBB, or angiographically documented new graft or native coronary artery occlusion, or imaging evidence of new loss of viable myocardium have been designated as defining CABG-related myocardial infarction.
- Pathologic findings of an acute myocardial infarction

Data from Thygesen K, Alpert J, White H: *J Am Coll Cardiol* 50:2173-2195, 2007.

CPK-MB is less specific than troponins and may increase in individuals with certain other conditions (e.g., muscular dystrophy, hypothermia, chronic obstructive pulmonary disease [COPD], pulmonary embolism, extensive third-degree burns, small bowel infarction). Elevation of troponin, CPK-MB, and LDH_1 may not increase immediately after infarction and laboratory confirmation that an infarction has occurred may be delayed up to 12 hours.

Myocardial infarction can occur in various regions of the heart wall and may be described as anterior, inferior, posterior, lateral, subendocardial, or transmural, depending on its location and extent of tissue damage from infarction. Twelve-lead ECGs help localize the affected area through identification of Q waves and changes in ST segments and T waves (Figure 30-23). The infarcted myocardium is surrounded by a zone of hypoxic injury, which may progress to necrosis or return to normal, and adjacent to this zone of hypoxic injury is a zone of reversible ischemia (Figure 30-24). If the thrombus breaks up before complete distal tissue necrosis has occurred, the infarction will involve only the myocardium directly beneath the endocardium. This type of myocardial infarction most often presents with no elevation of the ST segment on ECG and therefore is non-STEMI. In addition, this form of infarction will not be associated with the classic Q-wave tracing on the ECG (non–Q-wave MI). It is especially important to recognize this form of acute coronary syndrome because recurrent clot formation on the disrupted atherosclerotic plaque is likely, with resultant infarct expansion. If the thrombus lodges more permanently in the vessel, the infarction will extend through the myocardium from endocardium to epicardium resulting in severe cardiac dysfunction. This usually presents with significant ST-segment elevation on ECG (STEMI). A characteristic Q wave often develops on ECG some hours later (Q-wave MI). STEMI requires rapid intervention to prevent serious complications and sequelae.

Additional laboratory data may reveal leukocytosis and elevated sedimentation rate, both of which indicate inflammation. The individual's blood sugar is usually elevated and the glucose tolerance level may remain abnormal for several weeks. Hypoxemia may accompany heart failure.

Acute myocardial infarction requires admission to the hospital, often directly into a coronary care unit. The individual should be placed on supplemental oxygen and given an aspirin immediately (ticlopidine if allergic to aspirin).[156-158,166] Pain relief is of utmost importance and involves the use of sublingual nitroglycerin or morphine sulfate. Continuous monitoring of cardiac rhythms and biomarker changes is essential because the first 24 hours after onset of symptoms is the time of highest risk for sudden death. Both non-STEMI and STEMI are managed with the urgent administration of thrombolytics or by PCI along with antithrombotics.[156,166-169] Further management may include ACE inhibitors and beta-blockers. Individuals who are in shock require aggressive fluid resuscitation, ionotropic drugs, and possible emergent invasive procedures.

Bed rest, followed by gradual return to activities of daily living, reduces the myocardial oxygen demands of the compromised heart. Individuals not receiving thrombolytic or heparin infusion must receive DVT prophylaxis as long as their activity is significantly limited. Stool softeners are given to eliminate the need for straining, which can precipitate bradycardia and can be followed by increased venous return to the heart, causing possible cardiac overload.

Treatment of dyslipidemia with 3-hydroxy-3-methylglutaryl-CoA (HMG-CoA) reductase inhibitors (statins) can reduce the risk of cardiovascular events. The National Cholesterol Education Program (NCEP) Expert Panel[107] has recommended target total blood cholesterol levels of less than 200 mg/dl with LDLs less than 100 mg/dl and HDLs more than 40 mg/dl. Drugs that decrease lipidemia should be administered

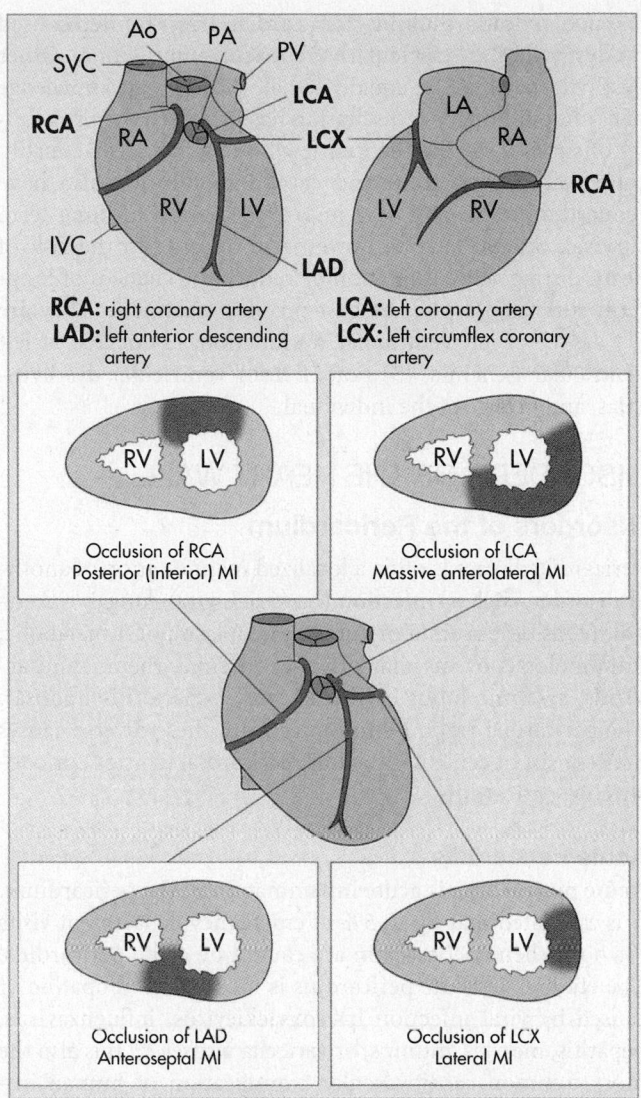

Figure 30-23 Site of myocardial infarction (MI) and vessel involvement. *Ao,* Aorta; *IVC,* inferior vena cava; *LA,* left atrium; *LV,* left ventricle; *PA,* pulmonary artery; *PV,* pulmonary vein; *RA,* right atrium; *RV,* right ventricle; *SVC,* superior vena cava. (Modified from Stevens A, Lowe J: *Pathology,* St Louis, 1995, Mosby.)

prior to discharge from the hospital.[169] Education on diet, caffeine, smoking cessation, exercise, and other aspects of risk factor reduction is crucial for secondary prevention of recurrent myocardial ischemia.

COMPLICATIONS The number and severity of postinfarction complications depend on the location and extent of necrosis, the individual's physiologic condition before the infarction, and the availability of swift therapeutic intervention.

Dysrhythmias (arrhythmias), which are disturbances of cardiac rhythm, are the most common complication of acute myocardial infarction, affecting more than 90% of individuals. Dysrhythmias can be caused by ischemia, hypoxia, autonomic nervous system (ANS) system imbalances, lactic acidosis, electrolyte abnormalities, alterations of impulse conduction pathways or conduction defects, drug toxicity, or hemodynamic abnormalities. Dysrhythmias may originate from the atria, ventricles, nodal regions, or conduction tissues. The seriousness of dysrhythmias depends on the hemodynamic consequences. For example, there is no ventricular contraction in ventricular fibrillation; consequently, there is no cardiac output. Atrial fibrillation, however, does not affect ventricular contraction and thus can be tolerated by most individuals. (Dysrhythmias are described in Table 30-12.) Prophylactic use of antiarrhythmics, such as lidocaine and amiodarone, do not improve mortality; however, individuals at high risk should be considered for implantable cardioverter-defibrillators (ICDs).

Acute MI usually is accompanied by a reduction in cardiac output and some degree of left ventricular failure (congestive heart failure), which is characterized by pulmonary congestion, reduced myocardial contractility, and abnormal heart wall motion (see p. 1171). Anterior infarction is associated with more severe left heart failure than is inferior infarction. If cardiac output is insufficient to maintain normal arterial pressure and to perfuse the kidneys and other organs adequately, cardiogenic shock develops. Cardiogenic shock characteristically develops if 40% or more of the left ventricular myocardium is infarcted. (Cardiogenic shock is discussed in Chapter 46.)

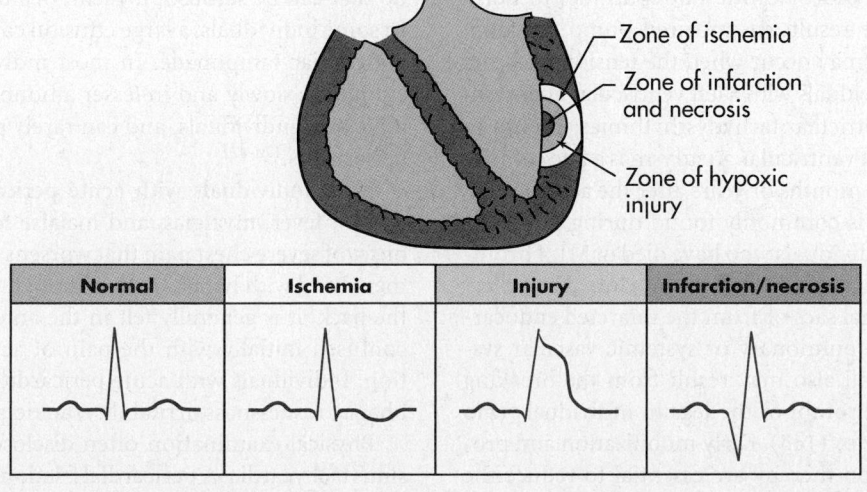

Figure 30-24 Electrocardiographic alterations associated with the three zones of myocardial infarction.

Inflammation of the pericardium (**pericarditis**) is a common complication of acute myocardial infarction. Pericardial friction rubs often are noted 2 to 3 days after MI and are associated with anterior chest pain that worsens with respiratory effort. Specific treatment is not required; however, corticosteroids dramatically relieve symptoms. **Dressler postinfarction syndrome**, which is a delayed form of acute pericarditis, can occur from 1 week to several months after acute myocardial infarction. Although poorly understood, the syndrome is thought to be an immunologic (antigen-antibody) response to the necrotic myocardium. Pain, fever, friction rub, pleural effusion, and arthralgias may accompany this syndrome. Steroids may alleviate symptoms.

Organic brain syndrome may occur in acute or chronic form if blood flow to the brain is impaired secondary to MI. Transient ischemic attacks or an outright cerebrovascular accident may result from thromboemboli that have broken loose from the wall of the left ventricle or from cardiac valves.

Cardiac complications of MI can include rupture of heart structures. Necrosis of tissue in or around the papillary muscles can cause rupture of these muscles or of the chordae tendineae. Factors that lead to rupture of the free wall of the infarcted ventricle include thinning of the wall, poor collateral flow, shearing effect of muscular contraction against the stiffened necrotic area, marked necrosis at the terminal end of the blood supply, and aging of the myocardium with laceration of the myocardial microstructure. Infarctions around septal structures that separate the heart chambers can lead to septal rupture. Ruptures are associated with audible, harsh cardiac murmurs; increased left ventricular end-diastolic pressure; and decreased systemic blood pressure.

Weakening of the wall of the infarcted ventricle can cause **ventricular aneurysm** formation. According to Laplace's law, with decreased muscle mass at the infarcted site, the wall is weakened and tension stretches the noncontracting infarcted heart muscle, thus producing infarct expansion or aneurysm formation (see p. 1144 for a discussion of aneurysm). Decreased muscle mass causes an increase in the radius of the ventricle, and because the radius is directly proportional to pressure and tension, both increase with time. The wall of the aneurysm becomes more fibrotic but continues to bulge with systole. The bulge results in impaired pump function. Although rare, rupture may occur when the tension becomes too great. Death in individuals with a left ventricular aneurysm is usually related to ventricular tachydysrhythmias and not to ventricular rupture. Left ventricular aneurysm is a late complication of MI, occurring months or years after the acute event.

Thromboembolism is commonly found during postmortem examinations of individuals who have died of MI. Thromboemboli may disseminate from debris and clots that collect inside dilated aneurysmal sacs or from the infarcted endocardium and travel to the pulmonary or systemic vascular systems. Pulmonary emboli also may result from the breaking loose of deep venous thrombi of the legs in individuals who are confined to bed (see p. 1143). Early mobilization and prophylactic anticoagulation therapy are essential to reduce the incidence of this complication.

Sudden death resulting from cardiac arrest is often caused by dysrhythmias, particularly ventricular fibrillation. Other dysrhythmias may be equally lethal. Widespread knowledge of cardiopulmonary resuscitation has increased the probability of survival during the first few hours after cardiac insult. Immediate intervention and careful monitoring also have reduced mortality and have improved chances for long-term survival. Several factors, however, contribute to the risk of death during acute infarction or reduce the chances of long-term survival, despite the best possible treatment. They are (1) degree of left ventricular dysfunction, (2) degree of left ventricular ischemia, (3) potential for ventricular dysrhythmias, and (4) age of the individual.

DISORDERS OF THE HEART WALL

Disorders of the Pericardium

Pericardial disease is often a localized manifestation of another disorder, such as infection (bacterial, viral, fungal, rickettsial, parasitic); trauma or surgery; neoplasm; or a metabolic, immunologic, or vascular disorder (uremia, rheumatoid arthritis, systemic lupus erythematosus, periarteritis nodosa). The pericardial response to injury from these diverse causes may consist of acute pericarditis, pericardial effusion, or constrictive pericarditis.

Acute Pericarditis

Acute pericarditis is acute inflammation of the pericardium. It is estimated that up to 5% of emergency department visits for nonischemic chest pain are caused by acute pericarditis. The etiology of acute pericarditis is most often idiopathic or caused by viral infection by coxsackievirus, influenzavirus, hepatitis, measles, mumps, or varicella viruses.[170] It is also the most common cardiovascular complication of human immunodeficiency virus (HIV) infection. Other causes include myocardial infarction, trauma, neoplasm, surgery, bacterial infection (especially tuberculosis), connective tissue disease, or radiation therapy. The pericardial membranes become inflamed and roughened, and a pericardial effusion may develop that can be serous, purulent, or fibrinous (Figure 30-25). In some individuals, a large effusion can develop rapidly causing cardiac tamponade. In most individuals an effusion accumulates slowly and in lesser amounts that can recur in up to 30% of individuals, and can rarely progress to constrictive pericarditis.[170-172]

Most individuals with acute pericarditis describe several days of fever, myalgias, and malaise followed by the sudden onset of severe chest pain that worsens with respiratory movements and with lying down. Although the pain may radiate to the back, it is generally felt in the anterior chest and may be confused initially with the pain of acute myocardial infarction. Individuals with acute pericarditis also may report dysphagia, restlessness, irritability, anxiety, and weakness.

Physical examination often discloses low-grade fever and sinus tachycardia. A pericardial friction rub—a short, scratchy, grating sensation similar to the sound of sandpaper—may be

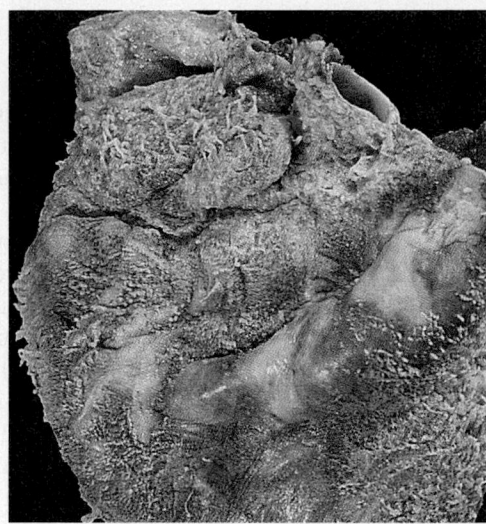

Figure 30-25 Acute pericarditis. Note shaggy coat of fibers covering surface of heart. (From Damjanov I, Linder J: *Pathology: a color atlas,* St Louis, 2000, Mosby.)

heard at the cardiac apex and left sternal border and is highly specific for pericarditis. The rub is caused by the roughened pericardial membranes rubbing against each other. Friction rubs are not always present and may be intermittently heard. ECG changes may reflect inflammatory processes through diffuse ST segment elevation that is concaved upward without Q waves.[173] The ECG may remain abnormal for days or even weeks. Echocardiography may reveal a pericardial effusion.

Treatment for uncomplicated acute pericarditis consists of relieving symptoms. Rest is helpful during episodes of acute pain. Salicylates and nonsteroidal anti-inflammatory drugs reduce inflammation.[170,174] Combined nonsteroidals and colchicine (prevents fibrosis) is a highly effective regimen.[170,174,175] Additional analgesics may be given to relieve pain. Exploration of the underlying cause is important. If pericardial effusion develops, aspiration of the excessive fluid may be necessary.

Pericardial Effusion

Pericardial effusion, the accumulation of fluid in the pericardial cavity, can occur in all forms of pericarditis.[170,171] The fluid may be a transudate, such as the serous effusion that develops with left heart failure, overhydration, or hypoproteinemia. More often, however, the fluid is an exudate, which indicates pericardial inflammation like that seen with acute pericarditis, heart surgery, some chemotherapeutic agents, infections, and autoimmune disorders, such as systemic lupus erythematosus. (Types of exudate are described in Chapter 6.) If the fluid is serosanguineous, the underlying cause is likely to be tuberculosis, neoplasm, uremia, or radiation. Idiopathic serosanguineous (cause unknown) effusion is possible, however. Effusions of frank blood are generally related to aneurysms, trauma, or coagulation defects. If chyle leaks from the thoracic duct, it may enter the pericardium and lead to cholesterol pericarditis.

Pericardial effusion, even in large amounts, is not necessarily clinically significant, except that it indicates an underlying disorder. The important consideration is whether the fluid creates sufficient pressure to cause cardiac compression, which is a serious condition known as **tamponade.**[171] If an effusion develops gradually, the pericardium can stretch to accommodate large quantities of fluid without compressing the heart. If the fluid accumulates rapidly, however, even a small amount (50 to 100 ml) may cause serious tamponade. The danger is that pressure exerted by the pericardial fluid eventually will equal diastolic pressure within the heart chambers, thus preventing chamber filling.[171] The first structures to be affected by tamponade are the right atrium and ventricle, where diastolic pressures are normally lowest. Compression by pericardial fluid interferes with right atrial filling during diastole, resulting in increased venous pressure, systemic venous congestion, and signs and symptoms of right heart failure (distention of the jugular veins, edema, hepatomegaly). Decreased atrial filling leads to decreased ventricular filling, decreased stroke volume, and reduced cardiac output. If the left atrium collapses because of lack of filling, life-threatening circulatory collapse may occur.[176]

Individuals with cardiac tamponade most often present with dyspnea, tachycardia, jugular venous distention, cardiomegaly, and pulsus paradoxus.[177] Pulsus paradoxus means that the arterial blood pressure during expiration exceeds arterial pressure during inspiration by more than 10 mmHg. This clinical finding reflects impairment of diastolic filling of the left ventricle plus reduction of blood volume within all four cardiac chambers. Presence of a large pericardial effusion or tamponade magnifies the normally insignificant effect of inspiration on intracardiac flow and volume.

Other clinical manifestations of pericardial effusion are distant or muffled heart sounds, poorly palpable apical pulse, dyspnea on exertion, and dull chest pain. A chest roentgenogram may disclose a "water-bottle" configuration of the cardiac silhouette. An echocardiogram can detect an effusion as small as 20 ml and is considered the most accurate and reliable method of diagnosis, although CT also is commonly used.[178]

Treatment of pericardial effusion or tamponade generally consists of pericardiocentesis (aspiration of excessive pericardial fluid). Pericardiocentesis is diagnostic and therapeutic: the fluid is analyzed to identify the cause of the effusion, and its removal alone may bring dramatic relief from symptoms. Persistent pain may be treated with analgesics, anti-inflammatory medications, or steroids. Surgery may be required if the underlying cause of tamponade is trauma or aneurysm. If an effusion is neoplasm induced, chemotherapeutic agents may be injected into the pericardial space.[179] If the effusion recurs, a pericardial "window" can be created or the individual may require pericardectomy.[180]

Constrictive Pericarditis

Constrictive pericarditis, or **restrictive pericarditis (chronic pericarditis),** was synonymous with tuberculosis years ago; tuberculosis continues to be an important cause of pericarditis in immunocompromised individuals.[181] In the United States, this form of pericardial disease is more often idiopathic or associated with radiation exposure, rheumatoid arthritis, uremia, or CABG. In constrictive pericarditis, fibrous scarring with occasional calcification of the pericardium causes the visceral and parietal pericardial layers to adhere, obliterating the pericardial cavity. The fibrotic lesions encase the heart in a rigid shell (Figure 30-26). Like tamponade, constrictive pericarditis compresses the heart and eventually reduces cardiac output. Unlike tamponade, however, constrictive pericarditis never develops suddenly.

Because the onset of constrictive pericarditis is gradual, clinical manifestations seldom include pulsus paradoxus. Symptoms tend to be exercise intolerance, dyspnea on exertion, fatigue, and anorexia. Clinical assessment shows weight loss, edema, distention of the jugular vein, and hepatic congestion. Restricted ventricular filling may cause a pericardial knock (early diastolic sound).

ECG findings include T wave inversions and atrial fibrillation. Chest roentgenograms often disclose prominent pulmonary vessels and calcification of the pericardium. An echocardiogram may suggest evidence of nonspecific pericardial thickening.[171] CT or MRI is best able to detect constrictive processes. Some individuals require diagnostic thoracotomy in order to make the diagnosis, especially in cases of postoperative restrictive pericarditis.

Initial treatment for constrictive pericarditis consists of dietary sodium restriction, digitalis glycosides, and diuretics to improve cardiac output. If these modalities are not successful, surgical excision of the restrictive pericardium is indicated.

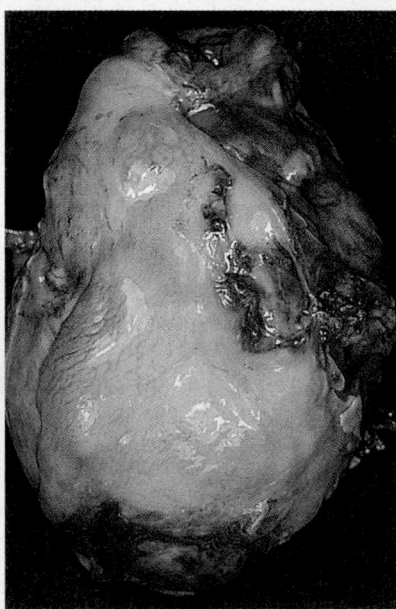

Figure 30-26 Constrictive pericarditis. The fibrotic pericardium encases the heart in a rigid shell. (From Damjanov I, Linder J: *Pathology: a color atlas,* St Louis, 2000, Mosby.)

Disorders of the Myocardium: The Cardiomyopathies

The **cardiomyopathies** are a diverse group of diseases that primarily affect the myocardium. Most are the result of underlying cardiovascular disorders, such as ischemic heart disease or hypertension. Cardiomyopathies also can be secondary to infectious disease, exposure to toxins, systemic connective tissue disease, infiltrative and proliferative disorders, or nutritional deficiencies. Despite this large number of possible causes, most cases of cardiomyopathy are idiopathic; that is, their cause is unknown. The cardiomyopathies are categorized as dilated, hypertrophic, or restrictive depending on their tissue characteristics, genomics, and hemodynamic effects[182] (Figure 30-27 and Table 30-8). An individual may display characteristics of more than one type.

Dilated Cardiomyopathy

Dilated cardiomyopathy (congestive cardiomyopathy) is characterized by ventricular dilation and grossly impaired systolic function, leading to dilated heart failure (Figure 30-28).

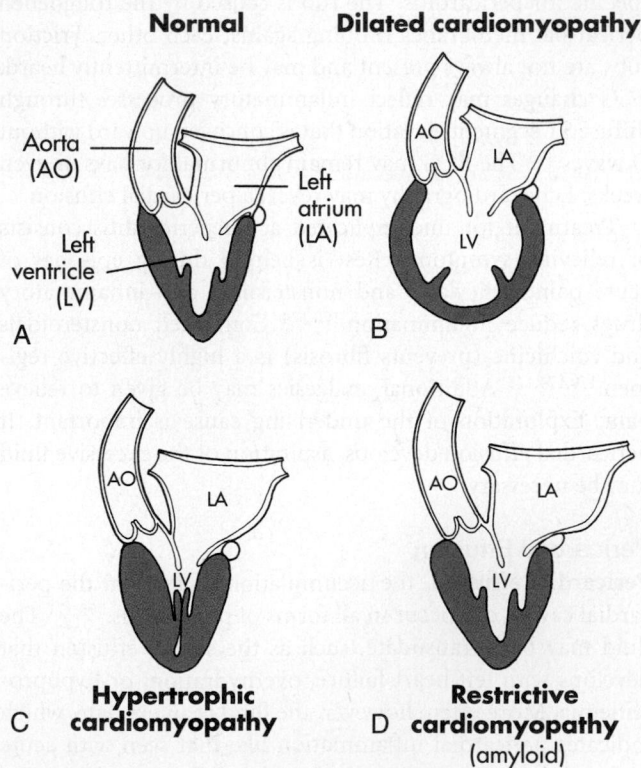

Figure 30-27 Diagram showing major distinguishing pathophysiologic features of the types of cardiomyopathy. **A,** The normal heart. **B,** In the dilated type of cardiomyopathy, the heart has a globular shape and the largest circumference of the left ventricle is not at its base but midway between apex and base. **C,** In the hypertrophic type of cardiomyopathy the wall of the left ventricle is greatly thickened; the left ventricular cavity is small, but the left atrium may be dilated because of poor diastolic relaxation of the ventricle. **D,** In the restrictive type the left ventricular cavity is of normal size, but again, the left atrium is dilated because of the reduced diastolic compliance of the ventricle. (From Kissane JM, editor: *Anderson's pathology,* ed 9, St Louis, 1990, Mosby.)

Table 30-8	Pathophysiologic Effects of the Cardiomyopathies		

| | Type of Cardiomyopathy | | |
Pathophysiology	Dilated	Hypertrophic	Restrictive
Major symptoms	Fatigue, weakness, palpitations	Dyspnea, angina pectoris, fatigue, dizziness (syncope), palpitations	Dyspnea, fatigue
Cardiomegaly	Moderate to marked	Mild to moderate	Mild
Hypertrophy	Left ventricular myocardium	Left ventricular myocardium and interventricular septum	Left ventricular myocardium
Alterations of chamber volume	Volume increased	Volume decreased, particularly in left ventricle	Volume normal to decreased
Alterations of chamber compliance	Compliance increased	Compliance decreased, particularly in left ventricle	Compliance decreased, particularly in left ventricle
Alterations of systolic function (myocardial contractility)	Contractility decreased in left ventricle	Contractility increased or vigorous	None
Valvular incompetence	Atrioventricular valves, particularly mitral	Mitral valve	Atrioventricular valve
Conduction defects	Intraventricular	Nonspecific	Atrioventricular
Dysrhythmias	Sinoatrial tachycardia; atrial and ventricular dysrhythmias	Atrial and ventricular dysrhythmias	Tachydysrhythmias
Thromboembolism	Systemic or pulmonary	Systemic or pulmonary	Systemic or pulmonary
Associated conditions	Alcoholism, pregnancy, infection, nutritional deficiency, exposure to toxins	Possible inherited defect of muscle growth and development	Infiltrative disease
Eventual cardiovascular event	Left heart failure	Left heart failure	Right heart failure

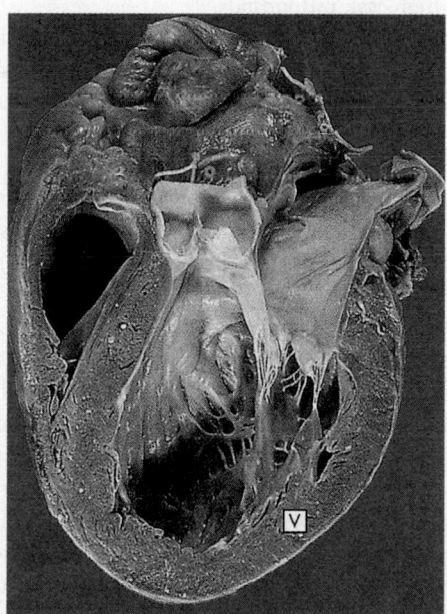

Figure 30-28 Dilated cardiomyopathy. The dilated left ventricle has a thin wall *(V)*. (From Stevens A, Lowe J: *Pathology*, St Louis, 1995, Mosby.)

The most common causes are ischemic heart disease or valvular heart disease. The basic problem is diminished myocardial contractility, which is reflected in diminished systolic performance of the heart. Abnormalities in myocardial energy metabolism are implicated.[183] Dilated cardiomyopathy causes decreased ejection fraction, increased end-diastolic and residual volumes, decreased ventricular stroke volume, and biventricular failure.

About two thirds of the cases of dilated cardiomyopathy are idiopathic; the remainder result from some underlying disease process. Secondary causes of dilated cardiomyopathy include ischemic heart disease, valvular heart disease, diabetes, renal failure, alcohol use, drug toxicity, nutritional deficiencies postpartum, postinfectious, and hyperthyroidism.

Idiopathic dilated cardiomyopathy has a familial origin in 20% to 30% of cases and genes coding for contractile proteins are implicated. In the majority of familial and sporadic idiopathic cases, cardiac-specific autoantibodies can be detected.[184]

Ischemic heart disease damages the ventricular myocardium both through necrosis and peri-infarct remodeling (see p. 1165). Valvular heart disease causes cardiac chamber volume and pressure overload that can result in long-term myocardial dysfunction (see p. 1181). Diabetes and uremia are associated with decreased myocardial contractility and dilated cardiomyopathy. Alcohol can be directly toxic to the myocardium,[185] as can many drugs such as some chemotherapeutic, inotropic, and antidysrhythmic agents. Many nutritional deficiencies can cause cardiomyopathy including niacin, vitamin D, and selenium. Peripartum cardiomyopathy usually develops in the first 3 to 4 months after completion of a pregnancy, after the period of maximum physiologic stress is thought to have ended. Dilated cardiomyopathies also may be the late consequences of previous viral (especially coxsackievirus), bacterial, or parasitic infections or an autoimmune process.

Inflammatory and immune responses include release of cytokines and interleukins resulting in significant myocarditis and contractile dysfunction.[186] Hyperthyroidism may present with atrial fibrillation as well as dilated cardiomyopathy, which may be reversible with treatment of the thyroid disorder. (Pathophysiologic effects of the cardiomyopathies are summarized in Table 30-8.)

The most common symptoms of dilated cardiomyopathy are dyspnea and fatigue. Pulmonary congestion is expected, although fulminant pulmonary edema is uncommon. Palpitations and associated dysrhythmias may cause dizziness (syncope). Systemic and pulmonary emboli are common complications. Chest pain may be present but it is usually nonspecific and unlike anginal pain.

In the presence of dilated heart failure, blood pressure may be elevated initially; however, hypotension indicates progressive decreases in contractility. Extra heart sounds and cardiac murmurs may be present as well. Dilated cardiomyopathy may be difficult to distinguish from acute myocarditis, valvular heart disease, CAD, and hypertensive heart disease. Echocardiography and MRI can confirm the diagnosis; however, careful evaluation for potentially reversible underlying causes is essential.

General treatment for dilated cardiomyopathy consists of salt restriction and the careful use of vasodilators, diuretics, and inotropic agents. Anticoagulants are given to prevent pulmonary and systemic embolism. Corticosteroids and immunosuppressants can benefit individuals with documented inflammatory disease. Myocardial pacemakers (pacing) can improve cardiac output in many individuals. Cardiac transplantation may be lifesaving. The use of cardiac stem cells to restore myocardial contractility is an area of promising research.[187]

Hypertrophic Cardiomyopathy

Hypertrophic cardiomyopathy refers to two major categories of thickening of the myocardium: (1) hypertrophic obstructive cardiomyopathy (asymmetric septal hypertrophic cardiomyopathy or subaortic stenosis) and (2) hypertensive or valvular hypertrophic cardiomyopathy. These two categories are very different in their etiology, pathophysiology, and clinical presentation.

Hypertrophic obstructive cardiomyopathy is the most commonly inherited cardiac disorder and is one of an autosomal dominant inheritance.[188,189] It is characterized by thickening of the septal wall (Figure 30-29), which may cause outflow obstruction to the left ventricle outflow tract.[190] Additional changes include abnormalities of collagen deposition and altered contractile proteins in the myocytes. The thickening of the septum results in a hyperdynamic state, especially with exercise. Diastolic relaxation also is impaired and ventricular compliance is decreased. Obstruction of left ventricular outflow can occur when heart rate is increased and intravascular volume is decreased. Individuals complain of angina, syncope, palpitations, and symptoms of myocardial infarction and left heart failure. Examination may reveal extra heart sounds and murmurs. Echocardiography and cardiac catheterization

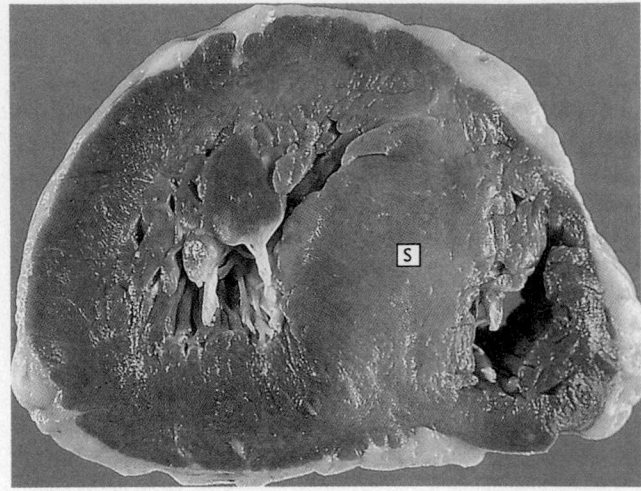

Figure 30-29 Hypertrophic cardiomyopathy. There is marked left ventricular hypertrophy. This often affects the septum *(S)*. (From Stevens A, Lowe J: *Pathology,* St Louis, 1995, Mosby.)

can confirm the diagnosis. This type of hypertrophic cardiomyopathy is a significant risk for serious ventricular arrhythmias and sudden death. Management includes beta-blockers to slow the heart rate, surgical resection of the hypertrophied myocardium, septal ablation, and prophylactic placement of an ICD in high-risk individuals.[190]

Hypertensive, or **valvular hypertrophic, cardiomyopathy** occurs because of increased resistance to ventricular ejection commonly seen in hypertension or in valvular stenosis (usually aortic). In this case, hypertrophy of the myocytes is an attempt to compensate for increased workload; however, long-term dysfunction of the myocytes develops over time, with diastolic dysfunction leading eventually to systolic dysfunction of the ventricle (see Heart Failure, p. 1189).

Restrictive Cardiomyopathies

Restrictive cardiomyopathy is characterized by restrictive filling and reduced diastolic volume of either or both ventricles with normal or near-normal systolic function and wall thickness.[191] It may occur idiopathically or as a cardiac manifestation of systemic diseases, such as scleroderma, amyloidosis, sarcoidosis, lymphoma, and hemochromatosis, or a number of inherited storage diseases.[191] The myocardium becomes rigid and noncompliant, impeding ventricular filling and raising filling pressures during diastole. The overall clinical and hemodynamic picture mimics and may be confused with that of constrictive pericarditis.

The most common clinical manifestation of restrictive cardiomyopathy is right heart failure with systemic venous congestion. Cardiomegaly and dysrhythmias are common. A thorough evaluation for the underlying cause should be initiated (and may include myocardial biopsy) because there is no effective therapy for restrictive cardiomyopathy other than treating the underlying disease process.[191] Death occurs as a result of heart failure or dysrhythmias.

Disorders of the Endocardium

Valvular Dysfunction

Disorders of the endocardium, the innermost lining of the heart wall, all damage the heart valves, which are made up of endocardial tissue. Endocardial damage can be either congenital or acquired. The acquired forms cause inflammatory, ischemic, traumatic, degenerative, or infectious alterations of valvular structure and function.[192] Structural alterations of the heart valves lead to stenosis, incompetence, or both. Although all four heart valves may be affected, those of the left heart (mitral and aortic semilunar valves) are far more commonly affected than those of the right heart (tricuspid and pulmonic semilunar valves).

In **valvular stenosis** the valve orifice is constricted and narrowed, impeding the forward flow of blood and increasing the workload of the cardiac chamber proximal to the diseased valve (Figure 30-30). Intraventricular or atrial pressure increases in the chamber to overcome resistance to flow through the valve. Increased pressure causes the myocardium to work harder, causing myocardial hypertrophy. In **valvular regurgitation** (also called *insufficiency* or *incompetence*) the valve leaflets, or cusps, fail to shut completely, permitting blood flow to continue even when the valve is supposed to be closed (see Figure 30-30). During systole or diastole some blood leaks back into the chamber proximal to the incompetent valve. Valvular regurgitation increases the volume of blood the heart must pump and increases the workload of the affected heart chamber. Increased volume leads to chamber dilation, and increased workload leads to hypertrophy.

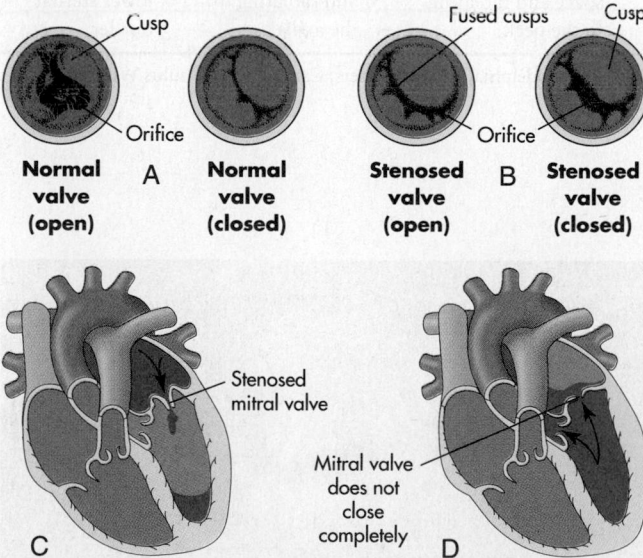

Figure 30-30 Valvular stenosis and regurgitation. **A,** Normal position of the valve leaflets, or cusps, when the valve is open and closed. **B,** Open position of a stenosed valve *(left)* and open position of a closed regurgitant valve *(right)*. **C,** Hemodynamic effect of mitral stenosis. The stenosed valve is unable to open sufficiently during left atrial systole, inhibiting left ventricular filling. **D,** Hemodynamic effect of mitral regurgitation. The mitral valve does not close completely during left ventricular systole, permitting blood to reenter the left atrium.

Valvular dysfunction stimulates chamber dilation and/or myocardial hypertrophy, both of which are compensatory mechanisms intended to increase the pumping capability of the heart. Eventually, myocardial contractility is diminished, the ejection fraction is reduced, diastolic pressure increases, and the ventricles fail from overwork. Depending on the severity of the valvular dysfunction and the capacity of the heart to compensate, valvular alterations cause a range of symptoms and some degree of incapacitation (Table 30-9). The effects of valvular dysfunction are treated with medications until surgical prosthetic valve replacement becomes necessary.

Stenosis

Aortic Stenosis. Aortic stenosis is the most common valvular abnormality affecting nearly 2% of adults older than 65 years of age. The three common causes are (1) congenital bicuspid valve, (2) degeneration with aging, and (3) inflammatory damage caused by rheumatic heart disease (less than 10% of cases). Numerous gene abnormalities have been associated with aortic stenosis.[192-194] Aortic stenosis is also associated with many risk factors for coronary artery disease.[195] Evidence suggests that degenerative aortic stenosis is linked to hyperlipidemia and that its prevalence might be decreased by more aggressive lipid lowering in adults.[193,196] Disorders in calcium transport, apoptosis of endocardial cells, and decreased nitric oxide synthesis also have been implicated.[193] Aortic valve degeneration with aging is associated with lipo protein deposition in the tissue with chronic inflammation and leaflet calcification.[197] The orifice of the aortic semilunar valve narrows, causing diminished blood flow from the left ventricle into the aorta (see Figures 30-30 and 30-31). Outflow obstruction increases pressure within the left ventricle as it tries to eject blood through the narrowed opening. Left ventricular hypertrophy develops to compensate for the increased workload. Eventually, hypertrophy increases myocardial oxygen demand that the coronary arteries may not be able to supply. If this occurs, ischemia may cause attacks of angina. Untreated aortic stenosis can lead to dysrhythmias, myocardial infarction, and heart failure.[195]

Aortic stenosis tends to develop gradually. The classic manifestations of aortic stenosis are angina, syncope, and heart failure.[192,195] These manifestations are attributable to diminished stroke volume that results in diminished tissue perfusion. Clinical manifestations include decreased stroke volume, reduced systolic blood pressure, and narrowed pulse pressure (difference between systolic and diastolic pressure). Heart rate is often slow, and pulses are faint. Resistance to flow through the stenotic valve gives rise to a crescendo-decrescendo systolic heart murmur heard best at the second intercostal space and may radiate to the neck.

Mitral Stenosis. Mitral stenosis impairs the flow of blood from the left atrium to the left ventricle. Mitral stenosis is most commonly caused by acute rheumatic fever (see p. 1185) and is two to three times more common in women than in men.[192] Autoimmunity in response to group A beta-hemolytic streptococcal M protein antigens leads to inflammation and scarring of the valvular leaflets (Figure 30-32).

Table 30-9	Clinical Manifestations of Valvular Stenosis and Regurgitation				
Manifestation	Aortic Stenosis	Mitral Stenosis	Aortic Regurgitation	Mitral Regurgitation	Tricuspid Regurgitation
Most common cause	Congenital bicuspid valve, degenerative (calcification) changes with aging, rheumatic fever	Rheumatic heart disease	Infective endocarditis; aortic root disease (connective tissue diseases, Marfan syndrome); dilation of the aortic root due to hypertension and aging	Myxomatous degeneration (mitral valve prolapse)	Congenital
Cardiovascular outcome (untreated)	Left ventricular hypertrophy followed by left heart failure; decreased coronary blood flow with myocardial ischemia	Left atrial hypertrophy and dilation with fibrillation, followed by right ventricular failure	Left ventricular hypertrophy and dilation, followed by heart failure	Left atrial hypertrophy and dilation, followed by left heart failure	Right heart failure
Pulmonary effects	Pulmonary edema: dyspnea on exertion	Pulmonary edema: dyspnea on exertion, orthopnea, paroxysmal, nocturnal dyspnea, predisposition to respiratory infections, hemoptysis, pulmonary hypertension, and edema	Pulmonary edema with dyspnea on exertion	Pulmonary edema with dyspnea on exertion	Dyspnea
Central nervous system effects	Syncope, especially on exertion	Neural deficits only associated with emboli (e.g., hemiparesis)	Syncope	None	None
Pain	Angina pectoris	Atypical chest pain	Angina pectoris	Atypical chest pain	Palpitations
Heart sounds	Systolic murmur heard best at the right parasternal second intercostal space and radiating to the neck	Low rumbling diastolic murmur heard best at the apex and radiating to the axilla, accentuated first heart sound, opening snap	Diastolic murmur heard best at the right parasternal second intercostal space and radiating to the neck	Murmur throughout systole heard best at the apex and radiating to the axilla	Murmur throughout systole heard best at the left lower sternal border

Data from Braunwald E, editor: *Heart disease: a textbook of cardiovascular medicine,* ed 7, Philadelphia, 2005, Saunders; Carabello BA, Paulus WJ: Valvular heart disease. In Crawford MH, DiMarco JP, editors: *Cardiology,* London, 2001, Mosby-Wolfe.

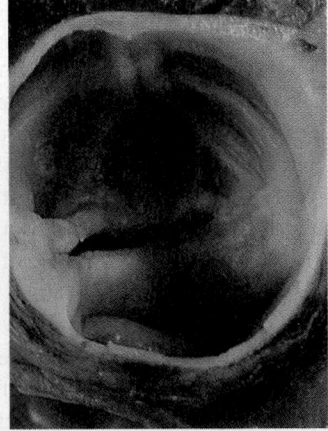

Figure 30-31 Aortic stenosis. Mild stenosis in valve leaflets of a young adult. (From Damjanov I, Linder J: *Pathophysiology: a color atlas,* St Louis, 2000, Mosby.)

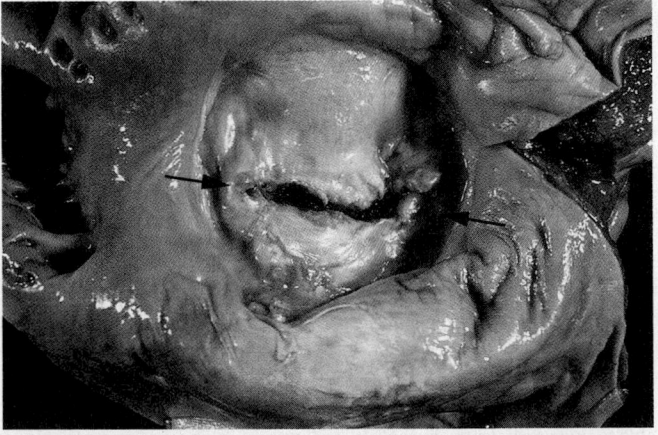

Figure 30-32 Mitral stenosis with classic "fish mouth" (*arrows*) orifice. (From Kumar: *Pathologic basis of disease,* ed 8, St Louis, 2010, Mosby.)

Scarring causes the leaflets to become fibrous and fused and the chordae tendineae cordis becomes shortened.

Clinical manifestations depend on the size of the valvular orifice. Impedance to blood flow results in incomplete emptying of the left atrium and elevated atrial pressure as the chamber tries to force blood through the stenotic valve. Continued increases in left atrial volume and pressure cause chamber dilation and hypertrophy. The risk of developing atrial dysrhythmias (especially fibrillation) and dysrhythmia-induced thrombi is high. As mitral stenosis progresses, symptoms of decreased cardiac output occur, especially during exertion. Continued elevation of left atrial pressure and volume causes pressure to rise in the pulmonary circulation. The outcomes of untreated chronic mitral stenosis are pulmonary hypertension, edema, and right ventricular failure.

Blood flow through the stenotic valve gives rise to a rumbling decrescendo diastolic murmur heard best over the cardiac apex and radiating to the left axilla. If the mitral valve is forced open during diastole, it may make a sharp noise called an *opening snap*. The first heart sound (S_1) is often accentuated and somewhat delayed because of increased left atrial pressure. Other signs and symptoms result from pulmonary congestion and right heart failure. Atrial enlargement is demonstrated by chest roentgenograms and electrocardiography.

Regurgitation

Aortic Regurgitation. **Aortic regurgitation** results from an inability of the aortic valve leaflets to close properly during diastole resulting from abnormalities of the leaflets or the aortic root and annulus, or both. It can be congenital (bicuspid valve) or acquired. Acquired aortic regurgitation can be caused by rheumatic heart disease, bacterial endocarditis, syphilis, hypertension, connective tissue disorders (e.g., Marfan syndrome and ankylosing spondylitis), appetite suppressing medications, trauma, or atherosclerosis.[192] In many cases dilation of the aortic root as a cause of regurgitation is idiopathic and more than a third of cases of aortic regurgitation have no known cause. The hemodynamic repercussions depend on the size of the "leak." During systole, blood is ejected from the left ventricle into the aorta. If the aortic semilunar valve fails to close completely, some of the ejected blood flows back into the left ventricle during diastole. Volume overload occurs in the ventricle because it receives blood from the left atrium and the aorta during diastole. Over time, the end-diastolic volume of the left ventricle increases and myocardial fibers stretch to accommodate the extra fluid. Compensatory dilation permits the left ventricle to increase its stroke volume and maintain cardiac output. Ventricular hypertrophy also occurs as an adaptation to the increased volume and increased afterload created by the high stroke volume and resultant systolic hypertension.[192] Ventricular dilation and hypertrophy eventually cease to compensate for aortic incompetence, and heart failure develops.[198]

Clinical manifestations include widened pulse pressure resulting from increased stroke volume and diastolic backflow. Turbulence across the aortic valve during diastole produces a decrescendo murmur heard best in the second, third, or fourth intercostal spaces parasternally and may radiate to the neck. Large stroke volume and rapid runoff of blood from the aorta cause prominent carotid pulsations and bounding peripheral pulses (Corrigan pulse). Other symptoms are usually associated with heart failure that occurs when the ventricle can no longer pump adequately. Dysrhythmias and endocarditis are common complications of aortic regurgitation.

Mitral Regurgitation. **Mitral regurgitation** has a variety of causes. The most common are mitral valve prolapse and rheumatic heart disease. Other causes include infective endocarditis, CAD, connective tissue diseases (Marfan syndrome), and congestive cardiomyopathy.[192] Mitral regurgitation permits backflow of blood from the left ventricle into the left atrium during ventricular systole, giving rise to a loud pansystolic (throughout systole) murmur heard best at the apex that radiates into the back and axilla. Because of increased volume in the left atrium entering the ventricle, the left ventricle becomes dilated and hypertrophied to maintain adequate cardiac output. The volume of backflow reentering the left atrium gradually increases, causing atrial dilation and associated atrial fibrillation. As the left atrium enlarges, the valve structures stretch and become deformed, leading to further backflow. As mitral valve regurgitation progresses, left ventricular function may become impaired to the point of failure. Eventually, increased atrial pressure also causes pulmonary hypertension and failure of the right ventricle. Mitral incompetence is usually well tolerated—often for years—until ventricular failure occurs. Most clinical manifestations are caused by heart failure.

Tricuspid Regurgitation. **Tricuspid regurgitation** is more common than tricuspid stenosis and usually is associated with cardiac failure and dilation of the right ventricle secondary to pulmonary hypertension. Rheumatic heart disease and infective endocarditis are less common causes. Tricuspid valve incompetence leads to volume overload in the right ventricle, increased systemic venous blood pressure, and right heart failure. Pulmonic semilunar valve dysfunction can have the same consequences as tricuspid valve dysfunction.

Mitral Valve Prolapse Syndrome

Mitral valve prolapse syndrome is a condition in which the anterior and posterior cusps of the mitral valve billow upward (prolapse) into the atrium during systole (Figure 30-33). The most common cause of mitral valve prolapse is myxomatous degeneration of the leaflets in which the cusps are redundant, thickened, and scalloped because of changes in tissue proteoglycans, increased proteinases, and infiltration by myofibroblasts.[192] The chordae tendineae may be elongated, permitting the valve cusps to stretch upward. Mitral regurgitation occurs if the ballooning valve permits blood to leak into the atrium.

Mitral valve prolapse is the most common valve disorder in the United States, with a prevalence of 1% to 3% in adults.[192,199] Mitral valve prolapse tends to be most prevalent in young women. Studies suggest an autosomal dominant and X-linked inheritance pattern.[199] Because mitral valve prolapse often is associated with other inherited connective tissue disorders (Marfan syndrome, Ehlers-Danlos

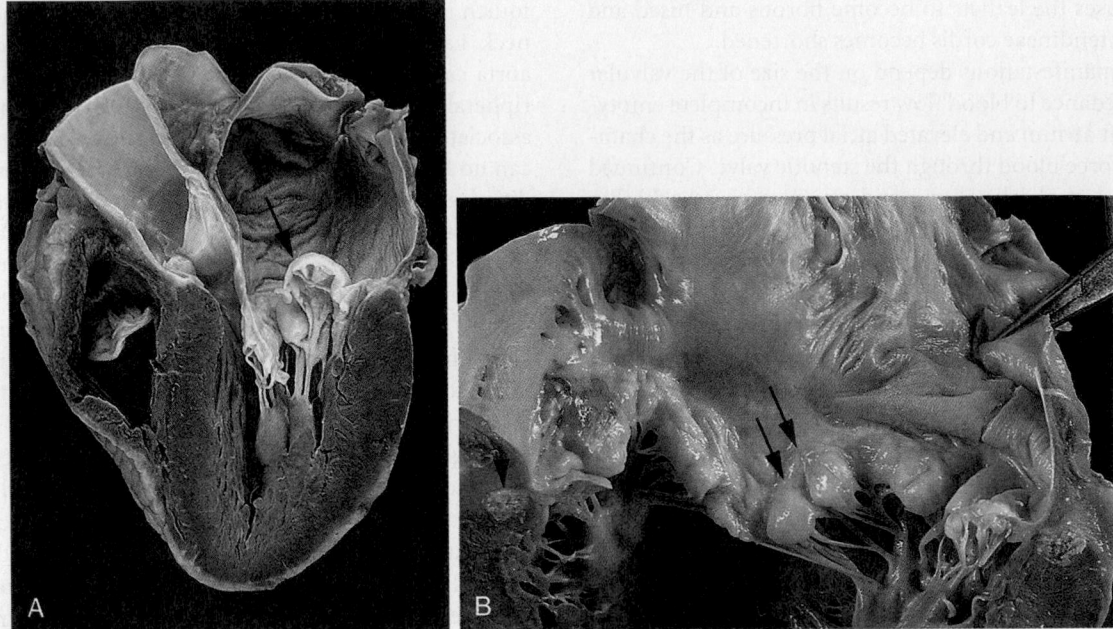

Figure 30-33 Mitral valve prolapse. **A,** Prolapsed mitral valve. Prolapse permits the valve leaflets to billow back *(arrow)* into the atrium during left ventricular systole. The billowing causes the leaflets to part slightly, permitting regurgitation into the atrium. **B,** Looking down into the mitral valve, the ballooning *(arrows)* of the leaflets is seen. (From Kumar V: *Pathologic basis of disease,* ed 8, St Louis, 2010, Mosby.)

syndrome, osteogenesis imperfecta), it is thought to result from a genetic or environmental disruption of valvular development during the fifth or sixth week of gestation. There may be a relationship between symptomatic mitral valve prolapse and hyperthyroidism. Other neuroendocrine abnormalities have been suggested, including polymorphisms of the angiotensin II type 1 (AT_1) receptor and alterations in ANS function.

Many cases of mitral valve prolapse are completely asymptomatic. Cardiac auscultation on routine physical examination may disclose a regurgitant murmur or midsystolic click in an otherwise healthy individual, or echocardiography may demonstrate the condition in the absence of auscultatory findings. Symptomatic mitral valve prolapse can cause palpitations related to dysrhythmias, tachycardia, lightheadedness, syncope, fatigue (especially in the morning), lethargy, weakness, dyspnea, chest tightness, hyperventilation, anxiety, depression, panic attacks, and atypical chest pain. Many symptoms are vague and puzzling and are unrelated to the degree of prolapse. Although severe sequelae—such as chordae rupture, ventricular failure, systemic emboli, and sudden death—are possible, the disorder is actually associated with minimal mortality and morbidity. Most individuals with mitral valve prolapse have an excellent prognosis, do not develop symptoms, and do not require any restriction in activity or medical management. However, a subset of individuals have an increased risk for complications such as infective endocarditis, cardioembolic stroke, and sudden death. These high-risk individuals can be identified by clinical and echocardiographic findings. Overall, the most

common complication of mitral valve prolapse is infective endocarditis.

EVALUATION AND TREATMENT The diagnosis of valvular heart disease is most often made by echocardiography. Cardiac catheterization is done prior to surgery to more directly evaluate valve structure and function as well as cardiac output.[200] Valvular heart disease can often be managed temporarily with careful fluid management and medications, such as diuretics and vasodilators. However, most significant valvular abnormalities eventually require surgical intervention either by repair of the valve or replacement with either a porcine or mechanical valve.[200] In the case of mechanical valve replacement, lifelong antibiotic prophylaxis prior to invasive procedures is required, as is lifelong anticoagulation to prevent clot formation on the valve with the possibility of embolization.

The majority of individuals with mitral valve prolapse have very few complications and require no treatment. Management is matched to the degree of mitral regurgitation. If regurgitation is present, antibiotic prophylaxis for infective endocarditis may be indicated before invasive procedures but physical activities are not restricted. Occasionally, beta-blockers are required to alleviate syncope, severe chest pain, or palpitations. Hypovolemia (resulting from diuretics or donating blood) is avoided because it can decrease ventricular volume, thereby increasing stress on the prolapsed mitral valve. Because surgical repair of redundant mitral valve tissue is safe and effective, some surgeons recommend operative treatment even in asymptomatic individuals who have prolapse and regurgitation to reduce the risk of stroke or sudden death.[201]

Acute Rheumatic Fever and Rheumatic Heart Disease

Rheumatic fever is a diffuse, inflammatory disease caused by a delayed immune response to infection by group A beta-hemolytic streptococci. In its acute form, rheumatic fever is a febrile illness characterized by inflammation of the joints, skin, nervous system, and heart.[202] If untreated, rheumatic fever can cause scarring and deformity of cardiac structures, resulting in **rheumatic heart disease (RHD).**

The incidence of acute rheumatic fever declined in the United States during the 1960s, 1970s, and early 1980s because of medical and socioeconomic improvements, as well as changes in the virulence of group A streptococci. More recent outbreaks in the United States and abroad corresponded to the reappearance of highly virulent strains. These virulent microorganisms have different M protein serotypes than the less pathogenic strains and can be identified as nephritogenic or rheumatogenic.[203] Because crowding and poor hygiene are environmental risk factors for acute rheumatic fever, the disease continues to be a major cause of death and disability for underprivileged populations.

The acute disease occurs most often in children between 5 and 15 years of age. Only 3% of those in whom pharyngeal streptococcal infection develops acquire acute rheumatic fever. Because beta-hemolytic streptococcus infection must persist for some time to cause acute rheumatic fever, appropriate antibiotic therapy given within the first 9 days of infection usually prevents rheumatic fever. Initiation of antibiotic therapy 2 weeks after the start of streptococcal infection does not prevent rheumatic fever in susceptible individuals.

Rheumatic fever tends to run in families, lending support to the concept of genetic predisposition, perhaps involving an abnormal immune response to antigens expressed by the bacterial membrane. Individuals who have experienced one attack of acute rheumatic fever are more susceptible than the general population to recurrent attacks.

PATHOPHYSIOLOGY Acute rheumatic fever can develop *only* as a sequel to pharyngeal infection by group A beta-hemolytic streptococci. Streptococcal skin infections do not progress to acute rheumatic fever because the strains of the microorganism that infect the skin do not have the same antigenic molecules in their cell membranes as do those that cause pharyngitis and therefore do not elicit the same kind of immune response. However, skin infections and pharyngeal infections can cause acute glomerulonephritis. Acute rheumatic fever affects the heart, joints, CNS, and skin through an abnormal humoral and cell-mediated immune response to the M proteins on the microorganisms that cross react with normal tissues[203,204] (Figure 30-34). These antigens can bind to receptors on cells in the heart, muscle, brain, and synovial joints.

Diffuse, proliferative, and exudative inflammatory lesions develop in the connective tissues, especially in the heart, joints, and skin. The inflammation may subside before treatment, leaving behind damage to the heart valves and increasing

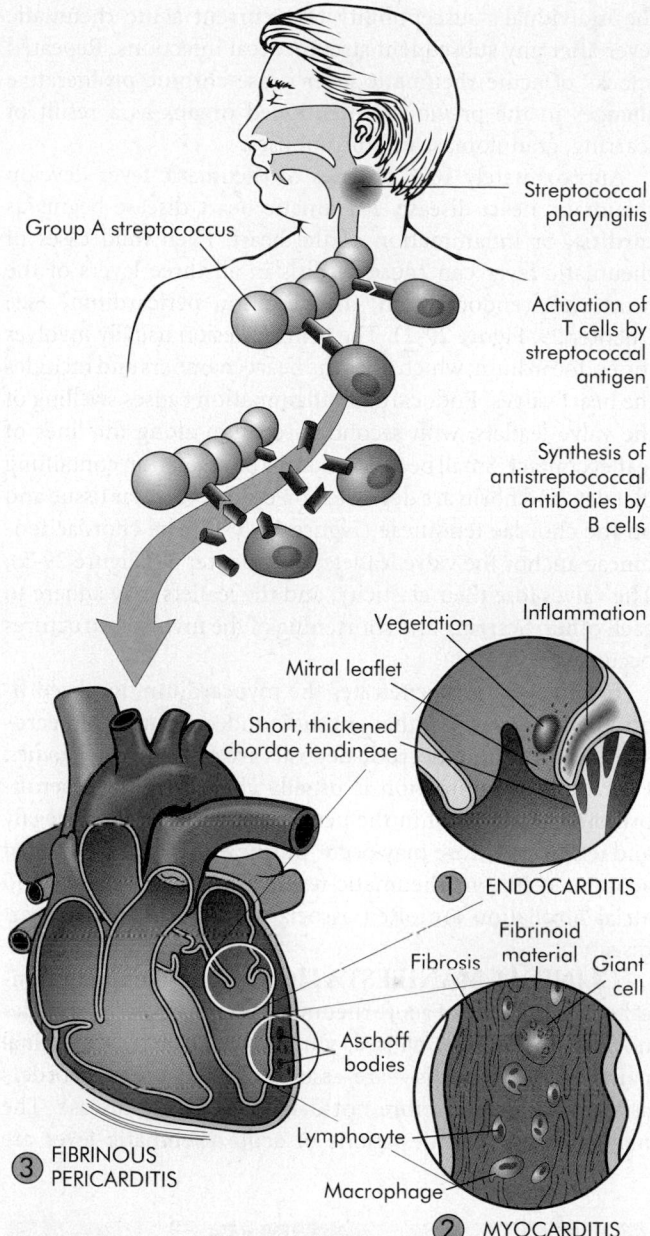

Figure 30-34 Pathogenesis and structural alterations of acute rheumatic heart disease. Beginning usually with a sore throat, rheumatic fever can develop only as a sequel to pharyngeal infection by group A beta-hemolytic streptococcus. Suspected as a hypersensitivity reaction, it is proposed that antibodies directed against the M proteins of certain strains of streptococci cross-react with tissue glycoproteins in the heart, joints, and other tissues. The exact nature of cross-reacting antigens has been difficult to define, but it appears that the streptococcal infection causes an autoimmune response against self-antigens. Inflammation is found in various sites including **(1)** endocardium, **(2)** myocardium, and **(3)** pericardium. The most distinctive inflammatory lesions within the heart are called *Aschoff bodies.* The chronic sequelae result from progressive fibrosis because of healing of the inflammatory lesions and the changes induced by valvular deformities. (From Damjanov I: *Pathology for the health-related professions,* ed 2, Philadelphia, 2000, Saunders.)

the individual's susceptibility to recurrent acute rheumatic fever after any subsequent streptococcal infections. Repeated attacks of acute rheumatic fever cause chronic proliferative changes in the previously mentioned organs as a result of scarring, granulomas, and thromboses.

Approximately 10% of cases of rheumatic fever develop rheumatic heart disease. Rheumatic heart disease begins as **carditis,** or inflammation of the heart. Even mild cases of rheumatic fever can cause carditis in all three layers of the heart wall (endocardium, myocardium, pericardium) (see Chapter 29, Figure 29-2). The primary lesion usually involves the endocardium, which lines the heart chambers and includes the heart valves. Endocardial inflammation causes swelling of the valve leaflets, with secondary erosion along the lines of leaflet contact. Small beadlike clumps of vegetation containing platelets and fibrin are deposited on eroded valvular tissue and on the chordae tendineae (Figure 30-35). (The chordae tendineae anchor the valve leaflets; see Chapter 29, Figure 29-3). The valves lose their elasticity, and the leaflets may adhere to each other. Scarring and shortening of the involved structures occur over time.

If inflammation penetrates the myocardium, localized fibrin deposits develop that are surrounded by areas of necrosis. These fibrinoid necrotic deposits are called *Aschoff bodies.* Pericardial inflammation is usually characterized by serofibrinous effusion within the pericardial cavity. Cardiomegaly and left heart failure may occur during episodes of untreated acute or recurrent rheumatic fever. Conduction defects and atrial fibrillation are often associated with rheumatic heart disease.

CLINICAL MANIFESTATIONS Many common clinical manifestations of acute rheumatic fever—fever, lymphadenopathy, arthralgia, nausea, vomiting, epistaxis, abdominal pain, and tachycardia—are associated with other disorders as well and are therefore not diagnostic of the disease. The major specific manifestations of acute rheumatic fever are

carditis, acute migratory polyarthritis, chorea, and erythema marginatum, which may occur singly or in combination after a latent period of 1 to 5 weeks after streptococcal infection of the pharynx.

Carditis. The earliest cardiac manifestation of acute rheumatic fever may be a previously undetected murmur caused by mitral or aortic semilunar valve dysfunction. Chest pain is caused by pericardial inflammation. Pericardial effusion produces an audible friction rub. Extra heart sounds, heart block (see p. 1199), atrial fibrillation, and a prolonged PR interval are often associated with chronic rheumatic heart disease. Endocardial inflammation may be manifested years later with serious valvular diseases (stenosis and regurgitation) and recurrent infective endocarditis.

Polyarthritis. The classic presenting manifestation of acute rheumatic fever is acute migratory polyarthritis (inflammation of more than one joint). Although all of the synovial joints may be involved, the large joints of the extremities are most often affected. Two or more joints are usually involved simultaneously or in succession, with each joint being symptomatic for approximately 2 to 3 days while the overall polyarthritis continues for up to 3 weeks. Exudative synovitis causes heat, redness, swelling, severe pain, and tenderness but no permanent disability. Palpable subcutaneous nodes often develop over bony prominences and along extensor tendons. They do not interfere with joint function and often go unnoticed.

Chorea. **Sydenham chorea,** or **St. Vitus dance,** is a disorder of the CNS characterized by sudden, aimless, irregular, involuntary movements. (Chorea is described in Chapter 16.) It is the most common acquired chorea in children and is more common in girls than in boys. It consists of psychologic and neurologic changes that occur 1 to 6 months after a streptococcal infection. The chorea is self-limiting, although severe cases may require the use of dopamine receptor blockers and antiepileptic medications.[205] It resolves within 1 to 6 months and has no permanent neural sequelae.

Erythema Marginatum. **Erythema marginatum** is a distinctive truncal rash that often accompanies acute rheumatic fever. It consists of nonpruritic, pink, erythematous macules that never occur on the face or hands. The rash is transitory and may change in appearance within minutes or hours. Heat (e.g., bathing) darkens the rash. The macules may fade in the center and be mistaken for ringworm.

EVALUATION AND TREATMENT Criteria for the diagnosis of rheumatic fever have been developed and updated by both the American Heart Association and the World Health Organization (Table 30-10).[206-208] No single laboratory test, sign, or symptom is pathognomonic of acute rheumatic fever but certain combinations of criteria indicate that acute disease is probably present.

When correlated with findings from physical assessment, laboratory values lend significant support to the diagnosis of acute rheumatic fever. A throat culture positive for group A beta-hemolytic streptococci can be an important finding when associated with certain physical signs. Cultures may be

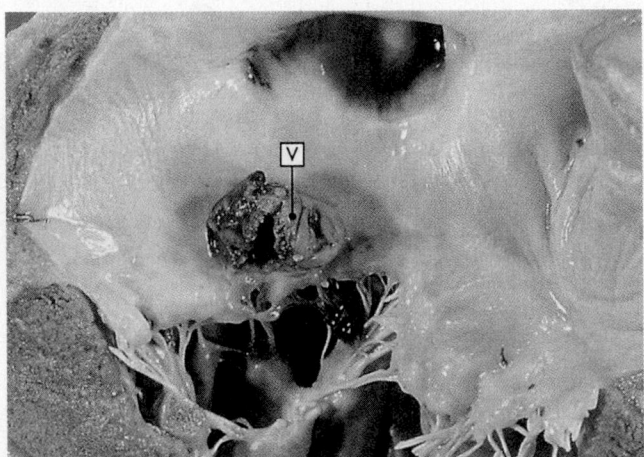

Figure 30-35 Mitral stenosis. Mitral stenosis and clumps of vegetation *(V)* containing platelets and fibrin. Mitral leaflets are thickened and fused and have clumps of vegetation containing platelets and fibrin. (From Stevens A, Lowe J: *Pathology,* St Louis, 1995, Mosby.)

Table 30-10	Jones Criteria (Revised) for Diagnosis of Rheumatic Fever	
Criteria	**Description**
Essential	Evidence of streptococcal infection (increased titer of streptococcal antibodies: antistreptolysin-O [ASO]; positive throat culture for group A streptococci; recent scarlet fever)
Major	Carditis, arthritis, chorea, erythema marginatum, subcutaneous nodules
Minor	*Clinical:* arthralgia, fever
	Laboratory: increased C-reactive protein, increased white blood cell count, increased erythrocyte sedimentation rate
	Electrocardiographic: prolonged PR interval

From Dajani AS, et al: Guidelines for the diagnosis of rheumatic fever: Jones criteria, updated 1992, *Circulation* 87: 302-307, 1993.

negative when the rheumatic attack begins, however. Documented recent scarlet fever is another potentially strong diagnostic aid to acute rheumatic fever, but diagnosis of scarlet fever also depends on a positive throat culture and may be difficult to distinguish from other disorders associated with a similar rash. Most strains of group A beta-hemolytic streptococcus produces a hemolytic factor called *streptolysin-O.* Antibodies against this hemolytic factor increase as an individual's immune system fights the disease. A high or rising antistreptolysin-O (ASO) antibody titer is an accurate means of diagnosing the presence of a streptococcal infection. ASO antibody titers higher than 250 Todd units in adults and 333 Todd units in children are considered elevated. Several other antibody tests are sensitive indicators of streptococcal infection. These include antideoxyribonucleotidase (anti-DNase B), antihyaluronidase, and antistreptozyme (ASTZ).

Elevated white blood cell count, erythrocyte sedimentation rate, and CRP indicate inflammation. All three are usually increased at the time cardiac or joint symptoms begin to appear. They are more useful in identifying an acute inflammatory process and suggesting prognosis than in diagnosing acute rheumatic fever. The levels of these tests decrease as the inflammatory process resolves.

Therapy for acute rheumatic fever is aimed at eradicating the streptococcal infection using a 10-day regimen of antibiotics. Nonsteroidal anti-inflammatory drugs (NSAIDs) are used as anti-inflammatory agents for rheumatic carditis and arthritis. Serious carditis may require that cardiac glycosides, corticosteroids, diuretics, and bed rest be added to the regimen. Surgical repair of damaged valves may be necessary in cases of chronic recurrent rheumatic fever or carditis. Active disease is considered resolved when (1) the murmur has disappeared or cardiac status becomes stable, (2) major manifestations are no longer present, (3) the individual is afebrile, and (4) the erythrocyte sedimentation rate is normal or stabilized. This may take 1 to 6 months.

A rheumatic recurrence will develop in 50% to 65% of children with known rheumatic fever if they have another group A streptococcal infection. Recurrence rates decline with the length of time elapsed since the last infection. Continuous prophylactic antibiotic therapy for as long as 5 years is necessary to prevent recurrence of acute rheumatic fever. Several group A streptococcus vaccines are in development.[209]

Infective Endocarditis

Infective endocarditis is a general term used to describe infection and inflammation of the endocardium—especially the cardiac valves. Bacteria are the most common cause of infective endocarditis, especially streptococci, staphylococci, or enterococci.[210,211] Other causes include viruses, fungi, rickettsiae, and parasites. Recognizing the likely mode of exposure is helpful in identifying the microorganism involved.[211] Untreated, infective endocarditis is a lethal disease but morbidity and mortality diminish significantly with the use of antibiotics and improved diagnostic techniques.

The American Heart Association has identified the cardiac disorders at highest risk for infective endocarditis.[212] These disorders are (1) the presence of prosthetic heart valves, (2) a history of infective endocarditis, (3) unrepaired or incompletely repaired congenital heart disease, (4) congenital heart disease repaired with prosthetic materials, and (5) cardiac transplant recipients who develop valvular disease. Other risk factors for infective endocarditis include acquired valvular heart disease, male gender, intravenous drug abuse, long-term indwelling catheterization (e.g., for pressure monitoring, hyperalimentation, or hemodialysis), and recent cardiac surgery.[212]

PATHOPHYSIOLOGY The pathogenesis of infective endocarditis is a complex process that requires at least three critical elements (Figure 30-36). First, the endocardium (e.g., heart valve) must be "prepared" (usually by endothelial damage) for microorganism colonization. Second, blood-borne microorganisms must adhere to the damaged endocardial surface. Third, the adherent microorganisms must proliferate and promote the propagation of infective endocardial vegetation.

The first critical element, endocardial damage, exposes the endothelial basement membrane. The basement membrane contains a type of collagen that attracts platelets and thereby stimulates thrombus formation on the membrane. Platelet activation and thrombus formation can cause an inflammatory reaction termed **nonbacterial thrombotic endocarditis.**[211,212]

Bacteremia and adherence constitute the second critical element. Infective endocarditis cannot develop unless microorganisms gain access to the bloodstream. Microorganisms may enter the bloodstream as a result of minor procedures, such as dental cleaning or bladder catheterization, or they may spread from uncomplicated upper respiratory or skin infections. Any time pathogens gain access to the bloodstream, the potential for endocardial infection exists. Adherence of microorganisms to the endocardial surface is facilitated by the coexistence of nonbacterial thrombotic endocarditis. It should be noted,

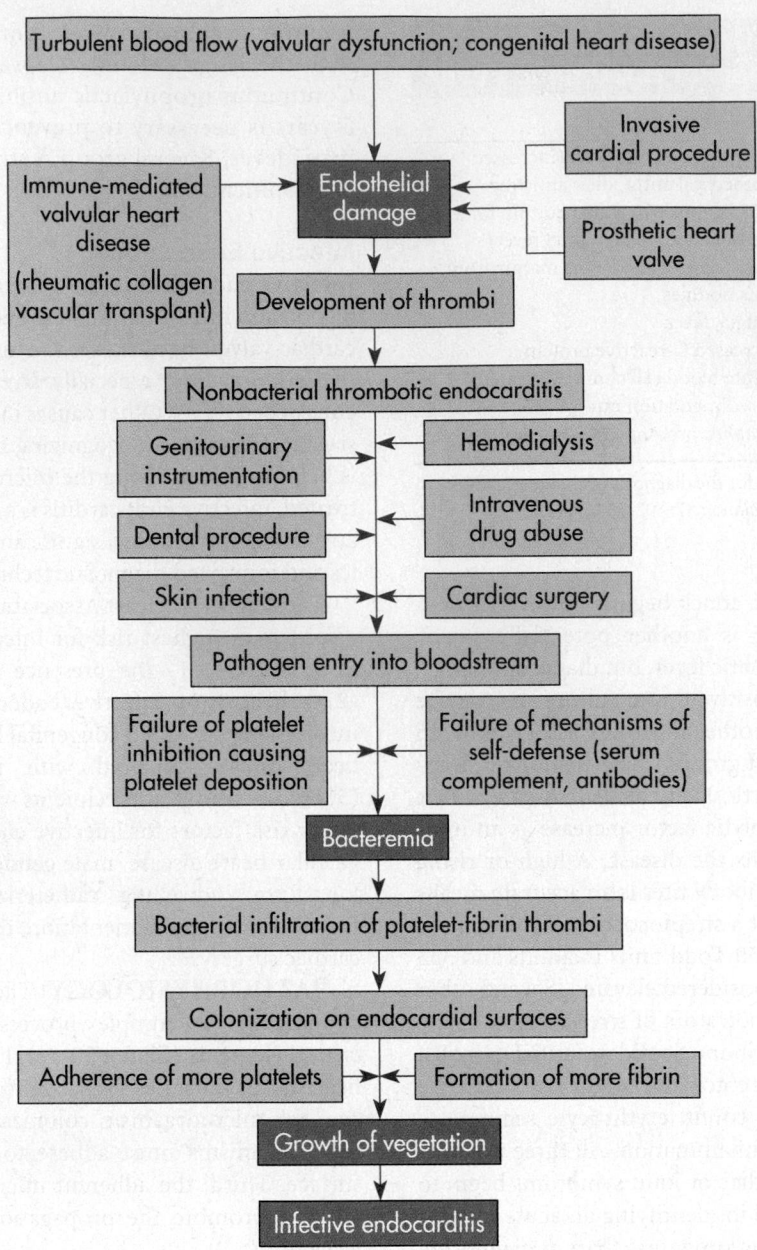

Figure 30-36 Pathogenesis of infective endocarditis.

however, that highly invasive organisms can cause infective endocarditis even on the healthy intact endocardium through bacterial virulence factors called adhesins.[212] Some bacteria are able to synthesize extracellular polysaccharides, such as dextran or fibronectin that promote stickiness on endocardial surfaces.

The third critical element, bacterial proliferation and vegetation formation, also is promoted by coexistent nonbacterial thrombotic endocarditis. Once the endocardial surface is colonized, formation of infected vegetation proceeds by a series of complex steps (Figure 30-37). Within 3 to 6 hours after infection, microbial replication occurs and bacterial colonies form within aggregates of fibrin and platelets. Within 24 hours, infected vegetation has increased in size, with colonies of microorganisms sandwiched between layers of fibrin and platelets. Bacteria may accelerate fibrin formation by activating the clotting cascade. As the growing bacterial colonies become progressively enmeshed in the tight fibrin network, which contains few phagocytic cells, they become less and less susceptible to the host's mechanisms of self-defense. Although endocardial tissue is constantly bathed in antibody-containing blood and is surrounded by scavenging monocytes and polymorphonuclear leukocytes, bacterial colonies are inaccessible to host defenses because they are embedded in the protective fibrin clots. The lesions can form anywhere on the endocardium but usually occur on the endocardial surfaces of heart valves and surrounding structures (see Figure 30-37).

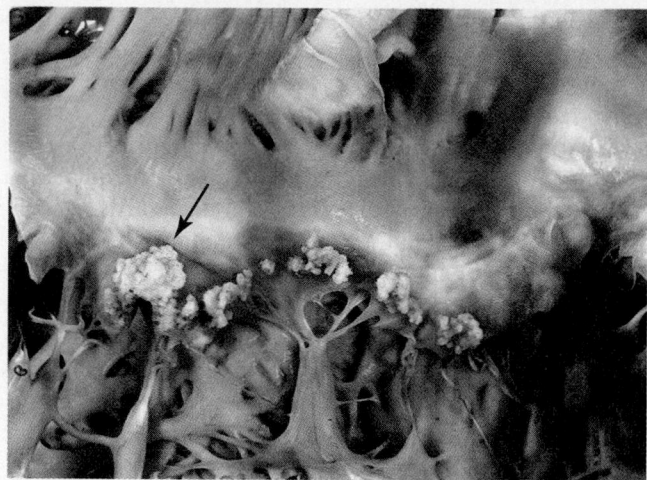

Figure 30-37 **Bacterial endocarditis of mitral valve.** Lesion (*see arrow*) in combination with old rheumatic valvulitis. (From Damjanov I, Linder J: *Pathology: a color atlas,* St Louis, 2000, Mosby.)

CLINICAL MANIFESTATIONS Infective endocarditis may be acute, subacute, or chronic. It causes varying degrees of valvular dysfunction and may be associated with manifestations involving several organ systems (lungs, eyes, kidneys, bones, joints, CNS), making diagnosis exceedingly difficult. Signs and symptoms of infective endocarditis are caused by infection and inflammation, systemic spread of microemboli, and immune complex deposition. The "classic" findings are fever; new or changed cardiac murmur; and petechial lesions of the skin, conjunctiva, and oral mucosa. Characteristic physical findings include Osler nodes (painful erythematous nodules on the pads of the fingers and toes) and Janeway lesions (nonpainful hemorrhagic lesions on the palms and soles).[213] Other manifestations include weight loss, back pain, night sweats, and heart failure. CNS, splenic, renal, pulmonary peripheral arterial, coronary and ocular emboli may lead to a wide variety of signs and symptoms. Sudden onset of severely debilitating symptoms indicates acute disease.

EVALUATION AND TREATMENT The criteria for the diagnosis of infective endocarditis include persistent bacteremia, new heart murmurs, vascular complications, and appropriate echocardiographic findings.[211,214] If infective endocarditis extends into the heart wall and invades the conduction system, electrocardiography may show a prolonged PR interval, left bundle branch block, or complete heart block (see Table 30-12). If emboli are suggested, organ scans can be performed to confirm their presence. Antimicrobial therapy is generally given for 4 to 6 weeks, beginning with intravenous and ending with oral administration.[215] In some cases two different antibiotics are given simultaneously to eliminate the offending microorganism and prevent the development of drug resistance. Other drugs may be necessary to treat left heart failure secondary to valvular dysfunction, and surgical intervention to repair or replace the valve may be required.[193]

Antibiotic prophylaxis is indicated for high-risk individuals (prosthetic valve, congenital heart disease, cardiac transplant recipients with valvular disease) prior to dental procedures that involve manipulation of gingival tissue or the periapical region of teeth or perforation of the oral mucosa.[212] Prophylaxis is no longer recommended for genitourinary or gastrointestinal procedures, although this has sparked controversy.[212,216]

Cardiac Complications in Acquired Immunodeficiency Syndrome

Individuals infected with the HIV and resultant acquired immunodeficiency syndrome (AIDS) are at risk for numerous cardiac complications. Pericardial effusion and left heart failure are the most common complications of HIV infection. Other conditions include cardiomyopathy, myocarditis, tuberculous pericarditis, infective and nonbacterial endocarditis, heart block, pulmonary hypertension, and non-antiretroviral drug-related cardiotoxicity. Malignancies, such as lymphoma and Kaposi sarcoma, are often seen in individuals with AIDS and can affect the heart. Furthermore, treatment with highly active antiretroviral therapy (HAART) can cause hyperlipidemia and atherosclerotic disease.[217,218]

MANIFESTATIONS OF HEART DISEASE

Heart Failure

Heart failure is defined as the pathophysiologic condition in which the heart is unable to generate an adequate cardiac output such that there is inadequate perfusion of tissues or increased diastolic filling pressure of the left ventricle, or both, so that pulmonary capillary pressures are increased. It is estimated that nearly 10% of Americans older than age 65 have symptomatic heart failure and approximately 20% of asymptomatic individuals older than age 40 have some evidence of myocardial dysfunction.[36] In the past three decades, hospitalizations for heart failure have increased 171%.[36] Mortality remains high with an estimated 8-year survival rate of only 15%, overall.[36] The most common risk factors for heart failure are increasing age, hypertension, ischemic heart disease, obesity, diabetes, and renal failure. Others include valvular heart disease, cardiomyopathies, myocarditis, congenital heart disease, and excessive alcohol use. Numerous genetic polymorphisms have been linked to an increased risk for heart failure, including genes for cardiomyopathies, myocyte contractility, and neurohumoral receptors. Genetic changes in kinases, phosphatases, and cellular calcium cycling are being explored.[219] Most causes of heart failure result in dysfunction of the left ventricle (systolic and diastolic heart failure). The right ventricle also may be dysfunctional, especially in pulmonary disease (right ventricular failure). Finally, some conditions cause inadequate perfusion despite normal or elevated cardiac output (high-output failure).

Types

Left Heart Failure (Congestive Heart Failure)

Left heart failure, commonly called **congestive heart failure,** is categorized as systolic heart failure or diastolic heart failure. Synonyms for these terms are systolic ventricular dysfunction and diastolic ventricular dysfunction. These two types of heart failure can occur together in one individual or singly.

Systolic Heart Failure. Systolic heart failure is defined as an inability of the heart to generate an adequate cardiac output to perfuse vital tissues. Cardiac output depends on the heart rate and stroke volume. Stroke volume is influenced by three major factors: contractility, preload, and afterload (see Chapter 29).

Contractility is reduced by diseases that disrupt myocyte activity. Myocardial infarction is the most common cause of decreased contractility; other causes include myocarditis and cardiomyopathies. Secondary causes of decreased contractility, such as myocardial ischemia and increased myocardial workload, contribute to inflammatory, immune, and neurohumoral changes that mediate a process called ventricular remodeling. **Ventricular remodeling** results in hypertrophy and dilation of the myocardium and causes progressive myocyte contractile dysfunction over time[220] (Figure 30-38). When contractility is decreased, stroke volume falls, and left ventricular end-diastolic volume (LVEDV) increases. This causes dilation of the heart and an increase in preload.

Preload, or LVEDV, increases with decreased contractility (see earlier) or when there is an excess of plasma volume (intravenous fluid administration, renal failure, mitral valvular disease). Increases in LVEDV can actually improve cardiac output to a certain point, but as preload continues to rise, it causes a stretching of the myocardium that eventually can lead to dysfunction of the sarcomeres and decreased contractility (Figure 30-39).

Increased afterload is most commonly a result of increased peripheral vascular resistance (PVR), such as that seen with hypertension (Figure 30-40). Although much less common, it also can be the result of aortic valvular disease. With increased PVR, there is resistance to ventricular emptying and more workload for the left ventricle, which responds with hypertrophy of the myocardium. Hypertrophy is mediated by angiotensin II and catecholamines and results in an increase in oxygen and energy demand by the thickened myocardium. The myocardium consumes a huge amount of metabolic energy and relies on the efficient production of ATP. This production of ATP depends on the myocytes getting enough fuel, having adequate mitochondrial function, and using an effective creatine kinase system. When demand for energy is greater than the ability of these systems to supply the necessary ATP, contractility of the myocardium is compromised.[221-223] An energy-starved state develops that further contributes to changes in the myocytes themselves and ventricular remodeling that significantly impairs contractility and, therefore, ventricular function (see Figure 30-38). Remodeling also results in the deposition of collagen between the myocytes, which can disrupt the integrity of the muscle,

decrease contractility, and make the ventricle more likely to dilate and fail. Weakness of the cardiac muscle due to hypertension-induced hypertrophy is called hypertensive hypertrophic cardiomyopathy.

As cardiac output falls, renal perfusion diminishes with activation of the RAAS, which acts to increase PVR and plasma volume, thus increasing afterload and preload further. In addition, baroreceptors in the central circulation detect the decrease in perfusion and stimulate the SNS to cause yet more vasoconstriction and to cause the hypothalamus to produce antidiuretic hormone. This vicious cycle of decreasing contractility, increasing preload, and increasing afterload causes progressive worsening of left heart failure (Figure 30-41).

In addition to these hemodynamic interactions, systolic congestive heart failure is characterized by a complex constellation of neurohumoral, inflammatory, and metabolic processes:

1. *Catecholamines.* Sympathetic nervous system activation initially compensates for a decrease in cardiac output by increasing heart rate and peripheral vascular resistance. However, catecholamines cause numerous deleterious effects on the myocardium, including direct toxicity to myocytes, induction of myocyte apoptosis, myocardial remodeling, down-regulation of adrenergic receptors, facilitation of dysrhythmias, and potentiation of autoimmune effects on the heart muscle.[223-225]

2. *RAAS*
   a. Angiotensin II (Ang II). Activation of the RAAS causes not only increases in preload and afterload but also direct toxicity to the myocardium (see Figure 30-38). Ang II mediates remodeling of the ventricular wall, contributing to sarcomere death, loss of the normal collagen matrix, and interstitial fibrosis. This leads to decreased contractility, changes in myocardial compliance, and ventricular dilation.
   b. Aldosterone. Aldosterone not only causes salt and water retention by the kidney but also contributes to myocardial fibrosis, autonomic dysfunction, and dysrhythmias. It also has been implicated in endothelial dysfunction and prothrombotic effects.[226,227]

3. *Arginine vasopressin.* Arginine vasopressin is also known as antidiuretic hormone and causes both peripheral vasoconstriction and renal fluid retention. These actions exacerbate hyponatremia and edema in heart failure.[228]

4. *Natriuretic peptides.* Atrial and brain natriuretic peptides (BNPs) are increased and may have some protective effect by decreasing preload; however, their compensatory mechanisms are inadequate in heart failure.[229-231]

5. *Inflammatory cytokines*
   a. Endothelial hormones. Endothelin is a potent vasoconstrictor and is associated with a poor prognosis in individuals with heart failure.[231]
   b. TNF-α and IL-6. TNF-α is elevated in heart failure and contributes to myocardial remodeling.[232] It

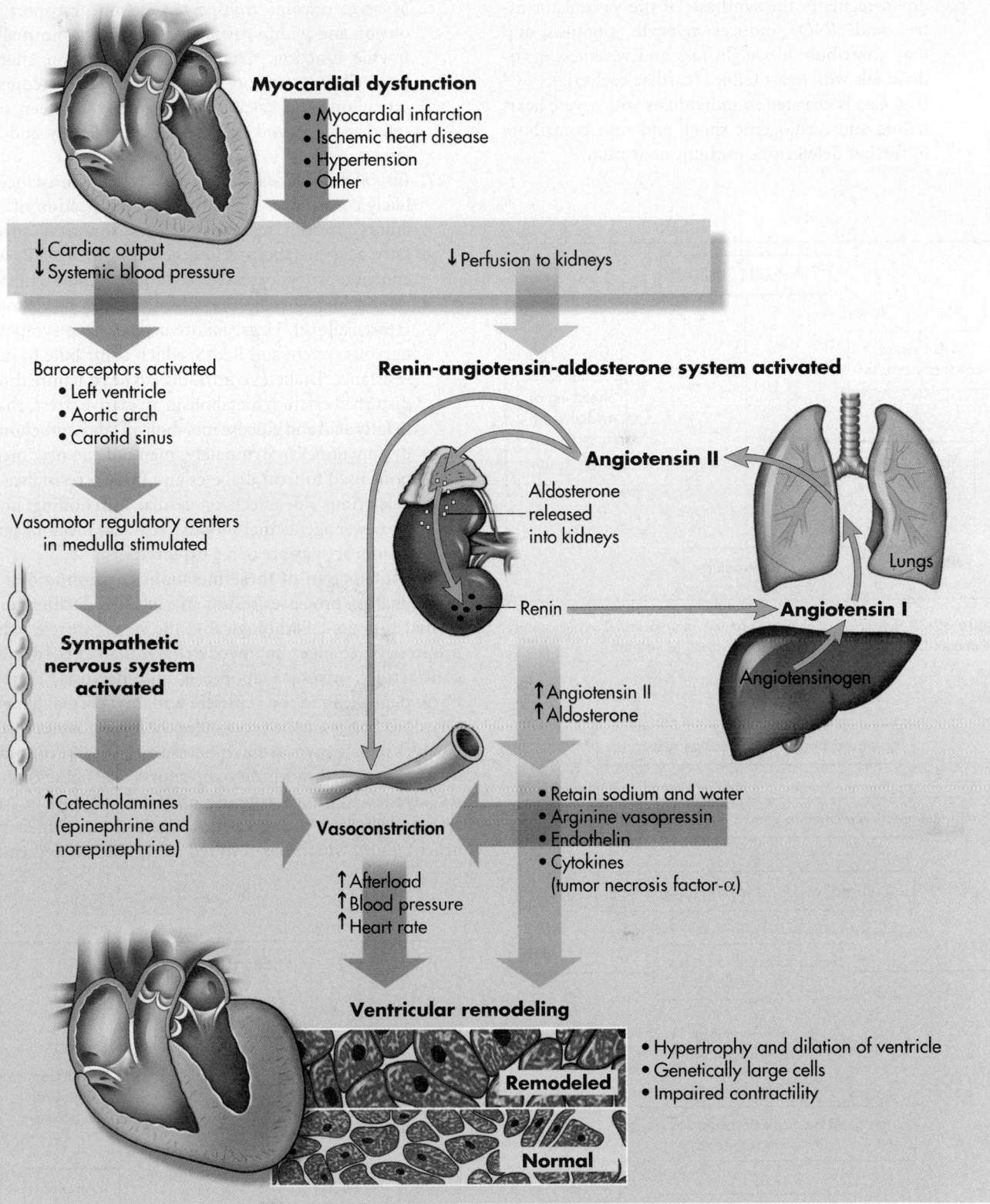

Myocardial dysfunction

- Myocardial infarction
- Ischemic heart disease
- Hypertension
- Other

↓ Cardiac output
↓ Systemic blood pressure

↓ Perfusion to kidneys

Baroreceptors activated
- Left ventricle
- Aortic arch
- Carotid sinus

Renin-angiotensin-aldosterone system activated

Angiotensin II

Aldosterone released into kidneys

Lungs

Vasomotor regulatory centers in medulla stimulated

Renin

Angiotensin I

Angiotensinogen

Sympathetic nervous system activated

↑ Angiotensin II
↑ Aldosterone

↑ Catecholamines (epinephrine and norepinephrine)

Vasoconstriction

- Retain sodium and water
- Arginine vasopressin
- Endothelin
- Cytokines (tumor necrosis factor-α)

↑ Afterload
↑ Blood pressure
↑ Heart rate

Ventricular remodeling

Remodeled

Normal

- Hypertrophy and dilation of ventricle
- Genetically large cells
- Impaired contractility

Figure 30-38 Pathophysiology of ventricular remodeling. Myocardial dysfunction activates the renin-angiotensin-aldosterone and sympathetic nervous systems, releasing neurohormones (angiotensin II, aldosterone, catecholamines, and cytokines). These neurohormones contribute to ventricular remodeling. (Redrawn from Carelock J, Clark AP: *Am J Nurs* 101[12]:27, 2001.)

down-regulates the synthesis of the vasodilator nitric oxide (NO), induces myocyte apoptosis, and may contribute to weight loss and weakness in individuals with heart failure (cardiac cachexia).[233,234] IL-6 also is elevated in individuals with severe heart failure and cardiogenic shock and may contribute to further deleterious immune activation.[232]

6. *Myocyte calcium transport.* Calcium transport into, out of, and within myocytes is critical to normal contractile function. Changes in calcium ion channels, intracellular transport mechanisms in the sarcoplasmic reticulum, and calcium cycling have all been implicated in decreased myocardial contractility and heart failure.[221,223,231]

7. *Insulin resistance and diabetes.* Insulin resistance is a likely contributor to, as well as complication of, heart failure. Insulin resistance causes abnormal myocyte fatty acid metabolism and generation of ATP, which contributes to decreased myocardial contractility and remodeling.[221] (see What's New? Metabolic Changes in Heart Failure). Heart failure activates the sympathetic nervous system and RAAS, which contribute to insulin resistance. Diabetes contributes to heart failure through disturbed calcium metabolism, oxidative stress, changes in fatty acid and glucose metabolism, and mitochondrial dysfunction. Unfortunately, many of the new medications used to treat diabetes and insulin resistance have deleterious side effects on cardiac functioning; however, newer agents that modify fatty acid metabolism and insulin activity are being explored.[221]

The interaction of these metabolic, neurohumoral, and inflammatory processes results in a gradual decline in myocardial function. Pathologically, the heart muscle exhibits progressive changes in myocyte myofilaments, decreased contractility, myocyte apoptosis and necrosis, abnormal fibrin deposition in the ventricle wall, myocardial hypertrophy, and changes in the ventricular chamber geometry. These changes reduce myocardial function and cardiac output and lead to increased morbidity and mortality. These discoveries have led to the routine use of ACE inhibitors or Ang II receptor blockers plus beta-blockers in the management of heart failure, which has resulted in significant decreases in

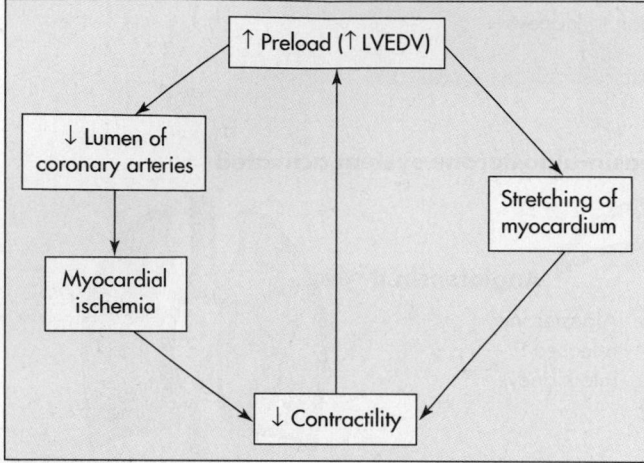

Figure 30-39 The effect of elevated preload on myocardial oxygen supply and demand. *LVEDV,* Left ventricular end-diastolic volume.

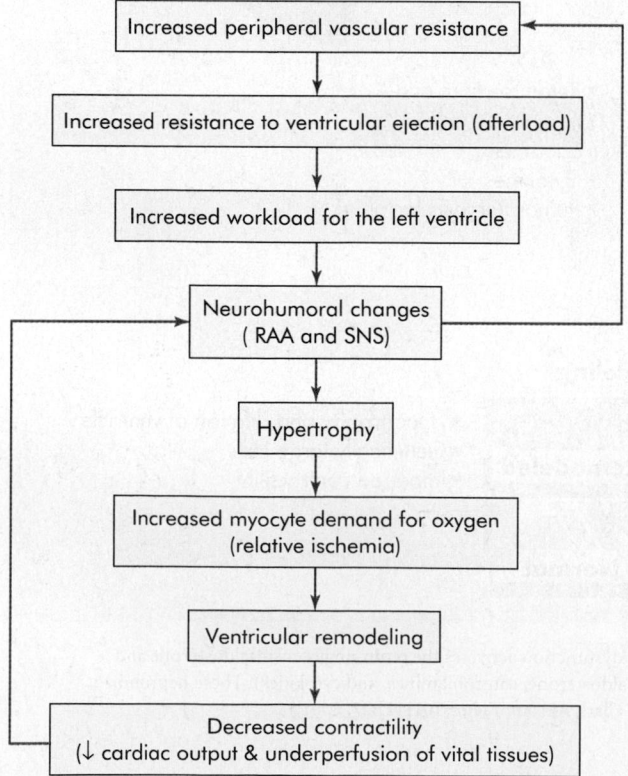

Figure 30-40 The role of increased afterload in the pathogenesis of heart failure.

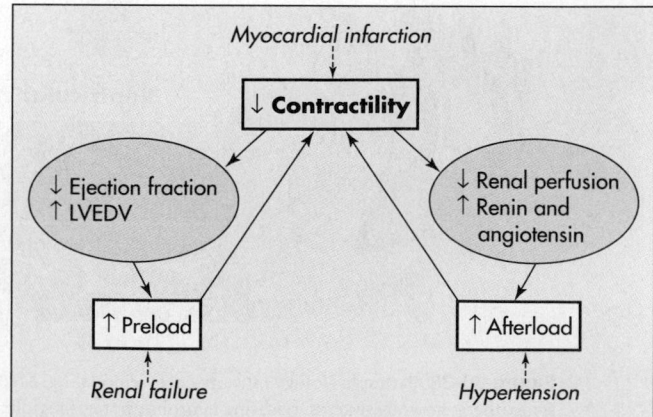

Figure 30-41 The vicious cycle of systolic heart failure. Although the initial insult may be one of primary decreased contractility (e.g., myocardial infarction), increased preload (e.g., renal failure), or increased afterload (e.g., hypertension), all three factors play a role in the progression of left heart failure. *LVEDV,* Left ventricular end-diastolic volume.

The heart is the largest consumer of energy in the body and relies on the efficient production of adenosine triphosphate (ATP). The heart has very little capacity for energy storage. In the failing heart, increased demand for oxygen and energy is coupled with a decreased ability to utilize fatty acids as an energy source. As a result, there is activation of several genes that alter the ability of myocytes to use lipids and glucose as fuel sources, the most studied of which are the peroxisome proliferator-activated receptor (PPAR) family of genes. These genes control fatty acid oxidation and are of particular importance in heart failure associated with insulin resistance and diabetes. Energy starvation and high levels of catecholamines associated with heart failure lead to altered fatty acid oxidation and decreased effective ATP generation and utilization. This results in decreased myocardial contractility and structural changes in the myocardium (remodeling). Increasing knowledge of these mechanisms has led to the exploration of potential new therapies for heart failure. For example, although currently available PPAR-gamma agonists (thiazolidinediones) are contraindicated in worsening heart failure because of increased fluid retention at the renal tubule, insulin sensitizers are being explored that may improve myocardial metabolic function. In addition, inhibitors of fatty acid oxidation (e.g., trimetazidine) have been tried in several small studies with some improvement in cardiac function. Many new potential pharmacologic interventions are under investigation, but in the meantime, most researchers agree that exercise and a healthy diet can improve myocardial metabolic function.

Data from Ashrafian H et al: *Circulation* 116(4):434-448, 2007; Boudina S et al: *Circulation* 115(25):3213-3223, 2007; Neubauer S: *N Engl J Med* 356(11):1140-1151, 2007; Mudd JO et al: *Nature* 451(7181):919-928, 2008; Tang WH et al: *Diabetes Obes Metab* 9(4):447-454, 2007.

Brain natriuretic peptide (BNP) is produced and released in response to pressure and volume overload of the cardiac chambers. This occurs in both systolic and diastolic heart failure (HF). BNP causes arterial and venous dilation, natriuresis, and suppression of the renin-angiotensin-aldosterone system and the sympathetic nervous system. BNP inhibits myocardial fibrosis and hypertrophy and enhances diastolic function. There are currently four uses for BNP: three are measures of serum levels of endogenous BNP and one is a therapeutic use for exogenous BNP:

1. *Diagnosis of heart failure:* significantly elevated serum levels of BNP have a sensitivity ranging from 93% to 98% in diagnosing heart failure in symptomatic patients, and negative predictive values ranging from 92% to 98%, demonstrating BNP ability to rule out heart failure. It also can be used for the diagnosis of diastolic heart failure.
2. *Prognosis in HF:* serum levels of BNP are correlated with the American Heart Association/American College of Cardiology class of heart failure morbidity and mortality, and risk for future acute exacerbations.
3. *Monitoring treatment of HF:* serum levels of BNP-guided treatment of heart failure reduced total cardiovascular events and delayed time to first event compared with intensive clinically guided treatment.
4. *Treatment of HF:* approved in August 2001 by the U.S. Food and Drug Administration, nesiritide is the first of a new class of drugs, human B-type natriuretic peptide (hBNP), and it is manufactured from *Escherichia coli* using recombinant deoxyribonucleic acid (DNA) technology. Nesiritide is an effective agent for improving hemodynamic profiles and symptoms of disease in individuals with acute severe decompensated heart failure; however, its overall safety continues to be evaluated.

Data from Bettencourt P et al: *Am J Cardiol* 101(3A):67-71, 2008; Elkayam U et al: *Crit Care Med* 36(1 Suppl):S95-S105, 2008; Hildebrandt P et al: *Am J Cardiol* 101(3A):25-28, 2008; Hunt SA et al: *Circulation* 112:E154-E235, 2005; Januzzi JL Jr et al: *Am J Cardiol* 101(3A):29-38, 2008; Shin DD et al: *Am J Cardiol* 99(2A):4A-23A, 2007.

morbidity and mortality.[235-237] Individuals selected for use of these medications may soon be facilitated through the use of pharmacogenetics that can identify those genotypes most likely to respond favorably to specific treatment options.[238] Aldosterone blockade with spironolactone is associated with a significant improvement in cardiac function and vasopressin blockade (e.g., tolvaptan) improve fluid balance.[226,227] Unfortunately, endothelin blockers and inflammatory cytokine blockers (e.g., etanercept) have not been effective.[235]

The clinical manifestations of left heart failure are the result of pulmonary vascular congestion and inadequate perfusion of the systemic circulation. Individuals experience dyspnea, orthopnea, cough of frothy sputum, fatigue, decreased urine output, and edema. Physical examination often reveals pulmonary edema (cyanosis, inspiratory crackles, pleural effusions), hypotension or hypertension, an S_3 gallop, and evidence of underlying CAD or hypertension. The diagnosis is made with echocardiography, revealing decreased cardiac output and cardiomegaly; some people may require invasive catheterization to document underlying coronary disease. Serum BNP levels should be measured to assist in diagnosing heart failure and to give some insight into its severity and response to treatment[239-241] (see What's New? Brain Natriuretic Peptide and Heart Failure).

Management of systolic left heart failure is aimed at interrupting the worsening cycle of decreasing contractility, increasing preload, and increasing afterload, as well as blocking the neurohormonal mediators of myocardial toxicity. The acute onset of left heart failure is most often the result of acute myocardial ischemia and must be managed in conjunction with the underlying coronary disease. Oxygen, nitrates, and morphine administration improve myocardial oxygenation and help relieve coronary spasm while lowering preload through systemic venodilation.[237] Diuretics reduce preload and are the mainstay of therapy.[237,242] Intravenous inotropic drugs, such as dopamine or dobutamine, increase contractility and can help raise the blood pressure in hypotensive individuals. New calcium-sensitizing inotropic drugs (e.g., levosimendan) have shown promise for acute heart failure in selected individuals.[231,243] ACE inhibitors (which reduce preload and afterload) and intravenous beta-blockers (which reduce myocardial demand) have been found to reduce mortality but must be used with caution in hypotensive individuals.[220,236,237,242,244] Intravenous administration of nesiritide (recombinant BNP) also improves preload and contractility; however, results of this therapy have been mixed.[231,237,244] Individuals with severe systolic failure because of myocardial ischemia may benefit from acute coronary bypass or PCI. Those with refractory hypotension may be supported with the intra-aortic balloon pump (IABP) until they can be taken safely to the operating room; the IABP is positioned in the aorta just distal to the aortic valve and is inflated during diastole to improve coronary perfusion and deflated during systole to reduce afterload.

Management of **chronic left heart failure** also relies on increasing contractility and reducing preload and afterload. The current standard of care for chronic heart failure includes diuretics, ACE inhibitors, and beta-blockers for all clinical stages. Salt restriction and diuretics (especially aldosterone-blockers such as spironolactone) are effective in reducing preload and improving outcomes.[226,235,236] ACE inhibitors (or Ang II receptor blockers) reduce preload and afterload and have been shown to significantly reduce mortality in chronic left heart failure.[235,236,245] Beta-blockers, especially some of the newer drugs such as bisoprolol, improve symptoms and increase survival.[235,236,246] The ionotropic drug digoxin may be considered in some individuals, especially those with atrial fibrillation.[236,247] Interestingly, statins have been associated with improved outcomes in some heart failure trials; however, their mechanism of action in heart failure is still being explored.[235,248,249] Anticoagulants and antithrombotics may be indicated in selected individuals, particularly those with intracardiac thrombi or atrial fibrillation.[236,248] Although many individuals with left heart failure die suddenly from dysrhythmias, prophylactic administration of antidysrhythmics has not been shown to improve survival. In individuals with sustained ventricular tachycardia, amiodarone or ICDs are indicated. Cardiac resynchronization therapy is proving to be an important modality in selected individuals.[250] Coronary bypass surgery or PCI may improve perfusion to ischemic myocardium (hibernating myocardium) and improve cardiac output. Other types of surgical intervention that improve ventricular geometry may be considered.[251,252] Finally, heart transplant may be the only remaining option. Experimental therapies, including gene and stem cell therapies, are being explored.[253,254]

Diastolic Heart Failure. **Diastolic heart failure** can occur singly or along with systolic heart failure. Isolated diastolic heart failure is defined as pulmonary congestion despite a normal stroke volume and cardiac output. It is the cause of approximately 50% of all cases of left heart failure and is more common in women.[255] The major causes of diastolic dysfunction include hypertension-induced myocardial hypertrophy and myocardial ischemia with resultant ventricular remodeling. Hypertrophy and ischemia cause a decreased ability

of the myocytes to actively pump calcium from the cytosol, resulting in impaired relaxation.[255,256] Other causes include aortic valvular disease, mitral valve disease, pericardial diseases, and cardiomyopathies. Diabetes also increases the risk for diastolic dysfunction.

Two areas of pathophysiologic changes in the ventricle have been identified in diastolic dysfunction: decreased compliance of the left ventricle and abnormal diastolic relaxation (lusitropy). Decreased ventricular compliance has been linked to changes in myocardial structure such as that seen with molecular alterations in collagen, which forms the extracellular matrix for myocytes. Another recently identified structural change is because of abnormalities in an intracellular protein component of the myocyte cytoskeleton called titin.[257] Abnormal lusitropy is caused by changes in calcium transport from myocytes and may be related to the activity of sarcoplasmic reticulum-calcium adenosine triphosphatase (ATPase).[257,258] The resultant noncompliant and poorly lusitropic ventricle cannot accept filling with blood without significant resistance and an increase in wall tension. Thus diastolic failure occurs because a normal LVEDV is associated with an increased left ventricular end-diastolic pressure (LVEDP), which is then reflected back into the pulmonary circulation and results in pulmonary edema. The increase in pressure is made worse when ventricular filling is rapid so symptoms worsen with tachycardia (e.g., with exercise).

Individuals with diastolic dysfunction most often present with dyspnea on exertion and fatigue. If diastolic dysfunction is severe, there may be evidence of pulmonary edema (crackles on auscultation, pleural effusions). Late in diastole, atrial contraction with rapid ejection of blood into the noncompliant ventricle may give rise to an S_4 gallop. Electrocardiography will often reveal evidence of left ventricular hypertrophy, and chest x-ray will show pulmonary congestion without cardiomegaly (Table 30-11). There also may be evidence of underlying coronary disease, hypertension, or valvular disease. Diagnosis is made initially by echocardiography, which demonstrates poor ventricular filling with normal ejection fractions. Management is aimed at improving ventricular relaxation and prolonging diastolic filling times to reduce diastolic pressure. Beta-blockers, ACE inhibitors, ARBs, and aldosterone blockers have been used with varying success.[256,257] Inotropic drugs are not indicated in isolated diastolic heart failure because contractility and ejection fraction are not affected.

Right Heart Failure

Right heart failure is defined as the inability of the right ventricle to provide adequate blood flow into the pulmonary circulation at a normal central venous pressure.[259] It most often results from left heart failure when the increase in left ventricular filling pressure that is reflected back into the pulmonary circulation is severe enough. As pressure in the pulmonary circulation rises, the resistance to right ventricular emptying increases.[259,260] The right ventricle is poorly prepared to compensate for this increased workload and will dilate and fail. When this happens, pressure will rise in

Table 30-11   Comparison of Systolic and Diastolic Heart Failure

Characteristic	Systolic Heart Failure	Diastolic Heart Failure
Gender	Male>female	Female>male
Left ventricular ejection fraction	Decreased	Normal
Left ventricular chamber size	Increased	Decreased
Left ventricular hypertrophy on electrocardiogram	Possible	Probable
Chest radiography	Pulmonary congestion with cardiomegaly	Pulmonary congestion without cardiomegaly
Gallop	S_3	S_4

Adapted from Jessup M, Brozena S: *N Engl J Med* 348(20):2007-2018, 2003.

the systemic venous circulation, resulting in jugular venous distension, peripheral edema, and hepatosplenomegaly. Treatment relies on management of the left ventricular dysfunction as just outlined. When right heart failure occurs in the absence of left heart failure, it is caused most commonly by diffuse hypoxic pulmonary disease such as COPD, cystic fibrosis, and ARDS (Figure 30-42). The mechanisms for this type of right ventricular dysfunction *(cor pulmonale)* are discussed in Chapter 33. Finally, right heart failure can result from right ventricular MI, cardiomyopathies, and pulmonic valvular disease.

High-Output Failure

High-output failure is the inability of the heart to adequately supply the body with blood-borne nutrients, despite adequate blood volume and normal or elevated myocardial contractility. In high-output failure the heart increases its output but the body's metabolic needs are still not met. Common causes of high-output failure are anemia, septicemia, hyperthyroidism, and beriberi (Figure 30-43).

Anemia decreases the oxygen-carrying capacity of the blood (see Chapter 26). Metabolic acidosis occurs as the body's cells switch to anaerobic metabolism (see Chapter 3). In response to metabolic acidosis, heart rate and stroke volume increase in an attempt to circulate blood faster. If anemia is severe, however, even maximum cardiac output does not supply the cells with enough oxygen for metabolism.

In septicemia, disturbed metabolism, bacterial toxins, and the inflammatory process cause systemic vasodilation and fever. Faced with a lowered systemic vascular resistance (SVR) and an elevated metabolic rate, cardiac output increases to maintain blood pressure and prevent metabolic acidosis. In overwhelming septicemia, however, the heart may not be able to raise its output enough to compensate for vasodilation. Body tissues show signs of inadequate blood supply despite a very high cardiac output.

Hyperthyroidism accelerates cellular metabolism through the actions of elevated levels of thyroxine from the thyroid gland. This may occur chronically (thyrotoxicosis) or acutely (thyroid storm). Because the body's demand for oxygen threatens to cause metabolic acidosis, cardiac output increases. If blood levels of thyroxine are high and the metabolic response to thyroxine is quite vigorous, even an abnormally elevated cardiac output may be inadequate.

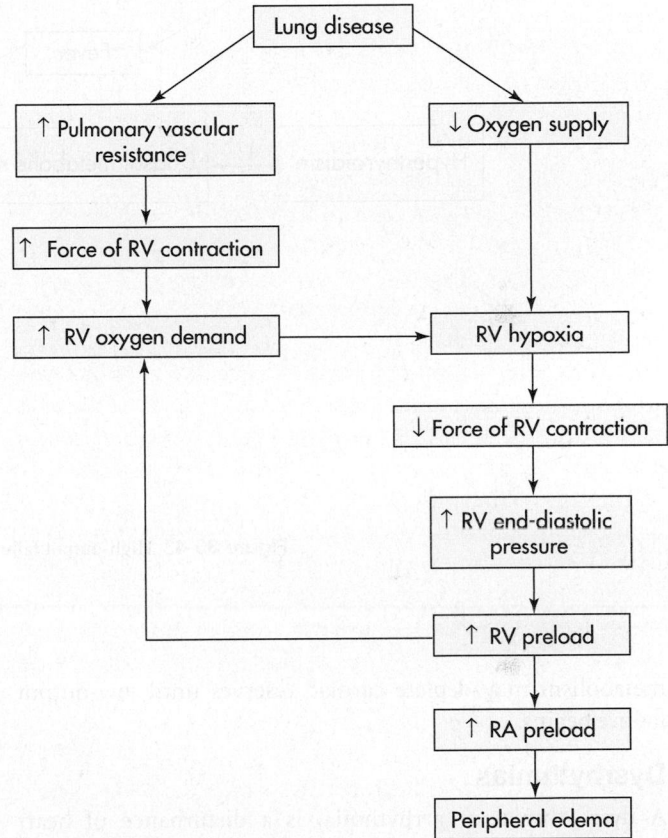

Figure 30-42 Right heart failure (cor pulmonale) caused by lung disease. *RA,* Right atrial; *RV,* right ventricular.

In the United States, beriberi (thiamine deficiency) usually is caused by malnutrition secondary to chronic alcoholism. Beriberi actually causes a mixed type of heart failure. Thiamine deficiency impairs cellular metabolism in all tissues, including the myocardium. In the heart, impaired cardiac metabolism leads to insufficient contractile strength. In blood vessels, thiamine deficiency leads mainly to peripheral vasodilation, which decreases SVR. Heart failure ensues as decreased SVR triggers increased cardiac output, which the impaired myocardium is unable to deliver. The strain of demands for increased output in the face of impaired

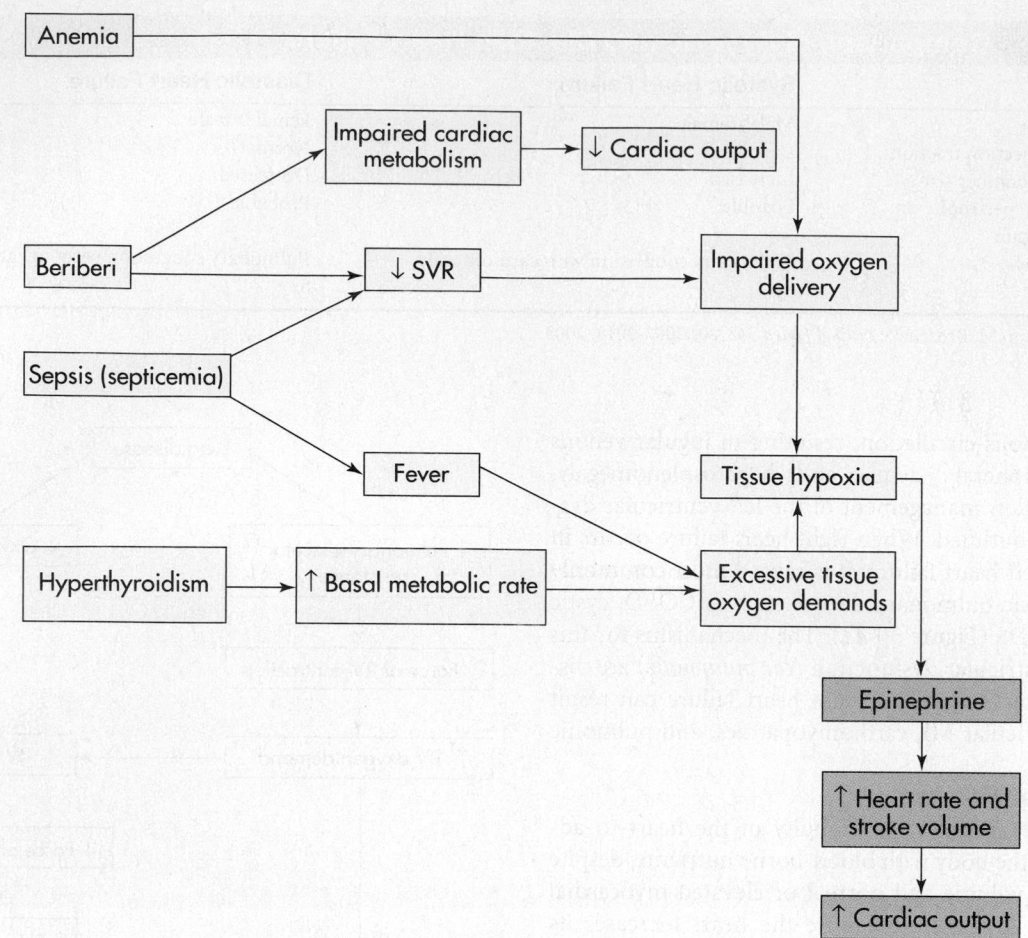

Figure 30-43 High-output failure. *SVR,* Systemic vascular resistance.

metabolism may deplete cardiac reserves until low-output failure begins.

Dysrhythmias

A dysrhythmia, or arrhythmia, is a disturbance of heart rhythm. Normal heart rhythms are generated by the SA node and travel through the heart's conduction system, causing the atrial and ventricular myocardium to contract and relax at a regular rate that is appropriate to maintain circulation at various levels of physical activity (see Chapter 29). Dysrhythmias range in severity from occasional "missed" or rapid beats to serious disturbances that impair the pumping ability of the heart, contributing to heart failure and death. Dysrhythmias can be caused by either an abnormal rate of impulse generation (Table 30-12) by the SA node or other pacemaker or the abnormal conduction of impulses (Table 30-13) through the heart's conduction system, including the myocardial cells themselves.

Table 30-12 Disorders of Impulse Formation

Type	Electrocardiogram	Effect	Pathophysiology	Treatment
Sinus bradycardia	P rate 60 or less PR interval normal QRS for each P	Increased preload Decreased mean arterial pressure	Hyperkalemia: slows depolarization Vagal hyperactivity: unknown Digoxin toxicity common Late hypoxia: lack of adenosine triphosphate (ATP)	If hypotensive, treat cause and support Follow with sympathomimetics, cardiotonics, and pacer Vagolytics
Simple sinus tachycardia	P rate 100-150 PR interval normal QRS for each P	Decreased filling times Decreased mean arterial pressure Increased myocardial demand	Catecholamines; rise in resting potential, calcium influx Fever: unknown Early failure and lung disease: hypoxic cell metabolism Hypercalcemia	Oxygen, bed rest Calcium channel blockers
Premature atrial contractions (PACs) or beats*	Early P waves that may have changed morphology PR interval normal QRS for each P	Occasional decreased filling time and mean arterial pressure	Electrolyte disturbances: decrease in all phases Hypoxia and elevated preload: cell membrane disturbances Hypercalcemia	Treat underlying cause Digoxin
Sinus dysrhythmias	Rate varies P-P regularly irregular, short with inspiration, long with exhalation PR interval normal QRS for each P	Variable filling times Variable mean arterial pressures Variable oxygen demand	Unknown Common in young children and young adults	None
Atrial tachycardia (includes premature atrial tachycardia if onset is abrupt)	P rate 151-250 P morphology may differ from sinus P PR interval normal P/QRS ratio variable	Decreased filling time Decreased mean arterial pressure Increased myocardial demand	Same as PACs: leads to increased atrial automaticity, atrial reentry Digoxin toxicity: common	Control ventricular rate Digoxin, calcium channel blockers, vagus stimulation Pace to override
Atrial flutter*	P rate 251-300, morphology may vary from sinus P PR interval usually not observable P/QRS ratio variable	Decreased filling time Decreased mean arterial pressure	Same as atrial tachycardia Aging	Same as atrial tachycardia Synchronous cardioversion
Atrial fibrillation*	P rate > 300 and usually not observable No PR interval QRS rate variable and rhythm irregular	Same as atrial flutter	Same as atrial tachycardia Aging	Same as atrial tachycardia
Idiojunctional rhythm	P absent or independent QRS normal, rate 41-59, regular	Decreased cardiac output from loss of atrial contribution to ventricular preload Decreased mean atrial pressure as a result of bradycardia	Atrial and sinus bradycardia, standstill, or block	Same as sinus bradycardia
Junctional bradycardia	P absent or independent QRS normal, rate 40 or less	Same as idiojunctional rhythm	Same as idiojunctional rhythm Vagal hyperactivity	Same as sinus bradycardia

*Most common in adults.
†Life threatening in adults.

Continued

Table 30-12   Disorders of Impulse Formation—cont'd

Type	Electrocardiogram	Effect	Pathophysiology	Treatment
Premature junctional contractions (PJCs) or beats	Early beats without P waves QRS morphology normal	Decreased cardiac output from loss of atrial contribution to ventricular preload for that beat	Hyperkalemia (6-5.4 mEq/L) Hypercalcemia, hypoxia, and elevated preload (see PACs)	Same as PAC
Accelerated junctional rhythm	P absent or independent QRS morphology normal, rate 60-99	Decreased cardiac output from loss of atrial contribution to ventricular preload	Same as PJCs	Same as PAC
Junctional tachycardia	P absent or independent QRS morphology normal, rate 100 or more	Decreased cardiac output from loss of atrial contribution to ventricular preload Increased myocardial demand because of tachycardia	Same as PJCs	Same as PAC
Idioventricular rhythm[†]	P absent or independent QRS >0.11 and rate 20-39	Same as idiojunctional rhythm	Sinus, atrial, and junctional bradycardia, standstill, or block	Same as sinus bradycardia
Ventricular bradycardia[†]	P absent or independent QRS >0.11 and rate 60-21	Same as idiojunctional rhythm	Same as idiojunctional rhythm	Same as sinus bradycardia
Agonal rhythm/electromechanical dissociation[†]	P absent or independent QRS >0.11 and rate 20 or less	Absent or barely present cardiac output and pulse Not compatible with life	Depolarization and contraction not coupled: electrical activity present with little or no mechanical activity Usually caused by profound hypoxia	Vigorous pharmacology aimed at restoring rate and force Usually ineffective May attempt to pace
Ventricular standstill or asystole[†]	P absent or independent QRS absent	No cardiac output Not compatible with life	Profound ischemia, hyperkalemia, acidosis	Same as agonal rhythm, including electrical defibrillation
Premature ventricular contractions (PVCs) or depolarizations*	Early beats with P waves QRS occasionally opposite in deflection from usual QRS	Same as premature junctional contractions	Same as PJCs, including aging and induction of anesthesia Impulse originates in cell outside normal conduction system and spreads through intercalated disks	Pharmacology to change thresholds, refractory periods; reduce myocardial demand, increase supply Removal of cause
Accelerated ventricular rhythm	P absent or independent QRS >0.11 and rate 41-99	Same as accelerated junctional rhythm	Same as PVCs	Same as PVCs
Ventricular tachycardia[†]	P absent or independent QRS >0.11 and rate 100 or more	Same as junctional tachycardia	Same as PVCs	Same as PVCs, including electrical cardioversion
Ventricular fibrillation[†]	P absent QRS >300 and usually not observable	Same as ventricular standstill	Same as PVCs Rapid infusion of potassium	Same as PVCs including electrical defibrillation

*Most common in adults.
[†]Life threatening in adults.

Table 30-13 Disorders of Impulse Conduction

Type	Electrocardiogram	Effect	Pathophysiology	Treatment
Sinus block	Occasionally absent P, with loss of QRS for that beat	Occasional decrease in cardiac output Increase in preload for the following beat	Local hypoxia, scarring of intra-atrial conduction pathways, electrolyte imbalances Increased atrial preload	Conservative Usually do not progress in severity Pharmacologic treatment includes vagolytics, sympathomimetics, pacing
First-degree block*	PR interval >0.2	None	Same as sinus block Hyperkalemia (>7 mEq/L) Hypokalemia (<3.5 mEq/L) Formation of myocardial abscesses in endocarditis	Conservative Discovery and correction of cause
Second-degree block, Mobitz I, or Wenckebach*	Progressive prolongation of PR interval until one QRS is dropped Pattern of prolongation resumes	Same as sinus block	Hypokalemia (<3.5 mEq/L) Faulty cell metabolism in atrioventricular (AV) node Severity increases as heart rate increases Supports theory that AV node is fatiguing Digoxin toxicity, beta-blockade Coronary artery disease (CAD), myocardial infarction (MI), hypoxia, increased preload, valvular surgery and disease, diabetes	Same as sinus block
Second-degree block or Mobitz II	Same as sinus block	Same as sinus block	Hypokalemia (<3.5 mEq/L) Faulty cell metabolism below AV node Antidysrhythmics, cyclic antidepressants CAD, MI, hypoxia, increased preload, valvular surgery and disease, diabetes	More aggressively than Mobitz I because block can progress to type III Pacemaker after pharmacologic treatment
Third-degree block†	P waves present and independent of QRS No observed relationship between P and QRS Always AV dissociation	Same as idiojunctional rhythm	Hypokalemia (<3.5 mEq/L) Faulty cell metabolism low in bundle of His MI, especially inferior wall, as nodal artery interrupted; results in ischemia of AV node	Pharmacologic until pacemaker inserted Temporary pacing if caused by inferior MI because ischemia usually resolves
Atrioventricular dissociation	P waves present and independent of QRS, but not always because of block (e.g., ventricular tachycardia) AV dissociation not always third-degree block	Decreased cardiac output from loss of atrial contribution to ventricular preload Variable effect on myocardial demand, depending on ventricular rate	May result from third-degree block or accelerated junctional or ventricular rhythm, or be caused by sinus, atrial, and junctional bradycardias	Treat according to cause Pacemaker or reducing rate of AV or ventricular discharge, or increasing rate of sinus or AV node discharge

Continued

Table 30-13   Disorders of Impulse Conduction—cont'd

Type	Electrocardiogram	Effect	Pathophysiology	Treatment
Ventricular block	QRS >0.11 R-S-R′ in V_1, V_2, V_5, V_6	None	Faulty cell metabolism in right and left bundle branches RBBB more common than LBBB because of dual blood supply to left bundle branch Congestive heart failure, mitral regurgitation, especially anterior MI, because of infarct of fascicles Left anterior hemiblock more common than left posterior hemiblock, since posterior fascicles have dual blood supply	Isolated right bundle branch block (RBBB) or left bundle branch block (LBBB) or hemiblock not treated If acute and/or associated with acute anterior MI, treated with permanent pacer and vigorous pharmacology
Aberrant conduction	QRS >0.11	None unless ventricular rate abnormalities present	Conduction of impulse through intercalated disks because conduction system transiently blocked because of hypoxia, electrolyte imbalances, digoxin toxicity, excessively rapid rates of discharge	Correct underlying cause
Preexcitation syndromes (Wolff-Parkinson-White and Lown-Ganong-Levine)	P present with QRS for each P PR interval >0.12 and QRS >0.11 because of presence of delta wave in PR interval	None	Congenital presence of accessory pathways (bundle of Kent and fiber of Mahaim) that conduct very rapidly and bypass the AV node, causing early ventricular depolarization in relation to atrial depolarization Prone (reason unknown) to tachycardias and atrial fibrillation that can result in very rapid ventricular rates	Aimed at lining up refractory periods of accessory pathway and AV node to prevent reentry May slow rate with pharmacology May surgically cut pathways

SUMMARY REVIEW

Diseases of the Veins

1. Varicosities are areas of veins in which blood has pooled, usually in the saphenous veins. Varicosities may be caused by damaged valves as a result of trauma to the valve or by chronic venous distention involving gravity and venous constriction.
2. Chronic venous insufficiency is inadequate venous return over a long period that causes pathologic ischemic changes in the vasculature, skin, and supporting tissues.
3. Venous stasis ulcers follow the development of chronic venous insufficiency and probably develop as a result of the borderline metabolic state of the cells in the affected extremities.
4. DVT occurs in individuals who have venous stasis (immobility, age, left heart failure), spinal cord injury, vein wall damage (trauma, intravenous medications), or hypercoagulable states (pregnancy, oral contraceptives, malignancy, genetic coagulopathies).
5. DVT is often asymptomatic but may lead to fatal pulmonary emboli; prevention and careful assessment in individuals at risk are crucial.

Diseases of the Arteries

1. An aneurysm is a localized dilation of a vessel wall to which the aorta is particularly susceptible.
2. A thrombus is a clot that remains attached to a vascular wall.

3. An embolus is a mobile aggregate of a variety of substances that occludes the vasculature. Sources of emboli include thrombi, air, amniotic fluid, bacteria, fat, and foreign matter.

4. The most common sources of arterial thrombotic emboli from the heart are mitral and aortic valvular disease and atrial fibrillation. Tissues affected include the lower extremities, the brain, and the heart.

5. Emboli to the central organs cause tissue death in lungs, kidneys, and mesentery.

6. The generation of air emboli requires a connection between the vascular compartment and a source of air. These emboli cause ischemia and necrosis when a vessel is totally blocked.

7. Amniotic fluid may be forced into the bloodstream and generate an embolus during the labor and delivery of pregnancy.

8. Aggregates of bacteria in the vasculature may be large enough to form an embolus.

9. Fat emboli are caused mainly by trauma to the long bones, either through defective fat metabolism after trauma or through the release of fat globules from bone marrow exposed by fracture.

10. The introduction of foreign matter into the vasculature can occur with trauma and also can occur in a hospital setting in which intravenous and intra-arterial lines are being used.

11. Vasospastic disorders include Raynaud disease, involving arterioles of the extremities; variant angina, involving coronary arteries; and Buerger disease, involving arteries of the hands and feet.

12. Hypertension is a sustained elevation of the systemic arterial blood pressure resulting from increases in cardiac output or total peripheral resistance or both. Hypertension can be primary (without known cause) or secondary (caused by disease or drugs). Systolic hypertension is the most significant factor in causing target organ damage.

13. The risk factors for hypertension include a positive family history; male gender; advanced age; black race; obesity; high sodium intake; low potassium, calcium, and magnesium intake; diabetes mellitus; labile blood pressure; cigarette smoking; and heavy alcohol consumption.

14. Primary hypertension is the result of extremely complicated interactions of genetics and the environment mediated by a host of neurohumoral effects. These genes interact with diet, smoking, age, and the other risk factors to cause chronic changes in vasomotor tone and blood volume.

15. The most frequently cited theories of the pathogenesis of primary hypertension include overactivity of the SNS; overactivity of the RAAS; alterations in other neurohumoral mediators of blood volume and vasomotor tone such as ANP, BNP, and adrenomedullin; inflammation; a complex interaction involving insulin resistance and endothelial function; and obesity-related hormonal changes.

16. Clinical manifestations of hypertension result from damage of organs and tissues outside the vascular system. These include heart disease, renal disease, CNS problems, and retinal changes.

17. Hypertension is managed pharmacologically, using diuretics, adrenergic blockers, calcium channel blockers, ACE inhibitors, and Ang II receptor blockers. Nonpharmacologic methods include cessation of smoking, dietary modifications, and exercise.

18. Orthostatic hypotension is a drop in blood pressure that occurs on standing. The compensatory vasoconstriction response to standing is altered by a marked vasodilation and blood pooling in the muscle vasculature.

19. Orthostatic hypotension may be acute or chronic. The acute form is caused by a delay in the normal regulatory mechanisms. The chronic forms are secondary to a specific disease or are idiopathic in nature.

20. The clinical manifestations of orthostatic hypotension include fainting and may involve cardiovascular symptoms, as well as impotence and bowel and bladder dysfunction.

21. Atherosclerosis is a form of arteriosclerosis and is the leading cause of coronary artery and cerebrovascular disease.

22. Atherosclerosis is an inflammatory disease that begins with endothelial tissue and progresses through several stages to become a fibrotic plaque.

23. Traditional risk factors include age, family history, gender, smoking, dyslipidemia, hypertension, and diabetes.

24. Novel risk factors include elevated CRP, increased serum fibrinogen, oxidative stress, infection, and periodontal disease.

25. Once a plaque has formed, it can rupture resulting in thrombosis and vasoconstriction leading to obstruction of the lumen and inadequate perfusion of distal tissues.

26. PAD is atherosclerosis of arteries that perfuse the limbs, especially the lower extremities.

27. PAD is often asymptomatic but can present with intermittent claudication (pain in leg on walking). Treatment includes risk factor reduction and antiplatelet therapy.

28. CAD is spasm or occlusion of the coronary arteries and is most often the result of atherosclerotic lesions that limit the flow of blood to the heart.

29. Many risk factors contribute to the onset and escalation of CAD, including advanced age, male gender (younger than age 60), hypertension, dyslipidemia (including elevated Lp[a]), diabetes mellitus, smoking, obesity, sedentary lifestyle, psychosocial factors, elevated CRP, and possibly infectious agents.

30. CAD results in an imbalance between coronary supply of blood and myocardial demand for oxygen and nutrients such that reversible myocardial ischemia or irreversible infarction may result.

31. Reversible myocardial ischemia presents clinically in several ways. Chronic coronary obstruction results in recurrent predictable chest pain called *stable angina*. Abnormal vasospasm of coronary vessels results in unpredictable chest pain called *Prinzmetal angina*. Myocardial ischemia that does not cause detectable symptoms is called *silent ischemia*.

32. Stable angina is evaluated by noninvasive techniques of assessing coronary flow with or without exercise (stress ECG, thallium, or SPECT). Management may include lifestyle changes, vasodilators, antithrombotics, PCI, or CABG surgery.

33. When there is sudden coronary obstruction because of thrombosis formation over a ruptured atherosclerotic plaque, the acute coronary syndromes result. Unstable angina causes reversible myocardial ischemia and is a harbinger of impending infarction. Myocardial infarction results when prolonged ischemia causes irreversible damage to the heart muscle. Sudden cardiac death can occur in any of the acute coronary syndromes.

34. Unstable angina occurs because of transient episodes of thrombotic vessel occlusion and vasoconstriction at the site of plaque damage, with return of perfusion before significant myocardial necrosis occurs. This must be managed aggressively with antithrombotic agents to prevent myocardial infarction.

35. When coronary blood flow is interrupted for an extended period, myocyte necrosis occurs; this is called MI. Pathologically, there are two major types of myocardial infarction: subendocardial infarction and transmural infarction. In addition to myocyte necrosis, other changes in the heart with MI include hibernating, stunning, and remodeling of the myocardium.

36. Acute coronary syndromes are assessed by measuring serum enzymes, such as creatinine kinase and troponins, as well as looking for characteristic changes in the ECG. Those individuals at highest risk for complications present with ST segment elevations on the ECG (STEMI) and require immediate intervention. Smaller subendocardial infarctions are not associated with ST segment elevations (non-STEMI) but suggest that additional myocardium is still at risk for recurrent ischemia and infarction. Management may include thrombolytic drugs, antithrombotic drugs, vasodilators, PCI, or immediate surgery.

37. Dysrhythmias, congestive heart failure, and sudden death are the most common complications of the acute coronary syndromes.

Disorders of the Heart Wall

1. Inflammation of the pericardium (pericarditis) may result from innumerable sources (infection, drug therapy, tumors). Pericarditis presents with symptoms that are physically troublesome, but in and of themselves they are not life threatening.

2. Fluid may collect within the pericardial sac (pericardial effusion). Cardiac function may be severely impaired if a large volume of fluid accumulates rapidly.

3. Cardiomyopathies are a diverse group of primary myocardial disorders that are poorly understood. The cardiomyopathies are categorized as dilated (congestive), restrictive (rigid and noncompliant), and hypertrophic (asymmetric). Size of the cardiac muscle walls and chambers may increase or decrease, depending on the type of cardiomyopathy, thereby altering contractile activity.

4. Hemodynamic integrity of the cardiovascular system depends to a great extent on properly functioning cardiac valves. Congenital or acquired disorders that result in stenosis or incompetence or both can structurally alter the valves.

5. Characteristic heart sounds, cardiac murmurs, and systemic complaints assist in determination of which valve is abnormal. If severely compromised function exists, a prosthetic heart valve may be surgically implanted to replace the faulty one.

6. Mitral valve prolapse is a common finding, especially in young women. Although not grossly abnormal, the mitral valve leaflets do not position themselves properly during systole. MVP may be a completely asymptomatic condition, or it may result in severe subjective symptoms. Afflicted valves may be at greater risk for developing infective endocarditis.

7. Rheumatic fever is an inflammatory disease that results from a delayed autoimmune response to a streptococcal infection. The disorder usually resolves without sequelae if treated early.

8. Severe or untreated cases of rheumatic fever may progress to rheumatic heart disease, a potentially disabling cardiovascular disorder.

9. Infective endocarditis is a general term for infection and inflammation of the endocardium, especially the cardiac valves. A wide range of conditions predisposes one to the development of this disorder. In the mildest cases, valvular function may be slightly impaired by vegetations that collect on the valve leaflets. If infective endocarditis is left unchecked, severe valve abnormalities, chronic bacteremia, and systemic emboli may occur as vegetations break off the valve surface and travel through the bloodstream. Antibiotic therapy can limit the extent of this disease.

10. HIV is associated with cardiac abnormalities, including myocarditis, endocarditis, pericarditis, and cardiomyopathy. Left heart failure is the most common clinical manifestation.

Manifestations of Heart Disease

1. Heart failure is an inability of the heart to supply the metabolism with adequate circulatory volume and pressure.

2. Left heart failure can be categorized as systolic heart failure or diastolic heart failure.

3. Systolic heart failure is defined as an inability of the heart to generate an adequate cardiac output to perfuse vital tissue.

4. Cardiac output depends on the heart rate and stroke volume. Stroke volume is influenced by contractility, preload, and afterload. Myocardial infarction is the most common cause of decreased contractility. Myocardial ischemia results in ventricular remodeling that causes progressive myocyte contractile dysfunction over time.

5. Preload LVEDV is increased when there is decreased contractility or excess plasma volume.

6. Increased afterload is most commonly the result of increased peripheral vascular resistance. This increase in resistance decreases ventricular emptying and makes more workload for the left ventricle, resulting in hypertrophy and ventricular remodeling. The vicious cycle of decreasing contractility, increasing preload, and increasing afterload causes progressive worsening.

7. Neurohumoral mechanisms of CHF include abnormalities in the SNS, RAAS, arginine vasopressin, natriuretic peptides, inflammatory cytokines, and in myocyte metabolism.

8. The clinical manifestations of left heart failure are the result of pulmonary vascular congestion and inadequate systemic perfusion.

9. Management of left heart failure relies on increasing contractility and reducing preload and afterload.

10. Diastolic heart failure can occur singly or with systolic heart failure. The major causes of diastolic dysfunction include hypertension-induced myocardial hypertrophy and ischemia with resultant ventricular remodeling.

11. Right heart failure can result from left heart failure and/or diffuse hypoxic pulmonary disease, such as COPD, cystic fibrosis, and ARDS. These mechanisms are discussed in Chapter 33.

12. High output failure is the inability of the heart to adequately supply the body with blood-borne nutrients despite adequate volume and normal or elevated myocardial contractility. Common causes are anemia, septicemia, hyperthyroidism, and beriberi.

13. A dysrhythmia (arrhythmia) is a disturbance of heart rhythm. Dysrhythmias range in severity from occasional missed beats or rapid beats to disturbances that impair myocardial contractility and are life threatening.

14. Dysrhythmias can occur because of an abnormal rate of impulse generation or the abnormal conduction of impulses.

KEY TERMS

Acute coronary syndrome, 1160
Acute orthostatic hypotension, 1157
Acute pericarditis, 1176
Aneurysm, 1144
Angina pectoris, 1166
Aortic dissection, 1146
Aortic regurgitation, 1183
Aortic stenosis, 1181
Arcus senilis, 1167
Atherosclerosis, 1157
Cardiomyopathy, 1178
Carditis, 1186
Chronic left heart failure, 1194
Chronic orthostatic hypotension, 1157
Chronic venous insufficiency (CVI), 1143
Chylomicrons, 1161
Complicated plaques, 1159
Constrictive pericarditis (restrictive
  pericarditis, chronic pericarditis), 1177
Coronary artery bypass graft, 1169
Coronary artery disease (CAD), 1160
Deep venous thrombosis (DVT), 1143
Diastolic heart failure, 1194
Dilated cardiomyopathy (congestive
  cardiomyopathy), 1178
Dressler postinfection syndrome, 1176
Dyslipidemia (dyslipoproteinemia), 1162
Dysrhythmia (arrhythmia), 1175
Embolism, 1147
Embolus, 1147
Erythema marginatum, 1186
Essential (or idiopathic) hypertension,
  1149
False aneurysm, 1146
Fatty streak, 1159
Fibrous plaque, 1159
Foam cell, 1159
Heart failure, 1189
Hibernating myocardium, 1172
High-density lipoprotein (HDL), 1162

Highly sensitive C-reactive protein
  (hs-CRP), 1165
High-output failure, 1195
Hyperhomocysteinemia, 1165
Hypertension, 1149
Hypertensive (valvular hypertrophic)
  cardiomyopathy, 1180
Hypertrophic cardiomyopathy, 1180
Hypertrophic obstructive cardiomyopathy,
  1180
Infarction, 1160
Infective endocarditis, 1187
Intermittent claudication, 1160
Ischemia, 1160
Ischemic preconditioning, 1172
Isolated systolic hypertension, 1149
Lanthanic (silent) disease, 1155
Left heart failure (congestive heart failure),
  1190
Lipoprotein, 1161
Lipoprotein (a) (Lp[a]), 1164
Low-density lipoprotein (LDL), 1162
Malignant hypertension, 1154
Metabolic syndrome, 1164
Minimally invasive direct coronary artery
  bypass (MIDCAB), 1169
Mitral regurgitation, 1183
Mitral stenosis, 1181
Mitral valve prolapse syndrome, 1183
Myocardial infarction (MI), 1169
Myocardial remodeling, 1172
Myocardial stunning, 1172
Nonbacterial thrombotic endocarditis, 1187
Non–ST elevation MI (non-STEMI), 1169
Organic brain syndrome, 1176
Orthostatic (postural) hypotension, 1156
Percutaneous coronary intervention (PCI),
  1169
Pericardial effusion, 1177
Pericarditis, 1176

Peripheral artery disease (PAD), 1160
Plaque, 1157
Post-thrombotic syndrome (PTS), 1144
Primary hypertension (essential hyperten-
  sion, idiopathic hypertension), 1149
Prinzmetal angina, 1165
Raynaud disease, 1149
Raynaud phenomenon, 1148
Restrictive cardiomyopathy, 1180
Rheumatic fever, 1185
Rheumatic heart disease (RHD), 1185
Right heart failure, 1194
Saccular aneurysm, 1146
Secondary hypertension, 1149
Silent ischemia, 1165
Stable angina, 1165
ST elevation MI (STEMI), 1169
Superior vena cava syndrome (SVCS),
  1144
Sydenham chorea (St. Vitus dance), 1186
Systolic heart failure, 1190
Tamponade, 1177
Thromboangiitis obliterans (Buerger
  disease), 1148
Thromboembolism, 1147
Thromboembolization, 1144
Thromboembolus, 1143
Thrombus, 1143
Tricuspid regurgitation, 1183
True aneurysm, 1146
Unstable angina, 1169
Valvular regurgitation, 1181
Valvular stenosis, 1181
Varicose vein, 1142
Venous stasis ulcer, 1143
Ventricular aneurysm, 1176
Ventricular remodeling, 1190
Very-low-density lipoprotein (VLDL),
  1162
Xanthelasma, 1167

REFERENCES

1. World Health Organization: *Fact sheet No 317, cardiovascular diseases*, February 2007. Available at www.who.int/mediacentre/factsheets/fs317/en/index.html. Accessed February 15, 2009.
2. Eberhardt RT, Raffetto JD: Chronic venous insufficiency, *Circulation* 111(18):2398-2409, 2005.
3. Meissner MH et al: The hemodynamics and diagnosis of venous disease, *J Vasc Surg* 46(Suppl S):4S-24S, 2007.
4. Dietzek AM: Endovenous radiofrequency ablation for the treatment of varicose veins. *Vascular* 15(5):255-261, 2007.
5. Cushman M: Epidemiology and risk factors for venous thrombosis, *Semin Hematol* 44(2):62-69, 2007.
6. Mackman N: Triggers, targets and treatments for thrombosis, *Nature* 451(7181):914-918, 2008.
7. Philbrick JT et al: Air travel and venous thromboembolism: a systematic review, *J Gen Intern Med* 22(1):107-114, 2007.
8. Baker WF Jr, Bick RL: The clinical spectrum of antiphospholipid syndrome. *Hematol Oncol Clin North Am* 22(1):33-52, v-vi, 2008.
9. Gatt A, Makris M: Hyperhomocysteinemia and venous thrombosis, *Semin Hematol* 44(2):70-76, 2007.
10. Lim W, Eikelboom JW, Ginsberg JS: Inherited thrombophilia and pregnancy associated venous thromboembolism, *BMJ* 334(7607): 1318-1321, 2007.
11. Bezemer ID et al: Gene variants associated with deep vein thrombosis, *JAMA* 299(11):1306-1314, 2008.
12. Wakefield TW, Myers DD, Henke PK: Mechanisms of venous thrombosis and resolution, *Arterioscler Thromb Vasc Biol* 28(3):387-391, 2008.
13. Tapson VF: Acute pulmonary embolism, *N Engl J Med* 358(10):1037-1052, 2008.
14. Meissner MH et al: Secondary chronic venous disorders, *J Vasc Surg* 46(Suppl S):68S-83S, 2007.
15. Frances C: Prophylaxis for thromboembolism in hospitalized medical patients, *N Engl J Med* 356:1438-1444, 2007.
16. Sjalander A et al: Efficacy and safety of anticoagulant prophylaxis to prevent venous thromboembolism in acutely ill medical inpatients: a meta-analysis, *J Intern Med* 263(1):52-60, 2008.
17. Hill J, Treasure T: Reducing the risk of venous thromboembolism (deep vein thrombosis and pulmonary embolism) in inpatients having surgery: summary of NICE guidance, *BMJ* 334(7602):1053-1054, 2007.
18. Blaivas M: Ultrasound in the detection of venous thromboembolism, *Crit Care Med* 35(5 Suppl):S224-S234, 2007.
19. Di Nisio M et al: Diagnostic accuracy of D-dimer test for exclusion of venous thromboembolism: a systematic review, *J Thromb Haemost* 5(2):296-304, 2007.
20. Thomas SM et al: Diagnostic value of CT for deep vein thrombosis: results of a systematic review and meta-analysis, *Clin Radiol* 63(3):299-304, 2008.

21. Sampson FC et al: The accuracy of MRI in diagnosis of suspected deep vein thrombosis: systematic review and meta-analysis, *Eur Radiol* 17(1):175-181, 2007.

22. McRae SJ, Eikelboom JW: Latest medical treatment strategies for venous thromboembolism, *Exp Opin Pharmacother* 8(9):1221-1233, 2007.

23. Agnelli G, Becattini C: Treatment of DVT: how long is enough and how do you predict recurrence, *J Thromb Thrombolysis* 25(1):37-44, 2008.

24. Wilson LD, Detterbeck FC, Yahalom J: Clinical practice. Superior vena cava syndrome with malignant causes, *N Engl J Med* 356(18):1862-1869, 2007.

25. Schifferdecker B et al: Nonmalignant superior vena cava syndrome: pathophysiology and management, *Cath Cardiovasc Interven* 65(3):416-423, 2005.

26. Kuivaniemi H, Platsoucas CD, Tilson MD 3rd: Aortic aneurysms: an immune disease with a strong genetic component, *Circulation* 117(2):242-252, 2008.

27. Thompson AR et al: Candidate gene association studies in abdominal aortic aneurysm disease: a review and meta-analysis, *Eur J Vasc Endovasc Surg* 35(1):19-30, 2008.

28. Raffetto JD, Khalil RA: Matrix metalloproteinases and their inhibitors in vascular remodeling and vascular disease, *Biochem Pharmacol* 75(2):346-359, 2008.

29. Rentschler ME, Baxter BT: Medical therapy approach for treating abdominal aortic aneurysm, *Vascular* 15(6):361-365, 2007.

30. Eliason JL, Upchurch GR Jr: Endovascular abdominal aortic aneurysm repair, *Circulation* 117(13):1738-1744, 2008.

31. Kamalakannan D, Rosman HS, Eagle KA: Acute aortic dissection, *Crit Care Clin* 23(4):779-800, vi, 2007.

32. Puechal X, Fiessinger JN: Thromboangiitis obliterans or Buerger's disease: challenges for the rheumatologist, *Rheumatol* 46(2):192-199, 2007.

33. Paraskevas KI et al: Thromboangiitis obliterans (Buerger's disease): searching for a therapeutic strategy, *Angiology* 58(1):75-84, 2007.

34. Gayraud M: Raynaud's phenomenon, *Joint Bone Spine* 74(1):e1-8, 2007.

35. Pope JE: The diagnosis and treatment of Raynaud's phenomenon: a practical approach, *Drugs* 67(4):517-525, 2007.

36. Rosamond W et al: Heart disease and stroke statistics—2008 update: a report from the American Heart Association Statistics Committee and Stroke Statistics Subcommittee, *Circulation* 117(4):e25-146, 2008.

37. Chobanian AV: The Seventh Report of the Joint National Committee on Prevention, Detection, Evaluation, and Treatment of High Blood Pressure. JNC Report, *JAMA* 289(19):2560-2572, 2003.

38. Elliott WJ: Systemic hypertension, *Curr Probl Cardiol* 32(4):201-259, 2007.

39. Puddu P et al: The genetic basis of essential hypertension, *Acta Cardiol* 62(3):281-293, 2007.

40. Weder AB: Genetics and hypertension, *J Clin Hypertens* 9(3):217-223, 2007.

41. Adrogue HJ, Madias NE: Sodium and potassium in the pathogenesis of hypertension, *N Engl J Med* 356(19):1966-1978, 2007.

42. Frohlich ED: The salt conundrum: a hypothesis, *Hypertension* 50(1):161-166, 2007.

43. Rodriguez-Iturbe B, Vaziri ND: Salt-sensitive hypertension—update on novel findings, *Nephrol Dial Transpl* 22(4):992-995, 2007.

44. Harding S et al: Overweight, obesity and high blood pressure in an ethnically diverse sample of adolescents in Britain: the Medical Research Council DASH study, *Int J Obesity* 32(1):82-90, 2008.

45. Schultz HD, Li YL, Ding Y: Arterial chemoreceptors and sympathetic nerve activity: implications for hypertension and heart failure, *Hypertension* 50(1):6-13, 2007.

46. Coffman TM, Crowley SD: Kidney in hypertension: Guyton redux, *Hypertension* 51(4):811-816, 2008.

47. Johnson RJ et al: Pathogenesis of essential hypertension: historical paradigms and modern insights, *J Hypertens* 26(3):381-391, 2008.

48. Hamming, I et al: The emerging role of ACE2 in physiology and disease, *J Pathol* 212(1):1-11, 2007.

49. Wysocki J, Gonzalez-Pacheco FR, Batlle D: Angiotensin-converting enzyme 2: possible role in hypertension and kidney disease, *Curr Hypertens Rep* 10(1):70-77, 2008.

50. Hernandez Schulman I, Zhou MS, Raij L: Cross-talk between angiotensin II receptor types 1 and 2: potential role in vascular remodeling in humans [comment], *Hypertension* 49(2):270-271, 2007.

51. Barri YM: Hypertension and kidney disease: a deadly connection, *Curr Hypertens Rep* 10(1):39-45, 2008.

52. Stowasser M, Gordon RD: Aldosterone excess, hypertension, and chromosome 7p22: Evidence continues to mount [comment], *Hypertension* 49(4):761-762, 2007.

53. Perkins JM, Davis SN: The renin-angiotensin-aldosterone system: a pivotal role in insulin sensitivity and glycemic control, *Curr Opin Endocrinol Diabetes Obes* 15(2):147-152, 2008.

54. Matchar DB et al: Systematic review: comparative effectiveness of angiotensin-converting enzyme inhibitors and angiotensin II receptor blockers for treating essential hypertension, *Ann Intern Med* 148(1):16-29, 2008.

55. Ostergren J: Renin-angiotensin-system blockade in the prevention of diabetes, *Diabetes Res Clin Pract* 76(Suppl 1):S13-S21, 2007.

56. Voors AA: Vascular benefits of angiotensin receptor blockers, *Exp Opin Invest Drugs* 16(7):987-997, 2007.

57. Woodard GE, Rosado JA: Natriuretic peptides in vascular physiology and pathology, *Rev Cell Mol Biol* 268:59-93, 2008.

58. Gardner DG et al: Molecular biology of the natriuretic peptide system: implications for physiology and hypertension, *Hypertension* 49(3):419-426, 2007.

59. de Sa DD, Chen HH: The role of natriuretic peptides in heart failure, *Curr Cardiol Rep* 10(3):182-189, 2008.

60. Xue H et al: Atrial natriuretic peptide gene promoter polymorphism is associated with left ventricular hypertrophy in hypertension, *Clin Sci.* 114(2):131-137, 2008.

61. Irzmanski R et al: The concentration of atrial and brain natriuretic peptide in patients with idiopathic hypertension, *Med Sci Monit* 13(10):CR449-CR456, 2007.

62. Hildebrandt P, Richards AM: Amino-terminal pro-B-type natriuretic peptide testing in patients with diabetes mellitus and with systemic hypertension, *Am J Cardiol* 101(3A):21-24, 2008.

63. Savoia C, Schiffrin EL: Vascular inflammation in hypertension and diabetes: molecular mechanisms and therapeutic interventions, *Clin Sci* 112(7):375-384, 2007.

64. Virdis A et al: C-reactive protein and hypertension: Is there a causal relationship? *Curr Pharm Design* 13(16):1693-1698, 2007.

65. Feldstein C, Romero C: Role of endothelins in hypertension, *Am J Ther* 14(2):147-153, 2007.

66. Kohan DE: Endothelin-1 and hypertension: from bench to bedside, *Curr Hypertens Rep* 10(1):65-69, 2008.

67. Lapu-Bula R, Ofili E: From hypertension to heart failure: role of nitric oxide-mediated endothelial dysfunction and emerging insights from myocardial contrast echocardiography, *Am J Cardiol* 99(6B):714, 2007.

68. Bian K et al: Vascular system: role of nitric oxide in cardiovascular diseases, *J Clin Hypertens* 10(4):304-310, 2008.

69. Heerkens EH, Izzard AS, Heagerty AM: Integrins, vascular remodeling, and hypertension, *Hypertension* 49(1):1-4, 2007.

70. Kakar P, Lip GY: Hypertension: endothelial dysfunction, the prothrombotic state and antithrombotic therapy, *Exp Rev Cardiovasc Ther* 5(3):441-450, 2007.

71. Boban M et al: Obesity-hypertension: emerging concepts in pathophysiology and treatment, *Am J Med Sci* 334(1):23-30, 2007.

72. Deedwania P, Srikanth S: Diabetes and vascular disease, *Exp Rev Cardiovasc Ther* 6(1):127-138, 2008.

73. Meeuwisse-Pasterkamp SH, van der Klauw MM, Wolffenbuttel BH: Type 2 diabetes mellitus: prevention of macrovascular complications, *Exp Rev Cardiovasc Ther* 6(3):323-341, 2008.

74. Grossman E, Messerli FH: Hypertension and diabetes, *Adv Cardiol* 45:82-106, 2008.

75. Sarafidis PA, McFarlane SI, Bakris GL: Antihypertensive agents, insulin sensitivity, and new-onset diabetes, *Curr Diabetes Rep* 7(3):191-199, 2007.

76. Rao MV et al: Hypertension and CKD: Kidney Early Evaluation Program (KEEP) and National Health and Nutrition Examination Survey (NHANES):1999-2004, *Am J Kidney Dis* 51(4 Suppl 2):S30-S37, 2008.

77. Takeda S et al: The renin-angiotensin system, hypertension and cognitive dysfunction in Alzheimer's disease: new therapeutic potential, *Front Biosci* 13:2253-2265, 2008.

78. van den Born BJ, Koopmans RP, van Montfrans GA: The renin-angiotensin system in malignant hypertension revisited: plasma renin activity, microangiopathic hemolysis, and renal failure in malignant hypertension, *Am J Hypertens* 20(8):900-906, 2007.

79. Feldstein C: Management of hypertensive crises, *Am J Ther* 14(2):135-139, 2007.

80. Pickering T et al: AHA scientific statement: recommendations for blood pressure measurement in humans and experimental animals part 1: blood pressure measurement in humans: a statement for professionals from the Subcommittee of Professional and Public Education of the American Heart Association Council on High Blood Pressure Research, *Hypertension* 45:142-161, 2005.

81. Ogedegbe G: White-coat effect: unraveling its mechanisms, *Am J Hypertens* 21(2):135, 2008.

82. Rosendorff C et al: Treatment of hypertension in the prevention and management of ischemic heart disease: a scientific statement from the American Heart Association Council for High Blood Pressure Research and the Councils on Clinical Cardiology and Epidemiology and Prevention, *Circulation* 115(21):2761-2788, 2007.

83. The Consensus Committee of the American Autonomic Society and the American Academy of Neurology: Consensus statement on the definition of orthostatic hypotension, pure autonomic failure, and multiple system atrophy, *Neurol* 46(5):1470, 1996.

84. Medow MS et al: Pathophysiology, diagnosis, and treatment of orthostatic hypotension and vasovagal syncope, *Cardiol Rev* 16(1):4-20, 2008.

85. Ejaz AA, Kazory A, Heinig ME: 24-hour blood pressure monitoring in the evaluation of supine hypertension and orthostatic hypotension, *J Clin Hypertens* 9(12):952-955, 2007.

86. Hansson GK: Inflammation, atherosclerosis, and coronary artery disease, *N Engl J Med* 352:1685-1695, 2005.

87. Packard RR, Libby P: Inflammation in atherosclerosis: from vascular biology to biomarker discovery and risk prediction, *Clin Chem* 54(1):24-38, 2008.

88. VanEpps J, Vorp D: Mechanopathobiology of atherogeneisis: a review, *J Surg Res* 142:202-217, 2007.

89. Jevon M, Dorling A, Hornick PI: Progenitor cells and vascular disease, *Cell Prolif* 41(Suppl 1):146-164, 2008.

90. Deanfield J, Hlacox J, Rabelink T: Endothelial function and dysfunction: testing and clinical relevance, *Circulation* 106:1285-1295, 2007.

91. Schafer A, Bauersachs J: Endothelial dysfunction, impaired endogenous platelet inhibition and platelet activation in diabetes and atherosclerosis, *Curr Vasc Pharmacol* 6(1):52-60, 2008.

92. Langer HF, Gawaz M: Platelet-vessel wall interactions in atherosclerotic disease, *Thromb Haemost* 99(3):480-486, 2008.

93. Liang CP et al: The macrophage at the crossroads of insulin resistance and atherosclerosis, *Circ Res* 100(11):1546-1555, 2007.

94. Doran AC, Meller N, McNamara CA: Role of smooth muscle cells in the initiation and early progression of atherosclerosis, *Arterioscler Thromb Vasc Biol* 28(5):812 819, 2008.

95. Dunn S et al: The lectin-like oxidized low-density-lipoprotein receptor: a pro-inflammatory factor in vascular disease, *Biochem J* 409(2):349-355, 2008.

96. Agius LM: Complicated atheromatous plaque as integral atherogenesis, *J Clin Pathol* 60(6):589-592, 2007.

97. Rodriguez JA et al: Metalloproteinases and atherothrombosis: MMP-10 mediates vascular remodeling promoted by inflammatory stimuli, *Front Biosci* 13:2916-2921, 2008.

98. Parahuleva MS et al: Factor seven activating protease (FSAP) expression in human monocytes and accumulation in unstable coronary atherosclerotic plaques, *Atherosclerosis* 196(1):164-171, 2008.

99. Ellahham S: Role of antiplatelet agents in the primary and secondary prevention of atherothrombotic events in high risk-patients, *South Med J* 101(3):273-283, 2008.

100. Stern S: Are we getting nearer to screening for atherosclerosis? *Circulation* 117(1):122-126, 2008.

101. Sanz J, Moreno PR, Fuster V: The year in atherothrombosis, *J Am Coll Cardiol* 49(16):1740-1749, 2007.

102. Schaar JA et al: Current diagnostic modalities for vulnerable plaque detection, *Curr Pharm Des* 13(10):995-1001, 2007.

103. Shamoun F, Sural N, Abela G: Peripheral artery disease: therapeutic advances, *Exp Rev Cardiovasc Ther* 6(4):539-553, 2008.

104. Damani SB, Topol EJ: Future use of genomics in coronary artery disease, *J Am Coll Cardiol* 50(20):1933-1940, 2007.

105. McGill HC Jr, McMahan CA, Gidding SS: Preventing heart disease in the 21st century: implications of the Pathobiological Determinants of Atherosclerosis in Youth (PDAY) study, *Circulation* 117(9):1216-1227, 2008.

106. Peng R et al: Course particulate matter air pollution and hospital admissions for cardiovascular and respiratory diseases among Medicare patients, *JAMA* 299(18):2172-2179, 2008.

107. Expert Panel on Detection: Evaluation and Treatment of High Blood Cholesterol in Adults: Executive summary of the third report of the National Cholesterol Education Program (NCEP) expert panel on detection, evaluation, and treatment of high blood cholesterol in adults (Adult Treatment Panel III), *JAMA* 285(19):2486-2497, 2001.

108. Garg A, Simha V: Update on dyslipidemia, *J Clin Endocrinol Metab* 92(5):1581-1589, 2007.

109. Brunzell JD et al: Lipoprotein management in patients with cardiometabolic risk: consensus conference report from the American Diabetes Association and the American College of Cardiology Foundation, *J Am Coll Cardiol* 51(15):1512-1524, 2008.

110. Glassberg H, Rader DJ: Management of lipids in the prevention of cardiovascular events, *Annu Rev Med* 59:79-94, 2008.

111. Grundy SM: Promise of low-density lipoprotein-lowering therapy for primary and secondary prevention, *Circulation* 117(4):569-573, 2008.

112. Tannock LR: Advances in the management of hyperlipidemia-induced atherosclerosis, *Exp Rev Cardiovasc Ther* 6(3):369-383, 2008.

113. Link JJ, Rohatgi A, de Lemos JA: HDL cholesterol: physiology, pathophysiology, and management, *Curr Probl Cardiol* 32(5):268-314, 2007.

114. Feig JE, Shamir R, Fisher EA: Atheroprotective effects of HDL: beyond reverse cholesterol transport, *Curr Drug Targets* 9(3):196-203, 2008.

115. Yu R et al: Proatherogenic high-density lipoprotein, vascular inflammation, and mimetic peptides, *Curr Atheroscler Rep* 10(2):171-176, 2008.

116. Garcia RA: Pharmacological therapies for raising HDL cholesterol beyond synthetic small molecules, *Curr Opin Invest Drugs* 9(3):274-280, 2008.

117. Miller M, Ginsberg HN, Schaefer EJ: Relative atherogenicity and predictive value of non-high-density lipoprotein cholesterol for coronary heart disease, *Am J Cardiol* 101(7):1003-1008, 2008.

118. Schmieder RE et al: Renin-angiotensin system and cardiovascular risk, *Lancet* 369(9568):1208-1219, 2007.

119. Rader DJ, Daugherty A: Translating molecular discoveries into new therapies for atherosclerosis, *Nature* 451(7181):904-913, 2008.

120. Basta G: Receptor for advanced glycation endproducts and atherosclerosis: from basic mechanisms to clinical implications, *Atherosclerosis* 196(1):9-21, 2008.

121. Kashyap SR, Defronzo RA: The insulin resistance syndrome: physiological considerations, *Diabetes Vasc Dis Res* 4(1):13-19, 2007.

122. Farmer JA: Diabetic dyslipidemia and atherosclerosis: evidence from clinical trials, *Curr Diabetes Rep* 8(1):71 77, 2008.

123. Grundy SM: Metabolic syndrome pandemic, *Arterioscler Thromb Vasc Biol* 28(4):629-636, 2008.

124. Rader DJ: Effect of insulin resistance, dyslipidemia, and intra-abdominal adiposity on the development of cardiovascular disease and diabetes mellitus, *Am J Med* 120(3 Suppl 1):S12-S18, 2007.

125. Fantuzzi G, Mazzone T: Adipose tissue and atherosclerosis: exploring the connection, *Arterioscler Thromb Vasc Biol* 27(5):996-1003, 2007.

126. Bays HE et al: Pathogenic potential of adipose tissue and metabolic consequences of adipocyte hypertrophy and increased visceral adiposity, *Exp Rev Cardiovasc Ther* 6(3):343-368, 2008.

127. Steffens S et al: Adiponectin and adaptive immunity: linking the bridge from obesity to atherogenesis, *Circ Res* 102(2):140-142, 2008.

128. Singh SK et al: The connection between C-reactive protein and atherosclerosis, *Ann Med* 40(2):110-120, 2008.

129. Virani SS, Polsani VR, Nambi V: Novel markers of inflammation in atherosclerosis, *Curr Atheroscler Rep* 10(2):164-170, 2008.

130. Rossi GP, Seccia TM, Pessina AC: Homocysteine, left ventricular dysfunction and coronary artery disease: is there a link? *Clin Chem Lab Med* 45(12):1645-1651, 2007.

131. Mallika V, Goswami B, Rajappa M: Atherosclerosis pathophysiology and the role of novel risk factors: a clinicobiochemical perspective, *Angiology* 58(5):513-522, 2007.

132. Lago F et al: The emerging role of adipokines as mediators of inflammation and immune responses, *Cytokine Growth Factor Rev* 18(3-4):313-325, 2007.

133. Selcuk MT et al: Impact of plasma adiponectin levels to the presence and severity of coronary artery disease in patients with metabolic syndrome, *Coron Artery Dis* 19(2):79-84, 2008.

134. Komura N et al: Clinical significance of high-molecular weight form of adiponectin in male patients with coronary artery disease with metabolic syndrome, *Circ J* 72(1):23-28, 2008.

135. Wang SS et al: Circulating *Chlamydia pneumoniae* DNA and advanced coronary artery disease, *Int J Cardiol* 118(2):215-219, 2007.

136. Vahdat K et al: Concurrent increased high sensitivity C-reactive protein and chronic infections are associated with coronary artery disease: a population-based study, *Indian J Med Sci* 61(3):135-143, 2007.

137. Madjid M et al: Systemic infections cause exaggerated local inflammation in atherosclerotic coronary arteries: clues to the triggering effect of acute infections on acute coronary syndromes, *Texas Heart Inst J* 34(1):11-18, 2007.

138. Foreman RD: Neurological mechanisms of chest pain and cardiac disease, *Cleve Clin J Med* 74(Suppl 1):S30-S33, 2007.

139. Li JJ et al: Inflammation in variant angina: is there any evidence? *Med Hypotheses* 68(3):635-640, 2007.

140. Yuksel UC et al: Polymorphic ventricular tachycardia induced by coronary vasospasm: a malignant case of variant angina, *Int J Cardiol* 121(2):210-212, 2007.

141. D'Antono B et al: Silent ischemia: silent after all? *Can J Cardiol* 24(4):285-291, 2008.

142. Rozanski A: Mental stress and the induction of silent myocardial ischemia in patients with coronary artery disease, *N Engl J Med* 318(16):1005-1012, 1988.

143. Kop WJ et al: Effects of acute mental stress and exercise on inflammatory markers in patients with coronary artery disease and healthy controls, *Am J Cardiol* 101(6):767-773, 2008.

144. Dimsdale JE: Psychological stress and cardiovascular disease, *J Am Coll Cardiol* 51(13):1237-1246, 2008.

145. Soufer R, Burg MM: The heart-brain interaction during emotionally provoked myocardial ischemia: implications of cortical hyperactivation in CAD and gender interactions, *Cleve Clin J Med* 74(Suppl 1):S59-S62, 2007.

146. Beller GA: Noninvasive screening for coronary atherosclerosis and silent ischemia in asymptomatic type 2 diabetic patients: is it appropriate and cost-effective? *J Am Coll Cardiol* 49(19):1918-1923, 2007.

147. Madsen JK et al: DANAMI study group. Revascularization compared to medical treatment in patients with silent vs. symptomatic residual ischemia after thrombolyzed myocardial infarction—the DANAMI study, *Cardiology* 108(4):243-251, 2007.

148. Cademartiri F et al: Non-invasive visualization of coronary atherosclerosis: state-of-art, *J Cardiovasc Med* 8(3):129-137, 2007.

149. Ben-Dor I, Battler A: Treatment of stable angina, *Heart* 93(7):868-874, 2007.

150. Fraker T, Fihn S: 2007 chronic angina. Focused update of the ACC/AHA 2002 guidelines for the management of patients with chronic stable angina: a report of the American College of Cardiology/American Heart Association Task Force on Practice Guidelines Writing Group to develop the focused update of the 2002 guidelines for the management of patients with chronic stable angina, *J Am Coll Cardiol* 50:2264-2274, 2007.

151. Akdim F et al: Pleiotropic effects of statins: stabilization of the vulnerable atherosclerotic plaque? *Curr Pharm Des* 13(10):1003-1012, 2007.

152. Clappers N et al: Antiplatelet treatment for coronary heart disease, *Heart* 93(2):258-265, 2007.

153. Kiernan TJ, Prasad A, Gersh BJ: Current indications for percutaneous coronary intervention for chronic stable angina: implications of the COURAGE Trial, *Rev Cardiovasc Med* 8(4):234-239, 2007.

154. Bravata DM et al: Systematic review: the comparative effectiveness of percutaneous coronary interventions and coronary artery bypass graft surgery, *Ann Intern Med* 147(10):703-716, 2007.

155. Klein LW: Clinical implications and mechanisms of plaque rupture in the acute coronary syndromes, *Am Heart Hosp J* 3(4):249-255, 2005.

156. Bhatheja R, Mukherjee D: Acute coronary syndromes: unstable angina/non-ST elevation myocardial infarction, *Crit Care Clin* 23(4):709-735, 2007.

157. Anderson J et al: ACC/AHA 2007 guidelines for the management of patients with unstable angina/non–ST-elevation myocardial infarction: a report of the American College of Cardiology/American Heart Association Task Force on Practice Guidelines, *J Am Coll Cardiol* 50:e1-e157, 2007.

158. Mukherjee D, Eagle KA: The use of antithrombotics for acute coronary syndromes in the emergency department: considerations and impact, *Prog Cardiovasc Dis* 50(3):167-180, 2007.

159. Bavry AA et al: Long-term benefit of statin therapy initiated during hospitalization for an acute coronary syndrome: a systematic review of randomized trials, *Am J Cardiovasc Drugs* 7(2):135-141, 2007.

160. Thygesen K, Alpert J, White H: ESC/ACCF/AHA/WHF expert consensus document: universal definition of myocardial infarction, *J Am Coll Cardiol* 50:2173-2195, 2007.

161. Burke AP, Virmani R: Pathophysiology of acute myocardial infarction, *Med Clin North Am* 91(4):553-572; 2007.

162. Bolli R: Preconditioning: a paradigm shift in the biology of myocardial ischemia, *Am J Physiol Heart Circ Physiol* 292(1):H19-H27, 2007.

163. Camici P, Prasad S, Rimoldi O: Stunning, hibernation and assessment of myocardial viability, *Circulation* 117:103-114, 2008.

164. Sun Y: Oxidative stress and cardiac repair/remodeling following infarction, *Am J Med Sci* 334(3):197-205, 2007.

165. Palardy M, Ducharme A, O'Meara E: Inhibiting the renin-angiotensin system with ACE Inhibitors or ARBs after MI, *Curr Heart Fail Rep* 4(4):190-197, 2007.

166. Antman E et al: Focused Update of the ACC/AHA 2004 Guidelines for the Management of Patients With ST-Elevation Myocardial Infarction, *J Am Coll Cardiol* 51:210-247, 2008.

167. Bogaty P et al: Primary PCI in ST-segment elevation myocardial infarction, *N Engl J Med* 358(16):1751-1752, 2008.

168. King S et al: 2007 focused update of the ACC/AHA/SCAI 2005 guideline update for percutaneous coronary intervention, *J Am Coll Cardiol* 51:172-209, 2008.

169. Vun Liew T, Ray KK: Aggressive statin therapy for acute coronary syndromes, *Curr Cardiol Rep* 9(4):298-302, 2007.

170. Tingle LE, Molina D, Calvert CW: Acute pericarditis, *Am Fam Physician* 76(10):1509-1514, 2007.

171. Hoit BD: Pericardial disease and pericardial tamponade, *Crit Care Med* 35(8 Suppl):S355-S364, 2007.

172. Marnejon T et al: The constricted heart, *Postgrad Med* 120(1):8-10, 2008.

173. Ariyarajah V, Spodick DH: Acute pericarditis: diagnostic cues and common electrocardiographic manifestations, *Cardiol Rev* 15(1):24-30, 2007.

174. Imazio M, Trinchero R, Shabetai R: Pathogenesis, management, and prevention of recurrent pericarditis, *J Cardiovasc Med* 8(6):404-410, 2007.

175. Saltzman H, Weitz HH: Should all patients with acute pericarditis be treated with colchicine? *Cleve Clin J Med* 74(5):385-386, 2007.

176. Mullens W, De Keyser J, Herregods MC: Collapse of three cardiac chambers due to a pericardial effusion, *Int J Cardiol* 123(3):e62-e63, 2008.

177. Roy CL et al: Does this patient with a pericardial effusion have cardiac tamponade? *JAMA* 297(16):1810-1818, 2007.

178. Wann S, Passen E: Echocardiography in pericardial disease, *J Am Soc Echocardiogr* 21(1):7-13, 2008.

179. Thai V, Oneschuk D: Malignant pericardial effusion treated with intrapericardial bleomycin, *J Palliat Med* 10(2):281-282, 2007.

180. Swanson N et al: Primary percutaneous balloon pericardiotomy for malignant pericardial effusion, *Catheter Cardiovasc Interv* 71(4):504-507, 2008.

181. Syed FF, Mayosi BM: A modern approach to tuberculous pericarditis, *Prog Cardiovasc Dis* 50(3):218-236, 2007.

182. Ohtsuki I, Morimoto S: Troponin: regulatory function and disorders, *Biochem Biophys Res Commun* 369(1):62-73, 2008.

183. Taha M, Lopaschuk GD: Alterations in energy metabolism in cardiomyopathies, *Ann Med* 39(8):594-607, 2007.

184. Caforio AL et al: Clinical implications of anti-heart autoantibodies in myocarditis and dilated cardiomyopathy, *Autoimmunity* 41(1):35-45, 2008.

185. Djousse L, Gaziano JM: Alcohol consumption and heart failure: a systematic review, *Curr Atheroscler Rep* 10(2):117-120, 2008.

186. Esfandiarei M, McManus BM: Molecular biology and pathogenesis of viral myocarditis, *Annu Rev Pathol* 3:127-155, 2008.

187. Strauer BE, Brehm M, Schannwell CM: The therapeutic potential of stem cells in heart disease, *Cell Prolif* 41(Suppl 1):126-145, 2008.

188. Keren A, Syrris P, McKenna WJ: Hypertrophic cardiomyopathy: the genetic determinants of clinical disease expression, *Nat Clin Pract Cardiovasc Med* 5(3):158-168, 2008.

189. van Spaendonck-Zwarts KY, van den Berg MP, van Tintelen JP: DNA analysis in inherited cardiomyopathies: current status and clinical relevance, *Pacing Clin Electrophysiol* 31(Suppl 1):S46-S49, 2008.

190. Fifer MA, Vlahakes GJ: Management of symptoms in hypertrophic cardiomyopathy, *Circulation* 117(3):429-439, 2008.

191. Stollberger C, Finsterer J: Extracardiac medical and neuromuscular implications in restrictive cardiomyopathy, *Clin Cardiol* 30(8):375-380, 2007.

192. Schoen FJ: Cardiac valves and valvular pathology: update on function, disease, repair, and replacement, *Cardiovasc Pathol* 14(4):189-194, 2005.

193. Rahimtoola SH: The year in valvular heart disease, *J Am Coll Cardiol* 51(7):760-770, 2008.

194. Bosse Y, Mathieu P, Pibarot P: Genomics: the next step to elucidate the etiology of calcific aortic valve stenosis, *J Am Coll Cardiol* 51(14):1327-1336, 2008.

195. Aronow WS: Aortic stenosis, *Compr Ther* 33(4):174-183, 2007.

196. Rosenhek R, Baumgartner H: Aortic sclerosis, aortic stenosis and lipid-lowering therapy, *Exp Rev Cardiovasc Ther* 6(3):385-390, 2008.

197. Ramaraj R, Sorrell VL: Degenerative aortic stenosis, *Br J Med* 336(7643):550-555, 2008.

198. Goldbarg SH, Halperin JL: Aortic regurgitation: disease progression and management, *Nat Clin Pract Cardiovasc Med* 5(5):269-279, 2008.

199. Grau JB et al: The genetics of mitral valve prolapse, *Clin Genet* 72(4):288-295, 2007.

200. Bonow RO et al: ACC/AHA 2006 guidelines for the management of patients with valvular heart disease: a report of the American College of Cardiology/American Heart Association Task Force on Practice Guidelines (Writing Committee to Revise the 1998 Guidelines for the Management of Patients With Valvular Heart Disease), *J Am Coll Cardiol* 48:e1-e148, 2006.

201. Fedak PW, McCarthy PM, Bonow RO: Evolving concepts and technologies in mitral valve repair, *Circulation* 117(7):963-974, 2008.

202. Carapetis JR, McDonald M, Wilson NJ: Acute rheumatic fever, *Lancet* 366(9480):155-168, 2005.

203. Cunningham MW: Pathogenesis of group A streptococcal infections and their sequelae, *Adv Exp Med Biol* 609:29-42, 2008.

204. Guilherme L et al: T cell response in rheumatic fever: crossreactivity between streptococcal M protein peptides and heart tissue proteins, *Curr Protein Pept Sci* 8(1):39-44, 2007.

205. Weiner SG, Normandin PA: Sydenham chorea: a case report and review of the literature, *Ped Emer Care* 23(1):20-24, 2007.

206. Djani AS et al: Guidelines for the diagnosis of rheumatic fever. Jones criteria, updated 1993, *Circulation* 87:302, 1993.

207. Ferrieri P: Jones Criteria Working Group: Proceedings of the Jones criteria workshop, *Circulation* 106(19):2521-2523, 2002.

208. World Health Organization: *Rheumatic fever and rheumatic heart disease: report of a WHO expert consultation*, Geneva, 2004, World Health Organization.

209. Dale JB: Current status of group A streptococcal vaccine development, *Adv Exp Med Biol* 609:53-63, 2008.

210. Prendergast M: The changing face of infective endocarditis, *Heart* 92:879-885, 2006.

211. Dandache P, Aronow WS, Sakoulas G: Clinical update on the diagnosis and treatment of bacterial endocarditis, *Compr Ther* 33(4):192-207, 2007.

212. Wilson W et al: Prevention of infective endocarditis: recommendations by the American Heart Association: a guideline from the American Heart Association Rheumatic Fever, Endocarditis and Kawasaki Disease Committee, Council on Cardiovascular Disease in the Young, and the Council on Clinical Cardiology, Council on Cardiovascular Surgery and Anesthesia, and the Quality of Care and Outcomes Research Interdisciplinary Working Group, *Circulation* 116:1736-1754, 2007.

213. Marrie TJ: Osler's nodes and Janeway lesions, *Am J Med* 121(2): 105-106, 2008.

214. Durack DT, Lukes AS, Bright DK: New criteria for diagnosis of infective endocarditis: utilization of specific echocardiographic findings. Duke Endocarditis Service, *Am J Med* 96(3):200-209, 1994.

215. Habib G: Management of infective endocarditis, *Heart* 92(1):124-130, 2006.

216. Kim A, Keys T: Infective endocarditis prophylaxis before dental procedures: new guidelines spark controversy, *Cleve Clin J Med* 75(2):89-92, 2008.

217. Pao V, Lee GA, Grunfeld C: HIV therapy, metabolic syndrome, and cardiovascular risk, *Curr Atheroscler Rep* 10(1):61-70, 2008.

218. Stein JH: Cardiovascular risks of antiretroviral therapy, *N Engl J Med* 356(17):1773-1775, 2007.

219. Nass RD et al: Mechanisms of disease: ion channel remodeling in the failing ventricle, *Nat Clin Pract Cardiovasc Med* 5(4):196-207, 2008.

220. Chatterjee K, Rame JE: Systolic heart failure: chronic and acute syndromes, *Crit Care Med* 36(1 Suppl):S44-S51, 2008.

221. Ashrafian H, Frenneaux MP, Opie LH: Metabolic mechanisms in heart failure, *Circulation* 116(4):434-448, 2007.

222. Neubauer S: The failing heart—an engine out of fuel, *N Engl J Med* 356(11):1140-1151, 2007.

223. Mudd JO, Kass DA: Tackling heart failure in the twenty-first century, *Nature* 451(7181):919-928, 2008.

224. Feldman DS et al: Mechanisms of disease: detrimental adrenergic signaling in acute decompensated heart failure, *Nat Clin Pract Cardiovas Med* 5(4):208-218, 2008.

225. Osadchii OE: Cardiac hypertrophy induced by sustained beta-adrenoreceptor activation: pathophysiological aspects, *Heart Fail Rev* 12(1):66-86, 2007.

226. Pitt B: Aldosterone blockade in patients with chronic heart failure, *Cardiol Clin* 26(1):15-21, v, 2008.

227. Selektor Y, Weber KT: The salt-avid state of congestive heart failure revisited, *Am J Med Sci* 335(3):209-218, 2008.

228. Rossi J, Orlandi C, Gheorghiade M: Vasopressin antagonists in the management of heart failure, *Exp Rev Cardiovasc Ther* 5(2):323-330, 2007.

229. Lee CY, Burnett JC Jr: Natriuretic peptides and therapeutic applications, *Heart Fail Rev* 12(2):131-142, 2007.

230. Onwuanyi A, Taylor M: Acute decompensated heart failure: pathophysiology and treatment, *Am J Cardiol* 99(6B):2530, 2007.

231. Tavares M et al: New pharmacologic therapies for acute heart failure, *Crit Care Med* 36(1 Suppl):S112-S120, 2008.

232. Chen D et al: Cytokines and acute heart failure, *Crit Care Med* 36 (1 Suppl):S9-S16, 2008.

233. Conraads VM, Hoymans VY, Vrints CJ: Heart failure and cachexia: insights offered from molecular biology, *Front Biosci* 13:325-335, 2008.

234. von Haehling S, Doehner W, Anker SD: Nutrition, metabolism, and the complex pathophysiology of cachexia in chronic heart failure, *Cardiovasc Res* 73(2):298-309, 2007.

235. Anand IS, Florea VG: Traditional and novel approaches to management of heart failure: successes and failures, *Cardiol Clin* 26(1):59-72, 2008:vi, 2008.

236. Hunt SA et al: ACC/AHA 2005 guideline update for the diagnosis and management of chronic heart failure in the adult: a report of the American College of Cardiology/American Heart Association Task Force on Practice Guidelines (Writing Committee to Update the 2001 Guidelines for the Evaluation and Management of Heart Failure) developed in collaboration with the American College of Chest Physicians and the International Society for Heart and Lung Transplantation, endorsed by the Heart Rhythm Society, *Circulation* 112:E154-E235, 2005.

237. Shin DD et al: Review of current and investigational pharmacologic agents for acute heart failure syndromes, *Am J Cardiol* 99(2A):4A-23A, 2007.

238. McNamara DM: Pharmacogenomics for neurohormonal intervention in heart failure, *Cardiol Clin* 26(1):127-135, viii, 2008.

239. Januzzi JL Jr, Chen-Tournoux AA, Moe G: Amino-terminal pro-B-type natriuretic peptide testing for the diagnosis or exclusion of heart failure in patients with acute symptoms, *Am J Cardiol* 101(3A):29-38, 2008.

240. Hildebrandt P, Collinson PO: Amino-terminal pro-B-type natriuretic peptide testing to assist the diagnostic evaluation of heart failure in symptomatic primary care patients, *Am J Cardiol* 101(3A):25-28, 2008.

241. Bettencourt P, Januzzi JL Jr: Amino-terminal pro-B-type natriuretic peptide testing for inpatient monitoring and treatment guidance of acute destabilized heart failure, *Am J Cardiol* 101(3A):67-71, 2008.

242. Onwuanyi A, Taylor M: Acute decompensated heart failure: pathophysiology and treatment, *Am J Cardiol* 99(6B):2530, 2007.

243. Lehtonen L, Poder P: The utility of levosimendan in the treatment of heart failure, *Ann Med* 39(1):2-17, 2007.

244. Elkayam U et al: Vasodilators in the management of acute heart failure, *Crit Care Med* 36(1 Suppl):S95-S105, 2008.

245. Kazi D, Deswal A: Role and optimal dosing of angiotensin-converting enzyme inhibitors in heart failure, *Cardiol Clin* 26(1):1-14, 2008.

246. Rosenberg J, Gustafsson F: Bisoprolol for congestive heart failure, *Exp Opin Pharmacother* 9(2):293-300, 2008.

247. Ahmed A et al: Effects of digoxin at low serum concentrations on mortality and hospitalization in heart failure: a propensity-matched study of the DIG trial, *Int J Cardiol* 123(2):138-146, 2008.

248. Farmakis D et al: Anticoagulants, antiplatelets, and statins in heart failure, *Cardiol Clin* 26(1):49-58, vi, 2008.

249. Lipinski MJ et al: Drug insight: statins for nonischemic heart failure—evidence and potential mechanisms, *Nat Clin Pract Cardiovasc Med* 4(4):196-205, 2007.

250. Anderson LJ et al: Patient selection and echocardiographic assessment of dyssynchrony in cardiac resynchronization therapy, *Circulation* 117(15):2009-2023, 2008.

251. Ailawadi G, Kron IL: New strategies for surgical management of ischemic cardiomyopathy, *Esp Rev Cardiovasc Ther* 6(4):521-530, 2008.

252. Kale P, Fang JC: Devices in acute heart failure, *Crit Care Med* 36 (1 Suppl):S121-S128, 2008.

253. Leri A et al: Myocardial regeneration and stem cell repair, *Curr Probl Cardiol* 33(3):91-153, 2008.

254. Mishra PK: Bone marrow-derived mesenchymal stem cells for treatment of heart failure: is it all paracrine actions and immunomodulation? *J Cardiovasc Med* 9(2):122-128, 2008.

255. Sanderson JE: Heart failure with a normal ejection fraction, *Heart* 93(2):155-158, 2007.

256. Kumar R, Gandhi SK, Little WC: Acute heart failure with preserved systolic function, *Crit Care Med* 36(1 Suppl):S52-S56, 2008.

257. Rapp JA, Gheorghiade M: Role of neurohormonal modulators in heart failure with relatively preserved systolic function, *Cardiol Clin* 26(1): 23-40, vi, 2008.

258. Periasamy M, Janssen PM: Molecular basis of diastolic dysfunction, *Heart Fail Clin* 4(1):13-21, 2008.

259. Greyson CR: Pathophysiology of right ventricular failure, *Crit Care Med* 36(1 Suppl):S57-S65, 2008.

260. Haddad F et al: Right ventricular function in cardiovascular disease, part II: pathophysiology, clinical importance, and management of right ventricular failure, *Circulation* 117(13):1717-1731, 2008.

ALTERATIONS OF CARDIOVASCULAR FUNCTION IN CHILDREN

NANCY L. McDANIEL

MEDIA RESOURCES

evolve **Evolve Website** (http://evolve.elsevier.com/McCance/)
- Review Questions and Answers
- Animations
- Glossary (with audio pronunciation for selected terms)
- WebLinks

CHAPTER OUTLINE

DEVELOPMENT OF THE CARDIOVASCULAR SYSTEM
Developmental Anatomy
Transitional Circulation
Postnatal Development
CONGENITAL HEART DEFECTS
Classification of Congenital Heart Defects and
    Associated Conditions
Hypoxemia

Defects Increasing Pulmonary Blood Flow
Defects Decreasing Pulmonary Blood Flow
Obstructive Defects
Mixing Defects
ACQUIRED CARDIOVASCULAR DISORDERS
Kawasaki Disease
Systemic Hypertension
Childhood Obesity

Cardiovascular disease in children can be classified as congenital or acquired heart disease. Congenital heart disease is the most common. The diagnosis and management of congenital heart defects continue to improve with the use of fetal echocardiography, early interventional catheterization, and refined surgical repair. Acquired heart defects in children continue to present challenges to the practitioner; although guidelines for diagnosing acquired defects are available, work is needed in developing standards of treatment and long-term follow-up.

DEVELOPMENT OF THE CARDIOVASCULAR SYSTEM

Developmental Anatomy

Embryology

Cardiogenesis begins at approximately 3 weeks of gestation; however, most cardiovascular development occurs between the fourth and seventh weeks.[1] The heart arises from the mesenchyme and begins development as an enlarged blood vessel with a large lumen and a muscular wall (Figure 31-1, A).

Initially, two lateral endocardial heart tubes fuse to form a single structure (Figure 31-1, B). During the fifth week of gestation, the midsection of this tube begins to grow faster than its ends. This single heart tube elongates and rotates to the right (D-loop formation), creating a bulboventricular loop by approximately the twenty-eighth day[1] (Figure 31-1, C). Also at this time the first fetal heart contractions occur. At this stage the primitive heart structures include a common atrium; common ventricle; the sinus venosus, which eventually evolves into the superior and inferior venae cavae; the bulbus cordis, which eventually evolves into the ventricular outflow tracts; and the truncus arteriosus, which eventually yields the main pulmonary artery (PA) and aorta (Figure 31-1, D). By the fourth week of gestation, cardiovascular septation, ventricular development, aortic arch evolution, and circulation begin.

Cardiac Septation

Separation first begins when collections of mesenchymal cells cause the endocardial lining of the heart to bulge into the internal lumen. These changes, known as **endocardial cushions,** are instrumental in closing the lower portion of the atrial septum, dividing the atrioventricular (AV) canals into the right and left

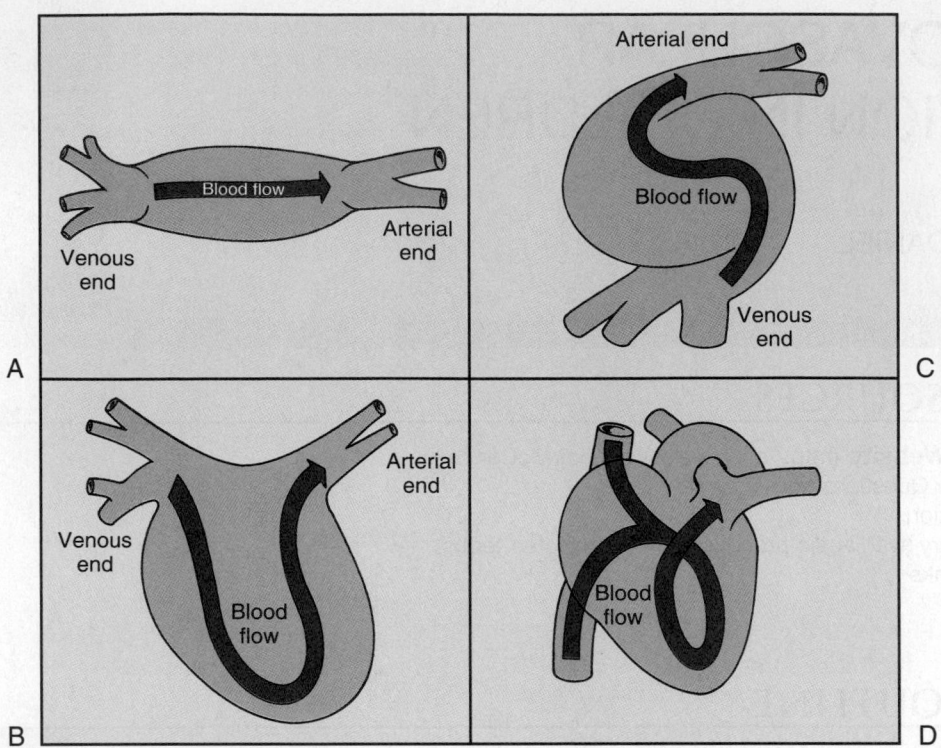

Figure 31-1 Embryologic development of the heart. A, The earliest heart structure consists of a muscular tube with a large lumen. About the fifth week of gestation, the tube, **B,** bulges and, **C,** twists until, **D,** the ends come together and fuse.

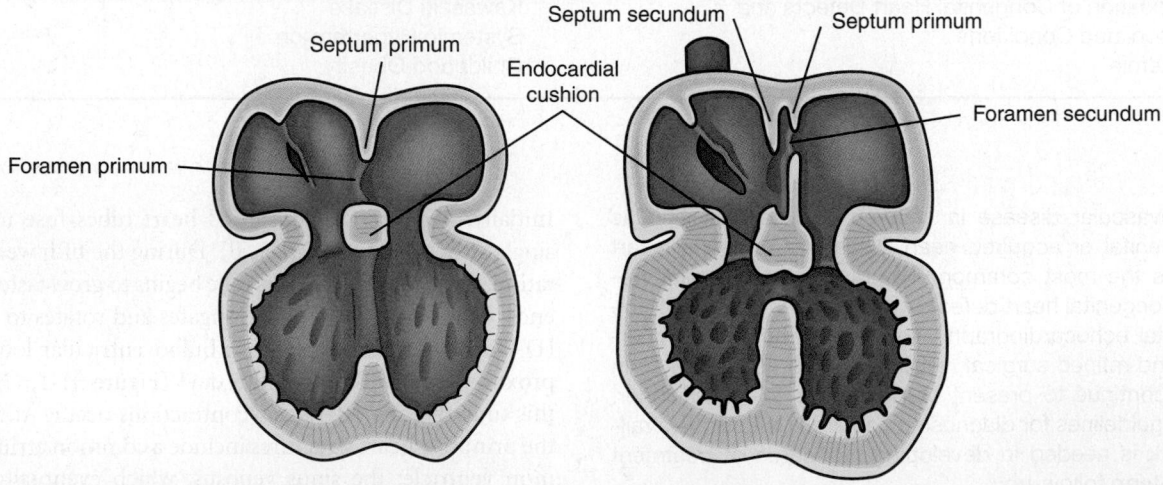

Figure 31-2 Development of the cardiac septa.

AV orifices, and forming the upper portion of the interventricular septum. Altered formation of the endocardial cushions can result in ostium primum atrial septal defects, inlet ventricular septal defects (VSDs), malformation of the AV valves, or a complete AV defect (also known as atrioventricular septal defect).[2]

Atrial septation begins when two thin membrane-like structures, known as the **septum primum** and the **septum secundum,** grow toward the area of the endocardial cushions (Figure 31-2). The septum primum forms along the posterior wall of the common atrium and grows downward toward the center

portion of the heart. The gap between the two structures, known as the **ostium primum,** normally closes by extensions from the endocardial cushions. At the time of closure, fenestrations or openings develop in the superior portion of the septum primum, creating the **ostium secundum.** Failure of the septum primum to fuse with the endocardial cushions results in an ostium primum defect in the atrial septum near the AV valve area.

The septum secundum is also a fenestrated, membrane-like structure located anteriorly that grows toward the endocardial cushions. During fetal development this structure

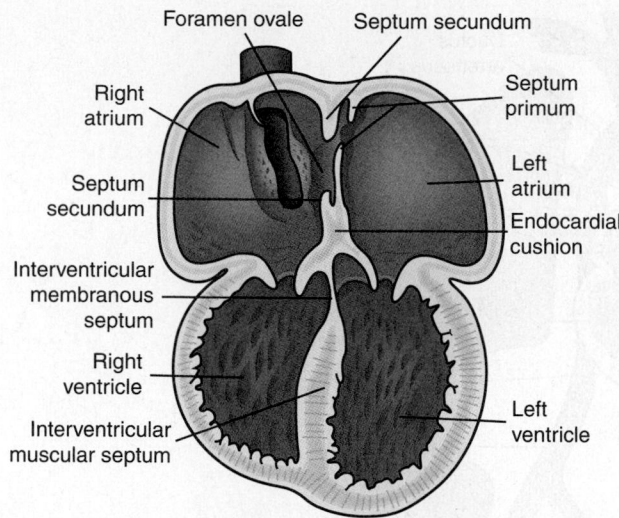

Figure 31-3 Septal development of the heart.

does not completely fuse with the endocardial cushions to achieve complete atrial septal closure. The nonfused septum secundum and ostium secundum result in the formation of a flapped orifice known as the **foramen ovale,** which allows the right-to-left shunting necessary for fetal circulation. Altered development in any of these structures can lead to an atrial septal defect.

Ventricular septation develops when the muscular ridge located at the apex, the endocardial tissue, and the bulbar ridges in the bulbus cordis fuse (Figure 31-3). Closure of the interventricular septum ensures communication between the right ventricle (RV) and the PA and between the left ventricle (LV) and the aorta. Further evolution of the endocardial tissue gives rise to the membranous ventricular septum and the AV valves. The conal portion of the ventricular septum that separates the aorta from the PA forms from the **bulbus cordis.**

When the single primitive heart tube begins to form the D-loop, the venous and arterial poles of the heart are fixed, resulting in torsion within the anterosuperior region of the loop, known as the *truncus arteriosus.* This torsion creates a spiral ridgelike structure or septum within the truncus arteriosus that divides it into the PA and the aorta. The semilunar valves evolve from tubercles after this division is complete.

Before this division occurs, however, two large arteries form at the distal end of the truncus arteriosus. Over time they give rise to a series of arterial vessels, collectively called the six aortic arches. By the fifth week of gestation, the first two pairs disappear and the third eventually evolves into the common carotid artery, the external carotid artery, and part of the internal carotid artery. The fourth pair of aortic arches will form part of the true aortic arch and the proximal segment of the right subclavian artery. The fifth pair disappears; however, the sixth pair yields the proximal and branch pulmonary arteries within the lung parenchyma and the ductus arteriosus.

Swellings in the conal region at the base of the main trunk separate the right ventricular outflow (pulmonary outflow) tract from the left ventricular outflow (aortic outflow) tract.

The conus also contributes to complete closure of the interventricular septum, and normal reabsorption of the subaortic conal region ensures rotation of the great arteries so that the aorta is posterior and to the right of the PA and the PA is anterior and to the left of the aorta. Despite division of the truncus arteriosus and separation of the right and left outflow tracts, a communication exists between the aorta and the PA known as the **ductus arteriosus.**

In order to deliver maximally oxygenated blood to the developing brain, fetal circulation differs from the adult pattern by the presence of alternate pathways known as fetal shunts (Figure 31-4). Fetal oxygenation occurs in the placenta instead of the fetal lungs. The fetal lungs are not aerated, although the fetus does make breathing motions.

In utero the fetus receives blood carrying oxygen and nutrients from the placenta through the umbilical vein. Fetal arterial oxygen tension is much lower than that found in the postnatal period—approximately 20 to 30 torr (mmHg pressure). Yet, despite this hypoxemic state, tissue hypoxia does not occur because of high fetal cardiac output and fetal hemoglobin. The blood travels to the liver, where a portion enters the portal and hepatic circulation; approximately half the flow is diverted away from the liver through the ductus venosus and into the inferior vena cava. Because the blood received from the inferior vena cava yields a higher pressure, blood entering the right atrium (RA) from the inferior vena cava is shunted through the foramen ovale and into the left atrium (LA) and is then pumped through the LV and into the aorta. Approximately two thirds of the blood flows to the head and upper extremities. Because this blood is mainly from the placenta, the brain and coronary arteries receive the blood with the highest oxygen concentration. The remaining blood flows into the descending aorta.

Less-saturated blood, with an oxygen tension of 15 to 19 torr, returns from the upper body, head, neck, and arms and travels from the superior vena cava into the RA. A small portion of this blood flows into the RV and out the PA and enters the nonfunctioning lungs. Most of the blood, however, bypasses the lungs by flowing through the ductus arteriosus and into the descending aorta. Blood from the descending aorta returns to the placenta through two umbilical arteries.[1]

The nonaerated lungs and low oxygen tension induce vasoconstriction, creating high pulmonary vascular resistance. This is transmitted to the right side of the heart and the PAs. Conversely, fetal systemic resistance is low because of the large-volume placenta and ductus arteriosus. Therefore, because blood flow follows the path of least resistance, high pulmonary resistance diverts most of the blood flow into the PA, through the ductus arteriosus, and into the aorta. From there it travels into the low-resistance placenta.

Transitional Circulation

At birth a series of circulatory changes occur that affect blood flow, vascular resistance, and oxygen tension. The most important change that takes place in the circulation is the shift of gas exchange from the placenta to the lungs. In addition, alterations

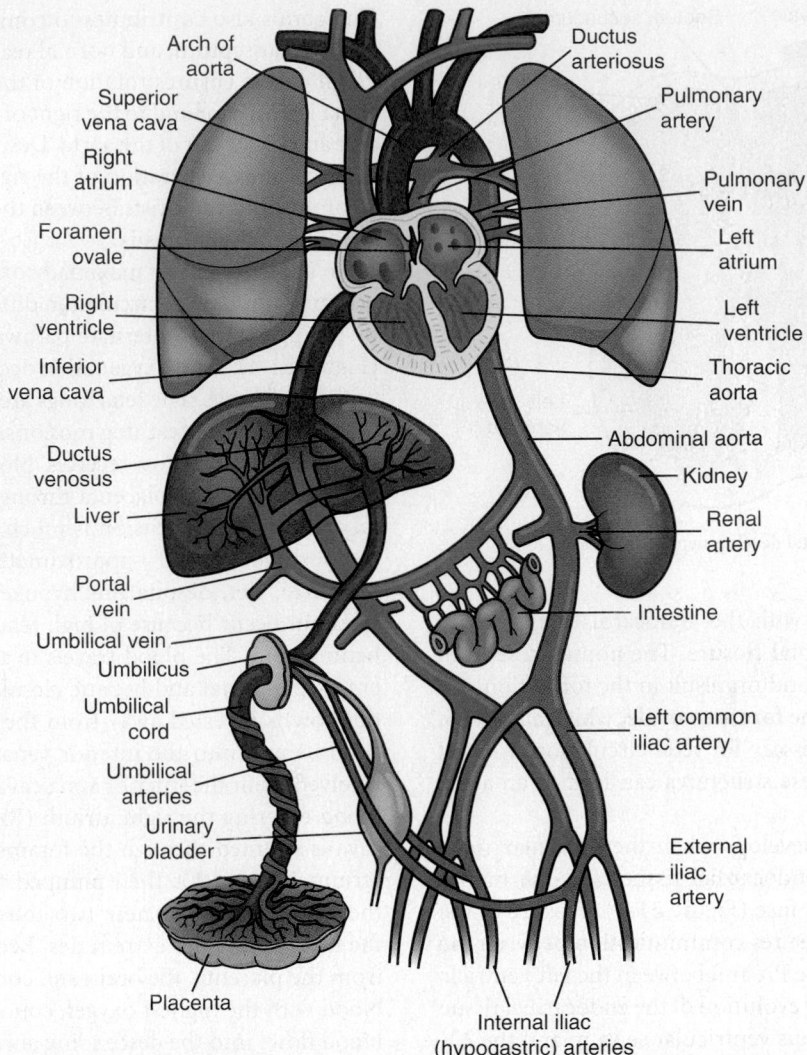

Figure 31-4 Fetal circulation. Circulation of the fetus reflects the fact that oxygenation of fetal blood does not take place in the lungs, but rather in the placenta. Therefore, the pulmonary circulatory system is essentially "bypassed." Instead of traveling from the right heart to the lungs, as occurs after birth, most blood entering the right heart passes through the ductus arteriosus and into the systemic circulation.

in pressure and volume of blood flowing through the heart chambers functionally close the ductus arteriosus, ductus venosus, and foramen ovale. A decrease of pulmonary vascular resistance and an increase of systemic vascular resistance lead to changes in the size and shape of the heart chambers.

Clamping of the umbilical cord and expansion of the lungs at birth shift gas exchange from the placenta to the lungs. Removal of the low-resistance placenta from circulation also causes an immediate increase in systemic vascular resistance to about twice that before birth. Conversely, pulmonary vascular resistance decreases because of expansion of the lungs that results from the infant's respirations and exposure to more oxygen-rich blood.

Closure of Fetal Shunts

Once the umbilical cord is clamped, the umbilical arteries and vein, which comprise the cord, vasoconstrict and undergo fibrous changes. Therefore, blood flow through the ductus

venosus falls instantly; absence of fetal shunting through this vessel usually occurs within the first 7 days of life. Once the ductus venosus closes, its remnants form the **ligamentum venosum,** or round ligament of the liver.

Increased pulmonary venous return and decreased inferior vena cava return cause functional closure of the foramen ovale within the first month of life. In the fetus the foramen ovale is held open by the blood flow from the high-pressure right side, reflecting pulmonary vascular resistance, to the lower-pressure area on the left side of the heart, reflecting systemic vascular resistance. At birth the pressure gradients reverse (left atrial pressure exceeds right atrial pressure by a small degree), causing the valve flaps of the foramen ovale to close. Functional closure occurs by the adherence of these flaps to the atrial septum. Anatomic closure occurs within the first month of life after deposition of fibrin tissue and cell products permanently seals the flaps closed. Until this occurs, any condition that stimulates an increase in the right-sided pressures or causes dilation of the RA can reopen the foramen ovale. Conditions in which a patent foramen ovale may continue past the first month of life include pulmonary hypertension, RV failure, and tricuspid atresia.

The ductus arteriosus closes more gradually. Increased oxygen saturation in the systemic arterial blood is thought to be the major stimulus causing vasoconstriction of the ductus arteriosus. In addition, a decrease in the amount of endogenous prostaglandins promoting dilation and the release of vasoactive substances stimulate further ductal closure. Vasoconstriction of the ductal medial smooth muscle shortens and thickens the intima of the ductal wall within 15 to 18 hours after birth. Permanent closure is complete 10 to 21 days after birth. Fibrous tissue adheres to the remaining structure, and the ductus arteriosus eventually evolves into the ligamentum arteriosum. Conditions that involve low arterial oxygen saturations, such as cyanotic heart disease, decreased medial muscle layer within the ductus, or increased levels of circulating vasodilating substances in the blood, may delay or prevent ductal closure.[3]

Postnatal Development

The infant's cardiopulmonary system is proportionally larger in relation to body surface area than the adult's. The infant's heart points at a transverse angle, but as the lungs and heart mature, the heart shifts lower in the chest and is rotated at a more oblique angle. Unlike the adult heart, the newborn heart has RV dominance with a thickened RV wall. This is because of the high pulmonary vascular resistance in the fetal circulation that subjects the RV to high afterload, which in turn causes the right ventricular myocardium to become as thick and strong as the left.

After birth the right ventricular myocardium becomes less dominant as pulmonary vascular resistance drops. As systemic vascular resistance increases, the left ventricular myocardium becomes thicker. By 1 month of age, the newborn's ventricles are approximately equal in weight. As the child grows, the heart size increases accordingly. The weight of the heart doubles during the first year of life and increases six times that by 9 years of age.[3]

Postnatal changes involve a rise in arterial oxygen tension and an increase in alveolar oxygenation that stimulates vasodilation, resulting in a decrease in pulmonary vascular resistance. During the first 2 to 9 weeks of life, the inner medial linings of the small pulmonary arterioles thin out in response to decreased pulmonary arterial pressure. This increased diameter of the pulmonary vessels, along with further development of the pulmonary bed in response to lung growth, results in a decrease in pulmonary vascular resistance. By 2 months of age, pulmonary resistance may approximate adult levels. During the neonatal period, however, care must be taken to maintain homeostasis because of hyperactivity of the pulmonary bed. Adverse conditions, such as alveolar hypoxia, acidosis, and hypothermia, may trigger pulmonary vasoconstriction and lead to pulmonary hypertension.

Postnatal Hemodynamics

As stated, systemic vascular resistance begins to rise once the placenta is removed from the circulation. Normal levels in the infant range from approximately 10 to 15 Wood units × body surface area (in square meters) and gradually increase to 15 to 30 Wood units × body surface area (in square meters) by childhood.[4] Likewise, the systolic pressure is low in the full-term newborn (approximately 39 to 59 mmHg), reflecting the decreased LV strength. As the systemic vascular resistance increases, the LV becomes more developed and the systolic pressure rises steadily until it equals adult levels once the child reaches puberty.

The heart rate of the newborn ranges from 100 to 180 beats/minute, which gradually decreases as the child grows. Similarly, the newborn's cardiac output is high, which is a reflection of the fetal circulation described earlier. Oxygen consumption doubles at birth; to maintain adequate oxygen delivery, the cardiac output also remains high. These changes, however, cause minimal cardiac reserve in the newborn. Additional stressors could increase oxygen demands and result in acute deterioration. By 2 months of age, oxygen consumption decreases by half. As the newborn grows, stroke volume steadily increases while the heart rate decreases.[2]

Postnatal Circulation

Postnatal circulation allows the lungs to oxygenate the venous blood and allows saturated blood to be delivered to the systemic circulation. Desaturated blood returning from the superior vena cava, inferior vena cava, and coronary veins enters the RA and is pumped to the RV through the tricuspid valve. The RV then pumps the blood through the pulmonic valve to the PA; the blood flows to the lungs, where it is oxygenated. The oxygenated blood returns from the lungs through the pulmonary veins and enters the LA, which pumps blood to the LV through the mitral valve. The LV then pumps blood through the aortic valve and into the aorta. The coronary arteries receive the saturated blood along with delivery to the systemic circulation.

CONGENITAL HEART DEFECTS

Congenital heart disease is the leading cause of death, excluding prematurity, during the first year of life.[5] It is estimated that as many as 35% of deaths caused by congenital heart defects occur in the first year of life and that one third of children born with congenital heart disease will die as a result of their cardiac disease (Box 31-1). There are more than 35 documented types of congenital heart defects, and the frequency of occurrence in the United States is on the rise. Although researchers have not determined the reason for this increase, one explanation is that it may be the result of improved methods of detection.[6]

The underlying cause of congenital heart disease is known in only 10% of cases. Several factors place the fetus at risk for

Box 31-1   Endocarditis Risk

Until 2007 it was common to prescribe an antibiotic to be given prior to dental, gastrointestinal, or genitourinary procedures for almost all children with congenital heart defects. This practice started in the 1950s and continued until a committee of the American Heart Association (AHA) reviewed all of the major literature related to infectious endocarditis (IE), a serious and sometimes fatal condition in which the heart valves become infected with bacteria. The AHA committee concluded that (1) IE is more likely to result from bacteremia from daily activities, such as brushing one's teeth than from procedures; (2) prophylaxis was not effective in preventing IE; (3) there are significant risks to giving antibiotics; and (4) good oral health and hygiene is most important in the prevention of IE. Current recommendations suggest giving prophylactic antibiotic prior to dental procedures only to the most high-risk children and adults: those with prosthetic cardiac valves, cyanotic congenital heart disease, repaired heart defects for the first 6 months after the procedure, repaired heart defects with certain residual defects, and those with previous IE. The best thing we as healthcare providers can teach our patients and their parents is to take excellent care of their teeth!

Data from Wilson W et al: *Circulation* 166:1737-1754, 2007.

Table 31-1   Environmental Factors and Associated Congenital Heart Defects

Cause	Type of Congenital Heart Defect
Infection	
Intrauterine	Patent ductus arteriosus (PDA), pulmonary stenosis, coarctation of aorta
Systemic viral	PDA, pulmonary stenosis, coarctation of aorta
Rubella	PDA, pulmonary stenosis, coarctation of aorta
Coxsackie B5	Endocardial fibroelastosis
Herpesvirus cytomegalovirus (HCMV)	Can infect endothelial cells and vascular endothelium
	Specific cardiovascular effect not known
Radiation	
Metabolic Disorders	
Diabetes	Ventricular septal defect (VSD), cardiomegaly, transposition of the great vessels
Phenylketonuria (PKU)	Coarctation of the aorta, PDA
Hypercalcemia	Supravalvular aortic stenosis, pulmonic stenosis; aortic hyperplasia
Drugs	
Thalidomide	No specific lesion
Alcohol	Tetralogy of Fallot, atrial septal defect, VSD
Lithium	Exact effect not known
Phenytoin	Embryonic dysrhythmia and valvular heart disease
Warfarin	Atrial septal defect (ASD) and PDA
Peripheral Conditions	
Increased maternal age	VSD, tetralogy of Fallot (relationship unclear)
Antepartal bleeding	Various defects (relationship unclear)
Prematurity	PDA, VSD
High altitude	PDA, ASD (increased incidence)

developing congenital heart disease, including prenatal, environmental, and genetic factors. Among the prenatal factors are maternal rubella, maternal insulin-dependent diabetes, maternal alcoholism, maternal age (older than 40 years), maternal phenylketonuria, and maternal hypercalcemia (Table 31-1). The use of some drugs during pregnancy is associated with an above-average incidence of congenital heart disease. Examples of these drugs include thalidomide, lithium, phenytoin (Dilantin), and warfarin. The incidence of heart defects also has been found to be higher in stillbirths, spontaneous abortions, and low-birth-weight or small-for-gestational-age infants.[2] In general, the likelihood of unaffected parents having a child with congenital heart disease is about 1% with a recurrence risk of 2% to 6%.

Genetic factors also have been implicated in the development of congenital heart disease, although the mechanism of causation is often multifactorial. Recent progress, accelerated through the Human Genome Project, has resulted in the rapid identification of some genes causing congenital heart disease.[5]

ETIOLOGY The etiology of congenital heart disease is unknown. Early epidemiologic studies report a multifactorial influence to be the cause of up to 90% of cardiac anomalies, with a recurrence rate of 2% to 6%.[2] Associated risk factors include maternal, gestational, and familial conditions. (Maternal risk factors are discussed in the previous section.) Exposure to teratogens in utero also may be a risk factor. Likewise, fetal exposure to active maternal infections, such as rubella, herpesvirus, coxsackievirus B5, and cytomegalovirus, may be a risk.

Chromosomal aberrations account for about 6% of all congenital heart defects (Table 31-2). Many genetic and hereditary diseases are associated with congenital heart defects, although the mechanism of causation is unknown (Table 31-3). As many as 50% of infants with trisomy 21 have a congenital heart defect, either an AV canal defect or a VSD. Extracardiac defects are noted in as many as 35% of infants with cardiac lesions. Prospective studies using chromosomal analysis have suggested that congenital cardiac malformations may be the result of a single gene defect.[5]

Because of improved screening methods, surgical interventions, and management, children with congenital heart defects are now surviving into adulthood and bearing children of their own. Studies report a 5% to 15% incidence of congenital heart disease in offspring of a parent having a congenital heart lesion. If two siblings have a congenital cardiac anomaly, the recurrence risk is 9%, and if three siblings have a congenital

Table 31-2	Genetic Factors and Congenital Heart Defects	
Chromosomal Aberrations or Syndrome	**Incidence of Defects**	**Type of Defect**
Trisomy 13	80%	Ventricular septal defect (VSD), atrial septal defect (ASD), patent ductus arteriosus (PDA), anomalous pulmonary venous connection, bicuspid aorta, overriding aorta
Trisomy 18	90%	VSD, PDA, patent foramen ovale, bicuspid aortic valve, dextrocardia
Down syndrome	12%-44%	Endocardial cushion defects, VSD, PDA, ASD, transposition of great vessels, tetralogy of Fallot, persistent truncus arteriosus, coarctation of aorta, endocardial fibroelastosis
Cri du chat syndrome	20%	PDA, mixed defects
Turner syndrome	20%-40%	Coarctation of aorta, pulmonary stenosis, subaortic and aortic stenosis, PDA, septal defects

Data from Doyle EF, Rutkowski M: Etiology of congenital heart disease, *Cardiovasc Clin* 2:1, 1970.

Table 31-3	Disorders Coexistent with Congenital Heart Defects
Disorder	**Associated Cardiovascular Defect**
Connective Tissue Disorders	
Marfan syndrome	Aortic or mitral regurgitation, aortic aneurysm
Hurler syndrome	Pseudoatherosclerosis
Hunter syndrome	Pseudoatherosclerosis, hypertension
Osteogenesis imperfecta	Incompetent aortic valve
Complex Syndromes	
Kartagener syndrome	Dextrocardia
Holt-Oram syndrome	Atrial septal defect (ASD), ventricular septal defect (VSD)
Ellis–van Creveld syndrome	Defect or absence of atrial septum
Laurence-Moon-Biedl syndrome	Tetralogy of Fallot, single ventricle, transposition of aorta
Inborn Errors of Metabolism	
Pompe disease	Cardiomegaly, left heart failure, supraventricular tachycardia
Homocystinuria	Thromboembolic episodes, pulmonic and aortic regurgitation
Phakomatosis	
Neurofibromatosis (von Recklinghausen disease)	Hypertension, pheochromocytoma
von Hippel–Lindau disease	Hypertension, pheochromocytoma
Sturge-Weber-Dimitri disease	Anomalies of carotid and meningeal arteries
Vascular Malformations	
Osler-Weber-Rendu disease (hereditary hemorrhagic telangiectasia)	Atrioventricular fistula, telangiectasia
Milroy disease (lymphedema)	Hypoplasia or lymphatic vessels

Data from Doyle EF, Rutkowski M: Etiology of congenital heart disease, *Cardiovasc Clin* 2:1, 1970.

cardiac anomaly, the rate jumps to a 50% chance that the next child also will have a cardiovascular malformation.

Classification of Congenital Heart Defects and Associated Conditions

There are more than 35 different types of congenital anomalies that can be classified into four categories based on blood flow pattern: (1) lesions increasing pulmonary blood flow; (2) lesions decreasing pulmonary blood flow; (3) obstructive lesions, in which right- or left-sided outflow tract obstructions curtail or prohibit blood flow out of the heart; and (4) mixing lesions, in which desaturated blood and saturated blood mix within the chambers or great arteries of the heart (Table 31-4).

By classifying lesions in this way, the clinical manifestations, as well as associated sequelae, are more predictable.

Associated conditions and their clinical manifestations are lesion dependent. The two most common conditions associated with congenital heart disease are heart failure (HF) and hypoxemia. Lesions increasing pulmonary blood flow include defects that allow blood flow to shunt from the high-pressure left side to the lower-pressure right side, resulting in pulmonary congestion. Lesions that cause decreased pulmonary blood flow are generally complex and result in cyanosis. Obstructive lesions increase the pressure needed to eject the blood from the ventricle. The two types of obstructive lesions are right-sided lesions that may result in hypoxemia

Table 31-4	Classification of Congenital Heart Defects		
Classification	**Shunt Direction**	**Presentation**	**Specific Defects**
Lesions increasing pulmonary blood flow	Left to right	Acyanotic congestive heart failure	Patent ductus arteriosus, atrial septal defect, ventricular septal defect, complete atrio-ventricular canal defect
Lesions decreasing pulmonary blood flow	Right to left	Cyanotic	Tetralogy of Fallot, tricuspid atresia
Obstructive lesions*	None	Low cardiac output Shock	Coarctation of the aorta, hypoplastic left heart syndrome, aortic stenosis, pulmonary stenosis
Mixed lesions†	Variable	Variable	Transposition of the great arteries, total anomalous pulmonary venous connection, truncus arteriosus

*If patent ductus arteriosus closes, newborns with hypoplastic left heart syndrome, coarctation of the aorta, or critical aortic stenosis will present with shock. Newborns with aortic stenosis or pulmonary stenosis may have only mild symptoms depending on severity of stenosis.
†Transposition of the great arteries and truncus arteriosus will present with cyanosis as patent ductus arteriosus closes. Total anomalous pulmonary venous connection usually presents with congestive heart failure.

and cyanosis, and left-sided lesions that may result in HF. Mixing lesions are variable in their physiology and clinical manifestation.

Heart Failure

Heart failure (HF), sometimes called congestive heart failure (CHF), is classified as an acquired condition. HF occurs when the heart is unable to maintain sufficient cardiac output to meet the metabolic demands of the body. HF can occur as the result of decreased myocardial function or excessive metabolic demands. The most common causes of HF in infancy and childhood are cardiomyopathy or the result of poor ventricular function. Table 31-5 lists the congenital heart defects that cause HF by age. Pulmonary overcirculation from large left-to-right shunts (mixing) is often called CHF but is not usually associated with decreased ventricular function and failure to meet metabolic demands. However the clinical manifestations are similar, such as failure to thrive (FTT), tachypnea, tachycardia, and respiratory infections.

PATHOPHYSIOLOGY In general, the pathophysiologic mechanisms of HF in infants and children are very similar to those in adults. The same compensatory mechanisms are activated in the face of inadequate cardiac output. An acute decrease in blood pressure stimulates stretch receptors and baroreceptors in the aorta and carotid arteries, which in turn stimulate the sympathetic nervous system. With the release of catecholamines and the stimulation of β-receptors, heart rate and the force of myocardial contraction increase. Venous smooth muscle tone also increases, which increases return of venous blood to the heart. Sympathetic stimulation also decreases blood flow to the kidneys, skin, spleen, and extremities so that maximum flow to the brain, heart, and lungs can be maintained. Decreased blood flow to the kidneys causes the release of renin, angiotensin, and aldosterone. If chronic, this cycle results in retention of sodium and fluid by the kidneys, which in turn increases volume in the circulatory system.

Table 31-5	Congenital Heart Defects Causing Heart Failure
Age	**Congenital Heart Defect**
Time of birth	Hypoplastic left heart syndrome
	Volume overload caused by tricuspid regurgitation (rare)
	Arteriovenous fistula
Birth to 1 week	Hypoplastic left heart syndrome
	Aortic atresia
	Transposition of the great vessels with ventricular septal defect (VSD)
	Coarctation of the aorta
	Total anomalous pulmonary venous connection (TAPVC) with obstruction
	Patent ductus arteriosus (PDA) in premature infants
First 4 weeks	Coarctation of the aorta
	TAPVC
	Large left-to-right shunt caused by VSD, PDA in premature infants
	Tricuspid atresia
	All previously mentioned defects
4 to 6 weeks	Transposition of the great vessels with VSD
	Large left-to-right shunt caused by endocardial cushion defect
6 weeks to 6 months	VSD
6 months	Endocardial fibroelastosis
	Persistent truncus arteriosus with large left-to-right shunt

These neurohumoral and hemodynamic changes create abnormal ventricular wall stress and cause the myocardium to hypertrophy. The myocardial fibers also stretch to accommodate the increased volume. Hypertrophy and fiber stretch temporarily increase contractility and hence the force of ventricular contraction. These mechanisms eventually fail to maintain cardiac output as HF progresses. A review of the Frank-Starling law of the heart (see Chapter 29) is useful for an understanding of the cycle of compensation and decompensation that occurs in HF.

CLINICAL MANIFESTATIONS Symptomatic HF in children has many causes. It is not usually necessary to determine if it is right- or left-sided HF. When assessing a child with HF, a combination of symptoms generally is present. Pulmonary overcirculation is the predominant cause associated with congenital defects.

HF in infants is manifested as poor feeding and sucking, often leading to FTT. Dyspnea, tachypnea, and diaphoresis may be accompanied by retractions, grunting, and nasal flaring. Wheezing, coughing, and rales are rare even with significant HF. Common skin changes, such as pallor or mottling, are often present.

Hepatomegaly (enlargement of the liver) is atypically attributable to systemic venous congestion. In infants the normal liver is soft, sharp-edged, and palpable 1 to 2 cm below the costal margin. However, the absence of hepatomegaly does not rule out HF.

Periorbital edema and weight gain without caloric increase are uncommon manifestations of right ventricular failure in infants. Peripheral edema, which is a common finding in adults, is rare in infants and young children and more often signifies renal disease rather than cardiac disease. The clinical manifestations of HF are listed in Box 31-2.

EVALUATION AND TREATMENT A thorough physical examination with an emphasis on cardiac and pulmonary findings often will reveal the degree of HF. Plotting the child's growth (height, weight, head circumference) is an important method for monitoring a child's health. Infants with HF and pulmonary overcirculation usually have low weight with normal length and head circumference. Failure to thrive (FTT) is usually the result of increased metabolic expenditure relative to caloric intake. An electrocardiogram (ECG) should be performed to determine the presence of dysrhythmias or hypertrophy. A chest radiograph is useful in assessing the presence of cardiomegaly and signs of increased pulmonary circulation.

Treatment is aimed at decreasing cardiac workload and increasing the efficiency of heart function. Medical management initially consists of diuretics, such as furosemide. Depending on the degree of HF, other diuretics can be used in combination with furosemide to counteract potassium losses. Agents that reduce afterload, such as angiotensin-converting enzyme (ACE) inhibitors and beta-blockers, have recently been used to further manage severe HF.[2,3] Caloric supplementation is routinely prescribed.

Hypoxemia

Heart defects that allow desaturated blood to enter the systemic system without passing through the lungs result in hypoxemia and cyanosis. Hypoxemia occurs when arterial oxygen tension is below normal and results in low oxygen arterial saturations and cellular function alteration. **Cyanosis,** a blue discoloration of the mucous membranes and nail beds, results from deoxygenated hemoglobin in a concentration of at least 5 g/dl of blood or from arterial saturations less than 85%.[2,4] Anemia may mask the signs of hypoxemia, whereas children who are polycythemic with a normal arterial saturation may appear cyanotic. Older children who have an unrepaired septal defect with a left-to-right shunt may become cyanotic because of pulmonary vascular changes secondary to increased pulmonary blood flow. Because of these progressive pulmonary vascular changes, pulmonary vascular resistance increases to exceed or equal vascular resistance, resulting in a reversal of shunting known as **Eisenmenger syndrome.** Three types of defects cause hypoxemia and cyanosis:

1. Lesions that cause right ventricular outflow tract obstruction and shunting from the right side of the heart to the left side, as in tetralogy of Fallot (see p. 1223)
2. Defects involving the mixing of saturated and unsaturated blood within the heart chambers, as in a univentricular heart (also referred to as a single ventricle)

Box 31-2   Clinical Manifestations of Heart Failure

Impaired Myocardial Function	Pulmonary Congestion	Systemic Venous Congestion
Tachycardia	Tachypnea	Weight gain
Sweating (inappropriately)	Dyspnea	Hepatomegaly
Decreased urinary output	Retractions (infants)	Peripheral edema (rare)
Fatigue	Flaring nares	Ascites
Weakness	Exercise intolerance	Neck vein distention (rare in children)
Restlessness	Orthopnea	
Anorexia	Cough, hoarseness	
Pale, cool extremities	Cyanosis	
Weak peripheral pulses	Wheezing (rare)	
Decreased blood pressure	Grunting	
Gallop rhythm		
Cardiomegaly		

From Hockenberry MJ et al: *Wong's nursing care of infants and children,* ed 8, St Louis, 2007, Mosby.

3. Defects in children with transposition of the great arteries (see p. 1231), in which two parallel circulations exist and survival depends on the existence of a patent ductus arteriosus or septal defect

CLINICAL MANIFESTATIONS Infants with mild hypoxemia may show signs of cyanosis only occasionally when stressed; otherwise they may exhibit near-normal age-projected growth and development. Infants with severe hypoxemia may display signs of feeding intolerance, poor weight gain, tachypnea, and dyspnea. Children with chronic hypoxemia are small for their age, may display cognitive and motor skill delays, experience shortness of breath with exertion, fatigue easily, and have exercise intolerance. Acute, severe hypoxemia will lead to tissue hypoxia, metabolic acidosis, hyperventilation, poor perfusion, and eventually shock.

In response to chronic hypoxemia, polycythemia occurs as the body generates additional red blood cells to increase the oxygen-carrying capacity of the blood. In some infants, however, microcytic anemia may result because of limited stores of iron. Polycythemia and the associated platelet dysfunction also places children at risk for thromboembolic events, especially infants with severe cyanosis and iron deficiency anemia. In addition to the 2% risk of cerebrovascular accidents, there is a small chance that children with right-to-left shunting will develop a brain abscess.[4] Clubbing of the nail beds occurs because of chronic tissue hypoxemia and polycythemia.

Defects Increasing Pulmonary Blood Flow

Cardiac lesions that increase pulmonary blood flow include defects that involve septal abnormalities or communications between the great arteries. These allow the shunting of blood from the high-pressure left side to the lower-pressure right side. Infants with left-to-right shunts are acyanotic and, depending on the degree of shunting, will often develop signs and symptoms of CHF. Children with significant left-to-right shunts left untreated are at risk for development of irreversible pulmonary hypertension.

Patent Ductus Arteriosus

The **patent ductus arteriosus (PDA)** is a vessel located between the junction of the main and left pulmonary arteries and the lesser curvature of the descending aorta, usually just distal to the left subclavian artery. During fetal circulation the PDA allows blood to shunt from the PA to the aorta. At birth, once the placenta is removed and the lungs are expanded, the PDA will start to constrict within the first hours of life. Closure of the PDA in full-term infants is usually noted between 15 hours of life and 2 weeks of age.[7] As an isolated defect, PDA occurs in 5% to 10% of all congenital cardiac defects. In premature infants, studies have shown that the incidence of PDA is as high as 45% in newborns less than 1750 g.[8]

PATHOPHYSIOLOGY Failure of the PDA to close results in persistent patency of the ductus arteriosus. The hemodynamic effects of PDA depend on the size of the lumen and the resistance in the pulmonary and systemic circulations. At birth the pulmonary and systemic vascular resistances are almost equal and are reflected in the PA and aorta, respectively; therefore, shunting is minimal. However, as pulmonary vascular resistance falls, a reversal of fetal shunting occurs. Blood now begins to shunt left to right, from the aorta to the PA. The hemodynamic effect is increased pulmonary blood flow, resulting in increased pulmonary venous return to the LA and LV with increased workload on the left side of the heart. The increased workload is caused by increased pulmonary venous return to the LA and, potentially, an increase in right ventricular pressure if pulmonary vascular changes occur in response to the increased blood flow, leading to an increase in pulmonary vascular pressure (Figure 31-5, C).

CLINICAL MANIFESTATIONS If pulmonary vascular resistance has fallen, infants with PDA will characteristically have a continuous-machinery type murmur heard best at the left upper sternal border throughout systole and diastole. If the PDA is significant, the infant also will have bounding pulses, an active precordium, a thrill upon palpation, and signs and symptoms of pulmonary overcirculation. Infants with a small PDA will usually remain asymptomatic.

EVALUATION AND TREATMENT Chest radiograph will reveal cardiomegaly and increased pulmonary vascular markings. An ECG may demonstrate ventricular enlargement, particularly on the left, but in most cases it is within the normal range. Echocardiography and auscultation confirm the diagnosis based on the characteristic continuous-machinery type of murmur.

PDA closure in asymptomatic children is recommended by 2 years of age because of the risk of subacute bacterial endocarditis. Premature infants who develop respiratory distress are initially given indomethacin, a prostaglandin inhibitor, to close the duct. If this is unsuccessful, surgical ligation and division may be warranted.

Historically the most widely used method for PDA closure is surgical closure involving ligation and division of the ductus with complete closure in nearly 100% of cases. Mortality associated with surgical intervention nears 0%; however, there continues to be some morbidity associated with the approach through a left thoracotomy incision.

Several other options for PDA closure are available depending on the size of the child and the PDA. Many specialists perform interventional closure of the PDA during catheterization. The catheter is advanced into the ductal opening whereby multiple coils or other devices are placed into the lumen that prohibit flow through the duct. The greatest advantages to this procedure are the avoidance of a surgical procedure and thoracotomy pain and a brief observation stay in the hospital.

Another option is closure through video-assisted thoracoscopic surgery. This procedure involves making three small incisions in the left lateral wall, through which a probe is inserted. A clip is then placed around the vessel to occlude it. An advantage of this procedure over surgery is that there is less associated morbidity because of the avoidance of a thoracotomy incision.[7]

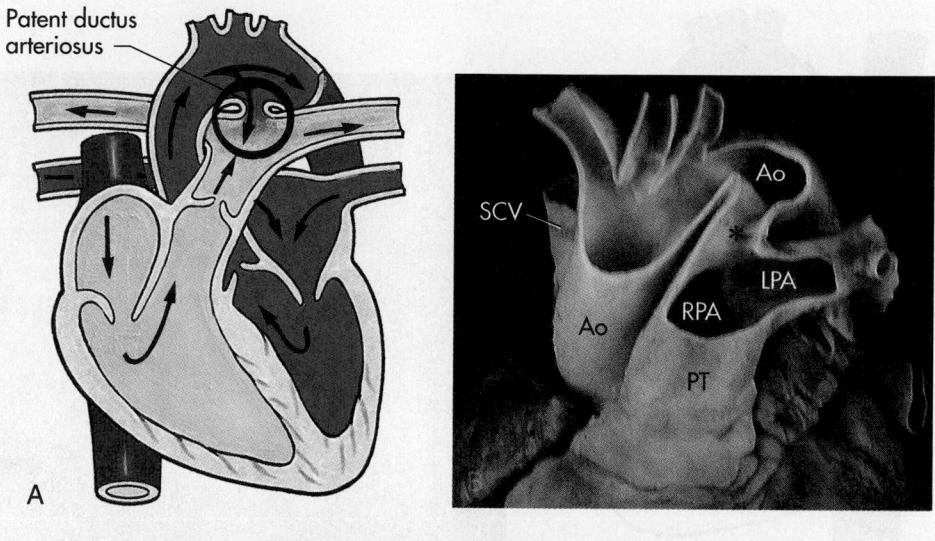

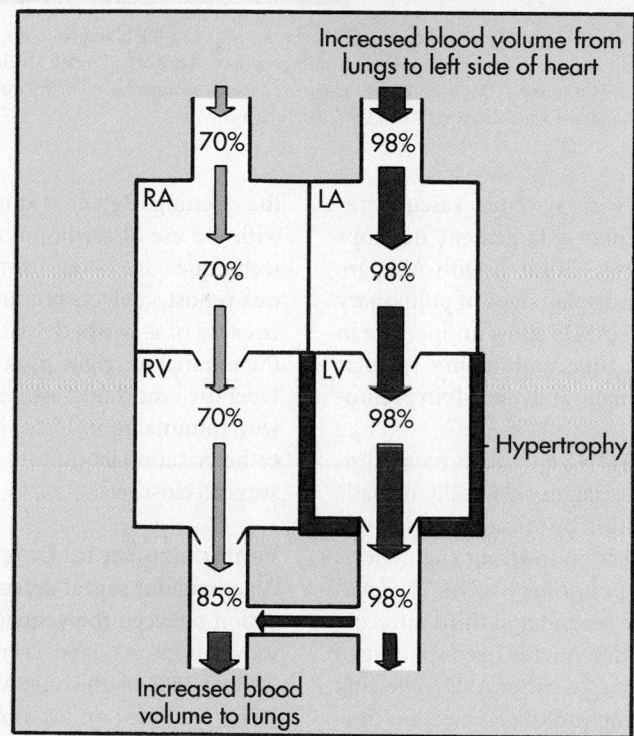

Figure 31-5 Patent ductus arteriosus (PDA). **A,** PDA with left-to-right shunt. **B,** PDA (*) in an adult with pulmonary hypertension. **C,** Changes in oxygen saturation, left ventricular volume, and the myocardium caused by left-to-right shunt through a PDA. *Ao,* Aorta; *LA,* left atrium; *LPA,* left pulmonary artery; *LV,* left ventricle; *PT,* pulmonary trunk; *RA,* right atrium; *RPA,* right pulmonary artery; *RV,* right ventricle; *SCV,* subclavian vein. (**A** from Hockenberry MJ et al: *Wong's essentials of pediatric nursing,* ed 8, St Louis, 2009, Mosby; **B** from Damjanov I, Linder J, editors: *Anderson's pathology,* ed 10, St Louis, 1996, Mosby.)

Atrial Septal Defect

An **atrial septal defect (ASD)** is an abnormal communication between the atria (Figure 31-6, *A* and *B*). Although it is an isolated lesion, it is the fourth most common congenital heart defect, occurring in 5% to 10% of all congenital cardiac defects. The three major types are an ostium primum defect, an opening found low in the septum that may be associated with AV valve abnormalities, especially mitral insufficiency; an ostium secundum defect, an opening in the center of the septum (this is the most common type of atrial defect); and a sinus venosus defect, an opening that occurs high up in the atrial septum near the superior vena cava and RA junction. This defect is often associated with partial anomalous pulmonary venous connection.

PATHOPHYSIOLOGY Although the pressure difference between the two atria is minimal, the ASD allows blood to be shunted from left to right because of the slightly higher pressure of the left atrial chamber and lower pulmonary

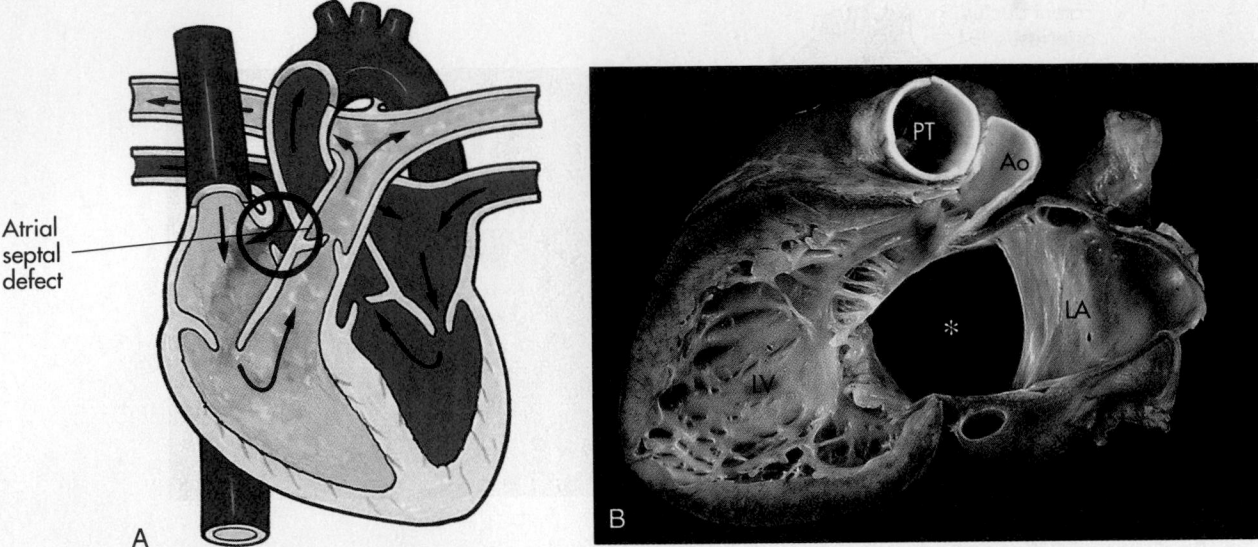

Figure 31-6 Atrial septal defect (ASD). **A,** Abnormal opening between the atria causing blood from the higher-pressure left atrium to flow into the lower-pressure right atrium. **B,** Complete ASD (*) form in children. *Ao,* Aorta; *LA,* left atrium; *LV,* left ventricle; *PT,* pulmonary artery trunk. (A from Hockenberry MJ et al: *Wong's essentials of pediatric nursing,* ed 8, St Louis, 2009, Mosby; B from Damjanov I, Linder J, editors: *Anderson's pathology,* ed 10, St Louis, 1996, Mosby.)

vascular resistance as compared with systemic vascular resistance. Right atrial and ventricular enlargement develops as a result of left-to-right shunting. Children with ASD are generally asymptomatic and rarely display signs of pulmonary overcirculation. Moderate to large ASDs allow an increase in pulmonary blood flow and, over time, pulmonary vascular changes can occur that may, although rarely, result in pulmonary hypertension.

CLINICAL MANIFESTATIONS Because most children with ASD are asymptomatic, diagnosis usually is made during a routine physical examination by the auscultation of a crescendo-decrescendo systolic ejection murmur that reflects increased blood flow through the pulmonary valve. The location of the murmur is between the second and third intercostal spaces along the left sternal border. A wide fixed splitting of the second heart sound is also characteristic of ASD, reflecting volume overload to the RV, causing prolonged ejection time and delay of pulmonic valve closure.

EVALUATION AND TREATMENT In most cases an echocardiogram is sufficient to confirm the diagnosis of an ASD. A chest radiograph may reveal cardiomegaly and increased pulmonary vascular markings in an asymptomatic child. An ECG may demonstrate right axis deviation and diastolic overload of the RV manifested as right ventricular hypertrophy.[2]

ASD closure, generally before the child reaches school age, results in improved health later in life. If left unrepaired, right ventricular compliance decreases with age, and pulmonary hypertension and right ventricular hypertrophy may occur, placing the person at risk for the development of HF, atrial dysrhythmias, or embolic events later in life. Surgical closure is the corrective method of choice and involves a pericardial patch or suture closure of the defect, depending on the size of the opening. Repair is done through a midsternal approach with the use of cardiopulmonary bypass. Minimally invasive techniques are being used on near-adult sized patients. Sinus venosus defects require a slightly different approach that consists of a synthetic patch to close the opening and baffle the anomalous right pulmonary venous drainage to the LA. Operative mortality associated with ASD closure is near 0%, with minimal morbidity.[7,9,10] Device closure performed in the catheterization laboratory is becoming a routine alternative to surgical closure.[7]

Ventricular Septal Defect

A **ventricular septal defect (VSD)** is an abnormal communication between the ventricles (Figure 31-7, *A*). VSDs are the most common type of congenital heart lesion and account for 25% to 33% of all congenital heart defects. The four types of VSDs are based on location in the septum. The perimembranous type, which occurs in the outflow tract on the LV immediately below the aortic valve, is the most common type, accounting for up to 80% of all VSDs that require treatment. Muscular VSDs, which occur low in the ventricular septum between the trabeculae, are most likely to close spontaneously and are difficult to close surgically because of their location low in the ventricular apex. Most muscular VSDs are hemodynamically insignificant and require no medical or surgical treatment. Supracristal VSDs occur in the right ventricular outflow tract or infundibulum, below the pulmonary valve. AV canal or inlet VSDs occur posterior and inferior to the membranous system, beneath the septal cusp of the tricuspid valve and inferior to the papillary muscles of the conus.

PATHOPHYSIOLOGY The direction of shunting in a child with a VSD is from the high-pressure left side to the lower-pressure right side. The amount of shunting depends

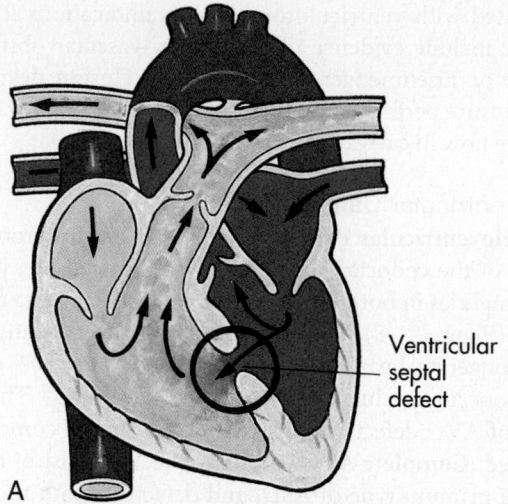

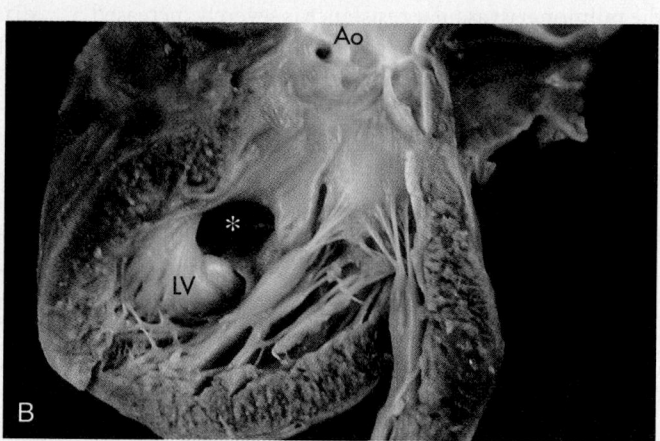

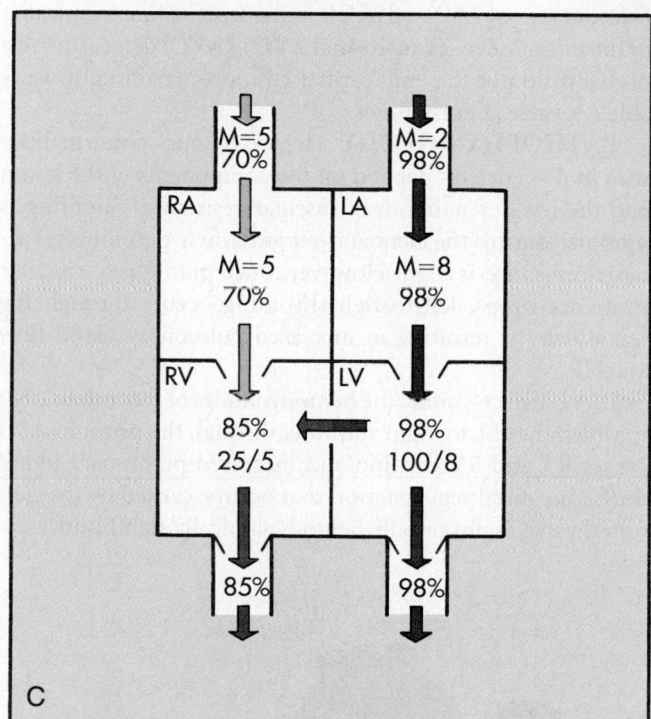

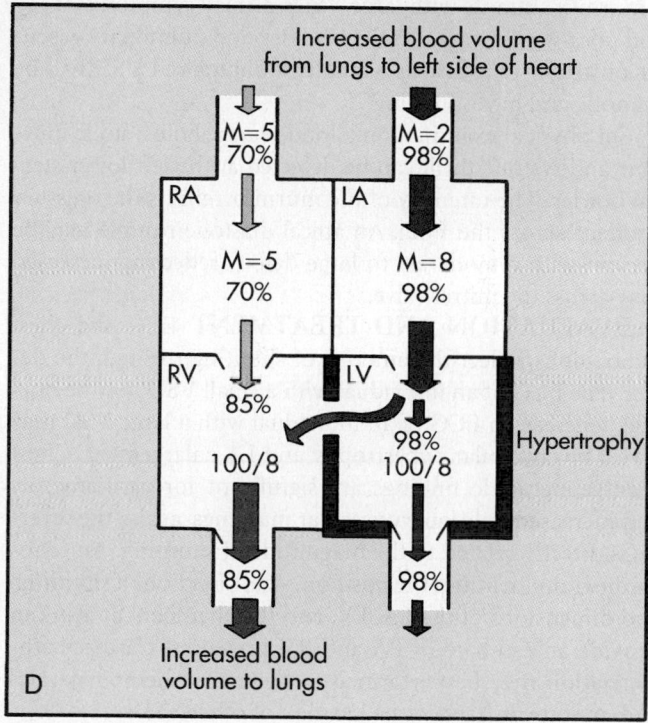

Figure 31-7 Ventricular septal defects (VSDs). **A,** VSD with left-to-right shunt. **B,** Muscular (*) defect (opened left ventricle). **C,** Hemodynamics of a small VSD with left-to-right shunt. Mean (M) indicates mean of pressure; systolic/diastolic pressures are in mmHg; and percentages indicate oxygen saturation. **D,** Hemodynamics of a large VSD with left-to-right shunt. Like the shunting that occurs in preductal coarctation of the aorta, the shunting pictured here causes left ventricular overload and hypertrophy. *Ao,* Aorta; *LA,* left atrium; *LV,* left ventricle; *RA,* right atrium; *RV,* right ventricle. (**A** from Hockenberry MJ et al: *Wong's essentials of pediatric nursing,* ed 8, St Louis, 2009, Mosby; **B** from Damjanov I, Linder J, editors: *Anderson's pathology,* ed 10, St Louis, 1996, Mosby.)

on the size of the defect and the degree of pulmonary vascular resistance. Small VSDs present increased resistance to shunting and limit blood flow through the defect; thus the degree of pulmonary vascular congestion and ventricular chamber enlargement is minimal (Figure 31-7, *C*).

After 1 to 2 weeks of life, when pulmonary vascular resistance has decreased, moderate-size to large VSDs allow a large amount of shunting from left to right. The shunted blood goes directly out the RV outflow tract and into the PA rather

than remaining in the RV cavity (Figure 31-7, *D*). Therefore, the main PA, LA, and LV all enlarge. LV hypertrophy occurs to effectively pump the additional volume. Pulmonary overcirculation accounts for the symptoms associated with a large VSD in most cases.

Over time the pulmonary bed also undergoes changes because of increased pulmonary blood flow caused by the left-to-right shunting. The smooth muscle layer in the arteriolar walls thickens and proliferation of the intimal layer occurs.

The effect of these changes is a decrease in the diameter of the pulmonary vessels, which increases the resistance to blood flow. If the pulmonary vascular resistance is severely increased these changes eventually become irreversible, and pulmonary vascular resistance continues to rise. In some cases it exceeds systemic vascular resistance, causing the shunt through the VSD to reverse direction. Deoxygenated blood now flows into the systemic circulation, and cyanosis occurs, a phenomenon known as *Eisenmenger syndrome.*

CLINICAL MANIFESTATIONS Clinical manifestations in children with VSDs depend on the age of the child, size of the defect, and level of pulmonary vascular resistance. Newborns with small VSDs are relatively asymptomatic. Initially no murmur is present because the newborn's high pulmonary vascular resistance causes equalization of the pressures between both ventricles. Once pulmonary vascular resistance has dropped, left-to-right shunting occurs, creating a murmur. Infants with large VSDs display symptoms of HF and poor weight gain. Adults who develop pulmonary vascular obstructive disease as a result of unrepaired VSD will be cyanotic and have clubbing.

On physical examination a loud, harsh, holosystolic murmur and systolic thrill can be detected at the left lower sternal border. The intensity of the murmur reflects the pressure gradient across the VSD. An apical diastolic rumble may be present with a moderate to large defect, reflecting increased flow across the mitral valve.

EVALUATION AND TREATMENT ECG and chest radiographs reflect the amount of shunting through the defect. The ECG of an individual with a small VSD may be normal, whereas an ECG of an individual with a large VSD may reveal biventricular hypertrophy and LA enlargement. Chest roentgenographic findings are significant for cardiomegaly and increased pulmonary vascular markings; again, the severity is directly related to the magnitude of shunting. An echocardiogram identifies the position, size, direction of shunting, and dimensions of the LA, LV, and RV chambers. It also can provide an estimate of PA and RV pressures. Cardiac catheterization may be performed to determine hemodynamics and, in some instances, the location of other VSDs.

Many VSDs spontaneously close during the first year of life.[2] Infants with symptoms of HF and poor weight gain despite medical management should have their VSD corrected as soon as possible. Left-to-right shunting with a pulmonary flow/systemic flow (Qp:Qs) ratio of greater than 2:1 or evidence of elevated pulmonary vascular resistance are indications for closure. Closure of the VSD at this time is to prevent the development of pulmonary vascular obstructive disease.

Placement of a PA band to decrease the amount of pulmonary blood flow was initially used as a palliative procedure but is now rarely used unless the presence of an additional lesion makes complete repair difficult. Patch closure, using a synthetic material such as Dacron, is accomplished through a sternotomy and with the use of cardiopulmonary bypass. A transatrial approach is preferable to a right ventriculotomy because of the increased incidence of conduction disturbances associated with ventriculotomy. Contraindications for VSD closure include evidence of pulmonary vascular obstructive disease or Eisenmenger syndrome.[2,7] Occlusion devices for VSD closure performed in the cardiac catheterization laboratory are now in early clinical use.[7,11]

Atrioventricular Canal Defect

An **atrioventricular canal (AVC) defect** results from nonfusion of the endocardial cushions during fetal life, yielding abnormalities in both the atrial and ventricular septa and AV valves (Figure 31-8). This defect accounts for as many as 5% of all congenital heart defects, and approximately 30% of AVC defects occur in children with Down syndrome.[7] The three types of AVC defects are based on the cardiac components involved. **Complete AVC (CAVC)** defects consist of an inlet VSD, a primum type of ASD, and defects in both the mitral and tricuspid valves. **Partial AVC (PAVC) defects** consist of a primum type of ASD and a cleft in the septal or anterior leaflet of the mitral valve. **Transitional AVC (TAVC)** defects involve partial fusion of the endocardial cushions, resulting in variable AV valve abnormalities.[7]

PATHOPHYSIOLOGY Hemodynamic abnormalities seen in AVC defects depend on the components of the lesion and the level of pulmonary vascular resistance. Shunting is minimal during the neonatal period when pulmonary vascular resistance is high. However, once pulmonary vascular resistance drops, left-to-right shunting occurs through the septal defects, resulting in increased pulmonary blood flow and HF.

PAVC defects mimic the hemodynamics of secundum ASD in which the left-to-right shunting through the primum ASD causes RA and RV dilation and increased pulmonary blood flow. The mitral regurgitation that occurs, caused by the cleft mitral valve, is not usually hemodynamically significant.

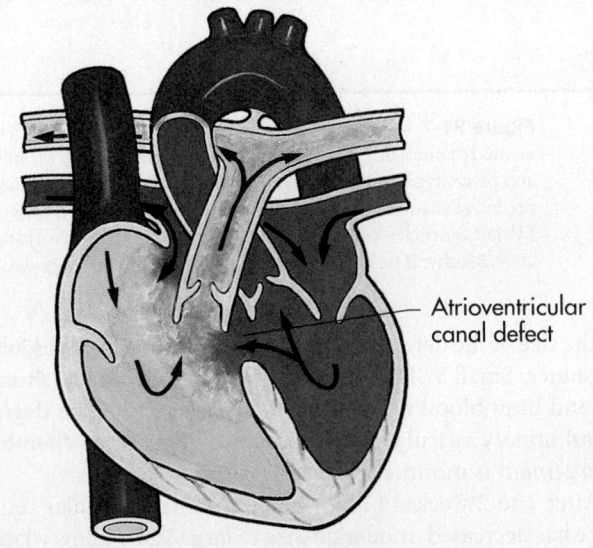

Figure 31-8 Atrioventricular canal defect. (From Hockenberry MJ et al: *Wong's essentials of pediatric nursing,* ed 8, St Louis, 2009, Mosby.)

CAVC defects reflect the hemodynamics of an ASD and a VSD, resulting in biatrial and biventricular enlargement. RA and RV volume overload occurs because of shunting through the primum ASD and tricuspid regurgitation. Likewise, LA and LV volume overload occurs because of shunting through the VSD, increased pulmonary venous return, and mitral regurgitation.

CLINICAL MANIFESTATIONS Children with PAVC defects are generally asymptomatic. Findings on physical examination are similar to those of secundum ASD except for the systolic regurgitant murmur of mitral regurgitation at the apex. At 4 to 12 weeks of age, when pulmonary vascular resistance drops, children with CAVC defects usually begin to show symptoms of HF. Physical findings are similar to those found in individuals with VSDs with the addition of a holosystolic murmur radiating to the back and apex, reflecting mitral regurgitation. A mid-diastolic rumble at the left lower sternal border or apex reflects relative stenosis of the mitral or tricuspid valve from increased flow. Infants with CAVC may have signs of HF and frequent respiratory infections.

EVALUATION AND TREATMENT The ECG generally demonstrates a superior left axis deviation, first-degree AV block, and RV hypertrophy or right bundle branch block. The ECG of CAVC defects also may show LV hypertrophy. Chest radiograph shows cardiomegaly, increased pulmonary vascular markings, and a prominent main PA. Echocardiography allows visualization of the components of the defect, including continuity between the AV valves, their sizes, and chordal attachments. Cardiac catheterization may be electively performed and can confirm the location of septal defects, AV valve abnormalities, degree of left-to-right shunting, and presence of pulmonary hypertension.

Timing of surgical repair depends on the severity of symptoms, degree of shunting, and level of pulmonary vascular resistance. The trend is to perform complete repair between 3 and 6 months of life to avoid the development of pulmonary vascular changes. Surgical repair is performed through a midsternotomy implementing a one- or two-patch repair to close the septal defects and repair the involved AV valves. Mortality has declined below 10% unless the child is a newborn, has severe AV valve incompetence, or has a small LV (unbalanced AV canal). Postoperative complications include heart block, dysrhythmias, or mitral regurgitation requiring further surgical intervention or valve replacement.[7,12]

Defects Decreasing Pulmonary Blood Flow

Defects decreasing pulmonary blood flow involve obstruction to pulmonary blood flow and septal communications. Because of RV outflow tract obstruction, right-sided pressures exceed left-sided pressures, resulting in right-to-left shunting. Children with these defects have hypoxemia and cyanosis.

Tetralogy of Fallot

Tetralogy of Fallot (TOF) consists of four defects: a large VSD that is high in the septum, an overriding aorta that straddles the VSD, pulmonary stenosis (PS), and RV hypertrophy (Figure 31-9, *A*). It is the most common cyanotic congenital heart defect and accounts for 10% of all defects.[2]

PATHOPHYSIOLOGY TOF develops during two phases of embryologic growth: (1) during the division of the truncus arteriosus by the spiral septum in the third or fourth week of gestation and (2) during the division of the ventricles between the fourth and eighth weeks of gestation. Normally as these events progress, the truncal septum fuses with the bulbar ridges and in turn with the endocardial cushions. The membranous portion of the interventricular septum grows upward to meet the endocardial cushions, and ultimately all of these tissues come together to complete the interventricular septum.

The embryologic error that causes TOF is not known for certain, but two theories have been proposed.[1] The first is that the truncus arteriosus divides unevenly, resulting in great vessels of unequal size. The second theory proposes that infundibular overgrowth in the RV is the major developmental anomaly. Defects in ventricular septation also occur, producing the large VSD, which allows the aorta to override the VSD.

The pathophysiology associated with TOF varies widely, depending primarily on the degree of pulmonary stenosis, the size of the VSD, and the pulmonary and systemic resistance to flow. Because the VSD is usually large, pressures are equal in the RV and LV. Therefore, the major determinant of shunt direction through the VSD is the difference between pulmonary and systemic vascular resistance (see Figure 31-9, *C*). Infants who have little or no right-to-left shunting are acyanotic and are known as "pink tets." They may have a net left-to-right shunt similar to a large VSD. If pulmonary vascular resistance is higher than systemic resistance, the shunt is from right to left. Because many factors can alter the balance between pulmonary and systemic resistance, shunt direction is not necessarily constant.

Pulmonary stenosis decreases blood flow to the lungs and, consequently, the amount of oxygenated blood that returns to the left heart. If blood also shunts from right to left through the VSD, deoxygenated blood mixes with the oxygenated blood returning from the lungs. The result is low oxygen saturation (hypoxemia) in the systemic circulation. The body attempts to compensate for chronic hypoxemia by producing more red blood cells (thereby causing polycythemia) and by increasing blood flow to the lungs through collateral bronchial vessels in long-standing cases.

CLINICAL MANIFESTATIONS In cases with decreased pulmonary flow through the right ventricular outflow tract as long as the ductus arteriosus remains open, the newborn's pulmonary blood flow may be adequate. As the ductus closes, however, cyanosis becomes apparent. Chronic hypoxemia causes clubbing of the fingers and toes (see Chapter 33).

A rare manifestation of TOF is the sudden onset of dyspnea, cyanosis, and restlessness, sometimes called a *hypercyanotic spell* or a *"tet spell,"* that generally occurs with crying and exertion. The cause of these episodes is unknown, but it is theorized that the RV outflow tract goes into spasm or the

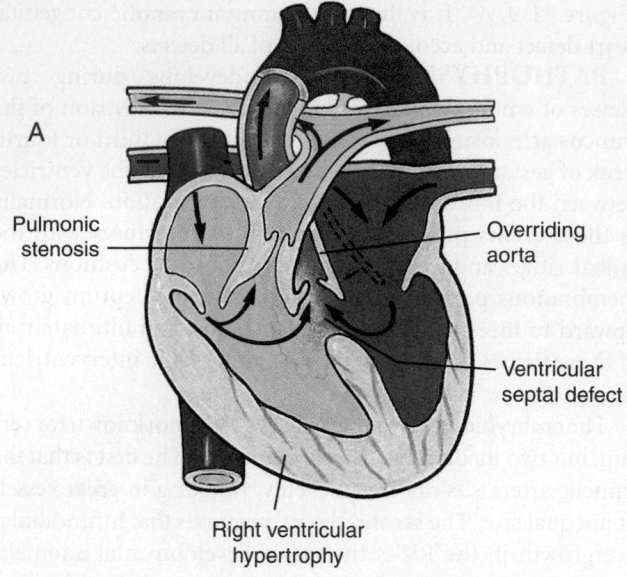

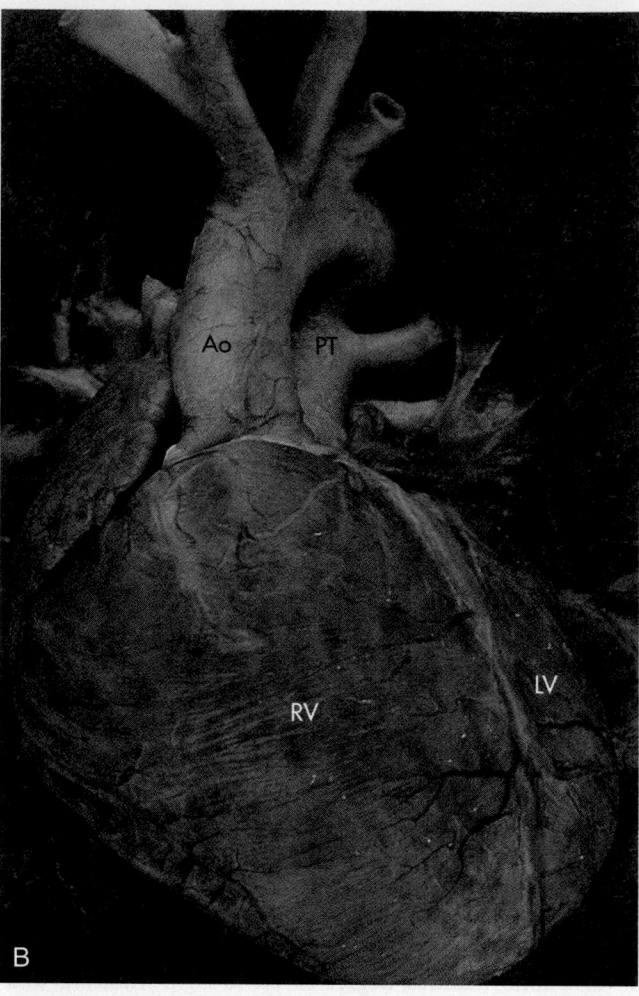

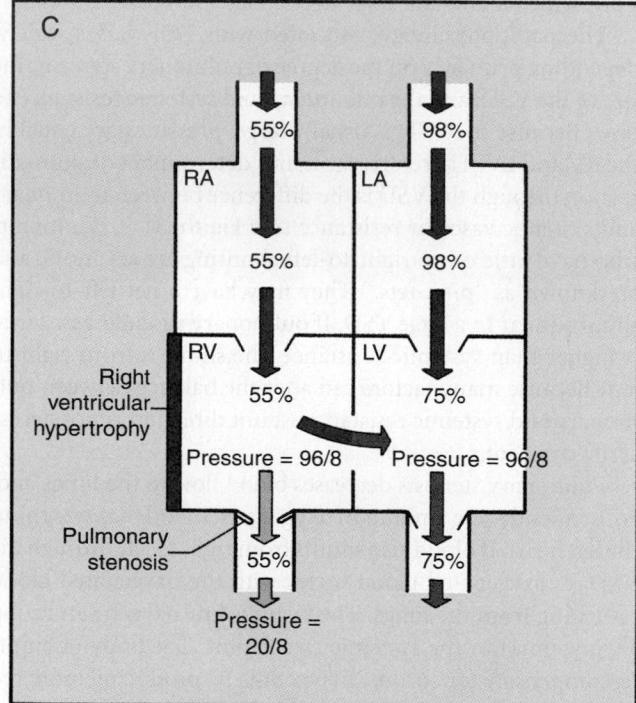

Figure 31-9 Tetralogy of Fallot. **A,** Anatomic defects in tetralogy of Fallot. **B,** Complete transposition of the aorta and pulmonary artery. **C,** Hemodynamics of tetralogy of Fallot with right-to-left shunt. *Ao,* Aorta; *LA,* left atrium; *LV,* left ventricle; *PT,* pulmonary artery trunk; *RA,* right atrium; *RV,* right ventricle. (A from Hockenberry MJ et al: *Wong's essentials of pediatric nursing,* ed 8, St Louis, 2009, Mosby; B from Damjanov I, Linder J, editors: *Anderson's pathology,* ed 10, St Louis, 1996, Mosby.)

systemic resistance drops suddenly. In either case the relative or actual increase in pulmonary vascular resistance increases the right-to-left shunt and the cyanosis. Hypercyanotic spells are often the event that initiates surgical intervention. If the spells are frequent or do not terminate spontaneously, they are considered a medical-surgical emergency.[7]

Infants with TOF may have difficulty with feeding because the exertion required increases hypoxia, and therefore they experience slow growth and FTT. Most infants with TOF grow normally.

Squatting is a spontaneous compensatory mechanism used by older children to alleviate hypoxic spells. Squatting and its variants increase systemic resistance while decreasing venous return to the heart from the inferior vena cava. The decrease of systemic return makes relatively more oxygenated blood available to the body. The increase of systemic resistance also reverses the shunt through the VSD to a left-to-right shunt, which has the effect of increasing pulmonary blood flow. Through both of these mechanisms, squatting temporarily decreases the degree of hypoxemia. It is uncommon to witness this because most cases are surgically corrected in early infancy.

The typical heart murmur of TOF is a pulmonary systolic ejection murmur caused by the obstruction in the outflow tract, which creates turbulence during systole. More obstruction to flow (e.g., smaller orifice for blood to flow through) produces a louder murmur. This explains why the murmur often disappears during a hypoxic spell, when obstruction increases and pulmonary blood flow decreases to a minimal amount. The second heart sound seems to be single, but in fact it is not. The pulmonary component is very soft and delayed and usually is not heard, although it is present. The enlarged RV may cause the left side of the chest to be more prominent, and a "heave" also may be palpated.

EVALUATION AND TREATMENT The ECG indicates RV hypertrophy. Chest radiographic examination shows that the heart is shaped like a boot (upturned apex because of a small main PA) and that pulmonary vascular markings are decreased. Echocardiograms and angiograms enable the clinician to see the size and position of the VSD, the stenotic pulmonary infundibulum or valve, the smaller-than-normal PA, and the overriding aorta. Measurements made during cardiac catheterization (electively done) demonstrate equal systemic pressure in the RV and LV, decreased pressure in the PA distal to the obstruction, and low oxygen saturation in the aorta if there is right-to-left shunting.

The current practice is to repair TOF before 1 year of life. Triggers for repair include increasing cyanosis and hypercyanotic spells. Palliative procedures include the placement of a pulmonary-to-systemic artery shunt known as the Blalock-Taussig shunt to increase pulmonary blood flow or

a modification of the shunt using prosthetic graft material placed from either the subclavian or innominate artery to the PA. These shunts may cause PA distortion but may be necessary in a very small symptomatic child. Corrective repair involves patch closure of the VSD, resection of infundibular or valvular stenosis, and patch augmentation of the RV outflow tract. The procedure is done through a median sternotomy on cardiopulmonary bypass. The operative mortality is less than 5%. Complications include dysrhythmias and occasionally heart block.[13]

Tricuspid Atresia

Tricuspid atresia consists of an imperforate tricuspid valve, resulting in no communication between the RA and RV (Figure 31-10). This defect accounts for 2% to 3% of congenital heart defects and is the third most common cyanotic heart defect. Tricuspid atresia is a combination of defects, including the imperforate tricuspid valve as well as a septal defect, hypoplastic or absent RV, enlarged mitral valve and LV, and varying degrees of pulmonic stenosis. Tricuspid atresia also may be associated with transposition of the great vessels. The most common type of tricuspid atresia involves a hypoplastic RA with decreased pulmonary blood flow, ASD, VSD, and normally related great vessels.[2]

PATHOPHYSIOLOGY Systemic blood returns through the superior and inferior venae cavae to the RA. Venous return flows through the ASD into the LA, mixing with blood returning from the pulmonary circulation. The blood then enters the LV. Most of this blood goes out into the systemic circulation through the aorta, but varying amounts pass through the VSD into the hypoplastic RV and to the lungs. Pulmonary circulation depends on the presence of a VSD and the presence of a functioning RV of reasonable capacity. If the RV is absent, the pulmonary valve is usually imperforate as

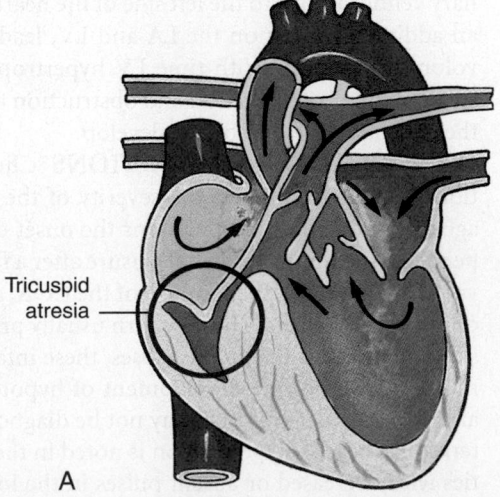

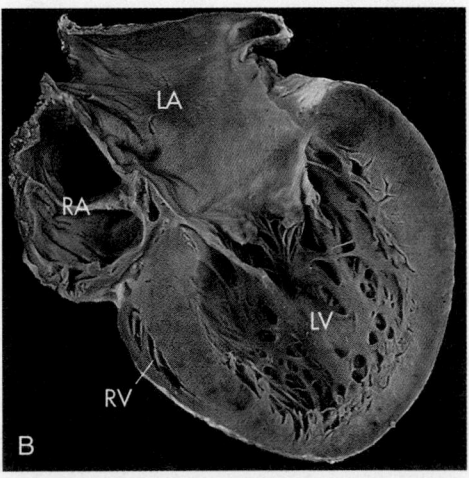

Figure 31-10 Tricuspid atresia. **A,** No communication from the right atrium to the right ventricle. **B,** Tricuspid atresia with absent right atrioventricular connection with a hypoplastic right ventricle (four-chamber view). *LA,* Left atrium; *LV,* left ventricle; *RA,* right atrium; *RV,* right ventricle. (**A** from Hockenberry MJ et al: *Wong's essentials of pediatric nursing,* ed 8, St Louis, 2009, Mosby; **B** from Damjanov I, Linder J, editors: *Anderson's pathology,* ed 10, St Louis, 1996, Mosby.)

well. If this is the case, a PDA is necessary to ensure that some blood flows into the pulmonary circulation.[7]

Pulmonary circulation also depends on the relationship between pulmonary and systemic vascular resistance. As long as pulmonary resistance is lower than systemic resistance, blood flows through the VSD from left to right, feeding the pulmonary circulation. If pulmonary resistance rises above systemic resistance, pulmonary blood flow will be significantly diminished.

CLINICAL MANIFESTATIONS Some degree of central cyanosis is common in tricuspid atresia, depending on the amount of pulmonary blood flow. Growth failure also is common. Children experience exertional dyspnea, tachypnea, and hypoxemia. Long-term effects of hypoxia are polycythemia and clubbing. These children also may display hypercyanotic spells. Hepatomegaly may be present if the ASD is restrictive or CHF occurs as a result of increased pulmonary blood flow.

The murmur heard with tricuspid atresia may have several components. The VSD causes a systolic regurgitant murmur; the larger the VSD, the softer and shorter the murmur is likely to be. A narrowly split second heart sound caused by decreased pulmonary blood flow may be present, or the second heart sound may be single if there is pulmonary atresia.

EVALUATION AND TREATMENT Chest radiographic examination shows a heart size that is normal or slightly increased. ECG usually shows RA, LA, and LV hypertrophy with left axis deviation. Echocardiography and cardiac catheterization, if performed, depict left-to-right shunting at the ventricular level, inability of blood flow to enter the RV, and the presence of associated defects.

Newborns with ductal dependent pulmonary blood flow are immediately given prostaglandins to maintain adequate pulmonary perfusion. Initial surgical intervention involves the placement of a Blalock-Taussig shunt (or its modification). If the ASD is restrictive, a Rashkind procedure (balloon atrial septostomy) may be performed during catheterization. Children who experience increased pulmonary blood flow may require the placement of a PA band. Corrective repair involves closing the septal defects, taking down the previous shunts or band, and connecting the superior and inferior venae cavae to the PA to separate the pulmonary systemic circulation (Fontan procedure and its modifications). Postoperative complications include pleural effusions, elevated pulmonary vascular resistance, LV dysfunction, and dysrhythmias.[13]

Obstructive Defects

Obstructive defects are conditions in which anatomic stenosis (narrowing) in either the right or left outflow tract causes obstruction to blood flow and results in a pressure load on the ventricles. The difference between the obstruction is the gradient that reflects the severity of the narrowing; the higher the gradient is the more obstruction to flow and increased afterload on the ventricle. The location is classified according to the location of the narrowing in relation to the valve. Valvular stenosis refers to stenosis of the valve itself; subvalvular

indicates that the stenotic area is below the valve or in the ventricular outflow tract; and supravalvular is the area above the valve in the great artery. The obstructive defects include coarctation of the aorta, aortic stenosis, pulmonary stenosis, and hypoplastic left heart syndrome. Symptoms associated with the defect depend on the site and severity of stenosis.

Coarctation of the Aorta

Coarctation of the aorta (COA) is a narrowing of the lumen of the aorta that impedes blood flow. This defect accounts for 8% to 10% of all congenital heart defects. COA is almost always in a juxtaductal position, although it can occur anywhere between the origin of the aortic arch and the bifurcation of the aorta in the lower abdomen. About 50% of individuals with COA have a bicuspid aortic valve (Figure 31-11).[2]

PATHOPHYSIOLOGY COA may develop because of an abnormal contractile ductal tissue that constricts at the time of ductal closure. COA causes a condition in which there are higher pressures proximal to the site of stenosis and lower pressures distal to the site. In preductal COA the RV acts as a systemic pump, sending unoxygenated blood through the ductus into the descending aorta below the coarctation (Figure 31-12). In postductal COA the RV cannot pump enough blood through the ductus to the descending aorta because of pressure caused by the narrowed aorta. Systolic pressures increases in the ascending aorta and LV and decreases in the descending aorta beyond the COA (Figure 31-13). Longstanding COA, collateral circulation, which involves small arteries arising from the subclavian arteries, joins intercostal arteries that flow into the descending aorta. These collateral vessels bypass the COA and supply blood to the lower extremities. The direction of shunting through the ductus, if present, depends on the pressure difference between the PA and aorta and the location of the ductus. When blood pressure is greater in the aorta than in the PA, blood flow through the ductus will be left to right toward the lungs, resulting in increased pulmonary venous return to the left side of the heart. This may place an additional strain on the LA and LV, leading to increased volume and work. With time LV hypertrophy develops because of increased afterload and obstruction to flow caused by the coarctation. HF also may develop.

CLINICAL MANIFESTATIONS Clinical manifestations vary depending on the severity of the coarctation and age of presentation. In newborns the onset of symptoms depends on the timing of ductal closure after a fall in pulmonary vascular resistance, the location of the COA, and the presence of associated defects. The newborn usually presents with CHF symptoms. Once the ductus closes, these infants will deteriorate rapidly from the development of hypotension, acidosis, and shock. Older children may not be diagnosed until hypertension is noted. Hypertension is noted in the upper extremities with decreased or absent pulses in the lower extremities. Children may have cool mottled skin and occasionally leg cramps during exercise. A systolic ejection murmur, heard best at the left interscapular area, is caused by rapid blood flow through the narrowed area.

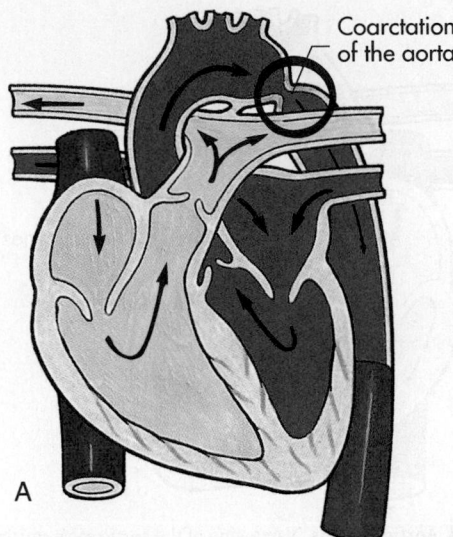

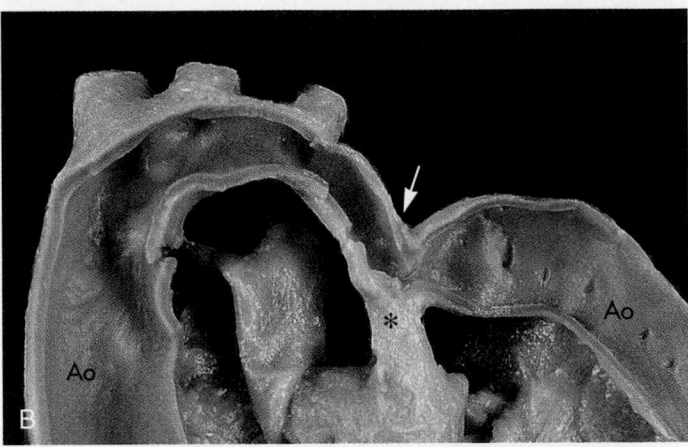

Figure 31-11 Postductal and preductal coarctation of the aorta. **A,** Postductal coarctation occurs distal to ("after") the insertion of the closed ductus arteriosus into the aortic arch. Preductal coarctation occurs proximal to ("before") insertion of the patent ductus arteriosus. The coarctation consists of a flap of tissue that protrudes from the tunica media of the aortic wall. **B,** Coarctation of the aorta with typical indentation of the aortic wall *(arrow)* opposite the ductal arterial ligament (*). *Ao,* Aorta. (**A** from Hockenberry MJ et al: *Wong's essentials of pediatric nursing,* ed 8, St Louis, 2009, Mosby; **B** from Damjanov I, Linder J, editors: *Anderson's pathology,* ed 10, St Louis, 1996, Mosby.)

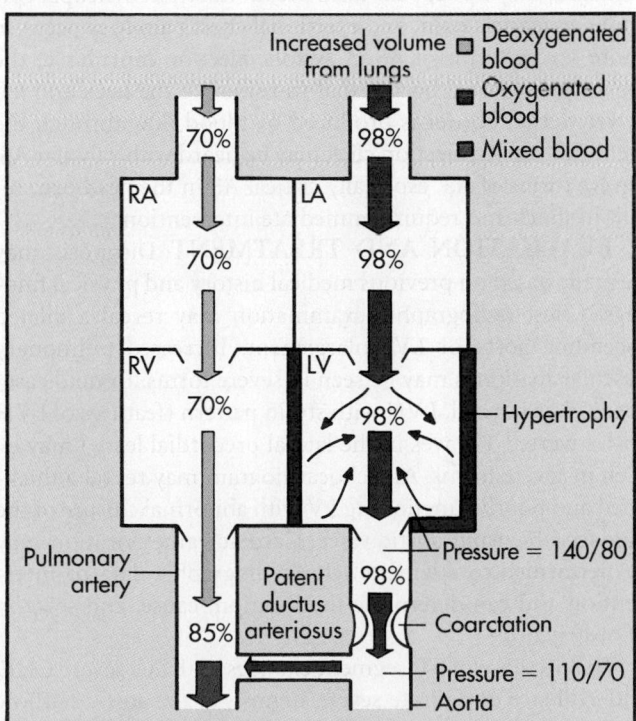

Figure 31-12 Hemodynamics of preductal coarctation of the aorta with a patent ductus arteriosus. The left-to-right shunt through the ductus arteriosus increases the volume of blood in the pulmonary circulation. Afterload *(small black arrows)* is increased in the left heart by *(1)* increased return from the lungs and *(2)* decreased ventricular outflow caused by the coarctation. The outcome is heart failure. *LA,* left atrium; *LV,* left ventricle; *RA,* right atrium; *RV,* right ventricle.

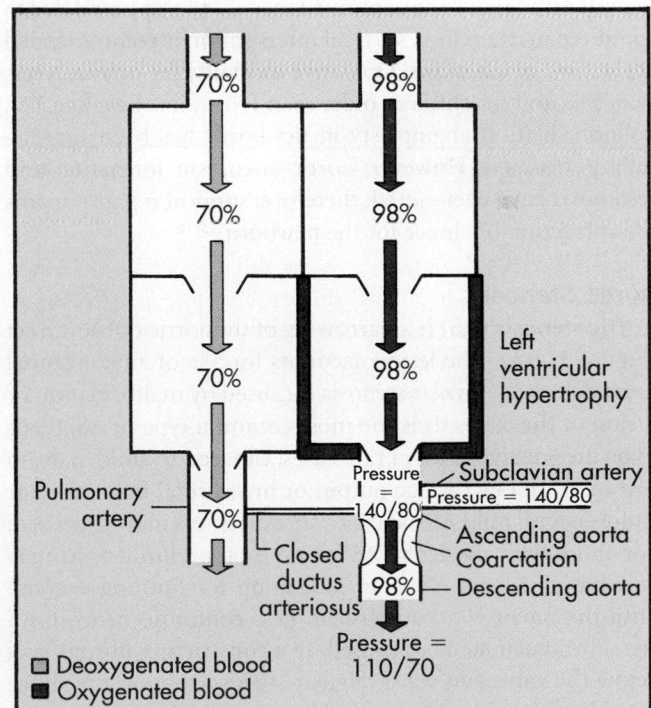

Figure 31-13 Hemodynamics of postductal coarctation of the aorta. Blood pressure increases in the ascending aorta and subclavian artery and decreases in the descending aorta. These pressure changes eventually occur in the parts of the systemic circulation served by arteries that branch from the aorta before and after the coarctation.

EVALUATION AND TREATMENT A chest radiograph shows an enlarged heart with congested lung fields in newborns. Rib notching between the fourth and eighth ribs may be seen in children older than 5 years, reflecting erosion of the ribs from enlarged collateral vessels from the ascending aorta to the descending aorta, bypassing the coarctation. An ECG may be normal or reveal LV hypertrophy. An echocardiogram will confirm the diagnosis and rule out other intracardiac defects. Cardiac catheterization and/or magnetic resonance imaging (MRI) is performed only if the echocardiogram is inconclusive.

The first step in treatment of the symptomatic infant is stabilization, which may require prostaglandin administration, mechanical ventilation, and inotropic support to maintain adequate cardiac output. Once this is achieved, surgical intervention is indicated. Surgical repair for infants younger than 1 year consists of either a subclavian flap aortoplasty technique to enlarge the constricted area or resection with end-to-end anastomosis of the arch segments. Depending on the arch morphology, a modification of this procedure enlarges the aorta beyond the area of constriction. For children older than 1 year, surgical repair consists of resection with end-to-end anastomosis.[13] Cardiopulmonary bypass is not required because of the extracardiac nature of the lesion, and the approach is accomplished through a left thoracotomy.

Postoperative complications include recoarctation and paradoxical postoperative hypertension. Residual permanent hypertension requiring continued medical therapy is related to age at repair; therefore, surgical intervention is recommended at the time of diagnosis. Operative mortality for infants is less than 5%, and for children older than 1 year, it is less than 1%. Balloon dilation angioplasty in newborns has been successfully performed. However, aortic aneurysm formation and restenosis have been noted; therefore, surgical repair remains the correction of choice for the newborn.[13-16]

Aortic Stenosis

Aortic stenosis (AS) is a narrowing of the aortic outflow tract (Figure 31-14). The lesion accounts for 5% of all congenital heart defects.[2] Valvular stenosis is caused by malformation or fusion of the cusps. It is the most common type of AS, tends to be progressive, and, in rare cases, can lead to sudden death as a result of low cardiac output or myocardial ischemia. For children with mild AS, no exercise restrictions may be needed. For those with moderate AS, some exercise limitations may be advised. Severe AS is an indication for limiting exercise until the repair is accomplished. Less common forms of AS are subvalvular stenosis caused by a constricting fibrous ring below the valve and supravalvular stenosis that occurs above the valve.[7]

PATHOPHYSIOLOGY Obstruction to blood flowing out of the aorta causes an increased workload on the LV, resulting in left ventricle hypertrophy (LVH). LV failure may develop, leading to an increase in LA pressure and a backup in the system, eventually resulting in pulmonary vascular congestion and pulmonary arterial hypertension. LVH can

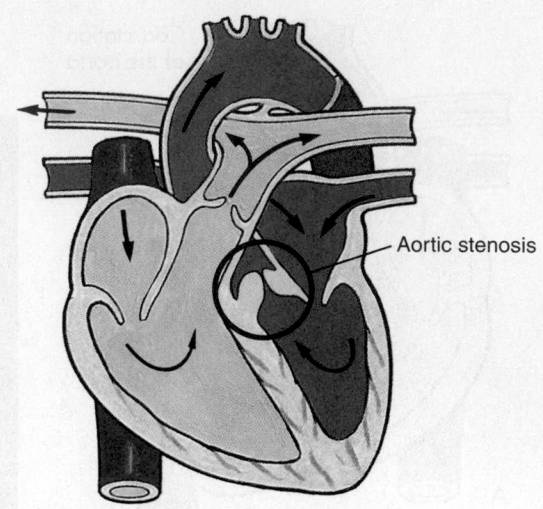

Figure 31-14 Aortic stenosis. Narrowing of the aortic valve causing resistance to blood flow in the left ventricle, decreased cardiac output, left ventricular hypertrophy, and pulmonary congestion. (From Hockenberry MJ et al: *Wong's essentials of pediatric nursing,* ed 8, St Louis, 2009, Mosby.)

decrease coronary artery perfusion, resulting in myocardial ischemia and it can alter the LV papillary muscle, causing mitral insufficiency.

CLINICAL MANIFESTATIONS Most children with mild to moderate AS are asymptomatic. Signs of exercise intolerance may not appear until preadolescence. Syncopal episodes, epigastric pain, and exertional chest pain may occur in more severe forms of AS. A systolic ejection murmur at the right upper sternal border that transmits to the neck and left lower sternal border is produced by blood flow through the stenotic area. An ejection click may be heard with valvular AS. Severe forms of AS, especially critical AS in the newborn, result in shock and require immediate intervention.

EVALUATION AND TREATMENT Diagnosis may be made based on previous medical history and physical findings. Chest radiographic examination may reveal a dilated ascending aorta or LV enlargement. Increased pulmonary vascular markings may be seen in severe forms. In mild cases the ECG is normal. LVH with strain pattern (features of LVH with inverted T waves in the lateral precordial leads) may be seen in severe forms. An echocardiogram may reveal a thickened and poorly functioning LV with abnormal closure of the damaged bicuspid aortic valve. Cardiac catheterization may be performed to augment echocardiographic data or intervention and can determine the location, cause, and severity of obstruction.

The presence of ST-segment changes on ECG, severe CHF, and evidence of discrete severe stenosis at the aortic outflow tract are indications for intervention. Balloon aortic valvuloplasty is a palliative procedure performed for valvular AS; however, it is associated with complications, including aortic insufficiency and dysrhythmia.[17] Aortic valvotomy, under inflow occlusion or cardiopulmonary bypass, is performed for valvular AS. Operative mortality remains high in infants (up to 20%), although older children have a mortality close to

0%.[13] As many as 25% of individuals require a second surgery within 10 years for restenosis, at which time valve replacement may be the procedure of choice.

Subvalvular AS and supravalvular AS require surgical repair involving excision of the area causing the constriction. For subvalvular AS involving a small LV outflow tract and aortic annulus, a Konno procedure may be done to enlarge the LV outflow tract and aortic annulus with a patch.[13,18]

Pulmonary Stenosis

Pulmonary stenosis (PS) is the narrowing of the pulmonary outflow tract. This may be in the form of abnormal thickening of the valve leaflets or narrowing of the arterial (supravalvular) or ventricular (subvalvular) side of the valve (Figure 31-15, *A*). **Pulmonary atresia** is the severe form of PS and involves complete fusion of the commissures, allowing no blood flow out of the RV to the PA. PS accounts for 5% to 8% of all congenital heart defects.[2]

PATHOPHYSIOLOGY PS creates resistance to blood flow from the RV to the PA. The narrowed orifice (valve) produces increased resistance (afterload) to ejection. In order for the RV to maintain adequate cardiac output, the myocardium hypertrophies. If the RV outflow tract obstruction is severe, blood may back up into the RA, causing dilation. This may result in reopening of the foramen ovale with resultant unoxygenated blood shunting to the LA, causing cyanosis (see Figure 31-15, *B*).

CLINICAL MANIFESTATIONS Clinical manifestations depend on the severity of PS. A systolic ejection murmur at the left upper sternal border reflects obstruction to flow through the narrowed pulmonary valve. A systolic ejection click is present with valvular stenosis at the upper left sternal border. A thrill also may be palpated at the upper left sternal border. Children with moderate PS may have exertional dyspnea and fatigability because of the inability of the body to increase pulmonary blood flow to meet demands for increased cardiac output. Severe PS will produce cyanosis and HF.

EVALUATION AND TREATMENT A chest radiograph shows a normal-size heart with a prominent main PA caused by poststenotic dilation. An ECG is usually normal but may reveal right axis deviation and RV hypertrophy with moderate PS. Echocardiography confirms the diagnosis and detects associated defects. Cardiac catheterization, if performed for interventional purposes, further demonstrates PA anatomy.

Mild to moderate PS will not likely require intervention but should be observed closely with prophylaxis for subacute bacterial endocarditis. Most mild PS is not progressive.

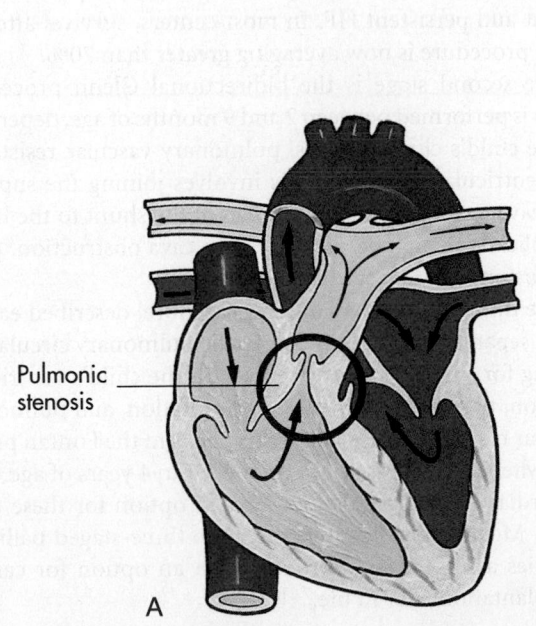

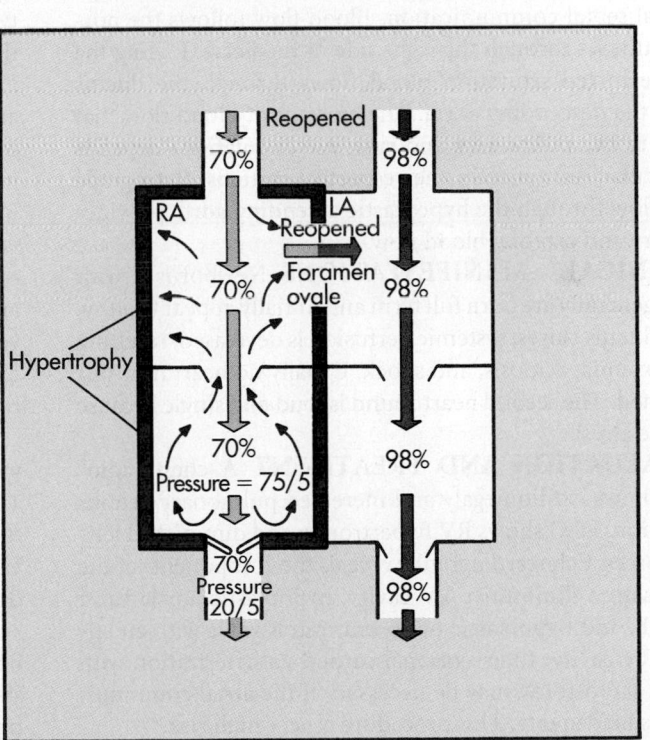

A

B

Figure 31-15 Pulmonary stenosis. **A,** Obstruction of right ventricular outflow caused by pulmonary stenosis. Pressure on the ventricular side of the pulmonic semilunar valve (pulmonary valve) is much greater than that on the pulmonary arterial side. This difference disrupts the normal pressure gradient across the valve. Pulmonary stenosis increases ventricular afterload by decreasing blood flow through the valve, which causes ventricular hypertrophy. **B,** The backup of ventricular afterload into the right atrium reopens the foramen ovale. Venous blood then flows from the area of higher pressure (the right atrium) to the area of lower pressure (the left atrium), causing a left-to-right shunt. Cyanosis occurs if enough venous blood shunts from right to left to reduce oxygen saturation in the systemic circulation by 3% to 5%. *LA,* left atrium; *RA,* right atrium. (A from Hockenberry MJ et al: *Wong's essentials of pediatric nursing,* ed 8, St Louis, 2009, Mosby.)

Treatment is indicated when a significant pressure gradient is detected across the RV outflow tract.

Critical (severe) PS must be addressed immediately. The treatment of choice is balloon angioplasty. This procedure is considered highly effective in decreasing the pressure gradient across the pulmonic valve and is noted to have few associated complications.[19] Surgical correction involves a pulmonary valvotomy incising the fused commissures. Operative mortality is less than 1%.[2] Both valvotomy and balloon angioplasty may result in some pulmonary valve incompetence, and long-term follow-up may reveal the need for further intervention.

Hypoplastic Left Heart Syndrome

Hypoplastic left heart syndrome (HLHS) refers to the abnormal development of the left-sided cardiac structures, resulting in obstruction to blood flow from the LV outflow tract. HLHS involves underdevelopment of the LV, aorta, and aortic arch, as well as mitral atresia or stenosis (Figure 31-16). Therefore, infants with HLHS must have a well-functioning RV and the presence of a PDA and atrial septal communication for survival. HLHS accounts for 1% of all congenital heart defects and is considered the most complex congenital defect.[3]

PATHOPHYSIOLOGY Because of the high pressures caused by LV outflow tract obstruction, saturated blood enters the LA and mixes with desaturated blood in the RA through an atrial septal communication. Blood flow follows the normal pathways through the right side of the heart. Exiting the PA, the mixed-saturation blood flows through the ductus and to the descending aorta. The amount of blood flow that travels to the pulmonary and systemic circulations depends on vascular resistance in the respective systems. Retrograde blood flow through the hypoplastic ascending aorta provides coronary and cerebral blood flow.

CLINICAL MANIFESTATIONS Newborns with HLHS generally are born full term and initially appear healthy. As the ductus closes, systemic perfusion is decreased, resulting in hypoxemia, acidosis, and shock. Usually no heart murmur is detected. The second heart sound is loud and single because of aortic atresia.

EVALUATION AND TREATMENT A chest radiograph shows cardiomegaly and increased pulmonary venous congestion. ECG shows RV hypertrophy and diminished left-sided forces. Echocardiography reveals the components of the defect with a diminutive LV cavity, hypoplastic aortic valve and arch, and hypoplastic or absent mitral valve with an enlarged RV cavity. Interventional cardiac catheterization with balloon septostomy may be necessary if the atrial communication is inadequate. This procedure is very high risk.[7]

Prostaglandin infusion to maintain patency of the ductus arteriosus is essential for newborn infant survival. Immediate correction of acidosis, inotropic support for adequate cardiac output, and ventilatory manipulation to balance systemic and pulmonary blood flow prevent further deterioration and achieve stabilization.

Surgical intervention includes a three-stage approach that classically begins with a Norwood procedure. The Norwood

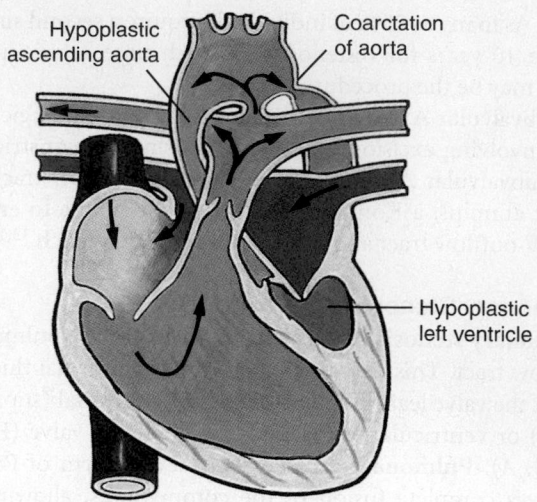

Figure 31-16 Hypoplastic left heart syndrome. (From Hockenberry MJ et al: *Wong's essentials of pediatric nursing*, ed 8, St Louis, 2009, Mosby.)

procedure consists of an atrial septectomy, placement of a pulmonary-to-systemic artery shunt to maintain adequate pulmonary blood flow, creation of a permanent communication between the RV and aorta, and patch augmentation of the hypoplastic aorta. The Sano modification utilizes a graft between the RV and the PA to provide stable pulmonary blood flow rather than a pulmonary to systemic arterial shunt.[20] Postoperative complications include imbalance of systemic and pulmonary blood flow, leading to inadequate cardiac output and persistent HF. In most centers, survival after the initial procedure is now averaging greater than 70%.

The second stage is the bidirectional Glenn procedure, which is performed between 2 and 9 months of age, depending on the child's clinical status, pulmonary vascular resistance, and ventricular function. This involves joining the superior vena cava to the PA and take-down of the shunt to the lungs. Complications include superior vena cava obstruction, pleural effusion, and low cardiac output.

The third stage is the Fontan procedure, described earlier, which separates the systemic from the pulmonary circulation. Timing for surgical repair depends on the child's ventricular function, presence of AV valve regurgitation, and pulmonary vascular resistance. Most surgeons perform the Fontan procedure when the child is approximately 2 to 4 years of age.[7,13]

Cardiac transplant also may be an option for these newborns. Most surgical centers offer the three-staged palliative surgeries as an initial approach, with an option for cardiac transplantation later in life.[7,21]

Mixing Defects

Many complex defects are classified as mixing defects because of their dependence on the mixing of pulmonary and systemic circulations for survival during the postnatal period. This mixing results in desaturated systemic blood flow and cyanosis. Pulmonary congestion occurs because of preferential pulmonary blood flow. Clinically each defect has varying degrees

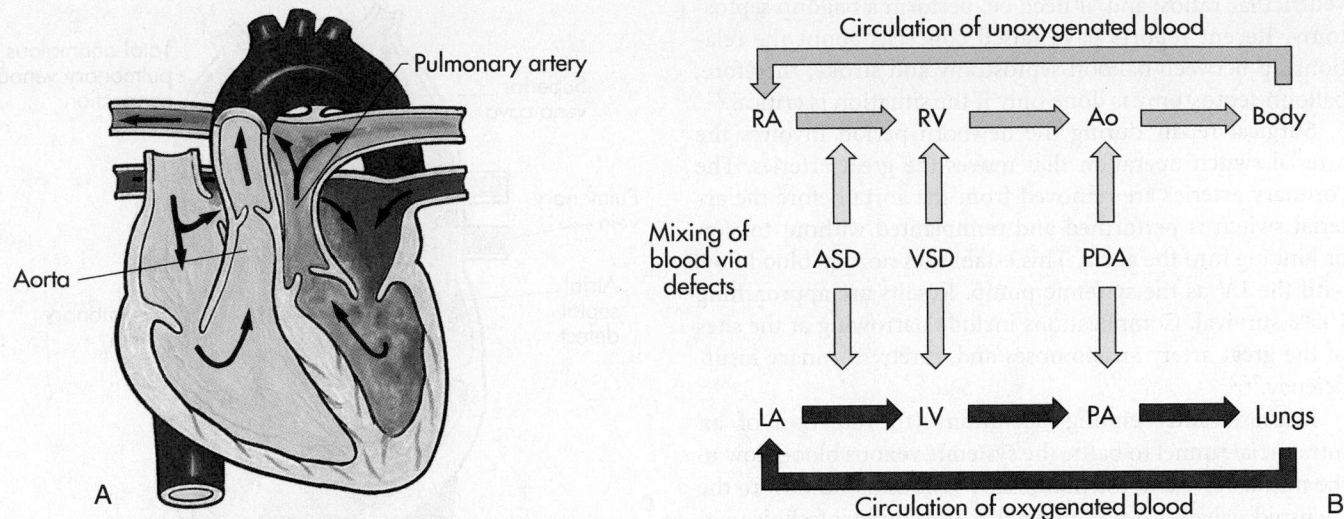

Figure 31-17 Hemodynamics in transposition of the great arteries (TGA). **A,** Complete transposition of the great vessels with an intact interventricular septum. The aorta arises from the right ventricle and the pulmonary artery from the left. **B,** Oxygen saturation in the two parallel circuits. *Ao,* Aorta; *ASD,* atrial septal defect; *LA,* left atrium; *LV,* left ventricle; *PA,* pulmonary artery; *PDA,* patent ductus arteriosus; *RA,* right atrium; *RV,* right ventricle; *VSD,* ventricular septal defect. (**A** from Hockenberry MJ et al: *Wong's essentials of pediatric nursing,* ed 8, St Louis, 2009, Mosby.)

of cyanosis and HF depending on the various components of the lesion.

Transposition of the Great Arteries

Transposition of the great arteries (TGA) refers to a condition in which the aorta arises from the RV and the PA from the LV (Figure 31-17, *A*). The result is two separate, parallel circuits in which unoxygenated blood circulates continuously through the systemic circulation and oxygenated blood circulates repeatedly through the pulmonary circulation. This condition is incompatible with extrauterine life unless a communication exists between the two circuits to provide the necessary oxygen to the body. Communication is accomplished through mixing of pulmonary and systemic circulations through a PDA, ASD, or VSD (see Figure 31-17, *B*). Dextro-transposition of the great arteries (d-TGA) is the most common cyanotic congenital heart defect and accounts for 10% of all congenital heart defects; "dextro" refers to the aorta remaining to the right of the PA.[2]

Two factors allow newborns with complete transposition to survive long enough to be treated. First, blood from the two closed systems can mix through the ductus arteriosus for a short time after birth if pulmonary vascular resistance remains high. Some mixing also may occur through the foramen ovale. If the child has a VSD, mixing occurs through that opening as well.

PATHOPHYSIOLOGY It is not known precisely which embryologic events lead to transposition, but researchers have proposed that the fault lies in the development of conal tissue in the fibrous skeleton of the heart.[1] The **conus** is a segment of muscle that separates the AV (tricuspid and mitral) valves from the semilunar (aortic and pulmonic) valves. (The

fibrous skeleton and heart valves are described and illustrated in Chapter 29; see Figure 29-4.) The interventricular septum is intact in about 60% of cases of transposition; a VSD is present in the remaining 40%. PS is associated with the transposition in about 4% to 6% of children with intact septa and in 28% to 31% of children with VSDs.[2,7]

The discussion that follows is limited to the pathophysiology of complete transposition with an intact interventricular septum.

CLINICAL MANIFESTATIONS The degree of mixing permitted by fetal structures determines the type and severity of clinical manifestations. Cyanosis may be mild shortly after birth and worsen during the first day because of functional closure of the ductus arteriosus. Low oxygen levels in the blood (hypoxemia) cause metabolic acidosis, tachycardia, and tachypnea. The presence of a PDA or large ASD allows for more mixing and results in only mild cyanosis, but the infant may develop CHF.

The first heart sound is normal, and the second sound may be heard as a single sound even though both the aortic and pulmonic valves are functioning. The single S_2 may occur because transposition places the aortic valve closer to the chest wall than the pulmonic valve. No murmur is noted with transposition of the great arteries with an intact ventricular septum.

EVALUATION AND TREATMENT On chest radiograph the heart has a characteristic shape—like an egg on its side—and pulmonary vascular markings are increased. The heart may be enlarged if the infant is a few weeks old and has a VSD. ECG findings reveal a right-axis deviation and some RV hypertrophy. Echocardiography confirms the diagnosis of transposition of the great arteries. Cardiac catheterization may be necessary to define the coronary anatomy; measure ventricular ratios; and, if need be, perform a balloon septostomy. Recent reports have raised concerns about the relationship between balloon septostomy and stroke; therefore, balloon septostomy is done only if the situation is critical.[22]

Surgical repair during the newborn period involves the arterial switch operation that moves the great arteries. The coronary arteries are removed from the aorta before the arterial switch is performed and reimplanted without torsion or kinking into the aorta. This establishes normal blood flow with the LV as the systemic pump. Results are approaching 100% survival. Complications include narrowing at the sites of the great artery anastomoses and, rarely, coronary insufficiency.[7,22]

Mustard and Senning operations (the creation of an intra-atrial tunnel to baffle the systemic venous blood flow to the mitral valve and the pulmonary venous blood flow to the tricuspid valve) are no longer the procedures of choice because the RV must perform as the systemic pump. Long-term follow-up of children with Mustard and Senning operations revealed significant rates of RV failure and dysrhythmias.[7]

The Rastelli procedure is used with children with transposition, VSD, and severe PS. This procedure involves closing the VSD with a baffle by rerouting LV blood through the VSD to the aorta. The pulmonary valve is closed, and an RV-to-PA prosthetic or homograft valve conduit is placed. This procedure requires prosthetic conduit replacement as the child grows and is associated with ventricular failure and dysrhythmias in the postoperative period.

Total Anomalous Pulmonary Venous Connection

Total anomalous pulmonary venous connection (TAPVC), or total anomalous pulmonary venous return, occurs when the pulmonary veins abnormally connect to the right side of the heart either directly or through one or more systemic veins that drain into the RA (Figure 31-18). An ASD generally is present also. This defect is extremely rare, accounting for only 1% of all congenital heart defects. The four types of TAPVC are based on the site of drainage. Supracardiac TAPVCs are the most common form (50%) and drain to the superior vena cava through the vertical or innominate vein. Cardiac TAPVCs (20%) drain directly into the RA or through the coronary sinus. Infracardiac TAPVCs (20%) traverse the diaphragm and drain into the portal or hepatic vein or the inferior vena cava. Mixed TAPVCs (10%) are a combination of the various types. Partial anomalous venous connection is a condition in which only one or a few of the pulmonary veins, usually the right-sided veins, drain into the RA or one of its tributaries.[2]

PATHOPHYSIOLOGY Physiologically TAPVC can be differentiated into two groups: nonobstructive and obstructive, depending on the absence or presence of obstruction to pulmonary venous drainage. The hemodynamics of the nonobstructive group involve the RA receiving the oxygenated blood that would normally flow into the LA. The amount of blood shunted into the LA versus the volume entering the RV depends on the size of the ASD and compliance of the RV.

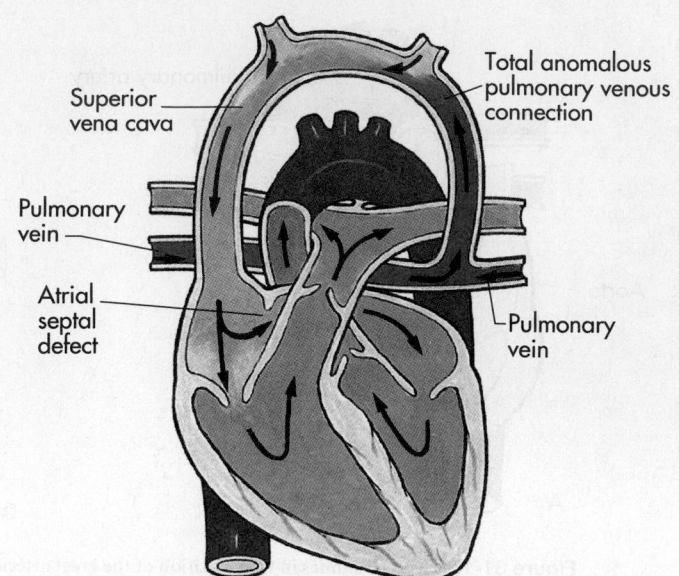

Figure 31-18 Hemodynamics of total anomalous pulmonary venous connection (TAPVC). In the form of TAPVC represented here, the pulmonary veins enter the left anomalous vertical vein instead of the left atrium. From the left anomalous vertical vein, the mixed blood from the lungs flows into the superior vena cava through an innominate vein (literally, a "vein without a name"). Oxygen saturation within the four heart chambers, the pulmonary artery, and the aorta is the same. Blood pressure in the right heart exceeds that in the left heart because the right heart is receiving blood from both the pulmonary and systemic circulatory systems. (Abnormal vessels are shaded.) (From Hockenberry MJ et al: *Wong's essentials of pediatric nursing*, ed 8, St Louis, 2009, Mosby.)

Therefore, if the ASD is restrictive and RV compliance approaches normal, more blood will enter the RV than the LA, resulting in RA and RV enlargement, as well as increased pulmonary blood flow. This causes increased pulmonary venous blood return and larger amounts of saturated blood. If the ASD is unrestrictive and the RV does not thin out to increase compliance, the majority of mixed saturated blood is shunted from the higher pressure RA to the LA.

The hemodynamics of obstructed TAPVC cause pulmonary venous hypertension because of resistance caused by the obstruction resulting in an elevation in pulmonary vascular and RV pressures. Pulmonary edema occurs from hydrostatic capillary pressure exceeding the osmotic pressure of the blood and eventually contributing to the development of HF. This group has a strong association with the infracardiac type of TAPVC and is a surgical emergency.

CLINICAL MANIFESTATIONS The predominant clinical manifestation in infants with TAPVC is cyanosis caused by mixture of oxygenated and deoxygenated blood entering the systemic circulation. The degree of cyanosis is inversely related to the amount of pulmonary blood flow. Children with unobstructed TAPVC may be asymptomatic until pulmonary vascular resistance drops, at which time pulmonary blood flow will increase, resulting in signs of pulmonary overcirculation, particularly growth retardation and frequent pulmonary infections, in addition to mild cyanosis.

Obstructed TAPVC results in cyanosis and rapid deterioration necessitating immediate surgical correction, or death will occur.

Physical examination may reveal a systolic murmur at the left upper sternal border and a mid-diastolic murmur at the left lower sternal border. A murmur may be absent in obstructed TAPVC. A characteristic quadruple rhythm, consisting of S_1, widely split S_2, and S_3 or S_4, or a gallop rhythm also is present.

EVALUATION AND TREATMENT The ECG shows a right-axis deviation, RV hypertrophy, and occasionally RA hypertrophy. The chest radiograph of unobstructed TAPVC reveals cardiomegaly, increased pulmonary vascular markings, and a snowman or figure-eight appearance in the supracardiac type. A chest roentgenogram of obstructed TAPVC shows a normal-size heart and a ground-glass appearance of the lung fields, reflecting pulmonary venous congestion or edema. The echocardiogram reveals the abnormal pulmonary venous connections.

Surgical repair varies with the type of TAPVC and whether the defect is obstructed or unobstructed. Obstructed lesions are repaired at the time of diagnosis, whereas the unobstructed type generally is repaired during infancy. The procedure is performed on cardiopulmonary bypass and involves anastomosis of the common pulmonary vein to the LA; ligating the common pulmonary vein; and closing the ASD, as in the supracardiac and infracardiac types. Repair of the supracardiac type involves baffling the pulmonary venous drainage to the LA. This repair has the highest success rate because of the low technical difficulty, whereas infracardiac repair is associated with a high mortality (up to 25%) and morbidity. Potential complications include reobstruction; atrial dysrhythmias, including sick sinus syndrome; PA hypertension; and LV dysfunction.[13]

Truncus Arteriosus

Truncus arteriosus is the failure of the large embryonic artery, the truncus arteriosus, to divide into the PA and the aorta. This results in a single vessel arising from both ventricles, providing blood flow to the pulmonary and systemic circulations (Figure 31-19, A). This common trunk straddles the VSD (always present) and has a single valve with three or four leaflets, which may result in stenosis or regurgitation, or both. The incidence is 2% of all congenital heart defects, and a right aortic arch is present 50% of the time. There are four types of truncus arteriosus. Type I is the most common (60%) and involves the main PA arising from the truncus and then dividing into the right and left PAs. Type II is less common (20%) and involves the PAs arising from the posterior aspect of the truncus. Type III is the least common (10%) and involves the PAs arising from the lateral aspect of the truncus. Type IV, also known as pseudotruncus, is now considered a

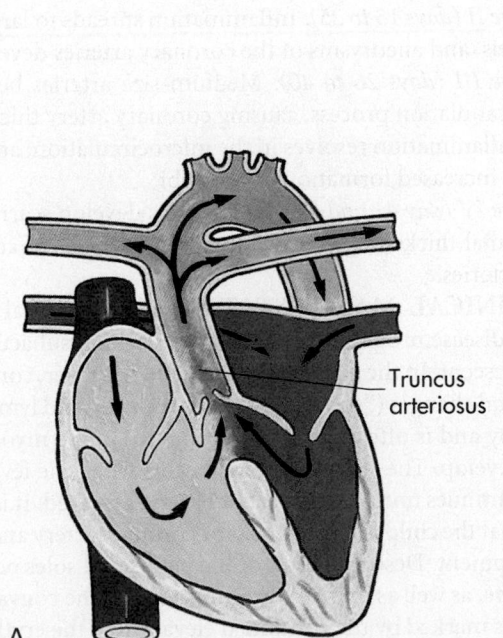

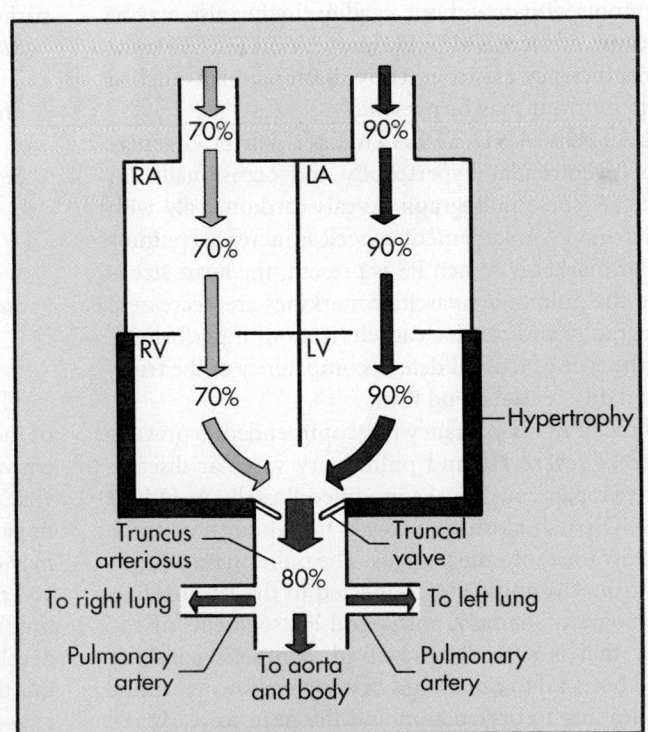

Figure 31-19 Truncus arteriosus. **A,** Persistent truncus arteriosus. The truncus arteriosus fails to divide into the pulmonary artery and aorta, and the interventricular septum fails to close at the top. Blood from both ventricles mixes in the truncus arteriosus and then enters the pulmonary and systemic circuits. **B,** Alterations of hemodynamics and oxygen saturation by persistent truncus arteriosus. *LA,* Left atrium; *LV,* left ventricle; *RA,* right atrium; *RV,* right ventricle. (A from Hockenberry MJ et al: *Wong's essentials of pediatric nursing,* ed 8, St Louis, 2009, Mosby.)

severe form of TOF with the bronchial arteries arising from the descending aorta to supply the lungs.[2]

PATHOPHYSIOLOGY Blood flow from the RV and LV is pumped into the main truncus, resulting in mixing of the pulmonary and systemic circulations (see Figure 31-19, *B*). The differential flow out to either the pulmonary bed or the systemic circulation depends on the pulmonary and systemic vascular resistances. Generally the pulmonary vascular resistance is less than the systemic vascular resistance, resulting in the majority of blood flow traveling to the lungs. This may be altered, however, because of PS, small pulmonary arteries, or increased pulmonary vascular resistance. Pulmonary vascular disease develops early with this defect because of increased pulmonary blood flow.

CLINICAL MANIFESTATIONS Physical findings depend on the amount of pulmonary blood flow and the presence of other cardiac anomalies. If PS is present, a newborn will present with cyanosis, caused by already elevated pulmonary vascular resistance, but no HF. Conversely, if PS is not present, the newborn initially will have mild to moderate cyanosis that worsens with activity. Once pulmonary vascular resistance drops, the pulmonary bed will receive preferential flow and the infant will have signs of HF. A wide pulse pressure with bounding pulses also may be present, caused by increased pulmonary blood flow. A harsh systolic regurgitant murmur is present along the left sternal border as a result of the VSD, and a systolic click at the apex and left upper sternal border may be present, reflecting opening of the truncal valve. An apical rumble with or without a gallop rhythm also may be present because of increased pulmonary blood flow. If truncal valve insufficiency exists, an early diastolic, high-pitched decrescendo murmur may be present.

EVALUATION AND TREATMENT An ECG generally reveals biventricular hypertrophy and occasionally LA enlargement. A chest radiograph reveals cardiomegaly with biventricular and LA enlargement, as well as increased pulmonary vascular markings. When PS is present, the heart size is normal and the pulmonary vascular markings are decreased. Echocardiography and cardiac catheterization, if performed, determine the type of truncal defect, competency of the truncal valve, and differential blood flow.

Surgical repair in early infancy is recommended to prevent the sequelae of severe HF and pulmonary vascular disease. The definitive repair consists of a modified Rastelli procedure involving VSD patch closure to divert the blood flow from the LV outflow tract into the truncus. The pulmonary arteries are excised from the aorta and connected to the RV through a tissue homograft—namely, aortic and PA segments or cadaver tissue that is specially preserved. Synthetic conduits may be used but tend to calcify and develop narrowing within the lumen, leading to obstruction and the need for early replacement. Mortality varies depending on the type of truncal anomaly (20% to 50%). Postoperative complications include HF, residual VSD, dysrhythmias, and pulmonary hypertension. The RV to PA homograft requires replacement because it becomes inadequate for somatic growth.[13]

ACQUIRED CARDIOVASCULAR DISORDERS

Acquired heart diseases are those disease processes or abnormalities that occur after birth. They result from various causes, such as infection, genetic disorders, autoimmune processes in response to infection, environmental factors, or autoimmune diseases. Examples of acquired heart diseases include Kawasaki disease, myocarditis, rheumatic heart disease, cardiomyopathy, and systemic hypertension. This chapter discusses Kawasaki disease and systemic hypertension. Myocarditis, rheumatic heart disease, and cardiomyopathy are discussed in Chapter 30.

Kawasaki Disease

Kawasaki disease, otherwise known as mucocutaneous lymph node syndrome, is an acute, self-limiting systemic vasculitis that may result in cardiac sequelae. Although Kawasaki disease occurs throughout the world, the greatest number of cases are reported in Japan.

Kawasaki disease is primarily a condition of young children: 80% of cases are seen in children younger than 5 years of age, with the incidence peaking in the toddler age group. Males are affected slightly more than females. Its peak incidence is in winter and spring.

The etiology of Kawasaki disease remains unknown. Theories center on an immunologic response to an infectious, toxic, or antigenic substance (including superantigen).[2,7,23]

PATHOPHYSIOLOGY Kawasaki disease progresses pathologically and clinically in the following stages:

Stage I (days 1 to 12): Small capillaries, arterioles, and venules become inflamed, as does the heart itself.

Stage II (days 13 to 25): Inflammation spreads to larger vessels, and aneurysms of the coronary arteries develop.

Stage III (days 26 to 40): Medium-size arteries begin the granulation process, causing coronary artery thickening; inflammation resolves in the microcirculation; and there is increased formation of thrombi.

Stage IV (day 41 and beyond): Vessels develop scarring, intimal thickening, calcification, and stenosis of coronary arteries.

CLINICAL MANIFESTATIONS The clinical course of the disease progresses in three stages: acute, subacute, and convalescent. In the acute phase the child has fever, conjunctivitis, oral changes ("strawberry" tongue), rash, and lymphadenopathy and is often irritable. During this phase myocarditis may develop. The subacute phase begins when the fever ends and continues until the clinical signs have resolved. It is at this time that the child is most at risk for coronary artery aneurysm development. Desquamation of the palms and soles occurs at this time, as well as marked thrombocytosis. The convalescent phase is marked by the continued elevation of the erythrocyte sedimentation rate and platelet count. Arthritis still may be present. This phase continues until all laboratory values return to normal—usually about 6 to 8 weeks after onset.

EVALUATION AND TREATMENT The diagnosis is based on the diagnosis criteria for Kawasaki disease, which state that the child must exhibit five of six criteria, including fever (Box 31-3). These children usually have leukocytosis, increased erythrocyte sedimentation rates, marked thrombocytosis, and elevated liver enzymes. An echocardiogram is obtained at the time of diagnosis as a baseline to assess for coronary aneurysms or inflammation. Serial echocardiograms are obtained after treatment to assess for future development of coronary aneurysms.

The use of aspirin and intravenous immunoglobulin during the acute phase has decreased the mortality of Kawasaki disease and has reduced the incidence of coronary abnormalities from approximately 20% to less than 2% at 6 to 8 weeks after initiation of therapy. Most children recover completely from Kawasaki disease, including the regression of aneurysms. The most common cardiovascular sequela is coronary thrombosis. Studies are investigating long-term results of the disease.[23]

Systemic Hypertension

Hypertension (HTN) in children differs from adult HTN in etiology and presentation. Children diagnosed with HTN are often found to have some underlying disease, such as renal disease or COA (Box 31-4). In recent years an increased prevalence of primary HTN in older children has been noted. Researchers are now focusing on primary HTN in older children in relation to morbidity and mortality and the presence of early atherosclerotic disease.[2,7,24,25]

Systemic hypertension in children is defined as systolic and diastolic blood pressure levels greater than the 95th percentile for age and gender on at least three occasions. The Fourth Task Force on Blood Pressure Control in Children uses height as an additional criterion to the blood pressure guide.[26]

PATHOPHYSIOLOGY Hypertension is classified as (1) primary (or essential) hypertension, in which a specific cause cannot be identified; or (2) secondary hypertension, in which a cause is secondary to another alteration (see Box 31-4). In infants and children a cause of HTN is almost always found.

Box 31-3   Diagnostic Criteria for Kawasaki Disease

The child must exhibit five of the following six criteria, including fever:

1. Fever for 5 or more days (often diagnosed with shorter duration of fever if other symptoms are present)
2. Bilateral conjunctival infection without exudation
3. Changes in the oral mucous membranes, such as erythema, dryness, and fissuring of the lips; oropharyngeal reddening; or "strawberry tongue"
4. Changes in the extremities, such as peripheral edema, peripheral erythema, and desquamation of palms and soles, particularly periungual peeling
5. Polymorphous rash, often accentuated in the perineal area
6. Cervical lymphadenopathy

Modified from Hockenberry MJ et al: *Wong's nursing care of infants and children,* ed 7, St Louis, 2003, Mosby.

Box 31-4   Conditions Associated with Secondary Hypertension in Children

Renal Disorders
Congenital defects
  Polycystic kidney, ectopic kidney, horseshoe kidney, etc.
  Obstructive anomalies
  Hydronephrosis
Renal tumor
  Wilms tumor
  Retrovascular tumor
Abnormalities of renal arteries
Renal vein thrombosis
Acquired disorders
  Glomerulonephritis—acute or chronic
  Pyelonephritis
  Nephritis associated with collagen disease

Cardiovascular Disease
Coarctation of the aorta
Arteriovenous fistulae
Patent ductus arteriosus
Aortic or mitral insufficiency

Metabolic and Endocrine Diseases
Adrenal tumors
  Adenoma
  Pheochromocytoma
  Neuroblastoma

Cushing syndrome
Adrenogenital syndrome
Hyperthyroidism
Aldosteronism
Hypercalcemia
Diabetes mellitus

Neurologic Disorders
Space-occupying lesions of cranium (increased intracranial pressure)
  Tumors, cysts, hematoma
  Cerebral edema
  Encephalitis (including Guillain-Barré and Reye syndromes)

Miscellaneous Causes
Drugs (corticosteroids, oral contraceptives, pressor agents, amphetamines)
Burns
Genitourinary surgery
Trauma (e.g., stretching of femoral nerve with leg traction)
Insect bites (e.g., scorpion)
Intravascular overload (blood, fluid)
Hypernatremia
Toxemia of pregnancy
Heavy metal poisoning

From Hockenberry MJ et al: *Wong's essentials of pediatric nursing,* ed 8, St Louis, 2009, Mosby.

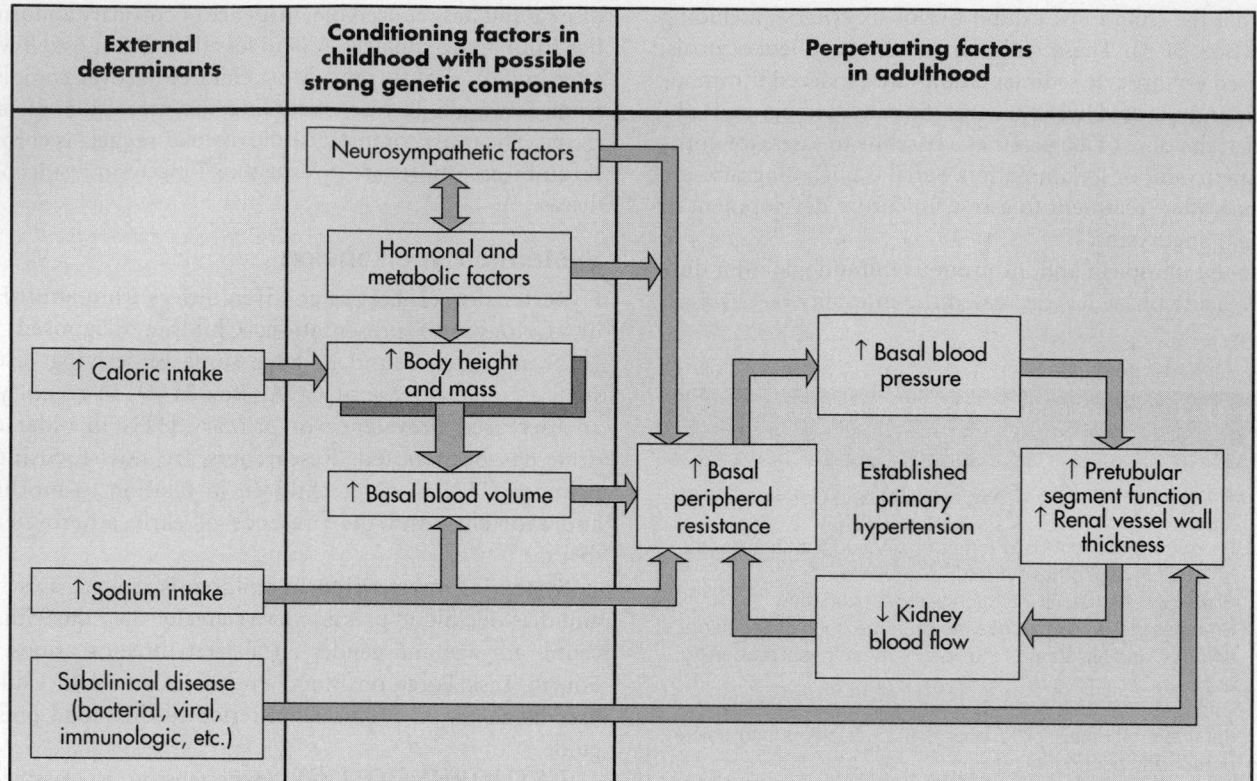

Figure 31-20 Mechanisms believed to influence blood pressure in children. According to this model, a critical factor in the development of hypertension is obesity during childhood. Increased body mass, coupled with excessive sodium intake, can cause primary hypertension in children or set the stage for its development later in life.

In general, the younger the child with significant hypertension, the more likely that a correctable cause can be found. Therefore, a thorough evaluation needs to be done.[27]

The pathophysiology of primary HTN in children is not clearly understood but may result from a complex interaction of a strong disposing genetic component with disturbances in sympathetic vascular smooth muscle tone, humoral agents (angiotensin, catecholamines), renal sodium excretion, and cardiac output (Figure 31-20). Ultimately these factors impair the ability of the peripheral vascular bed to adjust its own resistance to meet tissue perfusion needs.[24]

CLINICAL MANIFESTATIONS Most children with systemic HTN are asymptomatic. It is necessary that a thorough history and physical examination be obtained. The examination should include an accurate blood pressure measurement on three separate occasions using a cuff of appropriate size (Tables 31-6 and 31-7).

Certain factors influence blood pressure in children. Smoking is also associated with an increased risk for HTN. Obesity is emerging as one of the most important factors in the increasing prevalence of HTN in children.

EVALUATION AND TREATMENT In children the history and physical examination should be directed at determining the etiology of HTN, such as COA or renal disease (Table 31-8). If COA is found, surgical or interventional correction is initiated. A complete blood count, serum chemistry levels, urinalysis, urine culture, lipid profile, and renal

ultrasound are part of the routine evaluation for renal disease (Table 31-9).

Although the criteria for the diagnosis of hypertension are based on the use of a standard blood pressure cuff, some children have what is termed "white coat hypertension."

Table 31-6	Suggested Normal BP Values (mmHg) by Auscultatory Method (Systolic/Diastolic K5)		
Age (Years)	Mean BP Levels	90th Percentile	95th Percentile
6-7	104/55	114/73	117/78
8-9	106/58	117/76	120/82
11-11*	108/60	120/77	124/82
12-13*	112/62	124/78	128/83
14-15			
Boys	116/66	132/80	138/86
Girls	112/68	126/80	130/83
16-18			
Boys	121/70	136/82	140/86
Girls	110/68	125/81	127/84

From Park MK: *Pediatric cardiology for practitioners,* ed 4, St Louis, 2002, Mosby; modified from Goldring D et al: *J Pediatr* 91:884, 1977; Prineas RJ et al: *Hypertension* 1 (Suppl):18, 1980.
BP, Blood pressure; *K5,* phase V of Korotkoff sound.
*Values for ages 10 to 13 years have been extrapolated from these two studies using age-related increments from other studies.

Table 31-7	Normative BP Levels (Systolic/ Diastolic [Mean]) by Dinamap Monitor in Children 5 Years Old and Younger		
Age	Mean BP Levels (in mmHg)	90th Percentile	95th Percentile
1-3 days	64/41 (50)	75/49 (50)	78/52 (62)
1 month-2 years	95/58 (72)	106/68 (83)	110/71 (86)
2-5 years	101/57 (74)	112/66 (82)	115/68 (85)

From Park MK: *Pediatric cardiology for practitioners,* ed 4, St Louis, 2002, Mosby; modified from Park MK, Menard SM: *Am J Dis Child* 143:860, 1989.

BP, Blood pressure.

Table 31-8	Most Common Causes of Chronic Sustained Hypertension
Age Group	Causes
Newborn	Renal artery thrombosis, renal artery stenosis, congenital renal malformation, COA, bronchopulmonary dysplasia
<6 years	Renal parenchymal disease, COA, renal artery stenosis
6-10 years	Renal artery stenosis, renal parenchymal disease, primary hypertension
>10 years	Primary hypertension, renal parenchymal disease

From Park MK: *Pediatric cardiology for practitioners,* ed 4, St Louis, 2002, Mosby; modified from Report of the Second Task Force on Blood Pressure Control in Children. *Pediatrics* 79:1, 1987.

COA, Coarctation of the aorta.

Elevated blood pressure readings in these children occur only when measured in the clinic and may be caused by fear and anxiety. The use of ambulatory blood pressure monitoring (ABPM) records the blood pressure over a 24-hour period. In addition to identifying children with white coat hypertension, ABPM has been found to be useful in children with hypertension that is resistant to treatment (see What's New? Ambulatory Blood Pressure Monitoring in Children).[26]

If HTN is found to be essential, or primary, in nature, nonpharmacologic therapy is used initially. Moderate weight loss can decrease systolic and diastolic pressures in many children. Appropriate diet, regular physical activity, and avoidance of smoking have been shown to be effective in reducing blood pressure.[28]

Drug therapy is controversial in children with primary hypertension; however, when nonpharmacologic therapy fails, a staged approach with the use of diuretics and/or beta-blockers and afterload reduction is indicated. The emphasis on preventive cardiology, especially for children, is significant because many investigators believe signs of atherosclerosis and other cardiovascular risk factors are present from childhood.[29-32]

WHAT'S NEW? Ambulatory Blood Pressure Monitoring in Children

Ambulatory blood pressure monitoring (ABPM) records blood pressure over a 24-hour period. Its use in children was endorsed by the Fourth Report of the National High Blood Pressure Education Program Working Group on High Blood Pressure in Children primarily to help identify those children with "white coat hypertension." Paradoxically, some children have normal blood pressure readings in the clinic but are hypertensive during other parts of the day. This is called "masked hypertension" and also can be identified by ABPM. ABPM is useful in documenting what is called the "BP load," which is the total amount of time the blood pressure (BP) is elevated above normal limits during a 24 hour period. By measuring BP load, ABPM may be able to identify those children who are at greatest risk for target organ damage. It can also help with management of children who suffer hypotensive episodes in response to pharmacologic therapy for their hypertension. Finally, ABPM facilitates medication changes in those with hypertension resistant to medication.

Data from Flynn JT: *Am J Hypertens* 21(6):605-612, 2008; Kavey RE et al: *J Pediatr* 150:491-497, 2007; National High Blood Pressure Education Program Working Group on High Blood Pressure in Children: *Pediatr* 114:555-576, 2004.

Childhood Obesity

Childhood obesity is considered an epidemic in not only the United States but also in other countries such as Australia.[33-35] Despite attention from U.S. federal and state initiatives, the prevalence of obesity in children and young adults has steadily increased over the past four decades, with estimates as high as 25% of children considered obese.[33] Although not without controversy, percentile of body mass index (BMI) expressed as weight/height^2 (BMI; kg/m^2) is used to identify overweight and obesity in children and adolescents. The Centers for Disease Control and Prevention (CDC), the supplier of national growth charts and prevalence data, avoids characterizing children and adolescents as "obese"; instead, the CDC suggests two levels of overweight: (1) the 85th percentile, an "at risk" level; and (2) the 95th percentile, the more severe level.[36]

Causes of obesity in young children and adolescents are multivariable and multidimensional. Risk factors associated with developing childhood obesity include race, socioeconomic status, and lack of health insurance. Children of black and Hispanic race are at higher risk, as well as children with no insurance.[34] The presence of parental obesity also is associated with childhood obesity.[37] In addition, early childhood nutrition, level of physical activity, and engagement of sedentary activities, such as watching television and computer use, is associated with the development of overweight and obese children.[38-40]

Similar to obese adults, overweight and obese children are at risk for acquiring numerous other serious and potentially life-threatening illnesses such as asthma, sleep apnea, hypertension, type 2 diabetes, dyslipidemia, and cardiovascular

Table 31-9	Routine and Special Laboratory Tests for Hypertension
Laboratory Tests	**Significance of Abnormal Results**
Urinalysis, urine culture, blood urea nitrogen, and creatinine levels	Renal parenchymal disease
Serum electrolyte levels (hypokalemia)	Hyperaldosteronism, primary or secondary
	Adrenogenital syndrome
	Renin-producing tumors
Serum uric acid level	Elevations associated with systolic and diastolic levels and premetabolic syndrome
ECG, chest roentgenogram	Cardiac cause of hypertension, also baseline function
Renal (imaging; or ultrasonography, radionuclide studies, computed tomography of the kidney)	Renal parenchymal disease
	Renovascular hypertension
	Tumors (neuroblastoma, Wilms tumor)
Plasma renin activity, peripheral	High-renin hypertension
	Renovascular hypertension
	Renin-producing tumors
	Some caused by Cushing syndrome
	Some caused by essential hypertension
	Low-renin hypertension
	Adrenogenital syndrome
	Primary hyperaldosteronism
24-hour urine collection for 17-ketosteroids and 17-hydroxycorticosteroids	Cushing syndrome
	Adrenogenital syndrome
24-hour urine collection for catecholamine levels and vanillylmandelic acid	Pheochromocytoma
	Neuroblastoma
Aldosterone	Hyperaldosteronism, primary or secondary
	Renovascular hypertension
	Renin-producing tumors
Renal vein plasma renin activity	Unilateral renal parenchymal disease
	Renovascular hypertension
Abdominal aortogram	Renovascular hypertension
	Abdominal COA
	Unilateral renal parenchymal diseases
	Pheochromocytoma

Adapted from Park MK: *Pediatric cardiology for practitioners,* ed 4, St Louis, 2002, Mosby.
COA, Coarctation of the aorta; *ECG,* electrocardiogram.

disease.[7] Researchers also have reported a multitude of social and economic consequences in adolescents as a result of being overweight. Overweight adolescents are more likely to complete fewer years of education, are less likely to marry, and have a lower household income in adulthood, independent of familial socioeconomic status.[41]

As in other acquired diseases, efforts should be focused on prevention. The initial approach is a combined program of physical activity with nutritional improvements. Healthcare professionals play a vital role in recognizing the need for intervention, immediate referral, and support. Successful outcomes for most overweight and obese children require support, change in lifestyle at home, and involvement of family members. Researchers are involving school-based programs in promoting and preventing obesity in the young.[42]

SUMMARY REVIEW

Development of the Cardiovascular System

1. The heart arises from the mesenchyme and begins as an enlarged blood vessel with a large lumen and a muscular wall. By approximately the eighth week of gestation, all structures of the fetal heart and vascular system are present.

2. The endocardial cushions are instrumental in closing the atrial septum, dividing the AV canals into the right and left AV orifices, and closing the septum.

3. In the fetus the pulmonary and systemic circulatory systems are connected by the foramen ovale, an opening between the atria; by the ductus arteriosus, a fetal vessel that joins the PA to the aorta; and by the ductus venosus, a fetal vessel that connects the inferior vena cava to the umbilical vein.

4. Fetal circulation is different from postnatal circulation because of the presence of fetal shunts and altered metabolic needs of the various organs.

5. Fetal blood flow depends on resistance for its distribution through the body. Resistance in the pulmonary circulation is higher than resistance in the systemic circulation, so myocardial thickness is about the same in the right heart and the left heart.

6. After birth, systemic resistance increases and pulmonary resistance decreases.

7. Pulmonary vascular resistance drops suddenly at birth because the lungs expand and the pulmonary vessels dilate. It continues to decrease gradually during the first 6 to 8 weeks after birth. Decreased resistance causes the right myocardium to thin out.

8. Systemic vascular resistance increases markedly at birth because severance of the umbilical cord removes the low-resistance placenta from the systemic circulation. Increased systemic resistance causes the left myocardium to become dominant and thicken over time.

9. Changes in resistance cause the fetal connections between the pulmonary and systemic circulatory systems to disappear. The foramen ovale closes functionally at birth and anatomically several months later; the ductus arteriosus closes functionally 15 to 18 hours after birth and anatomically within 10 to 21 days; and the ductus venosus closes within 1 week after birth.

10. At birth a series of circulatory changes occur that affect blood flow, vascular resistance, and oxygen tension. The most important change is the shift of gas exchange from the placenta to the lungs.

11. After birth, significant postnatal changes occur, including thinning of the right ventricular myocardium as the pulmonary vascular resistance drops. As the systemic vascular resistance increases, the left ventricular myocardium becomes thicker and more dominant as it is in the adult heart.

Congenital Heart Defects

1. Most congenital cardiovascular defects have begun to develop by the eighth week of gestation, and most have many causes, both environmental and genetic.

2. Environmental risk factors associated with the incidence of congenital heart defects typically are maternal conditions. Among these are viral infections, diabetes, drug intake, alcohol intake, metabolic disorders, and advanced maternal age.

3. Genetic factors associated with congenital heart defects include but are not limited to Down syndrome, trisomy 13, trisomy 18, cri du chat syndrome, and Turner syndrome. It now appears, however, that most genetic mechanisms of causation are multifactorial.

4. Classification of congenital heart defects is based on whether they (a) cause blood flow to the lungs to increase or decrease, (b) obstruct ventricular blood flow patterns, or (c) cause mixing of unoxygenated and oxygenated blood.

5. Symptoms of HF are usually the result of congenital heart defects that increase blood volume and pressure in the pulmonary circulation. Clinical manifestations are almost the same as the manifestations of CHF in adults. A unique manifestation in children is FTT.

6. Cyanosis, a bluish discoloration of the skin, indicates that the tissues are not receiving normally adequate oxygenated blood. Cyanosis can be caused by defects that (a) reduce pulmonary blood flow; (b) overload the pulmonary circulation, causing pulmonary hypertension, pulmonary edema, and respiratory difficulty; and (c) cause large amounts of unoxygenated blood to shunt from the pulmonary to the systemic circulation.

7. Congenital defects that maintain or create direct communication between the pulmonary and systemic circulatory systems cause blood to shunt from one system to another, mixing oxygenated and unoxygenated blood and increasing blood volume and pressure on the receiving side of the shunt.

8. The direction of shunting through an abnormal communication depends on differences in pressure and resistance between the two systems. Flow is always from an area of high pressure to an area of low pressure. The resistance to flow determines the volume of the shunting.

9. Acyanotic congenital defects that increase pulmonary blood flow consist of abnormal openings (PDA, ASD, VSD, AVC defect, or truncus arteriosus) that permit blood to shunt from left (systemic circulation) to right (pulmonary circulation). Cyanosis does not occur because the left to right shunt does not interfere with the flow of oxygenated blood through the systemic circulation.

10. If the abnormal communication between the left and right circuits is large, volume and pressure overload in the pulmonary circulation leads to CHF.

11. In truncus arteriosus the main trunk fails to divide longitudinally into the aorta and PA. All blood from both ventricles enters the truncus, so that mixed blood is delivered by both circulatory systems, causing varying degrees of cyanosis and HF.

12. In heart defects that decrease pulmonary blood flow (TOF, tricuspid atresia), myocardial hypertrophy cannot compensate for restricted right ventricular outflow. Flow to the lungs decreases, and cyanosis is caused by mixing of systemic and pulmonary venous return.

13. Obstruction of ventricular outflow commonly is caused by PS, AS, COA, interrupted aortic arch, or hypoplastic left heart syndrome.

14. Despite obstruction, ventricular outflow remains normal because of compensatory ventricular hypertrophy stimulated by increased afterload and, in postductal COA, development of collateral circulation around the coarctation.

15. Signs of HF can occur with pulmonary overcirculation or myocardial failure.

16. Complex congenital defects that depend on mixing of the pulmonary and systemic circulations for survival during the postnatal period include complete transposition of the great arteries and total anomalous pulmonary venous connection. This mixing results in desaturated systemic blood flow and cyanosis.

SUMMARY REVIEW—cont'd

17. In complete transposition of the great vessels, the circulatory systems are not connected serially or through a shunt, so that oxygenated blood remains permanently in the pulmonary circulation and unoxygenated blood remains in the systemic circulation. Survival depends on patency of the ductus arteriosus; after that, surgical intervention is mandatory.

18. Total anomalous pulmonary venous connection is caused by the persistence of the fetal common PA and the lack of pulmonary venous return to the LA. All blood from the pulmonary and systemic circulations enters the RA. Mixed blood enters the LA through an ASD; it then flows into the systemic circulation and causes cyanosis.

19. Treatment for all hemodyamically severe congenital defects is surgical or interventional correction of the anomaly and management of cyanosis and HF.

Acquired Cardiovascular Disorders

1. The most common acquired cardiovascular disorders of childhood are Kawasaki disease, rheumatic heart disease, and hypertension.

2. Kawasaki disease is an acute systemic vasculitis that also may result in the development of coronary artery aneurysms and thrombosis.

3. Essential hypertension in children is the same as that in adults, except that it is more likely to be diagnosed in an early, asymptomatic stage. Most cases of hypertension in young children have an underlying cause.

4. Obesity in childhood is an epidemic in the United States and other countries.

5. Obese children are at risk for acquiring numerous other serious and potentially life-threatening illnesses, such as asthma, sleep apnea, hypertension, type 2 diabetes mellitus, and cardiovascular disease.

KEY TERMS

Aortic stenosis (AS), 1228
Atrial septal defect (ASD), 1219
Atrioventricular canal (AVC) defect, 1222
Bulbus cordis, 1211
Coarctation of the aorta (COA), 1226
Complete AVC (CAVC) defect, 1222
Conus, 1231
Cyanosis, 1217
Ductus arteriosus, 1211
Eisenmenger syndrome, 1217
Endocardial cushion, 1209
Foramen ovale, 1211

Heart failure (HF), 1216
Hypoplastic left heart syndrome (HLHS), 1230
Kawasaki disease, 1234
Ligamentum venosum, 1212
Ostium primum, 1210
Ostium secundum, 1210
Partial AVC (PAVC) defect, 1222
Patent ductus arteriosus (PDA), 1218
Pulmonary atresia, 1229
Pulmonary stenosis (PS), 1229
Septum primum, 1210

Septum secundum, 1210
Systemic hypertension, 1235
Tetralogy of Fallot (TOF), 1223
Total anomalous pulmonary venous connection (TAPVC), 1232
Transitional AVC (TAVC) defect, 1222
Transposition of the great arteries (TGA), 1231
Tricuspid atresia, 1225
Truncus arteriosus, 1233
Ventricular septal defect (VSD), 1220

REFERENCES

1. Clark EB, Nakazawa M, Takao A, editors: *Etiology and morphogenesis of congenital heart disease: twenty years of progress in genetics and developmental biology*, Mount Kisco, NY, 2000, Futura Publishing Company.

2. Park MK: *Pediatric cardiology for practitioners*, ed 5, Philadelphia, 2008, Mosby.

3. Wilson D, Hockenberry MJ: *Wong's clinical manual of pediatric nursing*, ed 7, St Louis, 2008, Mosby.

4. Hazinski MF: *Nursing care of the critically ill child*, ed 2, St Louis, 1991, Mosby.

5. Gelb DB: Genetic basis of congenital heart disease, *Curr Opin Cardiol* 19(2):110-115, 2004.

6. American Heart Association: *Heart disease and stroke statistics, 2004 update*, Dallas, 2004, Author.

7. Allen HD: *Moss and Adam's heart disease in infants, children, and adolescents: including the fetus and young adult*, ed 7, Philadelphia, 2008, Wolters Kluwer Health/Lippincott Williams & Wilkins.

8. Dimenna L et al: Management of the neonate with patent ductus arteriosus, *J Perinat Neonat Nurs* 20(4):333-340, 2006.

9. Bichell DP et al: Minimal access approach for the repair of atrial septal defect: the initial 135 patients, *Ann Thorac Surg* 70(1):115-118, 2000.

10. Moodie DS, Sterba R: Long-term outcomes excellent for atrial septal defect repair in adults, *Cleve Clin J Med* 67(8):591-597, 2000.

11. Knauth AL et al: Transcatheter device closure of congenital and postoperative residual ventricular septal defects, *Circulation* 110(5):501-507, 2004.

12. El-Najdawi EK et al: Operation for partial atrioventricular septal defect: a forty-year review, *J Thorac Cardiovasc Surg* 119(5):880-889, 2000.

13. Mavroudis C, Backer CL, editors: *Pediatric cardiac surgery*, ed 3, St Louis, 2003, Mosby.

14. Fawzy MR et al: Long-term outcome (up to 15 years) of balloon angioplasty of discrete native coarctation of the aorta in adolescents and adults, *J Am Coll Cardiol* 43(6):1062-1067, 2004.

15. Walhout RJ et al: Comparison of surgical repair with balloon angioplasty for native coarctation in patients from 3 months to 16 years of age, *Eur J Cardiothorac Surg* 25(5):722-727, 2004.

16. Ricci M: Repair of coarctation of the aorta, *J Thorac Cardiovasc Surg* 127(4):1224-1225, 2004.

17. Hasaniya N et al: Outcome of aortic valve repair in children with congenital aortic valve insufficiency, *J Thorac Cardiovasc Surg* 127(4):970-974, 2004.

18. Hrasja V et al: Ross and Ross-Konno procedure in children and adolescents: mid-term results, *Eur J Cardiothorac Surg* 25(5):742-747, 2004.

19. Poon LK, Menahem S: Pulmonary regurgitation after percutaneous balloon valvoplasty for isolated pulmonary valvar stenosis in childhood, *Cardiol Young* 13(5):444-450, 2003.

20. Wernovsky G: Hypoplastic left heart syndrome: consensus and controversies in 2007, *Cardiol Young* 17(Suppl 2):75-86, 2007.

21. Gutgesell HP, Massaro TA: Management of hypoplastic left heart syndrome in a consortium of university hospitals, *Am J Cardiol* 76(11):809-811, 2000.

22. McQuillen PS: Balloon atrial septostomy is associated with preoperative stroke in neonates with transposition of the great arteries, *Circulation* 113(2):280-285, 2006.

23. Newburger JW: Diagnosis, treatment, and long term management of Kawasaki disease: statement for health professionals from the Committee on Rheumatic Fever, Endocarditis and Kawasaki Disease, Council on Cardiovascular Disease in the Young, and American Heart Association, *Circulation* 110:2747–2271, 2004.

24. Sinha MD, Reid C: Evaluation of blood pressure in children, *Curr Opin Nephrol Hypertens* 16(6):577-584, 2007.

25. Munter R et al: Trends in blood pressure among children and adolescents, *JAMA* 291:2107-2113, 2004.

26. National High Blood Pressure Education Program Working Group on High Blood Pressure in Children: The fourth report on the diagnosis, evaluation, and treatment of high blood pressure in children and adolescents, *Pediatrics* 114:555-576, 2004.

27. Nguyen M, Mitsnefes M: Evaluation of hypertension by the general pediatrician, *Curr Opin Pediatr* 19(2):165-169, 2007.

28. Seikaly MG: Hypertension in children: an update on treatment strategies, *Curr Opin Pediatr* 19(2):170-177, 2007.

29. Feld LG, Corey H: Hypertension in childhood, *Pediatr Rev* 28(8): 283-298, 2007.

30. McNiece KL et al: Prevalence of hypertension and pre-hypertension among adolescents, *J Pediatr* 150(6):640-644, 2007:644e1, 2007.

31. Hansen ML et al: Underdiagnosis of hypertension in children and adolescents, *JAMA* 298(8):874-879, 2007.

32. Din-Dzietham R et al: High blood pressure trends in children and adolescents in national surveys, 1963-2002, *Circulation* 116(13):1488-1496, 2007.

33. Beilin L, Huang RC: Childhood obesity, hypertension, the metabolic syndrome and adult cardiovascular disease, *Clin Exp Pharmacol Physiol* 35(4):409-411, 2008.

34. Haas JS et al: The association of race, socioeconomic status, and health insurance status with the prevalence of overweight among children and adolescents, *Am J Public Health* 93(12):2105-2110, 2003.

35. Harding S et al: Overweight, obesity and high blood pressure in an ethnically diverse sample of adolescents in Britain: the Medical Research Council DASH study, *Int J Obesity* 32(1):82-90, 2008.

36. Kuczmarski RJ et al: CDC growth charts: United States, *Adv Data* (314):1-27, 2000.

37. Whitaker RC et al: Predicting obesity in young adulthood from childhood and parental obesity, *N Engl J Med* 337(13):869-873, 1997.

38. Crespo CJ et al: Television watching, energy intake, and obesity in US children: results from the third National Health and Nutrition Examination Study, 1988-1994, *Arch Pediatr Adolesc Med* 155(3): 360-365, 2001.

39. Gordon-Larsen P, McMurray RG, Popkin BM: Adolescent physical activity and inactivity vary by ethnicity: The National Longitudinal Study of Adolescent Health, *J Pediatr* 135(3):301-306, 1999.

40. Kimm SY et al: Racial divergence in adiposity during adolescence: the NHLBI Growth and Health Study, *Pediatrics* 107(3):E34, 2001.

41. Rome ES et al: Children and adolescents with eating disorders: the state of the art, *Pediatrics* 111(1):e98-e108, 2003.

42. Centers for Disease Control and Prevention: Guidelines for school health programs to promote lifelong healthy eating: Centers for Disease Control, *MMWR Recomm Rep* 45(RR-9):1-41, 1996.

STRUCTURE AND FUNCTION OF THE PULMONARY SYSTEM

VALENTINA L. BRASHERS

MEDIA RESOURCES

CHAPTER OUTLINE

STRUCTURES OF THE PULMONARY SYSTEM
  Conducting Airways
  Gas-Exchange Airways
  Pulmonary and Bronchial Circulation
  Chest Wall and Pleura
FUNCTION OF THE PULMONARY SYSTEM
  Ventilation

  Gas Transport
  Control of the Pulmonary Circulation
TESTS OF PULMONARY FUNCTION
  Aging and the Pulmonary System

The pulmonary system consists of upper and lower airways, the chest wall, and pulmonary circulation. In addition, the respiratory center of the central nervous system and the phrenic nerve participate in pulmonary function by providing the neurochemical control of breathing. The primary function of the pulmonary system is the exchange of gases between the environmental air and the blood. There are three steps in this process: (1) ventilation, the movement of air into and out of the lungs; (2) diffusion, the movement of gases between air spaces in the lungs and the bloodstream; and (3) perfusion, the movement of blood into and out of the capillary beds of the lungs to body organs and tissues. The first two functions are carried out by the pulmonary system and the third by the cardiovascular system (see Chapter 29). Normally the pulmonary system functions efficiently under a variety of conditions and with little energy expenditure.

STRUCTURES OF THE PULMONARY SYSTEM

The pulmonary system is made up of the upper airways, two lungs, the lower airways, and the blood vessels that serve them (Figure 32-1), and the chest wall, or thoracic cage. The lungs are divided into lobes: three in the right lung (upper, middle, lower) and two in the left lung (upper, lower). Each lobe is further divided into segments and lobules. The space between the lungs, which contains the heart, great vessels, and esophagus, is called the *mediastinum*. A set of conducting airways, called bronchi, deliver air to each section of the lung. The lung tissue that surrounds the airways supports them, preventing their distortion or collapse as gas moves in and out during ventilation.

The lungs are protected from a variety of exogenous contaminants by a series of mechanical barriers (Table 32-1). These defense mechanisms are so effective that in the healthy individual, contamination of the lung tissue itself is unusual. (Other mechanisms of self-defense are discussed in Chapters 6 and 7.)

Conducting Airways

The conducting airways are the portion of the pulmonary system that provides a passage for the movement of air into and out of the gas-exchange portions of the lung. They consist of upper and lower airways. The **nasopharynx, oropharynx,** and related structures often are called the *upper airway* (Figure 32-2). These structures are lined with a ciliated mucosa with

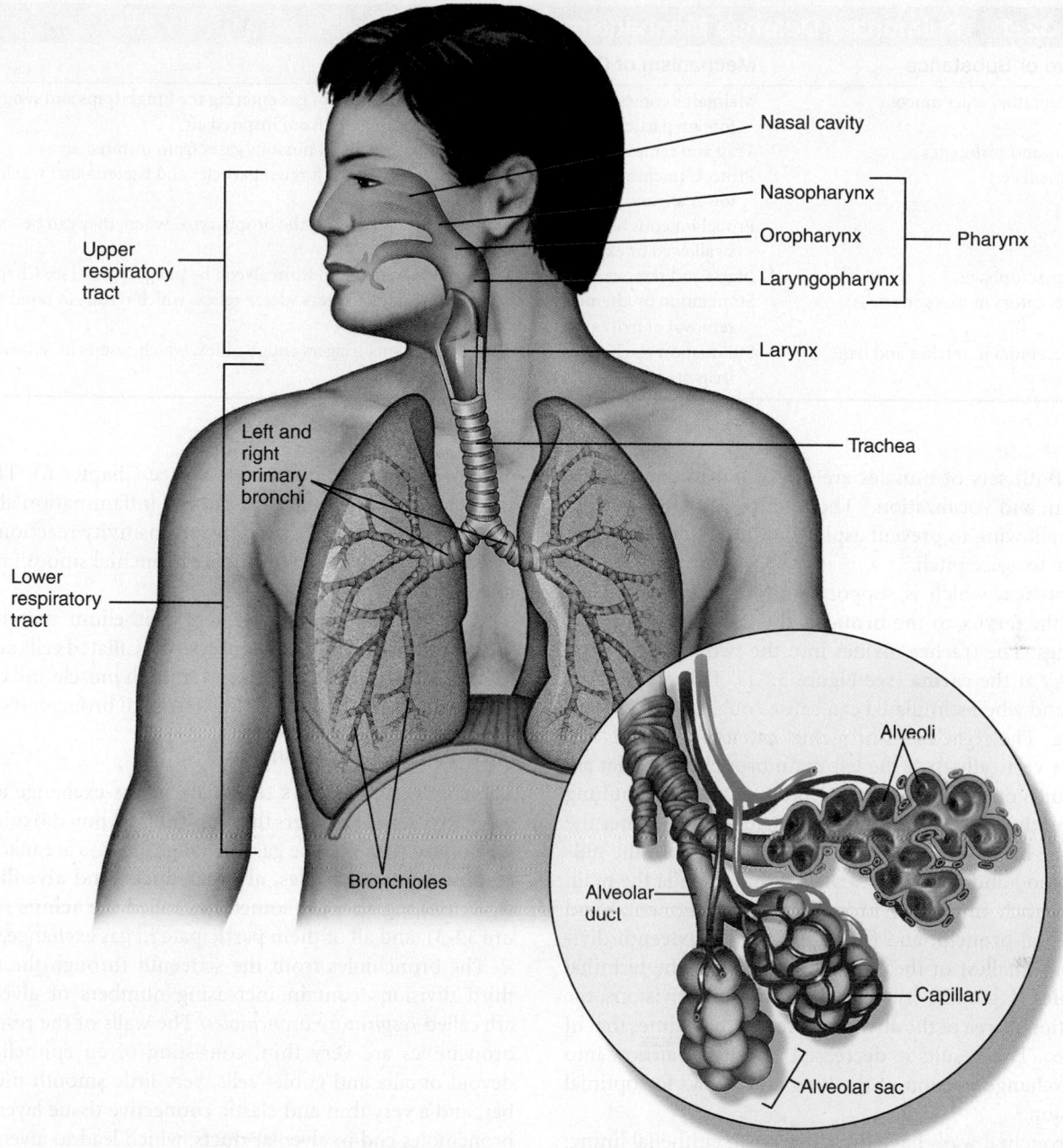

Figure 32-1 **Structural plan of the respiratory system.** *Inset* shows alveolar sacs where the interchange of oxygen and carbon dioxide takes place through the walls of the grapelike alveoli. Capillaries surround the alveoli. (From Patton KT, Thibodeau GA: *Anatomy & physiology*, ed 7, St Louis, 2010, Mosby.)

a very rich vascular supply. The mucosal lining warms and humidifies inspired air and removes foreign particles from it as it passes into the lungs. During quiet breathing, gas usually flows through the nose, nasopharynx, and oropharynx to the lower airways. The mouth and oropharynx provide for ventilation when the nose is obstructed or when increased flow is required, such as during exercise. Filtering and humidifying are not, however, as efficient with mouth breathing.

The **larynx** connects the upper and lower airways. The structure of the larynx consists of the endolarynx and its surrounding triangular-shaped bony and cartilaginous structures.

The endolarynx is formed by two pairs of folds that form the false vocal cords (supraglottis) and the true vocal cords. The slit-shaped space between the true cords forms the glottis (see Figure 32-2). The vestibule is the space above the false vocal cords. The laryngeal box is formed of three large cartilages—the epiglottis, thyroid, and cricoid—and three smaller cartilages—the arytenoid, corniculate, and cuneiform—that are connected by ligaments. The supporting cartilages prevent collapse of the larynx during inspiration and swallowing. The internal laryngeal muscles control vocal cord length and tension, and the external laryngeal muscles move the larynx as

Table 32-1	Pulmonary Defense Mechanisms
Structure or Substance	**Mechanism of Defense**
Upper respiratory tract mucosa	Maintains constant temperature and humidification of gas entering the lungs; traps and removes foreign particles, some bacteria, and noxious gases from inspired air
Nasal hairs and turbinates	Trap and remove foreign particles, some bacteria, and noxious gases from inspired air
Mucous blanket	Protects trachea and bronchi from injury; traps most foreign particles and bacteria that reach the lower airways
Cilia	Propel mucous blanket and entrapped particles toward the oropharynx, where they can be swallowed or expectorated
Alveolar macrophages	Ingest and remove bacteria and other foreign material from alveoli by phagocytosis (see Chapter 6)
Irritant receptors in nares (nostrils)	Stimulation by chemical or mechanical irritants triggers sneeze reflex, which results in rapid removal of irritants from nasal passages
Irritant receptors in trachea and large airways	Stimulation by chemical or mechanical irritants triggers cough reflex, which results in removal of irritants from the trachea and large airways

a whole. Both sets of muscles are important to swallowing, respiration, and vocalization.[1] The internal muscles contract during swallowing to prevent aspiration into the trachea and contribute to voice pitch.

The **trachea,** which is supported by U-shaped cartilage, connects the larynx to the **bronchi,** the conducting airways of the lungs. The trachea divides into the two main airways, or bronchi, at the **carina** (see Figure 32-1). This area is very sensitive and when stimulated can cause coughing and airway narrowing. The right main bronchus extends from the trachea more vertically than the left main bronchus, so that aspirated fluids or foreign particles tend to enter the right lung rather than the left. The right and left main bronchi enter the lungs at the **hila,** or "roots" of the lungs, along with the pulmonary blood and lymphatic vessels. From the hila the main bronchi branch into lobar bronchi, then to segmental and subsegmental bronchi, and finally end at the sixteenth division in the smallest of the conducting airways, the terminal **bronchioles** (Figure 32-3). With these multiple divisions, the cross-sectional area of the airways increases to 20 times that of the trachea. This results in decreased velocity or airflow into the gas-exchange portion of the lung and allows for optimal gas diffusion.[2]

The bronchial walls have three layers: an epithelial lining, a smooth muscle layer, and a connective tissue layer. In the large bronchi (to approximately the tenth division), the connective tissue layer contains cartilage. The epithelial lining of the bronchi contains single-celled exocrine glands—the mucus-secreting **goblet cells**—and ciliated cells. High columnar pseudostratified epithelium lines the larger airways, changing to columnar cuboidal epithelium in the bronchioles (types of epithelia are illustrated in Chapter 1). The submucosal glands of the bronchial lining also produce mucus, contributing to the mucous blanket that covers the bronchial epithelium. The ciliated epithelial cells rhythmically beat this mucous blanket toward the trachea and pharynx, where it can be swallowed or expectorated by coughing. Foreign particles and microorganisms that are not expelled by mucociliary clearance and coughing are attacked by cellular components of the inflammatory response and antibodies

of the secretory immune system (see Chapter 6). The biochemical mediators released early in inflammation also play a part in antibody-mediated hypersensitivity reactions, such as asthma, because they stimulate bronchial smooth muscles to constrict.

With branching, the layers of epithelium that line the bronchi become thinner (Figure 32-4). Ciliated cells and goblet cells become more sparse, and smooth muscle and connective tissue layers thin toward the terminal bronchioles.[2]

Gas-Exchange Airways

The conducting airways terminate in gas-exchange airways, where oxygen (O_2) enters the blood and carbon dioxide (CO_2) is removed from it. The gas-exchange airways are made up of **respiratory bronchioles, alveolar ducts,** and **alveoli.** These structures together are sometimes called the **acinus** (see Figure 32-3), and all of them participate in gas exchange.[3]

The bronchioles from the sixteenth through the twenty-third divisions contain increasing numbers of alveoli and are called *respiratory bronchioles.* The walls of the respiratory bronchioles are very thin, consisting of an epithelial layer devoid of cilia and goblet cells, very little smooth muscle fiber, and a very thin and elastic connective tissue layer. These bronchioles end in alveolar ducts, which lead to alveolar sacs made up of numerous alveoli.

The alveoli are the primary gas-exchange units of the lung, where oxygen enters the blood and CO_2 is removed (Figure 32-5). Tiny passages called *pores of Kohn* permit some air to pass through the septa from alveolus to alveolus, promoting collateral ventilation and even distribution of air among the alveoli. The lungs contain approximately 25 million alveoli at birth and 300 million by adulthood.

The alveolar septa consist of an epithelial layer and a thin, elastic basement membrane but no muscle layer (Figure 32-6). Two major types of epithelial cells appear in the alveolus. Type I alveolar cells provide structure, and type II alveolar cells secrete **surfactant,** a lipoprotein that coats the inner surface of the alveolus and facilitates its expansion during inspiration, lowers alveolar surface tension at end-expiration, and, thereby, prevents lung collapse.[1-4]

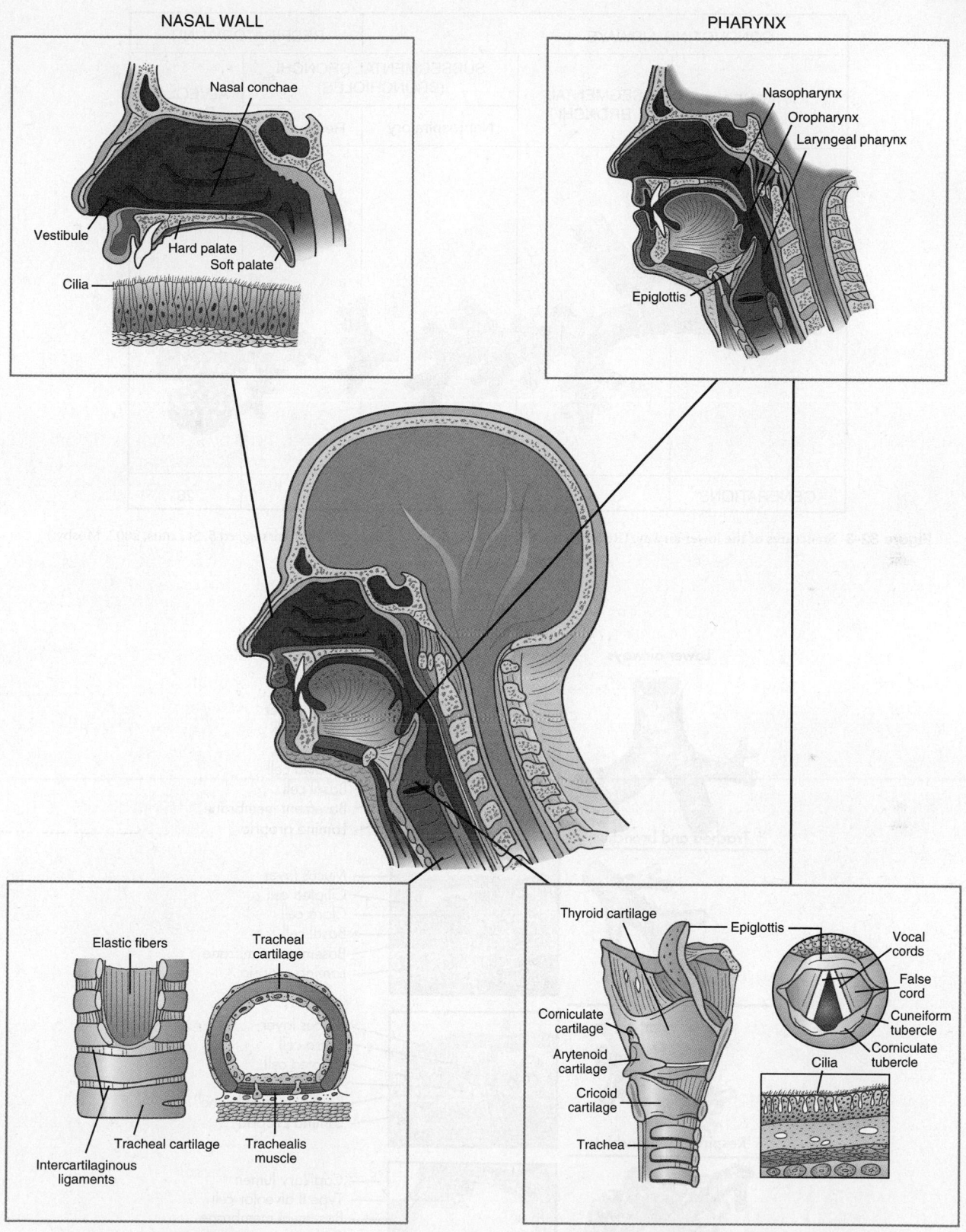

Figure 32-2 **Structures of the upper airway.** (Redrawn from Thompson JM et al: *Mosby's clinical nursing,* ed 5, St Louis, 2002, Mosby.)

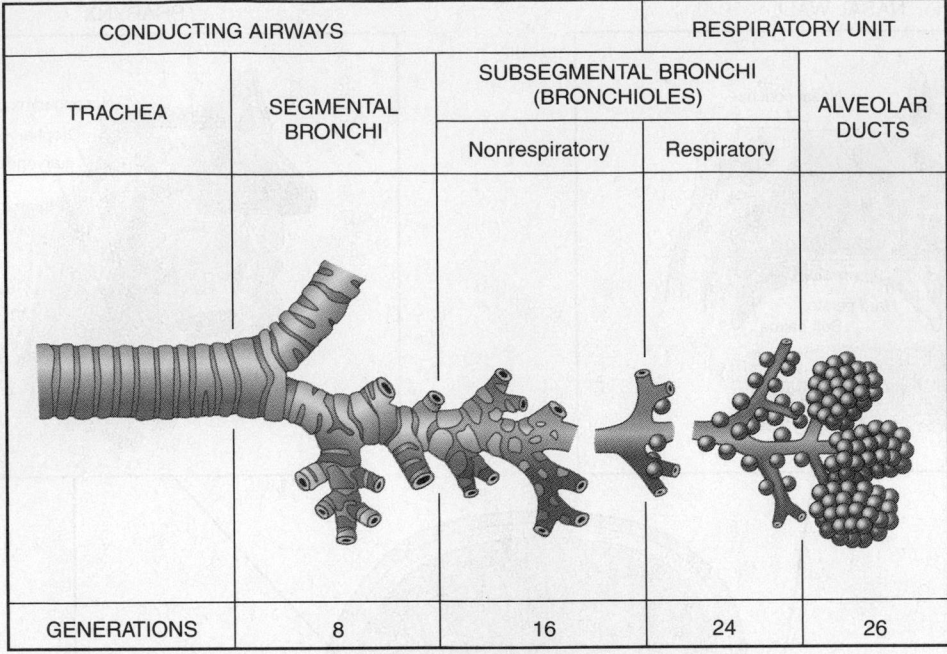

CONDUCTING AIRWAYS				RESPIRATORY UNIT
TRACHEA	SEGMENTAL BRONCHI	SUBSEGMENTAL BRONCHI (BRONCHIOLES)		ALVEOLAR DUCTS
		Nonrespiratory	Respiratory	
GENERATIONS	8	16	24	26

Figure 32-3 Structures of the lower airway. (Redrawn from Thompson JM et al: *Mosby's clinical nursing,* ed 5, St Louis, 2002, Mosby.)

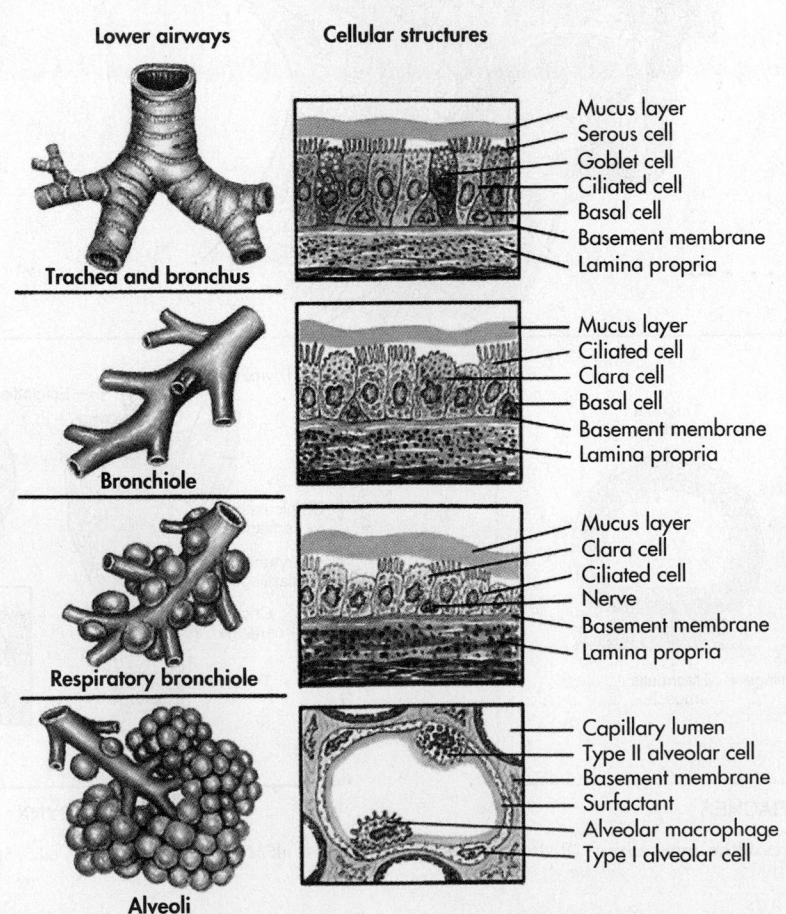

Figure 32-4 Changes in the bronchial wall with progressive branching. (From Wilson SF, Thompson JM: *Respiratory disorders,* St Louis, 1990, Mosby.)

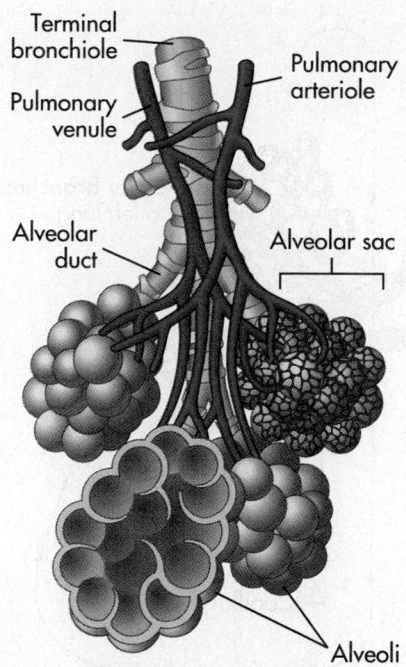

Figure 32-5 **Alveoli.** Bronchioles subdivide to form tiny tubes called *alveolar ducts* that end in clusters of alveoli called *alveolar sacs.* (From Patton KT, Thibodeau GA: *Anatomy & physiology,* ed 7, St Louis, 2010, Mosby.)

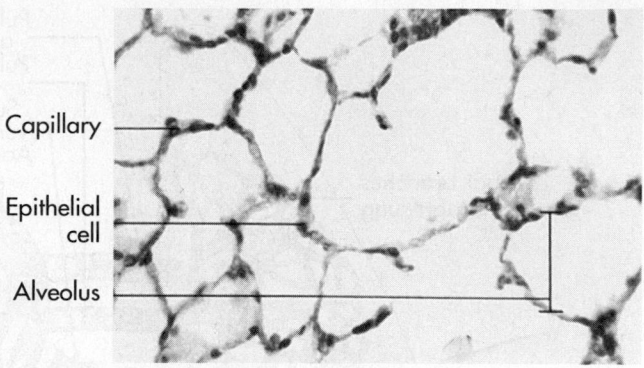

Figure 32-6 Photomicrograph of lung, showing several alveoli. Note the proximity of the capillary to the alveolar wall. (From Patton KT, Thibodeau GA: *Anatomy & physiology,* ed 7, St Louis, 2010, Mosby.)

Like the bronchi, alveoli contain cellular components of inflammation and immunity, particularly the mononuclear phagocytes. The mononuclear phagocytes of the lungs are called *alveolar macrophages.* These cells ingest foreign material that reaches the alveolus and prepare it for removal through the lymphatics.[1] (Phagocytosis and the mononuclear phagocyte system are described in Chapters 6 and 7.)

Pulmonary and Bronchial Circulation

The pulmonary circulation facilitates gas exchange, delivers nutrients to lung tissues, acts as a reservoir for the left ventricle, and serves as a filtering system that removes clots, air, and other debris from the circulation (Figure 32-7).

Although the entire cardiac output from the right ventricle goes into the lungs, the pulmonary circulation has a lower pressure and resistance than the systemic circulation. Pulmonary arteries are exposed to about one fifth the pressure of the systemic circulation and have a much thinner muscle layer. (Systemic vessels are described in Chapter 29.) Mean pulmonary artery pressure is 18 mmHg; mean aortic pressure is 90 mmHg. About one third of the pulmonary vessels are filled with blood (perfused) at any given time. More vessels become perfused when right ventricular cardiac output increases. Therefore, increased delivery of blood to the lungs does not normally increase mean pulmonary artery pressure.

The **pulmonary artery** divides and enters the lung at the hilus with each main bronchus and branches with the bronchus at every division so that every bronchus and bronchiole has an accompanying artery or arteriole. The arterioles, less

than 1 mm in diameter, regulate blood flow through their respective capillary beds.

The arterioles divide at the terminal bronchiole to form a network of **pulmonary capillaries** around the acinus. The capillaries are an integral part of the alveolar septa. Capillary walls consist of an endothelial layer and a thin basement membrane, which often fuses with the basement membrane of the alveolar septum (see Figure 32-6). This results in very little separation between blood in the capillary and gas in the alveolus.

The shared alveolar and capillary walls compose the **alveolocapillary membrane,** a very thin membrane made up of the alveolar epithelium, the alveolar basement membrane, an interstitial space, the capillary basement membrane, and the capillary endothelium (Figure 32-8). These extremely thin alveolar walls are easily damaged and can leak plasma and blood into the alveolar space. Gas exchange occurs across the alveolocapillary membrane. With normal perfusion approximately 100 ml of blood in the pulmonary capillary bed is spread very thinly over 70 to 100 m^2 of alveolar surface area. The alveolocapillary membrane efficiently exposes large quantities of blood to gas in the alveoli. Any disorder that thickens the membrane impairs gas exchange.

Each **pulmonary vein** drains several pulmonary capillaries. Unlike the pulmonary arteries, which follow the branching bronchi, pulmonary veins are dispersed randomly throughout the lung and then leave the lung at the hila and enter the left atrium. They are similar to veins in the systemic circulation, but they have no valves.

The bronchial circulation is part of the systemic circulation. It supplies nutrients to the conducting airways, nerves, lymph nodes, large pulmonary vessels, and membranes (pleurae) that surround the lungs.[2] The bronchial circulation is unique in that not all of its capillaries drain into its own venous system. Some of the bronchial capillaries empty into the pulmonary vein and contribute to the normal venous admixture (mixing of oxygenated and deoxygenated blood) or right-to-left shunt (right-to-left shunts are described in Chapter 33). The bronchial circulation does not participate in gas exchange.

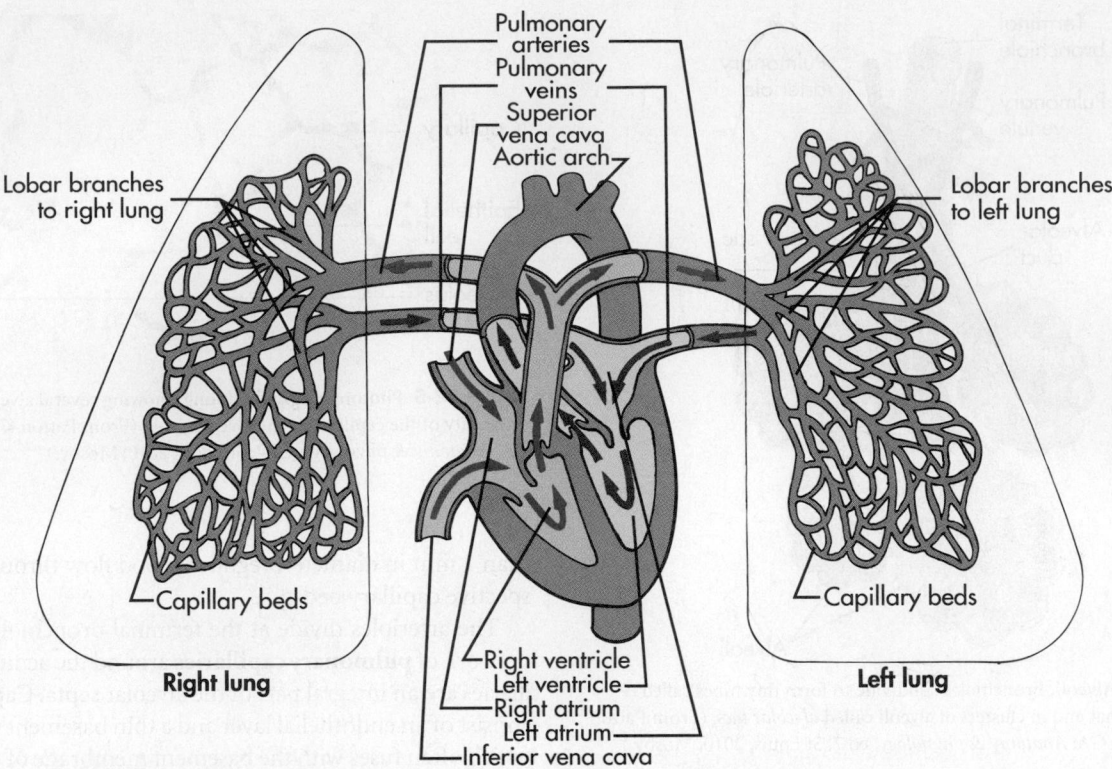

Figure 32-7 **The pulmonary circulation.** The right and left pulmonary veins and arteries and the branching capillaries are illustrated. Note the pulmonary artery carries venous blood, and the pulmonary vein carries arterial blood.

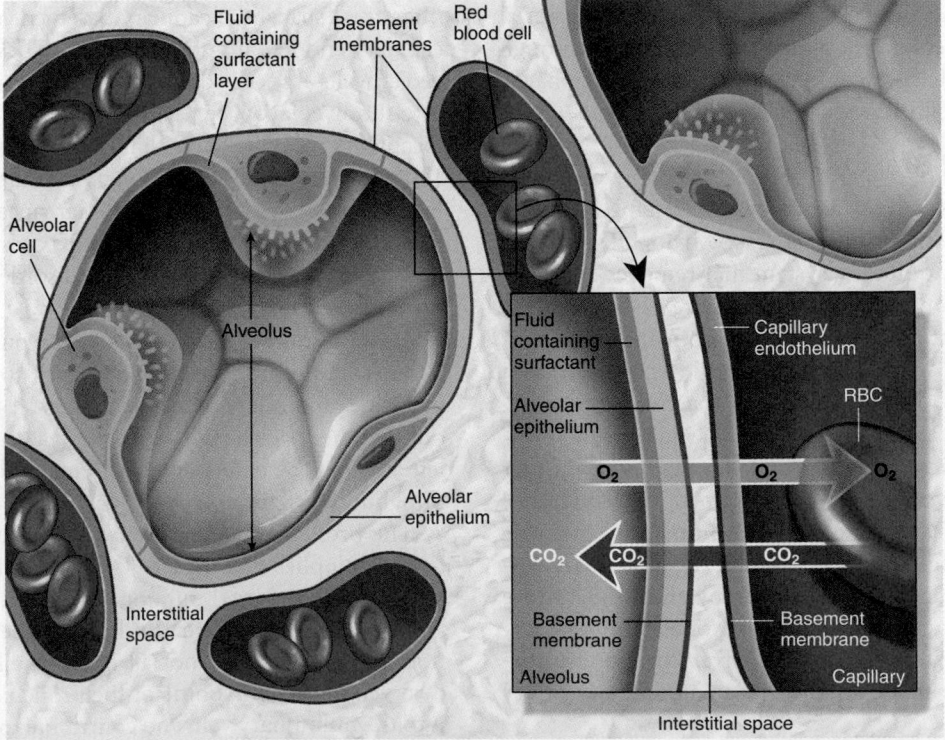

Figure 32-8 Section through the alveolar septum (gas-exchange membrane). *Inset* shows a magnified view of the respiratory membrane composed of the alveolar wall (fluid coating, epithelial cells, basement membrane), interstitial fluid, and wall of a pulmonary capillary (basement membrane, endothelial cells). The gases—carbon dioxide (CO_2) and oxygen (O_2)—diffuse across the respiratory membrane. (From Thibodeau GA, Patton KT: *Anatomy & physiology,* ed 6, St Louis, 2007, Mosby.)

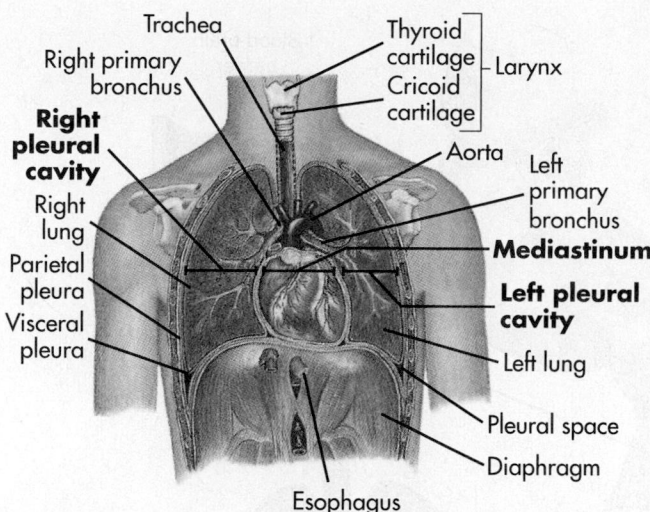

Figure 32-9 Thoracic (chest) cavity and related structures. The thoracic cavity is divided into three subdivisions (left and right pleural divisions and mediastinum) by a partition formed by a serous membrane called the *pleura*. (From Thibodeau GA, Patton KT: *Anatomy & physiology,* ed 3, St Louis, 1996, Mosby.)

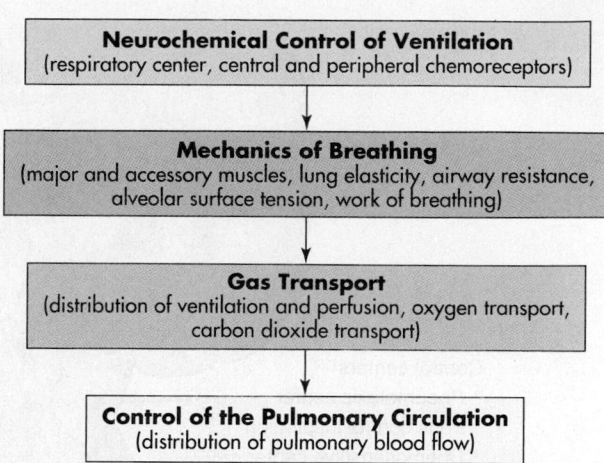

Figure 32-10 Functional components of the respiratory system. The central nervous system responds to neurochemical stimulation of ventilation and sends signals to the chest wall musculature. The response of the respiratory system to these impulses is influenced by several factors that affect the mechanisms of breathing and therefore affect the adequacy of ventilation. Gas transport between the alveoli and pulmonary capillary blood depends on a variety of physical and chemical activities. The control of the pulmonary circulation plays a role in the appropriate distribution of blood flow.

Lung vasculature also includes deep and superficial **lymphatic capillaries.** The deep lymphatic capillaries begin at the level of the terminal bronchioles; there are no lymphatic structures in the acinus. Fluid and alveolar macrophages migrate from the alveoli to the terminal bronchioles, where they enter the lymphatic system. The superficial lymphatic capillaries drain the membrane that surrounds the lungs. Both deep and superficial lymphatic vessels leave the lung at the hilus. The lymphatic system plays an important role in keeping the lung free of fluid. (The lymphatic system is described in Chapter 29.)

Chest Wall and Pleura

The chest wall (skin, ribs, intercostal muscles) protects the lungs from injury, and its muscles, in conjunction with the diaphragm, perform the muscular work of breathing. The **thoracic cavity** is contained by the chest wall and encases the lungs (Figure 32-9). A serous membrane called the **pleura** adheres firmly to the lungs. It then folds over itself and attaches firmly to the chest wall. The membrane covering the lungs is the visceral pleura; that lining the thoracic cavity is the parietal pleura. The area between the two pleurae is called the **pleural space,** or **pleural cavity.** Normally only a thin layer of fluid secreted by the pleura (pleural fluid) fills the pleural space. This lubricates the pleural surfaces, allowing the two layers to slide over each other without separating. Pressure in the pleural space is usually negative or subatmospheric (−4 to −10 mmHg).

FUNCTIONS OF THE PULMONARY SYSTEM

The pulmonary system functions to (1) ventilate the alveoli, (2) diffuse gases into and out of the blood, and (3) perfuse the lungs so that the organs and tissues of the body receive blood

that is rich in oxygen and low in CO_2. Each component of the pulmonary system contributes to one or more of these functions (Figure 32-10).

Ventilation

Ventilation is the mechanical movement of gas or air into and out of the lungs. Ventilation often is misnamed **respiration,** which is actually the exchange of O_2 and CO_2 during cellular metabolism. "Respiratory rate" is actually the ventilatory rate, or the number of times gas is inspired and expired per minute. The amount of effective ventilation is calculated by multiplying the ventilatory rate (breaths per minute) by the volume of air per breath (liters per breath, tidal volume). This is called the **minute volume** or minute ventilation and is expressed in liters per minute.

CO_2, the gaseous form of carbonic acid (H_2CO_3), is a product of cellular metabolism. The lung eliminates about 10,000 milliequivalents (mEq) of carbonic acid per day in the form of CO_2, which is produced at the rate of approximately 200 ml/minute. CO_2 elimination is necessary to maintain a normal arterial CO_2 ($Paco_2$) of 40 mmHg and normal acid-base balance (see Chapter 3 for a discussion of acid-base regulation).

The adequacy of **alveolar ventilation** *cannot* be accurately determined by observation of ventilatory rate, pattern, or effort. If a healthcare professional needs to determine the adequacy of ventilation, an arterial blood gas analysis must be performed to measure $Paco_2$.

Neurochemical Control of Ventilation

The mechanisms that control respiration are very complex.[1-5] Breathing is usually involuntary because homeostatic changes in the ventilatory rate and volume are adjusted automatically

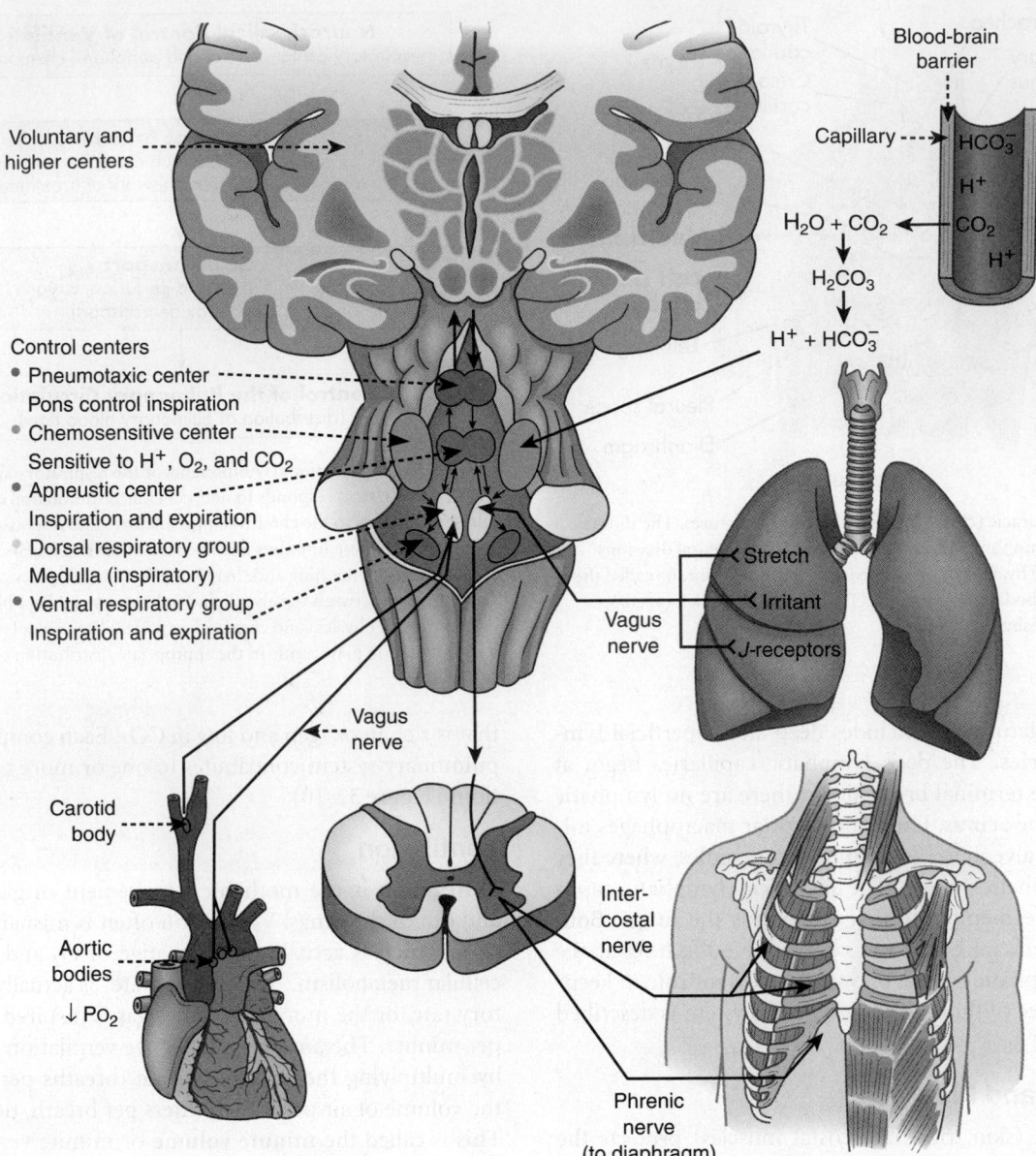

Voluntary and higher centers

Blood-brain barrier

Capillary

HCO_3^-

H^+

$H_2O + CO_2 \leftarrow CO_2$

H^+

H_2CO_3

$H^+ + HCO_3^-$

Control centers
- Pneumotaxic center
  Pons control inspiration
- Chemosensitive center
  Sensitive to H^+, O_2, and CO_2
- Apneustic center
  Inspiration and expiration
- Dorsal respiratory group
  Medulla (inspiratory)
- Ventral respiratory group
  Inspiration and expiration

Stretch

Irritant

Vagus nerve

J-receptors

Vagus nerve

Carotid body

Aortic bodies

$\downarrow PO_2$

Inter-costal nerve

Phrenic nerve (to diaphragm)

Figure 32-11 Neurochemical respiratory control system.

by the nervous system to maintain normal gas exchange. Voluntary breathing is necessary for talking, singing, laughing, and holding one's breath.

The **respiratory center** in the brainstem controls respiration by transmitting impulses to the respiratory muscles, causing them to contract and relax (Figure 32-11). The respiratory center is composed of several groups of neurons located bilaterally in the brainstem: the dorsal respiratory group (DRG), the ventral respiratory group (VRG), the pneumotaxic center, and the apneustic center.[1,4] The basic automatic rhythm of respiration is set by the DRG, a cluster of inspiratory nerve cells located in the medulla that sends efferent impulses to the diaphragm and inspiratory intercostal muscles. The DRG also receives afferent impulses from

peripheral chemoreceptors in the carotid and aortic bodies, which detect the Pa_{CO_2} and the amount of oxygen in the arterial blood (Pa_{O_2}). In addition, several different types of receptors in the lungs stimulate the VRG through afferent nerves. The VRG, also located in the medulla, contains inspiratory and expiratory neurons. It is almost inactive during normal, quiet respiration, becoming active when increased ventilatory effort is required. The pneumotaxic center and apneustic center, situated in the pons, do not generate primary rhythm but rather act as modifiers of the inspiratory depth and rate established by the medullary centers.[4] Breathing can be modified by input from the cortex, the limbic system, and the hypothalamus, and the pattern of breathing can be influenced by emotion and by disease.

$\uparrow CO_2 \rightarrow BBB \rightarrow CO_2 + H_2O = H^+ H_2CO_3$

Lung Receptors

Three types of lung receptors send impulses from the lungs to the dorsal respiratory group:

1. **Irritant receptors** are found in the epithelium of the conducting airways. They are sensitive to noxious aerosols (vapors), gases, and particulate matter (e.g., inhaled dusts), which cause them to initiate the cough reflex. When stimulated, irritant receptors also cause bronchoconstriction and increased ventilatory rate. These receptors are located primarily in the proximal larger airways and are nearly absent in the distal airways; thus it is possible for secretions to accumulate in the distal respiratory tree without initiating cough.

2. **Stretch receptors** are located in the smooth muscles of airways and are sensitive to increases in the size or volume of the lungs. They decrease ventilatory rate and volume when stimulated, an occurrence sometimes referred to as the *Hering-Breuer expiratory reflex*. This reflex is active in newborns and assists with ventilation. In adults, this reflex is active only at high tidal volumes (such as with exercise and mechanical ventilation) and may play a role in protecting against excess lung inflation.[6] Stretch receptors called **rapidly adapting receptors** have been found to be an important mediator of cough.[7]

3. **J-receptors** (juxtapulmonary capillary receptors) are located near the capillaries in the alveolar septa. They are sensitive to increased pulmonary capillary pressure, which stimulates them to initiate rapid, shallow breathing; hypotension; and bradycardia.[4]

The lung is innervated by the autonomic nervous system (ANS). Fibers of the sympathetic division of the ANS in the lung branch from the upper thoracic and cervical ganglia of the spinal cord. Fibers of the parasympathetic division of the ANS travel in the vagus nerve to the lung. (Structures and function of the ANS are discussed in detail in Chapter 14.) The parasympathetic and sympathetic divisions of the ANS control airway caliber (interior diameter of the airway lumen) by stimulating bronchial smooth muscle to contract or relax. The parasympathetic receptors cause smooth muscle to contract, whereas sympathetic receptors cause it to relax. Bronchial smooth muscle tone depends on equilibrium, that is, equal stimulation of contraction and relaxation. The parasympathetic division of the ANS is the main controller of airway caliber under normal conditions.[4] Constriction occurs if the irritant receptors in the airway epithelium are stimulated by irritants in inspired air, by endogenous substances (e.g., histamine, serotonin, prostaglandins), by many drugs, and by humoral substances.

Chemoreceptors

Chemoreceptors monitor pH, $Paco_2$, and Pao_2. **Central chemoreceptors** monitor arterial blood indirectly by sensing changes in the pH of cerebrospinal fluid (CSF).[5] They are located near the respiratory center and are sensitive to hydrogen ion concentration in the CSF. (Chapter 3 describes the relationship between ions and the pH, or acid-base status, of

body fluids.) The pH, or concentration of hydrogen ions in the CSF, reflects $Paco_2$ because, unlike H^+ ions, CO_2 in arterial blood diffuses across the blood-brain barrier (the capillary wall separating blood from cells of the central nervous system) into the CSF until the partial pressure of CO_2 (Pco_2) is equal on both sides. CO_2 that has entered the CSF combines with H_2O to form carbonic acid, which subsequently dissociates into hydrogen ions that are capable of stimulating the central chemoreceptors. In this way $Paco_2$ regulates ventilation through its effect on the pH (hydrogen ion content) of the CSF.[1,4]

If alveolar ventilation is inadequate, $Paco_2$ increases. CO_2 diffuses across the blood-brain barrier until Pco_2 in the blood and CSF reaches equilibrium. As the central chemoreceptors sense the resulting decrease in pH (increase in hydrogen ion concentration), they stimulate the respiratory center to increase the depth and rate of ventilation. Increased ventilation causes the $Paco_2$ to decrease below that of the CSF, and CO_2 diffuses back out of the CSF, returning its pH to normal.

$\uparrow CO_2$
$\uparrow H^+$
$\downarrow pH$

The central chemoreceptors are sensitive to very small changes in the pH of CSF (equivalent to a 1- to 2-mmHg change in Pco_2) and are able to maintain a normal $Paco_2$ under many different conditions, including strenuous exercise. If inadequate ventilation, or hypoventilation, is long term (e.g., in chronic obstructive pulmonary disease), these receptors become insensitive to small changes in $Paco_2$ and regulate ventilation poorly. In addition, prolonged increases in $Paco_2$ result in renal compensation through bicarbonate retention. This bicarbonate gradually diffuses into the CSF, where it normalizes the pH and negates the effect on ventilatory drive.[1,4]

The **peripheral chemoreceptors** are located in aortic bodies, the aortic arch, and carotid bodies at the bifurcation of the carotids, near the baroreceptors (see Chapter 29). Although the peripheral chemoreceptors are sensitive to changes in $Paco_2$ and pH, they are primarily sensitive to oxygen levels in arterial blood (Pao_2) and are responsible for all of the increase in ventilation that occurs in response to arterial hypoxemia.[4] As Pao_2 and pH decrease, peripheral chemoreceptors, particularly in the carotid bodies, send signals to the respiratory center to increase ventilation. The peripheral chemoreceptors are not as sensitive as the central chemoreceptors. The Pao_2 must drop well below normal (to approximately 60 mmHg) before the peripheral chemoreceptors have much influence on ventilation. If $Paco_2$ is elevated as well, however, ventilation increases much more than it would in response to either abnormality alone. The peripheral chemoreceptors become the major stimulus to ventilation when the central chemoreceptors are "reset" by chronic hypoventilation.

Mechanics of Breathing

The mechanical aspects of inspiration and expiration are known collectively as the *mechanics of breathing* and involve (1) major and accessory muscles of inspiration and expiration, (2) elastic properties of the lungs and chest wall, and (3) resistance to airflow through the conducting airways.

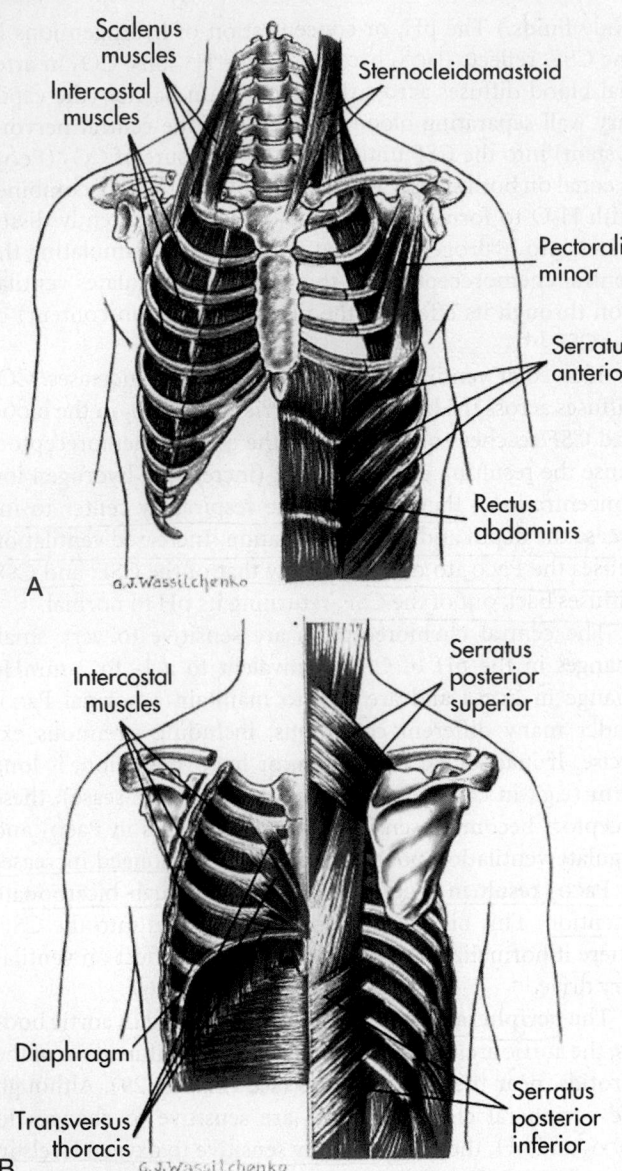

Figure 32-12 Muscles of ventilation. **A,** Anterior view. **B,** Posterior view. (From Wilson SF, Thompson JM: *Respiratory disorders,* St Louis, 1990, Mosby.)

Alterations in any of these properties increase the work of breathing, or the metabolic energy that must be exerted to achieve adequate ventilation and oxygenation of the blood.

Major and Accessory Muscles

The major muscles of inspiration are the **diaphragm** and the external intercostal muscles (muscles between the ribs) (Figure 32-12). The diaphragm is a dome-shaped muscle that separates the abdominal and thoracic cavities. When the diaphragm contracts, it flattens downward, increasing the volume of the thoracic cavity, and creates a negative pressure that draws gas into the lungs through the upper airways and trachea. Contraction of external intercostal muscles elevates the anterior portion of the ribs. This increases the volume of the thoracic cavity by increasing its front-to-back

(anteroposterior [AP]) diameter. Although the external intercostal muscles may contract during quiet breathing, inspiration at rest usually is assisted by the diaphragm only.

The accessory muscles of inspiration are the sternocleidomastoid and scalene muscles. Like the external intercostal muscles, these muscles enlarge the thorax by increasing its AP diameter. The accessory muscles of inspiration assist inspiration when minute volume (volume of air inspired and expired per minute) is very high, such as during strenuous exercise or when the work of breathing is increased because of disease. The accessory muscles do not increase the volume of the thorax as efficiently as the diaphragm does.

There are no major muscles of expiration because normal, relaxed expiration is passive and requires no muscular effort. The accessory muscles of expiration, the abdominal and internal intercostal muscles, assist expiration when minute volume is high, during coughing, or when airway obstruction is present. When the abdominal muscles contract, intra-abdominal pressure increases, pushing up the diaphragm and decreasing the volume of the thorax. The internal intercostal muscles pull down the anterior ribs, decreasing the AP diameter of the thorax.

Alveolar Surface Tension

Surface tension occurs at any gas-liquid interface and refers to the tendency for liquid molecules that are exposed to air to adhere to one another. This phenomenon can be seen, for example, in a glass of liquid that is about to overflow or in the way liquids "bead" when splashed on a waterproof surface. In both examples this phenomenon decreases the surface area exposed to the air.

Within a sphere, such as an alveolus, surface tension tends to make expansion difficult. According to the law of Laplace, the pressure (P) required to inflate a sphere is equal to two times the surface tension (2T) divided by the radius (r) of the sphere, or $P = (2T/r)$.[1] As the radius of the sphere (or alveolus) becomes smaller, more and more pressure is required to inflate it. If the alveoli were lined with a water-like fluid, taking breaths would be extremely difficult.

Alveolar ventilation, or distention, is made possible by surfactant, which lowers the surface tension by coating the air-liquid interface in the alveoli. Surfactant, a lipoprotein produced by type II alveolar cells (see Figure 32-4), has a detergent-like effect that separates the liquid molecules, thereby decreasing alveolar surface tension.

Surfactant lines the alveolar side of the alveolocapillary membrane and, in effect, reverses Laplace's law. As the radius of a surfactant-lined sphere (alveolus) grows smaller, the surface tension *decreases,* and as the radius grows larger, the surface tension *increases.* This occurs because the surfactant molecules have much weaker intermolecular attraction compared with the liquid molecules. The surfactant molecules occupy most of the air-fluid interface and disrupt the intermolecular forces that tend to collapse the alveoli. Therefore, the alveoli are much easier to inflate at low lung volumes (i.e., after expiration) than at high volumes (i.e., after inspiration). If surfactant production is disrupted or surfactant is not produced in adequate quantities, alveolar surface tension increases and results in alveolar collapse, decreased lung expansion, increased work of breathing, and severe gas-exchange abnormalities (see What's New? Update on Surfactant).

The decrease in surface tension caused by surfactant is also responsible for keeping the alveoli free of fluid. In the absence of surfactant, the surface tension tends to attract fluid into the alveoli. In addition, surfactant participates in host defense against respiratory pathogens.[1,8]

Elastic Properties of the Lung and Chest Wall

The lung and chest wall have elastic properties that permit expansion during inspiration and return to resting volume during expiration. The elasticity of the lungs is caused both by elastin fibers in the alveolar walls and surrounding the small airways and pulmonary capillaries and by surface tension at the alveolar air-liquid interface.[1] The elasticity of the chest wall is the result of the configuration of its bones and musculature.

Elastic recoil is the tendency of the lungs to return to the resting state after inspiration. Normal elastic recoil permits passive expiration, eliminating the need for major muscles of expiration. Passive elastic recoil may be insufficient during labored breathing (high minute volume), in which case the accessory muscles of expiration may be needed. The accessory muscles also are used if disease comprises elastic recoil (e.g., in emphysema) or blocks the conducting airways.

Normal elastic recoil depends on an equilibrium between opposing forces of recoil in the lungs and chest wall. Under normal conditions the chest wall tends to recoil by expanding outward. This can be observed readily during open heart surgery. When the sternum is split to open the thoracic cavity, the chest wall moves outward laterally. The tendency of the chest wall to recoil by expanding is balanced by the tendency of the lungs to recoil or collapse around the hila. This reaction is caused by elastic recoil and surface tension in the alveoli. The tendency of the lungs to collapse can be demonstrated if the chest is opened without mechanically ventilating the lungs (e.g., at postmortem examination). As the thorax is opened, the lungs immediately collapse, like inflated balloons that have been released. The opposing forces of the chest wall and lungs create, in part, the small negative intrapleural pressure.

Balance between the outward recoil of the chest wall and inward recoil of the lungs occurs at the resting level, at the end of expiration. During inspiration the diaphragm and intercostal muscles contract, air flows into the lungs, and the chest wall expands. Muscular effort is needed to overcome the resistance of the lungs to expansion. During expiration the muscles relax and the elastic recoil of the lungs causes the thorax to decrease in volume until, once again, balance between the chest wall and lung recoil forces is reached[1] (Figure 32-13).

Compliance is the measure of lung and chest wall distensibility. It represents the relative ease with which these structures can be stretched. Compliance is therefore the reciprocal of elasticity. Compliance is determined by alveolar surface tension and the elastic recoil of the lung and chest wall. It can be measured with the following formula:

$$C = \frac{\Delta V}{\Delta P}$$

where C = compliance in liters per centimeter of water, ΔV = volume change (usually tidal volume), and ΔP = pressure change (airway or pleural pressure) in centimeters of water.[1,9]

Increased compliance indicates that the lungs or chest wall is abnormally easy to inflate and has lost some elastic recoil. A decrease indicates that the lungs or chest wall is abnormally stiff or difficult to inflate. Compliance is increased in emphysema and decreased in acute respiratory distress syndrome, pneumonia, pulmonary edema, and fibrosis. (These disorders are described in Chapter 33.)

Airway Resistance

Airway resistance, which is similar to resistance to blood flow (described in Chapter 29), is determined by the length, radius, and cross-sectional area of the airways and density, viscosity, and velocity of the gas (Poiseuille's law). Resistance is computed by dividing change in pressure *(P)* by rate of flow *(F)*, or $R = \{P/F\}$ (Ohm's law) and can easily be measured in the pulmonary function laboratory.[5] Airway resistance is normally very low. One half to two thirds of total airway resistance occur in the nose. The next highest resistance is in the oropharynx and larynx. There is very little resistance in the conducting airways of the lungs because of their large cross-sectional area. Resistance increases as the diameter of the airways (total cross-sectional area) decreases; airway resistance

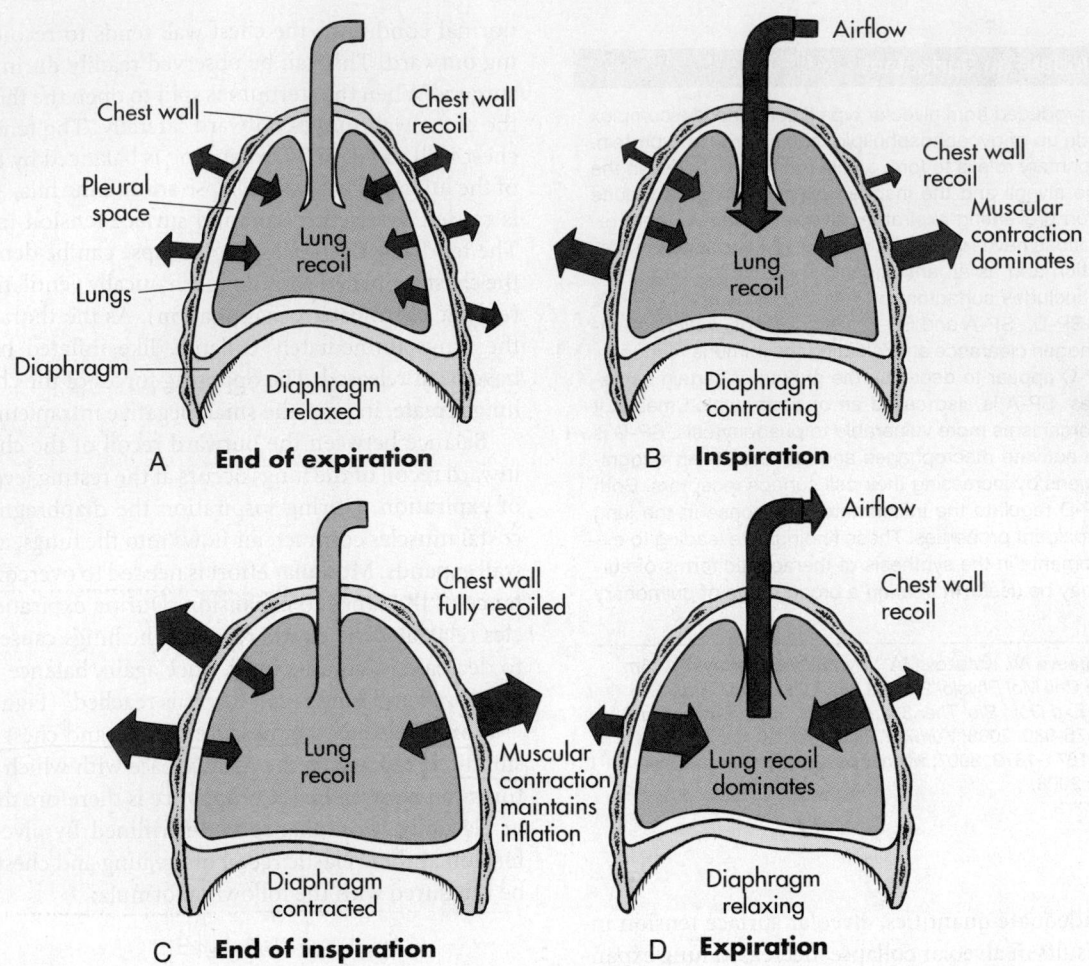

Figure 32-13 Interaction of forces during inspiration and expiration. **A,** Outward recoil of the chest wall equals inward recoil of the lungs at the end of expiration. **B,** During inspiration, contraction of respiratory muscles, assisted by chest wall recoil, overcomes tendency of lungs to recoil. **C,** At the end of inspiration, respiratory muscle contraction maintains lung expansion. **D,** During expiration, respiratory muscles relax, allowing elastic recoil of the lungs to deflate the lungs.

increases when the diameter of the airways decreases. **Bronchoconstriction**, which increases airway resistance, can be caused by stimulation of parasympathetic receptors in the bronchial smooth muscle and by numerous irritants and inflammatory mediators.[2] **Bronchodilation**, which decreases resistance to airflow, is caused by β_2-adrenergic receptor stimulation. Airway resistance also can be increased by edema of the bronchial mucosa and by airway obstructions such as mucus, tumors, or foreign bodies.

Work of Breathing

The **work of breathing** is determined by the muscular effort (and therefore oxygen and energy) required for ventilation. The work of breathing is normally very low but may increase considerably in disease states that disrupt the equilibrium between forces exerted by the lung and chest wall. More muscular effort is required when lung compliance is decreased (e.g., in pulmonary edema), chest wall compliance is decreased (e.g., in spinal deformity or obesity), or airways are obstructed by bronchospasm or mucous plugging (e.g., in asthma or bronchitis).[9] An increase in the work of breathing

can result in a marked increase in oxygen consumption and metabolic demand, which can cause significant morbidity in individuals with severe lung disease.

Measurement of Gas Pressure

A gas is made up of millions of molecules moving randomly. As they move, they collide with each other and the wall of the space in which they are contained. These collisions exert pressure. If more molecules are present in the space, the pressure, or number of collisions, increases (Figure 32-14). If the same number of gas molecules is contained in a small and a large container, the pressure is greater in the small container because more collisions occur in the smaller space. Heat increases the speed of the molecules, which increases the number of collisions. Therefore, pressure also increases at higher temperatures.

Barometric pressure (P_B) (atmospheric pressure) is the pressure exerted by gas molecules in air at specific altitudes. At sea level, barometric pressure is 760 mmHg. This number is the sum of the pressure exerted by each gas in the air at sea level. The portion of the total pressure exerted by any

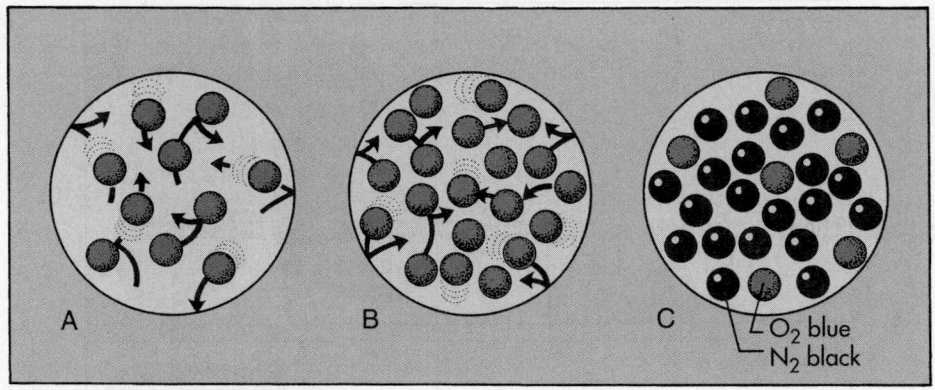

Figure 32-14 Relationship between number of gas molecules and pressure exerted by the gas in an enclosed space. *(A)*, Theoretically 10 molecules of the same gas exert a total pressure of 10 within the space. *(B)*, If the number of molecules is increased to 20, total pressure is 20. *(C)*, If there are different gases in the space, each gas exerts a partial pressure: here the partial pressure of nitrogen (N_2) is 18, that of oxygen (O_2) is 6, and total pressure is 24.

Table 32-2	Common Pulmonary Abbreviations
Symbol	**Definition**
V	Volume or amount of gas
Q	Perfusion or blood flow
P	Pressure (usually partial pressure) of a gas
Pa_{O_2}	Partial pressure of oxygen in arterial blood
PA_{O_2}	Partial pressure of oxygen in alveolar blood
Pa_{CO_2}	Partial pressure of carbon dioxide in arterial blood
PH_2O	Partial pressure water vapor
P_{N_2}	Partial pressure of nitrogen
$P\bar{v}_{O_2}$	Partial pressure of oxygen in mixed venous or pulmonary artery blood
$P(A-a)_{O_2}$	Difference between alveolar and arterial partial pressure of oxygen (A–a gradient)
P_B	Barometric or atmospheric pressure
Sa_{O_2}	Saturation of hemoglobin (in arterial blood) with oxygen
$S\bar{v}_{O_2}$	Saturation of hemoglobin (in mixed venous blood)
V_A	Alveolar ventilation
V_D	Dead-space ventilation
V_E	Minute capacity
V_T	Tidal volume or average breath
$\dot{V}/\dot{Q}$	Ratio of ventilation to perfusion
Fi_{O_2}	Fraction of inspired oxygen
FRC	Functional residual capacity
FVC	Forced vital capacity
FEV_1	Forced expiratory volume in one second

Subscripts identify the particular gas, volume, or pressure being discussed. A dot (·) means measurement over time, usually 1 minute.

individual gas is its **partial pressure** (see Figure 32-14). At sea level the air is made up of oxygen (20.9%), nitrogen (78.1%), and a few other trace gases. The partial pressure of oxygen is equal to the percentage of oxygen in the air (20.9%) times the total pressure (760 mmHg), or 159 mmHg (760 × 0.209 = 158.84). (Symbols used in the measurement of gas pressures and pulmonary ventilation are defined in Table 32-2.)

The amount of water vapor contained in a gas mixture is determined by the temperature of the gas and is unrelated to barometric pressure. Gas that enters the lungs becomes saturated with water vapor (humidified) as it passes through the upper airway. At body temperature (37° C, 98.6° F), water vapor exerts a pressure of 47 mmHg. Because this is true regardless of total (barometric) pressure, the partial pressure of water vapor (always 47 mmHg) must be subtracted from the barometric pressure before the partial pressure of other gases in the mixture can be determined. In saturated air at sea level, the partial pressure of oxygen is therefore (760 − 47) × 0.209 = 149. All pressure and volume measurements made in pulmonary function laboratories specify the temperature and humidity of a gas at the time of measurement.

Many pressure measurements are stated as variations from barometric pressure, rather than percentages of it. On such scales, barometric pressure is considered zero, and pressure varies up or down from zero. Physiologic pressure measurements that involve fluids, rather than gases, are measured as variations from barometric pressure. For example, a systolic blood pressure of 120 mmHg indicates that systolic pressure is 120 mmHg above barometric pressure.

Gas Transport

Gas transport, the delivery of oxygen to the cells of the body and the removal of CO_2, has four steps:
1. Ventilation of the lungs
2. Diffusion of oxygen from the alveoli into the capillary blood
3. Perfusion of systemic capillaries with oxygenated blood
4. Diffusion of oxygen from systemic capillaries into the cells

Steps in the transport of CO_2 occur in reverse order:
1. Diffusion of CO_2 from the cells into the systemic capillaries
2. Perfusion of the pulmonary capillary bed by venous blood

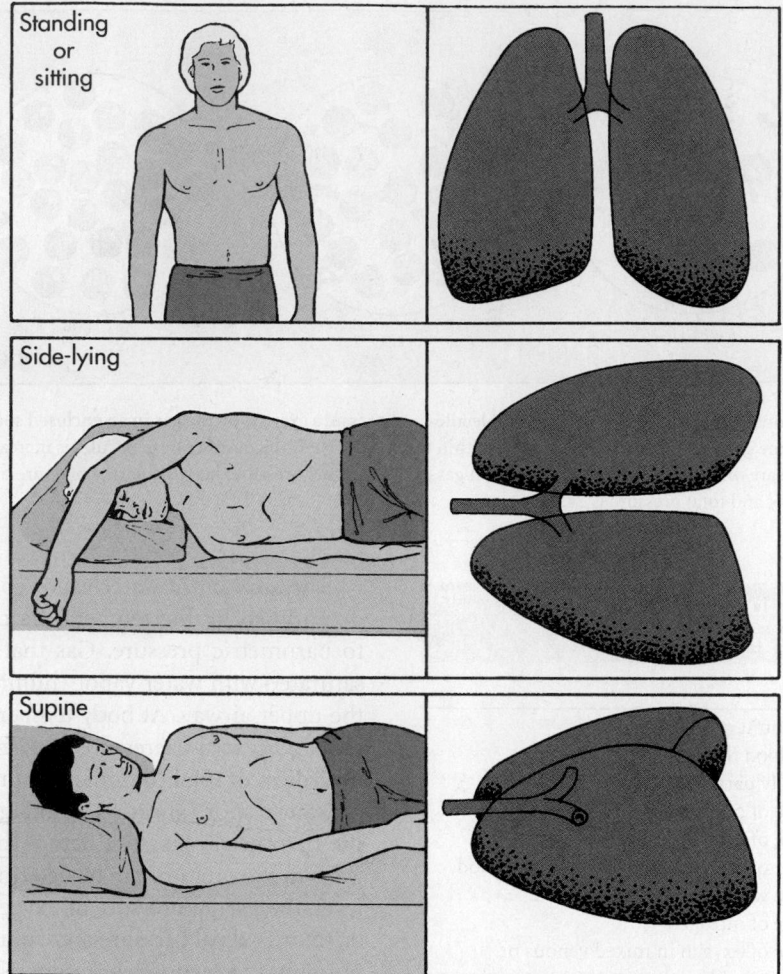

Figure 32-15 Pulmonary blood flow and gravity. The greatest volume of pulmonary blood flow will normally occur in the gravity-dependent areas of the lungs. Body position has a significant effect on the distribution of pulmonary blood flow.

3. Diffusion of CO_2 into the alveoli
4. Removal of CO_2 from the lung by ventilation

If any step in gas transport is impaired by a respiratory or cardiovascular disorder, gas exchange at the cellular level is compromised.

Distribution of Ventilation and Perfusion

Effective gas exchange depends on an approximately even distribution of gas (ventilation) and blood (perfusion) in all portions of the lungs. The lungs are suspended from the hila in the thoracic cavity. When the individual is in an upright position (sitting or standing), gravity pulls the lungs down toward the diaphragm and compresses their lower portions or bases. The alveoli in the upper portions, or apices, of the lungs contain a greater residual volume of gas and are larger and less numerous than those in the lower portions. Because surface tension increases as the alveoli become larger, the larger alveoli in the upper portions of the lung are more difficult to inflate (less compliant) than the smaller alveoli in the lower portions of the lung. Therefore, during ventilation most of

the tidal volume is distributed to the bases of the lungs, where compliance is greater.

The heart pumps against gravity to perfuse the pulmonary circulation. As blood is pumped into the lung apices of a sitting or standing individual, some blood pressure is dissipated in overcoming gravity. As a result, blood pressure at the apices is lower than that at the bases. Because greater pressure causes greater perfusion, the bases of the lungs are better perfused than the apices (Figure 32-15). Thus ventilation and perfusion are greatest in the same lung portions: the lower lobes. Ventilation and perfusion depend on body position. If a standing individual assumes a supine or side-lying position, the areas of the lungs that are then most dependent become the best ventilated and perfused.

Distribution of perfusion in the pulmonary circulation also is affected by alveolar pressure (gas pressure in the alveoli). The pulmonary capillary bed differs from the systemic capillary bed in that it is surrounded by gas-containing alveoli. If the gas pressure in the alveoli exceeds the blood pressure in the capillary, the capillary collapses and flow ceases. This is

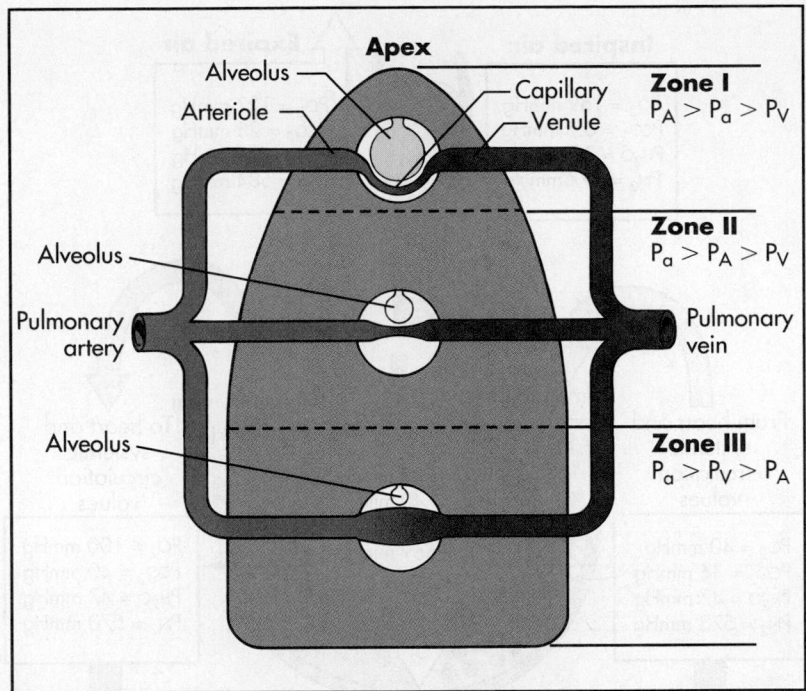

Figure 32-16 Gravity and alveolar pressure. Effects of gravity and alveolar pressure on pulmonary blood flow in the three lung zones. In zone I, alveolar pressure (P_A) is greater than arterial and venous pressure, and no blood flow occurs. In zone II, arterial pressure (P_a) exceeds alveolar pressure, but alveolar pressure exceeds venous pressure (P_V). Blood flow occurs in this zone, but alveolar pressure compresses the venules (venous ends of the capillaries). In zone III, both arterial and venous pressures are greater than alveolar pressure and blood flow fluctuates, depending on the difference between arterial and venous pressures.

most likely to occur in portions of the lung where blood pressure is lowest and alveolar gas pressure is greatest, that is, the apex of the lung.

The lungs are divided into three zones on the basis of the relationships among all the factors affecting pulmonary blood flow. Alveolar pressure plus the forces of gravity, arterial blood pressure, and venous blood pressure affect the distribution of perfusion (Figure 32-16).

Zone I is where alveolar pressure exceeds pulmonary arterial and venous pressures. The capillary bed collapses, and normal blood flow ceases. Normally zone I is a very small part of the lung at the apex. Zone II is the portion where alveolar pressure is greater than venous pressure but not greater than arterial pressure. Blood flows through zone II, but it is impeded to a certain extent by alveolar pressure. Zone II is normally above the level of the left atrium. In zone III arterial and venous pressures are greater than alveolar pressure and blood flow is not affected by alveolar pressure. Zone III is in the base of the lung. Blood flow through the pulmonary capillary bed increases in regular increments from the apex to the base.

Although blood flow and ventilation are greater at the base of the lungs than at the apices, they are not perfectly matched in any of the zones. Perfusion exceeds ventilation in the bases of the lungs, and ventilation exceeds perfusion in the apices of the lung. The relationship between ventilation and perfusion is expressed as a ratio called the **ventilation-perfusion ratio**, or $\dot{V}/\dot{Q}$.[1,4] The normal $\dot{V}/\dot{Q}$ ratio is 0.8. This is the amount by which perfusion exceeds ventilation under normal conditions.

Oxygen Transport

Approximately 1000 ml (1 L) of oxygen is transported to the cells each minute. Oxygen is transported in the blood in two forms. A small amount dissolves in plasma, and the remainder binds to hemoglobin molecules. Without hemoglobin, oxygen would not reach the cells in amounts sufficient to maintain normal metabolic function. (Hemoglobin is discussed in detail in Chapter 25; cellular metabolism is discussed in Chapter 1.)

Diffusion Across the Alveolocapillary Membrane

The alveolocapillary membrane is the ideal medium for oxygen diffusion because it has a large total surface area (70 to 100 m²) and is very thin (0.5 μm). In addition, the partial pressure of oxygen molecules (P_{O_2}) is much greater in alveolar gas than in capillary blood, a condition that promotes rapid diffusion down the concentration gradient from the alveolus into the capillary.

The amount of oxygen in the alveoli (P_{AO_2}) depends on the amount of oxygen in the inspired air (see p. 1255) and on the amount of air that remains in the alveoli and tracheobronchial tree between breaths (**physiologic dead space**).[1,4] This can be estimated by using the alveolar gas equation:

$$P_{AO_2} = 149 - Pa_{CO_2}/0.8 \text{ (the respiratory quotient)}$$

This value is approximately 104 with relaxed breathing; therefore a pressure gradient of approximately 60 mmHg

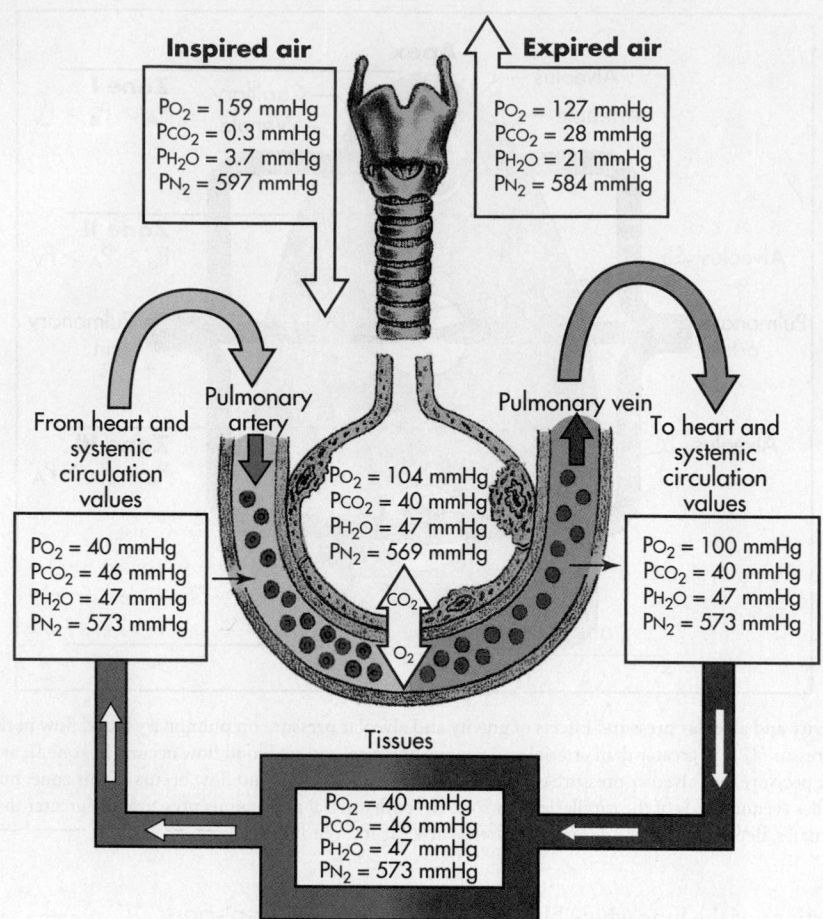

Figure 32-17 **Partial pressure of respiratory gases in normal respiration.** These are average values. The values of Po_2, Pco_2, and PN_2 fluctuate from breath to breath. CO_2, Carbon dioxide; H_2O, water; N, nitrogen; O_2, oxygen; Pco_2, partial pressure of carbon dioxide; PH_2O, partial *pressure* of water; PN_2, partial pressure of nitrogen; Po_2, partial pressure of oxygen.

facilitates the diffusion of oxygen from the alveolus into the capillary (Figure 32-17). Different values for Pao_2 can be calculated if there are changes in the inspired oxygen content or the $Paco_2$, which are common occurrences in clinical settings.

Blood remains in the pulmonary capillary for about 0.75 second, but only 0.25 second is required for oxygen concentration to equilibrate (equalize) across the alveolocapillary membrane. Therefore, oxygen has ample time to diffuse into the blood, even during increased cardiac output, which speeds blood flow, shortening the time the blood remains in the capillary.

Determinants of Arterial Oxygenation

As oxygen diffuses across the alveolocapillary membrane, it dissolves in the plasma, where it exerts pressure (the partial pressure of oxygen in arterial blood, or Pao_2). As the Pao_2 increases, oxygen moves from the plasma into the red blood cells (erythrocytes) and binds with hemoglobin molecules. Oxygen continues to bind with hemoglobin until the hemoglobin binding sites are filled or saturated. Oxygen then continues to diffuse across the alveolocapillary membrane until the Pao_2 and Pao_2 equilibrate, eliminating the pressure gradient across

the alveolocapillary membrane. At this point diffusion ceases (see Figure 32-17).

Normally approximately 20 ml of oxygen is transported per 100 ml of blood. Because oxygen is not very soluble in plasma, most of the oxygen molecules bind with hemoglobin. Plasma carries only about 0.3 ml of oxygen per 100 ml of blood (at sea level). Although the remaining 19.7 ml is carried by hemoglobin, it is the small amount of oxygen dissolved in plasma that is responsible for oxygen's partial pressure (Pao_2) in the blood.

Although Pao_2 is important in that it provides the driving pressure that loads the hemoglobin with oxygen, it gives little information about the *amount* of oxygen carried in the blood. This amount, which is measured in milliliters per deciliter (100 ml) of blood, is the **oxygen content** of the blood. The total oxygen content of the blood depends on the amount of oxygen chemically combined with hemoglobin, as well as that dissolved in the blood. To calculate the total arterial oxygen content, we must know (1) hemoglobin concentration, or the amount of hemoglobin that is available to bind with oxygen (hemoglobin [Hb] in grams per deciliter); (2) the oxygen saturation or percentage of available hemoglobin that is bound to oxygen (Sao_2); and (3) the partial pressure of oxygen (Pao_2). The maximum amount of oxygen that can be transported by hemoglobin is 1.34 ml/g. The amount of oxygen that can be physically dissolved in blood is 0.003 ml/dl per mmHg. If these specific values are known, the oxygen content of arterial blood can be calculated.[1]

$$O_2 \text{ content} = (Hb \times Sao_2 \times 1.34) + (Pao_2 \times 0.003)$$

To calculate the oxygen content of venous blood, the partial pressure of mixed venous blood (P_Vo_2) and venous oxygen saturation (Svo_2) are substituted for the arterial values in the basic formula. Normal venous oxygen content is 15 to 16 ml/dl.

Because hemoglobin transports all but a small fraction of the oxygen carried in arterial blood, increases in hemoglobin concentration affect the oxygen content of the blood. Decreases in hemoglobin concentration below the normal value of 15 ml/dl of blood reduce oxygen content, and increases in hemoglobin concentration may minimize the effect of impaired gas exchange. In fact, an increase in hemoglobin concentration is a major compensatory mechanism in pulmonary diseases that impair gas exchange. For this reason, measurement of hemoglobin concentration is important in assessing individuals with pulmonary disease. If cardiovascular function is normal, the body's initial response to low oxygen content is to speed up cardiac output. In individuals who also have cardiovascular disease, this compensatory mechanism does not work, making increased hemoglobin concentration an even more important compensatory mechanism. (Hemoglobin structure and function are described in Chapter 25.)

Oxyhemoglobin Association and Dissociation

When hemoglobin molecules bind with oxygen, **oxyhemoglobin (HbO_2)** is formed. Binding occurs in the lungs and is called *oxyhemoglobin association* or *hemoglobin saturation with oxygen* (Sao_2). The reverse process, in which oxygen is released from hemoglobin, occurs in the body tissues at the cellular level and is called *hemoglobin desaturation*. When hemoglobin saturation and desaturation are plotted on a graph, the result is a distinctive S-shaped curve known as the **oxyhemoglobin dissociation curve** (Figure 32-18).

Several factors can change the relationship between Pao_2 and Sao_2, causing the oxyhemoglobin dissociation curve to shift to the right or left (see Figure 32-18). A shift to the right depicts hemoglobin's decreased affinity for oxygen or an increase in the ease with which oxyhemoglobin dissociates and oxygen moves into the cells. A shift to the left depicts hemoglobin's increased affinity for oxygen, which promotes association in the lungs and inhibits dissociation in the tissues.

The oxyhemoglobin dissociation curve is shifted to the right by acidosis (low pH) and hypercapnia (increased $Paco_2$). In the tissues the increased levels of CO_2 and hydrogen ions produced by metabolic activity decrease the affinity of hemoglobin for oxygen. The curve is shifted to the left by alkalosis (high pH) and hypocapnia (decreased $Paco_2$). In the lungs, as CO_2 diffuses from the blood into the alveoli, the blood CO_2 level is reduced and the affinity of hemoglobin for oxygen is increased. The shift in the oxyhemoglobin dissociation curve caused by changes in CO_2 and hydrogen ion concentration in the blood is called the **Bohr effect.**

The oxyhemoglobin curve is shifted also by changes in body temperature and increased or decreased levels of 2,3-diphosphoglycerate (2,3-DPG), a substance normally present in erythrocytes. Hyperthermia and increased 2,3-DPG levels shift the curve to the right. Hypothermia and decreased 2,3-DPG levels shift the curve to the left.

Carbon Dioxide Transport

Approximately 200 ml of CO_2 is produced by the tissues per minute as a byproduct of cellular metabolism. This CO_2 equilibrates with carbonic acid ($H_2O + CO_2 \rightleftharpoons H_2CO_3 \rightleftharpoons H + HCO_3^-$) and must be eliminated continuously to prevent acidosis. The elimination of CO_2 by the lungs plays an important role in the regulation of acid-base balance (see Chapter 3).

CO_2 is carried in the blood in three ways: (1) dissolved in plasma, (2) as bicarbonate, and (3) as carbamino compounds. As CO_2 diffuses out of the cells into the blood, it dissolves in the plasma. Approximately 10% of the total CO_2 in venous blood and 5% of the CO_2 in arterial blood is carried dissolved in the plasma. As CO_2 moves into the blood, it diffuses into the red blood cells. Within the red blood cells, CO_2, with the help of the enzyme carbonic anhydrase, combines with water to form carbonic acid and then quickly dissociates into H^+ and HCO_3^-. As carbonic acid dissociates, the H^+ binds to hemoglobin, where it is buffered, and the HCO_3^- moves out of the red blood cell into the plasma. Approximately 60% of the CO_2 in venous blood and 90% of the CO_2 in arterial blood are carried in the form of bicarbonate. The remainder combines with blood proteins, hemoglobin in particular, to form carbamino compounds. Approximately 30% of the CO_2 in venous blood and 5% of the CO_2 in arterial blood are carried as carbamino compounds (see Figure 3-9).

CO_2 is 20 times more soluble than O_2 and diffuses quickly from the tissue cells into the blood. The amount of CO_2 that is able to enter the blood is enhanced by diffusion of oxygen out of the blood and into the cells. Reduced hemoglobin (hemoglobin that is dissociated from oxygen) is able to carry more CO_2 than hemoglobin that is saturated with O_2. Therefore, the drop in Sao_2 at the tissue level increases the ability of hemoglobin to carry CO_2 back to the lung.

The diffusion gradient for CO_2 in the lung is only approximately 6 mmHg (venous $Pvco_2$ = 46 mmHg; alveolar $Paco_2$ = 40 mmHg), yet CO_2 is so soluble in the alveolocapillary membrane that the CO_2 in the blood quickly diffuses into the alveoli, where it is removed from the lung with each expiration. Diffusion of CO_2 in the lung is so efficient that diffusion defects that cause hypoxemia (low oxygen content of the blood) do not cause hypercapnia (excessive CO_2 in the blood).

The diffusion of CO_2 out of the blood also is enhanced by oxygen binding with hemoglobin in the lung. As hemoglobin binds with O_2, the amount of CO_2 carried by the blood is decreased. Thus in the tissue capillaries, O_2 dissociation from hemoglobin facilitates the pickup of CO_2, and the binding of

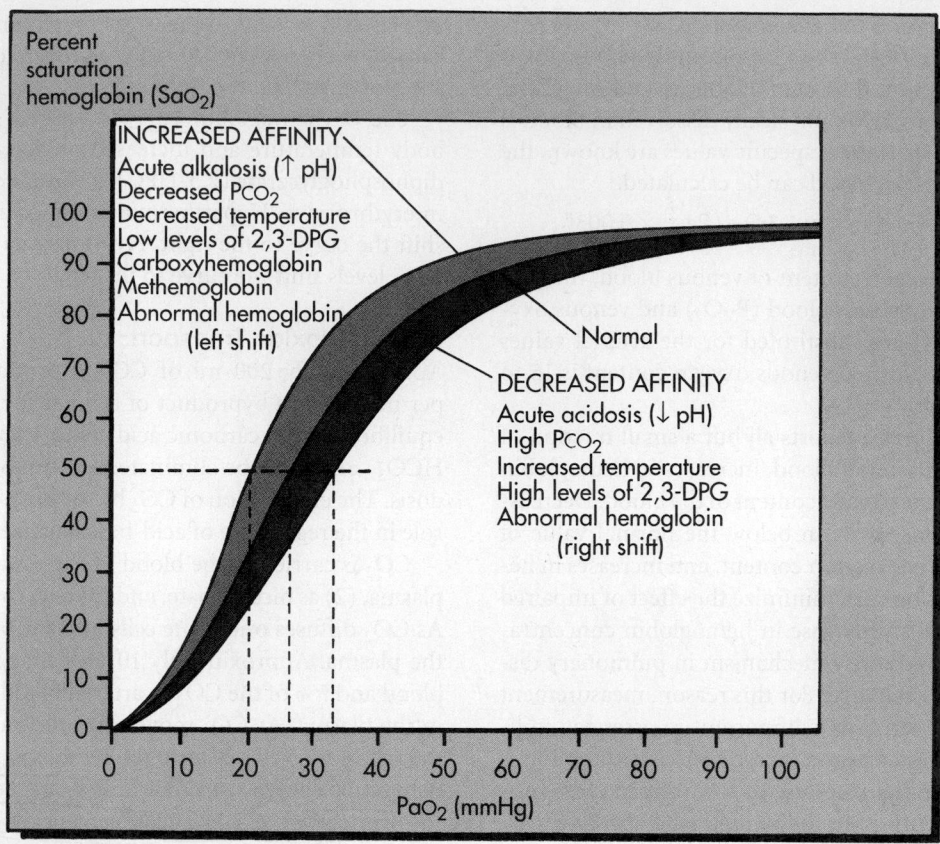

Figure 32-18 **Oxyhemoglobin dissociation curve.** The horizontal or flat segment of the curve at the top of the graph is sometimes called the *arterial portion*, or that part of the curve where oxygen is bound to hemoglobin. This portion of the curve is flat because partial pressure changes of oxygen between 60 and 100 mmHg do not significantly alter the percent saturation of hemoglobin with oxygen. The wide range of partial pressures of oxygen (Pao_2—60 to 100 mmHg), represented by the flat part of the curve—allows adequate hemoglobin saturation at a variety of *altitudes*. For example, a Pao_2 of 100 mmHg at sea level results in a hemoglobin saturation with oxygen of 98%. At an altitude of 5000 feet the Pao_2 is about 70 mmHg and hemoglobin saturation is 94%, only 4% less than at sea level. If the relationship between Sao_2 and Pao_2 were linear (in a downward-sloping straight line) instead of flat between 60 and 100 mmHg, there would be inadequate saturation of hemoglobin with oxygen. For example, with a Pao_2 of 70 mmHg the saturation would be only 70%, which is equivalent to normal venous oxygen saturation, and life could not be sustained at altitudes much above sea level. The steep part of the oxyhemoglobin dissociation curve occurs after the Pao_2 drops below 60 mmHg and represents the rapid dissociation of oxygen from hemoglobin. During this phase oxygen diffuses rapidly from the blood into tissue cells. Conditions associated with altered affinity of hemoglobin for O_2 are listed. P_{50} is the Pao_2 at which hemoglobin is 50% saturated, normally 26.6 mmHg. A lower than normal P_{50} represents increased affinity of hemoglobin for O_2; a high P_{50} is seen with decreased affinity. Note that variation from the normal is associated with decreased (low P_{50}) or increased (high P_{50}) availability of O_2 to tissues (*dotted lines*). The *shaded area* shows the entire oxyhemoglobin dissociation curve under the same circumstances. *2,3-DPG*, 2,3-diphosphoglycerate. (From Lane EE, Walker JF: *Clinical arterial blood gas analysis,* St Louis, 1987, Mosby.)

O_2 to hemoglobin in the lungs facilitates the release of CO_2 from the blood. This effect of oxygen on CO_2 transport is called the **Haldane effect** and can have significant clinical implications for the management of lung disease.[10,11]

Control of the Pulmonary Circulation

The caliber of pulmonary artery lumina decreases as smooth muscle in arterial walls contracts. Contraction increases pulmonary artery pressure. Caliber increases as these muscles relax, decreasing blood pressure. Contraction (vasoconstriction) and relaxation (vasodilation) apparently occur in response to local humoral conditions, even though the pulmonary circulation is innervated by the ANS in the same manner as the systemic circulation.

The most important cause of pulmonary artery constriction is a low alveolar partial pressure of oxygen (Pao_2). Vasoconstriction caused by alveolar and pulmonary venous hypoxia, often termed **hypoxic pulmonary vasoconstriction,** can affect only one portion of the lung or the entire lung. If only one segment of the lung is involved, the arterioles to that segment constrict, shunting blood to other, well-ventilated portions of the lung. This reflex improves the lung's efficiency by better matching ventilation and perfusion. If alveolar hypoxia affects all segments of the lung, however, vasoconstriction occurs throughout the pulmonary vasculature, and pulmonary hypertension (elevated pulmonary artery pressure) can result. The pulmonary vasoconstriction caused by low Pao_2 is reversible if the $Paco_2$ is corrected. Chronic alveolar hypoxia

Hypoxic pulmonary vasoconstriction is a physiologic response to changes in the environment and pulmonary pathologic conditions that affect alveolar oxygen content (Pao_2). Decreases in Pao_2 to less than 12% of normal induce constriction of preacinar arteriolar smooth muscle cells and therefore decrease blood flow through those vessels. When a pulmonary disorder is characterized by localized areas of acutely decreased alveolar oxygen content, vasoconstriction of the arterioles perfusing those areas is a positive compensatory mechanism that reduces shunt (wasted perfusion). However, in diffuse and chronic lung disorders (e.g., chronic obstructive pulmonary disease [COPD] or cystic fibrosis), widespread and persistent hypoxic pulmonary vasoconstriction creates resistance to pulmonary blood flow and raises the pressure in the pulmonary artery, causing a condition known as *secondary pulmonary artery hypertension*. Pulmonary hypertension can become severe enough to impede right ventricular ejection and eventually cause right heart failure known as *cor pulmonale*. In addition, lung hypoxia activates many hypoxia-dependent genes in pulmonary vascular endothelial cells to produce a variety of chemicals and growth factors. Recent studies have shown that alveolar hypoxia causes the production of reactive oxygen species (toxic oxygen radicals), vasoconstrictors, such as endothelin, and vascular endothelial growth factor that in conjunction with vascular fibroblasts cause deleterious changes in the pulmonary arteriolar walls called *remodeling*. Remodeling is a process by which the vascular wall becomes scarred and thickened, thus resulting in permanent decreases in luminal diameter, increased resistance to blood flow, and permanent pulmonary artery hypertension. Research is in progress to inhibit and potentially reverse this remodeling.

Data from Chan SY, Loscalzo J: *J Mol Cell Cardiol* 44(1):14-30, 2008; Girgis RE, Mathai SC: *Clin Chest Med* 28:219-232, 2007; Jain S, Ventura H, deBoisblanc B: *Semin Cardiothorasc Vasc Anesth* 11(2):104-109, 2007; Nozik-Grayck E, Stenmark K: *Adv Exp Med Biol* 61:101-112, 2007; Rhodes CJ et al: *Pharm Ther* 121(1):69-88, 2009; Tuder R et al: *J Mol Med* 85(12):1317-1324, 2007; Waypa GB, Schumacker PT: *Exp Physiol* 93(1):133-138, 2008.

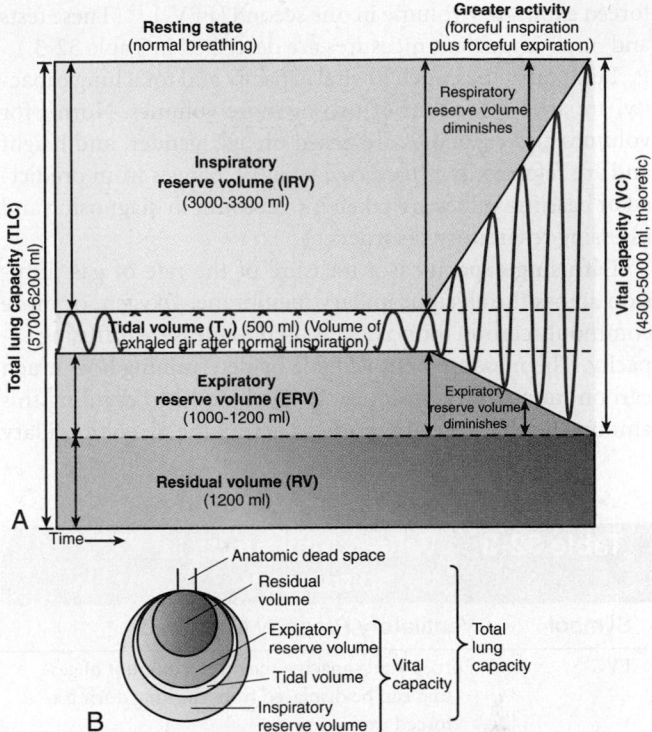

Figure 32-19 Pulmonary ventilation and lung capacities. A, Spirogram. During normal, quiet respirations the atmosphere and lungs exchange about 500 ml of air (V_T). With a forcible inspiration, about 3300 ml more air can be inhaled (IRV). After a normal inspiration and normal expiration, approximately 1000 ml more air can be forcibly expired (ERV). Vital capacity is the amount of air that can be forcibly expired after a maximal inspiration and indicates, therefore, the largest amount of air that can enter and leave the lungs during respiration. Residual volume is the air that remains trapped in the alveoli. B, Lung capacities. (From, Patton KT, Thibodeau GA *Anatomy & physiology*, ed 7, St Louis, 2010, Mosby.)

can result in permanent pulmonary artery hypertension, which eventually leads to cor pulmonale and heart failure (see What's New? Hypoxic Pulmonary Vasoconstriction).[12,13]

Acidemia also causes pulmonary artery constriction. If the acidemia is corrected, the vasoconstriction is reversed. (Respiratory acidosis and metabolic acidosis are described in Chapter 3.) It is important to note that an elevated $Paco_2$ without a drop in pH does not cause pulmonary artery constriction. Other biochemical factors that affect the caliber of vessels in pulmonary circulation are histamine, prostaglandins, endothelin, serotonin, nitric oxide, and bradykinin.

TESTS OF PULMONARY FUNCTION

Several laboratory tests aid in the diagnosis and evaluation of pulmonary system abnormalities. Most of them are easy to perform at hospitals and clinics. They provide valuable information as to the possible cause of a respiratory abnormality and evaluate the progression or resolution of disease.

Spirometry is used to measure forced expiration, which often is affected by diffuse pulmonary disease. Because the pulmonary system has remarkable reserves, disease may become well established before clinical manifestations appear. Spirometry enables clinicians to detect restrictive or obstructive deficits early in the course of disease. Restrictive lung diseases restrict the lungs' volume: the lungs are unable to expand normally, diminishing the amount of gas that can be inspired. Obstructive diseases affect gas flow: airflow into and out of the lungs is obstructed.

Spirometry measures both volume and flow. The test is performed with a spirometer, which is a water-filled cylinder into which an inverted cylinder or bell has been inserted. A length of tubing runs from the inverted bell to a mouthpiece through which a person breathes during testing. The bell is attached to a pen that writes on calibrated paper rotating at a constant speed. As a person performs various breathing maneuvers, the inverted bell moves up and down, causing the pen to move on the calibrated paper. This produces a spirogram, which is a record of the individual's ventilation in relation to time (Figure 32-19). Clinically the most important spirometric tests are the forced vital capacity (FVC) and the forced expiratory volume in one second (FEV_1).[13] (These tests and other important measures are described in Table 32-3.)

Lung capacities, such as vital capacity and total lung capacity, are always the sum of two or more volumes. Norms for volumes and capacities are based on age, gender, and height and are referred to as *predicted values*. Changes from predicted or baseline values are taken into account in diagnosing and assessing respiratory disorders.

Diffusing capacity is a measure of the rate of gas diffusion across the alveolocapillary membrane. Oxygen, or more commonly carbon monoxide, is used to measure diffusing capacity. The measurement is made by determining how much carbon monoxide is taken up by the blood and dividing this amount by the pressure gradient across the alveolocapillary membrane. Helium often is added to the gas mixture to obtain a simultaneous measurement of **residual volume (RV)**, **functional reserve capacity (FRC)**, and **total lung capacity (TLC)**. Individuals are asked to perform ventilatory maneuvers similar to those of spirometry. A decreased diffusing capacity can be the result of an abnormal ventilation-perfusion ratio or an actual diffusion defect. Diffusing capacity is decreased in individuals with emphysema.

Arterial blood gas analysis commonly is performed for individuals with suggested or diagnosed pulmonary disease. Direct analysis of the pH and gas concentrations in arterial blood provides valuable information about an individual's gas exchange and acid-base status. Acidosis (low pH), alkalosis (high pH), ventilatory alterations, and decreased Pao_2 can be diagnosed accurately only by arterial blood gas analysis. A blood gas report may be divided into an acid-base/ventilation portion and an oxygenation portion. (Normal values for arterial blood gases are given in Table 32-4; acid-base alterations are described in Chapter 3.) Oximetry can be used to monitor oxygen saturation once the arterial blood gas analysis has accurately measured the Pao_2, but it does not measure $Paco_2$ or pH.

Signs and symptoms of most respiratory abnormalities first appear when the system is stressed during exercise. Therefore, if pulmonary disease is suspected, the individual is evaluated at rest and during exercise. During exercise the usual procedures are spirometry and withdrawal of arterial blood for gas analysis. The exercise usually consists of riding a stationary bicycle or walking on a treadmill. Exercise testing enables clinicians to detect early changes in respiratory function and thus begin treatment. Exercise tests also are used in planning and evaluating exercise and rehabilitation programs.

Chest radiographs are among the most common examinations of the pulmonary system. A few of the abnormalities detected in chest radiographs are air trapping in the alveoli

Table 32-3 Values Measured by Spirometry

Symbol	Ventilatory Property Measured
FVC	Forced vital capacity: maximum amount of gas that can be displaced from the lung during a forced expiration
FEV_1	Forced expiratory volume in 1 second: maximum amount of air that can be expired from the lung in 1 second
FEV_1/FVC	Percentage of maximum inspiration that is expired in 1 second, usually 80% of FVC
FEV_3	Forced expiratory volume in 3 seconds; maximum amount of gas that can be expired in 3 seconds
FEV_3/FVC	Percentage of FVC that is expired in 3 seconds; usually 95% of FVC
$FEF_{25\%-75\%}$	Forced expiratory flow rate during the middle 50% of expiration; sometimes reported as maximum midexpiratory flow rate (MMFR)

Table 32-4 Normal Ranges for Arterial and Mixed Venous Blood Gases

Measurement	Arterial Blood	Mixed Venous Blood*	Clinical Notes
Acid-base status (pH)	7.35-7.45	7.33-7.43	Most important acid-base value; detects acidosis or alkalosis
Partial pressure of carbon dioxide (Pco_2)	35-45 mmHg	41-57 mmHg	Measures adequacy of ventilation and respiratory contribution of acid-base abnormality (respiratory acidosis)
Bicarbonate (HCO_3^-)	22-26 mEq/L	24-28 mEq/L	Measures metabolic contribution to acid-base abnormality (metabolic acidosis); calculated from pH and Pco_2
Base excess (BE)	−2 to +2	0 to +4	Reflects deviation of bicarbonate concentration from normal
Partial pressure of oxygen (Po_2) (sea level)	80-100 mmHg	35-40 mmHg	Indicates driving pressure that causes oxyhemoglobin binding; varies with age and barometric pressure
Saturation of hemoglobin with oxygen (So_2)	96%-98%	70%-75%	Indicates abnormalities of oxyhemoglobin association and dissociation; may be measured directly or calculated from Pco_2, pH, and body temperature
Concentration of hemoglobin in the blood	15 g/dl	15 g/dl	Detects alterations of gas transport caused by anemia

*Mixed venous (pulmonary artery) blood is analyzed for critically ill individuals and those undergoing cardiac catheterization (it is not practical to withdraw samples except from a pulmonary artery catheter). Mixed venous blood gas analysis, in conjunction with arterial analysis, provides important information about the adequacy of cardiac output and tissue oxygenation.

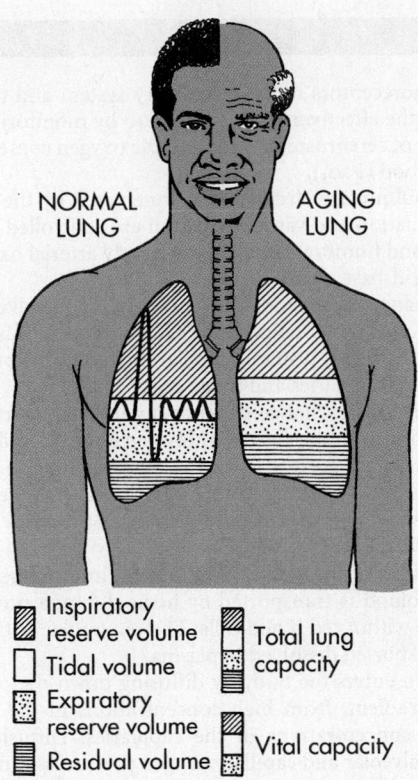

Inspiratory reserve volume

Tidal volume

Expiratory reserve volume

Residual volume

Total lung capacity

Vital capacity

Figure 32-20 Changes in lung volumes with aging. With aging, note particularly the decrease in vital capacity and the increase in residual volume.

and airways (e.g., in asthma or emphysema), consolidation of lung tissue (in pneumonia or pulmonary edema), cavities (abscesses or tuberculosis), and nodules (lung cancer). Often pulmonary abnormalities are detected in routine chest radiographs of asymptomatic individuals. Various radiographic techniques are available for the diagnosis and evaluation of respiratory disorders.

Aging and the Pulmonary System

Most knowledge about pulmonary structure and function is based on norms for the middle years. Less is known about structure and function in the very young (see Chapter 34) and older adults, but a few normal physiologic (developmental and degenerative) changes are known to occur from birth to old age. An understanding of these changes is needed to provide appropriate care and to differentiate between normal alterations and disease. Normal alterations include (1) loss of elastic

recoil, (2) stiffening of the chest wall, (3) alterations in gas exchange, and (4) increases in flow resistance (Figure 32-20). These changes are influenced by environmental factors, respiratory disease, body size, and race.[14]

During adulthood and as age advances, the alveoli tend to lose alveoli wall tissue and capillaries. This process diminishes alveolar surface area available for gas diffusion and decreases airway support provided by normal lung tissues. Mechanical changes involve elastic properties of the lungs and chest wall. Chest wall compliance decreases with age because the ribs become ossified (less flexible) and joints become stiffer. As a result the chest wall loses some of its ability to expand. In addition, respiratory muscle strength and endurance decrease by up to 20% by age 70.[14] These mechanical changes in the lung and chest wall, along with structural changes in the alveoli, reduce ventilatory capacity in older adults. Vital capacity decreases and residual volume increases; however, total lung capacity remains unchanged. These changes decrease ventilatory reserves and lead to decreased ventilation-perfusion ratios.[14] With advancing age there is also increased immune dysregulation, asymptomatic low-grade inflammation, and increased risk of infection.[14-16]

Alterations in gas exchange are reflected by blood gas analysis. With advancing age, pH and $Paco_2$ do not change much, even though it has been documented that the chemoreceptors become less sensitive to gas partial pressures with age. Older adults have a decreased compensatory response to hypercapnia and hypoxemia; however, the perception of dyspnea remains intact and is even enhanced. Pao_2 declines with age as a result of structural and mechanical changes, such as loss of alveolar surface area and increased ventilation-perfusion mismatch. The maximum Pao_2 in an older adult at sea level can be estimated by multiplying the person's age by 0.3 and subtracting the product from 100. For example, an 80-year-old individual would have an estimated maximum Pao_2 of 76 mmHg ($0.3 \times 80 = 24$; $100 - 24 = 76$).[17] There is also a decrease in the capillary network.

The decrease in Pao_2 and diminished ventilatory reserve in an older adult lead to a decrease in exercise tolerance. Respiratory muscle strength and endurance decrease with age.[17] Furthermore, older adults are at greater risk for respiratory depression caused by medications. Changes in respiratory function can vary considerably from person to person, however. Changes also are affected by activity and fitness earlier in life. A very active, physically fit individual will, all else being equal, have fewer changes in function at any age than one who has been sedentary.

SUMMARY REVIEW

Structures of the Pulmonary System

1. The pulmonary system consists of the lungs, airways, chest wall, and pulmonary and bronchial circulation.
2. Air is inspired and expired through the conducting airways, which include the nasopharynx, oropharynx, trachea, bronchi, and bronchioles to the sixteenth division.
3. Gas exchange occurs in structures beyond the sixteenth division: the respiratory bronchioles, alveolar ducts, and alveoli. Together these structures comprise the acinus.
4. The chief gas-exchange units of the lungs are the alveoli. The membrane that surrounds each alveolus and contains the pulmonary capillaries is called the *alveolocapillary membrane.*
5. The gas-exchange airways are served by the pulmonary circulation, a separate division of the circulatory system. The bronchi and other lung structures are served by a branch of the systemic circulation called the *bronchial circulation.*
6. The chest wall, which contains and protects the contents of the thoracic cavity, consists of the skin, ribs, and intercostal muscles, which lie between the ribs.
7. The chest wall is lined by a serous membrane called the *parietal pleura;* the lungs are encased in a separate membrane called the *visceral pleura.* The area where these two pleurae come into contact and slide over each another is called the *pleural space.*

Function of the Pulmonary System

1. The pulmonary system enables oxygen to diffuse into the blood and CO_2 to diffuse out of the blood.
2. Ventilation is the process by which air flows into and out of the gas-exchange airways.
3. Successful ventilation involves the mechanics of breathing: the interaction of forces and counterforces involving the muscles of inspiration and expiration, alveolar surface tension, elastic properties of the lungs and chest wall, and resistance to airflow.
4. The major muscle of inspiration is the diaphragm. When the diaphragm contracts, it moves downward in the thoracic cavity, creating a vacuum that causes air to flow into the lungs.
5. The alveoli produce surfactant, a lipoprotein that lines the alveoli. Surfactant reduces alveolar surface tension and permits the alveoli to expand more easily as air flows in.
6. Compliance is the ability of the lungs and chest wall to expand during inspiration. Lung compliance is ensured by adequate production of surfactant; chest wall expansion depends on flexibility.
7. Elastic recoil is the tendency of the lungs and chest wall to return to their resting state after inspiration. The elastic recoil forces of the lungs and chest wall are in opposition and pull on each other, creating the normally negative pressure of the pleural space.
8. Most of the time ventilation is involuntary. It is controlled by the sympathetic and parasympathetic divisions of the ANS, which adjust airway caliber (by causing bronchial smooth muscle to contract or relax) and control the rate and depth of ventilation.
9. Neuroreceptors in the lungs (lung receptors) monitor the mechanical aspects of ventilation. Irritant receptors sense the need to expel unwanted substances, stretch receptors sense lung volume (lung expansion), and *J*-receptors sense alveolar size.
10. Chemoreceptors in the circulatory system and brain stem sense the effectiveness of ventilation by monitoring the pH status of cerebrospinal fluid and the oxygen content of arterial blood (PaO_2).
11. The pulmonary circulation is innervated by the ANS, but vasodilation and vasoconstriction are controlled mainly by local and humoral factors, particularly arterial oxygenation and acid-base status.
12. Gas transport depends on ventilation of the alveoli, diffusion across the alveolocapillary membrane, perfusion of the pulmonary and systemic capillaries, and diffusion between systemic capillaries and tissue cells.
13. Efficient gas exchange depends on an even distribution of ventilation and perfusion within the lungs. Ventilation and perfusion are greatest in the bases of the lungs because the alveoli in the bases are more compliant (their resting volume is low), and perfusion is greater in the bases as a result of gravity.
14. Almost all of the oxygen that diffuses into pulmonary capillary blood is transported by hemoglobin, a protein contained within red blood cells. The remainder of the oxygen is transported dissolved in plasma.
15. Oxygen enters the body by diffusing down the concentration gradient, from high concentrations in the alveoli to lower concentrations in the capillaries. Diffusion ceases when alveolar and capillary oxygen pressures equilibrate.
16. Oxygen is loaded onto hemoglobin by the driving pressure exerted by PaO_2 in the plasma. As pressure decreases at tissue level, oxygen dissociates from hemoglobin and enters tissue cells by diffusion, again down the concentration gradient.
17. CO_2 is more soluble in plasma than oxygen is and diffuses readily from tissue cells into plasma. CO_2 returns to the lungs dissolved in plasma, as bicarbonate, or in carbamino compounds (e.g., bound to hemoglobin).
18. Vasoconstriction of the pulmonary arterial system is caused by alveolar hypoxia, acidemia, and inflammatory mediators—histamine, serotonin, prostaglandins, and bradykinin.

Tests of Pulmonary Function

1. Spirometry measures volume and flow rate during forced expiration.
2. The alveolar-arterial oxygen gradient is used to evaluate the cause of hypoxia.
3. Diffusing capacity is a measure of the gas diffusion rate at the alveolocapillary membrane.
4. Arterial blood gas analysis can be used to determine pH and oxygen and CO_2 concentrations.
5. Radiographic examination of the chest evaluates air trapping, consolidation, cavity formation, or presence of tumors.

Aging and the Pulmonary System

1. Aging affects the mechanical aspects of ventilation by decreasing chest wall compliance and elastic recoil of the lungs. Changes in these elastic properties reduce ventilatory reserve.
2. Aging causes the PaO_2 to decrease but does not affect the $PaCO_2$.

KEY TERMS

Airway resistance, 1253
Acinus, 1244
Alveolar duct, 1244
Alveolar ventilation, 1249
Alveoli (sing., alveolus), 1244
Alveolocapillary membrane, 1247
Arterial blood gas analysis, 1262
Bohr effect, 1259
Bronchiole, 1244
Bronchoconstriction, 1254
Bronchodilation, 1254
Bronchus (pl., bronchi), 1244
Carina, 1244
Central chemoreceptor, 1251
Chest radiograph, 1262
Compliance, 1253
Diaphragm, 1252
Diffusing capacity, 1262
Elastic recoil, 1253
Functional reserve capacity (FRC), 1262

Gas transport, 1255
Goblet cell, 1244
Haldane effect, 1260
Hilus (pl., hila), 1244
Hypoxic pulmonary vasoconstriction, 1260
Irritant receptor, 1251
J-receptor, 1251
Larynx, 1243
Lymphatic capillary, 1249
Minute volume, 1249
Nasopharynx, 1242
Oropharynx, 1242
Oxygen content, 1258
Oxyhemoglobin (HbO_2), 1259
Oxyhemoglobin dissociation curve, 1259
Partial pressure (of a gas), 1255
Peripheral chemoreceptor, 1250, 1251
Physiologic dead space, 1257
Pleura (pl., pleurae), 1249
Pleural space (pleural cavity), 1249

Pulmonary artery, 1247
Pulmonary capillary, 1247
Pulmonary vein, 1247
Rapidly adapting receptor (RAR), 1251
Residual volume (RV), 1262
Respiration, 1249
Respiratory bronchiole, 1244
Respiratory center, 1250
Spirometry, 1261
Stretch receptor, 1251
Surface tension, 1252
Surfactant, 1244
Thoracic cavity, 1249
Total lung capacity (TLC), 1262
Trachea, 1244
Ventilation, 1249
Ventilation-perfusion ratio ($\dot{V}/\dot{Q}$), 1257
Work of breathing, 1254

REFERENCES

1. Lumb AB: *Nunn's applied respiratory physiology*, ed 6, St Louis, 2005, Elsevier.
2. Ganong W: *Review of medical physiology*, ed 22, Philadelphia, 2005, McGraw-Hill.
3. Corrin B: *Pathology of the lungs*, London, 2000, Churchill Livingstone.
4. West JB: *Respiratory physiology: the essentials*, ed 8, Philadelphia, 2008, Lippincott Williams & Wilkins.
5. Benarroch EE: Brainstem respiratory chemosensitivity: new insights and clinical implications, *Neurology* 68(24):2140-2143, 2007.
6. Haberthur C, Guttmann J: Short-term effects of positive end-expiratory pressure on breathing pattern: an interventional study in adult intensive care patients, *Crit Care* 9(4):R407-R415, 2005.
7. Canning BJ: Anatomy and neurophysiology of the cough reflex, *Chest* 129:33s-47s, 2006.
8. Kuroki Y, Takahashi M, Nishitani C: Pulmonary collectins in innate immunity of the lung, *Cell Microbiol* 9(8):1871-1879, 2007.
9. Des Jardins T, Burton GC: *Clinical manifestations and assessment of respiratory disease*, ed 5, St Louis, 2006, Mosby.
10. Cavaliere F et al: Comparison of two methods to assess blood CO_2 equilibration curve in mechanically ventilated patients, *Resp Physiol Neurobiol* 146(1):77-83, 2005.
11. Chien JW et al: Uncontrolled oxygen administration and respiratory failure in acute asthma, *Chest* 117(3):728-733, 2000.
12. Pak O et al: The effects of hypoxia on the cells of the pulmonary vasculature, *Eur Resp J* 30(2):364-372, 2007.
13. Mason RJ et al, editors: *Murray and Nadel's textbook of respiratory medicine*, ed 4, St Louis, 2005, Elsevier.
14. Sharma G, Goodwin J: Effect of aging on respiratory system physiology and immunology, *Clin Interven Aging* 1(3):253-260, 2006.
15. Haas CF, Loik PS, Gay SE: Airway clearance applications in the elderly and in patients with neurologic or neuromuscular compromise, *Respir Care* 52(10):1362-1381, discussion 1381, 2007.
16. Ely KH et al: Aging and CD8+ T cell immunity to respiratory virus infections, *Exp Gerontol* 42(5):427-431, 2007.
17. Hardie JA et al: Reference values for arterial blood gases in the elderly, *Chest* 125(6):2053-2060, 2004.

ALTERATIONS OF PULMONARY FUNCTION

VALENTINA L. BRASHERS

MEDIA RESOURCES

 Evolve Website (http://evolve.elsevier.com/McCance/)
- Review Questions and Answers
- Animations
- Glossary (with audio pronunciation for selected terms)
- WebLinks

Online Course
- Module 16

CHAPTER OUTLINE

CLINICAL MANIFESTATIONS OF PULMONARY ALTERATIONS
Signs and Symptoms of Pulmonary Disease
Conditions Caused by Pulmonary Disease or Injury
DISORDERS OF THE CHEST WALL AND PLEURA
Disorders of the Chest Wall
Pleural Abnormalities

PULMONARY DISORDERS
Restrictive Lung Disorders
Obstructive Pulmonary Disease
Respiratory Tract Infections
Pulmonary Vascular Disease
Malignancies of the Respiratory Tract

Pulmonary disease is often classified as acute or chronic, obstructive or restrictive, and infectious or noninfectious. Because skillful and knowledgeable clinical care plays a major role in decreasing respiratory morbidity and mortality, the clinician with a clear understanding of the pathophysiology of common respiratory problems can greatly affect the outcome for each individual.

CLINICAL MANIFESTATIONS OF PULMONARY ALTERATIONS

Signs and Symptoms of Pulmonary Disease

Pulmonary disease is associated with many signs and symptoms. The most common of these are cough and dyspnea. Other manifestations include chest pain, abnormal sputum, hemoptysis, altered breathing patterns, cyanosis, clubbing of the digits, and fever. The signs and symptoms and their specific characteristics often help in identifying the underlying disorder.

Cough

Cough is an important reflex that helps clear the airways of large amounts of inhaled material, excessive secretions, or abnormal substances, such as edema or pus. Individuals with

an inability to cough normally are at greater risk for pneumonia. The cough reflex results from a complex interaction of sensory receptors in the upper and lower airways, including stimulation of mechanical and chemical "irritant" receptors.[1,2] There are few such receptors in the most distal bronchi and the alveoli; thus it is possible for significant amounts of secretions to accumulate in the distal respiratory tree without cough being initiated. Other cough receptors are located in the external auditory canal, diaphragm, pericardium, pleura, and stomach. Stimulation of cough receptors is transmitted centrally through the vagus nerve, and central modulation of the cough reflex can be influenced by opiates and serotonergic agents.[3]

Acute cough is cough that resolves within 2 to 3 weeks of the onset of illness or resolves with treatment of the underlying condition. It is most commonly the result of upper respiratory infections, allergic rhinitis, acute bronchitis, pneumonia, congestive heart failure, pulmonary embolus, or aspiration.[4] **Chronic cough** is defined as cough that has persisted for more than 3 weeks, although some researchers have suggested that 7 or 8 weeks is a more appropriate timeframe because acute cough and bronchial hyperreactivity can be prolonged in some cases of viral infection. In nonsmokers, chronic cough is almost always caused by postnasal drainage syndrome, nonasthmatic eosinophilic bronchitis, asthma, or gastroesophageal reflux disease.[4,5] In smokers, chronic bronchitis is the most common cause of chronic cough, although lung cancer must always be considered. Up to 33% of individuals taking angiotensin-converting enzyme inhibitors for cardiovascular disease develop chronic cough that resolves with discontinuation of the drug.

Dyspnea

Dyspnea is the subjective sensation of being unable to get enough air. It is often described as breathlessness, air hunger, shortness of breath, labored breathing, and preoccupation with breathing. Dyspnea is a common symptom of respiratory disease.

The severity of the sensation of dyspnea may not directly correlate with the severity of underlying pulmonary disease.[6,7] Either diffuse or focal disturbances of ventilation, gas exchange, or ventilation-perfusion relationships can cause dyspnea, as can increased work of breathing or diseases that damage lung tissue (lung parenchyma). Many mechanisms have been proposed to explain the complex sensation of dyspnea, but no single mechanism has been found to be responsible in all situations. One commonly accepted mechanism involves an impaired sense of effort. This is a situation in which the perceived work of breathing is greater than the actual motor response generated. Mechanoreceptors in the chest wall respond to the length and tension in muscles and can contribute to the sensation of dyspnea as can upper airway receptors that signal the brain through trigeminal nerve fibers.[7] A second explanation involves the stimulation of central and peripheral chemoreceptors. It has long been known that decreased pH, hypercapnia, and hypoxemia can cause dyspnea.[6,7] (The neurochemical control of ventilation is described in Chapter 32.) Stimulation of chemoreceptors causes dyspnea in many lung diseases in which oxygenation and gas exchange are impaired.

A third explanation is stimulation of the afferent receptors in the lung (the stretch receptors, irritant receptors, and J-receptors), which send impulses to the central nervous system through the vagus nerve.[6,7] Stretch receptors are stimulated in asthma and may be the primary cause of the sensation of dyspnea and chest tightness in that disorder. J-receptors also trigger dyspnea in individuals with pulmonary edema and pulmonary microemboli. Finally, the sensation of dyspnea also can be caused by increased work of breathing, respiratory muscle fatigue, decreased breathing reserve, and strong emotions, particularly anxiety and anger. There is general agreement that neurologic control and function of respiratory muscles are the common elements in most clinical experiences of dyspnea and that the sensation perceived is that of increased respiratory effort.

The signs of dyspnea include flaring of the nostrils, use of accessory muscles of respiration, and retraction (pulling back) of the intercostal spaces. In dyspnea caused by parenchymal disease (e.g., pneumonia), retractions of tissue between the ribs (subcostal and intercostal retractions) are observed more often than supercostal retractions (retractions of tissues above

the ribs), which predominate in upper airway obstruction. Retractions of any type are more commonly seen in children or in adults who are thin and have poorly developed thoracic musculature. Dyspnea can be quantified by the use of ordinal rating scales or visual analog scales.[7]

Dyspnea can occur transiently or can become chronic. The first episode commonly occurs with exercise and is called **dyspnea on exertion**. Dyspnea also can be associated with body positioning. **Orthopnea** is dyspnea that occurs when an individual lies flat and is common in individuals with heart failure. The recumbent position redistributes body water, causes the abdominal contents to exert pressure on the diaphragm, and decreases the efficiency of the respiratory muscles. Orthopnea is generally relieved by sitting up in a forward-leaning posture or supporting the upper body on several pillows. Another type of positional dyspnea is termed **paroxysmal nocturnal dyspnea (PND)** in which individuals with heart failure or lung disease wake up at night gasping for air and must sit up or stand to relieve the dyspnea.

Pain

Pain caused by pulmonary disorders originates in the pleurae, airways, or chest wall. Pleural pain is the most common pain caused by pulmonary disease and is usually sharp or stabbing in character. Infection and inflammation of the parietal pleura (pleuritis or pleurisy) cause pain when the pleura stretch during inspiration. The pain is usually localized to a portion of the chest wall, where a unique breath sound called a *pleural friction rub* may be heard over the painful area. Laughing or coughing makes pleural pain worse. Pleural pain is also common with pulmonary infarction (tissue death) caused by pulmonary embolism and emanates from the area around the infarction.

Pulmonary pain is central chest pain that is pronounced after coughing and occurs in individuals with infection and inflammation of the trachea or bronchi (tracheitis or tracheobronchitis). Central chest pain can be difficult to differentiate from cardiac pain (see Chapter 30). High blood pressure in the pulmonary circulation (pulmonary hypertension) can cause pain during exercise that is often mistaken for cardiac pain (angina pectoris).

Pain in the chest wall is muscle pain or rib pain. The common causes of chest wall pain are excessive coughing, which makes the muscles sore, and rib fractures. Inflammation of the costochondral junction (costochondritis) also can cause chest wall pain. Chest wall pain can often be reproduced by pressing on the sternum or ribs.

Abnormal Sputum

The color, consistency, odor, and amount of **sputum** vary with different pulmonary disorders. A distinctive color or odor may suggest infection by a specific microorganism. Changes in the amount and consistency of sputum provide information about progression of disease and effectiveness of therapy. The gross and microscopic appearances of sputum enable the clinician to identify cellular debris or microorganisms that aid in diagnosis and choice of therapy.

Hemoptysis

Hemoptysis is the coughing up of blood or bloody secretions. Hemoptysis is sometimes confused with hematemesis, which is the vomiting of blood. Blood that is coughed up is usually bright red, has an alkaline pH, and is mixed with frothy sputum, whereas blood that is vomited is dark, has an acidic pH, and is mixed with food particles.

The most common causes of hemoptysis are bronchiectasis, lung cancer, bronchitis, and pneumonia. Tuberculosis remains an important cause of hemoptysis but is less common in the United States than in many other parts of the world. Hemoptysis results from damage to the lung parenchyma with rupture of pulmonary vessels or from inflammation, injury, or cancer of the bronchial tree. The amount and duration of bleeding (i.e., a sudden large amount versus a persistent slight amount) provide important clues about the source of the bleeding.[8] Bronchoscopy, combined with chest computed tomography (CT), can identify the cause in the majority of cases of hemoptysis.

Abnormal Breathing Patterns

Normal breathing (eupnea) is rhythmic and effortless. Ventilatory rate is 8 to 16 breaths per minute, and tidal volume ranges from 400 to 800 ml. A short expiratory pause occurs with each breath, and the individual takes an occasional deeper breath or sigh. Sigh breaths, which help maintain normal lung function, are usually 1.5 to 2 times the normal tidal volume and occur approximately 10 to 12 times per hour.

The rate, depth, regularity, and effort of breathing undergo characteristic alterations in response to physiologic and pathophysiologic conditions. Patterns of breathing automatically adjust to minimize the work of respiratory muscles. Strenuous exercise or metabolic acidosis induces **Kussmaul respiration (hyperpnea)**. Kussmaul respiration is characterized by a slightly increased ventilatory rate, very large tidal volume, and no expiratory pause.

Labored breathing occurs whenever there is an increased work of breathing, especially if the airways are obstructed, as in chronic obstructive pulmonary disease (COPD). If the large airways are obstructed, a slow ventilatory rate, increased effort, prolonged inspiration or expiration, and stridor (high-pitched sounds made during inspiration) or audible wheezing (whistling sounds on expiration) are typical. In small airway obstruction, like that seen in asthma and chronic obstructive pulmonary disease, a rapid ventilatory rate, small tidal volume, increased effort, prolonged expiration, and wheezing are often present.

Restricted breathing is commonly caused by disorders such as pulmonary fibrosis that stiffen the lungs or chest wall and decrease compliance. Restricted breathing is characterized by small tidal volumes and rapid ventilatory rate (tachypnea).

Shock and severe cerebral hypoxia (insufficient oxygen in the brain) contribute to gasping respirations that consist of irregular, quick inspirations with an expiratory pause. Anxiety can cause sighing respirations that consist of irregular breathing characterized by frequent, deep sighing inspirations.

Cheyne-Stokes respirations are characterized by alternating periods of deep and shallow breathing. Apnea lasting 15 to 60 seconds is followed by ventilations that increase in volume until a peak is reached, after which ventilation (tidal volume) decreases again to apnea. Cheyne-Stokes respirations result from any condition that slows the blood flow to the brainstem, which in turn slows impulses sending information to the respiratory centers of the brainstem. Neurologic impairment above the brainstem is also a contributing factor (see Table 16-5).

Hypoventilation and Hyperventilation

Hypoventilation is inadequate alveolar ventilation in relation to metabolic demands. It is caused by alterations in pulmonary mechanics or in the neurologic control of breathing such that minute volume (tidal volume times respiratory rate) is reduced. When alveolar ventilation is normal, carbon dioxide (CO_2) is removed from the lungs at the same rate at which it is produced by cellular metabolism. This maintains arterial CO_2 (Pao_2) at normal levels (40 mmHg). With hypoventilation, CO_2 removal does not keep up with CO_2 production and $Paco_2$ increases, causing hypercapnia ($Paco_2$ greater than 44 mmHg). (Table 32-2 contains the definition of gas partial pressure and other pulmonary abbreviations.) This results in an increase in hydrogen ion in the blood, termed respiratory acidosis, which can affect the function of many tissues throughout the body.

Hypoventilation is often overlooked until it is severe because breathing pattern and ventilatory rate may appear normal. Blood gas analysis (i.e., measurement of the $Paco_2$ of arterial blood) reveals the hypercapnia. Pronounced hypoventilation can cause somnolence or disorientation. In addition, hypoventilation with hypercapnia results in secondary hypoxemia.

Hyperventilation is alveolar ventilation that exceeds metabolic demands. The lungs remove CO_2 at a faster rate than it is produced by cellular metabolism, resulting in decreased $Paco_2$ or **hypocapnia** ($Paco_2$ less than 36 mmHg). Hypocapnia results in a respiratory alkalosis that also can interfere with tissue function. Like hypoventilation, hyperventilation can be determined only by arterial blood gas analysis. Hyperventilation commonly occurs with severe anxiety, acute head injury, and conditions that cause insufficient oxygenation of the blood.

Cyanosis

Cyanosis is a bluish discoloration of the skin and mucous membranes caused by increasing amounts of desaturated or reduced hemoglobin (which is bluish) in the blood. Cyanosis generally develops when 5 g of hemoglobin is desaturated, regardless of hemoglobin concentration. For example, if total hemoglobin concentration is 15 g/dl of blood, 5 g/dl must be desaturated to cause cyanosis. If total hemoglobin is 11 g/dl, 5 g/dl must still be desaturated for cyanosis to occur.

Peripheral cyanosis is most often caused by poor circulation resulting from intense peripheral vasoconstriction, like that seen in Raynaud disease, cold environments, or severe stress.

Central cyanosis is caused by decreased arterial oxygenation (low Pa_{O_2}) from pulmonary diseases or pulmonary or cardiac right-to-left shunts. In adults, cyanosis is not evident until severe hypoxemia is present and therefore is an insensitive indicator of respiratory distress. Lack of cyanosis does not necessarily indicate that oxygenation is normal. For example, severe anemia (inadequate hemoglobin concentration) and carbon monoxide poisoning (in which hemoglobin binds to carbon monoxide instead of binding to oxygen) can cause inadequate oxygenation of tissues without causing cyanosis. Individuals with polycythemia (an abnormal increase in numbers of red blood cells), however, may have cyanosis when tissue oxygenation is adequate. Because polycythemia causes hemoglobin concentration to be greater than normal, 5 g/dl can be desaturated, causing cyanosis, without having much effect on oxygenation. Therefore, the significance of cyanosis as a clinical finding must be interpreted in relation to the underlying pathophysiology. Central cyanosis is best seen in buccal mucous membranes and lips. Peripheral cyanosis is best seen in nail beds. If cyanosis is suggested, the Pa_{O_2} should be measured.

Clubbing

Clubbing is the selective bulbous enlargement of the end (distal segment) of a digit (finger or toe) (Figure 33-1) whose severity can be graded from 1 to 5 based on the extent of nail bed hypertrophy and the amount of changes in the nails themselves. Usually it is painless. Clubbing is commonly associated with diseases that interfere with oxygenation, such as bronchiectasis, cystic fibrosis, pulmonary fibrosis, lung abscess, and congenital heart disease. It is usually reversible with treatment of the underlying pulmonary condition.

Clubbing—early

Clubbing—middle

Clubbing—severe

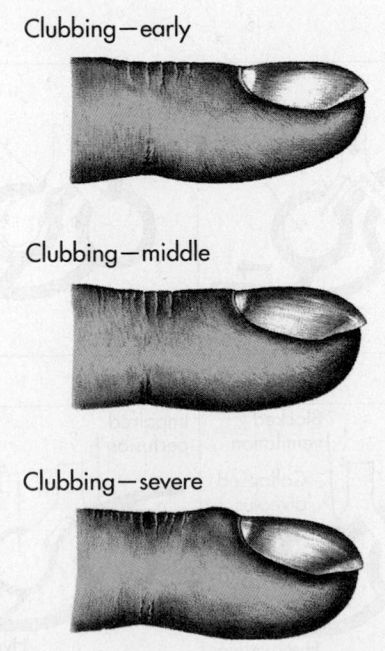

Figure 33-1 Clubbing of fingers caused by chronic hypoxemia. (From Seidel HM et al: *Mosby's guide to physical examination,* ed 6, St Louis, 2006, Mosby.)

Lung cancer is sometimes associated with clubbing even in the absence of significant hypoxemia. This syndrome is called *hypertrophic osteoarthropathy (HOA)* and its pathogenesis is unknown, although tumor-associated production of inflammatory cytokines and growth factors have been implicated.

Conditions Caused by Pulmonary Disease or Injury

Hypercapnia

Hypercapnia, or increased CO_2 in the arterial blood (increased Pa_{CO_2}), is caused by hypoventilation of the alveoli. As discussed in Chapter 32, CO_2 is easily diffused from the blood into the alveolar space; thus minute volume (respiratory rate × tidal volume) determines not only alveolar ventilation but also Pa_{CO_2}. Hypoventilation is often overlooked because breathing pattern and ventilatory rate may appear normal; it is important to obtain blood gas analysis to determine the severity of hypercapnia and resultant respiratory acidosis (acid-base balance is described in Chapter 3).

There are many causes of hypercapnia. Most are a result of decreased drive to breathe or an inadequate ability to respond to ventilatory stimulation. Causes include (1) depression of the respiratory center by drugs; (2) diseases of the medulla, including infections of the central nervous system or trauma; (3) abnormalities of the spinal conducting pathways, as in spinal cord disruption or poliomyelitis; (4) diseases of the neuromuscular junction or of the respiratory muscles themselves, as in myasthenia gravis or muscular dystrophy; (5) thoracic cage abnormalities, as in chest injury or congenital deformity; (6) large airway obstruction, as in tumors or sleep apnea; and (7) increased work of breathing or physiologic dead space, as in emphysema.

Hypercapnia and the associated respiratory acidosis can result in several important clinical manifestations. Of greatest concern are electrolyte abnormalities that occur in response to the low pH that may cause dysrhythmias. Individuals also may have somnolence and even be in a coma because of changes in intracranial pressure associated with high levels of arterial carbon dioxide, which causes cerebral vasodilation. Alveolar hypoventilation with increased alveolar carbon dioxide limits the amount of oxygen available for diffusion into the blood, leading to secondary hypoxemia.

Hypoxemia

Hypoxemia, or reduced oxygenation of arterial blood (reduced Pa_{O_2}), is caused by respiratory alterations, whereas **hypoxia,** or reduced oxygenation of cells in tissues, may be caused by alterations of other systems as well. Although hypoxemia can lead to tissue hypoxia, tissue hypoxia can result from other abnormalities, such as low cardiac output or cyanide poisoning, that have no relation to alterations of pulmonary function.

Hypoxemia results from problems with one or more of the major mechanisms of oxygenation:
1. Oxygen delivery to the alveoli
   a. Oxygen content of the inspired air (Fi_{O_2})

b. Ventilation of the alveoli
2. Diffusion of oxygen from the alveoli into the blood
   a. Balance between alveolar ventilation and perfusion ($\dot{V}/\dot{Q}$ march)
   b. Diffusion of oxygen across the alveolocapillary barrier
3. Perfusion of pulmonary capillaries

Table 33-1 lists some of the common clinical causes of these problems.

The amount of oxygen in the alveoli is called the P_{AO_2} and is dependent on two factors. The first factor is the presence of adequate oxygen content of the inspired air. The amount of oxygen in inspired air is expressed as the percentage or fraction of air that is composed of oxygen called the FiO_2. The FiO_2 of air at sea level is approximately 21% or 0.21. Anything that decreases the FiO_2 (such as high altitude) decreases the P_{AO_2}. The second factor is the amount of alveolar minute ventilation (tidal volume × respiratory rate). Hypoventilation results in an increase in P_ACO_2 and a decrease in P_{AO_2} such that there is less oxygen available in the alveoli for diffusion into the blood. This type of hypoxemia can be completely corrected if alveolar ventilation is improved by increases in the rate and depth of breathing. Hypoventilation causes hypoxemia in unconscious persons; in people with neurologic, muscular, or bone diseases that restrict chest expansion; and in individuals who have COPD.

Diffusion of oxygen from the alveoli into the blood is also dependent on two factors. The first is the balance between the amount of air getting into alveoli ($\dot{V}$) and the amount of blood perfusing the capillaries around the alveoli ($\dot{Q}$). An abnormal ventilation-perfusion ratio ($\dot{V}/\dot{Q}$) is the most common cause of hypoxemia (Figure 33-2). Normally, alveolocapillary lung units receive almost equal amounts of ventilation and perfusion. The normal $\dot{V}/\dot{Q}$ is 0.8 to 0.9 because perfusion is somewhat greater than ventilation in the lung bases and because some blood is normally shunted to the bronchial circulation. $\dot{V}/\dot{Q}$ mismatch refers to an abnormal distribution of ventilation and perfusion. Hypoxemia can be caused by inadequate ventilation of well-perfused areas of the lung (low $\dot{V}/\dot{Q}$). Mismatching of this type, called **shunting,** occurs in atelectasis, in asthma as a result of bronchoconstriction, and in pulmonary edema and pneumonia when alveoli are filled with fluid. When blood passes through portions of the pulmonary capillary bed that receive no ventilation, right-to-left shunt occurs, resulting in decreased systemic P_{aO_2} and hypoxemia. Hypoxemia also can be caused by poor perfusion of well-ventilated portions of the lung (high $\dot{V}/\dot{Q}$), resulting in wasted ventilation. The most common cause of high $\dot{V}/\dot{Q}$ is a pulmonary embolus that impairs blood flow to a segment of the lung. An area where alveoli are ventilated but not perfused is termed **alveolar dead space.**

The second factor affecting diffusion of oxygen from the alveoli into the blood is the alveolocapillary barrier. Diffusion of oxygen through the alveolocapillary membrane is impaired if the alveolocapillary membrane is thickened or the surface area available for diffusion is decreased. Abnormal thickness,

Table 33-1	Causes of Hypoxemia
Mechanism	**Common Clinical Causes**
Decrease in inspired oxygen (decreased FiO_2)	High altitude
	Low oxygen content of gas mixture
	Enclosed breathing spaces (suffocation)
Hypoventilation of the alveoli	Lack of neurologic stimulation of the respiratory center (oversedation, drug overdose, neurologic damage)
	Defects in chest wall mechanics (neuromuscular disease, trauma, chest deformity, air trapping),
	Large airway obstruction (laryngospasm, foreign body aspiration, neoplasm)
	Increased work of breathing (emphysema, severe asthma)
Ventilation-perfusion mismatch	Asthma
	Chronic bronchitis
	Pneumonia
	Acute respiratory distress syndrome
	Atelectasis
	Pulmonary embolism
Alveolocapillary diffusion abnormality	Edema
	Fibrosis
	Emphysema
Decreased pulmonary capillary perfusion	Intracardiac defects
	Intrapulmonary arteriovenous malformations

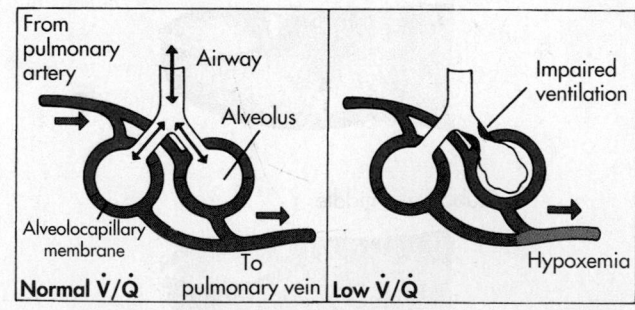
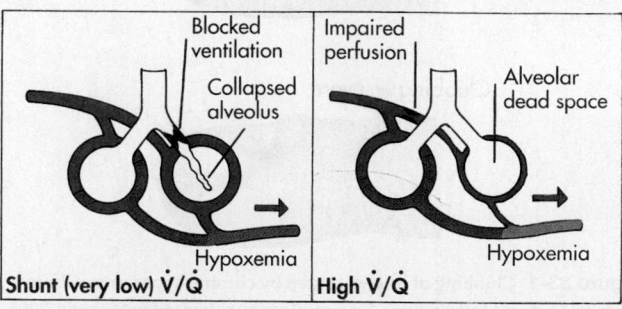

Figure 33-2 Ventilation-perfusion abnormalities.

as occurs with edema (tissue swelling) and fibrosis (formation of fibrous lesions), increases the time required for diffusion across the alveolocapillary membrane. If diffusion is slowed enough, the oxygen in the alveolar gas (P_{AO_2}) and capillary blood does not have time to equilibrate during the fraction of a second that blood remains in the capillary. Destruction of alveoli, such as that which occurs in emphysema, decreases the surface area available for diffusion. Hypercapnia is rarely produced by impaired diffusion because carbon dioxide diffuses so easily from capillary to alveolus that the individual with impaired diffusion would die from hypoxemia before hypercapnia could occur.

Hypoxemia most often is associated with a compensatory hyperventilation and resultant respiratory alkalosis (i.e., decreased Pa_{CO_2} and increased pH). However, in individuals with associated ventilatory difficulties, hypoxemia may be complicated by hypercapnia and respiratory acidosis. Hypoxemia results in widespread tissue dysfunction and, when severe, can lead to organ infarction. In addition, hypoxic pulmonary vasoconstriction can contribute to increased pressures in the pulmonary artery and lead to right-sided heart failure and cor pulmonale (see p. 1298). Clinical manifestations of acute hypoxemia may include cyanosis, confusion, tachycardia, edema, and decreased renal output.

Acute Respiratory Failure

Respiratory failure is defined as inadequate gas exchange, that is, hypoxemia, in which Pa_{O_3} is ≤50 mmHg, or hypercapnia, in which Pa_{CO_2} is ≥50 mmHg with a pH of ≤7.25. Respiratory failure can result from direct injury to the lungs, airways, or chest wall or indirectly because of injury to another body system such as the brain. It can occur in individuals who have an otherwise normal respiratory system or in those with underlying chronic pulmonary disease. Most pulmonary diseases can cause episodes of acute respiratory failure. If the respiratory failure is primarily hypercapnic, it is the result of inadequate alveolar ventilation (see Hypercapnia, p. 1269) and the individual must receive ventilatory support, such as with a bag-valve mask, noninvasive positive pressure ventilation, or intubation and placement on mechanical ventilation. If the respiratory failure is primarily hypoxemic, it is the result of inadequate exchange of oxygen between the alveoli and the capillaries (see Hypoxemia, p. 1269) and the individual must receive supplemental oxygen therapy. Many individuals have a combined hypercapnic and hypoxemic respiratory failure and require both kinds of support.

Respiratory failure is an important potential complication of any major surgical procedure, especially those that involve the central nervous system, thorax, or upper abdomen. Smokers are at risk, particularly if they have preexisting lung disease. Limited cardiac reserve, chronic renal failure, chronic hepatic disease, and infection also increase the tendency to develop postoperative respiratory failure. The most common postoperative pulmonary problems are atelectasis, pneumonia, pulmonary edema, and pulmonary emboli (these conditions are discussed later in this chapter).

Prevention of postoperative respiratory failure includes frequent turning, deep breathing, and early ambulation to prevent atelectasis and accumulation of secretions. Humidification of inspired air can help loosen secretions. Incentive spirometry gives individuals immediate feedback about tidal volumes, which encourages them to breathe deeply. Supplemental oxygen is given for hypoxemia, and antibiotics are given as appropriate to treat infection. If respiratory failure develops, the individual may require mechanical ventilation for a time.

DISORDERS OF THE CHEST WALL AND PLEURA

There are many conditions that can affect the chest wall and/or pleura that affect the function of the respiratory system. Chest wall disorders primarily affect tidal volume and therefore result in hypercapnia. Pleural diseases affect ventilation and oxygenation.

Disorders of the Chest Wall

Chest Wall Restriction

If the chest wall is deformed, traumatized, immobilized, or made heavy by fat, the work of breathing is increased and ventilation may be compromised because of a decrease in tidal volume. The degree of ventilatory impairment depends on the severity of the chest wall abnormality. Grossly obese individuals are often dyspneic on exertion or when recumbent. Individuals with severe kyphoscoliosis (lateral bending and rotation of the spinal column with distortion of the thoracic cage) often have dyspnea on exertion that can progress to respiratory failure. Such individuals are also susceptible to lower respiratory tract infections. Obesity and kyphoscoliosis are risk factors for respiratory disease in individuals admitted to a hospital for other problems, particularly those who require surgery. Other musculoskeletal abnormalities that can impair ventilation are ankylosing spondylitis and pectus excavatum (a deformity characterized by depression of the sternum) (see Chapters 42 and 43, respectively). Pain from chest wall injury, surgery, or disease is also an important cause of restriction and decreased tidal volume. This can cause significant hypoventilation, especially in those with underlying lung disease.

Impairment of respiratory muscle function caused by neuromuscular disease also can restrict the chest wall or impair pulmonary function. Muscle weakness can result in hypoventilation and hypercapnia, inability to remove secretions, and hypoxemia. The most common cause of hospital admission for individuals with neuromuscular diseases, such as poliomyelitis, muscular dystrophy, myasthenia gravis, and Guillain-Barré syndrome, is respiratory difficulty. (See Unit V for a more complete discussion of these disorders.)

Because chest wall restriction results in a decrease in tidal volume, an increase in respiratory rate can temporarily compensate and restore minute ventilation. However, many individuals will eventually progress to hypercapnic respiratory failure. Diagnosis of chest restriction is made by pulmonary function testing (reduction in forced vital capacity [FVC]), arterial blood gas measurement (hypercapnia), and radiographs. Treatment is aimed at any reversible underlying cause but is otherwise supportive. In severe cases, mechanical ventilation may be indicated.

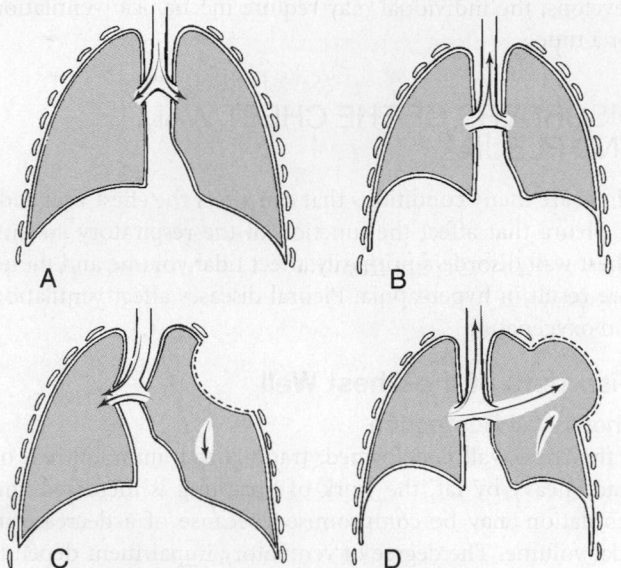

Figure 33-3 Flail chest. Normal respiration: A, inspiration; B, expiration. Paradoxical motion: C, inspiration, area of lung underlying unstable chest wall sucks in on inspiration; D, expiration, unstable area balloons out. Note movement of mediastinum toward opposite lung during inspiration.

Flail Chest

Flail chest results from the fracture of several consecutive ribs in more than one place, or the fracture of the sternum plus several consecutive ribs. These multiple fractures result in instability of a portion of the chest wall, causing paradoxical movement of the chest with breathing. During inspiration the unstable portion of the chest wall moves inward and during expiration it moves outward, impairing movement of gas in and out of the lungs (Figure 33-3). Flail chest is usually associated with significant underlying lung contusion.

The clinical manifestations of flail chest are pain, dyspnea, unequal chest expansion, hypoventilation, and hypoxemia. Treatment is internal fixation by controlled mechanical ventilation until the chest wall has stabilized.

Pleural Abnormalities

Pneumothorax

Pneumothorax is the presence of air or gas in the pleural space caused by a rupture in the visceral pleura (which surrounds the lungs) or the parietal pleura and chest wall (see Chapter 32). As air separates the visceral and parietal pleurae, it destroys the negative pressure of the pleural space. This disrupts the state of equilibrium that normally exists between elastic recoil forces of the lung and chest wall. No longer held in check by the recoil forces of the chest wall, the lung fulfills its tendency to recoil by collapsing toward the hilum (Figure 33-4).

Primary (spontaneous) pneumothorax, which occurs unexpectedly in healthy individuals (usually men) between ages 20 and 40 years, is most often caused by the spontaneous

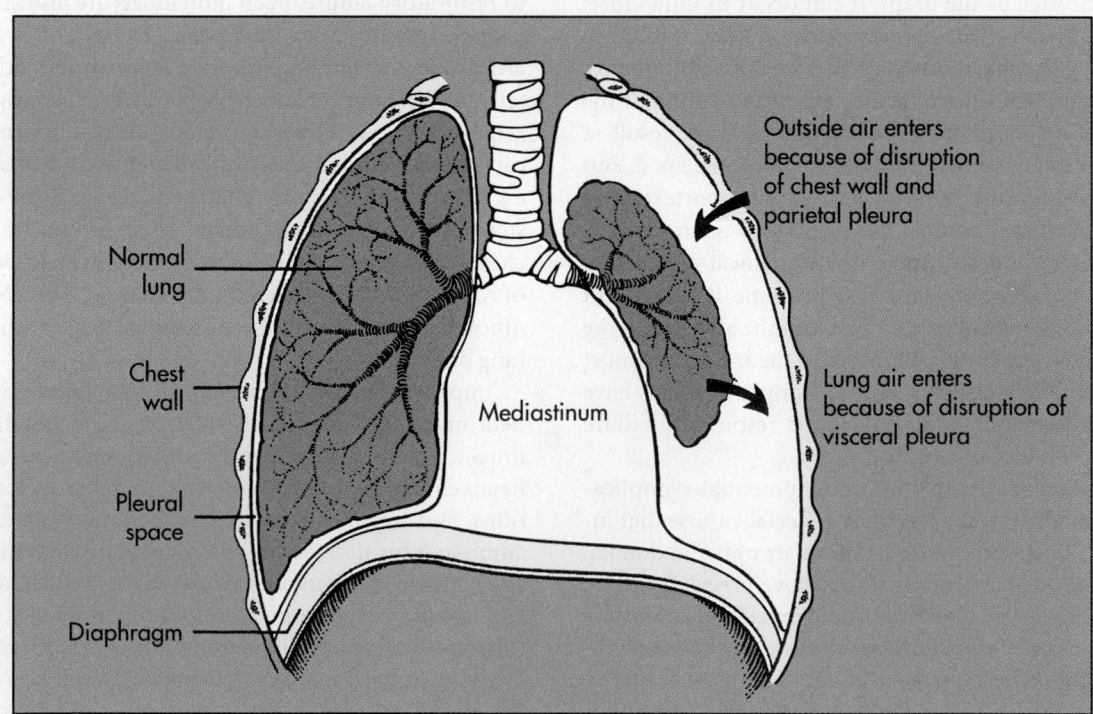

Figure 33-4 Pneumothorax. Air in the pleural space causes the lung to collapse around the hilus and may push mediastinal contents (heart and great vessels) toward the other lung.

rupture of blebs (blister-like formations) on the visceral pleura.[9,10] The cause of bleb formation is not known, although more than 80% of these individuals have been found to have emphysema-like changes in their lungs even if they have never smoked or have no known genetic disorder. Approximately 10% of affected individuals have a significant family history of primary pneumothorax that has been linked to mutations in the folliculin gene.[11] Bleb rupture can occur during sleep, rest, or exercise. The ruptured bleb or blebs are usually located in the apexes of the lungs. A **secondary pneumothorax** can be caused by chest trauma, such as a rib fracture, stab or bullet wounds, or surgical procedure that tears the pleura; rupture of a bleb or bulla (larger vesicle) as occurs in COPD; or mechanical ventilation, particularly if it includes positive end-expiratory pressure (PEEP).[10]

Spontaneous and secondary pneumothorax can present as either open or tension. In **open pneumothorax (communicating pneumothorax)**, air pressure in the pleural space equals barometric pressure because air that is drawn into the pleural space during inspiration (through the damaged chest wall and parietal pleura or through the lungs and damaged visceral pleura) is forced back out during expiration. In **tension pneumothorax**, however, the site of pleural rupture acts as a one-way valve, permitting air to enter on inspiration but preventing its escape by closing up during expiration. As more and more air enters the pleural space, air pressure in the pneumothorax begins to exceed barometric pressure. The pathophysiologic effects of tension pneumothorax are life threatening. Air pressure in the pleural space pushes against the already recoiled lung, causing compression atelectasis, and against the mediastinum, compressing and displacing the heart and great vessels.

Clinical manifestations of spontaneous or secondary pneumothorax begin with sudden pleural pain, tachypnea, and possibly mild dyspnea. The manifestations depend on the size of the pneumothorax. Physical examination may reveal absent or decreased breath sounds and hyperresonance to percussion on the affected side. Clinical manifestations of tension pneumothorax may also include severe hypoxemia, dyspnea, tracheal deviation away from the affected lung, and hypotension (low blood pressure).

Diagnosis of open pneumothorax is made with chest radiographs and CT. A thoracostomy (chest) tube is placed, and its efficacy in relieving the pneumothorax is documented on repeat chest radiograph. The diagnosis of tension pneumothorax is made on physical examination alone. It requires immediate treatment and a chest tube must be placed quickly. If a chest tube is not readily available, a large-bore needle is inserted into the pleural space to decompress it until a chest tube can be placed. An outward gush of air as the needle or chest tube is inserted confirms the presence of tension pneumothorax. For both open and tension pneumothorax, the chest tube is connected to a water-seal drainage and suction until the damaged pleura is healed.

In some situations, the pleural tear does not heal spontaneously and it is necessary to prevent recurrence of the pneumothorax by a process called *pleurodesis*. This procedure uses the chest tube to instill a caustic substance, such as talc, into the pleural space. The resultant inflammation and scarring as the pleura heals result in closure of the pleural tear. Some individuals require thoracotomy with pleurectomy.

Pleural Effusion

Pleural effusion is the presence of fluid in the pleural space. The source of the fluid is usually blood vessels or lymphatic vessels lying beneath either pleura, but occasionally an abscess or other lesion may drain into the pleural space. Because the pleura is a relatively permeable membrane, fluids that accumulate in the lung can cross into the pleural space.

The most common mechanism of pleural effusion is migration of fluids and other blood components through the walls of intact capillaries bordering the pleura. Pleural effusions that enter the pleural space from the intact blood vessels can be transudative or exudative. In **transudative effusion,** the fluid, or transudate, is watery and diffuses out of the capillaries as a result of disorders that increase intravascular hydrostatic pressure or decrease capillary oncotic pressure. Examples are congestive heart failure, in which venous and left atrial pressures are increased, and liver or kidney disorders that cause hypoproteinemia. Hypoproteinemia decreases capillary oncotic pressure, which promotes diffusion of water out of the capillaries. (This mechanism is discussed in Chapter 3).

Exudative effusion is less watery and contains high concentrations of white blood cells and plasma proteins. Exudative effusion occurs in response to inflammation, infection, or malignancy and involves inflammatory processes that increase capillary permeability (see Chapter 6). When stimulated by biochemical mediators of inflammation, junctions in the capillary endothelium separate slightly, enabling leukocytes and plasma proteins to migrate out into affected tissues. Other types of pleural effusion are characterized by the presence of pus **(empyema),** blood **(hemothorax),** or chyle **(chylothorax).** Mechanisms of pleural effusion are summarized in Table 33-2.

Small pleural effusions may not affect lung function and go undetected. Most will be removed by the lymphatic system once the underlying condition is resolved. Like pneumothorax, larger pleural effusions can cause compression atelectasis and displace mediastinal contents. Unlike pneumothorax, however, pleural effusion does not cause the lung to collapse. Because there is no communication between the pleural space and environmental air, pressure in the pleural space remains negative and atelectasis is caused solely by pressure exerted by the effusion.

The most common symptom associated with pleural effusion is dyspnea. Pleuritic chest pain may be present if the pleura is inflamed. Physical examination usually reveals decreased breath sounds and dullness to percussion on the affected side, and a pleural friction rub may be heard. In large, rapidly developing effusions, compression atelectasis may cause hypoxemia and mediastinal shift. Inability to expand the lungs may impair ventilation, leading to hypercapnia.

Table 33-2	Mechanisms of Pleural Effusion	
Type of Fluid/Effusion	**Source of Accumulation**	**Primary or Associated Disorder**
Transudate (hydrothorax)	Watery fluid that diffuses out of capillaries beneath the pleurae (i.e., capillaries in lung or chest wall)	Cardiovascular disease that causes high blood pressure; liver or kidney disease that disrupts plasma protein production, causing hypoproteinemia (decreased oncotic pressure in the blood vessels)
Exudate	Fluid rich in proteins (leukocytes, plasma proteins of all kinds; see Chapter 8) that migrates out of the capillaries	Infection, inflammation, or malignancy of the pleurae that stimulates mast cells to release biochemical mediators that increase capillary permeability
Empyema (pus)	Detritus of infection (microorganisms, leukocytes, cellular debris) dumped into the pleural space by blocked lymphatic vessels	Pulmonary infections, such as pneumonia; lung abscesses; infected wounds
Hemothorax (blood)	Hemorrhage into the pleural space	Traumatic injury, surgery, rupture, or malignancy that damages blood vessels
Chylothorax (chyle)	Chyle (milky fluid containing lymph and fat droplets) that is dumped by lymphatic vessels into the pleural space instead of passing from the gastrointestinal tract to the thoracic duct	Traumatic injury, infection, or disorder that disrupts lymphatic transport

NOTE: The principles of diffusion are discussed in Chapter 1; mechanisms that increase capillary permeability and cause exudation of cells and proteins are discussed in Chapter 8.

Diagnosis is confirmed by chest x-ray and thoracentesis (needle aspiration) with pleural fluid analysis, which can determine the type of effusion and provide symptomatic relief.[12] Small effusions will usually resolve with treatment of the underlying disorder. Large pleural effusions can contain several liters of fluid and require the placement of a thoracostomy (chest) tube.

Empyema

Empyema (infected pleural effusion) is the presence of pus in the pleural space. It is thought to develop when the pulmonary lymphatics become blocked, leading to an outpouring of contaminated lymphatic fluid into the pleural space. Empyema occurs most commonly in older adults and children and usually develops as a complication of pneumonia, surgery, trauma, or bronchial obstruction from a tumor.[13] Commonly documented infectious microorganisms include *Staphylococcus aureus*, *Escherichia coli*, anaerobic bacteria, and *Klebsiella pneumoniae*.

Individuals with empyema are usually quite ill and may have cyanosis, fever, tachycardia (rapid heart rate), cough, and pleural pain. Breath sounds are decreased directly over the empyema. Diagnosis is made by chest radiographs and thoracentesis. Identification of the causative microorganism by positive cultures from the pleural fluid is obtained only about 50% of the time, and empiric antibiotics may be needed. The treatment for empyema includes the administration of appropriate antimicrobials, and thoracentesis is performed to drain the pleural space. Continuous drainage with a chest tube may be required. In severe cases, instillation of fibrinolytic agents or deoxyribonuclease (DNase) into the pleural space may be required to mobilize the fluid and facilitate drainage. Surgical débridement of the pleural space also may be performed to prevent reaccumulation and achieve adequate drainage.

PULMONARY DISORDERS

Restrictive Lung Disorders

Restrictive lung disorders are characterized by decreased compliance of lung tissue. This means that it takes more effort to expand the lungs during inspiration, which increases the work of breathing. Individuals with lung restriction complain of dyspnea and have an increased respiratory rate and decreased tidal volume. Pulmonary function testing reveals a decrease in FVC. Restrictive lung diseases can cause ventilation and perfusion mismatch or can affect the alveolocapillary membrane. In both cases there is decreased diffusion of oxygen from the alveoli into the blood, resulting in hypoxemia. Some of the most common restrictive lung diseases in adults are aspiration, atelectasis, bronchiectasis, bronchiolitis, pulmonary fibrosis, inhalational disorders, pneumoconiosis, allergic alveolitis, pulmonary edema, and acute respiratory distress syndrome.

Aspiration

Aspiration is the passage of fluid and solid particles into the lung. It tends to occur in individuals whose normal swallowing mechanism and cough reflex are impaired by a decreased level of consciousness or central nervous system abnormalities. It has been estimated that more than 10% of all hospital admissions for community-acquired pneumonias and up to 30% of admissions for pneumonia in residents of long-term facilities are the result of aspiration.[13] Predisposing factors include altered level of consciousness caused by substance abuse, sedation, or anesthesia; seizure disorders; cerebrovascular accident; and neuromuscular disorders that cause dysphagia. In individuals who require enteral feeding (through a nasogastric feeding tube), aspiration is common and frequently leads to bacterial pneumonia.[14] The right lung, particularly the right lower lobe, is more susceptible to aspiration than the left lung because the branching angle of the right mainstem bronchus is straighter than the branching angle of the left mainstem bronchus.

The effects of aspiration depend on the material aspirated. The aspiration of large food particles or gastric fluid with pH of less than 2.5 has serious consequences. Solid food particles can obstruct a bronchus, resulting in bronchial inflammation and collapse of airways distal to the obstruction. If the aspirated solid is not identified and removed by bronchoscopy, a chronic, local inflammation develops that may lead to recurrent infection and bronchiectasis (permanent dilation of the bronchus). Once the pathologic process has progressed to bronchiectasis, surgical resection of the affected area is usually required.

Aspiration of oral or pharyngeal secretions can lead to aspiration pneumonia, especially if the oral cavity is colonized with bacteria (e.g., individuals with poor dentition). Intubation of the trachea also can cause aspiration and bacterial pneumonia. Aspiration of acidic gastric fluid may cause severe pneumonitis. Bronchial damage includes inflammation, loss of ciliary function, and bronchospasm. In the alveoli, acidic fluid damages the alveolocapillary membrane. This allows plasma and blood cells to move from capillaries into the alveoli, resulting in hemorrhagic pneumonitis. The lung becomes stiff and noncompliant as surfactant production is disrupted, leading to further edema and collapse. Hypoventilation may develop as this progresses, and systematic complications, such as hypotension, may occur.

The clinical manifestations of aspiration include the sudden onset of choking and intractable cough with or without vomiting, fever, dyspnea, and wheezing. Some individuals have no symptoms acutely; instead they have recurrent lung infections, chronic cough, or persistent wheezing over months and even years.

Preventive measures for individuals at risk are more effective than treatment of known aspiration. The most important preventive measures include a semirecumbent position, surveillance of enteral feeding, use of promotility agents, and avoidance of excessive sedation. Individuals undergoing general anesthesia should not receive food or fluid for several hours before or after surgery. Antacids are sometimes given to individuals at risk for aspiration to keep gastric pH greater than 2.5. Individuals who have difficulty swallowing are fed with extreme caution and positioned to minimize the likelihood of aspiration. Nasogastric tubes, which often are used to remove stomach contents and reduce the risk for aspiration, also can cause aspiration if fluid and particulate matter are regurgitated as the tube is being placed. For those who suffer from swallowing difficulties, speech-language pathologists can often improve swallowing abilities and prevent recurrence.

The rate of deaths resulting from aspiration-caused pneumonitis has been estimated to be as high as 50%. Treatment includes supplemental oxygen and may require mechanical ventilation with PEEP. Fluids are restricted to decrease blood volume and minimize pulmonary edema. Steroids often

are administered during the first 72 hours after aspiration, although their effectiveness is not well documented. Bacterial pneumonia may develop as a complication of aspiration pneumonitis and must be treated with broad-spectrum antibiotics.

Atelectasis

Atelectasis is the collapse of lung tissue. There are three types of atelectasis: compression, absorption, and surfactant impairment[15]:

1. **Compression atelectasis** is caused by the external pressure exerted on lung tissue, such as occurs with tumors, or by fluid or air in the pleural space. Atelectasis at the base of the lungs can be caused by abdominal distention pressing on a portion of the lung, causing the alveoli to collapse.
2. **Absorption atelectasis** results from gradual absorption of air from obstructed or hypoventilated alveoli or from inhalation of concentrated oxygen or anesthetic agents.
3. **Surfactant impairment** results from decreased production or inactivation of surfactant that is necessary to reduce surface tension in the alveoli and thus prevent lung collapse during expiration. Surfactant impairment can occur because of prematurity, acute respiratory distress syndrome, anesthesia, or mechanical ventilation.

Atelectasis tends to occur after surgery. Intraoperative high-dose supplemental oxygen in combination with general anesthesia increases the likelihood of postoperative atelectasis.[15] In addition, individuals are often in pain, breathe shallowly, are reluctant to change position, and produce viscous secretions that tend to pool in dependent portions of the lung after surgical procedures, especially those involving the thorax or upper abdomen.

Clinical manifestations of atelectasis are similar to those of pulmonary infection: dyspnea, cough, fever, and leukocytosis. Prevention and treatment of postoperative atelectasis usually include deep breathing (often with the aid of an incentive spirometer), frequent position changes, and early ambulation. Deep breathing is beneficial because it (1) promotes the ciliary clearance of secretions, (2) stabilizes the alveoli by redistributing surfactant, and (3) permits collateral ventilation of the alveoli through pores of Kohn in the alveolar septa. The pores of Kohn, which open only during deep breathing, allow air to pass from well-ventilated alveoli to obstructed alveoli, minimizing their tendency to collapse and facilitating expectoration of the bronchial obstruction (Figure 33-5).

Bronchiectasis

Bronchiectasis is persistent abnormal dilation of the bronchi. It usually occurs in conjunction with other respiratory conditions that are associated with chronic bronchial inflammation. Causes include obstruction of an airway with mucous plugs, atelectasis, aspiration of a foreign body, infection, cystic fibrosis, tuberculosis, congenital weakness of the bronchial wall, or impaired defense mechanisms. Bronchiectasis

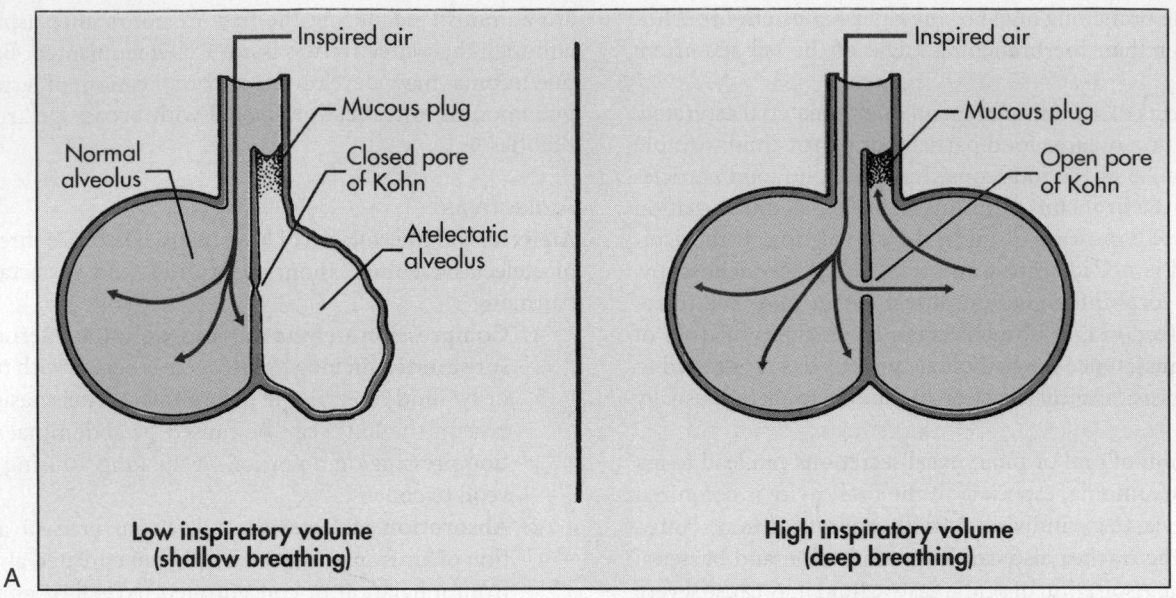

Figure 33-5 Pores of Kohn. **A,** Absorption atelectasis caused by lack of collateral ventilation through pores of Kohn. **B,** Restoration of collateral ventilation during deep breathing.

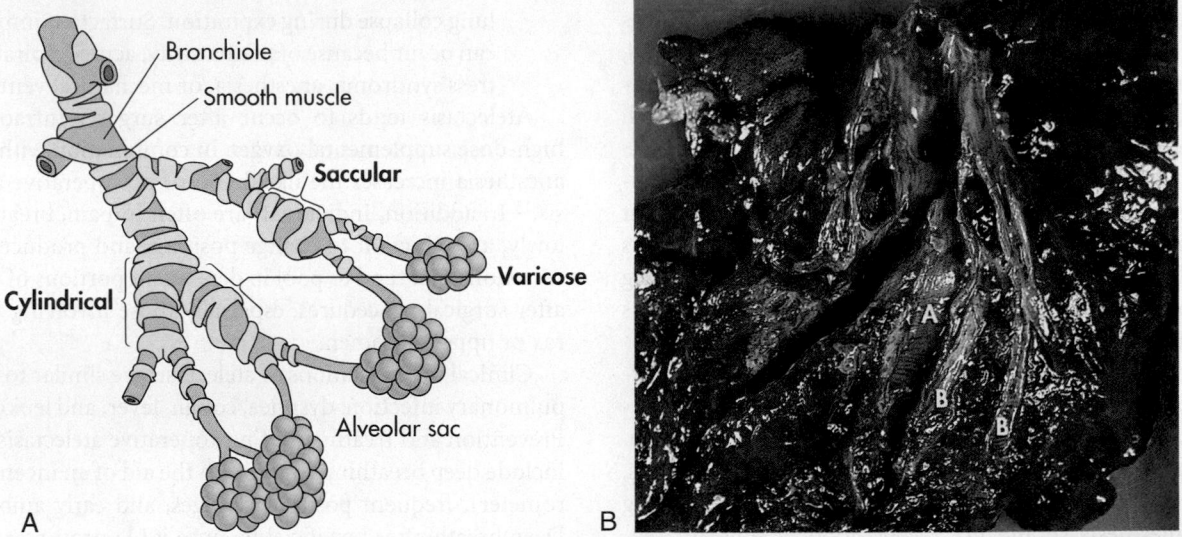

Figure 33-6 Bronchiectasis. **A,** Types of bronchiectasis. **B,** Cylindrical bronchiectasis. The dilated bronchi *(A)* and bronchioles *(B)* can be dissected almost to the pleural surface. **(B,** From Damjanov I, Linder J, editors: *Anderson's pathology,* ed 10, St Louis, 1996, Mosby.)

is also associated with a number of systemic disorders such as rheumatologic disease, inflammatory bowel disease, and immunodeficiency syndromes (e.g., acquired immunodeficiency syndrome [AIDS]).[16]

Chronic inflammation of the bronchi leads to destruction of elastic and muscular components of their walls and permanent dilation.[16] Bronchial dilation (Figure 33-6) may be *cylindrical* (**cylindrical bronchiectasis**), with symmetrically dilated airways as can be seen after pneumonia and is reversible; *saccular* (**saccular bronchiectasis**), in which the bronchi become large and balloon-like; or *varicose* (**varicose bronchiectasis**), in which constrictions and dilations

deform the bronchi. In both varicose and saccular bronchiectasis, the smaller bronchial divisions are plugged with secretions or obliterated by fibrosis. Large anastomoses (connections) develop between the bronchial and pulmonary blood vessels, increasing blood flow through the bronchial circulation. These anastomoses are thought to cause the hemoptysis experienced by individuals with bronchiectasis. Airway damage leads to bronchospasm and copious production of purulent mucus. Ventilation-perfusion abnormalities develop and result in hypoxemia. In severe cases, minute ventilation is also compromised and $Paco_2$ may become elevated.

The primary symptom of bronchiectasis is chronic productive cough. The symptoms of bronchiectasis may date back to a childhood illness or infection. The disease is commonly associated with recurrent lower respiratory tract infections and expectoration of voluminous amounts of purulent sputum (measured in cupfuls). If the individual is not receiving antibiotics, the sputum has a foul odor. Hemoptysis and clubbing of the fingers are common. Pulmonary function studies show decreases in FVC and expiratory flow rates. The diagnosis is usually confirmed by the use of high-resolution CT. Bronchiectasis is treated with antibiotics, bronchodilators, chest physiology, and supplemental oxygen.[16] In selected individuals with localized areas of involvement, surgery may be indicated to remove the affected portion of the lung.

Bronchiolitis

Bronchiolitis is inflammation of the small airways or bronchioles. It is most common in children (see Chapter 34). In adults it usually occurs with chronic bronchitis but can occur in otherwise healthy individuals in association with an upper or lower airway viral infection (e.g., respiratory syncytial virus [RSV]), or with inhalation of toxic gases. Atelectasis or emphysematous destruction of the alveoli may develop distal to the inflammatory lesion. Bronchiolitis is usually diffuse. The resulting decrease in the ventilation-perfusion ratio results in hypoxemia. A decrease in minute ventilation with resulting carbon dioxide retention also may occur as lung restriction worsens.

Clinical manifestations include a rapid ventilatory rate; marked use of accessory muscles; low-grade fever; dry, nonproductive cough; and hyperinflated chest. If bronchiolitis is caused by an inhalation injury, pulmonary edema occurs rapidly and then quickly clears. One to 2 weeks later, respiratory distress develops, and infiltrates are seen on chest radiographs. Bronchiolitis is treated with appropriate antibiotics, steroids, and chest physical therapy (humidified air, coughing and deep breathing, postural drainage).

Bronchiolitis obliterans is a late-stage fibrotic process that occludes the airways and causes permanent scarring of the lungs. This process can occur in all causes of bronchiolitis but is most common after lung transplantation. Bronchiolitis obliterans can be further complicated by the development of pneumonia (called **bronciolitis obliterans organizing pneumonia [BOOP]**) in which the alveoli and bronchioles become filled with plugs of connective tissue.[16] This complication of lung transplant has a high morbidity. Diagnosis is made by spirometry and bronchoscopy with biopsy. Treatment includes corticosteroids and other immunosuppressive agents.[17]

Pulmonary Fibrosis

Pulmonary fibrosis is an excessive amount of fibrous or connective tissue in the lung. When no specific cause for the development of fibrosis is known, it is called *idiopathic pulmonary fibrosis*. Although fibrosis can complicate healing after active pulmonary diseases, such as ARDS or tuberculosis, specific causes most often include inhalation of harmful substances, such as toxic gases, inorganic dusts, or organic dusts, and underlying autoimmune systemic disorders, such as rheumatologic disease. The fibrotic process results from chronic inflammation, alveolar epithelialization, and myofibroblast proliferation. Fibrosis causes a marked loss of lung compliance. The lung becomes stiff and difficult to ventilate, and the diffusing capacity of the alveolocapillary membrane may decrease, causing hypoxemia.

Idiopathic Pulmonary Fibrosis

Idiopathic pulmonary fibrosis (IPF) is the most common idiopathic interstitial lung disorder. It is more common in men than in women and most cases occur after age 60. The median survival is only 2 to 4 years after diagnosis. IPF is characterized by chronic inflammation and fibroproliferation of the interstitial lung tissue around the alveoli. This causes decreased oxygen diffusion across the alveolocapillary membrane and hypoxemia. As the disease progresses decreased lung compliance leads to increased work of breathing, decreased tidal volume, and resultant hypoventilation with hypercapnia. Acute exacerbations of IPF can occur with rapid decompensation and a mortality as high as 40%.[18] The primary symptom of IPF is increasing dyspnea on exertion; examination reveals diffuse inspiratory crackles and diagnosis is confirmed by pulmonary function testing (decreased FVC), high-resolution CT, and lung biopsy. Treatment with corticosteroids alone causes remission in approximately 50% of individuals. Combined treatment with cytotoxic drugs has a higher success rate but also higher toxicity. Newer therapies include antifibrotic drugs (such as *N*-acetylcysteine and pirfenidone), interferon, and anticoagulation.[19] Selected individuals may benefit from lung transplantation.

Exposure to Toxic Gases

Inhalation of gaseous irritants can cause significant respiratory dysfunction. Commonly encountered toxic gases include ammonia, hydrogen chloride, sulfur dioxide, chlorine, phosgene, and nitrogen dioxide. Inhalation injuries in burns can include toxic gases from household or industrial combustants, heat, and smoke particles. Inhaled toxic particles cause damage to the airway epithelium, mucus secretion, inflammation, mucosal edema, ciliary damage, pulmonary edema, and surfactant inactivation. The cellular effects of toxic gases are described in Chapter 2. Acute toxic inhalation is frequently complicated by the ARDS and pneumonia.[20] Initial symptoms include burning of the eyes, nose, and throat; coughing; chest tightness; and dyspnea. Hypoxemia is common. Treatment includes supplemental oxygen, mechanical ventilation with PEEP, and support of the cardiovascular system. Steroids sometimes are used, although their effectiveness has not been well documented. Most individuals respond quickly to therapy. Some, however, may improve initially and then deteriorate as a result of bronchiectasis or bronchiolitis.

Prolonged exposure to high concentrations of supplemental oxygen can result in a relatively rare iatrogenic condition known as **oxygen toxicity**. The basic underlying mechanism of injury is a severe inflammatory response mediated primarily by oxygen radicals. The result is damage to alveolocapillary membranes, disruption of surfactant production, interstitial and alveolar edema, and decrease in compliance. Treatment involves ventilatory support and reduction of inspired oxygen concentration to less than 60% as soon as tolerated.

Pneumoconiosis

Pneumoconiosis represents any change in the lung caused by inhalation of inorganic dust particles, which usually occurs in the workplace. As in all cases of environmentally acquired lung disease, the individual's history of exposure is important in determining the diagnosis. Pneumoconiosis often occurs after years of exposure to the offending dust, and manifestations are often difficult to differentiate from those resulting from smoking.

The dusts of silica, asbestos, and coal are the most common causes of pneumoconiosis. Others include talc, fiberglass, clays, mica, slate, cement, cadmium, beryllium, tungsten, cobalt, aluminum, and iron. Deposition of these materials in the lungs leads to chronic inflammation with scarring of the alveolar capillary membrane, leading to pulmonary fibrosis and progressive pulmonary deterioration (see p. 1277). Clinical manifestations with advancement of disease may include cough, sputum production, dyspnea, decreased lung volumes, and hypoxemia. In most cases, diagnosis is made by chest x-ray, CT, and careful occupational history.[21] Treatment is usually palliative and focuses on preventing further exposure and improving working conditions, along with pulmonary rehabilitation and management of associated hypoxemia and bronchospasm.

Silicosis is a type of pneumoconiosis resulting from the inhalation of free silica (silicon dioxide) and silica-containing compounds. Silica exposure occurs in mining and other industries involved with the extraction and processing of ores; preparation and use of sand; and manufacture of pipe, building, and roofing materials. Silica exposure activates innate and adaptive immune mechanisms and causes tissue injury and cellular apoptosis.[22] Acute inflammation contributes to bronchospasm and wheezing. Persistent alveolitis progresses to diffuse fibrosis and nodules within the lung. Release of proteolytic enzymes and toxic oxygen radicals increases the risk for lung cancer.[22] Exposed individuals may remain asymptomatic long after the nodules are visible on chest radiography. When clinical manifestations do appear, they include cough and dyspnea. There is no specific treatment for the disease, although corticosteroids may produce some improvement in the early, more acute stages.

Coal worker pneumoconiosis (coal miner lung, black lung) is caused by coal dust deposits in the lung. Although coal dust itself is relatively well tolerated by the lung, it is frequently inhaled as a mixture of coal, silica, and quartz, which is strongly inflammatory.[23] Its mild form is asymptomatic, except for possible chronic bronchitis. Its advanced form consists of severe pulmonary fibrosis. Individuals usually are seen with a productive cough and wheezing. Symptoms are more severe with advanced disease and mimic those of chronic bronchitis (see p. 1287). Diagnosis is made by history of exposure and characteristic chest radiographs. There is no specific treatment for coal worker pneumoconiosis. Individuals with the mild form of the disease usually do well. Those with more

complicated forms often develop marked cardiopulmonary dysfunction.

Asbestos exposure affects not only factory workers but also individuals who live in areas of asbestos emission. Asbestos exposure can result in a type of pulmonary fibrosis called **asbestosis**, but can also cause lung cancer; mesothelioma (cancer of the pleura); or pleural plaques, especially in those also exposed to cigarette smoke.[24] Asbestosis is caused by inhalation of hydrous silicates of various metals in fibrous form. Asbestos fibers cause inflammation, release of toxic oxygen radicals, and cellular apoptosis leading to both fibrosis and malignancy. The most prominent clinical manifestations of asbestosis with fibrosis are dyspnea on exertion, a nonproductive cough, diffuse inspiratory crackles on examination, hypoxemia, and decreased lung volume. Progressive disease may lead to respiratory failure and cardiac complications. Diagnosis is made by chest x-ray, pulmonary function testing, and CT. Therapy is supportive.

Allergic Alveolitis

Inhalation of organic dusts can result in an allergic inflammatory response called **allergic alveolitis (hypersensitivity pneumonitis).** Many allergens can cause this disorder, including grains, silage, bird droppings or feathers, wood dust (particularly redwood and maple), cork dust, animal pelts, coffee beans, fish meal, mushroom compost, and molds that grow on sugar cane, barley, and straw. The immune response to these allergens results in immunoglobulin G (IgG) antibody production and cellular immune activation with initiation of the inflammatory response.[25] Granuloma formation is common.

Allergic alveolitis can be acute, subacute, or chronic. The acute form causes a fever, cough, dyspnea, and chills a few hours after exposure that resolve without treatment in 1 to 3 days. With continued exposure, the disease becomes chronic and pulmonary fibrosis develops. (The mechanisms of hypersensitivity reactions are discussed in Chapter 8.) Chronic allergic alveolitis causes weight loss, fever, fatigue, and gradually progressive respiratory failure. Diagnosis is made by obtaining a history of allergen exposure and by serum antibody testing, chest x-ray, bronchoscopy, and CT.[26] Treatment consists of avoidance of the offending agent and corticosteroid administration.

Systemic Disorders

Several systemic diseases affect the airways, pleurae, or lung parenchyma, causing fibrosis, vasculitis, pulmonary hemorrhage, or granuloma formation. Clinical manifestations of lung involvement are usually nonspecific, and the diagnosis is based on involvement of other organs. There is usually no specific treatment, although corticosteroids often are used. Some of the systemic diseases affecting the lung are granulomatous disorders such as sarcoidosis, Wegener granulomatosis, lymphomatoid granulomatosis, and eosinophilic granuloma; connective tissue diseases such as rheumatoid arthritis, systemic lupus erythematosus, scleroderma, polymyositis or dermatomyositis, Sjögren syndrome, and polyarteritis nodosa; angioimmunoblastic or immunoblastic lymphadenopathy (a disease of the lymph nodes); cystic fibrosis (see Chapter 34); and Goodpasture syndrome (a pulmonary and renal disorder).

Pulmonary Edema

Pulmonary edema is excess water in the lung. The normal lung contains very little fluid. It is kept dry by lymphatic drainage and a balance among capillary hydrostatic pressure, capillary oncotic pressure, and capillary permeability. In addition, surfactant lining the alveoli repels water, keeping fluid from entering the alveoli. Predisposing factors for pulmonary edema include heart disease, ARDS, and inhalation of toxic gases. The pathogenesis of pulmonary edema is illustrated in Figure 33-7.

The most common cause of pulmonary edema is heart disease (see Chapter 30). When the left ventricle fails, filling pressures on the left side of the heart increase and cause a concomitant increase in pulmonary capillary hydrostatic pressure. When the hydrostatic pressure exceeds oncotic pressure, fluid moves out into the interstitium, or interstitial space (the space within the alveolar septum between alveolus and capillary). Fluid is initially picked up by lymphatic vessels and removed from the lung. When the flow of fluid out of the capillaries exceeds the lymphatic system's ability to remove it, pulmonary edema develops. Pulmonary edema usually begins to develop at a pulmonary capillary wedge pressure or left atrial pressure of 20 mmHg. If the capillary oncotic pressure is decreased for any reason (e.g., anemia or decreased plasma proteins), pulmonary edema develops at a lower hydrostatic pressure.

Another cause of pulmonary edema is capillary injury that increases capillary permeability. Capillary injury causes edema in cases of ARDS or inhalation of toxic gases, such as ammonia. Capillary injury causes water and plasma proteins to leak out of the capillary and move into the interstitium. When plasma proteins move into the lung interstitium, they increase the interstitial oncotic pressure, which is usually very low. As the interstitial oncotic pressure begins to equal capillary oncotic pressure, water moves out of the capillary and into the lung. (Mechanisms of edema are discussed in Chapter 3.)

Pulmonary edema also can result from obstruction of the lymphatic system. Drainage can be blocked by compression of lymphatic vessels caused by edema, tumors, and fibrotic tissue or by increased systemic venous pressure that elevates hydrostatic pressure of the large pulmonary veins into which the pulmonary lymphatic system drains. This can happen in left-sided heart failure.

Clinical manifestations of pulmonary edema include dyspnea, orthopnea, hypoxemia, and increased work of breathing. Physical examination may reveal inspiratory crackles (rales), dullness to percussion over the lung bases, and evidence of ventricular dilation (S_3 gallop and cardiomegaly). In severe edema, pink, frothy sputum is expectorated, hypoxemia worsens, and hypoventilation with hypercapnia may develop.

The treatment of pulmonary edema depends on its cause. If the edema is caused by increased hydrostatic pressure caused by heart failure, therapy is geared toward improving cardiac output and volume status with diuretics, vasodilators, and drugs that improve the contraction of the heart muscle. If edema is the result of increased capillary permeability resulting from injury, the treatment is focused on removing the offending agent and supportive therapy to maintain adequate oxygenation, ventilation, and circulation. Individuals with either type of pulmonary edema require supplemental oxygen. Mechanical ventilation may be needed if edema significantly impairs ventilation and oxygenation.

Acute Respiratory Distress Syndrome

Acute respiratory distress syndrome (ARDS) is a fulminant form of respiratory failure characterized by acute lung inflammation and diffuse alveolocapillary injury. In the United

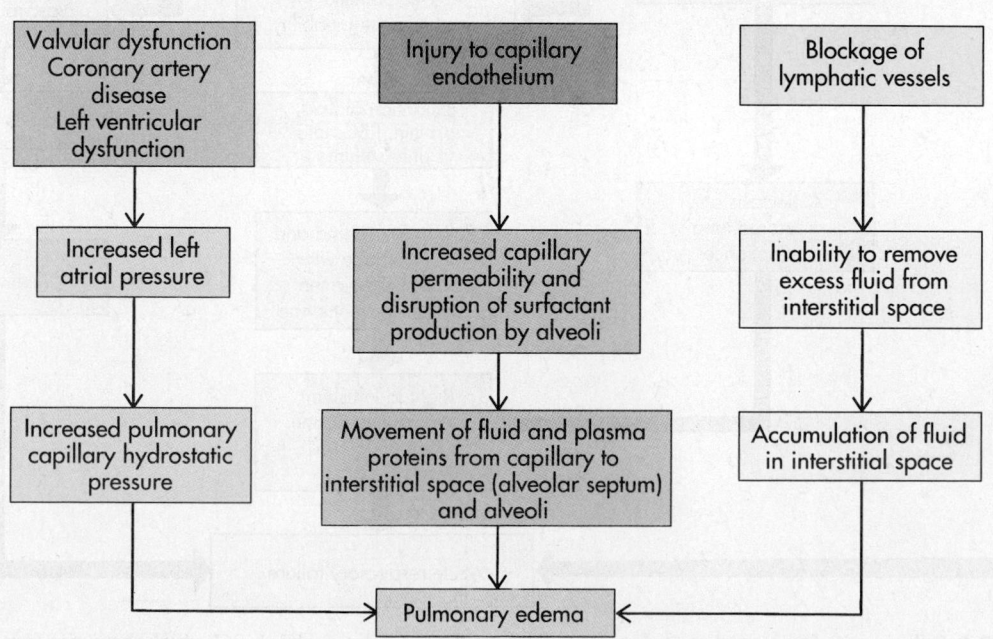

Figure 33-7 Pathogenesis of pulmonary edema.

States, acute lung injury (a slightly milder form of lung injury) and ARDS complicate more than 30% of all intensive care unit (ICU) admissions.[27] Advances in therapy have decreased the overall mortality rate to approximately 40%, although older people and those with severe infections or are immunocompromised continue to have a much higher mortality rate.[27] Most survivors, however, have almost normal lung function 1 year after the acute illness. ARDS is the result of injury to the lung by numerous unrelated causes. The most common predisposing factors are sepsis and multiple trauma (especially

when multiple transfusions are received); however, there are many other causes, including pneumonia, burns, aspiration, cardiopulmonary bypass surgery, pancreatitis, drug overdose, smoke or noxious gas inhalation, oxygen toxicity, radiation therapy, and disseminated intravascular coagulation.[27]

PATHOPHYSIOLOGY All disorders that result in ARDS cause massive pulmonary inflammation that acutely injures the alveolocapillary membrane and produces severe pulmonary edema (Figure 33-8). The alveolocapillary damage can occur directly, as with the aspiration of highly acidic

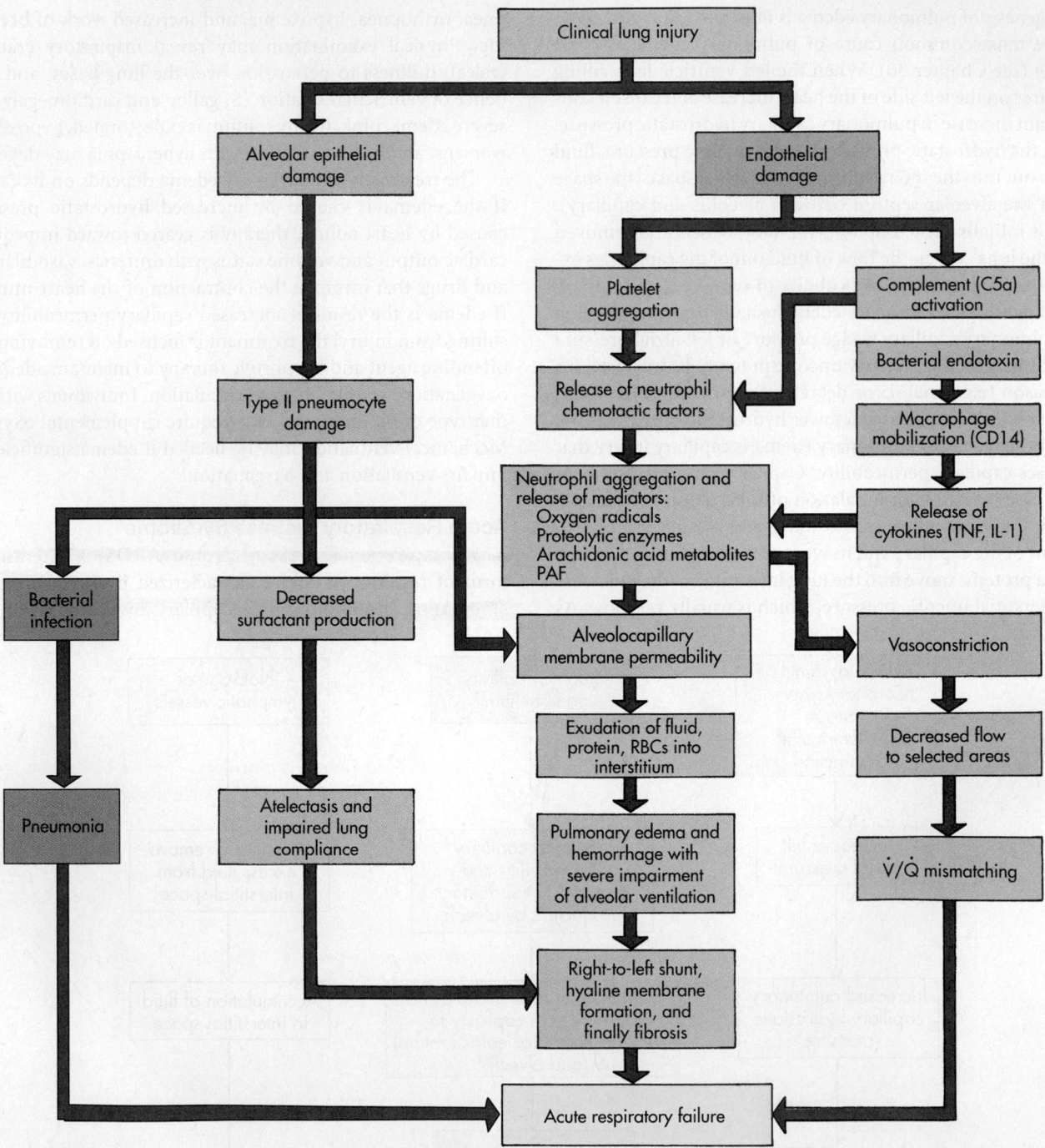

Figure 33-8 Pathogenesis of acute respiratory distress syndrome (ARDS). *IL-1*, Interleukin-1; *PAF*, platelet-activating factor; *RBCs*, red blood cells; *TNF*, tumor necrosis factor.

gastric contents or inhalation of toxic gases, or indirectly from chemical mediators released in response to systemic disorders, as with sepsis and trauma. Because the form of pulmonary edema is not secondary to heart failure, ARDS is often referred to as *noncardiogenic pulmonary edema.*

The initial injury to the lungs damages the pulmonary capillary endothelium, activating complement and stimulating platelet aggregation and intravascular thrombus formation. Platelets release substances that attract and activate neutrophils. In ARDS caused by sepsis, bacterial toxins are recognized by the CD14 receptors on macrophages and result in chemotaxis of large numbers of neutrophils to the lungs. A cascade of inflammatory mediators is released by the macrophages, including tumor necrosis factor (TNF), interleukin-1 (IL-1), alpha and beta chemokines, and other interleukins.[28,29] Complement is also activated and contributes to lung capillary damage.

The role of neutrophils is central to the development of ARDS. Activated neutrophils release a battery of inflammatory mediators, among them proteolytic enzymes, oxygen-free radicals (superoxide radicals, hydrogen peroxide, hydroxyl radicals), arachidonic acid metabolites (prostaglandins, thromboxanes, leukotrienes), and platelet-activating factor. These mediators cause extensive damage of the alveolocapillary membrane and greatly increase capillary membrane permeability.

Increased capillary permeability, a hallmark of ARDS, allows fluids, proteins, and blood cells to leak from the capillary bed into the pulmonary interstitium and alveoli. The resulting pulmonary edema and hemorrhage severely reduce lung compliance and impair alveolar ventilation (Figure 33-9).

Mediators released by neutrophils, and to a certain extent by macrophages, also cause pulmonary vasoconstriction. Pulmonary hypertension occurs early in the course of the disease secondary to vasoconstriction and to vascular occlusion by aggregated neutrophils, macrophages, and platelets. Because vasoconstriction occurs more in some vascular beds than others, blood flow to selected areas of the lungs is decreased, resulting in $\dot{V}/\dot{Q}$ mismatching.

Lung inflammation and injury damages the alveolar epithelium and the vascular endothelium. Surfactant is inactivated, and its production by type II alveolar cells is impaired as alveoli and respiratory bronchioles fill with fluid or collapse. The lungs become less compliant, resulting in increased work of breathing and decreased minute ventilation and hypercapnia.

Within 24 to 48 hours after the acute hemorrhagic phase of ARDS, hyaline membranes form, and after approximately 7 days, fibrosis progressively obliterates the alveoli, respiratory bronchioles, and interstitium. This leads to a decrease in functional residual capacity (FRC) and even more $\dot{V}/\dot{Q}$ mismatching with severe right-to-left shunting. The result of this overwhelming inflammatory response by the lungs is acute respiratory failure.

The same chemical mediators responsible for the alveolocapillary damage of ARDS often cause widespread inflammation, endothelial damage, and capillary permeability throughout the body, resulting in the systemic inflammatory response syndrome (SIRS), which then leads to multiple organ dysfunction syndrome (MODS). In fact, death may not be caused by respiratory failure alone but by MODS associated with ARDS. (MODS is discussed in Chapter 46.)

CLINICAL MANIFESTATIONS The primary symptom of ARDS is progressive dyspnea. The initial physical examination may only reveal tachypnea, followed by gradually increasing inspiratory crackles heard throughout the lungs. Over the first 24 to 48 hours after injury, interstitial and alveolar infiltrates appear on chest radiographs. Hypoxemia and respiratory alkalosis are common at this stage. As pulmonary edema worsens, hypoxemia becomes refractory to oxygen therapy, and hypoventilation develops with increasing $PaCO_2$. Worsening hypoxemia and hypercapnia lead to respiratory failure. Decreased oxygen delivery to tissues results in metabolic acidosis and organ dysfunction (e.g., decreased urine output and a decline in cognitive functioning). Decreased cardiac output and hypotension eventually lead to death. The clinical course of progressive ARDS can be summarized as follows: dyspnea and hypoxemia → hyperventilation and respiratory alkalosis → decreased tissue perfusion, organ dysfunction, and metabolic acidosis → decreased tidal volume and hypoventilation → respiratory acidosis and further hypoxemia → decreased cardiac output and hypotension → death.

EVALUATION AND TREATMENT Diagnosis is made on the basis of a history of systemic insult, physical examination, analysis of arterial blood gases, and chest x-ray. Initial physical examination may show fine inspiratory crackles, and the chest film may be clear or show a few scattered infiltrates. With progressive respiratory involvement, crackles are heard throughout the lungs and radiographs show extensive bilateral infiltrates. The criteria for diagnosis of ARDS include refractory hypoxemia, a chest x-ray with bilateral infiltrates, and the exclusion of cardiogenic pulmonary edema. Further diagnostic testing may include CT of the chest and bronchoscopy.

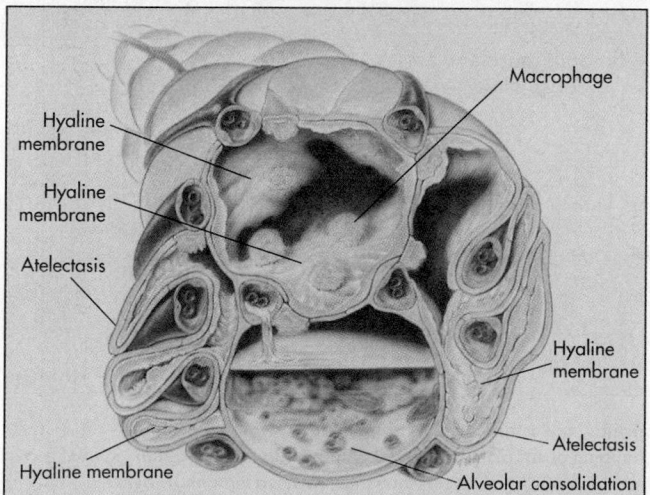

Figure 33-9 Acute respiratory distress syndrome (ARDS). Cross-sectional view of alveoli in ARDS. (Modified from Des Jardins T, Burton GG: *Clinical manifestations and assessment of respiratory disease,* ed 3, St Louis, 1995, Mosby.)

Treatment is based on early detection, supportive therapy, and prevention of complications such as pneumonia. Traditional therapy involves mechanical ventilation with PEEP and high oxygen concentrations. Numerous alternative modalities of ventilation are being tested, including low volume ventilation, noninvasive positive pressure ventilation, permissive hypercapnia, prone positioning, extracorporeal gas exchange, and partial liquid ventilation; some of these methods have shown apparent reductions in mortality rates.[30]

Many studies are investigating new ways to prevent or treat ARDS. Anticoagulant therapy with recombinant human-activated protein C improves outcomes in sepsis associated with ARDS and continues to be evaluated. Prophylactic immunotherapy, antibodies against endotoxins, antioxidants, surfactant replacement, nitric oxide inhalation, and inhibition of various inflammatory mediators are among other possibilities being

tested.[31] Steroid administration remains controversial but may improve overall outcomes when given in physiologic doses.[32]

Obstructive Pulmonary Disease

Obstructive pulmonary disease is characterized by airway obstruction that is worse with expiration. Either more force (i.e., use of accessory muscles of expiration) or more time is required to expire a given volume of air, or both. The unifying symptom of obstructive pulmonary disease is dyspnea; the unifying sign is wheezing. Individuals have an increased work of breathing, ventilation-perfusion mismatching, and a decreased forced expiratory volume in one second (FEV_1). The most common obstructive diseases are asthma, chronic bronchitis, and emphysema. Because many individuals have chronic bronchitis and emphysema, these diseases together are often called COPD (Figure 33-10).

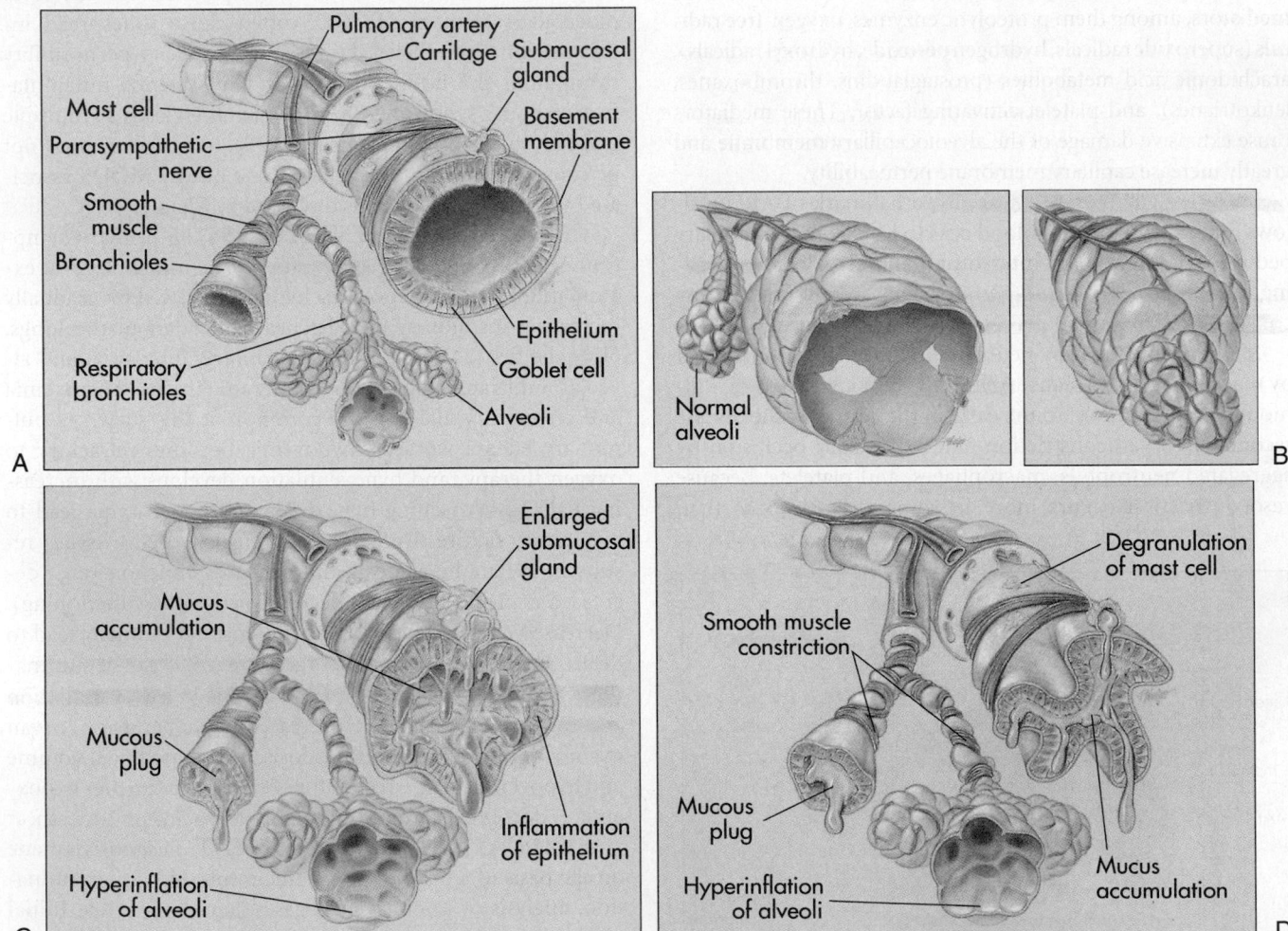

Figure 33-10 Airway obstruction caused by emphysema, chronic bronchitis, and asthma. **A,** The normal lung. **B,** Emphysema: enlargement and destruction of alveolar walls with loss of elasticity and trapping of air; *(left)* panlobular emphysema showing abnormal weakening and enlargement of all air spaces distal to the terminal bronchioles (normal alveoli shown for comparison only); *(right)* centrilobular emphysema showing abnormal weakening and enlargement of the respiratory bronchioles in the proximal portion of the acinus. **C,** Chronic bronchitis: inflammation and thickening of mucous membrane with accumulation of mucus and pus leading to obstruction; characterized by cough. **D,** Bronchial asthma: thick mucus, mucosal edema, and smooth muscle spasm causing obstruction of small airways; breathing becomes labored and expiration is difficult. (Modified from Des Jardins T, Burton GG: *Clinical manifestations and assessment of respiratory disease,* ed 3, St Louis, 1995, Mosby.)

Asthma

Asthma is defined as "a chronic disorder of the airways that involves a complex interaction of airway obstruction, bronchial hyperresponsiveness and an underlying inflammation."[33] Many cells and cellular elements contribute to the inflammatory response including mast cells, eosinophils, neutrophils, T lymphocytes, macrophages, and damaged epithelial cells (especially in sudden onset, fatal exacerbations, occupational asthma, and individuals who smoke). In susceptible individuals, this inflammation causes recurrent episodes of coughing (particularly at night or early in the morning), wheezing, breathlessness, and chest tightness. These episodes are usually associated with widespread but variable airflow obstruction that is often reversible either spontaneously or with treatment.[33]

Asthma occurs at all ages, with approximately half of all cases developing during childhood and another third before age 40. In the United States, asthma affects more than 22 million persons and is a major global health problem affecting more than 300 million people worldwide.[33,34] With the projected increase in the proportion of the world's population that lives in cities, it is estimated that there may be an additional 100 million people with asthma by 2025.[34] Mortality rates have declined since 1995 in the United States, but the incidence of asthma has increased over the past two decades, especially in urban areas.[33]

Asthma is a familial disorder and more than 100 genes have been identified that may play a role in the susceptibility and pathogenesis of asthma, including those that influence the production of IL-4, IL-5, and IL-13; IgE; eosinophils; mast cells; adrenergic receptors; leukotrienes; and bronchial hyperresponsiveness.[35-36] The *ADAM* 33 (a disintegrin and metalloprotease)[33] gene is particularly associated with asthma and bronchial hyperresponsiveness.[37] Furthermore, there is increasing understanding of the specific interactions of susceptibility genes with the environment that can guide prevention and treatment interventions.[38-40] Risk factors for asthma, in addition to family history, include allergen exposure, urban residence, exposure to air pollution and cigarette smoke, recurrent respiratory viral infections, and obesity.[33,41]

There is significant evidence that allergy and inflammation involving the upper airway (allergic rhinitis) can contribute to lower airway inflammation and bronchospasm ("one airway hypothesis") (see What's New? The Link Between the Upper and Lower Airways in Asthma and COPD).[42] Based on this understanding, it has been shown that prevention and treatment of allergic rhinitis may prevent the development of asthma.[43]

Of great interest in recent years has been the effect of recurrent allergen exposure during childhood on the subsequent development of asthma. A significant amount of evidence indicates that exposure to high levels of most allergens (e.g., dust mites) is correlated with an increased risk of asthma, although the age at the time of exposure may influence the risk.[33] It also has been noted that children who live on farms or have certain childhood infections may have a decreased

risk for asthma, theoretically because they become less immunologically "primed" to be allergic (see What's New? New Understandings of Gene and Environmental Interactions in Asthma).[33,41,44] These relationships have been described as the *hygiene hypothesis,* and many studies are being conducted to further elucidate the relationship between allergen exposure and infection and asthma risk and to see if asthma can be prevented through allergen reduction and exposure to probiotics.[33,41,44,45]

Inflammation resulting in hyperresponsiveness of the airways is the major pathologic feature of asthma. Airway epithelial cell irritation combined with exposure to antigens initiates both an innate and an adaptive immune response (see Chapter 8). In sensitized individuals, allergen exposure leads to activation of T-helper cells. These cells release what are called T-helper 2 cytokines, especially IL-4, IL-5, IL-8, and IL-13. IL-4 stimulates B-cell activation, proliferation, and production of antigen-specific IgE. IgE causes mast cell degranulation with the release of a large number of inflammatory

---

WHAT'S NEW? The Link Between the Upper and Lower Airways in Asthma and COPD

More than one third of individuals with allergic rhinitis have asthma, and those who do not yet have asthma have a three-fold increase in the probability of developing it over the next two decades. The majority of individuals with asthma also have allergic rhinitis. These epidemiologic findings led researchers to discover that rhinitis and asthma are the clinical manifestations of inflammation that involves the entire respiratory system. Biopsies of the upper and lower airways in individuals with asthma show chronic inflammatory changes throughout the respiratory system, including tissue infiltration with polymorphonucleocytes, eosinophils, and lymphocytes, and the presence of numerous inflammatory cytokines. The "unified airway" (or "one airway") hypothesis describes what has been called upper and lower airway "crosstalk" in which antigen stimulation of just the upper airway results in innate and adaptive immune responses in the lower airway. This suggests that there is a central regulatory process that may be triggered by stimulation of any component of the respiratory tract and involves immune and neurogenic pathways. Further evidence for this hypothesis is provided by the finding that treatment of the upper respiratory tract with appropriate anti-inflammatory medications (such as nasal corticosteroids and antileukotriene agents) can result in significant improvement in asthma symptoms and lung function. Recently the unified airway hypothesis also has been applied to chronic obstructive pulmonary disease (COPD). Individuals with COPD have been found to have more nasal symptoms than those without lung disease, and their nasal secretions contain higher levels of interferons, interleukins, eotaxin, and colony-stimulating factors. These findings may lead to new ways to help manage COPD by treating the upper airway.

Data from Butler CA, Heaney LG: *Inflamm Allergy Drug Targets* 6(2):127-132, 2007; Corren J: *Curr Opin Pulm Med* 13(1):13-18, 2007; Hens G et al: *Allergy* 63(3):261-267, 2008; Hurst JR et al: *Am J Respir Crit Care Med* 173(1):71-78, 2006; Jeffery PK, Haahtela T: *BMC Pulm Med* 6(Suppl 1):S5, 2006; Krouse JH et al: *Otolaryngol Head Neck Surg* 136(5 Suppl):S75-S106, 2007; Krouse JH: *Otolaryngol Clin North Am* 41(2):257-266, 2008; Palma-Carlos AG: *Eur Ann Allergy Clin Immunol* 39(6):195-199, 2007.

There are wide variations in symptom severity and responses to allergen exposures among individuals with asthma. This suggests a complex interaction of genetic susceptibility and environmental exposure. Although more than 100 asthma susceptibility genes have been identified, there remains only a limited understanding of gene-environment interactions and how to apply that knowledge to reduce the risk and symptoms of asthma. Linking gene polymorphisms with specific environmental exposures is key in tailoring allergen avoidance strategies to individuals. For example, the hygiene hypothesis suggests that exposure to farming environments and house dust endotoxin reduces the risk for asthma by modulating the immune response. However, this has not been found to be true for all individuals, suggesting different genetics among those persons. It has been found that some individuals who have a change in their cluster of differentiation (CD14) gene (codes for a receptor on the surface of macrophages that detects endotoxin) actually have an increased risk for asthma when exposed to high levels of endotoxin. Another type of CD14 polymorphism is associated with a decreased risk for asthma when exposed to tobacco smoke, as opposed to the increased risk seen in most individuals. In some people with asthma, polymorphisms of the tumor necrosis factor gene cause them to have increased susceptibility to environmental ozone exposure when compared with other persons with asthma. An improved understanding of gene-environment interactions in asthma may lead to more effective allergen avoidance techniques, individually tailored immunotherapy, and reductions in asthma risk and severity.

Data from Holloway JW, Koppelman, GH: *Curr Opin Allergy Clin Immunol* 7(1):69-74, 2007; Kiley J et al: *Curr Opin Pulm Med* 13(1):19-23, 2007; Le Souët PN: *Curr Opin Allergy Clin Immunol* 9(2):123-127, 2009; Miller RL, Ho SM: *Am J Respir Crit Care Med* 177(6):567-573, 2008; Scirica CV, Celedon JC: *Chest*, 132(5 Suppl):770S-781S, 2007; Schwartz DA: *Pediatrics* 123 (Suppl 3):s151-159, 2009; von Mutius E: *J Allergy Clin Immunol* 123 (1):3-11, 2009.

mediators, such as histamine, prostaglandins, and leukotrienes[33,41,46] (Figure 33-11; see Figure 34-14, p. 1331, for additional detail). IL-5 stimulates the activation, migration, and proliferation of eosinophils, which cause direct tissue injury and release toxic neuropeptides that contribute to increased bronchial hyperresponsiveness, fibroblast proliferation, and airway scarring.[33,47] IL-8 activates polymorphonucleocytes that contribute to a more exaggerated inflammatory response. IL-13 impairs mucociliary clearance, enhances fibroblast secretion, and contributes to bronchoconstriction. The resulting inflammatory process produces bronchial smooth muscle spasm, vascular congestion, increased vascular permeability, edema formation, production of thick tenacious mucus, impaired mucociliary function (see Figure 33-10), thickening of airway walls, and increased contractile response of bronchial smooth muscle.[48] Other inflammatory cytokines, such as TNF and IL-1, have been found to alter muscarinic receptor function, leading to increased levels of acetylcholine, which cause bronchial smooth muscle contraction and mucus secretion.[33,49,50] These changes, combined with the epithelial cell damage caused by eosinophil infiltration, produce acute airway hyperreponsiveness and obstruction. Recent studies have identified important roles for nitric oxide and reduced airway pH in the pathogenesis of asthma and airway inflammation.[51,52] Untreated inflammation can lead to long-term airway damage that is irreversible (airway remodeling).[33,49]

Airway obstruction increases resistance to airflow and decreases flow rates, especially expiratory flow. Impaired expiration causes air trapping, hyperinflation distal to obstructions, altered pulmonary mechanics, and increased work of breathing. Changes in resistance to airflow are not uniform throughout the lungs and the distribution of inspired air is uneven, with more air flowing to the less resistant portions. Continued air trapping increases intrapleural and alveolar gas pressures and causes decreased perfusion of the alveoli. Increased alveolar gas pressure, decreased ventilation, and decreased perfusion lead to variable and uneven ventilation-perfusion relationships within different lung segments. Hyperventilation is triggered by lung receptors responding to increased lung volume and obstruction. The result is early hypoxemia without CO_2 retention. Hypoxemia further increases hyperventilation through stimulation of the respiratory center, causing $Paco_2$ to decrease and pH to increase (respiratory alkalosis). As the obstruction becomes more severe, the number of alveoli being inadequately ventilated and perfused increases. As air trapping in the lungs because of obstruction of expiratory airflow progresses, the lungs and thorax become hyperexpanded putting the respiratory muscles at a mechanical disadvantage. This leads to CO_2 retention and respiratory acidosis. Respiratory acidosis signals respiratory failure.

CLINICAL MANIFESTATIONS Individuals are asymptomatic between attacks and pulmonary function tests are normal. No clinical symptoms are present during partial remission but pulmonary function tests are abnormal. At the beginning of an attack, the individual experiences chest constriction, expiratory wheezing, dyspnea, nonproductive coughing, prolonged expiration, tachycardia, and tachypnea. Severe attacks involve the use of accessory muscles of respiration, and wheezing is heard during both inspiration and expiration. A **pulsus paradoxus** (decrease in systolic blood pressure during inspiration of more than 10 mmHg) may be noted. Because the severity of blood gas alterations is difficult to evaluate by clinical signs alone, arterial blood gas tensions should be measured. In cases of significant allergen exposure, asthma symptoms can recur 4 to 12 hours after the initial attack because of persistent eosinophil and lymphocyte activation. This is called the *late asthma response* and it can be even more severe than the initial attack.

If bronchospasm is not reversed by usual measures, the individual is considered to have severe bronchospasm or **status asthmaticus.** If status asthmaticus continues, hypoxemia worsens, expiratory flows decrease further, and effective ventilation decreases. Acidosis develops as arterial $Paco_2$ begins to rise. Asthma becomes life threatening at this point. A silent chest (no audible air movement) and a $Paco_2$ greater than 70 mmHg are ominous signs of impending death.

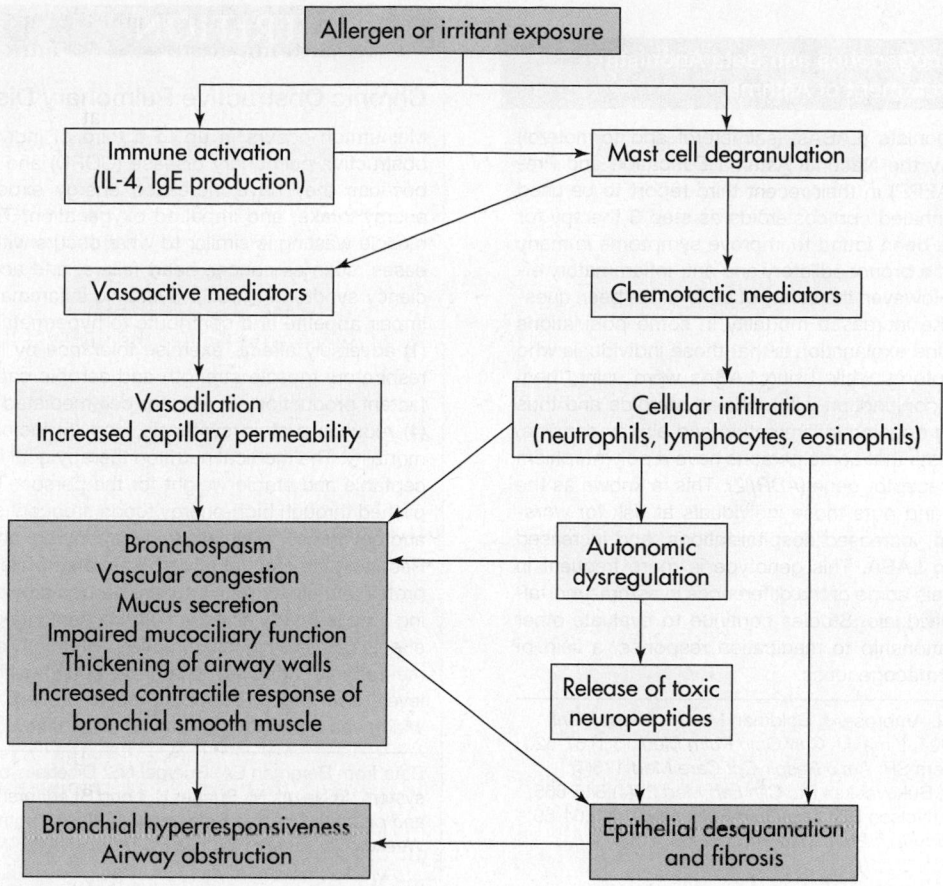

Figure 33-11 Pathophysiology of asthma. Allergen or irritant exposure results in a cascade of inflammatory events leading to acute and chronic airway dysfunction. *IgE,* Immunoglobulin E; *IL-4,* interleukin-4.

EVALUATION AND TREATMENT The evaluation of an acute asthma attack requires the rapid assessment of arterial blood gases, expiratory flow rates (using a peak flowmeter), and a search for underlying triggers, such as infection. The degree of decrease in peak expiratory flow is a useful indicator of the severity of the attack. Hypoxemia and respiratory alkalosis are expected early in the course of an acute attack. The development of hypercapnia with respiratory acidosis signals the need for mechanical ventilation. Repeated peak flow rates help to determine whether the individual is responding to treatment. Management of the acute asthma attack requires immediate administration of oxygen and inhaled beta-agonist bronchodilators. In addition, oral corticosteroids should be administered early in the course of management.[33,51,53] Careful monitoring of gas exchange and airway obstruction in response to therapy provides information necessary to determine whether hospitalization is necessary. Antibiotics are not indicated for acute asthma unless there is a documented bacterial infection.[33]

Further evaluation is indicated once the individual is stable. A careful family and personal history of allergies and other illness should be obtained. Pulmonary function testing (spirometry) will reveal decreases in expiratory flow rate as measured by the FEV_1 (see Chapter 32). FVC will also be reduced, but much less so relative to the FEV_1. FRC and total lung capacity (TLC) are increased. Responses to bronchodilator treatment also can be documented.

In 2007 the National Asthma Education and Prevention Program (NAEPP) classified asthma on clinical severity (intermittent, mild persistent, moderate persistent, and severe persistent). The NAEPP then offered six sequential guidelines for the management of chronic asthma based on this classification scheme. Chronic management of asthma begins with avoidance of allergens and other triggers. In the mildest form of asthma (intermittent), short acting beta-agonist inhalers are prescribed. However, individuals tend to underestimate the severity of their asthma and should receive extensive patient education, including the use of a peak flowmeter and the adherence to an action plan should symptoms worsen.[33,34] For all categories of persistent asthma, anti-inflammatory medications are essential and inhaled corticosteroids are the mainstay of therapy.[33,51] In individuals who are not adequately controlled on inhaled corticosteroids, leukotriene antagonists can be considered.[46] In more severe asthma, long-acting beta agonists can be used to control persistent bronchospasm; however, they can actually worsen asthma in some individuals with certain genetic polymorphisms (see What's New? Pharmacogenetics and Beta Agonists in the Treatment of Asthma).[33,49,54,55] For those persons who do not achieve adequate asthma control on inhaled corticosteroids and a beta agonist, a monoclonal antibody that

WHAT'S NEW?   Pharmacogenetics and Beta Agonists in the Treatment of Asthma

Long-acting beta agonists (LABAs) (salmeterol and formoterol) are recommended by the National Asthma Education and Prevention Program (NAEPP) in their recent third report to be used in conjunction with inhaled corticosteroids as step 3 therapy for asthma. LABAs have been found to improve symptoms in many individuals, and exert a bronchodilatory and anti-inflammatory effect on the airways. However, the safety of LABAs has been questioned because of the increased mortality in some populations using these drugs. One explanation is that those individuals who had worsening symptoms while using LABAs were using them instead of (rather in conjunction with) inhaled steroids and thus were simply masking ongoing inflammation and airway damage. New evidence suggests that some persons have a polymorphism of the β-adrenergic receptor gene ($ADR\beta2$). This is known as the Arg16Arg genotype and puts those individuals at risk for worsening bronchospasm, increased hospitalizations, and increased mortality when using LABA. This genotype is more frequent in blacks and may explain some of the differences in asthma mortality among these individuals. Studies continue to evaluate other genes and their relationship to medication response, a field of study known as pharmacogenetics.

Data from Lawrence R, Ambrose H, Goldman M: *Am J Respir Crit Care Med* 175:A59,2007; Lima JJ: *Curr Opin Pulm Med* 15(1):57-62, 2009; Moore WC, Peters SP: *Am J Respir Crit Care Med* 175(7): 649-654, 2007; Yu IW, Bukaveckas BL: *Clin Lab Med* 28(4):645-665, 2008; Oppenheimer J, Nelson HS: *Curr Opin Pulm Med* 14(1):64-69, 2008; Prenner BM: *Curr Opin Pulm Med* 14(1):57-63, 2008.

NUTRITION & DISEASE

Chronic Obstructive Pulmonary Disease

Malnutriton occurs in up to a third of individuals with chronic obstructive pulmonary disease (COPD) and is a major concern because they have increased energy expenditure, decreased energy intake, and impaired oxygenation. The disproportionate muscle wasting is similar to what occurs with other chronic diseases, such as cancer, heart failure, and acquired immunodeficiency syndrome (AIDS). Systemic inflammatory mediators may impair appetite and contribute to hypermetabolism. Malnutrition (1) adversely affects exercise tolerance by limiting skeletal and respiratory muscle strength and aerobic capacity, (2) limits surfactant production, (3) reduces cell-mediated immune responses, (4) reduces protein synthesis, and (5) increases morbidity and mortality. The medical nutrition therapy goal is to maintain an acceptable and stable weight for the person. This can be accomplished through high-energy foods, frequent snacking, soft foods and beverages, assistance with shopping, and meal preparation. Reducing the amount of carbohydrates while providing adequate protein and lipids may improve carbon dioxide balance. Increasing omega-3 fatty acids and antioxidant intake may modulate the effects of systemic inflammation. Vitamin D and calcium supplementation is indicated to improve bone health. Serum phosphate levels also should be monitored to prevent hypophosphatemia, which can contribute to muscle weakness.

Data from Bergman EA, Buergel NS: Diseases of the respiratory system. In Nelms M, Sucher K, Long S, editors: *Nutrition therapy and pathophysiology*, Belmont, CA, 2007, Thomson Brooks/Cole; Weekes CE, Emery PW: Elia M: *Thorax* 64(4):326-331, 2009.

---

blocks IgE (omalizumab) is recommended.[33] Long-term therapy with oral corticosteroids should be avoided if possible. Immunotherapy has been shown to be highly effective in selected allergic children in preventing and treating asthma.[56] Treatments, such as phosphodiesterase-4 inhibitors and specific cytokine blockers, are continually being developed and tested.[51]

Chronic Obstructive Pulmonary Disease

Chronic obstructive pulmonary disease (COPD) has been defined as pathologic lung changes consistent with emphysema or chronic bronchitis. A recent consensus report defines COPD as a "preventable and treatable disease with some significant extrapulmonary effects that may contribute to the severity in individual patients. Its pulmonary component is characterized by airflow limitation that is not fully reversible. The airflow limitation is usually progressive and associated with an abnormal inflammatory response of the lung to noxious particles or gases."[57] It is the fourth leading cause of death in the United States and is the sixth leading cause of death worldwide.[57] Overall mortality from COPD has increased 103% in the United States over the past 30 years; however, mortality in women has increased more than twice that much.[58] COPD is primarily caused by cigarette smoke, and active as well as passive smoking have been implicated. Other risks include occupational exposures, indoor and outdoor air pollution, and history of severe childhood respiratory infections. Genetic susceptibilities have been identified, including polymorphisms of genes that code

for TNF, surfactant, proteases, and antiproteases.[59,60] Gender differences in the genes that code for the breakdown and removal of cigarette smoke metabolites may explain the increased susceptibility of women smokers to COPD and lung cancer.[58] An inherited mutation in the α_1-antitrypsin gene results in the development of COPD at an early age, even in nonsmokers.

Chronic Bronchitis

Chronic bronchitis is defined as hypersecretion of mucus and chronic productive cough that continues for at least 3 months of the year (usually the winter months) for at least 2 consecutive years. Incidence is increased in smokers (up to 20-fold) and even more so in workers exposed to air pollution. It is a major health problem for older adults. Repeated infections are common.

PATHOPHYSIOLOGY Inspired irritants increase not only mucus production but also the size and number of mucous glands and goblet cells in airway epithelium. The mucus produced is thicker and more tenacious than normal. This sticky mucus coating makes it much more likely that bacteria, such as *Haemophilus influenzae* and *Streptococcus pneumoniae*, will become embedded in the airway secretions, where they reproduce rapidly. Ciliary function is impaired, reducing mucus clearance further. The lung's defense mechanisms are therefore compromised, which increases susceptibility to pulmonary infection and injury. As infection and injury increase mucus production further, the bronchial walls become inflamed and thickened from edema and accumulation

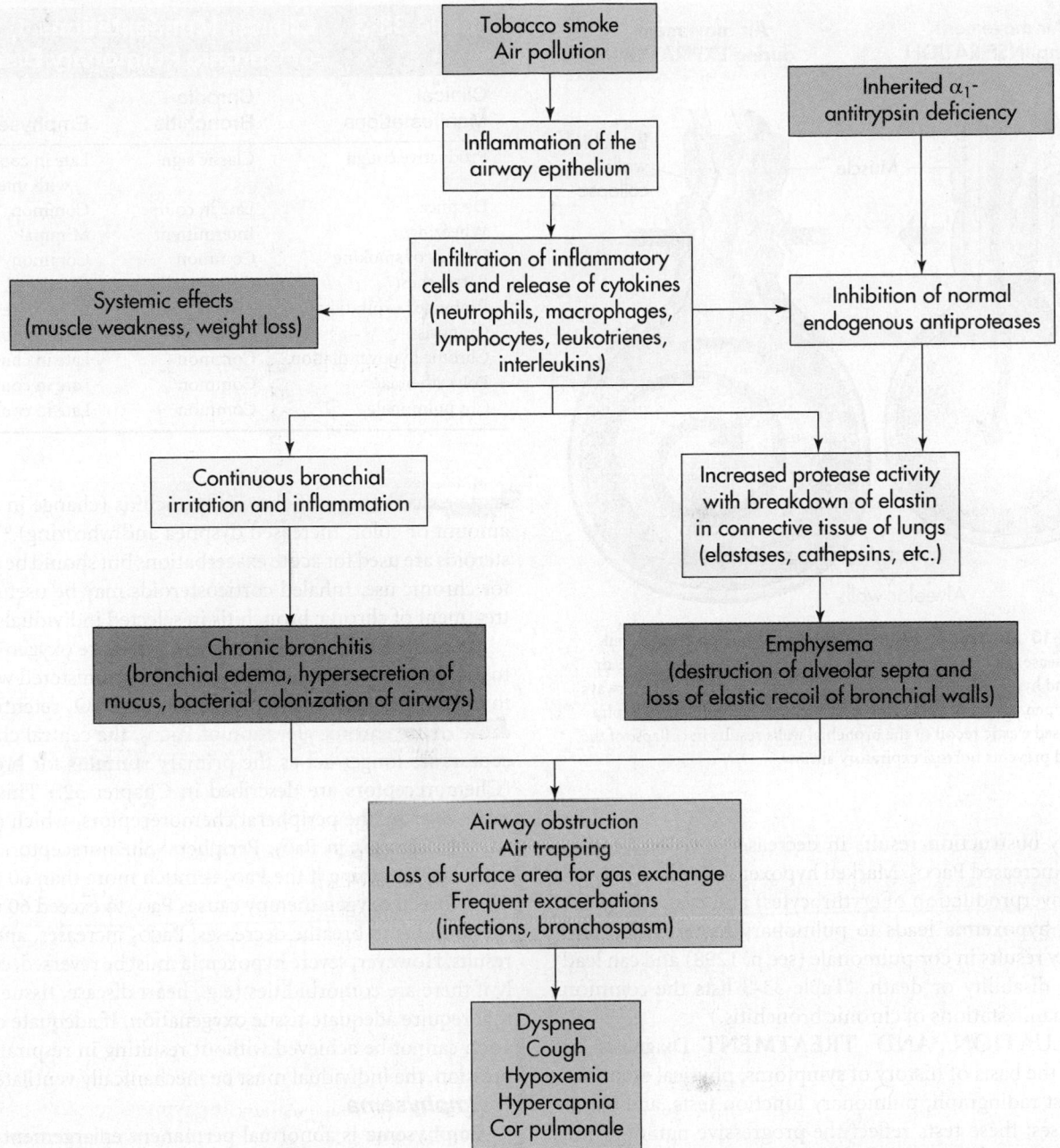

Figure 33-12 Pathogenesis of chronic bronchitis and emphysema (chronic obstructive pulmonary disease [COPD]).

of inflammatory cells. Persistent inflammation and recurrent infection lead to bronchospasm and eventual permanent narrowing of the airways.[61] (The pathogenesis of chronic bronchitis is shown in Figure 33-12.)

Initially chronic bronchitis affects only the larger bronchi, but eventually all airways are involved. The thick mucus and hypertrophied bronchial smooth muscle obstruct the airways and lead to obstruction, particularly during expiration when the airways are narrowed (Figure 33-13). Obstruction eventually leads to ventilation-perfusion mismatch with hypoxemia. The airways collapse early in expiration, trapping gas in the distal portions of the lung. Air trapping expands the thorax, putting the respiratory muscles at a mechanical

disadvantage. This leads to decreased tidal volume, hypoventilation, and hypercapnia.

CLINICAL MANIFESTATIONS The symptoms that lead individuals with chronic bronchitis to seek medical care include decreased exercise tolerance, wheezing, and shortness of breath. Individuals usually have a productive cough ("smoker's cough"), and evidence of airway obstruction (decreased FEV$_1$) is shown by spirometry. Hypoxemia may occur with exercise. As the disease progresses, copious amounts of sputum are produced, accompanied by frequent pulmonary infections.[62] FVC and FEV$_1$ become markedly reduced, and FRC and residual volume (RV) are increased as airway obstruction and air trapping become more pronounced.

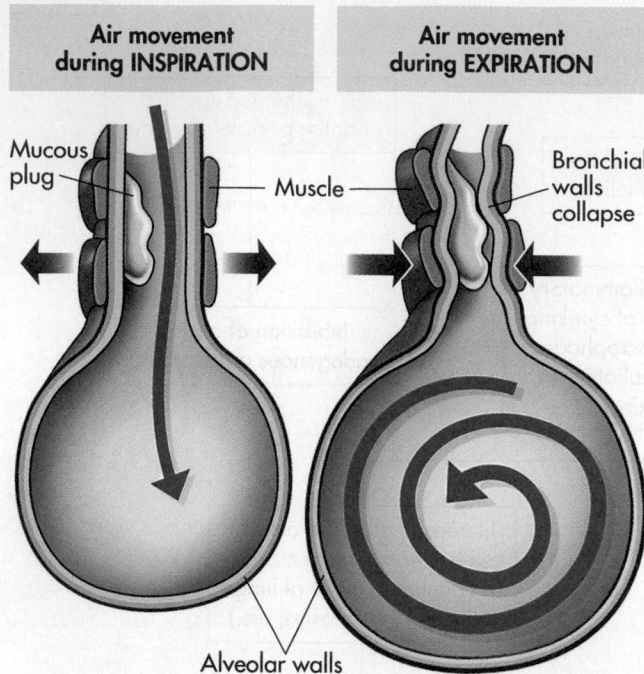

| Air movement during INSPIRATION | Air movement during EXPIRATION |

Figure 33-13 Mechanisms of air trapping in chronic obstructive pulmonary disease (COPD). Mucous plugs and narrowed airways cause air trapping and hyperinflation on expiration. During inspiration the airways are pulled open, allowing gas to flow past the obstruction. During expiration decreased elastic recoil of the bronchial walls results in collapse of the airways and prevents normal expiratory airflow.

Table 33-3	Clinical Manifestations of Chronic Pulmonary Disease	
Clinical Manifestations	Chronic Bronchitis	Emphysema
Productive cough	Classic sign	Late in course with infection
Dyspnea	Late in course	Common
Wheezing	Intermittent	Minimal
History of smoking	Common	Common
Barrel chest	Occasionally	Classic
Prolonged expiration	Always present	Always present
Cyanosis	Common	Uncommon
Chronic hypoventilation	Common	Late in course
Polycythemia	Common	Late in course
Cor pulmonale	Common	Late in course

Airway obstruction results in decreased alveolar ventilation and increased Pa_{CO_2}. Marked hypoxemia leads to polycythemia (overproduction of erythrocytes) and cyanosis. If not reversed, hypoxemia leads to pulmonary hypertension and eventually results in cor pulmonale (see p. 1298) and can lead to severe disability or death. (Table 33-3 lists the common clinical manifestations of chronic bronchitis.)

EVALUATION AND TREATMENT Diagnosis is made on the basis of history of symptoms, physical examination, chest radiograph, pulmonary function tests, and blood gas analyses; these tests reflect the progressive nature of the disease. The best "treatment" for chronic bronchitis is prevention because pathologic changes are not reversible. By the time an individual seeks medical care for symptoms, considerable airway damage is present. If the individual stops smoking, disease progression can be halted. If smoking is stopped before symptoms occur, the risk of chronic bronchitis decreases considerably and eventually reaches that of nonsmokers.

Bronchodilators and expectorants are prescribed to control cough and reduce dyspnea. Chest physical therapy may be helpful and includes deep breathing and postural drainage. Teaching of individuals includes nutritional counseling, respiratory hygiene, recognition of the early signs of infection, and techniques that relieve dyspnea, such as pursed-lip breathing.[57] The role of antibiotics in the management of acute exacerbations of chronic bronchitis has been controversial. Good evidence now indicates that antibiotics should be used for all acute exacerbations of chronic bronchitis (change in sputum amount or color, increased dyspnea and wheezing).[63,64] Oral steroids are used for acute exacerbations but should be avoided for chronic use. Inhaled corticosteroids may be useful in the treatment of chronic bronchitis in selected individuals.[57,65]

Individuals with severe hypoxemia require oxygen therapy to prevent cor pulmonale.[66] Oxygen is administered with care to individuals with severe hypoxemia and CO_2 retention. Because of the chronic elevation of Pa_{CO_2}, the central chemoreceptors no longer act as the primary stimulus for breathing. (Chemoreceptors are described in Chapter 32.) This role is taken over by the peripheral chemoreceptors, which are sensitive to changes in Pa_{O_2}. Peripheral chemoreceptors do not stimulate breathing if the Pa_{O_2} is much more than 60 mmHg. Therefore, if oxygen therapy causes Pa_{O_2} to exceed 60 mmHg, the stimulus to breathe decreases, Pa_{CO_2} increases, and apnea results. However, severe hypoxemia must be reversed, especially if there are comorbidities (e.g., heart disease, tissue injury) that require adequate tissue oxygenation. If adequate oxygenation cannot be achieved without resulting in respiratory depression, the individual must be mechanically ventilated.

Emphysema

Emphysema is abnormal permanent enlargement of gas-exchange airways (acini) accompanied by destruction of alveolar walls without obvious fibrosis. The major mechanism of airflow limitation in emphysema is loss of elastic recoil. Some degree of emphysema is considered normal in older adults but results in a slow and predictable decline in lung function with aging. When it occurs earlier in life, however, it is usually secondary to cigarette smoking or indoor and outdoor air pollution, although it may be primary emphysema in rare cases.

Primary emphysema, which accounts for 1% to 3% of all cases of emphysema, is commonly linked to an inherited deficiency of the enzyme α_1-antitrypsin.[67] Normally α_1-antitrypsin inhibits the action of many proteolytic enzymes (enzymes that break down proteins). Individuals who have α_1-antitrypsin deficiency (an autosomal recessive trait) have an increased likelihood of developing emphysema because proteolysis in lung tissues is not inhibited. Homozygous individuals have a 70%

to 80% likelihood of developing lung disease. (Mechanisms of genetic inheritance are described in Chapter 4.) Persons with α_1-antitrypsin deficiency who smoke are even more susceptible to emphysema than those with the deficiency alone. α_1-Antitrypsin deficiency is suggested in individuals who develop emphysema before age 40 years (or in their early 40s) and in nonsmokers who develop emphysema. (The principles of risk factor analysis are discussed in Chapter 5.)

Secondary emphysema also is caused by an inability of the body to inhibit proteolytic enzymes in the lung. It results from an insult to the lungs from inhaled toxins, such as cigarette smoke and air pollution. Not all smokers develop emphysema, but approximately 20% are especially susceptible and develop significant lung damage if they continue to smoke.[57]

PATHOPHYSIOLOGY Emphysema is characterized by destruction of alveoli through the breakdown of elastin within the septa by proteases.[60,68] In most individuals this process is initiated through the inhalation of inflammatory oxidants such as cigarette smoke. Toxins in smoke lead to airway epithelial inflammation with infiltration of numerous cells such as neutrophils, macrophages, and lymphocytes (see Figure 33-12). Inflammatory cytokines are released that increase protease activity and inhibit the normal endogenous antiproteases in the lung.[60,68] Some of the most important proteases activated in emphysema are elastases, cathepsins, and matrix metalloproteases. The imbalance between proteases and antiproteases leads to breakdown of elastin in the alveolar septa.[60,68] Septal destruction eliminates portions of the pulmonary capillary bed and results in ventilation-perfusion

mismatching and hypoxemia. In addition, destruction of elastin in the bronchial walls reduces elastic recoil of the airways. Expiration becomes difficult because loss of elastic recoil reduces the volume of air that can be expired passively. Hyperinflation of alveoli causes large air spaces within the lung parenchyma (bullae) and air spaces adjacent to pleura (blebs) to develop. Septal destruction also affects airway caliber because the force that normal alveoli exert on bronchiolar walls is diminished. The combination of increased RV in the alveoli and diminished caliber of the bronchioles causes part of each inspiration to be trapped in the acinus. Air trapping causes hyperexpansion of the chest, which puts the muscles of respiration at a mechanical disadvantage. This results in increased work of breathing so that many individuals will develop hypoventilation and hypercapnia late in the course of the disease. Persistent inflammation in the airways can result in hyperreactivity of the bronchi with bronchoconstriction, which may be partially reversible with bronchodilators. Chronic inflammation also can have significant systemic effects including weight loss, muscle weakness, and increased susceptibility to comorbidities, such as infection.[57]

Emphysema can be centriacinar (centrilobular) or panacinar (panlobular), depending on the site of involvement (Figure 33-14). In **centriacinar emphysema** septal destruction occurs in the respiratory bronchioles and alveolar ducts, usually in the upper lobes of the lung. The alveolar sac (alveoli distal to the respiratory bronchiole) remains intact. It tends to occur in smokers with chronic bronchitis. **Panacinar emphysema** involves the entire acinus, with damage more randomly

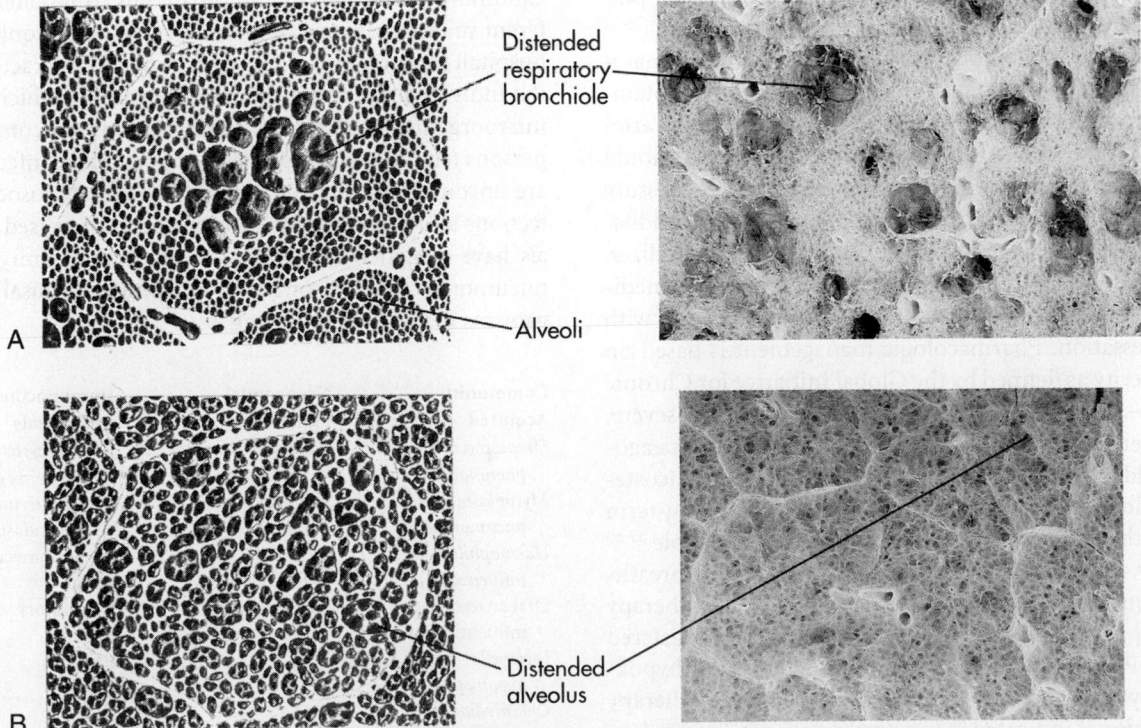

Figure 33-14 Types of emphysema. **A,** Centriacinar emphysema. **B,** Panacinar emphysema. (Micrographs from Damjanov I, Linder J, editors: *Anderson's pathology,* ed 10, St Louis, 1996, Mosby.)

distributed and involving the lower lobes of the lung. It tends to occur in older adults and in those with α_1-antitrypsin deficiency.

CLINICAL MANIFESTATIONS Individuals with emphysema usually have dyspnea on exertion that later progresses to marked dyspnea, even at rest (see Table 33-3). Little coughing and very little sputum are produced. The individual often is thin, has tachypnea with prolonged expiration, and must use accessory muscles for ventilation. The anteroposterior diameter of the chest is increased (barrel chest), and the chest has a hyperresonant sound with percussion. To increase lung capacity, the individual often leans forward with arms extended and braced on knees when sitting. In addition, people with emphysema often exhale through pursed lips, which helps prevent expiratory airway collapse.

EVALUATION AND TREATMENT Emphysema is usually diagnosed and staged by pulmonary function measures. In COPD, pulmonary function tests indicate obstruction to gas flow during expiration with a marked decrease in FEV_1. Airway collapse and air trapping in distal portions of the lung lead to a decrease in FVC (but less so than FEV_1) and an increase in FRC, RV, and TLC.[57] Diffusing capacity is decreased because of destruction of the alveolocapillary membranes. On radiographs the diaphragm appears flattened and the lung fields appear overdistended. In individuals for whom pulmonary function testing is not definitive for the diagnosis, high-resolution CT scanning may be indicated.[57,69] Arterial blood gas measurements reveal varying degrees of hypoxemia and/or hypercapnia. The disease course is usually prolonged, with increasing dyspnea and intermittent bouts of infection that culminate in failure of the right side of the heart (cor pulmonale) and death.

Management of acute exacerbations of emphysema is similar to that for chronic bronchitis and requires obtaining a chest radiograph, serum white blood cell count, arterial blood gas, and sputum sample.[57,63] Individuals should receive oxygen and may require noninvasive positive pressure ventilation or mechanical ventilation. Inhaled bronchodilators should be administered by either inhaler or nebulizer. Oral corticosteroids and antibiotics should begin immediately.[57,62,63] Chronic management of emphysema begins with smoking cessation. Pharmacologic management is based on clinical severity as defined by the Global Initiative for Chronic Obstructive Lung Disease (GOLD) as mild, moderate, severe, or very severe.[57] Inhaled anticholinergic agents and beta agonists should be prescribed.[57] A trial of inhaled corticosteroids should be used for severe COPD, although long-term therapy with oral steroids should be avoided if possible.[57,65] Pulmonary rehabilitation, improved nutrition, and breathing techniques all can improve symptoms.[70] Oxygen therapy is indicated in chronic hypoxemia but must be administered with care. Progressive pulmonary dysfunction with hypoxemia and hypercapnia may require long-term oxygen therapy and ventilation if indicated.[66] In selected patients, lung reduction surgery or transplantation can be considered.[57] A new class of drugs called phosphodiesterase E4 (PDE4) inhibitors is proving to be effective in selected patients with severe COPD.[71] α_1-Antitrypsin augmentation may be indicated for primary emphysema.[72]

Respiratory Tract Infections

Respiratory tract infections are the most common cause of short-term disability in the United States. Most of these infections—the common cold, pharyngitis (sore throat), and laryngitis—involve only the upper airways. Although the lungs have direct contact with the atmosphere, they remain sterile under most circumstances. Infections of the lower respiratory tract occur most often in the very young, the very old, or individuals with impaired immunity or underlying disease. In all cases the body's normal defense mechanisms are impaired.

Pneumonia

Pneumonia is infection of the lower respiratory tract caused by bacteria, viruses, fungi, protozoa, or parasites. It is the sixth leading cause of death in the United States and is responsible for more disease and death than any other infection.[73] More than half of those hospitalized for pneumonia are older than age 65; mortality from pneumonia is highest in older adults.[74,75] Risk factors for pneumonia include advanced age, immunocompromise, underlying lung disease (especially COPD), alcoholism, altered consciousness, impaired swallowing, smoking, endotracheal intubation, malnutrition, immobilization, underlying cardiac or liver disease, and residence in a nursing home. The causative microorganism influences the symptoms and signs with which the patient presents, how the pneumonia should be treated, and the prognosis.[73] Community-acquired pneumonia tends to be caused by different microorganisms than those infections acquired in the hospital (nosocomial).[76] In addition, the characteristics of the individual are important in determining which etiologic microorganism is likely; for example, immunocompromised persons tend to be susceptible to opportunistic infections that are uncommon in normal adults. In general, nosocomial infections and those affecting immunocompromised individuals have a higher mortality rate than community-acquired pneumonias.[77] Some of the most common causal microorganisms include the following[74-77]:

Community Acquired	Nosocomial Pneumonia	Immunocompromised Individuals
Streptococcus pneumoniae	*Pseudomonas aeruginosa*	*Pneumocystis jiroveci* (formerly *carinii*)
Mycoplasma pneumoniae	*Staphylococcus aureus*	*Mycobacterium tuberculosis*
Haemophilus influenzae	*Klebsiella pneumoniae*	Atypical mycobacteria
Oral anaerobic influenzavirus	*Escherichia coli*	Fungi
Legionella pneumophila		Respiratory viruses
Chlamydia pneumoniae		Protozoa
Moraxella catarrhalis		Parasites

The most common community-acquired pneumonia is caused by *S. pneumoniae* (also known as *pneumococcus*), which has a relatively high mortality in older adults.[74,75,78] *M. pneumoniae* and *C. pneumoniae* are common causes of pneumonia in young people, especially those living in group housing, such as dormitories and army barracks.[79] Influenza is the most common viral community-acquired pneumonia in adults and causes more than 200,000 hospitalizations and more than 30,000 deaths annually in the United States.[80] *Legionella* species can contaminate cooling systems and are an important cause of community-acquired pneumonia. Legionnaire disease has increased in incidence since it was first described in water supplies leading to outbreaks of disease, such as the 1976 incident at the American Legion convention in Philadelphia.[81] Nosocomial pneumonia is a frequent complication in the ICU, most often in individuals placed on mechanical ventilation (ventilator-associated pneumonia [VAP]). *P. aeruginosa*, other gram-negative microorganisms, and *S. aureus* (including methicillin-resistant *Staphylococcus aureus* [MRSA]) are the most common etiologic agents in nosocomial pneumonia.[82] Immunocompromised individuals are especially susceptible to *P. jiroveci*, other fungal infections, viruses, and mycobacterial infections of the respiratory tract.[83-85]

PATHOPHYSIOLOGY Aspiration of oropharyngeal secretions is the most common route of lower respiratory tract infection; thus the nasopharynx and oropharynx constitute the first line of defense for most infectious agents. Another route of infection is through the inhalation of microorganisms that have been released into the air when an infected individual coughs, sneezes, or talks, or from aerosolized water, such as that from contaminated respiratory therapy equipment. This route of infection is most important in viral and mycobacterial pneumonias and in *Legionella* outbreaks. Pneumonia also can occur when bacteria are spread to the lungs in the blood from bacteremia that can result from infection elsewhere in the body or from intravenous drug use.

In healthy individuals, pathogens that reach the lungs are expelled or held in check by mechanisms of self-defense (see Chapters 6, 7, and 32). If a microorganism gets past the upper airway defense mechanisms, such as the cough reflex and mucociliary clearance, the next line of defense is the airway epithelial cell. Airway epithelial cells can recognize some pathogens directly (e.g., *P. aeruginosa* and *S. aureus*).[73] However, the most important guardian cell of the lower respiratory tract is the alveolar macrophage. This phagocyte can recognize pathogens through its pattern-recognition receptors (e.g., Toll-like receptors) which then activates both innate and adaptive immune responses.[86] Release of TNF-α and IL-1 from macrophages contributes to widespread inflammation in the lung with recruitment of polymorphonuclear neutrophils (PMNs). PMNs migrate from the capillaries of the lungs into the alveoli. PMNs are critical phagocytes that kill microbes through the formation of phagolysosomes filled with degradative enzymes, antimicrobial proteins, and toxic oxygen radicals.[73] PMNs have also been found to extrude a

meshwork of proteins called a neutrophil extracellular trap (NET) that can capture and kill bacteria that have not yet been phagocytosed. Unfortunately many pathogens, such as the pneumococcus, can release a DNase that cleaves the NET and thus escape PMN defense. In addition to activating PMNs, macrophages also present infectious antigens to the adaptive immune system activating T cells and B cells with the induction of cellular and humoral immunity. The release of inflammatory mediators and immune complexes can damage bronchial mucous membranes and alveolocapillary membranes, causing the acini and terminal bronchioles to fill with infectious debris and exudate. In addition, some microorganisms release toxins from their cell walls that can cause further lung damage. The accumulation of exudate in the acinus leads to dyspnea and to $\dot{V}/\dot{Q}$ mismatching and hypoxemia.

Pneumococcal Pneumonia

The pathogenesis of pneumococcal pneumonia (*S. pneumoniae*) has been well documented and serves as a model for understanding other forms of bacterial pneumonia (Figure 33-15). *S. pneumoniae* microorganisms initiate innate and adaptive immune responses (see Chapters 6 and 7). The immune response includes complement activation and the production of antibodies, which are crucial for opsonizing the encapsulated bacterium. Rapid lysis of pneumococcal bacteria (as occurs with antibiotic treatment) results in the release of intracellular bacterial proteins that can be toxic. The best known of these proteins is pneumolysin, which is cytotoxic to virtually every cell in the lung and is partially responsible for the worsening in clinical symptoms sometimes seen in individuals immediately after they begin antibiotic treatment.[87] Inflammatory cytokines and cells are released that cause alveolar edema.[73] Edema creates a medium for the multiplication of bacteria and aids in the spread of infection into adjacent portions of the lung. The involved lobe undergoes consolidation (solidification of the tissue caused by filling with exudate). A stage of red hepatization follows in which alveoli fill with blood cells, fibrin, edematous fluid, and pneumococci, giving lung tissue a red appearance. This passes into the stage of gray hepatization, in which affected tissues become gray because of fibrin deposition over the pleural surfaces and the presence of fibrin and leukocytes (neutrophils) in the consolidated alveoli, where phagocytosis is rapidly taking place. With resolution, increasing numbers of macrophages appear in the alveolar spaces, the neutrophils degenerate, and the fibrin threads and remaining bacteria are digested by macrophages and removed by lymphatic vessels. Usually infection is limited to one or two lobes.

Viral Pneumonia

Viral pneumonia is usually mild and self-limiting, but it can set the stage for a secondary bacterial infection (especially by *S. aureus* microorganisms) by providing an ideal environment for bacterial growth and by damaging ciliated epithelial cells, which normally prevent pathogens from reaching the lower airways. Viral pneumonia can be a primary infection (e.g., influenza pneumonia) or a complication of another viral

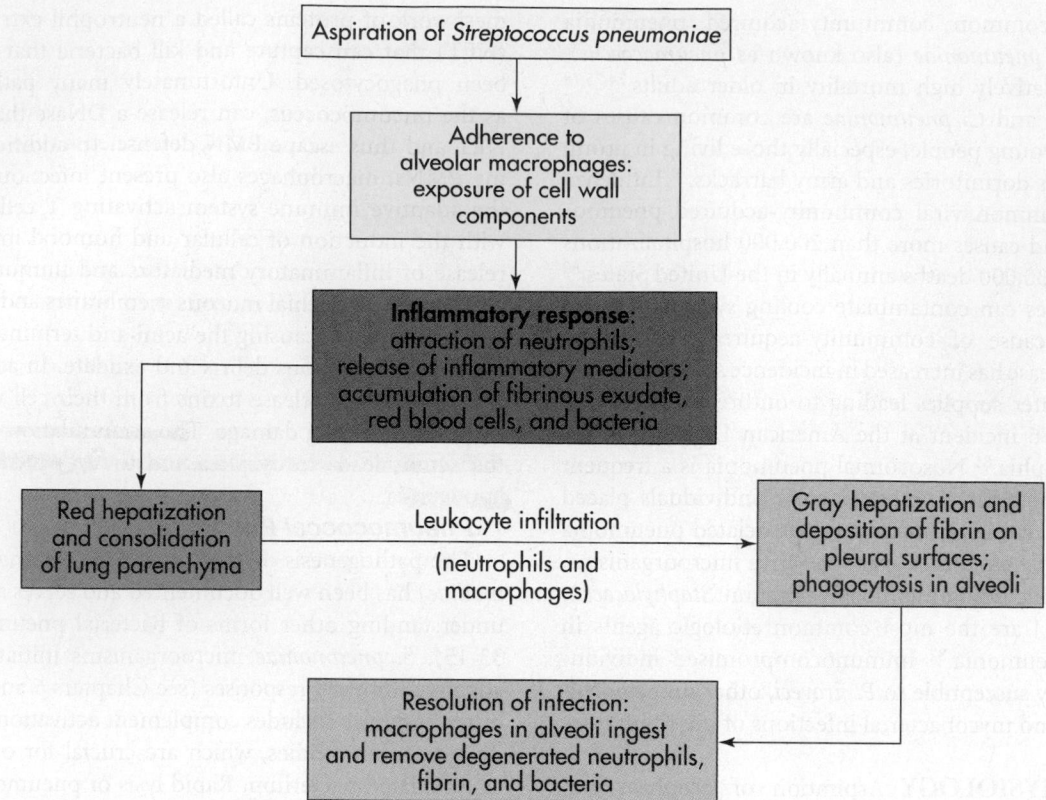

Figure 33-15 Pathophysiologic course of pneumococcal pneumonia.

[The flowchart in the figure reads:]

Aspiration of *Streptococcus pneumoniae*

↓

Adherence to alveolar macrophages: exposure of cell wall components

↓

Inflammatory response: attraction of neutrophils; release of inflammatory mediators; accumulation of fibrinous exudate, red blood cells, and bacteria

Red hepatization and consolidation of lung parenchyma

Leukocyte infiltration (neutrophils and macrophages)

Gray hepatization and deposition of fibrin on pleural surfaces; phagocytosis in alveoli

Resolution of infection: macrophages in alveoli ingest and remove degenerated neutrophils, fibrin, and bacteria

illness (e.g., chickenpox, measles). The virus not only destroys the ciliated epithelial cells but also invades the goblet cells and bronchial mucous glands. Sloughing of destroyed bronchial epithelium occurs throughout the respiratory tract, preventing mucociliary clearance. Bronchial walls become edematous and infiltrated with leukocytes.

Some forms of viral pneumonia can progress to severe systemic illness with many complications and a high morbidity and mortality. Severe viral pneumonia can include common types of influenza which can be fatal, especially in older adults. Other severe viral infections are considered opportunistic infections, such as cytomegalovirus pneumonia in immunocompromised individuals. New or atypical forms of viral infection, such as influenza A (H1N1) virus, avian influenza and the virus that causes the severe acute respiratory syndrome (SARS), are affecting previously healthy populations and pose a considerable threat for pandemics.[88-90]

CLINICAL MANIFESTATIONS Most cases of pneumonia are preceded by an upper respiratory infection, which is usually viral. This is then followed by the onset of cough, dyspnea, and fever. The cough is often productive but may be nonproductive, especially in viral pneumonia. Other symptoms include chills, malaise, and pleuritic chest pain. Physical examination may reveal signs of pulmonary consolidation, such as inspiratory crackles, increased tactile fremitus, egophony, and whispered pectoriloquy. Individuals also may demonstrate symptoms and signs of underlying systemic disease or sepsis.

EVALUATION AND TREATMENT Diagnosis is made on the basis of physical examination, white blood cell count, chest x-ray, stains and cultures of blood, cultures of respiratory secretions, and blood cultures.[91] The white blood cell count is usually elevated, although it may be low if the individual is debilitated or immunocompromised. Chest radiographs show infiltrates that may involve a single lobe of the lung or may be more diffuse. Once the diagnosis of pneumonia has been made, the pathogen is identified by means of sputum characteristics (Gram stain, color, odor) and cultures or, if sputum is absent, blood cultures.[91] Because many pathogens exist in the normal oropharyngeal flora, the specimen may be contaminated with pathogens from oral secretions. If sputum studies fail to identify the pathogen, the individual is immunocompromised, or the individual's condition worsens, further diagnostic studies may include molecular testing of blood or urine, bronchoscopy, or lung biopsy.[92-94]

Prevention of pneumonia includes prevention of aspiration, respiratory isolation of immunocompromised individuals, vaccination for appropriate populations, and reduction of ventilator-associated pulmonary infections through a variety of dental and endotracheal tube interventions.[95-97] The first step in the management of pneumonia is establishing adequate ventilation and oxygenation. Most individuals have hypoxemia and a respiratory alkalosis, although persons with underlying lung disease may require ventilation. Adequate hydration and good pulmonary hygiene (e.g., deep breathing, coughing, chest physical therapy) are also important.

Antibiotics are used to treat bacterial pneumonia; however, resistant strains of *Pneumococcus* are on the rise.[91,97] In individuals for whom a specific microorganism is not identified, empiric antibiotics are chosen based on the likely causative microorganism.[91,97,98] Viral pneumonia is usually treated with supportive therapy alone (unless secondary bacterial infection is present); however, antivirals may be needed in severe cases. Infections with opportunistic microorganisms may be polymicrobial and require multiple drugs, including antifungals.

Tuberculosis

Tuberculosis (TB) is an infection caused by *M. tuberculosis*, an acid-fast bacillus that usually affects the lungs but may invade other body systems. TB is the leading cause of death from a curable infectious disease throughout the world. TB cases increased greatly during the mid-1990s because of AIDS.[99] Many ambitious programs for prevention and treatment have been initiated worldwide and the World Health Organization (WHO) 2008 Global Tuberculosis Control Report indicates that global TB incidence and prevalence have declined in most regions of the world in recent years, although southern Africa continues to carry a huge portion of the burden of TB infection and mortality.[100] In the United States, the incidence of TB has reached its lowest level since 1953, but the rate of decline has begun to slow with more than half of new cases of TB occurring in foreign-born individuals, especially those from Mexico, the Philippines, India, and Vietnam.[101] Individuals with AIDS are highly susceptible to respiratory infections, including multidrug-resistant TB. Emigration of infected individuals from high-prevalence countries, transmission in crowded institutional settings, homelessness, substance abuse, and lack of access to medical care have contributed to the spread of TB.[100,101]

PATHOPHYSIOLOGY TB is highly contagious and is transmitted from person to person in airborne droplets. Host susceptibility to infection is influenced by genetic polymorphisms, including those that affect macrophages, tumor necrosis factor, and interleukins.[100] In immunocompetent individuals, the microorganism is usually contained by the inflammatory and immune response systems, and latent TB infection (LTBI) develops with no clinical evidence of disease.[102] Microorganisms lodge in the lung periphery, usually in the upper lobe. Once the bacilli are inspired into the lung, they multiply and cause nonspecific pneumonitis (lung inflammation). Some bacilli migrate through the lymphatics and become lodged in the lymph nodes, where they encounter lymphocytes and initiate the immune response.

Inflammation in the lung causes neutrophils and macrophages to migrate to the area. These cells are phagocytes that engulf the bacilli and begin the process by which the body's defense mechanisms isolate the bacilli, preventing their spread. However, the bacterium is successful as a pathogen because it can survive within macrophages, resist lysosomal killing, and multiply within the cell. In defense, macrophages and lymphocytes release interferon, which inhibits the replication

of the microorganism and stimulates more macrophages to attack the bacterium.[103] Apoptotic infected macrophages also can activate cytotoxic T cells (CD8). Neutrophils, lymphocytes, and macrophages seal off the colonies of bacilli, forming a granulomatous lesion called a *tubercle*.[104] Infected tissues within the tubercle die, forming cheeselike material called *caseation necrosis*. (Necrosis is described in Chapter 2.) Collagenous scar tissue then grows around the tubercle, completing isolation of the bacilli. The immune response is complete after 10 days or so, preventing further multiplication of the bacilli.

Once the bacilli are isolated in tubercles and immunity develops, TB may remain dormant for life.[102] If the immune system is impaired, however, or if live bacilli escape into the bronchi, active disease occurs and may spread through the blood and lymphatics to other organs. Infection with human immunodeficiency virus (HIV) is the single greatest risk factor for reactivation of tuberculosis infection. Other medical conditions that can cause reactivation include cancer, immunosuppressive medications, antirejection medications, and renal failure. Endogenous reactivation of dormant bacilli in older adults may be caused by poor nutritional status, insulin-dependent diabetes, long-term corticosteroid therapy, and other debilitating diseases.

CLINICAL MANIFESTATIONS Latent TB infection is asymptomatic. In some individuals, symptoms develop so gradually that they are not noticed until the disease is advanced. However, symptoms can appear in immunosuppressed individuals within weeks of exposure to the bacillus. Common clinical manifestations include fatigue, weight loss, lethargy, anorexia (loss of appetite), and a low-grade fever that usually occurs in the afternoon. (These are common signs and symptoms of all chronic infections.) A cough that produces purulent sputum develops slowly and becomes more frequent over several weeks or months. Night sweats and general anxiety are often present. Dyspnea, chest pain, and hemoptysis also may occur as the disease progresses. Extrapulmonary TB disease is common in HIV-infected individuals and may cause neurologic deficits, meningitis symptoms, bone pain, and urinary symptoms.

EVALUATION AND TREATMENT TB is diagnosed by a positive tuberculin skin test (TST; purified protein derivative [PPD]), sputum culture, immunoassays, and chest radiographs.[85,105] A positive tuberculin skin test indicates that an individual has been infected and has mounted an immune response against the bacillus; however, the skin test does not differentiate between past, latent, or active disease. In addition, those individuals who have received the TB vaccine with bacille Calmette-Guérin (BCG) will have a positive TST even if they have never had TB. Two immunoassays (enzyme-linked immunospot and quantitative blood interferon-gamma assay) are available.[85] These new tests are more sensitive and specific for the diagnosis of latent and active TB and are not confounded by previous BCG vaccination.[106]

When active pulmonary disease is present, the tubercle bacillus can be cultured from the sputum and may be seen with an acid-fast stain. However, sputum culture can take up to 6 weeks to become positive. Chest radiographs of individuals with current or previous active disease demonstrate characteristic changes. Nodules, calcifications, cavities, and hilar enlargement (enlarged mediastinal lymph nodes) commonly are seen in the upper lobes. A positive skin test indicates the need for yearly chest radiographs to detect active disease.

Prevention of tuberculosis infection is a complex challenge. Isolating individuals with active tuberculosis, limiting use of immunosuppressive medications, and treating underlying immunocompromising diseases, such as AIDs, are all critical steps. Development of an effective TB vaccine has been elusive. A recent report states that although eight new vaccines are in clinical trials, none are yet approved.[107]

Treatment consists of antibiotic therapy to control active disease or prevent reactivation of latent TB infection. The choice of drugs and the duration of treatment depend on the individual's health history, the likelihood of bacterial resistance to certain drugs, and the presence of active disease. The waxy coat of *M. tuberculosis* renders it impermeable to many common drugs. Today, with the increased numbers of immunosuppressed and susceptible individuals and drug-resistant bacilli, the recommended treatment for those with active infection is a combination of drugs to which the microorganism is susceptible, including isoniazid, rifampin, pyrazinamide, ethambutol, rifapentine, and streptomycin. Treatment must be continued for a minimum of 6 months.[85,108] Infection in immunocompromised individuals and multidrug-resistant strains of mycobacteria require the use of newer drugs for longer periods.[108,109] Newer drugs being tested include immune amplifiers.[110]

In the past, individuals with active TB were isolated from the community and their families in sanitariums. Today individuals remain at home or, rarely, in the hospital, until sputum cultures show that the active bacilli have been eliminated. This usually takes a few weeks to 2 months if the antibiotics are taken conscientiously. If the individual's cooperation is in question, it is advisable for the administration of the drugs to be supervised by healthcare workers.[111]

Abscess Formation and Cavitation

An **abscess** is a circumscribed area of suppuration and destruction of lung parenchyma. Abscess formation follows **consolidation** of lung tissue, in which inflammation causes alveoli to fill with fluid, pus, and microorganisms. Necrosis (death and decay) of consolidated tissue may progress proximally until it communicates with a bronchus. If this occurs, the abscess empties into the bronchus, leaving a cavity that has a radiographic appearance similar to that of a lesion of tuberculosis. **Cavitation** is the process of abscess emptying and cavity formation. Diagnosis is made by radiography.

Pneumonia caused by aspiration, *Klebsiella*, or *Staphylococcus* is the most common cause of abscess formation. Aspiration abscess is usually associated with alcohol abuse, seizure disorders, general anesthesia, and swallowing disorders.

Immunocompromised individuals also are at greater risk for lung abscesses and may be infected with opportunistic microorganisms, such as fungi and mycobacteria. The clinical manifestations of abscess formation are similar to those of pneumonitis: fever, cough, chills, sputum production, and pleural pain. Abscess communication with a bronchus causes a severe cough, copious amounts of often foul-smelling sputum, and occasionally hemoptysis.

Treatment includes the administration of appropriate antibiotics and chest physical therapy, including chest percussion and postural drainage. Bronchoscopy is sometimes performed to drain the abscess. Mortality rates are influenced by the severity of the primary disease that initially caused consolidation and by the virulence of the causative microorganism.

Acute Bronchitis

Acute bronchitis is acute infection or inflammation of the airways or bronchi. The vast majority of acute bronchitis is caused by viruses.[112] Many of the clinical manifestations are similar to those of pneumonia (i.e., fever, cough, chills, malaise), but physical examination does not reveal signs of pulmonary consolidation and chest radiographs do not show infiltrates. Individuals with viral bronchitis usually have a nonproductive cough that occurs in paroxysms and is aggravated by cold, dry, or dusty air. However, purulent sputum may be produced with some viral infections. Chest pain often develops from the effort of coughing. Treatment consists of rest, aspirin, humidity, and a cough suppressant, such as codeine.

Individuals with bacterial bronchitis have a productive cough, fever, and pain behind the sternum (breast bone) that is aggravated by coughing. It is rare in previously healthy adults except after viral infection but is common in those with COPD. Bacterial bronchitis is treated with rest, aspirin, humidity, and antibiotics.[112]

Pulmonary Vascular Disease

Blood flow through the lungs can be disrupted by a number of disorders that result in occlusion of the vessels, an increase in pulmonary vascular resistance, or destruction of the vascular bed. The consequences of altered pulmonary blood flow may be of no functional significance or can result in severe and life-threatening changes in ventilation-perfusion ratios. Major disorders include pulmonary embolism, pulmonary hypertension, and cor pulmonale.

Pulmonary Embolism

Pulmonary embolism (PE) is occlusion of a portion of the pulmonary vascular bed by an embolus that can be a thrombus (blood clot), a tissue fragment, lipids (fats), or an air bubble (Figure 33-16). The most common emboli are thrombi dislodged from deep veins in the thigh and pelvis, termed *venous thromboembolism*. Symptomatic pulmonary embolism occurs in approximately 50% of cases of untreated deep venous thrombosis (DVT).[113] PE has an incidence of nearly 300,000 cases per year in the United States, although it is estimated

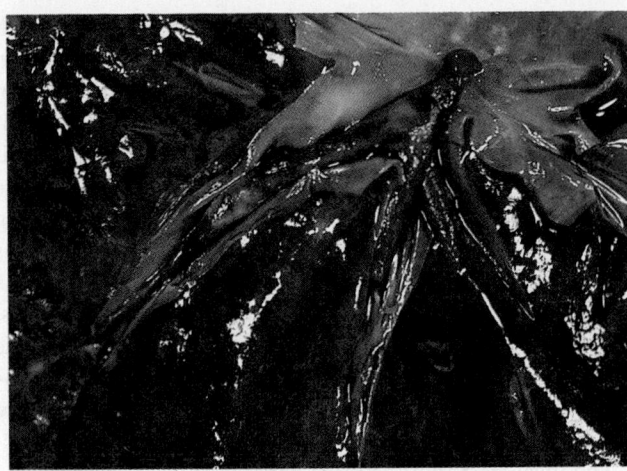

Figure 33-16 **Pulmonary embolus.** The embolus extends into major branches of the pulmonary artery. (From Damjanov I, Linder J, editors: *Anderson's pathology,* ed 10, St Louis, 1996, Mosby.)

that if undiagnosed cases also were counted, the number would be closer to 900,000. Many with PE die before reaching the hospital, and mortality at 3 months remains at 15% to 18% despite adequate anticoagulation therapy.[114]

Risk factors for **pulmonary thromboembolism** include many conditions and disorders that promote blood clotting (see Chapter 25). The three categories of pathologic risks are called the *Virchow triad* and include (1) venous stasis (slowing or stagnation of blood flow through the veins), (2) hypercoagulability (increased tendency of the blood to form clots), and (3) injuries to the endothelial cells that line the vessels. Venous stasis is usually caused by immobility with prolonged bed rest or sitting, for example, with air travel, neurologic disorders, advanced age, or immobilzer and cast use. Other causes of venous stasis include obesity, pregnancy, congestive heart failure, and sickle cell disease. Hypercoagulability can result from inherited or acquired conditions. Some of the most important acquired hypercoagulable states include malignancy, antiphospholipid antibody syndrome, heparin-induced thrombocytopenia, polycythemia vera, hyperhomocysteinemia, and hormone use (oral contraceptives or hormone replacement therapy).[113-115] Some of the most common inherited clotting disorders include factor V Leiden or prothrombin mutations and deficiencies of antithrombin III, protein C, protein S, or plasminogen.[113-115] Endothelial injury and clot formation also proceed if vessel damage occurs, as in traumatic injury, surgery (especially obstetric or orthopedic procedures), indwelling venous catheters, or caustic intravenous medication use. No matter what its source, a blood clot becomes an embolus when all or part of it breaks away from the site of formation and begins to travel in the bloodstream. (Thromboembolism is described further in Chapter 30.)

PATHOPHYSIOLOGY The effect of the embolus depends on the extent of pulmonary blood flow obstruction, the size of the affected vessels, the nature of the embolus, and the secondary effects. Pulmonary emboli can occur as any of the following:

1. *Embolus with infarction:* an embolus that causes infarction (death) of a portion of lung tissue
2. *Embolus without infarction:* an embolus that does not cause permanent lung injury (perfusion of the affected lung segment is maintained by the bronchial circulation)
3. *Massive occlusion:* an embolus that occludes a major portion of the pulmonary circulation (i.e., main pulmonary artery embolus)
4. *Multiple pulmonary emboli:* multiple emboli may be chronic or recurrent

As a result of the thrombus lodging in the pulmonary circulation, there is a release of neurohumoral substances, such as serotonin, histamine, catecholamines and angiotensin II, and inflammatory mediators, such as endothelin, leukotrienes, thromboxanes, and toxic oxygen radicals. This causes widespread vasoconstriction that further impedes blood flow to the lung. Hemodynamically, this results in increased pulmonary artery pressures and can lead to right heart failure.[114] Absent blood flow to a lung segment causes a ventilation-perfusion mismatch (increased dead space) and a decrease in surfactant production. The resulting atelectasis of the affected lung segments further contributes to hypoxemia. If the thrombus is large enough, infarction of lung tissue, dysrhythmias, decreased cardiac output, shock, and death are possible.[114] The pathogenesis of venous thromboembolism is summarized in Figure 33-17.

If the embolus does not cause infarction, the clot is dissolved by the fibrinolytic system (see Chapter 25) and pulmonary function returns to normal. If pulmonary infarction occurs, shrinking and scarring develop in the affected area of the lung. The risk of recurrent venous thromboembolism is 30% over the next 10 years, and is much higher in those individuals who have irreversible risk factors for the disease.[113]

CLINICAL MANIFESTATIONS In most cases the clinical manifestations of PE are nonspecific; therefore, evaluation of risk factors and predisposing factors is an important aspect of diagnosis. Consequently, the recognition of individuals at high risk for PE is crucial to assessing the clinical presentation.[113-117] A list of an individual's predisposing factors for venous thromboembolism can be inserted into one of several clinical prediction models (e.g., Wells Prediction Rule model) to obtain a prediction score that helps determine risk probability.[114,116,117]

In suspected PE, assessment for DVT may indicate the presence of a lower extremity source for the thromboembolism. Calf pain and tenderness, along with calf asymmetry when documented with a tape measure, are some of the most important findings in DVT. Unfortunately, DVT is often asymptomatic and clinical examination has low sensitivity for the presence of a clot, especially in the thigh and pelvis. Therefore, the lack of clinical indicators for DVT does not rule out the possibility for PE.

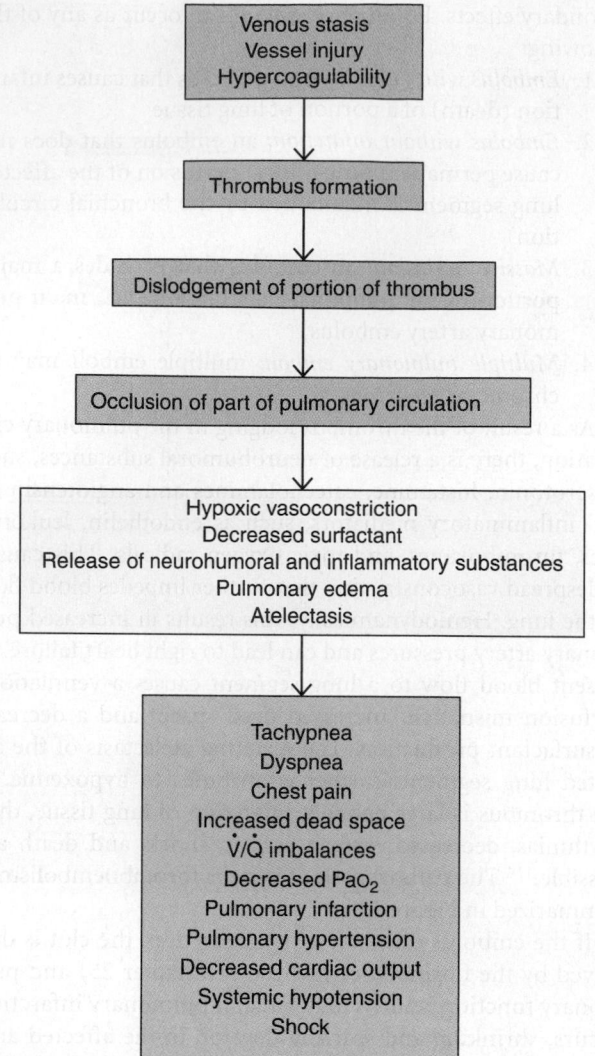

Venous stasis
Vessel injury
Hypercoagulability

↓

Thrombus formation

↓

Dislodgement of portion of thrombus

↓

Occlusion of part of pulmonary circulation

↓

Hypoxic vasoconstriction
Decreased surfactant
Release of neurohumoral and inflammatory substances
Pulmonary edema
Atelectasis

↓

Tachypnea
Dyspnea
Chest pain
Increased dead space
V̇/Q̇ imbalances
Decreased PaO$_2$
Pulmonary infarction
Pulmonary hypertension
Decreased cardiac output
Systemic hypotension
Shock

Figure 33-17 Pathogenesis of massive pulmonary embolism caused by a thrombus (pulmonary thromboembolism).

An individual with PE usually presents with the sudden onset of pleuritic chest pain, dyspnea, tachypnea, tachycardia, and unexplained anxiety. Occasionally syncope (fainting) or hemoptysis occurs. With large emboli, a pleural friction rub, pleural effusion, fever, and leukocytosis may be noted. Recurrent pulmonary emboli occur in individuals with a history of previous emboli. Recurrent small emboli may not be detected until progressive incapacitation, precordial pain, anxiety, dyspnea, and right ventricular enlargement are exhibited. Massive occlusion causes profound shock, hypotension, tachypnea, tachycardia, severe pulmonary hypertension, and chest pain.

EVALUATION AND TREATMENT When an individual is suspected of having a PE based on the presence of risk factors, symptoms, and physical findings, a chest x-ray, arterial blood gas, and ECG are obtained immediately.[114-117] Chest x-ray findings are nonspecific in PE and often can be normal for the first 24 hours until atelectasis occurs in the

lung. The arterial blood gas commonly reveals hypoxemia with a respiratory alkalosis (most individuals will hyperventilate in response to PE). The ECG may show evidence of strain on the right side of the heart. A serum D-dimer measures a product of thrombus degradation by the fibrinolytic system and, if normal, makes the presence of a PE highly unlikely.[118] If the D-dimer is elevated, further evaluation is conducted using single or multidetector spiral CT arteriography.[114,115,117] This highly sensitive and specific test has replaced the radionucleotide ventilation-perfusion scan in most hospitals. In rare cases, a pulmonary angiogram is necessary to confirm the diagnosis of PE. Recently, the measurement of elevated serum troponin levels has been useful in stratifying the risk and severity of PE.[114,115,117]

The ideal treatment of PE is prevention through risk factor recognition and elimination of predisposing factors. Venous stasis in hospitalized individuals is minimized by bed exercises, frequent position changes, early ambulation, and pneumatic calf compression.[119] Most at-risk individuals also will receive prophylactic anticoagulation with unfractionated heparin, low-molecular-weight heparin, warfarin, or fondaparinux.[119,120] In individuals who have contraindications to anticoagulation, the placement of a filter in the inferior vena cava can prevent emboli from reaching the lungs.[119,121]

Management of PE begins with administration of oxygen and hemodynamic stabilization with fluids, if needed, followed by rapid administration of anticoagulation, usually unfractionated or low-molecular-weight heparin.[114,115,117,122] This is usually followed by weeks or months of outpatient warfarin. Newer anticoagulants that target factor Xa or thrombin are showing considerable clinical promise and include fondaparinux, idraparinux, rivaroxaban, and apixaban.[123] If a massive life-threatening embolism occurs, a fibrinolytic agent, such as streptokinase, can be used and may be infused through a pulmonary artery catheter.[124] Some individuals require emergent percutaneous or surgical embolectomy.[124,125] Reversal of the underlying cause of the thrombus is important in preventing recurrent venous thromboembolism.

Pulmonary Artery Hypertension

Pulmonary artery hypertension (PAH) is defined as a mean pulmonary artery pressure above 25 mmHg at rest or 30 mmHg with exercise.[126] Pulmonary artery pressure is lower than systemic arterial pressure and is normally 15 to 18 mmHg. Box 33-1 contains the WHO[127] categories for PAH. Idiopathic PAH (IPAH) is rare with only one or two cases per million people. It is more common in women than in men and presents in women in the third decade of life and in men in the fourth decade.[126,127] Familial PAH (FPAH) describes those individuals with PAH who have a family history of the disorder, most often due to mutations in the gene encoding the bone morphogenetic protein receptor type II (BMPR2).[127,128] Associated PAH (APAH) is a leading cause of mortality in many connective tissue disorders and affects up to 1 in 200 individuals infected with HIV.[127] Diet drugs, amphetamines, and cocaine also have been linked to an increased risk for

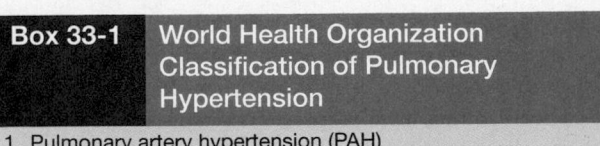

Box 33-1 World Health Organization Classification of Pulmonary Hypertension

1. Pulmonary artery hypertension (PAH)
   1.1 Idiopathic (IPAH)
   1.2 Familial (FPAH)
   1.3 Associated with (APAH)
      1.3.1 Connective tissue disease
      1.3.2 Congenital to systemic pulmonary shunts
      1.3.3 Portal hypertension
      1.3.4 HIV infection
      1.3.5 Drugs and toxins
      1.3.6 Other
   1.4 Associated with significant venous or capillary involvement
   1.5 Persistent pulmonary hypertension of the newborn
2. Pulmonary hypertension associated with left-sided heart diseases
   2.1 Left-sided atrial or ventricular heart disease
   2.2 Left-sided valvular heart disease
3. Pulmonary hypertension associated with lung respiratory disease and/or hypoxia
   3.1 Chronic obstructive pulmonary disease
   3.2 Interstitial lung disease
   3.3 Sleep-disordered breathing
   3.4 Alveolar hypoventilation disorders
   3.5 Chronic exposure to high attitude
   3.6 Developmental abnormalities
4. Pulmonary hypertension because of chronic thrombotic or embolic disease
5. Miscellaneous

Data from Heresi GA, Dweik RA: *Comp Ther* 33(3):150-161, 2007. *HIV*, Human immunodeficiency virus.

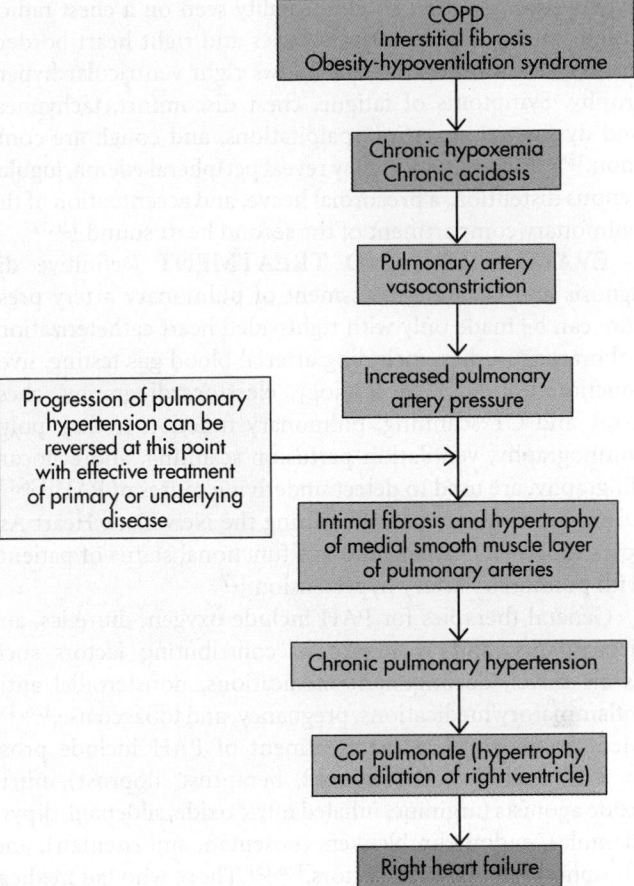

Figure 33-18 Pathogenesis of pulmonary hypertension and cor pulmonale caused by disease of the respiratory system or hypoxia. *COPD,* Chronic obstructive pulmonary disease.

PAH. Pulmonary artery hypertension associated with left heart failure or valvular disease is caused by increased pulmonary venous pressure and is discussed in Chapter 30. COPD is the most common lung disease associated with PAH, but any condition that causes chronic hypoxemia can result in pulmonary hypertension. Recurrent pulmonary embolism may be subclinical in its presentation and unrecognized until the signs and symptoms of PAH are detected.

PATHOPHYSIOLOGY PAH is characterized by endothelial dysfunction with overproduction of vasoconstrictors (e.g., thromboxane and endothelin) and decreased production of vasodilators (e.g., nitric oxide and prostacyclin).[126,128] In individuals with *BMPR2* gene mutations, intracellular signaling abnormalities result in vascular proliferation. This, along with release of vascular growth factors such as vascular endothelial growth factor, cause changes in the vascular smooth wall called *remodeling*.[128] Endothelial-derived nitric oxide is an important vasodilator that also reduces smooth muscle cell proliferation and vascular thrombosis, and dysfunction of nitric oxide pathways is considered an important component of PAH pathophysiology.[128,129] Other important mediators, including phosphodiesterases, serotonin, and adrenomedullin, also play a role in the pathogenesis of this disorder.[128,129] Together, this results in pathologic changes in the pulmonary vasculature characterized by fibrosis and thickening of the vessel wall with luminal narrowing and abnormal vasoconstriction. These changes cause resistance to pulmonary artery blood flow, thus increasing the pressure in the pulmonary arteries. As resistance and pressure increase, the workload of the right ventricle increases and subsequent right ventricular hypertrophy, followed by failure, may occur (cor pulmonale). This eventually results in the death of most individuals with PAH.

Pulmonary artery hypertension associated with lung respiratory diseases and hypoxia is usually mild to moderate; however, resultant cor pulmonale is a significant cause of morbidity and mortality in late-stage chronic lung disease. Chronic hypoxemia, especially in association with respiratory acidosis, results in vasoconstriction and in vascular remodeling with significant smooth muscle hypertrophy, fibrosis, and luminal narrowing.[130] The pathogenesis of pulmonary artery hypertension and cor pulmonale, resulting from disease of the respiratory system or hypoxia, is shown in Figure 33-18.

CLINICAL MANIFESTATIONS Pulmonary artery hypertension may not be detected until it is quite severe. The symptoms are often masked by primary pulmonary or cardiovascular disease. The first indication of pulmonary hypertension is often an abnormality seen on a chest radiograph (enlarged pulmonary arteries and right heart border) or an electrocardiogram that shows right ventricular hypertrophy. Symptoms of fatigue, chest discomfort, tachypnea, and dyspnea on exertion, palpitations, and cough are common.[126,127] Examination may reveal peripheral edema, jugular venous distention, a precordial heave, and accentuation of the pulmonary compartment of the second heart sound.[126,127]

EVALUATION AND TREATMENT Definitive diagnosis and accurate assessment of pulmonary artery pressure can be made only with right-sided heart catheterization. Laboratory studies, including arterial blood gas testing, liver function testing, HIV serology, electrocardiography, chest x-ray and CT scanning, pulmonary function testing, polysomnography, ventilation-perfusion scanning, and echocardiography, are used to detect underlying causes of PAH.[126,127] Disease severity is quantified using the New York Heart Association/WHO classification of functional status of patients with pulmonary artery hypertension.[127]

General therapies for PAH include oxygen, diuretics, anticoagulants, and avoidance of contributing factors such as air travel, decongestant medications, nonsteroidal antiinflammatory medications, pregnancy, and tobacco use.[126, 130] Medications used in the treatment of PAH include prostacyclin analogs (epoprostenol, beraprost, iloprost), nitric oxide agonists (arginine, inhaled nitric oxide, sildenafil, dipyridamole), endothelin blockers (bosentan, ambrisentan), and phosphodiesterase-5 inhibitors.[126,131] Those who fail medical therapy require lung transplantation to survive.

The most effective treatment for secondary pulmonary artery hypertension is treatment of the primary disorder. However, once pulmonary hypertension has persisted long enough for hypertrophy of the medial smooth muscle layer to develop (as it does with chronic hypoxemia), it is no longer reversible. Treatment relies on the use of supplemental oxygen to reverse hypoxic vasoconstriction.

Cor Pulmonale

Cor pulmonale is secondary to pulmonary artery hypertension and consists of right ventricular enlargement (hypertrophy, dilation, or both).

PATHOPHYSIOLOGY Cor pulmonale develops as pulmonary artery hypertension creates chronic pressure overload in the right ventricle similar to that created in the left ventricle by systemic hypertension. (Systemic hypertension is discussed in Chapter 30.) Pressure overload increases the work of the right ventricle and causes hypertrophy of the normally thin-walled heart muscle. Acute hypoxemia, such as might occur with pneumonia, can exaggerate pulmonary hypertension and dilate the ventricle as well. Right ventricular filling pressures are normal until failure occurs. The right ventricle usually fails when pulmonary artery pressure equals systemic blood pressure.

CLINICAL MANIFESTATIONS The clinical manifestations of cor pulmonale may be obscured by primary respiratory disease and appear only during exercise testing. The heart appears normal at rest, but with exercise, cardiac output falls. The electrocardiogram shows right ventricular hypertrophy. Chest pain is common. The pulmonary component of the second heart sound, which represents closure of the pulmonic valve, may be accentuated, and a pulmonic valve murmur also may be present. Tricuspid valve murmur may accompany the development of right ventricular failure. Peripheral edema, hepatic congestion, and jugular venous distention often may be detected.

EVALUATION AND TREATMENT Diagnosis is made on the basis of physical examination, radiologic examination, and electrocardiogram or echocardiogram, or both. The goal of treatment for cor pulmonale is to decrease the workload of the right ventricle by lowering pulmonary artery pressure. Treatment is the same as for pulmonary artery hypertension, and its success depends on reversal of the underlying lung disease.

Malignancies of the Respiratory Tract

Lip Cancer

Cancer of the lip is more prevalent in men, with 3100 new cases per year accounting for about 1% of all cancers in men.[132] Long-term exposure to sun, wind, and cold over a period of years results in dryness, chapping, hyperkeratosis, and predisposition to malignancy. The lower lip is the most common site.

PATHOPHYSIOLOGY The most common form of lower **lip cancer** is termed *exophytic*. The lesion usually develops in the outer part of the lip along the vermilion border. The lesion becomes thickened and evolves to an ulcerated center with a raised border (Figure 33-19). Verrucous-type lesions are less common. They have an irregular surface, follow cracks in the lip, and tend to extend toward the inner surface. Squamous cell carcinoma is the most common cell type. Basal cell carcinoma does not develop unless there is extension beyond the mucous membrane or vermilion border of the lip.

CLINICAL MANIFESTATIONS Malignant lesions often are preceded by the development of a blister that evolves into a superficial ulceration. In some cases there is a history of recurrent scales that precede development of a bleeding ulceration. Metastases to the cervical lymph nodes have a low rate of occurrence and are more likely when the primary lesion is thicker and exists for a longer period.

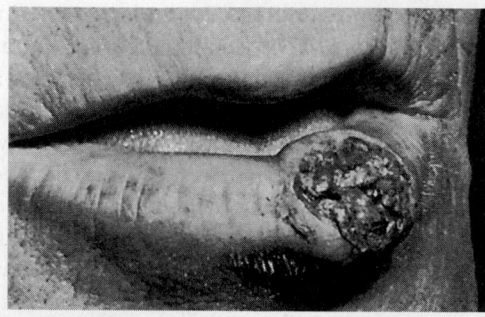

Figure 33-19 Lip cancer. Carcinoma of the lower lip with central ulceration and raised, rolled borders. (From del Regato JA, Spjut HJ, Cox JD: *Ackerman and del Regato's cancer,* ed 2, St Louis, 1985, Mosby.)

EVALUATION AND TREATMENT Diagnosis is commonly made by clinical history and presentation of the lesion. Biopsy confirms the presence of malignant cells. The staging for lip cancer is based on the size of the primary tumor, the extent of lymph node involvement, and the presence of metastases. Surgical excision, such as the Mohs micrographic surgery technique, is effective for smaller lesions. Larger lesions that require extensive resection may need subsequent cosmetic surgeries. Interstitial irradiation and radioactive implants have proved effective for control of primary lesions. The prognosis for recovery is excellent, and deaths are usually the result of delayed or inadequate treatment.

Laryngeal Cancer

Cancer of the larynx represents approximately 2% to 3% of all cancers in the United States. There were an estimated 12,290 new cases in 2009, 9920 of them in men.[132] The risk of **laryngeal cancer** is increased by the amount of tobacco smoked; risk is further heightened with the combination of smoking and alcohol consumption. Gastroesophageal reflux disease is also a risk factor.[133] The human papillomavirus (HPV) has been linked to both benign and malignant disease of the larynx.[134] The highest incidence is in men between 50 and 75 years of age.

PATHOPHYSIOLOGY Carcinoma of the true vocal cords (glottis) is more common than that of the supraglottic structures (epiglottis, aryepiglottic folds, arytenoids, and false cords). Tumors of the subglottic area are rare. Squamous cell carcinoma is the most common cell type, although small cell carcinomas also occur (Figure 33-20). Metastasis develops by spreading to the draining lymph nodes, and distant metastasis, usually to the lung, is rare.

CLINICAL MANIFESTATIONS The presenting symptoms of laryngeal cancer include hoarseness, dyspnea, and cough. Progressive hoarseness is the most significant symptom and can result in voice loss. Dyspnea is rare in the case of supraglottic tumors but can be severe in subglottic tumors. Cough occurs less commonly and may follow swallowing. Laryngeal pain or a sore throat is likely to be present with supraglottic lesions.

EVALUATION AND TREATMENT Evaluation of the larynx includes external inspection and palpation of the larynx and the lymph nodes in the neck. Indirect laryngoscopy provides a stereoscopic view of the structure and movement of the larynx. A biopsy also can be obtained during this procedure. Direct laryngoscopy provides specific visualization of the tumor. Plain films of the larynx and CT facilitate the identification of tumor boundaries and the degree of extension to surrounding tissue. Magnetic resonance imaging (MRI) and positron-emission tomography (PET) can be used for staging.

Combined chemotherapy and radiation can result in cure in selected cases; however, sequelae such as swallowing and speech difficulties may result.[135] Photodynamic therapy improves outcomes while preserving function in many individuals with early stage disease.[136] Partial laryngectomies are the preferred treatment for small supraglottic and subglottic malignancies.[137] Total laryngectomy is required when lesions are extensive and involve the cartilage. Swallowing and speech therapy after treatment can significantly improve recovery.

Lung Cancer

Lung cancers (bronchogenic carcinomas) arise from the epithelium of the respiratory tract. As such, the term *lung cancer* excludes other pulmonary tumors, including sarcomas, lymphomas, blastomas, hematomas, and mesotheliomas. Lung cancer is the number one cancer killer in the United States and the world. In the United States, there were an estimated 219,440 new cases and 159,390 deaths in 2009. It accounts for 15% of all cancers in men and 14% in women but is responsible for 31% of all cancer deaths in men and 26% of all cancer deaths in women (Box 33-2). Lung cancer is more common in blacks, for whom survival rates are lower.[132] Although the mortality rate for lung cancer has leveled off in men, it is still rising in women. Overall 5-year survival remains low at 20%.

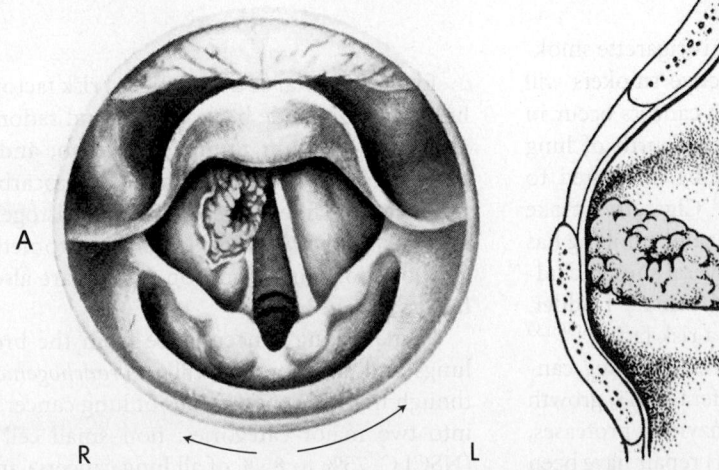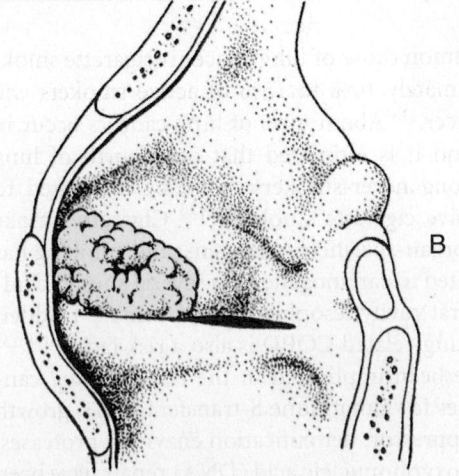

Figure 33-20 Laryngeal cancer. **A,** Mirror view of carcinoma of right false cord partially hiding true cord. **B,** Lateral view. (From del Regato JA, Spjut HJ, Cox JD: *Ackerman and del Regato's cancer,* ed 2, St Louis, 1985, Mosby.)

Box 33-2 Important Trends for Lung Cancer

Incidence
An estimated 219,440 new cases in 2009: 116,090 in men and 103,350 in women.

Mortality
An estimated 159,390 deaths in 2009: 88,900 in men and 70,490 in women. The death rate in men is declining but continues to rise for women, and lung cancer remains by far the greatest cancer killer of men and women.

Risk Factors
Cigarette smoking is the number one risk factor. Environmental smoke exposure (exposure to someone else's cigarette smoke) increases the risk of lung cancer. Occupational risk factors include exposure to asbestos dust, arsenic, chromium, nickel, ionizing radiation, chloromethyl methyl ether, coal products, mustard gas, and vinyl chloride.

Warning Signs
A persistent cough, sputum streaked with blood, chest pain, recurring attacks of pneumonia or bronchitis, weight loss, hard nodes in neck or axilla.

Early Detection and Prevention
Lung cancer is very difficult to detect early. Periodic chest x-ray films, sputum cytologic analysis, and computed tomography can detect presymptomatic, early stage lung cancers, particularly of the squamous cell type; however, no conclusive evidence of reduction in lung cancer mortality as a consequence of screening has been found.

Treatment
Surgical resection of the entire tumor is the only treatment that results in cure; however, the disease is often too advanced by the time of diagnosis for surgery to be indicated. Radiation therapy and chemotherapy can be used as adjunctive or palliative treatment modalities. New treatments include gene and immunotherapies.

Survival
Although the stage of cancer progression at the time of diagnosis greatly affects prognosis, overall only 20% of individuals live 5 or more years after diagnosis.

Data from American Cancer Society, Inc., Surveillance and Health Policy Research: Estimated New Cancer Cases and Deaths by Sex, U.S, 2009 available at http://www.cancer.org/downloads/stt/CFF2009_EstCD_3.pdf

WHAT'S NEW? The Genetics of Lung Cancer

Lung cancer is caused by repetitive insults to the bronchial mucosa that result in multiple mutations in the genome of susceptible cells. By far the most important causes of these changes are the carcinogens in cigarette smoke, although air pollution and occupational exposures also are culprits. Genetic studies can help determine which individuals are at greatest risk for the development of cancer and identify the common mutations that occur during tumor development. The sequential accumulation of genetic mutations includes formation of oncogenes that results in the secretion of tumor growth–supporting factors, an increase in the number of growth factor receptors on cancer cells, the loss of activity of tumor-suppressor genes, the reordering of chromosomal sequences that lead to unregulated cell division, and the increased production of angiogenesis and tumor invasion factors. The expanded understanding of the genetics of lung cancer and the effect genetic mutations have on bronchial cell function and morphology are leading toward more effective means of detection and treatment of this deadly disease. Examples of how genetics can help with lung cancer management include (1) identification of genetically high-risk individuals who are critical candidates for focused intensive smoking cessation interventions, (2) screening for early tumor formation through examination of sputum DNA changes, (3) determination of those steps in carcinogenesis that would likely be most responsive to chemoprevention therapies, (4) better determination of treatment and prognosis through molecular examination of individual tumors, and (5) gene-directed therapies. Examples of gene therapies being developed for the treatment of lung cancer include administration of antisense molecules and angiogenesis blockers, induction of tumor cell "suicide" genes, blockers of growth factor receptors on cancer cell surfaces, promotion of the immune response to the cancer cells (cancer vaccines and immunogene therapy), and intratumoral gene replacement therapy (e.g., replacement of the tumor suppressor gene *TP53*).

Data from Brock MV et al: *N Engl J Med* 358:1118-1128, 2008; Carlsten C et al: *Am J Epidemiol* 167(7):759-774, 2008; Chada S et al: *Front Biosc* 13:1959-1967, 2008; Ciardiello F, Tortora G: *N Engl J Med* 358(11):1160-1174, 2008; Daigo Y, Nakamura Y: *Gen Thorac Cardiovasc Surg* 56(2):43-53, 2008; D'Amico TA: *Ann Thorac Surg* 85(2):S737-S742, 2008; Eberhard DA et al: *J Clin Oncol* 26(6):983-994, 2008; Esteller M: *N Engl J Med* 358:1148-1159, 2008; Gutierrez M, Giaccone G: *Curr Opin Oncol* 20(2): 176-182, 2008; Hersh CP, DeMeo DL, Silverman EK: *Proc Am Thorac Soc* 5(4):486-493, 2008; Reck KM, Crino L: *Lung cancer* 63(1):1-9, 2009.

The most common cause of lung cancer is cigarette smoking, and approximately 10% to 15% of active smokers will develop lung cancer.[138] About 10% of lung cancers occur in never-smokers and it is estimated that one fourth of lung cancer cases among never-smokers could be attributed to exposure to passive cigarette smoke.[138,139] Cigarette smoke contains several organ-specific carcinogens, and smoking has been causally related to carcinogenesis at several sites, including the larynx, oral cavity, esophagus, and urinary bladder. Underlying smoking-related COPD is also a risk factor.[138,139] Many genes have been implicated in the risk for lung cancer including genes for glutathione S-transferase M1, growth factors, tumor suppressor, detoxification enzymes, proteases, addiction, and deoxyribonucleic acid (DNA) repair have been identified[138-141] (see What's New? The Genetics of Lung Cancer). Theories of carcinogenesis are discussed in Chapter 11.

Environmental or occupational risk factors associated with lung cancer include benzopyrene and radon particles associated with uranium mining, radiation, and nuclear bombs. Others are polycyclic aromatic hydrocarbons and arsenicals, asbestos fibers, diesel exhaust, nitrogen mustard gases, nickel, silica, vinyl chloride, and chloromethyl methyl ether. Air pollution, coal, and iron mining are also considered risk factors.[139]

Primary lung cancers arise from the bronchi within the lungs and are therefore called *bronchogenic carcinomas*. Although there are many types of lung cancer, they are divided into two major categories: non–small cell lung carcinoma (NSCLC, 75% to 85% of all lung cancers) and small cell lung carcinoma (SCLC, 15% to 20% of all lung cancers). The NSCLC can be subdivided into three common types of lung

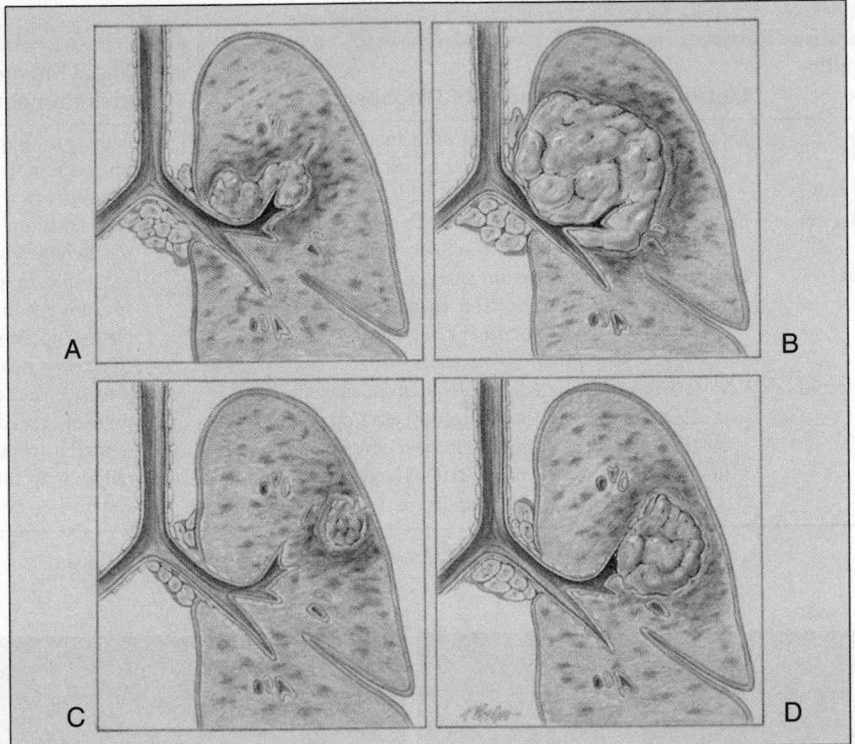

Figure 33-21 Cancer of the lung. A, Squamous (epidermoid) cell carcinoma. B, Small cell (oat cell) carcinoma. C, Adenocarcinoma. D, Large cell carcinoma. (From Des Jardins T, Burton GG: *Clinical manifestations and assessment of respiratory disease,* cd 3, St Louis, 1995, Mosby.)

cancer: squamous cell carcinoma, adenocarcinoma, and large cell undifferentiated carcinoma.[141] The clinical and pathologic features that most commonly characterize these cancer types are illustrated in Figure 33-21 and described in Table 33-4. Many cancers that arise in other organs of the body metastasize to the lungs; however, these are not considered lung cancers and are categorized by their primary site of origin.

Non–Small Cell Lung Cancer (NSCLC)

Squamous Cell Carcinoma. Squamous cell carcinoma accounts for about 30% of bronchogenic carcinomas, representing a sharp decline in incidence in the past two decades. These tumors are typically located centrally near the hilus and project into bronchi.

Because of the location in the central bronchi, obstructive manifestations are nonspecific and include nonproductive cough or hemoptysis. Pneumonia and atelectasis are often associated with squamous cell carcinoma (Figure 33-22, *A*). Chest pain is a late symptom associated with large tumors. These tumors can remain fairly well localized and tend not to metastasize until late in the course of the disease. The preferred treatment is surgical resection, although once metastasis has taken place, total surgical resection is difficult and survival rates dramatically decrease. Although chemotherapy has limited effectiveness, adjuvant treatment with newer agents has been shown to improve survival and quality of life.[142,143]

Adenocarcinoma. Adenocarcinoma (tumor arising from glands) of the lung constitutes 35% to 40% of all bronchogenic carcinomas (Figure 33-22, *B*). The recent increase in incidence of adenocarcinoma has been ascribed to the increasing frequency of lung cancer in women, environmental and occupational carcinogens, and changes in the histologic criteria for diagnosis. These tumors, which are usually smaller than 4 cm, more commonly arise in the peripheral regions of the pulmonary parenchyma. They may be asymptomatic and discovered by routine chest roentgenogram in the early stages, or the individual may seek treatment for pleuritic chest pain and shortness of breath from pleural involvement by the tumor.

Included in the category of adenocarcinoma is bronchoalveolar cell carcinoma. These tumors tend to arise from the terminal bronchioles and alveoli. They are slow-growing tumors with an unpredictable pattern of metastasis. Metastasis occurs through the pulmonary arterial system and mediastinal lymph nodes. This cell type has the weakest association with smoking.[144]

Surgical resection is possible in a high proportion of adenocarcinoma cases, but because metastasis occurs early, the 5-year survival rate remains below 15%. Newer chemotherapeutic agents are resulting in increased survival rates.[142,143]

Large Cell Carcinoma (Undifferentiated)

Large cell carcinomas constitute 10% to 15% of bronchogenic carcinomas. This cell type has lost all evidence of differentiation and is therefore commonly referred to as **undifferentiated large cell anaplastic cancer.** Because large cell carcinomas show none of the histologic findings of squamous cell carcinoma or adenocarcinoma, they are diagnosed by

Table 33-4   Characteristics of Lung Cancers

Tumor Type	Growth Rate	Metastasis	Means of Diagnosis	Clinical Manifestations and Treatment
Squamous cell carcinoma	Slow	Late; mostly to hilar lymph nodes	Biopsy, sputum analysis, bronchoscopy, electron microscopy, immunohisto-chemistry	Cough, sputum production, airway obstruction; treated surgically, chemotherapy adjunctive
Adenocarcinoma	Moderate	Early	Radiography, fiberoptic bronchoscopy, electron microscopy	Pleural effusion; treated surgically, chemotherapy adjunctive
Large cell carcinoma	Rapid	Early and widespread	Sputum analysis, bronchoscopy, electron microscopy (by exclusion of other cell types)	Chest wall pain, pleural effusion, cough, sputum production, hemoptysis, airway obstruction resulting in pneumonia (if airways involved); treated surgically
Small cell (oat cell) carcinoma	Very rapid	Very early; to mediastinum or distally in lung	Radiography, sputum analysis, bronchoscopy, electron microscopy, immunohistochemistry, and clinical manifestations (cough, chest pain, dyspnea, hemoptysis, localized wheezing)	Airway obstruction, signs and symptoms of excessive hormone secretion; treated by chemotherapy and ionizing radiation to thorax and central nervous system

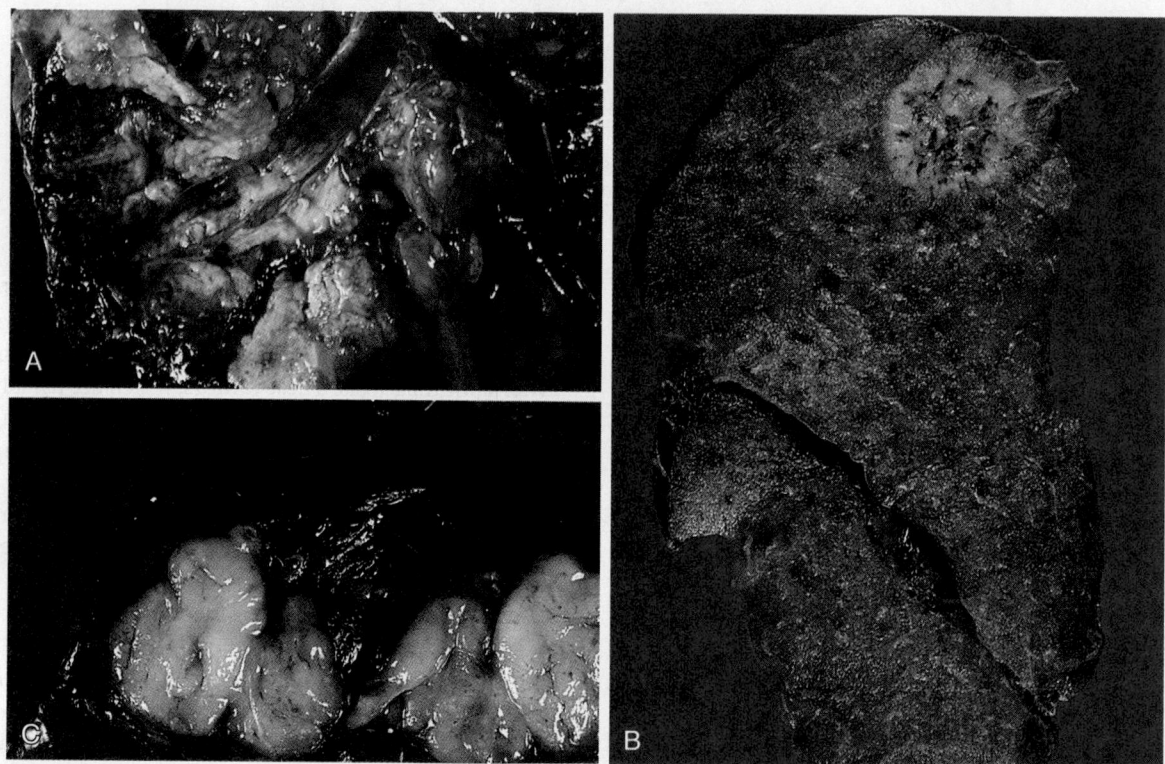

Figure 33-22 Lung cancer. A, Squamous cell carcinoma. This hilar tumor originates from the main bronchus. B, Peripheral adenocarcinoma. The tumor shows prominent black pigmentation, suggestive of having evolved in an anthracotic scar. C, Small cell carcinoma. The tumor forms confluent nodules. On cross sectioning, the nodules have an encephalid appearance. (From Damjanov I, Linder J, editors: *Anderson's pathology,* ed 10, St Louis, 1996, Mosby.)

a process of exclusion. The cells are generally larger than leukocytes and contain large, darkly stained nuclei. These tumors commonly arise peripherally but are found centrally and can grow to distort the trachea and cause widening of the carina.

Once metastasis has occurred, surgical therapy is limited to palliative procedures (comfort measures) designed to relieve obstructive pneumonitis or prevent recurrence of pleural effusion. Neither radiation therapy nor chemotherapy has been successful in increasing survival.

Small Cell Carcinoma

Small cell lung carcinomas (SCLC) constitute about 15% of bronchogenic carcinomas but cause 25% of lung cancer deaths.[145] Most tumors arise from the central part of the lung (see Figures 33-21 and 33-22, *C*). Cell sizes range from 6 to 8 μm.

This cell type has the strongest correlation with cigarette smoking. Because these tumors show a rapid rate of growth and tend to metastasize early and widely, this type of carcinoma has the worst prognosis of all lung cancers. Staging for small cell carcinoma is divided into only two categories: limited disease (20% to 30%) and extensive disease (70% to 80%).[145] Survival time for untreated small cell carcinoma is usually 1 to 3 months with treatment. With chemotherapy, radiation, or both, approximately 90% of individuals respond to treatment, but virtually all relapse within 2 years.[145]

Small cell carcinoma arises from neuroendocrine cells that contain neurosecretory granules and exist throughout the tracheobronchial tree. Thus small cell carcinoma is often associated with ectopic hormone production. Ectopic hormone production is important to the clinician because resulting signs and symptoms (called *paraneoplastic syndromes*) may be the first manifestation of the underlying cancer. The most common paraneoplastic syndrome associated with SCLC is the syndrome of inappropriate antidiuretic hormone secretion (see Chapter 21). Small cell carcinomas also commonly produce gastrin-releasing peptide, calcitonin, arginine vasopressin, and adrenocorticotropic hormone (ACTH). As a result of ACTH secretion, individuals with lung cancer secrete large quantities of 17-hydroxysteroids and 17-ketosteroids, leading to the development of Cushing syndrome. Signs and symptoms related to this condition include muscular weakness, facial edema, hypokalemia, alkalosis, hyperglycemia, hypertension, and increased pigmentation.

PATHOGENESIS Tobacco smoke contains as many as 20 documented lung carcinogens and is responsible for the vast majority of lung cancers. These carcinogens, along with probable inherited genetic predisposition to cancers, result in multiple genetic abnormalities in bronchial cells, including deletions of chromosomes, activation of oncogenes, and inactivation of tumor-suppressor genes.[138] The most common genetic abnormality associated with lung cancer is a mutation of the tumor-suppressor gene *TP53*. Mutations in this gene have been found in 45% to 55% of NSCLCs and 75% to 100% of small cell cancers.[146] Once lung cancer is initiated by these carcinogen-induced mutations, further tumor development is promoted by growth factors, such as epidermal growth factor, and by production of inflammatory mediators, such as toxic oxygen radicals.[146-148]

The bronchial mucosa suffers multiple carcinogenic "hits" because of repetitive exposure to cigarette smoke, and eventually epithelial cell changes begin to be visible on biopsy. These changes progress from metaplasia to carcinoma in situ and finally to invasive carcinoma.[141] Tumor progression includes invasion of surrounding tissues and, finally, metastasis to distant sites, including the brain, bone marrow, and liver.

CLINICAL MANIFESTATIONS Symptoms of early stage, localized disease are nonspecific and are likely to be attributed by the individual to the effects of smoking. The clinical manifestations are ambiguous and insidious; they include coughing, chest pain, sputum production, hemoptysis, pneumonia, airway obstruction, and pleural effusions. By the time manifestations are severe enough to motivate the individual to seek medical advice, the disease is usually advanced, and symptoms and signs of metastatic disease (e.g., neurologic deficits, bone pain) or paraneoplastic syndromes may be evident.

EVALUATION AND TREATMENT Although it is clear that diagnosing and treating lung cancer early in its development are crucial for long-term survival, screening for the presence of asymptomatic tumors in high-risk individuals remains controversial. The latest guidelines state that the evidence remains insufficient to recommend for or against screening asymptomatic individuals with sputum cytology, chest x-ray, or CT.[149,150] However, many clinicians and researchers continue to examine these and other modalities in an effort to find more effective ways of catching this deadly disease when it is still curable. The diagnosis of lung cancer relies on the history of risk factors and symptoms, a careful physical examination, and a constellation of diagnostic tests including sputum cytology, chest x-ray, CT scanning, PET scanning, bronchoscopy, biopsy, and search for potential metastatic disease.[151] The goal of these evaluations is to (1) establish the presence of a primary lung cancer, (2) determine its cell type, and (3) stage the tumor. As stated, SCLC is staged as either limited or extensive. The staging of NSCLC uses the **TNM classification system** in which T denotes the extent of the primary tumor, N indicates nodal involvement, and M describes the extent of metastasis and is illustrated in Figure 33-23. The use of biomarkers has been explored as a way of early detection and staging of lung cancer.[152,153]

The choice of treatment for lung cancer relies on an accurate description of the type of cancer cell and the stage of the tumor. In general, surgical removal of the entire tumor is the only certain cure. NSCLC is less responsive to chemotherapy than is small cell carcinoma, but chemotherapy and radiation are commonly used as adjuvant or palliative care.[138,142,143,154] Small cell carcinoma is usually widely metastasized by the time of diagnosis, and treatment, although palliative, can markedly extend survival. Small cell carcinoma is most often treated with chemotherapy or radiation.[145] Other therapies for lung cancer that can be used in selected individuals are laser phototherapy, photodynamic therapy, cryotherapy, and brachytherapy. New and exciting treatments for lung cancer are under investigation, including antiangiogenic therapy, targeting growth factor receptors, tumor sensitizing agents, gene therapy, and immunotherapy.[138,146,155-160]

Prevention of lung cancer relies primarily on reduction of exposure to carcinogens. For most individuals this means smoking cessation, and numerous governmental and private organizations are working toward the complete end of cigarette smoking. Other forms of prevention also are being explored.[161]

Other Lung Cancers

Bronchial carcinoid tumors represent about 1% of all lung tumors. The tumor cells have dense granules containing neuroendocrine-like hormones, but they rarely produce endocrine symptoms (carcinoid syndrome).[162]

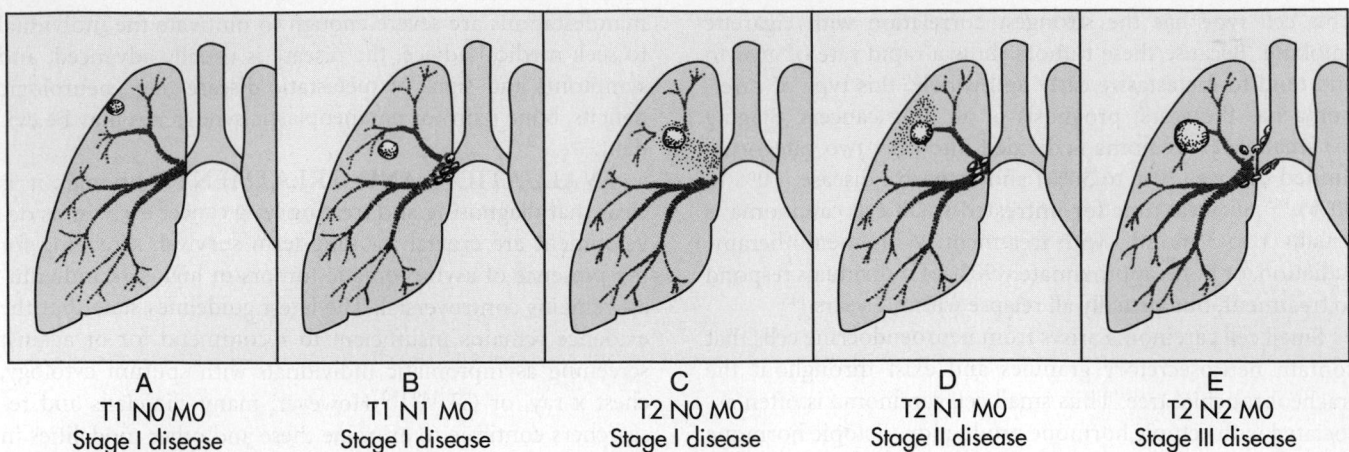

A	**B**	**C**	**D**	**E**
T1 N0 M0	T1 N1 M0	T2 N0 M0	T2 N1 M0	T2 N2 M0
Stage I disease	Stage I disease	Stage I disease	Stage II disease	Stage III disease

Figure 33-23 Staging of lung cancer by the TNM classification system. A, B, Stage I disease includes tumors classified as T1, with or without metastasis to the lymph nodes in the ipsilateral hilar region. C, Also included in stage I are tumors classified as T2 but having no nodal or distant metastases. D, Stage II disease includes those tumors classified as T2, with metastasis only to the ipsilateral hilar lymph nodes. E, Stage III includes all tumors more extensive than T2 or any tumor with metastasis to the lymph nodes in the mediastinum or with distant metastasis.

Carcinoid tumors tend to occur earlier in life than bronchogenic carcinoma, although they can occur through the seventh decade of life. The average age at diagnosis is about 45 years. Carcinoid tumors are not related to smoking. They arise more commonly in the main or segmental bronchi, are easily visualized bronchoscopically, and are found on routine chest radiographs. Cells are not recovered from bronchial washings because the tumor is covered with normal mucosa. These tumors are slow-growing cancers, and 50% of individuals with bronchial carcinoid tumors are asymptomatic. Local surgical resection is curative if metastasis has not occurred; this can often be done by bronchoscopic laser electrocautery. **Adenocystic tumors (cylindromas)** and **mucoepidermoid carcinomas** are rare bronchial gland tumors. They arise predominantly in the trachea or large airways and cause obstruction. They can be malignant and metastasize early, although distal pulmonary metastases are usually slow growing. Thus it is not unusual for an individual to survive 10 to 15 years after diagnosis.

Mesotheliomas can be benign but most often are aggressive malignant tumors arising from the epithelium covering the serous membranes.[163] Most arise from the pleural surface (80%). Benign pleural mesotheliomas have a slow clinical onset and are usually asymptomatic, but over a period of years they can cause dyspnea and mild pleuritic pain. These tumors can grow to be very large and fill the entire pleural cavity.

There is a clear association between asbestos exposure and malignant mesothelioma, especially in asbestos workers, although the minimum amount of exposure that constitutes risk has not been determined. A long latent interval between exposure to asbestos and appearance of mesothelioma usually occurs, and onset of symptoms may take 20 to 40 years. Clinical manifestations include dyspnea and chest pain that result from tumor-derived pleural fluid and invasion of the chest wall. Diagnosis is made by chest x-ray, CT scan, and thoracentesis with cytologic examination of the pleural fluid. Thoracoscopy also may be used for biopsy. Osteopontin and mesothelin are being explored as potential tumor markers for early diagnosis.[163] Current management of malignant mesothelioma includes a combination of pleuropneumonectomy, chemotherapy, radiation, and hyperthermia.[163,164]

SUMMARY REVIEW

Clinical Manifestations of Pulmonary Alterations

1. Dyspnea is a feeling of breathlessness and increased respiratory effort.
2. Abnormal breathing patterns are adjustments made by the body to minimize the work of respiratory muscles. They include Kussmaul, obstructed, restricted, gasping, and/or Cheyne-Stokes respirations, and sighing.
3. Hypoventilation is decreased alveolar ventilation caused by airway obstruction, chest wall restriction, or altered neurologic control of breathing. Hypoventilation causes increased $Paco_2$.
4. Hyperventilation is increased alveolar ventilation produced by anxiety, head injury, or severe hypoxemia. Hyperventilation causes decreased $Paco_2$.
5. Cyanosis is a bluish discoloration of the skin caused by desaturation of hemoglobin, polycythemia, or peripheral vasoconstriction.
6. Clubbing of the fingertips is associated with diseases that interfere with oxygenation of the tissues.
7. Coughing is a protective reflex that expels secretions and irritants from the lower airways.

continued

SUMMARY REVIEW—cont'd

8. Hemoptysis is expectoration of bloody mucus that can be caused by bronchitis, TB, abscess, neoplasms, and other conditions that cause hemorrhage from damaged vessels.

9. Chest pain can result from inflamed pleurae, trachea, bronchi, or respiratory muscles.

10. Hypercapnia is increased $Paco_2$ caused by a decrease in minute volume (respiratory rate × tidal volume).

11. Hypoxemia is a reduced Pao_2 caused by (1) decreased oxygen content of inspired gas, (2) hypoventilation, (3) diffusion abnormality, (4) ventilation-perfusion mismatch, or (5) shunting.

12. Acute respiratory failure is caused by inadequate gas exchange or ventilation (PaO_2 ≤50 mmHg or $Paco_2$ ≥50 mmHg and pH ≥7.25).

Disorders of the Chest Wall and Pleura

1. Chest wall compliance is diminished by obesity and kyphoscoliosis, which compress the lungs, and by neuromuscular diseases that impair chest wall muscle function.

2. Flail chest results from rib or sternal fractures that disrupt the mechanics of breathing.

3. Pneumothorax is the accumulation of air in the pleural space. It can be caused by spontaneous rupture of weakened areas of a pleura or can be secondary to pleural damage caused by disease, trauma, or mechanical ventilation.

4. Tension pneumothorax is a life-threatening condition caused by trapping of air in the pleural space.

5. Pleural effusion is the accumulation of fluid in the pleural space, usually resulting from disorders that promote transudation or exudation from capillaries underlying the pleura but occasionally resulting from blockage or injury that causes lymphatic vessels to drain into the pleural space.

6. Empyema is the presence of pus in the pleural space (infected pleural effusion). The source of the pus is usually lymphatic drainage from sites of bacterial pneumonia.

Pulmonary Disorders

1. Aspiration is passage of fluid and solid particles into the lung, usually from impaired swallowing and coughing. It frequently results in pneumonitis and pulmonary infection.

2. Atelectasis is the collapse of alveoli resulting from compression of the lung tissue or absorption of gas from obstructed alveoli.

3. Bronchiectasis is abnormal dilation of the bronchi secondary to another pulmonary disorder, usually infection or inflammation.

4. Bronchiolitis is the inflammatory obstruction of small airways. It is most common in children.

5. Pulmonary fibrosis is an excessive amount of connective tissue in the lung. It diminishes lung compliance and may be idiopathic or caused by disease.

6. Inhalation of noxious gases or prolonged exposure to high concentrations of oxygen can damage the bronchial mucosa or alveolocapillary membrane and cause inflammation or acute respiratory failure.

7. Pneumoconiosis, which is caused by inhalation of dust particles in the workplace, including coal dust, can cause pulmonary fibrosis, susceptibility to lower airway infection, and tumor formation.

8. Silicosis is a type of pneumoconiosis caused by inhalation of silica.

9. Allergic alveolitis is an allergic or hypersensitivity reaction to many allergens.

10. Pulmonary edema is excess water in the lung caused by disturbances of capillary hydrostatic pressure, capillary oncotic pressure, or capillary permeability. A common cause is left-sided heart failure that increases the hydrostatic pressure in the pulmonary circulation.

11. ARDS results from an acute, diffuse injury to the alveolocapillary membrane and decreased surfactant production, which increases membrane permeability and causes edema and atelectasis.

12. Obstructive pulmonary disease is characterized by airway obstruction that causes difficult expiration. Obstructive disease can be acute or chronic and includes asthma, chronic bronchitis, and emphysema.

13. In asthma, obstruction is caused by episodic attacks of bronchospasm, bronchial inflammation, mucosal edema, and increased mucus production.

14. COPD is the coexistence of chronic bronchitis and emphysema.

15. Chronic bronchitis causes airway obstruction resulting from bronchial smooth muscle hypertrophy and production of thick, tenacious mucus.

16. In emphysema, destruction of the alveolar septa and loss of passive elastic recoil lead to airway collapse and obstruct gas flow during expiration.

17. Emphysema in which septal deterioration is caused by α_1-antitrypsin deficiency or old age tends to be panacinar.

18. Emphysema in which septal deterioration results from smoking tends to be centriacinar.

19. Upper respiratory tract infections, which are the most common cause of short-term disability in the United States, include rhinitis (the common cold), pharyngitis, and laryngitis.

20. Serious lower respiratory tract infections, which occur most often in older adults and individuals with impaired immunity or underlying disease, include pneumonia and tuberculosis.

21. Pneumococcal pneumonia is an acute lung infection resulting in an inflammatory response with four phases: (1) consolidation, (2) red hepatization, (3) gray hepatization, and (4) resolution.

22. Viral pneumonia is an acute, self-limiting lung infection usually caused by the influenzavirus.

23. TB is a lung infection caused by *M. tuberculosis* (tubercle bacillus).

24. In TB the inflammatory response isolates colonies of bacilli by enclosing them in tubercles and surrounding the tubercles with scar tissue.

25. Bacilli may remain dormant within the tubercles for life or, if the immune system breaks down, cause recurrence of active disease.

26. Abscesses are circumscribed areas of destruction of lung parenchyma with suppuration usually resulting from aspiration pneumonia.

27. Pulmonary vascular diseases are caused by embolism or hypertension in the pulmonary circulation.

28. PE is occlusion of a portion of the pulmonary vascular bed by a thrombus (most common), a tissue fragment, or an air bubble. Depending on its size and location, the embolus can cause hypoxic vasoconstriction, pulmonary edema, atelectasis, pulmonary hypertension, shock, and even death.

SUMMARY REVIEW—cont'd

29. Pulmonary artery hypertension (pulmonary artery pressure 5 to 10 mmHg greater than normal) is caused by (1) elevated left ventricular pressure, (2) increased blood flow through the pulmonary circulation, (3) obliteration or obstruction of the vascular bed, or (4) active constriction of the vascular bed produced by hypoxemia or acidosis.

30. Cor pulmonale is right ventricular enlargement caused by chronic pulmonary hypertension. Cor pulmonale progresses to right ventricular failure if the pulmonary hypertension is not reversed.

31. Lip cancer is most common in men and represents about 1% of all cancers. In the most common cell type, squamous cell, metastasis is rare when lesions are diagnosed and treated early.

32. Laryngeal cancer occurs primarily in men and represents 2% to 3% of all cancers. Squamous cell carcinoma of the true vocal cords is most common and manifests with a clinical symptom of progressive hoarseness.

33. Lung cancer, the most frequent cause of cancer death in the United States, is commonly caused by cigarette smoking.

34. Cancer cell types include squamous cell carcinoma, small cell (oat cell) carcinoma, adenocarcinoma, large cell carcinoma, bronchial adenoma, and mesothelioma. Each type arises in a characteristic site or type of tissue, causes distinctive clinical manifestations, and differs in likelihood of metastasis and prognosis.

35. Bronchial carcinoid and adenocystic tumors are rare tumors of the bronchial airways.

KEY TERMS

Abscess, 1294
Absorption atelectasis, 1275
Acute cough, 1266
Acute respiratory distress syndrome (ARDS), 1279
Adenocarcinoma, 1301
Adenocystic tumor (cylindroma), 1304
Allergic alveolitis (hypersensitivity pneumonitis), 1278
Alveolar dead space, 1270
Asbestosis, 1278
Aspiration, 1274
Asthma, 1283
Atelectasis, 1275
Bronchial carcinoid tumor, 1303
Bronchiectasis, 1275
Bronchiolitis, 1277
Bronchiolitis obliterans, 1277
Bronchiolitis obliterans organizing pneumonia (BOOP), 1277
Cavitation, 1294
Centriacinar emphysema, 1289
Cheyne-Stokes respiration, 1268
Chronic bronchitis, 1286
Chronic cough, 1266
Chronic obstructive pulmonary disease (COPD), 1286
Chylothorax, 1273
Clubbing, 1269
Coal worker pneumoconiosis (coal miner lung, black lung), 1278
Compression atelectasis, 1275

Consolidation, 1294
Cor pulmonale, 1298
Cough, 1266
Cyanosis, 1268
Cylindrical bronchiectasis, 1276
Dyspnea, 1267
Dyspnea on exertion, 1267
Emphysema, 1288
Empyema (infected pleural effusion), 1273
Exudative effusion, 1273, 1274
Flail chest, 1272
Hemoptysis, 1268
Hemothorax, 1273
Hypercapnia, 1268
Hyperventilation, 1268
Hypocapnia, 1269
Hypoventilation, 1268
Hypoxemia, 1269
Hypoxia, 1269
Idiopathic pulmonary fibrosis (IPF), 1277
Kussmaul respiration (hyperpnea), 1268
Large cell carcinoma, 1301
Laryngeal cancer, 1299
Lip cancer, 1298
Lung cancer, 1299
Mesothelioma, 1304
Mucoepidermoid carcinoma, 1304
Obstructive pulmonary disease, 1282
Open pneumothorax (communicating pneumothorax), 1273
Orthopnea, 1267

Oxygen toxicity, 1277
Pain, 1267
Panacinar emphysema, 1289
Paroxysmal nocturnal dyspnea (PND), 1267
Pleural effusion, 1273
Pneumoconiosis, 1278
Pneumonia, 1290
Pneumothorax, 1272
Primary (spontaneous) pneumothorax, 1272
Pulmonary artery hypertension (PAH), 1296
Pulmonary edema, 1279
Pulmonary embolism (PE), 1294
Pulmonary fibrosis, 1277
Pulmonary thromboembolism, 1295
Pulsus paradoxus, 1284
Respiratory failure, 1271
Saccular bronchiectasis, 1276
Secondary pneumothorax, 1273
Shunting, 1270
Silicosis, 1278
Small-cell lung carcinoma, 1302
Sputum, 1267
Status asthmaticus, 1284
Surfactant impairment, 1275
Tension pneumothorax, 1273
TNM classification system, 1303
Transudative effusion, 1273
Tuberculosis (TB), 1293
Undifferentiated large cell anaplastic cancer, 1301
Varicose bronchiectasis, 1276

REFERENCES

1. Millqvist E, Bende M: Role of the upper airways in patients with chronic cough, *Curr Opin Allergy Clin Immunol* 6(1):7-11, 2006.
2. Canning BJ: Anatomy and neurophysiology of the cough reflex: ACCP evidence-based clinical practice guidelines, *Chest* 129:33S-47S, 2006.
3. Boulet LP: Future directions in the clinical management of cough: ACCP evidence-based clinical practice guidelines, *Chest* 129:287S-292S, 2006.
4. Brashers VL, Haden K: Differential diagnosis of cough: focus on lung malignancy, *Lippincott Prim Care Pract* 4(4):374-389, 2000.
5. Pratter MR: Overview of common causes of chronic cough: ACCP evidence-based clinical practice guidelines, *Chest* 129:59S-62S, 2006.
6. Lumb AB: *Nunn's applied respiratory physiology*, ed 6, St. Louis, 2005, Butterworth-Heinemann.
7. Spector N et al: Dyspnea: applying research to bedside practice, *AACN Adv Crit Care* 18(1):45-58:quiz 59-60, 2007.
8. Corder R: Hemoptysis, *Emerg Med Clin North Am* 21(2):421-435, 2003.
9. Noppen M, Baumann MH: Pathogenesis and treatment of primary spontaneous pneumothorax: an overview, *Respiration* 70(4):431-438, 2003.
10. Currie GP et al: Pneumothorax: an update, *Postgrad Med J* 83(981):461-465, 2007.
11. Chiu HT, Garcia CK: Familial spontaneous pneumothorax, *Curr Opin Pulm Med* 12(4):268-272, 2006.
12. Sahn SA: The value of pleural fluid analysis, *Am J Med Sci* 335(1):7-15, 2008.
13. Shigemitsu H, Afshar K: Aspiration pneumonias: under-diagnosed and under-treated, *Curr Opin Pulm Med* 13(3):192-198, 2007.
14. Metheny NA, Meert KL, Clouse RE: Complications related to feeding tube placement, *Curr Opin Gastroenterol* 23(2):178-182, 2007.
15. Duggan M, Kavanagh BP: Atelectasis in the perioperative patient, *Curr Opin Anaesthesiol* 20(1):37-42, 2007.
16. Drakopanagiotakis F, Polychronopoulos V, Judson MA: Organizing pneumonia, *Am J Med Sci* 335(1):34-39, 2008.
17. Gottlieb J et al: Long-term azithromycin for bronchiolitis obliterans syndrome after lung transplantation, *Transplantation* 85(1):36-41, 2008.
18. Hyzy R et al: Acute exacerbation of idiopathic pulmonary fibrosis, *Chest* 132(5):1652-1658, 2007.
19. Noth I, Martinez FJ: Recent advances in idiopathic pulmonary fibrosis, *Chest* 132(2):637-650, 2007.
20. Palmieri TL: Inhalation injury: research progress and needs, *J Burn Care Res* 28(4):549-554, 2007.
21. Chong S et al: Pneumoconiosis: comparison of imaging and pathologic findings, *Radiograph* 26(1):59-77, 2006.
22. Huaux F: New developments in the understanding of immunology in silicosis, *Curr Opin Allergy Clin Immunol* 7(2):168-173, 2007.
23. Cohen R, Velho V: Update on respiratory disease from coal mine and silica dust, *Clin Chest Med* 23(4):811-826, 2002.
24. O'Reilly KM et al: Asbestos-related lung disease, *Am Fam Physician* 75(5):683-688, 2007.
25. Greenberger PA: 7. Immunologic lung disease, *J Allergy Clin Immunol* 121(2 Suppl):S393-S397, quiz S418, 2008.
26. Madison JM: Hypersensitivity pneumonitis: clinical perspectives, *Arch Pathol Lab Med* 132(2):195-198, 2008.
27. Rubenfeld GD, Herridge MS: Epidemiology and outcomes of acute lung injury, *Chest* 131(2):554-562, 2007.
28. Ware LB, Matthay MA: The acute respiratory distress syndrome, *N Engl J Med* 342(18):1334-1349, 2000.
29. Bhatia M, Moochhala S: Role of inflammatory mediators in the pathophysiology of acute respiratory distress syndrome, *J Pathol* 202(2):145-156, 2004.
30. Girard TD, Bernard GR: Mechanical ventilation in ARDS: a state-of-the-art review, *Chest* 131(3):921-929, 2007.
31. Calfee CS, Matthay MA: Nonventilatory treatments for acute lung injury and ARDS, *Chest* 131(3):913-920, 2007.
32. Peter JV et al: Corticosteroids in the prevention and treatment of acute respiratory distress syndrome (ARDS) in adults: meta-analysis, *BMJ* 336:1006-1009, 2008.
33. National Heart, Lung, and Blood Institute. National Asthma Education and Prevention Program Expert Panel Report 3: *Guidelines for the diagnosis and management of asthma*, 2007, p.12. Available at www.nhlbi.nih.gov/guidelines/asthma/asthgdin.pdf.
34. Global Initiative for Asthma (GINA): Global strategy for asthma management and prevention, *2006*. Available from www.ginasthma.org.
35. Zhang J, Pare PD, Sandford AJ: Recent advances in asthma genetics, *Resp Res* 9:4, 2008.
36. Holloway JW, Koppelman GH: Identifying novel genes contributing to asthma pathogenesis, *Curr Opin Allergy Clin Immunol* 7(1):69-74, 2007.
37. Yang Y et al: Epigenetic mechanisms silence a disintegrin and metalloprotease 33 expression in bronchial epithelial cells, *J Allergy Clin Immunol* 121(6):1393-1399, 2008.
38. McLeish S, Turner SW: Gene-environment interactions in asthma, *Arch Dis Child* 92(11):1032-1035, 2007.
39. Miller RL, Ho SM: Environmental epigenetics and asthma: current concepts and call for studies, *Am J Respir Crit Care Med* 177(6):567-573, 2008.
40. Yang IA et al: Gene-environmental interaction in asthma, *Curr Opin Allergy Clin Immunol* 7(1):75-82, 2007.
41. Effros RM, Nagaraj H: Asthma: New developments concerning immune mechanisms, diagnosis and treatment, *Curr Opin Pulm Med* 13(1):37-43, 2007.
42. Corren J: The connection between allergic rhinitis and bronchial asthma, *Curr Opinin Pulm Med* 13(1):13-18, 2007.
43. Passalacqua G, Durham SR: Global Allergy and Asthma European Network: allergic rhinitis and its impact on asthma update: allergen immunotherapy, *J Allergy Clin Immunol* 119(4):881-891, 2007.
44. Kiechl-Kohlendorfer U et al: Neonatal characteristics and risk of atopic asthma in schoolchildren: results from a large prospective birth-cohort study, *Acta Paediatr* 96(11):1606-1610, 2007.
45. Cabana MD et al: Examining the hygiene hypothesis: the Trial of Infant Probiotic Supplementation, *Paediatr Perinat Epidemiol* 21(Suppl 3):23-28, 2007.
46. Peters-Golden M, Henderson WR Jr: Leukotrienes, *N Engl J Med* 357(18):1841-1854, 2007.
47. Trivedi SG, Lloyd CM: Eosinophils in the pathogenesis of allergic airways disease, *Cell Mol Life Sci* 64(10):1269-1289, 2007.
48. Tliba O, Amrani Y, Panettieri RA Jr: Is airway smooth muscle the "missing link" modulating airway inflammation in asthma? *Chest* 133(1):236-242, 2008.
49. Moore WC, Peters SP: Update in asthma 2006, *Am J Respir Crit Care Med* 175(7):649-654, 2007.
50. Frieri M: Advances in the understanding of allergic asthma, *Allergy Asthma Proc* 28(6):614-619, 2007.
51. Holgate ST, Polosa R: Treatment strategies for allergy and asthma, *Nat Rev Immunol* 8(3):218-230, 2008.
52. Stewart L, Katial R: Exhaled nitric oxide, *Immunol Allergy Clin North Am* 27(4):571-586:v, 2007.
53. Kaza V, Bandi V, Guntupalli KK: Acute severe asthma: recent advances, *Curr Opin Pulm Med* 13(1):1-7, 2007.
54. Oppenheimer J, Nelson HS: Safety of long-acting beta-agonists in asthma: a review, *Curr Opin Pulm Med* 14(1):64-69, 2008.
55. Taylor DR: Beta-adrenergic receptor polymorphisms: relationship to the beta-agonist controversy and clinical implications, *Exp Opin Pharmacother* 8(18):3195-3203, 2007.
56. Jacobsen L, Valovirta E: How strong is the evidence that immunotherapy in children prevents the progression of allergy and asthma? *Curr Opin Allergy Clin Immunol* 7(6):556-560, 2007.
57. Rabe KF et al: Global strategy for the diagnosis, management, and prevention of chronic obstructive pulmonary disease: GOLD executive summary, *Am J Respir Crit Care Med* 176(6):532-555, 2007:(Available at http://ajrccm.atsjournals.org/cgi/content/full/176/6/532).
58. Ben-Zaken Cohen S et al: The growing burden of chronic obstructive pulmonary disease and lung cancer in women: examining sex differences in cigarette smoke metabolism, *Am J Respir Crit Care Med* 176(2):113-120, 2007.
59. Molfino NA: Current thinking on genetics of chronic obstructive pulmonary disease, *Curr Opin Pulm Med* 13(2):107-113, 2007.
60. Hallberg J et al: Interaction between smoking and genetic factors in the development of chronic bronchitis, *Am J Resp Critical Care Med* 177:486-490, 2008.
61. Barnes PJ: Immunology of asthma and chronic obstructive pulmonary disease, *Nat Rev Immunol* 8(3):183-1892, 2008.
62. Braman SS: Chronic cough due to chronic bronchitis: ACCP evidence-based clinical practice guidelines, *Chest* 129(1 Suppl):104S-115S, 2006.

63. Quon BS, Gan WQ, Sin DD: Contemporary management of acute exacerbations of COPD: a systematic review and metaanalysis, *Chest* 133(3):756-766, 2008.

64. Martinez FJ, Anzueto A: Appropriate outpatient treatment of acute bacterial exacerbations of chronic bronchitis, *Am J Med* 118(Suppl 7A):39S-44S, 2005.

65. Sin DD, Man SF: Do chronic inhaled steroids alone or in combination with a bronchodilator prolong life in chronic obstructive pulmonary disease patients, *Curr Opin Pulm Med* 13(2):90-97, 2007.

66. O'Reilly P, Bailey W: Long-term continuous oxygen treatment in chronic obstructive pulmonary disease: proper use, benefits and unresolved issues, *Curr Opin Pulm Med* 13(2):120-124, 2007.

67. Stoller JK: Aboussouan LS:.Alpha 1-antitrypsin deficiency, *Lancet* 365(9478):2225-2236, 2005.

68. Taraseviciene-Stewart L, Voelkel NF: Molecular pathogenesis of emphysema, *J Clin Invest* 118(2):394-402, 2008.

69. Friedman PJ: Imaging studies in emphysema, *Proc Am Thorac Soc* 5(4):494-500, 2008.

70. Ries AL et al: Pulmonary rehabilitation: joint ACCP/AACVPR evidence-based clinical practice guidelines, *Chest* 131(5 Suppl):4S-42S, 2007.

71. Boswell-Smith V, Spina D: PDE4 inhibitors as potential therapeutic agents in the treatment of COPD-focus on roflumilast, *Int J COPD* 2(2):121-129, 2007.

72. Heresi GA, Stoller JK: Augmentation therapy in alpha-1 antitrypsin deficiency, *Exp Opin Biol Ther* 8(4):515-526, 2008.

73. Mizgerd JP: Acute lower respiratory tract infection, *N Engl J Med* 358(7):716-727, 2008.

74. Niederman MS, Brito V: Pneumonia in the older patient, *Clin Chest Med* 28(4):751-771:vi, 2007.

75. Donowitz GR, Cox HL: Bacterial community-acquired pneumonia in older patients, *Clin Geriatr Med* 23:515-534, 2007.

76. File TM: Community-acquired pneumonia, *Lancet* 362(9400): 1991-2001, 2003.

77. Kollef MH et al: Epidemiology and outcomes of health-care-associated pneumonia: results from a large US database of culture positive patients, *Chest* 128:3854-3862, 2005.

78. Ortqvist A, Hedlund J, Kalin M: *Streptococcus pneumoniae*: epidemiology, risk factors, and clinical features, *Semin Respir Crit Care Med* 26(6):563-574, 2005.

79. Blasi F et al: *Chlamydia pneumoniae* and *Mycoplasma pneumoniae*, *Semin Respir Crit Care Med* 26(6):617-624, 2005.

80. Lynch JP 3rd, Walsh EE: Influenza: evolving strategies in treatment and prevention, *Semin Respir Crit Care Med* 28(2):144-158, 2007.

81. Diederen BM: *Legionella* spp. and legionnaires' disease, *J Infect* 56(1):1-12, 2008.

82. Mueller EW et al: Repeat bronchoalveolar lavage to guide antibiotic duration for ventilator-associated pneumonia, *J Trauma* 63(6): 1329-1337, discussion 1337, 2007.

83. Davaro RE, Thirumalai A: Life-threatening complications of HIV infection, *J Intern Care Med* 22(2):73-81, 2007.

84. Morris A et al: Epidemiology and clinical significance of pneumocystis colonization, *J Infect Dis* 197(1):10-17, 2008.

85. Yew WW, Leung CC: Update in tuberculosis 2007, *Am J Respir Crit Care Med* 177(5):479-485, 2008.

86. Gerold G, Zychlinsky A, de Diego JL: What is the role of toll-like receptors in bacterial infections? *Semin Immunol* 19(1):41-47, 2007.

87. Shoma S et al: Critical involvement of pneumolysin in production of interleukin-1 alpha and caspase-1-dependent cytokines in infection with *Streptococcus pneumoniae* in vitro: a novel function of pneumolysin in caspase-1 activation, *Infect Immun* 76(4):1547-1557, 2008.

88. Rothberg MB, Haessler SD, Brown RB: Complications of viral influenza, *Am J Med* 121(4):258-264, 2008.

89. Writing Committee of the Second World Health Organization Consultation on Clinical Aspects of Human Infection with Avian Influenza(H5N1) virus A et al: update on avian influenza A (H5N1) virus infection in humans, *N Engl J Med* 358(3):261-273, 2008.

90. Centers for Disease Control and Prevention (CDC): Update: novel influenza A (H1N1) virus infections—worldwide, May 6, 2009, *MMWR Morb Mortal Wkly Rep* 58(17):453-458, 2009.

91. Mandell L et al: Infectious Diseases Society of America/American Thoracic Society Guidelines on the management for community-acquired pneumonia in adults, *Clin Infect Dis* 44(Suppl 2):S27-S72, 2007.

92. Chan YR, Morris A: Molecular diagnostic methods in pneumonia, *Curr Opin Infect Dis* 20(2):157-164, 2007.

93. Soto G: J: Diagnostic strategies for nosocomial pneumonia, *Curr Opin Infect Dis* 20(2):157-164, 2007.

94. Ramirez P, Valencia M, Torres A: Bronchoalveolar lavage to diagnose respiratory infections, *Semin Respir Crit Care Med* 28(5):525-533, 2007.

95. Oosterhuis-Kafeja F, Beutels P, Van Damme P: Immunogenicity, efficacy, safety and effectiveness of pneumococcal conjugate vaccines (1998-2006), *Vaccine* 25(12):2194-2212, 2007.

96. Ramirez P, Ferrer M, Torres A: Prevention measures for ventilator-associated pneumonia: a new focus on the endotracheal tube, *Curr Opin Infect Dis* 20(2):190-197, 2007.

97. Armitage K, Woodhead M: New guidelines for the management of adult community-acquired pneumonia, *Curr Opin Infect Dis* 20(2):170-176, 2007.

98. Aarts MA et al: Empiric antibiotic therapy for suspected ventilator-associated pneumonia: a systematic review and meta-analysis of randomized trials, *Crit Care Med* 36(1):108-117, 2008.

99. Dye C: Global epidemiology of tuberculosis, *Lancet* 367(9514):938-940, 2006.

100. WHO 2008 Report: *Global tuberculosis control—surveillance, planning, financing*. Available at www.who.int/tb/publications/global_report/2008/download_centre/en/index.html.

101. Centers for Disease Control and Prevention: Trends in tuberculosis—United States, 2007, *JAMA* 299(18):2142–2144, 2008.

102. Cardona PJ: New insights on the nature of latent tuberculosis infection and its treatment, *Inflamm Allergy Drug Targets* 6(1):27-39, 2007.

103. Bottasso O et al: The immuno-endocrine component in the pathogenesis of tuberculosis, *Scand J Immunol* 66(2-3):166-175, 2007.

104. Russell DG: Who puts the tubercle in tuberculosis? *Nat Rev Microbiol* 5(1):39-47, 2007.

105. Lalvani A: Diagnosing tuberculosis infection in the 21st century: new tools to tackle an old enemy, *Chest* 131(6):1898-1906, 2007.

106. Campbell IA, Bah-Sow O: Pulmonary tuberculosis: diagnosis and treatment, *BMJ* 332(7551):1194-1197, 2006.

107. Gupta UD, Katoch VM, McMurray DN: Current status of TB vaccines, *Vaccine* 25(19):3742-3751, 2007.

108. Zhang Y: Advances in the treatment of tuberculosis, *Clin Pharmacol Ther* 82(5):595-600, 2007.

109. Furin J: The clinical management of drug-resistant tuberculosis, *Curr Opin Pulm Med* 13(3):212-217, 2007.

110. Roy E, Lowrie DB, Jolles SR: Current strategies in TB immunotherapy, *Curr Mol Med* 7(4):373-386, 2007.

111. Volmink J, Garner P: Directly observed therapy for treating tuberculosis, *Cochrane Database Syst Rev* (4):CD003343, 2007.

112. Braman SS: Chronic cough due to acute bronchitis: ACCP evidence-based clinical practice guidelines, *Chest* 129(1 Suppl):95S-103S, 2006.

113. Tapson VF: Acute pulmonary embolism, *N Engl J Med* 358(10): 1037-1052, 2008.

114. Heit JA: The epidemiology of venous thromboembolism in the community, *Arterioscler Thromb Vasc Biol* 28(3):370-372, 2008.

115. Dimarsico L, Cymet T: Pulmonary embolism—a state of the clot review, *Comprehen Ther* 33(4):184-191, 2007.

116. Hunt D: Determining the clinical probability of deep venous thrombosis and pulmonary embolism, *South Med J* 100(10):1015-1021, 2007.

117. Minichiello T, Fogarty PF: Diagnosis and management of venous thromboembolism, *Med Clin North Am* 92(2):443-465, 2008.

118. Di Nisio M et al: Diagnostic accuracy of D-dimer test for exclusion of venous thromboembolism: a systematic review, *J Thromb Haemost* 5(2):296-304, 2007.

119. Francis CW: Clinical practice: prophylaxis for thromboembolism in hospitalized medical patients, *N Engl J Med* 356(14):1438-1444, 2007.

120. Sjalander A et al: Efficacy and safety of anticoagulant prophylaxis to prevent venous thromboembolism in acutely ill medical inpatients: a meta-analysis, *J Intern Med* 263(1):52-60, 2008.

121. Barral FG: Vena cava filters: why, when, what and how? *J Cardiovasc Surg* 49(1):35-49, 2008.

122. Segal JB et al: Management of venous thromboembolism: a systematic review for a practice guideline, *Ann Internal Med* 146(3):211-222, 2007.

123. Gross PL, Weitz JI: New anticoagulants for treatment of venous thromboembolism, *Arterioscler Thromb Vasc Biol* 28(3):380-386, 2008.

124. Carlbom DJ, Davidson BL: Pulmonary embolism in the critically ill, *Chest* 132(1):313-324, 2007.

125. Uflacker R, Schonholz C: Percutaneous interventions for pulmonary embolism, *J Cardiovasc Surg* 49(1):3-18, 2008.

126. Highland KB: Pulmonary arterial hypertension, *Am J Med Sci* 335(1):40-45, 2008.

127. Heresi GA, Dweik RA: Pulmonary hypertension: evaluation and management, *Comprehen Ther* 33(3):150-161, 2007.

128. Chan SY, Loscalzo J: Pathogenic mechanisms of pulmonary arterial hypertension, *J Mol Cell Cardiol* 44(1):14-30, 2008.

129. Jain S, Ventura H, deBoisblanc B: Pathophysiology of pulmonary arterial hypertension, *Sem Cardiothorac Vasc Anesth* 11(2):104-109, 2007.

130. Tuder R et al: Hypoxia and chronic lung disease, *J Molec Med* 85(12):1317-1324, 2007.

131. Driscoll JA, Chakinala MM: Medical therapy for pulmonary arterial hypertension, *Exp Opin Pharmacother* 9(1):65-81, 2008.

132. American Cancer Society, Inc., Surveillance and Health Policy Research: Estimated New Cancer Cases and Deaths by Sex, U.S. 2009 available at: http://www.cancer.org/downloads/stt/CFF2009_EstCD_3.pdf

133. Karamanolis G, Sifrim D: Developments in pathogenesis and diagnosis of gastroesophageal reflux disease, *Curr Opin Gastroenterol* 23(4):428-433, 2007.

134. Torrente MC, Ojeda JM: Exploring the relation between human papillomavirus and larynx cancer, *Acta Otolaryngol* 127(9):900-906, 2007.

135. Genden EM et al: Recent changes in the treatment of patients with advanced laryngeal cancer, *Head Neck* 30(1):103-110, 2008.

136. Biel MA: Photodynamic therapy treatment of early oral and laryngeal cancers, *Photochem Photobiol* 83(5):1063-1068, 2007.

137. Marioni G et al: Organ-preservation surgery following failed radiotherapy for laryngeal cancer. Evaluation, patient selection, functional outcome and survival, *Curr Opin Otolaryngol Head Neck Surg* 16(2):141-146, 2008.

138. Dubey S, Powell CA: Update in lung cancer 2007, *Am J Respir Crit Care Med* 177(9):941-946, 2008.

139. Alberg AJ et al: Epidemiology of lung cancer: ACCP evidence-based clinical practice guidelines (ed 2), *Chest* 132(3 Suppl):29S-55S, 2007.

140. Kiyohara C et al: Lung cancer susceptibility: are we on our way to identifying a high-risk group? *Future Oncol* 3(6):617-627, 2007.

141. Maitra A, Kumar V: The lung. In Kumar V, et al, editors: *Robbins basic pathology*, ed 8, Philadelphia, 2007, Saunders.

142. Malingam S, Belani C: Systemic chemotherapy for advanced non-small cell lung cancer: recent advances and future directions, *Oncologist* 13(Suppl 1):5-13, 2008.

143. Alberts WM: American College of Chest Physicians: Introduction: diagnosis and management of lung cancer: ACCP evidence-based clinical practice guidelines (2nd ed), *Chest* 132(3 Suppl):20S-22S, 2007.

144. Garfield DH, Cadranel J, West HL: Bronchioloalveolar carcinoma: the case for two diseases, *Clin Lung Can* 9(1):24-29, 2008.

145. Sher T, Dy GK, Adjei AA: Small cell lung cancer, *Mayo Clin Proc* 83(3):355-367, 2008.

146. Hudkinson PS, MacKinnin A, Sethi T: Targeting growth factors in lung cancer, *Chest* 133:1209-1216, 2008.

147. Krysan K et al: Inflammation, epithelial to mesenchymal transition, and epidermal growth factor receptor tyrosine kinase inhibitor resistance, *J Thorac Oncol* 3(2):107-110, 2008.

148. Azad N, Rojanasakul Y, Vallyathan V: Inflammation and lung cancer: roles of reactive oxygen/nitrogen species, *J Toxicol Environ Health B Crit Rev* 11(1):1-15, 2008.

149. Bach PB et al: Screening for lung cancer: ACCP evidence-based clinical practice guidelines (2nd ed), *Chest* 132(3 Suppl):69S-77S, 2007.

150. Aberle DR, Brown K: Lung cancer screening with CT, *Clin Chest Med* 29(1):1-14, 2008.

151. Rivera PM, Mehta AC: Initial diagnosis of lung cancer: ACCP evidence-based clinical practice guidelines (2nd ed), *Chest* 132 (3 Suppl):1315-1485, 2007.

152. Patz EF Jr et al: Panel of serum biomarkers for the diagnosis of lung cancer, *J Clin Oncol* 25:5578-5583, 2007.

153. D'Amico TA: Molecular biologic staging of lung cancer, *Ann Thorac Surg* 85(2):S737-S742, 2008.

154. de Marinis F, Grossi F: Clinical evidence for second- and third-line treatment options in advanced non-small cell lung cancer, *Oncologist* 13(Suppl 1):14-20, 2008.

155. Chada S et al: Cancer targeting using tumor suppressor genes, *Front Biosci* 13:1959-1967, 2008.

156. Deng WG et al: Enhancement of antitumor activity of cisplatin in human lung cancer cells by tumor suppressor FUS1, *Cancer Gene Ther* 15(1):29-39, 2008.

157. Gutierrez M, Giaccone G: Antiangiogenic therapy in nonsmall cell lung cancer, *Curr Opin Oncol* 20(2):176-182, 2008.

158. Ruttinger D et al: Current immunotherapeutic strategies in lung cancer, *Surg Oncol Clin North Am* 16(4):901-918:x, 2007.

159. Sequist LV, Lynch TJ: EGFR tyrosine kinase inhibitors in lung cancer: an evolving story, *Annu Rev Med* 59:429-442, 2008.

160. Wheatley-Price P, Shepherd FA: Epidermal growth factor receptor inhibitors in the treatment of lung cancer: reality and hopes, *Curr Opin Oncol* 20(2):162-175, 2008.

161. Omenn GS: Chemoprevention of lung cancers: lessons from CARET, the beta-carotene and retinol efficacy trial, and prospects for the future, *Eur J Cancer Prev* 16(3):184-191, 2007.

162. Garcia-Yuste M, Matilla JM, Gonzalez-Aragoneses F: Neuroendocrine tumors of the lung, *Curr Opin Oncol* 20(2):148-154, 2008.

163. Zervos MD, Bizekis C, Pass HI: Malignant mesothelioma 2008, *Curr Opin Pulm Med* 14(4):303-309, 2008.

164. Fennell DA et al: Advances in the systemic therapy of malignant pleural mesothelioma, *Nat Clin Pract Oncol* 5(3):136-147, 2008.

ALTERATIONS OF PULMONARY FUNCTION IN CHILDREN

KRISTI GOTT • DEBORAH K. FROH

MEDIA RESOURCES

⊛volve **Evolve Website** (http://evolve.elsevier.com/McCance/)
- Review Questions and Answers
- Animations
- Glossary (with audio pronunciation for selected terms)
- WebLinks

CHAPTER OUTLINE

STRUCTURE AND FUNCTION
Upper Airway
Lower Airways and Lung Parenchyma
Chest Wall Dynamics
Metabolic Characteristics
Immunologic Incompetence
Physiologic Control of Respiration

PULMONARY DISORDERS
Disorders of the Upper Airways
Disorders of the Lower Airways
SUDDEN INFANT DEATH SYNDROME

Alterations of respiratory function in children are influenced by age, development, gender, race, genetic dominance, and environmental conditions. Newborns are especially vulnerable to a variety of upper and lower airway infections caused by immunologic immaturity. Structural differences in infants and children also render them less competent to tolerate conditions that cause increased work of breathing. Access to healthcare and timeliness of immunizations influence the incidence and severity of pulmonary disorders.

STRUCTURE AND FUNCTION

A number of structural characteristics of the pulmonary system influence the way in which infants and children respond to respiratory disturbances. These include structural characteristics of the upper and lower respiratory tracts, chest wall and lung dynamics, metabolic requirements, immunologic immaturity, and physiologic control of respiration.

Upper Airway

All conducting airways (the portions of airway that do not participate in gas exchange) are present at birth and change only in size throughout childhood. Branching of the bronchial tree is in fact complete by the sixteenth week of fetal life.

Because infants and children naturally have smaller-diameter airways than do adults, they suffer exponentially more obstruction for a given degree of mucosal edema or secretion accumulation. The relative sizes of tonsils, adenoids, and epiglottis likewise are proportionately greater in the young child and with swelling can impose a significant site of obstruction. Infants up to 2 to 3 months of age are "obligatory nose breathers" and are unable to breathe in through their mouths. Nasal congestion is therefore a serious threat to a young infant.

Lower Airways and Lung Parenchyma

During fetal development the lung is transformed from a somewhat dense organ to one that is more delicately structured to facilitate air exchange. Beginning in the second trimester, there is loss of interstitial (mesenchymal) tissue with concomitant expansion of the future air spaces. Capillaries grow into the distal respiratory units that keep subdividing (alveolarization) to maximize surface area for gas exchange. In fact the number of alveoli continues to increase during the first 5 to 8 years of life, after which the alveoli increase in size

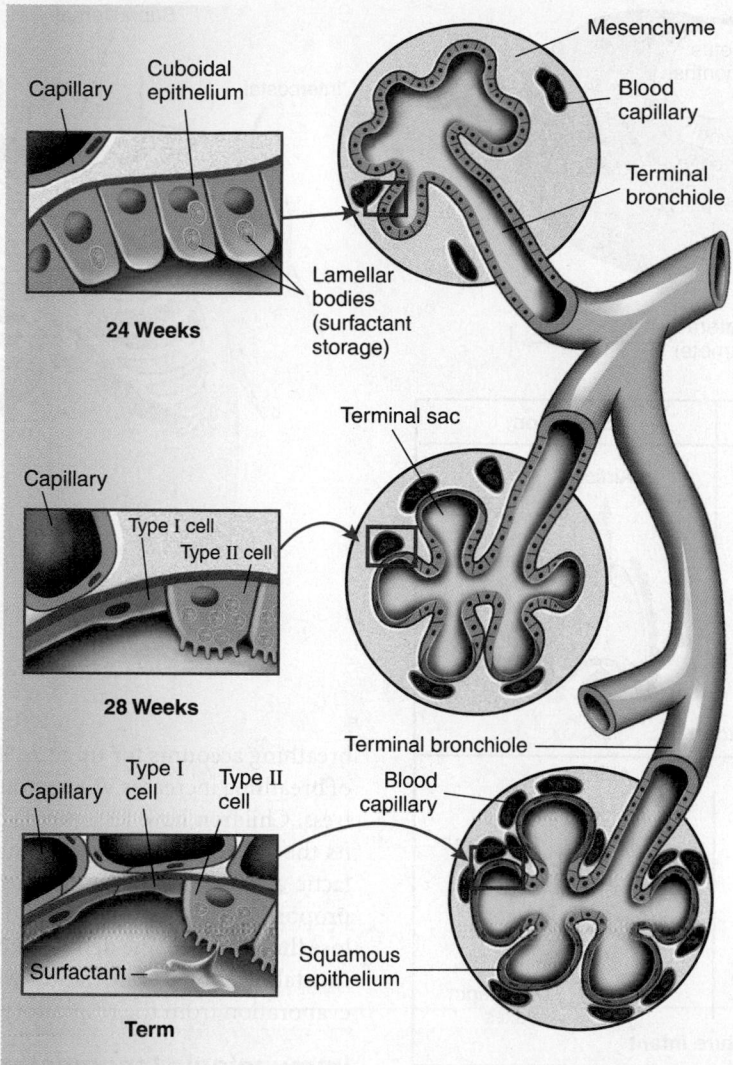

Figure 34-1 **Prenatal development of the alveolar unit.** Epithelial cells differentiate into type II and type I cells. Mature type II cells are cuboidal, have apical microvilli, and contain lamellar bodies for surfactant storage and secretion. Type I cells are derived from type II cells and consist of flattened epithelium overlying capillaries, thus forming part of the desired thin air-blood barrier. During fetal development the pulmonary capillaries initially are randomly distributed in mesenchyme. They progressively arrange around the epithelial tubes and establish close contacts to the lining epithelium. Overall the volume of mesenchyme decreases and that of the potential air space increases.

and complexity. In addition to the structural development of the lung in utero there is accompanying functional maturation, and specialized cell types, such as type II cells, become manifest (Figure 34-1).

Surfactant is a lipid-protein mix that is produced by type II cells and is critical for maintaining alveolar expansion (thus allowing normal gas exchange). It lines alveoli and reduces surface tension, preventing alveolar collapse at the end of each exhalation. Without surfactant the alveoli tend to stay closed, demanding greater inspiratory force and work of breathing to reexpand the alveoli on the next breath. Deficiency of surfactant is often seen in premature infants and causes respiratory distress syndrome (RDS), also known as hyaline membrane disease. Thus surfactant deficiency reflects developmental immaturity. Surfactant lipid is produced by 20 to 24 weeks

of gestation and is secreted into the fetal airways by 30 weeks. The more premature the infant, the higher the risk of RDS.

Chest Wall Dynamics

Chest wall compliance is high in infants, particularly premature infants. The cartilaginous structures of the thoracic cage are not yet well ossified (ossification continues to occur throughout childhood), and the chest wall is easily collapsible. During inspiration in the young child, air is drawn in by the downward movement of the diaphragm, but the resulting negative pressure causes the "soft" chest wall to be drawn *inward* (Figure 34-2); this produces so-called *paradoxic breathing*, or *diaphragmatic breathing*. Paradoxic breathing is especially seen during rapid eye movement (REM) sleep of premature infants. With pulmonary compromise the accessory muscles

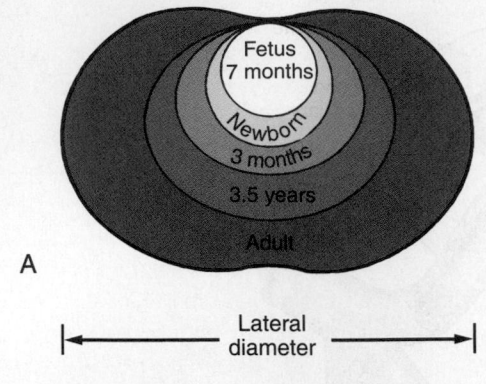

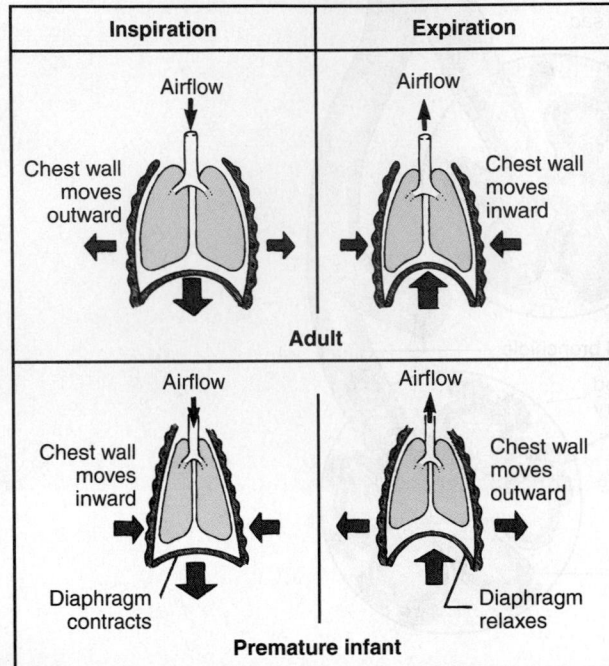

Figure 34-2 Developmental differences in the chest wall and lung mechanics. **A,** Changes in chest wall shape with age. **B,** Differences in lung mechanics caused by differences in chest wall compliance (degree of rigidity) in premature infants and adults. (Arrows indicate direction of airflow, chest wall movement, and diaphragm movement.)

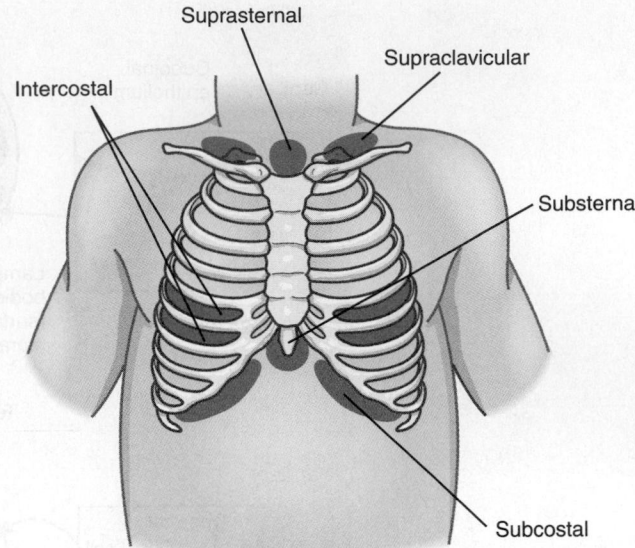

Figure 34-3 Areas of chest muscle retraction.

also are drawn inward, creating retraction of the intercostal and supraclavicular spaces (Figure 34-3).

Resting lung volume, or **functional residual capacity (FRC)**, represents the balance point between the natural elastic recoil of the lungs (to collapse) and the elastic recoil of the chest wall (to expand). In the face of an overly compliant chest wall, infants up to about 1 year of age are thought to maintain their FRC and avoid atelectasis by muscular "braking" of their expiration. This may occur either by active glottic narrowing or by increased activity of the inspiratory intercostal muscles.

Metabolic Characteristics

The basal metabolic rate of a child is greater than that of an adult, and thus oxygen consumption (VO_2) is greater per unit of body weight. The VO_2 of the child's normal

breathing accounts for up to 25% of the total VO_2. The work of breathing increases VO_2 exponentially with respiratory distress. Children have less muscle glycogen reserve, which limits the efficiency of accessory muscles such that fatigue with lactic acidosis can occur quickly. Children also have a high proportion of extracellular fluid and therefore more quickly lose fluid and become dehydrated as a result of fever, environmental heat, or in association with tachypnea (which causes evaporation from the respiratory tract).

Immunologic Incompetence

Passive immunity with immunoglobulin G (IgG) is normally conveyed transplacentally from the mother to the fetus beginning at 20 weeks of gestation; thus IgG levels are lower in preterm than term infants. Breast-feeding allows transfer of secretory IgA, IgG, and IgM after birth. Because IgG has a half-life of approximately 21 days, the placentally transferred antibodies are gone after just a few months. Babies are able to make IgG, IgM, and IgA, and levels of these increase slowly with age. Cell-mediated immunity is also not fully developed in the neonate, which creates a situation of enhanced susceptibility to viral and fungal infections.

Physiologic Control of Respiration

For up to 3 weeks, the newborn has a blunted ventilatory response to hypoxia compared with older children and adults. The mechanisms for this are not well understood but may reflect reduced activity of the peripheral chemoreceptors (in the carotid body) and nonadaptive responses in the respiratory center (in the brainstem). Ventilatory response to hypercarbia is normal in term infants but may be reduced in premature infants. Congenital or acquired lesions of the central nervous system may cause hypoventilation or apnea.

PULMONARY DISORDERS

Pulmonary dysfunction can be categorized into disorders of either the upper airway or lower airway. Signs of acute respiratory failure, however, are the same regardless of etiology. These include the following:

- Increased respiratory effort with retractions (see Figure 34-3) or gasping (apnea in some conditions)
- Cyanosis or pallor
- Agitation
- Decreased level of consciousness
- Cardiovascular signs: tachycardia, mottled color, or bradycardia
- Physiologic compromise reflected by hemoglobin desaturation, hypoxemia, hypercarbia, and acidosis

Disorders of the Upper Airways

The crucial issue in the upper airways is patency. The most common causes of *acute-onset* **upper airway obstruction (UAO)** in children are infections, foreign body aspiration, angioedema, and trauma. *Chronic UAO* has many etiologies, including congenital malformations affecting the airway, cartilaginous weakness, vocal cord paralysis, and subglottic stenosis. Chronic upper airway symptoms should prompt

referral to a pediatric pulmonologist or an otolaryngologist because specialized diagnostic studies may be needed. A list of causes of pediatric UAO can be found in Box 34-1.

The site and nature of the obstruction are often discernible by assessing the noise associated with breathing, the quality of the voice or cry, and presence of feeding difficulties. This assessment often can be made without even touching the patient. Likewise, the severity of the problem can to a great extent be judged by simple visual observation of signs, including retractions, nasal flaring, gasping or obstructed breaths, anxiety, restlessness, or need to maintain a specific head or body position. Agitation should be regarded as a likely sign of hypoxemia or obstruction. In acute UAO, increasing the child's anxiety by excessive physical examination can worsen the condition. The child should be kept as calm as possible. The clinician should never attempt a pharyngeal examination if there is any suspicion of epiglottitis or retropharyngeal abscess because this maneuver may precipitate acute obstruction of the airway.

The sounds of the child's breathing can provide key clues (Figure 34-4). A sonorous, snoring noise is typical for

Box 34-1	Causes of Upper Airway Obstruction in Children According to Site of Obstruction

Nose and Pharynx
Choanal atresia
Lingual thyroid or thyroglossal cyst
Macroglossia
Micrognathia
Hypertrophic tonsils/adenoids
Retropharyngeal or peritonsillar abscess

Larynx
Laryngomalacia
Laryngeal web, cyst, or laryngocele
Laryngotracheobronchitis (viral croup)
Acute spasmodic laryngitis (spasmodic croup)
Epiglottitis
Vocal cord paralysis
Laryngotracheal stenosis
Intubation
Foreign body
Cystic hygroma
Subglottic hemangioma
Laryngeal papilloma
Angioneurotic edema
Laryngospasm (hypocalcemic tetany)
Psychogenic stridor

Trachea
Tracheomalacia
Bacterial tracheitis
External compression

Adapted or reprinted with permission from 'Diagnosis of Stridor in Children,' November 15, 1999, American Family Physician. Copyright 1999 American Academy of Family Physicians. All Rights Reserved.

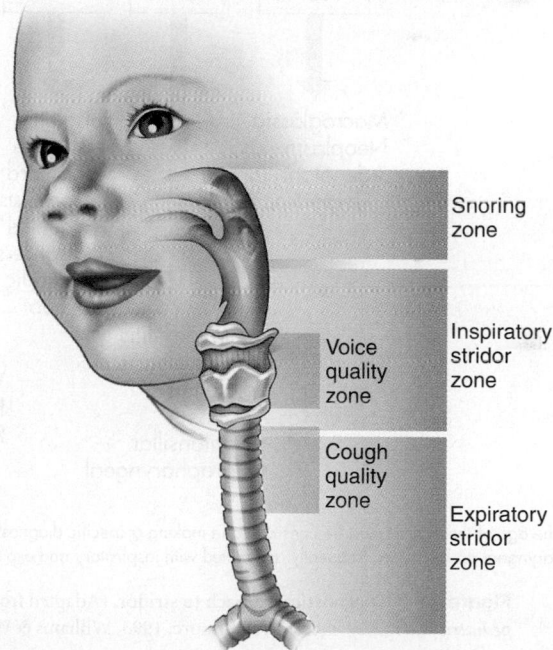

Figure 34-4 Listening can help locate the site of airway obstruction. A loud, gasping snore suggests enlarged tonsils or adenoids. Stridor during inspiration suggests the airway is compromised at the level of the supralaryngeal structures (epiglottis and arytenoid cartilages), vocal cords, subglottic region, or upper trachea. With forced inspiration, intrathoracic pressure becomes quite negative and is less than atmospheric pressure, promoting collapse at or just above the site of obstruction. Expiratory stridor or central wheeze results from narrowing or collapse of the lower trachea or bronchi. During forced exhalation, rising pleural pressure may exceed intratracheal pressure. Airway noise during both inspiration and expiration often represents a fixed obstruction of the vocal cords or subglottic space. Hoarseness or a weak cry is a byproduct of obstruction at the vocal cords. If a cough is croupy or low pitched, suspect tracheal pathology. (Redrawn from Eavey RD: *Contemp Pediatr* 3(6):78, 1986; used with permission; original illustration by Paul Singh-Roy.)

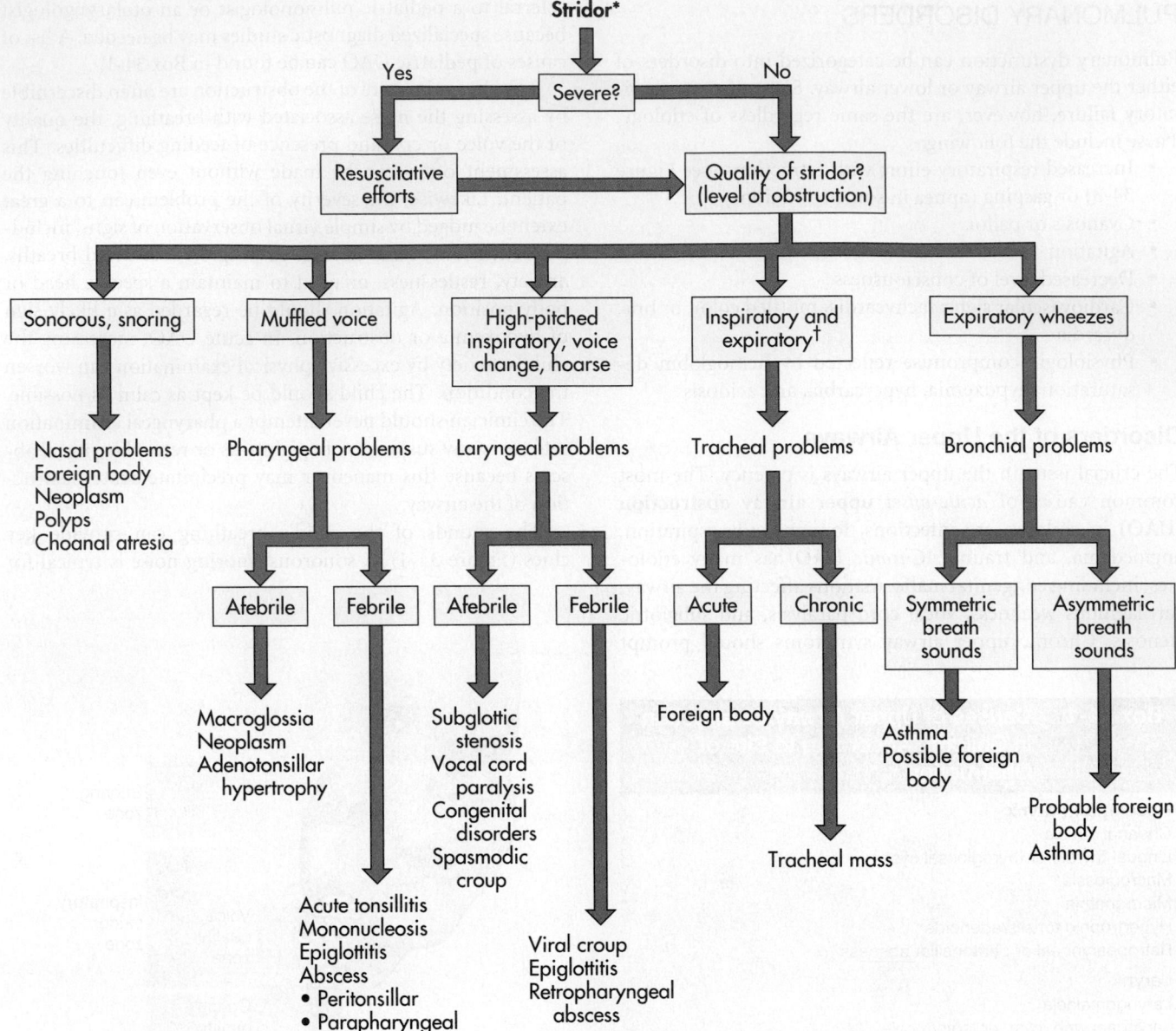

Figure 34-5 **Diagnostic approach to stridor.** (Adapted from Handler SD: Stridor. In Fleisher GR, Ludwig S, editors: *Textbook of pediatric emergency medicine,* Baltimore, 1993, Williams & Wilkins.)

nasopharyngeal obstruction, such as adenotonsillar hypertrophy. A common sign of pediatric UAO is **stridor,** a harsh, vibratory sound of variable pitch caused by turbulent flow through the partially obstructed airway. A diagnostic approach to stridor is outlined in Figure 34-5. Whether it is present in inspiration, expiration, or both reflects the site of the problem. In general, *inspiratory* stridor is generated with obstruction of the *extrathoracic* airway (above the thoracic inlet), which includes the supraglottic structures, the larynx, the subglottic space, and the upper trachea. *Expiratory* stridor or a monophonic wheeze may be generated by an obstruction in

the *intrathoracic* airway (the mid- to lower trachea and central bronchi). Biphasic stridor typically reflects obstruction at the glottis (e.g., vocal cord paralysis) itself or a *fixed* rather than a *dynamic* lesion in the subglottic space (e.g., hemangioma or subglottic stenosis). Biphasic noise may sometimes mean abnormalities of both extrathoracic and intrathoracic trachea (long-segment stenosis or malacia).

Abnormalities of voice or cry (weak or hoarse) suggest problems at the larynx, such as vocal cord paralysis. Muffling of the voice, especially in an acute condition, suggests supralaryngeal obstruction, such as epiglottitis or retropharyngeal abscess. Pronounced cough may be an irritative symptom, such as that produced by an aspirated foreign body, or may be a sign of tracheal obstruction. The cough associated with croup or tracheal foreign body is usually harsh and barking.

Airway obstruction occurs sooner in infants than in older children. Obviously, airway luminal size is smaller in accordance with smaller body size, but any decrease in luminal diameter will be much more significant. This is because airway resistance is proportional to the inverse of the *fourth* power of the radius; thus a decrease to half the original diameter increases resistance 16-fold. Furthermore, an infant's cartilaginous structures are more collapsible and thus are prone to creating or contributing to a situation of UAO.

Infections

Infections of the upper airway (Table 34-1) are common in children; some have the potential to cause life-threatening emergencies. Recognition and rapid evaluation of these problems are crucial pediatric care skills.

Other Acute Upper Airway Infections

Bacterial Tracheitis. **Bacterial tracheitis** can cause rapidly fatal airway obstruction. It accounts for 5% to 14% of UAO in children requiring intensive care.[1] The epidemiology of this illness has changed dramatically secondary to immunization against *Haemophilus influenzae*. Bacterial tracheitis is most often caused by *Staphylococcus aureus* (including methicillin-resistant *Staphylococcus aureus* [MRSA] strains), *H. influenzae* or group A beta-hemolytic *Streptococcus*

(GABHS).[2] A virus or a fungus is more likely to be seen as the source of tracheitis in immunocompromised children.[1] Treatment of viral croup with corticosteroids has increased the risk for serious bacterial tracheitis (especially by GABHS) placing mortality rates between 18% and 40%.[2] This makes it the most common potentially life-threatening upper airway infection in children. The presence of airway edema and copious purulent secretions leads to airway obstruction that can be worsened by the formation of a tracheal pseudomembrane and mucosal sloughing. Increased morbidity can occur because of respiratory and cardiopulmonary arrest, respiratory failure, pneumonia, septic shock, toxic shock syndrome, acute respiratory distress syndrome (ARDS), and multiple organ dysfunction syndrome (MODS). The onset of symptoms may be sudden or may be preceded by a preexisting viral upper respiratory infection or croup. The acute clinical presentation frequently includes tachypnea, stridor, hoarse voice, fever, cough, and/or increased secretions from the mouth and nose. There also may be evidence of concurrent infections, such as sinusitis, otitis, pneumonia or pharyngitis. Children with chronic gastroesophageal reflux are more likely to experience difficulty with these types of concurrent infections.[1] Management requires the rapid administration of broad-spectrum intravenous antibiotics. The majority of children with tracheitis require endotracheal intubation in order to prevent airway obstruction. Corticosteroids (parenteral and inhaled) are used to decrease tracheal inflammation. Many children recover adequately to be extubated within 72 to 96 hours.

Table 34-1	Comparison of Upper Airway Infections				
Condition	Age	Onset	Etiology	Pathophysiology	Symptoms
Acute laryngotracheobronchitis (croup)	6 mo-3 yr	Usually gradual	Viral (parainfluenza 1 and 3, influenza A, respiratory syncytial virus)	Inflammation from vocal cords to bronchial lumina	Harsh cough; stridor; low-grade fever; may have nasal discharge, conjunctivitis
Acute tracheitis	1-12 yr	Abrupt or following viral illness	*Staphylococcus aureus/* methicillin-resistant *Staphylococcus aureus* (MRSA) *Haemophilus influenzae* Group A streptococci	Inflammation of upper trachea	High fever; toxic appearance; thick harsh cough; purulent secretions; may prefer head elevation
Epiglottitis	2-6 yr	Abrupt	*Haemophilus influenzae* type B (Hib) Group A streptococci	Inflammation of supraglottic structures	Severe sore throat; high fever; toxic appearance; muffled voice; may drool; sits erect and quietly
Retropharyngeal abscess	>6 yr	Gradual, 2-5 days; may follow oral trauma	*S. aureus*/MRSA *Streptococcus pyogenes* Anaerobes Group A beta-hemolytic streptococci	Abscess in posterior pharyngeal wall	Similar to epiglottitis
Peritonsillar abscess	>9 yr	May be abrupt	Group A beta-hemolytic streptococci *S. aureus*/MRSA	Abscess within or around tonsil	Similar to epiglottitis; may have trismus

Retropharyngeal Abscess. Retropharyngeal abscess can be caused by aerobic, anaerobic, or polymicrobial infection. A change in the epidemiologic pattern has been noted in the past several years that is likely related to the use of corticosteroids in the treatment of influenza and croup. There also has been an increase in GABHS strains associated with this condition, and the emergence of MRSA as the offending microorganism is increasingly noted.[3-5] Retropharyngeal abscess usually occurs in children younger than 2 years of age and as a consequence of either nasopharyngeal infection or penetrating local injury. Clinical signs include fever, dysphagia, drooling, stridor, respiratory distress, and stiff neck. This condition requires intravenous antibiotics targeted at the suspected microorganism, and sometimes incision and drainage.

Tonsillar Infections. Tonsillar infections (tonsillitis) are occasionally severe enough to cause UAO.[6] As with other infections of the upper airway, the incidence of tonsillitis secondary to GABHS (group A streptococci) and MRSA has risen notably in the past 15 years. A classic example of UAO secondary to tonsillitis, now rare because of routine immunization, is **diphtheria,** which causes sore throat and dysphagia along with fever, malaise, headache, and nausea. Significant swelling of the tonsils and pharynx occurs, and a tenacious membrane may cover the mucosa. UAO because of tonsillitis is a well-known complication of infectious mononucleosis, especially in a young child. The development of UAO in tonsillar infections requires the use of appropriately selected antibiotics and may require the use of corticosteroids, especially in the case of mononucleosis.[5,7]

Peritonsillar abscess is usually unilateral and is most often a complication of acute tonsillitis.[7] The most common causative microorganism is GABHS. Children have fever, sore throat, dysphagia, trismus, pooling of saliva, and muffled voice. Peritonsillar bulging (Figure 34-6) and cervical adenopathy on the same side are usually visible. The abscess must be drained and the child given antibiotics. Death can occur from spontaneous abscess rupture with aspiration or airway obstruction.[8]

Croup

Classic **croup** is an acute **laryngotracheobronchitis** and is the most common cause of acute upper respiratory obstruction in young children.[9] It occurs most often in children from 6 months to 5 years of age, with peak incidence in the second year of life.[10] In 85% of cases, croup is caused by a virus, most commonly parainfluenza; however, other viruses such as influenza A or respiratory syncytial virus (RSV) also can cause croup.[9] Rhinovirus, adenovirus, measles, and the atypical bacteria *Mycoplasma pneumoniae* also have been associated with causation. The incidence of croup is highest in late autumn and winter, corresponding to the parainfluenza and RSV seasons, respectively. Croup is more common in boys than girls. In a significant portion of affected children, croup is a recurrent problem during childhood, and there is a family history of croup in about 15% of cases.

PATHOPHYSIOLOGY The pathophysiology of viral croup is caused primarily by subglottic edema from the infection. The mucous membranes of the larynx are tightly adherent to the underlying cartilage, whereas those of the subglottic space are looser and thus allow accumulation of mucosal and submucosal edema (Figure 34-7). Furthermore, the cricoid cartilage is structurally the narrowest point of the airway, making edema in this area critical. As illustrated in Figure 34-8, increased resistance to airflow leads to increased work of breathing, which generates more negative intrathoracic pressure, which in turn may exacerbate dynamic collapse of the upper airway.

CLINICAL MANIFESTATIONS Typically there is a prodrome of rhinorrhea, sore throat, and low-grade fever for a few days. The child then develops the characteristic harsh (seal-like) barking cough, hoarse voice, and inspiratory stridor. Most cases are mild and resolve spontaneously after several more days. Occasionally, however, UAO becomes severe and requires urgent management.

Spasmodic croup is another clinical entity that is characterized by similar hoarseness, barking cough, and stridor but is of sudden onset, usually at night and without viral prodrome. It often resolves as quickly as it develops. The etiology

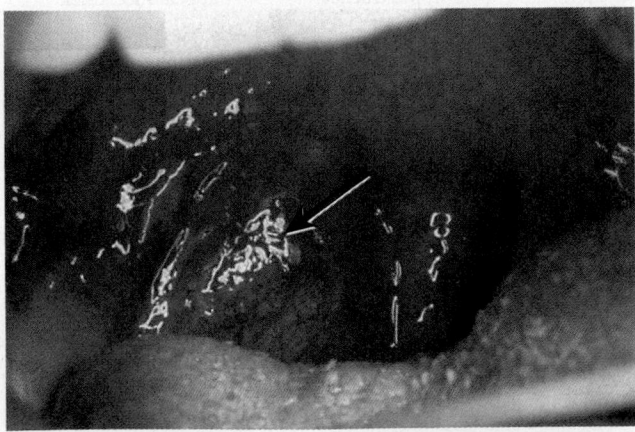

Figure 34-6 Peritonsillar abscess. Unilateral bulging of the tonsillar region is evident. (From Whiting JL, Chow AW: *J Crit Ill* 2[7]:36, 1987.)

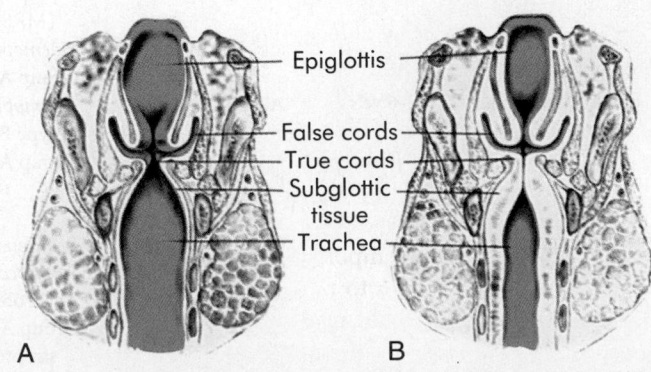

Figure 34-7 The larynx and subglottic trachea. A, Normal. B, Narrowing and obstruction from edema caused by croup. (From Hockenberry MJ et al: *Wong's nursing care of infants and children,* ed 8, St Louis, 2007, Mosby.)

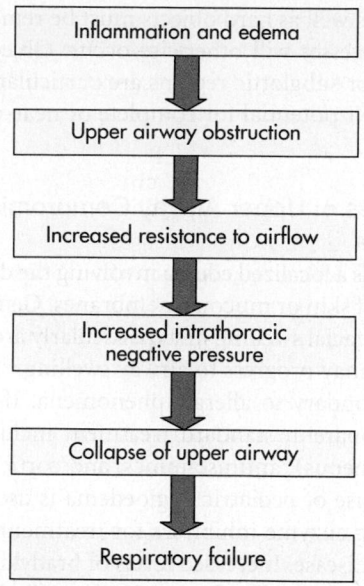

Figure 34-8 Upper airway obstruction with croup.

is unknown although an association with a history of atopy has been observed.[10]

EVALUATION AND TREATMENT The degree of symptoms determines the level of treatment. Most children have a barking cough and viral symptoms and may need no specific treatment. However, the presence of stridor (especially at rest), retractions, or agitation suggests a sicker child. A number of clinical tools are used to assess the severity of croup in children. The tool most often used is the Westley croup score, which provides a cumulative score for the degree of stridor, retractions, air entry, cyanosis, dyspnea, and level of consciousness in the child.[9] Severity also is classified into mild, moderate, and severe.

Croup therapy has been the subject of debate for years. Nonpharmacologic treatment options include steam inhalation, ice masks, and oxygen. The first two, however, lack scientific studies to support or refute their benefit. The consensus from numerous controlled studies is that oral, intravenous, or nebulized corticosteroids have a significant effect on croup-related hospitalizations and are cost effective.[9] Symptoms improve faster, less sleep is lost by children, less stress is experienced by parents, and fewer children have a need for return healthcare visits when corticosteroids are used.[11] The emergent use of nebulized epinephrine is indicated when significant respiratory distress is present. Epinephrine stimulates α- and β-adrenergic receptors and is thought to decrease airway secretions and mucosal edema. However, its effect lasts only 2 hours and should be considered a temporizing measure until concomitantly given steroids begin to take effect. Thus children who are given nebulized epinephrine should be observed for 2 to 3 hours to ensure that they will remain stable, and close follow-up is mandatory. Heliox (helium-oxygen mixture of 80:20 or 70:30) can be used for severe cases of croup, although this is not considered part of the routine treatment regimen.[9,10]

Acute Epiglottitis

Acute epiglottitis is a severe, life-threatening, rapidly progressive infection of the structures above the insertion point of the glottis, which include the epiglottis, aryepiglottic folds, arytenoid soft tissue, and the uvula. Historically, cases were nearly always caused by *H. influenzae* type B (Hib). Since the advent of Hib immunization, the overall incidence of acute epiglottitis has decreased to only 10% to 20% of previous levels.[9,12] Current pediatric cases usually represent vaccine failures or are caused by alternative pathogens, such as groups A, B, C, F, and G streptococci, *Streptococcus pneumoniae, Candida* species. *S. aureus,* and viral pathogens.[12] Hib still accounts for approximately 25% of the cases seen in children.[12] Thermal injuries, trauma, and posttransplant lymphoproliferative disorder also have been reported as causes of epiglottitis.[12]

CLINICAL MANIFESTATIONS In the classic form of the disease, a child between 2 and 6 years of age suddenly develops high fever, irritability, sore throat, a "hot potato voice," inspiratory stridor, and severe respiratory distress. The child appears ill and classically will adopt a forward-leaning position (tripod position) with drooling and dysphagia (inability to swallow). Examination of the throat may trigger laryngospasm and cause respiratory collapse. Death may occur in a few hours. Pneumonia, cervical lymph node inflammation, otitis, and, rarely, meningitis or septic arthritis may occur during the course of epiglottitis.

EVALUATION AND TREATMENT Despite its decreasing incidence, all pediatric practitioners must be familiar with epiglottitis and understand it is a life-threatening emergency. The essentials are recognition, avoidance of disturbing the child (which could worsen the obstruction), and securing the airway. Tracheal intubation should be accomplished by the most experienced personnel (usually an anesthesiologist and/or otolaryngologist) using fiberoptic laryngoscopy. Subsequent culture of the airway is obtained and intravenous broad-spectrum antibiotics are administered promptly. Therapy is reevaluated after culture results return. Corticosteroids also are generally used in treatment regimens although there are no published randomized trials to support this practice.[9,12,13] Despite the severe presentation of epiglottitis, resolution with treatment is usually rapid, with intubation rarely needed for more than a couple of days. When Hib epiglottitis is diagnosed, the American Academy of Pediatrics (AAP) recommends that postexposure prophylaxis with rifampin be administered to household contacts (specific to certain ages of children present).[13] When caused by microorganisms other than *H. influenzae*, as is now the usual situation, epiglottitis may present in ages outside the typical range and with more gradual rather than fulminant onset, thus making diagnosis less obvious. Such cases also may respond more slowly to treatment.

Aspiration of Foreign Bodies

Most children who aspirate a foreign object (**foreign body aspiration**) are between 1 and 3 years of age. More than 100,000 cases occur each year.[14] Often the aspiration either is not witnessed or does not seem significant to the parent, thus medical care is often not pursued until after the first 24 hours. At the time of aspiration, the child may cough, choke, gag, or wheeze, and stridor or cyanosis occasionally occurs. This may be followed by a quiescent interval of minutes to even weeks or months before symptoms reappear from resulting local irritation, granulation, bronchial obstruction, or infection (pneumonia or bronchiectasis). Pronounced inspiratory stridor, cough, and wheezing are typical symptoms that prompt the parents to seek medical attention. Examples of common aspirated objects include nuts, sunflower seeds, hot dog chunks, popcorn, coins, and small toys or toy parts. Meat or food impactions are more common in adolescents. Items of particular concern are batteries and multiple magnets. In general, foreign bodies require early intervention secondary to their propensity to cause respiratory symptoms and complications, including esophageal erosions or aortoesophageal fistula.

The symptom history is often the most critical aid in diagnosis.[14,15] Symptoms are determined by the size of the object and the site in which it is located, as well as the child's age and size (see Figure 34-4). Foreign bodies lodged in the upper trachea typically produce inspiratory stridor, whereas those located in the lower intrathoracic airways more commonly produce wheezing. About 75% of aspirated foreign bodies lodge in a bronchus. Children with an unexplained persistent cough and refractory parenchymal infiltrates also should be considered for unrecognized foreign body aspiration.[16] Many objects are not radiopaque; however, if the object has completely occluded a lung segment, atelectasis will be visible on a chest radiograph. Occasionally, air will accumulate distal to the obstruction if the object is causing a ball-valve effect. This effect can sometimes be documented by inspiratory and expiratory chest films (Figure 34-9). In a younger child, bilateral decubitus films may show failure to compress the obstructed lung when in the "down" position.

Most foreign bodies can be removed by bronchoscopy and only rarely is a pulmonary lobectomy required. Soft particles

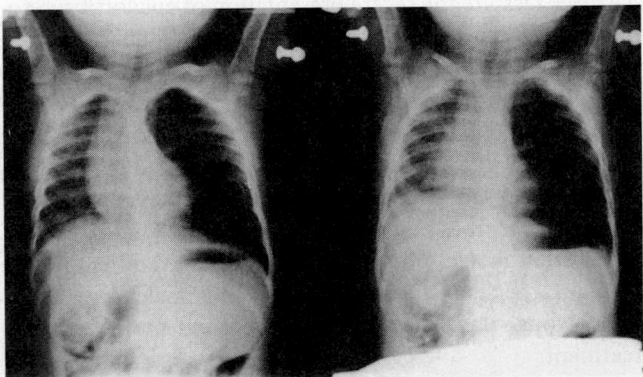

Figure 34-9 Foreign body aspiration. Inspiratory (*left*) and expiratory (*right*) chest radiographs of a child who aspirated a portion of a potato into the left mainstem bronchus. Left lung field is hyperaerated and the mediastinum is shifted to the right on expiration because of left-sided obstructive emphysema. (From Kenna MA, Bluestone CD: *Pediatr Rev* 10[1]:25, 1988.)

such as food as well as hard objects must be removed because infectious processes will otherwise occur. Objects lodged in the laryngeal or subglottic regions are particularly dangerous because of their potential for complete or near-complete airway occlusion.

Other Causes of Upper Airway Compromise
Angioedema
Angioedema is a localized edema involving the deep, subcutaneous layers of skin or mucous membranes. Generally, angioedema causes facial swelling first, particularly around the eyes and lips, and may progress to airway swelling.[17] Angioedema is usually secondary to allergic phenomena. If airway compromise is apparent, standard treatment includes epinephrine (subcutaneous), antihistamines, and corticosteroids. An occasional cause of pediatric angioedema is use of angiotensin-converting enzyme inhibitors for treatment of hypertension or heart disease. Increased levels of bradykinin appear to mediate this adverse effect by causing vasodilation, increased vascular permeability, and histamine release.[18]

An inherited deficiency of the plasma protein C-1 inhibitor (C-1 INH), causes *hereditary angioneurotic edema* (HAE), a rare but serious problem in children. This autosomal dominant trait has an estimated prevalence of 1 in 10,000 to 50,000 births, and a family history is positive in 75% of cases.[17] The mean age of onset of initial symptoms is 8 to 12 years but it also may occur as early as the first year of life. This condition is characterized by recurring attacks of angioedema involving subcutaneous tissues (especially limbs, genitalia, and face); abdominal and pelvic viscera; and, much less often, the airway. Laryngeal attacks in these individuals may be life threatening and do not respond reliably to standard measures for airway edema. The mortality of undiagnosed HAE can be as high as 50%. The mainstays of supportive care are airway monitoring, hydration, pain relief, and control of nausea.[19] Concentrates of C-1 INH appear to produce rapid improvement within 15 to 60 minutes. Short- and long-term prophylaxis can be instituted using antifibrinolytic agents, attenuated androgens, and C-1 INH concentrates.[20]

Subglottic Stenosis
Congenital subglottic stenosis is the third most common laryngeal anomaly and is defined as a subglottic airway diameter of less than 4 mm at the cricoid region in a full-term infant, and less than 3 mm in a premature infant.[21] Incomplete recanalization of the laryngotracheal tube during the third month of gestation results in this defect. Subglottic stenosis also is associated with eosinophilic esophagitis, Wegener granulomatosis, and neurofibromatosis.[22-24] Traumatic injury to the upper airway with development of **subglottic stenosis** is a well-described complication of endotracheal intubation.[25] Factors that contribute to subglottic stenosis include long-term assisted ventilation, use of an endotracheal tube that is too large, excessive movement of the tube, and individual susceptibility.[26] Neonates can tolerate long periods of endotracheal intubation; the overall rate of symptomatic subglottic stenosis in neonates is 0.2%.[26] The occurrence of

subglottic stenosis can be minimized by ensuring that the tube size allows a small air leak during inspiration (at a peak inspiratory force of approximately 25 mmHg) and that the tube is securely taped. Sedation is generally required to reduce head movement for children who are intubated. Because of the rapid growth of the lumen of the trachea and cricoid cartilage in the first year (which triples in size), infants may outgrow the obstruction, particularly if mild or moderate.[27] Clinical trials are underway to evaluate topical mitomycin C (an antineoplastic agent) as an adjunct in reducing scarring of the airways; this has met with mixed results in the adult population.[28] For significant subglottic stenosis, tracheostomy or tracheal reconstructive surgery may be needed.

Laryngomalacia and Tracheomalacia

Laryngomalacia is the most common cause of chronic stridor in infants. Boys are twice as likely to present with symptoms than girls. In laryngomalacia, the epiglottis or arytenoids, or both, fold inward with inspiration partially covering the glottis (Figure 34-10). The pathophysiology of these abnormalities is still not completely understood. Two primary hypotheses are anatomic or neuromuscular.[29] Anatomically there may be foreshortened or tight aryepiglottic folds or there may be redundant soft tissue in the supraglottis. The neuromuscular hypothesis suggests that there is an abnormality of the sensorimotor integrative function of the brainstem and peripheral reflexes are responsible for laryngeal tone and airway patency.[30] Laryngomalacia is frequently associated with gastroesophageal reflux disease (GERD).[27] Typical signs of laryngomalacia include inspiratory stridor beginning in the first days or weeks of life, accentuated with activity, and sometimes with positional changes (worse in supine or head-flexed positions). Feeding difficulties may be noted, but they are usually mild. Cry is normal. Laryngoscopy is used to confirm

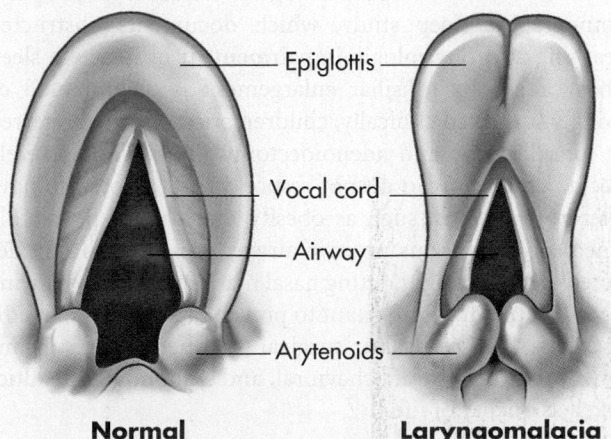

Epiglottis

Vocal cord

Airway

Arytenoids

Normal   **Laryngomalacia**

Figure 34-10 Laryngomalacia. In the normal larynx *(left)*, supralaryngeal structures maintain their upright orientation during inspiration. In contrast, in infants with laryngomalacia *(right)*, there is inward prolapse of the arytenoid masses, which include the prominent cuneiform tubercles and the arytenoid cartilages. The glottis becomes partially covered, and airflow is impeded. Sometimes the edges of the epiglottis curl inward, further exacerbating the obstruction. In expiration, these structures are "blown" aside passively.

the diagnosis. Laryngomalacia is usually mild and improves spontaneously over the first year of life as the supralaryngeal cartilage structures stiffen, thus most cases are managed with watchful waiting. A late-onset variant of this disease has been noted in the literature and should be suspected if the following occurs: potential cause of feeding difficulties in toddlers, sleep apnea in children, and exercise intolerance in teenagers.[31,32]

In **tracheomalacia,** or **tracheobronchomalacia,** the tracheobronchial cartilages tend to collapse during the respiratory cycle. This may be classified as primary (idiopathic) or secondary. When malacia is caused by a secondary source, it is usually related to extrinsic compression of the trachea from a vascular malformation.[27] Tracheobronchomalacia presents clinically as a spectrum of respiratory illnesses that range from life-threatening conditions to chronic cough and wheeze conditions.[33] In some cases symptoms may be more subtle than in laryngomalacia. Low-pitched inspiratory stridor may be a sign of malacia of the upper trachea or centrally located, single-pitch (monophonic) wheeze may be present in malacia of the mid- to distal trachea. Tracheomalacia can be suspected clinically and confirmed by bronchoscopy. Depending on the type and severity of the lesion, surgical approaches for repair may be indicated.

Vocal Cord Paralysis

The vocal cords should move apart to facilitate inspiration and move together to facilitate vocalization. Paralysis of one or both vocal cords may affect breathing, swallowing, and speech. Although it is classified as the second most common congenital laryngeal anomaly, vocal cord paralysis is a relatively uncommon condition. The etiology of the congenital abnormality is unclear but may be caused by immaturity of the vagus nerve or brainstem or both.[27] Iatrogenic injury is frequently cited as the major secondary cause of vocal cord paralysis, such as surgical trauma to the recurrent laryngeal nerve during cardiac surgery.[34] Other secondary causes include Arnold-Chiari malformation (the region of the brainstem in which the nucleus ambiguus acts as the "relay station" for laryngeal function), cerebral palsy, hydrocephalus, myelomeningocele, spina bifida, or hypoxia.[21] Other associations include infectious and neoplastic causes, trauma, and inflammatory conditions.[34] In older children and adolescents, exercise has been known to precipitate vocal cord dysfunction (VCD).[35]

Clinical findings of vocal cord paralysis in children less than 1 year include dysphonia, glottic incompetence, GERD, and stridor.[34] It sometimes resolves spontaneously (most often during the first year of life) or with correction of the underlying problem. Flexible laryngoscopy and chest x-ray are common evaluative tools that may help determine the cause. Medical therapy may include use of corticosteroids, proton pump inhibitors, and speech therapy. Recurrent pulmonary infections secondary to aspiration may occur and require treatment until the cords are repaired.[21] Severe cases may necessitate endotracheal intubation and tracheostomy. Tracheostomy may be used until the vocal cords are surgically repaired or can be used as a permanent measure for bilateral vocal cord paralysis.[21]

Congenital Malformations

Congenital malformations of the trachea and bronchial tree cause airway obstruction. Lesions include laryngeal atresias and webs, cysts, clefts, and subglottic hemangiomas. Webs and atresias are caused by failure of the larynx to recanalize during embryogenesis. Most of these disorders are in the area of the glottis with extension into the subglottis.[21] Structural abnormalities involving the great vessels also can result in tracheal compression, for example, absent pulmonary valve syndrome dilates the pulmonary artery, which can compress the trachea and bronchi.[36] Tracheal or bronchial compression results in airway symptoms or feeding difficulties, or both, ranging from dysphagia, recurrent respiratory infections, wheezing, and stridor to acute respiratory distress or "dying spells." Many older children are first thought to have gastroesophageal reflux or asthma as the principal problem. Surgical management is usually required for these conditions, and some infants may require mechanical ventilation while awaiting surgery.[36]

Obstructive Sleep Apnea

Obstructive sleep apnea syndrome (OSAS) is a breathing disorder defined by prolonged partial and/or intermittent complete UAO during sleep with disruption of normal ventilation and normal sleep patterns.[37] Childhood OSAS is common with an estimated prevalence of 2% to 3% among middle-school children and as many as 13% of children ages 3 to 6 years. Prevalence is estimated to be two to four times higher in vulnerable populations (blacks, Hispanics, and preterm infants).[38] Unlike adults, OSAS in children occurs equally among males and females. Possible influences early in life may include passive smoke exposure, socioeconomic status, and snoring together with genetic modifiers such as those that promote airway inflammation.

PATHOPHYSIOLOGY The pathophysiology of childhood OSAS is likely to be multifactorial in origin. In otherwise healthy children, the most common predisposing factor is adenotonsillar hypertrophy, which causes physical impingement on the nasopharyngeal airway. OSAS often occurs in overweight or obese children as well as in those with orthodontic/craniofacial anomalies or neurologic disorders. Allergy and asthma also may contribute to this condition. In addition to physical narrowing, other mechanisms have been suggested, such as abnormalities in the motor tone of the upper airways (frequently an issue in neurologically impaired children) or abnormal arousal mechanisms.[39] Recent studies have documented that children with sleep disordered breathing (SDB) have increased inflammation in the upper airway and elevated serum levels of C-reactive protein that are relationally proportional to the severity and frequency of UAO.[40] Lastly, genetic susceptibility likely plays a role in neurocognitive dysfunction associated with this condition.

CLINICAL MANIFESTATIONS OSAS may present with a history of snoring and labored breathing, restlessness, and sweating during sleep, which can be continuous or intermittent. There may be episodes of increased respiratory effort but no audible airflow, often terminated by snorting, gasping, repositioning, or arousal. Affected children are often chronic mouth breathers and have large tonsils. They also may exhibit nocturnal enuresis and intrusive nap habits.[41] Unlike adults, no correlation between OSAS and sleep position has been noted in children. Similar to adults, it appears that there also may be a correlation between OSAS and elevated blood pressure. This is further linked to increased body mass index (BMI) and episodes of desaturation and apnea/hypopnea.[42] Children who are overweight or obese often have severe OSAS and adopt the prone sleeping position to facilitate improved airway patency and are at a 4.6-fold increase for sleep apnea compared with healthy children.[38]

OSAS can result in chronic hypoxemia and hypercapnia affecting multiple organ systems. Significant morbidity is associated with OSAS including cognitive, neurobehavioral (inattention, hyperactivity, aggression, conduct problems, attention deficit/hyperactivity disorder [ADHD]/emotional [mood]) impairment, excessive daytime sleepiness, impaired school performance, and poor quality of life.[38] Left untreated it also can cause cardiovascular disease, particularly left ventricular hypertrophy, and insulin resistance, as well as pulmonary complications (upper and lower respiratory tract infections) and reduced somatic growth.[38,41,43-45]

EVALUATION AND TREATMENT All parents should be asked if their child exhibits snoring, a symptom that is often not spontaneously reported to a healthcare provider. The history and physical examination are the most effective means of diagnosis.[46] Screening tools and sleep questionnaires may be helpful in evaluating the presence of SDB.[41] Radiographic image of the upper airway may reveal upper airway narrowing caused by adenoidal hypertrophy and magnetic resonance imaging (MRI) and acoustic reflectometry may detect reduced upper airway dimensions.[38,41] The most definitive evaluation ("gold standard") is the polysomnographic sleep study, which documents obstructed breathing and physiologic impairment. If obstructive sleep apnea caused by tonsillar enlargement is documented or strongly suspected clinically, children are most often referred for tonsillectomy and adenoidectomy (T&A). For severely affected children who do not respond to T&A or who have different problems, such as obesity that cannot be rapidly remedied, continuous positive airway pressure (CPAP) delivered through a tight-fitting nasal mask may be used during sleep. Treatment is important to prevent associated morbidities. Successful medical or surgical treatment results in improvement in physical, behavioral, and emotional difficulties as well as quality of life.[41,47]

Disorders of the Lower Airways

Lower airway disease is one of the leading causes of morbidity in the first year of life and continues to be an important component of other illnesses. Pulmonary disorders commonly observed include perinatal conditions such as neonatal RDS, congenital malformations, asthma, cystic fibrosis, infections, aspiration syndrome, and ARDS.

| **Box 34-2** | Respiratory Distress Syndrome |

Epidemiology
Worldwide
Prematurity predisposes
Cesarean section without labor predisposes
Perinatal asphyxia predisposes
Male > female
White > black
Second-born twin at greater risk
PROM spares
IUGR spares
Maternal stress spares
Maternal diabetes predisposes if less than 37 weeks
Maternal hemorrhage predisposes

Clinical Signs
Onset near the time of birth
Retractions and tachypnea
Expiratory grunt
Cyanosis
Systemic hypotension
Characteristic chest film
Course to death or improvement in 3 to 5 days
Fine inspiratory rales
Hypothermia
Peripheral edema
Pulmonary edema

Pathophysiology
Reduced lung compliance
Reduced FRC
Poor lung distensibility

Poor alveolar stability
Right-to-left shunts
Reduced effective pulmonary blood flow
If hypotensive and hypoxic, poor peripheral perfusion, poor renal perfusion, myocardial malfunction
Patent ductus arteriosus contributes

Pathobiochemistry
Respiratory acidosis
Decreased saturated phospholipids
Low amniotic fluid L/S ratio
Low surfactant-associated proteins
Decreased total serum proteins
Decreased fibrinolysis
Low thyroxine levels

Pathology
Atelectasis
Injury to epithelial cells, edema
Membrane contains fibrin and cellular products
No tubular myelin
Osmiophilic lamellar bodies decreased early, increased later

Etiology
Surfactant deficiency during disease
Probable inadequate hormonal (corticoid) stimulus in utero
DPL synthesis impaired and/or destruction increased
Autonomic dysfunction

Prevention
Prenatal glucocorticoids for more than 24 hours
Surfactant replacement before 1 or 2 hours

From Welty S, Hansen TN, Corbet A: Respiratory distress in the preterm infant. In Taeusch HW, Ballard RA, Gleason CA, editors: *Avery's diseases of the newborn*, ed 8, Philadelphia, 2005, Saunders.
DPL, Dipalmitoyl lecithin; *FRC,* functional residual capacity; *IUGR,* intrauterine growth restriction; *L/S,* lecithin/sphingomyelin; *PROM,* prolonged rupture of membranes (>16 hours).

Neonatal Respiratory Distress Syndrome

Respiratory distress syndrome (RDS) of the newborn, also known as **hyaline membrane disease (HMD),** is a major cause of morbidity and mortality in premature newborns.[48] The epidemiology, pathophysiology, and clinical presentation of RDS are outlined in Box 34-2. The major predisposing factor is prematurity because the immature lung is not well structured for gas exchange and has not yet developed adequate surfactant production and secretion. Occasionally RDS is seen in other situations, most notably infants of diabetic mothers. An additional factor that increases risk is cesarean delivery. It is more common in boys than girls and in whites than nonwhites. The incidence of RDS (in the absence of preventive treatment) is approximately 50% to 60% at 29 weeks of gestation and decreases significantly by 36 weeks. Preterm births account for up to 12% of all births[49] and approximately 10% of newborns who require some assistance to begin breathing at birth.[50] Antenatal stress on the fetus may accelerate lung maturation and decrease RDS risk. In special circumstances, such as elective early delivery (e.g., for maternal health reasons), RDS risk is assessed by sampling amniotic fluid for quantification of secreted surfactant lipids, the basis of the lecithin/sphingomyelin (L/S) ratio (value of 2

or greater predicts low risk). Another common test looks for presence of the lipid phosphatidylglycerol, which also reflects lung maturity.

PATHOPHYSIOLOGY RDS is a state of pulmonary insufficiency that in its natural course commences at or shortly after birth. Severity tends to increase over the first 2 days of life.[51] It is caused primarily by surfactant deficiency and, secondarily, by a deficiency in alveolar surface area for gas exchange. Premature infants are born with many underdeveloped and small alveoli that are difficult to inflate. Those that are available for gas exchange do not have adequate surfactant, which is necessary at the air interface to maintain alveolar distention at end-expiration. The net effect is *atelectasis* (see Figure 34-11), which causes significant hypoxemia, and is difficult for the neonate to overcome because it requires a significant negative inspiratory pressure to open the alveoli with each breath. The chest wall is weak and highly compliant, making it difficult to overcome this increased work of breathing. This results in a decrease in tidal volume causing alveolar hypoventilation and hypercapnia. Hypoxia and hypercapnia cause pulmonary vasoconstriction, which increases intrapulmonary resistance and shunting (Figure 34-12). To make the situation more complex, prolonged hypoxemia activates

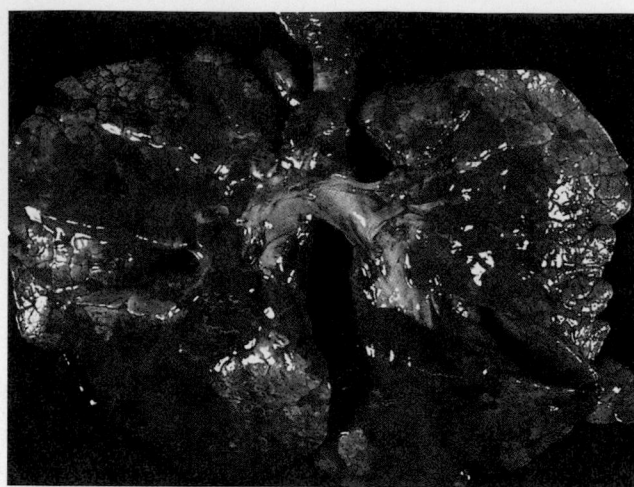

Figure 34-11 Patchy atelectasis of neonatal lungs with respiratory distress syndrome (RDS). (From Damjanov I, Linder J, editors: *Anderson's pathology,* ed 10, St Louis, 1996, Mosby.)

anaerobic glycolysis, which produces lactic acid and thus causes metabolic acidosis. Alveolar hypoventilation makes it impossible to get rid of excess carbon dioxide (CO_2), and combined metabolic and respiratory acidosis develops. Lowered pH causes further vasoconstriction. This results in hypoperfusion of the lung and a decrease in effective pulmonary blood flow. Increased pulmonary vascular resistance causes a partial return to fetal circulation, with right-to-left shunting of blood through the ductus arteriosus and foramen ovale (see Figures 34-11 and 34-12). With inadequate pulmonary circulation and alveolar perfusion, the oxygen content of the blood continues to decrease, pH decreases, and materials needed for surfactant production are not circulated to the alveoli. Capillary permeability increases, resulting in the leakage of plasma proteins. Fibrin deposits in the air spaces create the appearance of *hyaline membranes* for which the disorder is named. The plasma proteins leaked into the air space have the additional adverse effect of interfering with the function of surfactant that may be present. The pathogenesis of RDS is summarized in Figure 34-12.

CLINICAL MANIFESTATIONS Signs of RDS appear within minutes of birth. Some neonates require immediate resuscitation because of asphyxia or initial severe respiratory distress. Tachypnea (respiratory rate more than 60 breaths per minute), expiratory grunting or whining, intercostal and subcostal retractions, nasal flaring, and poor color are the most striking clinical manifestations of RDS. The natural course is characterized by progressive hypoxemia and dyspnea. Apnea and irregular respirations occur as the infant tires. The severity of the hypoxemia and the difficulty in providing adequate supplemental oxygenation give rise to the Vermont Oxford Neonatal Network definition of RDS as a Pao_2 less than 50 mmHg in room air, central cyanosis in room air, or a need for supplemental oxygen to maintain Pao_2 greater than 50 mmHg, as well as the classic chest film appearance.[51] Within the first 6 hours of life, a chest radiograph will reveal air-filled bronchi (air bronchograms) silhouetted against lung fields

that have a "ground glass" appearance associated with alveolar consolidation. RDS can progress to death in severe cases, but in most cases the clinical manifestations reach a peak within 3 days, after which there is gradual improvement with appropriate treatment.

EVALUATION AND TREATMENT Diagnosis is made on the basis of clinical manifestations, chest radiographs, and, occasionally, confirmatory analysis (e.g., L/S ratio) of amniotic fluid or tracheal aspirates. The ultimate treatment for RDS would be prevention of premature birth, but in the meantime other significant advances in treatment have been made.

The first is *antenatal treatment with glucocorticoids* for women in preterm labor. Glucocorticoids induce a significant and rapid acceleration of lung maturation and stimulation of surfactant production in the fetus, and there is extensive evidence that maternal steroid therapy significantly reduces the incidence of RDS, central nervous system hemorrhage, and neonatal mortality.[49,52] This treatment is currently recommended in the setting of preterm labor at 24 to 34 weeks of gestation unless delivery is imminent; ideally, dosing continues for 48 hours while attempts are made to halt labor. It remains unclear whether repeated courses of steroids are safe in this setting.[51]

The second major advance in RDS treatment has been *exogenous surfactant,* either synthetic or purified from animal sources and instilled down an endotracheal tube (ETT). This may be administered in prophylactic or rescue protocol. Unfortunately, liquid dosing down the ETT may result in peridosing adverse events like hypoxia, hypercapnia, and changes in cerebral blood flow. There has been recent progress in administering surfactant by less invasive methods such as through nebulization or nasal CPAP. These modalities result in more uniform distribution of the drug than through the ETT.[53] Current protocols recommend prophylactic administration of surfactant to infants weighing less than 1000 g beginning within 15 to 30 minutes of birth, after the infant is stabilized. Repeat dosing is usually given every 12 hours during the first few days. There is usually a dramatic improvement in oxygenation. For infants weighing more than 1000 g, surfactant replacement is based on clinical need. Because of concerns about intervention-induced lung injury, guidelines for surfactant administration are being reconsidered (see What's New? Pulmonary Resuscitation of the Newborn—Setting the Stage for Injury?).

Systematic reviews of randomized, controlled trials have confirmed that surfactant replacement improves oxygenation as well as reduces the incidence of RDS, death, pneumothorax, and pulmonary interstitial emphysema.[54] Therapy with surfactant should be considered complementary to antenatal glucocorticoids, which promote not only accelerated surfactant synthesis but also enhanced structural development of the lung and beneficial effects on mechanisms of fluid clearance from the lung. These two therapies together appear to have an additive effect on improving lung function. Supplemental inositol also may promote maturation of surfactant and prevent adverse neonatal outcomes in preterm infants.[55]

Newborns, especially those born prematurely, are exceptionally susceptible to harm from therapies intended to help them, starting as early as the delivery room resuscitation and the early hours afterward. For example, oxygen has known toxicities, and the standard use of 100% oxygen to resuscitate asphyxiated newborns (term or preterm), has come into question. Although current data have not been considered conclusive, even brief resuscitation with 100% oxygen has been reported to be associated with delayed initiation of breathing, increased mortality, and persistence of systemic markers of oxidative stress for as long as 28 days postpartum. Data from animal studies and from limited human studies suggest that initial resuscitation with room air appears to be similarly effective as 100% oxygen, and may carry reduced risk. A significant reduction in mortality (40%) was noted in these studies. Given strong evidence from these studies, current recommendations are to avoid exposure to 100% oxygen if possible provided that the infant's heart rate is greater than 100 beats per minute.

Similarly, mechanical ventilation with excessively large tidal volumes, perhaps even for just a few breaths given after birth, may be sufficient to damage the immature lung. Commonly used self-inflating bags do not allow monitoring of tidal volume or inspiratory pressure, nor can they deliver positive end-expiratory pressure (PEEP) or prolonged inflation (useful for establishing the baby's functional residual capacity). Other devices incorporate these features but require expertise to use. The use of nasal continuous positive airway pressure (CPAP) in the delivery room for spontaneously breathing premature infants has been reported to significantly reduce the need for subsequent mechanical ventilation and decreases the incidence of chronic lung disease. New consensus guidelines recommend that although extremely premature infants be considered for intubation and prophylactic surfactant therapy, more mature babies should have a CPAP trial with rescue surfactant only if respiratory distress progresses. Repeat doses of surfactant should be delivered as needed depending on the course of the infant's respiratory distress.

Data from American Heart Association (AHA): *Pediatrics*, 117(5): e1029-1038, 2005; Finer NN, Rich WD: *Curr Opin Pediatr* 16(2):157-162, 2004; Saugstad OD: *Acta Paediatr* 96(3):333-337, 2007; Sweet D et al: *J Perinatal Med* 35:175-186, 2007; Rojas MA et al: *Pediatrics* 123(1):137-142, 2009; Aski LM, Henderson Smart DJ, Ko H: *Cochrane Database Syst Rev* (1) CD001077, 2009.

The third advance in RDS treatment has been in *supportive care*. Newborns with RDS need oxygen and often ventilatory support such as CPAP or mechanical ventilation. Strategies that are lung protective, such as greater reliance on nasal CPAP, permissive hypercapnia, lower oxygen saturation targets, modulation of tidal volume (V_T) settings, use of nitric oxide, and use of high-frequency oscillation, are being evaluated.[56] Nitric oxide has found acceptance for treatment of persistent pulmonary hypertension of the newborn and for hypoxic respiratory failure in term and near-term infants although the precise mechanisms of how it may improve lung function are yet unclear.[57,58] The use of nitric oxide in moderately ill, ventilated premature infants appears safe in infants between 1000 and 1250 g birth weight. Benefits include decreased oxygen use and fewer days of ventilation,

prevention of bronchopulmonary dysplasia (BPD), and neurologic protection. Additional therapies, such as antioxidants, late surfactant doses, caffeine, and improved ventilatory strategies (including steroids surrounding the time of extubation), can provide additional benefit in these vulnerable infants.[59,60] Other key components of supportive care include prophylactic antibiotics, temperature control, fluid and nutritional management, maintenance of blood pressure, and management of patent ductus arteriosus.[51]

The extremely preterm lung is particularly vulnerable to injury. Mechanical ventilation may interfere with alveolarization and surfactant metabolism and may aggravate the proinflammatory state (as reflected by abnormal cytokine profiles) that is believed to accompany premature birth and RDS. Injury from oxygen toxicity also is a concern and is mediated through reactive oxygen species.[61] This combination of factors may lead to subsequent development of chronic lung disease or bronchopulmonary dysplasia.[62,63] The use of CPAP rather than intubation may reduce these complications.[64] Most infants with RDS survive with treatment. However, the incidence of subsequent chronic lung disease is significant among very low-birth-weight infants.

Bronchopulmonary Dysplasia

Bronchopulmonary dysplasia (BPD), often used synonymously with *chronic lung disease of infancy*, is the most common chronic lung disease of infancy in the United States. It is the term used for persisting lung disease following premature birth and perinatal respiratory support. When originally described by Northway and colleagues in 1967, the term was applied to premature infants (30 to 37 weeks' gestation) who had survived acute RDS but continued to have pulmonary dysfunction and oxygen dependence, which was attributed to injury from postnatal mechanical ventilation and oxygen therapy.[65] The terms of definition and evolution of disease have changed notably since the original description of the disease. Premature infants are now consistently surviving at 23 to 26 weeks and have different mechanisms of lung injury.[66]

In the current era of neonatology, the widespread use of antenatal glucocorticoids and postnatal surfactant has lessened the incidence and severity of RDS, and BPD is occurring almost exclusively in the smallest premature infants (23 to 28 weeks' gestation) who have received mechanical ventilation. Surprisingly, some of these tiny infants who develop BPD have had few or no clinical signs of RDS at birth or have initially received only low levels of supplemental oxygen or ventilatory support.[67] Nevertheless, a highly significant predictor of subsequent BPD remains the need for mechanical ventilation on the day of birth. The presence of antenatal chorioamnionitis, postnatal sepsis, or a patent ductus arteriosus may confer additive risk of developing BPD.

The reported incidence of BPD is widely variable because of the lack of consistent diagnostic criteria, but is most common in infants delivered at gestational ages less than 30 weeks or who have birth weights of less than 1500 g. There are approximately 60,000 infants born at less than 1500 g in the United States on an annual basis. About 20% to 30% of

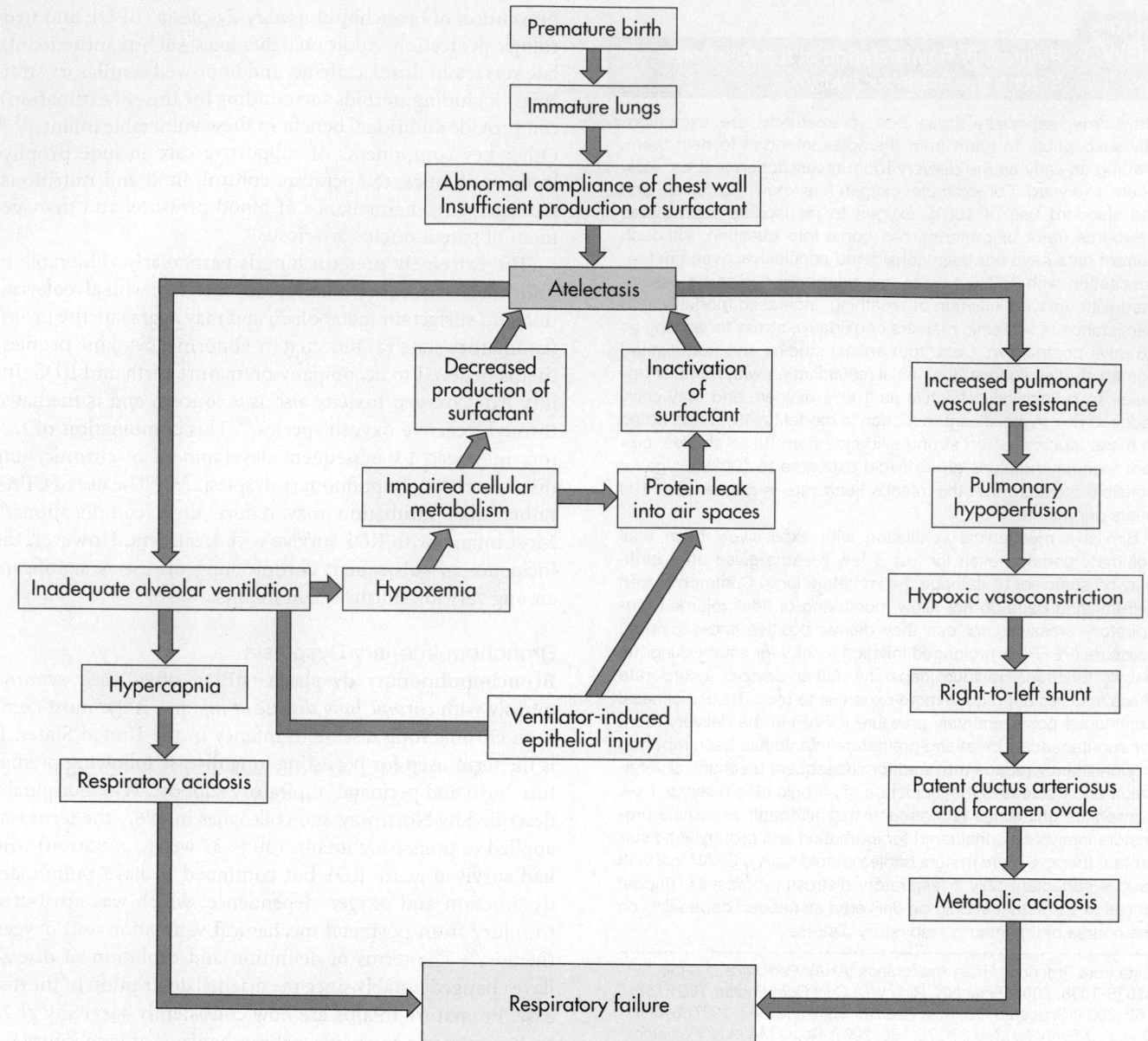

Figure 34-12 Pathogenesis of respiratory distress syndrome (RDS) of the newborn. RDS is also known as hyaline membrane disease.

these infants develop BPD. Because BPD is a multisystem condition, it also is associated with developmental disorders in other systems, such as growth retardation, pulmonary hypertension, neurodevelopmental delays (e.g., cerebral palsy), hearing defects, and retinopathy of prematurity.[66,68]

PATHOPHYSIOLOGY In preterm infants born at less than 28 weeks of gestation, the fetal lung is in the *canalicular stage* of development (16 to 28 weeks), a critical period during which type II epithelial cells appear, capillaries grow into the future distal alveolar regions, and the interstitium begins to condense. Ultimately the alveoli must have a very thin interface between the air space and the capillary for appropriate gas exchange. The extensive network of alveoli develop by septation within the terminal respiratory unit, beginning in the

saccular stage, which starts at approximately 26 to 28 weeks.

Prior to the widespread use of surfactant therapy, BPD was a disease characterized by airway injury, inflammation, and parenchymal fibrosis. Now, after the initiation of surfactant therapy, what is called *new BPD* is most often a form of arrested lung development.[69] The characteristic pathologic changes seen in new BPD are fewer and larger alveoli with less functional surface area, and reduced and dysplastic capillary ingrowth to the alveolar region. There may be accompanying pulmonary hypertensive changes, interstitial fibrosis, and smooth muscle hyperplasia, but certainly to a much lesser degree than that associated with *classic BPD.* Airway epithelial lesions are negligible. The pathophysiology of BPD is diagrammed in Figure 34-13.

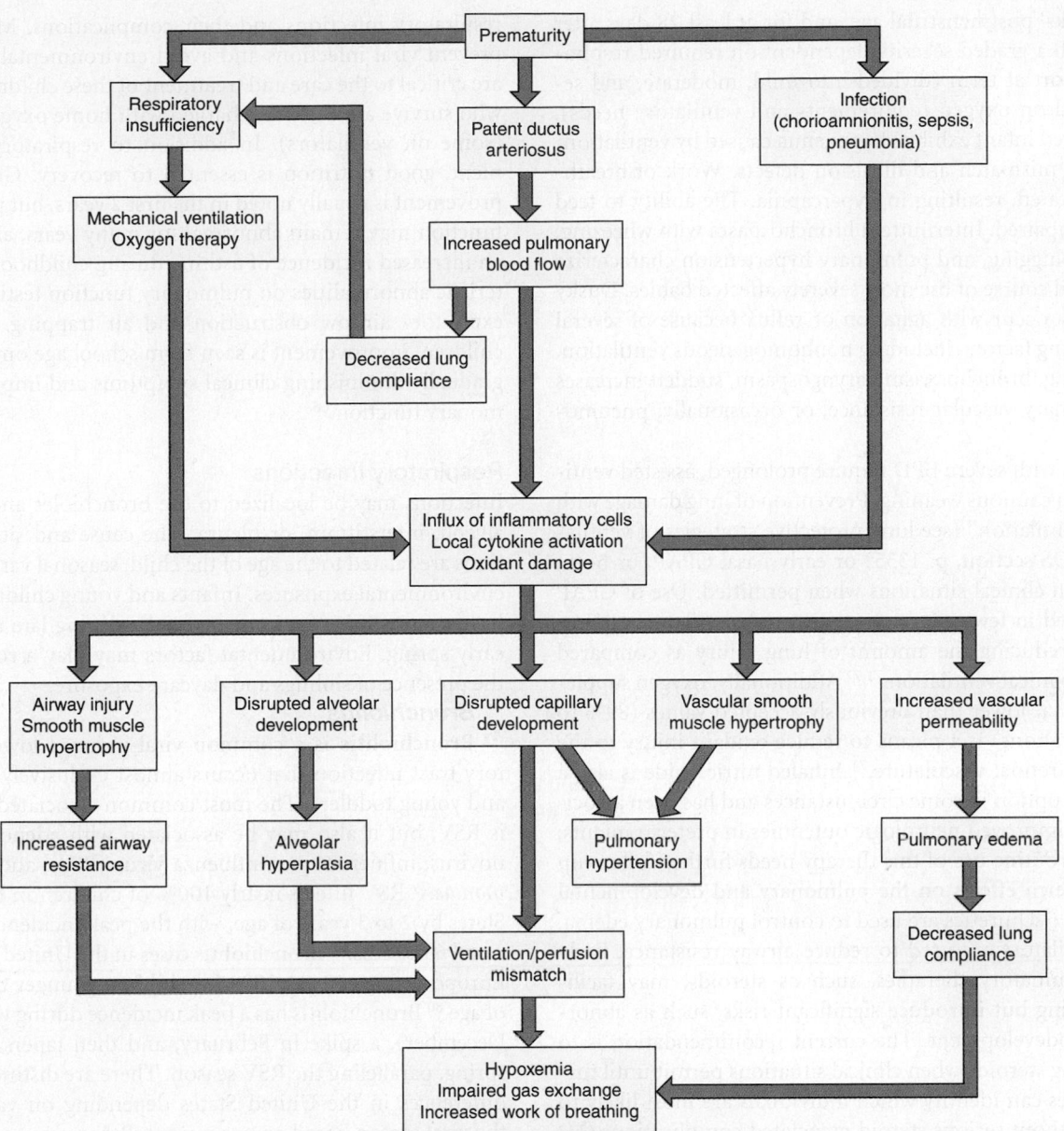

Figure 34-13 Pathophysiology of bronchopulmonary dysplasia (BPD).

Genetic susceptibility and hereditary influences on gene expression that are pivotal for surfactant synthesis, vascular development, and inflammatory regulation have been documented as being associated with new BPD.[66] To a significant extent, cytokines may mediate the abnormal alveolarization and injury response that lead to BPD, although this has not been directly proven. In the case of intrauterine infection, inflammatory mediators may prime the lung for an exaggerated path of injury after birth. Proinflammatory cytokines, such as tumor necrosis factor-alpha (TNF-α), interleukin-1 (IL-1), IL-6, and IL-8, are elevated in the amniotic fluid or tracheal aspirates of preterm infants who later develop BPD. Interestingly, the predominant mediators of *new BPD* are profibrotic and angiogenic cytokines rather than proinflammatory cytokines.[70] Antenatal and postnatal exposures also play into the

progression of this "developmental disorder." In the antenatal period, the use of steroids, chorioamnionitis, or the presence of intrauterine growth restriction influences the development and progression of BPD. Postnatally, administration of steroids, nutritional issues, as well as mechanical ventilator damage and pulmonary edema, influence progression of BPD.

Ventilation-perfusion matching is compromised as a result of structural underdevelopment, pulmonary hypertension, increased lung fluid content, airway injury, and smooth muscle hypertrophy, as well as adverse chest wall dynamics. Thus infants with BPD exhibit an increased oxygen requirement, increased work of breathing, and in the most severe cases, right-sided heart failure.

CLINICAL MANIFESTATIONS The current clinical definition of BPD includes the need for supplemental oxygen at 36 weeks' postmenstrual age, and for at least 28 days after birth, with a graded severity dependent on required respiratory support at term (divided into mild, moderate, and severe based on oxygen requirements and ventilatory needs). The affected infant exhibits hypoxemia caused by ventilation-perfusion mismatch and diffusion defects. Work of breathing is elevated, resulting in hypercapnia. The ability to feed may be impaired. Intermittent bronchospasm with wheezing, mucous plugging, and pulmonary hypertension characterize the clinical course of the most severely affected babies. Dusky spells may occur with agitation or reflux because of several contributing factors, including nonhomogeneous ventilation, air trapping, bronchospasm, laryngospasm, sudden increases in pulmonary vascular resistance, or occasionally, pneumothorax.

Infants with severe BPD require prolonged, assisted ventilation with cautious weaning. Prevention of lung damage with "gentle ventilation" (see lung protective strategies of ventilation in RDS section, p. 1335) or early nasal CPAP, or both, are used in clinical situations when permitted. Use of CPAP has resulted in fewer days of oxygen and ventilator requirement by reducing the amount of lung injury as compared with mechanical ventilation.[71,72] Additionally, oxygen supplementation at lower than previously accepted values (89% to 94% saturations) is a means to reduce oxidant injury to the lungs and retinal vasculature.[71] Inhaled nitric oxide is also a treatment option in some circumstances and has been associated with improved neurologic outcomes in preterm infants; however, routine use of this therapy needs further follow-up for long-term effects on the pulmonary and developmental systems.[73-75] Diuretics are used to control pulmonary edema. Bronchodilators are used to reduce airway resistance. Early anti-inflammatory therapies, such as steroids, may facilitate weaning but introduce significant risks, such as abnormal neurodevelopment. The current recommendation is to avoid using steroids when clinical situations permit until further studies can identify which individuals are most likely to benefit without serious steroid-associated complications.[75,76] Azithromycin also may have a role in controlling the inflammatory portion of this disease process as it does in other pulmonary diseases; however, research in this area is ongoing.[77] Caffeine citrate is commonly used and has been associated with decreased rates of BPD. Other therapies in the early stages of investigation include targeted cytokine and anticytokine therapies, antioxidants, and antiproteinases. Infection is a constant threat because of invasive lines, the endotracheal tube, and a compromised immune system. Nutritional needs are high and must be met to promote growth and healing. Most infants can be fed enterally. Early supplemental vitamin A and/or amino acids, which play a role in normal lung development, may be required in low-birth-weight infants and have resulted in as much as a 12% reduction in development of BPD.[71,75,78]

Death from BPD is usually caused by infection or respiratory failure. Recurrent cough and wheezing are frequent in survivors with BPD, as well as a high susceptibility to repeated respiratory infections and their complications. Measures to prevent viral infections and avoid environmental exposures are critical to the care and treatment of these children. Infants who survive are often discharged with home oxygen therapy (some on ventilators). In addition to respiratory management, good nutrition is essential to recovery. Gradual improvement is usually noted in the first 2 years, but pulmonary function may remain abnormal for many years, and there is an increased incidence of asthma during childhood. Characteristic abnormalities on pulmonary function testing include expiratory airflow obstruction and air trapping. For some children, improvement is seen from school age onward, with gradually diminishing clinical symptoms and improved pulmonary function.[66]

Respiratory Infections

Infections may be localized to the bronchioles and bronchi, alveoli, interstitium, or pleura. The cause and site of infections are related to the age of the child, seasonal variables, and environmental exposures. Infants and young children tend to have more viral infections, especially during late autumn to early spring. Environmental factors may play a role such as the presence of siblings and daycare exposure.

Bronchiolitis

Bronchiolitis is a common viral-induced lower respiratory tract infection that occurs almost exclusively in infants and young toddlers. The most common associated pathogen is RSV, but it also may be associated with adenovirus, rhinovirus, influenza, parainfluenza virus (PIV), and *M. pneumoniae*.[79] RSV infects nearly 100% of children in the United States by 2 to 3 years of age, with the peak incidence between 2 and 6 months.[79] Bronchiolitis cases in the United States and Europe average 30 per 1000 for children younger than 1 year of age.[80] Bronchiolitis has a peak incidence during winter (late December), a spike in February, and then tapers off in the spring, paralleling the RSV season. There are distinct regional differences in the United States depending on variation in the viral season based on geography. Other viruses, especially human metapneumovirus (hMPV), also follow a seasonal pattern and result in coinfection with RSV.[80] It is a major reason for hospital admission of children younger than 1 year, particularly children of lower socioeconomic status. Healthy infants usually make a full recovery from RSV bronchiolitis, but infants who are premature or who have underlying lung disease, heart disease, or immune deficiency may have a much more severe or even deadly course. Certain types of PIV and adenovirus are associated with more severe disease that can progress to bronchiolitis obliterans. Nonetheless, mortality rates are low at 2 per 100,000 live births.[80]

PATHOPHYSIOLOGY Viral infection causes necrosis of the bronchial epithelium and destruction of ciliated epithelial cells. There is infiltration with lymphocytes around the bronchioles and a cell-mediated hypersensitivity to viral antigens with release of lymphokines causing inflammation, as well as activation of eosinophils, neutrophils, and monocytes. The inflammatory process extends from the respiratory tract to the eustachian tubes and the middle ear. The submucosa becomes edematous, and cellular debris and fibrin form plugs within the bronchioles. Edema of the bronchiolar wall, accumulation of mucus and cellular debris, and possibly bronchospasm narrow or occlude many peripheral airways. Resultant uneven ventilation and atelectasis lead to perfusion mismatch and hypoxemia.

The mechanics of breathing are disrupted by bronchiolitis. Airway narrowing causes obstruction of airflow that is worse with expiration. This leads to air trapping, hyperinflation, and an increase in FRC. Airway resistance and hyperinflation result in a decrease in lung compliance and an increased work of breathing. This increased work of breathing leads to a decrease in alveolar ventilation with resultant hypercapnia.

CLINICAL MANIFESTATIONS Children with bronchiolitis generally have several of the following signs and symptoms, although there is no standard definition of the condition. They may have tachypnea, expiratory wheezing, cough, rhinorrhea, mild fever, and varying grades of respiratory distress. Mild conjunctivitis occurs in up to 33% of cases, and otitis media occurs in 16% to 50%.[79,80] Infants may have difficulty with apnea (8% to 20%). Chest radiographs often reveal hyperexpanded lungs, patchy or peribronchial infiltrates, and atelectasis. Severely affected infants appear anxious and distressed because of dyspnea or hypoxemia. The thoracic cage is overexpanded, particularly in its anteroposterior diameter. The infant takes rapid, short breaths, and wheezing and rales are often heard on auscultation. With overexpansion of the lungs, the diaphragm is flattened, causing downward displacement of the liver and spleen. Abdominal distention results from air swallowing. Some individuals have persistent high airway resistance and airway hyperresponsiveness, including increased risk for asthma, long after resolution of the viral process.[81] Genetic tendencies have been noted that correlate RSV bronchiolitis and long-term pulmonary sequelae.[77]

EVALUATION AND TREATMENT Diagnosis is made by review of signs and symptoms (e.g., rhinitis, cough, wheezing, crackles, chest retractions and/or hyperinflation, tachypnea) and radiologic examination. Nasal washings/swabbings may be tested for specific viral agents, such as RSV. RSV swabs are positive in 70% of cases of bronchiolitis. Routine chest films have fallen out of favor because they often reveal nonspecific findings (hyperinflation and patchy atelectasis) and are associated with an increase in antibiotic use that is unwarranted.[82] Treatment is determined by the severity of the disease and age of the child. Infants younger than 1 year are most at risk for acute respiratory failure and may require assisted ventilation. Supplemental oxygen is given as needed, and adequate hydration should be maintained. The use of nasal CPAP and heliox (mixture of helium and oxygen) is being explored, and studies to prove effectiveness are ongoing.[83] Bronchodilators have not been scientifically validated as consistently providing significant benefit, but are widely tried on an empiric basis. Likewise, steroids are not of proven benefit but have been associated with small decreases

in length of stay and improved symptoms in some cases.[82,84] Racemic epinephrine has shown promising results in small subsets of children.[82] Antiviral agents (ribavirin) for RSV are no longer widely used because of high cost and unclear efficacy; however, several new antiviral agents are being investigated for treatment and prophylaxis. Prophylactic treatment with RSV-specific monoclonal antibody is recommended for high-risk infants younger than 2 years old, although high cost is sometimes a barrier.[85] For those requiring hospitalization, length of stay is generally 3 to 4 days.

Pneumonia

Pneumonia is a process that results from infection and resultant inflammation in the terminal airways and alveoli. **Community-acquired pneumonia (CAP)** is one of the most common global infections in the pediatric age group, as well as one of the leading causes of hospital admission. Identification of the etiologic agent is often challenging because the range of pathogens is quite large.[86] The most common agents are viral, followed by bacteria and atypical microorganisms. The incidence of viral and bacterial pneumonia varies according to age, time of year, and geographic location. In children, fungal and anaerobic pneumonias are rare, and opportunistic infections occur only in the immunocompromised child (these unusual forms of pneumonia are not discussed further in this chapter).

The incidence of CAP in the developed world is 21 to 36 per 1000 with 40% of these cases requiring hospitalization.[87] Pneumonia is most common in children younger than the age of 2, with the highest frequency between 6 and 12 months.[88] Risk factors for bacterial and viral pneumonia include age younger than 2 years, overcrowded living conditions, winter season, recent antibiotic treatment, attendance at daycare centers, and passive smoke exposure. Nutritional status, age, and underlying disease process influence morbidity and mortality rates related to CAP.

PATHOPHYSIOLOGY Bacterial pneumonia in young children beyond the neonatal period is most commonly the result of infection with streptococcal and staphylococcal microorganisms (Table 34-2). *S. pneumoniae* (pneumococcal) pneumonia is the most common causative microorganism and manifests acutely and with variable severity. Pneumococci and many of the other bacteria that commonly cause pneumonia have specific virulence factors (such as capsules) that increase their survival and proliferation while causing insult to the host.[89] Infection usually begins with inhalation of microbes dispersed in ambient air or in secretion droplets (person-to-person spread) or by aspiration of one's own nasopharyngeal bacteria into the trachea. A preceding viral infection sometimes sets the stage for bacterial infection by causing epithelial damage and reduced mucociliary clearance in the trachea and major bronchi. Colonization of the trachea then ensues, with the microorganism, host, and environment all playing a role in the development of pneumonia. Once in the alveolar region, bacteria encounter local host defenses, such as antibodies, complement, phagocytes, and cytokines, that prepare bacteria for ingestion by alveolar macrophages.

Table 34-2	Common Types of Pneumonia in Children				
Type	Causal Agent	Age	Onset	Signs/Symptoms	Pathophysiology
Viral pneumonia	Respiratory syncytial virus (RSV), influenza (A and B), adenovirus, parainfluenza, human metapneumovirus (hMPV)	Infants for RSV All ages for others	Acute or gradual, winter and early spring	Mild to high fever, cough, rhinorrhea, malaise, rales, rhonchi, or wheezing, variable radiographic pattern	Edema, increased mucus, and interstitial pneumonia
Pneumococcal pneumonia	Pneumococci (Streptococcus pneumoniae)	1-4 yr	Acute, follows an upper respiratory infection, winter and early spring	High fever, productive cough, pleuritic pain, increased respiratory rate, decreased breath sounds in area of consolidation; lobar pattern or "round pneumonia" on radiograph	Inflammation of bronchial mucosa, alveolar exudate Early: red hepatization with WBCs, RBCs, and fibrin consolidation Late: gray hepatization with fibrin and neutrophils in alveoli Resolution: many phagocytic macrophages
Staphylococcal pneumonia	Staphylococcus aureus Methicillin-resistant Staphylococcus aureus (MRSA)	1 wk-2 yr	Acute, winter months	High fever, cough, respiratory distress, toxic appearance, sepsis, empyema, pneumatoceles are common; multilobar consolidation	Necrotizing patterns may occur in severe cases
Streptococcal pneumonia	Group A streptococci	All ages	Acute, any season	High fever, chills, respiratory distress sepsis or shock; empyema, pneumatoceles	Tracheobronchitis, interstitial pneumonia with ulcers, exudate edema, and localized hemorrhage
Mycoplasma and Chlamydophila pneumoniae	M. pneumoniae C. pneumoniae	School age and adolescents	Gradual	Low-grade fever; cough	Inflammation of bronchi with lymphocyte and chlamydia neutrophil recruitment

RBCs, Red blood cells; WBCs, white blood cells.

If these mechanisms fail, neutrophils will be recruited and an intense cytokine-mediated inflammation will ensue. Vascular engorgement, edema, and a fibrinopurulent exudate with tissue damage occur. Alveolar filling precludes gas exchange and, if extensive, can lead to respiratory failure. If sepsis occurs at the same time, shock and end-organ hypoperfusion may develop. Staphylococcal and group A streptococcal pneumonia can be particularly fulminant and necrotizing, with a high incidence of accompanying empyema, pneumatoceles, and sepsis. Empyema is increasingly associated with pneumococcal infections and with MRSA.[90,91]

The clinical presentation of bacterial pneumonia, particularly pneumococcal, may include a preceding viral illness followed by fever with chills and rigors, shortness of breath, and an increasingly productive cough. Occasionally there is blood streaking of the sputum. Respiratory rate and oxygen saturation also are important clinical indicators. Auscultation usually reveals such abnormalities as crackles or decreased breath sounds. Other less specific findings may include malaise,

emesis, abdominal pain, and chest pain. Chest film will usually present with a lobar pattern in older children and adolescents but may appear patchier with a bronchopneumonic pattern in younger children.[88]

Viral pneumonia is more common than bacterial pneumonia and is acquired by direct contact, droplet transmission, or aerosol. Children are two to three times more likely than adults to become infected with respiratory viruses, with the majority occurring in otherwise healthy children. Although mortality from respiratory viruses in developed countries is rare, they are a major source of morbidity. In less developed countries viral pneumonia results in nearly 5 million deaths in children younger than the age of 5 each year.[79] Viral infections often occur in epidemics, whereas others occur endemically; however, most tend to follow a seasonal pattern. The most common cause of viral pneumonia in infants and young children is RSV,[92] occurring most often in winter to early spring. A number of other viruses are important, including parainfluenza, influenza A and B, coronaviruses, rhinoviruses, enteroviruses, human metapneumovirus (hMPV), bocavirus, and adenoviruses.

Viral infection of the lower respiratory tract results in destruction of ciliated epithelium of the distal airway, with sloughing of cellular material. A mononuclear-predominant inflammatory response occurs first in the interstitium and may later involve the alveoli. Certain serotypes of adenovirus can cause necrotizing disease, sometimes leading to obliterative bronchiolitis and significant lung disability.

Early in the course of illness, it is often difficult to determine whether the pneumonia is of viral or bacterial origin. Differences that may be noted are elevated temperatures, absolute neutrophil counts, and percent of bands are consistently higher in bacterial pneumonias than with those of viral etiology.[93] Diagnosis of a viral etiology requires laboratory confirmation (immunofluorescence tests). Development of safe agents to treat viral pneumonias continues to be a priority, as is development of more effective vaccines.[79]

Atypical pneumonia *Chlamydophila pneumoniae* (previously *Chlamydia pneumoniae*) is clinically indistinguishable from, and is typically grouped with, *M. pneumoniae* as "atypical" pneumonia.[94,95] These microorganisms are the most common cause of CAP for school-age children (ages 5 and older) and young adults, accounting for nearly one fourth of all cases of bacterial pneumonia.[89] *Mycoplasma* is known to cause a wide spectrum of disease and has more extensive complications than previously recognized. Studies reveal that it is seen increasingly in infants and younger children.[96,97] Children experiencing recurrent respiratory tract infections often have been found to be infected with atypical bacteria.

Transmission of atypical microorganisms is person to person, with a 2- to 3-week incubation period. *Mycoplasma* microorganisms lack cell walls but have a limiting membrane and a specialized tip for attaching to ciliated respiratory epithelial cells. Local sloughing of cells occurs. Peribronchial lymphocytic infiltration develops, along with neutrophil recruitment to the airway lumen. The pattern resembles bronchitis or bronchopneumonia.

Onset of symptoms is usually gradual, resembling a typical upper respiratory infection with low-grade fever and prominent cough. There may be accompanying sore throat, myalgia, and headache. Cases are not usually clinically severe, and full recovery should be expected without complications. When complications do occur, they can include bronchopneumonia, parapneumonic effusions, and necrotizing pneumonitis.[96]

EVALUATION AND TREATMENT Diagnosis of pneumonia is based on clinical, laboratory and chest radiograph findings. Guidelines have been developed to improve and aid assessment and management, although consensus has not been reached in their clinical application. Identifying pathogens is very difficult in children, especially since there is often overlap between bacterial and viral pathogens. Some newer studies are recommending use of highly sensitive C-reactive protein (hs-CRP) as a tool to help discern between viral and bacterial pneumonias. hs-CRP in combination with clinical signs and symptoms and chest film may correlate to help the clinician more accurately diagnose the etiology of the pneumonia.[86] Other laboratory tests that may be helpful include a white cell–granulocyte count, procalcitonin, or erythrocyte sedimentation rate (ESR) but they do not indicate a specific etiology. Several microbiologic tests are available including polymerase chain reaction (PCR) and nucleic acid amplification tests (NAAT). On chest radiography, a bacterial pneumonia initially produces an alveolar infiltrate and later causes a segmental or lobar disease. A viral infection is more likely to be associated with an interstitial pattern.

Most pneumonias may be treated on an outpatient basis; however, some children require oxygen supplementation and, occasionally, assisted ventilation. This is particularly true with infants who have a viral interstitial pneumonia, such as RSV. In addition, adequate hydration, nutrition, and supportive pulmonary therapy are required to reduce the duration and severity of illness. Many hospitalized infants are markedly tachypneic and unable to coordinate their breathing with swallowing such that they may require enteral feeding. Aspiration is always a risk with infants in respiratory distress.

Appropriate antibiotic administration, whether oral or intravenous (IV), for bacterial pneumonias is usually instituted for a minimum of 10 days, although studies suggest that shorter courses of antibiotics may be adequate in children with mild to moderate to severe cases.[98] Local patterns of drug resistance must be considered as there is 20% to 40% pneumococcal resistance to penicillin and up to 40% resistance for macrolides in the United States. New antibacterials are under development for treatment of antibiotic-resistant pathogens.[96,99] Use of the heptavalent pneumococcal conjugate vaccine has led to a decrease in invasive infections.[100]

Aspiration Pneumonitis

Aspiration pneumonitis is caused by a foreign substance, such as food material, secretions (e.g., saliva or gastric contents), or chemical compounds entering the lung and causing inflammation. The aspiration of meconium from amniotic fluid can occur at birth. Meconium contains bile salts from the fetal intestinal tract that cause inflammation. Neurologically compromised children or children undergoing sedation or anesthesia may aspirate oral secretions (containing anaerobic bacteria) or stomach contents. Children with neurologic compromise, other underlying diseases such as chronic lung disease/BPD, anatomic tracheoesophageal, or craniofacial abnormalities may present with chronic pulmonary aspiration (CPA). Left unaddressed, CPA can result in progressive lung disease, bronchiectasis, and respiratory failure and is the leading cause of death in children with severe neurologic compromise.[101] The severity of lung injury after an acute aspiration incident is determined by the amount of material aspirated, the pH of the aspirated material, and the presence of pathogenic bacteria. Very low pH or very high pH causes a significant inflammatory response. With hydrocarbon ingestions, lung injury is determined by the volatility and viscosity of the aspirated substance. A low-viscosity substance, such as gasoline or lighter fluid, is the most toxic; high-viscosity hydrocarbons, such as petroleum jelly or mineral oil, are much less likely to cause pneumonitis. Treatment for aspiration pneumonitis depends on the material aspirated but generally includes broad-spectrum antibiotic therapy. Strategies for prevention of aspiration are an important part of the therapeutic plan at every well-child visit.

Bronchiolitis Obliterans

Bronchiolitis obliterans (BO), a relatively rare diagnosis in children, is fibrotic obstruction of the respiratory bronchioles and alveolar ducts secondary to intense inflammation. The inflammation leads to narrowing, complete obliteration, or both of the airway lumen. Pathologically, there are two forms: proliferative and constrictive; the latter results in the obliteration of the lumen and is the more common form. Most cases of bronchiolitis obliterans in children are associated with viral pulmonary infections, such as influenza, adenoviral infection, pertussis (whooping cough), measles, parainfluenza, RSV, human immunodeficiency virus (HIV) or *M. pneumoniae.* BO may occur after allograft transplantation (lung, heart-lung, and bone marrow) as a manifestation of graft-versus-host disease. It also is associated with collagen vascular disease, toxic fume inhalation, chronic hypersensitivity pneumonitis, Crohn disease, and Stevens-Johnson syndrome.[102,103] For reasons that are unclear, BO seems to occur more frequently in the Southern Hemisphere, although it is certainly noted in other parts of the world as well. Genetic factors influence susceptibility; however, these factors have yet to be clarified.[103] Initially cough, respiratory distress, and cyanosis occur, followed by a brief period of improvement. The progression of disease is then reflected by tachypnea, sputum production, increased anterior/posterior diameter, crackles, wheezing, and hypoxemia.[104]

There is no specific treatment for BO. Supportive care is usually given with mechanical ventilation, although there is evidence that this also may contribute to the progression of the disease. Use of antiviral agents may be warranted in managing those with viral infection. For transplant recipients, augmentation of immunosuppressive therapies and treatment with anti-inflammatory agents are showing promise in reducing airway inflammation, thus improving pulmonary function.[105] Clinical progression can be quite variable depending on the predisposing condition. Some children experience partial recovery, whereas others follow a course of steady decline in lung function.

Asthma

Asthma is an obstructive airway disease characterized by reversible airflow obstruction, bronchial hyperreactivity, and inflammation. The onset of asthma generally occurs early in life and is associated with identifiable risk factors.[106] The prevalence of asthma is significantly higher in children than adults and is the most prevalent chronic disease in childhood, affecting 5% to 13% of all children. In the prepubertal years, more boys than girls are affected. Although statistics suggest that asthma has become more prevalent in the past two decades, some of this increase may be related to improved awareness of the diagnosis of the condition.[107] Populations most affected include those living in an urban setting, ethnic minorities, and those of low-socioeconomic status.[108] There also may be associations between those children living with a single mother and having multiple siblings that result in reduction in treatment and worsened outcomes from asthma.[109] Asthma-related deaths almost always occur outside the hospital setting. The severity and persistence of asthma are influenced by age at disease onset, genetics, behavior, atopy, air pollution, level of allergen exposure, environmental tobacco smoke, gastroesophageal reflux, and respiratory infections.[106] Additional confounding variables that affect disparity in asthma morbidity and therapy are lack of health insurance, poor access to asthma specialists, inappropriate utilization of healthcare resources, and inadequate medical care.[108] Inner-city black and Hispanic children have higher morbidity and mortality rates than white children.[108] After decades of rising mortality rates, there has been a decrease in the number of children dying of this disease in recent years.[110]

The wide spectrum of clinical disease in asthma probably reflects a complex interaction between *genetic susceptibility* and *environmental factors,* including allergens (e.g., air pollution, dust mite and cockroach allergen, tobacco smoke) and infections, particularly viral respiratory infections (e.g., rhinovirus).[108,111] The genetics of asthma are complex. Population genomic screening has led to the identification of many candidate genes or chromosomal regions that are associated with asthma. Included in the long list of asthma-associated genes are those that code for increased levels of immune and inflammatory mediators (e.g., IL-4, IgE, and leukotrienes), nitric oxide, and transmembrane proteins in the endoplasmic reticulum.[111,112] In addition, genes may impart associated phenotypes, such as bronchial hyperresponsiveness (BHR), sensitization to allergens, and responsiveness to asthma therapies. For example, a specific polymorphism in the gene for the β-adrenergic receptor that is prevalent in black children is associated with poor response to β-adrenergic inhaled medication.[108]

Environmental exposures such as allergens, viruses, smoke, and air pollutants interact with an individual's genetic vulnerabilities to induce the onset of clinical asthma.[106,111,113,114] One hypothesis for the high prevalence of asthma in westernized cultures is called the "hygiene hypothesis." This theory suggests that certain early childhood respiratory viral infections could favor the Th2-predominant phenotype and contribute to inducing asthma in susceptible individuals. It also suggests that *lack* of sufficient early exposure to other types of infections (e.g., hepatitis) also favors the Th2 phenotype in the airways and permits induction of asthma.[115] Asthma develops because the Th2 response (in which CD4 T-helper [Th] cells produce specific cytokines, such as IL-4, IL-5, and IL-13) promotes an atopic/allergic response in the airways as opposed to a Th1 response characteristic of delayed-type hypersensitivity and phagocyte-mediated host defense. IL-4 and

IL-13 are particularly important for B-cell switching to favor IgE production, and IL-5 is crucial for local differentiation and enhanced survival of eosinophils within the airways. This theory about the origins of asthma is consistent with many of the epidemiologic and pathophysiologic features of childhood asthma, but is not yet proven.

PATHOPHYSIOLOGY The pathophysiology of asthma in children is similar to that for adults (see Chapter 33, Figure 33-11, p. 1285). However, good criteria for predicting adult asthma in persons with childhood asthma remains unclear.[116,117] For acute allergen-induced asthma, the paradigm of the *early asthmatic response* remains useful (Figure 34-14, *A*

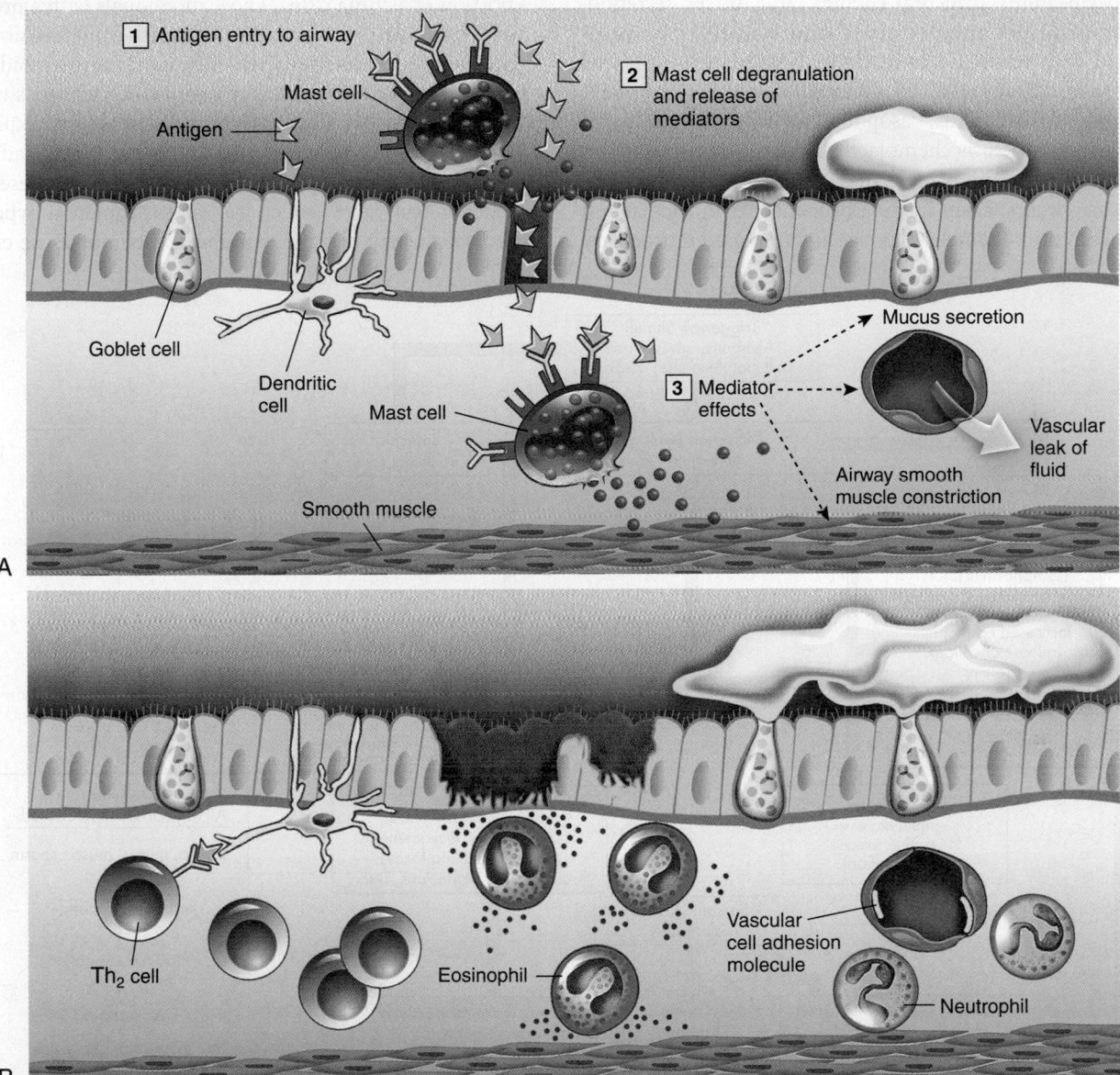

Figure 34-14 Asthmatic responses. A, In the early asthmatic response, inhaled antigen *(1)* binds to preformed IgE on mast cells. Mast cells degranulate *(2)* and release mediators such as histamine, leukotrienes, prostaglandin D_2, platelet-activating factor, and others. Acute inflammation opens intercellular tight junctions, allowing antigen to penetrate and activate submucosal mast cells. Secreted mediators *(3)* induce active bronchospasm, edema, and mucus secretion. Inflammatory responses are set in motion by chemotactic factors and upregulation of adhesion molecules (not shown). At the same time, as shown on the left, antigen may be received by dendritic cells that process and later present it, either in regional lymph nodes to naive (Th_0) T lymphocytes or locally to memory Th_2 cells in the airway mucosa (see **B**). **B,** In the late asthmatic response are areas of epithelial damage caused at least in part by toxicity of eosinophil products (major basic protein, eosinophilic cationic protein, eosinophil-derived neurotoxin, and eosinophil peroxidase). Many inflammatory cells have been recruited by chemokines and upregulation of vascular cell adhesion molecules. Local T lymphocytes display a predominant Th_2 cytokine profile. They produce interleukin-4 (IL-4) and IL-13, which promote switching of B cells to favor immunoglobulin E (IgE) production, and IL-3, IL-5, and granulocyte-macrophage colony-stimulating factor, which encourage eosinophil differentiation and survival.

and 34-15). This begins immediately after exposure and lasts up to 2 hours. The allergen binds to preformed IgE on the surface of mucosal mast cells, and crosslinking of these IgE molecules triggers degranulation of the mast cell, releasing mediators such as histamine, leukotrienes, prostaglandins, platelet-activating factor, chemotactic chemokines, and certain cytokines (e.g., IL-1).[106] These mediators cause airway smooth muscle constriction (bronchospasm), increased vascular permeability (mucosal edema), and mucus secretion. The *late asthmatic response* starts 4 to 8 hours after exposure and may persist up to 24 hours (Figure 34-14, *B*). The response is characterized by inflammatory cell recruitment (neutrophils, eosinophils, basophils, and T lymphocytes) that was triggered earlier by chemotactic factors and up-regulation of endothelial adhesion molecules. Another wave of mediator release occurs, again inciting bronchospasm, edema, and mucus secretion. Epithelial damage and impaired mucociliary

function may be seen because of direct toxic effects of cellular products such as major basic protein from eosinophils. This local injury stimulates local nerve endings, which may aggravate bronchoconstriction and mucus secretion through autonomic pathways (Figure 34-15).

Although allergen-associated immune and inflammatory processes are considered the primary etiologic processes in asthma, neutrophilic airway inflammation likely accounts for a portion of asthma cases. Those individuals with a predominance of inflammatory neutrophils (rather than eosinophils) have allergies less often and are less responsive to steroids.[106,111] As the inflammatory process continues, bronchospasm develops which narrows the airways especially during expiration. Mucous plugging, edema, and cellular infiltration lead to further airway narrowing. A partial obstruction is present that creates a "ball-valve" effect, leading to segmental hyperinflation, which may become extreme and compromise effective

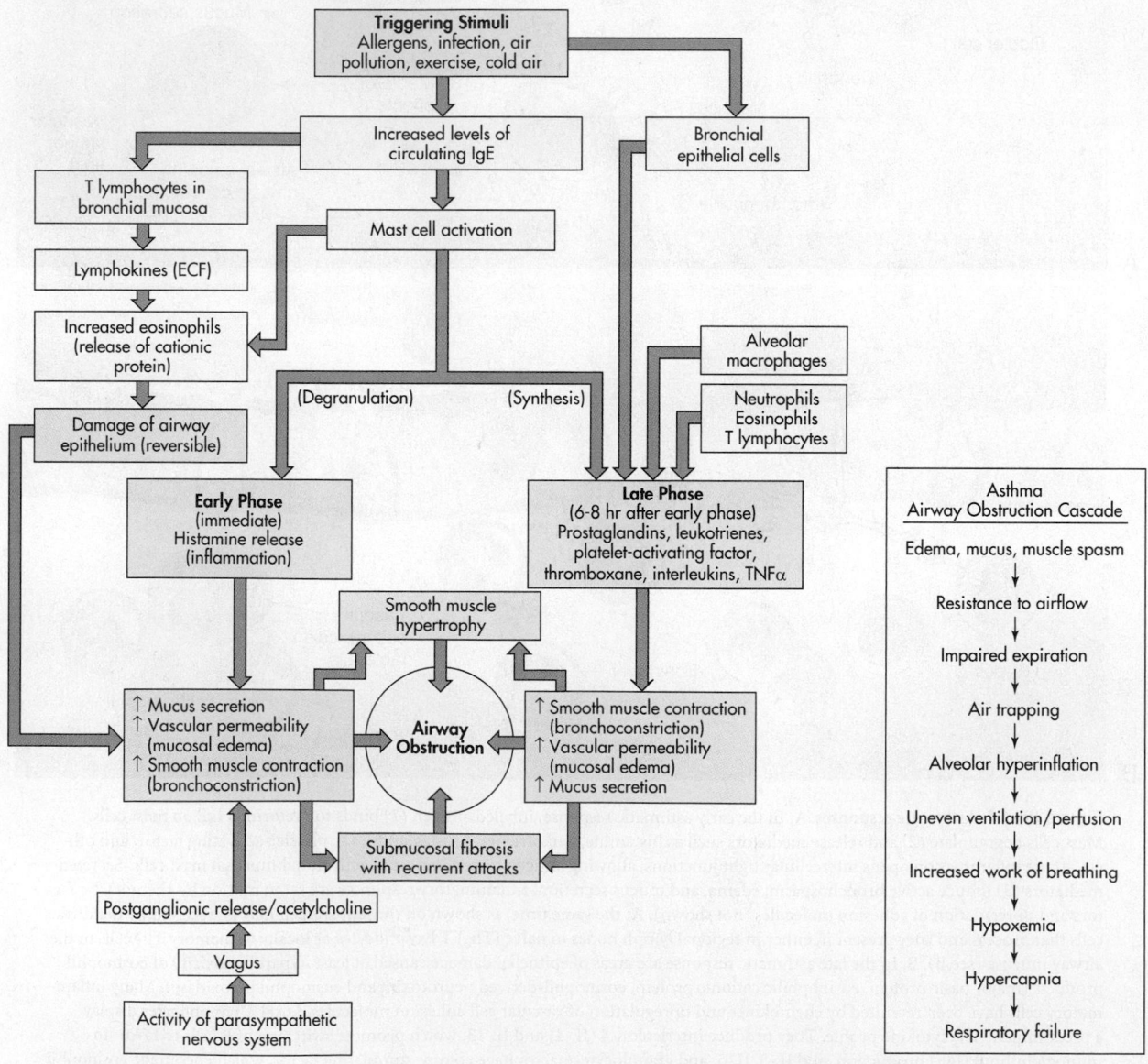

Figure 34-15 Pathophysiology of asthma. *ECF*, Eosinophil chemotactic factor; *IgE*, immunoglobulin E; *TNF*, tumor necrosis factor.

tidal volume. Measures of expiratory flow rates, such as forced expiratory volume in 1 second (FEV_1) and peak flow, are markedly reduced.

Examination of postmortem lung specimens of individuals who died from asthma reveals abnormalities consistent with acute and chronic changes in the airways. These include extensive mucous plugging, mucosal edema, and denudation of bronchial and bronchiolar epithelium. Eosinophilia is present in the submucosa, and a multicellular inflammatory infiltrate accumulates in the airways. Thickening of the basement membrane, airway smooth muscle hypertrophy, and mucous gland hypertrophy are often noted. In chronic asthma, chronically increased numbers of inflammatory cells may lead to long-term changes, such as goblet cell hyperplasia and airway wall remodeling (subepithelial fibrosis, smooth muscle hypertrophy).

The typical arterial blood gas abnormalities in acute asthma are hypoxemia, hypocarbia, and respiratory alkalosis. Because bronchial obstruction is nonuniform, ventilation is likewise uneven, causing ventilation mismatch and hypoxemia. The degree of hypoxemia is usually mild, however, and arterial saturations of less than 90% indicate severe airway obstruction. Pulmonary circulation may be altered by regional hypoxic vasoconstriction, as well as the effect of increased intra-alveolar pressure (caused by expiratory airway obstruction and alveolar hyperinflation) to decrease perfusion of alveolar capillaries. Typically, respiratory rate is elevated to compensate for hypoxemia and reduces arterial P_{CO_2} (respiratory alkalosis). If airway resistance and hyperinflation become severe, increased respiratory rate can no longer compensate for decreasing V_T causing a reduction in minute ventilation and a gradual rise in arterial P_{CO_2}, thus even a normal Pa_{CO_2} value should be of concern if respiratory distress is significant. Retention of CO_2 is a late finding, usually occurring only if FEV_1 falls to around 15% to 20% of predicted values, and reflects inadequate alveolar ventilation and increased functional dead space. With severe and prolonged airway obstruction (**status asthmaticus**), the end result of the pathophysiologic processes may be respiratory failure with acute CO_2 retention and respiratory acidosis. Metabolic acidosis may accompany life-threatening asthma, especially when left ventricular filling and thus cardiac output become compromised because of severe hyperinflation.

CLINICAL MANIFESTATIONS In a typical acute asthma attack, the major complaints are cough, wheeze, and shortness of breath. Signs of a preceding upper respiratory infection, such as rhinorrhea or low-grade fever, may be present. In children, 70% to 80% of acute wheezing episodes are associated with viral respiratory infections. In infants and toddlers younger than 2 years old, the most common of these is RSV. In older children and adults, the major viral trigger is rhinovirus. In fact, rhinovirus is reportedly associated with 60% to 80% of asthma exacerbations in school-age children.[118]

On physical examination, expiratory wheezing that is often described as high pitched and musical is found, along with prolongation of the expiratory phase of the respiratory cycle.

Sometimes hyperinflation is visible. Respiratory rate is elevated, as is heart rate. Nasal flaring and accessory muscle use are evident, with retractions in the substernal, subcostal, intercostal, suprasternal, or sternocleidomastoid areas. Infants may appear to be "head bobbing" because of sternocleidomastoid muscle use. Pulsus paradoxus (decrease in systolic blood pressure of more than 10mmHg during inspiration) may be present. The child may appear anxious or diaphoretic, important signs of respiratory compromise.

Findings in chronic asthma may include hyperinflation of the thorax (barrel chest) or pectus excavatum. Clubbing should not be seen in those with asthma and, if present, should trigger evaluation for other conditions, such as cystic fibrosis.

EVALUATION AND TREATMENT Asthma is often underdiagnosed and untreated, especially in preschool-age children. The fact that many of the symptoms overlap with other respiratory illness, like bronchitis or upper respiratory infections, may confuse the diagnosis. Because of the changing appearance of asthma in some children, tools to help confirm diagnosis are recommended. The modified asthma predictive index (API) is recommended by the National Institutes of Health (NIH) guidelines. Diagnosis is based on episodes of wheezing noted on an annual basis as well as concurrent risk factors. The major historical and physical factors that contribute to the diagnosis of asthma are parental history of asthma, physician-diagnosed atopic dermatitis, and evidence of sensitization to aeroallergens. Minor factors include evidence of sensitization to foods, 4% or greater peripheral blood eosinophilia, or wheezing not associated with upper respiratory illnesses.[106] To firmly establish the diagnosis, objective information is gathered by medical history, physical examination, and, when the child is 5 or older, pulmonary function testing (spirometry).

Characteristic abnormalities of spirometry would be reduced expiratory flow rates, namely FEV_1 and to an even greater extent, the midexpiratory flow rate (or forced expiratory flow rate between 25% and 75% [$FEF_{25\%-75\%}$] of total exhaled volume); also the ratio of FEV_1 to forced vital capacity (FVC) would be typically decreased. Unlike asthmatic adults, however, asthmatic children often have normal or near-normal spirometry between attacks. Other potentially useful supportive diagnostic findings would include evidence of air trapping on lung volume measurement (by plethysmography), documentation of bronchial hyperreactivity (in response to challenge such as exercise or inhaling methacholine) or increased expiratory flow rates in response to an inhaled bronchodilator. Often it is not feasible to obtain the above tests on children, so in practice an empiric trial of asthma-directed medications is commonly initiated, using clinical symptoms (wheeze, cough, exercise tolerance, handling of respiratory infections, etc.) as a guideline. During a significant asthma attack, individuals may be too dyspneic to perform spirometry, and it may precipitate excessive coughing.

For home management of asthma, peak flowmeters are often used. Peak flow measures are less reliable and less reproducible than those obtained by spirometry but can be helpful. For serial tracking, peak flow measurements should be obtained at consistent times of day because of the natural diurnal variation in peak flow, which is usually lowest at approximately 4 AM and highest at approximately 4 PM. Once a baseline value has been established on the basis of repeated measurements over a period of time, decreases in peak flow can be interpreted meaningfully to help assess the child and modify treatment in the face of increased symptoms or intercurrent illness.

The goal of asthma therapy is to achieve long-term control by reduction in impairment and risk.[106] Management of asthma medications in children is often difficult because remission is common. Care providers must periodically assess asthma control in children to decide if a "step up" (increase) or "step down" (decrease) is indicated in their asthma therapy. Algorithms can help assess asthma control and offer information about how to adjust therapy accordingly. Key features to assess include nighttime awakenings, interference with normal activities, use of short-acting beta$_2$ agonist, lung function, and exacerbations requiring oral steroids. Before therapy is augmented, reassessment of inhaler technique, adherence, environmental controls, and comorbidities should occur. For a reduction in therapy, the child's asthma should be well controlled for a minimum of 3 months.[106]

For management of intermittent (formerly called mild) asthma, rapid-acting bronchodilators, such as albuterol (a β_2-adrenergic agonist) or levalbuterol, may be sufficient with addition of oral systemic steroids for more significant attacks to decrease inflammatory responses in the lung.[106] Inhaled ipratropium bromide is an anticholinergic agent that contributes to bronchodilation by inhibiting vagal tone; it is sometimes used together with albuterol for acute treatment or sometimes as an alternative, though generally considered less potent for those who cannot tolerate β_2-adrenergic agonists because of side effects. Environmental controls and monitoring would also be included in the treatment plan for children as noted below.

There are a growing number of options for management of persistent asthma depending on chronicity and severity of symptoms, as well as on individual compliance issues. Guidelines have been outlined and widely distributed by an NIH expert panel.[106] In addition to medications, environmental controls are instituted. There also is a new focus on child-parent education and monitoring control of symptoms more closely and by a variety of methods. For individuals with persistent symptoms, daily "controller" medication is recommended. The most widely preferred controller therapy remains inhaled corticosteroids (ICS), although there is some debate about their safety in children younger than 2 years of age.[119] Montelukast (an oral leukotriene receptor antagonist) is frequently used as supplemental therapy or, for milder allergic or exercise-induced asthma, as monotherapy.[120] Inhaled cromolyn and nedocromil remain available anti-inflammatory therapies, but their use has declined in the United States in favor of other therapies. Long-acting β_2-adrenergic agonists,

such as salmeterol, also may be applied to pediatric asthma except in the youngest children. All classifications of asthma also require intermittent use of a short-acting bronchodilator during times of exacerbation or illness. Depending on the severity of symptoms, short courses of oral systemic corticosteroids also are prescribed. For allergic asthma, immunotherapy has been shown to be an important tool in reducing asthma symptoms and exacerbations, and can now be given sublingually.[121] Anti-IgE therapy is indicated for select individuals with severe asthma.[122] There also may be utility in using inhaled nitric oxide as an objective measure to determine asthma relapse after cessation of ICS.[123] Research in the area of pediatric asthma is targeted at evaluating the effects of vitamin D supplementation on wheezing; the associations between asthma and other underlying illnesses, such as sickle cell disease; the role of intermittent inhaled steroid use; and the effect of functional polymorphisms of antioxidant genes in regard to air pollution (in vitro).[111]

Regardless of the type of asthma, written asthma action plans and extensive child and family education is necessary for everyone. Asthma management education is necessary for children and their parents to ensure disease control and compliance. Follow-up care is needed every 3 to 6 months to evaluate control and need for change in the treatment plan.

Acute Respiratory Distress Syndrome

Acute respiratory distress syndrome (ARDS) is a condition that can result from either a direct or indirect pulmonary insult. It is defined as respiratory failure of acute onset characterized by severe hypoxemia that is refractory to treatment with supplemental oxygen, bilateral infiltrates on chest x-ray, and no evidence of heart failure.[124] Individuals with conditions such as pneumonia, aspiration, near-drowning, and smoke inhalation or a systemic insult such as sepsis, multiple trauma, or burns are susceptible to triggering this process. All of these clinical scenarios activate an inflammatory response that causes alveolocapillary injury. ARDS accounts for approximately 10% of total patient days and one third of all deaths in pediatric intensive care units. The overall mortality in children is less than that experienced by the adult population but can be as high as 40%, depending on age and associated conditions and complications.[125] Children younger than 5 years appear to have diminished mortality compared with those older than 5 years of age. Children with underlying disease processes, such as Down syndrome,[126] systemic lupus erythematosus, and those who have undergone lung transplantation have decreased survival. Genetic predisposition to developing ARDS has been documented in adults; however, this is less well characterized in the pediatric population.[127]

PATHOPHYSIOLOGY The hallmark of ARDS is lung inflammation. Destruction of the capillary-alveolar unit leads to activation of a number of systems and mediators (Figure 34-16), including complement, cytokines, arachidonic acid metabolites, platelet-activating factor, reactive oxygen species, and others (specifically TNF, interferon-alpha, and lipopolysaccharide).[128] Sources of these mediators include neutrophils,

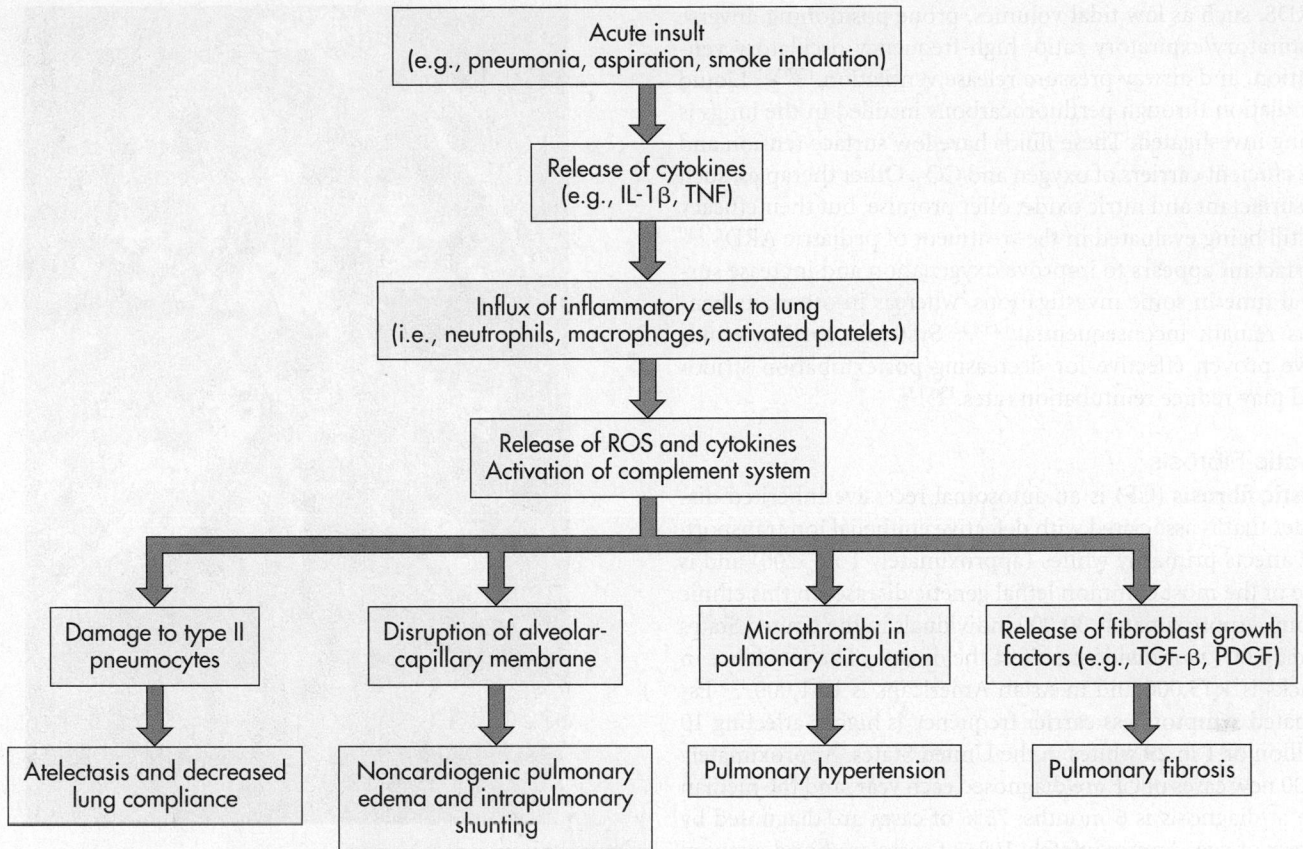

Figure 34-16 Proposed mechanisms for the pathogenesis of acute respiratory distress syndrome (ARDS). *IL-1β*, Interleukin-1β; *PDGF*, platelet-derived growth factor; *ROS*, reactive oxygen species; *TGF-β*, transforming growth factor-beta; *TNF*, tumor necrosis factor. (From Soubani AO, Pieroni R: *South Med J* 92[5]:452, 1999.)

activated platelets, macrophages, and injured endothelium. Early, during the *inflammatory* or *exudative phase* of ARDS, there is pulmonary neutrophil influx along with intraluminal fibrin and platelet aggregation. Injury to the endothelial barriers results in capillary leak and noncardiogenic pulmonary edema. The presence of inflammatory mediators and edema fluid in the alveoli inactivates surfactant, contributing further to alveolar collapse.[125] This fluid also has procoagulant activity, leading to fibrin clotting within air spaces. Similarly, the pulmonary microcirculation is compromised by the formation of thrombi composed of fibrin, platelets, and leukocytes.

The early accumulation of edema fluid in the air spaces results in decreased lung compliance, decreased functional residual volume, and increased dead space. Ventilation-perfusion mismatching, intrapulmonary shunting, and hypoxemia occur. Diffuse pulmonary thrombosis contributes further to the formation of pulmonary edema by increasing capillary hydrostatic pressure and may lead to pulmonary hypertension.

In the *fibroproliferative phase*, type II alveolar cells proliferate, and there is alveolar septal thickening and collagen deposition. Interstitial fibrosis can be evident as early as 10 days after the initial insult. Similarly, vascular changes may occur, including obliteration of the microcirculation and thickening

of the walls of pulmonary arterioles and arteries, which can lead to chronic pulmonary hypertension in survivors.

CLINICAL MANIFESTATIONS ARDS develops acutely after the initial insult, usually within 24 hours (although occasionally it is delayed up to a few days). There is progressive respiratory distress and severe hypoxemia with poor response to oxygen supplementation. Initially, hyperventilation occurs, but CO_2 retention may ultimately develop because of inadequate functional air space, atelectasis, decreased pulmonary compliance, and respiratory muscle fatigue. Severity of the clinical course is modified by comorbid factors, such as the presence of sepsis or multisystem organ failure, and whether complications develop, such as nosocomial pneumonia.

EVALUATION AND TREATMENT Treatment of ARDS remains supportive in nature. Any underlying condition, such as sepsis, must be treated. The goals of therapy are to preserve and restore oxygen delivery, minimize acute lung injury, and decrease mortality by avoiding iatrogenic pulmonary complications. Most individuals with ARDS require mechanical ventilation and often high levels of positive end-expiratory pressure to promote alveolar recruitment, stabilization, and redistribution of alveolar edema fluid into the interstitium. Various ventilation strategies may be used for

ARDS, such as low tidal volumes, prone positioning, inverse inspiratory/expiratory ratio, high-frequency oscillatory ventilation, and airway pressure release ventilation.[129-131] Liquid ventilation through perfluorocarbons instilled in the lungs is being investigated. These fluids have low surface tension and are efficient carriers of oxygen and CO_2. Other therapies, such as surfactant and nitric oxide, offer promise, but their efficacy is still being evaluated in the treatment of pediatric ARDS.[130] Surfactant appears to improve oxygenation and increase survival time in some investigations, whereas in others its benefits remain inconsequential.[125,132] Systemic corticosteroids have proven effective for decreasing postextubation stridor and may reduce reintubation rates.[130,131]

Cystic Fibrosis

Cystic fibrosis (CF) is an autosomal recessive inherited disorder that is associated with defective epithelial ion transport. CF affects primarily whites (approximately 1 in 3200) and is one of the most common lethal genetic diseases in this ethnic group. Approximately 30,000 individuals in the United States and 70,000 worldwide manifest the disease. The incidence in blacks is 1:15,000 and in Asian Americans is 1:31,000.[133] Estimated symptomless carrier frequency is higher affecting 10 million or 1 in 29 whites in the United States. Approximately 1000 new cases of CF are diagnosed each year, and the median age at diagnosis is 6 months; 75% of cases are diagnosed by 1 year of age. Approximately 10% of cases are not diagnosed until after age 10; however, these cases usually have milder symptoms. The median age of survival in the United States is 36.5 years of age (2005 data).[133]

PATHOPHYSIOLOGY On a simplistic level, CF is characterized by abnormal secretions that cause obstructive problems within the respiratory, digestive, and reproductive tracts. However, research suggests that there may be additional CF-associated primary defects, such as an intrinsic proinflammatory state and abnormal local immune defenses in the lungs. The CF gene *(CFTR)* has been located on chromosome 7. Its mutation results in the abnormal expression of **cystic fibrosis transmembrane conductance regulator (CFTCR) protein,** which is a cyclic adenosine monophosphate (cAMP)–activated chloride channel present on the surface of many types of epithelial cells, including those lining airways, bile ducts, pancreas, sweat ducts, and vas deferens. Despite knowing that chloride transport is a fundamental abnormality, the exact disease mechanisms in CF have still not been clearly defined at the cellular and end-organ levels.

Although CF is a multiorgan disease, the lungs are the most critical site of involvement, and respiratory failure is almost always the cause of death. The typical features of CF lung disease are mucous plugging, chronic inflammation, and infection. The abnormalities primarily involve the airways, with progressive bronchiectasis that becomes widespread. Parenchymal involvement occurs much later and includes microabscess formation, patchy consolidation and pneumonia, peribronchial fibrosis, and cyst formation (Figure 34-17). The pathophysiology for these changes is outlined in a simplified

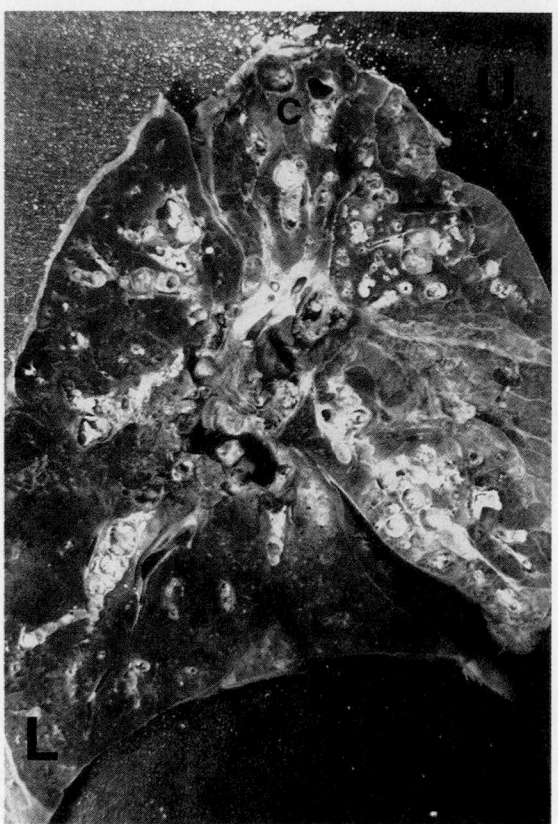

Figure 34-17 Pathology of the lung in end-stage cystic fibrosis. Key features are widespread mucus impaction of airways and bronchiectasis (especially in upper lobe, *U*), with hemorrhagic pneumonia in the lower lobe *(L)*. Small cysts *(C)* are present at the apex of the lung. (From Kleinerman J, Vauthy P: *Pathology of the lung in cystic fibrosis,* Atlanta, 1976, Cystic Fibrosis Foundation.)

form in Figure 34-18. Peripheral bullae may develop because of obstruction and airway wall weakening, and pneumothorax can occur. Hemoptysis, sometimes life threatening, may occur because of erosion of enlarged bronchial arteries that develop in response to the inflammation associated with bronchiectasis. Over a long period of time, pulmonary vascular remodeling occurs because of localized hypoxia and arteriolar vasoconstriction; pulmonary hypertension and cor pulmonale may develop with end-stage disease.

The mucus plugging seen in CF probably results from the combination of increased production of mucus, altered physicochemical properties of the mucus, and reduced mucociliary clearance.[134] Mucus-secreting airway cells (goblet cells and submucosal glands) are increased in number and size. Dysregulation of the airway epithelial sodium channel (ENaC) causes abnormal chloride secretion and exaggerated sodium absorption, resulting in depletion of the airway surface liquid volume and therefore dehydration of airway mucus.[135] This appears to facilitate mucus adherence to the epithelium, subsequent impairment of ciliary mobility, and retention of bacteria that can then form biofilms. Finally, after secretion, CF mucus becomes even more viscous because of deoxyribonucleic acid (DNA) and filamentous (F) actin released from

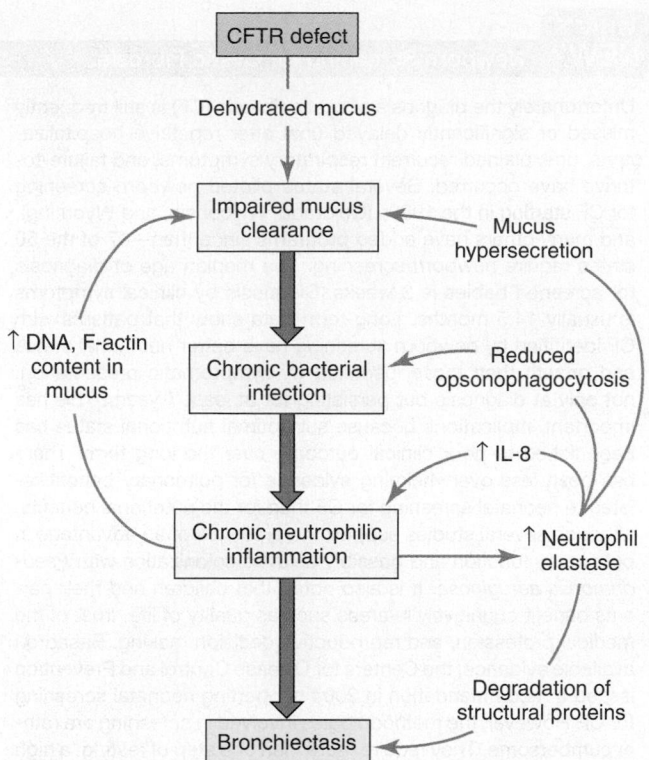

Figure 34-18 Pathogenesis of cystic fibrosis lung disease. *CFTR*, Cystic fibrosis transmembrane conductance regulator; *IL-8*, interleukin-8.

degraded neutrophils, which are present in very high numbers in CF airways.

Chronic, intense neutrophil-dominated inflammation occurs in CF airways, and plays a critical role in long-term damage.[136] Abnormal cytokine profiles have been documented in CF airway fluids, including deficient IL-10 and excessive IL-1, IL-8, and TNF-α, all changes conducive to promoting inflammation. Neutrophils are present in great excess in CF airways and release damaging oxidants, such as myeloperoxidase[136] and proteases in massive amounts that overwhelm local antiprotease defenses. One protease in particular, *neutrophil elastase,* has the following detrimental effects: (1) direct damage to lung structural proteins, such as elastin; (2) induction of airway cells to produce IL-8, a strong attractant for neutrophils and thus a means for augmenting a local "vicious cycle" of inflammation; (3) destruction of IgG and complement components important for opsonization and phagocytosis of pathogens; and (4) direct stimulation of mucus secretion by mucus-producing cells. Other contributors to CF pathogenesis are being explored including errant epithelial oxidant defense with exposure to airborne bacteria, major vault protein migration with pseudomonas infection, and antiprotease activity relating to the inflammatory process.[137]

Children with CF have a propensity for chronic endobronchial infection that remains poorly understood. It is likely that local factors in the CF airway microenvironment favor bacterial colonization because no systemic immune defect has been found. *Staphylococcus aureus* is common, and *Pseudomonas*

aeruginosa ultimately colonizes airways in 75% of children with CF. Infecting colonies of *Pseudomonas* appear to adopt a mucoid phenotype and organize themselves into adherent biofilms, making it difficult for antibiotics and local defenses to reach them. *Pseudomonas* acquisition has been linked with more rapid decline in pulmonary function.[138] Persistence of infection incites chronic local inflammation, airway damage, bronchiectasis, microabscess formation, and foci of hemorrhagic pneumonia. New evidence suggests that anaerobes present in the CF lung may contribute to the cycle of infection and ongoing inflammation. The amount of smooth muscle present in the airway in this group of children, increased from normal, is also a contributor to the chronic inflammatory process.[139,140]

CLINICAL MANIFESTATIONS The most common manifestations are respiratory and gastrointestinal, including the pancreas and biliary tract. Respiratory symptoms at presentation may include persistent (but not necessarily severe) cough or wheeze, sputum production, and recurrent or severe pneumonia. More subtle respiratory tract presentations of CF include chronic sinusitis and nasal polyps. With appropriate treatment, cough, sputum production, and exercise limitation do not usually reach debilitating levels during childhood. Digital clubbing may appear quite early and in the absence of significant pulmonary impairment. Development of barrel chest or persistent crackles occurs much later in the course of the disease.

Classic gastrointestinal manifestations include meconium ileus at birth, which is almost pathognomonic for CF. Approximately 15% to 20% of individuals with CF present with this. Another classic presentation is failure to thrive and malabsorptive symptoms, such as frequent loose and oily stools. Metabolic abnormalities, trace element deficiencies, fat-soluble vitamin alterations, and electrolyte imbalances may occur early in the course of disease.[137] Rectal prolapse is an occasional presenting sign that should always prompt testing for CF. About 10% of CF patients do not experience gastrointestinal problems and are termed "pancreatic sufficient." Several specific *CFTR* mutations are predictive of this milder phenotype. Males with CF are typically infertile (98%). Other complications of CF may include liver disease (approximately 5%), diabetes mellitus (10% to 25%), and decreased bone mineral density as early as preschool age.[137]

Overall severity of CF lung disease is highly variable. Even affected siblings may have disparate courses despite identical *CFTR* mutations, environment, and treatment strategy. We now know that some genetic variants significantly influence survival among children with the same mutations.[133] Mutations in the *CFTR* gene have been classified based on the type of defect. Classes 1 through 3 are associated with more severe disease and 4 and 5 with milder pulmonary disease (generally pancreatic sufficient). Mortality rates correlate respectively with the classes noted above. Researchers continue to explore identification of "gene modifiers," other than *CFTR*, that may serve to lessen or aggravate the degree of CF lung disease and increase or decrease the risk of developing other CF complications, such as severe liver disease.[141] Other variables that have long been associated with decline in pulmonary status for those with CF and, thus earlier demise, include colonization with *P. aeruginosa*, female sex, and poor nutritional status.[142]

EVALUATION AND TREATMENT The standard method of diagnosis has been the sweat test, which will reveal sweat chloride concentration in excess of 60 mEq/L. Genotyping for CFTR mutations is also available as an alternative or supplemental method but may fail to confirm up to 10% of cases because of a lack of ability to screen for every described CF-associated mutation. There are more than 1500 specific mutations, but most standard laboratory panels include fewer than 100 mutations.[133] Newborn screening for CF is currently mandated in 32 of the 50 states in the United States and will continue to expand, on a voluntary, state-by-state basis subsequent to recent recommendations developed by the Centers for Disease Control and Prevention (CDC) and an advisory panel of CF experts[143] (see What's New? Newborn Screening for Cystic Fibrosis).

Treatment is primarily focused on pulmonary health and nutrition. Because the pulmonary decline in CF is slow and insidious, and because of the early onset of chronic inflammation and infection, treatment strategies begin immediately at diagnosis and are modified over time as disease progresses. Pulmonary therapies include techniques to promote mucus clearance, such as chest physical therapy and related equipment (such as the high-frequency chest wall oscillation vest) and an assortment of handheld positive expiratory pressure (PEP) devices. Aerosol therapy includes bronchodilators and nebulized deoxyribonuclease (DNase), which acts to liquefy mucus and may even have anti-inflammatory effects.[144] Antibiotic practices vary, with prophylactic and treatment strategies being used. Increasing emphasis has been placed on delaying and controlling *Pseudomonas* colonization, such as the maintenance use of inhaled antibiotics.[145] Macrolide antibiotics, such as azithromycin, have been reported to improve pulmonary function through improvement in the airway inflammation process.[136] Hypertonic saline also has proven beneficial to improve airway surface water, thus improving mucus viscosity.[146] Ibuprofen has been shown to improve lung function in several clinical trials.[137,147] Intravenous antibiotics are used to treat major exacerbations of pulmonary infection, which may be either subacute or acute. Individuals with end-stage lung disease may consider double lung transplant as a life-lengthening measure.[148]

Nutritional problems are extremely common in CF, and poor nutrition is correlated with worse outcomes including progression of lung disease and onset of additional complications such as decreased bone mineral density.[149] Elements of aggressive nutritional support include meticulous monitoring of growth parameters, controlling fat malabsorption, ensuring adequate caloric intake, and keeping overall health stable. Approximately 90% of children with CF have pancreatic insufficiency. This is the result of abnormal ion transport causing decreased fluid and bicarbonate secretion from the pancreatic acinar cells, which leads to thickened secretions plugging the smaller pancreatic ducts, and eventual autodigestion or

atrophy of the acinar cells. Therefore, patients must take exogenous pancreatic enzymes with meals and snacks in order to absorb nutrients and control malabsorptive symptoms. Fat-soluble vitamins (A, D, E, and K) must be supplemented. Caloric needs are high, especially with advancing lung disease, and high-calorie supplements or even gastrostomy feeding may be warranted.

Future treatments for CF in trial phases are aimed at improving inhaled antibiotic therapy (duramycin, denufosol and dry powder tobramycin), a vaccine against *Pseudomonas*, and the use of growth hormone. Gene transfer and stem cell therapies also are being investigated.[150]

There is a growing contingent of adults with CF living into their 40s and 50s. Care for these individuals shifts away from a pediatric focus because their care needs are unique and often extremely complex. Challenges noted in this specialty area are

---

WHAT'S NEW?   Newborn Screening for Cystic Fibrosis

Unfortunately the diagnosis of cystic fibrosis (CF) is still frequently missed or significantly delayed until after repetitive hospitalizations, unexplained recurrent respiratory symptoms, and failure-to-thrive have occurred. Several states piloted newborn screening for CF starting in the 1980s (Colorado, Wisconsin, and Wyoming), and many others have added programs since then—47 of the 50 states require newborn screening. The median age of diagnosis for screened babies is 2 weeks. Diagnosis by clinical symptoms is usually 14.5 months. Long-term data show that patients with CF identified by newborn screening have better nutritional status and growth than those identified by symptomatic presentation, not only at diagnosis but persisting for at least 7 years. This has important implications because suboptimal nutritional status has been linked to poor clinical outcome over the long term. There has been less overwhelming evidence for pulmonary benefit related to neonatal screening for CF than for the nutritional benefits, although several studies support the presence of an advantage in pulmonary function and possibly delayed colonization with *Pseudomonas aeruginosa*. It is also noted that children and their parents benefit cognitively in areas such as quality of life, trust of the medical profession, and reproductive decision making. Based on available evidence, the Centers for Disease Control and Prevention issued a recommendation in 2004 supporting neonatal screening for CF. However, the methodologies involved in screening are rather cumbersome. They require more than one step of testing, a high level of support from CF centers and genetic counseling professionals, and education of primary physicians and the community. Difficult problems include handling initial false positives, ensuring appropriate information for those with select "mild" mutations that are not well understood, and making sure that the many CF gene carriers that will be identified do not misunderstand their status. States choosing to adopt screening will have to tailor the details of their programs to match available resources statewide.

Data from Balfour-Lynn I: *Arch Dis Child* 93(1):7-10, 2008; Castellani C: *Paediatr Respir Rev* 4(4):278-284, 2003; Centers for Disease Control and Prevention: *MMWR Morb Moral Wkly Rep* 53(RR-13): 1-36, 2004; Farrell PM et al: *Am J Respir Crit Care Med* 168(9):1100-1108, 2003; Farrell PM et al: *Pediatrics* 107(1):1-13, 2001; Lai HJ et al: *Am J Epidemiol* 159(6):537-546, 2004; Wang SS et al: *J Pediatr* 141(6):804-810, 2002; Cystic Fibrosis Foundation: Newborn screening for cystic fibrosis, 2009.

pregnancy and details about balancing disease management and adult life issues.

SUDDEN INFANT DEATH SYNDROME

Sudden infant death syndrome (SIDS) remains a disease of unknown cause and is the most common cause of unexplained infant death in Western countries.[151,152] It is defined as "sudden death of an infant under 1 year of age which remains unexplained after a thorough case investigation, including performance of a complete autopsy, examination of the death scene, and review of the clinical history."[152]

The incidence of SIDS is low during the first month of life but sharply increases in the second month of life, peaks at 2 to 4 months old, and is unusual after 6 months of age. The incidence of SIDS in the United States is 0.57 per 1000 live births.[153] It is more common in male (60%) than female (40%) infants. It almost always occurs during nighttime sleep, when infants are least likely to be observed. A seasonal variation has been noted, with higher frequencies during the winter months. This has been related to a higher rate of respiratory tract infection during those months, and such infections are often reported to have preceded the death, leading to speculation regarding etiology.

Clinical risk groups include babies who were preterm or low birth weight, multiple births, and siblings of prior SIDS victims (fourfold to sixfold increased risk). SIDS is more prevalent among infants of low or adverse socioeconomic status and occurs more frequently when family size is larger.[154] Nevertheless, about three quarters of all SIDS victims have no known predisposing clinical risk factor. Maternal factors that predict increased SIDS risk are maternal smoking, young maternal age (younger than 20 years), unmarried mother, less prenatal care, poverty, and illicit drug use or binge-drinking. Risk factors that relate to the baby's sleeping situation are prone positioning (and to a lesser extent, side sleeping), sleeping on soft bedding, and overheating. Prone sleeping was concluded to be a major and modifiable risk factor. Epidemiologic studies have shown that SIDS rates decreased by 50% to 90% in countries, including the United States, where massive public campaigns warned against prone sleeping for infants.[151-153] Other avoidable risk factors include loose bedding materials and sleeping on top of any soft surface (such as sheepskins, quilts, comforters, pillows, adult-type mattresses, or waterbeds). Bed sharing with parents increases risk in some situations.[155] Overwrapping the infant or overheating the room also appear to increase risk, particularly if the infant is sleeping prone.

The etiology of SIDS remains unknown, but probably involves a combination of predisposing factors along with external stressors.[151,154] There has been long-standing interest in hypotheses involving impaired autonomic regulation and failure of cardiovascular, ventilatory, and arousal responses to hypoxemia or hypercarbia, or to airway obstruction events.[156] This blunted responsiveness could be related to developmental immaturity, or may be inducible by external factors such as exposure to maternal smoking or recent infection.[157] Infection may be linked to SIDS on the basis of exaggerated inflammation, eosinophil degranulation, and massive cytokine release, causing pulmonary or airway edema in response to either bacterial pathogens from the nasopharynx or viral respiratory tract infections. Finally, there is growing evidence that genetic factors may predispose certain individuals to SIDS.[158] A number of candidate gene polymorphisms (16) have been proposed based on epidemiologic evidence, including defects in sodium and potassium cardiac ion channels; *5-HTT,* the serotonin transporter gene; and genes linked with the autonomic nervous system.[159] The complement components make up the many other gene polymorphisms: C4A and B, IL-6, IL-10, and vascular endothelial growth factor.[154,159] One study has also revealed a reduction in surfactant protein A (SP-A) expression in the first months after birth, which correlates with the peak age of SIDS.[160] Although still being elucidated, the responsiveness of the immune and inflammatory systems appears to be a causal mechanism to increased rates of SIDS.[159]

Currently, the best strategy to reduce SIDS is avoidance of all the controllable risk factors, particularly unsafe sleeping practices and maternal smoking. Parents of infants with clinical risk should be taught cardiopulmonary resuscitation as a precaution. Although home monitoring has not been proven to decrease the incidence of SIDS, some at-risk infants may warrant cardiorespiratory monitoring after careful consideration of the individual situation.[152] A number of challenges continue to face healthcare providers in continuing to lower the SIDS rate. There is a lack of testing available to identify and stratify the risk of SIDS and no universally accepted or proven intervention. Recent studies have shown that the epidemiology of this health issue is changing and that perhaps combined with the newer knowledge linking genetics to sudden infant death, identified risk factors can be used more effectively.[161]

SUMMARY REVIEW

Structure and Function

1. The airways of infants and children are narrower than those of adults, thus making them more prone to obstruction.
2. Infants and young children continue to form new alveoli for several years after birth.
3. Surfactant production is an important marker of developmental maturity of the fetal lung.
4. The immature chest wall is soft and compliant, contributing to inefficient mechanisms of breathing.
5. Children have greater oxygen consumption than adults.
6. Immune mechanisms are not fully developed at birth, making young infants more susceptible to infection.
7. Physiologic control of breathing may be impaired during the first few weeks of life.

SUMMARY REVIEW—cont'd

Pulmonary Disorders

1. Physical examination can provide important clues in assessing the location and nature of UAO.
2. Upper airway infections can pose serious threats, including bacterial tracheitis, retropharyngeal abscess, and peritonsillar infections. Recognition and rapid evaluation are crucial.
3. Viral croup (laryngotracheobronchitis) is the most common cause of acute upper airway obstruction in children and usually affects children ages 6 months to 5 years. Subglottic edema may be mild to severe. Parainfluenza is the most common cause.
4. Acute epiglottitis is a life-threatening emergency that is now rarely seen because of vaccination against *H. influenzae,* which had been the primary causative microorganism. Current cases usually represent vaccine failure or are caused by other bacteria, such as group A streptococci.
5. Aspiration of a foreign body should be considered whenever there is a sudden onset of stridor, coughing, wheezing, or hoarseness. This usually occurs in 1- to 3-year-olds. Occasionally diagnosis is delayed and symptoms may be attributed to asthma, bronchitis, or pneumonia without recognition of the underlying cause.
6. Chronic UAO may be manifested by stridor, abnormal cry, wheezing, or dyspnea. The most common cause of stridor in infants is laryngomalacia. Other causes include subglottic stenosis, vocal cord paralysis, and vascular rings.
7. Obstructive sleep apnea usually occurs in older children rather than infants and is underdiagnosed. Typical symptoms are snoring, gasping, and restless sleep. The most common cause in children is adenotonsillar hypertrophy.
8. RDS of the newborn usually occurs in premature infants who are born before surfactant production and alveolocapillary development are complete. Atelectasis and hypoventilation cause shunting, hypoxemia, and hypercapnia.
9. BPD is a chronic lung disease of infancy that is usually the consequence of acute respiratory disease in the newborn period. Almost always this occurs in infants who were premature and required ventilatory support. Contributing factors include structural immaturity, inflammation, and disordered lung repair processes.
10. Bronchiolitis occurs in infants and toddlers, usually in the winter and early spring. It is caused by viruses, most commonly RSV. There is extensive edema, inflammation, and damage to the bronchiolar epithelium. Injections of monoclonal antibody against RSV are recommended as a preventive measure for high-risk infants.
11. Childhood pneumonia can be caused by viruses, bacteria, or *Mycoplasma.* Lobar pneumonia is usually bacterial. Certain bacteria, such as *S. aureus* and group A streptococci, can cause particularly fulminant disease, as well as abscesses and empyema.
12. Aspiration pneumonitis can occur because of lung inflammation from entry of any foreign substance, including food, drink, or chemicals. Aspiration of oropharyngeal bacteria can occur because of loss of protective reflexes in neurologically impaired children, or during anesthesia.
13. ARDS is an acute life-threatening condition characterized by severe hypoxemia, poor lung compliance, and diffuse densities on chest radiograph. It can be triggered by acute pulmonary insults or major systemic illness (e.g., sepsis) or trauma. High-level ventilatory support is required, and mortality is significant.
14. Asthma is an obstructive airway disease with episodes of acute respiratory symptoms (cough, wheeze, dyspnea) and intermittent or chronic subacute symptoms. It is the most common chronic condition in children. It is a disease of local airway inflammation, with exacerbation in response to triggers, such as infections or allergens. Inflammatory cell infiltration, mucosal edema, mucus plugging of airways, and epithelial damage are seen, and there is evidence of long-term remodeling of airways.
15. CF is an autosomal recessive disease characterized by thick, tenacious mucus, plugging of airways, chronic pulmonary infection, and bronchiectasis. The other major manifestations are digestive and nutritional, related to pancreatic insufficiency. Median survival is currently 36.5 years, with mortality primarily related to lung disease.

Sudden Infant Death Syndrome

1. SIDS is a diagnosis of exclusion after thorough investigation and autopsy following sudden death of an infant less than 6 months of age. Usually the event occurs during nighttime sleep.
2. The cause is unknown. However, some known risk factors are avoidable, such as maternal smoking, prone sleeping, soft bedding surfaces, and overheating. The incidence of SIDS has decreased significantly since public health campaigns have encouraged the supine sleeping position for babies.

KEY TERMS

Acute epiglottitis, 1317

Acute respiratory distress syndrome (ARDS), 1334

Angioedema, 1318

Aspiration pneumonitis, 1329

Asthma, 1330

Atypical pneumonia, 1329

Bacterial pneumonia, 1327

Bacterial tracheitis, 1315

Bronchiolitis, 1326

Bronchiolitis obliterans (BO), 1330

Bronchopulmonary dysplasia (BPD), 1323

Community-acquired pneumonia (CAP), 1327

Croup, 1316

Cystic fibrosis (CF), 1336

Cystic fibrosis transmembrane conductance regulator (CFTCR) protein, 1336

Diphtheria, 1316

Foreign body aspiration, 1317

Functional residual capacity (FRC), 1312

Hyaline membrane disease (HMD), 1321

Laryngomalacia, 1319

Laryngotracheobronchitis, 1316

Obstructive sleep apnea syndrome (OSAS), 1320

Peritonsillar abscess, 1316

Pneumonia, 1327

Respiratory distress syndrome (RDS) of the newborn, 1321

Retropharyngeal abscess, 1316

Spasmodic croup, 1316

Status asthmaticus, 1333

Stridor, 1314

Subglottic stenosis, 1318

Sudden infant death syndrome (SIDS), 1339

Surfactant, 1311

Tracheomalacia (tracheobronchomalacia), 1319

Upper airway obstruction (UAO), 1313

Viral pneumonia, 1328

REFERENCES

1. Graf J, Stein F: Tracheitis in pediatric patients, *Sem Pediatric Infect Dis* 17:11-13, 2006.
2. Hopkins A et al: Changing epidemiology of life-threatening upper airway infections: the reemergence of bacterial tracheitis, *Pediatrics* 118(4):1418-1421, 2006.
3. Abdel-Haq N et al: Retropharyngeal abscess in children: the emerging role of group A beta hemolytic streptococcus, *South Med J* 99(9):927-931, 2006.
4. Ochoa T et al: Community-associated methicillin-resistant *Staphylococcus aureus* in pediatric patients, *Emerg Infect Dis* 11(6):966-968, 2005.
5. Ossowski K et al: Increased isolation of methicillin-resistant *Staphylococcus aureus* in pediatric head and neck abscesses, *Arch Otolaryngol Head Neck Surg* 132:1176-1181, 2006.
6. Hammer J: Acquired upper airway obstruction, *Paediatr Respir Rev* 5(1):25-33, 2004.
7. Cabrera C et al: Increased incidence of head and neck abscesses in children, *Otolaryngol Head Neck Surg* 136:176-181, 2007.
8. Brooke I: Microbiology and management of peritonsillar, retropharyngeal, and parapharyngeal abscesses, *J Oral Maxillofac Surg* 62(12):1545-1550, 2004.
9. Sobol SE, Zapata S: Epiglottitis and croup, *Otolaryngol Clin North Am* 41(3):551-566, ix, 2008.
10. Fitzgerald D: The assessment and management of croup, *Paediatr Respir Rev* 7:73-81, 2006.
11. Bjornson B et al: A randomized trial of a single dose of oral dexamethasone for mild croup, *N Engl J Med* 351:1306-1313, 2004.
12. Glynn F, Fenton J: Diagnosis and management of supraglottitis (epiglottitis), *Curr Infect Dis Rep* 10:200-204, 2008.
13. Alcaide M, Bisno A: Pharyngitis and epiglottitis, *Infect Dis Clin North Am* 21:449-469, 2007.
14. Kay M, Wyllie R: Pediatric foreign bodies and their management, *Curr Gastroenterol Rep* 7(3):212-218, 2005.
15. Lea E et al: Diagnostic evaluation of foreign body aspiration in children: a prospective study, *J Pediatr Surg* 40(7):1122-1127, 2005.
16. Chiu C et al: Factors predicting early diagnosis of foreign body aspiration in children, *Pediatr Emerg Care* 21(3):161-164, 2005.
17. Farkas H: Management of hereditary angioedema in pediatric patients, *Pediatrics* 120(3):e713-e722, 2007.
18. Zuran BL: Current and future therapy for hereditary angioedema, *Clin Immunol* 114(1):10-16, 2005.
19. Bracho FA: Hereditary angioedema, *Curr Opin Hematol* 12(6):493-498, 2005.
20. Frank MM: Hereditary angioedema, *J Allergy Clin Immunol* 121(2 Suppl):S398-S401, 2008.
21. Daniel S: The upper airway: congenital malformations, *Paediatr Respir Rev* 7S:S260-S263, 2006.
22. Alvarez-Neri H et al: Primary cricotracheal resection with thyrotracheal anastomosis for the treatment of severe subglottic stenosis in children and adolescents, *Ann Otol Rhinol Laryngol* 114(1 pt 1):2-6, 2005.
23. Dauer EH et al: Airway manifestations of pediatric eosinophilic esophagitis: a clinical and histopathologic report of an emerging association, *Ann Otol Rhinol Laryngol* 155(7):507-517, 2006.
24. Erickson VR, Hwang PH: Wegener's granulomatosis: current trends in diagnosis and management, *Curr Opin Otolaryngol Head Neck Surg* 15(3):170-176, 2007.
25. Khariwala S, Lee W, Koltai P: Laryngotracheal consequences of pediatric cardiac surgery, *Arch Otolaryngol Head Neck Surg* 131(4):336-339, 2005.
26. Sidman J, Jaguan A, Couser R: Tracheotomy and decannulation rates in a level 3 neonatal intensive care unit: a 12 year study, *Laryngoscope* 116:136-139, 2006.
27. Bluestone C: Humans are born too soon: impact on pediatric otolaryngology, *Int J Pediatr Otorhinolaryngol* 69:1-8, 2005.
28. Hueman E, Simpson B: Airway complications from topical mitomycin C, *Otolaryngol Head Neck* 133(6):831-835, 2005.
29. Smith JL et al: State-dependent laryngomalacia in sleeping children, *Ann Otol Rhinol Laryngol* 114(2):111-114, 2005.
30. Thompson DM: Abnormal sensorimotor integrative function of the larynx in congenital laryngomalacia: a new theory of etiology, *Laryngoscope* 117(6 pt 2 Suppl 114):1-33, 2007.
31. Richter G et al: Late-onset laryngomalacia, *Arch Otolaryngol Head Neck Surg* 134(1):75-80, 2008.
32. Weinberger M, Abu-Hasan M: Pseudo-asthma: when cough, wheezing and dyspnea are not asthma, *Pediatrics* 120(4):855-864, 2007.
33. Masters I et al: Quantified tracheobronchomalacia disorders and their clinical profiles in children, *Chest* 133(2):461-467, 2008.
34. Ishman S et al: Management of vocal paralysis: a comparison of adult and pediatric practices, *Otolaryngol Head Neck Surg* 135:590-594, 2006.
35. Doshi D, Weinberger M: Long-term outcome of vocal chord dysfunction, *Ann Allergy Asthma Immunol* 96:794-799, 2006.
36. McLaren C, Elliott M, Roebuck D: Vascular compression of the airway in children, *Paediatr Respir Rev* 9:85-94, 2008.
37. Tarasuik A et al: Elevated morbidity and health care use in children with obstructive sleep apnea syndrome, *Am J Respir Crit Care Med* 175:55-61, 2007.
38. Ievers-Landis C, Redline S: Pediatric sleep apnea, *Am J Respir Crit Care Med* 175:436-441, 2007.
39. Arens R, Marcus CL: Pathophysiology of upper airway obstruction: a developmental perspective, *Sleep* 27(5):997-1019, 2004.
40. Goldbart A et al: Inflammatory mediators in exhaled breath condensate of children with obstructive sleep apnea syndrome, *Chest* 130:143-148, 2006.
41. Fauroux B, Aubertin G, Clement A: What's new in paediatric sleep in 2007? *Paediatr Respir Rev* 9:139-143, 2008.
42. Leung L et al: Twenty-four-hour ambulatory BP in snoring children with obstructive sleep apnea syndrome, *Chest* 130:1009-1017, 2006.
43. American Academy of Pediatrics: Clinical practice guidelines: diagnosis and management of childhood obstructive sleep apnea, *Pediatrics* 109(4):704-712, 2002.
44. Gozal D, O'Brien LM: Snoring and obstructive sleep apnoea in children: why should we treat? *Paediatr Respir Rev* 5(Suppl A):S371-S376, 2004.
45. Rosen CL: Obstructive sleep apnea syndrome in children: controversies in diagnosis and treatment, *Pediatr Clin North Am* 51(1):153-167, vii, 2004.
46. Ray M, Bower C: Pediatric obstructive sleep apnea: the year in review, *Curr Opin Otolaryngol Head Neck Surg* 13(6):360-365, 2005.
47. Tran K et al: Child behavior and quality of life in pediatric obstructive sleep apnea, *Arch Otolaryngol Head Neck Surg* 131(1):52-57, 2005.
48. Fraser J, Walls M, McGuire W: Respiratory complications of preterm birth, *Br Med J* 329:962-965, 2004.
49. Dalziel S et al: Long term effects of antenatal betamethasone on lung function: 30 year follow up of a randomised controlled trial, *Thorax* 61:678-683, 2006.
50. American Heart Association (AHA): Guidelines for cardiopulmonary resuscitation (CPR) and emergency cardiovascular care (ECC) of pediatric and neonatal patients: neonatal resuscitation guidelines (2005), *Pediatrics,* 117(5):e1029-e1038, 2005.
51. Sweet D et al: European consensus guidelines on the management of neonatal respiratory distress syndrome, *J Perinatal Med* 35:175-186, 2007.
52. NIH Consensus Development Conference Statement: Effect of corticosteroids for fetal maturation on perinatal outcomes, *Am J Obstet Gynecol* 173:246, 1995.
53. Mazela J, Merritt T, Finer N: Aerolsized surfactants, *Curr Opin Pediatr* 19:155-162, 2007.
54. Engle W: Committee on Fetus and Newborn: Surfactant-replacement therapy for respiratory distress in the preterm and term neonate, *Pediatrics,* 121(2):419-432, 2008.
55. Howlett A, Ohlsson A: Inositol for respiratory distress syndrome in preterm infants, *Cochrane Database Syst Rev* (4):CD000366, 2005.
56. Shah S: Is elective high frequency oscillatory ventilation better than conventional mechanical ventilation in very low birth weight infants? *Arch Dis Child* 88(9):833-834, 2003.
57. Firer NN, Barrington KJ: Nitric oxide for respiratory failure in infants born at or near term, *Cochrane Database Syst Rev* :CD000399, (1), 2005.
58. Kinsella J et al: Early inhaled nitric oxide therapy in premature newborns with respiratory failure, *N Engl J Med* 355(4):354-364, 2006.
59. Ballard P et al: Plasma biomarkers of oxidative stress: relationship to lung disease and inhaled nitric oxide therapy in premature infants, *Pediatrics* 121(3):555-561, 2008.
60. Doyle L et al: Outcome at 2 years of age of infants from the DART study: a multicenter, international, randomized, controlled trial of low-dose dexamethasone, *Pediatrics* 119(4):716-721, 2007.

61. Asikainen TM, White CW: Pulmonary antioxidant defenses in the preterm newborn with respiratory distress and bronchopulmonary dysplasia in evolution: implications for antioxidant therapy, *Antioxid Redox Signal* 6(1):155-167, 2004.

62. Baier RJ et al: CC chemokine concentrations increase in respiratory distress syndrome and correlate with development of bronchopulmonary dysplasia, *Pediatr Pulmonol* 37(2):137-148, 2004.

63. Jobe AH: Antenatal factors and the development of bronchopulmonary dysplasia, *Semin Neonatol* 8(1):9-17, 2003.

64. Morley C et al: Nasal CPAP or intubation at birth for very preterm infants, *N Engl J Med* 358(14):700-708, 2008.

65. Northway WH Jr, Rosan RC, Porter DY: Pulmonary disease following respiratory therapy of hyaline-membrane disease: bronchopulmonary dysplasia, *N Engl J Med* 276(7):357-368, 1967.

66. Baraldi E, Filippone M: Chronic lung disease after premature birth, *N Engl J Med* 357(19):1946-1955, 2007.

67. Bancalari E, Claure N, Sosenko IRS: Bronchopulmonary dysplasia: changes in pathogenesis, epidemiology, and definition, *Semin Neonatol* 8(1):63-71, 2003.

68. Eichenwald E, Stark A: Management and outcomes of very low birth weight, *N Engl J Med* 358(16):1700-1711, 2008.

69. Mahut B et al: Chest computed tomography findings in bronchopulmonary dysplasia and correlation with lung function, *Arch Dis Child Fetal Neonatal Ed* 92(6):F459-F464, 2007.

70. Vento G et al: Serum levels of seven cytokines in premature ventilated newborns: correlations with old and new forms of bronchopulmonary dysplasia, *Intensive Care Med* 32(5):723-730, 2006.

71. Geary C et al: Decreased incidence of bronchopulmonary dysplasia after early management changes, including surfactant and nasal continuous positive airway pressure treatment at delivery, lowered oxygen saturation coals, and early amino acid administration: a historical cohort study, *Pediatrics*, 121:89-96, 2008.

72. Morley C et al: Nasal CPAP or intubation at birth for very preterm infants, *N Engl J Med* 358(7):700-708, 2008.

73. Ballard PL et al: Plasma biomarkers of oxidative stress: relationship to lung disease and inhaled nitric oxide therapy in premature infants, *Pediatrics*, 121(3):555-561, 2008.

74. Barrington K, Finer N: Inhaled nitric oxide for preterm infants: a systematic review, *Pediatrics* 120:1088-1099, 2007.

75. Bhandari A et al: Effect of a short course of prednisolone in infants with oxygen-dependent bronchopulmonary dysplasia, *Pediatrics* 121:e344-e349, 2008.

76. Kobaly K et al: Outcomes of extremely low birth weight (<1 kg) and extremely low gestational age (<28 weeks) infants with bronchopulmonary dysplasia: effects of practice changes in 2000 to 2003, *Pediatrics* 121:73-81, 2008.

77. Aghai Z et al: Azithromycin suppresses activation of nuclear factor-kappa B and synthesis of pro-inflammatory cytokines in tracheal aspirate cells from premature infants, *Pediatric Res* 62(4):483-488, 2007.

78. Mentro AM: Vitamin A and bronchopulmonary dysplasia: research, issues and related clinical practice, *Neonatal Netw* 23(4):19-21, 2004.

79. Kesson A: Respiratory virus infections, *Paediatr Respir Rev* 8:240-248, 2007.

80. Smyth R, Openshaw P: Bronchiolitis, *Lancet*, 368:312-322, 2006.

81. Piippo-Savolainen E, Korppi M: Wheezy babies—wheezy adults? Review on long-term outcome until adulthood after early childhood wheezing, *Acta Paediatr* 97(1):5-11, 2008.

82. Christakis D et al: Variation in inpatient diagnostic testing and management of bronchiolitis, *Pediatrics* 115(4):878-884, 2005.

83. Martinon-Torres F, Rodriguez-Nunez A, Martinon-Sanchez J: Nasal continuous positive airway pressure with heliox versus air oxygen in infants with acute bronchiolitis: a crossover study, *Pediatrics* 121:E1190-E1195, 2008.

84. Patel H et al: Glucocorticoids for acute viral bronchiolitis in infants and young children, *Cochrane Database Syst Rev* (3):CD004878, 2004.

85. Steiner RW: Treating acute bronchiolitis associated with RSV, *Am Fam Physician* 15(69):325-330, 2004.

86. Flood R, Badik J, Aronoff S: The utility of serum C-reactive protein in differentiating bacterial from nonbacterial pneumonia in children, *Pediatr Infect Dis J* 27(2):95-99, 2008.

87. Atkinson M et al: Comparison of oral amoxicillin and intravenous benzyl penicillin for community acquired pneumonia in children (PIVOT trial): a multicentre pragmatic randomized controlled equivalence trial, *Thorax* 62:1102-1106, 2007.

88. Wolf J, Daly A: Microbiological aspects of bacterial lower respiratory tract illness in children: typical pathogens, *Paediatr Respir Rev* 8:204-211, 2007.

89. Sandora T, Harper M: Pneumonia in hospitalized children, *Pediatr Clin North Am* 52:1059-1081, 2005.

90. Ozcelik C et al: Management of postpneumonic empyemas in children, *Eur J Cardiothorac Surg* 25(6):1072-1078, 2004.

91. Schultz KD et al: The changing face of pleural empyemas in children: epidemiology and management, *Pediatrics* 113(6):1735-1740, 2004.

92. Sinaniotis CA: Viral pneumoniae in children: incidence and aetiology, *Paediatr Respir Rev* 5(Suppl A):S197-S200, 2004.

93. Moreno L et al: Development and validation of a clinical predication rule to distinguish bacterial from viral pneumonia in children, *Pediatr Pulmonol* 41:331-337, 2006.

94. Hammerschlag MR: Pneumonia due to *Chlamydia pneumoniae* in children: epidemiology, diagnosis, and treatment, *Pediatr Pulmonol* 36(5):384-390, 2003.

95. Waites KB: New concepts of *Mycoplasma pneumoniae* infections in children, *Pediatr Pulmonol* 36(4):267-278, 2003.

96. Bradley J et al: Comparative study of levofloxacin in the treatment of children with community-acquired pneumonia, *Pediatr Infect Dis J* 26(10):868-878, 2007.

97. Klig J, Shah N: Office pediatrics: current issues in lower respiratory infections in children, *Curr Opin Pediatr* 17(1):111-118, 2005.

98. Moussaoui E, deBorgie C, van den Broek P: Short course antibiotics in community acquired pneumonia, *BMJ* 332:1355-1358, 2006.

99. Clark J et al: Children with pneumonia: how do they present and how are they managed? *Arch Dis Child* 92:394-398, 2007.

100. Posfay-Barbe KM, Wald ER: Pneumococcal vaccines: do they prevent infection and how? *Curr Opin Infect Dis* 17(3):177-184, 2004.

101. Boesch RP et al: Advances in the diagnosis and management of chronic pulmonary aspiration in children, *Eur Respir J* 28:847-861, 2006.

102. Kurland G, Michelson P: Bronchiolitis obliterans in children, *Pediatr Pulmonol* 39:193-208, 2005.

103. Smith K, Fan L: Insights into post-infectious bronchiolitis obliterans in children, *Thorax* 61:462-463, 2006.

104. Colom A et al: Risk factors for the development of bronchiolitis obliterans in children with bronchiolitis, *Thorax* 61:503-506, 2006.

105. Verleden G et al: Azithromycin reduces airway neutrophilia and interleukin-8 in patients with bronchiolitis obliterans syndrome, *Am J Respir Crit Care Med* 174:566-570, 2006.

106. National Heart, Lung, and Blood Institute: *National Asthma Education and Prevention Program Expert Panel Report 3: guidelines for the diagnosis and management of asthma*. 2007. Available at www.nhlbi.nih.gov/guidelines

107. Pearce N, Douwes J: The global epidemiology of asthma in children, *Int J Tuberc Lung Dis* 10(2):125-132, 2006.

108. Clement L, Jones C, Cole J: Health disparities in the United States: childhood asthma, *Am J Med Sci* 335(4):260-265, 2008.

109. Chen A, Escarce J: Family structure and the treatment of childhood asthma, *Med Care* 46(2):174-184, 2008.

110. Van Schayck C, Smit H: The prevalence of asthma in children: a reversing trend, *Eur Respir J* 26(4):647-650, 2005.

111. Grigg J: Asthma year in review 2006-7, *Paediatr Respir Rev* 9:134-138, 2008.

112. Zhang J, Pare PD, Sandford AJ: Recent advances in asthma genetics, *Respir Res* 9:4, 2008.

113. McLeish S, Turner SW: Gene-environment interactions in asthma, *Arch Dis Child* 92(11):1032-1035, 2007.

114. Morgenstern V et al: Atopic diseases, allergic sensitization, and exposure to traffic-related air pollution in children, *Am J Respir Crit Care Med* 177:1331-1337, 2008.

115. Kiechl-Kohlendorfer U et al: Neonatal characteristics and risk of atopic asthma in schoolchildren: results from a large prospective birth-cohort study, *Acta Paediatrica* 96(11):1606-1610, 2007.

116. Vonk JM, Boezen HM: Predicting adult asthma in childhood, *Curr Opin Pulm Med* 12(1):42-47, 2006.

117. Panettierri RA Jr: Natural history of asthma: persistence versus progression—does the beginning predict the end? *J Allergy Clin Immunol* 121(3):607-613, 2008.

118. Brownlee J, Turner R: New developments in the epidemiology and clinical spectrum of rhinovirus infections, *Curr Opin Pediatr* 20:67-71, 2008.

119. Lenney W: Pro-con debate: inhaled corticosteroids should not be prescribed in primary care to children under two years of age—the case against, *Prim Care Respir J* 17(3):181-184, 2008.

120. Bisgaard H et al: Montelukast reduces asthma exacerbations in 2 to 5 year old children with intermittent asthma, *Am J Respir Crit Care Med* 171:315-322, 2005.

121. Penagos M et al: Metaanalysis of the efficacy of sublingual immunotherapy in the treatment of allergic asthma in pediatric patients, 3 to 18 years of age, *Chest* 133(3):599-609, 2008.

122. Niven R et al: Effectiveness of omalizumab in patients with inadequately controlled severe persistent allergic asthma: an open-label study, *Respir Med* 102(10):1371-1378, 2008.

123. Pijnenburg M et al: Exhaled nitric oxide predicts asthma relapse in children with clinical asthma remission, *Thorax* 60:215-218, 2005.

124. Bernard GR et al: The American-European Consensus Conference on ARDS: definitions, mechanisms, relevant outcomes, and clinical trial coordination, *Am J Respir Crit Care Med* 149:818-824, 1994.

125. Willson DF, Chess PR, Notter RH: Surfactant for pediatric acute lung injury, *Pediatr Clin North Am* 55(3):545-575, ix, 2008.

126. Bruijn M et al: High incidence of acute lung injury in children with Down syndrome, *Intensive Care Med* 33(12):2179-2182, 2007.

127. Cincotta D et al: Fatal acute fibrinous and organizing pneumonia in an infant: the histopathologic variability of acute respiratory distress syndrome, *Pediatr Crit Care Med* 8(4):378-382, 2007.

128. Bhatia M, Moochhala S: Role of inflammatory mediators in the pathophysiology of acute respiratory distress syndrome, *J Pathol* 202(2):145-156, 2004.

129. Ferguson ND, Slutsky AS: Point: high-frequency ventilation is the optimal physiological approach to ventilate ARDS patients, *J Appl Physiol* 104(4):1230-1231, 2008.

130. Turner D, Arnold J: Insights in pediatric ventilation: timing of intubation, ventilatory strategies, and weaning, *Curr Opin Crit Care* 13:57-63, 2007.

131. Wunsch H, Mapstone J: High-frequency ventilation versus conventional ventilation for the treatment of acute lung injury and acute respiratory distress syndrome: a systematic review and Cochrane analysis, *Crit Care Trauma* 100:1765-72, 2005.

132. Been JV, Zimmerman LJ: What's new in surfactant? A clinical view on recent developments in neonatology and paediatrics, *Eur J Pediatr* 166(9):889-899, 2007.

133. Strausbaugh S, Davis P: Cystic fibrosis: a review of epidemiology and pathobiology, *Clin Chest Med* 28:279-288, 2007.

134. Rogers DF: Physiology of airway mucus secretion and pathophysiology of hypersecretion, *Respir Care* 52(9):1134-1146:discussion 1146-1149, 2007.

135. Donaldson SH, Boucher RC: Sodium channels and cystic fibrosis, *Chest* 132(5):1631-1636, 2007.

136. Elizur A, Cannon CL, Ferkol TW: Airway inflammation in cystic fibrosis, *Chest* 133(2):489-495, 2008.

137. Accurso F: Update in cystic fibrosis 2007, *Am J Respir Crit Care Med* 177:1058-1061, 2008.

138. Elkin S, Geddes D: Pseudomonal infection in cystic fibrosis: the battle continues, *Expert Rev Anti Infect Ther* 1(4):609-618, 2003.

139. Tunney M et al: Detection of anaerobic bacteria in high numbers in sputum from patients with cystic fibrosis, *Am J Respir Crit Care Med* 177:995-1001, 2008.

140. Regamey N et al: Increased airway smooth muscle mass in children with asthma, cystic fibrosis and non-cystic fibrosis bronchiectasis, *Am J Respir Crit Care Med* 177:837-843, 2008.

141. Sontag MK, Accurso FJ: Gene modifiers in pediatrics: application to cystic fibrosis, *Adv Pediatr* 51:5-36, 2004.

142. Konstan M et al: Risk factors for rate of decline in forced expiratory volume in one second in children and adolescents with cystic fibrosis, *J Pediatr* 151:134-139, 2007.

143. Grosse SD et al: Newborn screening for cystic fibrosis: evaluation of benefits and risks and recommendations for state newborn screening programs, *MMWR Morb Mortal Wkly Rep* 53(RR-13):1-36, 2004.

144. Paul K et al: Effect of treatment with dornase alpha on airway inflammation in patients with cystic fibrosis, *Am J Respir Crit Care Med* 169(6):719-725, 2004.

145. Rosenfeld M, Ramsey BW, Gibson RL: *Pseudomonas* acquisition in young patients with cystic fibrosis: pathophysiology, diagnosis, and management, *Curr Opin Pulmon Med* 9(6):492-497, 2003.

146. Boucher RC: Cystic fibrosis: a disease of vulnerability to airway surface dehydration, *Trends Mol Med* 13(6):231-240, 2007.

147. Konstan M: Ibuprofen theory for cystic fibrosis lung disease: revisited, *Curr Opin Pulmon Med* 14(6):567-573, 2008.

148. Aurora P: Lung transplantation for cystic fibrosis, *J Royal Soc Med* 100(Suppl 47):46-52, 2007.

149. Milla CE: Nutrition and lung disease in cystic fibrosis, *Clin Chest Med* 28(2):319-330, 2007.

150. Sueblinvong V, Suratt BT, Weiss DJ: Novel therapies for the treatment of cystic fibrosis: new developments in gene and stem cell therapy, *Clin Chest Med* 28(2):361-379, 2007.

151. Daley KC: Update on sudden infant death syndrome, *Curr Opin Pediatr* 16(2):227-232, 2004.

152. American Academy of Pediatrics Task Force on Sudden Infant Death Syndrome: The changing concept of sudden infant death syndrome: diagnostic coding shifts, controversies regarding the sleeping environment, and new variables to consider in reducing risk, *Pediatrics* 116(5):1245, 2005.

153. Moon R, Horne S, Hauck F: Sudden infant death syndrome, *Lancet* 370:1578-1587, 2007.

154. Blair P, Fleming P: Recurrence risk of sudden infant death syndrome, *Arc Dis Child* 93(4):269-270, 2008.

155. Berkowitz CD: Cosleeping: benefits, risks, and cautions, *Adv Pediatr* 51:329-349, 2004.

156. Horne RS, Parslow PM, Harding R: Respiratory control and arousal in sleeping infants, *Paediatr Respir Rev* 5(3):190-198, 2004.

157. Horne RS et al: Influences of maternal cigarette smoking on infant arousability, *Early Hum Dev* 79(1):49-58, 2004.

158. Hunt CE: Gene-environment interactions: implications for sudden unexpected deaths in infancy, *Arch Dis Child* 90(1):48-53, 2005.

159. Hunt C: Small for gestational age infants and sudden infant death syndrome: a confluence of complex conditions, *Arch Dis Child* 92:428-430, 2007.

160. Stray-Pedersen A et al: Post-neonatal drop in alveolar SP-A expression: biological significance for increase vulnerability to SIDS? *Pediatr Pulmonol* 43:160-168, 2008.

161. Leiter J, Bohm I: Mechanisms of pathogenesis in the sudden infant death syndrome, *Resp Physiol Neurobiol* 159(2):127-138, 2007.

STRUCTURE AND FUNCTION OF THE RENAL AND UROLOGIC SYSTEMS

SUE E. HUETHER

MEDIA RESOURCES

Evolve Website (http://evolve.elsevier.com/McCance/)
- Review Questions and Answers
- Animations
- Glossary (with audio pronunciation for selected terms)
- WebLinks

CHAPTER OUTLINE

STRUCTURES OF THE RENAL SYSTEM
   Structures of the Kidney
   Urinary Structures
RENAL BLOOD FLOW
   Autoregulation
   Neural Regulation
   Hormones and Other Factors
KIDNEY FUNCTION
   Nephron Function
   Concentration and Dilution of Urine
   Renal Hormones

TESTS OF RENAL FUNCTION
   The Concept of Clearance
   Blood Tests
   Urinalysis
Aging and Renal Function

The primary function of the kidney is to maintain a stable internal environment for optimal cell and tissue metabolism. The kidneys accomplish these life-sustaining tasks by balancing solute and water transport, excreting metabolic waste products, conserving nutrients, and regulating acids and bases. The kidney also has an endocrine function, secreting the hormones renin, erythropoietin, and 1,25-dihydroxyvitamin D_3 for regulation of blood pressure, erythrocyte production, and calcium metabolism, respectively. In times of severe fasting the kidney also can synthesize glucose from amino acids, performing the process of gluconeogenesis. The formation of urine is achieved through the processes of filtration, reabsorption, and secretion by the glomeruli and tubules within the kidney. The bladder stores the urine that it receives from the kidney by way of the ureters. Urine is then removed from the body through the urethra.

STRUCTURES OF THE RENAL SYSTEM

Structures of the Kidney

The **kidneys** are paired organs located on the posterior abdominal wall outside the peritoneal cavity. They lie on either side of the vertebral column with their upper and lower poles extending from the twelfth thoracic to the third lumbar vertebrae (Figure 35-1). Each kidney is approximately 11 cm long, 5 to 6 cm wide, and 3 to 4 cm thick. A tightly adhering capsule (the **renal capsule**) surrounds each kidney, and the kidney then is embedded in a mass of fat. The capsule and fatty layer are covered with a double layer of **renal fascia,** fibrous tissue that attaches the kidney to the posterior abdominal wall.

The cushion of fat and the position of the kidney between the abdominal organs and muscles of the back protect it from trauma. The right kidney is slightly lower than the

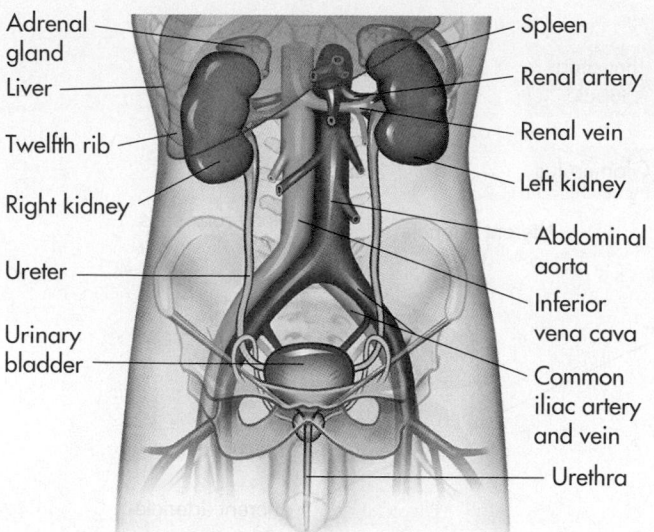

Figure 35-1 Organs of the urinary system. (From Patton KT, Thibodeau GA: *Anatomy & physiology*, ed 7, St Louis, 2010, Mosby.)

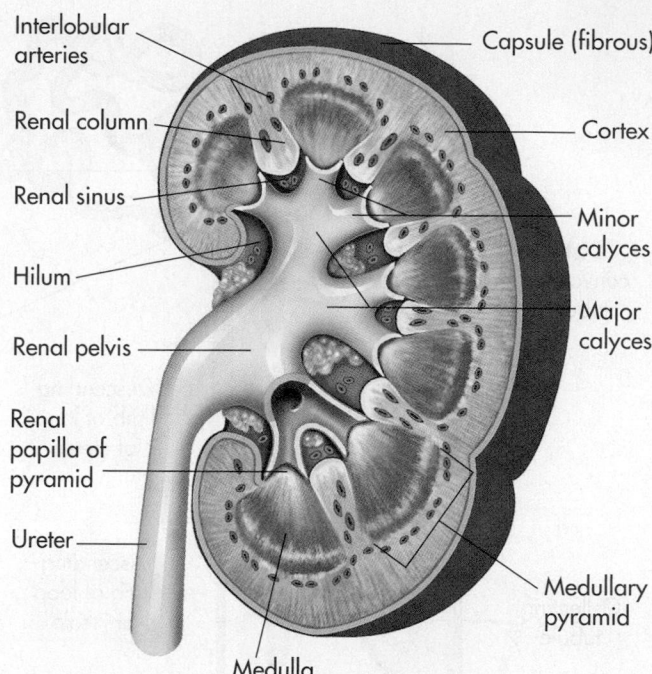

Figure 35-2 Kidney structure. (From Patton KT, Thibodeau GA: *Anatomy & physiology*, ed 7, St Louis, 2010, Mosby.)

left; it is displaced downward by the overlying liver. A medial indentation (the **hilum**) contains the entry and exit for the renal blood vessels, nerves, lymphatic vessels, and ureter.

The gross structure of the kidney can be identified when it is divided from top to bottom in a coronal plane (Figure 35-2). The major components are the outer **renal cortex** and the inner **renal medulla.** The cortex contains all the glomeruli and portions of the tubules. The medulla is formed by the straight segments of the proximal and distal tubules and the collecting ducts. It consists of a series of wedges, called **renal pyramids,** with an outer zone close to the cortex and an inner zone. **Renal columns** extend from the cortex down between the renal pyramids. The apexes of the pyramids project into a **minor calyx** (a cup-shaped cavity) that join together to form a **major calyx.** The calyces receive urine from the large collecting ducts. The major calyces join to form the **renal pelvis,** an extension of the upper end of the ureter. The walls of the calyces and ureters contain smooth muscles that contract to move urine to the bladder.

The structural unit of the kidney is the lobe. Each lobe is composed of a pyramid and the overlying cortex. There are about 14 lobes in each kidney.

Nephron

The **nephron** is the functional unit of the kidney. Approximately 1.2 million nephrons are contained in each kidney. The nephron is a tubular structure with subunits that include the renal corpuscle, proximal convoluted tubule, loop of Henle, distal convoluted tubule, and collecting duct, all of which contribute to the formation of final urine (Figure 35-3). The different structures of the epithelial cells lining various segments of the tubule facilitate the special functions of secretion and reabsorption (Figure 35-4).

The kidney has three kinds of nephrons: (1) **superficial cortical nephrons** (85% of all nephrons), which extend only

partially into the medulla; (2) **midcortical nephrons** with short or long loops; and (3) **juxtamedullary nephrons,** which lie close to and extend deep into the medulla and are important for the process of concentrating urine (Figure 35-5). The **glomerulus** (Figure 35-6; see also Figure 35-3) is a tuft of capillaries, the glomerular capillaries, that loop into a circular capsule, the **Bowman capsule,** like fingers pushed into bread dough. **Mesangial cells** (shaped like smooth muscle cells) and the **mesangial matrix** lie between and support the glomerular capillaries.[1] They have contractile and phagocytic properties, similar to monocytes, release inflammatory cytokines, and produce vasoactive substances that influence the glomerular filtration rate (GFR) by regulating glomerular capillary blood flow. The space inside the Bowman capsule is called the **Bowman space.** Together, the glomerulus, Bowman capsule, and mesangial cells are called the **renal corpuscle.**

The wall of the glomerular capillary serves as a filtration membrane (the **glomerular filtration membrane**) and has three layers: (1) an inner capillary endothelium, (2) a middle basement membrane, and (3) an outer layer of capillary epithelium (also called **podocytes** or *visceral epithelium*). Each layer has unique structural properties that allow all components of the blood to filter through, with the exception of blood cells and plasma proteins with a molecular weight greater than 70,000 (Figure 35-7; see also Figure 35-6). The **glomerular endothelium** is composed of cells in continuous contact with the basement membrane. Glomerular endothelial cells synthesize nitric oxide (a vasodilator) and endothelin-1 (a vasoconstrictor important to regulating glomerular blood flow). The glomerular endothelium is perforated by many small openings or windows, called *fenestrae*. The fenestrae are

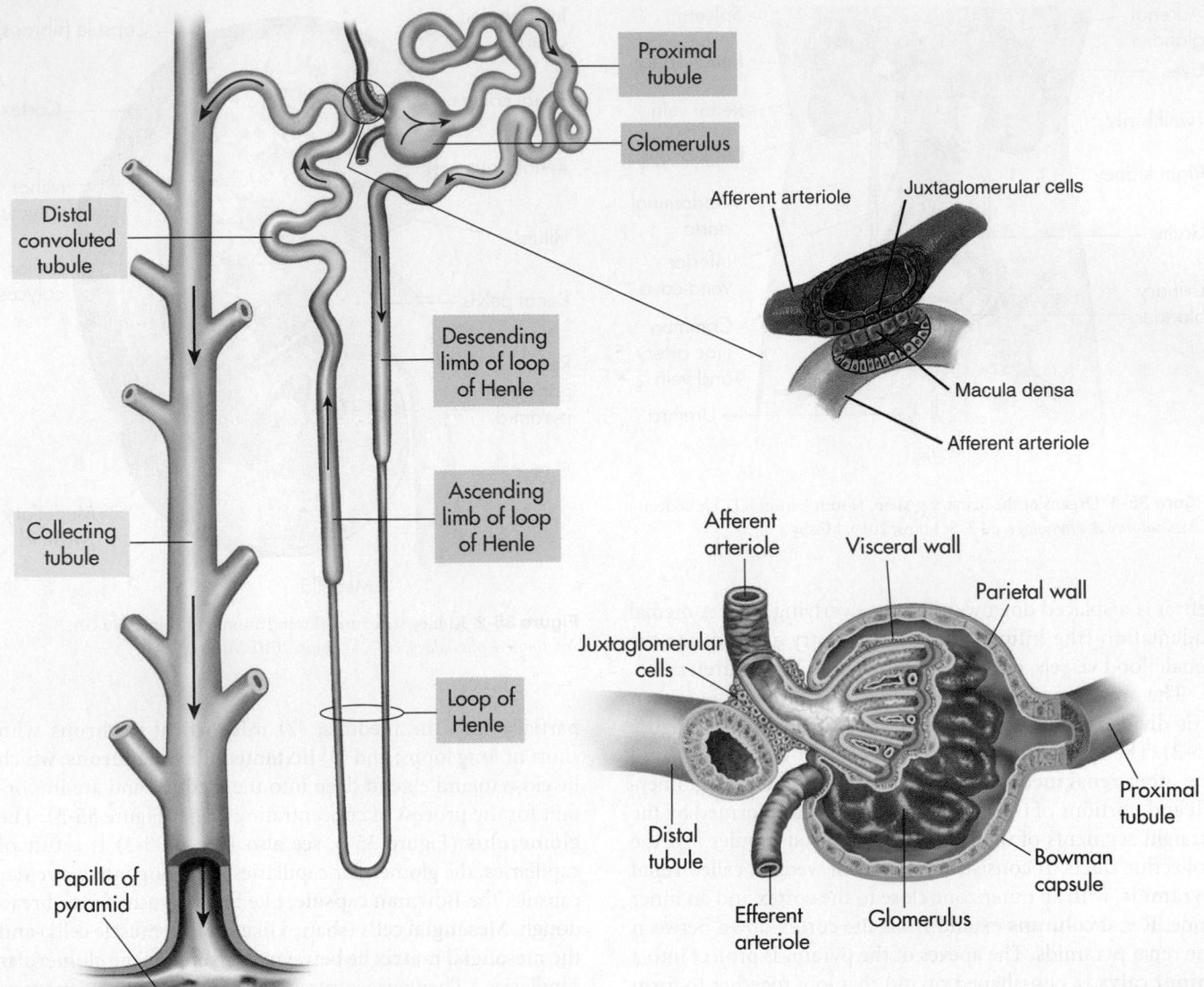

Figure 35-3 Components of the nephron. (From Patton KT, Thibodeau GA: *Anatomy & physiology*, ed 7, St Louis, 2010, Mosby; Damjanov: *Pathology for health professions*, St Louis, 2006, Mosby.)

maintained by vascular epithelial growth factor (VEGF) produced by visceral epithelium. The middle basement membrane is a negatively charged, selectively permeable network of glycoproteins and mucopolysaccharides and may be secreted and maintained by the epithelial cells.[2] The **visceral epithelium,** also called **podocytes,**[3] has footlike processes that radiate and adhere to the basement membrane covering the glomerular capillaries. The visceral epithelium is reflected back at the vascular pole to become the **parietal epithelium.** The space between the visceral and parietal epithelia is the Bowman space, which continues to become the proximal tubule. The foot processes of one podocyte interlock with the foot processes of adjacent podocytes, forming an elaborate network of intercellular clefts. These clefts are called **filtration slits** (see Figure 35-7), or slit membranes, and modulate filtration. *Nephrin, podocin, and CD2-associated protein* are proteins that are exclusively located in the slit membrane and are required for normal filtration.[4]

The podocytes are endocytic, which allow molecules to enter the cell without passing through the cell membrane, and they prevent leakage of proteins into the urine.

The glomerular filtration membrane separates the blood within the glomerular capillaries from the filtered fluid in the Bowman space. The glomerular filtrate passes through the three layers of the glomerular membrane and forms the primary urine. The endothelial cells and basement membrane of the filtration membrane express negatively charged glycoproteins and form a filtration barrier to anionic proteins.

The glomerulus is supplied by the afferent arteriole and drained by the efferent arteriole. A group of specialized cells known as **juxtaglomerular cells** are located around the afferent arteriole where it enters the glomerulus (see Figures 35-3 and 35-6). Between the afferent and efferent arterioles is a portion of the distal convoluted tubule with specialized sodium and chloride-sensing cells known as the **macula densa** (see

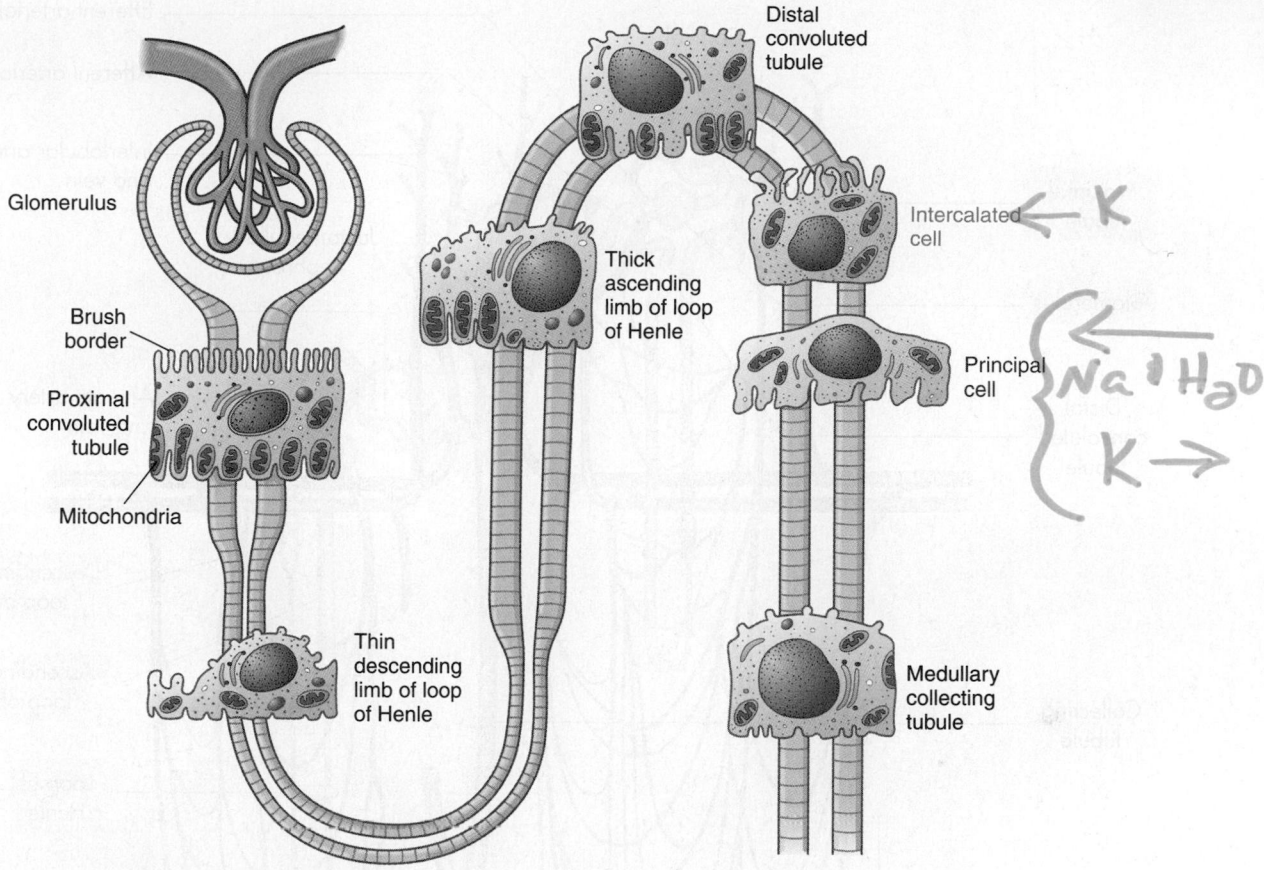

Figure 35-4 Epithelial cells of the various segments of nephron tubules. The brush border and high number of mitochondria in the cells of the proximal convoluted tubule permit reabsorption of 60% of the glomerular filtrate. *Intercalated cells* (blue) secrete either H^+ (reabsorb HCO_3^-) or HCO_3^- and reabsorb K^+. *Principal cells* (magenta) reabsorb Na^+ and water and secrete K^+.

Figure 35-6). Together the juxtaglomerular cells and macula densa cells form the **juxtaglomerular apparatus (JGA)** (see Figure 35-6). Control of renal blood flow, glomerular filtration, and renin secretion occurs at this site.

The **proximal tubule** continues from the Bowman space and has an initial convoluted segment (pars convoluta) and then a straight segment (pars recta) that descends toward the medulla (see Figure 35-3). The proximal tubular lumen consists of one layer of cuboidal cells with a surface layer of microvilli that increases reabsorptive surface area. This is the only surface inside the nephron where the cells are covered with microvilli (a brush border) (see Figure 35-4). The proximal tubule joins the **loop of Henle,** a hairpin-shaped loop composed of thick and thin portions of a descending segment that goes into the medulla. The tube then loops and becomes the thickening ascending segment that extends toward the cortex. The thin segment is composed of thin squamous cells with no active transport function. The cells of the thick segment are cuboidal and actively transport several solutes but not water.

The more numerous cortical nephrons have glomeruli originating close to the surface of the cortex or in the mid-cortex, unlike the juxtamedullary nephrons, whose glomeruli are located deep in the cortex close to the medulla. The major structural difference between the glomeruli in the two types of

nephrons is the length of the loop of Henle. In cortical nephrons the loop is short and may not extend into the medulla. The loop of Henle for the juxtamedullary nephrons, however, may extend the whole length of the medulla (40 mm). Juxtamedullary nephrons represent about 12% of the total number of nephrons and are important for the concentration and dilution of urine.

The **distal tubule** has convoluted and straight segments. It extends from the macula densa to the **collecting duct.** The collecting duct is a large tubule that descends down the cortex, through the renal pyramids of the inner and outer medullae, and into the minor calyx. The collecting duct is composed of two cell types: principal cells and intercalated cells (see Figure 34-4). **Principal cells** resorb sodium and water and secrete potassium. **Intercalated cells** secrete either hydrogen or bicarbonate and reabsorb potassium.

Blood Vessels

The blood vessels of the kidney closely parallel nephron structure. The **renal arteries** arise as the fifth branches of the abdominal aorta. At the renal hilum they divide into anterior and posterior branches and then subdivide into lobar arteries that supply blood to the lower, middle, and upper thirds of the kidney. The **interlobar arteries** are further subdivisions that

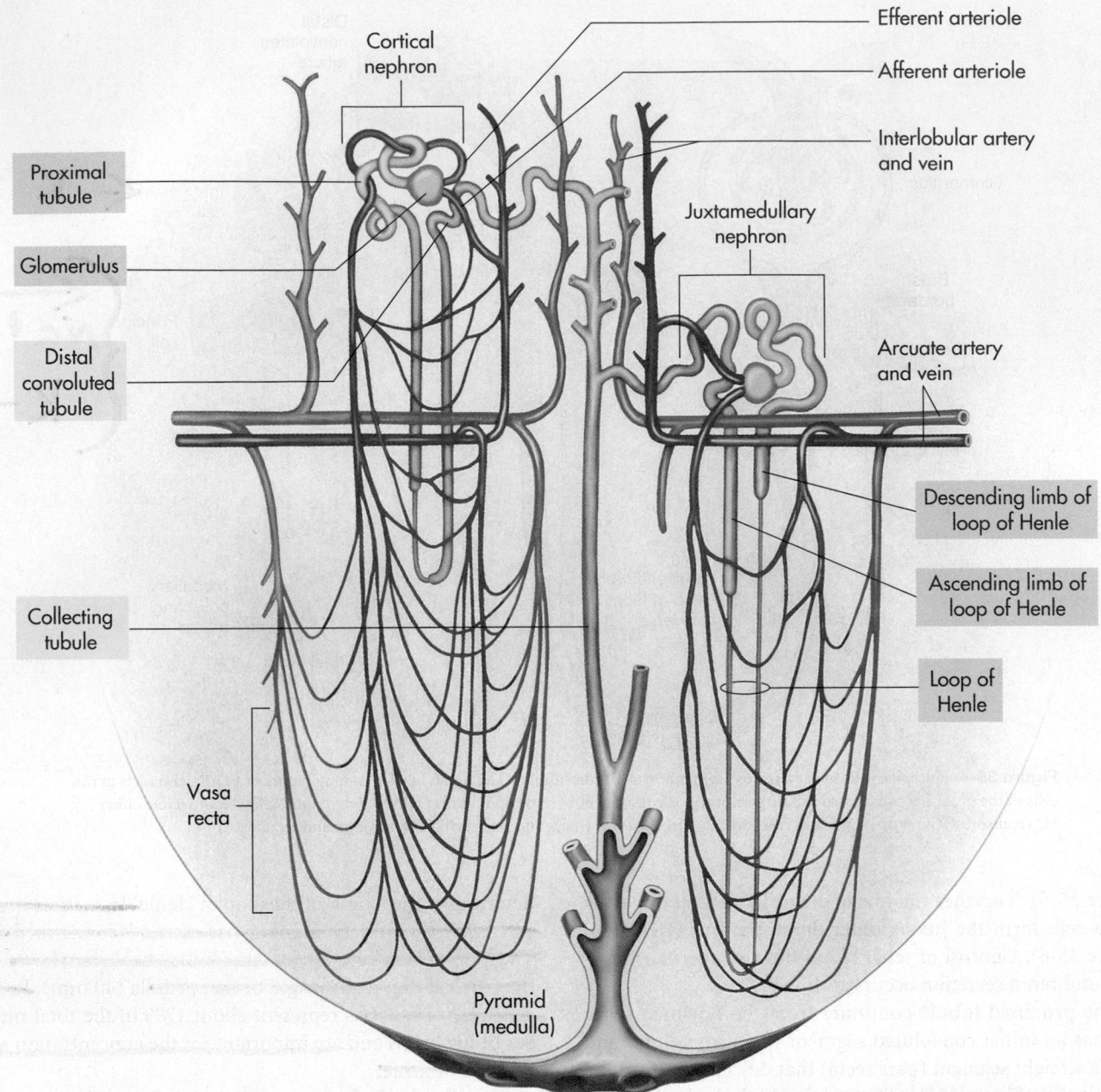

Figure 35-5 **The nephron unit with its blood vessels.** Blood flows through nephron vessels as follows: interlobular artery, afferent arteriole, glomerulus, efferent arteriole, peritubular capillaries (around the tubules), venules, interlobular vein. (From Patton KT, Thibodeau GA: *Anatomy & physiology,* ed 7, St Louis, 2010, Mosby.)

travel down the renal columns and between the pyramids. At the cortical medullary junction, interlobar arteries branch into the **arcuate arteries** that arch over the base of the pyramids and run parallel to the surface of the kidney.

The **interlobular arteries** arise from the arcuate arteries and extend through the cortex toward the periphery and form the afferent glomerular arterioles (see Figure 35-5). The afferent arterioles subdivide into a fistlike structure of four to eight **glomerular capillaries** (see Figure 35-6). The glomerular capillaries empty into the efferent arteriole, which conveys blood to a second capillary bed, the peritubular capillaries.

This is the only place in the body where an arteriole is positioned between two capillary beds. Increases or decreases in the resistance of the afferent and efferent arterioles increase or decrease glomerular filtration.

The **peritubular capillaries** surround the convoluted portions of the proximal and distal tubules and the loop of Henle (see Figure 35-5). The peritubular capillaries are adapted differently for the cortical and juxtamedullary nephrons. The peritubular capillaries surrounding the tubules of the cortical nephrons are similar to capillaries in other tissues. For the juxtamedullary nephrons a network of capillaries called the

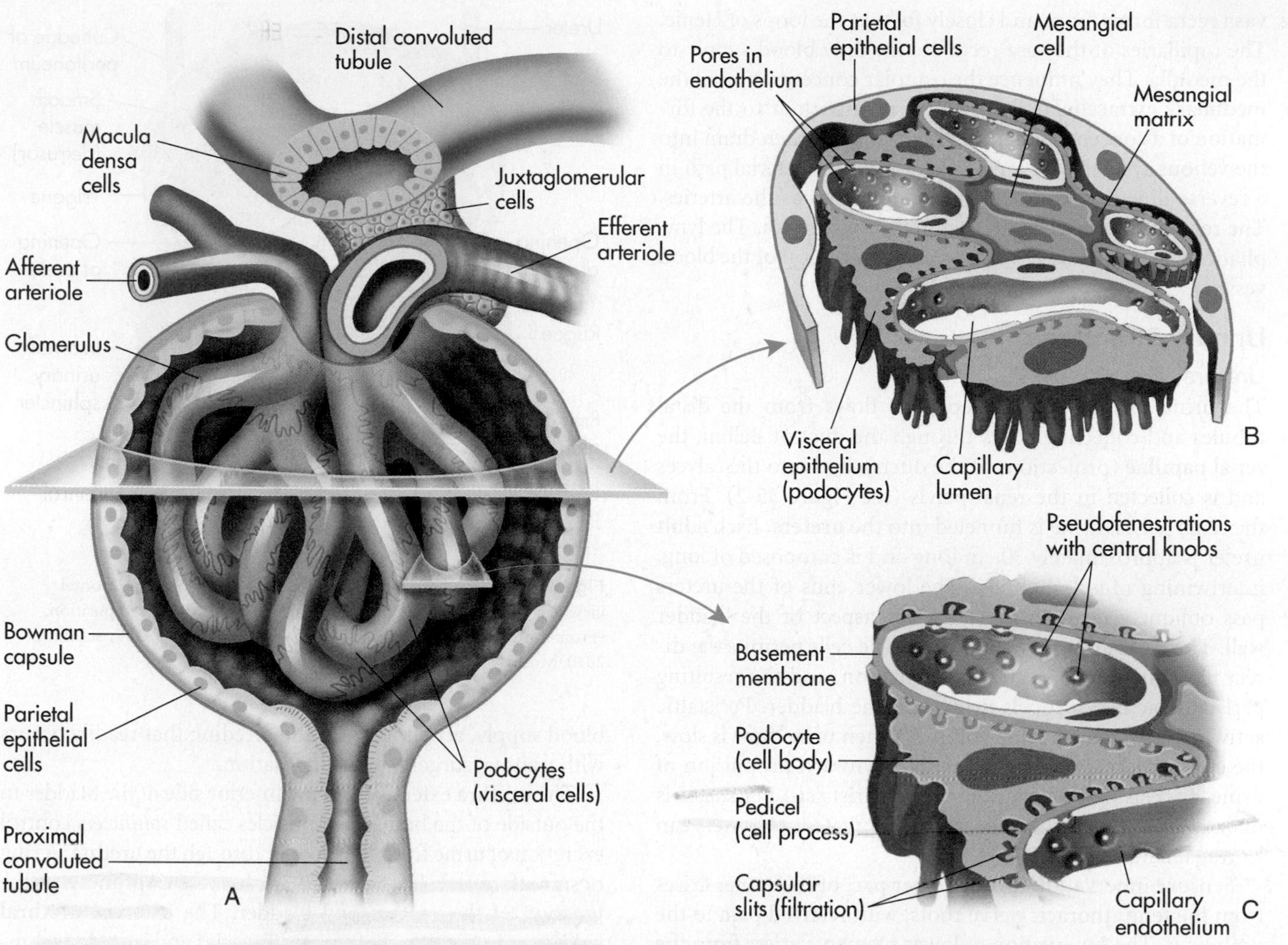

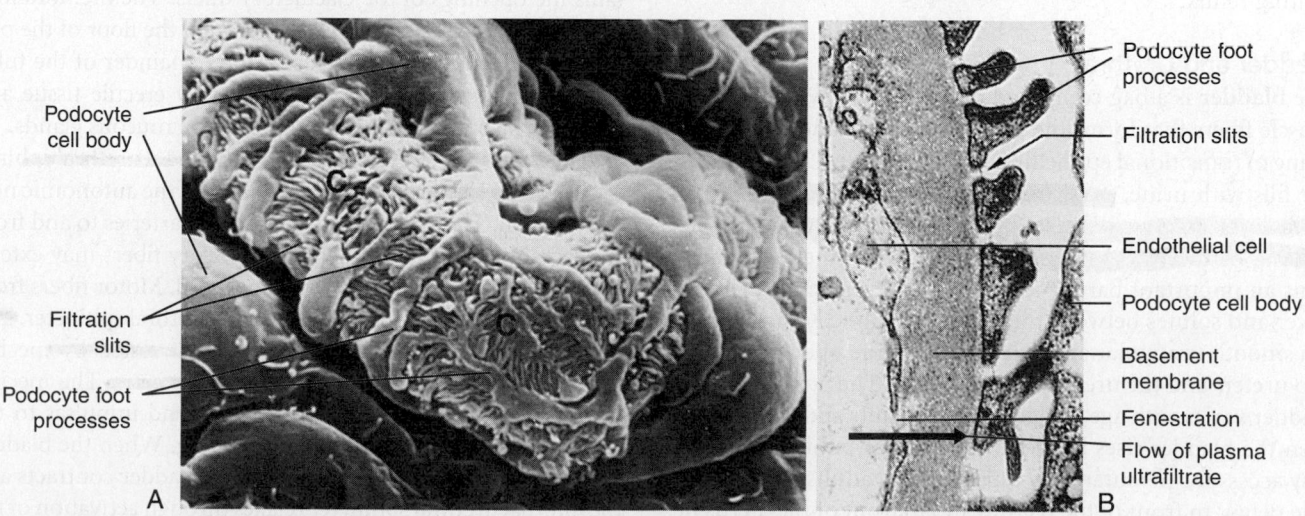

Figure 35-6 Anatomy of the glomerulus and juxtaglomerular apparatus. A, Longitudinal cross section of glomerulus and juxtaglomerular apparatus. B, Horizontal cross section of glomerulus. C, Enlargement of glomerular capillary filtration membrane.

Figure 35-7 Glomerular capillary. A, Scanning electron micrograph of normal glomerular capillary (C). B, Glomerular capillary wall (× 40,000.) (From Kissane JM, editor: *Anderson's pathology*, ed 9, St Louis, 1990, Mosby.)

vasa recta forms loops and closely follows the loops of Henle. The capillaries of the vasa recta are the only blood supply to the medulla. They influence the osmolar concentration of the medullary extracellular fluid, which is important to the formation of a concentrated urine. All capillaries then drain into the venous system. The renal veins follow the arterial path in a reverse direction and have the same names as the arteries. The renal vein empties into the inferior vena cava. The lymphatic vessels tend also to follow the distribution of the blood vessels.

Urinary Structures

Ureters

The urine formed by the nephrons flows from the distal tubules and collecting ducts through the duct of Bellini, the **renal papillae** (projections of the ducts), and into the calyces and is collected in the renal pelvis (see Figure 35-2). From the renal pelvis, urine is funneled into the **ureters.** Each adult ureter is approximately 30 cm long and is composed of long, intertwining muscle bundles. The lower ends of the ureters pass obliquely through the posterior aspect of the bladder wall. The close approximation of muscle cells permits the direct transmission of electrical stimulation, and the resulting peristaltic activity propels urine into the bladder. Peristaltic activity is affected by urine volume. When urine flow is slow, the contraction is segmented, with downward propulsion of urine. Increasing flow rates increase peristalsis. Peristalsis is maintained even when the ureter is denervated, so ureters can be transplanted.

Sensory innervation for the upper part of the ureter arises from the tenth thoracic nerve roots, with referred pain to the umbilicus. The innervation of lower segments arises from the sacral nerves with referred pain to the vulva or penis. The ureters have a rich blood supply. The primary arteries come from the kidney with contributions from the lumbar and superior vesical arteries. Contraction of the bladder during **micturition** (urination) compresses the lower end of the ureter, preventing reflux.

Bladder and Urethra

The **bladder** is a bag composed of a basket weave of smooth muscle fibers that forms the **detrusor muscle** and its smooth lining of transitional epithelium (uroepithelium). As the bladder fills with urine, it distends and the layers of transitional epithelium slide past each other and become thinner as the volume of the bladder increases. The uroepithelium maintains an important barrier function to prevent movement of water and solutes between the urine and blood.[5] The **trigone** is a smooth triangular area lying between the openings of the two ureters and the urethra (Figure 35-8). The position of the bladder varies with age and gender. In infants and young children the bladder rises above the symphysis pubis, providing easy access for percutaneous aspiration. In adults it lies in the true pelvis, in front of the rectum and in front of the uterus in women. Inferiorly, the bladder sits on the prostate in men and on the anterior vagina in women. The bladder has a profuse

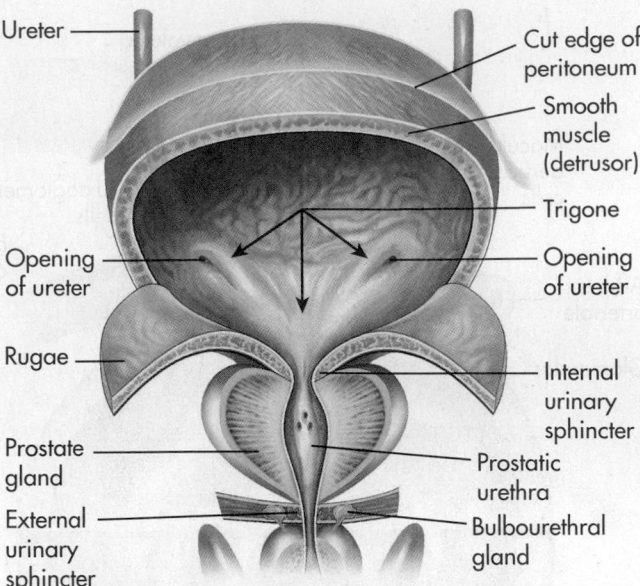

Figure 35-8 **Structure and location of the urinary bladder.** Frontal view of a dissected urinary bladder (male) in a fully distended position. (From Patton KT, Thibodeau GA: *Anatomy & physiology*, ed 7, St Louis, 2010, Mosby.)

blood supply, accounting for the bleeding that readily occurs with trauma, surgery, or inflammation.

The **urethra** extends from the inferior side of the bladder to the outside of the body. Two muscles called *sphincters* control excretion of urine from the bladder through the urethra. A ring of smooth muscle forms the **internal urethral sphincter** at the junction of the urethra and bladder. The **external urethral sphincter** is composed of striated muscles and is under voluntary control. The entire urethra is lined with mucus-secreting glands. The female urethra is short (3 to 4 cm). The male urethra is long (18 to 20 cm) and has three segments: prostatic, membranous, and cavernous. The prostatic urethra is closest to the bladder. It passes through the prostate gland and contains the openings of the ejaculatory ducts. The membranous urethra is the segment that passes through the floor of the pelvis. The cavernous segment forms the remainder of the tube. The cavernous segment is surrounded by erectile tissue and contains the openings of the bulbourethral mucous glands.

The innervation of the bladder and internal urethral sphincter is supplied by parasympathetic fibers of the autonomic nervous system. They primarily pass with the arteries to and from the sacral levels of the spinal cord. Sensory fibers may extend as high as the T6 portion of the spinal cord. Motor fibers from the pudendal nerve supply the external urethral sphincter. The reflex arc required for micturition is stimulated by mechanoreceptors that respond to stretching of tissue. The mechanoreceptors sense bladder fullness and send impulses to the sacral level of the cord with bladder filling. When the bladder accumulates 250 to 300 ml of urine, the bladder contracts and the internal urethral sphincter relaxes through activation of the spinal reflex arc (known as the *micturition reflex*). At this time a person feels the urge to void. In older children and adults, the reflex can be inhibited or facilitated by impulses coming from the brain, resulting in voluntary control of micturition.

RENAL BLOOD FLOW

The kidneys are highly vascular organs and usually receive 1000 to 1200 ml of blood per minute, or about 20% to 25% of the cardiac output. With a normal hematocrit of 45%, about 600 to 700 ml of blood flowing through the kidney per minute is plasma. From the renal plasma flow (RPF), 20% (approximately 120 to 140 ml/minute) is filtered at the glomerulus and passes into the Bowman capsule. The filtration of the plasma per unit of time is known as the **glomerular filtration rate (GFR)**, which is directly related to the perfusion pressure in the glomerular capillaries.

The remaining 80% (about 480 ml) of plasma flows through the efferent arterioles to the peritubular capillaries. The ratio of glomerular filtrate to RPF per minute (120/600 = 0.20) is called the *filtration fraction*. Normally all but 1 to 2 ml of the glomerular filtrate is reabsorbed and returned to the circulation by the peritubular capillaries.

The GFR is directly related to renal blood flow (RBF), which is regulated by intrinsic autoregulatory mechanisms, neural regulation, and hormonal regulation. In general, blood flow to any organ is determined by the arteriovenous pressure differences across the vascular bed. If mean arterial pressure decreases or vascular resistance increases, RBF decreases.

Autoregulation

In the kidney a local mechanism of **autoregulation** tends to keep the rate of glomerular blood flow and therefore the GFR fairly constant over a range of arterial pressures between 80 and 180 mmHg (Figure 35-9). This means that changes in afferent arteriolar resistance and arteriolar pressure occur in the same direction. For example, as systemic blood pressure increases, the afferent arterioles constrict, preventing an increase in glomerular blood flow and filtration pressure. Opposite processes occur with a decrease in systemic blood pressure. Therefore, RBF and GFR are relatively constant. This "constant" state is maintained by intrinsic autoregulatory mechanism mediating the arteriolar resistance changes. The purpose of renal autoregulation is to prevent wide fluctuations in systemic arterial pressure from being transmitted to the glomerular capillaries. In this way, large fluctuations in GFR are prevented and solute and water excretion is constantly maintained when arterial pressure changes.[6] Autoregulation may also protect the kidney from damage by hypertension.[7]

One mechanism responsible for the autoregulatory response in the kidney is probably a **myogenic mechanism.** As arterial pressure declines, the stretch on the afferent arteriolar smooth muscle decreases and the arteriole relaxes, with an increase in RBF; an increase in arteriolar pressure causes the arteriole smooth muscle to contract and decreases RBF. **Tubuloglomerular feedback** is a second mechanism for autoregulation of RBF and GFR. The macula densa cells of

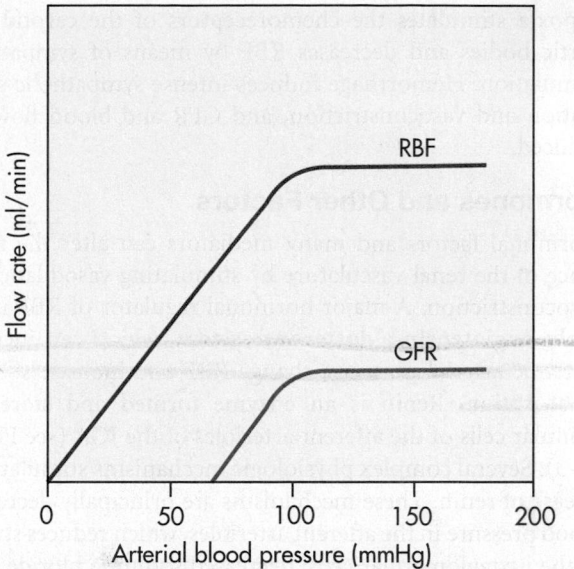

Figure 35-9 Renal autoregulation. Blood flow and glomerular filtration rate are stabilized in the face of changes in perfusion pressure. (From Berne RM, Levy MN, editors: *Principles of physiology,* ed 3, St Louis, 2000, Mosby.)

the distal tubule in the JGA sense changes in flow rate and sodium chloride content of the lumenal fluid. This information initiates a signal causing compensatory changes in afferent arteriolar resistance and GFR.[8]

Neural Regulation

The blood vessels of the kidney are innervated by the sympathetic noradrenergic fibers that cause arteriolar vasoconstriction and reduce renal blood flow. The innervation of the kidney comes primarily from the celiac ganglion and greater splanchnic nerve (see Figure 14-24). The afferent and efferent arterioles are richly innervated, but nerves have not been observed in the glomerular capillaries.

The RBF is reflexively related to the systemic arterial pressure. When systemic arterial pressure decreases, increased renal sympathetic nerve activity is mediated reflexively through the carotid sinus and the baroreceptors of the aortic arch. This stimulates renal arteriolar vasoconstriction and decreases RBF and GFR. Thus RBF still changes when systemic arterial pressure is significantly reduced, although autoregulatory processes dampen the response. The decreased RBF decreases the GFR and diminishes excretion of sodium and water, promoting an increase in blood volume and thus an increase in systemic pressure. The afferent and efferent arterioles are innervated by sympathetic nerves. Norepinephrine causes vasoconstriction by activation of α_1-adrenoreceptors on afferent arterioles. The nerves are stimulated by decreased blood volume and cause vasoconstriction and decreased glomerular filtration.

Exercise, body position, and hypoxia also influence RBF. Exercise and change of body position activate renal sympathetic neurons and cause mild vasoconstriction. Severe hypoxia stimulates the chemoreceptors of the carotid and aortic bodies and decreases RBF by means of sympathetic stimulation. Hemorrhage induces intense sympathetic stimulation and vasoconstriction, and GFR and blood flow are reduced.

Hormones and Other Factors

Hormonal factors and many mediators can alter the resistance of the renal vasculature by stimulating vasodilation or vasoconstriction. A major hormonal regulator of RBF is the **renin-angiotensin-aldosterone system,** which can increase systemic arterial pressure, change RBF and increase sodium reabsorption. Renin is an enzyme formed and stored in granular cells of the afferent arterioles of the JGA (see Figure 35-3). Several complex physiologic mechanisms stimulate the release of renin. These mechanisms are principally decreased blood pressure in the afferent arterioles, which reduces stretch of the juxtaglomerular cells; decreased sodium chloride concentration in the distal convoluted tubule; sympathetic nerve stimulation of β-adrenergic receptors on the juxtaglomerular cells and prostaglandins.[9]

When renin is released, it cleaves an α-globulin (angiotensinogen produced by liver hepatocytes) in the plasma to form angiotensin I, which is physiologically inactive. In the presence of **angiotensin-converting enzyme (ACE)** produced from pulmonary and renal endothelium, angiotensin I is converted to angiotensin II. **Angiotensin II** stimulates secretion of aldosterone by the adrenal cortex (see Chapter 20), is a potent vasopressor, inhibits renin release, and stimulates antidiuretic hormone (ADH) secretion and thirst. Vitamin D₃ is a potent negative endocrine regulator of renin gene expression.[10] Numerous physiologic effects of the renin-angiotensin-aldosterone system serve the purpose of stabilizing systemic blood pressure and preserving the extracellular fluid volume during hypotension or hypovolemia, including sodium reabsorption, potassium excretion, systemic vasoconstriction, sympathetic nerve stimulation, thirst stimulation, and drinking. (The combined effects of the renin-angiotensin-aldosterone system are summarized in Figure 35-10.) ACE inhibitors are drugs that decrease blood pressure.

Natriuretic peptides are a group of peptide hormones including **atrial natriuretic peptide (ANP)** secreted from cells in the right atrium, **brain natriuretic peptide (BNP)** secreted from the cardiac ventricles, **C-type natriuretic peptide** from vascular endothelium, and **urodilantin** secreted by the distal tubules and collecting ducts.[11] When the heart dilates during volume expansion or heart failure, ANP and BNP inhibit secretion of renin, inhibit angiotensin-induced secretion of aldosterone, vasodilate the afferent and constrict the efferent glomerular arterioles, and inhibit sodium and water absorption by kidney tubules. C-type natriuretic peptide is a vasodilator, and urodilantin promotes renal sodium chloride excretion. The result is increased urine formation and decreased blood volume and blood pressure.[12] Other hormones and mediators that influence renal blood flow are summarized in Table 35-1.

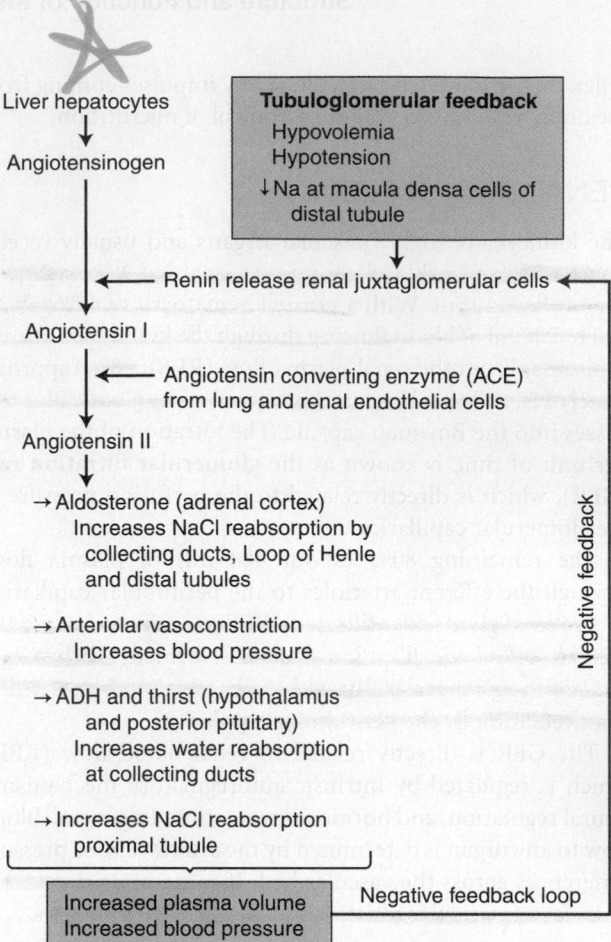

Figure 35-10   Renin-angiotensin-aldosterone system. Activation of tubuloglomerular feedback mechanisms stimulates the release of renin with activation of the renin-angiotensin-aldosterone system. Plasma volume and blood pressure are increased with the reabsorption of sodium chloride and water from the renal tubules. The restoration of plasma volume and blood pressure then decrease the release of renin, forming a negative feedback loop.

KIDNEY FUNCTION

Nephron Function

The nephron can perform many functions simultaneously. It filters the plasma at the glomerulus and reabsorbs and secretes different substances at various parts of its tubular structure (Figure 35-11). The function of the nephron is to form a filtrate of protein-free plasma. This process, known as **ultrafiltration,** occurs across the glomerular capillaries. The nephron then regulates the filtrate to maintain body fluid volume, electrolyte composition, and pH within narrow limits.

Regulation of the filtrate occurs through two processes: tubular reabsorption and tubular secretion. **Tubular reabsorption** is the movement of fluids and solutes from the tubular lumen to the peritubular capillary plasma. Transfer of substances from the plasma of the peritubular capillary to the tubular lumen is **tubular secretion.** The transport mechanisms are active as well as passive (processes defined in Chapter 1). The elimination of a substance in the final urine is known as **excretion** (Figure 35-12).

Table 35-1	Hormones, Mediators, and Renal Blood Flow
Hormone or Mediator	**Effect on Renal Blood Flow**
Adenosine	Produced within kidney; causes vasoconstriction of afferent arteriole; decreases RBF and GFR
Angiotensin II	Produced systemically and within kidneys; constricts afferent and efferent arterioles; decreases RBF and GFR
Atrial and brain natriuretic peptides	Produced by atria and ventricles of the heart with hypertension and increased blood volume; causes vasodilation of afferent arteriole and vasoconstriction of efferent arteriole; modest increase in GFR with little change in RBF
Bradykinin	Produced in kidney from kininogen and causes vasodilation by release of nitric oxide and prostaglandins; increases RBF and GFR
Dopamine	Produced by the proximal tubule; increases RBF; inhibits renin secretion
Endothelin	Produced by renal vessel endothelial cells, mesangial cells, and distal tubule cells in response to bradykinin, angiotensin II, epinephrine, and stretch; most active with renal disease; profound vasoconstriction of afferent and efferent arterioles; decreases RBF and GFR
Histamine	Produced locally within the kidney; modulates RBF in basal state and during inflammation; increases RBF by decreasing afferent and efferent arteriolar resistance and does not decrease GFR
Nitric oxide	Produced by renal vessel endothelial cells with increased stretch and by stimulation of acetylcholine, histamine, bradykinin, ATP; increases vasodilation of afferent and efferent arterioles
Prostaglandins, PGI$_2$, PGE$_2$	Produced locally within kidney with decreased RBF; dampen vasoconstriction caused by sympathetic nerves and angiotensin II; prevent harmful vasoconstriction and renal ischemia
Urodilantin (a natriuretic peptide)	Produced by distal tubule and collecting duct when there is increased circulating volume and increased blood pressure; inhibits sodium and water reabsorption from medullary part of collecting duct, thereby producing diuresis

ATP, Adenosine triphosphate; *GFR*, glomerular filtration rate; *RBF*, renal blood flow.

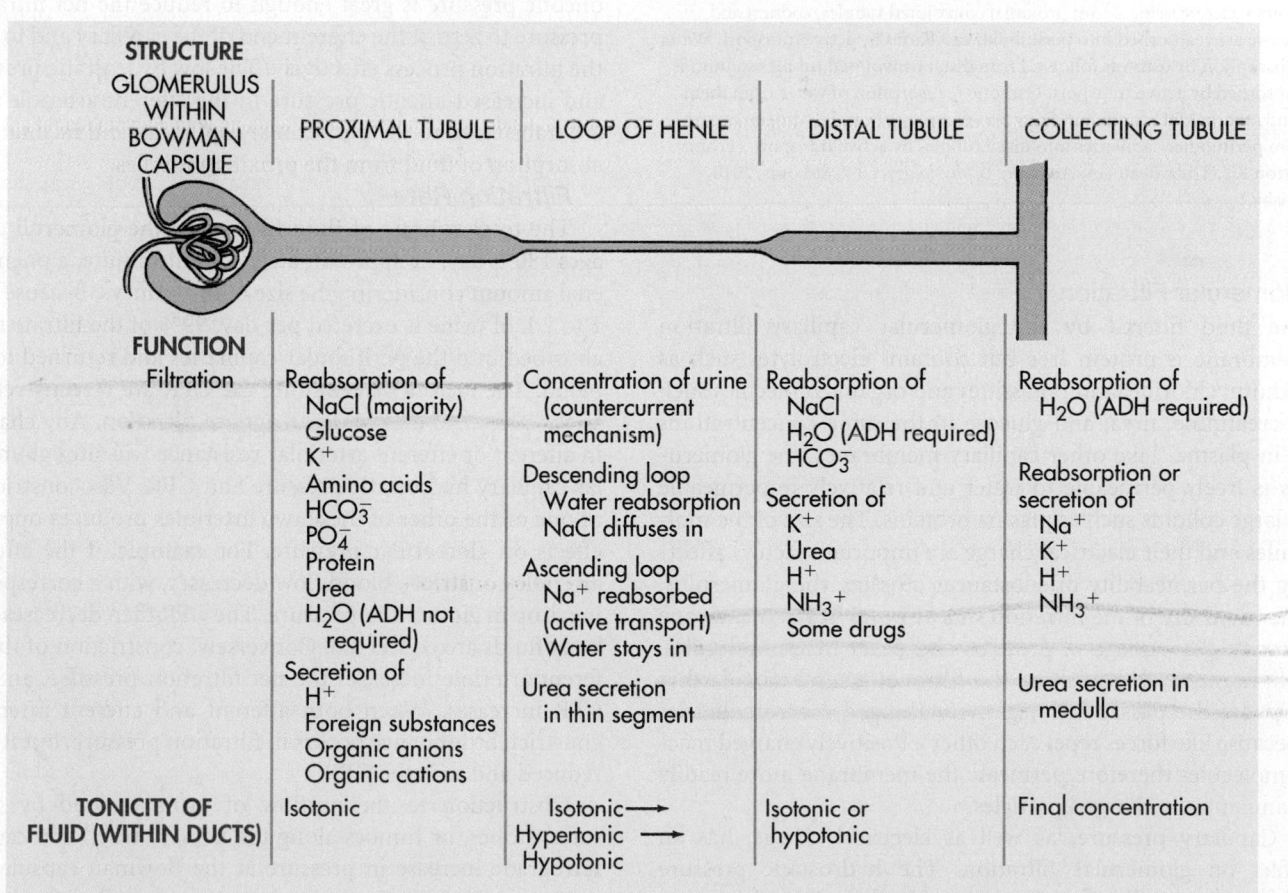

Figure 35-11 Major functions of nephron segments. *ADH*, Antidiuretic hormone. (Modified from Hockenberry MJ: *Wong's nursing care of infants and children*, ed 8, St Louis, 2007, Mosby.)

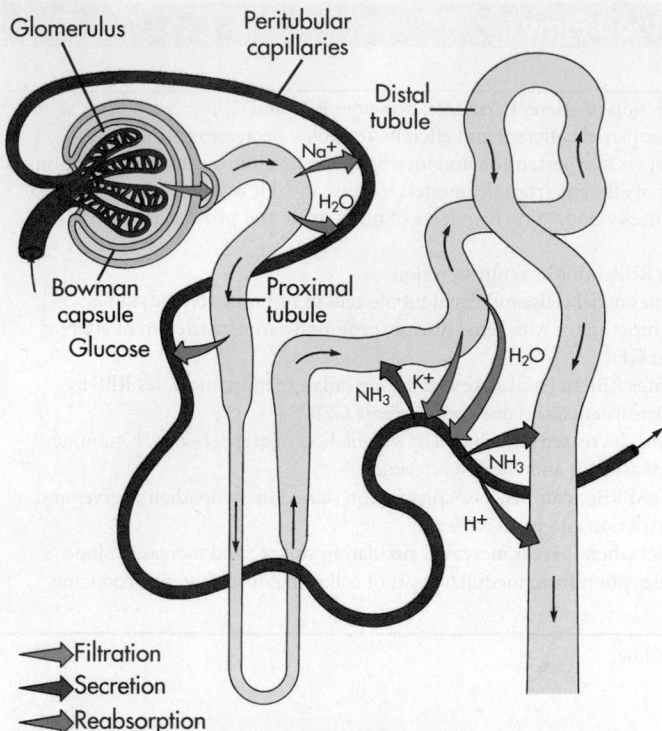

Figure 35-12 Urine formation: glomerular filtration, tubular reabsorption, and tubular secretion. The three processes by which the kidneys excrete urine. From proximal convoluted tubules, sodium and glucose are reabsorbed into peritubular capillaries by active transport. Water reabsorption by osmosis follows. From distal convoluted tubules sodium is reabsorbed by active transport. Osmotic reabsorption of water from them occurs when ADH is present. Secretion of ammonia and hydrogen occurs from peritubular capillaries into distal tubules by active transport. (From Patton KT, Thibodeau GA: *Anatomy & physiology*, ed 7, St Louis, 2010, Mosby.)

Glomerular Filtration

The fluid filtered by the glomerular capillary filtration membrane is protein free but contains electrolytes such as sodium, chloride, and potassium and organic molecules such as creatinine, urea, and glucose in the same concentrations as in plasma. Like other capillary membranes, the glomerulus is freely permeable to water and relatively impermeable to large colloids such as plasma proteins. The size of the molecules and their electrical charge are important factors affecting the permeability of substances crossing the glomerulus. The small size of the filtration slits or pores in the membrane restricts the passage of proteins and other macromolecules. The negative charge along the filtration membrane further impedes the passage of negatively charged macromolecules (because like forces repel each other). Positively charged macromolecules therefore permeate the membrane more readily than neutrally charged particles.

Capillary pressure, as well as electrical charge, has an effect on glomerular filtration. The hydrostatic pressure within the capillary is the major force for inducing water and solutes across the filtration membrane and into the Bowman capsule. This pressure is determined indirectly by the efficiency of cardiac contraction and directly by the systemic arterial pressure and the resistances to blood flow in the afferent and efferent arterioles. Two forces oppose the filtration effects of the glomerular capillary hydrostatic pressure (P_{GC}): (1) the hydrostatic pressure in the Bowman space (P_{BC}) and (2) the effective oncotic pressure of the glomerular capillary blood (π_{GC}). (As explained in Chapter 3, hydrostatic pressure is a pushing force in relation to water, and oncotic pressure is a pulling force.) Because the fluid in the Bowman space normally contains only minute amounts of protein, it normally does not have an oncotic influence on the plasma of the glomerular capillary (Figure 35-13).

The combined effect of forces favoring and forces opposing filtration determines the filtration pressure. The **net filtration pressure (NFP)** is the sum of forces favoring and opposing filtration and is expressed by the following equation:

$$NFP = (P_{GC} + \pi_{BC}) \text{ (forces favoring filtration)} - (P_{BC} + \pi_{GC})$$
$$\text{(forces opposing filtration)}$$

The estimated values contributing to the forces of net filtration are presented in Table 35-2.

As the protein-free fluid is filtered into the Bowman capsule, the plasma oncotic pressure increases and the hydrostatic pressure decreases. The increase in glomerular capillary oncotic pressure is great enough to reduce the net filtration pressure to zero at the efferent end of the capillary and to stop the filtration process effectively. The low hydrostatic pressure and increased oncotic pressure in the efferent arteriole then are transferred to the peritubular capillaries and facilitate reabsorption of fluid from the proximal tubules.

Filtration Rate

The total volume of fluid filtered by the glomeruli averages 180 L/day, or approximately 120 ml/minute, a phenomenal amount considering the size of the kidneys. Because only 1 to 2 L of urine is excreted per day, 99% of the filtrate is reabsorbed into the peritubular capillaries and returned to the blood. The factors determining the GFR are directly related to the pressures that favor or oppose filtration. Any changes in afferent or efferent arteriolar resistance will alter glomerular capillary hydrostatic pressure and GFR. Vasoconstriction of one or the other of these two arterioles produces opposite effects on glomerular pressure. For example, if the afferent arteriole constricts, blood flow decreases, with a corresponding drop in glomerular pressure. The GFR then decreases, and body fluids are conserved. Conversely, constriction of the efferent arteriole increases the net filtration pressure, and the GFR increases. When both afferent and efferent arterioles constrict, little change occurs in filtration pressure, but RBF is reduced and so is the GFR.

Obstruction to the outflow of urine (caused by strictures, stones, or tumors along the urinary tract) can cause a retrograde increase in pressure at the Bowman capsule and a decrease in GFR. Excessive loss of protein-free fluid from vomiting, diarrhea, use of diuretics, or excessive sweating can increase glomerular capillary oncotic pressure and decrease

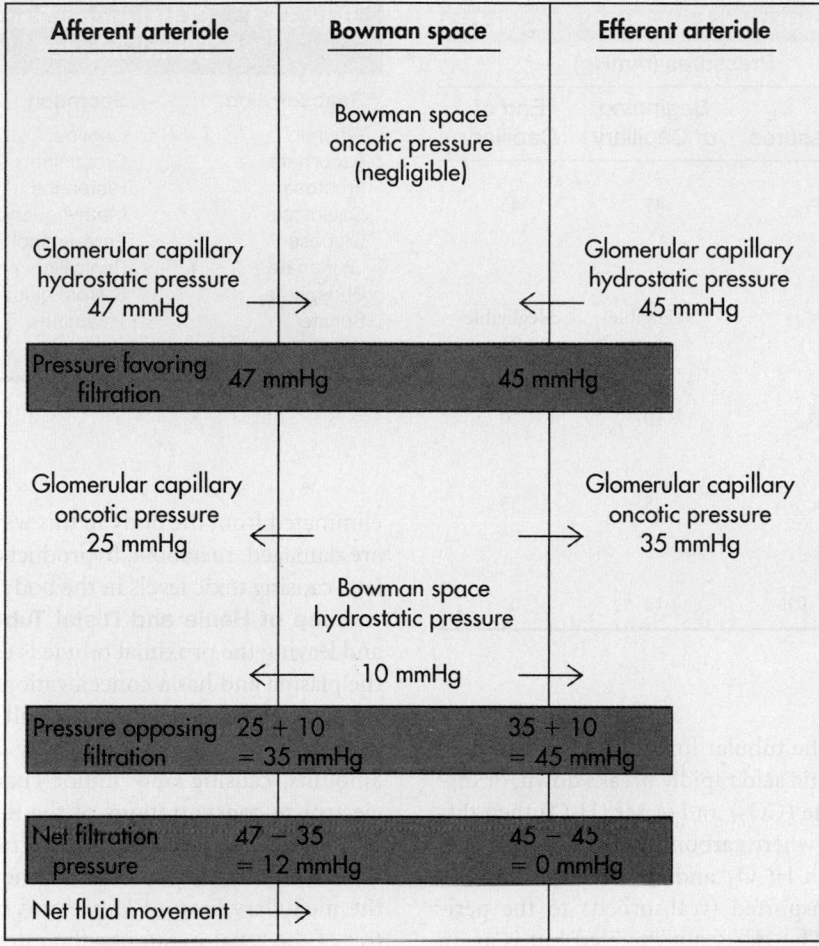

Figure 35-13 Glomerular filtration pressures.

the GFR. Renal disease also can cause changes in pressure relationships by altering capillary permeability and the surface area available for filtration (see Chapter 36).

Tubular Transport

By the time fluid reaches the end of the proximal tubule, approximately 60% to 70% of filtered sodium and water and about 50% of urea have been reabsorbed, along with 90% or more of potassium, glucose, bicarbonate, calcium, phosphate, amino acids, and uric acid. All this occurs by active transport. Chloride, water, and urea are reabsorbed passively but are linked to the active transport of sodium (cotransport). Active transport in the renal tubules can be limited as the carrier molecules become saturated, a phenomenon known as **transport maximum (T_m)**. Transport maximums exist for most substances actively transported by the tubular epithelium. The reabsorption of glucose is a significant example. Glucose is coupled to sodium transport and is almost completely reabsorbed in the proximal tubule. Like other actively transported substances, glucose has a maximal transport capacity, or renal threshold. This means that when the carrier molecules for glucose become saturated, the excess will be excreted in the urine. Normally the plasma level and filtered glucose load are not high enough to saturate the carrier mechanism. When the

plasma glucose reaches 180 mg/dl, however, as occurs in the individual with uncontrolled diabetes mellitus, the threshold for glucose is achieved. Any further increase in the plasma level causes loss of glucose in the urine.

Proximal Tubule. Active reabsorption of sodium is the primary function of the proximal tubule. Water, most electrolytes, and organic substances are cotransported with sodium. The osmotic force generated by active sodium transport promotes the passive diffusion of water out of the tubular lumen and into the peritubular capillaries. Passive transport of water is further enhanced by the elevated oncotic pressure of the blood in the peritubular capillaries. The reabsorption of water leaves an increased concentration of urea within the tubular lumen, creating a gradient for its passive diffusion to the peritubular plasma.

As the positively charged sodium ions leave the tubular lumen, negatively charged chloride ions passively follow to maintain electroneutrality. Because the luminal membrane (the inside of the tubule) of the proximal tubular cell has a limited permeability to chloride, however, chloride reabsorption lags behind sodium.

Hydrogen ions are actively exchanged for sodium ions in the tubular lumen. The hydrogen ions (H^+) then combine with

Table 35-2	Glomerular Filtration Pressures		
	Pressures (mmHg)		
Forces	Pressures	Beginning of Capillary	End of Capillary
Promoting Filtration			
Glomerular capillary hydrostatic pressure	P_{GC}	47	45
Bowman capsule oncotic pressure	π_{BC}	Negligible effect	Negligible effect
Opposing Filtration			
Bowman capsule hydrostatic pressure	P_{BC}	10	10
Glomerular capillary oncotic pressure	π_{GC}	25	35
NET FILTRATION PRESSURE		12	0

Box 35-1	Substances Transported by Renal Tubules
Reabsorption	**Secretion**
Albumin	Choline
Ascorbate	Creatinine
Fructose	Histamine
Galactose	Methyl guanidine
Glucose	Para-aminohippurate
Glutamate	Penicillin
Phosphate	Steroid glucuronides
Sulfate	Thiamine
Xylose	

bicarbonate (HCO_3^-) in the tubular lumen to form carbonic acid (H_2CO_3). The carbonic acid rapidly breaks down, or dissociates, to carbon dioxide (CO_2) and water (H_2O) then diffuse into the tubular cell, where carbonic anhydrase catalyzes the CO_2 and H_2O to form HCO_3^- and H^+. HCO_3^- combines with sodium and is transported (reabsorbed) to the peritubular capillary blood. The H^+ is not excreted but is again exchanged for sodium and reenters the lumen to recombine with HCO_3^-. Thus, in the proximal tubule, for every H^+ ion secreted into the tubular lumen, a HCO_3^- ion enters the blood (see Figure 3-10, page 117).

Bicarbonate is freely filtered at the glomerulus, but is not highly permeable at the peritubular capillary membrane. As described above it combines with H^+ and is reabsorbed as CO_2 and H_2O, which are readily diffusible. One of the unusual aspects of this process is that the bicarbonate molecule filtered at the glomerulus is not the same molecule that is reabsorbed (because it dissociates) and the hydrogen ion secreted by the proximal tubule is not excreted in the urine. Bicarbonate is thus conserved, and in this exchange, bicarbonate and hydrogen normally do not contribute to the urinary excretion of acid or the addition of acid to the blood. Approximately 90% of bicarbonate is reabsorbed by the proximal tubules.

In addition to the proximal tubular secretion of hydrogen ions, secretory transport mechanisms exist for creatinine, other organic bases, and endogenous and exogenous organic acids, including para-aminohippurate (PAH) and penicillin (Box 35-1). These secretory mechanisms are important for eliminating drugs and other exogenous chemical products from the body. Frequently, exogenous substances are conjugated with sulfate and glucuronic acid by the liver and then actively secreted by the renal tubules. This has important clinical implications because many drugs and their metabolites are

eliminated from the body in this way. When the renal tubules are damaged, metabolic byproducts and drugs may accumulate, causing toxic levels in the body.

Loop of Henle and Distal Tubule. The filtrate entering and leaving the proximal tubule is essentially isoosmotic with the plasma and has a concentration of about 285 mOsm. Although approximately 65% of salt and water is reabsorbed along the proximal tubule, they are reabsorbed in equal amounts, causing only minor changes in the osmotic and electrolyte concentrations of the fluid flowing into the loop of Henle. Therefore, any concentration or dilution of urine occurs at more distal sites of the nephron, principally in the medullary loop of Henle and collecting ducts. Near the top of the renal pyramids, the interstitial osmolality reaches 1200 mOsm/L.

These quantitative changes taking place in the loop of Henle are related to the length of the loop and its depth of penetration into the medulla. The structural features of the medullary hairpin loops provide the kidney with the ability to concentrate urine and conserve water for the body. The transition of the filtrate into urine is a function of the concentrating ability of the loops and final adjustments in urine composition made by the distal tubule and collecting duct.

The primary function of the loop of Henle is to establish a hyperosmotic state within the medullary interstitial fluid. This is achieved by reabsorbing more solute than water into the interstitium. The fluid leaving the ascending limb of the loop is therefore hypoosmotic, or more dilute than the fluid that entered. This dilution allows the distal tubule and collecting duct to make final adjustments in the concentration or dilution of the excreted urine according to body needs. The vasa recta act to maintain the high osmotic gradient established by the loop of Henle.

Different transport or permeability functions of the loop of Henle are important for dilution and concentration of urine. The thin, descending segment of the loop of Henle is highly permeable to water and moderately permeable to sodium, urea, and other solutes. The thin, ascending segment is more permeable to solutes and almost impermeable to water. The thick portion of the ascending segment is highly permeable

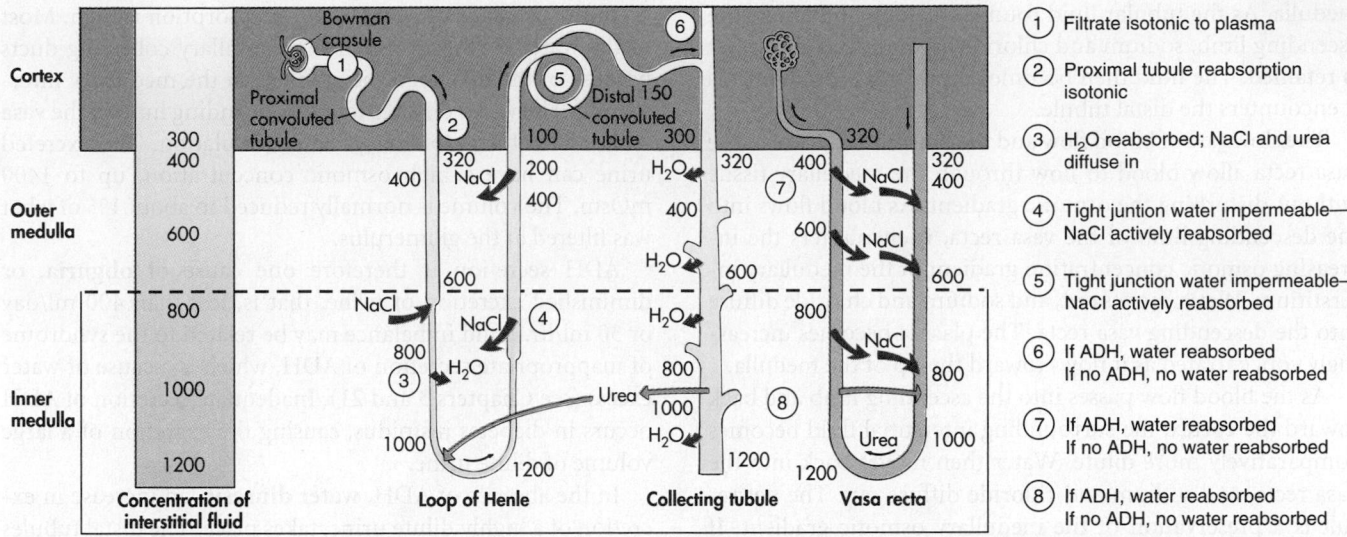

Figure 35-14 Countercurrent mechanism for concentrating and diluting urine. *ADH,* Antidiuretic hormone. (NOTE: Numbers on illustration represent milliosmoles [mOsm].)

to sodium, potassium, and chloride and significantly less permeable to water and urea. *Tamm-Horsfall glycoprotein,* also known as uromedulin, is formed on the epithelial surface of the thick ascending segment and the first segment of the distal tubule. It is the most abundant urinary protein and protects against bacterial adhesion and urolithiasis, and is a ligand for lymphokines.[13]

The convoluted portion of the distal tubule is poorly permeable to water but readily absorbs ions and contributes to the dilution of the tubular fluid. The later, straight segment of the distal tubule and the collecting duct are permeable to water as controlled by ADH. Sodium is readily absorbed by the later segment of the distal tubule and collecting duct under the regulation of the hormone aldosterone (see Chapter 20). Potassium is actively secreted by principal cells and is reabsorbed in lesser amounts by intercalated cells in these segments. Potassium also is controlled by aldosterone and other factors related to the concentration of potassium in body fluids.[14]

Hydrogen is also secreted by the distal tubule and combines with nonbicarbonate buffers (ammonium and phosphate) for the elimination of excess acids in the urine. The distal tubule thus contributes to the regulation of acid-base balance by excreting hydrogen ions into the urine and by adding new bicarbonate to the plasma (see Figure 3-10, page 117). The mechanism is similar to the conservation of bicarbonate by the proximal tubule, except that the hydrogen ion is excreted in the urine. (The specific mechanisms of acid-base balance and acid excretion are described in Chapter 3.)

Glomerulotubular Balance

To regulate body fluid balance, the kidney must not reabsorb or excrete too much sodium or water. Normally 99% of the glomerular filtrate is reabsorbed. When the GFR spontaneously decreases or increases, the renal tubules, primarily the proximal tubules, automatically adjust their rate of reabsorption of sodium and water to balance the change in

GFR. Thus a constant fraction of filtered sodium and water is reabsorbed from the proximal tubule. This prevents wide fluctuations in sodium and water excretion into the urine and maintains sodium and water balance.[15]

Concentration and Dilution of Urine

The production of a concentrated urine involves a **countercurrent exchange system,** in which fluid flows in opposite directions through parallel tubes. A concentration gradient causes fluid to be exchanged across the parallel pathways. In the nephron the fluid moves up and down the parallel sides of the hairpin loop of Henle in the medulla. The longer the loop, the greater the concentration gradient because the concentration gradient increases from the cortex to the tip of the medulla. The loops of Henle serve as multipliers of the concentration gradient, and the vasa recta act as a countercurrent exchanger for maintaining the gradient.[15]

Water, Sodium, and Chloride

The process is initiated in the thick ascending limb of the loop of Henle with the active transport of chloride and sodium out of the tubular lumen and into the medullary interstitium (Figure 35-14). Because the lumen of the ascending limb is impermeable to water, water cannot follow the sodium/chloride transport. This lack of luminal permeability causes the ascending tubular fluid to become hypoosmotic and the medullary interstitium to become hyperosmotic. The descending limb of the loop, which receives fluid from the proximal tubule, is highly permeable to water, but it is the only place in the nephron that does not actively transport either sodium or chloride. Sodium and chloride may, however, diffuse into the descending tubule from the interstitium. The hyperosmotic interstitium causes water to move out of the descending limb, and the remaining fluid in the descending tubule becomes increasingly concentrated as it flows toward the tip of the medulla. As the tubular fluid rounds the loop and enters the ascending limb, sodium and chloride are removed and water is retained. The fluid then becomes more and more dilute as it encounters the distal tubule.

The slow rate of blood flow and the hairpin structure of the vasa recta allow blood to flow through the medullary tissue without disturbing the osmotic gradient. As blood flows into the descending limb of the vasa recta, it encounters the increasing osmotic concentration gradient of the medullary interstitium. Water moves out, and sodium and chloride diffuse into the descending vasa recta. The plasma becomes increasingly concentrated as it flows toward the tip of the medulla.

As the blood flow passes into the ascending limb and back toward the cortex, the surrounding interstitial fluid becomes comparatively more dilute. Water then moves back into the vasa recta, and sodium and chloride diffuse out. The net result is a preservation of the medullary osmotic gradient. If blood were to flow rapidly through the vasa recta, as occurs in some renal diseases, the medullary concentration gradient would be washed away and the ability to concentrate urine and conserve water would be lost. The efficiency of water conservation is related to the length of the loops: the longer the loops, the greater the ability to concentrate the urine. Many desert animals have very long loops and can reabsorb water so efficiently that they rarely need to drink.

Urea

Urea is an end product of protein metabolism and is the major constituent of urine along with water. The glomerulus freely filters urea, and tubular reabsorption of urea depends on urine flow rate with less reabsorption at higher flow rates. Approximately 50% of urea is excreted in the urine, and 50% is recycled within the kidney. The recycling of urea from the tubules and collecting ducts contributes to the osmotic gradient within the medulla and is necessary for the concentration and dilution of urine. Because urea is an end product of protein metabolism, individuals with protein deprivation cannot maximally concentrate their urine.

Catecholamines

With hemorrhage or extracellular fluid depletion, sympathetic nerves are activated to release norepinephrine and dopamine, and the adrenal medulla releases epinephrine. Norepinephrine and epinephrine promote afferent arteriolar vasoconstriction and decrease GFR and RBF.[15] **Renalase** is a hormone produced by the kidney that degrades catecholamines and may be important in blood pressure regulation.[16]

Antidiuretic Hormone

The distal tubule in the cortex receives the hypoosmotic urine from the ascending limb of the loop of Henle. The concentration of the final urine is controlled by **antidiuretic hormone (ADH)**, which is secreted from the posterior pituitary, or neurohypophysis. ADH increases water permeability in the last segment of the distal tubule and along the entire length of the collecting ducts, which pass through the inner and outer zones of the medulla.

In the presence of ADH, water reabsorption is high. Most of the water is reabsorbed in the medullary collecting ducts because of the high osmotic gradient in the medullary interstitium. The water diffuses into the ascending limb of the vasa recta and returns to the systemic circulation. The excreted urine can have a high osmotic concentration, up to 1400 mOsm. The volume is normally reduced to about 1% of what was filtered at the glomerulus.

ADH secretion is therefore one cause of **oliguria,** or diminished excretion of urine, that is, less than 400 ml/day or 30 ml/hr. Fluid imbalance may be related to the syndrome of inappropriate secretion of ADH, which is a cause of water excess (see Chapters 3 and 21). Inadequate secretion of ADH occurs in diabetes insipidus, causing the excretion of a large volume of dilute urine.

In the absence of ADH, **water diuresis,** an increase in excretion of a highly dilute urine, takes place. The distal tubules and collecting ducts become impermeable to water. Water remains in the tubular lumen and is excreted as a dilute and large volume of urine. Because ADH has no effect on sodium reabsorption, it continues to be actively transported from the distal tubule. (The mechanism for the regulation of ADH and plasma osmolality is described in Chapter 3.)

Natriuretic Peptides

The natriuretic peptides (urodilantin, ANP, and BNP) promote diuresis and were described on p. 1352.

Diuretics as a Factor in Urine Flow

A **diuretic** is any agent that enhances the flow of urine. Clinically, diuretics interfere with renal sodium reabsorption and reduce extracellular fluid volume. Diuretics are commonly used to treat hypertension and edema caused by heart failure, cirrhosis, and nephrotic syndrome.

Different diuretics affect different sites of tubular function and may produce side effects that alter acid-base and electrolyte balance. Therefore, health professionals need to understand their indications for use, mechanisms of action, and toxic side effects. Diuretics are divided into five general categories: (1) osmotic diuretics, (2) carbonic anhydrase inhibitors (inhibitors of urinary acidification), (3) inhibitors of loop sodium or chloride transport, (4) aldosterone antagonists, and (5) aquaretics. (The physiologic mechanism related to each category is summarized in Table 35-3.)

Renal Hormones

Certain hormones are either activated or synthesized by the kidney. These hormones have significant systemic effects and include the active form of vitamin D, erythropoietin; renin-angiotensin and aldosterone and natriuretic hormones (see p. 1352).

Vitamin D

Vitamin D is a hormone that can be obtained in the diet or synthesized by the action of ultraviolet radiation on cholesterol in the skin. These forms of vitamin D (cholecalciferol) are

Table 35-3   Action of Diuretics

Diuretic	Site of Action	Action	Side Effects
Osmotic Diuretic			
Mannitol Glycerol Urea	Proximal tubule	Freely filtered but not reabsorbed; osmotically attracts water and diminishes sodium reabsorption	Hypokalemia, dehydration
Carbonic Anhydrase Inhibitors			
Acetazolamide	Proximal tubule	Inhibits carbonic anhydrase; blocks hydrogen ion secretion and reabsorption of sodium and bicarbonate	Hypokalemia, systemic acidosis, alkaline urine
Inhibitors of Sodium/Chloride Reabsorption			
Thiazides	Between end of ascending loop and beginning of distal tubule	Blocks sodium and chloride reabsorption; mildly suppresses carbonic anhydrase	Hypokalemia, metabolic alkalosis
Furosemide Ethacrynic acid Torsemide	Thick ascending limb of Henle loop	Blocks active transport of chloride, sodium, and potassium	Hypokalemia, uric acid retention
Bumetanide	Cortical vasodilation	Increased rate of urine formation	Hypokalemia, uric acid retention
Potassium Sparing			
Spironolactone	Distal tubule	Inhibits aldosterone, blocks sodium reabsorption, and results in potassium retention	Hyperkalemia, nausea, confusion, gynecomastia
Triamterene	Distal tubule	Blocks sodium reabsorption and inhibits potassium excretion	Nausea, vomiting, headache, and amiloride granulocytopenia, skin rash
Aquaretics			
Vasopressin (V2 receptor) blockers (i.e., conivaptan)	Distal tubule and collecting ducts	Blocks action of antidiuretic hormone	Dehydration

inactive and require two hydroxylations to establish a metabolically active form. The first step occurs in the liver with hydroxylation at the 25th carbon (calcifediol), and the second hydroxylation occurs at the first carbon position in the kidneys and is stimulated by parathyroid hormone. The end product is 1,25-dihydroxycholecalciferol, or 1,25-dihydroxyvitamin D_3 (1,25-OH_2D_3) (calcitriol), the active form of vitamin D.[17]

Calcitriol (vitamin D_3) is necessary for the absorption of calcium and phosphate by the small intestine. A decreased plasma calcium level (less than 10 mg/dl) stimulates the secretion of parathyroid hormone. Parathyroid hormone then stimulates a sequence of events that help restore plasma calcium back toward normal including:

- Calcium mobilization from bone
- Absorption of calcium and phosphate from the intestine by stimulating renal activation of vitamin D
- Increased renal calcium and phosphate reabsorption and decreased secretion

Serum phosphate fluctuations also influence the renal hydroxylation of vitamin D. Decreased levels stimulate active 1,25-OH_2D_3 formation, and increased levels inhibit formation. This results in compensatory changes in phosphate absorption from bone and the intestine. The clinical significance of the role of the kidney in calcium and phosphate metabolism

WHAT'S NEW?   Vitamin D and Immunity

The role of vitamin D in calcium and phosphorus metabolism, bone formation, and skeletal homeostasis is well known. Vitamin D, through its action on the vitamin D receptor (VDR), also has an immunoregulatory role that promotes innate and inhibits adaptive immunity and contributes to immune self-tolerance. Vitamin D deficiency is implicated in the etiology of autoimmune diseases, including multiple sclerosis, rheumatoid arthritis, systemic lupus erythematosus, type-1 diabetes mellitus, inflammatory bowel disease, Parkinson disease, and certain types of cancer including prostate, colon, and breast. Vitamin D_3 (calcitriol) inhibits expression of immunoglobulin E (IgE) by B cells, enhances expression of interleukin-10 (IL-10) by dendritic cells and T cells, and enhances T-regulatory cell function mediating a shift to a more antiinflammatory immune response. Vitamin D_3 also promotes immune protection against tuberculosis by enhancing macrophage defense against mycobacteria. Maintaining adequate levels of calcium and vitamin D is important to bone as well as immunologic health.

Data from Abbas S, Chang-Claude J, Linseisen J: *Int J Cancer*, 2008 Oct 6 (Epub ahead of print); Adams JS, Hewison M: *Nat Clin Pract Endocrinol Metab* 4(2):80-90, 2008; Evatt ML et al: *Arch Neurol* 65(10):1348-1352, 2008; Ralph AP, Kelly PM, Anstey NM: *Trends Microbiol* 16(7):336-344, 2008; Bikle D: *J Clin Endorinol Metab* 94(1): 26-34, 2009.

is evident in renal disease. Patients with renal disease have a deficiency of 1,25-OH₂D₃ and manifest symptoms of disturbed calcium and phosphate balance (see Chapter 36).

Erythropoietin

Erythropoietin (Epo) is produced by the fetal liver and in the adult kidney and is essential for normal erythropoiesis. Epo stimulates the bone marrow to produce red blood cells in response to tissue hypoxia (see Chapter 25). The stimulus for erythropoietin release is decreased oxygen delivery in the kidneys. The anemia of chronic renal failure and cancer chemotherapy is treated with recombinant human erythropoietin (rH-Epo). Epo also affects endothelium and promotes angiogenesis, mitogenesis, and antiapoptosis.[18]

TESTS OF RENAL FUNCTION

The Concept of Clearance

A number of specific renal functions can be measured by renal clearance. Renal clearance techniques determine how much of a substance can be cleared from the blood by the kidneys per given unit of time. The application of this principle permits an indirect measure of GFR, tubular secretion, tubular reabsorption, and renal blood flow.

Clearance and Glomerular Filtration Rate

The GFR provides the best estimate of functioning renal tissue. Loss or damage to nephrons leads to a corresponding decrease in GFR. The measurement of GFR requires use of a substance that has a stable plasma concentration; is not protein bound; is freely filtered at the glomerulus; does not influence GFR; and is not secreted, reabsorbed, or metabolized by the tubules. *Inulin* (a fructose polysaccharide) is one substance that meets the criteria for measurement of GFR.

The kidney "clears" inulin from the plasma by filtering it at the glomerulus, reabsorbing nearly all of the fluid, and excreting the inulin left behind in the urine. The amount of inulin filtered is equal to the volume of plasma filtered (GFR) multiplied by the plasma concentration of inulin (P_{IN}). The amount of inulin in the urine is equal to a volume of urine per unit of time ($\dot{V}$) (usually 24 hours) multiplied by the inulin concentration of urine (U_{IN}). Because all the inulin filtered is excreted in the urine,

$$GFR \times P_{IN} = U_{IN} = \dot{V}$$

GFR can be calculated by rearranging the formula:

$$GFR \text{ (ml/min)} = \frac{U_{IN} \times \dot{V}}{P_{IN}}$$

The accurate determination of **inulin clearance** requires constant infusion to maintain a stable plasma level. This is time consuming, inconvenient, and at risk for error. Therefore, the clearance of *creatinine*, a natural substance produced by muscle and released into the blood at a relatively constant rate, is commonly used clinically. It is freely filtered at the

glomerulus, but a small amount is secreted by the renal tubules. Therefore, creatinine clearance overestimates the GFR but within tolerable limits. **Creatinine clearance** provides a good measure of GFR because only one blood sample is required in addition to a 24-hour volume of urine. The GFR estimated by creatinine clearance is calculated as follows:

$$GFR \text{ (ml/min)} = \frac{U_{CR} \times \dot{V}}{P_{CR}}$$

Similar calculations can be made for all solutes excreted in the urine per unit of time. Substances freely filtered at the glomerulus but with a clearance less than inulin or creatinine have been reabsorbed along the tubules. For example, glucose is completely reabsorbed and has a clearance rate of nearly zero. Conversely, substances secreted by the tubules have a clearance rate greater than inulin or creatinine (i.e., greater than 1). Numerous formulas have been developed for estimating GFR using creatine and other indicators.[19]

Clearance and Renal Blood Flow

The standard clearance formula also can be used to estimate RPF and RBF. The substance used for this evaluation is para-aminohippuric acid (PAH). Some PAH is filtered at the glomerulus, and most of the remainder is secreted into the tubules in one circulation through the kidney. If all the PAH were removed from the plasma during a single pass through the kidney, total RPF could be determined. Because the supporting and nonsecreting structures of the kidney receive 10% to 15% of **effective renal blood flow** (**ERBF**), clearance of PAH measures only what is known as the **effective renal plasma flow** (**ERPF**), which is 85% to 90% of the true renal plasma flow:

$$ERPF = \frac{U_{PAH} \times \dot{V}}{P_{PAH}}$$

where C_{PAH} = renal clearance of PAH, U_{PAH} = PAH in urine, and P_{PAH} = PAH in plasma.

The estimation of ERBF can then be calculated by considering the hematocrit in the following formula

$$ERBF = ERPF \frac{1}{1-Hematocrit} \\ (1.0 - 0.45)$$

Blood Tests

Plasma Creatinine Concentration

A long-term decline in GFR over weeks or months is reflected in the **plasma creatinine** (**P_{CR}**) **concentration** (normal value = 0.7 to 1.2 mg/dl). The P_{CR} concentration has a stable value when the GFR is stable because creatinine has a constant rate of production as a product of muscle metabolism. The amount filtered is approximately equal to the amount excreted, and a small amount is secreted by kidney tubules. When the GFR declines, the P_{CR} increases proportionately. Thus the GFR and P_{CR} are inversely related. If the GFR were to decrease by 50%, the filtration and excretion of creatinine would be reduced by 50% and creatinine would accumulate in plasma to twice the normal value. Therefore, elevated P_{CR} values represent decreasing GFR. In the new steady state, however, the total amount of creatinine excreted in the urine would remain the same because of the proportionate decrease in GFR and increase in P_{CR}.

The application of this principle is simple and useful for monitoring progressive changes in renal function. The test is most valuable for monitoring the progress of chronic rather than acute renal disease because it takes 7 to 10 days for the plasma creatinine level to stabilize when GFR declines. Serial measures can be obtained over a long time and plotted as a curve of glomerular function. The P_{CR} also becomes elevated during trauma or breakdown of muscle tissue. In such instances the value is then not useful for estimating GFR.

Plasma Cystatin C Concentration

Serum concentrations of **cystatin C** have been proposed for estimations of GFR, particularly in children.[20] The reciprocal of the serum concentrations of cystatin C can be used as estimates of changes in GFR similar to measures of plasma creatinine concentration. The National Kidney Foundation publishes guidelines for estimating GFR for monitoring renal failure.[21]

Blood Urea Nitrogen

The concentration of urea nitrogen in the blood reflects glomerular filtration and urine-concentrating capacity. Because urea is filtered at the glomerulus, **blood urea nitrogen (BUN)** levels increase as glomerular filtration drops. Because urea is reabsorbed by the blood through the permeable tubules, the BUN rises in states of dehydration and acute and chronic renal failure when passage of fluid through the tubules is slowed. BUN also varies as a result of altered protein intake and protein catabolism and therefore is a poor measure of GFR. The normal range for BUN in the adult is 10 to 20 mg/dl of blood.

Urinalysis

Urinalysis is a noninvasive and relatively inexpensive diagnostic procedure. The best results are obtained from a fresh, cleanly voided specimen because decay permits changes in the composition of urine. Urinalysis includes evaluation of color, turbidity, protein, pH, specific gravity, sediment, and supernatant.

Urine color is normally a clear, light yellow because of urochrome and other pigments. When formed substances (crystals, blood cells, or casts) are in the urine, it appears turbid. Protein in the urine creates marked foaming when shaken, and the foam is yellow or orange when the urine contains bile pigments. Urine does not normally contain protein or bile.

Urine pH normally ranges between 5 and 6.5, but it may vary from 4.5 to 8. Urine is more alkaline after eating and then becomes less alkaline before the next meal. Because sleep is accompanied by intermittent hypoventilation, urine is more acidic on awakening.

Specific gravity is an estimated measure of the solute concentration of the urine. Specific gravity of any solution is measured by comparing the weight of the solution with an equal volume of distilled water. Hence specific gravity is not a true measure of the number or concentration of particles, but it correlates well with osmolality and is a useful clinical tool. Specific gravity usually is measured with a hydrometer in a cylinder of urine; the normal value is 1.016 to 1.022. Dipstick evaluations may be falsely high when urine pH is less than 6 and falsely low when the pH is more than 7.

The final urine osmolality is primarily a function of ADH, which controls water reabsorption in the collecting ducts. If the kidney is unable to concentrate or dilute urine, given a stimulus, the cause is usually a malfunction of the renal tubules or inappropriate ADH secretion by the posterior pituitary gland. The state of hydration also affects the urine specific gravity, so hydration status should be evaluated before making a diagnosis. This determination is helpful for differentiating oliguria caused by intrinsic renal disease from hypovolemia as a result of dehydration.

Urine Sediment

The urine sediment is examined microscopically and may contain cells, casts, crystals, and bacteria. Epithelial cells may be seen in the microscopic field because they are shed naturally throughout the urinary tract.

Red Blood Cells

Normal urine contains few or no red blood cells. If a large number of red cells are present, this is known as **hematuria,** and the sediment may be red. An alkaline or hypotonic urine causes lysis of red cells, however, so that the cells will not be seen. Urine then will be positive for hemoglobin, and the specific gravity will be elevated. Hematuria can occur with the administration of anticoagulants and with several renal diseases.

Casts

Casts (accumulations of cellular precipitates) originate in the renal tubules, from which they take their shape. They are cylindrical with distinct borders. All casts have a precipitated microprotein matrix and arise primarily from the ascending limb of the distal tubule. Red cell casts indicate bleeding into the tubules; white cell casts are associated with an inflammatory process. Epithelial cell casts indicate degeneration of the tubular lumen or necrosis of the renal tubules. The type of cast identified suggests the disease process occurring in the kidney.

Crystals

Numerous kinds of **crystals** can be observed in the urine. They may be composed of cystine, uric acid, calcium oxalate, or phosphate. They may not be initially observable, but as the urine cools, crystals will form. Crystals tend to form in a concentrated acidic or alkaline urine. Generally they are not clinically significant. Crystal formation is diagnostically significant, usually indicating inflammation, infection, or a metabolic disorder.

White Blood Cells

White blood cells (WBCs) in the urine (a condition termed **pyuria**) are indicative of urinary tract infection, particularly when bacteria are present. Glomerulonephritis and nephrotic syndrome also may demonstrate pyuria but usually in combination with proteinuria, red cells, and casts. The finding of WBC casts reflects a kidney infection because these casts are not formed in the bladder or prostate. If WBCs are present in the urine, a culture should be done for specific identification of bacteria and sensitivity of bacteria to antibiotics.

Other Measures

Dipsticks and reagent strips are available for detecting other substances in the urine, including glucose, bilirubin, urobilinogen, leukocyte esterase and nitrates, ketones, proteins, hemoglobin, and myoglobin.[2]

Aging and Renal Function

Throughout life the kidney responds to an increased workload by compensatory hypertrophy. This hypertrophy is marked in individuals who have donated a kidney for transplant or have lost functioning nephrons from trauma or disease. The glomeruli increase in diameter, and the tubules enlarge effectively to maintain the regulatory functions of the kidney. Hypertrophy occurs more rapidly and with a larger size increase in younger individuals and in those with high protein intake.

Changes in the kidneys occur throughout life, with decrease in size and a linear decrease in renal blood flow and GFR.[22,23] With aging the number of nephrons decreases and may be related to oxidative stress and inflammation.[24] The primary mechanism appears to be a change in the renal vasculature and perfusion pattern, which leads to a reduction in numbers of nephrons. The rate of nephron loss accelerates between 40 and 80 years of age. By 75 years of age the nephron population is reduced by 30% to 50%, with loss of renal mass occurring primarily in the cortex.[2] Degenerative changes within nephrons also occur with aging. The glomerular capillaries atrophy, with a reduction in the branching vessels. The glomeruli

then may disappear completely. The arcuate and interlobular arteries become tortuous, contributing to ischemia. The loss of the glomerular tuft may cause a shunt between the afferent and efferent arterioles. Although loss of juxtaglomerular nephrons still allows the vasa recta to be perfused, the combination of events contributes to a decreasing ability to excrete a concentrated urine. Thus the specific gravity of the urine in older individuals tends to be on the low side of normal.

Tubular transport changes with aging, although under normal conditions the tubules function adequately. Adaptation to stressful conditions is more difficult. Glucose, bicarbonate, and sodium are not as efficiently reabsorbed, and hyperkalemia is more common because of decreased secretion. Response to acid or base loads is delayed and prolonged. Sudden or large changes in pH or fluid load may lead to serious imbalances with increased risk of hypervolemia or hypovolemia. Acute losses or chronic fluid deficits can lead to renal insufficiency in the older adult. Administration of drugs eliminated by renal processes may require dose modifications and more astute observations for toxic side effects.[25] The T_m for glucose reabsorption decreases with age, contributing to a greater amount of glucose in the urine. This is an important consideration when glycosuria is used for screening or monitoring the process of diabetes mellitus in older adults. These changes occur independently of disease, however, indicating a normal process of aging. An age-related decline in renal activation of vitamin D decreases intestinal absorption of calcium, and older adults need more vitamin D to overcome diminishing renal function.[26] Previous or concurrent renal disease or urinary tract obstruction may amplify age-related changes in function.

Bladder symptoms are common among older adults and include frequency, urgency, and nocturia. Neurogenic and myogenic changes in bladder structure and function may contribute to some symptoms as well as influences outside the urinary tract. Changes in neurotransmission influence the micturition reflex and may lead to overactive bladder.[27] Obstruction related to prostate hypertrophy may lead to urine retention with frequency, urgency, nocturia, and slow or intermittent urinary stream.

SUMMARY REVIEW

Structures of the Renal System

1. The kidneys are paired structures lying bilaterally between the twelfth thoracic and third lumbar vertebrae.
2. The kidney is composed of an outer cortex containing the glomeruli and an inner medulla containing the tubules and collecting ducts.
3. The calyces join to form the renal pelvis, receive urine from the collecting ducts, and are continuous with the upper end of the ureter.
4. The nephron is the urine-forming unit of the kidney and is composed of the glomerulus, proximal tubule, hairpin loops of Henle, distal tubule, and collecting duct.
5. The glomerulus contains loops of capillaries. The capillary walls serve as a filtration membrane for the formation of the primary urine. The layers of the glomerular capillary include the endothelium, basement membrane, and epithelium.
6. Mesangial cells and matrix lie between and support the glomerular capillaries.
7. Juxtaglomerular cells secrete renin and are located around the afferent arteriole. They are contiguous with the sodium-sensing macula densa cells of the distal convoluted tubule.
8. The Bowman space is the space between the visceral and parietal epithelium.
9. The proximal tubule is lined with microvilli to increase surface area and enhance reabsorption.
10. The hairpin-shaped loops of Henle transport solutes and water, contributing to the hypertonic state of the medulla.
11. The distal tubule adjusts acid-base balance by excreting acid into the urine and forming new bicarbonate ions.
12. The collecting duct contains principal cells that resorb sodium and water and excrete potassium and intercalated cells that secrete hydrogen or bicarbonate and potassium.

Continued

13. The ureters extend from the renal pelvis to the posterior wall of the bladder. Urine flows through the ureters by means of peristaltic contraction of the ureteral muscles.
14. The bladder is a bag composed of the detrusor and trigone muscles and innervated by parasympathetic fibers. When accumulation of urine reaches 250 to 300 ml, mechanoreceptors, which respond to stretching of tissue, stimulate the micturition reflex.

Renal Blood Flow

1. Renal blood flows at about 1000 to 1200 ml/min, or 20% to 25% of the cardiac output.
2. Blood flow through the glomerular capillaries is maintained at a constant rate in spite of a wide range of arterial pressures (autoregulation).
3. The GFR is the filtration of plasma per unit of time and is directly related to the perfusion pressure of renal blood flow.
4. Autoregulation of RBF and sympathetic neural regulation of vasoconstriction maintain a constant GFR.
5. The renal blood vessels are innervated by the sympathetic noradrenergic nerves that regulate vasoconstriction.
6. Renin is an enzyme secreted from the juxtaglomerular apparatus; it causes the generation of angiotensin I, which is converted to angiotensin II by the action of ACE. Angiotensin II stimulates release of aldosterone from the adrenal cortex and is a potent vasoconstrictor. Thus the renin-angiotensin-aldosterone system is a regulator of renal blood flow and blood pressure.
7. Natriuretic peptides promote sodium and water loss by inhibiting aldosterone and increasing sodium chloride excretion.

Kidney Function

1. The major function of the nephron is urine formation, which involves the processes of glomerular filtration, tubular reabsorption, and tubular secretion and excretion.
2. Glomerular filtration is favored by capillary hydrostatic pressure and opposed by oncotic pressure in the capillary and hydrostatic pressure in the Bowman capsule. The balance of favoring and opposing filtration forces is the NFP.
3. The GFR is approximately 120 ml/minute, and 99% of the filtrate is reabsorbed.
4. The proximal tubule reabsorbs about 60% to 70% of the filtered sodium and water and 90% of other electrolytes.
5. Because most molecules are reabsorbed by active transport, the carrier mechanism can become saturated at the T_m. Molecules not reabsorbed are excreted with the urine.

6. The distal tubules actively reabsorb sodium and secrete potassium and hydrogen for the regulation of electrolyte and acid-base balance.
7. The concentration of the final urine is a function of the level of ADH that stimulates the distal tubules and collecting ducts to reabsorb water. The countercurrent exchange system of the long loops of Henle and their accompanying capillaries establishes a concentration gradient within the renal medulla to facilitate the reabsorption of water from the collecting duct.
8. The distal nephron regulates acid-base balance by excreting hydrogen ions and forming new bicarbonate.
9. The kidney secretes or activates a number of hormones that have systemic effects, including vitamin D_3 (1,25-OH_2D_3) and erythropoietin, which stimulates erythropoiesis when there is hypoxia.

Tests of Renal Function

1. Tests that measure renal clearance indicate how much of a substance can be cleared from the blood by the kidneys per given amount of time.
2. Creatinine, a substance produced by muscle, is measured in plasma and urine to calculate a commonly used clinical measurement of GFR (creatinine clearance).
3. The plasma creatinine concentration, cystatin C plasma concentration, and BUN levels indicate glomerular function. Plasma creatinine and cystatin C are measured to monitor progressive renal dysfunction; BUN is an indicator of hydration status.
4. PAH clearance is used to determine renal plasma flow and blood flow.
5. Urinalysis involves evaluation of color, turbidity, protein, pH, specific gravity, sediment, and supernatant.
6. Presence of bacteria, red blood cells, white blood cells, casts, or crystals in the urine sediment may indicate a renal disorder.

Aging and Renal Function

1. As a person grows older, a decrease occurs in the number of nephrons. Renal blood flow and glomerular filtration rate decline.
2. Tubular transport and reabsorption decrease with age. Response to acid-base changes and reabsorption of glucose are delayed. Drugs eliminated by the kidney can accumulate in the plasma, causing toxic reactions.
3. Neurogenic and myogenic changes in the bladder may lead to symptoms of urgency and frequency.

KEY TERMS

Angiotensin II, 1352
Angiotensin converting enzyme (ACE), 1352
Antidiuretic hormone (ADH), 1358
Arcuate arteries, 1348
Atrial natriuretic peptide (ANP), 1352
Autoregulation, 1351
Bladder, 1350
Blood urea nitrogen (BUN), 1361
Bowman capsule, 1345
Bowman space, 1345
Brain natriuretic peptide (BNP), 1352
Calcitriol, 1359

Cast, 1361
Collecting duct, 1347
Countercurrent exchange system, 1357
Creatinine clearance, 1360
Crystal, 1361
Cystatin C, 1361
C-type natriuretic peptide, 1352
Detrusor muscle, 1350
Distal tubule, 1347
Diuretic, 1358
Effective renal plasma flow (ERPF), 1360
Effective renal blood flow (ERBF), 1360

Excretion, 1352
External urethral sphincter, 1350
Filtration slit, 1346
Glomerular capillary, 1348
Glomerular endothelium, 1345
Glomerular filtration membrane, 1345
Glomerular filtration rate (GFR), 1351
Glomerulus, 1345
Hematuria, 1361
Hilum, 1345
Intercalated cell, 1347
Interlobar artery, 1347

KEY TERMS—cont'd

Interlobular arteries, 1348
Internal urethral sphincter, 1350
Inulin clearance, 1360
Juxtaglomerular apparatus (JGA), 1347
Juxtaglomerular cell, 1346
Juxtamedullary nephron, 1345, 1346
Kidney, 1344
Loop of Henle, 1347
Macula densa, 1346
Major calyx, 1345
Mesangial cell, 1345
Mesangial matrix, 1345
Micturition, 1350
Midcortical nephron, 1345
Minor calyx, 1345
Myogenic mechanism, 1351
Natriuretic peptide, 1352
Nephron, 1345
Net filtration pressure (NFP), 1354
Oliguria, 1358

Parietal epithelium, 1346
Peritubular capillary, 1348
Plasma creatinine (P_{CR}) concentration, 1360
Podocyte, 1345
Principal cell, 1347
Proximal tubule, 1347
Pyuria, 1362
Renal artery, 1347
Renalase, 1358
Renal capsule, 1344
Renal column, 1345
Renal corpuscle, 1345
Renal cortex, 1345
Renal fascia, 1344
Renal medulla, 1345
Renal papillae, 1348
Renal pelvis, 1345
Renal pyramid, 1345
Renin-angiotensin-aldosterone system, 1352
Specific gravity, 1361

Superficial cortical nephron, 1345
Transport maximum (T_m), 1355
Trigone, 1348
Tubular reabsorption, 1352
Tubular secretion, 1352
Tubuloglomerular feedback, 1351
Ultrafiltration, 1352
Urea, 1358
Ureter, 1348
Urethra, 1350
Urinalysis, 1361
Urine color, 1361
Urine pH, 1361
Urodilantin, 1352
Vasa recta, 1350
Vitamin D, 1358
Visceral epithelium, 1346
Water diuresis, 1358

REFERENCES

1. Vaughan MR, Quaggin SE: How do mesangial and endothelial cells form the glomerular tuft? *J Am Soc Nephrol* 19(1):24-33, 2008.
2. Brenner BM: *Brenner and Rector's the kidney*, ed 8, Philadelphia, 2008, Saunders.
3. Faul C et al: Actin up: regulation of podocyte structure and function by components of the actin cytoskeleton, *Trends Cell Biol* 17(9):438-437.
4. Marshall SM: The podocyte: a potential therapeutic target in diabetic nephropathy? *Curr Pharm Des* 13(26):2713-2720, 2007.
5. Wein AJ: Role of the urothelium in bladder function, *J Urol* 173(6):2199-2200, 2005.
6. Persson PB: Renal blood flow autoregulation in blood pressure control, *Curr Opin Nephrol Hypertens* 11(1):67-72, 2002.
7. Loutzenhiser R et al: Renal autoregulation: new perspectives regarding the protective and regulatory roles of the underlying mechanisms, *Am J Physiol Regul Integr Comp Physiol* 290(5):R1153-R1167, 2006.
8. Castrop H: Mediators of tubuloglomerular feedback regulation of glomerular filtration: ATP and adenosine, *Acta Physiol (Oxf)* 189(1): 3-14, 2007.
9. Schweda et al: *Renin release, Physiology (Bethesda)* 22:310-319, review, 2007.
10. Yuan et al: 1,25-dihydroxyvitamin D_3 suppresses renin gene transcription by blocking the activity of the cyclic AMP response element in the renin gene promoter, *J Biol Chem* 282(41):29821-29830, 2007.
11. Martinez-Rumayor A et al: Biology of the natriuretic peptides, *Am J Cardiol* 101(3A):3-8, 2008.
12. Cea LB: Natriuretic peptide family: new aspects, *Curr Med Chem Cardiovasc Hematol Agents* 3(2):87-98, 2005.
13. Zasloff M: Antimicrobial peptides, innate immunity, and the normally sterile urinary tract, *J Am Soc Nephrol* 18(11):2810-2816, 2007.
14. Goodfriend TL: Aldosterone—a hormone of cardiovascular adaptation and maladaptation, *J Clin Hypertens (Greenwich)* 8(2):133-139, 2006.

15. Koeppen BM, Stanton BA: *Renal physiology*, ed 4, pp 81-83, St Louis, 2007, Mosby.
16. Li G et al: Catecholamines regulate the activity, secretion, and synthesis of renalase, *Circulation* 117(10):1277-1282, 2008.
17. Lips R: Vitamin D physiology, *Prog Biophys Mol Biol* 92(1):4-8, 2006.
18. Johnson DW, Forman C, Vesey DA: Novel renoprotective actions of erythropoietin: new uses for an old hormone, *Nephrology (Carlton)* 11(4):306-312, 2006.
19. Israni AK, Kasiske BL: Laboratory assessment of kidney disease: clearance, urinalysis, and kidney biopsy. In Brenner BM, editor: *Brenner & Rector's the kidney*, ed 8, Philadelphia, 2008, Saunders.
20. Zaffanello M, Franchini M, Fanos V: Is serum cystatin-C a suitable marker of renal function in children? *Ann Clin Lab Sci* 37(3):233-240, 2007.
21. Prigent A: Monitoring renal function and limitations of renal function tests, *Semin Nucl Med* 38(1):32-46, 2008.
22. Fehrman-Ekholm I, Skeppholm L: Renal function in the elderly (>70 years old) measured by means of iohexol clearance, serum creatinine, serum urea and estimated clearance, *Scand J Urol Nephrol* 38(1):73-77, 2004.
23. Martin JE, Sheaff MT: Renal aging, *J Pathol* 211(2):198-205, 2007.
24. Csiszar A et al: The aging kidney: role of endothelial oxidative stress and inflammation, *Acta Physiol Hung* 94(1-2):107-115, 2007.
25. El Desoky ES: Pharmacokinetic-pharmacodynamic crisis in the elderly, *Am J Ther* 14(5):488-498, 2007.
26. Vieth R, Ladak Y, Walfish PG: Age-related changes in the 25-hydroxyvitamin D versus parathyroid hormone relationship suggest a different reason why older adults require more vitamin D, *J Clin Endocrinol Metab* 88(1):185-191, 2003.
27. Chu FM, Dmochowski R: Pathophysiology of overactive bladder, *Am J Med* 119(3 Suppl 1):3-8, 2006.

ALTERATIONS OF RENAL AND URINARY TRACT FUNCTION

SUE E. HUETHER • BETH A. FORSHEE

MEDIA RESOURCES

 Evolve Website (http://evolve.elsevier.com/McCance/)
- Review Questions and Answers
- Animations
- Glossary (with audio pronunciation for selected terms)
- WebLinks

Online Course
- Module 17

CHAPTER OUTLINE

URINARY TRACT OBSTRUCTION
  Upper Urinary Tract Obstruction
  Lower Urinary Tract Obstruction
  Tumors
URINARY TRACT INFECTION
  Causes of Urinary Tract Infection
GLOMERULAR DISORDERS
  Glomerulonephritis
  Nephrotic Syndrome

ACUTE KIDNEY INJURY
  Classification of Kidney Dysfunction
  Acute Kidney Injury
CHRONIC KIDNEY DISEASE
  Creatinine and Urea Clearance
  Fluid and Electrolyte Balance
  Calcium, Phosphate, and Bone

Renal and urinary function can be affected by a variety of disorders. The most common type of urinary dysfunction is infection. Stones or tumors also can obstruct the urinary tract. Renal function can be impaired by disorders of the kidney itself or by many other systemic diseases and ultimately may result in renal insufficiency or renal failure. Because the kidney filters the blood, it is directly linked to every other organ system. Renal failure, whether acute or chronic, is therefore a life-threatening condition.

URINARY TRACT OBSTRUCTION

Urinary tract obstruction is an interference with the flow of urine at any site along the urinary tract (Figure 36-1). An obstruction may be anatomic or functional; it impedes flow proximal to the blockage, dilates of the urinary system, increases risk for infection, and compromises renal function. Anatomic changes in the urinary system caused by obstruction are referred to as **obstructive uropathy.** The severity of an obstructive uropathy is determined by (1) the location of the obstructive lesion, (2) whether one or both upper urinary tracts are involved, (3) the severity (completeness) of the blockage, (4) its duration, and (5) the nature of the obstructive lesion.[1] Obstructions may be relieved or partially alleviated by correction of the obstruction, although permanent impairments occur if a complete or partial obstruction persists over weeks to months or longer.

Upper Urinary Tract Obstruction

Common causes of upper urinary tract obstruction include stricture or congenital compression of a calyx or the ureteropelvic or ureterovesical junction (i.e., stones [calculi]); compression from an aberrant vessel, tumor, or abdominal inflammation and scarring (retroperitoneal fibrosis); or ureteral blockage from stones or a malignancy of the renal pelvis or ureter.

Obstruction of the upper urinary tract causes dilation of the ureter, renal pelvis, calyces, and renal parenchyma proximal to the site of urinary blockage. Dilation of the ureter is referred to as **hydroureter** (accumulation of urine in the ureter), and dilation of the renal pelvis and calyces proximal to a blockage leads to **hydronephrosis** (enlargement of the

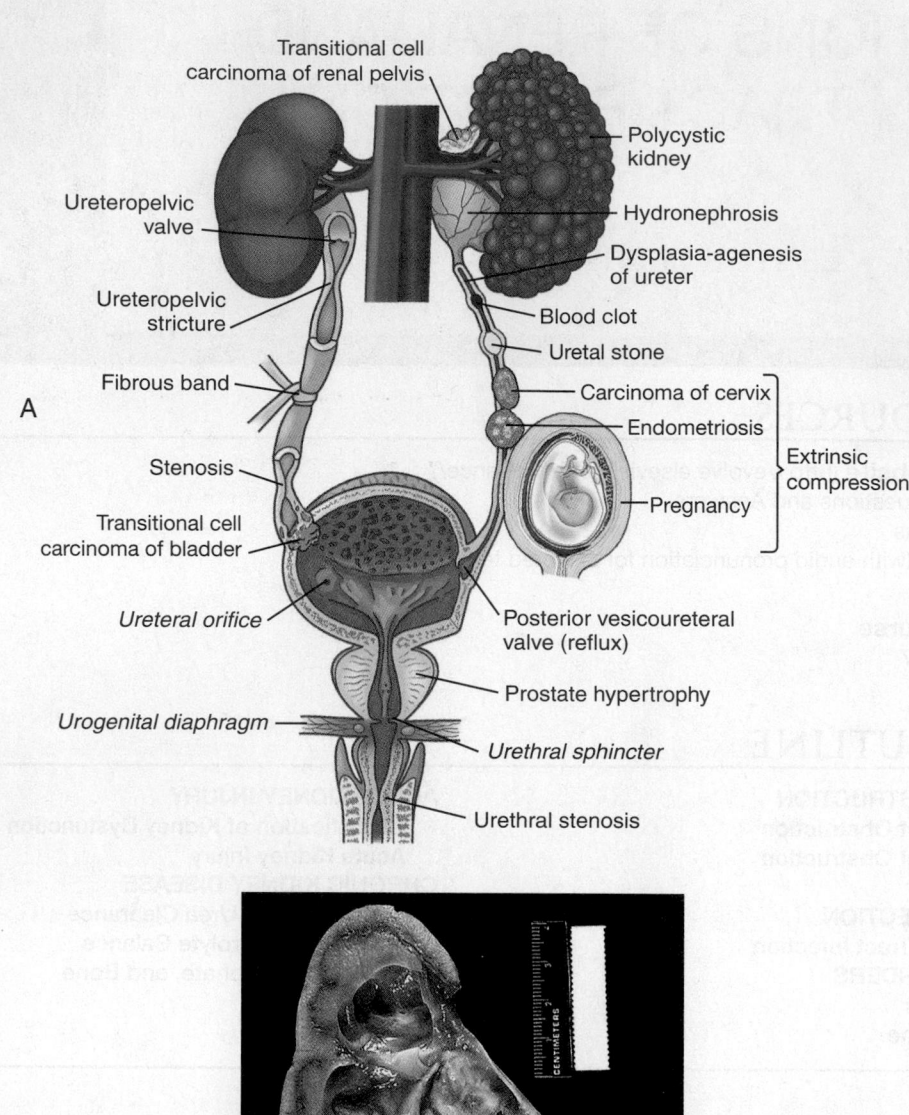

Figure 36-1 Urinary tract obstruction and hydronephrosis. **A,** Major sites of urinary tract obstruction. **B,** Hydronephrosis, marked dilation of renal pelvis and calyces with thinning of parenchyma.

renal pelvis and calyces) or **ureterohydronephrosis** (dilation of both the ureter and pelvicaliceal system) (Figure 36-2). Dilation of the upper urinary tract is an early response to obstruction and reflects smooth muscle hypertrophy and accumulation of urine above the level of blockage (urinary stasis/retention). The increased pressure is transmitted to the glomerulus, which decreases filtration. Unless the obstruction

is relieved, this dilation leads to enlargement with tubulointerstitial fibrosis and apoptosis affecting the distal nephron and renal function. **Tubulointerstitial fibrosis** is the deposition of excessive amounts of extracellular matrix (collagen and other proteins). Deposition of extracellular matrix is a normal process of organ repair and maintenance, and the deposition of extracellular matrix is balanced by its breakdown

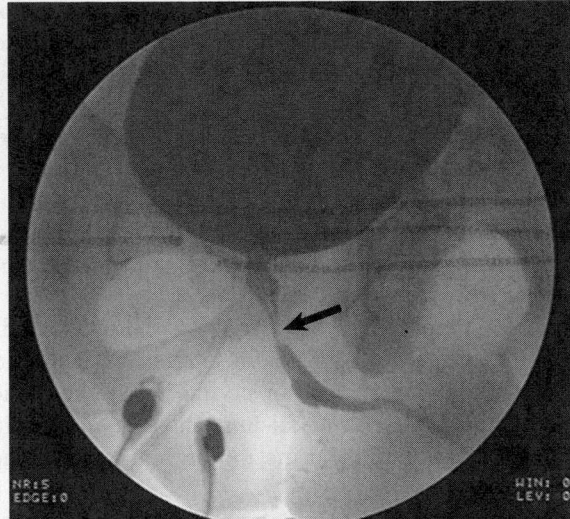

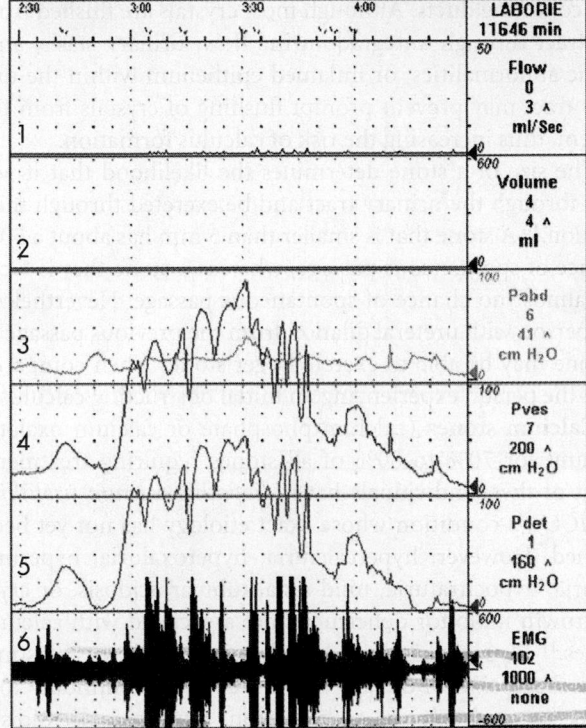

Figure 36-2 Neurogenic detrusor overactivity with vesicosphincter. The arrow indicates narrowing of the striated sphincter consistent with electromyographic activity *(Line 6)* noted on the urodynamic tracing. Note the characteristic poor flow pattern *(Line 1)* with elevated voiding pressures *(Lines 4 and 5)* indicating obstruction. Line 1 = Urine flow rate; Line 2 = urine volume; Line 3 = abdominal pressure (Pabd); Line 4 = intravesicular (inside) bladder) pressure (Pves); Line 5 = detrusor muscle pressure (Pdet); Line 6 = bladder electromyelogram (EMG).

under the influence of metalloproteinases. Multiple cytokines and growth factors have been implicated in the process of tubulointerstitial fibrosis and irreversible loss of kidney function, including transforming growth factor-beta-1 (TGF-β1), angiotensin II, and various tumor necrosis factors. **Apoptosis** is a normal process that the body uses to replace damaged or senescent cells with new ones, but the imbalance in growth

factors provoked by obstruction leads to excess cellular destruction and death, ultimately resulting in loss of functioning nephrons and kidney damage.

Tubulointerstitial fibrosis and apoptosis result in detectable damage to the distal renal tubules within approximately 7 days. By 14 days, obstruction has adversely affected both distal and proximal aspects of the nephron. Within 28 days the glomeruli of the kidney have been damaged and the renal cortex and medulla are reduced in size (thinned). Distal tubular damage occurs initially and decreases the kidney's ability to concentrate urine, causing an increase in urine volume despite a decrease in glomerular filtration rate (GFR). The affected kidney is unable to conserve sodium, bicarbonate, and water or to excrete hydrogen or potassium, leading to metabolic acidosis and dehydration. The magnitude of this damage, and the kidney's ability to recover normal homeostatic function, is affected by the severity and duration of the obstruction. With complete obstruction, damage to the renal tubules and compression of the renal vasculature occurs in a matter of hours, and irreversible damage occurs within 3 to 4 weeks. Nevertheless, even in the face of a complete obstruction, the human kidney may recover at least partial homeostatic function provided the blockage is removed within 56 to 69 days.[2] This recovery requires approximately 4 months. Partial obstruction, in the absence of renal infection, leads to subtler but ultimately permanent impairments including loss of the kidney's ability to concentrate urine, reabsorb bicarbonate, excrete ammonia, or regulate metabolic acid-base balance. Complete bilateral obstruction causes anuria.

The body is able to partially counteract the negative consequences of unilateral obstruction by a process called **compensatory hypertrophy** and **hyperfunction.**[3] The compensatory response is the result of two growth processes: **obligatory growth** occurs under the influence of somatomedins, and **compensatory growth** occurs under the influence of a yet-to-be-identified hormone or hormones. These processes cause the contralateral (unobstructed) kidney to increase the size of individual glomeruli and tubules but not the total number of functioning nephrons. The ability of the body to engage in compensatory hypertrophy and hyperfunction diminishes with age, and the process is reversible when relief of obstruction results in recovery of function by the obstructed kidney. Unilateral obstruction may remain silent for a long time.

Relief of bilateral, partial urinary tract obstruction, or complete obstruction of one kidney is usually followed by a brief period of diuresis (commonly called **postobstructive diuresis**).[4] It is a physiologic response and is typically mild, representing a restoration of fluid and electrolyte imbalance caused by the obstructive uropathy. Alterations in tubular transport and water reabsorption and volume expansion contribute to the diuresis. Occasionally relief of obstruction will cause rapid excretion of large volumes of water, sodium, or other electrolytes, resulting in a urine output of 10 L/day or more. Rapid postobstructive diuresis causes dehydration and fluid and electrolyte imbalances if not promptly corrected.

Risk factors for severe postobstructive diuresis include bilateral obstruction, impairment of one or both kidneys' ability to concentrate urine or reabsorb sodium (*nephrogenic diabetes insipidus*), hypertension, edema and weight gain, congestive heart failure, and uremic encephalopathy.

Kidney Stones

Calculi, or **urinary stones,** are masses of crystals, protein, or other substances that are a common cause of urinary tract obstruction in adults. The prevalence of stones in the United States is approximately 6% in women and 15% in men.[5] The recurrence rate is approximately 30% to 50% within 5 years.[6] The risk of urinary calculi formation is influenced by a number of factors, including age, gender, race, geographic location, seasonal factors, fluid intake, diet, occupation, genetic predisposition and other conditions including urinary tract infection, hypertension, and obesity.[7,8] Most persons develop their first stone before age 50 years. Geographic location influences the risk of stone formation because of indirect factors, including average temperature, humidity, and rain fall, and its influence on fluid and dietary patterns. Persons who regularly consume an adequate volume of water and those who are physically active are at reduced risk when compared with people who are inactive or consume lower volumes of fluid. Most renal stones are unilateral.

Urinary calculi can be classified according to the primary minerals (salts) that make up the stones. The most common stone types include calcium oxalate or phosphate (70% to 80%), struvite (magnesium, ammonium, and phosphate) (15%), and uric acid (7%). Cystine stones are rare, less than 1%. Less common stone elements include cystine, 2,8-dihydroxyadeninuria (a rare genetic disorder that increases risk of xanthine stones), triamterene (a diuretic), and indinavir (a protease inhibitor used in management of HIV infection).

PATHOPHYSIOLOGY The specific cascade of events that lead to stone formation is unknown. Stone formation requires (1) supersaturation of one or more salts in the urine, (2) precipitation of the salts from a liquid to a solid state, (3) growth through crystallization or agglomeration (sometimes called aggregation), and (4) the presence or absence of stone inhibitors.[9] Supersaturation is the presence of a higher concentration of a salt within a fluid (in this case, the urine) than the volume is able to dissolve to maintain equilibrium.

Human urine contains many positively and negatively charged ions capable of *precipitating* from solution and forming a variety of salts. The salts form crystals that are retained and grow into stones. *Crystallization* is the process by which crystals grow from a small *nidus* or nucleus to larger stones in the presence of supersaturated urine. Although supersaturation is essential for stone formation, the urine need not remain continuously supersaturated for a calculus to grow once its nidus has precipitated from solution. Intermittent periods of supersaturation after the ingestion of a meal or during times of dehydration are sufficient for stone growth in many individuals. In addition, the renal tubules and papillae have many surfaces that may attract a crystalline nidus and add biologic material (matrix) to the forming stone. *Matrix* is an organic material that is formed in the presence of urea-splitting pathogens and is high in stones associated with infection.[9]

Temperature and pH of the urine also influence the risk of precipitation and calculus formation—pH is more important. An alkaline urinary pH significantly increases the risk of calcium phosphate stone formation, whereas acidic urine increases the risk of a uric acid stone. Cystine and xanthine precipitate more readily in acidic urine.

Stone or *crystal growth inhibiting substances*, including Tamm-Horsfall protein, potassium citrate, pyrophosphate, and magnesium, are capable of crystal growth inhibition, thereby reducing the risk of calcium phosphate or calcium oxalate precipitation in the urine and preventing subsequent stone formation.

Retention of *crystal particles* occurs primarily at the papillary collecting ducts. Although most crystals are flushed from the tract through antegrade urine flow, urinary stasis, anatomic abnormalities, or inflamed epithelium within the urinary tract may prevent prompt flushing of crystals from the system, thus increasing the risk of calculus formation.

The size of a stone determines the likelihood that it will pass through the urinary tract and be excreted through micturition.[10] A stone that is smaller than 5 mm has about a 50% chance of spontaneous passage, whereas a stone that is 1 cm has almost no chance of spontaneous passage. Nevertheless, the person with ureteral dilation from the previous passage of a stone may be able to excrete larger stones when compared with the person experiencing an initial obstructing calculus.

Calcium stones (calcium phosphate or calcium oxalate) account for 70% to 80% of all stones requiring treatment. Most of these individuals have *idiopathic calcium urolithiasis (ICU)*, a condition whose exact etiology has not yet been defined. However, hypercalciuria, hyperoxaluria, hyperuricosuria, hypocitraturia, mild renal tubular acidosis, or crystal growth inhibitor deficiencies are associated with calcium stones.[11] Hypercalciuria is usually attributable to intestinal hyperabsorption of dietary calcium and less commonly to a defect in renal calcium reabsorption. Hyperparathyroidism and bone demineralization associated with prolonged immobilization are also known to cause hypercalciuria. An alkaline urine also promotes calcium stone formation.[12] Although oxalate in the diet influences the risk of calcium stones, primary hyperoxaluria is a rare, inherited disorder.

Struvite stones primarily contain magnesium-ammonium-phosphate as well as varying levels of matrix. Matrix forms in an alkaline urine and during infection with a urease-producing bacterial pathogen, such as a *Proteus, Klebsiella,* or *Pseudomonas*. Struvite calculi may grow quite large and branch into a staghorn configuration (**staghorn calculus**) that approximates the pelvicaliceal collecting system.[13] Women are at greater risk for struvite stones because they have an increased incidence of urinary tract infection.

Uric acid is primarily a product of biosynthesis of endogenous purines and is secondarily affected by consumption of purines in the diet. Persons who excrete excessive uric acid in the urine, such as those with gouty arthritis, are at particular risk for **uric acid stones.** A consistently acidic urine greatly increases this risk. Cystine and xanthine are amino acids that precipitate more readily in acidic urine. *Cystinuria* and *xanthinuria* are genetic disorders of amino acid metabolism, and their excess in urine can cause **cystinuric,** or **xanthine, stone** formation in the presence of a low urine pH of 5.5 or less.

CLINICAL MANIFESTATIONS Renal colic, described as moderate to severe pain often originating in the flank and radiating to the groin, usually indicates obstruction of the renal pelvis or proximal ureter.[14] Colic that radiates to the lateral flank or lower abdomen typically indicates obstruction in the midureter, and bothersome lower urinary tract symptoms (urgency, frequent voiding, urge incontinence) indicate obstruction of the lower ureter or ureterovesical junction. The pain can be severe and incapacitating and may be accompanied by nausea and vomiting. Gross or microscopic hematuria may be present.

EVALUATION AND TREATMENT The evaluation and diagnosis of urinary calculi are based on presenting symptoms and history combined with a focused physical assessment, imaging studies, and possibly a functional study of renal pelvic and ureteral pressures.[15] The history also queries dietary habits, the age of the first stone episode, stone analysis, and presence of complicating factors including hyperparathyroidism or recent gastrointestinal or genitourinary surgery. Urinalysis (including pH) is obtained and a 24-hour urine is completed to identify calcium oxalate, citrate, and other significant constituents. In addition, every effort is made to retrieve and analyze calculi that are passed spontaneously or retrieved through aggressive intervention. Additional tests are obtained in selected individuals, such as those with suspected hyperparathyroidism or cystine or uric acid stones, in order to diagnose and manage underlying metabolic disorders. An x-ray film of the kidneys, ureters, and bladder (KUB radiograph) is obtained to evaluate radiopaque stones (comprising more than 90% of all stones), and an ultrasound, intravenous pyelogram (IVP), or computed tomography (CT) scan or ultrasonography is obtained to determine the location of the calculi, the severity of obstruction, and associated obstructive uropathy.[16] CT urography is used for pre- and postoperative evaluation and fluoroscopy guides intraoperative imaging.[17]

The goals of treatment are to manage acute pain, promote stone passage, reduce the size of stones already formed, and prevent new stone formation. The components of treatment include (1) parenteral and/or oral analgesics for acute pain, (2) medical therapy promoting stone passage, (3) reducing the concentration of stone-forming substances by increasing urine flow rate with high fluid intake, (4) decreasing the amount of stone-forming substances in the urine by decreasing dietary intake or endogenous production or by altering urine pH,[18] and (5) removing stones using percutaneous nephrolithotomy, ureteroscopy, or ultrasonic or laser lithotripsy to fragment stones for excretion in the urine.[19,20]

Lower Urinary Tract Obstruction

Obstructive disorders of the lower urinary tract (LUT) are primarily related to storage of urine in the bladder or emptying of urine through the bladder outlet. The causes of the obstruction include neurogenic and anatomic alterations or, in some instances, a combination of both. Incontinence is a common symptom and types of incontinence are reviewed in Table 36-1.

Neurogenic Bladder

Neurogenic bladder is a general term for bladder dysfunction caused by neurologic disorders. The types of dysfunction are related to the sites in the nervous system that control sensory and motor bladder function (Figure 36-3). Lesions that develop in upper motor neurons of the brain and spinal cord result in **dyssynergia** (loss of coordinated neuromuscular contraction) and overactive or hyperreflexive bladder function. Lesions in the sacral area of the spinal cord or peripheral nerves result in underactive, hypotonic, or atonic (flaccid) bladder function, often with loss of bladder sensation.

Neurologic disorders that develop above the pontine micturition center result in **detrusor hyperreflexia,** also known as an uninhibited or reflex bladder. This is an upper

Table 36-1	Types of Incontinence
Type	**Description**
Urge incontinence (most common in older adults)	Involuntary loss of urine associated with an abrupt and strong desire to void (urgency) Often associated with involuntary contractions of the detrusor. When associated with a neurologic disorder this is called detrusor hyperreflexia. When no neurologic disorder exists this is called detrusor instability. May be associated with decreased bladder wall compliance.
Stress incontinence (most common in women younger than 60 years and men who have had prostate surgery)	Involuntary loss of urine during coughing, sneezing, laughing, or other physical activity associated with increased abdominal pressure
Overflow incontinence	Involuntary loss of urine with overdistention of the bladder Associated with neurologic lesions below S1, polyneuropathies and urethral obstruction (i.e., an enlarged prostate)
Mixed incontinence (most common in older women)	A combination of stress and urge incontinence
Functional incontinence	Involuntary loss of urine due to dementia or immobility

Data from Agency for Healthcare Research and Quality: *Overview: urinary incontinence in adults, clinical practice guideline update,* Rockville, MD, 1996. Available at www.ahrq.gov/clinic/uiovervw.htm.

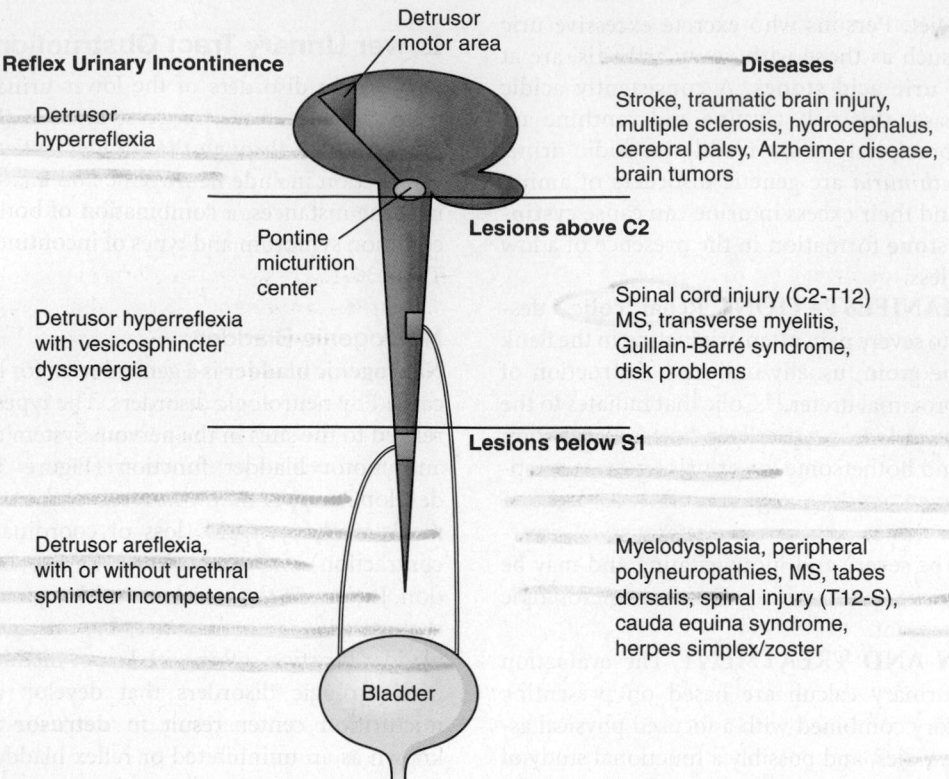

Reflex Urinary Incontinence

Detrusor
hyperreflexia

Detrusor hyperreflexia
with vesicosphincter
dyssynergia

Detrusor areflexia,
with or without urethral
sphincter incompetence

Detrusor
motor area

Pontine
micturition
center

Bladder

Lesions above C2

Lesions below S1

Diseases

Stroke, traumatic brain injury,
multiple sclerosis, hydrocephalus,
cerebral palsy, Alzheimer disease,
brain tumors

Spinal cord injury (C2-T12)
MS, transverse myelitis,
Guillain-Barré syndrome,
disk problems

Myelodysplasia, peripheral
polyneuropathies, MS, tabes
dorsalis, spinal injury (T12-S),
cauda equina syndrome,
herpes simplex/zoster

Figure 36-3 Causes of neurogenic bladder and reflex incontinence. (Adapted from Doughty DB: Urinary and fecal incontinence. In Doughty DB, editor: *Urinary and fecal incontinence: nursing management,* ed 2, St Louis, 2000, Mosby.)

motor neuron disorder in which the bladder empties automatically when it becomes full and the external sphincter functions normally. Because the pontine micturition center remains intact, there is coordination between detrusor muscle contraction and the relaxation of the urethral sphincter. Stroke, traumatic brain injury, dementia, and brain tumors are examples of disorders that result in detrusor hyperreflexia. Symptoms include urine leakage and incontinence.

Neurologic lesions that occur below the pontine micturition center but above the sacral micturition center (between C2 and S1) are also upper motor neuron lesions and result in **detrusor hyperreflexia with vesicosphincter dyssynergia.** There is loss of pontine coordination of detrusor muscle contraction and external sphincter relaxation, so both the bladder and the sphincter are contracting at the same time, causing a functional obstruction of the bladder outlet.[21] Spinal cord injury, multiple sclerosis, Guillain-Barré syndrome, and intervertebral disk problems are causes of this disorder. There is diminished bladder relaxation during storage with small urine volumes and high intravesicular (inside the bladder) pressures. This results in an overactive bladder syndrome with symptoms of frequency, urgency, and urge incontinence and increased risk for urethral turbulence and urinary tract infection.

Lesions that involve the sacral micturition center (below S1; may also be termed *cauda equina syndrome*) or peripheral nerve lesions result in **detrusor areflexia** (acontractile

detrusor), a lower motor neuron disorder. The result is an acontractile detrusor or atonic bladder with retention of urine and distention. If the sensory innervation of the bladder is intact, the full bladder will be sensed but the detrusor may not contract. This is an *underactive bladder syndrome* and may have symptoms of stress and overflow incontinence. Myelodysplasia, multiple sclerosis, tabes dorsalis, and peripheral polyneuropathies are associated with this disorder.

Overactive Bladder Syndrome

Overactive bladder syndrome (OAB) is a syndrome of detrusor overactivity characterized by urgency with involuntary detrusor contractions during the bladder filling phase that may be spontaneous or provoked.[22] There is coordination between the contracting bladder and the external sphincter, but the detrusor is too weak to empty the bladder, resulting in urinary retention with overflow or stress incontinence. Overactive bladder as defined by the International Continence Society as a *symptom syndrome* of urgency, with or without urge incontinence and usually associated with frequency and nocturia.[23] Overactive bladder syndrome affects millions of men, women, and children; adults are often reluctant to discuss this syndrome with their healthcare provider. Sexual dysfunction and bowel problems often accompany OAB.[24] Diagnosis is usually made by evaluation of symptoms. Urodynamic evaluation confirms the diagnosis. Antimuscarinics are the most common treatment and in intractable cases, surgery is recommended.[25] When left untreated, OAB is costly, impairs health and quality of life, causes depression, and leads to social isolation; in older adults it may cause risk for falls and urinary tract infection.[26]

Obstructions to Urine Flow

Anatomic causes of resistance to urine flow include urethral stricture, prostatic enlargement in men, and pelvic organ prolapse in women. Symptoms of obstruction are more common in men and include (1) frequent daytime voiding (urination more than every 2 hours while awake); (2) nocturia (awakening more than once each night to urinate for adults less than 65 years of age or more than twice for older adults); (3) poor force of stream; (4) intermittency of urinary stream; (5) bothersome urinary urgency, often combined with hesitancy; and (6) feelings of incomplete bladder emptying despite micturition.

A **urethral stricture** is a narrowing of its lumen. It occurs when infection, injury, or surgical manipulation produces a scar that reduces the caliber of the urethra.[27] The vast majority of urethral strictures occur in men; they are rare in women.[28] The severity of obstruction is influenced by its location within the urethra, its length, and the minimum caliber of urethral lumen within the stricture. Specifically, proximal urethral strictures cause more severe obstruction than do strictures of the distal urethra, longer strictures tend to be more obstructive, and the magnitude of blockage is in *reverse* proportion to the urethral caliber.

Prostate enlargement is caused by acute inflammation, benign prostatic hyperplasia, or prostate cancer (see Chapter 23). Each of these disorders can cause encroachment on the urethra with obstruction to urine flow and the symptoms summarized previously.

Severe **pelvic organ prolapse** (see Chapter 23) in a woman causes bladder outlet obstruction when a cystocele (the downward protrusion of the bladder into the vagina) descends below the level of the urethral outlet. Cystoceles that reach or protrude beyond the vaginal introitus create the greatest risk for obstruction, particularly if the bladder neck has been surgically repaired without simultaneous repair of the cystocele.[29] In men the bladder may rarely herniate into the scrotum, causing a similar type of obstruction.

Partial obstruction of the bladder outlet or urethra initially causes an increase in the force of detrusor contraction. If the blockage persists, afferent nerves within the bladder wall are adversely affected, leading to urinary urgency and, in some cases, overactive detrusor contractions (a myogenic cause of overactive bladder). When obstruction persists, there is an increased deposition of collagen within the smooth muscle bundles of the detrusor muscle (*trabeculation*), possibly in an attempt to increase the force of its contraction strength. Ultimately, the bladder wall loses its ability to stretch and accommodate urine, a condition called **low bladder wall compliance,** and the detrusor loses its ability to contract efficiently. Low bladder wall compliance chronically elevates intravesicular pressure, greatly increasing the problems of hydroureter, hydronephrosis, and impaired renal function.

EVALUATION AND TREATMENT Although the history and physical examination are critical to the evaluation of lower urinary tract disorders, it must be remembered that no symptom or cluster of symptoms has been identified that accurately differentiates the various causes of these disorders. For example, symptoms such as urgency, urge incontinence, frequent urination, and nocturia may develop because of overactive bladder or either increased or decreased bladder outlet resistance. Reduced resistance is associated with the symptom of stress incontinence (incontinence with coughing or sneezing) and symptoms of increased resistance are similar to bladder outlet obstruction, including poor force of urinary stream, hesitancy, and feelings of incomplete bladder emptying.

Various diagnostic tests assist with evaluation. The *postvoid urine* is measured by catheterization within 5 to 15 minutes of urination or through a bladder ultrasound machine that measures bladder height and width to provide an approximation of urine within the vesicle. This measurement may be combined with *uroflowmetry*, a graphic representation of the force of the urinary stream expressed as milliliters voided per second. Each of these measurements assesses the lower urinary tract's efficiency in evacuating urine through micturition but neither differentiates poor detrusor contraction strength from obstruction as a cause of urinary retention. Instead, *multichannel urodynamic testing* is used to identify obstruction, quantify its severity, and measure detrusor contraction strength (see Figure 36-2). *Video-urodynamic recordings* can also demonstrate overactive bladder and detrusor sphincter dyssynergia. An evaluation of renal function, including functional imaging studies and serum creatinine, is completed particularly when obstruction is severe and associated with elevated residuals or urinary tract infection.

Because the bladder neck consists of circular smooth muscle with adrenergic innervation, detrusor sphincter dyssynergia may be managed by α-adrenergic blocking (antimuscarinic) medications. Obstruction that is not adequately managed by pharmacotherapy may require bladder neck incision. Detrusor sphincter dyssynergia may be managed by intermittent catheterization in combination with higher dose antimuscarinic drugs to prevent overactive detrusor contractions and associated dyssynergia while ensuring regular, complete bladder evacuation through catheterization. Alternatively, men with dyssynergia may be managed by condom catheter containment, supplemented by an α-adrenergic blocking drug or transurethral sphincterotomy (surgical incision of the striated sphincter) in order to relieve obstruction. Low bladder wall compliance may be managed by antimuscarinic drugs and intermittent catheterization; however, more severe cases may require augmentation enterocystoplasty (enlargement of the low compliant bladder wall using a detubularized piece of small bowel), urinary diversion, or long-term indwelling catheterization.

Prostate enlargement is managed by treating the underlying cause of the prostate enlargement with medication or surgery. Acute prostatitis is initially managed by broad-spectrum antibiotics until the results of a urine culture are obtained. Urinary retention may require transient placement of a suprapubic catheter. The management of benign prostatic hyperplasia and treatment options for prostate cancer are presented in Chapter 23.

Urethral stricture is treated with urethral dilation accomplished by using a steel instrument shaped like a catheter (urethral sound) or a series of incrementally increasing catheter-like tubes (filiforms and followers). Long, dense strictures typically require surgical repair to prevent recurrence.

A pessary (rubber or silicone device designed to compensate for vaginal wall prolapse) may be inserted to mechanically reverse severe pelvic organ (bladder, uterus, or rectum) prolapse. Depending on the device, the woman may be able to remove, cleanse, and replace the pessary, or it may be changed during a clinic visit. Intravaginal hormone replacement therapy and regular follow-up are critical to the long-term success of a pessary. Alternatively, pelvic organ prolapse may be repaired surgically; the procedure may be combined with a urethral suspension to correct stress urinary incontinence or rectocele repair.

Tumors

Renal Tumors

Renal tumors account for about 57,760 (3.8%) new cancer cases and 12,980 (2.3%) deaths each year.[30] There are a number of different types of kidney tumors. **Renal adenomas** (benign tumors) are uncommon but are increasing in number. The tumors are solid, encapsulated and are usually located near the cortex of the kidney. Because they can become malignant, they are usually surgically removed. **Renal cell carcinoma (RCC)** is the most common renal neoplasm (85% of all renal neoplasms) and represents about 2% of cancer deaths (Figure 36-4). Renal cell carcinoma usually occurs in men (two times more often than in women) between 50 and 60 years of age.

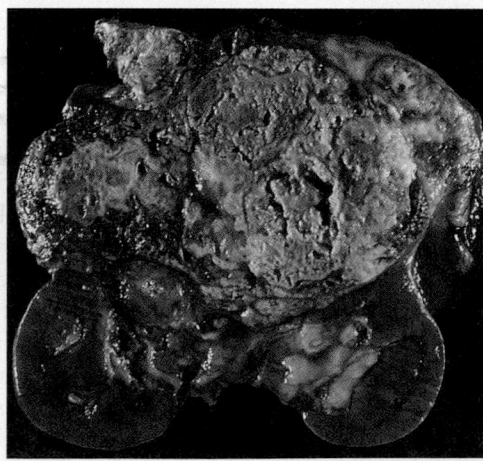

Figure 36-4 Renal cell carcinoma. Renal cell carcinomas usually are spheroidal masses composed of yellow tissue mottled with hemorrhage, necrosis, and fibrosis. (From Damjanov I, Linder J, editors: *Anderson's pathology,* ed 10, St Louis, 1996, Mosby.)

Risk factors include cigarette smoking, obesity and hypertension.[31] Five-year survival is 96% for stage I cancer and about 23% for stage V cancer.[30] Black Americans have shorter survival than their white counterparts and this may be related to extent of comorbid conditions and lower rate of surgical treatment.[32]

PATHOGENESIS Renal cell carcinomas are adenocarcinomas that usually arise from tubular epithelium commonly in the renal cortex. The etiology is unknown. They are classified according to cell type and extent of metastasis. *Clear cell tumors*, the most common, present a better prognosis than granular cell or spindle tumors. Confinement within the renal capsule, together with treatment, is associated with a better survival rate. The tumors usually occur unilaterally (see Figure 36-4). About 25% to 30% of individuals with RCC present with metastasis.[33]

CLINICAL MANIFSTATIONS The classic clinical manifestations of renal tumors are hematuria, dull and aching flank pain, and palpable flank mass in thinner individuals. Systemic manifestations usually represent an advanced stage of disease and include weight loss, fatigue, intermittent fever from tumor toxins, anemia from hematuria and lack of erythropoietin or polycythemia from tumor secretion of erythropoietin, hypertension from elevated renin levels, and alterations in liver function tests. All of these symptoms occur in less than 10% of cases. Further, they represent an advanced stage of disease, whereas earlier stages are often silent. The most common sites of distant metastasis are the lung, lymph nodes, liver, bone, thyroid, and central nervous system.[34]

EVALUATION AND TREATMENT Diagnosis is based on the clinical symptoms, plain x-ray films of the abdomen, intravenous pyelography, renal angiography, and CT. (Staging of renal cell carcinoma is presented in Table 36-2.) Staging systems using molecular tumor markers are rapidly advancing.[35] Treatment for localized disease is surgical removal of the affected kidney (radical nephrectomy) with combined use of chemotherapeutic agents. Smaller tumors may be removed by nephron-sparing surgery (partial nephrectomy).[36] Radiation therapy also may be used and new techniques using radiofrequency ablation, cryoablation and laparoscopy are promising.[37] Immunotherapy (i.e., interferon-alpha and interleukin-2) is promising in selected cases, and new targeted therapies are being developed.[38] Tumor obstruction is relieved by placing ureteral catheters, placement of nephrostomy tubes, or completion of urinary diversion procedures. Survival is related to tumor grade, tumor cell type, and extent of metastasis.

Bladder Tumors

Bladder tumors represent about 3% of all malignant tumors and are the fourth most common malignancy in men.[30,39] Approximately 70,980 (4.8%) people develop bladder cancer each year, and 14,430 (2.5%) die of it.[30,39] The development of bladder cancer is most common in men older than 60 years. *Urothelial carcinoma* previously known as *transitional cell*

Table 36-2   Staging of Renal Cell Carcinoma (TNM System)

Stage	Metastasis
I	Tumor confined within kidney capsule ≤7cm in size
II	Invasion through renal capsule and renal vein but within surrounding fascia ≥7 cm in size
III	Involvement of adrenal glands and vena cava and one nearby lymph node:
	T3a-T3c, N0, M0: The main tumor has reached the adrenal gland, the fatty tissue around the kidney, the renal vein, and/or the large vein (vena cava) leading from the kidney to the heart. It has not spread beyond Gerota's fascia. There is no spread to lymph nodes or distant organs.
	T1a-T3c, N1, M0: The main tumor can be any size and may be outside the kidney, but it has not spread beyond Gerota's fascia. The cancer has spread to 1 nearby lymph node but has not spread to distant lymph nodes or other organs.
IV	Distant metastases (e.g., liver and lung) and more than one lymph node:
	T4, N0-N1, M0: The main tumor has invaded beyond Gerota's fascia. It has spread to no more than 1 nearby lymph node. It has not spread to distant lymph nodes or other organs.
	Any T, N2, M0: The main tumor can be any size and may be outside the kidney. The cancer has spread to more than 1 nearby lymph node but has not spread to distant lymph nodes or other organs.
	Any T, Any N, M1: The main tumor can be any size and may be outside the kidney. It may or may not have spread to nearby lymph nodes. It has spread to distant lymph nodes and/or other organs.

Adapted from American Cancer Society: *Detailed guide: kidney cancer. How is kidney cancer (renal cell carcinoma) staged?* Available at www.cancer.org/docroot/CRI/content/CRI_2_4_3X_How_is_kidney_cancer_staged_22.asp (accessed April 2008).
T, Tumor; *N,* node; *M,* metastasis.

carcinoma is the most common bladder malignancy, appearing usually as a superficial tumor.

PATHOGENESIS The risk of primary bladder cancer is greater among people who smoke or are exposed to metabolites of aniline dyes or other aromatic amines or chemicals and with heavy consumption of phenacetin.[40] Oncogenes of the *ras* gene family and tumor-suppressor genes including *TP53* mutations and inactivation of *retinoblastoma gene (pRb)* are implicated in bladder cancer. The tumor is usually composed of uroepithelial cells (cells lining the bladder, ureters, urethra and renal pelvis) and most have a papillary growth pattern (a tuftlike lesion attached to a stalk). (Figure 36-5). Nonpapillary tumors (sessile or nodular represent 10% to 30% of bladder tumors) are not as common as papillary tumors, but they tend to be more invasive and have a poorer prognosis. Carcinoma in situ can present with papillary tumors. Worldwide squamous cell carcinoma is the most prevalent. Metastasis is usually to lymph nodes, liver, bones, or lungs. Staging for bladder carcinoma is presented in Table 36-3. Secondary bladder cancer develops by invasion of cancer from bordering organs, such as cervical carcinoma in women or prostatic carcinoma in men.

CLINICAL MANIFESTATIONS Gross painless hematuria is the archetypal clinical manifestation of bladder cancer. Episodes of hematuria tend to recur, and they are often accompanied by bothersome lower urinary tract symptoms including daytime voiding frequency, nocturia, urgency, and urge urinary incontinence. Flank pain may occur if tumor growth obstructs one or both ureterovesical junctions. Bothersome lower urinary tract symptoms are particularly intense in individuals with carcinoma in situ. Metastasis is the cause of death from bladder cancer.[41]

EVALUATION AND TREATMENT Urinalysis for evidence of hematuria in the absence of infection provides a useful screening tool for high-risk patients. Several bladder tumor antigen-testing systems have been developed for screening, but they have proved more useful in monitoring patients with known cancer as compared to being used for primary screening. Urine cytology (pathologic analysis of sloughed cells within the urine) is completed in individuals with evidence of hematuria from unknown causes; cystoscopy or fluorescence cystoscopy with tissue biopsy can confirm the diagnosis. Biologic markers for the diagnosis of bladder cancer are under investigation.[42] Transurethral resection or laser ablation, combined with intravesical chemotherapy or immunotherapy, is effective for superficial tumors.[43] Radical cystectomy with urinary diversion and adjuvant chemotherapy is required for locally invasive tumors, and radiation therapy may be used to support palliative or adjuvant treatment for muscle invasive tumors.[44]

URINARY TRACT INFECTION

Causes of Urinary Tract Infection

A **urinary tract infection** (UTI) is an inflammation of the urinary epithelium usually caused by bacteria from gut flora. A UTI can occur anywhere along the urinary tract including the urethra, prostate, bladder, ureter, or kidney. At risk are premature newborns; prepubertal children; sexually active and pregnant women; women treated with antibiotics that disrupt vaginal flora; spermicide users; estrogen-deficient postmenopausal women; individuals with indwelling catheters; and persons with diabetes mellitus, neurogenic bladder, or urinary tract obstruction. UTIs are commonly classified by their location or complicating factors: *cystitis* (bladder inflammation), *pyelonephritis* (inflammation of upper urinary tract), *uncomplicated UTI* (occur in a normally functioning urinary system) and *complicated UTI* (occur with defects in the urinary system or in individuals with other health problems).

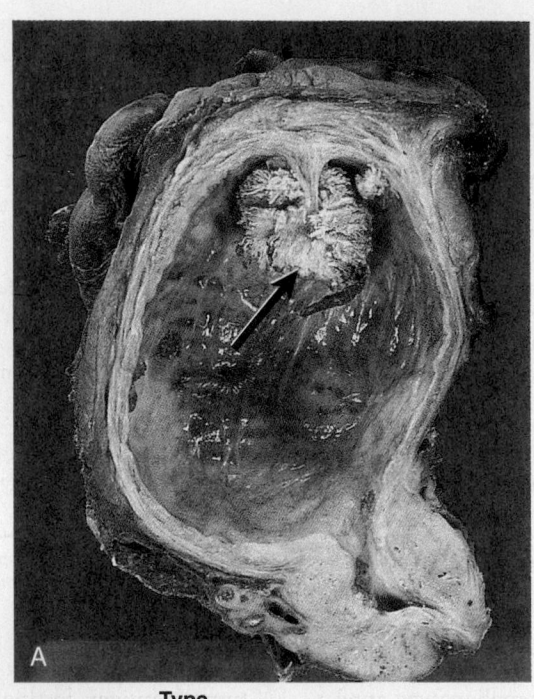

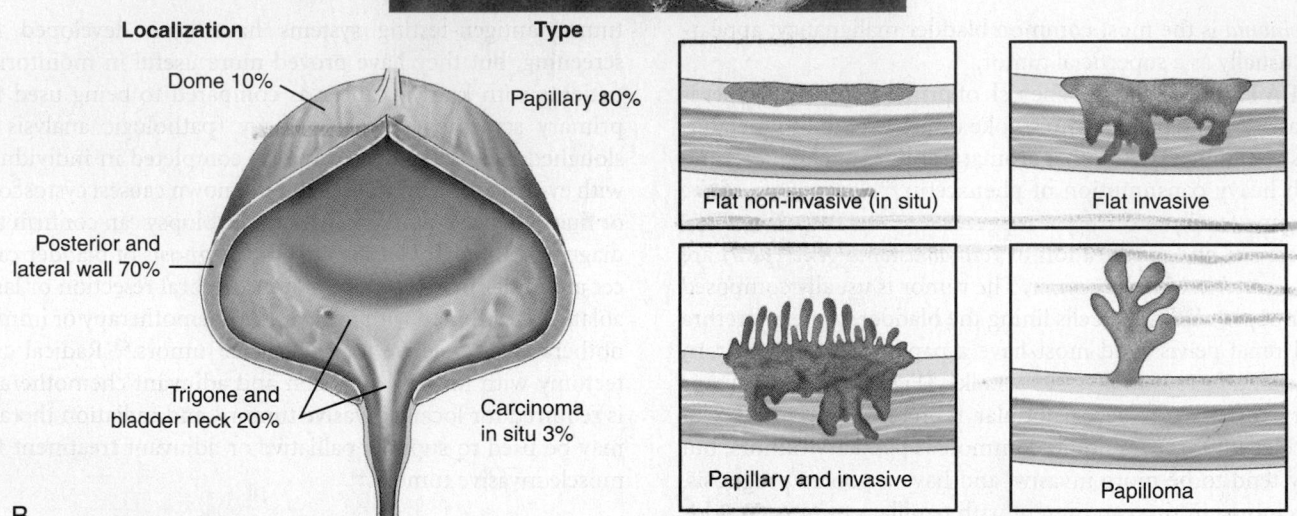

Figure 36-5 Carcinoma of the bladder. **A,** Bladder cancer with morphologic patterns of most common tumors. **B,** Papillary transitional cell carcinoma arising in the dome of the bladder as a cauliflower-like lesion *(arrow).* (**A** from Stevens A, Lowe J, editors: *Pathology,* ed 2, St Louis, 2008, Mosby; **B** from Kissane JM, editor: *Anderson's pathology,* ed 9, St Louis, 1990, Mosby.)

Cystitis is more common in women because of the shorter urethra and the closeness of the urethra to the anus (increasing the possibility of bacterial contamination). Up to 10% of women have an acute uncomplicated UTI in a year and up to 60% of women may have a lower UTI at some time in their life.[45] Several factors normally combine to protect against UTIs. Most bacteria are washed out of the urethra during micturition. The low pH and high osmolality of urea, the presence of Tamm-Horsfall protein, and secretions from the uroepithelium provide a bactericidal effect. The uretero-vesical junction closes during bladder contraction, preventing reflux of urine to the ureters and kidneys. Both the longer urethra and prostatic secretions decrease the risk of infection in men.

Types of Urinary Tract Infection
Cystitis
Acute cystitis is an inflammation of the bladder and is the most common site of UTI. The morphologic appearance of the bladder through cystoscopy describes different types of cystitis. With mild inflammation, the mucosa is hyperemic (red). More advanced cases may show diffuse hemorrhage (termed *hemorrhagic cystitis*), pus formation, or suppurative exudates (termed *suppurative cystitis*) on the epithelial surface of the bladder. Prolonged infection may lead to sloughing of the bladder mucosa with ulcer formation (termed *ulcerative cystitis*). The most severe infections may cause necrosis of the bladder wall (termed *gangrenous cystitis*). Generally infections are mild, without complications, and occur in individuals

Table 36-3	Staging of Bladder Carcinoma (TNM* System)
Stage	**Description**
Primary Tumor	
T0	No primary tumor identified
Ta	Noninvasive papillary carcinoma—not in bladder muscle
Tis	Carcinoma in situ (CIS)
T1	Tumor invades connective tissue
T2	Tumor invades detrusor muscle
T3	Invasion of fatty tissue around bladder
T4	Tumor has invaded adjacent structures
Region of Lymph Nodes	
N0	No lymph node involvement
N1 to N3	Lymph node metastasis to pelvic or adjacent region
Distant Metastasis	
M0	No metastasis
M1	Distant metastasis

Adapted from American Cancer Society: *Detailed guide: bladder cancer. How is bladder cancer staged?* 2006. Available at www.cancer.org/docroot/CRI_2_4_3X_How_is_bladder_cancer_staged_22.asp?sitearea= (accessed April, 2007).

*T, Tumor; N, node; M, metastasis.

with a normal urinary tract. Acute cystitis may occur alone or in association with pyelonephritis or prostatitis.

PATHOPHYSIOLOGY The most common infecting microorganisms are uropathic strains of *Escherichia coli (E. coli)* (80% to 85%) and the second most common is *Staphylococcus saprophyticus* (10%). Less common microorganisms include *Klebsiella, Proteus, Pseudomonas*, fungi, viruses, parasites, or tubercular bacilli. Bacterial contamination of the normally sterile urine usually occurs by retrograde movement of gram-negative bacilli into the urethra and bladder and then to the ureter and kidney.[46] Some women may be genetically susceptible to certain strains of *E. coli* attachment.[47]

Fungal infections are comparatively uncommon. The most common pathogen is *Candida*, but multiple fungal species may colonize the urinary tract or urinary catheters and produce symptomatic UTI particularly in those who are immunosuppressed.[48]

Hematogenous infections are uncommon and often preceded by septicemia. Infection initiates an inflammatory response and the symptoms of cystitis. The inflammatory edema in the bladder wall stimulates discharge of stretch receptors, initiating symptoms of bladder fullness with small volumes of urine and producing the urgency and frequency of urination associated with cystitis.

Schistosomiasis is the most common cause of parasitic invasion of the urinary tract on a global basis; it infects more than 200 million people.[49] Although rare among people living in the United States, the parasite dwells in waters of the various rivers of fresh water bodies in Africa, South America, and Pacific Rim countries. It usually enters the human by swimming up the urethra while the host swims or is partly submerged in an infected body of water. The parasite burrows into the walls of the urinary tract, causing inflammation and scarring of the urinary tract and an increased risk for urothelial malignancies.[50]

Two factors account for the presence of a UTI: the efficiency of defense mechanisms within the host (individual) and the virulence of the pathogen (bacterium, fungus, or parasite). In the healthy individual, host defense mechanisms maintain a sterile posterior urethra and bladder. Even if bacteria manage to enter the bladder, these defense mechanisms prevent it from clinging to the walls of the bladder or ascending to the upper urinary tracts.[51] Most people are able to rapidly rid the urinary tract of invading bacteria, but some show evidence of bacteria in the urine that does not provoke an infection. This condition is called **asymptomatic bacteriuria** and does not harm urinary function or require intervention except in pregnant women.[52] A UTI occurs when a pathogen circumvents or overwhelms the host's defense mechanisms and rapidly reproduces.

Virulence of Uropathogens
Virulence is a pathogen's ability to evade or overwhelm the host defense mechanisms and cause disease in a host (see Chapter 9). Several factors contribute to bacterial virulence within the urinary tract,[53] including the ability of uropathic bacteria to adhere (attach) to the uroepithelium.[54] Uropathic strains of *E. coli* have *type-1 fimbriae* that bind to latex catheters and to receptors on uroepithelium resisting flushing during normal micturition. Additionally they have pyelonephritis-associated fimbriae (*P fimbriae*) that bind to the uroepithelial P-blood group antigen that is present in most of the human population and readily ascend the urinary tract.[55] Strains of *E. coli* also produce *siderophores* for acquiring nutrient iron, are resistant to bactericidal effects of complement, and express toxins including *cytotoxin necrotizing factor-1* and *hemolysins*. Certain bacterial species also enhance their virulence by acting together to form a biofilm that enhances colonization and resists efficiency of innate host defense mechanisms and antimicrobial therapy.[56,57]

Host Defense Mechanisms
Opposing bacterial virulence are multiple host defense mechanisms including the immune system and the uroepithelium. Periurethral mucus-secreting glands surround the distal two thirds of the female urethra. Mucus from these glands traps bacteria before it can ascend from proximal urethra to the bladder. In men, the length of the male urethra and secretions from the prostate and accessory periurethral glands combine to form a protective barrier against infection. In addition, the urethral sphincter mechanism acts as a mechanical barrier to bacterial ascent from the distal urethra.

Bacteria that successfully ascend the urethra face detection and destruction by components of the body's immune system provided they come into contact with the bladder wall. Unfortunately, time is required for the immune system to respond to the potential threat, and this period may provide adequate time for bacteria or other pathogens to reproduce several times.

The efficiency of the bladder's defenses is also influenced by the person's Lewis blood group.[58] This taxonomy is based on recognition of inherited antigens associated with the ABO blood factors. Individuals with certain Lewis blood groups are more prone to UTI because they secrete fewer antigens capable of resisting bacterial adherence by pili formation.

The urine itself may contain components that enhance resistance to UTI. These include hydrogen ion concentration (pH), osmolarity (concentration of salts within the urine), glucose content, urea, and glycoproteins. Ideally, the urine should have a slightly acidic pH (6 or less), moderate to high urea concentration, and abundant glycoproteins (slimy substances that interfere with bacterial adherence). Dilute urine washes out bacteria, and urine with higher urea concentrations (high osmolarity) is more bacteriostatic. In contrast, glucose in the urine, a higher (alkaline) pH, or urine with high osmolarity but low urea concentration is less bacteriostatic.

CLINICAL MANIFESTATIONS Many individuals with bacteriuria are asymptomatic. Clinical manifestations of cystitis, however, usually include frequency, urgency, dysuria (painful urination), and suprapubic and low back pain. Hematuria, cloudy and foul-smelling urine, and flank pain are more serious symptoms. Approximately 10% of individuals with bacteriuria have no symptoms, and 30% of individuals with symptoms are abacteriuric. Older adults with cystitis may be asymptomatic or demonstrate confusion or vague abdominal discomfort. Older adults with recurrent UTI and other concurrent illness have a higher risk of mortality.[59]

EVALUATION AND TREATMENT Infections are diagnosed by urine culture of specific microorganisms with counts of 10,000/ml or more from freshly voided urine. Dipstick urinalysis and microscopy are adequate to diagnose an uncomplicated UTI, but urine culture is critical for complicated infections. Risk factors, such as a urinary tract obstruction, which are associated with a complicated UTI, should be identified and treated. Increased fluid intake and urinary analgesics can relieve symptoms. Evidence of bacteria from urine culture and antibiotic sensitivity warrants treatment with a microorganism-specific antibiotic to eradicate the underlying pathogen. A single large dose of antibiotic or a 3-day course may be effective when symptoms are of short duration and there are no complications. Three to 7 days of treatment is most common depending on antimicrobial selection; older adults with obstructive disorders may require 7 to 14 days of treatment. Frequent, recurrent, acute uncomplicated UTI requires low-dose antimicrobial therapy from 6 months to 2 years.[46] Follow-up urine cultures should be obtained 1 week after initiation of treatment and at monthly intervals for 3 months. Clinical symptoms are frequently relieved, but bacteriuria may still be present, particularly with the development of antimicrobial-resistant bacterial strains. Repeat cultures should be obtained every 3 to 4 months until 1 year after treatment for evaluation of recurrent infection.[60] Urosepsis and septic shock are medical emergencies that usually demand parenteral, broad-spectrum antibiotic therapy and may require hospitalization. A UTI caused by

WHAT'S NEW?   Urinary Tract Infection and Antibiotic Resistance

Uncomplicated urinary tract infection (UTI) occurs primarily in sexually active women with fewer cases among older and pregnant women and older men. The leading cause of UTI is *Escherichia coli*, and *E. coli* continues to evolve in response to antimicrobial use. Of major concern is the worldwide emergence of bacterial strains resistant to specific antibiotics in both hospital- and community-acquired infections. The resistance is caused in part by high human use of antibiotics and antibiotics in animal feed. Rates of resistance are highest in regions with the highest rates of prescription; ampicillin and trimethoprim-sulfamethoxazole (TMP-SMX) have a high rate of resistance and there is increasing resistance to fluoroquinolones. Risks for resistance include TMP-SMX treatment within the past 3 months, diabetes mellitus, recent hospitalization, and specific antibiotic resistance rates in a community of greater than 20%. However, reliable data regarding the true prevalence of resistance in a community are often lacking. Other factors to consider in choice of antibiotic treatment include infection severity, complicated or uncomplicated UTI, accuracy of diagnosis, broad-spectrum (i.e., TMP-SMX, ampicillin, and cephalothin) versus narrow-spectrum (i.e., nitrofurantoin and ciprofloxacin) antibiotic sensitivity, cost-effectiveness, and instructing consumers about the correct use of antibiotics.

Data from Chulain MN et al: *Ir J Med Sci* 174(4):6-9, 2005; Kahlmeter G: *J Antimicrob Chemother* 51:69-76, 2003; Nicolle LE: *Urol Clin North Am* 35(1):1-12, vi, 2008; Wagenlehner FM, Weidner W, Naber KG: *Urol Clin North Am* 35(1):69-79, vi, 2008; Alam MF et al: *Int J Antimicrob Agents* 33(3):255-257, 2009.

Schistosomiasis is treated with praziquantel, and vaccines are under development.[61]

Painful Bladder Syndrome/Interstitial Cystitis

Painful bladder syndrome/interstitial cystitis (PBS/IC) is a condition that includes **nonbacterial infectious cystitis** (viral, mycobacterial, chlamydial, fungal), and **noninfectious cystitis** (radiation, chemical, autoimmune, hypersensitivity).[62] It occurs most commonly in women ages 20 to 30 years who have symptoms of cystitis, such as frequency, urgency, dysuria, and nocturia, but with negative urine cultures and no other known etiology. Nonbacterial infectious cystitis is most common among those who are immunocompromised. Noninfectious cystitis is associated with radiation or chemotherapy treatment for pelvic and urogenital cancers.

The cause of PBS/IC is unknown, but an autoimmune reaction may be responsible for the inflammatory response, which includes mast cell activation, altered epithelial permeability, and increased sensory nerve sensitivity.[63] The inflammation is associated with a derangement of the bladder mucosa that makes it more susceptible to penetration by bacteria and noxious urinary solutes.[64] Inflammation and fibrosis of the bladder wall are accompanied by the presence of hemorrhagic ulcers (Hunner ulcers), and bladder volume may decrease as a result of fibrosis. More recently, the identification of antiproliferative factor (APF), a protein expressed by the bladder uroepithelium in those with IC, is important. APF appears to block the normal growth of cells that line the inside wall of the bladder and indirectly increases bladder sensation.[65] Characteristic symptoms of IC include bladder fullness, frequency (including nocturia), small urine volume, and chronic pelvic pain with symptoms lasting longer than 9 months. Diagnosis of IC requires the exclusion of other diagnoses, and extensive evaluations are completed.[66] No single treatment is effective, and different approaches are used for symptom relief.[67]

Acute Pyelonephritis

Pyelonephritis is an infection of one or both upper urinary tracts (ureter, renal pelvis, and interstitium). Common causes are summarized in Table 36-4. Urinary obstruction and reflux of urine from the bladder (vesicoureteral reflux) are the most common underlying risk factors. One or both kidneys may be involved. Most cases occur in women. The responsible microorganism is usually *E. coli*, *Proteus*, or *Pseudomonas*. The latter two microorganisms are more commonly associated with infections after urethral instrumentation or urinary tract surgery. These microorganisms also split urea into ammonia, making alkaline urine that increases the risk of stone formation.

PATHOPHYSIOLOGY The infection is probably spread by ascending uropathic microorganisms along the ureters, but spread also may occur by way of the bloodstream. The inflammatory process is usually focal and irregular, primarily affecting the pelvis, calyces, and medulla. The infection causes medullary infiltration of white blood cells with renal inflammation, renal edema, and purulent urine. In severe infections, localized abscesses may form in the medulla and extend to the cortex. Primarily affected are the tubules; the

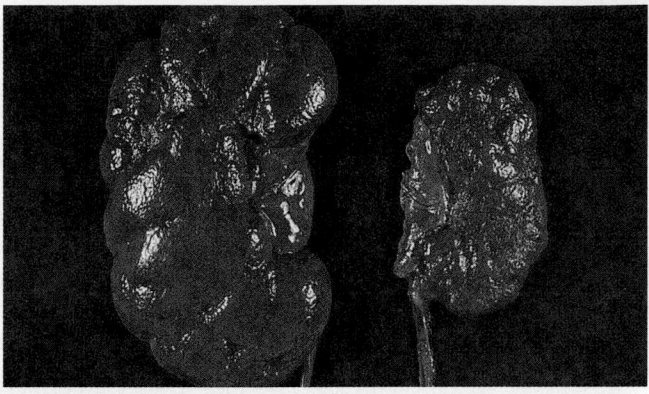

Figure 36-6 Pyelonephritis. *Right*: Small, shrunken, irregularly scarred kidney of an individual with chronic pyelonephritis. *Left*: Kidney is of normal size but also shows scarring on the upper pole. (From Damjanov I: *Pathology for the health professions*, ed 3, St Louis, 2006, Saunders.)

glomeruli usually are spared. Necrosis of renal papillae can develop. After the acute phase, healing occurs with deposition of scar tissue, fibrosis and atrophy of affected tubules (Figure 36-6). Acute pyelonephritis rarely causes renal failure.[68]

CLINICAL MANIFESTATIONS The onset of symptoms is usually acute, with fever, chills, and flank or groin pain. Symptoms characteristic of a UTI, including frequency, dysuria, and costovertebral tenderness, may precede systemic signs and symptoms. Older adults may have nonspecific symptoms, such as low-grade fever and malaise.

EVALUATION AND TREATMENT Differentiating symptoms of cystitis from those of pyelonephritis by clinical assessment alone is difficult. The specific diagnosis is established by urine culture, urinalysis, and clinical signs and symptoms. White blood cell casts indicate pyelonephritis, but they are not always present in the urine. Complicated pyelonephritis requires blood cultures and urinary tract imaging.[69,70]

Uncomplicated acute pyelonephritis responds well to 2 to 3 weeks of microorganism-specific antibiotic therapy. Follow-up urine cultures are obtained at 1 and 4 weeks after treatment if symptoms recur. Antibiotic-resistant microorganisms or reinfection may occur in cases of urinary tract obstruction or reflux. Intravenous pyelography and voiding cystourethrography identify surgically correctable lesions.

Chronic Pyelonephritis

Chronic pyelonephritis is a persistent or recurrent infection of the kidney leading to scarring of the kidney. One or both kidneys may be involved. The specific cause of chronic pyelonephritis may be unknown (idiopathic) or associated with versicoureteral reflux or renal stones. Recurrent infections from acute pyelonephritis may be associated with chronic pyelonephritis. Causes other than chronic pyelonephritis include drug toxicity from analgesics such as nonsteroidal anti-inflammatory drugs, ischemia, irradiation, and immune-complex diseases.

PATHOPHYSIOLOGY Chronic urinary tract obstruction prevents elimination of bacteria and starts a process of progressive inflammation, altered renal pelvis and calyces,

Table 36-4	Common Causes of Pyelonephritis
Predisposing Factors	**Pathologic Mechanisms**
Kidney stones	Obstruction and stasis of urine contributing to bacteriuria and hydronephrosis; irritation of epithelial lining with entrapment of bacteria
Vesicoureteral reflux	Chronic reflux of urine up the ureter and into kidney during micturition contributing to bacterial infection
Pregnancy	Dilation and relaxation of ureter with hydroureter and hydronephrosis; partly caused by obstruction from enlarged uterus and partly from ureteral relaxation caused by higher progesterone levels
Neurogenic bladder	Neurologic impairment interfering with normal bladder and urethral sphincter contraction with residual urine and ascending infection
Instrumentation	Introduction of organisms into urethra and bladder by catheters and endoscopes introduced into the urinary tract for diagnostic purposes
Female sexual trauma	Movement of organisms from the urethra into the bladder with infection and retrograde spread to kidney

destruction of the tubules, atrophy or dilation and diffuse scarring, and finally impaired urine-concentrating ability, leading to chronic kidney failure. The lesions of chronic pyelonephritis are sometimes termed *chronic interstitial nephritis* because the inflammation and fibrosis are located in the interstitial spaces between the tubules (see Figure 36-6).

CLINICAL MANIFESTATIONS The early symptoms of chronic pyelonephritis are often minimal and may include hypertension, frequency, dysuria, and flank pain. With loss of tubular function is an inability to conserve sodium, and development of hyperkalemia and metabolic acidosis. Risk for dehydration must be considered if there is loss of ability to concentrate the urine. Progression of disease leads to renal failure, particularly in the presence of other risk factors (i.e., obstructive uropathy or diabetes mellitus).[71]

EVALUATION AND TREATMENT Urinalysis, intravenous pyelography, and ultrasound are used diagnostically. Treatment is related to the underlying cause. Obstruction must be relieved. Antibiotics may be given, with prolonged antibiotic therapy for recurrent infection.

GLOMERULAR DISORDERS

Glomerular disease can be caused by primary injury within the glomulus or secondarily as a result of systemic disease including metabolic disorders such as diabetes mellitus, bacterial or viral infectious disease, or systemic immune disease such as systemic lupus erythematosus (lupus nephritis). Most primary and many secondary glomerular diseases are the result of immune injury (Figure 36-7). Immune injury includes (1) deposition of circulating antigen-antibody immune complexes in the glomulus (type III hypersensitivity reaction); (2) antibodies reacting in situ against planted antigens within the glomerulus (type III hypersensitivity); (3) action of antibodies directed against the glomerular capillary wall (antiglomerular basement membrane antibodies), the least common and most severe form of immune injury (type II hypersensitivity); and (4) cell-mediated immune injury (type IV hypersensitivity) (see Chapter 8). The severity of glomerular damage and decline in glomerular function are related to the size, number, location (focal or diffuse), duration of exposure, and type of antigen-antibody complexes.

Patterns of antigen-antibody complex deposition or formation within the glomerular capillary filtration membrane have been established using light, electron, and immunofluorescent microscopy for different disease processes (Table 36-5). Electron microscopy differentiates morphologic changes within the glomerular capillary wall. Staining with fluorescein identifies different antibodies (i.e., immunoglobulin G [IgG] or IgA) and their configurations when viewed under ultraviolet light with a microscope (see Figure 36-8, *C*, p. 1382).

Immune injury is caused by activation of mediators of inflammation (complement, leukocytes, fibrin) and begins after the antibody or antigen-antibody complexes have localized in the glomerular capillary wall. Complement is deposited with the antibodies, and its activation can cause cell lysis or serve as a chemotactic stimulus for attraction of neutrophils and monocytes.[72] These phagocytes further the inflammatory reaction by releasing lysosomal enzymes, reactive oxygen species, and cytokines, which damage glomerular cell walls and contribute to swelling and proliferation of mesangial cells and expansion of the extracellular matrix causing a decrease in glomerular blood flow, decreased GFR, and hypoxic injury.[73]

The inflammatory processes alter membrane permeability with injury to epithelial cells, the glomerular basement membrane (GBM) and endothelial cells (podocytes). Loss of the negative electrical charge across the glomerular filtration membrane enhances filtration of proteins into the urine, which are normally repelled because they also have a negative charge. Membrane damage can lead to platelet aggregation and degranulation, whereby platelets release substances that increase glomerular permeability, permitting the passage of protein molecules or red blood cells into the urine and causing **proteinuria** (excess protein in the urine, usually albumin), **hematuria** (blood in the urine), or both. The coagulation system also may be activated and lead to fibrin deposition in Bowman space, contributing to crescent formation (deposition of substances in the Bowman space forming the shape of a crescent moon).[74] Renal blood flow decreases, and glomerular filtration is reduced. Hematuria results from increased glomerular permeability or bleeding along the nephron.

Different causes of injury may cause more than one type of glomerular lesion, so lesions are not necessarily disease-specific (Table 36-6). The onset of glomerular disease may be sudden or insidious and significant loss of nephron function can occur before symptoms develop. Glomerular disease may be silent, mild, moderate, or severe in symptom presentation. Severe or progressive glomerular disease causes oliguria, hypertension, and renal failure.

Different types of glomerular disease may be associated with patterns of urinary sediment (Table 36-7). Urine in diseases associated with **nephrotic sediment** contains massive amounts of protein and lipids and either a microscopic amount of blood or no blood. Urine in diseases associated with **nephritic sediment** is characterized by the presence of blood in the urine with red cell casts, white cell casts, and varying degrees of protein, which usually is not severe. The sediment of chronic glomerular disease has waxy casts, granular casts, and less protein and blood than does nephrotic or nephritic sediment.

Reduced GFR during glomerular disease is evidenced by elevated plasma urea, creatinine concentration, or reduced renal creatinine clearance (see Chapter 35). Edema, caused by excessive sodium and water retention, may require the use of diuretics or dialysis. The volume expansion that accompanies salt and water retention leads to hypertension. During the first few weeks, the major life-threatening problems are acute renal insufficiency with fluid, electrolyte, and acid-base imbalances; acute hypertension that may cause hypertensive encephalopathy; circulatory failure; and pulmonary edema.

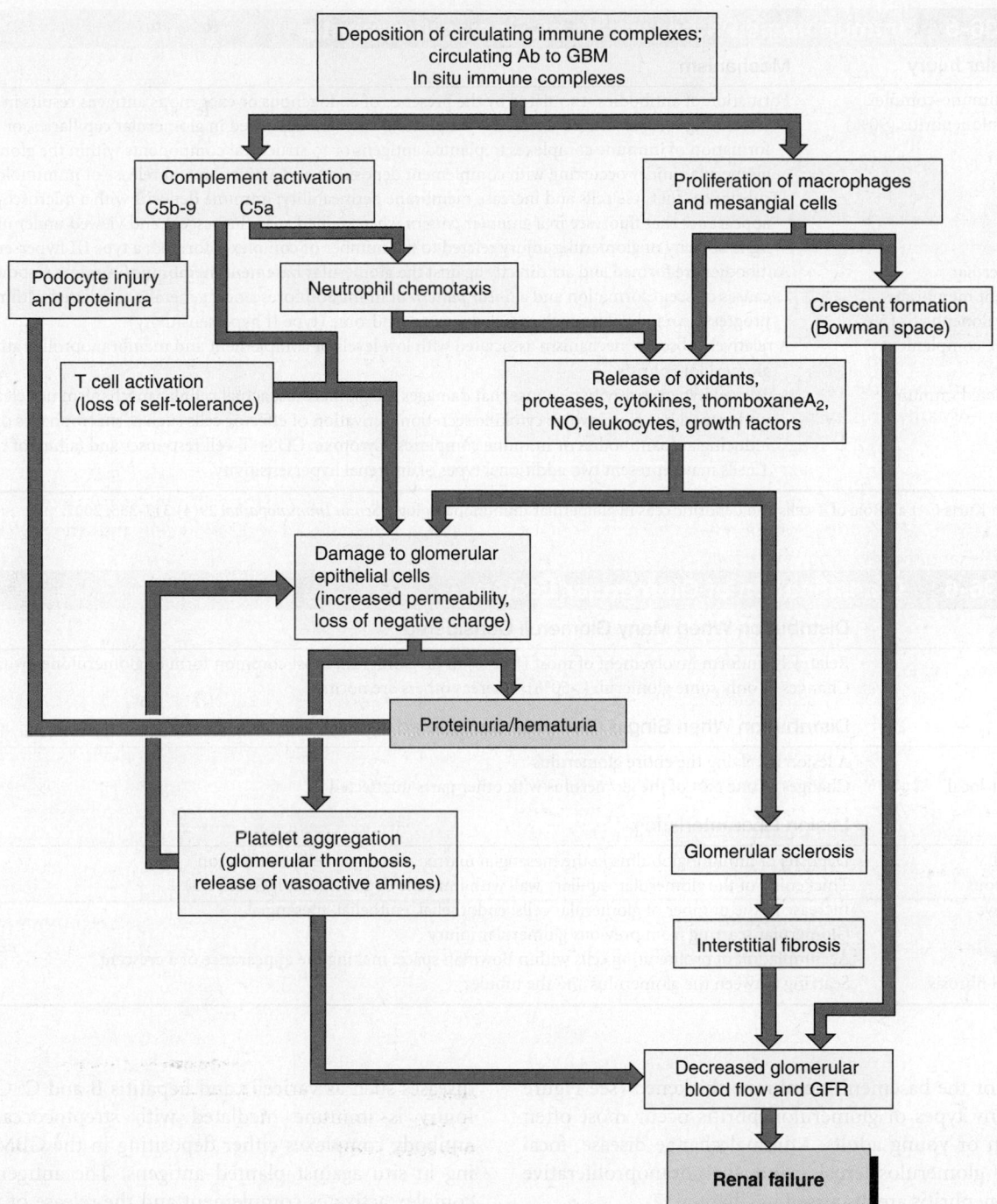

Figure 36-7 Mechanisms of glomerular injury. *Ab,* antibody; *GBM,* glomerular basement membrane; *GFR,* glomerular filtration rate; *NO,* nitric oxide.

Glomerulonephritis

Glomerulonephritis is an inflammation of the glomerulus caused by numerous factors, including infection, immunologic abnormalities (the most common cause), ischemia, free radicals, drugs, toxins, vascular disorders, and systemic diseases, including diabetes mellitus and lupus erythematosus. Glomerular disease is the most common cause of chronic kidney disease and end-stage renal failure.[75]

The classification of glomerulonephritis can be described according to cause, pathologic lesions, disease progression (acute, rapidly progressive, chronic), or clinical presentation (nephrotic syndrome, nephritic syndrome, acute or chronic kidney failure). In nearly all types of glomerulonephritis, the epithelial or podocyte layer of the glomerular capillary membrane is disturbed with loss of negative charges and changes in membrane permeability; the mesangial matrix may be

Table 36-5	Immunologic Pathogenesis of Glomerulonephritis
Glomerular Injury	**Mechanism**
Soluble immune-complex glomerulonephritis (90%)	Formation of antibodies stimulated by the presence of endogenous or exogenous antigens results in circulating soluble antigen-antibody complexes, which are deposited in glomerular capillaries, or the in situ formation of immune complexes to planted antigens or to structural components within the glomerulus; glomerular injury occurring with complement deposition and activation and release of immunologic substances that lyse cells and increase membrane permeability; immune deposits with a microscopic appearance that fluoresce in a *granular pattern* when stained with fluorescein and viewed under ultraviolet light; severity of glomerular injury related to the number of complexes formed; a type III hypersensitivity
Antiglomerular basement membrane glomerulonephritis (5%)	Antibodies are formed and act directly against the glomerular basement membrane; immune response that causes crescent formation and a *linear pattern* of immunofluorescence; generally associated with rapidly progressive renal failure such as Goodpasture syndrome (type II hypersensitivity)
Alternative complement pathway	A relatively obscure mechanism associated with low levels of complement and membranoproliferative glomerulonephritis
Cell-mediated immunity	A delayed hypersensitivity response that damages the glomerulus; actual cellular mechanism not clearly understood but may involve cytokine secretion, activation of effector cells such as macrophages or by inducing autoantibodies or immune complexes. Cytotoxic CD8+ T-cell responses and failure of regulatory T cells may represent two additional types of antirenal hypersensitivity*

*Data from Kurts C et al: Role of T cells and dendritic cells in glomerular immunopathology, *Semin Immunopathol* 29(4):317-335, 2007.

Table 36-6	Classification of Glomerular Lesions	
Lesion	**Distribution When Many Glomeruli Considered**	
Diffuse	Relatively uniform involvement of most (>50%) or all glomeruli; most common form of glomerulonephritis	
Focal	Changes in only some glomeruli (>50%), whereas others are normal	
Lesion	**Distribution When Single Glomeruli Considered**	
Global	A lesion involving the entire glomerulus	
Segmental-local	Changes in one part of the glomerulus with other parts unaffected	
Lesion	**Lesion Characteristics**	
Mesangial	Deposits of immunoglobulins in the mesangial matrix; mesangial cell proliferation	
Membranous	Thickening of the glomerular capillary wall with immune deposits (i.e., IgG and C3)	
Proliferative	Increase in the number of glomerular cells: endothelial, epithelial, mesangial	
Sclerotic	Glomerular scarring from previous glomerular injury	
Crescentic	Accumulation of proliferating cells within Bowman space, making the appearance of a crescent	
Interstitial fibrosis	Scarring between the glomerulus and the tubules	

expanded or the basement membrane thickened (see Figure 36-7). Many types of glomerulonephritis occur most often in children or young adults. Minimal change disease, focal segmental glomerulosclerosis, and membranoproliferative glomerulonephritis are discussed in Chapter 37.

Acute Postinfectious Glomerulonephritis

Acute postinfectious glomerulonephritis (PIGN) usually involves an immunologic mechanism that activates inflammation with damage to the glomerular basement membrane, capillary endothelium, and mesangium. Acute postinfectious glomerulonephritis is most often is associated with a streptococcal infection *(acute poststreptococcal glomerulonephritis)*. The disease begins abruptly and usually occurs 7 to 10 days after a streptococcal infection of the skin (impetigo) or of the throat (pharyngitis) and commonly affects children (see Chapter 37). Sporadic occurrences have been observed after bacterial endocarditis, which may be associated with streptococcal or staphylococcal microorganisms, or after viral diseases such as varicella and hepatitis B and C. Glomerular injury is immune mediated with streptococcal antigen-antibody complexes either depositing in the GBM or forming in situ against planted antigens. The antigen-antibody complex activates complement and the release of inflammatory mediators that damage endothelial and epithelial cells lying on the basement membrane and causes altered permeability and cellular proliferation.[76]

Symptoms may be insidious or sudden and usually occur 10 to 21 days after infection and include hematuria, red blood cell casts, proteinuria, decreased GFR, oliguria, hypertension, edema around the eyes or feet and ankles, and, occasionally, ascites or pleural effusions. Blood urea nitrogen (BUN) is elevated. Immunofluorescent findings from renal biopsy indicate immune complex deposits in the glomerulus (complement C3 and IgG), neutrophil and macrophage recruitment and activation, with diffuse mesangial cell and capillary endothelial cell proliferation of the entire glomeruli[77] (Figure 36-8). The thickened glomerular membrane contributes to the decreased

Table 36-7   Features of the Common Types of Glomerulonephritis

Type and Cause	Pathophysiology
Associated with Nephritic Syndrome	
Acute postinfectious glomerulonephritis (PIGN) (group A beta-hemolytic streptococci)	Subepithelial deposits of IgG and complement complexes; infiltration of neutrophils and monocytes; proliferation of mesangial and epithelial cells with occlusion of glomerular capillary blood flow and decreased glomerular filtration; usually diffuse lesions
Crescentic or rapidly progressive glomerulonephritis (a clinical syndrome): *Type I:* Formation of antiglomerular basement membrane antibodies (Goodpasture syndrome) *Type II:* Immune complex deposition (PIGN, SLE, IGA nephropathy) *Type III:* Pauci-immune, lack of anti-GBM antibodies or immune complexes; presence of serum antineutrophil cytoplasmic (ANC) antibodies associated with systemic vasculitides (usually idiopathic) Nonspecific response to glomerular injury; can occur in any severe glomerular disease	Accumulation of fibrin, macrophages, and epithelial cell proliferation into the Bowman space forms crescents and occludes glomerular capillary blood flow decreasing glomerular filtration; antiglomerular basement membrane antibodies lead to necrotizing, proliferative glomerulonephritis, and renal failure; diffuse lesions
Mesangial proliferative glomerulonephritis Can be associated with IgA nephropathy or lupus nephritis	Deposits of immune complexes in the mesangium with mesangial cell proliferation; results in decreased glomerular blood flow and glomerular filtration; leads to hematuria/proteinuria and nephrotic syndrome
Associated with Nephrotic Syndrome	
Minimal change disease (lipoid nephrosis) Glomerular basement membrane appears normal Most common cause of nephrotic syndrome in children (see Chapter 37) Usually idiopathic	Uniform diffuse effacement of epithelial (podocyte) foot processes; loss of negative charge in basement membrane and increased permeability lead to severe proteinuria and nephrotic syndrome
Focal segmental glomerulosclerosis Usually idiopathic (see Chapter 37) Can be associated with HIV infection or IgA nephropathy	Focal glomerulosclerosis from hyaline deposits in the glomerular membrane resulting in proteinuria and nephrotic syndrome
Membranous nephropathy (autoimmune response to unknown renal antigen) Usually idiopathic; can be associated with systemic diseases, i.e., hepatitis B virus, systemic lupus erythematosus, solid malignant tumors	Diffuse thickening of glomerular basement membrane and capillary wall from deposits of antibody, complement, and release of inflammatory cytokines; increased permeability with proteinuria and nephrotic syndrome
Membranoproliferative (MPGN) Usually idiopathic; associated with hypocomplementemia (see Chapter 37) *Type I:* Activation of classical complement pathway with nephrotic syndrome (hepatitis B and C, SLE) *Type II:* Activation of alternate complement pathway with hematuria (idiopathic) *Type III:* Activation of alternative complement pathway with nephrotic syndrome	Mesangial cell proliferation; thickening of basement membrane; subendothelial deposits of immune complex occlude glomerular capillary blood flow and decrease glomerular filtration; diffuse lesions
IgA nephropathy (Berger disease) Usually idiopathic (see Chapter 37) elevated IgA plasma levels	Mesangial deposition of IgA; release of inflammatory mediators with cellular proliferation; crescent formation, sclerosis, interstitial fibrosis, decreased GFR and hematuria; usually focal, some diffuse lesions
Chronic glomerulonephritis Can be a consequence of any of the types of glomerulonephritis; more common with crescentic or rapidly progressive glomerulonephritis	Glomerular fibrosis and scarring, interstitial and tubular fibrosis and vascular sclerosis; original glomerular lesions may not be definable; progression to end-stage kidney disease with uremia

GBM, Glomerular basement membrane; *GFR*, glomerular filtration rate; *HIV*, human immunodeficiency virus; *IgA*, immunoglobulin A; *IgG*, immunoglobulin G; *SLE*, systemic lupus erythematosus.

GFR. Activated complement, inflammatory cytokines, oxidants, proteases, and growth factors attack epithelial cells, alter membrane permeability, and cause proteinuria. More severe renal disease is observed after a prolonged infection and before antibiotic therapy. In acute poststreptococcal glomerulonephritis the streptococcal exoenzymes are elevated, such as antistreptolysin-O and antistreptokinase. Serum complement is decreased, and serum creatinine concentration and blood urea nitrogen are elevated.

There is no specific treatment for glomerulonephritis. Most individuals, especially children, recover without significant loss of renal function or recurrence of the disease. During

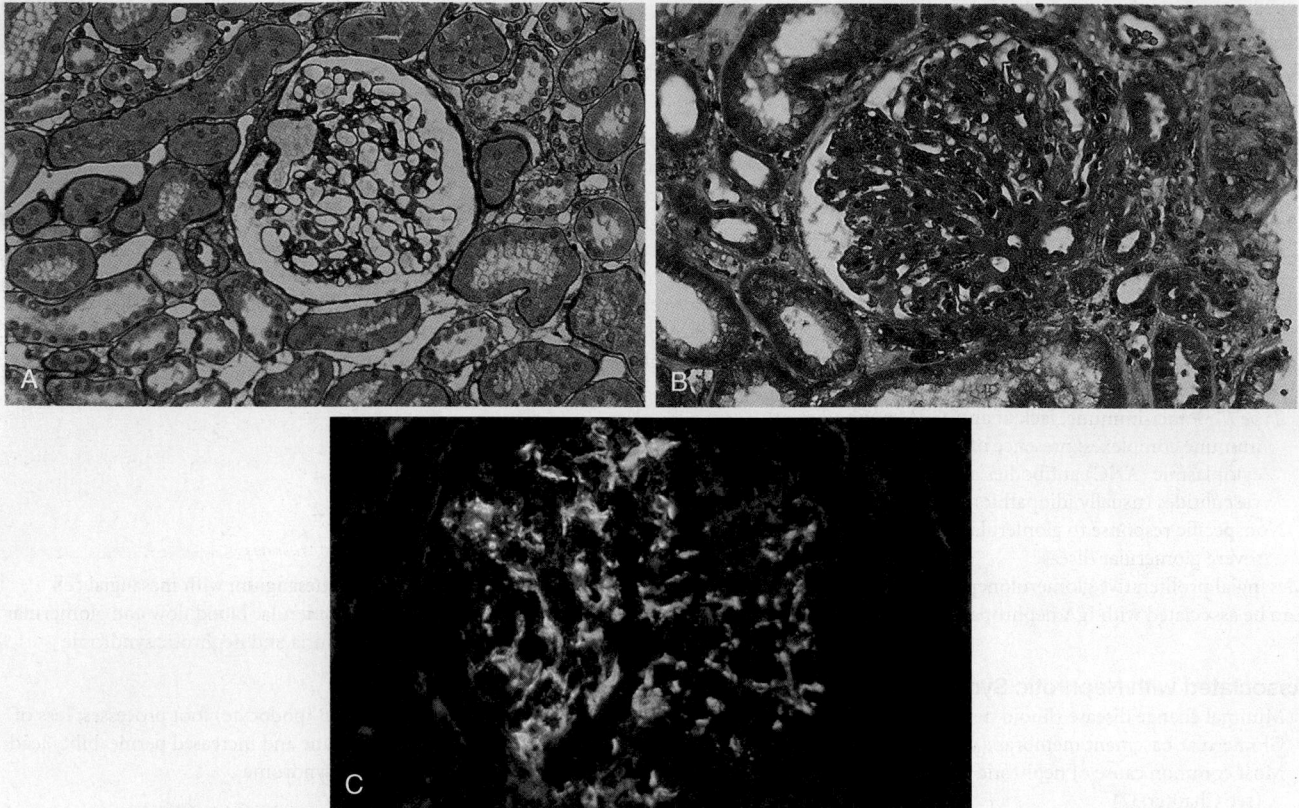

Figure 36-8 Glomerulonephritis. **A,** Normal glomerulus; note single-contoured walls, patent capillaries, inconspicuous mesangium, and degree of cellularity. (Periodic acid–methenamine silver stain.) **B,** Acute postinfectious glomerulonephritis. There is considerable increase in cellularity, mainly because of accumulation of numerous polymorphonuclear leukocytes in capillary lumina. Note numerous subepithelial hump-shaped fuchsinophilic deposits in many capillary walls. Protein precipitates (hyalinization) are in the arteriole. (Masson trichrome stain.) **C,** Postinfectious glomerulonephritis. Irregular mesangial and capillary wall immunostaining for C3. (From Damjanov I, Linder J, editors: *Anderson's pathology*, ed 10, St Louis, 1996, Mosby.)

the first few weeks the major life-threatening problems are acute renal insufficiency with fluid, electrolyte, and acid-base imbalances; acute hypertension may cause hypertensive encephalopathy. Death occurs in about 1% of all persons with PIGN, mostly in developing countries.[78]

Lupus Nephritis

Lupus nephritis is an inflammatory complication of the chronic autoimmune syndrome, systemic lupus erythematosus (see Chapter 8). The renal component of the disease is one of the more severe complications and is associated with autoantibodies against double-stranded deoxyribonucleic acid (dsDNA) and nucleosomes.[79] Complexes of these autoantibodies and complement accumulate in the glomerulus, causing cell proliferation, inflammation, and injury. Different glomerular lesion patterns are identifiable on biopsy including membranous, mesangial, membranoproliferative, and diffuse proliferative glomerulonephritis (see Table 36-6).[80] Symptom presentation is variable depending on lesion involvement and can include proteinuria, edema, and other signs of nephrotic syndrome (p. 1384). Disease progression may be silent or may progress to end-stage kidney failure over a period of years. Long-term management

includes corticosteroids, immunosuppressants, and renal replacement therapy.

IgA Nephropathy

IgA nephropathy (Berger disease) is the most common form of acute glomerulonephritis in developed countries, especially Asia. The cause is unknown and more commonly affects adults ages 20 to 30 years. Henoch-Schönlein purpura is a milder systemic form of the disease that presents with hematuria and occurs more often in children (see Chapter 37). Abnormal glycosylated IgA-1 (galactose-deficient IgA-1) produced by the bone marrow and complement molecules binds to glomerular mesangial cells, stimulating them to proliferate and release oxidants and proteases, thereby contributing to diffuse mesangioproliferative glomerular injury and glomerulosclerosis.[81] The disease manifests with gross or microscopic (30% to 40%) hematuria 24 to 48 hours after an upper respiratory or gastrointestinal viral infection. Proteinuria, edema, and hypertension are less common. Diagnosis is made by renal biopsy. Treatment may include angiotensin-converting enzyme (ACE) inhibitors, glucocorticoids, and cyclophosphamide. The prognosis is variable, with 14% to 39% of cases progressing to renal failure over a period of years.[82]

Crescentic or Rapidly Progressive Glomerulonephritis

Rapidly progressive (crescentic) glomerulonephritis (RPGN) is also known as subacute or extracapillary glomerulonephritis and develops over days to weeks. The disease affects primarily adults in their 50s and 60s and may be idiopathic or associated with a proliferative glomerular disease (diffuse proliferation of extracapillary cells), such as lupus or poststreptococcal glomerulonephritis. Antiglomerular basement membrane antibodies and antineutrophil cytoplasmic antibodies are associated with glomerular injury.[83] There is extensive proliferation of cells into the Bowman space with crescent formation (the shape of the Bowman capsule). Typically the glomerular injury is accompanied by a rapid decline in glomerular function, progressing to renal failure in a few weeks or months.[84] Hematuria is common and may or may not be accompanied by proteinuria, edema, or hypertension. There are three types of RPGN:

Type I: **Antiglomerular basement membrane disease (Goodpasture syndrome)** is a type of RPGN. The disease is rare and associated with IgG antibody formation against pulmonary capillary and glomerular basement membranes, with activation of complement and neutrophils that damage the basement membrane. The disease occurs most often in men 20 to 30 years of age, often accompanied by pulmonary hemorrhage and renal failure.

Type II: **Immune complex deposition** involves deposition of immune complexes in the mesangium and is often associated with lupus nephritis and PIGN.

Type III: **Pauci immune glomerulonephritis** involves the presence of serum antineutrophil cytoplasmic antibodies without immune complex deposition. It is usually idiopathic.

RPGN has a relatively poor prognosis if not diagnosed and treated early. Anticoagulants may be of some benefit in reducing the fibrin component of crescent formation. Plasmapheresis is usually combined with steroids and immunosuppression therapy, including plasma exchange. Dialysis or transplantation is required when failure is irreversible.[85]

Mesangial Proliferative Glomerulonephritis

Mesangial proliferative glomerulonephritis involves deposits of immune complex in the mesangium with mesangial cell proliferation. Mesangial expansion reduces blood flow and alters filtration membrane permeability with development of hematuria, proteinuria, hypertension, and uremia (nephritic syndrome).

Membranous Nephropathy

Membranous nephropathy, also known as **membranous glomerulonephritis,** is usually caused by deposition of circulating antibodies or antibodies formed in situ to antigens located in the glomerular basement membrane. The antigen-antibody complexes activate C5b-C9 fragments of complement (the membrane attack complex) on glomerular epithelial cells with injury and release of inflammatory mediators by mesangial and epithelial cells resulting in increased membrane permeability, thickening of the glomerular membrane, and ultimately glomerular sclerosis. Proteinuria and nephrotic syndrome are common manifestations.

Membranoproliferative Glomerulonephritis

Membranoproliferative glomerulonephritis (MPGN) is usually idiopathic, involves proliferation of mesangial cells, and the formation of crescents related to the deposition of complement. This disease occurs more commonly in children and young adults. Hypocomplementemia is associated with all types of MPGN. Immune complexes are deposited in the mesangium and subendothelial spaces in *type I MPGN,* activating complement and release of inflammatory cytokines that leads to mesangial and endothelial cell proliferation. In *type II MPGN* there are dense deposits that are also present in other organs, so it is a systemic disease. There are no circulating immune complexes. *Type III MPGN* can be familial and involves deposition and activation of complement in the capillary wall with subepithelial and subendothelial deposits. Injury to the glomerular capillary wall in all types of MPGN can cause proteinuria, hematuria, nephrotic syndrome, and acute or chronic kidney failure.

Chronic Glomerulonephritis

Chronic glomerulonephritis encompasses glomerular diseases with a progressive course leading to chronic kidney disease (see p. 1389). Immune injury may cause progressive glomerular destruction but in many cases the cause is unknown and there may be no history of renal disease before the diagnosis. Hypercholesterolemia and proteinuria have been associated with progressive glomerulosclerosis, tubulointerstitial fibrosis and tubular atrophy.[86] The primary cause may be difficult to establish because advanced pathologic changes may obscure specific disease characteristics (Figures 36-9 and 36-10). Diabetes mellitus and systemic lupus erythematosus are secondary causes of chronic glomerular injury.[87]

CLINICAL MANIFESTATIONS Injury to the glomeruli causes various signs and symptoms consequent to changes in glomerular capillary wall structure and GFR. Two major changes distinctive of more severe glomerulonephritis are (1) hematuria with red blood cell casts and (2) proteinuria exceeding 3 to 5 g/day with albumin as the major protein. Gross proteinuria is associated with nephrotic syndrome and a decrease in urine output accompanies a decreased GFR with elevations in plasma creatinine (see Chapter 35).

Several disorders may produce hematuria because bleeding can occur anywhere along the urinary tract. The characteristics of hematuria from red blood cells escaping through the glomerular membrane include a smoky brown–tinged urine, red blood cell casts, and accompanying proteinuria. Bleeding from sites lower in the urinary tract may produce a pink or red-tinged urine. Glomerular bleeding provides prolonged contact with the acidic urine and transforms hemoglobin to methemoglobin, which is brownish and has no blood clots. The history and physical examination may disclose findings

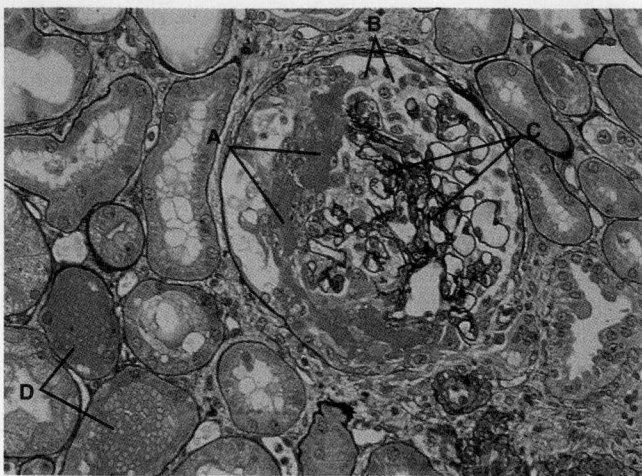

Figure 36-9 Antiglomerular basement membrane nephritis. Glomerulus with a fresh crescent consisting of fibrin and cells in the Bowman space *(A)*. There is disruption of the basement membrane of the Bowman capsule, with migration of cells from the interstitium into the Bowman space *(B)*. The capillary tufts *(C)* are distorted and compressed because of the crescent. Note the free erythrocytes in tubular lumina *(D)*. The interstitium is mildly edematous. (Periodic acid–methenamine silver stain.) (Modified from Damjanov I, Linder J, editors: *Anderson's pathology,* ed 10, St Louis, 1996, Mosby.)

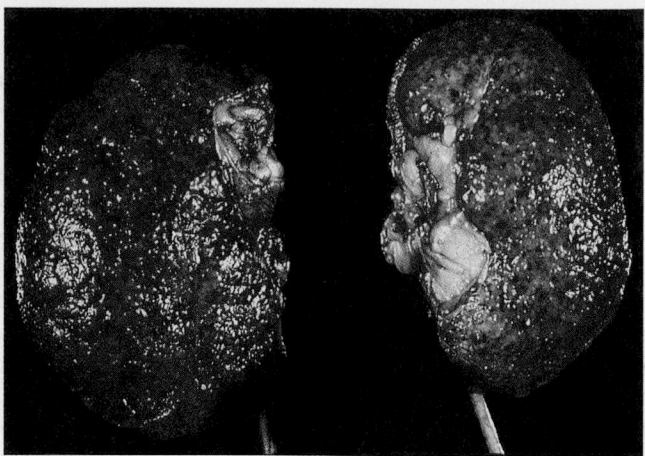

Figure 36-10 Chronic glomerulonephritis. The kidneys appear small, are uniformly shrunken, and have a finely granular external surface. (From Damjanov I: *Pathology for the health professions,* ed 3, St Louis, 2006, Saunders.)

that differentiate glomerular disease from another source of urinary tract bleeding.

The immune-mediated inflammatory response with cellular infiltration decreases GFR, which leads to fluid retention. Salt and water are also reabsorbed, contributing to fluid volume expansion, edema, and hypertension.

Microscopic proteinuria and hematuria may occur during the early years of the disease. Blood pressure may be normal. After 5 to 20 years, renal insufficiency usually begins to develop, followed by nephrotic syndrome and an accelerated progression to end-stage renal failure. Symptom patterns vary depending on the underlying cause. Biopsy may reveal the underlying glomerular lesion (see Table 36-6).

EVALUATION AND TREATMENT The diagnosis of glomerular disease is confirmed by the progressive development of clinical manifestations and laboratory findings of abnormal urinalysis with proteinuria, red blood cells, white blood cells, and casts. Microscopic evaluation from renal biopsy provides a specific determination of renal injury and type of pathologic condition (see Tables 36-6 and 36-7).

Management principles for treating glomerulonephritis are related to treating the primary disease, preventing or minimizing immune responses, and correcting accompanying problems, such as edema, hypertension, hyperlipidemia, hyperkalemia, and hyperglycemia in those with diabetes mellitus. Specific treatment regimens are necessary for particular types of glomerulonephritis. Antibiotic therapy is essential for the management of underlying infections that may be contributing to ongoing antigen-antibody responses. Corticosteroids may decrease antibody synthesis and suppress inflammatory responses. Cytotoxic agents (i.e., cyclophosphamide) may be used to suppress the immune response.

Anticoagulants may be useful for controlling fibrin crescent formation in RPGN. Dialysis or kidney transplantation ultimately may be needed.

Nephrotic Syndrome

Nephrotic syndrome is the excretion of 3.5 g or more of protein in the urine per day and is characteristic of glomerular injury. Lipoid nephrosis (minimal change disease), membranous glomerulonephritis, and focal glomerulosclerosis are directly related to nephrotic syndrome, although these conditions can occur with other types of glomerular disease.[88] Nephrotic syndrome is more common in children than adults (see Chapter 37). Secondary forms of nephrotic syndrome occur in systemic diseases, including diabetes mellitus, amyloidosis, systemic lupus erythematosus, and Henoch-Schönlein purpura. Nephrotic syndrome is also seen with certain drugs, infections, malignancies, and vascular disorders. Familial forms of nephrotic syndrome result from genetic defects that affect the function and composition of the glomerular capillary wall (i.e., Alport syndrome with alterations in basement membrane type IV collagen).[89] Nephrotic syndrome often signifies a more serious prognosis when present as a secondary complication.

PATHOPHYSIOLOGY Disturbances in the GBM and podocyte injury lead to increased permeability to protein and loss of electrical negative charge. Loss of plasma proteins, particularly albumin and some immunoglobulins, occurs across the injured glomerular filtration membrane (Figure 36-11).[88] Sustained proteinuria can result in the release of inflammatory mediators and cytokines by tubular cells with influx of leukocytes resulting in progressive glomerulosclerosis and renal fibrosis.[90] Hypoalbuminemia results from urinary loss of albumin combined with a diminished synthesis of replacement albumin by the liver. Albumin is lost in the greatest quantity because of its high plasma concentration and low molecular weight. Decreased dietary intake of protein from anorexia or malnutrition or accompanying liver disease may also contribute to lower levels of plasma

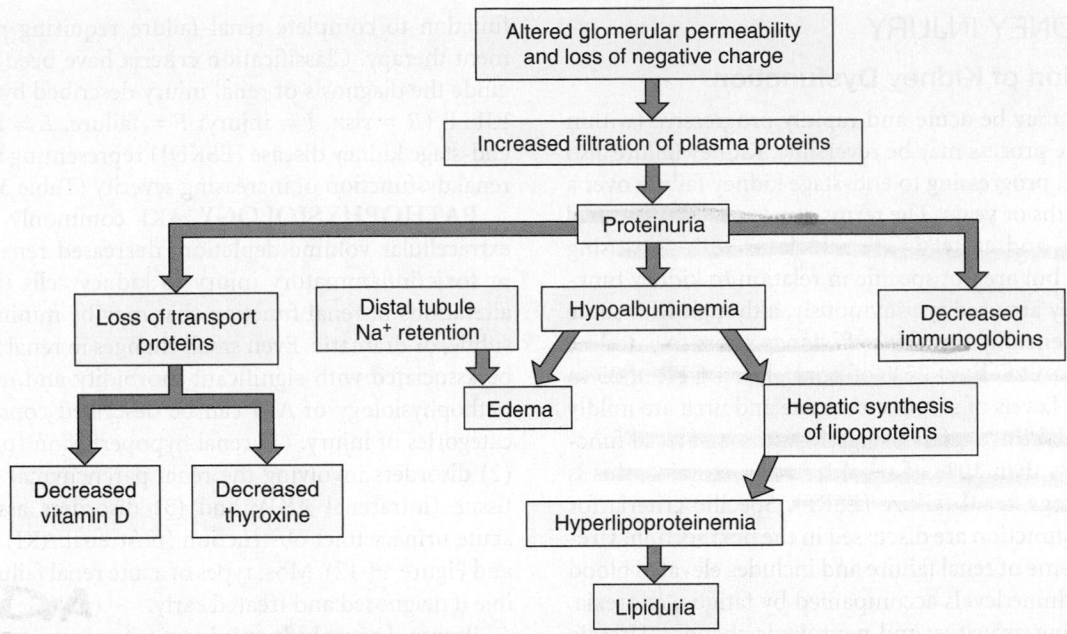

Figure 36-11 Pathophysiology of nephrotic syndrome.

Table 36-8	Clinical Manifestations of Nephrotic Syndrome	
Manifestations	**Contributing Factors**	**Result**
Proteinuria	Increased glomerular permeability, decreased proximal tubule reabsorption	Edema, increased susceptibility to infection from loss of immunoglobulins
Hypoalbuminemia	Increased urinary losses of protein	Edema
Edema	Hypoalbuminemia (decreased oncotic pressure, sodium and water retention, increased aldosterone and antidiuretic hormone [ADH] secretion), unresponsiveness to atrial natriuretic peptides	Soft, pitting, generalized edema
Hyperlipidemia	Decreased serum albumin; increased hepatic synthesis of very-low-density lipoproteins; increased cholesterol, phospholipids, triglycerides	Increased atherogenesis
Lipiduria	Sloughing of tubular cells containing fat (oval fat bodies); free fat from hyperlipidemia	Fat droplets that may float in urine
Decreased vitamin D	The globulin to which 1,25-vitamin D_3 is attached for transport passes through the glomerulus and is lost in the urine	Decreased absorption of calcium from gut Risk for osteodystrophies
Hypothyroidism	Loss of thyroid-binding globulin and other thyroid hormone transport proteins in the urine	May have no symptoms; may have elevated thyroid-stimulating hormone

albumin. Loss of albumin stimulates lipoprotein synthesis by the liver and hyperlipidemia. Loss of immunoglobulins may increase susceptibility to infections. Sodium retention also is associated with nephrotic syndrome contributing to the development of edema and ascites. The exact mechanism is unknown but the site of retention is the distal nephron tubules and collecting ducts.[91]

CLINICAL MANIFESTATIONS Many clinical manifestations of nephrotic syndrome are related to loss of serum proteins (Table 36-8) and sodium retention. They include edema, hyperlipidemia, lipiduria, vitamin D deficiency, and hypothyroidism.[92,93] Vitamin D deficiency is related to loss of serum transport proteins and decreased vitamin D activation by the kidney. Hypothyroidism can result from urinary loss of thyroid-binding protein and thyroxine. Alterations in coagulation factors cause hypercoagulability and may lead to thromboembolic events, particularly in young adults.[94]

EVALUATION AND TREATMENT Nephrotic syndrome is diagnosed when the protein level in a 24-hour urine collection is greater than 3.5 g. Serum albumin decreases (to less than 3 g/dl), and serum cholesterol, phospholipids, and triglycerides increase. Fat bodies may be present in the urine. The specific pathologic condition is identified by renal biopsy.

Nephrotic syndrome is commonly treated with a normal-protein (i.e., 1 g/kg body weight/day) low-fat diet, salt restriction, diuretics, immunosuppression, and heparinoids. When diuretics are used, care must be taken to observe for hypovolemia and hypokalemia or potassium toxicity in the presence of renal insufficiency. Aldactone may be combined with loop diuretics to suppress aldosterone activity to conserve potassium. Steroids may be particularly effective for the initial treatment of nephrotic syndrome in children.[95]

ACUTE KIDNEY INJURY

Classification of Kidney Dysfunction

Kidney injury may be acute and rapidly progressive (within hours), and the process may be reversible. Kidney failure also can be chronic, progressing to end-stage kidney failure over a period of months or years. The terms *renal insufficiency, renal failure, uremia,* and *azotemia* are associated with decreasing renal function but are not specific in relation to kidney function. Often they are used synonymously, although with some distinctions. Generally, **renal insufficiency** refers to a decline in renal function to about 25% of normal or a GFR of 25 to 30 ml/minute. Levels of serum creatinine and urea are mildly elevated. **Renal failure** refers to significant loss of renal function. When less than 10% of renal function remains, this is termed **end-stage renal failure (ESRF).** Specific criteria for acute renal dysfunction are discussed in the next section. **Uremia** is a syndrome of renal failure and includes elevated blood urea and creatinine levels accompanied by fatigue, anorexia, nausea, vomiting, pruritus, and neurologic changes. Uremia represents the numerous consequences related to renal failure, including retention of toxic wastes, deficiency states, and electrolyte disorders. **Azotemia** means increased serum urea levels and frequently increased creatinine levels as well. Renal insufficiency or renal failure causes azotemia. Both azotemia and uremia indicate an accumulation of nitrogenous waste products in the blood, a common characteristic that explains the overlap in definitions of terms.

Acute Kidney Injury

Acute kidney injury (AKI) is a sudden decline in kidney function with a decrease in glomerular filtration and accumulation of nitrogenous waste products in the blood as demonstrated by an elevation in plasma creatinine and blood urea nitrogen. The term *acute kidney injury* is preferred to the term *acute renal failure* as it captures the diverse nature of this syndrome ranging from minimal or subtle changes in renal function to complete renal failure requiring renal replacement therapy. Classification criteria have been developed to guide the diagnosis of renal injury described by the acronym RIFLE (*R* = risk, *I* = injury, *F* = failure, *L* = loss, and *E* = end-stage kidney disease [ESKD]) representing three levels of renal dysfunction of increasing severity (Table 36-9).[96]

PATHOPHYSIOLOGY AKI commonly results from extracellular volume depletion, decreased renal blood flow, or toxic/inflammatory injury to kidney cells that results in alterations in renal function that may be minimal or severe, subtle, or dramatic. Even small changes in renal function may be associated with significant morbidity and mortality. The pathophysiology of AKI can be described considering three categories of injury: (1) renal hypoperfusion (prerenal AKI); (2) disorders involving the renal parenchymal or interstitial tissue (intrarenal AKI); and (3) disorders associated with acute urinary tract obstruction (postrenal AKI) (Table 36-10 and Figure 36-12). Most types of acute renal failure are reversible if diagnosed and treated early.

Prerenal acute kidney injury is the most common cause of AKI and is caused by renal hypoperfusion that occurs rapidly over a period of hours with elevation of BUN and plasma creatinine levels. During the early phases of hypoperfusion protective autoregulatory mechanisms maintain GFR at a relatively constant level through afferent arteriolar dilation

Table 36-9	RIFLE Criteria for Acute Renal Dysfunction/Failure	
Category	**GFR Criteria**	**Urine Output (UO) Criteria**
Risk	Increased creatinine × 1.5 or GFR decrease >25%	UO <0.5ml/kg/hr × 6 hr
Injury	Increased creatinine × 2 or GFR decrease >50%	UO <0.5ml/kg/hr × 12 hr
Failure	Increased creatinine × 3 or GFR decrease >75%	UO <0.3ml/kg/hr × 24 hr or anuria
Loss	Persistent ARF = complete loss of kidney function >4 weeks	
ESKD	End-stage kidney disease (>3 months)	

Adapted from Bellomo R et al: *Curr Opin Crit Care* 8(6):505-508, 2002; Bellomo R et al: *Crit Care* 8(4):R204-R212, 2004. Available at www.medicalcriteria.com/criteria/neph_rifle.htm (accessed October, 2008). *ARF,* Acute renal failure; *GFR,* glomerular filtration rate.

Table 36-10	Classification of Acute Kidney Injury
Area of Dysfunction	**Possible Causes**
Prerenal	Hypovolemia
	Hemorrhagic blood loss (trauma, gastrointestinal bleeding, complications of childbirth)
	Loss of plasma volume (burns, peritonitis)
	Water and electrolyte losses (severe vomiting or diarrhea, intestinal obstruction, uncontrolled diabetes mellitus, inappropriate use of diuretics)
	Hypotension or hypoperfusion
	Septic shock
	Cardiac failure or shock
	Massive pulmonary embolism
	Stenosis or clamping of renal artery
Intrarenal	Acute tubular necrosis (postischemic or nephrotoxic)
	Glomerulopathies
	Acute interstitial necrosis (tumors or toxins)
	Vascular damage
	Malignant hypertension, vasculitis
	Coagulation defects
	Renal artery/vein occlusion
	Bilateral acute pyelonephritis
Postrenal	Obstructive uropathies (usually bilateral)
	Ureteral destruction (edema, tumors, stones, clots)
	Bladder neck obstruction (enlarged prostate)
	Neurogenic bladder

and efferent arteriolar vasoconstriction (mediated by angiotensin II). Tubuloglomerular feedback mechanisms also maintain GFR and distal tubular nephron flow (see Chapter 35). The GFR ultimately declines because of the decrease in filtration pressure. Poor perfusion can result from renal vasoconstriction, hypotension, hypovolemia, hemorrhage, or inadequate cardiac output. AKI may occur during chronic kidney failure if a sudden stress is imposed on already marginally functioning kidneys. Failure to restore blood volume or blood pressure and oxygen delivery can cause cell injury and acute tubular necrosis or acute interstitial necrosis, a more severe form of AKI.

Intrarenal (intrinsic) acute kidney injury (AKI) may result from ischemic acute tubular necrosis (ATN), nephrotoxic ATN (i.e., exposure to radiocontrast media), acute glomerulonephritis, vascular disease (malignant hypertension, disseminated intravascular coagulation, and renal vasculitis), allograft rejection, or interstitial disease (drug allergy, infection, tumor growth). **Acute tubular necrosis (ATN)** caused by ischemia is the most common cause of intrarenal AKI. It occurs most often after surgery (40% to 50% of cases) but is also associated with severe sepsis, obstetric complications, and severe trauma, including severe burns. A combination of events and predisposing factors leads to the greatest risk for acute renal failure. The terms *acute tubular necrosis* and *acute renal failure* are sometimes used interchangeably, but the conditions are not the same because acute renal failure can occur without ATN. ATN is generally described as postischemic or nephrotoxic or it can be a combination of both.[97] Postischemic ATN involves persistent hypotension, hypoperfusion, and hypoxemia producing ischemia, reduced ATP, and generate toxic oxygen-free radicals with loss of antioxidant protection that causes cell swelling, injury, and necrosis. The release of inflammatory cytokines contributes to tubular injury and increases neutrophil adhesion.[98] Transport of sodium and other molecules is disrupted with damage to the tubular epithelium and shedding of the brush border. Ischemic necrosis tends to be patchy and may be distributed along any part of the nephron tubules. Injury is most severe in the outer medulla with scattered necrosis in the cortex and loss of cells along the tubular epithelium. Severe disease of the glomeruli (i.e., acute or rapidly progressive glomerulonephritis) or renal microvascular disorders can also cause intrinsic kidney injury. Oliguria is common (urine output less than 30 ml/hour) with intrarenal AKI, but anuria is rare. Acute kidney failure associated with sepsis may involve different mechanisms of tubular injury including apoptosis (does not result in inflammation because there is no release of intracellular contents into the extracellular space) (see Chapter 2 for apoptosis) and tubular cell dysfunction. Urinalysis in septic renal injury may not reflect renal injury because elevated creatinine and oliguria may be physiologic responses to hypovolemia and decreased renal blood flow.[99,100]

Nephrotoxic ATN can be produced by numerous antibiotics, but the aminoglycosides (neomycin, gentamicin, tobramycin) are the major culprits. The drugs tend to accumulate in the renal cortex and may not cause renal failure until after treatment is complete. Radiocontrast media (x-ray media) and cisplatin also may be nephrotoxic. Dehydration, advanced age, concurrent renal insufficiency, and diabetes mellitus tend to enhance nephrotoxicity from either aminoglycosides or radiocontrast media. Other substances such as excessive myoglobin (oxygen-transporting substance in muscles), carbon tetrachloride, heavy metals (mercury, arsenic), methoxyflurane anesthesia, or bacterial toxins may promote renal failure. Necrosis and tubular cell apoptosis caused by nephrotoxins is usually uniform and limited to the proximal tubules. The high surface area of the brush border of the proximal tubular cells makes them more vulnerable to toxic injury.[101]

Postrenal acute kidney injury is rare and usually occurs with urinary tract obstruction that affects the kidneys bilaterally (e.g., bilateral ureteral obstruction, bladder outlet obstruction–prostatic hypertrophy, tumors or neurogenic bladder, and urethral obstruction). The obstruction causes an increase in intraluminal pressure upstream from the site of obstruction with a gradual fall in GFR. A pattern of several hours of anuria with flank pain followed by polyuria is a characteristic finding. This type of AKI can occur after diagnostic catheterization of the ureters, a procedure that may cause edema of the tubular lumen.

Oliguria can occur in AKI, and three mechanisms have been proposed to account for the decrease in urine output. All three mechanisms probably contribute to oliguria in varying combinations and degrees throughout the course of the disease (Figure 36-12). These mechanisms are as follows[102]:

1. *Alterations in renal blood flow.* Efferent arteriolar vasoconstriction may be produced by intrarenal release of angiotensin II or by redistribution of blood flow from the cortex to the medulla. Autoregulation of blood flow may be impaired, resulting in decreased GFR. Changes in glomerular permeability and decreased GFR also may result from the ischemia.

2. *Tubular obstruction.* Advanced injury with necrosis of the tubules causes sloughing of cells, cast formation, or ischemic edema that results in tubular obstruction, which in turn causes a retrograde increase in pressure and reduces the GFR. Renal failure can occur within 24 hours.

3. *Backleak.* Glomerular filtration remains normal, but tubular reabsorption or "leak" of filtrate is accelerated as a result of permeability caused by ischemia and increased tubular pressure from obstruction.

CLINICAL MANIFESTATIONS The clinical progression of acute renal failure, particularly acute tubular necrosis, occurs in three phases: the initiation phase, maintenance phase, and recovery phase. The *initiation phase* is the phase of reduced perfusion or toxicity in which renal injury is evolving. Prevention of injury is possible during this phase. The *maintenance phase* is the period of established renal injury and dysfunction after the initiating event has been resolved and may last from weeks to months. Urine output is lowest during this phase, and serum creatinine and blood urea nitrogen

↑ BUN/CC

Mechanisms of oliguria in acute kidney injury

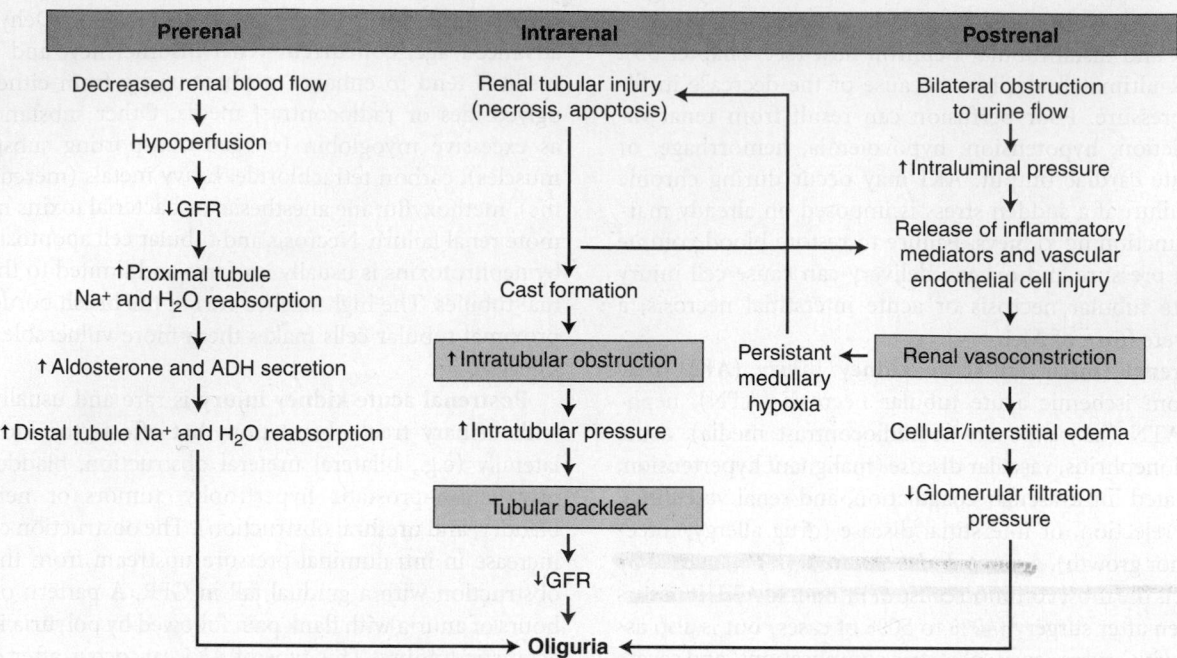

Figure 36-12 Acute kidney injury and mechanisms of oliguria. *ADH,* Antidiuretic hormone; *GFR,* glomerular filtration rate.

increase. The *recovery phase* is the interval when renal injury is repaired and normal renal function is reestablished. Diuresis is common during this phase, with a decline in serum creatinine and urea and an increase in creatinine clearance.

Oliguria begins within 1 day after a hypotensive event and lasts for 1 to 3 weeks, but it may regress in several hours or extend for several weeks, depending on the duration of ischemia or severity of toxic injury and the initiation of treatment. **Anuria** (urine output less than 50 ml/day) is uncommon in ATN, and 10% to 20% of cases have nonoliguric failure (decreased urine output but greater than 30 ml/hour). Anuria involves both kidneys and suggests bilateral renal artery occlusion, obstructive uropathy, or acute cortical necrosis. Nonoliguric failure usually represents less severe injury. The urine output may vary in volume, but the BUN and plasma creatinine concentrations increase (plasma creatinine is inversely proportional to the GFR). Urine sediment should be evaluated for casts, cells, and crystals.

Other early manifestations depend on the underlying cause of renal failure. Individuals who have experienced trauma or surgery or people in a catabolic state may have more rapid elevations in BUN. They are prone to hyperkalemia and hyperphosphatemia from cellular breakdown. Fluid retention may cause edema. Symptoms of congestive heart failure develop in persons with cardiac disease. Nausea, vomiting, and fatigue accompany uremia and electrolyte imbalances. Wound healing is delayed, and the risk of infection, particularly pneumonia, is greater. Nonoliguric renal failure generally has a better prognosis because of fewer complications. Oliguric patients may require maintenance dialysis to attenuate symptoms of renal failure.

As renal function improves during the recovery phase, increase in urine volume (diuresis) is progressive. During the early diuretic phase the tubules are still recovering secretory and reabsorptive function. Sodium and potassium are lost in the urine, and the risk for hypokalemia is greater. Volume depletion may ensue, with fluid losses of 3 to 4 L/day. Fluid and electrolyte balance must be carefully monitored and excessive urinary losses replaced. Return to normal status may take 3 to 12 months, and approximately 30% of individuals do not have full recovery of a normal GFR or tubular function.

EVALUATION AND TREATMENT The diagnosis of AKI is related to the cause of the disease. A history of surgery, trauma, or cardiovascular disorders is common, and exposure to nephrotoxins and obstructive uropathies (i.e., an enlarged prostate) must be considered. The diagnostic challenge is to differentiate prerenal acute renal injury from acute tubular necrosis. Urine composition may provide helpful diagnostic clues to changes in tubular function (Table 36-11).

The ratios of the BUN to plasma creatinine concentration and fractional excretion of sodium (the ratio of filtered sodium to excreted sodium) are helpful diagnostic indicators because the tests reflect renal tubular reabsorption ability. In prerenal AKI, tubular function is maintained and salt, water, and urea are reabsorbed. With ATN, reabsorption and urinary concentration abilities are compromised. Other causes of renal failure also may exhibit similar clinical findings. Serial measurements of plasma creatinine provide an index of renal function during the recovery phase. *Cystatin C,* a serum protein constantly produced by nucleated cells, is freely filtered by the glomerulus, and its concentration can serve as a measure of GFR and may be useful for detecting early changes

Table 36-11	Urine Characteristics of Prerenal and Intrinsic Acute Kidney Injury	
Diagnostic Index	Prerenal	ATN
Urine volume	<400 ml	<400 ml
Urine specificity	1.016-1.020	1.010-1.012
Urine osmolality	>500 mOsm	<300 mOsm
Urine sodium	<10 mEq/L	>30 mEq/L
BUN/plasma	>15:1	<15:1 creatinine
FE_{Na}	<1% (also seen in acute glomerulonephritis	>1% (also seen in urinary tract obstruction and renal parenchymal disease)
Urine sediment	Usually no cells, some hyaline casts	Brown granular casts, epithelial cells

ATN, Acute tubular necrosis; *BUN,* blood urea nitrogen; FE_{Na}, fractional excretion of sodium.

in glomerular filtration rate.[103] Biomarkers of AKI that detect injury very early are needed to prevent delay in initiating therapy. New diagnostic tests are being developed to provide more sensitive markers of AKI.[104,105]

Prevention of acute renal injury and maintenance of renal perfusion are major treatment factors and involve maintenance of fluid volume before and after surgery or diagnostic procedures or when nephrotoxic drugs or contrast agents are in use. The primary goal of therapy is to maintain the individual's life until renal function has recovered. There is no specific treatment for acute renal failure. Management principles directly related to physiologic alterations generally include (1) correcting fluid and electrolyte disturbances, (2) managing blood pressure, (3) treating infections, (4) maintaining nutrition, and (5) remembering that drugs or their metabolites are not excreted. Fluid and electrolyte replacement must be carefully calculated with consideration of urine losses, insensible losses (up to 1000 ml/day), and production of endogenous water by oxidation (450 ml/day). Overhydration of patients dilutes their plasma sodium concentration. Metabolic acidosis is usually not treated until serum HCO_3^- is less than 15 mEq/L.[106]

Hyperkalemia can be managed by restricting dietary sources of potassium, using non–potassium-sparing diuretics, or using cation-ion exchange resins, which may be administered orally or rectally. These resins exchange potassium for another cation, such as sodium in the bowel, and the potassium then is excreted attached to the resin. With severe hyperkalemia (more than 6.5 mEq/L), dialysis may be required or potassium can be driven back temporarily into the cells by administering glucose and insulin or by infusing sodium bicarbonate or albuterol. Glucose metabolism causes potassium to move to the intracellular fluid, and insulin infusions therefore can be effective in shifting potassium from the extracellular to intracellular space, along with the transport of glucose, within 30 minutes. (Glucose metabolism is discussed in Chapter 1 and Chapter 21.) Using sodium bicarbonate to cause alkalemia also shifts potassium into cells in exchange for hydrogen ions.

Careful monitoring of the electrocardiogram for peaking T waves is essential for individuals with hyperkalemia. Intravenous infusion of calcium is the most rapid method of treating cardiac effects of hyperkalemia. Calcium decreases the threshold potential and reduces the membrane excitability caused by hyperkalemia (see Chapter 3). Calcium should be used only in emergencies, however, because hypercalcemia also may cause cardiac arrest.

Azotemia is generally controlled and nutrition maintained with a low-protein, high-carbohydrate diet. Essential amino acid replacement can be given orally or parenterally. Adequate carbohydrate intake slows protein catabolism and helps prevent hyperkalemia. Because sepsis is a common serious or fatal complication of renal failure, observation for signs of infection and early treatment with antibiotics are necessary. Drug dosage levels may require adjustment if they are metabolized or excreted by the kidneys. Recovery may take up to 1 year.

Continuous renal replacement therapy (hemodialysis) (mechanical removal of water, electrolytes, and toxins from the blood) is indicated for uncontrollable hyperkalemia or acidosis or severe fluid overload. Continuous renal replacement therapy is particularly promising in critically ill patients with multiple organ dysfunction.[107]

CHRONIC KIDNEY DISEASE

Chronic kidney disease (CKD) is the progressive loss of renal function associated with systemic diseases such as hypertension and diabetes mellitus or intrinsic kidney disease including chronic glomerulonephritis, chronic pyelonephritis, obstructive uropathies or vascular disorders. The National Kidney Foundation (www.kidney.org/professionals/) defines kidney damage as a GFR less than 60 mL/min/1.73 m² for 3 months or more, irrespective of cause. Chronic kidney disease is the preferred terminology and is referenced to declining GFR. The terms *renal insufficiency* and *chronic renal failure* are still often used to describe declining renal function, but they do not have the specificity of the stages recommended by the National Kidney Foundation (Table 36-12). CKD decreases GFR and tubular functions with changes manifested throughout all organ systems (Table 36-13).[108]

PATHOPHYSIOLOGY The kidneys have a remarkable ability to adapt to loss of nephron mass.[109] Symptomatic changes resulting from increased creatinine, urea,

WHAT'S NEW? **Continuous Renal Replacement and Renal Tubule Therapy**

Continuous renal replacement therapy (CRRT) is a treatment that provides a form of continuous dialysis for acute renal failure. It is replacing intermittent hemodialysis (IHD), particularly for critically ill individuals. Generally, there are two forms of CRRT: hemofiltration and hemodiafiltration. Each may be further subdivided into arteriovenous or venovenous, depending on the site of vascular access. Hemofiltration removes excess fluid and solutes (urea, creatinine, sodium, potassium) by pumping blood through the semipermeable membranes of a hemofilter in a compartment of ultrafiltrate. Individuals must be carefully monitored for either volume excess or deficit and electrolyte imbalance. Hemodiafiltration is a combination of hemofiltration and hemodialysis with the removal of solutes by diffusion gradients from the blood across semipermeable membranes to a dialysis solution.

Advances are being made in the application of renal tubule assist devices that include a conventional hemodialysis filter with a bioreactor containing living renal proximal tubule cells. In addition to the solute and fluid management provided by hemofiltration, the renal tubule-assist device extends function to include reabsorptive and endocrine functions of the kidney. Progress also is being made in the development of nanofabrication technology to further improve the clearance function of the kidney to replicate glomerular permselectivity while retaining high rates of hydraulic permeability. Although mortality from acute renal failure remains high, there is hope these new devices will improve survival with earlier recovery of renal function and hospital discharge. Large randomized clinical trials are needed to determine outcomes and costs of these different renal replacement modalities.

Data from Ding F, Humes HD: *Nephron Exp Nephrol* 109(4):e118-e122, 2008; Pannu N et al: *JAMA* 299(7):793-805, 2008; Rauf AA et al: *J Intensive Care Med* 23(3):195-203, 2008; Tumlin J et al: *J Am Soc Nephrol* 19(5):1034-1040, 2008.

Table 36-12 **Stages of Chronic Kidney Disease**

Stage	Severity	GFR ml/min	Progression	Symptoms
1	Kidney damage: normal or increased GFR	≥90	None apparent	Usually none Hypertension common
2	Kidney damage: mild ↓GFR	60-89	Increasing PTH Early bone disease Increasing plasma creatinine and urea	Subtle Hypertension
3	Moderate: ↓GFR	30-59	Erythropoietin deficiency, anemia Increased plasma creatinine and urea	Mild Hypertension
4	Severe: ↓GFR	15-29	Increased triglycerides Metabolic acidosis Hyperkalemia Salt/water retention Increasing plasma creatinine and urea	Moderate Hypertension Hyperphosphatemia Anemia
5	End-stage kidney disease; kidney failure	<15	Uremia	Severe Hypertension Hyperphosphatemia Anemia

Adapted from National Kidney Foundation, Chronic Kidney Disease 2006: *A Guide to Select NKF KDOQI Guidelines and Recommendations,* 2006. Available at http://www.kidney.org/professionals/kls/pdf/Pharmacist_CPG.pdf
Normal glomerular filtration rate in a 70-kg male is about 120 ml/min.
GFR, Glomerular filtration rate; *PTH,* parathyroid hormone.

potassium, and alterations in salt and water balance usually do not become apparent until renal function declines to less than 25% of normal when adaptive renal reserves have been exhausted.

Different theories have been proposed to account for the adaptation to loss of renal function. The *intact nephron hypothesis* proposes that loss of nephron mass with progressive kidney damage causes the surviving nephrons to sustain normal kidney function. These nephrons are capable of a compensatory hypertrophy and expansion or hyperfunction in

their rates of filtration, reabsorption, and secretion and can maintain a constant rate of excretion in the presence of overall declining GFR. The intact nephron hypothesis explains adaptive changes in solute and water regulation that occur with advancing renal failure. Although the urine of an individual with chronic kidney failure may contain abnormal amounts of protein and red and white blood cells or casts, the major end products of excretion are similar to those of normally functioning kidneys until the advanced stages of renal failure when there is a significant reduction of functioning nephrons.[110,111]

Table 36-13   Systemic Effects of Chronic Kidney Disease and Uremia

System	Manifestations	Mechanisms	Treatment
Skeletal	Spontaneous fractures and bone pain; Deformities of long bones	Osteitis fibrosa: bone inflammation with fibrous degeneration related to hyperparathyroidism; Osteomalacia: bone resorption associated with vitamin D and calcium deficiency	Control of hyperphosphatemia to reduce hyperparathyroidism; administration of calcium and aluminum hydroxide antacids, which bind phosphate in the gut, together with a phosphate-restricted diet; vitamin D replacement; avoidance of magnesium antacids because of impaired magnesium excretion
Cardiopulmonary	Pulmonary edema, Kussmaul respirations	Fluid overload associated with pulmonary edema and metabolic acidosis leading to Kussmaul respirations	ACE inhibitors; combination of propranolol, hydralazine, and minoxidil for those with high levels of renin; bilateral nephrectomy with dialysis or transplantation
Cardiovascular	Left ventricular hypertrophy, cardiomyopathy, and ischemic heart disease; hypertension, dysrhythmias, accelerated atherosclerosis; pericarditis with fever, chest pain, and pericardial friction rub	Extracellular volume expansion and hypersecretion of renin associated with hypertension; anemia increases cardiac workload; hyperlipidemia promotes atherosclerosis; toxins precipitate into pericardium	Volume reduction with diuretics that are not potassium sparing (to avoid hyperkalemia); dialysis
Neurologic	Encephalopathy (fatigue, loss of attention, difficulty with problem solving); peripheral neuropathy (pain and burning in the legs and feet, loss of vibration sense and deep tendon reflexes); loss of motor coordination, twitching, fasciculations, stupor, and coma with advanced uremia	Progressive accumulation of uremic toxins associated with end-stage renal disease; Stroke or intracerebral hemorrhage associated with chronic dialysis	Dialysis or successful kidney transplantation
Endocrine	Restricted growth in children; Higher incidence of goiter; Osteomalacia	Elevated parathyroid hormone levels; Decreased thyroid hormone	Endogenous recombinant human growth hormone; thyroid hormone replacement; Same as skeletal above
Hematologic	Anemia, usually normochromic normocytic; platelet disorders with prolonged bleeding times	Reduced erythropoietin secretion and reduced red cell production; uremic toxins shorten red blood cell survival and alter platelet function	Dialysis; recombinant human erythropoietin and iron supplementation; conjugated estrogens; DDAVP (1-deamino[8-D-arginine] vasopressin); transfusion
Gastrointestinal	Anorexia, nausea, vomiting; mouth ulcers, stomatitis, urinous breath (uremic factor), hiccups, peptic ulcers, gastrointestinal bleeding, and pancreatitis associated with end-stage renal failure	Retention of metabolic acids and other metabolic waste products	Protein-restricted diet for relief of nausea and vomiting
Integumentary	Abnormal pigmentation and pruritus	Retention of urochromes, contributing to sallow, yellow color; high plasma calcium levels and neuropathy associated with pruritus	Dialysis with control of serum calcium and phosphate levels
Immunologic	Increased risk of infection that can cause death; increased risk of carcinoma	Suppression of cell-mediated immunity; reduction in number and function of lymphocytes, diminished phagocytosis	Routine dialysis
Reproductive	Sexual dysfunction: menorrhagia, amenorrhea, infertility, and decreased libido in women; decreased testosterone levels, infertility, and decreased libido in men	Dysfunction of ovaries and testes; presence of neuropathies	No specific treatment

With data from Keane WF: *Kidney Int Suppl* 75:S27-S31, 2000; Uribarri J: *Semin Dial* 13(4):232-234, 2000.

However, the continued loss of functioning nephrons and the adaptive hyperfiltration (increased glomerular pressure) can result in glomerulosclerosis contributing to uremia and end-stage renal failure.[111] This is known as the *trade-off hypothesis*.

The *particular location of kidney damage* can also influence loss of kidney function. For example, tubular interstitial diseases damage primarily the tubular or medullary parts of the nephron, producing problems such as renal tubular acidosis, salt wasting, and difficulty diluting or concentrating the urine. When the damage is primarily vascular or glomerular, proteinuria, hematuria, and nephrotic syndrome are more prominent. This theory is useful for planning treatment in early stages of renal failure when symptomatic differences in renal disease may be distinct. A summary of factors involved in the progression of chronic kidney disease is outlined in Table 36-14.

Progression of chronic kidney disease is thought to be associated with common pathogenic processes regardless of the initial disease (Figure 36-13).[112] These processes include the following:

- Glomerular hypertension, hyperfiltration, and hypertrophy
- Glomerulosclerosis
- Tubulointerstitial inflammation and fibrosis

The factors that contribute to the pathogenesis of chronic kidney disease are complex and involve the interaction of many cells, cytokines, and structural alterations. Two factors that have consistently been recognized to advance renal

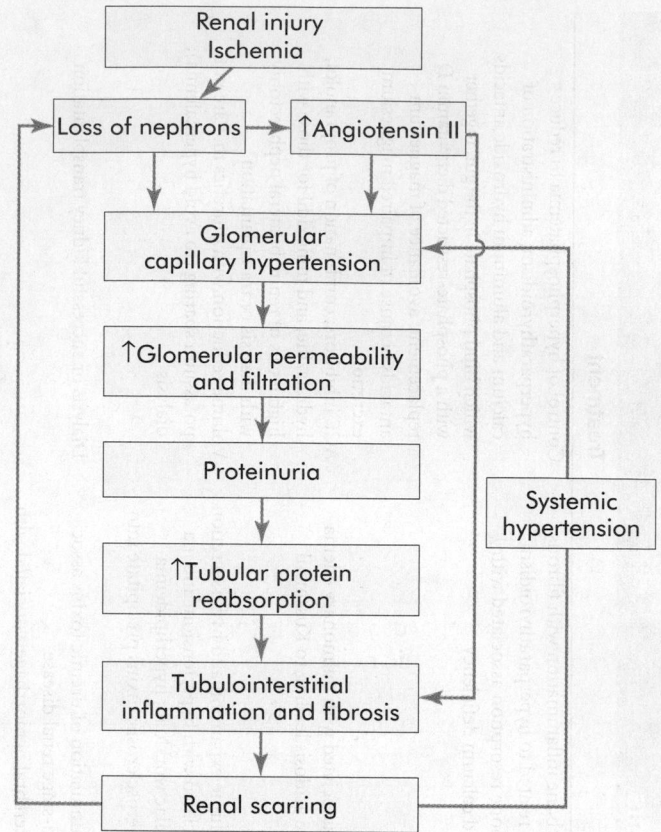

Figure 36-13 Mechanisms related to the progression of chronic kidney disease.

Table 36-14	Factors Representing Progression of Chronic Kidney Disease
Factor	**Characteristics**
Proteinuria	Glomerular hyperfiltration of protein contributes to tubular intestinal injury by accumulating in the interstitial space and promoting inflammation and progressive fibrosis.
Creatine and urea clearance	In chronic renal failure, the GFR falls and the plasma creatinine concentration increases by a reciprocal amount; because there is no regulatory adjustment for creatinine, plasma levels continue to rise and serve as an index of changing glomerular function.
	As GFR declines, urea clearance increases. (NOTE: Urea is filtered and reabsorbed and varies with the state of hydration.)
Sodium and water balance	In chronic renal failure, sodium load delivered to nephrons exceeds normal, so excretion must increase, thus less is reabsorbed. Obligatory loss occurs, leading to sodium deficits and volume depletion. As GFR is reduced, ability to concentrate and dilute urine diminishes.
Phosphate and calcium balance	Changes in acid-base balance affect phosphate and calcium balance. The major disorders associated with chronic renal failure are reduced renal phosphate excretion, decreased renal synthesis of 1,25-$(OH)_2$ vitamin D_3, and hypocalcemia.
	Hypocalcemia leads to secondary hyperparathyroidism, GFR falls, and progressive hyperphosphatemia, hypocalcemia, and dissolution of bone result.
Hematocrit	Lack of erythropoietin and anemia accompanies chronic renal failure. Lethargy, dizziness, and low hematocrit are common.
Potassium balance	In chronic renal failure, tubular secretion of potassium increases until oliguria develops. Use of potassium-sparing diuretics also may precipitate elevated serum potassium levels. As disease progresses, total body potassium levels can rise to life-threatening levels and dialysis is required.
Acid-base balance	In early renal insufficiency, acid excretion and bicarbonate reabsorption are increased to maintain normal pH. Metabolic acidosis begins when GFR reaches 30% to 40%. Metabolic acidosis and hyperkalemia may be severe enough to require dialysis when end-stage renal failure develops.
Dyslipidemia	Chronic hyperlipidemia may induce glomerular and tubulointerstitial injury contributing to the progression of chronic kidney disease.

GFR, Glomerular filtration rate.

disease are proteinuria and angiotensin II.[113,114] Glomerular hyperfiltration and increased glomerular capillary permeability lead to proteinuria. Proteinuria contributes to tubulointerstitial injury by accumulating in the interstitial space and activating complement proteins and other mediators and cells, such as macrophages, that promote inflammation and progressive fibrosis. Angiotensin II activity is elevated with progressive nephron injury. **Angiotension II** promotes glomerular hypertension and hyperfiltration caused by efferent arteriolar vasoconstriction and also promotes systemic hypertension. The chronically high intraglomerular pressure increases glomerular capillary permeability contributing to proteinuria. Angiotensin II also may promote the activity of inflammatory cells and growth factors that participate in tubulointerstitial fibrosis and scarring.

CLINICAL MANIFESTATIONS The clinical manifestations of chronic kidney disease are often described using the terms azotemia and uremia. Azotemia is increased levels of serum urea, serum creatinine and other nitrogenous compounds related to decreasing kidney function. **Uremic syndrome** is the systemic manifestations associated with the accumulation of urea and other nitrogenous compounds and toxins caused by decline in renal function. Sources of toxins include the accumulation of end products of protein metabolism, alterations in fluid and electrolytes, metabolic acidosis, intestinal absorption of toxins produced by gut bacteria and results of altered renal hormone synthesis (i.e., anemia, hyperphosphatemia, and hypocalcemia). Uremia represents a proinflammatory state with many systemic effects.[115] Generally, the symptoms include hypertension, anorexia, nausea, vomiting, diarrhea or constipation, weight loss, pruritus, edema, anemia, and neurologic, cardiovascular, and skeletal changes. The many systemic manifestations associated with uremia are summarized in Table 36-13, p. 1391 and Figure 36-14.

Creatinine and Urea Clearance

Creatinine is constantly released from muscle and excreted primarily by glomerular filtration. In CKD, as the GFR declines, the plasma creatinine level increases by a reciprocal amount to maintain a constant rate of excretion (Figure 36-15). Because no significant tubular adjustment occurs for creatinine (i.e., tubular secretion), the plasma levels continue to increase as the GFR decreases. Therefore, measures of plasma creatinine can serve as an index of changing glomerular function. The clearance of *urea* follows a similar pattern, but urea is filtered as well as reabsorbed and varies with the state of hydration and it is not a good index of GFR. However, as the GFR decreases, plasma urea concentration also increases.

Fluid and Electrolyte Balance

Fluid and electrolyte and acid-base balance are significantly disturbed with chronic kidney disease. A summary of electrolyte and acid-base balance alterations is presented in Table 36-15.

Levels of *sodium* must be regulated within narrow limits because sodium is the major extracellular solute. In CKD sodium and water balance is maintained very close to normal

until the development of stage V ESKD. This occurs because of the increased fractional excretion of sodium, particularly in the distal nephron, in relation to decreasing GFR. Hormones including aldosterone, prostaglandins, and natriuretic peptides also modulate sodium excretion and they are elevated with progressive renal failure. Individual variation in the underlying pathology of CKD must be considered in the management of sodium intake or restriction. Sodium wasting

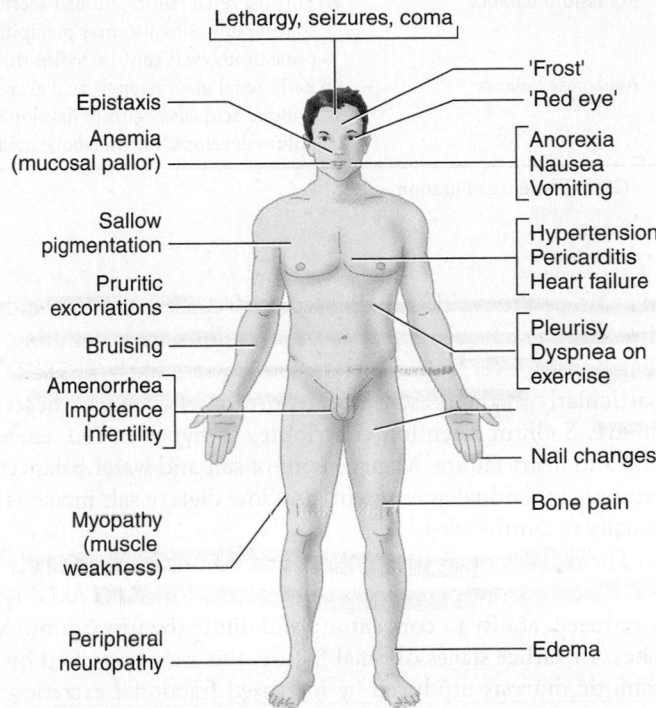

Figure 36-14 Common signs and symptoms of kidney failure (see text for reference site). (From Goldman L, Ausiello D: *Cecil medicine*, ed 23, Philadelphia, 2008, Saunders.)

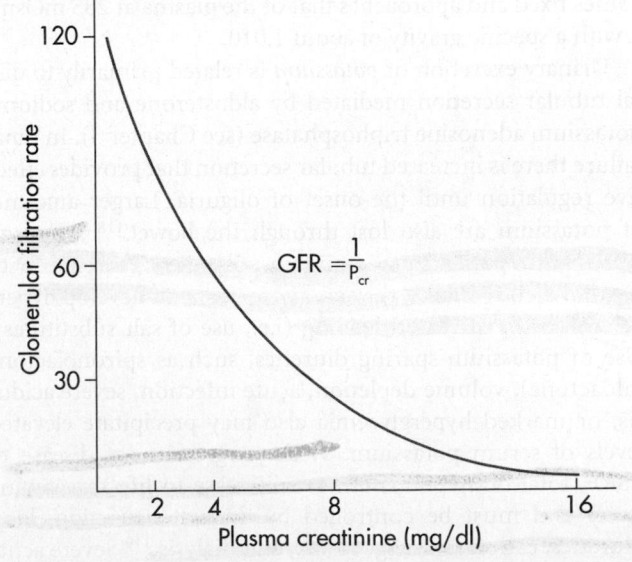

$$GFR = \frac{1}{P_{cr}}$$

Figure 36-15 Plasma creatinine (P_{cr}) and glomerular filtration rate (GFR).

Table 36-15	Electrolyte and Acid-Base Alterations of Chronic Kidney Failure
Factor	Characteristics
Sodium and water balance	In chronic renal failure, sodium load delivered to nephrons exceeds normal, so excretion must increase; thus less is reabsorbed. Obligatory loss occurs, leading to sodium deficits and volume depletion. As GFR is reduced, ability to concentrate and dilute urine diminishes.
Phosphate and calcium balance	Changes in acid-base balance affect phosphate and calcium balance.
	The major disorders associated with chronic renal failure are reduced renal phosphate excretion, decreased renal synthesis of 1,25-$(OH)_2$ vitamin D_3 (calcitriol), and hypocalcemia.
	Hypocalcemia leads to secondary hyperparathyroidism, GFR falls, and progressive hyperphosphatemia, hypocalcemia, and dissolution of bone result.
Potassium balance	In chronic renal failure, tubular secretion of potassium increases until oliguria develops. Use of potassium-sparing diuretics also may precipitate elevated serum potassium levels. As disease progresses, total body potassium levels can rise to life-threatening levels and dialysis is required.
Acid-base balance	In early renal insufficiency, acid excretion and bicarbonate reabsorption are increased to maintain normal pH.
	Metabolic acidosis begins to develop when GFR decreases to 30% to 40% of normal. When end-stage renal failure develops, the metabolic acidosis may be severe enough to require dialysis.

GFR, Glomerular filtration rate.

may be present with tubulointerstitial causes of CKD and there may also be extra renal losses of sodium from vomiting, diarrhea, or fever. Sodium retention is more likely in ESKD particularly in the presence of nephrotic syndrome or heart failure. Sodium retention contributes to hypertension, edema, and heart failure. Management of salt and water balance requires individual assessment, and low dietary salt intake is usually recommended.[116,117]

The regulation of *water balance* and osmolality is normally achieved by urinary concentration mediated by ADH. As GFR is reduced, ability to concentrate and dilute the urine diminishes. In earlier stages of renal failure, this may be caused by osmotic diuresis produced by increased fractional excretion of solutes by the remaining nephrons or by a decreased tubular response to ADH. Individual nephrons can maintain water balance until severe renal failure occurs and GFR declines to 15% to 20% of normal with extensive loss of nephron and tubular function. At this stage the urinary concentration becomes fixed and approaches that of the plasma at 285 mOsm/L with a specific gravity of about 1.010.

Urinary excretion of *potassium* is related primarily to distal tubular secretion mediated by aldosterone and sodium-potassium adenosine triphosphatase (see Chapter 3). In renal failure there is increased tubular secretion that provides effective regulation until the onset of oliguria. Larger amounts of potassium are also lost through the bowel.[118] Although nonoliguric patients can maintain potassium excretion with normal dietary intake, they are more prone to develop hyperkalemia with increased loading (i.e., use of salt substitutes). Use of potassium-sparing diuretics, such as spironolactone (aldactone), volume depletion, acute infection, severe acidosis, or marked hyperglycemia also may precipitate elevated levels of serum potassium. With progression of disease to ESRF, total body potassium can increase to life-threatening levels and must be controlled by dietary restriction, loop diuretics, cation exchange resins, and dialysis.[119] Severe acute hyperkalemia is treated with intravenous calcium, intravenous

glucose, and insulin and nebulized albuterol (sympathetic beta$_2$-agonist, promotes Na^+, K^+-ATPase pump and intracellular movement of potassium).[120]

The intake of a normal diet produces 50 to 100 mEq of hydrogen per day. These ions are secreted from the renal tubules and excreted in the urine combined with phosphate and ammonia buffers (buffering is described in Chapter 3). *Metabolic acidosis* develops when GFR decreases to less than 20% to 25% of normal.[121] The causes of acidosis are primarily related to decreased hydrogen ion elimination and decreased bicarbonate reabsorption. With end-stage renal failure, metabolic acidosis may be severe enough to require alkali therapy and dialysis.[122]

Calcium, Phosphate, and Bone

Bone and skeletal changes develop with alterations in **calcium** and **phosphate metabolism** (Table 36-16). These changes begin when GFR decreases to 25% or less. *Hypocalcemia* is accelerated by impaired renal synthesis of 1,25-vitamin D_3 (calcitriol) with decreased intestinal absorption of calcium. Renal phosphate excretion also decreases and the increased serum phosphate binds calcium, further contributing to hypocalcemia. Acidosis also contributes to a negative calcium balance. Decreased serum calcium stimulates parathyroid hormone secretion with mobilization of calcium from bone and may cause calcium levels to approach normal. The combined effect of *hyperparathyroidism* and *vitamin D deficiency* can result in renal osteodystrophies (i.e., *osteomalacia* and *osteitis fibrosa* with increased risk for fractures.[123] Other consequences of secondary hyperparathyroidism include soft tissue and vascular calcification, cardiovascular disease, and less commonly, calcific uremic arteriolopathy.[124]

Protein, Carbohydrate, and Fat Metabolism

Protein, carbohydrate, and fat metabolism are altered in chronic renal failure (CRF). *Proteinuria* and a catabolic state contribute to a negative nitrogen balance. Serum proteins

Table 36-16	Calcium and Phosphate Metabolism in Chronic Kidney Failure	
Kidney	**Plasma**	**Bone**
Decreased renal production of vitamin D_3	Decreased calcium absorption from gut Decreased ionized calcium Increased PTH secretion (secondary hyperparathyroidism)	Decreased calcium deposition
Decreased phosphate excretion	Elevated phosphate Formation of $CaHPO_4$	Release of calcium and phosphate Osteitis fibrosa, osteomalacia, calcium deposits in soft tissue (occurs when kidney fails to respond to PTH secretion because of loss of renal mass and calcium and phosphate continues to be absorbed from bone)

PTH, Parathyroid hormone.

diminish, including albumin, complement, and transferrin, and there is loss of muscle mass. Proteinuria may independently cause renal damage by promoting tubular inflammation and fibrosis.[125] The amount of proteinuria is also related to the extent of renal injury and predicts disease progression.[126] The effectiveness of a low-protein diet on progression of chronic kidney disease is inconclusive.[127,128]

Hyperinsulinemia and glucose intolerance related to insulin resistance are common and may be related to alterations in adipokines (high leptin and low adiponectin) that interfere with insulin action and oxidative stress that contribute to renal tubular and vascular injury in both nondiabetic and diabetic CKD.[129] Hyperparathyroidism also decreases insulin sensitivity and impairs glucose tolerance.

Dyslipidemia is common among individuals with CKD. There is a high ratio of low-density lipoprotein (LDL) to high-density lipoprotein (HDL), high triglycerides, accumulation of LDL particles with accelerated atherosclerosis and vascular calcification.[130] Uremia causes a deficiency in lipoprotein lipase and decreased hepatic triglyceride lipase. Decreased lipolytic activity results in a reduction in HDL. Apolipoprotein B is also elevated, thereby accelerating atherogenesis.[131]

Cardiovascular System

Cardiovascular disease is a major cause of morbidity and mortality in CKD. Proinflammatory mediators, oxidative stress, and metabolic derangements are significant contributors. Elevated renin stimulates the secretion of aldosterone, increasing sodium reabsorption. *Hypertension* is the result of excess sodium and fluid volume. *Dyslipidemia* occurs early in CKD. Arterial wall thickness increases with decreased elastic fibers and increased extracellular matrix. Atheromatous plaque and calcium deposits contribute to loss of vessel elasticity and obstruction and are accelerated by the oxidative stress of CKD.[132] Macrovascular disease is responsible for increased risk for ischemic heart disease, left ventricular hypertrophy, congestive heart failure, stroke, and peripheral vascular disease in individuals with uremia.

Endothelial cell dysfunction and calcium deposits lead to a loss of vessel elasticity and vascular calcification. The resulting vascular disease increases the risk for *ischemic heart disease, left ventricular hypertrophy, congestive heart failure, stroke,* and *peripheral vascular disease* in individuals with uremia. Declining erythropoietin production causes anemia, thereby increasing demands for cardiac output and adding to cardiac workload. *Pericarditis* can develop from inflammation caused by the presence of uremic toxins. Accumulation of fluid in the pericardial space can compromise ventricular filling and cardiac output.

Pulmonary System

Pulmonary complications are associated with fluid overload and congestive heart failure. Pulmonary edema develops and metabolic acidosis can cause Kussmaul respirations. *Dyspnea* is common in ESKD.

Hematologic System

Hematologic alterations include *normochromic normocytic anemia, impaired platelet function,* and *hypercoagulability.* Inadequate production of erythropoietin decreases red blood cell production and is the most significant factor in contributing to anemia. Chronic inflammation, iron deficiency, and decreased half-life of erythrocytes are also contributing factors. Anemia contributes to decreased tissue oxygenation and contributes to progression of kidney disease. Lethargy, dizziness, low hematocrit, and increased cardiac workload and increased risk for congestive heart failure are common findings. Treatment of anemia includes erythropoiesis stimulating agents (i.e., recombinant human erythropoietin) and intravenous iron.

Disorders of hemostasis in CKD and uremia are primarily related to defective platelet aggregation and impaired adhesion of platelets to the vascular endothelium. The consequence is an increased bleeding tendency and an increased risk for bruising, epistaxis, gastrointestinal bleeding, or cerebrovascular hemorrhage and cutaneous or submucosal hemorrhage.[133] Adequate dialysis improves platelet function. Alterations of individual clotting factors, fibrin, thrombin and fibrinolysis contribute to alterations of blood coagulation and can promote a hypercoagulable state and thrombosis with increased risk for myocardial infarction and stroke.[134,135]

Immune System

Immune system dysregulation with immune suppression, deficient response to vaccination, and increased risk for infection develops with CRF.[136] Chemotaxis, phagocytosis, antibody production, and cell-mediated immune responses are suppressed. Malnutrition, metabolic acidosis, hyperglycemia, or effects of hemodialysis may amplify immunosuppression.

Neurologic System

Neurologic symptoms are common and progressive with CRF and are related to uremic toxicity, chronic hyperkalemic depolarization, and anemia.[137] Symptoms may include headache, drowsiness, pain, sleep disorders, impaired concentration, memory loss, and impaired judgment. Neuromuscular irritation can cause hiccups, muscle cramps, and muscle twitching. In advanced stages of renal failure, symptoms may progress to seizures and coma. Peripheral neuropathies also develop with impaired sensations decreased tendon reflexes, muscle weakness and muscle atrophy, most commonly in the lower extremities.

Gastrointestinal System

Gastrointestinal complications are common in individuals with CRF. Uremic gastroenteritis can cause bleeding ulcer and significant blood loss. Nonspecific symptoms include anorexia, nausea, vomiting, and constipation or diarrhea. Uremic fetor is a form of bad breath caused by the breakdown of urea by salivary enzymes. Malnutrition is common.

Endocrine and Reproductive Systems

Endocrine and reproductive alterations develop with progression of CKD. Males and females have a decrease in circulating sex steroids. Males often experience a reduction in testosterone levels and may be impotent. Oligospermia and germinal cell dysplasia can result in infertility. Females have reduced estrogen levels, amenorrhea, and difficulty maintaining a pregnancy to term. A decrease in libido occurs in both genders.[138,139]

Insulin resistance is common in uremia. Low-grade systemic inflammation and oxidative stress may be contributing factors with increased risk for cardiovascular disease.[140] As CKD progresses the ability of the kidney to degrade insulin is reduced, and the half-life of insulin is prolonged. Individuals with diabetes mellitus and CKD need to carefully manage their insulin dosages. Low-protein diets and renal replacement therapy improve insulin sensitivity.[141]

CRF also causes alterations in thyroid hormone metabolism and low thyroid hormone levels and is known as nonthyroidal illness syndrome (euthyroid sick syndrome). Low-grade inflammation and oxidative stress may be contributing factors.[142] Uremia also reduces conversion of T_3 to T_4.[143] A low-protein, low-phosphorus diet may improve thyroid hormone function.[144]

Integumentary System

Skin changes are associated with other complications that develop with CKD. Anemia can cause pallor and bleeding into the skin and results in hematomas and ecchymosis. Retained urochromes manifest as a sallow skin color. Hyperparathyroidism and uremic skin residues (known as uremic frost) are associated with irritation and pruritus with scratching, excoriation, and increased risk for infection.[145]

EVALUATION AND TREATMENT Early screening and evaluation of chronic kidney disease are based on risk factors, history, presenting signs and symptoms, and diagnostic testing. Prediction equations are used for estimating GFR from serum creatinine values or creatinine clearance may be completed. Markers of kidney damage include urine protein, particularly albumin and examination of urine sediment. Ultrasound, CT scan, or plain x-ray films will show small kidney size. Renal biopsy confirms the diagnosis.

Management involves dietary control, including phosphate restriction, vitamin D supplementation, sodium and fluid maintenance, potassium restriction, adequate caloric intake, management of dyslipidemias, and erythropoietin as needed. ACE inhibitors or receptor blockers are often used to control systemic hypertension and provide renoprotection.[146] ESKD related to diabetic nephropathy can be significantly reduced with control of hyperglycemia by intense insulin therapy.[147] ESKD is treated with dialysis, supportive therapy, and renal transplantation.

NUTRITION & DISEASE

Acute and Chronic Kidney Failure

The malnutrition-inflammation-complex syndrome is a common condition associated with renal failure and leads to accelerated atherosclerosis and cardiovascular disease. Inflammatory cytokines, including interleukin-6, tumor necrosis factor-alpha, and interferon, suppress appetite and cause muscle proteolysis, decreased protein assimilation, and hypoalbuminemia. Reduced renal function, oxidative stress, decreased levels of antioxidants, infection, exposure to dialysis tubing and membranes during hemodialysis, and back-filtration of contaminants during hemodialysis contribute to inflammation. Acidosis also acts synergistically with inflammatory cytokines and insulin to promote protein catabolism. The provision of nutrients, including adequate calories along with protein supplementation that includes amino acids, in the form of intradialytic parenteral nutrition or enteral feeding during dialysis, assists a person to meet the metabolic requirement. Dietary supplements of antioxidants, such as vitamins A and C and carotenoids, are required. Low-protein, low-phosphorus, and low-sodium diets assist with reducing proteinuria, preventing hyperphosphatemia and secondary hyperparathyroidism and lowering blood pressure. The vegetarian nature of renal diets may improve lipid profiles. Adequate nutritional support promotes renal recovery and may prevent consequences of muscle weakness and immune dysfunction.

Data from Cano NJ, Leverve XM: *Curr Opin Clin Nutr Metab Care* 11(2):147-151, 2008; Cupisti A, Apariciio M, Barsotti G: *Ren Fail* 29(5):529-534, 2007; Ikizler TA: *Curr Opin Nephrol Hypertens* 17(2):162-167, 2008; Dukkipati R, Kopple JD: *Semin Nephrol* 29(1):39-49, 2009.

SUMMARY REVIEW

Urinary Tract Obstruction

1. Obstruction can occur anywhere in the urinary tract, and may be anatomic or functional, including renal stones, an enlarged prostate gland, or urethral strictures. The most serious complications are hydronephrosis, hydroureter, ureterohydronephrosis, and infection caused by the accumulation of urine behind the obstruction.
2. Compensatory hypertrophy and hyperfunction of the opposite kidney compensate for loss of function of the kidney with obstructive disease.
3. Relief of obstruction is usually followed by postobstructive diuresis and may cause fluid and electrolyte imbalance.
4. Persistent obstruction of the bladder outlet leads to residual urine volumes, low bladder wall compliance, and risk for vesicoureteral reflux and infection.
5. Kidney stones are caused by supersaturation of the urine with precipitation of stone-forming substances, changes in urine pH, or urinary tract infection. Most stones are unilateral.
6. The most common kidney stone is formed from calcium oxalate and most often causes obstruction by lodging in the ureter.
7. Obstructions of the bladder are a consequence of neurogenic or anatomic alteration of bladder or both.
8. A neurogenic bladder is caused by a neural lesion that interrupts innervation of the bladder.
9. Upper motor neuron lesions above the pontine micturition center result in detrusor hyperreflexia and uninhibited or reflex bladder.
10. Upper motor neuron lesions between C2 and S1 result in overactive or hyperreflexive bladder function and vesicosphincter dyssynergia (lack of coordinated neuromuscular contraction).
11. Lower motor neuron lesions result in detrusor areflexia with underactive, hypotonic, or atonic bladder function.
12. OAB syndrome is an uncontrollable or premature contraction of the bladder that results in urgency with or without incontinence, frequency, and nocturia.
13. Anatomic obstructions to urine flow include prostatic enlargement, urethral stricture, and pelvic organ prolapse in women.
14. Partial obstruction of the bladder can result in overactive bladder contractions with urgency. There is deposition of collagen in the bladder wall over time, resulting in decreased bladder wall compliance and ineffective detrusor muscle contraction.
15. Renal cell carcinoma is the most common renal neoplasm. The larger neoplasms tend to metastasize to the lung, liver, and bone.
16. Bladder tumors are commonly composed of transitional cells with a papillary appearance and a high rate of recurrence.

Urinary Tract Infection

1. UTIs are commonly caused by the retrograde movement of bacteria into the urethra and bladder. UTIs are uncomplicated when the urinary system is normal or complicated when there is a defect or abnormality.
2. Cystitis is an inflammation of the bladder commonly caused by bacteria and may be acute or chronic.
3. Painful bladder syndrome/interstitial cystitis includes nonbacterial infectious cystitis (viral, mycobacterial, chlamydial, fungal), noninfectious cystitis (i.e., radiation injury), and interstitial cystitis, which is probably related to autoimmune injury.
4. Pyelonephritis is an acute or chronic inflammation of the renal pelvis often related to ascending infection and obstructive uropathies and may cause abscess formation and scarring with an alteration in renal function.

Glomerular Disorders

1. Glomerular disorders are a group of related diseases of the glomerulus that can be caused by immune injury, toxins or drugs, vascular disorders, and other systemic diseases.
2. Acute glomerulonephritis commonly results from inflammatory damage to the glomerulus as a consequence of immune reactions including deposition of circulating immune complexes, antibodies reacting in-situ to planted antigens, and antibodies directed against the glomerular basement membrane.
3. The urine sediment may contain large amounts of protein (nephrotic sediment) or have red and white blood cells and protein (nephritic sediment).
4. Acute postinfectious glomerulonephritis is commonly associated with immune complex deposition in the glomerulus or forming in situ.
5. Lupus nephritis is caused by the formation of autoantibodies against dsDNA and nucleosomes in the glomerulus, causing inflammation and injury.
6. IgA nephropathy is the binding of abnormal IgA to mesangial cells in the glomerulus resulting in injury and mesangial proliferation.
7. RPGN is associated with injury that results in the proliferation of glomerular capillary endothelial cells and a rapid loss of renal function.
8. Mesangial proliferative glomerulonephritis involves deposits of immune complexes in the mesangium with mesangial proliferation leading to nephritic syndrome.
9. Membranous nephropathy is complement-mediated glomerular injury with increased glomerular permeability and glomerulosclerosis.
10. Membranoproliferative glomerulonephritis involves mesangial cell proliferation, complement deposition, and crescent formation.
11. Chronic glomerulonephritis is related to a variety of diseases that cause deterioration of the glomerulus and a progressive loss of renal function over a period of months to years.
12. Nephrotic syndrome is the excretion of at least 3.5 g protein (primarily albumin) in the urine per day primarily because of glomerular injury with increased capillary permeability and loss of membrane negative charge. The principal signs are hypoproteinuria, hyperlipidemia, and edema. The liver cannot produce enough protein to adequately compensate for urinary loss.

Acute Kidney Injury

1. AKI is the sudden decline in kidney function with decreased glomerular filtration and an increase in serum creatinine and BUN.
2. AKI is considered in three categories as prerenal, intrarenal, or postrenal and is usually accompanied by oliguria with elevated plasma BUN and plasma creatinine levels.
3. Prerenal acute renal failure is caused by decreased renal perfusion with a decreased GFR, ischemia, and tubular necrosis.
4. Intrarenal acute renal failure is associated with several systemic diseases but is commonly related to ATN.
5. Postrenal acute renal failure is associated with diseases that obstruct the flow of urine from the kidneys.

Chronic Kidney Disease

1. Chronic kidney disease is a progressive loss of renal function. Plasma creatinine levels gradually become elevated as GFR declines, sodium is lost in the urine, potassium is retained, acidosis develops, calcium metabolism and phosphate metabolism are altered, and erythropoietin production is diminished. All organs systems are affected by CRF.

SUMMARY REVIEW—cont'd

2. Symptomatic changes usually do not become evident until renal function declines to less than 25%.
3. Glomerular hypertension, hyperfiltration, and tubulointerstitial inflammation and fibrosis contribute to the progression of chronic kidney disease. Proteinuria and angiotensin II promote the pathologic changes of chronic renal injury.

4. Uremic syndrome is a proinflammatory state with the accumulation of solutes; toxins; and alterations in fluid, electrolyte and acid-base balance that result from chronic kidney failure. All organ systems are affected and contribute to disease symptoms.

KEY TERMS

Acute cystitis, 1374
Acute kidney injury (AKI), 1386
Acute postinfectious glomerulonephritis (PIGN), 1380
Acute renal failure, 1386
Acute tubular necrosis (ATN), 1387
Angiotensin II, 1393
Antiglomerular basement membrane disease (Goodpasture syndrome), 1383
Anuria, 1388
Apoptosis, 1367
Asymptomatic bacteriuria, 1375
Azotemia, 1386
Calcium metabolism, 1394
Calcium stone, 1368
Calculus (pl., calculi) (urinary stone), 1368
Chronic glomerulonephritis, 1383
Chronic kidney disease (CKD), 1389
Chronic pyelonephritis, 1377
Compensatory growth, 1367
Compensatory hypertrophy, 1367
Continuous renal replacement therapy (hemodialysis), 1389
Cystinuric (xanthine) stone, 1369
Detrusor areflexia, 1370
Detrusor hyperreflexia, 1369
Detrusor hyperreflexia with vesicosphincter dyssynergia, 1370
Dyssynergia, 1369

End-stage renal failure (ESRF), 1386
Glomerulonephritis, 1379
Hematuria, 1378
Hydronephrosis, 1365
Hydroureter, 1365
Hyperfunction, 1367
IgA nephropathy (Berger disease), 1382
Immune complex deposition, 1383
Intrarenal (intrinsic) acute kidney injury (AKI), 1387
Low bladder wall compliance, 1371
Lupus nephritis, 1382
Membranoproliferative glomerulonephritis (MPGN), 1383
Membranous nephropathy (membranous glomerulonephritis), 1383
Mesangial proliferative glomerulonephritis, 1383
Nephritic sediment, 1378
Nephrotic sediment, 1378
Nephrotic syndrome, 1384
Neurogenic bladder, 1369
Nonbacterial infectious cystitis, 1376
Noninfectious cystitis, 1376
Obligatory growth, 1367
Obstructive uropathy, 1365
Oliguria, 1388
Overactive bladder syndrome (OAB), 1370
Painful bladder syndrome/interstitial cystitis (PBS/IC), 1376

Partial obstruction of the bladder outlet or urethra, 1371
Pauci immune glomerulonephritis, 1383
Pelvic organ prolapse, 1371
Phosphate metabolism, 1394
Postobstructive diuresis, 1367
Postrenal acute kidney injury, 1388
Prerenal acute kidney injury, 1386
Prostate enlargement, 1371
Proteinuria, 1378
Pyelonephritis, 1377
Rapidly progressive (crescentic) glomerulonephritis (RPGN), 1383
Renal adenoma, 1372
Renal cell carcinoma (RCC), 1372
Renal colic, 1369
Renal insufficiency, 1386
Renal failure, 1386
Staghorn calculus (pl., calculi), 1368
Struvite stone, 1368
Tubulointerstitial fibrosis, 1366
Uremia, 1386
Uremic syndrome, 1393
Ureterohydronephrosis, 1366
Urethral stricture, 1371
Uric acid stone, 1369
Urinary tract infection (UTI), 1373
Virulence, 1375

REFERENCES

1. Selius BA, Subedi R: Urinary retention in adults: diagnosis and initial management, *Am Fam Physician* 77(5):643-650, 2008.
2. Gillenwater JY: Hydronephrosis. In Gillenwater JY et al, editors: *Adult and pediatric urology*, ed 4, Lippincott Williams & Wilkins, 2002, Philadelphia.
3. Maarten TW, Brenner BM: Adaptation to nephron loss. In Brenner BM, editor, *Brenner and Rector's the kidney*, ed 8, p 783, Saunders, 2008, Philadelphia.
4. Frokiaer J, Zeidel ML: Urinary tract obstruction. In Brenner BM, editor, *Brenner and Rector's the kidney*, ed 8, p 1260, Saunders, 2008, Philadelphia.
5. Porena M, Guggi P, Micheli C: Prevention of stone disease, *Urol Int* 79(Suppl 1):37-46, 2007.
6. Chandhoke PS: Evaluation of the recurrent stone former, *Urol Clin North Am* 34(3):315-322, 2007.
7. Miano R, Germani S, Vespasiani G: Stones and urinary tract infection, *Urol Int* 79(Suppl 1):32-36, 2007.

8. Obligado SH, Goldfarb DS: The association of nephrolithiasis with hypertension and obesity: a review, *Am J Hypertens* 21(3):257-264, 2008.
9. Miller NL, Evan AP, Lingeman JE: Pathogenesis of renal calculi, *Urol Clin North Am* 34(3):295-313, 2007.
10. JE Lingeman, DA Lifshitz, AP Evan: Surgical management of urinary lithiasis. In Walsh PC, et al, editors: *Campbell's urology*, ed 8, Saunders, 2002, Philadelphia.
11. Trinchieri A et al: Calcium stone disease: a multiform reality, *Urol Res* 33(3):194-198, 2005.
12. Park S, Pearle MS: Pathophysiology and management of calcium stones, *Urol Clin North Am* 34(3):323-334, 2007.
13. Healy KA, Ogan K: Pathophysiology and management of infectious staghorn calculi, *Urol Clin North Am* 34(3):363-374, 2007.
14. Ahmed HU et al: Diagnosis and management of renal (ureteric) colic, *Br J Hosp Med (Lond)* 67(9):465-469, 2006.
15. Pietrow PK, Karellas ME: Medical management of common urinary calculi, *Am Fam Physician* 74(1):86-94, 2006.
16. Asplin JR: Evaluation of the kidney stone patient, *Semin Nephrol* 28(2):99-110, 2008.

17. Park S, Pearle MS: Imaging for percutaneous renal access and management of renal calculi, *Urol Clin North Am* 33(3):353-364, 2006.

18. Taylor EN, Curhan GC: Diet and fluid prescription in stone disease, *Kidney Int* 70(5):835-839, 2006.

19. Steggall MJ, Omara M: Urinary tract stones: types, nursing care and treatment options, *Br J Nurs* 17(9):520-523, 2008.

20. Wen CC, Nakada SY: Treatment selection and outcomes: renal calculi, *Urol Clin North Am* 34(3):409-419, 2007.

21. Karsenty G et al: Understanding detrusor sphincter dyssynergia—significance of chronology, *Urology* 66(4):763-768, 2005.

22. Chu FM, Dmochowski R: Pathophysiology of overactive bladder, *Am J Med* 199(3 Suppl 1):3-8, 2006.

23. Abrams P et al: The standardisation of terminology of lower urinary tract function: report from the Standardisation Sub-committee of the International Continence Society, *Am J Obstet Gynecol* 187(1):116-126, 2002.

24. Franco I: Overactive bladder in children: Part 1: pathophysiology, *J Urol* 178(3 Pt 1):761-768, 2007.

25. Srikrishna S et al: Management of overactive bladder syndrome, *Postgrad Med J* 83(981):481-486, 2007.

26. Staskin DR, MacDiarmid SA: Pharmacologic management of overactive bladder: practical options for the primary care physician, *Am J Med* 119(3 Suppl 1):24-28, 2006.

27. Mundy AR: Management of urethral strictures, *Postgrad Med J* 82(970):489-493, 2006.

28. Valchanov K et al: An unusual cause of acute renal failure: urethral stricture in a female, *Nephron* 87(1):89-90, 2001.

29. Anger JU, Raz S, Rodriguez LV: Severe cystocele: optimizing results, *Curr Urol Rep* 8(5):394-398, 2007.

30. American Cancer Society, Inc., Surveillance and Health Policy Research: Estimated New Cancer Cases and Deaths by Sex, U.S. 2009 available at www.cancer.org/downloads/stt/CFF2009_EstCD_3.pdf.asp.

31. Setoawan VW et al: Risk factors for renal cell cancer: the multiethnic cohort, *Am J Epidemiol* 166(8):932-940, 2007.

32. Berndt SI et al: Disparities in treatment and outcome for renal cell cancer among older black and white patients, *J Clin Oncol* 24(25):3589-3595, 2007.

33. Gupta K et al: Epidemiologic and socioeconomic burden of metastatic renal cell carcinoma (mRCC): a literature review, *Cancer Treat Rev* 34(3):193-205, 2008.

34. Corgna E et al: Renal cancer, *Crit Rev Oncol Hematol* 64(3):247-262, 2007.

35. George S, Burkowski RM: Biomarkers in clear cell renal cell carcinoma, *Expert Rev Anticancer Ther* 7(12):1737-1747, 2007.

36. Pahernik S et al: Elective nephron sparing surgery for renal cell carcinoma larger than 4 cm, *J Urol* 179(1):71-74, 2008.

37. Lehman DS, Landman J: Cryoablation and radiofrequency for kidney tumor, *Curr Urol Rep* 9(2):128-134, 2008.

38. Costa LJ, Drabkin HA: Renal cell carcinoma: new developments in molecular biology and potential for targeted therapies, *Oncologist* 12(12):1404-1415, 2007.

39. Pelucchi C et al: Mechanisms of disease: the epidemiology of bladder cancer, *Nat Clin Pract Urol* 3(6):327-340, 2006.

40. Murta-Nascimento C et al: Epidemiology of urinary bladder cancer: from tumor development to patient's death, *World J Urol* 25(3): 285-295, 2007.

41. Madeb R et al: Current state of screening for bladder cancer, *Expert Rev Anticancer Ther* 7(7):981-987, 2007.

42. Mohammed A et al: Biological markers in the diagnosis of recurrent bladder cancer: an overview, *Expert Rev Mol Diag* 8(1):63-72, 2008.

43. Dalbagni G: The management of superficial bladder cancer, *Nat Clin Pract Urol* 4(5):254-260, 2007.

44. Barocas DA, Clark PE: Bladder cancer, *Curr Opin Oncol* 20(3): 307-314, 2008.

45. Foxman B et al: Urinary tract infection: self-reported incidence and associated costs, *Ann Epidemiol* 10:509-515, 2000.

46. Nicole LE: Uncomplicated urinary tract infection in adults including uncomplicated pyelonephritis, *Urol Clin North Am* 35(1):1-12, 2008.

47. Bouckaert J et al: Receptor binding studies disclose a novel class of high-affinity inhibitors of the *Escherichia coli* FimH adhesion, *Mol Microbiol* 55(2):441-455, 2005.

48. Malani AN, Kaufman CA: Candida urinary tract infections: treatment options, *Expert Rev Anti Infect Ther* 5(2):277-284, 2007.

49. Barsoum RS: Schistosomiasis and the kidney, *Semin Nephrol* 23(1): 24-46, 2003.

50. Vauhkonen H et al: Can bladder adenocarcinomas be distinguished from schistosomiasis-associated bladder cancers by using array comparative genomic hybridization analysis? *Cancer Genet Cytogenet* 177(2):153-157, 2007.

51. Hladunewich M, Rosenthal MH: Pathophysiology and management of renal insufficiency in the perioperative and critically ill patient, *Anesthesiol Clin North Am* 18(4):773-789, 2000.

52. Smaill F: Asymptomatic bacteriuria in pregnancy, *Best Pract Res Clin Obstet Gynaecol* 21(3):439-450, 2007.

53. Yamamoto S: Molecular epidemiology of uropathogenic *Escherichia coli*, *J Infect Chemother* 13(2):68-73, 2007.

54. Bricker NS, Morrin PA, Kime SW Jr: The pathologic physiology of chronic Bright's disease: an exposition of the "intact nephron hypothesis," *J Am Soc Nephrol* 8(9):1470-1476, 1997.

55. Neal DE: Complicated urinary tract infections, *Urol Clin North Am* 35(1):13-22, 2008.

56. Hancock V, Ferrieres L, Klemm P: Biofilm formation by asymptomatic and virulent urinary tract infectious *Escherichia coli* strains, *FEMS Microbiol Lett* 267(1):30-37, 2007.

57. Jacobsen SM et al: Complicated catheter-associated urinary tract infections due to *Escherichia coli* and *Proteus mirabilis*, *Clin Microbiol Rev* 21(1):26-59, 2008.

58. Sakallioglu O, Sakallioglu AE: The effect of ABO-Rh blood group determinants on urinary tract infections, *Int Urol Nephrol* 39(2):577-579, 2007.

59. Juthani-Mehta M: Asymptomatic bacteriuria and urinary tract infection in older adults, *Clin Geriatr Med* 23(3):585-594, 2007.

60. Czaja CA, Hooton TM: Update on acute uncomplicated urinary tract infection in women, *Postgrad Med* 119(1):39-45, 2006.

61. McManus DP, Loukas A: Current status of vaccines for schistosomiasis, *Clin Microbiol Rev* 21(1):225-242, 2008.

62. van de Merwe JP et al: Diagnostic criteria, classification, and nomenclature for painful bladder syndrome/intersitial cystitis: an ISSIC proposal, *Eur Urol* 53(1):60-67, 2008.

63. Nazif O, Teichman JM, Bebhart GF: Neural upregulation in interstitial cystitis, *Urology* 60(4 Suppl):24-30, 2007.

64. Teichman JM, Moldwin R: The role of the bladder surface in interstitial cystitis/painful bladder syndrome, *Can J Urol* 14(4):3599-3607, 2007.

65. Graham E, Chai TC: Dysfunction of bladder urothelium and bladder urothelial cells in interstitial cystitis, *Curr Urol Rep* 7(6):440-446, 2006.

66. Teichman JM, Parsons CL: Contemporary clinical presentation of interstitial cystitis, *Urology* 69(4 Suppl):41-47, 2007.

67. Dell JR: Interstitial cystitis/painful bladder syndrome: appropriate diagnosis and management, *J Womens Health (Larchmt)* 16(8):1181-1187, 2007.

68. Funfstuck R, Ott U, Naber KG: The interaction of urinary tract infection and renal insufficiency, *Int J Antimicrob Agents* 28(Suppl 1):S72-S77, 2006.

69. Craig WD, Wagner BJ, Travis MD: Pyelonephritis: radiologic-pathologic review, *Radiographics* 28(1):255-277, 2008.

70. Hsu CY et al: The clinical impact of bacteremia in complicated acute phylonephritis, *Am J Med Sci* 332(4):175-180, 2006.

71. Funfstuck R, Ott U, Naber KG: The interaction of urinary tract infection and renal insufficiency, *Int J Antimicrob Agents* 28(Suppl 1):S72-S77, 2006.

72. Berger SP, Daha MR: Complement in glomerular injury, *Semin Immunopathol* 29(4):375-384, 2007.

73. Norman JT, Fine LG: Intrarenal oxygenation in chronic renal failure, *Clin Exp Pharmacol Physiol* 33(10):989-996, 2006.

74. Lizakowski S et al: Plasma tissue factor and tissue factor pathway inhibitor in patients with primarily glomerulonephritis, *Scand J Urol Nephrol* 41(3):237-242, 2007.

75. Cattran DC: Outcomes research in glomerulonephritis, *Semin Nephrol* 23(4):340-354, 2003.

76. Naicker S et al: Infection and glomerulonephritis, *Semin Immunopathol* 29(4):397-414, 2007.

77. El-Husseini AA et al: Acute postinfectious crescentic glomerulonephritis: clinicopathologic presentation and risk factors, *Int Urol Nephrol* 37(3):603-609, 2005.

78. Carapetis JR et al: The global burden of group A streptococcal diseases, *Lancet Infect Dis* 5(11):685-694, 2005.

79. Mortensen ES, Fenton KA, Rekvig OP: Lupus nephritis: the central role of nucleosomes revealed, *Am J Pathol* 172(2):275-283, 2008.

80. Liapis H, Tsokos GC: Pathology and immunology of lupus glomerulonephritis: can we bridge the two? *Int Urol Nephrol* 39(1):223-231, 2007.

81. Novak J et al: IgA glycoslylation and IgA immune complexes in the pathogenesis of IgA nephropathy, *Semin Nephrol* 28(1):78-87, 2008.

82. Berthoux FC, Mohey H, Afiani A: Natural history of primary IgA nephropathy, *Semin Nephrol* 28(1):4-9, 2008.

83. Lionaki S, Jeannette JC, Falk RJ: Anti-neutrophil cytoplasmic (ANCA) and anti-glomerular basement membrane (GBM) autoantibodies in necrotizing and crescentic glomerulonephritis, *Semin Immunopathol* 29(4):459-474, 2007.

84. Little MA, Pusey CD: Rapidly progressive glomerulonephritis: current and evolving treatment strategies, *J Nephrol* 17(Suppl 8):S10-S19, 2004.

85. Papiris SA et al: Bench-to-bedside review: pulmonary-renal syndromes-an update for the intensivist, *Crit Care* 11(3):213, 2007.

86. Wolf G, Ziyadeh FN: Cellular and molecular mechanisms of proteinuria in diabetic nephropathy, *Nephron Physiol* 106(2):26-31, 2007.

87. Johnson DW: Evidence-based guide to slowing the progression of early renal insufficiency, *Intern Med J* 34(1-2):50-57, 2004.

88. Cho MH et al: Pathophysiology of minimal change nephritic syndrome and focal segmental glomerulosclerosis, *Nephrology (Carlton)* 12(Suppl 3):S11-S14, 2007.

89. Glubler MC: Inherited diseases of the glomerular basement membrane, *Nat Clin Pract Nephrol* 4(1):24-37, 2008.

90. Camici M: The nephrotic syndrome is an immunoinflammatory disorder, *Med Hypothesis* 68(4):900-905, 2007.

91. Kim SW, Frøkiaer J, Nielsen S: Pathogenesis of oedema in nephritic syndrome: role of epithelial sodium channel, *Nephrology (Carlton)* 12(Suppl 3):S8-S10, 2007.

92. Crew RJ, Radhakrishnan J, Appel G: Complications of the nephrotic syndrome and their treatment, *Clin Nephrol* 62(4):245-259, 2004.

93. Fehally J, Floege J, Johnson R, editors: *Comprehensive clinical nephrology*, Mosby, 2007, St Louis.

94. Zaffanello M, Franchini M: Thromboembolism in childhood nephritic syndrome: a rare but serious complication, *Hematology* 12(1):69-73, 2007.

95. Hodson EM, Willis NS, Craig JC: Corticosteroid therapy for nephritic syndrome in children, *Cochrane Database Syst Rev* (4):CD001533, 2007.

96. Bellomo R et al: Acute Dialysis Quality Initiative workgroup. Acute renal failure—definition, outcome measures, animal models, fluid therapy and information technology needs: the Second International Consensus Conference of the Acute Dialysis Quality Initiative (ADQI) Group, *Crit Care* 8(4):R204-R212, 2004.

97. Santos WJ et al: Patients with ischaemic, mixed and nephrotoxic acute tubular necrosis in the intensive care unit—a homogeneous population? *Crit Care* 10(2):R68, 2006.

98. Bonventre JV: Pathophysiology of acute kidney injury: roles of potential inhibitors of inflammation, *Contrib Nephrol* 156:39-46, review, 2007.

99. Kellum JA: Acute kidney injury, *Crit Care Med* 36(4 Suppl):S141-S145, 2008.

100. Wan L et al: Pathophysiology of septic acute kidney injury: what do we really know? *Crit Care Med* 36(4 Suppl):S198-S203, 2008.

101. Ortiz A et al: Targeting apoptosis in acute tubular injury, *Biochem Pharmacol* 66(8):1589-1594, 2003.

102. Clarkson MR et al: Acute kidney injury. In Brenner BM, editor: *Brenner and Rector's the kidney*, ed 8, Saunders, 2007, Philadelphia.

103. Bagshaw SM, Gibney RT: Convention markers of kidney function, *Crit Care Med* 36(4 Suppl):S152-S158, 2008.

104. Endre ZH, Westhuzyen J: Early detection of acute kidney injury: emerging new biomarkers, *Nephrology (Carlton)* 13(2):91-98, 2008.

105. Parikh CR, Devarajan P: New biomarkers of acute kidney injury, *Crit Care Med* 36(4 Suppl):S159-S165, 2008.

106. Kraut JA, Kurtz I: Metabolic acidosis of CKD: diagnosis, clinical characteristics, and treatment, *Am J Kidney Dis* 45(6):978-993, 2005.

107. Ronco C, Cruz D, Bellomo R: Continuous renal replacement in critical illness, *Contrib Nephrol* 156:309-319, 2007.

108. Snyder S, Pendergraph B: Detection and evaluation of chronic kidney disease, *Am Fam Physician* 72(9):1723-1732, 2005.

109. Mene P, Polci R, Festuccia F: Mechanisms of repair after kidney injury, *J Nephrol* 16(2):186-195, 2003.

110. Bricker NS, Morrin PA, Kime SW Jr: The pathologic physiology of chronic Bright's disease: an exposition of the "intact nephron hypothesis," *J Am Soc Nephrol* 8(9):1470-1476, 1997.

111. Tall MW, Luychx VA, Brenner BM: Adaptation to nephron loss. In Brenner BM, editor: *Brenner and Rector's the kidney*, ed 7, pp 1954, Saunders, 2004, Philadelphia.

112. Schieppati A, Pisoni R, Remuzzi G: Pathophysiology and management of chronic kidney disease. In Greenberg A, editor: *Primer on kidney diseases*, ed 4, pp 445-447, Saunders, 2005, St Louis.

113. Chang SS: Albuminuria and diabetic nephropathy, *Pediatr Endocrinol Rev* 5(Suppl 4):974-979, 2008.

114. Nangaku M, Jujita T: Activation of the renin-angiotensin system and chronic hypoxia of the kidney, *Hypertens Res* 31(2):175-184, 2008.

115. Vanholder R et al: Uremic toxins: do we know enough to explain uremia? *Blood Purif* 26(1):77-81, 2008.

116. Thijssen S, Kitzler TM, Levin NW: Salt: its role in chronic kidney disease, *J Ren Nutr* 18(1):18-26, 2008.

117. Weir MR, Fink JC: Salt intake and progression of chronic kidney disease: an overlooked modifiable exposure: a commentary, *Am J Kidney Dis* 45(1):176-188, review; 2005.

118. Kupin WL, Narins RG: The hyperkalemia of renal failure: pathophysiology, diagnosis, and therapy, In Bourke E, Mallick NP, Pollak BE, editors: *Moving points in nephrology*, Basel, 1993, Karger.

119. Giovannetti S, Cupisti A, Barsotti G: The mentabolic acidosis of chronic renal failure: pathophysiology and treatment. In Berlyn GM, editor: *The kidney today*, Basel, 1992, Karger.

120. Putcha N, Allon M: Management of hyperkalemia in dialysis patients, *Semin Dial* 20(5):431-439, 2007.

121. Kraut JA, Kurtz J: Metabolic acidosis of CKD: diagnosis, clinical characteristics, and treatment, *Am J Kidney Dis* 45(6):978-993, 2005.

122. Fehally J, Floege J, Johnson R: *Comprehensive clinical nephrology*, St Louis, 2007, Mosby.

123. Ferreira A: Development of renal bone disease, *Eur J Clin Invest* 36(Suppl 2):2-12, 2006.

124. Brancaccio D et al: Management of secondary hyperparathyroidism in uremic patients: the role of the new vitamin D analogs, *J Nephrol* 20(1):3-9, 2007.

125. Abbate M, Zoja C, Remuzzi G: How does proteinuria cause progressive renal damage? *J Am Soc Nephrol* 17(11):2974-2984, 2006.

126. Bakris GL: Slowing nephropathy progression: focus on proteinuria reduction, *Clin J Am Soc Nephrol* 3(Suppl 1):S3-S10, 2008.

127. Chaturvedi S, Jones C: Protein restriction for children with chronic renal disease, *Cochrane Database Syst Rev* (4):CD002181, 2007.

128. Levey AS et al: Effect of dietary protein restriction on the progression of kidney disease: long-term follow-up of Modification of Diet in Renal Disease (MDRD) study, *Am J Kidney Dis* 48(6):879-888, 2006.

129. Ikee R et al: Glucose metabolism, insulin resistance and renal pathology in non-diabetic chronic kidney disease, *Nephron Clin Pract* 108(2):c163-c168, 2008.

130. Chan DT et al: Dyslipidaemia and cardiorenal disease: mechanisms, therapeutic opportunities and clinical trials, *Atherosclerosis* 196(2):823-834, 2008.

131. Krane V, Wanner C: Dyslipidaemia in chronic kidney disease, *Minerva Urol Nefrol* 59(3):299-316, 2007.

132. Zanetti M et al: Vascular sources of oxidative stress: implications for uremia-related cardiovascular disease, *J Ren Nutr* 17(1):53-56, 2007.

133. Kaw D, Malhotra D: Platelet dysfunction and end-stage renal disease, *Semin Dial* 19(4):317-322, 2006.

134. Adams MJ et al: Hypercoagulability in chronic kidney disease is associated with coagulation activation but not endothelial function, *Thromb Res* 123(2):374-380, 2008.

135. Molino D et al: Coagulation disorders in uremia, *Semin Nephrol* 26:46-51, 2006.

136. Chonchol M: Neutrophil dysfunction and infection risk in end-stage renal disease, *Semin Dial* 19(4):291-296, 2006.

137. Krishnan AV, Kiernan MC: Uremic neuropathy: clinical features and new pathophysiological insights, *Muscle Nerve* 35(3):273-290, 2007.

138. Bellinghieri G, Savica V, Santoro D: Vascular erectile dysfunction in chronic renal failure, *Semin Nephrol* 26(1):42-45, 2006.

139. Kettas E et al: Sexual dysfunction and associated risk factors in women with end-stage renal disease, *J Sex Med* 5(4):872-877, 2007.

140. Zanetti M, Barazzoni R, Guarnieri G: Inflammation and insulin resistance in uremia, *J Ren Nut* 18(1):70-75, 2008.

141. Rigalleau V, Gin H: Carbohydrate metabolism in uraemia, *Curr Opin Clin Nutr Metab Care* 8(4):463-469, 2005.

142. Carrero JJ et al: Clinical and biochemical implication of low thyroid hormone levels (total and free forms) in euthyroid patients with chronic kidney disease, *J Intern Med* 262(6):690-701, 2007.

143. Adler S, Wartofsky L: The nonthyroidal illness syndrome, *Endocrinol Metab Clin North Am* 36(3):657-672, 2007.

144. Rosolowska-Huszcz D, Kozlowska L, Rydzewski A: Influence of low protein diet on nonthyroidal illness syndrome in chronic renal failure, *Endocrine* 27(3):283-288, 2005.

145. Patel TS, Freedman BI, Yosipovitch G: An update on pruritus associated with CKD, *Am J Kidney Dis* 50(1):11-20, 2007.

146. Kunz R et al: Meta-analysis: effect of monotherapy and combination therapy with inhibitors of the renin angiotensin system on proteinuria in renal disease, *Ann Intern Med* 148(1):30-48, 2008.

147. Schrijvers BF, De Vriese AS: Novel insights in the treatment of diabetic nephropathy, *Acta Clin Belg* 62(5):278-290, 2007.

ALTERATIONS OF RENAL AND URINARY TRACT FUNCTION IN CHILDREN

SUE E. HUETHER

MEDIA RESOURCES

*e*volve **Evolve Website** (http://evolve.elsevier.com/McCance/)
- Review Questions and Answers
- Animations
- Glossary (with audio pronunciation for selected terms)
- WebLinks

CHAPTER OUTLINE

STRUCTURE AND FUNCTION OF THE URINARY SYSTEM IN CHILDREN
Development of the Urinary System
Fluid and Electrolyte Balance in Children
ALTERATIONS IN RENAL AND BLADDER FUNCTION IN CHILDREN
Congenital Abnormalities

Glomerular Disorders
Renal Injury
Bladder Disorders
Wilms Tumor
Enuresis

Renal and urinary disorders occur in children as well as adults. In childhood, however, the kidney and genitourinary structures are continuing to develop, so renal dysfunction may be associated with mechanisms and manifestations that are different from those in adults. In addition, some renal and urinary disorders are congenital and involve structural anomalies of the kidney and urinary drainage system.

STRUCTURE AND FUNCTION OF THE URINARY SYSTEM IN CHILDREN

Development of the Urinary System

The embryonic urinary system develops as three sets of sequentially replaced organs, the pronephros, mesonephros and metanephros. The **pronephros** is a nonfunctional structure that arises at the level of the cervical and upper thoracic regions during the third fetal week and connects the primitive Wolffian duct to the cloaca as the foundation for male sexual development (Figure 37-1). The development of the **mesonephros** and **metanephros** are described in Figure 37-1.

The Wilms tumor 1 *(WT1)* gene plays an important role at all stages of kidney development and maintenance of kidney function.[1] The wingless type signaling (WNT signaling) transduction pathway also is important for mesenchyme growth and differentiation.[2]

After glomeruli and tubules form, the tissues organize and progressively differentiate over approximately 30 days. Initial glomerular development is staggered, so there are glomeruli in various stages. In fact, a few of the first glomeruli formed degenerate and disappear during the later stages of fetal development. Progressive development continues into the ninth fetal month, when all metanephrogenic tissue then disappears.

As the embryo develops and the vertebral column straightens, the kidneys appear to ascend to the sacral area at about 6 weeks, to the third lumbar area by the third month, and to the first lumbar area at term. The kidneys rotate 90 degrees as they ascend so that renal tissue is lateral and the collecting system is medial.

While the kidneys mature, the *cloaca* becomes the urogenital sinus. It then differentiates into the vesicourethral canal, which forms the bladder and the upper urethra, and the urogenital sinus, which forms the main part of the urethra.

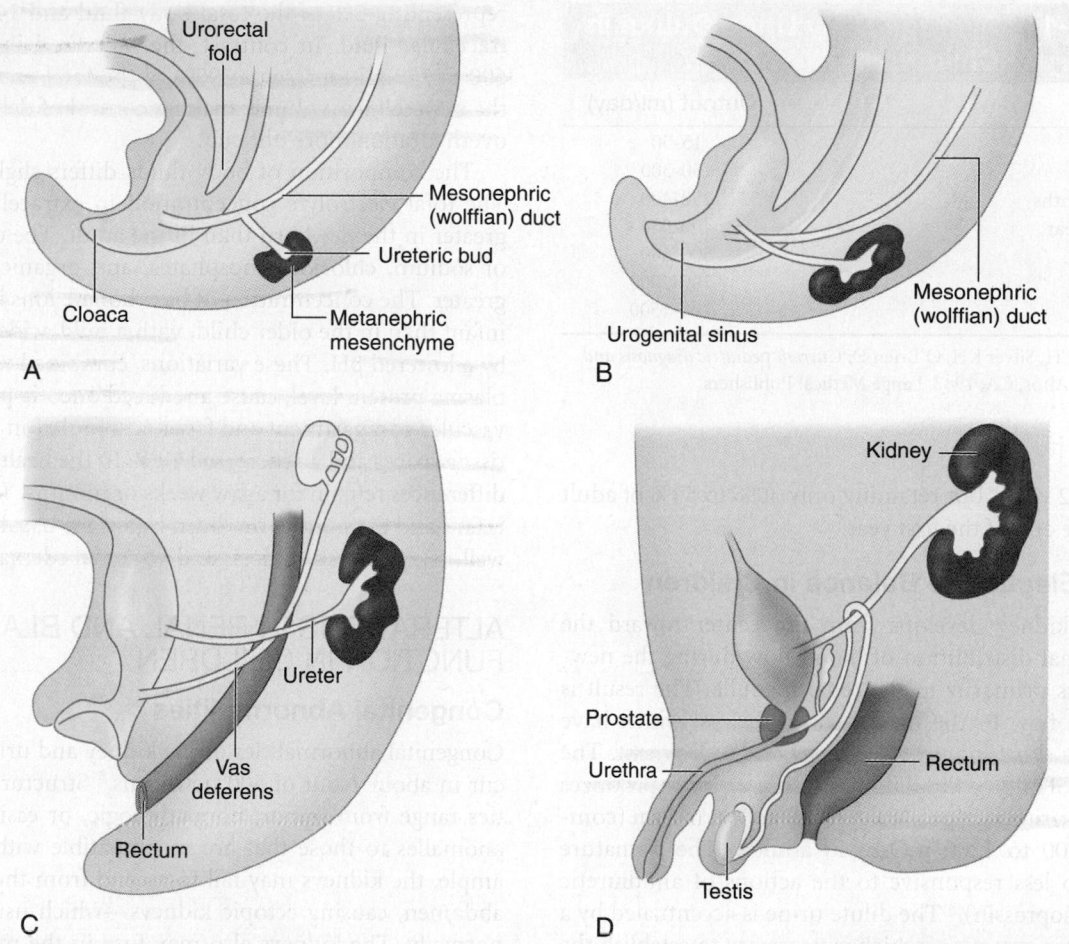

Figure 37-1 Embryonic development of the kidneys. The mesonephros begins development more caudally about the fourth fetal week and begins excretory function in the sixth week. Most of the mesonephros degenerates and disappears by the end of the embryonic period. The metanephros, the permanent kidney, arises distal to the bifurcation of the aorta and develops from two different sources: 1) the *ureteric bud* (metanephric duct) forms as an outgrowth of the mesonephritic (wolffian) duct and grows dorsocranially and starts subdividing to become the collecting system for the kidneys by forming the ureter, renal pelvis, and calyces; by the fifth fetal month it will have progressively branched into the collecting ducts, and 2) the *metanephrogenic mesenchyme* sits atop the terminal branches of the collecting ducts and develops into primitive glomeruli and uriniferous tubules (**A**). Genetic information from the metanephrogenic mesenchyme guides the development of the ureteric bud. Establishing the connection between the uriniferous tubules and the collecting ducts is a vital part of kidney development; errors in this stage can result in polycystic kidneys. As the embryo grows, the definitive kidneys migrate from the caudal position to the lumbar region and the ureters connect with the bladder (**B, C, D**). In the 8-week male embryo, the wolffian duct begins to give rise to the epididymis, the seminal vesicles, and the caudal part of the vas deferens (**C**). The external genitalia develop between 8 and 16 weeks, and testicular descent begins in month 7 of gestation (**D**). (From: Goldman L, Ausiello D: *Cecil Medicine,* ed 23, Philadelphia, 2008, Saunders.)

At birth the kidneys occupy a large portion of the posterior abdominal wall, and the ureters are proportionately shorter than those of an adult. All the nephrons are present at birth, and their number does not increase as the kidney grows and matures. The kidney reaches adult size by adolescence and, because of maturation of the tubular system, increases in weight 10-fold from the time of birth.

Urine formation and excretion begin by the third month of gestation, contributing to the amniotic fluid. In infancy the bladder lies close to the abdominal wall, making urinary bladder aspiration for diagnostic purposes a relatively simple procedure. The bladder descends into the pelvis with growth, changing from a cylindrical organ to the adult pyramidal shape. Although small amounts of urine are found in the bladder at birth, the newborn may not void for 12 to 24 hours. (The average daily urine output is shown in Table 37-1.)

Immediately at birth the renal blood flow and glomerular filtration rate (GFR) increase because of a decrease in vascular resistance and the need to perform excretory functions no longer performed by the placenta. Renal vascular resistance remains higher in newborns and infants, however, which may be attributed to increased levels of circulating renin. The resistance progressively declines during the first year of development, with an increasing fraction of the cardiac output going to the kidney. The GFR continues to increase, becoming

Table 37-1	Average Daily Urine Output in Children
Age	Output (ml/day)
1 and 2 days	15-50
3-10 days	50-300
10 days-2 months	250-400
2 months-1 year	400-500
1-3 years	500-600
5-8 years	700-1000
8-14 years	700-1500

From Kempe CH, Silver KH, O'Brien D: *Current pediatric diagnosis and treatment,* Los Altos, CA, 1982, Lange Medical Publishers.

stable at 1 or 2 years, but retaining only 30% to 50% of adult levels until the end of the first year.

Fluid and Electrolyte Balance in Children

Because the kidney develops from the center toward the periphery, renal distribution of blood flow during the newborn period is primarily to the renal medulla. The result is a preferential flow to the medullary nephrons, which have comparatively short loops at this stage of development. The combination of higher blood flow and shorter loops produces a more dilute urine—approximately 600 to 700 mOsm (compared with 800 to 1200 mOsm in adults). The immature kidney is also less responsive to the actions of antidiuretic hormone (vasopressin).[3] The dilute urine is accentuated by a low rate of urea excretion, which is necessary to establish the concentration gradient in the medulla. Urea excretion is low primarily because infants are in a high anabolic state and use their protein for growth.

Because of a high hydrogen ion concentration, limited ability to regulate the internal environment, and lowered osmotic pressure, the infant's renal system has a narrow chemical safety margin. The immaturity and smaller surface area of the tubules also may diminish the water reabsorption response to antidiuretic hormone (ADH). An immature tubular transport capacity means that the ability to excrete a potassium load, reabsorb bicarbonate, or buffer hydrogen with ammonia does not become efficient until approximately 2 years of age. Consequently, any disturbance such as diarrhea, infection, fasting for diagnostic tests, or improper feeding can rapidly lead to severe acidosis and fluid imbalance because the infant can rapidly develop overhydration, or edema.[4]

After birth the proportion of total body water to body weight does not change markedly. Considerable change occurs, however, in the location of that body water as the child matures (see Chapter 3). The percentage of extracellular fluid volume of the newborn infant is nearly double that of an adult's. Decrease in extracellular fluid volume occurs in two different periods of rapid growth—infancy and adolescence.

An infant has not only a greater content of extracellular fluid but also a greater rate of fluid exchange. The adult takes in and excretes approximately 2000 ml of water daily, representing 5% of the total body fluid and 14% of the extracellular fluid. In contrast, the infant's daily exchange of 600 to 700 ml represents 290% of the total or nearly 50% of the extracellular volume, making control of dehydration and overhydration more difficult.

The composition of body fluids differs slightly with age. The total electrolyte concentration in extracellular fluids is greater in the newborn than in the adult. The concentration of sodium, chloride, phosphates, and organic acids is also greater. The concentration of bicarbonate ions is lower in the infant than in the older child, with a mild acidosis evidenced by a lowered pH. These variations, combined with a lowered plasma protein level, cause a reduced oncotic pressure of the vascular compartment and favor accumulation of fluid in the tissue spaces and an increased GFR. In the healthy child these differences remain for a few weeks or months. The premature infant and the normal newborn infant are usually in a state of well-compensated acidosis and potential edema.

ALTERATIONS IN RENAL AND BLADDER FUNCTION IN CHILDREN

Congenital Abnormalities

Congenital abnormalities of the kidney and urinary tract occur in about 1 out of 500 newborns.[5] Structural abnormalities range from minor, nonpathologic, or easily correctable anomalies to those that are incompatible with life. For example, the kidneys may fail to ascend from the pelvis to the abdomen, causing ectopic kidneys—which usually function normally. The kidneys also may fuse in the midline as they ascend, causing a single U-shaped **horseshoe kidney** with an incidence of 1 per 600 births.[6] Approximately one third of individuals with horseshoe kidneys are asymptomatic, and the most common problems are hydronephrosis, infection, and stone formation.[7] Collectively, structural anomalies of the renal system account for approximately 45% of cases of renal failure in children.

Some anomalies are obvious at birth, whereas others remain latent. The following structural anomalies are commonly associated with urinary tract malformations[8]:

Low-set, malformed ears
Chromosomal disorders, especially trisomy 13 (Patau syndrome) and trisomy 18
Absent abdominal muscles (prune-belly syndrome)
Anomalies of the spinal cord and lower extremities
Imperforate anus or genital deviation
Wilms tumor
Congenital ascites
Cystic disease of the liver
Positive family history of renal disease (hereditary nephritis or cystic disease)

Hypospadias

Hypospadias is a congenital condition in which the urethral meatus is located on the ventral side or undersurface of the penis. The meatus can be located anywhere on the glans, the

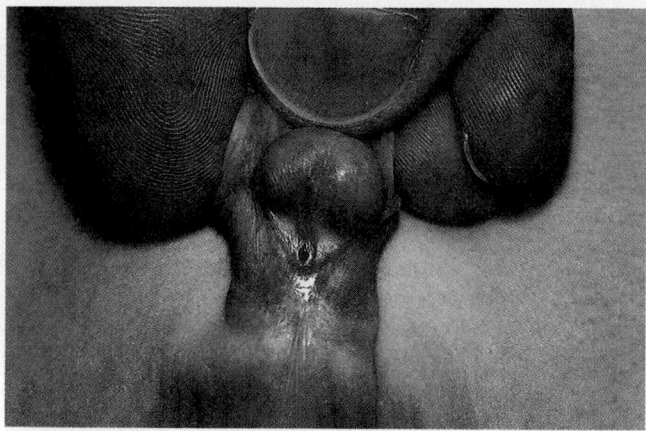

Figure 37-2 Hypospadias. (Courtesy H. Gil Rushton, MD, Children's National Medical Center, Washington, DC; from Hockenberry MJ: *Wong's nursing care of infants and children,* ed 7, St Louis, 2003, Mosby.)

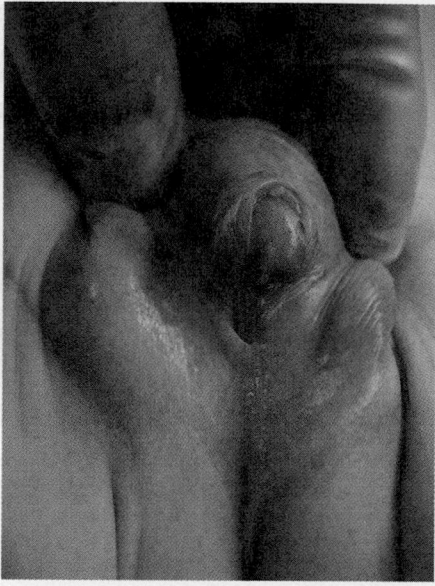

Figure 37-3 Perineal hypospadias with chordee and partial penoscrotal transposition. (From Kliegman RM et al, editors: *Nelson textbook of pediatrics,* ed 18, Philadelphia, 2007, Saunders.)

penile shaft, the base of the penis, the penoscrotal junction, or the perineum (Figure 37-2). This is the most common anomaly of the penis and occurs in about 1 in 300 infant boys. The etiology is multifactorial and related to disruptions in male hormones, including testosterone biosynthesis defects, 5alpha-reductase mutations, hormones administered for in vitro fertilization, advanced maternal age, and other environmental factors.[9] **Chordee,** or penile torsion, may accompany hypospadias. In chordee a shortage of skin on the ventral surface causes the penis to bend or to "bow" ventrally (Figure 37-3). *Penile torsion* is a counterclockwise twist of the penile shaft. Partial absence of the foreskin, inguinal hernia and cryptorchidism (undescended testes, see Chapter 23) are associated with the anomaly.[10]

The goals for corrective surgery on the child with hypospadias are (1) a straight penis when erect to facilitate sexual intercourse as an adult, (2) a uniform urethra of adequate caliber to prevent spraying during urinations, (3) a cosmetic appearance satisfactory to the individual, and (4) repair completed in as few procedures as possible. Formerly performed in two or more stages, hypospadias repairs are now done in one stage. Improvements in microsurgical techniques have enhanced outcomes and decreased complications. Surgery is usually performed between 6 and 12 months of age.[10]

Epispadias

Epispadias and exstrophy of the bladder are the same congenital defect but expressed to a different degree. In male epispadias the urethral opening is on the dorsal surface of the penis. In females a cleft along the ventral urethra usually extends to the bladder neck. The incidence of epispadias is about 1 in 40,000 to 118,000 births. About twice as many boys as girls present with this defect.

In boys the urethral opening may be small and situated behind the glans (anterior epispadias), or a fissure may extend the entire length of the penis and into the bladder neck (posterior epispadias). Children with anterior epispadias can

be continent with perhaps only stress incontinence, but those with posterior epispadias will experience constant dribbling of urine.[11] Surgical repair provides good structural and functional outcomes.

Exstrophy of the Bladder

Exstrophy of the bladder is a rare extensive congenital anomaly in which the bladder opens directly onto the abdominal wall (Figure 37-4). The posterior portion of the bladder mucosa is exposed and appears bright red through a fissure in the abdominal wall. The incidence of exstrophy of the bladder is about 1 in 400,000 live births. Boys are predominant by a ratio of 5:1.[12]

Exstrophy of the bladder is caused by intrauterine failure of the abdominal wall and the mesoderm of the anterior bladder to fuse. Urine seeps onto the abdominal wall from the ureters, causing a constant odor of urine and excoriation of the surrounding skin. The rectus muscles below the umbilicus are separated, and the pubic rami (bony projections of the pubic bone) are not joined. The clitoris in girls is divided into two halves with the urethra between them. The penis in boys is epispadic. In addition, the posterior aspect of the pelvis is externally rotated, which retroverts the acetabula and causes external rotation of the feet. This causes a waddling gait when the child first learns to walk, but most children quickly learn to compensate and surgical correction is helpful.[13]

Because the exposed bladder mucosa becomes hyperemic and edematous, it bleeds easily and is painful. It should be covered with Silastic or a plastic dressing (e.g., kitchen plastic wrap) for protection from diaper irritation while permitting urine drainage. The unrepaired exstrophic bladder is cosmetically unacceptable and prone to cancerous changes as soon as 1 year after birth. Ideally the bladder and pubic defect should

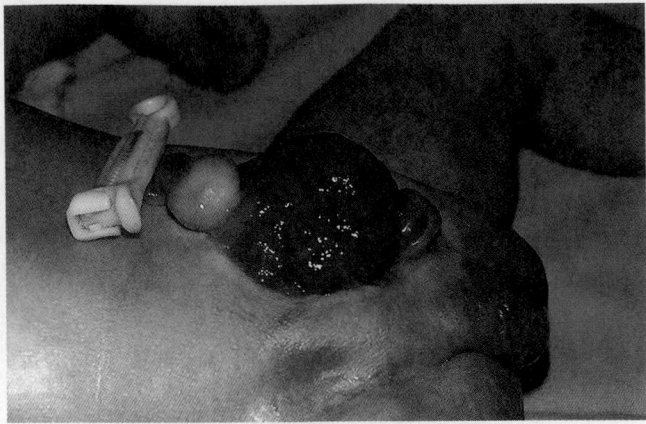

Figure 37-4 **Exstrophy of bladder.** (Courtesy H. Gil Rushton, MD, Children's National Medical Center, Washington, DC; from Hockenberry MJ: *Wong's nursing care of infants and children*, ed 7, St Louis, 2003, Mosby.)

WHAT'S NEW? Pediatric Urology and Robotics

Robotic-assisted, minimally invasive surgery for pediatric urology procedures is progressing rapidly. Robotic techniques bridge the gap between laparoscopy and open surgery. Robotic procedures are used for pyeloplasty for repair of ureteropelvic junction obstruction, including suturing with either a transperitoneal or retroperitoneal approach. Other procedures include ureteral reimplantation and partial or total nephrectomy. Cost and clinician skill are significant considerations, and advancements in the technique are promising.

Data from Muneer A et al: *Pediatr Surg Int* 24(9):973-977, 2008; Lee RS et al: *J Urol* 181(2):823-828, 2009; Casale P: *Curr Opin Urol* 19(1):97-101, 2009.

be closed before the infant is 48 hours old. Surgical reconstruction is performed usually within the first year as either a complete primary repair or as staged procedures. Staged procedures include bladder augmentation, bladder neck closure, or reconstruction of both bladder neck closures and reconstruction. Objectives of management include preservation of renal function, attainment of urinary control, prevention of infection, reconstructive repair of the defect, and improvement of sexual function and quality of life.

Cloacal exstrophy is the most rare and severe form of bladder exstrophy. The intestines, genitourinary tract, and spine may be involved, and reconstruction with restored urine and fecal control is difficult.[14]

Ureteropelvic Junction Obstruction

Ureteropelvic junction (UPJ) obstruction is a blockage of the tapered point where the renal pelvis transitions into the ureter.[15] An intrinsic malformation of smooth muscle hypertrophy and fibrosis produces obstruction in 90% of cases.[16] It is the most common cause of hydronephrosis in neonates.[17] Diagnosis can be made by ultrasound, and treatment is a surgical pyeloplasty or endopyelotomy.[18] During infancy or childhood, **secondary ureteropelvic junction (UPJ) obstruction** is caused by kinking or secondary scarring in the presence of high-grade vesicoureteral reflux. An increased risk of vesicoureteral reflux in children with UPJ obstruction affects the obstructed as well as contralateral kidneys. Other defects are sometimes associated with ureteral duplication including complete ureteral duplication (abnormal growth of two ureters and ureteral orifices draining a single kidney), incomplete duplication (bifurcation of the ureter terminates into one ureteral orifice and serves a single kidney), and ureterocele (cystic dilation of the intravesical ureter). Obstruction of the distant ureter causes dilation of the entire ureter, renal pelvis, and caliceal system.[19] It occurs when a short acontractile segment of the ureter develops just above the ureterovesical junction.

Bladder Outlet Obstruction

Congenital causes of bladder outlet obstruction are rare and include urethral valves, urethral polyps, and urethral atresia. A **urethral valve** is a thin membrane of tissue that occludes the urethral lumen and obstructs urinary outflow in males and it is the most common cause of congenital lower urinary tract obstruction and renal failure. Most valves occur in the posterior urethra, although a few arise from the embryologically distinct anterior urethra.[20] **Urethral polyps** rarely arise from the prostatic urethra. They often cause relatively severe obstruction and may impair renal embryogenesis and lead to urinary tract infection, vesicoureteric reflux, and renal failure.[21] **Urethral atresia** is absence of the urethra and is rare.

Congenital urethral valves or polyps can be diagnosed with prenatal ultrasound and treated with prenatal bladder shunting or with resection during the first days of life.[22] Infants with significant renal (and pulmonary) hypoplasia who are unable to undergo primary resection may be managed with a vesicostomy, a small opening created by pulling the bladder wall to the abdomen.[23]

Hypoplastic or Dysplastic Kidneys

During embryologic development the ureteric duct grows into the metanephric tissue, triggering the formation of the kidneys. If this growth does not occur, the kidney is absent—a condition called **renal aplasia.** Occasionally a **hypoplastic kidney,** a very small normal kidney, may develop. These aberrations may be unilateral or bilateral; the occurrence may be incidental or familial. Bilateral hypoplastic kidneys are a common cause of chronic renal failure in children. Segmental hypoplasia (the Ask-Upmark kidney) is not the result of developmental abnormalities but instead a deformity acquired secondary to vesicoureteral reflux.[24]

Renal dysplasia usually results from abnormal differentiation of the renal tissues; for example, primitive glomeruli and tubules, cysts, and nonrenal tissue (such as cartilage) are found in the dysplastic kidney. Dysplasia usually is associated also with a functional or organic obstruction of the collecting system. The obstruction may begin before birth, as in prune-belly syndrome (congenital absence of abdominal muscles), posterior urethral valves, or ureteroceles (dilation of the ureter where it enters the bladder).

Renal Agenesis

Renal agenesis (the absence of one or both kidneys) may be unilateral or bilateral, and it may occur randomly or be clearly hereditary. The condition may occur as an isolated entity or as a problem associated with anomalies in other organs.[25]

Unilateral renal agenesis occurs in approximately 1 of 1000 live births. Males are more often affected, and it is usually the left kidney that is absent. The single kidney is often completely normal so that the child can expect a normal, healthy life. The normal solitary kidney grows because of compensatory hypertrophy before and after birth, and by the time the child is several years older, the volume of this kidney may approach twice the normal size.[26]

In some instances the single kidney is abnormally formed and associated with abnormalities of its collecting system.[27] Extrarenal congenital abnormalities are relatively more common with unilateral renal agenesis.

Bilateral renal agenesis (also called **Potter syndrome**) occurs in about 1 to 4 in 10,000 live births,[28] and 75% of affected infants are male. Bilateral renal agenesis results from either an abnormal development of the normal progression from pronephros to mesonephros to metanephros or an isolated bilateral failure of development of the ureteral buds. The term *Potter syndrome* refers to the association with a specific group of facial anomalies (wide-set eyes, parrot-beak nose, low-set ears, and receding chin). Affected infants rarely live more than a few hours. Approximately 40% of affected infants are stillborn. Renal agenesis can be detected prenatally by ultrasound.

Polycystic Kidneys

Polycystic kidney disease (PKD) is an autosomal dominant inherited disorder that occurs in about 1 in 1000 live births. Mutations of two genes, *PKD-1* (chromosome 16) and *PKD-2* (chromosome 4) account for the disease most often found in adults. The gene products (polycystins) regulate growth and differentiation of the tubular epithelium.[29] Defects in the formation of epithelial cells and their cilium result in cyst formation and obstruction accompanied by destruction of renal parenchyma, interstitial fibrosis, and loss of functional nephrons. Other organs also may have cysts, including the liver and pancreas, and hypertension, heart valve defects, and cerebral and aortic aneurysms may develop. Other signs include urinary tract infection, hematuria, and flank pain. Diagnosis is usually confirmed by ultrasound. Individuals may live for decades before developing symptoms; PKD is often an adult disease. Up to 10% require renal replacement therapy.[30]

In children there is an autosomal recessive form of PKD (*ARPKD*) with cystic changes in the kidney and liver. The gene mutation for *ARPKD* encodes a protein important to maintaining structural integrity and cellular function of the kidneys and liver.[31]

Table 37-2	Primary Glomerulonephritis in Children
Classification	**Findings**
Cause	Poststreptococcal infection
	Related to other bacterial or viral infection
	Unknown
Immunologic mechanism	Antigen-antibody complex deposition
	Planted antigens with immune complex formed in situ
	Formation of antiglomerular basement membrane antibodies (rare)
	No immunologic cause established
Histopathology	No lesion
	Diffuse, focal, or segmented
	Membranous, proliferative, or combination of types
	Lobular, exudative, necrotizing, and other types
	Chronic with glomerular proliferation
Clinical manifestations of disease	Acute glomerulonephritis
	Persistent (chronic) glomerulonephritis
	Idiopathic nephrotic syndrome

Glomerular Disorders

The most common glomerular disorders in children are glomerulonephritis, nephrotic syndrome, and hemolytic uremic syndrome. Most glomerular diseases are acquired and immunologically mediated. The disease can be acute or chronic; renal failure is rare.

Glomerulonephritis

Glomerulonephritis includes a number of renal disorders in which proliferation and inflammation of the glomeruli are secondary to an immune mechanism (Table 37-2). (The major glomerulopathies and their histologic characteristics can be reviewed in Chapter 36.) Chronic glomerulonephritis is the causative factor for 30% to 50% of renal failure in children and is the condition responsible for most school-age and teenage children requiring dialysis and kidney transplantation.

Acute Poststreptococcal Glomerulonephritis

Acute poststreptococcal glomerulonephritis (PSGN) is one of the most common postinfectious renal diseases in children ages 5 to 15 years. It occurs after a throat (pharyngitis) or skin (impetigo) infection with nephritogenic strains of group A beta-hemolytic streptococci and is characterized by a sudden onset of gross hematuria, edema, hypertension, and renal insufficiency.

The pathophysiology of PSGN in children is similar to that occurring in adults (see Chapter 36). Antigen-antibody complexes of immunoglobulin G (IgG), IgA, and C_3 complement are deposited in the glomerulus or the antigen may be trapped within the glomerulus and immune complexes formed in situ. The exact mechanism of immune complex formation is unknown. The immune complexes initiate inflammation and glomerular injury. Immunofluorescence microscopy shows lumpy deposits of immunoglobulin and complement on the glomerular basement membrane (see Figure 36-8). Increased vascular permeability and loss of electrical negative charge along the glomerular vascular membrane leads to hematuria and proteinuria. Hypertension occurs with increased blood volume and release of endothelin-1, a potent vasoconstrictor.[32]

Typically a child is in good health until the onset of an upper respiratory or skin infection. Pharyngeal infections are most common during cold weather. Skin infections from impetigo, infected insect bites, or varicella sores usually occur during warm weather. One to 2 weeks later, mild proteinuria (less than 2 g per 4 hours), hematuria, and periorbital edema appear. The urine is usually smoky brown or cola colored because of the presence of red blood cells, and the volume is reduced. The onset of symptoms in the child is abrupt and consists of flank or midabdominal pain, irritability, general malaise, and fever. Acute hypertension may cause headache; vomiting; somnolence; and other central nervous system (CNS) manifestations, including seizures. Cardiovascular symptoms are related to circulatory overload and are compounded by hypertension. These include dyspnea, tachypnea, and an enlarged, tender liver. The most severely affected children develop acute renal failure with oliguria. As many as half the children affected are asymptomatic.

The disease is usually mild and runs its course in 1 month, but urine abnormalities may be found up to 1 year after the onset. Some children (less than 1%) become oliguric and develop rapidly progressive glomerulonephritis, whereas others slowly progress to chronic glomerulonephritis. Prolonged proteinuria and abnormal GFR indicate an unfavorable prognosis. More than 95% recover completely.

Acute glomerulonephritis (AGN) may be accompanied by a positive throat or skin culture for *Streptococcus*. Antistreptolysin-O titers confirm a recent streptococcal infection. Antihyaluronidase, antideoxyribonuclease B, and antistreptokinase antibody are other diagnostic markers. The urine usually contains red blood cells and proteins. Treatment is symptom specific. Because oliguria and hypertension are common, fluid, sodium, and potassium intakes are restricted. Antihypertensive medication and diuretic agents are indicated during the acute phase.

Immunoglobulin A Nephropathy

Immunoglobulin A (IgA) nephropathy (Berger nephropathy) is the most common type of childhood glomerulonephritis, occurs almost twice as often in males as in females, and is rare in blacks. It is characterized by deposition mainly of IgA, but also some IgM and complement proteins in the mesangium of the glomerular capillaries. There is no evidence of systemic immunologic disease such as systemic lupus erythematosus or anaphylactoid purpura (Henoch-Schönlein purpura). IgA may show decreased glycosylation that favors antibody formation and mesangial deposition.[33] Binding of the IgA to mesangial cells stimulates them to proliferate, secrete extracellular matrix proteins, and release inflammatory cytokines and chemokines (interleukin-6, tumor necrosis factor-alpha, and transforming growth factor beta 1) that cause injury. The damage to the glomerulus can progress to glomerulosclerosis and tubular interstitial involvement, which is usually reversible.[34]

The classic presentation of the disease is recurrent gross hematuria, often after a respiratory infection. Most continue to have microscopic hematuria between the attacks of gross hematuria. Many children also have a mild proteinuria in spite of otherwise normal renal function and may report flank pain caused by renal swelling. The diagnosis may be missed and specific diagnosis is made by renal biopsy.[35] Treatment is supportive with control of hypertension. Some studies report that tonsillectomy and use of corticosteroids reduces formation of IgA and reduces proteinuria.[36] Long-term follow-up consists of evaluating blood pressure, urinalysis, proteinuria levels, and renal function every 6 to 12 months. Approximately 25% of affected children develop the progressive form of the disease with hypertension, proteinuria, and decreasing renal function that extends into adulthood.[37] Hypertriglyceridemia and hyperuricemia are predictors of poor outcome.[38] These children eventually require dialysis and transplantation.

Henoch-Schönlein Purpura Nephritis—IgA Nephropathy

Henoch-Schönlein purpura nephritis, also known as **anaphylactoid purpura**, is an IgA nephropathy that affects the glomerular blood vessels causing inflammation and damage to the vessel wall. The disease also involves small vessels in the skin and gut. The most typical renal lesion is focal segmental glomerulonephritis (see Table 36-7 in Chapter 36) with IgA deposits in the mesangium. Transient hematuria and mild proteinuria without functional impairment are more common in children. Children also may exhibit signs of intestinal colic and arthralgia.[39] The development of interstitial fibrosis and crescent formation from subepithelial immune deposits along the glomeruli increases the risk of chronic renal failure.[40] Most children recover with supportive care. Severe symptoms require steroids and other immunosuppressant drugs.[41]

Hemolytic Uremic Syndrome

Hemolytic uremic syndrome (HUS) is an acute disorder characterized by microangiopathic hemolytic anemia and thrombocytopenia and is the most common cause of acute renal failure in young children.[42] The etiology remains unknown, although an association between HUS and both bacterial and viral agents has been established. The disease also occurs with cancer and use of chemotherapeutic agents. *Escherichia coli (E. coli)* O157:H7, a shiga toxin-producing bacterium, is the most commonly associated microorganism in the United States, usually found in undercooked meat and unpasteurized milk.[43] The disease occurs in infants and children younger than 4 years. The prognosis has improved dramatically in recent years, with more than 90% of children surviving and most regaining normal renal function.

PATHOPHYSIOLOGY In HUS, verotoxin from *E. coli* is absorbed from the intestines into the blood, binds to polymorphonuclear leukocytes, and is transported to the kidney, causing a cascade of effects including lysis of glomerular capillary endothelial cells, separation of endothelial cells from the basement membrane, activation and aggregation of platelets, and activation of the coagulation cascade. The glomerular arterioles becomes swollen and occluded with platelets and fibrin clots. There is decreased glomerular filtration, and the damaged glomerular membrane results in hematuria and proteinuria. Oliguria with renal failure occurs in up to 50% of children. Narrowed vessels damage erythrocytes as they pass through. These damaged red blood cells, identified as burr cells, helmet cells, and fragmented red blood cells, are removed by the spleen, causing acute hemolytic anemia. Fibrinolysis, the process of dissolution of a clot, acts on precipitated fibrin, causing the fibrin split products to appear in serum and urine. The platelet clustering within damaged vessels, combined with the damage and removal of platelets, produces thrombocytopenia. Fibrin-rich thrombi can be found throughout the microcirculation.[44] Other tissues, including the brain, liver, heart, and intestines, are often involved, which portends a poorer prognosis.

CLINICAL MANIFESTATIONS Typical HUS is preceded by a prodromal gastrointestinal (GI) illness with diarrhea and is known as D+ HUS. Less frequently atypical or sporadic HUS is preceded by an unknown event or an upper respiratory infection and is known as D- HUS. A rare familial form is associated with mutations in complement proteins. The onset of D+ HUS occurs about 1 to 2 weeks after a GI illness with a symptom-free 1- to 5-day period. There is sudden onset of pallor, bruising or purpura, irritability, and oliguria. Slight fever, anorexia, vomiting, diarrhea (with the stool characteristically watery and blood stained—hemorrhagic diarrhea), abdominal pain, mild jaundice, and circulatory overload are accompanying symptoms. Seizures and lethargy indicate CNS involvement. Renal failure is apparent within 2 days to 2 weeks of onset. The renal failure causes metabolic acidosis, uremia, hyperkalemia, and often hypertension.

EVALUATION AND TREATMENT Clinical evaluation includes history of preexisting illness, presenting symptoms, and urine and blood analysis. Antibiotics are not used in the initial treatment because they increase shiga toxin release and increase the risk of HUS. Management consists of maintaining nutrition and hydration (to dilute toxins) and controlling hypertension, hyperkalemia, and seizures.[45] When renal failure occurs, early and frequent dialysis is indicated. Blood transfusions with packed red blood cells are needed to maintain reasonable hemoglobin levels. The response to treatment is usually good and the disease is self-limiting. Death usually occurs from complications related to CNS or myocardial involvement.[46] Preventing shiga toxin–producing bacterial infection (i.e., *E. coli*) prevents HUS.

Nephrotic Syndrome

Nephrotic syndrome is a term used to describe a symptom complex characterized by proteinuria, hypoproteinemia, hyperlipidemia, and edema. The syndrome is more common in children than adults. When no other identifiable causes are found the condition is termed **primary (idiopathic) nephrotic syndrome.** If it results from a systemic disease or other causes (e.g., drugs, toxins, diabetes mellitus, lupus nephritis) it is called **secondary nephrotic syndrome.** Primary nephrotic syndrome is usually described by histopathology (i.e., minimal change nephropathy [MCN], focal segmental glomerulosclerosis [FSGS], membraneous nephropathy [MN], or membranoproliferative glomerulonephritis [MPGN]) (see Table 36-7). Secondary nephrotic syndrome has the same patterns of histopathology but is associated with an underlying cause.

Approximately 95% of cases of nephrotic syndrome in children occur in the absence of systemic or preexisting renal disease. Primary nephrotic syndrome is found predominantly in preschool children, with a peak incidence of onset between 2 and 3 years of age. It is rare after 8 years of age. Boys are affected more often than girls. No prevalent racial or geographic distributions are evident. The incidence is approximately 3 per 100,000 children per year.

PATHOPHYSIOLOGY The cause of nephrotic syndrome in children is usually idiopathic and includes minimal change nephropathy (85%), FSGS (10%), and mesangial proliferative nephropathy (MPN) (5%).[47] Secondary nephrotic syndrome may develop during the course of several different renal or systemic diseases. The pathophysiology (see Figure 36-11) and common clinical manifestations of nephrotic syndrome in adults are described in Chapter 36 (Table 36-8), and are similar in children. The most common causes of nephrotic syndrome in children are presented here.

Minimal change nephropathy (MCN), also known as *lipoid nephrosis,* is the most common cause of nephrotic syndrome in children. A systemic immune mechanism is a likely cause of the disease, but the true etiology is unknown. MCN is found in 85% of children with idiopathic nephrosis. The mechanism of increased glomerular permeability is unknown but is related, in part, to release of permeability factors from abnormal circulating T cells that injure the glomerular epithelial cells. The glomeruli appear normal, and immunoglobulin deposition is usually absent. The only change is *fusion of epithelial cell podocyte foot processes.*[47] There are few other renal structural abnormalities. Loss of the electrical negative charge and increased permeability within the glomerular capillary wall leads to albuminuria.[48,49] Hyperlipidemia leads to hyperlipiduria and primarily results from increased hepatic lipid synthesis and decreased plasma lipid catabolism.[50]

Focal segmental glomerulosclerosis (FSGS) is present in approximately 15% of children with nephrotic syndrome and is more common in blacks. The frequency of FSGS is increasing in children and adults.[51] The primary injury is effacement (thinning or deletion) of epithelial podocytes, with a significant increase in pore size leading to impairment of size selectivity and proteinuria. Progressive disease results in proliferation of endothelial and mesangial cells with occlusion and sclerosis of glomerular capillaries. The more severe the proteinuria, the more likely that end-stage renal disease will occur.

Edema is the classic symptom of nephrotic syndrome. Several factors contribute to edema formation with hypoalbuminemia (decreased plasma oncotic pressure) and sodium retention as major contributors. The movement of fluid from the vascular to the interstitial space can decrease blood volume and increase activity of aldosterone and antidiuretic hormone (vasopressin), and decrease atrial natriuretic peptide, all of which promote fluid retention.[52]

Hyperlipidemia occurs in inverse proportion to the decrease in plasma proteins, particularly albumin. There are high concentrations of triglycerides, low-density lipoprotein (LDL), and very low-density lipoprotein (VLDL) cholesterol. High-density lipoprotein (HDL) cholesterol concentration is decreased. Hypoalbuminemia leads to a deficiency in the carrier protein for the transport of fatty acids, and they remain elevated in the serum. There is hepatic compensation for hypoalbuminemia with increased synthesis of lipoproteins to maintain plasma oncotic pressure. Hypoalbuminemia also leads to an increased hepatic stimulus for synthesis of LDL and VLDL cholesterol by the liver. Serum lipids may remain elevated from 1 to 3 months after remission of proteinuria.

Hypercoagulation with risk for arterial or venous thrombosis results from abnormalities in the coagulation pathways during nephrotic syndrome. Although rare, thrombosis can occur in the brain or lung. Family history and predisposing risk factors should be evaluated. Anticoagulants may be required.[53]

Congenital nephrotic syndrome (Finnish type) is caused by an autosomal recessive mutation of the *NPHS1* gene that encodes an immunoglobulin-like protein, nephrin, at the podocyte slit membrane. Lack of nephrin causes heavy proteinuria.[54] The disease usually manifests within the first 3 months of life, and these babies do not respond to steroid treatment.[55]

CLINICAL MANIFESTATIONS Onset of nephrotic syndrome is insidious, with periorbital edema as the first sign. The edema is most noticeable in the morning but subsides during the day as fluid shifts to the abdomen and lower extremities (Figure 37-5). Parents become alerted to an abnormality when they notice diminished "frothy" or "foamy" urine and when edema becomes pronounced with ascites, respiratory difficulty from pleural effusion, and labial or scrotal swelling.

Edema of the intestinal mucosa may cause diarrhea, anorexia, and poor absorption. Edema often masks the malnutrition caused by malabsorption and protein loss. Because of protein deficiency, changes in the quality of hair indicate a malnourished state. Pallor, with shiny skin and prominent veins, is also common. Blood pressure is usually normal or slightly decreased. The child has an increased susceptibility to infection, especially pneumonia, peritonitis, cellulitis, and septicemia. Irritability, fatigue, and lethargy are common. Infants born with congenital nephrotic syndrome have large fontanels, have separated cranial sutures, and may show gingival hyperplasia.[56]

EVALUATION AND TREATMENT The diagnosis of nephrotic syndrome is evident from the clinical presentation and findings of proteinuria, hyperlipidemia, and lipiduria. Several diagnostic tests, including kidney biopsy, may be required to determine whether the cause is an intrinsic renal disease or a consequence of systemic disease.

The goals of treatment are to reduce the excretion of protein and to maintain a protein-free urine. Prevention or treatment of infection, control of edema, establishment of a balanced nutritional state, and restoration of normal metabolic processes also are important in managing the disorder and avoiding adverse aspects of treatment. Basic management of nephrotic syndrome includes activity as tolerated; a low-sodium, well-balanced diet; diuretics (furosemide [Lasix]); angiotensin-converting enzyme (ACE) inhibitors (inhibits formation of angiotensin II and aldosterone resulting in decreased blood pressure and decreased renal sodium reabsorption); paracentesis (for ascites); and skin care. Corticosteroids are the primary therapeutic agents, and outcomes in children are often described according to their response to steroid therapy (Table 37-3). Steroid-sensitive nephrotic syndrome usually results in complete remission without serious adverse

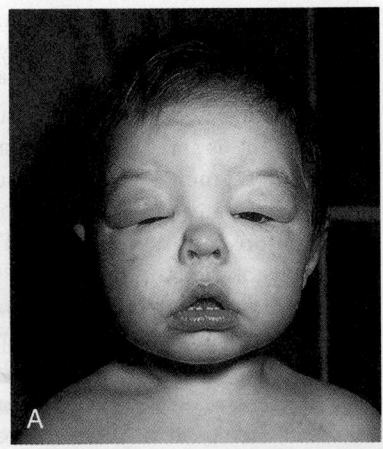
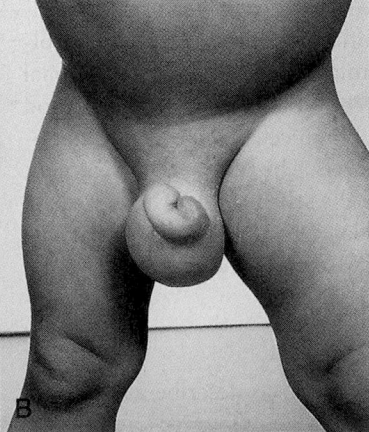

Figure 37-5 Nephrotic syndrome. **A,** Facial edema. **B,** Gross edema of scrotum and legs with abdominal distention from ascites. (From Lissauer T, Clayden G: *Illustrated textbook of pediatrics*, St Louis, 2001, Mosby.)

effects of therapy. Children who fail to respond to prednisone within 8 weeks are termed *steroid resistant* and may be treated with noncorticosteroid immunosuppressive agents or combinations of corticosteroids and noncorticosteroid immunosuppressives to prolong remission.[57,58] Renal transplant is performed for those children who progress to renal failure; those with FSGS are at greatest risk.[59]

Renal Injury

Renal injury, either acute or chronic, is rare in children. The pathophysiology and management are similar to renal injury in adults (see Table 36-9). A modification of the RIFLE criteria (R = risk, I = injury, F = failure, L = loss, and E = end-stage kidney disease [ESKD]) that was proposed to standardize the definition of acute kidney injury in adults has been used in critically ill children (pRIFLE criteria) (Table 37-4).[60]

The most common causes of *prerenal acute renal injury* are dehydration, hemorrhage, and sepsis. Glomerulonephritis, hemolytic uremic syndrome, and hypersensitivity reactions to drugs or infectious agents are the most common causes of *intrinsic acute renal injury*. Obstructive uropathies, such as posterior urethral valves and obstruction of the ureteropelvic junction, are associated with *postrenal acute renal injury*.[61] Chronic renal failure in very young children is commonly associated with congenital renal structural abnormalities. In older children the most common cause is glomerulonephropathies.[62,63] Renal transplants are successful in children.[64,65] The use of growth hormone before and after transplant has contributed to normal growth and development particularly in prepubertal children.[66]

Bladder Disorders

Urinary Tract Infections

Urinary tract infection (UTI) is the colonization of a pathogen anywhere along the urinary tract (urethra, bladder, ureter, kidney) and occurs commonly in children.[67] The incidence of UTI is greater in boys up to 1 year of age, particularly among those not circumcised.[68] Girls have a greater incidence after 1 year of age with an increasing incidence at adolescence. UTIs in girls occur as a result of perineal bacteria, especially *E. coli*, ascending the urethra. The incidence of UTI in neonates and infants is low, but the risk is high because of an immature immune system.

The pathophysiology of UTIs in children is similar to that of adults (see Chapter 36). However, UTIs in children are often clinically categorized as first or recurrent infection.[69] Individual susceptibility, bacterial virulence, and the host's anatomy (presence of reflux, obstruction, stasis, stones, or structural anomalies of the urinary tract) affect the severity of the disease. The recurrence rate is approximately 30% to 40%[70] and is highest in females. Sexually active female adolescents are more likely to have a UTI. Similar to adult women, susceptibility is increased when genetically controlled blood group antigens (P1 and Lewis blood group nonsecretor) are present on surface uroepithelial cells and act as receptors for bacterial attachment.[71]

Cystitis, or infection of the bladder, results in mucosal inflammation and congestion. This causes detrusor muscle hyperactivity and a resulting decrease in the bladder capacity. It also can lead to transient reflux of urine up the ureters, sending bacteria all the way to the kidney, causing acute or chronic pyelonephritis and renal abscesses or scarring.

Symptoms of UTI in children are nonspecific, and differentiating whether an infection is in the bladder or kidneys is difficult based on symptoms alone. Infants usually develop nausea, vomiting, diarrhea, or jaundice. Infants and young children may present only with fever of undetermined origin and others may present with urinary tract symptoms of frequency; urgency; enuresis or incontinence in a previously dry child; abdominal, flank, or back pain; foul-smelling urine; and sometimes hematuria. **Acute pyelonephritis** usually

Table 37-3	Corticosteroid Treatment in Children with Nephrotic Syndrome		
Response to Corticosteroid	**Incidence (%)**	**Outcomes**	
Steroid sensitive	>80	Single course of therapy, low recurrence rate	
Steroid dependent (frequently relapsing)	7	Intermittent exacerbations with remissions for several years	
Steroid resistant	Rare	Resistance to steroids, eventual development of chronic renal failure	

Data from Kim JS et al: *Kidney Int* 68(3):1275-1281, 2005.

Table 37-4	Pediatric-Modified RIFLE (pRIFLE) Criteria	
Risk Category	**Estimated CCl-GFR Criteria**	**Urine Output Criteria**
Risk	eCCl decrease by 25%	<0.5 ml/kg/hr for 8 hr
Injury	eCCl decrease by 50%	<0.5 ml/kg/hr for 16 hr
Failure	eCCl decrease by 75% or eCCl <35 ml/min/1.73 m^2	<0.3 ml/kg/hr for 24 hr or anuric for 12 hr
Loss (of kidney function)	Persistent failure >4 weeks	
End-stage	End-stage renal disease (persistent failure >3 months)	

Data from Akcan-Arikan A et al: *Kidney Int* 71(10):1028-1035, 2007.

eCCl, Estimated creatinine clearance; *GFR*, glomerular filtration rate, *pRIFLE*, pediatric risk, injury, failure, loss, and end-stage renal disease.

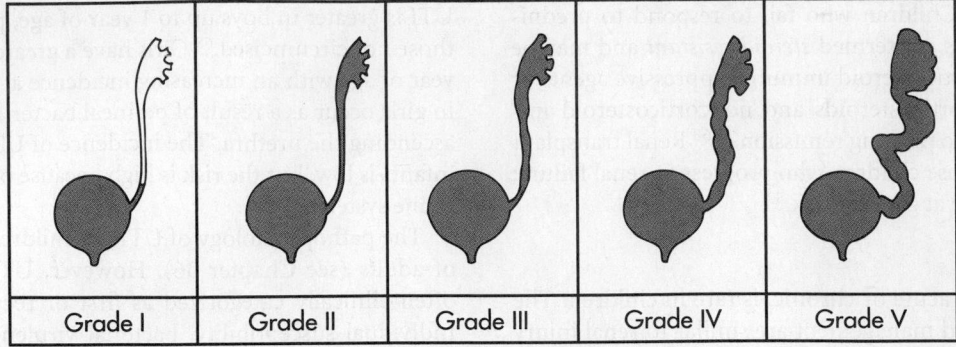

Figure 37-6 Grades of reflux. (From Retik A, Cukier J, editors: *Pediatric urology,* Baltimore, 1987, Williams & Wilkins.)

causes chills, fever, and flank or abdominal pain along with enlarged kidney(s) caused by edema. **Chronic pyelonephritis** may be asymptomatic.

Diagnosis of UTIs is by urine culture of a pathogen prior to antimicrobial treatment. An accompanying urinalysis can show pyuria and microscopic hematuria. The presence of casts in the urine can indicate pyelonephritis. Ultrasound, voiding cystourethrography (VCUG) or radionuclide cystography, computed tomography (CT) scan, or voiding cystourethrogram may be necessary to rule out obstructions, abscesses, or reflux, particularly in young children that do not respond to antimicrobial therapy.[72]

With treatment, UTI symptoms are usually relieved in 1 to 2 days and the urine becomes sterile. A 2- to 4-day course of oral antibiotics is effective for uncomplicated UTI.[73] More potent medications may be required if the child has a recurrent UTI, has a complicated UTI including congenital abnormalities of the urinary tract, or is immunosuppressed. About 3 to 6 weeks after treatment is completed, all children with a first UTI should have imaging done to rule out reflux and urinary tract abnormalities. Follow-up urine cultures should be done 2 to 3 weeks after the medication is completed and every 3 months for the next 1 to 2 years to monitor for recurrence, to prevent renal scarring, and for assessment of normal renal development and function, even if the child is asymptomatic.

Surgical correction of reflux or obstruction is necessary before the urinary tract can be sterilized. Children who develop frequent recurrences and who do not have surgically correctable anomalies may need prophylactic antibiotic therapy. These children also require regular cultures to rule out asymptomatic infections with resistant microorganisms.

Vesicoureteral Reflux

Vesicoureteral reflux (VUR) is the retrograde flow of bladder urine into the ureters. Reflux allows infected urine from the bladder to be repeatedly swept up into the kidneys. The reflux perpetuates infection by preventing complete emptying of the bladder, because infected, refluxed urine drains back into the bladder at the end of each voiding. In addition, the reflux allows the maximal intravesical pressure to be transmitted to the renal calyces and pyramids. The combination of reflux

and infection is an important cause of pyelonephritis, especially in children younger than 5 years.

Vesicoureteral reflux occurs more often in girls by a ratio of 10:1 and is uncommon in blacks. Its incidence is approximately 1 in 1000 children, and siblings of those affected have up to a 50% chance of developing reflux.[74] Although reflux is considered abnormal at any age, the shortness of the submucosal segment of the ureter during infancy and childhood renders the antireflux mechanism relatively inefficient and delicate. Thus reflux is seen commonly in association with infections during early childhood but rarely in older children and adults. (Among adults with UTIs, the incidence of reflux is approximately 5%.)

Reflux may be unilateral or bilateral, and it can be classified or graded (Figure 37-6) for comparative purposes:

Grade I—Reflux into a nondilated distal ureter

Grade II—Reflux into the upper collecting system without dilation

Grade III—Reflux into dilated ureter or blunting of calyceal fornices

Grade IV—Reflux into a grossly dilated ureter

Grade V—Massive reflux with ureteral dilation and tortuosity and effacement of the calyceal details; occurs almost exclusively in male infants[75]

PATHOPHYSIOLOGY Primary reflux results from a congenitally abnormal or ectopic insertion of the ureter into the bladder. In some infants VUR may be related to inadequate relaxation of the external urethral sphincter.[76] Occasionally the condition is hereditary. Secondary reflux is more serious and may be transient or persistent. It develops in association with infection, malformations of the ureterovesical (UV) junction, increased intravesical pressures, and surgery on the UV junction (Figure 37-7). Urinary tract infection associated with VUR may lead to permanent renal scarring, particularly when there is pyelonephritis.[77] The actual cause of renal cell damage and scarring is unknown but contributing factors include inflammatory cytokines activated by bacterial virulence factors.[78]

CLINICAL MANIFESTATIONS Children with reflux have recurrent UTIs or unexplained fever, poor growth and development, irritability, and feeding problems. Children and

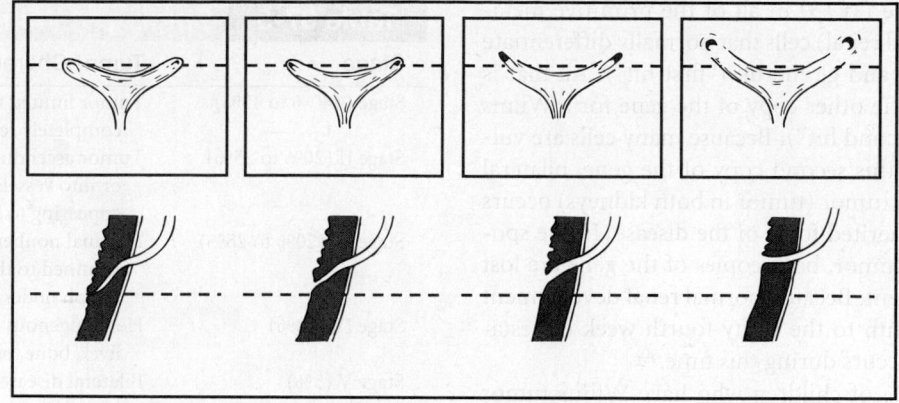

Figure 37-7 Normal and abnormal configuration of the ureteral orifices. *Left to right:* Progressive lateral displacement of the ureteral orifices and shortening of the intramural tunnels. *Top row:* Endoscopic appearance. *Bottom row:* Sagittal view through the intramural ureter. (From Behrman R et al, editors: *Nelson textbook of pediatrics,* ed 16, Philadelphia, 2000, Saunders.)

adults may have a family history of reflux or UTI, pain with voiding, and signs of urinary obstruction or nephropathy.

EVALUATION AND TREATMENT Early diagnosis of VUR in infants is critical to preventing renal scarring. Some infants may have renal scarring at birth from intrauterine damage caused by destruction or reflux.

In addition to the history of recurrent UTIs and other symptoms, imaging may be required for diagnosis and assessment of structural change, scarring, urinary tract function, and risk for future infection and renal damage.[78] Most children with vesicoureteral reflux respond to nonoperative management aimed at prevention and treatment of infection. Spontaneous remission of grades I and II reflux may occur in 30% to 60% of children younger than 5 years. Children with grades III and IV reflux need long-term monitoring and prophylactic antibiotics, but there are concerns regarding antibiotic resistance.[79] Endoscopic injection with biomaterials may be a treatment alternative.[80] Recurrent infection may require surgical intervention. In cases of grade V reflux, early surgical intervention is indicated to prevent renal scarring, although spontaneous resolution can occur during the first year. Siblings of children

with vesicoureteral reflux should be monitored for risk of developing vesicoureteral reflux.[81] Up to 50% have been found to have asymptomatic vesicoureteral reflux.[82,83]

Wilms Tumor

Wilms tumor is an embryonal tumor of the kidney arising from epigenetic and genetic changes that lead to abnormal proliferation of renal stem cells (metanephric blastema). It is also known by the histologic name of **nephroblastoma** and is the most common solid tumor occurring in children.

The incidence of Wilms tumor remains constant in the United States, with approximately 500 children diagnosed each year. Most children are between 1 and 5 years of age when they are diagnosed. The peak incidence occurs between 2 and 3 years of age. Wilms tumor is slightly more common in females and in black than in white children, and is less common in Asian children.[84,85]

Microscopically, Wilms tumor is composed of three cellular components: stromal, epithelial, and blastemic. This occurs because blastemic cells, which are primitive and undifferentiated, may have partially developed into epithelial or stromal tissue. With each of these three cellular components, varying stages of differentiation may be evident within the tumor.

PATHOGENESIS Wilms tumor has sporadic and inherited origins. The sporadic form occurs in children with no known genetic predisposition. Inherited cases, which are relatively rare (1% to 2% of cases), are transmitted in an autosomal dominant fashion.

The Wilms tumor suppressor gene *(WT1)* has been located at various chromosomal regions.[86,87] The deletion or inactivation of the *WT1* gene accounts for about 5% to 10% of Wilms tumor cases. The *WTX* gene located on the X chromosome is inactivated and found in 7% to 30% of cases; these tumors lack *WT1* mutations.[88,89]

The pathogenesis of the sporadic and inherited forms of Wilms tumor is similar to retinoblastoma (the "two hit" mutation) (see Figure 19-16). In the inherited form of the disease, the child inherits the loss of one copy of the Wilms

WHAT'S NEW? Procalcitonin and First Febrile Urinary Tract Infection

Procalcitonin (PCT) is the precursor of calcitonin synthesized by thyroid gland C cells. PCT has become a marker of bacterial infection with production by various cell types, including hepatocytes, nephrons, and monocytes, after exposure to bacterial endotoxin. The diagnosis of first febrile urinary tract infection (UTI) related to acute pyelonephritis and vesicoureteral reflux is associated with elevated levels of PCT. PCT can be used to identify severity of bacterial infection, children who are at low risk for renal scarring, and avoid unnecessary cystourethrographies with a first febrile UTI.

Data from Leroy S et al: *J Pediatr* 150(1):89-95, 2007; Pecile P, Romanello C: *Curr Opin Infect Dis* 20(1):83-87, 2007; Maniaci V et al: *Pediatrics* 122(4):701-710 2008; Kotoula A et al: *Urology* 73(4): 782-786, 2009.

tumor-suppressor gene *(WT3)* in all of the primitive meta-nephric blastemic (fetal renal) cells that normally differentiate into the renal tubules and glomeruli ("first hit"). All that is needed is the loss of the other copy of the gene for a Wilms tumor to develop ("second hit"). Because many cells are vulnerable to the loss of this second copy of the gene, bilateral presentation of Wilms tumor (tumor in both kidneys) occurs occasionally in the inherited form of the disease. In the sporadic form of Wilms tumor, both copies of the gene are lost during fetal development. Because normal renal development occurs during the eighth to the thirty-fourth week of gestation, gene loss likely occurs during this time.[90]

Approximately 10% of children who have Wilms tumor also have loss of other important genes and therefore have a number of congenital anomalies. These anomalies include aniridia (lack of an iris in the eye), hemihypertrophy (an asymmetry of the body), and genitourinary malformations (i.e., horseshoe kidneys, hypospadias, ureteral duplication, polycystic kidneys, uterine abnormalities).[91,92] Children with congenital anomalies as well as Wilms tumor are more likely to have the inherited bilateral form of the disease.

CLINICAL MANIFESTATIONS Most Wilms tumors (90%) present as an enlarging asymptomatic upper abdominal mass in a healthy, thriving child. Other presenting complaints include vague abdominal pain, hematuria, fever, and hypertension.[93]

EVALUATION AND TREATMENT On physical examination the tumor feels firm, nontender, smooth, and generally is a solitary mass of varying size confined to one side of the abdomen. Once an abdominal mass is detected, diagnostic imaging demonstrates a solid intrarenal mass.

Diagnosis is based on surgical biopsy. Additional laboratory and radiologic studies are used to evaluate the presence or absence of metastasis. The most common sites of metastasis are regional lymph nodes and the lungs and less commonly liver, brain, and bone.

Staging systems for Wilms tumor have been developed and serve as guides to treatment. The most widely accepted system was developed by the National Wilms Tumor Study Group (Table 37-5). The system is based on surgical findings and the extent of disease at diagnosis.[94] Children are further classified as either high or low risk according to favorable or unfavorable histology (anaplasia).

Surgical exploration and resection begin the treatment of Wilms tumor. In bilateral disease, surgical intervention may include heminephrectomy of the less involved kidney and nephrectomy of the other. Radiation therapy has been found to be most effective if begun 1 to 3 days after surgery for stages III and IV disease and metastases. Chemotherapy is specific to histology and stage of disease.[94]

The overall cure rate is as high as 95% for children with stage I through stage III disease (Table 37-6). Prognosis is improving for children with metastases, and this is one of the few tumors for which lung metastases have been cured. Recurrent disease is treated aggressively in children with favorable histology.

Table 37-5	Staging of Wilms Tumor
Stage	**Tumor Characteristics**
Stage I (40% to 45%)	Tumor limited to the kidney, completely resected
Stage II (20% to 25%)	Tumor ascending beyond the kidney or into vessels of renal sinus, but appearing to be totally resected
Stage III (20% to 25%)	Residual nonhematogenous tumor confined to the abdomen, positive lymph nodes in renal hila
Stage IV (10%)	Hematogenous metastases (e.g., lung, liver, bone, brain)
Stage V (5%)	Bilateral disease either at diagnosis or later, but need to stage each kidney

Data from American Cancer Society. Available at www.cancer.org/docroot/CRI/content/CRI_2_4_3X_How_is_Wilms_tumor_staged.asp.
NOTE: Staging system of the Third National Wilms Tumor Study Group (NWTS-3).

Table 37-6	National Wilms Tumor Study 4-Year Survival Rates	
Tumor Stage	**Favorable Histology**	**Unfavorable Histology (Anaplastic Wilms Tumor)**
I	96%	83%
II	91%	81%
III	91%	72%
IV	81%	38%
V	82%	55%

From National Wilms Tumor Studies, American Cancer Society. Available at www.cancer.org/docroot/CRI/content/CRI_2_4_3X_How_is_Wilms_tumor_staged.asp.

Enuresis

Enuresis refers to the voluntary or involuntary passage of urine by a child who is beyond the age when voluntary bladder control should have been acquired. Bladder control is accomplished by most children before the age of 4 years. Functional incontinence is urinary incontinence in which no structural or neurologic abnormality can be identified. The underlying mechanism may include disorders of both the storage and voiding phases of the bladder cycle.[95]

The incidence of enuresis is difficult to determine because it is not a problem that parents readily share with others and because definitions vary according to cultural norms and family practices. According to research data, the incidence of enuresis in children older than 5 years ranges from 15% to 20%. Boys are more enuretic than girls by a ratio of 3:2. Teenage and adult enuresis is usually a continuation of childhood bed-wetting in about 2% of individuals.[96,97]

PATHOGENESIS Multiple pathologic factors are likely responsible for enuresis. All or part of each one might be operating in a given child. A reasonable approach is to eliminate organic or physiologic causes for enuresis before exploring the psychologic ones.

Table 37-7	Classification of Incontinence
Types of Incontinence	**Definition**
Total incontinence	Inability to store any urine; indicates an anatomic or functional absence of urinary sphincters (e.g., epispadias, myelomeningocele) or a bypassing of urinary sphincters (e.g., vesicovaginal fistula)
Overflow incontinence	Frequent dribbling that relieves a constantly full bladder; occurs when urinary outlet is obstructed
Urge incontinence	Sudden and uncontrollable need to void that cannot be suppressed; suggests bladder irritation
Precipitate voiding	Voiding without a preceding urge to void; suggests neurologic origin
Stress incontinence	Uncontrollable voiding that occurs when intravesical pressure momentarily exceeds intravesical resistance, as in "giggle incontinence"
Paradoxical incontinence	Incontinence in spite of normal voiding; suggests an ectopic ureteral orifice outside the urinary sphincter mechanism (e.g., a girl who is constantly wet, yet voids normally)

Organic causes of enuresis account for 2% to 10% of cases. The causes include urinary tract infections; neurologic disturbances; congenital defects of the meatus, urethra, and bladder neck; allergies; or alteration in renal tubular ion and water transport related to prostaglandin secretion.[98] Disorders that increase the normal output of urine, such as diabetes mellitus and diabetes insipidus, or disorders that impair the concentrating ability of the kidney must be considered in the evaluation of enuresis.

Enuresis in children is possibly caused by a maturational lag. Studies have demonstrated that the child with enuresis has a smaller functional bladder capacity than a nonenuretic child.[99] A number of children show a general developmental delay along with elevated intravesical pressure and spikelike detrusor contractions during bladder filling. Enuresis may spontaneously disappear in these children as they get older. Other studies have shown that children with enuresis completely fill and empty their bladder several times each night because of a constant urine output and a stable level of ADH. Children who remain dry usually have elevated levels of ADH and thus a decreased urine output at night which may be combined with reduced bladder capacity.[100] Still other studies indicated loss of diurnal variation in ADH.[101]

Genetic factors as a cause of enuresis are being investigated. Linkages have been proposed between nocturnal enuresis and chromosomes 8, 12, 13, and 22.[102] Bed-wetting does occur with high frequency among parents, siblings, and other near relatives of symptomatic children. These observations are further supported by a high concordance rate in enuretic monozygotic twins.

Recent research studying sleep and nocturnal enuresis indicates that enuresis may be related to non–rapid eye movement (non-REM) sleep, and that those with enuresis may spend more time in stage 3 sleep and have a greater depth of sleep.[103,104] Enuresis may be a symptom of obstructive sleep apnea. Inspiratory effort against a closed airway increases intrathoracic negative pressure causing cardiac distention and release of atrial natriuretic hormone and decreased vasopressin and renin-angiotensin-aldosterone complex. Children with nocturnal polyuria and enuresis should be evaluated for sleep-disordered breathing.[105]

A variety of psychosocial factors also have been postulated as explanations of enuresis. Enuresis has been associated with temper tantrums, fear reactions, excitability, low birth weight, and minimal brain dysfunction.[106,107]

CLINICAL MANIFESTATIONS Primary enuresis refers to a condition in which the child has never been continent. **Secondary enuresis,** or **acquired enuresis**, occurs when a child who has experienced a period of dryness of at least 3 to 6 months after toilet training becomes incontinent again. Secondary enuresis may be diurnal, nocturnal, or a combination of both. (Types of incontinence are defined in Table 37-7.) In 80% of children, enuresis that occurs at night only and more frequently than once a month is called **nocturnal enuresis.** Wetting during the day is called **diurnal enuresis.**

EVALUATION AND TREATMENT Evaluation of enuresis includes use of questionnaires, drinking and voiding charts, physical examination, and urinalysis. Underlying pathology, including kidney disease, vesicoureteral reflux, urinary tract infection, or neurogenic bladder, is excluded. Radiologic and urodynamic evaluation may be required.[108]

Behavioral interventions—such as self-awakening techniques, enuresis alarms, and motivational therapy—have good results in treating enuresis.[96,97] Treatment with desmopressin (an antidiuretic hormone analog) and tricyclics has similar beneficial effects, but most children relapse when treatment is stopped.[109,110] Desmopressin acetate nasal spray, a synthetic ADH, is best used when other treatments have not worked, but children must be evaluated for hyponatremia.[111] Psychotherapy and behavior modification are recommended when enuresis is associated with psychologic stress. Stress is reduced when families and caregivers receive information and support.[112]

Structure and Function of the Urinary System in Children

1. The Wilms tumor 1 gene and WNT signaling are important for kidney development, growth, and differentiation.
2. The kidney develops from three sets of structures: the pronephros (nonfunctional by the end of the embryonic period), mesonephros (nonfunctional), and metanephros (the functional kidney).
3. All nephrons are present at birth. The number does not increase with maturation, but they do increase in weight and function.
4. Urine formation begins by the third gestational month and contributes to the amniotic fluid.
5. Infants have a narrow chemical safety margin because of high hydrogen ion concentration, limited ability to regulate the internal environment, and lowered osmotic pressure.
6. Any disturbance, such as diarrhea, infection, fasting, or feeding alterations, can lead rapidly to severe acidosis and fluid imbalance in infants.
7. The composition of body fluids differs with age, thus making children more vulnerable to pathophysiologic changes.
8. Because the kidney develops from the medulla to the cortex, blood flow to the medullary nephrons is limited in infancy, and infants thus have limited urine-concentrating capacity.

Alterations in Renal and Bladder Function in Children

1. Congenital renal disorders affect about 1 out of 500 newborns. These disorders range in severity from minor, easily correctable anomalies to those incompatible with life.
2. Horseshoe kidney is a single U-shaped kidney that develops from fusion of the kidneys as they descend from the midline. The kidney may be asymptomatic or associated with hydronephrosis, stone formation, or infection.
3. Hypospadias is a congenital condition in which the urethral meatus is located on the undersurface of the penis; epispadias is a congenital condition in which the urethral opening is located on the dorsal surface of the penis.
4. Exstrophy of the bladder is a congenital malformation in which the pubic bones are separated, the lower portion of the abdominal wall and anterior wall of the bladder are missing, and the back wall of the bladder is everted through the opening.
5. Ureteropelvic junction obstruction is blockage where the renal pelvis joins the ureter and is often caused by smooth muscle or urothelial malformation or scarring that leads to hydronephrosis.
6. Bladder outlet obstruction is usually caused by urethral valves or polyps.
7. A dysplastic kidney is the result of abnormal differentiation of renal tissues. The hypoplastic kidney is a very small but otherwise normal kidney.

8. Renal agenesis is the failure of a kidney to grow or develop. The condition may be unilateral or bilateral and may occur as an isolated entity or in association with other disorders.
9. Polycystic kidney disease is an autosomal dominant disorder in which the renal tubule or epithelium proliferates; excessive fluid transport causes cyst formation and obstruction.
10. Glomerulonephritis is an inflammation of the glomeruli secondary to immune mechanisms characterized by hematuria, edema, and hypertension. The cause is unknown but poststreptococcal glomerulonephritis may occur after infection, especially of the upper respiratory tract.
11. IgA nephropathies result from deposition of IgA immunoglobulins and other immune products in the mesangium of the glomerular capillaries. It is the most common type of childhood glomerulonephritis.
12. Henoch-Schönlein nephritis is an IgA nephropathy that affects glomerular blood vessels.
13. Hemolytic uremic syndrome is an acute disorder characterized by hemolytic anemia, acute renal failure, and thrombocytopenia and can be associated with *E. coli* verotoxin.
14. Nephrotic syndrome is a term used to describe a symptom complex characterized by proteinuria, hypoproteinemia, hyperlipidemia, and edema. Metabolic, biochemical, or physiochemical disturbance in the glomerular basement membrane leads to increased permeability to protein. The most common form is minimal change nephropathy.
15. Acute or chronic renal injury is rare in children and the most common cause is prerenal acute renal failure related to dehydration, sepsis, or hemorrhage.
16. Urinary tract infections can result from general sepsis in the newborn but are caused by bacteria ascending the urethra in older children. The bladder alone is infected in cystitis. The infection ascends to the kidney or kidneys in pyelonephritis. Urinary tract anomalies must be surgically corrected to prevent frequent recurrent infections.
17. Vesicoureteral reflux, which refers to the retrograde flow of bladder urine into the ureters, provides mechanisms for bladder infection in children whose ureters are shorter than those of adults. It can be unilateral or bilateral.
18. Wilms tumor is an embryonal tumor of the kidney that usually presents between birth and 5 years of age as an inherited (5% to 10%) or sporadic form. The tumor can be successfully treated by surgery, with a combination of drugs, and, sometimes, radiation therapy.
19. Enuresis refers to the involuntary passage of urine. Enuresis may occur during the day (diurnally) or night (nocturnally). The disorder tends to occur during non-REM sleep and can have a variety of organic and psychologic causes.

Acquired enuresis, 1415
Acute poststreptococcal glomerulonephritis (PSGN), 1407
Acute pyelonephritis, 1411
Anaphylactoid purpura, 1408
Chordee, 1405
Chronic pyelonephritis, 1412
Cloacal exstrophy, 1406

Congenital nephrotic syndrome (Finnish type), 1410
Cystitis, 1411
Diurnal enuresis, 1415
Edema, 1410
Enuresis, 1414
Epispadias, 1405
Exstrophy of the bladder, 1405

Focal segmental glomerulosclerosis (FSGS), 1409
Glomerulonephritis, 1407
Hemolytic uremic syndrome, 1408
Henoch-Schönlein purpura nephritis, 1408
Horseshoe kidney, 1404
Hypercoagulation, 1410
Hyperlipidemia, 1410

KEY TERMS—cont'd

Hypoplastic kidney, 1406
Hypospadias, 1404
Immunoglobulin A (IgA) nephropathy
   (Berger nephropathy), 1408
Mesonephros, 1402
Metanephros, 1402
Minimal change nephropathy (MCN), 1409
Nephroblastoma, 1413
Nephrotic syndrome, 1409
Nocturnal enuresis, 1415
Polycystic kidney disease (PKD), 1407
Potter syndrome, 1407

Primary enuresis, 1415
Primary (idiopathic) nephrotic
   syndrome, 1409
Pronephros, 1402
Renal agenesis, 1407
Renal aplasia, 1406
Renal dysplasia, 1406
Secondary enuresis, 1415
Secondary nephrotic syndrome, 1409
Secondary uteropelvic junction (UPJ)
   obstruction, 1406
Unilateral renal agenesis, 1407

Urethral atresia, 1406
Urethral polyp, 1406
Urethral valve, 1406
Urinary tract infection (UTI), 1411
Ureteropelvic junction (UPJ)
   obstruction, 1406
Vesicoureteral reflux (VUR), 1412
Wilms tumor, 1413

REFERENCES

1. Menke Al, Schedl A: WT1 and glomerular function, *Semin Cell Dev Biol* 14(4):233-240, 2003.
2. Merkel CE, Karner CM, Carroll TJ: Molecular regulation of kidney development: is the answer blowing in the Wnt? *Pediatr Nephrol* 22(11):1825-1838, 2007.
3. Bonilla-Felix M: Development of water transport in the collecting duct, *Am J Physiol Renal Physiol* 287(6):F1093-F1101, 2004.
4. Hartnoll G: Basic principles and practical steps in the management of fluid balance in the newborn, *Semin Neonatol* 8(4):307-313, 2003.
5. Schedl A: Renal abnormalities and their developmental origin, *Nat Rev Genet* 8(10):791-802, 2007.
6. Weizer AZ et al: Determining the incidence of horseshoe kidney from radiographic data at a single institution, *J Urol* 170(5):1722-1726, 2003.
7. McAninch JW: Disorders of the kidneys. In Taragho EA, McAninch JW, editors: *Smith's general urology*, Norwalk, CT, 1995, Appleton & Lange.
8. Kelalis PP, Lowell RK, Bellmam BA: *Clinical pediatric oncology*, ed 3, Philadelphia, 1992, Saunders.
9. Nelson CP et al: The increasing incidence of congenital penile anomalies in the United States, *J Urol* 174(4 Pt 2):1573-1576, 2005.
10. Leung AK, Robson WL: Hypospadias: an update, *Asian J Androl* 9(1):16-22, 2007.
11. Grady RW, Mitchell ME: Management of epispadias, *Urol Clin North Am* 29(2):349-360, vi, 2002.
12. Frimberger D, Gearhart JP, Mathews R: Female exstrophy: failure of initial reconstruction and its implications for continence, *J Urol* 170(6 PT 1):2428-2431, 2003.
13. Jones D, Parkinson S, Hosalkar HS: Oblique pelvic osteotomy in the exstrophy/epispadias complex, *J Bone Joint Surg Br* 88(6):799-806, 2006.
14. Thomas JC et al: First stage approximation of the exstrophic bladder in patients with cloacal exstrophy—should this be the initial surgical approach in all patients? *J Urol* 178(4 Pt2):1632-1635, 2007.
15. Zhang PL, Peters CA, Rosen S: Ureteropelvic junction obstruction: morphological and clinical studies, *Pediatr Nephrol* 14(8-9):820-826, 2000.
16. Rosen S et al: The kidney in congenital ureteropelvic junction obstruction: a spectrum from normal to nephrectomy, *J Urol* 179(4):1257-1263, 2008.
17. Fefer S, Ellsworth P: Prenatal hydronephrosis, *Pediatr Clin North Am* 53(3):429-447, 2006.
18. Stein RJ, Gill IS, Desai MM: Comparison of surgical approaches to ureteropelvic junction obstruction: endopyeloplasty versus endopyelotomy versus laparoscopic pyeloplasty, *Curr Urol Rep* 8(2):140-149, 2007.
19. Shokier AA, Nijman RJ: Primary megaureter: current trends in diagnosis and treatment, *BJU Int* 86(7):861-868, 2000.
20. Krishnan A et al: The anatomy and embryology of posterior urethral valves, *J Urol* 175(4):1214-1220, 2006.
21. Demircan M et al: Urethral polyps in children: a review of the literature and report of two cases, *Int J Urol* 13(6):841-843, 2006.

22. Baird JM et al: Long-term outcomes in children treated by prenatal vesicoamniotic shunting for lower urinary tract obstruction, *Obstet Gynecol* 106(3):503-508, 2005.
23. Narasimhan KL et al: Does mode of treatment affect the outcome of neonatal posterior urethral valves? *J Urol* 171(6 Pt 1):2423-2426, 2004.
24. Arant BS Jr, Sotelo-Avila C, Bernstein J: Segmental "hypoplasia" of the kidney (ask-upmark), *J Pediatr* 95(6):931-939, 1979.
25. Dursan H et al: Associated anomalies in children with congenital solitary functioning kidney, *Pediatr Surg Int* 21(6):456-459, 2005.
26. Glazebrook KN, McGrath FP, Steele BT: Prenatal compensatory renal growth: documentation with US, *Radiology* 189(3):733, 1993.
27. Cascio S, Paran S, Puri P: Associated urological anomalies in children with unilateral renal agenesis, *J Urol* 162(3 Pt 2):1081, 1999.
28. Parikh CR et al: Congenital renal agenesis: case-control analysis of birth characteristics, *Am J Kidney Dis* 39:689-694, 2002.
29. Sutters M: The pathogenesis of autosomal dominant polycystic kidney disease, *Nephron Exp Nephrol* 103(4):e149-e155, 2006.
30. Chang MY, Ong AC: Autosomal dominant polycystic kidney disease: recent advances in pathogenesis and treatment, *Nephron Physiol* 108(1):1-7, 2008.
31. Al-Bhalal L, Akhtar M: Molecular basis of autosomal recessive polycystic kidney disease (ARPKD), *Adv Anat Pathol* 15(1):54-58, 2008.
32. Richter CM: Role of endothelin in chronic renal failure-developments in renal involvement, *Rheumatology (Oxford)* 47(2):234-235, 2008.
33. Novak J et al: IgA glycosylation and IgA immune complexes in the pathogenesis of IgA nephropathy, *Semin Nephrol* 28(1):78-87, 2008.
34. Moura IC et al: The glomerular response to IgA deposition in IgA nephropathy, *Semin Nephrol* 28(1):88-95, 2008.
35. Berthoux FC, Mohey H, Afiani A: Natural history of primary IgA nephropathy, *Semin Nephrol* 28(1):4-9, 2008.
36. Kawamura T: treatment of IgA nephropathy: corticosteroids, tonsillectomy and mycophenolate mofetil, *Contrib Nephrol* 157:37-33, 2007.
37. Coppo R: Pediatric IgA nephropathy: clinical and therapeutic perspectives, *Semin Nephrol* 28(1):18-26, 2008.
38. Syrhanen J, Mustonen J, Pasternack A: Hypertriglyceridaemia and hyperuricaemia are risk factors for progression of IgA nephropathy, *Nephrol Dial Transplant* 15(1):34, 2000.
39. Delos Santos NM, Wyatt RS: Pediatric IgA nephropathies: clinical aspects and therapeutic approaches, *Semin Nephrol* 24(3):269-286, 2004.
40. Rieu P, Noel LH: Henoch-Schönlein nephritis in children and adults. Morphological features and clinicopathological correlations, *Ann Med Interne (Paris)* 150(2):151, 1999.
41. Zaffanello M, Brugnara M, Franchini M: Therapy for children with Henoch-Schönlein purpura nephritis: a systematic review, *Scientific World Journal* 7:20-30, 2007.
42. Miller DP et al: Incidence of thrombotic thrombocytopenic purpura/hemolytic uremic syndrome, *Epidemiology* 15(2):208-215, 2004.
43. Serna A 4th, Boedeker EC: Pathogenesis and treatment of Shiga toxin-producing *Escherichia coli* infections, *Curr Opin Gastroenterol* 24(1):38-47, 2008.
44. Franchini M, Zaffanello M, Veneri D: Advances in the pathogenesis, diagnosis and treatment of thrombotic thrombocytopenic purpura and hemolytic uremic syndrome, *Thromb Res* 118(2):177-184, 2006.

45. Iijima K, Kamioka I, Nozu K: Management of diarrhea-associated hemolytic uremic syndrome in children, *Clin Exp Nephrol* 12(1):16-19, 2008.

46. Repetto HA: Long-term course and mechanisms of progression of renal disease in hemolytic uremic syndrome, *Kidney Int Suppl* 8(97):S102-S106, 2005.

47. Behrman RE, Kliegman RM, Jenson HB, editors: *Nelson textbook of pediatrics*, ed 17, Philadelphia, 2004, Saunders.

48. Salomon R et al: NF-kappa B p65 antagonizes IL-4 induction by c-maf in minimal change nephrotic syndrome, *J Immunol* 172(1):688-698, 2004.

49. Tain YL, Chen TY, Yang KD: Implications of serum TNF-beta and IL-13 in the treatment response of childhood nephrotic syndrome, *Cytokine* 21(3):155-159, 2003.

50. Saland JM, Ginsberg H, Fisher EA: Dyslipidemia in pediatric renal disease: epidemiology, pathophysiology, and management, *Curr Opin Pediatr* 14(2):197-204, 2002.

51. Borges et al: Is focal segmental glomerulosclerosis increasing in patients with nephritic syndrome? *Pediatr Nephrol* 22(9):1309-1313, 2007.

52. Kim SW, Frokiaer J, Nielsen S: Pathogenesis of oedema in nephrotic syndrome: role of epithelial sodium channel, *Nephrology (Carlton)* 12(Suppl 3):8-10, 2007.

53. Zaffanello M, Franchini M: Thromboembolism in childhood nephrotic syndrome: a rare but serious complication, *Hematology* 12(1):69-73, 2007.

54. Simons M, Huber TB: It's not all about nephrin, *Kidney Int* 73(6):697-704, 2008.

55. Hinkes BG: Nephrotic syndrome in the first year of life: two thirds of cases are caused by mutations in four genes (NPHS1, NPHS2, WT1, and LAMB2), *Pediatrics* 119(4):Le907-Le919, 2007.

56. Mattoo TK: Gingival hyperplasia in congenital and infantile nephrotic syndrome, *Pediatr Nephrol* 11(3):388, 1997.

57. Hodson EM, Willis NS, Craig JC: Corticosteroid treatment for nephrotic syndrome in children, *Cochrane Database Syst Rev* 17(4):CD001533, 2007.

58. Hodson EM, Willis NS, Craig JC: Non-corticosteroid treatment for nephrotic syndrome in children, *Cochrane Database Syst Rev* 23(1):CD002290, 2008.

59. Crosson JT: Focal segmental glomerulosclerosis and renal transplantation, *Transplant Proc* 39(3):737-743, 2007.

60. Akcan-Arikan A et al: Modified RIFLE criteria in critically ill children with acute kidney injury, *Kidney Int* 71(10):1028-1035, 2007.

61. Andreoli SP: Acute renal failure in the newborn, *Semin Perinatol* 28(2):112-123, 2004.

62. Hari P et al: Chronic renal failure in children, *Indian Pediatr* 40(11):1035-1042, 2003.

63. Seikaly MG et al: Acute renal failure in the newborn, *Semin Perinatol* 28(2):112-123, 2004.

64. Magee JC et al: Pediatric transplantation, *Am J Transplant* 4(Suppl 9):54-71, 2004.

65. Magee JC et al: Pediatric transplantation in the United States, 1997-2006, *Am J Transplant* 8(4 Pt 2):935-945, 2008.

66. Seikaly MG et al: Use of rhGH in children with chronic kidney disease: lessons from NAPRTCS, *Pediatr Nephrol* 22(8):1195-1204, 2007.

67. Sedberry-Ross S, Pohl HG: Urinary tract infections in children, *Curr Urol Rep* 9(2):165-171, 2008.

68. Kanellopoulos TA et al: First urinary tract infection in neonates, infants and young children: a comparative study, *Pediatr Nephrol* 21(8):1131-1137, 2006.

69. Chang SL, Shortliffe LD: Pediatric urinary tract infections, *Ped Clin North Am* 53(3):379-400, 2006.

70. Le Saux N, Pham B, Moher D: Evaluating the benefits of antimicrobial prophylaxis to prevent urinary tract infections in children: a systemic review, *CMAJ* 163(5):523, 2000.

71. Jantausch BA et al: Association of Lewis blood group phenotypes with urinary tract infection in children, *J Pediatr* 124(6):863-868, 1994.

72. Bauer R, Kogan BA: New developments in the diagnosis and management of pediatric UTIs, *Urol Clin North Am* 35(1):47-58, 2008.

73. Michael M et al: Short versus standard duration oral antibiotic therapy for acute urinary tract infection in children, *Cochrane Database Syst Rev* (1):CD003966, 2003.

74. Mak RH, Kuo HJ: Primary urethral reflux: emerging insights from molecular and genetic studies, *Curr Opin Pediatr* 15(2):181-185, 2003.

75. Sillen U: Vesicoureteral reflux in infants, *Pediatr Nephrol* 13(4):355, 1999.

76. Chandra M, Maddix H: Urodynamic dysfunction in infants with vesicoureteral reflux, *J Pediatr* 136(6):754, 2000.

77. Jakobsson G, Jacobson SH, Hjalmas K: Vesico-ureteric reflux and other risk factors for renal damage: identification of high- and low-risk children, *Acta Pediatr Suppl* 88(431):31, 1999.

78. Smith EA: Pyelonephritis, renal scarring, and reflux nephropathy: a pediatric urologist's perspective, *Pediatr Radiol* 38(Suppl 1):S76-S82, 2008.

79. Koyle MA, Caldamone AA: Part 4: considerations regarding the medical management of VUR: what have we really learned? *Curr Med Res Opin* 23(Suppl 4):S21-S25, 2007.

80. Hensle TW et al: Part 2: examining pediatric vesicoureteral reflux: a real-world evaluation of treatment patterns and outcomes, *Curr Med Res Opin* 23(Suppl 4):S7-S13, 2007.

81. MacNeily AE, Afshar K: Screening asymptomatic siblings for vesicoureteral reflux sound science or religious rhetoric? *Can J Urol* 13(6):3309-3316, 2006.

82. Chertin B, Puri P: Familial vesicoureteral reflux, *J Urol* 269(5):1804-1808, 2003.

83. Peeden JN, Noe HN: Is it practical to screen for familial vesicoureteral reflux within a private pediatric practice? *Pediatrics* 89(4):758, 1992.

84. Fukuzawa R, Reeve AE: Molecular pathology and epidemiology of nephrogenic rests and Wilms tumors, *J Pediatr Hematol Oncol* 29(9):589-594, 2007.

85. National Cancer Institute: Wilms tumor and other childhood kidney tumors treatment (PDQ), 2009. Available from www.cancer.gov/cancertopics/pdq/treatment/wilms/HealthProfessional/page2

86. Brown KW, Malik KTA: The molecular biology of Wilms tumour, *Exp Rev Mol Med*. Available from www.expertreviews.org/010030227h.htm.

87. Peres EM et al: Chromosome analyses of 16 cases of Wilms tumor: different pattern in unfavorable histology, *Cancer Cenet Cytogenet* 148(1):66-70, 2004.

88. Perotti D et al: Functional inactivation of the WTX gene is not a frequent event in Wilms tumors, *Oncogene* 27(33):4625-4632, 2008.

89. Rivera MN et al: An X chromosome gene, WTX, is commonly inactivated in Wilms tumor, *Science* 315(5812):642-645, 2007.

90. Belasco J, Chatten J, D'Angio G: Wilms tumor. In Sutow W, Fernbach D, Vietti T, editors: *Clinical pediatric oncology*, ed 3, St Louis, 1984, Mosby.

91. Kurli M, Finger PT: The kidney, cancer, and the eye: current concepts, *Surv Ophthalmol* 50(6):507-518, 2005.

92. Nicholson HS et al: Uterine anomalies in Wilms' tumor survivors, *Cancer* 78(4):887, 1996.

93. Green DM: The diagnosis and management of Wilms' tumor, *Pediatr Clin North Am* 32:735, 1985.

94. Neville HL, Ritchey ML: Wilms' tumor: overview of National Wilms' Tumor Study Group results, *Urol Clin North Am* 27(3):435, 2000.

95. Djurhuus JC, Rittig S: Nocturnal enuresis, *Curr Opin Urol* 12(4):317-320, 2002.

96. Glazener CM, Evans JH: Simple behavioral and physical interventions for nocturnal enuresis in children, *Cocharane Database Syst Rev* (2):CD003637.

97. Glazener CM, Evans JH, Peto RE: Alarm interventions for nocturnal enuresis in children, *Cochrane Database Syst Rev* (2):CD002911.

98. Kamperis K et al: Nocturnal polyuria in monosymptomatic nocturnal enuresis refractory to desmopressin treatment, *Am J Physiol Renal Physiol* 291(6):F1232-F1240, 2006.

99. Troup CW, Hodgson NB: Nocturnal functional bladder capacity in enuretic children, *J Urol* 105:129, 1971.

100. Stark M: Assessment and management of the care of children with nocturnal enuresis: guidelines for primary care, *Nurs Pract Forum* 5(3):170, 1994.

101. Uygur MC, Ergen A, Remzi D: Enuresis nocturna: new concepts in pathophysiology, *Int Urol Nephrol* 27(4):439, 1995.

102. Gontard A et al: Molecular genetics of nocturnal enuresis: linkage to a locus on chromosome 22, *Scand J Urol Nephrol Suppl* 202:76, 1999.

103. Neveus T: The role of sleep and arousal in nocturnal enuresis, *Acta Pediatr* 92(10):1118-1123, 2003.

104. Neveus T et al: Sleep of children with enuresis: a polysomnographic study, *Pediatrics* 103(6 part 1):1193, 1999.

105. Firoozi F et al: Resolution of diurnal incontinence and nocturnal enuresis after adenotonsillectomy in children, *J Urol* 175(5): 1885-1888, 2006.

106. Backes M et al: Cognitive and behavioral profile of fragile X boys: correlations to molecular data, *Am J Med Genet* 95(2):150-156, 2000.

107. Von Gontard A, Hollmann E: Comorbidity of functional urinary incontinence and encoporesis: somatic and behavioral associations, *J Urol* 171(6 Pt 2):2644-2647, 2004.

108. Feldman AS, Gauer SB: Diagnosis and management of dysfunctional voiding, *Curr Opin Pediatr* 18(2):139-147, 2006.

109. Cutting DA, Pallant JF, Cutting FM: Nocturnal enuresis: application of evidence-based medicine in community practice, *J Paediatr Child Health* 43(3):167-172, 2007.

110. Zaffanello M et al: Therapeutic options in childhood nocturnal enuresis, *Minerva Urol Nefrol* 59(2):199-205, 2007.

111. Robson WL, Leung AK, Norgaard JP: The comparative safety of oral versus intranasal desmopressin for the treatment of children with nocturnal enuresis, *J Urol* 178(1):24-30, 2007.

112. Weaver A, Dobson P: Nocturnal enuresis in children, *J Fam Health Care* 17(5):159-161, 2007.

STRUCTURE AND FUNCTION OF THE DIGESTIVE SYSTEM

SUE E. HUETHER

MEDIA RESOURCES

CHAPTER OUTLINE

THE GASTROINTESTINAL TRACT
  Mouth and Esophagus
  Stomach
  Small Intestine
  Large Intestine
  Intestinal Bacteria
ACCESSORY ORGANS OF DIGESTION
  Liver
  Gallbladder
  Exocrine Pancreas

TESTS OF DIGESTIVE FUNCTION
  Gastrointestinal Tract
  Liver
  Gallbladder
  Exocrine Pancreas
Aging and the Gastrointestinal System

The digestive system breaks down ingested food, prepares it for uptake by the body's cells, provides body water, and eliminates wastes. This system consists of the gastrointestinal tract and accessory organs of digestion: the liver, gallbladder, and exocrine pancreas.

Food breakdown begins in the mouth with chewing and continues in the stomach, where food is churned and mixed with acid, mucus, enzymes, and other secretions. From the stomach, the fluid and partially digested food pass into the small intestine, where biochemicals and enzymes secreted by the liver and exocrine pancreas, and small intestinal epithelium break it down into absorbable components of proteins, carbohydrates, and fats. These nutrients pass through the walls of the small intestine into blood vessels and lymphatics that carry them to the liver via the portal circulation for further processing and storage.

Ingested substances and secretions that are not absorbed in the small intestine pass into the large intestine, where fluid continues to be absorbed. Fluid wastes travel to the kidneys and are eliminated in the urine. Solid wastes pass into the rectum and are eliminated from the body through the anus.

Except for chewing, swallowing, and defecation of solid wastes, the movements of the digestive system (gastrointestinal motility) are controlled by hormones and the autonomic nervous system. As ingested substances move through the gastrointestinal tract, they trigger the release of hormones that stimulate or inhibit (1) the muscular contractions that mix and propel food from the esophagus to the anus and (2) the timely secretion of substances that aid in digestion. The autonomic innervation, sympathetic and parasympathetic, is controlled by centers in the brain and by local stimuli that are mediated by neural plexuses within the gastrointestinal walls.

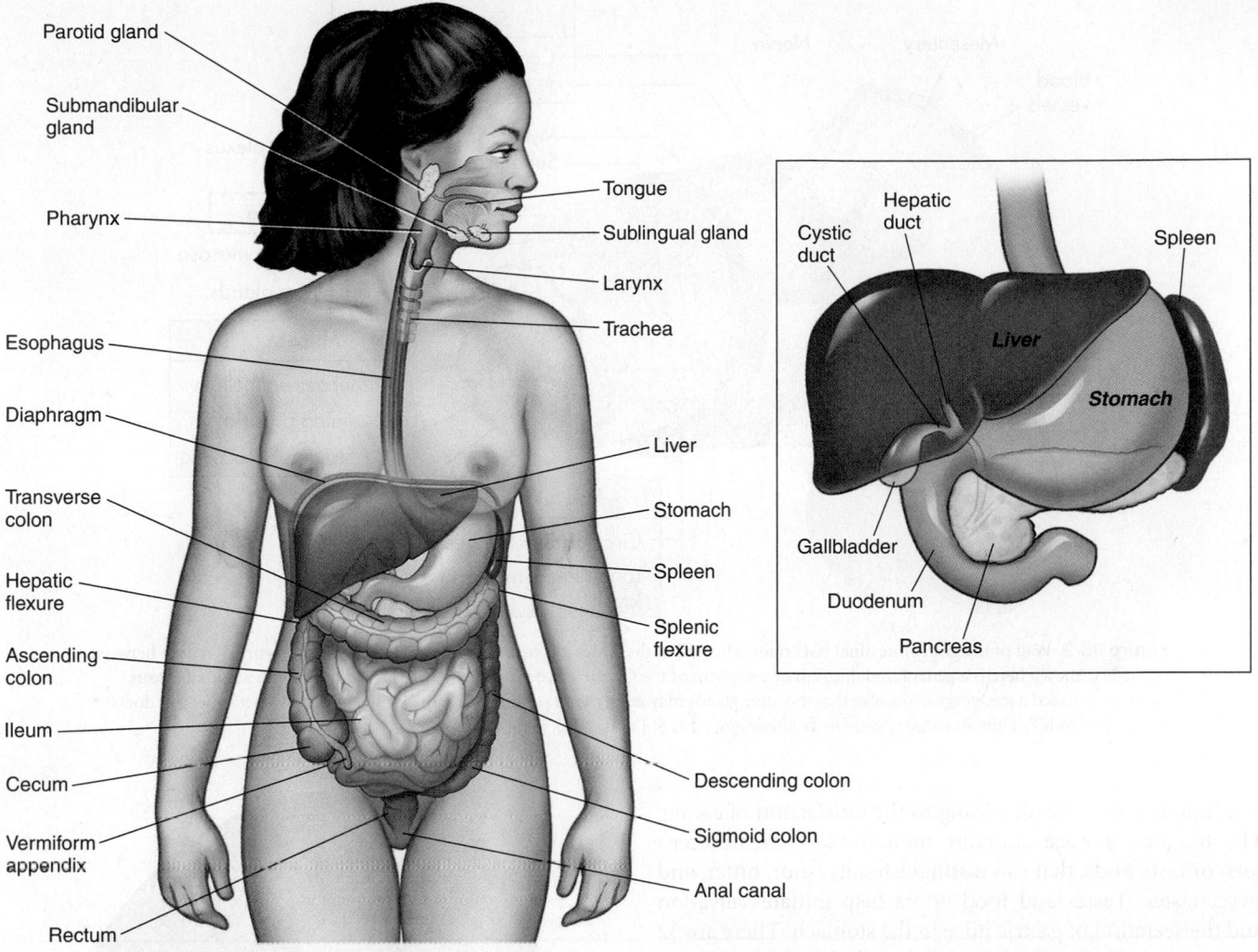

Figure 38-1 Structure and function of the digestive system. Digestion begins in the mouth with chewing, which breaks down food mechanically and mixes it with saliva. Swallowing propels chewed food through the esophagus to the stomach, where acids and stomach motility liquefy it further. Next the liquefied food enters the small intestine, where secretions of the intestinal walls, liver, gallbladder, and pancreas digest it into absorbable nutrients. Nutrients are absorbed through intestinal walls, and unabsorbed wastes enter the large intestine (colon), where fluids are removed. Solid wastes then enter the rectum and leave the body through the anus. (From Patton KT, Thibodeau GA: *Anatomy & physiology*, ed 7, St Louis, 2010, Mosby.)

THE GASTROINTESTINAL TRACT

The **gastrointestinal tract (alimentary canal)** consists of the mouth, esophagus, stomach, small intestine, large intestine, rectum, and anus (Figure 38-1). It carries out the following digestive processes:

1. Ingestion of food
2. Propulsion of food and wastes from the mouth to the anus
3. Secretion of mucus, water, and enzymes
4. Mechanical digestion of food particles
5. Chemical digestion of food particles
6. Absorption of digested food
7. Elimination of waste products by defecation

Histologically the gastrointestinal tract consists of four layers. From the inside out they are the mucosa, submucosa, muscularis, and serosa or adventitia. These concentric layers vary in thickness, and each layer has sublayers (Figure 38-2). Intrinsic nerves are located solely within the gastrointestinal tract and are controlled by local and autonomic nervous system stimuli through the **enteric plexus,** which comprises three nerve plexuses located in different layers of the gastrointestinal walls. The **submucosal plexus (Meissner plexus)** is located in the muscularis mucosae, the **myenteric plexus (Auerbach plexus)** between the inner circular and outer longitudinal muscle layers (tunica muscularis), and the **subserosal plexus** just beneath the serosa. These enteric nerve circuits regulate motility reflexes, blood flow, absorption, secretions, and immune response.[1]

Mouth and Esophagus

The **mouth** is a reservoir for the chewing and mixing of food with saliva. As food particles become smaller and move around in the mouth, the taste buds and olfactory nerves are

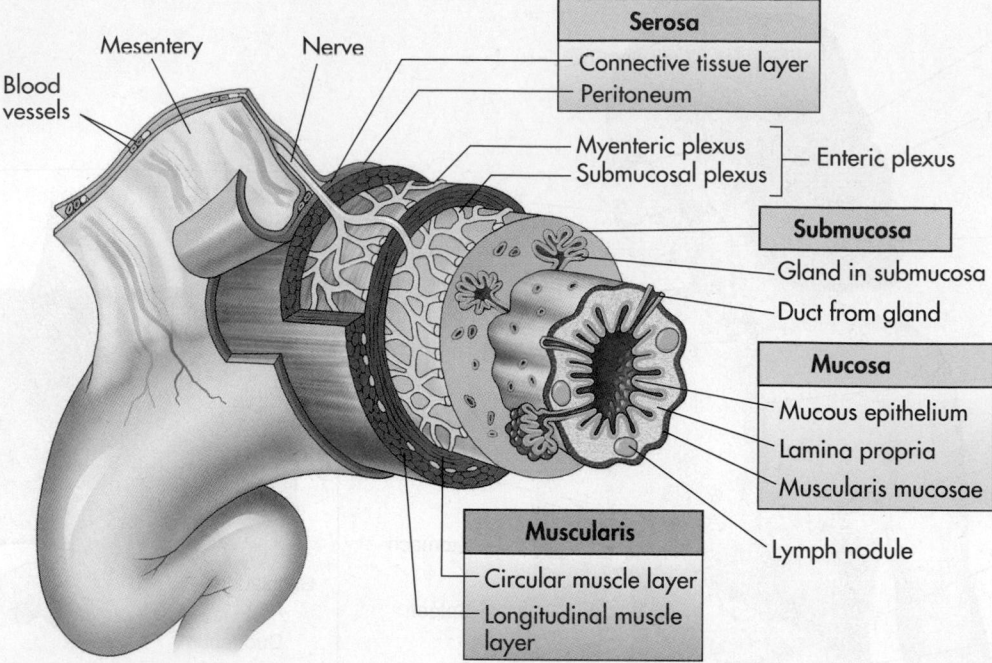

Figure 38-2 Wall of the gastrointestinal (GI) tract. The wall of the GI tract is made up of four layers with a network of nerves between the layers. Shown here is a generalized diagram of a segment of the GI tract. Note that the serosa is continuous with a fold of serous membrane called a *mesentery*. Note also that digestive glands may empty their products into the lumen of the GI tract by way of ducts. (From Patton KT, Thibodeau GA: *Anatomy & physiology*, ed 7, St Louis, 2010, Mosby.)

continuously stimulated, adding to the satisfaction of eating. The tongue's surface contains thousands of chemoreceptors, or taste buds, that can distinguish salty, sour, bitter, and sweet tastes. Tastes and food odors help initiate salivation and the secretion of gastric juice in the stomach. There are 32 permanent teeth in the adult mouth, and they are important for speech and mastication.

Salivation

The three pairs of **salivary glands** (the submandibular, sublingual, and parotid glands) (Figure 38-3) secrete about 1 L of saliva per day. **Saliva** consists mostly of water that contains varying amounts of mucus; sodium; bicarbonate; chloride; potassium; and **salivary α-amylase (ptyalin),** an enzyme that initiates carbohydrate digestion in the mouth and stomach.

The sympathetic and parasympathetic divisions of the autonomic nervous system control salivation. Because cholinergic parasympathetic fibers stimulate the salivary glands, atropine (an anticholinergic agent) inhibits salivation and makes the mouth dry. β-Adrenergic stimulation from sympathetic fibers also increases salivary secretion. The salivary glands are not regulated by hormones.

The composition of saliva depends on the rate of secretion (Figure 38-4). Aldosterone can increase an exchange of sodium for potassium, increasing sodium conservation and potassium excretion. The bicarbonate concentration of saliva sustains a pH of about 7.4, which neutralizes bacterial acids and prevents tooth decay. Saliva also contains immunoglobulin

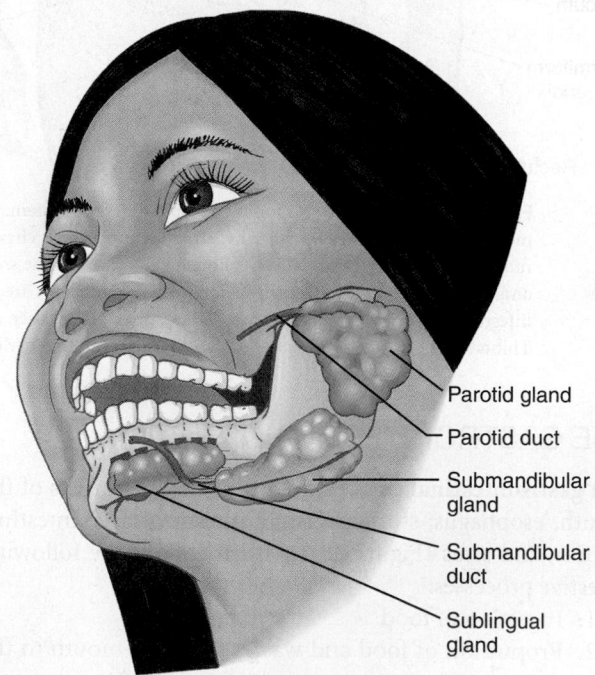

Figure 38-3 Salivary glands. (From Patton KT, Thibodeau GA: *Anatomy & physiology*, ed 7, St Louis, 2010, Mosby.)

A (IgA), which helps prevent infection. Exogenous fluoride (e.g., fluoride in drinking water) is absorbed and then secreted in the saliva, providing additional protection against tooth decay.

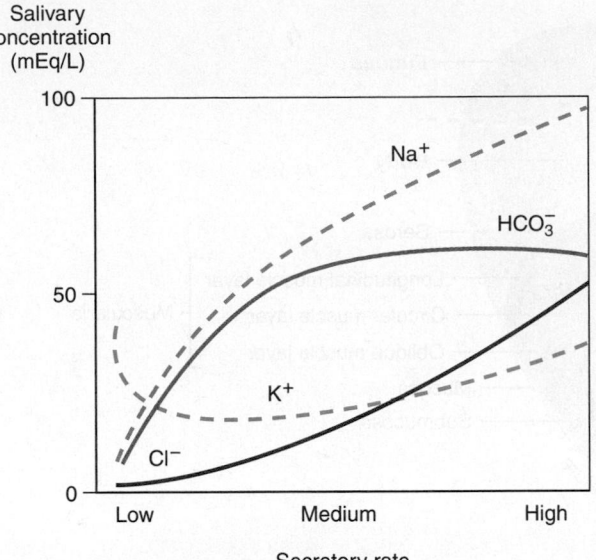

Figure 38-4 Salivary electrolyte concentrations and flow rate. Changes in concentration of sodium (Na^+), potassium (K^+), chloride (Cl^-), and bicarbonate HCO_3^- with increases in flow rate of saliva. *Green line,* Sodium; *orange line,* bicarbonate; *red line,* chloride; *blue line,* potassium.

Swallowing

The **esophagus** is a hollow muscular tube approximately 25 cm long that conducts substances from the oropharynx to the stomach (see Figure 38-1). Swallowed food is moved to the stomach by esophageal **peristalsis,** the coordinated sequential contraction and relaxation of outer longitudinal and inner circular layers of muscles. The upper third of the esophagus contains striated muscle that is directly innervated by motor neurons. The middle third contains a mix of striated and smooth muscle, and the lower third is smooth muscle that is innervated by preganglionic cholinergic fibers from the vagus nerve. The muscles are activated in a downward sequence. Peristalsis is stimulated when afferent fibers distributed along the length of the esophagus sense changes in wall tension caused by stretching as food passes. The greater the tension, the greater the intensity of esophageal contraction. Occasionally, intense contractions cause pain similar to "heartburn" or angina.

Each end of the esophagus is opened and closed by a sphincter. The **upper esophageal sphincter (cricopharyngeal muscle)** prevents entry of air into the esophagus during respiration.[2] The **lower esophageal sphincter (cardiac sphincter)** prevents regurgitation from the stomach. The lower esophageal sphincter is located near the esophageal hiatus—the opening in the diaphragm where the esophagus ends at the stomach.

Swallowing is a complex event mediated by the swallowing center, which is located in the reticular formation of the brainstem and also involves other brain regions, including the insula/claustrum and cerebellum.[3,4] Swallowing occurs in two phases: the oropharyngeal (voluntary) phase and the esophageal (involuntary) phase. During the **oral and pharyngeal phases of swallowing,** food is segmented into a bolus by the tongue and forced posteriorly toward the pharynx as the tongue pushes upward against the hard palate. The swallowing center and respiratory center provide the coordinating innervation. The superior constrictor muscle of the pharynx contracts, preventing movement of food into the nasopharynx. At the same time, respiration is inhibited and the epiglottis slides downward to prevent the bolus from entering the larynx and trachea. The movements of the tongue and pharyngeal constrictors propel the food into the esophagus in a series of coordinated events, taking less than 1 or 2 seconds.[5]

The **esophageal phase of swallowing** begins as the bolus of food enters the esophagus. The bolus is transported by peristalsis—the sequential waves of smooth muscle contractions that travel down the esophagus and are preceded by receptive waves of relaxation.[6] The wave of relaxation reduces resistance and allows food to pass, after which the wave of contraction pushes food farther along. The terminal 1 to 2 cm of musculature act as a lower esophageal sphincter and it relaxes just before the arrival of a peristaltic wave. The sphincter muscles return to their resting tone after the bolus of food passes into the stomach. The esophageal phase of swallowing takes 5 to 10 seconds, with the bolus moving 2 to 6 cm/second. Throughout swallowing, the sphincters and esophagus work in concert with the peristaltic wave that moves food from the mouth to the stomach.[7]

Peristalsis that immediately follows the oropharyngeal phase of swallowing is called **primary peristalsis.** If a bolus of food becomes stuck in the esophageal lumen, the distention of the esophageal wall stimulates **secondary peristalsis,** a wave of contraction and relaxation that is independent of voluntary swallowing. This is in response to stretch receptors that are stimulated by increased wall tension, causing an increase in impulses from the swallowing center of the brain.

When it is closed, the lower esophageal sphincter serves as a barrier between the stomach and esophagus. The muscle tone of the lower sphincter changes with neural and hormonal stimulation and relaxes with swallowing. Cholinergic vagal input and the digestive hormone gastrin increase sphincter tone. Nonadrenergic, noncholinergic vagal impulses relax the lower esophageal sphincter, as do the hormones progesterone, secretin, and glucagon. Relaxation during swallowing is mediated by the vagus.[8]

Stomach

The **stomach** is a hollow muscular organ that stores food during eating, secretes digestive juices, mixes food with these juices, and propels partially digested food, called **chyme,** into the duodenum of the small intestine. The anatomy of the stomach is presented in Figure 38-5. Its major anatomic boundaries are the lower esophageal sphincter, where food passes through the **cardiac orifice** (gastroduodenal junction) into the stomach; the greater and lesser curvatures; and the **pyloric sphincter,** which relaxes as food is propelled through the **pylorus** into the duodenum. Functional areas of

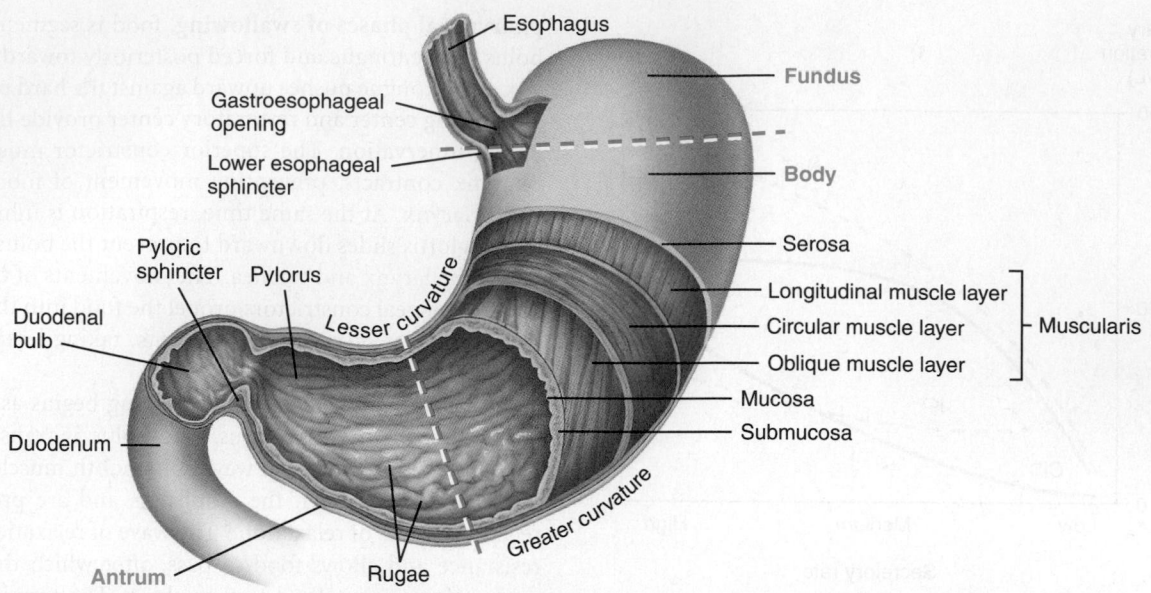

Figure 38-5 Stomach. A portion of the anterior wall has been cut away to reveal the muscle layers of the stomach wall. Note that the mucosa lining the stomach forms folds called *rugae*. The dotted lines distinguish the fundus, body, and antrum of the stomach. (Modified from Thibodeau GA, Patton KT: *Anatomy & physiology*, ed 6, St Louis, 2007, Mosby.)

the stomach are the **fundus** (upper portion), **body** (middle portion), and **antrum** (lower portion).

The stomach has three layers of smooth muscle: an outer, longitudinal layer; a middle, circular layer; and an inner, oblique layer (the most prominent) (see Figure 38-5). These layers become progressively thicker in the body and antrum, where food is mixed, churned, and pushed out into the duodenum. The circular layer is most prominent and the oblique layer is the least complete; the longitudinal layer is absent on the anterior and posterior surfaces. The glandular epithelium is discussed in the section about secretory functions of the stomach (see p. 1425).

Blood is supplied to the stomach by a branch of the celiac artery. The blood supply is so abundant that nearly all arterial vessels must be occluded before ischemic changes occur in the stomach wall. The splenic vein drains the right side of the stomach, and the gastric vein drains the left side.

The stomach is innervated by sympathetic and parasympathetic divisions of the autonomic nervous system. Some of the autonomic fibers are extrinsic; that is, they originate outside the stomach and are controlled by nerve centers in the brain: the vagus nerve and branches of the celiac plexus. Others are intrinsic, that is, they originate within the stomach and respond to local stimuli, such as the myenteric plexus, which lies between the longitudinal and circular muscle layer and within the circular layer. Extrinsic sympathetic fibers reach the stomach through the celiac plexus (solar plexus), whereas extrinsic parasympathetic fibers enter through the gastric branch of the vagus nerve.

Few substances are absorbed in the stomach. The stomach mucosa is impermeable to water, but the stomach can absorb alcohol and aspirin.

Gastric Motility

In its resting state the stomach is small and contains about 50 ml of fluid. There is little wall tension, and the muscle layers in the fundus contract very little. Swallowing causes the fundus to relax (receptive relaxation) to receive a bolus of food from the esophagus. Relaxation is coordinated by efferent, nonadrenergic, noncholinergic vagal fibers and is facilitated by gastrin and cholecystokinin, two polypeptide hormones secreted by the gastrointestinal mucosa. (The actions of digestive hormones are summarized in Table 38-1.) Food is stored in vertical or oblique layers as it arrives in the fundus, whereas fluids flow relatively quickly down to the antrum.

Gastric (stomach) motility increases with the initiation of peristaltic waves, which sweep over the body of the stomach toward the antrum. The rate of peristaltic contractions is approximately three per minute and is influenced by neural and hormonal activity. **Gastrin** and **motilin** (intestinal hormones), and the vagus nerve increase contraction by making the threshold potential of muscle fibers less negative. (The neural and biochemical mechanisms of muscle contraction are described in Chapter 41.) Sympathetic activity and **secretin** (another intestinal hormone) are inhibitory and make threshold potential more negative. The rate of peristalsis is mediated by pacemaker cells that initiate a wave of depolarization (basic electrical rhythm), which moves from the upper part of the stomach to the pylorus.

The mixing and emptying of food (chyme) from the stomach take several hours. Mixing occurs as food is propelled toward the antrum. As food approaches the pylorus, the velocity of the peristaltic wave increases, forcing the contents back toward the body of the stomach. This **retropulsion** effectively mixes food with digestive juices, and the oscillating

Table 38-1	Selected Hormones and Neurotransmitters of the Digestive System		
Source	**Hormone**	**Stimulus for Secretion**	**Action**
Mucosa of the stomach	Gastrin	Presence of partially digested proteins in the stomach	Stimulates gastric glands to secrete hydrochloric acid and pepsinogen; growth of gastric mucosa; promotes gastric motility
	Histamine	Gastrin	Stimulates acid secretion
	Somatostatin	Acid in the stomach	Inhibits acid and pepsinogen secretion and release of gastrin
	Acetylcholine	Vagus and local nerves in stomach	Stimulates release of pepsinogen and acid secretion
	Gastrin-releasing peptide (bombesin)	Vagus and local nerves in stomach	Stimulates gastrin and release of pepsinogen and acid secretion
Mucosa of the small intestine	Motilin	Presence of acid and fat in the duodenum	Increases gastrointestinal motility
	Secretin	Presence of chyme (acid, partially digested proteins, fats) in the duodenum	Stimulates pancreas to secrete alkaline pancreatic juice and liver to secrete bile; decreases gastrointestinal motility; inhibits gastrin and gastric acid secretion
	Cholecystokinin	Presence of chyme (acid, partially digested proteins, fats) in the duodenum	Stimulates gallbladder to eject bile and pancreas to secrete alkaline fluid; decreases gastric motility; constricts pyloric sphincter; inhibits gastrin; delays gastric emptying
	Enteroglucagon	Intraluminal fats and carbohydrates	Weakly inhibits gastric and pancreatic secretion and enhances insulin release, lipolysis, ketogenesis, and glycogenolysis; delays gastric emptying
	Entero-oxytin	Presence of chyme in duodenum	Delays gastric emptying
	Gastric inhibitory peptide (GIP)	Fat and glucose in small intestine	Inhibits gastric secretion and gastric emptying, stimulates insulin release
	Peptide YY	Intraluminal fat and bile acids	Inhibits postprandial gastric acid and pancreatic secretion and delays gastric and small bowel emptying
	Pancreatic polypeptide	Protein, fat and glucose in small intestine	Decreases pancreatic HCO_3^- and enzyme secretion
	Vasoactive intestinal peptide	Intestinal mucosa and muscle	Relaxes intestinal smooth muscle, increases blood flow

Modified from Johnson LR: *Gastrointestinal physiology*, ed 7, St. Louis, 2007, Mosby.
Data from Schubert ML, Peura DA: *Gastroenterology* 134(7):1842-1860, 2008; Wren AM, Bloom SR: *Gastroenterology* 132(6):2116-2130, 2007.
NOTE: The digestive hormones are not secreted into the gastrointestinal lumen but rather into the bloodstream, in which they travel to target tissues. There are more than 30 peptide hormone genes expressed in the gastrointestinal tract and more than 100 hormonally active peptides.

motion breaks down large food particles. With each peristaltic wave a small portion of the gastric contents (chyme) passes through the pylorus and into the duodenum. The pylorus is about 1.5 cm long and is always open about 2 mm. It opens wider during antral contraction. Normally there is no regurgitation from the duodenum into the antrum.

The rate of **gastric emptying** (movement of gastric contents into the duodenum) depends on the volume, osmotic pressure, and chemical composition of the gastric contents. Larger volumes of food increase gastric pressure, peristalsis, and rate of emptying. Solids, fats, and nonisotonic solutions delay gastric emptying.[9] (Osmotic pressure and tonicity are described in Chapters 1 and 3.) Products of fat digestion, which are formed in the duodenum by the action of bile from the liver and enzymes from the pancreas, stimulate the secretion of **cholecystokinin.** This hormone inhibits gastric motility and decreases gastric emptying so that fats are not emptied into the duodenum at a rate that exceeds the rate of bile and enzyme secretion. Osmoreceptors in the wall of the duodenum are sensitive to the osmotic pressure of duodenal contents. The arrival of hypertonic or hypotonic gastric contents activates the osmoreceptors, which delays gastric emptying to facilitate formation of an isoosmotic duodenal environment. The rate at which acid enters the duodenum also influences gastric emptying. Secretions from the pancreas, liver, and duodenal mucosa neutralize gastric acid in the duodenum. The rate of emptying is adjusted to the duodenum's ability to neutralize the incoming acidity.[10] Peristaltic activity in the stomach is also affected by blood glucose levels. Low blood glucose levels stimulate the vagus nerve and gastric smooth muscles. There is an increase in peristalsis but not gastric emptying, stimulating the sensation of "hunger pains."[11]

Gastric Secretion

Stimulated by eating, the stomach secretes large volumes of gastric juices or gastric secretions. Specialized cells located throughout the gastric mucosa produce mucus, acid, enzymes, hormones, intrinsic factor, and gastroferrin. Intrinsic factor is necessary for the intestinal absorption of vitamin B_{12} and gastroferrin facilitates small intestinal absorption of iron. The hormones are secreted into the blood and travel to target

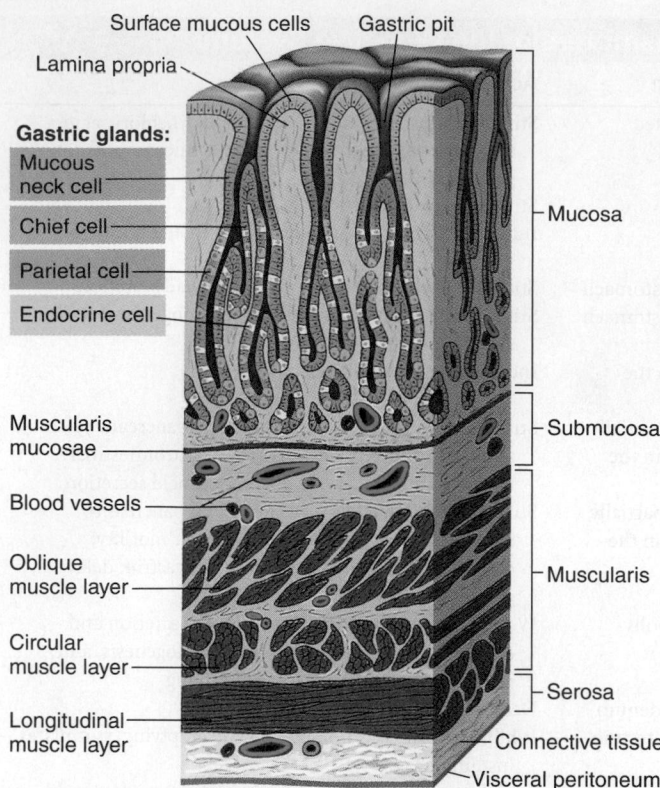

Figure 38-6 **Gastric pits and gastric glands.** Gastric pits are depressions in the epithelial lining of the stomach. At the bottom of each pit is one or more tubular gastric glands. Chief cells produce the enzymes of gastric juice, and parietal cells produce stomach acid. (From Patton KT, Thibodeau GA: *Anatomy & physiology,* ed 7, St Louis, 2010, Mosby.)

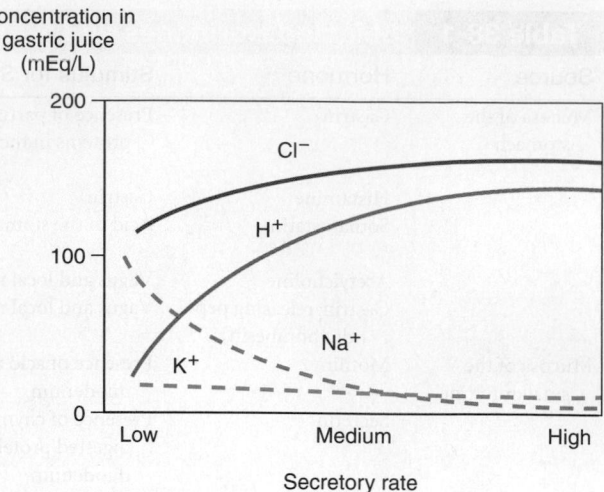

Figure 38-7 **Relationship between secretory rate and electrolyte composition of the gastric juice.** Sodium (Na^+) concentration is lower in the gastric juice than in the plasma, whereas hydrogen (H^+), potassium (K^+), and chloride (Cl^-) concentrations are higher. *Red line,* Chloride; *orange line,* hydrogen; *green line,* sodium; *blue line,* potassium.

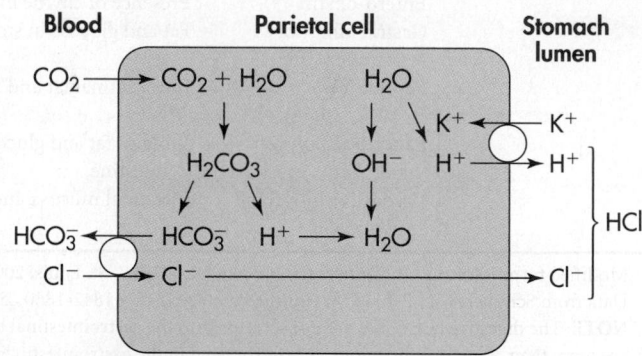

Figure 38-8 Hydrochloric acid secretion by parietal cell.

tissues in the bloodstream. The other gastric secretions are released directly into the stomach lumen under neural and hormonal regulation.[12] Mucus covering the entire mucosa, intercellular tight junctions, and submucosal acid sensors form a protective barrier against acid and proteolytic enzymes, which otherwise would damage the gastric lining.[13]

In the fundus and body of the stomach the **gastric glands** of the mucosa are the primary secretory units (Figure 38-6). Several of these glands (three to seven) empty into a common duct known as the **gastric pit.** The **parietal cells (oxyntic cells)** within the glands secrete hydrochloric acid and intrinsic factor. The **chief cells** within the glands secrete **pepsinogen,** an enzyme precursor that is readily converted to **pepsin** (a proteolytic enzyme) in the gastric juice. The pyloric gland mucosa in the antrum synthesizes and releases the hormone gastrin from **G cells. Enterochromaffin-like cells** secrete **histamine,** and **D cells** secrete **somatostatin.**

The composition of gastric juice depends on volume and flow rate (Figure 38-7). Potassium remains relatively constant, but its concentration is greater in gastric juice than in plasma. The rate of secretion varies with the time of day. Generally the rate and volume of secretion are lowest in the morning and highest in the afternoon and evening. Loss of gastric juices through vomiting, drainage, or suction may decrease body stores of sodium and potassium.

Gastric secretion is inhibited by unpleasant odors and tastes and by rage, fear, or pain. These sensations and emotions cause a discharge of sympathetic impulses and inhibit parasympathetic impulses. Increased secretions may be associated with feelings of aggression or hostility and may contribute to some forms of gastric pathology.

Acid

The major functions of **gastric acid** are to dissolve food fibers, act as a bactericide against swallowed organisms, and convert pepsinogen to pepsin. The production of acid by the parietal cells requires the transport of hydrogen and chloride from the parietal cells to the stomach lumen. Acid is formed in the parietal cells, primarily through the hydrolysis of water (Figure 38-8). At a high rate of gastric secretion, bicarbonate moves into the plasma, producing an "alkaline tide" in the venous blood, which also may result in a more alkaline urine.[14]

Acid secretion by parietal cells is stimulated by acetylcholine (a neurotransmitter), gastrin (a hormone), and histamine (a biochemical mediator). The vagus nerve also releases acetylcholine and stimulates the secretion of histamine.[12]

Histamine secretion is also stimulated by gastrin. Histamine is stored in enterochromaffin cells (mast cells; see Chapter 6) in the gastric mucosa. Histamine receptors in the gastric mucosa are histamine (H_2) receptors (unlike those in the bronchial mucosa, which are H_1 receptors). Gastric lipase is produced by glands in the fundus of the stomach and is most effective in an acid environment. Prostaglandins, enterogastrones, such as gastric inhibitory peptide, somatostatin, and secretin, inhibit acid secretion.[15]

Pepsin

Acetylcholine, through vagal stimulation during the cephalic and gastric phases, is the strongest stimulation for pepsin secretion. The precursor pepsinogen is quickly converted to pepsin at a pH of 2. Acid also stimulates a local cholinergic reflex and stimulates chief cells to secrete pepsin. Gastrin and secretin are weaker pepsinogen secretagogues. **Pepsin** is a proteolytic enzyme that breaks down protein-forming polypeptides in the stomach. Once chyme has entered the duodenum, the alkaline environment of the duodenum inactivates pepsin.

Mucus

The gastric mucosa is protected from the digestive actions of acid and pepsin by a coating of mucus called the **mucosal barrier.** Gastric mucosal blood flow is important to maintaining mucosal barrier function.[13] The quality and quantity of mucus and the tight junctions between epithelial cells make gastric mucosa relatively impermeable to acid. Prostaglandins and nitric oxide protect the mucosal barrier by stimulating the secretion of mucus and bicarbonate and by inhibiting secretion of acid. A break in the protective barrier may occur because of exposure to aspirin or other nonsteroidal anti-inflammatory drugs, *Helicobacter pylori,* ethanol, regurgitated bile, or ischemia. Breaks cause inflammation and ulceration.

Intrinsic factor (IF), a mucoprotein produced by parietal cells, combines with vitamin B_{12} in the stomach. It is required for the absorption of vitamin B_{12} by the ileum. Atrophic gastritis and failure to absorb vitamin B_{12} result in pernicious anemia (see Chapter 26).

Phases of Gastric Secretion

The secretion of gastric juice is influenced by numerous stimuli that together facilitate the process of digestion. The **phases of gastric secretion** are the cephalic phase, the gastric phase, and the intestinal phase (Figure 38-9).

Cephalic Phase. The anticipatory and sensory experiences of smelling, seeing, tasting, chewing, and swallowing food contribute to the **cephalic phase of secretion.**[16] The cephalic phase of gastric secretion is mediated by the vagus nerve through the myenteric plexus. Acetylcholine (ACh) is liberated and stimulates the parietal and chief cells to secrete acid and pepsinogen, respectively. The G cells in the antrum release gastrin into the bloodstream, through which it travels to the gastric glands and stimulates acid and pepsinogen secretion.

Insulin secretion by the endocrine pancreas, stimulated by hyperglycemia, also is a strong stimulus for gastric secretion and is mediated by the vagus nerve through sensors located in the hypothalamus. Maintenance of steady serum glucose levels suppresses the gastric response to insulin.

Gastric Phase. The **gastric phase of secretion** begins with the arrival of food in the stomach. Two major stimuli

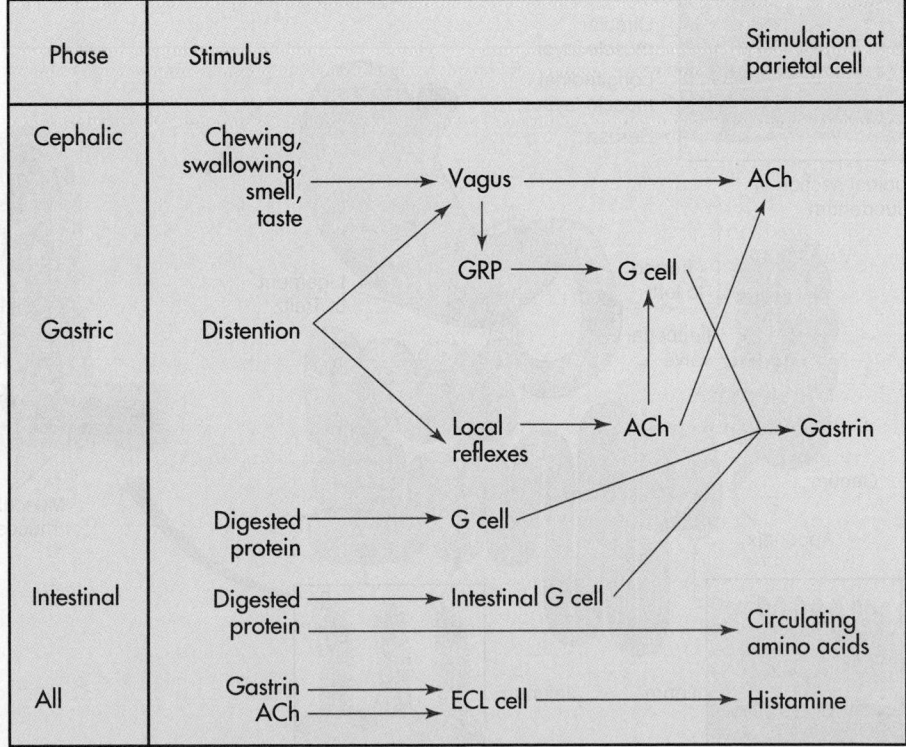

Phase	Stimulus	Stimulation at parietal cell

Cephalic — Chewing, swallowing, smell, taste → Vagus → ACh
Vagus → GRP → G cell
Gastric — Distention → Local reflexes → ACh → Gastrin
GRP → G cell
ACh → Gastrin
Digested protein → G cell → Gastrin
Intestinal — Digested protein → Intestinal G cell → Gastrin
Digested protein → Circulating amino acids
All — Gastrin, ACh → ECL cell → Histamine

Figure 38-9 Mechanisms for stimulating acid secretion. *ACh,* Acetylcholine; *ECL,* enterochromaffin-like cell; *GRP,* gastrin-releasing peptide. (From Johnson LR: *Gastrointestinal physiology,* ed 7, St Louis, 2007, Mosby.)

have a secretory effect: (1) distention of the stomach and (2) the presence of digested protein. The vagus and enteric nerve plexuses are stimulated by distention and contribute to gastric secretion through a local reflex. Both neural reflexes are mediated by acetylcholine and can be blocked by atropine. As digestion proceeds, products of protein break down, stimulating the release of gastrin from G cells in the antrum. Proteins in the stomach buffer the acid gastric juice and increase the gastric pH. Caffeine stimulates acid secretion, as does calcium.

Intestinal Phase. The movement of chyme from the stomach into the duodenum initiates the **intestinal phase of secretion.** This phase represents a slowdown of the gastric secretory response and appears to be hormonally mediated by a hormone called **entero-oxyntin. Gastric inhibitory peptide** decreases gastric motility and the secretion of acid and pepsin when chyme enters the duodenum. The intestinal absorption of some amino acids (products of protein breakdown) also stimulates gastric secretion. The intestinal phase of gastric secretion is limited by the fact that acidic chyme in the duodenum tends to inhibit gastric acid secretion and

gastric motility. Acid in the duodenum stimulates the release of hormones that inhibit acid secretion while stimulating pepsinogen secretion. One of these hormones, cholecystokinin, inhibits gastrin-stimulated acid production. Other intestinal hormones probably also act synergistically to regulate gastric secretion.

Small Intestine

The **small intestine** is about 5 to 6 m long and is functionally divided into three segments: the duodenum, jejunum, and ileum (Figure 38-10). The **duodenum** begins at the pylorus and ends where it joins the **jejunum** at a suspensory ligament called the *Treitz ligament*. The end of the jejunum and beginning of the **ileum** are not distinguished by an anatomic marker. These structures are not grossly different, but the jejunum has a slightly larger lumen. The **ileocecal valve (sphincter)** controls the flow of digested material from the ileum into the large intestine and prevents reflux into the small intestine.[17]

The **peritoneum** is the serous membrane surrounding the organs of the abdomen and pelvic cavity. It is analogous to the

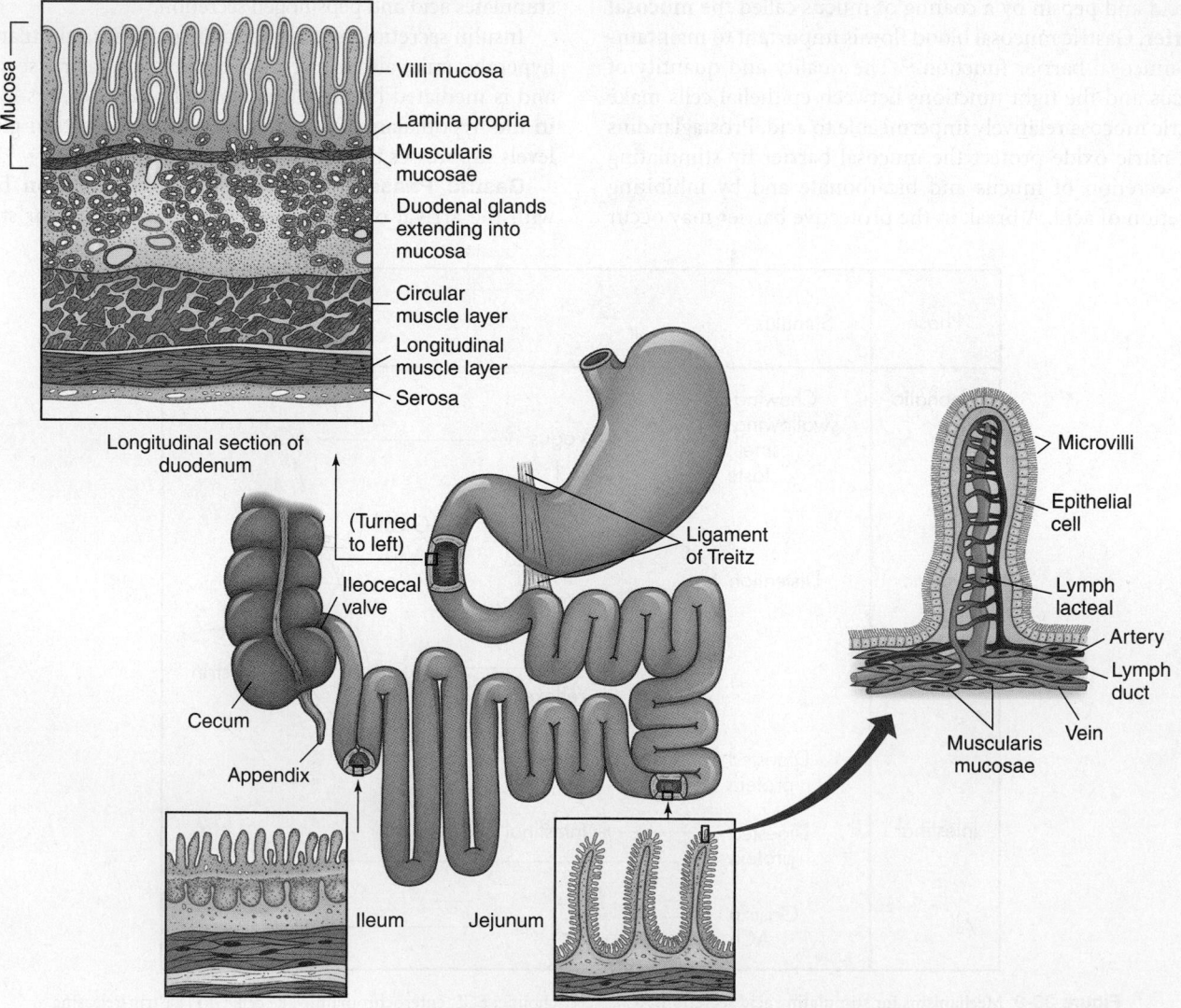

Figure 38-10 Small intestine.

pericardium and pleura that surround the heart and lungs, respectively. The *visceral peritoneum* lies over the organs, and the *parietal peritoneum* lines the wall of the abdominal cavity. The space between these two layers is called the **peritoneal cavity.** This cavity normally contains just enough fluid to lubricate the two layers and prevent friction during organ movement. Inflammation of the peritoneum, called *peritonitis,* may occur with perforation of the intestine or after abdominal surgery. As the inflammatory process resolves, adhesions may form and cause colonic obstruction.

The duodenum lies behind the peritoneum, or retroperitoneally, and is attached to the posterior abdominal wall and has an essential role in mixing food with digestive juices from the liver and pancreas. The ileum and jejunum are suspended in loose folds from the posterior abdominal wall by a peritoneal membrane called the **mesentery.** The mesentery facilitates intestinal motility and supports blood vessels, nerves, and lymphatics.

The arterial supply to the duodenum arises primarily from the gastroduodenal artery. The jejunum and ileum are supplied by branches of the superior mesenteric artery. Blood flow increases significantly during digestion. The superior mesenteric vein joins the splenic vein and empties into the portal circulation to the liver. The regional lymph nodes and lymphatics drain into the thoracic duct. Both divisions of the autonomic nervous system innervate the small intestine. Secretion, motility, pain sensation, and intestinal reflexes (e.g., relaxation of the lower esophageal sphincter) are mediated by parasympathetic nerves. Sympathetic activity inhibits motility and produces vasoconstriction. Intrinsic motor innervation is mediated by the myenteric plexus (Auerbach plexus) and the submucosal plexus (Meissner plexus).

The smooth muscles of the small intestine are arranged in two layers: a longitudinal, outer layer; and a thicker, inner circular layer (see Figure 38-10). Mucosal folds (plica) within the small intestine slow the passage of food, thereby providing more time for digestion and absorption. The folds are most numerous and prominent in the jejunum and upper ileum (see Figure 38-10).

Absorption occurs through **villi,** which cover the mucosal folds and are the functional units of the intestine (see Figure 38-10). Each villus also secretes some of the enzymes necessary for digestion and absorbs nutrients. A villus is composed of absorptive columnar cells (enterocytes) and mucus-secreting goblet cells of the mucosal epithelium. Near the surface, columnar cells closely adhere to each other at sites called *tight junctions*. Water and electrolytes are absorbed through these intercellular spaces. The surface of each columnar epithelial cell contains tiny projections called **microvilli** (see Figure 38-10). Together the microvilli create a mucosal surface known as the **brush border.** The villi and microvilli greatly increase the surface area available for absorption. Coating the brush border is an "unstirred" layer of fluid that is important for the absorption of substances other than water and electrolytes. The **lamina propria** (a connective tissue layer of the mucous membrane) lies beneath the epithelial cells of the

villi and contains lymphocytes; plasma cells, which produce immunoglobulins; and macrophages.

Central arterioles ascend within each villus and branch into a capillary array that extends around the base of the columnar cells and cascades down to the venules that lead to the portal circulation. The opposing ascending and descending blood flow provides a countercurrent exchange system for absorbed substances and blood gases. A central **lacteal,** or lymphatic channel, is also contained within each villus and is important for the absorption and transport of fat molecules. Contents of the lacteals flow to regional nodes and channels that eventually drain into the thoracic duct[18] (see Figure 38-10).

Between the bases of the villi are the **crypts of Lieberkühn,** which extend to the submucosal layer. Undifferentiated (**stem cells**) and secretory cells and Paneth epithelial cells are located here. The stem cells are precursors of columnar epithelial and goblet cells. These premature cells produce alkaline fluids containing electrolytes, mucus, and water. These cells arise from the base of the crypt and move toward the tip of the villus, maturing in shape and function as they progress. After becoming columnar cells and completing their migration to the tip of the villus, they function for a few days and then are sloughed into the intestinal lumen and digested. Sloughed epithelial cells are an important source of endogenous protein. The entire epithelial population is replaced about every 4 to 7 days. Many factors can influence this process of cellular proliferation. Starvation, vitamin B_{12} deficiency, and cytotoxic drugs or irradiation suppress cell division and shorten the villi. The decreased absorption that results can cause diarrhea and malnutrition. Nutrient intake and intestinal resection stimulate cell production. The **Paneth cells** produce defensins and other antibiotic peptides and proteins.[19] Other secretory cells produce digestive enzymes.[20]

Intestinal Digestion and Absorption

The process of intestinal digestion is initiated in the stomach by the actions of hydrochloric acid and pepsin, which break down food fibers and proteins. The chyme that passes into the duodenum is a liquid that contains small particles of undigested food. Digestion is continued in the proximal portion of the small intestine by the action of pancreatic enzymes, intestinal brush border enzymes, and bile salts (Box 38-1). Here carbohydrates are broken down to monosaccharides and disaccharides; proteins are degraded further to amino acids and peptides; and fats are emulsified and reduced to fatty acids and monoglycerides (Figure 38-11). These nutrients, along with water, vitamins, and electrolytes, are absorbed across the intestinal mucosa and into the blood by active transport, diffusion, or facilitated diffusion. Products of carbohydrate and protein breakdown move into villus capillaries and then to the liver through the portal vein. Digested fats move into the lacteals and eventually reach the liver through the systemic circulation. Intestinal motility exposes nutrients to a large mucosal surface area by mixing chyme and moving it through the lumen. Different segments of the gastrointestinal tract absorb different nutrients. Digestion and absorption of all major

Box 38-1	Sources of Digestive Enzymes

Salivary Glands
Amylase
Lingual lipase

Stomach
Pepsin
Gastric lipase

Pancreas
Amylase
Trypsin
Chymotrypsin
Carboxypeptidase
Elastase
Lipase-colipase
Phospholipase A_2
Cholesterol esterase–nonspecific lipase

Small Intestine
Enterokinase
Disaccharidases
  Maltase
  Sucrase
  Lactase
  α, α-Trehalase
Isomaltase
Peptidases
  Amino-oligopeptidase
  Dipeptidase

From Johnson LR: *Gastrointestinal physiology*, ed 6, St Louis, 2007, Mosby.

nutrients occur in the small intestine. Sites of absorption are shown in Figure 38-12.

Water and Electrolytes

The epithelial cell membranes of the small intestine are formed of lipids and therefore are hydrophobic, or tend to repel water. (The properties of cell membranes are described in Chapter 1.) Therefore, water and electrolytes are transported in both directions (toward the capillary blood or toward the intestinal lumen) through the tight junctions and intercellular spaces rather than across cell membranes. Water diffuses passively according to hydrostatic pressure and in relation to osmotic gradients established by the active transport of sodium and other substances. Approximately 85% to 90% of the water that enters the gastrointestinal tract each day is absorbed in the small intestine. The remaining water and electrolytes are absorbed at a constant rate in the colon.[21] Sodium passes through the tight junctions and is actively transported across cell membranes. The proximal part of the small intestine is more permeable to sodium than the distal part. Sodium is transported into the intestinal cells in exchange for hydrogen at the brush border, and chloride actively enters the cell in exchange for bicarbonate to maintain electroneutrality in the ileum. There is also a sodium pump at the basolateral membrane. Sodium and glucose share a common carrier mechanism, so that sodium absorption is enhanced by glucose transport (Figure 38-13). Potassium moves passively across the tight junctions with changes in the electrochemical

gradient. Net potassium secretion occurs in the colon. Because of potassium secretion in the colon and the exchange of chloride for bicarbonate, prolonged diarrhea results in hypokalemic metabolic acidosis.

Carbohydrates

Carbohydrate (starch, table sugar—sucrose, milk sugar—lactose, cereal sugar—maltose) accounts for at least 50% of the American diet. Because only monosaccharides (galactose, glucose, fructose) are absorbed by the intestinal mucosa, the complex carbohydrates (polysaccharides and oligosaccharides) must be hydrolyzed to their simplest form (see Figure 38-10). Ribose, a five-carbon sugar that forms part of ribonucleic acid (RNA), adenosine triphosphate (ATP), and deoxyribonucleic acid (DNA), is an important part of the diet. Salivary and pancreatic amylases break down starches to oligosaccharides by splitting α-1,4-glucosidic linkages of long-chain molecules. The major oligosaccharides are sucrose (glucose-fructose), maltose (glucose-glucose), and lactose (glucose-galactose). Approximately half of starch hydrolysis occurs in the stomach and about half in the duodenum. In the small intestine the oligosaccharides are hydrolyzed by brush-border enzymes, mainly sucrase, maltase, and lactase, to their respective monosaccharides (fructose, glucose, galactose). The sugars then pass through the unstirred layer by diffusion. At the cell membrane, glucose and galactose are actively transported with a sodium carrier (sodium-glucose transporter [SGLT-1]) and fructose absorption is facilitated by a glucose transporter (GLUT-5) (Figure 38-13). Consequently, glucose and galactose are absorbed more rapidly than fructose. Transport of all three hexoses from the cytosol of the bloodstream is facilitated by the GLUT-2 carrier.[22] Insulin is not required for the intestinal absorption of carbohydrates. The sugars are absorbed primarily in the duodenum and upper jejunum. Cellulose is a glucose polysaccharide found in plants. Humans lack enzymes to digest cellulose, and the undigested fiber contributes to stool volume and stimulates large intestine motility.

Proteins

Protein intake varies among different populations. Adults require 44 to 56 g of protein per day. Approximately 20 to 30 g of protein is derived endogenously from shed epithelial cells and small amounts of plasma proteins. Most protein is absorbed; only 5% to 10% is eliminated in the stool.

Gastric digestion of protein by pepsin and acid is not essential. Major protein hydrolysis is accomplished in the small intestine by the pancreatic enzymes: trypsin, chymotrypsin, and carboxypeptidase (see Figure 38-10). **Trypsin** and **chymotrypsin** (endopeptidase) hydrolyze the interior bonds of the large molecules, and **carboxypeptidases** break away the end amino acids (exopeptidase). Hydrolysis of proteins is also carried out by the brush-border enzymes and enzymes in the epithelial cytosol (intracellular fluid). The brush-border enzymes hydrolyze the large oligopeptides (proteins composed of three to six amino acids) into smaller peptides, which can cross cell membranes. The cytosol then breaks them down to amino acids. Amino acids are actively transported by a carrier

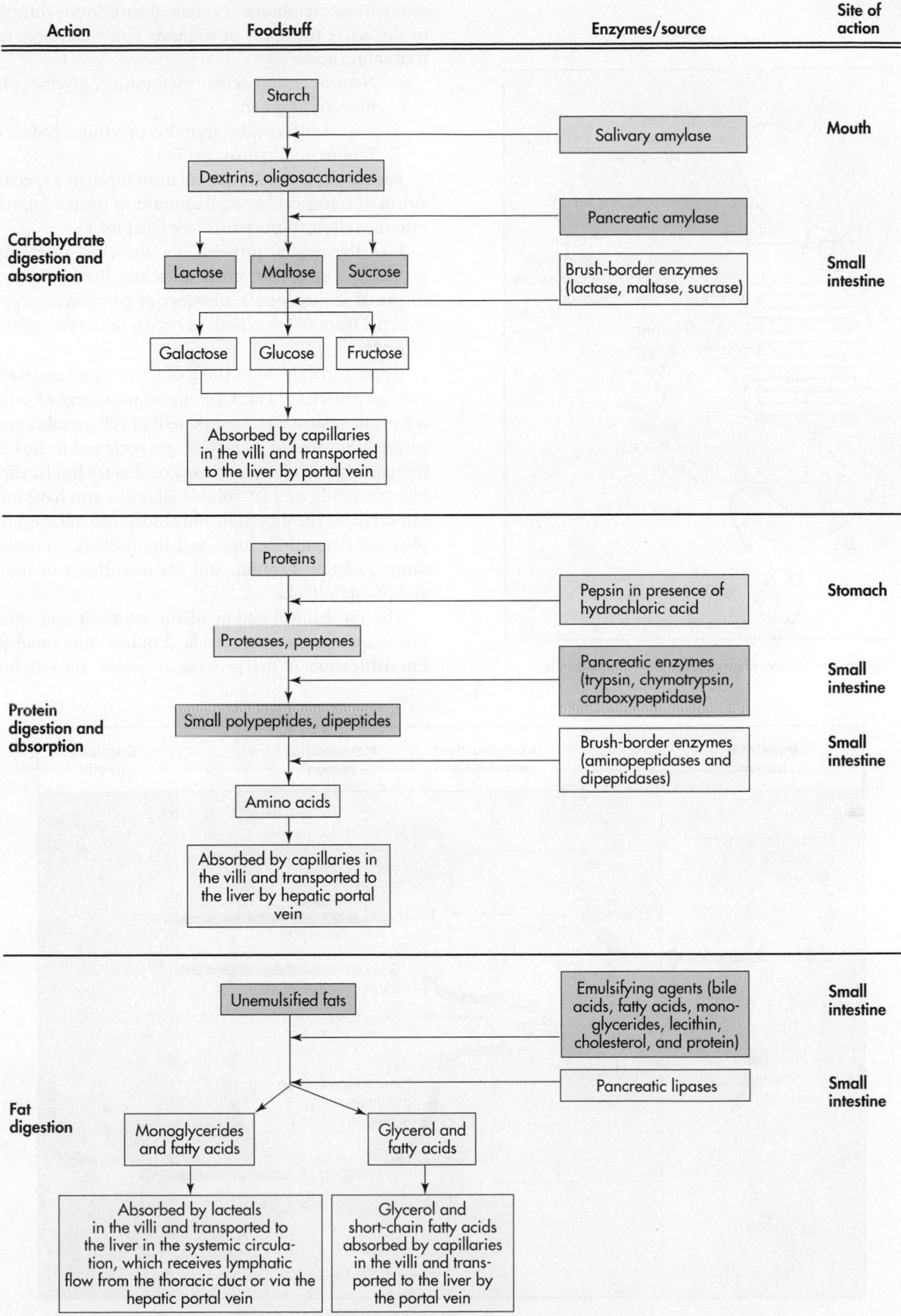

Figure 38-11 Digestion and absorption of foodstuffs.

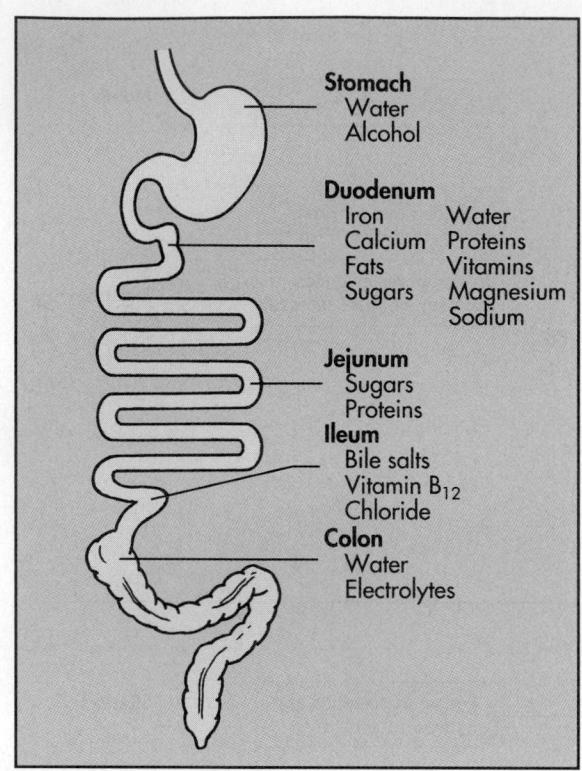

Figure 38-12 Sites of absorption of major nutrients.

at the basal membrane. Protein absorption is directly linked to the active transport of sodium. There are three groups of free amino acids:

1. Neutral amino acids (methionine, glycine, phenylalanine, tryptophan)
2. Basic amino acids (arginine, ornithine, lysine, cystine)
3. Proline and hydroxyproline

Each group enters the circulation through a specific mechanism of transport. A small amount of protein may be taken into the cells by pinocytosis (see Chapter 1).

Like the sugars, proteins are absorbed primarily in the proximal area of the small intestine. Protein absorption is impaired if inadequate amounts of proteolytic enzymes are secreted from the pancreas, as occurs with cystic fibrosis.

Fats

Approximately 90 to 100 g of fat is consumed daily by the average American. **Fat** is an important source of calories and is a primary structural component of cell membranes and organelles. Sources of dietary fat are reviewed in Box 38-2. Although triglycerides are the major dietary lipids, cholesterol, phospholipids, and fat-soluble vitamins also have nutritional importance. The digestion and absorption of fat occur in four phases: (1) emulsification and lipolysis, (2) micelle formation, (3) fat absorption, and (4) resynthesis of triglycerides and phospholipids.

The mechanical action of the stomach and small intestine disperses the triglyceride droplets into small particles. **Emulsification** is the process by which emulsifying agents

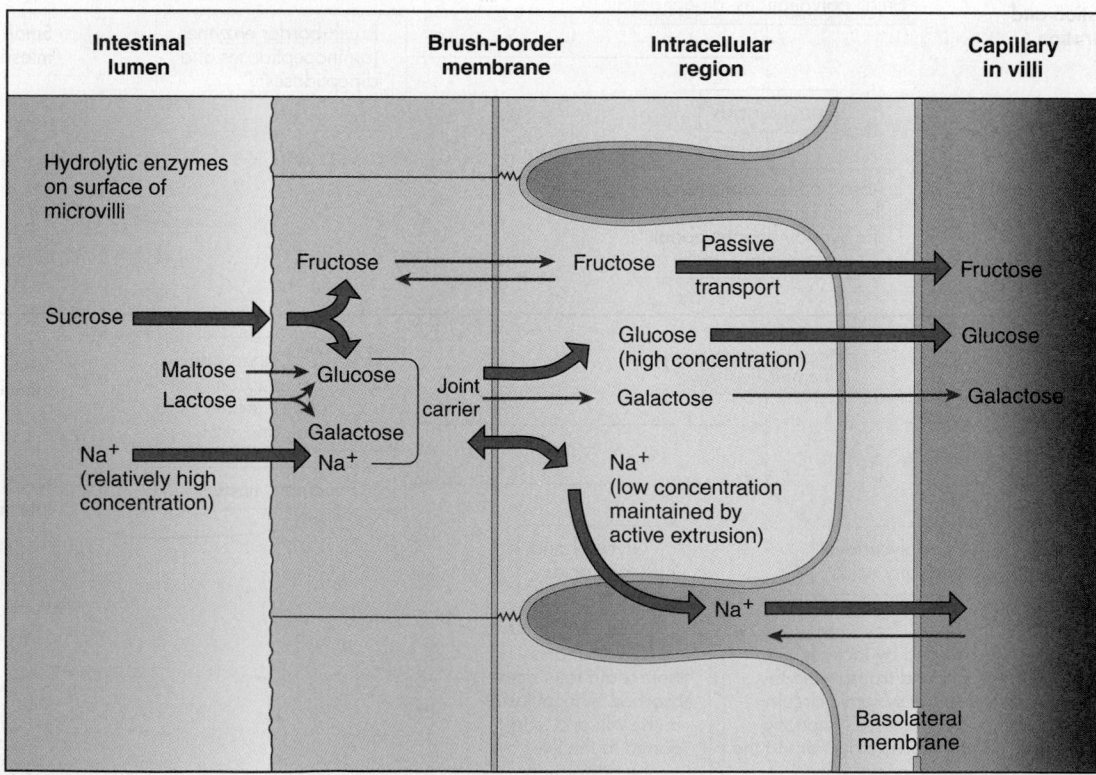

Figure 38-13 **Glucose and sodium transport.** Schematic showing glucose and sodium (Na^+) transport through the intestinal epithelium. Glucose and sodium are transported into the epithelial cell by a joint carrier.

Box 38-2   Dietary Fat

Saturated Fatty Acid (Palmitic Acid [$C_{16}H_{32}O_2$])
Each carbon atom in the chain is linked by single bonds to adjacent carbon and hydrogen atoms; atoms are solid at room temperature and found in animal fat and tropical oils (coconut and palm oil); they increase low-density lipoprotein (LDL) cholesterol ("bad" cholesterol) blood levels and increase the risk of coronary artery disease

Unsaturated Fatty Acid
Unsaturated fatty acids are soft or liquid at room temperature; omega-6 fatty acids are found in plants and vegetables (olive, canola, and peanut oils), and omega-3 fatty acids are found in fish and shellfish.
1. Monounsaturated fatty acids (oleic acid [$C_{18}H_{34}O_2$])
   Contain one double bond in the carbon chain and are found in plants and animals; may be beneficial in reducing blood cholesterol, glucose levels, and systolic blood pressure; do not lower high-density lipoprotein (HDL) cholesterol ("good" cholesterol) level; low HDL levels have been associated with coronary heart disease
2. Polyunsaturated fatty acids (linoleic acid [$C_{18}H_{32}O_2$])
   Contain two or more double bonds in the carbon chain and are found in plants and fish oils; omega-6 fatty acids lower total and LDL cholesterol blood levels; high levels of polyunsaturated fatty acids may lower LDL; omega-3 fatty acids lower blood triglyceride levels and reduce platelet aggregation and reduce blood clotting tendency; are necessary for growth and development and may prevent coronary artery disease, hypertension, cancer, inflammatory and immune disorders

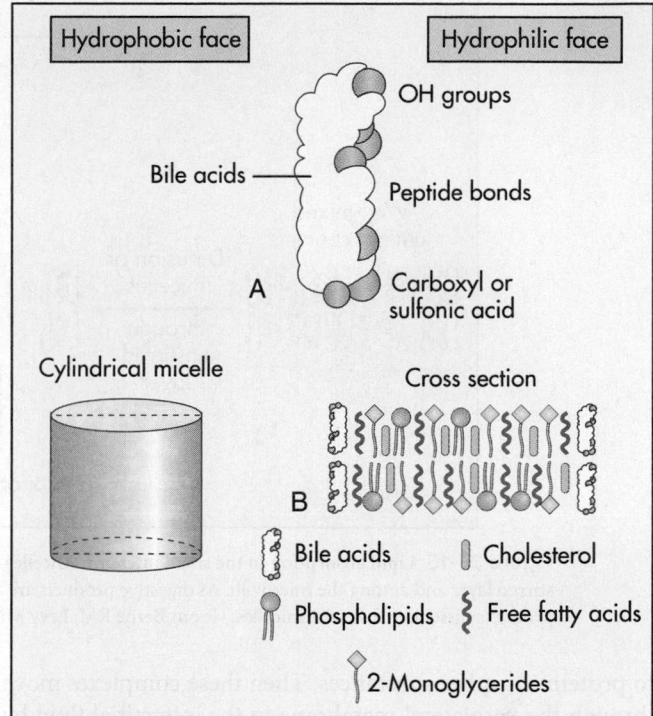

Figure 38-14 Structure of bile acid and micelle. **A,** A bile acid molecule in solution. The molecule is amphipathic in that it has a hydrophilic face and a hydrophobic face. The amphipathic structure is key in the ability of the bile acids to emulsify lipids and form micelles. **B,** A model of the structure of a bile acid–lipid mixed micelle, an emulsified fat. (From Berne RM, Levy MN, editors: *Principles of physiology,* ed 3, St Louis, 2000, Mosby.)

(fatty acids, monoglycerides, lecithin, cholesterol, protein, bile salts) in the intestinal lumen cover the small fat particles and prevent them from re-forming into fat droplets (decrease their surface tension). Emulsified fat is then ready for **lipolysis** (lipid hydrolysis) by pancreatic lipase, phospholipase, and hydrolase. **Lipase** breaks down triglycerides to diglycerides, monoglycerides, free fatty acids, and glycerol (see Figure 38-11). The action of lipase requires the presence of **colipase,** a pancreatic enzyme that allows lipase to penetrate the triglyceride molecule. **Phospholipase** cleaves fatty acids from phospholipids, and **cholesterol esterase** breaks cholesterol esters into fatty acids and glycerol.

The products of lipid hydrolysis must be made water soluble if they are to be absorbed efficiently from the intestinal lumen. This is accomplished by the formation of water-soluble molecules known as **micelles** (Figure 38-14). Micelles are formed of bile salts, the products of fat hydrolysis, fat-soluble vitamins, and cholesterol. The fats form the core of the micelle, and the polar bile salts form an outer shell, with the hydrophobic ("water-hating") side facing the interior and the hydrophilic ("water-loving") side facing the aqueous (water-like) content of the intestinal lumen. Because the unstirred layer of the brush border is aqueous, the micelles readily diffuse through it. The micelles maintain the fat molecules in the dissolved or solubilized form, which allows them to move more rapidly from the micelle toward the absorbing surface of the intestinal epithelium. The fat products of the micelle then readily diffuse through the epithelial cell membrane, while

the bile salts remain in the lumen and proceed to the ileum, where they are absorbed into the circulation and returned to the liver via the enterohepatic circulation (Figure 38-15 and Figure 38-21, p. 1440). Almost all of the bile salts are recycled in this way.

When the fat products reach the inside of the epithelial cell, they are resynthesized into triglycerides and phospholipids. The triglycerides are covered with phospholipids, lipoproteins, and cholesterol to become particles called **chylomicrons.** The chylomicrons travel to the basolateral membrane of the columnar epithelial cells, where they are extruded into the intercellular spaces of the villus. From here they enter the lacteals and lymphatic channels and, eventually, the systemic circulation.

Minerals and Vitamins

The recommended intake of calcium ranges from 1000 to 1500 mg/day. Between 500 and 600 mg is secreted or shed into the lumen with desquamated epithelial cells. Not all of this calcium is absorbed. Daily absorption of **calcium** is approximately 600 mg. This amount increases with increased intake. When its concentration in the lumen is greater than 5 mmol/L, calcium is absorbed by passive diffusion. At concentrations less than 5 mmol/L, calcium is transported actively across cell membranes, bound to a carrier protein. The carrier formation requires the presence of the active form of vitamin D_3 (1,25-dihydroxyvitamin D). The calcium-protein complex moves into the epithelial cell, where the calcium binds

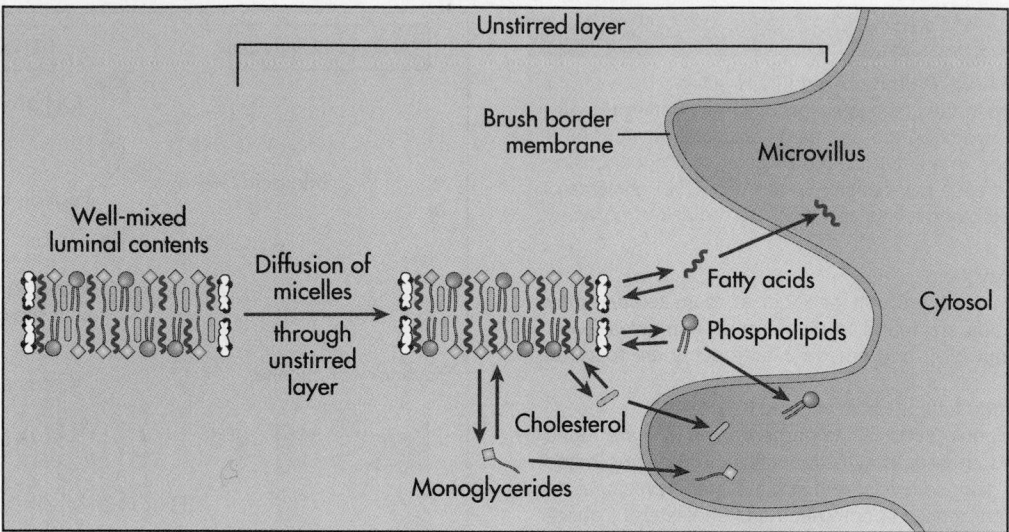

Figure 38-15 Lipid absorption in the small intestine. Micelles of bile salts and products of lipid digestion diffuse through the unstirred layer and among the microvilli. As digestive products are absorbed from free solution by epithelial cells of the villi, more digestive products dissociate from the micelles. (From Berne RM, Levy MN, editors: *Principles of physiology*, ed 3, St Louis, 2000, Mosby.)

to proteins or other substances. Then these complexes move through the basolateral membrane to the interstitial fluid by diffusion or active transport. Calcium is absorbed throughout the small intestine, but primarily in the ileum. Increased serum calcium inhibits parathyroid hormone, which in turn decreases the formation of vitamin D_3 by the kidney, thus regulating calcium absorption.

Increased demand for calcium results in increased uptake, as evidenced by the fact that calcium is absorbed more rapidly in children and pregnant or lactating women. Bile salts enhance calcium absorption indirectly by facilitating the absorption of vitamin D which is fat soluble. In addition, bile salts promote the absorption of free fatty acids that, at high concentrations, bind calcium and form soaps in the intestinal lumen. In older individuals calcium is absorbed less readily because of inadequate amounts of the active form of vitamin D.[23]

The recommended intake of **magnesium** for adults is 300 to 350 mg/day. Approximately 50% of it is absorbed by active transport or passive diffusion in the jejunum and ileum. **Phosphate** is also absorbed in the small intestine by passive diffusion and active transport.

The levels of **iron** in the body are regulated primarily by intestinal absorption and secretion. The average intake ranges from 15 to 30 mg/day. Of this amount, menstruating women absorb 1 to 1.5 mg and men absorb 0.15 to 1 mg. Generally the amount of iron absorbed is equal to the amount required. Iron is absorbed more rapidly if a deficiency exists. The primary source of iron is heme from animal protein. This iron is rapidly absorbed by the epithelial cells primarily in the duodenum. Inorganic iron (e.g., iron in fruits, cereals, eggs, vegetables) is also readily absorbed. The presence of vitamin C reduces ferric iron to ferrous iron, which is the form more easily absorbed. Calcium phosphate and phosphoproteins (milk and antacids) in the intestinal lumen bind iron and reduce absorption. Tea also binds iron by forming iron tannate complexes.

Iron is bound to *intestinal transferrin* in the small bowel and is absorbed and bound to the protein *ferritin* and to amino acid chelates in the cytosol of epithelial cells. Transport of iron across the basolateral membrane is determined by the amount of iron in the circulation. It is transported in the blood by *plasma transferrin* (a globulin protein) and is carried to body tissues. When there is less need for iron, it remains in the enterocyte as ferritin and is carried into the lumen when the cell is sloughed from the end of the villus. The intestinal cells require 3 days to increase their rate of iron absorption after hemorrhage. This is because the need for iron is perceived by the precursor stem cells in the crypts of Lieberkühn, and they take 3 days to mature and migrate to the tips of the villi, where they absorb more iron. **Hepcidin** is a protein synthesized by the liver that inhibits apical uptake of iron by enterocytes and modulates iron trafficking.[24]

The absorption of **vitamins** is summarized in Table 38-2. Most of the water-soluble vitamins are absorbed passively or by sodium-dependent active transport. Most vitamin B_{12} (cobalamin) is bound to intrinsic factor (making it resistant to digestion) and absorbed in the terminal ileum, although a small amount of the vitamin is absorbed in its free (unbound) form.

Intestinal Motility

The movements of the small intestine facilitate digestion and absorption. Chyme coming from the stomach stimulates intestinal movements that mix in secretions from the liver, pancreas, and intestinal glands. A churning motion brings the luminal content into contact with the absorbing cells of the villi. Propulsive movements then advance the chyme toward the large intestine.

Table 38-2	Intestinal Absorption of Vitamins	
Vitamin	Mechanisms of Absorption	State of Absorption
Fat-Soluble Vitamins		
A (retinal)	Micelle formation with bile salts	Upper small intestine
D$_3$ (1,25-dihydroxycholecalciferol)		
E (tocopherol)		
K		
Water-Soluble Vitamins		
B$_1$ (thiamine)	Active transport (sodium dependent)	Duodenum and jejunum
B$_2$ (riboflavin)	Unknown	Duodenum and jejunum
Niacin (nicotinic acid)	Passive diffusion	Jejunum
C (ascorbic acid)	Active transport (sodium dependent)	Ileum
Folic acid	Active transport (sodium dependent)	Jejunum
B$_{12}$ (cobalamin)	Active transport (intrinsic factor–dependent)	Terminal ileum
B$_6$ (pyridoxine, pyridoxamine, pyridoxal phosphate)	Passive diffusion	Jejunum
Pantothenic acid	Passive diffusion	Duodenum and jejunum
Biotin	Unknown	Unknown

Intestinal motility is regulated by the enteric nervous system and humoral substances (see p. 1421 and Table 38-1). Two movements promote motility: segmentation and peristalsis.[25] **Segmentation** consists of localized rhythmic contractions of the circular smooth muscles and occurs more frequently than peristalsis.[26] The contraction waves occur at different rates in different parts of the small intestine in segments of 1 to 4 cm. Frequency is greatest (12 per minute) in the upper small intestine and least (8 per minute) in the distal part of the ileum. Segmentation divides and mixes the chyme, bringing it into contact with the absorbent mucosal surface. It also helps to propel the chyme toward the large intestine. The frequency of the segmentation is regulated intrinsically by the frequency of the basic electrical rhythm (BER), which arises in the myenteric plexus of longitudinal smooth muscle. Although the basic rate of contraction is controlled intrinsically, the force of contraction can be enhanced by vagal stimulation (i.e., extrinsically).

Intestinal peristalsis involves short segments (about 10 cm) of longitudinal smooth muscle and propels chime through the intestine. The wave of contraction moves slowly (1 to 2 cm/second) to allow time for digestion and absorption.

Peptide hormones, including motilin, gastrin, secretin, and cholecystokinin, facilitate intestinal motility. Neural reflexes along the length of the small intestine facilitate motility, digestion, and absorption. Through reflex action, receptors in one part of the intestine transmit signals that influence the function of another part. The **ileogastric reflex** inhibits gastric motility when the ileum becomes distended. This prevents the continued movement of chyme into an already distended intestine. The **intestinointestinal reflex** inhibits intestinal motility when one part of the intestine is overdistended. Both of these reflexes require extrinsic innervation. The **gastroileal reflex,** which is activated by an increase in gastric motility and secretion, stimulates an increase in ileal motility and relaxation of the ileocecal sphincter. This empties the ileum and prepares it to receive more chyme. The gastroileal reflex is probably regulated by the hormones gastrin and cholecystokinin or through the autonomic nerves.

During prolonged fasting or between meals, particularly overnight, slow waves sweep along the entire length of the intestinal tract from the stomach to the terminal ileum. This is known as the *interdigestive myoelectric complex,* and it appears to propel residual gastric and intestinal contents, including bacteria, into the colon.

The intestinal villi move with contractions of the muscularis mucosae, a very thin layer of muscle that separates the mucosa and submucosa. Absorption is promoted by the swaying of villi in the luminal contents. Contractile activity also helps to empty the central lacteals, which contain products of fat digestion.

The **ileocecal valve (sphincter)** marks the junction between the terminal ileum and the large intestine. This valve is intrinsically regulated and is normally closed. The arrival of peristaltic waves from the last few centimeters of the ileum causes the ileocecal valve to open, allowing a small amount of chyme to pass through. Distention of the upper large intestine causes the sphincter to constrict, preventing further distention or retrograde flow of intestinal contents.

Large Intestine

The **large intestine** is approximately 1.5 m long and consists of the cecum, appendix, colon, rectum, and anal canal (Figure 38-16). The **cecum** is a pouch that receives chyme from the ileum. Attached to the cecum is the **vermiform appendix,** an appendage having little or no physiologic function. From the cecum, chyme enters the **colon,** a four-part length of intestine that loops upward, traverses the abdominal cavity, and descends to the anal canal. The four parts of the colon are the **ascending colon, transverse colon, descending colon,** and **sigmoid colon.** Two sphincters control the flow of intestinal contents through the cecum and colon: the ileocecal valve, which admits chyme from the ileum to the cecum, and the **O'Beirne sphincter,** which controls the movement of wastes

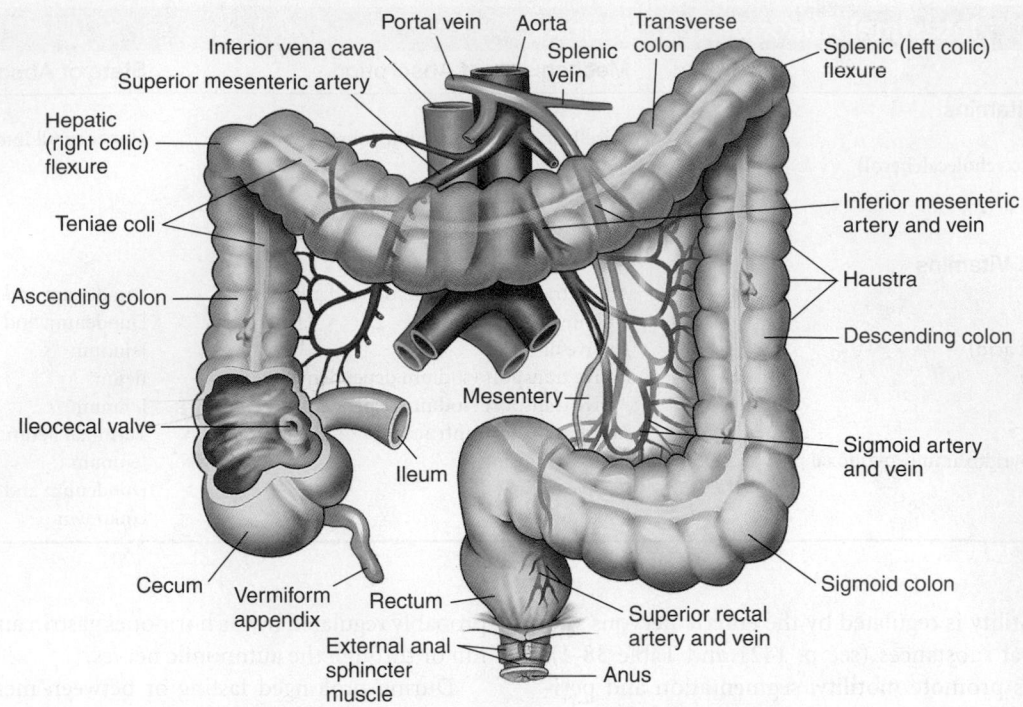

Figure 38-16 Large intestine. (Modified from Patton KT, Thibodeau GA: *Anatomy & physiology*, ed 7, St Louis, 2010, Mosby.)

from the sigmoid colon into the rectum. A thick (2.5 to 3 cm) portion of smooth muscle surrounds the anal canal, forming the **internal anal sphincter.** Overlapping it distally is the striated muscle of the **external anal sphincter.**

In the cecum and colon the longitudinal muscle layer consists of three longitudinal bands called **teniae coli** (Figure 38-16). The teniae coli are shorter than the colon, giving the colon its "gathered" appearance. The circular muscles of the colon separate the gathers into outpouchings called **haustra.** The haustra become more or less prominent with the contractions and relaxations of the circular muscles. The mucosal surface of the colon has rugae (folds), particularly between the haustra, and Lieberkühn crypts but no villi. Columnar epithelial cells and mucus-secreting goblet cells form the mucosa throughout the large intestine. The columnar epithelium absorbs fluid and electrolytes, and the mucus-secreting cells lubricate the mucosa.

The myenteric plexus regulates motor and secretory activity independently of the extrinsic system. Extrinsic parasympathetic innervation occurs through the vagus and extends from the cecum up to the first part of the transverse colon. Vagal stimulation increases rhythmic contraction of the proximal colon. Extrinsic parasympathetic fibers reach the distal colon through the pelvic nerves and can increase motility throughout the colon. The internal anal sphincter is usually in a state of contraction, and its reflex response is to relax when the rectum is distended. The intrinsic nerve plexuses provide the major innervation of the internal anal sphincter, which also receives sympathetic innervation to maintain contraction and parasympathetic innervation that facilitates relaxation when

the rectum is full. The external anal sphincter is innervated by branches of the sacral division of the spinal cord. Sympathetic innervation of this sphincter arises from the celiac and superior mesenteric ganglia and the sphincter nerve. The external anal sphincter is paralyzed after destruction of the lower spinal cord, but the internal sphincter is not. Sympathetic activity in the entire large intestine modulates intestinal reflexes, conveys somatic sensations of fullness and pain, participates in the defecation reflex, and constricts blood vessels. The blood supply of the large intestine and rectum is derived primarily from branches of the superior and inferior mesenteric artery.[27]

The primary type of colonic movement is segmental. The circular muscles contract and relax at different sites, shuttling the intestinal contents back and forth between the contracting and relaxing haustra, most commonly during fasting. The movements massage the intestinal contents, then called the **fecal mass,** and facilitate the absorption of water. Propulsive movement occurs with the proximal-to-distal contraction of several haustral units. **Peristaltic movements** also occur and promote the emptying of the colon. The **gastrocolic reflex** initiates propulsion in the entire colon, usually during or immediately after eating, when chyme enters from the ileum. The gastrocolic reflex causes the fecal mass to pass rapidly into the sigmoid colon and rectum, stimulating defecation. Gastrin and cholecystokinin participate in stimulating this reflex. Epinephrine inhibits contractile activity.

Approximately 500 to 700 ml of chyme flows from the ileum to the cecum per day. Most of the water is absorbed in the colon by diffusion and active transport. The electrochemical gradient established by sodium movement enhances the diffusion of serum potassium from the capillaries in the lumen. Aldosterone increases colon membrane permeability to sodium, thereby increasing both the diffusion of sodium into the cell and its active transport across the basolateral membrane to the interstitial fluid. (See Chapters 3, 20, and 35 for a discussion of aldosterone secretion.) This increases the cell-to-lumen diffusion gradient for potassium. Potassium moves outward, and chloride is absorbed with sodium as the complementary anion. Chloride also enters the cell in exchange for bicarbonate.

Absorption and epithelial transport occur in the cecum, ascending colon, transverse colon, and descending colon. By the time the fecal mass enters the sigmoid colon, the mass consists entirely of wastes and is called the feces. **Feces,** or excrement, consists of food residue, unabsorbed gastrointestinal secretions, shed epithelial cells, and bacteria.

The movement of feces into the sigmoid colon and rectum stimulates the **defecation reflex (rectosphincteric reflex).** The rectal wall stretches and the tonically constricted internal anal sphincter (smooth muscle with autonomic nervous system control) relaxes, creating the urge to defecate. The defecation reflex can be overridden voluntarily by contraction of the external anal sphincter and muscles of the pelvic floor. The rectal wall gradually relaxes, reducing tension, and the urge to defecate passes. Retrograde contraction of the rectum may displace the feces out of the rectal vault until a more convenient time for evacuation. Pain or fear of pain associated with defecation (e.g., rectal fissures or hemorrhoids) can inhibit the defecation reflex. The defecation reflex is regulated by parasympathetic and cholinergic fibers. Voluntary inhibition or facilitation of defecation is mediated from cortical projections onto the medulla and down to sacral segments of the cord.

Defecation is facilitated by squatting or sitting because these positions straighten the angle between the rectum and anal canal and increase the efficiency of straining (increasing intra-abdominal pressure). Intra-abdominal pressure is increased by initiating the **Valsalva maneuver.** This maneuver consists of inhaling and forcing the diaphragm and chest muscles against the closed glottis. This increases both intrathoracic and intra-abdominal pressure, which is transmitted to the rectum.

Intestinal Bacteria

The type and number of bacterial flora vary greatly throughout the normal gastrointestinal tract, with an increasing number of bacteria from the stomach to the distal colon. The stomach is relatively sterile because of the secretion of acid that kills ingested pathogens or inhibits bacterial growth. Bile acid secretion, intestinal motility, and antibody production suppress bacterial growth in the duodenum, and in the duodenum and jejunum there is a low concentration of aerobes (10^{-1} to 10^{-4}/ml), primarily streptococci, lactobacilli, staphylococci, enterobacteria, and *Bacteroides*.[28] There are no anaerobes proximal to the ileum. Anaerobes are found distal to the ileocecal valve. They constitute about 95% of the fecal flora in the colon and

contribute one third of the solid bulk of feces. *Bacteroides,* clostridia, anaerobic lactobacilli, and coliforms are the most common microorganisms from the ileum to the cecum.

The intestinal tract is sterile at birth but becomes colonized with *Escherichia coli, Clostridium welchii,* and *Streptococcus* within a few hours. Within 3 to 4 weeks after birth, the normal flora are established. The normal flora do not have the virulence factors associated with pathogenic microorganisms, thus permitting immune tolerances.[29] The intestinal mucosal environment also produces a broad spectrum of protective antimicrobial agents.[30] The intestinal bacteria do not have major digestive or absorptive functions. They do play a role in the metabolism of bile salts (contributing to the intestinal reabsorption of bile and the elimination of toxic bile metabolites); the metabolism of estrogens, androgens, and lipids and conversion of unabsorbed carbohydrates to absorbable organic acids; the synthesis of vitamin K_2; and metabolism of various nitrogenous substances and drugs.[31]

ACCESSORY ORGANS OF DIGESTION

The liver, gallbladder, and exocrine pancreas all secrete substances necessary for the digestion of chyme. These secretions are delivered to the duodenum through ducts (Figure 38-17). The liver produces bile, which contains salts necessary for fat digestion and absorption. Between meals bile is stored in the gallbladder. The exocrine pancreas produces enzymes needed for the complete digestion of carbohydrates, proteins, and fats. The exocrine pancreas also produces an alkaline fluid that neutralizes chyme, creating a duodenal pH that supports enzymatic action. The liver receives nutrients absorbed by the small intestine and metabolizes or synthesizes these nutrients

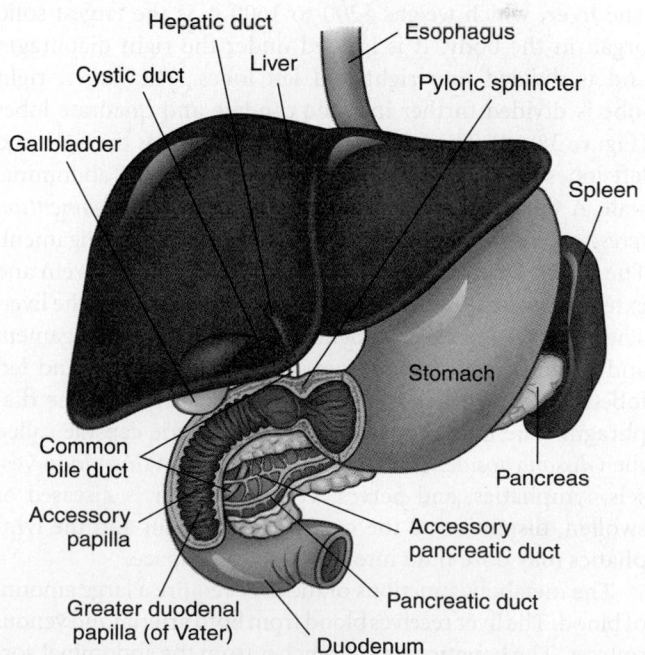

Figure 38-17 Location of the liver, gallbladder, and exocrine pancreas, which are the accessory organs of digestion.

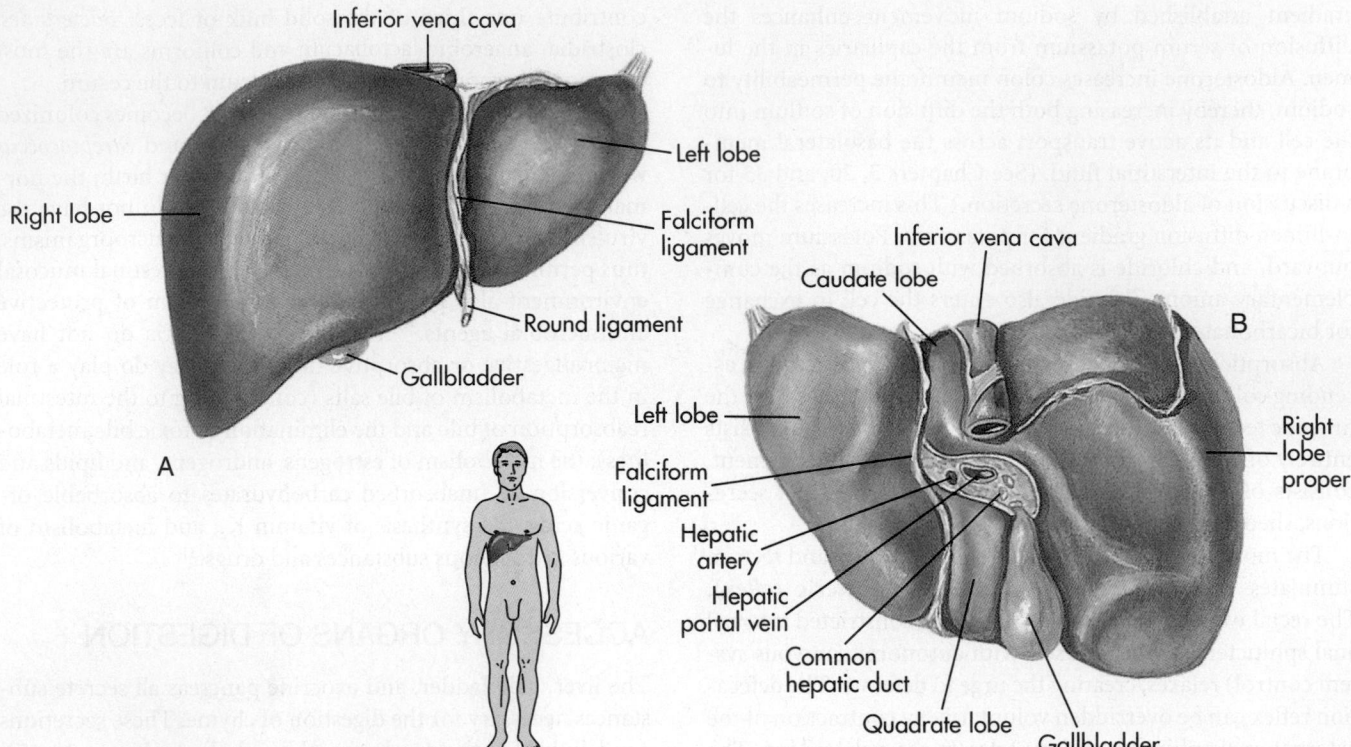

Figure 38-18 Gross structure of the liver. **A,** Anterior view. **B,** Inferior view. (From Thibodeau GA, Patton KT: *Anatomy & physiology,* ed 5, St Louis, 2003, Mosby.)

into forms that can be absorbed by the body's cells. It then releases the nutrients into the bloodstream or stores them for later use.

Liver

The **liver,** which weighs 1200 to 1600 g, is the largest solid organ in the body. It is located under the right diaphragm and is divided into right and left lobes. The larger, right lobe is divided further into the caudate and quadrate lobes (Figure 38-18). The *falciform ligament* separates the right and left lobes and attaches the liver to the anterior abdominal wall. A fibrous cord called the *round ligament (ligamentum teres)* extends along the free edge of the falciform ligament. The round ligament is the remnant of the umbilical vein and extends from the umbilicus to the inferior surface of the liver. The *coronary ligament* branches from the falciform ligament and extends over the superior surface of the right and left lobes, adhering the liver to the inferior surface of the diaphragm. The liver is covered by a fibroelastic capsule called the *Glisson capsule.* The **Glisson capsule** contains blood vessels, lymphatics, and nerves. When the liver is diseased or swollen, distention of the capsule causes pain and the lymphatics may ooze fluid into the peritoneal space.

The metabolic functions of the liver require a large amount of blood. The liver receives blood from both arterial and venous sources. The **hepatic artery** branches from the abdominal aorta and provides oxygenated blood at the rate of 400 to 500 ml/minute (about 25% of the cardiac output). The **hepatic portal**

vein, which receives deoxygenated blood from the inferior and superior mesenteric veins and the splenic vein, delivers about 1000 to 1200 ml/minute of blood to the liver. The **portal vein** carries 70% of the blood supply to the liver. This blood carries some oxygen and is rich in nutrients that have been absorbed from the digestive tract and transported through the mesenteric veins to the portal vein (Figure 38-19).

Within the liver lobes are multiple, smaller anatomic units called **liver lobules** (Figure 38-20). The lobules are formed of cords or plates of **hepatocytes,** which are the functional cells of the liver. These cells are capable of regeneration; therefore, damaged or resected liver tissue can regrow. Hepatocytes secrete electrolytes, lipids, lecithin, bile acids, and cholesterol into the canaliculi. Plasma proteins are also synthesized and released into the bloodstream. **Lipocytes** are star-shaped cells that store lipids, including vitamin A. Small capillaries, or **sinusoids,** are located between the plates of hepatocytes. The sinusoids receive a mixture of venous and arterial blood from branches of the hepatic artery and portal vein. Blood from the sinusoids drains into to a central vein in the middle of each liver lobule. Venous blood from all the lobules then flows into the **hepatic vein,** which empties into the inferior vena cava. The sinusoids of the liver lobules are lined with highly permeable endothelium. This permeability enhances the transport of nutrients from the sinusoids into the hepatocytes, where they are metabolized.[32] The sinusoids are also lined with phagocytic cells known as **Kupffer cells.** Kupffer cells are part of the mononuclear phagocyte system (see Chapter 25)

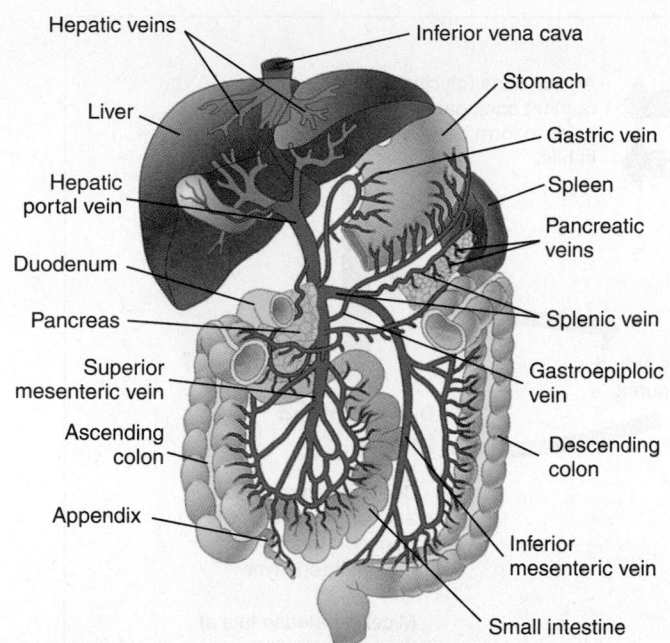

Figure 38-19 Hepatic portal circulation. In this unusual circulatory route, a vein is located between two capillary beds. The hepatic portal vein collects blood from capillaries in visceral structures located in the abdomen and empties into the liver for distribution to the hepatic capillaries. Hepatic veins return blood to the inferior vena cava. (Organs are not drawn to scale.) (From Thibodeau GA, Patton KT: *Anatomy & physiology,* ed 5, St Louis, 2003, Mosby.)

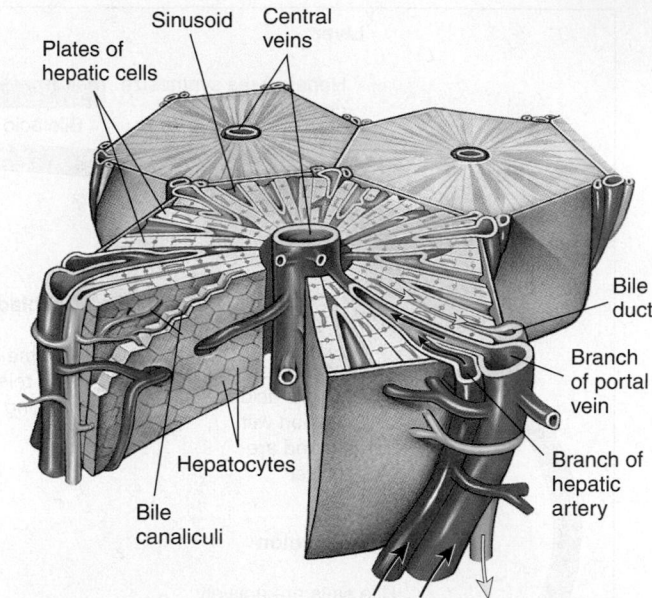

Figure 38-20 Diagrammatic representation of a liver lobule. A central vein is located in the center of the lobule, with plates of hepatocytes disposed radially. Branches of the portal vein and hepatic artery are located on the periphery of the lobule, and blood from both perfuse the sinusoids. Peripherally located bile ducts drain the bile canaliculi that run between the hepatocytes. (Modified from Patton KT, Thibodeau GA: *Anatomy & physiology,* ed 7, St Louis, 2010, Mosby.)

and are the largest population of tissue macrophages. They are bactericidal and are important for bilirubin production and lipid metabolism.[33] **Stellate cells** contain retinoids (vitamin A), are contractile in liver injury, regulate sinusoidal blood flow, and may proliferate into myofibroblasts.[34] They remove foreign substances from the blood and trap bacteria. **Pit cells** are natural killer cells found in the sinusoidal lumen; they produce interferon-γ and are important in tumor defense.[35] Between the endothelial lining of the sinusoid and the hepatocyte is the **Disse space,** which drains interstitial fluid into the hepatic lymph system.

Secretion of Bile
The liver assists intestinal digestion by secreting 700 to 1200 ml of bile per day. **Bile** is an alkaline, bitter-tasting yellowish green fluid that contains bile salts (conjugated bile acids), cholesterol, bilirubin (a pigment), electrolytes, and water. It is formed by hepatocytes and secreted into the canaliculi small channels adjacent to hepatocytes. **Bile salts,** which are conjugated bile acids, are required for the intestinal emulsification and absorption of fats. The **bile canaliculi** empty into bile ducts and eventually drain into the **common bile duct** (see Figure 38-20). The union of the common bile duct and pancreatic duct is at the papilla or **ampulla of Vater),**[32] which empties into the duodenum through an opening called the **major duodenal papilla (sphincter of Oddi).** Having facilitated fat emulsification and absorption in the small intestine, most bile salts are actively absorbed in the terminal ileum and returned to the liver through the portal circulation for resecretion. The recycling of bile salts is termed the **enterohepatic circulation** (Figure 38-21).[36]

Bile has two fractional components: the acid-dependent fraction and the acid independent fraction. Hepatocytes secrete the **bile acid–dependent fraction** of the bile. This fraction consists of bile acids, cholesterol, lecithin (a phospholipid), and bilirubin (a bile pigment). The **bile acid–independent fraction** of the bile, which is secreted by the hepatocytes and epithelial cells of the bile canaliculi, is a bicarbonate-rich aqueous fluid that gives bile its alkaline pH.

Bile salts are conjugated in the liver from primary and secondary bile acids. The **primary bile acids** are cholic acid and chenodeoxycholic (chenic acid or chenodiol) acid. These acids are synthesized from cholesterol by the hepatocytes. The **secondary bile acids** are deoxycholic acid and lithocholic acid. These acids are formed in the small intestine by the action of intestinal bacteria, after which they are absorbed and flow to the liver (see Figure 38-21). Both forms of bile acids are conjugated with amino acids (glycine or taurine) in the liver to form bile salts. Conjugation makes the bile acids more water soluble, thus restricting their diffusion from the duodenum and ileum. The primary and secondary bile acids together form the **bile acid pool.** Other components of bile include phospholipids and cholesterol.

Bile salts are planar molecules; that is, they are hydrophobic on one end and hydrophilic on the other. When the concentration of bile salts in the intestine is adequate or has reached the **critical micelle concentration,** the molecules

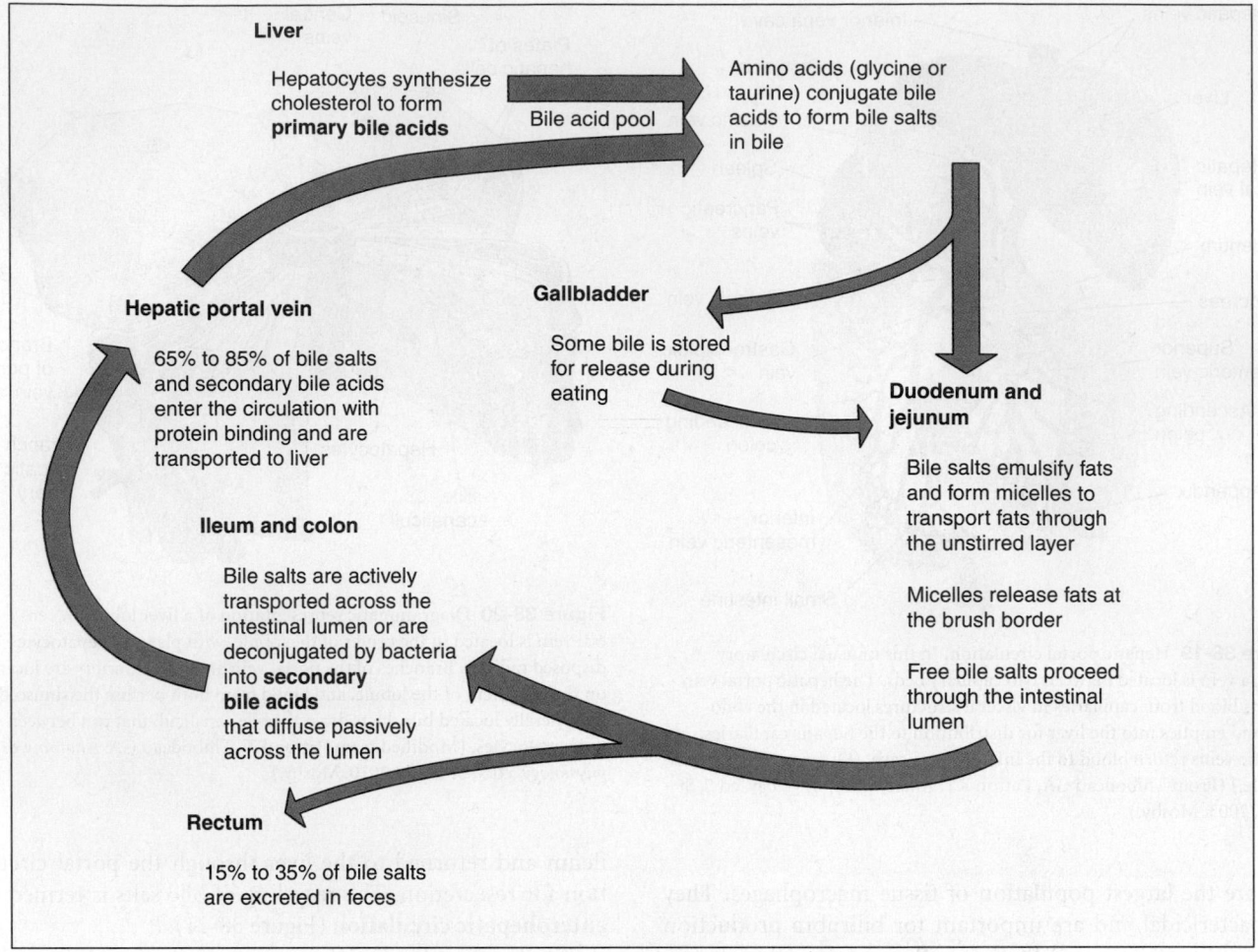

Liver

Hepatocytes synthesize
cholesterol to form
primary bile acids

Bile acid pool

Amino acids (glycine or
taurine) conjugate bile
acids to form bile salts
in bile

Hepatic portal vein

65% to 85% of bile salts
and secondary bile acids
enter the circulation with
protein binding and are
transported to liver

Gallbladder

Some bile is stored
for release during
eating

**Duodenum and
jejunum**

Bile salts emulsify fats
and form micelles to
transport fats through
the unstirred layer

Micelles release fats at
the brush border

Free bile salts proceed
through the intestinal
lumen

Ileum and colon

Bile salts are actively
transported across the
intestinal lumen or are
deconjugated by bacteria
into **secondary
bile acids**
that diffuse passively
across the lumen

Rectum

15% to 35% of bile salts
are excreted in feces

Figure 38-21 The enterohepatic circulation of bile salts.

form water-soluble micelles (aggregates) with their hydrophilic side toward the watery chyme of the intestine and their hydrophobic side surrounding fat molecules such as cholesterol, free fatty acids, and phospholipids (see Figure 38-14). Micelle formation facilitates the absorption of fat by the intestinal mucosa by promoting diffusion through the aqueous intestinal layer of the brush border.

Bile secretion is called **choleresis.** A **choleretic agent** is a substance that stimulates the liver to secrete bile. One strong stimulus is a high concentration of bile salts. Other choleretics include secretin, which increases the rate of bile flow by promoting the secretion of bicarbonate from canaliculi and other intrahepatic bile ducts; cholecystokinin; and vagal stimulation.

Metabolism of Bilirubin

Bilirubin is a byproduct of destruction of aged red blood cells. It gives bile a greenish black color and produces the yellow tinge of jaundice. Aged red blood cells are taken up and destroyed by macrophages of the mononuclear phagocyte system, primarily in the spleen and liver. (In the liver these macrophages are Kupffer cells.) Within these cells, hemoglobin is separated into its component parts—heme and globin (Figure 38-22). The globin component is further degraded into its constituent amino acids, which are recycled to form new protein. The heme moiety is converted to **biliverdin** by the enzymatic cleavage of iron. The iron attaches to transferrin in the plasma and can be stored in the liver or used by the bone marrow to make new red blood cells. The biliverdin is enzymatically converted to bilirubin in the macrophage of the mononuclear phagocytic system and then is released into the plasma. In the plasma, bilirubin binds to albumin and is known as **unconjugated bilirubin,** or free bilirubin, which is lipid soluble. Bilirubin also may have a role as an antioxidant and provide cytoprotection.[37,38] Elevated circulating bilirubin levels may protect against cancer and cardiovascular disease.[39]

In the liver, unconjugated bilirubin moves from plasma in the sinusoids into the hepatocyte. Within hepatocytes it joins with glucuronic acid to form **conjugated bilirubin,** which is water soluble. Conjugation transforms bilirubin from a lipid-soluble substance that can cross biologic membranes to a water-soluble substance that can be excreted in the bile. When conjugated bilirubin reaches the distal ileum and colon, it is deconjugated by bacteria and converted to **urobilinogen.** Urobilinogen is then excreted in the urine as urobilin; a small amount is recirculated back into the liver and eliminated in feces.

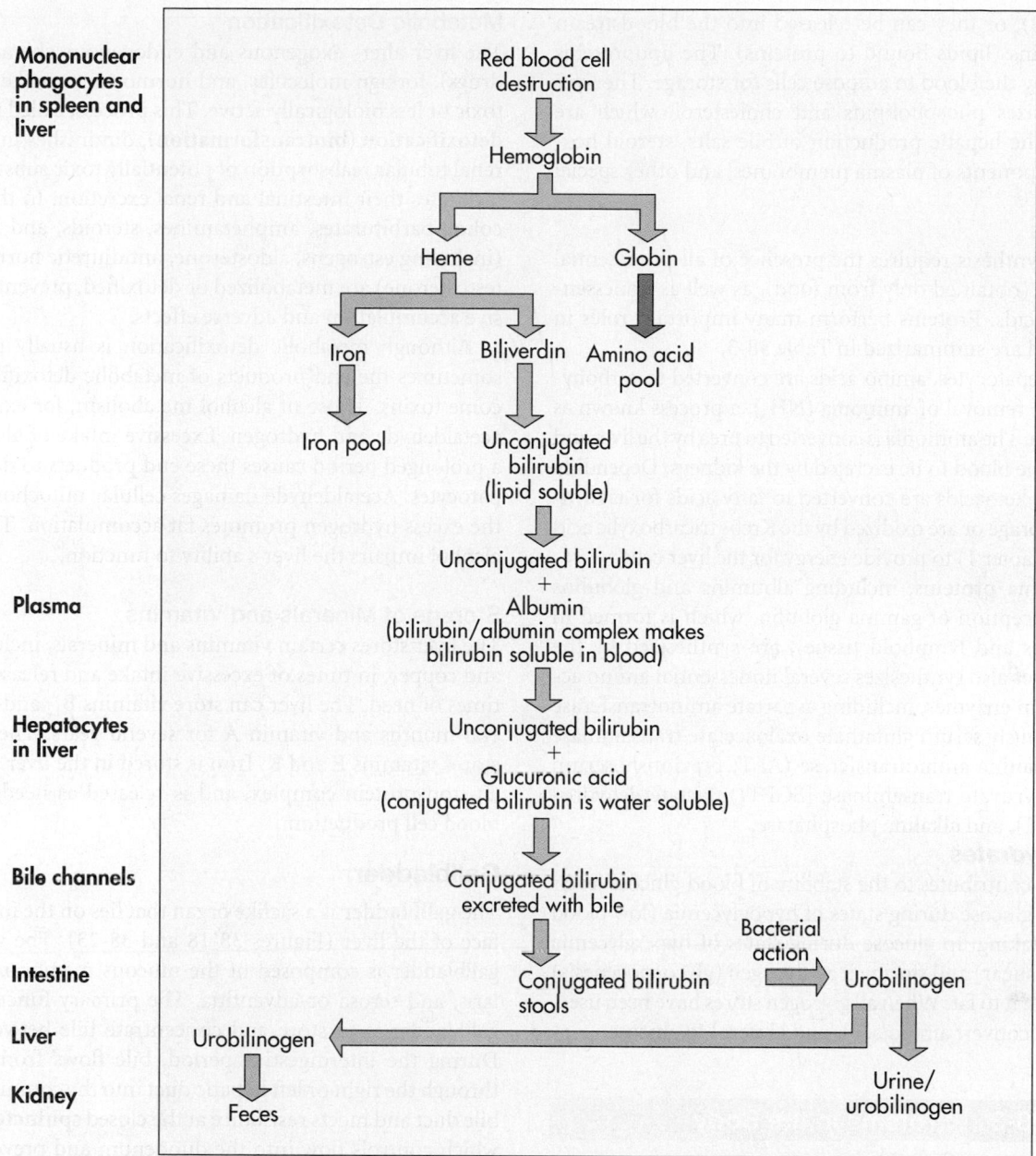

Figure 38-22 Bilirubin metabolism (see text).

Vascular and Hematologic Functions

Because of its extensive vascular network, the liver can store a large volume of blood. The amount stored at any one time depends on pressure relationships in the arteries and veins. The liver also can release blood to maintain systemic circulatory volume in the event of hemorrhage.

Kupffer cells (macrophages) in the sinusoids of the liver remove bacteria and foreign particles from the portal blood. Because the liver receives all of the venous blood from the gut and pancreas, the Kupffer cells play an important role in destroying intestinal bacteria and preventing infections.

The liver also has hemostatic functions. It synthesizes prothrombin; fibrinogen; and factors I, II, VII, IX, and X, all of which are necessary for effective clotting (see Chapter 25).

Vitamin K, a fat-soluble vitamin, is essential for the synthesis of other clotting factors. Because bile salts are needed for reabsorption of fats, vitamin K absorption depends on adequate bile production in the liver. Impairment of vitamin K absorption diminishes production of clotting factors and increases risk of bleeding.

Metabolism of Nutrients
Fats

Fat is synthesized from carbohydrate and protein, primarily in the liver. Ingested fat absorbed by lacteals in the intestinal villi enters the liver through the lymphatics, primarily as triglycerides. In the liver the triglycerides can be hydrolyzed to glycerol and free fatty acids and used to produce metabolic energy (ATP), or they can be released into the bloodstream as lipoproteins (lipids bound to proteins). The lipoproteins are carried by the blood to adipose cells for storage. The liver also synthesizes phospholipids and cholesterol, which are needed for the hepatic production of bile salts, steroid hormones, components of plasma membranes, and other special molecules.

Proteins

Protein synthesis requires the presence of all the essential amino acids (obtained only from food), as well as nonessential amino acids. Proteins perform many important roles in the body and are summarized in Table 38-3.

Within hepatocytes, amino acids are converted to carbohydrates by the removal of ammonia (NH_3), a process known as **deamination.** The ammonia is converted to urea by the liver and passes into the blood to be excreted by the kidneys. Depending on need, the ketoacids are converted to fatty acids for fat synthesis and storage or are oxidized by the Krebs tricarboxylic acid cycle (see Chapter 1) to provide energy for the liver cells.

The plasma proteins, including albumins and globulins (with the exception of gamma globulin, which is formed in lymph nodes and lymphoid tissue), are synthesized by the liver. The liver also synthesizes several nonessential amino acids and serum enzymes, including aspartate aminotransferase (AST; previously serum glutamate oxaloacetate transaminase [SGOT]), alanine aminotransferase (ALT; previously serum glutamate pyruvate transaminase [SGPT]), lactate dehydrogenase (LDH), and alkaline phosphatase.

Carbohydrates

The liver contributes to the stability of blood glucose levels by releasing glucose during states of hypoglycemia (low blood sugar) and taking up glucose during states of hyperglycemia (high blood sugar) and storing it as glycogen (glyconeogenesis) or converting it to fat. When all glycogen stores have been used, the liver can convert amino acids and glycerol to glucose.

Table 38-3	Proteins in the Body
Role	**Example**
Contraction	Actin and myosin enable muscle contraction
Energy	Proteins can be metabolized for energy
Fluid balance	Albumin, a major source of plasma oncotic pressure
Protection	Antibodies and complement protect against infection and foreign substances
Regulation	Enzymes control chemical reactions; hormones regulate many physiologic processes
Structure	Collagen fibers provide structural support to many parts of the body; keratin strengthens skin, hair, and nails
Transport	Hemoglobin transports oxygen and carbon dioxide in the blood; plasma proteins serve as transport molecules; proteins in cell membranes control movement of materials into and out of cells
Coagulation	Hemostasis is regulated by proteins that balance coagulation and anticoagulation

Metabolic Detoxification

The liver alters exogenous and endogenous chemicals (e.g., drugs), foreign molecules, and hormones to make them less toxic or less biologically active. This process, called **metabolic detoxification (biotransformation),** diminishes intestinal or renal tubular reabsorption of potentially toxic substances and facilitates their intestinal and renal excretion. In this way alcohol, barbiturates, amphetamines, steroids, and hormones (including estrogens, aldosterone, antidiuretic hormone, and testosterone) are metabolized or detoxified, preventing excessive accumulation and adverse effects.

Although metabolic detoxification is usually protective, sometimes the end products of metabolic detoxification become toxins. Those of alcohol metabolism, for example, are acetaldehyde and hydrogen. Excessive intake of alcohol over a prolonged period causes these end products to damage hepatocytes. Acetaldehyde damages cellular mitochondria, and the excess hydrogen promotes fat accumulation. This is how alcohol impairs the liver's ability to function.

Storage of Minerals and Vitamins

The liver stores certain vitamins and minerals, including iron and copper, in times of excessive intake and releases them in times of need. The liver can store vitamins B_{12} and D for several months and vitamin A for several years. The liver also stores vitamins E and K. Iron is stored in the liver as ferritin, an iron-protein complex, and is released as needed for red blood cell production.

Gallbladder

The **gallbladder** is a saclike organ that lies on the inferior surface of the liver (Figures 38-18 and 38-23). The wall of the gallbladder is composed of the mucous membrane, muscularis, and serosa or adventitia. The primary function of the gallbladder is to store and concentrate bile between meals. During the interdigestive period, bile flows from the liver through the right or left hepatic duct into the common hepatic bile duct and meets resistance at the closed **sphincter of Oddi,** which controls flow into the duodenum and prevents reflux of duodenal contents into the pancreatobiliary system.[40] Bile then flows into the gallbladder through the **cystic duct** where it is concentrated and stored. The mucosa of the gallbladder wall readily absorbs water and electrolytes, leaving a high concentration of bile salts, bile pigments, and cholesterol. The gallbladder holds about 90 ml of bile.

Within 30 minutes after eating, the gallbladder begins to contract forcing stored bile through the cystic duct and into the common bile duct. The sphincter of Oddi relaxes, and bile flows into the duodenum through the major duodenal papilla. During the cephalic and gastric phases of digestion, gallbladder contraction is mediated by cholinergic branches of the vagus nerve. Hormonal regulation of gallbladder contraction is derived primarily from the release of cholecystokinin secreted by the duodenal mucosa in the presence of fat. Vasoactive intestinal peptide, pancreatic polypeptide, and sympathetic nerve stimulation relax the gallbladder.

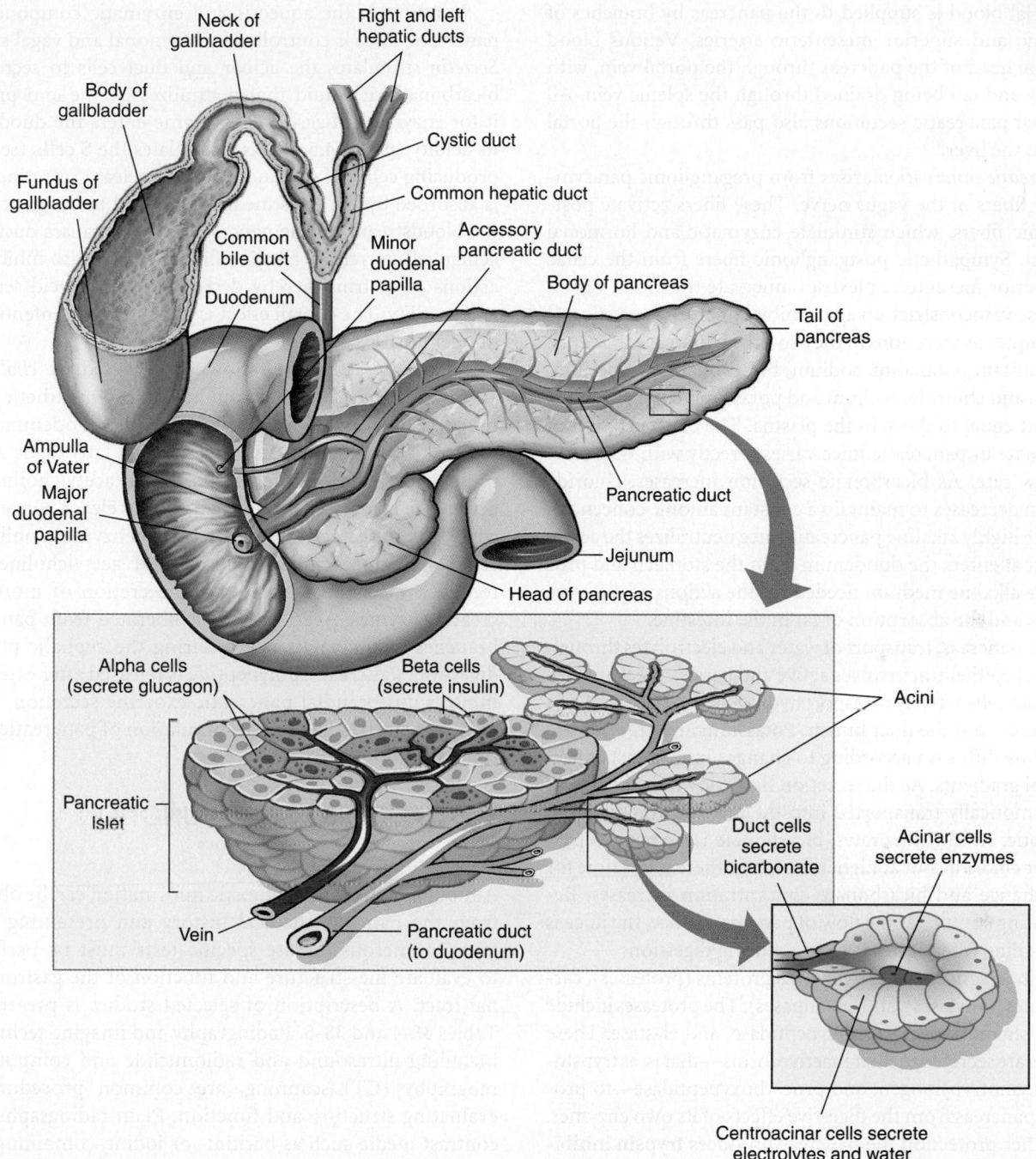

Figure 38-23 Associated structures of the gallbladder, pancreas, and pancreatic acinar cells and duct. (Modified from Thibodeau GA, Patton KT: *Anatomy & physiology,* ed 6, St Louis, 2007, Mosby.)

Exocrine Pancreas

The **pancreas** is approximately 20 cm long, with its head tucked into the curve of the duodenum and its tail touching the spleen. The body of the pancreas lies deep in the abdomen, behind the stomach (see Figure 38-23). The pancreas is unique in that it has endocrine as well as exocrine functions. The endocrine pancreas secretes insulin, glucagon, somatostatin, and pancreatic polypeptide (see Chapter 20).

The **exocrine pancreas** is composed of acinar cells that secrete enzymes and networks of ducts that secrete alkaline

fluids with important digestive functions. The acinar cells are organized into spherical lobules (acini) around small secretory ducts (see Figure 38-23). Secretions drain into a system of ducts that leads to the **pancreatic duct (Wirsung duct),** which empties into the common bile duct at the **ampulla of Vater** and then through the duodenal papilla into the duodenum. In some individuals an accessory duct (the duct of Santorini) branches off the pancreatic duct and drains directly into the duodenum at an opening called the *minor duodenal papilla* (see Figure 38-23).

Arterial blood is supplied to the pancreas by branches of the celiac and superior mesenteric arteries. Venous blood leaves the head of the pancreas through the portal vein, with the body and tail being drained through the splenic vein. All hormonal pancreatic secretions also pass through the portal vein into the liver.

Pancreatic innervation arises from preganglionic parasympathetic fibers of the vagus nerve. These fibers activate postganglionic fibers, which stimulate enzymatic and hormonal secretion. Sympathetic postganglionic fibers from the celiac and superior mesenteric plexuses innervate the blood vessels and cause vasoconstriction and inhibit pancreatic secretion.[41]

The aqueous secretions of the exocrine pancreas are isotonic and contain potassium, sodium, bicarbonate, magnesium, calcium, and chloride. Sodium and potassium concentrations are about equal to those in the plasma. The concentration of bicarbonate in pancreatic juice varies directly with the secretory flow rate. As bicarbonate secretion increases, chloride secretion decreases to maintain a constant anionic concentration. The highly alkaline pancreatic juice neutralizes the acidic chyme that enters the duodenum from the stomach and provides the alkaline medium needed for the actions of digestive enzymes and the absorption of fat in the intestine.

In the pancreas, transport of water and electrolytes through the ductal epithelium involves active and passive mechanisms. The ductal cells actively transport hydrogen into the blood and bicarbonate into the duct lumen. Potassium and chloride are secreted by diffusion according to changes in electrochemical potential gradients. As the secretion flows down the duct, water is osmotically transported into the juice until it becomes isoosmotic. At low flow rates, bicarbonate is exchanged passively for chloride, but at higher flow rates there is less time for this exchange and bicarbonate concentration increases. Because eating stimulates the flow of pancreatic juice, the juice is most alkaline when it needs to be—during digestion.

The *pancreatic enzymes* hydrolyze proteins (proteases), carbohydrates (amylases), and fats (lipases). The proteases include trypsin, chymotrypsin, carboxypeptidase, and elastase. These enzymes are secreted in their inactive forms—that is, as trypsinogen, chymotrypsinogen, and procarboxypeptidase—to protect the pancreas from the digestive effects of its own enzymes. For further protection the pancreas produces **trypsin inhibitor,** which prevents the activation of proteolytic enzymes while they are in the pancreas. Once in the duodenum, the inactive forms (proenzymes) are activated by **enterokinase,** an enzyme secreted by the duodenal mucosa. Trypsinogen is the first proenzyme to be activated. Its conversion to trypsin stimulates the conversion of chymotrypsinogen to chymotrypsin and procarboxypeptidase to carboxypeptidase. Each of these enzymes cleaves specific peptide bonds to reduce polypeptides to smaller peptides.

Pancreatic α-amylase is secreted in active form and digests carbohydrate by cleaving interior α-1,4-glucosidic bonds at an optimum pH of approximately 6.9. **Pancreatic lipases** hydrolyze triglycerides, cholesterol, and phospholipids to free fatty acids.

Secretion of the aqueous and enzymatic components of pancreatic juice is controlled by hormonal and vagal stimuli. *Secretin* stimulates the acinar and duct cells to secrete the bicarbonate-rich fluid that neutralizes chyme and prepares it for enzymatic digestion. As chyme enters the duodenum, its acidity (pH of 4.5 or less) stimulates the **S cells** (secretin-producing cells) of the duodenum to release secretin, which is absorbed by the intestine and delivered to the pancreas in the bloodstream. In the pancreas, secretin causes ductal and acinar cells to release alkaline fluid. Secretin also inhibits the actions of gastrin, thereby decreasing gastric acid secretion and motility. The overall effect is to neutralize contents of the duodenum.

Enzymatic secretion follows, stimulated by *cholecystokinin* and *acetylcholine* (from the parasympathetic vagus nerve). Cholecystokinin is released in the duodenum in response to the essential amino acids and fatty acids already present in chyme. Cholecystokinin and acetylcholine both act on the acinar cells, causing enzyme release. Once in the small intestine, activated pancreatic enzymes inhibit the release of more cholecystokinin and acetylcholine. This feedback mechanism inhibits the secretion of more pancreatic enzymes. Acetylcholine is liberated from pancreatic branches of the vagus nerve during the cephalic phase of digestion. Pancreatic polypeptide is released after eating and inhibits postprandial pancreatic exocrine secretion. (Table 38-1 summarizes hormonal stimulation of pancreatic secretions.)

TESTS OF DIGESTIVE FUNCTION

Gastrointestinal Tract

Although important diagnostic information can be obtained from the patient's medical history and presenting symptoms, numerous disease-specific tests must be performed to evaluate the structure and function of the gastrointestinal tract. A description of selected studies is presented in Tables 38-4 and 38-5. Radiography and imaging techniques, including ultrasound and radionuclide and computed tomography (CT) scanning, are common procedures for evaluating structure and function. Plain radiographs using contrast media such as barium- or iodine-containing compounds can be used to outline the gastrointestinal lumen, biliary tree and pancreatic ducts, fistulae, and arteriovenous systems. CT scanning is particularly useful for diagnosis of pancreatic or hepatic tumors or cysts. Ultrasonic scanning is a safe, simple, and relatively inexpensive technique used to detect liver-related jaundice and intra-abdominal masses, particularly abscesses.

Fiberoptic endoscopy, using flexible endoscopes, allows direct visualization of the gastrointestinal tract. A biopsy channel allows tissue sampling, and suction can be applied to remove gastrointestinal secretions or blood. Analysis of stool, gastric secretions, and plasma provides important clues to infection, malabsorption syndromes, ulcerative lesions, and tumor growth.

Table 38-4   Selected Studies of Gastrointestinal Structure

Test	Description	Application
Plain roentgenograms	Use of high-energy electromagnetic radiation to evaluate tissue structure by radiopacity or radiolucency	Visualization of the position, size, and structure of abdominal contents
Air or barium contrast roentgenograms	Introduction of radiopaque substances into the upper or lower gastrointestinal tract	Enhanced visualization of the contours, position, and size of the gastrointestinal tract to detect umbilical hernia, ulcers, diverticula, congenital anomalies, polyps, tumors, strictures, obstructions
Endoscopy Esophagoscopy (esophagus) Gastroscopy (stomach) Duodenoscopy (duodenum) Colonoscopy (large intestine) Sigmoidoscopy (sigmoid colon)	Passage of rigid or flexible (fiberoptic) endoscope into the gastrointestinal tract for visualization or biopsy	Visualization or biopsy of inflamed hernias, polyps, ulcers, strictures, varices, tumors, sites of bleeding, mucosal or neoplastic lesions and for culture of *Helicobacter pylori* from stomach
Ultrasound	Use of piezoelectric crystal to generate sound waves that are reflected from tissue interfaces to provide an image	Imaging of abdominal organs (gallbladder, liver, pancreas, spleen), masses, stones, abscesses, structural abnormalities
Computed tomography (CT)	Use of a computer to integrate differences in absorption of a large number of x-rays to produce a cross-sectional image; may be done with contrast agents	Imaging of gallbladder, liver, pancreas, spleen, cysts, hematomas, abscesses, stones, extrahepatic bile ducts, and portal vein
Magnetic resonance imaging (MRI)	Projection of differences in magnetic properties of molecules within different cells and tissues, using the field of a large magnet	Same applications as CT scan; also can detect blood flow and vessel patency

Table 38-5   Selected Tests of Gastrointestinal Function

Test	Normal Findings	Clinical Significance of Abnormal Findings
Stool studies	Resident microorganisms: clostridia, enterococci, *Pseudomonas,* a few yeasts	Detection of *Salmonella typhi* (typhoid fever), *Shigella* (dysentery), *Vibrio cholerae* (cholera), *Yersinia* (enterocolitis), *Escherichia coli* (gastroenteritis), *Staphylococcus aureus* (food poisoning), *Clostridium botulinum* (food poisoning), *Clostridium perfringens* (food poisoning), *Aeromonas* (gastroenteritis)
	Fat: 2-6 g/24 hr	Steatorrhea (increased values) can result from intestinal malabsorption or pancreatic insufficiency
	Pus: none	Large amounts of pus are associated with chronic ulcerative colitis, abscesses, and anorectal fistula
	Occult blood: none (orthotolidin or guaiac test)	Positive tests associated with bleeding
	Ova and parasites: none	Detection of *Entamoeba histolytica* (amebiasis), *Giardia lamblia* (giardiasis), and worms
D-Xylose absorption	5-Hr urinary excretion: 4.5 g/L Peak blood level: >30 mg/dl	Differentiation of pancreatic steatorrhea (normal D-xylose absorption) from intestinal steatorrhea (impaired D-xylose absorption)
Gastric acid stimulation	11-20 mEq/hr after stimulation	Detection of duodenal ulcers, Zollinger-Ellison syndrome (increased values), gastric atrophy, gastric carcinoma (decreased values)
Manometry (use of water-filled catheters connected to pressure transducers passed into the esophagus, stomach, colon, or rectum to evaluate contractility)	Values vary at different levels of the intestine	Inadequate swallowing, motility, sphincter function
Culture and sensitivity of duodenal contents	No pathogens	Detection of *Salmonella typhi* (typhoid fever)
Breath tests		
Glucose or D-xylose breath test	Negative for hydrogen or CO_2	May indicate intestinal bacterial overgrowth
Urea breath test	Negative for isotopically labeled CO_2	Presence of *Helicobacter pylori* infection
Lactose breath test	Negative for exhaled hydrogen	Lactose intolerance

Liver

A variety of diagnostic tests can be performed to evaluate liver function[42,43] (Table 38-6). Imaging techniques similar to those described for the gastrointestinal tract are also useful for evaluating liver structure and function. Plasma chemistry findings are also altered with many liver diseases because of release of cytoplasmic enzymes into the circulation when there is damage to the hepatocyte. Of particular importance are elevations of aminotransferases and LDH. Obstruction of bile canaliculi or ducts results in regurgitation of bile back into the hepatic sinusoids and into the circulation, with elevation of bilirubin levels. Prothrombin times are often prolonged with both hepatitis and chronic liver disease. In severe disease, other plasma proteins, such as albumin and globulins, may be diminished as a result of hepatocyte damage. Liver biopsies are often performed to evaluate the extent of liver involvement or degeneration with cirrhosis or hepatitis.

Gallbladder

Evaluation of structural alterations in the gallbladder may be achieved by the use of various imaging techniques. Table 38-7 summarizes these techniques. Obstruction of the common ducts from stones, tumors, or inflammation prevents the flow of bile from the liver and gallbladder from reaching the gastrointestinal tract. Both the conjugated and total serum bilirubin values are elevated, urine urobilinogen is increased, stools are clay colored, and jaundice develops. Fat absorption can be impaired and the prothrombin time prolonged if vitamin K is not absorbed. With inflammation of the gallbladder, the white cell count is elevated.

Exocrine Pancreas

Tests of pancreatic function are summarized in Table 38-8. Evaluation of plasma and urinary amylase provides particularly significant measures of pancreatic function. Inflammation or obstruction of the pancreas results in an increase in serum

Table 38-6   Common Liver Function Tests

Test	Normal Value	Interpretation
Serum Enzymes		
Alkaline phosphatase	13-39 units/L	Increases with biliary obstruction and cholestatic hepatitis
Gamma-glutamyl transpeptidase (GGT)	Male 12-38 units/L Female 9-31 units/L	Increases with biliary obstruction and cholestatic hepatitis
Aspartate aminotransferase (AST; previously serum glutamate oxaloacetate transaminase [SGOT])	5-40 units/L	Increases with hepatocellular injury (and injury in other tissues, i.e., skeletal and cardiac muscle)
Alanine aminotransferase (ALT; previously serum glutamate pyruvate transaminase [SGPT])	5-35 units/L	Increases with hepatocellular injury and necrosis
Lactate dehydrogenase (LDH)	90-220 units/L	Isoenzyme LD_5 is elevated with hypoxic and primary liver injury
5′-Nucleotidase	2-11 units/L	Increases with increase in alkaline phosphatase and cholestatic disorders
Bilirubin Metabolism		
Serum bilirubin		
Indirect (unconjugated)	<0.8 mg/dl	Increases with hemolysis (lysis of red blood cells)
Direct (conjugated)	0.2-0.4 mg/dl	Increases with hepatocellular injury or obstruction
Total	<1.0 mg/dl	Increases with biliary obstruction
Urine bilirubin	0	Increases with biliary obstruction
Urine urobilinogen	0-4 mg/24 hr	Increases with hemolysis or shunting of portal blood flow
Serum Proteins		
Albumin	3.5-5.5 g/dl	Reduced with hepatocellular injury
Globulin	2.5-3.5 g/dl	Increases with hepatitis
Total	6-7 g/dl	
Albumin/globulin (A/G) ratio	1.5:1 to 2.5:1	Ratio reverses with chronic hepatitis or other chronic liver disease
Transferrin	250-300 mcg/dl	Liver damage with decreased values, iron deficiency with increased values
Alpha fetoprotein (AFP)	6-20 ng/ml	Elevated values in primary hepatocellular carcinoma
Blood-Clotting Functions		
Prothrombin time (PT)	11.5-14 sec or 90%-100% of control	Increases with chronic liver disease (cirrhosis) or vitamin K deficiency
Partial thromboplastin time (PTT)	25-40 sec	Increases with severe liver disease or heparin therapy
Bromsulphalein (BSP) excretion	<6% retention in 45 min	Increased retention with hepatocellular injury

Table 38-7	Diagnostic Evaluation of the Gallbladder
Test	Application
Plain roentgenogram of the abdomen	Visualization of calcified gallstones
Oral cholecystogram (use of an oral contrast medium such as iodopanoic acid, which is excreted with bile and concentrated in the gallbladder for visualization by radiography; may be administered as a double dose)	Visualization of gallstones; evaluation of filling and emptying of gallbladder
Intravenous cholangiography (use of intravenous contrast agents for visualization of gallbladder and bile ducts)	Diagnosis of acute gallbladder inflammation (cholecystitis) or disease of bile ducts
Cholecystonography (ultrasound imaging of gallbladder and bile ducts)	Preferred method for detecting gallstones; differentiation of hepatic disease from biliary obstruction; diagnosis of chronic cholecystitis
Cholescintigraphy (radioisotope imaging of gallbladder)	Diagnosis of cholecystitis in individuals allergic to iodine-containing contrast agents; diagnosis of cystic duct obstruction
Endoscopic retrograde cholangiography (instillation of contrast medium through cannulation of ampulla of Vater with a duodenoscope)	Differentiation of intrahepatic or extrahepatic obstructive jaundice
Computed tomography (CT)	Diagnosis of biliary obstruction or malignancy when ultrasound is not successful

Table 38-8	Selected Tests of Pancreatic Function	
Test	Normal Value	Clinical Significance
Serum amylase	60-180 Somogyi units/ml	Elevated levels with pancreatic inflammation
Serum lipase	1.5 Somogyi units/ml	Elevated levels with pancreatic inflammation (may be elevated with other conditions; differentiates with amylase isoenzyme study)
Urine amylase	35-260 Somogyi units/hr	Elevated levels with pancreatic inflammation
Secretin test	Volume 1.8 ml/kg/hr Bicarbonate concentration: >80 mEq/L Bicarbonate output: >10 mEq/L/30 sec	Decreased volume with pancreatic disease as secretin stimulates pancreatic secretion
Stool fat	2-5 g/24 hr	Measures fatty acids; decreased pancreatic lipase increases stool fat

amylase levels. Decreased renal absorption of amylase results in increased urine amylase levels. Increased stool fat can reflect pancreatic insufficiency caused by decreased lipase secretion when biliary function is normal.

Aging and the Gastrointestinal System

Age-related changes in gastrointestinal function begin to occur before 50 years of age. Tooth enamel and dentin wear down, making the teeth vulnerable to cavities. Teeth are lost, often as a result of periodontal (gum) disease, recession of the gums, osteoporotic bone changes, and more brittle roots that fracture easily. Taste buds decline in number, and the sense of smell diminishes. Together these losses decrease the sense of taste. Salivary secretion decreases and contributes to dry mouth.[44] In very old adults these oral and sensory changes make eating less pleasurable and reduce appetite. Food may not be chewed or lubricated sufficiently, making swallowing difficult. The esophagus develops decreased motility, and changes in the upper esophageal sphincter may affect swallowing.[45]

Age also diminishes gastric motility and volume, including secretion of bicarbonate and gastric mucus.[46] Acid content

of gastric juice is related to gastric atrophy, which results in hypochlorhydria (insufficient hydrochloric acid) and delayed gastric emptying, best managed with frequent and small meals. Decreased production of intrinsic factor leads to inadequate small intestinal absorption of vitamin B_{12} and pernicious anemia. Aging also is associated with a change in the composition of the microflora and increased susceptibility to disease. There is greater frequency of *H. pylori* infection[47] and compromise of the gastric mucosal barrier. The villi of the small intestine become broader and shorter, perhaps because of a decrease in cell turnover. Intestinal absorption, motility, and blood flow decrease, impairing nutrient absorption.[48] Proteins, fats, minerals (including iron and calcium), and vitamins are absorbed more slowly and in lesser amounts, and absorption of carbohydrates, particularly lactose, is decreased.[49,50] Intestinal transit time is delayed. Constipation is often described as a condition of old age, but it is probably caused by lifestyle factors rather than physiologic decline although recent studies demonstrate there can be alterations in intestinal innervation.[51] Lifelong bowel habits, current diet, lack of fluid intake, pelvic floor dysfunction, and immobility contribute to constipation in older adults.[52]

The liver decreases in size and weight with advancing age, cell numbers, and their regeneration decrease, and there is reduced sinusoidal perfusion.[53] Alterations in liver function in older individuals are usually a sign of a pathologic condition. Liver blood flow and enzyme activity decreases with age and can influence efficiency of drug and alcohol metabolism. Oxidative metabolism of drugs may be decreased.[54] However, liver function test results often remain within relatively normal ranges. The pancreas undergoes structural changes, such as fibrosis, fatty acid deposits, and atrophy. Pancreatic secretion decreases, but there is usually no observable dysfunction.[50,55] Aging does not cause apparent changes in the structure and function of the gallbladder and bile ducts, but incidence of gallstones increases.

SUMMARY REVIEW

The Gastrointestinal Tract

1. The major functions of the gastrointestinal tract are the mechanical and chemical breakdown of food and the absorption of digested nutrients.
2. The gastrointestinal tract is a hollow tube that extends from the mouth to the anus.
3. The walls of the gastrointestinal tract have several layers: mucosa, muscularis mucosae, submucosa, tunica muscularis (circular muscle and longitudinal muscle), and serosa.
4. Except for swallowing and defecation, which are controlled voluntarily, the functions of the gastrointestinal tract are controlled by extrinsic and intrinsic autonomic nerves (enteric plexus) and intestinal hormones.
5. Digestion begins in the mouth, with chewing and salivation. The digestive component of saliva is α-amylase, which initiates carbohydrate digestion.
6. The esophagus is a muscular tube that transports food from the mouth to the stomach. The tunica muscularis in the upper part of the esophagus is striated muscle, and that in the lower part is smooth muscle.
7. Swallowing is controlled by the swallowing center in the reticular formation of the brain. The two phases of swallowing are the oropharyngeal phase (voluntary swallowing) and the esophageal phase (involuntary swallowing).
8. Food is propelled through the gastrointestinal tract by peristalsis: waves of sequential relaxations and contractions of the tunica muscularis.
9. The lower esophageal sphincter opens to admit swallowed food into the stomach and then closes to prevent regurgitation of food back into the esophagus.
10. The stomach is a baglike structure that secretes digestive juices, mixes and stores food, and propels partially digested food (chyme) into the duodenum. The smooth muscles of the stomach include the outer longitudinal, middle circular, and internal oblique.
11. The vagus nerve stimulates gastric (stomach) secretion and motility.
12. The hormones gastrin and motilin stimulate gastric emptying; the hormones secretin and cholecystokinin delay gastric emptying.
13. Gastric glands in the fundus and body of the stomach secrete intrinsic factor, which is needed for vitamin B_{12} absorption, and hydrochloric acid, which dissolves food fibers, kills microorganisms, and activates the enzyme pepsin.
14. Chief cells in the stomach secrete pepsinogen, which is converted to pepsin in the acid environment created by hydrochloric acid.
15. Acid secretion is stimulated by the vagus nerve, gastrin, and histamine and inhibited by sympathetic stimulation and cholecystokinin. Acetylcholine stimulates pepsin secretion.
16. Mucus is secreted throughout the stomach and protects the stomach wall from acid and digestive enzymes.
17. The three phases of acid secretion by the stomach are the cephalic phase (anticipation and swallowing), the gastric phase (food in the stomach), and the intestinal phase (chyme in the intestine).
18. The small intestine is 5 m long and has three segments: the duodenum, jejunum, and ileum. Digestion and absorption of all major nutrients and most ingested water occur in the small intestine.
19. The peritoneum is a double layer of membranous tissue. The visceral layer covers the abdominal organs, and the parietal layer extends along the abdominal wall.
20. Blood flow to the small intestine is primarily provided by the superior mesenteric artery.
21. The duodenum receives chyme from the stomach through the pyloric valve. The presence of chyme stimulates the liver and gallbladder to deliver bile and the pancreas to deliver digestive enzymes and alkaline secretions. Bile and enzymes flow through an opening guarded by the sphincter of Oddi.
22. Bile is produced by the liver and is necessary for fat digestion and absorption. Bile's alkalinity helps neutralize chyme, thereby creating a pH that enables the pancreatic enzymes to digest proteins, carbohydrates, and sugars.
23. Enzymes secreted by the small intestine (maltase, sucrose, lactase), pancreatic enzymes (proteases, amylase and lipase), and bile salts act in the small intestine to digest proteins, carbohydrates, and fats.
24. Digested substances are absorbed across the intestinal wall and then transported to the liver through the portal vein, where they are metabolized further.
25. The ileocecal valve connects the small and large intestines and prevents reflux into the small intestine.
26. Villi are small finger-like projections that extend from the small intestinal mucosa and increase its absorptive surface area.
27. Sugars, amino acids, and fats are absorbed primarily by the duodenum and jejunum; bile salts and vitamin B_{12} are absorbed by the ileum. Vitamin B_{12} absorption requires the presence of intrinsic factor.
28. Bile salts emulsify and hydrolyze fats and incorporate them into water-soluble micelles that transport them through the unstirred layer to the brush border of the intestinal mucosa. The fat content of the micelles readily diffuses through the epithelium into lacteals (lymphatic ducts) in the villi. From there fats flow into lymphatics and into the systemic circulation, which delivers them to the liver.
29. Minerals and water-soluble vitamins are absorbed by active and passive transport throughout the small intestine.
30. Peristaltic movements created by longitudinal muscles propel the chyme along the intestinal tract, whereas contractions of the circular muscles (segmentation) mix the chyme and promote digestion.
31. The ileogastric reflex inhibits gastric motility when the ileum is distended.
32. The intestinointestinal reflex inhibits intestinal motility when one intestinal segment is overdistended.

continued

33. The gastroileal reflex increases intestinal motility when gastric motility increases.
34. The large intestine consists of the cecum, appendix, colon (ascending, transverse, descending, and sigmoid), rectum, and anal canal.
35. The teniae coli are three bands of longitudinal muscle that extend the length of the colon.
36. Haustra are pouches of colon that are formed with alternating contraction and relaxation of the circular muscles.
37. The mucosa of the large intestine contains mucus-secreting cells and mucosal folds, but no villi.
38. The large intestine massages the fecal mass and absorbs water and electrolytes.
39. Distention of the ileum with chyme causes the gastrocolic reflex, or the mass propulsion of feces to the rectum.
40. Defecation is stimulated when the rectum is distended with feces. The conically contracted internal anal sphincter relaxes and, if the voluntarily regulated external sphincter relaxes, defecation occurs.
41. The largest numbers of intestinal bacteria are in the colon. They are anaerobes consisting of *Bacteroides,* clostridia, coliforms, and lactobacilli.
42. The intestinal tract is sterile at birth and becomes totally colonized within 3 to 4 weeks.
43. Endogenous infections of the gastrointestinal tract occur by excessive proliferation of bacteria, perforation of the intestine, or contamination from neighboring structures.

Accessory Organs of Digestion

1. The liver is the largest organ in the body. It has digestive, metabolic, hematologic, vascular, and immunologic functions.
2. The liver is divided into the right and left lobes and is supported by the falciform, round, and coronary ligaments.
3. Liver lobules consist of plates of hepatocytes, which are the functional cells of the liver.
4. The hepatic artery supplies blood to the liver. The portal vein receives blood from the inferior and superior mesenteric veins.
5. Hepatocytes synthesize 700 to 1200 ml of bile per day and secrete it into the bile canaliculi, which are small channels between the hepatocytes. The bile canaliculi drain bile into the common bile duct and then into the duodenum through an opening called the *major duodenal papilla (sphincter of Oddi).*
6. Sinusoids are capillaries located between the plates of hepatocytes. Blood from the portal vein and hepatic artery flows through the sinusoids to a central vein in each lobule and then into the hepatic vein and inferior vena cava.
7. Kupffer cells, which are part of the mononuclear phagocyte system, line the sinusoids and destroy microorganisms in sinusoidal blood.
8. The primary bile acids are synthesized from cholesterol by the hepatocytes. The primary acids are then conjugated to form bile salts. The secondary bile acids are the product of bile salt deconjugation by bacteria in the intestinal lumen.
9. Most bile salts and acids are recycled. The absorption of bile salts and acids from the terminal ileum and their return to the liver are known as the enterohepatic circulation of bile.
10. Bilirubin is a pigment liberated by the lysis of aged red blood cells in the liver and spleen. Unconjugated bilirubin is fat soluble and can cross cell membranes. Unconjugated bilirubin is converted to water-soluble, conjugated bilirubin by hepatocytes and is secreted with bile.
11. Fats are synthesized by the liver from protein and carbohydrates and include glycerol, free fatty acids, phospholipids, and cholesterol. Fat absorbed by intestinal lacteals is primarily triglyceride, which is hydrolyzed to glycerol and free fatty acid.
12. Proteins synthesis by the liver requires all essential amino acids. The liver synthesizes albumin, globulin, and several serum enzymes and can convert amino acids to carbohydrates by removal of ammonia.
13. Carbohydrates can be released as glucose, stored as glycogen, or converted to fat.
14. The liver performs many metabolic functions including detoxification of exogenous and endogenous chemicals and hormones.
15. The gallbladder is a saclike organ located in the inferior surface of the liver. The gallbladder stores bile between meals and ejects it when chyme enters the duodenum.
16. Stimulated by cholecystokinin, the gallbladder contracts and forces bile through the cystic duct and into the common bile duct. The sphincter of Oddi relaxes, enabling bile to flow through the major duodenal papilla into the duodenum.
17. The pancreas is a gland located behind the stomach. The endocrine pancreas produces hormones (glucagon and insulin) that facilitate the formation and cellular uptake of glucose. The exocrine pancreas secretes an alkaline solution and the enzymes (trypsin, chymotrypsin, carboxypeptidase, α-amylase, lipase) that digest proteins, carbohydrates, and fats.
18. Secretin stimulates pancreatic secretion of alkaline fluid, and cholecystokinin and acetylcholine stimulate secretion of enzymes. Pancreatic secretions originate in acini and ducts of the pancreas and empty into the duodenum through the common bile duct or an accessory duct that opens directly into the duodenum.

Tests of Digestive Function

1. Numerous diagnostic tests can evaluate structure and function (digestion, secretion, absorption) of the gastrointestinal tract. Radiographs and scans are most commonly used to evaluate structure, in addition to direct observation by endoscopy. Gastric and stool analysis and blood studies provide important information about digestion, absorption, and secretion.
2. Plasma chemistry levels and imaging procedures are commonly used to diagnose alterations in liver function. Of particular importance are the enzymes LDH, AST, and ALT. Plasma bilirubin levels reflect alterations in bilirubin and bile metabolism, and prothrombin times are prolonged in hepatitis and chronic liver disease.
3. Obstructive diseases of the gallbladder are evident by elevated serum bilirubin, elevated urine urobilinogen, and increased stool fat. The serum leukocytes become elevated with inflammation of the gallbladder.
4. The most significant indicators of pancreatic dysfunction are serum amylase and stool fat. Both values are increased with diseases of the pancreas.

Aging and the Gastrointestinal System

1. Advancing age is often associated with the loss or wearing down of teeth, diminished senses of taste and smell, and diminished salivary secretions, all of which may make eating difficult and reduce appetite.
2. Aging reduces gastric motility and secretions, particularly of hydrochloric acid. These changes slow gastric digestion and emptying.
3. Intestinal motility and absorption of carbohydrates, proteins, fats, and minerals decrease with age.
4. Efficiency of drug and alcohol metabolism decreases with age and can be related to decreased liver perfusion and decreased liver enzymes.

KEY TERMS

Ampulla of Vater, 1439, 1443
Antrum of stomach, 1424
Ascending colon, 1435
Bile, 1439
Bile acid–dependent fraction, 1439
Bile acid–independent fraction, 1439
Bile acid pool, 1439
Bile canaliculi, 1439
Bile salt, 1439
Bilirubin, 1440
Biliverdin, 1440
Body of stomach, 1424
Brush border, 1429
Calcium, 1433
Carboxypeptidase, 1430
Cardiac orifice, 1423
Cecum, 1435
Cephalic phase of secretion, 1427
Chief cell, 1426
Cholecystokinin, 1425
Choleresis, 1440
Choleretic agent, 1440
Cholesterol esterase, 1433
Chylomicron, 1433
Chyme, 1423
Chymotrypsin, 1430
Colipase, 1433
Colon, 1435
Common bile duct, 1439
Conjugated bilirubin, 1440
Critical micelle concentration, 1439
Crypts of Lieberkühn, 1429
Cystic duct, 1442
D cell, 1426
Deamination, 1442
Defecation reflex (rectosphincteric reflex), 1437
Descending colon, 1435
Disse space, 1439
Duodenum, 1428
Emulsification, 1432
Enteric plexus, 1421
Enterochromaffin-like cell, 1426
Enterohepatic circulation, 1439
Enterokinase, 1444
Entero-oxyntin, 1428
Esophageal phase of swallowing, 1423
Esophagus, 1423
Exocrine pancreas, 1443
External anal sphincter, 1436
Fat, 1432
Fecal mass, 1436
Feces, 1437
Fundus of stomach, 1424
G cell, 1426

Gallbladder, 1442
Gastric acid, 1426
Gastric emptying, 1425
Gastric gland, 1426
Gastric inhibitory peptide, 1428
Gastric phase of secretion, 1427
Gastric pit, 1426
Gastrin, 1424
Gastrocolic reflex, 1436
Gastroileal reflex, 1435
Gastrointestinal tract (alimentary canal), 1421
Glisson capsule, 1438
Haustrum (pl., haustra), 1436
Hepatic artery, 1438
Hepatic portal vein, 1438
Hepatic vein, 1438
Hepatocyte, 1438
Hepcidin, 1434
Histamine, 1426
Ileocecal valve (sphincter), 1428
Ileogastric reflex, 1435
Ileum, 1428
Internal anal sphincter, 1436
Intestinal peristalsis, 1435
Intestinal phase of secretion, 1428
Intestinointestinal reflex, 1435
Intrinsic factor (IF), 1427
Iron, 1434
Jejunum, 1428
Kupffer cell, 1438
Lacteal, 1429
Lamina propria, 1429
Large intestine, 1435
Lieberkühn crypt, 1429
Lipase, 1433
Lipocyte, 1438
Lipolysis, 1433
Liver, 1438
Liver lobule, 1438
Lower esophageal sphincter (cardiac sphincter), 1423
Magnesium, 1434
Major duodenal papilla, 1439
Mesentery, 1429
Metabolic detoxification (biotransformation), 1442
Micelle, 1433
Microvillus (pl., microvilli), 1429
Motilin, 1424
Mouth, 1421
Mucosal barrier, 1427
Myenteric plexus (Auerbach plexus), 1421
O'Beirne sphincter, 1435
Oral phase of swallowing, 1423

Pancreas, 1443
Pancreatic α-amylase, 1444
Pancreatic duct (Wirsung duct), 1443
Pancreatic lipase, 1444
Paneth cells, 1429
Parietal cell (oxyntic cell), 1426
Pepsin, 1426, 1427
Pepsinogen, 1426
Peristalsis, 1423
Peristaltic movement, 1436
Peritoneal cavity, 1429
Peritoneum, 1428
Pharyngeal phase of swallowing, 1423
Phases of gastric secretion, 1427
Phosphate, 1434
Phospholipase, 1433
Pit cell, 1439
Portal vein, 1439
Primary bile acid, 1439
Primary peristalsis, 1423
Pyloric sphincter, 1423
Pylorus, 1423
Retropulsion, 1424
S cell, 1444
Saliva, 1422
Salivary α-amylase (ptyalin), 1422
Salivary gland, 1422
Secondary bile acid, 1439
Secondary peristalsis, 1423
Secretin, 1424
Segmentation, 1435
Sigmoid colon, 1435
Sinusoid, 1438
Small intestine, 1428
Somatostatin, 1426
Sphincter of Oddi, 1439, 1442
Stellate cell, 1439
Stem cell, 1429
Stomach, 1423
Submucosal plexus (Meissner plexus), 1421
Subserosal plexus, 1421
Swallowing, 1423
Teniae coli, 1436
Transverse colon, 1435
Trypsin, 1430
Trypsin inhibitor, 1444
Unconjugated bilirubin, 1440
Upper esophageal sphincter (cricopharyngeal muscle), 1423
Urobilinogen, 1440
Valsalva maneuver, 1437
Vermiform appendix, 1435
Villus (pl., villi), 1429
Vitamin, 1434

REFERENCES

1. Mazzone A, Farrugia G: Evolving concepts in the cellular control of gastrointestinal motility: neurogastroenterology and enteric sciences, *Gastroenterol Clin North Am* 36(3):499-513, vii, 2007.
2. Lang IM, Shaker R: An overview of the upper esophageal sphincter, *Curr Gastroenterol Rep* 2(3):185-190, 2000.
3. Zald DH, Pardo JV: The functional neuroanatomy of voluntary swallowing, *Ann Neurol* 46(3):281-286, 1999.
4. Ertekin C, Aydogdu I: Neurophysiology of swallowing, *Clin Neurophysiol* 114(2):2226-2244, 2003.
5. Logemann JA: Swallowing disorders, *Best Pract Res Clin Gastroenterol* 21(40):563-573, 2007.
6. Ludlow CL: Sensorimotor control for voice, speech and swallowing, *Curr Opin Otolaryngol Head Neck Surg* 12(3):160-165, 2004.
7. Nguyen HN et al: Relationship between bolus transit and LES-relaxation studies with concurrent impedance and manometry, *Hepatogastroenterology* 53(68):218-223, 2007.
8. Goyal RK, Chaudhury A: Physiology of normal esophageal motility, *J Clin Gastroenterol* 42(5):610-619, 2008.
9. Hellström PM, Grybäck P, Jacobsson H: The physiology of gastric emptying, *Best Pract Res Clin Anaesthesiol* 20(3):397-407, 2006.
10. Lee KJ et al: Influence of duodenal acidification on the sensorimotor function of the proximal stomach in humans, *Am J Physiol Gastrointest Liver Physiol* 286(2):G278-G294, 2004.
11. Smith ME, Morton DG: *The digestive system*, St Louis, 2001, Mosby
12. Schubert ML: Gastric secretion, *Curr Opin Gastroenterol* 23(6):595-601, 2007.
13. Ham M, Kaunitz JD: Gastroduodenal defense, *Curr Opin Gastroenterol* 23(6):607-616, 2007.
14. Helander HF, Keeling DJ: Cell biology of gastric acid secretion, *Baillieres Clin Gastroenterol* 7(1):1-21, 1993.
15. Wolfe MM, Soll AH: The physiology of gastric acid secretion, *N Engl J Med* 319(26):1707-1715, 1988.
16. Zafra MA, Molina F, Puerto A: The neural/cephalic phase reflexes in the physiology of nutrition, *Neurosci Biobehav Rev* 30(7):1032-1044, 2006.
17. Thompson AB et al: Small bowel review: part 1, *Can S Gastroentrol* 12(7):487, 1998.
18. Kvietys PR, Barrowman JA, Granger ND: *Pathophysiology of the splanchnic circulation*, Boca Raton, FL, 1987, CRC Press.
19. Salaman NL, Undersood MA, Bevins CL: Paneth cells, defensins, and the commensal microbiota: a hypothesis on intimate interplay at the intestinal mucosa, *Semin Immunol* 19(2):70-83, 2007.
20. Bevins CL: The Paneth cell and the innate immune response, *Curr Opin Gastroenterol* 20(6):572-580, 2004.
21. Ashton KA et al: Basal and meal-stimulated colonic absorption, *Dis Colon Rectum* 39(8):865-870, 1996.
22. Leturque A, Brot-Laroche E: Sugar sensing by enterocytes combines polarity, membrane bound detectors and sugar metabolism, *J Cell Physiol* 213(3):834-843, 2007.
23. Dawson-Hughes B, Bischoff-Ferrari HA: Therapy of osteoporosis with calcium and vitamin D, *J Bone Miner Res* 22(Suppl 2):V59-V63, 2007.
24. Sharp P, Srai SK: Molecular mechanisms involved in intestinal iron absorption, *World J Gastroenterol* 13(35):4716-4724, 2007.
25. Bornstein JC, Costa M, Grider JR: Enteric motor and interneuronal circuits controlling motility, *Neurogastroenterol Motil* 16(Suppl 1):34-38, 2004.
26. Husebye E: The patterns of small bowel motility: physiology and implications in organic disease and functional disorders, *Neurogastroenterol Motil* 11(3):141-161, 1999.
27. Jeays AD et al: A framework for the modeling of gut blood flow regulation and postprandial hyperaemia, *World J Gastroenterol* 13(9):1393-1398, 2007.
28. Mims CA et al: *Medical microbiology*, ed 2, St Louis, 1998, Mosby.
29. Kelly D, Conway S, Aminov R: Commensal gut bacteria: mechanisms of immune modulation, *Trends Immunol* 26(6):26-33, 2005.
30. Magalhaes JG, Tattoli J, Girardin SE: The intestinal epithelial barrier: how to distinguish between the microbial flora and pathogens, *Semin Immunol* 19(2):106-115, 2007.
31. Ridlon JM, Kang DJ, Hylemon PB: Bile salt biotransformations by human intestinal bacteria, *J Lipid Res* 47(2):241-259, 2006.
32. Johnson LR: *Gastrointestinal physiology*, ed 7, St Louis, 2007, Mosby, p 102.
33. Bilzer M, Roggel F, Gerbes AL: Role of Kupffer cells in host defense and liver disease, *Liv Int* 26(10):1175-1186, 2006.
34. Friedman SL: Hepatic stellate cells: protean, multifunctional, and enigmatic cells of the liver, *Physiol Rev* 88(1):125-172, 2008.
35. Swain MG: Hepatic NKT cells: friend or foe? *Clin Sci (Lond)* 114(7):457-466, 2008.
36. Alrefai WA, Gill RK: Bile acid transporters: structure, function, regulation and pathophysiological implications, *Pharm Res* 24(10):1803-1823, 2007.
37. Ollinger R et al: Therapeutic applications of bilirubin and biliverdin in transplantation, *Antioxid Redox Signal* 9(12):2175-2185, 2007.
38. Stocker R: Antioxidant activites of bile pigments, *Antioxid Redox Signal* 6(5):841-849, 2004.
39. Bulmer AC et al: The anti-mutagenic properties of bile pigment, *Mutat Res* 658(1-2):28-41, 2008.
40. Woods CM, Saccone CT: Neurohomornal regulation of the sphincter of Oddi, *Curr Gastroenterol Rep* 9(2):165-170, 2007.
41. Love JA, Yi E, Smith TG: Autonomic pathways regulating pancreatic exocrine secretion, *Auton Neurosci* 133(1):19-34, 2007.
42. Johnston DE: Special considerations in interpreting liver function tests, *Am Fam Physician* 59(8):2223-2230, 1999.
43. Aranda-Michel J, Sherman KE: Tests of the liver: use and misuse, *Gastroenterologist* 6(1):34-43, 1998.
44. Gupta A, Epstein JB, Sroussi H: Hyposalivation in elderly patients, *J Can Dent Assoc* 72(9):841-846, 2006.
45. Achem SR, Devault KR: Dysphagia in aging, *J Clin Gastroenterol* 39(5):357-371, 2005.
46. Guslandi M, Pellegrini A, Sorghi M: Gastric mucosal defenses in the elderly, *Gerontology* 45(4):206-208, 1999.
47. Pilotto A: Aging and upper gastrointestinal disorders, *Best Pract Res Clin Gastroenterol* 18(Suppl):73-81, 2004.
48. Drozdowski L, Thomson AB: Aging and the intestine, *World J Gastroenterol* 12(47):7578-7584, 2006.
49. Timiras PS: *Physiological basis of aging and geriatrics*, ed 3, Boca Raton, FL, 2003, CRC Press.
50. Saltzman JR, Russell RM: The aging gut. Nutritional issues, *Gastroenterol Clin North Am* 27(2):309-324, 1998.
51. Phillips RJ, Rowley TL: Innervation of the gastrointestinal tract: patterns of aging, *Auton Neurosci* 136(1-2):1-19, 2007.
52. McCrea GL et al: Pathophysiology of constipation in the older adult, *World J Gastroenterol* 14(17):2631-2638, 2008.
53. Le Couteur DG et al: Old age and the hepatic sinusoid, *Anat Rec (Hoboken)* 291(6):672-683, 2008.
54. Kinirons MT, O'Mahony MS: Drug metabolism and ageing, *Br J Clin Pharmacol* 57(5):540-544, 2004 May.
55. Glaser J, Stienecker K: Pancreas and aging: a study using ultrasonography, *Gerontology* 46(2):93, 2000.

ALTERATIONS OF DIGESTIVE FUNCTION

SUE E. HUETHER

MEDIA RESOURCES

 Evolve Website (http://evolve.elsevier.com/McCance/)
- Review Questions and Answers
- Animations
- Glossary (with audio pronunciation for selected terms)
- WebLinks

Online Course
- Module 18

CHAPTER OUTLINE

DISORDERS OF THE GASTROINTESTINAL TRACT
Clinical Manifestations of Gastrointestinal Dysfunction
Disorders of Motility
Gastritis
Peptic Ulcer Disease
Malabsorption Syndromes
Inflammatory Bowel Disease
Appendicitis
Irritable Bowel Syndrome
Vascular Insufficiency
Disorders of Nutrition

DISORDERS OF THE ACCESSORY ORGANS OF DIGESTION
Clinical Manifestations of Liver Disorders
Disorders of the Liver
Disorders of the Gallbladder
Disorders of the Pancreas
CANCER OF THE DIGESTIVE SYSTEM
Cancer of the Gastrointestinal Tract
Cancer of the Accessory Organs of Digestion

The gastrointestinal tract is a continuous hollow organ that extends from the mouth to the anus. It includes the esophagus, stomach, small intestine (duodenum, jejunum, ileum), large intestine (ascending, transverse, descending, and sigmoid colon), and rectum. The accessory organs of digestion include the salivary glands, liver, gallbladder, and pancreas.

Disorders of the gastrointestinal tract disrupt one or more of its functions. Structural and neural abnormalities can slow, obstruct, or accelerate the movement of chyme at any level of the gastrointestinal tract. Inflammatory and ulcerative conditions of the gastrointestinal wall disrupt secretion, motility, and absorption. Inflammation or obstruction of the liver, pancreas, or gallbladder can alter metabolism and result in local or systemic symptoms, or both. Many clinical manifestations of gastrointestinal tract disorders are nonspecific and they can be caused by a variety of impairments. These manifestations are described in the next section.

DISORDERS OF THE GASTROINTESTINAL TRACT

Clinical Manifestations of Gastrointestinal Dysfunction

Anorexia

Anorexia is lack of a desire to eat despite physiologic stimuli that would normally produce hunger. Anorexia is a nonspecific symptom that is often associated with nausea, abdominal pain, diarrhea, and psychologic distress. Disorders of other organ systems, including cancer, heart disease, and renal disease, are often accompanied by anorexia (see p. 1480 for a discussion of anorexia nervosa).

Vomiting

Vomiting is the forceful emptying of stomach and intestinal contents (chyme) through the mouth. In the brain stimulation of receptors (e.g., dopamine (D_2), serotonin, opioid, acetylcholine and substance P) in the chemoreceptor trigger zone of the area postrema in the fourth ventricle leads to vomiting. The vestibular system initiates vomiting (motion sickness) via the eighth cranial nerve. Several types of intestinal, vagal, or sympathetic stimuli also initiate the vomiting reflex, including the presence of ipecac or copper salts in the duodenum; severe pain; distention of the stomach or duodenum; torsion or trauma affecting the ovaries, testes, uterus, bladder, or kidney; and activation of the chemoreceptor trigger zone in the medulla. 5-Hydroxytryptamine (5-HT, i.e., serotonin) stimulates the vomiting center and appears to be released from enterochromaffin cells in the intestinal wall and possibly from neurons in the brainstem.[1-3] 5-HT type 3 receptor antagonists are effective antiemetics and have been used to treat nausea and vomiting associated with postoperative vomiting and cancer chemotherapy. Apomorphine, levodopa, and bromocriptine are dopamine D_2 agonists that cause nausea and vomiting. Metoclopramide, domperidone, and haloperidol are D_2 antagonists and are effective antiemetics.

Nausea and retching usually precede vomiting. **Nausea** is a subjective experience that is associated with many different conditions, including visceral pain, labyrinthine stimulation (i.e., motion) and use of opiate medications. Specific neural pathways have not been identified for nausea. Hypersalivation and tachycardia are common associated symptoms. **Retching** begins with deep inspiration. The glottis closes, intrathoracic pressure falls, and the esophagus becomes distended. Simultaneously the abdominal muscles contract, creating a pressure gradient from abdomen to thorax. The lower esophageal sphincter and body of the stomach relax, but the duodenum and antrum of the stomach go into spasm. The reverse peristalsis and pressure gradient force chyme from the stomach and duodenum up into the esophagus. Because the upper esophageal sphincter is closed, chyme does not enter the mouth. As the abdominal muscles relax, the contents of the esophagus drop back into the stomach. This process may be repeated several times before vomiting occurs. A diffuse sympathetic discharge causes the tachycardia, tachypnea, and sweating that accompany retching and vomiting. The parasympathetic system mediates copious salivation, increased gastric motility, and relaxation of the upper and lower esophageal sphincters.

Vomiting is usually associated with nausea and follows retching. The duodenum and antrum of the stomach produce retrograde peristalsis while the body of the stomach and esophagus relax. When the stomach is full of gastric contents, the diaphragm is forced high into the thoracic cavity by strong contractions of the abdominal muscles. The higher intrathoracic pressure forces the upper esophageal sphincter to open, and chyme is expelled from the mouth. Then the stomach relaxes and the upper part of the esophagus contracts, forcing the remaining chyme back into the stomach. The lower esophageal sphincter then closes. The cycle is repeated if there is a volume of chyme remaining in the stomach.

Spontaneous vomiting that is not preceded by nausea or retching is called **projectile vomiting**. Projectile vomiting is caused by direct stimulation of the vomiting center by neurologic lesions (e.g., increased intracranial pressure, tumors, or aneurysms involving the brain stem [see Chapter 16]). The metabolic consequences of vomiting are fluid, electrolyte, and acid-base disturbances (see Chapter 3).

Constipation

Constipation is difficult or infrequent defecation and is estimated to affect 2% to 28% of the population.[4,5] Constipation must be individually defined because patterns of bowel evacuation differ greatly among individuals. Constipation usually means a decrease in the number of bowel movements per week, hard stools, and difficult evacuation. Normal bowel habits range from two or three evacuations per day to one per week. Constipation is not significant until it causes health risks or impairs quality of life.

PATHOPHYSIOLOGY Chronic constipation can be caused by neurogenic disorders of the large intestine in which neurotransmitters are altered or neural pathways are absent or degenerated and colon transit time is delayed.[6] An example is Hirschsprung disease (congenital megacolon)—the absence of ganglion cells in the myenteric plexus of the large intestine causes loss of propulsive movements that move feces into the rectum (see Chapter 40). Other disorders associated with constipation include acquired megacolon (enlarged or dilated colon), hypothyroidism, pelvic hiatal hernia, multiple sclerosis, spinal cord trauma, cancer, cerebrovascular disease, and irritable bowel disease with constipation (Box 39-1).

Many functional or mechanical conditions can slow intestinal transit time. Muscle weakness or pain caused by abdominal surgery can impair or inhibit defecation. Normally the abdominal muscles are used to create the intra-abdominal pressure required to evacuate the rectum. Weakness or pain can interfere with the generation of adequate intra-abdominal pressure. Lesions of the anus, such as inflamed hemorrhoids, fissures, or fistulae, make defecation painful because of stretching. With the urge to defecate, the sphincter becomes hypertonic, and the stool is not eliminated.

Box 39-1	Causes of Constipation

Megacolon (enlarged or dilated colon)
Pelvic floor dyssynergia
Abdominal muscle weakness
Painful anal lesions
Low-residue diet
Sedentary lifestyle
Dehydration
Delayed spontaneous defecation
Emotional depression
Cancer and cancer treatment
Selected drugs
   Opiates
   Anticholinergics
   Antacids (calcium carbonate, aluminum hydroxide)
Systemic diseases
   Hypothyroidism
   Diabetic neuropathy

A low-residue diet (the habitual consumption of highly refined foods) decreases the volume and number of stools and causes constipation. A sedentary lifestyle, lack of regular exercise, and insufficient hydration are common causes of constipation. Lack of access to toilet facilities and consistent suppression of the urge to empty the bowel are other causes. Depression often impairs bowel evacuation, partly because depressed individuals tend to be sedentary and lack the motivation to eat a healthy diet. The problem is made worse if antidepressant drugs (e.g., anticholinergics) are used to treat the depression. Anticholinergics block parasympathetic impulses in the gastrointestinal tract, thereby impairing motility. Aging may result in changes in neuromuscular function, causing constipation or use of medications that cause constipation.[7]

Excessive use of antacids containing calcium carbonate or aluminum hydroxide often results in constipation. Opiates, particularly codeine, tend to inhibit bowel motility.[8]

CLINICAL MANIFESTATIONS Changes in bowel evacuation patterns—such as less frequent defecation, smaller stool volume, difficulty in evacuating the rectum, or a feeling of bowel fullness and discomfort—require investigation.

EVALUATION AND TREATMENT The individual's medical history, physical examination, and stool diaries provide precise clues regarding the nature of constipation. Functional constipation (i.e., constipation resulting from lifestyle or bowel habits) usually has a long history. Dysfunctional constipation is more likely to be sudden. Sudden-onset constipation can accompany the development of organic lesions and requires careful evaluation.

The Rome III criteria for constipation includes two of the following that occur for 12 weeks (consecutive not required) in the previous 12 months[9]:

1. Straining during 25% of defecations
2. Lumpy or hard stool in at least 25% of defecations
3. Sensation of incomplete evacuation in at least 25% of defecations
4. Manual maneuvers to facilitate at least 25% of defecations
5. Sensation of anorectal blockage/obstruction in at least 25% of defecations
6. Fewer than three bowel movements per week

The individual's description of frequency, stool consistency, associated pain, and presence of blood is significant. Blood may be present as a result of bleeding hemorrhoids or a neoplastic lesion of the colon. Cramping abdominal pain may be symptomatic of partial bowel obstruction. In assessing frequency, it is important to discover whether evacuation was stimulated by enemas or cathartics (laxatives). Palpation discloses colonic distention, masses, and tenderness. Stool transit time is evaluated. Digital examination of the rectum is performed to assess sphincter tone and detect anal lesions. Proctosigmoidoscopy is used to visualize the lumen directly. A barium enema may be required if no lesions are directly visualized and symptoms continue after simple treatment. Colonic transit studies and anal manometry may be useful.

The treatment for dysfunctional constipation is to manage the underlying lesion or disease. Management of functional constipation likewise depends on its cause. Irritable bowel syndrome with constipation is presented on p. 1476. Treatment usually consists of bowel retraining, in which the individual establishes a satisfactory bowel evacuation routine without becoming preoccupied with bowel movements. Biofeedback training can be effective for dyssynergic defecation (failure to relax the pelvic floor).[10] Moderate exercise, increased fluid and fiber intake, bulk supplements (e.g., Metamucil, Konsyl), stool softeners, and laxative agents are useful for some individuals. Enemas can be used to establish bowel routine, but they should not be used habitually. Lubiprostone is a drug used for the treatment of chronic constipation.[9]

Diarrhea

Diarrhea is an increase in the frequency of defecation and the fluidity, volume, and weight of feces and is often a protective response. Three or more stools per day are considered abnormal. Many factors determine stool volume and consistency, including water content of the colon and the presence of unabsorbed food, unabsorbable material, and intestinal secretions. Stool volume in the normal adult averages less than 200 g/day. Stool volume in children depends on age and size. An infant may pass up to 100 g/day. The adult intestine processes approximately 9 L of luminal content per day; 2 L is ingested, and the remaining 7 L consists of intestinal secretions. Of this volume, 99% of the fluid is absorbed—90% (7 to 8 L) in the small intestine and 9% (1 to 2 L) in the colon. Normally, approximately 150 ml of water is excreted daily in the stool.

PATHOPHYSIOLOGY Diarrhea in which the volume of feces is increased is called *large-volume diarrhea*. Large-volume diarrhea generally is caused by excessive amounts of water or secretions or both in the intestines. *Small-volume diarrhea*, in which the volume of feces is not increased, usually results from excessive intestinal motility. The three major mechanisms of diarrhea are osmotic, secretory, and motility.[11] (Specific mechanisms of diarrhea in children are described in Chapter 40.)

In **osmotic diarrhea** a nonabsorbable substance in the intestine draws water into the lumen by osmosis. The excess water and the nonabsorbable substance cause large-volume diarrhea. Magnesium, sulfate, and phosphate are poorly absorbed ions and can increase intraluminal osmotic pressure. *Lactase deficiency* is the most common cause of osmotic diarrhea and loss of pancreatic enzymes can be a contributing factor. In this condition the nonabsorbable substance is milk sugar, or lactose. Lactose remains in the intestinal lumen because it is not digested or absorbed (see p. 1470). Excessive ingestion of synthetic, nonabsorbable sugars (e.g., sorbitol) has a similar effect. Osmotic diarrhea disappears when ingestion of the osmotic substance stops. Malabsorption related to bile salt deficiency, small intestine bacterial overgrowth, and celiac disease also cause diarrhea.[12]

Secretory diarrhea is a form of large-volume diarrhea caused by excessive mucosal secretion of chloride- or bicarbonate-rich fluid or inhibition of net sodium absorption. Primary causes are bacterial enterotoxins (particularly those released by cholera or strains of *Escherichia coli*) and neoplasms (such as gastrinoma or thyroid carcinoma). These tumors produce hormones that stimulate intestinal secretion.

Large-volume diarrhea also can result from excessive motility of the intestine. The cause is usually a lesion that impairs autonomic control of motility, such as diabetic neuropathy. Excessive motility decreases transit time, mucosal surface contact, and opportunities for fluid absorption. Therefore, a larger volume of stool reaches the rectum, producing urgency and frequency of elimination.

Small-volume diarrhea usually is caused by an inflammatory disorder of the intestine, such as ulcerative colitis or Crohn disease. Inflammation of the colon causes cramping pain, urgency, and frequency. Small-volume diarrhea also can be caused by fecal impaction, a severe form of constipation. This diarrhea consists of secretions (mucus and fluid) produced by the colon to lubricate the impacted feces and move it toward the anal canal. These secretions flow around the impaction and cause low-volume, secretory diarrhea.

Motility diarrhea is caused by resection of the small intestine (short bowel syndrome), surgical bypass of an area of the intestine, or fistula formation between loops of intestine. Food is not mixed properly, and there is impaired digestion and increased motility.

CLINICAL MANIFESTATIONS Diarrhea can be acute or chronic, depending on its cause. Systemic effects of prolonged diarrhea are dehydration, electrolyte imbalance, metabolic acidosis, and weight loss. Manifestations of acute bacterial or viral infection include fever, with or without cramping pain. Fever, cramping pain, and bloody stools accompany diarrhea caused by inflammatory bowel disease. Steatorrhea (fat in the stools) and diarrhea are common signs of malabsorption syndromes.

EVALUATION AND TREATMENT A thorough history is taken to document the onset and frequency of diarrhea. Exposure to contaminated food or water is indicated if the individual has traveled in foreign countries or areas where drinking water might be contaminated. Iatrogenic diarrhea is suggested if the individual has undergone abdominal radiation therapy, intestinal resection, or treatment with selected drugs (e.g., antibiotics, diuretics, antihypertensives, laxatives). Physical examination helps the clinician to identify underlying systemic disease. Stool culture, examination of stool specimens for blood, abdominal roentgenograms, and intestinal biopsies provide more specific data.[13]

Treatment for diarrhea includes restoration of fluid and electrolyte balance, management of distressing symptoms, and treatment of causal factors. In older adults and children, dehydration and electrolyte imbalance may be severe and require intravenous fluid therapy. Nutritional deficiencies need to be corrected in cases of chronic diarrhea or malabsorption. Substances that solidify stools decrease frequency and water content. Natural bran and commercial preparations of psyllium, such as Konsyl and Metamucil, are inexpensive and effective treatments for mild diarrhea. Loperamide (an opiate) or diphenoxylate and atropine (Lomotil) suppress motility, relieve cramping, and reduce stool volume and frequency.

Abdominal Pain

Abdominal pain is the presenting symptom of a number of gastrointestinal diseases and can be acute or chronic; it is usually associated with tissue injury. (The physiology of pain is described in Chapter 15.) Abdominal pain may be generalized to the abdomen or localized to a particular abdominal quadrant. The pain is often described as sharp, dull, or colicky. The causal mechanisms of abdominal pain are mechanical, chemical mediators of inflammation, or ischemic. Generally the abdominal organs are not sensitive to mechanical stimuli, such as cutting, tearing, or crushing. These organs are, however, sensitive to stretching and distention, which activate nerve endings in hollow as well as solid structures. The onset of pain is associated with rapid distention; gradual distention causes little pain. Traction on the peritoneum caused by adhesions, distention of the common bile duct, or forceful peristalsis resulting from intestinal obstruction causes pain because of increased tension. Capsules that surround solid organs, such as the liver and gallbladder, contain pain fibers that are stimulated by stretching if these organs swell.

Biochemical mediators of the inflammatory response, such as histamine, bradykinin, and serotonin, stimulate pain nerve endings and produce abdominal pain. The edema and vascular congestion that accompany chemical, bacterial, or viral inflammation also cause painful stretching. Obstruction of blood flow from the distention of bowel obstruction or mesenteric vessel thrombosis produces the pain of ischemia, and increased concentrations of tissue metabolites stimulate pain receptors.

Abdominal pain can be parietal (somatic), visceral, or referred. **Parietal pain** arises from the parietal peritoneum. This pain is more localized and intense than visceral pain, which arises from the organs themselves. Nerve fibers from the parietal peritoneum travel with peripheral nerves to the spinal cord, and the sensation of pain corresponds to skin dermatomes T6 and L1. Parietal pain lateralizes because, at any particular point, the parietal peritoneum is innervated from only one side of the nervous system.

Visceral pain arises from a stimulus (distention, inflammation, ischemia) acting on an abdominal organ.[14] Chronic low-grade inflammation can cause pain hypersensitivity with involvement of neurokinins, serotonin, and voltage-gated ion channels.[15] Pain is usually felt near the midline in the epigastrium (upper midabdomen), midabdomen, or lower abdomen. The pain is poorly localized, is dull rather than sharp, and is difficult to describe. Its location is generally related to the corresponding skin dermatomes of the affected organ and may be referred pain. Visceral pain is diffuse and vague because nerve endings in abdominal organs are sparse and multisegmented. Pain arising from the stomach, for example, is experienced as a sensation of fullness, cramping, or gnawing in the midepigastric area.

Referred pain is visceral pain felt at some distance from a diseased or an affected organ. Referred pain is usually well localized and is felt in skin or deeper tissues that share a central afferent pathway with the affected organ. Generally referred pain develops as the intensity of a visceral pain stimulus increases. Intense gallbladder pain is, for example, referred to the back between the scapulae (shoulder blades). The pain may begin as a vague discomfort in the right epigastric region and then, as inflammation worsens, progress to a sharp, localized, referred pain between the shoulder blades.

Gastrointestinal Bleeding

Numerous disorders cause bleeding in the gastrointestinal tract, and the bleeding can occur from more than one site. **Upper gastrointestinal bleeding,** which is defined as bleeding in the esophagus, stomach, or duodenum, is commonly caused by bleeding peptic ulcers. Other causes include esophageal or gastric varices, a Mallory-Weiss tear at the esophageal gastric junction from severe retching, cancer, or angiodysplasias.[16] **Lower gastrointestinal bleeding**—bleeding below the ligament of Treitz or bleeding from the small bowel (jejunum or ileum), colon, or rectum—can be caused by polyps, inflammatory disease, diverticulosis, cancer, vascular ectasias, or hemorrhoids.[17] Acute, severe gastrointestinal bleeding is life threatening. Mortality depends on the volume and rate of blood loss, associated disease, age, and effectiveness of treatment.

The presentation of gastrointestinal bleeding is summarized in Table 39-1. Acute blood loss is usually characterized by **hematemesis** (the presence of blood in the vomitus), **hematochezia** (bright red or burgundy blood from the rectum), or **melena** (dark, tarry stools). **Occult bleeding** is usually caused by slow, chronic blood loss that is not obvious and results in iron deficiency anemia as iron stores in the bone marrow are slowly depleted. Physiologic response to gastrointestinal bleeding depends on the amount and rate of the loss (Figure 39-1). Changes in blood pressure and heart rate are the best indicators of massive blood loss in the gastrointestinal tract. Blood losses of 1000 ml or more over a short

time cause a decrease in cardiac output, a decrease in systolic and diastolic blood pressure, and an increase in pulse rate. With losses of 1000 ml or more, the heart rate is greater than 100 beats/minute and systolic blood pressure is less than 100 mmHg. During the early stages of blood volume depletion, the peripheral vascular compartment constricts to shunt blood to vital organs, including the brain (see Chapters 30 and 46). Signs that this is happening are postural hypotension (a drop in blood pressure that occurs with a change from the recumbent position to a sitting or upright position), lightheadedness, and loss of vision. If blood loss continues, hypovolemic shock progresses. Diminished blood flow to the kidneys causes decreased urine output and may lead to oliguria (low urine output), tubular necrosis, and renal failure. Ultimately, insufficient cerebral and coronary blood flow causes irreversible anoxia and death.

The accumulation of blood in the gastrointestinal tract is irritating and increases peristalsis, causing vomiting or diarrhea, or both. If bleeding is from the lower gastrointestinal tract, the diarrhea is frankly bloody. Bleeding from the upper gastrointestinal tract also can be rapid enough to produce bright red stools, but generally some digestion of the blood components will have occurred, producing melena. The digestion of blood proteins originating from massive upper gastrointestinal bleeding is reflected by an increase in blood urea nitrogen (BUN) levels (see Figure 39-1).

The hematocrit and hemoglobin values are not the best indicators of acute gastrointestinal bleeding because plasma and red cell volume are lost proportionately. As the plasma volume is replaced, the hematocrit and hemoglobin values begin to reflect the extent of blood loss. The interpretation of these values is modified to account for exogenous replacement of fluids and the hydration status of the tissues. Iron deficiency anemia is associated with obscure bleeding.[18]

Disorders of Motility

Dysphagia

PATHOPHYSIOLOGY Dysphagia is difficulty swallowing. It can result from mechanical obstruction of the esophagus or a functional disorder that impairs esophageal motility. *Mechanical obstructions* can be intrinsic or extrinsic. Intrinsic obstructions originate in the wall of the esophageal lumen. Tumors, strictures, and diverticular herniations (outpouchings) are all causes of intrinsic mechanical obstruction. Extrinsic mechanical obstructions originate outside the esophageal lumen and narrow the esophagus by pressing inward on the esophageal wall. The most common cause of extrinsic mechanical obstruction is tumor.

Functional dysphagia is caused by neural or muscular disorders that interfere with voluntary swallowing or peristalsis. Disorders that affect the striated muscles of the upper esophagus interfere with the oropharyngeal (voluntary) phase of swallowing. Typical causes of functional dysphagia in the upper esophagus are dermatomyositis (a muscle disease) and neurologic impairments caused by cerebrovascular accidents, Parkinson disease, or achalasia.[19]

Table 39-1	Presentations of Gastrointestinal Bleeding
Presentation	**Definition**
Acute bleeding	
Hematemesis	Bloody vomitus; either fresh, bright red blood or dark, grainy, digested blood with "coffee grounds" appearance
Melena	Black, sticky, tarry, foul-smelling stools caused by digestion of blood in the gastrointestinal tract
Hematochezia	Fresh, bright red blood passed from the rectum
Occult bleeding	Trace amounts of blood in normal-appearing stools or gastric secretions; detectable only with a guaiac test

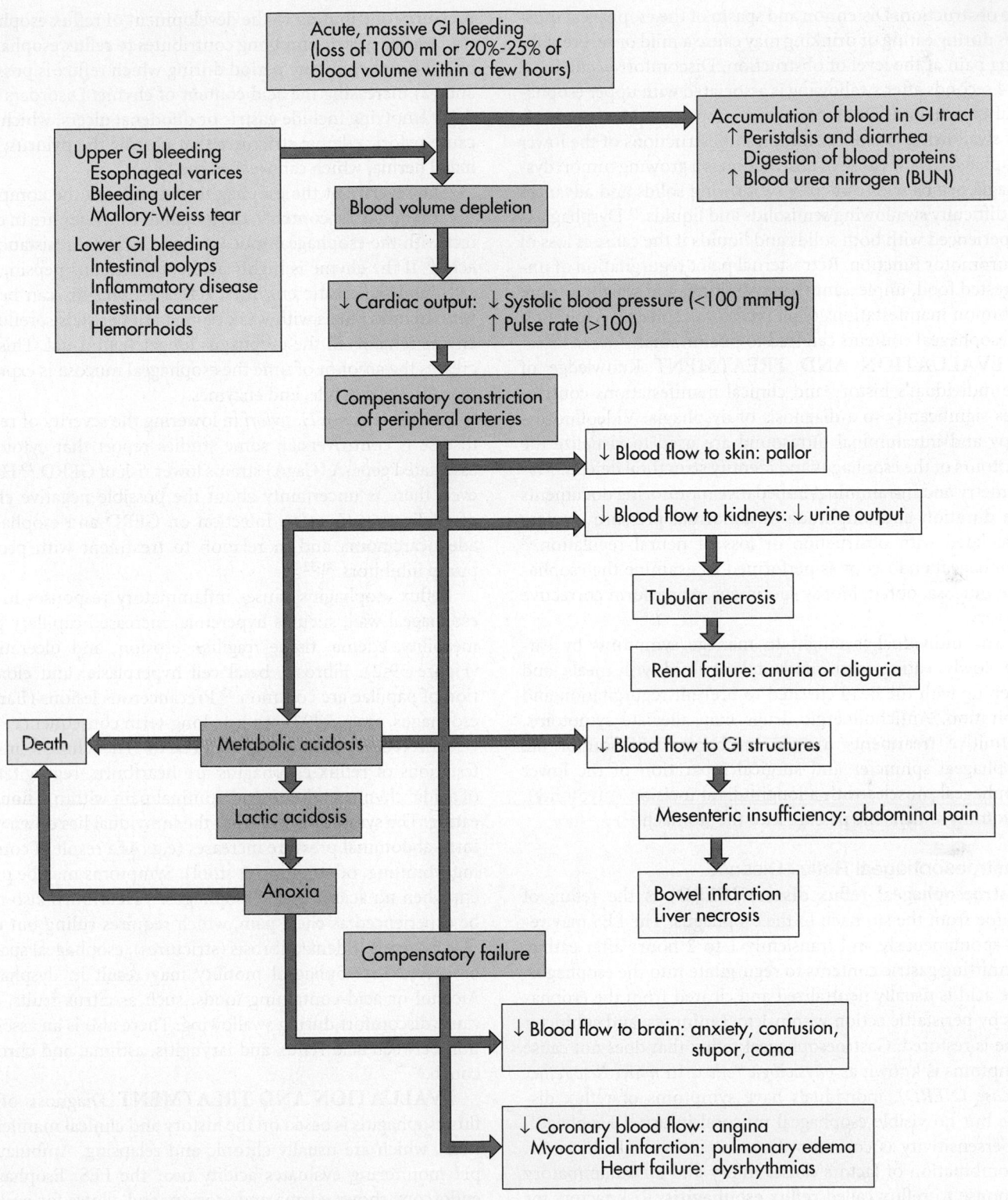

Figure 39-1 Pathophysiology of gastrointestinal (GI) bleeding.

Achalasia is a rare disorder related to (1) denervation of smooth muscle in the middle and lower portions of the esophagus, and (2) failure of the lower esophageal sphincter (LES) to relax causing functional obstruction of the lower esophagus.[20] Achalasia results from an unknown cause of an autoimmune destruction of myenteric ganglion cells and atrophy of smooth muscle cells. Food accumulates above the obstruction, distends the esophagus, and causes dysphagia. As hydrostatic pressure increases, food is slowly forced past the obstruction into the stomach.

CLINICAL MANIFESTATIONS Clinical manifestations of dysphagia vary according to the cause and location of the obstruction. Distention and spasm of the esophageal muscles during eating or drinking may cause a mild or severe stabbing pain at the level of obstruction. Discomfort occurring 2 to 4 seconds after swallowing is associated with upper esophageal obstruction. Discomfort occurring 10 to 15 seconds after swallowing is more common in obstructions of the lower esophagus. If the cause of obstruction is a growing tumor, dysphagia begins with difficulty swallowing solids and advances to difficulty swallowing semisolids and liquids.[21] Dysphagia is experienced with both solids and liquids if the cause is loss of neuromotor function. Retrosternal pain, regurgitation of undigested food, unpleasant taste, vomiting, and weight loss are common manifestations of all types of dysphagia. Aspiration of esophageal contents can lead to pneumonia.

EVALUATION AND TREATMENT Knowledge of the individual's history and clinical manifestations contributes significantly to a diagnosis of dysphagia. Videofluoroscopy and intraluminal ultrasound are used to visualize the contours of the esophagus and identify structural defects. Manometry and intraluminal impedance monitoring documents the duration and amplitude of abnormal pressure changes associated with obstruction or loss of neural regulation.[22] Esophageal endoscopy is performed to examine the esophageal mucosa, obtain biopsy specimens, or perform corrective surgery.

The individual is taught to manage symptoms by eating slowly, eating small meals, taking fluid with meals, and sleeping with the head elevated to prevent regurgitation and aspiration. Anticholinergic drugs may alleviate symptoms. Definitive treatments include mechanical dilation of the esophageal sphincter and surgical separation of the lower esophageal muscles with a longitudinal incision (myotomy). Myotomy widens the passage into the stomach.[23]

Gastroesophageal Reflux Disease

Gastroesophageal reflux disease (GERD) is the reflux of chyme from the stomach to the esophagus. The LES may relax spontaneously and transiently 1 to 2 hours after eating, permitting gastric contents to regurgitate into the esophagus. The acid is usually neutralized and cleared from the esophagus by peristaltic action within 1 to 3 minutes, and sphincter tone is restored. Gastroesophageal reflux that does not cause symptoms is known as *physiologic reflux*. In *nonerosive reflux disease (NERD)*, individuals have symptoms of reflux disease but no visible esophageal mucosal injury.[24] Esophageal hypersensitivity is common. In some individuals, however, a combination of factors causes injury and an inflammatory response to reflux called **reflux esophagitis.** Risk factors for GERD include obesity and *Helicobacter pylori*.[25] GERD may be a trigger for asthma or chronic cough.[26]

PATHOPHYSIOLOGY Normally the resting tone of the LES maintains a zone of high pressure that prevents gastroesophageal reflux. In individuals who develop reflux esophagitis, this pressure tends to be lower than normal from either transient relaxation or weakness of the sphincter. Vomiting, coughing, lifting, bending, or obesity increases abdominal

pressure contributing to the development of reflux esophagitis. Delayed gastric emptying contributes to reflux esophagitis by (1) lengthening the period during which reflux is possible and (2) increasing the acid content of chyme. Disorders that delay emptying include gastric or duodenal ulcers, which can cause pyloric edema; strictures that narrow the pylorus; and hiatal hernia, which can weaken the LES.[27]

The severity of the esophagitis depends on the composition of the gastric contents, the length of time they are in contact with the esophageal mucosa, and epithelial resistance to acid.[28] If the chyme is highly acidic, or contains pepsin, bile salts, and pancreatic enzymes, reflux esophagitis can be severe. In individuals with weak esophageal peristalsis, refluxed chyme remains in the esophagus longer than usual. This increases the amount of time the esophageal mucosa is exposed to acids, pepsin, bile, and enzymes.

The presence of *H. pylori* in lowering the severity of reflux disease is controversial; some studies report that cytotoxin associated gene-A (CagA) strains lower risk of GERD.[29] However, there is uncertainty about the possible negative effect of eradicating *H. pylori* infection on GERD and esophageal adenocarcinoma and in relation to treatment with proton pump inhibitors.[30-32]

Reflux esophagitis causes inflammatory responses in the esophageal wall, such as hyperemia, increased capillary permeability, edema, tissue fragility, erosion, and ulcerations (Figure 39-2). Fibrosis, basal cell hyperplasia, and elongation of papillae are common.[33] Precancerous lesions (Barrett esophagus, see p. 1497) can be a long-term consequence.[34]

CLINICAL MANIFESTATIONS The clinical manifestations of reflux esophagitis are heartburn, regurgitation of acidic chyme, and upper abdominal pain within 1 hour of eating. The symptoms worsen if the individual lies down or if intra-abdominal pressure increases (e.g., as a result of coughing, vomiting, or straining at stool). Symptoms may be present when no acid is in the esophagus.[33] Heartburn also may be experienced as chest pain, which requires ruling out cardiac ischemia. Edema, fibrosis (strictures), esophageal spasm, or decreased esophageal motility may result in dysphagia. Alcohol or acid-containing foods, such as citrus fruits, can cause discomfort during swallowing. There also is an association between acid reflux and laryngitis, asthma, and chronic cough.[35,36]

EVALUATION AND TREATMENT Diagnosis of reflux esophagitis is based on the history and clinical manifestations, which are usually chronic and relapsing. Ambulatory pH monitoring evaluates acidity near the LES. Esophageal endoscopy shows edema and erosion, and allows for evaluation of dysplastic changes (Barrett esophagus) and the development of esophageal carcinoma. It also identifies associated conditions, such as hiatal hernia, gastric ulcers, and abnormal contours of the esophageal lumen.[37]

Proton pump inhibitors are the most effective monotherapy. Other therapies include histamine-2 (H_2) receptor antagonists or prokinetics, antacids, and alginate-antacids.[38] Elevation of the head of the bed 6 inches prevents reflux. Weight reduction and cessation of smoking also help to alleviate symptoms. Laparoscopic fundoplication is the most common surgical intervention when medical treatment fails.[39]

Eosinophilic esophagitis is a rare, idiopathic inflammatory disease of the esophagus characterized by esophageal infiltration of eosinophils associated with atopic disease, including asthma and food allergies. It occurs in adults and children. Complex molecular mechanisms and gene and environmental interactions contribute to the pathogenesis of this disease.[40] Dysphagia and food impaction in the esophagus are common symptoms in the adult that can result from chronic inflammation and fibrosis. Diagnosis includes

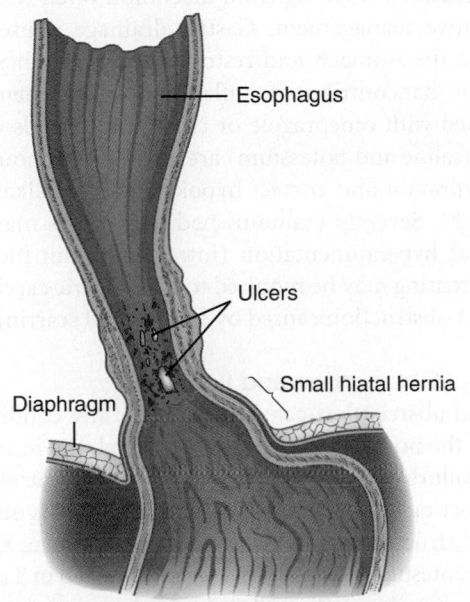

Figure 39-2 Esophagitis with esophageal ulcerations.

differentiation from GERD.[41] Treatment is symptomatic including elimination diets and steroids.

Hiatal Hernia

PATHOPHYSIOLOGY **Hiatal hernia,** a type of diaphragmatic hernia, is the protrusion (herniation) of the upper part of the stomach through the diaphragm and into the thorax. The two types of hiatal hernia are (1) sliding (direct) hiatal hernia, and (2) paraesophageal (rolling) hiatal hernia (Figure 39-3). In **sliding hiatal hernia** (the most common type, 90%) the stomach slides or moves into the thoracic cavity through the esophageal hiatus, an opening in the diaphragm for the esophagus and vagus nerves. A congenitally short esophagus, trauma, or weakening of the diaphragmatic muscles at the gastroesophageal junction contributes to the hernia. While the individual is in the supine position, the lower esophagus and stomach are pulled into the thorax. Standing causes the stomach to "slide" back into the abdomen. Sliding hiatal hernia is exacerbated by factors that increase intra-abdominal pressure. Therefore, coughing, bending, tight clothing, ascites, obesity, or pregnancy accentuates the hernia. This type of hernia is associated with gastroesophageal reflux and esophagitis because the hernia diminishes the resting pressure of the LES. In pregnant women with sliding hiatal hernia, progesterone and estrogen may lower the resting pressure of the LES further.

Paraesophageal hiatal hernia (rolling hiatal hernia) is herniation of the greater curvature of the stomach through a secondary opening in the diaphragm (see Figure 39-3). The entire stomach can pass into the thorax. As the stomach protrudes through the opening into the thorax, it lies alongside the esophagus. The gastroesophageal junction remains below the diaphragm. With paraesophageal hernia, reflux is uncommon. The position of a portion of the stomach above the diaphragm, however, causes congestion of mucosal blood

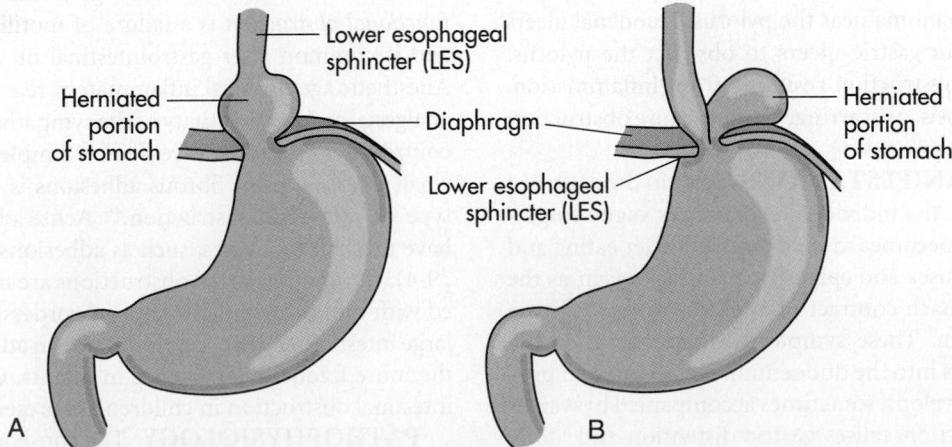

Figure 39-3 Types of hiatal hernia. **A,** In sliding hiatal hernia the visceral peritoneum remains intact and restrains the size of the hernia. **B,** In paraesophageal hernia the membrane becomes thinned out or defective, allowing a true peritoneal sac to protrude into the posterior mediastinum, where negative intrathoracic pressure causes it to enlarge. (From Monahan FD et al: *Phipps' Medical-surgical nursing: concepts and clinical practice,* ed 8, St Louis, 2007, Mosby.)

flow and can lead to gastritis and ulcer formation. A mechanical strangulation of the hernia is a major complication, and surgical correction is required. Strangulation occludes blood vessels and causes vascular engorgement, edema, ischemia, and hemorrhage. Hiatal hernias of both types tend to occur in conjunction with several other diseases, including reflux, peptic ulcer, cholecystitis (gallbladder inflammation), cholelithiasis (gallstones), chronic pancreatitis, and diverticulosis.

CLINICAL MANIFESTATIONS Hiatal hernias are often asymptomatic. Generally a wide variety of symptoms develop later in life and are associated with other gastrointestinal disorders as well. Manifestations of the various types of hiatal hernia are difficult to distinguish and include gastroesophageal reflux, dysphagia, heartburn, vomiting, and epigastric pain.[42] Regurgitation and substernal discomfort after eating are common.

EVALUATION AND TREATMENT Diagnostic procedures include barium roentgenogram and endoscopy. A chest roentgenogram often will show the protrusion of the stomach into the thorax, indicating paraesophageal hiatal hernia.

Treatment for sliding hiatal hernia is usually conservative. The individual can diminish reflux by eating small, frequent meals and avoiding the recumbent position after eating. Abdominal supports and tight clothing are avoided, and weight control is recommended for obese individuals. Antacids alleviate reflux esophagitis. Anticholinergic drugs are contraindicated because they relax the LES and delay gastric emptying. Individuals who are uncomfortable at night benefit from sleeping in a semi-Fowler position. Surgery (i.e., fundoplication) may be performed for paraesophageal hiatal hernia or if medical management fails to control symptoms.[43]

Pyloric Obstruction
PATHOPHYSIOLOGY **Pyloric obstruction** is the narrowing or blocking of the opening between the stomach and the duodenum. This condition can be congenital (see Chapter 40) or acquired. Acquired obstruction is caused by peptic ulcer disease or carcinoma near the pylorus. Duodenal ulcers are more likely than gastric ulcers to obstruct the pylorus. Ulceration causes obstruction resulting from inflammation, edema, spasm, fibrosis, or scarring. Tumors cause obstruction by growing into the pylorus.

CLINICAL MANIFESTATIONS Early in the course of pyloric obstruction, the individual experiences vague epigastric fullness, which becomes more distressing after eating and later in the day. Nausea and epigastric pain may occur as the muscles of the stomach contract in attempts to force chyme past the obstruction. These symptoms disappear when the chyme finally moves into the duodenum. As obstruction progresses, anorexia develops, sometimes accompanied by weight loss. Severe obstruction causes gastric distention and atony (lack of muscle tone and gastric motility). Gastric distention stimulates gastric secretion, which increases the feeling of fullness. Rolling or jarring of the abdomen produces a sloshing sound called the *succussion splash*. At this stage, vomiting is a cardinal sign of obstruction. It is usually copious and occurs several hours after eating. The vomitus contains undigested food but no bile. Prolonged vomiting leads to dehydration, which is accompanied by a hypokalemic and hypochloremic metabolic alkalosis caused by loss of potassium and gastric acid. Because food does not enter the intestine, stools are infrequent and small. Prolonged pyloric obstruction causes malnutrition, dehydration, and extreme debilitation.

EVALUATION AND TREATMENT Diagnosis is based on clinical manifestations, a history of ulcer disease, and examination of residual gastric contents. Endoscopy is performed if gastric carcinoma is the suggested cause of pyloric obstruction. Barium studies are contraindicated because the barium may harden and be retained in the stomach.

Obstructions resulting from ulceration often resolve with conservative management. Gastric drainage is used to decompress the stomach and restore normal motility. Gastric secretions that contribute to inflammation and edema can be suppressed with omeprazole or cimetidine. Fluids and electrolytes (saline and potassium) are given intravenously to effect rehydration and correct hypokalemia and alkalosis (see Chapter 3). Severely malnourished individuals may require parenteral hyperalimentation (intravenous nutrition). Surgery or stenting may be required to treat gastric carcinoma or persistent obstruction caused by fibrosis and scarring.[44]

Intestinal Obstruction and Ileus
Intestinal obstruction can be caused by any condition that prevents the normal flow of chyme through the intestinal lumen or failure of normal intestinal motility in the absence of an obstructing lesion (ileus). The small intestine is more commonly obstructed because of its narrower lumen. Common causes of intestinal obstruction are summarized in Table 39-2. More specific causes of small and large bowel obstruction are summarized in Table 39-3. Criteria for classifying intestinal obstruction are summarized in Table 39-4. Intestinal obstruction is classified by cause as simple or functional. *Simple obstruction* is mechanical blockage of the lumen by a lesion; *functional obstruction* is a failure of motility (**paralytic ileus**) and is common after gastrointestinal or abdominal surgery. Anesthetic agents, local inflammatory reactions, use of opioid analgesia, and hyperactivity of the sympathetic nervous system contribute to postoperative ileus.[45] Simple obstruction of the small intestine from fibrous adhesions is the most common type of intestinal obstruction.[46] Acute obstructions usually have mechanical causes, such as adhesions or hernias (Figure 39-4). Chronic or partial obstructions are more often associated with tumors or inflammatory disorders, particularly of the large intestine. Intussusception is rare in adults compared with the more frequent occurrence in infants. Common causes of intestinal obstruction in children are presented in Chapter 40.

PATHOPHYSIOLOGY The consequences of intestinal obstruction are related to its onset and location, the length of intestinal tract proximal to the obstruction, and the presence and severity of ischemia. The major pathophysiologic alterations are presented in Figure 39-5. The most common

Table 39-2 Common Causes of Intestinal Obstruction

Cause	Pathophysiology
Herniation	Protrusion of the intestine through a weakness in the abdominal muscles or through the inguinal ring
Intussusception	Telescoping of one part of the intestine into another; this usually causes strangulation of the blood supply; more common in the ileocecal area in infants 10 to 15 months of age than in adults
Torsion (volvulus)	Twisting of the intestine on its mesenteric pedicle, with occlusion of the blood supply; often associated with fibrous adhesions in the small intestine; occurs most often in the large intestine in older adults
Diverticulosis	Inflamed saccular herniations (diverticula) of the mucosa and submucosa through the tunica muscularis of the colon; diverticula are interspersed between thick, circular, fibrous bands; most common in obese individuals older than 60 years
Tumor	Tumor growth into the intestinal lumen; adenocarcinoma of the colon and rectum is the most common tumoral obstruction; most common in individuals older than 60 years
Paralytic (adynamic) ileus	Loss of peristaltic motor activity in the intestine; associated with abdominal surgery, peritonitis, hypokalemia, ischemic bowel, spinal trauma, pneumonia, neuropathies, or myopathies; affects small and large intestines
Fibrous adhesions	Peritoneal irritation from surgery or trauma leads to formation of fibrin and adhesions that attach to intestine, omentum, or peritoneum and can cause traction and obstruction; most common in small intestine

Table 39-3 Large and Small Bowel Obstruction

Cause	Pathogenesis
Small bowel obstruction	Adhesions: secondary to previous abdominal surgeries: 50%-70%
	Hernia: inguinal, ventral, or femoral: 20%-25%
	Tumors: may be associated with intussusception: 10%
	Mesenteric ischemia 3%-5%
Large bowel obstruction	Colon/rectal cancer 90%
	Colonic volvulus 4%-5%
	Diverticular disease 3%-5%
	Other causes (inflammatory bowel disease, adhesions, hernia, adynamic ileus)

Adapted from Feldman M et al: *Sleisenger & Fordtran's gastrointestinal liver disease,* ed 8, Philadelphia, 2006, Saunders.

causes of **small intestine obstruction** are intra-abdominal adhesions, hernias, and neoplasms.[47] Obstruction leads to accumulation of fluid and gas inside the lumen proximal to the obstruction. Fluids accumulate from impaired water and electrolyte absorption and enhanced secretion with net movement of fluid from the vascular space to the intestinal lumen. Gas from swallowed air, and to a lesser extent from bacterial overgrowth, contributes to the distention. Distention begins almost immediately, as gases and fluids accumulate proximal to the obstruction. Distention decreases the intestine's ability to absorb water and electrolytes and increases the net secretion of these substances into the lumen. Within 24 hours, up to 8 L of fluid and electrolytes enters the lumen in the form of saliva, gastric juice, bile, pancreatic juice, and intestinal secretions. Copious vomiting or sequestration of fluids in the intestinal lumen prevents their reabsorption and produces severe fluid and electrolyte disturbances. Extracellular fluid volume and plasma volume decrease, causing dehydration. Hemoconcentration (decreased plasma volume) elevates hematocrit,

decreases central venous pressure, and causes tachycardia. Severe dehydration leads to hypovolemic shock.

If the obstruction is at the pylorus or high in the small intestine, metabolic alkalosis develops initially as a result of excessive loss of hydrogen ions that normally would be reabsorbed from the gastric juice. With prolonged obstruction or obstruction lower in the intestine, metabolic acidosis is more likely to occur because bicarbonate from pancreatic secretions and bile cannot be reabsorbed. Hypokalemia can be extreme, promoting acidosis and atony of the intestinal wall. Metabolic acidosis also may be accentuated by ketosis, the result of declining carbohydrate stores caused by starvation. If pressure from the distention is severe enough, it occludes the arterial circulation and causes ischemia, necrosis, perforation, and peritonitis. Fever and leukocytosis are often associated with loss of intestinal motility, overgrowth of bacteria, strangulation, and bowel necrosis. Lack of circulation permits the buildup of significant amounts of lactic acid, which worsen the metabolic acidosis. Bacterial proliferation and translocation across the mucosa to the mesenteric lymph nodes or systemic circulation cause peritonitis or sepsis. The release of inflammatory mediators into the circulation causes remote organ failure.[48]

The most common causes of **large bowel obstruction** are malignancy, volvulus (twisting), and strictures related to diverticulitis. Consequences of colonic or large bowel obstruction are related to the competence of the ileocecal valve, which normally prevents reflux of colonic contents into the small intestine. When the ileocecal valve is competent, the cecum cannot decompress into the small intestine resulting in distention. Ischemia occurs when the intraluminal pressure exceeds capillary pressure in the lumen. Acute colonic pseudo-obstruction (Ogilvie syndrome) is a massive dilation of the large bowel that occurs in critically ill patients, and immobilized older adults. It is characterized by significant dilation of the cecum and absence of mechanical obstruction.

CLINICAL MANIFESTATIONS Signs and symptoms of *small intestine obstruction* are consistent with the pathophysiology. Colicky pains caused by distention followed by

Table 39-4   Classification of Intestinal Obstruction

Criteria for Classification	Definition
Onset	
Acute	Sudden onset; often caused by torsion, intussusception, or herniation
Chronic	Protracted onset; more commonly from tumor growth or progressive formation of strictures
Extent of Obstruction	
Partial	Incomplete obstruction of intestinal lumen
Complete	Complete obstruction of intestinal lumen
Location of Obstructing Lesion	
Intrinsic	Obstruction develops within intestinal lumen; examples: luminal edema or hemorrhage, foreign bodies (gallstones), tumors, or intraluminal fibrosis
Extrinsic	Obstruction originates outside the intestine; examples: tumors, torsion, fibrosis, hernia, intussusception
Effects on Intestinal Wall	
Simple	Luminal obstruction without impairment of blood supply
Strangulated	Luminal obstruction with occlusion of blood supply
Closed loop	Obstruction at each end of a segment of the intestine
Causal Factors	
Mechanical	Blockage of the intestinal lumen by intrinsic or extrinsic lesions; usually treated surgically
Functional (paralytic ileus)	Paralysis of the intestinal musculature as a result of accidental or surgical trauma, peritonitis, electrolyte imbalances, or spasmolytic agents; usually treated medically

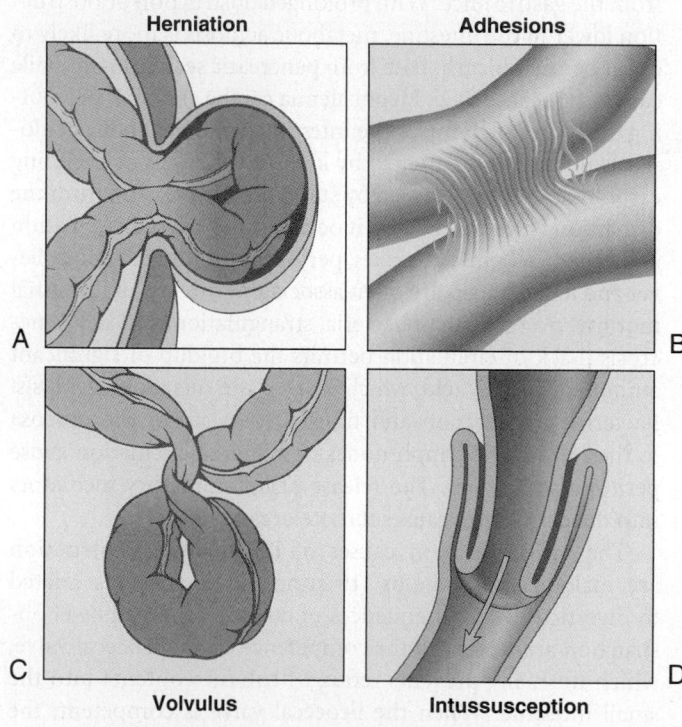

Figure 39-4 Intestinal obstructions. A, Hernia. B, Constriction from adhesions. C, Volvulus. D, Intussusception. (From Kumar V et al: *General pathology*, ed 8, Philadelphia, 2010, Saunders.)

vomiting are the cardinal symptoms. Typically the pain occurs intermittently. Pain intensifies for seconds or minutes as a peristaltic wave of muscle contraction meets the obstruction. The passing of the wave is followed by a pain-free interval. Pain may be continuous with severe distention and then diminish in intensity. If strangulation occurs, the pain loses its colicky character, becoming more constant and severe as ischemia progresses to necrosis or perforation. Sweating, nausea, and hypotension occur as an autonomic nervous system response.

Vomiting and distention vary, depending on the level and completion of the obstruction. Obstruction at the pylorus causes early, profuse vomiting of clear gastric fluid. Obstruction in the proximal small intestine causes mild distention and vomiting of bile-stained fluid. Obstruction lower in the small intestine causes more pronounced distention because a greater length of intestine is proximal to the obstruction. In this case, vomiting may not occur or may occur later and contain fecal material. Partial obstruction can cause diarrhea or constipation, but complete obstruction usually causes constipation only. Complete obstruction increases the number of bowel sounds, which may be tinkly and accompanied by peristaltic rushes and crampy, abdominal pain. Signs of dehydration, hypovolemia, and metabolic acidosis may be observed as early as 24 hours after the occurrence of complete obstruction. Distention may be severe enough to push against the diaphragm and decrease lung volume. This can lead to atelectasis and pneumonia, particularly in debilitated individuals.

Colonic obstruction usually presents as hypogastric pain and abdominal distention. Pain can vary from vague to excruciating, depending on the degree of ischemia and the development of peritonitis. Colon cancer is the most common cause, followed by diverticular strictures or volvulus.

EVALUATION AND TREATMENT Evaluation is based on clinical manifestations and includes ultrasound and radiography.[49,50] Successful management requires early identification of the site and type of obstruction. Replacement of fluid and electrolytes and decompression of the lumen with gastric or intestinal suction are essential forms of therapy.

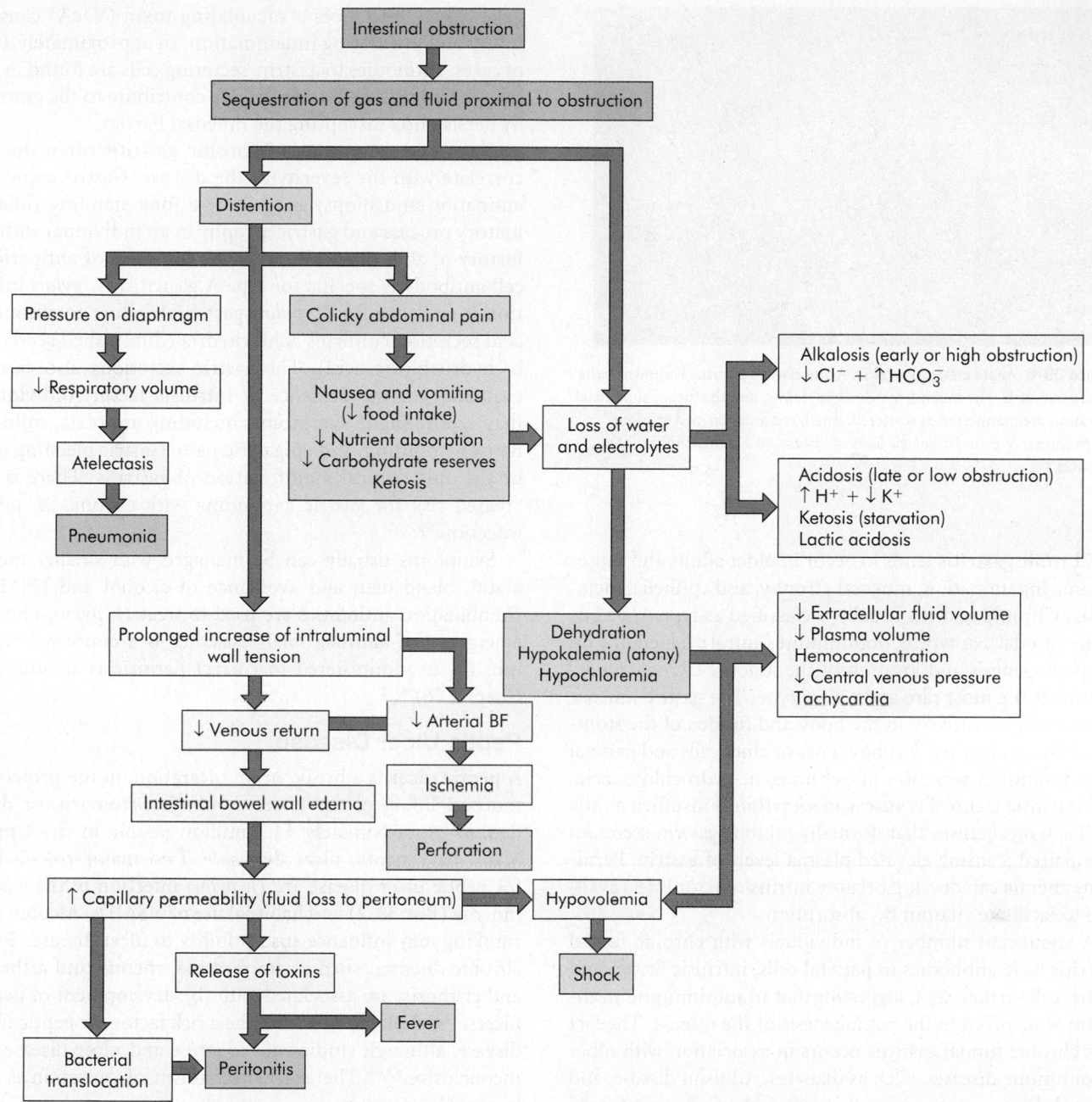

Figure 39-5 Pathophysiology of intestinal obstruction. *BF,* blood flow.

Immediate surgical intervention is required for strangulation and complete obstruction. Neostigmine is used for colonic pseudo-obstruction.[51]

Gastritis

Gastritis is an inflammatory disorder of the gastric mucosa. It can be acute or chronic and can affect the fundus or antrum or both. Acute gastritis erodes the surface epithelium in a diffuse or localized pattern. The erosions are usually superficial.

Acute gastritis is usually injury of the protective mucosal barrier by drugs, chemicals, or *H. pylori* infection (Figure 39-6). Nonsteroidal anti-inflammatory drugs (NSAIDs), such as

aspirin, ibuprofen, naproxen, and indomethacin, are known to cause erosive gastritis because they inhibit prostaglandins, which normally stimulate the secretion of mucus.[52] Alcohol, histamine, digitalis, and metabolic disorders such as uremia are contributing factors. *H. pylori* infection causes inflammation, pain, nausea, and vomiting.[53] The clinical manifestations of acute gastritis can include vague abdominal discomfort, epigastric tenderness, and bleeding. Healing usually occurs spontaneously within a few days. Discontinuing injurious drugs, using antacids, or decreasing acid secretion with a histamine H_2 receptor antagonist and proton pump inhibitor also promote healing.

Figure 39-6 **Acute erosive gastritis.** Acute erosive gastritis is shown in the opened stomach. The mucosa appears hyperemic, and the foci of superficial ulceration are manifested as scattered, small, red areas termed erosions. (From Kumar V et al: *Pathologic basis of disease,* ed 7, Philadelphia, 2006, Saunders.)

Chronic gastritis tends to occur in older adults and causes chronic inflammation, mucosal atrophy, and epithelial metaplasia. Chronic gastritis usually is classified as type A, or immune (fundal), or type B, nonimmune (antral), depending on the pathogenesis and location of the lesions. *Chronic fundal gastritis* is the most rare and severe type. The gastric mucosa degenerates extensively in the body and fundus of the stomach, leading to gastric atrophy. Loss of chief cells and parietal cells diminishes secretion of pepsinogen, hydrochloric acid, and intrinsic factor. Because acid secretion is insufficient, the feedback mechanism that normally inhibits gastrin secretion is impaired, causing elevated plasma levels of gastrin. Pernicious anemia can develop because intrinsic factor is less available to facilitate vitamin B_{12} absorption.

A significant number of individuals with chronic fundal gastritis have antibodies to parietal cells, intrinsic factor, and gastric cells in their sera, suggesting that an autoimmune mechanism is involved in the pathogenesis of the disease. The fact that chronic fundal gastritis occurs in association with other autoimmune diseases, such as diabetes, Addison disease, and thyroid disease, strengthens this association. Chronic fundal gastritis is a risk factor for gastric carcinoma, particularly in individuals who develop pernicious anemia.[54,55]

Chronic antral gastritis generally involves the antrum only and is approximately four times more common than fundal gastritis. It is not associated with decreased hydrochloric acid secretion, pernicious anemia, or presence of parietal cell antibodies. Several factors are associated with chronic antral gastritis, including use of alcohol, tobacco, and NSAIDs. *H. pylori* is a major causative factor associated with chronic atrophic antral gastritis and peptic ulcer disease. The host response to *H. pylori* infection is activation of T and B lymphocytes with infiltration of neutrophils. Release of inflammatory cytokines (e.g., tumor necrosis factor-α [TNF-α]; interleukin-1 [IL-1], IL-6, IL-8, IL-10; and leukotrienes) damage the gastric epithelium.[56-58] An *H. pylori*

gene *(CagA)* produces a vacuolating toxin (VacA) causing injury and promoting inflammation. In approximately 10% of cases, antibodies to gastrin-secreting cells are found in the serum. Chronic reflux of bile may contribute to the gastritis by persistently disrupting the mucosal barrier.

Signs and symptoms of chronic gastritis often do not correlate with the severity of the disease. Gastroscopic examination and biopsy may show a long-standing inflammatory process and gastric atrophy in an individual with no history of abdominal distress. The presence of antiparietal cell antibody is specific for type A gastritis. *H. pylori* infection is evidence for *H. pylori* gastritis. Failure to stimulate acid secretion confirms achlorhydria (diminished secretion of hydrochloric acid). The gastric secretions also can be evaluated for the presence of intrinsic factor. Individuals may report vague symptoms, including anorexia, fullness, nausea, vomiting, and epigastric pain. Gastric bleeding may be the only clinical manifestation of gastritis. There is increased risk for gastric carcinoma with chronic *H. pylori* infection.[59]

Symptoms usually can be managed with smaller meals; a soft, bland diet; and avoidance of alcohol and NSAIDs. Combination antibiotics are used to treat *H. pylori,* and the emergence of antimicrobial resistance is a concern.[60] Vitamin B_{12} is administered to correct pernicious anemia (see Chapter 26).[61]

Peptic Ulcer Disease

A **peptic ulcer** is a break, or an ulceration, in the protective mucosal lining of the lower esophagus, stomach, or duodenum. Approximately 14.5 million people in the United States have peptic ulcer disease.[62] Two major risk factors for peptic ulcer disease are *H. pylori* infection of the gastric mucosa (Box 39-2) and habitual use of NSAIDs. Alcohol and smoking may influence susceptibility to ulcer disease. Some chronic diseases, such as emphysema, rheumatoid arthritis, and cirrhosis, are associated with the development of peptic ulcers. Psychologic stress may be a risk factor for peptic ulcer disease, although studies of life stress and ulcer disease are inconclusive.[63,64] The exact mechanism of causation is not known.[65]

Peptic ulcers can be acute or chronic, and superficial or deep. Superficial ulcerations are called *erosions* because they erode the mucosa but do not penetrate the muscularis mucosae (Figure 39-7). True ulcers extend through the muscularis mucosae and damage blood vessels causing hemorrhage or perforate the gastrointestinal wall.

Gastric mucosal infection with *H. pylori* is a major cause of peptic ulcers (Box 39-2).[66] Chronic use of NSAIDs suppresses mucosal prostaglandin synthesis resulting in decreased bicarbonate secretion and mucin production and increased secretion of hydrochloric acid. The interaction of NSAIDs and *H. pylori* in the pathogenesis of peptic ulcer is not clear.[67] Disruption of the mucosa exposes submucosal areas to gastric secretions and autodigestion causing erosion and ulceration.

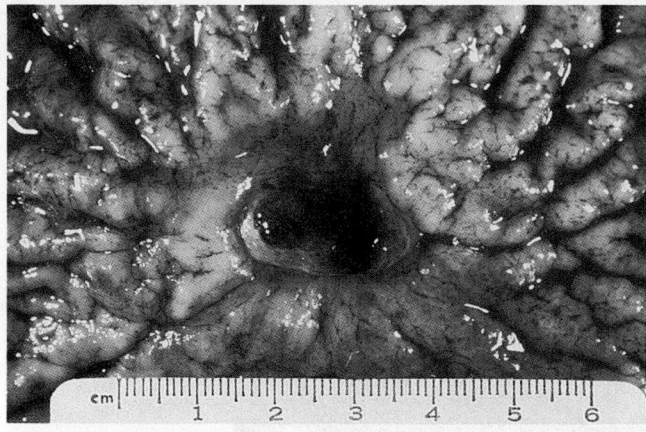

Figure 39-7 Chronic peptic ulcer. Gross photograph of a chronic peptic ulcer located in the lesser curvature, straddling the antrum and corpus of the stomach. (From Damjanov I, Linder J, editors: *Anderson's pathology,* ed 10, St Louis, 1996, Mosby.)

Duodenal Ulcers

Duodenal ulcers occur with greater frequency than other types of peptic ulcers and affect 10% to 15% of the population.[68] The incidence of duodenal ulcers is approximately the same among men and women in the United States.[69] Duodenal ulcers tend to develop in younger persons, and there may be an association with type O blood.[70,71]

PATHOPHYSIOLOGY Factors other than *H. pylori* and use of NSAIDs that may be associated with duodenal ulcer include:

1. Increased mass of gastric parietal cells
2. Serum gastrin levels that remain high longer than normal after eating and continue to stimulate secretion of acid and pepsin (may be caused by *H. pylori* in gastric antrum)
3. Failure of the feedback mechanism whereby acid in the gastric antrum inhibits gastrin release
4. Rapid gastric emptying, which overwhelms the buffering capacity of the bicarbonate-rich pancreatic secretions
5. Acid production stimulated by cigarette smoking
6. Decreased duodenal mucosal bicarbonate secretion

All these factors, singly or in combination, cause acid and pepsin concentrations in the duodenum to penetrate the mucosal barrier and lead to ulceration[72,73] (Figure 39-8).

CLINICAL MANIFESTATIONS The characteristic manifestation of a duodenal ulcer is chronic intermittent pain in the epigastric area. The pain begins 30 minutes to 2 hours after eating, when the stomach is empty. It is not unusual for pain to occur in the middle of the night and disappear by morning. The pain results from sensorineural stimulation by acid, muscle spasm, or both. Pain is relieved rapidly by ingestion of food or antacids, creating a typical "pain-food-relief" pattern. Some individuals with duodenal ulcer have no symptoms, particularly older adults; the first manifestation may be hemorrhage or perforation, particularly with a history of NSAID or anticoagulant use.

Duodenal ulcers often heal spontaneously but recur within months. Exacerbations tend to develop in the spring and fall.

| Box 39-2 | Pathogenesis of *Helicobacter pylori*–related disease |

H. pylori is a gram-negative spiral bacterium with a flagella and is a major cause of acute and chronic gastritis, peptic ulcer disease in the duodenum and stomach, gastric adenocarcinoma, and gastric mucosa-associated lymphoid tissue (MALT) (see p. 1499). *H. pylori* is transmitted through the fecal-oral route and is usually acquired in childhood. Infection is asymptomatic in about 70% of cases. In other cases, inflammation and immune responses promote mucosal ulcerations or prevent healing of injured tissue. Gene-environment interaction and different pathogenic strains of *H. pylori* increase risk for disease. Patterns of gastritis and disease progression vary by site of infection and strain of *H. pylori*. Pathogenic and virulence factors include:

1. An ability to colonize and adhere to gastric epithelial cells.
2. The possession of flagella that allows movement through the luminal mucous layer to a site of higher pH.
3. An ability of adherent strains to suppress acid secretion to improve their survival.
4. Secretion of urease that produces ammonia results in a more alkaline environment.
5. Release of vacuolating cytotoxin (VacA) that promotes bacterial survival and causes epithelial injury.
6. The presence of cytotoxin-associated gene (CagA) strains that can escape normal immune responses and cause inflammation with release of inflammatory cytokines and reactive oxygen metabolites that damages mucosal epithelial cells and loss of the protective mucosal barrier.
7. Recruitment and activation of neutrophils, macrophages, and mast cells with release of inflammatory cytokines (tumor necrosis factor-alpha [TNF-α], interleukin [IL]-1, IL-6, IL-8, histamine) that promote cellular injury.
8. Down-regulation of antral somatostatin leading to increased gastrin, increased acid, impaired mucosal bicarbonate production, and increased mucosal exposure to acid and pepsin.
9. Activation or inhibition of T- and B-cell immune responses that may contribute to mucosal injury.
10. Release of cytokines and chemokines that promote gastric epithelial cell death (apoptosis) and cell proliferation that can result in atrophy, ulcers, or malignant growth.

Data from Allen LA: *Cell Microbiol* 9(4):817-828, 2008; McNamara D, El-Omar E: *Dig Liver Dis* 40(7):504-509, 2008; Wessler S, Backert S: *Trends Microbiol* 16(8):397-405, 2008.

Healing is accompanied by relief of pain. Constant, unremitting pain may be caused by complications, such as intestinal obstruction or perforation. Bleeding from duodenal ulcers causes hematemesis or melena. It is not clear why individuals infected with *H. pylori* do not develop duodenal cancer.[74]

EVALUATION AND TREATMENT Several diagnostic approaches are used to differentiate duodenal ulcers from gastric ulcers or gastric carcinoma. Endoscopic evaluation allows visualization of lesions and biopsy. Radioimmune assays of gastrin levels are evaluated to identify ulcers associated with gastric carcinomas. The urea breath test, serum antibodies, stool and serum antigen, and positive findings from gastric biopsy detect *H. pylori* infection.[75]

Management of duodenal ulcers is aimed at relieving the causes and effects of hyperacidity. Antacids neutralize gastric

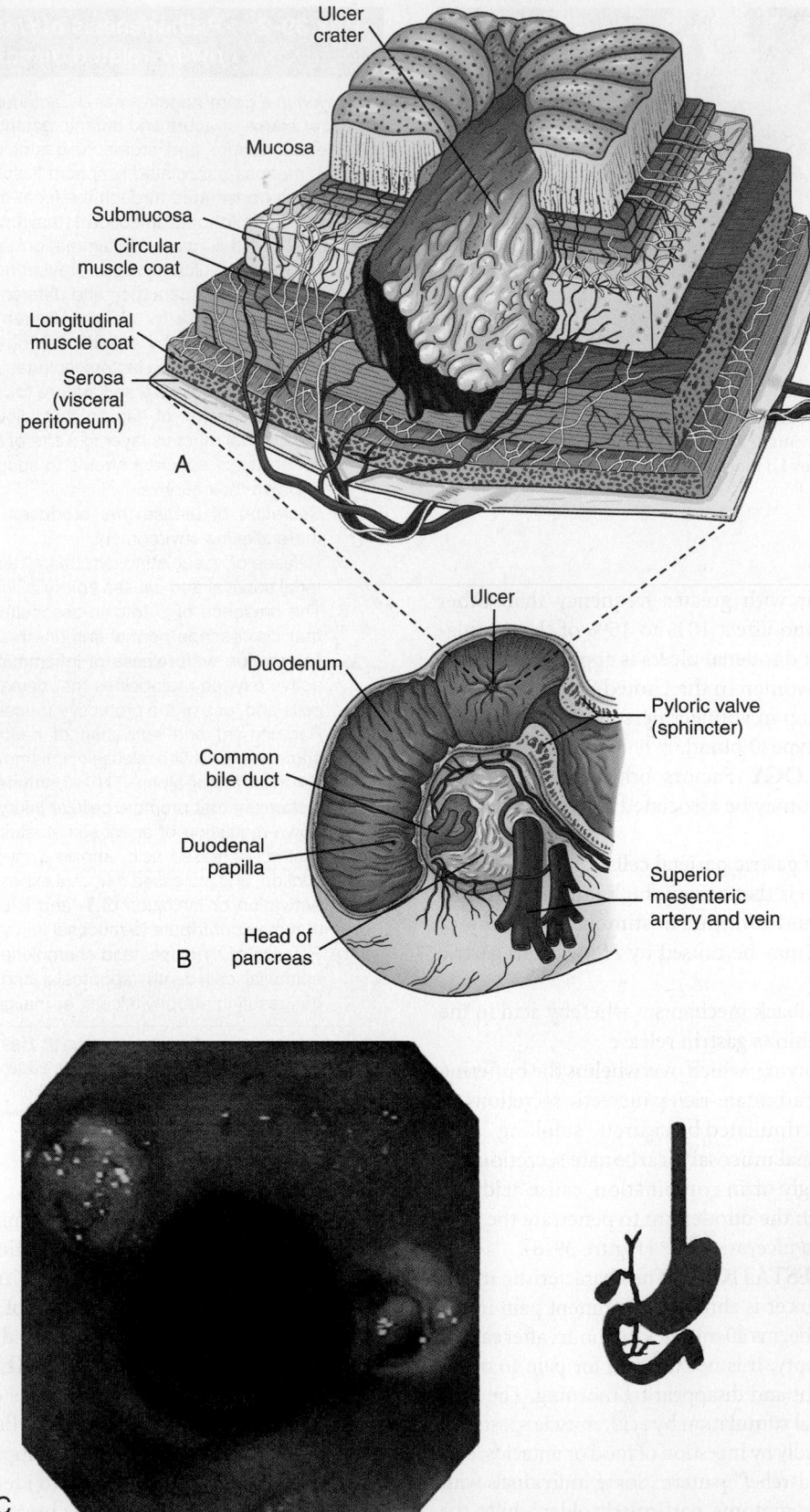

Figure 39-8 Duodenal ulcer. A, A deep ulceration in the duodenal wall extending as a crater through the entire mucosa and into the muscle layers. **B,** Duodenal ulcer. **C,** Bilateral (kissing) duodenal ulcers in a person using nonsteroidal anti-inflammatory drugs (NSAIDs). (C Courtesy David Bjorkman, MD, University of Utah School of Medicine, Department of Gastroenterology.)

contents, elevate pH, inactivate pepsin, and relieve pain. Acid secretion can be suppressed with drugs that block H_2 receptors and inhibit the secretion of acid. Proton pump inhibitors inhibit acid production. Eradication of *H. pylori* with bismuth and combinations of antibiotics supplemented with vitamin C usually prevents relapse, although there is increasing drug resistance.[76] Ulcer-coating agents, such as sucralfate and colloidal bismuth, promote healing. Anticholinergic drugs may be used to inhibit gastric secretion, suppress gastric motility, and delay gastric emptying. Surgical resection may be required for bleeding or perforating ulcers, obstruction, or peritonitis.[77] Risk of duodenal ulcer may be reduced with a diet high in vitamin A and fiber.[78] Clinical trials are in progress for a vaccine against *H. pylori*.[79]

Gastric Ulcers

Gastric ulcers are ulcers of the stomach. They occur with about equal frequency in males and females, usually between the ages of 55 and 65 years, and are about one fourth as common as duodenal ulcers (Table 39-5 and Figure 39-9).

PATHOPHYSIOLOGY Generally gastric ulcers develop in the antral region, adjacent to the acid-secreting mucosa of the body, and are frequently caused by *H. pylori* (see Box 39-2).[80] The primary defect is an abnormality that increases the mucosal barrier's permeability to hydrogen ions. Gastric secretion may be normal or less than normal and there may be a decreased mass of parietal cells. Chronic pangastritis is often associated with development of gastric ulcers and may precipitate ulcer formation by limiting the mucosa's ability to secrete a protective layer of mucus (Figure 39-10).

Duodenal reflux of bile is associated with gastric ulcer (alkaline reflux gastritis, p. 1469) and may occur after cholescystectomy, pyloroplasty, or gastrojejunostomy.[81] The pyloric sphincter also may fail to respond to stimuli that normally increase resting tone, such as entry of acid, protein, and fat into the duodenum. An increased concentration of bile salts disrupts the gastric mucosa. The break damages the mucosal barrier by permitting hydrogen ions to diffuse into the mucosa, where they disrupt permeability and cellular structure. A vicious cycle can be established as the damaged mucosa liberates histamine, which stimulates the increase of acid and pepsinogen production, blood flow, and capillary permeability. The disrupted mucosa becomes edematous and loses plasma proteins. Destruction of small vessels causes bleeding.

Zollinger-Ellison syndrome is associated with peptic ulcers related to increased secretion of gastrin, which causes excess secretion of gastric acid. A gastrinoma (a gastrin-secreting neuroendocrine tumor or multiple tumors) of the pancreas or duodenum stimulates a proliferation of gastric parietal cells and chronic secretion of gastric acid. The resulting excess acid causes gastric and duodenal ulcers, gastroesophageal reflux with abdominal pain, and diarrhea. Diagnosis includes secretin- or calcium-stimulated measures of gastrin levels, gastric pH levels less than 2, and symptomatic evidence of peptic ulcer disease. Proton pump inhibitors reduce gastric acid secretion, and surgical removal of tumors limits metastasis.[82,83]

CLINICAL MANIFESTATIONS The clinical manifestations of gastric ulcers are similar to those of duodenal ulcers (see Table 39-5). The pattern of pain, food, and relief is common, but the pain of gastric ulcers also occurs immediately after eating. Gastric ulcers also tend to be chronic rather than alternate between periods of remission and exacerbation and cause more anorexia, vomiting, and weight loss than duodenal ulcers. The evaluation and treatment of gastric ulcers are similar to the evaluation and treatment of duodenal ulcers.

Stress-Related Mucosal Disease

A **stress ulcer (stress-related mucosal disease)** is an acute form of peptic ulcer that tends to accompany the physiologic stress of severe illness; multisystem organ failure; or major trauma, including severe burns or head injury. Usually, multiple sites of ulceration are distributed within the stomach or duodenum. Stress ulcers may be classified as ischemic ulcers or Cushing ulcers.

Ischemic ulcers develop within hours of an event—such as hemorrhage, multisystem trauma, severe burns, heart failure, or sepsis—that causes ischemia of the stomach and duodenal mucosa. Stress ulcers that develop as a result of burn injury are often called **Curling ulcers**.

The shock, anoxia, and sympathetic responses produced by the precipitating event decrease mucosal blood flow, leading to gastric ischemia. In intensive care units, use of positive-pressure mechanical ventilation can induce splanchnic hypoperfusion and contribute to stress-related mucosal injury.[84] Because the metabolism of the mucosal cells declines as a result of ischemia, the mucosal lining degenerates. Acid diffuses back into the mucosa, causing inflammation, ulceration, hemorrhage, and necrosis. The ulcerative process is accelerated if bile or pancreatic enzymes are regurgitated from the duodenum. Bleeding occurs more readily with the presence of coagulopathy.[85]

Cushing ulcer is a stress ulcer associated with severe head trauma or brain surgery. This ulcer results from decreased mucosal blood flow and hypersecretion of acid caused by overstimulation of the vagal nuclei. Excessive acid damages the mucosal barrier, initiating the processes summarized in Figure 39-10.

The primary clinical manifestation of stress-related mucosal disease is bleeding. Other symptoms may not be present. The bleeding may be slight or, if a small vessel is perforated, amount to hundreds of milliliters. Prophylactic treatment regimens are used to prevent this disease.[86] Stress ulcers seldom become chronic.

Surgical Treatment of Ulcer

Advances in the medical treatment of peptic ulcer disease with proton pump inhibitors and eradication of *H. pylori*, and laparoscopic and endoscopic repair techniques have significantly reduced the number of cases requiring surgery.[87] The indications for ulcer surgery are recurrent or uncontrolled bleeding and complicated perforation of the stomach or duodenum.[88]

Table 39-5   Characteristics of Gastric and Duodenal Ulcers

Characteristics	Gastric Ulcer	Duodenal Ulcer
Incidence		
Age at onset	50-70 years	20-50 years
Family history	Usually negative	Positive
Gender (prevalence)	Equal in women and men	Equal in women and men
Stress factors	Increased	Average
Ulcerogenic drugs	Normal use	Increased use
Cancer risk	Increased	Not increased
Pathophysiology		
Helicobacter pylori infection	Often present (60%-80%)	Often present (95%-100%)
Abnormal mucus	May be present	May be present
Parietal cell mass	Normal or decreased	Increased
Acid production	Normal or decreased	Increased
Serum gastrin	Increased	Normal
Serum pepsinogen	Normal	Increased
Associated gastritis	More common	Usually not present
Clinical Manifestations		
Pain	Located in upper abdomen	Located in upper abdomen
	Intermittent	Intermittent
	Pain-antacid-relief pattern	Pain-antacid or food-relief pattern
	Food-pain pattern	Nocturnal pain common
Clinical course	Chronic ulcer without pattern of remission and exacerbation	Pattern of remissions and exacerbations for years

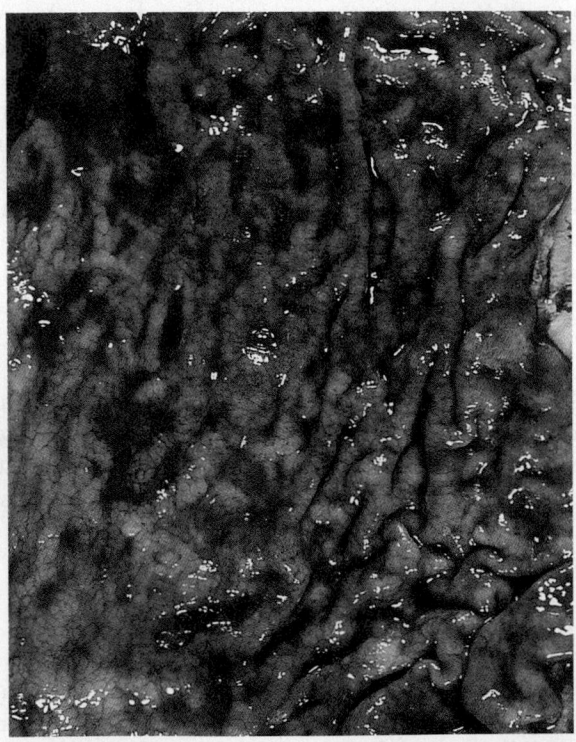

Figure 39-9 Macroscopic appearance of benign gastric ulcers. (From Damjanov I, Linder J, editors: *Anderson's pathology,* ed 10, St Louis, 1996, Mosby.)

Different types of gastric resection may be performed to treat gastric cancer.

Acute complications of gastrectomy or anastomosis, such as poor wound healing, abscess formation, or suture failure, are relatively uncommon except in the debilitated person. Chronic complications, however, occur more often and are likely to develop if a large portion of the stomach has been removed. These complications and their pathophysiologic mechanisms are described in the next section.

Postgastrectomy Syndromes

Postgastrectomy syndromes are a group of signs and symptoms that occur after gastric resection. They are caused by changes in motor and control functions of the stomach and upper small intestine.[89]

Dumping Syndrome

Dumping syndrome is the rapid emptying of hypertonic chyme from the surgically created, residual stomach into the small intestine 10 to 20 minutes after eating (early dumping syndrome). It occurs with varying severity in 5% to 10% of individuals who have undergone partial gastrectomy or pyloroplasty.[90] It is not common in individuals who have undergone a Billroth II anastomosis (gastrojejunostomy) accompanied by vagotomy. Factors that promote *early dumping syndrome* include (1) loss of gastric capacity, (2) loss of emptying control

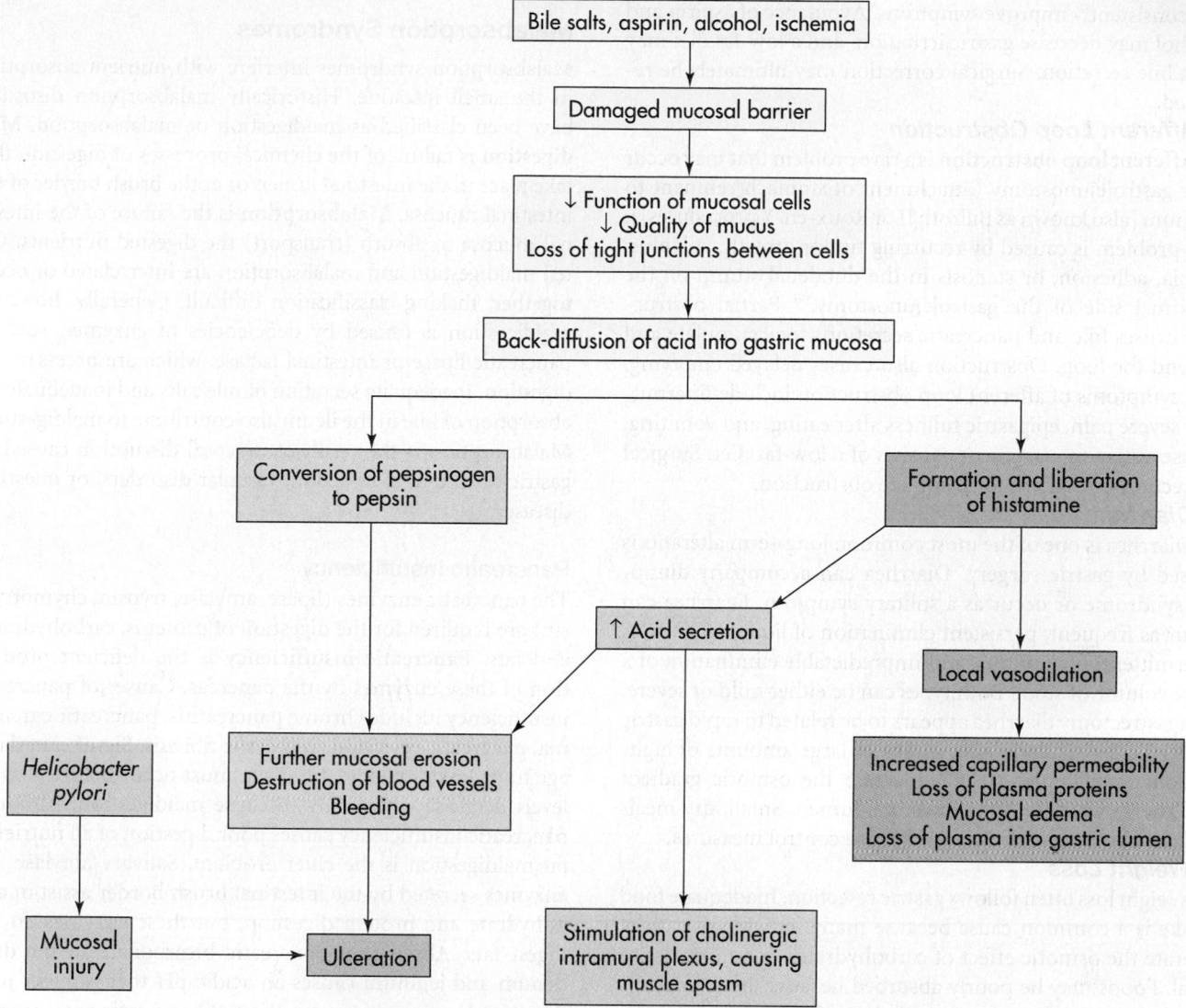

Figure 39-10 Pathophysiology of gastric ulcer formation.

when the pylorus is removed, and (3) loss of feedback control by the duodenum when it is removed. Rapid gastric emptying and creation of a high osmotic gradient within the small intestine cause a sudden shift of fluid from the vascular compartment to the intestinal lumen. Plasma volume decreases, causing vasomotor responses, such as increased pulse rate, hypotension, weakness, pallor, sweating, and dizziness. Rapid distention of the intestine produces a feeling of epigastric fullness, cramping, nausea, vomiting, and diarrhea.[91]

A less common form of dumping syndrome, *late dumping syndrome*, occurs 1 to 3 hours after eating. The symptoms include weakness, diaphoresis, and confusion, but they cannot be explained by rapid gastric emptying. After a high-carbohydrate meal, individuals who have undergone gastrectomy may develop hypoglycemia, which causes the symptoms. The hypoglycemia is caused by an increase in insulin secretion stimulated by the hyperglycemia that follows eating. Other hormonal responses may also participate in the development of hypoglycemia.

Most cases of dumping syndrome respond well to dietary management.[92] Frequent small meals that are high in protein and low in carbohydrates relieve symptoms. Other measures include drinking fluids between meals instead of at mealtime and reclining on the left side after eating. Some cases require surgical intervention, including reconstruction of the pylorus or a gastrojejunostomy.[93] Octreotide reduces abdominal and vasomotor symptoms of dumping syndrome by unknown mechanisms.[94]

Alkaline Reflux Gastritis

Alkaline reflux gastritis is a stomach inflammation caused by reflux of bile and alkaline pancreatic secretions that contain proteolytic enzymes and disrupt the mucosal barrier. This form of gastritis occurs in 5% to 20% of individuals who have undergone gastrectomy or pyloroplasty. Clinical manifestations include nausea, bilious vomiting (vomiting in which the vomitus contains bile), and sustained epigastric pain that worsens after eating and is not relieved by antacids.[95] Endoscopy shows a hemorrhagic and friable gastric mucosa. Conservative management is often difficult because antacids do not consistently improve symptoms. Avoidance of aspirin and alcohol may decrease gastric irritation, and a low-fat diet may limit bile secretion. Surgical correction may ultimately be required.

Afferent Loop Obstruction

Afferent loop obstruction is a rare problem that may occur after gastrojejunostomy (attachment of stomach remnant to jejunum [also known as Billroth II or Roux-en-Y procedures]). The problem is caused by recurring tumor growth, volvulus, hernia, adhesion, or stenosis in the duodenal stump on the proximal side of the gastrojejunostomy.[96] Partial obstruction causes bile and pancreatic secretions to accumulate and distend the loop. Obstruction also causes delayed emptying. The symptoms of afferent loop obstruction include intermittent severe pain, epigastric fullness after eating, and vomiting. Conservative management consists of a low-fat diet. Surgical correction is required for complete obstruction.

Diarrhea

Diarrhea is one of the most common long-term alterations caused by gastric surgery. Diarrhea can accompany dumping syndrome or occur as a solitary symptom. Diarrhea can occur as frequent, persistent elimination of liquid stool or as intermittent, precipitous, and unpredictable elimination of a large volume of stool. Both types can be either mild or severe. Postgastrectomy diarrhea appears to be related to rapid gastric emptying, particularly after intake of large amounts of high-carbohydrate liquids, which increase the osmotic gradient and attract water into the intestinal lumen. Small, dry meals and anticholinergic drugs are effective control measures.

Weight Loss

Weight loss often follows gastric resection. Inadequate food intake is a common cause because many individuals cannot tolerate the osmotic effect of carbohydrates or a normal-size meal. Foods may be poorly absorbed because the stomach is less able to mix, churn, and break down food particles. Vomiting, diarrhea, and malabsorption of fats also contribute to weight loss.

Anemia

Anemia after gastrectomy results from iron, vitamin B_{12}, or folate deficiency. Iron malabsorption may be caused by decreased acid secretion. Acid changes iron from a trivalent to a divalent molecule, making it easier to absorb. Iron absorption is also compromised in individuals who have undergone a Billroth II procedure because the duodenum is no longer available to absorb iron.

Vitamin B_{12} deficiency may occur several years after gastrectomy. Contributing factors include loss of parietal cells, which secrete intrinsic factor. (Intrinsic factor facilitates absorption of vitamin B_{12}; see Chapter 38.) Vitamin B_{12} absorption is also compromised if gastric contents are not mixed adequately with pancreatic enzymes, such as may occur after a Billroth II anastomosis.

Folate deficiency is related to poor intake or malabsorption. Management of deficiencies consists of replacement of iron and folate with supplements. Vitamin B_{12} can be administered monthly by injection or oral supplements.[97]

Malabsorption Syndromes

Malabsorption syndromes interfere with nutrient absorption in the small intestine. Historically malabsorption disorders have been classified as maldigestion or malabsorption. **Maldigestion** is failure of the chemical processes of digestion that take place in the intestinal lumen or at the brush border of the intestinal mucosa. **Malabsorption** is the failure of the intestinal mucosa to absorb (transport) the digested nutrients. Often maldigestion and malabsorption are interrelated or occur together, making classification difficult. Generally, however, maldigestion is caused by deficiencies of enzymes, such as pancreatic lipase or intestinal lactase, which are necessary for digestion. Inadequate secretion of bile salts and inadequate reabsorption of bile in the ileum also contribute to maldigestion. Malabsorption is the result of mucosal disruption caused by gastric or intestinal resection, vascular disorders, or intestinal disease.

Pancreatic Insufficiency

The pancreatic enzymes (lipase, amylase, trypsin, chymotrypsin) are required for the digestion of proteins, carbohydrates, and fats. **Pancreatic insufficiency** is the deficient production of these enzymes by the pancreas. Causes of pancreatic insufficiency include chronic pancreatitis, pancreatic carcinoma, pancreatic resection, and cystic fibrosis. Significant damage to or loss of pancreatic tissue must occur before enzyme levels decrease sufficiently to cause maldigestion. Although pancreatic insufficiency causes poor digestion of all nutrients, fat maldigestion is the chief problem. Salivary amylase and enzymes secreted by the intestinal brush border assist in carbohydrate and protein digestion, but these enzymes do not digest fats. Absence of pancreatic bicarbonate in the duodenum and jejunum causes an acidic pH that worsens maldigestion by preventing activation of pancreatic enzymes that are present. Maldigestion, a large amount of fat in the stool (steatorrhea), and weight loss are the most common signs of pancreatic insufficiency. Lipase supplementation is usually successful.[98]

Lactase Deficiency

Deficiency of disaccharidase at the villus brush border of the small intestine is caused by a congenital defect in the lactase gene.[99] **Lactase deficiency** inhibits the breakdown of lactose (milk sugar) into monosaccharides and therefore prevents lactose digestion and absorption across the intestinal wall. Lactase deficiency is most common in blacks. Congenital lactase deficiency causes watery diarrhea in breast milk or lactose-containing formulas in infants. Lactase expression is lost before adulthood in adult-type lactose intolerance and is genetically determined.[100] Secondary (acquired) lactase deficiency can be caused by several diseases of the intestine, including gluten-sensitive enteropathy (see Chapter 40), enteritis, and bacterial overgrowth.

The undigested lactose remains in the intestine, where bacterial fermentation causes gases to form. Undigested lactose also increases the osmotic gradient in the intestine, causing irritation and osmotic diarrhea. Clinical manifestations of lactase deficiency are bloating, crampy pain, diarrhea, and flatulence. The disorder is diagnosed by a lactose-hydrogen breath test, dietary lactose withdrawal, or small intestinal biopsy.[101] Avoiding milk products and adhering to a lactose-free diet relieve symptoms. Maintaining an adequate calcium intake with restricted intake of milk products decreases risk of osteoporosis.[102]

Bile Salt Deficiency

Conjugated bile acids (bile salts) are necessary for the digestion and absorption of fats. Bile salts are conjugated in the bile that is synthesized from cholesterol and secreted from the liver.[103] When bile enters the duodenum, the bile salts aggregate with fatty acids and monoglycerides to form micelles. Micelle formation solubilizes fat molecules and allows them to pass through the unstirred layer at the brush border (see Chapter 38). A minimum concentration of bile salts, termed the *critical micelle concentration,* is required to allow micelles to form. Therefore, conditions that decrease the production or secretion of bile result in decreased micelle formation and fat malabsorption. These conditions include advanced liver disease, which decreases production of bile salts; obstruction of the common bile duct, which decreases flow of bile into the duodenum; intestinal stasis (lack of motility), which permits overgrowth of intestinal bacteria that deconjugate bile salts; and diseases of the ileum, which prevent the reabsorption and recycling of bile salts (enterohepatic circulation).

Clinical manifestations of bile salt deficiency are related to poor intestinal absorption of fat and fat-soluble vitamins (A, D, E, K). Increased fat in the stools (steatorrhea) leads to diarrhea and decreased plasma proteins. The losses of fat-soluble vitamins and their effects include the following:

1. Vitamin A deficiency results in night blindness.
2. Vitamin D deficiency results in decreased calcium absorption with bone demineralization (osteoporosis), bone pain, and fractures.
3. Vitamin K deficiency prolongs prothrombin time, leading to spontaneous development of purpura (bruising) and petechiae.
4. Vitamin E deficiency has uncertain effects but may cause testicular atrophy and neurologic defects in children.

The most effective treatment for fat-soluble vitamin deficiency is to increase medium-chain triglycerides in the diet, for example, by using coconut oil for cooking. Vitamins A, D, and K are given parenterally.

Inflammatory Bowel Disease

Ulcerative colitis and Crohn disease are chronic relapsing inflammatory bowel diseases (IBDs) of unknown origin that affect about 1 million people in the United States.[104] Both diseases are associated with genetic factors, alterations in epithelial cell barrier functions, and immunopathology related to abnormal T-cell reactions to commensal microflora and other luminal antigens.[105,106] Ulcerative colitis is limited to the mucosa of the colon and rectum. Crohn disease can involve any part of the gastrointestinal tract from the mouth to the anus and involves transmural granulomatous inflammatory lesions (Figure 39-11).

Ulcerative Colitis

Ulcerative colitis (UC) is a chronic inflammatory disease that causes ulceration of the colonic mucosa and extends proximally from the rectum into the colon. The lesions appear in susceptible individuals between 20 and 40 years of age. Risk factors include family history of disease or Jewish descent, and the disease is more prevalent among white populations and Northern Europeans. UC is less common in smokers.[107]

Although the cause of UC is unknown, dietary, infectious, genetic, and immunologic factors are all suggested causes.[108] Inflammation may be caused by commensal or pathogenic enteric microogansims with increased mucosal adherence and invasion and persistent activation of T cells. The familial tendency to develop ulcerative colitis and the occurrence of disease in identical twins supports a genetic theory of causation. Perhaps most significant are the humoral and cellular immunologic factors associated with the disease. Colonic epithelial antibodies of the immunoglobulin G (IgG) class have been identified in the sera of individuals with ulcerative colitis and a large number of plasma cells are found in the inflamed colon. Lymphocytes (T cells) in individuals with ulcerative colitis may have cytotoxic effects on the epithelial cells of the colon, as well as damage caused by inflammatory cytokines (IL-1, IL-2, IL-6, IL-8, IL-10, TNF-α), toxic oxygen radicals, and interferon-gamma (IFN-γ).[109] Activated macrophages also contribute cytokines that cause fever and the acute phase response. Furthermore, autoimmune disorders, such as systemic lupus erythematosus and erythema nodosum, may accompany ulcerative colitis.

PATHOPHYSIOLOGY The primary lesions of UC are continuous with no skip lesions, limited to the mucosa, and not transmural. The mucous layer is thinner than normal and there is impairment of the epithelial barrier. The rectum is almost always involved. Inflammation begins at the base of the crypt of Lieberkühn in the large intestine, primarily the left colon, with infiltration and release of inflammatory cytokines from neutrophils, lymphocytes, plasma cells, macrophages, eosinophils, and mast cells.[110] The disease is most severe in the rectum and sigmoid colon. With milder inflammation, the mucosa is hyperemic, edematous, and may appear dark red and velvety (Figure 39-12). In more severe inflammation, the mucosa becomes hemorrhagic, and small erosions form and coalesce into ulcers. Abscess formation occurs in the crypts. Necrosis and ragged ulceration of the mucosa ensue. Edema and thickening of the muscularis mucosae may narrow the lumen of the involved colon. In chronic disease, inflammatory polyps (pseudopolyps) develop in the colon from rapidly regenerating epithelium.

CLINICAL MANIFESTATIONS The course of UC consists of intermittent periods of remission and exacerbation. Clinical manifestations vary with the severity and extent of

CROHN DISEASE

ULCERATIVE COLITIS

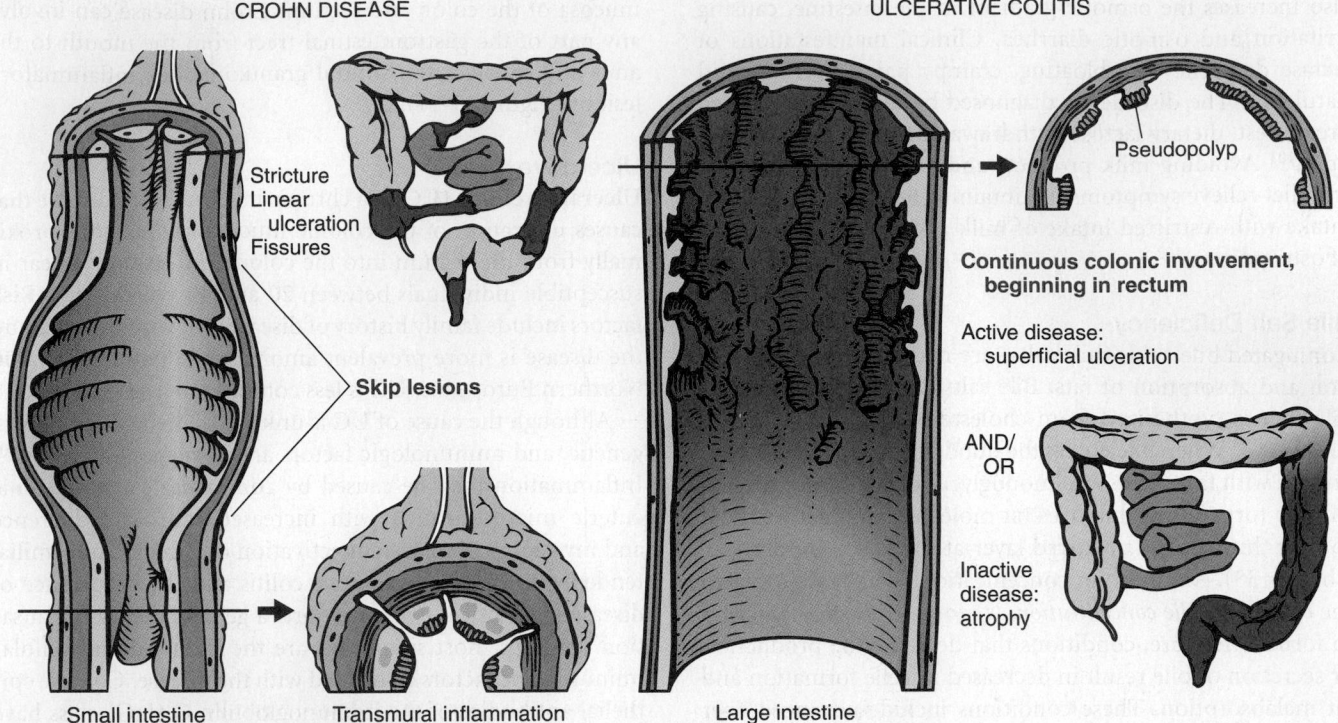

Figure 39-11 Distribution patterns of Crohn disease and ulcerative colitis. Comparison of distribution patterns of Crohn disease and ulcerative colitis as well as different conformations of ulcers and wall thickenings. (From Kumar V et al, editors: *Robbins basic pathology*, ed 7, St Louis, 2003, Mosby.)

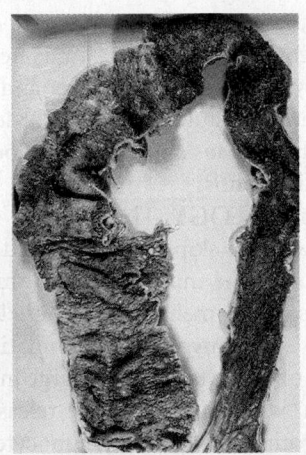

Figure 39-12 Acute ulcerative colitis. Colitis with extensive mucosal ulceration involving the entire colon. (From Damjanov I, Linder J, editors: *Anderson's pathology*, ed 10, St. Louis, 1996, Mosby.)

disease. Loss of the absorptive mucosal surface and decreased colonic transit time can cause large volumes of watery diarrhea. Mucosal destruction causes bleeding, cramping pain, and an urge to defecate. Frequent diarrhea, with passage of small amounts of blood and purulent mucus, is common.[111]

Mild UC involves less mucosa and may be limited to proctitis, so that frequency of bowel movements, bleeding, and pain is minimal. Severe forms may involve the entire colon (pancolitis) and are characterized by fever; elevated

pulse rate; frequent diarrhea (10 to 20 movements per day); urgency; obviously bloody stools; and continuous, crampy pain. Dehydration, weight loss, anemia, and fever result from fluid loss, bleeding, and inflammation. Complications include toxic megacolon, anal fissures, hemorrhoids, and perirectal abscess. Severe hemorrhage is rare, but chronic blood loss may precipitate hypotension and shock. Edema, strictures, or fibrosis can obstruct the colon. Perforation is an unusual but possible complication. The risk of left-sided colon cancer increases significantly after many years of ulcerative colitis and the presence of primary sclerosing cholangitis.[112]

Extraintestinal manifestations of UC and Crohn disease occur in 20% to 40% of cases and include cutaneous lesions (erythema nodosum and pyoderma gangrenosum), migratory polyarthritis and sacroiliitis, osteopenia and osteoporosis, mouth ulcers, episcleritis or anterior uveitis of the eye, and primary sclerosing colangitis in the liver.[113] Gallstones are common. Alterations in coagulation can cause life-threatening microthrombi and deep vein thrombosis.[114,115]

EVALUATION AND TREATMENT Diagnosis of ulcerative colitis is based on the medical history, clinical manifestations, imaging procedures, and histologic criteria.[116] Endoscopic evaluation shows an inflamed and hemorrhagic mucosa. Radiologic assessment may show loss of haustra, ulceration, and irregular mucosa. The laboratory data include low hemoglobin values, hypoalbuminemia, and low serum potassium levels. Infectious causes are ruled out by stool culture. The symptoms of ulcerative colitis can be very similar to those of Crohn disease, making differential diagnosis difficult.[110]

Treatment depends on the severity of symptoms and the extent of mucosal involvement. First line therapy is 5-aminosalicylic acid (mesalazine). Steroids and salicylates suppress the inflammatory response and help alleviate the cramping pain. Immunosuppressive agents (e.g., 6-mercaptopurine or azathioprine), cyclosporine, tacrolimus, and infliximab (a monoclonal anti-TNF-α antibody) are used for chronic active disease[117]. Broad-spectrum antibiotics or probiotics, or both, can modulate intestinal flora[111] (see What's New? Inflammatory Bowel Disease and Probiotics). For unknown reasons, nicotine may have a protective effect in ulcerative colitis but not in Crohn disease.[118,119] Severe, unremitting disease can require hospital admission and administration of intravenous fluids. Extreme malnutrition may require intravenous hyperalimentation. Surgical resection of the colon or a colostomy may be performed if other forms of therapy are unsuccessful.[120,121]

Crohn Disease

Crohn disease (CD) (granulomatous colitis, ileocolitis, or regional enteritis) is an idiopathic inflammatory disorder that affects any part of the gastrointestinal tract from the mouth to the anus. The distal small intestine and proximal large colon are most commonly affected by the disease. In a small percentage of cases, CD is difficult to differentiate from ulcerative colitis (Table 39-6). Risk factors include family history, tobacco use, Jewish ethnicity, urban residency, and the *CARD15/ NOD2* (nucleotide-binding-oligomerization-domains) gene mutations (10% to 15% of cases).[122] The *CARD15/NOD2*

WHAT'S NEW?   Inflammatory Bowel Disease and Probiotics

The etiology of inflammatory bowel disease (IBD) remains uncertain but the pathogenesis includes abnormal cell-mediated and humoral immune responses to commensal microflora in genetically susceptible individuals. There may be disturbances in mucosal permeability and the number and type of microflora. Probiotics are living microorganisms in food or dietary supplements that survive in stomach acid and bile and are safe for human ingestion. Their beneficial properties include altering the composition of bacterial flora, improvement of intestinal epithelial barrier function, and modulation of the mucosal immune system. The results of research using probiotics to treat IBD are controversial because there are few randomized controlled clinical trials. A multiagent mixture of probiotic strains appears to be more useful for treating pouchitis and ulcerative colitis than for Crohn disease and for maintaining remission in pediatric ulcerative colitis. There is a need for further research and controlled clinical trails to evaluate efficacy of probiotics for the remission of IBD.

Data from: Butterworth AD, Thomas AG, Akobeng AK: *Cochrane Database Syst Rev* (3):CD006634, 2008; Heilpern D, Szilagyi A: *Rev Recent Clin Trials* 3(3):167-184, 2008; Miele E et al: *Am J Gastroenterol* 104(2):437-443, 2009.

---

gene codes for a protein (a Toll-like receptor; see Chapter 9) involved in the recognition of gram-negative and gram-positive bacteria. Mutations in this gene are linked to the pathogenesis of CD, particularly ileal disease. Other candidate gene mutations are located on chromosomes 5 *(IBD5)*, 6 *(IBD3)*, and 10 *(IBD10)*.[123] The colony-stimulating factor IR gene, which is involved in monocyte to macrophage differentiation, also may be a susceptibility gene for CD.[124] The pathogenesis of CD may be associated with an overly aggressive response to normal flora bacteria in genetically predisposed individuals.[125,126] Th$_1$-mediated inflammation with activation of leukocytes and cytokines (TNF-α, IFN-γ, and interleukins) causes injury. Recruited leukocytes release proinflammatory substances, including prostaglandins, leukotrienes, proteases, reactive oxygen species, and nitric oxide, which cause further injury and inflammation. Elevations in IgG are associated with severity of disease.[127]

PATHOPHYSIOLOGY The inflammatory process of CD begins in the intestinal submucosa and spreads across the intestinal wall to involve the mucosa and serosa in areas overlying lymphoid tissue. Progression of the disease involves neutrophil infiltration of the crypts resulting in abscess formation and crypt destruction. The most common site of the disease is the ileocolon, but both the large and small intestines may be involved. The inflammation can affect some haustral segments but not others, creating a pattern called *skip lesions*. One side of the intestinal wall may be affected but not the other.

The ulcerations of CD produce longitudinal and transverse fissures that extend inflammation into lymphoid tissue. The typical chronic lesion is a granuloma having cobblestone projections of inflamed tissue surrounded by areas of ulceration (Figure 39-13). (Granulomas are described in Chapter 6.) The lumen can narrow with inflammation, edema, and fibrotic strictures. Fistulae may form in the perianal area between loops of intestine or extend into the bladder.

CLINICAL MANIFESTATIONS Individuals with CD may have no specific symptoms other than an "irritable bowel" for several years. Symptoms vary and are associated with disease location. Abdominal pain and diarrhea are the most common signs (more than five stools per day), with passage of blood and mucus. Diarrhea can result from decreased colonic absorption, bypass fistulae, medications, bacterial overgrowth, and the presence of bile in the colon that inhibits water absorption.[128] Other manifestations are related to the location and extent of intestinal involvement. Inflammation of the ileum, for example, causes tenderness in the lower right side of the abdomen. If the ileum is involved, the individual may be anemic as a result of malabsorption of vitamin B$_{12}$. There also may be deficiencies in folic acid, vitamin D absorption, and calcium leading to bone disease. Proteins may be lost, leading to hypoalbuminemia. Weight loss is common. Anal manifestations occur in about 30% of cases, including anal fissure, perianal abscess, and fistula.[129] Individuals with CD of long duration are also at risk for intestinal adenocarcinoma.[130] Complications include obstruction, fistulae, abscess

Table 39-6 Features of Ulcerative Colitis and Crohn Disease

Feature	Ulcerative Colitis	Crohn Disease
Incidence		
Age at onset	Any age; 10-40 years most common	Any age; 10-30 years most common
Family history	Less common	More common
Gender (prevalence)	Equal in women and men	About equal in women and men
Cancer risk	Increased	Increased
Pathophysiology		
Location of lesions	Colon and rectum, no "skip" lesions	All of GI tract: mouth to anus, "skip" lesions common
Inflammation and ulceration	Mucosal layer involved	Entire intestinal wall involved
Granulomas	Rare	Common
Friable mucosa	Common	Less common
Fistulas and abscesses	Rare	Common
Strictures and possible obstruction	Rare	Common
Clinical Manifestations		
Abdominal pain	Occasional	Common
Diarrhea	Common	Common
Bloody stools	Common	Less common
Abdominal mass	Rare	Common
Small intestinal malabsorption	Rare	Common
Steatorrhea	Rare	Common
Potential for malignancy	Common	Common
Antineutrophil cytoplasmic antibodies	Common	Rare
Antisaccharomyces cerevisiae antibodies	Rare	Common
Clinical course	Remissions and exacerbations	Remissions and exacerbations

GI, Gastrointestinal.

formation, and chronic blood loss. Extraintestinal manifestations are similar to those described for UC.

EVALUATION AND TREATMENT The diagnosis and treatment of CD are similar to the diagnosis and treatment of ulcerative colitis. Treatment with immunomodulatory agents can be effective. TNF-α–blocking agents are used for treatment of fistulas and to maintain remission.[131] Surgery is generally performed to manage complications such as strictures, fistula, abscess, and perforation, or to relieve obstruction.[132]

When treatment involves surgical resection of small intestinal segments, complications related to **short bowel syndrome** can occur, including malabsorption, diarrhea and nutritional deficiencies. Symptoms are related to the extent and location of resection.

Diverticular Disease of the Colon

Diverticula are herniations or saclike outpouchings of mucosa through the muscle layers of the colon wall. **Diverticulosis** is asymptomatic diverticular disease. The cause is unknown but is associated with decreased dietary fiber and increased intracolonic pressure. **Diverticulitis** represents inflammation. Diverticular disease is most common in individuals older than 60 years of age, particularly those who live in developed countries where much of the diet consists of refined foods.[133]

PATHOPHYSIOLOGY Although diverticula can occur anywhere in the gastrointestinal tract, the most common site is the left colon.[134] The diverticula form at weak points

in the colon wall, usually where arteries penetrate the tunica muscularis to nourish the mucosal layer. Abnormal colonic motility with intraluminal hypertension also may be contributing factors. The colonic mucosa herniates through the smooth muscle layers (Figure 39-14). A common associated finding is thickening of the circular and longitudinal (teniae coli) muscles surrounding the diverticula. Hypertrophy and contraction of these muscles increase intraluminal pressure and degree of herniation. Habitual consumption of a low-residue diet reduces fecal bulk, thus reducing the diameter of the colon. According to Laplace's law (see Chapter 29), wall pressure increases as the diameter of a cylindrical structure decreases. Therefore, pressure within the narrow lumen can increase enough to rupture the diverticula. Insoluble dietary fiber deficiency also may change the intestinal microflora, decreasing the immune response in the colon and permitting low-grade inflammation.[135,136] Diverticulitis can cause abscess formation, fistula formation, peritonitis, or obstruction.[137]

CLINICAL MANIFESTATIONS Symptoms of diverticular disease are usually vague or absent. Cramping pain of the lower abdomen can accompany constriction of the hypertrophied colonic muscles. Diarrhea, constipation, distention, or flatulence may occur. Diverticula with an obstructed opening become inflamed or abscesses form, and the individual develops fever, leukocytosis (increased white blood cell count), and tenderness of the lower left quadrant. Right lower

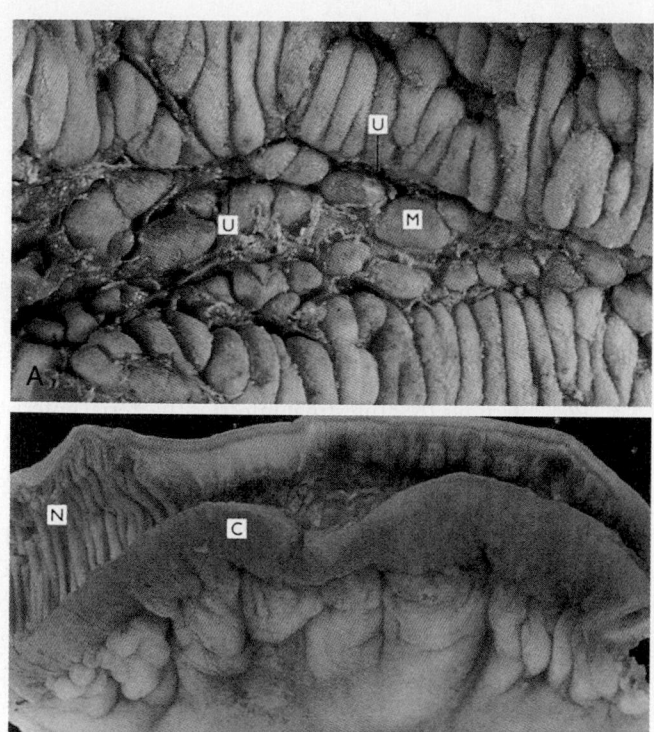

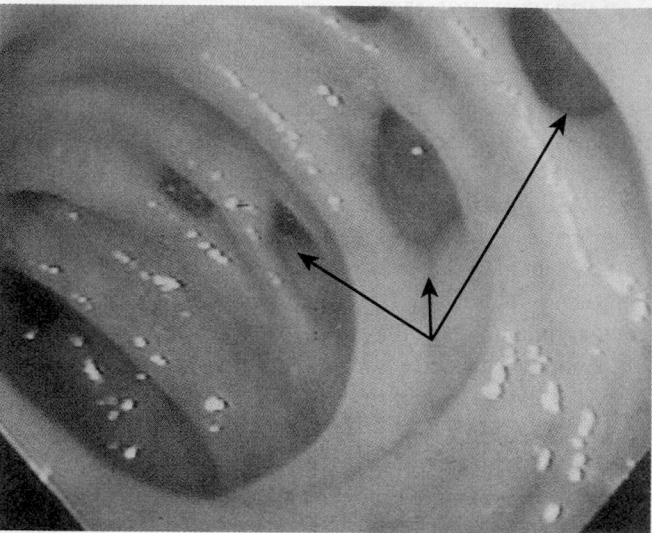

Figure 39-14 Diverticular disease. In diverticular disease, the outpouches *(arrows)* of mucosa seen in the sigmoid colon appear as slitlike openings from the mucosal surface of the opened bowel. (From Townsend C *Sabiston textbook* of surgery, ed 18, Philadelphia 2008, Saunders.)

Figure 39-13 Crohn disease. **A,** The mucosa in Crohn disease demonstrates a cobblestone pattern as a result of fissured ulcers *(U)* with intervening areas of edematous mucosa *(M)*. **B,** Compared with normal small bowel wall *(N),* the Crohn segment *(C)* shows wall thickening that has caused a stenosis. (From Kumar V et al: *Pathologic basis of disease,* ed 7, Philadelphia, 2006, Saunders.)

quadrant pain and severe complications, such as hemorrhage, perforation with peritonitis, bowel obstruction, and fistula formation, are rare.

EVALUATION AND TREATMENT Diverticula are often discovered during diagnostic procedures performed for other problems. Ultrasound, sigmoidoscopy, or barium enema is used for diagnosis of uncomplicated diverticula. Abdominal computed tomography (CT) is used for complicated cases.

An increase of dietary fiber intake increases stool weight, lowers colonic pressures, improves transit times, and often relieves symptoms (see Nutrition & Disease: Diverticular Disease and Diet). Probiotics combined with salicylates are effective in arresting infection. Diverticulitis with small abscesses is treated with antibiotics and reestablishing the microflora.[134] Surgical resection may be required if there are severe complications.[138]

Appendicitis

Appendicitis is an inflammation of the vermiform appendix, which is a projection from the apex of the cecum. It is the most common surgical emergency of the abdomen and affects 7% to 12% of the population. The most common occurrence is between 20 and 30 years of age, although it may develop at any age.[139]

NUTRITION & DISEASE

Diverticular Disease and Diet

Daily consumption of fiber-enriched foods is recommended for the prevention of diverticula. A high-fiber diet increases fecal bulk, decreases transit time, lowers intracolonic pressures, and eases stool elimination. The recommendation for fiber is 20 to 35 g/day. Some examples of high-fiber choices are whole wheat bread and other grain products, baked potato with skin, fresh fruit with skins, raw vegetables, beans, peas, legumes, wheat bran, and brown rice. Side effects may include flatulence, intestinal rumbling, cramps, and diarrhea. A gradual increase in dietary fiber over a month or two helps to avoid these problems. Other potential problems with an excessively high fiber diet (greater than 40 to 45 g) might include a decrease in nutrient absorption because of the increased volume of intestinal contents, which in turn decreases the ability of the digestive enzymes to come into contact with the food. An increase of water (eight 8-ounce glasses) is important so intestinal blockage will not occur. For small children and older adults a high-fiber diet increases the volume of food needed to meet energy requirements, and that increase may be difficult to obtain. Although some doctors recommend restricting nuts, seeds, and foods containing seeds such as berries, kiwi, and tomatoes that might lodge in the pouches, there is no evidence that this happens. If the diverticula become inflamed, a low-fiber, low-residue (no milk products), or elemental diet, or in complicated cases, total parenteral nutrition (TPN), is required to prevent continued irritation of the inflamed tissue. Controlled clinical trials are needed to evaluate the effectiveness of high-fiber diets in preventing diverticular disease.

Data from Floch MH, Bina I: *J Clin Gastroenterol* 38(5 Suppl):S2-S7, 2004; Commane DM et al: *World J Gastroenterol* 15(20): 2479-2488, 2009; Tan KY, Seow-Choen F: *World J Gastroenterol* 13(310):4161-4167, 2007.

PATHOPHYSIOLOGY The exact cause of appendicitis is controversial. Obstruction of the lumen with stool, tumors, or foreign bodies with consequent, increased, intraluminal pressure, ischemia, bacterial infection, and inflammation is a common theory. The obstructed lumen does not allow drainage of the appendix, and as mucosal secretion continues, intraluminal pressure increases. The resultant increased pressure decreases mucosal blood flow, and the appendix becomes hypoxic. The mucosa ulcerates, promoting bacterial or other microbial invasion with further inflammation and edema. Inflammation may involve the distal or entire appendix. Gangrene develops from thrombosis of the luminal blood vessels, followed by perforation.[140]

CLINICAL MANIFESTATIONS Epigastric or periumbilical pain is the typical symptom of an inflamed appendix. The pain may be vague at first, increasing in intensity over 3 to 4 hours. It may subside and then recur with a shift of location to the right lower quadrant with rebound tenderness. Right lower quadrant pain is associated with extension of the inflammation to the surrounding tissues. Nausea, vomiting, and anorexia follow the onset of pain, and fever is common. Diarrhea occurs in some individuals, particularly children; others have a sensation of constipation. Perforation, peritonitis, and abscess formation are the most serious complications of appendicitis.

EVALUATION AND TREATMENT In addition to clinical manifestations, the clinician can usually locate the painful site with one finger. Rebound tenderness is usually referred to the right lower quadrant. The white blood cell count ranges from 10,000 to 16,000 cells/mm³, with increased neutrophils. C-reactive protein is elevated.[141] Roentgenograms of the abdomen, CT scans, and ultrasound assist diagnostic accuracy. The combined information provides the best discriminating diagnosis.[142]

Antibiotics and appendectomy is the treatment for simple or perforated appendicitis. Laparoscopic surgery provides quick recovery for simple appendicitis. Recovery is more complicated in cases of perforation or abscess formation.[143]

Irritable Bowel Syndrome

Irritable bowel syndrome (IBS) is a functional gastrointestinal disorder characterized by abdominal pain and altered bowel habits that affects approximately 7 to 20 percent of individuals throughout the world and is more common in women, with a higher prevalence in youth and middle age. Individuals with IBS are more likely to have anxiety and depression. Subtypes of IBS are described on the basis of predominant symptoms—diarrhea, constipation, or pain. Symptoms of IBS can negatively affect quality of life and present a significant economic burden.

PATHOPHYSIOLOGY There are no specific structural or biochemical alterations as a cause of IBS but there is increasing evidence to explain the varying symptom presentations and they are summarized below.[144-146]

1. *Abnormal gastrointestinal motility and secretion:* Individuals with diarrhea-type IBS have more rapid colonic transit times, whereas those with bloating and constipation have delayed transit times. The mechanism may be related to visceral hypersensitivity as well as dysregulation of the brain-gut axis or to the role of serotonin in the function of the enteric nervous system.

2. *Visceral hypersensitivity or hyperalgesia particularly with distention of the rectum but also other areas of the gut:* The mechanism may be related to a dysregulation of the "brain-gut-axis," the role of serotonin in the enteric nervous system, infiltration and activation of mast cells and T lymphocytes, or alterations in autonomic or central nervous system processing of information in contributing to increased sensitivity to visceral pain.

3. *Post infectious IBS:* Intestinal infection (bacterial enteritis) has been associated with symptoms of IBS and may be related to ongoing low-grade inflammation and an abnormal immune response in gut tissues.

4. *Overgrowth of intestinal flora:* Overgrowth of normal gut bacteria may precipitate IBS symptoms and it is proposed that methane gas may slow intestinal transit time, resulting in constipation and bloating.

5. *Food allergy or food intolerance:* Food antigens may activate the mucosal immune system mediating hypersensitivity reactions and IBS symptoms. Food elimination approaches are helpful in some cases.

6. *Psychosocial factors:* Psychosocial factors including emotional stress influence brain-gut interaction including neuroendocrine, autonomic nervous system, and pain modulatory responses contributing to the symptoms of IBS.

CLINICAL MANIFESTATIONS IBS is characterized by lower abdominal pain, diarrhea-predominant, constipation-predominant, or alternating diarrhea/constipation, gas, bloating, and nausea. Individuals may also describe fecal urgency and incomplete evacuation. Symptoms are usually relieved with defecation and usually to not interfere with sleep.

EVALUATION AND TREATMENT The diagnosis of IBS is based on signs and symptoms and includes the exclusion of structural or biochemical causes of disease. In the absence of "alarm symptoms" such as fever, weight loss, gastrointestinal bleeding, anemia, or abdominal mass only limited diagnostic tests are needed. The individual may be evaluated for food allergies, lactose intolerance, parasites, or bacterial growth. The Rome III criteria for diagnosing IBS have been released to guide evaluation (Box 39-3).

There is no cure for IBS, and treatment is individualized. Treatment of symptoms may include laxatives and fiber, antidiarrheals, antispasmodics, low-dose antidepressants, visceral analgesics, and serotonin agonists or antagonists. For more severe constipation, 5-hydroxytryptomine 4 agonist (e.g tegaserod) may be used (not approved for use in North America as of 2007) or CIC-2 chloride channel activators (e.g., lubiprostone). For more severe diarrhea 5-hydroxytryptomine 3 receptor antagonists (e.g., alosetron) may be used to normalize bowel habits. Alternative therapies including probiotics, hypnosis, and psychotherapy are treatment options. Research continues to advance the management of this complex syndrome.[147-148]

Vascular Insufficiency

The stomach and intestines are supplied by three branches of the abdominal aorta: the celiac axis and the superior and inferior mesenteric arteries. Because of the rich collateral circulation, at least two of the supplying vessels must be compromised to cause ischemia. Atherosclerotic lesions, thrombi, and emboli can develop in these vessels, occluding blood flow and causing ischemia or necrosis in the gastrointestinal tract.[149]

Mesenteric venous thrombosis is the least common of the causes of mesenteric vascular insufficiency. Malignancies, right-sided heart failure, and deep vein thrombosis are risk factors.

Acute occlusion of mesenteric artery blood flow (acute mesenteric ischemia) results in a significant reduction in mucosal blood flow from the arteries supplying the large and small intestine. Dissecting aortic aneurysms, thrombi, or emboli can be causes. Embolic obstruction is associated with atrial fibrillation, mitral valve disease, heart valve prostheses, or myocardial infarction. The superior mesenteric artery has a more direct line of flow from the aorta; therefore, emboli enter it more readily than the inferior branch, causing ischemia and necrosis of the small intestine.[150] Ischemia and necrosis alter membrane permeability. There is initially increased motility, nausea and vomiting, urgent bowel evacuation, and severe abdominal pain. Ischemia leads to decreased motility and distention. The damaged intestinal mucosa cannot produce enough mucus to protect itself from digestive enzymes.[151] Mucosal alteration causes fluid to move from the blood vessels into the bowel wall and peritoneum. Fluid loss causes hypovolemia and further decreases in intestinal blood flow. As intestinal infarction progresses, shock, fever, bloody diarrhea, and leukocytosis develop. Bacteria invade the necrotic intestinal wall, causing gangrene and peritonitis.

Chronic mesenteric insufficiency, or nonocclusive mesenteric insufficiency, can develop secondary to atherosclerosis, congestive heart failure, acute myocardial infarction, dysrhythmias, hemorrhage, stenosis, thrombus formation, aortic aneurysm, or any condition that decreases arterial blood flow. Older adults with arteriosclerosis are particularly susceptible. Chronic occlusion is often accompanied by formation of collateral circulation that may be able to nourish the resting intestine. After eating, however, when the intestine requires more blood, the arterial supply may be insufficient. Ischemia develops, causing a cramping abdominal pain, called *abdominal angina*, after meals. Progressive vascular obstruction eventually causes continuous abdominal pain and necrosis of the intestinal tissue. Reperfusion injury related to reactive oxygen metabolites and inflammatory mediators contributes to further tissue damage.

Colicky abdominal pain after eating is a cardinal symptom of chronic mesenteric insufficiency. Some individuals suffer significant weight loss because they stop eating to control the pain. Chronic segmental ischemia may lead to strictures and destruction.

Diagnosis of mesenteric artery occlusion is based on clinical manifestations, laboratory findings, mesenteric artery angiography, and abdominal radiography and ultrasonography. Bruit often can be heard over the occluded artery. With angiography a vasodilating agent may be injected into the vessels to improve the circulation. Heparin may be used if there are no contraindications. Medical management includes antibiotics, anticoagulation, vasodilators, and inhibitors of reperfusion injury. Surgery is required to remove necrotic tissue, repair sclerosed vessels, and for revascularization. Mortality is high (60% to 100%) for individuals with acute occlusion and compromised cardiac output. Early diagnosis and aggressive treatment result in the best survival rates.[152]

Disorders of Nutrition

Obesity

Obesity is an increase in body fat mass and a metabolic disorder that has increased significantly over the past two decades. Obesity is an energy imbalance, with energy intake exceeding energy expenditure, and is defined as a body mass index (BMI) greater than 30.[153] It is a major cause of morbidity, death, and high healthcare cost in the United States and worldwide.[154] Three leading causes of death in the United States are associated with obesity: cardiovascular disease, type 2 diabetes mellitus, and cancer (colon, breast in postmenopausal women, endometrium, prostate, kidney, and esophagus.[155] Obesity is also a risk factor for hypertension, stroke, hepatobiliary disease (gallstones and nonalcoholic steatohepatitis), osteoarthritis, and sleep apnea. Obesity is increasing in children and obese children tend to become obese adults.[156]

The causes and consequences of obesity are multiple and complex with rapidly advancing research regarding causal mechanisms and complications. Genotype and environmental-gene interactions are important predisposing factors.[157] Single gene defects are rare and obesity is usually polygenic and associated with other phenotypes such as endocrine disorders (i.e., diabetes and hypothyroidism) and mental retardation (i.e., Down and Prader-Willi syndromes). Single gene defects include the melanocortin-receptor gene, leptin gene (also known as the *obesity gene*), and leptin-receptor-gene. All single-gene defects are directly or indirectly-related to leptin and melanocortin pathways.[158] Metabolic abnormalities contributing to obesity include Cushing syndrome, Cushing disease, polycystic ovary syndrome, hypothyroidism, and hypothalamic injury. Environmental factors include culture, socioeconomic status, food intake, and exercise. Obesity is associated with adverse social and psychologic consequences.[159]

PATHOPHYSIOLOGY The pathophysiology of obesity is complex and involves the interaction of numerous cytokines, hormones, and neurotransmitters. Mechanisms contributing to the imbalance of energy intake in relation to energy expenditure and the multiple pathogenic effects of excess adipose tissue are not completely understood. Adipocytes secrete a number of hormones and cytokines known as adipokines (Box 39-4). These adipokines participate in regulation of food intake, lipid storage and metabolism, insulin sensitivity, the alternative complement system, vascular homeostasis, blood pressure regulation, angiogenesis, the inflammatory and immune responses, female reproduction, and regulation of energy metabolism.[160] Visceral fat accumulation causes dysfunction of adipocytes and results in alterations in the regulation and interaction of these hormones and cytokines contributing to the causes and complications of obesity, particularly cardiovascular disease.[161]

Regulation of appetite and satiety occurs through neuroendocrine regulation of eating behavior, energy metabolism, and body fat mass. The system is complex and controlled by a dynamic circuit of signaling molecules from the periphery acting on central controls including the brain stem, hypothalamus, and autonomic nervous system. An imbalance in this system is usually associated with excessive caloric intake in relation to exercise with the consequence of weight gain and obesity.

The arcuate nucleus (ARC) in the hypothalamus has two sets of neurons with opposing effects that interact to regulate and balance food intake and energy metabolism. One set of neurons produces neuropeptide Y (NPY) and agouti-related protein (AGRP), which stimulates eating and decreases metabolism (anabolic). Another set of neurons synthesizes pro-opiomelanocortin (POMC)-producing peptide and cocaine-and-amphetamine-regulated transcript (CART), collectively known as POMC/CART neurons. They inhibit eating and increase metabolism (catabolic). Both sets of neurons express their effects by activating second-order neurons in the hypothalamus, which increases or decreases appetite and energy metabolism (Figure 39-15). Molecules that stimulate eating are called *orexins* (i.e., hypocretins [from the hypothalamus], a peptide family that acts as neurotransmitters for stimulating eating). Molecules that inhibit eating are called *anorexins* (Box 39-5). Peripheral effects of these signaling pathways are transmitted through the

---

Box 39-4   Hormones and Adipokines Secreted by Adipose Tissue

Hormones (Adipokines)
Leptin
  Satiety (hunger/appetite suppression) and regulation of eating behavior by hypothalamus
  Sympathoactivation
  Insulin sensitizing
  Modulating role in reproduction, angiogenesis, immune response, blood pressure control, and osteogenesis
Adiponectin
  Insulin sensitizing
  Anti-inflammatory
  Anti-atherogenic
Resistin
  Promotes insulin resistance and increased blood glucose levels
  Inhibits adipocyte differentiation and may function as a feedback regulator of adipogenesis
Visfatin (from visceral fat)
  Mimics insulin and binds to insulin receptors in rats
Vaspin—may be insulin sensitizing

Regulators of Lipoprotein Metabolism
Lipoprotein lipase
Apolipoprotein E
Cholesterol ester transfer protein

Inflammatory Cytokines
Tumor necrosis factor-alpha
Interleukins (IL-6, IL-8, IL-10)
Plasminogen activator inhibitor-1
Monocyte chemoattractant protein-1

Other Hormones and Cytokines
Estrogen
Angiotensinogen
Tissue factor
Transforming growth factor-beta
Insulin-like growth factor
Nitric oxide synthase
Acylation stimulating protein
Adipophilin
AdipoQ
Monobutyrin
Agouti protein

Data from Fonesca-Alaniz MH et al: *J Pediatr (Rio J)* 83(5 Suppl): S192-S303, 2007; Halberg N, Wenstedt-Asterholm I, Scherer PE: *Endocrinol Metab Clin North Am* 37(3):753-768, x-xi, 2008; Youn BS et al: *Diabetes* 57(2):372-377, 2008.

Box 39-5   Examples of Neuropeptides that Influence Eating Behavior

Orexins (Appetite Stimulants)
Neuropeptide Y (NPY)
Melanin-concentrating hormone (MCH)
Agouti-related protein (AGRP)
Ghrelin
Galanin
Orexins A and B
Peptide YY (PYY)
Cortisol

Anorexins (Appetite Suppressants)
Leptin
Insulin
Cholecystokinin (CCK)
Corticotropin-releasing hormone (CRF)
Urocortin (a CRF satiety signaling hormone)
Cocaine- and amphetamine-regulated transcript (CART)
Alpha-melanocyte-stimulating hormone (α-MSH)
Bombesin
Serotonin
Calcitonin

autonomic nervous and endocrine systems to regulate appetite, food intake, and energy metabolism.[162]

Many different hormones control appetite, satiety, and body weight. Their sources include ghrelin from the stomach; peptide YY, cholecystokinin (CCK), and glucagon-like peptide (GLP-1) from the intestines; insulin from pancreatic beta cells; and leptin, adiponectin, and resistin from adipose tissue. These hormones circulate in the blood at concentrations proportional to body fat mass, and serve as *peripheral signals* to the ARC in the hypothalamus, where appetite (food intake) and metabolism (energy expenditure) are regulated. Leptin and insulin normally decrease appetite by inhibiting NPY/AGRP neurons (anabolic circuits) and stimulating POMC/CART neurons (catabolic circuits) (Figure 39-15). Ghrelin, CCK, and other hormones stimulate appetite by activating NPY/AGRP-expressing neurons. Peptide YY (PYY) and other hormones inhibit these neurons and decrease appetite. Other peripheral hormones and neurotransmitters

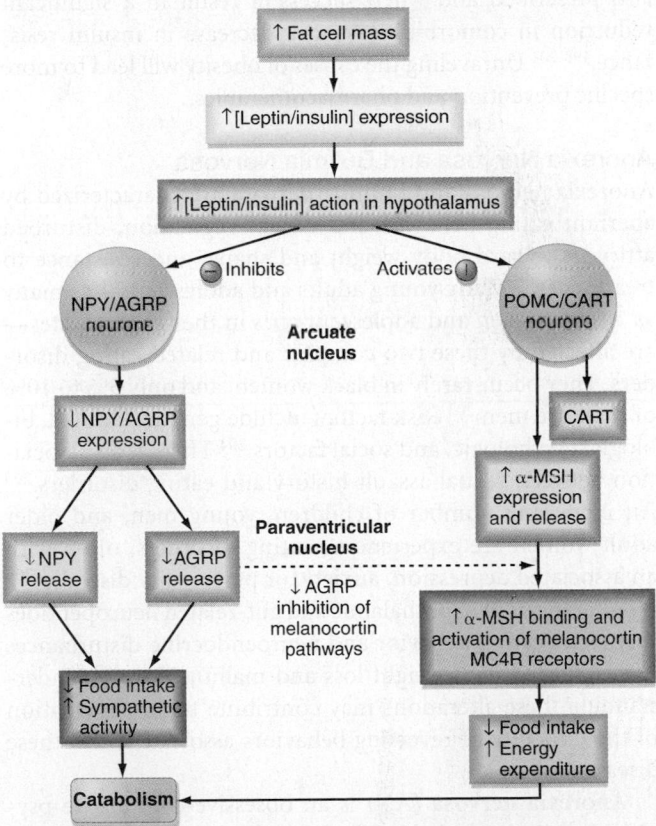

Figure 39-15 Neuroendocrine control of food intake and energy expenditure. Leptin and insulin normally decrease appetite, increase satiety, and increase energy expenditure (catabolism). Leptin/insulin inhibits NPY/AGRP gene expression resulting in decreased appetite and food intake; and stimulates POMC/CART gene expression with resulting α-MSH release and decrease in appetite and food intake. With leptin resistance as occurs in obesity, these effects are depressed and food intake increases in excess of energy expenditure. *AGRP,* agouti-related peptide; *α-MSH,* alpha-melanocyte stimulating hormone; NPY, neuropeptide Y; *POMC/CART,* proopiomelanocortin/cocaine-and-amphetamine-related transcript. (Reprinted with permission from Schwartz MW et al, Central nervous system control of food intake, *Nature* 404:661-671, 2000.)

also can influence the hypothalamus and affect appetite and energy expenditure (see Box 39-4).

Obesity is associated with increased circulating plasma levels of leptin, insulin, ghrelin, and PYY. Interaction among these hormones at the level of the hypothalamus may be an important determinant of excessive fat mass. *Leptin receptors* in the hypothalamus function to regulate satiety and body weight within a fairly narrow range or set point. Low leptin levels during fasting normally stimulate food intake and reduce energy expenditure and high leptin levels in the fed state inhibit food intake and increase energy expenditure. Leptin secretion increases as adipocytes increase in size or number (hyperleptinemia). The high levels of leptin in obesity are ineffective at decreasing appetite and increasing energy expenditure—this is known as **leptin resistance.** Leptin resistance disrupts hypothalamic satiety signaling and promotes overeating and excessive weight gain.[163]

The cause of leptin resistance is unknown. It may be related to a defect in leptin transport,[164] an inability of leptin to cross the blood-brain barrier[165]; an alteration in the permissive effect of leptin on urocortin (a satiety-signaling molecule)[166]; or a defect in the leptin receptor.[167] *Hyperleptinemia* also stimulates the sympathetic nervous system, chronic inflammation, oxidative stress, and ventricular hypertrophy and may contribute to the pathogenesis of hypertension, atherosclerosis, and cardiovascular disease associated with obesity.[168,169]

Ghrelin is produced by the stomach in response to hunger and stimulates food intake and induces metabolic changes leading to an increase in body weight and body fat mass. Ghrelin also stimulates release of growth hormone (GH) from anterior pituitary cells, the release of gastric acid and gastric motility, and affects pancreatic functions. It has vasodilatory, cardioprotective, and antiproliferative effects.[170,171] Leptin and ghrelin are complementary, yet antagonistic signals reflecting acute and chronic changes in energy balance the effects of which are mediated by hypothalamic neuropeptides, such as NPY and AGRP. Plasma ghrelin is decreased in obesity, and its role in contributing to obesity is yet to be defined. Leptin may regulate ghrelin levels.[172] Endocrine and vagal afferent pathways are also involved in the actions of ghrelin and leptin, adding to the complexity of mechanisms that can affect obesity.[173]

Adiponectin has insulin-sensitizing properties and plasma levels decrease with visceral obesity, contributing to insulin resistance, cardiovascular disease, and metabolic syndrome.[174] Obese individuals, particularly those with expansion of visceral adipose tissue, are at increased risk for coronary artery disease resulting from hyperlipidemia, hypertension, and factors that promote thrombosis and inflammation (see Chapter 30). Decreased adiponectin levels are associated with increased levels of inflammatory markers, such as IL-6 and TNF-α. Adiponectin may serve as an anti-inflammatory and anti-atherogenic plasma protein and may have an important role in vascular remodeling that is limited with obesity.[175]

Obesity is associated with *insulin resistance,* which predisposes an individual to type 2 diabetes mellitus (see Chapter 21). The insulin resistance may be related to an insulin receptor defect or to postreceptor effects with alteration in glucose transporter functions. Excess insulin also may be a response to excessive caloric intake.[176] *Resistin* is greatly increased in those with obesity and may be an antagonist to insulin action and a mediator of inflammation.[177]

CLINICAL MANIFESTATIONS Increased visceral fat is associated with *metabolic syndrome* (hypertriglyceridemia, reduced high-density lipoprotein, increased low-density lipoproteins, hypertension, and insulin resistance), a complex of traits that increase risk for ischemic heart disease and type 2 diabetes mellitus[178,179] (see Chapters 21 and 30).

The *hypertension* of obesity is complex and may be related to insulin resistance, activation of the sympathetic nervous system, activation of renin-angiotensin, leptin resistance, physical compression of the kidneys, and alterations in vascular structure and function.[180,181]

Pulmonary function can be compromised by a large amount of adipose tissue overlying the chest cage. Work of breathing increases, and gas exchange, vital capacity, and expiratory volume all decrease causing low oxygen tension and high carbon dioxide tension. The hypoventilation causes daytime hypercapnia and sleep-disordered breathing. Hypoxemia causes pulmonary hypertension contributing to right ventricular hypertrophy and heart failure.[182] Asthma is also associated with obesity, particularly among females, but the exact mechanisms of airway hyperresponsiveness are unknown. Obesity-related factors include airway narrowing, low-grade inflammation, gastroesophageal reflux, leptin resistance, and decreased adiponectin.[183]

Obstructive sleep apnea syndrome (OSAS) is a consequence of obesity and obesity hypoventilation syndrome. It involves episodic partial or complete obstruction of the upper airway, hypoventilation, and hypercapnia (see Chapters 15, 33, and 34). The hypoventilation also may be caused by leptin resistance, which has respiratory stimulant effects independent of the amount of visceral fat mass.[184] OSAS results in fragmentation of sleep with daytime sleepiness and further complications of hypoxia and heart disease.

The development of *osteoarthritis* occurs as a function of mechanical stress and limb malalignment on weight-bearing joints. Exercise intolerance and pain in the weight-bearing joints, particularly the hips and knees, are common. Inflammation may cause erosion of cartilage.[185]

Obesity also increases the risk for *cancer* including adenocarcinoma of the esophagus and the gastric cardia, colorectal cancer, postmenopausal breast cancer, endometrial cancer, and renal-cell carcinoma. Less commonly associated cancers include thyroid, gallbladder, pancreatic, leukemia, multiple myeloma, and non-Hodgkin lymphoma. The pathophysiologic mechanisms that increase cancer risk are not clear, but insulin resistance and other factors, including insulin-like growth factors, sex steroids, adipokines, obesity-related inflammatory markers, the nuclear factor kappa beta system, and oxidative stresses, are being evaluated.[186,187]

EVALUATION AND TREATMENT There are several methods for measuring or estimating body fat mass, including CT and magnet resonance imaging (MRI) techniques; bioimpedance analysis; underwater weighing; and anthropometric measurements, such as skinfold thickness, circumferences, and various body diameters (i.e., waist-to-hip ratios and waist circumference, and BM-kg/m² tables).[188] The BMI and waist-to-hip ratios are most commonly used because they are the easiest to measure. Overweight is defined as a BMI greater than 25 and obesity is a BMI greater than 30. BMI charts are available for children ages 2 to 20 years; these can be used for comparison during adulthood because obese children generally become obese adults.[153,189,190] No specific diagnostic criteria for obesity have been established.

Obesity is a chronic disease for which various treatment approaches have been used, including correction of metabolic abnormalities, individually tailored weight-reduction diets, and exercise programs.[191-196] A combination of weight reduction and exercise is the most effective.[197] Self-motivation and support systems are critical aspects of treatment. Additional treatments, such as psychotherapy, behavioral modification, medications, bariatric surgery (i.e., the Roux-en-Y gastric bypass or gastric banding), and liposuction are also prescribed and when successful result in a significant reduction in comorbidities and a decrease in insulin resistance.[198-201] Unraveling the causes of obesity will lead to more specific prevention and pharmacotherapies.

Anorexia Nervosa and Bulimia Nervosa

Anorexia nervosa and bulimia nervosa are characterized by aberrant eating behavior and weight regulation, disturbed attitudes toward body weight and shape, and resistance to treatment.[202] Many young adults and adolescents—as many as 1% of women and adolescent girls in the United States—are affected by these two complex and related eating disorders. They occur rarely in black women, and only 5% to 10% of cases are men.[203] Risk factors include genetic, familial, biologic, psychologic, and social factors.[204] There is an association between sexual assault history and eating disorders.[205] An increasing number of children, young men, and older adult women are experiencing eating disorders, often with an associated depression, anxiety, or personality disorder.[206]

Alterations in hypothalamic and gut-related neuropeptides that effect eating behavior and neuroendocrine disturbances are associated with weight loss and malnutrition.[207] Understanding these alterations may contribute to an explanation of the difficulty of reversing behaviors associated with these diseases.[208]

Anorexia nervosa (AN) is an obsessive-compulsive psychiatric disorder and physiologic syndrome that affects 1% to 3% of U.S. women. It has the highest mortality rate of any psychiatric disease and has a familial tendency.[209] AN is characterized by the following[210,211]:

1. A fear of becoming obese despite progressive weight loss
2. A distorted body image: the perception that the body is fat when it is actually underweight
3. Body weight 15% less than normal for age and height because of refusal to eat
4. In women and girls, absence of three consecutive menstrual periods

Persons with AN frequently deny they have any eating problem. Two types of eating behavior are distinguished in AN and both involve subnormal body weight and ongoing malnutrition. *Restrictive AN* entails unremitting food avoidance. *Binge eating/purging AN* includes binge eating followed by self-induced vomiting or laxative abuse. AN usually emerges during adolescence and in females who have a history of childhood abuse.[212]

As the disease progresses, multiple organs are affected.[213] Muscle and fat depletion gives the individual a skeleton-like appearance and increases the risk for osteopenia and osteoporosis. Iron deficiency anemia promotes fatigue, and low white blood cell count increases risk of infection. Reproductive functioning is affected, including ovarian function, menstruation, fertility, and pregnancy. Sodium, potassium, phosphate, and magnesium are depleted. Postural hypotension, edema, bradycardia, hypothermia, constipation, and sleep disturbances may ensue. The loss of 25% to 30% of ideal body weight can eventually lead to death caused by starvation-induced cardiac failure.[214] Diagnosis of AN involves a thorough medical history, physical and psychologic examination, and ruling out other causes of anorexia and malnutrition.[215]

There are no universally accepted treatments. Treatment objectives for AN include reversing the compromised physical state, promoting insights and knowledge about the disorder, mutual goals, interaction with family members, restoring development growth, and modifying food habits.[216 218] Correction of nutritional status may require intensive treatment, including total parenteral nutrition. When the individual demonstrates the willingness to eat food for nourishment, dietary protein, carbohydrate, and fat are introduced in tolerable amounts. Care must be taken to prevent refeeding syndrome, which can result in fluid and electrolyte, cardiac, neurologic, and hematologic complications during nutritional rehabilitation.[219] Behavioral intervention begins as soon as physical symptoms are stabilized and may continue for several years. Family therapy is helpful for adolescents. Formal genetic studies are in progress and results may advance specificity of treatment.[209]

Bulimia nervosa is more common than anorexia, and body weight remains near normal but with aspirations for weight loss. The group at risk is the same as that for AN except that bulimia tends to occur in slightly older, less affluent women. Diagnosis of bulimia is based on the following findings[220]:

1. Recurrent episodes of binge eating during which the individual fears not being able to stop
2. Self-induced vomiting, use of laxatives (purging type)
3. Two binge-eating episodes per week for at least 3 months (purging type)
4. Fasting to oppose the effect of binge eating or excessive exercise (nonpurging type)

Because of negative connotations associated with self-stimulated vomiting and purging, individuals who have bulimia binge and purge secretly. Bulimic individuals may binge and purge as often as 20 times each day. Weight will fluctuate by about 10 pounds. Continual vomiting of acidic chyme can cause pitted teeth, pharyngeal and esophageal inflammation, and tracheoesophageal fistulae. Overuse of laxatives can cause rectal bleeding. Secret binge eating isolates the bulimic individual and leads to depression and anger that is turned inward. A vicious cycle of depression, overeating to try to feel better, vomiting and purging to maintain a normal weight, and returning depression perpetuates this eating disorder. Mood symptoms are often worse in the winter.[221]

Because persons with bulimia are usually older than individuals with AN and usually have separated from a family core, individual or group cognitive behavior change is the treatment focus. Fluoxetine may be beneficial.[222] Individuals with bulimia rarely have physical problems requiring hospital care and respond to treatment more readily than those with AN.[223]

Starvation

Starvation is a reduction in energy intake leading to weight loss. Short-term and long-term starvation have different effects. Therapeutic short-term starvation is part of many weight-reduction programs because it causes an initial rapid weight loss that reinforces the individual's motivation to diet. Therapeutic long-term starvation is used in medically controlled environments to facilitate rapid weight loss in morbidly obese individuals. Pathologic long-term starvation can be caused by poverty; chronic diseases of the cardiovascular, pulmonary, hepatic, and digestive systems; malabsorption syndromes; human immunodeficiency virus (HIV) infection; and cancer. In-hospital starvation primarily affects individuals with functional and cognitive deficits and inadequate caloric intake.[224]

Short-term starvation, or extended fasting, consists of several days of total dietary abstinence or deprivation. The body responds with protective mechanisms.[225] For 4 to 6 hours after the last meal, the body is in a well-fed state and its energy requirements are supplied by glucose from recently ingested carbohydrates. Once all available energy has been absorbed from the intestine, glycogen in the liver is converted to glucose through **glycogenolysis,** the splitting of glycogen into glucose. This process peaks within 4 to 8 hours, and gluconeogenesis begins. **Gluconeogenesis** is the formation of glucose from noncarbohydrate molecules: lactate, pyruvate, amino acids, and the glycerol portion of fats. Like glycogenolysis, gluconeogenesis takes place within the liver. Both of these processes deplete stored nutrients and thus cannot meet the body's energy needs indefinitely. Proteins continue to be catabolized to a minimal degree, providing carbon for the synthesis of glucose.[225]

Long-term starvation begins after several days of dietary abstinence and eventually causes death. Absolute deprivation of food causes **marasmus** or protein energy malnutrition. Protein deprivation in the presence of carbohydrate intake is called **kwashiorkor.** Marasmic kwashiorkor (edematous, severe childhood malnutrition) is a combination of chronic energy deficiency and chronic or acute protein deficiency.[226] The major characteristic of long-term starvation is a decreased dependence on gluconeogenesis and an increased use of ketone bodies (products of lipid and pyruvate metabolism) as a cellular energy source. During long-term starvation, depressed insulin levels and increased glucagon, cortisone, epinephrine, and growth hormones promote lipolysis in adipose tissue. Lipolysis liberates fatty acids, which supply energy to cardiac and skeletal muscle cells, and ketone bodies, which sustain brain tissue. Fatty acid, or ketone body, oxidation meets most of the energy needs of the cells. (Some glucose is still needed as fuel for brain tissue.) Once the supply of adipose tissue is depleted, proteolysis begins. The breakdown of muscle and visceral protein is the last process the body engages to supply energy for life. Death results from severe alterations in electrolyte balance and loss of renal, pulmonary, and cardiac function.[227]

Adequate ingestion of appropriate nutrients is the obvious treatment for starvation. In medically induced starvation the body is maintained in a ketotic state until the desired amount of adipose tissue has been lysed. Starvation imposed by chronic disease, long-term illness, or malabsorption is treated with enteral or parenteral nutrition. Perioperative management of nutrition is necessary to prevent unnecessary starvation.[228]

DISORDERS OF THE ACCESSORY ORGANS OF DIGESTION

The accessory organs of digestion (liver, gallbladder, pancreas) secrete substances necessary for digestion and, in the case of the liver, carry out metabolic functions needed to maintain life. Inflammatory disease is a common cause of accessory organ dysfunction. Inflammation disrupts secretory function and prevents secretions from flowing into the duodenum. Lack of accessory organ secretions is a major cause of maldigestion and malabsorption in the small intestine. Other causes of accessory organ dysfunction are obstruction of ducts by aggregates in the secretions themselves (e.g., obstruction of bile flow by gallstones) or by tumors. (Cancers of the digestive tract are described at the end of this chapter.)

Clinical Manifestations of Liver Disorders

Of all the accessory organ disorders, acute or chronic liver disease leads to the most systemic, life-threatening complications. These complications include portal hypertension, ascites, hepatic encephalopathy, jaundice, and hepatorenal syndrome.

Portal Hypertension

Portal hypertension is abnormally high blood pressure in the portal venous system primarily caused by resistance to portal blood flow. Pressure in this system is normally 3 mmHg; portal hypertension is an increase to at least 10 mmHg. The portal veins carry blood from the gastrointestinal tract, pancreas, and spleen to the liver. In the liver the blood flows through the sinusoids and empties into the hepatic veins, which carry it into the inferior vena cava. The inferior vena cava delivers blood to the right atrium. The portal veins, sinusoids, and hepatic veins comprise the portal venous system (see Chapter 38).

PATHOPHYSIOLOGY Portal hypertension is caused by disorders that obstruct or impede blood flow through any component of the portal venous system or vena cava. *Intrahepatic* causes result from vascular remodeling with intrahepatic shunts, thrombosis, inflammation, or fibrosis of the sinusoids, as occurs in cirrhosis of the liver, viral hepatitis, or schistosomiasis (a parasitic infection). *Posthepatic* causes occur from hepatic vein thrombosis or cardiac disorders—such as failure of the right side of the heart or constrictive pericarditis—that impair the pumping ability of the right heart. This causes blood to back up and increase pressure in the portal system. Thrombosis or narrowing of the portal vein is the major *prehepatic* cause. The most common cause of portal hypertension is obstruction caused by cirrhosis of the liver (see p. 1491), the formation of intrahepatic arteriovenous shunts, and increased portal blood flow from anterior splanchnic vasodilation.[229]

High pressure in the portal veins causes collateral vessels to open between the portal veins and the systemic veins, in which blood pressure is considerably lower (Figure 39-16). This enables blood to bypass the obstructed portal vessels. The collateral veins develop in the esophagus, anterior abdominal wall, and rectum. High pressure and increased flow volume are transmitted through these veins from the portal to the systemic venous circulation.

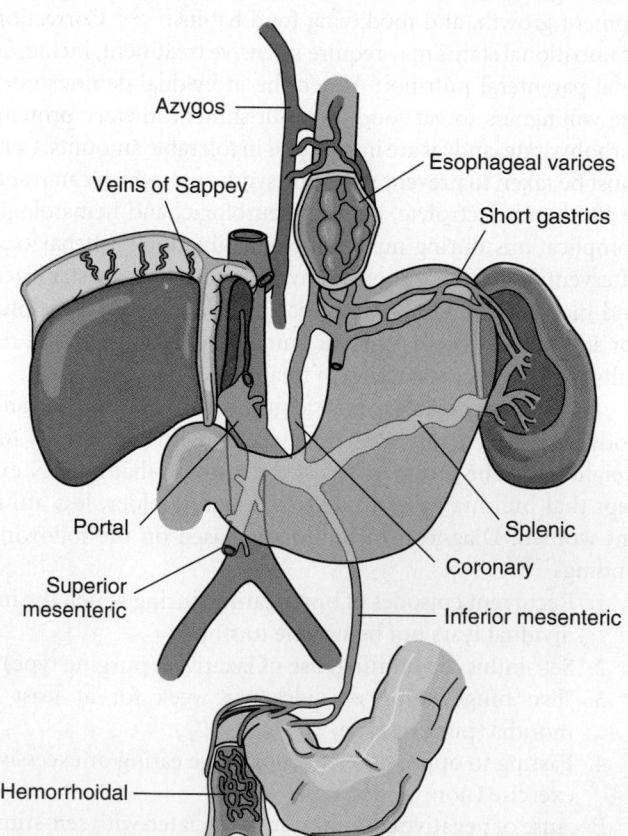

Figure 39-16 Varices related to portal hypertension. Portal vein, its major tributaries, and the most important shunts (collateral veins) between the portal and caval systems. (From Monahan FD et al: *Phipps' Medical-surgical nursing: concepts and clinical practice*, ed 8, St Louis, 2007, Mosby.)

Hepatopulmonary syndrome and portopulmonary hypertension are common complications of portal hypertension. Arterial pulmonary hypertension develops as a result of microvascular intrapulmonary vasodilation caused by release of nitric oxide and carbon monoxide in the presence of liver injury.[230] There are no specific clinical manifestations, although dyspnea, cyanosis, and digital clubbing may occur. Diagnosis is made by contrast echocardiography and right heart catheterization when pulmonary artery pressure is 730 mmHg by echocardiography. Treatment may include systemic vasodilators and endothelin receptor antagonists, which can reduce pulmonary and portal hypertension[231] and improve outcome of liver transplant.

Long-term portal hypertension causes several problems that are difficult to treat and can be fatal:

1. *Varices* (distended, tortuous, collateral veins): prolonged elevation of pressure in collateral veins causes their transformation into varices, particularly in the lower esophagus and stomach but also in the rectum.
2. *Splenomegaly* (enlargement of the spleen): caused by increased pressure in the splenic vein, which branches from the portal vein.
3. *Ascites* (the accumulation of fluid in the peritoneal cavity, which is the space between the visceral peritoneum and the parietal peritoneum): caused in part by increased pressure in the mesenteric tributaries of the portal vein. Hydrostatic pressure forces water out of these vessels and into the peritoneal cavity. (This process, termed *transudative effusion*, is described in Chapter 33.)
4. *Hepatic encephalopathy* (also called *portosystemic encephalopathy*): characterized by central nervous system disturbances with astrocyte changes that lead to alterations of consciousness.

CLINICAL MANIFESTATIONS The vomiting of blood from bleeding **esophageal varices** is the most common clinical manifestation of portal hypertension.[232] Slow, chronic bleeding from varices causes anemia or melena. Usually the bleeding is from varices that have developed slowly over a period of years.

Rupture of esophageal varices causes hemorrhage and voluminous vomiting of dark blood. The ruptured varices are usually painless. Rupture is caused by a combination of erosion by gastric acid and elevated venous pressure. Hemorrhoidal varices present as hematochezia and copious rectal bleeding. Mortality from ruptured esophageal varices ranges from 30% to 60%. Recurrent bleeding of esophageal or gastric varices indicates a poor prognosis. Most individuals die within 1 year.

EVALUATION AND TREATMENT Diagnosis of portal hypertension is often made at the time of variceal bleeding and confirmed by endoscopy and evaluation of portal venous pressure. Distended collateral veins may radiate over the abdomen, giving rise to caput medusae (Medusa's head) from opening of the paraumbilical veins. The individual usually has a history of jaundice, hepatitis, or alcoholism.

Beta-blockers can be effective in preventing variceal bleeding. Emergency management of bleeding varices includes fluid resuscitation, prophylactic antibiotics, vasoactive drugs,

endoscopic variceal band ligation, compression of the varices with an inflatable tube or balloon, and injection of a sclerosing agent.[233,234] Surgical construction of transjugular intrahepatic portosystemic shunts (TIPS) (anastomosis of the portal vein to the inferior vena cava) may decompress the varices, but this treatment can precipitate encephalopathy or liver failure resulting from reduced hepatic blood flow. There is no effective, definitive treatment for portal hypertension. Liver transplant is the most successful option for liver failure.[235]

Splenomegaly

Splenomegaly is an enlargement of the spleen. Portal hypertension contributes to congestive splenomegaly by increasing intrasplenic blood pressure. Thrombocytopenia (decreased platelet count) is the most common manifestation of congestive splenomegaly and can contribute to an increased bleeding tendency. Splenomegaly also can be predictive of esophageal varices severity.[236]

Ascites

Ascites is the accumulation of fluid in the peritoneal cavity. Ascites traps body fluid in a "third space" from which it cannot escape. The effect reduces the amount of fluid available for normal physiologic functions. Cirrhosis is the most common cause of ascites; ascites is the most common complication of cirrhosis. Other diseases associated with ascites include heart failure, constrictive pericarditis, abdominal malignancies, nephrotic syndrome, and malnutrition. Twenty-five percent of individuals who develop ascites caused by cirrhosis die within 1 year. Continued heavy drinking of alcohol is associated with this mortality rate.

PATHOPHYSIOLOGY Several factors contribute to the development of ascites, including portal hypertension, splanchnic vasodilation, hepatocyte failure, and sodium retention. Impaired excretion of sodium by the kidneys promotes water retention, but the initiating event is not clear. The *overflow theory* proposes that renal sodium retention is stimulated by portal hypertension with intravascular hypervolemia and overflow into the peritoneal cavity. Portal hypertension also increases the production of hepatic lymph, which "weeps" into the peritoneal cavity. The *underfill theory* proposes an increase in hepatic sinusoidal hydrostatic pressure and decreased plasma oncotic pressure with weeping of lymph fluid from the surface of the liver. There is a decrease in effective circulating plasma volume activating the renin-angiotensin-aldosterone system and stimulating the kidney to retain more sodium and water, leading to intravascular volume overload.[237] The *arterial vasodilation theory* proposes that circulating nitric oxide or release of endotoxin from translocation of intestinal bacteria triggers arterial vasodilation of the splanchnic organs early in the course of cirrhosis and stimulates renal sodium retention through renin-angiotensin-aldosterone, increased sympathetic tone, and changes in the intrarenal blood flow.[238,239]

In cases of cirrhosis, both portal hypertension and decreased production of albumin by hepatocytes contribute to the

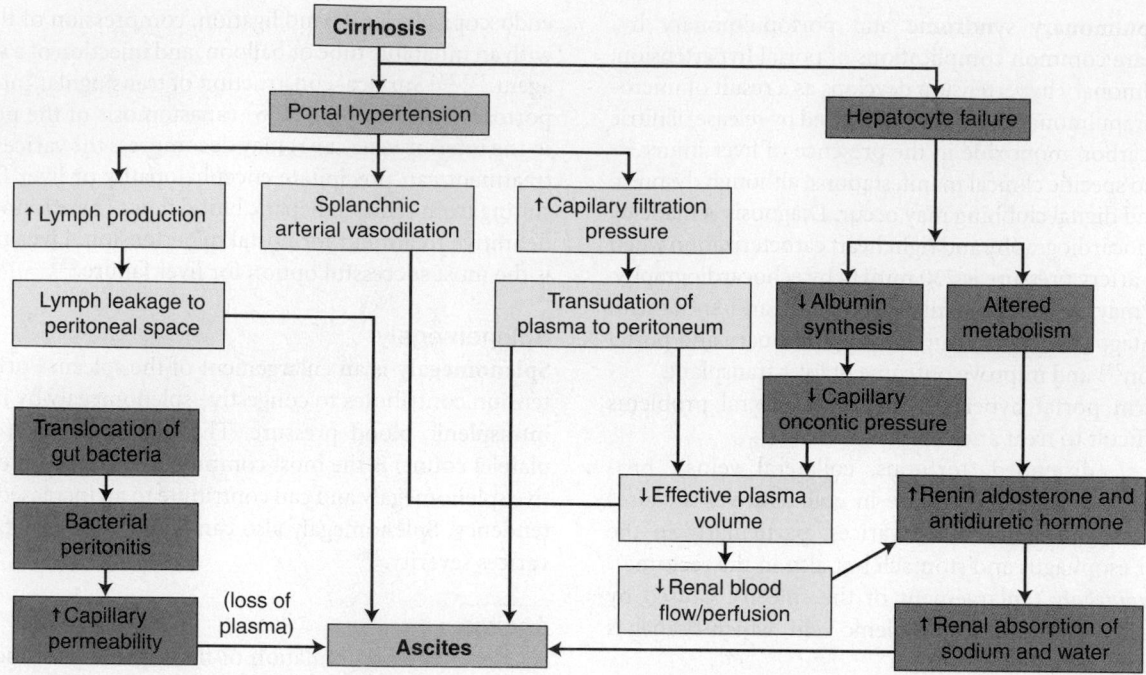

Figure 39-17 Mechanisms of ascites caused by cirrhosis.

ascites. Deranged liver metabolism also permits the accumulation of hormones that regulate sodium and water balance. Excessive amounts of aldosterone and antidiuretic hormone remain in the blood, stimulating the kidneys to retain sodium and water. High aldosterone levels can be attributed also to increased secretion mediated by excessive plasma renin activity. The increased plasma renin activity may develop because of decreased metabolic function of the liver, increased renal secretion stimulated by low blood flow, or both.

As ascites sequesters more and more body fluid, the kidneys respond by retaining sodium and water in amounts exceeding intake. Retention of sodium and water expands plasma volume, thereby accelerating portal hypertension and ascites formation.

Ascites can be complicated by bacterial peritonitis. Peritonitis involves an inflammatory response that worsens ascites by increasing mesenteric capillary permeability. As plasma seeps out of the permeable mesenteric capillaries, it adds to the volume of ascitic fluid. Figure 39-17 summarizes the mechanisms by which cirrhosis of the liver causes ascites.

CLINICAL MANIFESTATIONS The accumulation of ascitic fluid causes weight gain, abdominal distention, and increased abdominal girth (Figure 39-18). Large volumes of fluid (10 to 20 L) displace the diaphragm and cause dyspnea by decreasing lung capacity. Respiratory rate increases, and the individual assumes a semi-Fowler position to relieve the dyspnea. Some peripheral edema is usually present. Dilutional hyponatremia is a consequence of excess fluid volume. Approximately 10% of individuals with ascites develop bacterial peritonitis, either spontaneously or as a result of paracentesis (needle aspiration of ascitic fluid). Peritonitis

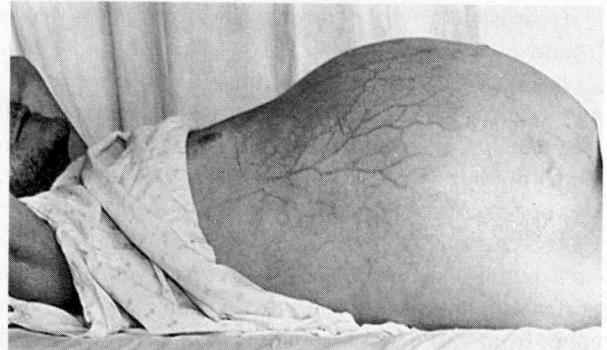

Figure 39-18 Massive ascites in an individual with cirrhosis. Distended abdomen, dilated upper abdominal veins, and inverted umbilicus are classic manifestations. (From Prior JA, Silberstein JS, Stang JM: *Physical diagnosis: the history and examination of the patient,* ed 6, St Louis, 1981, Mosby.)

causes fever, chills, abdominal pain, decreased bowel sounds, and cloudy ascitic fluid.

EVALUATION AND TREATMENT Diagnosis of ascites is usually based on clinical manifestations and identification of liver disease. The serum-ascites albumin gradient (SAAG) is the most specific diagnostic indicator for portal hypertension-related ascites.[240] Paracentesis is used to aspirate ascitic fluid for bacterial culture, biochemical analysis, and microscopic examination. The goal of treatment is to relieve discomfort. If the restoration of liver function is possible (e.g., in ascites caused by viral hepatitis), the ascites diminishes spontaneously. In the meantime, dietary salt restriction and potassium-sparing diuretics can reduce ascites. Strong diuretics, such as furosemide or ethacrynic acid, may be used and vasopressin receptor 2 antagonists are effective for dilutional hyponatremia.[241] Albumin may be given.[242] Serum electrolytes are monitored carefully because the individual is at risk for hyponatremia and hypokalemia.

Palliative measures include paracentesis to remove 1 or 2 L of ascitic fluid and relieve respiratory distress. This procedure can have serious complications, however. The removal of too much fluid too fast relieves pressure on blood vessels causing arteriolar vasodilation and carries the risk of hypotension, shock, or death.[243] Despite repeated paracentesis, ascitic fluid reaccumulates in individuals with irreversible disease, drawing more albumin and electrolytes out of the vascular compartment. Paracentesis is also likely to cause peritonitis. Peritonitis is treated with long-term antibiotics. A transjugular intrahepatic portosystemic shunt or peritoneovenous shunt may be used to treat refractory ascites.[237] Individuals with ascites and portal hypertension have a poor prognosis, and liver transplant is the best treatment option.

Hepatic Encephalopathy

Hepatic encephalopathy (portosystemic encephalopathy) is a complex neurologic syndrome characterized by impaired cognitive function, flapping tremor (asterixis), and electroencephalogram (EEG) changes. The syndrome may develop rapidly during acute fulminant hepatitis or slowly during the course of chronic liver disease. Risk factors in the presence of advanced liver disease include gastrointestinal bleeding, increased dietary protein, electrolyte imbalance, and hypoxia.

PATHOPHYSIOLOGY Hepatic encephalopathy probably results from a combination of biochemical alterations that affect neurotransmission. Liver dysfunction and collateral vessels that shunt blood around the liver to the systemic circulation permit neurotoxins and other harmful substances absorbed from the gastrointestinal tract to circulate freely to the brain. Also, permeability of the blood-brain barrier may be increased. The most hazardous substances are end products of intestinal protein digestion, particularly ammonia.[244] The digestion of blood from leaking or ruptured varices adds to the amount of ammonia present in systemic blood, as does the action of ammonia-forming bacteria in the colon. The astrocyte is the most vulnerable because it is the site of ammonia detoxification.[245] Ammonia that reaches the brain is metabolized to glutamine with osmotic disturbances and alterations in cerebral blood flow that interfere with neurotransmitters, cause astrocyte edema and oxidation, and can result in brain herniation and death.[246,247]

Blood levels of ammonia do not account for all symptoms associated with hepatic encephalopathy. The accumulation of short-chain fatty acids, serotonin, tryptophan, and false neurotransmitters probably contributes to neural derangement. Excessive gamma-aminobutyric acid (GABA), an inhibitory neurotransmitter, may contribute to reduced levels of consciousness.[248] Infection, hemorrhage, inflammation, electrolyte imbalance, sedatives, and analgesics also can precipitate stupor and coma in the presence of liver disease.

CLINICAL MANIFESTATIONS Subtle changes in personality, memory loss, irritability, lethargy, and sleep disturbances are common initial manifestations of hepatic encephalopathy. Symptoms then can progress to confusion, flapping tremor of the hands, stupor, convulsions, and coma. Coma is usually a sign of liver failure and ultimately results in death.

EVALUATION AND TREATMENT Diagnosis of hepatic encephalopathy is based on a history of liver disease and clinical manifestations. Electroencephalography and blood chemistry tests, including blood ammonia levels, provide supportive data. There is no specific diagnostic test.

Correction of fluid and electrolyte imbalances and withdrawal of depressant drugs metabolized by the liver are the first steps in the treatment of hepatic encephalopathy. Reduction of blood ammonia levels is a major objective. This is accomplished by restricting dietary protein intake and eliminating intestinal bacteria. Neomycin is effective in sterilizing the bowel, but it can be nephrotoxic. Lactulose may be administered to prevent ammonia absorption in the colon.[244] Antibiotics appear superior to nonabsorbable disaccharides in improving hepatic encephalopathy by reducing bacterial production of ammonia but adverse effects are a concern.[249] Sodium benzoate and L-ornithine-L-aspartate also detoxify ammonia.

Jaundice

Jaundice (icterus) is a yellow or greenish pigmentation of the skin caused by **hyperbilirubinemia** (total plasma bilirubin concentrations greater than 2.5 to 3 mg/dl). Hyperbilirubinemia and jaundice can result from (1) extrahepatic obstruction to bile flow (gallstones), (2) intrahepatic obstruction (hepatocellular disease such as cirrhosis or hepatitis), or (3) excessive production of bilirubin (excessive hemolysis of red blood cells) (Figure 39-19). Jaundice in newborns is caused by impaired bilirubin uptake and conjugation (see Chapter 40).

PATHOPHYSIOLOGY **Obstructive jaundice** can result from extrahepatic or intrahepatic obstruction.[250] *Extrahepatic obstructive jaundice* develops if the common bile duct is occluded by a gallstone, tumor, or compression from edema of pancreatitis. Because the bile duct is obstructed, bilirubin is conjugated by the hepatocytes but cannot flow into the duodenum. (Conjugated bilirubin is soluble in water and is then soluble in aqueous bile.) Therefore, it accumulates in the liver and enters the bloodstream, causing hyperbilirubinemia. Because conjugated bilirubin is water soluble, it appears in the urine. The stools may be light colored or clay colored because they lack bile pigments. The stools also lack urobilinogen because bile is not available for conversion to urobilinogen.

Intrahepatic obstructive jaundice involves disturbances in hepatocyte function and obstruction of *bile canaliculi*. The uptake, conjugation, and excretion of bilirubin are affected with elevated levels of both conjugated and unconjugated bilirubin. Hepatocellular damage increases plasma concentrations of unconjugated bilirubin. The major disorder, however, is

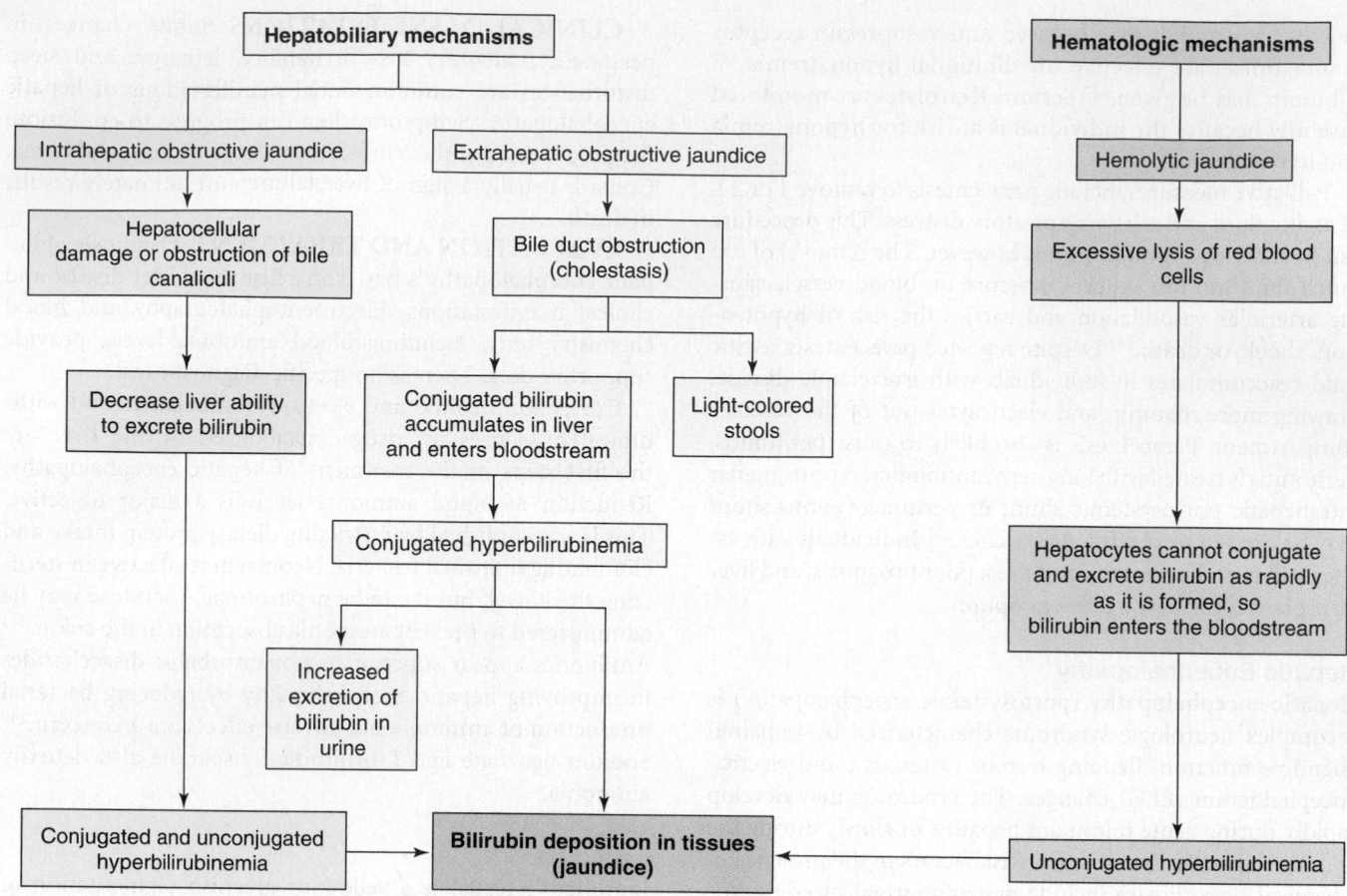

Figure 39-19 Mechanisms of jaundice.

obstruction of bile canaliculi, which diminishes flow of conjugated bilirubin into the common bile duct with elevations in the plasma. In mild cases, some of the bile canaliculi open. Consequently, the amount of bilirubin in the intestinal tract may be only slightly decreased. The stools may appear normal or light colored.

Excessive hemolysis (breakdown) of red blood cells or absorption of hematoma can cause **hemolytic jaundice (prehepatic** or **nonobstructive jaundice).** An increased amount of unconjugated bilirubin is formed through metabolism of the heme component of destroyed red blood cells. The extra amount of unconjugated bilirubin exceeds the conjugation ability of the liver, causing blood levels of unconjugated bilirubin to rise. Unconjugated hyperbilirubinemia is the major cause of hemolytic jaundice. Because unconjugated bilirubin is not water soluble, it is not excreted in the urine. The reserve conjugation ability of the liver usually prevents long-term unconjugated hyperbilirubinemia greater than 4 to 5 mg/dl. Severe hemolytic crisis, as occurs with sickle cell disease (see Chapter 28), is a cause of hemolytic jaundice. Hemolytic drugs also can cause jaundice. If unconjugated hyperbilirubinemia exceeds 5 mg/dl, both hemolytic and liver disorders are indicated.

Hyperbilirubinemia and jaundice can be caused also by metabolic defects that impair the uptake or conjugation of unconjugated bilirubin in the liver. *Gilbert disease,* for example, causes an elevation of unconjugated bilirubin in the plasma but no other symptoms of liver disease. Gilbert disease is probably caused by an inherited deficiency of glucuronyl transferase enzyme, which is required for the hepatic uptake of unconjugated bilirubin. The causes of jaundice are summarized in Table 39-7.

CLINICAL MANIFESTATIONS The clinical manifestations of jaundice vary and are related to the underlying pathology. Conjugated hyperbilirubinemia may cause the urine to darken several days before the onset of jaundice. The complete obstruction of bile flow from the liver to the duodenum causes light-colored stools. With partial obstruction, stool color is normal and bilirubin is present in the urine. Extrahepatic biliary obstruction is associated with increased intestinal permeability and bacterial translocation, and may contribute to the pathogenesis of sepsis and renal failure.[251]

Fever, chills, and pain often accompany jaundice resulting from viral or bacterial inflammation of the liver (e.g., viral hepatitis). Manifestations of liver injury from any cause commonly include anorexia, malaise, and fatigue. Yellow discoloration may first occur in the sclera of the eye and then progress to the skin. Skin xanthomas (cholesterol deposits) and pruritus commonly accompany jaundice with an elevation of serum alkaline phosphatase.[252]

Table 39-7	Three Common Types of Jaundice	
Type	Mechanism	Causes
Hemolytic jaundice (predominantly unconjugated bilirubin)	Excessive destruction of erythrocytes	Membrane defect of erythrocytes Hemolytic anemias Immune reaction Severe infection Toxic substances in the circulation (e.g., snake venom) Transfusion of incompatible blood
Obstructive (cholestatic) jaundice (predominantly conjugated bilirubin)	Obstruction to passage of conjugated bilirubin from liver to intestine	Obstruction of bile duct by gallstones or tumor (extrahepatic obstructive jaundice) Obstruction of bile flow through the liver (intrahepatic obstructive jaundice) Drugs
Hepatocellular jaundice (both conjugated and unconjugated bilirubin)	Failure of liver cells (hepatocytes) to conjugate bilirubin and of bilirubin to pass from liver to intestine	Genetic defect of hepatocyte (decreased enzymes), such as occurs in premature infants (see Chapter 40) Hepatitis or biliary cirrhosis

EVALUATION AND TREATMENT Laboratory evaluation of serum establishes whether elevated plasma bilirubin is conjugated or unconjugated or both. Unconjugated bilirubinemia results from hemolysis or hereditary disorders of bilirubin metabolism. Elevations of conjugated bilirubin indicate liver injury or extrahepatic obstruction. The history, physical examination and laboratory tests identify underlying disorders, such as alcoholism, exposure to hepatitis virus, or gallbladder disease. The treatment for jaundice consists of correcting the cause.

Hepatorenal Syndrome

Hepatorenal syndrome (HRS) is a complication of advanced liver disease characterized by functional renal failure with oliguria, sodium and water retention (with or without ascites and peripheral edema), hypotension, and peripheral vasodilation. There are two types of HRS: type 1 involves rapid and progressive renal failure, and type 2 is more chronic and stable accompanied by refractory ascites.[253] Renal disorders associated with liver disease can have numerous causes, but HRS is usually associated with alcoholic cirrhosis and fulminant hepatitis. The renal failure is not caused by primary renal disease or other extrinsic factors, but rather by arterial vasodilation of the splanchnic vasculature and renal vasoconstriction with decreased blood flow (prerenal renal failure) and it is reversible.[254]

PATHOPHYSIOLOGY Oliguric hepatic failure generally accompanies a sudden decrease in blood volume secondary to massive gastrointestinal bleeding or hypotension caused by failing liver function. Hypotension also can be caused by the excessive use of diuretics to treat ascites with decreased renal blood flow, decreased glomerular filtration rate, and oliguria. The hypotension results in decreased glomerular filtration; however, the ability to concentrate and dilute urine is usually maintained. A significant number of individuals with advanced liver disease develop oliguria unrelated to any precipitating event. Inappropriate constriction of renal arterioles is proposed as the causative mechanism. Intrarenal vasoconstriction may result from the selective effects of vasoactive substances that accumulate in the blood because of liver failure. The diseased liver fails to remove excessive angiotensin, vasopressin, prostaglandins, and catecholamines from the blood. These substances travel to the kidneys and cause vasoconstriction. Vasoconstriction also may be a compensatory response to portal hypotension and vasodilation in the splanchnic circulation. The exact reason for the renal vasoconstriction is unknown but is related to vasoconstrictive mediators and sympathetic nerve stimulation. Systemic vasodilation caused by increases in nitric oxide and other substances also may contribute to vascular alterations and renal failure in advanced liver disease.[255]

CLINICAL MANIFESTATIONS The onset of hepatorenal manifestations may be gradual or acute. Oliguria and complications of advanced liver disease, including jaundice, ascites, and gastrointestinal bleeding, are usually present. Systolic blood pressure is usually less than 100 mmHg. Nonspecific symptoms of hepatorenal syndrome include anorexia, weakness, and fatigue.

EVALUATION AND TREATMENT Diagnosis of HRS is made by excluding all other causes of renal failure. Despite oliguria, serum potassium levels do not become dangerously elevated until the terminal stages of the hepatorenal syndrome. Blood urea increases, followed by an increase in serum creatinine concentration. Urine osmolality is increased, but urine sodium concentrations are below normal (unlike acute tubular necrosis). Urine specific gravity is greater than 1.015. The prognosis for hepatorenal syndrome is usually poor and is related to liver function. Secondary problems, including fluid and electrolyte disorders, bleeding, infections, and encephalopathy, are vigorously treated. Treatment may include systemic vasoconstrictors (α-adrenergic agonists). Pentoxifylline is used to treat HRS in severe alcoholic hepatitis.

Table 39-8	Characteristics of Viral Hepatitis					
Characteristic	**Hepatitis A**	**Hepatitis B**	**Hepatitis D**	**Hepatitis C**	**Hepatitis E**	**Hepatitis G**
Size of virus	27 nm RNA virus	47 nm DNA virus	36 nm RNA virus, defective virus with HbsAg coat	30-60 nm RNA virus	32 nm RNA virus	30-60 nm RNA virus
Incubation phase	30 days	60-180 days	30-180 days; dependent on HBV for multiplication	35-72 days	15-60 days	Unknown
Route of transmission	Fecal-oral, parenteral, sexual	Parenteral, sexual	Parenteral, fecal-oral, sexual	Parenteral	Fecal-oral	Parenteral, sexual
Onset	Acute with fever	Insidious	Insidious	Insidious	Acute	Unknown
Carrier state	Negative	Positive	Positive	Positive	Negative	Positive
Severity	Mild	Severe; may be prolonged or chronic	Severe	Mild to severe	Severe in pregnant women	Unknown
Chronic hepatitis	No	Yes	Yes	Yes	No	Unknown
Age-group affected	Children and young adults	Any	Any	Any	Children and young adults	Any
Prophylaxis	Hygiene, immune serum globulin HAV vaccine	Hygiene, HBV vaccine	Hygiene, HBV vaccine	Hygiene, screening blood, interferon-alpha or combined with ribavirin	Hygiene, safe water	

DNA, Deoxyribonucleic acid; *HbsAg*, hepatitis B surface antigen; *HBV*, hepatitis B virus; *RNA*, ribonucleic acid.

Symptoms improve with TIPS and extracorporeal albumin dialysis (ECAD). Liver transplant reverses symptoms.[256]

Disorders of the Liver

Viral Hepatitis

Viral hepatitis is a relatively common systemic disease that affects primarily the liver. Six strains of viruses cause various types of hepatitis: hepatitis A virus (HAV), hepatitis B virus (HBV), hepatitis D virus (HDV), hepatitis C virus (HCV), and hepatitis E virus (HEV). Hepatitis A was previously known as infectious hepatitis, and hepatitis B as serum hepatitis. Coinfection of HBV, HCV, HDV, and HIV occurs because these viruses share the same routes of transmission with more rapid progression of liver disease.[257] Hepatitis G virus is a blood-borne virus and is usually not a significant cause of liver disease.[258] Characteristics of the various types are presented in Table 39-8.

Types

Hepatitis A. HAV can be recovered from the feces, bile, and sera of infected individuals. The usual mode of transmission is the fecal-oral route (contaminated food or water), but the virus can be spread also by the transfusion of infected blood. Approximately 45% of adults in urban areas have HAV antibodies in their blood. The disease spreads readily in crowded, unsanitary conditions, usually through contaminated food or water. Person-to-person spread is more likely to occur in settings such as daycare centers or institutions for the mentally retarded, where there is contact between clients and caregivers who are not vaccinated.[259]

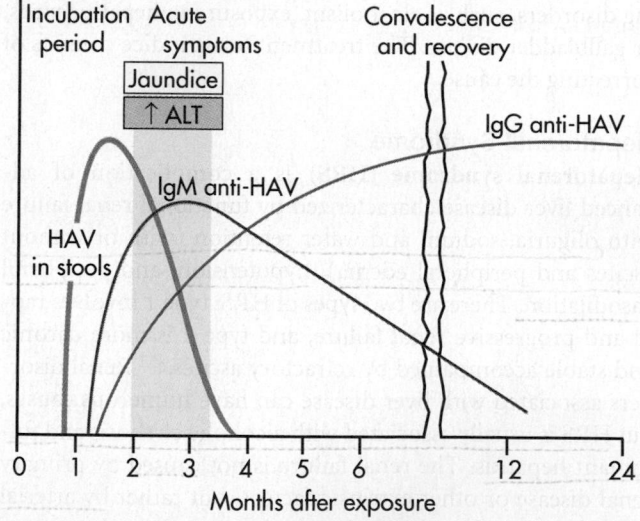

Figure 39-20 Course of infection with the hepatitis A virus (HAV). *ALT*, Alanine transaminase; *IgG*, immunoglobulin G; *IgM*, immunoglobulin M.

The incubation period (the time between exposure and onset of symptoms) for HAV is 4 to 6 weeks (Figure 39-20). Fecal shedding of the virus is greatest for 10 to 14 days before the onset of symptoms and during the first week of symptoms and up to 3 months after onset of symptoms. The disease is most contagious during this time. Antibodies to HAV (anti-HAV) develop about 4 weeks after infection. The serum immunoglobulin M (IgM) concentration increases initially and

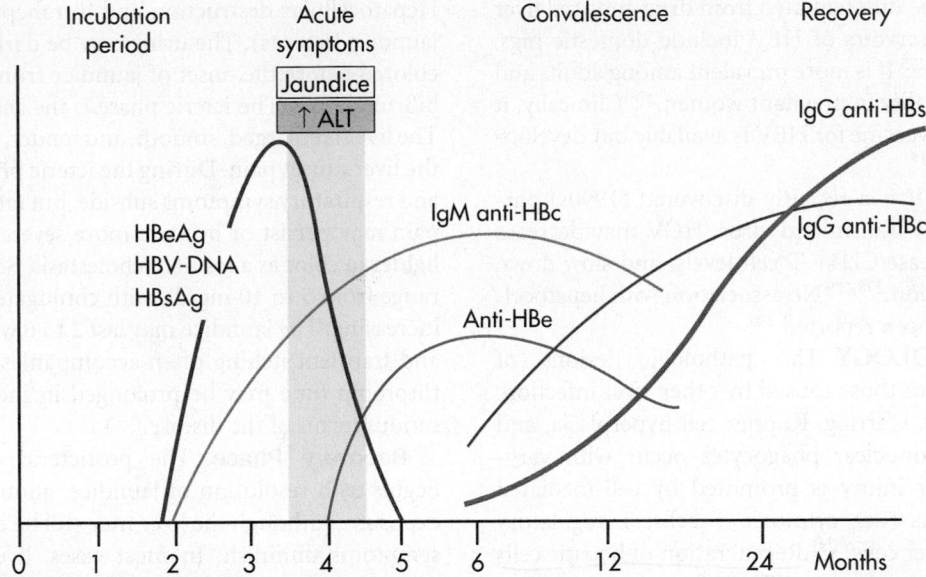

Figure 39-21 Course of infection with the hepatitis B virus (HBV). *HbsAg*, Hepatitis B surface antigen; *anti-HBs*, antibody to HBsAg; *HbeAg*, hepatitis B e-antigen; *anti-Hbe*, antibody to HBeAg; *anti-HBc*, antibody to hepatitis B core antigen. The antibody to HBs (anti-HBs) is IgG, the immunoglobulin that creates immunity. *ALT*, Alanine transaminase; *DNA*, deoxyribonucleic acid; *IgG*, immunoglobulin G; *IgM*, immunoglobulin M.

is followed by an increase of serum IgG, whose levels remain elevated for several years after infection, creating immunity to the disease. (See Chapters 6 and 7 for a description of immune functions.) Immunization is effective in preventing the disease and confers long-term immunity.[260] A combined HAV and HBV vaccine is available and effective.[261]

Hepatitis B. Hepatitis B is transmitted through contact with infected blood, body fluids, or contaminated needles. Hepatitis B is also a sexually transmitted disease (see Chapter 24). Transmission among homosexual men may be by oral or genital contact with bleeding lesions in the rectal mucosa. People receiving hemodialysis, multiple blood transfusions, or immunosuppressive drugs have a greater risk of exposure or less resistance to HBV. Coinfection with HCV, HDV, and HIV is common because these viruses share the same routes of transmission.[257,262] Mother-infant transmission of HBV occurs if the mother becomes infected during the third trimester of pregnancy. Approximately 0.3% of adults in the United States and up to 400 million worldwide carry the hepatitis B surface antigen (HBsAg) marker for active HBV.[263] HBV is a major cause of chronic hepatitis, cirrhosis, and hepatocellular carcinoma.[264]

Three types of viral particles are involved in HBV infection. The larger (47 nm) Dane particle probably represents the intact HBV. The Dane particle has a double-layered outer coat and carries HBsAg, which was originally called the *Australia antigen*. HBsAg can be identified in the serum by radioimmunoassay. Hepatitis B core antigen (HBcAg) usually is not detected in the serum. The HBeAg is a derivative of HBcAg and is a marker of HBV replication. The HBV has an incubation period of 6 to 8 weeks. The initial serologic change is a transient increase in IgM. Levels of IgG antibodies to HBsAg

rise more slowly and remain elevated for years (Figure 39-21). Chronic infection develops in 15% to 30% of those with acute infection with increased risk for cirrhosis and hepatocellular carcinoma.[265] Antiviral and immunomodulatory treatment for chronic hepatitis B includes combination therapy and prevention of drug resistance.[266] Vaccine prevents transmission of hepatitis B and the development of acute or chronic hepatitis B, particularly in high-risk populations.[267]

Hepatitis C. HCV (previously known as non-A, non-B hepatitis) is a parenterally transmitted flavivirus with six genotypes. About 40% of HCV cases involve intravenous drug users, who also have a high incidence of HIV infection.[268] Coinfection with HBV also is prevalent.[269] It is the most common cause of chronic liver disease and HCV in the Western world. The variants of HCV make vaccine development difficult and resistance to drug therapy is common.[270] Persistent infection with recurring acute symptoms and elevated aminotransferase levels represent the clinical presentation. Half of infected individuals have a viral response to treatment.[271]

Hepatitis D. HDV occurs in individuals with hepatitis B. The delta virus depends on the HBV for its replication because the coat of the delta virus consists of HBsAg molecules that are on the surface of HBV. Hepatitis D has been shown to suppress replication of HBV.[272] Parenteral drug users have a high incidence of HDV infection. The clinical course of HDV is similar to that of hepatitis A and B, although it is sometimes more severe. Treatment for chronic HDV may best be treated with antiviral drugs (i.e., pegylated interferon alpha and ribavirin).[273]

Hepatitis E. Hepatitis E is most common in developing countries and is transmitted by the fecal-oral route, usually by way of contaminated water. It is also found in developed countries and must be differentiated from drug-induced liver injury.[274] Animal reservoirs of HEV include domestic pigs, wild boars, and deer.[275] It is more prevalent among adults and has the highest mortality in pregnant women.[276] Clinically, it resembles HAV. No vaccine for HEV is available but development is in progress.[277]

Hepatitis G. HGV is a recently discovered (1990s) parenterally and sexually transmitted virus. HGV may decrease HIV viral load, increase CD4+ T cell levels, and slow down HIV disease progression.[278,279] No association with hepatocellular carcinoma has been reported.[280]

PATHOPHYSIOLOGY The pathologic lesions of hepatitis are similar to those caused by other viral infection. Hepatic cell necrosis, scarring, Kupffer cell hyperplasia, and infiltration by mononuclear phagocytes occur with varying severity. Cellular injury is promoted by cell-mediated immune mechanisms (i.e., cytotoxic T cells, T regulatory cells, and natural killer cells).[281] Regeneration of hepatic cells begins within 48 hours of injury. The inflammatory process can damage and obstruct bile canaliculi, leading to cholestasis and obstructive jaundice. In milder cases the liver parenchyma is not damaged. Damage tends to be most severe in cases of hepatitis B and hepatitis C. Hepatitis B is also associated with *acute fulminating hepatitis,* a rare form of the disease that is characterized by massive hepatic necrosis (see p. 1491). Acute fulminating hepatitis causes severe encephalopathy, which is manifested as confusion, stupor, and coma. Liver failure can occur, leading to intestinal bleeding, cardiorespiratory insufficiency, and renal failure. Mortality is high, but recovery can be complete.

CLINICAL MANIFESTATIONS The clinical manifestations of the various types of hepatitis are very similar. The spectrum of manifestations ranges from absence of symptoms to fulminating hepatitis, with rapid onset of liver failure and coma. Acute viral hepatitis causes abnormal liver function test results. The serum aminotransferase values, aspartate transaminase (AST) and alanine transaminase (ALT), are elevated, but their elevation may not be consistent with the extent of cellular damage. The clinical course of hepatitis usually consists of four phases: incubation, prodromal, icteric, and recovery phases. The **incubation phase** is reviewed in Table 39-8.

Prodromal Phase. The **prodromal (preicteric) phase** of hepatitis begins about 2 weeks after exposure and ends with the appearance of jaundice. Fatigue, anorexia, malaise, nausea, vomiting, headache, hyperalgia, cough, and low-grade fever are prodromal symptoms that precede the onset of jaundice. About 10% of individuals may develop extrahepatic symptoms including rash, arthralgias, and purpura. HBV and HCV may cause nephritis related to glomerular immune complex deposition.[282] Food odors often cause nausea, and changes in taste suppress the desire to smoke and drink alcohol. Right upper abdominal pain is common, and a weight loss of 2 to 4 kg is not unusual. The infection is highly transmissible during this phase.

Icteric Phase (Jaundice). The **icteric phase** begins about 1 to 2 weeks after the prodromal phase and lasts 2 to 6 weeks.

Hepatocellular destruction and intrahepatic bile stasis cause jaundice (icterus). The urine may be dark and the stools clay colored before the onset of jaundice from conjugated hyperbilirubinemia. The icteric phase is the actual phase of illness. The liver is enlarged, smooth, and tender, and percussion over the liver causes pain. During the icteric phase, gastrointestinal and respiratory symptoms subside, but fatigue and abdominal pain may persist or become more severe. The stools may be lighter in color as a result of cholestasis. Serum bilirubin levels range from 5 to 10 mg/dl, with conjugated bilirubin fraction increasing. The jaundice may last 2 to 6 weeks or longer. Mild and transient itching often accompanies jaundice. The prothrombin time may be prolonged in individuals with more serious forms of the disease.

Recovery Phase. The posticteric or **recovery phase** begins with resolution of jaundice, about 6 to 8 weeks after exposure. Although the liver may still be enlarged and tender, symptoms diminish. In most cases, liver function test results return to normal within 2 to 12 weeks after the onset of jaundice.

Chronic hepatitis may begin at this point and is associated with HBV and HCV infection. **Chronic active hepatitis** is the persistence of clinical manifestations and liver inflammation after acute stages of HBV, HCV, and HDV. Liver function tests remain abnormal for longer than 6 months, and HBsAg persists. Chronic, active HBV is a predisposition to cirrhosis and primary hepatocellular carcinoma. Chronic active hepatitis constitutes a carrier state, and hepatitis C can be transmitted from mothers to infants.[283]

EVALUATION AND TREATMENT Diagnosis of type A hepatitis is based on the presence of anti-HAV, as is the diagnosis of HCV. The most specific diagnostic test for HBV is serologic analysis for HBsAg, which is the marker for HBV. The assay for HDV is the total antibody to HDV and antigen (anti-HDV). A test for HEV has not been developed. Liver enzyme levels and function tests also can indicate other viral liver diseases, drug toxicity, or alcoholic hepatitis.

Specific treatments are previously described for the different types of hepatitis viruses. Physical activity may be restricted. A low-fat, high-carbohydrate diet is beneficial if bile flow is obstructed.

To prevent transmission of hepatitis A, handwashing and use of gloves for disposing of fecal matter are imperative. Molecular procedures are available for direct surveillance of HAV in food and environmental samples should be used for the prevention of food-borne infections.[284] There should be no direct contact with blood or body fluids of individuals with hepatitis B or hepatitis C. The administration of immunoglobulin before exposure or early in the incubation period can prevent hepatitis A. A combined vaccine for HAV and HBV is available. Hepatitis B immunoglobulin provides passive prophylactic immunity against HBV. Prophylaxis is recommended for healthcare workers, liver transplant recipients, and others who are at risk for contact with infected body fluids.[285]

WHAT'S NEW?   Acetaminophen and Acute Liver Failure

Acetaminophen toxicity from chronic use or intentional overdose is the leading cause of acute liver failure in the United States. Liver injury may occur with doses of 4 to 10 g and hepatotoxicity should be suspected when doses exceed 4 g/day. The onset is sudden and unpredictable accompanied by coagulopathy and encephalopathy. Elevated serum aminotransferase accompanied by hypoprothrombinemia, metabolic acidosis, and renal failure support a diagnosis of acute liver failure caused by acetaminophen. Complications of cerebral edema and infection are difficult to diagnose and treat and may lead to multiorgan failure and irreversible brain damage. Early treatment with correct dosing with N-acetylcysteine provides a 66% chance of recovery and there is 70% survival at 1 year after liver transplant.

Data from Fontana RJ: *Med Clin North Am* 92(4):761-794, viii, 2008; Khashab M Tector AJ, Kwo PY: *Curr Gastroenterol Rep* 9(1):66-73, 2007; Sandlands EA, Bateman DN: Adverse reaction associated with acetylcysteine, *Clin Toxicol (Phila)* 47(2):81-88, 2009.

Fulminant Hepatitis

Fulminant hepatitis is a clinical syndrome resulting in severe impairment or necrosis of liver cells and potential liver failure. The disorder may occur as a complication of hepatitis C or hepatitis B, particularly HBV infection compounded by infection with the delta virus. Toxic reactions to drugs and congenital metabolic disorders also can cause fulminant hepatitis.[286] Acetaminophen overdose is the leading cause of acute liver failure in the United States (see What's New? Acetaminophen and Acute Liver Failure).

Causative mechanisms of fulminant hepatic failure are poorly understood. Hepatocytes become edematous, and patchy areas of necrosis and inflammatory cell infiltrates disrupt the parenchyma. The death of hepatocytes may be caused by toxic, viral, or immunologic damage.

Fulminant hepatitis usually develops 6 to 8 weeks after the initial symptoms of viral hepatitis or a metabolic liver disorder. Anorexia, vomiting, abdominal pain, and progressive jaundice are initial signs, followed by ascites and gastrointestinal bleeding. Hepatic encephalopathy is manifested as lethargy, altered motor functions, and coma. Liver function tests show elevations of both direct and indirect serum bilirubin, serum transaminases, and blood ammonia. Prothrombin time is prolonged.

Treatment of fulminant hepatitis is supportive. The hepatic necrosis is irreversible, and 60% to 90% of affected children die. Liver transplantation may be lifesaving.[287] Survivors usually do not develop cirrhosis or chronic liver disease. Artificial liver support systems are continuing to be developed for use as a bridge to transplant or recovery from acute or acute on chronic liver failure[288] (see What's New? Artificial Liver Support).

Cirrhosis

Cirrhosis is an irreversible inflammatory disease that disrupts liver structure and function and is a leading cause of death in the United States. Disorganization of hepatic tissues is caused

WHAT'S NEW?   Artificial Liver Support

During the past several years, advances have been made in the development of materials and methods to artificially support liver function. Because of the shortage of donor organs there is a high incidence of mortality related to acute or chronic liver failure. Bioartificial liver devices have demonstrated temporary support of liver function in animal studies and are encouraging in early clinical trials in humans. Bioartificial livers can serve as a bridge to liver transplantation or support liver function long enough to allow regeneration of normal liver function. One type of bioartificial liver (BAL) circulates the individual's blood around the outside of a system of hollow fibers packed with pig hepatocytes. The fiber membrane allows toxins to be removed and nutrients to be replaced but does not allow cells to be exchanged. Another type of liver support is the molecular absorbents recirculating system (MARS), an extracorporeal albumin dialysis technique that uses an albumin-impregnated membrane to remove protein-bound and water-soluble toxins from the blood. Prometheus is a system being evaluated for removal of albumin bound toxins. Clinical trials are in progress for the development of internal devices, strategies that promote hepatic regeneration, and ways to enhance replacement of pig hepatocytes with human hepatocytes, including stem cell research and other tissue engineering techniques, with continuing evaluation of safety and biochemical outcomes.

Data from Gerlach JC, Zeilinger K, Patzer Li JF: *Regen Med* 3(4):575-595, 2008; Sussman NL, McGuire BM, Kelly JH: *Curr Gastroenterol Rep* 11(1):64-68, 2009, Montejo Gonzaliz JC et al: *Hepatogastroenterology* 56(90):456-461, 2009. McKenzie TJ et al: *Semin Liver Dis* 28(2):210-217, 2008; Phau J, Lee KH: *Curr Opin Crit Care* 14(2):208-215, 2008.

by nodular regeneration forming fibrous bands, giving the liver a cobbly appearance.[289] The liver may be larger or smaller than normal, and usually it is firm or hard when palpated. A variety of disorders can cause cirrhosis. Therefore, it is often classified by cause (Table 39-9).

The precise process of cellular injury depends on the cause of cirrhosis, and the causes are not all clearly understood. Structural changes result from fibrosis, which is a consequence of leukocyte release, inflammatory cytokines, and chemokines with activation of fibrogenic fibroblasts.[290] The parenchyma of the liver becomes distorted, and biliary channels may be altered or obstructed, producing jaundice. Obstruction caused by cirrhosis can cause portal hypertension (see p. 1482). New vascular channels can form shunts, and blood from the portal vein bypasses the liver. These vascular changes compromise liver function further, and the process of regeneration is replaced by hypoxia; necrosis; atrophy; and ultimately, liver failure.

Cirrhosis develops slowly over a period of years. Its severity and rate of progression depend on the cause. If toxins, such as alcohol, are involved, the rate of cell death and the severity of inflammation depend on the amount of toxin present.[291]

Alcoholic Liver Disease

Deaths from alcohol-related liver disease have increased over the past decade and the amount and duration of alcohol consumption are positively related to the extent of liver

Table 39-9	Cirrhosis of the Liver	
Type and Disease Name	**Causal Mechanisms**	**Pathophysiology**
Alcoholic cirrhosis, Laennec cirrhosis, portal cirrhosis, fatty cirrhosis	Toxic effects of chronic, excessive alcohol intake; acetaldehyde formed by alcohol metabolism damages hepatocytes	Fatty liver, inflammation (alcoholic steatohepatitis), and derangement of the lobular architecture by necrosis and fibrosis (cirrhosis) with obstruction of biliary and vascular channels
Biliary cirrhosis (intrahepatic or extra hepatic obstruction of bile flow)		
Primary biliary cirrhosis	Unknown; possible an autoimmune mechanism	Inflammation and scarring of lobular bile ducts
Secondary biliary cirrhosis	Obstruction by neoplasms, strictures, or gallstones	Inflammation and scarring of bile ducts proximal to the obstruction
Postnecrotic cirrhosis	Viral hepatitis caused by hepatitis A, B, or C virus; drugs or other toxins; autoimmune destruction	Replacement of necrotic tissue with cirrhotic tissue, particularly fibrous, nodular scar tissue
Metabolic cirrhosis	Metabolic defects and storage disease, such as α_1-antitrypsin deficiency, glycogen storage disease, hemochromatosis, Wilson disease, galactosemia	Inflammation and scarring with specific morphologic changes related to cause

damage. Abuse of any type of alcoholic beverage can cause cirrhosis. Malnutrition may add to the risk of cirrhosis in alcohol abusers. The incidence of alcoholic cirrhosis is greatest in middle-aged men. In the United States, mortality resulting from cirrhosis is highest among non-white individuals. Although alcoholic cirrhosis is the most prevalent of the various types of cirrhosis, the occurrence of cirrhosis among persons with alcoholism is relatively low (approximately 25%).

PATHOPHYSIOLOGY Chronic alcoholic hepatitis is a precursor of cirrhosis characterized by inflammation, degeneration, and necrosis of hepatocytes, infiltration of polymorphonuclear leukocytes and lymphocytes, immunologic alterations, and lipid peroxidation. The injured hepatocytes contain Mallory bodies (hyaline endoplasmic reticulum). The presence of Mallory bodies indicates the onset of fibrosis. Neutrophils infiltrate and surround degenerating hepatocytes. The mechanism of hepatocyte injury is not clearly understood, but inflammatory mediators, acetaldehyde, reactive oxygen and nitrogen species, and genetic factors are involved.[292,293] Serum IgA is often elevated in individuals with alcoholic hepatitis, and liver antigens and antibodies have been identified in persons with progressive alcoholic liver disease. The inflammation and necrosis caused by alcoholic hepatitis stimulate the fibrosis characteristic of the cirrhotic stage of disease.[294]

Alcoholic cirrhosis is a complex process that begins with fatty infiltration (hepatic steatosis). Fatty infiltration can occur without subsequent hepatitis or cirrhosis. Fat deposition (deposition of triglycerides) within the liver hepatocytes is caused primarily by increased lipogenesis and decreased fatty acid oxidation by hepatocytes. Cessation of alcohol intake reverses fat accumulation. Lipids mobilized from adipose tissue or dietary fat intake may contribute to fat accumulation.

Alcoholic cirrhosis is caused by the toxic effects of alcohol metabolism on the liver, immunologic alterations, lipid peroxidation, and malnutrition.[295] Alcoholic cirrhosis is more severe when associated with HCV.[296] The oxidative metabolism of alcohol occurs primarily in the liver (see Chapter 2). Alcohol is

transformed to acetaldehyde. Excessive amounts of acetaldehyde induce lipid peroxidation, oxidative stress, and disrupt cytoskeleton and membrane function. Acetaldehyde inhibits export of proteins from the liver, alters metabolism of vitamins and minerals, promotes liver fibrosis, and induces malnutrition.[297] Mitochondrial function is impaired, decreasing oxidation of fatty acid. Enzyme and protein synthesis may be depressed or altered, and hormone and ammonia degradation is diminished. Alcohol also may stimulate the formation of autoantibodies specific to hepatic cells. Bacterial endotoxin from the intestine contributes to progressive injury and inflammation.[298,299] Cellular damage initiates an inflammatory response. Inflammatory cytokines, including TNF-α and IL-6, IL-8, and IL-18, are associated with alcoholic liver disease. Inflammation and necrosis result in excessive collagen formation. Transforming growth factor-beta (TGF-β) contributes to fibrosis and is produced in part by activated Kupffer cells.[300] TGF-β activates hepatic stellate cells to produce excess collagen.[301] Dense bands of fibrosis surround regenerative hepatocellular nodules. Fibrosis and scarring alter the structure of the liver and obstruct biliary and vascular channels.[302] Examples of liver damage are shown in Figure 39-22.

CLINICAL MANIFESTATIONS Fatty infiltration causes no specific symptoms or abnormal liver function test results. The liver is usually enlarged, however, and the individual has a history of continuous alcohol intake during the previous weeks or months. Anorexia, nausea, jaundice, and edema develop with advanced fatty infiltration or the onset of alcoholic hepatitis (Figure 39-23).

The clinical manifestations of alcoholic hepatitis can be mild or severe. Nonspecific symptoms include fatigue, weight loss, and anorexia.[303] Manifestations of acute illness include nausea, anorexia, fever, abdominal pain, and jaundice. Toxic effects of alcohol also can cause testicular atrophy, reduced libido, azoospermia, and decreased testosterone in men.[304] Cirrhosis is a multiple-system disease and causes hepatomegaly, splenomegaly, ascites, gastrointestinal hemorrhage, portal hypertension, hepatic encephalopathy,

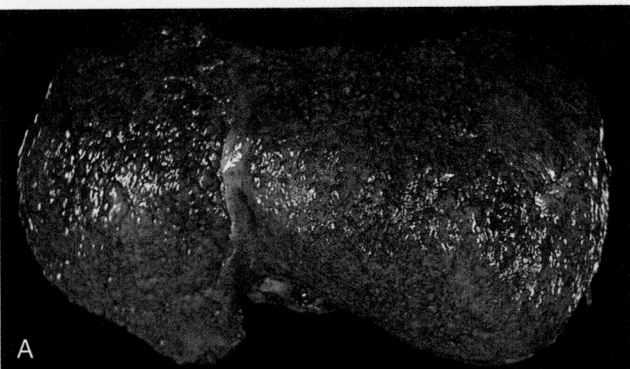

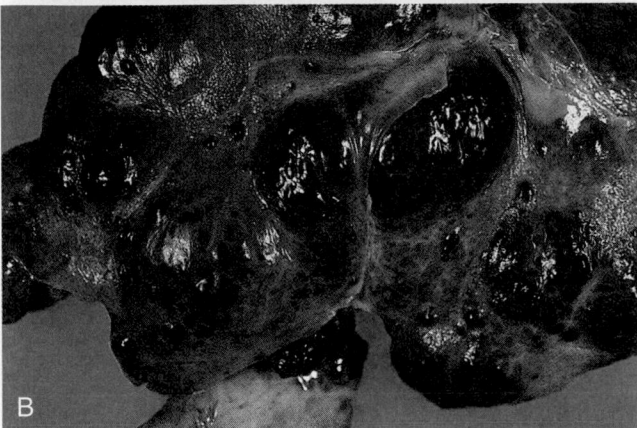

Figure 39-22 Cirrhosis. **A,** Micronodular cirrhosis. The nodular appearance develops from regeneration of hepatocytes projecting through fibrous bands of tissue. **B,** Macronodular cirrhosis. (From Damjanov I, Linder J, editors: *Anderson's pathology,* ed 10, St Louis, 1996, Mosby.)

and esophageal varices. Anemia results from blood loss, poor nutrition, and hypersplenism. Risk for infection is greater, in part because of altered macrophage function.[305] The presence of numerous and severe manifestations increases the risk of death. The clinical features of alcoholic cirrhosis depend on the duration of the disease and the severity of liver damage.

EVALUATION AND TREATMENT The diagnosis of alcoholic hepatitis is based on the individual's history and clinical manifestations. The results of liver function tests are abnormal, and serologic studies show elevated serum enzymes and bilirubin and decreased serum albumin. Prolonged prothrombin time cannot easily be corrected with vitamin K therapy. Liver biopsy can confirm the diagnosis of cirrhosis, but biopsy is not necessary if clinical manifestations of cirrhosis are evident.

There is no specific treatment for alcoholic cirrhosis, but many of the complications are treatable. Rest, a nutritious diet, corticosteroids, antioxidants, drugs that slow fibrosis, and management of complications such as ascites, gastrointestinal bleeding, infection, and encephalopathy slow disease progression. Cessation of alcohol consumption slows the progression of liver damage, improves clinical symptoms, and prolongs life. Although the liver damage is irreversible, measures that halt the inflammation and destruction of liver cells prolong life. Liver transplant is the treatment for liver failure[289,306] and artificial liver support systems are being developed (see What's New? Artificial Liver Support).

Biliary Cirrhosis

Biliary cirrhosis differs from alcoholic cirrhosis in that the damage and inflammation leading to cirrhosis begin in bile canaliculi and bile ducts, rather than in the hepatocytes. The two types of biliary cirrhosis are *primary* and *secondary*. Although both involve bile duct pathology, they differ with respect to cause, risk factors, and mechanisms of obstruction and inflammation.

Primary Biliary Cirrhosis. Primary biliary cirrhosis is an autoimmune disease of unknown etiology leading to destruction of small intrahepatic bile ducts. Mitochondrial autoantibodies are a hallmark of the disease and may be triggered by xenobviotics of infectious agents in genetically susceptible individuals.[307] The disease is characterized by inflammation and destruction of small intrahepatic bile ducts with portal inflammation and, ultimately, fibrosis. Women are affected more commonly (90%) than men. Symptoms rarely develop before the age of 30 years. Primary biliary cirrhosis often accompanies the autoimmune diseases.[308]

Primary biliary cirrhosis develops insidiously. It begins with inflammation, destruction, fibrosis, and obstruction of the intrahepatic bile ducts. Nodular regeneration and cirrhosis follow. Portal hypertension develops during the later stages of the disease.[309]

Individuals with primary biliary cirrhosis may be asymptomatic or symptomatic at diagnosis.[308] The earliest manifestations are pruritus, fatigue, and abdominal pain. Jaundice and light-colored stools are later symptoms. These symptoms are caused by intrahepatic obstruction of bile flow. Steatorrhea and fat-soluble vitamin deficiencies are present in some cases. The malabsorption can lead to osteomalacia and osteoporosis. Cirrhosis, symptoms of portal hypertension and encephalopathy, and ultimately liver failure develop.

Serologic tests show elevated alkaline phosphatase levels, hyperbilirubinemia, and hyperlipidemia, with or without other clinical manifestations. Most individuals have a circulating IgG antimitochondrial antibody that is not found in other types of liver disease. Evaluation involves ruling out biliary obstruction caused by gallstones, tumor, or inflammation of the common bile duct (i.e., secondary biliary cirrhosis). The presence of positive cholestatic liver test for 6 months' duration, positive serum antimitochondrial antibody, and liver biopsy confirms the diagnosis of primary biliary cirrhosis.[310]

Corticosteroids or azathioprine may be used to suppress the immune response. No specific treatment is available. The distressing pruritus may be relieved by cholestyramine, which binds bile salts in the intestine. Intramuscular injections of vitamins D and K alleviate the vitamin deficiency. The other symptoms of cirrhosis are managed as they develop. Long-term treatment with ursodeoxycholic acid slows disease progression.[308] Life expectancy is about 8 to 10 years after symptom onset.[311] Liver transplant is the only definitive therapy.

Secondary Biliary Cirrhosis. Secondary biliary cirrhosis develops when there is prolonged partial or complete obstruction of the common bile duct or its branches. The

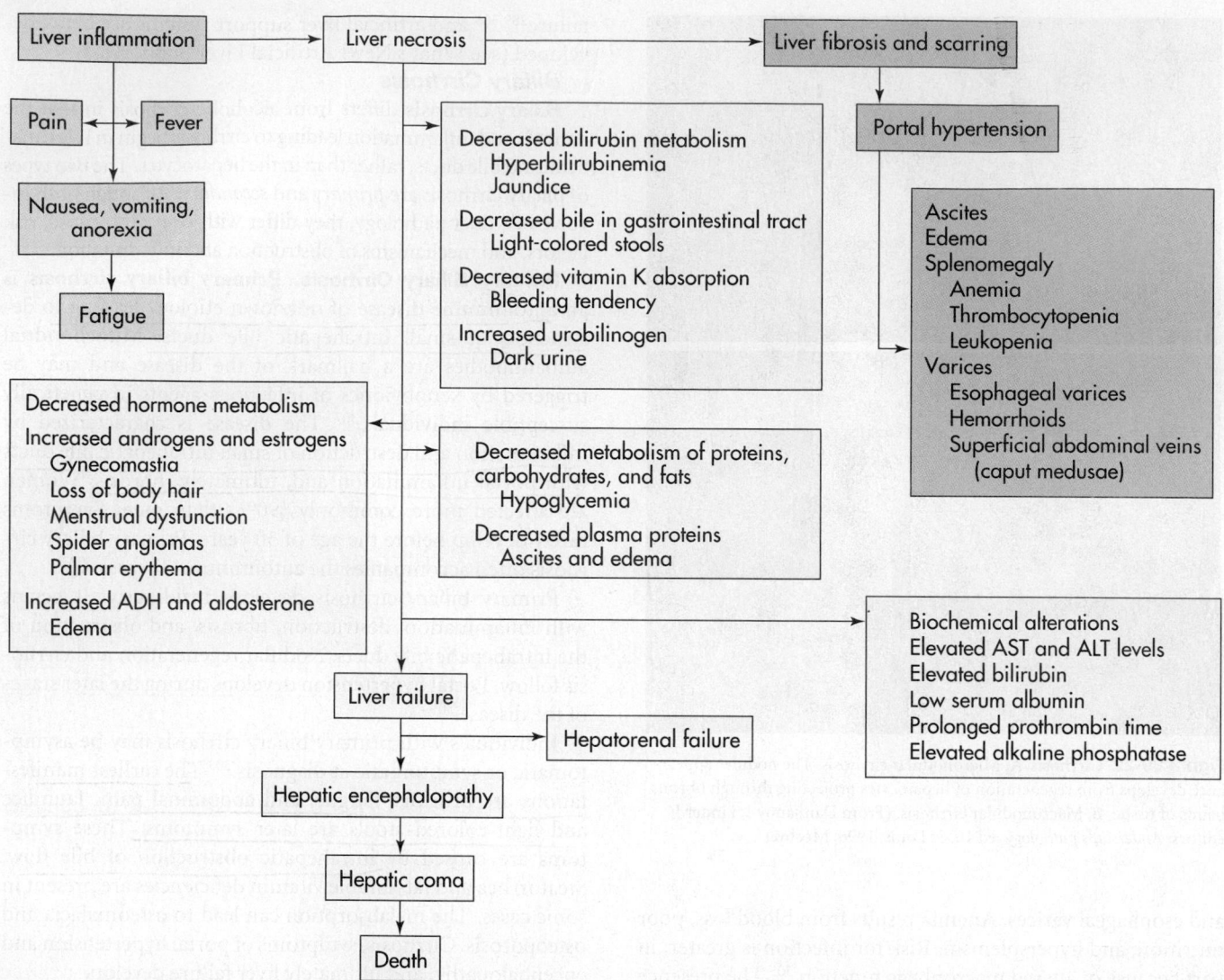

Figure 39-23 Clinical manifestations of cirrhosis. *ADH,* Antidiuretic hormone; *ALT,* alanine transaminase; *AST,* aspartate transaminase.

obstruction may be caused by gallstones, tumors, fibrotic strictures, or chronic pancreatitis. Biliary atresia and cystic fibrosis cause secondary biliary cirrhosis in children.

Chronic obstruction to bile flow increases pressure in the hepatic bile duct and results in the accumulation of bile in the centrilobular spaces. Necrotic areas develop and are followed by proliferation and inflammation of the portal ducts that result in edema and fibrosis. Pools of bile form when the portal ducts rupture into surrounding necrotic areas. Injury is accompanied by regeneration of hepatic cells with the development of finely nodular cirrhosis.

Clinical manifestations are similar to those of primary biliary cirrhosis, with jaundice and pruritus the most distressing symptoms. Right upper quadrant pain is common, and a low-grade fever may be present from bile duct inflammation (cholangitis).

Cholangiography provides the most definitive diagnosis. Laboratory tests usually show elevated conjugated bilirubin and alkaline phosphatase levels. Aminotransferase increases if there is an accompanying cholangitis. Surgery or endoscopy relieves obstruction, prolongs survival, and diminishes or resolves symptoms. Continued obstruction leads to advanced cirrhosis and liver failure.

Disorders of the Gallbladder

Obstruction and inflammation are the most common disorders of the gallbladder. Obstruction is caused by **gallstones** (cholelithiasis), which are aggregates of substances in the bile. The gallstones may remain in the gallbladder or be ejected, with bile, into the cystic duct. Gallstones that become lodged in the cystic duct obstruct the flow of bile into and out of the gallbladder and cause inflammation. Gallstone formation is termed *cholelithiasis.* Inflammation of the gallbladder or cystic duct is known as *cholecystitis.*

Cholelithiasis (Gallstones)

Cholelithiasis is a prevalent disorder in developed countries, where incidence is 10% to 20%. The actual incidence is unknown because many individuals who have gallstones are

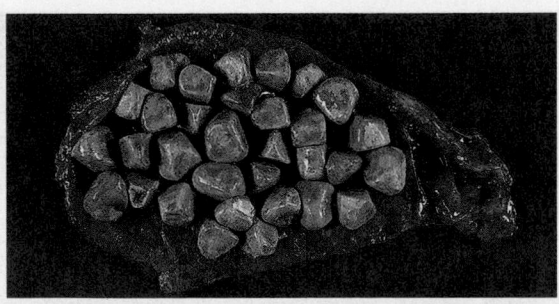

Figure 39-24 Resected gallbladder containing mixed gallstones. (From Kissane JM, ed: *Anderson's pathology, ed 9,* St Louis, 1990, Mosby.)

asymptomatic. Risk factors include obesity; rapid weight loss in obese individuals; middle age; female gender; oral contraceptives; American Indian ancestry; gallbladder, pancreatic, or ileal disease; high dietary cholesterol; and gene-environmental interactions.[312]

PATHOPHYSIOLOGY Gallstones are commonly of two types: cholesterol and pigmented.[313] Cholesterol stones are the most common. Pigmented stones, which are less common, occur later in life and are associated with cirrhosis. *Cholesterol gallstones* form in bile that is supersaturated with cholesterol produced by the liver. Supersaturation sets the stage for cholesterol crystal formation, or the formation of "microstones." More crystals then aggregate on the microstones, which grow to form "macrostones." This process usually occurs in the gallbladder, which may have decreased motility. The stones may lie "silent" or become lodged in the cystic or common duct, causing pain and cholecystitis. Gallstone formation may be such that the stones accumulate and fill the entire gallbladder (Figure 39-24). Impaired gallbladder motility and gallbladder stasis also may contribute to stone formation.[314]

It is not known why the hepatocytes secrete bile that is supersaturated with cholesterol. Proposed mechanisms include (1) an enzymatic defect that increases the hepatocytes' synthesis of cholesterol; (2) diminished secretion of bile acids, which normally promote cholesterol solubility; (3) decreased resorption of bile salts from the ileum, which decrease the bile acid pool; (4) gallbladder smooth muscle hypomotility and stasis; (5) genetic predisposition; and (6) some combination of these mechanisms.[315] In obese individuals the mechanism appears to involve cholesterol synthesis, whereas in nonobese individuals, it appears to involve decreased secretion of bile acids.

Pigmented stones are created by cholesterol, calcium bilirubinate, or pigmented polymers. The formation of pigmented stones is associated with biliary tract obstruction and bacterial degradation and precipitation of biliary lipids.[316]

CLINICAL MANIFESTATIONS Epigastric and right hypochondrium pain and intolerance to fatty foods are the cardinal manifestations of cholelithiasis. Vague symptoms include heartburn, flatulence, epigastric discomfort, pruritus, jaundice, and food intolerances, particularly to fats and cabbage. The pain, often called *biliary colic,* is most characteristic and is caused by the lodging of one or more gallstones in the cystic or common duct.[317] The pain can be intermittent or steady.

It usually is located in the right upper quadrant and radiates to the mid-upper back. Jaundice indicates that the stone is located in the common bile duct. Abdominal tenderness and fever indicate cholecystitis. Complications can include pancreatitis.

EVALUATION AND TREATMENT Diagnosis is based on the individual's medical history, physical examination, and radiographic evaluation. An oral cholecystogram usually outlines the stones. Intravenous cholangiography is used to differentiate cholelithiasis from other causes of extrahepatic biliary obstruction if the cholecystogram is negative. Endoscopic or percutaneous cholangiography and endoscopic or transabdominal ultrasonography are diagnostic options.[318]

Laparoscopic cholecystectomy is the preferred treatment for gallstones that cause obstruction or inflammation. Use of transluminal endoscopic surgery is advancing rapidly.[319] Endoscopic retrograde cholangiopancreatography and sphincterotomy with stone retrieval is used for the treatment of bile duct stones. Large stones may be managed with lithotripsy.[320] An alternative treatment is the administration of drugs that dissolve smaller stones. For example, the bile acid chenodeoxycholic acid (CDCA) can completely or partially dissolve cholesterol gallstones. Ursodeoxycholic acid (UDCA), which is structurally similar to CDCA, is also effective, is less toxic to hepatocytes, and does not cause fatty diarrhea, as does CDCA.

Cholecystitis

Cholecystitis can be acute or chronic. Both forms are almost always caused by the lodging of a gallstone in the cystic duct. Obstruction causes the gallbladder to become distended and inflamed. The pain is similar to that caused by gallstones. Pressure against the distended wall of the gallbladder decreases blood flow. Ischemia, necrosis, and perforation of the gallbladder are possible. Fever, leukocytosis, rebound tenderness, and abdominal muscle guarding are common findings. Serum bilirubin and alkaline phosphatase levels may be elevated. Nevertheless, the acute abdominal pain of cholecystitis must be differentiated from the pain caused by other disorders, such as pancreatitis, myocardial infarction, and acute pyelonephritis of the right kidney. Cholangiography or radioactive scan can confirm a diagnosis of cholecystitis.

Treatment includes pain control, replacement of fluid and electrolytes, and fasting. Antibiotics are often prescribed to manage bacterial infection in severe cases. Immediate cholecystectomy is required for complications such as peritonitis from gallbladder perforation. Persistent symptoms or development of chronic cholecystitis punctuated by recurrent acute attacks usually requires cholecystectomy. If pancreatic abscesses develop, they usually are resected.[321]

Disorders of the Pancreas

Pancreatitis, or inflammation of the pancreas, is a relatively rare and potentially serious disorder. Incidence is about equal in men and women and is more common between 50 and 60 years of age. Pancreatitis can be acute or chronic. It is associated with several other clinical conditions, including alcoholism, obstructive biliary tract disease (particularly

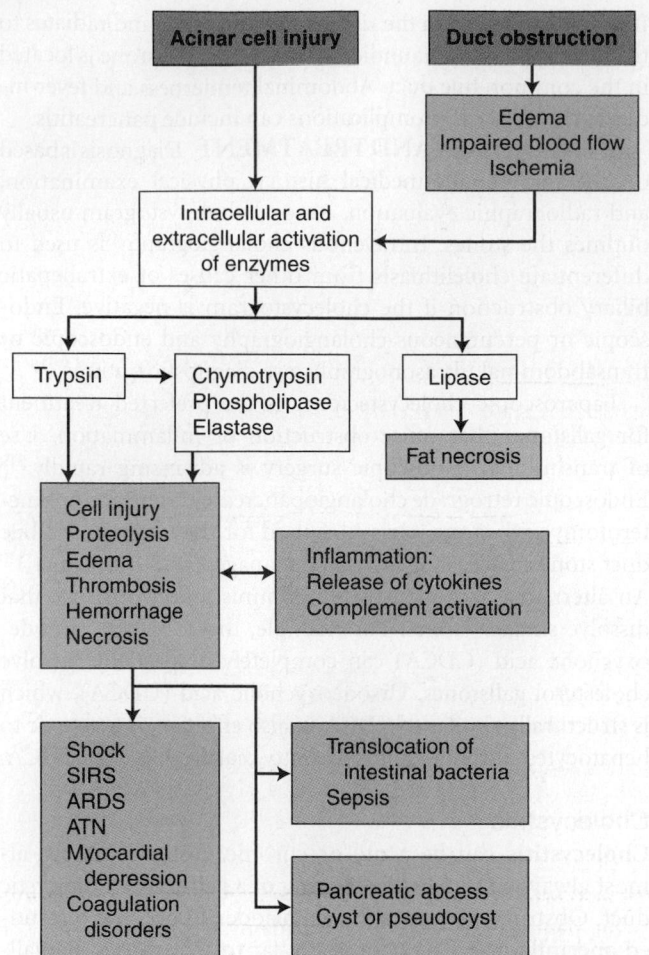

Figure 39-25 Pathophysiology of acute pancreatitis. *ARDS*, Acute respiratory distress syndrome; *ATN*, acute tubular necrosis; *SIRS*, systemic inflammatory response syndrome.

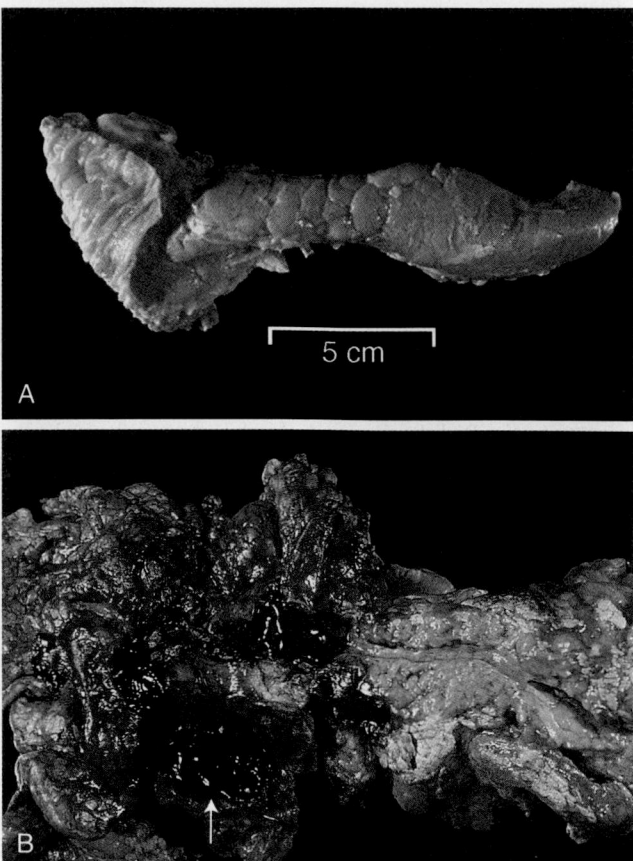

Figure 39-26 Normal and acute hemorrhagic pancreatitis. **A,** Normal pancreas. **B,** Acute hemorrhagic pancreatitis. The pancreas has hemorrhage, fat necrosis *(white patches)*, and a pseudocyst filled with blood *(white arrow)*. (A from Klatt EC, editor: *Robbins and Cotran atlas of pathology*, Philadelphia, 2006, Saunders. B from Damjanov I, Linder J, editors: *Pathology: a color atlas*, St Louis, 2000, Mosby.)

cholelithiasis), peptic ulcers, trauma, hyperlipidemia, and certain drugs. The cause is unknown in 15% to 25% of cases.[322]

Acute Pancreatitis

PATHOPHYSIOLOGY Acute pancreatitis (acute hemorrhagic pancreatitis) is initiated by intrapancreatic activation of proteases (Figure 39-25). It is usually a mild disease, but about 20% of those afflicted develop a severe pancreatic inflammation requiring hospital care. Although the precise pathogenic mechanism or sequence of events often is unknown, alcoholism and biliary tract obstruction are commonly associated. Bile reflux into the pancreas occurs if gallstones obstruct the common bile duct and bile contributes to attacks of acute pancreatitis.[323] The pancreatic acinar cell metabolizes ethanol with the generation of toxic metabolites.[324] The most common theory is that pancreatitis develops because of an injury or disruption of pancreatic acinar cells, which permit leakage of pancreatic enzymes (trypsin, chymotrypsin, and elastase) into pancreatic tissue.[325] Activated proteolases (trypsin and elastase) and lipases break down tissue and cell membranes, causing inflammation, edema, vascular damage, hemorrhage,

necrosis, and fibrosis (Figure 39-26).[326] (Fatty necrosis is described in Chapter 2.) Toxic enzymes, infiltration of macrophages and leukocytes with release of inflammatory mediators (TNF-α, IL-1β, IL-6, IL-8, IL-10, C5a, intercellular-adhesion molecule [ICAM], and substance P) into the bloodstream cause injury to vessels and other organs, such as the lungs, heart, and kidneys. Translocation of bacteria occurs with gut barrier dysfunction resulting in local or systemic infection.[327]

CLINICAL MANIFESTATIONS Epigastric or midabdominal pain is the cardinal symptom of acute pancreatitis. The pain may radiate to the back because of the retroperitoneal location of the pancreas. The pain is caused by edema, which distends the pancreatic ducts and capsule; chemical irritation and inflammation of the peritoneum; and irritation or obstruction of the biliary tract. Fever and leukocytosis accompany the inflammatory response. Nausea and vomiting are caused by hypermotility or paralytic ileus secondary to the pancreatitis or peritonitis.

Abdominal distention accompanies bowel hypermotility and the accumulation of fluids in the peritoneal cavity. Hypotension and shock occur frequently because enzymes and kinins released into the circulation increase vascular permeability and dilate vessels. Hypovolemia, hypotension, and myocardial insufficiency result. A small percentage of individuals develop tachypnea and hypoxemia secondary to pulmonary edema, atelectasis, or pleural effusions caused by circulating pancreatic enzymes and inflammatory mediators. In severe cases, hypovolemia decreases renal blood flow sufficiently to impair renal function.[328] Pancreatic encephalopathy and coagulation abnormalities are complications of severe pancreatitis and often occur with multiple organ failure.[329] Tetany may develop as a result of calcium deposition in areas of fat necrosis or as a decreased response to parathyroid hormone. Transient hyperglycemia also can occur if glucagon is released from damaged A cells in the pancreatic islets. A systemic inflammatory response and multiple organ failure account for most deaths with severe pancreatitis.[330] In hemorrhagic pancreatitis, some individuals develop flank or periumbilical ecchymosis, a sign of poor prognosis.

EVALUATION AND TREATMENT Diagnosis of pancreatitis is based on clinical findings, identification of associated disorders, and laboratory studies. Elevated serum amylase and lipase are characteristic diagnostic features and serum lipase is more specific and sensitive. The amylase level usually rises within 12 hours after the onset of symptoms and returns to normal within 3 to 5 days in most cases. Serum lipase levels increase within 4 to 8 hours of clinical symptom onset and decrease within 8 to 14 days. Serum trypsin levels are very specific for pancreatitis but may not be readily available. Urine trypsinogen-2 and urine amylase also are elevated. C-reactive protein elevates within 48 hours and is a marker of severity.[331,332] The ratio of amylase clearance to creatinine clearance by the kidney can be diagnostic because, in cases of pancreatitis, amylase clearance increases significantly compared with creatinine clearance. Serum transferrin is a diagnostic marker for alcoholic acute pancreatitis.[333] Acute pancreatitis is difficult to diagnose because several other disorders can cause similar clinical and laboratory findings. These disorders include perforating duodenal ulcer, acute cholecystitis, small-bowel obstruction, and kidney stones. Ultrasound and CT scan are used in more severe cases to evaluate extent of involvement and complications. Intra-abdominal pressure monitoring assesses risk for abdominal compartment syndrome[334] (see What's New? Abdominal Compartment Syndrome).

The goal of treatment for acute pancreatitis is to stop the process of autodigestion and prevent systemic complications. Narcotic medications may be needed to relieve pain. Meperidine hydrochloride (Demerol) is used instead of morphine because it causes less spasm of the sphincter of Oddi than morphine. Nasogastric suction may not be necessary with mild pancreatitis but may help relieve pain and prevent paralytic ileus in individuals who are nauseated and vomiting. Enteral nutrition with use of nasogastric or jejunal tube feedings is often effective, but an effort is made to maintain normal enteral nutrition.[335] Probiotics may be helpful. Parenteral fluids are essential to restore blood volume and prevent hypotension and shock. Parenteral hyperalimentation should be initiated

---

WHAT'S NEW? Abdominal Compartment Syndrome

Abdominal compartment syndrome (ACS), also known as *intra-abdominal hypertension,* develops when there is abnormally high intra-abdominal pressure associated with organ dysfunction. ACS is associated with abdominal injury, including trauma, ruptured aortic aneurysm, acute pancreatitis, and massive fluid volume replacement. Increased intra-abdominal pressure increases intrathoracic, intracardiac, and intracranial filling pressures and results in decreased cardiac output, atelectasis, pulmonary edema, oliguria, compromise of splanchnic and hepatic blood flow, and translocation of bacteria from the gut. The end consequence is multiple organ failure.

Normally intra-abdominal pressure is slightly greater than atmospheric pressure. Organ dysfunction develops at pressures greater than 20 mmHg and lasting for more than 6 hours. Automated serial or continuous monitoring of pressure inside the bladder provides an estimate of intra-abdominal pressure. New techniques of measurement, identification of risk factors, and standards of care are emerging. Treatment is decompressive laparotomy, which may be performed at the bedside if the individual is too unstable to move.

Data from Dambrausk Z et al: *World Gastroenterol* 15(6):717-721, 2009; Maerz L, Kaplan LJ: *Crit Care Med* 36(4 Suppl):S212-S215, 2008; Zengerink I et al: *J Trauma* 64(5):1159-1164, 2008; World Society of the Abdominal Compartment Syndrome: *WSACS Resuscitation Algorithms*, 2007. Available at www.wsacs.org/algorithms.php.

when enteral feeding is not tolerated. Drugs that decrease gastric acid production (e.g., cimetidine) can decrease stimulation of the pancreas by secretin. Necrotizing pancreatitis requires surgical resection, and antibiotics may control infection. The risk of mortality increases significantly with the development of pulmonary, cardiac, and renal complications.

Chronic Pancreatitis

Chronic alcohol abuse is the most common cause of **chronic pancreatitis.** Obstruction from gallstones, autoimmune disease, gene mutations, smoking, and obesity can be contributing factors.[336] The disease is idiopathic in about 25% of cases.[337] Toxic metabolites and chronic release of inflammatory cytokines contribute to the destruction of acinar cells and islets of Langerhans. Fibrosis, strictures, calcification, ductal obstruction, and pancreatic cysts are the common lesions of chronic pancreatitis. The cysts are walled-off areas or pockets of pancreatic juice, necrotic debris, or blood within or adjacent to the pancreas. Continuous or intermittent abdominal pain, weight loss, and less commonly, steatorrhea and diabetes mellitus accompany disease progression. Pain is associated with increased intraductal pressure, increased tissue pressure, ischemia, neuritis, ongoing injury, and changes in central pain perception.[338] Preventing disease progression includes lifestyle modification to stop alcohol use and smoking. Pain management is complex with use of analgesics. A fat-free diet and oral enzyme replacements prevent malabsorption and weight loss. Surgical drainage or partial resection of the pancreas may be required to relieve pain and prevent cystic rupture.[339] Chronic pancreatitis is a risk factor for pancreatic cancer.[340]

Table 39-10	Cancer of the Gut, Liver, and Pancreas			
Organ	Percentage of Deaths of All Cancers	Risks	Cell Type	Common Manifestations
Esophagus	2%	Malnutrition Alcohol Tobacco Chronic reflux	Squamous cell Adenocarcinoma	Chest pain Dysphagia
Stomach	2%	Salty food Nitrates and nitrosamines Gastric atrophy	Adenocarcinoma Squamous cell	Anorexia Malaise Weight loss Upper abdominal pain Vomiting Occult blood
Colorectal	9%	Polyps Ulcerative colitis Diverticulitis High–refined-carbohydrate, low-fiber, high-fat diet	Adenocarcinoma (left colon grows in ring; right colon grows as mass)	Pain Mass Anemia Bloody stool Obstruction Distention
Liver	3%	Hepatitis B, C, and D viruses Cirrhosis Intestinal parasite Aflatoxin from moldy peanuts	Hepatomas Cholangiomas	Pain Anorexia Bloating Weight loss Portal hypertension Ascites ± jaundice
Pancreas	6%	Chronic pancreatitis Cigarette smoking Alcohol (?) Diabetic women	Adenocarcinoma (exocrine part of gland, ductal epithelium)	

NOTE: Esophageal (men), colorectal, liver, and pancreatic cancers are within the top 10 causes of death from cancer.
Amended with permission from the American Cancer Society. *Cancer Facts and Figures 2009.* Atlanta: American Cancer Society, Inc.

CANCER OF THE DIGESTIVE SYSTEM

Cancer occurs throughout the alimentary tract and the accessory organs of digestion (liver, gallbladder, and pancreas) (Table 39-10). A genetic predisposition is being evaluated.[341]

Cancer of the Gastrointestinal Tract

Cancer of the Esophagus

Carcinoma of the esophagus is a rare disease with 16,470 new cases and 14,530 deaths each year. Adenocarcinoma is increasing in white men and women in the United States.[342] Squamous cell carcinoma is more prevalent in China, Iran, South America, and South Africa and is more common in black men in the United States.[343] The incidence in the United States and Europe is less than 1% of new cancers per year.[344] The U.S. incidence is higher in blacks than in whites and peaks at about 60 years of age.

Squamous cell carcinoma is associated with malnutrition caused by poor economic conditions, dietary habits, alcoholism, tobacco use, obesity, radiation exposure, and chronic gastroesophageal reflux.[345] Adenocarcinoma is associated with reflux esophagitis and sliding hiatal hernia. Both of these conditions can cause erosive esophagitis and ulceration that can eventually lead to metaplasia (Barrett esophagus) and neoplastic changes.

PATHOGENESIS Carcinomas of the esophagus are often secondary to infiltration by a gastric carcinoma or to the presence of Barrett (dysplastic) epithelium (columnar rather than squamous epithelium in the lower esophagus), which is associated with chronic gastroesophageal reflux. The disease progresses from Barrett metaplasia, to dysplasia, to adenocarcinoma, and then metastasis. Carcinomas can occur at any level of the esophageal tract but are most common at the gastroesophageal junction.[346]

The pathogenesis of esophageal carcinoma is facilitated by (1) alterations of esophageal structure and function that permit food and drink to remain in the esophagus for prolonged periods; (2) ulceration and metaplasia caused by esophageal reflux; and (3) long-term exposure to irritants, such as alcohol and tobacco, that cause neoplastic transformation (see Chapter 11). *H. pylori* do not colonize the intestinal epithelium of Barrett esophagus and may be a protection against esophageal adenocarcinoma.[347] Chronic inadequate nutrition can impair structure and function of the esophagus. Mutation of the *TP53* gene is an early event in Barrett adenocarcinoma.[348]

CLINICAL MANIFESTATIONS Early stages of esophageal carcinoma are asymptomatic. The two main manifestations of esophageal carcinoma are chest pain and dysphagia. The most common type of pain is heartburn (pyrosis). It is initiated by eating spicy or highly seasoned foods and by lying down. Dysphagia (pain on swallowing), another common symptom, is usually pressure-like and may radiate posteriorly between the scapulae. Some individuals with esophageal cancer complain of a constant retrosternal pain that radiates to the back. Dysphagia usually progresses rapidly.

EVALUATION AND TREATMENT Individuals who present with dysphagia undergo endoscopy so that specimens can be obtained and examined for neoplastic change and type of carcinoma. CT studies of the thorax also are used for diagnosis. Prevention and treatment of gastroesophageal reflux are essential to the management of Barrett esophagus. Untreated esophageal cancer metastasizes rapidly and has a poor prognosis. The cancer has often metastasized by the time of diagnosis. The lymphatic vessels of the esophagus are continuous with vital mediastinal structures and drain to the lymph nodes from the neck of the celiac axis, making it impossible to remove all the lymph nodes with the tumor. Removal of the primary lesion and the local lymph nodes, however, can benefit the individual with esophageal cancer and cure is likely if there is not malignancy. If spread has occurred, treatment is combined radiation, chemotherapy, and palliative care.[346]

Cancer of the Stomach

Although the incidence of gastric cancer has declined in the United States, it still represents about 2% (21,130 cases) of all new cancer cases and 10,620 deaths annually.[344] The incidence of gastric cancer is greater in men than in women. In countries such as Japan, the British Isles, and Iceland, the incidence of stomach cancer has remained high consistently. Gastric cancer is the second most common cause of death from cancer in Asia.[349] These data illustrate the importance of environmental factors, such as diet, to carcinogenesis.

Nonenvironmental risk factors include a family history of gastric adenocarcinoma; blood type (blood group A); type A atrophic gastritis; and pernicious anemia, which is associated with atrophy of the gastric mucosa in the same locations where gastric tumors arise.[350]

The most important environmental risk factors in causing gastric cancer are (1) infection with *H. pylori* that carries the *CagA* gene product cytotoxin-associated antigen A; (2) salt added to food; (3) food additives (e.g., nitrates) in pickled or salted foods (e.g., bacon); and (4) low intake of fruits and vegetables. Infection with *H. pylori* and severe chronic gastritis change the mucosal cell proliferation pattern, increasing the risk for gastric and duodenal carcinoma.[351,352] *H. pylori* also is causatively linked to **mucosa-associated lymphoid tissue (MALT) lymphoma** (a low-grade B-cell lymphoma) that originates in the stomach.[353] Vitamin C and carotenoids are possible protective factors.[354] Dietary salt enhances the conversion of nitrates to carcinogenic nitrosamines in the stomach. Salt is also caustic to the stomach and can cause chronic atrophic gastritis. Finally, hypertonic salt solutions delay gastric emptying. Delayed emptying increases the time during which carcinogenic nitrosamines can exert their effects on the stomach mucosa.

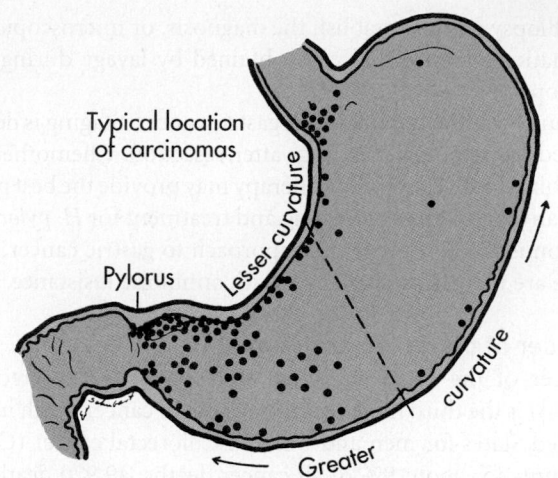

Figure 39-27 Typical sites of stomach cancer. (From del Regato JA, Spjut HJ, Cox JD: *Cancer: diagnosis, treatment, and prognosis*, ed 2, St Louis, 1985, Mosby.)

The metabolism of nitrates and nitrites is very complex. Nitrates interact with amino acids in the stomach to form nitrosamines. The conversion of these carcinogenic nitrosamines is enhanced at a low pH by iodides and thiocyanates. Nitrates are thought to be active only when converted to nitrites and to cause stomach cancer once atrophic gastritis has occurred.

PATHOGENESIS Gastric cancer usually begins in the glands of the stomach mucosa. Approximately 50% of all gastric cancers develop in the prepyloric antrum (Figure 39-27). Atrophic gastritis and intestinal metaplasia are strongly linked to the development of gastric cancer.[355] Insufficient acid secretion by the atrophic mucosa creates a relatively alkaline environment that permits bacteria to multiply and act on nitrates. The resulting increase in nitrosoamines damages the deoxyribonucleic acid (DNA) of mucosal cells further, promoting metaplasia and neoplasia. Duodenal reflux also may contribute to intestinal metaplasia. The reflux contains caustic bile salts that destroy the mucosal barrier that normally protects the stomach. Alterations in *TP53* and *p21* gene expression and DNA ploidy occur in gastric carcinomas.[356]

CLINICAL MANIFESTATIONS The early stages of gastric cancer are generally asymptomatic or produce vague symptoms such as loss of appetite (especially for meat), malaise, and "indigestion." Later manifestations include unexplained weight loss, upper abdominal pain, vomiting, change in bowel habits, and anemia caused by persistent occult bleeding. The prognosis is poor because symptoms usually do not occur until the tumor has penetrated the muscle layers of the stomach; spread to surrounding tissues; and entered the draining lymph nodes and veins, causing distant metastases. Generally the first manifestations of carcinoma are caused by distant metastases.

EVALUATION AND TREATMENT The choice of diagnostic tests depends on the clinical manifestations at the time of presentation. Most symptoms suggest a problem in the upper gastrointestinal tract. Direct endoscopic visualization and biopsy usually establish the diagnosis, or microscopic examination of exfoliated cells obtained by lavage during endoscopy.

Surgery is the treatment for gastric cancer. Staging is determined by pathologic findings after resection. Chemotherapy combined with chemoradiotherapy may provide the best postoperative outcomes. Screening and treatment for *H. pylori* infection is the best preventive approach to gastric cancer, and there are increasing challenges with antibiotic resistance.[357]

Cancer of the Colon and Rectum

Cancer of the lower intestinal tract (colon [78%] rectum [28%]) is the third most common cause of cancer death in the United States for men and women. Colorectal cancer (CRC) accounts for about 9% of all cancer deaths; 49,920 deaths in 2009.[339] Cancer of the colon tends to occur in individuals older than 50 years with 146,970 new cases in 2009. It is more common in African Americans and is rare in children.[344] Worldwide, the prevalence of colorectal cancer is highest in populations with high socioeconomic standards, possibly because of dietary and lifestyle habits.[358,359]

Small intestine carcinoma is rare and represents less than 1% of gastrointestinal cancers (6230 new cases in 2009).[344,360] Carcinoma occurs more frequently in familial adenomatous polyposus and Crohn disease. Long term management includes frequent screening and endoscopic surveillance.[361] **Anal carcinioma** is rare (5290 cases in 2009).[344] The most common risk factor is infection with human papillomavirus (93%), and less commonly, anal involvment in Crohn disease.[361]

PATHOGENESIS Genetic and environmental factors are associated with the development of CRC (Figure 39-28). Alterations in the tumor-suppressor *TP53* gene are present in 75% to 85% of colorectal cancers.[362,363] Allelic deletion on chromosomes 5, 17, and 18 appears to promote transition from normal to malignant colon mucosa. Progression from adenomas to colon cancer involves a multistep cascade of genetic mutations involving the *DCC* (deleted in colorectal cancer gene) and *TP53* (protein 53) tumor-suppressor genes; *k-ras* (retrovirus-associated DNA sequence) gene mutations that are more common in hyperplastic polyps; loss of heterozygosity in which cells lose one allele of some genes with loss of genetic stability and tumor suppressor function; and DNA methylation that can silence DNA expression and inactivate tumor suppression. Cyclooxygenase-2 (COX-2) is variably expressed in right-sided and left-sided colorectal cancer, and COX-2 may participate in regulation of apoptosis, angiogenesis, and invasiveness of adenomatous polyposis coli.[364] Numerous environmental factors can increase the risk of colon cancer, presumably by modulating these molecular pathways.[365]

The adenomatous polyposis coli (*APC*) gene was first identified as the gene mutated (chromosome 5q) in an autosomal dominant inherited syndrome of colon cancer known as *familial adenomatous polyposis (FAP)* coli. These cancers are more common in the left colon. Hereditary nonpolyposis colon cancer (HNPCC), also known as Lynch syndrome, is

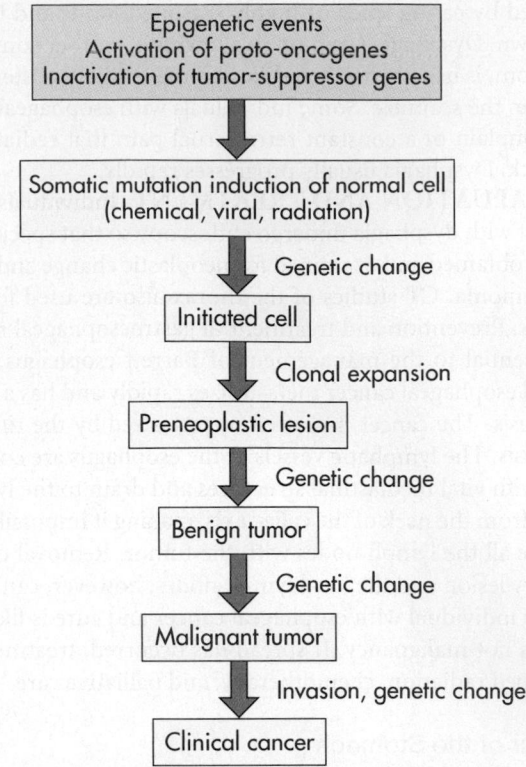

Figure 39-28 Multistage development of colonic cancer.

less common and caused by an inherited mutation in a DNA mismatch repair (*MMR*) gene.[366] These tumors are more common in the right colon and occur in other organs.[367] Hereditary colon cancers have a high risk of occurrence and represent about 3% to 5% of all colon cancers[368]; most colon cancers are sporadic and caused by somatic mutations.

Most CRC develops from polyps. A **polyp is** a finger-like projection arising from the mucosal epithelium. Most polyps are benign. The two types of neoplastic polyps are hypoplastic and adenomatous. Most colon cancers arise from adenomatous polyps (Figure 39-29). *Hypoplastic polyps* generally lack atypia but when they are large (greater than 1 cm), numerous (more than 20), and located in the right colon they are associated with cancer. The two major types of *adenomatous polyps* are pedunculated (stalk or tubular), the most common, and sessile (papillary, villous or serrated) (Figure 39-30). Once the adenoma traverses the muscularis mucosae, it becomes invasive and highly malignant. Adenomas can be detected early, however, and the submucosa may not be penetrated for several years. The larger the polyp is, the greater the risk of colorectal cancer. Although lesions larger than 1.5 cm occur less often, they are more likely to be malignant than those smaller than 1 cm. The adenomatous polyp forms in an area of epithelial cell hyperproliferation and crypt dysplasia. Table 39-11 gives other conditions commonly confused with colorectal cancer.

Most colorectal cancers are moderately differentiated adenocarcinomas. These tumors have a long preinvasive phase,

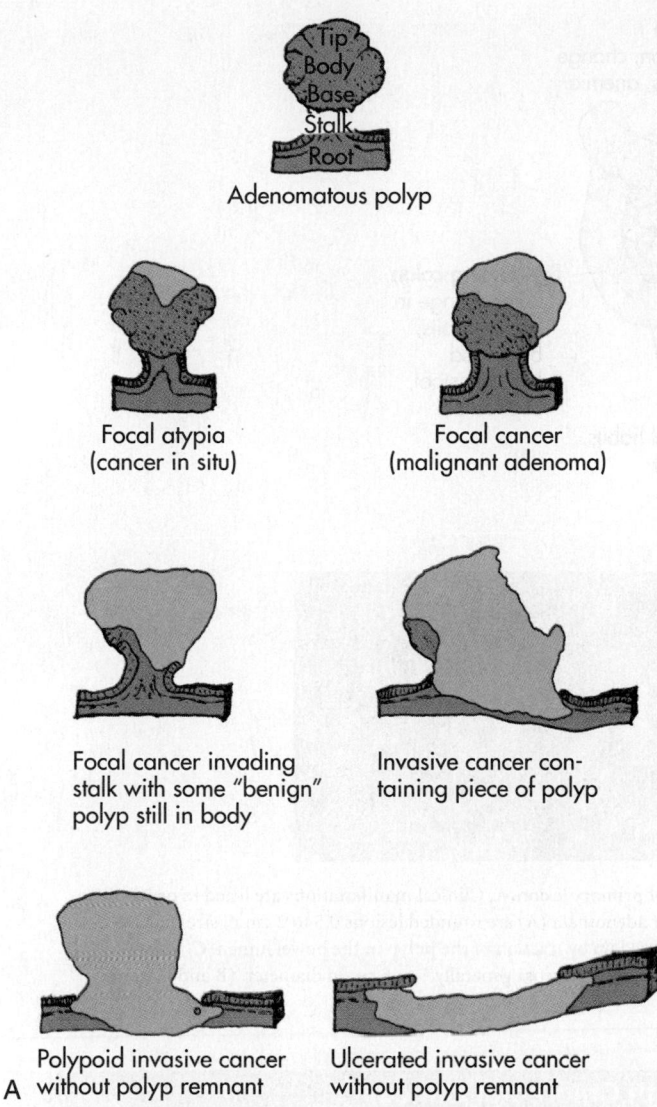

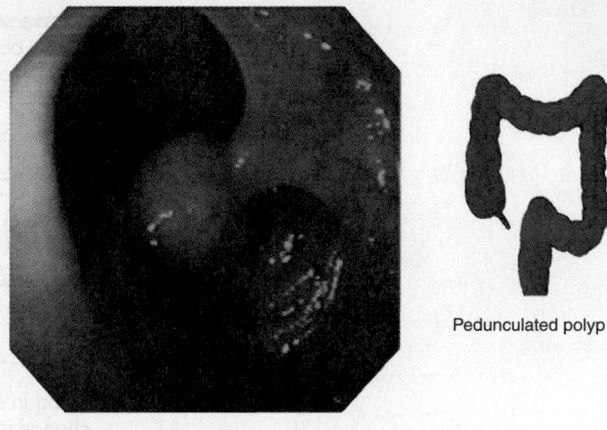

Figure 39-29 Development of cancer of the colon from adenomatous polyps. **A**, The tumor becomes invasive if it penetrates the muscularis mucosae and enters the submucosal layer. **B**, Endoscopic image of pedunculated polyp in descending colon. (**A** from del Regato JA, Spjut HJ, Cox JD: *Cancer: diagnosis, treatment, and prognosis,* ed 2, St Louis, 1985, Mosby. **B** courtesy David Bjorkman, MD, University of Utah School of Medicine, Department of Gastroenterology, Salt Lake City.)

and when they invade they tend to grow slowly. Because the lymphatic channels are located underneath the muscularis mucosae, the lesions must traverse this layer before metastasis can occur. Systemic lymphatic spread occurs along the aorta to the mesenteric and pancreatic lymph nodes. Liver metastasis follows invasion of the mesenteric veins (left colon) or superior veins (right colon), which drain into the portal circulation.

Lower risk for colon cancer may be associated with diets high in cereal grains, vegetables, folic acid, calcium, and vitamin D; hormone replacement therapy; physical activity; and use of NSAIDs.[369,370] Cancer-promoting mechanisms are related to prolonged contact of the fecal mass with colon mucosa, including processed red meats, and substances produced by microflora of the sigmoid colon.[371,372]

CLINICAL MANIFESTATIONS Tumors of the right (ascending) and left (descending) colon evolve into two distinct types. On the right side the lesions are polypoid and extend along one wall of the cecum and ascending colon.

Clinical manifestations include pain, a palpable mass in the lower right quadrant, anemia, and dark red or mahogany-colored blood mixed with the stool (see Figure 39-30). These large, bulky tumors become necrotic and ulcerated, contributing to persistent blood loss and anemia. Obstruction is unusual because the feces are more liquid.

Tumors of the left, or descending, colon start as small, elevated, button-like masses. They grow circumferentially and spread along the entire bowel wall, eventually ulcerating in the middle as the tumor penetrates the blood supply. Obstruction is common but occurs slowly. Manifestations include progressive abdominal distention, pain, vomiting, constipation, need for laxatives, cramps, and bright red blood on the surface of the stool.

Rectal carcinomas are defined as tumors occurring up to 15 cm from the anal opening. Tumors of the rectum can spread through the rectal wall to nearby structures: the prostate in men and the vagina in women. Penetration occurs more readily in the lower third of the rectum because it has no serosal covering. Systemic and pulmonary metastases occur through the hemorrhoidal plexus, which drains into the vena cava.

EVALUATION AND TREATMENT Individuals with hereditary polyposis should begin screening at an early age (10 to 12 years) using colonoscopy with a consideration of prophylactic surgery.[367] Genetic markers in stool and blood are being developed.[373] Screening for nonhereditary CRC in asymptomatic individuals older than age 50 includes fecal occult blood and immunochemical tests, and sigmoidoscopy or colonoscopy.[374,375] A diet rich in vegetables, grains, fruit, and calcium and low in fat and red meat may modify cancer risk. Uncertainties remain in the dietary modulation of colon cancer.[376,377] In 8% to 29% of cases, bowel obstruction is the primary symptom at diagnosis.[378]

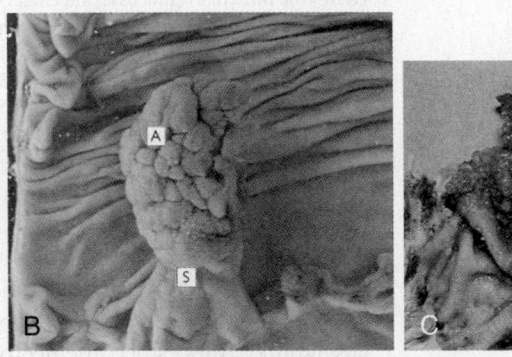

Transverse colon
Pain, obstruction, change
in bowel habits, anemia

**Ascending
colon**
Pain, mass,
change in
bowel habits,
anemia

Descending colon
Pain, change in
bowel habits,
bright red
blood in stool,
obstruction

Rectum
Blood in stool,
change in bowel habits,
rectal discomfort

A

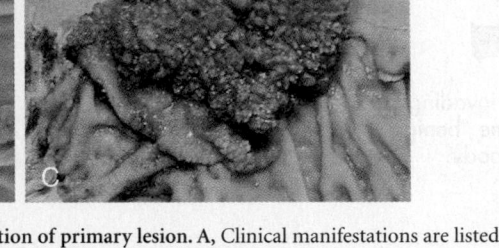

Figure 39-30 Signs and symptoms of colorectal cancer by location of primary lesion. **A,** Clinical manifestations are listed in order of frequency for each region (lymphatics of colon also shown). **B,** Tubular adenomata *(A)* are rounded lesions 0.5 to 2 cm in size that are generally red and sit on a stalk *(S)* of normal mucosa that has been dragged up by traction of the polyp in the bowel lumen. **C,** Villous adenomata are frondlike lesions about 0.6 cm thick that occupy a broad area of mucosa generally 1 to 5 cm in diameter. (B and C from Stevens A, Lowe J: *Pathology,* ed 2, London, 2000, Mosby.)

Table 39-11	Conditions Commonly Confused with Colorectal Cancer
Condition	**Significant Characteristics**
Diverticulitis	Left-sided pain similar to that of appendicitis; tender lower left quadrant. Associated findings: nausea, vomiting, fever, obstruction, anorexia, and leukocytosis; mucosa is intact, and perforation, peritonitis, and abscesses occur more often than in cancer; ultrasound, CT scan, MRI, and proctosigmoidoscopy are used to distinguish from cancer
Ulcerative colitis	Younger people with chronic attacks of bloody diarrhea, crampy abdominal pain, fever, malnutrition, and dehydration; usually involves the left colon and rectum; endoscopy, barium enema, and biopsy performed for definitive diagnosis
Crohn disease (granulomatous colitis)	Generally involves the right colon; chronic diarrhea with abdominal cramps, fever, weight loss, and often a palpable abdominal mass; difficult at times to distinguish Crohn disease from ulcerative colitis; endoscopic examination and CT scan used to distinguish from cancer
Appendicitis	Vague abdominal symptoms, often with a tender or nontender mass in the lower right quadrant; associated symptoms: mild fever and leukocytosis; CT scan used to distinguish cancer of the cecum from appendiceal abscess
Thrombosed hemorrhoids	Examination shows a tender, swollen, bluish painful mass in the anus; individual has a history of hemorrhoids

The staging of colorectal cancer involves preoperative testing and operative exploration. Preoperative testing begins with physical examination of the abdomen to detect liver enlargement and ascites and palpation of appropriate lymph nodes. Elevations of carcinoembryonic antigen (CEA) are often detected in the sera of individuals with colorectal carcinoma. The amount of CEA in the serum is a function of the stage of the disease and the type of tumor. Operative staging consists of careful exploration during surgery and biopsy of possible metastases. The National Cancer Institute[379] classification is widely used for staging of colorectal cancer and is as follows:

Stage 0 (carcinoma in situ): involves only the mucosal lining, also known as carcinoma in-situ

Stage I: extension of cancer to the middle layers of the colon wall, no spread to lymph nodes. Stage I colon cancer is sometimes called Dukes' A colon cancer.

Stage II: extension beyond the colon wall to nearby tissues around the colon or *rectum*, and/or through the *peritoneum*. Stage II colon cancer is sometimes called Dukes' B colon cancer.

Stage III: spread beyond the colon into lymph nodes and nearby organs and/or through the *peritoneum*. Stage III colon cancer is sometimes called Dukes' C colon cancer.

Stage IV: spread to nearby *lymph nodes* and has spread to other parts of the body, such as the *liver* or *lungs*. Stage IV colon cancer is sometimes called Dukes' D colon cancer.

Treatment for cancer of the colon is always surgical. The location and amount of colon resected depend on the site of the cancer. Resection and anastomosis can be performed for cancer of the ascending, transverse, descending, or sigmoid colon and upper rectum. These surgeries are performed through abdominal incisions, and natural defecation is preserved.

Growths in the lower portion of the rectum require removal of the entire rectum with formation of a permanent colostomy. Prognosis after surgery depends on the stage and location of the tumor.

Radiation therapy is often given before surgery in the hope that it will shrink the tumor, alter the malignant cells, or both so that these cells will not survive after surgery. Adjuvant chemotherapy is used to treat metastatic disease and cases with a high risk of recurrence. New chemotherapeutic agents are improving first line treatment.[380] Immunotherapy can boost the immune response.[381] Recombinant vaccines for colon cancer are in clinical trials.[382,383] Molecular prognostic markers are being developed.[384]

Cancer of the Accessory Organs of Digestion

Cancer of the Liver

Cancer of the liver is the fifth most common cause of cancer and the third leading cause of cancer death worldwide; however, the incidence is increasing as a result of chronic hepatitis B and C infection.[385] Cancer in the liver is usually caused by metastatic spread from a primary site elsewhere in the body. Liver cancer is relatively rare in the United States but is common in densely populated parts of the Far East, southern Africa, China, and Greece. The number of deaths in the United States from liver cancer is greatest among Asians and Pacific Islanders (the third leading cause of cancer deaths) and is higher in blacks and Hispanics compared with whites. For reasons not understood, incidence is higher in men than in women.[386] Primary liver cancer is rare before the age of 40 years and most common during the sixth decade. Together, primary and secondary liver cancer accounts for about 3% of all cancer deaths in the United States.[344] The incidence of hepatocellular carcinoma is increasing from dissemination of hepatitis B and, particularly, C infection.[387]

Risk factors for primary liver cancer include the following:

1. Infection with HBV, HCV, and HDV, particularly in conjunction with cirrhosis, acts either as a carcinogen or as a co-carcinogen in chronically infected hepatocytes.[388]
2. Chronic liver disease, especially cirrhosis.[389]
3. Exposure to mycotoxins. The most significant mycotoxins are the aflatoxins, particularly those produced by *Aspergillus flavus,* a mold found on spoiled corn, peanuts, and grain. Aflatoxins cause mutation of the *TP53* suppressor gene and activation of WNT signal transduction pathway.[390]
4. Heavy smoking and heavy drinking of alcohol.[391,392]
5. The presence of liver flukes (ingestion of raw fish) in Southeast Asia.[393]

PATHOGENESIS Primary carcinomas of the liver are hepatocellular or cholangiocellular. Hepatocellular carcinoma develops in the hepatocytes, whereas cholangiocellular carcinoma (cholangiocarcinoma) develops in the bile ducts. **Hepatocellular carcinoma (hepatocarcinoma) (HCC)** can be nodular (consisting of multiple, discrete nodules), massive (consisting of a large tumor mass having satellite nodules), or diffuse (consisting of very small nodules distributed throughout most of the liver). HCC is the type of primary liver cancer that is closely associated with cirrhosis (Figure 39-31). Chronic hepatitis and cirrhosis give rise to HCC repetitive cellular proliferation that occurs in the inflamed liver in response to growth factor and cytokine stimulation. Numerous genetic and epigenetic alterations, including failure of tumor-suppressor genes and signaling pathways, combine to promote carcinogenesis.[394,395] Because carcinoma of the liver invades the hepatic and portal veins, it often spreads to the heart and lungs. Other sites of metastases are the brain, kidney, and spleen.

Cholangiocellular carcinomas (cholangiocarcinoma) occur less often than hepatocellular carcinomas in the United States. This type of primary liver cancer is most common in areas where liver fluke infestation is prevalent in many parts of Southeast Asia. The mechanism by which fluke infestation causes cholangiocellular carcinoma is multifactorial and

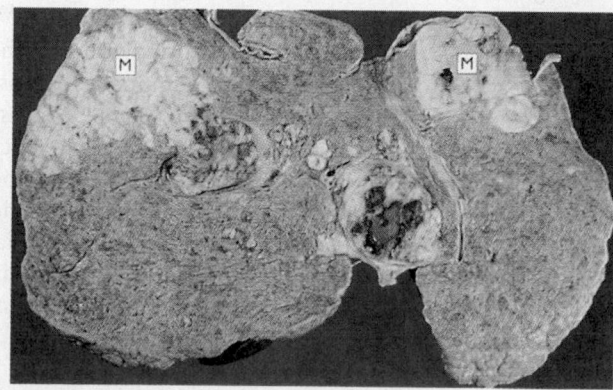

Figure 39-31 Hepatocellular carcinoma. Macroscopically, hepatocellular carcinomas may be single or multifocal. They usually develop in a liver already affected by cirrhosis. Tumor appears as an abnormal mass *(M)* within the liver. (From Stevens A, Lowe J: *Pathology,* ed 2, London, 2000, Mosby.)

includes parasite secretions, immunopathology, and mechanical damage.[388] Other risk factors include primary sclerosing cholangitis, hepatolithiasis, and choledochal cysts. However, most individuals diagnosed with cholangiocellular carcinoma do not have an identifiable risk factor.[396] Cholangiocellular carcinoma can occur anywhere along the bile duct and extend directly into the liver, usually as a solitary lesion. It is difficult to distinguish an invasion of cholangiocellular carcinoma from a metastatic adenocarcinoma except by neoplastic changes found in nearby ducts.

CLINICAL MANIFESTATIONS The clinical presentation of liver cancer in adults is characterized by vague abdominal symptoms, such as nausea and vomiting, fullness, pressure, dull ache in the right hypochondrium, and weight loss. Manifestations of hepatocellular carcinoma can occur slowly or abruptly. In individuals with cirrhosis, deepening jaundice or abrupt lack of appetite is a sign of hepatocellular carcinoma. Obstruction by the tumor can cause sudden worsening of portal hypertension and development of ascites. As the tumor enlarges, it causes pain. Cholangiocellular carcinoma more commonly presents insidiously as pain, loss of appetite, weight loss, and gradual onset of jaundice. Some carcinomas of the liver rupture spontaneously, causing hemorrhage. Others are discovered accidentally during evaluation of a bone fracture or surgical exploration.

EVALUATION AND TREATMENT There is no specific test for the diagnosis of liver cancer. For high-risk individuals alpha fetoprotein and abdominal ultrasound are common screening tools. The diagnosis is based on additional laboratory findings, radiologic examination, biopsy findings, and exploratory laparotomy.[397] Serum levels of alkaline phosphatase, aspartate aminotransferate (AST), and alanine aminotransferase (ALT) are commonly elevated in individuals with hepatocellular carcinoma. Excessive levels of alpha fetoprotein (>400 ng/ml) have been correlated with hepatitis B antigen, rapid tumor growth, and poor tumor differentiation. Erythrocytosis is secondary to erythropoietin production. Hepatitis B vaccination and antiviral treatment of hepatitis C will advance prevention of HCC.[398]

Staging of the tumor is important to guiding treatment but does not accurately predict postoperative outcome.[399] Surgical resection is possible in noncirrhotic individuals if the tumor is localized to a removable lobe. Tumors of the posterior segment of the right lobe are not resectable, because this segment contains the right hepatic vein. Radiofrequency (thermal) ablation has emerged as the most effective method for local tumor destruction.[400] Tyrosine kinase inhibitors and monoclonal antibodies are improving survival. Transarterial embolization and radiation is used for management of pain and to reduce tumor size. Surgical resection or liver transplant is the only alternative for cure.[401]

Cancer of the Gallbladder

Cancer of the gallbladder and biliary tract is a rare but lethal disease. It is more common in women than in men by a ratio of about 2 to 1.[344] It occurs rarely before age 40 and is most common between the ages of 50 and 60 years. Obesity is a risk factor. Native populations in North and South America have greater risk of gallbladder cancer, and it is more common in Chile, Poland, India, Japan, and Israel.[402,403] Most gallbladder cancer is caused by metastasis. Primary carcinoma of the gallbladder is rare and is usually associated with chronic cholecystitis and cholelithiasis.

PATHOGENESIS Most primary carcinomas of the gallbladder are adenocarcinomas. A few are squamous cell carcinomas; *TP53* gene mutation, altered expression of P-glycoprotein, COX-2, epidermal growth factor receptor, and *K-ras* gene mutation occur.[404] Invasion of the liver occurs early. Spreading progresses to the cystic and periportal lymph nodes with invasion of the pancreas and retroperitoneal lymph nodes. Direct invasion of the stomach and the duodenum can cause pyloric obstruction. Infection often accompanies cancer of the gallbladder. Generalized peritonitis, gangrene, perforation, and liver abscesses are potential complications of infection.

CLINICAL MANIFESTATIONS A typical presentation of carcinoma of the gallbladder is steady upper-right-quadrant pain for about 2 months. Other manifestations include diarrhea, belching, weakness, loss of appetite, weight loss, and vomiting. Obstructive jaundice can occur if an enlarging tumor presses on the extrahepatic ducts.

EVALUATION AND TREATMENT Early diagnosis of cancer of the gallbladder is not possible because of lack of symptoms, and individuals present with an advanced stage of disease. Individuals with gallstones, especially older women, are evaluated carefully. Inflammatory disorders, such as cholangitis (bile duct inflammation) and peritonitis, often obscure an underlying malignancy. The most specific diagnostic procedures include ultrasonography, CT, and MRI.

Complete surgical resection of the gallbladder is the only effective treatment. Because advanced malignancies cannot be resected, gallbladders containing stones are removed as a preventive measure. Palliative chemotherapy provides symptom improvement but does not improve survival.[405] The prognosis of gallbladder cancer is extremely poor; most individuals die within 1 to 2 years after surgery.[406]

Cancer of the Pancreas

Pancreatic cancer now ranks fourth in men in as a cause of cancer deaths in the United States. The incidence of pancreatic cancer rises steadily with age. Men are affected slightly more often than women and blacks more often than whites. Pancreatic cancer accounts for about 35,240 deaths annually in the United States.[344] Mortality is about 95% within 12 months. Pancreatic cancer is a disease of inherited and acquired mutation in cancer-related genes.[407] With the exception of an association of risk with cigarette smoking, no external risk factors have been identified.[408] Pancreatitis is associated with 50% of pancreatic cancers.[409]

PATHOGENESIS Cancer of the pancreas can arise from exocrine or endocrine cells. Most pancreatic tumors arise from exocrine cells in the ducts and are called *ductal adenocarcinomas*. Tumors arising in small ducts invade nearby glandular

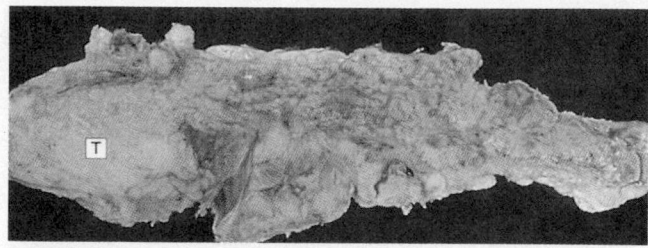

Figure 39-32 Hepatocellular carcinoma. Tumors appear as gritty, gray, hard nodules *(T)* irregularly invading the adjacent gland and local structures. (From Stevens A, Lowe J: *Pathology,* ed 2, London, 2000, Mosby.)

tissue, penetrate the covering of the pancreas, and extend into surrounding tissues.[410] A *K-ras* mutation is the most common genetic alteration; tumor suppressor gene alterations are also found, including *TP53, p16,* and *DCC.* Growth factors are overexpressed in ductal cancer.[411]

Ductal adenocarcinomas can occur in the head, body, or tail of the pancreas. Tumors of the head quickly spread to obstruct the common bile duct and portal vein (Figure 39-32). These tumors can then infiltrate the superior mesenteric artery, the vena cava, and the aorta. Cancer cells that enter the blood vessels can form emboli. Tumors of the body and tail infiltrate the posterior abdominal wall. Lymphatic invasion occurs early and rapidly and involves local and regional lymph nodes. Venous invasion causes metastases to the liver. Tumor implants on the peritoneal surface can obstruct veins and promote development of ascites.

Ductal adenocarcinomas arising in the head of the pancreas cause biliary obstruction somewhat early in the disease. Individuals with such tumors survive slightly longer than those with cancer of the body and tail, presumably because they seek medical attention earlier.

Tumors of the endocrine pancreas are rare neoplasms of the islets of Langerhans known as *apudomas.* The first four letters in *apudoma* derive from *amine precursor uptake* and *decarboxylation.* The apudomas are so named because they contain neurosecretory granules. Endocrine neoplasms secrete abnormal amounts of hormones, such as insulin.

CLINICAL MANIFESTATIONS Cancer of the body and tail of the pancreas is generally asymptomatic until there is intraductal obstruction or the tumor invades adjacent tissue. Often vague back pain is an initial symptom.[412] Jaundice develops in most cases, usually caused by obstruction of the bile duct. Because obstruction impairs enzyme secretion and flow to the duodenum, pancreatic cancer causes fat and protein malabsorption, resulting in weight loss. Distant metastases are found in the neck nodes, the lungs, and the brain. Most individuals die of hepatic failure, malnutrition, or systemic diseases.

EVALUATION AND TREATMENT Pancreatic cancer is usually at an advanced stage at the time of diagnosis and has a poor prognosis.[413] A laparotomy is often performed, particularly if jaundice is present. Ultrasonography, CT, or endoscopic retrograde cholangiopancreatography may be needed to confirm the need for a laparotomy, especially in individuals without jaundice. Laparotomy is used to establish a definitive diagnosis, evaluate the extent of disease, and determine whether palliative bypass surgery (i.e., cholecystojejunostomy and gastrojejunostomy) is needed. Most individuals require palliative double bypass of the blocked bile ducts, as well as gastrojejunostomy to prevent duodenal obstruction.

Many surgeons recommend a total pancreatectomy because cancer of the pancreas seldom consists of a single lesion.[414] Adjuvant chemotherapy and new systemic agents are improving survival.[415] Radiochemotherapy may produce favorable controls in locally advanced cancer.[416]

SUMMARY REVIEW

Disorders of the Gastrointestinal Tract

1. Anorexia (loss of appetite), vomiting, constipation, diarrhea, abdominal pain, and evidence of gastrointestinal bleeding are clinical manifestations of many disorders of the gastrointestinal tract.

2. Vomiting is the forceful emptying of the stomach effected by gastrointestinal contraction and reverse peristalsis of the esophagus. It is usually preceded by nausea and retching with the exception of projectile vomiting, which is associated with direct stimulation of the vomiting center in the brain.

3. Constipation is often caused by unhealthy dietary and bowel habits combined with lack of exercise. Constipation also can result from a neurogenic disorder, a disorder that impairs intestinal motility, or a disorder that obstructs the intestinal lumen.

4. Diarrhea can be caused by excessive fluid drawn into the intestinal lumen by osmosis (osmotic diarrhea), excessive secretion of fluids by the intestinal mucosa (secretory diarrhea), or excessive gastrointestinal motility.

5. Abdominal pain is caused by stretching, inflammation, or ischemia. Abdominal pain originates in the organs themselves (visceral pain) or in the peritoneum (parietal pain). Visceral pain is often referred to the back.

6. Gastrointestinal bleeding can occur in the upper or lower gastrointestinal tract. Obvious manifestations of gastrointestinal bleeding are hematemesis (vomiting of blood), melena (dark, tarry stools), and hematochezia (frank bleeding from the rectum). Occult bleeding can be detected only by testing stools or vomitus for the presence of blood.

7. Dysphagia is difficulty in swallowing. It can be caused by a mechanical or functional obstruction of the esophagus. Functional obstruction is an impairment of esophageal motility.

8. Achalasia is a form of functional dysphagia caused by loss of esophageal innervation or relaxation of the lower esophageal sphincter.

9. Gastroesophageal reflux is the regurgitation of chyme from the stomach into the esophagus. An inflammatory response (reflux esophagitis) ensues if the esophageal mucosa is repeatedly exposed to acids and enzymes in the regurgitated chyme.

10. Hiatal hernia is the protrusion of the upper part of the stomach through the hiatus (esophageal opening in the diaphragm) at the gastroesophageal junction. Hiatal hernia can be sliding or paraesophageal.

11. Pyloric obstruction is the narrowing or blockage of the pylorus, which is the opening between the stomach and the duodenum. It can be caused by a congenital defect, inflammation and scarring secondary to a gastric ulcer, or tumor growth.

12. Intestinal obstruction prevents the normal movement of chyme through the intestinal tract. It is usually mechanical—that is, caused by torsion, herniation, or tumor. Functional obstruction is caused by paralytic ileus.

13. The most severe consequences of intestinal obstruction are fluid and electrolyte losses, hypovolemia, shock, intestinal necrosis, and perforation of the intestinal wall.

14. Gastritis is an acute or a chronic inflammation of the gastric mucosa.

15. Regurgitation of bile, use of anti-inflammatory drugs or alcohol, H. pylori infection, and some systemic diseases are associated with gastritis.

16. Chronic fundal gastritis is rare and associated with autoantibodies to parietal cells and intrinsic factor resulting in gastric atrophy and pernicious anemia.

17. Chronic antral gastritis is the most common and is associated with H. pylori and NSAIDs.

18. A peptic ulcer is a circumscribed area of mucosal inflammation and ulceration caused by excessive secretion of gastric acid, disruption of the protective mucosal barrier, or both.

19. The three types of peptic ulcers are duodenal, gastric, and stress ulcers and they are usually caused by H. pylori infection or NSAIDs.

20. Duodenal ulcers, the most common peptic ulcers, are associated with increased numbers of parietal (acid-secreting) cells in the stomach, elevated gastrin levels, and rapid gastric emptying. Pain occurs when the stomach is empty, and pain is relieved with food or antacids. Duodenal ulcers tend to heal spontaneously and recur frequently.

21. Gastric ulcers develop near parietal cells, generally in the antrum, and tend to become chronic. Gastric secretions may be normal or decreased, and pain may occur after eating.

22. Zollinger-Ellison syndrome is associated with a gastrinoma, chronic secretion of gastric acid, and gastric and duodenal ulcers.

23. Ischemic stress ulcers develop suddenly after severe illness, systemic trauma, or neural injury. Ulceration follows mucosal damage caused by ischemia (decreased blood flow to the gastric mucosa).

24. Cushing ulcer is a stress ulcer caused by head trauma. Ulceration follows hypersecretion of hydrochloric acid caused by overstimulation of the vagal nuclei.

25. Postgastrectomy syndromes are long-term complications that follow gastrectomy—the resection of all or part of the stomach. The postgastrectomy syndromes include dumping syndrome, alkaline reflux gastritis, afferent loop obstruction, diarrhea, weight loss, and anemia.

26. Dumping syndrome is the rapid emptying of hypertonic chyme from the surgically created residual stomach into the small intestine. It causes an osmotic shift of fluid from the vascular compartment to the intestinal lumen, which decreases plasma volume.

27. Alkaline reflux gastritis is stomach inflammation caused by the reflux of bile and pancreatic secretions from the duodenum into the stomach. These substances disrupt the mucosal barrier and cause inflammation.

28. Afferent loop obstruction is an obstruction of the duodenal stump on the proximal side of a gastrojejunostomy. Biliary and pancreatic secretions accumulate in the stump, causing distention, intermittent pain, and vomiting.

29. Malabsorption syndromes result in impaired digestion or absorption of nutrients.

30. Pancreatic insufficiency causes malabsorption associated with insufficient amounts of the enzymes that digest protein, carbohydrates, and fats into components that can be absorbed by the intestine.

31. Deficient lactase production in the brush border of the small intestine inhibits the breakdown of lactose. This prevents lactose absorption and causes osmotic diarrhea.

32. Bile salt deficiency causes fat malabsorption, including fat soluble vitamins, and steatorrhea (fatty stools). Bile salt deficiency can result from inadequate secretion of bile, excessive bacterial deconjugation of bile, or impaired reabsorption of bile salts caused by ileal disease.

33. Ulcerative colitis is an inflammatory disease that causes ulceration, abscess formation, and necrosis of the colonic and rectal mucosa. Cramping pain, bleeding, frequent diarrhea, dehydration, and weight loss accompany severe forms of the disease. A course of frequent remissions and exacerbations is common.

34. Crohn disease is similar to ulcerative colitis, but it affects the large and small intestines, and ulceration tends to involve all the layers of the lumen. "Skip lesion" fissures and granulomas are characteristic of Crohn disease. Abdominal tenderness, nonbloody diarrhea, and weight loss are the usual symptoms.

35. Diverticula are outpouchings of colonic mucosa through the muscle layers of the colon wall. Diverticulosis is the presence of these outpouchings; diverticulitis is inflammation of the diverticula.

36. Appendicitis is the most common surgical emergency of the abdomen. Obstruction of the lumen leads to increased pressure, ischemia, and inflammation of the appendix. Without surgical resection, inflammation may progress to gangrene, perforation, and peritonitis.

37. Vascular insufficiency in the intestine is associated most often with acute or chronic occlusion or obstruction of the mesenteric vessels or insufficient arterial blood flow. The resulting ischemia and necrosis produce abdominal pain, fever, bloody diarrhea, hypovolemia, and shock.

38. Obesity is defined as a BMI greater than 30 from energy intake exceeding expenditure.

39. Single gene and polygenetic disorders are associated with obesity, as well as social, cultural, economic, exercise, and metabolic factors.

40. Increases in body fat mass are associated with increases in the adipokines leptin and resistin, as well as other hormones including insulin, ghrelin, and PYY. Adiponectin is decreased. Obesity may be associated with alterations in the expression and action of peripheral hormones and neurotransmitters that affect appetite and metabolic rate at the level of the hypothalamus.

41. Anorexia nervosa, or self-imposed starvation, is a psychogenic disorder primarily of adolescent and young women. It causes significant weight loss and developmental delays and can be fatal.

42. Bulimia nervosa (binge eating and purging) involves eating normal or large amounts of food and then purging by inducing vomiting or abusing laxatives. Severe weight loss is rare, but frequent vomiting causes tooth decay, pharyngitis, and esophagitis.

Continued

43. Short-term starvation, or lack of dietary intake for 3 or 4 days, stimulates mobilization of stored glucose by two metabolic processes: glycogenolysis (splitting of glycogen into glucose) and gluconeogenesis (formation of glucose from noncarbohydrate molecules).

44. Long-term starvation triggers the breakdown of ketone bodies and fatty acids. Eventually proteolysis (protein breakdown) begins, and death ensues if nutrition is not restored.

Disorders of the Accessory Organs of Digestion

1. Portal hypertension, ascites, hepatic encephalopathy, jaundice, and hepatorenal syndrome are complications of many liver disorders.

2. Portal hypertension is an elevation of portal venous pressure to at least 10 mmHg. It is caused by increased resistance to venous flow in the portal vein and its tributaries, including the sinusoids and hepatic vein.

3. Portal hypertension is the most serious complication of liver disease because it can cause fatal complications, such as bleeding varices, ascites, hepatic encephalopathy, and renal failure.

4. Hepatopulmonary syndrome is pulmonary hypertension associated with the release of vasodilators that effect pulmonary arterioles and is associated with portal hypertension and severe liver disease.

5. Splenomegaly is an enlargement of the spleen caused by increased splenic vein pressure caused by portal hypertension.

6. Ascites is the accumulation and sequestration of fluid in the peritoneal cavity, often as a result of portal hypertension, decreased concentrations of plasma proteins, and sodium retention.

7. Hepatic encephalopathy (portosystemic encephalopathy) is impaired cerebral function caused by blood-borne toxins (particularly ammonia) not metabolized by the liver.

8. Jaundice (icterus) is a yellow or greenish pigmentation of the skin or sclera of the eyes caused by increases in plasma bilirubin concentration (hyperbilirubinemia).

9. Obstructive jaundice is caused by obstructed bile canaliculi (intrahepatic obstructive jaundice) or obstructed bile ducts outside the liver (extrahepatic obstructive jaundice). Bilirubin accumulates proximal to sites of obstruction, enters the bloodstream, and is deposited in the skin and other connective tissues.

10. Hemolytic jaundice is caused by destruction of red blood cells at a rate that exceeds the liver's ability to metabolize unconjugated bilirubin.

11. Hepatorenal syndrome is functional kidney failure caused by advanced liver disease, particularly cirrhosis with portal hypertension. Renal failure is caused by a sudden decrease in blood flow to the kidneys, usually as a result of massive gastrointestinal hemorrhage or liver failure. Its chief clinical manifestation is oliguria.

12. Viral hepatitis is an infection of the liver caused by strains of the hepatitis virus: HAV, HBV, HCV, HDV, HEV, and HGV. HAV and HEV are transmitted via the fecal-oral route. The hepatitis viruses are blood-borne and can cause hepatic cell necrosis, Kupffer cell hyperplasia, and infiltration of liver tissue by mononuclear phagocytes. These changes obstruct bile flow and impair hepatocyte function.

13. The clinical manifestations of viral hepatitis depend on the stage of infection. Fever, malaise, anorexia, and liver enlargement and tenderness characterize the prodromal phase (stage 1). Jaundice and hyperbilirubinemia mark the icteric phase (stage 2). During the recovery phase (stage 3), symptoms resolve. Recovery takes several weeks.

14. Chronic active hepatitis can occur with HBV and HCV with predisposition to cirrhosis and hepatocellular carcinoma.

15. Fulminant hepatitis is a complication of hepatitis B (with or without hepatitis D infection) or hepatitis C. It causes widespread hepatic necrosis and is often fatal.

16. Cirrhosis is an inflammatory disease of the liver that causes disorganization of lobular structure, fibrosis, and nodular regeneration. Cirrhosis can result from hepatitis or exposure to toxins, such as acetaldehyde (a product of alcohol metabolism). The disease causes progressive irreversible liver damage, usually over a period of years.

17. Alcoholic cirrhosis impairs the hepatocytes' ability to oxidize fatty acids, synthesize enzymes and proteins, degrade hormones, and clear portal blood of ammonia and toxins. The inflammatory response includes excessive collagen formation, fibrosis, and scarring, which obstruct bile canaliculi and sinusoids. Bile obstruction causes jaundice. Vascular obstruction causes portal hypertension, shunting, and varices.

18. Primary biliary cirrhosis is an autoimmune disease with inflammatory destruction of intrahepatic bile ducts. Mitochondrial autoantibodies are found in this disease.

19. Secondary biliary cirrhosis develops from prolonged obstruction of bile flow with increased pressure in the hepatic bile ducts that causes pooling of bile and necrosis of tissue. Relief of obstruction relieves symptoms of jaundice and pruritus. Continued obstruction causes cirrhosis and liver failure.

20. Cholelithiasis (the formation of gallstones) is a common disorder of the gallbladder. Gallstones form in the bile as a result of the aggregation of cholesterol crystals (cholesterol stones) or precipitates of unconjugated bilirubin (pigmented stones). Gallstones that fill the gallbladder or obstruct the cystic, or common, bile duct cause abdominal pain and jaundice.

21. Cholecystitis is an inflammation of the gallbladder. It is usually associated with obstruction of the cystic duct by gallstones.

22. Acute pancreatitis (pancreatic inflammation) is a serious but relatively rare disorder associated with biliary obstruction and alcoholism. Injury permits leakage of digestive enzymes into pancreatic tissue, where they become activated and begin the process of autodigestion, inflammation, and destruction of tissues. Release of pancreatic enzymes into the bloodstream or abdominal cavity causes damage to other organs.

23. Chronic pancreatitis results from structural or functional impairment of the pancreas usually related to alcoholism. It causes recurrent abdominal pain and digestive disorders.

Cancer of the Digestive System

1. Cancer of the esophagus is rare and tends to occur in people older than 60 years. Alcohol and tobacco use, reflux esophagitis, radiation exposure, and nutritional deficiencies are associated with esophageal carcinoma.

2. Dysphagia and chest pain are the primary manifestations of esophageal cancer. Early treatment of tumors that have not spread into the mediastinum or lymph nodes results in a good prognosis.

3. Gastric carcinoma is associated with *H. pylori* (CagA), high salt intake, food preservatives (nitrates and nitrites), and atrophic gastritis.

4. Approximately 50% of all gastric cancers are located in the prepyloric antrum. Clinical manifestations (weight loss, upper abdominal pain, vomiting, hematemesis, anemia) develop only after the tumor has penetrated the wall of the stomach.

Continued

SUMMARY REVIEW—cont'd

5. Cancer of the colon and rectum (colorectal cancer) is the second most common cancer death in the United States. Small intestinal cancers are rare. Familial adenomatous polyposis coli is an inherited form of colon cancer. Preexisting large and numerous polyps are highly associated with sporadic adenocarcinoma of the colon.

6. Tumors of the right (ascending) colon are usually large and bulky; tumors of the left (descending, sigmoid) colon develop as small button-like masses. Manifestations of colon tumors include pain, bloody stools, and change in bowel habits.

7. Rectal carcinoma is located up to 15 cm from the opening of the anus. The tumor spreads transmurally to the vagina in women or to the prostate in men.

8. Metastatic invasion of the liver is more common than primary cancer of the liver.

9. Primary liver cancers are associated with chronic liver disease (cirrhosis and hepatitis B and C). Hepatocellular carcinomas arise from the hepatocytes, whereas cholangiocellular carcinomas arise from the bile ducts. Primary liver cancer spreads to the heart, lungs, brain, kidney, and spleen through the circulation.

10. Cancer of the gallbladder is relatively rare and tends to occur in women older than 50 years. Adenocarcinoma is most common. Because clinical manifestations occur late in the disease, metastases to lymph channels have usually occurred by the time of diagnosis, and the prognosis is poor.

11. Cancer of the pancreas ranks fifth as a cause of cancer deaths. The one known risk factor is heavy cigarette smoking. Most tumors are adenocarcinomas that arise in the exocrine cells of ducts in the head, body, or tail of the pancreas. Symptoms may not be evident until the tumor has spread to surrounding tissues. Treatment is palliative, and mortality is nearly 100%.

KEY TERMS

Achalasia, 1457
Acute gastritis, 1463
Acute occlusion of mesenteric artery blood flow (acute mesenteric ischemia), 1477
Acute pancreatitis (acute hemorrhagic pancreatitis), 1496
Afferent loop obstruction, 1470
Alcoholic cirrhosis, 1492
Alcoholic hepatitis, 1492
Alkaline reflux gastritis, 1469
Anal carcinoma, 1500
Anorexia, 1452
Anorexia nervosa (AN), 1480
Appendicitis, 1475
Ascites, 1483
Biliary cirrhosis, 1493
Bulimia nervosa, 1481
Cholangiocellular carcinoma (cholangiocarcinoma), 1503
Cholecystitis, 1495
Cholelithiasis, 1494
Chronic active hepatitis, 1490
Chronic alcoholic hepatitis, 1492
Chronic gastritis, 1464
Chronic mesenteric insufficiency, 1477
Chronic pancreatitis, 1497
Cirrhosis, 1491
Constipation, 1453
Crohn disease (CD), 1473
Curling ulcer, 1467
Cushing ulcer, 1467
Diarrhea, 1454
Diverticula (sing., diverticulum), 1474
Diverticulitis, 1474
Diverticulosis, 1474
Dumping syndrome, 1468
Duodenal ulcer, 1465
Dysphagia, 1456
Eosinophilic esophagitis, 1459
Esophageal varices, 1483

Fulminant hepatitis, 1491
Gallstone, 1494
Gastric ulcer, 1467
Gastritis, 1463
Gastroesophageal reflux disease (GERD), 1458
Gluconeogenesis, 1481
Glycogenolysis, 1481
Hematemesis, 1456
Hematochezia, 1456
Hemolytic jaundice (prehepatic jaundice, nonobstructive jaundice), 1486
Hepatic encephalopathy, 1485
Hepatocellular carcinoma (hepatocarcinoma; HCC), 1503
Hepatopulmonary syndrome, 1483
Hepatorenal syndrome (HRS), 1487
Hiatal hernia, 1459
Hyperbilirubinemia, 1485
Icteric phase (jaundice), 1490
Incubation phase of hepatitis, 1490
Intestinal obstruction, 1460
Irritable bowel syndrome (IBS), 1476
Ischemic ulcer, 1467
Jaundice (icterus), 1485
Kwashiorkor, 1481
Lactase deficiency, 1470
Large bowel obstruction, 1461
Leptin resistance, 1479
Long-term starvation, 1481
Lower gastrointestinal bleeding, 1456
Malabsorption, 1470
Maldigestion, 1470
Marasmus, 1481
Melena, 1456
Mesenteric venous thrombosis, 1477
Motility diarrhea, 1455
Mucosa-associated lymphoid tissue (MALT) lymphoma, 1499
Nausea, 1453

Obesity, 1477
Obstructive jaundice, 1485
Occult bleeding, 1456
Osmotic diarrhea, 1454
Polyp, 1500
Pancreatic insufficiency, 1470
Pancreatitis, 1495
Paraesophageal hiatal hernia, 1459
Paralytic ileus, 1460
Parietal pain, 1455
Peptic ulcer, 1464
Polyp, 1500
Portal hypertension, 1482
Primary biliary cirrhosis, 1493
Prodromal (preicteric) phase, 1490
Projectile vomiting, 1453
Pyloric obstruction, 1460
Recovery phase, 1490
Rectal carcinoma, 1501
Referred pain, 1456
Reflux esophagitis, 1458
Retching, 1453
Secondary biliary cirrhosis, 1493
Secretory diarrhea, 1454
Short bowel syndrome, 1474
Short-term starvation, 1481
Sliding hiatal hernia, 1459
Small intestine carcinoma, 1500
Small intestine obstruction, 1461
Splenomegaly, 1483
Starvation, 1481
Stress ulcer (stress-related mucosal disease), 1467
Ulcerative colitis (UC), 1471
Upper gastrointestinal bleeding, 1456
Viral hepatitis, 1488
Visceral pain, 1455
Vomiting, 1452
Zollinger-Ellison syndrome, 1467

REFERENCES

1. Meadows N: The central control of vomiting, *J Pediatr Gastroenterol Nutr* 21(Suppl 1):S20-S21, 1995.
2. Navari RM: Prevention of emesis from multiple-day and high-dose chemotherapy regimens, *J Natl Compr Canc Netw* 5(1):51-59, 2007.
3. Santucci G, Mack JW: Common gastrointestinal symptoms in pediatric palliative care: nausea, vomiting, constipation, anorexia, cachexia, *Pediatr Clin North Am* 54(5):673-689, 2007.
4. Talley NJ: Definitions, epidemiology, and impact of chronic constipation, *Rev Gastroenterol Disord* 4(Suppl 2):S3-S10, 2004.
5. Loening-Baucke V: Prevalence rates for constipation and faecal and urinary incontinence, *Arch Dis Child* 92(6):486-489, 2007.
6. Mitolo-Chieppa D et al: Cholinergic stimulation and nonadrenergic, noncholinergic relaxation of human colonic circular muscle in idiopathic chronic constipation, *Dig Dis Sci* 43(12):2719-2726, 1998.
7. Spinzi GC: Bowel care in the elderly, *Dig Dis* 25(2):160-165, 2007.
8. Panchal SJ, Muller-Schwefe P, Wurzelmann JI: Opioid-induced bowel dysfunction: prevalence, pathophysiology and burden, *Int J Clin Pract* 61(17):1181-1187, 2007.
9. Rao SS: Constipation: evaluation and treatment of colonic and anorectal motility disorders, *Gastroenterol Clin North Am* 36(3):686-711, 2007.
10. Chiarioni G, Heymen S, Whitehead WE: Biofeedback therapy for dyssnergic defecation, *World J Gastroenterol* 12(44):7069-7074, 2006.
11. Feldman M, Friedman LS, Brandt LJ: *Sleisenger & Fordtran's Gastrointestinal and Liver Diseases*. vol. 1, ed 8, Philadelphia, 2006, Saunders.
12. Spiller R: Role of motility in chronic diarrhoea, *Neurogastroenterol Motil* 18(12):1045-1055, 2006.
13. Sellin JH: A practical approach to treating patients with chronic diarrhea, *Rev Gastroenterol Disord* 7(Supp l3):S19-S26, 2007.
14. Al-Chaer ED, Traub RJ: Biological basis of visceral pain: recent developments, *Pain* 96(3):221-225, 2002.
15. Vergnolle N: Postinflammatory visceral sensitivity and pain mechanisms, *Neurogastroenterol Motil* 20(Suppl 1):73-80, 2008.
16. DiMaio CJ, Stevens PD: Nonvariceal upper gastrointestinal bleeding, *Gastrointest Endosc Clin North Am* 17(2):253-272, 2007:v, 2007.
17. Edelman DA, Sugawa C: Lower gastrointestinal bleeding: a review, *Surg Endosc* 21(4):514-520, 2007.
18. Killip S, Bennett JM, Chambers MD: Iron deficiency anemia, *Am Fam Physician* 75(5):671-678, 2007.
19. Vela MF, Vaezi MF: Cost-assessment of alternative management strategies for achalasia, *Expert Opin Pharmacother* 4(11):2019-2025, 2003.
20. Boeckxstaens GE: Achalasia, *Best Pract Res Clin Gastroenterol* 21(4):595-608, 2007.
21. Nellemann H et al: Bread and barium: diagnostic value in patients with suspected primary esophageal motility disorders, *Acta Radiol* 41(2):145-150, 2000.
22. Smout AJ: Advances in esophageal motor disorders, *Curr Opin Gastroenterol* 24(4):485-489, 2008.
23. Pohl D, Tutuian R: Achalasia: an overview of diagnosis and treatment, *J Gastrointestin Liver Dis* 16(3):297-303, 2007.
24. Long JD, Orlando RC: Nonerosive reflux disease, *Minerva Gastroenterol Dietol* 53(2):127-141, 2007.
25. Richter JE: Gastroesophageal reflux disease, *Best Pract Res Clin Gastroenterol* 21(4):609-631, 2007.
26. Havemann BD, Henderson CA, El-Serag HB: The association between gastro-oesphageal reflux disease and asthma: a systematic review, *Gut* 56(12):1654-1664, 2007.
27. Johanson JF: Epidemiology of esophageal and supraesophageal reflux injuries, *Am J Med* 108(Suppl 41):99S, 2000.
28. Orlando RC: Mechanisms of reflux-induced epithelial injuries in the esophagus, *Am J Med* 108(Suppl 4a):104S, 2000.
29. Rajendra S et al: *Helicobacter pylori*, ethnicity, and the gastroesophageal reflux disease spectrum: a study from the East, *Helicobacter* 12(2):177-183, 2007.
30. Holmes RS, Vaughan TL: Epidemiology and pathogenesis of esophageal cancer, *Semin Radiat Oncol* 17(1):2-9, 2007.
31. Anderson LA et al: Relationship between *Helicobacter pylori* infection and gastric atrophy and the stages of the oesophageal inflammation, metaplasia, adenocarcinoma sequence: results from the FINAR case-control study, *Gut* 57(6):734-739, 2008.
32. Sqouros SN, Mantides A: Refractory heartburn to proton pump inhibitors: epidemiology, etiology and management, *Digestion* 73(4):218-227, 2006.
33. Haggitt RC: Histopathology of reflux-induced esophageal and supraesophageal injuries, *Am J Med* 108(Suppl 4a):109S, 2000.
34. Hornick JL, Odze RD: Neoplastic precursor lesions in Barrett's esophagus, *Gastroenterol Clin North Am* 36(4):775-796, 2007.
35. Holmes RL, Fadden CT: Evaluation of the patient with chronic cough, *Am Fam Physician* 69(9):2159-2166, 2004.
36. Vaezi MF: Extraesophageal manifestations of gastroesophageal reflux disease, *Clin Cornerstone* 5(4):32-38, 2003:discussion 39-40, 2003.
37. Levine MS, Rubesin SE, Laufer I: Barium esophagography: a study for all seasons, *Clin Gastroenterol Hepatol* 6(1):11-25, 2008.
38. Tytgat GN et al: New algorithm for the treatment of gastro-oesphageal reflux disease, *Aliment Pharmacol Ther* 27(3):249-256, 2008.
39. Vakil N: Review article: the role of surgery in gastro-oesophageal reflux disease, *Aliment Pharmacol Ther* 25(12):1365-1372, 2007.
40. Blanchard C, Rothenberg ME: Basic pathogenesis of eosinophilic esophagitis, *Gastrointest Endosc Clin North Am* 18(1):133-143, 2008.
41. Straumann A: The natural history and complications of eosinophilic esophagitis, *Gastrointest Endosc Clin North Am* 18(1):99-118, 2008.
42. Boushey RP et al: Laparoscopic repair of paraesophageal hernias: a Canadian experience, *Can J Surg* 51(5):355-360, 2008.
43. Karmali S et al: Primary laparoscopic and open repair of paraesophageal hernias: a comparison of short-term outcomes, *Dis Esophagus* 21(1):63-68, 2008.
44. Stawowy M et al: Endoscopic stenting for malignant gastric outlet obstruction, *Surg Laparosc Endosc Percutan Tech* 17(1):5-9, 2007.
45. Maron DF, Fry RD: New therapies in the treatment of postoperative ileus after gastrointestinal surgery, *Am J Ther* 15(1):59-65, 2008.
46. Attard JA, MacLean AR: Adhesive small bowel obstruction: epidemiology, biology and prevention, *Can J Surg* 50(4):291-300, 2007.
47. Tumage RH, Heldmann M, Cole P: Intestinal obstruction and ileus. In Feldman M, Friedman LS, Lawrence BL, editors: *Sleisenger & Fordtran's gastrointestinal and liver disease*, ed 8, Saunders, 2006, Philadelphia.
48. Cappell MS, Batke M: Mechanical obstruction of the small bowel and colon, *Med Clin North Am* 92(3):575-577, 2008:viii, 2008.
49. Cerro P et al: Sonographic diagnosis of intussusceptions in adults, *Abdom Imaging* 25(1):45, 2000.
50. Maglinte DD et al: Small-bowel obstruction: state-of-the-art imaging and its role in clinical management, *Clin Gastroenterol Hepatol* 6(2):130-139, 2008.
51. McNamara R, Mihalakis MJ: Acute colonic pseudo-obstruction: rapid correction with neostigmine in the emergency department, *J Emerg Med* 35(2):167-170, 2008.
52. Parfitt JR, Driman DK: Pathological effects of drugs on the gastrointestinal tract: a review, *Hum Pathol* 38(4):527-536, 2007.
53. Yardley JH, Hendrix TR: Gastritis and gastropathy. In Yamada T, Alpers DH, Laine L, editors: *Atlas of gastroenterology*, ed 3, Philadelphia, 1999, Lippincott Williams & Wilkins.
54. Neesse A et al: Multifiocal early gastric cancer in a patient with autoimmune atrophic gastritis and iron defciency anaemia, *Z Gastroenterol* 47(2):223-227, 2009.
55. Kapadia CR: Gastric atrophy, metaplasia, and dysplasia: a clinical perspective, *J Clin Gastroenterol* 36(5 Suppl):S29-S36, 2003:discussion S61-S62, 2003.
56. D'Elios MM et al: Gastric autoimmunity: the role of *Helicobacter pylori* and molecular mimicry, *Trends Mol Med* 10(7):316-323, 2004.
57. Oksanen A et al: Atrophic gastritis and *Helicobacter pylori* infection in outpatients referred for gastroscopy, *Gut* 46(4):460, 2000.
58. Presotto F et al: *Helicobacter pylori* infection and gastric autoimmune disease: is there a link? *Helicobacter* 8(6):578-584, 2003.
59. Annibale B, Laqhner E: Assessing the severity of atrophic gastritis, *Eur J Gastroenterol Hepatol* 19(12):1059-1063, 2007.
60. Boyanova L et al: Prevalence and evolution of *Helicobacter pylori* resistance to 6 antibacterial agents over 12 years and correlation between susceptibility testing methods, *Diagn Microbiol Infect Dis* 60(4):409-415, 2008.
61. Erkurt MA et al: Effects of cyanocobalamin on immunity in patients with pernicious anemia, *Med Princ Pract* 17(2):131-135, 2008.
62. Lethbridge-Cejku M, Vickerie J: Summary health statistics for U.S. adults: National Health Interview Survey, 2003, *Vital Health Stat* 10(225), 2005.

63. Goodwin RD, Stein MB: Generalized anxiety disorder and peptic ulcer disease among adults in the United States, *Psychosom Med* 64:862-866, 2002.

64. Razvodovsky YE: Suicide and stomach ulcer mortality rate in Russia, *Psychiatr Danub* 19(1-2):35-41, 2007.

65. Levenstein S: The very model of a modern etiology: a biopsychosocial view of peptic ulcer [review], *Psychosom Med* 62(2):176, 2000.

66. Hobsley M, Tovey FI, Holton J: Precise role of *H. pylori* in duodenal ulceration, *World J Gastroenterol* 12(40):6413-6419, 2006.

67. Ji KY, Hu FL: Interaction or relationship between *Helicobacter pylori* and non-steroidal anti-inflammatory drugs in upper gastrointestinal diseases, *World J Gastroenterol* 12(24):3789-3792, 2006.

68. Kurata JH: Epidemiology of peptic ulcer disease. In Swabb EA, Szabo S, editors: *Investigation and basis for therapy*, New York, 1991, Marcel Dekker.

69. Schineller BA, Ramchandani D: Psychologic factors associated with peptic ulcer disease, *Med Clin North Am* 75(4):865, 1991.

70. Kuyvenhoven JP, Veenendaal RA, Vandenbroucke JP: Peptic ulcer bleeding: interaction between non-steroidal anti-inflammatory drugs, *Helicobacter pylori* infection, and the ABO blood group system, *Scand J Gastroenterol* 34(11):1082-1086, 1999.

71. Sharara AI et al: Association of gastroduodenal disease phenotype with ABO blood group and *Helicobacter pylori* virulence-specific serotypes, *Dig Liver Dis* 38(11):829-833, 2006.

72. Gisbert JP et al: *H. pylori*-negative duodenal ulcer prevalence and causes in 774 patients, *Dig Dis Sci* 44(11):2295, 1999.

73. Tovey FI, Hobsley M: Is *Helicobacter pylori* the primary cause of duodenal ulceration? *J Gastroenterol Hepatol* 14(11):1053, 1999.

74. Axon AT: Relationship between *Helicobacter pylori* gastritis, gastric cancer and gastric acid secretion, *Adv Med Sci* 52:55-60, 2007.

75. Hirschi AM, Makristathis A: Methods to detect *Helicobacter pylori*: from culture to molecular biology, *Helicobacter* 12(Suppl 2):6-11, 2007.

76. Chuang CH et al: Adjuvant effect of vitamin C on omeprazole-amoxicillin-clarithromycin triple therapy for *Helicobacter pylori* eradication, *Hepatogastroenterology* 54(73):320-324, 2007.

77. Ramakrishna K, Salinas RC: Peptic ulcer disease, *Am Fam Physician* 76(7):1005-1012, 2007.

78. Aldoori WH et al: Prospective study of diet and the risk of duodenal ulcer in men, *Am J Epidemiol* 145(1):42, 1997.

79. Agarwal K, Agarwal S: *Helicobacter pylori* vaccine: from past to future, *Mayo Clin Proc* 83(2):169-175, 2008.

80. Kamada T et al: endoscopic characteristics and *Helicobacter pylori* infection in NSAID-associated gastric ulcer, *J Gastroenterol Hepatol* 21(1 Pt 1):98-102, 2006.

81. Vere CC et al: Endoscopical and histological features in bile reflux gastritis, *Rom J Morphol Embryol* 46(4):269-274, 2005.

82. Anlauf M et al: Sporadic versus hereditary gastrinomas of the duodenum and pancreas: distinct clinico-pathological and epidemiological features, *World J Gastroenterol* 12(34):5440-5446, 2005.

83. Campana D et al: Zollinger-Ellison syndrome: Diagnosis and therapy, *Minerva Med* 96(3):187-206, 2005.

84. Stollman N, Metz DC: Pathophysiology and prophylaxis of stress ulcer in intensive care unit patients, *J Crit Care* 20(1):35-45, 2005.

85. Yang YX, Lewis JD: Prevention and treatment of stress ulcers in critically ill patients, *Semin Gastroenterol Dis* 14(1):11-19, 2003.

86. Klebl FH, Scholmerich J: Therapy insight: prophylaxis of stress-induced gastrointestinal bleeding in critically ill patients, *Nat Clin Pract Gasteroenterol Hepatol* 4(10):562-570, 2007.

87. Lipof T, Shapiro D, Kozol RA: Surgical perspectives in peptic ulcer disease and gastritis, *World J Gastroenterol* 12(20):3248-3252, 2006.

88. Martin RF: Surgical management of ulcer disease, *Surg Clin North Am* 85(5):907-929, 2005.

89. Tack J: Gastric motor disorders, *Best Pract Res Clin Gastroenterol* 21(4):633-644, 2007.

90. Ukleja A: Dumping syndrome: pathophysiology and treatment, *Nutr Clin Pract* 20(5):517-525, 2005.

91. Carvajal SH, Mulvihill SJ: Postgastrectomy syndromes: dumping and diarrhea, *Gastroenterol Clin North Am* 23(2):261, 1994.

92. Karamanolis G, Tack J: Nutrition and motility disorders, *Best Pract Res Clin Gastroenterol* 20(3):485-505, 2006.

93. Pedrazzani C et al: Postoperative complications and functional results after subtotal gastrectomy with Billroth II reconstruction for primary gastric cancer, *Dig Dis Sci* 52(8):1757-1763, 2007.

94. Didden P, Penning C, Masclee AA: Octreotide therapy in dumping syndrome: analysis of long-term results, *Aliment Pharmacol Ther* 24(9):1367-1375, 2006.

95. Zobolas B et al: Alkaline reflux gastritis: early and late results of surgery, *World J Surg* 30(6):1043-1049, 2006.

96. Kim HC et al: Afferent loop obstruction after gastric cancer surgery: helical CT findings, *Abdom Imaging* 28(5):624-630, 2003.

97. Beyan C et al: Post-gastrectomy anemia: evaluation of 72 cases with post-gastrectomy anemia, *Hematology* 12(1):81-84, 2007.

98. Ferrone M, Raimondo M, Scolapio JS: Pancreatic enzyme pharmacotherapy, *Pharmacotherapy* 27(6):910-920, 2007.

99. Kuokkanen M et al: Mutation in the translated region of the lactase gene (LCT) underlie congenital lactase deficiency, *Am J Hum Genet* 78(2):339-344, 2006.

100. Troelsen JT: Adult-type hypolactasia and regulation of lactase expression, *Biochem Biophys Acta* 1723(1-3):19-32, 2005.

101. Heyman MB et al: Lactose intolerance in infants, children, and adolescents, *Pediatrics* 118(3):1279-1286, 2006.

102. Obermayer-Pietsch BM et al: Adult-type hypolactasia and calcium availability: decreased calcium intake or impaired calcium absorption? *Osteoporosis Int* 18(4):445-451, 2007.

103. Norlin M, Wikvall K: Enzymes in the conversion of cholesterol into bile acids, *Curr Mol Med* 7(2):199-218, 2007.

104. Loftus CG et al: Update on the incidence and prevalence of Crohn's disease in ulcerative colitis in Olmstead County, Minnesota, 1940-2000, *Inflamm Bowel Dis* 13(3):254-261, 2007.

105. Baumgart DC: What's new in inflammatory bowel disease in 2008? *World J Gastroenterol* 14(3):329-330, 2008.

106. Scaldaferri F, Fiocchi C: Inflammatory bowel disease: progress and current concepts of etiopathogenesis, *J Dig Dis* 8(4):171-178, 2007.

107. Karban A, Eliakim R: Effect of smoking on inflammatory bowel disease: is it disease or organ specific? *World J Gastroenterol* 13(15):2150-2152, 2007.

108. Packey CD, Sartor RB: Interplay of commensal and pathogenic bacteria, genetic mutations, and immunoregulatory defects in the pathogenesis of inflammatory bowel diseases, *J Intern Med* 263(6):597-606, 2008.

109. Zhong W et al: Chemokines orchestrate leukocyte trafficking in inflammatory bowel disease, *Front Biosci* 13:1654-1664, 2008.

110. Thoreson R, Cullen JJ: Pathophysiology of inflammatory bowel disease, *Surg Clin North Am* 87(3):575-585, 2007.

111. Baumgart DC, Sandborn WJ: Inflammatory bowel disease: clinical aspects and established and evolving therapies, *Lancet* 369(9573):1641-1657, 2007.

112. Xie J, Itzkowitz SH: Cancer in inflammatory bowel disease, *World J Gastroenterol* 14(3):378-389, 2008.

113. Agrawal D, Rukkannagari S, Kethu S: Pathogenesis and clinical approach to extraintestinal manifestations of inflammatory bowel disease, *Minerva Gastroenterol Dietol* 53(3):233-248, 2007.

114. Denese S et al: Inflammation and coagulation in inflammatory bowel disease: the clot thickens, *Am J Gastroenterol* 102(1):174-186, 2007.

115. Freeman HJ: Venous thromboembolism with inflammatory bowel disease, *World J Gastroenterol* 14(7):991-993, 2008.

116. Nikolaus S, Schreiber S: Diagnostics of inflammatory bowel disease, *Gastroenterology* 133(5):1670-1689, 2007.

117. Hanauer SG: Risks and benefits of combining immunosuppressives and biological agents in inflammatory bowel disease: is the synergy worth the risk? *Gut* 56(9):1181-1183, 2007.

118. Lakatos PL, Szamosi T, Lakatos L: Smoking in inflammatory bowel disease: good, bad or ugly? *World J Gastroenterol* 13(46):6134-6139, 2007.

119. McGilligan VE et al: Hypothesis about mechanisms through which nicotine might exert its effect on the interdependence of inflammation and gut barrier function in ulcerative colitis, *Inflamm Bowel Dis* 13(1):108-115, 2007.

120. Ba'ath ME et al: Surgical management of inflammatory bowel disease, *Arch Dis Child* 92(4):312-316, 2007.

121. Caprilli R, Viscido A, Latella G: Current management of severe ulcerative disease, *Nat Clin Pract Gastroenterol Hepatol* 4(2):92-101, 2007.

122. Brant SR et al: A population-based case-control study of CARD15 and other risk factors in Crohn's disease and ulcerative colitis, *Am J Gastroenterol* 102(2):313-323, 2007.

123. de Mesquita MB, Cvitelli F: Levine A: Epidemiology, genes and inflammatory bowel diseases in childhood, *Dig Liver Dis* 40(1):3011, 2007.

124. Ng AZ-VS-S et al: Associate of the T allele of an intronic single nucleotide polymorphism in the colony stimulating factor 1 receptor with Crohn's disease: a case-control study, *J Immune Based Ther Vaccines* 2:6, 2004.

125. Bruzzese E et al: Microflora in inflammatory bowel diseases: a pediatric perspective, *J Clin Gastroenterol* 38(6 Suppl):S91-S93, 2004.

126. Darfeuille-Michaud A et al: High prevalence of adherent-invasive *Escherichia coli* associated with ileal mucosa in Crohn's disease, *Gastroenterology* 127(2):412-421, 2004.

127. Shinzaki S et al: IgG oligosaccharide alterations are a novel diagnostic marker for disease activity and the clinical course of inflammatory bowel disease, *Am J Gastroenterol* 103(5):1173-1181, 2008.

128. Shah SB, Hanauer SB: Treatment of diarrhea in patients with inflammatory bowel disease: concepts and cautions, *Rev Gastroenterol Disord* 7(Suppl 3):S3-S10, 2007.

129. Allison MC et al: *Inflammatory bowel disease*, St Louis, 1998, Mosby.

130. Friedman S: Cancer in Crohn's disease, *Gastroenterol Clin North Am* 35(3):621-639, 2006.

131. Behm BW, Bickston SJ: Tumor necrosis factor-alpha for maintenance of remission in Crohn's disease, *Cochrane Database Syst Rev* (1):CD006893, 2008.

132. Casillas S, Delaney CP: Larparoscopic surgery for inflammatory bowel disease, *Dig Surg* 22(3):135-142, 2005.

133. Tursi A: New physiopathological and therapeutic approaches to diverticular disease of the colon, *Expert Opin Pharmacother* 8(3):299-307, 2007.

134. Petruzziello L et al: Review article: uncomplicated diverticular disease of the colon, *Aliment Pharmacol Ther* 23(10):1379-1391, 2006.

135. Colecchia A et al: Diverticular disease of the colon: new perspectives in symptom development and treatment, *World J Gastroenterol* 9(7):1385-1389, 2003.

136. Floch MH, Bina O: The natural history of diverticulitis: fact and theory, *J Clin Gastroenterol* 38(5 Suppl):S2-S7, 2004.

137. Bogardus ST: Jr: What do we know about diverticular disease? A brief overview, *Clin Gastroenterol* 40(7 Suppl 3):S108-S111, 2006.

138. Szojda MM et al: Review article: management of diverticulitis, *Aliment Pharmacol Ther* 226(Suppl 2):67-76, 2007.

139. Addiss DG et al: The epidemiology of appendicitis and appendectomy in the United States, *Am J Epidemiol* 132(5):910-925, 1990.

140. Brennan GD: Pediatric appendicitis: pathophysiology and appropriate use of diagnostic imaging, *CJEM* 8(6):425-432, 2006.

141. Birchley D: Patients with clinical acute appendicitis should have pre-operative full blood count and C-reactive protein assays, *Ann R Coll Surg Engl* 88(1):27-32, 2006.

142. Kosaka N et al: Difficulties in the diagnosis of appendicitis: review of CT and US images, *Emerg Radiol* 14(5):289-295, 2007.

143. Ditillo MF, Dziura JD, Rabinovici R: Is it safe to delay appendectomy in adults with acute appendicitis? *Ann Surg* 244(5):656-660, 2006.

144. Parkes GC et al: Gastrointestinal microbiota in irritable bowel syndrome: their role in its pathogenesis and treatment, *Am J Gastroenterol* 103(6):1557-1567, 2008.

145. De Giorgio R, Barbara G: Is irritable bowel syndrome an inflammatory disorder? *Curr Gastroenterol Rep* 10(4):385-390, 2008.

146. Spiller R, Garsed K: Postinfectious irritable bowel syndrome, *Gastroenterology* 136(6):1979-1988, 2009.

147. Hammerle CW, Surawicz CM: Updates on treatment of irritable bowel syndrome, *World J of Gastroenterol* 14(17):2639-2649, 2008.

148. American College of Gastroenterology Task Force on Irritable Bowel Syndrome: An evidence-based review on the management of irritable bowel syndrome, *Am J Gastroenterol* 104(Supplement 1):1-40, 2009.

149. Sreenarasimhaiah J: Chronic mesenteric ischemia, *Best Pract Res Clin Gastroenterol* 19(2):283-295, 2005.

150. Herbert GS, Steele SR: Acute and chronic mesenteric ischemia, *Surg Clin North Am* 87(5):1115-1134, 2007:ix, 2007.

151. Kvietys PR, Barrowmand A, Granger ND: *Pathophysiology of the splanchnic circulation*, Boca Raton, FL, 1987, CRC Press.

152. Berland T, Oldenburg WA: Acute mesenteric ischemia, *Curr Gastroenterol Rep* 10(3):341-346, 2008.

153. National Heart, Lung, and Blood Institute, National Institutes of Health: *Clinical guidelines on the identification, evaluation, and treatment of overweight and obesity in adults—executive summary*, 1998. Available at www.nhlbi.nih.gov/guidelines/obesity/sum_intr.htm.

154. James WP: The epidemiology of obesity: the size of the problem, *J Intern Med* 263(4):336-352, 2008.

155. Wolin KY, Colditz GA: Can weight loss prevent cancer? *Br J Cancer* 99(7):995-999, 2008.

156. Barness LA, Opitz JM, Gilbert-Barness E: Obesity: genetic, molecular and environmental aspects, *Am J Med Genet A* 143A(24):3016-3034, 2007.

157. Korner A et al: Polygenic contribution to obesity: genome-wide strategies reveal new targets, *Front Horm Res* 36:12-36, 2008.

158. Farooqi S, O'Rahilly S: Genetics of obesity in humans, *Endocr Rev* 27(7):710-718, 2006.

159. Rosengren A, Lissner L: The sociology of obesity, *Front Horm Res* 36:260-270, 2008.

160. Rocha VZ, Libby P: The multiple facets of the fat tissue, *Thyroid* 18(2):175-183, 2008.

161. Bays HE et al: Pathogenic potential of adipose tissue and metabolic consequences of adipocyte hypertrophy and increased visceral adiposity, *Expert Rev Cardiovasc Ther* 6(3):343-368, 2008.

162. Coll AP, Farooqui IS, O'Rahilly S: The hormonal control of food intake, *Cell* 129(2):251-262, 2007.

163. Myers MG, Cowley MA, Munzberg H: Mechanisms of leptin action and leptin resistance, *Annu Rev Physiol* 70:537-556, 2008.

164. Levin BE, Dunn-Meynell AA, Banks WA: Obesity-prone rats have normal blood-brain barrier transport but defective central leptin signaling before obesity onset, *Am J Physiol Regul Integr Comp Physiol* 286(1):R143-R150, 2004.

165. Banks WA: The blood-brain barrier as a cause of obesity, *Curr Pharm Des* 14(16):1606-1614, 2008.

166. Pan W: Modulation of feeding-related peptide/protein signals by the blood-brain barrier, *J Neurochem* 90(2):455-461, 2004.

167. Scarpace PJ, Zhang Y: Elevated leptin: consequence or cause of obesity? *Front Biosci* 12:3531-3544, 2007.

168. Martin SS, Qasim A, Reilly MP: Leptin resistance: a possible interface of inflammation and metabolism in obesity-related cardiovascular disease, *J Am Coll Cardiol* 52(15):1201-1210, 2008.

169. Calabro P, Yeh ET: Intra-abdominal obesity, inflammation and cardiovascular risk: new insight into global cardiometabolic risk, *Curr Hypertens Rep* 10(1):32-38, 2008.

170. Leite-Moreira AF, Rocha-Sousa A, Henriques-Coelho T: Cardiac, skeletal and smooth muscle regulation by ghrelin, *Vitam Horm* 77:207-238, 2008.

171. Wu JT, Kral JG: Ghrelin: Integrative neuroendocrine peptide in health and disease, *Ann Surg* 239(4):464-474, 2004.

172. Williams J, Mobarhan S: A critical interaction: leptin and ghrelin, *Nutr Rev* 61(11):391-393, 2003.

173. Klok MD, Jakobsdottir S, Drent ML: The role of leptin and ghrelin in the regulation of food intake and body weight in humans, a review, *Obes Rev* 8(1):21-34, 2007.

174. Fantuzzi G: Adiponectin and inflammation: consensus and controversy, *J Allergy Clin Immunol* 121(2):326-330, 2008.

175. Guerre-Millo M: Adiponectin: an update, *Diabetes Metab* 34(1):12-18, 2008.

176. Zick Y: Molecular basis of insulin action, *Novartis Found Symp* 262(36-50):265-268, 2004:discussion 50-55, 2004.

177. Lazar MA: Resistin-and obesity-associated metabolic diseases, *Horm Metab Res* 39(10):710-716, 2007.

178. Hamdy O, Porramatikul S, Al-Ozairi E: Metabolic obesity: the paradox between visceral and subcutaneous fat, *C urr Diabetes Rev* 2(4):367-373, 2006.

179. Kong AP, Chan NN, Chan JC: The role of adipocytokines and neurohormonal dysregulation in metabolic syndrome, *Curr Diabetes Rev* 2(4):397-407, 2006.

180. Damjanovi M, Barton M: Fat intake and cardiovascular response, *Curr Hypertens Rep* 10(1):25-31, 2008.

181. Yanai H et al: The underlying mechanisms for development of hypertension in the metabolic syndrome, *Nutr J* 7:10, 2008.

182. Mokhlesi B, Tulaimat A: Recent advances in obesity hypoventilation syndrome, *Chest* 132(4):1322-1336, 2007.

183. Shore SA: Obesity and asthma: possible mechanisms, *J Allergy Clin Immunol* 121(5):1087-1093, 2008.

184. Shimura R et al: Fat accumulation, leptin, and hypercapnia in obstructive sleep apnea-hypopnea syndrome, *Chest* 127(2):543-549, 2005.

185. Wearing SC et al: Musculoskeletal disorders associated with obesity: a biomechanical perspective, *Obes Rev* 7(3):239-250, 2006.

186. Pischon T, Nothlings U, Boeing H: Obesity and cancer, *Proc Nutr Soc* 67(2):128-145, 2008.

187. Renehan AG, Roberts DL, Dive C: Obesity and cancer: pathophysiological and biological mechanisms, *Arch Physiol Biochem* 114(1):71-83, 2008.

188. Sweeting HN: Measurement and definitions of obesity in childhood and adolescence: a field guide for the uninitiated, *Nutr J* 6:32, 2007.

189. Centers for Disease Control and Prevention: *BMI—body mass index: BMI calculator for children and teens*, 2004. Available at www.cdc.gov/growthcharts.

190. Jaski CB, Lustig RH: Adolescent obesity and puberty: the "perfect storm,", *Ann N Y Acad Sci* 1135:265-279, 2008.

191. Hensrud DD: Diet and obesity, *Curr Opin Gastroenterol* 20(2):119-124, 2004.

192. Ruser CB, Federman DG, Kashaf SS: Whittling away at obesity and overweight: small lifestyle changes can have the biggest impact, *Postgrad Med* 117(1):37-40, 2005:31-34, 2005.

193. Teixeira PJ et al: A review of psychosocial pre-treatment predictors of weight control, *Obes Rev* 6(1):43-65, 2005.

194. Tsai AG, Wadden TA: Systematic review: an evaluation of major commercial weight loss programs in the United States, *Ann Intern Med* 142(1):56-66, 2005.

195. Volek JS, Vanheest JL, Forsythe CE: Diet and exercise for weight loss: a review of current issues, *Sports Med* 35(1):1-9, 2005.

196. Wynne K et al: Appetite control, *J Endocrinol* 184(2):291-318, 2005.

197. Kruger J, Blanck HM, Gillespie C: Dietary practices, dining out behavior, and physical activity correlates of weight loss maintenance, *Prev Chronic Dis* 5(1):A11, 2008.

198. Aylwin S, Al-Zamin Y: Emerging concepts in the medical and surgical treatment of obesity, *Front Horm Res* 36:229-259, 2008.

199. Powell LH, Calvin JE 3rd, Calvin JE Jr: Effective obesity treatments, *Am Psychol* 62(3):234-246, 2007.

200. Suastika K: Update in the management of obesity, *Acta Med Indones* 38(4):231-237, 2006.

201. Waseem T et al: Pathophysiology of obesity: why surgery remains the most effective treatment, *Obes Surg* 17(10):1389-1398, 2007.

202. Kaye W: Neurobiology of anorexia and bulimia nervosa, *Physiol Behav* 94(1):121-235, 2008.

203. National Institute of Mental Health: *Eating disorders, NIH Pub 93-3477*, Washington, DC, 1993, US Government Printing Office.

204. Berkman ND, Lohr KN, Bulik CM: Outcomes of eating disorders: a systematic review of the literature, *Int J Eat Disord* 40(4):293-309, 2007.

205. Law SA, Golding JM: Sexual assault history and eating disorder among White, Hispanic, and African-American women and men, *Am J Public Health* 86(14):579, 1996.

206. Emous SJ: Eating disorders in adolescent girls, *Pediatr Int* 42(1):107, 2000.

207. Hebebrand J et al: The role of leptin in anorexia nervosa: clinical implications, *Mol Psychiatry* 12(1):23-35, 2007.

208. Mantzoros C et al: Cerebrospinal fluid leptin in anorexia nervosa: correlation with nutritional status and potential role in resistance to weight gain, *J Clin Endocrinol Metab* 82(6):1845-1851, 1997.

209. Bulik CM et al: The genetics of anorexia nervosa, *Annu Rev Nutr* 27:263-275, 2007.

210. American Psychiatric Association: *Diagnostic and statistical manual of mental disorders*, ed 4, Washington, DC, 1994, Academic Press.

211. Seidenfeld ME, Sosin E, Rickert VI: Nutrition and eating disorders in adolescents, *Mt Sinai J Med* 71(3):155-161, 2004.

212. Rayworth BB, Wise LA, Harlow BL: Childhood abuse and risk of eating disorders in women, *Epidemiology* 15(3):271-278, 2004.

213. Mitchell JE, Crow S: Medical complications of anorexia nervosa and bulimia nervosa, *Curr Opin Psychiatry* 29(4):438-443, 2006.

214. Casiero D, Frishman WH: Cardiovascular complications of eating disorders, *Cardiol Rev* 14(5):227-231, 2006.

215. Kohn M, Golden NH: Eating disorders in children and adolescents: epidemiology, diagnosis, and treatment, *Paediatr Drugs* 3(2):91-99, 2001.

216. Gowers SG: management of eating disorders in children and adolescents, *Arch Dis Child* 93(4):331-334, 2008.

217. Guarda AS: Treatment of anorexia nervosa: insights and obstacles, *Physiol Behav* 94(1):113-120, 2008.

218. Williams PM, Goodie J, Motsinger CD: Treating eating disorders in primary care, *Am Fam Physician* 77(2):187-195, 2008.

219. Yantis MA, Velander R: How to recognize and respond to refeeding syndrome, *Nursing* 38(5):34-39, 2008.

220. Mehler PA: Eating disorders: bulimia nervosa, *Hosp Pract (Off Ed)* 31(2):107, 1996.

221. Lam RW, Golder EM, Gerwal A: Seasonality of symptoms in anorexia and bulimia nervosa, *Int J Eat Disord* 19(1):35, 1996.

222. Shapiro JR et al: Bulimia nervosa treatment: a systematic review of randomized controlled trials, *Int J Eat Disord* 40(4):321-336, 2007.

223. Williamson DA, Martin CK, Stewart T: Psychological aspects of eating disorders, *Best Pract Res Clin Gastroenterol* 18(6):1073-1088, 2004.

224. Incalzi RA et al: Energy intake and in-hospital starvation, *Arch Intern Med* 156(4):425, 1996.

225. Finn PF, Dice JF: Proteolytic and lipolytic responses to starvation, *Nutrition* 22(7-8):830-844, 2006.

226. Jahoor F et al: Protein metabolism in severe childhood malnutrition, *Ann Trop Paediatr* 28(2):87-101, 2008.

227. Berkley JA et al: Prognostic indicators of early and late death in children admitted to district hospital in Kenya: cohort study, *BMJ* 326(7385):361, 2003.

228. Lidder PG, Lewis S: Perioperative and postoperative nutrition, *Hosp Med* 65(12):717-720, 2004.

229. Zipprich A: Hemodynamics in the isolated cirrhotic liver, *J Clin Gastroenterol* 41(10 Suppl 3):S254-S258, 2007.

230. Varghese J et al: Hepatopulmonary syndrome—past to present, *Ann Hepatol* 6(3):135-142, 2007.

231. Colle I et al: Hepatopulmonary syndrome and portopulmonary hypertension: what's new? *Acta Gastroenterol Belg* 70(2):203-209, 2007.

232. Habib A, Sanyal AJ: Acute variceal hemorrhage, *Gastrointest Endosc Clin North Am* 17(2):223-252, 2007:v, 2007.

233. Abraldes JG, Bosch J: The treatment of acute variceal bleeding, *J Clin Gastroenterol* 41(10 Suppl 3):S312-S317, 2007.

234. Thabut D, Bernard-Chabert B: Management of acute bleeding from portal hypertension, *Best Pract Res Clin Gastroenterol* 21(1):19-29, 2007.

235. Ravindra KV, Eng M, Marvin M: Current management of sinusoidal portal hypertension, *Am Surg* 74(1):4-10, 2008.

236. Poordad F: Review article: thrombocytopenia in chronic disease, *Aliment Pharmacol Ther* 26(Suppl 1):5-11, 2007.

237. Kashani A et al: Fluid retention in cirrhosis: pathophysiology and management, *QJM* 101(2):71-85, 2008.

238. Iwakiri Y: The molecules: mechanisms of arterial vasodilation observed in the splanchnic and systemic circulation in portal hypertension, *J Clin Gastroenterol* 41(10 Suppl 3):S288-S294, 2007.

239. LaVilla G, Gentillini P: Hemodynamic alterations in liver cirrhosis, *Mol Aspects Med* 29(1-2):112-118, 2008.

240. McGibbon A et al: An evidence-based manual for abdominal paracentesis, *Dig Dis Sci* 52(12):3307-3315, 2007.

241. Gines P, Cardenas A: The management of ascites and hyponatremia in cirrhosis, *Semin Liver Dis* 28(1):43-58, 2008.

242. Gentilini P et al: Albumin improves the response to diuretics in patients with cirrhosis and ascites: results of a randomized, controlled trial, *J Hepatol* 30(4):639, 1999.

243. Coll S et al: Mechanisms of early decrease in systemic vascular resistance after total paracentesis: influence of flow rate of ascites extraction, *Eur J Gastroenterol Hepatol* 16(3):347-353, 2004.

244. Av SP: Hepatic encephalopathy: pathophysiology and advances in therapy, *Trop Gastroenterol* 28(1):4-10, 2007.

245. Wright G, Jalan R: Management of hepatic encephalopathy in patients with cirrhosis, *Best Pract Res Clin Gastroenterol* 21(1):95-110, 2007.

246. Haussinger D, Schliess F: Pathogenetic mechanisms of hepatic encephalopathy, *Gut* 57(8):1156-1165, 2008.

247. Vaquero J, Butterworth RF: Mechanisms of brain edema in acute liver failure and impact of novel therapeutic interventions, *Neurol Res* 29(7):683-690, 2007.

248. Ahboucha S, Butterworth RF: The neurosteroid system: an emerging therapeutic target for hepatic encephalopathy, *Metab Brain Dis* 22(3-4):291-308, 2007.

249. Bass NM: Review article: the current pharmacological therapies for hepatic encephalopathy, *Aliment Pharmacol Ther* 25(Suppl 1):23-31, 2007.

250. Roche SP, Kobos R: Jaundice in the adult patient, *Am Fam Physician* 69(2):299-304, 2004.

251. Assimakopoulos SF, Scopa CD, Vagianos CE: Pathophysiology of increased intestinal permeability in obstructive jaundice, *World J Gastroenterol* 13(48):6458-6464, 2008.

252. Raiford DS: Pruritus of chronic cholestasis, *QJM* 88(9):603, 1995.

253. Fabrizi F, Martin P, Messa P: Recent advances in the management of hepato-renal syndrome (HRS), *Acta Clin Belg Suppl* (2):393-396, 2007.

254. Turban S, Thuluvath PJ, Atta MG: Hepatorenal syndrome, *World J Gastroenterol* 13(30):4046-4055, 2007.

255. Angeli P, Merkel C: Pathogenesis and management of hepatorenal syndrome in patients with cirrhosis, *J Hepatol* 48(Suppl 1):S93-S103, 2008.

256. Barve A et al: Treatment of alcoholic liver disease, *Ann Hepatol* 7(1):5-15, 2008.

257. Sukowski MS: Viral hepatitis and HIV coinfection, *J Hepatol* 48(2):353-367, 2008.

258. Kumar D et al: Occurrence & nucleotide sequence analysis of hepatitis G virus in patients with acute viral hepatitis and fulminant hepatitis, *Indian J Med Res* 125(6):752-755, 2007.

259. Ciocca M: Clinical course and consequences of hepatitis A infection, *Vaccine* 18(Suppl 1):S71, 2000.

260. Brundage SC, Fitzpatrick AN, Hepatitis A: *Am Fam Physician* 73(12):2162-2168, 2006.

261. Keystone JS, Hershey JH: The underestimated risk of hepatitis A and hepatitis B: benefits of an accelerated vaccination schedule, *Int J Infect Dis* 12(1):3-11, 2007.

262. McGovern BH: The epidemiology, natural history and prevention of hepatitis B: implications of HIV coinfection, *Antivir Ther* 12(Suppl 3):H3-H13, 2007.

263. Kumar R, Agrawal B: Novel treatment options for hepatitis B virus infection, *Curr Opin Investig Drugs* 5(2):171-178, 2004.

264. Lin CL, Kao JH: Hepatitis B viral factors and clinical outcomes of chronic hepatitis B, *J Biomed Sci* 15(2):137-145, 2008.

265. Ayoub WS, Keeffe EB: Review article: current antiviral therapy of chronic hepatitis B, *Aliment Pharmacol Ther* 28(2):167-177, 2008.

266. Balsano C, Alisi A: Viral hepatitis B: established and emerging therapies, *Curr Med Chem* 15(9):930-939, 2008.

267. Oldfield EC 3rd, Keeffe EB: The A's and B's of vaccine-preventable hepatitis: improving prevention in high-risk adults, *Rev Gastroenterol Disord* 7(1):1-21, 2007.

268. Balasubramanian A, Groopman JE, Ganju RK: Underlying pathophysiology of HCV infection in HIV-positive drug users, *J Addict Dis* 27(2):75-82, 2008.

269. Cheruvu S, Marks K, Talal AH: Understanding the pathogenesis and management of hepatitis B/HIV and hepatitis B/hepatitis C virus coinfection, *Clin Liv Dis* 11(4):917-943, 2007:ix-x, 2007.

270. Koev G, Kati W: The emerging field of HCV drug resistance, *Expert Opin Investig Drugs* 17(3):303-319, 2008.

271. Yuan HJ, Lee WM: Nonresponse to treatment for hepatitis C: current management strategies, *Drugs* 68(1):27-42, 2008.

272. Tong MJ, Terrault NA, Klintmalm G: Hepatitis B transplantation: special conditions, *Semin Liver Dis* 20((Suppl 1):25, 2000.

273. Berg T: Tailored treatment for hepatitis C, *Clin Liver Dis* 12(3):507-528, 2008.

274. Dalton HR et al: The role of hepatitis E virus testing in drug-induced liver injury, *Aliment Pharmacol Ther* 26(10):1429-1435, 2007.

275. Okamomo H: Genetic variability and evolution of hepatitis E virus, *Virus Res* 127(2):216-228, 2007.

276. Panda SK, Thakral D, Rehman S: Hepatitis E virus, *Rev Med Virol* 17(3):151-180, 2007.

277. Mushahwar IK, Hepatitis E: molecular virology, clinical features, diagnosis, transmission, epidemiology, and prevention, *J Med Virol* 80(4):646-658, 2008.

278. Baggio-Zappia GL, Hernandes Granato CL: HIV-GB virus C co-infection an overview, *Clin Chem Lab Med* 47(1):12-19, 2009.

279. Reshetnyak VI, Karlovich TI, Hehenko LU: Hepatitis G virus, *World J Gastroenterol* 14(30):4725-4734, 2008.

280. Leao-Filho GC: Hepatitis G virus infection in patients with hepatocellular carcinoma in Recife, Brazil, *Jpo J Clin Oncol* 37(8):632-636, 2007.

281. Billerbeck E, Bottler T, Thimme R: Regulatory T cells in viral hepatitis, *World J Gastroenterol* 13(36):4858-4864, 2007.

282. Naicker S et al: Infection and glomerulonephritis, *Semin Immunopathol* 29(4):397-414, 2007.

283. Ohto H et al: Transmission of hepatitis C from mothers to infants, *N Engl J Med* 330(11):744, 1994.

284. Sánchez G, Bosch A, Pintó RM: Hepatitis A virus detection in food: current and future prospects, *Lett Appl Microbiol* 45(1):1-5, 2007.

285. Habib S, Shaikh OS: Hepatitis B immune globulin, *Drugs Today (Barc)* 43(6):379-394, 2007.

286. Gotthardt D et al: Fulminant hepatic failure: etiology and indications for liver transplant, *Nephrol Dial Transplant* 22(Suppl 8):viii5-viii8, 2007.

287. Khashab M, Tector AJ, Kwo PY: Epidemiology of acute liver failure, *Gastroenterol Rep* 9(1):66-73, 2007.

288. Phau J, Lee KH: Liver support devices, *Curr Opin Crit Care* 14(2):208-215, 2008.

289. Schuppan D, Afdhal NH: Liver cirrhosis, *Lancet* 371(9615):838-851, 2008.

290. Wallace K, Burt AD, Wright MC: Liver fibrosis, *Biochem J* 411(1):1-18, 2008.

291. Hill DB, Kugelmas M: Alcoholic liver disease: treatment strategies for the potentially reversible stages, *Postgrad Med* 103(4):261, 1998.

292. Arteel G et al: Advances in alcoholic liver disease, *Best Pract Res Clin Gastroenterol* 17(4):625-647, 2003.

293. Bradbury MW, Berk PD: Lipid metabolism in hepatic steatosis, *Clin Liver Dis* 8(3):639-671, 2004.

294. Savolainen V et al: Early perivenular fibrosis —precirrhotic lesions among moderate alcohol consumers and chronic alcoholics, *J Hepatol* 23(5):524, 1995.

295. Zetterman RZ: Alcoholic liver disease. In Gitnick G, editor: *Current hepatology*, vol. 16, St Louis, 1996, Mosby.

296. Singal AK, Anand BS: Mechanisms of synergy between alcohol and hepatitis C virus, *J Clin Gastroenterol* 41(8):761-772, 2007.

297. Greenwel P: Acetaldehyde-mediated collagen regulation in hepatic stellate cells, *Alcohol Clin Exp Res* 23(5):930, 1999.

298. Nagata K, Suzuki H, Sakaguchi S: Common pathogenic mechanism in development progression of liver injury caused by non-alcoholic or alcoholic steatohepatitis, *J Toxicol Sci* 32(5):453-468, 2007.

299. Paik YH et al: Toll-like receptor 4 mediates inflammatory signaling by bacterial lipopolysaccharide in human hepatic stellate cells, *Hepatology* 37(5):1043-1055, 2003.

300. Kolios G, Valatas V, Kouromalis E: Role of Kupffer cells in the pathogenesis of liver disease, *World J Gastroenterol* 12(46):7413-7420, 2006.

301. Parsons CJ, Takashima M, Rippe RA: Molecular mechanisms of hepatic fibrogenesis, *J Gastroenterol Hepatol* 22(Suppl 1):S79-S84, 2007.

302. Yip WW, Burt AD: Alcoholic liver disease, *Semin Diagn Pathol* 23(3-4):149-160, 2006.

303. O'Shea RS, McCullough AJ: Treatment of alcoholic hepatitis, *Clin Liver Dis* 9(1):103-134, 2005.

304. Gavaler JS, van Thiel DH: Ethanol: its adverse effects upon the hypothalamic pituitary-gonadal axis, *J Lab Clin Med* 101:21, 1983.

305. Gomez F, Ruiz P, Schreiber AD: Impaired function of macrophage Fc gamma receptors and bacterial infection in alcoholic cirrhosis, *N Engl J Med* 331(17):1122-1128, 1994.

306. Brave A et al: Treatment of alcoholic liver disease, *Ann Hepatol* 7(1):5-15, 2008.

307. Gershwin ME, Mackay IR: The causes of primary biliary cirrhosis: convenient and inconvenient truths, *Hepatology* 47(2):737-745, 2008.

308. Kumagi T, Heathcote EJ: Primary biliary cirrhosis, *Orphanet J Rare Dis* 23(3):1, 2008.

309. Heathcote EJ: Management of primary biliary cirrhosis. The American Association of the Study of Liver Disease practice guidelines, *Hepatology* 31(4):1005, 2000.

310. Lazaridis KN, Talwalkar JA: Clinical epidemiology of primary biliary cirrhosis: incidence, prevalence, and impact of therapy, *J Clin Gastroenterol* 41(5):494-500, 2007.

311. Prince MI et al: Asymptomatic primary biliary cirrhosis: clinical features, prognosis, and symptom progression in a large population based cohort, *Gut* 53(6):865-870, 2004.

312. Attasaranya S, Fogel EL, Lehman GA: Choledocholithiasis, ascending cholangitis, and gallstone pancreatitis, *Med Clin North Am* 92(4):925-960, 2008.

313. Carey MC: Pathogenesis of gallstones, *Am J Surg* 165(4):410, 1993.

314. Portincasa P, Di Ciaula A, vanBerge-Henegouwen GP: Smooth muscle function and dysfunction in gallbladder disease, *Curr Gastroenterol Rep* 6(2):151-162, 2004.

315. Wang HH, Portincasa P, Wang DQ: Molecular pathophysiology and physical chemistry of cholesterol gallstones, *Front Biosci* 13:401-423, 2008.

316. Donovan JM: Physical and metabolic factors in gallstone pathogenesis, *Gastroenterol Clin North Am* 28(1):75, 1999.

317. Berger MY et al: Abdominal symptoms: do they predict gallstones? A systemic review, *Scand J Gastroenterol* 35(1):70, 2000.

318. Williams EJ et al: Guidelines on the management of common bile duct stones (CBDS), *Gut* 57(7):1004-1021, 2008.

319. Lammert F, Miquel JF: Gallstone disease: from genes to evidence-based therapy, *J Hepatol* 48(Suppl 1):S124-S135, 2008.

320. Hochberger J et al: Management of difficult common bile duct stones, *Gastrointest Endosc Clin North Am* 13(4):623-634, 2003.

321. Venu RP et al: Endoscopic transpapillary drainage of pancreatic abscess: technique and results, *Gastrointest Endosc* 51(4 Pt 1):391, 2000.

322. Frossard JL, Steer ML, Pastor CM: Acute pancreatitis, *Lancet* 37(9618):1072, 2008.

323. Arendt T et al: Gallstones, the choledochoduodenal junction and initiation of acute pancreatitis: are two stones the culprit rather than one stone? *Med Hypotheses* 54(4):570, 2000.

324. Vonlaufen A et al: Role of alcoholic metabolism in chronic pancreatitis, *Alcohol Res Health* 30(1):48-54, 2007.

325. Bhatia M: Apoptosis versus necrosis in acute pancreatitis, *Am J Physiol Gastrointest Liver Physiol* 286(2):G189, 2004.

326. Apte MV, Wilson JS: Alcohol-induced pancreatic injury, *Best Pract Res Clin Gastroenterol* 17(4):593-612, 2003.

327. Elfar M et al: The inflammatory cascade in acute pancreatitis: relevance to clinical disease, *Surg Clin North Am* 87(6):1325-1340, 2007:vii, 2007.

328. Zhang XP, Wang L, Zhou YF: The pathogenic mechanism of severe acute pancreatitis complicated with renal injury: a review of current knowledge, *Dig Dis Sci* 53(2):297-306, 2008.

329. Kakafika A et al: Coagulation, platelets, and acute pancreatitis, *Pancreas* 34(1):15-20, 2007.

330. Lytras D et al: Persistent early organ failure: defining the high-risk group of patients with severe acute pancreatitis? *Pancreas* 36(3):249-254, 2008.

331. Kemppainen EA et al: Advances in the laboratory diagnostics of acute pancreatitis, *Ann Med* 30(2):169, 1998.

332. Papachristou GI, Whitcomb DC: Predictors of severity and necrosis in acute pancreatitis, *Gastroenterol Clin North Am* 33(4):871-890, 2004.

333. Methuen T et al: Disialotransferrin, determined by capillary electrophoresis, is an accurate biomarker for alcoholic cause of acute pancreatitis, *Pancreas* 34(4):405-409, 2007.

334. Rosas JM et al: Intra-abdominal pressure as a marker of severity in acute pancreatitis, *Surgery* 141(2):173-178, 2007.

335. Curtis CS, Kudska KA: Nutrition support in pancreatitis, *Surg Clin North Am* 87(6):1403-1415, 2007:viii, 2007.

336. Spanier BW, Dijkgraaf MG, Bruno MJ: Epidemiology, aetiology and outcome of acute and chronic pancreatitis: an update, *Best Pract Res Clin Gastroenterol* 22(1):45-63, 2008.

337. Keller J, Layer P: Idiopathic chronic pancreatitis, *Best Pract Res Clin Gastroenterol* 22(1):105-113, 2008.

338. Fregni F, Pascual-Leone A, Freedman SD: Pain in chronic pancreatitis: a salutogenic mechanism or a maladaptive brain response? *Pancreatology* 7(5-6):409-410, 2007.

339. Gachago C, Draganov PV: Pain management in chronic pancreatitis, *World J Gastroenterol* 14(2):3137-3148, 2008.

340. Martin RF, Marion MD: Resectional therapy for chronic pancreatitis, *Surg Clin North Am* 87(6):1461-1475, 2007:ix, 2007.

341. Robertson EV, Jankowski JA: Genetics of gastroesophageal cancer: paradigms, paradoxes, and prognostic utility, *Am J Gastroenterol* 103(2):443-449, 2008.

342. Brown LM, Devesa SS, Chow WH: Incidence of adenocarcinoma of the esophagus among white American by sex, stage and age, *J Natl Cancer Inst* 100(16):1184-1187, 2008.

343. Shimizu M, Ban S, Odze RD: Squamous dysplasia and other precursor lesions related to esophagesl squamous cell carcinoma, *Gastroenterol Clin North Am* 36(4):787-811, 2007:v-vi, 2007.

344. American Cancer Society, Inc., Surveillance and Health Policy Research: Estimated New Cancer Cases and Deaths by Sex, U.S., 2009 Available at: http://www.cancer.org/downloads/stt/CFF2009_EstCD_3.pdf

345. Holmes RS, Vaughan TL: Epidemiology and pathogenesis of esophageal cancer, *Semin Radiat Oncol* 17(1):2-9, 2007.

346. Gee DW, Rattner DW: Management of gastroesophageal tumors, *Oncologist* 19(1):79-88, 2007.

347. Rokkas T et al: Relationship between *Helicobacter pylori* infection and esophageal neoplasia: a meta-analysis, *Clin Gastroenterol Hepatol* 5(12):1413-1417, 2007:e1–2, 2007.

348. Lin J, Beerm DC: Molecular biology of upper gastrointestinal malignancies, *Semin Oncol* 31(4):476-486, 2004.

349. Leung WK et al: Screening for gastric cancer in Asia: current evidence and practice, *Lancet Oncol* 9(3):279-287, 2008.

350. Ye W, Nyren O: Risk of cancers of the oesophagus and stomach by histology or subsite in patients hospitalized for pernicious anemia, *Gut* 52(7):938-941, 2003.

351. Cheung TK, Xia HH, Wong BC: *Helicobacter pylori* eradication for gastric cancer prevention, *J Gastroenterol* 42(Suppl 17):10-15, 2007.

352. Lochhead P, El-Omar EM: *Helicobacter pylori* infection and gastric cancer, *Best Pract Res Clin Gastroenterol* 21(2):281-297, 2007.

353. Du Mq: MALT lymphoma: recent advances in aetiology and molecular genetics, *J Clin Exp Hematop* 47(2):31-42, 2007.

354. Tsugane S, Sasazuki S: Diet and risk of gastric cancer: review of epidemiological evidence, *Gastric Cancer* 10(2):75-83, 2007.

355. Houben GM, Stockbrugger RW: Bacteria in the aetio-pathogenesis of gastric cancer: a review, *Scand J Gastroenterol* 212(Suppl):13, 1995.

356. Wilksten JP et al: Comparison of the prognostic value of a panel of tissue tumor markers and established clinicopathological factors in patients with gastric cancer, *Anticancer Res* 28(4C):2279-2287, 2008.

357. Fuccio L et al: Systematic review: *Helicobacter pylori* eradication for the prevention of gastric cancer, *Aliment Pharmacol Ther* 25(2):133-141, 2007.

358. Pufulete M: Intake of diary products and risk of colorectal neoplasia, *Nutr Res Rev* 21(1):56-67, 2008.

359. Sharma S, O'Keefe SJ: Environmental influences on the high mortality from colorectal cancer in African Americans, *Postgrad Med J* 83(983):583-589, 2007.

360. Kam MH et al: Small bowel malignancies: a review of 20 patients at a single centre, *Colorectal Dis* 6(3):195-197, 2004.

361. Will OC et al: Familial adenomatous polyposis and the small bowel: a loco-regional review and current management strategies, *Pathol Res Pract* 204(7):449-458, 2008.

362. Ahnen JD: The genetic basis of colorectal cancer risk, *Adv Intern Med* 41:531-532, 1996.

363. Jen J et al: Allelic loss of chromosome 18q and prognosis in colorectal cancer, *N Engl J Med* 331(4):213-221, 1994.

364. Eisinger AL et al: The role of cyclooxygenase-2 and prostaglandins in colon cancer, *Prostaglandins Other Lipid Mediat* 82(1-4):147-154, 2007.

365. Cappell MS: Pathophysiology: Clinical presentation and management of colon cancer, *Gastroenterol Clin North Am* 37(1):1-24, 2008:v, 2008.

366. Evans DG et al: Strategies for identifying hereditary nonpolyposis colon cancer, *Semin Oncol* 34(5):411-417, 2007.

367. Al-Sukhni W, Aronson M, Gallinger S: Hereditary colorectal cancer syndromes: familial adenomatous polyposis and Lynch syndrome, *Surg Clin North Am* 88(4):819-844, 2008.

368. Rustgi AK: The genetics of hereditary colon cancer, *Genes Dev* 21(20):2525-2538, 2007.

369. Antonakopoulos N: The role of NSAIDs in colon cancer prevention, *Hepatogastroenterology* 54(78):1694-1700, 2007.

370. Ryan-Harshman M, Aldoori W: Diet and colorectal cancer: Review of the evidence, *Can Fam Physician* 53(11):1913-1920, 2007.

371. Kuhnle GG, Bingham SA: Dietary meat, endogenous nitrosation and colorectal cancer, *Biochem Soc Trans* 36(Pt 5):1355-1357, 2007.

372. Rescigno M: The pathogenic role of intestinal flora in IBD and colon cancer, *Curr Drug Targets* 9(5):395-403, 2008.

373. Gupta AK, Brenner DE, Turgeon DK: Early detection of colon cancer: new tests on the horizon, *Mol Diagn Ther* 12(2):77-85, 2008.

374. Bonanno E et al: Stool test for colorectal cancer screening: what is going on? *Surg Oncol* 16(Suppl 1):S43-S45, 2007.

375. Cappell MS: From colonic polyps to colon cancer: pathophysiology, clinical presentation, screening and colonoscopic therapy, *Minerva Gastroenterol Dietol* 53(4):351-373, 2007.

376. Kim YS, Milner JA: Dietary modulation of colon cancer risk, *J Nutr* 137(Suppl 11):2576S-2579S, 2007.

377. Weingarten MA, Zalmanovici A, Yaphe J: Dietary calcium supplementation for preventing colorectal cancer and adenomatous polyps, *Cochrane Database Syst Rev* (1):CD003548, 2008.

378. De Salvo GL et al: Curative surgery for obstruction from primary left colorectal carcinoma: primary or staged resection? *Cochrane Database Syst Rev* (2):CD002101, 2004.

379. National Cancer Institute: *Stages of colon cancer, 4/28/2008*. Available at: http://cancerweb.ncl.ac.uk/cancernet/200008.html#2_STAGESOFCOLONCANCER

380. Braun AH et al: New systemic frontline treatment for metastatic colorectal carcinoma, *Cancer* 100(8):1558-1577, 2004.

381. Midgley RS, Kerr DJ: Immunotherapy for colorectal cancer, *Expert Rev Anticancer Ther* 3(1):63-78, 2003.

382. Schlom J et al: Strategies in the development of recombinant vaccines for colon cancer, *Semin Oncol* 26(6):672-682, 1999.

383. Sobrero A et al: New directions in the treatment of colon cancer: a look to the future, *Eur J Cancer* 36(5):559-566, 2000.

384. Lurje G, Zhang W, Lenz HJ: Molecular prognostic markers in locally advanced colon cancer, *Clin Colorectal Cancer* 6(10):683-690, 2007.

385. El-Serag HB, Rudolph KL: Hepatocellular carcinoma: epidemiology and molecular carcinogenesis, *Gastroenterology* 132(7):2557-2576, 2007.

386. Wong R, Corley DA: Racial and ethnic variations in hepatocellular carcinoma incidence within the United States, *Am J Med* 121(6):525-531, 2008.

387. But DY, Lai CL, Yuen MF: Natural history of hepatitis-related hepatocellular carcinoma, *World J Gastroenterol* 14(11):1652-1656, 2008.

388. Barazani Y et al: Chronic viral hepatitis and hepatocellular carcinoma, *World J Surg* 31(6):1243-1248, 2007.

389. Okuda H: Hepatocellular carcinoma development in cirrhosis, *Best Pract Res Clin Gastroenterol* 21(1):161-173, 2007.

390. Hussain SP et al: *TP53* mutations and hepatocellular carcinoma: insights into the etiology and pathogenesis of liver cancer, *Oncogene* 26(15):2166-2176, 2007.

391. Hara M et al: Case-control study on cigarette smoking and the risk of hepatocellular carcinoma among Japanese, *Cancer Sci* 99(1):93-97, 2008.

392. Zhu K et al: Cigarette smoking and primary liver cancer: a population-based case control study in US men, *Cancer Causes Control* 18(3):315-321, 2007.

393. Kaewpitoon N et al: Opisthorchis viverrini: the carcinogenic human liver fluke, *World J Gastroenterol* 14(5):666-674, 2008.

394. Rougier P et al: Hepatocellular carcinoma (HCC): an update, *Semin Oncol* 34(2 Suppl 1):S12-S20, 2007.

395. Tommasi S et al: Molecular pathways and related target therapies in liver carcinoma, *Curr Pharm Des* 13(32):3279-3287, 2007.

396. Ben-Menachem T: Risk factors for cholangiocarcinoma, *Eur J Gastroenterol Hepatol* 19(8):615-617, 2007.

397. El-Serag HB et al: Diagnosis and treatment of hepatocellular carcinoma, *Gastroenterology* 134(6):1752-1763, 2008.

398. Tan A et al: Viral hepatocarcinogenesis: from infection to cancer, *Liver Int* 28(2):175-188, 2008.

399. Cho CS et al: A novel prognostic nomogram is more accurate than conventional staging systems for predicting survival after resection of hepatocellular carcinoma, *J Am Coll Surg* 206(2):281-291, 2008.

400. Lencioni R, Crocetti L: Image-guided thermal ablation of hepatocellular carcinoma, *Crit Rev Oncol Hematol* 66(3):200-207, 2008.

401. Volk ML, Marrero JA: Early detection of liver cancer: diagnosis and management, *Curr Gastroenterol Rep* 10(1):60-66, 2008.

402. Lowenfels AB et al: Epidemiology of gallbladder cancer, *Hepatogastroenterology* 46(27):1529, 1999.

403. Pandy M: Risk factors for gallbladder cancer: a reappraisal, *Eur J Cancer Prev* 12(1):15-24, 2003.

404. Malik IA: Gallbladder cancer: current status, *Expert Opin Pharmacother* 5(6):1271-1277, 2004.

405. Thomas MB: Targeted therapies for cancer of the gallbladder, *Curr Opin Gastroenterol* 24(3):372-376, 2008.

406. Foster JM et al: Gallbladder cancer: defining the indications for primary radical resection and radical re-resection, *Ann Surg Oncol* 14(2):833–340, 2007.

407. Koorstra JB et al: Pancreatic carcinogenesis, *Pancreatology* 8(2):110-125, 2008.

408. Hart AR, Kennedy H, Harvey I: Pancreatic cancer: a review of the evidence on causation, *Clin Gastroenterol Hepatol* 6(3):275-282, 2008.

409. Lowenfels AB, Maisonneuve P, Lankisch PG: Chronic pancreatitis and other risk factors for pancreatic cancer, *Gastroenterol Clin North Am* 28(3):673-685, 1999.

410. Kloppel G, Luttges J: The pathology of ductal-type pancreatic carcinomas and pancreatic intraepithelial neoplasia: insights for clinicians, *Curr Gastroenterol Rep* 6(2):111-118, 2004.

411. Pryczynicz A et al: Expression of EGF and EGFR strongly correlates with metastasis of pancreatic ductal carcinoma, *Anticancer Res* 28(2B):1399-1404, 2008.

412. Lomberk G: Pain management, *Pancreatology* 8(6):542-543, 2008.

413. Chari ST: Detecting early pancreatic cancer: problems and prospects, *Semin Oncol* 34(4):284-294, 2007.

414. Koliopanos A et al: Radical resection of pancreatic cancer, *Hepatobiliary Pancreat Dis Int* 7(1):11-18, 2008.

415. von Wichert G, Seufferlein T, Adler G: Palliative treatment of pancreatic cancer, *J Dig Dis* 9(1):1-7, 2008.

416. Wilkowski R, Wolf M, Heinemann V: Primary advanced unresectable pancreatic cancer, *Recent Results Cancer Res* 177:79-93, 2008.

ALTERATIONS OF DIGESTIVE FUNCTION IN CHILDREN

SUE E. HUETHER

MEDIA RESOURCES

*e*volve **Evolve Website** (http://evolve.elsevier.com/McCance/)
- Review Questions and Answers
- Animations
- Glossary (with audio pronunciation for selected terms)
- WebLinks

CHAPTER OUTLINE

DISORDERS OF THE GASTROINTESTINAL TRACT
Congenital Impairment of Motility
Esophageal Malformations
Acquired Impairment of Motility
Impairment of Digestion, Absorption, and Nutrition
Diarrhea

DISORDERS OF THE LIVER
Disorders of Biliary Metabolism and Transport
Inflammatory Disorders
Portal Hypertension
Metabolic Disorders

Disorders of the gastrointestinal tract, liver and pancreas in children include congenital anomalies with structural and functional alterations, enzyme deficiencies, and infections. These disorders lead to impairment of motility, digestion, nutrition and normal growth and development

DISORDERS OF THE GASTROINTESTINAL TRACT

Congenital Impairment of Motility

Cleft Lip and Cleft Palate

Cleft lip (harelip) and **cleft palate** are developmental anomalies of the first branchial arch (Figure 40-1). The incidence of cleft lip with or without cleft palate is estimated at 10.48 per 10,000 live births; the incidence of cleft palate only is 6.39 per 10,000 live births.[1] Incidence is lower in black populations and higher in Asian populations.[2] Cleft lip, with or without cleft palate, is more common in females. Both anomalies can be unilateral or bilateral, partial or complete and may also be associated with other malformations.[3] *Nonsyndromic cleft lip and/or palate* is a malformation with an incomplete separation between nasal and oral cavities without any associated anomaly and is associated with a number of different genes.[4]

In most cases, cleft lip and cleft palate are caused by multiple gene-environmental interactions, including maternal deficiency of B vitamins (B_6, folic acid, and B_{12}), maternal tobacco[5] and alcohol use, maternal diabetes mellitus, and genetic variations of several biomolecules including transforming growth factor, interferon regulatory factor-6, fibroblast growth factor, and other growth factors.[6-9] (This phenomenon, called *multifactorial inheritance,* is discussed in Chapter 4.) Maternal hyperhomocysteinemia also may be a factor associated with orofacial clefts.[10] Together these factors reduce the amount of neural crest mesenchyme that migrates into the area that will develop into the face of the embryo. If the amount is sufficiently reduced, clefting occurs.

PATHOPHYSIOLOGY
Cleft Lip

Cleft lip is caused by the incomplete fusion of the nasomedial or intermaxillary process beginning during the fourth week of embryonic development,[3] a period of very rapid fetal growth. The cleft causes structures of the face and mouth to develop without the normal restraints of encircling lip muscles. A characteristic depression or flattening of the infant's midfacial contour may occur because normal antagonistic forces across the midline are absent, and growth of the involved facial segments is disturbed. The facial cleft may affect not

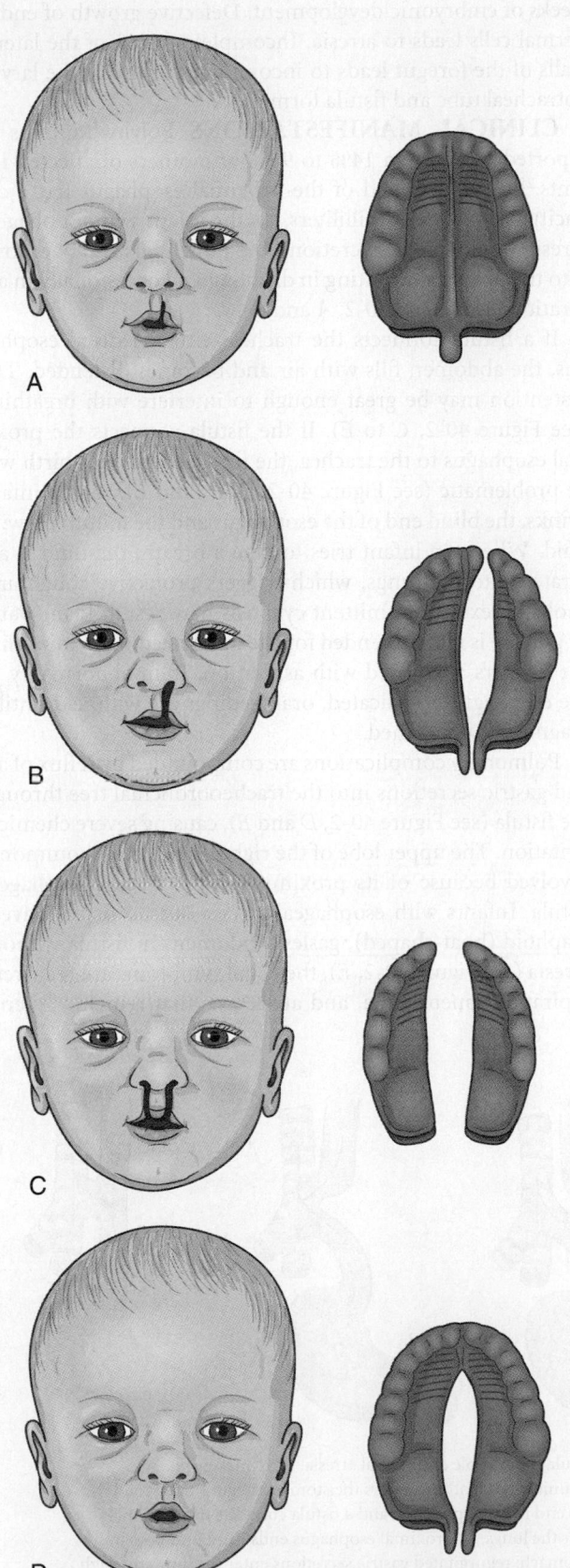

Figure 40-1 Variations in clefts of the lip and palate. **A,** Notch in vermilion border. **B,** Unilateral cleft lip and palate. **C,** Bilateral cleft lip and cleft palate. **D,** Cleft palate.

only the lip but also the external nose, the nasal cartilages, the nasal septum, and the alveolar processes (bony ridge of maxilla that contains the tooth sockets).

The cleft is usually just beneath the center of one nostril. The defect may occur bilaterally and may be symmetric or asymmetric. The cleft can range in severity from a slight indentation of the lip to a fissure that extends to the nostril, causing a sagging and flattening of the nose. The failure of lip fusion by 35 days of gestation may impair closure of the palatal shelves. The more complete the cleft lip, the greater the chance that teeth in the line of the cleft will be missing or malformed.

Cleft Palate

Cleft palate is often associated with cleft lip but may occur without it. Cleft palate results from the failure of the primary palatal shelves, or processes, to fuse during the third month of gestation. The fissure may affect only the uvula and soft palate, or it may extend forward to the nostril and involve the hard palate and the maxillary alveolar ridge. It may be unilateral or bilateral, with the cleft occupying the midline posteriorly and as far forward as the alveolar process, where it deviates to the involved side. Clefts involving the palate only are usually but not necessarily in the midline. In some cases the vomer and nasal septum are partly or completely undeveloped. When these facial bones are involved, the nasal cavity may freely communicate with the oral cavity.

CLINICAL MANIFESTATIONS Feeding the infant with cleft lip usually presents no difficulty if the cleft lip is simple and the palate intact. Nursing at breast or bottle depends on suction developed by pressing the nipple against the hard palate with the tongue. Closure of the lips is not necessary, but the tongue must work harder if the lips cannot be pursed. A baby with cleft palate usually requires large, soft nipples with cross-cut openings. Although most infants with cleft palate can be successfully breast-fed, it may be impossible for some because of an unproductive suck.[11,12] An orthodontic prosthesis for the roof of the mouth may facilitate sucking for some infants.[13]

EVALUATION AND TREATMENT Facial x-ray films confirm the extent of bone deformity. Soft tissue alterations are evaluated by history and physical examination. Prenatal ultrasound has aided early diagnosis of orofacial clefting.[14]

The nature and extent of the cleft, the infant's condition, and the method of surgical correction proposed determine the course of treatment.[15] The lip is united first. Although this can be done within a few weeks of birth, most surgeons prefer to wait until the infant is 3 months old to allow sufficient growth to occur. The initial repair may be revised when the child is 4 to 5 years old.

Repair of a cleft lip that is accompanied by bilateral cleft palate is technically more difficult, so the procedure is often performed in two steps. The lip is repaired when the infant is a few weeks old. Surgical correction of the cleft palate is often planned in stages with the soft palate closed first. Presurgical nasoalveolar molding can reduce the severity of the initial cleft.[16] The palate is closed after the child is weaned from the nipple but before beginning to talk, usually at about 10 to 12 months of age. The aim of surgery is to obtain an airtight closure of the palatal cleft and to preserve the mobility and length of the soft palate. Even with early closure, the child may experience difficulty sealing off the nasopharynx from the buccal cavity during swallowing and while pronouncing certain consonants. Speech training and special attention by a prosthodontist and orthodontist are almost always required.[3]

Before and after surgery, children with cleft lip and palate tend to have recurrent infections of the paranasal sinuses and middle ear. Parents should be alerted to this increased risk so that otitis media can be detected and treated earlier to decrease the chance of long-term scarring and subsequent hearing loss.[17] Breast-milk feedings have been associated with a lower incidence of otitis media in these infants.[18] Hypertrophy of the tonsils and adenoids is common. Children with an orofacial cleft are at an increased risk of being infected by *Streptococcus mutans* and *Lactobacillus* at a very early age. Such colonization indicates a high risk for caries in the primary dentition.[19,20] Displacement of the maxillary arches and malposition of the teeth usually require orthodontic correction.

Esophageal Malformations

Congenital malformations of the esophagus are rare and occur in 1 of 3000 to 5000 live births. **Esophageal atresia** is a condition in which the esophagus ends in a blind pouch. Esophageal atresia is usually accompanied by a fistula between the esophagus and the trachea. This connection is called a **tracheoesophageal fistula (TEF).** Either defect can occur alone (Figure 40-2).

PATHOPHYSIOLOGY The esophageal abnormalities are thought to arise from defective differentiation as the trachea separates from the esophagus during the fourth to sixth weeks of embryonic development. Defective growth of endodermal cells leads to atresia. Incomplete fusion of the lateral walls of the foregut leads to incomplete closure of the laryngotracheal tube and fistula formation.[21]

CLINICAL MANIFESTATIONS Polyhydramnios is reported to occur in 14% to 90% of mothers of affected infants.[22] The blind end of the proximal esophagus has a capacity of only a few milliliters. As the infant with esophageal atresia swallows oral secretions, the pouch fills and overflows into the pharynx, resulting in drooling and occasionally in aspiration (see Figure 40-2, *A* and *C*).

If a fistula connects the trachea with the distal esophagus, the abdomen fills with air and becomes distended. The distention may be great enough to interfere with breathing (see Figure 40-2, *C* to *E*). If the fistula connects the proximal esophagus to the trachea, the first feeding after birth will be problematic (see Figure 40-2, *B, D,* and *E*). As the infant drinks, the blind end of the esophagus and the mouth fill with fluid. When the infant tries to take a breath, the fluid is aspirated into the lungs, which triggers protective cough and choke reflexes. Intermittent cyanosis may result. Plain water or glucose is recommended for the initial feeding to minimize the dangers associated with aspiration. If an abnormality of the esophagus is indicated, oral feedings are withheld until a diagnosis is confirmed.

Pulmonary complications are compounded by reflux of air and gastric secretions into the tracheobronchial tree through the fistula (see Figure 40-2, *D* and *E*), causing severe chemical irritation. The upper lobe of the right lung is most commonly involved because of its proximity to the tracheoesophageal fistula. Infants with esophageal atresia but no fistula have a scaphoid (boat-shaped), gasless abdomen. In fistula without atresia (see Figure 40-2, *E*), the usual symptoms are recurrent aspiration, pneumonia, and atelectasis that remains "silent"

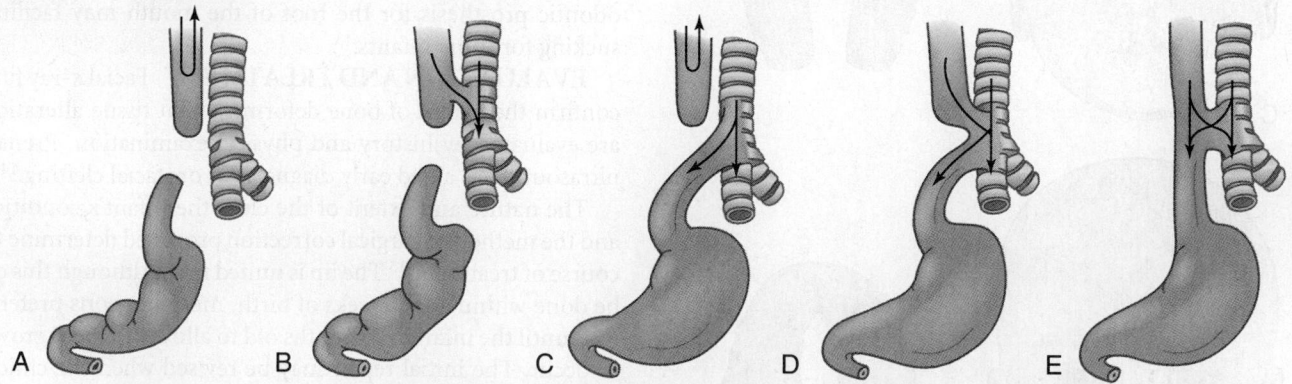

Figure 40-2 Five types of esophageal atresia and tracheoesophageal fistulae. **A,** Simple esophageal atresia. Proximal esophagus and distal esophagus end in blind pouches, and there is no tracheal communication. Nothing enters the stomach; regurgitated food and fluid may enter the lungs. **B,** Proximal and distal esophageal segments end in blind pouches, and a fistula connects the proximal esophagus to the trachea. Nothing enters the stomach; food and fluid enter the lungs. **C,** Proximal esophagus ends in a blind pouch, and a fistula connects the trachea to the distal esophagus. Air enters the stomach; regurgitated gastric secretions enter the lungs through the fistula. **D,** Fistula connects proximal and distal esophageal segments to the trachea. Air, food, and fluid enter the stomach and the lungs. **E,** Simple tracheoesophageal fistula between otherwise normal esophagus and trachea. Air, food, and fluid enter the stomach and the lungs. Between 85% and 90% of esophageal anomalies are type C; 6% to 8% are type A; 3% to 5% are type E; and less than 1% are type B or D. **NOTE:** Type F, esophageal stenosis is not shown.

for days or even months. Late complication of esophageal atresia or tracheal esophageal fistula include stricture, reflux, and dysphagia.[23]

In at least 50% of infants with esophageal defects, other congenital anomalies are present as well. Cardiovascular anomalies are the most common, but other digestive tract, urinary, vertebral, and central nervous system defects can accompany esophageal atresia and tracheoesophageal fistula.

EVALUATION AND TREATMENT Esophageal atresia is usually diagnosed at birth, when attempts to pass a small-bore orogastric or nasogastric tube into the stomach fail.[24] X-ray films show the catheter coiled in the upper esophageal pouch. Prenatal ultrasound reveals defects in some cases.[25]

Treatment is surgical and may include esophageal replacement for long-gap atresia. Esophageal continuity is restored, and the fistula is eliminated. Surgery is usually undertaken after birth, sometimes in stages. The child may continue to have problems with aspiration, gastroesophageal reflux, and esophagitis after surgical repair.[21] The overall survival rate for infants with esophageal defects exceeds 90%.[25]

Pyloric Stenosis

Pyloric stenosis is an obstruction of the pyloric sphincter caused by hypertrophy of the sphincter muscle. It is one of the most common disorders of early infancy and affects infants between the ages of either 1 and 2 weeks or 3 and 4 months.[26] The incidence of pyloric stenosis among males is approximately 5 in 1000, whereas among females it is only 1 in 1000. Whites are affected more often than blacks or Asians, and full-term infants are affected more often than premature infants.[27] The cause is unknown but increased gastrin secretion by the mother in the last trimester of pregnancy increases the likelihood of pyloric stenosis in the infant. The overproduction of gastric secretions in the infant may be caused by stress-related factors in the mother. Exogenous administration of prostaglandin E is associated with an increased incidence of pyloric stenosis. There is an increased incidence of pyloric stenosis in children with Down syndrome; 6.9% of children have a parent who had pyloric stenosis, and 4.9% have a close relative that is affected.[28,29] Pyloric stenosis occurs in approximately 20% of male and 10% of female descendants of mothers who had pyloric stenosis.[30]

PATHOPHYSIOLOGY The circular muscle of the pylorus is grossly enlarged because of an increase in cell size (hypertrophy) and an increase in cell number (hyperplasia).[31] Research has shown that transforming growth factor-alpha plays a role in stimulating this increase in muscle mass.[32] The mucosal lining of the pyloric opening is folded and the lumen is narrowed by the encroaching muscle. Because of the extra peristaltic effort necessary to force the gastric contents through the narrow pylorus, the muscle layers of the stomach may become hypertrophied as well.

CLINICAL MANIFESTATIONS Between 2 and 3 weeks after birth, an infant who has fed well and gained weight begins to vomit without apparent reason. The vomiting gradually becomes more forceful. In some cases, stomach contents may shoot out 3 or 4 feet. Food is often regurgitated through the nose. The forceful, or projectile, vomiting usually occurs immediately after eating, and the vomitus consists of the bulk of the feeding plus some food retained from previous feedings but is almost always free of bile. Usually infants are hungry and want to eat again after vomiting.[33]

Prolonged retention of food in the stomach is a characteristic feature of pyloric stenosis and food is present after 4 hours unless vomiting has occurred. Constipation is the rule because not much food reaches the intestine.

In severe untreated cases, increased gastric peristalsis and vomiting lead to severe fluid and electrolyte imbalances (hypochloremic metabolic alkalosis), chronic malnutrition, and weight loss that can be fatal within 4 to 6 weeks. Infants with pyloric stenosis are irritable because of hunger, and they may have esophageal discomfort caused by repeated vomiting and esophagitis. The vomitus may be blood streaked because of rupture of gastric and esophageal vessels.

EVALUATION AND TREATMENT Diagnosis is based on the history of clinical manifestations. Occasionally, gastric peristalsis is observable over the abdomen. A firm, small, movable mass, approximately the size of an olive, is felt in the right upper quadrant in 70% to 90% of infants with pyloric stenosis. A visible gastric peristaltic wave after eating is observed in some infants. Sonography is routinely done because this clearly shows the hypertrophied pyloric muscles and narrowed pyloric channel.[34]

The standard treatment for hypertrophic pyloric stenosis is a pyloromyotomy, in which the muscles of the pylorus are split and separated. The procedure can be completed with an open technique or with laparoscopy.[35] The mortality rate associated with surgical correction is less than 0.5%.

Intestinal Malrotation

During the tenth week of embryonic development, the emerging ileum and cecum normally rotate, so that the cecum moves into the lower right quadrant of the abdomen and is fixed there by the mesentery. **Intestinal malrotation** is a condition in which rotation does not occur and the colon remains in the upper right quadrant, where an abnormal membrane may press on and obstruct the duodenum. The obstructing band over the duodenum, called a **periduodenal band,** is one of the most significant findings in malrotation. Associated abnormalities are seen in 30% to 62% of children in a reported series; 50% of children with duodenal atresia and 33% of those with jejunal atresia have associated malrotation.[36]

PATHOPHYSIOLOGY The small intestine lacks a normal posterior fixation in malrotation because it has only a rudimentary attachment near the origin of the superior mesenteric artery. Therefore, the entire mass can twist when the mobile loops of intestine from the duodenojejunal junction to the middle of the transverse colon twist on themselves. The twisting is termed *volvulus*. Intestinal twisting around the rudimentary mesentery angulates and obstructs the intestinal lumen and partly or completely occludes the superior mesenteric artery, causing infarction and necrosis of the entire midgut.

CLINICAL MANIFESTATIONS Although most cases of malrotation-associated volvulus and infarction develop during the neonatal period (50%) or infancy (85% are younger than 1 year), some develop during childhood or even adulthood.[37] In infants the obstruction causes intermittent or persistent bile-stained vomiting after feedings. Abdominal distention is limited initially to the epigastrium because only the stomach and duodenum are dilated. The degree of distention depends on the pressure of swallowed air and the degree of obstruction caused by the volvulus. Dehydration and electrolyte imbalance may occur rapidly because large amounts of pancreatic juice, bile, and gastric secretions are lost through vomiting. Fever usually ensues. Pain, scanty stools, diarrhea, and bloody stools are associated with progressive volvulus, vascular compression, and infarction of the intestine in infants. Intermittent or partial volvulus may be seen in older children and adults. This may be asymptomatic (25% to 50% of the time) and discovered during unrelated abdominal surgery, or it may cause minor abdominal complaints, such as nausea after meals, recurrent episodes of vomiting, or abdominal pain.[38]

EVALUATION AND TREATMENT Diagnosis of malrotation with volvulus and infarction is based on a review of the clinical manifestations. X-ray films of the abdomen show gas bubbles and distention proximal to the site of obstruction.

Treatment consists of opening the abdomen and reducing the volvulus manually. Necrotic bowel is resected and a primary anastomosis performed. An enterostomy may be created. In cases of malrotation without duodenal obstruction, the operative survival rate is 80%. The operative survival rate is 40% to 50% in cases of malrotation complicated by obstruction caused by periduodenal bands or other intra-abdominal anomalies. Resection of large segments of the small intestine results in short-bowel syndrome and its long-term sequelae.

Meconium Ileus

Meconium is a substance that fills the entire intestine before birth. It consists of intestinal gland secretions and some amniotic fluid. Normally, meconium is passed from the rectum during the first 12 to 72 hours after birth.

Meconium ileus is intestinal obstruction caused by meconium formed in utero that is abnormally sticky and adheres firmly to the mucosa of the small intestine, resisting passage beyond the terminal ileum. The cause is usually a lack of digestive enzymes during fetal life. This meconium is also found to contain albumin, which is not normally found in meconium. The detection of albumin in meconium has been used as a screening test for cystic fibrosis.[39] Neonatal meconium ileus occurs in 15% of newborns with cystic fibrosis.[40] Partial aplasia of the pancreas is an associated factor, however, and one fifth of infants with meconium ileus are premature or have a history of maternal hydramnios (excessive amniotic fluid). After intestinal atresia and malrotation with volvulus,

meconium ileus is the most common cause of small intestinal obstruction in newborns.

PATHOPHYSIOLOGY The terminal ileum is plugged with thick, viscous meconium resulting from the formation of an insoluble, calcium-glycoprotein compound in abnormal mucus. The segment of the ileum proximal to the obstruction is distended with liquid contents, and its walls may be hypertrophied. The segment distal to the obstruction is collapsed and filled with small pellets of pale-colored stool. Meconium in the obstructed segment has the consistency of thick syrup or glue. Peristalsis fails to propel this viscous material through the ileum, so it becomes impacted. Volvulus, atresia, or perforation of the bowel sometimes accompanies meconium ileus.

CLINICAL MANIFESTATIONS Abdominal distention usually develops during the first few days after birth. The infant does not pass meconium and begins to vomit within hours or days of birth. Infants with cystic fibrosis may have signs of pulmonary involvement, such as tachypnea, intercostal retractions, and grunting respirations. The distended abdomen shows patterns of dilated intestinal loops that feel doughlike when palpated. Some of the loops contain scattered, firm, movable masses. Despite hyperactive peristalsis, the rectal ampulla is empty.

EVALUATION AND TREATMENT Radiologic examination is used to confirm the presence of meconium ileus.[41] The sweat test, which is accurate in 90% of infants, is performed to detect or rule out cystic fibrosis. The treatment of choice for cases not complicated by volvulus or perforation is a hyperosmolar enema done using fluoroscopy to evacuate the meconium. Although the success of this technique has not correlated with osmolality of the enema, the overall success rate is higher when metglutamine diatrizoate (Gastrografin) is used or when additives, such as polysorbate 80 (Tween 80) and acetylcysteine (Mucomyst), are used.[42] Enterotomy and irrigation are reserved for complicated cases and enema failures.

Survival of infants with meconium ileus is improving, with a 97% to 98% survival rate at 1 year.[43] The mortality rate increases to 70% if obstruction is complicated by peritonitis. After recovery from neonatal meconium ileus, the long-term outlook depends on the severity and progression of pulmonary disease. Recent research demonstrates a clear association of meconium ileus with poor long-term nutritional outcomes in children with cystic fibrosis related to surgical treatment for the ileus and poor essential fatty acid status.[44]

Distal Intestinal Obstruction Syndrome

Distal intestinal obstruction syndrome (DIOS), formerly called *meconium ileus equivalent,* affects approximately 15% of children and adults with cystic fibrosis.[45] Intestinal contents may become abnormally thick and impact the intestinal lumen, particularly after episodes of dehydration or lack of pancreatic enzymes. Use of high-strength pancreatic enzymes has been implicated in formation of strictures of the ascending colon in children with cystic fibrosis and resultant chronic DIOS.[46] The child displays signs and symptoms of intestinal obstruction. In most cases the obstruction is relieved by hypertonic enemas. Meconium ileus and DIOS have been shown to be risk factors for the development of liver disease and other abdominal manifestations in those with cystic fibrosis.[47]

Obstructions of the Duodenum, Jejunum, and Ileum

Congenital obstruction of the duodenum can be caused by intrinsic malformations or external pressure. Intrinsic obstruction is caused by failure of the duodenum to become patent. The obstruction may be partial or complete and usually is located at or near the major duodenal papilla. Extrinsic obstructions can be caused by peritoneal bands that constrict the duodenum. The duodenum can be obstructed by an annular pancreas—a defect in which the head of the pancreas surrounds part of the duodenum. Congenital obstructions of the jejunum and ileum can be attributable to atresia, stenosis, meconium ileus, megacolon (Hirschsprung disease), intussusception, Meckel diverticulum, intestinal duplication, or strangulated hernia.

In ileal atresia or jejunal atresia, the intestine ends blindly proximal and distal to an interruption in its continuity, with or without a gap in the mesentery. Stenosis (narrowing of the lumen) causes dilation proximal to the obstruction and luminal collapse distal to it.

Congenital Aganglionic Megacolon

Congenital aganglionic megacolon (Hirschsprung disease) is a functional obstruction of the colon caused by the absence of the enteric ganglia along a variable length of the colon with inadequate motility. The incidence is 1 in 5000 live births with an increased incidence in males, siblings of children with Hirschsprung disease, and children with Down syndrome.[48] The exact cause is unknown but multiple interacting factors and a complex inheritance pattern that involves the RET proto-oncogene have been found.[49]

PATHOPHYSIOLOGY Congenital aganglionic megacolon is caused by a malformation of the parasympathetic nervous system. It is characterized by abnormalities of the basement membrane and extracellular matrix and absence of the intramural ganglion cells in the enteric nerve plexuses (Meissner and Auerbach plexuses) along variable lengths of the colon.[50] Lacking neural stimulation, the muscle layers of the colon wall fail to propel feces through the colon, leading to functional obstruction. In 80% of cases the aganglionic segment is limited to the rectal end of the sigmoid colon; in 3% the entire colon lacks ganglion cells. The abnormally innervated colon impairs fecal movements, causing the proximal colon to become distended, hence the term *megacolon* (Figure 40-3).

The ganglia normally develop from an advancing neural crest between the muscle layers (tunica muscularis) in the submucosal area (muscularis mucosae) of the intestinal wall. In cases of congenital megacolon, neurologic development is blocked and large, nonmyelinated fibers develop in place of these ganglion cells.[50] The segment of colon that lacks ganglion cells has a relatively normal lumen caliber and wall

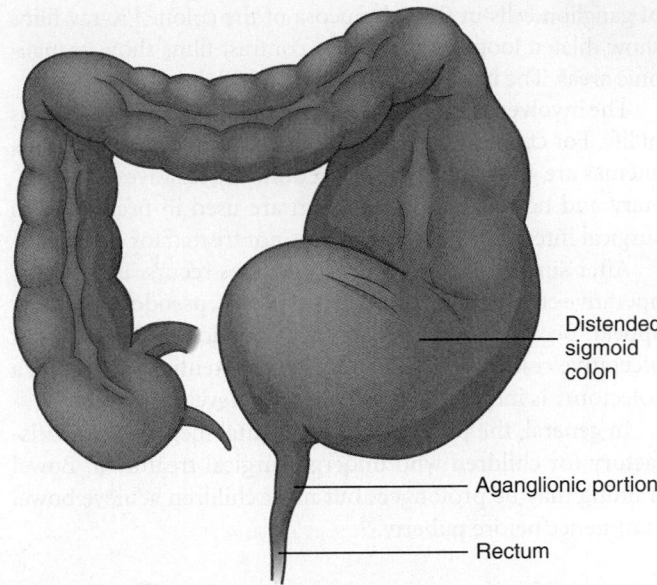

Figure 40-3 Congenital aganglionic megacolon (Hirschsprung disease).

thickness. In the segment of the colon proximal to it, the lumen is dilated and the muscle hypertrophied. Therefore, the abnormal portion of the colon appears to be normal and the normal portion appears to be diseased.

CLINICAL MANIFESTATIONS The extent of the aganglionic portion of the colon determines the severity of the symptoms of congenital aganglionic megacolon. The most distal part of the rectum is always involved. This is the extent of the aganglionic portion in some children, and the child is said to have "ultrashort-segment" Hirschsprung disease and generally has only mild constipation as a symptom. These individuals may not be diagnosed until adulthood.[51] Symptoms of constipation, poor feeding, poor weight gain, and progressive abdominal distention increase in severity as the aganglionic portion extends proximally. Diarrhea may be the first sign, however, because only water can travel around the impacted feces.

The most serious complication in the neonatal period is enterocolitis related to fecal impaction. Bowel dilation stretches and partly occludes the encircling blood and lymphatic vessels, causing edema, ischemia, infarction of the mucosa, and significant outflow of fluid into the bowel lumen. Copious, liquid stools result. Infarction and destruction of the mucosa enable enteric microorganisms to penetrate the bowel wall. Frequently, gram-negative sepsis occurs, accompanied by fever and vomiting. Severe and rapid electrolyte changes may take place, causing collapse and rapid death.

EVALUATION AND TREATMENT Anorectal manometry and rectal suction biopsy are the most reliable screening tools for the diagnosis of Hirschsprung disease. Serial manometry measurements may be required in neonates.[52] This test has uncovered ultrashort-segment Hirschsprung disease in older children with a history of constipation.[53] The definitive diagnosis is made by rectal suction biopsy showing an absence of ganglion cells in the submucosa of the colon.[54] X-ray films show dilated loops of colon, and contrast films show aganglionic areas. The infant usually cannot expel the barium.

The involved segment is resected within the first few months of life. For children with short-segment Hirschsprung disease, enemas are given to relieve impaction, and laxatives with a dietary and bowel training program are used in preference to surgical intervention.[53] The child is not treated for diarrhea.

After surgery, enterocolitis sometimes recurs. If the postoperative enterocolitis is allowed to persist, pseudopolyps may appear. Because these are essentially identical to the lesions of ulcerative colitis, they have malignant potential. Therefore, a colectomy is indicated if pseudopolyps develop.

In general, the prognosis of congenital megacolon is satisfactory for children who undergo surgical treatment. Bowel training may be prolonged, but most children achieve bowel continence before puberty.[55]

Anorectal Malformations

Several congenital malformations of anorectal structures can obstruct the passage of feces. The incidence of minor abnormalities is approximately 1 in 500 and that of major anomalies is approximately 1 in 5000.

Congenital anorectal malformations range from mild anal stenosis, which is corrected by simple dilation, to complex deformities, such as anal or rectal agenesis, atresia, and rectourethral fistula (Figure 40-4). Deformities that cause complete obstruction are known collectively as **imperforate anus.**

Approximately 40% of infants with anorectal malformations have other developmental anomalies as well. The most commonly associated major anomalies are Down syndrome, congenital heart disease, renal and urologic abnormalities, cryptorchidism, esophageal atresia, and malformations of the spine.[56]

Imperforate anus may not be obvious. It can be detected by gentle insertion of a rectal tube. X-ray films show dilations throughout the intestinal tract. Anal stenosis can be treated by dilations, but all other anorectal malformations require surgical correction. The overall mortality rate is approximately 10%. More than 90% of children with a low (anal) anomaly and intact sacrum achieve bowel continence; however, less than 30% of those with very high anomalies or anomalies associated with genitourinary fistulae achieve continence.[57]

Acquired Impairment of Motility

Intussusception

The most common cause of acquired intestinal obstruction in infants is intussusception. **Intussusception** is the telescoping or invagination of one portion of the intestine into another. Usually, the ileum invaginates the cecum and part of the

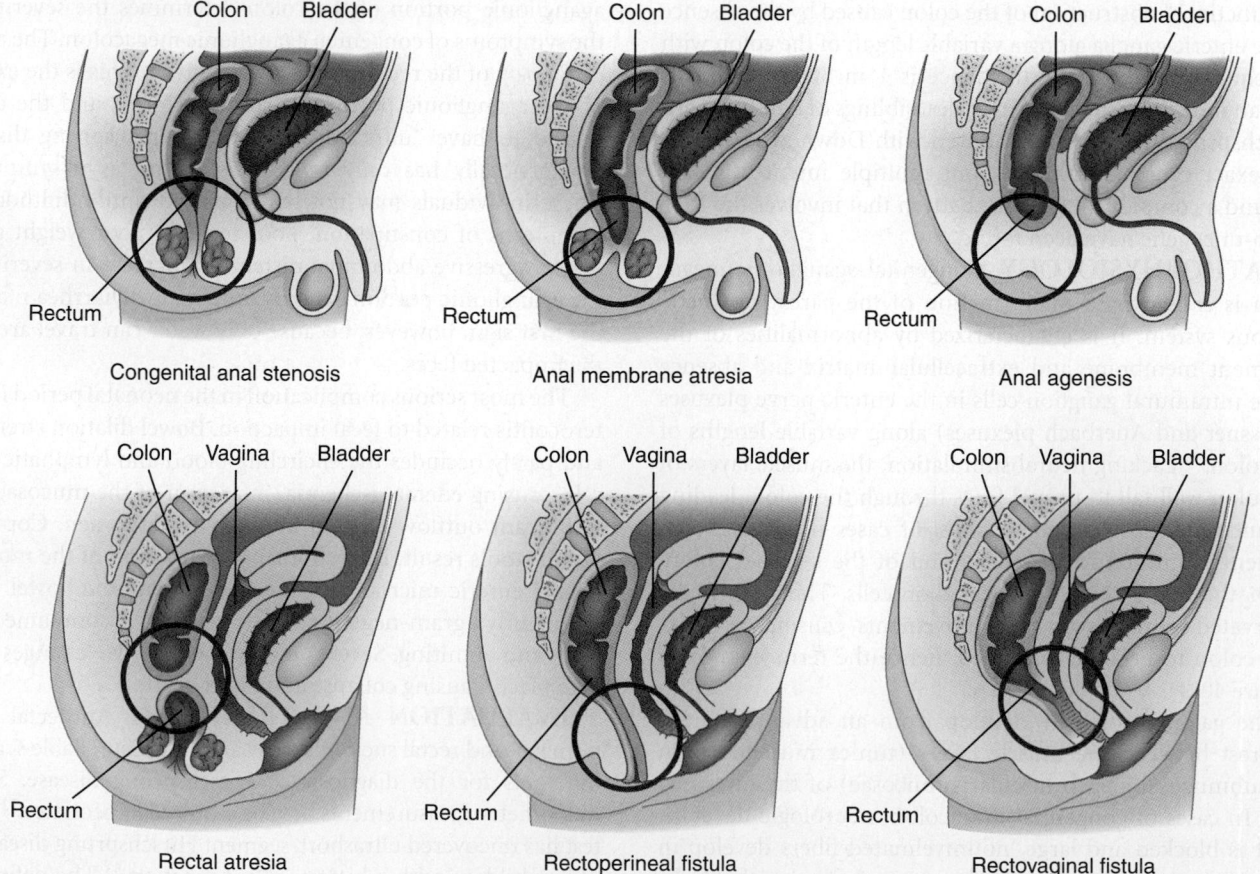

Figure 40-4 Anorectal stenosis and imperforate anus.

ascending colon by collapsing through the ileocecal valve. Intussusception involving the ileum and colon (ileocolic intussusception) accounts for 80% to 90% of intestinal obstructions in infants and is two to three times more common in males than in females.[58] Most intussusceptions occur before 1 year of age, most commonly between 4 and 7 months. Intussusception is rare in infants younger than 3 months and is infrequent after 36 months. Intussusception has occurred in children of all ages recovering from abdominal surgery; intussusception has been found in children with cystic fibrosis and symptoms of bowel obstruction that were initially misdiagnosed as having distal intestinal obstruction syndrome (meconium ileus equivalent).[59,60]

PATHOPHYSIOLOGY Most commonly, the proximal portion of the intestine, the intussusceptum, collapses into the distal portion, the intussuscipiens, in the direction of peristaltic flow (Figure 40-5). As it does so, the intussusceptum drags its mesentery into the enveloping lumen. Initially, the mesentery is constricted, obstructing venous return. Compression of the mesenteric vessels between the two layers of intestinal wall and at the U-shaped angle at either end of the intussusceptum leads within hours to venous stasis, engorgement, edema, exudation, and further vascular compression. Unless the intussusception is treated, bleeding and gangrene ensue. The tension of the mesentery on the intussusceptum tends to arch the bowel in a curve with its center at the mesenteric root. Edema and compression obstruct the flow of chyme through the intestine.

CLINICAL MANIFESTATIONS The affected infant suddenly develops *abdominal pain*, becomes irritable (colicky), and draws up the knees. *Vomiting* occurs soon afterward. A single normal stool may be passed, evacuating the colon distal to the apex of the intussusception. After that, 60% of infants pass *"currant jelly" stools*, which appear dark and gelatinous because of their blood and mucus content. In one study, less than one third of children had this clinical triad of vomiting, colicky abdominal pain, and bloody stools.[61] Most infants have a tender, sausage-shaped *abdominal mass*. Abdominal tenderness and distention develop as intestinal obstruction becomes more acute.[62]

EVALUATION AND TREATMENT Diagnosis is based on clinical manifestations and onset of symptoms. Ultrasound of the abdomen, computed tomography (CT) and magnetic resonance imaging (MRI) are commonly completed for diagnosis.[63] More than 82% of children have positive ultrasound results in ileocolic and jejunointestinal intussusception. Reduction is an emergency procedure involving hydrostatic pressure generated by an air or a barium enema given using fluoroscopic guidance.[64] This technique is successful 45% to 90% of the time. A potential complication of enema reduction is bowel perforation, and for this reason the use of air rather than barium is favored.[65] Surgical reduction is done on children who fail or are not candidates for hydrostatic reduction. Untreated intussusception in infants is nearly always fatal. Most infants recover if the intussusception is reduced within 24 hours.[66] Spontaneous reduction of

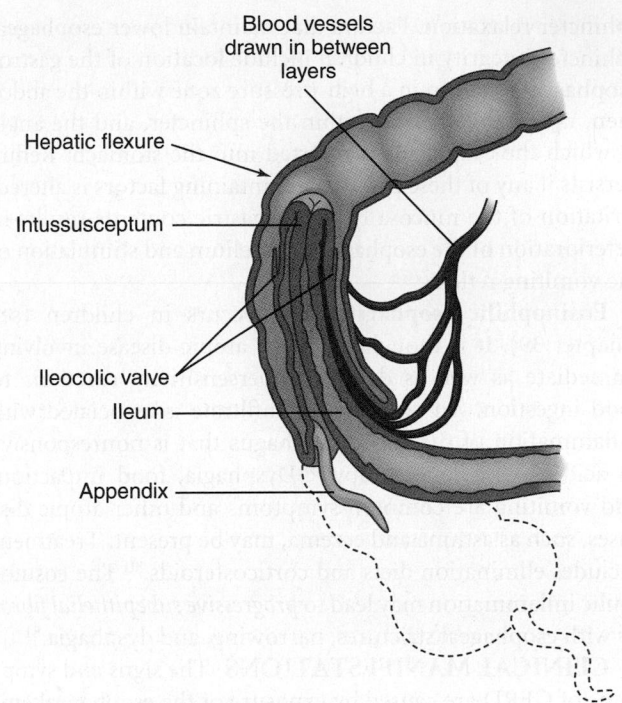

Figure 40-5 Ileocolic intussusception.

intussusception may occur in symptomatic or asymptomatic children and occurs more commonly than previously reported. These intussusceptions are usually short-segment, small-bowel intussusceptions with no recognizable lead point.[67] Recurrent intussusception is more common after nonsurgical reduction than after surgical reduction. Risk of recurrence cannot be predicted by initial features or symptoms, and children with recurrent intussusception may exhibit fewer symptoms with a shorter interval to bowel necrosis and perforation.[68]

Gastroesophageal Reflux Disease

Gastroesophageal reflux disease (GERD) is common in children and involves dilation of the esophagus and intrusion of acid contents into it; GERD is believed to be related to relaxation or incompetence of the lower esophageal sphincter (see Chapter 39). In newborns, reflux is normal because neuromuscular control of the gastroesophageal sphincter is not fully developed. The frequency of reflux is highest in premature infants and decreases during the first 6 to 12 months of life.

GERD is thought to be a factor in the stimulation of reactive airway disease and otitis media with effusion in some children.[69,70] Reflux also is thought to be a contributing cause in apparent life-threatening events and a significant problem for children with cerebral palsy and cystic fibrosis.[71-74] The relationship between apnea of prematurity and GERD is controversial.[75,76]

PATHOPHYSIOLOGY Delayed maturation of the lower esophageal sphincter or impaired hormonal or neurotransmitter response mechanisms (i.e., vasoactive intestinal peptide and nitric oxide) are possible causes of inappropriate sphincter relaxation. Factors that maintain lower esophageal sphincter integrity in children include location of the gastroesophageal junction in a high-pressure zone within the abdomen, mucosal gathering within the sphincter, and the angle at which the esophagus is inserted into the stomach. Reflux persists if any of these pressure-maintaining factors is altered. Irritation of the mucosa by acidic gastric contents results in deterioration of the esophageal epithelium and stimulation of the vomiting reflex.[77,78]

Eosinophilic esophagitis also occurs in children (see Chapter 39). It is thought to be an atopic disease involving immediate as well as delayed hypersensitivity reactions to food ingestion. An eosinophilic infiltrate is associated with inflammation of the entire esophagus that is nonresponsive to acid-suppression therapy.[79] Dysphagia, food impaction, and vomiting are common symptoms and other atopic diseases, such as asthma and eczema, may be present. Treatment includes elimination diets and corticosteroids.[80] The eosinophilic inflammation may lead to *progressive subepithelial fibrosis* with esophageal strictures, narrowing, and dysphagia.[81]

CLINICAL MANIFESTATIONS The signs and symptoms of GERD are caused by exposure of the esophageal epithelium to refluxed gastric contents. Eighty-five percent of affected infants vomit excessively during the first week of life and usually have other symptoms by 6 weeks.

Vomiting may be forceful and must be differentiated from pyloric stenosis. Aspiration pneumonia develops in one third of infants with gastroesophageal reflux (GER). In cases that persist into childhood, chronic cough, wheezing, and recurrent pneumonia are common.[82,83] Repeated vomiting leads to inadequate retention of nutrients, adversely affecting growth and weight gain. Esophagitis from exposure of the esophageal mucosa to acidic gastric contents is manifested by pain, bleeding, and eventually stricture formation and abnormal motility. Approximately 10% to 25% of children with GERD also have iron deficiency anemia caused by frank or occult blood loss.

EVALUATION AND TREATMENT The clinical manifestations are often adequate to confirm a diagnosis of GERD. Esophageal pH monitoring with a probe for 24 hours and endoscopy are routinely used for diagnosis.[84]

Mild GER resolves without treatment. Maintaining infants in a flat prone or a left lateral position, particularly during and for the first hour after a feeding, results in fewer or shorter episodes of GER.[85] Infants with GER are excepted from the Academy of Pediatrics recommended sleep position for healthy infants to decrease the risk of sudden infant death syndrome (SIDS).[86] Older infants and children achieve better results in an upright (sitting or standing) position while awake, with prone positioning used for sleeping.[87] Thickened feedings may help some infants[88]; however, this has not been shown to be consistently helpful. For some infants, thickened feedings may actually worsen reflux by causing a delay in gastric emptying time. Small, frequent feedings and frequent burping are generally universally accepted strategies for managing reflux.[29] Medications to increase motility,

increase lower esophageal sphincter pressure, or decrease gastric acid production have been used to treat GERD. If no improvement is seen with medical management or the child has life-threatening events with reflux, an antireflux surgical procedure, including gastropexy and fundoplication, is performed. A fundoplication re-creates a valve by wrapping the fundus of the stomach around the lower esophagus.[89]

Impairment of Digestion, Absorption, and Nutrition

Cystic Fibrosis

Cystic fibrosis (CF) of the pancreas, which is also called *mucoviscidosis* or *fibrocystic disease* of the pancreas, is a genetically transmitted disease (mutation of the long arm of chromosome 7) that involves many organs and systems and usually causes death in childhood or young adulthood. It is the most common cause of chronic suppurative lung disease in children and is the most common life-threatening inherited disease in the white population. This section focuses on the deficiency of pancreatic enzymes. (Chapter 34 discusses the pulmonary consequences of cystic fibrosis.)

PATHOPHYSIOLOGY The pathophysiologic triad that is the hallmark of CF includes (1) pancreatic enzyme deficiency, which causes maldigestion; (2) overproduction of mucus in the respiratory tract and inability to clear secretions, which cause progressive chronic obstructive pulmonary disease; and (3) abnormally elevated sodium and chloride concentrations in sweat. Exocrine secretions tend to be abnormally thick and precipitate in the glandular ducts, obstructing flow. Almost all clinical manifestations of CF are a result of overproduction of extremely viscous mucus and pancreatic enzyme deficiency. The full spectrum of involvement is summarized in Table 40-1.

Pancreatic function may range from normal to completely ablated. Approximately 85% of patients have pancreatic insufficiency. Obstruction of the pancreatic ducts with thick mucus blocks the flow of pancreatic enzymes and causes degenerative and fibrotic changes in the pancreas. Pancreatic damage eventually can affect the beta cells, resulting in diabetes mellitus in some children. The incidence of diabetes mellitus and cirrhosis in this population has increased as larger numbers of people with cystic fibrosis have moved into young and middle adulthood. Severe problems with maldigestion of proteins, carbohydrates, and fats occur because of insufficient secretion of pancreatic enzymes.[90]

CLINICAL MANIFESTATIONS Clinical manifestations are presented in Table 40-1.

EVALUATION AND TREATMENT To determine the extent of pancreatic function 72-hour stool fat measurements are used. Stools also may be examined for absence of pancreatic enzymes, particularly fecal elastase, trypsin, and chymotrypsin. To optimize treatment, the carbon-13 (^{13}C) mixed triglyceride breath test offers a simple, noninvasive way of assessing the need for pancreatic enzyme supplementation in children with cystic fibrosis.[91] Pancreatic replacement enzymes are administered before or with meals and high-calorie,

Table 40-1	Pathophysiology, Clinical Manifestations, and Complications of Cystic Fibrosis		
Organ Involved	Secretory Dysfunction	Clinical Manifestations	Complications
Sweat glands	Elevated concentration of sodium and chloride in sweat	Hyponatremia; hypochloremia	Heat prostration; shock
Intestine			
Newborn	Viscid meconium	Meconium ileus with intestinal obstruction	Meconium peritonitis
Older child and adult	Inspissated (dried out) mucofecal masses (intestinal sludging)	Partial intestinal obstruction with severe cramping pains	Volvulus (obstruction), intussusception (prolapse)
			Distal intestinal obstruction syndrome
Pancreas (enzyme deficiency)	Inspissation and precipitation of pancreatic secretions, causing obstruction of pancreatic ducts	Absence of pancreatic enzymes, causing malabsorption of food and fatty, bulky stools	Hypoproteinemia; iron deficiency anemia; malnutrition
		Decreased vitamins A, D, E, and K absorption	Vitamins A, D, E, and K deficiency and rectal prolapse
	Insulin deficiency	Glucose intolerance	Diabetes mellitus
Liver	Inspissation and precipitation of bile in biliary system	Focal biliary cirrhosis; shrunken, "hobnail" liver	Portal hypertension with esophageal varices, hematemesis and hypersplenism
Salivary glands	Inspissation and precipitation of secretions in small ducts of submaxillary and sublingual salivary glands	Mild patchy fibrosis of salivary glands	None
Paranasal structures	Viscid mucus	Retention of mucus; clouding seen on sinus roentgenograms	Mucopyoceles (pus accumulations) with nasal deformity or orbital cavity extension
Nose	Nasal polyps	Obstruction of nasal airflow	None
Lungs	Viscid mucus in bronchioles and bronchi	Obstruction of bronchioles causing bronchiolectasis, bronchiectasis, and chronic lung infection	Hemoptysis; pneumothorax; cor pulmonale; atelectasis; respiratory failure
Reproductive tract			
Male	Viscid genital tract secretions during embryologic development, causing failure of formation of normal vas deferens	Sterility	None
Female	Distention of endocervical epithelial cells with cytoplasmic mucin	Decreased fertility	Polypoid cervicitis (cervical inflammation) while taking oral contraceptives

Data from Rudolph CD et al: *Rudolph's pediatrics,* ed 21, New York, 2003, McGraw-Hill.

high-protein diets with frequent snacks and vitamin supplements are used to treat the malnutrition. However, anorexia is not uncommon in this group secondary to pulmonary disease and frequently large sputum output. To combat the worsening problem of growth failure in children with cystic fibrosis, nasogastric or gastrostomy tube feedings are used to supplement oral intake and promote weight gain. Monitoring of growth and body mass index is critical to treatment evaluation.[92,93]

Gluten-Sensitive Enteropathy

Gluten-sensitive enteropathy, formerly called *celiac sprue* or *celiac disease,* is an autoimmune disease that damages the small intestinal villous epithelium when there is ingestion of gluten (gliadin), the protein component of cereal grains. The gluten in wheat, rye, barley, and oats is toxic to the intestinal epithelial cells of genetically susceptible individuals.[94] The disease occurs largely in whites and has been documented in Asians from India and Pakistan, but it is almost nonexistent in native Africans, Japanese, and Chinese. Prevalence rates in Europe range from 1 in 1000 to 1 in 3000. Recent data suggest that gluten-sensitive enteropathy, traditionally considered rare in the United States, occurs in about 1% of the population or 1 in 100 children.[95] Other autoimmune diseases have been associated with gluten-sensitive enteropathy including type 1 diabetes mellitus and autoimmune thyroiditis.[96]

The pathogenesis appears to require interaction between a number of intrinsic factors (genetic susceptibility, activation of the immune system) and extrinsic factors (gluten and possibly other environmental factors). Cellular immunity as well as humoral immunity are implicated. There are increases in the percentages of T cells, immunoglobulin, and complement in the mucosa of active celiac disease. Immunoglobulin A (IgA) and immunoglobulin M (IgM) antigliadin antibodies have been found in jejunal fluid of persons with untreated disease.[97] Autoantibody reactivity to transglutaminase-2 (TG-2) has been shown to closely correlate with the acute phase of the disease.[98] Although gluten-sensitive enteropathy is widely perceived as a malabsorption syndrome of childhood, the diagnosis is increasingly being made for the first time in adult life.[99]

PATHOPHYSIOLOGY The major pathophysiologic characteristics of the disease are atrophy and flattening of villi in the upper small intestine and malabsorption of most nutrients in the presence of cereal gluten (Figures 40-6 and 40-7). The atrophy is caused by accelerated shedding of epithelial cells from the villi. To compensate for this loss, epithelial cell production increases, causing hypertrophy of the crypts of Lieberkühn.[100] Increased cell production is not sufficient to keep pace with cell loss, however. Inflammation and edema develop around the enlarged cysts. The villi shorten and atrophy, and their surface cells are not mature enough to sustain absorptive functions. The microvilli and brush border disappear, leaving patches of bald mucosa. The loss of mucosal surface area and brush-border enzymes leads to severe malabsorption. The pathologic process is most pronounced in the duodenum and jejunum. The ileum may be spared. The severity of disease correlates with the length of the small intestinal mucosa involved.

Damage to the mucosa of the duodenum and jejunum has secondary effects that exacerbate malabsorption. The secretion of intestinal hormones, such as secretin and cholecystokinin, may be diminished. Because these chemical messengers are scarce, secretion of pancreatic enzymes and expulsion of bile from the gallbladder decrease.

Destruction of mucosal cells causes inflammation, and water and electrolytes are secreted, leading to watery diarrhea. In addition, absorption that normally occurs by sodium-dependent active transport or facilitated diffusion is impaired. Carbohydrates, amino acids, dipeptides, water-soluble vitamins, bile salts, and cations are not absorbed from the intestinal lumen. Potassium loss, which is more severe than sodium loss, leads to muscle weakness. Magnesium and calcium malabsorption can cause seizures or tetany. Unabsorbed fatty acids combine with calcium, and secondary hyperparathyroidism increases phosphorus excretion, resulting in bone reabsorption. Calcium is no longer available to bind oxalate in the intestine and is absorbed, which causes hyperoxaluria. Gallbladder function may be abnormal, and bile salt conjugation may be decreased.

Fat malabsorption in the jejunum is the major cause of steatorrhea (fatty stools). Malabsorption may be mild early in the disease. Fecal nitrogen is elevated because peptidase deficiencies impair protein absorption. Pancreatic function is decreased, not only because of decreased hormonal levels but also because of malnutrition.

Deficiencies of fat-soluble vitamins are common in children with gluten-sensitive enteropathy. Vitamin K malabsorption leads to hypoprothrombinemia. In one third of cases, iron and folic acid malabsorption is manifested as cheilosis; anemia; and a smooth, red tongue. Vitamin B_{12} absorption

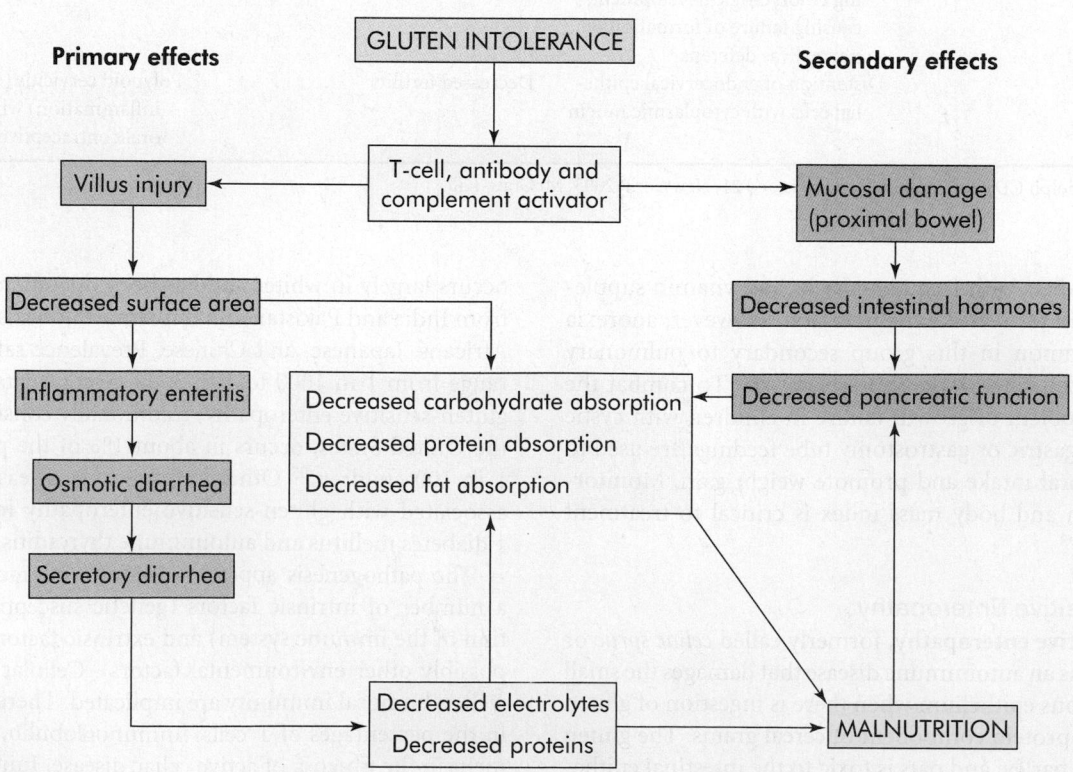

Figure 40-6 Pathophysiology of gluten-sensitive enteropathy.

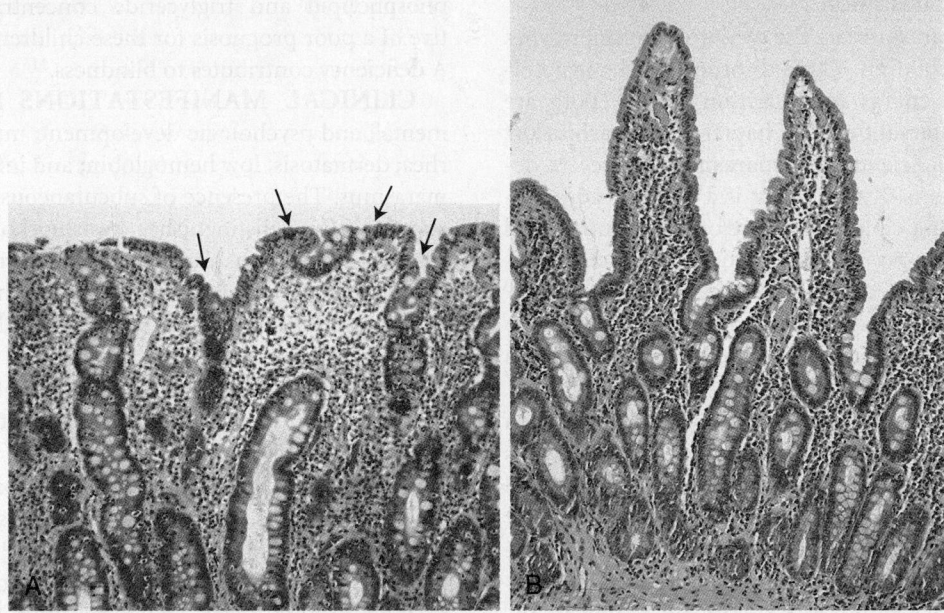

Figure 40-7 Gluten-sensitive enteropathy. **A,** Atrophy of villi and elongation of crypts that result in malabsorption *(arrows)*. **B,** Recovery of normal villus structure after 6 months of gluten-free diet. (From Damjanov I, Linder J: *Pathology: a color atlas,* St Louis, 2000, Mosby.)

is impaired in those with extensive ileal disease. Because the absorption of folate and iron is greatest in the proximal small intestine, deficiencies of these substances are common.

CLINICAL MANIFESTATIONS The onset of clinical manifestations of gluten-sensitive enteropathy depends on the age of the infant when gluten-containing substances are added to the diet. In 50% of affected children, onset occurs by 18 months of age, with latent intervals varying from months to years. Severity of symptoms can vary tremendously, and many children older than 3 years of age present with non-gastrointestinal symptoms.[101]

Diarrhea is an early sign in most infants accompanied by failure to thrive and anemia. The stools are pale, bulky, greasy, and foul smelling, and may contain oil droplets. Three to five such movements occur daily. As early as 3 or 4 months of age, growth failure, anorexia, and constipation can begin. In older children constipation is occasionally seen despite steatorrhea. Vomiting and abdominal pain are prominent in infants but unusual in older children. Anorexia is prevalent. The classic physical manifestations of organic failure to thrive, such as abdominal protuberance, wasted buttocks and limbs, and hypotonia, occur in less than 50% of infants with gluten-sensitive enteropathy. Growth is usually diminished.[102]

Manifestations of malabsorption, such as rickets, tetany, frank or occult bleeding, or anemia, may be obvious. Some children urinate more at night. The tongue is smooth and red, and the child may bruise and bleed easily. Hypomagnesemia and hypocalcemia cause irritability, tremor, convulsions, tetany, bone pain, osteomalacia, and dental abnormalities. If vitamin D deficiency is prolonged, rickets and clubbing of the terminal phalanges are likely. Eighty-six percent of older children have fingerprint changes (ridge atrophy). In older

children, delayed puberty and infertility may be a manifestation of otherwise subtle gluten-sensitive enteropathy.[103] Osteomalacia may be severe.[104] Small intestinal lymphoma is also associated with gluten-sensitive enteropathy.[105]

A rare complication of gluten-sensitive enteropathy in infancy is celiac crisis. Celiac crisis is characterized by severe diarrhea, dehydration, and hypoproteinemia as a result of malabsorption and protein loss and requires aggressive treatment.

EVALUATION AND TREATMENT Diagnosis includes confirmation with serologic antiendomysial or antitransglutaminase IgA antibodies as well as an intestinal biopsy to detect the classic mucosal changes caused by gluten-sensitive enteropathy.[106] The initial biopsy may be followed by a second intestinal biopsy to demonstrate regeneration of intestinal villi after treatment with a gluten-free diet. Most children with celiac disease remain undiagnosed.

Treatment consists of the immediate and permanent institution of a diet free of cereal grains (wheat, rye, barley, oats, malt). Lactose intolerance is presumed because of damage to the villi; therefore, lactose (milk sugar) is excluded from the diet. Tolerance to lactose improves with removal of gluten and healing of the mucosa and may be reintroduced at a later point.[107] Infants are routinely given vitamin D, iron, and folic acid supplements to treat deficiencies. Breast-feeding at the time of gluten introduction in the diet delays the appearance of celiac disease.[108]

Approximately 25% of children experience recurrent relapses that interfere with growth. For most children, however, the long-term prognosis is excellent. There is an increased incidence of malignant disease, particularly T-cell lymphoma, in individuals who fail to respond to gluten-free diets.[109]

Protein Energy Malnutrition

Kwashiorkor and marasmus are the two most common types of malnutrition in children. These disorders are known collectively as **protein energy malnutrition (PEM)**. Both are states of long-term starvation (see Chapter 39). **Kwashiorkor** is a severe protein deficiency, and **marasmus** is a severe deficiency of all nutrients. Kwashiorkor is a widespread nutritional problem among children in developing countries and economically destitute populations particularly when associated with human immunodeficiency virus (HIV) infection.[110] The disease usually occurs in infants or children from 1 to 4 years of age who have been weaned from breast milk to a high-starch, protein-deficient diet.

Marasmus can occur at any age, but it is common in children younger than 1 year. In marasmus, starvation is attributable to lack of protein and carbohydrates. One third of the world's children suffer from PEM, with the highest concentrations in, Asia, Africa, Latin America, and the Carribbean.[111,112] The mortality risk for children in developing countries has been found to be inversely related to anthropometric indicators (height, weight, head circumference, skinfold thickness, midarm muscle circumference). There is elevated risk even in the mild to moderate range of malnutrition.[113] Poor sanitation, early weaning of breast-fed infants, use of overdiluted commercial formulas, and infection (measles, malaria, pneumonia, HIV, and diarrheal disease) are major risk factors for PEM.

PEM is a complication of some diseases, such as chronic fever, tuberculosis, malignancy, digestive and malabsorptive disorders, and psychogenic illness. Radiation therapy and chemotherapy also can contribute to PEM. Acute and chronic malnutrition is common in hospitalized children in the United States and Europe.[114]

PATHOPHYSIOLOGY In kwashiorkor, the deficit of dietary amino acids reduces protein synthesis in all tissues. Physical growth and mental growth are stunted, and maintenance of minimal life processes is in jeopardy. The lack of sufficient plasma proteins, particularly albumin, causes systemic pressure changes that result in generalized edema. The volume of total body water and extracellular fluid increases, causing a substantial loss of potassium. The liver swells with stored fat because no hepatic proteins are synthesized to form and release lipoproteins. Pancreatic atrophy and fibrosis may be present. Kwashiorkor also causes malabsorption, reduced bone density, and impaired renal function. If the condition is not reversed, the prognosis is very poor.

Because the intake of all dietary nutrients is reduced to a minimum in marasmus, metabolic processes, including liver function, are preserved but growth is severely retarded. Caloric intake is too low to support protein synthesis for growth or the storage of fat. If more protein is needed than is ingested, muscle wasting occurs. Fat wasting and anemia are common and can be severe. The volume of total body water is high. Serum triglyceride and phospholipid levels increase with increasing severity of malnutrition, but other serum values, such as cholesterol, are normal or slightly reduced. High fasting phospholipid and triglyceride concentrations are predictive of a poor prognosis for these children.[115] Severe vitamin A deficiency contributes to blindness.[116]

CLINICAL MANIFESTATIONS Retarded physical, mental, and psychologic development; muscle wasting; diarrhea; dermatosis; low hemoglobin; and infection characterize marasmus. The presence of subcutaneous fat, hepatomegaly, and fatty liver distinguishes kwashiorkor from marasmus. These manifestations are missing in marasmus because caloric intake is not sufficient to support fat synthesis and storage.[117]

EVALUATION AND TREATMENT Evaluation of PEM is based on nutritional history and clinical manifestations. Providing deficient nutrients resolves clinical symptoms in 4 to 6 weeks. Physical and mental retardation may not be reversible, however. Nutritional rehabilitation with appropriate environmental stimulation for infants and young children resolves or improve cerebral shrinkage, physical growth, and psychomotor development.[118,119] Advances are being made in the local preparation of ready-to-use therapeutic food for both home- and community-based malnutrition management.[120]

Failure to Thrive

Failure to thrive (FTT) is the inadequate physical development of an infant or a child. It is manifested as a deceleration in weight gain, a low weight/height ratio, or a low weight/height/head circumference ratio. FTT is a common problem and can present at any time in childhood.

PATHOPHYSIOLOGY **Organic FTT** has a pathophysiologic cause, such as GERD, pyloric stenosis, gastroenteritis, malabsorption syndromes, infection by intestinal parasites, congenital anomalies, very low birth weight, or chronic diseases of major body systems. All these factors either reduce the availability of nutrients for maintenance and growth or increase nutrient requirements, particularly when there is chronic infection. A chronic disease or congenital anomaly that causes weakness or reduced stature can create developmental, psychosocial, and emotional problems for the child.[121]

Nonorganic FTT occurs in the absence of any gastrointestinal, endocrine, or other chronic diseases. It is usually associated with psychosocial deprivation, although behavior problems may contribute to its occurrence in the absence of maternal pathologic findings. Behavioral and psychosocial problems may be compounded by inadequate economic resources and lack of knowledge. Generally the problem in nonorganic FTT is ineffective nurturing by parents and primary caregivers. A variety of parental stressors may be involved and include the following:

- Lack of nurturance in the parents' own childhood
- Unwanted pregnancy
- Inability to bond with the infant because of health or other problems
- Postpartum or maternal depression
- Family crisis, such as a death or marital problems
- Stress caused by single parenthood or social isolation
- Mental, emotional, or physical illness

The first few postnatal months appear to be a sensitive period in the relationship between growth and mental development, suggesting a critical need for early diagnosis and aggressive interventions.[122,123]

CLINICAL MANIFESTATIONS Clinical manifestations of organic FTT are restricted growth accompanied by manifestations of the underlying disease. Manifestations of nonorganic FTT are restricted growth plus reduced energy level, reduced responsiveness and interaction with the environment, social isolation, spasticity or rigidity when held or touched, inability to make eye contact or smile, refusal to eat, and rejection of foods. Weight loss and decelerated growth are accompanied by restricted development in many areas. Nonorganic FTT is a complex syndrome involving psychosocial, emotional, and parent-child problems that compound the pathophysiologic abnormalities.[124,125] Children with primarily organic FTT have been found to have lower developmental skills, and their parents have been found to have higher emotional distress. Infant stress, vomiting, feeding disorders, and psychosocial factors have been noted in children with organic and inorganic FTT making the distinction between the two complex.[126]

EVALUATION AND TREATMENT Failure to thrive is suggested if a child falls below the third percentile on the growth curve or is falling off a previously established growth curve. Organic FTT is manifested in infancy by weight, height, and head circumference growth that may be parallel to but below the normal ranges. If no genetic, endocrine, or other systemic disorder is identified and if the physical and laboratory examinations show no abnormalities other than delayed growth, an environmental cause is indicated.

Hospital admission is recommended if the diagnosis is unclear or the child is in nutritional or emotional jeopardy. Eating patterns, food preferences, caloric intake, and family interactions can be assessed during the hospital stay. If the cause is environmental, the hospitalized child with FTT usually begins to gain weight.

If an organic problem has been identified, management of FTT consists of treating the cause. Management of nonorganic FTT involves the immediate total care of the child and measures to address (1) the psychosocial and emotional problems of the caregivers and (2) parent-child interactions. Counseling, parental modeling, and long-term family support are sometimes required.[127,128] Clinical manifestations of organic FTT have inorganic components in the majority of children. The most successful interventions not only treat the underlying organic cause but also address assisting parents with feeding practices and management of psychosocial symptoms.[129,130]

Necrotizing Enterocolitis

Necrotizing enterocolitis (NEC) is an ischemic, inflammatory condition of the bowel that causes necrosis, perforation, and death if untreated. It is the most common gastrointestinal emergency in the newborn. The overall mortality rate is between 12% and 30% and is higher for infants requiring surgery.[131] The incidence of NEC is increasing, causing 1500 to 2000 infant deaths every year in the United States.[132] Premature very-low-birth-weight infants are the most likely victims; it rarely occurs in full-term infants, but when it does it usually is a result of other complications.[133] The risk of NEC decreases as the gastrointestinal tract matures.

PATHOPHYSIOLOGY The exact etiology of NEC is unclear. Multiple factors probably contribute to the development of NEC including premature birth, immature immunity, immature intestinal motility and barrier function, abnormal bacterial colonization, infections, maternal age greater than 35 years, perinatal stress, effects of medications, feeding practices, and genetic predisposition.[131,134] The intestinal mucosal barrier in premature infants is scanty, which delays digestion. Motility is slower, allowing for the accumulation of noxious substances that damage the intestine and increase the risk for infection. Immaturity of the intestinal mechanical and biochemical barrier contributes to increased permeability resulting in translocation of bacteria and other substances, causing injury, inflammation, and development of systemic inflammatory disease.[135] Preterm infants also may have immature intestinal innate immunity and an unfavorable balance between commensal and pathogenic bacteria, promoting intestinal inflammation and release of proinflammatory mediators.[136]

Reduced mucosal blood flow leading to hypoxic injury to intestinal mucosa is thought to be a cause. Normally there is a balance between vasodilator and vasoconstrictor inputs with a tendency toward vasodilation because of the copious production of endothelium-derived nitric oxide. With endothelial injury the balance is shifted toward endothelin-1–mediated vasoconstriction leading to ischemia, injury, and inflammation.[137] This injury allows bacterial invasion of the bowel wall and release of inflammatory mediators. Accumulation of gas in the mucosa and submucosa also can lead to ischemic inflammation and necrosis of intestinal segments. The terminal ileum and proximal colon are most often involved.[138]

CLINICAL MANIFESTATIONS Manifestations of NEC usually appear within 2 weeks of birth, with earlier symptoms in full-term infants (5.3 days compared with 15.3 days in premature infants).[139] They range from mild abdominal distention to bowel perforation, sepsis, and death. Abdominal pain, unstable temperature, bradycardia, and apnea are nonspecific signs. Affected infants have abdominal distention, occult or grossly bloody stools, retained gastric contents, and septicemia with elevated white blood cell and falling platelet counts. The more premature the infant, the greater the incidence of NEC and related diseases of prematurity, such as respiratory distress syndrome and immunocompromise.

EVALUATION AND TREATMENT Diagnosis is based on clinical manifestations, laboratory results, and plain films of the abdomen that show gas accumulation in the intestine. Preventive strategies include breast milk feeding, judicious fluid management to prevent patent ductus arteriosus, administration of arginine and glutamine supplements and epidermal growth facor to support intestinal epithelial cell growth, and enteral probiotics to support commensal gut bacteria.[140,141] Treatments include cessation of feeding, gastric suction to decompress the intestines, fluid and electrolyte maintenance, and administration of antibiotics to control sepsis.[142] Surgical resection is the treatment of choice for intestinal perforation, and the mortality rate is high. For very ill infants weighing less than 1000 g, peritoneal drainage may used as an adjunct to laparotomy.[143] Following treatment of NEC, infants treated by medical and surgical management are at risk for intestinal obstruction related to the development of strictures.[144] Infants who have extensive resection of necrotic bowel may develop short-bowel syndrome, requiring chronic total parenteral nutrition. Intestinal lengthening procedures and intestinal transplantation are available as a lifesaving option for these children.[145]

Diarrhea

Diarrhea is a common gastrointestinal problem during infancy and early childhood, and infectious diarrhea is the leading cause of death worldwide, primarily in young children in developing countries. Severe diarrhea occurs one to three times during the first 3 years of life. Most episodes are self-limiting and resolve within 72 hours.

The pathophysiologic mechanisms of diarrhea in children are similar to those for adults described in Chapter 39. Prolonged diarrhea is more dangerous in children, however, because they have much smaller fluid reserves than adults. Therefore, dehydration can develop rapidly if any disturbance increases fluid secretion into the gastrointestinal lumen (secretory diarrhea), draws fluid into the lumen by osmosis (osmotic diarrhea), or prevents fluid absorption in the intestine.

Infant diarrhea is of special concern because its cause may be a congenital or metabolic anomaly. Infants have low fluid reserves and relatively rapid peristalsis and metabolism. Therefore, the danger of dehydration is great.

Common causes of acute diarrhea in infants include infections, congenital aganglionic megacolon, milk-protein allergies, and NEC. Less common causes are adrenogenital syndrome, impaired chloride-bicarbonate exchange, congenital lactase deficiency, glucose-galactose malabsorption, and sucrase-isomaltase deficiency.

Acute Diarrhea in Children

Infectious diarrhea in newborns is usually associated with nursery epidemics involving such pathogens as *Escherichia coli*, *Klebsiella*, staphylococci, *Salmonella*, and *Shigella*. Diarrhea caused by these agents has a rapid onset, and acidosis and shock can occur quickly. *Clostridium difficile*, often associated with previous antibiotic therapy, can cause acute, profuse, watery diarrhea and symptoms of colitis.[146] Viral causes of diarrhea include rotaviruses, noroviruses, astroviruses, and certain types of adenoviruses. Causes of diarrhea in young children are unknown in about 40% of cases.[147] True milk-protein allergy, which is uncommon, causes bloody, explosive stools after the introduction of milk into the diet.

Acute diarrhea in children is almost synonymous with acute viral or bacterial gastroenteritis. Viral gastroenteritis tends to be self-limiting. Bacterial gastroenteritis is treated with antibiotics if the causal pathogen can be identified. Other causes of acute diarrhea in the older child include antibiotic therapy, appendicitis, chemotherapy, inflammatory bowel disease, parasitic infestation, and ingestion of toxic substances.

Rotavirus, the leading cause of severe diarrhea in infants and young children, invades enterocytes of the intestinal mucosa and releases an enterotoxin that damages these cells. Damage decreases viable absorptive surface causing an imbalance of secretion and absorption and increases motility resulting in diarrhea and dehydration. Recovery from mucosal damage may take several weeks. Rotavirus is transmitted by the fecal-oral route among humans.[148] Two new live, oral, attenuated rotavirus vaccines were licensed in 2006 and appear safe to use for prevention of rotavirus infection without any increased risk of intussusception as occurred with the first rotavirus vaccine.[149] By 5 years of age most children have developed resistance to rotavirus infection.

Chronic Diarrhea in Children

Children with acute gastroenteritis often remain mildly symptomatic for up to 4 weeks; therefore, diarrhea that persists longer than 4 weeks is considered to be chronic. Children with **chronic diarrhea** can be divided into two groups: (1) otherwise well children whose growth is normal and (2) ill children whose growth is restricted. Causes of chronic diarrhea in the first group include abnormal colonic motility, lactose intolerance, encopresis, parasitic infestation, and antibiotic use.[150,151] Chronic diarrhea in the second group is usually caused by a disease that impairs absorption.

Chronic Nonspecific Diarrhea

Chronic nonspecific diarrhea of childhood is a condition in which uncoordinated colonic motility causes forceful expulsion of feces in otherwise healthy children. It affects children between 1 and 5 years of age. Apparently, the lower sigmoid colon remains in a tonically contracted state. Defecation occurs when pressure in the upper sigmoid colon and distal descending colon becomes great enough to force feces through the nonmotile, contracted segment. Prostaglandin synthesis is increased in the jejunum, and there are bile salts in the stools that may act as secretagogues.

In some instances there is a family history of bowel complaints. As an infant the child is likely to have experienced colic and diarrhea associated with teething and immunizations. In more than 90% of cases, chronic nonspecific diarrhea resolves by 40 to 50 months of age. The cure often accompanies toilet training. Many children with chronic nonspecific diarrhea develop irritable bowel syndrome (which is also called *mucous colitis*) as adults.[152] Children with chronic nonspecific diarrhea usually do well with normal food and fluid intake with a balance of fluid, fiber, fat, and fruit juices without high amounts of sorbitol (sorbitol content is higher in pear, apple, and prune juices and may cause diarrhea in children 1 to 3 years of age).

Primary Lactose Intolerance

Lactose intolerance is the inability to digest milk sugar. It is caused by inadequate production of lactase and is a common cause of diarrhea in children, particularly nonwhite children, younger than 7 years of age. The malabsorption of lactose results in osmotic diarrhea, in which fluids move by osmosis from the vascular compartment into the intestinal lumen. The undigested sugar is acted on by the colonic bacteria, and intestinal gas is produced. The diarrhea is accompanied by abdominal pain, bloating, and flatulence. Diagnosis includes elimination of dietary lactose or hydrogen breath testing. Treatment consists of lactase-treated dairy products, lactase supplements, or reducing dairy product consumption. Other sources of dietary calcium or supplements need to be provided if dairy products are eliminated. Some children can tolerate lactose in fermented forms, such as cheese and yogurt. Complete restriction of lactose-containing foods is rarely necessary in young infants.[153]

DISORDERS OF THE LIVER

Disorders of Biliary Metabolism and Transport

Neonatal Jaundice

Physiologic jaundice of the newborn is usually a transient, benign icterus that occurs during the first week of life in otherwise healthy full-term infants. Physiologic jaundice is caused by mild unconjugated (indirect-reacting) hyperbilirubinemia. Total serum bilirubin greater than 20 mg/dl or an indirect bilirubin greater than 15 mg/dl is considered **pathologic jaundice.** Risk factors include fetal-maternal blood type incompatibility (ABO and Rh incompatibility), prematurity, exclusive breast-feeding, maternal age greater than or equal to 25 years, male sex, delayed meconium passage, and excessive birth trauma such as bruising or cephalhematomas.[154] Hyperbilirubinemia is a risk with early hospital discharge (within 48 hours) because hyperbilirubinemia may not be evident prior to this time.[155]

PATHOPHYSIOLOGY Physiologic jaundice results from the complex interaction of factors that cause (1) increased bilirubin production (e.g., hemolysis), (2) impaired hepatic uptake or excretion of unconjugated bilirubin, and (3) delayed maturation of liver conjugating mechanisms.[155] Unconjugated bilirubin is lipid soluble, bound to albumin in the blood, and in the free form readily crosses the blood-brain barrier in infants. Chronic bilirubin encephalopathy (**kernicterus**) is caused by the deposition of toxic, unconjugated bilirubin in brain cells and usually does not occur in healthy full-term infants. Elevated conjugated bilirubin in a sign of underlying disease. A late rising indirect bilirubin level also may be a manifestation of **glucose-6-phosphate dehydrogenase deficiency,** a hereditary X-linked genetic defect.[156,157] Elevated unconjugated bilirubin levels also can cause hemolysis, further increasing neonatal jaundice.[158]

CLINICAL MANIFESTATIONS Physiologic jaundice develops during the second or third day after birth and usually subsides in 1 to 2 weeks in full-term infants and 2 to 4 weeks in premature infants. After this, increasing bilirubin values and persistent jaundice indicate pathologic hyperbilirubinemia. Manifestations include yellowing skin, dark urine, light-colored stools, and weight loss. Premature infants with respiratory distress, acidosis, or sepsis are at greater risk for encephalopathy. The resulting disabilities include athetoid cerebral palsy and speech and hearing impairment.[159,160]

EVALUATION AND TREATMENT Total and direct (conjugated) bilirubin levels are monitored and the bilirubin/albumin ratio is being evaluated.[161, 161a] Pathologic jaundice should be suspected with serum bilirubin values that increase greater than 5 mg/dl per day, persistent jaundice (greater than 7 to 10 days in the full-term infant), or conjugated bilirubin greater than 2 mg/dl. Other causes of jaundice must be eliminated to confirm physiologic jaundice. Treatment depends on the degree of hyperbilirubinemia. Physiologic jaundice is usually treated by phototherapy (ultraviolet light) with good eye protection.[162] Pathologic jaundice requires an exchange transfusion and treatment of the underlying cause.

Biliary Atresia

Biliary atresia is a rare congenital malformation characterized by the absence or obstruction of intrahepatic or extrahepatic bile ducts. Extrahepatic ducts may end in a blind pouch. The cause of the intrauterine injury to the ducts is not clear, but is thought to be related to a chromosomal abnormality or active agents, such as infection or drugs or an autoimmune response.[163] The disease expression is a continuum in which the principal process is one of bile duct destruction. The points of destruction are influenced by the stage of intrauterine development in which injury occurs.[161]

The atresia or obstruction of the bile ducts leads to plugging, inflammation, and fibrosis of the bile canaliculi and extrahepatic biliary tree. Progressive obstruction may lead to biliary cirrhosis (see Chapter 39), portal hypertension, or liver failure.[164]

Jaundice is the primary clinical manifestation of biliary atresia. Other signs are hepatomegaly and acholic (clay-colored) stools. Fat absorption is impaired for lack of bile salts, and the infant may fail to gain weight. Cirrhosis and liver failure lead to death within 2 years if untreated.

Early diagnosis of biliary atresia is mandatory and is based on clinical manifestations and liver biopsy. Liver function test results are abnormal. Serum transaminase and alkaline phosphatase values are elevated, and conjugated (direct) serum bilirubin levels rise progressively.

Extrahepatic atresia can be relieved by surgical drainage and correction in approximately 10% of cases. Some infants benefit from the Kasai procedure, in which a hepatic duct remnant is anastomosed to the jejunum or a jejunal segment is anastomosed to the porta hepatis if the patent hepatic duct remnant is not available (Figure 40-8). Even with initial restoration of bile flow, however, fibrosis and obliteration of intrahepatic bile ducts continue and cirrhosis

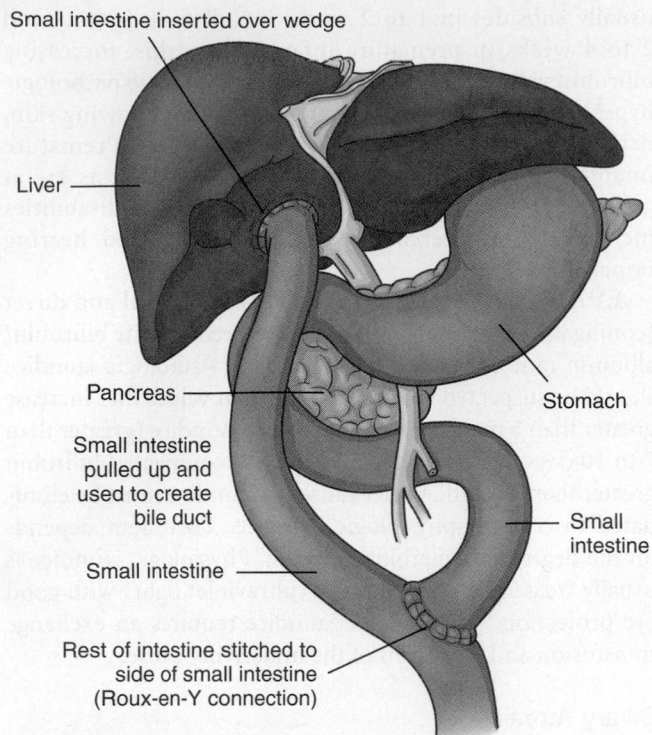

Small intestine inserted over wedge

Liver

Pancreas

Stomach

Small intestine pulled up and used to create bile duct

Small intestine

Small intestine

Rest of intestine stitched to side of small intestine (Roux-en-Y connection)

Figure 40-8 Kasai procedure. Surgical correction for extrahepatic biliary atresia. The jejunal segment between the liver and the bowel may be externalized, creating a double-barrel portoenterostomy.

results. Liver transplantation is the long-term therapy for biliary atresia. Approximately 40% of children with biliary atresia are immediate candidates for transplantation. Approximately 90% of children transplanted for biliary atresia become long-term survivors with good physical and mental development.[165] The use of reduced and split livers from living, related donors has increased the number of children who survive after transplantation.[166]

Inflammatory Disorders

Hepatitis

The pathophysiology of viral and fulminant hepatitis is described in Chapter 39.

Hepatitis A

Approximately one third to one half of the reported cases of **hepatitis A virus (HAV)** occur in children.[167] Incidence is highest among young children of preschool age. Outbreaks tend to occur in daycare centers with large numbers of children who are not toilet trained and staff members who practice poor handwashing techniques.[168] HAV replicates in the liver and is excreted through the biliary system into the stool. HAV in young children is usually mild and asymptomatic. Clinical manifestations, however, may include nausea, vomiting, and diarrhea. Because jaundice is absent, infected children appear to have the "flu." Almost all children recover from hepatitis A without residual liver damage.[169] Vaccination for hepatitis A should begin at 12 to 23 months of age.[170]

Hepatitis B

Infants of mothers who are chronic **hepatitis B surface antigen (HBsAg)** carriers, hemophiliacs who receive frequent blood transfusions, children who abuse parenteral drugs, and children who live in institutions for the mentally retarded are all at risk for **hepatitis B virus (HBV)** infection. Of newborns infected by their mothers, 90% develop chronic hepatitis and become carriers. The risk of chronic hepatitis is more than 25% to 90% for children younger than 6 years who contract HBV; HBV leads to chronic hepatitis in only 5% to 10% of cases among adults.[171] Chronic hepatitis may develop more often in young children because of their immature immune systems. Infected infants and children are at risk for cirrhosis and hepatocellular carcinoma. The most serious consequence of HBV infection is fulminant hepatitis, which occurs in 1% of cases. Hepatitis D infection (HDV) depends on active infection with HBV. There is evidence that the risk of fulminant hepatitis is higher in individuals with combined infection of HBV and HDV than in those with HBV infection alone.[172] The most effective approach to the treatment of hepatitis B is prevention. The American Academy of Pediatrics has added immunization for hepatitis B to those immunizations recommended for infants. Efforts are under way to immunize children and adolescents who did not receive this series as infants.

Hepatitis C

Hepatitis C virus (HCV) in children is most commonly transmitted vertically and is enhanced with maternal coinfection with HIV.[173] It also is transmitted with blood transfusions. Between 10% and 50% of affected children develop chronic liver disease. Antivirals are effective in the treatment of both hepatitis B and hepatitis C.[174]

Chronic Hepatitis

The cause of **chronic hepatitis** is unknown in most cases, but an autoimmune mechanism is suggested because inflammatory findings are commonly seen in biopsy specimens of the liver. Manifestations of chronic hepatitis include malaise, anorexia, fever, gastrointestinal bleeding, hepatomegaly, edema, and transient joint pain. Serum transaminase and bilirubin levels are elevated. There may be evidence of impairment of synthetic functions of the liver: prolonged prothrombin time and hypoalbuminemia. Diagnosis is based on the clinical manifestations and liver biopsy.

Symptoms are often absent in children. Treatment has variable efficacy and differs by the causative pathogen. The goals are to suppress the virus and prevent cirrhosis and hepatocellular carcinoma. Treatment includes interferon-alpha, ribavirin, and lamivudine.[175]

Cirrhosis

Cirrhosis is the excessive formation of fibrous tissue in response to inflammation and tissue damage (see Chapter 39). Most forms of chronic liver diseases in children can progress to cirrhosis, but they seldom do. Nonalcoholic fatty liver disease (steatohepatitis) is increasing in children in correlation with an increase in childhood obesity and it can progress to cirrhosis and liver cancer[176] (see What's New? Childhood Obesity and Nonalcoholic Fatty Liver Disease).

The complications of cirrhosis in children are the same as those in adults: portal hypertension, the opening of collateral vessels between the portal and systemic veins, and varices. In addition, children with cirrhosis experience growth failure caused by nutritional deficits and developmental delay, particularly in gross motor function because of ascites and weakness. The cause of cirrhosis may influence its severity and course. Some types of cirrhosis can be stabilized if the cause is identified and treated early.

Portal Hypertension

The two basic causes of **portal hypertension** in children are (1) increased resistance to blood flow within the portal system and (2) increased volume of portal blood flow. Increased resistance to flow can occur anywhere in the portal circulatory system. Portal hypertension can accompany cirrhosis, intra-abdominal infections, portal vein thrombosis, congenital anomalies of the portal vein, and congenital hepatic fibrosis.

Types

Extrahepatic Portal Hypertension

Extrahepatic (prehepatic) portal venous obstruction causes 50% to 70% of extrahepatic portal hypertension in children. For at least half of these children, no specific cause can be found. Obstruction is almost always in the portal vein and is usually caused by thrombosis. Umbilical infection with or without a history of catheterization of the umbilical vein may be a cause in neonates. Portal vein thrombosis can occur as a complication of intra-abdominal infections, pancreatitis, and blunt abdominal trauma. It also has been associated with neonatal dehydration, inflammatory bowel disease, and hypercoagulable states, such as protein C and protein S deficiencies.[161] The liver is usually normal in cases of extrahepatic portal hypertension.

Intrahepatic Portal Hypertension

Cirrhosis is the primary cause of **intrahepatic portal hypertension.** The most common finding is fibrosis, which increases resistance to portal blood flow by constricting and reducing the compliance of the hepatic sinusoids.

CLINICAL MANIFESTATIONS The clinical manifestations of portal hypertension are splenomegaly, upper gastrointestinal variceal bleeding, ascites, and hepatic encephalopathy. Severe liver disease is characterized by hypoalbuminemia, prolonged prothrombin times, hyperbilirubinemia, electrolyte imbalance, and hypoglycemia. **Splenomegaly** is the most common sign of portal hypertension in children. The spleen may be firm or hard, depending on the duration of portal hypertension. Hematemesis, possibly associated with abdominal pain, often accompanies sudden pallor. Melena is observed, either at the time of hematemesis or soon afterward. In children most episodes of gastrointestinal bleeding are caused by rupture of esophageal varices. Clotting abnormalities caused by altered liver function promote the bleeding. If plasma volume is increased, esophageal varices readily rupture during activities, such as coughing, that increase blood pressure. Acetylsalicylic acid (aspirin), which should not be administered to children, can trigger bleeding, but its exact mechanisms of action are not known. Severe bleeding episodes can cause hypovolemic shock and death. Symptoms of ascites include weight gain, protruding abdomen, and reduced tidal volumes if the ascites is severe. **Hepatic encephalopathy** in children can be acute or chronic. Acute encephalopathy is characterized by major disorders of consciousness, which may progress to coma. This may follow an acute episode of variceal bleeding as the impaired liver attempts to metabolize the large protein (nitrogenous) load from the blood. Chronic, or minimal, encephalopathy is characterized by emotional or psychiatric disorders, decreased intellectual functioning, personality disorders caused by minimal brain dysfunction, and spatial disorientation.

EVALUATION AND TREATMENT Assessment of portal hypertension in children must be thorough because the cause dictates the management. The objectives of the clinical investigation are to locate the site of the venous block and identify the disease responsible for the portal hypertension. Thorough physical examination, laboratory tests of liver function, imaging procedures, and biopsy may be included in the diagnostic evaluation (see Chapter 38). Sclerotherapy is the initial treatment of choice for severe esophageal varices in children.[177]

The indications for surgical shunting include gastrointestinal hemorrhage not responsive to sclerotherapy. Surgical venous shunts rarely have been performed on small children because of the high failure rate secondary to vessel occlusion, but they may be an alternative in older children, with some success.[161,178] Surgical shunts are no longer a contraindication

---

> **WHAT'S NEW?** Childhood Obesity and Nonalcoholic Fatty Liver Disease
>
> Nonalcoholic fatty liver disease (NAFLD) is the most common cause of liver disease in children and is associated with abdominal obesity, insulin resistance and features of metabolic syndrome. The rise in childhood obesity worldwide is associated with excessive consumption of saturated fats and refined sugars and is contributing to the increasing prevalence of NALFD. The disease usually presents in prepubertal children, with predominance in males and children of Hispanic origin. Diagnosis is made by exclusion of other disease causes. Liver biopsy is required for definitive diagnosis, and there are differences in the extent of fat, inflammation, and fibrosis in children compared with adults. There is no consensus regarding treatment. Exercise and slow, consistent weight loss with a low glycemic index diet have been shown to be more effective than a low-fat diet in lowering body weight. Pharmacologic agents are being evaluated to control insulin resistance and prevent progression of liver disease. Research is in progress to define the pathophysiology, noninvasive diagnostic procedures, and prevention of this disease.
>
> Data from: Barshop NJ et al: *Aliment Pharmacol Ther* 28(1):13-24, 2008; Dunn W, Schwimmer JB: *Curr Gastroenterol Rep* 10(1):67-72, 2008; Maneo M et al: *J Am Coll Nutr* 27(6):667-676, 2008.

for subsequent liver transplantation, although the shunt does make the transplantation technically more difficult. The transjugular intrahepatic portosystemic shunt (TIPS) procedure is performed for some children. This is a therapeutic option in which a stent is placed between the right hepatic vein and the right or left portal vein to allow shunting of blood without surgical intervention.[179]

The outcome of portal hypertension depends almost entirely on its cause. Children with extrahepatic disease are expected to recover with little morbidity. For children with intrahepatic disease, the prognosis varies.

Metabolic Disorders

More than 5000 genetically determined metabolic pathways have been identified in liver tissue. The earliest possible identification of metabolic disorders is essential because (1) early treatment may prevent permanent damage to vital organs, such as the liver or brain; (2) precise genetic counseling may be possible with prenatal diagnosis; and (3) complications can be minimized, even if cure is not possible. Galactosemia,[180] fructosemia, and Wilson disease are rare treatable metabolic disorders that have hepatic clinical manifestations. These disorders are summarized in Table 40-2 and Wilson disease is discussed next.

Wilson Disease

Wilson disease (hepatolenticular degeneration) is an autosomal recessive defect of copper metabolism that causes toxic amounts of copper to accumulate in the liver, brain, kidneys, and corneas. The gene *ATP7B* is localized on chromosome 13 and encodes copper-transporting P-type adenosine triphosphatase (ATPase) membrane-spanning protein. It is highly expressed in the liver, kidney, and placenta and is expressed in lower levels in the brain, heart, muscle, and pancreas.[181] This defect in the uptake and excretion of copper by hepatocytes is an important cause of progressive liver disease in children and young adults. Wilson disease is very rare, with an incidence of 1 in 30,000 live births worldwide.[182] Between 1 in 200 and 1 in 500 persons are carriers.[161]

PATHOPHYSIOLOGY Two major abnormalities in copper metabolism have been identified: (1) diminished biliary excretion of copper and (2) failure to insert copper into ceruloplasmin (a glycoprotein that transports copper in the blood). A positive copper balance is present from birth in children with Wilson disease, despite increased excretion of copper in the urine. Copper toxicity with accumulation in the liver and brain is the major abnormality. Excesses of copper generate free radicals that disrupt cellular organelles, deoxyribonucleic acid (DNA), microtubules, enzymes, and proteins. Copper overload is related to impaired biliary excretion of copper and may be related to failure of hepatocyte lysosomes to eliminate copper by exocytosis.[183]

Early in the disease, intestinal absorption of copper is normal, as is hepatic clearance of albumin-bound absorbed copper. As copper-binding proteins in the liver become saturated, hepatic uptake of copper diminishes, with elevated serum copper levels and biochemical and clinical evidence of liver damage caused by copper accumulation. In later stages of the disease copper accumulates in extrahepatic tissues, including the eyes, brain, and kidneys.

Table 40-2	Galactosemia, Fructosemia, and Wilson Disease		
	Galactosemia	**Fructosemia**	**Wilson Disease**
Mechanism of disease	Deficiency of galactose and phosphate, uridyl transferase	Deficiency of fructose-1-phosphate aldolase	Probably autosomal recessive: defect on chromosome 13
	An autosomal recessive trait	An autosomal recessive trait	Defect in copper excretion by liver
	Cannot convert galactose to glucose	Cannot metabolize fructose, sucrose, or honey; occurs when breast milk is replaced with cow's milk	Impaired transport of copper in blood caused by diminished transport protein (ceruloplasmin)
	Toxic accumulation of galactose in body tissues, liver, and brain	Toxic accumulation of fructose in body tissues	Toxic accumulations of copper in liver, brain, kidney, corneas
Clinical manifestations	High levels of blood galactose	High levels of blood fructose	Intention tremors
	Vomiting	Vomiting	Indistinct speech
	Hypoglycemia	Hypoglycemia	Dystonia
	May have failure to thrive	May have failure to thrive	Greenish-yellow rings in cornea
	Symptoms of cirrhosis at 2 to 6 months—jaundice	Hepatomegaly	Hepatomegaly
	Mental retardation if not treated	Jaundice	Jaundice
	Cataracts if not treated	Seizures	Anorexia
			Renal tubular defects
Evaluation	Presence of reducing substances in urine when infant is receiving lactose	Detailed dietary history	Low plasma ceruloplasmin
		Liver or intestinal mucosa biopsy	
Treatment	Galactose-free diet	Fructose-, sucrose-, honey-free diet	Chelation therapy to remove copper from body
		Vitamin C supplementation	Decreased dietary intake of copper
			Liver transplant

When cerebral copper-binding proteins become saturated, a characteristic pattern of brain damage develops, particularly in the basal ganglia. Neural effects include intention tremor, unsteady gait, dystonia, and behavioral changes. Manifestations of renal tubular injury usually appear simultaneously. The uptake of copper by red blood cells is thought to cause hemolytic anemia, a condition sometimes seen early in the clinical course of Wilson disease.

CLINICAL MANIFESTATIONS The clinical manifestations of Wilson disease may begin as young as 4 years of age, when control mechanisms responsible for copper homeostasis and biliary excretion should have matured. The mean age at diagnosis in one large study was 15.5 years.[184]

The classic clinical presentation of Wilson disease is a triad of neuromuscular abnormalities, intention tremors, dysarthria (indistinct speech), and dystonia (disordered muscular tonicity): (1) Kayser-Fleischer rings (accumulation of copper in the limbus of the cornea, causing a greenish-yellow ring), (2) cirrhosis associated with elevated serum copper, and (3) low ceruloplasmin levels.[185] Initial symptoms vary from malaise and abdominal pain to jaundice. Changes in mental and motor performance may develop at age 6 years or into adult life. The earliest signs of liver involvement include enlargement of the liver and spleen, jaundice, and anorexia. Edema and ascites may develop suddenly, or gastrointestinal hemorrhage may be the initial sign of the disease. Occasionally

Wilson disease begins with a hemolytic crisis caused by the toxic effects of copper on the red blood cells. Cirrhosis develops in all untreated cases. Copper deposition in the kidneys causes a proximal renal tubular defect that results in losses of glucose, amino acids, phosphate, and uric acid in the urine and renal tubular acidosis. All untreated individuals will develop behavioral or psychiatric disorders.

EVALUATION AND TREATMENT Because Wilson disease is rare, it may not be diagnosed until clinical manifestations develop in older childhood or adulthood. Laboratory tests detect a serum ceruloplasmin concentration less than 30 mg/dl. Serum copper values may be normal or high, and urine copper values are elevated. Liver biopsy is used to assess structural changes and measure copper concentrations. The goal of therapy is to decrease copper accumulation by decreasing intestinal absorption and increasing renal excretion. Medical treatments include D-penicillamine, trientine, zinc, and ammonium tetrathiomolybdate.[186] Copper intake is reduced by eliminating organ meats, nuts, legumes, shellfish, and chocolate from the diet. Physiotherapy may accelerate the recovery of gait and muscular coordination. Liver transplantation is the sole resolutive therapy for Wilson disease and is the treatment of choice for persons who develop fulminant hepatic failure or end-stage cirrhosis.[187] Children with untreated Wilson disease die of neural, hepatic, renal, or hematologic complications.

SUMMARY REVIEW

Disorders of the Gastrointestinal Tract

1. Most alterations of digestive function in children are caused by congenital anomalies of the intestinal tract; disorders of digestion, absorption, or nutrition; or liver disease.
2. Cleft lip (harelip) and cleft palate (failure of the bony palate to fuse in the midline) may occur separately or together and is associated with deficiency of B vitamins. The fissure may affect the uvula, soft palate, hard palate, nostril, and maxillary alveolar ridge.
3. Esophageal atresia, a condition in which the esophagus ends in a blind pouch, may occur with or without tracheoesophageal fistula, a connection between the esophagus and the trachea. As the infant swallows oral secretions or ingests milk, the pouch fills, causing either drooling or aspiration into the lungs.
4. Pyloric stenosis, an obstruction of the pyloric outlet caused by hypertrophy and hyperplasia of circular muscles in the pyloric sphincter, is more common in male infants and may require surgical correction.
5. Intestinal malrotation occurs with failure of the colon to rotate during fetal development and an obstructing band or volvulus (twisting of the bowel on itself) may partly or completely occlude the gastrointestinal tract and its blood vessels.
6. Meconium ileus is a condition in the newborn in which intestinal secretions and amniotic waste products produce a thick tarry plug that obstructs the intestine, usually from lack of fetal digestive enzymes. From 10% to 15% of children with CF have meconium ileus as neonates.
7. DIOS, formerly called *meconium ileus equivalent,* can occur when intestinal contents become abnormally thick and impact the intestinal lumen. CF and dehydration are common causes.

8. Duodenal, jejunal, and ileal obstructions can be caused by meconium ileus, atresia, congenital aganglionic megacolon, or acquired obstructive disorders.
9. Congenital aganglionic megacolon (Hirschsprung disease) is caused by a malformation of the parasympathetic nervous system in a segment of the colon, resulting is inadequate colon motility and functional obstruction.
10. Malformations of the anus and rectum range from mild congenital stenosis of the anus to complex deformities, all of which are classified as imperforate anus.
11. The most common cause of acquired intestinal obstruction in infants is intussusception, a condition in which one portion of the bowel telescopes or invaginates into another. It occurs most commonly in the area of the ileocecal junction.
12. GERD is caused by the relaxation or incompetence of the lower esophageal sphincter. Infants are susceptible to reflux because the sphincter is not fully mature, their diet consists of liquids, and they are seldom in an upright position.
13. Eosinophilic esophagitis involves an inflammation of the esophagus with dysphagia and vomiting that can be associated with asthma and eczema.
14. CF is an inherited disease with a pathophysiologic triad that includes pancreatic enzyme deficiency (which causes maldigestion), overproduction of mucus in the respiratory tract, and abnormally elevated sodium and chloride concentrations in sweat.
15. Gluten-sensitive enteropathy is an immune-mediated lifelong disease characterized by the loss of mature villous epithelium in the presence of a gluten-containing diet. It results in malabsorption and growth failure.

SUMMARY REVIEW—cont'd

16. Protein energy malnutrition is a group of disorders resulting from a severe dietary deficiency of proteins (kwashiorkor), carbohydrates, or both (marasmus). Starvation causes stunted mental and physical development. Kwashiorkor occurs most often in toddlers who have stopped breastfeeding and subsist on a high-carbohydrate diet.

17. Failure to thrive is inadequate physical growth of a child. Organic failure to thrive is caused by genetic, anatomic, or pathophysiologic factors that restrict normal growth and development. Nonorganic failure to thrive is caused by nutritional deficits associated with inadequate nurturing.

18. Necrotizing enterocolitis is a disorder in neonates, particularly premature infants, thought to result from stress and anoxia of an immature bowel wall. Bacteria invade the mucosa and submucosa resulting in colitis, necrosis, and even perforation of the intestinal wall.

19. Acute diarrhea in infants and children is often caused by infection and can rapidly cause dehydration and electrolyte imbalances because fluid reserves are relatively small. The most common cause of acute diarrhea in children is bacterial or viral enterocolitis.

20. Chronic diarrhea (diarrhea persisting longer than 4 weeks) can be caused by a wide variety of underlying conditions and often leads to growth failure and slow development.

21. Lactose intolerance causes diarrhea when failure to produce lactase results in osmotic diarrhea with ingestion of lactose-containing dairy products.

Disorders of the Liver

1. Physiologic jaundice of the newborn is caused by mild hyperbilirubinemia that subsides in 1 to 2 weeks. Pathologic jaundice is caused by severe hyperbilirubinemia and can cause brain damage.

2. Biliary atresia is a congenital malformation of the bile ducts that obstructs bile flow. Atresia causes jaundice, cirrhosis, and liver failure. Biliary atresia is the most common reason for liver transplantation in children.

3. Acute hepatitis has the same clinical course in children and adults but children have milder cases of the disease. Hepatitis A is the most common form of childhood hepatitis.

4. Cirrhosis is rare in children but can develop from most forms of chronic liver disease.

5. Portal hypertension in children usually is caused by extrahepatic obstruction. Thrombosis of the portal vein is the most common cause of portal hypertension in children and splenomegaly is the most common sign.

6. The three most common metabolic disorders that cause liver damage in children are galactosemia, fructosemia, and Wilson disease. All are rare, inherited as genetic traits, and permit the accumulation of toxins in the liver.

7. Wilson disease causes defective copper uptake and metabolism. Unexcreted copper accumulates in the liver, brain, kidney, and corneal cells. Damage from accumulated copper is gradual; the disease is usually not diagnosed before age 4 or 5 years.

KEY TERMS

Acute diarrhea, 1530
Biliary atresia, 1531
Chronic diarrhea, 1530
Chronic hepatitis, 1532
Chronic nonspecific diarrhea, 1530
Cirrhosis, 1532
Cleft lip (harelip), 1516
Cleft palate, 1516
Congenital aganglionic megacolon (Hirschsprung disease), 1521
Cystic fibrosis (CF), 1524
Diarrhea, 1530
Distal intestinal obstruction syndrome (DIOS), 1520
Eosinophilic esophagitis, 1524
Esophageal atresia, 1518
Extrahepatic (prehepatic) portal venous obstruction, 1533

Failure to thrive (FTT), 1528
Gastroesophageal reflux disease (GERD), 1523
Glucose-6-phosphate dehydrogenase deficiency, 1531
Gluten-sensitive enteropathy, 1525
Hepatic encephalopathy, 1533
Hepatitis A virus (HAV), 1532
Hepatitis B surface antigen (HBsAg), 1532
Hepatitis B virus (HBV), 1532
Hepatitis C virus (HCV), 1532
Imperforate anus, 1522
Infant diarrhea, 1530
Infectious diarrhea, 1530
Intestinal malrotation, 1519
Intrahepatic portal hypertension, 1533
Intussusception, 1522
Kernicterus, 1531

Kwashiorkor, 1528
Lactose intolerance, 1531
Marasmus, 1528
Meconium, 1520
Meconium ileus, 1520
Necrotizing enterocolitis (NEC), 1529
Nonorganic FTT, 1528
Organic FTT, 1528
Pathologic jaundice, 1531
Periduodenal band, 1519
Physiologic jaundice of the newborn, 1531
Portal hypertension, 1533
Protein energy malnutrition (PEM), 1528
Pyloric stenosis, 1519
Rotavirus, 1530
Splenomegaly, 1533
Tracheoesophageal fistula (TEF), 1518
Wilson disease, 1534

REFERENCES

1. Centers for Disease Control and Prevention: Improved national prevalence estimates for 18 selected major birth defects—United States, 1999-2001, *MMWR* 54(51,52):1301-1305, 2006.

2. Cooper ME, Tatay JS, Marazita ML: Asian oral-facial cleft birth prevalence, *Cleft Palate Craniofac J* 43(5):580-589, 2006.

3. Arosarena OA: Cleft lip and palate, *Otolaryngol Clin North Am* 4(1):27-60, 2007.

4. Carinci F et al: Human genetic factors in nonsyndromic cleft lip and palate: an update, *Int J Pediatr Otorhinolaryngol* 71(20):1509-1519, 2007.

5. Honein MA et al: Maternal smoking, environmental tobacco smoke, and the risk of oral clefts, *Epidemiology* 18(2):226-330, 2007.

6. Shi M, Wehby GL, Murray JC: Review on genetic variants and maternal smoking in the etiology or oral clefts and other birth defects, *Birth Defects Res C Embryo Today* 84(1):16-29, 2008.

7. Spilson SV, Kim HJ, Chung KC: Association between maternal diabetes mellitus and newborn oral clefts, *Ann Plast Surg* 47(5):477-481, 2001.

8. Vieira AR: Unraveling human cleft lip and palate research, *J Dent Res* 87(2):119-125, 2008.

9. Zucchero TM et al: Interferon regulating factor 6 (IRF6) gene variants and the risk of isolated cleft lip or palate, *N Engl J Med* 351(8):769-780, 2004.

10. Verkleij-Hagoort A et al: Hyperhomocysteinemia and MTHFR polymorphisms in association with orofacial clefts and congenital heart defects: a meta-analysis, *Am J Med Genet A* 143A(9):952-960, 2007.

11. da Silva Dalben G et al: Breastfeeding and sugar intake in babies with cleft lip and palate, *Cleft Palate Craniofac J* 40(1):84-87, 2003.

12. Redford-Badwal DA, Mabry K, Frassinelli JD: Impact of cleft lip and/or palate on nutritional health and oral-motor development, *Dent Clin North Am* 47(2):305-317, 2003.

13. Turner L et al: The effects of lactation education and a prosthetic obturator appliance of feeding efficiency in infants with cleft lip and palate, *Cleft Palate Craniofac J* 38(5):519-524, 2001.

14. Ramos GA et al: Diagnostic evaluation of the fetal face using 3-dimensional ultrasound, *Ultrasound Q* 24(4):215-253, 2008.

15. Weinfeld AB et al: International trends in the treatment of cleft lip and palate, *Clin Plas Surg* 32(1):19-23, 2005.

16. Barillas I et al: Nasoalveolar molding improves long-term nasal symmetry in complete unilateral cleft lip-palate patients, *Plast Reconst Surg* 123(3):1002-1006, 2009.

17. Sheahan P et al: Incidence and outcome of middle ear disease in cleft lip and/or cleft palate, *Int J Pediatr Otorhinolaryngol* 67(7):785-793, 2003.

18. Aniansson G et al: Otitis media and feeding with breast milk of children with cleft palate, *Scan J Plast Reconstr Surg Hand Surg* 36(1):9-15, 2002.

19. Ahluwalia M et al: Dental caries, oral hygiene, and oral clearance in children with craniofacial disorders, *J Dent Res* 83(2):175-179, 2004.

20. Kirchberg A, Treide A, Hemprich A: Investigation of caries prevalence in children with cleft lip, alveolus, and palate, *J Craniomaxillofac Surg* 32(4):216-219, 2004.

21. Achildi O, Grewal H: Congenital anomalies of the esophagus, *Otolaryngol Clin North Am* 40(1):219-244, viii, 2007.

22. Langer JC et al: Prenatal diagnosis of esophageal atresia using sonography and magnetic resonance imaging, *J Pediatr Surg* 36(5):804-807, 2001.

23. Kovesi T, Rubin S: Long-term complications of congenital esophageal atresia and/or tracheoesophageal fistula, *Chest* 126(3):915-925, 2004.

24. Spitz L: Oesophageal atresia, *Orphanet J Rare Dis* 2:24, 2007.

25. Houben CH, Curry H: Current status of prenatal diagnosis, operative management and outcome of esophageal atresia/tracheo-esophageal fistula, *Prenat Diagn* 28(7):667-675, 2008.

26. Hernanz-Schulman M: Infantile hypertrophic pyloric stenosis, *Radiology* 227(2):319-331, 2003.

27. Phillips JD: Abdominal surgical emergencies. In Wyllic R, Hyams J, editors: *Pediatric gastrointestinal diseases*, ed 2, Philadelphia, 1999, Saunders.

28. Armstrong M: The child with a cognitive deficit. In McKinney ES, et al, editors: *Maternal-child nursing*, ed 2, St. Louis, 2005, Saunders.

29. Sams CA: The child with a gastrointestinal alteration. In McKinney ES, et al, editors: *Maternal-child nursing*, ed 2, St. Louis, 2005, Saunders.

30. Kliegman R, et al: *Nelson textbook of pediatrics*, ed. 18, Philadelphia, 2007, Saunders.

31. Spinelli C et al: Muscle thickness in infantile hypertrophic pyloric stenosis, *Pediatr Med Chir* 25(2):148-150, 2003.

32. Shima H, Puri P: Increased expression of transforming growth factor-alpha in hypertrophic pyloric stenosis, *Pediatr Surg Intern* 15(3-4):198-200, 1999.

33. Blumer SL et al: The vomiting neonate: a review of the ACR appropriateness criteria and ultrasound's role in the work-up of such patients, *Ultrasound Q* 20(3):78-89, 2004.

34. Boneti C et al: Ultrasound as a diagnostic tool used by surgeons in pyloric stenosis, *J Pediatr Surg* 43(1):87091, 2008.

35. Aspelund G, Langer JC: Current management of hypertrophic pyloric stenosis, *Semin Pediatr Surg* 16(1):27-33, 2007.

36. Sweeney B, Surana R, Puri P: Jejunoileal atresia and associated malformations: correlation with the timing of in utero insult, *J Pediatr Surg* 36(5):774-776, 2001.

37. Durkin ET et al: Age-related differences in diagnosis and morbidity of intestinal malrotation, *J Am Coll Surg* 206(4):658-663, 2008.

38. Cohen Z et al: How much of a misnomer is "asymptomatic" intestinal malrotation? *Israel Med Assoc J* 5(3):172-174, 2003.

39. Lai HC: Nutritional status of patients with cystic fibrosis with meconium ileus: a comparison with patients without meconium ileus and diagnosed early through neonatal screening, *Pediatrics* 105(1 Pt 1):53, 2000.

40. Blackman SM et al: Relative contribution of genetic and nongenetic modifiers to intestinal obstruction in cystic fibrosis, *Gastroenterology* 131(4):1030-1039, 2006.

41. McAlister WH, Kronemer KA: Emergency gastrointestinal radiology of the newborn, *Radiol Clin North Am* 34(4):819-844, 1996.

42. Kao SC, Franken EA Jr: Nonoperative treatment of simple meconium ileus: a survey of the Society for Pediatric Radiology, *Pediatr Radiol* 25(2):97-100, 1995.

43. Evans AK, Fitzgerald DA, McKay KO: The impact of meconium ileus on the clinical course of children with cystic fibrosis, *Eur Respir J* 18(5):784-789, 2001.

44. Oliveira MC et al: Effect of meconium ileus on the clinical prognosis of patients with cystic fibrosis, *Braz J Med Biol Res* 35(1):31-38, 2002.

45. Dray X et al: Distal intestinal obstruction syndrome in adults with cystic fibrosis, *Clin Gastroenterol Hepatol* 2(6):498-502, 2004.

46. Schibli S, Dune PR, Tullis ED: Proper usage of pancreatic enzymes, *Curr Opin Pulm Med* 8(6):542-546, 2002.

47. Chaudry G et al: Abdominal manifestations of cystic fibrosis in children, *Pediatr Radiol* 36(3):233-240, 2006.

48. Hackam DJ et al: The influence of Down syndrome in the management and outcome of children with Hirschsprung disease, *J Pediatr Surg* 38(6):946-949, 2003.

49. Amiel J et al: Hirschsprung disease, associated syndromes and genetics: a review, *J Med Genet* 45(1):1-14, 2008.

50. Dasgupta R, Langer JC: Hirschsprung disease, *Curr Probl Surg* 41(12):942-988, 2004.

51. Kessmann J: Hirschsprung's disease: diagnosis and management, *Am Fam Physician* 74(8):1319-1322, 2006.

52. de Lorijn F et al: Diagnostic test in Hirschsprung disease: a systematic review, *J Pediatr Gastroenterol Nutr* 42(5):496-505, 2006.

53. Khan AR, Vujanic GM, Huddart S: The constipated child: how likely is Hirschsprung disease? *Pediatr Surg Int* 19(6):439-442, 2003.

54. de Lorijn F et al: Diagnostic tests in Hirschsprung disease: a systematic review, *Pediatr Gastroenterol Nutr* 42(5):496-505, 2006.

55. Bai Y et al: Long-term outcome and quality of life after the Swenson procedure for Hirschsprung disease, *J Pediatr Surg* 37(4):639-642, 2002.

56. Levitt MA, Pena A: Anorectal malformations, *Orphanet J Rare Dis* 2:33, 2007.

57. Rintala RJ: Fecal incontinence in anorectal malformations, neuropathy, and miscellaneous conditions, *Semin Pediatr Surg* 11(2):75-82, 2002.

58. Waseem M, Rosenberg HK: Intussusception, *Pediatr Emerg Care* 24(11):793-800, 2008.

59. de Vries S, Sleeboom C, Aronson DC: Postoperative intussusception in children, *Br J Surg* 13(4):81-83, 1999.

60. Eggermont E, De Boeck K: Small-intestinal anomalies in cystic fibrosis patients, *Eur J Pediatr* 150(12):824-828, 1991.

61. Fischer TK et al: Intussusception in early childhood: a cohort study of 1.7 million children, *Pediatrics* 114:782-785, 2004.

62. Blanch AJ, Perel SB, Acworth JP: Paediatric intussusception: epidemiology and outcome, *Emerg Med Australas* 19(1):45-50, 2007.

63. Byrne AT et al: The imaging of intussusception, *Clin Radiol* 60(3):412, 2005.

64. Kaiser AD, Applegate KE, Ladd AP: Current success in the treatment of intussusception in children, *Surgery* 142(4):469-477, 2007.

65. Navarro OM, Daneman A, Chae A: Intussusception: the use of delayed, repeated reduction attempts and the management of intussusception due to pathological lead points in pediatric patients, *Am J Roentgenol* 182(5):1169-1176, 2004.

66. Daneman A, Navarro O: Intussusception Part 1: a review of diagnostic approaches, *Pediatr Radiol* 33(2):79-85, 2003.

67. Kim JH: Ultrasound features of transient small bowel intussusception in pediatric patients, *Korean J Radiol* 5(3):178-184, 2004.

68. Bajaj L, Roback MG: Postreduction management of intussusception in a children's hospital emergency department, *Pediatrics* 112(6 Pt 1):1302-1307, 2003.

69. Crapko M et al: Role of extra-esophageal reflux in chronic otitis media with effusion, *Laryngoscope* 117(8):1419-1423, 2007.

70. Slocum C et al: Infant apnea and gastroesophageal reflux: a critical review and framework for further investigation, *Curr Gastroenterol Rep* 9(3):219-224, 2007.

71. Brodzicki J, Trawinska-Bartnicka M, Korzon M: Frequency, consequences and pharmacological treatment of gastroesophageal reflux in children with cystic fibrosis, *Med Sci Monit* 8(7):529-537, 2002.

72. Campanozzi A et al: Impact of malnutrition on gastrointestinal disorders and gross motor abilities in children with cerebral palsy, *Brain Dev* 29(8):534, 2007.

73. Maggio AB et al: Increased incidence of apparently life-threatening events due to supine position, *Paediatr Perinat Epidemiol* 20(6):491-496, 2006.

74. Tieder JS et al: Variation in inpatient resource utilization and management of apparent life-threatening events, *J Pediatr* 152(5):629-635, 2008.

75. Bhat RY et al: Acid gastroesophageal reflux in convalescent preterm infants: effect of posture and relationship to apnea, *Pediatr Res* 62(5):620-623, 2007.

76. Magista AM et al: Multichannel intraluminal impedance to detect relationship between gastroesophageal reflux and apnoea of prematurity, *Dig Liver Dis* 39(3):216-221, 2007.

77. Simanovsky N, Buonomo C, Nurko S: The infant with chronic vomiting: the value of the upper GI series, *Pediatr Radiol* 32(8):549-550, 2002.

78. Spitz L, McLeod E: Gastroesophageal reflux, *Semin Pediatr Surg* 12(4):237-240, 2003.

79. Chang F, Anderson F: Clinical and pathological features of eosinophilic oesophagitis: a review, *Pathology* 40(1):3-8, 2008.

80. Ireland-Jenkin K et al: Oesophagitis in children: reflux or allergy? *Pathology* 40(2):188-195, 2008.

81. Chehade M et al: Esophageal subepithelial fibrosis in children with eosinophilic esophagitis, *J Pediatr Gastroenterol Nutr* 45(3):3119-3128, 2007.

82. Ciorba A et al: Gastroesophageal reflux and its possible role in the pathogenesis of upper aerodigestive tract disorders, *Minerva Gastroenterol Dietol* 53(2):171-180, 2007.

83. Rohen R, Nurko S: The importance of multichannel intraluminal impedence in the evaluation of children with persistent respiratory symptoms, *Am J Gastroenterol* 99(12):2452-2458, 2004.

84. Dalby K et al: Reproducibility of 24-hour combined multiple intraluminal impedance (MII) and pH measurements in infants and children. Evaluation of a diagnostic procedure for gastroesophageal reflux disease, *Dig Dis Sci* 52(9):219-265, 2007.

85. Omari T: Gastroesophageal reflux in infants: can a simple left side positioning strategy help this diagnostic and therapeutic conundrum? *Minerva Pediatr* 60(2):193-200, 2008.

86. Rerksuppaphol S, Barnes G: Guidelines for the evaluation and treatment of gastroesophageal reflux in infants and children:recommendations of the North American Society for Pediatric Gastroenterology and Nutrition, *J Pediatr Gastroenterol Nutr* 35(4):583, 2002.

87. Arguin AL, Swartz MK: Gastroesophageal reflux in infants: a primary care perspective, *Pediatr Nurs* 30(1):45-51, 71, 2004.

88. Craig WR et al: Metoclopramide, thickened feedings, and positioning for gastro-oesophageal reflux in children under two years, *Cochrane Database Syst Rev* (4):CDC003502, 2004.

89. Lobe TE: The current role of laparoscopic surgery for gastroesophageal reflux disease in infants and children, *Surg Endosc* 21(2):167-174, 2007.

90. Konstan MW et al: Ultrase MT12 and Ultrase MT20 in the treatment of exocrine pancreatic insufficiency in cystic fibrosis: safety and efficiency, *Aliment Pharmacol Ther* 20(11-12):1365-1371, 2004.

91. Borowitz D: Update on the evaluation of pancreatic exocrine status in cystic fibrosis, *Curr Opin Pulm Med* 11(6):524-527, 2005.

92. Dodge JA, Turck D: Cystic fibrosis: nutritional consequences and management, *Best Pract Res Clin Gastroenterol* 20(3):531-546, 2006.

93. Stallings VA et al: Evidence-based recommendations for nutrition-related management of children and adults with cystic fibrosis and pancreatic insufficiency: results of a systematic review, *J Am Diet Assoc* 108(5):832-839, 2008.

94. Losowsky MS: A history of celiac disease, *Dig Dis* 26(2):112-120, 2008.

95. Rodrigues AF, Jenkins HR: Investigation and management of celiac disease, *Arch Dis Child* 93(3):251-254, 2008.

96. Di Sabatino A, Corazza GR: Coeliac disease, *Lancet* 373(9673):1480-1493, 2009.

97. Abdulkarim AS, Murray JA: Review article: the diagnosis of celiac disease, *Aliment Pharmacol Ther* 17(8):987-995, 2003.

98. Alaedini A, Green PH: Autoantibodies in celiac disease, *Autoimmunity* 41(1):19-26, 2008.

99. Gasbarrini G et al: Celiac disease in the 21st century: issues of under- and over-diagnosis, *Int J Immunopathol Pharmaco* 22(1):1-7, 2009.

100. Rossi T: Celiac disease, *Adolesc Med Clin* 15(1):91-103, 2004.

101. Telega G, Bennet TR, Werlin S: Emerging new clinical patterns in the presentation of celiac disease, *Arch Pediatr Adolesc Med* 162(2):164-168, 2008.

102. Catassi C, Fasano A: Celiac disease as a cause of growth retardation in children, *Curr Opin Pediatr* 16(4):445-449, 2004.

103. Eliakim R, Sherer DM: Celiac disease: fertility and pregnancy, *Gynecol Obstet Invest* 51(1):3-7, 2001.

104 Mora S: Celiac disease in children: impact on bone health, *Rev Endocr Metab Disord* 9(2):123-130, 2008.

105. Freeman HJ: Free perforation due to intestinal lymphoma in biopsy-defined or suspected celiac disease, *J Clin Gastroenterol* 37(4):299-302, 2003.

106. Scherer KR: Celiac disease, *Drugs Today (Barc)* 44(1):75-88, 2008.

107. Ojetti V et al: Regression of lactose malabsorption in celiac patients after receiving a gluten-free diet, *Scand J Gastroenterol* 43(2):174-177, 2008.

108. Guandalini S: The influence of gluten: weaning recommendations for healthy children and children at risk for celiac disease, *Nestle Nutr Workshop Ser Pediatr Program* 60:139-151, 2007.

109. Bernardo D et al: Decreased circulating iNKT cell numbers in refractory celiac disease, *Clin Immunol* 126(2):172-179, 2008.

110. Saloojee H et al: What's new: investigating risk factors for severe childhood malnutrition in a high HIV prevalence South African setting, *Scand J Public Health Suppl* 69:96-106, 2007.

111. Bern C et al: Assessment of potential indicators for protein-energy malnutrition in the algorithm for integrated management of childhood illness, *Bull WHO* 75(Suppl 1):87-96, 1997.

112. World Health Organization: *Water related diseases: malnutrition*. Available at www.who.int/water_sanitation_health/diseases/malnutrition/en.

113. Pelletier DL: The relationship between child anthropometry and mortality in developing countries: implications for policy, programs and future research, *J Nutr* 123(Suppl 10):2047S-2081S, 1994.

114. Joosten KF, Hulst JM: Prevalence of malnutrition in pediatric hospial patients, *Curr Opin Pediatr* 20(5):590-596, 2008.

115. Ogumkeye OO, Ighogboja IS: Increase in total serum triglyceride and phospholipids in kwashiorkor, *Ann Trop Pediatr* 12(4):463-466, 1992.

116. Maida JM, Mathers K, Alley CL: Pediatric ophthalmology in the developing world, *Curr Opin Ophthalmol* 19(5):403-408, 2008.

117. Latham MC: The dermatosis of kwashiorkor in young children, *Semin Dermatol* 10(4):270-272, 1991.

118. Ahmed T et al: Management of severe malnutrition and diarrhea, *Indian J Pediatr* 68(1):45-51, 2001.

119. Greco L et al: Effect of a low-cost food on the recovery and death rate of malnourished children, *J Pediatr Gastroenterol Nutr* 43(4):512-517, 2006.

120. Linneman Z et al: A large-scale operational study of home-based therapy with ready to use therapeutic food in childhood malnutrition in Malawi, *Matern Child Nutr* 3(3):206-215, 2007.

121. Steward DK, Moser DK, Ryan-Wenger NA: Behavioral characteristics of infants with failure to thrive, *J Pediatr Nurs* 16(3):162-171, 2003.

122. Stewart RC: Maternal depression and infant growth: a review of recent evidence, *Matern Child Nutr* 3(2):94-107, 2007.

123. Krugman SD, Dubowitz H: Failure to thrive, *Am Fam Physician* 68(5):879-884, 2003.

124. Piazza CC et al: Functional analysis of inappropriate mealtime behaviors, *J Appl Behav Anal* 36(2):187-204, 2003.

125. Steward DK: Behavioral characteristics of infants with nonorganic failure to thrive during a play interaction, *MCN Am J Matern Child Nurs* 26(2):79-85, 2001.

126. Bergman P, Graham J: An approach to "failure to thrive," *Aust Fam Physician* 34(9):725-729, 2005.

127. Marino R, Weinman ML, Soudelier K: Social work intervention and failure to thrive in infants and children, *Health Soc Work* 26(2):90-97, 2001.

128. Robinson JR, Drotar D, Boutry M: Problem-solving abilities among mothers of infants with failure to thrive, *J Pediatr Psychol* 26(1):21-32, 2001.

129. Black MM et al: Early intervention and recovery among children with failure to thrive: follow-up at age 8, *Pediatrics* 120(1):59-69, 2007.

130. Stewart RC: Maternal depression and infant growth: a review of recent evidence, *Matern Child Nutr* 3(2):94-107, 2007.

131. Lin PW, Stoll BJ: Necrotizing enterocolitis, *Lancet* 368(9543):1271-1283, 2006.

132. Lee JS, Polin RA: Treatment and prevention of necrotizing enterocolitis, *Semin Neonatol* 8(6):449-459, 2003.

133. Lambert DK et al: Necrotizing enterocolitis in term neonates: data from a multihospital health-care system, *J Perinatol* 27(7):437-443, 2007.

134. Hunter CJ et al: Understanding the susceptibility of the premature infant to necrotizing enterocolitis (NEC), *Pediatr Res* 63(2):117-123, 2008.

135. Anand RJ et al: The role of the intestinal barrier in the pathogenesis of necrotizing enterocolitis, *Shock* 27(2):124-133, 2007.

136. Frost BL, Jilling T, Caplan MS: The importance of pro-inflammatory signaling in neonatal necrotizing enterocolitis, *Semin Perinatol* 32(2):100-106, 2008.

137. Nankervis CA, Giannone PJ, Reber KM: The neonatal intestinal vasculature: contributing factors to necrotizing enterocolitis, *Semin Perinatol* 32(2):83-91, 2008.

138. Chardot C et al: Surgical necrotizing enterocolitis: are intestinal lesions more severe in infants with low birth weight? *J Pediatr Surg* 38(2):167-172, 2003.

139. Kabeer A, Gunnlaugsson S, Coren C: Neonatal necrotizing enterocolitis: a 12-year review at a county hospital, *Dis Colon Rectum* 38(8):866-872, 1995.

140. Alfaleh K, Bassler D: Probiotics for prevention of necrotizing enterocolitis in preterm infants, *Cochrane Database Syst Rev* (1):CD005496, 2008.

141. Embleton ND, Yates R: Probiotics and other preventative strategies for necrotizing enterocolitis, *Semin Fetal Neonatal Med* 13(1):35-43, 2008.

142. Srinivasan PS, Brandler MD, D'souza A: Necrotizing enterocolitis, *Clin Perinatol* 35(1):251-272, 2008.

143. Nguyen H, Lund CH: Exploratory laparotomy or peritoneal drain? Management of bowel perforation in the neonatal intensive care unit, *Perinat Neonatal Nurs* 21(1):50-60, 2007.

144. Butter A, Flageole H, Laberge JM: The changing face of surgical indications for necrotizing enterocolitis, *J Pediatr Surg* 37(3):496-499, 2002.

145. Nucci A et al: Interdisciplinary management of pediatric intestinal failure: a 10 year review of rehabilitation and transplantation, *J Gastrointest Surg* 12(3):429-435, 2008.

146. Bartlett JG, Gerding DN: Clinical recognition and diagnosis of *Clostridium difficile* infection, *Clin Infect Dis* 46(Suppl 1):S12-S18, 2008.

147. Finkbeiner SR et al: Metagenomic analysis of human diarrhea: vial detection and discovery, *PLoS Pathol* 4(2):e1000011, 2008.

148. Colbere-Garapin F et al: Prevention and treatment of enteric viral infections: possible benefits of probiotic bacteria, *Microbes Infect* 9(14-15):1623-1631, 2007.

149. Bernstein DI: Rotavirus overview, *Pediatr Infect Dis J* 28(3 Suppl):S50-S53, 2009.

150. Turck D et al: Incidence and risk factors of oral antibiotic-associated diarrhea in an outpatient pediatric population, *J Pediatr Gastroenterol Nutr* 37(1):22-26, 2003.

151. Lee SD, Surawicz CM: Infectious causes of chronic diarrhea, *Gastroenterol Clin North Am* 30(3):679-692, 2001.

152. Besedovsky A, Li BU: Across the developmental continuum of irritable bowel syndrome: clinical and pathophysiologic considerations, *Curr Gastroenterol Rep* 6(3):247-253, 2004.

153. Heyman MB: Committee on Nutrition: lactose intolerance in infants, children and adolescents, *Pediatrics* 118(3):1279-1286, 2006.

154. Chou SC et al: Management of hyperbilirubinemia in newborns: measuring performance by using a benchmarking model, *Pediatrics* 112(6):1264-1273, 2003.

155. Colletti JE et al: An emergency medicine approach to neonatal hyperbilirubinemia, *Emerg Med Clin North Am* 25(4):1117-1135, vii, 2007.

156. Cappellini MD, Fiorelli G: Glucose-6-phosphate dehydrogenase deficiency, *Lancet* 371(9606):64-74, 2008.

157. Iranpour R, Akbar MR, Haghshenas I: Glucose-6-phosphate dehydrogenase deficiency in neonates, *Indian J Pediatr* 70(1):855-857, 2003.

158. Alexandra Brito M, Silva RF, Brites D: Bilirubin toxicity to human erythrocytes: a review, *Clin Chim Acta* 374(1-2):46-56, 2006.

159. Blackmon LR, Fanaroff AA, Raju TN: Research on prevention of bilirubin-induced brain injury and kernicterus: National Institute of Child Health and Human Development conference executive summary, *Pediatrics* 114(1):229-233, 2004.

160. Bhutani VK, Johnson LH: Newborn jaundice and kernicterus—health and societal perspectives, *Indian J Pediatr* 70(5):407-416, 2003.

161. Behrman RE, Kliegman R, Jenson HB: *Nelson textbook of pediatrics*, ed 18, Philadelphia, 2007, Saunders.

161a. Hulzebos CV et al: Usefulness of the bilirubin/albumin ratio for predicting bilirubin-induced neurotoxicity in premature infants, *Arch Dis Child Fetal Neonatal Ed* 93(5):F84-F88, 2008.

162. Moerschel SK, Cianciaruso LB, Tracy LR: A practical approach to neonatal jaundice, *Am Fam Physician* 77(9):1255-1262, 2008.

163. Mack CL: The pathogenesis of biliary atresia: evidence for a virus-induced autoimmune disease, *Semin Liver Dis* 27(3):233-242, 2007.

164. de Carvalho E, Ivantes CA, Bezerra JA: Extrahepatic biliary atresia: current concepts and future directions, *J Pediatr (Rio J)* 83(2):105-120, 2007.

165. Chardot C: Biliary Atresia, *Orphanet J Rare Dis* 1:28, 2006.

166. Karakayali H et al: Liver transplantation for biliary atresia, *Transplant Proc* 40(1):231-233, 2008.

167. Armstrong GL, Bell BP: Hepatitis A virus infections in the United States: model-based estimates and implications for childhood immunizations, *Pediatrics* 109(5):839-845, 2002.

168. Muecke CJ et al: Hepatitis A seroprevalence and risk factors among day care educators, *Clin Invest Med* 27(5):259-264, 2004.

169. Koslap-Petraco MB, Shub M, Judelsohn R, Hepatitis A: disease burden and current childhood vaccination strategies in the United States, *J Pediatr Health Care* 22(1):3-11, 2008.

170. Centers for Disease Control and Prevention: Prevention of hepatitis A through active or passive immunization: recommendations of the Advisory Committee on Immunizations Practices, *MMWR* 55 (RR-7):1-23, 2006.

171. Chang MH: Hepatitis B virus infection, *Semin Fetal Neonatal Med* 12(3):160-167, 2007.

172. Shukla NB, Poles MA: Hepatitis B virus infection: co-infection with hepatitis C virus, hepatitis D virus, and human immunodeficiency virus, *Clin Liver Dis* 8(2):445-460, 2004.

173. Zein NN: Hepatitis C in children: recent advances, *Curr Opin Pediatr* 19(5):570-574, 2007.

174. Hsu EK, Murray KF: Hepatitis B and C in children, *Nat Clin Pract Gastroenterol Hepatol* 5(6):311-320, 2008.

175. Heller S, Valencia-Mayoral P: Treatment of viral hepatitis in children, *Arch Med Res* 38(6):702-710, 2007.

176. Roberts EA: Non-alcoholic steatohepatitis in children, *Clin Liver Dis* 11(1):155-172, 2007.

177. Sokucu S et al: Long-term outcomes after sclerotherapy with or without a beta blocker for variceal bleeding in children, *Pediatr Int* 45(4):388-394, 2003.

178. Ryckman FC, Alonso MH: Causes and management of portal hypertension in the pediatric population, *Clin Liver Dis* 5(3):789-818, 2001.

179. Rossle M, Grandt D: TIPS: an update, *Best Pract Res Clin Gastroenterol* 18(1):99-123, 2004.

180. Berry GT: Galactosemia and amenorrhea in the adolescent, *Ann N Y Acad Sci* 1135:112-117, 2008.

181. Ala A et al: Wilson's disease, *Lancet* 369(9559):397-408, 2008.

182. Brewer GJ: Recognition, diagnosis, and management of Wilson disease, *Proc Soc Exp Biol Med* 233(1):39-46, 2000.

183. Ferenci P: Pathophysiology and clinical features of Wilson disease, *Metab Brain Dis* 19(3-4):229-239, 2004.

184. Stremmel W et al: Wilson disease: clinical presentation, treatment, and survival, *Ann Intern Med* 115(9):720-726, 1991.

185. Mak CM, Lam CW: Diagnosis of Wilson's disease: a comprehensive review, *Crit Rev Clin Lab Sci* 45(3):263-290, 2008.

186. Medici V, Rossaro L, Sturniolo GC: Wilson disease—a practical approach to diagnosis, treatment and follow-up, *Dig Liver Dis* 39(7):601-609, 2007.

187. Sevmis S et al: Liver transplantation for Wilson's disease, *Transplant Proc* 40(1):228-230, 2008.

STRUCTURE AND FUNCTION OF THE MUSCULOSKELETAL SYSTEM

CHRISTY L. CROWTHER-RADULEWICZ

MEDIA RESOURCES

evolve **Evolve Website** (http://evolve.elsevier.com/McCance/)
- ■ Review Questions and Answers
- ■ Animations
- ■ Glossary (with audio pronunciation for selected terms)
- ■ WebLinks

CHAPTER OUTLINE

STRUCTURE AND FUNCTION OF BONES
  Elements of Bone Tissue
  Types of Bone Tissue
  Characteristics of Bone
  Maintenance of Bone Integrity
STRUCTURE AND FUNCTION OF JOINTS
  Fibrous Joints
  Cartilaginous Joints
  Synovial Joints
STRUCTURE AND FUNCTION OF SKELETAL MUSCLES
  Whole Muscle
  Components of Muscle Function

TESTS OF MUSCULOSKELETAL FUNCTION
  Tests of Bone Function
  Tests of Joint Function
  Tests of Muscular Function
Aging and the Musculoskeletal System
  Aging of Bones
  Aging of Joints
  Aging of Muscles

The way an individual functions in daily life, moves about, or manipulates objects physically depends on the integrity of the musculoskeletal system. The musculoskeletal system is actually composed of two systems: (1) the skeleton proper, which is composed of bones and joints; and (2) skeletal muscles. Each of the systems contributes to mobility. The skeleton supports the body and provides leverage to the skeletal muscles so that movement of various parts of the body is possible. This movement is accomplished by contraction of the skeletal muscles and bending or rotation at the joints.

STRUCTURE AND FUNCTION OF BONES

Bones give form to the body, support tissues, and permit movement by providing points of attachment for muscles. Many bones meet in movable joints that determine the type and extent of movement possible. Bones also protect many of the body's vital organs. For example, the bones of the skull,

thorax, and pelvis are hard exterior shields that protect the brain, heart, lungs, and reproductive and urinary organs.

The marrow cavities within certain bones serve as sites of blood cell formation. In adults, blood cells originate exclusively in the marrow cavities of the skull, vertebrae, ribs, sternum, shoulders, and pelvis. Bones also have a crucial role in mineral homeostasis, and storing and releasing minerals (i.e., calcium, phosphate, carbonate, magnesium) that are essential for the proper working of many delicate cellular mechanisms.

Elements of Bone Tissue

Mature bone is a rigid yet flexible connective tissue consisting of cells, fibers, a gelatinous material termed **ground substance,** and large amounts of crystallized minerals, mainly calcium, that give bone its rigidity. The structural elements of bone are summarized in Table 41-1.

Bone cells enable bone to grow, repair itself, change shape, and continuously synthesize new bone tissue and resorb (dissolve or digest) old tissue. The fibers in bone are made

Table 41-1   Structural Elements of Bone

Structural Element	Function
Bone Cells	
Osteoblasts	Synthesize collagen and proteoglycans; stimulate bone formation and are also involved in some osteoclast resorptive activity
Osteocytes	Maintain bone matrix; act as mechanoreceptors, influence osteoblasts and osteoclasts
Osteoclasts	Resorb bone; assist with mineral homeostasis
Bone Matrix	
Collagen fibers	Lend support and tensile strength
Proteoglycans	Control transport of ionized materials through matrix
Bone morphogenic proteins (BMPs)*	Induce cartilage and bone formation
BMP-2	Induces osteoblast differentiation in mesenchymal stem cells
BMP-6	Accelerates bone repair
BMP-9	Induces osteogenesis in mature osteoblasts
Glycoproteins	
Sialoprotein	Promotes calcification
Osteocalcin	Inhibits calcium-phosphate precipitation; promotes bone resorption
Laminin	Stabilizes basement membranes in bones
Osteonectin	Binds calcium in bones
Albumin	Transports essential elements to matrix; maintains osmotic pressure of bone fluid
α-Glycoprotein	Promotes calcification
Minerals (elements)	Crystallizes to lend rigidity and compressive strength
Calcium	Regulates vitamin D and thereby promotes mineralization
Phosphate	

*Data from Caetano-Lopes J, Canhão H, Fonseca JE: *Arthritis Res Ther* 9(Suppl 1):S1, 2007.

of collagen, which gives bone its tensile strength (the ability to hold itself together). Ground substance acts as a medium for the diffusion of nutrients, oxygen, metabolic wastes, biochemicals, and minerals between bone tissue and blood vessels.

Bone formation begins during embryonic development when mesenchymal stem cells begin differentiating into either chondrocytes or preosteoblasts. Endochondral ossification and intramembranous bone formation are the two major mechanisms responsible for normal bone development.

Endochondral ossification occurs when mesenchymal (**mesenchyme,** or loose tissue found during embryonic development) stem cells begin differentiating into chondrocytes (Figure 41-1), which in turn develop a mineralized cartilage scaffold that allows formation of osteoblasts. Most bone elements are formed this way. With the second mechanism, **intramembranous bone formation**, mesenchymal stem cells differentiate into a preosteoblast line that then forms osteoblasts without any cartilage framework.[1,2]

One of the major genetic factors influencing normal bone development and growth is a signaling family called Wnts. Wnt signaling of chondrocytes and osteoblasts affects bone mass and density, joint formation, fracture repair, and bone remodeling, as well as some bone diseases.[3] Osteoblasts are the principal cellular targets of Wnt signaling in bone.[4]

Wnt genes belong to a large family of protein-signaling factors that are required for the development of body systems, including the musculoskeletal system. They play a significant role in bone formation, developing bone mass, remodeling, and fracture healing. Wnt signaling regulates production and differentiation of osteoblasts and osteoclasts.[1,3,5]

Another major influence on bone and cartilage development is bone morphogenic proteins (BMPs). BMPs are multifunctional growth factors that belong to the transforming growth factor-beta (TGF-β) superfamily and affect several systems, including embryonic and postnatal cartilage and bone development. BMP activities are regulated at different molecular levels. Table 41-2 summarizes the role of several important BMP proteins.

In mature bone the formation of new tissue begins with the production of an organic matrix by the bone cells. This **bone matrix** consists of ground substances, collagen, and other proteins (see Table 41-1) that take part in bone formation and maintenance.

The next step in bone formation is **calcification,** when minerals are deposited and crystallize. Minerals bind tightly to collagen fibers, producing tensile and compressional strength in bone, and withstand pressure and weightbearing.

Bone Cells

Bone contains three types of cells: osteoblasts, osteocytes, and osteoclasts (Figure 41-2). Osteoblasts are the bone-forming cells, whose primary function is to lay down new bone. Once this function is complete, osteoblasts become osteocytes. Osteocytes are the most plentiful cells in bone. Osteocytes are osteoblasts that have become imprisoned within the mineralized bone matrix. They help maintain bone by signaling osteoblasts and osteoclasts to form and resorb bone.[6]

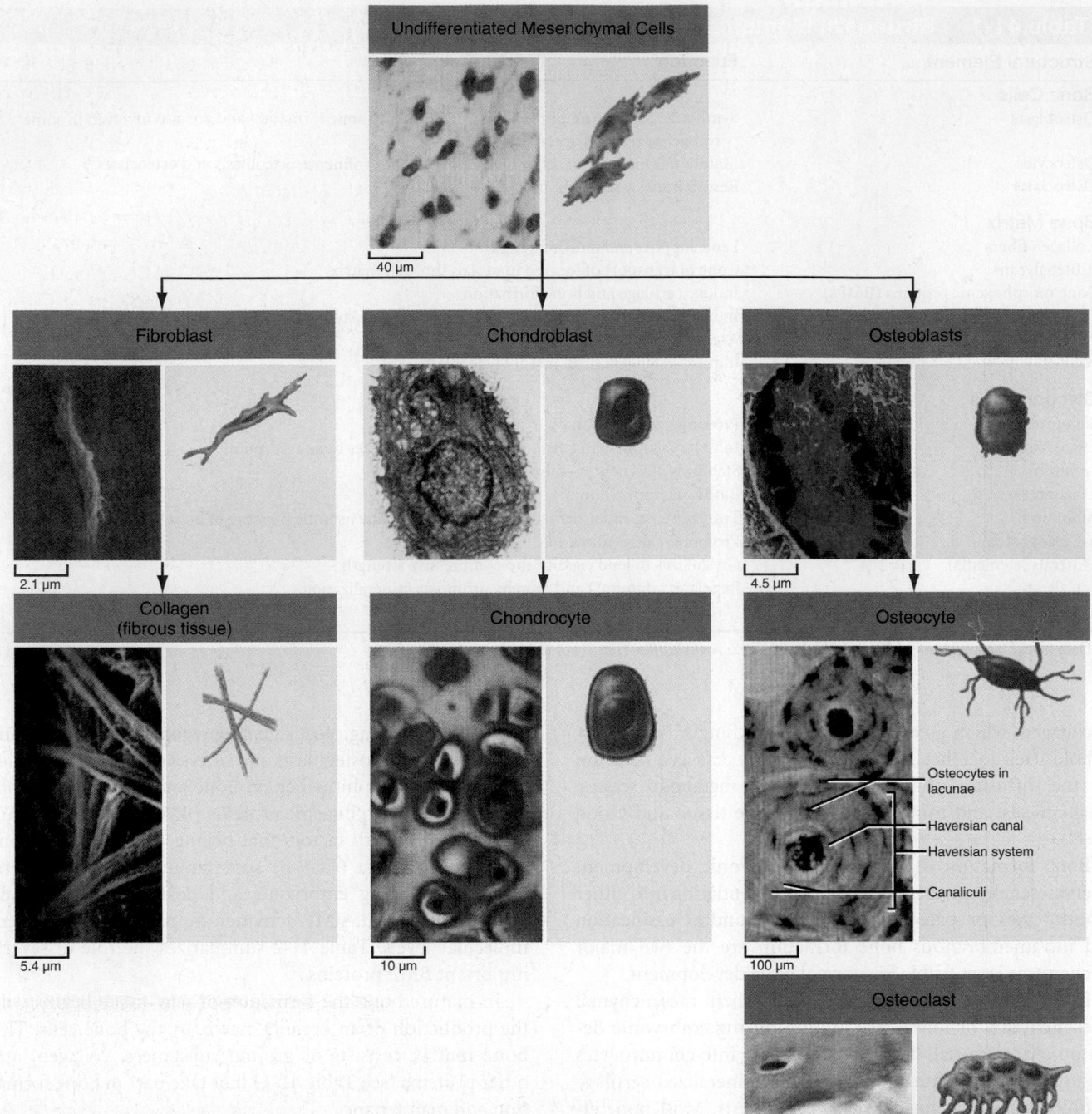

Figure 41-1 Mesenchymal stem cells. Undifferentiated mesenchymal cells give rise to a variety of cell types with distinct functions. (From Raven PH et al, editors: *Biology*, ed 8, New York, 2008, McGraw-Hill.)

Osteoblasts

Osteoblasts are cells derived from mesenchymal stem cells. Osteoblasts produce several substances, including osteocalcin, TGF-β (a growth inhibitor for many cells), macrophage colony-stimulating factor, receptor activator of nuclear factor κB-ligand, **osteoprotegerin** (OPG), and bone matrix[7] and osteocalcin when stimulated by 1,25-dihydroxyvitamin D. Osteoblasts are active on the outer surface of bones, where they form a single layer of cells. They bring about the formation of new bone by their synthesis of **osteoid** (nonmineralized bone matrix). The mechanism of osteoblast stimulation is reported to be the production of so-called coupling factors generated during the resorption process. Osteoblasts bring about the formation of new bone and the orderly mineralization of bone matrix by concentrating some of the plasma proteins (growth factors) found in the bone matrix and by facilitating the deposit and exchange of calcium and other ions at the site. Osteoblasts alter levels of receptor activator of nuclear factor κB-ligand (RANKL) and OPG. The balance of these two cytokines determines overall osteoclast formation[8] (see Figure 42-11). **RANKL** is part of a ligand-receptor system that assists in regulating osteoclastic bone remodeling. As new bone is formed it is shaped and remodeled through TGF-β, as well as other plasma proteins (growth factors) found in the bone marrow (Table 41-3).

Osteocytes communicate with other cells and appear to instruct both osteoclasts and osteoblasts about when and where to resorb and form bone.[6] In contact with bone mineral, osteoclasts use adhesive structures, called *podosomes*, to attach themselves to the bone surface. They then seal their cytoplasm with the underlying bone and dissolve the bone and matrix while protecting the surrounding tissue.[9] Thus the cells of the osteoblastic lineage (osteoblasts and osteocytes) form a network of cells in bone that sense the shape and structure of bone and determine where it is appropriate that bone be formed or resorbed, according to Wolfe's law (bone is shaped according to its function).

Table 41-2	Bone Morphogenic Proteins (BMPs) and Their Functions
BMP	**Known Function**
BMP1	Cartilage development; is actually a metalloprotease
BMP2	Induces bone and cartilage formation
BMP3	Induces bone formation
BMP4	Regulates formation of teeth, limbs, and bone
BMP5	Involved in cartilage development
BMP6	Helps maintain adult joint integrity
BMP7	Major role in osteoblast differentiation; important in renal development and repair
BMP8a	Bone and cartilage development
BMP8b	Found in hippocampus
BMP10	May play role in development of the heart

Osteoblasts have an active state and a resting state. When active, osteoblasts synthesize and secrete osteoid. When in the resting state, they appear dormant. If appropriately stimulated, however, the resting osteoblasts are capable of resuming activity.

Osteocytes

An **osteocyte** is a transformed osteoblast that is trapped or surrounded in osteoid as it hardens from minerals that enter during ossification (see Figure 41-2, *B*). It is the final differentiation stage for an osteoblast. The osteocyte is within a space in the hardened bone matrix called a **lacuna.** Each osteocyte has a high nucleus/cytoplasm ratio with a thin layer of nonmineralized osteoid around it, similar to the egg white surrounding an egg yolk. Osteocytes secrete proteins, such as sclerostin (a Wnt antagonist that binds BMPs), that result in reduced bone formation.[4,7]

The function of osteocytes is not fully known, but they communicate with each other and help concentrate nutrients in the matrix. Osteocytes obtain nutrients from capillaries in the canaliculi, which contain nutrient-rich fluids. Osteocytes also help synthesize and replace needed elements of the matrix by signaling both osteoclasts and osteoblasts to resorb and form new bone. Through exchanges between these cells, hormone catalysts, and minerals, optimal levels of calcium, phosphorus, and other minerals are maintained in blood plasma. The osteocyte also aids in modifying bone matrix through release of enzymes to dissolve the mineralized walls of the lacunae to prepare the bone for remodeling. (Remodeling is described on p. 1547.)

Osteoclasts

Osteoclasts are the major resorptive cells of bone. They are large multinucleated cells with a short life span. Osteoclasts develop from the hematopoietic stem cell in the bone marrow stroma[8] and adjacent vessels and from mononuclear phagocytic cells. Osteoclasts contain lysosomes (digestive vacuoles)

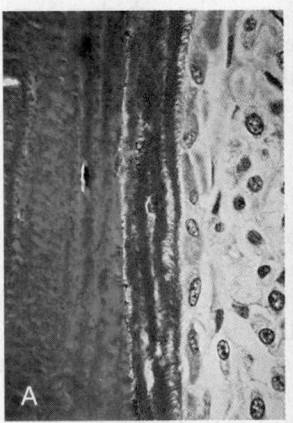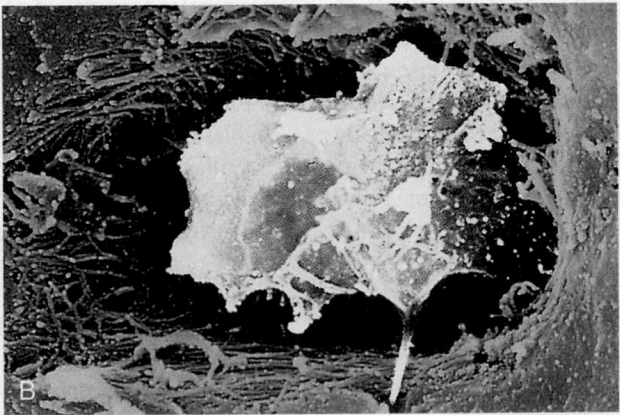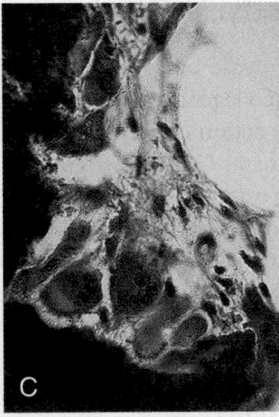

Figure 41-2 Bone cells. **A,** Osteoblasts are responsible for the production of collagenous and noncollagenous proteins that compose osteoid. Active osteoblasts are lined up on the osteoid. Note the eccentrically located nuclei. **B,** Osteocyte. Scanning electron micrograph showing an osteocyte within a lacuna. The cell is surrounded by collagen fibers and mineralized bone. **C,** Osteoclasts actively resorb mineralized tissue. The scalloped surface in which the multinucleated osteoclasts rest is termed the *Howship lacuna.* (**A** and **C** from Damjanov I, Linder J, editors: *Anderson's pathology,* ed 10, St Louis, 1996, Mosby. **B** from Erlandsen S, Magney J: *Color atlas of histology,* St Louis, 1992, Mosby.)

Table 41-3	Effects of Selected Cytokines (Growth Factors) on Skeletal Tissues			
Cytokine (Growth Factor)	**Target Tissue**	**Formation**	**Resorption**
Transforming growth factor–beta	Bone	+, −	+, −
	Cartilage	+, −	−
Transforming growth factor–alpha or epidermal growth factor	Bone	+, −	+
	Cartilage	+	0
Insulin-like growth factor	Bone	−	?
	Cartilage	−	0
Fibroblast growth factor	Bone	+, −	?
	Cartilage	+	0
Platelet-derived growth factor	Bone	0	+
Colony-stimulating factors	Bone	?	?
	Cartilage	−	?
Interferon-gamma	Bone	−	?
	Cartilage	−	+
Tumor necrosis factor	Bone	−	+
	Cartilage	+, −	+
Interleukins 1, 3, and 6	Bone	−	+
	Cartilage		

+, −, Both stimulatory and inhibitory properties on the specific cell listed; 0, no effects presently known; ?, possible effects on cell listed.

filled with hydrolytic enzymes. Fine projections, or micro-villi, fan out from the osteoclast cell's surface and are known as **ruffled borders;** these projections result from extensive infoldings of the cell membrane adjacent to the resorptive surface.[10] Osteoclasts in regions of bone resorption lie in pits called *Howship lacunae,* where the infolded, ruffled borders of the osteoclasts greatly increase the surface area of the plasma membrane. The infolds end in numerous channels and vesi-cles in the cell cytoplasm, permitting them to resorb the bone under their ruffled, infolded borders.

Osteoclasts bind to the bone surface of cell attachment proteins called **integrins.**[10] They bring about resorption of bone by secretion of hydrochloric acid (HCl) and cathepsin K (a protease enzyme),[9] which help dissolve bone miner-als and collagenase, which aids in digesting collagen, along with the action of cytokines (see Table 41-3). Matrix metal-loproteinases (MMPs), a group of proteolytic enzymes, help control osteoclast-matrix interactions necessary for bone resorption.[11] Once resorption is completed, the osteoclast disappears by degeneration, either by reverting back to its parent cell or by leaving the site through the process of cell mobility, wherein the osteoclast then becomes an inactive, or "resting," osteoclast.

Bone Matrix

Bone matrix is made of the extracellular elements of bone tissue, composed of about 35% organic and 65% inorganic materials. The major organic components are collagen fibers, and the major inorganic components are the calcium and phosphate minerals. Other parts of the bone matrix are the

proteins, carbohydrate-protein complexes, and ground sub-stances. Water makes up 5% to 8% of the matrix.

Collagen Fibers

Collagen fibers are the major organic component of bone matrix. The fibers are approximately 90% type I collagen, which is synthesized and secreted by osteoblasts. Collagen-I is essential for bone strength. Once secreted, the collagen molecules assemble into thin chains called α-*chains,* which combine in threes to form **fibrils.** The fibrils form a staggered pattern, overlapping nearby fibrils by approximately one fourth their length. This staggered, overlapping pattern cre-ates regular gaps, called *hole zones,* into which mineral crystals are deposited. After mineral deposition the fibrils link togeth-er and twist to form ropelike fibers. Collagen fibers then join to form a framework that gives bone its tensile strength and enables it to bear weight.

Collagen is the most abundant macromolecule in the body, accounting for approximately one third of all protein and providing the structural framework for nearly all tis-sues. Collagen is one of the extracellular components, along with proteoglycans and noncollagenous matrix proteins, of articular cartilage. To date, several types of collagen have been identified. Cartilage-specific collagens include types II (the principal component), VI, IX, X, and XI. Type IX col-lagen is thought to be the "glue" that holds together the type II collagen scaffold of articular cartilage, helps maintain the structural integrity of cartilage, and resists tensile forces on the joint cartilage. Type XI regulates the fibril diameter of type II cartilage. Degradation of type IX collagen by proteo-lytic enzymes has been seen in the early stages of osteoarthritis

Table 41-4	Types of Collagen in Musculoskeletal Tissues
Type of Collagen	**Distribution in Musculoskeletal Tissues**
I	Bone, tendon, ligament, intervertebral disk
II	Cartilage, intervertebral disk
IV	Basement cell membrane
V	Codistributed with type I
VI	Ubiquitous
IX	Codistributed with type II
X	Cartilage growth plate
XI	Cartilage
XII	Codistributed with type I
XIII	Molecule has not been isolated in connective tissues to date
XIV	Codistributed with type I

Table 41-5	Sequence of Calcium and Phosphate Compound Formation and Crystallization	
Formula	**Name**	**Abbreviation**
$Ca(HPO_4) \times 2H_2O$	Dicalcium phosphate dihydrate	DCPD
$Ca_4H(PO_4)_3$	Octacalcium phosphate	OCP
$Ca_9(PO_4)_6$ (var.)	Amorphous calcium phosphate	ACP
$Ca_3(PO_4)_2$	Tricalcium phosphate	TCP
$Ca_5(PO_4)_3OH$	Hydroxyapatite	HAP

NOTE: Compounds are listed in the order in which precipitation and crystal formation occur.

and rheumatoid arthritis. Researchers have proposed that this degradation, or "unplugging," may be the mechanism for the degenerative changes seen in osteoarthritic and rheumatoid cartilage. Table 41-4 gives the musculoskeletal distribution of other types of collagen.

Proteoglycans

Proteoglycans are large complexes of numerous polysaccharides attached to a common protein core. Hyaline cartilage is primarily composed of the glycosaminoglycans chondroitin sulfate and keratin sulfate. They strengthen bone by forming compression-resistant networks between the collagen fibrils. Proteoglycans also control the transport and distribution of electrically charged particles (ions), particularly calcium, through the bone matrix, thereby playing a role in bone calcium deposition and calcification.

Glycoproteins

Glycoproteins are also carbohydrate-protein complexes of bone. Glycoproteins control the collagen interactions that lead to fibril formation. They also may play a role in calcification.

Some of the glycoproteins in bone matrix include bone sialoprotein, osteocalcin, osteonectin, laminin, albumin, and α-glycoprotein. Other proteins found in bone matrix are the compounds currently called **bone morphogenic proteins (BMPs)** (see Table 41-1). **Sialoprotein (osteopontin)** makes up about 8% of the noncollagenous matrix of bone and easily binds with calcium.

Osteocalcin is also a calcium-binding protein that binds preferentially to calcium that has already crystallized. The roles of osteocalcin may be to inhibit calcium phosphate precipitation and play a part in bone resorption by recruiting osteoclasts.

Osteonectin is also thought to bind calcium in bones, and laminin stabilizes basement membranes in bones. **Laminin** is an abundant bone matrix protein in humans that is most effective in neurite and axon growth.

Bone albumin is identical to serum albumin. In calcified matrix, bone albumin is permanently fixed to bone mineral crystals and remains so until the bone is resorbed. Researchers believe bone albumin transports essential elements such as hormones, ions, and other metabolites to and from the bone cells and maintains the osmotic pressure of **bone fluid** (fluid surrounding mineral crystals and osteoblasts).

α-Glycoprotein is thought to be synthesized in the liver, to be released into blood plasma, and to circulate to bone matrix, where it accumulates. α-Glycoprotein's affinity for calcium is 40 times greater than that of albumin. Therefore, it probably plays an important role in the calcification of growing bone. α-Glycoprotein also may facilitate bone resorption by activating osteoclasts.

Bone Minerals

Mineralization is the final step in bone formation, after collagen synthesis and fiber formation. Mineralization has two distinct phases: (1) formation of the initial mineral deposit (initiation), and (2) proliferation or accretion of additional mineral crystals on the initial mineral deposits (growth).[10] The majority of the mineral content in the body is an analog of the naturally occurring mineral *hydroxyapatite*.

Table 41-5 lists the sequence in which calcium and phosphate form amorphous (fluid) calcium phosphate compounds that are converted, in stages, to solid hexagonal crystals of **hydroxyapatite (HAP)**. As the calcium and phosphorus concentrations increase in the bone matrix, the first precipitate to form is dicalcium phosphate dihydrate (DCPD). Once DCPD precipitation begins, the remaining phases of bone crystal formation proceed until insoluble HAP is produced, with approximately 80% to 90% of the HAP being incorporated into the collagen fibers. Amorphous calcium phosphate is distributed throughout the bone matrix.

Types of Bone Tissue

Bone is made up of two types of bony (osseous) tissue: **compact bone (cortical bone)** and **spongy bone (cancellous bone)** (Figure 41-3). Compact bone makes up approximately 85% of the skeleton; spongy bone makes up the remaining 15%. Both types of bone tissue contain the same structural elements, and, with a few exceptions, both compact tissue and spongy tissue are present in every bone. The major difference

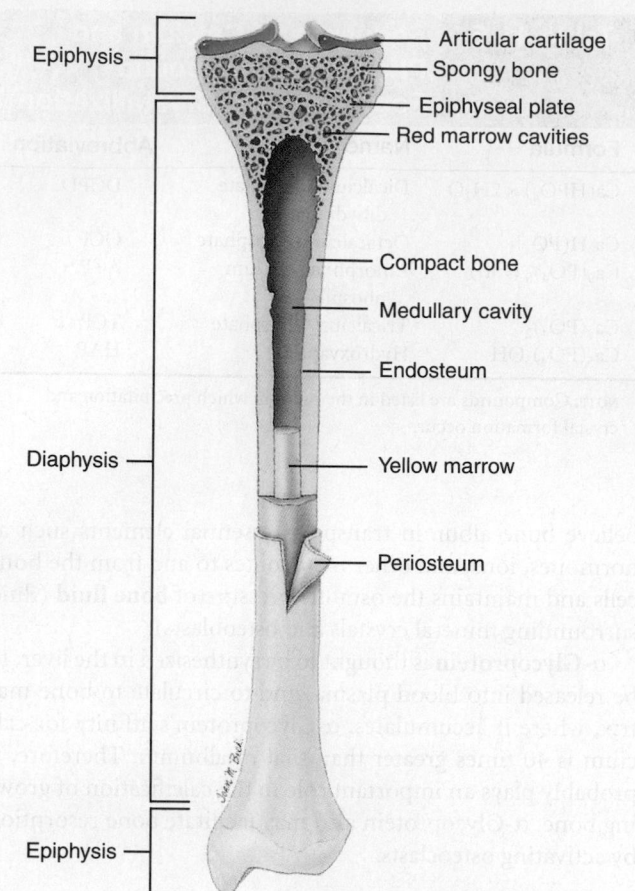

Epiphysis

Diaphysis

Epiphysis

— Articular cartilage
— Spongy bone
— Epiphyseal plate
— Red marrow cavities

— Compact bone

— Medullary cavity

— Endosteum

— Yellow marrow

— Periosteum

Figure 41-3 Cross section of bone. Longitudinal section of long bone (tibia) showing cancellous and compact bone. (From Patton KT, Thibodeau GA: *Anatomy & physiology*, ed 7, St Louis, 2010, Mosby.)

between the two types of tissue is the organization of the elements.

Compact bone is highly organized, solid, and extremely strong. The basic structural unit in compact bone is the haversian system (Figure 41-4). Each **haversian system** is made up of the following:

1. A central canal called the **haversian canal**
2. Concentric layers of bone matrix called **lamellae**
3. Tiny spaces (lacunae) between the lamellae
4. Bone cells (osteocytes) within the lacunae
5. Small channels or canals called **canaliculi**

Each haversian system is a separate cylindrical entity that looks like a set of concentric rings. In the center of the haversian system is the haversian canal. The haversian canal runs through the long axis of bone and contains one or two blood vessels and nerve fibers. The blood vessels in the canal communicate with blood vessels in the periosteum (surface cover) and marrow cavity to transport nutrients and wastes to and from the osteocytes contained within the lacunae. Surrounding each haversian canal are the concentric lamellae. Between the lamellae are the lacunae, each of which contains one osteocyte. The lacunae are connected to each other and to the haversian canal by the canaliculi, which run parallel to the

horizontal axis of the bone. Each canaliculus encloses a small extension (cytoplasmic process) from the osteocyte contained in the lacuna. The canaliculi transport both nourishment and molecular signals into the lacunae, a mechanism essential for osteocyte survival.

Spongy bone is less complex and lacks haversian systems. In spongy bone the lamellae are not arranged in concentric layers but in plates or bars termed **trabeculae** that branch and unite with one another to form an irregular meshwork. The pattern of the meshwork is determined by the direction of stress on the particular bone. The spaces between the trabeculae are filled with red bone marrow. The osteocyte-containing lacunae are distributed between the trabeculae and interconnected by canaliculi. Capillaries pass through the marrow to nourish the osteocytes.

All bones are covered with a double-layered connective tissue called the **periosteum.** The outer layer of the periosteum contains blood vessels and nerves, some of which penetrate to the inner structures of the bone through channels called Volkmann canals (see Figure 41-4). The inner layer of the periosteum is anchored to the bone by collagenous fibers (Sharpey fibers) that penetrate the bone. Sharpey fibers also help hold or attach tendons and ligaments to the periosteum of bones.[10]

Characteristics of Bone

The human skeleton consists of 206 bones that constitute the axial skeleton and the appendicular skeleton (Figure 41-5). The **axial skeleton** consists of 80 bones that make up the skull, vertebral column, and thorax. The **appendicular skeleton** consists of 126 bones that make up the upper and lower extremities, the shoulder girdle (pectoral girdle), and the pelvic girdle. The skeleton contributes about 14% of the weight of the adult body.

Bones can be classified by shape as long, flat, short (cuboidal), or irregular. **Long bones** are longer than they are wide and consist of a narrow tubular midportion (**diaphysis**) that merges into a broader neck (**metaphysis**) and a broad end (**epiphysis**) (see Figure 41-3).

The diaphysis consists of a shaft of thick, rigid compact bone that can tolerate bending forces. Contained within the diaphysis is the elongated marrow (medullary) cavity. The marrow cavity of the diaphysis contains primarily fatty tissue, which is referred to as *yellow marrow.* The yellow marrow assists red bone marrow in hematopoiesis only during times of stress. The yellow marrow cavity of the diaphysis is continuous with marrow cavities in the spongy bone of the metaphysis and diaphysis. The marrow contained within the epiphysis is red because it contains primarily blood-forming tissue (see Chapter 25). A layer of connective tissue, the **endosteum,** lines the outer surfaces of both types of marrow cavity.

The broadness of the epiphysis allows weightbearing to be distributed over a wide area. The epiphysis is made up of spongy bone covered by a very thin layer of compact bone. In a child the epiphysis is separated from the metaphysis by a cartilaginous **growth plate,** the **epiphyseal plate.** After puberty the epiphyseal plate calcifies and

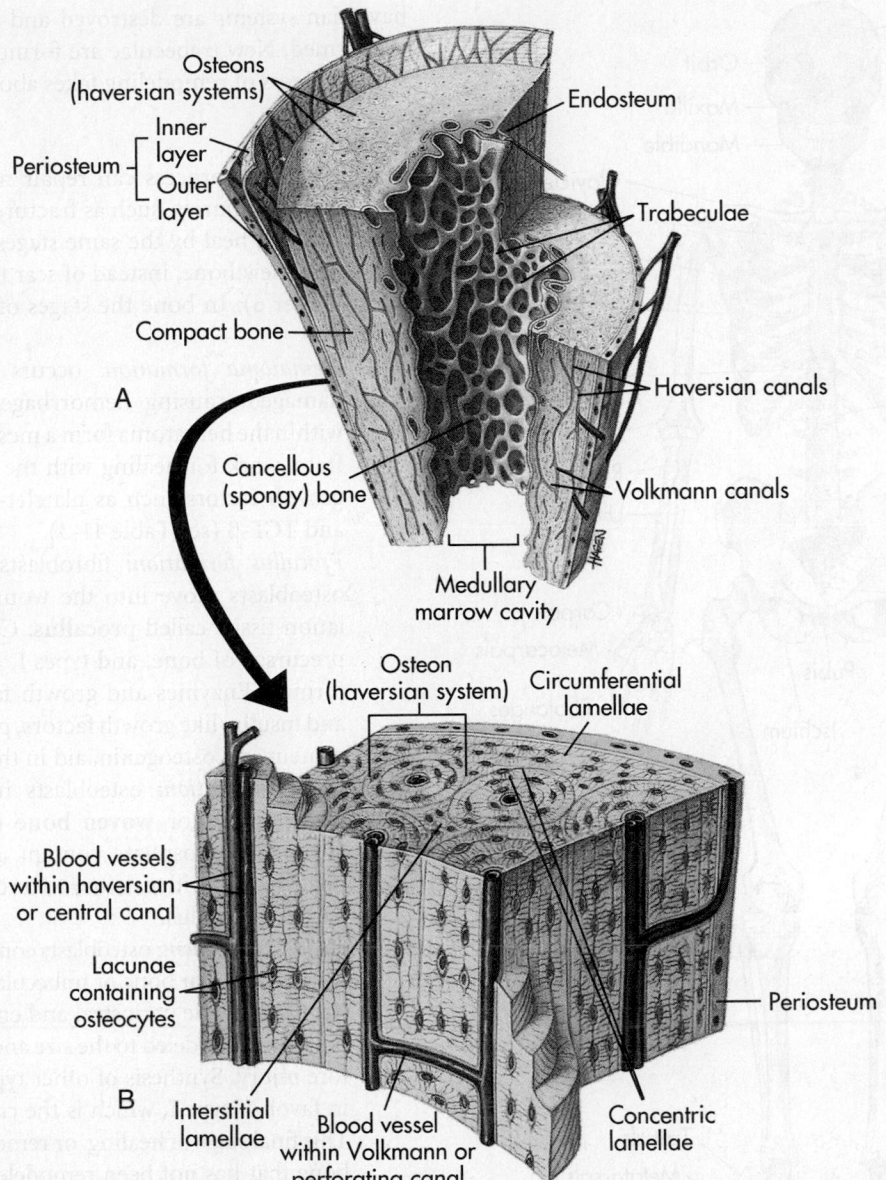

Figure 41-4 Structure of compact and cancellous bone. **A,** Longitudinal section of a long bone showing cancellous and compact bone. **B,** A magnified view of compact bone. (From Patton KT, Thibodeau GA: *Anatomy & physiology,* ed 7, St Louis, 2010, Mosby.)

the epiphysis and metaphysis merge. By adulthood the line of demarcation between the epiphysis and metaphysis is undetectable.

In **flat bones,** such as the ribs or scapulae, two plates of compact bone are roughly parallel to each other. Between the compact bone plates is a layer of spongy bone. **Short bones (cuboidal bones),** such as the bones of the wrist or ankle, are often cuboidal in shape. They consist of spongy bone covered by a thin layer of compact bone.

Irregular bones, such as the vertebrae, mandibles, or other facial bones, have various shapes that include thin and thick segments. The thin part of an irregular bone consists of two plates of compact bone with spongy bone between the plates. The thick part consists of spongy bone surrounded by a layer of compact bone.

Maintenance of Bone Integrity

Remodeling

The internal structure of bone is maintained by **remodeling,** a three-phase process in which existing bone is resorbed and new bone is laid down to replace it. Remodeling is carried out by clusters of bone cells termed **bone-remodeling units.** The bone remodeling units are made up of bone precursor cells that differentiate into osteoclasts and osteoblasts. Precursor cells are located on the free surfaces of bones and along the vascular channels (especially the marrow cavities).

In phase 1 (activation) of the remodeling cycle, a stimulus (e.g., hormone, drug, vitamin, physical stressor) activates programmed osteocyte cell death (apoptosis). The distribution of these apoptotic osteocytes provides osteoclasts with

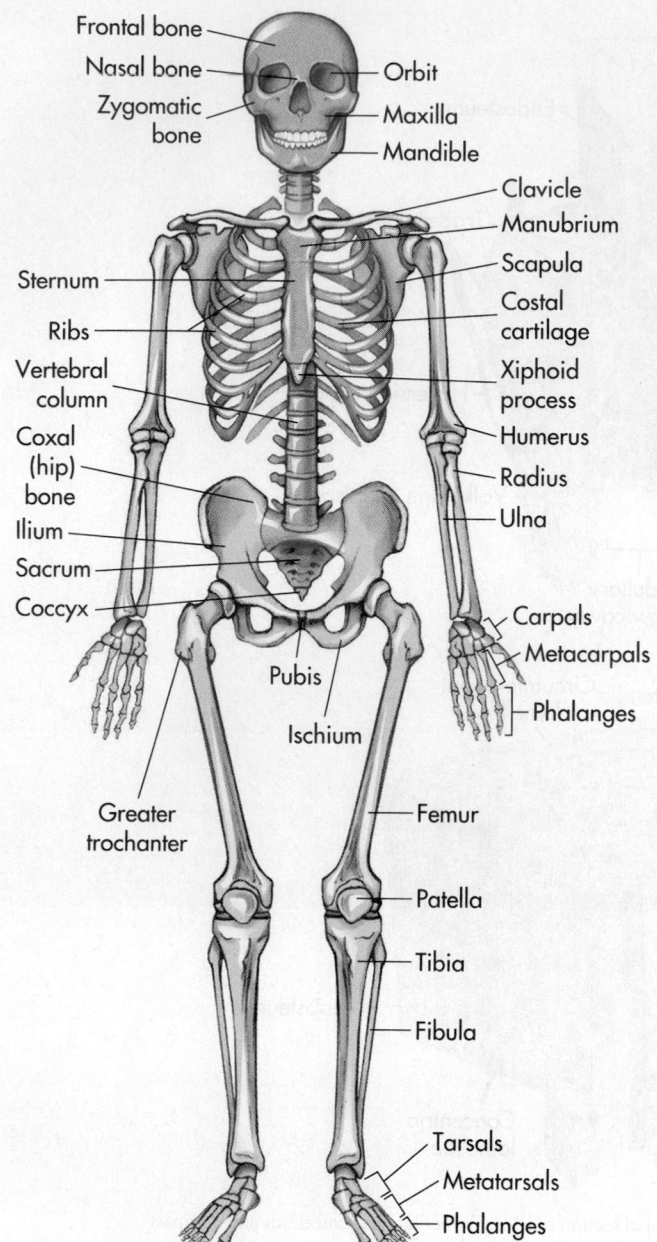

Figure 41-5 *Anterior view of skeleton.* Axial skeleton in blue; appendicular skeleton in tan. (From Patton KT, Thibodeau GA: *Anatomy & physiology,* ed 7, St. Louis, 2010, Mosby.)

information about where to begin resorbing damaged bone.[12] In phase 2 (resorption), the osteoclasts form a "cutting cone," which gradually resorbs bone, leaving behind an elongated cavity termed a *resorption cavity.* The resorption cavity in compact bone follows the longitudinal axis of the haversian system, and the resorption cavity in spongy bone parallels the surface of the trabeculae.

Phase 3 (formation) is the laying down of new bone, termed *secondary bone,* by osteoblasts lining the walls of the resorption cavity. Successive layers (lamellae) in compact bone are laid down until the resorption cavity is reduced to a narrow haversian canal around a blood vessel. In this way, old

haversian systems are destroyed and new haversian systems are formed. New trabeculae are formed in spongy bone. The entire process of remodeling takes about 3 to 4 months.

Repair
The remodeling process can repair microscopic bone injuries, but gross injuries, such as fractures and surgical wounds (osteotomies), heal by the same stages as soft tissue injuries, except that new bone, instead of scar tissue, is the final result (see Chapter 6). In bone the stages of wound healing are as follows:

1. *Hematoma formation:* occurs if vessels have been damaged, causing hemorrhage. Fibrin and platelets within the hematoma form a meshwork that is the initial framework for healing with the help of hematopoietic growth factors such as platelet-derived growth factor and TGF-β (see Table 41-3).
2. *Procallus formation:* fibroblasts, capillary buds, and osteoblasts move into the wound to produce granulation tissue called **procallus.** Cartilage is formed as a precursor of bone, and types I, II, and III collagen are formed. Enzymes and growth factors, such as insulin and insulin-like growth factors, plus bone morphogenic protein and osteogenin, aid in this stage of healing.
3. *Callus formation:* osteoblasts in the procallus form membranous or **woven bone (callus).** Enzymes increase the phosphate content and permit the phosphate to join with calcium to be deposited as mineral to harden the callus.
4. *Callus replacement:* osteoblasts continue to replace the callus with lamellar bone or trabecular bone (Figure 41-6).
5. *Remodeling:* the periosteal and endosteal surfaces of the bone are remodeled to the size and shape of the bone before injury. Synthesis of other types of collagen recedes in favor of type I, which is the collagen found in bone. This final stage of healing, or remodeling, is vital because bone that has not been remodeled does not have good mechanical properties for weightbearing and mobility.

The speed with which bone heals depends on the severity of the bone disruption; the type and amount of bone tissue that must be replaced (spongy bone heals faster); blood supply and oxygen to the site; presence of growth and thyroid hormones, insulin, vitamins, and other nutrients; presence of systemic disease; effects of aging; and effective treatment, including immobilization and the prevention of complications such as infection. In general, however, hematoma formation occurs within hours of fracture or surgery; formation of procallus by osteoblasts occurs within days; callus formation occurs within weeks; and replacement and contour modeling occur within years—up to 4 years in some cases.

STRUCTURE AND FUNCTION OF JOINTS

The site where two or more bones meet is called a **joint (articulation)** (Figure 41-7). The primary function of joints is to provide stability and mobility to the skeleton. Whether

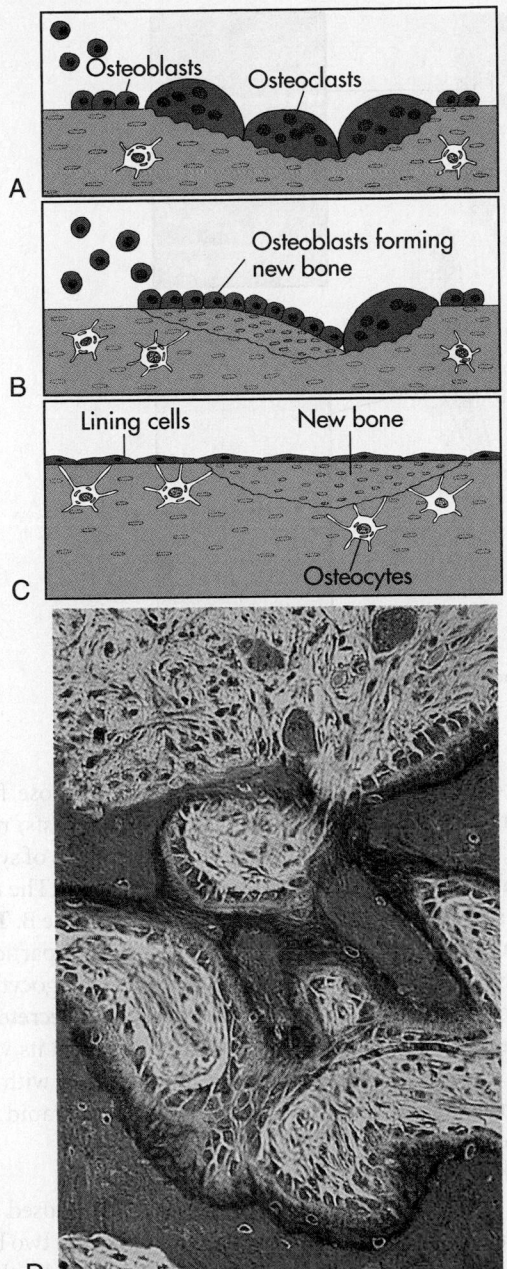

Figure 41-6 Bone remodeling. In the remodeling sequence, bone sections are removed by the bone-resorbing cells (osteoclasts) and replaced with a new section laid down by bone-forming cells (osteoblasts). The cells work in response to signals generated in that environment. The first phase of remodeling is mediated only by the multinucleated osteoclastic cells. They are activated, scoop out bone (A), and resorb it; then the work of the osteoblasts begins (B). Osteoblasts form new bone that replaces bone removed by the resorption process (C). The sequence takes 4 to 5 months. D, Active bone remodeling seen in the settings of primary or secondary hyperparathyroidism. Note the active osteoblasts surmounted on red-stained osteoid. Marrow fibrosis is present. (A to C from Mundy GR: *Bone remodeling and its disorders*, St Louis, 1995, Mosby. D from Damjanov I, Linder J, editors: *Anderson's pathology*, ed 10, St Louis, 1996, Mosby.)

a joint provides stability or mobility depends on its location and its structure. Generally, joints that stabilize the skeleton have a simpler structure than those that enable the skeleton to move. Most joints provide stability and mobility to some degree (Figure 41-8).

Joints are classified based on the degree of movement they permit or on the connecting tissues that hold them together. Based on movement, a joint is classified as a **synarthrosis (immovable joint)**, an **amphiarthrosis (slightly movable joint)**, or a **diarthrosis (freely movable joint)**. On the basis of connective structures, joints are classified broadly as fibrous, cartilaginous, and synovial. Each of these three structural classifications can be subdivided according to the shape and contour of the articulating surfaces (ends) of the bones and the type of motion the joint permits.

Fibrous Joints

A joint in which bone is united directly to bone by fibrous connective tissue is called a **fibrous joint**. Generally, fibrous joints are synarthroses (immovable), but many fibrous joints allow some movement. The degree of movement depends on the distance between the bones and the flexibility of the fibrous connective tissue.

Fibrous joints are further subdivided into three types: sutures, syndesmoses, and gomphoses. A **suture** has a thin layer of dense fibrous tissue that binds together interlocking flat bones in the skulls of young children. Sutures form an extremely tight union that permits no motion. By adulthood the fibrous tissue has been replaced by bone. A **syndesmosis** is a joint in which the two bony surfaces are united by a ligament or membrane. The fibers of ligaments are flexible and stretch, permitting a limited amount of movement. The paired bones of the lower arm (radius and ulna) and the lower leg (tibia and fibula) and their ligaments are syndesmotic joints. A **gomphosis** is a special type of fibrous joint in which a conical projection fits into a complementary socket and is held there by a ligament. The teeth held in the maxilla or mandible are gomphosis joints.

Cartilaginous Joints

The two types of cartilaginous joints are symphyses and synchondroses. A **symphysis** is a cartilaginous joint in which bones are united by a pad or disk of fibrocartilage. The articulating surfaces of the two bones are usually covered by a thin layer of hyaline cartilage, and the thick pad of fibrocartilage acts as a shock absorber and stabilizer. Examples of symphyses are the symphysis pubis, which joins the two pubic bones, and the intervertebral disks, which join the bodies of the vertebrae. A **synchondrosis** is a joint in which hyaline cartilage, rather than fibrocartilage, connects the two bones. The joints between the ribs and the sternum are synchondroses. The hyaline cartilage of these joints is called *costal cartilage*. Slight movement at the synchondroses between the ribs and the sternum allows the chest to move outward and upward during breathing.

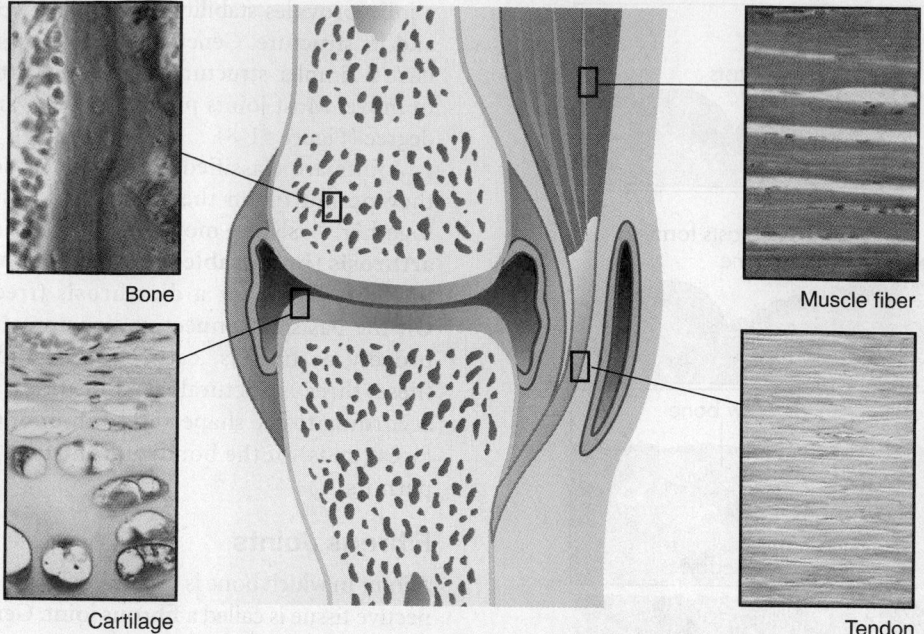

Bone

Muscle fiber

Cartilage

Tendon

Figure 41-7 Main tissues of a joint. (Micrographs from Erlandsen SL, Magney JE: *Color atlas of histology,* St Louis, 1992, Mosby.)

Synovial Joints

Structure

Synovial joints (diarthroses) are the most movable and the most complex joints in the body (Figure 41-9). A synovial joint consists of the following parts:

1. A fibrous joint capsule (articular capsule)
2. A synovial membrane that lines the inner surface of the joint capsule
3. A joint cavity (synovial cavity), a space formed by the capsule
4. Synovial fluid, which fills the joint cavity and lubricates the joint surface
5. Articular cartilage, which covers and pads the articulating bony surfaces

Joint Capsule

The fibrous **joint capsule (articular capsule)** is connective tissue that covers the ends of the bones where they meet in the joint. Sharpey fibers firmly attach the proximal and distal capsules to the periosteum and ligaments and tendons, which also reinforce the capsule. The joint capsule is made up of parallel, interlacing bundles of dense, white fibrous tissue. It is richly supplied with nerves, blood vessels, and lymphatic vessels. The nerves in and around the joint capsule are sensitive to the rate and direction of motion, compression, tension, vibration, and pain.

Synovial Membrane

The **synovial membrane (synovium)** is the smooth, delicate inner lining of the joint capsule (Figure 41-10). It lines the nonarticular portion of the synovial joint and any ligaments or tendons that traverse the joint cavity. It is made up of two layers—a vascular layer (**subintima**) and a thin cellular layer (**intima**). The vascular subintima merges with

the fibrous joint capsule and is composed of loose fibrous connective tissue, elastin fibers, fat cells, fibroblasts, macrophages, and mast cells. The intima consists of rows of synovial cells embedded in a fiber-free intercellular matrix. The intima contains two types of synovial cells: type A and type B. **Type A synovial cells** ingest and remove bacteria and particles of debris by phagocytosis in the joint cavity. (Phagocytosis is described in Chapter 6.) **Type B synovial cells** secrete **hyaluronate,** a binding agent that gives synovial fluid its viscous quality. The synovial membrane is richly supplied with blood and lymphatic vessels; therefore, it is capable of rapid repair and regeneration.

Joint Cavity

The **joint cavity (synovial cavity)** is an enclosed fluid-filled space between the articulating surfaces of the two bones. This small cavity, often called the *joint space,* enables the two bones to move "against" one another. The synovial cavity is surrounded by the synovial membrane and filled with a clear, viscous, slick fluid called the *synovial fluid.*

Synovial Fluid

Synovial fluid is superfiltrated plasma from blood vessels in the synovial membrane. Synovial fluid lubricates the joint surfaces, nourishes the pad of the articular cartilage that covers the ends of the bones, and contains free-floating synovial cells and various leukocytes that phagocytose joint debris and microorganisms. Loss of synovial fluid leads to rapid deterioration of articular cartilage.

Articular Cartilage

Articular cartilage is a layer of hyaline cartilage that covers the end of each bone (Figure 41-11). It ranges from 2 to 5 mm thick, depending on the size of the joint, the fit of the two bone ends, and the amount of weight and shearing

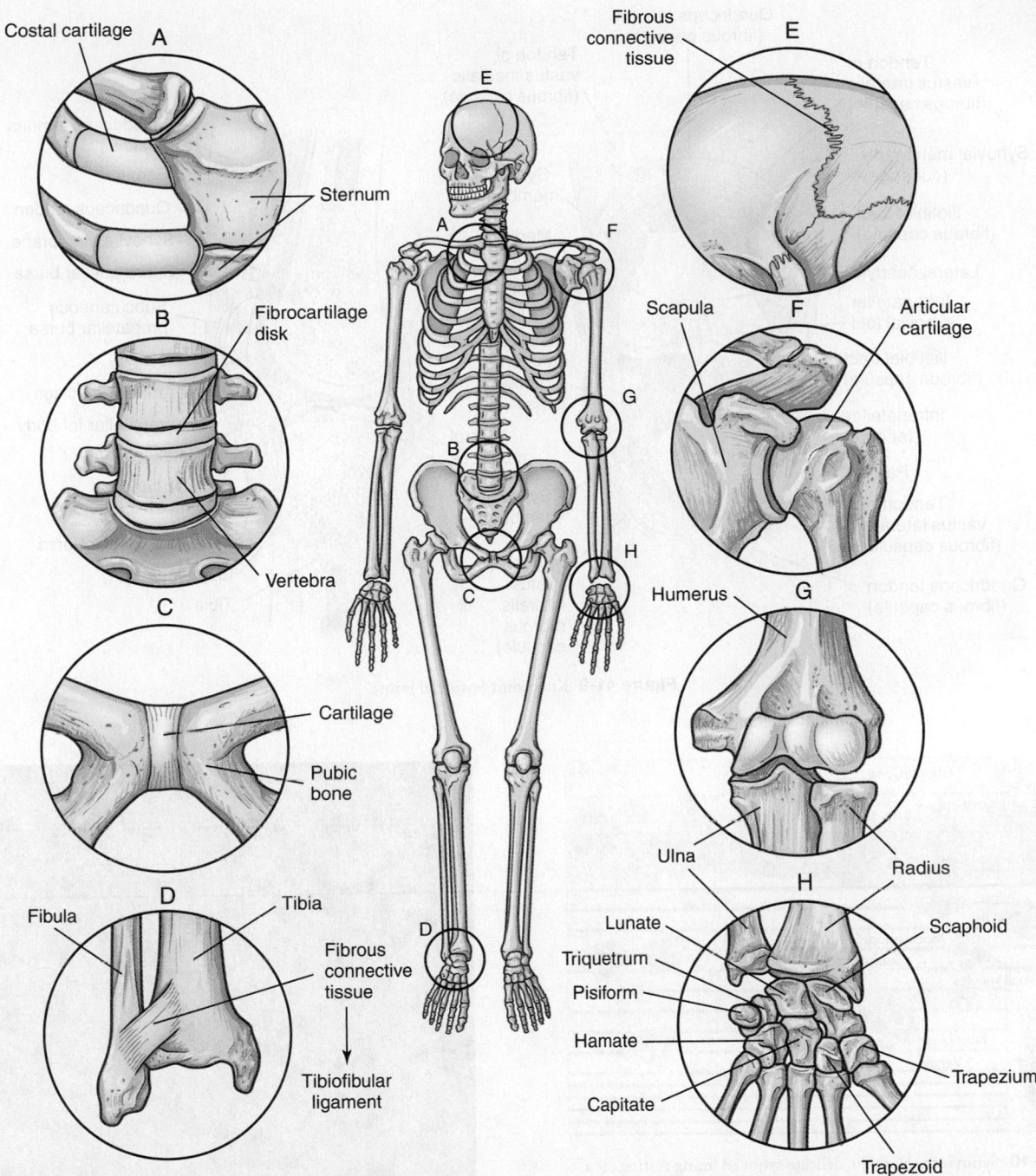

Figure 41-8 **Types of joints.** Cartilaginous (amphiarthrodial) joints, which are slightly movable, include (**A**) a synchondrosis that attaches ribs to costal cartilage; (**B**) a symphysis that connects vertebrae; and (**C**) the symphysis that connects the two pubic bones. Fibrous (synarthrodial) joints, which are immovable, include (**D**) the syndesmosis between the tibia and fibula; (**E**) sutures that connect the skull bones; and the gomphosis (not shown), which holds teeth in their sockets. The synovial joints include (**F**) the spheroid type at the shoulder; (**G**) the hinge type at the elbow; and (**H**) the gliding joints of the hand.

force the joint normally withstands. Cartilage strength and its biologic properties are due to an extensive network of cross-linked collagen fibers.[13] Figure 41-12 illustrates how collagen cross-links from cartilage. The function of articular cartilage is to reduce friction in the joint and to distribute the forces of weightbearing. Articular cartilage is composed of **chondrocytes** (cartilage cells) (making up about 2% of the tissue) and an intercellular matrix made up of collagen (making up about 10% to 30% of weight), protein polysaccharides (making up 5% to 10% of weight), and water. The water content ranges from 60% to almost 80% of the net weight of the cartilage, and individual molecules rapidly enter or exit the articular cartilage to contribute to the resiliency of the tissue.

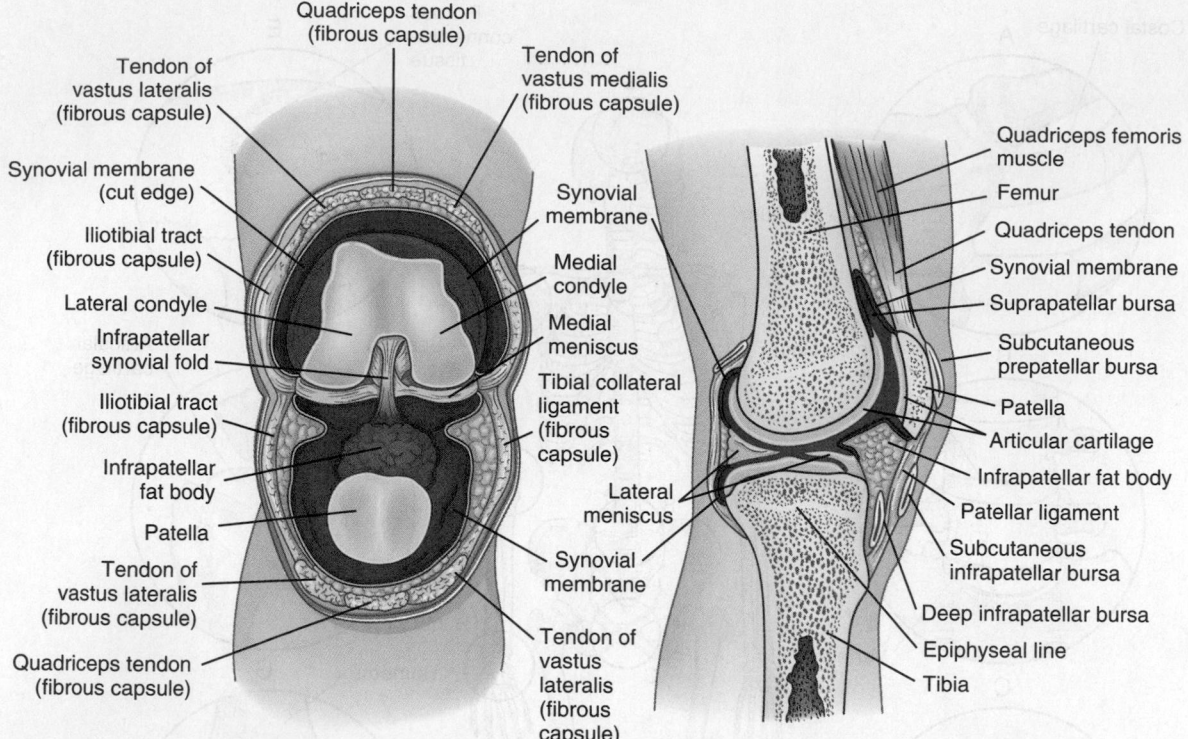

Figure 41-9 Knee joint (synovial joint).

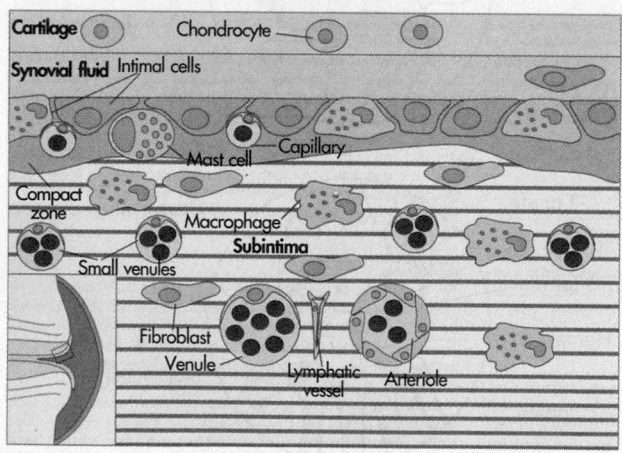

Figure 41-10 **Synovium.** Note the delicate synovial lining resting on a fibroadipose subintimal lining rich in capillaries, lymphatics, and nerve endings. (Modified from Klippel JH, Dieppe PA: *Rheumatology,* ed 2, London, 1998, Mosby-Wolfe.)

The intercellular matrix is produced by the chondrocytes, which synthesize and extrude collagen that, like the collagen produced by bone cells, is distributed throughout the cartilage in a highly organized system of fibers. Collagen fibers in cartilage are made up of many fine fibrils that, like bone fibrils, are assembled in an orderly fashion that makes them resistant to physical, metabolic, or chemical breakdown. The main differences between bone collagen and cartilage collagen are the amino acid content of the α-chains and the composition of the

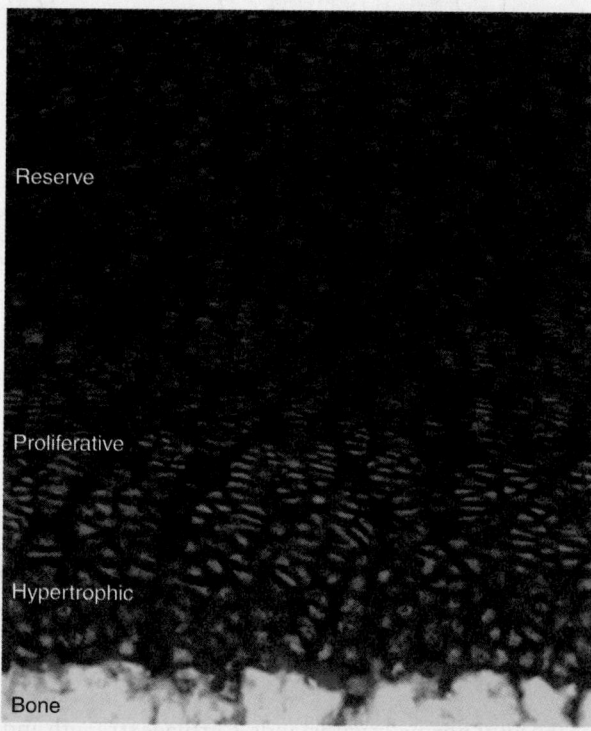

Figure 41-11 **Collagen zones.** The three collagen zones (reserve, proliferative, and hypertrophic) are distinctly shown in a growth plate. (From Hjorten R et al: *Bone* 41[4]:535, 2007.)

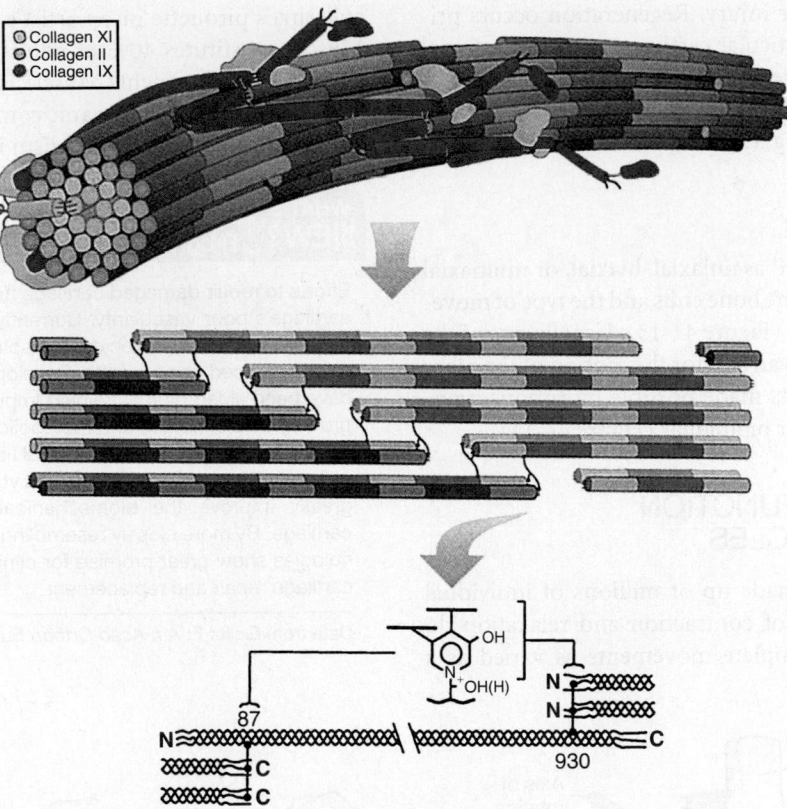

Figure 41-12 **Heterotypic collagen fibril.** Hierarchical depiction of heterotypic collagen fibril, emphasizing the internal axial relationships required for mature cross-link formation. *Upper drawing*: Three-dimensional concept of the type II/IX/XI heterotypic fibril of developing cartilage matrix. *Middle drawing*: Detail illustrating required nearest neighbor axial relationships for trifunctional intermolecular cross-links to form in collagens of cartilage, bone, and other high-tensile strength tissue matrices. The exact 3D spatial pattern of cross linking bonds is still unclear for any tissue. *Lower drawing*: Detail of the axial stagger of individual collagen molecules required for pyridinoline cross-linking. (From Eyre DA, Weiss MA, Wu JJ: *Methods* 4[1]:65, 2008.)

fibrils. Bone collagen fibrils are made up of two type I chains and one type II chain. Approximately 90% of the cartilage collagen fibrils is made up of three identical type II chains, with the remaining 10% made up of types V, VI, IX, X, and XI.

At the surface of articular cartilage, the collagen fibers run parallel to the joint surface and are closely compacted into a dense, protective mat. (Loss of this dense, compacted configuration at the surface subjects the underlying fibers to splitting and thinning, in which case the cartilage is unable to tolerate weightbearing.) In the middle layer (the proliferative zone) of the cartilage, the fibers are arranged tangential to the surface, which allows them to deform and absorb some of the force of weightbearing. In the bottom layer (the hypertrophic zone) of the cartilage, the fibers are perpendicular to the joint surface, allowing them to resist shear forces, and are embedded in a calcified layer of cartilage called the **tidemark.** The tidemark anchors the collagen fibers to the underlying (subchondral) bone and represents the zone between calcified and uncalcified cartilage. Collagen fibers are important components of the cartilage matrix because they account for approximately 60% of the dry weight and because they (1) anchor the cartilage securely to underlying bone, (2) provide a taut framework for the cartilage, (3) control the loss of fluid

from the cartilage, and (4) prevent the escape of protein polysaccharides (proteoglycans) from the cartilage.

The proteoglycans are macromolecules consisting of proteins, carbohydrates (**glycosaminoglycans),** and hyaluronic acid. The glycosaminoglycans (keratan sulfate and chondroitin sulfate) are attached to the **protein core,** and several protein cores (with their attached glycosaminoglycans) are bound to a hyaluronic acid chain by a special protein called **link protein.** The proteoglycans give articular cartilage its stiff quality and regulate the movement of synovial fluid through the cartilage. Without proteoglycans, normal weightbearing would rapidly and completely press all the synovial fluid out of the cartilage. The proteoglycans act as a pump, permitting enough fluid to be pressed out to ensure that a fluid film is always present on the surface of the cartilage, even after hours of weightbearing. The pumping action of proteoglycans also draws synovial fluid back into the cartilage after a weightbearing load is released. Mobility and weightbearing are necessary for the pumping action of proteoglycans to occur. Nonuse of a joint quickly reduces the pumping action, which changes the composition of the matrix and interferes with the nutrition of the chondrocytes.

Articular cartilage has no blood vessels, lymph vessels, or nerves. Therefore, it is insensitive to pain and regenerates slowly and minimally after injury. Regeneration occurs primarily at sites where the articular cartilage meets the synovial membrane, where blood vessels and nutrients are available. In general, it has been difficult to enhance cartilage repair, but that may be changing (see What's New? Progress in Rebuilding Cartilage).

Movement

Synovial joints are described as uniaxial, biaxial, or multiaxial according to the shapes of the bone ends and the type of movement occurring at the joint (Figure 41-13). Usually one of the bones is stable and serves as an axis for the motion of the other bone. The body movements made possible by various synovial joints are either circular or angular (Figure 41-14).

STRUCTURE AND FUNCTION OF SKELETAL MUSCLES

The skeletal muscles are made up of millions of individual fibers that by the process of contraction and relaxation do the work necessary to complete movements as varied as a

ballerina's pirouette or an artist's deft stroke (Figure 41-15). Muscle constitutes 40% of adults' body weight and 50% of children's body weight. Muscle is 75% water, 20% protein, and 5% organic and inorganic compounds; 32% of all protein stores for energy and metabolism is contained in muscle.

WHAT'S NEW? Progress in Rebuilding Cartilage

Efforts to repair damaged cartilage have been difficult because of cartilage's poor vascularity. Currently available techniques, such as autologous chondrocyte transplantation, have not consistently produced good results. Developments in tissue engineering have been aided by maintaining improved biologic control of cell growth, differentiation, and metabolic activity.

Techniques known as "functional tissue engineering" should not only provide a network of chondrocyte cell growth but also should greatly improve the biomechanical properties of engineered cartilage. By more closely resembling native cartilage, these technologies show great promise for clinically improved outcomes in cartilage repair and replacement.

Data from Guilaf F: *Am Acad Orthop Surg* 16(1):58, 2008.

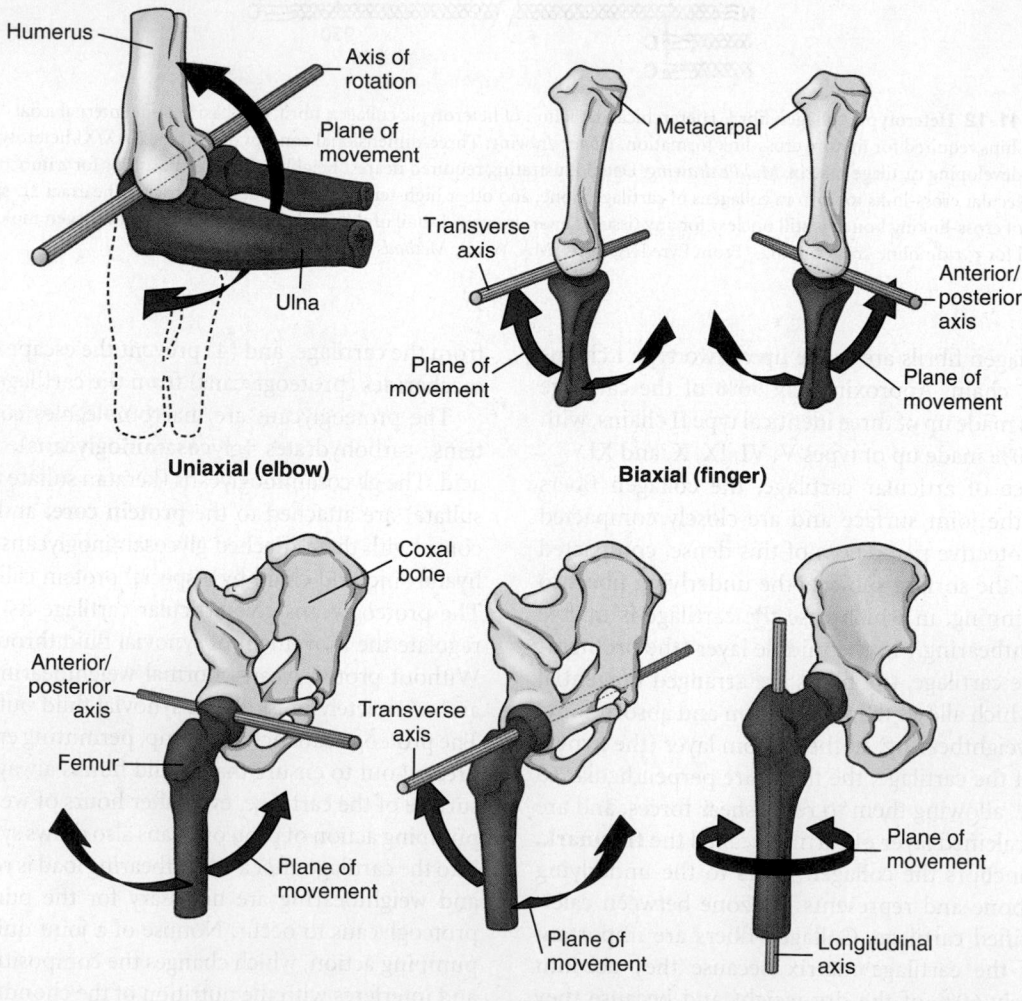

Figure 41-13 Movements of synovial (diarthrodial) joints.

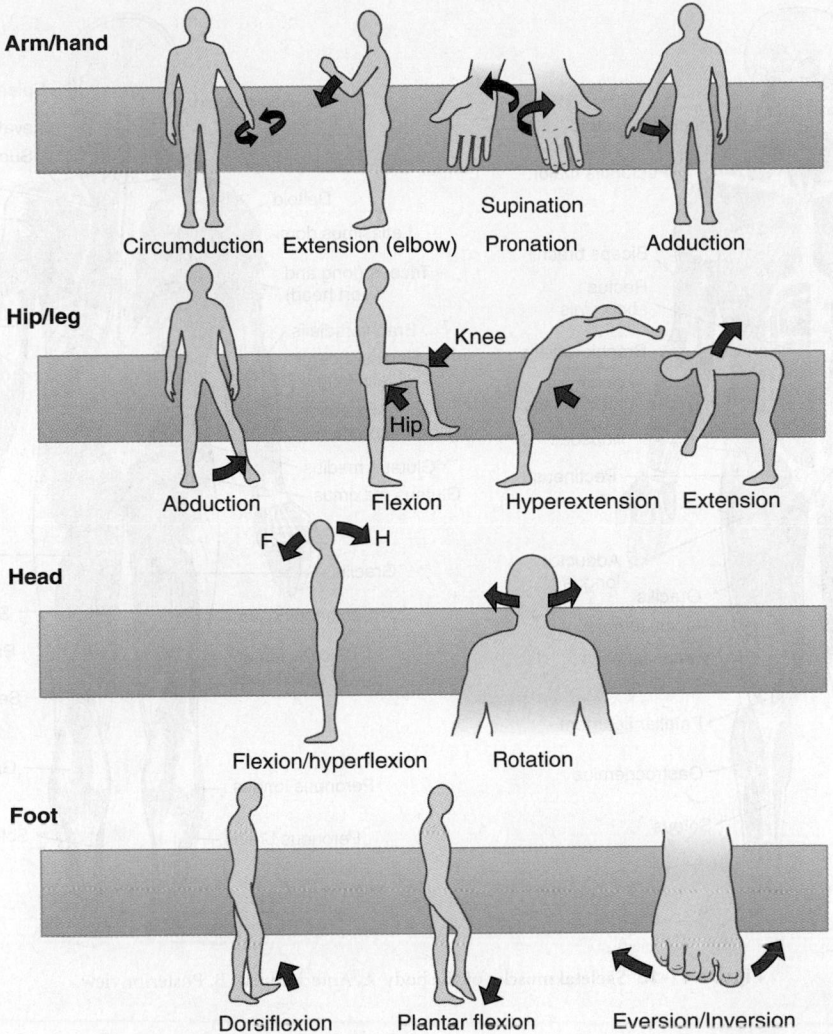

Arm/hand

Circumduction   Extension (elbow)   Supination / Pronation   Adduction

Hip/leg

Knee

Hip

Abduction   Flexion   Hyperextension   Extension

F   H

Head

Flexion/hyperflexion   Rotation

Foot

Dorsiflexion   Plantar flexion   Eversion/Inversion

Figure 41-14 Body movements provided by synovial (diarthrodial) joints.

Whole Muscle

There are more than 350 named muscles; almost all are paired. The body's muscles vary dramatically; they range from 2 to 60 cm in length and are shaped according to function. **Fusiform muscles** are elongated muscles shaped like straps and can run from one joint to another. **Pennate muscles** are broad, flat, and slightly fan shaped, with fibers running obliquely to the muscle's long axis. The multipennate deltoid muscle, which flexes and extends the arm, is a good example of a muscle shaped according to its function.

Each skeletal muscle is a separate organ encased in a three-part connective tissue framework called **fascia.** The layers of connective tissue protect the muscle fibers, attach the muscle to bony prominences, and provide a structure for a network of nerve fibers, blood vessels, and lymphatic channels.

The outermost layer, the **epimysium,** is located on the surface of the muscle and tapers at each end to form the **tendon** (Figure 41-16). Tendons allow a short muscle to exert power on a distant joint, whereas a thick muscle interferes with joint mobility. The next layer, the **perimysium,** further subdivides the muscle fibers into bundles of connective tissue, or **fascicles.** The **endomysium** surrounds the muscle fascicles, the smallest unit of muscle fibers visible without a microscope. The ligaments, tendons, and fascia are made up of connective tissue that also serves to buffer the limbs from the effects of sudden strains or changes in speed. The rapid recovery necessary for strenuous exercise is supported by the elastic property of muscle and its connective tissue.

Skeletal muscle is described, almost interchangeably, as **voluntary, striated,** or **extrafusal.** "Voluntary" indicates that the muscle is controlled directly by the central nervous system. "Striated" describes the striated, or striped, pattern of skeletal muscle viewed under a light microscope. The striations result from the organization of the muscle fibers into the contractile units called *sarcomeres.* "Extrafusal" distinguishes the skeletal muscle fibers from other contractile fibers located within the sensory organs of the muscle.

Other components that are visible on gross inspection of the whole muscle include the motor and sensory nerve fibers. These function together with the muscle, innervating portions of it and providing the electrical impulses needed for motor function.

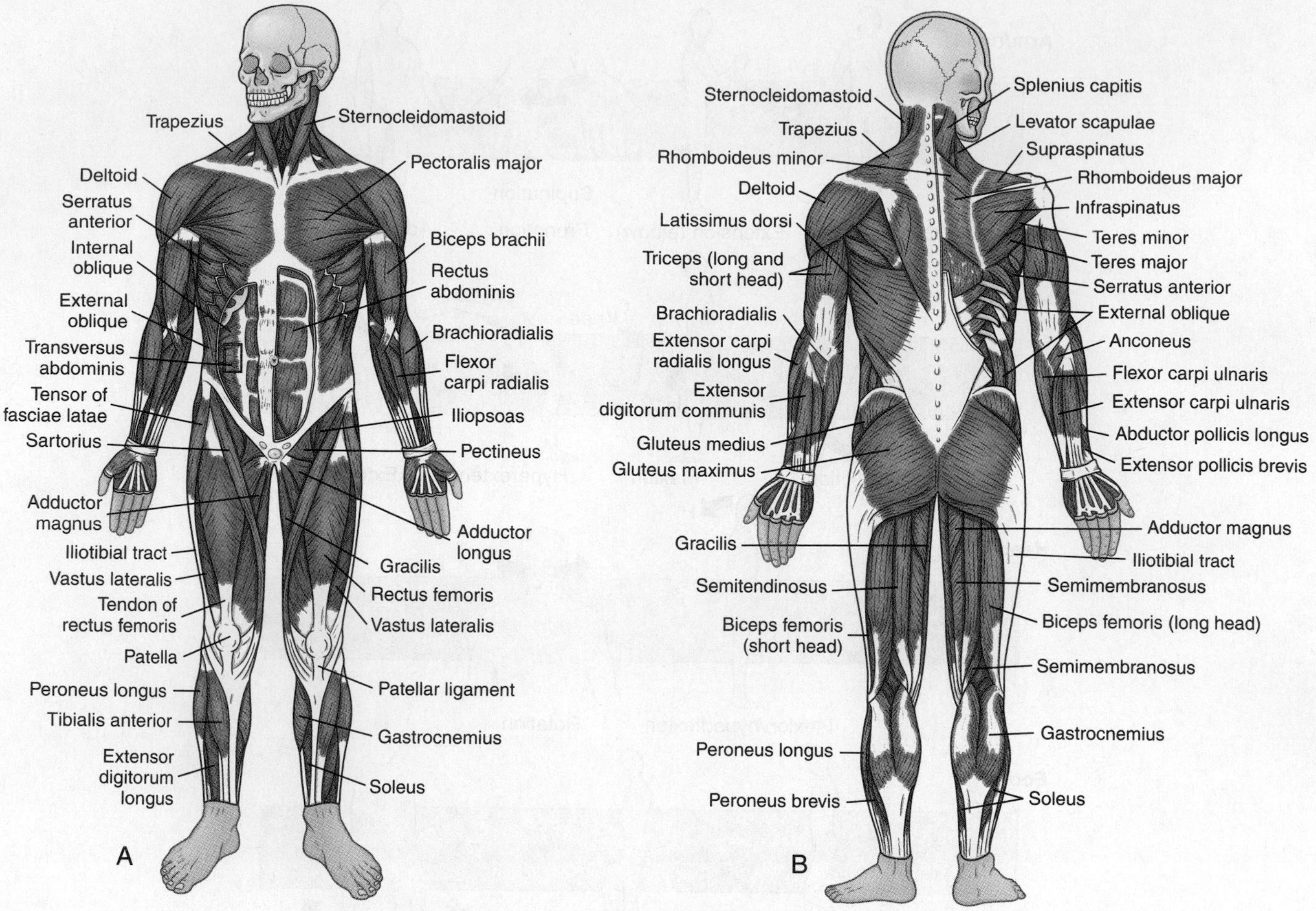

A (Anterior view)

Trapezius
Sternocleidomastoid
Deltoid
Serratus anterior
Internal oblique
External oblique
Transversus abdominis
Tensor of fasciae latae
Sartorius
Adductor magnus
Iliotibial tract
Vastus lateralis
Tendon of rectus femoris
Patella
Peroneus longus
Tibialis anterior
Extensor digitorum longus

Pectoralis major
Biceps brachii
Rectus abdominis
Brachioradialis
Flexor carpi radialis
Iliopsoas
Pectineus
Adductor longus
Gracilis
Rectus femoris
Vastus lateralis
Patellar ligament
Gastrocnemius
Soleus

B (Posterior view)

Sternocleidomastoid
Trapezius
Rhomboideus minor
Deltoid
Latissimus dorsi
Triceps (long and short head)
Brachioradialis
Extensor carpi radialis longus
Extensor digitorum communis
Gluteus medius
Gluteus maximus
Gracilis
Semitendinosus
Biceps femoris (short head)
Peroneus longus
Peroneus brevis

Splenius capitis
Levator scapulae
Supraspinatus
Rhomboideus major
Infraspinatus
Teres minor
Teres major
Serratus anterior
External oblique
Anconeus
Flexor carpi ulnaris
Extensor carpi ulnaris
Abductor pollicis longus
Extensor pollicis brevis
Adductor magnus
Iliotibial tract
Semimembranosus
Biceps femoris (long head)
Semimembranosus
Gastrocnemius
Soleus

Figure 41-15 Skeletal muscles of the body. **A,** Anterior view. **B,** Posterior view.

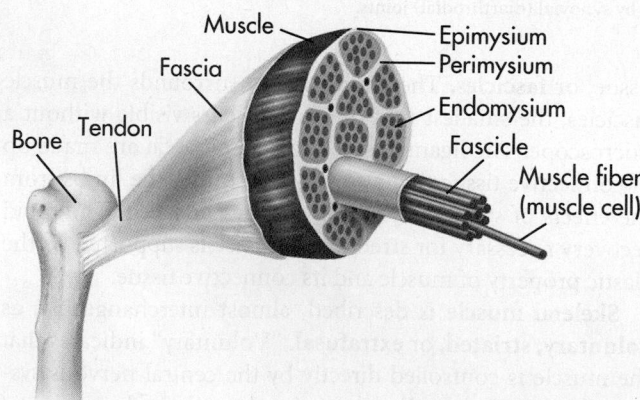

Muscle
Fascia
Bone
Tendon
Epimysium
Perimysium
Endomysium
Fascicle
Muscle fiber (muscle cell)

Figure 41-16 Cross section of skeletal muscle showing muscle fibers and their coverings. (From Thibodeau GA, Patton KT: *Anatomy & physiology,* ed 5, St Louis, 2003, Mosby.)

Motor Unit

From the anterior horn cell of the spinal cord, the axons of motor nerves branch out to innervate a specific group of muscle fibers. Each anterior horn cell, its axon (part of a lower motor neuron; see Chapter 14), and the muscle fibers innervated by

it are called a **motor unit** (Figure 41-17). The motor units are composed of lower motor neurons, which extend to skeletal muscles. Often termed the *functional unit* of the neuromuscular system, the motor unit behaves as a single entity and contracts as a whole when it receives an electrical impulse.

The whole muscle may be controlled by several motor nerve axons. These branch to innervate many motor units within the muscle. The whole muscle then may be made up of many motor units. The number of motor units per individual muscle varies greatly. In the calf, for example, one motor axon will innervate approximately 2000 muscle fibers, out of a total of 1,200,000 muscle fibers. This is a high innervation ratio of muscle fibers to axons, and it contrasts markedly with the low innervation ratio in the laryngeal muscles. There, two or three muscle fibers constitute each motor unit, and the innervation ratio can be of great functional significance. The greater the innervation ratio of a particular organ, the greater its endurance. Higher innervation ratios prevent fatigue, and lower innervation ratios allow for precision of movement.

Sensory Receptors

Although muscles function as effector organs, they also contain sensory receptors and are involved in sending different signals to the central nervous system. Among these

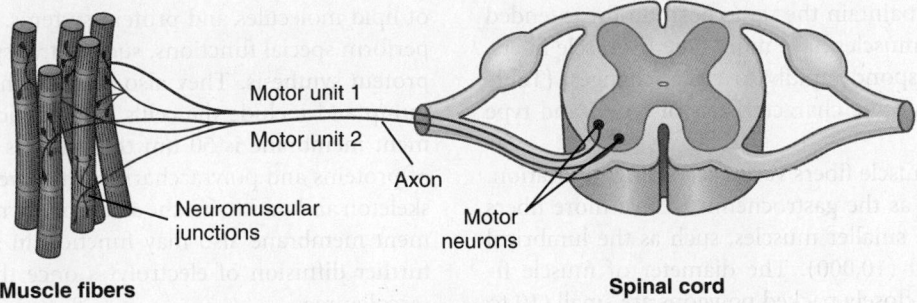

Figure 41-17 Motor units of a muscle. Each motor unit consists of a somatic motor neuron and all the muscle fibers (cells) supplied by the neuron and its axon branches.

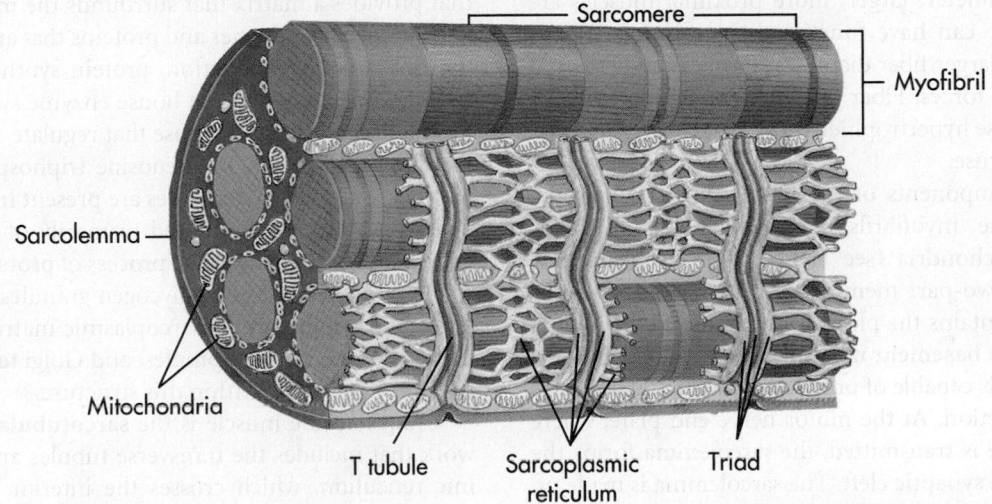

Figure 41-18 Myofibrils of a skeletal muscle fiber (cell) and overall organization of skeletal muscle. (From Thibodeau GA, Patton KT: *Anatomy & physiology,* ed 5, St Louis, 2003, Mosby.)

are the muscle spindles and Golgi tendon organs. **Spindles** are mechanoreceptors that lie parallel to muscle fibers and respond to muscle stretching. **Golgi tendon organs** are dendrites that terminate and branch to tendons near the neuromuscular junction. Motor and sensory neurons secrete a proteoglycan called *neuroregulin (NRG)* that increases acetylcholine receptors and helps in the formation of muscle spindle fibers.[14] The muscle spindles, Golgi tendon organs, and free nerve endings provide a means of reporting changes in length, tension, velocity, and tone in the muscle. This system of afferent signals is responsible for the muscle stretch response and maintenance of normal muscle tone.

Muscle Fibers

Each **muscle fiber** is a single **muscle cell.** This long cell is cylindrical and surrounded by a membrane capable of excitation and impulse propagation. The muscle fiber contains bundles of **myofibrils,** the fiber's functional subunits, in a parallel arrangement along the longitudinal axis of the muscle (Figure 41-18). At birth the muscle fibers have completed development from precursor cells called **myoblasts.** All voluntary muscles are derived from the mesodermal layer of the embryo.

The type of peripheral nerve influences the muscle fiber and motor unit considerably. Whether motor nerves are fast or slow determines the type of muscle fibers in the motor unit. Type II fibers, also called *white fast-motor fibers,* are innervated by relatively large type II alpha motor neurons with fast conduction velocities. These fibers rely on a short-term anaerobic glycolytic system for rapid energy transfer, whereas type I fibers depend on aerobic oxidative metabolism. Histochemical stains are now routinely used to describe the structure of muscle fibers and contractile elements of muscle biopsy specimens. White muscle (**type II fibers**) stains dark in the enzyme stain adenosine triphosphatase (ATPase) at a pH of 9.4. Red muscle (**type I fibers**) appears lightly stained.

The overlap of muscle fibers that appear with staining gives the checkerboard appearance of muscle biopsy specimens and provides an equal distribution of fiber types throughout the muscle. This overlap also helps compensate for muscle fiber loss and fatigue of individual motor units during activity. In spite of this, some muscles contain proportionally more of one fiber type than another. The postural muscles have more type I fibers, allowing them the high resistance to fatigue that is necessary to maintain the same position for extended periods. The ocular muscles have more type II muscle fibers, allowing them to respond rapidly to visual changes. (Table 41-6 describes the specific characteristics of type I and type II fibers.)

The number of muscle fibers varies according to location. Large muscles, such as the gastrocnemius, have more fibers (1,200,000) than the smaller muscles, such as the lumbrical muscles in the hand (10,000). The diameter of muscle fibers also varies. The closely packed polygons are small (10 to 20 μm) until puberty, when they attain the normal adult diameter of 40 to 80 μm. Women usually have smaller-diameter fibers than men. Small muscles, such as the ocular muscles, are 15 μm in diameter; larger, more proximal muscles are 40 μm. Fiber size can have functional significance. Studies have shown that larger fiber diameter is associated with generation of greater forces. Fiber diameter can be increased by activities that cause hypertrophied muscle, such as exercise or occupational overuse.

The major components of the muscle fiber include the muscle membrane, myofibrils, sarcotubular system, sarcoplasm, and mitochondria (see Figure 41-18). The **muscle membrane** is a two-part membrane. It includes the **sarcolemma,** which contains the plasma membrane of the muscle cell, and the cell's **basement membrane.** The sarcolemma is 7.5 nm thick and is capable of propagating electrical impulses to initiate contraction. At the motor nerve end plate, where the nerve impulse is transmitted, the sarcolemma forms the highly convoluted synaptic cleft. The sarcolemma is made up of lipid molecules and protein systems. The protein systems perform special functions, such as transport of nutrients and protein synthesis. They also provide the sodium-potassium pump and include the cell's cholinergic receptor. The basement membrane is 50 nm thick and is composed primarily of proteins and polysaccharides. It serves as the cell's microskeleton and maintains the shape of the muscle cell. The basement membrane also may function in some way to restrict further diffusion of electrolytes once they have crossed the sarcolemma.

The **sarcoplasm** is the cytoplasm of the muscle cell and contains the intracellular components that are common to all cells (see Chapter 1). The sarcoplasm is an aqueous substance that provides a matrix that surrounds the myofibrils. It contains numerous enzymes and proteins that are responsible for the cell's energy production, protein synthesis, and oxygen storage. The mitochondria house enzyme systems for energy production, particularly those that regulate such processes as the citric acid cycle and adenosine triphosphate (ATP) formation. Many other structures are present in the sarcoplasm. The ribosomes are composed primarily of ribonucleic acid (RNA) and participate in the process of protein synthesis. The cell nucleus, satellite cells, glycogen granules, and lipid droplets are suspended in the sarcoplasmic matrix. Blood vessels, nerve endings, muscle spindles, and Golgi tendon organs are also directly located within this structure.

Unique to the muscle is the **sarcotubular system,** a network that includes the transverse tubules and the sarcoplasmic reticulum, which crosses the interior of the cell. The

Table 41-6	Characteristics of Muscle Fibers	
Characteristic	Type I (Red)	Type II (White)
Anatomic location	Deep axial portion of surface muscle	Surface portion of surface muscle
Contraction speed	Slow	Fast
Motor neuron type	Type I, small alpha	Type II, large alpha
Firing frequency	Low, long duration	Rapid, short duration
Resistance to fatigue	High	Low
Myoglobin	High	Low
Capillary supply	Profuse	Intermediate to sparse
Metabolism	Oxidative	Glycolysis
Mitochondria	Many	Few
Enzymes	Lactate dehydrogenase, types 1 to 3	Lactate dehydrogenase, types 4 and 5
Creatine kinase	Cardiac type	Fast, skeletal
Example (most muscles are mixed)	Greater proportion of slow-contracting fibers in soleus	Greater proportion of fast-contracting fibers in laryngeal and ocular muscles
Glycogen content	Low	High
Intensity of contraction	Low	High
Aerobic metabolic capacity	High	Low
Fiber diameter	Small	Large
Myosin-adenosine triphosphatase (ATPase) activity	Low	High

From Spence AP, Mason EE: *Human anatomy and physiology,* ed 4, St Paul, MN, 1992, West Publishing.

sarcoplasmic reticulum is made in the same manner as the endoplasmic reticulum in other cells. In the muscle cells the sarcoplasmic reticulum is involved in calcium transport, which initiates muscle contraction at the **sarcomere,** a portion of the myofibril. The sarcoplasmic reticulum is composed of tubules that run parallel to the myofibrils. The longitudinal tubules are termed **sarcotubules.** The **transverse tubules,** which are closely associated with the sarcotubules, run across the sarcoplasm and communicate with the extracellular space. Together, the tubules of this membrane system allow for intracellular calcium uptake, regulation, release during muscle contraction, and storage of calcium during muscle relaxation.

Myofibrils. The myofibrils are the functional units of muscle contraction. Each myofibril contains sarcomeres,

which appear at intervals (see Figure 41-18). The sarcomeres are composed of two contractile proteins, **actin** and **myosin.** The sarcomere is responsible for converting chemical energy into movement.

The myofibrils are the most abundant subcellular muscle component, equaling 85% to 90% of the total volume. On cross section they are irregular polygons with a mean diameter of less than 1 μm. Each myofibril is composed of serially repeating sarcomeres, separated by Z lines that give the muscle its striped, cross-striated appearance. Each sarcomere has a dark A band and is flanked by two light I bands (Figure 41-19). Within the sarcomere is the giant muscle protein, titin. Titin functions as a molecular spring that plays a significant role in determining muscle stiffness and elasticity.[15]

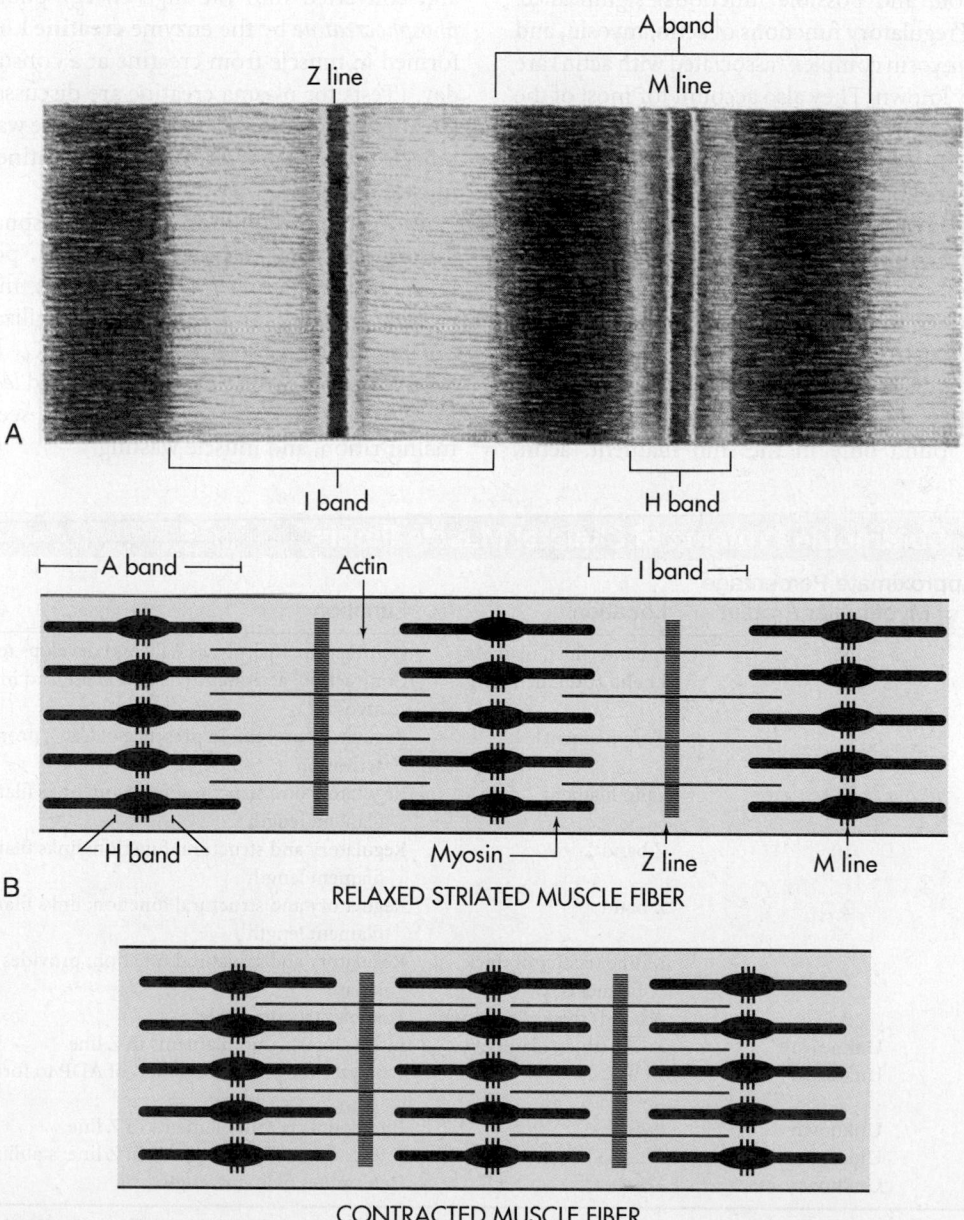

Figure 41-19 Muscle fibers. A, Lines and bands in striated muscle. B, Relationships of bands, actin, myosin, and lines in relaxed and contracted muscle fibers. (A modified from Thompson JM et al: *Mosby's clinical nursing,* ed 5, St Louis, 2002, Mosby.)

The A band is 1.5 to 1.6 μm long and contains thick myosin filaments. Included in the A band is a lighter zone called the H band, and in the center of the H band is the dark M band, or M line. The I band, which contains actin, is divided at the midpoint of each sarcomere by the Z line. Its length varies with the start of muscle contraction.

Myofibrils are composed of myofilaments. Each myofilament is structured in a closely packed hexagonal arrangement, with two thin filaments for every thick filament. The thick filament, along with C protein and M line protein, is made up of myosin. Myosin has two subunits, heavy and light meromyosin, which resemble twisted golf club shafts. The thin filaments are twisted double strands made up of actin, troponin, and tropomyosin (see Chapter 29 and Figure 28-15).

Muscle Proteins. Table 41-7 summarizes muscle protein distribution, location, and possible functional significance. The contractile and regulatory functions of actin, myosin, and the troponin-tropomyosin complex (associated with actin) are the most commonly known. They also account for most of the protein found in the myofibril. The structural and regulatory processes of muscle proteins are less well understood. Alpha actin and beta actin are known to link the filaments. M protein contains the enzyme creatine kinase (CK). Creatine is released when muscle cells are damaged, making serum creatine an important test of pathologic conditions of muscles.

The most abundant proteins, actin and myosin, are also found in other cells, particularly motile cells such as platelets. The complete amino acid sequences of actin and myosin have been identified. Noteworthy is the presence of the amino 3-methylhistidine, found only in the thin filament, actin; 85% to 90% of 3-methylhistidine is found in skeletal muscle. Because it is excreted unchanged (in the urine) after release from muscle and other tissue, 3-methylhistidine has been used to gauge muscle protein degradation. The amino acids lysine and histidine, in addition to leucine, have been used to study protein synthesis by means of stable isotope infusion and muscle biopsy analysis.

Nonprotein Constituents of Muscle. Nitrogen, creatine, creatinine, phosphocreatine, purines, uric acid, and amino acids serve in the complex process of muscle metabolism. Phosphocreatine concentration is an extremely sensitive indicator of muscle fiber activity.[16] Glycogen and its derivatives are present as energy sources.

Creatine and creatinine metabolism have been used to measure muscle mass. Plasma creatine is taken up by muscle and converted into the high-energy phosphate compound *phosphocreatine* by the enzyme **creatine kinase.** Creatinine is formed in muscle from creatine at a constant rate of 2% per day. (Tests for plasma creatine are discussed in Chapter 35.) Creatine excretion is increased in muscle wasting. This change reflects the reduction in total body creatine stores and loss of muscle mass.

Inorganic compounds, anions (phosphate, chloride), and cations (calcium, magnesium, sodium, potassium) are important in regulating protein synthesis, muscle contraction, enzyme systems, and membrane stabilization. Total body potassium (TBK), measured by the K_{40} method, has been used to measure muscle mass, also called *lean body mass.* TBK levels reflect changes in muscle mass seen during growth, malnutrition, and muscle wasting.

Table 41-7	Contractile Proteins of Skeletal Muscle Fibrils		
Name	Approximate Percentage of Myofibrillar Protein	Location	Function
Myosin	55	A band (thick filament)	Contraction; hydrolyzes ATP and develops tension
Actin	20	I band (thin filament)	Contraction; activates myosin ATPase and interacts with myosin
Troponin	7	Thin filament	Regulatory protein; in presence of Ca^{++}, promotes actin-myosin activation
Tropomyosin	5-7	Thin filament	Regulatory and structural function; links filaments, controls filament length
Alpha (α) actin	10	Z band	Regulatory and structural function; links filaments, controls filament length
Beta (β) actin	2	Z band	Regulatory and structural function; links filaments, controls filament length
M protein	2	M line (center of thick filaments)	Regulatory and structural function; provides enzyme creatine kinase
C protein	2	A band (thick filaments)	Possible structural role
Titin	Unknown	Z line (thick filament)	Interconnects thin filaments in Z line
Creatine kinase	Unknown	M line	Catalyzes the phosphorylation of ADP to form ATP
Desmin	Unknown	Z line	Interconnects thin filaments in Z line
*Filamin	Unknown	Z line	Interconnects thin filaments in Z line; stabilizes membrane
*Nebulin	Unknown	Z line	Determines filament length

*Data from Ma K, Wang K: *Fed Eur Biochem Soc Lett* 532(3):273-278, 2002; Sampson LJ, Leyland ML, Dart D: *J Biol Chem* 278(43):41988-41997, 2003.
ADP, adenosine diphosphate; *ATP,* Adenosine triphosphate; *ATPase,* adenosine triphosphatase.
Modified from Simon SR, editor: *Orthopaedic basic science,* Chicago, 1994, American Academy of Orthopaedic Surgeons.

Components of Muscle Function

The ultimate function of muscle is to accomplish work. Although variously expressed in such measures as foot-pounds or kilogram-meters, work usually refers to the amount of energy liberated or force exerted over a distance (work = force × distance). Muscles usually contract or tense while doing work. Muscle contraction occurs on the molecular level and leads to the observable phenomenon of muscle movement.

Muscle Contraction at the Molecular Level

Muscle contraction is a four-step process: excitation, coupling, contraction, and relaxation. The initial contraction process is the excitation-contraction coupling (ECC) series, which involves the electrical properties of all cells and the movement of ions across the plasma membrane (see Chapter 1). The muscle fiber is an excitable tissue. At rest an electric charge of −90 mV is continually maintained across the sarcolemma. This resting potential, generated by the separation of positive and negative charges on either side of the membrane, creates an electrochemical equilibrium caused by the selective permeability of the sarcolemma to electrolytes in the intracellular and extracellular fluids, particularly potassium and sodium.

Excitation, the first step of muscle contraction, begins with the spread of an action potential from the nerve terminal to the neuromuscular junction. The rapid depolarization of the membrane initiates an electrical impulse in the muscle fiber membrane called the **muscle fiber action potential.** As the action potential advances along the sarcolemmal membrane, it spreads to the transverse tubules. (The velocity of conduction is much slower in muscle fibers than in myelinated nerve fibers—only 3 to 5 m/second compared with 54 to 90 m/second in nerve fibers.)

The second stage, **coupling,** follows the depolarization of the transverse tubules. This stage consists of the migration of calcium ions, which are stored in the sarcoplasmic reticulum, to the myofilaments. Calcium affects troponin and tropomyosin, muscle proteins that bind with actin when the muscle is at rest. In the presence of calcium, however, both of these proteins are attracted to calcium ions, leaving the actin free to bind with myosin.

Contraction begins as the calcium ions combine with troponin, a reaction that overcomes the inhibitory function of the troponin-tropomyosin system. The thin filament *actin* then slides toward the thick filament, myosin. The two ends of the myofibril shorten after contraction when the myosin heads attach to the actin molecules, forming a cross-bridge that constitutes an actin-myosin complex. ATP, located on the actin-myosin complex, is released when the cross-bridges attach. This is the **sliding filament theory** described by A.F. Huxley in the 1950s, but it is now called the **cross-bridge theory** because of the formation of the actin-myosin cross-bridges. The process is so named because the actin actually slides onto the myosin, causing the sarcomere to shorten. The useful distance of contraction of a skeletal muscle is approximately 25% to 35% of the muscle's length.

The last step, **relaxation,** begins as the sarcoplasmic reticulum absorbs the calcium molecules, removing them from interaction with troponin. Calcium is pumped back into the sarcoplasmic reticulum by means of an active transport process. The cross-bridges detach, and the sarcomere lengthens. (The cross-bridge theory of muscle contraction is discussed in Chapter 29.)

Muscle Metabolism

Skeletal muscle requires a constant supply of ATP and phosphocreatine. These substances are necessary to fuel the complex processes of muscle contraction, driving the cross-bridges of actin and myosin together and transporting calcium from the sarcoplasmic reticulum to the myofibril. Other internal processes of the muscular system that require ATP include protein synthesis, which replenishes muscle constituents and accommodates growth and repair. The rate of protein synthesis is related to hormone levels (particularly insulin), amino acid substrates, and overall nutritional status. At rest the rate of ATP formation by oxidation of glucose or acetoacetate is sufficient to maintain internal processes, given normal nutritional status. During activity the need for ATP increases 100-fold. The metabolic pathways for muscle activity in Table 41-8 show reactions to the immediate need for increased ATP caused by contraction. Activity lasting longer than 5 seconds expends the available stored ATP and phosphocreatine.

Stored glycogen and blood glucose are converted anaerobically to sustain brief activity without increasing the demand for oxygen. Anaerobic glycolysis is much less efficient than aerobic glycolysis, using six to eight times more glycogen to

Table 41-8	Energy Sources for Muscular Activity
Sources	**Reactions**
Short-term (anaerobic) sources	Adenosine triphosphate (ATP) → adenosine diphosphate (ADP) + Inorganic phosphate (P_1) + Energy
	Phosphocreatine + ADP ⇌ Creatine + ATP
	Glycogen/glucose + P_1 + ADP → Lactate + ATP
Long-term (aerobic) sources	Glycogen/glucose + ADP + P_1 + O_2 → H_2O + CO_2 + ATP
	Free fatty acids + ADP + P_1 + O_2 → H_2O + CO_2 + ATP
	Creatine kinase catalyzes the reversible reaction of ATP to ADP: Creatine phosphate + ADP $\overset{\text{Creatine kinase}}{\rightleftharpoons}$ Creatine + ATP

From Spence AP, Mason EE: *Human anatomy and physiology,* ed 4, St Paul, MN, 1992, West Publishing.

produce the same amount of ATP. With increased activity, such as intense exercise, or ischemia, an increase in lactic acid occurs because of the breakdown of glycogen, thus causing a shift in muscle pH (see Table 41-8). This short-term mechanism "buys time" by allowing ATP formation in spite of inadequate energy stores or oxygen supply. When the anaerobic threshold is reached and more oxygen is required, physiologic changes occur, including an increase in lactic acid and increases in oxygen consumption, heart rate, respiratory rate, and muscle blood flow.

Strenuous exercise requires oxygen, which activates the aerobic glycogen pathway for ATP formation. During maximal exercise, free fatty acid mobilization and the aerobic glycogen pathways provide ATP over an extended time. These pathways require oxygen to maintain maximal activity and return the muscle to the resting state. Maximal exercise increases oxygen uptake 15 to 30 times over the resting state.[17] When this system becomes exhausted or inadequate to respond to the need for ATP, fatigue and weakness finally force the muscle to reduce activity, with a resultant buildup of lactic acid in muscle fibers.

The ability to sustain maximal muscular activity leads to the accumulation of oxygen debt. **Oxygen debt** is the amount of oxygen needed to convert the buildup of lactic acid to glucose and replenish ATP and phosphocreatine stores. For example, after running at maximal speed for 10 seconds, the average person has consumed 1 L of oxygen. At rest, oxygen consumption for the same period is approximately 40 ml. As the person recovers, the measured oxygen debt is 4 L greater than the amount used during activity.

Oxygen consumption is measured to calculate the metabolic cost of activity in normal and diseased muscle. It is an indirect measure of energy expenditure, along with timed tests of activity, heart rate, and respiratory quotient (ratio of carbon dioxide to expired oxygen consumed). Energy expenditure is measured directly by heat production because heat is released whenever work is accomplished.

Another factor that changes energy requirements is muscle fiber type. Type II fibers rely on anaerobic glycolytic metabolism and fatigue readily. Type I fibers can resist fatigue for longer periods because of their capacity for oxidative metabolism.

Muscle Mechanics

Muscle contraction cannot be viewed in isolation. Several factors determine how force is transmitted from the crossbridges on individual muscle fibers to accomplish wholemuscle contraction. First, when a motor unit responds to a single nerve stimulus, it develops a phasic contraction, also called *twitch.* Because the motor unit contracts in an "all or nothing" manner, the contraction that is generated will be a maximal contraction. The central nervous system smoothly grades the force generated by "recruiting" additional motor units and varying the discharge frequency of each active motor unit. This adding of motor units within the muscle is called **repetitive discharge.**

Recruitment and repetitive discharge of motor units allow the muscle to activate the number of motor units needed to generate the desired force. The total force developed is the sum of the force generated by each motor unit. As the strength, speed, and duration of stimuli increase, the summation of contractions reaches a critical frequency called **tetanus.** When tetanus is reached, no further increase in force can be achieved.

Other variables, such as fiber type, innervation ratio, muscle temperature, and muscle shape, influence the efficiency of muscular contraction. The two muscle fiber types differ in their responses to electrical activity. Tetanus and duration of phasic contractions, which take microseconds to accomplish, are achieved more rapidly in type II than in type I muscle fibers. Low-innervation ratios promote control and coordination, whereas high ratios promote strength and endurance. Muscles work best at normal body temperature, 37° C (98.6° F). Finally, muscles with a large cross-sectional area, such as the fan-shaped pennate muscles, develop greater contractile forces than smaller-diameter muscles. The initial length of a muscle and the range of shortening that occur when the muscle contracts also determine the forces it can generate. The long fusiform muscles have a greater range of shortening and can contract up to 57% of their resting length. A certain amount of elongation is necessary to generate sufficient tension and muscular force. The elongation that occurs during the swing of a golf club or tennis racquet is an example of how stretch improves contractile force.

Types of Muscle Contraction

During **isometric contraction (static or holding contraction),** the muscle maintains constant length as tension is increased. Isometric contraction occurs, for example, when the arm or leg is pushed against an immovable object. The muscle contracts, but the limb does not move.

During **isotonic contraction (lengthening or shortening contraction),** the muscle maintains a constant tension as it moves. The terms "eccentric" for lengthening and "concentric" for shortening are technically inaccurate descriptions of muscle movement; the terms "lengthening" and "shortening" are more precise. Positive work is accomplished during shortening, and energy is released to exert force or lift a weight. In contrast, during lengthening the muscle lengthens and absorbs energy. Negative work is accomplished on the muscle by the load. Lengthening requires less energy to accomplish and may result in the development of pain and stiffness after unaccustomed exercise.

Movement of Muscle Groups

Muscles do not act alone but rather in groups, often under automatic control. When a muscle contracts and acts as a "prime mover," or **agonist,** its reciprocal muscle, or **antagonist,** relaxes. This is easily tested by holding the right arm in the horizontal position in front of the body and then bending the elbow while feeling the upper arm, biceps in the front and the triceps in the back, with the other hand. The biceps is firm, and the triceps is soft. As the arm is extended, the muscles change. When the elbow is completely extended, the biceps is soft and the triceps firm. Completing this movement causes the agonist and antagonist to change automatically; only the movement is commanded, not the alternate contraction and relaxation of the specific muscle groups.

Other associated actions may be seen during walking; as the foot leaves the ground, the paravertebral and gluteal muscles on the opposite sides of the body contract to maintain balance. One notices the loss of the associated muscle's action when paralysis offsets this process and decreases balance. If a person is paralyzed, difficulty in maintaining balance is noticeable.

TESTS OF MUSCULOSKELETAL FUNCTION

Tests of Bone Function

Diagnostic procedures to evaluate bone function include gait analysis, serum calcium and phosphorus, and imaging studies. Most imaging techniques provide morphologic rather than functional information about bone. Roentgenograms visualize bone structure, because bone absorbs x-ray beams better than soft tissue. Magnetic resonance imaging (MRI) is useful for evaluating primary or metastatic bone lesions, infection, marrow edema, bony erosions, osteonecrosis, fractures, and other pathologic changes of bone. Bone scanning is used to evaluate bone metabolism. After a small amount of radioactive tracer is injected, a special camera is used to identify bone absorption of the tracer. Single- or dual-photon absorptiometry is often used to measure density of bones in the extremities (single-photon absorptiometry) and fracture risk of vertebral bodies and the femoral neck (dual-photon absorptiometry). Dual-photon absorptiometry allows the soft tissue component to be subtracted. New technology promises more accurate evaluation of bone (see What's New? Quantitative Assessment of Macro- and Microstructural Features of Bone).

Bone resorption is evaluated with urinary and serum measurements of cross-linked N-terminal telopeptides (NTx), a product of osteoclast bone resorption. NTx is specific for bone because the cross-links assessed are characteristic of bone collagen alone. Urine NTx is a more sensitive and specific biochemical marker of bone resorption than serum Ntx.[18,19]

WHAT'S NEW? Quantitative Assessment of Macro- and Microstructural Features of Bone

Quantitative assessment of macro- and microstructural features of bone may improve our ability to estimate its strength. Imaging techniques, including volumetric quantitative CT (vQCT), high-resolution CT (hrCT), micro-CT (mCT), high-resolution MRI (hrMRI), and micro-MRI (mMRI), can provide more detailed information about bone quality than plain radiographs or CTs.

Tests of Joint Function

Procedures used to diagnose joint function include arthrography, arthroscopy, magnetic resonance imaging, and synovial fluid analysis. **Arthrography** (the injection of dye into the joint) is particularly useful to diagnose tears in the fibrocartilage of the knee (meniscus) and the rotator cuff of the shoulder. **Arthroscopy** is the direct visualization of a joint through an arthroscope. **Magnetic resonance imaging (MRI)** produces images of body tissues through the use of electromagnetic (radio) waves that alter the atoms (hydrogen ions) in the nuclei of cells being examined. When the polarized radio waves are stopped, the nuclear atoms return to their original positions, emitting energy as signals as they move back. The signals produce visible images for examination and diagnosis. MRI produces excellent contrast of soft tissues for evaluation of musculoskeletal conditions.

Analysis of synovial fluid may reveal inflammatory, septic, and noninflammatory joint diseases, which cause characteristic changes in the color, clarity, viscosity, and cellular elements of the fluid. The presence of blood in the joint fluid (hemarthrosis) usually indicates joint trauma. Normal synovial fluid is sterile, so the presence of bacteria in the fluid always indicates disease. Cell fragments and fibrous tissue in the fluid are the result of inflammation or wear and tear on the articular surfaces.

Tests of Muscular Function

When the individual's history and physical examination disclose abnormalities, such as weakness, atrophy, muscle tenderness, cramps, and stiffness, specific tests of muscle function are in order. One of the most useful tests is the serum CK concentration. CK is found in large quantities in the muscle fibers, and when these are diseased or damaged, CK leaks into the serum. Myoglobin is also detectable in the urine after acute muscle damage caused by crush injury, ischemic disorders, extreme exertion, and some inherited diseases.

Because the muscle membrane tissue is excitable and carries an electrical charge, its capacity to function can be assessed by electromyography. Using sensitive needle electrodes, the **electromyogram (EMG)** records the summation of action potentials of the muscle fibers in each motor unit. The EMG is often compared with the electrocardiogram (ECG), but the activity recorded on the EMG is on a much smaller scale. The amplitude of the ECG is measured in volts, the duration of impulse is recorded in seconds, and both are recorded as the heart rate (e.g., 80 V/60 second). EMG amplitude is recorded in millivolts and the duration is measured in milliseconds, with a frequency of about 5 to 50 action potentials per second. Motor unit potentials are measured to determine rate of firing, duration, and amplitude. Abnormalities in EMG and nerve conduction velocities help differentiate muscle diseases (myopathy) from peripheral nerve (neuropathy) and neuromuscular junction disorders. The muscle biopsy (using histologic, histochemical, and electron microscopic studies) is used to further define the presence of myopathic and neuropathic disorders, many of which can be diagnosed only by muscle biopsy. Complex myography, a relatively new technique, allows a noninvasive way to gather information on the mechanical characteristics of muscle.[20]

A new area of evaluation is genetics. Recent advances in molecular genetics, deoxyribonucleic acid (DNA) libraries, genetic probes, and gene localization techniques have enhanced our knowledge of neuromuscular diseases, including types of muscular dystrophy, Charcot-Marie-Tooth disease, and familial amyotrophic lateral sclerosis.

Aging and the Musculoskeletal System

Aging of Bones

Aging is accompanied by the loss of bone tissue. Bones become less stiff, less strong, and more brittle with aging. The bone remodeling cycle takes longer to complete, and the rate of mineralization also slows down. Studies have shown that an individual's bone mass at the end of their growth period helps determine the significance of bone loss as they age.[12] With aging, women experience loss of bone density, accelerated by rapid bone loss during early menopause from increased osteoclastic bone resorption. By age 70, susceptible women have lost an average of 50% of their peripheral cortical bone mass. Extensive loss of bone mass leads to deformity, pain, stiffness, and a high risk for fractures. Men also experience bone loss but at later ages and much slower rates than women. Also, initial bone masses in men are approximately 30% higher than in women. However, the absolute risk for fracture is the same in men and women of the same age, and bone density is similar.[12] Men's peak bone mass is related to their race, heredity, hormonal factors (testosterone and estradiol), physical activity, and calcium intake during childhood. Bone loss in both sexes is related to smoking, calcium deficiency, magnesium deficiency, vitamin D deficiency, high protein intake, excess phosphorus intake, overly vigorous exercise, certain prescription and over-the-counter drug use, alcohol intake, and physical inactivity.[21]

Bone mass can be gained in healthy young women up to the third decade through physical activity, intake of dietary calcium, and magnesium. The positive effects of exercise in older adult women on bone mineral density (BMD) are not yet clear,[22] but exercise has been shown to improve balance, coordination, muscle strength, lean body mass, and mobility, all of which may decrease the incidence of falls (also see Figure 2-22, p. 71). The use of oral contraceptives for maintaining bone mass is controversial. Height is also lost with aging because of increased spinal curvature, often because of asymptomatic vertebral fractures.

Aging of Joints

With aging, cartilage becomes more rigid, fragile, and susceptible to fibrillation because of more cross-linking of collagen and elastin, decreasing water content in the cartilage ground substance, and decreasing concentrations of glycosaminoglycans. Decreased range of motion of the joint is related to the changes in ligaments and muscles. Bones in joints develop evidence of osteoporosis with fewer trabeculae and thinner, less dense bones, making them prone to fractures. Intervertebral disk spaces decrease in height.

Aging of Muscles

The function of skeletal muscle depends on many factors that are affected by aging, including the nervous, vascular, and endocrine systems. In the young child the development of muscle tissue is highly dependent on continuing neurodevelopmental maturation. Muscle function remains trainable even into advanced age. Muscle diseases have a definite association with specific age groups. Muscular dystrophies occur in children, and muscle disabilities related to rheumatic diseases usually occur in advancing age.

Age-related loss in skeletal muscle is referred to as **sarcopenia** and is a direct cause of the age-related decrease in muscle strength. As the body ages, muscle bulk and strength decline slowly; thus strength is maintained into the 50s, with a slow decline in dynamic and isometric strength evident after age 70. Type II fibers decrease to a greater extent than the slower-acting type I fibers. Loss of satellite cells appears to play a major role in the development of sarcopenia.[23] There is reduced RNA synthesis, loss of mitochondrial volume, and reduction in the size of motor units. The regenerative function of muscle tissue remains normal in aging persons. As much as 30% to 40% of skeletal muscle mass and strength may be lost from the third to ninth decades.

Maximal oxygen intake decreases with age. Reduced basal metabolic rate and decreased lean body mass are also seen in the older adult population.

SUMMARY REVIEW

Structure and Function of Bones

1. Bones provide support and protection for the body's tissues and organs and are important sources of minerals and blood cells.
2. Bone formation begins in utero with the differentiation of mesenchymal cells into either chondrocytes or osteoblasts. Bone minerals then either crystallize on a cartilage framework or become bone-forming cells without cartilage.
3. Bone tissue is continuously being resorbed and synthesized by bone-remodeling units of osteoclasts and osteoblasts.
4. RANKL induces osteoclast activation and bone resorption. OPG, a protein, binds to a protein called OPG ligand. This attachment serves as a decoy receptor for RANKL and blocks osteoclast activity, thus decreasing bone resorption. The balance between RANKL and OPG determines the quality of bone.
5. Bones in the body are made up of compact bone tissue and spongy bone tissue. Compact bone is highly organized into haversian systems that consist of concentric layers of crystallized matrix surrounding a central canal that contains blood vessels and nerves. Dispersed throughout the concentric layers of crystallized matrix are small spaces containing osteocytes. Smaller canals, called *canaliculi*, interconnect the osteocyte-containing spaces. The crystallized matrix in spongy bone is arranged in bars or plates. Spaces containing osteocytes are dispersed between the bars or plates and interconnected by canaliculi.
6. BMPs are part of the TGF-β superfamily and involved in nearly all aspects of bone formation.
7. There are 206 bones in the body, divided into the axial skeleton and the appendicular skeleton. Bones are classified by shape as long, short, flat, or irregular. Long bones have a broad end (epiphysis), broad neck (metaphysis), and narrow midportion (diaphysis) that contains the medullary cavity.
8. Bone injuries are repaired in stages. Hematoma formation provides the fibrin framework for formation and organization of granulation tissue. The granulation tissue provides a cartilage model for the formation and crystallization of bone matrix. Remodeling restores the original shape and size to the injured bone.

Structure and Function of Joints

1. A joint is where two or more bones attach. Joints provide stability and mobility to the skeleton.
2. Joints are classified as synarthroses, amphiarthroses, or diarthroses, depending on the degree of movement they allow. Joints are classified also by the type of connecting tissue holding them together. Fibrous joints are connected by dense fibrous tissue, ligaments, or membranes. Cartilaginous joints are connected by fibrocartilage or hyaline cartilage. Synovial joints are connected by a fibrous joint capsule. Within the capsule is a small fluid-filled space. The fluid in the space nourishes the articular cartilage that covers the ends of the bones meeting in the synovial joint.
3. Articular cartilage is a highly organized system of collagen fibers and proteoglycans. The fibers firmly anchor the cartilage to the bone, and the proteoglycans control the loss of fluid from the cartilage.
4. Joints help move bones and muscle.

Structure and Function of Skeletal Muscles

1. Skeletal muscle is the largest organ in the body and is made up of millions of individual fibers.
2. Whole muscles vary in size (2 to 60 cm) and shape (fusiform and pennate). They are encased in a three-part connective tissue framework. The fundamental concept of muscle function is the *motor unit*, defined as all muscle fibers innervated by a single motor nerve.
3. Muscle fibers contain bundles of myofibrils arranged in parallel along the longitudinal axis and include the muscle membrane, myofibrils, sarcotubular system, aqueous sarcoplasm, and mitochondria. There are two types of muscle fibers, type I and type II, determined by motor nerve innervation.
4. Myofibrils and myofilaments contain the major muscle proteins, actin and myosin, which interact to form cross-bridges during muscle contraction. The nonprotein muscle constituents provide an energy source for contraction and regulate protein synthesis, enzyme systems, and membrane stabilization.
5. Muscle contraction includes excitation, coupling, contraction, and relaxation.
6. Muscle strength is graded by the "all or nothing" phenomenon and recruitment. Speed of contraction is affected by several factors: muscle fiber type, temperature, stretch, and weight of the load.
7. The two types of muscle contraction are isometric and isotonic. Muscle shortening occurs during contraction but can be seen also during pathologic and physiologic contracture.
8. Actin and myosin filaments form cross-bridges that cause the sarcomere to shorten, a process now known as the *cross-bridge theory of muscle contraction.*
9. Skeletal muscle requires a constant supply of ATP and phosphocreatine to fuel muscle contraction and for growth and repair. ATP and phosphocreatine can be generated aerobically or anaerobically. Phosphocreatine concentration is an extremely sensitive indicator of muscle fiber activity.
10. Several factors determine how force is transmitted from the actin-myosin cross-bridges on individual muscle fibers to accomplish whole-muscle contraction. When a motor unit responds to a single nerve stimulus, it develops a phasic contraction. The central nervous system smoothly grades the force generated by "recruiting" additional motor units and varying the discharge frequency of each active motor unit.

Tests of Musculoskeletal Function

1. Various diagnostic procedures are used to evaluate bone function, including gait analysis, serum calcium and phosphorus, x-ray films, angiography, bone scanning, and MRI.
2. Procedures used to evaluate joint function include arthrography, arthroscopy, MRI, and synovial fluid analysis.
3. Tests of muscular function include physical examination, serum creatine kinase, myoglobin, electromyogram, muscle biopsy, myometers, and the forearm ischemic exercise test.
4. Genetic evaluation is useful in detecting, diagnosing, and developing specific treatment for certain inheritable muscle diseases such as muscular dystrophy.

Aging and the Musculoskeletal System

1. Muscle bulk and strength slowly decline with aging, although not to a pathologic degree. The bone remodeling cycle takes longer to complete, and the rate of mineralization slows down.
2. Exercise in older adults does little to increase bone mineral density, but exercise has been shown to improve balance, coordination, muscle strength, lean body mass, and mobility.
3. Age-related loss in skeletal muscle is referred to sarcopenia. Loss of satellite cells appears to play a major role in the development of sarcopenia.

KEY TERMS

α-Glycoprotein, 1545
Actin, 1559
Agonist, 1562
Amphiarthrosis (slightly movable joint), 1549
Antagonist, 1562
Appendicular skeleton, 1546
Arthrography, 1563
Arthroscopy, 1563
Articular cartilage, 1550
Axial skeleton, 1546
Basement membrane, 1558
Bone albumin, 1545
Bone fluid, 1545
Bone matrix, 1541
Bone morphogenic protein (BMP), 1545
Bone-remodeling unit, 1547
Calcification, 1541
Canaliculi (sing., canaliculus), 1546
Chondrocyte, 1551
Collagen fiber, 1544
Compact bone (cortical bone), 1545
Contraction, 1561
Coupling, 1561
Creatine, 1560
Creatine kinase, 1560
Cross-bridge theory, 1561
Diaphysis, 1546
Diarthrosis (freely movable joint), 1549
Electromyogram (EMG), 1563
Endochondral ossification, 1541
Endomysium, 1555
Endosteum, 1546
Epimysium, 1555
Epiphyseal plate (growth plate), 1546
Epiphysis, 1546
Excitation, 1561
Fascia, 1555
Fascicle, 1555
Fibril, 1544
Fibrous joint, 1549
Flat bone, 1547
Fusiform muscle, 1555
Glycoprotein, 1545
Glycosaminoglycan, 1553

Golgi tendon organ, 1557
Gomphosis, 1549
Ground substance, 1540
Growth plate, 1546
Haversian canal, 1546
Haversian system, 1546
Hyaluronate, 1550
Hydroxyapatite (HAP), 1545
Integrin, 1544
Intima, 1550
Intramembranous bone formation, 1541
Irregular bone, 1547
Isometric contraction (static or holding contraction), 1562
Isotonic contraction (lengthening or shortening), 1562
Joint (articulation), 1548
Joint capsule (articular capsule), 1550
Joint cavity (synovial cavity), 1550
Lacuna, 1543
Lamellae, 1546
Laminin, 1545
Link protein, 1553
Long bone, 1546
Magnetic resonance imaging (MRI), 1563
Mesenchyme, 1541
Metaphysis, 1546
Motor unit, 1556
Muscle cell, 1557
Muscle fiber, 1557
Muscle fiber action potential, 1561
Muscle membrane, 1558
Myoblast, 1557
Myofibril, 1557
Myosin, 1559
Osteoblast, 1542
Osteocalcin, 1545
Osteoclast, 1543
Osteocyte, 1543
Osteoid, 1542
Osteonectin, 1545
Osteoprotegerin, 1542
Oxygen debt, 1562

Pennate muscle, 1555
Perimysium, 1555
Periosteum, 1546
Procallus, 1548
Protein core, 1553
Proteoglycan, 1545
RANKL (receptor activator of nuclear factor κB-ligand), 1543
Relaxation, 1561
Remodeling, 1547
Repetitive discharge, 1562
Ruffled border, 1544
Sarcolemma, 1558
Sarcomere, 1549
Sarcopenia, 1564
Sarcoplasm, 1558
Sarcoplasmic reticulum, 1559
Sarcotubular system, 1558
Sarcotubule, 1559
Short bone (cuboidal bone), 1547
Sialoprotein (osteopontin), 1545
Skeletal (voluntary, striated, or extrafusal) muscle, 1555
Sliding filament theory, 1561
Spindle, 1557
Spongy bone (cancellous bone), 1545
Subintima, 1550
Suture, 1549
Symphysis, 1549
Synarthrosis (immovable joint), 1549
Synchondrosis, 1549
Syndesmosis, 1549
Synovial fluid, 1550
Synovial joint (diarthrose), 1550
Synovial membrane (synovium), 1550
Tendon, 1555
Tetanus, 1562
Tidemark, 1553
Trabeculae (sing., trabecula), 1546
Transverse tubule, 1559
Type A synovial cell, 1550
Type B synovial cell, 1550
Type I fiber, 1557
Type II fiber, 1557
Woven bone (callus), 1548

REFERENCES

1. Hartmann C: Skeletal development—Wnts are in control, *Mol Cell* 24(2):177, 2007.
2. Shapiro F: Bone development and its relation to fracture repair. The role of mesenchymal osteoblasts and surface osteoblasts, *Eur Cell Mater* 15:53, 2008.
3. Glass DA, Karsenty G: Minireview: in vivo analysis of Wnt signaling in bone, *Endocrinol* 148(6):2630, 2007.
4. Baron R, Rawadi G: Targeting the Wnt/beta-catenin pathway to regulate bone formation in the adult skeleton, *Endocrinol* 148(6):2635, 2007.
5. Issack PS, Helfet DL, Lane JM: Role of Wnt signaling in bone remodeling and repair, *HSS J* 4(1):66, 2008.
6. Caetano-Lopes J, Canhão H, Fonseca JE: Osteoblasts and bone formation, *Acta Reum Port* 32:103, 2007.
7. Yavropoulou MR, Yovos JG: The role of the Wnt signaling pathway in osteoblast commitment and differentiation, *Hormones* 6(4):279, 2008.

8. Zaudi M et al: Osteoclastogenesis, bone resorption, and osteoclast-based therapeutics, *J Bone Mineral Res* 18(4):599-609, 2003.
9. Boyce BF, Xing L: Biology of RANK, RANKL, and osteoprotegerin, *Arthritis Res Ther* 9(Suppl 1):S1, 2007.
10. Buckwalter JA, Einhorn TA, Simon SR, editors: *Orthopaedic basic science*, Rosemont, IL, 1999, American Academy of Orthopaedic Surgeons.
11. Delaisse JM et al: Matrix metalloproteinases (MMPs) and cathepsin K contribute differently to osteoclastic activities, *Microsci Res Tech* 61(6):504-513, 2003.
12. Seeman E: Structural basis of growth-related gain and age-related loss of bone strength, *Rheumatol* 47:iv2, 2008.
13. Eyre DR, Weis MA, Wu JJ: Articular cartilage collagen: an irreplaceable framework? *Eur Cell Mater* 12:57, 2006.
14. Jacobson C, Duggan D, Fishbach G: Neuregulin induces the expression of transcription factors and myosin heavy chains typical of muscle spindles in cultured human muscle, *Proc Natl Acad Sci U S A* 101(33):12218-12223, 2004.

15. Labiet D et al: Calcium-dependent molecular spring elements in the giant protein titin, *Proc Natl Acad Sci U S A* 100(23):13716-13721, 2003.

16. Sargeant AJ: Structural and functional determinants of human muscle power, *Exp Physiol* 92(2):323, 2007.

17. Richardson RS: Oxygen transport and utilization: an integration of the muscle systems, *Adv Physiol Edu* 27(1-4):183-191, 2003.

18. Abe Y, Ishikawa H, Fukao A: Higher efficacy of urinary bone resorption marker measurements in assessing response to treatment for osteoporosis in postmenopausal women, *Tohoku J Exp Med* 214(1):51, 2008.

19. Ulrich-Vinther M et al: Articular cartilage biology, *J Am Acad Orthoped Surg* 11(6):421-430, 2003.

20. Rahe-Meyer N et al: Complex myograph allows the examination of complex muscle contractions for the assessment of muscle force, shortening, velocity, and work in vivo, *Biomed Eng Online* 7:20, 2008.

21. Karlsson M: Does exercise reduce the burden of fractures? *Acta Orthop Scand* 73(6):691-705, 2002.

22. Moayyeri A: The association between physical activity and osteoporotic fracture: a review of the evidence and implications for future research, *Ann Epidemiol* 18(11):827-835, 2008.

23. Verdijk LB et al: Satellite cell content is specifically reduced in type II skeletal muscle fibers in the elderly, *Am J Physiol Endocrinol Metab* 292(1):E151, 2007.

ALTERATIONS OF MUSCULOSKELETAL FUNCTION

CHRISTY L. CROWTHER-RADULEWICZ • KATHRYN L. McCANCE

MEDIA RESOURCES

 Evolve Website (http://evolve.elsevier.com/McCance/)
- Review Questions and Answers
- Animations
- Glossary (with audio pronunciation for selected terms)
- WebLinks

Online Course
- Module 19

CHAPTER OUTLINE

MUSCULOSKELETAL INJURIES
  Skeletal Trauma
  Support Structures
DISORDERS OF BONES
  Metabolic Bone Diseases
  Infectious Bone Disease: Osteomyelitis
  Bone Tumors
DISORDERS OF JOINTS
  Osteoarthritis
  Classic Inflammatory Joint Disease

DISORDERS OF SKELETAL MUSCLE
  Secondary Muscular Dysfunction
  Muscle Membrane Abnormalities
  Metabolic Muscle Diseases
  Inflammatory Muscle Diseases: Myositis
  Myopathy
  Muscle Tumors

Musculoskeletal injuries include fractures, dislocations, sprains, and strains. Fractures are the most serious. Alterations in bones, joints, and muscles may be caused by metabolic disorders, infections, inflammatory or noninflammatory diseases, or tumors. Trauma is the leading cause of death of people ages 1 to 44 years of all races and socioeconomic levels.

MUSCULOSKELETAL INJURIES

Skeletal muscles can withstand many penetrating injuries without permanent loss of function. For example, studies of soldiers with severe combat injuries showed that muscle function was preserved after the removal of large portions of muscle tissue. Successful regeneration of skeletal muscle fibers depends primarily on the extent of injury, preservation of vascular supply (and source of nutrition), and the availability of terminal axons for reinnervation.

Skeletal Trauma

Fractures

A **fracture** is a break in the continuity of a bone. A break occurs when force is applied that exceeds the tensile or compressive strength of the bone. The incidence of fractures varies for individual bones according to age and gender. The highest incidence of fractures occurs in young males (between ages 15 and 24 years) and in adults 65 years of age and older. Fractures of healthy bones, particularly the tibia, clavicle, and lower humerus, tend to occur in young persons and tend to be the result of trauma. Fractures of the hands and feet are usually caused by accidents in the workplace. The incidence of fractures of the upper femur, upper humerus, vertebrae, and pelvis is highest in older or older adults and is often associated with osteoporosis (see p. 1576). In 1990, an estimated

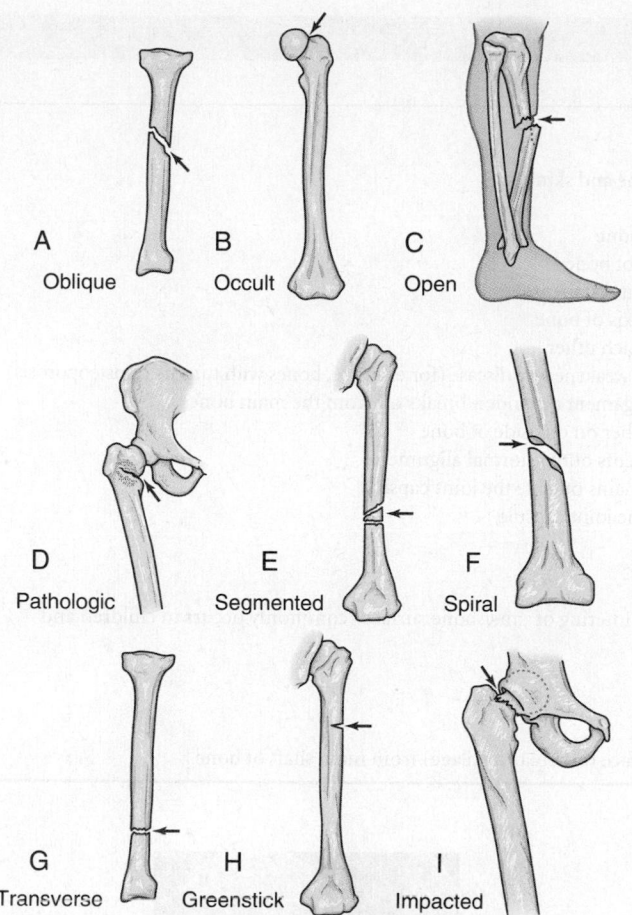

Figure 42-1 Examples of types of bone fractures. **A,** Oblique: fracture at oblique angle across both cortices. *Cause:* direct or indirect energy, with angulation and some compression. **B,** Occult: fracture that is hidden or not readily discernible. *Cause:* minor force or energy. **C,** Open: skin broken over fracture; possible soft tissue trauma. *Cause:* moderate to severe energy that is continuous and exceeds tissue tolerances. **D,** Pathologic: transverse, oblique, or spiral fracture of bone weakened by tumor pressure or presence. *Cause:* minor energy or force, which may be direct or indirect. **E,** Segmented: fracture with two or more pieces or segments. *Cause:* direct or indirect moderate to severe force. **F,** Spiral: fracture that curves around cortices and may become displaced by twist. *Cause:* direct or indirect twisting energy or force with distal part held or unable to move. **G,** Transverse: horizontal break through bone. *Cause:* direct or indirect energy toward bone. **H,** Greenstick: break in only one cortex of bone. *Cause:* minor direct or indirect energy. **I,** Impacted: fracture with one end wedged into opposite end of inside fractured fragment. *Cause:* compressive axial energy or force directly to distal fragment. (Redrawn from Mourad L: Musculoskeletal system. In Thompson JM et al, editors: *Mosby's clinical nursing,* ed 7, St Louis, 2002, Mosby.)

1.66 million hip fractures occurred worldwide; that number is expected to increase to 6.3 million by the year 2050.[1]

Classification

Fractures can be classified as complete or incomplete and open or closed (Figure 42-1). In a **complete fracture** the bone is broken all the way through, whereas in an **incomplete fracture** the bone is damaged but still in one piece. Complete or incomplete fractures also can be classified as **open** (formerly referred to as *compound*) if the skin is broken or as **closed** (formerly called *simple*) if it is not. A fracture in which a bone

breaks into more than two fragments is termed a **comminuted fracture.** Fractures are classified also according to the direction of the fracture line. A **linear fracture** runs parallel to the long axis of the bone. An **oblique fracture** is a slanted fracture of the shaft of the bone. A **spiral fracture** encircles the bone, and a **transverse fracture** occurs straight across the bone.

Incomplete fractures tend to occur in the more flexible, growing bones of children. The three main types of incomplete fractures are greenstick, torus, and bowing. A **greenstick fracture** perforates one cortex and splinters the spongy bone. The name is derived from the damage sustained by a young tree branch (a green stick) when it is bent sharply. The outer surface is disrupted, but the inner surface remains intact. Greenstick fractures typically occur in the metaphysis or diaphysis of the tibia, radius, and ulna. In a **torus fracture** the cortex buckles but does not break. **Bowing fractures** usually occur when longitudinal force is applied to bone. This type of fracture is common in children and usually involves the paired radius-ulna or fibula-tibia. A complete diaphyseal fracture occurs in one of the bones of the pair, which disperses the stress sufficiently to prevent a complete fracture of the second bone, which bows. A bowing fracture resists correction (reduction) because the force necessary to reduce it must be equal to the force that bowed it. Treatment of bowing fractures is difficult also because the bowed bone interferes with reduction of the fractured bone. A fracture that results from a low-level trauma (one that would not normally cause a fracture) is called a **fragility fracture,** which is often seen in osteoporosis. Types of fractures are summarized in Table 42-1.

Fractures may be further classified by cause as pathologic, stress, or transchondral. A **pathologic fracture** is a break at the site of a preexisting abnormality, usually by force that would not fracture a normal bone. Any disease process that weakens a bone (especially the cortex) predisposes the bone to pathologic fracture, commonly associated with tumors, osteoporosis, infections, and metabolic bone disorders.

Stress fractures occur in normal or abnormal bone that is subjected to repeated stress, such as occurs during athletics. The stress is less than the stress that usually causes a fracture. Two types of stress fractures are **fatigue fractures,** caused by abnormal stress or torque applied to a bone with normal ability to deform and recover (e.g., joggers, dancers, military recruits), and **insufficiency fractures,** stress fractures that occur in bones lacking normal ability to deform and recover (i.e., normal weight bearing or activity fractures the bone).

A **transchondral fracture** consists of fragmentation and separation of a portion of the articular cartilage that covers the end of a bone at a joint. (Joint structures are defined in Chapter 41.) The fragments may consist of cartilage alone or cartilage and bone. Typical sites of transchondral fracture are the distal femur, the ankle, the kneecap, the elbow, and the wrist. Transchondral fractures are most prevalent in adolescents.

Table 42-1   Types of Fractures

Type	Definition
Typical Complete Fractures	
Closed fracture	The skin overlying the bone is intact
Open fracture	Communicating wound between bone and skin
Comminuted fracture	Multiple bone fragments
Linear fracture	Fracture line parallel to long axis of bone
Oblique fracture	Fracture line at an angle to long axis of bone
Spiral fracture	Fracture line encircling bone (as a spiral staircase)
Transverse fracture	Fracture line perpendicular to long axis of bone
Impacted	Fracture fragments are pushed into each other
Pathologic	Fracture occurs at a point in the bone weakened by disease (for example, bones with tumors or osteoporosis)
Avulsion	A fragment of bone connected to a ligament or tendon breaks off from the main bone
Compression	Fracture is wedged or squeezed together on one side of bone
Displaced	Fracture with one, both, or all fragments out of normal alignment
Extracapsular	Fragment is close to the joint but remains outside the joint capsule
Intracapsular	Fragment extends into or is within the joint capsule
Fragility	Fracture caused by low-level trauma
Typical Incomplete Fractures	
Greenstick fracture	Break on one cortex of bone with splintering of inner bone surface (commonly occurs in children and older adults)
Torus fracture	Buckling of cortex
Bowing fracture	Bending of the bone
Stress fracture	Microfracture
Transchondral fracture	Separation of cartilaginous joint surface (articular cartilage) from main shaft of bone

PATHOPHYSIOLOGY When a bone is broken the periosteum and blood vessels in the cortex, marrow, and surrounding soft tissues are disrupted. Bleeding occurs from the damaged ends of the bone and from the neighboring soft tissue. A clot (hematoma) forms within the medullary canal, between the fractured ends of the bone, and beneath the periosteum. Bone tissue immediately adjacent to the fracture dies. This necrotic tissue (along with any debris in the fracture area) stimulates an intense inflammatory response characterized by vasodilation, exudation of plasma and leukocytes, and infiltration by inflammatory leukocytes and mast cells. Within 48 hours after the injury, vascular tissue invades the fracture area from surrounding soft tissue and the marrow cavity, and blood flow to the entire bone is increased. Bone-forming cells in the periosteum, endosteum, and marrow are activated to produce subperiosteal procallus along the outer surface of the shaft and over the broken ends of the bone (Figure 42-2). Osteoblasts within the procallus synthesize collagen and matrix, which becomes mineralized to form callus. As the repair process continues, remodeling occurs, during which unnecessary callus is resorbed and trabeculae are formed along lines of stress. Except for the liver, bone is unique among all body tissues in that it will form new bone, not scar tissue, when it heals after a fracture.

CLINICAL MANIFESTATIONS The clinical manifestations of a fracture vary according to the type of fracture, site of the fracture, and associated soft tissue injury. In general, the signs and symptoms of a fracture include impaired function, unnatural alignment (deformity), swelling, muscle spasm, tenderness, pain, and impaired sensation.

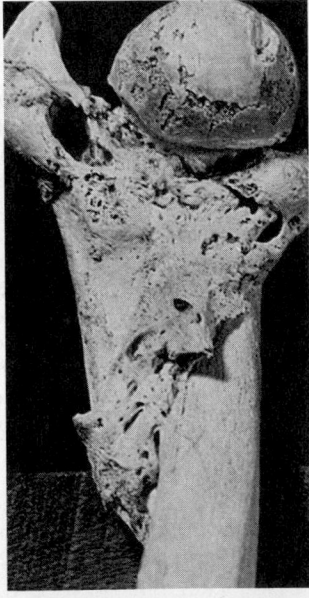

Figure 42-2 Exuberant callus formation following fracture. (From Rosai J: *Ackerman's surgical pathology,* ed 8, St Louis, 1996, Mosby.)

The position of the bone segments is determined by the pull of attached muscles, gravity, and the direction and magnitude of the force that caused the fracture. One or both segments may be rotated inward or outward on the bone's long axis (rotation), be misaligned at an angle (angulation), slide over the other segment (overriding), or be out of normal position (displaced).

The immediate pain of a fracture is severe and usually caused by trauma. Subsequent pain may be produced by muscle spasm, overriding of the fracture segments, or damage to adjacent soft tissues. Numbness is common and is caused by swelling, by the pinching or severing of a nerve, by the trauma, or by bone fragments. Pathologic fractures usually cause angular deformity, painless swelling, or generalized bone pain. Pathologic fractures are not usually associated with trauma or trauma-related pain. Stress fractures are painful, not because of trauma, but because of accelerated remodeling. The pain occurs during activity and is usually relieved by rest. Stress fractures also cause local tenderness and soft tissue swelling. Transchondral fractures may be entirely asymptomatic or painful during movement. Range of motion in the joint is limited, and movement may evoke audible clicking sounds (crepitus).

EVALUATION AND TREATMENT Treatment of a displaced fracture involves realigning the bone fragments (reduction) close to their normal or anatomic position and holding the fragments in place (immobilization) so that bone union can occur. Several methods are available to reduce a fracture: closed manipulation, traction, and open reduction. Many fractures heal without manipulation—they require only adequate immobilization. A fracture that is malaligned, however, requires more aggressive treatment.

Many fractures can be reduced by closed manipulation: the skin is not opened, and the bone is moved or manipulated into place. Closed manipulation is used when the contour of the bone is in fair alignment and can be maintained well with immobilization.

Traction is used to accomplish or maintain reduction. When bone fragments are displaced (not in their anatomic position), weights are used to apply firm, steady traction (pull) and countertraction to the long axis of the bone. Traction stretches and fatigues muscles that pull the bone fragments out of place, allowing the distal fragment to align with the proximal fragment. Traction can be applied to the skin (skin traction), directly to the involved bone, or distal to the involved bone (skeletal traction). Skin traction is used when only a few pounds of pulling force are needed to realign the fragments or when the traction will be used for brief times only, such as before surgery or, for children with femoral fractures, for 3 to 7 days before applying a cast. In skeletal traction, a pin or wire is drilled through the bone below the fracture site, and a traction bow, rope, and weights are attached to the pin or wire to apply tension and to provide the pulling force needed to overcome the muscle spasm and help realign the fracture fragments.

External fixation is used to reduce and immobilize significantly displaced open fractures. Pins are placed in the bone proximal and distal to the break and then stabilized by an external frame of clamps and rods (Figure 42-3).

Open reduction is a surgical procedure that exposes the fracture site; the fragments are brought into alignment under direct visualization. Some form of prosthesis, screw, plate, nail, or wire usually is used to maintain the reduction (internal fixation).

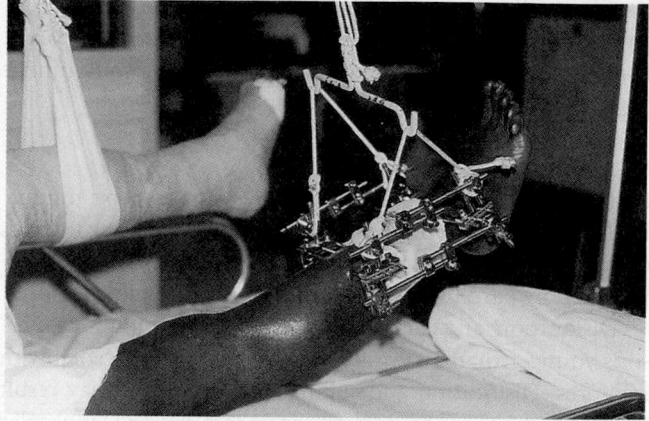

Figure 42-3 Example of an external fixation device on the right leg. The left leg is in a splint.

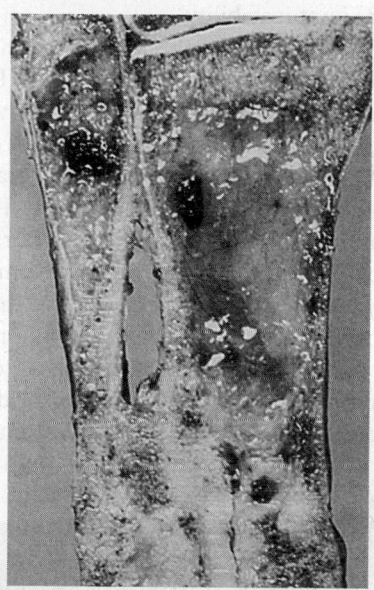

Figure 42-4 Nonunion of old fracture of tibia and fibula in a 53-year-old man. Multiple fractures had occurred in 2 years previous and necessitated bone grafting. (From Rosai J: *Ackerman's surgical pathology,* ed 8, St Louis, 1996, Mosby.)

Splints and casts are used to immobilize and hold a reduction in place. Improper reduction or immobilization of a fractured bone may result in nonunion, delayed union, or malunion. **Nonunion** is failure of the bone ends to grow together (Figure 42-4). The gap between the broken ends of the bone fills with dense fibrous and fibrocartilaginous tissue instead of new bone. Occasionally the fibrous tissue contains a fluid-filled space that resembles a joint and is termed a *false joint,* or *pseudoarthrosis.* **Delayed union** is union that does not occur until approximately 8 to 9 months after a fracture. **Malunion** is the healing of a bone in a nonanatomic position. Treatment of delayed union and nonunion includes use of various modalities designed to stimulate new bone formation. Physical modalities, such as implantable or external electric current devices, electromagnetic field generations, and low-density ultrasound, have been effective in stimulating bone formation. Gene therapy also shows promise in promoting formation of new bone. Large defects in bone can be filled with bone graft or synthetic materials, such as calcium phosphate cement.[2]

Dislocation and Subluxation

Dislocation and subluxation are usually caused by trauma. **Dislocation** is the temporary displacement of a bone from its normal position in a joint. If the contact between the two surfaces is only partially lost, the injury is called a **subluxation.**

Dislocation and subluxation are most common in persons younger than 20 years and are generally associated with fractures. Dislocation and subluxation, however, may result from congenital or acquired disorders that cause (1) muscular imbalance, as occurs with congenital dislocation of the hip or neurologic disorders; (2) incongruities in the articulating surfaces of the bones, as occurs with rheumatoid arthritis (see p. 1596); or (3) joint instability.

Most often dislocated or subluxated are the joints of the shoulder, elbow, wrist, finger, hip, and knee (Figure 42-5). The shoulder's glenohumeral joint is a relatively unstable joint because the articular surface of the glenoid cavity is only one third as large as the surface of the humeral head. As a result, the glenohumeral joint is often injured. Physical trauma to the shoulder can cause anterior, posterior, superior, or inferior dislocation. Anterior dislocation is the most common and is usually the result of an indirect force that places the shoulder in extreme external rotation. Posterior dislocations usually occur as a result of trauma. A superior dislocation is rare and usually the result of an extreme forward and upward force on an adducted arm. Inferior displacement is often seen

in persons with neurologic injuries of the brachial plexus and is believed to be caused by stretching of the supporting muscles or by joint effusion.

Traumatic dislocation of the elbow joint is common in the immature skeleton. In adults an elbow dislocation is usually associated with a fracture of the ulna or head of the radius. Posterior dislocations occur when the individual falls on an outstretched hand with the elbow extended. Anterior dislocations are usually the result of a direct blow to the flexed elbow.

Traumatic dislocation of the wrist usually involves the distal ulna and carpal bones. Any one of the eight carpal bones can be dislocated after an injury. The most common cause is a fall on the hyperextended hand.

Dislocation in the hand usually involves the metacarpophalangeal and interphalangeal joints. Dislocation of the metacarpophalangeal joint is often the result of a fall on the outstretched hand that forces the joint into hyperextension. Dislocation of the interphalangeal joint occurs as a result of injury to the fingers in a hyperextended position.

Considerable trauma is needed to dislocate the hip. Anterior hip dislocation is rather rare and is caused by forced abduction, for example, when an individual lands on the feet from a high fall. Posterior dislocation of the hip can occur in an automobile accident in which the flexed knee strikes the dashboard.

The knee is an unstable joint that depends heavily on the soft tissue structures around it for support. Because the knee is an unstable weight-bearing joint exposed to many different types of motion (flexion, extension, rotation), it is one of the most commonly injured joints. A knee dislocation can be anterior, posterior, lateral, medial, or rotary. It is usually the result of a hyperextension injury that occurs during sports activities.

PATHOPHYSIOLOGY Dislocations and subluxations are often accompanied by fracture because stress is placed on areas of bone not normally subjected to stress. In addition, as the bone separates from the joint, it may bruise or tear adjacent nerves, blood vessels, ligaments, supporting structures, and soft tissue. Dislocation of the shoulder may damage the shoulder capsule and the axillary nerve. Damage to the axillary nerve causes anesthesia in the sensory distribution of the nerve and paralysis of the deltoid muscle. Elbow dislocations are accompanied by torn periosteum, ligaments, and muscle. Bleeding from the damaged periosteum and muscle puts pressure on adjacent arteries that shuts off circulation to and from the forearm and hand. If the pressure is not promptly relieved, ischemic paralysis develops. Dislocations of the hand often result in permanent disability because of damage to the tendons and intricate mechanisms that allow smooth gliding in the joints. Avascular necrosis of the femoral head is a complication seen in hip dislocations. Knee dislocation usually tears both the collateral and cruciate ligaments.

CLINICAL MANIFESTATIONS Signs and symptoms of dislocations or subluxations include pain, swelling, limitation of motion, and joint deformity. Pain may be caused

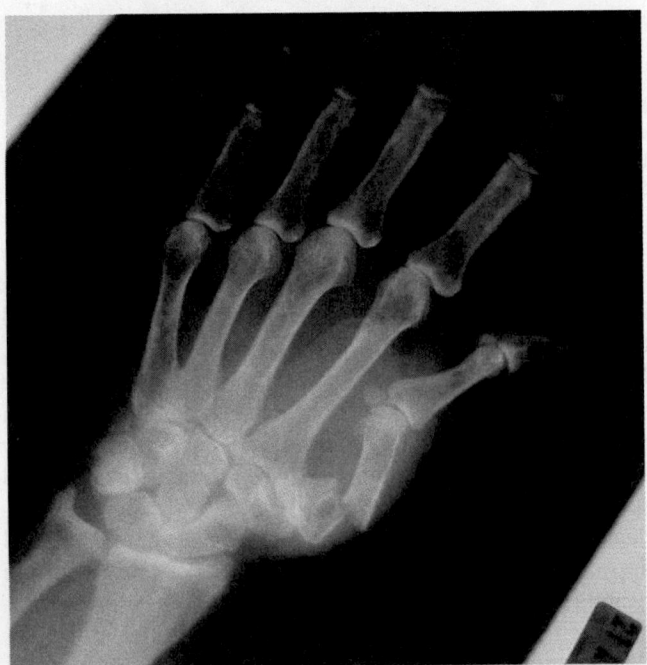

Figure 42-5 Displaced fracture. X-ray showing a displaced fracture of the base of the first metacarpal, also known as a Bennett fracture.

by effusion of inflammatory exudate into the joint or associated tension and ligament injury. Joint deformity is usually caused by muscle contractions that exert pull on the dislocated or subluxated joint or fluid within the joint. Limitation of motion may be a result of effusion into the joint or the displacement of bones.

Tenderness and deformity are prominent in dislocations of the fingers. Unusual muscle pull and pain often result in abnormal posturing of the fingers; for example, the fingers or thumb may be abnormally flexed. A dislocated elbow is often held in a flexed position, and the joint resists active or passive movement. Pain is the key symptom of shoulder injuries. Attempts to lift the arm aggravate the pain. In most shoulder dislocations, the ability to elevate the arm is minimal and the individual supports the injured arm with the opposite hand. Pain and an abnormal gait or limp or inability to bear full weight usually accompany traumatic dislocation of the hip. The pain is constant and severe and is often felt in the inguinal region or thigh. The thigh and leg may assume a position of inward rotation, adduction, or flexion and appear shortened. In a rare anterior dislocation, the limb is not shortened and the joint is fixed in abduction, outward rotation, and flexion.

EVALUATION AND TREATMENT Evaluation of dislocations and subluxations is based on clinical manifestations and roentgenograms. Treatment consists of reduction and immobilization for 2 to 6 weeks and exercises to maintain normal range of motion in the joint. Depending on the joint, healing is usually complete within months to years.

Support Structures

Sprains and Strains of Tendons and Ligaments

Tendon and ligament injuries can accompany fractures and dislocations. A **tendon** is fibrous connective tissue that attaches skeletal muscle to bone. A **ligament** is a band of fibrous connective tissue that connects bones where they meet at a joint. Tendons and ligaments support the bones and joints and either facilitate or limit motion. Tendons and ligaments can be torn, ruptured, or completely separated from bone at their points of attachment.

A tear in a tendon is commonly known as a **strain.** Major trauma can tear or rupture a tendon at any site in the body. Most often injured are the tendons of the hands and feet, the knee (patellar), the upper arm (biceps and triceps), the thigh (quadriceps), the ankle, and the heel (Achilles). Lifting excessive weight with the arms can cause traumatic rupture of the biceps tendon. Rupture of the Achilles tendon occurs when forced dorsiflexion is applied to the foot when it is in plantar flexion. Spontaneous tendon ruptures can occur in individuals receiving local corticosteroid injections, fluoroquinolones, and persons with rheumatoid arthritis or systemic lupus erythematosus.

Ligament tears are commonly known as **sprains.** Ligament tears and ruptures can occur at any joint but are most common in the wrist, ankle, elbow, and knee joints. A complete separation of a tendon or ligament from its bony attachment site is known as an **avulsion.** An avulsion is the result of abnormal stress on the ligament or tendon and is commonly seen in young athletes, especially sprinters, hurdlers, and runners.

Strains and sprains are classified as first degree (least severe), second degree, and third degree (most severe).

PATHOPHYSIOLOGY When a tendon or ligament is torn, an extensive cascade of inflammatory processes begins. An inflammatory exudate develops between the torn ends. Later, granulation tissue containing macrophages, fibroblasts, and capillary buds grows inward from the surrounding soft tissue and cartilage to begin the repair process. Within 4 to 5 days after the injury, collagen formation begins. At first, collagen formation is random and disorganized. As the collagen fibers interweave and connect with preexisting tendon fibers, they become organized parallel to the lines of stress. Eventually vascular fibrous tissue fuses the new and surrounding tissues into a single mass. As reorganization takes place, the healing tendon or ligament separates from the surrounding soft tissue. Usually a healing tendon or ligament lacks sufficient strength to withstand strong pull for 4 to 5 weeks after the injury. If strong muscle pull does occur during this time, the tendon or ligament ends may separate again, which causes the tendon or ligament to heal in a lengthened shape with an excessive amount of scar tissue that renders the tendon or ligament functionless. Scar remodeling may take months to years before it is complete.[3]

CLINICAL MANIFESTATIONS Tendon and ligament injuries are painful and are usually accompanied by soft tissue swelling, changes in tendon or ligament contour, and dislocation or subluxation of bones. The pain is generally sharp and localized, and tenderness persists over the distribution of the tendon or ligament. Painful joint swelling usually can be seen in finger and elbow sprains. Flexion deformities of the fingers and thumb occur in injuries to the extensor tendons. Crepitus may accompany tendon injury in the wrist. Pain in the elbow may be accentuated by flexion, supination, and extension of the elbow or by extension of the wrist. Lifting small objects requires extension of the wrist and therefore aggravates the pain. Tendon injuries in the upper arm cause weakness when the individual tries to flex the forearm. Pain is often the key symptom of shoulder injuries. It may be referred to the deltoid muscle or extend down the arm. The pain is usually aggravated by attempts to lift the arms. Depending on the ligament or tendon involved, tendon and ligament injuries in the knee may produce pronounced immobility, lost lateral movement, instability when walking down stairs, semiflexion, crepitus, or an upward or downward shift of the patella.

EVALUATION AND TREATMENT Evaluation is based on clinical manifestations, stress radiography, arthroscopy, or arthrography. When possible, treatment consists of protecting the involved structures (splinting), early motion, and rehabilitation. Suturing the tendon or ligament ends in close approximation may be necessary to treat complete rupture. If this is not possible because of the extent of damage, tendon or ligament grafting may be necessary. Prolonged rehabilitation exercises help ensure that the patient regains nearly normal functions.

Table 42-2	Histopathologic Classification of Tendon Disorders	
Pathologic Diagnosis	**Macroscopic Pathology**	**Histopathologic Findings**
Tendinosis	Intratendinous degeneration (commonly due to aging, microtrauma, muscular compromise)	Collagen disorientation, disorganization and fiber separation by an increase in mucoid ground substance, increased preponderance of cells and vascular spaces with or without neovascularization and focal necrosis or calcification
Tendinitis	Symptomatic degeneration of the tendon with vascular disruption and inflammatory repair response	Degenerative changes as noted above with superimposed evidence of tear, including fibroblastic and myofibroblastic proliferation, hemorrhage, and organizing granulation tissue
Paratenonitis	"Inflammation" of the outer layer of the tendon (paratenon) alone, whether or not the paratenon is lined by synovium	Mucoid degeneration if the areolar tissue is seen. A scattered mild mononuclear infiltrate with or without focal fibrin deposition and fibrinous exudate
Paratenonitis with tendinosis	Paratenonitis associated with intratendinous degeneration	Degenerative changes as noted in tendinosis with mucoid degeneration with or without fibrous and scattered inflammatory cells in the paratenon alveolar tissue

From Maffulli N, Wong J, Almekinders LC: *Clin Sports Med* 22(4):675-692, 2003.

Tendinopathy and Bursitis

Trauma and repetitive stress can cause painful degradation of collagen fibers (**tendinosis**), inflammation of tendons (**tendinitis**), or inflammation in bursal sacs (**bursitis**). The term *tendinopathy* includes tendinitis, tendinosis, and paratendinitis.[4] Other causes of tendinopathy include crystal deposits, postural misalignment, and hypermobility in a joint. Table 42-2 summarizes classes of tendinopathies.

Epicondylitis is inflammation of a tendon where it attaches to a bone (at its origin). Most tendon pathology, however, is caused by tissue degeneration rather than inflammation. Epicondylar areas of the humerus, radius, or ulna and the area around the knee are most often involved. **Lateral epicondylopathy,** commonly called **tennis elbow,** is the result of tissue degeneration or irritation of the extensor carpi radialis brevis tendon at its origin. **Medial epicondylopathy,** referred to as **golfer's elbow,** is a degenerative process of the pronator teres, flexor carpi radialis, and palmaris longus tendons at the medial humeral condyle[5] (Figure 42-6). Epicondylopathy is also related to smoking, obesity, and work activities that involve forceful or repetitive cyclic flexion and extension of the elbow, or cyclic pronation, supination, extension, and flexion of the wrist that generates loads to the elbow and forearm region.[6]

Bursae are small sacs lined with synovial membrane and filled with synovial fluid; they are located between tendons, muscles, and bony prominences. Their primary function is to separate, lubricate, and cushion these structures. Acute bursitis occurs primarily in the middle years and is caused by trauma. Chronic bursitis can result from repeated trauma. Septic bursitis is caused by wound infection or bacterial infection of the skin overlying the bursae. Bursitis commonly occurs in the shoulder, hip, knee, and elbow.

PATHOPHYSIOLOGY In tendinitis, fluid from inflammation accumulates, causing swelling of the tendon and its enclosing sheath. Inflammatory changes cause thickening of the sheath, which limits movements and causes pain. Microtears cause bleeding, edema, and pain in the involved tendons or surrounding structures. At times, after repeated

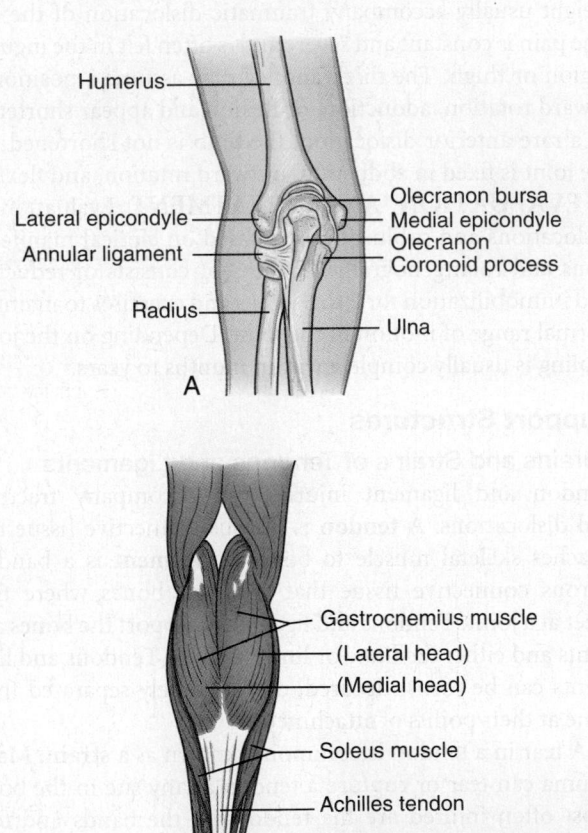

Figure 42-6 Tendinitis and epicondylitis. **A,** Medial or lateral epicondyles of humerus, site of epicondylitis. **B,** Achilles tendon, site of commonly occurring tendinitis.

inflammations, calcium may be deposited in the tendon origin area, causing a calcific tendinitis.

The usual bursitis is an inflammation that is reactive to overuse or excessive pressure. The inflamed bursal sac becomes engorged, and the inflammation can spread to adjacent

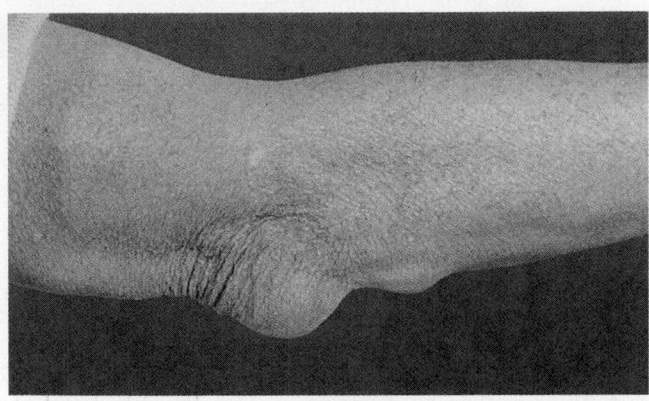

Figure 42-7 Olecranon bursa. A case of olecranon bursitis in a patient with rheumatoid arthritis. A rheumatoid nodule is also shown. (From Klippel JH, Deippe PA, editors: *Rheumatology,* ed 2, London, 1998, Mosby-Wolfe.)

Table 42-3	Common Sites and Causes of Bursitis
Site	**Common Causes**
Shoulder (subacromial)	Repetitive overhead activities
Elbow (olecranon)	Rheumatoid arthritis (RA), gout, tuberculosis, leaning on elbow
Hip (greater trochanter)	Acute trauma, chronic stress
Ischial (weaver's bottom)	Overuse (runner, ballet dancers), lumbosacral disease, RA, osteoarthritis (OA)
Knee	
Prepatellar (housemaid's knee)	Trauma, frequent kneeling, infection
Pes anserine (medial knee)	Obesity, long-distance runner, OA, type 2 diabetes
Heel (calcaneal)	Poorly fitting footwear, Achilles tendinitis

tissues (Figure 42-7). The inflammation may decrease with rest, heat, and aspiration of the fluid. (Inflammation is discussed in Chapter 6.)

CLINICAL MANIFESTATIONS Tendinopathy may be asymptomatic, but generally there is localized pain that worsens with active more than passive motion. With symptomatic tendinopathy, the pain is localized over the involved tendon and movement in the affected joint is limited. In bursitis, onset of pain may be gradual or sudden, and movement in the joint is, itself, normal. Shoulder bursitis impairs arm abduction because of pain and swelling of the bursa. Bursitis in the knee produces pain when climbing stairs, and crossing the legs is painful in bursitis of the hip. Lying on the side of the inflamed trochanteric bursa is also very painful. Table 42-3 summarizes common sites of bursitis. Signs of infectious bursitis may include the presence of a puncture site, prior corticosteroid injection, severe inflammation, or an adjacent source of infection.

EVALUATION AND TREATMENT Evaluation of tendinopathy, epicondylopathy, and bursitis is based on clinical manifestations, physical examination, arthroscopy, arthrography, ultrasound, and possibly magnetic resonance imaging (MRI). Treatment includes systemic analgesics, ice or heat applications, or local injection of an anesthetic and a corticosteroid to reduce inflammation. Physical therapy to prevent loss of function begins after acute symptoms subside.

Muscle Strains

Mild injury such as **muscle strain** is usually seen after traumatic or sports injuries. *Muscle strain* is a general term for local muscle damage. It is often the result of sudden, forced motion causing the muscle to become stretched beyond normal capacity. Strains often involve the tendon as well. Muscles are ruptured more often than tendons in young people; the opposite is true in older adults. Muscle strain may be chronic when the muscle is repeatedly stretched beyond its usual capacity. There is evidence of tissue disruption with subsequent signs of muscle regeneration and connective tissue repair when a biopsy is performed. Hemorrhage into the surrounding tissue and signs of inflammation also may be present. Knife and gunshot wounds also cause traumatic rupture. Regardless of the cause of trauma, muscle cells usually can regenerate. Regeneration may take up to 6 weeks, and the affected muscle should be protected during this time. Types of muscle strain, together with their manifestations and treatment, are summarized in Table 42-4.

A late complication of localized muscle injury is **myositis ossificans.** Its true etiology is usually unknown.[7] This condition is thought to be caused by scar tissue calcification and subsequent ossification. Examples include "rider's bone," in which the adductor muscle of the thigh of equestrians becomes calcified, as well as in football players after muscle injury to thigh muscles; and "drill bone," in which the same complication is seen in the deltoid and pectoral muscles of fencers and infantry soldiers.

Rhabdomyolysis

Rhabdomyolysis, or **myoglobinuria,** can be a life-threatening complication of severe muscle trauma with muscle cell loss. Myoglobinuria is named for the principal manifestation of the condition—an excess of **myoglobin** (an intracellular muscle protein) in the urine. Muscle cell damage releases the myoglobin. The most severe form is often called *crush syndrome.* Less severe and more localized forms of muscle damage are called **compartment syndromes,** which can lead to **Volkmann ischemic contracture** in the forearm or leg. Crush syndrome first gained notoriety in the reports of injuries seen after the London air raids in World War II. More recently it has been reported in individuals found unresponsive and immobile for long periods, often after a drug or alcohol overdose. Other causes of rhabdomyolysis include malignant hyperthermia, infection, herbal medicines, snakebite, cowfish ingestion, cocaine inhalation, hypernatremia, fire ant bites, and venlafaxine.[8-10] Rhabdomyolysis also can be seen after viral infections, administration of certain anesthetic agents, or some cholesterol-lowering agents known as "statins," strychnine poisoning, tetanus, heat stroke, electrolyte disturbances, and fractures. Strains themselves may

Table 42-4	Muscle Strain	
Type	Manifestations	Treatment
First degree (e.g., bench press in untrained athlete)	Muscle overstretched, painful	Ice should be applied 5 or 6 times in the first 24-48 hours; complete rest for up to 2 weeks, followed by weightbearing 3 times per week and range of motion daily
Second degree (e.g., any muscle strain with bruising and pain)	Muscle intact with some tearing pain, mild bruising; fascia is intact	Treatment similar to that for first-degree strains, with added mild analgesia; cryokinetics (a treatment system of alternating applications of cold with progressive exercise)
Third degree (e.g., traumatic injury)	Caused by tearing of fascia; muscle rupture palpable, bleeding present	Surgery to approximate ruptured edges; immobilization and rest for 6 weeks, followed by an individualized rehabilitation regimen of strengthening exercises

or may not lead to rhabdomyolysis, but drug interactions involving statins have been implicated.[11-12] Excessive muscular activity also has been implicated in reports of myoglobinuria in athletes, such as long-distance runners, ice skaters, skiers, military recruits, and those subjected to fraternity hazing. Status epilepticus, electroconvulsive therapy, and high-voltage electrical shock are also associated with severe and sometimes fatal myoglobinuria. Box 42-1 summarizes some of these risk factors for rhabdomyolysis.

If the myoglobinuria is caused by fulminant malignant hyperthermia, severe muscle spasm and rhabdomyolysis can lead to renal failure. Other complications include intraoperative rigidity, tachycardia, cardiac dysrhythmias, metabolic and respiratory acidosis, and temperature elevations up to 43° C (109.4° F), which can occur very rapidly. Cerebral edema, cardiogenic and hypovolemic shock, pulmonary edema, and disseminated intravascular clotting can contribute to the death of an individual with malignant hyperthermia.

PATHOPHYSIOLOGY The weight of a limp extremity can generate enough pressure to produce muscle ischemia (Figure 42-8). This causes edema, rising compartment pressure, and tamponade that leads to muscle infarction and neural injury and, finally, results in cell loss. Physical interruptions in the sarcolemmal membrane, called *holes* or *delta lesions,* suggest that the sarcolemmal membrane may be the route by which muscle constituents are released. (The sarcolemmal membrane, the plasma membrane [including creatine kinase, myoglobin, and phosphate] of the muscle cell, is described in Chapter 41.)

CLINICAL MANIFESTATIONS When myoglobin is released from the muscle cells into the circulation, it can cause a visible, dark reddish brown pigmentation of the urine. The renal threshold for myoglobin is low, approximately 0.5 mg/dl of urine, so that only 200 g of muscle need be damaged to cause visible changes in the urine. Along with the release of myoglobin, creatine kinase (CK) and other serum enzymes are released in massive quantities. The CK level is often 100 times greater than normal (5 to 25 units/ml for women and 5 to 35 units/ml for men). The efflux of proteins and enzymes also includes loss of potassium, phosphate, nucleotides, creatinine, and creatine. Serum hypocalcemia is seen early in the course of myoglobinuria and is followed by late hypercalcemia.

EVALUATION AND TREATMENT Careful and thorough preoperative assessment should alert the anesthesiologist to the possibility of a susceptible individual. A family history of anesthetic problems and previous untoward anesthetic experiences (muscle cramping, unexplained fevers, dark urine) are criteria that require further clarification before administration of a volatile anesthetic.

Priorities in treatment of myoglobinuria include identifying and treating the underlying disorder and preventing life-threatening renal failure. Malignant hyperthermia and myoglobinuria caused by succinylcholine or volatile anesthetic agents can be treated by halting the anesthetic administration and infusing dantrolene sodium (Dantrium). Diluting myoglobin using intravenous fluids and administration of diuretics to "flush" the kidney have been advocated to prevent renal failure. Correction of any electrolyte imbalance also is important. Other secondary problems include electrolyte imbalance, volume depletion, acidosis, hyperuricemia, hyperkalemia, and calcium imbalance. These require specific treatment. Short-term dialysis also may be necessary.

Compartment syndromes may require emergency treatment when blood flow to the affected extremity is compromised because of increased venous pressure, leading to decreased arterial inflow, ischemia, and edema. When clinical evaluation is inconclusive, the rising compartment pressure can be directly measured by inserting a wick catheter, needle, or slit catheter into the muscle. Immediate fasciotomy and débridement have been advocated for elevated intracompartmental pressures.[13] Compartments frequently affected are the compartments of the leg, the volar compartment of the hand, and the gluteal compartments.

DISORDERS OF BONES
Metabolic Bone Diseases

Metabolic bone disease is characterized by abnormal bone structure that is caused by altered or inadequate biochemical reactions. The altered or inadequate biochemical reactions may be attributable to genetics, diet, or hormones.

Osteoporosis

Osteoporosis, or porous bone, is a disease in which bone tissue is normally mineralized but the mass—*density of bone*—is decreased and the structural integrity of trabecular bone is impaired. There are two types of osteoporosis. Type 1,

Box 42-1	Causes of Rhabdomyolysis

Medications and Toxic Substances That Increase the Risk of Rhabdomyolysis
Direct Myotoxicity
HMG-CoA reductase inhibitors, (statins), especially in combination with fibrate-derived lipid-lowering agents such as niacin (nicotinic acid; Nicolar)
Cyclosporine (Sandimmune)
Itraconazole (Sporanox)
Erythromycin
Colchicine
Zidovudine (Retrovir)
Corticosteroids

Indirect Muscle Damage
Alcohol
Central nervous system depressants
Cocaine
Amphetamine
Ecstasy (MDMA)
LSD
Neuromuscular-blocking agents

Traumatic, Heat-Related, Ischemic, and Exertional Causes
Traumatic Causes
Lightning strike
Immobilization
Extensive third-degree burn
Crush injury

Heat-Related Causes
Heat stroke
Malignant hyperthermia
Neuroleptic malignant syndrome

Ischemic Causes
Ischemic limb injury

Exertional Causes
Marathon running
Physical overexertion in untrained athletes
Pathologic muscle exertion
Heat dissipation impairment
Physical overexertion in persons with sickle cell disease

Genetic Causes
Lipid Metabolism
Carnitine palmitoyltransferase deficiency
Carnitine deficiency

Short-chain and long-chain acetyl-coenzyme A dehydrogenase deficiency

Carbohydrate Metabolism
Myophosphorylase deficiency (McArdle disease)
Phosphorylase kinase deficiency
Phosphofructokinase deficiency
Phosphoglycerate mutase deficiency
Lactate dehydrogenase deficiency (characteristic elevation of creatine kinase level with normal lactate dehydrogenase level)

Purine Metabolism
Myoadenylate deaminase deficiency
Duchenne muscular dystrophy

Infectious, Inflammatory, Metabolic, and Endocrinologic Causes
Infectious Causes
Viruses: influenza virus B, parainfluenza virus, adenovirus, coxsackievirus, echovirus, herpes simplex virus, cytomegalovirus, Epstein-Barr virus, human immunodeficiency virus
Bacteria: *Streptococcus, Salmonella, Legionella, Staphylococcus,* and *Listeria* species

Inflammatory Causes
Polymyositis
Dermatomyositis
Capillary leak syndrome
Snake bites (mostly in South America, Asia, and Africa)

Metabolic and Endocrinologic Causes
Electrolyte imbalances: hyponatremia, hypernatremia, hypokalemia, hypophosphatemia, hypocalcemia
Hypothyroidism
Thyrotoxicosis
Diabetic ketoacidosis
Nonketotic hyperosmolar syndrome

Herbal Supplements
Red yeast rice (monaseus, purpureus)
Compounds containing ma huang, guarana, and garcinia cambogia
Ephedra-based compounds, especially weight-loss supplements

HMG-CoA, 3-hydroxy-3-methylglutaryl coenzyme A; *LSD,* lysergic acid diethylamide; *MDMA,* 3,4-methylenedioxymethamphetamine.
From Sauret JM, Marinides G, Wang GK: *Am Fam Physician* 65(3):907, 2002.

or primary osteoporosis, can be further subdivided into postmenopausal or senile types. Senile osteoporosis occurs after age 70. Type 2, or secondary osteoporosis, is caused by other etiologies, such as disease or drugs. Cortical bone becomes more porous and thinner, making bone weaker and prone to fractures (Figure 42-9). The World Health Organization (WHO) has defined osteoporosis based on bone density:

1. Normal bone is greater than 833 mg/cm^2
2. **Osteopenia,** or decreased bone mass, is 833 to 648 mg/cm^2
3. Osteoporosis is less than 648 mg/cm^2

Severe or established osteoporosis is identified when there has been a fragility fracture. The disease can be (1) generalized, involving major portions of the axial skeleton, or (2) regional, involving one segment of the appendicular skeleton.

Throughout a lifetime, old bone is removed (resorption) and new bone is added (formation) to the skeleton. During childhood and teenage years, new bone is added faster than old bone is removed. Consequently, bones become larger, heavier, and denser. Bone formation continues at a pace faster than resorption until **peak bone mass,** or maximum bone density and strength, is reached, around age 30, after which bone resorption slowly exceeds bone formation. In women, bone loss is most rapid in the first years after menopause but persists throughout the postmenopausal years. Bone loss in women begins before menopause. The WHO recently

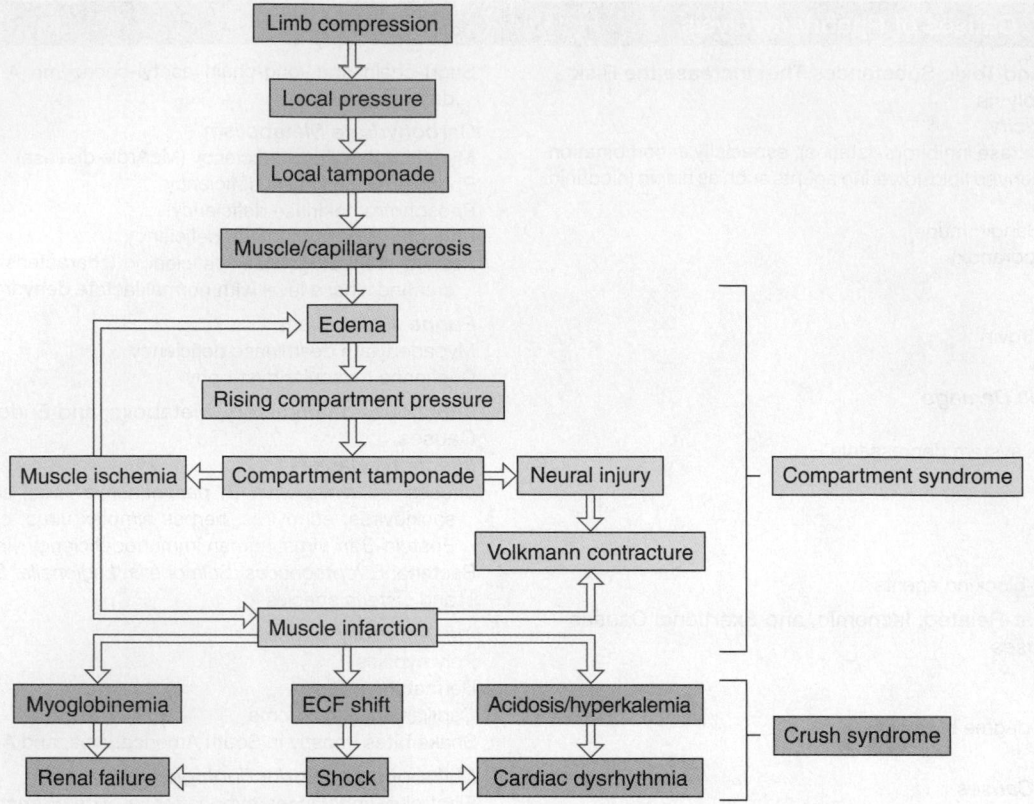

Figure 42-8 Pathogenesis of compartment syndrome and crush syndrome caused by prolonged muscle compression. *ECF,* Extracellular fluid.

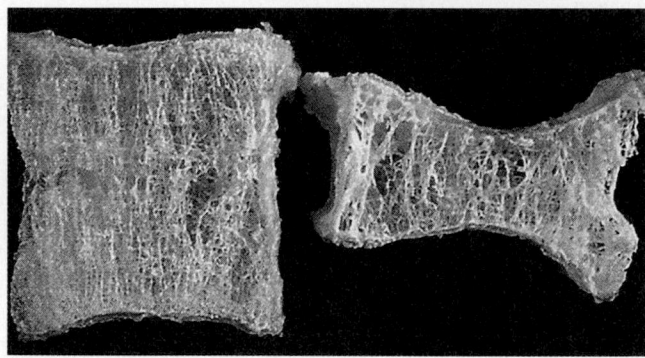

Figure 42-9 **Vertebral body.** Osteoporotic vertebra *(right)* shortened by compression fractures compared with normal vertebral body *(left).* Note that the osteoporotic vertebra has characteristic loss of horizontal trabeculae and thickened vertebral trabeculae. (From Kumar et al: *Robbins & Cotran pathologic basis of disease,* ed 7, Philadelphia, 2005, Saunders.)

redefined the approach to evaluating, treating, and preventing fractures associated with low bone density. Rather than diagnosing osteoporosis solely on low bone mass, worldwide efforts are being directed toward individualized assessment of a 10-year fracture risk.[14] An estimated 10 million Americans older than age 50 have osteoporosis, and 34 million are at risk.[15] The major risks for persons with osteoporosis are fractures. Men lose bone density with aging but because they begin with a higher bone density, they reach osteoporotic levels at

an older age than do women. Osteoporotic fractures affect 1 in 2 women and 1 in 5 men older than the age of 50.[16]

Vertebral fractures are the most common osteoporotic fracture but may be asymptomatic.[17] Even if the fracture does not cause pain, vertebral fractures can cause deformity, reduced pulmonary function, and loss of height. The degree of compression necessary to define a vertebral fracture has not been standardized. Thus the true prevalence is unknown, but fractures do increase in frequency by the sixth and seventh decades. Vertebral fracture prevalence in men is close to that in women.[18]

Osteoporosis is most common in white and Asian women, but affects all races. Whites are more susceptible than other races to osteoporosis caused by loss of bone density with age. Blacks have only about half the fracture of whites, probably related to their higher peak bone mass.[19,20] The cause of generalized osteoporosis remains uncertain but is probably multifactorial (see following).

Bone quality is not just bone mass (as measured by bone density) but also the microarchitecture of the bone. Thus other variables include crystal size and shape, brittleness, vitality of the bone cells, structure of the bone proteins, integrity of the trabecular network, and the ability to repair tiny cracks.[18] Because bone density relates to *quantity* of bone, *quality* of the bone is not accurately identified by bone density testing. Therefore, bone density testing may or may not accurately identify those who will go on to develop a fracture.

Box 42-2	Risk Factors for Osteoporosis

Genetic
Family history of osteoporosis
White/Asian race
Increased age
Female sex

Anthropometric
Small stature
Fair or pale skinned
Thin build

Hormonal and Metabolic
Early menopause (natural or surgical)
Late menarche
Nulliparity
Obesity
Hypogonadism
Gaucher disease
Cushing syndrome
Weight below healthy range
Acidosis

Dietary
Low dietary calcium and vitamin D
Low endogenous magnesium
Excessive protein*
Excessive sodium intake
High caffeine intake
Anorexia
Malabsorption

Lifestyle
Sedentary
Smoker
Alcohol consumption (excessive)

Concurrent
Hyperparathyroidism

Illness and Trauma
Renal insufficiency, hypocalciuria
Rheumatoid arthritis
Spinal cord injury
Systemic lupus

Liver Disease
Marrow disease (myeloma, mastocytosis, thalassemia)

Drugs
Corticosteroids
Dilantin
Gonadotropin-releasing hormone agonists
Loop diuretics
Methotrexate
Thyroid
Heparin
Cyclosporine
Depo-medroxyprogesterone acetate
Retinoids

*Low levels of protein intake also have been reported.

Osteoporosis is a complex, multifactorial chronic disease that often progresses silently for decades until fractures occur. It is the most common disease that affects bone. It is not necessarily a consequence of the aging process because some older adults retain strong, relatively dense bones.[21] In osteoporosis, the old bone is being reabsorbed faster than new bone is being made, causing the bones to lose density, becoming thinner and more porous. A progressive loss of bone mass may continue until the skeleton is no longer strong enough to support itself. Eventually, bones can fracture spontaneously. As bone becomes more fragile, falls or bumps that would not have caused fracture previously at that point do cause a fracture.

Postmenopausal osteoporosis—which occurs in middle-aged and older women is probably caused by changes in osteoprotegerin, (see Pathophysiology) insulin-like growth factor (IGF), a combination of inadequate dietary calcium intake and lack of vitamin D, possibly decreased magnesium, lack of exercise, decreased levels of estrogen, and family history. IGF is known to help in fracture healing and collagen synthesis and improves conditions for bone mineralization. IGF levels significantly decline by age 60. Excessive phosphorus intake, chiefly through the intake of sodas and junk foods interferes with the calcium-phosphorus balance, resulting in an increased risk of brittle bones.

Sex hormones, especially estrogen and testosterone, are significant in premenopausal bone maintenance; however, when estrogen levels drop after menopause, it appears that circulating androgens become significant effectors on bone metabolism. In clinical studies of women, data have suggested that serum androgens influence bone density in pre-, peri-, and postmenopausal women.[22,23] Androgens (i.e., testosterone and dihydrotestosterone) have long been recognized to stimulate bone formation. Testosterone is converted to estradiol by the enzyme aromatase. Increasing age in men and women is associated with declining levels of estrogen. In addition, progesterone deficiency may be related to osteoporosis. Decreases in weight-bearing exercise are associated with osteoporosis. Other risk factors are identified in Box 42-2.

Poor nutrition and insufficient intake or malabsorption of dietary minerals, particularly calcium, are factors in the development of osteoporosis.[24] Calcium absorption from the intestine decreases with age, and studies of individuals with osteoporosis show that their calcium intake is lower than that of age-matched controls. Deficiencies of vitamins, particularly vitamins C and D, also contribute to bone loss.

Skeletal homeostasis depends on a very narrow range of plasma calcium and phosphate concentrations, which are maintained by the endocrine system. Therefore, endocrine dysfunction ultimately can cause metabolic bone disease. In addition to declining levels of sex steroids, the hormones most commonly associated with osteoporosis are parathyroid hormone, cortisol, thyroid hormone, and growth hormone. Excessive intakes of caffeine, alcohol, and nicotine along with

NUTRITION & DISEASE

Trace Elements and Their Effects on Skeletal Tissue*

Fluoride accumulates in new bone formation sites and results in a net gain in bone mass; however, at higher doses the new bone may be structurally abnormal.

Magnesium enhances bone turnover by stimulating osteoclastic function and may help with regulation of calcium.

Zinc regulates secretion of calcitonin from the thyroid gland and influences bone turnover; it is essential for enzymes in osteoblasts responsible for collagen synthesis and alkaline phosphatase and is required for osteoblasts.

Iodine enhances bone turnover as hormonal forms of thyroxine and triiodothyronine.

Aluminum induces impairment of bone formation by inhibiting osteoblastic function.

Copper induces low bone turnover by suppressing osteoblastic and osteoclastic function.

Boron may be used by osteoblasts for bone formation and may be related to magnesium in its effect on bone.

Iron functions in mitochondrial oxidative phosphorylation in osteoblasts and osteoclasts.

Manganese is required for biosynthesis of mucopolysaccharides in bone matrix formation.

Data from Mahan LK, Escott-Stump S: *Krause's food, nutrition, and diet therapy*, ed 10, Philadelphia, 2000, Saunders; Okano T: *Nippon Rinsho* 54(1):148, 1996 (non-English).
*The exact involvement of these trace elements in osteoporosis has not been clarified.

low body fat have been considered risk factors. In addition, significant differences in the trace elements (zinc, copper, manganese) were noted in the bones and hair of unaffected individuals compared with those with osteoporosis[25] (see Nutrition & Disease: Trace Elements and Their Effects on Skeletal Tissue). Development of selective androgen receptor modulators (SARMs) promises novel treatment for osteoporosis through increasing bone formation and building more muscle mass. By selectively affecting bone, muscle mass, and other desired sites while not affecting lipid or estrogen levels or blood pressure, side effects can be controlled.[26]

Secondary osteoporosis sometimes develops temporarily in individuals receiving large doses of heparin, perhaps because heparin promotes bone resorption by decreasing collagen synthesis or by increasing collagen breakdown. Osteoporosis caused by heparin therapy usually resolves when therapy ceases. Treatment with other medications may lead to development of osteoporosis, such as the use of glucocorticoid treatment for rheumatoid arthritis. Other medications increasing risk of osteoporosis include lithium, methotrexate, anticonvulsants, cyclophosphamide, and cyclosporine.

One form, transient osteoporosis of the hip, is associated with the third trimester of pregnancy or the immediate postpartum period. However, most transient osteoporosis is a typically self-limiting syndrome affecting the lower extremity joints of middle-aged men. The etiology is unknown and although most cases spontaneously resolve, some occurrences of bone demineralization may be related to osteonecrosis.[27-29]

Regional osteoporosis—osteoporosis confined to a region or segment of the appendicular skeleton—usually has a known cause. Classic regional osteoporosis is associated with disuse or immobilization of a limb because of fractures, motor paralysis, or bone or joint inflammation (see Figure 42-13). A negative calcium balance develops early and continues throughout the period of immobilization. After 8 weeks of immobilization, significant osteoporosis is present, although it may develop earlier in persons younger than 20 years or older than 50 years. A uniform distribution of osteoporosis also has been observed in astronauts and in individuals treated with air suspension therapy as a result of weightlessness and lack of mechanical strain.

PATHOPHYSIOLOGY Whatever the cause, osteoporosis develops when the remodeling cycle—the process of bone resorption and bone formation—is disrupted, leading to an imbalance in the coupling process. Osteoclasts are differentiated cells that function to resorb bone. The explosion of new information in the field of bone biology has led to new understanding of osteoclast biology and bone pathophysiology. The osteoclast differentiation pathway is directed by a series of processes that include proliferation, differentiation, fusion, and activation.[30] These processes are controlled by hormones and cytokines and paracrine stromal-cell microenvironment interactions. Thus the intercellular communication in bone and the key molecular regulators are necessary for bone homeostasis. Interleukins (IL-1, IL-4, IL-6, IL-7, IL-11, IL-17), tumor necrosis factor (TNF), transforming growth factor-beta (TGF-β), prostaglandin E_2, and hormones interact to control osteoclasts[30] (Figure 42-10). Staggering in its importance is the recent identification of the cytokine **receptor activator of nuclear factor $\kappa\beta$ ligand (RANKL),** its receptor **RANK,** and its decoy receptor **osteoprotegerin (OPG);** this has led to a tremendously increased understanding of osteoclast biology and pathogenesis of bone diseases.

RANKL, a member of the TNF family, is expressed by osteoblasts and their immature precursors and is necessary for osteoclast development. RANKL activates the receptor RANK, which is expressed on osteoclasts and their precursors and suppresses apoptosis, which leads to activation and prolongation of osteoclast survival.[31] The effects of RANKL are blocked by OPG, which is a glycoprotein that acts as a decoy or soluble receptor antagonist for RANKL that prevents it from binding and activating RANK (see Figure 42-10). The balance between RANKL and OPG is regulated by cytokines and hormones, and alterations of the RANKL/RANK/OPG system can lead to dysregulation and pathologic conditions including osteoporosis, immune-mediated bone diseases, malignant bone disorders, and inherited skeletal diseases (see Figure 42-10).

Postmenopausal osteoporosis is characterized by increased bone resorption relative to the rate of bone formation, leading to sustained bone loss resulting from estrogen deficiency. Bone loss resulting from estrogen deficiency also contributes to

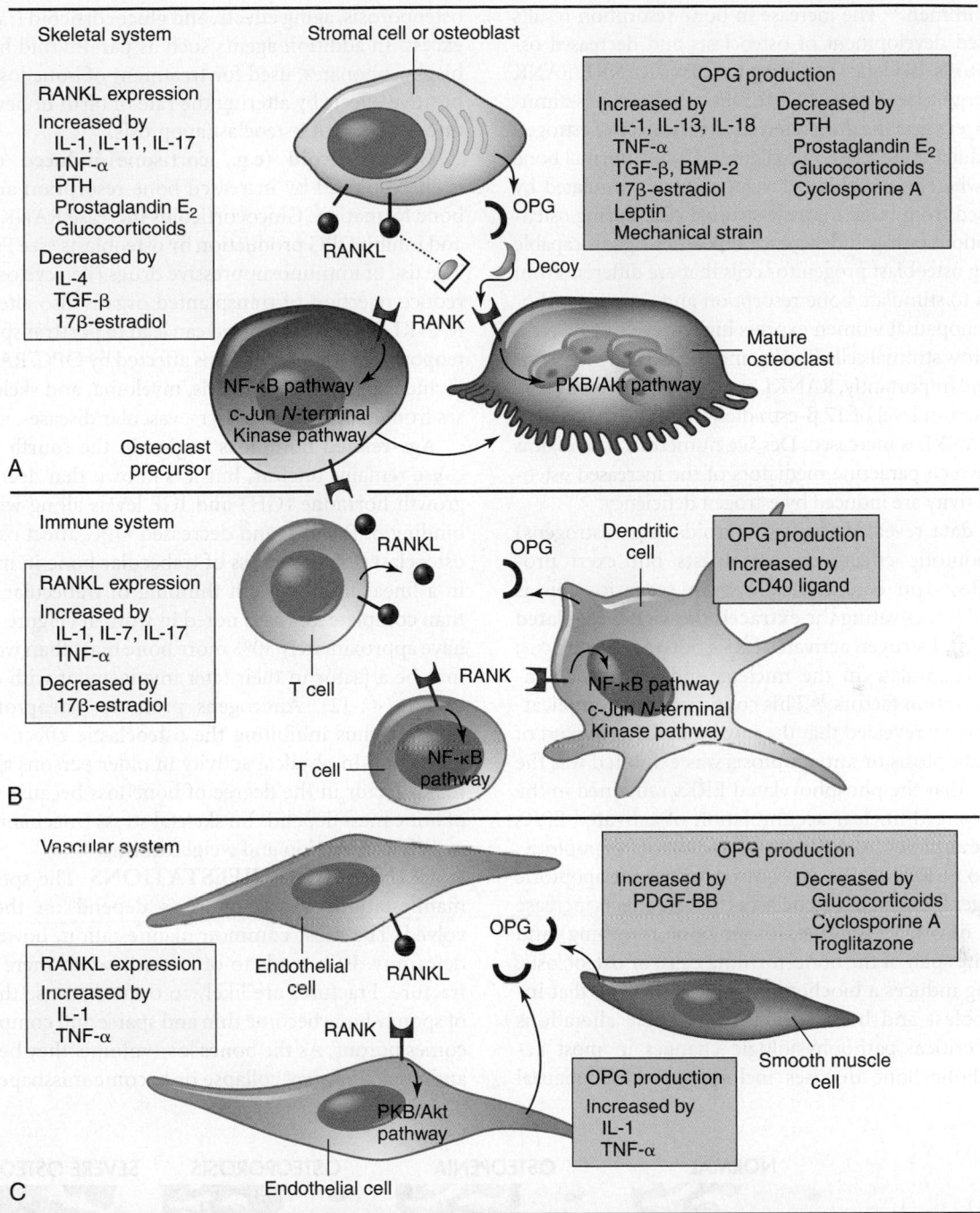

Figure 42-10 OPG/RANKL/RANK system. Receptor activator of nuclear factor κβ ligand (RANKL), a cytokine and part of the tumor necrosis factor (TNF) family, expression and osteoprotegerin (OPG), a glycoprotein receptor antagonist, are modulated by various cytokines, hormones, drugs, and mechanical strains *(see inserts)*. **A,** In bone, RANKL is expressed by both stromal cells and osteoblasts. RANKL stimulates the receptor RANK on osteoclast precursor cells and mature osteoclasts, activates intracellular signaling pathways to promote osteoclast differentiation and activation and cytoskeletal reorganization and survival (PKB/Akt pathway) that increases resorption and bone loss. OPG, secreted by stromal cells and osteoblasts, acts as a "decoy" receptor and blocks RANKL binding to and activating RANK. **B,** In the immune system, RANKL is expressed and secreted by T cells. T-cell–derived RANKL also can activate RANK on osteoclasts, T cells, and dendritic cells (antigen-presenting cells), which enhances bone loss that occurs in inflammatory bone diseases such as rheumatoid arthritis. Dendritic cells may regulate these processes by secreting OPG. **C,** In the vascular system, endothelial cells express RANKL and the RANK receptor. RANKL/RANK interactions contribute to endothelial and smooth muscle cells and can block RANKL binding. The physiologic significance of the OPG/RANKL/RANK system in endothelial and smooth muscle cells is being studied. *BMP-2,* Bone morphogenic protein 2; *IL,* interleukin, *PDGF-BB,* platelet-derived growth factor beta polypeptide; *PTH,* parathyroid hormone; *TGF-β* transforming growth factor-beta. (Adapted from Hofbauer LC, Schoppet M: *JAMA* 292[4]:490-495, 2004.)

osteoporosis in men.[32] The increase in bone resorption results from increased development of osteoclasts and decreased osteoclast apoptosis. Evidence involving the OPG/RANKL/RANK system is emerging (see Figure 42-10). OPG production is stimulated by estrogens and the drug referred to as a selective estrogen receptor modulator (SERM), raloxifene.[30] Unlike normal bone remodeling whereby osteoblast development is stimulated by factors released from bone marrow stromal cells during osteoclastic resorption, estrogen deficiency unleashes signals capable of stimulating osteoblast progenitor cells that are different from those needed to stimulate bone resorption and thus are pathologic. Postmenopausal women express higher levels of RANKL on bone marrow stromal cells, T cells, and B cells than premenopausal women. Importantly, RANKL expression is inversely correlated with serum level of 17 β-estradiol, that is, with estradiol deficiency, RANKL is increased. Despite numerous studies, it is still unclear which paracrine mediators of the increased osteoclastogenic activity are induced by estrogen deficiency.

Recently, data revealed that sex steroids (e.g., estrogens) exert antiapoptotic effects on osteoblasts but exert proapoptotic effects on osteoclasts; in both scenarios this is accomplished by activating the **extracellular signal regulated kinases (ERKs).** Estrogen activates ERKs outside the nucleus; ERKs then accumulate in the nucleus and activate downstream transcription factors.[33] This confusing and complicated data eventually revealed that the important determinant of whether proapoptosis or antiapoptosis was exhibited was the *length of time* that the phosphorylated ERKs remained in the nucleus. Prolonged nuclear accumulation of activated ERKs converted the antiapoptotic effect of estradiol to proapoptotic. In addition to ERKs, RANKL is required for the antiapoptotic and thus longer life span of osteoclasts.[34] These effects increase the life span of osteoclasts (i.e., longer bone resorbing) and shorten the life span of the bone-forming cells, or osteoblasts. Wnt signaling induces a biochemical series of events that increases osteoblast and bone formation.[31] These alterations account for critical pathophysiologic changes in most acquired metabolic bone diseases including postmenopausal

osteoporosis, aging effects, and glucocorticoid (i.e., cortisone) excess. In addition agents such as parathyroid hormone and bisphosphonates, used for treatment of bone loss, exert their positive effects by altering the rate of birth of new osteoblasts or osteoclasts or osteoclast apoptosis.

Glucocorticoid (e.g., cortisone)-induced osteoporosis is characterized by increased bone resorption and decreased bone formation. Glucocorticoids increase RANKL expression and inhibit OPG production by osteoblasts (see Figure 42-10). The use of immunosuppressive drugs (i.e., cyclosporine A) to reduce rejection of transplanted organs also alters the OPG/RANKL/RANK system and can lead to posttransplantation osteoporosis. Other conditions affected by OPG/RANKL/RANK include rheumatoid arthritis, myeloma, and skeletal metastases from neoplastic disorders, vascular diseases, and others.

Age-related bone loss begins in the fourth decade. The cause remains unclear, but it is known that decreased serum growth hormone (GH) and IGF levels along with increased binding of RANKL and decreased OPG affect osteoblast and osteoclast function. Loss of trabecular bone in men proceeds in a linear fashion, with thinning of trabecular bone rather than complete loss as is noted in women (Figure 42-11). Men have approximately 30% more bone mass than women, which may be a factor in their later involvement with osteoporosis (Figure 42-12). Androgens promote osteoprotegerin production, thus inhibiting the osteoclastic effect of RANKL.[35] Reduction in physical activity in older persons also may be a major factor in the degree of bone loss because preservation of bone mass depends on skeletal stress (mechanical) through muscle contraction and weightbearing.[36]

CLINICAL MANIFESTATIONS The specific clinical manifestations of osteoporosis depend on the bones involved. The most common manifestation, however, is bone deformity. Pain tends to occur only when there is a fragility fracture. Fractures are likely to occur because the trabeculae of spongy bone become thin and sparse and compact bone becomes porous. As the bones lose volume, they become brittle and weak and may collapse or become misshapen. Vertebral

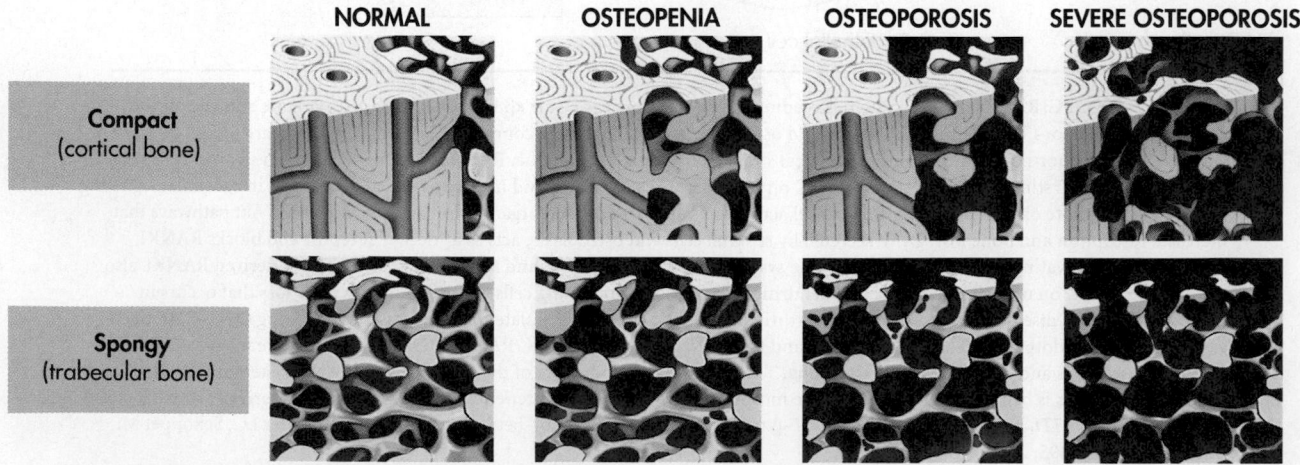

Figure 42-11 Osteoporosis in cortical and trabecular bone.

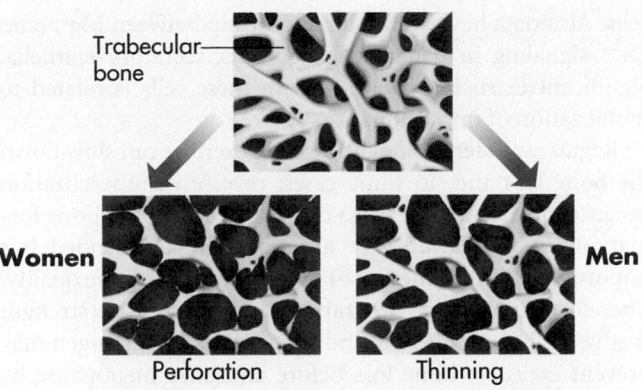

Figure 42-12 Mechanism of loss of trabecular bone in women and trabecular thinning in men. Bone thinning predominates in men because of reduced bone formation. Loss of connectivity and complete trabecular loss predominates in women.

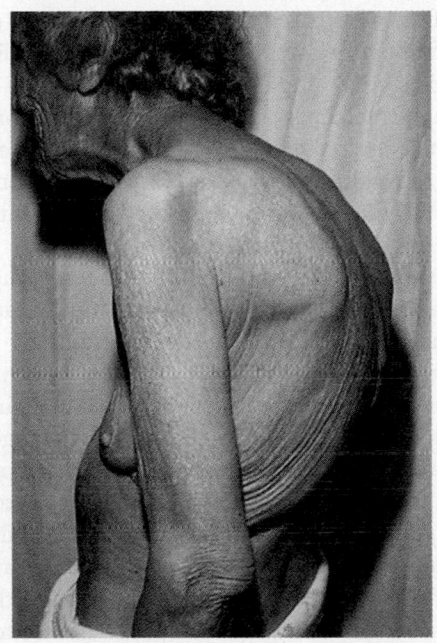

Figure 42-13 Kyphosis. This older adult woman's condition was caused by a combination of spinal osteoporotic vertebral collapse and chronic degenerative changes in the vertebral column. (From Kamal A, Brocklehurst JC: *Color atlas of geriatric medicine,* ed 2, St Louis, 1992, Mosby.)

collapse causes kyphosis (hunchback) and diminished height (Figure 42-13). Fractures of the long bones (particularly the femur and humerus), distal radius, ribs, and vertebrae are most common. Fracture of the neck of the femur—the so-called broken hip—tends to occur in older or older adult women with osteoporosis. Fatal complications of fractures include fat or pulmonary embolism, hemorrhage, and shock. Approximately 20% of persons with a hip fracture may die as a result of surgical complications.

EVALUATION AND TREATMENT Generally, osteoporosis is detected radiographically as increased radiolucency of bone. By the time abnormalities are detected by x-ray

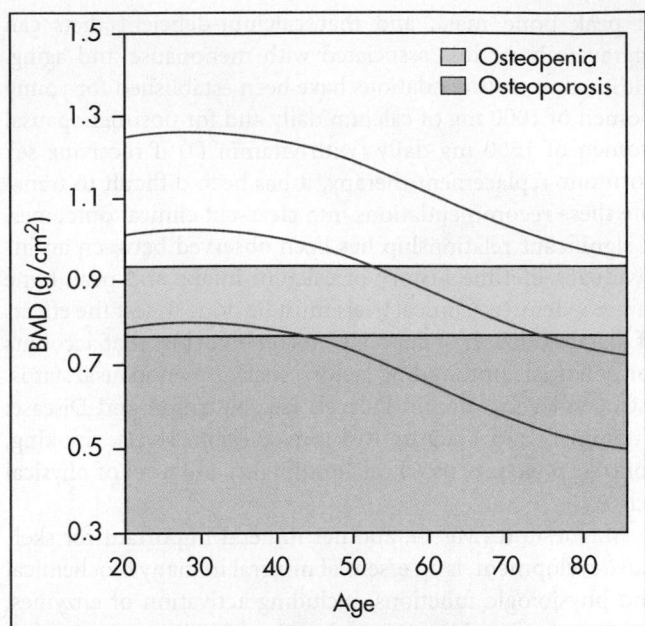

Figure 42-14 Lumbar spine bone mass density (BMD). The normal female reference curves for lumbar spine BMD are plotted in this graph to include the World Health Organization definitions of osteopenia and osteoporosis. (Redrawn from Collier BD, Fogelman I, Rosenthall L: *Skeletal nuclear medicine,* St Louis, 1996, Mosby.)

examination, as much as 25% to 30% of bone tissue may have been lost.

Types of radiologic examinations include single- or dual-photon absorptiometry (SXA, DXA) and computed tomography (CT) scans (Figure 42-14). Because osteoporosis is asymptomatic unless a fracture occurs, diagnosis is often delayed. At present, DXA is the current examination of choice for diagnosis. Unfortunately, DXA does not provide information about bone strength or fracture risk.[37]

Because fractures are the problem with osteoporosis, the WHO has developed an assessment tool to estimate an individual's 10-year risk of fracture. The WHO's Fracture Risk Assessment (FRAX) is a downloadable computer-drive questionnaire that has been developed for use in Europe, North America, Asia, and Australia. Once completed, the imbedded algorithms predict the 10-year probability of hip, spine, forearm, or shoulder fractures. This tool can be downloaded from www.shef.ac.uk/FRAX. Other evaluation procedures include tests for levels of serum calcium, phosphorus, and alkaline phosphatase and protein electrophoresis. Body calcium levels also can be measured by neuron activation analysis, a procedure involving use of radioactive calcium-49, whose gamma activity can be measured with a whole-body counter.

The goals of osteoporosis treatment are to slow down the rate of calcium and bone loss and to stop the disease before it progresses too far. Controversial is the role of calcium intake to prevent and treat osteoporosis. It is well accepted that oral calcium intake sufficient to maintain normal calcium balance is necessary during adolescence to ensure development of peak bone mass, and that calcium-deficient diets can aggravate bone loss associated with menopause and aging. Although recommendations have been established for young women of 1000 mg of calcium daily and for postmenopausal women of 1500 mg daily (with vitamin D) if receiving sex hormone replacement therapy, it has been difficult to translate these recommendations into clear-cut clinical outcomes. A significant relationship has been observed between an individual's lifetime history of calcium intake and peak bone mineral density. Clinical trials must be done to test the effects of dietary calcium or supplements on bone loss that accounts for potential confounding factors, such as menopausal status, estrogen levels, vitamin D levels (see Nutrition and Disease: Vitamin D and Fracture Risk), magnesium levels, smoking, contraceptive use, usual calcium intake, and level of physical activity.

Magnesium (Mg^{++}), another mineral important for skeletal development, is an essential mineral in many biochemical and physiologic functions, including activation of enzymes, involvement in adenosine triphosphate (ATP) synthesis, protein synthesis, regulation of membrane channels, and muscle contraction. New evidence suggests that large fluxes of magnesium can cross the cell plasma membrane in either direction following a variety of stimuli, resulting in a modification of activity for several cellular enzymes. Mg^{++} is important to bone quality because it controls hydroxyapatite crystal growth and thereby prevents formation of brittle bones. It seems reasonable that Mg^{++} is required for normal calcium (Ca^{++}) absorption because severe Mg^{++} deficiency results in hypocalcemia. Elevation of plasma Mg^{++} or Ca^{++} concentration inhibits Mg^{++} and Ca^{++} resorption, leading to hypermagnesiuria and hypercalciuria. An extracellular Ca^{++}/Mg^{++} sensing receptor has been found located on distal tubule

cells. Also data have shown a relationship between Mg^{++} and Ca^{++} signaling in pancreatic and other secretory epithelia. Significant extrusion of Mg^{++} from these cells is related to mobilization of intracellular Ca^{++}.[38]

Regular, moderate weight-bearing exercise can slow down the bone loss and, in some cases, reverse demineralization because the mechanical stress of exercise stimulates bone formation. Vitamin D and Mg^{++} also may be recommended. It is important to reduce the risk of falls and enhance bone quality. Therefore, an exercise program to enhance muscle strength is advised. Important new findings suggest that estrogen may prevent excessive bone loss before and after menopause by limiting osteoclast life span through promotion of apoptosis. Hormone replacement therapy helps maintain bone density but it is not routinely recommended because of the increased risk of stroke and breast cancer and no significant cardioprotective effects.

SERMs and SARMs have been developed to provide the positive effects of estrogen on bone but minimize estrogen's negative effect on breast and endometrial tissues. Raloxifene and tamoxifen are examples of SERMs.

The bisphosphonates alendronate and risedronate have been effective in reducing hip and vertebral fractures in glucocorticoid-induced osteoporosis and in women with osteoporosis by inhibiting bone resorption. Recent evidence reveals the bisphosphonates activate a previously unknown signaling pathway that is triggered by the opening of connexin 43, a protein that forms a gap junction important for intercellular communication. After opening of connexin 43, activation of ERKs (see p. 1582) occurs, which mediates osteocyte survival. Osteocyte viability possibly maintains the effectiveness of bisphosphonates as well as other agents (e.g., estrogen, and daily parathyroid injections) by preventing apoptosis of osteocytes and osteoblasts.[33] Two recombinant bone morphogenic proteins (BMPs), BMP-2 and BMP-7, have been used to improve fracture healing and spinal fusions.[39] Teriparatide, a biosynthetic form of parathormone, is injected subcutaneously. However, use is limited to a period of 24 months because of the risk of developing osteosarcoma. Men with osteoporosis are treated with bisphosphonates and testosterone. Controversial is testosterone treatment for women. Restoration of a balanced RANKL/OPG ratio (see p. 1580) or inhibiting RANK responsiveness is known to prevent osteoclast activation and bone resorption. Anti-RANKL therapy significantly reduces bone resorption. Denosumab, a monoclonal antibody, is the first of these compounds.[34,40]

Osteomalacia

Osteomalacia is a metabolic disease characterized by inadequate and delayed mineralization of osteoid in mature compact and spongy bone. In osteomalacia the remodeling cycle proceeds normally through osteoid formation, but mineral calcification and deposition do not occur. Bone volume remains unchanged, but the replaced bone consists of soft osteoid instead of rigid bone. The result is abnormal bone matrix mineralization. Rickets is similar to osteomalacia in

---

NUTRITION & DISEASE

Vitamin D and Fracture Risk

The beneficial effects of vitamin D on fracture risk are attributed to two explanations: (1) the decrease in bone loss in older adults and (2) the increase in muscle strength and balance mediated through vitamin D receptors in muscle tissue.

In addition, vitamin D has been correlated with a significant (22%) reduction in the risk of falling in older adults. Pooled analyses reveal that higher doses (700 to 800 international units/day) are better for reducing fractures than 400 international units/day. Previously the recommendation for vitamin D in middle-aged and older adults was 400 to 600 international units/day. With new data and the uncertainty of intake recommendations, higher doses may be more effective (700 to 800 international units/day).

Because calcium was administered in combination with vitamin D in all but one of the higher-dose vitamin D trials, the independent effects of vitamin D alone could not be determined. Still needing further research is whether and in what dose calcium adds value to fracture prevention with vitamin D.

Data from Bischoff-Ferrari HA et al: *JAMA* 293:2257-2264, 2005. (Also see p. 70.)

pathogenesis, but it occurs in the growing bones of children, whereas osteomalacia occurs in adult bone. Chronically low-serum phosphate level is a major cause of osteomalacia. Fibroblast growth factor-23 (FGF-23) plays a significant role in maintaining normal serum phosphate.[41] Primarily produced by osteocytes, FGF-23 functions to inhibit reabsorption of phosphate in the renal proximal tubule.[42] (Rickets is described in Chapter 43.)

Osteomalacia and rickets are rare in the United States and Western Europe but are significant health problems in Great Britain, Ethiopia, Pakistan, Iran, and India. In the United States these diseases occur in older adults, in premature infants of very low birth weight, and in individuals adhering to rigid macrobiotic vegetarian diets.

Certain forms of osteomalacia are caused by genetic abnormalities; other forms can be caused by tumors. Many factors contribute to the development of osteomalacia, but the most important is a deficiency of vitamin D. The major risk factors in vitamin D deficiency are diets deficient in vitamin D, decreased endogenous production of vitamin D, intestinal malabsorption of vitamin D, renal tubular diseases, and anticonvulsant therapy. Classic vitamin D deficiency is rare in the United States because of the addition of synthetic vitamin D to dairy products and bread.

However, disorders of the small bowel, hepatobiliary system, and pancreas are common causes of vitamin D deficiency in the United States. In malabsorptive disease of the small bowel, vitamin D and calcium absorption are decreased, so vitamin D is lost in feces. Liver disease interferes with the metabolism of vitamin D to its more active form, and diseases of the pancreas and biliary system cause a deficiency of bile salts, which are necessary for normal intestinal absorption of vitamin D.

The mechanism by which anticonvulsant drug therapy results in vitamin D deficiency is not completely understood, but researchers think that the anticonvulsants phenobarbital and phenytoin interfere with calcium absorption and increase degradation of vitamin D metabolism in the liver.

PATHOPHYSIOLOGY Crystallization of minerals in osteoid requires adequate concentrations of calcium and phosphate. When the concentrations are too low, crystallization (and hence ossification) does not proceed normally.

Vitamin D deficiency disrupts mineralization because vitamin D normally regulates and enhances the absorption of calcium ions from the intestine. A lack of vitamin D causes the plasma calcium concentrations to fall. Low plasma calcium levels stimulate increased synthesis and secretion of parathyroid hormone (PTH). Although the increase in circulating PTH raises the plasma calcium concentration, it also stimulates increased renal clearance of phosphate. When the concentration of phosphate in the bone decreases below a critical level, mineralization cannot proceed normally.

Abnormalities occur in spongy as well as compact bone. Trabeculae in spongy bone become thinner and fewer, whereas haversian systems in compact bone develop large channels and become irregular. Because osteoid continues to be produced but not mineralized, abnormal quantities of osteoid build up, coating the trabeculae and the linings of the haversian canals. Excessive osteoid also can accumulate in areas beneath the periosteum. The excess of osteoid leads to gross deformities of the long bones, spine, pelvis, and skull.

CLINICAL MANIFESTATIONS Osteomalacia causes varying degrees of diffuse skeletal pain and tenderness. Pain is noted particularly in the hips, and the individual may be hesitant to walk. Muscular weakness is common and may contribute to a waddling gait. Bone fractures and vertebral collapse occur with minimal trauma. Low back pain may be an early complaint, but pain also may involve ribs, feet, other areas of the vertebral column, and other sites. Uremia may be present in renal osteodystrophy.

EVALUATION AND TREATMENT Laboratory data may include elevated blood urea nitrogen (BUN) and creatinine levels, normal or low serum calcium levels, and a serum inorganic phosphate level that is usually higher than 5.5 mg. Alkaline phosphatase and PTH levels are usually elevated. Radiographic findings show pseudofractures and radiolucent bands perpendicular to the surface of involved bones. Diagnosis of certain types of osteomalacia is becoming easier because of the ability to measure an individual's serum FGF-23. Elevated FGF-23 levels are common in X-linked hypophosphatemic and tumor-induced osteomalacia.[43,44]

Treatment of osteomalacia includes the following:

1. Adjusting serum calcium and phosphorus levels to normal
2. Suppressing secondary hyperthyroidism
3. Chelating bone aluminum if needed
4. Administering calcium carbonate to decrease hyperphosphatemia
5. Dietary supplements of vitamin D
6. Renal dialysis
7. Renal transplant for renal osteodystrophy

Paget Disease

Paget disease (osteitis deformans) is a state of increased metabolic activity in bone characterized by abnormal and excessive bone remodeling, both resorption and formation. Genetic manipulations involving the RANK-NF-κβ signaling pathway are significant in the development of Paget disease.[45] Chronic accelerated remodeling eventually enlarges and softens the affected bones.

Paget disease most often affects the axial skeleton, especially the vertebrae, skull, sacrum, sternum, pelvis, and femur. The disease process may occur in one or more bones without causing significant clinical manifestations.

The disease is seldom found before age 40 years, but its incidence almost doubles each decade from age 50. It affects men more than women in a proportion of 1.8:1.[46] Because it is often symptomless and can be diagnosed only by invasive procedures, few epidemiologic data are available. Autopsy data from England and Germany indicate that approximately 3% to 4% of persons older than 40 years have Paget disease. It is most prevalent in Australia, Great Britain, New Zealand, and the United States.

The cause of Paget disease is unknown, but there appears to be a strong genetic component. A viral connection (slow virus infection) to Paget disease also has been proposed.[45] Classic Paget disease arises as a consequence of disorderly bone resorption and formation.

PATHOPHYSIOLOGY Paget disease begins with excessive resorption of spongy bone. The trabeculae diminish, and bone marrow is replaced by extremely vascular fibrous tissue.

The resorption phase of Paget disease is followed by the formation of abnormal new bone at an accelerated rate. The collagen fibers are disorganized, and glycoprotein levels in the matrix decrease. Mineralization may extend into the bone marrow. Bone formation is excessive around partially resorbed trabeculae, causing them to thicken and enlarge. Eventually, Paget disease progresses to an inactive phase, in which abnormal remodeling is minimal or absent. Osteoclasts of individuals with Paget disease have increased responses to RANKL.[45]

CLINICAL MANIFESTATIONS In the skull, abnormal remodeling is first evident in the frontal or occipital regions, then encroaches on the outer and inner surfaces of the entire skull. The skull thickens and assumes an asymmetric shape (Figure 42-15). Thickened segments of the skull may compress areas of the brain, producing altered mentality and dementia. Impingement of new bone on cranial nerves causes

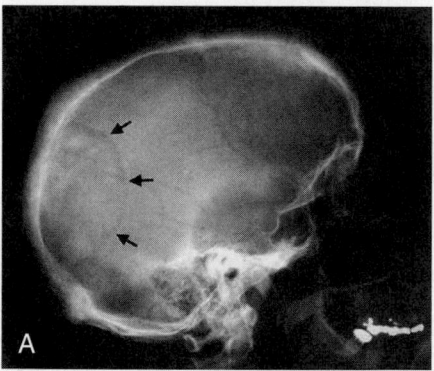
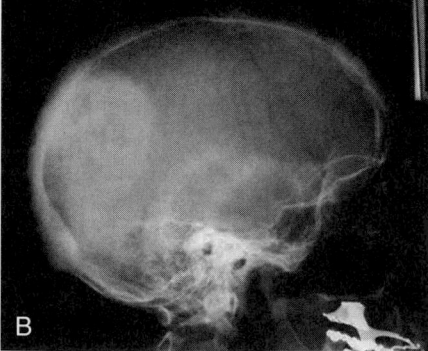

Figure 42-15 Paget disease of the skull. **A,** Active Paget disease of the skull, with marked cortical thickening and an area of osteoporosis circumscripta *(arrows)*. **B,** The same individual some years later (after bisphosphonate treatment), with the lytic lesion largely replaced by sclerotic bone. (From Walsh JP: *Med J Aust* 181[5]:263, 2004.)

sensory abnormalities, impaired motor function, deafness, atrophy of the optic nerve, and obstruction of the lacrimal duct. Headache is commonly noted.

Extensive alterations of the facial bones are rare except in the jaw, where sclerosis and thickening of the maxilla and mandible displace teeth and produce malocclusion. In long bones, resorption begins in the subchondral regions of the epiphysis and extends into the metaphysis and diaphysis. Warmth over the affected area, bone and joint pain, and bone deformity may occur. Occasionally, Paget disease affects both ends of a tubular bone. In the femur, Paget disease produces an exaggerated lateral curvature. In the tibia, anterior curvature is also exaggerated. Stress fractures are common in the lower extremities.

Clinical manifestations of Paget disease in the vertebral column depend on the level of involvement and are caused by compression of adjacent structures. In the cervical spine, cord compression can lead to spastic quadriplegia. Approximately 1% of persons with Paget disease develop osteogenic sarcoma. Paget-related sarcoma has a poor prognosis.

EVALUATION AND TREATMENT Evaluation of Paget disease is made on the basis of radiographic findings of irregular bone trabeculae with a thickened and disorganized pattern. Early disease is detected by bone scanning that shows increased uptake of bone radionuclides. Alkaline phosphatase and urinary hydroxyproline are elevated.

Most individuals require no treatment because the disease is localized and does not cause symptoms. Treatment during active disease is for pain relief, prevention of deformity, or fracture. Bisphosphonates (alendronate, risedronate, and pamidronate) and calcitonin (salmon and human) are the mainstays of treatment. Surgery is indicated if there are neurologic complications or severe bony deformities.

Infectious Bone Disease: Osteomyelitis

Infectious bone disease is expensive and difficult to treat and often culminates in extensive physical disability. The following factors contribute to the difficulty in treating bone infection:

1. Bone contains multiple microscopic channels that are impermeable to the cells and biochemicals of the body's natural defenses. Once bacteria gain access to these channels, they are able to proliferate unimpeded.
2. The microcirculation of bone is highly vulnerable to damage and destruction by bacterial toxins. Vessel damage causes local thrombosis (blockage) of the small vessels, which leads to ischemic necrosis (death) of bone.
3. Bone cells have a limited capacity to replace bone destroyed by infections. Initially, osteoclasts are stimulated by infection to resorb bone, which opens up isolated bone channels so that cells of the inflammatory and immune system can gain access to the infected bone. At the same time, however, resorption weakens the structural integrity of the bone. New bone formation usually lags behind resorption, and the haversian systems in the new bone are incomplete.

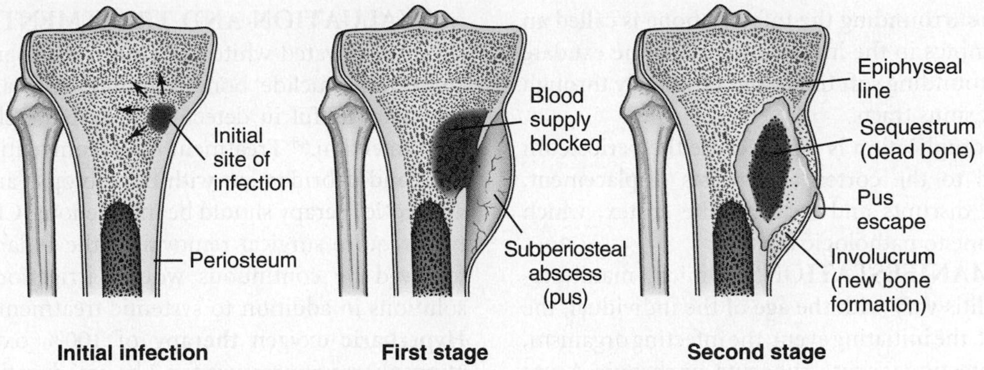

Figure 42-16 Osteomyelitis showing sequestration and involucrum.

Osteomyelitis is a bone infection most often caused by bacteria; however, fungi, parasites, and viruses also can cause bone infection (Figure 42-16). **Exogenous osteomyelitis** is an infection that enters from outside the body, for example, through open fractures, penetrating wounds, or surgical procedures. In exogenous osteomyelitis, the infection spreads from soft tissues into adjacent bone. **Endogenous (hematogenous) osteomyelitis** is caused by pathogens carried in the blood from sites of infection elsewhere in the body. In hematogenous osteomyelitis, the infection spreads from bone to adjacent soft tissues. Hematogenous osteomyelitis is commonly found in infants, children, and older adults. (Osteomyelitis in children is discussed in Chapter 43.) In infants, incidence rates among males and females are approximately equal. In children and older adults, however, males are most commonly affected. Osteomyelitis is a common complication of sickle cell anemia and low oxygen tension.

Staphylococcus aureus is the usual cause of hematogenous osteomyelitis. Other microorganisms include group B streptococci, *Haemophilus influenzae*, *Salmonella*, and gram-negative bacteria. Group B streptococci and *H. influenzae* tend to infect young children; *Salmonella* infection is associated with sickle cell anemia; and gram-negative infections are most common in older adults and individuals with impaired immunity. Mycobacterial and fungal infections occur in immunocompromised individuals.

Cutaneous, sinus, ear, and dental infections are the primary sources of bacteria in hematogenous bone infections. Soft tissue infections, disorders of the gastrointestinal tract, infections of the genitourinary system, and respiratory infections are also sources of bacterial contamination. In addition, infections contracted after total joint replacements can be causes of osteomyelitis. The vulnerability of specific bone depends on the anatomy of its vascular supply.

In adults, hematogenous osteomyelitis is more common in the spine, pelvis, and small bones. Microorganisms reach the vertebrae through arteries, veins, or lymphatic vessels. The spread of infection from pelvic organs to the vertebrae is well documented. Vaginal, uterine, ovarian, bladder, and intestinal infections can lead to iliac or sacral osteomyelitis.

Exogenous osteomyelitis can be caused by human bites or fist blows to the mouth. Superficial animal or human bites inoculate local soft tissue with bacteria that later spread to underlying bone. Deep bites can introduce microorganisms directly onto bone. The most common infecting organism in human bites is *S. aureus*. In animal bites the most common infecting organism is *Pasteurella multocida*, which is part of the normal mouth flora of cats and dogs.

Direct contamination of bones with bacteria also can occur in open fractures or dislocations with an overlying skin wound. Intervertebral disk surgery and operative procedures involving implantation of large foreign objects, such as metallic plates or artificial joints, are associated with exogenous osteomyelitis. Local injections and venous punctures are significant causes of exogenous osteomyelitis. Exogenous osteomyelitis of the arm and hand bones tends to occur in drug abusers. *S. aureus* is the most common pathogen. In general, persons who are chronically ill, have diabetes or alcoholism, or are receiving large doses of steroids or immunosuppressive drugs are particularly susceptible to exogenous osteomyelitis or recurring episodes of this disease.

PATHOPHYSIOLOGY Regardless of the source of the pathogen, the pathologic features of bone infection are similar to those in any other body tissue (see Chapter 9). First, the invading pathogen provokes an intense inflammatory response. Inflammation in bone is characterized by vascular engorgement, edema, leukocyte activity, and abscess formation. Once inflammation is initiated, the small terminal vessels thrombose and exudate seals the bone's canaliculi. Inflammatory exudate extends into the metaphysis and the marrow cavity and through small metaphyseal openings into the cortex. In children, exudate that reaches the outer surface of the cortex forms abscesses that lift the periosteum off underlying bone. Lifting of the periosteum disrupts blood vessels that enter bone through the periosteum, which deprives underlying bone of its blood supply; this leads to necrosis and death of the area of bone infected, producing **sequestrum,** an area of devitalized bone (see Figure 42-16). Lifting of the periosteum also stimulates an intense osteoblastic response. Osteoblasts lay down new bone that can partially or completely surround the infected bone. This layer of new bone surrounding the infected bone is called an **involucrum.** Openings in the involucrum allow the exudate to escape into surrounding soft tissue and ultimately through the skin by way of sinus tracts.

In adults this complication is rare because the periosteum is firmly attached to the cortex and resists displacement. Instead, infection disrupts and weakens the cortex, which predisposes the bone to pathologic fracture.

CLINICAL MANIFESTATIONS Clinical manifestations of osteomyelitis vary with the age of the individual, the site of involvement, the initiating event, the infecting organism, and whether the infection is acute, subacute, or chronic. Acute osteomyelitis causes an abrupt onset of inflammation. If an acute infection is not completely eliminated, the disease may become subacute or chronic. In subacute osteomyelitis, signs and symptoms are usually vague. In the chronic stage, infection is indolent or silent between exacerbations. The microorganisms persist in small abscesses or fragments of necrotic bone and produce occasional flare-ups of acute osteomyelitis. The progression from acute to subacute osteomyelitis may be the result of inadequate or inappropriate therapy or the development of drug-resistant microorganisms.

In the adult, hematogenous osteomyelitis has an insidious onset. The symptoms are usually vague and include fever, malaise, anorexia, and weight loss. Recent infection (urinary, respiratory, skin) or instrumentation (catheterization, cystoscopy, myelography, diskography) usually precedes onset of symptoms.

The primary symptom of acute osteomyelitis in the spine is back pain.[47] The pain may be intermittent or constant, aggravated by motion, and throbbing at rest. It may radiate in a radicular distribution and is commonly accompanied by spinal tenderness and rigidity. Hip contracture can occur in the presence of soft tissue inflammation as a result of irritation of the psoas muscle.

The signs and symptoms of sacroiliac osteomyelitis are generally severe and include local pain, tenderness, and a limp. The pain may radiate to the buttock or the abdomen.

Single or multiple abscesses (Brodie abscesses) characterize subacute or chronic osteomyelitis. Brodie abscesses are circumscribed lesions 1 to 4 cm in diameter, usually in the ends of long bones and surrounded by dense ossified bone matrix. The abscesses are thought to develop when the infectious microorganism has become less virulent or the individual's immune system is resisting the infection somewhat successfully.

In exogenous osteomyelitis, signs and symptoms of soft tissue infection predominate. Inflammatory exudate in the soft tissues disrupts muscles and supporting structures and forms abscesses. Low-grade fever, lymphadenopathy, local pain, and swelling usually occur within days of contamination by a puncture wound. Osteomyelitis in the hand causes exquisite tenderness over the course of tendon sheaths. The fingers are usually in a semiflexed position, and extension usually causes severe pain. Palmar swelling or symmetric swelling of the fingers may be present.

EVALUATION AND TREATMENT Laboratory data show an elevated white cell count. Radiographic studies include radionuclide bone scanning, CT, and MRI. MRI is especially useful in detecting early bone changes associated with infection.[48] Treatment of osteomyelitis includes antibiotics and débridement with bone biopsy and culture. Initial antibiotic therapy should be intravenous. Chronic conditions may require surgical removal of the inflammatory exudate followed by continuous wound irrigation with antibiotic solutions in addition to systemic treatment with antibiotics. **Hyperbaric oxygen therapy** of 100% oxygen, given at 2 atmospheres of pressure for 2 hours' duration per day for 30 treatments, is also beneficial for chronic refractory osteomyelitis. Implants for total joint replacements may be removed to treat the infected joint more thoroughly.

Bone Tumors

Many different types of tumors involve the skeleton. Bone tumors may originate from bone cells, cartilage, fibrous tissue, marrow, or vascular tissue. Based on the tissue of origin, bone tumors are classified as osteogenic, chondrogenic, collagenic, and myelogenic. Each of the four types arises from one of the four stem cells that are ultimately derived from the primitive mesoderm (Figure 42-17). In addition, bone tumors may be classified as being of histiocytic, notochordal, lipogenic, and neurogenic origins.

The mesoderm contributes the primitive fibroblast and reticulum cells. The fibroblast is the progenitor of the osteoblast and the chondroblast. Each cell synthesizes a specific type of intercellular ground substance, and the tumor derived from the cell is generally characterized by the type of ground substance produced by the cell. For example, osteogenic tumors usually contain cells that have the appearance of osteoblasts and produce an intercellular substance that can be recognized as osteoid. Chondrogenic tumors contain chondroblasts and produce an intercellular substance similar to chondroid (cartilage). Collagenic tumors contain fibrous tissue cells and produce an intercellular substance similar to the type of collagen found in fibrous connective tissue.

Tumors are also classified as benign or malignant. The criteria used to identify tumor cells as malignant are (1) an increased nuclear/cytoplasmic ratio, (2) an irregular nuclear border, (3) excess chromatin, (4) a prominent nucleolus, and (5) an increase in the number of cells undergoing mitosis. However, many young, rapidly growing, normal cells and cells subjected to inflammation and change in their blood supply also exhibit many of these same characteristics. (Tumor characteristics in general are described in Chapter 11.)

Epidemiology

The incidence of bone tumors varies with age. In children younger than 15 years, the rate of bone tumors is relatively low, constituting approximately 3% of all malignancies. Adolescents have the highest incidence of bone tumors, and adults between 30 and 35 years of age have the lowest incidence. After age 35, the incidence slowly increases until, at age

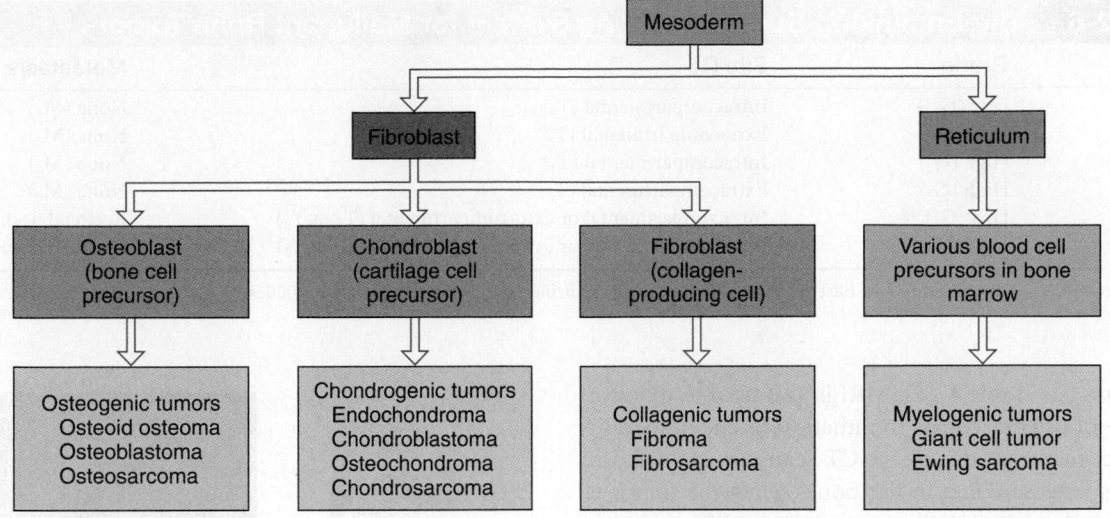

Figure 42-17 Derivation of bone tumors.

60, it equals the incidence in adolescents, primarily related to metastatic tumors.

Patterns of Bone Destruction

The general pathologic features of bone tumors include bone destruction, erosion or expansion of the cortex, and periosteal response to changes in underlying bone. The least amount of pathologic damage occurs with benign bone tumors that push against neighboring tissue. Because they usually have a symmetric, controlled growth pattern, benign bone tumors tend to compress and displace neighboring normal bone tissue, which weakens the bone's structure until it is incapable of withstanding the stress of ordinary use, leading to pathologic fracture. Other tumors invade and destroy adjacent normal bone tissue by producing substances that promote resorption by increasing osteoclast activity or by interfering with a bone's blood supply.

Three patterns of bone destruction by bone tumors have been identified: (1) the geographic pattern, (2) the moth-eaten pattern, and (3) the permeative pattern (Table 42-5).

Tumors that erode the cortex of the bone usually stimulate a periosteal response, that is, new bone formation at the interface between the surface of the bone and the periosteum. Slow erosion of the cortex usually stimulates a uniform periosteal response. Additional layers of bone are added to the exterior surface of the bone to buttress the cortex. Eventually the additional layers expand the bone's contour. Aggressive penetration of the cortex usually elevates the periosteum and stimulates erratic patterns of new bone formation. Examples of erratic patterns include concentric layers of new bone; a sunburst pattern, in which delicate rays of new bone radiate toward the periosteum from a single focus on the underlying surface; and rays of new bone that grow perpendicularly, creating a brush or bristle pattern.

Diagnosis

Malignant bone tumors account for less than 0.2% of all cancers. A tumor must be identified early to allow survival

Table 42-5	Patterns of Bone Destruction by Bone Tumors
Type of Destruction	**Pattern Seen**
Geographic	Well-defined margins separated from surrounding normal bone; well-defined lytic area in affected bone
Moth-eaten	Less-defined margin not easily separated from normal bone; areas of partially destroyed bone adjacent to completely lytic areas
Permeative	Poorly demarcated margins; abnormal lytic bone merges imperceptibly with surrounding normal bone

of the individual and the preservation of the affected limb. However, individuals often have only vague symptoms that may be attributed to minor trauma, degenerative changes, or inflammatory conditions. In addition, other conditions may obscure the diagnosis.

Thorough diagnostic studies are needed to determine the exact type and extent of bone tumor present, which also helps determine the optimal treatment regimen. Staging of any bone tumor is critical to determine future treatment and results. The Enneking staging system is the most commonly used arrangement (Table 42-6). This system classifies tumors as to grade (G), tumor site (T), and metastasis (M). Benign tumors are given a numeric value of zero, whereas malignant tumors are low grade (G_1) or high grade (G_2).

Serum alkaline phosphatase levels are elevated in bone lytic tumors, and they are significantly elevated in osteosarcoma and Ewing sarcoma. Radiologic studies include plain radiologic films, technetium-99 bone scan, CT scan, and MRI, which has become the examination of choice for the local staging of bone tumors, especially the staging of peripheral

Table 42-6	The Ennenking Surgical Staging System for Malignant Bone Tumors		
Stage	**Grade**	**Site (T)**	**Metastasis (M)**
IA	Low (G_1)	Intracompartmental (T_1)	None (M_0)
IB	Low (G_1)	Extracompartmental (T2)	None (M_0)
IIA	High (G_2)	Intracompartmental (T_1)	None (M_0)
IIB	High (G_2)	Extracompartmental (T_2)	None (M_0)
IIIA	Low (G_1)	Intracompartmental or extracompartmental (T_1 or T_2)	Regional or distant (M_1)
IIIB	High (G_2)	Intracompartmental or extracompartmental (T_1 or T_2)	Regional or distant (M_1)

Data from Rosen G et al: Bone tumors. In Bast RC et al, editors: *Cancer medicine*, ed 5, Hamilton, Ontario, 2000, B.D. Decker.

osteosarcomas (see Table 42-5). MRI is also used to monitor the response of osteosarcomas to radiation or chemotherapy and to detect recurrent disease. A CT scan can evaluate involvement of osteosarcoma in flat bones when the tumor is not well defined on a plain film, can assist in differentiating the tumor, and can locate pulmonary metastases. Radionucleotide bone scans show an increased uptake at the tumor site.

Additional diagnostic studies performed for specific bone tumors include a complete blood count and erythrocyte sedimentation rate (to rule out infection, myeloma, or Ewing sarcoma) and serum levels of calcium and phosphorus to detect hypercalcemia. Serum glucose levels may be elevated in chondrosarcoma. Acid phosphatase may show moderate elevations in bone metastases, multiple myeloma, and advanced Paget disease. Serum protein electrophoresis and immunoelectrophoresis are done to rule out multiple myeloma. Fine-needle biopsy is done, usually at the time of surgery, to determine the exact tumor type.

Types

A very large number of lesions are classified as bone tumors. The bone tumors most representative of the four derivative types (see Figure 42-17)—osteogenic, chondrogenic, collagenic, and myelogenic tumors—are described here.

Osteogenic Tumors: Osteosarcoma

Osteogenic (bone-forming) tumors are characterized by the formation of bone or osteoid tissue with a sarcomatous tissue. The tissue can have the appearance of compact or spongy bone. The most common malignant primary bone tumor is osteosarcoma. **Osteosarcomas** account for 38% of bone tumors. The male/female ratio is 3:2, and osteosarcoma occurs predominantly in adolescents and young adults; 60% of osteosarcomas occur in persons younger than 20 years. A secondary peak incidence for osteosarcoma occurs in the 50- to 60-year-old age group, primarily in individuals with a history of radiation therapy several years previously for pelvic or other malignancies (Figure 42-18).

An osteosarcoma is a malignant bone-forming tumor. It is aggressive and most often found in bone marrow; it has a moth-eaten pattern of bone destruction. The borders of the tumor are indistinct and merge into adjacent normal bone. Osteosarcomas always contain osteoid and callus (osteoblastic sarcoma), produced by anaplastic stromal cells, which are atypical, abnormal cells not seen in normal developing bone; they are neither normal nor embryonal. The osteosarcoma

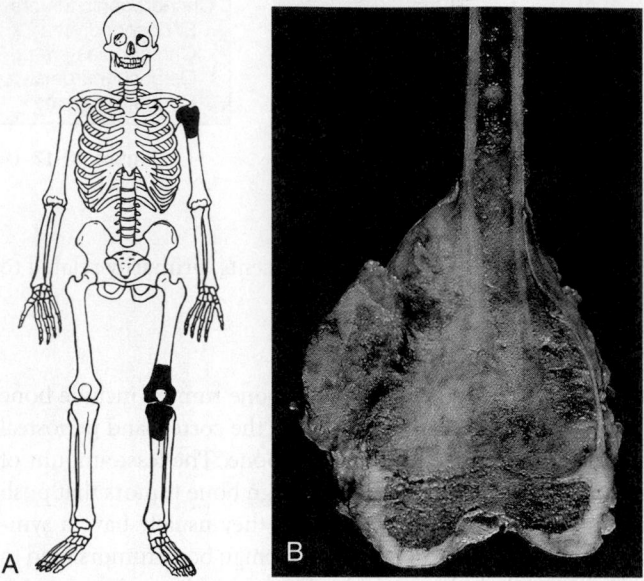

Figure 42-18 Osteosarcoma. **A,** Common locations of osteosarcoma. **B,** Femur has a large mass involving the metaphysis of the bone; the tumor has destroyed the cortex, forming a soft tissue component. (From Damjanov I, Linder J, editors: *Anderson's pathology,* ed 10, St Louis, 1996, Mosby.)

also may contain chondroid (cartilage) (chondroblastic sarcoma) and fibrinoid tissue (fibroblastic sarcoma) that may form the bulk of the tumor. The osteoid is deposited in thick masses or "streamers" between the trabeculae of callus, which infiltrate the normal compact bone, destroy it, and replace it with dense callus and masses of osteoid. Demonstrating the presence of osteoid aids in the diagnosis of osteosarcoma. Bone tissue produced by osteosarcomas never matures to compact bone.

Ninety percent of osteosarcomas are located in the metaphyses of long bones, especially the distal femur and proximal tibia, with 50% around the knee area.[49] The tumor typically breaks through the cortex, lifts the periosteum, and forms a soft tissue mass that is *not* covered by a smooth shell of new bone. Lifting of the periosteum stimulates bizarre patterns of new bone formation called a *periosteal reaction*. Distinct osteosarcomas occur on the surface of long bones, called parosteal, periosteal, or high-grade surface osteosarcomas; dedifferentiated parosteal and central osteosarcomas also occur.

The most common initial symptoms are pain and swelling. Initially the pain is slight and intermittent, but within a short time it increases in severity and duration. Pain is usually worse at night and gradually requires medication. Systemic symptoms are uncommon. Usually a coincidental history of trauma is noted. Occasionally the individual may have a pathologic fracture.

Systemic chemotherapy and surgery are the treatments of choice, with the location of the tumor, its size, malignancy grade, and evidence of metastasis dictating the type and extent of surgery. Preoperative chemotherapy has greatly increased the number of individuals qualifying for limb salvage surgery. Limb salvaging procedures have been made possible by advances in reconstructive techniques and endoprosthetics. Limb salvage ultimately may be successful in as many as 80% of persons. Individuals must have achieved most of their bone growth to be candidates for limb salvage procedures, which are preferred to amputation. Skeletally immature individuals may have a limb salvage operation, referred to as a *rotationplasty,* in which the major portions of the thigh, the tumor, and contaminated knee are resected while preserving the nerve supply (sciatic) to the leg and foot. The proximal tibia is internally fixed to the stump of the proximal femur after it has been rotated 180 degrees. The foot is positioned at a desired spot or direction, allowing the ankle joint to function as a knee joint with the foot supplying the traditional role of the tibial stump in a below-knee amputation.

If an amputation is done, individuals are monitored closely with chest roentgenograms and CT. Pulmonary metastases are surgically resected, and chemotherapy is now a common therapy given both before and after operation, using combinations of chemotherapeutic agents. Promising agents under investigation include monoclonal antibodies, hormone antagonists, gene therapy, and other biologic agents that may dramatically improve survival.[49]

Chondrogenic Tumors: Chondrosarcoma

Chondrogenic (cartilage-forming) tumors produce cartilage or **chondroid,** a primitive cartilage or cartilage-like substance. The most common chondrogenic tumor is chondrosarcoma, accounting for 20% of bone tumors.

Chondrosarcoma, the second most common primary malignant bone tumor, is a tumor of middle-age and older adults. Most cases of primary chondrosarcoma are found in persons between 50 and 70 years of age. Secondary chondrosarcoma (a chondrosarcoma derived from an **endochondroma**) occurs most often in young adults between 20 and 30 years of age. The tumor is found more commonly in men than in women.

A chondrosarcoma is a large ill-defined malignant tumor that infiltrates trabeculae in spongy bone. It occurs most often in the metaphysis or diaphysis of long bones, especially the femur, and in the bones of the pelvis (Figure 42-19). The tumor contains large lobules of hyaline cartilage that are separated by bands of fibrous tissue and anaplastic cells. Chondrosarcomas typically implant in surrounding tissue ("seeding").

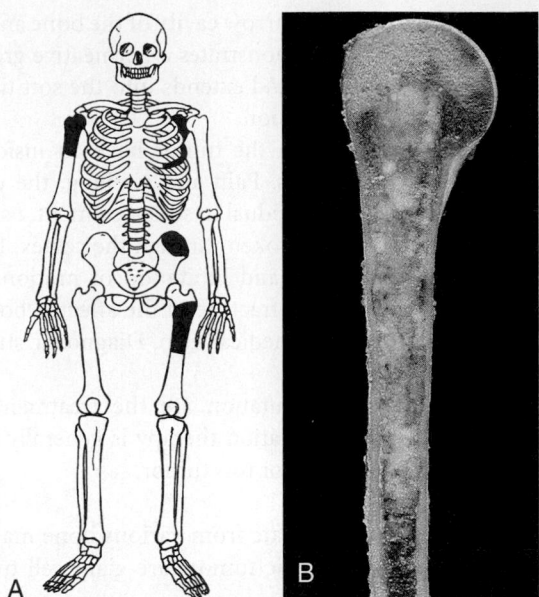

Figure 42-19 Chondrosarcoma. **A,** Common locations of chondrosarcoma. **B,** Chondrosarcoma of humerus. (From Damjanov I, Linder J, editors: *Anderson's pathology,* ed 10, St Louis, 1996, Mosby.)

Symptoms associated with chondrosarcoma have an insidious onset. Local swelling and pain are the usual symptoms that cause a person to seek treatment. At first the pain is dull and intermittent, then gradually intensifies and becomes constant. It may waken the person at night.

Diagnostic studies include radiographs, which must be reviewed carefully for an accurate diagnosis. Biopsy is done at the time of surgery. (If biopsy is done before scheduled surgical incision, seeding of tumor cells could occur.) Sufficient tumor material must be obtained to facilitate an accurate diagnosis.

Surgical excision is generally regarded as the treatment of choice because chemotherapy and radiation seem to have little effect. Many surgically treated individuals demonstrate recurrences, however, so amputation is becoming one treatment of choice. Therefore, individuals with tumors located in the limbs have a better prognosis than those with pelvic lesions.

Collagenic Tumors: Fibrosarcoma

Collagenic (collagen-forming) tumors produce fibrous connective tissue. The most typical collagenic tumor is the fibrosarcoma.

Fibrosarcomas represent 4% of primary malignant bone tumors, with a broad age distribution. They may occur at any age but are most common in adults between 30 and 50 years of age. The incidence is slightly greater in females. Fibrosarcoma also may be a secondary complication of radiation therapy, Paget disease, and long-standing osteomyelitis.

Fibrosarcoma is a solitary tumor that most often affects the metaphyseal region of the femur or tibia. The tumor is composed of a firm fibrous mass of tissue that contains collagen, malignant fibroblasts, and occasional osteoclast-like giant cells.

The tumor begins in the marrow cavity of the bone and infiltrates the trabeculae. It demonstrates a permeative growth pattern, destroys the cortex, and extends into the soft tissue. Metastasis to the lung is common.

Symptoms associated with the tumor have an insidious onset, which delays diagnosis. Pain and swelling, the usual symptoms that cause the individual to seek treatment, usually indicate that the tumor has broken through the cortex. Local tenderness, a palpable mass, and limitation of motion also may be present. A pathologic fracture in the affected bone is often the reason for seeking medical help. Diagnostic studies include radiographs and MRI.

Radical surgery and amputation are the treatments of choice for fibrosarcoma. Radiation therapy is generally considered ineffective treatment for this tumor.

Myelogenic Tumors

Myelogenic tumors originate from various bone marrow cells. Two types of myelogenic tumors are giant cell tumor and myeloma.

Giant Cell Tumor. Giant cell tumor is the sixth most common of the primary bone tumors, accounting for 4% to 5% of bone tumors. Giant cell tumors have a wide age distribution; however, they are rare in persons younger than 10 years or older than 70 years. Most giant cell tumors are found in persons between 20 and 40 years of age. Unlike most other bone tumors, giant cell tumors affect females more often than males.

The giant cell tumor is generally a benign, solitary, circumscribed tumor that causes extensive bone resorption because of its osteoclastic origin (Figure 42-20). Giant cell tumor has a high rate of recurrence but rarely metastasizes. The tumor is rich in osteoclast-like giant cells and anaplastic stromal cells. It also may contain osteoid, callus, and collagen. Overexpression of several genes, including osteoprotegerin ligand (OPGL), occurs in giant cell tumors. The giant cell tumor is typically located in the center of the epiphysis in the femur, tibia, radius, or humerus. The tumor has a slow, relentless growth rate and is usually contained within the original contour of the affected bone. Tumors are often associated with pathologic fractures. It may, however, extend into the articular cartilage. When the tumor extends, it is usually covered by periosteum or periosteal bone growth.

The most common symptoms associated with giant cell tumor are pain, local swelling, and limitation of movement. Diagnostic studies include radiographs, CT, and MRI. Cryosurgery and resection of the tumor with the use of adjuvant polymethyl methacrylate (PMMA) for bone grafts decrease recurrence and are more successful treatments than curettage and radiation.[50] Amputation may be necessary but is not common.

DISORDERS OF JOINTS

The American College of Rheumatology (ACR) recognizes 13 groups of joint disease—**arthropathies.** Most of these disorders can be placed into two major categories: noninflammatory joint disease and inflammatory joint

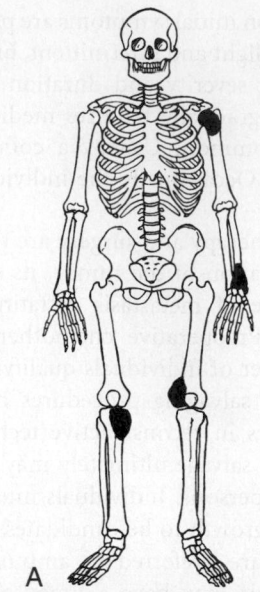

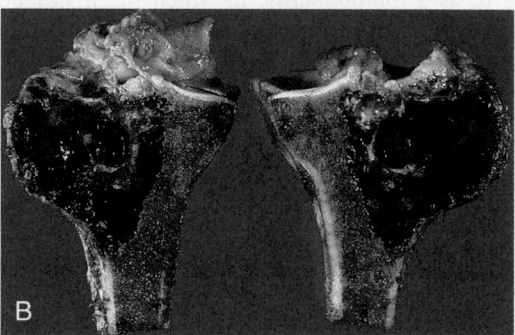

Figure 42-20 Giant cell tumor of bone. **A,** Common skeletal locations. **B,** Gross picture of cell tumor of bone (epimetaphysis). (From Damjanov I, Linder J, editors: *Anderson's pathology,* ed 10, St Louis, 1996, Mosby.)

disease. With recent improvements in detection methods, conditions such as osteoarthritis that were previously classified as noninflammatory have now had inflammatory pathways identified.

Osteoarthritis

Osteoarthritis (OA) has been commonly classified as **noninflammatory joint disease.** However, new information has made it clear that specific markers of inflammation are present in OA.[51-53] The discovery of inflammation in the joints also has emerged as an important feature of OA. The use of MRI and arthroscopy has made it clear that osteoarthritic changes are not defined by changes noted on x-ray films alone. Consequently OA has been reclassified as inflammatory joint disease (Figure 42-21).

Medical clinicians are somewhat divided about use of the terms *degenerative joint disease* and *osteoarthritis.* The term *osteoarthritis* has been used in most recent communications and appears to be the more accepted term in the European literature.

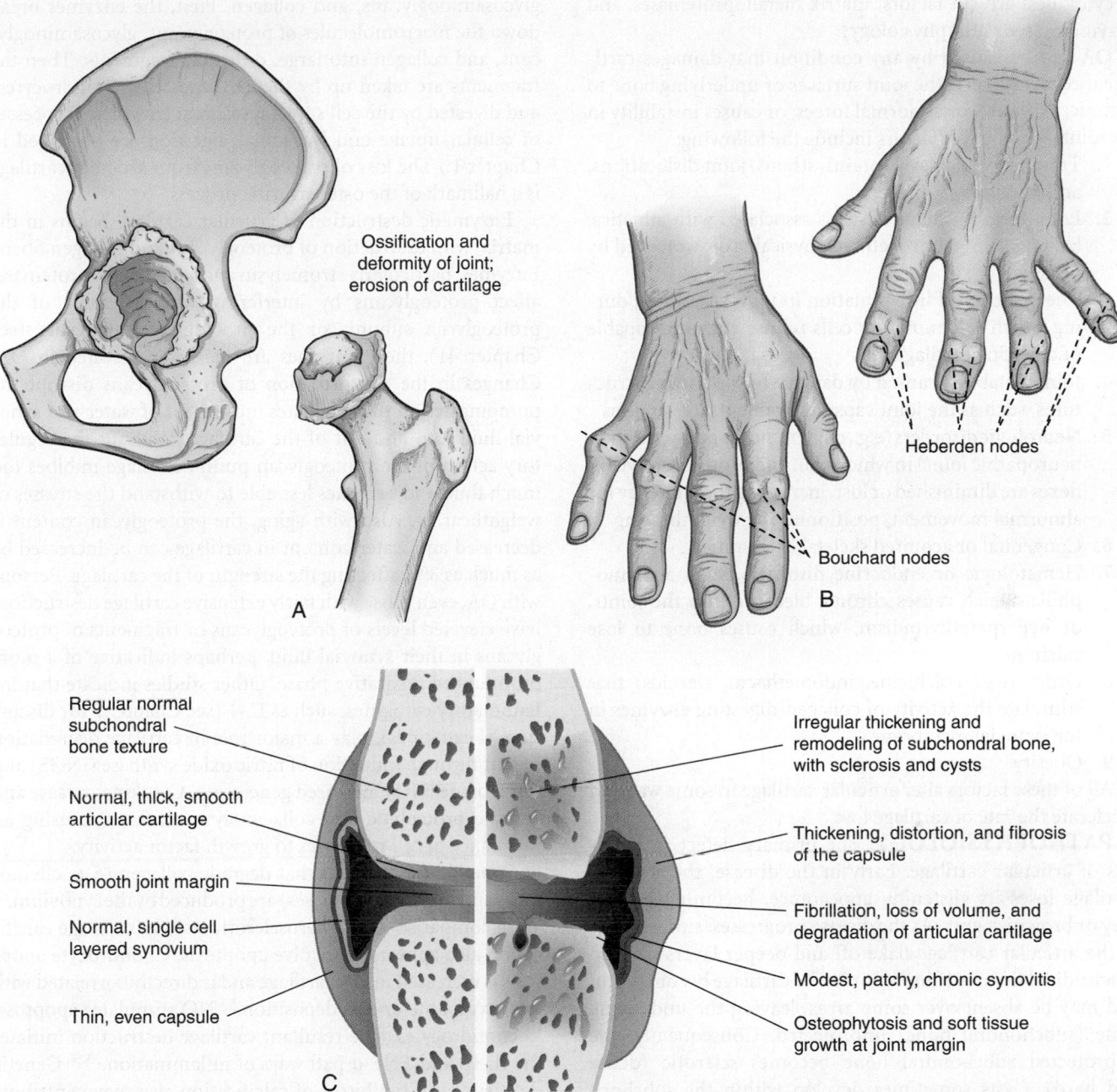

Ossification and
deformity of joint;
erosion of cartilage

A

Heberden nodes

Bouchard nodes

B

Regular normal
subchondral
bone texture

Normal, thick, smooth
articular cartilage

Smooth joint margin

Normal, single cell
layered synovium

Thin, even capsule

C

Irregular thickening and
remodeling of subchondral bone,
with sclerosis and cysts

Thickening, distortion, and fibrosis
of the capsule

Fibrillation, loss of volume, and
degradation of articular cartilage

Modest, patchy, chronic synovitis

Osteophytosis and soft tissue
growth at joint margin

Figure 42-21 Osteoarthritis (OA). A, Cartilage and degeneration of the hip joint resulting from osteoarthritis. B, Heberden nodes and Bouchard nodes. C, Characteristics of OA. Normal versus osteoarthritic synovial joint.

Osteoarthritis (OA) is a common age-related disorder of synovial joints. It is characterized by local areas of loss and damage of articular cartilage, new bone formation of joint margins (osteophytosis), subchondral bone changes, variable degrees of mild synovitis and thickening of the joint capsule (see Figure 42-21). Pathology centers on load-bearing areas. Advancing disease reveals narrowing of the joint space because of cartilage loss, bone spurs (**osteophytes**), and sometimes changes in the subchondral bone. OA can arise in any synovial joint but is commonly found in the hands, knees, hips, and spine. It is less common in people younger than 40 years

but rises in incidence with age. OA is a multifactorial disease involving environmental-lifestyle factors and genetics.

OA is generally distributed throughout the peripheral and central joints of the body and affects adult men more than women until after age 55. Although the exact causes of OA are unclear, they involve low-grade inflammation, calcification of articular cartilage, genetic alterations, and metabolic disorders.[54]

With aging, the quality and quantity of the proteoglycans in cartilage decrease in direct proportion to the severity of OA. Evidence also suggests that OA involves a complex interaction of cytokines, growth factors, matrix metalloproteinases, and enzymes[25] (see Pathophysiology).

OA can be caused by any condition that damages cartilage directly; subjects the joint surfaces or underlying bone to chronic, excessive, or abnormal forces; or causes instability in the joint. Specific risk factors include the following:

1. Trauma, particularly sprains, strains, joint dislocations, and fractures
2. Long-term mechanical stress associated with athletics, ballet dancing, or repetitive physical tasks worsened by obesity
3. The presence of inflammation in joint structures, during which inflammatory cells release enzymes capable of digesting cartilage cells
4. Joint instability caused by damage to supporting structures, such as the joint capsule, ligaments, or tendons
5. Neurologic disorders (e.g., diabetic neuropathy, Charcot neuropathic joint) in which pain and proprioceptive reflexes are diminished or lost, increasing the tendency for abnormal movement, positioning, or weightbearing
6. Congenital or acquired skeletal deformities
7. Hematologic or endocrine disorders, such as hemophilia, which causes chronic bleeding into the joints, or hyperparathyroidism, which causes bone to lose calcium
8. Drugs (e.g., colchicine, indomethacin, steroids) that stimulate the activity of collagen-digesting enzymes in the synovial membrane
9. Obesity

All of these factors alter articular cartilage in some way and accelerate the rate of cartilage loss.

PATHOPHYSIOLOGY The primary defect in OA is loss of articular cartilage. Early in the disease, the articular cartilage loses its glistening appearance, becoming yellow-gray or brownish gray. As the disease progresses, surface areas of the articular cartilage flake off and deeper layers develop longitudinal fissures (fibrillation). The cartilage becomes thin and may be absent over some areas, leaving the underlying bone (subchondral bone) unprotected. Consequently, the unprotected subchondral bone becomes sclerotic (dense and hard). Cysts sometimes develop within the subchondral bone and communicate with the longitudinal fissures in the cartilage. Pressure builds in the cysts until the cystic contents are forced into the synovial cavity, breaking through the articular cartilage on the way. As the articular cartilage erodes, cartilage-coated osteophytes may grow outward from the underlying bone and alter the bone contours and joint anatomy. These spur-like bony projections enlarge until small pieces, called *joint mice,* break off into the synovial cavity. If osteophyte fragments irritate the synovial membrane, synovitis and joint effusion result. The joint capsule also becomes thickened and at times adheres to the deformed underlying bone, which may contribute to the limitation of movement (see Figure 42-21).

Articular cartilage is probably lost through enzymatic breakdown of the cartilage matrix—the proteoglycans, glycosaminoglycans, and collagen. First, the enzymes break down the macromolecules of proteoglycans, glycosaminoglycans, and collagen into large, diffusible fragments. Then the fragments are taken up by the cartilage cells (chondrocytes) and digested by the cell's own lysosomal enzymes. (Processes of cellular uptake and lysosomal digestion are described in Chapter 1.) The loss of proteoglycans from articular cartilage is a hallmark of the osteoarthritic process.

Enzymatic destruction of articular cartilage begins in the matrix, with destruction of proteoglycans and collagen fibers. Enzymes, particularly stromelysin and acid metalloproteinase, affect proteoglycans by interfering with assembly of the proteoglycan subunit or the proteoglycan aggregate (see Chapter 41); these enzymes are markedly elevated in OA. Changes in the conformation of proteoglycans disrupt the pumping action that regulates movement of water and synovial fluid into and out of the cartilage. Without the regulatory action of the proteoglycan pump, cartilage imbibes too much fluid and becomes less able to withstand the stresses of weightbearing. Also with aging, the proteoglycan content is decreased and water content in cartilage can be increased by as much as 8%, affecting the strength of the cartilage. Persons with OA, even those with fairly extensive cartilage destruction, have elevated levels of proteoglycans or fragments of proteoglycans in their synovial fluid, perhaps indicative of a more pronounced reparative phase. Other studies indicate that inflammatory cytokines, such as IL-1 (see Chapter 7 for discussion of cytokines), play a major role in cartilage degradation in part through induction of nitric oxide synthase (iNOS) and nitric oxide (NO) increased generation. Cytokines release and activate proteolytic and collagenolytic enzymes, causing an imbalance of cell responses to growth factor activity.

Some of the enzymes that degrade collagen (e.g., chemokines and metalloproteinases) are produced by the synovium.[53] With comparisons to atherosclerotic lesions, cartilage calcification also appears to involve apoptosis. Chondrocyte apoptosis is increased in OA cartilage and is directly correlated with hydroxyapatite crystal deposition.[55] NO stimulates apoptosis in chondrocytes. The resultant cartilage destruction initiates the IL-1β and TNF-α pathways of inflammation.[53,56] Genetic deficiencies of inhibitors of calcification also may contribute to "run away" calcification (Figure 42-22). Collagen breakdown destroys the fibrils that give articular cartilage its tensile strength and exposes the chondrocytes to mechanical stress and enzyme attack. Thus a cycle of destruction begins that involves all the components of articular cartilage—proteoglycans, collagen fibers, and chondrocytes.

CLINICAL MANIFESTATIONS Clinical manifestations of OA typically appear during the fifth or sixth decade of life, although asymptomatic articular surface changes are common after age 40. Pain and stiffness in one or more joints, usually weightbearing or load-bearing joints, are the first symptoms of the disease. Use-related joint pain relieved by rest is a key feature. Examination usually shows general involvement of peripheral and central joints. Peripheral joints most often involved are in the hands, wrists, knees, and feet.

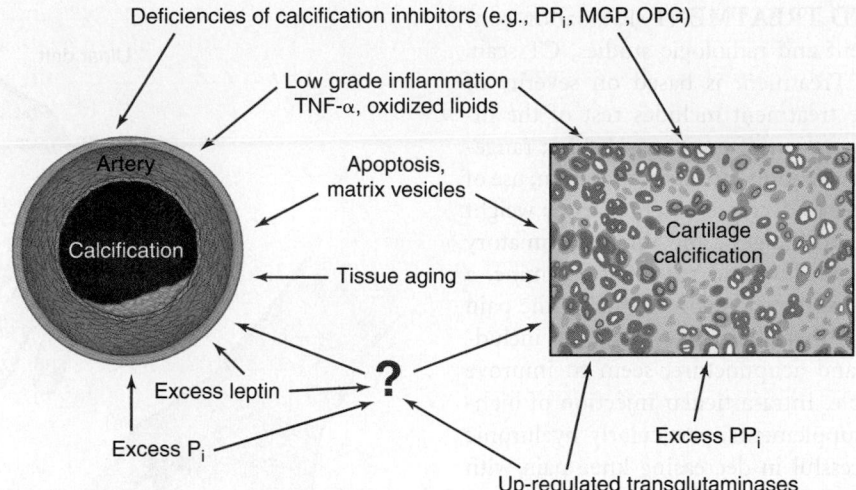

Figure 42-22 Mechanisms driving artery and cartilage calcification. All specified factors have been demonstrated to promote calcification in either arteries and/or cartilage (see text). *MGP,* (matrix GLA-protein): *OPG,* osteoprotegerin; *PP_i,* inorganic pyrophosphate. (From Rutsch F, Terkeltaub R: *Joint Bone Spine* 72:110-118, 2005.)

Central joints most often affected are in the lower cervical spine, lumbosacral spine, shoulders, and hips.

Joint structures are capable of generating a limited number of signs and symptoms. The primary signs and symptoms of joint disease are pain, stiffness, enlargement or swelling, tenderness, limited range of motion, muscle wasting, partial dislocation, and deformity.

Pain and stiffness are the predominant symptoms of OA. They are usually aggravated by weightbearing or use of the joint and relieved by resting the joint. Nocturnal pain is usually not relieved by rest and may be accompanied by paresthesias (numbness, tingling, prickling). Sometimes pain is referred to another part of the body. For example, osteoarthritis of the lumbosacral spine may mimic sciatica, causing severe pain in the back of the thigh along the course of the sciatic nerve. OA in the lower cervical spine may cause brachial neuralgia (pain in the arm) aggravated by movement of the neck. Osteoarthritic conditions in the hip cause pain that may be referred to the lower thigh and knee area.

The actual mechanisms of joint pain are complex and poorly understood, but several explanations are possible. The pain could be caused by articular distention and stretching of the fibrous joint capsule, which has an abundant nerve supply. In addition, inflammation of the joint capsule causes fibrous shrinking, so that movement of the joint in any direction causes painful stretching. Pain also can arise from the subchondral or periarticular bone (Figure 42-23).

The origin of joint stiffness is unknown. **Joint stiffness** is generally defined as difficulty in initiating joint movement, immobility, or a loss of range of motion. The stiffness usually occurs as joint movement begins and dissipates within 30 minutes. Enlargement and bulging of joint contour, commonly described as swelling, may be caused by bone enlargement or the proliferation of osteophytes around the margins of the joint. Swelling also occurs if inflammatory exudate or blood enters the joint cavity, thereby increasing

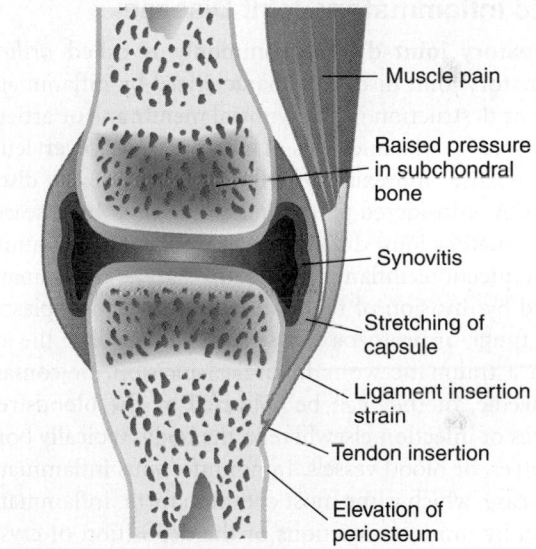

Figure 42-23 Possible causes of pain in osteoarthritis.

the volume of synovial fluid. This condition, termed **joint effusion,** is caused by (1) the presence of osteophyte fragments in the synovial cavity, (2) drainage of cysts from diseased subchondral bone, or (3) acute trauma to joint structures, resulting in hemorrhage and inflammatory exudation into the synovial cavity.

Range of motion is limited to some degree, depending on the extent of cartilage degeneration. Frequently, joint motion is accompanied by sounds of crepitus, creaking, or grating. Hypermobility and subluxation of joints occur in OA secondary to a neurologic disorder.

As OA of the lower extremity progresses, the person may begin to limp noticeably. Having a limp is distressing because it affects the person's independence and ability to do activities of daily living. The affected joint is also more symptomatic after use, such as at the end of the day.

EVALUATION AND TREATMENT Evaluation consists of clinical assessment and radiologic studies, CT scan, arthroscopy, and MRI. Treatment is based on severity of symptoms. Conservative treatment includes rest of the involved joint until inflammation, if present, subsides; range-of-motion exercise to prevent joint capsule contraction; use of a cane, crutches, or walker to decrease weightbearing; weight loss if obesity is present; and analgesic and anti-inflammatory drug therapy to reduce swelling and pain. Glucosamine, a nutraceutical, has shown some success in reducing the pain and progression of OA. Other alternative therapies, including magnetic bracelets and acupuncture, seem to improve symptoms in some people. Intra-articular injection of high-molecular-weight viscosupplements, particularly hyaluronic acid, also has been successful in decreasing knee pain with OA.[57] Surgery is used to improve joint movement, correct deformity or malalignment, or create a new joint with artificial implants. There are nearly 250,000 total hip replacements yearly in the United States, most of which are related to OA.

Classic Inflammatory Joint Disease

Inflammatory joint disease commonly is called *arthritis.* Inflammatory joint disease is characterized by inflammatory damage or destruction in the synovial membrane or articular cartilage and by systemic signs of inflammation (fever, leukocytosis, malaise, anorexia, hyperfibrinogenemia). See discussion on OA (considered part of inflammatory joint disease).

Inflammatory joint disease can be infectious or noninfectious. In infectious inflammatory joint disease, inflammation is caused by invasion of the joint by bacteria, mycoplasmas, viruses, fungi, or protozoa. These agents can invade the joint through a traumatic wound, surgical incision, or contaminated needle, or they can be delivered by the bloodstream from sites of infection elsewhere in the body, typically bones, heart valves, or blood vessels. In noninfectious inflammatory joint disease, which is the most common form, inflammation is caused by immune reactions or the deposition of crystals of monosodium urate in and around the joint. Rheumatoid arthritis and ankylosing spondylitis are noninfectious inflammatory diseases caused by disturbances in immune reactions[58]; gouty arthritis is a noninfectious inflammatory disease caused by crystal deposition.

Rheumatoid Arthritis

Rheumatoid arthritis (RA) is a systemic inflammatory autoimmune disease associated with swelling and pain in multiple joints. (Autoimmune disease is described in Chapter 8.) The first joint tissue to be affected is the synovial membrane, which lines the joint cavity (see Chapter 41 and Figure 42-9). Multiple immunoregulatory cytokines (such as interleukins, B-cells, and matrix metalloproteinases) contribute to joint damage. Eventually, inflammation may spread to the articular cartilage, fibrous joint capsule, and surrounding ligaments and tendons, causing pain, joint deformity, and loss of function (Figure 42-24). The joints most commonly affected are in the fingers, feet, wrists, elbows, ankles, and knees, but the

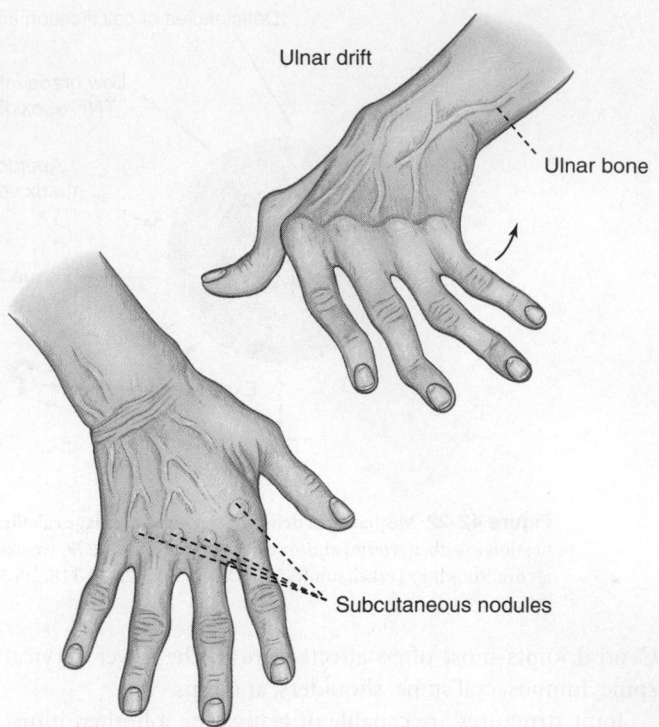

Figure 42-24 Rheumatoid arthritis of the hand. Note swelling from chronic synovitis of metacarpophalangeal joints, marked ulnar drift, subcutaneous nodules, and subluxation of metacarpophalangeal joints with extension of proximal interphalangeal joints and flexion of distal joints. Note also deformed position of thumb. Hand has wasted appearance. (From Mourad L: *Orthopedic disorders,* St Louis, 1991, Mosby.)

shoulders, hips, and cervical spine also may be involved, as well as the tissues of the lungs, heart, kidneys, and skin.

RA affects 1% to 2% of adults and, like most autoimmune diseases, develops most often in women, with a female/male ratio of 3:1. The frequency of RA increases from the third decade on, affecting 5% or more of the population ages 70 years and older. Besides inflammation of the joints, RA can cause fever, malaise, rash, lymph node or spleen enlargement, and Raynaud phenomenon (transient lack of circulation to the fingertips and toes).

Despite intensive research, the cause of RA remains obscure. Proposals of the initiating event include an infectious agent or other environmental exposure but genetic, hormonal, and reproductive factors may contribute to developing RA. The initiating event unleashes an immune response that results in inflammation of the lining of the joint—the synovial membrane. RA probably occurs in a genetically susceptible person because of an aberrant immune response to an unidentified antigen. A key genetic element has been localized to the human leukocyte antigen-death receptor 4 (HLA-DR4), HLA-DRB1 (death receptor beta), and HLA-DP genes of the major histocompatibility complex. Infectious microorganisms that may play a role in the cause of RA include bacteria, mycoplasmas, and viruses (especially Epstein-Barr virus) (Table 42-7). With long-term or intensive exposure to the antigen, normal antibodies (immunoglobulins [Ig])

Table 42-7   Types of Infectious Arthritis

Type and Microorganism	Comments
Lyme arthritis	Initial infection of skin followed by spreading to other sites including joints in days or weeks
Spirochete *Borrelia burgdorferi* Transmitted via ticks (*Ixodes scapularis* or *I. pacificus*)	Arthritis is a predominant feature involving mainly large joints; possibly caused by immune reactions against *Borrelia* antigens (such as Osp A) that cross-react with tissue antigens in joints
Tuberculous arthritis Complication of osteomyelitis or visceral, usually pulmonary, infection	Weight-bearing joints most susceptible Fibrous ankylosis and destruction of joint space; onset is insidious and gradual
Suppurative arthritis	Classic is a sudden onset of symptoms—painful, hot, swollen joint with decreased range of motion
Bacterial infections with *Gonococcus, Staphylococcus, Streptococcus, Haemophilus influenzae,* and gram-negative bacilli; *H. influenzae* arthritis more common in children younger than 2 years; *Staphylococcus aureus* in older children and adults	Prompt therapy prevents joint destruction
Viral arthritis	Symptoms vary from acute to subacute
Many viruses including parvovirus B19, rubella, hepatitis C virus, human immunodeficiency virus	Unclear if effects are from direct invasion of the virus or an autoimmune reaction

become autoantibodies—antibodies that attack host tissues (self-antigens). Because they are usually present in individuals with rheumatoid arthritis, the transformed antibodies are termed **rheumatoid factors (RFs)**. The RFs usually consist of two classes of immunoglobulin antibodies (antibodies for IgM and IgG) but occasionally involve antibodies for IgA. Their main antigenic targets are portions of the immunoglobulin molecules. RFs bind with their target self-antigens in blood and synovial membrane, forming immune complexes (antigen-antibody complexes) (see Chapter 7).

RA has a higher incidence in women, with evidence of hormonal involvement because disease symptoms lessen during pregnancy and exacerbate in the postpartal period. Evidence for endocrine involvement in RA tissues and cells includes (1) presence of androgen and estrogen receptors, (2) high concentrations of biologically active steroids, (3) key enzymes of steroid metabolism, and (4) significant changes of estrogen to androgen ratio. These data strongly suggest that individual immune cells, including synovial macrophages, may behave as steroid-sensitive cells. Most studies on the influence of exogenous hormones and risk of RA have focused on oral contraceptive pills, with inconsistent findings. Fewer studies have been done with hormone replacement; however, interest has emerged on the role of estrogen and autoimmunity. RA also has seasonal variations, being worse in winter months.

PATHOPHYSIOLOGY The pathogenesis of rheumatoid arthritis is summarized in Figure 42-25.

Cartilage damage in RA is the result of several processes:

1. CD4 T helper cells, and other cells in the synovial fluid become activated, promoting cytokine release and activating B lymphocytes
2. Recruitment and retention of inflammatory cells in the joint sublining region
3. Vicious cycle of altered cytokine and signal transduction pathways

4. Possible immune complex deposition and resultant inflammatory molecule release
5. RANKL release and osteoclast activation
6. Angiogenesis, or growth of new blood vessels in the synovium

Several types of leukocytes are attracted out of the circulation and into the synovial membrane. The phagocytes of inflammation (neutrophils and macrophages) ingest the immune complexes and, in the process of doing so, release powerful enzymes that degrade synovial tissue and articular cartilage (Figure 42-26). The immune system's B and T lymphocytes are also activated. The B lymphocytes are stimulated to produce more RFs, and the T lymphocytes eventually cause release of enzymes that amplify and perpetuate the inflammatory response.[59] Destruction of the extracellular matrix possibly leads to significant disability in individuals with RA.[60] Cartilage destruction is mediated by processes from the synovium and cellular invasion into the matrix. These processes may be facilitated by oxidative stress and alterations in deoxyribonucleic acid (DNA) repair mechanisms, causing mutation in key genes.[60] In addition RANKL is expressed by various cells in the synovium and induces osteoclast maturation and activation, thus producing increased bone resorption (see p. 1580).

Inflammatory and immune processes have several damaging effects on the synovial membrane. Along with the swelling caused by leukocyte infiltration, the synovial membrane undergoes hyperplastic thickening as its cells proliferate and enlarge abnormally. As synovial inflammation progresses to involve its blood vessels, small venules become occluded by the hypertrophied endothelial cells, fibrin, platelets, and inflammatory cells, which decrease vascular flow to the synovial tissue. Compromised circulation, coupled with increased metabolic needs because of hypertrophy and hyperplasia, causes hypoxia and metabolic acidosis. Acidosis stimulates the release of hydrolytic enzymes from synovial cells into the

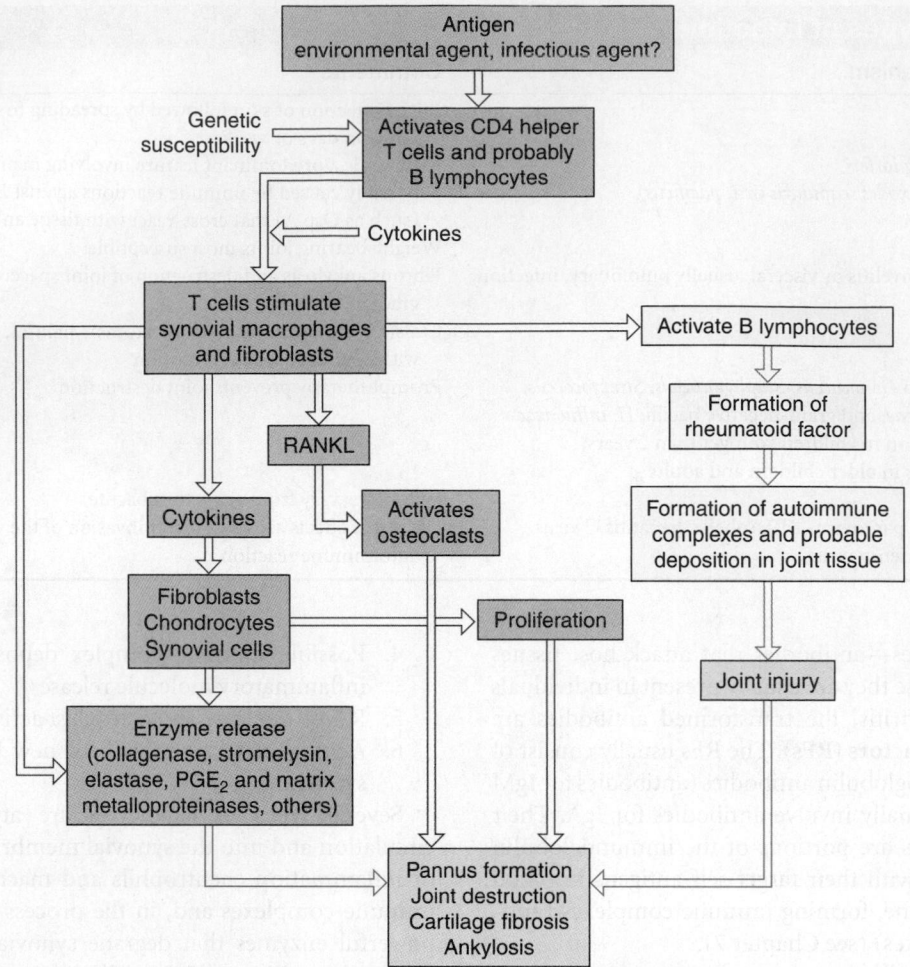

Figure 42-25 Emerging model of pathogenesis of rheumatoid arthritis. Rheumatoid arthritis is an autoimmune disease of a genetically susceptible host triggered by an unknown antigenic agent. Chronic autoimmune reaction with activation of CD4+ helper T cells and possibly other lymphocytes and the local release of inflammatory cytokines and mediators eventually destroys the joint. T cells stimulate cells in the joint to produce cytokines that are key mediators of synovial damage. Apparently immune complex deposition also plays a role. Tumor necrosis factor (TNF) and interleukin-1 (IL-1), as well as some other cytokines, stimulate synovial cells to proliferate and produce other mediators of inflammation, such as prostaglandins (PGE₂) matrix metalloproteinases, and enzymes that all contribute to destruction of cartilage. Activated T cells and synovial fibroblasts also produce receptor activator of nuclear factor κβ ligand (RANKL), which activates the osteoclasts and promotes bone destruction. Pannus is a mass of synovium and synovial stroma with inflammatory cells, granulation tissue, and fibroblasts that grows over the articular surface and causes its destruction.

surrounding tissue, initiating erosion of the articular cartilage and inflammation in the supporting ligaments and tendons.

Inflammation causes hemorrhage, coagulation, and fibrin deposition on the synovial membrane, in the intracellular matrix, and in the synovial fluid. Over denuded areas of the synovial membrane, fibrin develops into granulation tissue called **pannus.** Pannus is composed of several different cells; however, the two types primarily responsible for joint damage are osteoclasts and synovial fibroblasts.[61] (Granulation tissue is the tissue produced earliest in the process of healing; see Chapter 6.) Synovial fibroblasts also produce additional proinflammatory cells, cytokines, matrix metalloproteinases, and other cells involved in cartilage damage (Figure 42-27, *B*).

CLINICAL MANIFESTATIONS The onset of RA is usually insidious, although as many as 15% of cases have an acute onset. RA begins with general systemic manifestations

of inflammation, including fever, fatigue, weakness, anorexia, weight loss, and generalized aching and stiffness. Local manifestations also appear gradually over weeks or months. Typically the joints become painful, tender, and stiff. Pain early in the disease is caused by pressure from swelling; later it is caused by sclerosis of subchondral bone and new bone formation. Stiffness usually lasts for about 1 hour after arising in the morning and is thought to be related to synovitis. Initially most commonly involved are the metacarpophalangeal (MCP) joints, proximal interphalangeal (PIP) joints, and wrists, with later involvement of larger weight-bearing joints.

Joint swelling, which is widespread and symmetric, is caused by increasing amounts of inflammatory exudate (leukocytes, plasma, plasma proteins) in the synovial membrane, hyperplasia of inflamed tissues, and formation of new bone. On palpation, the swollen joint feels warm and the synovial

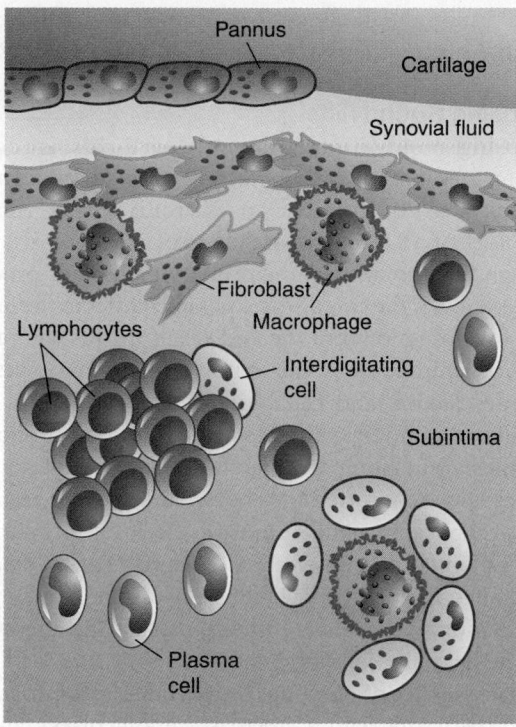

Figure 42-26 Synovitis. Inflamed synovium showing typical arrangements of macrophages and fibroblastic cells.

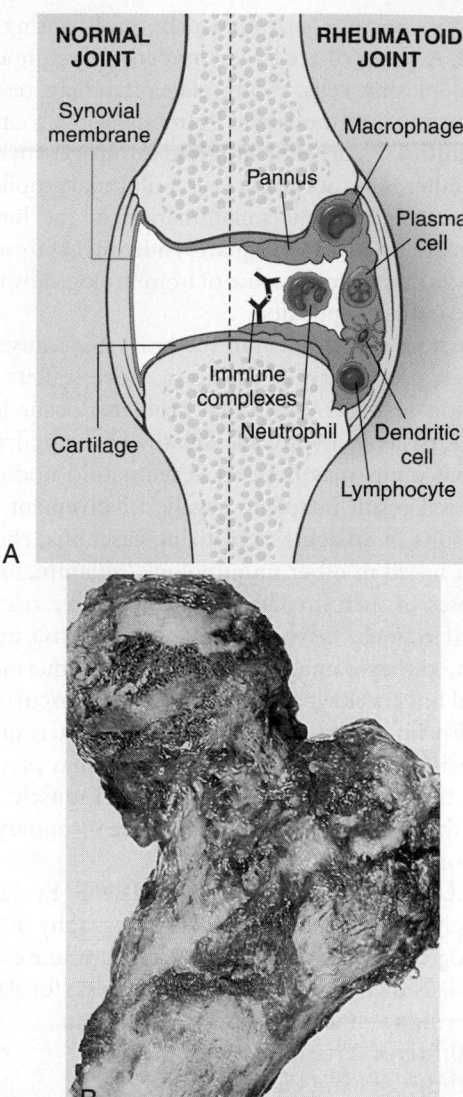

Figure 42-27 Rheumatoid arthritis. A, Schematic view of the joint lesion. B, Advanced rheumatoid arthritis involving femur. There is prominent proliferation of synovium and almost complete destruction of overlying articular cartilage. (A modified from Feldmann M: *Nat Rev Immunol* 2:364, 2002; B from Rosai J: *Ackerman's surgical pathology,* ed 8, St Louis, 1996, Mosby.)

membrane feels "boggy." The skin over the joint may have a ruddy, cyanotic hue and may look thin and shiny.

An inflamed joint may lose some of its mobility. Even mild synovitis can lead to loss of range of motion, which becomes evident after inflammation subsides. Extension becomes limited and is eventually lost if flexion contractures form. Loss of range of motion can progress to permanent deformities of the fingers, toes, and limbs, including ulnar deviation of the hands, boutonnière and swan-neck deformities of the finger joints, plantar subluxation of the metatarsal heads of the foot, and hallux valgus (angulation of the great toe toward the other toes). Flexion contractures of the knees and hips are also common.

Joint deformities cause the physical limitations experienced by persons with RA. Loss of joint motion is quickly followed by secondary atrophy of the surrounding muscles. With secondary muscle atrophy the joint becomes unstable, which further aggravates joint pathology.

Two complications of chronic RA are caused by an excessive amount of inflammatory exudate in the synovial cavity. One complication is the formation of cysts in the articular cartilage or subchondral bone. Occasionally these cysts communicate with the skin surface (usually the sole of the foot) and can drain through passages called fistulae. The second complication is rupture of a cyst or of the synovial joint itself, usually caused by strenuous physical activity that places excessive pressure on the joint. Rupture releases inflammatory exudate into adjacent tissues, thereby spreading inflammation.

Extrasynovial **rheumatoid nodules,** or swellings, are observed in areas of pressure or trauma in 20% of individuals with RA. Each nodule is an aggregate of inflammatory cells surrounding a central core of fibrinoid and cellular debris. T lymphocytes are the predominant leukocytes in the nodule; B lymphocytes, plasma cells, and phagocytes are found around the periphery. Nodules are found most often in subcutaneous tissue over the extensor surfaces of elbows and fingers. Less common sites are the scalp, back, feet, hands, buttocks, and knees.

Rheumatoid nodules also may invade the skin, cardiac valves, pericardium, pleura, lung parenchyma, and spleen. These nodules are identical to those encountered in some individuals with rheumatic fever and are characterized by central tissue necrosis surrounded by proliferating connective tissue. Also noted are large numbers of lymphocytes and occasional plasma cells. Acute glaucoma may result, with nodules forming on the sclera. Pulmonary involvement may result in diffuse pleuritis or multiple intraparenchymal nodules. Together, the occurrence of pulmonary nodules and pneumoconiosis (chronic inflammation of the lungs from inhalation of dust) creates **Caplan syndrome.** Diffuse pulmonary fibrosis may occur because of immunologically mediated immune complex deposition.

Rheumatoid nodules within the heart may cause valvular deformities, particularly of the aortic valve leaflets. Pericardial effusion or other pericardial problems occur in almost 50% of RA patients. Lymphadenopathy of the nodes close to the affected joints may develop. Rheumatoid nodules within the spleen result in splenomegaly. Involvement of blood vessels results in an acute necrotizing vasculitis, characteristic of that noted in other immunologic/inflammatory states. Thromboses of such involved vessels may give rise to myocardial infarctions, cerebrovascular occlusions, mesenteric infarction, kidney damage, and vascular insufficiency in the hands and fingers (Raynaud phenomenon). Vascular changes are noted primarily in individuals receiving steroid therapy; thus there is some concern that the therapy may play a role in initiating these lesions. Changes in skeletal muscle are often noted in the form of nonspecific atrophy secondary to joint dysfunction.

EVALUATION AND TREATMENT Evaluation of RA is by physical examination, roentgenography of the joint, and serologic tests for RF and circulating immune complexes. The ACR lists the following diagnostic criteria for RA:

1. Morning stiffness for longer than 1 hour
2. Arthritis of three or more joint areas
3. Arthritis of hand joints
4. Symmetric arthritis
5. Rheumatoid nodules over extensor surfaces or bony prominences
6. Serum RF present in abnormal amounts
7. Radiographic changes

The presence of four or more of the criteria is diagnostic of RA. Criteria 1 through 4 with joint signs or symptoms must be present for 6 weeks.

Treatment is conservative or surgical. Conservative treatment includes rest of the inflamed joint and whole-body rest for several hours daily, use of hot and cold packs, physical therapy, antineoplastic medications, a diet high in calories and vitamins, corticosteroids, anti-inflammatory drugs, immunosuppressants, and disease-modifying antirheumatic drugs (DMARDs) taken orally or by injection. Biologic agents that target cytokines have demonstrated significant improvement in outcomes for both adult and juvenile RA.[62] Surgical synovectomy may be done early in the disease to decrease inflammatory effusion and remove pannus. Surgery is used to correct deformity or mechanical deficiency in intermediate or late stages of the disease and includes arthrodesis, arthroplasty, or total joint replacement. Interestingly, total fasting induces a substantial reduction in joint pain, swelling, morning stiffness, and other symptoms in individuals with RA.

Ankylosing Spondylitis

Ankylosing spondylitis (AS) (spondyloarthritis) is a chronic, inflammatory joint disease characterized by stiffening and fusion (ankylosis) of the spine and sacroiliac joints. Although the etiology of AS is unknown, it is associated with HLA-B27. Although inflammation is the primary pathologic process in both RA and AS, the two diseases possibly differ in the primary site of inflammation and the end result. In RA the primary site of inflammation is the synovial membrane, resulting in the destruction and instability of synovial joints. In AS, the primary pathologic site has classically been proposed as the **enthesis** (the point at which ligaments, tendons, and the joint capsule are inserted into bone) and the end results are fibrosis, ossification, and fusion of the joint, primarily the sacroiliac joints and the vertebral column.[63] Recent data from MRI studies, however, show that synovitis and bone marrow inflammation, rather than enthesis, explain the alteration of AS in the sacroiliac joints.[64,65]

The prevalence of AS in the United States is approximately 0.5% to 1% among whites, 3% to 4% among blacks, and 18% to 50% in various nations of American Indians. Worldwide, the disease appears to be most prevalent in whites. The prevalence of AS in males is at least 10 times greater than previously considered. It affects men three times as often as women. In women, AS may affect the peripheral joints of the appendicular skeleton rather than the axial skeleton, progress less rapidly, and cause less dramatic spinal changes. Many individuals with AS remain undiagnosed.

Primary AS usually develops in late adolescence or young adulthood, with peak incidence at about 20 years of age. Secondary AS affects older age groups and is often associated with other inflammatory diseases (e.g., psoriatic arthropathy, inflammatory bowel disease, Reiter syndrome).

The cause of AS is unknown, but the disease is strongly associated with the presence of histocompatibility antigen HLA-B27 on the chromosomes of affected individuals, suggesting a genetic predisposition to the disease. Not all HLA-B27 subtypes, however, are associated with AS. *Klebsiella,* chlamydia-delivered peptides, or other "triggers" may perpetuate the inflammatory response.[66]

PATHOPHYSIOLOGY AS has a strong association with HLA-B27. Several hypotheses have been proposed to explain this association including the arthritogenic peptide theory that proposes that certain B-27 alleles bind certain arthritogenic peptides because of their specific anchoring proteins. Cartilage antigens are proposed as the targets for the immune response and the presentation of such antigens to CD8+ T cells. In the early phases of AS, T cells and macrophages invade and cause erosion of the cartilage at different sites. Based on these observations, it has recently been proposed that the cartilage is the primary target for the immune response.[67] **Aggrecan,** a proteoglycan, forms a major part of the extracellular matrix of cartilage and helps maintain its stability. A specific CD4+ T cell response to proteins derived from aggrecan has been found in animals and humans. Although these T cells have been found in AS, their role as a causative agent in AS remains unclear and necessitates future study.

AS involves inflammation of fibrocartilage in cartilaginous joints, primarily the vertebrae. The fibrous tissue of the joint capsule, the cartilage that surrounds intervertebral disks, the entheses, and periosteum are infiltrated by inflammatory cells. As inflammatory cells (chiefly macrophages) and lymphocytes infiltrate and erode bone and fibrocartilage in joint structures, repair begins. Repair of cartilaginous structures begins with the proliferation of fibroblasts. Fibroblasts synthesize and secrete collagen. The collagen becomes organized into fibrous scar tissue that eventually undergoes calcification and ossification. With time, all the cartilaginous structures of the joint are replaced by ossified scar tissue, causing the joint to fuse, or lose flexibility.

Repair of eroded bone begins with osteoblast activation and proliferation. Osteoblasts lay down new bone (callus), which is remodeled and replaced by compact, lamellar bone. Bone repair changes the contour of the bone's surface because the new bone grows outward to form a new enthesis with the end of the eroded ligament. The new enthesis, which forms on top of the old one, is called a **syndesmophyte.** As calcification of the spinal ligaments progresses, the vertebral bodies lose their concave anterior contour and appear square. On radiographs the spine assumes the classic "bamboo spine" appearance of AS.

CLINICAL MANIFESTATIONS The most common signs and symptoms of early AS are low back pain and stiffness. Typically the individual with primary disease develops low back pain during the early 20s. The pain is at first insidious but progressively becomes persistent. It is often worse after prolonged rest and is alleviated by physical activity. Early morning stiffness usually accompanies the low back pain, and the individual typically has difficulty sitting up or twisting the spine. Forward flexion, rotation, and lateral flexion of the spine are restricted and painful. Early pain and resultant loss of motion are caused by the underlying inflammation and reflex muscle spasm rather than by soft tissue or bony fusion.

As the disease progresses, the normal convex curve of the lower spine (lumbar lordosis) diminishes and concavity of the upper spine (kyphosis) increases. The individual becomes increasingly stooped. The thoracic spine becomes rounded, the head and neck are held forward on the shoulders, and the hips are flexed (Figure 42-28).

Inflammation in the tendon insertions of the many costosternal and costovertebral muscles can cause pleuritic chest pain and restricted chest movement. The pain is usually worse on inspiration. Movement in the diaphragm is normal and full. Pressure on the anterior chest wall over the sternum, ribs, and costal cartilages may cause tenderness. Tenderness over the pelvic brim may cause discomfort at night and interfere with sleep because turning onto the iliac crests causes pain. Tenderness over the ischial tuberosities may make

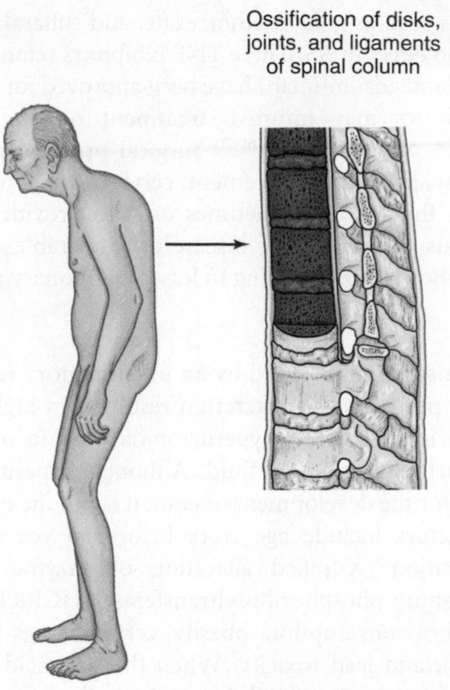

Ossification of disks, joints, and ligaments of spinal column

Figure 42-28 **Ankylosing spondylitis.** Characteristic posture and primary pathologic sites of inflammation and resulting damage.

sitting on hard seats unbearable. Tenderness in the heels may contribute to a limp or the cautious placement of the feet during walking.

Along with low back pain, many individuals have peripheral joint involvement, uveitis, fibrotic changes in the lungs, cardiomegaly, aortic incompetence, amyloidosis, and Achilles tendinitis. Symptoms may include fatigue, weight loss, low-grade fever, hypochromic anemia, and an increased erythrocyte sedimentation rate.[68]

EVALUATION AND TREATMENT Diagnosis of AS is made from the history and physical examination, roentgenograms, MRI, and serum analysis for the presence of the histocompatibility antigen HLA-B27. Erythrocyte sedimentation rate is elevated throughout the disease (normal is 0 to 9 mm/hr in males, 0 to 2 mm/hr in females). Alkaline phosphatase levels often are elevated. Treatment of individuals with AS consists of physical therapy to maintain skeletal mobility and prevent the natural progression of contractures. Prevention of deformity and maintenance of mobility require a continuous program of physical therapy. Exercises are performed several times each day to maintain chest expansion, full extension of the spine, and complete range of motion in the proximal joints. The long-term morbidity of AS has been previously underestimated.

Nonsteroidal anti-inflammatory drugs (NSAIDs) often provide relief of symptoms within 48 hours. Analgesic medications are prescribed to suppress some of the pain and stiffness and to facilitate exercise. The medications do not prevent disease progression, but they do provide relief from symptoms (see What's New? Cox II Inhibitors and Side Effects).

DMARDs such as gold, methotrexate, and sulfasalazine have little or no effect in AS. Three TNF inhibitors (etanercept, infliximab, and adalimumab) have been approved for severe AS.

Antibiotics may improve treatment outcomes in AS but results are conflicting.[69,70] Surgical procedures, such as osteotomy, total hip replacement, cervical spinal fusion, and radiation therapy are sometimes used to provide relief for individuals with end-stage disease or intolerable deformity. Persons should stop smoking to lessen pulmonary problems.

Gout

Gout is a syndrome caused by an inflammatory response to uric acid production or excretion resulting in high levels of uric acid in the blood (hyperuricemia) and in other body fluids, including synovial fluid. Although hyperuricemia is essential for the development of gout, it is not the only factor. Other factors include age (rare before 30 years), genetic predisposition (X-linked alteration of enzyme hypoxanthine-guanine phosphoribosyltransferase [HGPRT]), excessive alcohol consumption, obesity, certain drugs (especially thiazides), and lead toxicity. When the uric acid reaches a certain concentration in fluids, it crystallizes, forming insoluble precipitates that are deposited in connective tissues throughout the body. Crystallization in synovial fluid causes acute, painful inflammation of the joint, a condition known as **gouty arthritis.** With time, crystal deposition in subcutaneous tissues causes the formation of small, white nodules, or **tophi,** that are visible through the skin. Crystal aggregates deposited in the kidneys can form urate renal stones and lead to renal failure.

In classic gouty arthritis, monosodium urate crystals form and cause joint inflammation. **Pseudogout** is caused by the formation of calcium pyrophosphate dihydrate (CPPD) crystals. The effect of either crystal is the same—the onset of a cytokine-mediated acute inflammatory response (see Chapter 6).

Gout is rare in children and premenopausal women and is uncommon in males younger than 30 years. The peak age of onset in males is between 40 and 50 years, whereas it is somewhat later in females. The risk of developing gouty arthritis is similar in males and females for a particular urate concentration. The plasma urate concentration is an important determinant of the risk of developing gout (Table 42-8).

Uric acid is a byproduct of protein metabolism that normally assists with removal of nitrogen waste from the body.[71] When ionized, uric acid can form salts with various cations, but 98% of extracellular uric acid is in the form of monosodium urate (uric acid salt). At any time the proportion of uric acid or urate is pH dependent, so the ratio of these two forms varies considerably in urine (Figure 42-29).

The solubility of urate and uric acid is critical to the development of crystals. Urate is more soluble in plasma, synovial fluid, and urine than in aqueous solutions. The solubility of uric acid in urine rises dramatically as the pH increases to more than 4. There is little change, however, in the solubility of urate within the normal pH range that exists in the plasma, synovial fluid, and other tissues. Decreasing

Table 42-8	Mean Urate Concentrations by Age and Gender
Characteristic	**Mean Urate Levels**
Prepuberty	3.5 mg/dl
Males (at puberty)	Steep rise to 5.2 mg/dl
Females (puberty to premenopause)	Slow rise to ≅4 mg/dl
Females (after menopause)	4.7 mg/dl
Hyperuricemia	
Men	7 mg/dl
Women	6 mg/dl

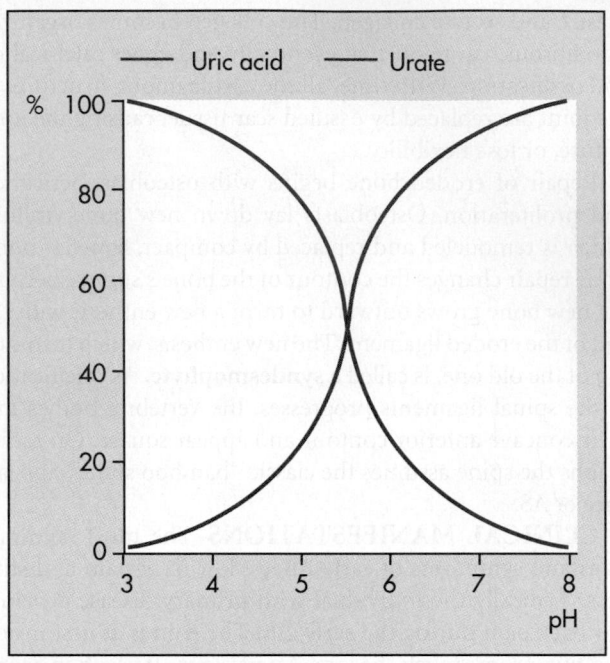

Figure 42-29 Effect of pH on uric acid and urate equilibrium. At pH 5.7, equal amounts of uric acid and urate are present in the solution. (Redrawn from Klippel JH, Dieppe PA, editors: *Rheumatology,* ed 2, London, 1998, Mosby-Wolfe.)

temperatures cause both urate and uric acid solubility to fall. The pathways of production of uric acid are shown in Figure 42-30.

PATHOPHYSIOLOGY The pathophysiology of gout is closely linked to purine metabolism (or cellular metabolism of purines) and kidney function. At the cellular level, purines are synthesized to purine nucleotides, which are used in the synthesis of nucleic acids, adenosine triphosphate, cyclic adenosine monophosphate (cAMP), and cyclic guanosine monophosphate (GMP). Uric acid is a breakdown product of purine nucleotides (uric acid synthesis and elimination are illustrated in Figure 42-31). Some individuals with gout have an accelerated rate of purine synthesis accompanied by an overproduction of uric acid. Other individuals break down purine nucleotides at an accelerated rate that also results in an overproduction of uric acid. Production of uric acid can be the result of an increased turnover of nucleic

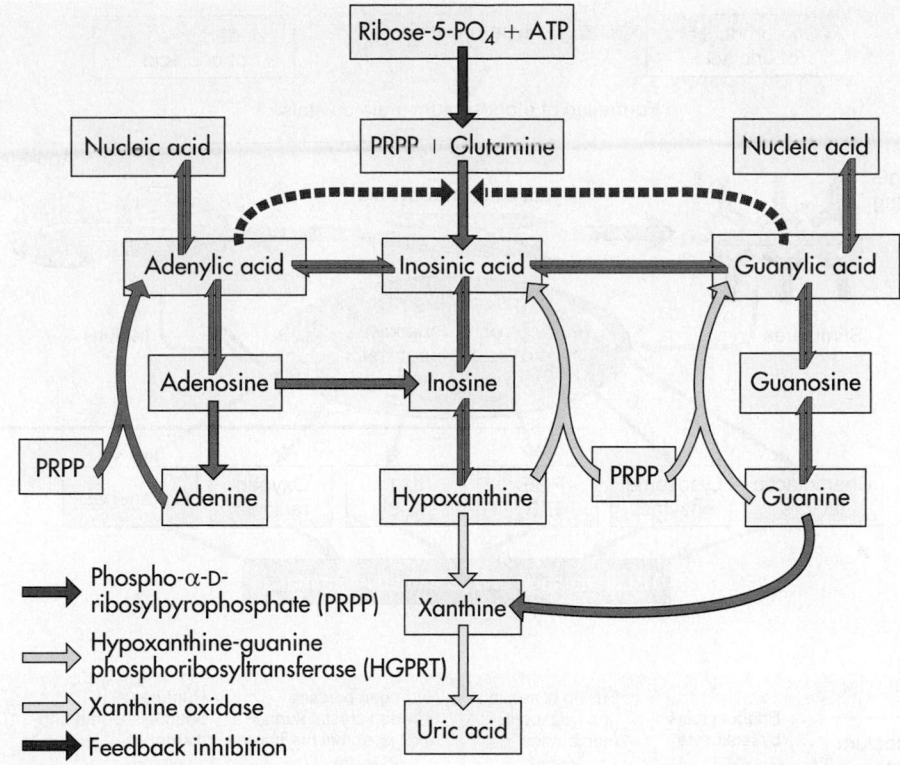

Figure 42-30 Production of uric acid. The major pathways involved in purine nucleotide synthesis. (Redrawn from Klippel JH, Dieppe PA, editors: *Rheumatology*, ed 2, London, 1998, Mosby-Wolfe.)

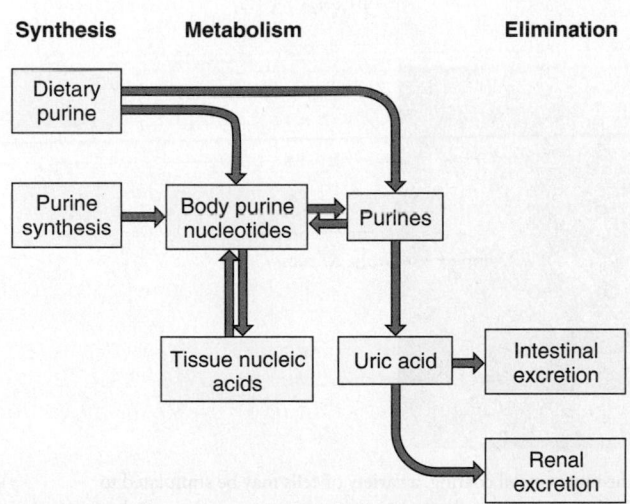

Figure 42-31 Uric acid synthesis and elimination. Uric acid is derived from ingested purines or synthesized from ingested foods, as well as being recycled following cell breakdown. Uric acid is then eliminated through the kidneys and gastrointestinal tract. (Redrawn from Klippel JH, Dieppe PA, editors: *Rheumatology*, ed 2, London, 1998, Mosby-Wolfe.)

acids, which is associated with an increased turnover of cells at other body sites. The increased turnover of nucleic acids leads to increased levels of uric acid with a compensatory increase in purine synthesis. A deficiency of the enzyme HGPRT (see earlier) can lead to an increased production of uric acid.

A complete absence of HGPRT is uncommon but can occur in the X-linked Lesch-Nyhan syndrome, with males at risk for hyperuricemia, neurologic alterations, and sometimes gouty arthritis.[72] The majority of individuals with gout, however, have an unknown metabolic defect, which is referred to as **primary gout.** When the etiology is known, it is referred to as **secondary gout.**

Most uric acid is eliminated from the body through the kidneys. Urate is filtered at the glomerulus and undergoes reabsorption and excretion within the renal tubules. In primary gout, urate excretion by the kidneys is sluggish. The sluggish excretion may be the result of a decrease in glomerular filtration of urate or an acceleration in urate reabsorption. In addition, monosodium urate crystals are deposited in renal interstitial tissues, causing impaired urine flow. (Kidney function is described in Chapter 35.)

The exact process by which crystals of monosodium urate are deposited in joints and induce gouty arthritis is unknown. However, several mechanisms may be involved, including the following:

1. Monosodium urate precipitates at the periphery of the body, where lower body temperatures may reduce the solubility of monosodium urate
2. Decreased albumin or glycosaminoglycan levels, which cause decreased urate solubility
3. Changes in ion concentration and decreases of pH that enhance urate deposition
4. Trauma that promotes urate crystal precipitation

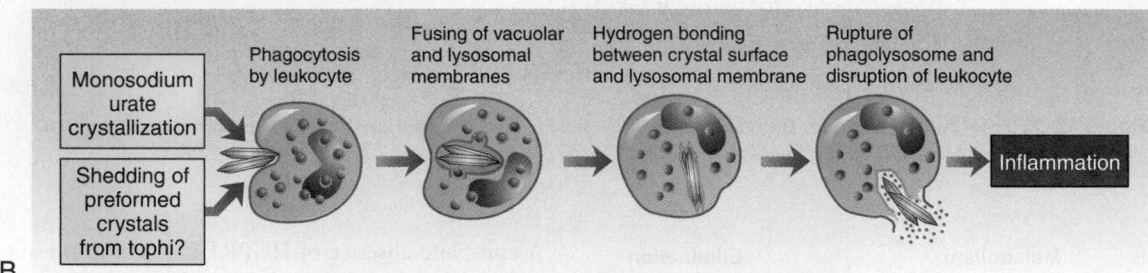

Figure 42-32 and diagram content:

A (top diagram)

Overproduction of uric acid → Hyperuricemia ← Underexcretion of uric acid

Formation of monosodium urate crystals

Crystals in synovial fluid

IgG coating — Stimulates →

Apo-E coating — Inhibits

Responding cell
Neutrophil, leukocyte, monocyte, fibroblast, synoviocyte, renal cell

Chemotactic factors | Lysosomal enzymes | PGE_2 LTB_4 | IL-1 IL-6 | Oxygen radicals | Collagenase

Tissue damage and continued inflammation

A

B

Monosodium urate crystallization / Shedding of preformed crystals from tophi?

Phagocytosis by leukocyte → Fusing of vacuolar and lysosomal membranes → Hydrogen bonding between crystal surface and lysosomal membrane → Rupture of phagolysosome and disruption of leukocyte → Inflammation

B

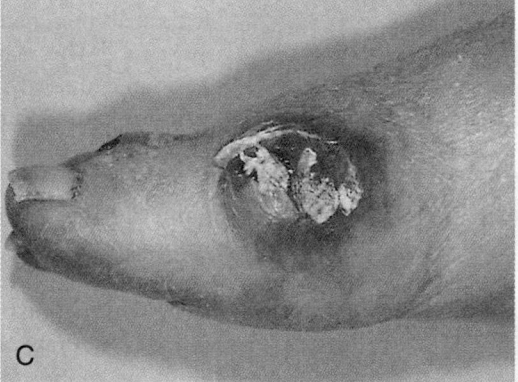

C

Figure 42-32 **Pathogenesis of acute gouty arthritis. A,** Depending on the urate crystal coating, a variety of cells may be stimulated to produce a wide range of inflammatory mediators. **B,** Sequence of events in the production of inflammation response to urate crystals. **C,** Gouty tophus on right foot. *Apo-E,* Apolipoprotein E; *IgG,* immunoglobulin G; *IL,* interleukin; *LTB₄,* leukotriene B₄; *PGE,* prostaglandin E. (C from Dieppe P et al: *Arthritis and rheumatism in practice,* London, 1991, Gower.)

The monosodium urate crystals may form in the synovial fluid or in the synovial membrane, cartilage, or other connective tissues in joints and elsewhere, such as in the heart, earlobes, and kidneys. Evidence suggests that an acute attack of gout is the result of the *formation* of crystals rather than the *releasing* of the crystals from connective tissues into the synovial fluid.

Monosodium urate crystals can stimulate and perpetuate the inflammatory response (Figure 42-32). The presence of the crystals triggers the acute inflammatory response. Initiation of the complement system activates cytokines and produces other substances, called chemoattractants, that draw neutrophils out of the circulation to begin phagocytizing (ingesting) the crystals.

Crystals coated with IgG are thought to react with crystallizable fragment (Fc) receptors on the surface of the responding cell (see Figure 42-32), thereby promoting phagocytosis with the formation of a phagolysosome. When the phagolysosomal enzymes strip the IgG from the surface of the crystal, the hydrogen bands on the surface of the crystal can induce membrane breakdown of the phagolysosome and cause rupture of the cell within. Recent evidence indicates that apolipoprotein-E coating of urate crystals will inhibit phagocytosis and the cellular response (see Figure 42-32, *A*).

A variety of inflammatory mediators are released during the crystal/cell response, including chemotactic factors, lysosomal enzymes, eicosanoids, prostaglandin E (PGE_2), IL-1 and IL-6, reactive oxygen species, and collagenase (see Figure 42-32, *B*). Some of these mediators stimulate the influx of neutrophils, monocytes, and lymphocytes. (Acute inflammation and phagocytosis are described in Chapter 6.)

Within the joint fluid, urate crystals react particularly with neutrophils and monocytes. Tissue damage begins to occur, principally when the neutrophils release the contents of their phagolysosomes. These contents also perpetuate inflammation. At an early phase of an acute gouty attack, synovial microtophi have been demonstrated. As the process continues, numerous microtophi may be present on the synovial membrane (see Figure 42-32, *C*).

CLINICAL MANIFESTATIONS Gout is manifested by (1) an increase in serum urate concentration (hyperuricemia), (2) recurrent attacks of monoarticular arthritis (inflammation of a single joint), (3) deposits of monosodium urate monohydrate (tophi) in and around the joints, (4) renal disease involving glomerular, tubular, and interstitial tissues and blood vessels, and (5) the formation of renal stones. These manifestations appear in three clinical stages:

1. **Asymptomatic hyperuricemia:** the serum urate level is elevated but arthritic symptoms, tophi, and renal stones are not present; may persist throughout life.
2. **Acute gouty arthritis:** attacks develop with increased serum urate concentrations; tends to occur with sudden or sustained increases of hyperuricemia but also can be triggered by trauma, drugs, and alcohol.
3. **Tophaceous gout:** the third and chronic stage of disease; can begin as early as 3 years or as late as 40 years after the initial attack of gouty arthritis. Progressive inability to excrete uric acid expands the urate pool until urate crystal deposits (tophi) appear in cartilage, synovial membranes, tendons, and soft tissue.

Trauma is the most common aggravating factor. The great toe is subject to chronic strain in walking, and subsequently an acute gout attack may follow long walks. Trauma associated with occupations, such as truck driving, also may precipitate an attack.

Attacks of gouty arthritis occur abruptly, usually in a peripheral joint. The primary symptom is severe pain. Approximately 50% of the initial attacks occur in the metatarsophalangeal joint of the great toe. The other 50% involve the heel, ankle, instep of the foot, knee, wrist, or elbow. The pain is usually noticed at night. Within a few hours the affected joint becomes hot, red, and extremely tender and may be slightly swollen. Lymphangitis and systemic signs of inflammation (leukocytosis, fever, elevated sedimentation rate) occasionally are present. Untreated, mild attacks usually subside in several hours but may persist for 1 or 2 days. Severe attacks may persist for several days or weeks. After recovery, the symptoms resolve completely. Intervals between acute attacks of gouty arthritis are called *intercritical periods.* Some individuals never have a second attack; others experience subsequent attacks within days to as long as 5 to 10 years after the first.

The helix of the ear is the most common site of tophi, which are the characteristic diagnostic lesions of chronic gout. Each tophus consists of a deposit of urate crystals, surrounded by a granuloma made up of mononuclear phagocytes (macrophages) that have developed into epithelial and giant cells. (Granuloma formation is described in and illustrated in Chapter 6.)

Tophaceous deposits produce irregular swellings of the fingers, hands, knees, and feet. Tophi commonly form lumps along the ulnar surface of the forearm, the tibial surface of the leg, the Achilles tendon, and the olecranon bursa. Tophi may produce marked limitation of joint movement and eventually cause grotesque deformities of the hands and feet. Although the tophi themselves are painless, they often cause progressive stiffness and persistent aching of the affected joint. Tophi in the upper extremities may cause nerve compressions such as carpal tunnel syndrome. Tophi in the lower extremities may cause tarsal tunnel syndrome. They also may erode and drain through the skin.

Renal stones are 1000 times more prevalent in individuals with primary gout than in the general population. The stones can be the size of a grain of sand or a piece of gravel, or they can accumulate in massive deposits called *staghorn calculi.* They range from pale yellow to brown to reddish black, depending on their composition. Some stones consist of pure monosodium urate; others are calcium oxalate or calcium phosphate. Renal stones can form in the collecting tubules, pelvis, or ureters, causing obstruction, dilation, and atrophy of the more proximal tubules and leading eventually to acute renal failure. Stones deposited directly in renal interstitial tissue initiate an inflammatory reaction that leads to chronic renal disease and progressive renal failure.

TREATMENT The aims of gout treatment are to terminate the acute gouty attack as promptly as possible, prevent recurring attacks, prevent or reverse complications associated with urate deposits in the joints and kidneys, and prevent formation of kidney stones. Acute gouty arthritis is treated with antiinflammatory drugs. The drugs of choice are NSAIDs and xanthine oxidase inhibitors, such as allopurinol and febuxostat. Colchicine is used in individuals unable to tolerate NSAIDs. Hydrocortisone may be injected into the joint to relieve pain. Drugs that block IL-1 have shown promise.[73] Ice also may relieve some of the inflammation of the joint. Weightbearing on the involved joint is avoided until the acute attack subsides. The individual is put on a low-purine diet, with high fluid intake to increase urinary output. Antihyperuricemic drugs are given to reduce serum urate concentrations.

DISORDERS OF SKELETAL MUSCLE

The common symptoms of disorders of skeletal muscle are muscle weakness and fatigue. In many cases, neural, traumatic, and psychogenic causes provide an adequate explanation for the failure to generate force (weakness) or sustain force (fatigue) seen in myopathies. The pathophysiologic mechanisms in some of the metabolic and inflammatory muscle diseases have been explored, but the cause of many of the myopathies remains obscure. The complex interaction between muscles and nerves affects muscular function as well. Only inherited and acquired disorders of skeletal muscles are discussed here.

Secondary Muscular Dysfunction

Muscular symptoms arise from a variety of causes unrelated to the muscle itself. Secondary muscular phenomena (contracture, stress-related muscle tension, immobility) are common disorders that influence muscular function.

Contractures

Contractures can be pathologic or physiologic. A physiologic muscle contracture occurs in the absence of a muscle action potential in the sarcolemma. Muscle shortening is explained on the basis of failure of the calcium pump in the presence of ATP. A physiologic contracture is seen in McArdle disease (muscle myophosphorylase deficiency) and malignant hyperthermia. The contracture is usually temporary if the underlying pathology is reversed.

A pathologic contracture is a permanent muscle shortening caused by muscle spasm or weakness. Heel cord (Achilles tendon) contractures are examples of pathologic contractures. They are associated with plentiful ATP and occur in spite of a normal action potential. The most common form of contracture is seen in such conditions as muscular dystrophy (see Chapter 43) and central nervous system (CNS) injury. Contractures also may develop secondary to scar tissue contraction in the flexor tissues of a joint, for example, contracture of burned tissues in the antecubital area of the forearm leading to a flexion contracture.

Stress-Induced Muscle Tension

Abnormally increased muscle tension has been associated with chronic anxiety, as well as a variety of stress-related muscular symptoms, including neck stiffness, back pain, and headache.[74,75] Abnormalities in the CNS, reticular activating system, and autonomic nervous system (ANS) have been implicated. For example, as an individual progressively relaxes, the amplitude of the knee-jerk reflex diminishes. Conversely, individuals with absent reflexes increase tension by such maneuvers as teeth clenching or hand grip. The underlying pathophysiology may be related to the fact that as a muscle contracts, the muscle spindle is activated. This gamma-feedback system produces a series of impulses that are transmitted to the brain by the sensitive 1A afferent fibers. Unconscious tension is thought to increase the activity of the reticular activating system as well. This influences increasing firing of the efferent loop of the gamma fibers and produces further muscle contraction and increases muscle tension. ANS function that regulates increased blood flow to the muscle during sympathetic activity may be related to increased muscle contraction tension.

Various forms of treatment have been used to reduce the muscle tension associated with stress. Progressive relaxation training, yoga, meditation, and biofeedback are examples of stress reduction therapies. **Biofeedback** uses an integrated electromyogram (EMG) to make recordings from the skin surface. The goal is to teach the individual to control tension that has been functioning maladaptively. It is particularly useful in individuals who have a connection between skeletal muscle tension and pain.

Progressive relaxation training emphasizes the individual's ability to perceive the difference between tension and relaxation. This technique involves sequential tensing and a relaxing environment. The individual is taught to practice this routine daily, often with the use of audiotaped instructions. By teaching the individual to recognize excessive contraction of skeletal muscle, one hopes to enhance the ability to relax specific muscle groups to relieve tension and thus reduce CNS as well as ANS arousal.

Fibromyalgia

Fibromyalgia is a chronic musculoskeletal syndrome characterized by widespread joint and muscle pain, fatigue, and tender points. Increased sensitivity to touch (i.e., tender points), the absence of systemic or localized inflammation, and fatigue and sleep disturbances are common. Because the symptoms are vague and the etiology unknown, fibromyalgia has been primarily diagnosed by exclusion. More recently, however, fibromyalgia has become a diagnosis based on specific criteria. A common misdiagnosis has been chronic fatigue syndrome but there is overlap of symptoms between these two conditions.[76] From 80% to 90% of individuals affected are women, and the peak age is 30 to 50 years. Although the incidence is unknown, the prevalence is reported to be 2% to almost 6% and increases with age. The ACR classification criteria include diffuse soft tissue pain of at least 3 months' duration and pain on palpation of at least 11 of 18 tender points (Figure 42-33). It is more common than RA, but its cause is still unknown.

The etiology of fibromyalgia has been debated for more than a century. It is unlikely that it is caused by a single factor. The most common precipitating factors include the following:

- Flulike viral illness
- Chronic fatigue syndrome
- Human immunodeficiency virus (HIV) infection
- Lyme disease
- Physical trauma
- Emotional trauma
- Medications, especially steroid withdrawal

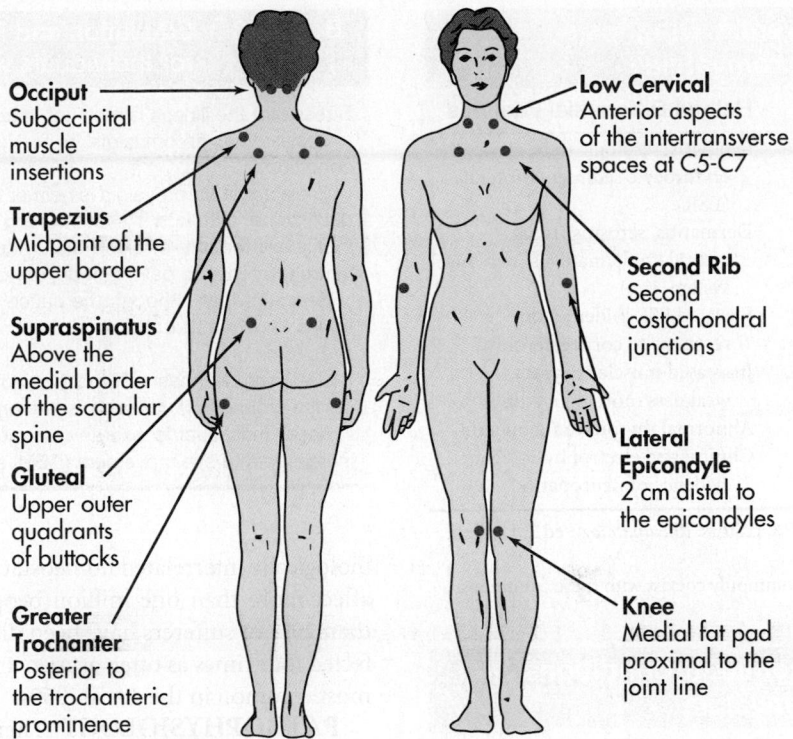

Occiput
Suboccipital muscle insertions

Trapezius
Midpoint of the upper border

Supraspinatus
Above the medial border of the scapular spine

Gluteal
Upper outer quadrants of buttocks

Greater Trochanter
Posterior to the trochanteric prominence

Low Cervical
Anterior aspects of the intertransverse spaces at C5-C7

Second Rib
Second costochondral junctions

Lateral Epicondyle
2 cm distal to the epicondyles

Knee
Medial fat pad proximal to the joint line

Figure 42-33 Location of specific tender points for diagnostic classification of fibromyalgia. (Redrawn from Freundlich B, Leventhal L: The fibromyalgia syndrome. In Schumacher HR Jr, Klippel JH, Koopman WJ, editors: *Primer on the rheumatic diseases,* ed 11, Atlanta, 1997, Arthritis Foundation. Copyright 1997. Reprinted with permission of the Arthritis Foundation.)

Table 42-9	Comparison of Fibromyalgia and Myofascial Pain Syndromes	
Variable	Fibromyalgia	Myofascial Pain
Location	Generalized	Regional
Examination	Tender points	Trigger points
Response to local therapy	Not sustained	Curative
Gender	Female/male ratio: 10:1	Equal or unknown
Systemic features	Characteristic	Unknown

Certain rheumatic diseases, such as RA or systemic lupus erythematosus, may coexist if not initially manifest with fibromyalgia. In addition, fibromyalgia may overlap with myofascial pain syndromes[77] (Table 42-9).

PATHOPHYSIOLOGY Fibromyalgia as a chronic pain syndrome is defined by subjective symptoms and not unique pathophysiologic characteristics. Individuals with fibromyalgia have lowered mechanical and thermal pain thresholds, high pain ratings for provoking stimuli, and altered temporal summation of pain stimuli.[77,78] These data provide some evidence of altered pain processing. Aggregation of fibromyalgia within families and other coexisting conditions such as irritable bowel syndrome, chronic fatigue, and mood disorders suggest a major role for neuroendocrine and stress-response alterations (see Chapter 10). Altered circadian activity of several neuroendocrine axes and ANS dysfunction have been reported.[79] Corticotropin-releasing hormone (CRH) locus ceruleus–norepinephrine (LC/NE), their peripheral effectors as well as the hypothalamic-pituitary-adrenal (HPA) axis are the main components of the stress system. Impaired functioning of the HPA axis and LC/NE system may be associated with fibromyalgia.

CLINICAL MANIFESTATIONS The prominent symptom of fibromyalgia is diffuse, chronic pain. The locations of nine pairs of tender points for diagnostic classification of fibromyalgia are shown in Figure 42-33. The pain often begins in one location, especially the neck and shoulders, but then becomes more generalized. People describe the pain as *burning* or *gnawing*. Fatigue is profound. The effect on everyday life is considerable.[80] Some investigators have found that the majority of women experienced pain and fatigue for more than 90% of their time awake.[81] Fatigue is most notable when arising from sleep and during the midafternoon. Headaches, symptoms of irritable bowel syndrome, and excess sensitivity to cold (Raynaud-like) are reported in 50% of individuals.

Almost 25% of individuals seek psychologic support for depression. Anxiety, particularly in regard to their diagnosis and future, is almost universal. Again, the only reliable finding on examination is the presence of multiple tender points.

EVALUATION AND TREATMENT Because the manifestations of chronic, generalized pain and fatigue are present in many musculoskeletal (e.g., rheumatic) disorders,

Table 42-10	Differential Diagnosis of Fibromyalgia
Differential Diagnosis	Helpful Differential Features
Rheumatoid arthritis*	Synovitis, serologic tests, elevated erythrocyte sedimentation rate (ESR)
Systemic lupus	Dermatitis, serositis (renal, central erythematosus* nervous system, etc.)
Polymyalgia rheumatica*	Elevated ESR, older adults, response to corticosteroids
Myositis	Increased muscle enzymes, weakness more than pain
Hypothyroidism*	Abnormal thyroid function tests
Neuropathies	Clinical and electrophysiologic evidence of neuropathy

Data from Klippel JH, Dieppe PA, editors: *Rheumatology*, ed 2, London, 1998, Mosby-Wolfe.
*Fibromyalgia may also more commonly coexist with these conditions.

Table 42-11	Concomitant Conditions with Fibromyalgia
Concomitant Condition	Relationship to Fibromyalgia
Depression	Present in 25%-60% of fibromyalgia cases
Irritable bowel	Present in 50%-80% of fibromyalgia cases
Migraine	Present in 50% of fibromyalgia cases
Chronic fatigue syndrome (CFS)	70% of CFS cases meet criteria for fibromyalgia
Myofascial pain	May be a localized form of fibromyalgia

Data from Klippel JH, Dieppe PA, editors: *Rheumatology*, ed 2, London, 1998, Mosby-Wolfe.

these disorders should be considered in the diagnosis of fibromyalgia (Tables 42-10 and 42-11).

No one regimen of medication has proved successful for fibromyalgia. Medications that improve sleep may be helpful as well as Vitamin D supplementation. Anti-inflammatories have been used despite the fact there is no evidence of tissue inflammation, but these medications have not been effective. Certain CNS-active medications, most notably pregabalin, were significantly better than placebo in controlled trials.[82] Treatment consists of a combination of patient education, medication, exercise, and cognitive therapy. Box 42-3 illustrates some of these modalities.

Chronic Fatigue Syndrome

Chronic fatigue syndrome (CFS) is a debilitating and complex disorder characterized by profound fatigue lasting six months or longer that is not improved by bed rest and may worsen with physical and mental activity. CFS is thought to be the result of alterations of multiple ecologically and

Box 42-3	Education and Reassurance for Individuals with Fibromyalgia

Stress that the illness is real, not imagined.
Explain that fibromyalgia is not a deforming or deteriorating condition.
Explain that fibromyalgia is neither life threatening nor markedly debilitating, although it is an irritating presence.
Discuss the role of sleep disturbances and the relationship of neurohormones to pain, fatigue, abnormal sleep, and mood.
Reassure that although the cause is unknown, some information is known about the physiologic changes responsible for the symptoms.
Use muscle "spasms" and perhaps low muscle blood flow to lay the groundwork for exercise recommendations.
Assist individual to use aerobic exercise to reduce stress and increase rapid eye movement (REM) sleep.

biologically interrelated homeostatic mechanisms.[83] CFS may affect more than one million people in the U.S., but fewer than 20% of sufferers have been diagnosed.[84] Women are affected four times as often as men and rarely in children and is most common in the 40s and 50s.

PATHOPHYSIOLOGY There are numerous hypotheses regarding the cause of CFS and research has implicated a number of contributory factors. To date, no specific etiologic factor has been identified. The Centers for Disease Control (CDC) recently instituted a public health research program for a 5-year strategic plan to explore neurologic, psychiatric, and biologic connections to CFS.

Functional MRI (fMRI) has shown lower blood perfusion to the brain stem in CFS individuals.[85] Other researchers have shown apparent central nervous system abnormalities, immunologic dysregulation, and higher-than-normal proinflammatory cytokines.[86, 87] Certain points in skeletal muscle may be affected by oxidative stress reactions (see Chapter 2), accounting for the muscle pain and fatigue associated with CFS.[88]

CLINICAL MANIFESTATIONS Unrestful sleep is a hallmark of CFS. Defining symptoms include debilitating fatigue made worse by physical or mental exercise (postexertional fatigue), muscle pain, noninflammatory joint pain, headaches, flu-like symptoms, and memory or concentration problems. Other common symptoms include bloating, morning joint stiffness, chest or jaw pain, chills and night sweats, visual disturbances, sore throat and tender axillary or cervical lymph nodes. In order to diagnose CFS, these symptoms need to be present for at least 6 months. Symptoms and their consequences can be severe.

EVALUATION AND TREATMENT Diagnosis of CFS is often delayed or missed because there is no biologic marker or specific laboratory test for CFS, many CFS symptoms are shared with other illnesses, individuals with CFS do not necessarily look sick, and symptoms typically have a variable course. The CDC recommends considering a diagnosis of CFS if the following two criteria are met[89]:

1. Unexplained, persistent fatigue that is not due to ongoing exertion, is not substantially relieved by rest, is

of new onset (not lifelong) and results in a significant reduction of previous levels of activity.

2. Four or more of the following symptoms are present for six months or more:
   - Impaired memory or concentration
   - Postexertional malaise (extreme, prolonged exhaustion and exacerbation of symptoms following physical or mental exertion)
   - Unrefreshing sleep
   - Muscle pain
   - Multijoint pain without swelling or redness (adults)
   - Headaches of a new type or severity
   - Sore throat that's frequent or recurring
   - Tender cervical or axillary lymph nodes

Treatment of CFS is primarily based on the person's individual needs and involves consideration of psychosocial factors as well as symptomatic and supportive care. Acknowledging the validity of the person's symptoms is important. Collaborative decision-making between patient and healthcare provider with regard to treatment, professional counseling, medication, diet and activity helps CFS sufferers deal with the limitations imposed by the disease. Alternative therapies such as acupuncture, massage, and therapeutic touch can relieve patient anxiety.

Disuse Atrophy

The term **disuse atrophy** describes the pathologic reduction in normal size of muscle fibers after prolonged inactivity from bed rest, trauma (casting), or local nerve damage. The effects of muscular deconditioning associated with lack of physical activity may be apparent in a matter of days. Oxidative stress from lack of muscle activity causes decreased protein synthesis and increased proteolysis, leading to muscle atrophy.[90] The normal individual on bed rest loses muscle strength from baseline levels at a rate of 3% per day. Bed rest also is associated with cardiovascular, skeletal, and other organ system changes.

Certain genes and transcription factors play a role in muscle atrophy. Measures to prevent atrophy include frequent forceful isometric muscle contractions and passive lengthening exercises. If reuse is not restored within 1 year, regeneration of muscle fibers becomes impaired.

Muscle Membrane Abnormalities

Two defects of the muscle membrane (plasma membrane of the muscle fiber) have been linked to clinical syndromes: the hyperexcitable membrane seen in the myotonic disorders and the intermittently unresponsive membrane seen in periodic paralyses. Although these are infrequent disorders, research into the pathologic processes has led to an improved understanding of the cell membrane.

Myotonia

Myotonia is a delayed relaxation after such voluntary muscle contractions as grip, eye closure, or muscle percussion. The distinctive "dive-bomber" noise, audible on needle EMG, is caused by the prolonged depolarization of the muscle membrane. Because the depolarization is not terminated by neuromuscular-blocking agents, such as curare, the abnormality has been localized at the muscle membrane; the basic defect is due to ion channel dysfunction. (These structures are described in Chapter 1.)

Myotonia can be reproduced by removing extracellular chloride, thus reducing chloride conductance across the plasma membrane. The delicate balance in which sodium diffuses into the intracellular fluid, potassium diffuses out of the intracellular fluid, and chloride is in flux is thus interrupted. Because the normal diffusion processes (described in Chapter 3) stabilize the membrane, the shift in chloride ions is thought to increase membrane excitability. The chloride abnormality may explain the resting membrane hyperexcitability, but it does not explain the delayed relaxation present in myotonia and has not been detected in human myotonia.

Myotonia is seen in several disorders: myotonia congenita, paramyotonia congenita, myotonic muscular dystrophy, and some forms of periodic paralysis. Most are inherited disorders and are mild in symptomatology, with the exception of myotonic muscular dystrophy (see p. 1633). Myotonia is treated by drugs that reduce muscle fiber excitability, such as procaine, procainamide, phenytoin, and quinine preparations. Recent treatments include acetazolamide and dichlorphenamide; both are carbonic anhydrase inhibitors.

Periodic Paralysis

During an attack of **periodic paralysis** the muscle membrane is unresponsive to neural stimuli and the resting membrane potential is reduced from −90 to −45 mV. Periodic paralysis can be either hyper- or hypokalemic. The disorder is often inherited in an autosomal dominant pattern, although it can be seen in hyperthyroidism.

The paralysis, which leaves the individual flaccid and weak, does not affect the respiratory muscles. Many individuals exhibit myotonia on examination. In most cases the weakness is accompanied by a change in serum potassium, although in some individuals the change may be negligible. Cardiac dysrhythmias have been present during attacks. Although the biochemical defect remains unknown, changes in the muscle membrane and sarcoplasmic reticulum have been described.

Hypokalemic periodic paralysis is triggered by high-carbohydrate meals, prolonged bed rest, or emotional stress. (The effect of potassium on the resting membrane potential is discussed in Chapter 3.) Glucose and insulin infusions and oral potassium loading are used as provocative tests; oral and intravenous potassium can relieve acute attacks. Treatment includes potassium-sparing diuretics and a high-salt diet. Acetazolamide, dichlorphenamide, and a low-salt diet are useful for long-term therapy. **Hyperkalemic periodic paralysis** is caused by a genetic mutation. Attacks are usually less severe than with the hypokalemic form. Treatment includes small carbohydrate-rich meals, light exercise, and intravenous calcium gluconate.

Metabolic Muscle Diseases

Disorders in muscle metabolism can be caused by endocrine abnormalities or diseases of energy metabolism, such as glycogen storage disease, enzyme deficiencies, and abnormalities in lipid metabolism and mitochondrial function.

Endocrine Disorders

Often the systemic effects of hormonal imbalance overshadow the individual's muscular symptoms. For example, individuals with thyrotoxicosis may have signs of proximal weakness, paresis of the extraocular muscles (exophthalmic ophthalmoplegia), and rarely, hypokalemic periodic paralysis. Hypothyroidism is often associated with a decrease in muscle mass and strength, with weak, flabby skeletal muscles and sluggish movements.

Thyroid hormone is believed to regulate muscle protein synthesis and electrolyte balance. Changes in muscle protein synthesis and electrolyte balance may therefore explain the changes in muscle mass and contractility seen in endocrine disorders. The muscle symptoms subside with appropriate treatment of the primary hormonal disorder.

Diseases of Energy Metabolism

Muscle relies on carbohydrates, such as glycogen and lipids (free fatty acids), for energy. When stored glycogen or lipids cannot be used because of a lack of the enzyme necessary to convert energy for contraction, the individual experiences cramps, fatigue, and exercise intolerance. Disorders of muscle metabolism can be self-limiting, such as is seen in McArdle disease and some lipid disorders, or cause widespread irreparable muscle destruction, as in acid maltase deficiency.

McArdle Disease

McArdle disease, or glycogen myophosphorylase deficiency, was the first myopathy in which a single enzyme defect was identified (Figure 42-34). Individuals with McArdle disease lack muscle phosphorylase, which is responsible for the breakdown of glycogen in muscle. Normally after the body uses the short-term ATP and phosphocreatine stores,

intramuscular lactic acid accumulates as glycogen is used (see Chapter 41). The individual with McArdle disease is not able to break down glycogen or produce lactic acid.

The altered energy production manifests itself in exercise intolerance, fatigue, and painful muscle cramps. When exercise is carried to an extreme, painful muscle contracture and myoglobinuria develop. Some individuals describe a "second wind" phenomenon, in which exercise tolerance increases if they slow their pace once the initial sensation of fatigue commences. This may be caused by the use of free fatty acids as a secondary source of energy. As the disease progresses, some individuals have pronounced muscle weakness and wasting. Other organs are not involved because the absence of phosphorylase is limited to muscle. Generally, individuals with McArdle disease learn to adapt their daily routine to avoid muscle symptoms. Usually the diagnosis of McArdle disease is made by the histochemical evaluation of myophosphorylase activity in frozen sections. There is no staining of myofibrils in affected individuals.

Acid Maltase Deficiency

Acid maltase deficiency is an uncommon glycogen storage disease associated with an accumulation of glycogen in the lysosomes of muscle cells and the cells of other tissues. The usual pathways of glycogen degradation are preserved. The absence of the enzyme acid maltase is responsible for the abnormality in glycogen metabolism, although the exact mechanism is unknown. It is an autosomal recessive disorder, with the gene located on the long arm of chromosome 17.

The infantile form, **Pompe disease,** is an autosomal recessive disease that causes lysosomal glycogen accumulation. The adult form tends to be less dramatic than the infantile type. The infantile form is recognized shortly after birth by hypotonia, dysreflexia, and an enlarged heart, tongue, and liver. Hypertrophy of these tissues is thought to be the result of glycogen deposition. Children die of cardiac or respiratory failure within 1 year of diagnosis. Recombinant human acid alpha-glucosidase administration has been shown to decrease mortality.[91,92] The adult variety becomes evident subacutely. The muscular symptoms resemble those of muscular

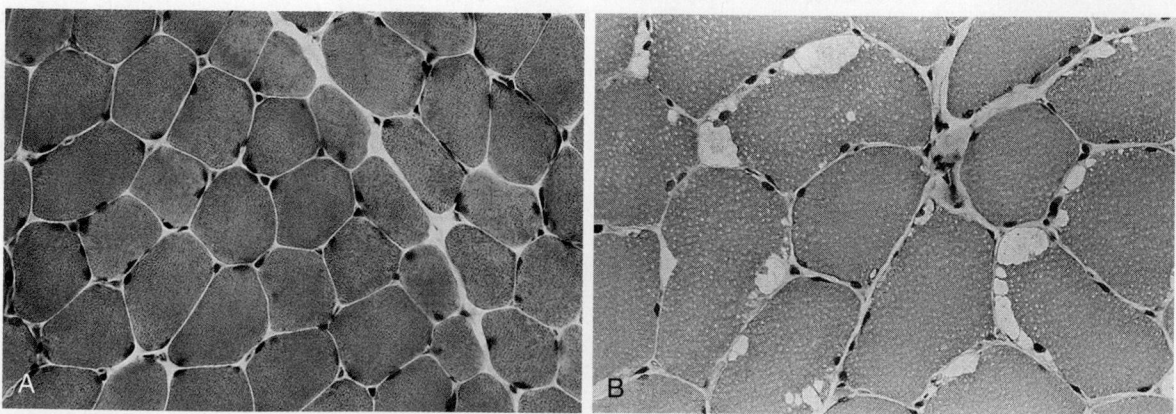

Figure 42-34 McArdle disease. A, Normal muscle fibers. B, Muscle fibers of McArdle disease. Note the enlarged (*white*) peripheral vacuoles. (From Damjanov I, Linder J, editors: *Anderson's pathology*, ed 10, St Louis, 1996, Mosby.)

dystrophy or polymyositis. A distinguishing feature in adults may be severe respiratory muscle weakness.

Myoadenylate Deaminase Deficiency

An enzyme deficiency that produces changes in skeletal muscle and is associated with exercise intolerance is **myoadenylate deaminase deficiency (MDD)**. Because these individuals lack myoadenylate deaminase, they have a poor capacity for sustained energy production. Myoadenylate deaminase is the catalytic enzyme that forms phosphocreatine and ATP during exercise through a metabolic pathway that binds the purine and phosphate molecules that constitute ATP. Persons with MDD differ from those with McArdle disease in that during the ischemic exercise test, lactate production is normal when ATP and phosphocreatine are synthesized. The enzyme defect has been reported to be common, but in practice it may rarely be recognized as a cause of exercise intolerance.

Lipid Deficiencies

Disorders of lipid metabolism are uncommon but account for severe changes in muscle metabolism. The lipid content of muscle cells consists of the free fatty acids, which are oxidized in the mitochondria. These acids require carnitine and the enzyme carnitine palmityl transferase (CPT) to transport metabolic byproducts and energy to the myofibrils. Individuals with CPT deficiency have mild muscular symptoms but can experience bouts of renal failure caused by myoglobinuria. Individuals with a deficiency of carnitine alone have progressive muscle weakness and can experience sudden exacerbations.

Measuring the CPT and carnitine content in muscle aids in the diagnosis. Cells in the muscle biopsy show vacuoles and lipid deposits. Treatments with riboflavin, medium-chain triglycerides, oral carnitine, and prednisone have been suggested.

Inflammatory Muscle Diseases: Myositis

Viral, Bacterial, and Parasitic Myositis

Viral, bacterial, and parasitic infections of varying severity are known to produce inflammatory changes in skeletal muscle, a group of conditions collectively described by the term **myositis.** In tuberculosis and sarcoidosis, chronic inflammatory changes and granulomas are found in muscle, as well as in other affected tissues. In trichinellosis, *Trichinella* larvae reside in infected pork and, after ingestion, migrate to the intestinal mucosa and from there to the lymphatics. Symptoms include severe pain, rash, and muscle stiffness. Treatment includes administration of corticosteroids and antiparasitic agents, such as mebendazole or albendazole. Unfortunately, once trichinella larvae are established they may reside for years in the muscles. Toxoplasmosis, a common parasitic infection, is also associated with a generalized polymyositis that responds rapidly to therapy.

In the tropics, more prevalent disorders include bacterial infections with *S. aureus* and parasites such as cysticercus, the larva of the tapeworm *Taenia solium*. Viral infections can be associated with an acute myositis. Muscle pain, tenderness, signs of inflammation, and CK elevation are common

manifestations of viral myositis. The self-limiting symptoms of muscle aches and pains during a bout of influenza may actually be a subacute form of viral myopathy.

Polymyositis and Dermatomyositis

Polymyositis (generalized muscle inflammation) and **dermatomyositis** (polymyositis accompanied by skin lesions) are the most common inflammatory muscle diseases requiring long-term care. Prevalence rates may be about 6 per 1 million persons.

PATHOPHYSIOLOGY Polymyositis and dermatomyositis are characterized by inflammation of connective tissue and muscle fibers that presumably causes the extensive necrosis and destruction of muscle fibers. The agent that causes the muscle inflammation has not been identified, but recent findings strongly suggest an autoimmune connection[93, 94] (Figure 42-35). Innate and adaptive immune responses are activated in these myopathies. There appears to be a genetic component in symptom manifestation.[95] This family of diseases is now designated as autoimmune because of the presence of autoantibodies in the serum of many individuals. Studies have shown that the inflammatory cells that surround the perimysial and perivascular sites are selectively enriched in B cells and helper

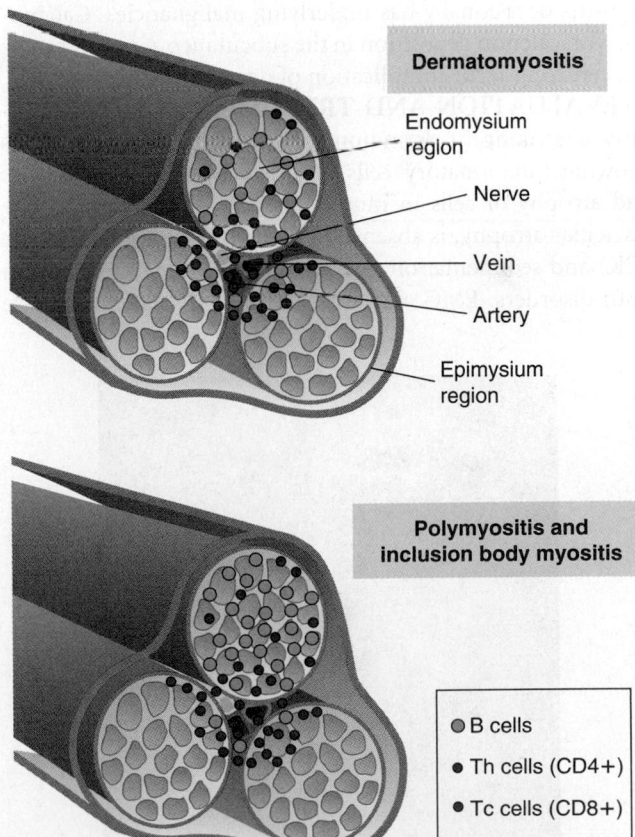

Figure 42-35 Distribution of CD4+ and CD8+ lymphocytes in different clinical forms of myositis. Dermatomyositis shows perivascular and CD4+ T cells (helper T-cells). Polymyositis shows mostly CD8+ T cells (cytotoxic T-cells).

T cells in those with dermatomyositis.[96] There is less vascular involvement in polymyositis, and most of the inflammatory cells, including B cells, T cells, and macrophages, surround the muscle fibers and fascicles.

CLINICAL MANIFESTATIONS The acute symptoms include many of those seen in any inflammatory process: malaise, fever, muscle swelling, pain and tenderness, lethargy, and listlessness. In adults, weakness of the shoulder and pelvic girdle muscles is a primary manifestation of polymyositis. Both illnesses are usually associated with a symmetric proximal muscle weakness and initially can be confused with other myopathies. A thorough evaluation is required to exclude other disorders. Clinical features common in both polymyositis and dermatomyositis are dysphagia, reduced esophageal motility, vasculitis, Raynaud phenomenon, cardiomyopathy, and interstitial pulmonary fibrosis. Some patients have other coexisting collagen vascular disorders, such as RA, systemic lupus erythematosus (SLE), and progressive systemic sclerosis (formerly called *scleroderma*).

The presence of skin rash, calcinosis, and eyelid edema most often suggests dermatomyositis (Figure 42-36). The skin rash is purple (heliotrope) and involves the eyelids, face, chest, and extensor surfaces of the extremities. Dermatomyositis is slightly more common in children and older adults, with an onset before age 15 or after age 50. The adult with dermatomyositis occasionally has underlying malignancies. Calcinosis, with calcium deposition in the subcutaneous tissue, can be a severe long-term complication of dermatomyositis.

EVALUATION AND TREATMENT The muscle biopsy is striking in dermatomyositis, with most individuals showing inflammatory cells grouped around blood vessels and atrophy of cells in muscle fascicles. This change, perifascicular atrophy, is absent in polymyositis. Creatine kinase (CK) and sedimentation rate are often extremely elevated in both disorders. EMG abnormalities include signs of muscle irritability and myopathic changes—usually large numbers of low-amplitude action potentials of brief duration. The EMG also shows a typical "myopathic" pattern, with short, low-amplitude polyphasic potentials, as well as signs of marked muscle irritability. Muscle biopsy is indispensable for determining a diagnosis of polymyositis or dermatomyositis as opposed to other myotonic diseases. MRI reveals inflammation and edema of the muscles.

Treatment primarily includes immunosuppressive drugs, although they are not always successful if uniformly applied. Most clinicians choose corticosteroids initially, usually prednisone on a daily or alternating-day schedule, tapering the dosage as the symptoms subside. Successful treatment with azathioprine, methotrexate, and cyclophosphamide also has been reported. Creatine supplements and physical therapy may improve muscle strength.[97]

Myopathy

Myopathy is the term applied to a primary muscle disorder. Many pathologic processes affect muscles and cause loss of functional muscle cells. Myopathies affect muscle strength, tone, and bulk. Primary muscle disease is invariably associated with weakness—usually marked weakness. The distribution of the weakness in myopathy is usually symmetric and proximal, although occasionally the weakness is predominantly distal, such as in myotonic dystrophy. The weakness is associated with mild fatigue. Tone is decreased, as are the tendon reflexes. Atrophy may be present. Some myopathies are associated with muscle hypertrophy as in cretinism and the familial progressive muscular dystrophies of childhood, in which hypertrophied muscles are rubbery and weak. Fasciculations are not present with myopathy because no denervation is present. No sensory changes are found. (Specific neurologic-associated myopathies are discussed in Chapter 16.)

Toxic Myopathies

A number of agents, including corticosteroids, chloroquine, alcohol, phenytoin, azathioprine, organophosphates, and reverse transcriptase inhibitors, have been shown to cause **toxic myopathy**.[98] The incidence of acute alcoholic myopathy has been estimated at up to 20% of individuals admitted with acute alcoholic withdrawal.

The pathologic abnormalities include necrosis of individual muscle fibers, particularly type II fibers; whole segments can be found in the same stage of degeneration. The mechanisms by which alcohol affects the muscle include disturbances of energy cell turnover, gene dysregulation, and initiation of apoptosis.[99]

Acute alcoholic myopathy can range from benign cramps and pain resolving in a matter of hours to severe weakness and markedly increased CK associated with myoglobinuria and renal failure. Individuals are prone to repeated attacks following recovery. The only treatment is abstinence from alcohol and improved nutrition. The individual with chronic alcoholic myopathy often has a coexisting peripheral neuropathy that complicates the diagnosis.

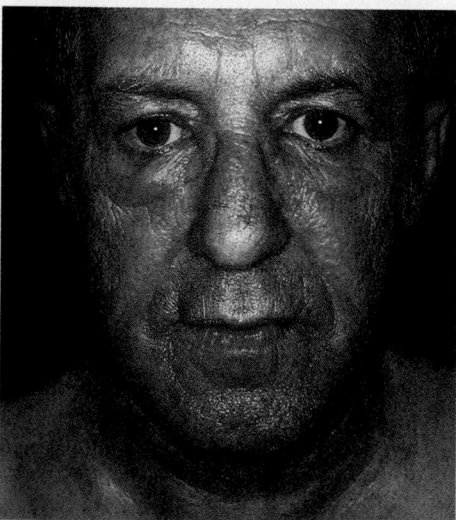

Figure 42-36 Dermatomyositis. Heliotrope (violaceous) discoloration around the eyes and periorbital edema. (From Habif TP: *Clinical dermatology*, ed 3, St Louis, 1996, Mosby.)

Rhabdomyolysis and myoglobinuria are often caused by sedatives and narcotics, particularly street heroin, clofibrate (a hypolipidemic agent), and the antifibrinolytic aminocaproic acid. Drugs that induce hypokalemia, such as amphotericin B, licorice, and azathioprine, also have been reported to cause myalgia and myopathy.

Repeated intramuscular injections have been associated also with changes in muscle fibers. Local necrosis of muscle fiber and elevated CK have been reported after intramuscular injections of certain cephalosporins, lidocaine, diazepam, and digoxin; these effects were not produced with injections of saline. When drugs are injected over long periods, a chronic focal myopathy develops. Proliferation of connective tissue in both the muscle fiber and overlying skin and subcutaneous tissue has been reported. Over time, segments of the muscles, particularly the deltoid and quadriceps, are converted into fibrotic bands. Pathophysiologic mechanisms for these changes include repeated needle trauma and infection, along with the nonphysiologic acidity and alkalinity of the injected material.

Muscle Tumors

Rhabdomyoma

Rhabdomyoma is an extremely rare benign tumor of muscle that generally occurs in the tongue, neck muscles, larynx, uvula, nasal cavity, axilla, vulva, and heart. These tumors are usually treated by surgical excision and do not recur.

Rhabdomyosarcoma

The malignant tumor of striated muscle is called **rhabdomyosarcoma.** These tumors are highly malignant, with rapid metastasis. They are located in the muscle tissue of the head,

neck, and genitourinary tract in 75% of cases. The remainder are in the trunk and extremities.

Three types of rhabdomyosarcoma are differentiated on pathologic section: pleomorphic, embryonal, and alveolar. The pleomorphic, or spindle cell, type is considered to be one of the most highly malignant tumors of the extremities seen in adulthood. Embryonal tumors are most commonly seen in childhood and appear on biopsy to be shaped like a tadpole or tennis racquet. Alveolar-type tumors appear lattice-like and look like lung tissue alveoli.

The diagnosis of rhabdomyosarcoma is made by history, physical examination, serologic testing, CT, and MRI, and is confirmed by incisional biopsy and examination of the specimen by a pathologist. On electron microscopy the tissue demonstrates myofilaments and Z-band material; CT scan helps define the tissue borders. Staging is based on pathologic grade of the tumor and is helpful in determining prognosis and treatment.

Treatment consists of a combination of surgical excision, radiation therapy, and systemic chemotherapy. Overall survival of childhood rhabdomyosarcoma has improved over the past decades but adult survival remains poor (see Chapter 43).

Other Tumors

Metastatic deposits of tumors in muscles are rare in spite of the extensive vascular supply of skeletal muscles. It is suggested that local pH or metabolic changes prevent metastatic involvement from other tumors. When adjacent carcinomas do cause muscle damage, it is usually related to the compression of tissue and resultant muscle atrophy.

SUMMARY REVIEW

Musculoskeletal Injuries

1. The most serious skeletal injury is a fracture. A bone can be completely or incompletely fractured. A closed fracture leaves the skin intact. An open fracture has an overlying skin wound. The direction of the fracture line can be linear, oblique, spiral, or transverse. Greenstick, torus, and bowing fractures are examples of incomplete fractures that occur in children. Stress fractures occur in normal or abnormal bone that is subjected to repeated stress. Fatigue fractures occur in normal bone subjected to abnormal stress. Normal weightbearing can cause an insufficiency fracture in abnormal bone.
2. Dislocation is complete loss of contact between the surfaces of two bones. Subluxation is partial loss of contact between two bones. As a bone separates from a joint, it may damage adjacent nerves, blood vessels, ligaments, tendons, and muscle.
3. Tendon tears are called *strains,* and ligament tears are called *sprains.* A complete separation of a tendon or ligament from its attachment is called an *avulsion.*
4. Epicondylitis is inflammation of a tendon where it attaches to a bone. Bursitis is inflammation of the bursae or small sacs lined with synovial membrane and filled with synovial fluid.

5. Muscle strain is a mild injury of local muscle damage.
6. Rhabdomyolysis, or myoglobinuria, can be a life-threatening complication of severe muscle trauma wherein muscle cell contents are released into the circulation. It may result in myoglobinuria, the filtration of myoglobin into the urine, and is often associated with acute renal failure.

Disorders of Bones

1. Metabolic bone diseases are characterized by abnormal bone structure. In osteoporosis bone tissue is normally mineralized, but the density or mass of bone is reduced because the bone remodeling cycle is disrupted. Osteoporosis is a complex, multifactorial, chronic disease that often progresses silently for decades until fractures occur. It is the most common bone disease. Multiple factors are involved including alternation in the OPG/RANKL/RANK system.
2. Postmenopausal osteoporosis occurs in middle-aged and older women and is probably caused by changes in osteoprotegerin, IGF, a combination of inadequate dietary calcium intake and lack of vitamin D, possibly decreased magnesium, lack of exercise, decreased levels of estrogen, and family history.
3. Glucocorticoids increase RANKL expression and inhibit OPG production by osteoblasts, thus leading to lower bone density.

Continued

4. Osteomalacia is a metabolic bone disease characterized by inadequate bone mineralization.

5. Excessive and abnormal bone remodeling occurs in Paget disease. Sporadic Paget disease involves overexpression of RANKL.

6. Osteomyelitis is a bone infection caused most often by bacteria (e.g., *S. aureus*) that can enter bone from outside the body (exogenous osteomyelitis) or from infection sites within the body (hematogenous osteomyelitis).

7. Bone tumors originate from bone cells, cartilage cells, fibrous tissue cells, or vascular marrow cells. Each cell produces a specific type of ground substance that is used to classify the tumor as osteogenic (bone cell), chondrogenic (cartilage cell), collagenic (fibrous tissue cell), or myelogenic (vascular marrow cell). Malignant bone tumors are large, aggressively destroy surrounding bone, invade surrounding tissue, and initiate independent growth outside the site of origin. Benign bone tumors are less destructive, limit their growth to the anatomic confines of the bone, and have a well-demarcated border.

Disorders of Joints

1. Noninflammatory joint disease is differentiated from inflammatory joint disease by the absence of synovial membrane inflammation, the absence of systemic signs and symptoms, and the presence of normal synovial fluid.

2. OA, now known as inflammatory joint disease, is characterized by the degeneration and loss of articular cartilage, sclerosis of underlying bone, and formation of bone spurs (osteophytes).

3. RA is an inflammatory joint disease characterized by inflammatory destruction of the synovial membrane, articular cartilage, joint capsule, and surrounding ligaments and tendons. RA involves an aberrant immune response and the transformed antibodies are called *rheumatoid factors*. The OPG/RANKL/RANK system is also involved. Rheumatoid nodules may also invade the skin, lung, and spleen and involve small and large arteries. RA is a systemic disease that affects the heart, lungs, kidneys, and skin, as well as the joints.

4. AS is a chronic inflammatory joint disease characterized by stiffening and fusion of the spine and sacroiliac joints. Recent data show that synovitis and bone marrow inflammation, rather than solely enthesis involvement, explain the alteration in sacroiliac joints.

5. Gout is a metabolic disorder associated with high levels of uric acid in the blood and body fluids. Uric acid crystallizes in the connective tissue of a joint, where it initiates inflammatory destruction of the joint.

Disorders of Skeletal Muscle

1. A pathologic contracture is permanent muscle shortening caused by muscle spasticity, as seen in CNS injury or severe muscle weakness.

2. Stress-induced muscle tension is presumably caused by increased activity in the reticular activating system and gamma loop in the muscle fiber. Progressive relaxation training and biofeedback has been advocated to reduce muscle tension.

3. Fibromyalgia is a chronic musculoskeletal syndrome characterized by diffuse pain and tender points. Unknown but suspected is that muscle is the end organ responsible for the pain and fatigue of the disease. Comorbidities (e.g., irritable bowel syndrome, mood disorders and chronic fatigue) suggest a major role for neuroendocrine and stress-response alterations.

4. Chronic fatigue syndrome (CFS) is a debilitating and complex disorder with profound fatigue lasting 6 months or more and is not improved by bed rest. The actual cause of CFS is unknown and hypotheses include central nervous system alterations, immunologic disruptions and chronic pro-inflammatory cytokines.

5. Atrophy of muscle fibers and overall diminished size of the muscle are seen after prolonged inactivity. Isometric contractions and passive lengthening exercises decrease atrophy to some degree in immobilized patients.

6. Hyperexcitable membranes cause the physical and electrical phenomenon of myotonia. The disorder is treated with drugs that reduce fiber excitability. Periodic paralysis is caused by an unresponsive muscle membrane and is accompanied by changes in serum potassium. The biochemical defect is possibly related to changes in the muscle membrane and sarcoplasmic reticulum.

7. Metabolic muscle diseases are caused by endocrine disorders, glycogen storage disease, enzyme deficiencies, and abnormal lipid function. The muscle depends on a complex system of carbohydrates and fats converted by enzymes to produce energy for the muscle cell. Abnormalities in these pathways can inhibit function or cause damage to the muscle fiber. These illnesses are rare, yet they account for significant functional abnormalities.

8. Viral, bacterial, and parasitic infections of muscles produce the characteristic clinical and pathologic changes associated with inflammation. These are usually treatable and self-limiting disorders.

9. Polymyositis (generalized muscle inflammation) and dermatomyositis (polymyositis accompanied with skin rash) are characterized by inflammation of connective tissue and muscle fibers, and muscle fiber necrosis. Cell-mediated and humoral immune factors have been implicated. Treatment with immunosuppressive agents is effective in many cases.

10. Primary disorders with weakness and atrophy are known as myopathies.

11. The most common toxic myopathy is caused by alcohol abuse. Direct toxic effects of alcohol-producing necrosis of muscle fibers and nutritional deficiency have been suggested. The only treatment is abstinence and improved nutrition. The toxic effects of many drugs on muscle fibers cause local trauma to the muscle fibers from direct effects of the needle, secondary infection, and changes caused by nonphysiologic acidity and alkalinity in the fibers.

12. Sarcomas of muscle tissue are rare. Rhabdomyosarcoma has a uniformly poor prognosis because of an aggressive invasion and early, widespread dissemination. The usual treatment includes surgical excision, radiation therapy, and systemic chemotherapy.

KEY TERMS

Acid maltase deficiency, 1610
Acute gouty arthritis, 1605
Age-related bone loss, 1582
Aggrecan, 1600
Ankylosing spondylitis (AS) (spondylo-
    arthritis), 1600
Arthropathy, 1592
Asymptomatic hyperuricemia, 1605
Avulsion, 1573
Biofeedback, 1606
Bowing fracture, 1569
Bursae, 1574
Bursitis, 1574
Caplan syndrome, 1600
Chondrogenic (cartilage-forming)
    tumor, 1591
Chondroid, 1591
Chondrosarcoma, 1591
Chronic fatigue syndrome, 1608
Closed (simple) fracture, 1569
Collagenic (collagen-forming) tumor, 1591
Comminuted fracture, 1569
Compartment syndrome, 1575
Complete fracture, 1569
Contracture, 1606
Delayed union, 1571
Dermatomyositis, 1611
Dislocation, 1572
Disuse atrophy, 1609
Enchondroma, 1591
Endogenous (hematogenous) osteomyelitis,
    1587
Enthesis, 1600
Epicondylitis, 1574
Exogenous osteomyelitis, 1587
Extracellular signal regulated kinases
    (ERKS), 1582
Fatigue fracture, 1569
Fibromyalgia, 1606
Fibrosarcoma, 1591
Fracture, 1568
Fragility fracture, 1569

Giant cell tumor, 1592
Glucocorticoid (e.g., cortisone)-induced
    osteoporosis, 1582
Gout, 1602
Gouty arthritis, 1602
Greenstick fracture, 1569
Hyperbaric oxygen therapy, 1588
Hyperkalemic periodic paralysis, 1609
Hypokalemic periodic paralysis, 1609
Incomplete fracture, 1569
Inflammatory joint disease (arthritis), 1596
Insufficiency fracture, 1569
Involucrum, 1588
Joint effusion, 1595
Joint stiffness, 1595
Lateral epicondylopathy (tennis elbow), 1574
Ligament, 1573
Linear fracture, 1569
Malunion, 1571
McArdle disease, 1610
Medial epicondylopathy
    (golfer's elbow), 1574
Muscle strain, 1675
Myelogenic tumor, 1592
Myoadenylate deaminase deficiency
    (MDD), 1611
Myoglobin, 1575
Myoglobinuria, 1575
Myopathy, 1612
Myositis, 1611
Myositis ossificans, 1575
Myotonia, 1609
Noninflammatory joint disease, 1592
Nonunion, 1571
Oblique fracture, 1569
Open (compound) fracture, 1569
Osteoarthritis (OA), 1593
Osteogenic (bone-forming) tumor, 1590
Osteomalacia, 1584
Osteomyelitis, 1587
Osteopenia, 1577
Osteophyte, 1593

Osteoporosis, 1576
Osteoprotegerin (OPG), 1580
Osteosarcoma, 1590
Paget disease (osteitis deformans), 1585
Pannus, 1598
Pathologic fracture, 1569
Peak bone mass, 1577
Periodic paralysis, 1609
Polymyositis, 1611
Pompe disease, 1610
Postmenopausal osteoporosis, 1579
Primary gout, 1603
Progressive relaxation training, 1606
Pseudogout, 1602
RANK, 1580
Receptor activator of nuclear factor $\kappa\beta$
    ligand (RANKL), 1580
Regional osteoporosis, 1580
Rhabdomyolysis, 1675
Rhabdomyosarcoma, 1613
Rheumatoid arthritis (RA), 1596
Rheumatoid factor (RF), 1597
Rheumatoid nodule, 1599
Secondary gout, 1603
Secondary osteoporosis, 1580
Sequestrum, 1587
Spiral fracture, 1569
Sprain, 1573
Strain, 1573
Stress fracture, 1569
Subluxation, 1572
Syndesmophyte, 1601
Tendinitis, 1574
Tendinosis, 1574
Tendon, 1573
Tophaceous gout, 1605
Tophi (sing., tophus), 1602
Torus fracture, 1569
Toxic myopathy, 1612
Transchondral fracture, 1569
Transverse fracture, 1569
Volkmann ischemic contracture, 1575

REFERENCES

1. Dennison E, Mohamed MA, Cooper C: Epidemiology of osteoporosis, *Rheum Dis Clin North Am* 32(4):617, 2006.
2. Bielby R, Jones E, McGonagle D: The role of mesenchymal stem cells in maintenance and repair of bone, *Injury* 38(Suppl 1):S26, 2007.
3. Soma IL, Messer TM: Complications after treatment of flexor tendon injuries, *J Am Acad Orthop Surg* 14:387-396, 2006.
4. Jaworski C: Current understanding of tendinopathies and treatment options, *Am Fam Physician* 76(6):773, 2007.
5. Nirschl RP, Ashman ES: Elbow tendinopathy: tennis elbow, *Clin Sports Med* 22(4):813-836, 2003.
6. Shiri R et al: Prevalence and determinants of lateral and medial epicondylitis: a population study, *Am J Epidemiol* 164:1065, 2006.
7. Sirvanci M et al: Myositis ossificans of psoas muscle: magnetic resonance imaging findings, *Acta Radiol* 45(5):523-525, 2004.
8. Koya S, Crenshaw D, Agarwal A: Rhabdomyolysis and acute renal failure after fire ant bites, *J Gen Intern Med* 22(1):145, 2007.
9. Shinzato T et al: Cowfish (Umisuzume, *Lactoria diaphana*) poisoning with rhabdomyolysis, *Intern Med* 47(9):853, 2008.

10. Yasue H et al: Severe hypokalemia, rhabdomyolysis, muscle paralysis, and respiratory impairment in a hypertensive patient taking herbal medicine containing licorice, *Intern Med* 46(9):575, 2007.
11. Kashani A et al: Risks associated with statin therapy: a systematic overview of randomized clinical trials, *Circulation* 19:114, 2006.
12. Molokhia M et al: Statin induced myopathy and myalgia: time trend analysis and comparison of risk associated with statin class from 1991-2006, *PLoS ONE* 3(6):E2522, 2008.
13. Gourgiotis S et al: Acute limb compartment syndrome: a review, *J Surg Educ* 64(3):178, 2007.
14. Czerwiński E et al: Current understanding of osteoporosis according to the position of the World Health Organization (WHO) and International Osteoporosis Foundation, *Orthop Traumatol Rehabil* 9(4):337, 2007.
15. *Bone health and osteoporosis: a report of the surgeon general 2004.* Available online at: www.surgeongeneral.gov/library/bonehealth/.
16. Poole KE, Compston JE: Osteoporosis and its management, *BMJ* 333(7581): 2006.
17. Lewiecki EM, Laster AJ: Clinical review: clinical applications of vertebral fracture assessment by dual-energy x-ray absorptiometry, *J Clin Endocrinol Metab* 91(11):4215-4222, 2006.

18. Ott S: *Osteoporosis.* Available online: http://courses.washington.edu/bonephys/oprisk.html.
19. Barrett-Connor E et al: Osteoporosis and fracture risk of women of different ethnic groups, *J Bone Min Res* 20:185, 2005.
20. Hochberg MC: Racial differences in bone strength, *Trans Am Clin Climatol Assoc* 118:305, 2007.
21. Ngyuen TV et al: Bone loss, physical activity, and weight change in elderly women: the Dubbo Osteoporosis Epidemiology Study, *J Bone Miner Res* 13(9):1458-1467, 1998.
22. Brown M: Skeletal muscle and bone: effect of sex steroids and aging, *Adv Physiol Educ* 32(2):120, 2008.
23. Fogle RH et al: Ovarian androgen production in postmenopausal women, *J Cin Endocrinol Metab* 92(8):3040, 2007.
24. Kin CF et al: Experience of famine and bone health in post-menopausal women, *Int J Epidemiol* 36(5):1143, 2007.
25. Moskowitz RW, Kelly MA, Lewallen DG: Understanding osteoarthritis of the knee—causes and effects, *Am J Orthop* 33(2 Suppl):5-9, 2004.
26. Gao W, Dalton JT: Expanding the therapeutic use of androgens via selective androgen receptor modulators (SARMs), *Drug Discov Today* 12(5-6):241, 2007.
27. Korompilias AV et al: Transient osteoporosis, *J Am Acad Orthop Surg* 16(8):480, 2008.
28. Niimi R et al: Changes on bone mineral density in transient osteoporosis of the hip, *J Bone Joint Surg Br* 88(11):1438, 2006.
29. Xyda A et al: Postpartum bilateral transient osteoporosis of the hip: MR imaging findings in three cases, *Radiol Med* 113(5):689, 2008.
30. Hofbauer LC, Schoppet M: Clinical implications of the osteoprotegerin/RANKL/RANK System for bone and vascular diseases, *JAMA* 292(4):490-495, 2004.
31. Shoback D: Update in osteoporosis and metabolic bone disorders, *J Clin Endocrinol Metab* 92(3):747, 2007.
32. Khosla S, Melton LJ, Riggs BL: Clinical review 144: estrogen and the male skeleton, *J Clin Endocrinol Metab* 87(4):1443-1450, 2002.
33. Plotkin LI et al: Bisphosphonates and estrogens inhibit osteocyte apoptosis via distinct molecular mechanisms downstream of extracellular signal-regulated kinase activation, *J Biol Chem* 280(8):7317-7325, 2005.
34. Schwartz EM, Ritchlin CT: Clinical development of anti-RANKL therapy, *Arthritis Res Ther* 9(Suppl 1):S7, 2007.
34. ŽofkováI: Hormonal aspects of the muscle-bone unit, *Physiol Res* 57(Suppl 1):S159, 2008.
36. Seeman E: Structural basis of growth-related gain and age-related loss of bone strength, *Rheumtology (Oxford)* 47:iv2, 2008.
37. Genant HK, Engelke K, Prevrhal S: Advanced CT bone imaging in osteoporosis, *Rheumatology (Oxford)* 47(Suppl 4):iv9, 2008.
38. Yago MD et al: Intracellular magnesium: transport and regulation in epithelial secretory cells, *Front Biosci* 5:D602, 2000.
39. Khosla S, Westendorf JJ, Oursler MJ: Building bone to reverse osteoporosis and repair fractures, *Clin Invest* 118(2):431, 2008.
40. Gallagher JC: Advances in bone biology and new treatments for bone loss, *Maturitas* 60(1):65, 2008.
41. Fukumoto S: Physiological regulation and disorders of phosphate metabolism—pivotal role of fibroblast growth factor 23, *Intern Med* 47(5):337, 2008.
42. Emmett M: What does serum fibroblast growth factor 23 do in hemodialysis patients? *Kidney Inter* 73:3, 2008.
43. Endo I et al: Clinical usefulness of measurement of fibroblast growth factor 23 (FGF 23) in hypophosphatemic patients: proposal of diagnostic criteria using FGF 23 measurement, *Bone* 42(6):1235, 2008.
44. Lewiecki EM, Urig EL Jr, Williams RC Jr: Tumor-induced osteomalacia: lessons learned, *Arthritis Rheum* 58(3):773, 2008.
45. Layfield R: The molecular pathogenesis of Paget disease of bone, *Expert Rev Mol Med* 9(27):1, 2007.
46. Walsh JP: Paget's disease of bone, *Med J Aust* 181(5):262, 2004.
47. Chen WC et al: Spinal epidural abscess due to *Staphylococcus aureus*: clinical manifestations and outcomes, *J Microbiol Immunol Infect* 41(3):215, 2008.
48. Kapoor A et al: Magnetic resonance imaging for diagnosing foot osteomyelitis: a meta-analysis, *Arch Intern Med* 167(2):125, 2007.
49. Marina N et al: Biology and therapeutic advances for pediatric osteosarcoma, *Oncologist* 9(4):422-441, 2004.
50. Kivioja AH et al: Cement is recommended in intralesional surgery of giant cell tumors: a Scandinavian Sarcoma Group study of 294 patients followed for a median time of 5 years, *Acta Orthop* 9(2):86, 2008.
51. Abramson SB: Inflammation in osteoarthritis, *J Rheumatol* (Suppl) 70:70, 2004.
52. Alturfan AA et al: Increased serum sialic acid levels in primary osteoarthritis and inactive rheumatoid arthritis, *Tohoku J Exp Med* 213(3):241, 2007.
53. Krasnokutsky S, Samuels J, Abramson SB: Osteoarthritis in 2007, *Bull NYU Hosp Jt Dis* 65(3):222, 2007.
54. Rutsch F, Terkeltaub R: Deficiencies of physiologic calcification inhibitors and low grade inflammation in arterial calcification: lessons for cartilage calcification, *Joint Bone Spine* 72(2):110-118, 2005.
55. Hashimoto S et al: Chondrocyte-derived apoptotic bodies and calcification of articular cartilage, *Proc Natl Acad Sci* 95(6):3094-3099, 1998.
56. Fan Z et al: Activation of interleukin-1 signaling cascades in normal and osteoarthritic articular cartilage, *Am J Pathol* 171(3):938, 2007.
57. Barron MC, Rubin BR: Managing osteoarthritic knee pain, *J Am Osteopath Assoc* 107(10 Suppl 6):ES21, 2007.
58. Otero M, Goldring MB: Cells of the synovium in rheumatoid arthritis. Chondrocytes, *Arthritis Res Ther* 9(5):220, 2007.
59. Mauri C, Ehrenstein MR: Cells of the synovium in rheumatoid arthritis. B cells, *Arthritis Res Ther* 9(2):205, 2007.
60. Sweeney SE, Firestein GS: Rheumatoid arthritis: regulation of synovial inflammation, *Int J Biochem Cell Biol* 36(3):372-378, 2004.
61. Abeles AM, Pillinger MH: The role of the synovial fibroblast in rheumatoid arthritis: cartilage destruction and the regulation of matrix metalloproteinases, *Bull NYU Hosp Jt Dis* 64(1-2):20, 2006.
62. Alonso-Ruiz A et al: Tumor necrosis factor alpha drugs in rheumatoid arthritis: systematic review and meta-analysis of efficacy and safety, *BMC Musculoskelet Disord* 9:52, 2008.
63. Davis JC et al: Definition of disease duration in ankylosing spondylitis: reassessing the concept, *Ann Rheum Dis* 65(11):1518, 2006.
64. Tuite MJ: Sacroiliac joint imaging, *Semin Musculoskelet Radiol* 12(1):72, 2008.
65. Zochling J et al: Magnetic resonance imaging in ankylosing spondylitis, *Curr Opin Rheumatol* 19(4):346, 2007.
66. Ikbal M et al: Association of chromatid exchange frequencies in patients with ankylosing spondylitis with and without HLA-B27, *Ann Rheum Dis* 62(8):775, 2003.
67. Samji MF, Bafaquh M, Tsai E: The pathogenesis of ankylosing spondylitis, *Neurosurg Focus* 24(1):E3, 2008.
68. Katana RK, Brent LJ: Spondyloarthropathies, *Am Fam Physican* 60(12):3853, 2004.
69. Inman RD: Mechanisms of disease: infection and spondyloarthritis, *Nat Clin Pract Rheumatol* 2(3):163, 2006.
70. Ogrendik M: Treatment of ankylosing spondylitis with moxifloxacin, *South Med J* 100(4):366, 2007.
71. Pillinger MH, Rosenthal P, Abeles AM: Hyperuricemia and gout: new insights into pathogenesis and treatment, *Bull NYU Hosp Jt Dis* 65(3):215, 2007.
72. Nyhan WL: Lesch-Nyhan disease, *J Hist Neurosci* 14(1):1-10, 2005.
73. So A et al: A pilot study of IL-1 inhibition by anakinra in acute gout, *Arthritis Res Ther* 9(2):R28, 2007.
74. Leistad RB et al: Similarities in stress physiology among patients with chronic pain and headache disorders: evidence for a common pathophysiological mechanism? *J Headache Pain* 9(3):165, 2008.
75. Nilsen KB et al: Autonomic and muscular responses and recovery to one-hour laboratory mental stress in healthy subjects, *BMC Musculoskelet Disord* 8:81, 2007.
76. Meeus M, Nijs J: Central sensitization: a biopsychosocial explanation for chronic widespread pain in patients with fibromyalgia and chronic fatigue syndrome, *Clin Rheumatol* 26(4):46, 2007.
77. Bennett R: Myofacial pain syndromes and their evaluation, *Best Pract Res Clin Rheumatol* 21(3):427, 2007.
78. Dannecker EA, Knoll V, Robinson ME: Sex differences in muscle pain: self-care behaviors and effects on daily activities, *J Pain* 9(3):200, 2008.
79. Martinez-Lavin M: Biology and therapy of fibromyalgia. Stress, the stress response system, and fibromyalgia, *Arthritis Res Ther* 9(4):216, 2007.
80. Verbunt JA, Pernot DH, Smeets RJ: Disability and quality of life in patients with fibromyalgia, *Health Qual Life Outcomes* 6:8, 2008.
81. Buckwalter JA, Lappin DR: The disproportionate impact of chronic arthralgia and arthritis among women, *Clin Orthop* (372):159, 2000.
82. Mease PJ et al: A randomized, double-blind, placebo-controlled, phase III trial of pregabalin in the treatment of patients with fibromyalgia, *J Rheumatol* 35(3):502, 2008.

83. Centers for Disease Control: www.cdc.gov/cfs/draft_5yr_research_plan. htm. Accessed 6/2/2009.

84. Centers for Disease Control:http://www.cdcgov/cfs/cfsatrisk.htm. Accessed 6/2/2009.

85. Meeus M, Nijs J: Central sensitization: a biopsychosocial explanation for chronic widespread pain in patients with fibromyalgia and chronic fatigue syndrome, *Clin Rheumatol* 26(4):465, 2007.

86. Gur A, Oktayoglu P: Central nervous abnormalities in fibromyalgia nad chronic fatigue syndrome: new concepts in treatment, *Curr Pharm Des* 14(13):1274, 2008.

87. Lorusso L et al: Immunological aspects of chronic fatigue syndrome, *Autoimmun Rev* 8(4):287, 2009.

88. Fulle S et al: Specific correlations between muscle oxidative stress and chronic fatigue syndrome: a working hypothesis, *J Muscle Res Cell Motil* 28(6):355, 2007.

89. Centers for Disease Control: Toolkit: Fact sheets for healthcare professionals: basic CFS overview. www.cdc.gov/cfs/toolkit.htm, Accessed 06/02/09.

90. Powers SK, Kavazis AN, McClung JM: Oxidative stress and disuse muscle atrophy, *J Appl Physiol* 102(6):2389, 2007.

91. Koeberl DD, Kishnani PS, Chen YT: Glycogen storage disease type I and II: treatment updates, *J Inherit Metab Dis* 320:159, 2007.

92. Pereira SJ, Berditchevisky CR, Suely KNM: Report of the first Brazilian infantile Pompe disease patient to be treated with recombinant human acid alpha-glucosidase, *J Pediatr (Rio J)* 84(3):272, 2008.

93. Dorph C et al: Signs of inflammation in both symptomatic and asymptomatic muscles from patients with polymyositis and dermatomyositis, *Ann Rheum Dis* 65(12):1565, 2006.

94. Koenig M et al: Heterogeneity of autoantibodies in 100 patients with autoimmune myositis: insights into clinical features and outcomes, *Arthritis Res Ther* 9(4):R78, 2007.

95. Walsh RJ et al: Type 1 interferon-inducible gene expression in blood is present and reflects disease activity in dermatomyositis and polymyositis, *Arthritis Rheum* 56(11):3784, 2007.

96. Bradshaw EM et al: A local antigen-driven humoral response is present in the inflammatory myopathies, *J Immunol* 178(1):547, 2007.

97. Chung YL et al: Creatine supplements in patients with idiopathic inflammatory myopathies who are clinically weak after conventional pharmacologic treatment: six-month, double-blind, randomized, placebo-controlled trial, *Arthritis Rheum* 57(4):694, 2007.

98. Scola RH et al: Toxic myopathies: muscle biopsy features, *Arg Neuropsiquiatr* 65(1):82, 2007.

99. Urbano-Marquez A, Fernandez-Sola J: Effects of alcohol on skeletal and cardiac muscle, *Muscle Nerve* 30(6):689-707, 2004.

ALTERATIONS OF MUSCULOSKELETAL FUNCTION IN CHILDREN

KRISTEN LEE CARROLL

43

MEDIA RESOURCES

evolve **Evolve Website** (http://evolve.elsevier.com/McCance/)
- Review Questions and Answers
- Animations
- Glossary (with audio pronunciation for selected terms)
- WebLinks

CHAPTER OUTLINE

MUSCULOSKELETAL DEVELOPMENT IN CHILDREN
  Bone Formation
  Bone Growth
  Skeletal Development
  Muscle Growth
MUSCULOSKELETAL ALTERATIONS IN CHILDREN
  Congenital Defects
  Abnormal Density or Modeling of the Skeleton

Bone Infection: Osteomyelitis
Juvenile Rheumatoid Arthritis
Avascular Diseases of the Bone: Osteochondrosis
Cerebral Palsy
Muscular Dystrophy
Musculoskeletal Tumors in Children
NONACCIDENTAL TRAUMA

Musculoskeletal alterations in children are very common. They may be congenital, such as clubfoot; hereditary, such as muscular dystrophy; or acquired, such as Legg-Calvé-Perthes disease. Some of these disorders are acute, and the child will recover completely; other disorders are chronic or, in some cases, terminal. An understanding of the pathophysiology of these alterations will aid in providing the best care possible for these children.

MUSCULOSKELETAL DEVELOPMENT IN CHILDREN

Bone Formation

Bone formation, which begins at about the sixth week of gestation, involves two phases: (1) the delivery of bone cell precursors to sites of bone formation and (2) the aggregation of these cells at **primary centers of ossification,** where they mature and begin to secrete osteoid (see Chapter 41). Some of the bone cell precursors are present in fetal connective tissues, whereas others migrate in blood to sites of bone formation after blood vessels have grown into the tissue.

Cellular aggregation and maturation occur in two types of fetal tissue, depending on which bones are being formed. The cranium, facial bones, clavicles, and parts of the jawbone (classically called "flatbones") arise from a fetal membrane termed the *mesenchyme.* Bones that develop on or within the mesenchyme grow by the process of **intramembranous formation of bone.** As the mesenchyme becomes vascularized, the immature bone cells aggregate and mature into osteoblasts, which form the centers of ossification. Osteoblasts secrete osteoid, which surrounds them and quickly ossifies, forming the lacunae and canaliculi of compact bone. Spicules of bone radiate from the ossification centers to form the primary trabeculae characteristic of spongy bone. Later, some of the spongy bone is replaced by compact bone.

Endochondral formation of bone is the development of new bone from cartilage (Figure 43-1). First, mesenchymal tissue forms a **cartilage anlage,** which defines the shape of the bone. This is usually found by 6 weeks of gestation. Blood vessel invasion to the inside the anlage brings osteoprogenitor cells leading to primary centers of calcification by 8 weeks. Endochondral bone formation begins in the outer layer of the cartilage model, which consists of a layer of dense connective tissue called **perichondrium.** The perichondrium contains cells that develop into osteoblasts, forming a collar of bone,

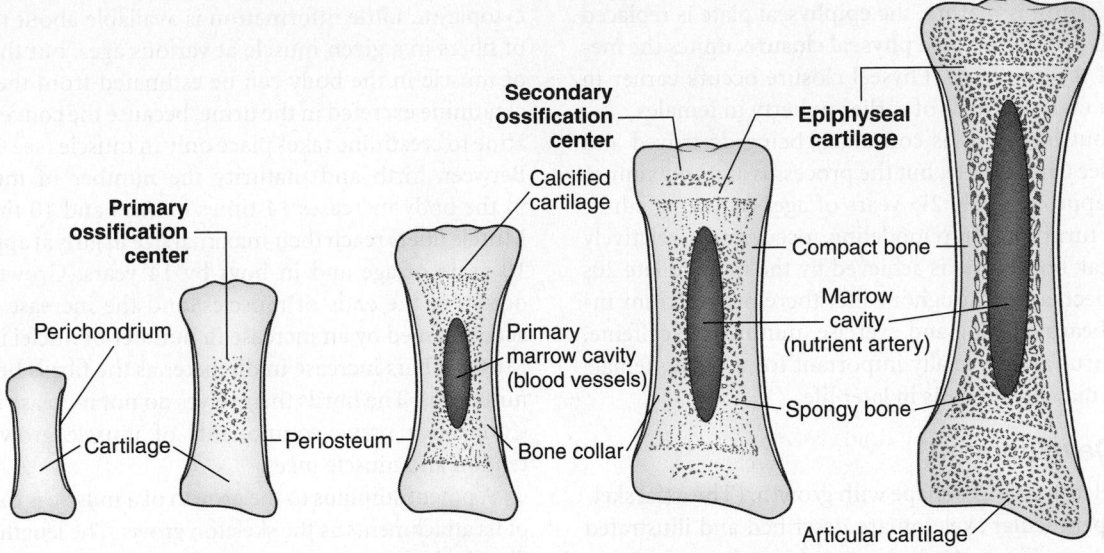

Figure 43-1 Stages of endochondral bone formation and centers of ossification in long bone.

termed the **periosteal collar,** around the cartilage model. Cartilage enclosed within the periosteal collar degenerates, and capillaries from outside the perichondrium invade the degenerating cartilage cells, carrying with them osteoblast precursors from the inner layer of the perichondrium and osteoclast precursors from the blood itself.

Endochondral bone formation progresses at the primary center of ossification in the middle of the cartilage model and extends toward either end of the developing bone. At the same time, the periosteal collar thickens and becomes wider toward the epiphyses. By the end of gestation **secondary centers of ossification** (i.e., the epiphyseal centers) begin to lay down bone at both ends of the cartilage model. Here, too, cartilage within the periosteal collar degenerates, and blood vessels grow inward, delivering bone cell precursors. Once the osteoblasts begin to secrete osteoid, ossification spreads from the secondary centers in all directions until all the cartilage within the model is replaced by bone.

Two regions of cartilage remain at the ends of long bones: (1) articular cartilage over the free ends of the bone and (2) the physeal plate, a layer of cartilage between the metaphysis and epiphysis. (These structures are described and illustrated in Chapter 41; see Figure 41-3.) The physeal plate retains the ability to form and calcify new cartilage and deposit bone until the skeleton matures roughly 1 year after sexual maturity (11 to 15 years of age in females, 15 to 18 in males).

Bone Growth

Until adult stature is reached, growth in the length of bone occurs at the physeal plate through endochondral ossification. Cartilage cells at the epiphyseal side of the physeal plate multiply and enlarge. As rapidly as new cartilage cells form, cartilage cells at the metaphyseal side of the plate are destroyed and replaced by bone.

In the shaft of new bone, where growth is relatively slow, the bone produced by accretion is compact and dense. The compact bone is thickest where it has to withstand the maximal stresses, which generally occur in the middle of the shaft.

The two physes of the long bone often have varying activity rates. For example, the distal physis in the femur contributes 80% of the overall length, whereas the proximal physis at the hip contributes only 20%. The more active of the two has more power to remodel deformity but also can be more sensitive to injury. The architecture of the physis also dictates its sensitivity to injury. The distal femur, for example, has an undulating pattern that increases its resistance to sheer force; when injured, however, growth disturbance is highly likely, whereas the distal radius, which contributes 80% of overall radial length, is a flat, smooth physis that is far more resistant to traumatic injury.

Growth in the diameter of bone occurs by deposition of new bone on an existing bone surface. Bone matrix is laid down by osteoblasts on the periosteal surface and subsequently becomes calcified. At the same time, bone resorption occurs on the endosteal surface. Endosteal resorption increases the diameter of the medullary cavity, which contains marrow and spongy bone.

Many factors affect the development, physiology, and rate of growth of the epiphyseal plate. Growth hormone must be secreted by the pituitary gland at a constant rate to stimulate the growth plate consistently. Other known factors affecting growth include peptide regulatory factors (e.g., fibroblast growth factor [FGF]); changes in cell-to-cell interactions through cell adhesion molecules (CAMs) and cell junctions; and complex interactions or changes in extracellular matrix (ECM), nutrition, general health, and other hormones (e.g., thyroid hormone, adrenal and gonadal androgens, estrogens). These factors influence both the rate of bone growth and the time of appearance of the secondary ossification centers.

When the skeleton is mature, the epiphyseal plate is replaced by bone. This process, termed **physeal closure,** unites the metaphysis and the epiphysis. Physeal closure occurs earlier in females than males because of earlier puberty in females.

Throughout life, bone is constantly being destroyed and re-formed (see Chapter 41), but the process is at its maximum in children approximately 2½ years of age. By young adulthood, bone turnover, or remodeling, occurs at a relatively slow rate. Peak bone mass is achieved by the mid- to late 20s and slowly decreases throughout life; therefore, calcium intake, weightbearing lifting and exercise, minimizing caffeine, and phosphorus are especially important for a young female if she is to avoid osteoporosis in later life.

Skeletal Development

The axial skeleton changes shape with growth. (The axial skeleton and appendicular skeleton are described and illustrated in Chapter 41; see Figure 41-5). In a newborn the entire spine is concave anteriorly, or **kyphosed.** In the first 3 months of life, with the infant's ability to control the head, the upper (cervical) spine begins to arch, or become **lordotic.** The normal lordotic curve of the lower (lumbar) spine begins to develop with sitting.

The appendicular skeleton (the extremities) grows faster during childhood than does the axial skeleton (see Figure 41-5). The newborn has a relatively large head and long spine with disproportionately shorter limbs than an adult. By 1 year of age, 50% of the total growth of the spine has occurred and is more than 70% complete by age 8.[1] Therefore, failure of the spine to grow (e.g., spinal fusion) does not limit eventual height as much as the premature fusion of the growth plates of the lower extremities. In children with congenital curvature of the spine, growth tends to worsen the deformity rather than to increase the length of the spine.

Besides getting longer, growing bones of the extremities undergo changes in rotation and alignment. In the newborn the proximal femur is rotated forward up to 40 degrees and the tibia is rotated inward. With growth the femur assumes its normal alignment (by 8 years of age) and tibial rotation neutralizes at 5 years of age. Bowlegs and knock knees are normal at certain stages of growth. At birth the newborn's legs are bowed because of stresses in utero. **Genu varum (bowleg)** reaches a peak by 30 months of age, whereas **genu valgum (knock knee)** maximizes by 5 to 6 years of age. If genu varum or genu valgum persists past these ages, a pathologic process rather than a physiologic phase may be present. Pathologic causes of genu varum are Blount disease, rickets, skeletal dysplasias (such as achondroplastic dwarfism), and traumatic injury. Genu valgum may persist also as a result of skeletal dysplasia or genetic predisposition.

Muscle Growth

The composition and size of muscles vary with age. In the fetus, muscle tissue contains a large amount of water and much intercellular matrix. After birth, both are reduced considerably as the muscle fibers (cells) enlarge by accumulating cytoplasm. Little information is available about the numbers of fibers in a given muscle at various ages, but the total mass of muscle in the body can be estimated from the amount of creatinine excreted in the urine, because the conversion of creatine to creatinine takes place only in muscle (see Chapter 41). Between birth and maturity the number of muscle nuclei in the body increases 14 times in boys and 10 times in girls. Muscle fibers reach their maximal size in girls at approximately 10 years of age and in boys by 14 years. Growth in length occurs at the ends of muscles, and the increase in length is accompanied by an increase in number of nuclei in the fibers. Muscle fibers increase in diameter as the fibrils become more numerous. The fibrils themselves do not increase in diameter. Connective tissue components of muscle grow where the tendon and muscle meet.

A potent stimulus to the growth of a muscle is the separation of its attachments as the skeleton grows. The length of a muscle fiber is the direct consequence of the range of movement it is called on to perform. The stimulus for the formation of a tendon is probably the pull of the muscle rudiment on undifferentiated connective tissue. The repair of a tendon from which a segment has been removed does not occur if the muscle is prevented from exercising tension on the damaged tendon. Replacement of muscle by bone (myositis ossificans) sometimes is the result of limitation of movement. If the normal opponents of a muscle are paralyzed, the muscle fails to grow properly, and it may be that the full development of a muscle depends on the progressive rise in the tension exerted on it by its antagonists.

Muscle growth during adolescence is a major factor in weight gain. Gender differences in muscle size and weight are minor in childhood but become considerable with the onset of puberty.

In the infant, muscle accounts for approximately 25% of total body weight, compared with 40% in the adult. In the adult, approximately 55% of muscle weight is in the lower limb muscles, whereas in the infant the majority of the weight is axial musculature. The respiratory and facial muscles are well developed at birth so that the infant can perform the vital functions of breathing and sucking. Other muscle groups, such as the pelvic muscles, take several years to develop fully. Throughout life the weight of the skeletal muscles can be increased by exercise. Less is known about the development of visceral and cardiac muscle. Visceral muscle fibers increase in number and size, but the increase in fiber size is most important. Fiber enlargement alone can increase the bulk of visceral muscle by as many as eight times. Cardiac muscle also grows mainly by enlargement of existing fibers.

MUSCULOSKELETAL ALTERATIONS IN CHILDREN

Congenital Defects

Syndactyly

The most common congenital defect of the upper extremity is **syndactyly,** or webbing of the fingers (Figure 43-2). Simple webbing involves the soft-tissue envelope alone and is best released surgically when the child is 1 to 2 years of age. Complex syndactyly involves fusion of the bones and nails as well as the soft tissues; it may be associated with absence or anomaly of bony or neurovascular units. The primary goal in surgical correction of these defects is to achieve maximal function and appearance. Ideally, corrective surgery is deferred until the child is 6 to 12 months of age and completed before the child enters school. **Vestigial tabs,** such as an extra digit, however, are best removed during the immediate neonatal period. Anomalies on the medial or radial aspect of the arm are often associated with abnormalities of blood, heart, or kidneys. Lateral or ulnar-sided defects are less often associated with systemic anomalies and are far more rare.

Developmental Dysplasia of the Hip

Developmental dysplasia of the hip (DDH), formerly known as congenital dislocation of the hip, is an abnormality in the development of the proximal femur, acetabulum, or both. Although most often present at birth, it may occur at any time in the newborn or infant period.

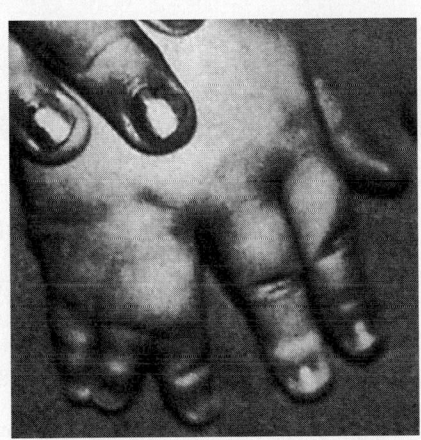

Figure 43-2 Syndactyly with polydactyly.

The incidence of true dislocation of the hip or a dislocatable hip is 1 in 1000 live births. Some degree of instability of the hip is present in approximately 10 per 1000 live births. The left hip is affected in 60% of cases, whereas the right hip alone is affected only 20% of the time. Bilateral DDH occurs 20% of the time.

Risk factors for DDH include family history, female sex (6:1), metatarsus adductus (20%), torticollis (10%), oligohydramnios, first pregnancy, and breech presentation. First pregnancies and oligohydramnios (deficient volume of amniotic fluid) are thought to limit fetal movement, and breech presentation not only limits movement but also places the hips in a position of flexion and adduction. Although only 2% of births have breech history, as many as 40% of infants with DDH had a breech birth. Maternal hormones that reportedly increase joint laxity also have an effect on DDH, although the exact mechanism is unknown. DDH also is more common in whites and those cultures that swaddle infants with the hips in extension and adduction. It is almost unknown in African cultures where infants are carried, with legs abducted, on the back.

PATHOPHYSIOLOGY The hip can be described as subluxated, dislocatable, or dislocated (Figure 43-3). The subluxated hip maintains contact with the acetabulum but is not well seated within the hip joint. The acetabulum is often dysplastic (or shallow) and the femur is often normal. The dislocatable hip is sometimes located but can be dislocated easily. The dislocated hip has no contact between the femoral head and the acetabulum. Some degree of acetabular dysplasia is present in almost all cases. Typically the acetabulum is shallow or sloping rather than cup shaped.

By approximately 10 weeks of gestation, the femur, acetabulum, and hip joint capsule are well developed. It appears that most dysplasias occur within the second and third trimesters and are often the result of positioning factors. Experimentally, DDH can be produced in laboratory animals by placing the developing hip in adduction and extension, replicating the breech position. There is, however, a genetic component that is poorly understood. In addition, 2% of DDH

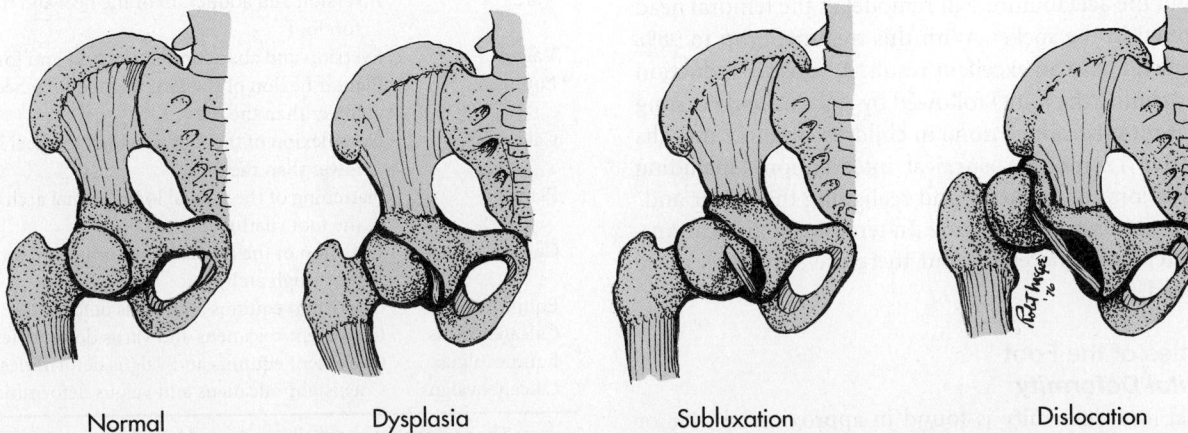

Normal   Dysplasia   Subluxation   Dislocation

Figure 43-3 Configuration and relationship of structures in developmental dysplasia of the hip. (From Hockenberry MJ: *Wong's nursing care of infants and children,* ed 8, St Louis, 2007, Mosby.)

cases are teratologic or caused by a systemic syndrome, such as arthrogryposis or spina bifida, in which muscle contracture or imbalance leads to DDH.

If DDH is left untreated in the growing child, secondary changes occur. If the hip is left subluxated or dislocated, the acetabulum becomes increasingly shallow and the soft tissues shorten about the proximal femur. If the hip is dislocated, the bone acetabulum fills with soft tissue and a false acetabulum forms where the femoral head contacts the iliac crest. An apparent limb length inequity and hip muscle weakness occurs, leading to a waddling gait. The subluxation leads to early osteoarthritis (OA), and it is now estimated that at least 60% of all OA of the hip is related to DDH.[2]

CLINICAL MANIFESTATIONS The clinical manifestations of DDH vary with the severity of the condition and the age of the child. Signs and symptoms that should be noted include the following:

1. Asymmetry of gluteal or thigh folds
2. Limb length discrepancy (Galeazzi sign)
3. Limitation of hip abduction
4. Positive Ortolani sign (clunk of dislocation)
5. Positive Barlow test (clunk of reduction)
6. Positive Trendelenburg gait (waddling)
7. Pain (very late)

The child also should be examined for other anomalies, such as torticollis or metatarsus adductus, which can be associated with DDH.

EVALUATION AND TREATMENT In the newborn period clinical examination is the most important diagnostic tool. Real-time ultrasound, in which the hip is examined while the ultrasound is performed, also is extremely valuable in the newborn period, especially in high-risk infants. The use of ultrasound allows visualization of the cartilaginous structures of the hip (the femoral head and the outer lip of the acetabulum), which are not seen on plain roentgenogram. Radiographs are used after age 6 months.[3]

Treatment depends on the age of the child, severity of dysplasia, and duration of dysplasia. The earlier that treatment is begun, the better the result. In children less than 4 months of age, a Pavlik harness can brace the hip in abduction and flexion, and the acetabulum will remodel as the femoral head rests centered in the socket. With this treatment, up to 98% of children will have an excellent result. A "closed" reduction (without opening the joint) followed by spica or body casting for up to 3 months can be done in children up to 12 months of age. After 12 months, surgical intervention—including opening the joint and cutting and realigning the femur and/or acetabulum—may be required. In teratologic dislocations, bracing often is unsuccessful and therefore surgery is more often needed.

Deformities of the Foot
Congenital Deformity

Congenital foot deformity is found in approximately 4% of all newborns, and metatarsus adductus accounts for 75% of these deformities (Table 43-1). **Metatarsus adductus** is a forefoot adduction deformity associated with a normal, plantigrade hindfoot and is believed to be secondary to intrauterine positioning. Metatarsus adductus is usually classified by two criteria: flexibility (passively correctable or rigid) and degree of deformity. The degree of deformity (mild, moderate, severe) is ascertained by the heel bisection line. A mild deformity is one in which the heel bisection line passes medial to the third toe; moderate, through the third or fourth toes; and severe, lateral to the fourth toe. It should be emphasized that a majority of children are well served by expectant treatment rather than early surgical intervention. Serial casts during the first 6 months of life are suggested for moderate to severe deformities and those deformities that appear less flexible. Casts are changed weekly for 6 to 12 weeks. Eighty-seven percent of children usually correct spontaneously by 6 years of age and 95% by 15 years of age. Even in those children with some residual deformity and an oblique medial cuneiform, they are rarely symptomatic.

Equinovarus Deformity

There are three types of equinovarus (clubfoot): positional equinovarus, idiopathic congenital equinovarus, and teratologic equinovarus (Figure 43-4). The true positional

Table 43-1	Terms Used to Describe Foot Abnormalities
Term	**Definition**
Position	
Abduction	Lateral deviation away from the midline of the body
Adduction	Lateral deviation toward the midline of the body
Eversion	Twisting of the foot outward along its long axis
Inversion	Twisting of the foot inward on its long axis
Dorsiflexion	Bending the foot upward and backward
Plantar flexion	Bending of the foot downward and forward
Abnormality	
Talipes	Congenital abnormality of the foot (clubfoot)
Pes	Acquired deformity of the foot
Varus	Inversion and adduction of the heel and the forefoot
Valgus	Eversion and abduction of the heel and forefoot
Equinus	Plantar flexion of the foot in which the heel is lower than the toes
Calcaneus	Dorsiflexion of the foot in which the heel is lower than the toes
Planus	Flattening of the medial longitudinal arch of the foot (flatfoot)
Cavus	Elevation of the medial longitudinal arch of the foot (high arch)
Equinovarus	Coexistent equinus and varus deformities
Calcaneovarus	Coexistent calcaneus and varus deformities
Equinovalgus	Coexistent equinus and valgus deformities
Calcaneovalgus	Coexistent calcaneus and valgus deformities

NOTE: The position listed can all be achieved by voluntary movement of the normal foot; an abnormality exists if the foot is fixed in one or more of the positions while at rest.

equinovarus lends itself to rapid correction by application of serial casts. The idiopathic variety is treated by attempting cast correction, followed by surgical intervention of resistant deformities. Teratologic equinovarus nearly always requires surgical correction and/or muscle balancing procedures.

Positional Equinovarus. **Positional equinovarus** is a deformity in which an infant's foot is in equinovarus position but does not have a deep posterior or plantar medial crease. It appears to be secondary only to intrauterine position. The foot can be passively brought to a plantigrade position and is amenable to casting. In general, 1 to 3 months of serial above-knee casting corrects this foot without the need for surgical intervention.

Idiopathic Congenital Equinovarus. The etiology of idiopathic equinovarus (clubfoot) is unknown. In one human fetal study, all clubfeet were associated with identifiable anterior horn cell changes in L5 and S1. Enterovirus infection, known to cause anterior horn cell damage if intrauterine, reaches a peak prevalence in the summer or fall of temperate climates. These two seasons correlate with the peaks of conception in children with clubfeet. Muscle biopsies of both the anterior tibialis long flexors and peroneus brevis muscles in clubfoot reveal that at least 50% of cases show a decreased number of muscle fibers and/or abnormal fiber histology. The soleus often has an increase in type 1 fibers, whereas the peroneus brevis has a fiber type disproportion. The more abnormal the histopathology is, the more severe the deformity, and the greater the chance of recurrent deformity after treatment. In addition to neurologic causes, positional abnormalities (e.g., oligohydramnios) have been implicated. The genetic component is unclear and studies are ongoing.

Idiopathic equinovarus occurs in approximately 1 of every 1000 live births, with males being affected twice as often as females. Although these deformities have been historically treated nonoperatively, surgical intervention became much more common after 1950. Over the past 10 years, nonoperative management has again become the mainstay. Ignacio Ponseti developed a casting technique that has been used for more than 50 years. Although used in Iowa since 1950, it was not well accepted nationally until recently. The technique involves six casts, left on for 5 to 7 days each, followed by a percutaneous tendoachilles lengthening procedure performed with local anesthesia in the clinic. The child then uses braces until 3 years of age. Noncompliance with braces leads to increased recurrence. Nearly 20% of children may need an anterior tibialis transfer around age 3.[4] Studies comparing operative posteromedial release with Ponseti techniques show better long-term results with the less invasive Ponseti method[5] (see What's New? Ponseti Casting).

Teratologic Equinovarus. The most common causes of **teratologic equinovarus** are either neuromuscular (such as spina bifida) or syndromic, as in arthrogryposis or osteochondrodysplasia (such as diastrophic dwarfism). The teratologic clubfoot, unlike the idiopathic type, usually fails to be corrected with casting protocols and requires operative intervention. The surgery is often more extensive than that for an idiopathic clubfoot, and revision surgery is also more common.

Pes Planus (Flatfoot) Deformity. **Pes planus** (flatfoot) commonly raises parental concern. Despite medical evidence to the contrary, it can be very difficult to convince families that a flexible flatfoot is as functional as the one with a "normal" arch. The majority of babies are born with flat (or "fat") feet, with the arch becoming more apparent with age. The relatively benign natural history, however, should not overshadow the importance of accurate diagnosis. Significant ankle valgus, vertical talus, tarsal coalition, and skewfoot must be accurately differentiated from flexible pes planus.

Flexible flatfoot deformity appears to be familial, with occasional association of generalized ligamentous laxity. Careful evaluation of possible occult Achilles contracture is done by holding the hindfoot in varus position and dorsiflexing the ankle. Achilles contracture can signify a more severe flatfoot variant. The flexibility of the hindfoot is evaluated by having the child stand on his or her toes or by dorsiflexing the first toe passively with the child in a non-weightbearing position. This "windlass mechanism" tightens the plantar fascia, thereby reconstituting an arch and hindfoot varus if the foot is indeed flexible. If hindfoot flexibility and an "underlying" arch are present, then flexible flatfoot is diagnosed.

By all recent data, the surgical or orthotic treatment of *asymptomatic* flexible pes planus is unnecessary. Custom orthotics, Helfet heel cups, and corrective orthopedic shoes may

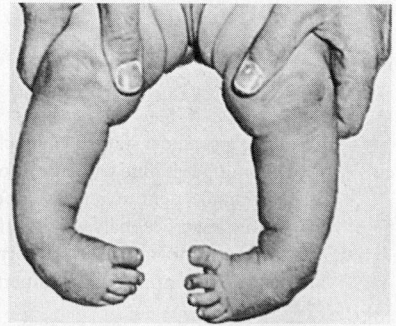

Figure 43-4 Infant with bilateral congenital talipes equinovarus. (From Brashear HR, Raney RB: *Shand's handbook of orthopedic surgery*, ed 9, St Louis, 1978, Mosby.)

WHAT'S NEW? Ponseti Casting

Ponseti casting implements toe-to-groin casts changed weekly for 6 weeks. Casting begins as early as possible after birth and culminates in a percutaneous tendoachilles lengthening in the clinic, followed by a final cast worn for 3 weeks. In recalcitrant cases, a full surgical posteromedial release (PMR) still may be required. The need for PMR in idiopathic clubfoot has decreased from 90% to less than 20% of infants when this casting technique is used. Long-term results, presumably because of less scarring and more long-term flexibility, are better with Ponseti casting than the PMR method.

relieve discomfort but will have no influence over the natural history (clinically or radiographically) of flat feet. Adult studies on army recruits have shown that soldiers with flat feet perform just as well as their counterparts without "fallen" arches.

There is a small subset of children with painful flexible flat feet. For these children careful attention to the possibility of Achilles contracture or tarsal coalition (congenital union of the hindfoot bones) must be made. This small group of children is best treated with inexpensive shoe inserts and then expectantly watched. If pain continues into adolescence, requiring more aggressive treatment, calcaneal lengthening will correct the pes planus without decreasing hindfoot motion. In rigid flat feet, a computed tomographic (CT) scan often will reveal coalition—if painful, this can be resected. Heel cord contractures can be surgically lengthened because stretching alone is often inadequate. All surgery carries risk; if a foot is flat but nonpainful, treatment is not required. The painless flatfoot should be viewed as a variation of normal feet.

Abnormal Density or Modeling of the Skeleton

Osteogenesis Imperfecta

Osteogenesis imperfecta (OI) (brittle bone disease) is a genetic disorder of connective tissues that affects primarily bone. The disorder was first described in 1840 as a syndrome in newborns that consisted of osteoporosis with fractures and skeletal deformities. The Sillence classification is based on both models of inheritance and clinical findings (Table 43-2). In the most severe form of this disorder, the child is usually stillborn or dies soon after birth, although some survive into childhood. OI in its more severe forms is evident at birth because fractures and deformity have occurred in utero. The less severe forms may not become evident until the child begins to walk. Some children with this milder form then experience numerous fractures and can be mistaken for battered children until the diagnosis is made.

The prevalence rate of the most common form is about 1 in 30,000. Inheritance is usually autosomal dominant but can be autosomal recessive. At least four syndromes have been identified that have various clinical manifestations and prognoses (see Table 43-2).

PATHOPHYSIOLOGY The major errors in OI lie in the synthesis of collagen. Genetic studies have shown that the gene responsible for the encoding of collagen easily mutates. These mutations cause osteogenesis imperfecta. The large range of phenotypes includes all mutants of the two collagen structural genes. (Genes are discussed in Chapter 4.) Abnormalities in collagen include (1) an increase in collagen hydroxylysine residue in bones; (2) a decrease in hydroxylysine-norleucine in skin collagen; and (3) absence of α-polypeptide production in cultured skin fibroblasts.[6]

A number of metabolic abnormalities have been reported. Some individuals have increased serum thyroxine levels, suggesting hyperthyroidism. This is consistent with the findings of

Type	Transmission	Main Biochemical Defect	Orthopedic	Miscellaneous
IA	AD	Decreased production of type I collagen	Mild to moderate bone fragility, osteoporosis, normal stature	Blue sclera, hearing loss, easy bruising, dentinogenesis imperfecta absent
IB	AD		Short stature	More severe in IA with dentinogenesis imperfecta
II	AD, AR, and mosaic	Substitutions of glycyl residue in X1 or X2 chains in triple helix	Multiple intrauterine fractures, extreme bone fragility	Usually lethal in perinatal period, delayed ossification of skull, intrauterine growth restriction
IIA			Long bones broad, crumpled; ribs broad with continuous beading	
IIB			Long bones broad, crumpled, ribs discontinuous or beading	
IIC			Long bones thin, fractured; ribs thin, beaded	
IID			Severely osteoporotic with generally well-formed skeleton; normal-shaped vertebrae and pelvis	
III	AD and AR (rare)	Abnormal type I collagen	Progressive deforming phenotype, severe bone fragility with fractures	Hearing loss, short stature, blue sclerae becoming less blue with age, shortened life expectancy, dentinogenesis imperfecta, relative macrocephaly with triangular facies
IVA	AD	Shortened pro–α (I)-chains	Mild to moderate bone fragility, osteoporosis, bowing of long bones, scoliosis	Light sclerae, normal hearing, normal dentition, dentinogenesis imperfecta absent
IVB	AD			Dentinogenesis imperfecta present

Table 43-2   Sillence Classification of Osteogenesis Imperfecta Syndromes

Reproduced with permission from Vaccaro AR (ed): *Orthopaedic knowledge update 8.* Rosemont IL, American Academy of Orthopaedic Surgeons, 2005.
AD, Autosomal dominant; *AR,* autosomal recessive.

increased sweating, heat intolerance, increased body temperature, a resting tachycardia, and tachypnea. The hyperthyroid findings, however, are not consistent in all individuals with OI. Studies of leukocyte metabolism suggest an uncoupling of oxidative phosphorylation. Reports of alterations of platelet function with defects in adhesion and clot retraction also exist.

CLINICAL MANIFESTATIONS The classic clinical manifestations of OI are osteoporosis and increased rate of fractures, possible bony deformation, triangular facies, possible vascular weakness (i.e., aortic aneurysm), possible blue sclera, and poor dentition. The Sillence classification designated types I through IV based on severity. The most severe, types II and III, are comparable to *osteogenesis imperfecta congenita*. These two types are characterized by autosomal recessive inheritance and early onset of manifestations. Both can cause stillbirth or severe neonatal deformity and a short life expectancy. Less severe are types I and IV, which are comparable to *osteogenesis imperfecta tarda*. Type I is slightly more common than types II and III, and type IV is quite rare. Types I and IV are inherited as autosomal dominant traits and vary in age of onset from birth to adulthood. Type IV, especially when the sclera are white, is the least deforming type and is often confused with nonaccidental trauma (child abuse).

EVALUATION AND TREATMENT Evaluation of OI is based on clinical manifestations and serologic tests. Serum alkaline phosphatase is elevated in all forms of the disease. Osteogenesis imperfecta can be diagnosed prenatally by ultrasound or chorionic villi sampling. Quantitative analysis of cultured skin fibroblast collagen by electrophoresis shows a decreased quantity of collagen in the affected individual.

Type II OI is often terminal in the perinatal period, and therefore little is known about appropriate treatment for the few children who survive. For other types of OI, careful positioning and handling of the newborn may prevent fractures. Beyond the neonatal period, various orthopedic measures are applied, such as prompt splinting of fractures and correction of deformities arising from the progressive bowing or bending of the skeleton by intermedullary rodding of the bones (Figure 43-5). Newer, telescoping rods, which grow with the child, have been shown to reduce the reoperative rate by 30%.[7] Scoliosis is present in up to 50% of Sillence III and often requires surgery. A multicenter study of a bisphosphonate therapy showed promising results in type III OI, with marked improvements of bone density (up to 30%). Despite these results, there is concern that the healing of fractures and surgical intervention can be more difficult. More study is needed to address the efficacy and safety of these types of drugs. Genetic counseling for affected families should aim at primary prevention.

Rickets

Rickets is a disorder in which growing bone fails to become mineralized (ossified), resulting in "soft" bones and skeletal deformity. Rickets results from either insufficient vitamin D, insensitivity to vitamin D, wasting of vitamin D by the kidney, or inability to absorb vitamin D and calcium in the gut. In industrialized nations the most common X-linked dominant form is hypophosphatemic rickets. Although in the past few years, as exclusive breast-feeding for a lengthy period has been encouraged, vitamin D deficiency has been increasing. This is especially problematic when the mother is vitamin D deficient.[8] Although unprotected exposure to ultraviolet rays is not suggested, children still need 15 to 20 minutes per week of true sun exposure to activate vitamin D, the mineral necessary for absorption and metabolism of calcium and phosphate. Rickets in the immature skeleton leads to broad, irregular growth plates because the rows of cells in the growth plate that are intended to ossify fail to do so as they reach the metaphysis (Figure 43-6).

Children with rickets are often listless and irritable. They have hypotonia and muscle weakness and may be unable to walk without support. Abnormal parietal flattening and frontal bossing occur in the skull. The calvaria become soft, and the sutures may widen. Cartilaginous attachments of the ribs become prominent, and the long bones of the extremities (tibia, femur, radius, ulna) may be bowed. Growth is restricted, and fractures are common.

Like osteogenesis imperfecta, surgical treatment of bony deformity is often required. However, medical management of calcium, phosphorus, and vitamin D levels must be optimized before surgical intervention. Deformity often improves with normalization of bone metabolism.

Scoliosis

Scoliosis is a rotational curvature of the spine most obvious in the anteroposterior plane (Figure 43-7). It can be classified as nonstructural or structural. **Nonstructural scoliosis** results from a cause other than the spine itself, such as posture, leg length discrepancy, or pain. **Structural scoliosis** is curvature of the spine associated with vertebral rotation. Nonstructural scoliosis can become structural if the underlying cause is not found and treated.

Structural scoliosis can be caused by a great variety of conditions. It can result from congenital skeletal abnormalities (15%), neuromuscular diseases (15%), trauma, extraspinal contractures, bone infections that involve the vertebrae, metabolic bone disorders (e.g., rickets, osteoporosis, osteogenesis imperfecta), joint disease, and tumors. Most cases of structural scoliosis, however, have no known cause, although genetic factors are suggested. Structural scoliosis with no known cause, termed **idiopathic scoliosis**, accounts for at least 65% of cases.

Idiopathic scoliosis is classified as infantile, juvenile, or adolescent, depending on the child's age at the time of onset. In infantile scoliosis, spinal curvature develops during the first 3 years of life; in juvenile scoliosis, curvature develops between the skeletal age of 4 years and the onset of adolescence; and in adolescent scoliosis, it develops after the skeletal age of 10. Adolescent idiopathic scoliosis is the most common. Scoliosis in its milder forms occurs equally in boys and girls once curves measure more than 15 degrees; however, girls are 5 times more likely to have scoliosis than boys.

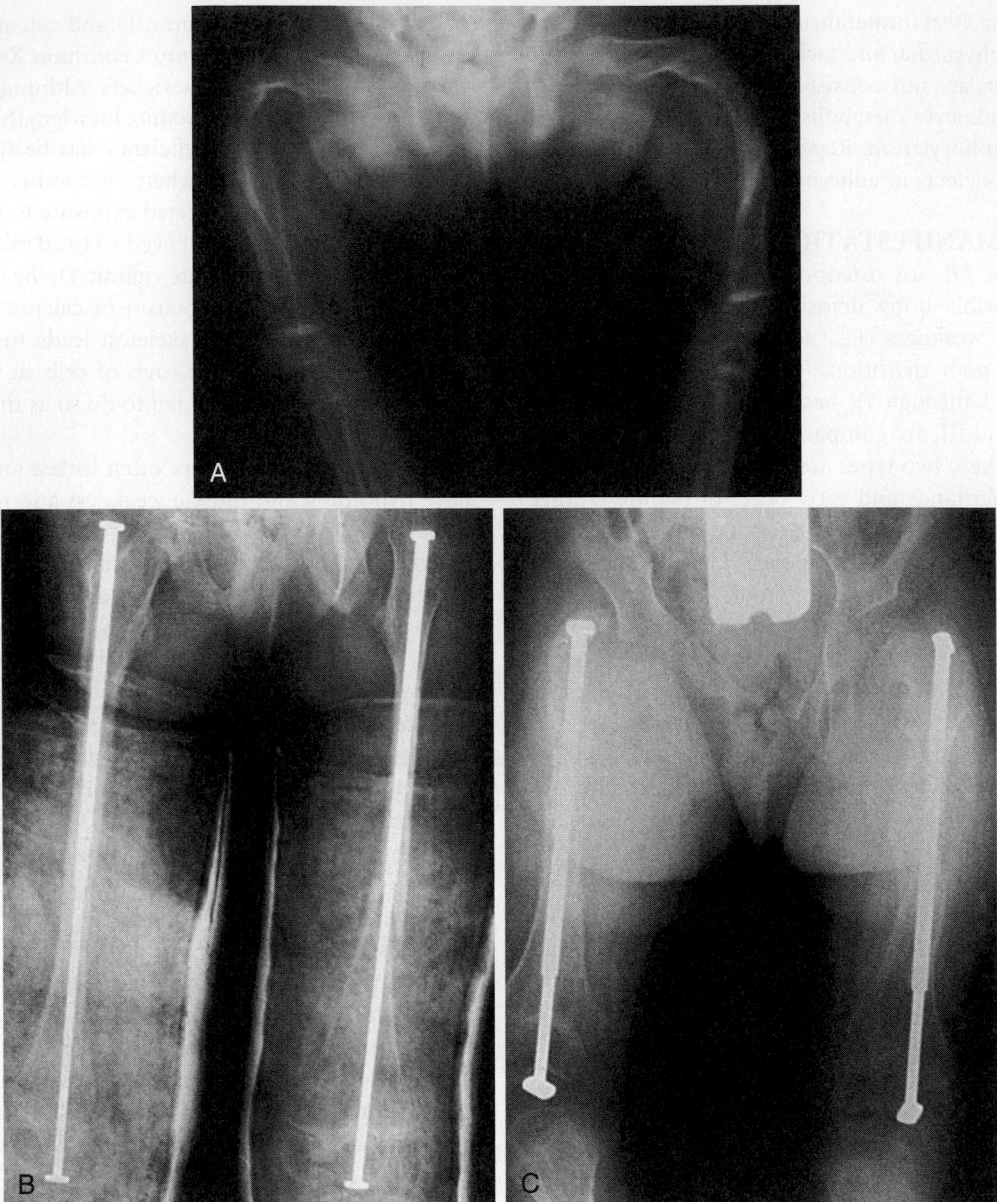

Figure 43-5 Osteogenesis imperfecta treated with osteotomies and telescoping medullary rods. **A,** Severe deformity of both femurs. **B,** Same individual after multiple osteotomies with telescoping medullary rod fixation. **C,** Same individual 4 years later demonstrating growth of femurs, no recurrence of deformity, and elongation of rods. (Plaster casts are in place for immobilization of tibial osteotomies.) (From Crenshaw AH, editor: *Campbell's operative orthopaedics*, ed 8, vol 3, St Louis, 1992, Mosby.)

PATHOPHYSIOLOGY It has been hypothesized that in individuals with adolescent scoliosis, there is an abnormality of the central nervous system involving the balance mechanism (reticular system) in the midbrain. A genetic component is also suggested because 30% occur within families. A recent study is making exciting gains in this area.

Experimentally it also has been shown that individuals with adolescent idiopathic scoliosis have an abnormality in the function of the posterior columns of the spinal cord. This results in abnormal proprioception and is not evident clinically except in the presence of scoliosis. The exact cause of scoliosis, however, remains elusive.[9,10]

The earliest pathologic changes, which are probably secondary changes, occur in the soft tissues. The muscles, ligaments, and other soft tissues become shortened on the concave side of the curve. With time, progressive deformities of the vertebral column and ribs develop. In growing children, lateral deviation of the spinal column ceases, and one-sided compression of the vertebral bodies on the concave side of the curve begins. Vertebral deformity occurs as asymmetric forces are applied to the epiphyseal center of the ossification by shortened and tight soft tissues on the concave side of the curve. The degree of compression and twisting varies according to the position of the vertebrae in the curve. The compressive force is greatest on the vertebrae in the apex of the concavity, so that the apical vertebrae become most deformed.

The curves increase most rapidly during periods of rapid skeletal growth. If the curve is less than 40 degrees at skeletal maturity, the risk of progression is quite small. In curves greater than 50 degrees, the spine is biomechanically unstable, and the curve will in all likelihood continue to progress even after the cessation of growth at an average rate of 1 degree per year. Curves in the thoracic spine greater than 80 degrees result in decreased pulmonary function, whereas the most common complication of large curves in the lumbar spine is back pain.

CLINICAL MANIFESTATIONS The clinical manifestations of nonstructural scoliosis are mild spinal curvature with prominence of one hip or rounded shoulders. The curvature disappears with forward flexion of the spine, lying down, or traction of the head. Treatment for nonstructural scoliosis is correction of the underlying disorder. The clinical manifestations of structural scoliosis include asymmetry of hip height, asymmetry of shoulder height, shoulder and scapular (shoulder blade) prominence, and rib prominence.

EVALUATION AND TREATMENT Spinal curvature is usually visible or palpable, and muscles on one side of the lower back (the convex side) may be prominent or bulging. Most cases of idiopathic scoliosis are noticed during school screening programs. In girls the deformity may be noticed because clothing does not "hang" properly on the body. Diagnosis is made by roentgenographic examinations.

Treatment of curves between 25 and 35 degrees in the skeletally immature child is with bracing. In most cases the low-profile brace is used. A brace used only at night, the Charleston bending brace, has shown it to be less effective than the traditional low-profile braces in preventing progression of curves. Occasionally a Milwaukee brace, which has a metal upper structure and neck ring, is needed for curves with an apex higher than midthoracic level. Low-profile and Milwaukee braces are worn for 23 hours daily until skeletal maturity. Bracing will only prevent progression of the curve; it will not correct the curvature. Bracing is not effective in curves greater than 40 degrees or in skeletally mature individuals; the most effective time for bracing is in a young child (less than 12 years of age) with a small curve.[11] Extensive chiropractic

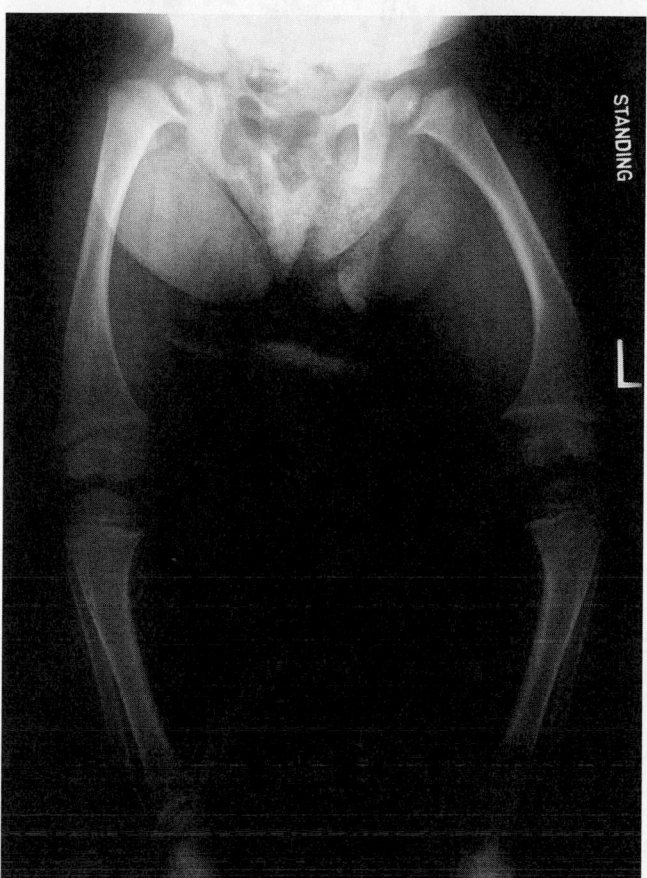

Figure 43-6 Rickets. This standing radiograph of an 8-year-old female with hypophosphatemic rickets shows cupping and widening of the growth plates throughout the lower extremities. Also note the bowing femoral deformity and hip deformity.

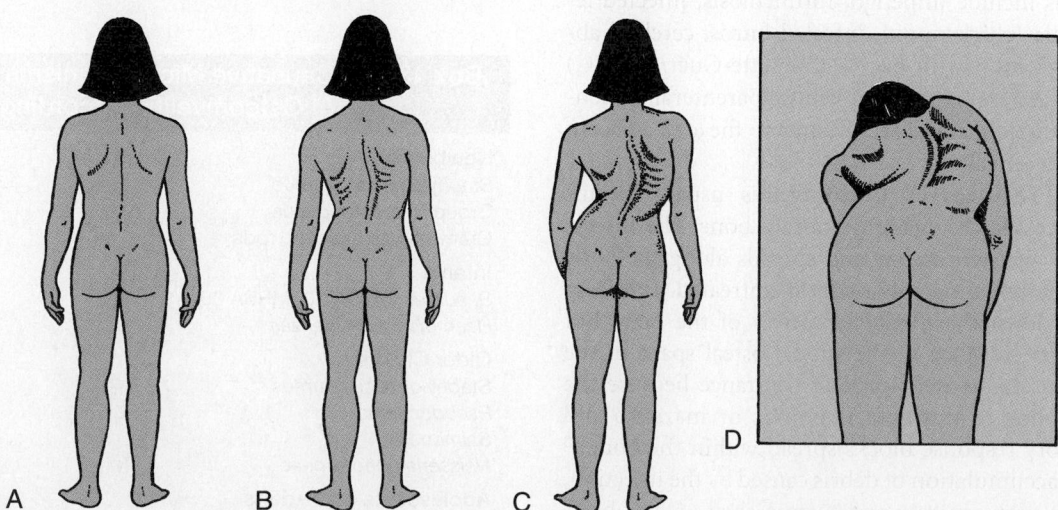

Figure 43-7 Scoliosis in children. Normal spinal alignment and abnormal spinal curvatures associated with scoliosis. A, Normal. B, Mild. C, Severe. D, Rotation and curvature of scoliosis.

manipulations and electrical stimulation have not been shown to change natural history. Surgical treatment with spinal fusion with instrumentation is recommended for curves greater than 40 to 50 degrees. If surgery is indicated, it is better performed during the adolescent years while there is greater flexibility of the curves and less risk of complications.

Bone Infection: Osteomyelitis

Osteomyelitis is an infection of the bone. Occurring twice as often in males as females, acute osteomyelitis may affect infants and children of any age, but it occurs most often between 3 and 12 years of age.

Bacteria enter the bone through the bloodstream and lodge in the medullary cavity, where a rich phagocytic mechanism often prevents most of the bacteria from establishing an infectious state. In some cases, however, the bacteria may lodge at the end of the venous loops beneath the epiphyseal plate, and infection then develops because there are no phagocytic cells present to remove the bacteria[12-14] (Figure 43-8).

The microorganism responsible for osteomyelitis varies and is related to the age of the child (Box 43-1). Osteomyelitis in the newborn is caused primarily by *Staphylococcus aureus*. Group B streptococcus and *Escherichia coli* infections are responsible for some cases, especially those of multiple bone involvement and in high-risk infants.[14]

S. aureus is the responsible microorganism in 80% to 90% of osteomyelitis cases in older children. *Haemophilus influenzae*, a previously common cause of osteomyelitis in children less than 5 years of age, has become rare with the improvements in immunization. However, cases of methicillin-resistant *Staphylococcus aureus* (MRSA) have risen alarmingly in the past 5 years. Once an infrequent cause of childhood osteomyelitis, MRSA now causes up to 30% of new cases.[15] Gram-negative microorganisms account for an increasing number of infections of the vertebrae,[16,17] whereas *Salmonella* infections are associated with sickle cell disease.

Factors that predispose an individual to the development of osteomyelitis include impetigo, furunculosis, infected lesions of varicella (chickenpox), infected burns, cerebral abscesses, immunization with bacille Calmette-Guérin (BCG) vaccine, prolonged intravenous or central parenteral alimentation, drug addiction, and direct trauma to the area adjacent to the site of osteomyelitis.

PATHOPHYSIOLOGY Osteomyelitis usually begins as a bloody abscess in the metaphysis of the bone. The abscess ruptures under the periosteum and spreads along the bone shaft or into the bone marrow cavity if untreated. Infection rarely spreads down the medullary cavity of the bone but rather first gains entrance to the subperiosteal space in the metaphysis. This is the path of least resistance because the cortex of the bone in this area is porous or mazelike and the inflammatory response blocks spread within the bone.[18] Because of the accumulation of debris caused by the infection, the periosteum may separate and form a shell of new bone around the infected portion of the shaft. Because the periosteum is separated from an adequate blood supply, sections of

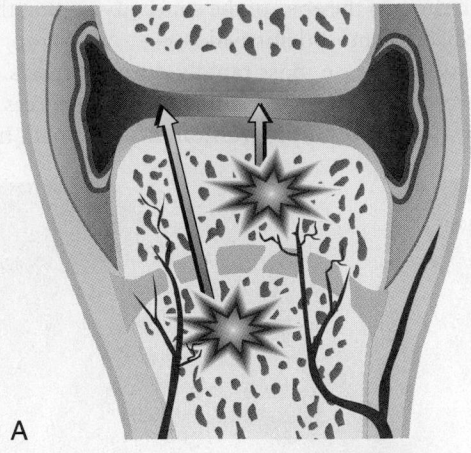

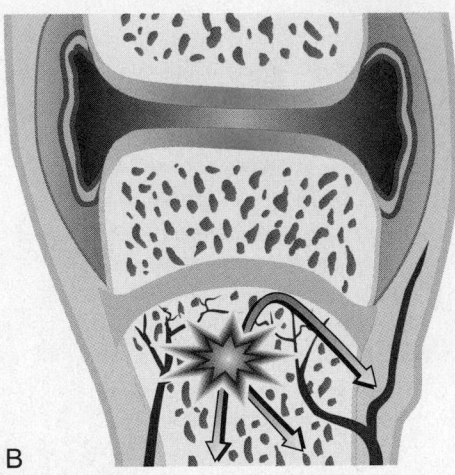

Figure 43-8 Pathogenesis of acute osteomyelitis differs with age. **A,** In infants younger than 1 year the epiphysis is nourished by penetrating arteries through the physis, allowing development of the condition within the epiphysis. **B,** In children up to 15 years of age the infection is restricted to below the physis because of interruption of the vessels.

Box 43-1	**Causative Microorganisms of Osteomyelitis According to Age**

Newborns
Staphylococcus aureus
Group B streptococcus
Gram-negative enteric rods

Infants
S. aureus (MSSA 70, MRSA 30)
Haemophilus influenzae

Older Children
Staphylococcus aureus
Pseudomonas
Salmonella
Neisseria gonorrhoeae

Adolescents and Adults
Pseudomonas
Mycobacterium tuberculosis

the bone die; these pieces of dead bone are called **sequestra.** The periosteum that maintains a blood supply generates new bone and is responsible for the appearance of the periosteal new bone, or **involucrum.** The presence of the sequestra and involucrum indicates that the disease has progressed to subperiosteal abscess formation.

In cases in which the infection in the metaphysis occurs near the joint, the accumulating pus (bacteria, white blood cells, fluid) creates increasing pressure that may cause a rupture into the joint cavity. If rupture into the joint occurs, the pus causes inflammation and a condition called **secondary septic arthritis.**[16] Although thought uncommon, a recent study shows 40% of children will have adjacent joint involvement with osteomyelitis. The most common joint to be affected is the knee. Osteomyelitis is most commonly caused by bacteria that reach the metaphysis through the bloodstream but may occur through secondary inoculation of microorganisms caused by trauma or contagious spread of infection from cellulitis in adjacent soft tissue.

Osteomyelitis in infants is often associated with septic arthritis because the infant's bone has blood vessels that perforate the growth plate. Because of the unique nature of blood supply to an infant's bones, osteomyelitis and septic arthritis commonly occur together. Normal anatomic variations in infants allow infection to spread directly to the epiphysis, which causes both joint disease and permanent epiphyseal disease. Multiple sites of osteomyelitis are also more common in children younger than 2 years, necessitating bone scan to check other bones when infants are infected. This can then lead to other areas of osteomyelitis and possibly septic arthritis.[19]

Children are susceptible to joint involvement for several reasons (Figure 43-9). In the immature infant, there is no epiphyseal plate or an ossific nucleus at the end of the bone and the cartilage precursor of bone is penetrated by vascular channels. In these infants the infection begins in the vulnerable cartilage precursor of the end bone itself and results in rapid destruction of the joint and arrested growth of the bone. For this reason the early detection and treatment of osteomyelitis are crucial if the infant's joint is to be saved from destruction. As the child matures and the epiphyseal plate forms, a temporary barrier is established against infection because the arterioles end beneath the epiphyseal plate.[18]

In children older than 2 years, the epiphyseal plate prevents the spread of a metaphyseal abscess into the epiphysis and the cortex of the metaphysis is thicker. These anatomic differences increase the likelihood that the metaphyseal abscess will extend into the diaphysis, and the blood supply of the bone will be disrupted. The periosteum is also more difficult to perforate in older children; this may lead to a larger subperiosteal abscess that could endanger the periosteal blood supply as well. This process commonly results in extensive sequestrum formation and chronic osteomyelitis.[18]

Osteomyelitis is much less common after the physeal plates are closed, except in the vertebral body. Infection may

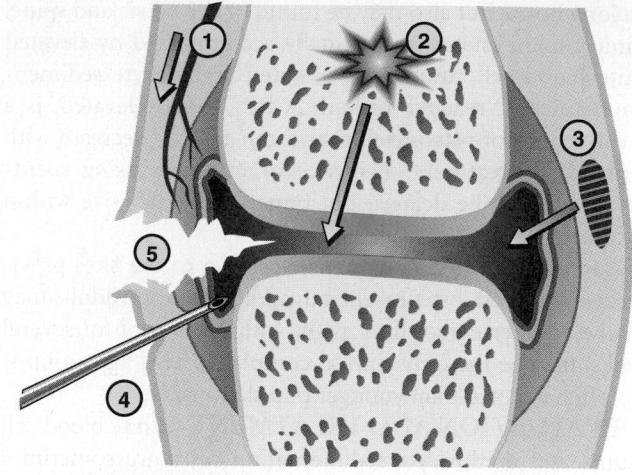

1. The hematogenous route
2. Dissemination from osteomyelitis
3. Spread from an adjacent soft tissue infection
4. Diagnostic or therapeutic measures
5. Penetrating damage by puncture or cutting

Figure 43-9 Routes of infection to the joint.

develop in any part of a bone, and abscesses spread slowly. Destruction of the cortex in a localized area may result in a pathologic fracture.[16,17]

Spread of infection to contiguous joints is related to the child's age. Metaphyseal infection may spread to contiguous joints if the fibrous joint capsule includes the metaphysis and epiphysis. This special situation exists at the hip joint, distal femur, proximal humerus and radius, and lateral ankle. Recent studies have shown, however, that like infants older children may demonstrate up to 42% of contiguous joint involvement. Even in areas where the involved osteomyelitis was extra-articular, joint involvement occurred; this differs from previous reports in the literature.[19]

CLINICAL MANIFESTATIONS The clinical manifestations of osteomyelitis are age dependent and are related to the differing vascular patterns found in the skeletal system at various ages. Three distinct groups may be identified: (1) infants younger than 1 year, (2) children from 1 year of age to puberty, and (3) adolescents after cessation of bone growth and adults.

Infants. Osteomyelitis may be an acute illness characterized by fever and failure to move the affected limb (pseudoparalysis). Infantile osteomyelitis is characterized by involvement of multiple sites within the same bone or in multiple bones. If untreated, involvement of the adjacent growth plate can result in growth arrest.

Children. Osteomyelitis in children between the ages of 1 year and puberty is characterized by fever and systemic signs of toxicity. The illness is sometimes subacute, with the child complaining of swelling, redness, tenderness, and decreasing ability to bear weight on or move the affected area. Onset can be abrupt. Osteomyelitis during childhood most often affects the long bones but also may be found in the pelvis and spine. Clinical manifestations are usually accompanied by elevated white blood cell counts and elevated erythrocyte sedimentation rates. C-reactive protein (CRP), when elevated, is a sensitive sign of osteomyelitis and can rapidly decrease with appropriate treatment. Evidence of infection using roentgenograms can be delayed but bone scan is positive within 48 hours.

Adolescents and Adults. In addition to the sites previously mentioned, osteomyelitis in adolescents and adults may involve the vertebrae. Back pain, with a duration of several weeks, may be the only clinical complaint. This age group is less often affected than younger populations.

EVALUATION AND TREATMENT White blood cell counts and erythrocyte sedimentation rates are sometimes elevated, but this is not a consistent finding. Monitoring of erythrocyte sedimentation rates is an indication of response to management but can be delayed. CRP is more quickly responsive to appropriate treatment. Blood cultures (positive in 30% to 40%) and aspiration of the soft tissue or bone, or both, should be done to identify the causative microorganism. Appropriate antibiotics should be prescribed *after* culture and sensitivity studies have been completed. A tuberculin test also is administered because *Mycobacterium tuberculosis* is sometimes responsible and has had a slight resurgence in incidence. Bone scans can be quite helpful with diagnosis and in children younger than 1 year are absolutely required to define whether multiple sites are involved.

Treatment includes intravenous (IV) antibiotics or, in highly reliable children and families, a combination of IV and oral antibiotics for 6 weeks. Drainage and margination of bone is required if changes are present on radiographs signifying abscess. Immobilization may help with pain control. If a joint is also infected (termed "septic arthritis"), the situation becomes a *surgical emergency*; surgery on the affected joint can help prevent damage to the articular cartilage by lysozymes released from the involved neutrophils.

Death is rare, but serious sequelae may occur. The course of the disease and prognosis depend on the age of the child, the rapidity with which the diagnosis is established, the initiation of early treatment, and maintenance of the treatment for an adequate time. The most serious complications are growth arrest, osseous necrosis, and recurrence.

Recurrence with presently available antibiotic regimens is less than 10%.

Juvenile Rheumatoid Arthritis

The rheumatic diseases are a group of diverse conditions having in common the inflammation of connective tissues. They include rheumatoid arthritis (RA), systemic lupus erythematosus, dermatomyositis, scleroderma, and polyarthritis. Incidence of these disorders in children is estimated in Table 43-3.

Juvenile rheumatoid arthritis (JRA) is the childhood form of rheumatoid arthritis (see Chapter 42). Like adult-onset RA, JRA is a syndrome that is often accompanied by systemic manifestations. Approximately 5% of all cases of RA begin in childhood. An estimated quarter of a million children in the United States have JRA.

The basic pathophysiology of JRA is the same as that of adult RA. The clinical manifestations of JRA may differ, however, beginning with mode of onset. Unlike adult RA, which begins insidiously with systemic signs of inflammation and generalized aches, JRA has three distinct modes of onset: arthritis in fewer than five joints (pauciarticular arthritis), arthritis in more than five joints (polyarticular arthritis), and systemic disease. Onset is less gradual in JRA than in adult RA. JRA also differs from the adult form in the following respects[20,21]:

1. Predominantly the large joints are affected.
2. Subluxation and ankylosis of the cervical spine are common if the disease progresses.
3. Joint pain may not be severe as in the adult type.
4. Serologic tests often detect antinuclear antibody (ANA).
5. Chronic uveitis is common, especially if ANA positive.
6. Serologic tests seldom detect rheumatoid factor.
7. Rheumatoid nodules are not limited to subcutaneous tissue but are found in the heart, lungs, eyes, and other organs.

Treatment for children with JRA is supportive but not curative. Many children with pauciarticular arthritis who are seronegative for ANA will resolve their symptoms over time. However, with systemic onset (Stills disease) or seropositivity, JRA may progress to true adult RA. The aims of treatment are

Table 43-3	Incidence of Connective Tissue Diseases in Children				
Disease	Annual Rate/10^5	Gender Ratio (Female/Male)	Race Ratio (White/Black)	Peak Age Group at Risk (yr)	Childhood Onset (%)
Rheumatoid arthritis	40	3:1	Equal	Increases with age (20-50)	5
Systemic lupus erythematosus	6	8:1	1:4	15-45	18
Dermatomyositis	0.8	2:1	1:3	45-65	20
Scleroderma	0.4	3:1	Equal	Increases with age (30-50)	3
Polyarteritis	0.2	1:3	Equal	Midadult	Rare

Data from Hollingworth P. In Klippel JH, Dieppe PA, editors: *Rheumatology,* St Louis, 1994, Mosby.

to control inflammation and other clinical manifestations of the disease and to minimize deformity.

Avascular Diseases of the Bone: Osteochondrosis

The avascular diseases of the bone, collectively termed **osteochondroses,** are caused by insufficient blood supply to growing bones. Disturbances of blood supply to primary and secondary centers of ossification during periods of rapid bone growth results in a variety of skeletal abnormalities.

The cause of the osteochondroses remains obscure. In the past, infection, nutritional deficiencies, and hormonal imbalances were blamed, but these causes have been largely disproved. Currently, vascular impairment and trauma, coupled with an underlying developmental or genetic predisposition, have been identified as probable causes of osteochondroses. The most common osteochondroses are Osgood-Schlatter disease (tibial tubercle), Sinding-Larsen-Johansson syndrome (distal patellar pole), Panner disease (radial head), Kohler disease (the navicular bone of the foot), and Sever disease (calcaneus). All are associated with activity-related pain of the affected region that improves with rest. All are more common in boys than girls and in athletes more than nonathletes.

The osteochondroses involve areas of significant tensile or compressing stress that undergo partial osseous necrosis, progressive bony weakness, and then microfracture. Most of these are associated with trauma and overuse and improve with rest. Anti-inflammatories, modification of activities, and even immobilization are used during active disease. Reparative correction by revascularization is the rule, although this may be a lengthy process.

Legg-Calvé-Perthes Disease

Legg-Calvé-Perthes disease, commonly called Perthes disease, is classically thought to be an osteochondroses like those previously described. This self-limited disease of the hip is presumably produced by recurrent interruption of the blood supply to the femoral head. The ossification center first becomes necrotic, collapses, and then is gradually remodeled by live bone.

Legg-Calvé-Perthes disease is relatively common (1 in 5000 children), usually occurring in children between 3 and 10 years of age, with a peak incidence at 6 years. It is more common in boys than in girls by a ratio of about 5:1. The condition is bilateral in approximately 10% of affected children; in 80% of these children, the effect on the second side is less severe.[22]

The cause of decreased blood supply to the head of the femur is unknown. Several theories have been proposed, including trauma, infection, and protein C and S deficiencies, which cause a hypercoagulable state or vascular anamolies.[23] A plausible theory is that acute synovitis (infection of the synovial membrane) and increased hydrostatic pressure in the hip joint compress blood vessels that supply the femoral head.

Constitutional factors definitely play a role. Skeletal maturation is delayed an average of 2 years in children with Legg-Calvé-Perthes disease, and affected children are between 2.5 and 7 cm shorter than unaffected children of the same age. Familial occurrence is 30% to 40%. The disease is rare in blacks, and it is frequent in children of Japanese and central European ancestry.

PATHOPHYSIOLOGY Legg-Calvé-Perthes disease runs its natural course in 2 to 5 years. In the incipient stage the soft tissues of the hip (synovial membrane and joint capsule) are swollen, edematous, and hyperemic, often with fluid present in the joint (Figure 43-10). The joint space widens, and the joint capsule bulges. The first stage lasts only a few weeks. In the second (or active avascular necrotic) stage, the entire epiphysis or the anterior half of the epiphysis of the femoral head loses blood supply and the metaphyseal bone at the junction of the femoral neck and capital epiphyseal plate is softened because of decalcification. Soon granulation tissue (procallus) and blood vessels invade the dead bone. This stage lasts several months to 1 year.

The third (or regenerative healing) stage ordinarily lasts 2 to 4 years. The dead femoral head is replaced by procallus, and new bone is laid down. Collapse and flattening of the femoral head occur, and the femoral neck becomes short and wide (see Figure 43-10).

In the fourth (or residual) stage, remodeling takes place and the newly formed bone is organized into a live spongy bone. Children less than 6 years of age at onset have more time to remodel the damage Perthes has caused and have the best outcome. Recent multicenter studies, using the Herring

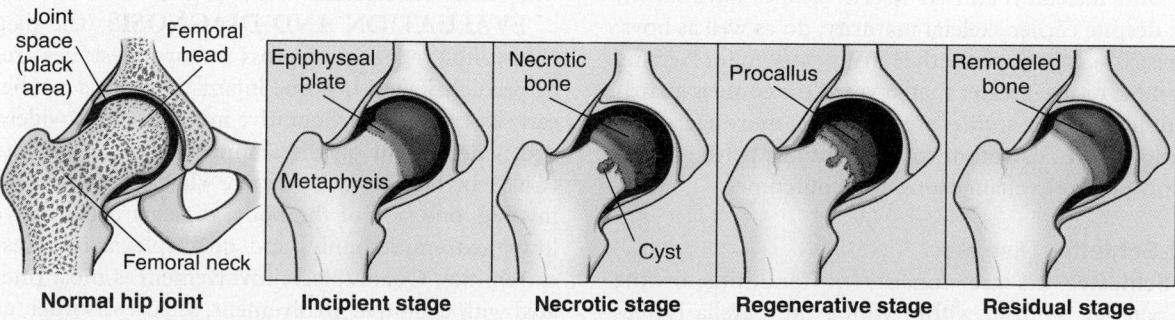

Figure 43-10 Stages of Legg-Calvé-Perthes disease, a form of osteochondrosis.

"lateral pillar" classification,[24] have shown that hips younger than 6 years with *no* involvement of the lateral femoral head (type A) do better than those with involvement of the lateral femoral head. Those children with complete collapse of the lateral femoral head (type C) have the worst prognosis. Long-term studies of type C hips show that 70% to 90% progress to osteoarthritis by 40 years of age.[25]

CLINICAL MANIFESTATIONS Injury or trauma precedes the onset of clinical manifestations in approximately one third of children with Legg-Calvé-Perthes disease. Onset of symptoms is insidious unless trauma aggravates the disease process. The child often complains of a limp or pain for several months. The pain usually is referred to the knee, inner thigh, and groin, following the path of the obturator nerve. In some children, pain may be absent or minimal. If pain is present, it is usually aggravated by activity and relieved by rest.

The typical physical findings include spasm on inward rotation of the hip and a limitation of internal rotation flexion and adduction. If the child is walking, an abnormal gait, termed a Trendelenburg gait or abductor lurch, is apparent. The child moves the trunk toward the affected side with stance to compensate for weak abductor musculature. If the hip pain or limp has been present for a prolonged period, muscles of the hip and thigh atrophy. A limb length inequity may be present if the proximal femoral physis is involved.

EVALUATION AND TREATMENT Diagnosis is confirmed by radiographic examination. Principles of treatment are *containment* (keeping the ball completely in the socket) and *motion* to maintain the articular cartilage. In the past, children were treated with bed rest and a variety of braces, which have now been shown to be ineffective.[26] Currently, most children can be managed with anti-inflammatory medications and crutches for episodes of synovitis and activity modification (avoidance of jumping activities that place increased stress on the hip) during the active phase of the disease. Serial roentgenograms monitor the progress of the disease and ensure that the hip remains congruent. Surgery may be necessary if the femoral head becomes subluxated or incongruent with the acetabulum before the reparative process. The ball must be congruent to take on the shape of the socket as remodeling occurs.

Factors affecting the outcome of Legg-Calvé-Perthes disease are the age of the child, the extent of necrosis, the stage of disease at the time treatment is begun, and congruence of the joint with skeletal maturity. Recent studies have shown that girls, despite earlier skeletal maturity, do as well as boys. Outcome is 70% satisfactory with Herring stage A; for Herring stages B and C or age greater than 8 years, outcome is guarded. Present prospective studies are evaluating more aggressive early treatment (i.e., osteotomy of the femur or pelvis) on the more involved hips to change long-term outcome.

Osgood-Schlatter Disease

Osgood-Schlatter disease consists of tendinitis of the anterior patellar tendon, within which the patella (kneecap) is embedded, and associated osteochondrosis of the tubercle of the tibia. Osgood-Schlatter disease occurs most often in preadolescents and adolescents who participate in sports. The incidence is higher in boys than in girls, many of whom have increased outward tibial fusion compared to controls.[27]

PATHOPHYSIOLOGY The severity of the lesion varies from mild tendinitis to a complete separation of the anterior extension of the tibial epiphysis, which is the part of the epiphysis that contributes to growth of the tibial tubercle. The underlying pathologic alterations also vary. The mildest form of Osgood-Schlatter disease causes ischemic (avascular) necrosis in the region of the bony tibial tubercle, with hypertrophic cartilage formation during the stages of repair. In more severe cases the abnormality involves a true epiphyseal separation of the tibial tubercle, with the characteristics of avascular necrosis that are described in the section on Legg-Calvé-Perthes disease.

CLINICAL MANIFESTATIONS The child experiences pain and swelling in the region of the patellar tendon and tibial tubercle, which becomes prominent and is tender to direct pressure. The pain is most severe after physical activity that involves vigorous quadriceps contraction or direct local trauma to the tibial tubercle area. Often the child experiences sudden acute discomfort referable to the affected region. Sudden onset of pain is caused by a pathologic fracture through an area of ischemic necrosis.

EVALUATION AND TREATMENT Diagnosis is confirmed by roentgenographic examination. The goal of treatment for Osgood-Schlatter disease is to decrease the stress at the tubercle. Often a period of 4 to 8 weeks of restriction from strenuous physical activity, especially activities requiring deep-knee bending, is sufficient. If pain relief is not achieved, a cast or brace is required to immobilize the knee, a situation that is particularly difficult if the condition is bilateral.

Gradual resumption of activity is permitted after 8 weeks, but return to unrestricted athletic participation requires an additional 8 weeks to allow for revascularization, healing, and ossification of the tibial tubercle.

Cerebral Palsy

Cerebral palsy (CP) is a static disorder of muscle tone and balance caused by an ischemic insult to the brain, usually perinatally. The incidence is presently 3% to 5% but is increasing with successful resuscitation of premature infants.

EVALUATION AND DIAGNOSIS The diagnosis of CP is often made when gross motor milestones are not met by predicted ages. In some infants, diagnosis can be made as early as 4 months.[28] Cognitive involvement is widely variable and is dependent on the amount of central nervous system (CNS) involvement. There are classic patterns: hemiplegia involves one side of the body, diplegia usually involves the lower extremities only, and quadriplegia involves all four extremities. Quadraplegic involvement is most often associated with cognitive involvement, seizure disorder, and aphasia. Many quadriplegics, however, are of normal intelligence and are "trapped" within aphasia. When given communication devices, these children are sometimes "discovered," as is their normal intelligence.

TREATMENT Treatment of cerebral palsy is multifaceted and undergoing constant evolution. The use of physical and occupational treatments, orthotics, spasticity reduction (by selected dorsal rhizotomy, oral, or intrathecal baclofen), botulinum-A (Botox) toxin injections, and surgery are often used to maximize a child's function. In many centers, a multispecialty approach at "CP clinics" occurs so that a family may, within one clinic visit, see neurology, pediatrics, orthotics, orthopedic surgery, and rehabilitation clinicians.

Children with CP should be carefully followed and given all possible opportunities to flourish. Although CP is a static disorder, progressive deformity because of increased muscle tone can occur. Monitoring these children as they grow with a multispecialty approach is essential to their optimal outcome.

Muscular Dystrophy

The **muscular dystrophies** are a group of familial disorders that cause degeneration of skeletal muscle fibers. The muscular dystrophies are the most prevalent of the muscle diseases in childhood and are characterized by progressive, symmetric weakness and wasting of skeletal muscle groups, with increasing disability and deformity.

Classification of the muscular dystrophies is based on age of onset, rate of progression, distribution of muscular involvement, and inheritance patterns. The major clinically and genetically distinct types are the pseudohypertrophic (Duchenne), facioscapulohumeral, limb girdle, and oculopharyngeal

dystrophies (Figure 43-11). Because the clinical findings and genetic inheritance patterns are consistent for each type, some researchers believe that each involves a separate biochemical defect. Genetic research has focused on identifying the site of abnormal gene function for each defect. This will permit more accurate carrier detection and, eventually, description of the biochemical aberration. (Table 43-4 summarizes the types of muscular dystrophy.)

Duchenne Muscular Dystrophy

In 1868 the French neurologist G.B.A. Duchenne described a pseudohypertrophic muscular paralysis associated with large amounts of fat and connective tissue. Today this form of muscular dystrophy, called **Duchenne muscular dystrophy,** is the most common of the muscular dystrophies. Its incidence is approximately 1 in 3500 male births.[29] Classic Duchenne muscular dystrophy occurs only in boys and has a history of X-linked inheritance in half of the cases.

PATHOPHYSIOLOGY The X-linked inherited type of Duchenne muscular dystrophy is thought to be caused by a deletion of a segment of deoxyribonucleic acid (DNA)[29] or a single-gene defect on the short arm of the X chromosome. A protein encoded by the Duchenne muscular dystrophy gene, called **dystrophin,** has been identified.

Dystrophin is present in normal muscle cells and absent in Duchenne muscular dystrophy. Dystrophin mediates anchorage of the actin cytoskeleton of skeletal muscle fibers to the basement membrane through a membrane glycoprotein complex. The complete lack of dystrophin in severe Duchenne dystrophy means that poorly anchored fibers tear themselves apart under the repeated stress of contraction. Free

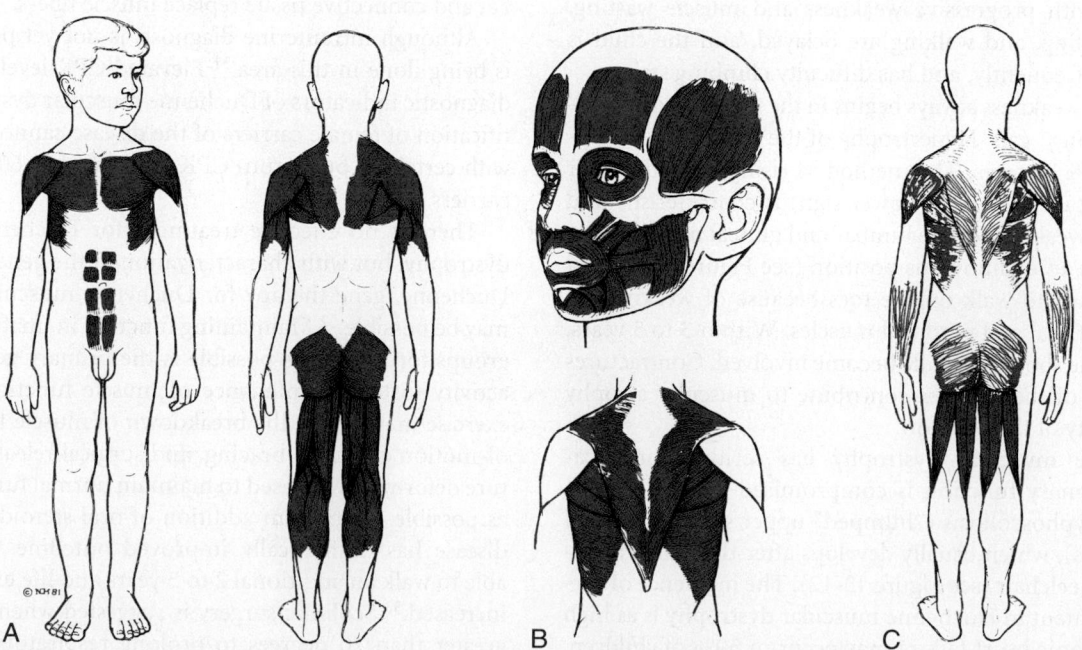

Figure 43-11 Initial muscle groups involved in three types of muscular dystrophy. A, Pseudohypertrophic. B, Facioscapulohumeral. C, Limb girdle. (From Hockenberry MJ: *Wong's nursing care of infants and children,* ed 8, St Louis, 2007, Mosby.)

Table 43-4   Major Muscular Dystrophy Syndromes

Disease	Mode of Inheritance	Age at Clinical Onset	Usual Distribution	Rate of Progression	Mental Retardation	Distinguishing Findings
Duchenne muscular dystrophy (DMD)	X-linked recessive	About 3 years	Hips and shoulders, quadriceps femoris, gastrocnemius (pseudohypertrophy)	Rapid	Frequent	Elevated serum enzymes (CPK, LDH, SGOT, aldolase)
Facioscapulohumeral dystrophy	Autosomal dominant	In first or second decade	Shoulder girdle, neck, face, pelvic girdle (late)	Moderate	Occasional	Several distinct muscle pathologic findings
Limb girdle (LG) dystrophy	Poorly defined or recessive	Variable	Pelvic and shoulder girdles	Variable	Variable	Collection of several diseases
Myotonic dystrophy (MyD)	Autosomal dominant	Variable—birth to fifth decades	Distal extensor muscle, eyelids, face, neck, hands, pharynx	Slow, related to age at clinical onset, faster with younger patients	Frequent	Percussion myotonia, cataracts, diabetic GTT despite increased insulin, testicular atropy, decreased IgG

CPK, Creatine phosphokinase; *GTT,* glucose tolerance test; *IgG,* immunoglobulin G; *LDH,* lactate dehydrogenase; *SGOT,* serum glutamic oxaloacetic transaminase.

calcium then enters the muscle cells, causing cell death and fiber necrosis[30] (Figure 43-12).

There is increased endomysial connective tissue and fat; loss of striations; and concomitant hyaline, granular, and fatty degeneration of fibers. Disorganization of tendinous insertions is associated with fat accumulation in these areas. Although fibers regenerate in the younger child, they are abnormal in many ways and become nonfunctional with time.

CLINICAL MANIFESTATIONS Duchenne muscular dystrophy is usually identified in children at approximately 3 years of age, when the parents first notice slow motor development with progressive weakness and muscle wasting. Sitting, standing, and walking are delayed, and the child is clumsy, falls frequently, and has difficulty climbing stairs.

Muscular weakness always begins in the pelvic girdle, causing a "waddling" gait. Hypertrophy of the calf muscles is apparent in 80% of cases. The method of rising from the floor by "climbing up the legs" (Gower sign) is characteristic and is caused by weakness of the lumbar and gluteal muscles. The foot assumes an equinovarus position (see Figure 43-4), and the child tends to walk on the toes because of weakness of the anterior tibial and peroneal muscles. Within 3 to 5 years, muscles of the shoulder girdle become involved. Contractures and wasting of the muscles contribute to muscular atrophy and deformity of the skeleton.

Duchenne muscular dystrophy has serious complications. Pulmonary function is compromised greatly because of marked kyphoscoliosis ("humped" upper spine combined with scoliosis), which usually develops after the child is confined to a wheelchair (see Figure 43-12). The incidence of cardiac involvement in Duchenne muscular dystrophy is as high as 95%. Chronic heart failure may occur in 50% of children. A moderate degree of mental retardation causes these children to have a mean IQ of approximately 80. Smooth muscle

dysfunction may cause megacolon, volvulus, cramping pain, and malabsorption in the gastrointestinal tract. The children usually succumb to other pulmonary or cardiac causes and death ensues by the late teens. Only 25% live to age 21.

EVALUATION AND TREATMENT Diagnosis is confirmed by measurement of serum enzymes, electromyography (EMG), and muscle biopsy. The serum enzymes, especially creatine phosphokinase (CPK), are increased to more than 10 times normal, even during infancy and before the onset of weakness. Histologic changes in muscle include degeneration of muscle fibers, with variation in fiber size and central nuclei. Fat and connective tissue replace muscle fibers.

Although intrauterine diagnosis is not yet possible, work is being done in this area.[31] Elevated CPK levels at birth are diagnostic indicators of Duchenne muscular dystrophy. Identification of female carriers of the disease cannot be achieved with certainty, but serum CPK is elevated in 60% to 80% of carriers.

There is no effective treatment for Duchenne muscular dystrophy, but with characterization of the genetic deficit for Duchenne, gene therapy for Duchenne muscular dystrophy may be possible.[32] Maintaining function in unaffected muscle groups for as long as possible is the primary goal. Although activity fosters maintenance of muscle function, strenuous exercise may hasten the breakdown of muscle fibers. Range-of-motion exercises, bracing, and surgical release of contracture deformities are used to maintain normal function as long as possible. The recent addition of oral steroids early in the disease has dramatically improved outcome. Children are able to walk an additional 2 to 5 years and life expectancy has increased.[33] Scoliotic surgery is suggested when curves reach greater than 20 degrees to prolong respiratory function or walking ability or both. Genetic counseling is recommended. With X-linked inheritance, male siblings of an affected child

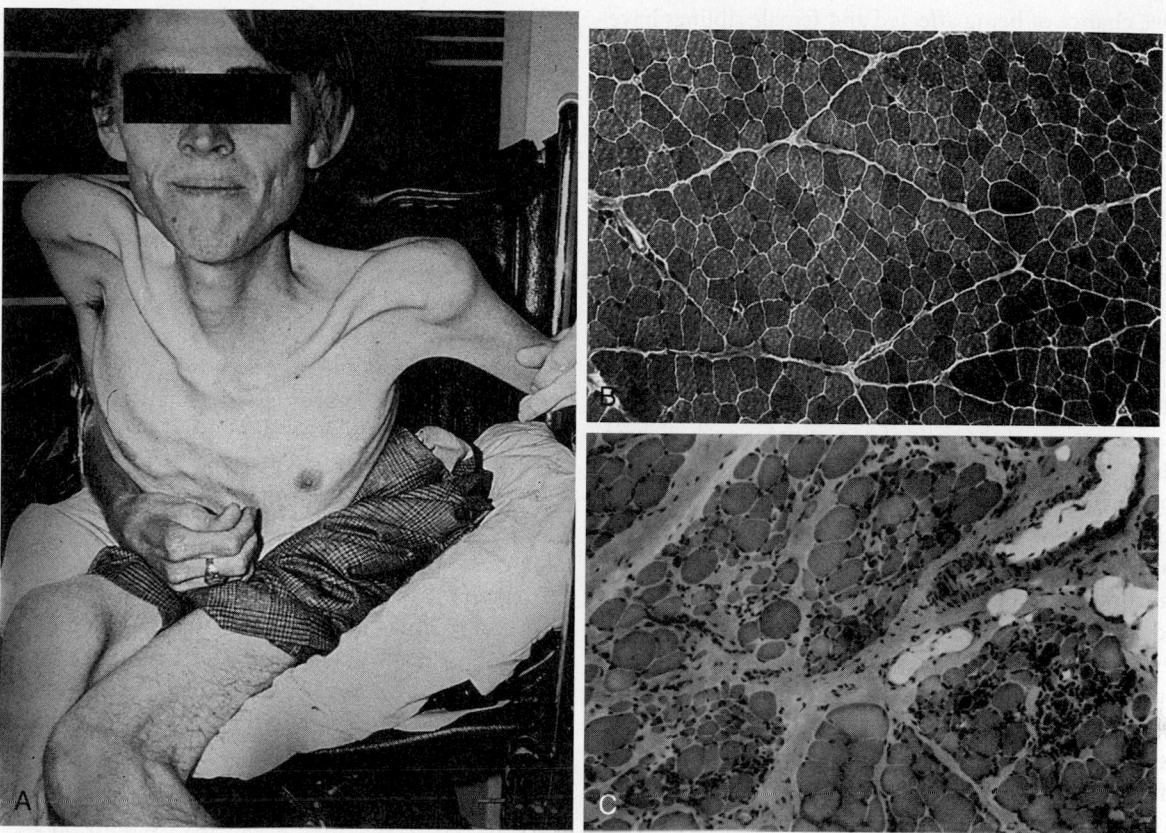

Figure 43-12 Duchenne muscular dystrophy. **A,** Patient with late-stage Duchenne muscular dystrophy showing severe muscle loss. **B,** Transverse section of gastrocnemius muscle from a normal boy. **C,** Transverse section of gastrocnemius muscle from a boy with Duchenne muscular dystrophy. Normal muscle fiber is replaced with fat and connective tissue. (From Jorde LB et al: *Medical genetics,* ed 3, St Louis, 2003, Mosby.)

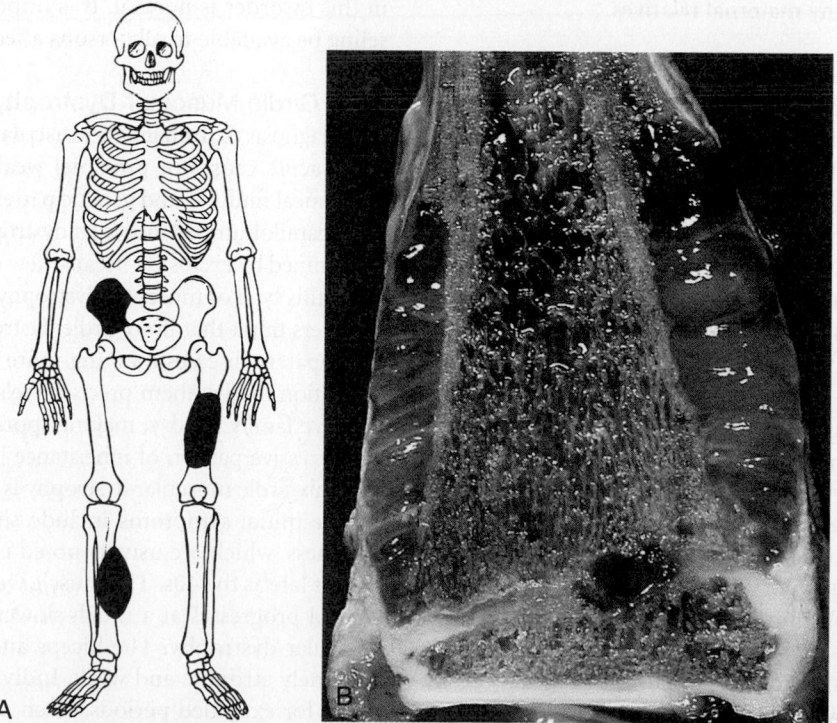

Figure 43-13 Ewing sarcoma. **A,** Most common anatomic sites. **B,** Close-up view of Ewing sarcoma of the distal end of the tibia. Tumor extends into the soft tissue. (From Damjanov I, Linder J, editors: *Anderson's pathology,* ed 10, St Louis, 1996, Mosby.)

have a 50% chance of being affected and female siblings have a 50% chance of being carriers.

Becker Muscular Dystrophy

Becker muscular dystrophy is often called *benign Duchenne muscular dystrophy* because it shares the X-linked inheritance pattern and similar but milder clinical features. The incidence of Becker dystrophy is one tenth that of Duchenne dystrophy. In Becker dystrophy, mutations in the middle rod region of dystrophin still allow anchorage of muscle to basement membrane. Clinical symptoms often begin between 5 and 15 years of age. Children with Becker muscular dystrophy remain ambulatory into their teens and early 20s; in one study the average age at the time of necessity for a wheelchair was 25 years.

The pattern of muscle weakness for both dystrophies is almost identical, but scoliosis and contractures are rare until the child with Becker muscular dystrophy is permanently wheelchair bound. The changes in creatine kinase levels and EMG and electrocardiogram (ECG) readings are the same as those seen in Duchenne muscular dystrophy. Many individuals live well into middle age. Heart failure is infrequent but can be a cause of premature death and disability.

Maintaining ambulation and careful follow-up for evidence of cardiopulmonary complications are essential for long-term care. Children with Becker muscular dystrophy rarely show the mental changes seen in Duchenne dystrophy. The accurate diagnosis of Becker muscular dystrophy is important. If the affected individual marries and has children, all daughters will be carriers of this X-linked recessive disorder. Genetic counseling should be offered to the mother, female siblings, offspring, and any maternal relatives.

Facioscapulohumeral Muscular Dystrophy

Facioscapulohumeral muscular dystrophy is a mild form of progressive, autosomal dominant muscular dystrophy. Age at onset varies from early childhood to adulthood, and the disease affects males and females equally. As the name implies, clinical manifestations begin with weakness and atrophy of facial and shoulder girdle (scapulohumeral) muscles. The illness progresses slowly. Inability to close the eyes completely may be noted from early childhood. The face is expressionless, and pouting of the lips makes whistling impossible. The first symptoms usually include drooping of the shoulders with difficulty in raising the arms above the head. Onset of weakness in the lower limbs often is delayed for 20 to 30 years, and pseudohypertrophy of muscles is rare. Contractures and skeletal deformities develop less often and are less prominent than in Duchenne muscular dystrophy.

Treatment includes supportive physiotherapy to prevent contractures and prolong ambulation. Lightweight plastic ankle-foot orthoses (AFOs) for footdrop are extremely helpful. Surgery to stabilize the shoulder is sometimes advised.

Some individuals with facioscapulohumeral muscular dystrophy improve with steroid therapy, particularly if the clinical picture includes rapidly progressive weakness. The

disease may be arrested for prolonged periods; however, most individuals remain active and have a normal life expectancy. Vocational training and genetic counseling are important to provide the information necessary to plan their future.

Scapuloperoneal Muscular Dystrophy

Scapuloperoneal muscular dystrophy is considered a variant of facioscapulohumeral muscular dystrophy, but distal muscles in the lower extremity are involved early instead of the facial and shoulder muscle weakness that is the early sign in facioscapulohumeral dystrophy. Many individuals seek initial treatment for troublesome footdrop and shoulder weakness. Analysis of inheritance patterns shows that the disease can be inherited either as an autosomal dominant trait or as an X-linked recessive trait.

The initial symptoms may resemble those of several other illnesses, including nemaline myopathy (a congenital muscle disease) and early hypertrophic peripheral neuropathy. A careful diagnostic evaluation therefore is in order. Other clinical findings include hypertrophy of the muscle that extends the toes, brought about by a futile attempt to overcome footdrop, and depressed or absent muscle stretch reflexes. Creatine kinase is elevated 2 to 20 times the normal level; EMG readings show myopathy.

Treatment is directed toward relieving symptoms and preserving ambulation and functional ability. Footdrop is easily treated with AFOs. Individuals with scapuloperoneal muscular dystrophy remain ambulatory for 40 or more years. Occasionally, walking may be hampered by paraspinal muscle contractures; in that case a wheelchair may assist the individual when it is necessary to cover long distances. The life span in this disorder is normal. It is important that genetic counseling be available to all persons affected.

Limb Girdle Muscular Dystrophy

The diagnosis of **limb girdle muscular dystrophy** is considered when acute causes of proximal weakness are eliminated and the clinical findings and genetic pattern exclude Duchenne and facioscapulohumeral muscular dystrophy. The diagnosis is often determined by exclusion because few consistent clinical features make this type of muscular dystrophy unique. In fact, some researchers think that limb girdle dystrophy actually may be several separate diseases awaiting more sophisticated methods of evaluation to give them precise labels. Most individuals have a negative family history, making sporadic disease or an autosomal recessive pattern of inheritance likely. The prevalence rate for limb girdle muscular dystrophy is set at 20 per million.

The initial symptoms include shoulder and pelvic girdle weakness, which are usually noted in the early 20s but can be seen as late as the 40s. The muscle weakness is often asymmetric and progresses at a much slower pace than in Duchenne muscular dystrophy. The biceps and deltoid muscles can be extremely atrophic and weak. Individuals can remain ambulatory for extended periods, often up to 20 years after initial diagnosis. When confined to wheelchairs, they show few of the severe effects of other dystrophies, such as contractures and scoliosis. Heart involvement and mental retardation also are rare.

The individual will have mild elevation in creatine kinase levels and a myopathic pattern on EMG. Muscle biopsy is often more characteristic, with fiber splitting and fibers that appear profusely "moth-eaten" and whorled. Treatment includes supportive measures to maintain ambulation and functional ability and frequent follow-up to eliminate secondary complications such as cardiopulmonary disease.

Musculoskeletal Tumors in Children

Bone Tumors

Bone tumors are uncommon childhood tumors and comprise less than 5% of all childhood malignancies. Of the malignant tumors, osteosarcoma and Ewing sarcoma are the most common. Fortunately, the majority of pediatric tumors are benign, most commonly nonossifying fibroma, chondroma, simple bone cyst, aneurysmal bone cyst, osteoid osteoma, and fibrous dysplasia.

Benign Bone Tumors

Nonossifying Fibroma. The **nonossifying fibroma (fibrous cortical deficit)**, which is believed to be a defect in ossification rather than a true tumor, makes up approximately 50% of benign bone tumors. Most fibrous cortical defects resolve spontaneously or are obliterated by reparative ossification or remodeling. In some cases, however, the fibrous cortical defect persists and proliferates, becoming a fibroma. Fibromas are found primarily in children and adolescents. Ninety percent of these tumors occur in persons younger than 20 years.

The nonossifying fibroma is a sharply demarcated cortical-based tumor surrounded by a dense border of hardened bone. The tumor itself consists of fibrocytes arranged in whorled bundles, fibroblastic tissue, and osteoclast-like giant cells. As the tumor evolves the fibrocytes imbibe lipids and assume a foamy appearance, known as *foam cells*. The tumor also contains extensive deposits of hemosiderin pigment. The long axis of the tumor parallels the long axis of the bone.

The nonossifying fibroma is usually asymptomatic and is found incidentally on radiographs. In the 1950s, when fluoride was added to drinking water, random skeletal surveys were done on hundreds of children. Nonossifying fibromas were discovered in 20% to 30% of children and were distributed in nearly every bone of the body. The fibroma is generally not treated until it occupies more than 50% of the diameter of the bone or extends more than 3 to 4 cm into the cortex. When the tumor grows to this size, a pathologic fracture may occur, and curettage and bone grafting of the defect is undertaken.

Simple Bone Cyst. **Simple bone cysts (SBCs)** are cystic lesions of the central region of the metaphyseal region in skeletally mature children. With growth these lesions may appear within the diaphysis. These children are usually asymptomatic until pathologic fracture or incidental discovery occurs. Lesions often heal after a fracture, but large lesions may require treatment. A large prospective, randomized study is comparing steroid injection (the classical treatment for these lesions) with bone marrow injection for treatment. Very large lesions in weightbearing areas may require internal fixation and bone grafting.

Aneurysmal Bone Cyst. **Aneurysmal bone cysts (ABCs)** are typically eccentric, metaphyseal lesions that occur in a slightly older population than SBCs. The etiology remains controversial; many consider ABC a lesion secondary to another process, such as giant cell tumor. This lesion must be differentiated from telangiectatic sarcoma, thus biopsy is necessary. Once diagnosed, curettage with complete removal of the "pseudolining" must be done with chemical or electrocautery to minimize recurrence. Bone graft is placed in the defect. Even with modern techniques, recurrence can be as high as 21%.[34]

Osteoid Osteoma. **Osteoid osteoma,** or the larger counterpart osteoblastoma, presents as painful lesions of the diaphysis or metadiaphysis of long bones. Involvement of the posterior elements of the spine—with resultant "splinting" scoliosis—can occur. Night pain is common, as is relief from symptoms with nonsteroidal anti-inflammatory drugs (NSAIDs), because these tumors release prostaglandins. When pain is too extreme to be controlled medically, resection of the "nidus," or central portion, of the lesion is uniformly successful. CT guidance to the lesion is often used and, if possible, CT-guided laser ablation can be done.

Fibrous Dysplasia. **Fibrous dysplasia (FD)** can occur in one bone (monostotic) or in multiple bones (polyostotic). Polyostotic fibrous dysplasia can occur with a triad of Albright syndrome that also includes precocious puberty and cutaneous pigmentation. Although any bone can be affected, the long bones, ribs, and skull are the most common. A radiographic "ground glass" appearance is present primarily in the metaphyseal or metadiaphyseal areas. Deformity can be marked and necessitate operative intervention. When allograft is used to replace fibrous dysplasia bone, it can become involved in the fibrous dysplasia as well. The majority of individuals are simply observed; however, endocrinology management also will be involved if Albright syndrome is present.

Malignant Bone Tumors

Osteosarcoma. **Osteosarcoma** is the most common bone tumor that occurs during childhood; it originates from bone-producing mesenchymal cells. Osteosarcoma occurs most commonly in the metaphysis of long bones, especially near active physes, such as the distal femur and proximal tibia. It accounts for 60% of all malignant bone tumors and strikes between the ages of 10 and 18.

Molecular analysis has demonstrated deletion of genetic material on the long arm of chromosome 13, leading to the identification of a tumor-suppressor gene as part of the mechanism for tumor development. The oncogene *src* also has been associated with osteosarcoma.

PATHOPHYSIOLOGY Osteosarcoma occurs mainly in the metaphyses of long bones. Most tumors arise in bones involved with the knee joint at the distal end of the femur or proximal end of the tibia. As a tumor of mesenchymal cells, osteosarcoma demonstrates production of osteoid tissue.

Osteosarcoma is a bulky tumor that extends beyond the bone into the soft tissues. It may encircle the bone and destroy the trabeculae of the diseased bone. Osteosarcoma disseminates through the bloodstream, usually to the lung. As many as 25% of children diagnosed with osteosarcoma exhibit lung metastases at diagnosis. Other sites of metastatic spread include other bones and visceral organs.

CLINICAL MANIFESTATIONS The most common presenting complaint is pain. There may be swelling, warmth, and redness caused by the vascularity of the tumor. Symptoms also may include cough, dyspnea, and chest pain if lung metastasis is present. If a lower extremity is involved, a limp or even pathologic fracture may be present.

Initial evaluation includes roentgenographic examination that shows the osteosarcoma's characteristic osteoblastic and osteolytic changes. "Staging" studies to determine not only local extent of the tumor but also possible metastatic spread must be done. These include bone scan (to assess bony spread), magnetic resonance imaging (MRI) of the lesion (to plan surgical resection and to compare with postchemotherapy studies), and chest roentgenograms or CT or both. The chest roentgenogram must be done *before* biopsy because the general anesthetic required for biopsy can give false-positive results on the roentgenogram.

EVALUATION AND TREATMENT Tissue biopsy confirms the diagnosis, although needle biopsy is often sufficient to establish the diagnosis. There are five histologic types of osteosarcoma, each determined by the predominant cell type. The tumor is then graded according to degree of malignancy; the higher the number, the worse the prognosis.

Surgery and chemotherapy are the primary treatments for osteosarcoma. Radiation is occasionally used. The 5-year survival rate with modern protocols is 70% to 80%.[35]

Chemotherapy is an important component of treatment because as many as 80% of children treated with surgery alone eventually develop metastatic disease. Chemotherapy is used preoperatively to shrink the size of the tumor and minimize metastatic growth. Following chemotherapy, the child is given a short "rest period" to regain strength for surgery. Following adjunctive chemotherapy, the majority of children undergo "limb salvage" rather than amputation procedures. Using preoperative MRI, the extent of the lesion is mapped and a tumor-free margin is left and reconstructed either with allograft bone or arthroplasty (artificial joint). The long-term survival rate of children treated with limb salvage and chemotherapy is now near equal to amputation in 5- and 10-year survival.[36]

A number of approaches have been used to treat pulmonary metastases. Because pulmonary metastases are generally solitary, thoracotomy with wedge resection has proved the most effective. Investigators have searched for adjuvant treatment to prevent pulmonary metastases, but nothing has proved useful.

Ewing Sarcoma. **Ewing sarcoma** is a malignant round cell tumor of bone and soft tissue that has a poor prognosis. It is the second most common and most lethal malignant bone tumor that can occur during childhood. This tumor is named after James Ewing, who first identified it as a separate clinical diagnosis in 1921. The most common period of diagnosis is between 5 and 15 years of age, and rare after 30 years of age; however, it may be seen in children younger than 3 years. Like osteosarcoma, Ewing sarcoma is slightly more common in males than females and is linked with periods of rapid bone growth. The incidence of Ewing sarcoma is less than 2% in blacks.[37]

PATHOPHYSIOLOGY Ewing sarcoma commonly occurs in the midshaft or diaphysis of long bones or in flat bones. The most common sites include the pelvis, femur, and tibia. The femur is involved in most cases, with the pelvis being the second most common site. It can occur in any bone.

Arising from bone marrow, Ewing sarcoma can break through the cortex of the bone to form a soft-tissue mass. It does not form bone, but abundant reactive bone may be present in an attempt to contain this quickly growing lesion. Metastasis occurs early and is usually apparent at diagnosis or within 1 year. The most common sites are the lung, other bones, lymph nodes, bone marrow, liver, spleen, and central nervous system, although invasion of any organ is possible.

CLINICAL MANIFESTATIONS Like osteosarcoma, the most common complaint is pain about the diaphysis that increases in severity. A soft-tissue mass is often present. Additional symptoms may include fever, malaise, and anorexia. Known as "the great imitator," Ewing sarcoma can appear radiographically identical to infection or even benign lesions such as Langerhans cell granulomatosis. Any pervasive diaphyseal or rib lesion must be regarded with a high index of suspicion.

EVALUATION AND TREATMENT In addition to plain roentgenogram, CT and MRI are needed to help establish the diagnosis and extent of the tumor. Bone scan, chest roentgenogram, and chest CT scan are also used to detect metastases. No specific laboratory test is diagnostic; however, the sedimentation rate will be elevated and lactic dehydrogenase (LDH) often is elevated. An elevated LDH level is a poor prognostic sign. Biopsy is used to conclusively establish the diagnosis. The identification of an 11:22 chromosomal translocation within the tumor cells confirms the diagnosis of Ewing sarcoma.

The use of multidrug chemotherapy has improved survival rates. Treatment protocols call for preoperative chemotherapy followed by radiation or surgical resection or both, with continuation of chemotherapy for 12 to 18 months afterward. Amputation is avoided when possible but may be considered in lower limb tumors of children younger than 8 years because of the serious discrepancy in bone growth that results if the primary treatment used is radiation, which can damage the physis. Secondary malignancies caused by high-dose radiation are also a concern.[38]

Historically, Ewing sarcoma had a dismal prognosis, with 5-year survival rates no better than 5% to 10%. Combinations of aggressive radiation, chemotherapy, and surgical resection have, however, improved the survival rate for localized disease to more than 60%.[39] The major predictor of prognosis appears to be the location of the primary tumor and whether metastases are present at diagnosis. The most favorable sites of involvement are the extremities; the worst prognosis involves tumors of the trunk, particularly the pelvis.

Muscle Tumors

Most soft-tissue tumors in children are benign. Only two malignant soft-tissue tumors occur with any frequency—rhabdomyosarcoma in the younger child and synovial cell sarcoma in the teenager. Both of these occur rarely. The annual incidence is 8 cases per million for white children and 7.7 per million for black children. About 230 U.S. children are diagnosed with a soft-tissue tumor each year. Soft-tissue tumors originate from the primitive mesenchymal cells that normally give rise to muscle, tendons, blood vessels, lymphatic structures, fibrous and connective tissue, and bursa and fascia. Table 43-5 identifies the classification of soft-tissue tumors according to origin. All malignant soft-tissue tumors are characterized as highly aggressive tumors that invade surrounding structures and metastasize early.

Rhabdomyosarcoma (RMS) is the most common soft-tissue sarcoma of childhood and accounts for more than 50% of soft-tissue tumors but less than 3% of all childhood cancers. RMS arises from embryonal rhabdomyoblasts that normally differentiate into mature striated muscle.

RMS can develop anywhere striated muscle is located. The primary locations and percentage range of incidence are the head and neck (including the orbit), 36% to 61%; the trunk, 8% to 33%; the extremities, 14% to 24%; and the genitourinary tract, 10% to 17%. Two age ranges (2 to 6 years and 15 to 19 years) are associated with RMS. More than two thirds of children with RMS are diagnosed by 10 years of age, and RMS is slightly more common in males than females.

Recent studies demonstrate an association between *TP53* (a tumor-suppressor gene) mutations and sporadic rhabdomyosarcoma.[40] Three oncogenes (*src, ras,* and *c-myb*) have been associated with this tumor.[41]

PATHOPHYSIOLOGY RMS generally appears as a firm, fleshy, grayish white mass. It sometimes exhibits variations that appear as a cystic polypoid mass. RMS has various appearances, depending on the phase of differentiation of the rhabdomyoblast. The cells may be round, spindle shaped, tadpole shaped, or multinucleated giant cells.

At least 20% of children with RMS have metastatic disease at diagnosis. The preferred sites of metastases include the lungs, lymph nodes, bone marrow, liver, brain, and bone. Another 30% have disease that is unresectable, although not widely spread. This also becomes a grave prognosis.

CLINICAL MANIFESTATIONS The signs and symptoms of RMS depend on the anatomic location of the primary tumor and presence of symptomatic metastases. The tumors are usually painless, and early detection of RMS is facilitated by the presence of a palpable or visible mass. Deep-seated tumors may cause functional impairment but can be silent until they are very large. The clinical manifestations of RMS are outlined in Table 43-6.

EVALUATION AND TREATMENT Diagnostic studies during the pretreatment phase are used to determine the extent of the primary tumor and presence or absence of distant metastases. Specific diagnostic studies depend on the primary site, but a combination of radiographic, nuclear, and

Table 43-5	Classification of Tumors by Origin
Tissue	**Tumor**
Muscle	
Striated	Rhabdomyosarcoma
Smooth	Leiomyosarcoma
Adipose	Liposarcoma
Fibrous	Fibrosarcoma
Synovial mesothelium	Synovial sarcoma
Lymphatic structures	Lymphangiosarcoma
Blood vessels	Hemangiopericytoma
Nerve sheath	Neurogenic sarcoma

Table 43-6	Clinical Manifestations of Rhabdomyosarcoma
Location	**Manifestation**
Head and Neck	
Orbit	Ptosis
	Exophthalmos
	Proptosis
Paranasal sinuses	Nasal obstruction
	Epistaxis
	Swelling
	Chronic sinusitis
Nasopharynx	Hypernasal speech
	Nasal discharge
	Visible polypoid mass
Oropharyngeal	Dysphagia
	Painful mastication
Middle ear	Chronic serous otitis media
	Discharge from affected ear
	Facial nerve palsy
	Conduction hearing loss
	Visible polypoid mass
Extremities	
All locations	Deep-seated, fixed palpable mass
Retroperitoneal	
All locations	Usually asymptomatic
	May have vague abdominal pain
	Bowel or genitourinary obstruction (late)
	Possible palpable mass
Genitourinary	
Vaginal	Abnormal vaginal bleeding
	Protruding polypoid mass
Prostate	Urinary tract obstruction
Bladder	Urinary retention
	Straining to void
	Hematuria
Paratesticular	Mass in scrotum that may be painful

CT scanning or MRI technology and blood studies is used. A biopsy of the primary tumor is necessary to confirm the diagnosis. Chromosomal abnormalities are being investigated for RMS. Although not widely incorporated into clinical management, identification of the DNA content has value as a prognostic factor and a determinant of treatment.

RMS is treated by a combination of surgery, radiation, and chemotherapy. Complete surgical resection provides the greatest assurance that cure can be achieved; however, cure occurs in only 16% of children. If surgical resection leads to serious disfigurement or functional disability (e.g., enucleation for orbital tumors or cystectomy for bladder tumors), chemotherapy and radiation serve as the primary treatment, and surgery is avoided or minimized. For all tumors except stage I disease, local radiation therapy is given. A variety of combination chemotherapies are used for RMS. Chemotherapy for stage I or II disease is given for 1 year if disease does not recur. For stage III or IV, treatment (combined with radiation therapy) continues an additional year. Intrathecal chemotherapy is given to children whose tumor locations favor CNS spread.

The primary prognostic factor in RMS is the degree of residual disease after surgical resection. Children with localized disease (stages I and II) have long-term survival rates of 70% to 80%. With widespread disease, long-term survival rates drop to 20%. Orbital tumors have an overall favorable prognosis, probably because of the lack of lymphatics in the area and early physical signs of disease.

NONACCIDENTAL TRAUMA

Abuse is estimated to occur in more than 1.5 million U.S. children per year. The maltreatment may be psychologic, sexual, or physical. Of children who suffer physical abuse, 30% are initially seen by an orthopedist. Accurate and appropriate referrals to child protection are not only legally mandated but also essential for the well-being of the child; an abused child who returns unmonitored to an abusive situation has a 15% chance of mortality.

ETIOLOGY Children who are not yet ambulatory and present with a long bone fracture have a greater than 75% chance of that fracture being caused by nonaccidental trauma. **"Corner" metaphyseal fractures,** caused by a twisting force, are *nearly pathognomonic* of abuse but occur only 25% of the time (Figure 43-14). Fractures at multiple stages of healing are also suggestive; however, osteogenesis imperfecta must be ruled out. The most common presentation is a transverse tibia fracture.[42] After walking age, only 2% of long bone fractures are the result of nonaccidental trauma.[43]

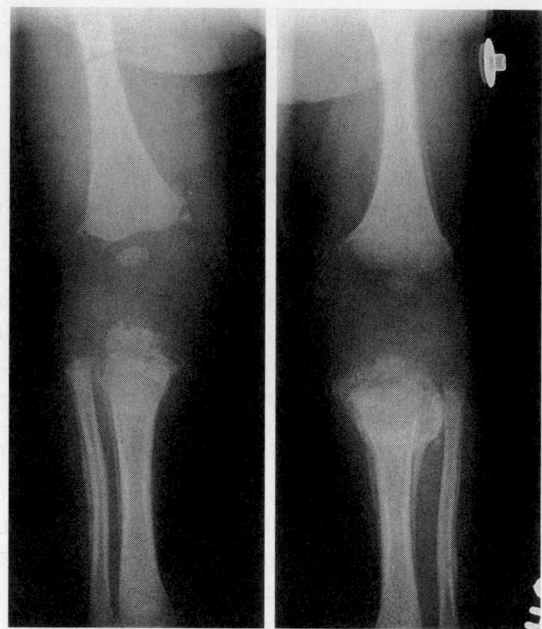

Figure 43-14 Corner fracture. Bilateral knee radiograph showing healing corner fractures of bilateral proximal tibias and distal femurs. Note the varying amount of callus formation signifying fractures at different stages of healing.

EVALUATION If suspected, nonaccidental trauma necessitates early consultation with child protective services. The child should undergo skeletal radiographic survey, especially if less than 2 years of age, and have a complete physical examination to evaluate for patterned bruising, burns, or multiple soft-tissue injuries. Ophthalmologic examination should be used to evaluate for retinal hemorrhage caused by shaking. A thorough history must be obtained for all identified injuries. It is important to remember that social isolation can lead to increased likelihood of abuse, but no social stratum is immune.

When cause is unclear, bone scan can be helpful in diagnosing subtle injuries, especially rib fractures. Posterior rib fractures are especially likely to be caused by abuse. MRI and CT of the brain can help diagnose injuries caused by shaking.

TREATMENT A nonjudgmental attitude on the part of the treating healthcare provider is essential. The child and family involved in nonaccidental trauma are delicate and require not only physical but emotional care. Social workers need to be involved early to ensure appropriate medical care to the child. Fortunately, fractures heal quickly in young children; neurologic injury and social disease, however, are much more difficult to cure.

SUMMARY REVIEW

Musculoskeletal Development in Children

1. Skeletal growth and development consists of two phases: (1) delivery of bone cell precursors to sites of bone formation, and (2) the aggregation of these cells at primary centers of ossification where they mature to secrete osteoid.
2. Ossification takes place in two centers in long bones: (1) the primary center, or the diaphysis (the long, central portion of the bone); and (2) the secondary center, or the epiphysis (the end portions of the bone).
3. Peak bone mass is achieved by the mid- to late 20s.
4. By 1 year of age 50% of the total growth of the spine has occurred, and most children have achieved 50% of their adult height by 2 years of age.
5. The appendicular skeleton (extremities) grows faster during childhood than does the axial skeleton.
6. Muscle fibers reach their maximal size in females at 10 years of age and at 14 years of age in males.

Musculoskeletal Alterations in Children

1. The most common congenital defect of the upper extremities is syndactyly (webbing of the fingers).
2. Developmental dysplasia of the hip is a serious and disabling condition in children if not diagnosed and treated.
3. Congenital muscle disorders (myopathies) include absence of muscles, hypoplasia, hyperplasia, and faulty intrinsic development.
4. Osteogenesis imperfecta (brittle bone disease) is a genetic disorder of collagen that affects primarily bones and results in serious fractures of many bones.
5. Rickets is a condition caused by deficiencies in vitamin D, calcium, and usually phosphorus that is characterized by the failure of bones to become mineralized (ossified) and results in skeletal deformity.
6. Scoliosis is a lateral curvature of the spinal column that can be caused by congenital malformations of the spine, neuromuscular disease, trauma, extraspinal contractures, bone infections, metabolic bone disorders, joint disease, and tumors.
7. Osteomyelitis is a local or generalized bacterial infection of bone and bone marrow. Bacteria are usually introduced by direct extension from a nearby infection, through the bloodstream, or by trauma.
8. JRA is an inflammatory joint disorder characterized by pain and swelling.
9. Avascular diseases of the bone are collectively referred to as osteochondroses and are caused by an insufficient blood supply to growing bones.
10. Legg-Calvé-Perthes disease is one of the most common osteochondroses. This disorder is characterized by epiphyseal necrosis or degeneration of the head of the femur followed by regeneration or recalcification.
11. Osgood-Schlatter disease is characterized by inflammation or partial separation of the tibial tubercle caused by chronic irritation, usually as a result of overuse of the quadriceps muscles. The condition is seen primarily in muscular, athletic adolescent males.

12. The muscular dystrophies are a group of genetically transmitted diseases characterized by progressive atrophy of symmetric groups of skeletal muscles without evidence of involvement or degeneration of neural tissue. There is an insidious loss of strength in all forms of the disorder with increasing disability and deformity.
13. Benign bone tumors include nonossifying fibroma, simple bone cysts, aneurysmal bone cysts, osteoid osteoma, and fibrous dysplasia.
14. The two main types of malignant childhood bone tumors are osteosarcoma and Ewing sarcoma.
15. Osteosarcoma, the most common malignant childhood bone tumor, originates in bone-producing mesenchymal cells and is most often located in the distal end of the femur or proximal end of the tibia.
16. Most childhood osteosarcoma tumors occur between the ages of 10 and 18 years.
17. Ewing sarcoma originates from cells within the bone marrow space and is located most often in the midshaft of long bones or in flat bones.
18. Ewing sarcoma is more common in males and is diagnosed most often between the ages of 5 and 15 years.
19. Pain is the usual presenting symptom for either osteosarcoma or Ewing sarcoma.
20. The primary treatments for osteosarcoma are surgery and chemotherapy. The primary treatment for Ewing sarcoma is a combination of chemotherapy, radiation, and surgery.
21. The most common type of childhood soft-tissue tumor is rhabdomyosarcoma.
22. Rhabdomyosarcoma originates from embryonal rhabdomyoblasts that normally differentiate into mature striated muscle.
23. Clinical manifestations of rhabdomyosarcoma depend on the anatomic location; superficial tumors exhibit a painless palpable mass, whereas deep-seated tumors cause functional impairment.
24. Rhabdomyosarcoma is treated with a combination of surgery, radiation, and chemotherapy.

Nonaccidental Trauma

1. Nonaccidental trauma must be considered with any long bone injury in a preambulatory child.
2. Evidence of soft tissue injury, corner fractures, and fractures at different stages of healing are extremely helpful in making a diagnosis of nonaccidental trauma.
3. When nonaccidental trauma is suspected, a child must be evaluated radiographically for other fractures, head trauma, and retinal hemorrhage.
4. All social strata are at risk.
5. The healthcare provider is legally responsible to report suspected nonaccidental trauma.

KEY TERMS

Aneurysmal bone cyst (ABC), 1637
Becker muscular dystrophy, 1636
Cartilage anlage, 1618
Cerebral palsy (CP), 1632
"Corner" metaphyseal fracture, 1640
Developmental dysplasia of the hip (DDH), 1621
Duchenne muscular dystrophy, 1633
Dystrophin, 1633
Endochondral formation of bone, 1618
Ewing sarcoma, 1638
Facioscapulohumeral muscular dystrophy, 1636
Fibrous dysplasia (FD), 1637
Genu valgum (knock knee), 1620
Genu varum (bowleg), 1620
Idiopathic equinovarus, 1623
Idiopathic scoliosis, 1625
Intramembranous formation of bone, 1618

Involucrum, 1629
Juvenile rheumatoid arthritis (JRA), 1630
Kyphosed, 1620
Legg-Calvé-Perthes disease, 1631
Limb girdle muscular dystrophy, 1636
Lordotic, 1620
Metatarsus adductus, 1622
Muscular dystrophy, 1633
Nonossifying fibroma (fibrous cortical deficit), 1637
Nonstructural scoliosis, 1625
Osgood-Schlatter disease, 1632
Osteochondrosis, 1631
Osteogenesis imperfecta (OI) (brittle bone disease), 1624
Osteoid osteoma, 1637
Osteomyelitis, 1628
Osteosarcoma, 1637
Perichondrium, 1618

Periosteal collar, 1619
Pes planus (flatfoot), 1623
Physeal closure, 1620
Positional equinovarus, 1623
Primary centers of ossification, 1618
Rhabdomyosarcoma (RMS), 1639
Rickets, 1625
Scapuloperoneal muscular dystrophy, 1636
Scoliosis, 1625
Secondary centers of ossification, 1619
Secondary septic arthritis, 1629
Sequestra (*sing.,* sequestrum), 1629
Simple bone cyst (SBC), 1637
Structural scoliosis, 1625
Syndactyly, 1620
Teratologic equinovarus, 1623
Vestigial tab, 1621

REFERENCES

1. Simkin P: The musculoskeletal system. In Klippel JH, Dieppe PA, editors: *Rheumatology,* ed 2, London, 1998, Mosby-Wolfe.
2. Weinstein SL: Congenital hip dislocation: long range problems, residual signs, and symptoms after successful treatments, *Clin Orthop Relat Res* Aug (281):69-74, 1992.
3. Weintraub S, Grill F: Ultrasonography in developmental dysplasia of the hip, *J Bone Joint Surg Am* 82-A(7):1004, 2000.
4. Ippolito E et al: Long-term comparative results in patients with congenital clubfoot treated with two different protocols, *Arch Gynecol Obstet* 268(4):331-332, 2003.
5. Dobbs MB et al: Factors predictive of outcome after use of the Ponseti method for the treatment of idiopathic clubfeet, *J Bone Joint Surg Am* 86-A(1):22-27, 2004.
6. Zaleske DJ, Doppelt SH, Mankin HJ: Endocrine abnormalities of the immature skeleton. In Lovell WW, Winter RB, editors: *Pediatric orthopedics,* ed 2, Philadelphia, 1986, Lippincott.
7. Zeitlin L, Fassier F, Glorieux FH: Modern approach to children with osteogenesis imperfecta, *J Pediatr Orthop B* 12(2):77-87, 2003.
8. Wharton B, Bishop N: Rickets, *Lancet* 362(9393):1389-1400, 2003.
9. Barrack R et al: Vibratory hypersensitivity in idiopathic sclerosis, *J Pediatr Orthop* 8(4):389, 1988.
10. Byrd JA: III: Current theories on the etiology of idiopathic scoliosis, *Clin Orthop Relat Res Apr* (299):114-119, 1988.
11. Vijermans V et al: Factors determining the final outcome of treatment of idiopathic scoliosis with the Boston brace: a longitudinal study, *J Pediatr Orthop B* 13(3):143-149, 2004.
12. Caksen H et al: Septic arthritis in childhood, *Pediatr Int* 42(5):534, 2000.
13. Gillespie WJ et al: Aspects of the microbe: host relationship in staphylococcal hematogenous osteomyelitis, *Orthopedics* 10(3):475, 1987.
14. Hedström SA, Lidgren L: Septic arthritis and osteomyelitis. In Klippel JH, Dieppe PA, editors: *Rheumatology,* ed 2, London, 1998, Mosby-Wolfe.
15. Stanitski C: Changes in pediatric acute hematogenous osteomyelitis management, *J Pediatr Orthop* 24(4):444-445, 2004.
16. Przybylski GJ, Sharan AD: Single-stage autogenous bone grafting and internal fixation in the surgical management of pyogenic discitis and vertebral osteomyelitis, *J Neurosurg* 94(1 Suppl):1, 2001.
17. Ray NJ, Basset RL: Pyogenic vertebral osteomyelitis, *Orthopedics* 8(4):504, 1985.
18. Mader JT et al: The host and skeletal infection: classification and pathogenesis of acute bacterial bone and joint sepsis, *Baillieres Best Pract Res Clin Rheumatol* 13(1):1, 1999.
19. Perlman M et al: The incidence of joint involvement of adjacent osteomyelitis in pediatric patients, *J Pediatr Orthop* 20(1):40, 2000.
20. Cassidy JT: *Textbook of pediatric rheumatology,* New York, 1982, Wiley & Sons.
21. Hollingworth P: Juvenile chronic arthritis. In Klippel JH, Dieppe PA, editors: *Rheumatology,* ed 2, London, 1998, Mosby-Wolfe.
22. Guille JT et al: Bilateral Legg-Calvé-Perthes disease: presentation and outcome, *J Pediatr Orthop* 22(4):458-463, 2002.
23. Glueck CJ et al: Association of antithrombotic factor deficiencies and hypofibrinolysis with Legg-Perthes disease, *J Bone Joint Surg Am* 78(1):3-13, 1996.
24. Herring JA et al: The lateral pillar classification of Legg-Calvé-Perthes disease, *J Pediatr Orthop* 12(2):143-150, 1992.
25. Schoenecker PL et al: Legg-Perthes disease in children under 6 years old, *Orthop Rev* 22:201, 1993.
26. Askoy MC et al: Comparison between braced and non-braced Legg-Calvé-Perthes-disease: a radiological outcome study, *J Pediatr Orthop B* 13(3):153-157, 2004.
27. Gigante A et al: What is the best treatment for Osgood-Schlatter disease? *J Fam Pract* 53(2):153-156, 2004.
28. Swanson MW et al: Identification of neurodevelopmental abnormality at 4 and 8 months by the movement assessment of infants, *Dev Med Child Neurol* 34(4):321-337, 1992.
29. Scott MO et al: Duchenne muscular dystrophy gene expression in normal and diseased human muscle, *Science* 239:1418, 1988.
30. Stevens A, Lowe J: *Pathology,* London, 1995, Mosby-Wolfe.
31. Nevo Y et al: Fetal muscle biopsy as a diagnostic tool in Duchenne muscular dystrophy, *Prenat Diag* 19(10):921, 1999.
32. Kapsa R et al: Novel therapies for Duchenne muscular dystrophy, *Lancet Neurol* 2(5):299-310, 2003.
33. Moxley RT 3rd et al: Practice parameter: corticosteroid treatment of Duchenne dystrophy: report of the Quality Standards Subcommittee of the American Academy of Neurology and the Practice Committee of the Child Neurology Society, *Neurology* 64(1):13-20, 2005.
34. Campanacci M, Capanna R, Picci P: Unicameral and aneurysmal bone cysts, *Clin Orthop Relat Res Mar* (204):25-36, 1986.
35. Glasser DB et al: Survival, prognosis, and therapeutic response in osteogenic sarcoma: the Memorial Hospital experience, *Cancer* 69(3):698-708, 1992.
36. Rougraff BT et al: Limb salvage compared with amputation for osteocarcoma of the distal end of the femur, *J Bone Joint Surg Am* 76(5):649-656, 1994.
37. Ayala AG, Ro JY, Raymond AK: Bone tumors. In Damjanov I, Linder J, editors: *Anderson's pathology,* ed 10, St Louis, 1996, Mosby.

38. Smith LM, Cox RS, Donaldson SS: Second cancers in long term survivors of Ewing's sarcoma, *Clin Orthop Relat Res Jan* (274):275-281, 1992.

39. Ruyman FB, Grovas AC: Progress in the diagnosis and treatment of rhabdomyosarcoma and related soft tissue sarcomas, *Cancer Invest* 18(3):223, 2000.

40. Lugo-Vicente H: Molecular biology and genetics affecting pediatric solid tumors, *Bol Asoc Med P R* 92(4-8):72-82, 2000.

41. Israel MA: Molecular and cellular biology in pediatric malignancies. In Pizzo PA, editor: *Principles and practice of pediatric oncology*, Philadelphia, 1989, Lippincott.

42. King J et al: Analysis of 429 fractures in 189 battered children, *J Pediatr Orthop* 8(5):585-589, 1988.

43. Thomas SA et al: Long-bone fracture in young children: distinguishing accidental injuries from child abuse, *Pediatrics* 88(3):471-476, 1991.

STRUCTURE, FUNCTION, AND DISORDERS OF THE INTEGUMENT

NOREEN HEER NICOL • SUE E. HUETHER

MEDIA RESOURCES

℮volve **Evolve Website** (http://evolve.elsevier.com/McCance/)
- Review Questions and Answers
- Animations
- Glossary (with audio pronunciation for selected terms)
- WebLinks

CHAPTER OUTLINE

STRUCTURE AND FUNCTION OF THE SKIN
Layers of the Skin
Subcutaneous Layer
  Aging and Skin Integrity
Tests of Skin Function
Clinical Manifestations of Skin Dysfunction
DISORDERS OF THE SKIN
Inflammatory Disorders
Papulosquamous Disorders
Vesiculobullous Disorders
Infections

Vascular Disorders
Insect Bites
Benign Tumors
Cancer
Frostbite
DISORDERS OF THE HAIR
Alopecia
Hirsutism
DISORDERS OF THE NAIL
Paronychia
Onychomycosis

The skin covers the entire body and is the body's largest organ accounting for approximately 20% of the body's weight. Combined with the accessory structures of hair, nails, and glands, it forms the *integumentary system*. The primary function of the skin is to protect the body from the environment by serving as a barrier against microorganisms, ultraviolet (UV) radiation, loss of body fluids, and the stress of mechanical forces. The skin also regulates body temperature within a very narrow range and is involved in the production of vitamin D. Touch and pressure receptors provide important protective functions and pleasurable sensations.

STRUCTURE AND FUNCTION OF THE SKIN

Layers of the Skin

The skin consists of three layers: the outer layer of epidermis, a deeper layer of dermis, and the subcutaneous layer (Figure 44-1 and Table 44-1). This underlying subcutaneous layer

of connective tissue contains macrophages, fibroblasts, and fat cells.

Epidermis

The **epidermis** grows continually by shedding the superficial layer of **stratum corneum,** which is formed primarily of keratinocytes and melanocytes. These cells are named for the substances they produce. **Keratinocytes** produce **keratin,** a scleroprotein that provides protection from mechanical stress. Keratin is the main constituent of skin, hair, and nail cells. The thickness of the epidermis varies from 0.3 mm on the eyelids to 1.5 mm on the palms of the hands and soles of the feet. New cells (keratinocytes) formed in the **basal layer (stratum basale)** move upward and differentiate, forming the **spinous layer (stratum spinosum).** Together they form the **germinative layer (stratum germinativum).** The cells enlarge and then become flattened, stacked, and cornified (stratum corneum) as they ascend to the skin surface. Cornification, or keratinization, prevents dehydration of deeper skin layers. The average turnover of the epidermis is about 30 days.

The epidermis has three additional types of cells that facilitate its functional characteristics: melanocytes, Langerhans cells, and Merkel cells. The **melanocytes** are usually located near the base of the epidermis. They synthesize and secrete the pigment melanin with exposure to UV light in response to melanocyte-stimulating hormone (MSH). Melanin in the epidermis provides a shield against UV radiation and determines

skin color. **Langerhans cells** migrate to the epidermis from the bone marrow. Langerhans cells (a type of dendritic cell) and dermal dendritic cells initiate an immune response by presenting processed antigen to T cells, thus providing a defense against environmental antigens.[1] **Merkel cells** are associated with touch receptors and function as slowly adapting mechanoreceptors when stimulated by deformation of the epidermis.

Dermis

The **dermis** is 1 to 4 mm thick and is composed of three types of connective tissue: (1) collagen, (2) elastin and reticulin, and (3) a gel-like ground substance. The haphazard arrangement of connective tissue allows the skin to be mobile and to stretch and contract with body movement. Hair follicles, sebaceous glands, sweat glands, blood vessels, lymphatic vessels, and nerves are contained in the dermis. The conelike projections of the papillary dermis interface with the epidermis. The papillae provide texture to the surface of the skin by forming *rete pegs*.

The cells of the dermis include fibroblasts, mast cells, and macrophages. Fibroblasts secrete the connective tissue matrix and collagen. Mast cells release histamine and play a role in hypersensitivity reactions in the skin. Macrophages are phagocytic and participate in immune responses. Histiocytes are macrophages that reside in loose connective tissue and phagocytize pigments and the debris of inflammation.

Subcutaneous Layer

The third layer of the skin is subcutaneous tissue and consists of fat cells or adipocytes. The lobules are separated by fibrous walls (septa) of collagen and large blood vessels. Dermal collagen is continuous with the collagen found in the subcutaneous tissue.[2]

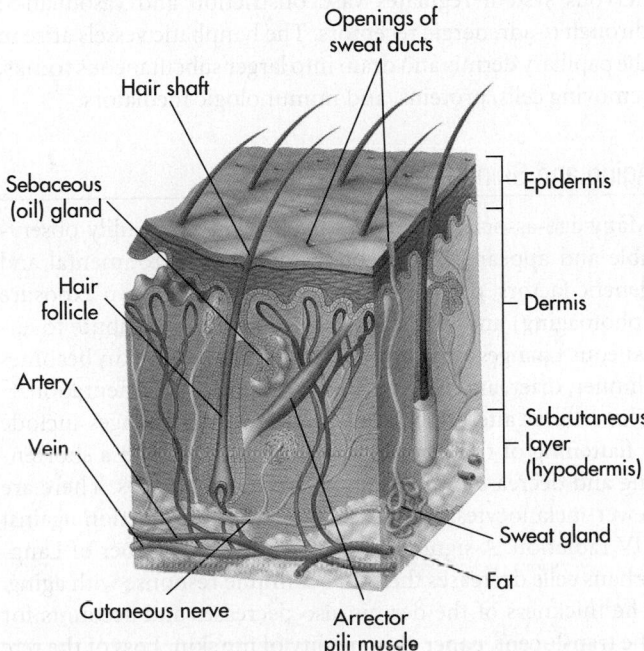

Figure 44-1 Structure of the skin. (From Thibodeau GA, Patton KT: *Anatomy and physiology,* ed 5, St Louis, 2003, Mosby.)

Image labels: Openings of sweat ducts; Hair shaft; Sebaceous (oil) gland; Hair follicle; Artery; Vein; Cutaneous nerve; Arrector pili muscle; Epidermis; Dermis; Subcutaneous layer (hypodermis); Sweat gland; Fat

Table 44-1		Layers of the Skin
Layer	**Cell Types**	**Characteristics**
Epidermis		Most important layer of skin; normally very thin (0.12 mm) but can thicken and form corns or calluses with constant pressure or friction
Stratum corneum	Keratinocytes	Tough superficial sheets of cornified cells
Stratum lucidum	Keratinocytes	Clear layers of cells containing eleidin, which becomes keratin as cells move up to the corneum layer; *found only in palmoplantar skin*
Stratum granulosum	Keratinocytes	Lose their nuclei
		Keratohyalin gives a granular appearance to this layer
Stratum spinosum	Keratinocytes	Polygonal-shaped with spinous processes projecting between adjacent keratinocytes
	Langerhans cells	Cell with dendrite process and immune function
Stratum basale (germinativum)	Keratinocytes	Basal layer where keratinocytes divide and move upward to replace cells shed from the surface
	Melanocytes	Originate in neural crest and migrate to stratum basale and produce melanin
	Merkel cells	The function of Merkel cells is not clearly known—may have role in sensation
Dermis	Macrophages	Irregular connective tissue layer with rich blood, lymphatic, and nerve supply; contains sensory receptors and special glands
Papillary layer (thin)	Mast cells	
Reticular layer (thick)	Histiocytes	Histiocytes are wandering macrophages that collect pigments and inflammatory debris
	Fibroblasts	
Subcutaneous		Subcutaneous tissue or superficial fascia of varying thickness that connects the overlying dermis to underlying muscle

Dermal Appendages

The **dermal appendages** include the nails, hair, sebaceous glands, and the eccrine and apocrine sweat glands. The **nails** are protective keratinized plates that appear at the ends of fingers and toes. Each nail is composed of four structural units: (1) the proximal nail fold, (2) the matrix from which the nail grows, (3) the hyponychium (nail bed), and (4) the nail plate (Figure 44-2). Nail growth is continuous throughout life at a rate of 1 mm or less per day.

Hair follicles and sebaceous glands are integrated units (see Figure 44-1). Hair color, density, grain, and pattern of distribution have considerable variability and depend on age, gender, and race. **Hair follicles** arise from the matrix (or bulb) located deep in the dermis. They extend from the dermis at an angle and have an erector pili muscle attached near the mid-dermis that straightens the follicle when contracted, causing the hair to stand up. Hair growth begins in the bulb, with cellular differentiation of stem cells occurring as the hair progresses up the follicle.[3,4] Hair is fully hardened, or cornified, by the time it emerges at the skin surface. Hair growth is cyclic, with periods of growth and rest that vary over different body surfaces.

The **sebaceous glands** open onto the surface of the skin through a canal. They are found in greatest numbers on the face, chest, and back; modified glands are found on the eyelids, lips, nipple, glans penis, and prepuce. Sebaceous glands secrete sebum that is composed primarily of lipids; sebum oils the skin and hair and prevents drying. Growth of sebaceous glands is stimulated by androgens, and their enlargement is one of the early signs of puberty.

The **eccrine sweat glands** are distributed over the body, with the greatest numbers in the palms of the hands, soles of the feet, and forehead. These secretions are important in thermoregulation and cooling of the body through evaporation. The **apocrine sweat glands** are fewer in number and are located in the axillae, scalp, face, abdomen, and genital area and have very limited proven function.

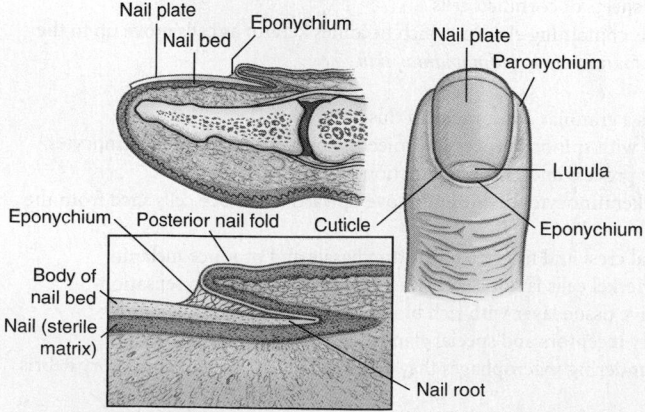

Figure 44-2 Structures of the nail. (Redrawn from Thompson JM et al: *Mosby's clinical nursing*, ed 5, St Louis, 2002, Mosby.)

Blood Supply and Innervation

The blood supply to the skin is limited to the **papillary capillaries,** or plexus, of the dermis. These capillary loops arise from a subpapillary plexus that is supplied by a deeper horizontal cutaneous arterial plexus. Branches from the deep plexus supply hair follicles and sweat glands. A subpapillary network of veins drains the capillary loops. Arteriovenous anastomoses in the dermis facilitate the regulation of body temperature. Heat loss can be regulated by varying blood flow through the skin by opening and closing the arteriovenous anastomoses in conjunction with evaporative heat loss of sweat. The sympathetic nervous system regulates vasoconstriction and vasodilation through α-adrenergic receptors. The lymphatic vessels arise in the papillary dermis and drain into larger subcutaneous trunks, removing cells, proteins, and immunologic mediators.

Aging and Skin Integrity

Many age-associated changes in the skin are readily observable and appear over the body surface. Environmental and genetic factors, particularly UV radiation from sun exposure (photoaging) and inflammatory responses, contribute to cutaneous changes with aging.[4,5] Structurally the skin becomes thinner, drier, and wrinkled with a change in pigmentation.[6,7] The cellular alterations contributing to the changes include a flattening of the dermoepidermal junction with a shortening and decrease in the number of capillary loops. There are fewer melanocytes, resulting in decreased protection against UV radiation. A significant decrease in the number of Langerhans cells decreases the skin's immune response with aging. The thickness of the dermis also decreases and accounts for the translucent, paper-thin quality of the skin. Loss of the rete pegs gives the skin a smooth, shiny appearance.[8]

The decreased vasculature and lymphatic drainage contribute to loss of barrier protection and the atrophy of eccrine, apocrine, and sebaceous glands that causes dry skin.[9] Loss of elastin fibers is associated with wrinkling. Collagen fibers become fragmented, and fibroblasts decrease in number, resulting in a decreased ability of the skin to stretch and regain shape. Decreased cell proliferation, decreased blood supply, and depressed immune responses also delay wound healing in aging skin.[10] Changes in hair color and distribution also occur. Graying is caused by loss of melanocytes from hair bulbs, and thinning occurs from a gradual decline in the number of hair follicles and growth of finer hair.

Epidermal cells change shape, and the barrier function of the stratum corneum is reduced. There is increased permeability and decreased clearance of substances from the dermis. The accumulation of such substances is related to decreased vascularity and can cause skin irritation. Temperature regulation is compromised in older adults, with an increased risk for heat stroke and hypothermia. Loss of cutaneous vasomotion and subcutaneous fat, decreased vascularity, and decreased eccrine sweat production are contributing factors. The pressure and touch receptors and free nerve endings decrease in number and reduce sensory perception. With aging many of the protective functions of the skin decrease, whereas infection and delay in wound healing increase.[11]

Tests of Skin Function

Diagnostic evaluations of skin disorders often can be completed by gathering historical information, performing a physical examination, and observing the distribution and characteristics of the presenting lesions. Additional diagnostic studies are summarized in Table 44-2.

Clinical Manifestations of Skin Dysfunction

Lesions

Lesions of the skin are readily observable and easily assessed for distribution and structure. Identification of the morphologic structure and appearance of the skin in combination with a health history is necessary to identify the underlying pathophysiology. Table 44-3 describes and illustrates the basic lesions of the skin. Special skin lesions are described in Table 44-4.

Pressure Ulcers

Pressure ulcers are lesions caused by unrelieved pressure resulting in damage of underlying tissue. Four factors contribute to the development of pressure ulcers: pressure, shearing forces, friction, and moisture. Pressure that consistently interrupts arterial and venous blood flow to and from the skin or deeper tissue is the most significant cause.[12,13] The term *decubitus ulcer* refers to an ulcer or pressure sore that results when an individual lies in the recumbent position for a long time. The more general terms of *pressure sore* or *ulcer* are used here. Factors associated with greatest risk are as follows[14]:

1. Older adults in hospitals and nursing homes
2. Neurologic disorders that result in loss of mobility and/or sensation (spinal cord injuries, dementia, or cerebrovascular disease)

3. Immobilization
4. Incontinence
5. Debilitation
6. Lying in bed without changing position or relieving pressure over an extended period
7. Lying for hours on hard imaging and operating tables
8. Chronic diseases accompanied by anemia, edema, renal failure, malnutrition, sepsis, and urinary or fecal incontinence
9. Coarse bed sheets used for turning by dragging, which produces a shearing force

Additional risk factors for the critically ill include the following[15,16]:

1. Norepinephrine infusion
2. Acute Physiology and Chronic Health Evaluation (APACHE II) score
3. Fecal incontinence
4. Anemia
5. Age greater than 60 years
6. Renal insufficiency
7. Length of hospital stay

Most individuals with darkly pigmented skin are at greater risk for developing pressure ulcers because early signs of skin damage may not be clearly visible.[17,18] Pressure sores usually develop over bony prominences: the sacrum, heels, ischia, and greater trochanters are the most common sites. Continuous pressure on tissue between the bony prominence and a resistant outside surface distorts capillaries and occludes the blood flow and oxygen supply. If the pressure is relieved within a few hours, a brief period of reactive hyperemia (redness) occurs with no lasting tissue damage. If the pressure continues unrelieved, the endothelial cells lining the capillaries become disrupted with platelet aggregation, forming microthrombi

Text continued on p. 1653.

Table 44-2	Summary of Skin Diagnostic Procedures
Test	**Purpose**
Skin biopsy	Histologic examination of tissue to determine differential diagnosis of cellular structure (i.e., benign growths vs. carcinoma, chronic infections, blistering diseases, and vasculitis)
Microscopic immunofluorescence	Identification of antibodies, immunoglobulins, and complement components for diseases such as pemphigus, vasculitis, and discoid lupus erythematosus using fluorescent light on slide-mounted biopsy specimens
Gram stain	Differentiation of gram-positive from gram-negative bacteria according to stain absorption
Culture	Identification of chronic bacterial and fungal infections by incubating skin specimens in culture media
Wood lamp examination	Examination of skin or hair to identify fungus that fluoresces bright yellow-green under ultraviolet light
Patch and scratch tests	Application of suspected allergens to skin by patch or scratch for evaluation of immune system responses to known allergens and evaluation of cell-mediated immune function (*Candida albicans*, skin fungus, chemicals, aeroallergens, and foods)
Skin scrapings	Application of potassium hydroxide and low heat to skin scrapings on a glass slide to identify dermatophytes and *C. albicans*
Side lighting	Indirect lighting of the skin using light to the side of the lesions to evaluate patterns of depression and elevation of skin lesions
Diascopy	Use of glass or clear plastic pressed on the skin to differentiate erythema caused by dilated capillaries (blanching) from extravasation of blood (no blanching)
Tzanck smear	A microscopic examination of cellular material from skin lesions to help diagnose vesicular diseases, including herpes simplex virus and varicella zoster

Table 44-3   Primary and Secondary Skin Lesions

Primary Skin Lesions	Examples		
Macule A flat, circumscribed area that is a change in the color of the skin; less than 1 cm in diameter	Freckles, flat moles (nevi), petechiae, measles, scarlet fever	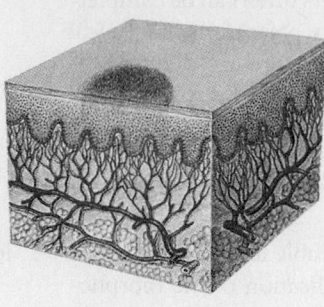	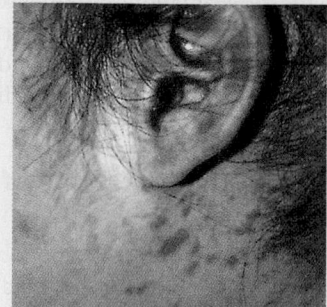 Macules[a]
Papule An elevated, firm, circumscribed area less than 1 cm in diameter	Wart (verruca), elevated moles, lichen planus	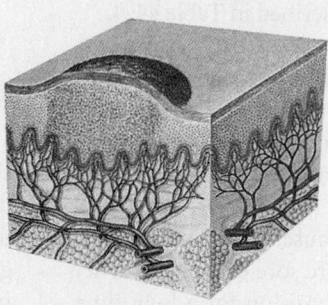	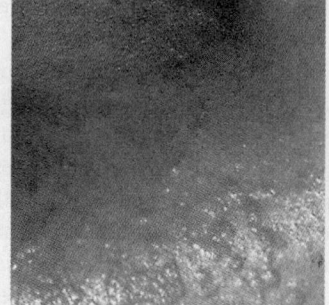 Flat warts[a] (Courtesy Dr. E. Sahn)
Patch A flat, nonpalpable, irregular-shaped macule more than 1 cm in diameter	Vitiligo, port-wine stains, mongolian spots, café-au-lait spots	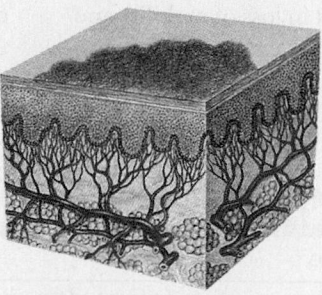	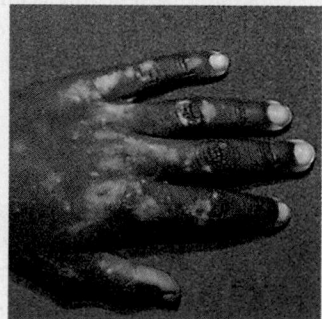 Vitiligo[b]
Plaque Elevated, firm, and rough lesion with flat top surface greater than 1 cm in diameter	Psoriasis, seborrheic and actinic keratoses	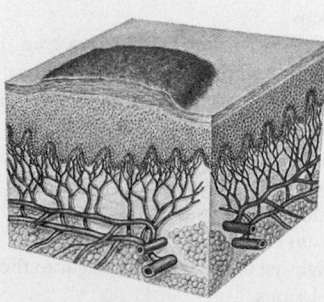	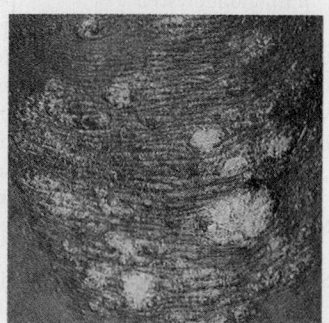 Plaque[f]

From Thompson JM, Wilson SF: *Health assessment for nursing practice*, St Louis, 2002, Mosby.

Table 44-3	Primary and Secondary Skin Lesions—cont'd

Primary Skin Lesions	Examples		
Wheal Elevated, irregular-shaped area of cutaneous edema; solid, transient; variable diameter	Insect bites, urticaria, allergic reaction	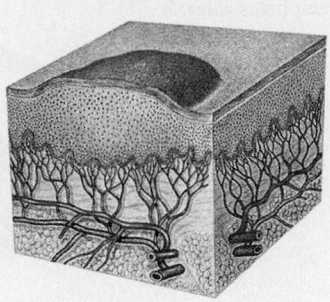	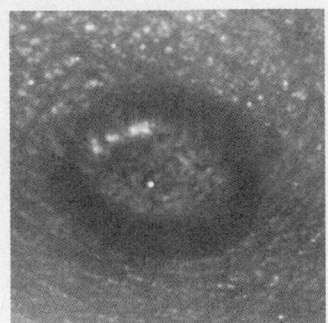 Wheal[a]
Nodule Elevated, firm, circumscribed lesion; deeper in dermis than a papule; 1-2 cm in diameter	Erythema nodosum, lipomas	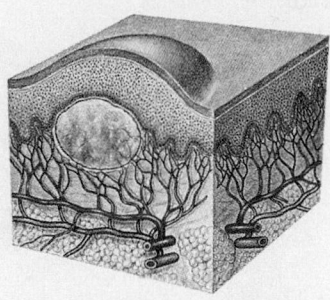	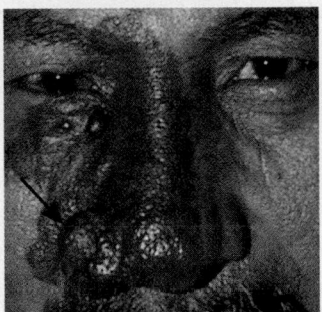 Hypertrophic nodule[c]
Tumor Elevated, solid lesion; may be clearly demarcated; deeper in dermis; greater than 2 cm in diameter	Neoplasms, benign tumor, lipoma, hemangioma	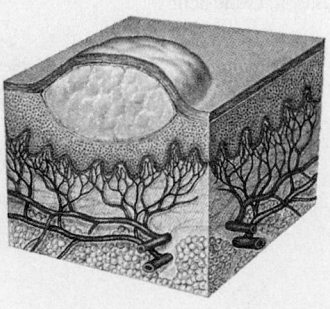	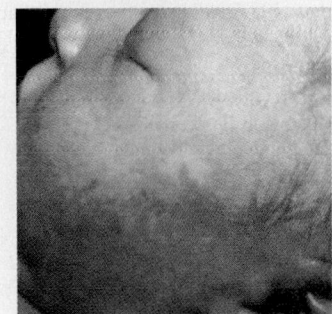 Hemangioma[b]
Vesicle Elevated, circumscribed, superficial, does not extend into dermis; filled with serous fluid; less than 1 cm in diameter	Varicella (chickenpox), herpes zoster (shingles)	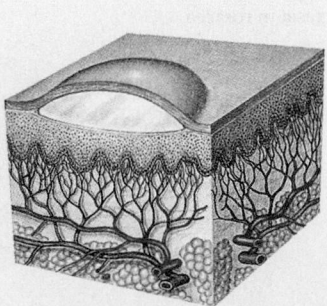	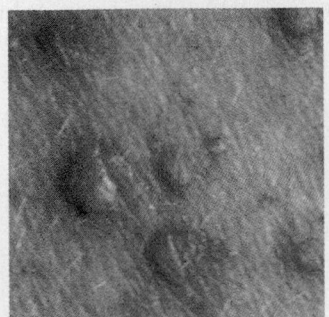 Vesicles[a]

Photo credits on p. 1653.

Continued

Table 44-3 Primary and Secondary Skin Lesions—cont'd

Primary Skin Lesions	Examples

Bulla

Vesicle greater than 1 cm in diameter

Blister, pemphigus vulgaris

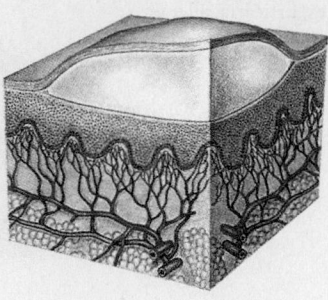

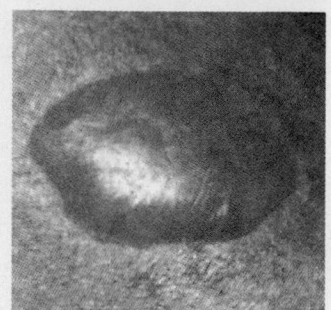

Bulla[a] (Courtesy Dr. K.A. Riley)

Pustule

Elevated, superficial lesion; similar to a vesicle but filled with purulent fluid

Impetigo, acne

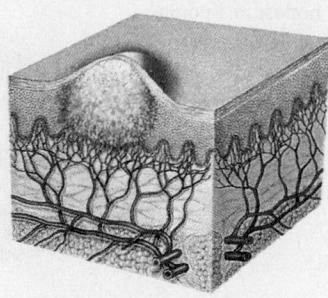

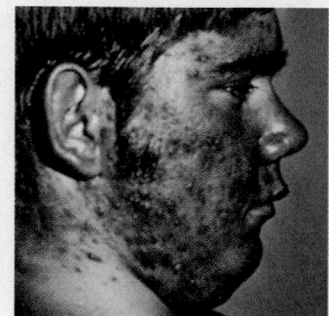

Acne[b]

Cyst

Elevated, circumscribed, encapsulated lesion; in dermis or subcutaneous layer; filled with liquid or semisolid material

Sebaceous cyst, cystic acne

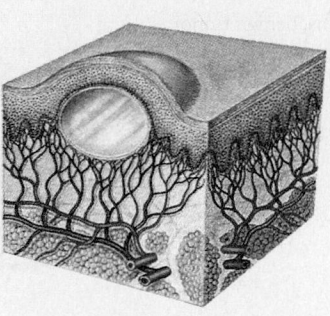

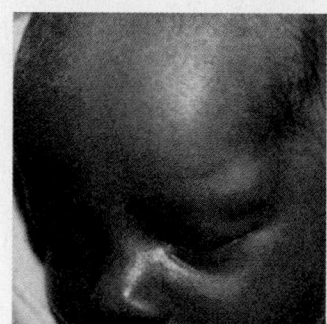

Sebaceous cyst[b]

Telangiectasia

Fine, irregular red lines produced by capillary dilation

Telangiectasia in rosacea

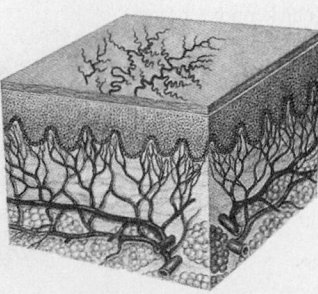

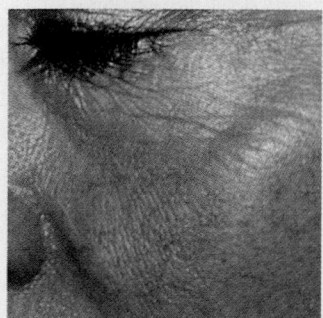

Telangiectasia[c]

Table 44-3　Primary and Secondary Skin Lesions—cont'd

Secondary Skin Lesions	Examples		
Scale Heaped-up, keratinized cells; flaky skin; irregular-shape; thick or thin; dry or oily; variation in size	Flaking of skin with seborrheic dermatitis following scarlet fever, or flaking of skin following a drug reaction; dry skin	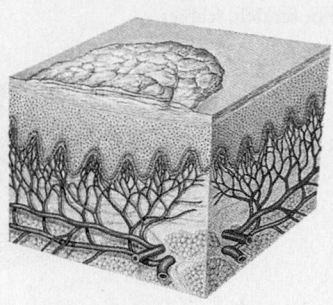	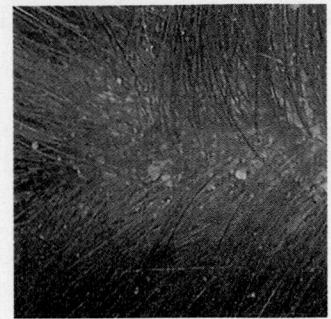 Fine scaling[d]
Lichenification Rough, thickened epidermis secondary to persistent rubbing, itching, or skin irritation; often involves flexor surface of extremity	Chronic dermatitis	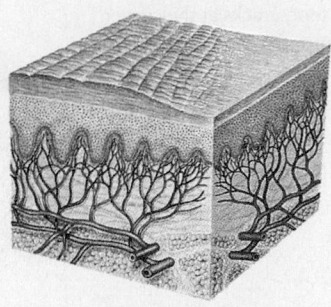	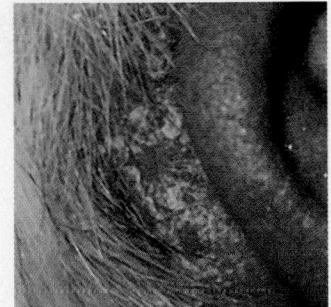 Stasis dermatitis in early stage[e]
Keloid Irregular-shaped, elevated, progressively enlarging scar; grows beyond the boundaries of the wound; caused by excessive collagen formation during healing	Keloid formation following surgery	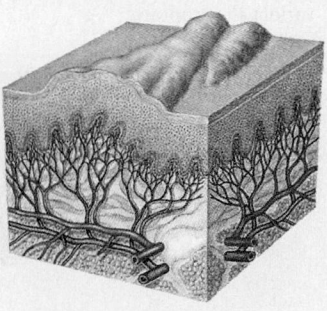	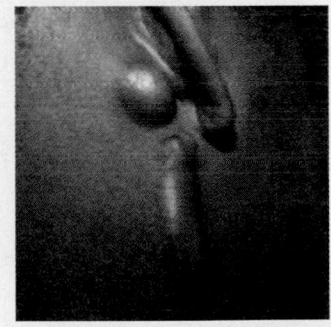 Keloid[b]
Scar Thin to thick fibrous tissue that replaces normal skin following injury or laceration to the dermis	Healed wound or surgical incision	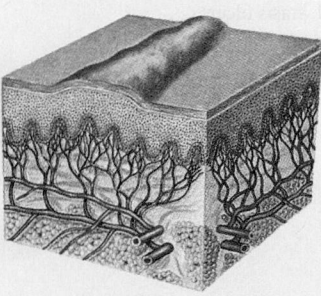	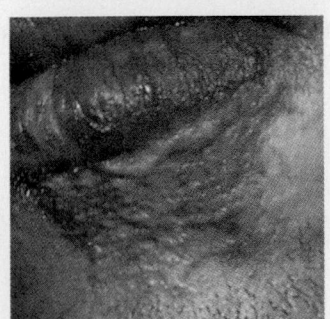 Hypertrophic scar[c]

Photo credits on p. 1653.

Continued

Table 44-3   Primary and Secondary Skin Lesions—cont'd

Secondary Skin Lesions	Examples

Excoriation

Loss of the epidermis; linear, hollowed-out, crusted area

Abrasion or scratch, scabies

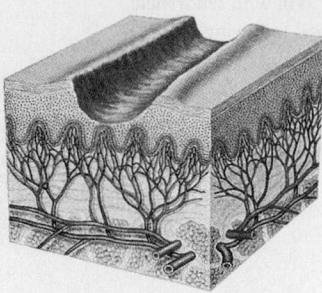
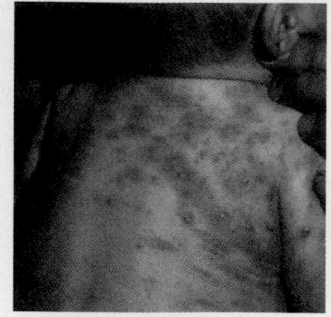

Scabies[b]

Fissure

Linear crack or break from the epidermis to the dermis; may be moist or dry

Athlete's foot, cracks at the corner of the mouth

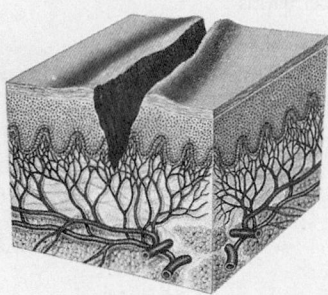
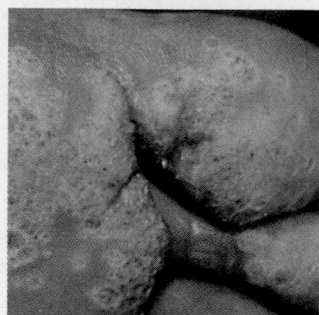

Fissures[c]

Erosion

Loss of part of the epidermis; depressed, moist, glistening; follows rupture of a vesicle or bulla

Varicella, variola after rupture

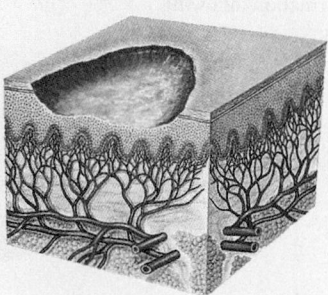
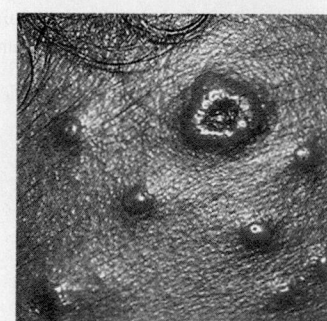

Erosion[g]

Ulcer

Loss of epidermis and dermis; concave; varies in size

Decubital, stasis ulcers

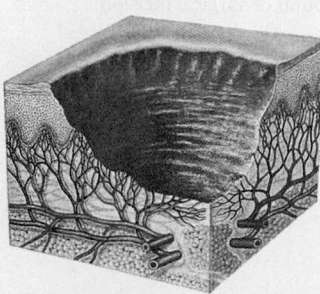
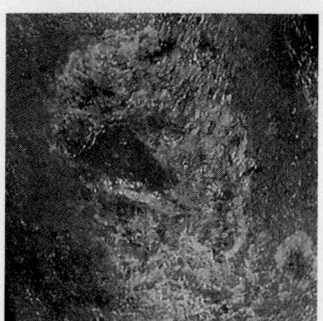

Stasis ulcer[f]

Table 44-3   Primary and Secondary Skin Lesions—cont'd

Secondary Skin Lesions   Examples

Atrophy

Thinning of the skin surface and loss of skin markings	Aged skin, striae

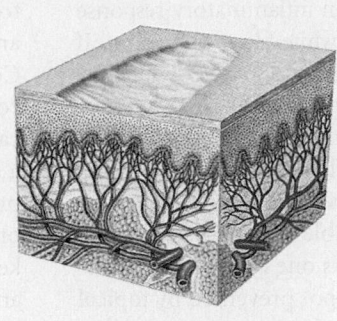
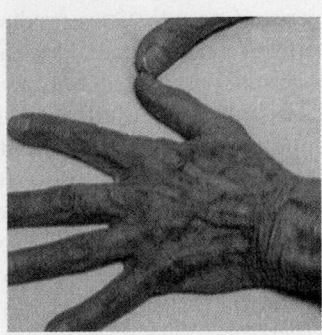

Aged skin[h]

[a]Farrar WE et al: *Infectious diseases,* ed 2, London, 1992, Gower.

[b]Weston WL, Lane AT: *Color textbook of pediatric dermatology,* ed 3, St Louis, 2002, Mosby.

[c]Goldman MP, Fitzpatrick RE: *Cutaneous laser surgery: the art and science of selective photo thermolysis,* ed 2, St Louis, 1998, Mosby.

[d]Baran R, Dawber RR, Levene GM: *Color atlas of the hair, scalp, and nails,* St Louis, 1991, Mosby.

[e]Marks JG Jr, DeLeo VA: *Contact and occupational dermatitis,* St Louis, 1991, Mosby.

[f]Habif TP: *Clinical dermatology,* ed 4, St Louis, 2004, Mosby.

[g]Cohen BA: *Pediatric dermatology,* London, 1993, Mosby-Wolfe.

[h]Seidel HM et al: *Mosby's guide to physical examination,* ed 5, St Louis, 2003, Mosby.

Table 44-4   Special Skin Lesions

Type	Clinical Manifestations
Comedone	A plug of sebaceous and keratin material lodged in the opening of a hair follicle; an open comedone has a dilated orifice (blackhead), and a closed comedone has a narrow opening (whitehead)
Burrow	A narrow, raised, irregular channel caused by a parasite
Petechiae	A circumscribed area of blood less than 0.5 cm in diameter
Purpura	A circumscribed area of blood greater than 0.5 cm in diameter

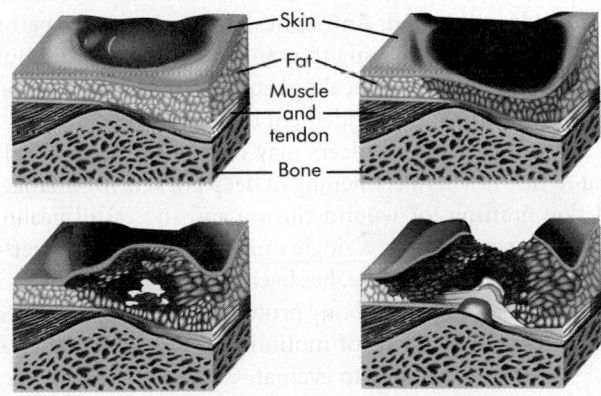

Figure 44-3 Progression of decubitus ulcer. Sustained pressure over a bony prominence compresses the tissue and reduces blood flow resulting in progressive ischemia and necrosis of tissue.

that block blood flow and cause anoxic necrosis of surrounding tissues. Pressure ulcers can be classified by stages[19]:

Suspected deep tissue injury: localized area of purple or maroon discolored intact skin or blood-filled blister caused by underlying soft tissue damage from pressure and/or shear.

I. Nonblanchable erythema of intact skin usually over bony prominence; darkly pigmented skin may not have visible blanching

II. Partial-thickness skin loss involving epidermis or dermis presenting as a shallow open ulcer with a red-pink wound bed, without slough; May also present as an intact or open/ruptured serum-filled blister

III. Full-thickness skin loss involving damage or necrosis of subcutaneous tissue that may extend to, but not through, underlying fascia; may include undermining and tunneling

IV. Full-thickness skin loss with extensive destruction, tissue necrosis, or damage to muscle, bone, or supporting structures

Unstageable: full-thickness tissue loss with base of ulcer covered by slough and/or eschar in the wound bed

A layer of dead tissue forms that appears as a blister when there is superficial damage or as a reddish blue discoloration when there is deeper tissue damage. Superficial sores are more common on the sacrum as a result of shearing or friction forces (forces parallel to the skin). Deep sores develop closer to the bone as a result of tissue distortion and vascular occlusion from pressure that is perpendicular to the tissue (over the heels, trochanter, and ischia) (Figure 44-3).

The necrotic tissue initiates an inflammatory response, with pain, fever, and leukocytosis. Although bacteria colonize the dead tissue, the infection is usually localized and self-limiting. Proteolytic enzymes from bacteria and macrophages dissolve necrotic tissues and cause a foul-smelling discharge that resembles, but is not, pus.

Pressure sores are often painful in individuals who do not have loss of sensation from spinal cord trauma or neuropathy. The presence of necrotic tissue produces an inflammatory response with hyperemia, fever, and increased white blood cell count. If the ulceration is large, toxicity and pain lead to loss of appetite, debility, and renal insufficiency. Individuals who are immunosuppressed or have diabetes mellitus may develop infection and inflammation of adjacent tissues (cellulitis) or septicemia.

The primary goal for those at risk for pressure ulcers is prevention. Several scales are available for predicting pressure sore risk, and the Braden Scale is one of those most frequently used. [20,21] Pressure sores are not prevented by topical agents because they do not relieve the pressure. Frequent skin assessment with repositioning and turning; use of pressure reduction surfaces; elimination of incontinence, moisture, and drainage; and maintenance of fluid, protein, and caloric intake are effective preventive techniques.[22,23] Nutrition, oxygenation, and fluid balance must be maintained.

Superficial ulcers should be covered with flat, nonbulky dressings that cannot wrinkle and cause increased pressure or friction. Spontaneous healing will occur more quickly when the ulcer is kept moist with an occlusive dressing.[24] Antibiotics are seldom required. Antiseptics, such as hydrogen peroxide or iodine, are damaging to granulation tissue and should not be used.[25] Successful healing requires continued adequate relief of pressure and débridement of dead tissue.[26]

Large, deep pressure ulcers may require surgical débridement of necrotic tissue, opening of deep pockets for drainage, and skin grafting for wound closure and successful healing. The myocutaneous flap, a single unit of skin with its underlying muscle and vasculature, has been an effective treatment in large avascular areas over bony prominences.[27] Application of wound tension by range of motion may also promote healing.[28] Tools are available to evaluate and document progress of healing and further research is needed to advance clinical assessment and interdisciplinary communication regarding the management of pressure ulcers.

Keloids and Hypertrophic Scars

Keloids are elevated, rounded, and firm with irregular clawlike margins that extend beyond the original site of injury. In contrast **hypertrophic scars** are elevated erythematous fibrous lesions that do not expand beyond the border of injury. Both lesions are caused by abnormal wound healing with excessive fibroblast activity and collagen formation during dermal connective tissue repair.[29] Many genes are involved.[30] Keloids are most common in darkly pigmented skin types and burn scars (see Chapter 46). Excessive or poorly aligned tension on a wound, introduction of foreign material into the skin, and certain types of trauma (e.g., burns) are provocative factors. At risk are the shoulders, back, chin, ears, and lower legs. Most keloids appear within 1 year of trauma. Individuals 10 to 30 years of age develop lesions much more commonly than do children before puberty or older adults. Hypertrophic scars usually regress within a year.

Type III collagen is increased with keloids. The increased synthesis of collagen is associated with interleukin-6 (IL-6) signaling and dermal fibroblasts that have high metabolic and mitotic rates and aberrant expression of various growth factors.[31] **Myofibroblasts,** cells with characteristics of fibroblasts and smooth muscle cells, are the principal cells in keloids. Collagenase activity in keloids is normal or increased, but the collagen may be protected from degradation by **proteoglycan,** a glycoprotein present in connective tissue that serves as a binding (cementing) material, and by specific inhibitors of proteolytic enzymes. Genes regulating fibroblasts may be up- or down-regulated in keloid tissue.[32] A familial tendency for keloid formation has been found, with autosomal recessive and autosomal dominant inheritance patterns reported.[33]

Keloids start as pink or red, firm, well-defined rubbery plaques that persist for several months after trauma. Later, uncontrolled overgrowth causes extension beyond the site of the original wound and the tumor becomes smoother, irregularly shaped, hyperpigmented, harder, and more symptomatic. Keloids typically send out **clawlike prolongations** (Figure 44-4).

Keloids are the most extreme example of cutaneous scarring and the most difficult to treat. Preventive measures such as avoiding unnecessary, elective surgeries are of paramount importance. Various treatments are available for the management of keloids and hypertrophic scars, and there is a need for research to improve treatment outcome.[34,35]

Pruritus

Pruritus, or itching, is the most common symptom associated with many primary skin disorders, such as eczema, psoriasis, or lice infestations, or it can be a manifestation of systemic disease (e.g., xerosis, chronic renal failure, cholestatic liver disease, thyroid disorders, iron deficiency) or drug reactions. Pruritus may be localized or generalized and may move from one location to another.[36] Central and peripheral nerve pathways are activated.[37]

Significant progress has been made in understanding the pathophysiology of itch. Studies show that peripheral itch mediators include neuropeptides, serotonin, prostaglandins, bradykinin, histamine, substance P, and acetylcholine and that the itch sensation is carried by specific unmyelinated

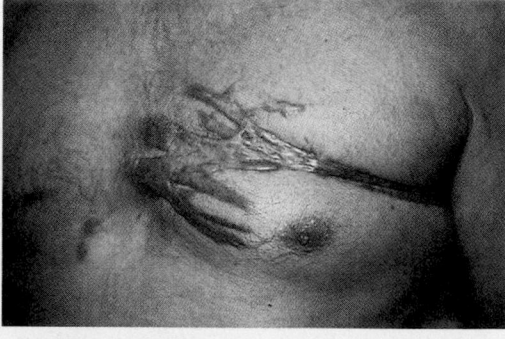

Figure 44-4 Keloid. (Courtesy Department of Dermatology, School of Medicine, University of Utah.)

C-nerve fibers.[38,39] These nerve fibers may also interact with dermal mast cells.[40]

Itching also has been linked to pain because many stimuli that induce pain produce itching at lower intensities. Central nervous system mechanisms also can modulate itching, which is less perceptible when the mind is concentrating on other things. How the central nervous system influences the itch sensation is unclear. *Neuropathic itch* is related to pathology along an afferent pathway (i.e., postherpetic neuropathy). *Psychogenic itch* is associated with psychologic disorders (i.e., depression and obsessive-compulsive disorder).[41]

Chronic itching is an unpleasant sensation relieved by scratching—often done so intensely that trauma to the skin occurs, resulting in infection and scarring. Some individuals become so distraught with the constant irritation that they apply heat with enough intensity and duration to produce burns.

Management of localized itching depends on the cause, and the primary condition must be treated. Symptomatic relief may be obtained from antihistamines, which also have a sedative effect. Minor tranquilizers, such as promethazine, may be effective for some causes of pruritus. Itching related to dry, rough skin (xerosis) can be managed with applications of emollients and increased environmental humidity. Topical steroids are immediately effective with some occurrences of pruritus; however, in some instances, pruritus is resistant to any type of therapy. New topical treatment therapies are being developed, as are the use of phototherapy treatment with narrow band UVB and vagal nerve stimulation[42] and cutaneous field stimulation.[43] Analgesics used to treat neuropathic pain also can be effective for treating pruritus.[44]

DISORDERS OF THE SKIN

Disruptions in skin integrity may be precipitated by trauma, abnormal cellular function, infection and inflammation, and systemic diseases. Many skin disorders are benign and self-limiting, whereas others are severe and life threatening.

Inflammatory Disorders

The most common inflammatory disorder of the skin is **eczema,** or dermatitis. Eczema and dermatitis are general terms that describe a particular type of inflammatory response in the skin—the terms can be used interchangeably. Diseases considered eczematous are generally characterized by pruritus, lesions with indistinct borders, and epidermal changes. These lesions can appear as either erythema, papules, or scales, and they can present in an acute, subacute, or chronic phase. Atopic dermatitis, contact dermatitis (whether nonallergic [irritant] or allergic), lichen simplex chronicus, nummular eczema, and seborrheic dermatitis are examples of specific types of eczema or dermatitis.[45] Edema, serous discharge, and crusting occur with continued irritation and scratching. In chronic eczema the skin becomes thickened, leathery, and hyperpigmented from recurrent irritation and scratching. The location of eczema is related to the underlying cause.

Eczematous inflammations need to be differentiated from other rashes and dermatoses, particularly psoriasis.

Allergic Contact Dermatitis

Allergic contact dermatitis is a common form of T-cell mediated or delayed hypersensitivity (type IV).[46] (See Chapter 8 for various types of allergic responses.) Allergens (e.g., microorganisms, chemicals, foreign proteins, drugs, metals, latex) can form the sensitizing antigen; contact with poison ivy is a common example (Figure 44-5). The response is a reaction to irritants with release of cytokines, chemokines, and cytotoxins from keratinocytes, dendritic cells (Langerhans cells), and natural killer cells. When the allergen comes into contact with the skin the allergen is bound to a carrier protein, forming a hapten-specific sensitizing antigen. Langerhans cells process the antigen and carry it to T cells that then become sensitized to the antigen releasing cytokines and chemokines leading to leukocyte infiltration and inflammation.[47] Latex allergy can be either a type IV hypersensitivity to chemicals used in latex rubber processing or a type I immediate hypersensitivity with IgE antibodies formed in response to latex rubber protein.[48]

In delayed hypersensitivity, several hours pass before an immunologic response is apparent. The T cells play an important role because they differentiate and secrete lymphokines that affect macrophage movement and aggregation, coagulation, and other inflammatory responses (see Chapter 8). Sensitization usually develops with first exposure to the antigen, and symptoms of dermatitis occur with reexposure.

The manifestations of allergic contact dermatitis include erythema and swelling with pruritic (itching) vesicular lesions

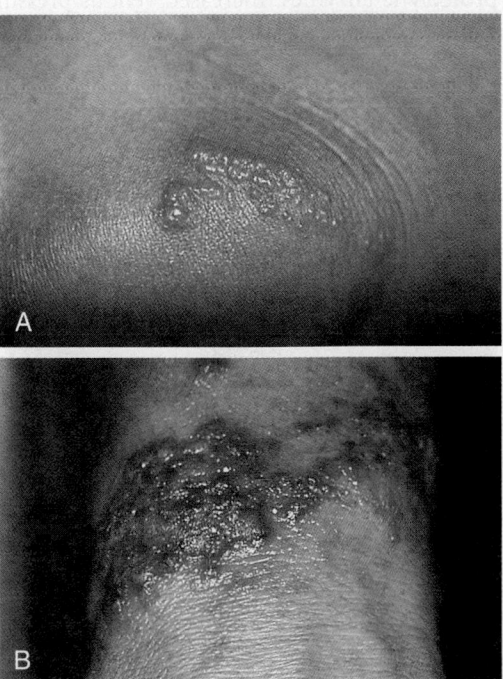

Figure 44-5 Poison ivy. A, Poison ivy on knee. B, Poison ivy dermatitis. (Courtesy Department of Dermatology, School of Medicine, University of Utah.)

in the areas of allergen contact. The pattern of distribution provides clues to the source of the antigen (e.g., hands exposed to chemical solutions or boundaries from rings and bracelets). Patch tests with specific antigens may assist with diagnosis. Removal of the allergen is necessary for resolution of the inflammatory response and tissue repair. Topical or systemic steroids, as well as other symptomatic treatment, may be required depending on the severity of the lesion.[47]

Atopic Dermatitis

Atopic dermatitis (allergic dermatitis) is more common in infancy and childhood; however, some individuals are affected throughout life. A family history of asthma, allergic rhinitis, dry skin, food allergy, and eczema often accompanies this disorder. During adolescence and childhood the lesions are usually localized to the hands and feet or flexor surfaces (i.e., antecubital fossa, popliteal space) of the arms and legs (Figure 44-6). The erythema, scaling, and lichenification (thickened and leather-like skin) are exacerbated by scratching because the lesions manifest by itching. The scratching increases susceptibility to infections from *Staphylococcus aureus* and predisposition to cutaneous dissemination of viruses, particular herpes simplex. The pathogenesis and treatment of atopic dermatitis in adults are similar to that in children[49] and are discussed in detail in Chapter 45.

Stasis Dermatitis

Stasis dermatitis usually occurs on the legs as a result of venous stasis and edema. The disorder is associated with varicosities (incompetent venous valves), phlebitis, and vascular trauma. Pooling of venous blood traps leukocytes that may release proteolytic enzymes. Increased venous pressure widens interendothelial pores with deposition of fibrin and other macromolecules making them unavailable for repair.[50] Edema evolves to erythema and pruritus and progression to scaling, petechiae, and hyperpigmentation. Progressive lesions become ulcerated (stasis ulcers), particularly around the ankles and tibia (Figure 44-7).

Treatment includes elevating the legs as often as possible, not wearing tight clothes around the legs, and not standing for long periods. Defined infections are treated with antibiotics. Chronic lesions with ulceration are treated with moist dressings, external compression, and vein ablation surgery.[51,52]

Irritant Contact Dermatitis

Irritant contact dermatitis is a common nonimmunologically mediated inflammation of the skin. The intensity of the inflammation is related to the concentration of the irritant, exposure time, and disruption of the skin barrier.[53] Irritation can occur from almost anything, especially if the epidermal barrier is compromised in any way (Box 44-1). The skin lesions are similar in appearance to allergic contact dermatitis. Removing the source of irritation and use of topical agents (i.e., corticosteroids and petroleum-based emollients) and non-irritating soaps constitute effective treatment.

Seborrheic Dermatitis

Seborrheic dermatitis is a common chronic inflammation of the skin involving the scalp, eyebrows, eyelids, ear canals, nasolabial folds, axillae, chest, and back (Figure 44-8). In infants it is known as *cradle cap*. The cause is unknown, but genetic predisposition an immunologic response to yeasts from the genus *Malassezia* have been implicated.[54] The lesions appear from infancy to old age, with periods of remission and exacerbation. The lesions appear as greasy, scaly, white, or yellowish inflammatory plaques in sebaceous areas with mild pruritus. Mild cases are treated with shampoos containing sulfur, salicylic acid, or tar. Ketoconazole has antifungal and anti-inflammatory effects and has been used with success.[55] Topical calcineurin inhibitors have also been effective and corticosteroid applications are useful for suppression of severe symptoms but should not be used for maintenance therapy.[54a]

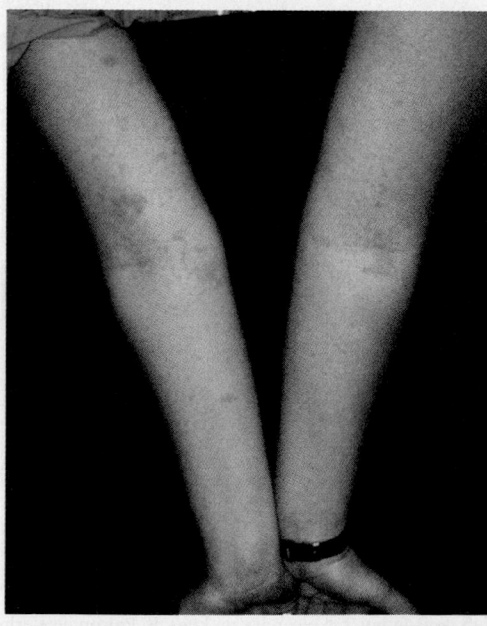

Figure 44-6 Atopic dermatitis. (Courtesy Department of Dermatology, School of Medicine, University of Utah.)

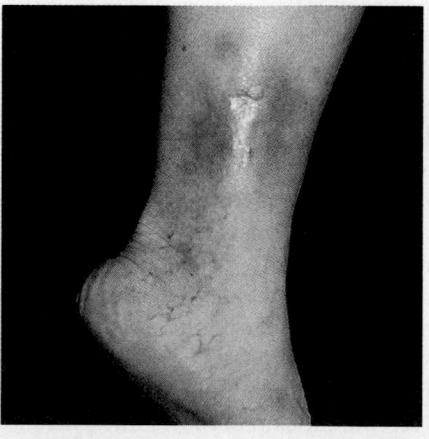

Figure 44-7 Stasis ulcer. (Courtesy Department of Dermatology, School of Medicine, University of Utah.)

Papulosquamous Disorders

Psoriasis, pityriasis rosea, and lichen planus are disorders characterized by inflammatory processes associated with papules, scales, plaques, and erythema. Collectively they are described as **papulosquamous disorders.**

Psoriasis

Psoriasis is a chronic, relapsing, proliferative skin disorder that involves the skin, scalp and nails and can occur at any age. The disease affects about 2% of the population.[56] Psoriasis is a T-cell mediated autoimmune disease. Inflammatory cytokines (i.e., tumor necrosis factor [TNF], interferon-gamma [IFN-γ], IL-6, IL-12, IL-15, IL-17, IL-22, IL-23) from activated T cells, B cells, and macrophages cause the skin changes

---

Box 44-1	Substances Known to Cause Contact Dermatitis

Alkalis
  Soaps
  Detergents
  Ammonia preparations
  Lye
  Drainpipe cleaners
  Toilet bowl cleaners
  Oven cleaners
Acids
Metal salts
  Cyanides of calcium, copper, mercury, nickel, silver, zinc
  Chlorides of calcium and zinc
Bromine, chlorine, iodine, fluorine
Insecticides
Dusts of lime, zinc, arsenic
Dyes and fragrances
Wood dust from teak, cinchona bark, quinine, pyrethrum
Tobacco dust from cigars
Explosive powders
Hydrocarbons
  Crude petroleum, lubricating oil, cutting oil
  Paraffins, mineral oils
  Asphalt, other tar products
Soot, peat
Preservatives

---

and comorbidities occurring in psoriasis.[57] The onset is generally established by 20 years of age. A family history of psoriasis is common. The genetic mechanisms are complex and the human leukocyte antigen (HLA)-Cw6 allele (PSORS1) is a major susceptibility gene.[58]

The dermis and epidermis are thickened, with cellular hyperproliferation, altered keratinocyte differentiation, expanded dermal vasculature, infiltration of neutrophils and lymphocytes, and inflammation.[59] The turnover time for shedding the epidermis is decreased from the normal 26 to 30 days to 3 to 4 days. There are increased numbers of germinative cells and an increase in transit time of cells through the dermis. The rapid cellular proliferation does not allow time for cell maturation and keratinization to occur, resulting in a thickened epidermis and plaque formation. The loosely cohesive keratin gives the lesion a silvery, scaly appearance. There is often capillary dilation and increased vascularization to accommodate the increased cell metabolism. The increased vascularity causes erythema.

The types of psoriasis include plaque (psoriasis vulgaris), inverse, guttate, pustular, and erythrodermic. **Plaque psoriasis** is the most common and affects 80% to 90% of individuals with psoriasis. The disease can be mild, moderate, or severe, depending on the size, distribution, and inflammation of the lesions. Early onset psoriasis is an inflammatory lesion with epidermal hyperproliferation and the presence of activated T lymphocytes.[57] The typical lesion of plaque psoriasis is a well-demarcated, thick, silvery, scaly, erythematous plaque surrounded by normal skin (Figure 44-9). Initial lesions usually develop insidiously as small erythematous papules that enlarge and coalesce into larger inflammatory lesions. The lesions are commonly located on the scalp, elbows, and knees and at sites of trauma. The scales are usually loosely adherent and may cause small bleeding points when removed. **Inverse psoriasis** involves lesions that develop in skinfolds (i.e., axilla or groin). They are large, smooth, dry, and deep red. The progress of psoriasis is characterized by remissions and exacerbations. Antimalarial drugs, lithium, nonsteroidal

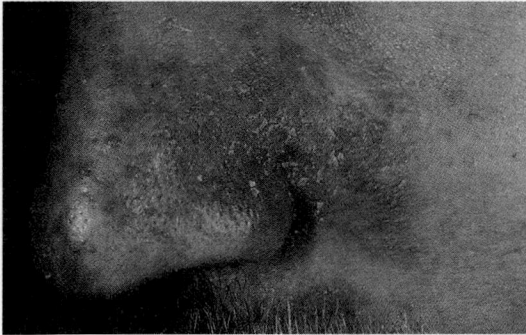

Figure 44-8 Seborrheic dermatitis. (Courtesy Department of Dermatology, School of Medicine, University of Utah.)

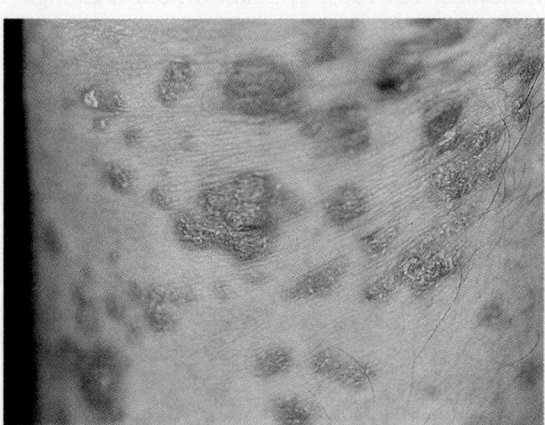

Figure 44-9 Psoriasis. Typical oval plaques with well-defined borders and silvery scale. (Courtesy Department of Dermatology, School of Medicine, University of Utah.)

anti-inflammatory drugs, and beta-blockers, tend to exacerbate existing psoriasis.

In **guttate psoriasis,** small papules (1 to 10 mm) appear suddenly on the trunk and extremities (Figure 44-10). The lesions may appear a few weeks after a streptococcal respiratory infection and are more common in children. Guttate psoriasis may resolve spontaneously in weeks or months. **Pustular psoriasis** appears as blisters of noninfectious pus (collections of neutrophils) that develop over areas of plaque psoriasis. **Erythrodermic (exfoliative) psoriasis** is often accompanied by itching or pain with widespread red, scaling lesions that cover a large area of the body.

Psoriatic arthritis and ankylosing spondylitis are associated with the proinflammatory cytokines that cause psoriatic skin lesions. Joints of the hands, feet, knees, and ankles are involved, and 5% to 50% of individuals with psoriasis have seronegative joint involvemment.[60] **Psoriatic nail disease** can occur in all psoriasis subtypes with pitting, onycholysis, subungual hyperkeratosis, and nail plate dystrophy. Psoriasis is also a risk factor for a number of comorbidities including inflammatory bowel disease, metabolic syndrome, including hypertension, insulin resistance, dyslipidemias, and abdominal obesity, and increased risk for atherosclerosis and myocardial infarction that is independent of traditional risk factors for these diseases.

Treatment is individualized and related to reducing epidermal cell turnover. Mild lesions are usually treated with emollients, keratolytic agents, and corticosteroids. Moderate lesions may respond to UV light, tar preparations, or a combination of both, and to methotrexate, cyclosporine A, and acitretin. Vitamin D₃ (calcitriol) is used to reduce epidermal proliferation. Moderate to severe disease is the indication for biologic treatment, including drugs that inhibit the activation and number of T lymphocytes (alefacept), drugs that block T-cell adhesion (efalizumab), or TNF-α inhibitors (adalimumab, etanercept, infliximab).[56]

Pityriasis Rosea

Pityriasis rosea is a benign self-limiting inflammatory disorder that occurs more often in young adults, usually during winter months. The cause is unknown but is thought to be associated with a virus because of the timing and clustering of the outbreaks.[61] Pityriasis rosea begins as a single lesion known as a **herald patch** (Figure 44-11) that is circular, demarcated, salmon-pink, approximately 3 to 4 cm in diameter, and usually located on the trunk. Early lesions are macular and papular; secondary lesions develop within 14 to 21 days and extend over the trunk and upper part of the extremities. Lesions are rarely located on the face. They emerge as small erythematous papules that expand into characteristic oval lesions. There may be few or hundreds of lesions. The pattern of distribution follows the skin lines around the trunk and resembles a drooping pine tree. As scales flake off from the margin of the lesions, a collarette pattern is formed. Itching is the most common symptom. Headache, fatigue, or sore throat may precede the development of the lesions.[62]

The diagnosis of pityriasis rosea is made by the clinical appearance of the lesion. It can be confused with secondary syphilis, psoriasis, or seborrheic dermatitis. The disorder is usually self-limiting and resolves in a few months with symptomatic treatment for pruritus. UV light, antihistamines, or topical corticosteroids may be used to control itching, and erythromycin may control the rash.[63] Sun exposure facilitates resolution of the lesions.

Lichen Planus

Lichen planus is a benign, autoimmune inflammatory disorder of the skin and mucous membranes. The cause is unknown, but T cells, adhesion molecules, inflammatory cytokines, perforin, and antigen-presenting cells are involved.[64] The infiltrate of T cells mediates immunoreactivity against basal layer keratinocytes, which have altered surface antigens and adhesion molecules.[65] Lichen planus is also linked to hepatitis C virus.[66] Some individuals develop lichenoid lesions after exposure to drugs or film-processing chemicals. The age of onset is usually between 30 and 70 years. The disorder begins with nonscaling, violet-colored pruritic papules, 2 to 4 mm in size, usually located on the wrists, ankles, lower legs, and genitalia (Figure 44-12). The papules are flat topped and have a polygonal shape. New lesions are pale pink and evolve into a dark violet. Persistent lesions may be thickened and red,

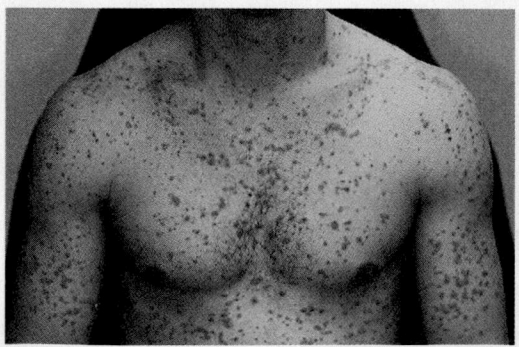

Figure 44-10 Guttate psoriasis after streptococcal infection. Numerous uniformly small lesions may abruptly occur after streptococcal pharyngitis. (Courtesy Department of Dermatology, School of Medicine, University of Utah.)

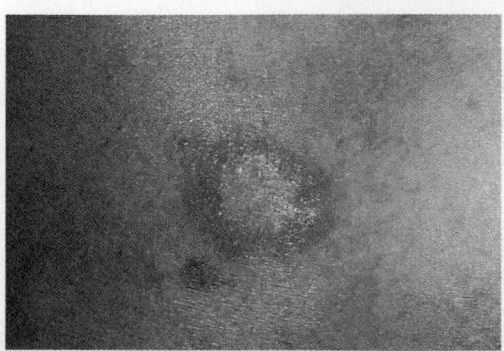

Figure 44-11 Pityriasis rosea herald patch. A collarette pattern has formed around the margins. (Courtesy Department of Dermatology, School of Medicine, University of Utah.)

forming hypertrophic lichen planus. The lesions often involve the oral mucous membranes, appearing as lacy white rings that must be differentiated from leukoplakia or oral candidiasis.[67] Fine white lines, known as Wickham striae, can be seen throughout the oral lesions on magnification. These lesions also can develop on the penis and vulvovaginal area. More commonly, oral lesions do not ulcerate, but localized or extensive painful ulcerations do, and frequently occur. Chronic ulcerated lesions become malignant in 1% of individuals with the disease. Thinning and splitting of nails are common, and part or all of the nail may be shed.

Pruritus is the most distressing symptom. The lesions are self-limiting and may last for months or years, with an average duration of 6 to 18 months. Postinflammatory hyperpigmentation is a common consequence of the lesion. Approximately 20% of individuals have a recurrence. Diagnosis is commonly made by the clinical appearance of the lesion. Treatment is individualized. Antihistamines are given for itching, and topical or systemic corticosteroids may be used to control inflammation. Mucous membrane lesions are treated with topical steroids, topical tacrolimus, or pimecrolimus.[68]

Acne Vulgaris

Acne vulgaris is an inflammatory disorder of the pilosebaceous follicle (the sebaceous gland contiguous with a hair follicle). It occurs most commonly during adolescence. Details of this disorder are presented in Chapter 45.

Acne Rosacea

Acne rosacea is an inflammation of the skin that develops in middle-age adults. The disease is chronic with episodes of exacerbation. The most common lesion types are erythematotelangiectatic, papulopustular, phymatous, and ocular.[69] They occur in the middle third of the face, including the forehead, nose, cheeks, and chin (Figure 44-13). The cause is unknown, but immune-mediated inflammation may be a factor.[70] The lesions are associated with chronic, inappropriate vasodilation resulting in flushing and sensitivity to the sun. Sebaceous hypertrophy, fibrosis, and telangiectasia may be severe enough to produce an irreversible bulbous appearance of the nose, known as *rhinophyma*. Disorders of the eye often accompany

rosacea, particularly conjunctivitis and, more rarely, keratitis, which can result in visual impairment.[71] Facial application of fluorinated topical steroids may precipitate rosacea-like lesions that are difficult to treat. There is controversy regarding the association between *Demodex folliculorum* (mites), *Helicobacter pylori* infection, and rosacea.[72,73]

Hot drinks or alcohol should be taken cautiously because the heat and vasodilation accentuate erythema. Tetracycline, though photosensitizing, continues to be the drug of choice for treatment, and a low-maintenance dose may be required after the most severe lesions are controlled. Daily use of photoprotection, including sunscreens, is recommended; 1% topical metronidazole and 15% azelaic acid gel may be effective.[74,75] Surgical excision of excessive tissue may be required for rhinophyma.

Lupus Erythematosus

Lupus erythematosus is an inflammatory, autoimmune, systemic disease with cutaneous manifestations. Discoid (or cutaneous) lupus erythematosus (DLE) is limited to the skin and can lead to systemic lupus erythematosus (SLE) in approximately 5% of individuals. DLE may be described as a subset of SLE, with cutaneous manifestations as the only symptom[76] (Figure 44-14). (SLE, a diffuse, multisystem disease, is discussed in Chapter 8.)

Discoid (Cutaneous) Lupus Erythematosus

Discoid (cutaneous) lupus erythematosus (DLE) usually occurs in genetically susceptible adults, particularly in women in their late 30s or early 40s. There are three forms of the disease: acute, subacute, and chronic. The lesions may be single or multiple and of various sizes. Often the lesions are located on light-exposed areas of the skin, and photosensitivity is common. The face is the most common site of lesion involvement; a butterfly pattern of distribution is found over the nose and cheeks.[77]

The cause is thought to be an altered immune response to an unknown antigen or response to UV wavelengths with the development of self-reactive T and B cells, decreased number

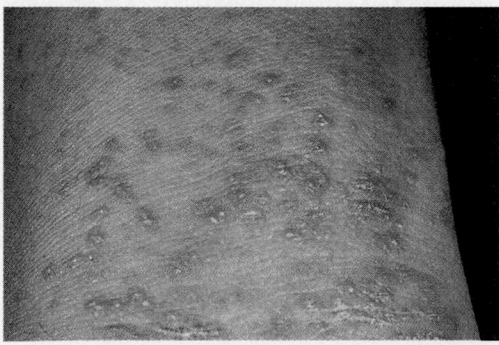

Figure 44-12 Hypertrophic lichen planus on arms. (Courtesy Department of Dermatology, School of Medicine, University of Utah.)

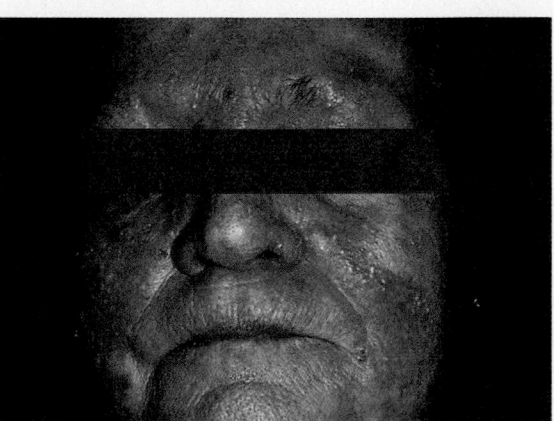

Figure 44-13 Granulomatous rosacea. Pustules and erythema occur on the forehead, cheeks, and nose. (Courtesy Department of Dermatology, School of Medicine, University of Utah.)

of regulatory T cells, and increased proinflammatory cytokines.[78] Autoantibodies and immune complexes cause tissue damage.[79]

The lesions of DLE usually begin as red macules or papules with an adherent scale that resolve with residual atrophy, scarring, or pigment changes. The characteristic manifestations of the different categories of DLE are summarized in Table 44-5.

Diagnosis of DLE is made from the presenting symptoms, biopsy of skin lesions with direct immunofluorescence, as well as histology. Skin biopsy with immunofluorescent observation reveals lumpy deposits of immunoglobulins, especially

IgM, in some individuals. Individuals with DLE must use sunscreen and limit direct exposure to the sun because this initiates or exacerbates lesions. Initial treatment with potent topical steroids relieves symptoms. Calcineurin inhibitors have been used with some success.[80] Antimalarial drugs (e.g., hydroxychloroquine sulfate) provide first-line systemic therapy and usually lead to clinical improvement within 1 to 3 months.[81] These medications must be used with caution to prevent serious side effects.

Vesiculobullous Disorders

Vesiculobullous skin disorders represent a group of diseases that have different causes and clinical courses but share a common characteristic of vesicle, or blister, formation. Two such diseases are pemphigus and erythema multiforme.

Pemphigus

Pemphigus (meaning to blister or bubble) is a rare autoimmune blistering disease of the skin and oral mucous membranes caused by circulating autoantibodies directed against the cell surface adhesion molecule, desmoglein, at the desmosomal cell junction in the suprabasal layer of the epidermis. Immunoglobulin G (IgG) autoantibodies and C3 complement bind to the desmoglein adhesion molecules resulting in the destruction of cell-to-cell adhesion (acantholysis) in the epidermis with fluid accumulation and the resulting symptom of blister formation. A subset of autoantibodies may block keratinocyte acetylcholine receptors, disrupting keratinocyte cohesion.[82] IgA autoantibodies have been found in some individuals.[83] Pemphigus can occur in all age groups but is more prevalent between 40 and 50 years of age. There is a genetic predisposition as well as environmental triggers.[84]

Pemphigus presents in varying forms. *Pemphigus vulgaris* is the most common form with acantholysis at the suprabasal level. Oral lesions precede the onset of skin blistering, which is more prominent on the face, scalp, and axilla. The blisters rupture easily because of the thin, fragile overlying portion of epidermis. *Pemphigus vegetans* is a variant of pemphigus vulgaris with large blisters occurring in tissue folds of the axilla and groin. *Pemphigus foliaceus* is a milder form of the disease

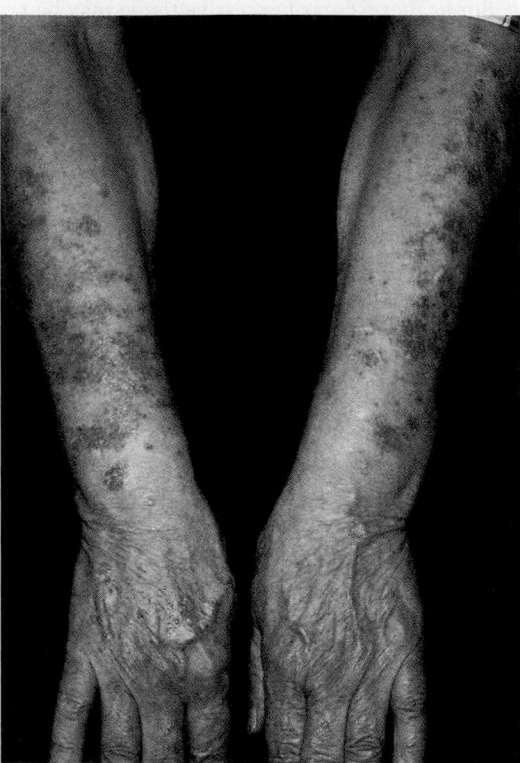

Figure 44-14 Subacute cutaneous lupus (discoid lupus erythematosus). (Courtesy Department of Dermatology, School of Medicine, University of Utah.)

Table 44-5	Categories and Manifestations of Discoid Lupus Erythematosus (DLE)
Category of DLE	**Clinical Manifestations**
Acute	
Localized	Butterfly pattern of erythema over bridge of nose and malar areas of face; may have fine surface scales and underlying edema; scalp areas may develop alopecia; lasts for hours to days
Generalized	Diffuse or papular erythema of face, upper trunk or extremities; develops quickly and lasts hours to days
Subacute	Erythematous macules and papules that evolve into *papulosquamous* or *annular* plaques developing on sun-exposed areas of the upper body (V area of neck, upper chest, back, shoulders, extensor surface of arms and hands); can be associated with reaction to drugs; may be accompanied by mild systemic disease
Chronic	Classic discoid lupus erythematosus is the most common form; lesions are red to purple macules or papules with a superficial brownish scale; scale can penetrate hair follicle leaving a carpet-tack appearance when removed; may have residual scarring, dermal atrophy hypopigmentation, alopecia, and telangiectasia; Raynaud phenomenon occurs in some individuals

Data from: Kuhn A, Biji M: *Lupus* 17(5):389-393, 2008; Rothfield N, Sontheimer RD, Bernstein M: *Clin Dermatol* 24(5):348-362, 2006.

and involves acantholysis at the subcorneal level with blistering, erosions, scaling, crusting, and erythema usually of the face and chest. Oral mucous membranes are rarely involved. *Pemphigus erythematosus* is a subset of pemphigus foliaceus often associated with systemic lupus erythematosus with positive antinuclear antibodies. The lesions are generally less widely distributed.

The diagnosis of pemphigus is made from the clinical manifestations and histologic examination of the skin. Immunofluorescence demonstrates the presence of antibodies at the site of blister formation. The clinical course of the disease may range from rapidly fatal to relatively benign. The primary treatment for pemphigus is systemic corticosteroids, usually in high doses during acute episodes or when there is widespread involvement. Adjuvant immunosuppressive therapy also may be used and decreases the steroid dosage requirement. Newer methods of treatment and a clearer understanding of the pathogenesis have improved the prognosis and decreased mortality.[85]

Bullous Pemphigoid

Bullous pemphigoid (BP) is a more benign disease than pemphigus vulgaris, with the presence of serum and bound IgG and blistering of the subepidermal skin layer.[86] Autoantibodies have been found to hemidesmosomal proteins designated BP 180 and BP 230. Loss of dermal-epidermal adhesion is caused by proteinases released by granulocytes.[87] The lesions of pemphigoid begin with localized erythema or as pruritic plaques that extend and become edematous. The plaques turn reddish-purple by 2 to 3 weeks, with vesicles and bullae emerging on the surface (Figure 44-15). The bullae do not extend with pressure. The blisters rupture within 1 week and heal rapidly. BP occurs more commonly after 60 years of age.

Diagnosis is by skin biopsy and immunofluorescent examination. The presence of subepidermal blistering and eosinophils distinguishes pemphigoid from pemphigus. Treatment usually includes hydroxyzine (Atarax) for itching and prednisone with an immunosuppressive drug to control blistering. Individuals who respond to treatment with sulfapyridine or dapsone do not require prednisone.

Erythema Multiforme

Erythema multiforme is not a single disease but rather a syndrome characterized by inflammation of skin and mucous membranes. It often is associated with a T-cell mediated immunologic reaction to microorganisms (e.g., *Mycoplasma pneumoniae,* herpes simplex virus) or a toxic reaction to drugs in which TNF-α causes tissue damage.[88] Overall, it is relatively rare and can occur at any age but is more common between 20 and 40 years of age. Immune complex formation and deposition of complement (C3), IgM, and fibrinogen around the superficial dermal blood vessels, basement membrane, and keratinocytes are found in most individuals with erythema multiforme. Edema develops in the superficial dermis, leading to the formation of vesicles and bullae. The lesions vary in clinical presentation and may involve the skin or mucous membranes or both. The characteristic "bull's-eye" or "target" lesions occur on the skin surface with a central dusky region surrounded by concentric rings or alternating edema and inflammation.[89] The lesions usually occur suddenly in groups over 2 to 3 weeks. Urticarial plaques, 1 to 2 cm in diameter, can develop without the target lesion. A vesiculobullous form is characterized by mucous membrane lesions and erythematous plaques over elbows and knees. Single or multiple vesicles or bullae may arise on a part of the plaque, accompanied by pruritus and burning. In the minor form there may be ten to hundreds of lesions.[90] The lesions heal within 3 to 4 weeks (Figure 44-16).

The most common severe forms in children and young adults are **Stevens-Johnson syndrome** (severe bullous form) and **toxic epidermal necrolysis,** in which there are numerous erythematous bullous lesions on the skin and mucous membranes. These diseases may have a different etiology than erythema multiforme.[91] The cause is unknown, but an immune mechanism related to drug administration is involved.[92] Bursts of nitric oxide formation have been proposed as the cause of epidermal apoptosis and necrosis.[93] There is destruction of the epidermis in toxic epidermal necrolysis. Cytotoxic lymphocytes (early) and monocytes-macrophages (late) are involved in this severe blistering disease.[94]

Prodromal symptoms of fever, headache, malaise, sore throat, and cough develop in approximately one third of cases.

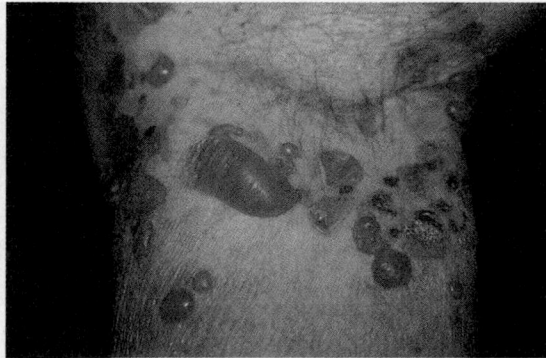

Figure 44-15 Bullous pemphigoid. Generalized eruption with blisters arising from an edematous, erythematous annular base. (Courtesy Department of Dermatology, School of Medicine, University of Utah.)

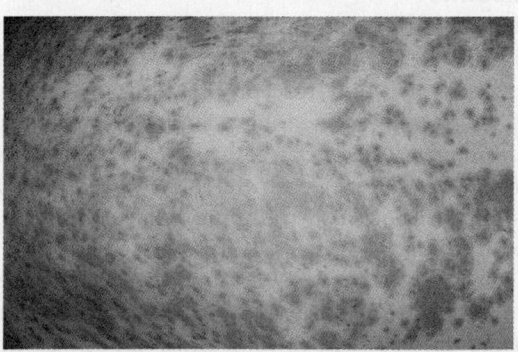

Figure 44-16 Erythema multiforme caused by doxepin. (Courtesy Department of Dermatology, School of Medicine, University of Utah.)

The bullous lesions form erosions and crusts when they rupture. The mouth, air passages, esophagus, urethra, and conjunctiva may be involved. Blindness can result from corneal ulcerations. Difficulty with eating, breathing, and urinating may develop with severe manifestations. The disease can involve the kidneys and extend from the upper respiratory passages into the lungs. Severe forms of the disease can be fatal.

Diagnosis is made by medication history, recognition of the target lesion, or by skin biopsy if the target lesion is absent. Mild acute forms of the disease last 10 to 14 days. Mild forms of the disease, usually self-limiting, require no treatment. Any ongoing drug therapy should be withdrawn or reevaluated and underlying infections treated. Fluid and electrolyte balance should be monitored in severe forms of the disease, and mucous membranes must be carefully managed with a bland diet, warm saline eyewashes, topical anesthetics, or corticosteroids to maintain comfort and prevent infection. Use of systemic steroids is controversial.[95] Cutaneous blisters can be treated with wet compresses of nanocrystalline silver. Ophthalmic, kidney, and lung involvement requires special care. Resolution occurs in 8 to 10 days, usually without scarring. Mucosal lesions may take 6 weeks to heal.

Infections

Cutaneous infections are common forms of skin disease. They generally remain localized; however, serious complications can develop with systemic involvement. The types of skin infection include bacterial, viral, and fungal. Most infections occur superficially; however, systemic signs and symptoms occasionally develop and rarely become life threatening. Aerobes, yeast, and anaerobes comprise the normal flora of the skin and often provide protection against pathogens that cause skin infections, including *Staphylococcus* and *Streptococcus*.[96]

Bacterial Infections

Most bacterial infections of the skin are caused by local invasion of pathogens. Coagulase-positive *S. aureus* and, less often, beta-hemolytic streptococci are the common causative microorganisms.[97] Community-acquired methicillin-resistant *Staphylococcus aureus* (C-MRSA) is also a cause of serious skin infection (Box 44-2).

Folliculitis

Folliculitis is usually caused by a bacterial infection of the hair follicle. *S. aureus* is a common causative organism. The infection develops from proliferation of the organism around the opening of the follicle and then spreads into the follicle. Inflammation is caused by the release of chemotactic factors and enzymes from the bacteria. The lesions appear as pustules with a surrounding area of erythema. They are most prominent on the scalp and extremities and rarely cause systemic symptoms. Prolonged skin moisture, skin trauma, and poor hygiene are associated contributing factors to the development of folliculitis. Cleaning with soap and water and topical application of antibiotics are effective forms of treatment.

Furuncles and Carbuncles

A **furuncle**, or "boil," is an inflammation of the hair follicles that may develop from a preceding folliculitis and spread through the follicular wall into the surrounding dermis. The invading organism is usually *S. aureus*. The infecting strain may spread to the skin from the anterior nares. Any skin area with hair can be infected, and one or several lesions may be present. The precipitating events are similar to folliculitis. The initial lesion is a deep, firm, red, painful nodule 1 to 5 cm in diameter (Figure 44-17). Within a few days the initial erythematous nodule changes to a large fluctuant and tender

Box 44-2	Community-Acquired Methicillin-Resistant *Staphylococcus aureus* (C-MRSA)

C-MRSA is a serious skin and soft tissue infection that includes abscesses, cellulitis, and necrotizing fasciitis. Infections are documented among healthy individuals who have no known risk factors, that is, no recent hospitalization, surgical procedures, or prolonged antibiotic treatment. Outbreaks have been documented among athletic teams, prisoners, and in daycare centers. C-MRSA strains are epidemiologically and clonally unrelated to hospital- or nursing home–acquired MRSA. Genotyping for the staphylococcal chromosomal cassette mec (SCCmec) type IV and Panton-Valentine leukocidin genes are the most common tests. C-MRSAs are more sensitive to antibiotic treatment and there is a wider choice of antibiotic treatment options for C-MRSA compared with hospital-acquired MRSA. C-MRSA is usually susceptible to a variety of oral non–beta-lactam antibiotics, including trimethoprim-sulfamethoxazole, clindamycin, tetracyclines, and linezolid. Parenteral therapy with vancomycin or daptomycin also can be considered. Mupirocin may be used to clear MRSA from nasal secretions if cultures show contamination in the nose. New drugs are under investigation. Preventive measures include good hand hygiene, applying antiseptics and covering cuts and abrasions, use of antibacterial soaps for showers after contact sports, avoidance of sharing towels and razors, and frequent towel washing.

Data from May TJ, Safranek S: *J Fam Pract* 58(5):276, 278, 2009; McConeghy KW, Mikolich DJ, LaPlante KL: *Pharmacotherapy* 29(3): 263-280, 2009; Miller LG; Kaplan SL: *Infect Dis Clin North Am* 23(1): 35-52, 2009.

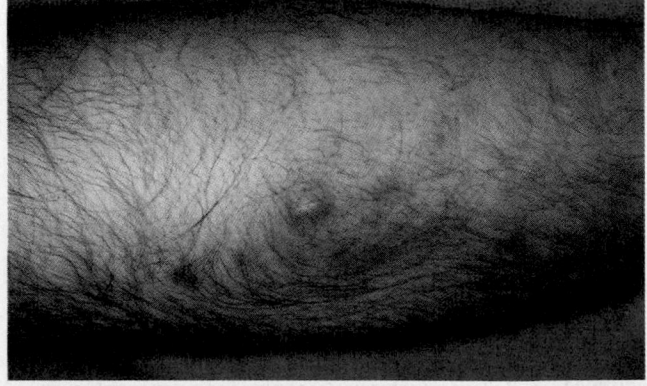

Figure 44-17 Furuncle on the forearm. (Courtesy Department of Dermatology, School of Medicine, University of Utah.)

cystic nodule that may be accompanied by cellulitis. No systemic symptoms are present, and the lesion may drain large amounts of pus and necrotic tissue.

A **carbuncle** is a collection of infected hair follicles occurring most often on the back of the neck, the upper back, and the lateral thighs. The lesion begins in the subcutaneous tissue and lower dermis as a firm mass that evolves into an erythematous, painful, swollen mass that drains through many openings. Abscesses may develop. Chills, fever, and malaise are systemic symptoms that can occur during the early stages of lesion development.

Furuncles and carbuncles are treated with warm compresses to provide comfort and promote localization and spontaneous drainage. Abscess formation requires incision and drainage, and recurrent infections are treated with systemic antibiotics.

Cellulitis

Cellulitis is an infection of the dermis and subcutaneous tissue usually caused by *Staphylococcus* or group B streptococci.[98] Cellulitis can occur as an extension of a skin wound, an ulcer, or from furuncles or carbuncles. Risk factors include diabetes mellitus, edema, peripheral vascular disease, tinea pedis, insect bites, and immune suppression.[99] The infected area is erythematous, warm, swollen, and painful and can extend to lymph nodes and the blood. The infection responds to systemic antibiotics, and Burow soaks can be used to relieve pain.

Erysipelas

Erysipelas is an acute superficial infection of the upper dermis (a superficial form of cellulitis) most often caused by group A streptococci. The face, ears, and lower legs are common sites of involvement, and the site of initial infection may not be identified. Chills, fever, and malaise precede the onset of lesions by 4 hours to 20 days. The initial lesions appear as firm, red spots that enlarge and coalesce to form a clearly circumscribed, advancing, bright red, hot lesion with a raised border. Vesicles may appear over the lesion and at the border, producing a bullous form of the disease. Itching, burning, and tenderness accompany the development of the lesion. Cold compresses provide symptomatic relief, and systemic antibiotics are required to arrest the infection.[100]

Impetigo

Impetigo is a superficial lesion of the skin caused by coagulase-positive *Staphylococcus* or alpha-hemolytic streptococci. It may complicate atopic dermatitis.[101] The disease occurs in adults but is more common in children (see Chapter 45).

Viral Infections
Herpes Simplex Virus

There are eight types of **herpes simplex virus (HSV),** a group of deoxyribonucleic acid (DNA) viruses: HSV-1 (type 1), HSV-2 (type 2), cytomegalovirus (CMV), varicella-zoster virus (VZV; type 3), Epstein-Barr virus, and human herpesviruses 6, 7, and 8 (Kaposi sarcoma–associated) cause substantial neurologic morbidity among infants and children.[102] A "cold sore" or "fever blister" is a type of HSV-1 infection and is the most common manifestation of HSV.[103] HSV-1 usually causes infection of the cornea (herpes keratitis), mouth (gingivostomatitis), and labia (labialis). Individuals receiving cytotoxic therapy for cancer are at risk.

The lesions of HSV-1 appear as a rash or clusters of inflamed and painful vesicles within the mouth, over the tongue, or on the lips and around the nose (Figure 44-18). Increased sensitivity, paresthesias, and mild burning may occur before onset of the lesion. The vesicles rupture, forming a crust. Lesions may last 2 to 6 weeks. Occasionally there is associated upper respiratory infection. HSV-1 is transmitted by contact with infected saliva. Treatment is symptomatic, and the lesions usually resolve within 2 weeks.

Genital infections are more commonly caused by HSV-2. The virus is spread by skin-to-skin mucous membrane contact during viral shedding. Risk of infection is high after sexual contact with infected individuals and when there is immunosuppression. Vertical transmission from mother to neonate is associated with significant neonatal morbidity and mortality.[104] After penetrating the skin, HSV is established in the sensory nerve ganglion innervating the primary site. Infection in one area does not protect other areas from subsequent infection. The primary infection is asymptomatic and can be determined only by a rising antibody titer.[105]

The incubation period ranges from 2 to 14 days, and clinical symptoms last 1 to 3 weeks. An individual then continues to shed the virus for 2 to 6 weeks. The virus remains dormant within sensory or autonomic nerve ganglia and can lead to recurrence of the disease. A number of factors stimulate

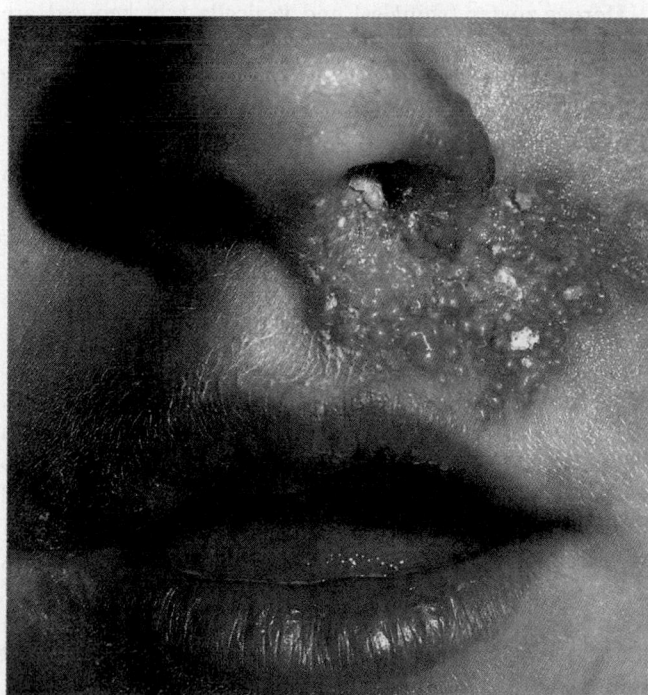

Figure 44-18 Herpes simplex labialis. Typical presentation with tense vesicles appearing on the lips and extending onto the skin. (From Habif TP: *Clinical dermatology: a color guide to diagnosis and therapy,* ed 4, St Louis, 2004, Mosby.)

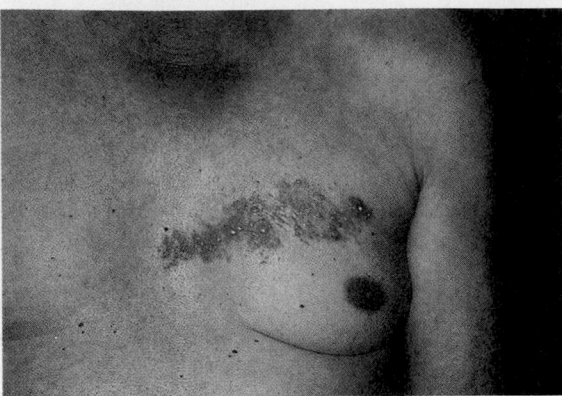

Figure 44-19 Herpes zoster. Diffuse involvement of a dermatome. (Courtesy Department of Dermatology, School of Medicine, University of Utah.)

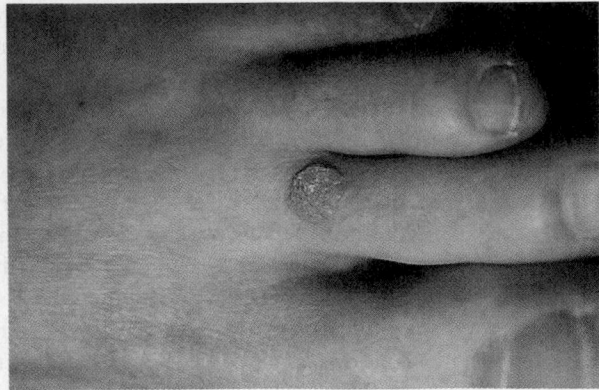

Figure 44-20 Verruca vulgaris. (Courtesy Department of Dermatology, School of Medicine, University of Utah.)

recurrence, including sun exposure, fever, or stress, and lesions are usually located at or near the primary site. Because anti-HSV antibodies develop in response to infection, recurrence is also related to the titer or amount of antibodies present.

Genital herpes (HSV-2) also may occur in primary or recurrent forms, and a large number of infections are sexually transmitted, usually within 3 to 14 days after exposure (see Chapter 24). The lesions begin as small vesicles that progress to ulceration within 3 to 4 days with pain, itching, and weeping. Treatment includes oral or topical administration of an antiviral drug that decreases new lesion formation and promotes healing. Progress is being made with development of both therapeutic and prophylactic vaccines.[106]

Herpes Zoster and Varicella

Herpes zoster (shingles) and **varicella** (chickenpox) are caused by the same herpesvirus—VZV. Varicella is a primary infection followed years later by herpes zoster, particularly among those who are immunosuppressed.[107] Chickenpox usually occurs in children (see Chapter 45).

Herpes zoster, or shingles, has initial symptoms of pain and paresthesia localized to the affected dermatome (the cutaneous area innervated by a single spinal nerve; see Chapter 14), followed by vesicular eruptions along a facial, cervical, or thoracic lumbar dermatome (Figure 44-19). Some individuals have vesicles scattered outside the area of the dermatome but lesions do not usually cross the midline. Local symptoms are alleviated with compresses, calamine lotion, or baking soda. Persistent pain is a debilitating complication, particularly in older adults and requires treatment.[108] Approximately 20% of individuals experience postherpetic neuralgias.[109] Antiviral drugs are useful if used within the first 72 hours.[110] Treatment includes a topical lidocaine patch, anti-convulsant medication, controlled-release narcotics, and tricyclic antidepressants.[108] Topical capsaicin may be used to relieve post-herpetic neuralgia. The varicella vaccine is safe and effective and may boost humoral and cellular immunity in older adults.[111]

Warts

Warts (verrucae) are benign lesions of the skin caused by the human papillomavirus (HPV). There are many different types of HPV, and specific viruses are associated with specific kinds and locations of lesions. An oncoprotein expressed by HPV is thought to inactivate growth controls regulated by *p53* tumor-suppressor protein.[112] The lesions are round and elevated with a rough, grayish surface; can occur anywhere on the skin[113]; and are transmitted by touch. *Common warts* (verrucae vulgaris) occur most often in children and are usually on the fingers, although they may be located on any skin surface or mucous membrane. Warts vary in shape, size (flat, round, or fusiform), and location (Figure 44-20). Plantar warts are usually located at pressure points on the bottom of the feet.

Diagnosis of warts is by visualization. Treatment considers age of the individual and size and location of the lesion. Warts can be removed by freezing with liquid nitrogen, electrocautery, vaporization with lasers, application of keratolytics, or application of irritants and corrosives such as salicylic acid, formaldehyde, interferons, or podophyllum.[114,115] Many warts resolve spontaneously but often recur.

Condylomata acuminata (venereal warts) are highly contagious and sexually transmitted. The cauliflower-like lesions occur in moist areas, along the glans of the penis, vulva, and anus (see Chapter 24). Oncogenic HPV is a primary cause of cervical cancer[116] (see Chapter 23).

Fungal Infections

The fungi causing superficial skin infections are called *dermatophytes,* and they thrive on keratin (stratum corneum, hair, nails). Fungal disorders are known as *mycoses;* when caused by dermatophytes, the mycoses are termed *tinea* (dermatophytosis or ringworm).

Tinea Infections

Tinea infections are fungal infections of the skin and are classified according to their location on the body.[117] The most common sites are summarized in Table 44-6. These infections are common in children (see Chapter 45). **Tinea pedis** is a chronic, superficial fungal infection of the skin of the foot common in adults (Figure 44-21). In prepubertal children, most scaling disorders of the toes and feet are eczema. **Tinea corporis** (**ringworm**) and **tinea capitis** (a fungal infection of the scalp) are much more common in children than

Table 44-6	Common Sites of Tinea Infections
Site	**Clinical Manifestations**
Tinea capitis (scalp)	Scaly, pruritic scalp with bald areas; hair breaks easily
Tinea corporis (skin areas, excluding scalp, face, hands, feet, groin)	Circular, clearly circumscribed, mildly erythematous scaly patches with a slightly elevated ringlike border; some forms are dry and macular, and other forms are moist and vesicular
Tinea cruris (groin, also known as "jock itch")	Small erythematous and scaling vesicular patches with a well-defined border that spreads over the inner and upper surfaces of the thighs; occurs with heat and high humidity
Tinea pedis (foot, also known as "athlete's foot")	Occurs between the toes and may spread to the soles of the feet, nails, and skin of toes; slight scaling, macerated painful skin, occasionally with fissures and vesiculation
Tinea manus (hand)	Dry, scaly, erythematous lesions, or moist vesicular lesions that begin with clusters of intensely itching, clear vesicles; often associated with fungal infection of the feet
Tinea unguium or onychomycosis (nails)	A superficial or deep inflammation of the nail that develops yellow-brown accumulations of brittle keratin over all or portions of the nail

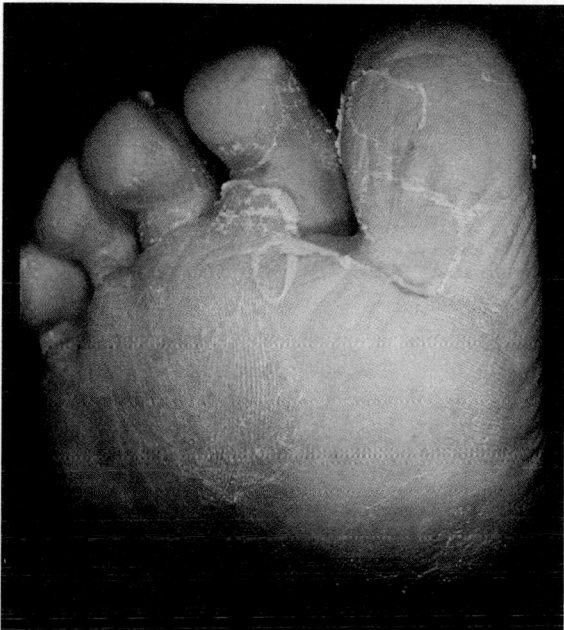

Figure 44-21 Tinea pedis. Inflammation has extended from the web area onto the dorsum of the foot. (Courtesy Department of Dermatology, School of Medicine, University of Utah.)

adults. (See Chapter 45 for a discussion of fungal infections in children.)

Tinea is diagnosed by culture, microscopic examination of skin scrapings prepared with potassium hydroxide wet mount, or observation of the skin with a UV light (Wood lamp). Cultures establish the particular type of fungus and are necessary for hair and nail infections. Fungi have characteristic spores and filaments known as **hyphae** that are more prominent when prepared in potassium hydroxide. The spores fluoresce blue-green when exposed to UV light. Treatment is related to the type of fungi and includes both topical and systemic antifungal medication.

Candidiasis

Candidiasis is caused by the yeastlike fungus *Candida albicans* and normally can be found on mucous membranes, on the skin, in the gastrointestinal tract, and in the vagina.

C. albicans can, under certain circumstances, change from a commensal organism to a pathogen, particularly in the critically ill and those who are immunosuppressed.[118] Factors that predispose to infection include (1) a local environment of moisture, warmth, maceration, or occlusion; (2) the systemic administration of antibiotics; (3) pregnancy; (4) diabetes mellitus; (5) Cushing disease; (6) debilitated states; (7) age younger than 6 months (more likely to get an infection because of decreased immune reactivity); (8) immunosuppression; and (9) certain neoplastic diseases of the blood and monocyte-macrophage system. The resident bacteria on the skin, mainly cocci, inhibit proliferation of *C. albicans*. Cell-mediated immunity plays a major role in the defense against monilial infections. *C. albicans* can activate the complement system by the alternative pathway and can include small abscesses. Candidiasis affects only the outer layers of mucous membranes and skin and occurs in the mouth, vagina, uncircumcised penis, and large skinfolds (under breast, in arm folds and abdominal creases). Table 44-7 lists the different sites of candidiasis. Innate and adaptive immune responses are required for elimination of *C. albicans*.[119,120]

The initial lesion is a thin-walled pustule that extends under the stratum corneum with an inflammatory base that may burn or itch. The accumulation of inflammatory cells and scale produces a whitish yellow curdlike substance over the infected area. The lesion ceases to spread when it reaches dry skin.[121] Antifungal medication is used for treatment.

Vascular Disorders

Vascular abnormalities are commonly associated with skin diseases, or they may be present as congenital vascular malformations (see Chapter 45) or as vascular responses to local or systemic vasoactive substances. Blood vessels may increase in number, dilate, constrict, or become obliterated by disease processes.

Cutaneous Vasculitis

Vasculitis (angiitis) is an inflammation of the blood vessels of the skin. The vasculitis is often idiopathic or can be triggered by infection, decreased blood flow (i.e., venous stasis), drugs, or autoimmune disorders. The initiating site of inflammation

Table 44-7	Sites of Candidiasis		
Site	**Risk Factors**	**Clinical Manifestations**	**Treatment**
Vagina (vulvovaginitis)	Heat, moisture, occlusive clothing Pregnancy Systemic antibiotic therapy Diabetes mellitus Sexual intercourse with infected male	Vaginal itching; white, watery, or creamy discharge Red and swollen vaginal and labial membranes with erosions Lesions may spread to anus and groin	Miconazole cream Clotrimazole tablets or cream Nystatin tablets Ketoconazole cream Loose cotton clothing
Penis (balanitis)	Uncircumcised Sexual intercourse with infected female	Pinpoint, red, tender papules and pustules on glans and shaft of penis	Any of creams listed above Topical steroids for severe inflammation
Mouth	Diabetes mellitus Immunosuppressive therapy Inhaled steroids	Red, swollen, painful tongue and oral mucous membranes Localized erosions and plaques appear with chronic infection	Nystatin oral suspension Clotrimazole troches Ketoconazole

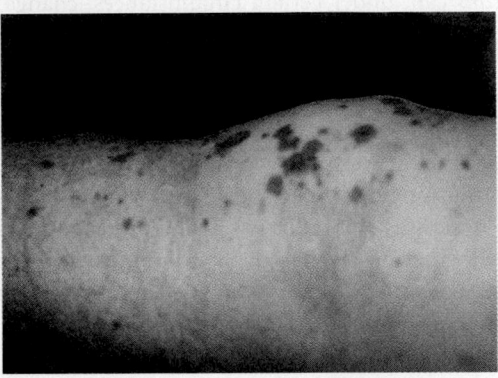

Figure 44-22 Vasculitis of the leg. (Courtesy Department of Dermatology, School of Medicine, University of Utah.)

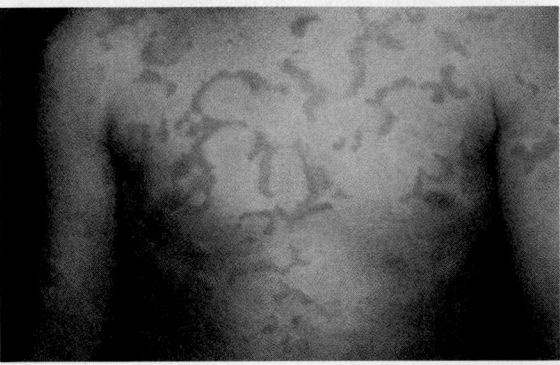

Figure 44-23 Urticaria. (Courtesy Department of Dermatology, School of Medicine, University of Utah.)

may be the blood, the vessel wall, or the adjacent tissue. Small vessels are usually affected. Immune complexes, which initiate an uncontrolled inflammatory response, are often the cause of damage, and the lesions are often polymorphic.

Cutaneous vasculitis develops from the deposit of immune complexes in small blood vessels as a toxic response to drugs (phenothiazines, barbiturates, sulfonamides) or allergens as a response to streptococcal or viral infection or as a component of systemic vasculitic syndromes. The precise mechanism is not known, but the deposit of immune complex activates complement, which is chemotactic for polymorphonuclear leukocytes and other mediators of inflammation which disrupt adhesion molecules and the vessel wall. The cutaneous form usually resolves in a few weeks and is treated with steroids.

The disorder is also known as *allergic vasculitis* and occurs primarily in adults. A systemic form (cutaneous systemic vasculitis) can involve other organs, including the kidneys, lungs, and gastrointestinal tract.[122] The extremities are the chief sites, primarily the lower legs and feet. The lesions appear as palpable purpuras (from the leakage of blood from damaged vessels) and progress to hemorrhagic bullae with necrosis and ulceration from occlusion of the vessel (Figure 44-22). Lesions appear in clusters and remain from 1 to 4 weeks. Recurrences are common. Biopsy may disclose the presence of complement or immunoglobulins in the vessel walls.

Identifying and removing the antigen (chemical, drug, or source of infection) is the first step of treatment. Corticosteroids and other drugs may be used when symptoms are severe.[123]

Urticaria

Urticaria (hives) is a circumscribed area of raised erythema and edema of the superficial dermis. **Urticarial lesions** are most commonly associated with type I hypersensitivity reactions to drugs (e.g., penicillin, aspirin), certain foods (e.g., strawberries, shellfish), systemic diseases (e.g., intestinal parasites, lupus erythematosus), physical agents (e.g., heat, cold), or complement-mediated reactions (see Chapter 8). The lesions are mediated by IgE-stimulated release of histamine, bradykinin, kallikrein from mast cells or basophils, or both, which causes the endothelial cells of skin blood vessels to contract.[124] Other inflammatory mediators such as serotonin, leukotrienes, prostaglandins and kinins may also be mediators of urticaria. The leakage of fluid from the vessels appear as wheals, welts, or hives and may be a few leaks or many leaks distributed over the entire body (Figure 44-23). Most lesions resolve spontaneously within 24 hours, but new lesions may appear. All possible causes should be removed. Antihistamines (H_1 antagonists) usually reduce hives and provide relief of itching. Epinephrine or corticosteroids and

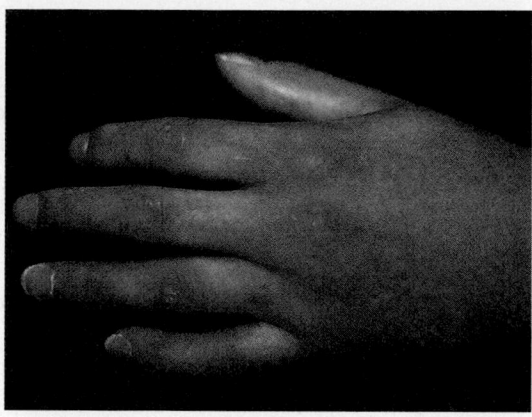

Figure 44-24 Scleroderma (acrosclerosis). Note inflammation and shiny skin. (Courtesy Department of Dermatology, School of Medicine, University of Utah.)

α-adrenergic agonists may be required for treatment of severe attacks (i.e., angioderma). Chronic urticaria (recurrent wheals for more than 6 weeks) is either an autoimmune or idiopathic disease.[125]

Scleroderma

Scleroderma means sclerosis of the skin, and the disease is associated with immune dysregulation and several autoantibodies.[126] The disease is more prominent in women. Genetic predisposition, autoimmunity, and an immune reaction to a toxic substance are possible initiating mechanisms of the disease. Impaired regulation of growth factors, collagen gene expression by fibroblasts, probably underlies the persistent fibrosis.[127] **Systemic scleroderma (sclerosis)** involves the connective tissues of many organs, including the kidney, heart, peripheral nervous system, gastrointestinal tract, and lungs.[128] Only a few organs are involved in some individuals. The cutaneous lesions are most often on the face and hands, neck, and upper chest. The entire skin can be involved, however.

There are massive deposits of collagen with fibrosis, accompanied by inflammatory reactions, vascular changes in the capillary network with a decrease in the number of capillary loops, dilation of the remaining capillaries, enhanced expression of adhesion molecules, endothelial injury and dysfunction, perivascular infiltrates, and ischemia.[129] Fibrosis occurs in the papillary and reticular dermis and in the subcutaneous tissue and deep fascia. The skin is hard, hypopigmented, taut, shiny, and tightly connected to the underlying tissue. The tightness of the facial skin projects an immobile masklike appearance, and the mouth may not open completely. The nose may assume a beaklike appearance. The hands are shiny and sometimes red and edematous (Figure 44-24). The fingers become tapered and flexed, often with depressed scars and loss of fingertips from atrophy. Raynaud phenomenon with episodic arteriolar vasoconstriction of the fingers contributes to ulcer formation and gangrene.[130] The nails may be shed. Calcium deposits develop in the subcutaneous tissue and erupt through the skin. Progression to body organs may

occur, and death is caused by subsequent respiratory failure, renal failure, cardiac dysrhythmias, or esophageal or intestinal obstruction or perforation.

Suitable clothing and a warm environment are essential to protecting the hands. Trauma and smoking should be avoided. Vasodilator drugs (i.e., angiotensin-converting enzyme inhibitors) or sympathectomy rarely has lasting effects. Symptomatic treatment is required for involved organs (e.g., intestinal resection for obstruction, antibiotics for pneumonitis, and regulation of hypertension).[131] There is no specific treatment, and progression of the disease is variable. Broad-spectrum immunosuppression and hematopoietic bone marrow or stem cell transplantation may be used early in the disease.[128,132] Fifty percent of individuals die within 5 years of the onset of scleroderma.

Insect Bites

Ticks

Ticks are significant vectors of transmitted diseases, including Rocky Mountain spotted fever and other rickettsial diseases, tularemia, and Lyme disease.[133] Ticks vary from 1 cm to about the size of a comma on this printed page. They embed their heads in the skin to obtain blood. As they gorge themselves on blood, they enlarge to many times their normal size and may release toxins or transmit microorganisms during feeding. In most instances, there is no consequence from a tick bite, with the exception of papular urticaria at the site of the bite. If mouthparts remain in the skin when the tick is removed, a persistent nodule remains that may require excision; ideally the tick should be removed completely intact. Irritant substances, such as camphor, soft wax, or heat from a match, may stimulate the tick to withdraw its head. Wearing protective clothing and applying tick repellant, such as diethyltoluamide (DEET), butopyronoxyl (Indalone), or benzylbenzoate, helps prevent tick bites.

Lyme disease is a multisystem inflammatory disease caused by the spirochete *Borrelia burgdorferi* transmitted by tick bites and is the most frequently reported vector-borne illness.[134] The highest incidence is among children (50% of infected individuals are symptom free). An immune response to *B. burgdorferi* may contribute to the pathogenesis of the disease.[135] The microorganism is difficult to culture and it escapes immunodefenses through antigenetic diversity, blocks complement-mediated killing, and hides in tissue.[136,137]

Symptoms of the disease occur in three stages.[134] *Localized infection* occurs soon after the bite with erythema migrans (rash), fever, fatigue, malaise, myalgias, and arthralgias. Within days to weeks after the onset of the illness, there is *disseminated infection* with secondary erythema migrans, arthralgias, meningitis, neuritis, or cardiovascular symptoms. *Late persistent infection* can continue for years with arthritis, encephalopathy, or polyneuropathy (see Chapter 16). The diagnosis of Lyme disease is based on the clinical presentation and history of tick bite, if known. Serologic tests often are used to confirm the diagnosis.[138] Antibiotics (i.e., doxycycline [not used in children younger than 8 years] or amoxicillin) are used for treatment.[134]

Reinfection can occur. Vaccines are in development, and personal protection is important to disease prevention.[139]

Mosquitoes and Flies

There are thousands of species of **mosquitoes** throughout the world. Species from the Culicidae family are responsible for malaria, yellow fever, dengue fever, filariasis, and St. Louis encephalitis. Several different species of mosquitoes can carry the West Nile virus which causes encephalitis (see Chapters 9 and 17). Mosquitoes can bite through thin, loose clothing and are attracted by warmth and sweat. The edema, pruritus, and papular lesions of the mosquito bite are caused by the disruption of the skin from the insertion of a blood tube by a female mosquito. Irritating salivary secretions also contain anticoagulants. Reactions vary depending on the sensitivity of the victim.

Several species of **flies** are blood suckers. The black fly (Simuliidae) is usually found in swarms—near moving bodies of water in the late spring and early summer—and is a vicious biter. The initial bite is painless because the fly injects an anesthetic with the bite. Subsequent lesions are painful and accompanied by significant swelling of surrounding tissues. Systemic reactions, such as fever, headache, and nausea, are common.

Very small flies of the Ceratopogonidae family, also known as "no-see-ums," "midges," "punkies," or sand fleas, are also blood suckers. The bite of the female is particularly miserable and produces immediate pain, erythema, and vesicles. Itching and vesicular reactions may persist for weeks.

The fiercest blood-sucking flies are the Tabanidae, or horseflies, deerflies, gadflies, greenheads, and clegs. These flies vary in size from 1 to 5 cm and produce painful, bleeding bites because of their large mouthparts. The bites produce urticaria that may be accompanied by weakness, dizziness, and wheezing.

Wounds produced by biting insects should be cleansed with soap and water, and a local antiseptic should be applied. Local applications of steroid creams or antihistamine will reduce symptoms. Systemic reactions may require more specific medical care.

Benign Tumors

Most benign tumors of the skin are associated with aging. Benign tumors include seborrheic keratosis, keratoacanthoma, actinic keratosis, and moles.

Seborrheic Keratosis

Seborrheic keratosis is a benign proliferation of cutaneous basal cells that produces smooth or warty elevated lesions. The pathogenesis is unknown. They are usually seen in older people and occur as multiple lesions on the chest, back, and face. The color varies from tan to waxy yellow, flesh colored, or dark brown-black. Lesion size varies from a few millimeters to several centimeters, and they are often oval and greasy appearing with a hyperkeratotic stuck-on scaly appearance (Figure 44-25). Cryotherapy with liquid nitrogen or electrocautery are effective treatments, and the lesions usually slough 2 to 3 weeks after treatment.

Keratoacanthoma

A **keratoacanthoma** is a benign self-limiting tumor of squamous cell differentiation arising from hair follicles. It usually occurs on sun-damaged skin of older adults and smokers; the incidence is high in males. The most commonly affected sites are the face, back of the hands, forearms, neck, and legs (Figure 44-26). The lesion develops over a period of 1 to 2 months and has a histology resembling a well-differentiated squamous cell carcinoma as follows[140]:

Proliferative stage: lesion develops as a rapidly growing, dome-shaped nodule with central crust.

Mature stage: Lesion fills with whitish keratin and requires differentiation from squamous cell carcinoma.[141]

Involution stage: Occurs over a 3- to 4-month period with regression of the lesion.

Although the lesions resolve spontaneously, they can be removed by curettage or excision to improve cosmetic appearance. Intralesional methotrexate also has been effective.[142]

Actinic Keratosis

Actinic keratosis is a premalignant lesion found on skin surfaces exposed to the UV radiation of the sun. The prevalence is highest in individuals with unprotected light-colored skin.

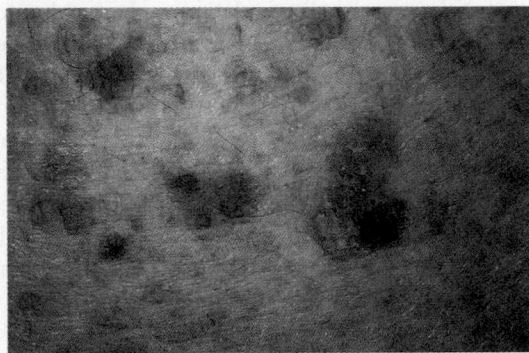

Figure 44-25 Seborrheic keratosis. Typical lesion that is broad, flat, and comparatively smooth surfaced. (Courtesy Department of Dermatology, School of Medicine, University of Utah.)

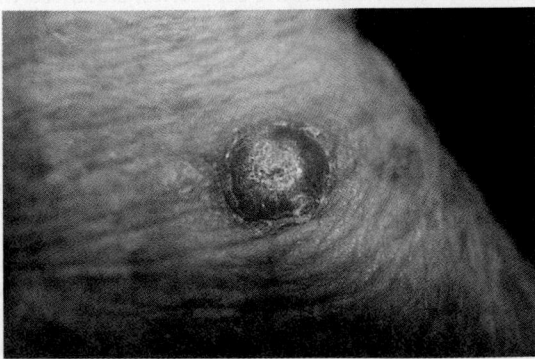

Figure 44-26 Keratoacanthoma. Classic presentation of a fully developed tumor. Round, smooth, dome-shaped mass with a central keratin-filled crater. (Courtesy Department of Dermatology, School of Medicine, University of Utah.)

Actinic keratosis is rare in black skin. The lesions appear as rough or scaly, poorly defined pink to reddish or reddish-brown papules that are felt more than seen (Figure 44-27) and are considered an early in situ squamous cell carcinoma.[143] Surrounding areas may have telangiectasia. Treatment options include ablative and topical therapies. The lesions should continue to be evaluated for progressive squamous cell carcinoma.[144] Protection from the sun with clothing or a sunblock to prevent lesions from developing elsewhere is advised.

Nevi

Nevi (moles) are pigmented or nonpigmented lesions that form from melanocytes beginning at ages 3 to 5 years. During the early stages of development, the cells accumulate at the junction of the dermis and epidermis and are macular lesions. Over time the cells move down into the dermis and the nevi become nodular and palpable. Nevi may appear on any part of the skin, and vary in size. They occur singly or in groups and are not considered disfiguring. Nevi may undergo transition to malignant melanomas (see p. 1670). Nevi irritated by clothing can be excised.

Cancer

Skin cancers account for about 5% of all cancers, and their incidence is increasing.[145] Basal cell carcinoma and squamous cell carcinoma are the most common. Incidence of these carcinomas is greater in men than in women, and increases steadily with age. Malignant melanoma is the most serious: an estimated 11,590 people die of skin cancer each year, 8650 of which are from malignant melanoma.[145] Important trends related to skin cancer are presented in Box 44-3.

UV solar radiation causes most skin cancers by inducing mutations in the *TP53* tumor-suppressor gene.[146] Protection from the sun during the childhood years of life significantly reduces the risk of skin cancer in later years.[147] Areas widely exposed to the sun's rays—face, neck, and hands—are highly vulnerable for such lesions. Outdoor workers (farmers, sailors, fishermen) are high-risk populations. Like other cancers, skin cancers progress through stages of initiation, progression, and metastasis.

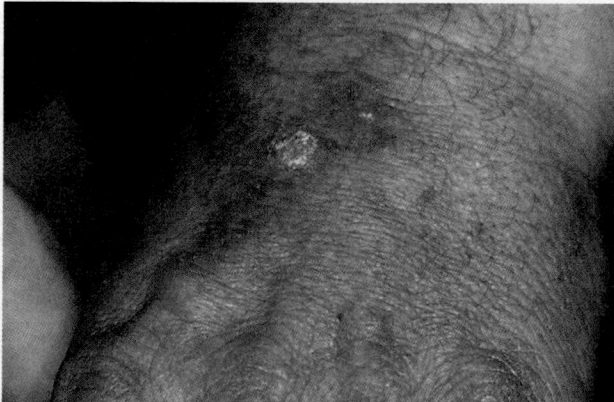

Figure 44-27 Actinic keratosis. (Courtesy Department of Dermatology, School of Medicine, University of Utah.)

Basal Cell Carcinoma

Basal cell carcinoma is a surface epithelial tumor of the skin originating from undifferentiated basal or germinative cells. The tumors grow upward and laterally or downward to the dermal epidermal junction (Figure 44-28). They usually have depressed centers and rolled borders. Early tumors are so small that they are not clinically apparent.

Basal cell carcinoma is the most common type of skin cancer in whites and is thought to be caused by UV radiation exposure.[148] Lesions are seen most often on people who live in regions with intense sunlight and on those areas of the skin most exposed—namely, the face and neck. Dark-skinned

---

Box 44-3	Important Trends for Skin Cancer Incidence

More than 1 million cases per year with likely underreporting because of lack of a nonmelanoma skin cancer registry

The majority are highly curable **basal** or **squamous** cell cancers and the most serious is **malignant melanoma** with an estimated 68,720 new cases in 2009, it represents 4% of all skin cancer cases but causes about 79% of all skin cancer deaths.

Mortality
Total estimated deaths in 2009 were 8650 from melanoma and approximately 2940 from other non-epithelial types of skin cancer.

Risk Factors
- Excessive exposure to ultraviolet radiation from the sun
- Fair complexion
- Occupational exposure to coal tar, pitch, creosote, arsenic compounds, and radium
- Exposure to human papillomavirus and human immunodeficiency virus
- Skin cancer is negligible in blacks because of heavy skin pigmentation

Warning Signals*
Any change on the skin, especially a change in the size or color of a mole or other darkly pigmented growth or spot.

Prevention and Early Detection
Avoidance of sun when ultraviolet light is strongest (e.g., 10 AM to 3 PM); use sunscreen preparations, especially those containing ingredients such as para-aminobenzoic acid (PABA); basal and squamous cell cancers often form a pale, waxlike pearly nodule or a red, scaly, sharply outlined patch; melanomas are usually dark brown or black pigmentation; they start as small molelike growths that increase in size, change color, become ulcerated, and bleed easily from a slight injury.

Treatment
There are four methods of treatment: surgery, electrodesiccation (tissue destruction by heat), radiation therapy, or cryosurgery (tissue destruction by freezing); for malignant melanomas, wide and often deep excisions and removal of nearby lymph nodes are required.

Survival*
For basal cell and squamous cell cancers, cure is highly likely with early detection and treatment; malignant melanoma, however, metastasizes quickly; this accounts for a lower 5-year survival rate, particularly for white individuals with this disease.

*Data from American Cancer Society: *Cancer facts and figures 2009*, Atlanta, 2009, The Society.

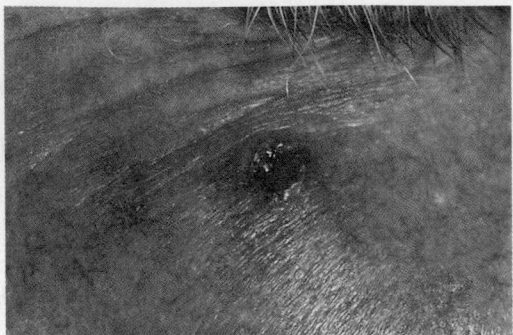

Figure 44-28 Basal cell carcinoma. Center has ulcerated. (Courtesy Department of Dermatology, School of Medicine, University of Utah.)

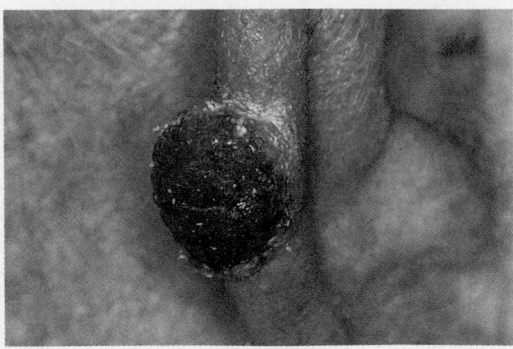

Figure 44-29 Squamous cell carcinoma. The sun-exposed ear is a common site for squamous cell carcinoma. (Courtesy Department of Dermatology, School of Medicine, University of Utah.)

persons and those avoiding sunlight are significantly less likely to develop these malignant tumors. In dark-skinned persons, basal cells contain the pigment melanin, a protective factor against sun exposure. Basal cell carcinoma arises as a consequence of UV-associated mutation in the *TP53* tumor-suppressor gene, leading to loss of keratinocyte repair functions and apoptosis resistance of DNA-damaged cells.[149] Other factors also are implicated: arsenic from groundwater wells[150] (alters DNA repair and causes mutation in *TP53* tumor-suppressor gene), autosomal dominant nevoid basal cell carcinoma syndrome with mutation in the *PTCH1* gene that has tumor-suppressor activity, and alteration in the Sonic Hedgehog signaling pathway genes (important for cell growth and differentiation).[151,152]

The lesion starts as a nodule (greater than 5 mm across) that is pearly or ivory in appearance and slightly elevated above the skin surface; it has small blood vessels on the surface. As the lesion grows, it often ulcerates, develops crusting, and becomes firm to the touch. If left untreated basal cell lesions invade surrounding tissues and, over months or years, can destroy a nose, an eyelid, or an ear (for treatment, see Box 44-3). Metastatic spread is rare because these tumors do not invade blood or lymph vessels.

Squamous Cell Carcinoma

Squamous cell carcinoma is a tumor of the epidermis characterized by two types: in situ (Bowen disease) and invasive. Areas affected are the head and neck (75%) and the hands (15%), with 10% of squamous cell carcinomas occurring elsewhere on the body. These tumors are more predominant in countries where arsenic is found in higher rates in drinking water. Gamma rays and x-rays are also associated with squamous cell carcinoma. In addition, patients who are immunosuppressed experience a greater occurrence of this carcinoma.

UV exposure causes squamous cell carcinoma, particularly with mutation of the *TP53* gene.[153] It is unclear how UV light produces alterations in DNA, and DNA repair.[154] Invasive squamous cell carcinoma can arise from premalignant lesions of the skin. It rarely arises from normal-appearing skin or de novo. The premalignant lesions include sun-damaged skin or dysplasias (actinic dermatitis); leukoplakia, or whitish, discolored areas; scars; radiation-induced keratosis; tar and oil keratosis; and chronic ulcers and sinuses. The invasive type grows more rapidly than basal cell carcinomas and can spread to regional lymph nodes with metastasis. These tumors are firm and increase in elevation and diameter. The surface may be granular and bleed easily (Figure 44-29).

In situ squamous cell carcinoma is usually confined to the epidermis (intraepidermal) but may extend into the dermis. Common premalignant skin lesions associated with in situ squamous cell carcinomas are actinic (solar) keratosis and Bowen disease. Actinic keratosis is a white, scaly, keratotic (horny) lesion on the exposed areas of the body (see p. 1668). Bowen disease is a dysplasia of the basal layer of the dermis or carcinoma in situ. It often is found on unexposed areas of the body and is demonstrated by flat, reddish, scaly patches. These lesions may enlarge to more than 1 cm in diameter, rarely invading surrounding tissue and almost never metastasizing. Other cellular components in the skin (sweat glands, hair follicles, etc.) can give rise to skin cancer, but these cancers are relatively uncommon.

Malignant Melanoma

Melanoma is a malignant tumor of the skin originating from melanocytes, or cells that synthesize the pigment melanin. The incidence of melanoma is increasing, and young to middle-age adults are at highest risk. Risk factors implicated in melanoma induction include genetic predisposition, exposure to ultraviolet light (solar and artificial), steroid hormone activity, fair hair, light skin with a propensity to sunburn, moles, and susceptibity genes[155,156] (see What's New? Melanoma, UVA Exposures and Cutaneous Vitamin D_3).

Melanomas arise as a result of malignant degeneration of melanocytes located either along the basal layer of the epidermis or in a benign melanocytic nevus. The pathogenesis of malignant melanoma is complex and a number of proto-oncogenes have been identified.[157]

A nevus, or mole, is an aggregation of melanocytes (Figure 44-30). These clusters of cells may not be apparent until puberty, when the pigmentation process is initiated by steroid

WHAT'S NEW?   Melanoma, UVA Exposures and Cutaneous Vitamin D₃

The incidence of cutaneous malignant melanoma (CMM) has been increasing over the past decades among those with white skin, primarily among indoor workers and those living in Australia, North America, and Europe; however, the mortality rate is stable or decreasing. Although intermittent, intense overexposures to the sun with sunburns can initiate CMM, sun exposure, particularly exposure to ultraviolet B (UVB) wavelengths (290-320 nm) may also have a protective action or an action that improves survival. One theory proposes that indoor workers are overexposed to ultraviolet A (UVA) wavelengths (321-400 nm) because UVA passes through glass windows whereas UVB does not. UVB promotes formation of vitamin D_3 in the skin which is then converted by the liver and kidney to its active form calcitriol which kills melanoma cells in-vitro and reduces tumor growth in-vivo. Melanoma cells can also convert skin vitamin D_3 to the active form. The action of UVA causes mutations in melanocytes and breaks down vitamin D_3. Inadequately maintained vitamin D_3 decreases its protective effects of reducing the promotion of melanoma. Thus, although intermittent overexposure to UVB can cause melanoma, overexposure to UVA and inadequate calcitriol may promote melanoma. Continuing research is needed to determine the actual UV exposures and levels of calcitriol needed to prevent melanoma.

Data from: Godar DE, Landry RJ, Lucas AD: *Med Hypotheses* 72(4):434-443, 2009; Moan J, Porojnicu AC, Dahlback A: *Adv Exp Med Biol* 624:104-116, 2008; Leiter U, Garbe C: *Adv Exp Med Biol* 624:89-103, 2008; Bennett DC: *Pigment Cell Melanoma Res* 21(5):520 524, 2008.

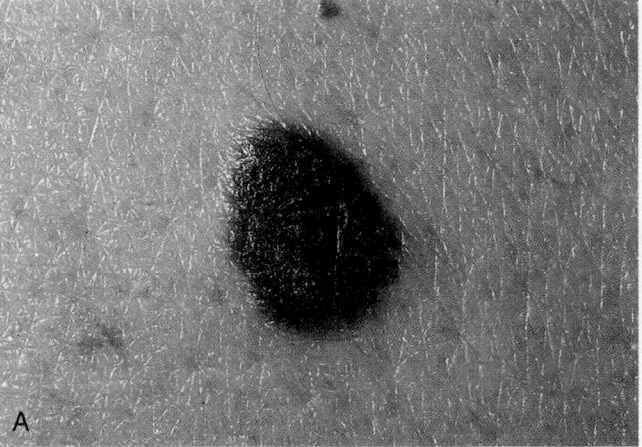

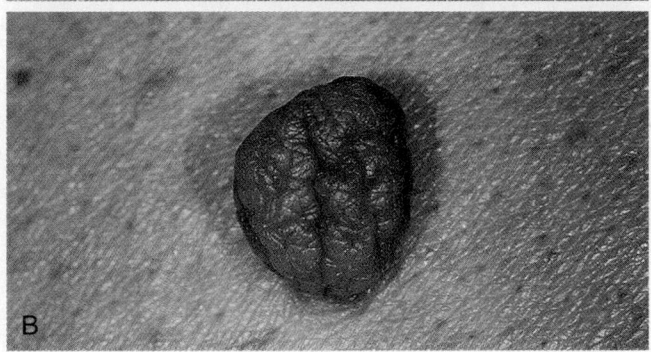

Figure 44-30 Nevi. A, Junction nevus: slightly raised, dark, and uniform. B, Dermal nevus: pedunculated with a soft, flabby, wrinkled surface. (From Habif TP: *Clinical dermatology: a color guide to diagnosis and therapy,* ed 4, St Louis, 2004, Mosby.)

hormones. The relationship between nevi and melanoma makes it important for the clinician to understand the various neval forms (Table 44-8). Most nevi never become suspicious; however, suspicious pigmented nevi should be removed.[158] Indications for biopsy include color change, size change, irregular notched margin, itching, bleeding or oozing, nodularity, scab formation, ulceration, or an unusual pattern of presentation. The ABCDE rule is used as a guide: **A**symmetry, **B**order irregularity, **C**olor variation, **D**iameter larger than 6 mm, and **E**levation which includes raised appearance or rapid enlargement.[158] Clinical characteristics are summarized in Table 44-9.

Staging of melanoma is determined from tissue biopsy, by assessing the thickness of the lesion using the Breslow microstage, and the Clark levels of tumor invasion[159] (Figure 44-31). The clinical classifications of cutaneous melanoma include lentigo malignant melanoma (LMM) (Figure 44-32), superficial spreading melanoma (SSM) (Figure 44-33), primary nodular melanoma (PNM), and acral lentiginous melanoma. A melanotic melanoma is the rarest subtype and is a nonpigmented melanoma.[160] Efforts are in progress to refine the morphologic classifications by adding subgroups that include molecular markers for proto-oncogene mutations and specific signaling pathways.[161,162] Early recognition of cutaneous melanomas can have a major effect on surgically curing this disease.

Table 44-8	Classification of Nevi
Nevi	**Common Characteristics**
Junctional nevus	Flat, well circumscribed, vary in size up to 2 cm, dark color, hairs may be present; originate in basal layer of epidermis and can eventually reach the cutaneous surface; rarely develop into a melanoma
Compound nevus	Most common in adolescents; the majority of pigmented lesions are in children; rarely develops into melanoma; usually 1 cm in size; hairs may be present; surface is elevated and smooth
Intradermal nevus	Small (less than 1 cm) with regular edges and bristle-like hairs; color ranges from skin tone to light brown; has a slight likelihood of developing into a melanoma

Treatment of melanoma with no evidence of metastatic disease involves surgical excision to the primary site and regional lymph nodes. The extent of surgery is determined by the staging of disease. Lesions of the extremities have the best prognosis; head and neck lesions and trunk lesions have the poorest prognosis. Survival rate for advanced disease is very low. Immunotherapy is advancing and vaccines and gene therapy are under investigation.[163,164]

Table 44-9   Clinical Characteristics of Varieties of Cutaneous Melanoma

Characteristic	Description
Lentigo Malignant Melanoma	
Frequency	10% to 15% of cutaneous melanomas
Age at diagnosis	50 to 80 years old
Primary location	Head, neck, dorsum of hands
Pigmentation according to thickness	
<1.5 mm (levels I and II)	Tan and brown
>1.5 mm (level III)	Tan, brown, and blue-black
>1.5 mm (levels IV and V)	Nodule formation
Superficial Spreading Melanomas	
Frequency	70% of cutaneous melanomas
Age at diagnosis	20 to 60 years old
Primary location	Legs of females; upper back of both genders
Pigmentation according to thickness	
<1.5 mm (levels I and II)	Tan and brown
>1.5 mm (level III)	Tan, brown, and blue-black
>1.5 mm (levels IV and V)	Nodule formation
Primary Nodular Melanoma	
Frequency	12% of cutaneous melanomas
Age at diagnosis	20 to 60 years old
Primary location	No specific site preference
Pigmentation according to thickness	
>1.5 mm (level III)	Small nodule (any hue)
>1.5 mm (levels IV and V)	Large nodule (any hue)
Acral-Lentiginous Melanoma	
Frequency	2% to 8% in whites; 30% to 75% in blacks, Hispanics, Asians
Age at diagnosis	20 to 60 years old
Primary location	Palms, soles of feet, mucous membranes
Pigmentation at any thickness	Blue-black

Kaposi Sarcoma

Kaposi sarcoma (KS) is a vascular malignancy with four different presentations:

1. In association with drug-induced immunosuppressions, for example, after kidney transplantation
2. An endemic form in equatorial Africa
3. A classic form presenting on the lower legs of older men
4. In association with acquired immunodeficiency syndrome (AIDS)

Kaposi-associated herpesvirus 8 is found in all four forms of KS and may be a common etiology for all types of KS through the development of an angiogenic-inflammatory state.[165] Immunosuppression allows for opportunistic infections and malignancy. Proliferation of the tumor depends on the presence of platelet-derived and other growth factors.[166]

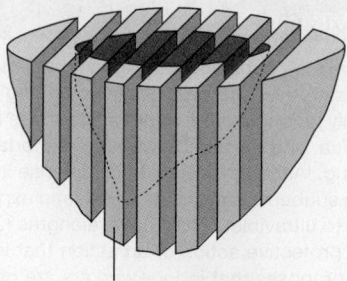

Biopsy specimen
Sections cut by pathologist

Section with deepest penetration of tumor; this section used to report Breslow microstage and Clark level

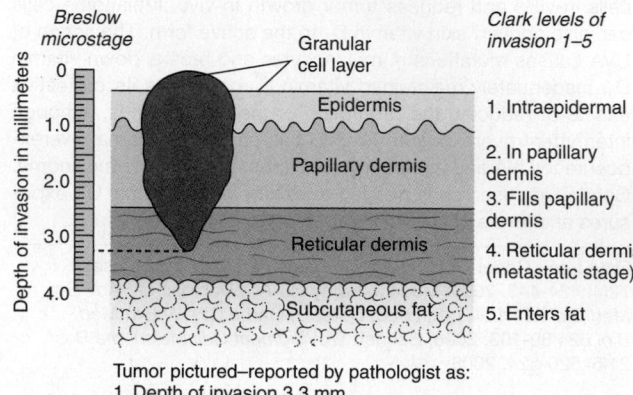

Tumor pictured—reported by pathologist as:
1. Depth of invasion 3.3 mm
2. Clark level 4

Figure 44-31 Melanoma staging using Breslow and Clark levels of invasion. (From Habif TP: *Clinical dermatology: a color guide to diagnosis and therapy,* ed 4, St Louis, 2004, Mosby.)

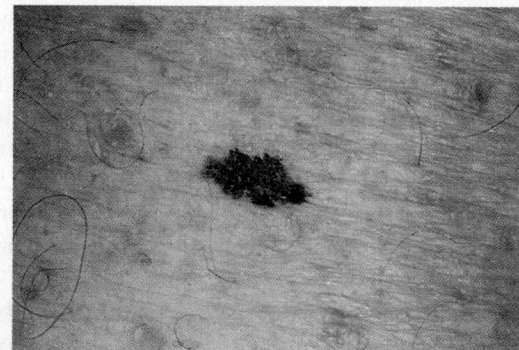

Figure 44-32 Lentigo malignant melanoma. (Courtesy Department of Dermatology, School of Medicine, University of Utah.)

The human immunodeficiency virus (HIV) and CMV have been proposed as cofactors in the development of KS.[167] The endothelial cell is thought to be the progenitor of KS but the specific origin is elusive. The lesions emerge as purplish-brown macules and develop into plaques and nodules. They tend to be multifocal rather than spreading by metastasis. The lesions initially appear over the lower extremities in the classic form (Figure 44-34). The rapidly progressive form associated

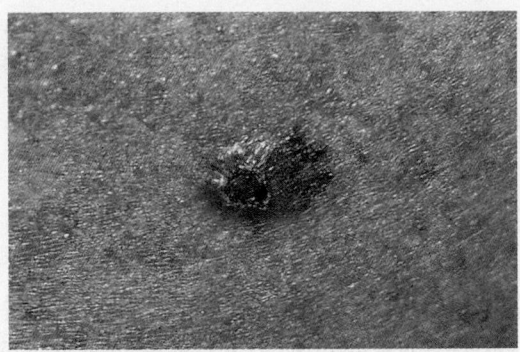

Figure 44-33 Level IV melanoma. (Courtesy Department of Dermatology, School of Medicine, University of Utah.)

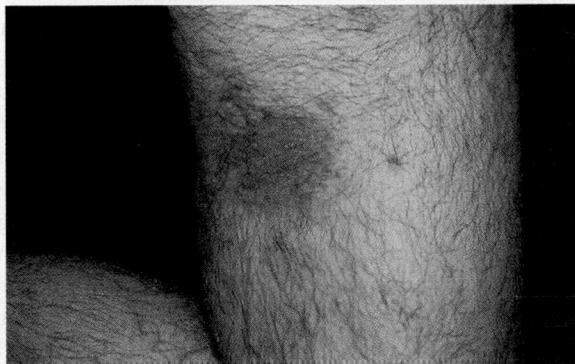

Figure 44-34 Kaposi sarcoma. The purple lesion commonly seen on the skin. (Courtesy Department of Dermatology, School of Medicine, University of Utah.)

with AIDS tends to spread symmetrically over the upper body, particularly the face and oral mucosa. The lesions are often pruritic and painful. About 75% of individuals with epidemic KS have involvement of lymph nodes, particularly in the gastrointestinal tract and lungs. Organ involvement is much less common in the classic form. The rapidly progressive form has a poor prognosis and shorter survival rates than the classic form. (See Chapter 9 for a further discussion on AIDS.)

Diagnosis is by skin biopsy, with a high index of suspicion for those with immunodeficiency. The disease is incurable. Local lesions can be excised. Multiple disseminated lesions may be treated with a combination of immunomodulator, cytotoxic, and antiviral drugs. The new, highly active antiretroviral therapy (HAART) for AIDS treatment is decreasing the incidence of KS, but new treatments are needed.[168]

Frostbite

Frostbite is injury to the skin caused by exposure to extreme cold. The areas most commonly affected are fingers, toes, ears, nose, and cheeks. Initially the body responds with alternating cycles of vasoconstriction and vasodilation—"the burning reaction." The mechanism of injury is complex but appears to be related to direct cold injury to cells, indirect injury and cell death from extracellular and intracellular ice crystal formation, and impaired circulation with anoxia

because of thrombosis in the exposed area.[169] The inflammatory mediators of frostbite are similar to burns and include prostaglandins, thromboxanes, bradykinin, and histamine. Reperfusion injury is part of the pathophysiology.[170] Frozen skin becomes white or yellowish and is waxy. There is numbness and no sensation of pain.

Skin damage can range from mild to severe. With mild frostbite, redness and discomfort occur during rewarming, followed by a return to normal in a few hours. In more severe cases, cyanosis and mottling develop, followed by redness, swelling, and burning pain on rewarming. Within 24 to 48 hours, vesicles and bullae appear and resolve into crusts that eventually slough off, leaving thin, newly formed skin. The most severe cases result in gangrene with loss of the affected part. Frostbite may be classified by depth of injury after rewarming as follows[171]:

First degree: Superficial, characterized by a numb central white area surrounded by erythema and edema and including partial skin freezing without blistering
Second degree:. Full-thickness skin freezing with blistering surrounded by edema and hyperemia
Third degree: Deep, characterized by full-thickness skin and subcutaneous freezing with tissue necrosis and hemorrhagic vesicles
Fourth degree: Deep tissue freezing with full-thickness necrosis and gangrene

Immediate treatment of frostbite is to cover affected areas with other body surfaces and warm clothing. The area should not be rubbed or massaged. Local, dry heat should be avoided. Immersion in a warm water bath (40° to 42° C 104° to 107.6° F]) until frozen tissue is thawed is the best treatment. Aspirin is used to inhibit prostaglandins, and aloe vera is a topical inhibitor of thromboxane.[172] Thrombolytic therapy reduces the incidence of amputation when administered with 24 hours.[173] Pain during the thawing period is severe and should be treated with potent analgesics. Gentle cleansing and no pressure on the skin should be maintained during healing. Amputation of necrotic tissue is delayed until a clear line of demarcation is established.

DISORDERS OF THE HAIR

Alopecia

Male-Pattern Alopecia (Androcentric Alopecia)

Alopecia means loss of hair. Localized hair loss in men is not a disease but rather a genetically predisposed response to androgens. The mechanism of inheritance is unknown. Within the distribution of hair over the scalp, androgen-sensitive hair follicles are on top and androgen-insensitive follicles are on the sides and back. In genetically predisposed men, the androgen-sensitive follicles are transformed into vellus follicles. The normal hair is shed and replaced by fine, light, short hair. Male-pattern baldness begins with frontotemporal recession and progresses to loss of hair over the top of the scalp. Minoxidil may be used to stimulate hair growth and finasteride may decrease the effect of androgens on hair follicles.[174] Affected men may choose to wear wigs or have hair transplants.

Female-Pattern Alopecia

Some women in their 20s and 30s experience progressive thinning and loss of hair over the central part of the scalp.[175] Contrary to male-pattern baldness, no loss of hair occurs along the frontal hairline. Many of these women have elevated levels of serum adrenal androgen dehydroepiandrosterone sulfate (DHEAS), and treatment with antiandrogens can be effective.[176,177] In rare instances a male-pattern baldness develops. Laboratory evaluation of serum androgenic hormones shows elevations, and some women have decreased hair loss when treated with daily doses of spironolactone.

Alopecia Areata

Alopecia areata is an autoimmune T-cell–mediated chronic inflammatory disease directed at hair follicles that results in baldness.[178] Hair loss occurs in multiple areas of the scalp, usually in round patches.[179] The eyebrows, eyelashes, beard, and other areas of the body are rarely involved. The cause is unknown, but stressful events, cell-mediated immune factors, and genetic susceptibility are linked to hair loss. Metabolic disorders, such as Addison disease, thyroid disease, and lupus erythematosus, also are associated with alopecia areata.[180]

The affected areas of skin are smooth or may have short shafts of hair. The hair shaft is poorly developed and breaks at the surface. Regrowth occurs within 1 to 3 months, but hair loss may recur at the same site. Permanent regrowth of hair usually occurs. Total loss of hair (alopecia totalis) occurs in some young people; the long-term prognosis for total hair regrowth is poor.

Diagnosis is made by observation of the pattern of hair loss. Biopsy may show a lymphocytic infiltrate around the follicle. There are several treatments for alopecia areata including corticosteroids and topical immunotherapy.[181]

Hirsutism

Hirsutism is the abnormal growth and distribution of hair on the face, body, and pubic area in a male pattern that occurs in women. There is also frontotemporal hair recession. These areas of hair growth are androgen sensitive.[182] Variations of hair growth in women are great, and a male pattern can be normal. Women who develop hirsutism may be secreting hormones associated with ovarian or adrenal disease, and such women should be evaluated for polycystic ovaries, adrenal hyperplasia, or adrenal tumors.[183] If no hormonal pathologic conditions exist undesirable hair can be mechanically removed.[184] Medical treatments are available by prescription.[185]

DISORDERS OF THE NAIL

Paronychia

Paronychia is an acute or chronic infection of the cuticle.[186] Acute paronychia is manifest by the rapid onset of painful inflammation of the cuticle, usually after minor trauma. An abscess may develop, requiring incision and drainage for relief of pain. The most common causative organisms are staphylococci, streptococci, and occasionally *Candida*.

Chronic paronychia develops slowly, with tenderness and swelling around the proximal or lateral nail folds. One or more fingers or toes may be involved. Individuals whose hands are frequently exposed to moisture are at greatest risk. Manipulation of the cuticle can be predisposing because it opens the space between the proximal nail fold and nail plate, leaving a moist, warm medium for pathogenic organisms to incubate. The skin around the nail becomes more edematous and painful with progressive infection. Pus may be expressed from the proximal nail fold. The nail plate is usually not affected, although it can become discolored and develop ridges.

Treatment includes keeping the hands dry. Oral antifungals are not very effective because they do not penetrate the affected tissues. Topical application of steroid creams can be effective.

Onychomycosis

Onychomycosis is a fungal or dermatophyte infection of the nail plate that occurs in 2% to 18% of the population.[187] The most common pattern is a nail plate that turns yellow or white (infection develops from the dorsal surface) and becomes elevated as a result of the accumulation of hyperkeratotic debris within the plate. Fungal infections of the nail may require culture and microscopy. In psoriasis, pitting often is found on the nail surface.[188] Treatment includes débridement and systemic antifungal therapy.[189] Surgical excision of the nail may be required. New systemic and topical antifungals are being investigated.[190]

SUMMARY REVIEW

Structure and Function of the Skin

1. Skin is the largest organ of the body and equals about 20% of body weight.
2. The skin has three layers: the dermis, epidermis, and subcutaneous layer.
3. Keratinocytes produce keratin to form the superficial layer of the epidermis. The underlying epidermis contains a basal and a spinous layer with melanocytes, Langerhans cells, and Merkel cells.
4. The dermis is composed of connective tissue elements, hair follicles, sweat glands, sebaceous glands, blood vessels, nerves, and lymphatic vessels.
5. The subcutaneous layer contains fat cells and connective tissue.
6. The papillary capillaries provide the major blood supply to the skin, arising from deeper arterial plexuses. The sympathetic nervous system regulates skin blood flow.
7. Heat loss and heat conservation are regulated by arteriovenous anastomoses that lead to the papillary capillaries.

Aging and Skin Integrity

1. Older skin is thinner and drier with less collagen; has fewer capillary loops and changes in pigmentation.
2. Loss of melanocytes and hair follicles leads to gray and thinner hair.
3. The skin of older adults is more permeable; there is decreased sweating and loss of thermal regulation and decreased protective functions.
4. Pressure ulcers develop from continuous pressure and shearing forces that occlude capillary blood flow with resulting ischemia and necrosis. Areas at greatest risk are pressure points over bony prominences, such as the greater trochanter, sacrum, ischia, and heels. Immobilized individuals with fractures and neurologic deficits are most likely to develop pressure ulcers.
5. Keloids are scars that extend beyond the border of injury and result from abnormal fibroblast activity and excess collagen formation.
6. Pruritus (itching) is associated with many skin disorders. Itch mediators, peripheral polymodal C-nerve fibers, and central processes contribute to itching. Scratching can cause skin trauma, infection, and scarring.

Disorders of the Skin

1. Allergic contact dermatitis is a form of delayed hypersensitivity that develops with sensitization to allergens, such as metals, chemicals, or poison ivy.
2. Atopic or allergic dermatitis is associated with a family history of allergies, hay fever, elevated IgE levels, and increased histamine sensitivity. Pruritus and scratching predispose the skin to infection, scaling, and thickening.
3. Stasis dermatitis occurs on the legs and results from venous stasis and edema.
4. Irritant contact dermatitis develops as an inflammatory response to prolonged exposure to chemicals, such as acids or soaps.
5. Seborrheic dermatitis involves scaly, yellowish, inflammatory plaques of the scalp, eyebrows, eyelids, ear canals, chest, axillae, and back. The cause is unknown.
6. Papulosquamous disorders are characterized by papules, scales, plaques, and erythema.
7. Psoriasis is a chronic autoimmune T-cell–mediated inflammatory skin disease with thickening of the epidermis and dermis characterized by scaly, erythematous pruritic plaques. The forms of psoriasis are plaque, guttate, pustular, and erythrodermic. Systemic complications can accompany the disease including arthritis and cardiovascular disease.
8. Pityriasis rosea is a self-limiting disease characterized by oval lesions with scales around the edges located along skin lines of the trunk.
9. Lichen planus is a papular violet-colored autoimmune inflammatory lesion involving T cells and inflammatory cytokines manifest by severe pruritus.
10. Acne vulgaris is a facial inflammation of the pilosebaceous follicles with hypertrophy of sebaceous glands and telangiectasia, particularly of the nose.
11. Acne rosacea develops on the middle third of the face with hypertrophy and inflammation of the sebaceous glands that may be the result of infection or immune-mediated inflammation.
12. Lupus erythematosus is an inflammatory autoimmune disease that can affect only the skin (discoid) or have a systemic presentation. The inflammatory lesions usually occur in sun-exposed areas with a butterfly distribution over the nose and cheeks.
13. Pemphigus is a chronic, autoimmune, blistering disease that begins in the mouth or on the scalp and spreads to other parts of the body, often with a fatal outcome. There are two major forms: pemphigus vulgaris and pemphigus foliaceus. Bullous pemphigoid is a blistering disease that resolves rapidly.
14. Erythema multiforme is an acute inflammation of the skin and mucous membranes with lesions that appear target-like with alternating rings of edema and inflammation; it is often associated with allergic reactions to drugs. Stevens-Johnson syndrome and toxic epidermal necrolysis are severe forms that also involve the mucous membranes.
15. Folliculitis is a bacterial infection of the hair follicle.
16. A furuncle is an infection of the hair follicle that extends to the surrounding tissue.
17. A carbuncle is a collection of infected hair follicles that forms a draining abscess.
18. Cellulitis is a diffuse infection of the dermis and subcutaneous tissue.
19. Erysipelas is a superficial streptococcal infection of the skin commonly affecting the face, ears, and lower legs.
20. Impetigo may have a bullous or an ulcerative form and is caused by *Staphylococcus or Streptococcus*.
21. HSV-1 causes cold sores but can infect the cornea, mouth, and labia. HSV-2 causes genital lesions and is usually spread by sexual contact.
22. Herpes zoster and varicella are both caused by the same herpesvirus, with herpes zoster manifesting years after the initial infection.
23. Warts (verrucae) are benign, rough, elevated lesions caused by papillomavirus. Venereal warts (*Condylomata acuminata*) are spread by sexual contact.
24. Tinea skin infections (fungal infections) can occur anywhere on the body and are classified by location (i.e., tinea pedis, tinea corporis, tinea capitis).
25. Candidiasis is a yeastlike fungal infection caused by *C. albicans* occurring on skin, mucous membranes, and in the gastrointestinal tract.
26. Cutaneous vasculitis is an immune-mediated inflammation of skin blood vessels with purpura, ischemia, and necrosis resulting from vessel necrosis.
27. Urticarial lesions are associated with type I hypersensitivity responses and appear as wheals, welts, or hives.
28. Scleroderma is an immune-mediated sclerosis of the skin that also may affect systemic organs and cause renal failure, bowel obstruction, or cardiac dysrhythmias.

SUMMARY REVIEW—cont'd

29. Ticks cause a local reaction on the skin of humans and can cause systemic disease when mouthparts pierce the skin and remain embedded in the tissue.

30. Lyme disease is a multisystem inflammatory disease caused by *B. burgdorferi* transmitted by tick bites. Complications may persist for years.

31. Mosquitoes can transmit infectious diseases, and the saliva from their bite produces the characteristic itching and wheal formation.

32. Blood-sucking flies are represented by many species, including Ceratopogonidae ("no-see-ums"), Tabanidae (horseflies), or Simuliidae (blackflies). Their bites are usually painful and produce bleeding; the itching and local reactions may last for days, and systemic symptoms of fever and malaise may develop.

33. Seborrheic keratosis is a proliferation of squamous cells that produce elevated, smooth, or warty lesions of varying size usually in sun-damaged skin. They are most common among older adults.

34. Keratoacanthoma arises from hair follicles on sun-exposed areas. There are three stages of development that result in a dome-shaped, crusty lesion filled with keratin that resolves in 3 to 4 months.

35. Actinic keratosis is a pigmented scaly lesion that develops in sun-exposed individuals with fair skin. The lesion may become malignant in the form of squamous cell carcinoma.

36. Nevi arise from melanocytes and may be pigmented or fleshy pink. They occur singly or in groups and may undergo transition to malignant melanoma.

37. Basal cell carcinoma is the most common skin cancer and occurs most often on sun-exposed areas.

38. Squamous cell carcinoma is a tumor of the epidermis associated with sun exposure and can be localized (in situ) or invasive.

39. Malignant melanoma arises from melanocytes; if it is not excised early, metastasis occurs through the lymph nodes.

40. KS is a vascular malignancy associated with immunodeficiency states and is associated with herpesvirus 8.

41. Frostbite usually occurs on cheeks and digits, causing direct injury to cells and impaired circulation.

Disorders of the Hair

1. Male-pattern alopecia is an inherited form of irreversible baldness with hair loss in the central scalp and recession of the temporofrontal hairline.

2. Female-pattern alopecia is a thinning of the central hair of the scalp beginning in women at 20 to 30 years of age.

3. Alopecia areata is patchy loss of hair associated with an autoimmune process and triggered by stress or metabolic diseases; it is usually reversible.

4. Hirsutism is a male pattern of hair growth in women that may be normal or the result of excessive secretion of androgenic hormones.

Disorders of the Nail

1. Paronychia is an inflammation of the cuticle that can be acute or chronic and is usually caused by staphylococci or streptococci.

2. Onychomycosis is a fungal infection of the nail plate.

KEY TERMS

Acne rosacea, 1659
Acne vulgaris, 1659
Actinic keratosis, 1668
Allergic contact dermatitis, 1655
Alopecia, 1673
Alopecia areata, 1674
Apocrine sweat gland, 1646
Atopic dermatitis, 1656
Basal cell carcinoma, 1669
Basal layer (stratum basale), 1644
Bullous pemphigoid, 1661
Candidiasis, 1665
Carbuncle, 1663
Cellulitis, 1663
Clawlike prolongation, 1654
Condylomata acuminata, 1664
Cutaneous vasculitis, 1666
Dermal appendage, 1646
Dermis, 1645
Discoid (cutaneous) lupus erythematosus (DLE), 1659
Eccrine sweat gland, 1646
Eczema, 1655
Epidermis, 1644
Erysipelas, 1663
Erythema multiforme, 1661
Erythrodermic (exfoliative) psoriasis, 1658
Flies, 1668
Folliculitis, 1662
Frostbite, 1673
Furuncle, 1662

Germinative layer (stratum germinativum), 1644
Guttate psoriasis, 1658
Hair follicle, 1646
Herald patch, 1658
Herpes simplex virus (HSV), 1663
Herpes zoster, 1664
Hirsutism, 1674
Hypertropic scar, 1654
Hyphae, 1665
Impetigo, 1663
Inverse psoriasis, 1657
Irritant contact dermatitis, 1656
Kaposi sarcoma (KS), 1672
Keloid, 1654
Keratin, 1644
Keratinocytes, 1644
Keratoacanthoma, 1668
Langerhans cell, 1645
Lichen planus, 1658
Lupus erythematosus, 1659
Lyme disease, 1667
Melanocyte, 1645
Melanoma, 1670
Merkel cell, 1645
Mosquito, 1668
Myofibroblast, 1654
Nail, 1646
Nevi (*sing.*, nevus; also known as a mole), 1669
Onychomycosis, 1674

Papillary capillary, 1646
Papulosquamous disorder, 1657
Paronychia, 1674
Pemphigus, 1660
Pityriasis rosea, 1658
Plaque psoriasis, 1657
Proteoglycan, 1654
Pruritus, 1654
Psoriasis, 1657
Psoriatic arthritis, 1658
Psoriatic nail disease, 1658
Pustular psoriasis, 1658
Scleroderma, 1667
Sebaceous gland, 1646
Seborrheic dermatitis, 1656
Seborrheic keratosis, 1668
Spinous layer (stratum spinosum), 1644
Squamous cell carcinoma, 1670
Stasis dermatitis, 1656
Stevens-Johnson syndrome, 1661
Stratum corneum, 1644
Systemic scleroderma (sclerosis), 1667
Tinea capitis, 1664
Tinea corporis (ringworm), 1664
Tinea infection, 1664
Tinea pedis, 1664
Toxic epidermal necrolysis, 1661
Urticaria, 1666
Urticarial lesion, 1666
Varicella, 1664
Wart, 1664

REFERENCES

1. Loser K, Beissert S: Dendritic cells and T cells in the regulation of cutaneous immunity, *Adv Dermatol* 23:307-333, 2007.
2. Nicol NH: Anatomy and physiology of the skin. In Hill MJ, editor; *Dermatologic nursing essentials: a core curriculum*, ed 2, Pitman, NJ, 2003, Anthony J. Jannetti, Inc.
3. Blanpain C, Fuchs E: Epidermal stem cells of the skin, *Ann Rev Cell Dev Biol* 22:339-373, 2006.
4. Landau M: Exogenous factors in skin aging, *Curr Probl Dermatol* 35: 1-13, 2007.
5. Thornfeldt CR: Chronic inflammation is etiology of extrinsic aging, *J Cosmet Dermatol* 7(1):78-82, 2008.
6. Baumann L: Skin aging and its treatment, *J Pathol* 211(2):241-251, 2007.
7. Imokawa G: Recent advances in characterizing biological mechanisms underlying UV-induced wrinkles: a pivotal role of fibroblast derived elastase, *Arch Dermatol Res* 300(Suppl 1):s7-s20, 2008.
8. Gilchrist BA: *Skin and aging processes*, Boca Raton, FL, 1984, CRC Press.
9. Ryan T: The ageing of the blood supply and the lymphatic drainage of the skin, *Micron* 35(3):161-171, 2004.
10. Bennett MF et al: Skin immune systems and inflammation: protector of the skin or promoter of aging? *J Investig Dermatol Symp Proc* 13(1):15-19, 2008.
11. Farage MA et al: Clinical implications of aging skin: cutaneous disorders in the elderly, *Am J Clin Dermatol* 10(2): 73-86, 2009. doi: 10.2165/00128071-200910020-00001.
12. Cannon BC, Cannon JP: Management of pressure ulcers, *Am J Health Syst Pharm* 61(18):1895-1905, 2004.
13. Stekelenburg A et al: Deep tissue injury: how deep is our understanding, *Arch Phys Med Rehabil* 89(7):141-143, 2008.
14. Berlowitz DR et al: Predictors of pressure ulcer healing among long-term care residents, *J Am Geriatric Soc* 45(1):30-34, 1997.
15. Theaker C et al: Risk factors for pressure sores in the critically ill, *Anesthesia* 55(3):221, 2000.
16. Frankel H, Sperry J, Kaplan L: Risk factors for pressure ulcer development in a best practice surgical intensive care unit, *Am Surg* 73(12):1215-1217, 2007.
17. Baumgarten M et al: Black/white differences in pressure ulcer incidence in nursing home residents, *J Am Geriatr Soc* 19(6):339-341, 2004.
18. Scanlon E, Stubbs N: Pressure ulcer risk assessment in patients with darkly pigmented skin, *Prof Nurse* 19(5):339-341, 2004.
19. National Pressure Ulcer Advisory Panel: *Pressure ulcer stages revised by NPUAP*, 2007. Available at www.npuap.org/pr2.htm.
20. Ayello EA: How and why to do pressure ulcer risk assessment, *Advances in Skin & Wound Care*. FindArticles.com. 28 May, 2009. Available at: http://findarticles.com/p/articles/mi_qa3977/is_200205/ai_n9033549/
21. Royal College of Nursing: *The management of pressure ulcers in primary and secondary care*, Royal College of Nursing, London, 2005, Available at www.nice.org.uk/nicemedia/pdf/cg029fullguideline_appendices.pdf.
22. Butler F: Essence of care and the pressure ulcer benchmark-an evaluation, *J Tissue Viabil* 17(2):44-59, 2008.
23. Reddy M, Gill SS, Rochon PA: Preventing pressure ulcers: a systematic review, *J Am Med Assoc* 296(8):974-984, 2006.
24. Smith DM: Pressure ulcers in the nursing home, *Ann Intern Med* 123(6):433, 1995.
25. Fine NA, Mustoe TA: Wound healing. In Greenfield LJ et al, editors: *Surgery: scientific principles and practice*, ed 2, Philadelphia, 1997, Lippincott-Raven.
26. Bauer J, Phillips LG: MOC-PSSM CME article: pressure sores, *Plast Reconstr Surg* 121(1Suppl):1-10, 2008.
27. Lee JT et al: A new technique of transferring island pedicled anterolateral thigh and vastus lateralis myocutaneous flaps for reconstruction of recurrent ischial pressure sores, *J Plast Reconstr Aesthet Surg* 60(9):1060-1066, 2007.
28. Sorenson JL, Jorgensen B, Gottrup F: Surgical treatment of pressure ulcers, *Am J Surg* 188(Suppl 1A):42-51, 2004.
28a. George-Saintilus E et al: Pressure ulcer PUSH score and traditional nursing assessment in nursing home residents: do they correlate? *J Am Med Dir Assoc* 10(2):141-144, 2009.
29. Köse O, Waseem A: Keloids and hypertrophic scars: are they two different sides of the same coin? *Dermatol Surg* 34(3):336-346, 2008.
30. Seifert O et al: Identification of unique gene expression patterns within different lesional sites of keloids, *Wound Repair Regen* 16(2):254-265, 2008.
31. Ghazizadeh M et al: Functional implications of the IL-6 signaling pathway in keloid pathogenesis, *J Invest Dermatol* 127(1):98-105, 2007.
32. Satish L et al: Gene expression patterns in isolated keloid fibroblasts, *Wound Repair Regen* 14(4):463-467, 2006.
33. Bayat A et al: Genetic susceptibility to keloid disease: transforming growth factor beta receptor gene polymorphisms are not associated with keloid disease, *Exp Dermatol* 13(2):120-124, 2004.
34. Durani P, Bayat A: Levels of evidence for the treatment of keloid disease, *J Plast Recontr Aesthet Surg* 61(1):4-17, 2008.
35. Robles DT et al: Keloids: pathophysiology and management, *Dermatol Online J* 13(3):9, 2007.
36. Greaves MW, Wall PD: Pathophysiology of itching, *Lancet* 348(9032):938, 1996.
37. Pogatzki-Zahn F et al: Chronic pruritus: targets, mechanisms and future therapies, *Drug News Perspect* 21(10):541-551, 2008.
38. Ständer S, Weisshaar E, Luger TA: Neurophysiological and neurochemical basis of modern pruritus treatment, *Exp Dermatol* 17(3):161-169, 2008.
39. Weldon D: What lies beneath the surface of the itch in adults, *Allergy Asthma Proc* 28(2):153-162, 2007.
40. Greaves MW: Recent advances in pathophysiology and current management of itch, *Ann Acad Med Singapore* 36(9):788-792, 2007.
41. Yosipovitch G, SamuelLS: Neuropathic and psychogenic itch, *Dermatol Ther* 21(1):32-41, 2008.
42. Langner MD, Maibach HI: Pruritus measurement and treatment, *Clin Exp Dermatol* 34(3):285-288, 2009.
43. Nilsson HJ et al: Profound inhibition of chronic itch induced by stimulation of thin cutaneous nerve fibres, *J Eur Acad Dermatol Venereol* 18(1):37-43, 2004.
44. Ständer S, Weisshaar E, Luger TA: Neurophysiological and neurochemical basis of modern pruritus treatment, *Exp Dermatol* 17(3):161-169, 2008.
45. Nicol NH: Dermatitis/eczema. In Hill MJ, editor: *Dermatologic nursing essentials: a core curriculum*, ed 2, Pitman, NJ, 2003, Anthony J. Jannetti, Inc.
46. Gober MD, Gaspari AA: Allergic contact dermatitis, *Curr Dir Autoimmun* 10:1-26, 2008.
47. Fyhrquist-Vanni N, Alenius H, Lauerma A: Contact dermatitis, *Dermatol Clin* 25(4):613-623, 2007.
48. Rolland JM, O'Hehir RE: Latex allergy: a model for therapy, *Clin Exp Allergy* 38(6):898-912, 2008.
49. Chan LS: Atopic dermatitis in 2008: *Curr Dir Autoimmun* 10:76-118, 2008.
50. Trent JT et al: Venous ulcers: pathophysiology and treatment options, *Ostomy Wound Manage* 51(5):38-54, 2005.
51. Howard DP et al: The role of superficial venous surgery in the management of venous ulcers: a systematic review, *Eur J Vasc Endovasc Surg* 36(4):458-465, 2008.
52. Palfreyman SJ et al: Dressings for healing venous leg ulcers, *Cochrane Database Syst Rev* 3:CD001103, 2006.
53. Fluhr JW et al: Skin irritation and sensitization: mechanisms and new approaches for risk assessment. 1. Skin irritation, *Skin Pharmacol Physiol* 21(3):124-135, 2008.
54. Dawson TL Jr: *Malassezia globosa* and *restricta*: breakthrough understanding of the etiology and treatment of dandruff and seborrheic dermatitis through whole-genome analysis, *J Investig Dermatol Symp Proc* 12(2):15-19, 2007.
54a. Cook BA, Warshaw EM: Role of topical calcineurin inhibitors in the treatment of seborrheic dermatitis: a review of pathophysiology, safety and efficacy, *Am J Clin Dermatol* 10(2):103-118, 2009.
55. Borgers M, Degreef H: The role of ketoconazole in seborrheic dermatitis, *Cutis* 80(4):359-363, 2007.
56. Menter A et al: Guidelines of care for the management of psoriasis and psoriatic arthritis: Section 1. Overview of psoriasis and guidelines of care of the treatment of psoriasis with biologics, *J Am Acad Dermatol* 58(5):826-850, 2008.
57. Hueber AJ, McInnes IB: Immune regulation in psoriasis and psoriatic arthritis—recent developments, *Immunol Lett* 114(2):59-65, 2007.
58. Duffin KC, Krueger GG: Genetic variations in cytokines and cytokine receptors associated with psoriasis found by genome-wide association, *J Invest Dermatol* 129(4):827-833, 2009.
59. Murphy M, Kerr P, Grant-Kels JM: The histopathologic spectrum of psoriasis, *Clin Dermatol* 25(6):624-628, 2007.
60. Kleinert S et al: Psoriatic arthritis: clinical spectrum and diagnostic procedures, *Clin Dermatol* 25(6):519-523, 2007.

61. Chuh A, Chan H, Zawar V: Pityriasis rosea—evidence for and against an infectious aetiology, *Epidemiol Infect* 132(32):381-390, 2004.

62. Stulberg DL, Wolfrey J: Pityriasis rosea, *Am Fam Physician* 69(1): 87-91, 2004.

63. Chuh AA et al: Interventions for pityriasis rosea, *Cochrane Database Syst Rev* (2):CD005068, 2007.

64. Prpic Massari L et al: Perforin expression in peripheral blood lymphocytes and skin-infiltrating cells in patients with lichen planus, *Br J Dermatol* 151(2):433-439, 2005.

65. Shiohara T et al: Pathomechanisms of lichen planus autoimmunity elicited by cross-reactive T cells, *Curr Dir Autoimmun* 10:206-226, 2008.

66. Carrozzo M: Oral diseases associated with hepatitis C virus infection. Part 2: lichen planus and other diseases, *Oral Dis* 14(3):217-228, 2008.

67. DeRossi SS, Ciarrocca KN: Lichen planus, lichenoid drug reactions, and lichenoid mucositis, *Dent Clin North Am* 49(1):77-89, 2005.

68. Gorruhi F et al: Randomized trial of pimecrolimus cream versus triamcinolone acetonide paste in the treatment of oral lichen planus, *J Am Acad Dermatol* 57(5):806-813, 2007.

69. Marks R: The enigma of rosacea, *J Dermatol Treat* 18(6):326-328, 2007.

70. Millikan LE: Rosacea as an inflammatory disorder: a unifying theory? *Cutis* 73(1 Suppl):5-8, 2004.

71. Stone DU, Chodosh J: Ocular rosacea: an update on pathogenesis and therapy, *Curr Opin Ophthalmol* 15(6):499-502, 2004.

72. Crawford GH, Pelle MT, James WD: Rosacea: I, etiology, pathogenesis, and subtype classification, *J Am Acad Dermatol* 51(3):327-341, 2004.

73. Lacey N et al: Mite-related bacterial antigens stimulate inflammatory cells in rosacea, *Br J Dermatol* 157(3):474-481, 2007.

74. Conde JF et al: Managing rosacea: a review of the use of metronidazole alone and in combination with oral antibiotics, *J Drugs Dermatol* 6(5):495-498, 2007.

75. Gooderham M: Rosacea and its topical management, *Skin Therapy Lett* 14(2):1-3, 2009.

76. Panjwani S: Early diagnosis and treatment of discoid lupus erythematosus, *J Am Board Fam Med* 22(2):206-213, 2009.

77. Pramatarov KD: Chronic cutaneous lupus erythematosus—clinical spectrum, *Clin Dermatol* 22(2):113-120, 2004.

78. Kuhn A, Biji M: Pathogenesis of cutaneous lupus erythematosus, *Lupus* 17(5):389-393, 2008.

79. Rothfield N, Sontheimer RD, Bernstein M: Lupus erythematosus: systemic and cutaneous manifestations, *Clin Dermatol* 1495:348-362, 2006.

80. Sárdy M, Ruzicka T, Kuhn A: Topical calcineurin inhibitors in cutaneous lupus erythematosus, *Arch Dermatol Res* 301(1):93-98, 2009.

81. Fabbri P et al: Cutaneous lupus erythematosus: diagnosis and management, *Am J Clin Dermatol* 4(7):449-465, 2003.

82. Baroni A et al: Vesicular and bullous disorders: pemphigus, *Dermatol Clin* 25(4):597-603, 2007.

83. Hashimoto T: Recent advances in the study of the pathophysiology of pemphigus, *Arch Dermatol Res* 395(Suppl 1):S2-11, 2003.

84. Tron F et al: Immunogenetics of pemphigus: an update, *Autoimmunity* 39(7):531-539, 2006.

85. Prajapati V, Mydlarski PR: Advances in pemphigus therapy, *Skin Therapy Lett* 13(3):4-7, 2008.

86. Olasz EF, Yancey KB: Bullous pemphigoid and related subepidermal autoimmune blistering diseases, *Curr Dir Autoimmun* 10:141-166, 2008.

87. Kasperkiewicz M, Zillikens D: The pathophysiology of bullous pemphigoid, *Clin Rev Allergy Immunol* 33(1-2):67-77, 2007.

88. Scully C, Bagan J: Oral mucosal diseases: erythema multiforme, *Br J Oral Maxillofac Surg* 46(20):90-95, 2008.

89. Katta R: Taking aim at erythema multiforme. How to spot target lesions and less typical presentations, *Postgrad Med* 107(1):87, 2000.

90. Provost TT, Weston WL: *Bullous diseases*, St Louis, 1993, Mosby.

91. Parrillo SJ: Stevens-Johnson syndrome and toxic epidermal necrolysis, *Curr Allergy Asthma Rep* 7(4):243-247, 2007.

92. Roujeau JC: Stevens-Johnson syndrome and toxic epidermal necrolysis are severity variants of the same disease which differs from erythema multiforme, *J Dermatol* 24(11):726, 1997.

93. Paquet P, Pierard GE: Toxic epidermal necrolysis: revisiting the tentative link between early apoptosis and late necrosis, *Int J Mol Med* 19(1):3-10, 2007.

94. Pereira FA, Mudgil AV, Rosmarin DM: Toxic epidermal necrolysis, *J Am Acad Dermatol* 56(2):181-200, 2007.

95. Mukasa Y, Craven N: Management of toxic epidermal necrolysis and related syndromes, *Postgrad Med J* 84(988):60-65, 2008.

96. Singh G, Marples RR, Klingman AM: Staphylococcus infections in humans, *J Invest Dermatol* 57(3):149-162, 1971.

97. Hirschmann JV: Antimicrobial therapy for skin infections, *Cutis* 79(Suppl):26-36, 2007.

98. Bernard P: Management of common bacterial infections of the skin, *Curr Opin Infect Dis* 21(2):122-128, 2008.

99. Koutkia P, Mylonakis E, Boyce J: Cellulitis: evaluation of possible predisposing factors in hospitalized patients, *Diagn Microbiol Infect Dis* 34(4):325, 1999.

100. Gabillot-Carré M, Roujeau JC: Acute bacterial skin infections and cellulites, *Curr Opin Infect Dis* 20(2):118-123, 2007.

101. Kiken DA, Silverberg NB: Atopic dermatitis in children, part 1: epidemiology, clinical features, and complications, *Cutis* 78(4):241-247, 2006.

102. Baringer JR: Herpes simplex infections of the nervous system, *Neurol Clin* 26(3):657-674, viii, 2008.

103. Hobbs MR et al: Identification of a herpes simplex labialis susceptibility region on human chromosome 21, *J Infect Dis* 197(3):340-346, 2008.

104. Brown Z: Preventing herpes simplex virus transmission to the neonate, *Herpes* 11(Suppl 3):175A-186A, 2004.

105. Gupta R, Warren T, Wald A: Genital herpes, *Lancet* 370(9605):2127-2137, 2007.

106. Koelle DM, Corey L: Herpes simplex: insights on pathogenesis and possible vaccines, *Annu Rev Med* 59:381-395, 2008.

107. Ahmed AM et al: Managing herpes zoster in immunocompromised patients, *Herpes* 14(2):32-36, 2007.

108. Johnson RW et al: Postherpetic neuralgia: epidemiology, pathophysiology and management, *Exp Rev Neurother* 7(11):1581-1595, 2007.

109. Ragozzino MW et al: Population based study of herpes zoster and its sequelae, *Medicine (Baltimore)* 5(61):310, 1982.

110. Dworkin RH et al: Recommendations for the management of herpes zoster, *Clin Infect Dis* 44(Suppl 1):S1-S26, 2007.

111. Oxman MN, Levin MJ: Shingles Prevention Study Group: vaccination against herpes zoster and postherpectic neuralgia, *J Infect Dis* 197(Suppl 2):S228-S236, 2008.

112. Lassus J, Ranki A: Simultaneously detected aberrant p53 tumor-suppressor protein and HPV-DNA localized mostly in separate keratinocytes in anogenital and common warts, *Exp Dermatol* 5(2):72, 1996.

113. Prasad CJ: Pathobiology of human papillomavirus, *Clin Lab Med* 15(3):685, 1995.

114. Gibbs S, Harvey I: Topical treatments for cutaneous warts, *Cochrane Database Syst Rev* 3:CD001781, 2006.

115. Lipke MM: An armamentarium of wart treatments, *Clin Med Res* 4(4):273-293, 2006.

116. Steben M, Duarte-Franco E: Human papillomavirus infection: epidemiology and pathophysiology, *Gynecol Oncol* 107(2 Suppl 1):A2-A5, 2007.

117. Woodfolk JA: Allergy and dermatophytes, *Clin Microbiol Rev* 18(1):30-43, 2005.

118. Armstron-James D: Invasive *Candida* species infection: the importance of adequate empirical antifungal therapy, *J Antimicrob Chemother* 60(3):459-460, 2007.

119. Ashman RB: Protective and pathologic immune responses against *Candida albicans* infection, *Front Biosci* 13:3334-3351, 2008.

120. Netea MG et al: An integrated model of the recognition of *Candida albicans* by the innate immune system, *Nat Rev Microbiol* 6(1):67-78, 2008.

121. Levitz SM: Overview of host defenses in fungal infections, *Clin Infect Dis* 14(Suppl 1):537, 1992.

122. Lotti TM, Comacchi C, Ghersetich I: Cutaneous necrotizing vasculitis. Relation to systemic disease, *Adv Exp Med Biol* 455:115, 1999.

123. Chen KR, Carlson JA: Clinical approach to cutaneous vasculitis, *Am J Clin Dermatol* 9(2):71-92, 2008.

124. Kapp A, Wedi B: Chronic urticaria: clinical aspects and focus on a new antihistamine, levocetirizine, *Drugs Dermatol* 3(6):632-639, 2004.

125. Brodell LA, Beck LA, Saini SS: Pathophysiology of chronic urticaria, *Ann Allergy Asthma Immunol* 100(4):291-297, 2008.

126. Steen VD: The many faces of scleroderma, *Rheum Dis Clin North Am* 34(1):1-15, v, 2008.
127. Varga JA, Trojanowska M: Fibrosis in systemic sclerosis, *Rheum Dis Clin North Am* 34(1):115-143, cii, 2008.
128. Gilliam AC: Scleroderma, *Curr Dir Autoimmun* 10:258-279, 2008.
129. Kahaleh B: Vascular disease in scleroderma: mechanisms of vascular injury, *Rheum Dis Clin North Am* 34(1):57-71, 2008.
130. Herrick A: Diagnosis and management of scleroderma peripheral vascular disease, *Rheum Dis Clin North Am* 34(1):89-114, vii, 2008.
131. Shah AA, Wigley FM: Often forgotten manifestations of systemic sclerosis, *Rheum Dis Clin North Am* 34(1):221-238, ix, 2008.
132. Nihtyanova SI, Denton CP: Current approaches to the management of early active diffuse scleroderma skin disease, *Rheum Dis Clin North Am* 34(1):161-179, 2008.
133. Amsden JR, Warmack S, Gubbins PO: Tick-borne bacterial, rickettsial, spirochetal, and protozoal infectious disease in the United States: a comprehensive review, *Pharmacotherapy* 25(2):191-210, 2005.
134. Bratton RL et al: Diagnosis and treatment of Lyme disease, *Mayo Clin Proc* 83(5):566-571, 2008.
135. Cruz AR et al: Phagocytosis of *Borrelia burgdorferi*, the Lyme disease spirochete, potentiates innate immune activation and induces apoptosis in human monocytes, *Infect Immun* 76(1):56-70, 2008.
136. Rupprechi TA et al: The pathogenesis of lyme neuroborreliosis: from infection to inflammation, *Mol Med* 14(3-4):205-212, 2008.
137. Hovius JW, van Dan AP, Fikrig E: Tick-host-pathogen interactions in Lyme disease, *Trends Parasitol* 23(9):434-438, 2007.
138. Aguero-Rosenfeld ME: Lyme disease: laboratory issues, *Infect Dis Clin North Am* 22(2):301-313, vii, 2008.
139. Vázquez M et al: Effectiveness of personal protective measures to prevent Lyme disease, *Emerg Infect Dis* 14(2):210-216, 2008.
140. Magalhães RF et al: Diagnosis and follow-up of keratoacanthoma-like lesions: clinical-histologic study of 43 cases, *J Cutan Med Surg* 12(4):163-173, 2008.
141. Kossard S, Tan KB, Choy C: Keratoacanthoma and infundibulocystic squamous cell carcinoma, *Am J Dermatopathol* 30(2):127-134, 2008.
142. Annest NM et al: Intralesional methotrexate treatment for keratoacanthoma tumors: a retrospective study and review of the literature, *J Am Acad Dermatol* 56(6):989-993, 2007.
143. Roewert-Huberj J, Stockfleth E, Kerl H: Pathology and pathobiology of actinic (solar) keratosis—an update, *Br J Dermatol* 157(Suppl 2):18-20, 2007.
144. McIntyre WJ, Downs MR, Bedwell SA: Treatment options for actinic keratoses, *Am Fam Physician* 76(5):667-671, 2007.
145. American Cancer Society: *Cancer facts and figures 2009*, Atlanta, 2009, The Society.
146. Benjamin CL, Meinikova VO, Ananthaswamy HN: P53 protein and pathogenesis of melanoma and nonmelanoma skin cancer, *Adv Exp Med Biol* 624:265-282, 2008.
147. Kyle JW et al: Economic evaluation of the US Environmental Protection Agency's SunWise program: sun protection education for young children, *Pediatrics* 121(5):e1074-e1084, 2008.
148. Lear JT et al: Basal cell carcinoma: from host response and polymorphic variants to tumour suppressor genes, *Clin Exp Dermatol* 30(1):49-55, 2005.
149. Erb P et al: Apoptosis and pathogenesis of melanoma and nonmelanoma skin cancer, *Adv Exp Med Biol* 624:283-295, 2008.
150. Zakl-Prelich M, Narbutt J, Sysa-Jedrzejowska A: Environmental risk factors predisposing to the development of basal cell carcinoma, *Dermatol Surg* 30(2 Pt 2):248-252, 2004.
151. Lindström E et al: PTCH mutations: distribution and analyses, *Hum Mutat* 27(3):215-219, 2006.
152. Lupi O: Correlations between the Sonic Hedgehog pathway and basal cell carcinoma, *Int J Dermatol* 46(11):1113-1117, 2007.
153. Rigel DS: Cutaneous ultraviolet exposure and its relationship to the development of skin cancer, *J Am Acad Dermatol* 58(5 Suppl 2):S129-S132, 2008.
154. Rass K, Reichrath J: UV damage and DNA repair in malignant melanoma and nonmelanoma skin cancer, *Adv Exp Med Biol* 624:162-178, 2008.
155. Berwick M, Erdei E, Hay J: Melanoma epidemiology and public health, *Dermatol Clin* 27(2):205-214, viii, 2009.
156. Rodenas JM et al: sun exposure, pigmentary traits, and risk of cutaneous maligant melanoma: a case-control study in a Mediterranean population, *Cancer Control* 7(2):275, 1996.
157. Dahl C, Guldberg P: The genome and epigenome of malignant melanoma, *APMIS* 115(10):1161-1176, 2007.
158. O'Conner KM, Chien AJ: Management of melanocytic lesions in the primary care setting, *Mayo Clin Proc* 83(2):208-213, 2008.
159. Habif TB: *Clinical dermatology: a color guide to diagnosis and therapy*, St Louis, 2004, Mosby.
160. Bishop JA: Melanoma, *Hosp Med* 61(2):103, 2000.
161. Fetcher LA et al: Toward a molecular classification of melanoma, *J Clin Oncol* 25(12):1606-1620, 2007.
162. Viros A et al: Improving melanoma classification by integrating genetic and morphologic features, *PLoS Med* 5(6):e120, 2008.
163. Kirkwood JM et al: Next generation of immunotherapy for melanoma, *J Clin Oncol* 26(20):3445-3455, 2008.
164. Lejeune FJ, Rimoldi D, Speiser D: New approaches in metastatic melanoma: biological and molecular targeted therapies, *Expert Rev Anticancer Ther* 7(5):701-713, 2007.
165. Szajerka T, Jablecki J: Kaposi's sarcoma revisited, *AIDS Rev* 9(4):230-236, 2007.
166. Dezube BJ, Sullivan R, Koon HB: Emerging targets and novel strategies in the treatment of AIDS-related Kaposi's sarcoma: bidirectional translations science, *J Cell Physiol* 209(3):659-662, 2006.
167. Goopman J: Neoplasms in the acquired immune deficiency syndrome: the multidisciplinary approach, *Semin Oncol* 14(2 Suppl 3):1, 1987.
168. Nguyen HQ et al: Persistent Kaposi sarcoma in the era of highly active antiretroviral therapy: characterizing the predictors of clinical response, *AIDS* 22(8):937-945, 2008.
169. Grandberg PO: Freezing cold injury, *Arctic Med Res* 50(Suppl 6):76, 1991.
170. Murphy JV et al: Frostbite: pathogenesis and treatment, *J Trauma* 48(1):171, 2000.
171. Greenfield LJ et al: *Surgery: scientific principles and practice*, ed 2, Philadelphia, 1997, Lippincott-Raven.
172. Raine TJ, London MD, Goluch L: Antiprostaglandins and antithromboxanes for treatment of frostbite, *Surg Forum* 31:557, 1980.
173. Bruen KJ et al: Reduction of the incidence of amputation in frostbite injury with thrombolytic therapy, *Arch Surg* 142(6):546-551, 2007.
174. Savin RC, Atton AV: Minoxidil: update on its clinical role, *Dermatol Clin* 11(1):55, 1993.
175. Norwood OT, Lehr B: Female androgenetic alopecia: a separate entity, *Dermatol Surg* 26(7):679, 2000.
176. Dinh QQ, Sinclair R: Female pattern hair loss: current treatment concepts, *Clin Interven Aging* 2(2):189-199, 2007.
177. Rushton DH: Management of hair loss in women, *Dermatol Clin* 11(1):47, 1993.
178. King LE Jr, McElwee KJ, Sundberg JP: Alopecia areata, *Curr Dir Autoimmun* 10:280-312, 2008.
179. Callen JP et al: *Color atlas of dermatology*, Philadelphia, 2000, Saunders.
180. Gilhar A, Paus R, Kalish RS: Lymphocytes, neuropeptides and genes involved in alopecia areata, *J Clin Invest* 117(8):2019-2027, 2007.
181. Avgerinou G et al: Alopecia areata: topical immunotherapy treatment with diphencyprone, *J Eur Acad Dermatol Venereal* 22(3):320-323, 2008.
182. Somani N, Harrison S, Bergfeld WF: The clinical evaluation of hirsutism, *Dermatol Ther* 21(5):376-391, 2008.
183. Archer JS, Chang RJ: Hirsutism and acne in polycystic ovary syndrome, *Best Pract Res Clin Obstet Gynaecol* 18(5):737-754, 2004.
184. Elghblawi E: idiopathic hirsutism: excessive bodily and facial hair in women, *Br J Nurs* 17(3):192-197, 2008.
185. Martin KA et al: Evaluation and treatment of hirsutism in premenopausal women: an endocrine society clinical practice guideline, *J Clin Endocrinol Metab* 93(4):1105-1120, 2008.
186. Rigopoulos D et al: Acute and chronic paronychia, *Am Fam Physician* 77(3):339-346, 2008.
187. Scher RK: Onychomycosis: therapeutic update, *J Am Acad Dermatol* 40(6 Pt 2):S21, 1999.
188. Elewski BE: Diagnostic techniques for confirming onychomycosis, *J Am Acad Dermatol* 35(3 Pt 2):S6, 1996.
189. Baran R, Hay RJ, Garduno JI: Review of antifungal therapy and the severity index for assessing onychomycosis: part 1, *J Dermatolog Treat* 19(2):72-81, 2008.
190. Nunley KS, Cornelius L: Current management of onychomycosis, *J Hand Surg Am* 33(7):1211-1214, 2008.

ALTERATIONS OF THE INTEGUMENT IN CHILDREN

NOREEN HEER NICOL • SUE E. HUETHER

MEDIA RESOURCES

e‍volve **Evolve Website** (http://evolve.elsevier.com/McCance/)
- Review Questions and Answers
- Animations
- Glossary (with audio pronunciation for selected terms)
- WebLinks

CHAPTER OUTLINE

ACNE VULGARIS
DERMATITIS
  Atopic Dermatitis
  Diaper Dermatitis
INFECTIONS OF THE SKIN
  Bacterial Infections
  Fungal Infections
  Viral Infections
INSECT BITES AND PARASITES
  Scabies
  Pediculosis (Lice Infestation)

  Fleas
  Bedbugs
HEMANGIOMAS AND VASCULAR MALFORMATIONS
  Hemangiomas
  Vascular Malformations
OTHER SKIN DISORDERS
  Miliaria
  Erythema Toxicum Neonatorum
  Toxic Epidermal Necrolysis and Stevens-Johnson
    Syndrome

Children often develop alterations in the skin that may be minor or severe and localized or generalized. Unfortunately the skin is often underrated in regard to its vital roles as a barrier, foundation, and calorie reservoir, as well as temperature regulation, sensation, grasp, insulation, psychosocial impact, and self-image. Manifestation of skin diseases in children may differ from those in adults, although the causative mechanisms may be similar. Some diseases resolve spontaneously and require no treatment. Diagnosis is commonly made from the history, appearance, and distribution of the lesion or lesions. Common skin diseases of childhood are presented here.

ACNE VULGARIS

Acne vulgaris is the most common skin disease and affects 85% of the population between the ages of 12 and 25 years. Genetic influences may determine an individual's susceptibility

and severity of disease. Severe acne tends to run in families. The incidence of acne is the same in both genders, although severe disease affects males more often.

Distinctive pilosebaceous units, known as *sebaceous follicles,* are the sites for development of acne lesions. The follicles are located primarily on the face and upper parts of the chest and back. These follicles have many large sebaceous glands, a small vellus hair, and a dilated follicular canal that is visible as a "pore" on the skin surface. Acne lesions may be divided into inflammatory lesions (pustules, papules, nodules) and noninflammatory lesions (closed and open comedones).[1] In **noninflammatory acne** the comedones are open (blackheads) and closed (whiteheads), with the accumulated material causing distention of the follicle and thinning of follicular canal walls. **Inflammatory acne** develops in closed comedones when the follicular wall ruptures, expelling sebum into the surrounding dermis and initiating inflammation. Pustules form when the inflammation is close to the surface; papules and cystic nodules can develop when the inflammation is deeper, causing mild to severe scarring (Figure 45-1). Both types of lesions may exist in the same individual.

The exact cause of acne is unknown and various pathophysiologic factors contribute to the development of acne. The principal factors are follicular hyperkeratinization, excessive sebum production, blockage of sebaceous glands, increased colonization of *Propionibacterium acnes,* and inflammation secondary to the action of extracellular inflammatory products produced by *P. acnes.* An excessive production and accumulation of sebum appear to be directly related to androgenic hormones and the pathogenesis of acne. Testosterone is converted to dihydrotestosterone in the skin, which increases the size and productivity of the sebaceous glands.[2] Acne begins with sebum accumulation that obstructs the pilosebaceous unit. The mass of accumulated keratinous sebaceous material and bacteria within the pilosebaceous follicle (see Figure 45-1) causes inflammation when it is exposed to the dermis with rupture of a follicle.

The *P. acnes* anaerobic bacteria produce extracellular porphyrins and proinflammatory molecules, including chemotactic factors and lipolytic and proteolytic enzymes. The hydrolytic action of the enzymes converts triglycerides into free fatty acids that stimulate inflammation and edema that result in breakdown of the follicle wall. Chemotactic substances also may be released that involve mediation of inflammation by attraction of polymorphonuclear leukocytes.

Acne conglobata is a highly inflammatory form of severe, disfiguring acne that involves the formation of communicating cysts and abscesses beneath the skin and requires referral and aggressive treatment. Remissions tend to occur during the summer, perhaps from more exposure to sunlight. External factors, such as cosmetics, use of oral and topical medications, mechanical friction, and occupation, may be etiologic factors. Abuse of anabolic-androgenic steroids is associated with acne conglobata.[3] Stress does not cause acne but can make it worse.

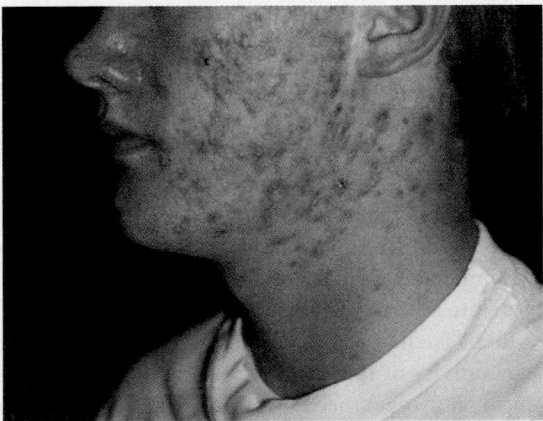

Figure 45-1 Cystic acne. Multiple pustules (erythematous papules and pustules) are present, and several have become confluent. Note areas of scarring. (Courtesy Department of Dermatology, School of Medicine, University of Utah.)

Self-manipulation of acne must be discouraged because it leads to increased inflammation and potential scarring.

Treatment of acne should address the causative factors and be individualized. Diet has not been proven to cause acne in spite of common lay opinion that there are acne-related foods; dietary restrictions are generally not effective.[4] Topical treatment, including topical antibiotics in combination with benzoyl peroxide (reduces bacterial resistance by disrupting the biofilm and increasing local oxygen tension), azelaic acid, and tretinoin should be the first line of therapy because it is the least invasive.[5] Systemic therapies, including oral antibiotics, sex hormones, corticosteroids, and isotretinoin, should be pursued when first-line therapy fails. Acne surgery, including comedo extraction, intralesional steroids, and cryosurgery, may be useful. Severe scarring may be treated with dermabrasion or subincision. Special consideration must be given to treatment for those with darker skin because they have greater risk for hyperpigmentation and keloidal scarring.[6]

DERMATITIS

Atopic Dermatitis

Atopic dermatitis (AD) is the most common cause of eczema with a prevalence rate of about 10% to 20% in children and 1% to 3% in adults. AD is increasing throughout the world.[7] Onset is usually from 2 to 6 months of age, and 85% of cases occur within the first 5 years of life; 75% to 80% of individuals with AD have a personal or family history of asthma, allergic rhinitis (hay fever), or food allergy. The cause of this chronic relapsing form of pruritic eczema involves an interplay of genetic predisposition, altered skin barrier function associated with filaggrin gene mutations (proteins that bind keratin in the epidermis), reduced ceramide (a stratum corneum lipid) levels, altered innate immunity, and altered immune responses to allergens, irritants, and microbes.[8] There is debate as to whether the pathophysiology favors an "inside-out" explanation with immunologic dysregulation leading to the skin barrier abnormality or an "outside-in" explanation with the primary barrier dysfunction causing the immunologic perturbations.[9] Positive immediate skin tests to a variety of common food and inhalant allergens are seen in approximately 80% of individuals with immunoglobulin E (IgE) sensitization and children are more likely to develop asthma.[10] Eosinophilia is common in both forms of AD.

In AD, memory T cells in the blood express cutaneous lymphocyte antigen (CLA), which leads to the homing of lymphocytes to the skin. In the acute phase of AD, inflammation is associated with activation of Th-1 cells with over-expression of cytokines (interleukin 4 [IL-4], IL-5, and IL13) and chemokines (CCL1 [chemotactic cytokine ligand 1] and CCL 18) with increases in IgE, eosinophils, and macrophages. In the chronic phase, there is activation of Th-1 cells with expression of interferon-gamma (IFN-γ), IL-12, and granulocyte-macrophage colony-stimulating factor (GM-CSF). There is activation of macrophages, dendritic cells (with high affinity for IgE), and mast cells with release of proinflammatory cytokines.[11] Th-2 cytokine expression also contributes to reduction in antimicrobial peptides and reduced filaggrin expression; however, the mechanisms leading to this effect are unknown.[12] Alterations in filaggrin protein lead to a defect of the epidermal barrier that causes transepidermal water loss and allows easy penetration of pathogens and allergens through the skin and a systemic hyperactive immune response.[13,14] Filaggrin gene mutations also are associated with increased risk for asthma in AD and ichthyosis vulgaris (dry, scaly skin).[15] In AD keratinocytes are deficient in their ability to express Toll-like antimicrobial peptides (see Chapter 6), including beta defensins and cathelicidins, and may predispose such individuals to skin colonization and infection with *Staphylococcus aureus*, viruses, and fungi.

AD has a long-term course with frequent exacerbations, severe pruritus, and characteristic eczematoid appearance with redness, edema, and scaling (Figure 45-2). The skin becomes increasingly dry, sensitive, itchy, and easily irritated because the barrier function is impaired. Microscopic epidermal cracks that let water out and irritants, allergens, and microbes in leads to further inflammation, drying, and cracking. Itching is the hallmark of atopic dermatitis, and rubbing and scratching to relieve the itch are responsible for many of the clinical changes of AD. Unlike its role in urticaria, histamine is not considered a major pruritogen in AD. Peripheral and central nerve sensitization, crosstalk among keratinocytes, immune

cells and nerve fibers, and release of mediators including serine proteases, IL-31, nerve growth factor, and the epidermal opioid system may contribute to pruritus of AD.[16,17]

In infants, the rash appears primarily on the face, scalp, trunk, and extensor surfaces of the arms and legs. In older children and adults, the rash tends to be found on the neck, antecubital and popliteal fossae, and hands and feet. Lichenification (thickening of the epidermis from constant scratching) is more common in adults with chronic eczema. Individuals with AD tend to develop viral, bacterial, and fungal skin infections in the areas with eczema. The irritation and itching interfere with sleep and cause irritability.

There are no specific laboratory features of AD that can be used for diagnostic purposes, and diagnosis is based on clinical history and presentation of symptoms.[18] Management of AD requires a systematic, multipronged approach. The approach includes parent education; identification and elimination of triggers or exacerbating factors, such as irritants, allergens, and emotional stressors; and incorporates skin moisturization, and pharmacologic and nonpharmacologic therapies. Hydration of the skin is the key to good therapy but is often difficult to achieve. Topical therapy can include baths, skin moisturizers, and wet wraps.[9] Anti-inflammatory agents, such as topical corticosteroids, topical calcineurin inhibitors, or tar preparations, are applied during active flares of eczema. Topical calcineurin inhibitors (tacrolimus and pimecrolimus) have an important role in the management of AD. Phototherapy may be beneficial. Systemic therapy includes the use of sedating antihistamines and antibiotics for treatment of infection. Systemic corticosteroids usually are not warranted. Treatment plans should be individualized to address the individual's skin reaction pattern and acuity of the rash.[19,20]

Diaper Dermatitis

Diaper dermatitis is probably the most common skin disorder of infancy and early childhood. It is a contact dermatitis (see Chapter 44) caused by chemical irritation. This form of irritant contact dermatitis is initiated by a combination of factors that include prolonged exposure to and irritation by urine and feces, maceration by wet diapers, airtight plastic diaper covers, and possibly increased association with intercurrent illnesses and early introduction of cereals. Diaper designs have decreased diaper dermatitis in infants.[21] Frequently, the infant with diaper dermatitis is secondarily infected with *Candida albicans*.

The lesions vary from mild erythema to erythematous papular lesions. Candidal (monilial) diaper dermatitis is usually very erythematous, with sharp margination and pustulovesicular satellite lesions (Figure 45-3).

Treatment is changing the diaper frequently to keep the area clean and dry or frequently exposing the perineal area to air. Topical antifungal medication is used to treat *C. albicans* when present. Short-term use of low-potency topical steroids alternately with antifungals at each diaper change helps reduce inflammation. Various topical agents provide a barrier from the irritating agents and promote healing.

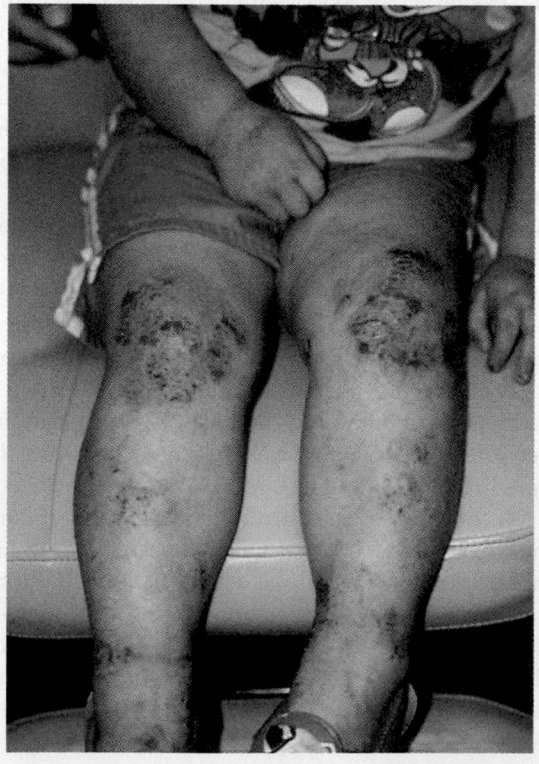

Figure 45-2 Atopic dermatitis. Characteristic lesions with crusting from irritation and scratching over knees and around ankles. (Courtesy Department of Dermatology, School of Medicine, University of Utah.)

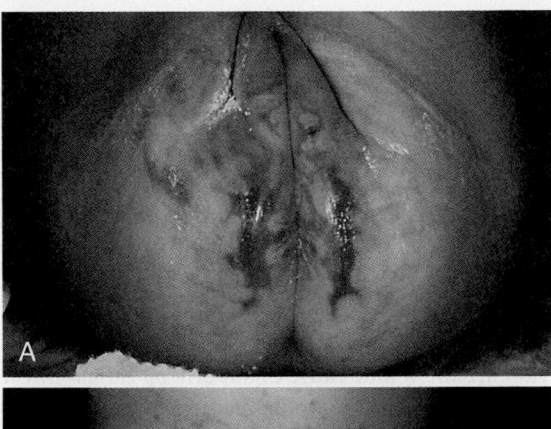

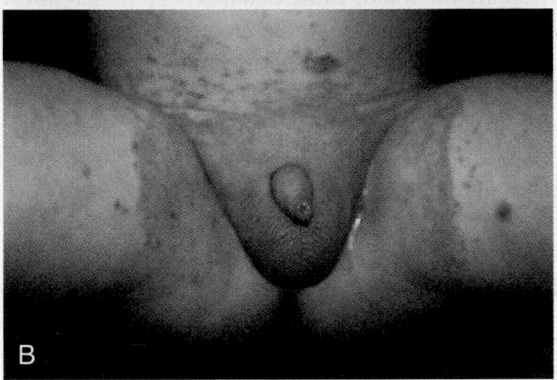

Figure 45-3 Diaper dermatitis. A, Diaper dermatitis with erosions. **B,** Diaper dermatitis with *Candida albicans* secondary infection. (Courtesy Department of Dermatology, School of Medicine, University of Utah.)

INFECTIONS OF THE SKIN

Infectious diseases caused by bacteria, viruses, and fungi constitute the major forms of skin disease. Breaks in the skin integrity, particularly those that inoculate pathogens into the dermis and epidermis, may cause or exacerbate infections. Most infections tend to occur superficially; however, systemic signs and symptoms do develop occasionally and rarely may be life threatening.

Bacterial Infections

Impetigo Contagiosum
Impetigo is a common bacterial skin infection in infants and children, usually caused by *S. aureus* or group A streptococcus. The disease is more common in midsummer to late summer, with a higher incidence in hot, humid climates. Impetigo is particularly infectious among people living in crowded conditions with poor sanitary facilities. It affects children in good health, but conditions such as anemia and malnutrition are predisposing factors. There are two common types of impetigo: bullous and vesicular.[22] Both start as vesicles with a very thin vesicular roof composed of stratum corneum.

Bullous Impetigo
Bullous impetigo is a rarer variant of impetigo caused by *S. aureus.* The staphylococci produce a bacterial toxin called *exfoliative toxin (ET)* that causes a disruption in desmosomal adhesion molecules with blister formation.[23] This form characteristically occurs in newborns and is highly contagious.

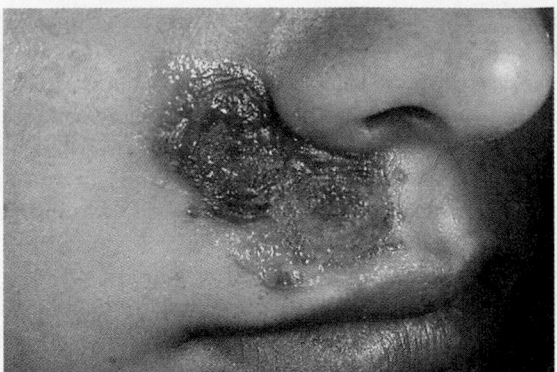

Figure 45-4 Impetigo and herpes simplex virus (HSV) of upper lip. Note weeping and crusting lesions. (Courtesy Department of Dermatology, School of Medicine, University of Utah.)

The source of the infection is usually a staff member in a newborn nursery or a family member with a pustule or who is an asymptomatic carrier. The pathogen is often carried in the anterior nares, perineal region, or fingernails and is transmitted by contact with the individual or contaminated equipment.[24]

The exfoliative toxin stimulates the formation of vesicles that enlarge or coalesce to form superficial bullae. There may be a few localized lesions or many lesions scattered over the skin. As the bullae rupture, a thin, flat, honey-colored crust appears. The crust is the hallmark of impetigo. A moist, inflamed serum-weeping base is revealed when the crust is removed. The lesions are often located on the face around the nose and mouth, but the hands and other exposed areas are also involved. Regional lymphadenitis is uncommon.

Vesicular Impetigo
Vesicular impetigo is a contagious, acute, superficial, vesiculopustular form of impetigo caused by group A *Streptococcus pyogenes* (alone or in combination with *S. aureus*). The microorganisms are disseminated by direct physical contact from other infected individuals or through insect bites. The lesions begin as small vesicles with a honey-colored serum. Yellow to white-brown crusts form as the vesicles rupture and extend radially (Figure 45-4). Untreated lesions may last for weeks and extend to cover a large area. In contrast to bullous impetigo, regional lymphadenitis is common.

The risk of nephritogenic strains of streptococci varies considerably in North America.[25] Aggressive treatment of infected individuals and their contacts significantly reduces the chance of acute glomerulonephritis, which is clearly the most serious complication of streptococcal impetigo.

Treatment of choice for both types of impetigo is topical mupirocin and topical fusidic acid or oral antibiotics.[22] Antibiotic therapy should be determined by bacterial culture and drug sensitivity because antimicrobial resistance is increasing.[26] Removal of crusts and scrubbing the lesions with antibacterial soaps have not been shown to be effective.[27] Good handwashing techniques and isolation of the infected child's washcloth, towels, drinking glass, and linen are important to control this highly contagious disease.

Staphylococcal Scalded-Skin Syndrome

Staphylococcal scalded-skin syndrome (SSSS) is the most serious staphylococcal infection that affects the skin and usually is seen in infants and children younger than 5 years.[28] SSSS is caused by virulent group II staphylococci, which produce an exfoliative toxin that attacks desmoglein and adhesion molecules and causes a separation of the skin just below the granular layer of the epidermis.[29] The toxins are usually produced at body sites other than the skin and arrive at the epidermis through the circulatory system. Staphylococci typically are not found in the skin lesions themselves. Adults have circulating antistaphylococcal antibodies and are better able to metabolize and excrete the toxin. Newborns are at the highest risk because of their lack of immunity (not having prior exposure to the toxin).

The clinical symptoms begin with fever, malaise, rhinorrhea, and irritability followed by generalized erythema with exquisite tenderness of the skin. There may be an associated impetigo, but the infection often begins in the throat or chest. The erythema spreads from the face and trunk to cover the entire body except the palms, soles, and mucous membranes. Within 48 hours, blisters and bullae may form, causing severe pain (Figure 45-5). Fluid loss from ruptured blisters and water evaporation from denuded areas may cause dehydration. Perioral and nasolabial crusting and fissures develop. In severe cases the skin of the entire body may slough. When secondary infection can be prevented, healing of the involved skin occurs in 10 to 14 days, usually without scarring.

Before medical intervention is begun, culture, histology, or exfoliative cytology must be done to differentiate SSSS from toxic epidermal necrolysis (TEN) (see p. 1692). When the infection is confirmed, treatment with oral or intravenous antibiotics is begun.[30] Topical antibiotics are ineffective. The skin should be treated the same as that with a severe burn—with meticulous aseptic technique. Special care is required in serious cases and when the lips and eyelids are involved.[28]

Fungal Infections

Fungal disorders are known as *mycoses* and, when caused by dermatophytes (fungi that thrive on keratin), the mycoses are termed *tinea* (dermatophytosis or ringworm).[31] **Tinea pedis** (a chronic, superficial fungal infection of the skin of the foot) occurs in children but is rare. Scaling disorders of the toes and feet in prepubertal children are usually eczema. Tinea capitis (infection of the scalp) and tinea corporis (infection of the body) are much more common in children than adults. (The different types of tinea are described in Chapter 44.) *Epidermophyton* are the major cause of superficial fungal infections in children.[32] These dermatophytes invade the stratum corneum and not the remainder of the epidermis or dermis. The inflammatory response is thought, in part, to be secondary to the toxins released by the dermatophyte. It is important to confirm by culture which microorganism is causing the fungal infection before commencing therapy.

Tinea Capitis

Tinea capitis, a fungal infection of the scalp, is the most common fungal infection of childhood. It rarely affects infants and is seen in children younger than age 12. Primary microorganisms responsible for the disease are *Microsporum canis* and *Trichophyton tonsurans. M. canis* is found on cats, dogs, and certain rodents. Humans appear to be a terminal host for *M. canis,* and children who handle such animals are possible hosts. Human-to-human transmission does not occur. *T. tonsurans* conversely *is* transmitted by human-to-human contact. Areas of crowding are the most prevalent environments for this microorganism, which frequently affects inner-city children. *T. tonsurans* is often the predominant dermatophyte found on inner-city children, and many of these infections are not symptomatic. The prevalence of asymptomatic carriers among household contacts of a child with active *T. tonsurans* disease is high.[33] Treatment of household contacts with a sporicidal shampoo should be considered and

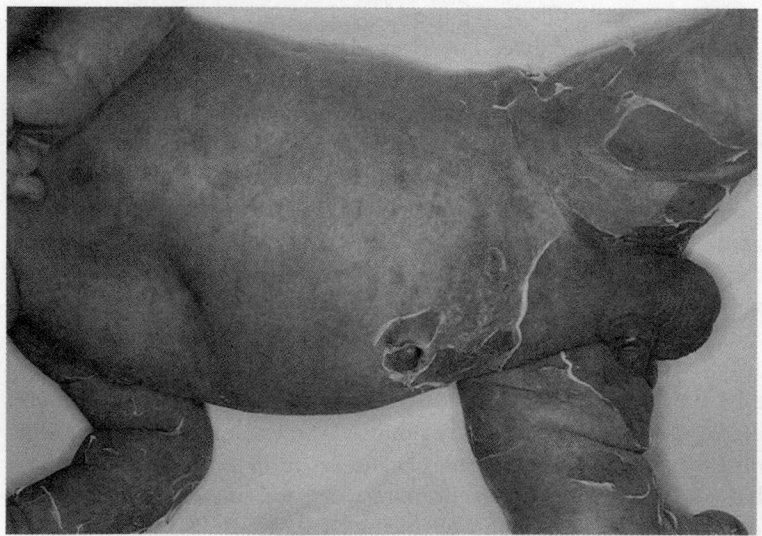

Figure 45-5 Staphylococcal scalded-skin syndrome (SSSS). The skin lesions, showing desquamation and wrinkling of the skin margins, appeared 1 day after drainage of a staphylococcal abscess. (From Habif TP: *Clinical dermatology: a color guide to diagnosis and therapy,* ed 5, St Louis, 2010, Mosby.)

co-sleeping and comb sharing must be discouraged. When symptoms are present, the clinical presentations vary, depending on the microorganism. Often the lesions are circular and manifest by broken hairs 1 to 3 mm above the scalp, leaving a partial alopecia 1 to 5 cm in diameter[34] (Figure 45-6). Slight erythema and scaling with raised borders can be observed.

Diagnosis is best confirmed by performing Wood light examination, potassium hydroxide (KOH) examination, and fungal culture, in that order. *T. tonsurans* does not fluoresce with Wood light examination. Oral griseofulvin is the treatment of choice because topical fungicides do not penetrate to the hair bulb. Terbinafine, itraconazole, and fluconazole are effective alternatives.[35] Adjunct therapy includes 2% ketoconazole and 1% selenium sulfide shampoos.[36]

Tinea Corporis

Tinea corporis is a common superficial dermatophyte infection in children. The microorganisms most commonly responsible for this disease are *M. canis* and *Trichophyton mentagrophytes*. As in tinea capitis, contact with kittens and puppies is a common source of the disorder. Tinea corporis preferentially affects the nonhairy parts of the face, trunk, and limbs. Lesions are often erythematous, round or oval scaling patches that spread peripherally with clearing in the center, creating the ring appearance, which is why this disease is commonly referred to as *ringworm*. The lesions are distributed asymmetrically, and multiple lesions (when present) overlap. KOH examination of the scale from the border of the lesions confirms the diagnosis for most lesions. Most lesions respond well to applications of appropriate topical antifungal medications.[32]

Thrush

C. albicans infection is a superficial fungal infection that commonly occurs in children. *C. albicans* is part of the normal skin flora in certain individuals and invades susceptible tissue sites if the predisposing factors are not eliminated. *C. albicans* penetrates the epidermal barrier more easily than other microorganisms because of its keratolytic proteases and other enzymes. *C. albicans* attracts neutrophils to skin sites of invasion and generates inflammation by activation of the complement system within the skin.

Thrush is the term used to describe the presence of *Candida* in the mucous membranes of the mouth of infants and, less commonly, adults. Thrush is characterized by the formation of white plaques or spots in the mouth that lead to shallow ulcers. The tongue may have a dense, white covering. The underlying mucous membrane is red and tender and may bleed when the plaques are removed. The disease is often accompanied by fever and gastrointestinal irritation. The infection commonly spreads to the groin, buttocks, and other parts of the body. Treatment may be difficult and may include oral antifungal washes, such as nystatin oral suspension. Gentian violet can also be effective. Simultaneous treatment of a *Candida* nipple infection or vaginitis in the mother is helpful in reducing the *C. albicans* surface colonization of the infant. Feeding bottles and nipples should be sterilized to prevent reinfection. The diaper area should be kept clean and dry.

Viral Infections

Viral infections of the skin in children are caused by poxvirus, papovavirus, and herpesvirus. The most common infections are described here.

Molluscum Contagiosum

Molluscum contagiosum is a common highly contagious poxvirus infection of the skin and occasionally conjunctiva that affects primarily children. It is transmitted by skin-to-skin contact, autoinoculation, and fomites, such as clothing, wash devices, and towels. This disease appears to be more common in individuals with atopic dermatitis and a variety of immunodeficient states, including human immunodeficiency virus (HIV).[37] The poxvirus induces epidermal cell proliferation and blocks immune responses that would control the virus. The epidermis grows down into the dermis to form saccules containing clusters of virus. The characteristic molluscum body is composed of mature, immature, and incomplete viruses and cellular debris.[38]

The lesions of molluscum are discrete, slightly umbilicated, dome-shaped papules 1 to 5 mm in diameter that appear anywhere on the skin or conjunctiva. The skin distribution in children is mainly on the trunk, face, and extremities (Figure 45-7). The pubic, genital, and perineal areas are favored in adults (see Chapter 24). Usually no inflammation surrounds molluscum lesions unless they are traumatized or secondary infection occurs. Scarring occurs with healing.

The best three diagnostic procedures are: (1) staining smears of the expressed molluscum body, (2) examining a biopsy, and (3) inoculating a molluscum suspension into cell cultures to demonstrate the cytotoxic reactions. Most lesions are self-limiting and clear in 6 to 9 months if not manipulated. However, because children often do manipulate these

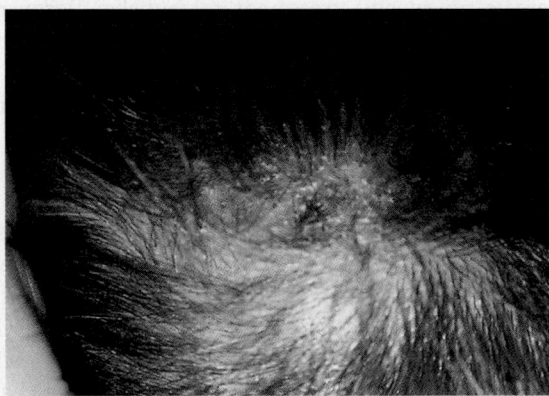

Figure 45-6 Tinea capitis. (Courtesy Department of Dermatology, School of Medicine, University of Utah.)

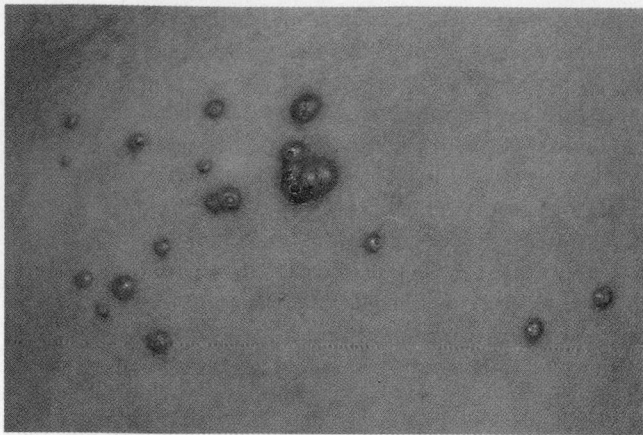

Figure 45-7 Molluscum contagiosum. Waxy pink globules with umbilicated centers. (From Habif TP: *Clinical dermatology: a color guide to diagnosis and therapy*, ed 3, St Louis, 1996, Mosby.)

lesions, spontaneous involution may take 2 to 4 years without therapy.

Treatment options include topical, oral, and surgical approaches (cryotherapy, curettage or laser ablation), and no treatment is universally effective. Destructive therapy is poorly tolerated by children.[39] Measures to prevent spread of infection must be taken and recurrences are common. Children must be taught not to manipulate or scratch these lesions.

Rubella (German or 3-Day Measles)

Rubella is a common communicable disease of children and young adults caused by a ribonucleic acid (RNA) virus that enters the bloodstream through the respiratory route. This disease is mild in most children. The incubation period ranges from 14 to 21 days. Prodromal symptoms are few but may include enlarged cervical and postauricular lymph nodes, low-grade fever, headache, sore throat, runny nose, and cough. A faint-pink to red, coalescing maculopapular rash develops on the face, with spread to the trunk and extremities 1 to 4 days after the onset of initial symptoms (Figure 45-8). The rash is thought to be the result of virus dissemination to the skin. The rash subsides after 2 to 3 days, usually without complications. Children are generally not contagious after development of the rash. There is lifelong immunity to rubella—as there is for measles, chickenpox, and roseola—after contracting the disease. Differential presentations of viral diseases producing rashes are given in Table 45-1.

Vaccination for rubella is usually combined with vaccines for mumps and measles (rubeola) (MMR). A quadravalent vaccine MMRV, combining the attenuated virus MMR vaccine with the addition of varicella (chickenpox), has been approved in the United States and Europe for children ages 1 to 12 years. Vaccine recommendations are presented in Chapter 9, Table 9-13. In the past, parents chose not to give the vaccine because of the misbelief that it would cause the disease. Studies have confirmed that measles or rubella-like illnesses in MMR-vaccinated children are often caused by

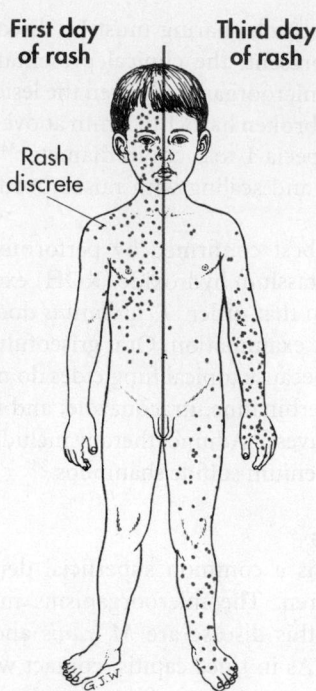

Figure 45-8 Measles. Full-blown maculopapular rash with tendency to coalesce. (From Wehrle PF, Top FH Sr: *Communicable and infectious diseases*, ed 9, St Louis, 1981, Mosby.)

other viruses.[40] Measles is known to occur in previously immunized children.[41]

More recently parental concern has focused on the belief that MMR vaccination may cause autism. Although MMR vaccine may rarely be associated with adverse neurologic events, studies conclude that MMR immunization does not cause autism.[42] Lack of vaccination, however, leads to significant morbidity and mortality,[43,44] with pneumonia, croup, and encephalitis being causes of death worldwide.[45,46]

Women of childbearing age are immunized if their rubella hemagglutination-inhibition titer is low. Pregnancy should be avoided for 3 months after vaccination because the attenuated virus in the vaccine may remain for this period. Pregnant women who have rubella early in the first trimester have an 80% risk of congenital defects.[47]

There is no specific treatment for rubella. Recovery is spontaneous, although lymph nodes may remain enlarged for weeks. Supportive therapy includes rest, fluids, and use of a vaporizer. In rare cases a mild encephalitis or peripheral neuritis may follow rubella.

Rubeola (Red Measles)

Rubeola is a highly contagious, acute viral disease of children. It is transmitted by direct contact with droplets from infected persons and is caused by an RNA-containing paramyxovirus with an incubation period of 7 to 12 days, during which time no symptoms manifest. Prodromal symptoms include high fever (up to 40.5° C [104.9° F]), malaise, enlarged lymph nodes, runny nose, conjunctivitis, and "barking" cough. Within 3 to 4 days, an erythematous maculopapular rash

Table 45-1	Differential Presentation of Viral Diseases Producing Rashes			
Viral Disease	Incubation	Prodromal Symptoms	Duration/Characteristics	Clinical Symptoms
Rubella (German measles)	14-21 days	1-2 days Mild fever Malaise Respiratory symptoms	1-3 days Pink-red maculopapular Face and trunk	Enlarged and tender occipital and periauricular nodes
Rubeola (measles)	7-12 days	2-5 days Fever Cough Respiratory symptoms	3-5 days Purple-red to brown maculopapular papules Face, trunk, extremities	Koplik spots 1-3 days before rash Rash develops when fever subsides
Roseola (exanthema subitum)	5-15 days	2-5 days High fever	1-3 days Red macular papules Neck and trunk	
Varicella (chickenpox)	11-20 days	1-2 days Low-grade fever Cough May be asymptomatic	Red papules, vesicles, pustules in clusters	Eruption of new lesions for 4-5 days Occasional ulcerative lesion in the mouth

develops over the head and spreads distally over the trunk, extremities, hands, and feet. Early lesions blanch with pressure, followed by a brownish hue that does not blanch as the rash fades. Characteristic pinpoint white spots surrounded by an erythematous ring develop over the buccal mucosa and are known as *Koplik spots*. These spots precede the rash by 1 to 2 days. The rash then subsides within 3 to 5 days.

Complications associated with measles may be caused by the primary infection or a secondary bacterial infection. Measles encephalitis occurs in about 1 of 800 cases, and most children recover completely. Only a small minority develop permanent brain damage or die. Bacterial complications include otitis media and pneumonia, usually caused by group A hemolytic streptococcus, *Haemophilus influenzae*, or *S. aureus* infection.

Measles is prevented by a single vaccination of live attenuated measles virus. There is no specific treatment for measles, and supportive therapy is the same as for rubella. Antibiotic therapy is initiated if secondary bacterial infections develop.

Roseola (Exanthema Subitum)

Roseola is a presumed viral infection of infants between 6 months and 2 years of age, but it can be seen in children as old as 4 years. The incubation period is 5 to 15 days, followed by the sudden onset of fever (38.9° to 40.5° C [102° to 104.5° F]) that lasts for 3 to 5 days. After the fever an erythematous macular rash that lasts about 24 hours develops primarily over the trunk and neck. Children usually feel well, eat normally, and have few other symptoms. Usually no treatment is required.

Chickenpox and Herpes Zoster

Chickenpox (varicella) and herpes zoster (shingles) are produced by the varicella-zoster virus (VZV). VZV is a complex herpes group deoxyribonucleic acid (DNA) virus. The incubation period is 10 to 27 days, averaging 14 days. Productive infection occurs within keratinocytes such that the vesicular lesions occur in the epidermis, and an inflammatory infiltrate is often present. Histologically, VZV lesions form

intraepidermal vesicles. Infected keratinocytes degenerate, swell, detach from each other, and often contain inclusions surrounded by a clear halo and a circle of darkly staining chromatin. As the vesicle evolves, polymorphonuclear cells enter the vesicle and can lead to a pustular appearance. The vesicle eventually ruptures and is followed by crust formation. On mucous membranes the vesicles rupture and leave superficial, transient ulcers. Varicella occurs in people not previously exposed to VZV, whereas herpes zoster occurs in partially immune individuals who have had varicella.[48]

Chickenpox (Varicella)

Chickenpox is a disease of early childhood, with 90% of children contracting the disease during the first decade of life. It is a highly contagious virus that is spread by person-to-person contact and airborne droplets. Introduction of an infected person into a household results in a 90% possibility of susceptible persons in the household developing the disease within the incubation period—usually 14 days. Children are contagious for at least 1 day before development of the rash. Transmission of the virus may occur until approximately 5 to 6 days after the onset of the first skin lesions in normal children. In immunocompromised children the virus is recoverable for a longer period, but these children must be considered contagious for at least 7 to 10 days. Chickenpox occurs most commonly in the late winter and early spring. Transmission occurs more readily in temperate climates than in tropical climates.

Healthy children who develop chickenpox have no prodromal symptoms. The first sign of illness may be itching or the appearance of vesicles, usually on the trunk, scalp, or face. The rash later spreads to the extremities. Characteristically, lesions can be seen in various stages of maturation with macules, papules, and vesicles present in a particular area at the same time (Figure 45-9). The vesicular lesions are superficial and can be easily ruptured. New lesions will erupt for 4 to 5 days, until there are approximately 100 to 300 in different stages of development. The vesicles become crusted, with only the crust remaining. Occasionally a vesicle may appear on the

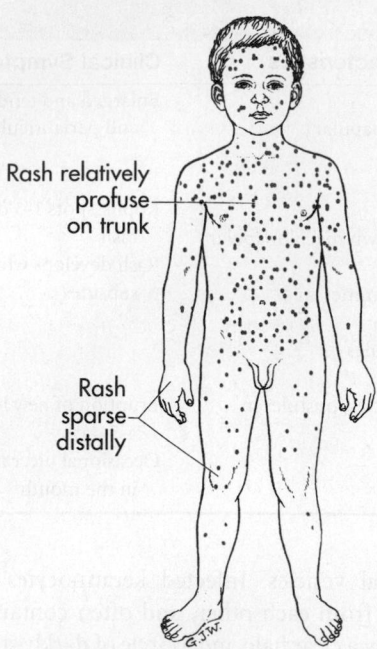

Rash relatively profuse on trunk

Rash sparse distally

Figure 45-9 Chickenpox. Generalized, polymorphous eruption. (From Wehrle PF, Top FH Sr: *Communicable and infectious diseases*, ed 9, St Louis, 1981, Mosby.)

palm later in the disease. Although uncommon, ulcerative lesions are sometimes seen in the mouth and, less commonly, on the conjunctiva and pharynx. Fever usually lasts 2 to 3 days and ranges from 38.5° to 40° C [101.3° to 104° F]).

Complications are rare in children but more common in adults. They can include transient hematuria (from rupture of vesicles in the bladder), epistaxis, laryngeal edema, and varicella pneumonia. One case of chickenpox produces almost complete immunity against a second attack. Rarely, the fetus may be malformed (congenital varicella syndrome) if chickenpox develops in the mother in the first trimester of pregnancy.[49,50] Infants whose mothers have chickenpox at any stage of pregnancy have a higher risk of developing herpes zoster during the first few years of life.

Uncomplicated chickenpox requires no specific therapy. Baths, wet dressings, and oral antihistamines are occasionally helpful to relieve itching and to prevent secondary infection as a result of scratching. Oral antistaphylococcal drugs should be given if secondary bacterial infection is present. Zoster immune globulin may be administered to immunodeficient individuals if given within 72 hours after exposure to chickenpox. Oral antiviral drugs may be valuable in reducing symptoms in otherwise healthy children as well as in immunosuppressed or other select groups of children.[51]

Chickenpox can be prevented with a safe and effective vaccine (see Chapter 9, Table 9-13).

Herpes Zoster

Although herpes zoster (shingles) occurs mainly in adults, approximately 5% of cases are in children younger than 15 years.[52] A wild-type VZV (a type not included in the vaccine strains) can cause herpes zoster. The course of the disease in children with an immune defect is more complicated and requires treatment with antiviral agents.[53] The chickenpox virus persists for life in sensory nerve ganglia and reactivates to cause herpes zoster. The eruption of **zoster** consists of groups of vesicles situated on an inflammatory base and following the course of a sensory nerve. Common dermatomal distribution in young children is cervical and sacral.[54] The base of the lesions often appears hemorrhagic, and some of the lesions may become necrotic and ulcerative. In addition to the localized eruption, there are commonly a few scattered lesions resembling chickenpox. Therapy is similar to that for chickenpox unless it is ophthalmic or disseminated zoster, for which systemic antiviral treatment and (when the eye is involved) a referral to an ophthalmologist are indicated. The herpes zoster vaccine has been approved for use in persons 60 years of age and older.[55] A tetravalent vaccine against measles, mumps, rubella, and varicella-zoster viruses (MMRV) is available for infants and children.[56]

Smallpox

Smallpox (variola) is a highly contagious and deadly but preventable disease. It is caused by poxvirus variolae. Because of worldwide mass immunization, the world is now virtually free of smallpox.[57] Concerns regarding smallpox as a weapon of bioterrorism have led to vaccination programs for the military and for selected civilian populations. The U.S. government has an adequate supply of smallpox vaccine to vaccinate the population in the event of an emergency.[58]

INSECT BITES AND PARASITES

Insect bites and infestations are common causes of skin disorders in children and adults. Skin damage occurs by various mechanisms, including trauma of bites and stings, allergic reactions, transmission of disease, injection of substances that cause local or systemic reactions, and inflammatory reactions from retained mouthparts.

Scabies

Scabies is a contagious disease caused by the itch mite, *Sarcoptes scabiei* (Figure 45-10, *A*). It is transmitted by personal contact (see Chapter 24) and by infected clothing and bedding. Scabies is often epidemic in areas of overcrowded housing, poor sanitation, or in long-term care institutions. Scabies is often associated with immunocompromised individuals, such as those with human T-cell leukemia/lymphoma virus I (HTLV-1) and HIV.[59] Infestation is initiated by a female mite that tunnels into the stratum corneum, depositing eggs and creating a burrow several millimeters to 1 cm long. Over a 3-week period, the eggs mature into adult mites, which sometimes can be recognized as tiny dots at the end of intact burrows.

Symptoms appear 3 to 5 weeks after infestation. The primary lesions are burrows, papules, and vesicular lesions, with severe itching that worsens at night. Two or three bites

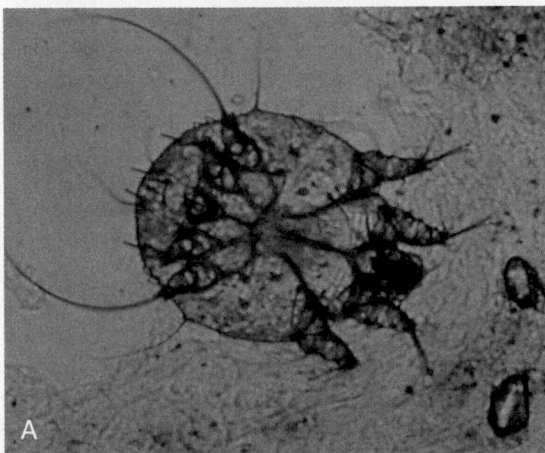

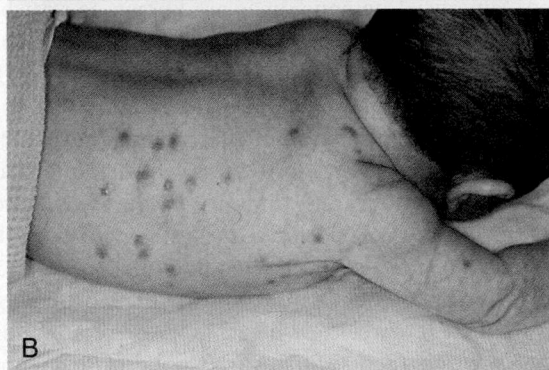

Figure 45-10 Scabies. A, Scabies mite, as seen clinically when removed from its burrow. **B,** Characteristic scabies bites. (Courtesy Department of Dermatology, School of Medicine, University of Utah.)

(commonly referred to as "breakfast, lunch, and dinner") usually appear in a line on exposed areas of the skin. Itching is thought to be related to sensitization to the larval stages of the parasite. In older children and adults the lesions occur in the webs of fingers, axillae, and creases of the arms and wrists; along the belt line; and around the nipples, genitalia, and lower buttocks. Infants and young children have a different pattern of distribution, with involvement of the palms, soles, head, neck, and face (see Figure 45-10, *B*). Secondary infections and crusting develop from scratching and eczematous changes.

Norwegian scabies (crusted scabies) is a relatively rare widespread scabetic infestation with an affinity for severely mentally retarded persons, those who are unable to effectively scratch, or in immunocompromised individuals. It is highly contagious and is characterized by heavily crusted lesions on the scalp, elbows, knees, palms, soles, and buttocks.[60]

Diagnosis of scabies is made by observation of the tunnels and burrows and scraping of the skin with microscopic examination of the mite or its eggs or feces. Treatment is the application of permethrin cream, a scabicide. Generalized scabies is treated with oral ivermectin.[61] Even with elimination of all viable scabies microorganisms, itching may persist for 10 days or longer. All clothing and linens should be washed and dried in hot cycles or dry-cleaned.

Pediculosis (Lice Infestation)

The three known types of human lice are: (1) the head louse *(Pediculus capitis)*, (2) the body louse *(Pediculus corporis)*, and (3) the crab or pubic louse *(Phthirus pubis)*. They are highly contagious parasites that survive by sucking blood. The female louse reproduces every 2 weeks, producing hundreds of nits as newly hatched lice mate with old lice. The mouthparts are shaped for piercing and sucking and attach to the skin while feeding. When piercing the skin, the louse secretes a toxic saliva; the mechanical trauma and toxin produce a pruritic dermatitis. Head and body lice are acquired by personal contact, combs, or brushes. Crab lice are spread by body contact, such as contact with an infected adult (see Chapter 24). Sharing clothing is also a common source of transmission.[62]

Itching is the major symptom of lice infestation. In head lice infestation the ova attach to hairs above the ears and in the occipital region. The primary lesion of the body louse is a pinpoint red macule, papule, or wheal with a hemorrhagic puncture site. The primary lesion often is not seen because it is masked by excoriations, wheals, and crusts. The crab louse is found on pubic hairs but also may involve other body hair such as eyelashes, mustache, beard, and axillae. Young children particularly may become infected with crab lice on their eyebrows or eyelashes.

The live louse, 2 to 3 mm long, is rarely observed, although the ova, or nits, can be observed as oval, yellowish pinpoint specks fastened to a hair shaft. The ova fluoresce under an ultraviolet light (Wood lamp) and can be best observed with a microscope. Infestations can be treated with a topical pediculicide (i.e., permethrin) or oral ivermectin.[63] All clothes, towels, bedding, combs, and brushes should be washed and dried in hot air or boiled, or the clothes should be ironed. Individuals who have personal contact also should be treated.

Fleas

Young children are very susceptible to **flea bites,** and the most common are the bites of cat, dog, and human fleas.[64] Bites occur in clusters along the arms and legs or where clothing fits tightly. The bite produces an urticarial wheal with a central hemorrhagic puncture (Figure 45-11). An immune response to flea bite proteins causes a chronic papular urticaria.[65] Tungiasis, caused by sand fleas, causes chronic morbidity in impoverished communities in Latin America, the Caribbean, and Sub-Saharan Africa.[66] Treatment includes spraying carpets, crevices, and furniture with malathion or lindane powder. Infected animals should be treated, and clothes and bedding should be washed in hot water. There is no specific treatment for tungiasis, but topical pesticides can reduce the number of lesions from embedded fleas.

Bedbugs

The common bedbug, *Cimex lectularius,* is a blood-sucking nocturnal parasite of man. Chickens, bats, and some domestic animals are the other hosts for this bug.[67] **Bedbugs** live in the crevices and cracks of floors, walls, and furniture and in

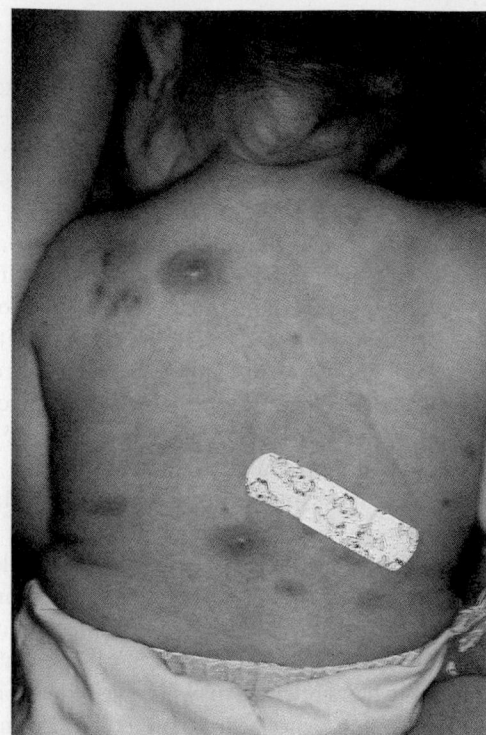

Figure 45-11 Flea bites. Flea bite producing an urticarial wheal with central puncture.

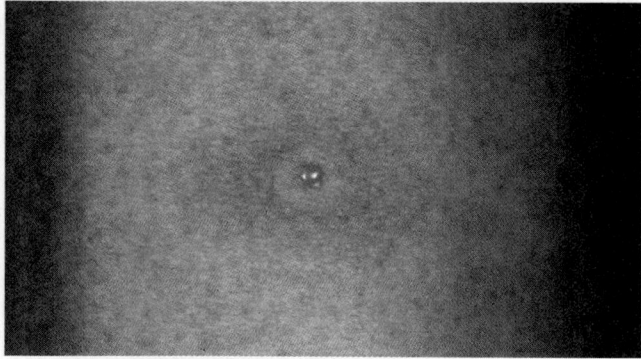

Figure 45-12 Bullous bedbug bites. (Courtesy Department of Dermatology, School of Medicine, University of Utah.)

bedding or furniture stuffing. They are 3 to 5 mm long and reddish brown. Bedbugs emerge to feed in darkness and attach to the skin to suck blood. Feeding occurs for 5 to 15 minutes, then the bedbug leaves. It will move long distances to search for food and can travel from house to house.

If the host has not been previously sensitized, the only symptom is a red macule that develops into a nodule, lasting up to 14 days. In sensitized children and adults, pruritic wheals, papules, and vesicles may form (Figure 45-12). These lesions respond to antihistamines or corticosteroids. Secondary infections require antibiotic treatment. Bedbugs are eliminated by inspecting and cleaning or disposing of bedding, mattresses, furniture and other contaminated items, and by

using applications of approved insecticides, usually by a professional.[68]

HEMANGIOMAS AND VASCULAR MALFORMATIONs

Vascular anomalies are frequent tumors of early infancy and can be categorized as either hemangiomas or vascular malformations.[69,70]

Hemangiomas

Hemangiomas are benign tumors that form from the rapid growth of vascular endothelial cells, which results in formation of extra blood vessels. Hemangiomas can be superficial or deep. Superficial hemangiomas are known as strawberry hemangiomas and deep lesions are known as cavernous hemangiomas. The etiology may be related to embolization of fetal placental endothelial cells related to placental trauma or loss of placental angiogenic inhibitor of placental and maternal origin.[71] There is proliferation of mast cells that are thought to promote the angiogenesis. Infiltration of fat cells, fibrosis, and the rich vascular network give the lesions a firm, rubbery feel. Females are affected more often than males. About 30% of hemangiomas are apparent at birth, with most emerging during the first few weeks of life; they grow rapidly during the first few years, then shrink or involute during childhood years. With involution the lesions become darker in color and then gradually turn to a flesh color. There may be some residual telangiectasia. Most require no treatment depending on location. Hemangiomas located over the eye, ear, nose, mouth, urethra, or anus may require treatment because they interfere with function and have a higher risk for infection or injury. Systemic or intralesional steroids are the treatment of choice. Interferons, vincristine, cyclophosphamide, and radiotherapy can suppress angiogenesis. Cryosurgery, laser surgery, sclerotherapy, and embolization are also alternative treatment options.[71-73]

Strawberry hemangiomas are distinct superficial hemangiomas that may be present at birth but usually emerge 3 to 5 weeks after birth. They proliferate and become bright red and elevated with minute capillary projections that give them a strawberry appearance. Only one lesion is usually present, and it is located on the head and neck area or trunk (Figure 45-13). After the initial growth, the lesion grows at the same rate as the child and then starts to involute at 12 to 16 months of age. Approximately 90% of strawberry hemangiomas involute by 5 to 6 years of age, usually without scarring.[71]

Cavernous (congenital) hemangiomas are present at birth and have larger and more mature vessels within the lesion than strawberry hemangiomas. Some lesions, however, are composed of a mixture of strawberry and cavernous hemangiomas. They appear primarily on the head and neck, are bluish red, and have less distinct borders (Figure 45-14). Cavernous hemangiomas grow rapidly up to 6 months of age and mature by 1 year of age. A period of involution begins and

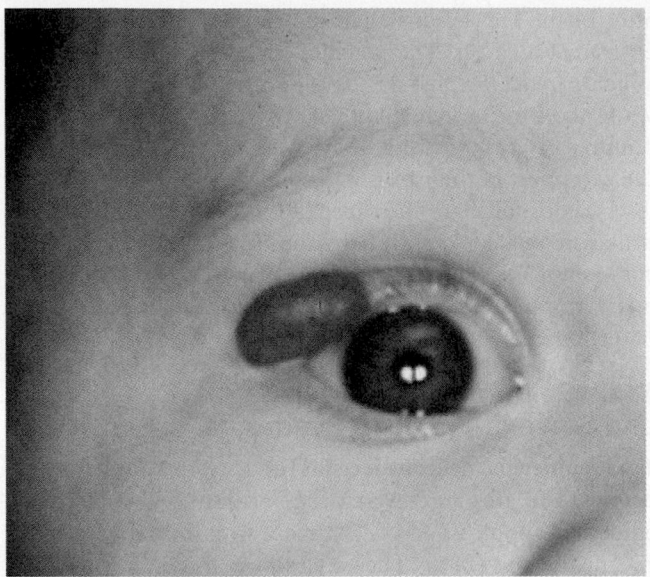

Figure 45-13 Strawberry hemangioma. (Courtesy Department of Dermatology, School of Medicine, University of Utah.)

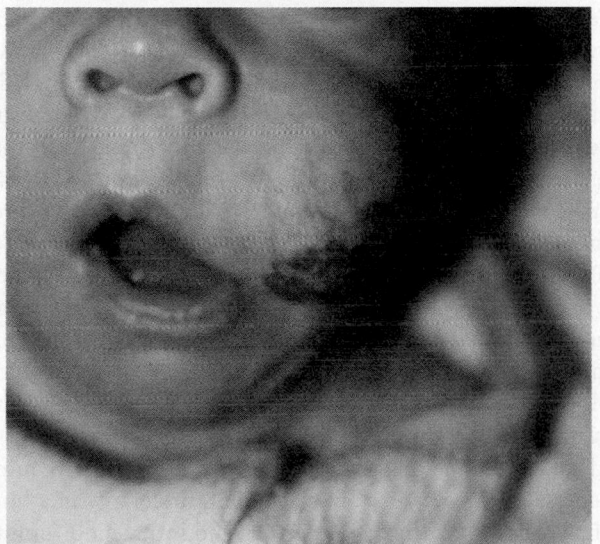

Figure 45-14 Cavernous hemangioma. (Courtesy Department of Dermatology, School of Medicine, University of Utah.)

proceeds for 6 to 12 months, with complete involution by 2 to 3 years in 30% of children and by 9 years of age in 90% of children.

Vascular Malformations

Vascular malformations are congenital anomalies of blood vessels present at birth but may not be apparent for several years. They grow proportionately with the child and never regress.[70] The malformations occur equally among males and females. Occasionally they expand rapidly, particularly during the hormonal changes of puberty or pregnancy and in association with trauma. Vascular malformations are classified as low flow or high flow. *Low-flow malformations* involve capillaries,

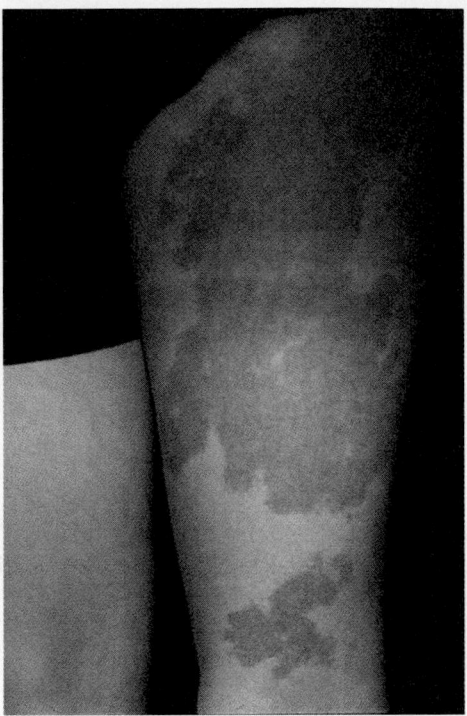

Figure 45-15 Capillary malformation in a child. (Courtesy Department of Dermatology, School of Medicine, University of Utah.)

veins, and lymphatics. *High-flow malformations* involve arteries. In addition to locations within the skin they may involve the gastrointestinal tract, bone (Maffucci syndrome or Sturge-Weber syndrome), facial capillary malformation, skin, vascular malformation of the eye, and vascular malformation of the brain (leptomeningeal hemangioma).[74] *Overgrowth syndromes* can occur with either high- or low-flow malformations, with overgrowth of the underlying structures (i.e., legs, arms, facial bones). The most common vascular malformation is nevus flammeus (port-wine stain) and salmon patches (stork bite, angel kiss).

Port-wine (nevus flammeus) stains are congenital malformations of the dermal capillaries. The lesions are flat, and their color ranges from pink to dark reddish purple. They are present at birth or within a few days after birth and do not fade with age. Involvement of the face and other body surfaces is common, and the lesions may be large (Figure 45-15). During adolescence and later adult years, the port-wine stain may become papular and cavernous. Treatments using cryosurgery or tattooing are not very satisfactory. The pulsed dye laser is the treatment of choice to successfully lighten the color and flatten the more nodular and cavernous lesions.[75] Waterproof cosmetics may be used to cover the lesions.

Salmon patches are macular pink lesions present at birth and located on the nape of the neck, forehead, upper eyelids, or nasolabial fold. They are a more superficial variant of nevus flammeus and one of the most common congenital malformations in the skin. The pink color results from distended

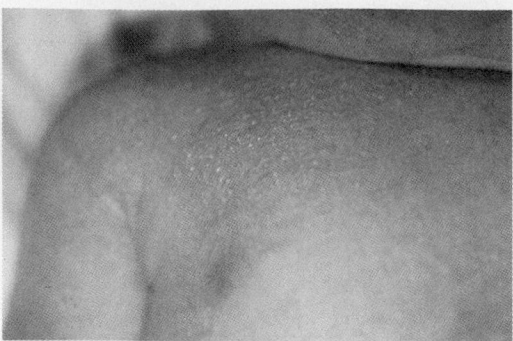

Figure 45-16 Miliaria rubra. Note discrete erythematous papules or papulovesicles. (Courtesy Department of Dermatology, School of Medicine, University of Utah.)

dermal capillaries, and 95% fade by 1 year of age. Those located at the nape of the neck may persist for a lifetime, but generally do not present a cosmetic problem.

OTHER SKIN DISORDERS

Miliaria

Miliaria is a dermatosis commonly seen in infants. It is characterized by a vesicular eruption after prolonged exposure to perspiration, with subsequent obstruction of the eccrine ducts. There are two forms of miliaria: miliaria crystallina and miliaria rubra. In **miliaria crystallina,** ductal rupture occurs within the stratum corneum and appears as 1- to 2-mm clear vesicles without erythema. They rupture within 24 to 48 hours and leave a white scale. In miliaria rubra the ductal rupture occurs in the lower epidermis, with inflammatory cells attracted to the site of the rupture. **Miliaria rubra** (prickly heat) is characterized by 2- to 4-mm discrete erythematous papules or papulovesicles (Figure 45-16). Both forms may become secondarily infected, requiring treatment with systemic antibiotics. The key to management is avoidance of excessive heat and humidity, which cause sweating. Light clothing, cool baths, and air conditioning assist in keeping the skin surface dry and cool.

Erythema Toxicum Neonatorum

Erythema toxicum neonatorum (toxic erythema of the newborn) is a benign, erythematous accumulation of macules, papules, or pustules that appear at birth or 3 to 4 days

after birth. The lesions first appear as a blotchy, macular erythematous rash. The macules vary from 1 mm to 1 cm. When papules or pustules develop, they are light yellow or white and 1 to 3 mm in diameter. There may be few or several hundred lesions, and any body surface can be affected, with the exception of the palms and soles, where there are no pilosebaceous follicles. The cause of the lesion is unknown but it may be related to an innate immune response to the first commensal microflora with release of mast cell mediators.[76] It is self-limiting and resolves spontaneously within a few weeks of birth. No treatment is required.

Toxic Epidermal Necrolysis and Stevens-Johnson Syndrome

Toxic epidermal necrolysis (TEN) and **Stevens-Johnson syndrome (SJS)** are rare, severe drug reactions with widespread epidermal apoptosis and detachment with mortality rates between 20% and 60%.[77] They are more common in adults but their incidence is increasing in children. The hypersensitivity to drugs includes sulfonamides, nonsteroidal anti-inflammatory agents, and anticonvulsants (i.e., phenytoin). Drug-specific cytotoxic T cells are involved in the immunopathology.[78] The onset of skin eruptions is preceded by malaise, anorexia, fever, and mild inflammation of the eyelids, conjunctiva, mouth, or genitalia. Erythema with tenderness is first described in the axillae and groin, extending over the body surface. Blisters and bullae form, and the entire epidermis may be shed, leaving open, weeping, painful areas of underlying skin. Complications include dehydration, protein loss, altered temperature regulation, and organ failure. About one third of children have pulmonary complications.[79] A severity of illness score for toxic epidermal necrolysis (SCORTEN) syndrome guides treatment and predicts mortality.[80] TEN must be confirmed by skin biopsy to differentiate from staphylococcal scalded skin syndrome (SSSS) and acute graft-versus-host disease. Skin biopsy shows full-thickness epidermal necrosis and subepidermal blister formation.[81] Treatment requires intensive burn equivalent management, preferably in a burn unit. Treatment with corticosteroids and intravenous immunoglobulin need further study, which is difficult because the disease is so rare.[82] Intravenous immunoglobulin may protect keratinocytes from apoptosis and oncosis from pathogenic autoantibodies.[83] The offending drug must be discontinued.

SUMMARY REVIEW

Acne Vulgaris

1. Acne vulgaris is the most common skin disease, affecting 85% of the population between the ages of 12 and 25 years.
2. Acne is characterized by noninflammatory and inflammatory lesions related to follicular hyperkeratinization, excessive sebum production, plugging of sebaceous glands, and *P. acnes* colonization. Acne conglobata is a severe form of acne with communicating cysts and abcesses.

Dermatitis

1. Atopic dermatitis is associated with elevated IgE levels, a family history of asthma and hay fever, and altered skin barrier function. Red, scaly lesions commonly occur on the face, cheeks, and flexor surfaces of the extremities in infants and young children.
2. Diaper dermatitis is a type of irritant contact dermatitis initiated by a combination of factors that include prolonged exposure to urine and feces; frequently the infant becomes infected secondarily with *C. albicans*.

Infections of the Skin

1. Impetigo is a contagious bacterial disease that occurs in two forms: bullous and vesicular (contagious). The toxins from the bacteria produce a weeping lesion with a honey-colored crust.
2. SSSS is a staphylococcal skin infection that occurs more commonly in young children with low titers of antistaphylococcal antibody. Painful blisters and bullae form over large areas of the skin, requiring systemic antibiotics for treatment.
3. Tinea capitis (infection of the scalp) and tinea corporis (infection of the body) are fungal infections caused by dermatophytes.
4. *C. albicans* infection is a superficial fungal infection of the mouth (thrush).
5. Molluscum contagiosum is a poxvirus of the skin that produces pale papular lesions filled with viral and cellular debris.
6. Rubella (also known as *German* or *3-day measles*) is a communicable disease characterized by fever, sore throat, enlarged cervical and postauricular nodes, and a generalized maculopapular rash that lasts 1 to 4 days.
7. Rubeola is a highly contagious disease of children. Symptoms include high fever, enlarged lymph nodes, conjunctivitis, and a red rash that begins on the head and spreads to the trunk and extremities and lasts 3 to 5 days. Bacterial and viral complications may accompany rubeola.
8. Roseola is a benign disease of infants with a sudden onset of fever that lasts 3 to 5 days, followed by a rash that lasts 24 hours.
9. Chickenpox (varicella) is a highly contagious disease caused by the VZV. Vesicular lesions occur on the skin and mucous membranes. Individuals are contagious from 1 day before the development of the rash until about 6 days after the rash develops.
10. Herpes zoster (shingles) is a viral eruption of vesicles on the skin along the distribution of a sensory nerve caused by latent activation of the VZV. Children with immune suppression develop more serious complications.
11. Smallpox (variola) is a highly contagious, deadly disease that has been eradicated worldwide by vaccination.

Insect Bites and Parasites

1. Scabies is an itching lesion caused by the itch mite that burrows into the skin, forming papules and vesicles. The mite is very contagious and is transmitted by direct contact.
2. Pediculosis (lice infestation) is caused by blood-sucking parasites that secrete a toxic saliva and damage the skin to produce a pruritic dermatitis. Lice are spread by direct contact and are recognized by the ova, or nits, that attach to the shaft of body hairs.
3. Flea bites produce a pruritic wheal with a central puncture site and occur as clusters in areas of tight-fitting clothing.
4. Bedbugs are blood-sucking parasites that live in cracks of floors, furniture, or bedding and feed at night. They produce pruritic wheals and nodules.

Hemangiomas and Vascular Malformations

1. Hemangiomas are benign vascular tumors that emerge at birth and resolve spontaneously through the childhood years. Strawberry hemangiomas (distinct, raised vascular lesions) are more superficial, and cavernous hemangiomas, with larger and more mature vessels, are deeper lesions.
2. Vascular malformations are congenital anomalies of blood vessels. Low-flow malformations involve capillaries, veins, and lymphatics; high-flow malformations involve arteries.
3. Nevus flammeus (port-wine stain) is a deeper congenital malformation of the dermal capillaries, and salmon patches are more superficial vascular malformations.

Other Skin Disorders

1. Miliaria is characterized by small pruritic papules or vesicles that result from prolonged exposure to perspiration and subsequent obstruction of the eccrine ducts in infants.
2. Erythema toxicum neonatorum is a benign, erythematous, accumulation of macules, papules, and pustules that appear at birth or 3 to 4 days after birth and then spontaneously resolve within a few weeks.
3. TEN and SJS are similar to SSSS with a blistering skin reaction; the causative agent is usually a drug.

KEY TERMS

Acne conglobata, 1681
Acne vulgaris, 1680
Atopic dermatitis (AD), 1681
Bedbugs, 1689
Bullous impetigo, 1683
Cavernous (congenital) hemangiomas, 1690
Chickenpox, 1687
Diaper dermatitis, 1682
Erythema toxicum neonatorum, 1692
Flea bites, 1689
Impetigo, 1683
Inflammatory acne, 1680

Miliaria, 1692
Miliaria crystallina, 1692
Miliaria rubra, 1692
Molluscum contagiosum, 1685
Noninflammatory acne, 1680
Norwegian scabies, 1689
Port-wine (nevus flammeus) stains, 1691
Roseola, 1687
Rubella, 1686
Rubeola, 1686
Salmon patches, 1691
Scabies, 1688

Smallpox (variola), 1688
Staphylococcal scalded-skin syndrome (SSSS), 1684
Stevens-Johnson syndrome (SJS), 1692
Strawberry hemangiomas, 1690
Thrush, 1685
Tinea capitis, 1684
Tinea corporis, 1685
Tinea pedis, 1684
Toxic epidermal necrolysis (TEN), 1692
Vesicular impetigo, 1683
Zoster, 1688

REFERENCES

1. Pochi PE et al: Report of the consensus conference on acne classification, *J Am Acad Dermatol* 24(3):495, 1991.
2. Zouboulis CC et al: Sexual hormones in human skin, *Horm Metab Res* 39(2):85-95, 2007.
3. Melnik B, Jansen T, Grabbe S: Abuse of anabolic-androgenic steroids and bodybuilding acne: an underestimated health problem, *J Dtsch Dermatol Ges* 5(2):110-117, 2007.
4. Strauss JS et al: Guidelines for acne vulgaris management, *J Am Acad Dermatol* 56(4):651-663, 2007.
5. Krakowski AC, Stendardo S, Eichenfield LF: Practical considerations in acne treatment and the clinical impact of topical combination therapy, *Pediatr Dermatol* 25 (Suppl 1):1-14, 2008.
6. Callender VD: Acne in ethnic skin: special considerations for therapy, *Dermatol Ther* 17(2):184-195, 2004.
7. Horii KA et al: Atopic dermatitis in children in the United States, 1997-2004: visit trends, patient and provider characteristics, and prescribing patterns, *Pediatrics* 120(3):e527-e534, 2007.
8. Bonness S, Bieber T: Molecular basis of atopic dermatitis, *Curr Opin Allergy Clin Immunol* 7(5):382-386, 2007.
9. Nicol NH, Boguniewicz M: Successful strategies in atopic dermatitis management, *Dermatol Nurs* :3-18, 2008.
10. Elias PM: Skin barrier function, *Curr Allergy Asthma Rep* 8(4):299-305, 2008.
11. Boguniewicz M, Leung DY: Atopic Dermatitis, *J Allergy Clin Immunol* 117(Suppl 2 Mini-Primer):S475-S480, 2006.
12. Howell MD et al: Th2 cytokines act on S11/A11 to downregulate keratinocyte differentiation, *J Invest Dermatol* 128(9):2248-2258, 2008.
13. Chan LS: Atopic dermatitis in 2008, *Curr Dir Autoimmun* 10:76-118, 2008.
14. Lipozenci J, Wolf R: Atopic dermatitis: an update and review of the literature, *Dermatol Clin* 25(4):605-12, x, 2007.
15. McGrath JA: Filaggrin and the great epidermal barrier grief, *Australas J Dermatol* 49(2):67-73, 2008.
16. Tominaga M, Ogawa H, Takamori K: Possible roles of epidermal opioid systems in pruritus of atopic dermatitis, *J Invest Dermatol* 127(9):2228-2235, 2007.
17. Yosipovitch G, Papolu AD: What causes itch in atopic dermatitis? *Curr Allergy Asthma Rep* 8(4):306-311, 2008.
18. Brenninkmeijer EE et al: Diagnostic criteria for atopic dermatitis: a systematic review, *Br J Dermatol* 158(4):754-765, 2008.
19. Boguniewicz M et al: A multidisciplinary approach to evaluation and treatment of atopic dermatitis, *Semin Cutan Med Surg* 27:115-127, 2008.
20. Ong PY, Boguniewicz M: Atopic dermatitis, *Prim Care* 35(1):105-117, vii, 2008.
21. Runeman B: Skin interaction with absorbent hygiene products, *Clin Dermatol* 26(1):45-51, 2008.
22. Cole C, Gazewood J: Diagnosis and treatment of impetigo, *Am Fam Physician* 75(6):859-864, 2007.
23. Nishifuji K, Sugai M, Amagai M: Staphylococcal exfoliative toxins: "molecular scissors" of bacteria that attack the cutaneous defense barrier in mammals, *J Dermatol Sci* 49(1):21-31, 2008.
24. Rudy SJ: Superficial fungal infections in children and adolescents, *Nurse Prac Forum* 19(2):56, 1999.
25. Ilyas M, Tolaymat A: Changing epidemiology of acute post-streptococcal glomerulonephritis in Northeast Florida: a comparative study, *Pediatr Nephrol* 23(7):1101-1106, 2008.
26. Bernard P: Management of common bacterial infections of the skin, *Curr Opin Infect Dis* 21(2):122-128, 2008.
27. Hacker SM: Common infections of the skin: characteristics, causes, and cures, *Postgrad Med* 96(2):43, 1994.
28. Blyth M, Estela C, Young AE: Severe staphylococcal scalded skin syndrome in children, *Burns* 34(1):98-103, 2008.
29. Nishifuji K, Sugai M, Amagai M: Staphylococcal exfoliative toxins: "molecular scissors" of bacteria that attack the cutaneous defense barrier in mammals, *J Dermatol Sci* 49(1):21-31, 2008.
30. Patel GK: Treatment of staphylococcal scalded skin syndrome, *Expert Rev Anti Infect Ther* 2(4):575-587, 2004.
31. Elewski BE: Cutaneous mycoses in children, *Br J Dermatol* 134(Suppl 46):7, 1996.
32. Andrews MD, Burns M: Common tinea infections in children: *Am Fam Physician* 77(1):1415-1420, 2008.
33. White JM, Higgins EM, Fuller LC: Screening for asymptomatic carriage of *Trichophyton tonsurans* in household contacts of patients with tinea capitis: results of 209 patients from South London, *J Eur Acad Dermatol Venereol* 21(8):1061-1064, 2007.
34. Williams JV et al: Semiquantitative study of tinea capitis and the asymptomatic carrier state in inner-city school children, *Pediatrics* 96(2 Pt 1):265, 1995.
35. Gonzalez U et al: Systemic antifungal therapy for tinea capitis in children, *Cochrane Database Syst Rev* (4):CD004685, 2007.
36. Chan YC, Friedlander SF: New treatments for tinea capitis, *Curr Opin Infect Dis* 17(2):97-103, 2004.
37. Pereira B et al: Exuberant molluscum contagiosum as a manifestation of the immune reconstitution inflammatory syndrome, *Dermatol Online J* 13(2):6, 2007.
38. Prasad SM: Molluscum contagiosum, *Pediatr Rev* 17(4):118, 1996.
39. Scheinfeld N: Treatment of molluscum contagiosum: a brief review and discussion of a case successfully treated with adapelene, *Dermatol Online* 13(3):15, 2007.
40. Davidkin I et al: Etiology of measles- and rubella-like illnesses in measles, mumps, and rubella-vaccinated children, *J Infect Dis* 178(6):1567, 1998.
41. Egami T, Egami K, Tanoue A: Study of antibody titres after measles vaccination: fever within 7 days of vaccination and efficacy of booster doses, *Arch Dis Child* 93(4):319-320, 2008.
42. DeStefano F: Vaccines and autism: evidence does not support a causal association, *Clin Pharmacol Ther* 82(6):756-759, 2007.
43. DeStefano F, Thompson WW: MMR vaccine and autism: an update of the scientific evidence, *Expert Rev Vaccines* 3(1):19-22, 2004.
44. Kennedy RC, Byers VS, Marchalonis JJ: Measles virus infection and vaccination: potential role in chronic illness and associated adverse events, *Crit Rev Immunol* 24(2):129-156, 2004.
45. Centers for Disease Control and Prevention (CDC): Progress in global measles control and mortality reduction, *MMWR Morb Mortal Wkly Rep* 56(47):1237-1241, 2007.
46. Update: global measles control and mortality reduction—worldwide, 1991-2001, *MMWR* 52(20):471-475, 2003.
47. Best JM: Rubella, *Semin Fetal Neonatal Med* 12(3):182-192, 2007.
48. Johnson R et al: Prevention of herpes zoster and its painful and debilitating complications, *Int J Infect Dis* 11(Suppl 2):S43-S48, 2007.
49. Daley AJ, Thrope S, Garland SM: Varicella and the pregnant woman: prevention and management, *Aust N Z J Obstet Gynaecol* 48(1):26-33, 2008.
50. Pastuszak AL et al: Outcome after maternal varicella infection in the first 20 weeks of pregnancy, *N Engl J Med* 330(13):901, 1994.
51. Breuer J, Whitley R: Varicella zoster virus: natural history and current therapies of varicella and herpes zoster, *Herpes* 14(Suppl 2):25-29, 2007.
52. Feder HM Jr, Hoss DM: Herpes zoster in otherwise healthy children, *Pediatr Infect Dis J* 23(5):451-457, 2004.
53. Ahmed AM et al: Managing herpes zoster in immunocompromised patients, *Herpes* 14(2):32-36, 2007.
54. Leung AK, Robson WL, Leong AG: Herpes zoster in childhood, *J Pediatr Health Care* 20(5):300-303, 2006.
55. Woolery WA: Herpes zoster vaccine, *Geriatrics* 63(10):6-9, 2008.
56. Dhillon S, Curran MP: Live attenuated measles, mumps, rubella, and varicella zoster virus vaccine, *Paediatr Drugs* 10(5):337-347, 2008.
57. Kman NE, Nelson RN: Infectious agents of bioterrorism: a review for emergency physicians, *Emerg Med Clin North Am* 26(2):517-547, 2008.
58. Metzger W, Mordmueller BG: Vaccines for preventing smallpox, *Cochrane Database Syst Rev* (3):CD004913, 2007.
59. Chosidow O: Scabies and pediculosis, *Lancet* 355(9206):819, 2000.
60. Walton SF et al: New insights into disease pathogenesis in crusted (Norwegian) scabies: the skin immune resonse in crusted scabies, *Br J Dermatol* 158(6):1247-1255, 2008.
61. Mounsey KE et al: Scabies: molecular perspectives and therapeutic implications in the face of emerging drug resistance, *Future Microbiol* 3(1):57-66, 2008.
62. Burkhart CN, Burkhart CG: Fomite transmission in head lice, *J Am Acad Dermatol* 56(6):144-147, 2007.
63. Strong M, Johnstone PW: Interventions for treating scabies, *Cochrane Database Syst Rev* (3):CD000320, 2007.
64. Howard R, Frieden IJ: Papular urticaria in children, *Pediatr Dermatol* 13(3):246, 1996.
65. Cuéllar A et al: Functional dysregulation of dendritic cells in patients with popular urticaria caused by fleabite, *Arch Dermatol* 143(11):1415-1419, 2007.

66. Kehr JD et al: Morbidity assessment in sand fleas disease (tungiasis), *Parasitol Res* 100(2):413-421, 2007.

67. Cestari TF, Martignago BF: Scabies, pediculosis, bedbugs, and stinkbugs: uncommon presentations, *Clin Dermatol* 23(6):545-554, 2005.

68. Ter Poorten MC: Prose NS The return of the common bedbug, *Pediatr Dermatol* 22(3):183-187, 2005.

69. Buckmiller LM: Update on hemangiomas and vascular malformations, *Curr Opin Otolaryngol Head Neck Surg* 12(6):476-487, 2004.

70. Willenberg T, Baumgartener T: Vascular birthmarks, *Vasa* 37(1):5-17, 2008.

71. Atherton DJ: Infantile haemangiomas, *Early Hum Dev* 82(12):789-795, 2006.

72. Musumeci ML et al: Management of cutaneous hemangiomas in pediatric patients, *Cutix* 81(4):315-322, 2008.

73. Song JK, Niimi Y, Berenstein A: Endovascular treatment of hemangioma, *Neuroimaging Clin N Am* 17(2):165-173, 2007.

74. Comi AM: Update on Sturge-Weber syndrome: diagnosis, treatment, quantitative measures, and controversies, *Lymphat Res Biol* 5(4): 257-264, 2007.

75. Bernstein EF: Treatment of a resistant port-wine stain with a new variable pulse-duration pulsed-dye laser, *J Cosmet Dermatol* 7(2):139-142, 2008.

76. Nelson A et al: Urticaria neonatorum: accumulation of tryptase-expressing mast cells in the skin lesions of newborns with erythema toxicum, *Pediatr Allergy Immunol* 18(8):652-658, 2007.

77. Dorafshar AH et al: Antishear therapy for toxic epidermal necrolysis: an alternative treatment approach, *Plast Reconstr Surg* 122(1):154-160, 2008.

78. Borchers AT et al: Stevens-Johnson syndrome and toxic epidermal necrolysis, *Autoimmun Rev* 7(8):598-605, 2008.

79. Kim MJ, Lee KY: Bronchiolitis obliterans in children with Stevens-Johnson syndrome: follow-up with high resolution CT, *Pediatr Radiol* 26(1):22, 1996.

80. Basuji-Garin S et al: SCORTEN: a Severity-of-Illness Score for Toxic Epidermal Necrolysis, *Inves Dermatol* 115(5):149-153, 2000.

81. Rzany B et al: Histopathological and epidemiological characteristics of patients with erythema exudativum multiforme major, Stevens-Johnson syndrome and toxic epidermal necrolysis, *Br J Dermatol* 135(1):6, 1996.

82. Abood GJ, Nickoloff BJ, Gamelli RL: Treatment strategies in toxic epidermal necrolysis syndrome: where are we at? *J Burn Care Res* 29(1):269-276, 2008.

83. Michael D, Grando SA: Novel mechanism for therapeutic action of IVIg in autoimmune blistering dermatoses, *Curr Dir Autoimmun* 10:333-343, 2008.

SHOCK, MULTIPLE ORGAN DYSFUNCTION SYNDROME, AND BURNS IN ADULTS

DENNIS J. CHEEK • LINDA L. MARTIN • STEPHEN E. MORRIS

MEDIA RESOURCES

 Evolve Website (http://evolve.elsevier.com/McCance/)
- Review Questions and Answers
- Animations
- Glossary (with audio pronunciation for selected terms)
- WebLinks

Online Course
- Module 20

CHAPTER OUTLINE

SHOCK
  Cellular Alterations
  Impairment of Cellular Metabolism
  Types of Shock
  Treatment for Shock

MULTIPLE ORGAN DYSFUNCTION SYNDROME
BURNS
  Epidemiology and Etiology
  Burn Wound Depth

Shock occurs when the cardiovascular system fails to perfuse tissues adequately, resulting in widespread impairment of cellular metabolism. Because tissue perfusion can be disrupted by any factor that alters heart function, blood volume, or blood pressure, shock has many causes and various clinical manifestations. Ultimately, however, shock from any cause progresses to organ failure and death, unless compensatory mechanisms reverse the process or clinical intervention succeeds. Untreated severe shock overwhelms the body's compensatory mechanisms through positive-feedback loops that initiate and maintain a downward physiologic spiral.

Multiple organ dysfunction syndrome (MODS) is progressive and often involves the ultimate failure of two or more organ systems after a severe illness or injury. The disease process is initiated and perpetuated by uncontrolled systemic inflammatory and stress responses and is characterized by a hypermetabolic and hyperdynamic state that persists as organ dysfunction develops. For many years the syndrome was referred to as *multiple organ failure* or *multiple systems organ failure*. Gradually it was recognized that the term *organ dysfunction* more accurately describes the syndrome as a process of physiologic deterioration.

Major burns result in extensive immediate tissue injury and thus are a form of trauma with wide-reaching effects on all organ systems. The cause of injury may be thermal contact, flame, chemical agents, or electrical agents; each cause requires a different approach in diagnosis and treatment. Closely associated with thermal burns is smoke inhalation injury, which accounts for about 25% of all burn unit admissions. As a multiorgan problem, thermal injuries can have an overwhelming effect on survival of the burned individual. Regardless of the cause of burns, the result is a final common pathway of physiologic response dependent on the extent of burn surface involvement and depth of tissue destruction.

SHOCK

Shock can be classified by type, principal pathophysiologic process, or clinical manifestations. Classification by type is perhaps the most useful because it suggests the cause and pathophysiologic process of the underlying disorder, which must be treated to prevent the irreversible impairment of cellular metabolism. **Shock** is classified as cardiogenic (caused by heart failure); neurogenic or vasogenic (caused by alterations in vascular smooth muscle tone); anaphylactic (caused by hypersensitivity); septic (caused by infection); or hypovolemic (caused by insufficient intravascular fluid volume). An additional type, traumatic shock, has components of hypovolemic and septic shock.[1]

Cellular Alterations

Because the body is made up of many cells that may function or malfunction at different stages of metabolic impairment, shock causes many signs and symptoms. Subjective complaints are usually nonspecific and may not be particularly helpful to the clinician attempting diagnosis and treatment. The individual may report feeling sick, weak, cold, hot, nauseated, dizzy, confused, afraid, thirsty, and short of breath.

Impairment of Cellular Metabolism

The common pathway in all types of shock is impairment of cellular metabolism, which is a complex concept. Figure 46-1 illustrates the pathophysiology of shock at the cellular level.

Impairment of Oxygen Use

In all types of shock the cell either is not receiving an adequate amount of oxygen or is unable to use oxygen (see Figure 46-1). In cardiogenic shock, cardiac output is too low to deliver adequate oxygen to the cell. In hypovolemic shock, oxygen delivery is impaired by inadequate numbers of red cells or inadequate volume of intravascular fluid. In neurogenic, anaphylactic, and septic shock, systemic vascular resistance (SVR) is too low and perfusion pressure in the capillaries is inadequate to drive oxygen across cell membranes. In septic shock, hypoxia is made worse by fever, which increases the cell's oxygen consumption rate, and by endotoxic and inflammatory chemical disruption of cell metabolism, which impairs the cells' ability to use oxygen.

Without oxygen the cell shifts from aerobic to anaerobic metabolism. Anaerobic metabolism is a less efficient method of extracting energy from carbon bonds, and the cell begins to use adenosine triphosphate (ATP) faster than it can be replaced. Without ATP the cell loses its ability to maintain an electrochemical gradient across its selectively permeable membrane. Specifically, the cell cannot operate the sodium-potassium pump. Sodium and chloride accumulate inside the cell, and potassium exits. Cells of the nervous system and myocardium are profoundly and immediately affected. The resting potentials of these cells are reduced, and action potentials decrease in amplitude (see Chapter 1). Myocardial depressant factor also decreases the contractility of the heart. A variety of clinical manifestations of impaired central nervous system and myocardial function result.

As sodium moves into the cell, water follows. Throughout the body, the water drawn from the interstitium into the cells is "replaced" by water that is in turn drawn out of the vascular space, often called "third spacing" of fluid. This decreases circulatory volume. Within the cells, water causes cellular edema that disrupts cellular membranes, releasing lysosomal enzymes that injure the cells internally and leak into the interstitium.

Three positive-feedback loops then begin that further impair oxygen use: (1) activation of the clotting cascade, (2) decreased circulatory volume, and (3) lysosomal enzyme release. First, enzymatic processes are disrupted by the change in the normal ionic and osmotic levels in the cell, as are those processes governed by the physical laws of diffusion. Diffusion of nutrients and wastes into and out of the cell takes longer, and cellular metabolism is further altered. At the same time, diffusion across capillary membranes occurs more slowly as blood flow in the capillary beds becomes sluggish. Sluggish capillary flow decreases tissue perfusion further and activates the clotting cascade (see Chapter 25). The clotting cascade accounts for common complications of shock, such as acute tubular necrosis, acute respiratory distress syndrome (ARDS), and disseminated intravascular coagulation (DIC). It also may activate or be activated by the inflammatory response.[2]

Intravascular fluid loss into the intracellular and interstitial spaces, described as "third spacing" earlier, is amplified when serum albumin and other plasma proteins are consumed for fuel, which results in decreased intravascular osmotic pressure, shift of fluid to the interstitial or extracellular spaces, and decreased circulation volume. Decreased circulatory volume magnifies decreased tissue perfusion in all types of shock. Decreased intravascular volume causes decreased cardiac output in septic shock and further decreases cardiac output in cardiogenic shock. In individuals with anaphylactic, neurogenic, or septic shock and an already dilated vasculature, hypotension worsens as a result of decreased circulatory volume. New data on additional mechanisms for hypotension (vasodilation) are illustrated in Figure 46-7 (p. 1706).

Lysosomal enzymes released during shock injure the cell that released them and injure adjacent cells. By damaging the mechanisms of surrounding cells, lysosomal enzymes extend areas of impaired metabolism and cellular injury.

In addition to decreasing ATP stores, anaerobic metabolism affects the pH of the cell, and metabolic acidosis develops. A compensatory mechanism is initiated that enables cardiac and skeletal muscles to use lactic acid as a fuel source, but only for a limited time. The decreasing pH of the cell that is functioning anaerobically has serious consequences. Enzymes necessary for cellular function dissociate under acid conditions. Enzyme dissociation stops cell function, repair, and division. As lactic acid is released systemically, blood pH drops, reducing the oxygen-carrying capacity of the blood (see Chapter 2). Therefore, less oxygen is delivered to the cells. Further acidosis triggers the release of more lysosomal enzymes because the low pH disrupts lysosomal membrane integrity.

Impairment of Glucose Use

Impaired glucose use can be caused by either impaired glucose delivery or impaired glucose uptake by the cells (see Figure 46-1). The reasons for inadequate glucose delivery are the same as those enumerated for inadequate oxygen delivery. In addition, in septic and anaphylactic shock, glucose

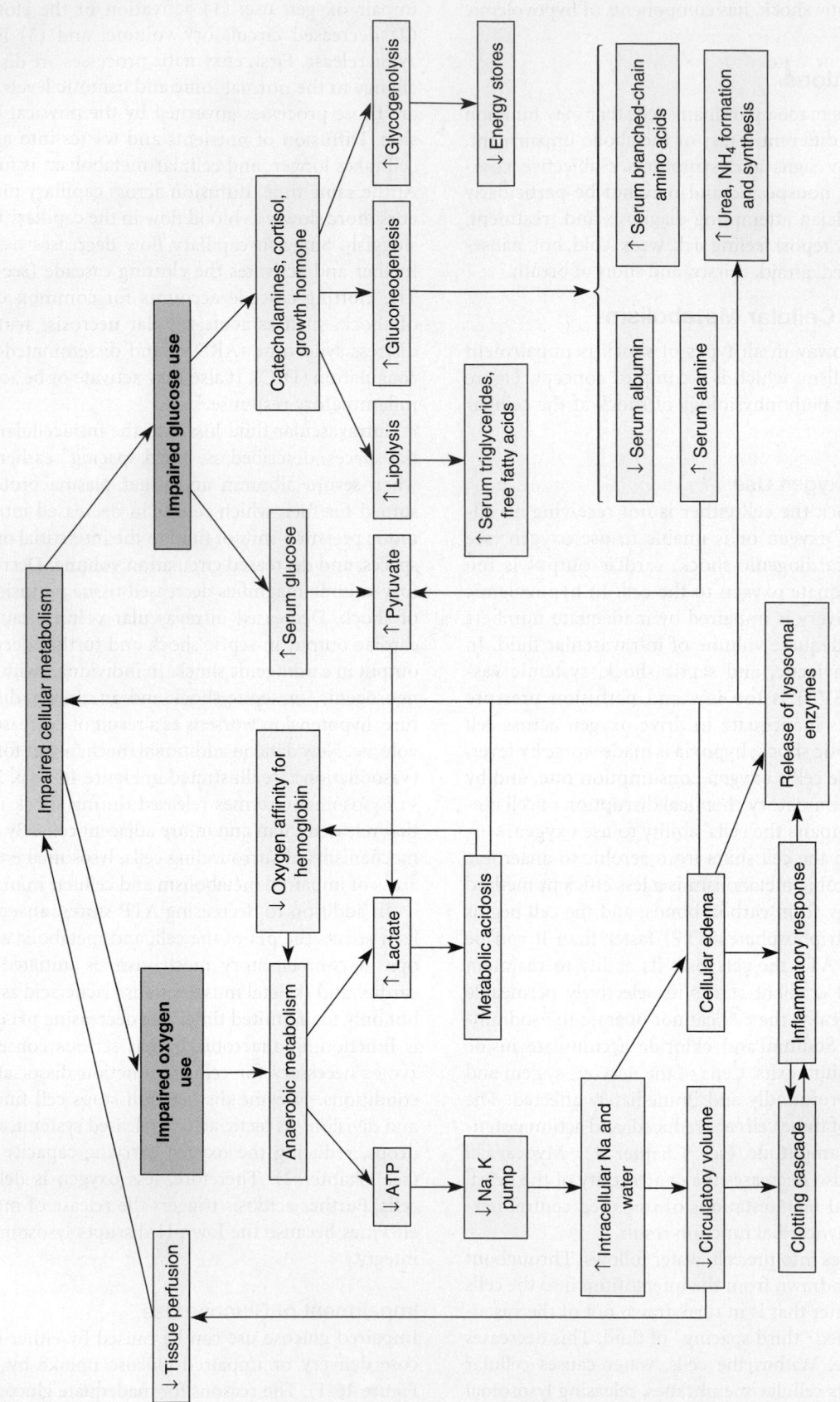

Figure 46-1 Impairment of cellular metabolism by shock. ATP, Adenosine triphosphate.

metabolism may be increased or disrupted because of fever or bacteria, and glucose uptake can be prevented by the presence of vasoactive toxins, endotoxins, histamine, and kinins.

Some of the compensatory mechanisms activated by shock contribute to decreased glucose uptake by the cells. High serum levels of cortisol, growth hormone, and catecholamines account for hyperglycemia and insulin resistance, tachycardia, increased SVR, and increased cardiac contractility. Cells shift to glycogenolysis, gluconeogenesis, and lipolysis to generate fuel for survival (see Chapter 1). Except in the liver, kidneys, and muscles, the body's cells have extremely limited stores of glycogen. In fact, total body stores can fuel the metabolism for only about 10 hours. The depletion of fat and glycogen stores is not itself a cause of organ failure, but the energy costs of glycogenolysis and lipolysis are considerable and contribute to the cells' failure.

The depletion of protein is, however, a cause of organ failure. When gluconeogenesis causes proteins to be used for fuel, these proteins are no longer available to maintain cellular structure, function, repair, and replication. The breakdown of protein occurs in starvation states, hyperdynamic metabolic states, and septic shock. Under anaerobic metabolism, protein breakdown liberates alanine, which is converted to pyruvate. In sepsis, pyruvic acid is changed into lactic acid and a positive-feedback loop is formed.

As proteins are broken down anaerobically, ammonia and urea are produced. Ammonia is toxic to living cells. Uremia develops, and uric acid further disrupts cellular metabolism. Proteins are broken down preferentially. Serum albumin and other plasma proteins are consumed for fuel first. Serum protein consumption decreases capillary osmotic pressure and contributes to the development of interstitial edema, creating another positive-feedback loop that decreases circulatory volume. In septic shock, plasma protein breakdown includes breakdown of immunoglobulins, thereby impairing immune system function when it is most needed.

Muscle wasting caused by protein breakdown weakens skeletal and cardiac muscle. Skeletal muscle wasting impairs the muscles that facilitate breathing. Muscle wasting therefore alters the actions of both heart and lungs. The delivery of oxygen and glucose to the cells is directly reduced, as is the removal of waste products, forming another positive-feedback loop.

A final outcome of impaired cellular metabolism is the buildup of metabolic end products in the cell and interstitial spaces. Waste products are toxic to the cells and further disrupt cellular function and membrane integrity. In septic shock, for example, a deficiency in cellular metabolism and the buildup of toxins may precede and cause decreased tissue perfusion.

Types of Shock

Each type of shock (cardiogenic, hypovolemic, neurogenic, anaphylactic, septic) involves numerous clinical manifestations that also characterize many other conditions, making diagnosis difficult. In addition, the body's many compensatory mechanisms can mask, for a time, many definitive signs of shock.

Cardiogenic Shock

Cardiogenic shock results from the inability of the heart to pump adequate blood to tissues and end organs from any cause, the most common being within hours of an acute myocardial infarction or severe episode of myocardial ischemia. **Cardiogenic shock** is defined as persistent hypotension and tissue hypoperfusion caused by cardiac dysfunction in the presence of adequate intravascular volume and left ventricular filling pressure.[3] Pathologic conditions that reduce contractility, impair diastolic filling, or cause obstruction can lead to cardiogenic shock. The decreased contractility can result from (1) acute myocardial infarction (AMI), cardiomyopathy, sepsis, myocarditis, dysrhythmias, metabolic abnormalities, papillary muscle rupture; (2) impaired diastolic filling related to arrhythmias; and (3) obstruction due to pulmonary embolism, cardiac tamponade, valvular disorders, and wall rupture or defects.[4] Although mortality rates have been estimated between 50% and 80%, there is some indication that overall hospital mortality is decreasing because of early recognition and interventional treatment advancements.[5] Mortality improves with early revascularization, cardio-supportive drug regimens, and mechanical assistive devices.

Reperfusion and revascularization can be achieved with treatment of fibrinolytic therapies (medications that disintegrate the coronary thrombus), percutaneous interventions (balloon angioplasty, stent placement, and thrombectomies), or surgery (coronary artery bypass, ventriculoplasty or heart transplant) to open the coronary vessels during an acute myocardial infarction (AMI) or replace irreparable heart muscle. Cardio-supportive drug and fluid regimens are initiated to maintain adequate blood pressure, and essential fluid and electrolyte balance, and optimize coronary perfusion to the myocardium. Mechanical assist devices, specifically intra-aortic balloon pumps and percutaneous or ventricular assist devices (VADS), are used to support cardiac output temporarily until the individual improves or transplantation is possible. Implantable VADS, pacemakers, or internal defibrillator devices are sometimes used as permanent treatment for those who survive cardiogenic shock. Continuous hemodynamic monitoring should be used to evaluate vascular volume and pressures, optimize fluid, and monitor drug administration with the goal of improving cardiac output and tissue perfusion.[6]

As cardiac output decreases, compensatory adaptive responses are activated, such as the renin-angiotensin, neurohormonal, and sympathetic nervous systems, that lead to fluid retention, systemic vasoconstriction, and tachycardia.[7] Blood pressure is maintained through vasoconstriction in response to catecholamine release from the adrenals. Catecholamines also increase contractility and heart rate. Increases in blood volume and vascular resistance succeed in normalizing blood pressure and increasing cardiac performance but at the cost of increasing myocardial demands for oxygen and nutrients. Increasing myocardial requirements further strain the already failing heart, which can no longer pump an adequate volume of blood with sufficient force to perfuse the tissues. Thus increased coronary, tissue, and cellular ischemia progressively deteriorate myocardial dysfunction and the shock state (see What's New? Cardiogenic Shock).

The clinical manifestations of cardiogenic shock are caused by inadequate perfusion to the heart and end organs (Figure 46-2). Subjective complaints of chest pain, dyspnea, and faintness, along with feelings of impending doom, are often revealed. Classic observable signs and symptoms of tachycardia, tachypnea, hypotension, jugular venous distention, and low measured cardiac output are hallmarks. Cyanosis; skin mottling; rapid, faint, or irregular pulses; low urine output; and occasional peripheral edema are additional signs and symptoms of end-organ hypoperfusion. Myocardial dysfunction from fluid overload may result in extra heart sounds and elevated laboratory values. Pulmonary edema is evidenced by audible crackles, wheezes, and abnormal vascular congestion on chest radiography. Metabolic abnormalities involving electrolyte imbalances and elevated inflammatory markers may result from or concur with the cardiac cascade of shock (see What's New? Interleukin-6 [IL-6]).

WHAT'S NEW?
Cardiogenic Shock

The "Should We Emergently Revascularize Occluded Coronaries for Cardiogenic Shock" (SHOCK) trial demonstrated that strategies of early revascularization versus initial medical stabilization showed greater reduction in mortality with the latter. However, a relative overall 67% improvement in survival at 6 years was found in the cohort of survivors sustaining acute myocardial infarction with complication of cardiogenic shock who had received early revascularization.

Data from Hochman J et al: *JAMA* 295(21):2511-2515, 2006.

WHAT'S NEW?
Interleukin-6 (IL-6)

Inflammation plays an important role in the pathogenesis and prognosis of cardiogenic shock. IL-6 concentrations are an independent predictor of 30-day mortality in individuals with acute myocardial infarction complicated by cardiogenic shock.

Data from Geppert A et al: *Crit Care Med* 34(8):2035-2042, 2006.

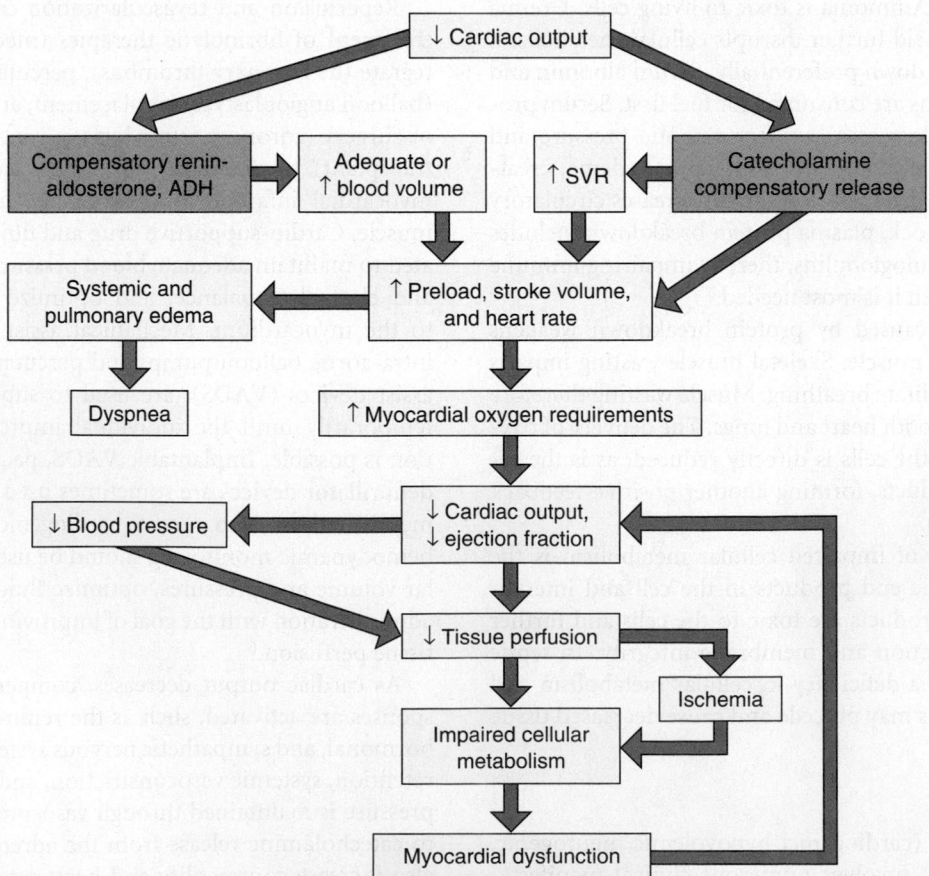

Figure 46-2 **Cardiogenic shock.** Shock becomes life threatening when compensatory mechanisms *(orange boxes)* cause increased myocardial oxygen requirements. *ADH,* Antidiuretic hormone; *SVR,* systemic vascular resistance.

Hypovolemic Shock

Hypovolemic shock is caused by loss of whole blood (hemorrhage), plasma (burns), or interstitial fluid (diaphoresis, diabetes mellitus, diabetes insipidus, emesis, or diuresis) in large amounts. Loss of whole blood or plasma causes hypovolemia directly. Loss of interstitial fluid causes an indirect "relative" hypovolemia by promoting diffusion of plasma from the intravascular to the extravascular space. Hypovolemic shock begins to develop when intravascular volume has decreased by about 15%.

Hypovolemia is offset initially by compensatory mechanisms (Figure 46-3). Heart rate and SVR increase as a result of catecholamine release by the adrenals. This boosts cardiac output and tissue perfusion pressures. Compelled by a decrease in capillary hydrostatic pressures, interstitial fluid moves into the vascular compartment. The liver and spleen add to blood volume by disgorging stored red blood cells and plasma. In the kidneys, renin (through several intermediaries) stimulates aldosterone release and the retention of sodium (and hence water), whereas antidiuretic hormone (ADH, or vasopressin) from the posterior pituitary gland increases water retention. Data on the compensation of ADH, however, show that as

shock worsens, ADH in plasma decreases. Hypovolemic shock results in compensatory vasoconstriction, increased SVR, and afterload in order to improve blood pressure and perfusion to core organs of the body.

These compensatory mechanisms are, however, finite. If the initial fluid or blood loss is great or if loss continues, compensation fails, resulting in decreased tissue perfusion. Nutrient delivery to the cells is impaired, and cellular metabolism

WHAT'S NEW?   Hypovolemic Shock

Research of fluid resuscitation is more focused on reducing the immune response that is part of the pathology of organ failure versus the frequent debate of ideal fluid for replacement. Timing and treatment with hypertonic saline in individuals with massive traumatic injury, especially blunt trauma, have shown benefit in those with severe injury requiring massive transfusions. This is speculated to be related to altering and reducing the early inflammatory response that often leads to organ injury.

Data from Bulger EM et al: *Arch Surg* 43(2):139-149, 2008.

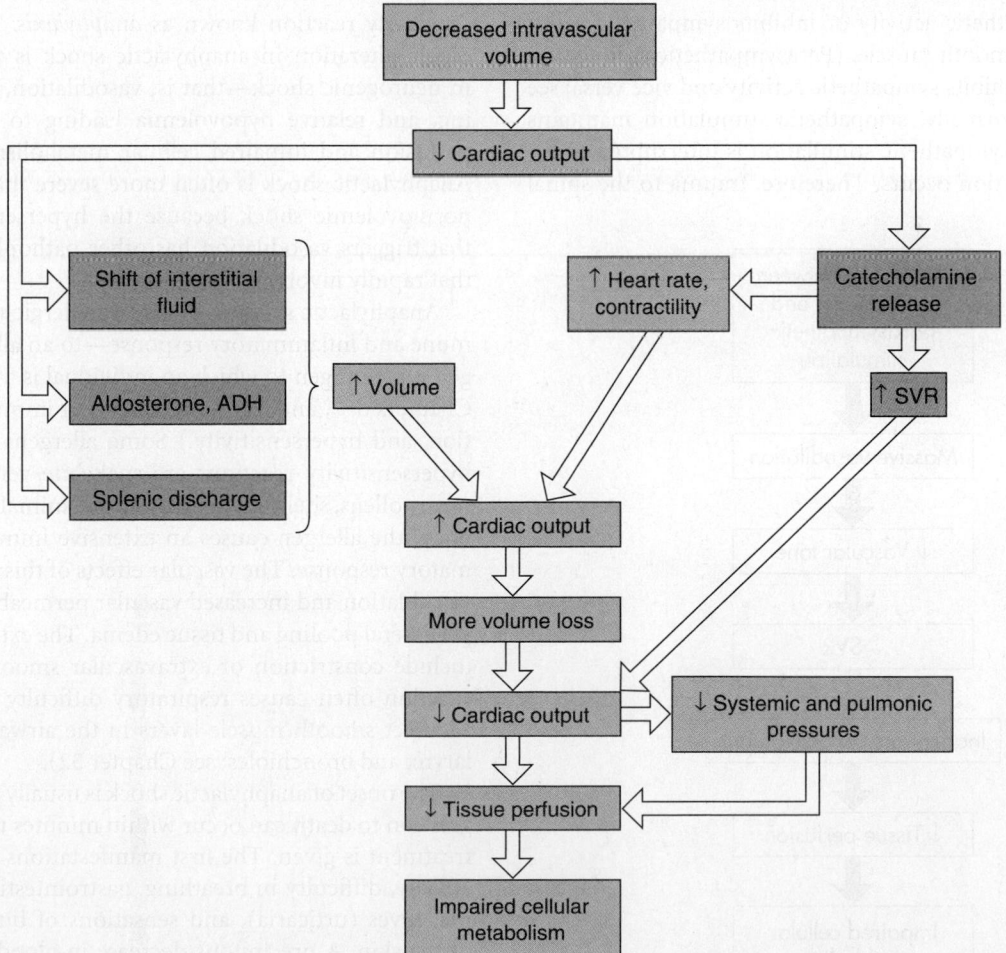

Figure 46-3 Hypovolemic shock. This type of shock becomes life threatening when compensatory mechanisms (*orange boxes*) are overwhelmed by continued loss of intravascular volume. *ADH,* Antidiuretic hormone; *SVR,* systemic vascular resistance.

fails. Mortality from traumatic hemorrhagic shock ranges from 10% to 31%. Prompt control of hemorrhage is the treatment of choice. Fluid replacement is also important, but the type of fluid to be used and the rate of replacement are controversial.[8,9] The clinical manifestations of hypovolemic shock include high SVR, poor skin turgor, thirst, oliguria, low systemic and pulmonary preloads, and rapid heart rates.

Neurogenic Shock

Neurogenic shock is sometimes called **vasogenic shock.** Both terms refer to a widespread and massive vasodilation that results from an imbalance between parasympathetic and sympathetic stimulation of vascular smooth muscle (see Chapter 29). Occasionally, parasympathetic overstimulation or sympathetic understimulation persists, causing vasodilation for an extended period. Extreme, persistent vasodilation leads to neurogenic shock (Figure 46-4). Neurogenic shock creates "relative hypovolemia." Blood volume has not changed, but the amount of space containing the blood has increased, so that SVR decreases drastically; thus pressure in the vessels is inadequate to drive nutrients across capillary membranes, and nutrient delivery to the cells is impaired. As with other types of shock, this leads to impaired cellular metabolism.

Neurogenic shock can be caused by any factor that stimulates parasympathetic activity or inhibits sympathetic activity of vascular smooth muscle. (Parasympathetic stimulation automatically inhibits sympathetic activity and vice versa; see Chapter 29.) Normally, sympathetic stimulation maintains muscle tone. If sympathetic stimulation is interrupted or inhibited, vasodilation occurs. Therefore, trauma to the spinal

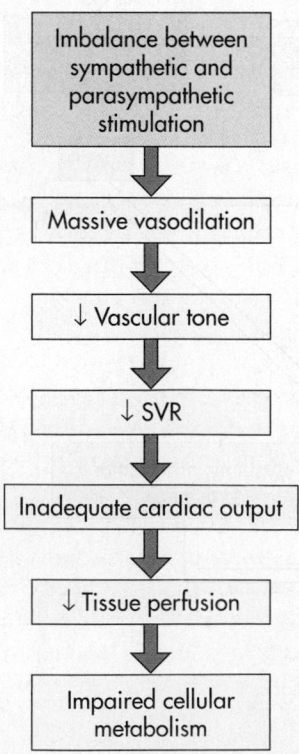

Figure 46-4 Neurogenic shock. *SVR,* Systemic vascular resistance.

cord or medulla, conditions that interrupt the supply of oxygen to the medulla, or conditions that deprive the medulla of glucose (e.g., insulin reactions) can cause neurogenic shock by interrupting sympathetic activity. Depressive drugs, anesthetic agents, and severe emotional stress and pain are other causes of neurogenic shock.

The clinical hallmark of neurogenic shock is a very low SVR, along with other indicators of excessive parasympathetic activity. Bradycardia is the most obvious manifestation, especially in the early stages. Bradycardia may cease when compensatory mechanisms, particularly an increase in sympathetic system activity, have been initiated. The ejection fraction remains high, indicating a healthy myocardium, whereas central venous pressure decreases as the veins dilate. Neurogenic shock causes fainting if blood pressure decreases to the point that cerebral metabolism is not sufficient to support consciousness. Most episodes of fainting are *not* shock, however; for such episodes to progress to shock is rare. By allowing the blood pressure to equalize from head to toe as the individual becomes prone, fainting can actually prevent shock.

Anaphylactic Shock

Anaphylactic shock is the outcome of a widespread hypersensitivity reaction known as *anaphylaxis.* The basic physiologic alteration in anaphylactic shock is the same as that in neurogenic shock—that is, vasodilation, peripheral pooling, and relative hypovolemia leading to decreased tissue perfusion and impaired cellular metabolism (Figure 46-5). Anaphylactic shock is often more severe than other types of normovolemic shock because the hypersensitivity reaction that triggers vasodilation has other pathophysiologic effects that rapidly involve the entire body.

Anaphylactic shock begins as an allergic reaction—an immune and inflammatory response—to an allergen. (An allergen is an antigen to which an individual is hypersensitive; see Chapters 6, 7, and 8 for discussions of immunity, inflammation, and hypersensitivity.) Some allergens known to cause hypersensitivity reactions are snakebite venom, insect venoms, pollens, shellfish, penicillin, and animal sera. Once in the body, the allergen causes an extensive immune and inflammatory response. The vascular effects of this response include vasodilation and increased vascular permeability, resulting in peripheral pooling and tissue edema. The extravascular effects include constriction of extravascular smooth muscle. Constriction often causes respiratory difficulty because it tends to affect smooth muscle layers in the airway walls (e.g., the larynx and bronchioles; see Chapter 32).

The onset of anaphylactic shock is usually sudden, and progression to death can occur within minutes unless emergency treatment is given. The first manifestations of shock may be anxiety, difficulty in breathing, gastrointestinal cramps, edema, hives (urticaria), and sensations of burning or itching of the skin. A precipitous decrease in blood pressure occurs and is followed by impaired mentation. Other signs include decreased SVR (with high or normal cardiac output) and

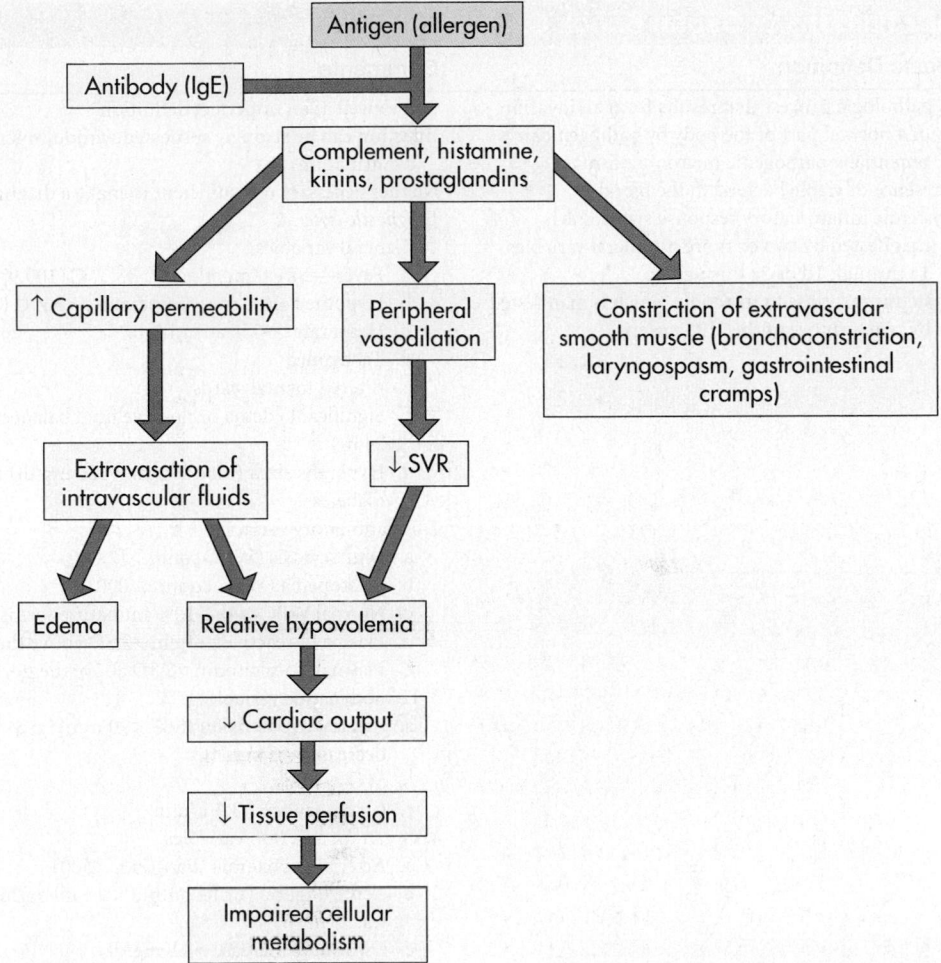

Figure 46-5 Anaphylactic shock. *IgE,* Immunoglobulin E; *SVR,* systemic vascular resistance.

oliguria. Treatment begins with removal of the antigen (if possible). Epinephrine is administered to decrease mast cell and basophil degranulation, cause vasoconstriction, and reverse airway constriction. Volume expanders (e.g., lactated Ringer solution) are given intravenously to reverse the relative hypovolemia, and antihistamines and steroids are given to stop the inflammatory reaction.

Septic Shock

Septic shock is the endpoint of a continuum of progressive dysfunction.[10] The syndrome begins with systemic inflammatory response syndrome (SIRS), then sepsis, then severe sepsis, and then septic shock. Consensus on definitions of each component was updated at an international sepsis conference in 2001 (Table 46-1).[10,11] The International Sepsis Forum reviewed research for sepsis to identify and define the six most common infection sites (pneumonia, bloodstream, intravascular catheter, intra-abdominal, urosepsis, and surgical wound infection) associated with sepsis in the intensive care setting.[12]

Severe sepsis is the eleventh most common cause of death in the United States. Mortality ranges from 28% to 60%.[13]

Septic shock is caused by gram-negative bacteria, gram-positive bacteria, and fungi. Advances in antibiotic therapy for gram-negative sepsis have made gram-positive bacteria the leading cause of sepsis.[14] Even when properly treated with available therapies, it carries a high mortality rate. Prognosis is significantly affected by the source and virulence of the infectious microorganism.

Septic shock begins with a nidus of infection that may be readily discernible or extremely difficult to locate (Figure 46-6). Bacteria then enter the bloodstream to produce bacteremia in one of two ways: (1) directly from the site of infection or (2) from toxic substances released by the bacteria directly into the bloodstream. These toxic substances, which act as triggering molecules in the septic syndrome, include endotoxins released by gram-negative microorganisms, lipoteichoic acids and peptidoglycan released by gram-positive microorganisms, and superantigens.[14]

The triggering molecules cause the host to initiate a proinflammatory response. Proinflammatory cells released include polymorphonuclear leukocytes, macrophages, monocytes, and platelets. Proinflammatory mediators released include cytokines (interleukins [IL]-1, IL-2, IL-6, IL-8, and

Table 46-1	Definitions of Septic Shock Components	
Term	**Basic Definition**	**Comments**
Infection	A pathologic process that results from an invasion of a normal part of the body by pathogenic or potentially pathogenic microorganisms	Still viewed as an imperfect definition Infection can be strongly suspected without microbiologic confirmation
Bacteremia	Presence of viable bacteria in the blood	Neither necessary nor sufficient to make a diagnosis of sepsis
SIRS	Systemic inflammatory response syndrome is manifested by two or more of general variables: 1a through 1d or 2a through 2c	*Diagnostic criteria:*

Sepsis	Systemic response to infection, which is manifested by two or more of the SIRS criteria	1. General variables
		  a. Fever—core temperature >38.3° C (100.9° F)
		  b. Hypothermia—core temperature <36° C (96.8° F)
		  c. Heart rate >90 beats/minute
		  d. Tachypnea
		  e. Altered mental status
		  f. Significant edema or positive fluid balance (>20 ml/kg over 24 hr)
		  g. Hyperglycemia (blood sugar >120 mg/dl) in the absence of diabetes
		2. Inflammatory variables
		  a. Leukocytosis (WBC count >12,000)
		  b. Leukopenia (WBC count <4000)
		  c. Normal WBC with >10% immature forms
		  d. Plasma C-reactive protein >2 SD above the normal value
		  e. Plasma procalcitonin >2 SD above the normal value
		3. Hemodynamic variables
		  a. Arterial hypotension (SBP <90 mmHg; MAP <70, or an SBP decrease >40 mmHg)
		  b. $S\bar{v}O_2$ >70%
		  c. Cardiac index >3.5 L/min
		4. Organ dysfunction variables
		  a. Arterial hypoxemia (Pao_2/Fio_2 <300)
		  b. Acute oliguria (urine output <0.5 ml/kg/hr or 45 ml for at least 2 hr)
		  c. Creatinine increase >0.5 mg/dl
		  d. Coagulation abnormalities (INR >1.5 or a PTT >60)
		  e. Ileus
		  f. Thrombocytopenia (platelet count <100,000)
		  g. Hyperbilirubinemia (plasma total bilirubin >4 mg/dl or 70 mmol/L)
		5. Tissue perfusion variables
		  a. Hyperlactatemia (>3 mmol/L)
		  b. Decreased capillary refill or mottling

Severe sepsis	Sepsis complicated with one or more organ system dysfunctions	May be difficult to differentiate underlying organ dysfunction from sepsis-related organ dysfunction
Septic shock	Severe sepsis complicated by persistent hypotension refractory to early fluid therapy	Persistent systolic blood pressure <90 mmHg

Data from Levy MM et al: *Crit Care Med* 312:1250, 2003; Opal SM, *Scand J Infect Dis* 35:529, 2003.

INR, International normalized ratio; *MAP*, mean arterial pressure; *Pao₂/Fio₂*, partial pressure of oxygen in arterial blood/fraction of inspired oxygen; *PTT*, partial thromboplastin time; *SD*, standard deviation; *SBP*, systolic blood pressure; *SṽO₂*, saturation of hemoglobin with oxygen; *WBC*, white blood cell.

IL-15; tumor necrosis factor-alpha [TNF-α]; and granulocyte cell–stimulating factor), complement and complement cascade activation, kinins, arachidonic acid metabolites (prostaglandins, prostacyclin, leukotrienes, and thromboxane), soluble adhesion molecules, platelet-activating factor, endorphins, vasoactive neuropeptides, histamine, serotonin, monocyte chemoattractant proteins 1 and 2, proteolytic enzymes (e.g., elastase and lysosomal enzymes), protein kinase, tyrosine kinase, CD14, toxic oxygen metabolites (e.g., superoxide, hydroxyl radical, hydrogen peroxide, peroxynitrite), neopterin, and clotting cascade activation.[2,15,16] Proinflammatory cytokines enhance tissue factors, which initiates coagulation. Diminished thrombomodulin (cell surface glycoprotein of endothelial cells) inhibits the conversion of protein C and activated protein C. A compensatory anti-inflammatory response syndrome is presumed to follow this response.[2,15,16] Anti-inflammatory mediators released include lipopolysaccharide-binding protein; IL-1 receptor antagonist; soluble CD-14; type 2 IL-1 receptor; leukotriene B₄ receptor antagonist; IL-4, IL-10, and IL-13; soluble tumor necrosis factor

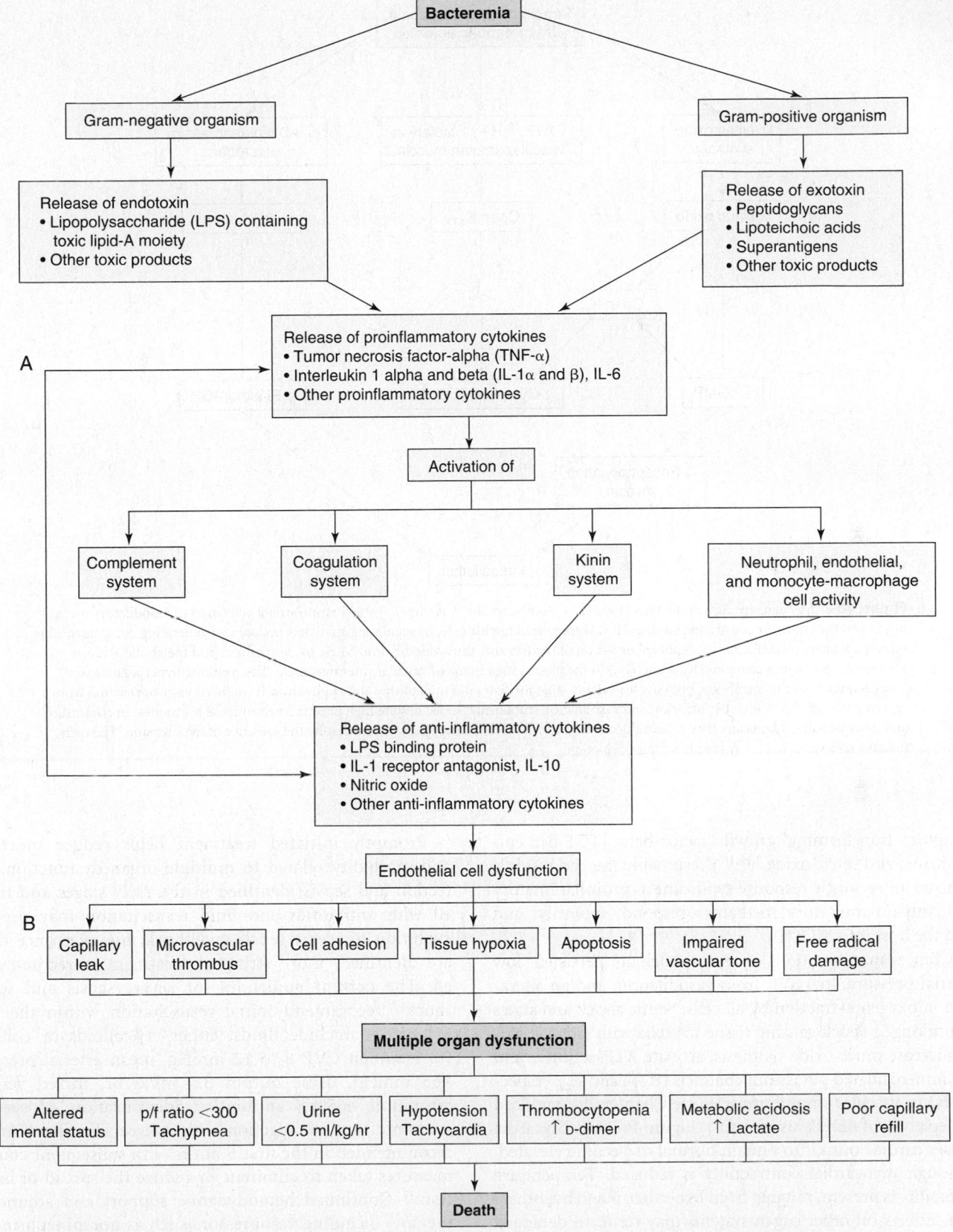

Figure 46-6 Summary of sepsis pathology. *p/f (Pao₂/Fio₂)*, oxygenation ratio. (A from Larson V, Barke RA: *Urol Clin North Am* 26[4]:687, 1999. B copyright © 2003, Eli Lilly and Company. All rights reserved. Reprinted with permission from Eli Lilly and Company.)

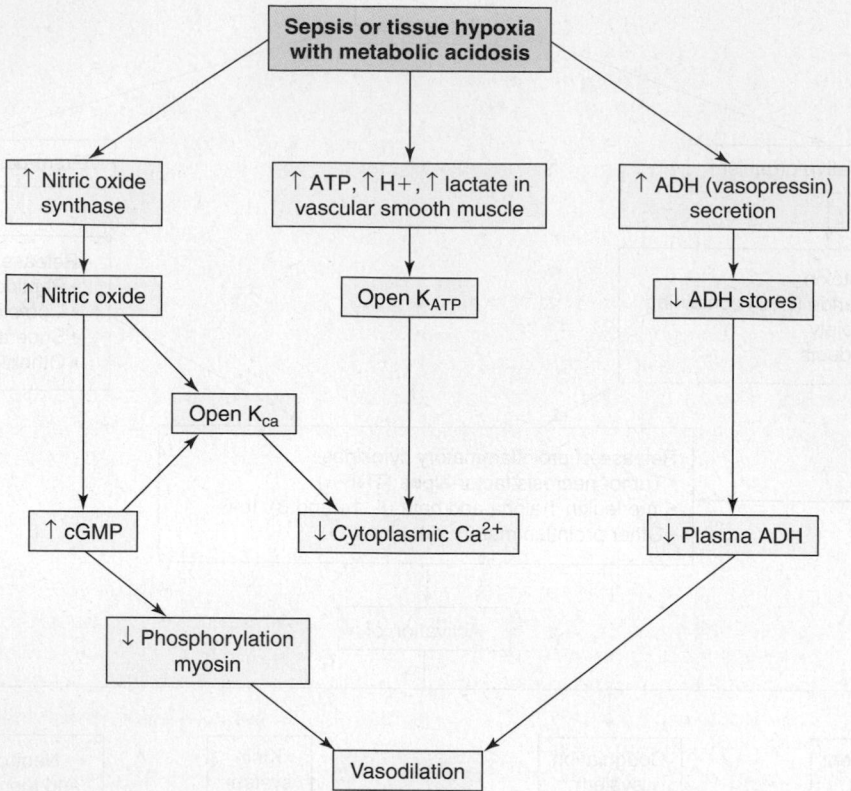

Figure 46-7 **Mechanisms of vasodilation in shock.** Vasodilatory shock is caused by the inappropriate activation of vasodilatory mechanisms and the failure of constrictor mechanisms. Unregulated nitric oxide, by regulating guanylate cyclase and generating cyclic guanosine monophosphate (cGMP), causes dephosphorylation of myosin and, thus, vasodilation. Nitric oxide synthesis and metabolic acidosis activate the potassium channels (K_{ATP} and K_{Ca}) in the plasma membrane of vascular smooth muscle. The resulting hyperpolarization (see Chapter 3) of the membrane presents the calcium that mediates norepinephrine and angiotensin II–induced vasoconstriction from entering the cell. Therefore, hypotension and vasodilation stubbornly persist despite high plasma levels of these hormones. In contrast, and unexpectedly, the plasma level of antidiuretic hormone (ADH) (vasopressin) is low despite the presence of hypotension. The early, massive release of ADH may result in future depletion.

receptor; transforming growth factor-beta [TGF-β]; epinephrine; and nitric oxide.[2,15,16] Presumably the end result is a mixed antagonistic response syndrome as proinflammatory and anti-inflammatory mediators respond, intensify, and lead the host into MODS.

Clinical manifestations of septic shock are persistent low arterial pressure, low SVR from vasodilation, and an alteration in oxygen extraction by all cells. Septic shock and states of prolonged shock causing tissue hypoxia with lactic acidosis increase nitric oxide synthesis, activate ATP-sensitive and calcium-regulated potassium channels (K_{ATP} and K_{ca}, respectively) in vascular smooth muscle (see Chapter 29), and lead to depletion of ADH (vasopressin) (Figure 46-7). Tachycardia causes cardiac output to remain normal or become elevated, although myocardial contractility is reduced. Temperature instability is present, ranging from hyperthermia to hypothermia. Effects on other organ systems may result in deranged renal function, gastrointestinal mucosa changes that result in release of bacteria from the gut, jaundice, clotting abnormalities, deterioration of mental status, and tachypnea that often progresses to ARDS.

Promptly initiated treatment helps reduce mortality and morbidity related to multiple organ dysfunction. Infection and sepsis identified in the early stages and treated with antibiotics and fluid resuscitation may prevent evolution to severe sepsis and shock; however once these are identified, more stringent treatment is recommended. The current guidelines for severe sepsis and septic shock[17] recommend initial resuscitation within the first 6 hours to include fluids, either crystalloids or colloids (to maintain CVP 8 to 12 mmHg, mean arterial pressure ≥65 mmHg, urine output 0.5 ml/kg/hr, mixed venous saturation ≥65%); antibiotics; identification of specific anatomic sites of infection with source identification are recommended in the first 6 hours with subsequent control measures taken to eliminate or reduce the spread of infection.[17] Continued hemodynamic support and adjunctive therapy, including vasopressors such as norepinephrine or dopamine, as initial vasopressor of choice with epinephrine, phenylephrine and vasopressin as alternatives, inotropic agents, such as dobutamine, if needed because of myocardial dysfunction, and intravenous hydrocortisone for adult septic shock if an individual remains hypotensive despite fluids and vasopressors. Adrenocorticotropic hormone (ACTH or corticotropin) stimulation test is not recommended and administration of recombinant human-activated protein C should be initiated if indicated.[17] Other supportive therapies in the treatment of severe sepsis include blood product administration to maintain hemoglobin between 7 and 9 g/dl, targeted tidal volume (6 ml/kg) when mechanically ventilated with plateau pressure less than 30 cm H_2O, utilization of sedation and analgesia protocols when needed, and avoidance of neuromuscular blockers if possible. Glucose is to be maintained at less than 150 mg/dl. If renal dialysis is required, intermittent hemodialysis and continuous venovenous hemofiltration are considered equivalent. Bicarbonate therapy is contraindicated for the purpose of treating hypoperfusion lactic acidemia. Use deep vein thrombosis prophylaxis, such as low-dose unfractionated heparin or low-molecular-weight heparin, or mechanical compression prophylaxis if heparin is contraindicated. Stress ulcer prophylaxis with H_2-receptor antagonist or proton pump inhibitors is indicated. It is important to discuss advanced directives with the individual and family.[17] Gaps in the current understanding of sepsis have led to research using experimental treatment such as immunomodulating therapies, including monoclonal antibodies and vaccines.[18-20]

Treatment for Shock

The first treatment for shock is to discover and correct or remove the underlying cause. Although this seems a simple tenet, it is one that is not always remembered. Thus treatment for cardiogenic shock begins with treatment of heart failure or at least enhancement of cardiac output. If hypovolemia is the cause of shock, hemorrhage and other causes of fluid loss must be stopped. In neurogenic shock as a result of spinal cord trauma, stabilization of the spine and surrounding tissue is a beginning, and pain usually can be decreased to a level at which neurally mediated decreases of SVR cease. The initial treatment for anaphylactic shock is to remove or neutralize the antigen. Treatment for septic shock begins with eradication of the infective agent, usually with antimicrobials (see preceding discussion).

After the underlying cause or condition is corrected as much as possible, treatment thereafter is supportive. Intravenous fluid is administered to expand intravascular volume, except in cases of cardiogenic shock, which require diuresis to reduce preload. Supplemental oxygen is always given. Cardiotonic drugs are given early in cardiogenic shock and given later in other forms of shock. Steroid use in septic shock remains unproven, although there is evidence that low-dose therapy improves mortality. Stress ulcer prophylaxis and gastric tonometry, to measure splanchnic blood flow, are imperative because the gut is one of the drivers of the septic syndrome.[17]

Once positive-feedback loops are established, intervention in shock is difficult. Prevention and early treatment offer the best prognosis.

MULTIPLE ORGAN DYSFUNCTION SYNDROME

Multiple organ dysfunction syndrome (MODS) is the progressive dysfunction of two or more organ systems resulting from an uncontrolled inflammatory response to a severe illness or injury. The organ dysfunction can progress to organ failure and death. MODS occurs during severe sepsis. In 2001, an international consensus conference developed a set of definitions for sepsis and related disorders (see Table 46-1), and a predisposition-infection-response-organ (PIRO) dysfunction staging system was proposed as a template for staging sepsis (Table 46-2). MODS is the end stage of a variety of injuries that terminate in severe, generalized inflammation.

MODS was first recognized as a distinct clinical syndrome in the mid-1970s,[21,22] when advances in resuscitation and support technologies allowed many individuals to survive life-threatening illness or trauma only to die of complications of their disease. Today MODS is a leading cause of mortality in surgical intensive care units (ICUs). Mortality for individuals with MODS increases progressively from 54% with two failing organ systems to 100% with five failing organ systems. Moreover, mortality has not improved much over the past 15 to 20 years.[23,24]

Although sepsis and septic shock are the most common causes, MODS can be initiated by any severe injury or disease process that activates a massive systemic inflammatory response by the host. Documented clinical infection is not necessary for its development. Other common triggers are severe trauma, major surgery, burns, circulatory shock, acute pancreatitis, acute renal failure, ARDS, blood transfusion, heat stroke, liver failure, mesenteric ischemia, Propofol infusion syndrome, persistent inflammatory foci, and necrotic tissue (Box 46-1). MODS is the major cause of death following septic shock, trauma, burn injuries, and ARDS. People at greatest risk for developing MODS are older adults and persons with significant tissue injury or preexisting disease.[11]

The PIRO system (see Table 46-2), a clinically useful sepsis staging system, stratifies individuals with disease by baseline risk of adverse outcomes and potential to respond to therapy.[11]

PATHOPHYSIOLOGY In **primary MODS** the organ injury is directly associated with a specific insult, most often ischemia or impaired perfusion from an episode of shock or trauma, thermal injury, soft tissue necrosis, or invasive infection.[25] This decreased perfusion is local (in the injured organs themselves) and generalized. The generalized hypoperfusion in primary MODS usually cannot be detected clinically. As a result of the insult, a stress response is initiated and stress hormones—in particular, catecholamines—are released. The inflammatory and stress responses are not as evident as they are in secondary MODS. In primary MODS during the inflammatory response, presumably neutrophils and macrophages are "primed" by cytokines.[25] Any second insult, such as additional tissue injury, infection, or organ ischemia, may then activate the primed cells to produce an exaggerated response of secondary MODS[25,26] (Figure 46-8).

Table 46-2   Predisposition-Infection-Response-Organ (PIRO) Dysfunction System for Staging Sepsis

Domain	Present	Future	Rationale
Predisposition	Premorbid illness with reduced probability of short term survival Cultural or religious beliefs Age Sex	Genetic polymorphisms in components of inflammatory response Enhanced understanding of specific interactions between pathogens and host diseases	Premorbid factors affect the potential attributable morbidity and mortality of an acute insult Deleterious consequences of insult heavily dependent on genetic predisposition (future)
Infection	Culture and sensitivity of infecting pathogens Detection of disease amenable to source control	Assay of microbial products Gene transcription profiles	Specific therapies directed against inciting insult require demonstration of characterization of that insult
Response	SIRS Other signs of sepsis Shock C-reactive protein	Nonspecific markers of activated inflammation or impaired host responsiveness Detection of specific target of therapy	Mortality risk and potential to respond to therapy vary with nonspecific measures of disease severity Specific mediator-targeted therapy is predicated on presence and activity of mediator
Organ dysfunction	Organ dysfunction as number of organs or composite score	Dynamic measures of cellular response to insult—apoptosis, cytopathic hypoxemia, cell stress	Response to preemptive therapy not possible if damage already present Therapies targeting the injurious cellular process require that it be present

From Levy MM et al: *2001 Intensive Care Med* 29:530, 2003, reproduced with kind permission of Springer Science + Business Media.
SIRS, Systemic inflammatory response syndrome.

Box 46-1   Other Common Triggers of MODS

Severe trauma
Major surgery
Burns
Circulatory shock
Acute pancreatitis
Acute renal failure
ARDS
Blood transfusion
Heat stroke
Liver failure
Mesenteric ischemia
Propofol infusion syndrome
Persistent inflammatory foci
Necrotic tissue

Data from Oeckler RA, Hubmayr RD: *Eur Resp J* 30(6):1216-1226, 2007; Ciesla DJ, Moore EE, Johnson JL, Burch JM, Cothren CC, Sauaia A: *Arch Surg* 140(5):432-440, 2005; Broessner G, Beer R, Franz G, Lackner P, Engelhard K, Brenneis C, Pfausler B, Schmutzhard E: *Crit Care* 9(5):R498-R501, 2006; Bouchama A, Knochel JP: *N Engl J Med* 346:1978-1988, 2002; Varghese GM, John G, Thomas K, Abraham OC, Mathai D: *Emerg Med J* 22:185-187, 2005; Adukauskien D, Dockien I, Naginien R, K velaitis E, Pundzius J, Kup inskas L: *Medicina (Kaunas)* 44(7):536-540, 2008; Abboud B, Daher R, Boujaoude J: *World J Gastroenterol* 14(35):5361-5370, 2008; Beger HG, Rau BM: *World J Gastroenterol* 13(38):5043-5051, 2007; Carnovale A, Rabitti PG, Manes G, Esposito P, Pacelli L, Uomo G: *J Pancreas (Online)* 6(5):438-444, 2005; Shaheen MA, Akhtar AJ: *J Nat Med Assoc* 99(12):1402-1406, 2007; Kam PCA, Cardone D: *Anesthesia* 62(1):690-701, 2007; Zaccheo MM, Bucher DH: *Crit Care Nurse* 28(3):18-26, 2008.

The progressive organ dysfunction of **secondary MODS** is the result of an excessive inflammatory reaction, after a latent period following the initial injury, in organs distant from the site of the original injury. It is postulated that the resulting organ trauma is caused by the host response to a second insult rather than being a direct result of the primary injury. Often the second insult is mild but produces an immense disproportionate response because of the previous priming of leukocytes. The interaction of injured organs then leads to a self-perpetuating inflammation.

Secondary MODS is initiated by the delayed postinjury insult as primed macrophages release a barrage of mediators, particularly the cytokines TNF and IL-1. These mediators damage the endothelium throughout the body. If a gram-negative bacterial infection is present, endotoxin released from the bacteria also causes severe damage to endothelial cells. Normal endothelial cells have little interaction with leukocytes, but when stimulated by TNF, IL-1, IL-6, or endotoxin, they change to a proinflammatory state and express adhesion molecules that mediate adhesion of neutrophils. The adhered neutrophils then migrate through the endothelium, aggregate in the area of damaged tissue, and amplify the inflammation.[2] The activated endothelial cells increase production and release of nitric oxide (endothelium), a potent vasodilator that is considered an important factor in the blood flow changes and loss of vascular tone noted in systemic inflammation.[27] The injured endothelium also becomes much more permeable, allowing fluid and protein to leak into the interstitial spaces. An important function of normal endothelium is anticoagulation. When damaged, the endothelium

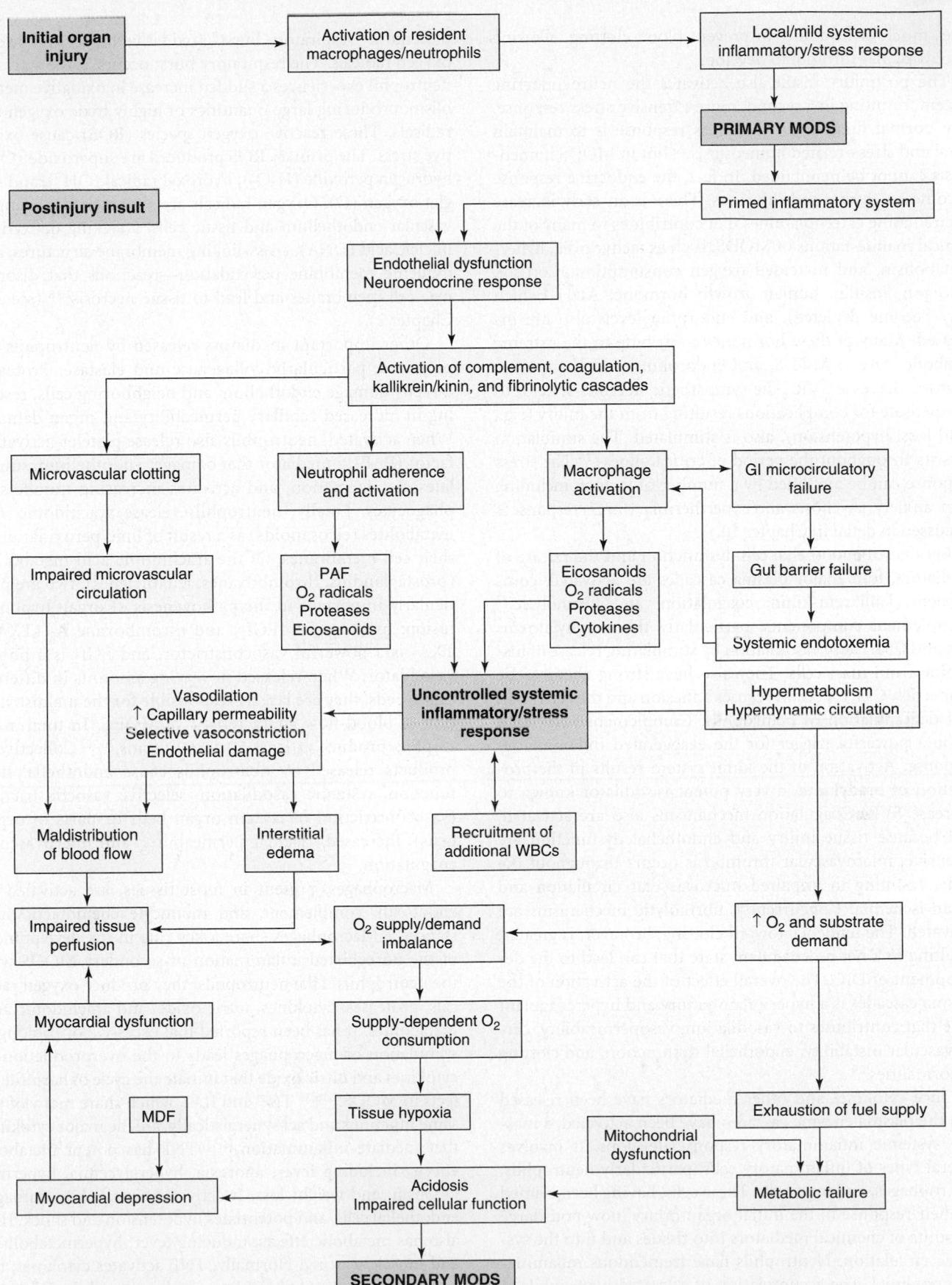

Figure 46-8 Pathogenesis of multiple organ dysfunction syndrome. *GI,* Gastrointestinal; *MDF,* myocardial depressant factor; *MODS,* multiple organ dysfunction syndrome; *PAF,* platelet-activating factor; *WBCs,* white blood cells.

loses much of its ability to prevent blood clotting, allowing microvascular thrombi to develop.

The postinjury insult also activates the neuroendocrine system, resulting in a second, more extensive stress response. The normal function of the stress response is to maintain basal and stress-related homeostasis,[28] but in MODS homeostasis cannot be maintained. In fact, the endocrine response becomes excessive and injurious. There is an early increase in circulating catecholamines that contributes to many of the clinical manifestations of MODS, such as tachycardia, hypermetabolism, and increased oxygen consumption. Cortisol, glucagon, insulin, human growth hormone, ADH (which may become depleted), and endorphin levels also are increased. Many of these hormones contribute to the extreme catabolic state of MODS, and endorphins, which are vasodilators, decrease SVR. The sympathetic nervous system, to compensate for complications resulting from the injury (e.g., fluid loss, hypotension), also is stimulated. The stimulation persists throughout the period of critical illness.[28] The stress response can be amplified by a number of factors, including pain, anxiety, psychosis, and hyperthermia. (Stress response is discussed in detail in Chapter 10.)

Because of endothelial cell dysfunction and the release of mediators, four major plasma cascades are activated: complement, kallikrein-kinin, coagulation, and fibrinolytic.[27] Complement components, particularly the anaphylatoxins C3a and C5a, cause vasodilation by stimulating release of histamine from mast cells. They also have strong chemotactic properties. C5a, especially, causes adhesion and the activation and degranulation of neutrophils. Complement is thought to be a powerful trigger for the exaggerated inflammatory response. Activation of the kinin system results in the production of bradykinin, a very potent vasodilator known to decrease SVR. Coagulation mechanisms also are activated, and because tissue injury and endothelial dysfunction are extensive, microvascular thrombosis occurs throughout the body, resulting in impaired microvascular circulation and organ ischemia. Concurrently, fibrinolytic mechanisms are activated. The tendency toward clotting, however, is greater, resulting in a net procoagulant state that can lead to the development of DIC. The overall effect of the activation of the plasma cascades is a hyperinflammatory and hypercoagulant state that contributes to vasodilation, vasopermeability, cardiovascular instability, endothelial dysfunction, and clotting abnormalities.[29]

Once cytokines and other mediators have been released and the plasma enzyme cascades have been activated, a massive systemic inflammatory response develops. It involves several types of inflammatory cells, particularly neutrophils, macrophages, and mast cells. These cells, having been primed by their response to the initial organ injury, now pour large amounts of chemical mediators into tissues and into the systemic circulation. Neutrophils have tremendous inflammatory potential. The accumulation of activated neutrophils in organs is thought to play a key role in the pathogenesis of MODS.[30] When neutrophils adhere to the endothelium, they undergo a "respiratory burst" (oxidative burst) and release oxygen radicals. The respiratory burst occurs as the activated neutrophil experiences a sudden increase in oxidative metabolism, producing large quantities of highly toxic oxygen free radicals. These reactive oxygen species (ROS) cause oxidative stress. The primary ROS produced are superoxide (O_2^-), hydrogen peroxide (H_2O_2), hydroxyl radical (OH^-), and singlet oxygen (O). Oxygen radicals are extremely damaging to vascular endothelium and tissue cells, attacking deoxyribonucleic acid (DNA), cross-linking membrane structures, and inducing membrane peroxidation—reactions that disorganize cell membranes and lead to tissue necrosis[2,16] (see also Chapter 2).

Other important mediators released by neutrophils are proteases, particularly collagenase and elastase. Proteases directly damage endothelium and neighboring cells, resulting in increased capillary permeability and organ damage. When activated, neutrophils also release platelet-activating factor (PAF), a mediator that damages endothelium, stimulates clot formation, and activates increasing numbers of phagocytes. Finally, neutrophils release arachidonic acid metabolites (eicosanoids) as a result of lipid peroxidation of their cell membranes. Of the arachidonic acid metabolites (prostaglandins, thromboxanes, leukotrienes), two are particularly important in the pathogenesis of organ hypoperfusion: prostacyclin (PGI_2) and thromboxane A_2 (TXA_2). TXA_2 is a powerful vasoconstrictor, and PGI_2 is a potent vasodilator. When released in varying amounts in different organ beds, they are largely responsible for the maldistribution of blood flow characteristic of MODS. In total, neutrophils produce at least 50 to 60 toxins.[30,31] Collectively, products released by neutrophils cause endothelial dysfunction, systemic vasodilation, selective vasoconstriction (vasoconstriction of certain organ beds or parts of organ beds), increased vascular permeability, and microvascular coagulation.

Macrophages, present in most tissues, are activated by endotoxin, complement, and monocyte chemotactic substances.[32] Macrophages share a key role in the development of the unregulated inflammation of secondary MODS with the neutrophils. Like neutrophils, they produce oxygen radicals, proteases, cytokines, nitric oxide, and arachidonic acid metabolites. It has been reported that excessive or prolonged stimulation of macrophages leads to the overproduction of cytokines and nitric oxide that initiate the cycle of harmful effects in MODS.[2,16,32] TNF and IL-1, which share many of the same functions and act synergistically, are the major cytokines that mediate inflammation.[32,33] TNF has potent metabolic effects, including fever, anorexia, hyperglycemia, hypermetabolism, and weight loss. It activates neutrophils, damages endothelial cells, and potentiates hypotension and shock. IL-1 also has metabolic effects, inducing fever, hypermetabolism, and muscle wasting. Normally, TNF activates cytokines, the coagulation system, fibrinolysis, and neutrophils. With the exception of neutrophil activation, IL-1 causes similar activation in individuals with cancer.[34] In the pathogenesis of

MODS, the cytokines are linked to all cellular, hemodynar[ ]
and metabolic alterations.

The gastrointestinal mucosa is particularly vulnerable[ ]
inflammatory mediators released by macrophages and n[ ]
trophils. Under normal circumstances the gut mucosa ser[ ]
as a barrier to prevent bacteria from the gastrointestinal t[ ]
from entering the systemic circulation. Damage to the muc[ ]
results in microcirculatory failure of the gut and consequ[ ]
loss of the gut barrier function. The loss of intestinal barr[ ]
function leads to the systemic spread of bacteria and/or [ ]
dotoxin from the gut (systemic endotoxemia). This pheno[ ]
enon is called *translocation of bacteria*. The idea that the g[ ]
acts as a reservoir of bacteria and endotoxin that can initi[ ]
or perpetuate the development of MODS is known as the **g**[ ]
hypothesis. The gut hypothesis provides a possible explar[ ]
tion for the fact that an infectious focus is not always fou[ ]
in individuals with MODS. Although this hypothesis has be[ ]
substantiated by animal studies and has much support, t[ ]
evidence from human studies is inconclusive.[35,36]

The numerous inflammatory processes operating [ ]
MODS cause maldistribution of blood flow and hyperm[ ]
tabolism. **Maldistribution of blood flow** refers to the uneve[ ]
distribution of flow to various organs and between the lar[ ]
vessels and capillary beds of the body. It is caused by generalized vasodilation, increased capillary permeability, selective vasoconstriction, endothelial dysfunction, and impaired
microvascular circulation. It is a major factor in the pathophysiology of MODS.[27] The alterations in blood flow—which
can occur at the cellular, organ, or regional level—lead to impaired tissue perfusion and a decreased supply of oxygen to
the cells. The organs most severely affected by hypoperfusion
are the lungs, splanchnic bed, liver, and kidneys. Despite su-
pernormal systemic blood flow, oxygen delivery to the tissues
decreases. Several factors contribute to the problem. First,
blood is shunted past selected regional capillary beds. Shunting, caused by loss of autoregulation in some organs, may be
an early indicator of progression of sepsis into MODS.[37] This
occurs because inflammatory mediators, particularly TXA_2,
override the normal vascular control to cause selective vasoconstriction and because injured endothelial cells are unable
to respond to normal vasodilator mediators. Second, interstitial edema, resulting from microvascular permeability, contributes to decreased oxygen delivery to cells by increasing the
distance oxygen must travel to reach the cells. Third, capillary
obstruction occurs because of the formation of microvascular
thrombi and the aggregation of leukocytes.[2,16]

Hypermetabolism, with accompanying alterations in
carbohydrate, fat, and lipid metabolism, is initially a compensatory measure to meet the body's increased demands
for energy. Eventually, however, hypermetabolism becomes
detrimental, placing enormous demands on the heart. Hypermetabolism is the result of (1) the neuroendocrine response
to stress with the release of catecholamines and cortisol, and
(2) the action of TNF and IL-1. With increased metabolism the
calorie requirements are markedly increased,[23] and the cardiac output increases 1.5 to 2 times normal.[38] The alterations in

Box 46-2 Clinical Manifestations of Organ[ ]

Pulmonary
- Acute respiratory distress syndrome (ARDS) pat[ ]
  failure (dyspnea, patchy infiltrates, refractory[ ]
  tory acidosis, abnormal O_2 indices)
- Pulmonary hypertension

Gastrointestinal
- Abdominal distention and ascites
- Intolerance to enteral feeding[ ]
- Paralytic ileus
- Upper and lower gastroi[ ]
- Diarrhea
- Ischemic colitis
- Mucosal ulcera[ ]
- Decreased b[ ]
- Bacterial [ ]

Liver
- Inc[ ]

has been exhausted and the amount of oxygen consumed becomes dependent on the amount the circulation is able to deliver. Because the amount is inadequate in MODS, the tissues
become hypoxic. Compounding the hypoxic damage to cells
is a phenomenon called *reperfusion injury* (see Chapter 2).
Much of the organ damage in MODS occurs with the reestab-
lishment of blood flow after a period of ischemia. During the
ischemic episode, energy stores and ATP are depleted and the
enzyme *xanthine dehydrogenase* is converted to *xanthine oxidase.* With reperfusion of the ischemic tissue, oxygen radicals
are formed from oxygen by the action of xanthine oxidase,
and they attack the already damaged tissues. Consequently,
although reperfusion is necessary to restore oxygen supply to
ischemic organs, it can increase the extent of injury. Therefore, because of supply-dependent oxygen consumption and
reperfusion injury, tissues become increasingly hypoxic. The
result is cellular acidosis, impaired cellular function, and ultimately multiple organ failure.

CLINICAL MANIFESTATIONS In MODS the organs
that show clinical manifestations of failure are not always the
organs involved as part of the initial injury, and there is usually a lag time between the initial insult and the development of
systemic organ failure. The development of primary MODS
is difficult to monitor, but there is a well-established general
pattern in the clinical development of secondary MODS.[25,26]
Following the inciting event and aggressive resuscitation of the
individual for approximately 24 hours, the individual develops low-grade fever, tachycardia, tachypnea, dyspnea, altered
mental status, and a general hyperdynamic and hypermetabolic state (Box 46-2). Following this, the lungs begin to fail
and ARDS may appear within 24 to 72 hours (see discussion
of ARDS, Chapter 33). Between days 7 and 10, the hypermetabolic and hyperdynamic state intensifies; bacteremia with

tern of respiratory
hypoxemia, respira-

ntestinal bleeding (guaiac-positive stools)

owel sounds
overgrowth in stool

eased serum bilirubin level (hyperbilirubinemia)
- ncreased liver enzyme levels (serum aspartate transaminase [SAST], serum alanine aminotransferase [SALT], lactic dehydrogenase [LDH], alkaline phosphatase)
- Increased serum ammonia level
- Decreased serum transferrin level
- Jaundice
- Hepatomegaly

Gallbladder
- Right upper quadrant tenderness or pain
- Abdominal distention
- Unexplained fever
- Decreased bowel sounds

Metabolic/Nutritional
- Decreased lean body mass
- Muscle wasting
- Severe weight loss
- Negative nitrogen balance
- Hyperglycemia
- Hypertriglyceridemia

- Increased serum lactate levels
- Decreased serum albumin, serum transferrin, prealbumin, retinol-binding protein

Renal
- Increased serum creatinine level and blood urea nitrogen
- Oliguria, anuria, or polyuria consistent with prerenal azotemia or acute tubular necrosis
- Urinary indices consistent with prerenal azotemia or acute tubular necrosis

Cardiovascular
Hyperdynamic
- Decreased pulmonary capillary wedge pressure
- Decreased systemic vascular resistance
- Decreased right atrial pressure
- Decreased left ventricular stroke work index
- Increased oxygen consumption
- Increased cardiac output, cardiac index, heart rate

Hypodynamic
- Increased systemic vascular resistance
- Increased right atrial pressure
- Increased left ventricular stroke work index
- Decreased oxygen delivery and consumption
- Decreased cardiac output and cardiac index

Central Nervous System
- Lethargy
- Altered level of consciousness
- Fever
- Hepatic encephalopathy

Coagulation and Hematologic
- Thrombocytopenia
- Disseminated intravascular coagulation

Immune
- Infection
- Decreased lymphocyte count
- Anergy

Modified from Thelan LA et al: *Critical care nursing: diagnosis and management*, ed 5, St Louis, 2006, Mosby.

---

enteric organisms is common; and signs of hepatic, intestinal, and renal failure develop. During days 14 to 21, the renal failure and liver failure become more severe. Hematologic failure and myocardial failure are usually later manifestations. Encephalopathy, characterized by mental status changes ranging from confusion to deep coma, may occur at any time. This sequence can evolve rapidly, with death occurring between 14 and 21 days later, or it can evolve over weeks. Individuals can recover from either the slowly or rapidly evolving course.

The clinical manifestations of failure of individual organs in MODS are caused by inflammatory mediator damage, tissue hypoxia, and hypermetabolism. Respiratory failure progresses early to ARDS and is characterized by tachypnea, pulmonary edema with crackles and diminished breath sounds, use of accessory muscles, and hypoxemia. Liver failure, although early in its development, is not clinically detectable until the later stages of MODS, when jaundice, abdominal distention, liver tenderness, muscle wasting, and hepatic encephalopathy

appear. All aspects of metabolism, substance detoxification, and immune response are impaired. Albumin and clotting factor synthesis decreases, protein wastes accumulate, and liver tissue macrophages (Kupffer cells) no longer function effectively.

The gastrointestinal system is very sensitive to ischemic and inflammatory injury. Clinical manifestations of bowel involvement are hemorrhage, ileus, stress ulcers, malabsorption, diarrhea or constipation, vomiting, anorexia, abdominal pain, and pancreatitis. Intolerance to enteral feeding may develop. Adding to damage caused by injury to the bowel is bacterial translocation into the bloodstream resulting from the loss of the gut barrier function. The overwhelmed liver is unable to clear the bacteria from the systemic circulation. Thus, regardless of whether infection or some other injury was the precipitating cause of MODS, once intestinal bacteria enter the systemic circulation, it is likely that sepsis will be a problem. Renal failure develops at about the same time and is marked by progressive oliguria, azotemia, and edema. If renal shutdown is severe, anuria, hyperkalemia, and metabolic acidosis occur.

The first manifestations of cardiac failure are similar to those of septic shock: tachycardia, bounding pulse, increased cardiac output, fall in SVR, hypotension, warm skin, and supraventricular dysrhythmias. In the terminal stages, profound hypotension and ventricular dysrhythmias may develop. Changes in central nervous system function may be noted. Ischemia and inflammation are responsible for the changes, which include apprehension, confusion, disorientation, restlessness, agitation, headache, decreased cognitive ability and memory, and decreased level of consciousness. When ischemia is severe, seizures and coma can occur.

EVALUATION AND TREATMENT Because there is no specific therapy for MODS, early detection or prevention is extremely important so that supportive measures are initiated instantly.[23] Frequent assessment of the clinical status of individuals at known risk is essential. Unfortunately, there is no way to determine with certainty when an organ is failing. Indicators of organ dysfunction are presented in Table 46-1.

Several systems for scoring severity of illness also have been developed. Commonly used systems are the **Acute Physiology and Chronic Health Evaluation II and III (APACHE II and APACHE III)**, sequential organ failure assessment (SOFA), MODS score, and the PIRO staging system.[41] Once organ failure develops, monitoring of laboratory values and hemodynamic parameters is necessary to assess the degree of clinical impairment.

The therapeutic management of MODS consists of prevention and support. Prevention of the syndrome is essential! First, if possible, the initial source of inflammation must be eliminated or controlled. Next, a second insult must be avoided. It is paramount to remove any potential site of infection by débriding necrotic tissue, draining abscesses, reducing the numbers of invasive procedures performed, and removing hematomas. Nosocomial infections from contaminated lines and catheters are of concern and must be prevented. Nosocomial infection rates of 15% to 25% have been reported in critically ill individuals.[42] Early reduction of long-bone fractures and surgical repair of injured tissues are also important preventive measures.

The goals of therapy are to control infection, provide adequate tissue oxygenation, restore intravascular volume, and support the function of individual organs.[43] After the initial injury has been aggressively treated and sources of infection have been removed, antibiotics generally are administered. The choice of agents is based on the individual's disease process, but the regimen is usually a combination of antibiotics that covers both gram-negative and gram-positive organisms.

Because oxygen is not stored in the tissues, it must be continuously delivered. Maintaining an arterial oxygen saturation of 88% to 92% is recommended,[43] and hemoglobin levels should be kept above 9 g/dl.[43] Mixed venous oxygen greater than or equal to 70% is recommended. Blood transfusions may be necessary to ensure an adequate hemoglobin level. To deliver oxygen to the organs in the face of profound systemic vasodilation, fluid volume must be restored. Therefore, aggressive fluid therapy is initiated early. Usually large volumes of isotonic crystalloid solutions are administered, although colloids (often albumin) also may be added to maintain adequate preload and circulation volume.[43]

Finally, support for individual organ systems must be provided. Respiratory failure is treated with mechanical ventilation with low tidal volumes, high oxygen concentrations, and positive end-expiratory pressures (PEEP).[44] To provide adequate nutrition and metabolic support, the failing gastrointestinal system is supported with enteral feedings (see Nutrition & Disease: Olive Oil). It is now well recognized that enteral feedings help preserve gut microbial barrier function, thus are preferred to parenteral feedings.[36] However, if the individual is unable to tolerate the amount of enteral feeding required to meet the enormous metabolic demands, hyperalimentation may be added. Ideally the feeding formula is carefully calculated to meet the individual's nutritional requirements. Tight glucose control (80 to 110 mg/dl) is recommended.[45] Once renal failure is established, dialysis or continuous hemofiltration may be required to maintain fluid and electrolyte balance. To support the failing cardiovascular system, inotropic drugs, such as low-dose dopamine and dobutamine, or vasopressors, such as norepinephrine, may be required to maximize cardiac contractility and maintain cardiac output. Although steroids have anti-inflammatory effects, use of them is controversial because they have been shown to be effective in adults with septic shock. Obtaining

NUTRITION & DISEASE

Olive Oil

The effects exerted by polyunsaturated fatty acids (PUFAs) on immune system functions have been investigated in recent years. These studies have reported the important role that n-3 PUFAs play in the diminution of incidence and severity of inflammatory disorders. Nevertheless, less attention has been paid to the action of monounsaturated fatty acids (MUFAs) on the immune system. The administration of a diet containing a high amount of olive oil in experimental animals produces a suppression of lymphocyte proliferation, an inhibition of cytokine production, and a reduction in natural killer (NK) cell activity. Despite these alterations in immune functions, it has been reported that olive oil–rich diets are not as immunosuppressive as fish oil diets. An important aspect in immunonutrition is focused on the relationship between fats, the immune system, and host resistance to infection, particularly when these nutrients are supplied to persons at risk of sepsis. Different studies have determined that olive oil–rich diets do not impair the host resistance to infection. Therefore, olive oil constitutes a suitable fat that may be applied in clinical nutrition and administered to critically ill persons.

Data from Puertollano MA et al: *Br J Nutr* 98(Suppl 1):S54-S58, 2007.

an ACTH level is not recommended. Deep vein thrombosis prophylaxis is also important.[3]

Scientific knowledge gained about MODS and inflammatory mediators has led to many investigational therapies. Recombinant human-activated protein C has been found to be effective in the treatment of severe sepsis.[17] Novel molecular approaches targeting a variety of interdependent mediators of MODS are being investigated.[34]

BURNS

Major thermal injury is a source of massive tissue injury and destruction that has wide-reaching effects on virtually all organ systems. **Burn** is a generic term used to describe cutaneous injury resulting from thermal, chemical, or electrical environmental causes. In addition to cutaneous injury, burns are often associated with smoke inhalation injury or other traumatic injuries that aggravate the local and systemic problems of burns. Pulmonary injury, both primary and secondary, is common and often calls for ventilator support. The use of tracheostomy also has been examined.[46,47] This model of multisystem injury provides an opportunity to examine the interaction of shock, inflammation, and immunocompromise in a clinical setting.

Epidemiology and Etiology

The incidence of burns in the United States has dropped from 4.2 cases per 100,000 from 1961 through 1964 to 1.5 per 100,000 from 1993 through 1996.[48] Deaths from fire-related injuries are estimated to be 5000 annually in the United States. Deaths from burn injuries decreased more than 50% from 9000 in 1971[49] to 4000 in 2005.[50] This remarkable progress is the result of several factors, including an increased national focus on fire safety and burn prevention, the establishment of regional burn centers, the use of smoke detectors, regulation of consumer product safety, and occupational safety mandates. A decrease in hospitalization reflects a shift to outpatient care and improved prehospital and emergency treatment. Burn assessment and delivery of care can be improved[51] to reduce medical transport and treatment costs.

The causes of burn injury may be **thermal** or **nonthermal,** such as chemical, electrical, or radioactive. Thermal burns may result from thermal contact, flame, or scald. Adherent materials (e.g., asphalt, tar, or plastic) may likewise produce a serious contact burn. Chemical injuries are a result of contact with substances that are directly toxic to skin or the lining of the respiratory or alimentary tract. Such chemicals are often acid, alkali, or organic agents, termed **vesicants,** that cause blistering of the epithelial surfaces. Electrical burns may be the result of the conduction of electrical current through the body and the resultant heating of tissue, or flash over the body surface associated with an electrical discharge. Quality of life can be affected but, by self-reports, may exceed normal population averages with proper intervention.[52]

Burn Wound Depth

The classification of **burn wound depth** is usually based on the physical appearance and the symptoms associated with the affected skin. The definitive diagnosis is determined by the histologic depth of tissue necrosis. Such evaluation, unfortunately, necessitates a skin biopsy. Because of the invasive nature of biopsy, clinical depth assessment is used, and the ultimate fate of the wound determines final diagnosis. Advances in laser Doppler technology have resulted in extensive exploration of noninvasive means for burn wound depth assessment.[53-65]

First-degree burns are a **partial-thickness injury** involving only the epidermis and no injury to the underlying dermal or subcutaneous tissue (Table 46-3). The skin maintains water vapor and bacterial barrier functions. Many sunburns are first-degree injuries caused by exposure of skin to ultraviolet radiation from the sun. Initially there is local pain and erythema, but no blisters appear until after about 24 hours. An extensive first-degree burn may cause systemic responses such as chills, headache, localized edema, and nausea or vomiting. Therapy consists of intravenous hydration until the nausea and vomiting subside 24 to 72 hours after burn injury. Comfort measures for previously healthy children or adults with extensive first-degree burns consist of aspirin for adults or acetaminophen (controversial) for children every 4 hours in age-appropriate doses and frequent application of a water-soluble lotion. First-degree burns heal in 3 to 5 days without scarring.

Second-degree burns describe two categories of burn depth with markedly different characteristics. Both of these are partial-thickness injuries, but they evoke vastly different responses. The hallmark of **superficial partial-thickness injury** is the appearance of thin-walled, fluid-filled blisters that develop within just a few minutes after injury. Another dominant characteristic of superficial injury is pain. As blisters break or are removed, nerve endings are exposed to air (Figure 46-9). Tactile and pain sensors remain intact throughout healing, with each wound care procedure causing substantial pain. Wounds heal in 3 to 4 weeks if the individual is adequately nourished and no complications develop (Figure 46-10). Scar formation is unusual with this injury. The amount of scarring that develops is a genetically determined trait and is not predictable during the early course of treatment.

Deep partial-thickness burns involve the entire dermis, sparing skin appendages such as hair follicles and sweat glands (see Table 46-3). The burn often looks waxy white and is surrounded by margins of superficial partial-thickness injury. The injury is often clinically indistinguishable from a full-thickness injury (Figure 46-11), but by 7 to 10 days after burn injury, skin buds and hair will appear from hair follicles, indicating that skin appendages remain. These wounds take weeks to heal, and therapy consists of surgical removal of the burn wound (excision) followed by application of the person's own unburned skin from another body area (autograft). Wounds that heal slowly produce more scar tissue and continue to be a potential source of infection until closed. In the presence of relative surgical contraindications, such as cardiopulmonary failure,

Table 46-3	Depth of Burn Injury			
		Second Degree		**Third Degree**
Characteristic	**First Degree**	**Superficial Partial Thickness**	**Deep Partial Thickness**	**Full Thickness**
Morphology	Destruction of epidermis only	Destruction of epidermis and some dermis	Destruction of epidermis and dermis, leaving only skin appendages	Destruction of epidermis, dermis, and underlying subcutaneous tissue
Skin function	Intact	Absent	Absent	Absent
Tactile and pain sensors	Intact	Intact	Intact but diminished	Absent
Blisters	Present only after first 24 hr	Present within minutes, thin walled and fluid filled	May appear as fluid-filled blisters; often is layer of flat, dehydrated "tissue paper" that lifts off in sheets	Blisters rare; usually is a layer of flat, dehydrated "tissue paper" that lifts off easily
Appearance of wound after initial débridement	Skin peels at 24-48 hr, normal or slightly red underneath	Red to pale ivory, moist surface	Mottled with areas of waxy white, dry surface	White, cherry red, or black; may contain visible thrombosed veins; dry, hard leathery surface
Healing time	3-5 days	21-28 days	30 days to many months	Will not heal; may close from edges as secondary healing if wound is small
Scarring	None	May be present; low incidence influenced by genetic predisposition	Highest incidence because of slow healing rate promoting scar tissue development; also influenced by genetic predisposition	Skin graft; scarring minimized by early excision and grafting; influenced by genetic predisposition

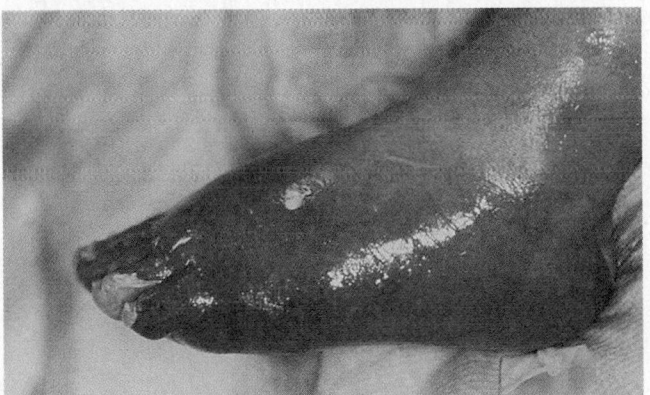

Figure 46-9 Superficial partial-thickness injury. Scald injury following débridement of overlying blister and nonadherent epithelium. (Courtesy Intermountain Burn Center, University of Utah.)

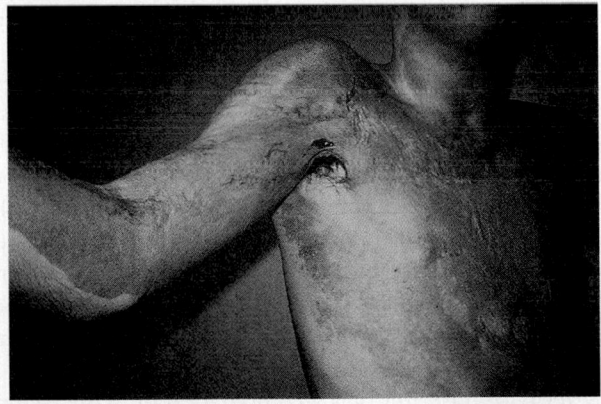

Figure 46-10 Axillary burn scar contracture. Note the blanching of the anterior axillary fold and small ulceration, both indicating the diminished range of motion. (Courtesy Intermountain Burn Center, University of Utah.)

deep partial-thickness wounds are not surgically treated but are allowed to heal from primary intention. The ultimate healing of deep partial-thickness burns commonly results in hypertrophic scarring with poor functional and cosmetic results.

Third-degree burns, or **full-thickness injuries,** involve destruction of the entire epidermis, dermis, and often the underlying subcutaneous tissue (see Table 46-3). On occasion, all underlying subcutaneous tissue is destroyed and muscle or bone may be involved. Full-thickness wounds often appear

relatively innocuous when their color is white and the delineation between normal and burned skin is not accompanied by a marked color change. Elasticity of the dermis is absent, leaving the wound dry and leathery in appearance and texture (Figure 46-12). As marked edema forms, distal circulation may be compromised in areas of circumferential burns. An **escharotomy** (cutting through burned skin) is performed to release underlying pressure. Full-thickness burns are painless because all nerve endings have been destroyed by the injury.

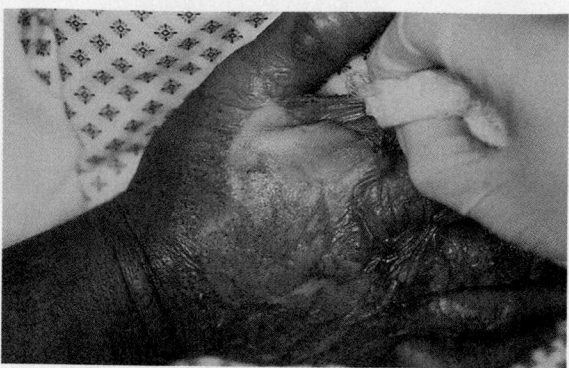

Figure 46-11 **Deep partial-thickness wound.** Note pale appearance and minimal exudate. (Courtesy Intermountain Burn Center, University of Utah.)

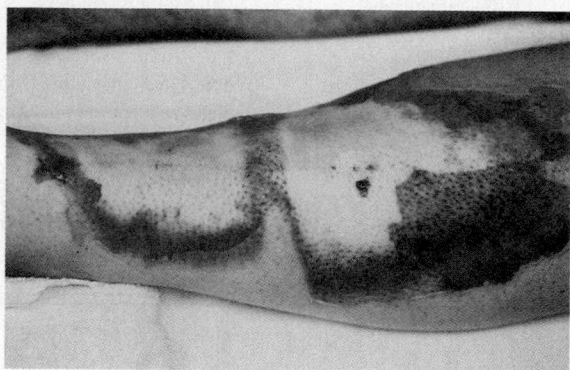

Figure 46-12 **Full-thickness thermal injury.** The wound is dry and insensate. (Courtesy Intermountain Burn Center, University of Utah.)

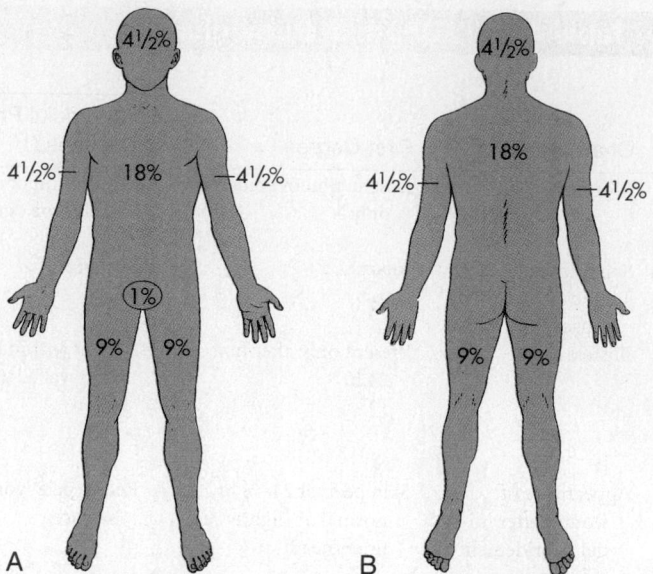

Figure 46-13 **Rule of nines.** A commonly used assessment tool with estimates of the percentages (in multiples of 9) of the total body surface area burned. A, Adults (anterior view). B, Adults (posterior view).

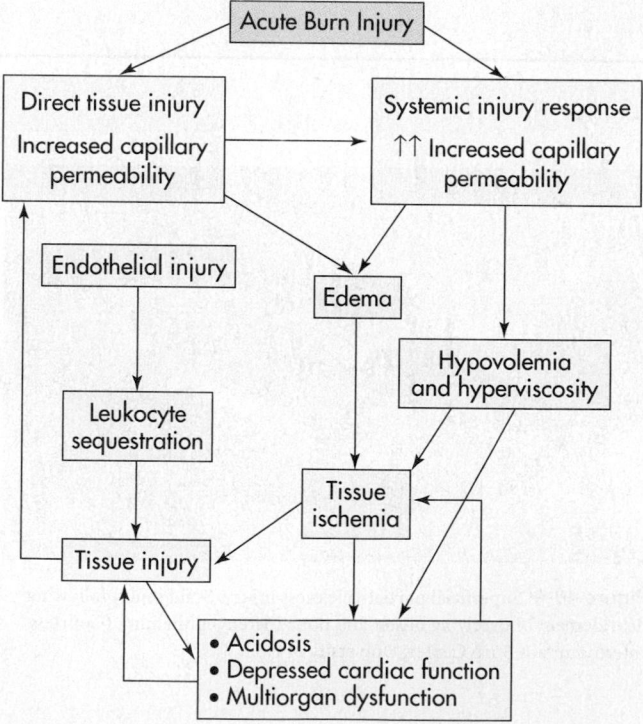

Figure 46-14 Immediate cellular and immunologic alterations of burn shock.

The extent of the **total body surface area (TBSA)** burn is estimated using the "rule of nines" (Figure 46-13). Areas of partial-thickness and full-thickness injury are marked on the diagram in Figure 46-14. First-degree burns are not included in the TBSA estimate. The surface area of the palm, including palmar finger surface, averages 1% of the body surface area over a wide range of ages; thus it can be used to estimate burn areas of irregular size and shape.[66]

Severity of burn injury is a combination of many factors, including age, medical history, extent and depth of injury, and body area involved. The American Burn Association has defined criteria to assist healthcare professionals in identifying individuals who require care at a specialized burn center (Box 46-3). The multidisciplinary burn center is recommended for those persons who are at high risk for morbidity, mortality, or permanent functional loss.

PATHOPHYSIOLOGY AND CLINICAL MANIFESTATIONS Burn injury results in dramatic changes in many physiologic functions of the body within the first few minutes after the event. The effect of burn depends on two factors: first, the extent of body surface involved and, second, the depth of cutaneous injury. Body surface burn extent is described by the percentage of TBSA injured. Burns exceeding

20% of TBSA in most adults are major burn injuries and are associated with massive evaporative water losses and flux of large amounts of fluid and electrolytes in the tissues, manifested as generalized edema and circulatory hypovolemia. Depth of cutaneous injury has been categorized in many ways but always depends on the severity of injury of epidermal and dermal elements of the skin and whether the alteration is a permanent or reversible injury.

With a major burn injury, a systemic pathophysiology ensues that requires therapeutic intervention to sustain life. The immediate (acute) physiologic consequences of major burn injury centers around the profound, life-threatening hypovolemic shock occurring in conjunction with cellular and immunologic disruption within a few hours of injury (see Figure 46-14). **Burn shock** consists of a hypovolemic cardiovascular component and a cellular component.

Hypovolemia associated with burn shock results from massive fluid losses from the circulating blood volume. The losses are caused by an increase in capillary permeability that persists for approximately 24 hours after burn injury. **Fluid resuscitation** is the administration of intravenous fluids, such as lactated Ringer solution, in an effort to restore the circulating blood volume during the period of increasing capillary permeability. In addition to hypovolemia, most other organ systems are affected. Cardiac contractility is diminished during the initial 24-hour resuscitation period with shunting of blood away from the liver, kidney, and gut. This is often termed the *ebb phase* of the response to trauma and can be seen with other severe injuries. Normal blood volume does not result in restoration of normal cardiac output because of a phenomenon known as *myocardial depression* (see MODS). The decrease in perfusion of viscera results in a decrease in

their function. This may be an explanation for decreased gut barrier function seen in thermal injury.[67]

There also is evidence that cellular metabolism is disrupted when the burn wound is created resulting in altered cell membrane permeability and loss of normal electrolyte homeostasis. This cellular defect may be the pathophysiologic process responsible for the genesis of burn shock. Numerous circulating factors in burn serum may play a role in these cellular processes. Although the cardiovascular and systemic response is intricately interwoven into the cellular response, these responses are presented here as discrete entities.

Cardiovascular and Systemic Response to Burn Injury

The clinical manifestations of burn shock are the result of more than simple loss of extracellular fluid at the burn wound site. Hypovolemia and numerous local mediators in the burn wound,[68] as well as systemic signals, result in alteration of cellular function throughout the body. The restoration of normal intravascular volume with either saline solutions or colloid materials (e.g., albumin, blood, or dextrans) does not reverse changes such as increases in pulmonary vascular resistance or myocardial contractility.[69-71] This is reflected in cardiac output with precipitous decreases that often result in inadequate perfusion of most tissues at the capillary level, which is the hallmark of burn shock. Fluid infusion does not return cardiac output to preburn levels.[72,73] These findings led to the postulation of a specific MDF.[74,75] Other causes also have been suggested, such as reactive oxygen radicals that attack cell membranes and other subcellular organelles as a result of first ischemia and then reperfusion of tissues during burn shock and resuscitation.[76] A third factor may be the level of nitric oxide after burn injury, which could have a direct myocardial depressant effect.[77,78] The relationship of nitric oxide and myocardial function is not yet totally clear. Gamelli and colleagues[79] found nitric oxide production to be significantly depressed in burned individuals who did not survive their injuries. They postulate that nitric oxide may scavenge reactive oxygen radicals and protect tissues from oxidative injury.

Regardless of the contribution of these mechanisms, fluid resuscitation eventually results in improved outcome of a massively burned person. This resuscitation involves infusion of intravenous fluid at a rate faster than the loss of circulation vascular volume for about 24 hours from the time of burn injury and may require up to 30 L in a major burn. Resuscitation from burn shock can be accomplished using any of a number of infusion protocols, most frequently the Parkland formula.[80] Lactated Ringer solution is used because it closely approximates extracellular fluid, the repository of fluid leaving the circulatory system during this phase of extensive edema formation (Table 46-4). The use of electrolyte-free fluids, such as D_5W, results in life-threatening hypovolemia and hyponatremia. Resuscitation with hypertonic saline has been used in some medical centers but is reserved for special circumstances; its use can result in adverse outcomes.[81]

Box 46-3 Burn Unit Referral Criteria

A burn unit may treat adults or children or both.

Burn injuries that should be referred to a burn unit include the following:

1. Partial-thickness burns greater than 10% total body surface area (TBSA)
2. Burns that involve the face, hands, feet, genitalia, perineum, or major joints
3. Third-degree burns in any age group
4. Electrical burns, including lightning injury
5. Chemical burns
6. Inhalation injury
7. Burn injury in individuals with preexisting medical disorders that could complicate management, prolong recovery, or affect mortality
8. Any patients with burns and concomitant trauma (such as fractures) in which the burn injury poses the greatest risk of morbidity or mortality. In such cases, if the trauma poses the greater immediate risk, the patient's condition may be initially stabilized in a trauma center before being transferred to a burn center; physician judgment will be necessary in such situations and should be in concert with the regional medical control plan and triage protocols.
9. Burned children in hospitals without qualified personnel or equipment for the care of children
10. Burn injury in patients who will require special social, emotional, or long-term rehabilitative intervention

From *Resources for Optimal Care of the Injured Patient*: "Guidelines for the Operation of Burn Centers." Chicago, IL, 2006, Committee on Trauma, American College of Surgeons.

The massive edema associated with burn shock is inevitable with fluid resuscitation, and failure to administer resuscitation fluid results in irreversible hypovolemic shock and death. The edema occurs in unburned as well as burned areas (Figure 46-15). Edema often leads to mechanical airway obstruction, necessitating tracheal intubation, and increased severity of the interstitial pulmonary edema associated with inhalation injury.

The most reliable criterion for adequate resuscitation of burn shock is urine output. The individual in hypovolemic shock will, as a compensatory mechanism, decrease or stop urine output in an effort to preserve circulation volume. The adult receiving sufficient intravenous fluids will excrete urine amounting to 30 to 50 ml/hr; children produce 1 ml/kg/hr. If the individual does not have adequate urine output, it often indicates inadequate fluid resuscitation. The massive amount of intravenous fluid required by burned individuals during the shock phase is often intimidating to the person unfamiliar with burns. One common concern is that massive fluid administration will result in pulmonary edema. It should be remembered that the individual is in hypovolemic shock and that fluid is lost dramatically during the resuscitation period from movement to the interstitium, exudation, and evaporation.

Table 46-4	Electrolyte Content of Ringer Lactate Solution and Extracellular Fluid	
Electrolyte	**Extracellular Fluid* (mEq/L)**	**Lactated Ringer Solution† (mEq/L)**
Sodium	135-145	130
Potassium	3.2-4.5	4
Chloride	95-105	109
Lactate (bicarbonate)	24-28	28

*Normal values may vary slightly between laboratories.

†Plus 80-100 ml free water per liter.

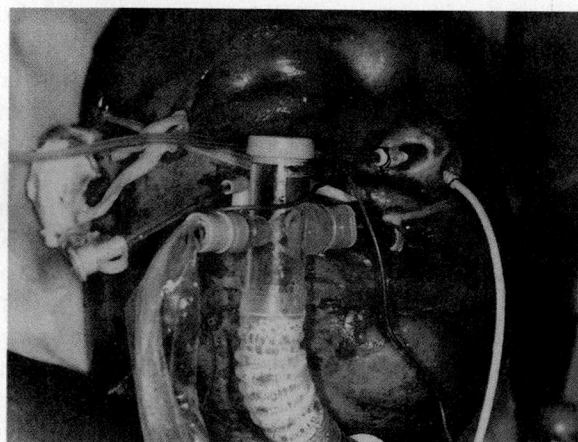

Figure 46-15 Edema related to burn injury. Superficial facial burns can result in marked swelling, requiring prompt endotracheal intubation to maintain the airway. (Courtesy Intermountain Burn Center, University of Utah.)

The endpoint of burn shock is defined as the state in which the individual is able to maintain adequate urine output for 2 hours with the intravenous fluid administration rate equal to the individual's calculated maintenance rate (Box 46-4). As burn shock ends, fluid administered remains in the circulating volume and is reflected as an increase in urine output. The mechanism whereby capillary integrity is restored is unknown but usually occurs about 24 hours after burn injury (Figure 46-16). After the individual has reached the endpoint of burn shock, the term used to describe the vascular status of the individual is **capillary seal.** In individuals with large burns, colloid-containing fluids may be given to help maintain oncotic pressure during the resuscitation phase and afterward to enhance the mobilization of interstitial fluid and diuresis.[82]

Cellular Response to Burn Injury

In addition to capillary endothelial permeability changes resulting in vascular fluid losses, transmembrane potential changes occur in cells not directly damaged by heat. The normal potential of −90 mV decreases to nearly −70 mV, with an increase in intracellular sodium and water. Such membrane potential changes may be caused by a circulating shock factor.[83] Other changes can be categorized as (1) a metabolic response to the burn injury or (2) an immunologic response to the burn injury.

Metabolic Response

The metabolic changes after a burn injury were described in 1967 by Welt and associates as "sick cell syndrome."[84] This was considered to be a cell membrane transport defect related to an alteration in the steady-state composition characterized by high intracellular concentrations of sodium. Trunkey and colleagues[85] found a marked decrease in primate muscle extracellular water and an increase in intracellular sodium and water during hypovolemic shock. In addition, other researchers demonstrated an associated decrease in resting membrane

Box 46-4	Maintenance Fluid Replacements After Major Burn Injury*

1. *Basal fluid* replacements per day
   1500 ml/day/m² body surface area = 24-hour requirements
2. Evaporative water loss from burn wound
   a. Adults: 25 + % total body surface area burn (m² body surface area) = ml/hr
   b. Children: 35 + % total body surface area burn (m² body surface area) = ml/hr
3. Total hourly maintenance fluids
   Basal fluid requirements per day ÷ 24 hours + evaporative water loss per hour = ml/hr maintenance fluids

Example: A 70-kg adult with a 50% total body surface area burn and a body surface area of 2 m requires the following:
   Basal = (1500 ml/day) (2 m² body surface area) = 3000 ml/24 hr, or 125 ml/hr
   Evaporative = (25 + 50% total body surface burn) (2m² total body surface area) = (75) (2) = 150 ml/hr
   Total maintenance fluids = 125 ml + 150 ml = 275 ml/hr

*From end of burn shock until wound closure is achieved.

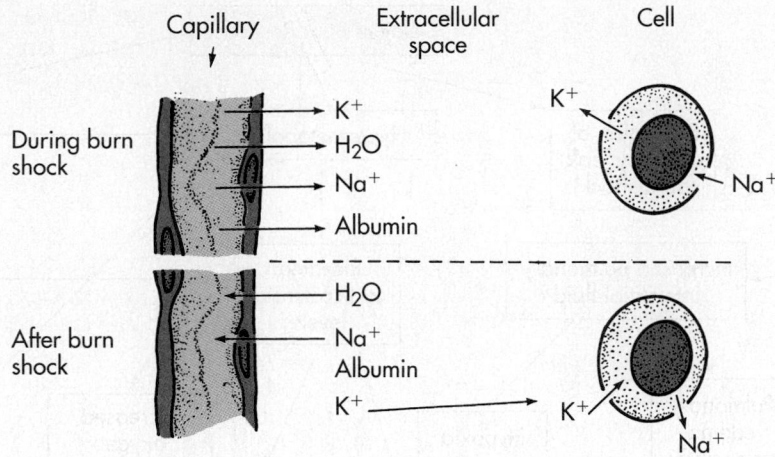

Figure 46-16 Direction of fluid and electrolyte shifts associated with burn shock. (Courtesy Intermountain Burn Center, University of Utah.)

potential, a decrease in amplitude of the action potential, and a prolongation of the repolarization and depolarization times in association with a decreased intracellular potassium concentration.[86,87] The cellular dysfunction of burn injury extends beyond the transmembrane potential disruption and the sodium-potassium pump impairment to include a loss of intracellular magnesium and phosphate[88] and elevated serum lactic dehydrogenase (LDH) levels.[89] Thus impairment of basic cellular function may be the underlying cause of the diminished membrane potentials. The data suggest a decrease in the efficiency of membrane pumps. The failure of rapid intravascular volume repletion to restore membrane potential completely suggests other pathways for cellular metabolic derangement.[90]

Metabolic reactions to the stress of a major burn injury involve the response of the sympathetic nervous system and other homeostatic regulators. Catecholamines are found in elevated amounts in both the serum and urine of burned individuals. Cortisol, glucagon, and insulin levels are elevated, with a corresponding increase in gluconeogenesis, lipolysis, and proteolysis. Changes in lipid metabolism are reflected as an elevation in plasma free fatty acids (FFA) and a decrease in plasma cholesterol and phospholipids.[91] Jeschke and colleagues[92] found that the use of propranolol, a nonselective beta$_1$- and beta$_2$-blocker, could decrease symptoms of the hypermetabolic response, including a decrease in heart rate and lipolysis. Glucose and lactate kinetics are altered after burn injury. Although tissue hypoxia produces lactic acidosis, its persistence in the presence of adequate tissue perfusion suggests an increased rate of glycogenolysis.[93]

Burn injury induces a hypermetabolic state that persists until wound closure. Wilmore and colleagues[94] described the hypermetabolic state of 20 burned individuals as unrelated to ambient temperatures, with persistent elevation of core body temperatures. The metabolic rate increased with burn size in a curvilinear relationship, with oxygen consumption rarely exceeding two times basal levels. Evaporative water loss and surface cooling are not the primary stimulus for the hypermetabolic state; rather, the hypermetabolism is related to an increase and resetting of the thermal regulatory set point. A core body temperature of 38.5° C (101.3° F) is typical. A reflex arc mobilizes neural or hormonal afferent stimuli to the hypothalamus, producing a catecholamine response clinically manifested as hypermetabolism, hyperthermia, and hyperglycemia.

Evidence also exists that the burn wound itself directly mediates the response to injury at both the local and system levels. Cytokines, oxygen radicals, chemotactic substances, and eicosanoids contribute to the systemic inflammatory response and hypermetabolic state. The inflammatory response to the wound level is magnified into a generalized systemic inflammatory response that is often deleterious.[95-97] Vasodilation, increased capillary permeability, and edema occur to facilitate healing of the local area. The distribution of the peripheral circulation after burn injury transports heat and glucose preferentially to the wound. The energy cost of these reparative and transport processes is reflected in the increased metabolism and hyperdynamic circulation.

The extensive evaporative water loss that occurs in burn tissue is a heat-consuming process, and the energy of evaporation is provided by increased visceral heat production. The signal for the response is unknown because individuals whose wounds have been denervated continue to have a **posttraumatic hypermetabolic response.** Hypothalamic function alterations result in the elevation of human growth hormone (hGH) serum levels in the presence of hyperglycemia, a finding opposite that in normal states.[94] Further, the hypermetabolic rate is not decreased during rest, sleep, or warmth.

Evidence of hepatic response to burn injury is characterized by alterations in the clotting factors.[98] A hypercoagulable state develops as manifested by an elevated plasma fibrinogen concentration in the presence of shortened prothrombin time (PT) and activated partial thromboplastin time (PTT).[99]

In summary, extensive burn injury initiates the most marked alterations in body metabolism associated with any

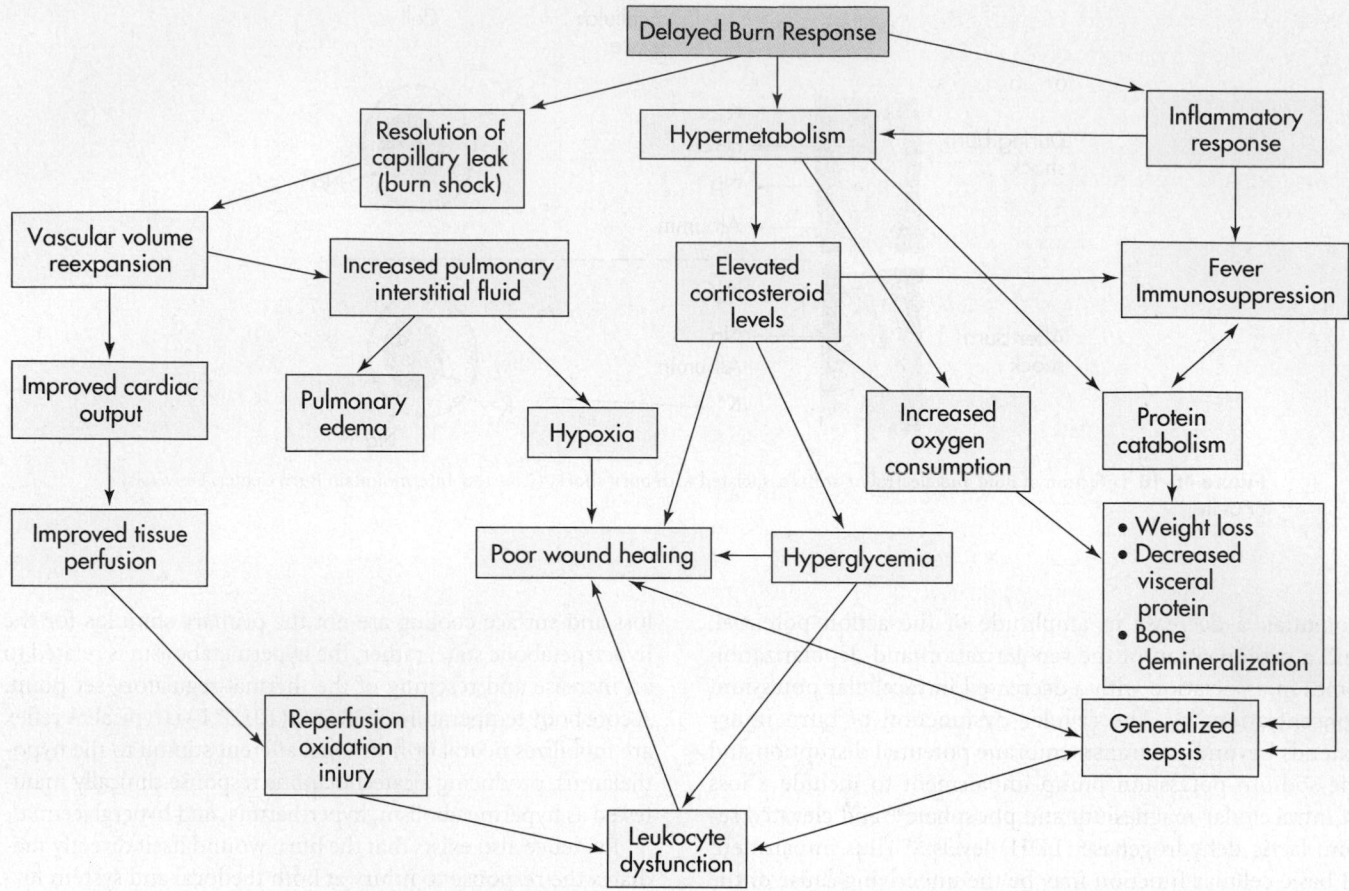

Figure 46-17 Physiologic alterations in inflammatory burn injury response.

illness (Figure 46-17). Much of the work explaining this response has been conducted by Wilmore,[100,101] who reported that the persistent tachycardia, hyperpnea, hyperpyrexia, and marked body wasting seen in burn injury reflect heightened metabolic activity and accelerated body catabolism. The development of decreased bone density can last long after discharge from the hospital.[102] These system alterations occur as a result of the cutaneous inflammatory process and are thought to facilitate wound repair. The neural component of this alteration is in response to a sympathetic reaction that releases catecholamines in large amounts.

Immunologic Response

The immunologic response to burn injury is immediate, prolonged, and severe. The result in individuals surviving burn shock is immunosuppression with increased susceptibility to potentially fatal systemic burn wound sepsis.

Several cytokines have been identified in the immediate postburn period. IL-1 is detected in the serum of burned individuals. The level of IL-1 correlates inversely with burn survival; low levels may be associated with a higher mortality.[103] Fatal burn injury has often shown decreased levels of IL-2, which may result in decreased T helper 1 (Th-1) lymphocytes. Th-1 cells produce IL-2, interferon-gamma, and TNF, which help to initiate cellular immunity and immunoglobulin G (IgG) production. IL-4 is elevated after burn injuries

and causes a shift in the T helper cell production from Th-1 to Th-2 lymphocytes. Th-2 cells secrete IL-4, which promotes further conversion of nonspecific Th cells to Th-2 cells. Th-2 cells also produce other cytokines and antibodies.[104] IL-6 levels increase quickly after burn injury and remain elevated for several weeks. The level of IL-6 correlates with the extent of burn injury.[105] IL-6, together with platelet-activating factor, activates polymorphonuclear neutrophils (PMNs), causing infiltration of neutrophils into burned tissue and adhesion to vascular endothelial surfaces.[106,107] IL-8 levels are elevated after burn injury, with significantly greater elevations in individuals with a TBSA burn of 40% or higher. IL-8 activity may play a role in the strong and persistent activation of neutrophils noted in people with large burns.[108] Burn blister fluid contains large amounts of IL-6 and IL-8 in addition to substances such as epidermal growth factor, platelet-derived growth factor, and TGF.[109]

Macrophages, platelets, neutrophils, and vascular endothelial cells release prostaglandins and leukotrienes, which are the byproducts of arachidonic acid metabolism. These chemical mediators cause peripheral vasodilation, pulmonary vasoconstriction, increased capillary permeability, and local tissue ischemia in the burn wound.

A host of chemicals found in burn plasma in altered concentrations also may play a role in burn shock. These include vasoactive amines (histamine, serotonin), products of complement activation (C3a, C5a), prostaglandins, kinins, endotoxin, and metabolic hormones (catecholamines, glucocorticoids). A decrease in complement components C3a and C5a in the circulation after burn injury suggests a nonspecific activation of the complement system.[110] Activation of the complement system in injured tissue results in an inflammatory response caused by release of histamine and serotonin by C3a and C5a, because histamine and serotonin alter capillary permeability and participate in the mechanism of burn shock along with kinin polypeptides and other chemical mediators. Prostaglandins function in the inflammatory process by regulating metabolism of cells of inflammation (see Chapter 6).

Burn shock can induce changes in the integrity of the intestinal wall, facilitating bacterial translocation and endotoxemia.[111] Bacterial translocation from the gut may be a mechanism of infection leading to septic shock after burn injury and other major trauma.[112] Circulating endotoxin is correlated with the development of MODS and death after major burn injury.[113]

White blood cells are also altered at this time, when their need to inhibit sepsis is vital. Natural resistance to infection in burn wounds is a function of the nonspecific immune system; that is, resistance to microorganisms that infect wounds rests almost solely on the ability of phagocytic cells (i.e., granulocytes, macrophages) to leave the bloodstream, migrate to the site of infection, and ingest and kill microorganisms.[114] Normally, opsonins render bacteria susceptible to phagocytosis, but the burn injury triggers a consumptive opsoninopathy. Burn serum contains an inhibitor of C3 conversion that leads to decreased opsonization and PMN dysfunction.[115,116]

Individuals with altered immunocompetence before burn injury are at additional risk for complications. Opportunistic infections, such as fungal sepsis, can increase hospital stay and ICU costs.[117] At risk individuals are those at the extremes of age and those with cardiac disease, malnutrition, immunodeficiency disease, and a history of alcohol or drug abuse.[118,119] Additional risk factors include diabetes mellitus and pulmonary or renal dysfunction.

Evaporative Water Loss

One of the major purposes of intact skin is to serve as a barrier to evaporative water loss (EWL) from the body. With major burn injury, this ability of the skin to regulate evaporative water loss is totally disrupted. In a classic study done in 1962, Moncrief and Mason[120] attempted to determine the magnitude of such a loss and determined that daily evaporative water loss was in the range of 20 times normal in the early phase of injury, with gradual decreases as wound closure is achieved. Further studies indicated that insensible water loss through burned skin is not from evaporation of water from sweat glands but rather from water vapor formed within the body and lost through the skin.[121,122]

Calculation of the amount of fluid lost by evaporative water loss includes losses from all sources. Normally the skin is the major source of insensible loss (75%) and the lungs

are minor sources of loss (25%), with a total loss of only approximately 600 to 800 ml/day. This changes dramatically with burns, because not only does skin loss increase but also lung loss increases by hypermetabolism and hyperventilation, especially in an intubated individual. Total evaporative losses exceed many liters per day in an adult with large burn wounds. Replacement of the loss is mandatory to prevent volume deficit.

EVALUATION AND TREATMENT Burn recovery is long and stormy, with complications the rule rather than the exception. The goal of burn management is wound closure in a manner that promotes survival. Scar formation with contractures is often a consequence of healing in deep partial-thickness and full-thickness burns (Figure 46-18). Assessment of tissue viability can be difficult in complex extremity injury; pyrophosphate nuclear scanning can assist in evaluation.[123]

The three essential elements of survival of major burn injury are (1) meticulous wound management, (2) adequate fluids and nutrition, and (3) early surgical excision and grafting. Therapy for deep partial- and full-thickness burn injury includes surgical removal of the burn tissue (excision) followed by grafting of the person's unburned skin (autograft) onto the excised wound. Satisfactory wound closure with cultured epithelial autograft (Figure 46-19) has been

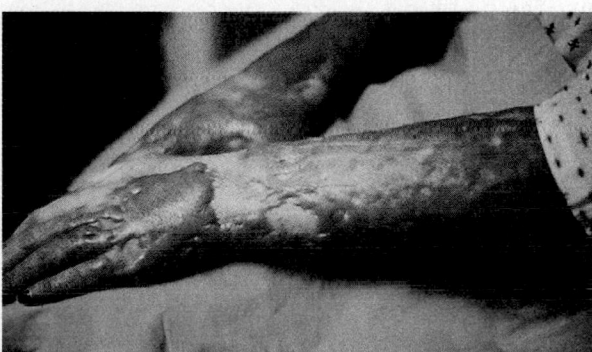

Figure 46-18 Hypertrophic scarring. Deep partial-thickness thermal injury can result in extensive hypertrophic scarring. (Courtesy Intermountain Burn Center, University of Utah.)

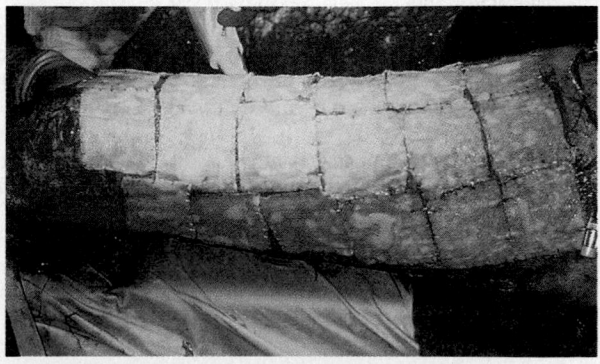

Figure 46-19 Application of cultured epithelial autografts. The thin sheets of keratinocytes are attached to gauze backing to allow application onto the clean, excised thigh. (Courtesy Intermountain Burn Center, University of Utah.)

Much of the effort in the management of individuals with massive burn wounds focuses on closure of the wound to diminish infection risks and decrease hypermetabolism associated with burns. Cadaveric allograft skin grafting, dermal matrix development, and cultured keratinocyte technology have become tools to promote this strategy. Fibrin sealant has become widely used to improve graft take, decrease blood loss, and improve cosmetic appearance. The cost and efficacy are under clinical evaluation but show promise. The traditional fibrin sealant is an aerosolized fibrin and thrombin that mixes in the aerosol and provides a hemostatic layer that adheres within a few seconds. The more recent applications for skin grafts use a mixture with one tenth the concentration of thrombin, thus affording the surgeon time to position the graft and improve the technical application in the operating room. Such advances may prove cost-effective and provide improved outcomes.

Data from Achauer BM, Miller SR, Lee TE: *J Burn Care Rehabil* 15(1):24-28, 1994; Chakravorty RC, Sosnowski KM: *Ann Plast Surg* 23(6):488-491, 1989; de Moraes AM, Annichino-Bizzacchi JM, Rossi AB: *Sao Paulo Med J* 116(4):1747-1752, 1998; Dean M, Nicholls M, Wedderburn C: *Med J Aust* 160(8):526-527, 1994; Foster K: *Surgery* 142(4 Suppl):S50-S54, 2007; Foster K et al: *J Burn Care Res* 29(2):293-303, 2008; Jeschke MG et al: *Plast Reconstr Surg* 113(2):525-530, 2004; McGill V et al: *J Burn Care Rehabil* 18(5):429-434, 1997; Ofodile FA, Sadana MK: *J Natl Med Assoc* 83(5):416-418, 1991; Ronfard V et al: *Burns* 17(3):181-184, 1991; Saltz R et al: *J Burn Care Rehabil* 10(6):504-507, 1989; Saltz R et al: *Plast Reconstr Surg* 88(6):1005-1015, 1991; Schumacher J et al: *Can J Vet Res* 60(2):158-160, 1996.

inconsistent and costly.[124,125] Early enthusiasm for synthetic dermal replacement has been tempered by a high rate of dermal graft loss and slow epidermal engraftment.[126,127] Such advancements in skin replacement technology include sheets of acellular dermal matrix that can be used with thin, meshed autografts or cultured epithelial autografts.[128,129] This concept is also being used on the donor site, and glycosaminoglycan hydrogels may supplement donor site wound dressings[130] (see What's New? Improving Skin Graft Success). Scar reduction or prevention is a challenging problem that is being addressed with pulsed-dye laser treatment.[131] Research is also directed toward therapies to modulate hypermetabolic and inflammatory responses. Nutritional therapy is focused on early enteral feeding to reduce the potential of gut-mediated sepsis. Ongoing clinical trials using anabolic agents (e.g., recombinant human growth hormone) and pharmacologic agents that modulate inflammatory and endocrine mediators (e.g., ibuprofen, propranolol) show promise in the treatment of severe burn injuries.[80] Burn pain is almost always acute, and treatment strategies usually differ from strategies for chronic pain. In addition to opioid-based agents, newer treatment approaches may include antianxiety agents, hypnosis, and relaxation techniques.[132]

SUMMARY REVIEW

Shock

1. Shock is a widespread impairment of cellular metabolism involving positive-feedback loops that places an individual on a downward physiologic spiral that, if not reversed, can lead to MODS.
2. Types of shock are cardiogenic, hypovolemic, neurogenic, anaphylactic, and septic. A newly identified type of shock, traumatic shock, combines features of hypovolemic shock and septic shock.
3. The final common pathway in all types of shock is impaired cellular metabolism—cells switch from aerobic to anaerobic metabolism. Energy stores drop, and cellular mechanisms relative to membrane permeability, action potentials, and lysozyme release fail.
4. Anaerobic metabolism results in activation of the inflammatory response, decreased circulatory volume, and decreasing pH.
5. Impaired cellular metabolism results in cellular inability to use glucose because of impaired glucose delivery or impaired glucose intake, resulting in a shift of glycogenolysis, gluconeogenesis, and lipolysis for fuel generation.
6. Glycogenolysis is affected for up to 10 hours. Gluconeogenesis results in the use of proteins necessary for structure, function, repair, and replication that leads to more impaired cellular metabolism. Lipolysis is ineffective because of a lack of transport serum proteins.
7. Gluconeogenesis contributes to lactic acid, uric acid, and ammonia buildup; interstitial edema; and impairment of the immune system, as well as general muscle weakness leading to decreased respiratory function and cardiac output.
8. Cardiogenic shock is attributable to heart failure and is characterized by a decrease in cardiac output and impaired cellular metabolism.
9. Hypovolemic shock is caused by loss of blood or fluid in large amounts. The use of compensatory mechanisms may be vigorous, but tissue perfusion ultimately decreases and results in impaired cellular metabolism.
10. Neurogenic (vasogenic) shock results from massive vasodilation, causing a relative hypovolemia (even though cardiac output may be high), and results in impaired cellular metabolism.
11. Anaphylactic shock is caused by physiologic recognition of a foreign substance. The inflammatory response is triggered, and a massive vasodilation with fluid shift into the interstitium follows. The relative hypovolemia leads to impaired cellular metabolism.
12. Septic shock begins with impaired cellular metabolism caused by uncontrolled septicemia. The infecting agent triggers the inflammatory and immune responses. It is part of a continuum known as SIRS. Mortality for septic shock is very high.

Multiple Organ Dysfunction Syndrome

1. MODS is the progressive dysfunction of two or more organ systems resulting from a systemic inflammatory response after a severe illness or injury. The inflammatory response can be triggered by sepsis, necrotic tissue, trauma, burns, ARDS, acute pancreatitis, major surgery, circulatory shock, acute renal failure, blood transfusion, heat stroke, liver failure, mesenteric ischemia, propofol infusion syndrome, persistent inflammatory foci, and other severe injuries.

2. Primary MODS is the immediate local or mild systemic response to the triggering event or illness. It primes the inflammatory system.

3. Secondary MODS is the uncontrollable, excessive systemic inflammatory response that develops after a latent period and results in organ dysfunction.

4. People at greatest risk for developing MODS are older adults, those with significant tissue injury or preexisting disease, and those in whom resuscitation from the initiating illness or injury has been delayed or inadequate.

5. Mortality from MODS is very high: 45% to 55% for failure of two organ systems, 80% for failure of three or more organ systems, and nearly 100% if the failure of three or more organs persists longer than 4 days.

6. Multiple organ dysfunction involves the stress response; release of complement, coagulation, and kinin proteins; changes in the vascular endothelium; and numerous inflammatory processes mediated by substances released by activated neutrophils and macrophages.

7. The consequences of the release of inflammatory mediators in MODS are vasodilation, increased vasopermeability, and selective vasoconstriction resulting in maldistribution of blood flow; hypermetabolism; myocardial depression; and hypoxic injury to cells. Cellular hypoxia and acidosis impair cellular metabolism, leading to organ dysfunction.

8. Clinical manifestations of the development of MODS are general during the first 24 hours: low-grade fever, tachycardia, tachypnea, dyspnea, and altered mental status. Over the next several days, beginning with the lungs, individual organ systems show signs of failure.

9. Because there is no specific therapy for MODS, early detection is extremely important so that supportive measures can be initiated as soon as possible.

10. At present the therapeutic management of MODS consists of prevention or removal of triggering mechanisms and support of individual organs. Recent scientific knowledge about inflammatory mediators has led to many promising future therapies for MODS.

Burns

1. Burns are classified according to depth and extent of injury.

2. First-degree burns involve the superficial skin without loss of protective function.

3. Second-degree burns are superficial (blister formation) or superficial involving partial skin thickness with a waxy white appearance and no involvement of dermal appendages.

4. Third-degree burns involve full skin thickness and often underlying tissues. They are painless and can be life threatening as a result of hypovolemic shock and metabolic and immunologic responses.

5. The TBSA burned is estimated using either the rule of nines or the Lund and Browder chart. Burns exceeding 20% TBSA are considered major burns.

6. Hypovolemia associated with burn shock is caused by increased capillary permeability with massive fluid losses from blood volume.

7. Altered cell membrane permeability and loss of electrolyte homeostasis contribute to burn shock.

8. Cardiac contractility is decreased during the first 24 hours with shunting of blood away from the liver, kidney, and gut.

9. Fluid resuscitation, such as with lactated Ringer solution, involves infusion of fluid at a rate faster than the loss of circulating volume.

10. The most reliable criterion for adequate resuscitation of burn shock is urine output.

11. Capillary seal is the term used to indicate the end of burn shock.

12. Transmembrane potentials are altered in cells not directly damaged by heat, with impairment of the sodium-potassium pump and loss of magnesium and phosphate.

13. The stress of a major burn activates the sympathetic nervous system with release of catecholamines, cortisol, glucagon, and insulin.

14. Burn injury produces a hypermetabolic state that persists until wound closure and is related to a higher thermal regulatory set point.

15. The local inflammatory response at the burn site releases cytokines, oxygen radicals, chemotactic factors, and eicosanoids, which leads to a systemic inflammatory response and contributes to hypermetabolism.

16. A posttraumatic hypermetabolic response is associated with increased visceral heat production.

17. Alterations in clotting factors produce a hypercoagulable state following major burns.

18. The immune response following a burn is immediate, prolonged, and severe.

19. Numerous alterations in inflammatory cytokines are evident in the immediate burn period, affecting cellular immunity, antibody production, and attraction of neutrophils and contributing to the vasodilation and increased capillary permeability associated with burn shock.

20. White blood cells are altered, and there is decreased opsonization and phagocytosis, contributing to the development of sepsis.

21. Changes in intestinal wall integrity lead to translocation of bacteria, endotoxemia, and septic shock.

22. Loss of intact skin with a major burn results in significant evaporative water loss contributing to hypovolemia.

23. Treatment of major burns involves meticulous wound management, adequate fluids and nutrition, early surgical excision and grafting, modulation of the hypermetabolic state, and pain management.

KEY TERMS

Acute Physiology and Chronic Health Evaluation II and III (APACHE II and APACHE III), 1713
Anaphylactic shock, 1702
Burn, 1714
Burn shock, 1717
Burn wound depth, 1714
Capillary seal, 1718
Cardiogenic shock, 1699
Deep partial-thickness burn, 1714
Escharotomy, 1715
First-degree burn, 1714

Fluid resuscitation, 1717
Full-thickness injury, 1715
Gut hypothesis, 1711
Hypermetabolism, 1711
Hypovolemic shock, 1701
Maldistribution of blood flow, 1711
Multiple organ dysfunction syndrome (MODS), 1707
Myocardial depression, 1711
Neurogenic shock (vasogenic shock), 1702
Nonthermal injury, 1714
Partial-thickness injury, 1714

Posttraumatic hypermetabolic response, 1719
Primary MODS, 1707
Secondary MODS, 1708
Second-degree burn, 1714
Septic shock, 1703
Shock, 1696
Superficial partial-thickness injury, 1714
Supply-dependent oxygen consumption, 1711
Thermal injury, 1714
Third-degree burn, 1715
Total body surface area (TBSA), 1716
Vesicants, 1714

REFERENCES

1. Garcia A: Critical care issue in the early management of severe trauma, *Surg Clin North Am* 86(6):1359-1387, 2006.
2. Cunneen J, Cartwright M: The puzzle of sepsis: fitting the pieces of the inflammatory response with treatment, *AACN Clin Issues* 15(1):18-44, 2004.
3. Topalian S, Ginsberg F, Parrillo J: Cardiogenic shock, *Crit Care Med* 36(1):S66-S77, 2008.
4. Jackson C, Boenau IB: How to recognize cardiogenic shock, *Emerg Med* 39(10):11-19, 2007.
5. Babaev A et al: Trends in management and outcomes of patients with acute myocardial infarction complicated by cardiogenic shock, *JAMA* 294(4):448-454, 2005.
6. Hochman J et al: Early revascularization and long-term survival in cardiogenic shock complicating acute myocardial infarction, *JAMA* 295(21):2511-2515, 2006.
7. Omland T: Advances in congestive heart failure management in the intensive care unit: b-type natriuretic peptides in evaluation of acute heart failure, *Crit Care Med* 36(1):S17-S27, 2008.
8. Russell J: Vasopressin versus norepinephrine infusion in patients with septic shock, *N Engl J Med* 358(9):877-887, 2008.
9. Holmes CL, Walley KR: The evaluation and management of shock, *Clin Chest Med* 24(4):775-789, 2003.
10. Bone RC et al: Definitions for sepsis and organ failure and guidelines for the use of innovative therapies in sepsis. The ACCP/SCCM Consensus Conference Committee, *Chest* 101(6):1644-1655, 1992.
11. Levy MM et al: 2001 SCCM/ESICM/ACCP/ATS/SIS International Sepsis Definition Conference, *Crit Care Med* 31(4):1250-1256, 2003.
12. Calandra T, Cohen J: The international sepsis forum consensus conference on definitions of infection in the intensive care unit, *Crit Care Med* 33(7):1538-1548, 2005.
13. Wenzel RP: Health care-associated infections: major issues in the early years of the 21st century, *Clin Infect Dis* 15(45-Suppl 1):S85-S88, 2007.
14. Albrecht SJ et al: Reemergence of gram-negative health care-associated bloodstream infections, *Arch Intern Med* 166(12):1289-1294, 2006.
15. Kleinpell RM, Graves BT, Ackerman MH: Incidence, pathogenesis, and management of sepsis: an overview, *AACN Adv Crit Care* 17(4): 385-393, 2006.
16. Papathanassoglou ED et al: Association of proinflammatory molecules with apoptotic markers and survival in critically ill multiple organ dysfunction patients, *Biol Res Nurs* 5(2):129-141, 2003.
17. Dellinger RP et al: Surviving sepsis campaign: international guidelines for management of severe sepsis and septic shock: 2008, *Intensive Care Med* 31(1):17-60, 2008.
18. Cross AS et al: Development of an anti-core lipopolysaccharide vaccine for the prevention and treatment of sepsis, *Vaccine* 22(7):812-817, 2004.
19. Cinel I, Dellinger RP: Advances in pathogenesis and management of sepsis, *Curr Opin Infect Dis* 20(4):345-352, 2007.
20. Honoré PM, Joannes-Boyau O, Gressens B: Blood and plasma treatments: the rationale of high-volume hemofiltration, *Contrib Nephrol* 156:387-395, 2007.
21. Baue AE: Multiple, progressive or sequential system failure: a syndrome for the 70's, *Arch Surg* 110(7):779-781, 1975.

22. Tilney NL, Bailey GL, Morgan AP: Sequential system failure after rupture of abdominal aortic aneurysm: an unsolved problem in postoperative care, *Ann Surg* 178(2):117-122, 1973.
23. Awad SS: State-of-the-art therapy for severe sepsis and multisystem organ dysfunction, *Am J Surg* 186(Suppl):23S-30S, 2003.
24. Cook R et al: Multiple organ dysfunction: baseline and serial component scores, *Crit Care Med* 29(11):2046-2050, 2001.
25. Rotstein OD: Modeling the two-hit hypothesis for evaluating strategies to prevent organ injury after shock/resuscitation, *J Trauma* 54(5 Suppl):S203-S206, 2003.
26. Brown MJ et al: The systemic inflammatory response syndrome, organ failure, and mortality after abdominal aortic aneurysm repair, *J Vasc Surg* 37(3):600-606, 2003.
27. Aird WC: The role of the endothelium in severe sepsis & MODS, *Blood* 101:3756-3777, 2003.
28. Vanhorebeek I, Van den Berghe G: The neuroendocrine response to critical illness is a dynamic process, *Crit Care Clin* 22(1):1-15, 2006.
29. van Meurs M et al: Early organ-specific endothelial activation during hemorrhagic shock and resuscitation, *Shock* 29(2):291-299, 2008.
30. Brown KA et al: Neutrophils in development of multiple organ failure in sepsis, *Lancet* 8(368):157-169, 2006.
31. Baue AE: Mediators or markers of injury, inflammation, and infection (harbingers of doom or predictors of disaster) and biologic puzzles or ambiguities, *Arch Surg* 142(1):89-93, 2007.
32. Maier RV: Pathogenesis of multiple organ dysfunction syndrome—endotoxin, inflammatory cells, and their mediators: cytokines and reactive oxygen species, *Surg Infect (Larchmt)* 1(3):197-204, 2000.
33. Rankin JA: Biological mediators of acute inflammation, *AACN Clin Issues* 15(1):3-17, 2004.
34. Matsuda N, Hattori Y: Systemic inflammatory response syndrome (SIRS): molecular pathophysiology and gene therapy, *J Pharmacol Sci* 101(3):189-198, 2006.
35. Deitch EA, Xu D, Kaise VL: Role of the gut in the development of injury- and shock-induced SIRS and MODS: the gut-lymph hypothesis, a review, *Front Biosci* 1(11):520-528, 2006.
36. Magnotti LJ, Deitch EA: Burns, bacterial translocation, gut barrier function, and failure, *J Burn Care Rehabil* 26(5):383-391, 2005.
37. Dixon B: The role of microvascular thrombosis in sepsis, *Anaesth Intensive Care* 32(5):619-629, 2004.
38. Di Giantomasso D, May CN, Bellomo R: Vital organ blood flow during hyperdynamic sepsis, *Chest* 124(3):1053-1059, 2003.
39. Merx MW, Weber C: Sepsis and the heart, *Circulation* 116(7):793-802, 2007.
40. Kumar A et al: Myocardial dysfunction in septic shock: part II. role of cytokines and nitric oxide, *J Cardiothorac Vasc Anesth* 15(4):485-511, 2001.
41. Pettila V et al: Comparison of multiple organ dysfunction scores in the prediction of hospital mortality in the critically ill, *Crit Care Med* 30(8):1705-1711, 2002.
42. Blot SI et al: Clinical and economic outcomes in critically ill patients with nosocomial catheter-related bloodstream infections, *Clin Infect Dis* 41(11):1591-1598, 2005.
43. Rivers EP et al: Early goal-directed therapy in the treatment of severe sepsis and septic shock, *N Engl J Med* 345:1368-1377, 2001.

44. The Acute Respiratory Distress Syndrome Network: Ventilation with lower tidal volumes as compared with traditional tidal volumes for acute lung injury and the acute respiratory distress syndrome, *N Engl J Med* 342:1301-1308, 2000.

45. Van den Berghe G et al: Intensive insulin therapy in the critically ill patients, *N Engl J Med* 345:1359-1367, 2001.

46. Caruso DM et al: Rationale for "early" percutaneous dilatational tracheostomy in patients with burn injuries, *J Burn Care Rehabil* 18(5):424-428, 1997.

47. Saffle JR, Morris SE, Edelman L: Early tracheostomy does not improve outcome in burn patients, *J Burn Care Rehabil* 23(6):431-438, 2002.

48. Clark DE, Dainiak CN, Reeder S: Decreasing incidence of burn injury in a rural state, *Ing Prev* 6(40):259-262, 2000.

49. Brigham PA, McLoughlin E: Burn incidence and medical care use in the United States: estimates, trends, and data sources, *J Burn Care Rehabil* 17(2):95-107, 1996.

50. American Burn Association: *Burn incidence and treatment in the U.S.: 2007 Fact Sheet,* 2007. Available at www.ameriburn.org/resources_factsheet.php. Accessed September 28, 2008.

51. Saffle JR, Edelman L, Morris SE: Regional air transport of burn patients: a case for telemedicine? *J Trauma* 57(1):57-64, 2004.

52. Cochran A et al: Self-reported quality of life after electrical and thermal injury, *J Burn Care Rehabil* 25(1):61-66, 2004.

53. Altintas MA et al: Differentiation of superficial-partial vs. deep-partial thickness burn injuries in vivo by confocal-laser-scanning microscopy, *Burns* 35(1):80-86, 2009.

54. Braue EH Jr et al: Noninvasive methods for determining lesion depth from vesicant exposure, *J Burn Care Res* 28(2):275-285, 2007.

55. Chiu T, Burd A: Laboratory assessment of burn depth, *Plast Reconstr Surg* 119(2):751-752, 2007.

56. Cross KM et al: Clinical utilization of near-infrared spectroscopy devices for burn depth assessment, *Wound Repair Regen* 15(3):332-340, 2007.

57. Devgan L et al: Modalities for the assessment of burn wound depth, *J Burns Wounds* 5:c2, 2006.

58. Hoeksema H et al: Accuracy of early burn depth assessment by laser Doppler imaging on different days post burn, *Burns* 35(1):36-45, 2009.

59. Kassira W, Namias N: Outpatient management of pediatric burns, *J Craniofac Surg* 19(4):1007-1009, 2008.

60. Mandal A: Burn wound depth assessment—is laser Doppler imaging the best measurement tool available? *Int Wound J* 3(2):138-143, 2006.

61. McGill DJ et al: Assessment of burn depth: a prospective, blinded comparison of laser Doppler imaging and videomicroscopy, *Burns* 33(7):833-842, 2007.

62. Monstrey S et al: Assessment of burn depth and burn wound healing potential, *Burns* 34(6):761-769, 2008.

63. Ng D et al: The use of laser Doppler imaging for burn depth assessment after application of flammacerium, *Burns* 33(3):396-397, 2007.

64. Renkielska A et al: Burn depths evaluation based on active dynamic IR thermal imaging—a preliminary study, *Burns* 32(7):867-875, 2006.

65. Tehrani H et al: Spectrophotometric intracutaneous analysis: a novel imaging technique in the assessment of acute burn depth, *Ann Plast Surg* 61(4):437-440, 2008.

66. Sheridan RL et al: Planimetry study of the percent of body surface represented by the hand and palm: sizing irregular burns is more accurately done with the palm, *J Burn Care Rehabil* 16(6):605-606, 1995.

67. Morris SE, Navaratnam N, Herndon DN: A comparison of effects of thermal injury and smoke inhalation on bacterial translocation, *J Trauma* 30(6):639-643, 1990.

68. Arturson G: Forty years in burns research—the postburn inflammatory response, *Burns* 26(7):599-604, 2000.

69. Baxter CR, Cook WA, Shires GT: Serum myocardial depressant factor of burn shock, *Surg Forum* 17:1-2, 1966.

70. Demling RH, Will JA, Belzer FO: Effect of major thermal injury on the pulmonary microcirculation, *Surgery* 83(6):746-751, 1978.

71. Horton JW et al: Calcium antagonists improve cardiac mechanical performance after thermal trauma, *J Surg Res* 87(1):39-50, 1999.

72. Aikawa N, Martyn JA, Burke JF: Pulmonary artery catheterization and thermodilution cardiac output determination in the management of critically burned patients, *Am J Surg* 135(6):811-817, 1978.

73. Dobson EL, Warner GF: Factors concerned in the early stages of thermal shock, *Circ Res* 5(1):69-74, 1957.

74. Lefer AM, Martin J: Origin of myocardial depressant factor in shock, *Am J Physiol* 218(5):1423-1442, 1970.

75. Rosenthal SR, Hawley PL, Hakim AA: Purified burn toxic factor and its competition, *Surgery* 71(4):527-536, 1972.

76. Horton JW, Burton KP, White DJ: The role of toxic oxygen metabolites in a young model of thermal injury, *J Trauma* 39(3):563-569, 1995.

77. Onuoha G, Alpar K, Jones I: Vasoactive intestinal peptide and nitric oxide in the acute phase following burns and trauma, *Burns* 27(1):17-21, 2001.

78. Ungureanu-Longrois D et al: Myocardial contractile dysfunction in the systemic inflammatory response syndrome: role of a cytokine-inducible nitric oxide synthase in cardiac myocytes, *J Mol Cell Cardiol* 27(1):155-167, 1995.

79. Gamelli RL et al: Burn-induced nitric oxide release in humans, *J Trauma* 39(5):869-877, discussion 77-78, 1995.

80. Baxter CR: Fluid volume and electrolyte changes of the early postburn period, *Clin Plast Surg* 1(4):693-703, 1974.

81. Huang PP et al: Hypertonic sodium resuscitation is associated with renal failure and death, *Ann Surg* 221(5):543-554, 1995.

82. Herndon DN, Spies M: Modern burn care, *Semin Pediatr Surg* 10(1):28-31, 2001.

83. Evans JA, Darlington DN, Gann DS: A circulating factor(s) mediates cell depolarization in hemorrhagic shock, *Ann Surg* 213(6):549-556, 1991.

84. Welt LG: Membrane transport defect: the sick cell, *Trans Assoc Am Physicians* 80:217-226, 1967.

85. Trunkey DD et al: The effect of hemorrhagic shock on intracellular muscle action potentials in the primate, *Surgery* 74(2):241-250, 1973.

86. Cunningham JN Jr, Shires GT, Wagner Y: Changes in intracellular sodium and potassium content of red blood cells in trauma and shock, *Am J Surg* 122(5):650-654, 1971.

87. Rosenthal SR, Tabor H: Electrolyte changes and chemotherapy in experimental burn and traumatic shock and hemorrhage, *Arch Surg* 51:244, 1945.

88. Turinsky J, Gonnerman WA, Loose LD: Impaired mineral metabolism in postburn muscle, *J Trauma* 21(6):417-423, 1981.

89. Deets DK, Glaviano VV: Plasma and cardiac lactic dehydrogenase activity in burn shock, *Proc Soc Exp Biol Med* 142(2):412-416, 1973.

90. Button B: Evidence of circulating membrane depolarization factor(s) in hemorrhagic shock, *Shock* 1(Suppl):15, 1994.

91. Okamoto R, Glaviano VV, Pindok M: Myocardial lipases and catecholamines in burn shock, *Proc Soc Exp Biol Med* 137(1):347-353, 1971.

92. Jeschke MG et al: Propranolol does not increase inflammation, sepsis, or infectious episodes in severely burned children, *J Trauma* 62(3):676-681, 2007.

93. Wilmore DW, Aulick HL, Goodwin CW: Glucose metabolism following severe injury, *Acta Chir Scand Suppl* 498:43-47, 1980.

94. Wilmore DW et al: Alterations in hypothalamic function following thermal injury, *J Trauma* 15(8):697-703, 1975.

95. Gump FE, Price JB Jr, Kinney JM: Blood flow and oxygen consumption in patients with severe burns, *Surg Gynecol Obstet* 130(1):23-28, 1970.

96. Wilmore DW et al: Influence of the burn wound on local and systemic responses to injury, *Ann Surg* 186(4):444-458, 1977.

97. Wilmore DW et al: Effect of injury and infection on visceral metabolism and circulation, *Ann Surg* 192(4):491-504, 1980.

98. Holder IA, Neely AN: Hageman factor dependent activation and its relationship to lethal *Pseudomonas aeruginosa* burn wound infections, *Agents Actions Suppl* 38(Pt 3):329-342, 1992.

99. McManus WF, Eurenius K, Pruitt BA Jr: Disseminated intravascular coagulation in burned patients, *J Trauma* 13(5):416-422, 1973.

100. Wilmore DW, editor: *The metabolic management of the critically ill,* ed 2, New York, 1990, Plenum.

101. Wilmore DW, Aulick LH: Metabolic changes in burned patients, *Surg Clin North Am* 58(6):1173-1187, 1978.

102. Edelman LS et al: Sustained bone mineral density changes after burn injury, *J Surg Res* 114(2):172-178, 2003.

103. Wright K et al: Burn-activated neutrophils and tumor necrosis factor-alpha alter endothelial cell actin cytoskeleton and enhance monolayer permeability, *Surgery* 128(2):259-265, 2000.

104. Goebel A et al: Injury induces deficient interleukin-12 production, but interleukin-12 therapy after injury restores resistance to infection, *Ann Surg* 231(2):253-261, 2000.

105. Nishiura T et al: Gene expression and cytokine and enzyme activation in the liver after a burn injury, *J Burn Care Rehabil* 21(2):135-141, 2000.

106. Biffl WL et al: Interleukin-6 delays neutrophil apoptosis via a mechanism involving platelet-activating factor, *J Trauma* 40(4): 575-578, 1996.

107. Choi M et al: Preventing the infiltration of leukocytes by monoclonal antibody blocks the development of progressive ischemia in rat burns, *Plast Reconstr Surg* 96(5):1177-1185, 1995.

108. Iocono JA et al: Interleukin-8 levels and activity in delayed-healing human thermal wounds, *Wound Repair Regen* 8(3):216-225, 2000.

109. Ortega MR, Ganz T, Milner SM: Human beta defensin is absent in burn blister fluid, *Burns* 26(8):724-726, 2000.

110. Heideman M, Kaijser B, Gelin LE: Complement activation and hematologic, hemodynamic, and respiratory reactions early after soft-tissue injury, *J Trauma* 18(10):696-700, 1978.

111. Grzybowski J et al: Antidietary antigen antibodies in the sera of patients with burns as a potential marker of gut mucosa integrity failure, *J Burn Care Rehabil* 13(2 Pt 1):194-197, 1992.

112. Deitch EA, Berg R: Bacterial translocation from the gut: a mechanism of infection, *J Burn Care Rehabil* 8(6):475-482, 1987.

113. Yao YM et al: The association of circulating endotoxaemia with the development of multiple organ failure in burned patients, *Burns* 21(4):255-258, 1995.

114. Benhaim P, Hunt TK: Natural resistance to infection: leukocyte functions, *J Burn Care Rehabil* 13(2 Pt 2):287-292, 1992.

115. Alexander JW et al: Consumptive opsoninopathy: possible pathogenesis in lethal and opportunistic infections, *Ann Surg* 184(6):672-678, 1976.

116. Bjornson AB, Altemeier WA, Bjornson HS: Changes in humoral components of host defense following burn trauma, *Ann Surg* 186(1):88-96, 1977.

117. Cochran A et al: Systemic Candida infection in burn patients: a case-control study of management patterns and outcomes, *Surg Infect (Larchmt)* 3(4):367-374, 2002.

118. Goff DR et al: Cardiac disease and the patient with burns, *J Burn Care Rehabil* 11(4):305-307, 1990.

119. McGill V et al: The impact of substance use on mortality and morbidity from thermal injury, *J Trauma* 38(6):931-934, 1995.

120. Moncrief JA, Mason AD Jr: Water vapor loss in the burned patient, *Surg Forum* 13:38-41, 1962.

121. Moncrief JA: Burns. In Schwartz SI, editor: *Principles of surgery*, ed 2, New York, 1974, McGraw-Hill.

122. Roe CF, Kinney JM: Water and heat exchange on third-degree burns, *Surgery* 56:212-220, 1964.

123. Affleck DG et al: Assessment of tissue viability in complex extremity injuries: utility of the pyrophosphate nuclear scan, *J Trauma* 50(2): 263-269, 2001.

124. Ronfard V et al: Long-term regeneration of human epidermis on third degree burns transplanted with autologous cultured epithelium grown on a fibrin matrix, *Transplantation* 70(11):1588-1598, 2000.

125. Williamson JS et al: Cultured epithelial autograft: five years of clinical experience with twenty-eight patients, *J Trauma* 39(2):309-319, 1995.

126. Fitton AR, Drew P, Dickson WA: The use of a bilaminate artificial skin substitute (Integra) in acute resurfacing of burns: an early experience, *Br J Plast Surg* 54(3):208-212, 2001.

127. Peck MD et al: A trial of the effectiveness of artificial dermis in the treatment of patients with burns greater than 45% total body surface area, *J Trauma* 52(5):971-978, 2002.

128. Carsin H et al: Cultured epithelial autografts in extensive burn coverage of severely traumatized patients: a five year single-center experience with 30 patients, *Burns* 26(4):379-387, 2000.

129. Wainwright D et al: Clinical evaluation of an acellular allograft dermal matrix in full-thickness burns, *J Burn Care Rehabil* 17(2):124-136, 1996.

130. Kirker KR et al: Glycosaminoglycan hydrogels as supplemental wound dressings for donor sites, *J Burn Care Rehabil* 25(3):276-286, 2004.

131. Liew SH, Murison M, Dickson WA: Prophylactic treatment of deep dermal burn scar to prevent hypertrophic scarring using the pulsed dye laser: a preliminary study, *Ann Plast Surg* 49(5):472-475, 2002.

132. Jellish WS et al: Effect of topical local anesthetic application to skin harvest sites for pain management in burn patients undergoing skin-grafting procedures, *Ann Surg* 229(1):115-120, 1999.

SHOCK, MULTIPLE ORGAN DYSFUNCTION SYNDROME, AND BURNS IN CHILDREN

MARY FRAN HAZINSKI • MARY A. MONDOZZI • ROSE A. URDIALES BAKER

MEDIA RESOURCES

CHAPTER OUTLINE

SHOCK AND MULTIPLE ORGAN DYSFUNCTION SYNDROME
Types of Shock
Reperfusion and Inflammatory Injury
Evaluation and Treatment of Shock
BURNS
Severity of Injury

This chapter reviews shock, multiple organ dysfunction syndrome, and burns in children. It summarizes the differences between these conditions in children and adults. These differences are noted not only in the pathophysiology section, but also in the epidemiology, clinical manifestations, and treatment and evaluation sections.

SHOCK AND MULTIPLE ORGAN DYSFUNCTION SYNDROME

Shock is a condition of acute and progressive circulatory dysfunction that results in inadequate delivery of oxygen and nutrients to the tissues. Shock in children typically results from hemorrhage, severe dehydration, progressive heart failure, or sepsis. It may also complicate the care of the child with pulmonary hypertension (cor pulmonale), drug toxicity, electrolyte or acid-base imbalance, dysrhythmias, or multiple organ failure. (The physiology of shock is discussed in Chapter 46.)

Shock in children is present when there are signs of poor systemic perfusion, regardless of the blood pressure—shock may be present with normal, high, or low blood pressure.

When the systolic blood pressure is appropriate for age, but there are signs of inadequate tissue perfusion, the child is in **compensated shock.** In such cases, although the systolic blood pressure may be normal, the diastolic and mean blood pressures are typically low. If systolic hypotension is associated with inadequate tissue perfusion, the child is in **hypotensive** (formerly called decompensated) **shock.**[1,2]

Shock causes ischemia and reperfusion injury may follow. **Ischemia** (or **hypoxia**) is inadequate oxygen delivery to the tissues. Oxygen delivery may be inadequate because arterial oxygen content or cardiac output is low, or because there are increased metabolic requirements or impaired cellular utilization of oxygen. The ischemia causes a primary insult and restoration of adequate blood flow, and oxygen delivery may trigger the development of *reperfusion injury*, a secondary problem characterized by an exaggerated inflammatory response that may produce cellular death and organ failure.

Multiple organ dysfunction syndrome (MODS) is the simultaneous failure of at least two organs that results from a single cause. MODS may be either primary or secondary. Primary MODS typically occurs soon after an insult and is directly attributable to the insult. Secondary MODS typically occurs later and may be associated with more sequential development of organ dysfunction. In most cases, MODS develops 3 to 7 days after the causative event, although secondary MODS may appear even later. Risk factors for MODS include sepsis, trauma, cardiopulmonary arrest, congenital heart disease, and liver and bone marrow transplantation.[3,4] Children with chronic diseases have an increased risk for MODS and increased mortality.[4]

Types of Shock

Shock is categorized by type as follows[2]:

1. *Hypovolemic shock:* caused by inadequate intravascular volume relative to the vascular space
2. *Cardiogenic shock:* results from impairment of myocardial function
3. *Distributive shock* (including neurogenic, anaphylactic, and septic): associated with inappropriate distribution of blood flow and increased capillary permeability (e.g., septic shock) or central nervous system injury (e.g., neurogenic or spinal shock)
4. *Obstructive shock:* caused by a mechanical obstruction to blood flow into and through the heart and great vessels (e.g., cardiac tamponade, pulmonary embolus, obstructive congenital heart lesions such as critical aortic stenosis) resulting in low cardiac output

An etiologic classification of shock is helpful because it indicates the major therapy required (Box 47-1). However, such a classification is inadequate for describing individuals with late or progressive shock because they are likely to demonstrate widespread cardiovascular dysfunction, including inappropriate intravascular volume relative to the vascular space, severe myocardial dysfunction, and maldistribution of blood flow. Severe shock of any kind may be followed by complications such as reperfusion injury or MODS. An etiologic classification is also incomplete for those with septic shock, because sepsis produces elements of hypovolemic and cardiogenic shock in addition to the complications of maldistribution of blood flow. Finally, anyone in shock is likely to develop some myocardial dysfunction and some compromise in organ perfusion and function. Thus healthcare providers must support all aspects of cardiovascular function and oxygen delivery during the treatment of any form of shock.

Hypovolemic Shock

Hypovolemic shock, the most common type of shock in children, is associated with a reduction in the intravascular volume relative to the vascular space. Dehydration and trauma are the most common causes of hypovolemic shock in children. A relative hypovolemia may result from a redistribution of blood volume or increased capillary permeability, such as develops following burns or sepsis.

When hypovolemia is mild or moderate, such as with 5% to 10% dehydration or mild hemorrhage, compensatory vasoconstrictive adrenergic responses redistribute blood from the mesenteric, renal, and skin circulations to maintain blood flow to the heart and brain. The child with mild hypovolemic shock typically maintains systolic blood pressure through vasoconstriction; hypotension may not develop unless intravascular volume loss is rapid or severe.[5] Severe volume loss is typically present with greater than 10% dehydration in the infant or child or greater than 6% dehydration in the adolescent.[6] A 20% to 25% acute hemorrhage is usually required to produce hypotension in the child with trauma. Thus a normal blood pressure is often observed in the child with hypovolemic shock. Hypotension is a sign of severe, decompensated shock.

Relative hypovolemia may be caused by an increase in the vascular space relative to intravascular volume. This may be associated with the vasodilation of sepsis, anaphylaxis, or neurogenic shock (see below) or with β-adrenergic drug toxicity. A relative hypovolemia also may be caused by increased

---

Box 47-1   Classification and Causes of Shock

Hypovolemic
1. Hemorrhage
   a. External: laceration
   b. Internal: ruptured spleen or liver, vascular injury, fracture (newborn: intracerebral/intraventricular hemorrhage)
   c. Gastrointestinal: bleeding ulcer, ruptured viscus, mesenteric hemorrhage
2. Plasma loss
   a. Burn
   b. Inflammation or sepsis: capillary leak syndrome
   c. Nephrotic syndrome
   d. Third spacing: intestinal obstruction, pancreatitis, peritonitis
3. Fluid and electrolyte loss
   a. Acute gastroenteritis
   b. Excessive evaporative loss (including burns)
   c. Renal disease
4. Endocrine
   a. Adrenal insufficiency, adrenogenital syndrome
   b. Diabetes mellitus
   c. Diabetes insipidus
   d. Hypothyroidism (myxedema coma)

Cardiogenic
1. Myocardial insufficiency
   a. Cardiomyopathy: myocarditis, ischemia, hypoxia, hypoglycemia, acidosis
   b. Drug intoxication or acid-base or electrolyte imbalance
   c. Hypothermia
   d. Congenital heart disease, including ductal-dependent lesion such as coarctation of the aorta or critical pulmonary stenosis
2. Dysrhythmia: bradycardia, atrioventricular (AV) block, ventricular tachycardia, supraventricular tachycardia

Distributive (Vasogenic)
1. High or normal resistance (increased venous capacitance)
   a. Septic shock
   b. Anaphylaxis
   c. Barbiturate intoxication
2. Low resistance, vasodilation: central nervous system injury (i.e., spinal cord transection)

Modified from Hazinski MF: Shock. In Barkin RM, editor: *Pediatric emergency medicine: concepts and clinical practice,* ed 2, St Louis, 1997, Mosby.

capillary permeability with a redistribution of intravascular volume, such as with burns, anaphylaxis, or sepsis. The translocation of extravascular fluid to a location that is neither intravascular nor intracellular, as in edema, is termed **"third spacing" of fluids.**

With **distributive (neurogenic, anaphylactic, and septic) shock,** a normal cardiac output will likely be inadequate to maintain sufficient blood flow to all tissue beds. Aggressive volume administration is necessary to ensure that the intravascular volume is adequate relative to the vascular space, and cardiac output must be supported at a level that is higher than normal. **Neurogenic shock** is a form of hypovolemic and vasogenic (maldistributive) shock. It is caused by loss of vasomotor tone after severe head or spinal cord injury. Massive vasodilation and loss of sympathomimetic tone result in a relative hypovolemia, but the loss of sympathetic tone prevents a compensatory tachycardia.

In **obstructive shock,** low cardiac output is caused by mechanical obstruction to blood flow, such as cardiac tamponade, tension pneumothorax, critical left heart or aortic obstruction, or pulmonary embolus. Obstructive shock is difficult to distinguish from cardiogenic shock because both may present with signs of low cardiac output and evidence of systemic or pulmonary venous congestion. Prompt detection and treatment are critical to survival.

Compensatory Responses

Significant dehydration, hypovolemia, and low cardiac output stimulate adrenergic and renal compensatory mechanisms characterized by the "fight or flight" response. These include tachycardia and redistribution of blood from the skin, gut, and kidney to the brain and heart. Reduced renal perfusion stimulates the renin-angiotensin-aldosterone system, resulting in renal sodium and water retention. Decreased atrial stretch stimulates the secretion of antidiuretic hormone (ADH, also known as *arginine vasopressin [AVP]*) and produces free water retention by the kidneys. These mechanisms are similar in adults and children and may help restore or maintain intravascular volume over time. Neonatal and young infant kidneys, however, are incapable of excreting concentrated urine, so these compensatory mechanisms are relatively ineffective during the first weeks of life.

Compensatory mechanisms cannot be maintained indefinitely. Systemic vasoconstriction increases left ventricular afterload and myocardial oxygen consumption. Prolonged tachycardia produces impaired subendocardial blood flow and increased myocardial oxygen consumption, which may ultimately contribute to myocardial ischemia. Extreme tachypnea increases oxygen demand and reduces effective ventilation. A severe compromise in blood flow and systemic perfusion contributes to cerebral, renal, or hepatic ischemia and possible organ failure.

CLINICAL MANIFESTATIONS The child with inadequate cardiac output demonstrates signs of inadequate blood flow to some tissue beds and some evidence of organ system dysfunction. When hypovolemic or cardiogenic shock is present, the extremities may feel cool (they cool in a peripheral to proximal fashion). Capillary refill time is often prolonged, despite a warm ambient temperature, and the skin may be pale or mottled. Excessive skin blood flow with instantaneous ("flash") capillary refill may be present in children with anaphylaxis, neurogenic shock, or severe sepsis or septic shock. Urine output decreases if renal perfusion is compromised and is less than 2 ml/kg/hr in infants, less than 1 ml/kg/hr in children, and less than 0.5 ml/kg/hr in adolescents despite adequate fluid intake. Liver enzymes may be elevated if hepatic perfusion is reduced. The development of a metabolic acidosis and a rise in serum lactate indicate that blood flow to some tissues is inadequate to support total aerobic metabolism. As noted, systolic hypotension is often not present unless or until shock is severe.

The child's level of consciousness and responsiveness may provide valuable information about the severity of illness. The healthy infant should orient to faces, make eye contact, and track bright objects across a visual field. The healthy child is alert and the toddler is reluctant to be separated from parents or examined by strangers. By comparison, the critically ill infant or child is often extremely irritable; lethargy indicates severe deterioration in the child's level of consciousness. A decreased response to painful stimulation is abnormal in the child of any age and usually indicates severe cardiorespiratory or neurologic compromise.[7]

Hypoglycemia may be observed in seriously ill or injured infants and may be associated with cardiovascular or neurologic deterioration. Infants have high glucose needs and low glycogen stores that may be rapidly depleted during stress. However, *hyperglycemia* (glucose greater than 150 mg/dl) may develop as the result of a relative insulin-resistant state associated with high levels of endogenous catecholamines and hydrocortisone secretion.[8] Hyperglycemia has been linked with poor survival in critically ill children, such as those with head injury or shock.[9,10]

Providers should evaluate the child's vital signs in light of the child's clinical condition. Normal vital signs are not always appropriate in the seriously ill or injured child[7] (Box 47-2). The clinical manifestations observed in the child with hypovolemic shock are those of inadequate systemic

---

Box 47-2	Estimating Blood Pressure in Children

The typical "normal" (i.e., median, or 50th percentile) systolic blood pressure for a child 1 to 10 years of age may be estimated by adding 90 mmHg to twice the child's age in years (90 mmHg + [2 × age in years]); this corresponds to the 50th percentile systolic blood pressure for the child's age. A systolic pressure equal to or less than 70 mmHg plus twice the child's age in years (70 mmHg + [2 × age in years]) is considered hypotensive beyond 1 year of age because this blood pressure corresponds to the 5th percentile systolic blood pressure for age (i.e., only 5% of normal, healthy children will demonstrate a systolic blood pressure lower than that number).

Data from Chameides L, Hazinski MF, editors: *Textbook of pediatric advanced life support,* Dallas, 1997, American Heart Association.

Table 47-1   Normal Pediatric Vital Signs

Age	Awake Heart Rate* (per min)	Sleeping Heart Rate (per min)
Newborn	100-180	80-160
Infant (6 mo)	100-160	75-160
Toddler	80-110	60-90
Preschooler	70-110	60-90
School-age child	65-110	60-90
Adolescent	60-90	50-90

Age	Respiratory Rate (breaths per min)
Infant	30-60
Toddler	24-40
Preschooler	22-34
School-age child	18-30
Adolescent	12-16

Age	Systolic Blood Pressure† (mmHg)	Diastolic Blood Pressure (mmHg)
Birth (12 hr, <1000 g)	39-59	16-36
Birth (12 hr, 3-kg weight)	50-70	25-45
Newborn (96 hr)	60-90	20-60
Infant (6 mo)	87-105	53-66
Toddler (2 yr)	95-105	53-66
School-age child (7 yr)	97-112	57-71
Adolescent (15 yr)	112-128	66-80

Modified from Hazinski MF: *Manual of pediatric critical care*, St Louis, 1999, Mosby.

NOTE: Always consider patient's normal range and clinical condition. Heart and respiratory rates will normally increase with fever or stress.

*Heart rate ranges from Gillette PC, Garson A Jr: *Pediatric cardiac dysrhythmias*, New York, 1982, Grune & Stratton.

†Blood pressure ranges taken from the following sources:

Neonate: Versmold H et al: *Pediatrics* 67:107, 1981 (10th-90th percentile ranges used).

Others: Horan MJ, chairman, Task Force on Blood-Pressure Control in Children: *Pediatrics* 79:1, 1987 (50th-90th percentile ranges used); National High Blood Pressure Education Program Working Group in Hypertension Control in Children and Adolescents. Update on the 1987 Task Force Report on High Blood Pressure in Children and Adolescents: a working group report from the National Blood Pressure Education Program. *Pediatrics* 98:649, 1996.

perfusion associated with intravascular volume loss and/or expansion of the vascular space. Adrenergic compensatory mechanisms produce tachycardia and redistribution of blood flow, including signs of peripheral vasoconstriction, cool extremities, delayed capillary refill, and oliguria. Hypotension is often only a late, and preterminal, sign of shock in the child. Table 47-1 contains normal vital signs in children.

The child's heart rate should be appropriate for age and clinical condition. The child in shock is often tachycardic. The **tachycardia** may be primary (dysrhythmia) or secondary to stress (sinus tachycardia). If the heart rate is extremely rapid or if it is present in the child with decreased myocardial function,

the tachycardia may be the cause rather than the symptom of the shock. In general, if the ventricular rate exceeds 200 to 220 beats/minute in the infant or 160 to 180 beats/minute in the child, ventricular diastolic filling time and coronary artery perfusion time are significantly reduced and stroke volume falls. As a result, cardiac output falls and signs of congestive heart failure or shock develop. Once supraventricular or ventricular tachycardia produces signs of shock, urgent treatment is required.[8]

Bradycardia, an abnormally low heart rate, can cause a fall in cardiac output or can be a symptom of deterioration. In young animal models a fall in heart rate produces a commensurate fall in cardiac output.[2,11] The most common cause of bradycardia in young children is hypoxia. Therefore, if the infant or child develops bradycardia with poor perfusion, the provider should immediately assess and support the child's airway, oxygenation, and ventilation. Bradycardia often indicates impending cardiovascular collapse or cardiac arrest and is the most common terminal cardiac rhythm observed in children.[12]

The child's stroke volume may be altered by conditions affecting ventricular preload, compliance, contractility, and afterload (Table 47-2). Evaluate and optimize each of these variables in the treatment of shock (see Chapter 46).

If the ambient temperature is warm, the child's capillary refill is normally brisk. A prolonged capillary refill time may indicate a compromise in systemic perfusion. Capillary refill time of less than 1.5 to 2 seconds is normal and may be observed in infants and children with minimal fluid deficit (less than 5% dehydration). If the capillary refill time is 1.5 to 3 seconds in a warm room, a 5% to 10% dehydration is likely to be present, and a refill time more than 3 seconds is associated with greater than 10% dehydration.[5,13] However, these findings may be subtle and difficult to detect.[14] Metabolic or lactic acidosis also may be present.

The central venous pressure (CVP) is normally 0 to 5 mmHg and the pulmonary artery wedge pressure (PAWP) (also called *pulmonary artery occlusion pressure [PAOP]*) is normally 5 to 8 mmHg or less. The cardiac silhouette is normally less than 50% of the width of the chest on chest radiograph.

Clinically significant dehydration is associated with weight loss (Table 47-3). Fluid intake and output records (or reports from parents or primary caretakers) reveal a history of inadequate fluid intake or excessive fluid losses. The child with significant dehydration demonstrates dry mucous membranes, a sunken fontanel (in infants), and poor skin turgor[5] (Table 47-4). The blood urea nitrogen (BUN) and urine specific gravity are usually elevated. The serum sodium concentration and osmolality are affected by the type and severity of dehydration present.

Hemorrhage is another potential cause of hypovolemic shock. To appreciate the significance of any blood lost or drawn for laboratory analysis, the total blood loss should be considered as a percentage of the child's circulating blood volume (Table 47-5).

Table 47-2	Factors Affecting Cardiovascular Performance in Children
Factor	Comments
Heart rate	Normally more rapid in children than in adults. Because the *stroke volume* is smaller than in adults, the *cardiac output* of the child is more closely related to heart rate than stroke volume. *Tachycardia* is expected in the seriously ill or injured child. The most common cause of *bradycardia* in young children is hypoxia and is an ominous sign if present in association with poor perfusion. Urgent treatment is required once bradycardia or supraventricular or ventricular tachycardia produces signs of shock.
Stroke volume	Averages 1.5 ml/kg; affected by conditions altering ventricular preload, compliance, contractility, and afterload.
Ventricular end-diastolic pressure (VEDP)	Optimal pressure for children in shock is unknown. Aggressive fluid administration is linked to improved survival in children with *septic* shock.
Ventricular compliance or distensibility	Can be affected by congenital heart defects such as atrial septal defects (ASDs). If compliance is low, such as in newborns and infants, volume administration may increase VEDP. Hypoplastic ventricles are often noncompliant. Hypertrophied ventricles, noted in children with severe pulmonary stenosis or aortic stenosis, may become fibrotic and noncompliant. Increased compliance may be present in early septic shock.
Contractility	No evidence exists that contractility is significantly lower in newborns, infants, and children than adults. Newborn myocardium does have fewer contractile proteins and higher water content than adult myocardium, but the clinical significance of this is probably minimal.
Afterload	Newborn myocardium *can* adapt to mild, nonacute increases in afterload. Afterload may be increased in children with systemic vasoconstriction or pulmonary hypertension (constrictors include alveolar hypoxia, acidosis, hypothermia, and alveolar distention). Some uncorrected congenital heart defects may increase afterload. Coarctation of the aorta and aortic stenosis increase left ventricular afterload. Pulmonary stenosis increases right ventricular afterload. Afterload may be decreased in septic shock.
Oxygen delivery and consumption	Highest per kilogram body weight during the neonatal period and infancy. Oxygen reserve is smaller in infants and children than in adults, and the young child requires a higher cardiac output and oxygen delivery per kilogram than the adult. Increased oxygen consumption occurs in critically ill newborns exposed to cold because they cannot shiver to generate heat. Other causes of increased oxygen consumption in children and infants include fever, sepsis, pain, and seizures.

Table 47-3	Dehydration and Hypovolemia
Type of Dehydration	Clinical Indicators
Isotonic dehydration	Fluid output exceeds intake. Loss of free water is proportional to loss of sodium, so serum sodium concentration remains normal. Fluid loss is from intravascular and extravascular compartments. Compromises peripheral perfusion when the young child has lost approximately 10% (100 ml/kg) of body weight. Compromises systemic perfusion in the adolescent with acute fluid loss equivalent to 5% to 6% of body weight.
	Produces hypotension (decompensated shock) when the young child has lost 15% (150 ml/kg) of body weight. Produces hypotension in the adolescent with a fluid loss equivalent to 7% to 9% of body weight because body water constitutes a smaller percentage of body weight in older children and adults than in young children.
Hypotonic/hyponatremic dehydration	Associated with a proportionally greater loss of sodium than free water; thus the serum sodium falls. Resultant acute fall in serum osmolality produces an acute extravascular fluid shift and further loss of extravascular volume. Fluid loss in hypotonic dehydration is primarily from the intravascular compartment; thus a compromise in systemic perfusion will be observed after even small quantities of fluid loss.
	Poor peripheral perfusion occurs in a child with a fluid loss equivalent to 5% (50 ml/kg) of body weight. Adolescents with hyponatremic dehydration may demonstrate a compromise in peripheral perfusion with a fluid loss equivalent to approximately 3% of body weight.
	Hypotension will often be observed when fluid loss is equal to approximately 10% (100 ml/kg) of body weight. Hypotension in an adolescent is observed when the fluid loss equals approximately 5% to 6% of body weight.
Hypertonic/hypernatremic dehydration	Free water deficit is proportionately greater than the deficit of sodium, so serum sodium concentration rises, increasing serum osmolality and producing an intravascular shift of free water. For this reason the child with hypernatremic dehydration is likely to maintain intravascular volume and systemic perfusion until relatively large quantities of fluid are lost.
	Compromise in systemic perfusion is not likely to be observed in the *child* with hypernatremic dehydration until *severe* dehydration is present with a fluid loss equivalent to 10% of body weight (or 5% to 6% of body weight in the adolescent).
	Hypotension may not be observed until the fluid loss approximates 15% or more of body weight (7% to 9% or more of body weight in the adolescent).
	Hypotension in the child with hypertonic/hypernatremic dehydration indicates a substantial fluid deficit. However, the deficit must be replaced carefully to correct shock and avoid rapid lowering of serum sodium concentrations.

Data in part from Roberts KB: *Pediatr Rev* 22:380-386, 2001.

Table 47-4	Assessment of Degree of Dehydration in Isotonic Fluid Losses*		
Clinical Parameters	Mild	Moderate	Severe
Body weight loss			
Infant	5% (50 ml/kg)	10% (100 ml/kg)	15% (150 ml/kg)
Adolescent	3% (30 ml/kg)	5%-6% (50-60 ml/kg)	7%-9% (70-90 ml/kg)
Skin turgor	Slightly ↓	↓↓	↓↓↓
Fontanel	May be flat or depressed	Depressed	Significantly depressed
Mucous membranes	Dry	Very dry	Parched
Skin perfusion	Warm, normal color	Extremities cool	Extremities cold
		Pale color	Mottled or gray color
Heart rate	Mild tachycardia	Moderate tachycardia	Extreme tachycardia
Peripheral pulses	Normal	Diminished	Absent
Blood pressure	Normal	Normal	Reduced
Sensorium	Normal or irritable	Irritable or lethargic	Unresponsive
Urine output	Slightly ↓	Mild oliguria	Marked oliguria or anuria
Azotemia	Absent	Present	Present and severe

Modified from Hazinski MF: Renal disorders. In Hazinski MF, editor: *Manual of pediatric critical care*, St Louis, 1999, Mosby.
*The interpretation of the assessments must be appropriately modified for age and *type* of dehydration (hypotonic or hypertonic).

Table 47-5	Estimation of Pediatric Circulating Blood Volume
Age of Child	Blood Volume (ml/kg body weight)
Newborn	85-90
Infant	75-80
Child	70-75
Adolescent	65-70

From Hazinski MF: Cardiovascular Disorders, In Hazinski MF, editor: *Manual of pediatric critical care*, St Louis, 1999, Mosby.

Acute blood loss (hemorrhage) typically is not thought to compromise peripheral perfusion until an estimated 25% to 30% of intravascular volume is lost (an acute intravascular or blood loss of 16 to 24 ml/kg). Tachycardia, peripheral vasoconstriction, and altered level of consciousness may be the only early evidence of hemorrhage in the child with trauma (Table 47-6). Once hypotension develops, cardiovascular collapse is imminent and rapid intravascular volume expansion is required immediately.

Redistribution of blood volume associated with systemic vasodilation, high capillary pressure or transudative fluid losses or capillary leak may produce signs of poor systemic perfusion in the absence of evidence of absolute volume loss. For example, children with end-stage hepatic failure may demonstrate a relative hypovolemia associated with ascites and hepatorenal syndrome. Children demonstrate increased capillary permeability and loss of intravascular volume immediately after a burn. The septic child also may demonstrate systemic edema associated with capillary leak and further intravascular volume loss. In these children, some evidence of extravascular fluid movement (ascites, systemic edema, or fluid loss to dressings over burns) is usually observed.

Signs of neurogenic shock in the child with recent, severe spinal cord injury include warm skin and hypotension with a low diastolic blood pressure. Signs of poor systemic perfusion also are observed (see Clinical Manifestations following), although loss of sympathetic nervous system tone prevents the typical tachycardic response.

Cardiogenic Shock

Cardiogenic shock is present when impaired myocardial function compromises cardiac output. This form of shock is observed:

1. Following cardiovascular surgery or with inflammatory disease of the heart, such as cardiomyopathy and myocarditis
2. With drug toxicity or severe electrolyte or acid-base imbalances
3. As a complication of any form of shock and early in septic shock

Compensatory Responses

In the early stages of cardiogenic shock, adrenergic compensatory responses produce tachycardia, peripheral vasoconstriction, and constriction of the splanchnic arteries to divert blood flow from the skin, kidneys, and gut and maintain flow to the heart and brain.[2,14] These compensatory mechanisms may be sufficient to maintain the child's systolic blood pressure and effective coronary artery and cerebral blood flow. However, tachycardia and systemic arterial constriction increase myocardial oxygen consumption. In addition, reduction in gut and kidney blood flow may produce hepatic, mesenteric, or renal ischemia or failure. Decreased renal perfusion stimulates the renin-angiotensin-aldosterone system, as described for hypovolemic shock on p. 1728.

If the mean arterial pressure or pulse pressure falls, stimulation of the baroreceptors in the carotid sinuses and aortic arch is reduced. This reduced baroreceptor activity removes inhibition from the vasomotor center in the medulla, resulting in increased adrenergic stimulation. If myocardial dysfunction progresses, cardiac output and systemic blood pressure ultimately fall. Myocardial ischemia then exacerbates myocardial

Table 47-6	Classification of Pediatric Hemorrhagic Shock in Trauma Patients Based on Clinical Evaluation		
System	Mild Hemorrhage, Compensated Shock, Simple Hypovolemia (<30%)	Moderate Hemorrhage, Decompensated Shock, Marked Hypovolemia (30%-45%)	Severe Hemorrhage, Cardiopulmonary Failure, Profound Hypovolemia (>45%)
Cardiovascular	Tachycardia	Moderate tachycardia	Severe tachycardia
	Weak peripheral pulses, strong central pulses	Thready peripheral pulses, weak central pulses	Absent peripheral pulses, thready central pulses
	Low to normal blood pressure (systolic BP >70 mmHg + [2 × (age in years)])	Frank hypotension (systolic BP <70 mmHg + [2 × (age in years)])	Profound hypotension (systolic BP <50 mmHg)
	Mild acidosis	Moderate acidosis	Severe acidosis
Respiratory	Mild tachypnea	Moderate tachypnea	Severe tachypnea
Central nervous system	Irritable, confused	Agitated or lethargic	Obtunded, comatose
Skin	Cool extremities, mottling	Cool extremities, pallor	Cool extremities, cyanosis
	Poor capillary refill (72 sec)	Delayed capillary refill (72 sec)	Prolonged (>5 sec) capillary refill
Kidneys	Mild oliguria, increased specific gravity	Marked oliguria, increased blood urea nitrogen (BUN)	Anuria

From Soud T, Pieper P, Hazinski MF: Pediatric Trauma. In Hazinski MF, editor: *Nursing care of the critically ill child*, ed 2, St Louis, 1992, Mosby.

dysfunction, and multisystem organ failure may result from persistent or severe organ ischemia.

CLINICAL MANIFESTATIONS The child with cardiogenic shock demonstrates signs of inadequate systemic perfusion despite adequate intravascular volume or even relative hypervolemia. This form of shock is generally associated with low cardiac output. The child's extremities are cool to touch (will cool peripherally to proximally), with delayed capillary refill despite a warm, ambient temperature.[2,7,14] The skin may be mottled (Figure 47-1).

Evidence of an adequate or high central venous pressure, including hepatomegaly and periorbital edema, is typically present in uncomplicated cardiogenic shock, particularly if right ventricular failure is involved. Evidence of pulmonary edema may be noted on chest radiograph or clinical assessment (including signs of respiratory distress, reduced lung compliance during hand ventilation, or frothy pink sputum suctioned from the endotracheal tube). The cardiac silhouette is usually enlarged on the chest radiograph, unless concurrent hypovolemia is present. If myocardial function is severely compromised, peripheral pulses may be diminished in intensity (dampened) or they may vary in intensity (pulsus alternans).

If a pulmonary artery catheter is in place, the cardiac output may be calculated through thermodilution technique, continuous monitoring of the mixed venous oxygen saturation, or continuous monitoring of cardiac output. A low cardiac output may be detected.

Signs of low cardiac output and cardiogenic shock may be identical to signs of cardiac tamponade. Although some classic signs of tamponade, including muffled heart tones or pulsus paradoxus may be observed, these signs may be difficult to appreciate if cardiac output and blood pressure are severely compromised. Therefore, if cardiogenic shock is suspected in a child after cardiovascular surgery or in any child at risk for

the development of pericardial effusion, tamponade should be ruled out through an echocardiogram.

Septic Shock

Sepsis and its complications result from activation of biochemical and physiologic cascades that lead to the formation or activation of cytokines and protein systems that result in vasodilation, increased capillary permeability, maldistribution of blood flow, and cardiovascular dysfunction. Sepsis and its complications may result in organ system dysfunction and are leading causes of death in noncoronary intensive care units. An estimated 42,000 pediatric cases of sepsis are reported annually in the United States and result in approximately 4400 deaths per year.[15]

Much information about the pathophysiology, clinical progression, and outcome of sepsis has been extrapolated from adult clinical studies and adult animal models of sepsis. However, it appears that some information gleaned from adult experience is applicable to children. In adults and children approximately 40% of all nosocomial infections are linked to gram-negative infections; 40% to gram-positive infections; and 20% to viruses, fungi, or rickettsial microorganisms.[16] Prevention of these infections can reduce the risk of sepsis.

The most common nosocomial infections reported in pediatric critical care units in the United States are primary bloodstream infections (28%) and pneumonia (21%)[17]; almost two thirds of infections causing severe sepsis are either respiratory (most common in older children) and bacteremias (particularly common in neonates).[16] Such infections may be prevented with proper handwashing by healthcare providers before and after patient contact, appropriate sterile and aseptic technique during catheter insertion and tubing changes, and use of protocols to reduce ventilator-associated pneumonias (including head-of-bed elevation, oral hygiene,

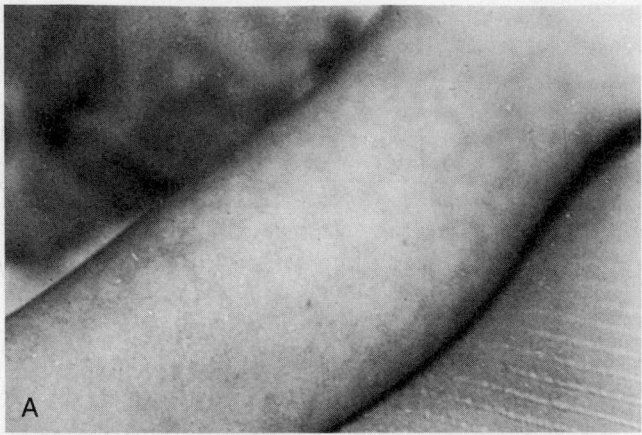

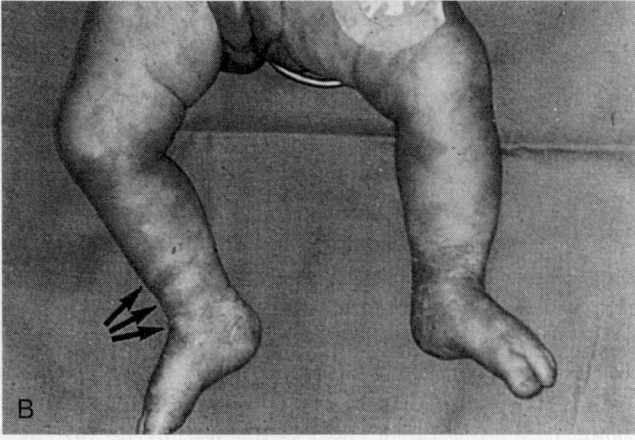

Figure 47-1 Mottling of skin caused by poor systemic perfusion.
A, Mottling of skin color often indicates inadequate tissue oxygenation; this may result from hypoxemia or poor systemic perfusion. This child developed myocardial dysfunction and signs of cardiogenic shock.
B, Mottled skin color is often associated with other signs of compromise of skin perfusion, including delayed capillary refill. The skin over this infant's right ankle was blanched using three fingers *(arrows)*, and the skin failed to perfuse for more than 5 seconds. This infant suffered from septic shock. (From Hazinski MF: Cardiovascular disorders. In Hazinski MF, editor: *Nursing care of the critically ill child,* ed 2, St Louis, 1992, Mosby.)

in-line suctioning, hand hygiene, and staff education).[18,19] More pediatric data is needed to develop evidence-based recommendations to reduce nosocomial infections and sepsis.

Factors associated with risk for the development of sepsis include extremes of age (infants, young children and older adults)[15]; invasive catheters, surgical incisions, or wounds or burns; immunocompromise; and long-term antibiotic therapy.[15-17,20] Many of these risk factors are present in any seriously ill or injured child or any child with a chronic disease. In fact, more than 50% of children with severe sepsis have underlying comorbidity.[15]

Both proinflammatory and anti-inflammatory cytokines serve an essential protective function in fighting infection and modulating the immune response. It is now clear that sepsis represents a disruption in the balance between *proinflammatory* mediators (including tumor necrosis factor-alpha [TNF-α], interleukins [IL]-1, IL-6, and IL-8; platelet-activating factor;

arachidonic acid metabolites; nitric oxide; and many kinins) and *anti-inflammatory* mediators (IL-4, IL-10, IL-11, and IL-13; transforming growth factor-beta; colony-stimulating factors; soluble tumor necrosis factor receptor; IL-1 receptor antagonist; and activated protein C). Extremely high levels of proinflammatory mediators, such as TNF, nitric oxide, and platelet-activating factor can become destructive.[21,22] High proinflammatory cytokine levels have been implicated in the development of sepsis-induced pulmonary injury and microcirculatory disruptions, such as are observed in burns, severe trauma, shock reperfusion syndromes, and MODS.[21] Tumor necrosis factor levels are directly related to mortality in newborns and children with meningitis and sepsis.[22] Increased nitric oxide concentrations are thought to be responsible for vasodilation, hypotension, and some of the decreased myocardial function that develop during sepsis. Children with sepsis, particularly those with hypotension, have increased total serum nitrite concentrations that probably reflect increased endogenous production of nitric oxide.[23]

During sepsis, endotoxin stimulates the endothelium to become a secretory organ. The endothelium changes from profibrinolytic and anticoagulant to antifibrinolytic and precoagulant, leading to the ultimate development of microthrombin in some areas of the microcirculation, further contributing to maldistribution of blood flow.[24] Mediators (e.g., activated protein C) that regulate coagulation pathways have been implicated in the sepsis process.[25-27] Low levels of activated protein C are present in children who develop coagulopathies during sepsis; activated protein C deficiency is a marker for severe sepsis in all ages,[28] and administration of activated protein C improved survival in adults with severe sepsis.[27] However, the study of activated protein C administration in children was halted because recipients developed excessive bleeding complications.

There is clear interaction among catecholamines, adrenoreceptors, and glucocorticoids. Endogenous glucocorticoids have an anti-inflammatory effect (they decrease activation of proinflammatory mediators), and they modulate vasomotor tone by enhancing cardiovascular and vasomotor response to catecholamines.[29] Septic children may have an actual adrenal insufficiency (caused by adrenal hemorrhage, decreased renal perfusion, inhibition of corticosteroid production by TNF, or actual adrenal disease) or a relative adrenal insufficiency (with inadequate adrenal stress response or decreased response to circulating glucocorticoids).[30] Although high-dose steroids have not improved survival from sepsis, a recent meta-analysis of the effect of steroids on survival showed that a 5- to 7-day course of physiologic doses of hydrocortisone increased survival in adults with severe sepsis.[31] A wide range of plasma cortisol levels have been reported in children with sepsis, and low plasma cortisol levels have been associated with the highest mortality in meningococcemia.[30] For these reasons, when sepsis is present, providers should rule out adrenal insufficiency and consider hydrocortisone administration if risk of adrenal insufficiency is present and the child does not respond to volume and inotropes.[32]

CLINICAL MANIFESTATIONS Sepsis and its complications produce a cascade of physiologic and biochemical changes. The clinical progression of sepsis produced by these changes was described and defined for adults by a consensus panel of physicians.[33] Consensus terms also have been proposed for children by several authors. In 2005, international pediatric consensus definitions were published[34] (Table 47-7).

Systemic inflammatory response syndrome (SIRS) represents a nonspecific response to a variety of insults, including trauma, burns, pancreatitis, or infection. SIRS is present when the child demonstrates two or more of the following as an acute change from baseline: fever (greater than 38.5° C [101.3° F]) or hypothermia (less than 36° C [96.8° F]), tachycardia, tachypnea, respiratory alkalosis, and alterations in white blood cell (WBC) count (including leukocytes, leukopenia, or an increase in the percentage of immature or band forms of WBCs). These clinical signs also may be altered by age, immune function, and clinical condition. For example, the newborn often develops hypothermia rather than fever as a sign of infection and may develop bradycardia rather than tachycardia.[34] The child with chronic lung disease and chronic hypercarbia or the child receiving controlled mechanical ventilatory support may not demonstrate tachypnea or a respiratory alkalosis. Because neutrophils are required for the development of fever and many of the local signs of infection, the neutropenic child may demonstrate normothermia despite infection.

Sepsis is a systemic response to infection. It is present when manifestations of SIRS are observed in conjunction with suspected infection; positive blood or other cultures are not necessary for the diagnosis, but suspicion of infection is required. For example, if the child with trauma develops a high fever or pulmonary congestion several days after injury, it is highly likely that an infection is present.

Severe sepsis is present when the child demonstrates evidence of sepsis (SIRS with suspected infection) and signs of cardiovascular or pulmonary organ dysfunction or if the child has sepsis and evidence of two or more other organ dysfunctions (see Table 47-7, Part 2). Altered organ perfusion is signaled by signs of organ system dysfunction. The dysfunctional organ system should be separate from the site of suspected infection and not explained by effects of drug therapy or other acute effects. This important distinction will enable separation of signs of severe sepsis from signs of pneumonia and associated respiratory failure.

Septic shock is heralded in the child with sepsis by the development of cardiovascular dysfunction. This may be characterized by hypotension despite adequate fluid resuscitation or by the need for vasopressors to maintain blood pressure. Because children tend to develop hypotension only late in the course of any shock, septic shock should be identified when the child develops more subtle signs of poor perfusion despite adequate fluid resuscitation. When the child with sepsis develops hypotension, hypotensive septic shock is present. Mortality from septic shock associated with hypotension may be as high as 46%.[35]

Children with septic shock may have a high, normal, or low cardiac output. In reports of adults with sepsis, low cardiac output was usually associated with poor survival.[35-37] However, in reports of children with sepsis, low cardiac output and low oxygen delivery are often present and they do not necessarily predict a poor outcome. This low cardiac output may be associated with vasoconstriction ("cold shock") or vasodilation ("warm shock").[32]

Low cardiac output responds to aggressive fluid administration[38, 38a] and titration of inotropes, vasopressors, and vasodilators with a therapeutic goal of restoring blood pressure, normalizing heart rate and capillary refill and maintaining high cardiac index (3.3 to 6 L/min/m^2) and oxygen delivery (more than 200 ml/min/m^2).[32, 38a]A In fact, in a small but seminal report of outcomes of septic shock in children, aggressive fluid resuscitation (more than 40 ml/kg administered within the first hour of therapy and more than 200 ml/kg administered during the first 8 hours of therapy) was associated with significantly higher survival than less aggressive fluid resuscitation.[38] In the most recent consensus statement regarding therapy for pediatric septic shock, the experts noted the reduction in mortality (from about 35%-40% to about 2%-8%) associated with the implementation of the 2002 consensus therapy recommendations and lower survival if such therapy is delayed.[38a] In fact, for every hour delay in the restoration of normal blood pressure for age and a capillary refill less than 3 seconds, the child's mortality doubles.[38a]

The ultimate goal of treatment of septic shock is to support adequate organ perfusion and function. This requires careful titration of fluid administration, inotropic support, and vasoconstrictors or vasodilators to maximize systemic and organ perfusion (and function).

The terms *warm* versus *cold* septic shock are imprecise terms and should be used only in conjunction with other descriptions of systemic perfusion and cardiovascular function. **Warm shock** is characterized by peripheral vasodilation (warm skin) and was thought to be associated with hyperdynamic cardiovascular function with high cardiac output. **Cold shock** is characterized by peripheral vasoconstriction (cold skin) and thought to be associated with low cardiac output. However, cardiac output may be low, normal, or high regardless of skin temperature, and skin temperature alone will not identify the cardiovascular support required. When systemic perfusion is inadequate, the child likely needs more aggressive fluid administration and titration of vasoactive drug therapy.

Many adults and some children with sepsis generate a cardiac output that is higher than normal despite a fall in ventricular ejection fraction. This high cardiac output may be associated with temporary adaptive ventricular dilation and an increase in ventricular end-diastolic volume, an increase in heart rate, and a fall in systemic vascular resistance.

Table 47-7 Definitions and Clinical Criteria for Sepsis and Septic Shock, Including 2005 International Pediatric Definitions

Clinical Stage	Clinical Criteria
Part 1	
Systemic inflammatory response syndrome (SIRS)	Two or more of the following as acute change (one must be abnormal temperature or leukocyte count): Core fever (>38.5° C [101.3° F]) or hypothermia (<36° C [96.8° F]) Tachycardia* (or bradycardia in infants) _Adults:_ >90 beats/min _Newborns:_ 180 or <100 beats/min _Infants:_ 180 or <90 beats/min _Children:_ 130 beats/min Tachypnea* or hypocarbic respiratory alkalosis ($Paco_2$ <32 mmHg with spontaneous breathing) _Adults:_ rate >20 breaths/min _Infants:_ rate 34-50 breaths/min _Children:_ rate 14-21 breaths/min Leukocytosis* (white blood cell count >11,000-19,500/mm³) Leukopenia* (white blood cell count <4500-6000/mm³) or >10% band forms
Sepsis	SIRS (two or more of above) _plus_ suspected or proven infection
Severe sepsis	Sepsis _plus_ signs of cardiovascular organ dysfunction, or respiratory distress syndrome, or two or more organ dysfunctions (see Part 2 below)
Septic shock	Sepsis plus cardiovascular organ dysfunction (see Part 2 below)
Part 2	
Cardiovascular dysfunction	Despite administration of isotonic intravenous fluid bolus ≥40 ml/kg in 1 hour: Decrease in BP (hypotension) <5th percentile for age or systolic BP <2 SD below normal for age _OR_ Need for vasoactive drug to maintain BP in normal range (dopamine >5 mcg/kg/min or dobutamine, epinephrine, or norepinephrine at any dose) _OR_ Two of the following: Unexplained metabolic acidosis: base deficit >5 mEq/L Increased arterial lactate two or more times upper limit or normal Oliguria: urine output >0.5 ml/kg/hr Core to peripheral temperature gap >3° C (37.4° F)
Respiratory†	Pao_2/Fio_2 <300 in absence of cyanotic heart disease of preexisting lung disease _OR_ $Paco_2$ >65 torr or 20 mmHg over baseline Pao_2 _OR_ Proven need‡ or >50% Fio_2 to maintain saturation ≥92% _OR_ Need for nonelective invasive or noninvasive mechanical ventilation§
Neurologic	Glasgow coma score ≤11 (57) _OR_ Acute change in mental status with a decrease in Glasgow Coma Scale score ≥3 points from abnormal baseline
Hematologic	Platelet count <80,000/mm³ or a decline of 50% in platelet count from highest value recorded over the past 3 days (for chronic hematology/oncology patients) _OR_ International normalized ratio >2
Renal	Serum creatinine two or more times upper limit of normal for age or twofold increase in baseline creatinine
Hepatic	Total bilirubin ≥4 mg/dl (not applicable for newborn) _OR_ ALT two times upper limit of normal for age

Part 1 data from Carcillo JA et al: _Crit Care Med_ 30(6):1365-1378, 2002; Hayden WR: _J Pediatr_ 124:657-658, 1994; Goldstein B et al: _Pediatr Crit Care Med_ 6(1):2-8, 2005; Hazinski MF et al: _Am J Crit Care_ 2:224, 1993. Part 2 from Goldstein B et al: _Pediatr Crit Care Med_ 6(1):2-8, 2005.

*Some age-related differences in these ranges apply; the abnormal limits are generally defined as more than 2 standard deviations above or below normal ranges for age.

†Acute respiratory distress syndrome must include a Pao_2/Fio_2 ratio ≤200 mmHg, bilateral infiltrates, acute onset, and no evidence of left heart failure; acute lung injury is defined identically except the Pao_2/Fio_2 ratio must be 300 mmHg.

‡Proven need assumes oxygen requirement was tested by decreasing flow.

§In postoperative persons, this requirement can be met if the patient has developed an acute inflammatory or infectious process in the lungs that prevent him or her from being extubated.

ALT, Alanine transaminase; _BP_, blood pressure; _SD_, standard deviation.

The child may maintain a high cardiac output if intravascular volume is supported with aggressive fluid resuscitation. Echocardiography may reveal the reduction in ventricular ejection fraction and left ventricular dilation. If the mixed venous oxygen saturation is monitored continuously (through use of a pulmonary artery catheter), the mixed venous oxygen saturation ($S\bar{v}O_2$) may initially be high because oxygen extraction is low.[37,38]A When the child with sepsis improves in response to therapy, the $S\bar{v}O_2$ may initially fall as oxygen extraction increases.

Reperfusion and Inflammatory Injury

Reperfusion (reoxygenation) injury is cellular injury caused by the restoration or reperfusion of physiologic concentrations of oxygen to cells that have been exposed to injurious but nonlethal hypoxic conditions.[39] Reperfusion injury is stimulated by the generation of highly reactive oxygen intermediates (e.g., free oxygen radicals and superoxide) that damage cell membranes, denature proteins, and disrupt chromosomes[40] (see Chapter 2). The amount of free oxygen radical produced is directly related to the severity and duration of the ischemic period. The process is most likely to affect endothelial cells of the microvasculature, causing MODS, and is likely to contribute to the compromise of organ perfusion after shock resuscitation.[40]

An ischemic insult activates white blood cells, priming monocytes and macrophages and contributing to the release of inflammatory mediators or cytokines, including TNF, IL-1, IL-6, IL-8, and platelet activating factor. These cytokines in turn contribute to vasodilation, increased capillary permeability, and altered platelet function. The ultimate result is a maldistribution of blood flow and a compromise in organ perfusion.[40] The role of these mediators is summarized in Table 7-5. Chapter 46 includes a more comprehensive discussion of MODS.

Signs of organ dysfunction include but are not limited to lactic acidosis, oliguria, and an acute alteration in level of consciousness (e.g., decrease in Glasgow Coma Scale score of 1 point or more); hypoxemia, hypotension, poor capillary refill, or shock plus signs of coagulopathy, respiratory, renal, or hepatic dysfunction or neurologic dysfunction.[41] Box 47-3 lists other potential signs of organ system failure in children.

Evaluation and Treatment of Shock

Acidosis and a rise in serum lactate may be the most sensitive indicator of inadequate systemic perfusion in children. Evaluation of trends in serum lactate are typically more helpful than evaluation of any single measurement. Systolic hypotension is a late sign of shock in infants and children and often indicates cardiovascular collapse.

Providers should evaluate and support the child's oxygenation and ventilation whenever shock is present. In addition, the child's electrolytes, glucose, BUN, creatinine, liver function, calcium, phosphorus, and cardiac enzyme concentrations should be evaluated in an attempt to identify the cause of the shock or treatment needed.

Box 47-3	Proposed Signs of Organ System Dysfunction*

Central Nervous System
Acute change in mental status (confusion, agitation, lethargy)
Glasgow Coma Scale score 15 (previously normal) or decreased by 1

Pulmonary (ARDS)
Unexplained hypoxemia with suspected sepsis (Pao_2/Fio_2 175-280 mmHg)
Bilateral pulmonary infiltrates with PAOP 18 mmHg
Deterioration from baseline

Renal (Not Prerenal)
Oliguria (urine output 0.5 ml/kg/hr) despite adequate fluid administration
Increase in serum creatinine from normal with urine sodium 40 mmol/L
Rise in serum creatinine by 2 mg/dl in presence of preexisting renal insufficiency

Hepatobiliary
Elevation in liver function enzymes to twice normal
Serum bilirubin 2 mg/dl

Gastrointestinal
Paralytic ileus
Gastrointestinal bleeding

Coagulation
Confirmatory test for DIC (FDP >1:40 or d-dimers >2)
Thrombocytopenia or fall in platelet count by 25%
Elevated prothrombin time (PT) and partial thromboplastin time (PTT)
Clinical evidence of bleeding

From Hazinski MF et al: *Am J Crit Care* 2:224, 1993.
*Clinical criteria indicating organ system failure. These signs are consistent with organ system dysfunction or failure in the absence of other attributable causes.
ARDS, Adult respiratory distress syndrome; *DIC,* disseminated intravascular coagulation; *FDP,* fibrin degradation products; *PAOP,* pulmonary artery occlusion pressure.

Hematologic evaluation is necessary if hemorrhage or disseminated intravascular coagulation (DIC) is apparent. Hemoglobin and hematocrit may be artificially normal in the face of an acute hemorrhage; unless volume resuscitation is provided with whole blood, the child's hematocrit ultimately falls during fluid resuscitation. Evaluation for nontraumatic hemorrhage or potential DIC includes a complete blood count, platelets, coagulation tests (prothrombin time [PT], partial thromboplastin time [PTT], bleeding time), and DIC screen (fibrinogen, fibrin split products).

Obtain a chest roentgenogram to evaluate cardiac size and exclude pneumonia, pneumothorax, and pulmonary edema. An arterial blood gas (ABG) measurement monitors progression of acidosis and evidence of oxygenation or ventilation problems associated with respiratory distress. Oximetry enables evaluation of hemoglobin saturation and may indicate the loss of peripheral pulses; however, oximetry should never be used as a "pulse check." Electrocardiogram (ECG) and echocardiogram should be selectively used to evaluate cardiac function and rule out dysrhythmias, effusion, and failure as contributing factors to low cardiac output.

Microbiologic evaluation should be performed when infection is suspected. Blood and urine cultures should be obtained as needed; a Gram stain should be available immediately with these cultures. Evaluation of spinal fluid, stool, and joints also may be required.

Early recognition and aggressive antimicrobial and fluid therapy are the keys to survival for children in septic shock. Therefore, signs of poor systemic perfusion must be identified as soon as they appear. Supportive therapy then is required to optimize each aspect of cardiovascular and pulmonary function. Throughout therapy it is important to evaluate the child's response to therapy and to monitor for evidence of further deterioration and development of MODS. If signs of MODS develop, organ function must be supported.

The goals of treatment of shock are maximization of oxygen delivery and minimization of oxygen demand. The airway, oxygenation, and ventilation must be supported. Reduction of oxygen demand requires the treatment for fever and pain. In addition, the child should be kept warm and shivering should be prevented. Blood components and, perhaps, intravenous fluids should be warmed before administration to young infants and children with hypothermia. Fear and pain increase oxygen consumption, so care must be taken to reassure the child and treat pain as indicated.

When signs of shock are detected, immediate resuscitation is required. Hemodynamic monitoring should be instituted and volume and inotropic support provided as needed. The warmth of the child's extremities, capillary refill, quality of peripheral pulses, level of consciousness and responsiveness, urine output, oxygenation, ventilation, and acid-base status (including trends in serum lactate) should be assessed throughout shock therapy. Once systemic perfusion is restored, transfer to a pediatric intensive care unit is advised.

Initial therapy for any unstable person requires evaluation and support of airway patency and ventilation. Position the child in a manner that supports maximal airway patency, and evaluate the effectiveness of ventilation. Administer supplementary oxygen as needed at up to 10 to 15 L/minute by nonrebreathing mask or bag-mask ventilation. Children in shock should be intubated *before* respiratory deterioration or arrest complicates shock management.

The child's heart rate must be adequate to support effective cardiac output and systemic perfusion. The most common pediatric dysrhythmias are listed in Box 47-4. Treat bradydysrhythmias and extreme tachydysrhythmias promptly. Pharmacologic therapy, pacing, or synchronized direct current (DC) cardioversion may be required.

The rhythms associated with loss of pulses ("arrest" rhythms) include asystole, electromechanical dissociation (EMD), pulseless ventricular tachycardia, and ventricular fibrillation. Regardless of ECG findings, provide cardiopulmonary resuscitation—including cardiac compression—when pulses are lost or if, despite support of oxygenation and ventilation, the child demonstrates a heart rate less than 60/min with poor perfusion.

Box 47-4	Most Common Pediatric Dysrhythmias

Heart (QRS) Rate Too Slow for Clinical Condition
QRS duration (width) normal
Sinus bradycardia
Junctional rhythm
Heart block
QRS duration (width) prolonged
Supraventricular tachycardia (SVT) with aberrant ventricular conduction
Ventricular rhythm
Heart block

Heart (QRS) Rate Too Fast for Clinical Condition
QRS duration (width) normal
Sinus tachycardia
SVT
QRS duration (width) prolonged
SVT with aberrant ventricular conduction
Ventricular tachycardia

Collapse (Pulseless) Rhythms
Electromechanical dissociation
Ventricular tachycardia
Ventricular fibrillation
Asystole

From Hazinski MF: Cardiovascular disorders. In Hazinski MF, editor: *Manual of pediatric critical care*, St Louis, 1999, Mosby.

Volume resuscitation is designed to restore intravascular volume relative to the vascular space and optimize ventricular preload. The specific fluid selected and route of administration are determined by the child's clinical condition. In general, however, isotonic **crystalloids** (salt-containing solutions, such as normal saline or lactated Ringer solution) or **colloids** (protein-containing fluids, such as albumin or blood) are administered in boluses of 20 ml/kg. Hypotonic fluids should not be administered.[42] Children in septic shock require a large volume of intravenous fluid to restore and maintain systemic perfusion. More than 40 ml/kg will likely be required during the first hour of volume resuscitation, and a total of 100 to 200 ml/kg or more may be required during the first several hours of therapy.[32,37] In fact, rapid volume administration, particularly during the first hour of therapy, has been linked with improved survival in hypotensive children in septic shock. If intravenous access cannot be achieved, an intraosseous needle should be inserted and intraosseous fluid and drug administration provided through that route.[2]

Unless shock is mild or responds immediately to volume therapy, insertion of a central venous (monitoring) catheter is advisable. Several multilumen catheters are available in pediatric sizes that enable simultaneous monitoring of central venous pressure and administration of fluids.

Monitoring of the volume of urine output and specific gravity is useful in determining the child's response to fluid therapy. A urinary catheter should be inserted if shock is present unless the child has sustained pelvic trauma or a urethral tear is suspected. All sources of fluid intake and output should be monitored and recorded hourly or more frequently if needed.

An intra-arterial line should be inserted if shock persists. This enables reliable, continuous evaluation of arterial pressure. Noninvasive oscillometric blood pressure–monitoring devices may not accurately measure low or rapidly falling blood pressures and may *overestimate* the blood pressure,[43] particularly in trauma patients.[44] Sphygmomanometry also may yield inaccurate blood pressure measurement; cuff pressure measurement of a person in shock typically *underestimates* the systolic blood pressure (cuff measurements are lower than intra-arterial pressure).[45]

Insertion of a pulmonary artery catheter should be considered if the child demonstrates shock that is unresponsive to volume and vasoactive drug support. A pulmonary artery catheter with thermodilution cardiac output thermistor, a fiberoptic pulmonary artery catheter, or both can enable continuous monitoring of mixed venous oxygen saturation or continuous monitoring of cardiac output. Quantification of these variables can be particularly helpful if precise tracking of hemodynamic measurements is desired.[32] This may be necessary in the care of the child with septic shock or MODS.

The optimal hemoglobin threshold for transfusion in critically ill children is unknown. In a multicenter trial of stable critically ill children, a hemoglobin red-cell transfusion threshold of 7 g/dl decreased transfusion requirements without increasing adverse outcomes.[46] However, there has been no similar study to guide transfusion therapy in premature infants or in children with severe hypoxemia, hemodynamic instability, active blood loss, or cyanotic heart disease.

Administration of blood or blood component therapy is needed to treat hemorrhage or severe coagulopathies. A "normal" hematocrit does not rule out the possibility of hemorrhage; the hematocrit typically falls in a person who has sustained whole blood loss after replacement of the blood loss with crystalloids or colloids. In general, 10 ml/kg boluses of packed red blood cells are administered to treat significant blood loss.

Transfusion for the child with chronic anemia and shock must be accomplished slowly to prevent hypervolemia and further deterioration in myocardial function. Administration of packed red blood cells at a rate averaging 3 to 5 ml/kg/hr over several hours may be well tolerated, particularly if it is preceded and followed by administration of diuretics. If severe anemia is associated with severe hypervolemia and myocardial dysfunction, an exchange transfusion may be required. If a coagulopathy is present, administer specific blood component therapy necessary to prevent or treat hemorrhage.

Hypoxemia, metabolic acidosis, and electrolyte imbalances depress myocardial function and must be corrected when shock is present. Administer oxygen during resuscitation of the child in shock and be prepared to institute mechanical ventilatory support when needed.

Hypoglycemia may develop rapidly in the critically ill or injured infant because infants have high glucose needs and low glycogen stores. If glucose is needed, however, continuous infusion is preferred to intermittent bolus therapy. In fact, hyperglycemia has been linked to poor outcome in some children with head injury,[9] although it is unclear whether the poor outcome is caused by idiopathic hyperglycemia or excessive glucose administration.[10] Careful glucose monitoring and treatment of hyperglycemia is now recommended for critically ill children to maintain blood glucose levels between 80 mg/dl and 120 mg/dl.[10]

Acute or severe alterations in the serum sodium concentration during fluid therapy should be avoided.[42] Acute changes in serum sodium produce changes in serum osmolality that result in fluid shifts into and out of the vascular spaces. Such fluid shifts can be associated with neurologic complications, including seizures, cerebral edema, and intracranial hemorrhage.[6,47]

Alterations in serum potassium concentration may affect myocardial contractility and conduction. However, children are far less sensitive than adults to minor changes in serum potassium concentration. Hypokalemia may result from inadequate potassium administration during volume therapy or from excessive potassium losses caused by drug therapy (e.g., furosemide). The serum potassium concentration falls in the presence of alkalosis; this represents an intracellular shift of potassium and is corrected when the pH is normalized. Treat true hypokalemia with an infusion of potassium chloride at a dose equivalent to 0.5 to 1 mEq/kg administered over several hours.

Hyperkalemia may result from excessive potassium administration, reduced potassium excretion (e.g., in renal failure), or massive cell lysis (e.g., tumor lysis syndrome). Serum potassium concentration also rises when acidosis develops; the rise in serum potassium is caused by a shift of potassium from the intracellular to the vascular space (e.g., exchange with vascular H^+) and falls when the serum pH is corrected.

Both ionized and total calcium concentration should be monitored, and documented hypocalcemia must be treated. Note that the ionized serum calcium falls with alkalosis and rises with acidosis. Serum ionized calcium concentration is often low (less than 4.5 mEq/L) in children with septic shock.[48]

Hypercalcemia may be observed in children with some malignancies, including acute lymphocytic leukemia, lymphomas, and soft tissue sarcomas. Malignant cells often secrete a parathormone-like substance that stimulates bone reabsorption, release of calcium, and rapid cell turnover.[49] Although mild hypercalcemia is not life threatening, extreme hypercalcemia (total serum calcium approaching 19 to 20 mEq/L) may produce renal and cardiovascular complications. Table 47-8 summarizes additional drug therapy for children in shock. If oxygenation, ventilation, heart rate, and intravascular volume are appropriate and myocardial function and systemic perfusion remain poor, vasoactive drug therapy with inotropes is indicated.

Table 47-8	Drug Therapies for Children in Shock	
Type	**Indications**	**Comments**
Vasoactive (inotropes)	If oxygenation, ventilation, and intravascular volume are appropriate but myocardial function and systemic perfusion remain poor or heart rate is low	Useful in the treatment of cardiogenic and distributive shock or any shock with impaired myocardial function; goals include increased heart rate (if it is low), increased cardiac output, redistribution of cardiac output, and increased cardiac contractility
Sympathomimetic	To stimulate particular adrenergic receptors	Receptors targeted will be determined by the child's heart rate, peripheral perfusion, blood pressure, and urine output
Dopamine	To improve renal, coronary artery, mesenteric, and cerebral circulation at low doses and increase heart rate or myocardial function at moderate doses; vasoconstriction may occur at high doses	Popular drug used especially in the presence of oliguria; provides dopaminergic effects (renal, coronary artery, mesenteric, cerebral vasodilation) and β- and α-adrenergic effects at higher doses
Epinephrine	For resuscitation from cardiopulmonary arrest or cardiovascular collapse; to treat symptomatic bradycardia unresponsive to oxygen therapy and adequate ventilation or in the treatment of hypotension	Effective in increasing mean arterial pressure and improving myocardial function in children with septic shock
Vasopressin	To improve blood pressure	May be useful in the treatment of shock associated with vasodilation
Vasodilators	To reduce impedance to ventricular ejection	Because they dilate both arteries and veins, they may reduce ventricular preload and afterload
Antibiotics	For treatment of bacterial infection	Broad spectrum used until a specific causative microorganism is identified
Steroids	For meningitis or septic shock that is unresponsive to initial volume administration and vasopressors	Given 20 to 30 min before first dose of antibiotics, steroids may be associated with improvement in auditory function

Emerging Therapies for Shock and Sepsis

Prevention of shock is important. Prevention of trauma (injury prevention) and treatment of dehydration can eliminate the two leading causes of hypovolemic shock in children. *Haemophilus influenzae* sepsis and meningitis have been nearly eradicated in the United States since the introduction and widespread use of *H. influenzae* vaccine for infants, and immunization against *Neisseria meningitidis* (the causative microorganism of meningococcal sepsis) may similarly reduce the incidence of meningococcal sepsis. Administration of colony-stimulating factors to increase white blood cell count in immunosuppressed persons has been shown to decrease infection and sepsis in this high-risk population.[49] Septic shock also may be prevented with good handwashing technique, early detection of infection, use of protocols to reduce ventilator-assisted pneumonias, and appropriate antimicrobial therapies for infection and sepsis.

Several advances in shock therapy have been made in recent years and several show promise for continued improvement in treatment. First, there is a better understanding of resuscitation goals with an appreciation of the need to target high, rather than normal, cardiac output and oxygen delivery during resuscitation.

Trauma resuscitation has become more targeted in adults and children. In the prehospital setting, aggressive fluid resuscitation may delay transport and increase bleeding, particularly in those with penetrating trauma, so prehospital fluid resuscitation is reserved for children with signs of shock. If penetrating trauma is associated with hypovolemic shock, the child requires urgent surgical intervention, thus prehospital providers should minimize delays during transport.

Colloids or isotonic crystalloids can be used for resuscitation in the case of hypovolemic shock. Recent studies have documented the efficacy of prehospital administration of hypertonic saline for adults with head trauma[50] and hypertonic saline is used during resuscitation of children. Because massive transfusions can produce immunologic and coagulation complications, the surgical approach to trauma has changed to include staged surgical repair of significant trauma injuries (e.g., liver and bowel injuries). The initial surgery is performed to stabilize and the second surgery repairs the injury. This two-stage approach typically reduces the amount of blood products required. Although initial experience with artificial blood products was discouraging, new products are being tested that show promise.[51]

We now have a better understanding of the pathophysiology of septic shock in children,[32] appreciating the critical role that early and aggressive fluid resuscitation and vasoactive therapy play in the outcome of pediatric sepsis. Children are far more likely to survive an episode of septic shock if they receive 40 to 60 ml/kg or more of fluid in the first hour of resuscitation and 200 to 240 ml/kg or more during the first 8 hours of therapy.[32] During fluid resuscitation, the healthcare provider should expect that the child will develop both systemic and pulmonary edema because capillary permeability is increased. For this reason, providers should plan for intubation and mechanical ventilatory support. Vasoactive therapy is needed if hypotension persists despite aggressive fluid resuscitation. Dopamine or dobutamine can be administered by peripheral intravenous access if central access is not established.

Goals of therapy for pediatric septic shock are to restore the child's heart rate and blood pressure to normal for age, to achieve targeted perfusion pressure (mean arterial pressure – CVP of about 55-65 mmHg), to reduce capillary refill to less than 2 seconds, and to support a cardiac index of 3.3 to 6.0 L/m/m^2 body surface area, and to maintain the mixed venous oxygen saturation ($S\bar{v}O_2$) above 70%.

The 2005 publication of international consensus definitions for sepsis and organ dysfunction in children[34] and the 2007 update of recommendations for hemodynamic support of children with septic shock[38a] will enable better standardization of care. Consistency in patient description and therapy will enable improvement in outcomes and accurate comparison of therapies.

In the 1980s and 1990s, mediator-specific therapies did improve survival in laboratory animals and in subsets of patients but failed to improve survival in large clinical trials. Activated protein C was the first mediatory-specific therapy shown to improve survival in a large, randomized controlled trial of adults with severe sepsis.[27] However, the trial with children was halted because of excessive bleeding complications.

Continuous plasma filtration improves organ function and blood pressure in septic adults and children but has not yet improved survival rates.[52] Glucocorticoid administration has been successful for treatment of infants and children with actual or relative adrenal insufficiency.[30] High doses of steroids do not improve adult survival from sepsis.[29] A recent meta-analysis showing that administration of physiologic doses to adults with septic shock improved survival but many of the patients that demonstrated improvement had been treated with etomidate.[31] Administration of low doses of glucocorticoids should be considered for the treatment of pediatric septic shock that is unresponsive to volume and inotropes, if adrenal insufficiency is suspected; routine use of glucocorticoids is not recommended.[8,32, 38a] The outcome of large, prospective, randomized controlled pediatric trials of glucocorticoids in fluid- and catecholamine-refractory septic shock in children are needed.

Therapeutic hypothermia suppresses proinflammatory mediators and may enhance anti-inflammatory mediators.[53] Moderate induced hypothermia (to 32° to 34° C [89.6° to 93.2° F]) has been shown to increase survival in neurologic outcome in neonates with hypoxic-ischemic encephalopathy[54] and in comatose, hemodynamically stable adults following resuscitation from cardiac arrest.[55] It is possible that such therapy may be helpful for victims of shock, particularly those with MODS.

It soon may be possible to tailor sepsis and other critical therapies through the use of genetic profiling.[56] Mannose-binding lectin (MBL) is a substance that plays a role in stimulating phagocytosis of microorganisms and in reducing production of inflammatory cytokines. One third of the population has genetic changes on the MBL gene that causes reduced MBL levels in the blood; this genotype has been shown to increase risk of SIRS in children[57] and in adults, although this has not been linked to increased mortality.[56] Prospective identification of genetic markers for risk of sepsis and responsiveness to therapy may enable individual tailoring of surveillance and therapy with the hope of improving outcome.

BURNS

Management of pediatric burn injuries requires an understanding of the differences that exist in this population related to etiology of injury, growth and development, physiology, and clinical course. In 1988 the American Burn Association established criteria to guide transfer of a patient to a specialized burn center. These recommendations are based on complex management issues related to treatment of acute burns and the long-term rehabilitation needs of children.[58]

Burn injuries in children often are preventable and often are the result of inadequate supervision, curiosity, inability to escape the burning agent, or intentional abuse. **Scald injuries** (i.e., hot water, grease, other) are most common among young children whereas flame burns are more prevalent among older children.[59] A child exposed to hot tap water at 60° C (140° F) for 3 seconds will sustain a third-degree burn.[60]

A child's skin is thinner and thus more susceptible to injury than an adult's. The extent of injury is determined by the temperature of the burning agent and the duration of exposure. Because very young children may be unable to escape the heat source, the depth of the injury is likely to be greater. The kitchen is also a common site of burn injury and often involves pulling over dishes or appliances containing hot liquids. These are common burn injury sources for children 2 years of age and younger.

Although **child abuse** can occur at any age, young children are particularly vulnerable to serious injury. Approximately 5% to 22% of all physical abuse cases in the United States are caused by burning.[61] Burns that may suggest physical maltreatment include (1) patterned burns, (2) classic forced emersion burn pattern with sharp stocking or glove demarcation and sparing of flexed protected areas, (3) splash/spill burn patterns not consistent with history or developmental level, and (4) cigarette burns. Abuse is suggested with (1) incompatible history and physical examination; (2) incompatible burn and developmental level; (3) bilateral or mirror image burns; (4) localized burns to genitals, buttocks, and perineum (especially at toilet-training stage); (5) evidence of excessive delay in seeking treatment; and (6) presence of other forms of injury.[62] Forced immersion in hot water typically presents with deep symmetric injuries lacking any evidence of splash wounds (Figure 47-2). **Contact burns** also may be intentionally inflicted by contact with cigarettes or other hot objects such as curling irons. Young children may inadvertently grasp a hot object. However, the pattern of injury will be confined to the palm. Burns to the dorsum of the hand are viewed with suspicion.[61]

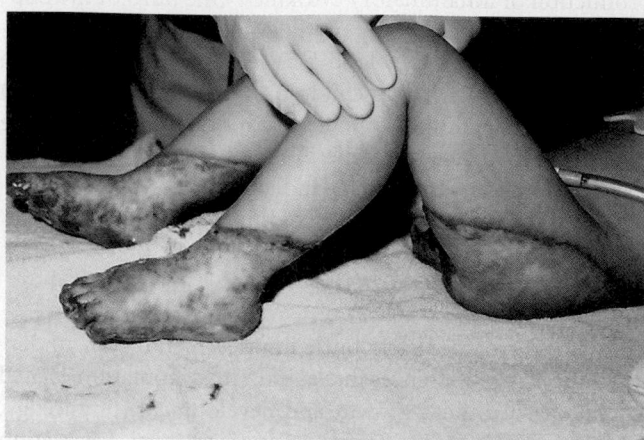

Figure 47-2 Burn pattern typically seen after forced emersion in hot water.

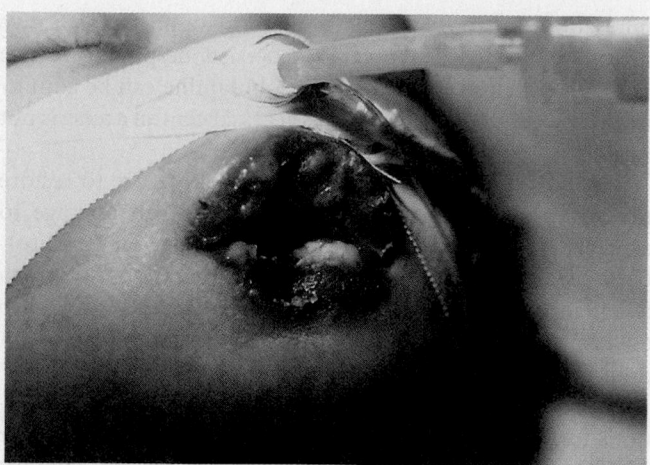

Figure 47-3 Commissure burn resulting from biting an electrical wire.

Children 3 to 8 years of age are most often injured by flame during fire play. Lighters and matches ignite clothing and cause house fires. Inhalation injury is the main cause of death in up to 80% of fire-related fatalities in the United States. Young children may run when clothing ignites and increase the severity of injury. Escape from a burning residence or motor vehicle is often delayed because young children cannot cognitively comprehend the circumstances or physically remove themselves from the danger. **Flame burns** involving flammable liquids, especially gasoline, are more common in older children.

Although flame and scald burns account for the majority of thermal injuries in children, **electrical burns** result from direct contact with high- or low-voltage current. Most commonly these injuries occur as a result of risk-taking behavior on the part of young males. Trauma from contact with electrical energy results from the passage of current through vital organs, muscle compartments, and nerve or vascular pathways. Very young children are at risk for injury from chewing on electrical cords or inserting objects into electrical outlets (Figure 47-3). Lightning strikes also account for some electrical burns. **Chemical burns** occur most often in an industrial setting for the adult. At home, children may be burned by swallowing corrosive agents. The type of causative agent has important implications for the evaluation, treatment, and prognosis of the child.

Severity of Injury

The severity of burn injury is assessed based on the percentage of the total body surface area (TBSA) involved. Use of the standard rule of nines results in inaccurate calculation of the percentage of TBSA involved in children. Although the infant's trunk and arms are of roughly the same proportion as the adult's, the head and neck make up 18% of TBSA and each lower extremity is 14% of TBSA. A modified rule of nines deducts 1% from the head and adds 0.5% to each leg for each year of life after 2 years.[63] Various charts are available that assign body proportions to children of different ages. These are

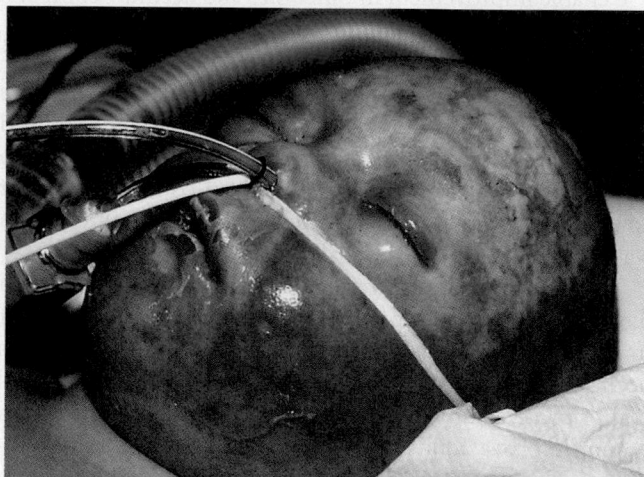

Figure 47-4 Areas of indeterminant depth of injury in a young child.

generally used in pediatric burn facilities and do accurately compute the extent of burn injury.

Because burn trauma represents a three-dimensional wound, the severity of injury is assessed also in relation to the **depth of injury.** The etiology of the burn and the duration of contact with the burning agent are important considerations in determining the depth of injury. In general, the more intense the heat source and the longer the contact, the deeper the resulting injury. However, infant skin is extremely fragile and more likely to sustain a deeper burn. This makes the estimation of the depth of burn difficult in very young children, especially following scald injuries (Figure 47-4). Intentionally inflicted burns tend to be more severe because contact with the burning agent is prolonged. Electrical injuries also may mask the extent of damage on initial assessment. Visible tissue damage may appear minimal despite severe injury to underlying structures.

Another important factor in assessing the severity of injury is the victim's age. Children younger than 2 years have a significantly higher risk for associated morbidity and mortality after sustaining burn injury. They have not achieved maturity of the immune system and are at increased risk for infection and sepsis. In addition, very young children are intolerant of rapid fluid shifts and demonstrate immature renal function, which negatively affects their ability to retain sodium and water (see the Shock section).

The areas of the body injured are another consideration when assessing the severity of the burn. Burns of the hands, feet, and perineum and burns across joints carry the potential for scar formation and contracture that may interfere with function as well as growth and development. Specialized care is required to preserve maximal function. In addition, burns to the face and neck may result in airway compromise as well as deformity caused by damage to delicate cartilage of the nose and ears.

Concomitant injuries may be suggested by the circumstances of the burn and should always be investigated; for example, initially burns do not bleed. Bloody drainage suggests another source of trauma. Fractures may result from jumping from a window to escape a house fire. Electrical injuries and motor vehicle accidents often result in associated trauma. Any suspicion of intentionally inflicted burns should alert the burn team to assess for other injuries.

PATHOPHYSIOLOGY Major burn trauma involves all body systems, and the consequences of injury include shock, infection, hypermetabolism, organ failure, and functional limitations. These effects can be magnified in the pediatric population as a result of physiologic immaturity and age-related variation in treatment modalities.

Integument

The local response manifested in the area of trauma includes cellular destruction and damage. Progressive injury caused by **dermal ischemia** may result from ineffective initial management, especially inadequate or delayed resuscitation. An increase in the permeability and hydrostatic pressure of the capillaries results in the loss of fluid, proteins, and electrolytes into the interstitial spaces. A diminishing intravascular oncotic pressure further enhances these losses and results in edema formation. Marked edema can result not only in the area of injury but also in unburned areas. Loss of substantial areas of skin has immediate and profound physiologic effects. Direct and evaporative fluid losses are seen immediately.[64] Although these losses are maximal in the immediate postburn period, they persist until wound closure.

Circulatory alterations also occur in the area of injury. Reduced blood flow and capillary stasis result from **hemoconcentration,** the release of thromboplastin and clot-activating factors from heat-damaged cells, reduced cardiac output, and edema formation. Circulation in the area of partial-thickness wounds ceases for 24 to 48 hours after injury, after which it is usually restored. Vascular supply in the area of full-thickness injuries is completely occluded and is not restored until granulation tissue forms or the wound is surgically repaired. The dry, leathery **eschar** provides an ideal environment for bacterial growth. Infection, trauma, or applying ice to the burn

area may convert a partial-thickness injury to a full-thickness one, especially in young children, who have thinner, more delicate skin.

Vitamin D, an essential factor for proper formation of bone during growth and development, is an important nutrient in children to facilitate intestinal absorption of calcium. Vitamin D deficiency has been associated with adverse effects on the skeletal system, as well as the immune system. Vitamin D production may be compromised in burned children demonstrated by a high incidence of low-serum vitamin D levels. Burn wound scarring and lack of sunlight may limit cutaneous vitamin D biosynthesis.[65]

Cardiovascular System

The marked reduction in cardiac output immediately following injury is accompanied by an initial increase in systemic vascular resistance. As fluid is lost into the interstitial spaces, a further reduction in cardiac output occurs, accompanied by vasodilation. Because the infant maintains cardiac output by increasing heart rate preferentially to stroke volume, extremely elevated heart rates result in a decreased filling time and a further reduction in cardiac output.[63] Adequate resuscitation returns cardiac output to normal levels in approximately 24 to 36 hours. Without fluid replacement, cardiac output continues to decrease and results in organ failure and death.

The inefficient and labile peripheral circulation of the infant further complicates management of the burn shock phase of treatment. The rapid fluid shift to the interstitial space and drying of the eschar result in compromised circulation and a resultant tourniquet effect in the extremities. Blood vessels and nerves become entrapped because the fascia cannot expand to accommodate the massive edema. Release of pressure is required to restore blood flow and preserve nerve function (Figure 47-5).

Constriction of the chest and impairment of respiratory excursion also may result, especially in the very young child, because of the increased pliability of the rib cage. Excessive fluid volume can contribute to a serious complication

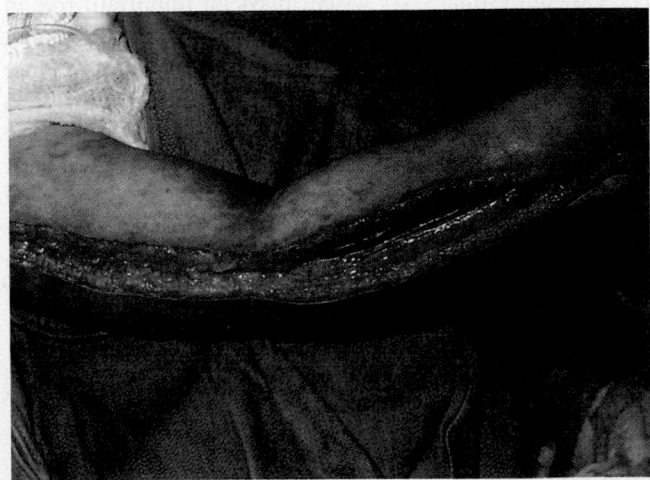

Figure 47-5 Escharotomy/fasciotomy in a severely burned arm.

(increased intra-abdominal pressure) that may have an underestimated incidence in burned individuals. Although children with increased intra-abdominal pressure readings tended to be younger, larger TBSA injuries and full-thickness components were significantly associated with elevated pressures.[66] Increased **intra-abdominal pressure** has the potential to impair hemodynamics, renal function, hepatic malperfusion, and pulmonary dysfunction. Despite maintaining cardiac output with fluid replacement, renal function remains impaired in the presence of increased intra-abdominal pressure. Increases in the production and release of the hormones norepinephrine, dopamine, epinephrine, angiotensin, and renin support the clinical finding of profoundly altered renal, pulmonary, and cardiovascular function.

Renal System

Loss of circulating volume into the interstitial spaces results in reduced renal blood flow and decreased glomerular filtration. An important measure of the adequacy of volume replacement is urine excretion. Sufficient volume replacement maintains urine output during resuscitation. Approximately 36 hours after injury, edema fluid begins to mobilize and output increases.

Evidence of pigment in the urine results from the hemolysis of red blood cells. This is especially common after extensive electrical injuries and destroyed muscle from deep thermal injury. The release of **myoglobin** may occlude the kidney tubules and result in renal failure.

Children younger than 2 years lack the ability to concentrate urine because of the immaturity of the renal system and are therefore at increased risk for dehydration. In addition, the child has a relatively larger TBSA in relation to weight than the adult. Combined with limited physiologic reserves, increased fluid requirements are necessary for children during burn shock resuscitation and to compensate for evaporative water losses.[67]

Gastrointestinal System

The gastrointestinal (GI) system plays an important role in the pathophysiology of burns. Alterations in blood flow result in decreased perfusion to the GI tract. Ischemia may cause erosion and necrosis of GI tissue. The GI response to a burn injury often includes mucosal atrophy, changes in digestive absorption, and increased intestinal permeability. Depending on the proportion of burn size, atrophy of small bowel mucosa occurs within 12 hours of injury. The atrophy may also result in a reduced uptake of glucose and amino acids, as well as decreased absorption of fatty acids and a reduction of brush border lipase activity.[68]

Paralytic ileus occurs often after major burn injuries. Although digestion ceases in the stomach and the large bowel, the small intestine maintains motility and absorptive capacity. Intestinal motility returns as fluid losses are replaced unless irreversible necrosis of the bowel has occurred as a result of insufficient perfusion.

Metabolism

Complex metabolic alterations are observed after burn injury. The extent of metabolic derangement is proportional to the magnitude of TBSA burn sustained. Wilmore[69] demonstrated the linear increase in metabolic rate up to 2½ times normal resting energy expenditure. As burn injury approaches 50% of TBSA, a plateau is reached, limiting further physiologic response to the trauma or other challenges such as infection.

A biphasic pattern of physiologic response is evident in thermally injured children. The initial **ebb phase** occurs during the immediate postburn period and continues for 3 to 5 days. This phase is characterized by reduced oxygen consumption, impaired circulation, and cellular shock. After the resolution of the shock and the restoration of circulating volume, the metabolic response shifts to a **catabolic (flow) phase** (Table 47-9). A state of **hypermetabolism** ensues, characterized by increased oxygen consumption and elevation of catecholamines, glucocorticoids, and glucagon.

Increased blood flow to the wound supplies additional glucose necessary for tissue repair. Insulin levels are usually normal or even elevated but are inappropriately low in relation to glucagon. Catecholamines and glucocorticoids act as antagonists to insulin. This effect combined with a tissue resistance to insulin stimulates glycogenolysis and gluconeogenesis, thus increasing glucose flow from the liver.[70] In the child, glycogen stores for meeting the increased energy demands of the burn are limited. The initiation of protein and lipid catabolism for glycogenesis is accelerated. This prolonged metabolic dysfunction may lead to loss of lean body mass and increased morbidity.[67]

Metabolic rates slowly return to normal with wound closure. However, a reactivation of the hypermetabolic response may occur with sepsis or organ failure.

Immune Function

Burn trauma–induced immunosuppression results in increased susceptibility to infection and sepsis. Although the exact mechanisms responsible for this immunosuppression remain obscure, it is clear that complex interactions of the hypermetabolic response, nutritional support, bacterial translocation, and defects in both innate and acquired immune function are involved (Figure 47-6). In addition, young children are at increased risk for microbial invasion caused by an immature immune system and limited antibody production.

Deitch reported that wound- or gut-derived endotoxemia may be one of the mediators of the hypermetabolic response observed after thermal injury.[71] When bacteria translocate from the gut or from the burn wound, endotoxin may affect immunologic response as inflammatory mediators are released. A further complication in the activation of inflammatory mediators is the release of toxic metabolites, such as oxygen free radicals.[72]

Circulating immunoglobulins may be affected by several factors, including age and the severity of injury.[73] Therapeutic interventions such as multiple transfusions, surgical

Table 47-9	Metabolic Alterations Following Injury	
Response	**Dominant Factors**	**Clinical Findings**
Ebb response	Loss of plasma volume Shock Low plasma insulin levels	Hyperglycemia Decreased oxygen consumption Depressed resting energy expenditure Decreased blood pressure Cardiac output below normal Decreased body temperature
Flow response Acute phase	Elevated catecholamines Elevated glucagons Elevated glucocorticoids Normal or elevated insulin levels High glucagon/insulin ratio	Catabolic Hyperglycemia Increased respiratory rate Increased oxygen consumption Increased body temperature Redistribution of polyvalent cations such as zinc and iron Mobilization of metabolic reserves Increased urinary excretion of nitrogen, sulfur, magnesium, phosphorus, potassium Accelerated gluconeogenesis
Adaptive phase	Stress hormone response subsiding	Anabolic Normoglycemia Energy turnover diminished Convalescence

From Gottschlich M, Alexander JW, Bower RH. In Rombeau JL, Caldwell MD, editors: *Enteral and tube feeding,* Philadelphia, 1990, Saunders.

procedures, and antibiotic and anesthetic administration also introduce elements that confound the evaluation of immunosuppressive effects. The immune system is activated systemically after a large burn injury with extensive tissue necrosis and may become ineffective or even self-destructive. Infections in burns may result in the loss of some components of innate immune function.[74]

Scar Maturation

In normal epidermal healing, minimal disruption in skin color, texture, and thickness occurs. However, burn wounds that extend into the dermis are repaired through **scar formation** and may result in an overgrowth of dermal constituents (Figure 47-7). Accelerated collagen synthesis most likely begins with high levels of activity in granulation tissue. The **hypertrophic scar** consists of hypercellular and disorganized connective tissue that is erythematous, raised, and pruritic. Normal dermis contains thick fibers and fiber bundles running parallel to the surface. In the hypertrophic scar, the collagen is arranged in whorls and nodules that account for its inelasticity and increased turgor.[75] As the hypertrophic scar matures, collagen begins to orient in a more parallel fashion and vascularity decreases (Figure 47-8). Collagen synthesis is very active soon after wound closure, and alteration of the scar can be accomplished before strong cross-linking of the collagen is established.

Although duration of wound healing varies among individuals, the length of time required to achieve wound closure is the most reliable predictor of hypertrophic scarring. Deeper burns demonstrate increased scarring caused by the formation of granulation tissue and prolonged healing time. Generally,

darker-pigmented races are more susceptible to hypertrophic scarring.[76] Although age has not been found to be a predictor of hypertrophic scar formation, younger individuals are more susceptible to trauma and have greater skin tension and an accelerated rate of collagen synthesis. Increased tension with resultant trauma stimulates inflammation, which in turn results in the formation of additional collagen.

CLINICAL MANIFESTATIONS The clinical manifestations of burn injuries are apparent in all organ systems. Although the cutaneous trauma is the initiator of the chain of responses, it is important to consider all of the likely consequences of the injury. An awareness of the changing patterns of convalescence and the development of complications assists in the identification and early treatment of potential sequelae.

Burn Shock

The pathophysiologic responses of burn injury result in **hypovolemia** and extracellular sodium depletion in the burn-injured individual. These manifestations are discussed in Chapter 46. Hypotension is a late sign of shock in the child. A complete circulatory assessment, including heart rate and peripheral parameters, is a more reliable measure. The urine output is a reflection of end-organ perfusion and is therefore the most accurate monitor of the adequacy of fluid resuscitation. A urine output of 30 to 50 ml/hr in adults and 1 ml/kg/hr in children weighing less than 30 kg are the suggested endpoints associated with many resuscitation formulas. Fluid is titrated to maintain the output within these parameters.[66]

The fluid of choice for burn shock resuscitation should approximate the fluid lost from the circulating volume—for example, lactated Ringer solution. Children require fluid

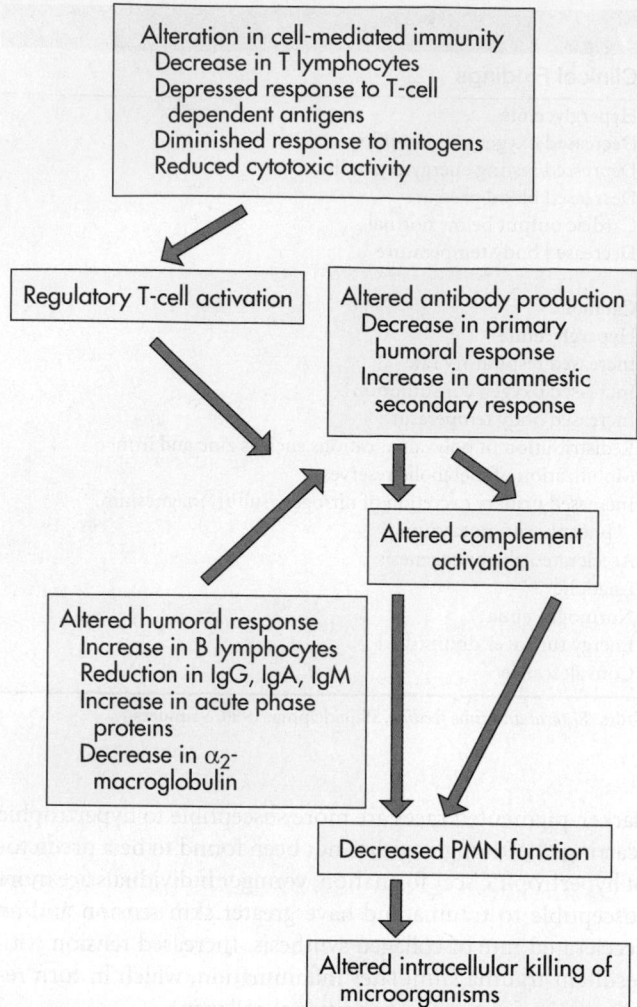

Alteration in cell-mediated immunity
  Decrease in T lymphocytes
  Depressed response to T-cell
    dependent antigens
  Diminished response to mitogens
  Reduced cytotoxic activity

Regulatory T-cell activation

Altered antibody production
  Decrease in primary
    humoral response
  Increase in anamnestic
    secondary response

Altered complement
  activation

Altered humoral response
  Increase in B lymphocytes
  Reduction in IgG, IgA, IgM
  Increase in acute phase
    proteins
  Decrease in α_2-
    macroglobulin

Decreased PMN function

Altered intracellular killing of
  microorganisms

Figure 47-6 Altered immune function after thermal injury. Cell-mediated immunity, antibody production, humoral response. *PMN*, polymorphonuclear leukocyte.

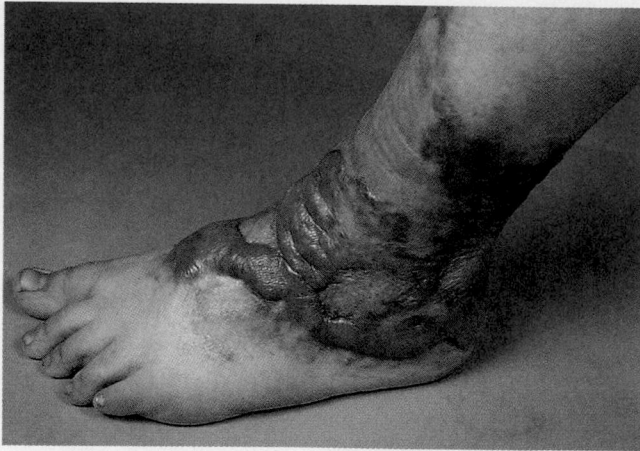

Figure 47-7 Immature hypertrophic scar.

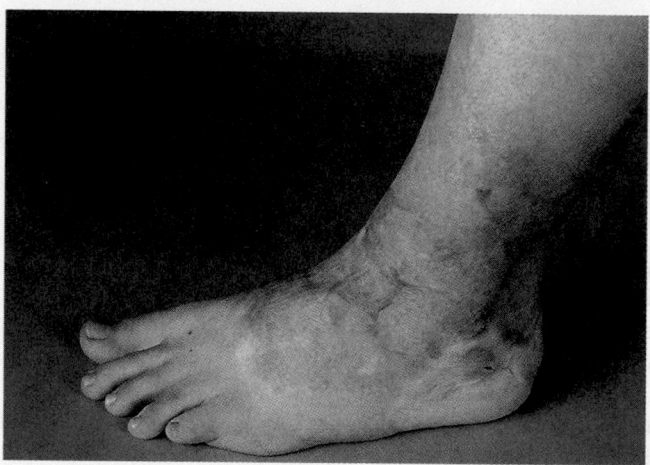

Figure 47-8 Flat, mature scar after pressure therapy.

resuscitation for smaller burns than do adults as a result of their limited physiologic reserves. The child's relatively greater ratio of body surface area to weight results in increased evaporative water losses and proportionately more fluid during resuscitation. Although **colloid replacement** during burn shock resuscitation remains controversial, replacement may be required in the very young child who fails to respond to fluid replacement.[77] A component for **maintenance fluid** *must* be included in the calculation of fluid needs during resuscitation. Maintenance fluids represent the body requirements in the absence of burn injury.

Successful resuscitation depends on establishment of intravenous access. Although this is usually accomplished by peripheral or central venous cannulation, circulatory collapse may preclude timely administration of fluid replacement. Cannulation of veins in the pediatric population is further complicated by small vessels and increased subcutaneous fat. Children are good candidates for **intraosseous cannulation** when traditional venous access techniques fail. Blood, drugs,

and fluid are readily absorbed by red marrow that drains into medullary venous channels and thus to the systemic circulation. This technique is most effective in children younger than 5 years, because red marrow is steadily replaced by yellow marrow in the limbs, making infusion more difficult, hence decreasing the infusion rate.[78] With proper care and removal as soon as other access is available, complications are minimal.

Pulmonary System

The clinical manifestations of burn injury related to the pulmonary system include a variety of complications ranging from inhalation injury, pulmonary edema, and respiratory failure to aspiration of gastric contents and pneumonia. Inhalation injury remains a major determinant of morbidity and mortality.[79]

Anatomic differences in the pediatric airway affect the response to pulmonary complications as well as therapeutic interventions. The infant airway is positioned anteriorly, making visualization of the cords more difficult. The difficult visualization is further compounded by the relatively large

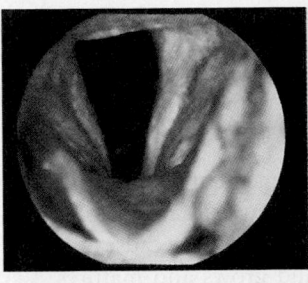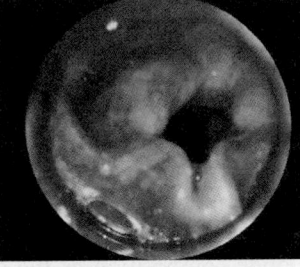

Figure 47-9 Airways. Adult airway *(left)*; smaller pediatric airway *(right)*.

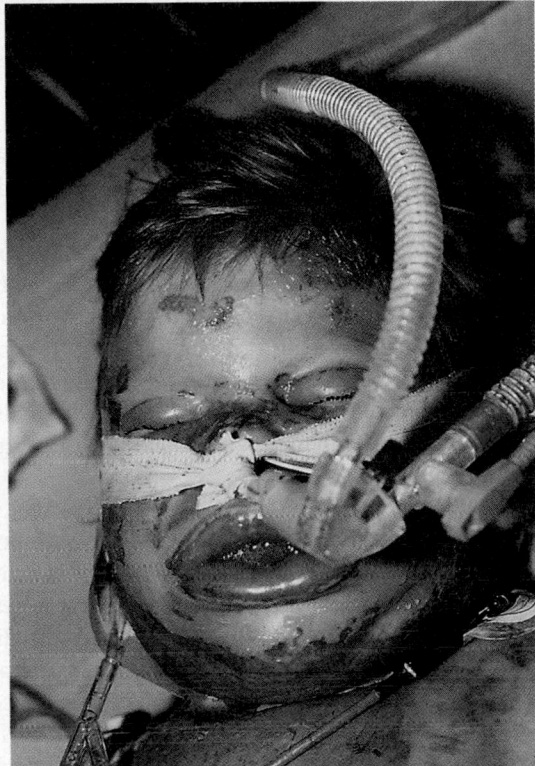

Figure 47-10 Severe facial edema during burn shock.

tongue and slanting vocal cords. A small degree of edema results in greatly increased work of breathing in the child (Figure 47-9). These considerations are particularly important during the resuscitation phase, when progressive edema threatens to obstruct the airway. Significant edema results in impairment of respiratory function unless an artificial airway is inserted (Figure 47-10). Malposition of an endotracheal tube may result in inadvertent extubation, intubation of the bronchi, and atelectasis. Because of the relatively short length of the infant trachea, alterations of the position of the head and neck can affect tube position despite maintenance of the tube position at the teeth.[80-82]

Infants compensate for pulmonary compromise by increasing the respiratory rate. However, because the child possesses fewer type I muscle fibers, fatigue related to the increased work of breathing results in more rapid desaturation than in adults. The soft cartilage of the pediatric airway is prone to

collapse in the presence of partial obstruction. Children with burns are at increased risk for these events because of underlying respiratory disease or injury.

Therapeutic interventions required for maintenance of pulmonary function also have been implicated in postextubation stridor and barotrauma. A mixture of helium and oxygen has been successfully used to decrease airway resistance and increase the volume of gas exchange after extubation.[83] Evidence suggests barotrauma from mechanical ventilation may be minimized by protocols based on permissive hypercapnia. Moderate respiratory acidosis was well tolerated and ventilating pressures maintained below 40 cm.[84] The low incidence of mortality associated with this strategy suggests a reduction in ventilator-induced lung injury.

The consequences of metabolic and physiologic changes occurring during the acute phase of injury remain apparent during convalescence. Severe burns result in a decrease in pulmonary function from restrictive and obstructive pulmonary disease evidenced by a reduction in pulmonary volumes and maximum voluntary ventilation lasting up to 8 years. At times, chest wall scarring in children caused by burns severely limits thoracic cage excursion.

Hypermetabolism

The hypermetabolic response after burn injury profoundly alters the production and use of nutrients. As a consequence of these phenomena, caloric requirements increase dramatically. Advances in burn care have allowed the performance of indirect calorimetry and assessment of metabolic rate at the bedside. Nutritional support must have an increased metabolic rate factored in (increased by 10% to 20%) because of fluctuations in energy use associated with activity. Current recommendations suggest 1.5 to 2 g protein/kg/day for adults and up to 3 g protein/kg/day for children.[85]

In addition to age, body composition has been found to significantly affect the postburn course. Preexisting obesity has been associated with increased clinical sepsis and associated morbidity.[86] However, the heightened nutrient requirements of the burned child preclude a reduction in nutritional support during the acute phase of recovery. Aggressive nutritional therapy is critical to the recovery of these children, and programs designed to achieve ideal body weight should not be instituted until wound healing is achieved.

Metabolism of many micronutrients are greatly affected by burn injury.[85] Hypermetabolism results in a rapid turnover in vitamins and trace minerals important in the wound healing and immune response. A deficiency of specific nutrients interferes with carbohydrate and nucleic acid metabolism, collagen formation, and immune function.

The **thermoregulatory response** after burn injury results in an elevation in core body temperature. Burned individuals strive for temperatures of about 38° C (100.4° F). Depressed or "normal" temperature may be indicative of overwhelming sepsis, or an exhausted physiologic capability to maintain temperature, and should be viewed as an ominous sign. Routine methods of heat conservation after a major burn injury are inadequate because of excessive heat loss through convection and evaporation.[85] Therapeutic intervention, such as operative procedures and dressing changes, and transport present situations requiring increased diligence to prevent inadvertent cooling.[85,87] Infants are at increased risk for a precipitous drop in core body temperature caused by an inability to regulate heat loss by shivering. Heat is also lost because of evaporation of water from damaged skin surfaces. Infants and children are especially vulnerable because of the large surface area relative to metabolically active tissue.

Infection

Whereas shock and pulmonary compromise present the most immediate threat after burn trauma, local as well as systemic infections become the primary complication during healing. The burn wound initially is relatively free of pathogens; however, dead, avascular tissue and wound exudate provide a fertile environment for bacterial growth. Colonization of the wound is apparent by the fifth postburn day. Gram-positive microorganisms are usually recovered from cultures first, followed by opportunistic gram-negative bacteria. The impaired vascular supply to burned tissue enhances the proliferation of pathogenic microorganisms. Bacterial invasion results in thrombosis and a further impairment of circulation sufficient to convert a partial-thickness injury to a full-thickness wound (see What's New? Innate Lymphocyte Subsets and Their Immunoregulatory Roles in Burn Injury and Sepsis).

Improvements in treatment have resulted in a reduction in wound infection. Aggressive excision and grafting of the wounds, improved nutritional support, and the development of microorganism-specific topical antimicrobials have contributed to this trend. However, the incidence of septicemia remains relatively constant. This is perhaps explained by the survival of children with burns of increasingly large body surface area. The burn wound serves as the site of primary invasion for the majority of instances of local or generalized infection. Because the burned child is immunosuppressed for many

WHAT'S NEW? Innate Lymphocyte Subsets and Their Immunoregulatory Roles in Burn Injury and Sepsis

Because overall immune alteration is a consequence of burn injury, research with innate lymphocyte subsets is particularly important. Innate regulatory lymphocytes are central to protective immunity and immunopathology. Most interesting is research regarding four cell types (natural killer cells [NK], natural killer T cells (NKT), gamma-delta T cells ($\gamma\delta$), and regulatory T cells (Treg). Convincing evidence in research studies indicates that these cells control the adaptive and innate arms of immunity after injury and sepsis. Research demonstrates a common mechanism by which regulatory subsets control immune responses through the production of immunomodulatory cytokines. Continued research will allow development of new perspectives on the immunopathologic consequences of trauma and infection.

Data from Schneider DF, Glenn CH, Faunce DE: *J Burn Care Res* 28(3):365-379, 2007.

weeks after injury, maintaining wounds at low contamination levels by meticulous wound care decreases the frequency and duration of septic episodes caused by wound flora.[88]

Functional Limitations

Children require specialized management to ensure optimal functional and cosmetic results. Scar and contracture management is necessary for prolonged periods because of changes in body composition as the child grows and matures. Very young children present unique challenges because the small body size can be difficult to fit with pressure garments and splints, growth is rapid, and cooperation with the rehabilitation program is limited. Children are reluctant to move when doing so causes pain, and they are likely to assume a position of comfort. Unfortunately this position often results in contracture formation and loss of function. Proper positioning and splint application are necessary to maintain body alignment. Physical therapy and occupational therapy provide exercise to maintain range of motion and function.

Infant skin is thinner, and the epidermis is more loosely connected to the dermis. This increases the risk of blistering, chafing, and rash formation. The infant also produces less sebum and sweat, which further exacerbates the propensity to skin irritation. Because scar tissue contains no sweat glands, these characteristics of the skin in growing children compound the difficulty in maintaining pressure on maturing scars while cooling the body.

Scar tissue is metabolically active and highly vascular. Collagen is deposited in random patterns, and contraction of the scar can result in disabling deformities. The scar is active as long as it is raised, red, and firm. **Scar maturation** requires 1 to 2 years and depends on individual differences and compliance with the rehabilitation program. The mature scar is characterized by increased suppleness, flattening, and pigmented color.

Scar tissue does not grow and expand like normal tissue. Although massage therapy offers some benefit in stretching, functional limitation may develop as the child grows. This is particularly evident over joints. Reconstructive surgery is often necessary to restore anatomic integrity and to promote independent function.

Itching may occur at any time during burn wound healing. As a complication, healed skin may be scratched away in an effort to obtain relief. The combination of H_1 and H_2 antagonists may be used to control itching.[89]

EVALUATION AND TREATMENT The initial assessment conducted on admission to the burn center includes maintenance of an adequate airway, fluid resuscitation to manage burn shock, and the evaluation and treatment of the wound itself. Other therapies are initiated throughout the course of treatment. Nutritional support is essential to ensure an optimal outcome. Positioning and splinting to prevent contracture formation as well as rehabilitative aspects of therapy are instituted on admission and continue throughout the hospitalization. Psychosocial support is very important for the child and the family. The information provided should be consistent and honest to allow clarification of concerns.

Fluid Resuscitation

Fluid resuscitation is generally required for children after thermal injuries in excess of 15% to 20% of the TBSA. Fluid is administered to compensate for the fluid and electrolytes extravasating into the interstitial spaces. This replacement restores circulating volume, improves perfusion, and alleviates organ dysfunction associated with impaired circulation.

Various protocols have been proposed as guidelines for fluid administration. It is important to remember that any regimen serves merely as a guideline and will require adjustment based on the individual response of each child. Because the linear relationship between weight and surface area does not exist in children (surface area varies to weight as a two-thirds function), use of adult formulas result in under- or over-resuscitation.[67] A commonly used protocol is a modification of the Parkland formula. Children also tend to require relatively more fluids than adults because they have higher evaporative losses because of their body surface area/weight ratio. **Evaporative fluid loss** can be a significant contributor to hypovolemia in the burned child. This evaporative fluid loss continues until the burn wounds are closed. As in adults, inhalation injury also continues until burn wounds are closed. And, as in adults, inhalation injury increases the magnitude of total body surface area injury; therefore, children with burn injuries require more fluids.[66]

Wound Management

The goals of wound management include prevention of infection, removal of devitalized tissue, and closure of the wound. Burns that are clearly deep dermal or full-thickness injuries are surgically excised as soon as the child is hemodynamically stable after resuscitation. Early excision reduces the incidence of wound infection and systemic sepsis.[90] Coverage of the excised wound is necessary to achieve wound closure. The choice of a coverage technique depends on the availability of donor skin.

Split-thickness sheet grafts are selected for areas of maximal functional and cosmetic results (Figure 47-11). Children with very large burn injuries often do not have sufficient unburned skin available to facilitate use of the sheet graft. In these cases the surgeon uses a meshing technique to expand the available skin and increase the size of the graft. The pattern created heals by migration of epithelium from the meshed edges. Scar formation is increased, and the mesh pattern will remain clearly visible (Figure 47-12). The color, texture, vascularity, thickness, and hair-bearing nature of the skin vary from one area to another. Site selection and depth of donor sites require careful consideration. Skin grafts for the face should be taken, if possible, from above the nipple line for best color match and "blush" ability.[91] Ongoing research and further refinement of tissue engineering by cultured epithelial autografts provide more therapeutic options with major wounds.[92]

Pulmonary Support

Smoke inhalation has a negative, prolonged effect on pulmonary function that has been associated with increased morbidity and mortality for the burned individual. Mechanical ventilation of severe inhalation injury is a dynamic and complex task.[93,94] In order to avoid barotrauma from high ventilating pressures and concentrations of oxygen, current management attempts to support pulmonary function through permissive hypercapnia and high-frequency percussive ventilation.[95] Current literature continues to support interest in this old technique as a means to prevent volutrauma.[96] *Volutrauma* refers to fluid compartment shifts in which intracellular and interstitial volumes increase at the expense of plasma volume and blood volume.[77] When this therapy fails, improvements in intrapulmonary shunt and pulmonary artery pressures may be realized by the inhalation of nitric oxide. This pulmonary vasodilator has been shown to offer short-term benefit in this population. However, long-term effect on survival remains controversial.[97] Use of extracorporeal membrane oxygenation (ECMO), another technique available for children resistant to conventional support, allows cardiopulmonary rest by a prolonged bypass. Maximal benefit is associated with a careful balance between improvement of pulmonary function and life-threatening complications.[98]

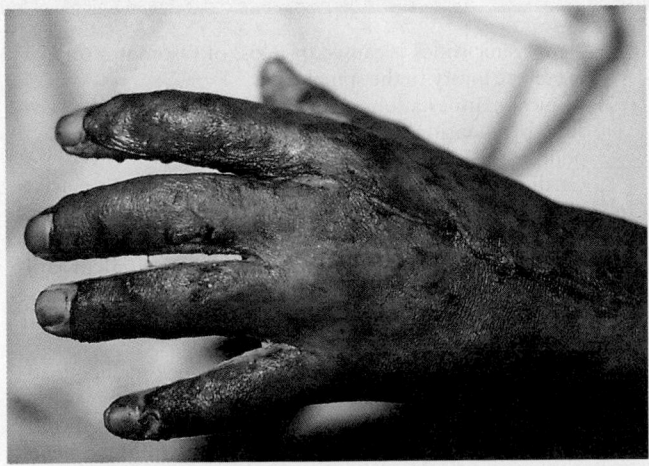

Figure 47-11 Split-thickness sheet graft.

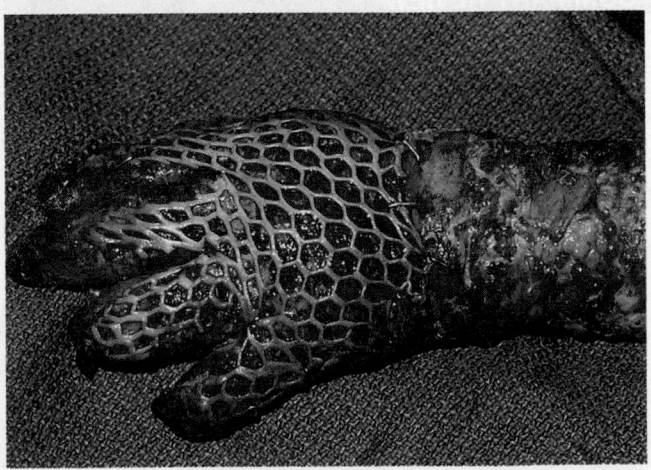

Figure 47-12 Meshed autograft.

Nutritional Support

The heightened metabolic demands after burn injury combined with a poor appetite often necessitate supplementation of oral intake. Children with burns in excess of 25% of TBSA often require supplementation with tube feeding. Feeding does not need to be delayed pending resolution of paralytic ileus and the resumption of bowel sounds because the small bowel maintains motility and absorptive capability. A small-bore feeding tube placed in the duodenum provides a safe route for the delivery of essential nutrients.[99] Parenteral hyperalimentation is reserved for those children who are unable to tolerate enteral support because of attendant risks of catheter sepsis and loss of intestinal integrity.[100] Early enteral supplementation preserves gut mucosal integrity and improves intestinal blood flow, as well as motility.[67] Early initiation of enteral supplementation along with aggressive management of complications permits successful enteral alimentation in most burned children.

Severe burn injury causes exaggerated muscle protein catabolism, contributing to weakness and delayed healing. Many therapeutic strategies have been used to avert the hypermetabolic response and improve clinical outcomes. Pharmacologic agents, such as recombinant growth hormone, low-dose insulin, and testosterone, have been shown to improve muscle kinetics and wound healing. However, these can cause serious side effects. Recently investigators found that anabolic steroid agents, along with nutritional support, improve muscle protein metabolism through enhanced protein synthesis efficiency in children and adults.[101] Outpatient follow-up should include regular weighing of the child and nutritional assessment to identify children at risk for further weight loss.

Comfort Management

Pain management presents a significant challenge in the pediatric population. In addition to procedural pain, there is a component of background pain that is present without actitity. Pain perception is also affected by the degree of emotional overlay or affective experience.[102] The measurement of pain is particularly challenging in young infants, who lack the language skills to express pain. A variety of tools, from physiologic monitors to behavioral analyses and analog scales, have been developed to measure pediatric pain. The quality of pain control in burn centers has improved along with the ability to assess pain in the pediatric population. Studies have documented pharmacologic as well as nonpharmacologic interventions that have improved the quality of pain control.[103]

Recovery from Burn Injury

Rehabilitation becomes the major focus of care once wound coverage has been achieved and continues until all reconstructive procedures have been completed. This phase may extend over many years in the pediatric population. In addition to the functional aspects of rehabilitation, attention must be directed to psychosocial needs and community reintegration. Children are increasingly surviving massive burn injuries because of advances in care in the past 20 years. Active participation by the child and family in rehabilitation is important. Early encouragement of the child to do as much as possible assists with loss of control and perceived helplessness. Most parents feel overwhelming guilt whether or not the guilt is justified. They feel responsible for the burn injury.[104] Post-traumatic stress symptoms are highly prevalent in parents of burned children.[105] Severe burn injuries tax the capabilities of children of all ages, which may result in regression of developmental milestones. Very young children with acute injuries suffer from separation anxiety. School-age children and adolescents may become more dependent, and a change in body image can impede social reintegration whether at school or in the community.[104] A method to facilitate the transition from the hospital to the community is the school reentry program offered by many burn centers. These programs provide education for teachers and peers about the injury, appearance, and abilities of the returning child.

SUMMARY REVIEW

Shock and Multiple Organ Dysfunction Syndrome

1. Shock in children is present when there are signs of poor systemic perfusion, regardless of blood pressure.
2. Hypovolemic shock is the most common type of shock in children. Dehydration and trauma are the most common causes of hypovolemic shock.
3. Hypotension is a sign of severe, decompensated shock, referred to as "hypotensive shock.".
4. Hypovolemia can be caused by volume loss, an increase in the vascular space relative to the amount of volume, or a redistribution of intravascular volume.
5. Clinical manifestations of hypovolemic shock include inadequate systemic perfusion associated with intravascular fluid loss. Adrenergic compensatory mechanisms can produce tachycardia, redistribution of blood flow, peripheral vasoconstriction, cool extremities, delayed capillary refill, and oliguria.
6. Neurogenic shock is caused by a loss of vasomotor tone after severe injury to the spinal cord.
7. Clinical manifestations of neurogenic shock include warm skin, hypotension with a low diastolic blood pressure, and poor systemic perfusion.
8. Cardiogenic shock, with decreased cardiac output, is observed most commonly after cardiovascular surgery or with inflammatory diseases of the heart, such as cardiomyopathy and myocarditis. It is also found in children with obstructive congenital heart disease and those with drug toxicity or severe electrolyte or acid-base imbalances.
9. Clinical manifestations of cardiogenic shock include inadequate systemic perfusion despite adequate intravascular volume. Cardiac output is typically low. Adrenergic compensatory mechanisms are similar to those found in hypovolemic shock.

10. Once septic shock is present, immediate treatment is necessary, including aggressive fluid resuscitation (typically 60-80 mL/kg administered in first hour of therapy, and approximately 200 to 240 ml/kg in the first 8 hours of therapy). Vasoactive support is typically needed early in the resuscitation (during the first minutes, and certainly within the first hour of treatment). Goals of therapy should be to rapidly normalize the heart rate and blood pressure for age, to rapidly reduce capillary refill to less than 2 seconds. Fluid and vasoactive therapy should support high cardiac output and oxygen delivery, maintaining the $S\bar{v}O_2$ at approximately 70%.

11. Altered cytokine levels are associated with septic shock in children. TNF levels are directly related to mortality in newborns and children with meningitis and sepsis.

12. Sepsis is a systemic response to infection. It is present when manifestations of SIRS are observed. SIRS is present when the child demonstrates two or more of the following as an acute change from baseline values: fever or hypothermia, altered heart rate, tachypnea with respiratory alkalosis, and alteration in the white blood cell count. The newborn often develops hypothermia rather than fever as a sign of infection and may develop bradycardia instead of tachycardia.

13. Severe sepsis is present when there is evidence of SIRS and signs of organ dysfunction, hypoperfusion, or hypotension.

14. The development of septic shock is heralded when the child with severe sepsis develops signs of cardiovascular dysfunction. The child may become hypotensive despite adequate fluid resuscitation or require vasopressors to maintain blood pressure.

15. Reperfusion and inflammatory injury stimulate free oxygen radicals that can damage cell membranes, denature proteins, and disrupt chromosomes. This process likely affects endothelial cells and the microvasculature, causing MODS.

16. Acidosis may be the most sensitive indicator of inadequate systemic perfusion in children. Hypotension is a late sign of shock in infants and children.

17. The goals of treatment for shock are maximization of oxygen delivery and minimization of oxygen demand. Airway, oxygenation, and ventilation must be supported. The child should be kept warm, and shivering should be prevented. Monitor the warmth of the child's extremities, capillary refill, quality of peripheral pulses, level of consciousness and responsiveness, urine output, oxygenation, ventilation, and acid-base status throughout shock therapy.

18. Treatment consists of immediate resuscitation, including fluid resuscitation as needed (must be aggressive in septic shock), ventilation, pharmacologic support (e.g., vasopressors), ECG analysis, hemodynamic monitoring, administration of blood or blood component therapy, and management of electrolyte and acid-base imbalances.

Burns

1. Burns in children are often the result of inadequate supervision, curiosity, inability to escape the burning agent, or intentional abuse.

2. Scald injuries are commonly seen in young children and result from exposure to hot water, grease, or other hot liquids, whereas flame burns are more prevalent among older children.

3. A child's skin is thinner and thus more susceptible to injury than adult skin. The kitchen and bathroom are common sites of burn injury.

4. It is estimated that from 5% to 22% of all child abuse cases in the United States result from burn injury.

5. Flame burns involving flammable liquids, most notably gasoline, are more common in older children. Risk-taking behaviors in young males can lead to electrical burns. Children may be exposed to chemical injury by swallowing caustic agents at home.

6. Use of the standard rule of nines results in inaccurate calculation of the percentage of TBSA in children. A modified rule of nines deducts 1% from the head and adds 0.5% to each leg for each year of life after 2 years of age.

7. Major burn trauma involves all body systems, and the consequences of injury include shock, infection, hypermetabolism, organ failure, and functional limitations. These effects can be magnified in the pediatric population as a result of physiologic immaturity and age-related variation in treatment modalities.

8. Infection, trauma, or applying ice to the burn area may convert a partial-thickness injury to a full-thickness one, especially in young children, who have thinner, more delicate skin.

9. Marked reduction in cardiac output occurs immediately after injury and is accompanied by an initial increase in systemic vascular resistance. The inefficient and labile peripheral circulation of the infant complicates management of the burn shock phase of treatment. Constriction of the chest and impairment of respiratory excursion may occur in the very young child because of the increased pliability of the rib cage. Younger children are also more susceptible to increased intra-abdominal pressure.

10. Children younger than 2 years lack the ability to concentrate urine because of the immaturity of the renal system and are therefore at increased risk for dehydration. Because children have a relatively larger body surface area in relation to weight than adults, they require proportionately increased fluid during burn shock resuscitation to compensate for evaporative water losses.

11. A biphasic pattern of physiologic responses is evident in the burn injured child. The initial ebb phase occurs during the immediate postburn period and continues for 3 to 5 days. This phase is characterized by reduced oxygen consumption, impaired circulation, and cellular shock. After this phase and the restoration of volume, the metabolic response shifts to a catabolic, or flow, phase. This phase is characterized by hypermetabolism with an increased oxygen consumption and elevation of catecholamines, glucocorticoids, and glucagon.

12. Glycogen stores are limited in children, making it hard for them to meet the increased energy demands of the burn. This prolonged metabolic dysfunction may lead to loss of lean body mass, delayed healing, and increased morbidity.

13. Some children exhibit immunosuppression for a prolonged period after wound closure.

14. Although age was not found to be a predictor of hypertrophic scarring, children have greater skin tension and an accelerated rate of collagen synthesis.

15. Children require fluid resuscitation for smaller burns than does the adult population as a result of limited physiologic reserves. Colloid replacement may be required in the very young child who fails to respond to fluid replacement.

16. The leading cause of death in children after burn injury, as in adults, is inhalation injury.

17. Children require specialized management to ensure optimal functional and cosmetic results. Long-term scar and contracture management is necessary because of changes in body composition as the child grows and matures.

KEY TERMS

Bradycardia, 1730
Cardiogenic shock, 1732
Catabolic (flow) phase, 1744
Chemical burn, 1741
Child abuse, 1741
Cold shock, 1735
Colloid, 1738
Colloid replacement, 1746
Compensated shock, 1727
Contact burn, 1741
Crystalloid, 1738
Depth of injury, 1742
Dermal ischemia, 1743
Distributive (neurogenic, anaphylactic, septic) shock, 1729
Ebb phase, 1744
Electrical burn, 1742

Eschar, 1743
Evaporative fluid loss, 1749
Flame burns, 1742
Fluid resuscitation, 1749
Hemoconcentration, 1743
Hypermetabolism, 1744
Hypertrophic scar, 1745
Hypotensive (decompensated) shock, 1727
Hypovolemia, 1745
Hypovolemic shock, 1728
Intra-abdominal pressure, 1744
Intraosseous cannulation, 1746
Ischemia (hypoxia), 1727
Maintenance fluid, 1746
Multiple organ dysfunction syndrome (MODS), 1727
Myoglobin, 1744

Neurogenic shock, 1729
Obstructive shock, 1729
Rehabilitation, 1750
Reperfusion (reoxygenation) injury, 1737
Scald injury, 1741
Scar formation, 1745
Scar maturation, 1748
Sepsis, 1733
Shock, 1727
Split-thickness sheet graft, 1749
Systemic inflammatory response syndrome (SIRS), 1735
Tachycardia, 1730
Thermoregulatory response, 1747
"Third spacing" of fluid, 1729
Warm shock, 1735

REFERENCES

1. Haque IU, Zaritsky AL: Analysis of the evidence for the lower limit of systolic and mean arterial blood pressure in children, *Pediatr Crit Care* 8:138-144, 2007.
2. Ralston M et al: Recognition of shock. In American Heart Association, editor: *PALS provider manual*, Dallas, 2006, American Heart Association.
3. Goldstein B, Giroir B, Randolph A: International Pediatric Sepsis Consensus Conference: definitions for sepsis and organ dysfunction in pediatrics, *Pediatr Crit Care Med* 6:2-8, 2005.
4. Proulx F et al: The pediatric multiple organ dysfunction syndrome, *Pediatr Crit Care* 2008, Dec 2, [Epub ahead of print].
5. Gorelick MH, Shaw KN, Murphy KO: Validity and reliability of clinical signs in the diagnosis of dehydration in children, *Pediatrics* 99(5):E6, 1997.
6. Roberts KB: Fluid and electrolytes: parenteral fluid therapy, *Pediatr Rev* 22(11):380-387, 2001.
7. Hazinski MF: Children are different. In Hazinski MF, editor: *Manual of pediatric critical care*, St Louis, 1999, Mosby.
8. Ralston M et al: Management of shock. In American Heart Association, editor: *PALS provider manual*, Dallas, 2006, American Heart Association.
9. Michaud LJ et al: Elevated initial blood glucose levels and poor outcome following severe brain injuries in children, *J Trauma* 31(10):1356-1362, 1991.
10. Faustino EV, Apkon M: Persistent hyperglycemia in critically ill children, *J Pediatr* 146(1):30-34, 2005.
11. Rudolph AM: *Congenital diseases of the heart*, Chicago, 1974, Year Book Medical.
12. Ralston M et al: Recognition of bradyarrhythmias and tachyarrhythmias. In American Heart Association, editor: *PALS provider manual*, Dallas, 2006, American Heart Association.
13. Sevedra JM et al: Capillary refill (skin turgor) in the assessment of dehydration, *Am J Dis Child* 145:296, 1991.
14. Otieno H et al: Are bedside features of shock reproducible between different observers? *Arch Dis Child* 89(10):977-979, 2004.
15. Watson RS et al: The epidemiology of severe sepsis in children in the United States, *Am J Respir Crit Care Med* 167(5):695-701, 2003.
16. Singh-Naz N et al: Risk factors for nosocomial infections in critically ill children; a prospective cohort study, *Crit Care Med* 24(5):875-878, 1996.
17. Richards MJ et al: Nosocomial infections in pediatric intensive care units in the United States, *Pediatrics* 103(4e39):1-7, 1999.
18. Foglia E, Meier MD, Elward A: Ventilator-associated pneumonia in neonatal and pediatric intensive care unit patients, *Clin Microbiol Rev* 20(3):409-425, 2007.
19. Principi N, Esposito S: Ventilator-associated pneumonia (VAP) in pediatric intensive care units, *Pediatr Infect Dis J* 26:841-844, 2007.

20. Hazinski MF et al: Epidemiology, pathophysiology, and clinical presentation of gram-negative sepsis, *Am J Crit Care* 2(3):224-235, 1993.
21. Wheeler AP, Bernard GR: Treating patients with severe sepsis, *N Engl J Med* 340(3):207-214, 1999.
22. Sullivan JS et al: Correlation of plasma cytokine elevation with mortality rate in children with sepsis, *J Pediatr* 120(4 Pt 1):510-515, 1992.
23. Wong HR et al: Nitric oxide production in critically ill patients, *Arch Dis Child* 74(6):482-489, 1996.
24. Glauser MP: Pathophysiologic basis of sepsis: considerations for future strategies of intervention, *Crit Care Med* 28(9 Suppl):S4-S8, 2000.
25. Decker T: Sepsis: avoiding its deadly toll, *J Clin Invest* 113(10):1387-1389, 2004.
26. Haley M et al: Activated protein C in sepsis: emerging insights regarding its mechanism of action and clinical effectiveness, *Curr Opin Infect Dis* 17(3):205-211, 2004.
27. Bernard GR et al: Efficacy and safety of recombinant human activated protein C for severe sepsis, *N Engl J Med* 344(10):699-709, 2001.
28. Fisher CJ Jr, Yan SB: Protein C levels as a prognostic indicator of outcome in sepsis and related diseases, *Crit Care Med* 28(9 Suppl):S49-S56, 2000.
29. Matot I, Sprung CL: Corticosteroids in septic shock: resurrection of the last rites? *Crit Care Med* 26(4):627-630, 1998.
30. Riordan FA et al: Admission cortisol and adrenocorticotrophic hormone levels in children with meningococcal disease: evidence of adrenal insufficiency? *Crit Care Med* 27(10):2257-2261, 1999.
31. Minneci PC et al: Meta-analysis: the effect of steroids on survival and shock during sepsis depends on the dose, *Ann Intern Med* 141(1):47-51, 2004.
32. Carcillo JA, Fields AI: Task Force Committee Members: Clinical practice parameters for hemodynamic support of pediatric and neonatal patients in septic shock, *Crit Care Med* 30(6):1365-1378, 2002.
33. American College of Chest Physicians/Society of Critical Care Medicine Consensus Conference: Definitions for sepsis and organ failure and guidelines for the use of innovative therapies in sepsis, *Crit Care Med* 20(6):864-874, 1992.
34. Goldstein B, Giroir B, Randolph A: Members of the International Consensus Conference on Pediatric Sepsis: International pediatric sepsis consensus conference: Definitions for sepsis and organ dysfunction in pediatrics, *Pediatr Crit Care Med* 6(1):2-8, 2005.
35. Barriere SL, Lowry SF: An overview of mortality risk prediction in sepsis, *Crit Care Med* 23(2):376-393, 1995.
36. Parker MM et al: Serial cardiovascular variables in survivors and nonsurvivors of human septic shock: heart rate as an early predictor of prognosis, *Crit Care Med* 15(10):923-929, 1987.
37. Dantzker D: Oxygen delivery and utilization in sepsis, *Crit Care Med* 5:81, 1989.

38. Carcillo JA, Davis AL, Zaritsky A: Role of early fluid resuscitation in pediatric septic shock, *JAMA* 266(9):1242-1245, 1991.

38a. Brierley, J, Carcillo JA, Choong K et al: Clinical practice parameters for hemodynamic support of pediatric and neonatal septic shock: 2007 update from American College of Critical Care Medicine, *Crit Care Med* 37:666-688, 2009.

39. Damjanov I, Linder J: *Anderson's pathology*, ed 10, St Louis, 1996, Mosby.

40. Waxman D: Shock: ischemia, reperfusion, inflammation, *New Horiz* 4:153, 1996.

41. Johnston JA et al: Importance of organ dysfunction in determining hospital outcomes in children, *J Pediatr* 144(5):595-601, 2004.

42. Armon K et al: Hyponatremia and hypokalemia during intravenous fluid administration, *Arch Dis Child* 93:285-287, 2008.

43. Hutton P et al: An assessment of the Dinamap 845, *Anesthesiology* 39:261, 1984.

44. Davis JW et al: Are automated blood pressure measurements accurate in trauma patients? *J Trauma* 55(5):860-863, 2003.

45. Cohn JN: Blood pressure measurement in shock: mechanisms of inaccuracy in auscultatory and palpatory methods, *JAMA* 199:188, 1967.

46. Lacroix J et al: Transfusion strategies for patients in pediatric intensive care units, *N Engl J Med* 356:1609-1619, 2007.

47. Oh MS, Carroll HJ: Electrolyte and acid-base disorders. In Chernow B, editor: *The pharmacologic approach to the critically ill patient*, ed 3, Baltimore, 1994, Williams & Wilkins.

48. Zaritsky A et al: CPR in children, *Ann Emerg Med* 16(10):1107-1111, 1987.

49. Whitlock D, Whitlock J, Coates TD: Hematologic and oncologic emergencies requiring critical care. In Hazinski MF, editor: *Nursing care of the critically ill child*, ed 2, St Louis, 1992, Mosby.

50. Cooper DJ et al: Prehospital hypertonic saline resuscitation of patients with hypotension and severe traumatic brain injury: a randomized controlled study, *JAMA* 291(11):1350-1357, 2004.

51. Moore FA, McKinley BA, Moore EE: The next generation in shock resuscitation, *Lancet* 363(9425):1988-1996, 2004.

52. Reeves JH et al: Continuous plasma filtration in sepsis syndrome, *Crit Care Med* 27(10):2096-2104, 1999.

53. Couzin J: News focus: the big chill, *Science* 317:743-745, 2007.

54. Shankaran S et al: Whole body hypothermia for neonates with hypoxic-ischemic encephalopathy, *N Engl J Med* 353:1574-1584, 2005.

55. Hypothermia After Cardiac Arrest Study Group: Mild therapeutic hypothermia to improve the neurologic outcome after cardiac arrest, *N Engl J Med* 346(8):549-556, 2002.

56. Carcillo JA: Mannose-binding lectin deficiency provides a genetic basis for the use of SIRS/sepsis definitions in critically ill patients, *Intensive Care Med* 30(7):1263-1265, 2004.

57. Fidler KJ et al: Increased incidence and severity of the systemic inflammatory response syndrome in patients deficient in mannose-binding lectin, *Intensive Care Med* 30(7):1438-1445, 2004.

58. Committee on Trauma: *Resource for optimal care of the injured patient* [pamphlet], 1999, American College of Surgeons.

59. Safe Kids Worldwide (SKW): *Burn and scalds safety 2007*. Available at www.usa.sfekids.org/content_documents/2007_Fact_Sheet_Burn_Scalds.doc. Accessed April 14, 2008.

60. American Burn Association: Pediatric burn injuries. *In Advanced burn life support course*, Chicago, 2001, American Burn Association.

61. Kos L, Shwayder T: Cutaneous manifestations of child abuse, *Pediatr Dermatol* 23(4):311-320, 2006.

62. Giardino AP: Child abuse and neglect: physical abuse. In Johnson C et al, editors: *eMedicine, 2005*. Available online at www.emedicine.com/PED/topic2648.htm.

63. Helvig E: Pediatric burn injuries, *AACN Clin Issues Crit Care Nurs* 4(2):433-442, 1993.

64. Sheridan RL, Tompkins RG: Alternative wound coverings. In Herndon DN, editor: *Total burn care*, Philadelphia, 2007, Saunders.

65. Gottschlich MM: Hypovitaminosis D in acutely injured pediatric burn patients, *J Am Diet Assoc* 104(6):931-941, 2004.

66. Ahrns KS: Trends in burn resuscitation: shifting the focus from fluids to adequate end-point monitoring, edema control, and adjuvant therapies, *Crit Care Nurs Clin North Am* 16(1):75, 2004.

67. Lee JO, Herndon DH: The pediatric burn patient. In Herndon DH, editor: *Total burn care*, Philadelphia, 2007, Saunders.

68. Wolf SE, Prough DS, Herndon DH: Critical care in the severely burned: organ support and management of complications. In Herndon DH, editor: *Total burn care*, Philadelphia, 2007, Saunders.

69. Wilmore DW: Nutrition and metabolism following thermal injury, *Clin Plast Surg* 1(4):603-619, 1974.

70. Gottschlich MM, Mayes T: Nutrition for the pediatric burn patient. In Samour PQ, Kind K, editors: *Handbook of pediatric nutrition*, Sudbury, MA, 2005, Jones & Bartlett.

71. Deitch EA: Nutritional support of the burn patient, *Crit Care Med* 11(3):735, 1995.

72. Supple KG: Physiologic response to burn injury, *Crit Care Nurs Clin North Am* 16(1):119, 2004.

73. Stratta RJ et al: Immunologic parameters in burned patients: effect of therapeutic interventions, *J Trauma* 26(1):7, 1986.

74. Murphy ED, Sherwood ER, Tolliver-Kinsky T: The immunological response and strategies for intervention. In Herndon DN, editor: *Total burn care*, Philadelphia, 2007, Saunders.

75. Scott PG et al: Molecular and cellular basis of hypertrophic scarring. In Herndon DN, editor: *Total burn care*, Philadelphia, 2007, Saunders.

76. Hawkins HK, Pereira CT: Pathophysiology of the burn scar. In Herndon DN, editor: *Total burn care*, Philadelphia, 2007, Saunders.

77. Warden GD: Fluid resuscitation and early management. In Herndon DN, editor: *Total burn care*, Philadelphia, 2007, Saunders.

78. Tintinalli JE et al: *Emergency medicine: a comprehensive study guide*, New York, 2004, McGraw-Hill.

79. Ryan CM et al: Objective estimates of the probability of death from burn injuries, *N Engl J Med* 338(6):362-366, 1998.

80. Conrardy PA et al: Alteration of endotracheal tube position, *Crit Care Med* 4(2):8, 1976.

81. Sharar SR: Endotracheal tube tip position in an infant with severe burns, *J Burn Care Rehabil* 16(6):654, 1995.

82. Trout S et al: Influence of head and neck position on endotracheal tube tip position on chest x-ray examination: a potential problem in the infant undergoing intubation, *J Burn Care Rehabil* 15(5):405-407, 1994.

83. Rodeberg DA et al: Use of a helium-oxygen mixture in the treatment of postextubation stridor in pediatric patients with burns, *J Burn Care Rehabil* 16(5):476-480, 1995.

84. Sheridan RL et al: Permissive hypercapnia as a ventilatory strategy in burned children: effect on barotrauma, pneumonia, and mortality, *J Trauma* 39(5):854, 1995.

85. Saffle JR, Graves C: Nutritional support of the burned patient. In Herndon DN, editor: *Total burn care*, Philadelphia, 2007, Saunders.

86. Gottschlich MM et al: Significance of obesity on nutritional, immunologic, hormonal, and clinical outcome parameters in burns, *J Am Diet Assoc* 93(11):1261, 1993.

87. Kagan R, Jenkins M: Transport and management of children with burns and inhalation injuries. In Jaimovich DG, Vidyasagar D, editors: *Handbook of pediatric and neonatal transport medicine*, Philadelphia, 1996, Hanley & Belfus.

88. Gallagher JJ et al: Treatment of infection in burns. In Herndon DN, editor: *Total burn care*, Philadelphia, 2007, Saunders.

89. Baker RU et al: Burn wound itch control using H_1 and H_2 antagonists, *J Burn Care Rehabil* 22(4):263, 2001.

90. Petersen SR, Umphred E, Warden GD: The incidence of bacteremia following burn wound excision, *J Trauma* 22(4):274-279, 1982.

91. Muller M, Gahankari D, Herndon DN: Operative wound management. In Herndon DN, editor: *Total burn care*, Philadelphia, 2007, Saunders.

92. Wood FM, Kolybaba ML, Allen P: The use of cultured epithelial autograft in the treatment of major burn wounds: a critical review of literature, *Burns* 32(4):395-401, 2006.

93. Merrel P, Mayo D: Inhalation injury in the burn patient, *Crit Care Nurs Clin North Am* 16(1):27, 2004.

94. Park GY et al: Prolonged airway and systemic inflammatory reactions after smoke inhalation, *Chest* 123(2):475, 2003.

95. Cortiella J, Mlcak R, Herndon D: High frequency percussive ventilation in pediatric patients with inhalation injury, *J Burn Care Rehabil* 20(3):232-235, 1999.

96. Schmidt GA, Hall JB: Management of the ventilated patient. In Hall JB, Schmidt GA, Wood LDH, editors: *Principles of critical care*, New York, 2005, McGraw-Hill.

97. Sheridan RL et al: Low-dose inhaled nitric oxide in acutely burned children with profound respiratory failure, *Surgery* 126(5):856-862, 1999.

98. Cedidi C et al: Survival of severe ARDS with five-organ failure following burns and inhalation injury in a 15-year-old patient, *Burns* 29(4):389-394, 2003.

99. Gottschlich MM: Early and perioperative support. In Matarese L, Gottschlich MM, editors: *Contemporary nutrition support practice: a clinical guide*, Philadelphia, 2003, Saunders.

100. Herndon DN et al: Failure of TPN to improve liver function, immunity, and mortality in thermally injured patients, *J Trauma* 2(2):195-204, 1987.

101. Wolf SE et al: Effects of oxandrolone on outcome measures in the severely burned: a multicenter prospective randomized double-blind trial, *J Burn Care Res* 25(2):131-139, 2006.

102. Gordon M et al: Use of pain assessment tools: is there a preference? *J Burn Care Rehabil* 19(5):451-454, 1998.

103. Martin-Hertz SP et al: Pediatric pain control practices of North American burn centers, *J Burn Care Rehabil* 24(1):26, 2003.

104. Baker RAU, Mondozzi MA, Hockenberry MJ: Complications that produce fluid and electrolyte imbalance. In Hockenberry MJ, Wilson D, editors: *Wong's nursing care of infants and children*, St Louis, 2007, Mosby.

105. Hall E et al: Posttraumatic stress symptoms in parents of children with acute burns, *J Pediatr Psychol* 31(4):402-412, 2006.

GLOSSARY*

BETH A. FORSHEE

Achalasia failure of a sphincter, usually the esophageal sphincter, to relax completely. Reducing the ability to move food down the esophagus.

Acidosis an acid-base imbalance characterized by reduction in arterial blood pH less than 7.4.

Acne rosacea a chronic form of dermatitis of the face in which the middle portion of the face appears red with small red lines caused by dilation of capillaries.

Acne vulgaris an inflammatory eruption of the sebaceous follicles usually occurring on the face, upper back, and chest that consists of blackheads, cysts, papules, and pustules.

Acromegaly a condition of excessive growth hormone secreted from the anterior pituitary often caused by a benign pituitary adenoma; it is manifested by organomegaly and progressive enlargement of the face, hands, and feet.

ACTH deficiency a condition characterized by decreased or absent production of adrenocorticotropic hormone (ACTH) by the pituitary gland, resulting in a reduction in the secretion of adrenal hormones and subsequent weight loss, lack of appetite, weakness, nausea, vomiting, and low blood pressure.

Actinic keratosis a condition in which a premalignant small, reddish, rough spot appears on skin chronically exposed to the sun.

Active transport movement of a substance across a membrane by a carrier protein that requires expenditure of energy for activation.

Acute epiglottitis an infection that causes inflammation of the epiglottis and surrounding tissues and may lead to upper airway blockage.

Acute kidney injury (ARI) rapid loss of renal function resulting in retention of waste products that may lead to metabolic disturbances, fluid imbalance, or oliguria.

Acute lymphoblastic leukemia (ALL) excessive production and continuous multiplication of malignant and immature white blood cells (lymphoblasts) in the bone marrow that progresses rapidly if left untreated.

Acute myelogenous leukemia (AML) excessive number of immature myeloid cells (myeloblasts) in the blood and bone marrow crowding out the marrow and decreasing other cell line functions.

Acute rejection rejection of a graft within days to months after transplantation.

Acute respiratory distress syndrome (ARDS) capillaries or alveoli of the lungs are damaged as a result of infection, injury, blood loss, or inhalation injury causing fluid to leak from the capillaries into the alveoli and causing pulmonary edema and collapse of some alveoli.

Acute tubular necrosis (ATN) the kidney undergoes ischemic or nephrotoxic injury because of severe hypotension, aminoglycosides, or radiocontrast agents and produces granular and epithelial cell casts in urine.

Acute urethral syndrome the bladder is irritated and the typical symptoms of a urinary tract infection are present in the absence of an infection.

Adaptive immunity called the immune response; develops more slowly than the inflammatory response because it is specific to antigen and has memory; involves many cells and systemic processes and is produced after natural exposure to an antigen or after immunization.

Adhesion molecule *see* **Cell adhesion molecule.**

Adrenal gland either of two small endocrine glands located above the kidney and functions to secrete several steroid hormones and epinephrine and norepinephrine.

Adrenergic transmission transmission of a nerve impulse using epinephrine or norepinephrine as a neurotransmitter.

Adrenomedullin (ADM) a protein hormone secreted by the adrenal medulla gland discovered in human pheochromocytoma that functions as a vasodilator and a regulator of growth cytokines and neurotransmission.

Afterload the tension or pressure that must be generated by a chamber of the heart in order to contract, such as that required to eject blood into the aorta.

Agnosia loss of comprehension of sensory stimuli, such as sounds or images, usually secondary to brain damage or dementia.

Aldosterone mineralocorticoid that is synthesized and secreted by the adrenal cortex and acts to regulate sodium and potassium balance by altering reabsorption in the kidney.

Alkalosis an acid-base imbalance characterized by elevated pH greater than 7.4.

Allergy hypersensitivity and immunologic protective reactions caused by exposure to an antigen that is usually a harmless environmental substance.

Alloimmunity immune reaction in which individuals of the same species have incompatible antigens, preventing them from receiving an organ transplant from each other.

Alveolar ventilation the volume of gas that reaches the alveoli per minute or the difference between tidal volume and dead space multiplied by ventilation rate.

Alzheimer disease (dementia of Alzheimer type [DAT]), senile disease complex a degenerative disease characterized by amyloid plaques and fibrillary tangles in the cortex and atrophy and widened sulci in the frontal and temporal lobes.

Amebiasis an infection by a protozoan that is usually contracted by ingesting contaminated water or food or by oral-anal sexual activity and may be asymptomatic or may cause diarrhea, vomiting, abdominal pain or discomfort, and fever.

Amyotrophy progressive wasting of muscle tissue frequently caused by diabetes mellitus or motor neuron disease.

Anabolism a cellular process that uses energy to synthesize complex molecules from simpler molecules.

---

*Items highlighted in red appear on the audio glossary, and a more comprehensive glossary appears on evolve (http://evolve.elsevier.com/McCance).

Anaerobic glycolysis the process of adenosine triphosphate (ATP) formation in the absence of oxygen, during which carbohydrate-derived pyruvate is reduced to form lactic acid.

Anaphase third phase of mitosis during which centromeres are separated and sister chromatids are moved to opposite poles.

Anaphylactic shock a state of shock caused by a severe allergic reaction that lowers blood pressure and results in urticaria, breathing difficulties, and possibly death.

Anaphylatoxin fragments of C3a, C5a, and C4a that degranulate mast cells, resulting in the release of histamine that vasodilates and increases capillary permeability.

Anaphylaxis a potentially life-threatening immediate hypersensitivity response caused by exposure of a sensitized individual to a specific antigen.

Anaplasia Loss of structural differentiation often with increased cellular proliferation as with tumor cells.

Anemia hemoglobin concentration is below normal because of a deficiency in red blood cells, a low level of hemoglobin in cells, or both; it manifests as pallor of the skin and mucous membranes, weakness, dizziness, easy fatigability, and drowsiness caused by oxygen deficiency.

Aneurysm a localized dilation or ballooning of a blood vessel.

Angina pectoris chest pain caused by reduced cardiac blood flow and myocardial ischemia.

Angiogenesis the formation of new blood vessels.

Anion gap (serum) the difference between unmeasured plasma cations and anions that is used to distinguish different causes of metabolic acidosis.

Ankylosing spondylitis (AS; spondyloarthritis) chronic inflammation of the spine and sacroiliac joints with gradual fusion of the vertebrae that immobilizes the spine.

Anoikis apoptosis caused by inappropriate cell adhesion to the extracellular matrix.

Anorexia nervosa (AN) a disorder with both psychologic and physiologic components that begins with dieting to lose weight and manifests into an inappropriate self-control behavior; continued restrictive eating may lead to starvation and eventually death.

Anoxia lack of oxygen caused by vascular obstruction.

Antigenic variation the process by which antigens change appearance by altering surface molecules, making it difficult for the immune response to maintain specificity.

Antimicrobial peptide protein released by epithelial cells that is toxic to some bacteria, fungi, and viruses and is capable of activating cells involved in innate and acquired immunity.

Antithrombin III (ATIII) deficiency an autosomal dominant disease that decreases the levels of antithrombin III, resulting in abnormal blood clots that may damage organs.

Aortic stenosis aortic valves do not open completely, thereby increasing afterload so that more pressure must be generated in the left ventricle to eject blood, a condition that results in ventricular hypertrophy.

Aphasia inability to articulate ideas or comprehend spoken or written language.

Aplastic anemia the bone marrow does not produce adequate amounts of new cells to replenish the blood cells lost during insults such as an autoimmune disorder or exposure to radiation or substances such as benzene or certain drugs.

Aplastic crisis temporary loss of bone marrow causes erythropoiesis, resulting in an acute fall in hemoglobin levels and subsequent anemia.

Apoptosis active process by which cells self-destruct in normal and pathologic tissues.

Appendicitis inflammation of the appendix as a result of blockage of the opening from the appendix into the cecum; the appendix wall becomes infected and ruptures, allowing the infection to spread throughout the abdomen and cause pain, anorexia, fever, nausea, vomiting, and diarrhea.

Arteriosclerosis blood vessel walls, mainly small arteries and arterioles thicken, harden, and lose elasticity, resulting in elevated blood pressure, and decreased perfusion to tissues and organs.

Ascites accumulation of fluid in the peritoneal cavity because of liver disease, portal hypertension, tuberculosis, or nephrotic syndrome, resulting in abdominal distention and para-umbilical herniations of the abdominal wall.

Asphyxial injury suffocation, strangulation, or chemical or drowning injury resulting from oxygen deprivation in cells.

Aspiration the removal of a gas or fluid by suction or the sucking of fluid or a foreign body into the airway when breathing.

Aspiration pneumonitis a condition caused by the abnormal entry of fluids, particulate matter, or secretions into the lower airways that can lead to chemical pneumonitis from entry of toxic material such as gastric acid, bacterial infection, or by mechanical obstruction of the lower airways.

Asthma a chronic inflammatory disorder of the airways involving bronchial hyper-responsiveness and airway obstruction marked by periodic attacks of wheezing, shortness of breath, a tight feeling in the chest, and a cough that produces mucus due to an allergic reaction triggered by certain drugs, irritants, viral infection, exercise, or emotional stress.

Astrocyte neuroglial cell of the central nervous system that branches into many processes and functions to fill spaces between neurons and surrounding blood vessels.

Atelectasis part of or a whole lung collapses and the alveoli deflate as a result of surgery, smoking, or blockage of a bronchiole.

Atherosclerosis a type of arteriosclerosis in which the inflammatory changes of thickening and hardening of the walls of large and medium-sized arteries caused by an atheroma or plaque of lipids, cells, and connective tissue in the tunica intima; it does not affect veins.

Atopic dermatitis (AD) a chronic hereditary skin disease characterized by intense itching and inflamed skin that causes redness, swelling, cracking, crusting, and scaling.

Atrial natriuretic peptide (ANP or factor) a protein hormone that is synthesized and released from the atria in response to high sodium concentration, high extracellular fluid volume, or high blood volume and functions to promote sodium excretion and to cause vasodilation in the circulatory system.

Atrial septal defect (ASD) a congenital heart disease involving the interatrial septum of the heart that separates the right and left atria, which results in misdirected blood flow between the two sides of the heart.

Atrioventricular canal (AVC) defect a large hole is present in the center of the heart where the wall between the atria joins the wall between the ventricles, and the tricuspid and mitral valves are formed into a single large valve that crosses the defect.

Atrioventricular node (AV node) the tissue between the atria and the ventricles that contains pacemaker cells and is capable of setting the heart rate but mainly functions to slowly conduct the normal electrical impulse from the atria to the ventricles.

Autocrine stimulation the ability of a cell to secrete a substance that can feed back and provide continued stimulation or inhibition of that cell.

Autoimmune hemolytic anemia (AIHA) a form of hemolytic anemia involving autoantibodies against red blood cell antigens.

Autoimmunity a condition in which the immune system considers an individual's own body tissues to be foreign antigens and initiates an immune response against the tissues.

Autonomic hyperreflexia (dysreflexia) a syndrome resulting from afferent stimuli which causes intense sympathetic discharge originating with spinal cord injury above the major splanchnic outflow characterized by hypertension, bradycardia, sweating of the forehead, severe headache, and piloerection on distention of the bladder and rectum.

Autoregulation The intrinsic ability of an organ to regulate local blood flow independent of changes in systemic arterial pressure.

Bacterial pneumonia an acute or chronic disease marked by inflammation of the lungs caused by bacterial infection.

Bacterial tracheitis a condition in which the larynx, trachea, and bronchi are inflamed and present with signs similar to epiglottitis and croup; may result in airway obstruction secondary to subglottic edema or sloughing of the epithelial lining or the mucopurulent membrane within the trachea.

Bacterial vaginosis a condition caused by an overgrowth of normal vaginal bacteria causing vaginal discharge with a foul odor.

Balanitis inflammation of the glans penis caused by irritation by environmental substances, physical trauma, or infection.

Baroreceptor reflex a homeostatic mechanism consisting of baroreceptors that maintain blood pressure, a negative feedback loop in which an elevated blood pressure reflexively causes blood pressure to decrease; similarly, decreased blood pressure inhibits the baroreflex, causing blood pressure to rise.

Baroreceptors stretch-sensitive mechanoreceptors located in the heart, aortic arch, and carotid sinuses that respond to changes in blood pressure and volume.

Basopenia the number of basophils decreases because of thyrotoxicosis, acute hypersensitivity reactions, or infection.

Basophilia the number of basophils in the blood elevates as a result of hypothyroidism.

Benign febrile seizure a condition that produces a tonic-clonic or tonic seizure that lasts less than 20 minutes in a 6-month-old to 5-year-old febrile child.

Benign prostatic hyperplasia (BPH) enlargement of the prostate gland that may press against the urethra and bladder, interfering with urine flow.

Benign tumor noncancerous but abnormal overgrowth or mass of cells that is typically cured after complete excision.

Biliary atresia a condition in newborn children in which the biliary tract is blocked or absent, causing bile accumulation and progressive liver failure.

Bipolar disorder psychiatric disorder characterized by alternating mania or hypomania and depression, often with periods of normal mood in between, and changes in energy and behavior according to mood.

Bladder neck dyssynergia the bladder contracts but the external sphincter does not open, thereby preventing urination and causing urine reflux into the bladder and kidneys.

Blast injury tissue damage from compressive waves of air against the body followed by waves of decreased pressure.

Blood group antigens antigens present on the surface of erythrocytes that determine blood groups.

Blunt force injuries tearing, shearing, or crushing of tissues caused by blows, impacts, or a combination of both.

Brain death (brainstem death) irreversible brain damage that renders an individual unresponsive to all stimuli and lacking in muscle activity such as that required for respiration and heart activity.

Brainstem gliomas a group of tumors located in the brainstem that is usually classified as high grade and results in the sudden onset of symptoms including headaches, vomiting, and visual disturbances.

Bronchial carcinoid tumor an obstructing tumor of the trachea or large bronchi that may cause paraneoplastic symptoms.

Bronchiectasis dilation of the bronchi in response to obstruction, necrotizing pneumonias, cystic fibrosis, or Kartagener syndrome.

Bronchiolitis inflammation of the bronchioles usually caused by viral infection.

Bronchiolitis obliterans partial or complete obliteration of bronchioles and some bronchi by granulation and fibrotic tissue masses.

Bronchopulmonary dysplasia (BPD) a condition most often found in premature infants in which chronic pulmonary insufficiency occurs because of long-term artificial pulmonary ventilation.

Bubo an inflamed, tender swelling of a lymph node, especially in the area of the armpit or groin, that is characteristic of infections such as syphilis.

Bulimia nervosa a psychologic disorder in which recurrent binge eating is followed by intentional vomiting; inappropriate use of laxatives, enemas, diuretics, or other medication; excessive exercising; and fasting—behavior intended to compensate for overeating that has become uncontrollable.

Burkitt lymphoma a malignant lymphoma, particularly of the B lymphocytes characterized by a large osteolytic lesion in the facial bones and is associated with the Epstein-Barr virus.

Cachexia illness and malnutrition seen in individuals with cancer that results in wasting and eventual death.

Calcification hardening of tissue caused by the incorporation of calcium or calcium salts.

Calculi stones usually formed of mineral salts and most commonly found in the gallbladder, kidney, or urinary bladder.

Candidiasis a fungal infection caused by an overgrowth of normal bacteria that usually occurs in the skin and mucous membranes of the mouth, respiratory tract, or vagina.

Carbuncles a condition in which a bacterial infection of the hair follicle or sebaceous gland ducts becomes painful and discharges pus through various openings.

Carcinoma epithelial cell tumor and if arises from a gland or duct is called adenocarcinoma.

Cardiogenic shock a condition resulting from decreased cardiac output caused by heart disease in which the heart is unable to pump blood through the body, usually because of myocardial infarction.

Cardiomyopathy(ies) a diverse group of diseases primarily affecting the myocardium resulting from tissue remodeling caused by myocardial and neurohumeral responses to ischemic and hypertensive alterations.

Carrier an individual that possesses genes for a disease but does not show phenotypical characteristics of the disease.

Caseous necrosis a combination of coagulative and liquefactive necrosis in which dead cells disintegrate but are not completely digested, resulting in soft granular clumped cellular debris.

Cast a mass comprised of fibrous material, coagulated protein, or exudate that takes the shape of the region in which it has been molded, such as the bronchial, renal, or intestinal structures or the vaginal cavity, and is usually found in urine or sputum.

Catabolism cellular process that provides energy by breaking down complex molecules into simpler molecules.

Cavernous hemangioma a birthmark that is similar to the strawberry hemangioma but is more deeply rooted and may appear as a red-blue spongy mass of tissue filled with blood.

Cell adhesion molecule (CAM) protein that aids in maintaining cell shape by allowing cells to join and attach to the cytoskeleton.

Cell cycle alternation between interphase and mitosis in all tissues with cellular turnover during which nuclear material of a parent cell is duplicated and divided to form two daughter cells.

Cell lysis cell dissolution and destruction.

Cellular accumulation (infiltration) accumulation of normal cellular substances in the cytoplasm or nucleus as a result of cellular injury or inefficient cell function.

Cellular immunity an arm of the immune response known as T cells or T lymphocytes and can develop into several subpopulations of effector T cells to protect against infection.

Cellular receptor protein molecule that can be embedded in the membrane or located within the cell in the cytoplasm or on the nucleus. This protein contains binding sites for a specific chemical (ligand) that when bound initiates a biological response.

Cellulitis a subcutaneous or connective tissue becomes infected and inflamed, causing tenderness, swelling, and redness that spreads to other regions of the body.

Central tolerance a state in which autoreactive T cells in the thymus with receptors against self-antigens are eliminated, thereby preventing an immunologic reaction to an individual's own tissues.

Cerebellar astrocytoma brain tumor of the right or left cerebellar hemisphere and cause symptoms on the same side as the tumor including head tilt, limb ataxia, and nystagmus.

Cerebral death irreversible brain damage that renders an individual unresponsive to all stimuli but able to maintain the necessary respiratory and cardiovascular functions of life.

Cerebral palsy (CP) a developmental brain injury that occurs before or shortly after birth that causes muscular impairment that affects motor function and also may alter speech and learning abilities.

Cerebrovascular accident (CVA, stroke) localized brain infarction that may result in facial, arm, or leg numbness and weakness, confusion, difficulty speaking or understanding, visual disturbances, dizziness, loss of balance, difficulty walking, and headache, are classified according to pathophysiology.

Cervical dysplasia a condition, also known as cervical intraepithelial neoplasia (CIN), that is characterized by the appearance of abnormal cervical cells that are considered precancerous.

Cervicitis inflammation of the mucous membrane of the uterine cervix caused by infection, typically by chlamydia, genital herpes, or gonorrhea.

Chancre a firm, painless skin ulceration localized at the point of initial exposure to the bacteria that causes syphilis, often on the penis, vagina, or rectum.

Chemical asphyxiant chemical or gas that prevents the delivery of oxygen to tissues or blocks its use.

Chemotaxis directional movement and attraction of microorganisms or phagocytes to substances released in the environment or tissues.

Cheyne-Stokes respiration an abnormal pattern of breathing in which tidal volume gradually increases followed by a gradual decrease and a period of apnea before returning to a normal respiratory pattern.

Chickenpox an infectious viral disease that is spread by direct contact or through the air by coughing or sneezing; it causes a blister-like rash that first affects the face and trunk and then can spread over the rest of the body; symptoms include severe itching, fatigue, and fever.

Chlamydia a sexually transmitted bacterial infection that can cause infertility and blindness.

Cholecystitis inflammation of the gallbladder commonly caused by impaction of a gallstone that causes right upper quadrant pain and possibly a rupture and abscess in the gallbladder.

Cholelithiasis the presence or formation of gallstones in the gallbladder or bile ducts.

Chondrosarcoma a cancer of the cartilage that usually occurs in the pelvic bones, shoulder bones, and the upper part of the arms and legs.

Chronic lymphocytic leukemia (CLL) malignant transformation and progressive accumulation in the marrow of monoclonal B lymphocytes rarely are CLL malignancies of T cell origin.

Chronic myelogenous leukemia (CML) a cancer of heterogenous myeloid cell production in the bone marrow is increased, majority involve the Philadelphia chromosome, CML is considered a myeloproliferative disorder.

Chronic obstructive pulmonary disease (COPD) any of a group of irreversible respiratory diseases (chronic bronchitis, emphysema, alpha-1-antitrypsin deficiency) that are characterized by airflow obstruction or limitation.

Chronic rejection rejection of a graft months to years after transplantation because of a gradual loss of organ function.

Chronic renal failure a slowly developing condition that can result as a complication of a large number of kidney diseases, such as IgA nephritis, glomerulonephritis, chronic pyelonephritis, and urinary retention, and leads to end-stage renal failure for which dialysis is generally required while a donor kidney is being sought.

Cirrhosis degeneration of liver tissue resulting in fibrosis with nodule and scar formation that compromises liver function.

Cleft lip (harelip) a deformity of the lip caused by abnormal maxillary and or mandible fusion during fetal development.

Classic cerebral concussion diffuse brain injury with cerebral disconnection from the brainstem reticular activating system and is a phenomenon of physiologic, neurologic dysfunction without substantial anatomic disruption.

Cluster headache headache characterized by unilateral severe pain over the eye and forehead that lasts 15 minutes to an hour, occurs in clusters, and is capable of waking the patient.

Coagulation cascade the clotting system formed by a group of plasma proteins that act to create a fibrinous meshwork at the injured or inflamed site to prevent spread of infection, stop bleeding by formation of a clot, and provide a framework for future repair and healing.

Coagulative necrosis a type of necrosis with denaturing and coagulation of proteins within the cytoplasm and loss of nuclei.

Coarctation of the aorta (COA) a condition in which the aorta narrows in the area where the ductus arteriosus inserts; narrowing usually occurs preductal in children and postductal in adults.

Codon a triplet of nucleotides located in the mRNA that determines which amino acids will be formed during translation.

Collectin surfactant protein produced by the lungs that provides a form of innate resistance by promoting phagocytosis and interacting with the acquired immune system.

Coma a state of unresponsiveness in which an individual cannot be aroused by verbal, physical, or powerful painful stimuli.

Comedo a yellowish or blackish plug of keratin and sebaceous gland secretions, also known as a blackhead, that accumulates in the duct of a sebaceous gland and creates an acne lesion.

Communicating (extraventricular) hydrocephalus a disorder in which the cerebrospinal fluid pathways are intact but cerebrospinal fluid absorption is impaired.

Compensation adjustment of acid or base content by removal or addition in response to changes in pH; for example, a decrease in pH is accompanied by an increase in carbon dioxide removal by the lungs, causing pH to increase.

Compensatory hyperplasia increased rate of cell division that compensates for absent or dysfunctional cells of the same tissue.

Complement deficiency a condition in which complement proteins are absent or suboptimal, resulting in either inhibition or activation of the complement system.

Compliance a measure of the ease with which a structure such as the lungs or chest wall may be deformed or stretched.

Compound fracture a broken bone that is protruding from the overlying skin.

Concordant trait a trait shared by both twins.

Condylomata lata warty, plaque-like lesions found in the perianal area and other moist body sites; commonly associated with secondary syphilis.

Congenital aganglionic megacolon (Hirschsprung disease) a congenital defect in which the nerves that innervate the anus through the wall of the bowel are absent, resulting in enlargement of the bowel above the point where the nerves are missing and a subsequent decrease in peristalsis that results in chronic constipation.

Congestive heart failure (left heart failure) a condition in which the heart cannot expel sufficient blood to satisfy the metabolic demands of the body as a result of diseases such as coronary artery disease, hypertension, valvular insufficiency, or rheumatic heart disease, is categorized as systolic or diastolic heart failure.

Connexon channel composed of six protein subunits that form a hollow center through the plasma membrane at a gap junction; when two connexons in adjacent cells are aligned, chemical and electrical communication can occur between the cells.

Contact dermatitis an allergic response to an environmental antigen binding to specific carrier proteins contained in an individual's skin.

Contracture a permanent shortening of muscle or scar tissue that distorts or deforms affected joints.

Contrecoup brain injury resulting from the brain hitting the inside of the skull on the side opposite the site of blunt force trauma.

Contusion bruise produced by bleeding into the skin or underlying tissues from an insult that did not break the skin but did rupture blood vessels.

Cor pulmonale right-sided heart failure caused by prolonged pulmonary hypertension.

Coup brain injury that occurs on the same side of blunt force to the head.

Craniopharyngioma a brain tumor that develops in the pituitary gland and most often affects children, causing headache, seizure, diabetes insipidus, early onset of puberty, and delayed growth.

Craniosynostosis premature ossification of the skull and closure of the sutures, resulting in abnormal skull expansion and asymmetric skull growth.

Crohn disease (CD) an autoimmune condition in which the intestines and possibly other regions of the digestive system are chronically inflamed and ulcerated, causing chronic diarrhea, disrupted digestion, and subsequent difficulty eating and digesting food.

Croup a viral infection that involves the larynx, trachea, and the airways leading to the lungs and that can result in serious breathing difficulties, hoarseness, sore throat, and a hacking cough.

Cryoglobulin an immunoglobulin that precipitates at low body temperatures.

Cryptorchidism the scrotum of one or both testes is absent because of failure of the testis to descend from the abdominal position during fetal development.

Cushing syndrome increased synthesis of secretion of cortisol from a tumor of the adrenal cortex or by taking glucocorticoid drugs or from an ACTH secreting tumor of the anterior lobe of the pituitary gland (Cushing disease), resulting in weight gain, glucose intolerance, and muscle wasting.

Cutaneous vasculitis a type of vasculitis that affects the skin and frequently other organs and is characterized by a polymorphonuclear infiltrate of the small vessels.

Cyanosis skin, mucous membranes, and nail beds appear blue because of a lack of oxygenated hemoglobin in the blood secondary to congenital heart defects, slowed circulation, or possibly poison.

Cyclooxygenase (COX) an enzyme responsible for formation of prostaglandins, prostacyclin, and thromboxane and subsequent inflammatory response.

Cystic fibrosis (CF) a genetic disorder of the exocrine glands caused by a mutation in the CF transmembrane regulator gene, resulting in impairment in chloride transfer across cell membranes and subsequent chloride and water accumulation in organs and in thickened secretions that block ducts and form cysts.

Cystitis a condition characterized by acute or chronic inflammation of the urinary bladder, usually caused by bacterial infection of the urethra; symptoms include frequent burning urination, blood in the urine, pain in the pubic area, chills and fever, back pain, and nausea.

Cystocele the muscle between a woman's bladder and vagina weakens and allows the bladder to descend into the vagina causing discomfort, urine leakage, and incomplete emptying of the bladder.

Cytokine molecule produced by cells of the immune system that mediates interactions between cells to kill bacteria and during the inflammatory response.

Cytomegalovirus (CMV) a type of herpesvirus that is transmitted by exchange of body fluids during sexual contact, kissing, or sharing of foods and beverages and may cause mild symptoms such as enlarged lymph nodes, low fever, and fatigue that may not be noticed but also can cause severe symptoms such as blindness in immunologically compromised individuals.

Cytoskeleton network of microtubules and microfilaments located in the eukaryotic cytosol that provides structure and organization to the cell and is involved in movement of substances within the cell and movement to structures outside the cell.

Cytotoxic (metabolic) edema cerebral edema resulting from tissue hypoxia and impairment of the Na^+,K^+-ATP pump, causing a loss of intracellular potassium and a gain of intracellular sodium and water.

Cytotoxic T lymphocyte (Tc-cell or CTL) killer lymphocyte that binds to and lyses specific cells containing particular antigen receptors.

Decompression sickness (caisson disease) gas embolism created when a person underwater returns to the surface too quickly, resulting in cellular hypoxia, joint and muscle pain, and tissue necrosis.

Deep venous thrombosis (DVT) a blood clot or thrombus in a deep vein usually of the leg.

Degenerative disk disease (DDD) intervertebral disk tissue is replaced by fibrocartilage during aging; functional capacity is rarely altered.

Dementia chronic long-term intellectual difficulties in areas such as memory, concentration, and judgment, resulting from a disease or disorder of the brain.

Depolarization the movement of sodium across the membrane, resulting in a change in membrane charge from a negative to positive potential.

Dermal ischemia lack of oxygen reaches a region of skin causing tissue destruction and damage.

Dermatome an area of skin that is innervated by a specific spinal nerve and usually displays a band pattern, such as that seen with reactivation of varicella zoster (shingles).

Dermoid cyst a benign tumor resulting from congenital malformation of the skin or ovary.

Desmosome region of tight adhesion between neighboring cells that provides structural strength to the tissue and allows the cells of the tissue to function as a unit.

Developmental dysplasia of the hip (DDH) a condition in which the hip joint of babies or young children is malformed, with the ball being completely out of the socket or the socket being too shallow to support the ball.

Diabetes insipidus a disease caused by a deficiency in or resistance to antidiuretic hormone that is characterized by excretion of large amounts of dilute urine due to a decrease in water reabsorption in the kidney.

Diabetic ketoacidosis (DKA) a complication of diabetes mellitus, DKA is caused by the buildup of byproducts of fat metabolism that occurs when glucose is not available as a fuel source for the body because of insulin deficiency.

Diabetic nephropathy a progressive kidney disease caused by diabetes-induced angiopathy of capillaries in the glomeruli that causes nodular glomerulosclerosis.

Diabetic neuropathy combined sensory and motor disorder often seen in older diabetic patients as a result of microvascular injury involving small blood vessels that supply nerves.

Diabetic retinopathy damage to the retina caused by an overaccumulation of glucose or fructose that damages the blood vessels in the retina; in advanced stages, lack of oxygen in the retina causes fragile blood vessels to grow along the retina and in the vitreous fluid of the eye that may bleed and cause blurred vision.

Diaper dermatitis a type of dermatitis characterized by inflammation of the skin in the diaper area in infants caused by exposure of the skin to feces and urine.

Diarrhea an increase in the frequency of watery bowel movements or a greater looseness of stools resulting from disease, excessive consumption of alcohol or other liquids or foods that irritate the stomach or intestine, allergy to certain food products, poisoning, hyperactivity of the nervous system, or viral or bacterial infection.

Diastolic heart failure a condition in which heart contractions are normal but the ventricle does not relax completely so less blood enters the heart.

Diffuse brain injury (diffuse axonal injury) injury to neuronal axons in many areas of the brain caused by stretching and shearing forces received during brain injury.

DiGeorge syndrome a genetic disorder caused by deletion of a piece of chromosome 22 that results in cardiac defects, abnormal facies, thymic aplasia, cleft palate, and hypocalcemia.

Dilated cardiomyopathy (congestive cardiomyopathy) a condition in which all four chambers of the heart are enlarged and weakened, resulting in progressive congestive heart failure and the need for heart transplantation.

Diphtheria a contagious upper respiratory bacterial disease in which the bacteria have been infected by a bacteriophage and become lodged in the mucous membranes of the throat, where they produce a toxin that destroys the tissue and causes the formation of a tough membrane that can spread to the larynx and lead to suffocation.

Disseminated intravascular coagulation (DIC) blood coagulation throughout the entire body after the uncontrolled activation of clotting factors and fibrinolytic enzymes in small blood vessels, resulting in platelet and coagulation factor depletion and increased bleeding.

Diverticulosis multiple bulging sacs pushing outward from the wall of the large intestine and may become infected and rupture, causing abdominal pain, tenderness, and fever.

Down-regulation the process by which a cell decreases its sensitivity to a hormone or neurotransmitter by decreasing the number of receptors in response to a high concentration of that particular hormone or neurotransmitter.

Drowning breathing in of fluid that causes airway obstruction, thereby decreasing oxygen delivery to tissues and leading to asphyxia.

Dry gangrene process by which the skin dries and shrinks because of coagulative necrosis.

Duchenne muscular dystrophy an X-linked genetic disorder in which fat and fibrous tissue infiltrate and weaken muscle tissues such as in the legs and pelvis, lungs, and heart and usually results in death before adulthood.

Dumping syndrome rapid emptying of hypertonic chyme from a surgically created residual stomach causing nausea, vomiting, bleeding, and diarrhea about 20 minutes after a meal.

Dysmnesia impaired memory similar to that seen in amnesia.

Dyspareunia a reversible condition in which sexual intercourse is painful.

Dysphasia impairment of speech that manifests as the inability to arrange words in logical order.

Dyspnea shortness of breath and difficulty in breathing usually caused by lung or heart disease.

Ebb phase early posttrauma period of hypotension and decreased energy consumption that serves as a protective response to preserve blood flow to essential organs.

Ectopic testis testis has descended but is located in an abnormal position.

Eisenmenger syndrome a progressively developing condition in which a congenital heart defect such as ventricular septal defect is left untreated and causes a reversed right-to-left shunt secondary to increased pressures on the right side of the heart because of pulmonary hypertension.

Electron-transport chain series of transfer reactions that includes transferring electrons from a donor to an acceptor, resulting in the release of energy during each transfer.

Embolic stroke stroke caused by blockage of cerebral vessels.

Embolus an air bubble, a detached blood clot, or a foreign body that travels in the bloodstream and gets stuck in a blood vessel, resulting in obstruction of vessels supplying the lungs, brain, or heart; and possibly gangrene and the need for amputation of extremities.

Embryonic tumor a tumor originating in the gestational period that contains predominantly immature blast cells that cannot differentiate into mature functional cells.

Empyema (infected pleural effusion) a condition in which purulent fluid is persistently discharged into the pleural space as a result of complications of bacterial infections.

Encephalitis inflammation of the brain usually caused by a virus.

Encephalocele congenital abnormality in which a gap in the skull results in a protrusion of brain material.

Encephalopathy any of the various diseases or syndromes of the brain.

End-diastolic volume the amount of blood found in the ventricle before a cardiac contraction; used as a measure of diastolic function.

Endocytosis a process by which extracellular substances are trapped in a section of the membrane that folds inward and separates from the membrane to form an intracellular vesicle.

Endogenous cryogen a substance capable of lowering body temperature.

Endometrial polyp a typically benign mass protruding from the mucous membrane of the endometrium.

Endometriosis a condition that is common in women of reproductive age in which the tissue lining the uterus is found outside of the uterus, resulting in pain and infertility.

Endoplasmic reticulum an organelle located in the cytoplasm that synthesizes, processes, and transports proteins.

Endothelial cell a cell of the endothelial layer that lines heart, blood, and lymph vessels and the lung cavity.

Endotoxin lipopolysaccharide that is released during cell lysis from the bacterial outer membrane and causes fever, leucopenia, and possibly diarrhea and hemorrhagic shock.

Enteritis an infection of the small intestine caused by eating or drinking contaminated food or water.

Enuresis a condition in which urination is uncontrolled or involuntary.

Eosinopenia a reduction in the number of eosinophils present in the blood.

Eosinophil a phagocyte that destroys antigen-antibody complexes, allergens, and inflammatory chemicals and is important in fighting parasitic infections.

Eosinophilia the number of eosinophils in the blood elevates because of diseases such as parasitic infections, allergies, cholesterol emboli, chronic myeloid leukemia, and some drug reactions.

Ependymoma intracranial tumor that is most commonly found in children and typically arises from the inner lining of the fourth ventricle and the spinal canal.

Epididymitis a painful condition in which the epididymis becomes inflamed, usually as a result of a secondary bacterial infection that is brought about by a variety of underlying conditions such as urinary tract or sexually transmitted infections.

Epidural hematoma collection of blood between the inner surface of the skull and the dura caused by torn arteries secondary to skull fracture.

Epigenetic mechanism by which changes in gene function can be inherited without alteration of gene sequence.

Epilepsy any of a group of syndromes characterized by recurring seizures of an unknown cause.

Epiphyseal plate a plate of hyaline cartilage at the end of long bones that provides a site for lengthening of the bone.

Epispadias a birth defect in which the urethra opens on the upper penile surface.

Epstein-Barr virus (EBV) a herpesvirus that causes mononucleosis and is associated with a number of cancers, such as lymphomas in immunosuppressed persons.

Erysipelas a highly contagious bacterial infection that produces shiny, red swollen areas and fever and can lead to blood poisoning and pneumonia.

Erythema marginatum an early symptom of rheumatic fever in which pink circular lesions appear on the skin, then fade in the center to leave raised margins.

Erythema multiforme a skin disease that is caused by allergies, seasonal changes, or drug sensitivities, resulting in the formation of red macules, papules, or subdermal vesicles on the skin and mucous membranes.

Erythema toxicum neonatorum a temporary eruption of redness of the skin, small papules, and occasionally pustules in newborns that is associated with contact dermatitis or hypersensitivity to milk or other allergens.

Erythromyalgia chronic disorder characterized by warmth, pain, and redness, occurring primarily in the feet and lower legs.

Eschar a scab of dead tissue on the skin caused by a burn or by the action of a corrosive or caustic substance.

Escharotomy an incision made into a burn or scar to decrease the amount of tension on the surrounding tissue.

Esophageal varices dilation of submucosal veins of the esophagus resulting from portal hypertension; varices may ulcerate and cause severe hemorrhage.

Exotoxin protein synthesized by a specific species of bacteria that is found outside the bacterial wall.

Exstrophy of the bladder a congenital defect in which the lower abdominal wall is malformed and ruptures.

Extracellular matrix (basement membrane) fibrous proteins embedded in a carbohydrate-rich liquid that is secreted by the cell and functions as a pathway for diffusion of nutrients, wastes, and other substances between the blood and tissues.

Extrinsic allergic alveolitis (hypersensitivity pneumonitis) an inflammation of the lung caused by an immune reaction to small airborne particles such as bacteria, mold, and fungi that causes fever, chills, coughing, shortness of breath, and body aches.

Exudate fluid with cells and proteins that has leaked from blood vessels.

Facioscapulohumeral muscular dystrophy an autosomal dominant genetic disorder that begins in childhood and causes muscle wasting and weakness, primarily in the face, shoulder, and arms.

Fanconi anemia a genetic disease affecting bone marrow that is characterized by pancytopenia, hypoplasia of the bone marrow, congenital anomalies, and pigment changes of the skin and that predisposes the individual to myelodysplasia and to acute myeloid leukemia or cancers of the mouth, esophagus, intestinal and urinary tracts, and the reproductive organs.

Fat necrosis lipase-induced cellular dissolution of triglycerides in breast, pancreas, and other abdominal structures.

Fibromyalgia muscles, tendons, and joints are painful, stiff, and tender; often accompanied by restless sleep, fatigue, anxiety, depression, and disturbances in bowel function.

Fibrosarcoma a malignant tumor of fibrous connective tissue that usually is derived from immature proliferating fibroblasts.

Fibrous dysplasia (FD) a genetic disorder in which tumor-like growths or lesions form in one or more bones and replace the medullary bone with fibrous tissue, resulting in expansion and weakening of the bone.

First-degree burn a mild burn that produces redness and tenderness of the skin but no blistering, such as that seen in a minor sunburn.

Focal segmental glomerulosclerosis (FSGS) a condition in which glomerular capillaries with thickened basement membranes and increased mesangial matrix collapse in segments. Usually presents as nephrotic syndrome.

Follicular cyst a cyst caused by the retention of secretions in a follicular structure because of the blockage of a duct, resulting in the failure of the dominant follicle to rupture or failure of the nondominant follicles to regress.

Folliculitis infection and inflammation of a hair follicle.

Frailty physiologic and immune changes that result in wasting of the body during aging and leave the affected person susceptible to falls, functional decline, disease, and death.

Frank-Starling law of the heart the idea that changes in the volume of blood filling the heart will change the volume that is ejected by the same amount because the force of the contraction will increase as the heart is filled with more blood.

Free radical highly reactive and destructive particle that has an unpaired electron and is produced from an atom or molecule.

FSH deficiency a condition characterized by decreased or absent production of follicle-stimulating hormone, resulting in a decline in spermatogenesis/oogenesis and associated infertility.

Fulminant hepatitis a type of viral hepatitis that has a high mortality rate and causes fatigue, nausea, jaundice, dark urine, flu-like symptoms, hepatomegaly, and eventually encephalopathy.

Furuncles staphylococcal infection produces painful pus-filled inflamed hair follicles and involves surrounding skin and subcutaneous tissue.

Fusiform aneurysm (giant aneurysm) large aneurysm that stretches to affect the entire circumference of the arterial wall.

G protein an intracellular protein that is activated by the binding of a hormone or neurotransmitter to an extracellular receptor and in turn activates adenylyl cyclase, which produces cAMP.

Galactorrhea inappropriate lactation; a condition in which milk-like fluid is secreted from the breast because of hormonal alterations that are not associated with childbirth or nursing.

Ganglia (ganglion) cells a relay point between different neurologic structures such as the peripheral and central nervous systems; two major groups are dorsal root ganglia that contain cell bodies of sensory afferent neurons and autonomic ganglia that interconnect to form a plexus.

Ganglioneuroma a benign neoplasm composed of mature ganglionic neurons scattered within a stroma of neurofibrils and collagenous fibers.

Gangrenous necrosis tissue death typically found in the lower leg as a result of severe hypoxic injury secondary to arteriosclerosis or blockage of major arteries.

Gap junction tunnel or connexon that joins two adjacent cells and allows for the passage of molecules and electrical signals between the cells.

Gas gangrene the formation of gas bubbles and subsequent destruction of connective tissue and cell membranes resulting from the hydrolytic enzymes produced by bacterium of the *Clostridium* species.

Gastritis the lining of the stomach becomes inflamed because of bacterial infection, bile reflux, or excessive consumption of alcohol or certain foods.

Gastroesophageal reflux (GER) a type of injury to the esophagus caused by chronic exposure of the esophagus to stomach liquid reflux composed of acid and pepsin that creates inflammation of the esophageal lining, strictures, heartburn, dysphagia, and chronic chest pain.

Gastroileal reflex a process by which food entering an empty stomach increases ileal motility and causes the opening of the ileocecal valve.

Gate control theory a proposal that a pain gate is present in the spinal cord that allows or blocks pain signals to the brain depending on whether the impulse is traveling on a large or small afferent fiber.

Gating calcium-induced decrease in permeability of a junctional complex that may aid in protecting uninjured cells from the increased calcium levels released by injured cells.

Gene-environmental interaction the multifactorial mechanism for developing a disease that includes genes as well as environment and lifestyle.

Generalized neuropathy a functional disturbance or pathologic change in the cell body of one type of peripheral neuron.

Generalized anxiety disorder (GAD) an anxiety disorder characterized by an excessively anxious mood lasting at least 1 month that interferes with daily functioning and may be accompanied by jitteriness, sweating, feelings of catastrophe concerning one's family or self, and irritability.

Generalized seizure a seizure occurring bilaterally with no local focal point that involves the entire body, resulting in muscle rigidity, violent muscle contractions, and impaired or lost consciousness.

Generalized symmetric polyneuropathy an apparent symmetric disturbance of function or pathologic change in several sensory, motor, or autonomic fibers.

Genital herpes a sexually transmitted viral infection that is caused primarily by herpes simplex virus type 2 and is characterized by painful lesions in the genital and anal regions.

Germline mosaicism mechanism by which a child can inherit a genetic disease even though the parents do not express the disease; the mechanism is believed to involve a mutation during the embryonic development of the parent germ cells.

GH deficiency a condition characterized by decreased or absent production of growth hormone, resulting in a decline in insulin-like growth factor-1 and dwarfism if the deficiency is prepubertal.

Giant cell tumor a benign tumor that usually occurs near the end of a bone close to a joint in the arm or leg, in the knee, and in flat bones.

Giantism severely increased long bone growth caused by excessive growth hormone secretion before and during puberty.

Glomerulonephritis an autoimmune or infectious disease characterized by inflammation of the glomeruli that may not produce symptoms or may present with hematuria and proteinuria.

Glucose-6-phosphate dehydrogenase (G6PD) deficiency an inherited condition that is asymptomatic in the absence of exposure to particular substances such as certain medicines, mothballs, or severe infections, but with exposure the red blood cells undergo destruction, producing excessive bilirubin that overloads the liver and causes jaundice.

Gluten-sensitive enteropathy (celiac sprue) this condition is characterized by mucosal inflammation and villous atrophy in the gastrointestinal tract formed in response to a genetic predisposition for an immune response to gluten and similar proteins.

Goiter a noncancerous enlargement of the thyroid gland that is visible as a swelling at the front of the neck.

Gonorrhea a sexually transmitted disease caused by the bacteria gonococci that invade the mucous membranes of the genitals and urinary tract and in women the cervix, fallopian tubes, and ovaries, causing chronic pelvic pain or infertility.

Gout a disorder of uric-acid metabolism that causes painful inflammation of the joints, commonly the big toe, and arthritic attacks resulting from elevated levels of uric acid in the blood and the deposition of negatively birefringent urate crystals around the joints.

Granulation tissue vascularized tissue that replaces the fibrin clot during the reconstructive phase of wound healing.

Granulocytopenia a decrease in the number of granular white blood cells in the blood.

Granulocytosis an increase in the number of granulocytes, usually neutrophils, in blood secondary to bacterial infection, leukemia, or autoimmune disease.

Granuloma a tumor-like mass containing macrophages and fibroblasts that forms as a result of chronic inflammation and isolation of the infected area.

Granuloma inguinale a bacterial-induced disease, also called Donovanosis, that is thought to be transmitted primarily by anal rather than vaginal intercourse and causes painless genital ulcers like syphilis but progresses to destruct the internal and external genital tissue.

Graves disease autoimmune hyperthyroidism caused by antibodies that continuously activate TSH receptors and characterized by an enlarged thyroid gland, protrusion of eyeballs, a rapid heartbeat, and nervous excitability.

Ground substance fluid or semisolid gel found in the extracellular matrix of bone that contains fibroblasts that produce collagenous, elastic, and reticular tissue fibers.

Gynecomastia abnormal breast tissue develops on adolescent boys or men as a result of an imbalance in hormones.

Hageman factor (factor XII) component of the kinin system that activates the clotting system, prekallikrein and C1 in the complement system and converts plasminogen proactivator to plasminogen activator.

Haploid cell cell that contains one copy of each chromosome, giving each cell 23 chromosomes.

Haplotype a group of alleles of closely linked genes located on one chromosome that are inherited together.

Hemachromatosis an iron overload disease, excess absorption of iron from the diet and can increase in vital organs such as the heart, joints, pancreas, and pituitary gland leading to dysfunction, has a genetic origin.

Hematoma collection of blood in soft tissue or an enclosed space.

Hemolytic anemia a condition in which red blood cells are destroyed in response to certain toxic or infectious agents or in certain inherited blood disorders and the rate of breakdown exceeds the body's ability to compensate.

Hemolytic disease of the newborn (HDN) a condition that affects a fetus or newborn in which red blood cells break down because of antibodies made by the mother that are directed against the infant's red cells, potentially resulting in anemia, heart failure, jaundice, and brain damage if left untreated.

Hemolytic-uremic syndrome a condition in which platelets aggregate within the kidney's small blood vessels, resulting in reduced blood flow to the kidney and subsequent kidney failure and destruction of the red blood cells usually after exposure to Shiga like toxin from a strain of E. coli.

Hemophilia A (classic hemophilia) a genetic disorder in which a mutation in factor VIII causes prolonged clotting time, decreased formation of thromboplastin, and diminished conversion of prothrombin.

Hemophilia B (Christmas disease) a genetic disorder similar to hemophilia A in terms of symptoms but with a mutation in the factor IX gene.

Hemophilia C (factor XI deficiency) a genetic disorder characterized by a deficiency in factor XI, resulting in a mild form of hemophilia.

Hemoptysis a manifestation of various respiratory, neoplastic, or hemolytic conditions in which blood or blood-stained sputum is spit or coughed from bronchi, larynx, trachea, or lungs.

Hemorrhagic stroke (intracranial hemorrhage) stroke usually caused by hypertension that results in bleeding in the brain and typically increases intracranial pressure and may lead to death.

Henoch-Schönlein purpura nephritis the blood vessels are inflamed causing bleeding into the skin, mucous membranes, internal organs, and other tissues; pain and inflammation in the joints; abdominal pain; gastrointestinal bleeding; inflammation of the kidneys; subcutaneous edema; encephalopathy; and inflammation of the testis.

Hepatic encephalopathy a condition that is usually caused by liver cirrhosis and portal hypertension in which toxins produced by the gut pass into the systemic circulation and damage brain cells, resulting in impaired cognition, tremor, and a decreased level of consciousness.

Hepatitis A a virus that is spread by the fecal-oral route through contaminated food and water or by close and intimate contact and results in liver inflammation, flu-like symptoms, nausea, poor appetite, abdominal pain, fatigue, yellow eyes and skin, and dark urine that can last weeks to months.

Hepatitis B virus (HBV) a DNA virus that is transmitted by contaminated blood or blood derivatives in transfusions, by sexual contact, or by the use of contaminated needles and instruments and may become chronic and cause long-term damage including hepatocellular carcinoma in the liver.

Hepatitis C an RNA virus that is transmitted primarily by blood and blood products and sometimes through sexual contact and may become chronic with few to no symptoms while causing long-term damage to the liver, such as cirrhosis and hepatocellular carcinoma.

Hepatorenal syndrome (HRS) acute renal failure occurs because of a decrease in renal blood flow secondary to liver disease.

Hereditary spherocytosis a defect in the cell membrane of red blood cells that causes thickened, fragile red blood cells that are susceptible to spontaneous hemolysis and results in chronic anemia, jaundice, fever, and abdominal pain.

Herpes simplex virus (HSV) a contagious sexually transmitted viral infection of the genital and anal or mouth regions that produces recurrent small clusters of painful lesions.

Hiatal hernia an anatomic abnormality in which the esophageal hiatus is larger than normal, causing part of the stomach to protrude through the diaphragm and up into the esophagus or chest.

Histamine an active amine produced by mast cells that dilates capillaries causing abnormal permeability, regulates gastric acid production in the gastrointestinal tract, causes many symptoms of the allergic reaction.

Hodgkin lymphoma (HL) a cancer of lymphoid tissue in which the lymph nodes, spleen, and liver become enlarged and is often accompanied by anemia, fever, and eventually death if not treated at an early stage; also referred to as Hodgkin disease.

Human papillomavirus (HPV) one of several viruses that are considered sexually transmitted infections and are characterized by internal or external plantar warts and genital warts and are a causal factor for cervical cancer and associated with oral cancer.

Humoral immunity an arm of the immune response consisting of B lymphocytes, immune protection afforded by the presence of antibodies in blood.

Huntington disease (HD) an autosomal dominant disease causing a progressive increase in involuntary, jerky, diskinetic movements, mental deterioration, and premature death.

Hydrocele serous fluid accumulates in a body cavity such as the testis.

Hydrops fetalis edema formation in the fetal subcutaneous tissue because of an enzyme deficiency or any one of several other disorders.

Hyperacute rejection rejection of a graft immediately after transplantation because of the prior formation of cytotoxic antibodies against the antigens on the graft.

Hyperaldosteronism excessive secretion of aldosterone and subsequent muscle weakness, cardiac irregularities, and abnormally high blood pressure.

Hyperchloremic metabolic acidosis anion gap is normal but bicarbonate is lost, whereas chloride is retained to maintain ionic balance, resulting in a drop in pH.

Hyperemia an increase in the quantity of blood flow to a body part.

Hyperhemolytic crisis an increased rate of destruction of red blood cells, resulting in decreased hemoglobin levels, increased reticulocyte count, elevated bilirubin, and elevated lactate dehydrogenase caused by infections, hemolytic transfusion reactions, sickle cell crisis, or a combination of glucose-6-phosphodisterase deficiency with oxidant stress.

Hyperhomocysteinemia an elevated plasma homocysteine concentration because of diet, vitamin B_6 or B_{12} deficiency, congenital enzyme deficiency, or renal failure, increasing the risk of developing atherosclerosis and venous thromboembolism.

Hypermetabolism an extreme elevation in metabolic rate.

Hyperpolarized the state of a membrane when the membrane potential is more negative than the resting membrane potential, thereby increasing the stimulus required to elicit an action potential.

Hyperprolactinemia excessive prolactin secretion, usually the result of a pituitary tumor, which can lead to anovulation or impaired spermatogenesis related to the inhibiting effects of prolactin on hypothalamic gonadotropin-releasing hormone and infertility.

Hypersensitivity a state in which the body undergoes an exaggerated immune response to an antigen.

Hyperthermic injury injury caused by excessive heat that includes heat cramps, heat exhaustion, and heat stroke.

Hypertonic hyponatremia increased plasma lipids, proteins, or glucose displace water balance and thus decrease sodium concentration.

Hypertrophic cardiomyopathy a genetic disorder caused by various mutations that thicken the heart muscle, possibly leading to obstruction of blood flow and heart dysfunction; this is a common cause of sudden death in young athletes.

Hyperventilation a condition in which breathing faster and deeper than necessary reduces carbon dioxide concentration, resulting in respiratory alkalosis with numbness or tingling in the hands, feet, and lips, lightheadedness, dizziness, headache, chest pain, and sometimes fainting.

Hypochloremic metabolic alkalosis acid loss caused by vomiting with depletion of extracellular fluid and chloride; to compensate the kidneys increase sodium and bicarbonate reabsorption with excretion of hydrogen.

Hypocortisolism a decrease in cortisol synthesis and release that may be related to deficiency at the adrenal, pituitary, or hypothalamic level.

Hypoglycemia a state of low blood glucose that stimulates epinephrine and glucagon secretion, resulting in mobilization of stored glycogen and fat and their conversion into glucose.

Hypoparathyroidism a condition marked by decreased function of the parathyroid glands, resulting in hypocalcemia and hyperphosphatemia and associated tremor, tetany, and convulsions.

Hypoplastic anemia a condition in which anemia results from greatly depressed, inadequately functioning bone marrow and smaller than normal erythrocytes.

Hypoplastic left heart syndrome (HLHS) a condition in which the left side of the heart, including the aorta, aortic valve, left ventricle, and mitral valve, is underdeveloped and blood returning from the lungs flows through an opening in the atrial septum and the right ventricle pumps the blood into the pulmonary artery and then into the aorta.

Hypospadias a birth defect in which the urethral opening is abnormally placed, opening anywhere from the tip of the glans of the penis to the shaft or the junction of the penis and scrotum or

perineum in males and usually opening in the vagina in females.

Hypothermic injury chilling or freezing of tissues, resulting in disturbances in ion balance and homeostasis.

Hypothyroidism a condition caused by insufficient thyroid hormone synthesis and secretion, resulting in impaired memory, increased sensitivity to heat and cold, slow heart rate, depression, weight gain, slowed metabolism, and several other systemic alterations.

Hypoventilation a condition in which ventilation is inadequate for proper gas exchange, causing an increase in carbon dioxide concentration and subsequent respiratory acidosis.

Hypovolemia decreased blood volume capable of causing hypotension, tachycardia, and decreased urine output.

Hypovolemic shock a state of shock caused by a decrease in blood volume secondary to dehydration, bleeding, and drugs such as diuretics or vasodilators.

Hypoxemia insufficient oxygenation of arterial blood.

Hypoxia a state in which the oxygen level reaching cells is insufficient, resulting in tissue injury; may be caused by a reduction in oxygen content of inspired air, a decrease in hemoglobin available for oxygen binding, or cardiovascular or respiratory disease.

Icterus neonatorum (neonatal jaundice) jaundice in newborn infants caused by functional immaturity of the liver and usually subsides within the first few days of life.

Immune thrombocytopenic purpura (ITP) a condition in which the number of platelets in the blood is reduced by the production of antibodies against platelets, resulting in ecchymoses and hemorrhages from mucous membranes, anemia, and extreme weakness.

Immunohemolytic anemia an acquired hemolytic anemia in which isoantibodies or autoantibodies are produced in response to drugs, toxins, or other antigens.

Imperforate anus a congenital defect in which the anal opening is absent because of the presence of a membranous septum or of complete absence of the anal canal.

Impetigo a contagious bacterial infection that produces superficial red blisters that rupture and produce thick yellow crusts that commonly occur on the face but can spread to other regions of the body easily.

Infectious mononucleosis (IM) a disease that is caused by the Epstein-Barr virus or the cytomegalovirus that is transmitted by exchanging saliva or blood or by coughing and sneezing and acts by infecting the B cells and atypical T cells resulting in fever, sore throat, and fatigue.

Inflammatory acne a condition characterized by comedones that appear as red, swollen, and inflamed blemishes and by larger, deeper, swollen tender lesions that become inflamed and rupture under the skin.

Inflammatory joint disease a disease in which inflammation affects joint structures and often leads to structural derangement of the joint, structural joint problems, and pain at rest and with motion.

Inflammatory response nonspecific response to tissue damaging irritants in which pain, heat, redness, and swelling rapidly occur at the site of injury.

Innate immunity (inflammation) natural, native, or innate resistance and protection conferred by inflammation

Innate resistance (immunity) protection or resistance to infection by nonimmune mechanisms such as natural physical, mechanical, and biochemical barriers.

Inotropic agent a substance that affects muscle contraction, especially contraction of the heart muscle.

Insulin protein hormone that is secreted by the beta cells of the islets of Langerhans and functions in carbohydrate and fat metabolism by increasing glucose uptake into and subsequent glycogen production in muscle and by activating adipose cells to form fat.

Insulin resistance a diminished response of liver, muscle, and adipose tissues to insulin, causing hyperglycemia and normal to elevated insulin levels.

Interstitial cystitis/painful bladder syndrome symptoms of cystitis with frequency and dysuria without bladder infection. Inflammation and fibrosis of the bladder may be evident with the development of Hunner ulcers. Occurs most commonly in women.

Interstitial edema fluid accumulation occurring in the space surrounding cells of a tissue.

Intracerebral hematoma (intraparenchymal hemorrhages) blood accumulation that partially clots inside the brain, usually in the frontal and temporal lobes.

Intramembranous formation the process responsible for the development of flat bones in which ossification of the collagenous matrix is direct and cartilage is not present.

Intrarenal acute renal injury a type of acute renal failure characterized by renal parenchymal damage that disrupts glomerular filtration and disrupts renal tubular function.

Intrinsic factor (IF) a small protein secreted by the parietal cells of gastric glands and required for adequate absorption of vitamin B_{12}.

Intrinsic pathway a component of the coagulation cascade that causes blood clotting in response to contact with a foreign substance.

Intussusception an infolding or prolapse of a segment of the small intestine into the adjacent but more distal segment of the intestine.

Ion positively or negatively charged molecule.

Iron deficiency anemia (IDA) an insufficient dietary intake or absorption of iron, resulting in decreased incorporation of hemoglobin into red blood cells and subsequent feelings of fatigue, weakness, and shortness of breath as well as pale earlobes, palms, and conjunctivae.

Ischemia inadequate blood supply in the circulation and can cause a decrease in blood flow to local vessels that may result in hypoxia and subsequent cell injury or death.

Islets of Langerhans the endocrine region of the pancreas that contains four cell types: alpha cells that secrete glucagon, beta cells that secrete insulin, delta cells that secrete somatostatin, and PP cells that secrete pancreatic polypeptide.

Isohemagglutinin an immunoglobulin that is capable of agglutinating erythrocytes of individuals within the same species.

Isolated systolic hypertension loss of elasticity of the arteries resulting in an increase in cardiac output or stroke volume, a systolic blood pressure consistently greater than 160 mmHg, and a diastolic pressure less than 90 mmHg.

Isthmus a narrow passage connecting two larger parts of an anatomic structure such as that seen in the thyroid gland.

Jaundice (icterus) yellowish brown staining of the skin and the conjunctiva caused by high bilirubin levels in blood secondary to excessive erythrocyte breakdown, obstruction in or around the liver, or liver disease.

Juvenile myoclonic epilepsy a type of epilepsy that occurs in adolescents and young adults, usually on awakening, and is characterized by jerks of the neck, shoulders, and arms and by clonic-tonic-clonic seizures.

Juvenile rheumatoid arthritis (JRA) a condition in which children younger than the age of 16 develop rheumatoid arthritis and experience swelling, tenderness, and pain in one or more joints and lymph node and splenic enlargement.

Kaposi sarcoma (KS) a rare cancer of connective tissue caused by the herpesvirus 8 (HHV8) in which many bluish red nodules appear on the skin, especially skin of the lower extremities; occurs in a particularly virulent form in individuals with AIDS.

Kawasaki disease a vascular disease characterized by inflamed heart and vessels, coronary artery aneurysm, thickening and stenosis, a fever that lasts at least 5 days, and at least four of the following: inflammation with reddening of the whites of the eyes; red, swollen hands or feet or peeling skin; rash; swollen lymph gland in the neck; inflamed lips or throat; or red "strawberry" tongue.

Keloid a red, raised overgrown fibrous scar formed by excessive cell growth during tissue repair after trauma or surgical incision.

Keratocanthoma a skin tumor that contains a central keratin mass and usually occurs on exposed skin areas and heals spontaneously but may leave a scar.

Kernicterus a fatal form of jaundice in the newborn caused by elevated levels of unconjugated bilirubin in the blood secondary to an increase in red blood cell number and breakdown and by jaundice-induced lesions in the cerebral gray matter.

Kussmal respiration (hyperpnea) deep, rapid respiration commonly seen in conditions causing acidosis.

Kwashiorkor a condition in which children do not receive enough protein in their diet, resulting in a swollen and severely bloated abdomen secondary to decreased albumin in the blood, skin changes resulting in a reddish discoloration of the hair and skin in dark-skinned children, severe diarrhea, fatty liver, muscle atrophy, and restricted development.

Lactase deficiency a condition in which not enough lactase is present in the small intestine to digest lactose, resulting in lactose intolerance characterized by diarrhea, bloating, and gas in response to exposure to lactose.

Lactose intolerance a condition caused by lactase deficiency in which lactose is not broken down, making it impossible for the small intestine to absorb it and causing excessive gas production and diarrhea when exposed to lactose-containing foods.

Langerhans cell immature dendritic cell that captures, takes up, and processes antigens in response to infection, then travels to the T-cell areas of the lymph node and matures into fully functional antigen-presenting cells.

Laryngomalacia a congenital anomaly caused by a developmental delay in the laryngeal cartilage and supporting structures of the larynx that causes the cartilage to be floppy and fold in on itself during inspiration, producing high-pitched, coarse, and low-pitched sounds.

Legg-Calvé-Perthes disease blood supply to the head of the femur near the hip joint is interrupted, resulting in osteonecrosis of the corresponding epiphysis.

Leiomyoma a benign smooth muscle mass that can occur in any organ, but most commonly occurs in the myometrium of the uterus or in the esophagus.

Lennox-Gastaut syndrome a generalized myoclonic epilepsy that occurs in children between 1 and 5 years of age as a result of various cerebral afflictions such as perinatal hypoxia, hemorrhage, encephalitis, and metabolic disorders of the brain and is characterized by mental retardation, personality disorders, and generalized tonic seizures.

Leptin a protein hormone that is produced by adipose tissue and provides the brain with an assessment of adipose mass and regulates appetite and metabolism by altering the actions of neuropeptide Y.

Leukemia an acute or chronic malignant disease of the bone marrow and blood-forming organs, an excessive proliferation of white blood cells occurs and is usually accompanied by dysfunctional blood cells, anemia, impaired blood clotting, and enlargement of the lymph nodes, liver, and spleen.

Leukemoid reaction a form of leukocytosis that is similar or mimics that occurring in leukemia but results from some other cause.

Leukocytosis an increase in the number of leukocytes in the blood as a result of fever, inflammation, hemorrhage, infection, etc.

Leukopenia a condition in which the number of white blood cells in the blood is decreased, resulting in an increased risk for infection.

Leukotriene a mediator of the prolonged inflammatory response that acts to contract smooth muscle, increase vascular permeability, and attract neutrophils.

LH deficiency a condition characterized by decreased or absent production of luteinizing hormone, resulting in a decline

in sex steroid production in testes/ovaries and associated infertility.

Liability distribution prediction of the probability of an individual having a specific disease based on exposure to genetic and environmental factors known to cause the disease.

Lichen planus a recurrent rash of small, flat-topped bumps and rough scaly patches appearing on the skin, in the lining of the mouth and in the vagina in response to inflammation or an allergy to a specific medication.

Ligand molecule including hormone, neurotransmitter, antigen, complement components, lipoproteins, infectious agent, drug, metabolite and others that binds to a specific cellular receptor, resulting in the initiation of cellular events specific to that receptor.

Limb girdle muscular dystrophy a progressive genetic disorder that usually begins before adolescence and presents similar to facioscapulohumeral muscular dystrophy but with the hips and shoulders being the most severely affected muscles.

Lipofuscin yellow-brown pigment produced by breakdown of damaged blood cells in heart and smooth muscle.

Liquefactive necrosis a type of necrosis with liquefaction of neurons and glial cells in the brain as a result of ischemic injury or bacterial infection.

Loss of heterozygosity with inheritance of two chromosomes, one from each parent, one is normally heterozygous for nearby genetic markers; thus loss of a chromosome region of one of the chromosomes is loss of heterozygosity a biological trait of tumor development.

Lupus erythematosus any of a group of autoimmune connective tissue disorders that commonly produce red scaly lesions and are accompanied by fever, malaise, myalgias, fatigue, and weight loss.

Lyme disease (borreliosis) tick-borne spirochete bacterial infection that is characterized by a rash in the area of the bite, headache, neck stiffness, chills, fever, myalgia, arthralgia, malaise, fatigue, and possible development of arthritis in large joints.

Lymphadenopathy swelling of one or more lymph nodes because of diseases such as bacterial or viral infection, Hodgkin lymphoma, non-Hodgkin lymphoma, or unknown causes.

Lymphocyte nonphagocytic leukocyte of the adaptive immune response that is immunologically competent and serves as the precursor for B and T lymphocytes.

Lymphocytopenia a decrease in the number of lymphocytes in the blood because of diseases and conditions such as human immunodeficiency virus, severe stress, or the administration of corticosteroids, chemotherapy, or radiation therapy.

Lymphocytosis an increase in the number of lymphocytes in the blood because of infection, inflammation, or leukemia.

Lymphogranuloma venereum (LGV) a sexually transmitted bacterial infection that enters the body through breaks in the skin or across the epithelial cell layer of mucous membranes and primarily targets the lymphatics and lymph nodes.

Lymphoma cancer arising from cell proliferation in lymphoid tissue.

Lysosomal storage diseases a group of more than 30 disorders that result from impaired lysosomal function, leading to mucopolysaccharidoses, lipid storage disorders, mucolipidoses, leukodystrophies, and glycoprotein storage disorders.

Macrocytic anemia (megaloblastic anemia) a condition characterized by a deficiency of vitamin B_{12} or folic acid caused by inadequate intake or insufficient absorption secondary to alcoholism or drugs that inhibit DNA replication.

Macrophage phagocyte that is produced from a monocyte and is important in cellular initiation of the inflammatory response.

Major (unipolar) depression severely depressed mood and loss of pleasure that may begin suddenly or slowly, persists for at least 2 weeks, and may recur throughout life.

Major histocompatibility complex (MHC) a set of glycoproteins found on the surface of all cells except red blood cells and serve as markers of cell recognition for the immune system by distinguishing self from non-self.

Malignant hypertension a complication of hypertension in which blood pressure is severely elevated and organ damage occurs in the eyes, brain, lung, and/or kidneys.

Malignant hyperthermia an inherited life-threatening disorder that causes muscle rigidity, a hypermetabolic state, tachycardia, and increased body temperature in response to administration of general anesthesics.

Malignant tumor cancerous mass of cells that grows, invades, and metastasizes to distant organs, usually causing death.

Marasmus a childhood disorder characterized by protein and energy malnutrition, resulting in dry skin, loss of adipose tissue from normal areas of fat deposits such as buttocks and thighs, and behavior that is fretful and irritable.

Margination (pavementing) a process by which leukocytes adhere better to endothelial cells of the capillary walls and venules by the reciprocal change in adhesion molecules on leukocytes.

Mast cell a cell of the connective tissue that produces substances that cause activation of the inflammatory response, vasoconstriction, and muscle contraction.

Mastocytosis a condition characterized by the abnormal proliferation of mast cells that results in an increase in mast cell–derived chemicals being released, subsequently causing changes in the immune system that produce typical allergy symptoms such as itching, abdominal cramping, and even anaphylaxis.

McArdle disease a metabolic disorder involving an enzyme defect that causes deficiency of muscle phosphorylase, which helps break down glycogen, and consequently this disorder causes an energy deficit in the muscles, resulting in muscle pain and cramping.

Meconium a dark green fecal material that accumulates in the fetal intestines and is discharged at or near the time of birth.

Meconium ileus obstruction with thickened meconium in the intestine of a newborn child as a result of a lack of trypsin and associated with cystic fibrosis of the pancreas.

Mediated transport the transport of inorganic ions and some organic compounds across the cell membrane by way of integral membrane or transmembrane proteins that contain specific receptors.

Medulloblastoma a malignant cerebellar tumor near the fourth ventricle that is most often found in children and consists of neoplastic cells that resemble the undifferentiated cells of the neural tube.

Megacalycosis a congenital condition in which enlarged calyces are present with a normal pelvis and ureter, possibly caused by previous obstruction or reflux.

Membranous glomerulonephritis a slowly progressive disease of unknown origin or that occurs secondary to autoimmune conditions, infections, specific drugs, or malignant tumors that is caused by a circulating immune complex formed from the binding of antibodies to antigens of the glomerular basement membrane (GBM) or antigens transported from the systemic circulation and implanted in the GBM.

Memory cell T or B lymphocyte that "remembers" a specific antigen after the initial exposure and initiates a more efficient immunologic response in response to subsequent exposures to the same antigen.

Meningioma a slow-growing mass of the meninges that is usually benign but increases intracranial pressure.

Meningocele neural tube defect in the skull or spinal column that forms a cyst filled with cerebrospinal fluid through which the meninges of the brain protrude.

Mental retardation impaired intellectual development as a result of congenital causes, brain injury, or disease, resulting in impaired learning, social, and vocational ability.

Mesenteric venous thrombosis a condition in which a blood clot blocks off one of the mesenteric veins and compromises the intestinal blood supply and can result in intestinal gangrene and tissue death.

Mesodermal germ layer tissue located between the ectoderm and endoderm that gives rise to an epithelial component of genital and urinary structures, striated muscle, connective tissue, cartilage, bone, smooth muscle, and blood cells.

Mesothelioma a type of cancer that is usually associated with previous exposure to asbestos, which affects the pleura, the lining of the abdominal cavity, the pericardium, and most internal organ coverings.

Metabolic acidosis decrease in pH caused by an increase in noncarbonic acids or a decrease in bicarbonate.

Metabolic alkalosis increase in pH caused by an increase in bicarbonate ions secondary to an increase in metabolic acid loss.

Metabolic syndrome a condition of unknown cause that presents with symptoms of insulin resistance, obesity, hypertension, dyslipidemia, and systemic inflammation.

Metastasis occurs when cancer cells break away from the original tumor, enter the systemic circulation, and invade distant tissues and organs.

Metatarsus adductus a foot deformity in which the front half of the foot bends inward, possibly because of the infant's position in the uterus.

Microcephaly defect in which failure of normal brain growth causes a delayed skull growth and production of a small head.

Microcytic-hypochromic anemia a condition in which red blood cells are smaller than normal due to iron deficiency.

Microglia neuroglial cell that migrates and functions as a phagocyte for nerve tissue waste products.

Microtubules small protein tubules located in the cytosol that add strength to the cell structure, facilitate intracellular organelle and cell movement and nerve transmission, and play a role in immune and inflammatory actions and hormone secretion.

Migraine headache headache that usually begins in the temporal region unilaterally after vascular changes of cranial arteries and may cause irritability, nausea, vomiting, constipation or diarrhea, and photophobia.

Mild concussion temporary axonal disturbances without the loss of consciousness in response to a violent blow, jarring, shaking, or other closed head injury.

Miliaria a skin disease caused by partially obstructed sweat glands that results in small and itchy rashes usually located in skinfolds and on areas of the body that may rub against clothing, such as the back, chest, and stomach.

Minimal change nephropathy (MCN) the foot processes of the renal capillary basement membrane are fused and deformed because of a T-cell disorder that reduces the anion component of the basement membrane and allows proteins to leak into the renal tubule.

Minimally conscious state (MCS) a condition in which a severely brain-damaged patient is capable of deliberate behavior distinguishable from unconscious reflexive actions.

Mitochondrion large organelle where most of the cell's ATP is generated by oxidative phosphorylation.

Mitosis the process of nuclear division during which two identical nuclei are produced from one parent cell after chromosomal replication.

Mitral valve a valve in the heart that lies between the left atrium and left ventricle and functions to allow blood to flow into the left ventricle during ventricular diastole and to prevent regurgitation from the ventricle to the left atrium during systole.

Mitral valve prolapse syndrome the mitral valve cannot close properly because of one or both flaps being too large, possibly resulting in mitral valve regurgitation.

Molluscum contagiosum a viral infection of the skin occuring in young children that affects the body, arms, and legs and is spread through direct contact, saliva, or shared articles of clothing and is considered a sexually transmitted disease in adults, affecting the genitals, lower abdomen, buttocks, and inner thighs.

Monoclonal gammopathy of undetermined significance (MGUS) production of monoclonal antibodies by noncancerous plasma cells that accumulate in the blood.

Monocyte immature white blood cell produced in bone marrow, circulates in blood, and migrates to the inflammatory site where they develop into macrophages.

Monocytopenia a decreased number of monocytes in the blood because of the release of toxins into the blood by bacteria or by administration of chemotherapy or corticosteroids.

Monocytosis an increased number of monocytes in the blood because of chronic infection, autoimmune disorder, blood disorder, or cancer.

Mononuclear phagocyte system (MPS) a collection of free and fixed macrophages derived from bone marrow cells whose phagocytic activity is primarily mediated by immunoglobulin and by the serum complement system.

Moyamoya disease an abnormality of the blood vessels that supply the frontal region of the brain in which vessels constrict or become completely occluded resulting in diminished blood flow. The body attempts to compensate by growing new vessels at the base of the brain, which appear as a puff of smoke on an angiography.

Mucoepidermoid carcinoma a tumor of the main or lobar bronchi lumen that may extend into the peribronchial tissue.

Mucopurulent cervicitis (MPC) inflammation of the cervix with purulent endocervical exudate that may be asymptomatic or cause abnormal vaginal discharge and vaginal bleeding.

Multifactorial trait a trait that is affected by genes and environment or lifestyle.

Multinucleated giant cells a cell mass formed by union of several cells in response to infection.

Multiple sclerosis chronic demyelinating disease of the central nervous system that causes inflammation and scarring of myelin sheaths.

Myasthenia gravis neuromuscular disorder caused by an autoimmune response in which antibodies to acetylcholine receptors impair neuromuscular transmission.

Mycotic aneurysm aneurysm that is caused by bacterial or fungal growth in the vessel wall or infection of a arteriosclerotic aneurysm.

Myelodysplasia abnormal formation of the spinal cord.

Myelodysplastic syndrome (MDS) a group of hematologic conditions characterized by ineffective production of blood cells, resulting in anemia that requires chronic blood transfusion.

Myeloma a tumor composed of cells derived from hemopoietic tissue of the bone marrow.

Myoadenylate deaminase deficiency (MDD) a genetic disorder in which an enzyme deficiency prevents the conversion of adenosine monophosphate (AMP) to inosine monophosphate, resulting in increased AMP loss and the inability to synthesize adenosine triphosphate for energy.

Myocardial infarction a heart condition of sudden onset in which muscle tissue dies because of a lack of blood flow, resulting in varying degrees of chest pain or discomfort, weakness, sweating, nausea, and vomiting, and possibly loss of consciousness.

Myositis inflammation of a muscle, usually a voluntary muscle, resulting in pain, tenderness, and sometimes spasm in the affected area.

Myositis ossificans a condition in which bone is deposited in muscle tissue, causing pain and swelling.

Myotonia a neuromuscular disorder in which muscle relaxation after voluntary contraction is delayed.

Myxedema cutaneous edema caused by deposition of connective tissue (e.g. glycosaminoglycans and hyaluronic acid) and associated with hypothyroidism and Graves' disease, characterized by dry skin, pretibial myxedema, swellings around the lips and nose, mental deterioration, and a decrease in basal metabolic rate.

Natural killer (NK) cell lymphocyte capable of killing target cells by binding specific receptors with or without the aid of antibodies and by releasing chemicals toxic to the targeted cells.

Necrotizing enterocolitis (NEC) a condition of extensive ulceration and necrosis of the ileum and colon in premature infants during the neonatal period.

Neonatal alloimmune thrombocytopenic purpura (NATP) a condition in which fetal platelets have an antigen from the father that is absent in the mother, and the mother forms antibodies that cross the placenta and destroy the fetal platelets.

Neovascularization growing new microvascular networks that are functional and perfused.

Nephritic syndrome a disorder of the glomerular filtration membrane in which plasma proteins and red blood cells pass into the urine resulting in mild proteinuria, hematuria, and mild hypertension.

Nephroblastoma a condition, also known as Wilms tumor, that is characterized by a malignant renal tumor that compresses the normal kidney parenchyma, causing an abdominal mass, blood in the urine, and fever and may be associated with anorexia, vomiting, and malaise.

Nephrotic syndrome a disorder of the glomerular filtration membrane which permits proteins to pass into the urine resulting in proteinuria, hypoalbuminemia, hyperlipidemia and systemic edema.

Neuroblastoma a malignant tumor containing neuroblast cells that originate in the autonomic nervous system or the adrenal medulla and is most common in infants and young children.

Neurofibrillary tangles protein aggregates formed by hyperphosphorylation of the tau protein within neurons, as seen in Alzheimer disease.

Neurogenic bladder dysfunction the underactivity or overactivity of the bladder caused by nervous system damage that prevents the bladder muscles from contracting to empty the bladder completely or that causes rapid bladder contraction that causes too rapid or frequent emptying.

Neurogenic detrusor overactivity a neurologic abnormality that impairs communication between the bladder and the central nervous system, preventing the brain from inhibiting the detrusor muscles that controls urination.

Neurogenic shock a type of shock caused by the sudden loss of the sympathetic nervous system signals to the smooth muscle in vessel walls, causing the vessels to relax and a decrease in peripheral vascular resistance and blood pressure.

Neuropathic pain chronic pain associated with nerve injury that is perceived as burning or pins and needles or electric shock that is produced by the stimulation of pain, touch, and temperature receptors in the same area.

Neutropenia the absence of neutrophils in the blood.

Neutrophil (polymorphonuclear neutrophil) (PMN) phagocyte that destroys bacteria by phagocytosis, digestion, and secretion of bacteria-killing chemicals.

Neutrophilia a condition in which the number of neutrophils, especially the younger, less mature cells in the blood is increased.

Nissl substances structures, also known as Nissl bodies, that are located in the cell bodies of neurons and are involved in protein synthesis.

Nonbacterial prostatitis prostatitis causes chronic pain that goes away and comes back without warning but shows no signs of bacterial infection in the prostatic fluid even though the semen and other fluids from the prostate contain immune cells that the body produces in response to infection.

Nonbacterial thrombotic endocarditis fibrin deposition on the valve leaflets of the heart, especially on the left side, as a result of cancer, rheumatic fever, or arteriosclerosis.

Noncommunicating hydrocephalus cerebrospinal fluid accumulation within the skull caused by obstruction of the cerebrospinal fluid pathways.

Non-Hodgkin lymphoma (NHL) a malignancy of lymphoid tissue classified as B-cell, T-cell, and NK-cell lymphomas that mimics Hodgkin lymphoma but does not produce the cells characteristic of Hodgkin lymphoma and does not have a definitive cause other than association with latent Epstein-Barr virus, AIDS, or Agent Orange exposure.

Noninflammatory acne open comedones caused by the enlargement and dilation of a plug resulting from the accumulation of oil and dead skin cells inside the hair follicle and by closed comedones that form if the hair follicle pore remains closed and appear as a tiny, sometimes pink bump in the skin.

Noninflammatory joint disease a disease in which alterations in the structure or mechanics of the joint results in pain during motion.

Nonossifying fibroma (fibrous cortical deficit) a benign fibrous tissue tumor forms in the metaphysis of any of the long bones but usually occurs in the thigh and shin bones in children and adolescents.

Non-REM (slow wave) sleep period of sleep during which dreams do not occur and brain waves are slow and high voltage.

Nonvolatile a substance that does not have a vapor form.

Normocytic-normochromic anemia (NNA) erythrocytes are of normal size and hemoglobin content but of insufficient number usually caused by hereditary spherocytosis, drug-induced anemia, and anemia secondary to other malignancies.

Nucleolus a small structure in the nucleus that contains the DNA of the cell and the associated binding proteins and where RNA subunits of ribosomes are assembled.

Nucleotide DNA subunit containing one deoxyribose molecule, one phosphate group, and one nitrogenous base.

Nucleus a large membrane-bound organelle that contains the cellular DNA and is usually located in the center of the cell.

Nystagmus involuntary, rapid, rhythmic movements of the eyeball in the horizontal, vertical, or rotational direction.

Obsessive-compulsive disorder (OCD) an anxiety disorder characterized by obsessive thoughts and repetitive compulsive actions, such as cleaning, checking, or counting.

Obstructive sleep apnea syndrome (OSAS) a disorder of sleep characterized by airway obstruction and episodes of apnea accompanied by snoring.

Obstructive uropathy the blockage of urine flow, often by ureteral or kidney stones, resulting in the reflux of urine and subsequent injury to kidneys.

Occult bleeding blood in the feces or vomit that is not visible upon gross inspection but is detected in tests used to screen for colon cancer.

Oligodendroglioma a slow-growing mass of oligodendrogliocytes that is usually benign.

Oncogene tumor-causing gene that increases the rate of cell proliferation if mutated.

Oncotic pressure (colloid osmotic pressure) pressure that is created by large molecules such as plasma proteins that cannot penetrate the membrane and pulls water toward the proteins.

Onychomycosis a fungal infection of the fingernails or toenails that causes thickening, roughness, and splitting of the nails.

Opsonin a molecule (e.g C3b complement, IgG and IgA) that attach to antigens and promotes binding to phagocytes.

Orchitis swelling of the testicles that can result in ejaculation of blood, blood in the urine, and pain and visible swelling of a testicle or testicles.

Organ tropism growth of a tissue or organism in response to external stimuli.

Orthostatic (postural) hypotension a sudden fall in blood pressure when a person assumes a standing position, resulting in dizziness, lightheadedness, blurred vision, and temporary loss of consciousness.

Osmotic pressure the hydrostatic pressure that results from the difference in solute concentration within solutions that are separated by a semi-permeable membrane.

Osteoarthritis (OA) previously classified as noninflammatory, inflammation is now known to be involved; degenerative joint disease in which synthesis and degradation of the articular cartilage in the movable joints is altered, resulting in wearing and destruction of cartilage.

Osteochondrosis a condition in children, also known as Osgood-Schlatter disease, that results from the tendons pulling on the epiphysis of long bones, causing pain just below the knee, irritation and swelling, and possibly abnormal bone growth.

Osteogenesis imperfecta (brittle bone disease) a genetic disease in which collagen production is deficient, making the bones abnormally fragile and causing recurring fractures with only minimal trauma, deformity of long bones, a bluish coloration of the sclerae, and often the development of otosclerosis.

Osteoid osteoma a benign tumor in one of the bones of the lower extremities that is painful and is characterized by vascularized connective tissue and osteoid material that is surrounded by a large zone of thickened bone.

Osteomalacia a disease in which vitamin D or calcium deficiency or excessive renal phosphate loss causes a softening of the bones with accompanying pain and weakness.

Osteomyelitis a bacterial infection of the bone and bone marrow that occurs through open fractures, penetrating wounds, surgical operations, or by entering via the bloodstream and causes pain, high fever, and formation of an abscess at the site of infection.

Osteonectin a protein in bone that binds collagen and hydroxyapatite and links collagen to minerals in the bone matrix.

Osteoporosis a disease in which the bones become porous and weakened, making them easily fracture and slow to heal.

Ovarian torsion a condition in which an ovary twists or turns on its supporting ligament to the point that its blood supply is compromised.

Oxidative stress tissue injury induced by free radicals that are produced during metabolic reactions and with exposure to some environmental agents.

Oxyhemoglobin dissociation curve a sigmoid plot of the percent hemoglobin bonding sites occupied by oxygen versus the partial pressure of oxygen, which illustrates the affinity of hemoglobin for oxygen.

Paget disease (osteitis deformans) a bone disorder in which excessive bone remodeling causes enlarged, deformed bones that can weaken the bone integrity and result in bone pain, arthritis, deformities, or fractures.

Pancreatic insufficiency a condition in which the pancreas does not secrete enough hormones and digestive enzymes for normal digestion to occur, resulting in malabsorption, malnutrition, vitamin deficiencies, and weight loss.

Pancreatitis inflammation of the pancreas usually resulting in abdominal pain.

Panic disorder a psychologic disorder that is characterized by recurrent attacks of anxiety or terror and usually results in the development of one or more phobias.

Papilloma a benign nodular breast lesion consisting of hyperplastic distorted ductal cells.

Paraneoplastic syndrome a condition in which a tumor, usually of the lung, breast, ovaries, or lymphatics, releases hormones or cytokines into the circulation that cause some biologic response.

Paraphimosis a condition in which the foreskin becomes trapped behind the glans penis and cannot return to its normal flaccid position covering the glans penis.

Parathyroid hormone (PTH) a protein hormone secreted by the parathyroid glands that regulates calcium and phosphate levels in the body by promoting the absorption of calcium by the intestine, mobilizing calcium and phosphate from bones, and increasing the tendency of the kidney to reabsorb calcium and excrete phosphate.

Parenchyma tissue that is responsible for the physiologic function of an organ.

Parkinson disease degeneration of the basal ganglia dopaminergic nigrostriatal pathway that causes hypokinesia, tremor, and muscular rigidity.

Paronychia inflammation of the tissue surrounding a fingernail or toenail.

Partial seizure (focal seizure) a seizure caused by focused excessive electrical activity secondary to a lesion in a particular brain region.

Passive acquired immunity (passive immunity) a form of acquired immunity in which the antibody or lymphocyte is provided by a donor.

Pathogen-associated molecular pattern (PAMP) molecular patterns on infectious agents or their products that allow recognition by specific receptors.

Pattern recognition receptor (PRR) a receptor involved in innate resistance that recognizes cellular damage or specific patterns on infectious agents.

Pediculosis pubis a contagious condition, also known as crabs or crab lice, that is an infestation of the pubic hair in which the louse feeds on human blood and multiplies rapidly.

Pelvic inflammatory disease (PID) inflammation of the female genital tract caused by microorganisms, typically those that are sexually transmitted such as chlamydia and gonococci, and is characterized by severe abdominal pain, high fever, vaginal discharge, and possibly infertility.

Pemphigus a group of autoimmune skin diseases marked by groups of itching blisters and raw sores on the skin and mucous membranes.

Peptic ulcer a nonmalignant stomach or duodenal wall ulceration, commonly caused by the bacterium *Helicobacter pylori* that thrives in the acidic environment of the stomach.

Pericarditis the pericardium is infected by a virus, bacteria, parasite, or fungus and becomes inflamed, resulting in pain and fluid and blood components entering into the pericardial space.

Perihepatitis a condition, also known as Fitz-Hugh-Curtis syndrome, that is a complication of pelvic inflammatory disease secondary to gonococci bacteria traveling up the peritoneum to the upper abdomen and causing inflammation.

Periodic paralysis one of a group of diseases in which muscular weakness or flaccid paralysis occurs without loss of consciousness, speech, or sensation.

Peripheral artery disease (PAD) any of a group of diseases caused by the obstruction of large peripheral arteries secondary to atherosclerosis, inflammatory processes, embolism, or thrombus formation that causes ischemia.

Peripheral tolerance a state in which peripheral lymphoid organs control autoreactive T cells to prevent an immunologic reaction to an individual's own tissues.

Pernicious anemia an autoimmune disorder that causes a deficiency in intrinsic factor resulting in the inability to absorb vitamin B_{12} and a subsequent increase in the production of abnormal erythrocytes.

Pes planus (flatfoot) a condition in which the arch of the foot never develops or it collapses and contacts the ground.

Peyronie disease (bent nail syndrome) a condition in which fibrous plaques grow in the soft tissue of the penis because of injury of the internal cavity of the penis that is accompanied by bleeding and scar

tissue formation at the tunica albuginea of the corpora cavernosa.

Phagocytosis a type of endocytosis sometimes referred to as "cell eating" in which substances such as bacteria and cell particulate are incorporated into large vesicles or vacuoles and digested.

Phantom limb pain pain experienced in an amputated limb after the stump has healed that may be caused by spontaneous firing of afferent pain fibers in the spinal cord that were previously associated with the limb.

Phenylketonuria (PKU) a genetic disorder in which the body lacks the enzyme necessary to metabolize the amino acid phenylalanine to tyrosine, resulting in accumulation of phenylalanine and subsequent brain damage and progressive mental retardation.

Pheochromocytoma a tumor of the adrenal medulla that causes the chromaffin cells to secrete increased amounts of epinephrine or norepinephrine.

Philadelphia chromosome a specific genetic abnormality that is associated with chronic myelogenous leukemia, acute lymphoblastic leukemia, and occasionally acute myelogenous leukemia.

Phimosis the foreskin of the penis of an uncircumcised male cannot be fully retracted.

Physiologic dead space the volume of air that does not participate in gas exchange or the sum of anatomic and alveolar dead space.

Pityriasis rosea a skin disorder, thought to be caused by a virus, in which patches of ovular pink rash appear primarily on the trunk and extremities.

Plasma cell a B lymphocyte that secretes antibodies in response to local cytokines released during the primary immune response.

Plasma kinin cascade a series of events that activates the kinin system to produce bradykinin.

Plasmin a degrading enzyme associated with fibrinolysis of many proteins of blood but primarily of fibrin clots.

Plasticity the ability of nervous system pathways to change function, sensitivity, and so forth in response to changes in the neural environment.

Platelet-activating factor (PAF) a mast cell–derived substance that increases vascular permeability, leukocyte adhesion to endothelial cells, and platelet activation.

Pleural effusion a medical condition in which fluid accumulates in the pleural cavity surrounding the lungs and thereby makes breathing difficult.

Pneumoconiosis a chronic disease of the lungs typically seen in miners, sandblasters, and metal grinders that is caused by repeated inhalation of dust particles, including iron oxides, silicates, and carbonates, that collect in the lungs and become sites for the formation of fibrous nodules that eventually replace lung tissue.

Pneumonia an infection of one or both lungs caused by a bacterium, virus, fungus, or other organism that enters the body through respiratory passages and causes high fever, chills, pain in the chest, difficulty in breathing, cough with sputum, and possibly bluish skin from insufficiently oxygenated blood.

Pneumothorax the collapse of a lung and subsequent escape of air into the pleural cavity between the lung and the chest wall that is caused by trauma, environmental factors, or spontaneous occurrence and results in a sudden pain in the chest.

Polycystic kidney disease (PKD) a condition in which several fluid-filled cysts grow in the kidneys and may reduce kidney function and result in kidney failure as well as damage to the liver, pancreas, and possibly the heart and brain.

Polycystic ovary syndrome (PCOS) a hormonal condition in which multiple ovarian cysts form because of elevated androgens, resulting in hirsutism, obesity, menstrual abnormalities, infertility, and enlarged ovaries.

Polycythemia an increase in red blood cell mass because of a defect in the erythroid progenitor cells or an increase in circulating serum factors such as erythropoietin.

Polycythemia vera a chronic, progressive disease that is characterized by overgrowth of the bone marrow, excessive red blood cell production, and an enlarged spleen and causes headache, inability to concentrate, and pain in the fingers and toes.

Portal hypertension an increase in blood pressure in the veins of the hepatic portal system resulting from obstruction in the liver, such as that seen in cirrhosis, that causes enlargement of the spleen and collateral veins.

Port-wine (nevus flammeus) stain a birthmark caused by superficial and deep dilated capillaries in the skin that produce a reddish to purplish discoloration of the skin, usually the face, but can occur anywhere on the body.

Posthemorrhagic anemia a type of normocytic-normochromic anemia that is caused by sudden blood loss in an individual with normal iron stores and triggers a compensatory response in which water and electrolytes from tissues and interstitial spaces are used to expand plasma volume and accelerate the formation and development of blood cells.

Postmortem change diffuse physiologic changes that occur within minutes after death.

Postobstructive diuresis elevated urine output occurring after surgery to remove an obstruction that causes the inability of the renal tubules to reabsorb water and electrolytes normally.

Postganglionic neuron nerve fibers that begin at the ganglia and terminate on the effector organ.

Postrenal acute renal injury a condition characterized by an obstruction that affects the normal flow of urine out of both kidneys and causes pressure to build in the nephrons that eventually shuts them down.

Posttraumatic stress disorder (PTSD) a psychologic disorder that may develop in individuals who have experienced or witnessed traumatic events and is characterized by recurrent flashbacks of the traumatic event, nightmares, irritability, anxiety, fatigue, forgetfulness, and social withdrawal.

Poverty of content a disorder, also called poverty of speech content, that is characterized by disorganized speech that conveys little information and may be vague or contain repetitive or obscure phrases.

Precocious puberty a condition in which a boy or girl undergoes the changes associated with puberty at an unexpectedly early age; often caused by a pathologic process that increases the secretion of estrogens or androgens.

Preload the volume of blood in the ventricle after atrial contraction and ventricular filling.

Premenstrual syndrome (PMS) a group of symptoms that occur in many women from 2 to 14 days before menstruation begins, such as abdominal bloating, breast tenderness, headache, fatigue, irritability, depression, and emotional distress.

Prerenal acute kidney injury rapid development of renal hypoperfusion with elevation of serum creatinine and urea.

Presbyopia a form of farsightedness usually accompanying advanced age in which the lens loses elasticity and becomes unable to accommodate and focus light for near vision.

Priapism a painful condition in which the erect penis maintains an erection in the absence of physical and psychologic stimulation.

Primary dysmenorrhea painful menstruation because of a functional disturbance rather than because of inflammation, growths, or anatomic factors.

Primary hyperparathyroidism usually the result of a benign parathyroid tumor that secretes parathyroid horomone and increases circulating calcium levels; this condition is accompanied by hypercalcemia, nausea, vomiting, lethargy, depression, muscular weakness, and an altered mental state.

Primary hypertension elevated blood pressure of unknown etiology accompanied by increased total peripheral vascular resistance by vasoconstriction, increased cardiac output, or both.

Primary immune response time interval between the first and second exposures to an antigen, during which antibodies against the antigen are produced.

Primary lysosome a lysosome that possesses hydrolytic enzymes but has a high pH and is therefore inactive and not yet involved in digestive activity.

Primary syphilis a stage of syphilis infection that occurs after an incubation period of 10 to 90 days and is characterized by a primary sore or chancre that develops at the point of initial exposure and lasts 4 to 6 weeks.

Prolactinoma the most common type of anterior pituitary tumor; produces visual disturbances and prolactin excess that results in infertility and changes in menstruation in females and impotence, loss of libido, and infertility in males.

Prostaglandin a mast cell–derived substance that increases vascular permeability, muscle contraction, and neutrophil chemotaxis, as well as induces pain, and potentially inhibits some aspects of inflammation.

Prostatitis inflammation of the prostate gland caused by urinary tract infection.

Protein C deficiency a disorder characterized by a lack of anticoagulant activity and an increased tendency to form blood clots because of decreased degradation of factor Va and factor VIIIa secondary to thrombosis, deep vein thrombosis, pulmonary embolism, thrombophlebitis, neonatal purpura fulminans, and disseminated intravascular coagulation.

Protein S deficiency a disorder characterized by a lack of anticoagulant activity and an increased tendency to form blood clots because of decreased degradation of factor Va and factor VIIIa.

Prothrombin time (PT) a test that measures the amount of time required for plasma to clot and is diagnostic for disorders of the extrinsic and common coagulation pathways.

Protopathic sensation of pain, heat, cold, or pressure without the ability to localize the stimulus.

Pruritus a condition characterized by a severe itching sensation usually on undamaged skin.

Psammoma bodies calcium salt layers present in calcified tissues.

Pseudothrombocytopenia an artificially low platelet count in anticoagulated blood caused by cooling of the blood and autoagglutination of platelets.

Psoriasis a noncontagious autoimmune skin disorder in which the skin becomes scaly and inflamed when cells in the outer layer of skin reproduce faster than normal and accumulate as plaques on the skin surface.

Pulmonary embolism (PE) dislodgement of a blood clot from its site of origin and embolization to the arterial blood supply of one of the lungs, resulting in shortness of breath and difficulty breathing, rapid breathing that is painful, cough, and in severe cases, hypotension, shock, loss of consciousness, and death.

Pulmonary fibrosis scarring of the lungs caused by any of several conditions such as sarcoidosis, hypersensitivity pneumonitis, rheumatoid arthritis, lupus, asbestosis, and certain medications and causing shortness of breath, coughing, and diminished exercise tolerance.

Pulmonary stenosis a condition in which the opening into the pulmonary artery from the right ventricle narrows.

Pulmonary thromboembolism obstruction of the pulmonary artery or one of its branches by a blood clot that originated in the deep venous system.

Pure red cell aplasia (PRCA) an acquired or congenital condition in which the bone marrow lacks red blood cell precursors even though megakaryocytes and white blood cell precursors are usually present at normal levels.

Pyelonephritis a condition in which a bacterial infection of the urinary system has extended through the urethra, bladder, ureters and into the renal pelvis causing abdominal or back pain, fever, malaise, nausea, and vomiting.

Pyloric stenosis a congenital abnormality in which the pylorus is narrow, resulting in poor feeding, weight loss, and progressively worsening vomiting.

Pyuria the presence of white blood cells in the urine that is usually the result of a urinary tract infection.

Quantitative trait multifactorial trait that is measured on a continuous numeric scale and tends to follow a bell-shaped curve among populations.

Rapid eye movement (REM) sleep period of sleep during which dreams occur, autonomic activities are irregular, and brain waves are fast and of low voltage.

Raynaud disease a condition in which the blood vessels spasm because of inadequate blood supply, resulting in discoloration of the fingers and/or toes after exposure to changes in temperature or emotional events.

Reactive response the secretion of stress hormones in response to a psychologic stressor.

Reagin antibody that is found in blood in response to several diseases and is involved in anaphylaxis and skin allergies.

Recombination physical exchange of genetic information between homologous chromosomes that results in the creation of new genotypes.

Relative polycythemia a relative increase in the number of red blood cells caused by loss of the fluid portion of the blood.

Remodeling a process in which bone is resorbed and then replaced without changing shape in order to release calcium and repair mildly damaged bones.

Renal adenoma a benign tumor originating in the renal tubules of the cortex that is similar in appearance to a renal cell carcinoma.

Renal agenesis only one functional kidney is present at birth.

Renal cell carcinoma (RCC) a malignancy arising from the renal tubule that produces hematuria, flank pain, and an abdominal mass.

Renal colic a condition in which a tiny stone passing through the ureter produces intermittent but very severe abdominal pain that begins in the flank or upper abdomen and travels down to the lower abdomen and possibly radiating into the pubic region or into the penis or testis in men.

Renal dysplasia abnormal tissue development in one or both kidneys.

Renin an enzyme secreted by the juxtaglomerular cells of the kidney that is released in response to decreased blood pressure in the kidney and sympathetic nerve stimulation.

Renin-angiotensin-aldosterone system a mechanism by which sodium and water levels are regulated in the body, including the release of renin, conversion of angiotensinogen into angiotensin I,

conversion of angiotensin I into angiotensin II, the release of aldosterone and its actions on the kidney that increase water and sodium reabsorption.

Reperfusion (reoxygenation) injury tissue injury resulting from the restoration of oxygen after an interval of hypoxia or anoxia because of generation of highly reactive oxygen intermediates or oxidative stress.

Residual volume (RV) the volume of air left in the lungs after maximal expiratory effort.

Respiratory acidosis decrease in pH caused by elevated carbon dioxide secondary to depressed ventilation.

Respiratory alkalosis increase in pH caused by alveolar hyperventilation and hypocapnia.

Respiratory distress syndrome (RDS) of the newborn a condition, also known as hyaline membrane disease (HMD), that is a type of respiratory distress in newborns, most often in prematurely born infants, those born by cesarean section, or those having a diabetic mother; the immature lungs do not produce enough surfactant to retain air so the air spaces empty completely and collapse after exhalation.

Resting membrane potential the difference in electrical charge across the membrane of an unstimulated cell.

Restrictive cardiomyopathy any of a group of disorders in which the heart chambers are unable to fill with blood completely because of stiffness of the heart and the inability of heart muscle to relax during diastole.

Retinoblastoma an autosomal dominant or sporadic disorder in which a malignant tumor forms in the retina of one or both eyes; typically found in infants.

Rectocele a condition caused by childbirth or hysterectomy in which the region between the rectum and vagina bulges toward the vagina, resulting in a sense of pressure or protrusion within the vagina, the feeling of incomplete emptying of the rectum, difficulty passing stool, discomfort or pain during evacuation or intercourse, constipation, vaginal bleeding, fecal incontinence, the prolapse of the bulge through the opening of the vagina, or rectal prolapse through the anus.

Reye syndrome a type of encephalopathy that occurs primarily in children that were given aspirin for a viral infection such as chickenpox or influenza and is characterized by fever, vomiting, fatty liver, disorientation, and coma.

Rhabdomyolysis a potentially fatal condition in which skeletal muscle breaks down as a result of injury such as physical damage to the muscle, high fever, metabolic disorders, excessive exertion, convulsions, or anoxia of the muscle for several hours; large amounts of myoglobin are usually excreted.

Rhabdomyosarcoma (RMS) a cancer that differentiates so that it resembles normal skeletal muscle.

Rheumatic fever an inflammatory disease that is associated with recent streptococcal infection and causes inflammation of the joints, fever, jerky movements, nodules under the skin, and skin rash and often is followed by serious heart damage or disease.

Rheumatoid arthritis an autoimmune disease that causes chronic inflammation of the joints and the tissue around the joints and other organs.

Rickets a bone disease that is caused by a deficiency of vitamin D or calcium and manifests in children as softening of bones, abnormal bone growth, and enlargement of cartilage at the ends of long bones.

Right heart failure inability of the right side of the heart to pump blood efficiently because of left-sided heart failure, lung disease, congenital heart disease, clots in pulmonary arteries, pulmonary hypertension, or heart valve disease.

Ringed sideroblast an erythroblast in which one third or more of the nucleus is encircled by 10 or more siderotic granules that may be caused by antituberculous drugs and alcohol abuse.

Roseola a viral disease in infants and young children that causes fever and a spotty rash that appears shortly after the fever has subsided.

Rotovirus a viral infection seen in young children that causes diarrhea by attacking the lining of the small intestine, resulting in the inability to absorb fluid and electrolytes.

Rubella an infectious viral disease of children and young adults that is spread by a droplet spray from the respiratory tract of an infected individual; the disease causes a rash that lasts about 3 days with tender and swollen lymph nodes behind the ears.

Rubeola an infectious viral disease of young children, also known as measles, that is spread by a droplet spray from the nose, mouth, and throat of individuals in the infective stage and causes a rash, white spots in the mouth, a rash on the face that spreads to the rest of the body, and fever.

Saccular aneurysm (berry aneurysm) a localized, progressively growing sac that affects only a portion of the circumference of the arterial wall and may be the result of congenital anomalies or degeneration.

Salmon patches (nevus simplex) patches, also known as stork bites, of small, pink, flat spots that are small dilated blood vessels visible through the skin and are usually found on the forehead, eyelids, upper lip, between the eyebrows, and the back of the neck.

Salpingitis inflammation of one of the two fallopian tubes caused by infection spreading from the vagina or uterus.

Sarcoma tumor of the connective tissue cells.

Sarcopenia loss of muscle mass and strength because of advanced age and decreased activity, resulting in impaired sense of balance.

Scabies skin infestation with the itch mite, *Sarcoptes scabiei,* acquired through close contact with an infected person or contaminated clothing that produces intense itching.

Schizophrenia a psychotic disorder characterized by delusions, hallucinations, loosening of associations, disturbances in mood and sense of self and relationship to the external world, and bizarre, purposeless behavior.

Sclerosing adenosis a condition in which the number of acini per terminal duct is more than twice the number of normal terminal ducts and is associated with a significantly increased risk of subsequent breast carcinoma.

Scoliosis a condition in which the spine is curved sideways to varying degrees due to either physiologic curvature or functional curvature in which contraction of the paraspinal muscles of the back creates a vertebral curve.

Seborrheic dermatitis scaly, flaky, itchy, and red skin on the scalp, face, and trunk because of a yeast infection.

Secondary (anamnestic) immune response production of great amounts of antibodies in response to the second exposure to an antigen.

Secondary amenorrhea menstruation begins at puberty but then is subsequently suppressed for three or more cycles or for 6 months in women that previously menstruated.

Secondary dysmenorrhea altered menstruation because of inflammation, infection, tumor, or anatomic factors.

Secondary generalization the process by which a simple partial seizure involving one hemisphere becomes a generalized seizure involving the second hemisphere.

Secondary hyperparathyroidism a condition of elevated parathyroid hormone resulting from disease such as renal failure in which parathyroid hormone is elevated in response to vitamin D deficiency.

Secondary hypertension a condition of elevated blood pressure that is associated with other conditions primarily with renal disease by a renin-dependent mechanism or a fluid volume–dependent mechanism.

Secondary septic arthritis a bacterial infection in the joints, causing them to become inflamed and the bacteria to proliferate.

Secondary syphilis the most contagious stage of syphilis infection, characterized by a skin rash that appears on the trunk and extremities 1 to 6 months after the primary infection and possibly mucous patches on the genitals or inside the mouth.

Second-degree burn a burn that blisters the skin and is more severe than a first-degree burn, causing intense pain.

Seizure a transient event of excessive neurologic activity that is disorderly and results in disturbances of motor, sensory, and autonomic function and alters behavior and the state of consciousness.

Senile plaque the excessive accumulation of proteins that forms neurofibrillary tangles and prevents intracellular transport and neurotransmission.

Sentinel nodes lymph nodes that are the first to receive drainage and are the first targets during cancer metastasis.

Septic shock a condition caused by systemic infection that causes decreased tissue perfusion and oxygenation and can result in multiple organ dysfunction syndrome and death.

Sequestration crisis a condition in which the cardiovascular system collapses, causing blood to pool in the spleen and liver.

Serum sickness a form of hypersensitivity caused by injection of soluble antigen such as antiserum that activates a type III hypersensitivity response (formation of soluble circulating antigen-antibody [IgG or IgM] complexes) that activates the complement system.

Severe pelvic organ prolapse weakened or damaged pelvic floor muscles that can no longer support the pelvic organs, causing the uterus to fall into the vagina.

Sheehan syndrome a condition characterized by decreased functioning of the pituitary gland caused by necrosis resulting from blood loss and hypovolemic shock during and after childbirth.

Shigellosis a potentially sexually transmitted bacterial disease that is transmitted by contaminated water or by anal-oral contact and causes diarrhea, fever, nausea, vomiting, and cramps within 1 to 3 days after contact with the bacteria.

Shock a condition in which the circulatory system is unable to provide adequate circulation to the body tissues due to inadequate pumping by the heart, a reduction in blood volume, or a reduction in blood pressure and results in slowing of vital functions and possibly death.

Sialoprotein (osteopontin) a glycoprotein that may play a role in maintaining or reconfiguring tissues during the inflammatory process and is required for stress-induced bone remodeling and cell-mediated immunity.

Sickle cell anemia an inherited disorder of the blood caused by abnormal hemoglobin that distorts red blood cells and makes them fragile and prone to rupture and can cause anemia, joint pain, fever, leg ulcers, and jaundice.

Sickle cell trait an inherited condition in which an individual carries only one gene for sickle cell disease and is without symptoms.

Sideroblastic anemia (SA) refractory anemia of varying severity that is caused by altered mitochondrial metabolism and is marked by sideroblasts in the bone marrow.

Signal transduction transmission of signals from an extracellular chemical to the intracellular region where cellular activity is affected. Signal transduction occurs when environmental stimuli are translated into electrical signals in the body as well as when a signal is transmitted between extracellular and intracellular domains.

Silencing epigenetic mechanism of inheritance from parent to child or single cell to progeny whereby gene expression is passed during cell division and does not require mutations or changes in the DNA sequence, abnormal silencing is emerging as a major cause of cancer.

Smallpox (variola) an infectious viral disease that is caused by a poxvirus and causes high fever, aches, and widespread eruption of large sores that leave scars.

Smoldering myeloma a condition in which abnormal plasma cells produce a monoclonal protein, but no symptoms or complications of myeloma are present and may not be present for several years.

Spermatocele a cyst of the rete testis or the head of the epididymis that is distended with a milky fluid that contains spermatozoa.

Spina bifida a congenital defect in which the spinal column is not closed correctly, causing protrusion of that part of the meninges or spinal cord.

Spinal stenosis narrowing of the spinal canal as a result of congenital anomaly or spinal degeneration, resulting in pain, paresthesias, and neurogenic caudication.

Stable angina a condition in which ischemic attacks occur at predictable frequencies and duration after activities that increase myocardial oxygen demands such as exercise and stress.

Stage a term used to describe the extent of tumor spread, ranging from local tumor with little to no invasion to metastasis to distant tissues.

Staphylococcal scalded-skin syndrome (SSSS) a disease in infants that is caused by an upper respiratory staphylococcal infection with release of an exfoliative toxin that results in peeling of large areas of skin.

Starling hypothesis proposal that net filtration is equal to the forces favoring filtration such as capillary hydrostatic pressure and interstitial oncotic pressure minus the forces opposing filtration such as capillary oncotic pressure and interstitial hydrostatic pressure.

Stasis dermatitis the skin appears brown and ulcerative because of blood pooling in the leg secondary to insufficient venous return.

Status epilepticus occurrence of multiple consecutive seizures without intervals of consciousness.

Stem cell precursor cell that can differentiate into multiple cell types.

Stevens-Johnson syndrome an inflammatory eruption of circular lesions that can cover the majority of the skin and mucous membranes and usually occurs after a respiratory infection or as an allergic reaction to drugs or other substances.

Strangulation cerebral hypoxia or anoxia caused by compression and closure of the blood vessels and air passages accomplished by applying external pressure on the neck.

Strawberry hemangioma a red birthmark caused by densely packed blood vessels that usually appears on the face, scalp, back, and chest and disappear during childhood.

Stress stimuli that when exposed to the human body cause a physiologic response characterized by sympathetic nervous system activity and the release of hypothalamic, pituitary, and adrenal hormones.

Stress response the mechanism by which the endocrine and central nervous systems increase the amount of energy available to combat stress when confronted with a physical or psychologic stressor.

Stress ulcer acute peptic ulcer that occurs in association with various other pathologic conditions, including burns, cor pulmonale, intracranial lesions, and surgical operations.

Stridor a harsh, shrill sound produced during inhalation or exhalation that indicates obstruction of the trachea or larynx.

Struvite stone a urinary stone, also called an infection stone, that develops when a urinary tract infection neutralizes the urine, enabling the resident bacteria to grow more rapidly and facilitate creation of a jagged ammoniomagnesium phosphate stone.

Subdural hematoma collection of blood between the inner surface of the dura mater and the surface of the brain caused by rupture of bridging veins of the subdural region.

Subglottic stenosis narrowing of the airway below the larynx caused by a congenital anomaly or acquired narrowing secondary to injury, possibly resulting in respiratory distress, cyanotic episodes, or recurrent lung infections.

Sudden infant death syndrome (SIDS) a syndrome, also known as crib death, that is characterized by the sudden, unexpected, and unexplained death of an apparently healthy infant less than 1 year of age.

Suffocation failure of oxygen to reach the blood because of a lack of oxygen in the environment or blockage of external airways.

Syndactyly two or more fused or webbed digits.

Syndenham chorea (St. Vitus dance) a nervous condition most commonly occurring in children or in fetuses during pregnancy that is associated with rheumatic fever and causes rapid, uncoordinated jerky, involuntary movements of the body, particularly the face, feet, and hands.

Syndrome of inappropriate secretion of ADH (SIADH) a condition in which the release of ADH is elevated relative to serum sodium levels, resulting in increased water reabsorption by the kidneys.

Syphilis a chronic infectious disease that is transmitted by direct contact, usually in sexual intercourse, or passed from mother to child in utero, and progresses through three stages characterized by chancres, ulcerous skin eruptions, and systemic infection that leads to damage to the cardiovascular and nervous systems.

Systole the period of time during which the chambers of the heart contract and force blood out of the chambers.

Systolic heart failure a condition in which the heart muscle contracts so weakly that not enough oxygenated blood is pumped throughout the body.

Tamponade blockage or compression of a body part such as heart compression caused by collection of blood or fluid.

Tay-Sachs disease an autosomal recessive disorder in which an enzyme deficiency leads to the accumulation of gangliosides in the brain and nerve tissue, resulting in mental retardation, convulsions, blindness, and premature death.

Telomere the ends of a chromosome that are shortened during each cycle of DNA replication; this shortening of the telomere is proposed to be a component of cellular aging because it deletes vital genetic information over time.

Tension headache headache caused by emotional strain or overwork that tends to be focused in the occipital region and can be continuous for months.

Termination (nonsense) codon a codon, also known as a stop codon, that signals the end of translation.

Tertiary syphilis the most severe stage of syphilis, which can begin as early as 1 year after the initial infection but can take up to 10 years to manifest and is characterized by gummas—soft, tumor-like growths found in the skin and mucous membranes and often in the skeleton—joint deformity, neurosyphilis, and cardiovascular syphilis.

Tetanus sustained muscle contraction resulting from maximal stimulation of a motor unit.

Tetralogy of Fallot a congenital condition that is characterized by four malformations including ventricular septal defect, misplacement of the origin of the aorta, narrowing of the pulmonary artery, and enlargement of the right ventricle.

Thalassemia a potentially fatal genetic disorder in which hemoglobin molecules are abnormal, resulting in severe anemia, enlarged heart, liver, and spleen, and skeletal deformation.

Therapeutic index a ratio of the median lethal dose to the median effective dose for a drug.

Third-degree burn a burn in which the skin and nerve endings die and the skin becomes charred and a scab forms over the burnt region.

Thrombin time a diagnostic test that measures the rate of fibrinogen to fibrin conversion when thrombin has been introduced.

Thromboangiitis obliterans (Buerger disease) inflammation of the medium-sized arteries and veins because of thrombotic occlusion, resulting in ischemia and gangrene.

Thrombocythemia a chronic disorder of sustained megakaryocyte proliferation that increases the number of circulating platelets and results in megakaryocytic hyperplasia, splenomegaly, and complications by hemorrhagic and thrombotic episodes.

Thrombocytopenia a decrease in the number of platelets in the blood is severely decreased.

Thrombophilia abnormal coagulation system and increased risk for thrombosis.

Thrombophlebitis a condition in which veins become inflamed because of a blood clot or thrombus secondary to prolonged sitting or clotting disorders.

Thrombotic stroke (cerebral thrombosis) stroke symptoms caused by thrombosis that is typically secondary to atherosclerosis.

Thrombotic thrombocytopenic purpura (TTP) altered blood coagulation caused by an enzymatic deficiency that is characterized by a reduced number of platelets in the blood, the formation of blood clots in tissue arterioles and capillaries, and neurologic damage.

Thrombus a fibrinous blood clot formed in a vessel or in a chamber of the heart that remains attached at its site of origin.

Thrush a yeast infection of the mouth and throat that presents as creamy white curd-like patches on the tongue, inside the mouth, and on the back of the throat and that is commonly associated with yeast infection of the esophagus.

Thyrotoxicosis excessive concentrations of thyroid hormones in the body that are marked by increased metabolic rate, heat intolerance, goiter, reproductive disorders, excessive sweating, and other alterations in systemic function.

Tinea infection one of a group of fungal skin infections that include athlete's foot, folliculitis, jock itch, ringworm, and pityriasis versicolor.

Tissue remodeling tissue changes or remodels, protein enzyme systems involved in remodeling include matrix-degrading plasminogen activators (PAs) and matrix metalloproteinases (MMPs) cause destruction and remodeling in a variety

of normal and pathologic states including ovulation, angiogenesis, implantation, tumor invasion and inflammatory diseases like rheumatoid arthritis.

Toll-like receptor (TLR) receptors expressed on the surface of many cells that interact with many pathogens to increase resistance and that bridge innate resistance and acquired immune response through cytokine production.

Toxic epidermal necrolysis (TEN) a rare adverse reaction to certain drugs in which a large portion of the skin becomes intensely red, may develop blisters, and peels off.

Tracheoesophageal fistula (TEF) a connection formed between the esophagus and the trachea because of esophageal atresia or laryngectomy.

Tracheomalacia a congenital or acquired condition characterized by weakness of the tracheal support cartilage, resulting in tracheal collapse when increased airflow is needed.

Transferrin a protein that is loaded with iron and transports iron into the cell by binding a transferring surface receptor and entering the cell where it releases iron ions.

Transposition of the great arteries (TGA) the aorta arises from the right ventricle and the pulmonary artery arises from the left ventricle.

Traumatic aneurysm aneurysm caused by weakening of arterial walls, penetrating missile, or after neurosurgery or neuroimaging following an injury.

Trichomoniasis a sexually transmitted bacterial infection of the urethra in males and vagina in females that can cause urinary tract infection and a painful, malodorous vaginitis in women and urethral and bladder infection in males.

Truncus arteriosus a congenital defect in which a large great vessel arises from a ventricular septal defect and does not divide into the aorta and pulmonary artery, resulting in one vessel carrying blood both to the body and to the lungs.

TSH deficiency a condition characterized by decreased or absent production of thyroid stimulating hormone, resulting in a decline in thyroid hormone and subsequent symptoms such as fatigue, cold intolerance, weakness, depression, muscle aches, weight gain, and constipation.

Tuberculosis (TB) an infectious disease of humans caused by *Mycobacterium tuberculosis* that results in the formation of tubercles on the lungs and other tissues of the body.

Tuberculosis (TB) meningitis severe form of bacterial meningitis that usually originates from a *Mycobacterium tuberculosis* infection in the lungs.

Tuberous sclerosis complex (TSC) an inherited disease caused by mutation of the hamartin and tuberin genes and resulting in malformation of the brain, retina, and viscera and the development of epileptic seizures, mental retardation, and skin nodules of the face.

Tubulointerstitial fibrosis accumulated extracellular matrix proteins, indicating chronic renal disease, normal aging of the kidney, or chronic allograft nephropathy.

Tumor a growth of tissue caused by the uncontrolled replication of cells.

Tumor marker a biochemical marker that is sensitive to specific types of tumors and is used to screen, diagnose, assess prognosis and treatment, and monitor recurrence.

Tumor protein 53 (p53) a transcription factor that inhibits the development of cancer by opposing oncogene action and promoting DNA repair.

Tumor-suppressor gene a gene whose protein product terminates cell proliferation, thereby inhibiting tumor formation.

Type 1 diabetes mellitus a disorder of carbohydrate metabolism characterized by a decrease in insulin production, resulting in hyperglycemia, ketoacidosis and eventually renal failure and coronary artery disease.

Type 2 diabetes mellitus a condition of glucose intolerance that normally appears first in adulthood and is exacerbated by obesity and an inactive lifestyle.

Type I fibers slow twitch fibers that are used primarily during aerobic metabolism and function during activities that require high endurance.

Type 1 (IgE-mediated) hypersensitivity reaction a rapid response to subsequent exposure to an allergen in which IgE molecules are cross-linked on mast cells, basophils and eosinophils, resulting in release of several chemical mediators.

Type II (tissue-specific) hypersensitivity reaction a condition in which antibodies are formed against cell or matrix antigens in a specific tissue, leading to tissue damage by opsonization of cells, activation of the complement system, recruitment of neutrophils and macrophages, or binding to normal cellular receptors and altering function.

Type III (immune complex-mediated) hypersensitivity reaction a process where self or foreign antigens complexed with antibodies are filtered out of the circulation in the small vessels to cause tissue damage.

Type IV (cell-mediated) hypersensitivity reaction a disease process caused by T-cell–induced delayed-type hypersensitivity or direct killing of the target cells by cytokines and macrophages in the inflammatory response.

Ulcerative colitis chronically inflamed and ulcerated mucosal and submucosal lining of the large intestine, resulting in abdominal pain, diarrhea, and rectal bleeding.

Ultrafiltration the process of filtering blood across a barrier between the capillary of the glomerulus and the Bowman capsule of the nephron at a rate that is determined by hydrostatic and oncotic pressures.

Unstable angina a condition in which unprovoked ischemic attacks occur at unpredictable frequencies and may increase in severity.

Upper airway obstruction obstruction at sites of anatomic narrowing such as the hypopharynx at the base of the tongue and the false and true vocal cords at the laryngeal opening.

Up-regulation the process by which a cell increases the number of receptors for a given ligand such as hormone or neurotransmitter to improve sensitivity in response to low hormone concentration.

Urethritis inflammation of the urethra that is usually caused by a sexually transmitted microorganism and results in painful urination.

Uric acid stone elevated uric acid levels in urine, preventing the uric acid from dissolving, causing uric acid stones to form.

Urinary tract infection an infection of the urinary tract that may occur anywhere from the kidneys to the urethra and is much more common in females because of the short distance between the urethra and the anus.

Urticaria (hives) allergic reaction in which capillaries become dilated and permeability increases, causing localized edema.

Uterine prolapse descent or herniation of the uterus into or beyond the vagina because of weakness of the pelvic musculature, ligaments, and fascia or obstetric trauma and lacerations sustained during labor and delivery.

Uterine sarcoma cancer of the muscle and supporting tissues of the uterus, usually developing from cells of the uterine lining.

Vacuolar myelopathy HIV-induced loss of myelin and spongy degeneration of the spinal cord that may cause spastic paraparesis, sensory ataxia in lower limbs, and unsteady gait.

Vaginismus a form of sexual dysfunction that is caused by a psychologic disorder or vaginal inflammation in which the muscles at the entrance to vagina contract and prevent sexual intercourse.

Vaginitis infection of the vagina usually caused by a fungus that may cause itching or burning and a discharge.

Valvular regurgitation a condition in which one or more of the heart's valves does not close properly causing blood to leak in the wrong direction.

Valvular stenosis one or more of the heart valves becomes narrow, stiff, thickened, fused, or blocked and blood does not flow through it smoothly.

Varicocele a painful condition in which the veins in the scrotum that develop in the spermatic cord enlarge, and if the valves that regulate blood flow from these veins become dysfunctional, blood does not leave the testis, thereby causing swelling in the veins above and behind the testis.

Vasogenic edema an accumulation of fluid in the cerebrum that is typically caused by an increase in capillary endothelial cell permeability and usually occurs near a tumor.

Vasogenic shock a form of shock caused by dilation of the blood vessels, usually a result of medication.

Vasomotor flush a sudden, brief sensation of heat, typically occurring over the entire body that is caused by a transient dilation of the blood vessels of the skin and possibly alterations in the temperature-regulating center of the hypothalamus secondary to decreased estrogen levels.

Vasoocclusive crisis (thrombotic crisis) obstruction of the microcirculation by sickled red blood cells, resulting in ischemic injury to the organ supplied in addition to pain and possibly irreversible organ damage.

Vegetative state transition of severely brain damaged patients from a coma to wakefulness without awareness; if this condition lasts for four weeks it is termed persistent vegetative state and after one year it is called permanent vegetative state.

Venous angioma abnormal veins, usually near the ventricular wall, that form as a congenital anomaly.

Venous stasis ulcer a condition affecting the lower leg in which leaky valves, obstructions, or regurgitation in veins impairs blood flow back to the heart, resulting in pooling of blood in the lower leg and subsequent tissue damage.

Ventricular septal defect (VSD) a congenital malformation in which the wall between the left and right ventricles has a hole that allows blood to travel between the left and right ventricles, potentially leading to congestive heart failure.

Vesicoureteral reflux (VUR) reflux of urine from the bladder into the ureter.

Volatile a substance such as carbonic acid that can evaporate rapidly.

Volkmann ischemic contracture a condition in which the distal humerus is fractured and disrupts the radial artery and median nerve, resulting in necrosis of the extensor muscles, contracture of elbow flexion, and claw hand.

von Willebrand disease an inherited disease in which the von Willebrand factor proteins that are made in the blood vessel walls and function to control platelet activity are abnormal or absent, resulting in a tendency to hemorrhage.

Wart (verruca) an outgrowth of the skin caused by a virus (human papilloma virus) that is easily transmitted by close contact and may persist for years.

Wet gangrene liquefactive necrosis resulting from neutrophil invasion usually occurring in internal organs.

Wheal and flare reaction a condition caused by an allergic reaction in which the area of skin around the site of antigen contact becomes flattened and red with fluid-filled blisters.

Wilson disease a genetic disease in which the ability to metabolize copper is impaired, resulting in an accumulation of copper deposits in organs such as the brain, liver, and kidneys and subsequent organ dysfunction and failure.

Window period a period during which a virus is replicating inside an organism and the organism may be infectious but the virus and/or antibodies to the virus are undetectable.

X-linked inheritance genetic conditions caused by genes located on sex chromosomes also termed sex linked.

INDEX

13q syndrome, and associated childhood cancers, 438
47 XYY karyotype, 141–142

A

A bands, of myocardial muscle, 1106
a wave, 1096
Aβ fibers, 486
ABCDE rule, 1670–1671
Abdominal angina, 1477
Abdominal compartment syndrome, 1497b
Abdominal pain, 1455–1456
  parietal, 1455
  referred, 1456
  visceral, 1455
Abducens nerve (CN VI), 466f
  origins, course, functions, and testing of, 468t
Aberrant conduction, 1199t–1200t
Aberrant methylation, epigenetic, 403. *See also* Epigenetic silencing.
Abnormal breathing patterns, 1268
Abnormal skeletal remodeling, 1618–1620
  in osteogenesis imperfecta, 1618–1619
  in rickets, 1625
  in scoliosis, 1625
Abnormal sputum, 1267
Abnormal uterine bleeding, 822–823, 823t
ABO alloimmunization, maternal hypersensitivity in, 271
ABO blood groups, 272, 273f
ABO transfusion reactions, 272
Abrasion, 64, 64f
Abscess(es), 205
  brain and spinal cord, 624
  Brodie, 1588
  peritonsillar, 1316
  pulmonary, 1294
  retropharyngeal, 1316
Abscess formation, 1294
Absolute polycythemia, 1009
Absolute refractory period, 33
Absorption atelectasis, 1275
Acanthosis nigricans,
  paraneoplastic, 389t
Accelerated junctional rhythm, 1197t–1198t
Accelerated ventricular rhythm, 1197t–1198t
Accessory muscles, of inspiration, 1252
Accessory organs of digestion, 1437–1444, 1437f. *See also* Exocrine pancreas; Gallbladder; Liver.
  cancer of, 1503
  disorders of, 1482

Accidental hyperthermia, 500
Accidental hypothermia, 501
  complications of rewarming in, 502t
Accidental injuries, and temperature regulation disorders, 502
Accommodative visual dysfunction, 511
Accumulative injuries, 75
Acetaminophen, and acute liver failure, 1491b
Acetazolamide, diuretic action of, 1359t
Acetylcholine, 447–448
  in digestive enzymatic stimulation, 1425t, 1444
  functions of, 448t–449t
  release of, in autonomic nervous transmission, 467–469
Achalasia, 1457
Achondroplasia, pedigree chart for, 147f
Acid-base balance
  cellular, 114–117
    buffering systems in, 115
    normal values in, 1262t
Acid-base imbalance, 117, 118f
  in chronic kidney disease, 1392t, 1393–1394, 1394t
Acid maltase deficiency, 1610–1611
Acidemia, 117
  and pulmonary artery constriction, 1261
Acidosis, 117. *See also* Metabolic acidosis; Respiratory acidosis.
  in rewarming in accidental hypothermia, 502t
Acids, body, 114
Acinus, 1244, 1247
Acne, inflammatory and noninflammatory, 1680–1681
Acne conglobata, 1681
Acne pustules, 1648t–1653t
Acne rosacea, 1659, 1659f
Acne vulgaris, 1659, 1680–1681
Acoustic nerve. *See* Vestibulocochlear nerve.
Acoustic neuroma, 617, 617f
Acquired hypercoagulability, 1056–1059
Acquired immune deficiencies, 275, 284–286. *See also* Secondary immune deficiencies.
Acquired immunity. *See* Immune response (adaptive immunity).
Acquired immunodeficiency syndrome (AIDS), 318–325
  and associated cancers, 378t
  cardiac complications in, 1189
  central nervous system involvement in, 324–325

Acquired immunodeficiency syndrome (AIDS) *(Continued)*
  clinical manifestations of, 321–322, 324f
  currently accepted definition of, 322
  major immunologic damage in, 319
  neurologic complications in, 626–630, 627b
  opportunistic infections and neoplasms characteristic of, 323b, 629
  pathogenesis of, 319–321
Acquired sideroblastic anemia, 998
Acrania, 672
Acromegaly, 733, 734f
ACTH. *See* Adrenocorticotropic hormone.
Actin, 1559, 1560t
  myocardial, 1106, 1106f
Actin filament(s), 9–10
Actinic keratosis, 1668–1669, 1669f
Action potential(s), 32–33
  cardiac, 1099
  skeletal muscle fiber, 1561
Activated partial thromboplastin time (aPTT), 1080
Active acquired immunity, 220
Active immunity, 220
Active transport, 25–26, 29
  sodium-potassium pump and, 29–30, 29f
Activin, 794
Acute alcoholic myopathy, 1612
Acute alcoholism, 60
Acute bacterial conjunctivitis, 506–507
Acute brain failure, 548
Acute bronchitis, 1294
Acute cerebral failure, 548
Acute chest syndrome, in sickle cell disease, 1074
Acute confusional states, 548
  clinical manifestations of, 551
  evaluation and treatment of, 551–553, 552t
  pathophysiology of, 548–551
Acute coronary syndrome(s), 1160, 1169–1170
  pathophysiology of, 1169–1170, 1170f. *See also* Myocardial infarction; Unstable angina.
Acute cough, 1266–1267
Acute cystitis, 1374–1375
Acute diarrhea, in children, 1530
Acute encephalopathies, 681
  drug induced, 682
  meningitis in, 682
  Reye syndrome in, 681
  viral meningitis in, 684

Acute epiglottitis, 1315t, 1317
Acute gouty arthritis, 1605
Acute graft rejection, 274, 274f
Acute hemorrhage, clinical manifestations of, 1003, 1003t
Acute hemorrhagic pancreatitis, 1496, 1496f
Acute hydrocephalus, 560
Acute inflammatory demyelinating polyneuropathy, 636, 637t
Acute kidney injury, 1386, 1386t
  classification of, 1386t
  clinical manifestations of, 1387–1388
  evaluation and treatment of, 1388–1389
  nutrition in, 1396b
  oliguria in, mechanisms of, 1387, 1388f
  pathophysiology of, 1386–1387
  prevention of, 1389
Acute leukemia(s), 1019, 1021–1022
  clinical manifestations of, 1024
  evaluation and treatment of, 1024–1025
  immunophenotypes of, 1023, 1024t
  incidence and prevalence of, 1021–1022
  pathophysiology of, 1022–1024
  survival rate in, 1025
Acute liver failure, acetaminophen and, 1491b
Acute lymphoblastic leukemia. *See* Acute lymphocytic leukemia.
Acute lymphocytic leukemia (ALL), 1021–1022
  cellular morphology in, 1029f
  in children, 1083–1084
  chromosomal translocation frequencies in, 1026f
  immunophenotypes of, 1023, 1024t
Acute mesenteric ischemia, 1477
Acute motor and sensory axonal neuropathy, 636, 637t
Acute motor axonal neuropathy, 636, 637t
Acute myelocytic leukemia. *See* Acute myelogenous leukemia(s).
Acute myelogenous leukemia(s) (AML), 365–366, 1021–1022
  cellular morphology in, 1029f
  in children, 1083–1084
  classification of, 1027b
  pathophysiology of, 1023–1024
Acute myeloid leukemia. *See* Acute myelogenous leukemia(s).
Acute orthostatic hypotension, 1157
Acute otitis media, 515

Page numbers followed by f, t, or b indicate figures, tables, or boxes, respectively. Syndromes and disorders appear in boldface.

Acute pain, 490–491
  chronic pain and, comparison of, 491t
  classifications of, 491
Acute pancreatitis, 1496
  clinical manifestations of, 1496–1497
  evaluation and treatment of, 1497
  pathophysiology of, 1496, 1496f
Acute pericarditis, 1176–1177, 1177f
Acute phase inflammation, chemical mediators of, 203f
Acute phase reactants, 206, 206t
Acute phase response, 499f
Acute Physiology and Chronic Health Evaluation II, III, 1713
Acute postinfectious glomerulonephritis, 1380–1382
  clinical manifestations of, 1380–1381
  pathophysiology of, 1381t
  treatment of, 1381–1382
Acute poststreptococcal glomerulonephritis, 1372–1373
Acute pyelonephritis, 1377
  in children, 1411–1412
  clinical manifestations of, 1377
  evaluation and treatment of, 1377
  pathophysiology of, 1377
Acute renal failure. *See* Acute kidney injury.
Acute respiratory distress syndrome (ARDS), 1279–1280
  in children, 1334
    clinical manifestations of, 1335
    evaluation and treatment of, 1335–1336
    fibroproliferative phase of, 1335
    inflammatory (exudative) phase of, 1334–1335
    pathophysiology of, 1334–1335, 1335f
  clinical manifestations of, 1281
  evaluation and treatment of, 1281–1284
  pathogenesis of, 1280–1281, 1280f–1281f
Acute respiratory failure, 1271
Acute tracheitis, 1315t
Acute tubular necrosis, 1387
  nephrotoxins causing, 1387
Acute urethral syndrome, 936
Aδ fibers (nociceptors), 483, 483f
ADAMTS13 plasma metalloprotease, 1046–1047, 1049–1050
Adaptive changes, in cellular biology, 47–50, 47f
Adaptive immunity. *See* Immune response (adaptive immunity).
Addison disease, 770
  clinical manifestations of, 770–771, 771t
  evaluation and treatment of, 771–772
  idiopathic, 770
  pathophysiology of, 770, 771t
Adenine, 129
Adenocarcinoma(s), 364t
  bronchogenic, 1301, 1302t
  definition of, 361
Adenocystic tumors, 1304

Adenohypophysis. *See* Anterior pituitary.
Adenomatous polyposal cancer, familial, 375–377, 377f
Adenomatous polyposis coli (*APC*) gene, 1500
Adenomatous polyps, of colon, 1500, 1501f
Adenomyosis, 839
Adenosine deaminase deficiency, 280
Adenosine triphosphate (ATP), in cellular metabolism, 22–23
S-Adenosyl-L-methionine (SAMe), 60–61
Adenovirus, 314t
ADH. *See* Antidiuretic hormone.
Adhesion molecules, 198–199
Adipokines, 750
  and coronary artery disease, 1165
Adiponectin, 1478b
  decreased plasma, in obesity, 1479
Adipose tissue, hormones and adipokines secreted by, 713–714, 714b, 1478b
Adjuvant chemotherapy, 388
Adjuvants, 222
Adopted children, studies of environmental factors in disease, 170–171
Adrenal(s), 715–720, 716f
  aging and effects on, 722
Adrenal cortex, 716–718, 716f
  aldosterone secretion by, 717–718
  glucocorticoid secretion by, 716–717
  mineralocorticoid secretion by, 717–718
  sex steroids secreted by, 718
Adrenal cortical disorders, 765
  androgen and estrogen hypersecretion in, 771–772
  hyperfunctional, 765. *See also* Cushing disease; Hyperaldosteronism.
  hypofunctional, 770. *See also* Addison disease.
Adrenal medulla, 716, 716f, 719–720
  catecholamine synthesis by, 719, 720f
  epinephrine release by, 719
Adrenal medullary hyperfunction, 772
Adrenal medullary hypofunction, 772
Adrenaline. *See* Norepinephrine.
Adrenarche, 784
Adrenergic receptor function, cardiac, 1105
Adrenergic receptors, four types of, 1105
Adrenergic thermogenesis, 496
Adrenergic transmission, 467–469
  neuroreceptors in, 472t
Adrenocortical hyperfunction, 765. *See also* Cushing disease; Hyperaldosteronism.
Adrenocortical hypofunction, 770. *See also* Addison disease.
Adrenocorticotropic hormone (ACTH), 707, 1706–1707
  physiologic effects of, 704f, 708t, 718b
  as tumor marker, 368t

Adrenocorticotropic hormone (ACTH) deficiency, 731–732
Adrenocorticotropic hormone (ACTH) secretion, 707
  hypothalamic regulation of, 717
  stimulation of adrenal cortisol by, 717
  target cells of, 704f, 708t
Adrenomedullin (ADM), cardiovascular effects of, 1128
Adult growth hormone deficiency syndrome, 732
Adult stem cells, 363–365
Advanced glycosylation end product, 759
Adventitia, 1113
Affective flattening, 651
Affective states, 652
Afferent loop obstruction, 1470
Afferent lymphatic vessels, 1133
Afferent (sensory) neurons, 444, 457, 567f
Afferent (ascending) pathways, 442–443
Affinity maturation, 242–243
Afterload, 1109
  cardiac output and, 1111
Agammaglobulinemia, 278
  and associated childhood cancer, 438t
Age-dependent penetrance, 148
Age-related macular degeneration, 510–511
Ageusia, 516
Agglutination, 244
  erythrocyte, in transfusion reaction, 273f
Aggrecan, 1600–1601
Aging, 86
  biology of, emerging focus on, 87b–88b
  body fluid distribution and, 97
  cancer as disease of, 367–368, 368f
  cardiovascular system in, 1136–1140
  cellular, 88–89
  endocrine system in, 720–725
    specific effects of, 721–725
  extracellular changes in, 88
  fever response in, 500
  frailty in, 90
  gastrointestinal tract in, 1447–1451
  hearing alterations in, 514–516, 514t
  hematologic system in, 982–987
  immune response depression in, 251, 284–285
  innate immunity in, 213
  musculoskeletal system in, 1564–1566
  nervous system changes in, 471–474
    cellular, 471–474
    functional, 474
    structural, 471–474
  olfaction and taste in, 516
  osteoporosis in, 1582, 1583f
  pain perception in, 495–496
  proprioceptive alterations in, 517
  pulmonary system in, 1263–1265
  renal function in, 1362–1364
  reproductive system changes in, 807–814

Aging (*Continued*)
  skin integrity in, 1646–1655
  sleep patterns in, 504–506
  stress and, 337, 355
  temperature regulation in, 498–502
  theories and mechanisms of, 87, 88t
  tissue and systemic, 86, 89–90
  vision in, 508–514, 509t
Agnosia, 543–544, 546
  types of, 548t
Agonal rhythm, 1197t–1198t
Agonist, in muscle movement, 1562–1563
Agoraphobia, 659
Agranulocytes, 956–957
Agranulocytosis, 1015
AIDS (acquired immunodeficiency syndrome), 318–325
  and associated cancers, 378t
  cardiac complications in, 1189
  central nervous system involvement in, 324–325
  clinical manifestations of, 321–322, 324f
  currently accepted definition of, 322
  major immunologic damage in, 319
  neurologic complications in, 626–630, 627b
  opportunistic infections and neoplasms characteristic of, 323b, 629
  pathogenesis of, 319–321
AIDS pandemic, 297t, 318
Air embolism, 1147–1148
Air pollutants, in cancer epidemiology, 426–431
Airway(s)
  adult and pediatric, 1747f
  conducting, 1242–1244, 1243f
  lower, 1244–1247, 1246f. *See also* Gas exchange, pulmonary.
  upper, 1242–1243, 1243f, 1245f
Airway maintenance, in burn injury in children, 1746–1747, 1747f
Airway obstruction, caused by obstructive pulmonary disease, 1282, 1282f
Airway resistance, 1253–1254
Akathisia, 568t–569t
Akinesia, 571
Akinetic mutism, 535
Alar plate, 666
Alarm stage, of general adaptation syndrome, 338
Albinism, 78–79
Albumin, 953
Alcoholic cirrhosis, 1492, 1492t
Alcoholic liver disease, 1491–1492
  clinical manifestations of, 1492–1493
  evaluation and treatment of, 1493–1495
  pathophysiology of, 1492, 1493f
Alcoholism
  in cancer epidemiology, 415–416
  cellular injury in, 59–61
  chronic, 60–61
  congenital heart defects associated with, 1214t
  genes and environmental interaction in, 179

Aldose reductase, 758
Aldosterone, 101, 717–718
  cardiovascular effects of, 1127–1128
  metabolism of, 718
  physiologic effects of, on kidney epithelium, 718
  in sodium-potassium pump regulation, 107, 717
  synthesis and secretion of, in adrenal cortex, 717–718, 719f
Aldosteronism
  in cardiovascular and renal toxicity, 769b
  primary, 768
    pathophysiology of, 768, 769f
  secondary, 768, 768t
    pathophysiology of, 769
Alendronate, and postmenopausal osteoporosis, 1584
Algor mortis, 90
Alimentary canal, 1421–1437. *See also* Gastrointestinal tract.
Alkalemia, 117
Alkaline phosphatase, serum, in bone tumor diagnosis, 1589–1590
Alkaline reflux gastritis, 1469–1470
Alkalosis, 117. *See also* Metabolic alkalosis; Respiratory alkalosis.
Allele(s), 143–145
  dominant and recessive, 145
  expression of, 145
  homozygous and heterozygous, 145
  penetrance and expressivity of, 148–149
  recombinant, 156, 156f
Allergen(s), 264, 266t
  desensitization to, 267
  sensitization to, 258
Allergic alveolitis, 267, 1278
Allergic conjunctivitis, 507
Allergic contact dermatitis, 1655–1656, 1655f
Allergic dermatitis, 1656
Allergic purpura, 1083
Allergic vasculitis, 1666
Allergy, 256, 257t, 264–265
  genetic predisposition to, 265
  tests of IgE-mediated, 265–267
  type I, 258–259, 259t
    allergy and symptoms associated with, 265–267, 266f, 266t
    mechanism of, 259, 260f
    tests of, 265–267
  type II, 258–261, 259t
    allergy and symptoms associated with, 266t, 267
    mechanisms of, 260, 262f
  type III, 258, 259t, 261–264, 263f
    allergy and symptoms associated with, 266t, 267
  type IV, 258, 259t, 264, 264f
    allergy and symptoms associated with, 266t, 267
Allodynia, 488
Alloimmune disorders
  graft rejection in, 274–275
  transfusion reactions in, 272–274
Alloimmune neutropenia, maternal hypersensitivity in, 271

Alloimmunity, 256–258, 257t, 270–271
  definition of, 270
  transient neonatal, 270–271
Alogia, 651
Alopecia, 1673–1674
  resulting from cancer therapy, 391–392
Alopecia areata, 1674
Alpha (α)-adrenergic receptors, 469–470, 1105
  cardiac, 1105
  in central stress response, 340
  physiologic actions of, 342t, 471f, 469–470
  specific tissues with, and physiologic actions of neurotransmitters, 472t
Alpha-1 (α-1) antitrypsin, destructive enzyme neutralization by, 201
Alpha-1 (α-1) antitrypsin deficiency
  gene and lifestyle interaction, 171b
  pulmonary effects of, 201, 1288–1289
Alpha cells, of pancreas, 714
  glucagon production in, 752
Alpha-fetoprotein (AFP), 367, 368t
Alpha (α) globulins, 953–954
Alpha (α) glycoprotein, 1545
Alpha granules, of platelets, 976
Alpha motor neurons. *See* Lower motor neuron(s).
Alpha-thalassemia, 1076–1077
  four forms of, 1077
Alpha-thalassemia major, 1077
Alpha-thalassemia minor, 1077
Alpha-trait thalassemia, 1077
Altered cellular biology, 46
  adaptive changes in, 47–50, 47f
  in aging, 86. *See also* Aging.
  in cancer and cell proliferation, 360–395. *See also* Cancer; Cancer epidemiology.
  cell death and, 81–90
  cell injuries and, 50–76. *See also* Cellular injury.
  cellular environment in, 96–125. *See also* Cellular environment.
  genetic and environmental interaction in, 164–182. *See also* Environmental factors; Multifactorial disorder(s).
  genetics in, 126–163. *See also* Genetic disorders; Genetics.
  infections and infectious disease in, 293–335. *See also* Infection(s); Infectious disease(s).
  inflammatory and immune response alterations in, 256-202. *See also* Allergy; Alloimmune disorders; Autoimmune disorders; Primary immune deficiencies; Secondary immune deficiencies.
  key terms of, 92b–93b
  manifestations of, 76–81
    systemic, 81, 81t
  references on, 93

Altered cellular biology (*Continued*)
  in shock, 1697
    glucose metabolic impairment in, 1697–1699
    oxygen metabolic impairment in, 1697
  in somatic death, 90
  stress and, 336–359. *See also* Stress.
  summary review of, 91b–92b
  tissue injury and, 62–69. *See also* Tissue injury.
Alternative pathway, of complement cascade activation, 188–189, 190f
Aluminum, and effect on bone tissue physiology, 1580b
Alveolar cells, types of, 1244, 1253b
Alveolar dead space, 1270
Alveolar ducts, 1244
Alveolar macrophage(s), 1247, 1291
Alveolar sacs, 1243f
Alveolar surface tension, 1252–1253
Alveolar ventilation, 1249, 1252
Alveoli, pulmonary, 1244, 1246f–1247f
  in aging, 1263
  immune cells of, 1247
  prenatal development of, 1310–1311, 1311f
Alveolitis, allergic, 1278
Alveolocapillary barrier, 1270–1271
Alveolocapillary membrane, 1247, 1248f
  oxygen diffusion across, 1257–1258
  surfactant and surface tension at, 1252–1253
Alzheimer disease, 553–554
  clinical manifestations of, 556, 556f
  diet and, 556b
  differential diagnosis of, 554t
  evaluation and treatment of, 556–557
  genetic-environmental interaction in, 178–179
  genetic-molecular basis of, 526t–527t, 553t
  pathophysiology of, 554–556, 555f
    altered cerebral blood flow in, 555f
    histologic changes in, 555f
  progression of, 556t
  risk factors for, 554, 555f
Amblyopia, 509
Ambulatory blood pressure monitoring, in children, 1236–1237, 1237b
Amebiasis, sexually transmitted, 946
Amenorrhea, 820
  evaluation and treatment of, 820–821, 821f
  pathophysiology of, 820
  primary, 820
Amine hormones, 697t
  receptors for, and mechanism of action, 700t
Amino acid(s), 129
Amino acid metabolism disorders, 677–678
Amino acid precursors
  in excitatory neurotransmission, 488
  neurologic functions of, 448t–449t

Amino acid transport systems, 30t
Ammonia, as renal buffer, 117, 117f
Amnesia, anterograde and retrograde, 543
Amnesic dysphasia, 549t–550t
Amniotic fluid embolism, 1148
Amoeboid protozoa, 310, 310t
AMPA/kinate receptors, 488
Amphiarthrosis, 1549
Amphipathic molecule, 11
Amphiregulin, 881–882
Ampulla of Vater, 1439, 1443
Amusia, 548t
Amygdala, 452–453
Amylin, 714, 752
Amyloid-beta (Aβ) peptide, 554
Amyotrophic lateral sclerosis (ALS), 633–634
  clinical manifestations of, 634
  evaluation and treatment of, 634–635
  pathophysiology of, 634
Amyotrophies, 567–568
Anabolism, 21
Anaerobic glycolysis, 24
Anaerobic metabolism, in shock, 1697
Anal gonococcal infection, 926
Anal herpes lesions, in AIDS, 324f
Anal sphincters, internal and external, 1435–1436
Anamnestic immune response, 240–241. *See also* Secondary immune response.
Anaphase, 35
Anaphylactic shock, 1702–1703, 1728
  pathophysiology of, 1702, 1703f, 1728b, 1729
Anaphylatoxins, 189
Anaphylaxis, 259
Anaplasia, 361–363, 363f, 365f
Anastomose, 208–210
Anchorage independency, of cancer cells, 362
Androcentric alopecia, 1673–1674
Androgen hypersecretion, adrenal, 771–772
Androgens
  adiposity and, 409
  physiologic effects of, 352
    in females, 792
  secreted by adrenal cortex, 718
Anemia(s), 989
  cancer associated, 391
  in children, 1065
  classification of
    etiologic (pathologic), 989, 990b
    morphologic, 991t
  clinical manifestations of, 989–993, 993f
  definition of, 989
  heart failure in, 1195
  hemodynamic alterations in, 990
  macrocytic-normochromic, 990–993
  microcytic-hypochromic, 995–996
  normocytic-normochromic, 1000–1002
  paraneoplastic, 389t
  in postgastrectomy syndromes, 1470
  progression of, 993f
  secondary to drug effects, 1001t

Anemia of chronic disease,
1007–1008
clinical manifestations of, 1008
evaluation and treatment of, 1008
laboratory findings in, 999t
pathophysiology of, 1008, 1009f
Anemia of infectious disease, of
newborn, 1068
Anencephaly, 168b, 167, 169f, 669
Anesthesia, and secondary immune
deficiencies, 286
Aneuploid cell, 136–137
Aneuploidy, 136–142
autosomal, 137–138
sex chromosome, 138–142
Aneurysm(s), 1144–1147, 1145f
abdominal aortic atherosclerotic,
1145f
apical, 1145f
clinical manifestations of, 1146
evaluation and treatment of, 1146
intracranial, 606
types of, 1146, 1146f
Aneurysmal bone cyst, 1637
Angelman syndrome, 150,
526t–527t
Angina
Prinzmetal, 1165–1166
stable, 1165–1166
unstable, 1169–1170
Angioedema, in children, 1318
Angiogenesis, 1097
tumor induced, 369, 372f
Angiogenesis factors
in tumor growth, 369
in wound healing, 210
Angiography
cerebral, 476
coronary, 1135
Angioma, 612t
Angiotensin-converting enzyme
(ACE), 1352
Angiotensin I, 101–102
cardiovascular effects of,
1125–1126
organs affected by, 1129f
Angiotensin II, 101–102, 1352
aldosterone synthesis stimulation
by, 718, 719f
cardiovascular effects of,
1125–1127
in chronic kidney disease,
1392–1393
organs affected by, 1129f
receptors of, 1127, 1130f
release of, in myocardial ischemia,
1168–1169
vascular endothelial effects of,
1119b
Anhedonia, 651
Anion(s), 26
extracellular and intracellular,
101, 101t
Anion gap, 118
Aniridia, and associated childhood
cancer, 438–439, 438t
Anisotropic bands, of myocardial
muscle, 1106
Ankylosing spondylitis, 1600
clinical manifestations of, 1601,
1601f
evaluation and treatment of,
1601–1602
pathophysiology of, 1600–1601

Anoikis, 382
Anomalous viscosity, 1119
Anomic dysphasia, 549t–550t
Anorectal malformations, 1522,
1522f
Anorexia, 1452
Anorexia nervosa, 1480
Anorexins, 1478–1479, 1478b
Anorgasmia, 849
Anosmia, 516
Anovulation, 821
Anoxia, 52–53, 68
ANP. *See* Atrial natriuretic peptide.
Antagonist, in muscle movement,
1562–1563
Anterior cerebral artery, 462, 463t,
464f
Anterior cerebral artery occlusion,
stroke syndromes resulting
from, 604t–605t
Anterior column (ventral column),
456–457
Anterior cord syndrome, 594t–595t
Anterior fossa, 459
Anterior horn (ventral horn), 456
Anterior interatrial myocardial
band, 1102
Anterior pituitary, 707–708
embryonic development and
function of, 783–784
hormones released by, 704f, 707
hypothalamic regulatory
hormones targeting,
703–704, 707t
Anterior pituitary disorders, 731
acromegaly in, 733
hypopituitarism in, 731
primary adenoma in, 733
prolactinoma in, 735
Anterior spinal arteries, 463–465
Anterior spinothalamic tract, 457f,
458–459
Anterolateral tract system, 459
Anti-anxiety medications, 657, 657b
Anti-inflammatory agents, 203f
Anti-inflammatory steroids, 211
**Antibiotic resistant
microorganisms,** 294, 306–307,
327–328
development of, 328
genetics and, 327–328
gonococcal, 927
phage therapy against, 328b
in urinary tract infections, 1376b
Antibiotics, 327–329
bacteriostatic, 327
in shock therapy for children,
1740t
Antibody(ies), 217–218, 222–225.
See also Immune response.
antigen binding by, 225
antigen binding region of, 225,
225f
biological properties of, 225t
classes of, 222–224
clinical uses of, 218t
cross-reactive, 269
functions of, 244–247, 245f
indirect, 246
physicochemical properties of,
224t
structure of, 224–225, 224f
therapeutic use of, 245b
valence of, 225

Antibody dependent cell-mediated
cytotoxicity (ADCC), 249f,
250, 261
**Antibody mediated hemorrhagic
disease,** 1081
Antibody screen, 983t–985t
Antibody titer, 244–245
Anticipatory response(s), 339
Anticoagulant replacement clinical
trials, 1054
Anticoagulants
in preventing stroke, 606
in pulmonary emboli
management, 1296
in stroke management, 603
Anticodon, 134
Antidepressants, 657–658, 657b
and neurotransmitter levels, 653,
655f
Antidiuretic hormone (ADH), 102,
102f, 705–707
altered secretion of, 729–730.
See also Diabetes insipidus;
Syndrome of inappropriate
antidiuretic hormone.
aging and, 722–725
systolic heart failure and, 1190
cardiovascular effects of, 1125
feedback mechanisms affecting
secretion of, 706
hypothalamic regulation of,
703–704, 706
physiologic effects of, 704f,
706–707
renal effects of, 1358
Antigen(s), 217–218, 221–222
blood group, 272–274
clinical uses of, 218t
exogenous and endogenous, 236
human leukocyte, 226–228.
See also Human leukocyte
antigens (HLAs).
sensitization to, 258
Antigen-antibody complex, 188–189
Antigen binding fragment (Fab), 224
Antigen binding molecules, 222–226,
223f. *See also* Antibody(ies); B
cell receptor; T cell receptors.
Antigen neutralization, 244
Antigen presentation, 226
Antigen-presenting cells (APCs),
345, 345f
helper T (Th) cell interaction
with, 238–239
processing pathways in, 226,
236–237
in clonal selection, 235–237
Antigen presenting molecules,
226–228. *See also* CD1; Major
histocompatibility complex
(MHC).
genetics of, 226–228, 227f
Antigen processing, 236, 238f
Antigenic determinant, 221–222, 221f
Antigenic drift, 316–317
Antigenic shifts, in influenza viruses,
317–318, 317f
Antigenic targets, of hypersensitivity
reactions, 264–271
Antigenic variation
bacterial mechanisms of, 304
fungal mechanisms of, 309
protozoan mechanisms of, 311
viral mechanisms of, 315–316

**Antiglomerular basement
membrane nephritis,** 1383,
1384f
Antigravity posture, 575
Antigrowth signals, alterations in
cellular, 368–369
Antihemophilic factor (clotting
factor VIII), 977t
disorders associated with, 1079t
Antimicrobial(s), 327–329
Antimicrobial lectins, 186
Antimicrobial peptides, 185–186
Antioxidant(s), 57t
and cancer risk, 410t–413t
Antioxidant mechanisms, in biologic
systems, 56f
Antiphospholipid syndrome,
arterial thrombosis associated
with, 1057, 1057f
Antiplatelet therapy, in preventing
stroke, 606
Antiport, 28
Antipsychotic drugs
atypical, 651
in schizophrenia treatment,
651–652, 651b
Antipyretics, 498
Antisperm antibody fertility test, 808t
Antithrombin III (AT-III), 978–979,
1080
**Antithrombin III (AT III)
deficiency,** 1081
Antithrombin III-heparan
sulfate system, in vascular
endothelium, 973f
Antithrombotic molecules, 972
Antithymocyte gobulin (ATG),
1002–1003
Antitoxins, 245, 301
Antrum, gastric, 1423–1424
Anuria, 1388
Anxiety disorders, 658–662
Aortic aneurysms, 1145, 1145f
complications of, 1146–1147
Aortic bodies, 1250–1251
Aortic dissection, 1146–1147
Aortic mechanoreceptors, 1112
Aortic regurgitation, 1183
clinical manifestations of, 1182t
Aortic semilunar valves, 1094
Aortic stenosis, 1181, 1182f, 1228,
1228f
clinical manifestations of, 1182t,
1228
evaluation and treatment of,
1228–1229
pathophysiology of, 1228
Aortic valve calcification, 80f
APACHE II, APACHE III, 1713
APC gene, 375t. *See also*
Adenomatous polyposal cancer.
Aphasia, 546
Aplastic anemia, 1000–1002
and associated childhood cancer,
438t
bone marrow in, 1000f
bone marrow transplantation in,
1002
clinical manifestations of, 1002
evaluation and treatment of,
1002–1004
laboratory findings in, 999t
pathophysiology of, 1002
secondary to drug effects, 1001t

Aplastic crisis, in sickle cell disease, 1074
Apneusis, 530t, 531f
Apocrine sweat glands, 1646
Apoferritin, 969, 1008
Apoproteins, 55
Apoptosis, 19, 81b, 82f, 84–86, 84f, 1365–1367
  gene mutations and dysfunction of, 369
  mechanisms of, 85f
Apotransferrin, 971
Appendicitis, 1475
  clinical manifestations of, 1476
  evaluation and treatment of, 1476–1478
  pathophysiology of, 1476
Appendicular skeleton, 1546
Appetite, and satiety, 1478
  regulation of, 1478–1479, 1478b
Apraxias, 576t, 577
Apudoma, 1505
Aquaporins, 97–98
Aquaretics, diuretic effect of, 1359t
Aqueduct of Sylvius, 455
Aqueous humor, 508
Arachidonic acid derivative hormones, 697t
Arachnoid membrane, 460
Arachnoid villi, 461
Arcuate arteries, 1347–1348
Arcus senilis, and dyslipidemia, 1167
Areflexia, 566
Areola, 803
Arginine vasopressin. *See* Antidiuretic hormone.
Arnold-Chiari type II malformation, 670, 671f
Aromatase inhibitors, 884–885
Aromatic amines, in cancer epidemiology, 397t
Arousal disorders, sleep, 505
Arrested state, of cell cycle, 35
Arrhythmias. *See* Dysrhythmias.
Arsenic, in cancer epidemiology, 426–428
Arterial blood gas analysis, 1262
  normal ranges in, 1262t
Arterial blood vessels, 1113–1114, 1114f
  endothelium of, 1116
  structure of, 1116f
Arterial chemoreceptors, 1125
Arterial circle, 462, 463f
Arterial disorders, 1144–1150
  acute coronary syndromes in, 1169–1170
  aneurysms in, 1144–1147
  atherosclerotic, 1157
  coronary, 1160–1165
  embolic, 1147–1148
  hypertensive, 1149–1150
  myocardial ischemic, 1165
  orthostatic hypotensive, 1156–1157
  peripheral, 1148–1149, 1160
  thrombus formation in, 1147
Arterial embolism, 1147–1148
Arterial oxygenation, determinants of, 1258–1259
Arterial plasma, organic and inorganic components of, 953t
Arterial pressure, 1122–1130. *See also* Blood pressure.

Arterial stiffening, 1136
Arterial thrombi, 1055
Arterial thrombosis, 1147
Arteries, 1113–1114, 1114f
  of brain, 462–463, 463f, 463t
  diseases of, 1144–1150
  endothelium of, 1116
  of head and neck, 462–463, 462f
  of spinal cord, 463–465, 465f
  structure of, 1116f
Arteriogenesis, 1097
Arteriography, 1136
Arterioles, 1113
  hypertensive changes in, 1154f
Arteriovenous malformation (AVM), 607
  clinical manifestations of, 608
  evaluation and treatment of, 608
  pathophysiology of, 607–608
Arthritis, 1596–1597
  gouty, 1602–1605, 1604f
  infectious, 1597t
  juvenile rheumatoid, 1630–1631
  rheumatoid, 1596–1597, 1596f
  secondary septic, 1629
Arthrography, 1563
Arthropathies, 1592. *See also* Joint disorders.
Arthropod-borne encephalitis, 625–626, 626t
Arthroscopy, 1563
Arthus reaction, 264, 267
Articular capsule, 1550
Articular cartilage, 1550–1554
  degeneration of, 1594
Articulation, of bones, 1548–1549. *See also* Joint(s).
Asbestos, 426
Asbestos exposure, and development of mesothelioma, 1304
Asbestosis, 1278
  and associated cancer, 378t
Ascaris lumbricoides, 310t
  tissue damage caused by, 312
Ascending colon, 1435–1436
Ascending pathways. *See* Afferent (ascending) pathways.
Ascites, 1483, 1484f
  clinical manifestations of, 1484
  evaluation and treatment of, 1484–1485
  pathophysiology of, 1483–1484
Ascorbic acid. *See* Vitamin C.
Aseptic meningitis, 620–622, 682
  AIDS associated, 629
Aspartate
  in excitatory neurotransmission, 488
  neurologic functions of, 448t–449t
Aspergillus spp., 307, 308t
  toxins of, 309
Asphyxial injuries, 68–69
Asphyxiants, chemical, 68
Aspiration, 1274–1275
  preventive measures for individuals at risk of, 1275
Aspiration pneumonitis, 1329–1330
Aspirin
  in reducing platelet activation, 976
  in reducing risk of breast cancer, 877b
  in stroke management, 603
Association fibers, 452
Associational neurons, 444

Associative movement, loss of, 572
Asterixis, 568t–569t
Asthma, 1283–1284
  airway obstruction in, 1282, 1282f
  allergic component of, 1283
  in children, 1330–1331. *See also* Childhood asthma.
  clinical manifestations of, 1284
  evaluation and treatment of, 1285–1286
  genetic and environmental interaction in, 1283, 1284b, 1330–1331
  genetic component of, 1283
  incidence and prevalence of, 1283
  inflammatory response in, 1283–1284, 1332–1333
    upper and lower airway, 1283, 1283b
  NAEPP classification of clinical severity of, 1285–1286
  pathophysiology of, 1283–1284, 1285f
  pharmacogenetics and beta agonists in treatment of, 1285–1286, 1286b
Astigmatism, 511
Astrocytes, 444–445, 445f
  functions of, 446t, 446b
Astrocytoma(s), 612t, 614–615, 614f
  in children, 686, 686t
    clinical manifestations of, 687
    treatment strategies for, 687t, 688
  infiltrating, 615f
  intramedullary spinal cord, 619
Asymptomatic bacteriuria, 1375
Asymptomatic hyperuricemia, 1605
Ataxia telangiectasia, 281
  and associated childhood cancers, 438t
Ataxia-telangiectasia mutation, 896, 896f
Ataxic breathing, 530t, 531f
Ataxic cerebral palsy, 676
Atelectasis, 1275
  in neonatal respiratory distress syndrome, 1321–1322, 1322f
Atherosclerosis, 1157
  clinical manifestations of, 1160
  of coronary artery, 1161f
  development of, in chronic diabetes mellitus, 763, 764f
  evaluation and treatment of, 1160–1165
  pathophysiology of, 1157–1160, 1158f
  and platelet adhesion, 1055
Atherosclerotic plaque rupture, and tissue factor in thrombus formation, 979f
Athetosis, 568t
Atmospheric pressure changes, in cell injury, 72
Atopic dermatitis, 267, 1656, 1656f
  in children, 1681–1682
  clinical signs and course of, 1682, 1682f
  evaluation and treatment of, 1682
  pathophysiology of, 1681–1682
Atopic state, 265
  genes associated with, 265
ATP (adenosine triphosphate), in cellular metabolism, 22–23

Atria, cardiac, 1093
Atrial fibrillation, 1197t
Atrial flutter, 1197t
Atrial natriuretic peptide (ANP), 48, 102
  cardiovascular effects of, 1128
  physiologic roles of, 1128b
  renal effects of, 1352
Atrial receptors, and effects on heart rate, 1112–1113
Atrial septal defect, 1219, 1220f
  clinical manifestations of, 1220
  evaluation and treatment of, 1220
  pathophysiology of, 1219–1220
Atrial septation, 1210
Atrial tachycardia, 1197t
Atrioventricular bundle, 1100–1101
Atrioventricular canal defect, 1222, 1222f
  clinical manifestations of, 1223
  evaluation and treatment of, 1223
  pathophysiology of, 1222–1223
Atrioventricular dissociation, 1199t–1200t
Atrioventricular node, 1100–1101
  innervation of, 1101
Atrioventricular valves, 1094
Atrophy, 47, 47f
  of human brain tissue, 48f
  skin, 1648t–1653t
Attention deficit, selective, 543, 547t
Attenuated viruses, 244–245, 330–331
Atypical antidepressants, 657b
Atypical antipsychotic drugs, 651
Atypical dysplasia, 49
Atypical hyperplasia, of breast, 875, 876f
Atypical lobular hyperplasia, 875, 876f
Auditory agnosia, 548t
Auditory dysfunction, 515
  conductive hearing loss in, 515
  functional hearing loss in, 515
  mixed hearing loss in, 515
  sensorineural hearing loss in, 515
Auditory function. *See* Hearing.
Auditory/positional receptors, 445b
Auerbach plexus, 1421
Aura, 542
Autoantibody model, of drug induced hemolytic anemia, 1006
Autocrine signaling, 18–19
Autocrine stimulation, 368
Autodigestion, 6
Autografts, cultured epithelial, 1721f
Autoimmune disorders, 256, 257t–258t, 271–275
  development of, 267–270
    defective peripheral tolerance in, 269
    forbidden clones in, 269
    genetic factors in, 270, 270t
    infectious disease in, 269
    maternal microchimerism in, 269b
    neoantigens in, 269
    sequestered antigen in, 268–269
  systemic lupus erythematosus in, 271–272
Autoimmune hemolytic anemia(s), 274, 1005
  in children, 1066t

Autoimmune neonatal thrombocytopenia, 1082
Autoimmune pernicious anemia, 993–994
Autoimmune polyendocrine syndrome, 770
Autoimmune thrombocytopenic purpura, 1081
Autoimmune thyroiditis, 741
Autoimmune vascular purpura, 1083
Autoimmunity, 256, 257t, 267–270
definition of, 267–268
development of, 267–269
Autolysosome(s), 6
Automatic cells, 1103
Automaticity, of cardiac cycle, 1103
Autonomic hyperreflexia, 595, 596f
Autonomic nervous system (ANS), 443, 467–471
functions of, 470–471
neurotransmitters and neuroreceptors of, 467–470, 471f, 472t
parasympathetic division of, 467–470, 470f. See also Parasympathetic nervous system.
preganglionic and postganglionic components of, 467
sympathetic division of, 467, 469f. See also Sympathetic nervous system.
Autonomy, of cancer cells, 362
Autophagic cell death, 82f
Autophagic vacuoles, 47
Autophagosome(s), 6
Autophagy, 6, 47
Autoreactive B lymphocytes, 235
Autoreactive T lymphocytes, 233
Autoregulation, 1131
of blood pressure, 558
of renal blood flow, 1351, 1351f
Autosomal agammaglobulinemia, 278
Autosomal aneuploidy, 137–138
Autosomal dominant inheritance, 146–150, 147f
pedigree characteristics in, 146
recurrence risk in, 148
Autosomal hyper-IgM syndrome, 278–279
Autosomal recessive inheritance, 151–152
pedigree characteristics in, 151–152
recurrence risk in, 152
Autosomes, 134
Avascular diseases of bone, 1631
Avian flu, 317b
Avolition, 651
Avulsion, 64, 64f, 1573
Awareness alterations, 542–544
clinical manifestations of, 545, 547t
evaluation and treatment of, 545–548
pathophysiology of, 544–545, 545f–546f
Axial skeleton, 1546
Axillary breast tissue, 876t
Axon(s), 443
divergence and convergence of, 443
wallerian degeneration in, 445

Axon hillock, 443
Axonal degeneration, 635
Azotemia, 1386, 1393
management of, 1389

B
B cell lymphoma(s), 1033
classification of, 1030b
B-cell receptor (BCR) complex, 226
B-cell receptors (BCR), 222–226
gene recombination in producing, 233–234, 235f
B lymphocyte deficiencies, 278–279
gene defects in, 276t, 277f
B lymphocytes (B cells), 218
activation of, 240–243, 241f
autoreactive, 235
differentiation and maturation of, 219–220, 220f, 233–235, 234f, 242–243
hematopoietic differentiation of, 964f
immunoglobulin class switching in, 242, 242f
interaction of, in immune response, 241–242, 241f
surface marker changes on, 234–235
B7-1. See CD80.
Bachmann bundle, 1102
Bacille Calmette-Guérin (BCG) vaccine, 1293
Bacillus spp., 299t–300t
Bacteremia, 300–301
Bacteria, 297–307, 298t, 301f
cancer and, 380–381
chemical from, as human defense mechanisms, 186
Bacterial conjunctivitis, acute, 506–507
Bacterial culture, of gastrointestinal contents, 1445t
Bacterial embolism, 1148
Bacterial infections, 297–307. See also Bacterial pathogens.
causative agents in, 299t–300t
congenital heart defects associated with, 1214t
cutaneous, 1662–1663, 1683–1684
evasion of immune mechanisms in, 301, 303t
human immunodeficiency virus infection and, 323b
tissue invasion and injury in, 300–305
example of, 305–307
transmission of, 298–300
urogenital, 924–925. See also Bacterial urogenital infections.
Bacterial meningitis, 620, 682
in children, 682
clinical manifestations of, 684
evaluation and treatment of, 684
pathophysiology of, 682–684
clinical manifestations of, 623–624
evaluation and treatment of, 624
pathophysiology of, 623, 623f
Bacterial myositis, 1611

Bacterial pathogens, 297–307, 298t, 301f
evasion mechanism(s) of, 301, 303t
antigenic variation, 304
complement evasion, 305
immune molecule degradation, 304
immune molecule neutralization, 304–305
immune suppression, 305
intracellular survival, 302–303
protection against phagocytosis, 303–304
rapid division, 302
self-protein coating, 304
tissue injury by, 305
example of, 305–307
tissue invasion by, 300–305
transmission and colonization by, 298–300
Bacterial pneumonia, 1290–1291
in children, 1327–1329, 1328t
Bacterial prostatitis, 862–863
chronic, 862
Bacterial skin infections, 1662–1663
agents causing, 299t–300t
in children, 1683–1684
Bacterial superantigens, 305
Bacterial tracheitis, 1315
Bacterial translocation, 1711, 1721
Bacterial urogenital infections, 924–925
chancroid in, 932
gonorrhea in, 924–925
granuloma inguinale in, 933
syphilis in, 927–928
vaginosis in, 934
Bacterial vaginosis
clinical manifestations of, 934
evaluation and treatment of, 934–935
pathophysiology of, 934
as risk factor in preterm delivery, 934b
Bactericidal antibiotics, 327
Bactericidal/permeability-inducing (BPI) protein, 186
Bacteriostatic antibiotics, 327
Baden-Walker Halfway System, 834b
Bainbridge reflex, 1112, 1112f
Balanitis, 852, 852f, 1666t
Balantidium coli, 310t
Ballism, 568t–569t
Bare lymphocyte syndrome, 280–281
Barometric pressure, 1254–1255
Baroreceptor(s), 102
Baroreceptor reflex, cardiovascular effects of, 1112, 1124–1125, 1126f
Barret esophagus, and associated cancer, 378t
Bartholin cyst, 832
Bartholin glands, 785–786
Bartholinitis, 832–833, 833f
Bartter syndrome, 768
pathophysiology of, 769
Basal cell carcinoma, 1669–1670, 1670f
ultraviolet radiation and, 422–423
Basal ganglia, 450t, 452–453
motor pathway of, 458

Basal ganglia motor syndromes, 577
Basal ganglia system, 452
Basal ganglion, 661–662, 662f
Basal ganglion gait, 576
Basal ganglion posture, 576
Basal layer, 1644–1645
Basal plate, 666, 666f
Base excess, normal values, 1262t
Base pair substitution, 129–132
Basement membrane, 15–16, 16f
of muscle fiber, 1558
Basic fibroblast growth factor (bFGF), 369
Basilar artery, 462
Basilar artery occlusion, stroke syndromes resulting from, 604t
Basilar skull fracture, 584
Basis pedunculi, 455
Basopenia, 1016t, 1017
Basophil count, 983t–985t
Basophilia, 1016t, 1017
Basophils, 956
hematopoietic differentiation of, 964f
in inflammatory response, 202
Batten disease, genetic basis and pathophysiology of, 526t–527t
BCG (bacille Calmette-Guérin) vaccine, 1293
Bcl-2 gene, 896
Becker muscular dystrophy, 1636–1637
Beckwith-Wiedemann syndrome, 149–150
and associated childhood cancer, 438–439, 438t
Bedbug bites, 1689–1690, 1690f
Bee sting allergy, 265
Bence-Jones protein, 1038
urinary, 368t
Benign breast disease, 872–875
evaluation and treatment of, 875–896
nonproliferative, 873–874
proliferative
with atypia, 875
without atypia, 874–875
tissue histology in, 873f
tumor types in, 874t
Benign febrile seizures, 680
clinical manifestations of, 681
evaluation and treatment of, 681
pathophysiology of, 680–681
Benign prostatic hyperplasia (BPH), 860–861, 860f
clinical manifestations of, 861–865
management of, 861
pathogenesis of, 861
Benign prostatic hypertrophy, 860–861
Benign tumor(s), 360–361
characteristics of, 361t
histology of, 362–363, 363f
naming, 361
nomenclature and classification of, 364t
Bent nail syndrome, 851–852
Berger disease or nephropathy. See IgA nephropathy.
Beriberi, heart failure in, 1195
Bernard-Soulier syndrome, 1048

Berry aneurysms, 606, 606f
Beta cell dysfunction,
  pathophysiology of, 746t
  in type 2 diabetes mellitus, 751
Beta cells, of pancreas, 713,
  751–752
  immunologic destruction of,
  746–748
Beta-thalassemia, 1076–1077
Beta-thalassemia major, 1077,
  1078b
Beta-thalassemia minor, 1077
β-adrenergic blockers, for
  myocardial ischemia, 1169
β-adrenergic receptors, 469–470,
  1105
  cardiac, 1105
  in central stress response, 340
  physiologic actions of, 342t,
  469–470, 471f
  specific, and physiologic actions
  of neurotransmitters,
  472f
β-endorphins, 708t
β-globulins, 953–954
β-human chorionic gonadotropin
  (β-HCG), 368t
β-lactamase, 306–307, 328
β-lipoprotein, 707
β-lipotropin, 708t
Bevacizumab (Avastin), 387t,
  907–908
Bicarbonate
  blood gas, normal values, 1262t
  and carbonic acid, in
  compensated maintenance,
  115–116, 116f
  renal conservation of, 117, 117f
BIER V (Fifth Biological Effects
  of Ionizing Radiation Panel),
  419–420
Bilateral acoustic neurofibromatosis.
  See Neurofibromatosis type 2.
Bilateral renal agenesis, 1407
Bile
  fractional components of, 1439
  secretion of, 1439–1440
Bile acid(s)
  and formation of micelles, 1433,
  1433f, 1439–1440
  primary, 1439
  secondary, 1439
Bile acid pool, 1439
Bile canaliculi, 1439
Bile salt(s), 1439–1440
  enterohepatic circulation of,
  1440f
Bile salt deficiency, 1471
Biliary atresia, 1531–1532
Biliary cancer, environmental
  factors in, 397t–400t
Biliary cirrhosis, 1492t, 1493–1494
Bilirubin, 79, 1440
Bilirubin metabolism, 1440, 1441f
  assessments of, 1446t
Biliverdin, 1440
Bioartificial liver, 1491b
Bioassay, 720
Biofeedback, 1606
Biofilm, 296
Biopsy, tissue, 385t
Biotin deficiency, and associated
  disorders, 70t
Biotransformation, 1442

Bipolar disorder, 652
  clinical manifestations of,
  656–657
  genetic predisposition and
  environmental factors in,
  179–180, 652–653
  treatment of, 657–658
Bipolar neurons, 444, 445f
Bisphosphonates, and
  postmenopausal osteoporosis,
  1584
Black lung, 1278
Bladder, urinary, 1350–1351, 1350f
Bladder cancer, 1372–1373
  clinical manifestations of, 1373
  environmental factors in,
  397t–400t, 401
  evaluation and treatment of, 1373
  incidence of, 1372–1373
  pathogenesis of, 1373
  staging of, 1375t
  types of, 1374f
Bladder disorders
  in children, 1411–1412
  infectious, 1374–1375
  neurogenic, 1369–1370
Bladder extrophy, 1405–1406, 1406f
Bladder outlet obstruction, 1406
Blalock-Taussig shunt, 1225–1226
Blast cell(s), 437
  in acute leukemia, 1085, 1085f
Blast injury, 72
Blastomyces dermatitidis, 307, 308t
Bleb rupture, 1272–1273
Bleeding time, 983t–985t
Blepharitis, 506
Blocking antibody, 267
Blood, 952–957
  cellular components of, 954–957.
  See also Erythrocytes;
  Leukocytes; Platelet(s).
  physiologic functions of, 952
  plasma and plasma proteins of,
  952–954
  postnatal changes in, 1063–1064
Blood-brain barrier, 465b
Blood cells, 954–957. *See also*
  Erythrocytes; Leukocytes;
  Platelet(s).
  autoimmunity to, 257t–258t
  development of, 961–972. *See also*
  Hematopoiesis.
Blood clot, 976
Blood clotting assessments, 1446t
Blood clotting mechanism, 974f
Blood flow, 1117–1122
  blood pressure and, 1125
  calculation of, through blood
  vessel, 1118
  factors regulating, 1124f
  blood velocity, 1120–1121
  fluid viscosity, 1118
  pressure and resistance,
  1117–1120
  vascular compliance, 1122
  laminar and turbulent, 1121,
  1124f
Blood group antigens, 272–274
Blood oxygen content, 1258–1259
Blood pressure
  in children, 1729
  estimating, 1729b
  mechanisms influencing, 1236f
  normal values for, 1236t–1237t

Blood pressure *(Continued)*
  classification of adult, 1149t
  in infants and toddlers, normal
  values, 1237t
  regulation of, 1122–1130
  arterial chemoreceptors in,
  1125
  baroreceptors in, 1124–1125
  blood volume and, 1123–1130
  cardiac output and, 1123
  hormones in, 1125–1130
  hyperemia in, 1125
  total peripheral resistance and,
  1123–1130
Blood sample evaluation, 982
Blood tests, 982, 983t–985t
  pediatric, and values, 985t
Blood transfusion
  in children in shock, 1739
  in immune deficiency therapies,
  288
Blood transfusion reactions,
  272–274
  agglutinated red blood cells in,
  273f
Blood urea nitrogen (BUN), 1361
Blood vessels, 1113–1131
  arterial, 1113–1114, 1114f
  calculation of blood flow through,
  1118. *See also* Blood flow.
  parallel and series arrangement
  of, 1123f
  physiology of, in hemostasis, 972
  ruptured, 1117f
  structure of, 1113–1117, 1116f
  vascular compliance of, 1122
  venous, 1114f, 1117
Blood volume. *See also* Fluid and
  electrolyte balance; Fluid
  resuscitation.
  blood pressure and, 1123–1130
Bloom syndrome, and associated
  childhood cancers, 438–439,
  438t
Blow back, 66
Blunt brain trauma, 583–584
Blunt force injuries, 62–65
BMI (body-mass index), 406
  WHO classification of, 408t
BMPR2 (bone morphogenetic
  protein receptor type II),
  1296–1297
BMPs. *See* Bone morphogenic
  proteins.
BNP. *See* Brain natriuretic peptide.
Body, gastric, 1423–1424, 1426
Body acids, 114
Body fluids, 96–98
  aging and distribution of, 97
  alterations in, 98–99. *See also*
  Edema.
  distribution of, 96–98, 97t
  electrolyte concentrations in, 107t
  pH of, 114
  water movement between
  intracellular and extracellular
  compartments, 97–98
  water movement between plasma
  and interstitial fluid, 98
Body image agnosia, 548t
Body-mass index (BMI), 406
  WHO classification of, 408t
Bohr effect, 1259
Bombesin, 1425t

Bone(s), 39t–40t
  aging of, 1564
  characteristics of, 1546–1547,
  1547f
  cross section of, 1546f
  formation of, 1545–1546, 1618–
  1619. *See also* Bone tissue.
  function testing of, 1563
  growth of, 1619–1620
  homeostasis of, 1579–1580
  maintenance of, 1547–1548
  structural assessment of, 1563,
  1563b
Bone albumin, 1545
Bone cancer, and tumors,
  1588–1592
  benign and malignant, 1588
  in children, 1637
  malignant, 1637
  diagnosis of, 1589–1590
  environmental factors in,
  397t–400t, 401
  epidemiology of, 1588–1589
  origins and types of, 1588, 1589f
  pathophysiology of, 1589, 1589t
  staging of malignant, 1589, 1590t
  type(s) of, 1590–1592
  chondrogenic, 1591
  collagenic, 1591–1592
  myelogenic, 1592
  osteogenic, 1590–1591
Bone cells, 1541–1544, 1541t, 1543t
Bone cysts, benign, 1637
Bone density testing, reliability of,
  for fracture risk, 1578
Bone destruction patterns, 1589,
  1589t
Bone disorders, 1576–1580
  cancer and tumors in, 1588–1592
  infectious, 1586–1587
  metabolic, 1576–1580
Bone fluid, 1545
Bone fracture(s), 65, 1568–1569
  clinical manifestations of,
  1570–1571
  evaluation and treatment of,
  1571–1572
  pathophysiology of, 1570
  types and classification of, 1569,
  1569f
  definitions of, 1570t
Bone healing, alterations in,
  1571–1572
Bone infection, 1586–1587, 1628.
  See also Osteomyelitis.
Bone marrow
  B cell maturation in, 233–235,
  234f
  cell types found in, 963
  hematopoiesis in, 962–963
  stromal cell and progenitor cell
  interaction in, 963
  structure and vasculature of,
  962–963, 962f
Bone marrow aspiration, 980–981
  in childhood T cell lymphoma,
  1088f
  in pernicious anemia, 994f
  results of, 981–982
Bone marrow fibroblasts, cytokines
  secreted by, 961t, 963
Bone marrow iron stores, 980–981
Bone marrow pool, 963–965, 965f
Bone marrow samples, 981f

Bone marrow tests, 980–982
Bone marrow transplantation
  in aplastic anemia, 1002
  in thalassemia, 1078, 1078b
Bone matrix, 1541, 1541t, 1544–1545
Bone minerals, 1541t, 1545
Bone morphogenetic protein
  receptor type II (BMPR2),
  1296–1297
Bone morphogenic proteins (BMPs),
  1541, 1543t, 1545
  recombinant, 1584
Bone remodeling, 1547–1548, 1549f
  stages of, 1548
Bone remodeling units, 1547
Bone resorption evaluation, 1563,
  1563b
Bone structure, and function,
  1540–1548
Bone tissue, 1545–1546, 1618–1619
  elements of, 1540–1545, 1541t
  remodeling, 1547–1548
  types of, 1545–1546
Bordatella pertussis, 298–300,
  299t–300t
  protective mechanisms of, against
    phagocytes, 303–304
Boron, and effect on bone tissue
  physiology, 1580b
Borrelia burgdorferi, 298, 299t–300t,
  629, 1667
Borrelia recurrentis, 298
  antigenic variation of, 304
Borrelia spp., complement evasion
  by, 305
Botulinum toxin therapy, for
  spasmodic torticollis, 575b
Bowing fracture, 1569
Bowman capsule, 1345
Bowman space, 1345
BPI (bactericidal/permeability-
  inducing) protein, 186
Brachial plexus, 465–467
Brachycephaly, 672f
Brachytherapy, 388
Bradycardia, 1197t–1198t
  in children, 1730
Bradykinesia, 571–572
  Parkinsonian, 529–531, 573
Bradykinin, 191, 203f
Bradyphrenia, 574
Brain. See also central nervous system
  entries., 449–456
  blood-brain barrier of, 465b
  blood supply of, 462–463, 463f,
    463t
  cerebrospinal fluid and
    ventricular system of, 461
  changes in aging, 471–474, 474t
    cellular, 471–474
    functional, 474
    structural, 471–474
  liquefactive necrosis of, 83f
  pain perception and processing in,
    484–486, 485f
  protective coverings of, 459, 460f
  region(s) of, 449–450, 450t, 451f
    forebrain, 452–455
    functional assignment to,
      450–452, 451f
    hindbrain, 455–456
    midbrain, 455
    reticular activating, 449–450,
      450f

Brain (Continued)
  reinforcement center of, 475b
  thermal sensory perception and
    processing in, 485f
  venous system of, 462, 464f
Brain abscess, 624, 625f
  clinical manifestations of, 625
  evaluation and treatment of,
    625–626
  extradural, 625
  pathophysiology of, 624–625
Brain cancer, and tumors, 611–618,
  612t
  AIDS associated, 629
  in children, 685, 686t
    clinical manifestations of,
      686–688
    pathophysiology of, 685–686
    treatment strategies for, 687t,
      688
    types of, 686, 686f, 686t
  common sites of, 613f
  extracerebral, 616–618
  metastatic, 618
  primary, 613–616
Brain death, 534
Brain dysfunction. See Cerebral
  hemodynamic alterations;
  Cognitive dysfunction; Motor
  function alterations.
Brain injury, traumatic, 583–591
  categories of, 583–584
  causes of, 584–591
  common types of, 584
  diagnostic tools in, 591
  diffuse, 588–591. See also Diffuse
    brain injury.
  focal, 585–588. See also Focal
    brain injury.
  genetics of, 484
  incidence of, 583
  penetrating focal, 588
  primary and secondary, 584–585
  severity of, and clinical
    manifestations, 584t
  temperature regulation disorders
    in, 502
Brain metastases, 618
Brain natriuretic peptide (BNP),
  48, 102
  cardiovascular effects of, 1128
  heart failure and, 1193b
  physiologic roles of, 1128b, 1193b
  renal effects of, 1352
Brain scan, 475–476
Brainstem, 449–450
Brainstem breathing patterns, 530t
Brainstem death, 534
  medical criteria for, 534
Brainstem glioma, 686, 686t
  clinical manifestations of, 687
  treatment strategies for, 687t,
    688
Brainstem injury, 591. See also
  Diffuse axonal injury.
Branched chain ketoaciduria,
  genetic basis and
  pathophysiology of, 526t
BRCA1, BRCA2. See Breast cancer
  susceptibility genes.
Breast(s)
  female, 802–805
    anatomy of, 802–805, 803f, 898f
    changes in

Breast(s) (Continued)
    during menopause, 810–811
    during menstrual cycle,
      803–804
    development of, 803
    examination of, 807
    function of, 804–805
    lymphatic drainage of, 803,
      804f
  male, 805
Breast biopsy tissue, classification of,
  873, 873b
Breast cancer, 175, 880–896. See
  also Ductal carcinoma in situ;
  Invasive breast carcinoma;
  Lobular carcinoma in situ.
  clinical manifestations of,
    905–906, 906f, 907t
  cyclooxygenase enzymes (COX-1,
    COX-2) in, 877b–878b
  estrogen receptor positive, 883,
    884f
  evaluation and treatment of,
    906–908
  gene expression profiling in
    evaluation of, 906–907
  histologic and anatomic locations
    of, 896–905, 898f
  incidence of, 880–881
  inherited, 375–377, 895–896
  male, 909
  metastasis of, 384t
  pathogenesis of, 896–905
    conceptual model of, 900f
    inflammatory stroma in,
      900–901
    mammary tissue
      transformation in, 904f
  pregnancy and protective effects
    against, 881–882, 881b
  progesterone receptor positive,
    883
  risk factors associated with, 880t
    adiposity, 409
    cyclooxygenase enzymes
      (COX-1, COX-2),
      877b–878b
    environmental, 397t, 401,
      888–895
    genetic, 895–896
    hormonal, 883–886, 883f
    hormonal therapies, 886–887
    lobular involution, 882–883
    mammographic breast density,
      887–888
    risk of, 880t
  staging of, 907b
  types of, 896–905
Breast cancer susceptibility genes
  (BRCA1, BRCA2), 375t,
  895–896. See also Breast cancer.
  association of, with ovarian
    cancer, 846–847
Breast disorders, 871
  female, 871. See also Female breast
    disorders.
  male, 908
Breast examination, 807
Breast inflammation, 876t
  in breast disorders and
    carcinogenesis, 877b–878b
Breast pain, medications for, 879t
Breast reconstruction, 876t
Breast sarcoma, 897t

Breath tests, of gastrointestinal
  function, 1445t
Breathing, mechanics of, 1251–1254,
  1254f
  in children, 1311–1312, 1312f
Breathing patterns, in brain
  dysfunction evaluation,
  529–531, 530t, 531f
Breathing sounds, in locating upper
  airway obstruction in children,
  1313–1314, 1313f
Brittle bone disease, 1618–1619
Broca dysphasia, 549t–550t
Broca speech area, 452
Brodie abscesses, 1588
Bronchi, 1244, 1246f
Bronchial carcinoid lung cancers,
  1303–1304
Bronchial circulation, 1247–1249
Bronchial epithelium, metaplastic
  and dysplastic changes in,
  50–51, 51f
Bronchial malformations,
  congenital, 1320
Bronchiectasis, 1275–1277, 1276f
Bronchioles, 1244, 1246f
  respiratory, 1244, 1246f
Bronchiolitis, 1277, 1326
  clinical manifestations of, 1327
  evaluation and treatment of, 1327
  pathophysiology of, 1326–1327
Bronchiolitis obliterans, 1277, 1330
Bronchiolitis obliterans organizing
  pneumonia, 1277
Bronchitis
  acute, 1294
  and associated cancer, 378t
  chronic, 1286
Bronchoconstriction, 1253–1254
Bronchodilation, 1253–1254
Bronchogenic carcinoma, 1299–
  1301. See also Lung cancer.
Bronchopulmonary dysplasia,
  1323–1324
  clinical manifestations of,
    1325–1326
  pathophysiology of, 1324–1325,
    1325f
  treatment of, 1326
Brown-Séquard syndrome,
  594t–595t, 619
Brucella abortus, 299t–300t
  intracellular survival of, 302–303
Brudzinski sign, 609
Brugia malayi, tissue damage caused
  by, 312
Brush border, 1429
Bruton's agammaglobulinemia, 278
Buboes, inguinal, 932
Bubonic plague, 297t
Buerger disease, 1148
Buffer(s), 115
Buffer systems, 115, 115t
  carbonic acid-bicarbonate,
    115–116
  protein, 116
  renal, 116–117
Buffering, 115
Bulbar palsy, 567–568
Bulbourethral glands, 800
Bulbus cordis, 1211
Bulimia nervosa, 1481
Bulla, 1648t–1653t
Bullous impetigo, 1683

Bullous pemphigoid, 1661, 1661f
Bumetanide, diuretic action of,
  1359t
Bundle branches, 1100–1101
Bundle of His, 1100–1102
Burkitt lymphoma, 1035
  clinical manifestations of,
    1035–1036, 1036f
  evaluation and treatment of, 1036
  pathophysiology of, 1035, 1036f
Burn injury, 72, 1714–1716
  in children, 1741–1743, 1742f,
    1745t. *See also* Pediatric burn
    injury.
  depth of, 1714–1716, 1715t, 1742
  evaluation and treatment of,
    1721–1724
  extent and severity of, 1716,
    1742–1743
  fluid resuscitation in, 1717, 1718t,
    1718b
  incidence of, 1714
  lymphocyte subsets and
    immunoregulation in, 1748,
    1748b
  pathophysiology of, 1714,
    1716–1721, 1716f
    cardiovascular and systemic,
      1717–1718, 1743–1744
    cellular, 1718–1721, 1743
    gastrointestinal, 1744
    immunologic, 1720–1721,
      1744–1745, 1746f
    integumentary, 1743
    metabolic, 1718–1720, 1744
    renal, 1744
  and secondary immune
    deficiencies, 285–286
  water loss in, 1721
Burn shock, 1717
  in children, 1745–1748. *See also*
    Pediatric burn injury.
  electrolyte movement in,
    1717–1718, 1719f
  endpoint of, 1718
  immunologic response in,
    1720–1721, 1720f
  metabolic response in, 1718–1720
  urine output in, 1718
Burn unit referral criteria, 1717b
Burning hand syndrome, 594t
Burrow, 1653t
Bursae, 1574
Bursitis, 1574
  common sites of, and causes, 1575t
Bystander effects, of ionizing
  radiation, 417–418, 420–422
  in gap junction communication,
    422
  signaling pathways of, 422f

C

C cells, 709
C fibers (nociceptors), 483, 483f
c-myc gene, 896
C-peptide, 414, 749
C-reactive protein, highly sensitive,
  and coronary artery disease,
  1164b, 1165
C-type natriuretic peptide
  cardiovascular effects of, 1119b,
    1128
  physiologic roles of, 1128b
  renal effects of, 1352

c wave, 1096
C1 deficiency, 281
C1 esterase inhibitor (C1 inh), 192
C2 deficiency, 281
C3, 188
C3 convertase, 188–189
C3 deficiency, 281
C3 receptor deficiency, 282
C4 deficiency, 281
C5 convertase, 188–189
C9 deficiency, 281
Ca⁺⁺, Ca²⁺. *See* Calcium.
Cachectin, 305
Cachexia, 390–391, 390f
Cadherin(s), dysfunctional, in
  melanoma, 424
Caisson disease, 72
Calcification, in bone tissue, 1541
Calcitonin, 112, 709
  physiologic effects of, 710t
Calcitonin gene-related peptide
  (CGRP), in stress response,
  348t
Calcitriol (vitamin D3), 1359, 1359b
Calcium, 111–112
  in bone, 1541t
  in bone homeostasis, 1579–1580
  cellular accumulation of, 79–81,
    80f
  clotting function of, 977t
  intake of, and postmenopausal
    osteoporosis, 1579
  intestinal absorption of,
    1433–1434
  in myocardial excitation-
    contraction coupling,
    1108–1109, 1169
  in second messenger signaling
    pathways, 23t, 702, 702t
Calcium channel blocking drugs,
  1108–1109
Calcium intake, 1433–1434
  and cancer risk, 410t
Calcium level regulation, by
  parathyroid hormone, 711–712,
  712f
Calcium-phosphate
  metabolism, 111–112.
    See also Hypercalcemia;
    Hyperphosphatemia;
    Hypocalcemia;
    Hypophosphatemia.
  in chronic kidney disease, 1392t,
    1394–1396, 1395t
  hormonal regulation of, 111, 112f
Calcium second messenger system,
  20, 22f, 702, 702t
Calcium sensitizing inotropic drugs,
  1193–1194
Calcium stones, 1368
Calcium-troponin complex, 1109
California encephalitis, 625–626,
  626t
California encephalitis virus, 621t
Callus, 49
  bone, 1548
Callus formation, post-fracture,
  1570, 1570f
Calymmatobacterium granulomatis,
  933–934
cAMP. *See* Cyclic adenosine
  monophosphate.
Campylobacter enteritis, sexually
  transmitted, 946

Campylobacter jejuni, 299t–300t, 946
CAMs. *See* Cellular adhesion
  molecules.
Canalicular state, of lung
  development, 1324
Cancer, 360–361
  bacteria-associated, 380–381
  bladder, 1372–1373
  bone, 1588–1592
    in children, 1637
  breast, 175
  cellular biology of, 362–366
  cervical, 841
  in children, 436–441
    environmental factors
      associated with, 439
    etiology of, 437–439
    genetics of, 438–439, 438t
    incidence and types of, 436–437
    prognosis for, 440–441
  chronic inflammation and,
    377–378, 378t
  chronic pain in, 493
  classification and nomenclature
    in, 361–362, 362f
  clinical manifestations of, 384
  colon and rectal, 175–176, 1500
  definition of, 360–361
  diagnosis and staging of, 384,
    386f, 387t
    biopsy of tissue in, 385t
    mammograms in, 384–387
  endometrial, 845–846
  epidemiology of, 396–435. *See also*
    Cancer epidemiology.
  epigenetics of, 373–377
  esophageal, 1498
  familial, 375–377
  female reproductive, 841
  gallbladder, 1504
  gastric, 1499
  genes and environmental
    interaction in, 174–176
  genetic basis of, 367–381, 401–404
    clonal selection in, 368
    gene mutations in, 367–368
    oncogenes and tumor-
      suppressor genes in,
      370–375
  genetic mutations causing,
    367–368, 370–375
    types of, 373, 368–370, 371b
  incidence of, in United States,
    401, 402t. *See also* Cancer
    epidemiology.
  kidney, 1372
  laryngeal, 1299
  lip, 1298
  liver, 1503
  lung, 1299–1303
  metastasis of, 381–384. *See also*
    Metastasis.
  ovarian, 846
  penile, 853–854
  prostate, 863–865
  radiation induced, 73–74
  references on, 394
  six hallmarks of, 370f
  skeletal muscle, 1613
  skin, 1669–1673
  staging of, 384, 386f, 387t
  summary review of, 393b
  testicular, 857
  treatment of, 387–394

Cancer *(Continued)*
  alopecia in, 391–392
  antinausea therapy in, 391
  chemotherapeutic, 387–388
  complications in, 388–394
  radiation therapy in, 388
  reproductive changes in,
    392–394
  surgical, 388
  vaginal, 844–845
  viral associated, 378–380
  vulvar, 845
Cancer cells, 362–366
  transformation and differentiation
    of, 362–363, 363f, 365f
  tumor markers of, 367, 368t
Cancer epidemiology, 396
  and cancers that have increased in
    United States, 401
  environmental factor(s) in,
    396–431, 397t
    air pollution as, 426–431
    alcohol consumption as,
      415–416
    chemical and occupational, 426
    in children, 439
    dietary, 404–415, 407t, 410t
    electromagnetic radiation as,
      424–425
    genetic and epigenetic,
      401–404, 896
    ionizing radiation as, 73–74,
      416–422
    obesity as, 406–415
    prenatal, 401, 403–404, 439
    risk for, 401b
    sexual and reproductive
      behaviors as, 425
    tobacco-related, 404
    ultraviolet radiation as,
      422–424
    viral and microbial, 425
  physical activity and, 426–431
  references on, 431
  summary review of, 429b
Cancer stem cells, 365–366, 367f
Candida albicans, 307, 308t, 309f,
  1665
  adhesion capability of, 308
Candidiasis, 1665
  chronic mucocutaneous, 279
  oral, 309f
  pathogenesis of, 309–310
  sites of, 1666t
Capillaries, 1113
  lymphatic, 1132, 1132f
  pulmonary, 1247, 1248f. *See also*
    Alveolocapillary membrane.
  renal, 1345–1346. *See also*
    Glomerular filtration
    membrane.
Capillary endothelium, 1113
Capillary filtration forces, 98–99,
  99f, 1114
Capillary flow, factors affecting,
  1125t
Capillary network, 1113, 1118f
Capillary permeability, increased,
  100
Capillary refill, in children, 1730
Capillary seal, 1718
Capillary telangiectasis, 607
Capillary wall, 1113, 1117f
Caplan syndrome, 1599

Capsules, bacterial, 304, 304f
Carbohydrate metabolism, in chronic kidney disease, 1394–1395
Carbohydrates, 1430
    and cancer risk, 410t
    cellular accumulation of lipids and, 76–77
    dietary intake of, 1430
    digestion and absorption of, 1430, 1431f
    hepatic metabolism of, 1442
    plasma membrane, 13
Carbon dioxide partial pressure, normal values, 1262t
Carbon dioxide transport, pulmonary, 1259–1260
    molecular forms of carbon dioxide in, 1259
Carbon monoxide affinity, to hemoglobin, 968
Carbon monoxide poisoning, 59
Carbon tetrachloride poisoning, 55, 58f
Carbonic acid, 114–115, 1249
Carbonic acid-bicarbonate buffer system, 115–116, 115t
Carbonic anhydrase inhibitors, diuretic action of, 1359t
Carboxyhemoglobin, 59
Carboxypeptidase(s), 189–190, 1430–1432
Carbuncle, 1662–1663
Carcinoembryonic antigen (CEA), 368t
Carcinogenesis, 420–422, 421f
    theoretic scheme of, 423f
Carcinogens, 396
    chemical, 426, 427b
Carcinoid lung cancers, 1303–1304
Carcinoid syndrome, paraneoplastic, 389t
Carcinoma(s), 364t
    definition of, 361
Carcinoma-associated fibroblasts, 866–867
Carcinoma in situ (CIS), 361, 362f
Cardiac action potential(s), 1099–1109, 1103f
    cardiac excitation and, 1102
    generation of, 1100–1103
    propagation of, 1102–1103, 1102t
Cardiac autoimmune disorders, 257t
Cardiac catheterization, and angiography, 1135
Cardiac cycle
    action potential propagation in, 1102–1103, 1103f
    automaticity of, 1103
    blood flow during, 1095–1096
        parameters of, 1097f
    phases of, 1095, 1098f
    cardiac excitation in, 1102
    conduction system in, 1100–1103
    electrical impulse generation in, 1099–1109
    electrocardiogram of, 1103, 1104f
    myocardial function in, 1108–1109. See also Myocardium.
    rhythmicity of, 1103
Cardiac excitation, 1102

Cardiac function, 1133–1136
    in aging, 1137t
    in children, 1731t
    coronary artery evaluation in, 1133–1135
    evaluation of, 1133–1135
        cardiac catheterization and angiography in, 1135
        chest radiographic examination in, 1134
        computed tomography and magnetic resonance imaging in, 1134–1135
        echocardiography in, 1134
        electrocardiography in, 1133–1134
        electrophysiologic studies of, 1135
        stress testing in, 1134
        technetium scanning in, 1135
    indicators of, 1133t
Cardiac index (CI), 1133t
Cardiac muscle. See also myocardial entries, 41t, 1105–1108
    length-tension relationship of, 1110
Cardiac orifice, of stomach, 1423–1424
Cardiac output (CO), 1109–1113, 1109f, 1133t
    afterload and, 1111
    blood pressure and, 1123
    Frank-Starling law of heart in, 1109–1110, 1110f
    heart rate and, 1111–1113
    Laplace's law in, 1110
    myocardial contractility and, 1111
    preload and, 1110–1111
Cardiac plexus, 1104
Cardiac septation, 1209–1211, 1210f–1211f
Cardiac sphincter, 1423
Cardiac troponins, 1173–1174
Cardiac valve(s), 1094, 1095f
Cardiac valve dysfunction, 1181–1184
Cardinal signs of inflammation, 186
Cardioembolism, 601
Cardioexcitatory center, 1112
Cardiogenic shock, 1175, 1728
    in children, 1732–1733
        clinical manifestations of, 1733–1735, 1734f
        compensatory responses in, 1732–1733
    clinical manifestations of, 1700
    compensatory responses in, 1699–1700
    pathogenesis of, 1699–1701, 1700b, 1700f, 1728b
    treatment of, 1699, 1700b
Cardiography, 1133–1134
Cardioinhibitory center, 1112
Cardiomyopathy(ies), 1178–1180
    dilated, 1178–1180
    pathophysiology of, 1178f
        and major symptoms, 1179t
Cardiovascular control center, 1111–1112
Cardiovascular disease, 1142, 1143t
    aging and, 1136
    AIDS associated, 629, 1189
    in aldosteronism, 769b
    arterial, 1144–1150

Cardiovascular disease (Continued)
    childhood, 1209
    acquired, 1234. See also Childhood obesity; Hypertension; Kawasaki disease.
    congenital, 1213–1214. See also Congenital heart defects.
        references on, 1240
    heart wall disorders in, 1176–1184
    manifestations of, 1189–1203
        dysrhythmias in, 1196–1203. See also Dysrhythmias.
        heart failure in, 1189–1196. See also Heart failure.
    references on, 1203
    summary review of, 1200b
    venous, 1142–1144
Cardiovascular function, 1133–1136
    in aging, 1137t
    in children, 1731t
    coronary artery evaluation in, 1133–1135
    indicators of, 1133t
Cardiovascular system, 1091–1093, 1092f
    aging and, 1136–1140, 1137t
    autonomic innervation of, 1100–1103, 1101f
    blood flow function in, 1117–1122
    blood pressure regulation in, 1122–1130. See also Blood pressure.
    cardiac anatomy and function in, 1093–1096. See also Heart.
    chronic kidney disease and effects on, 1391t, 1395
    coronary circulation of, 1130–1131
    development of, 1209–1213
        embryologic, 1209
        fetal, 1209–1211
        in infant, 1213
        in neonate, 1211–1213
    functional assessment of, 1133–1136. See also Cardiac function; Vascular evaluation.
    great vessels of, 1095. See also Heart.
    references on, 1140
    summary review of, 1137b
    vascular anatomy and function in, 1113–1131. See also Blood vessels.
Carditis, 1186
Caretaker genes, 375–377
    inherited mutations of, 375
Carina, 1244
Carotenoids, and cancer risk, 410t
Carotid arteries, internal, 462
Carotid bodies, 1250–1251
Carotid endarterectomy, in preventing stroke, 606
Carotid mechanoreceptors, 1112
Carrier(s)
    of genetically transmitted disease, 145
        obligate, 148
        Punnett square for heterozygous, 152, 152f
    of haptens, 222
Carrier detection tests, 152

Carrier protein. See Transport protein.
Cartilage, 39t
    articular, 1550–1554
    repair techniques for, 1554b
Cartilage anlage, 1618–1619
Cartilaginous joints, 1549
Caseation necrosis, 1293
Caseous necrosis, 82, 83f
Caspases, 85
Casts
    in fractured bone immobilization, 1571–1572
    in urine analysis, 1361
Catabolic (flow) phase, of burn injury, 1745
Catabolism, 21
    phases of, 24f
    of proteins, lipids, and polysaccharides, 23–24
Catalase, 7
Catalytic plasma membrane receptors, 15, 15t
Cataract(s), 509–510
Catechol-O-methyltransferase (COMT), 649
Catecholamines. See also Epinephrine; Norepinephrine.
    autonomic neurotransmission and action of, 469–470
    central stress response and release of, 339–343
    extracellular fluid potassium regulation and, 107
    immunologic effects of, 342–343
    physiologic effects of, 342t, 719–720
    synthesis of, in adrenal medulla, 719
    in systolic heart failure, 1190
    as tumor markers, 368t
    urine formation and, 1358
Cathelicidins, 185–186
Cation(s), 26
    extracellular and intracellular, 101, 101t
Cat's eye reflex, 691
Cauda equina, 456
Cauda equina syndrome, 594t, 1370
Causalgia, 494
Caveolae, 32
Cavernous angiomas (malformations), 607
Cavernous (congenital) hemangiomas, 1690–1691, 1691f
Cavernous sinus, 462
Cavitation, 1294
CC-chemokines, 205
CD (cluster of differentiation), 220–221
    selected, and associated function(s), 221t
CD1, 221t, 228, 237
CD2, 221t, 228, 228b, 231–233, 231f
CD2-associated protein, 1345–1346
CD3, 221t, 226, 233
    in TCR complex, 231–233, 231f, 243
CD4, 221t, 228, 228b, 233
    in TCR complex, 231–233, 231f, 243
CD4+ T cells, 238–239
    depletion of, in HIV infection, 319, 321–322, 323f

CD8, 221t, 228, 228b, 233
CD8+ T cells, 231–233, 231f, 243–244, 243f
CD19, 221t, 241–242
CD20, 221t, 245b
CD21, 221t, 241–242, 241f
CD25, 221t, 250
CD28, 221t, 228, 228b, 241–242, 241f, 244
CD40, 221t, 241–242, 241f
CD40-CD40L interaction, 242
CD45, 221t
CD45R, 233, 234f
CD58, 221t
CD80, 221t
CD154, 221t, 228, 228b, 241–242, 241f
Cecum, 1435–1436
Celiac crisis, 1527
Celiac ganglia, 467
Celiac sprue. *See* Gluten-sensitive enteropathy.
Cell adhesion molecules (CAMs), 12
Cell cycle, 33–35, 34f
phases of, 34
Cell death, 81–90, 82f
aging and, 88–89
necrotic, 81–84, 82f
programmed (apoptotic), 81b, 84–85
Cell killing mechanisms, 247–250, 249f
Cell lysis, 189
Cell-mediated hypersensitivity reactions, 258, 259t, 264, 264f
allergy and symptoms associated with, 266t, 267
Cell-mediated immunity, 219–220, 219f, 243–244. *See also* T lymphocytes (T cells), activation of.
Cell phones, electromagnetic emissions from, 424–425
Cell surface receptors. *See* Plasma membrane.
Cell-to-cell adhesions, 15–18
extracellular matrix in, 15–16
specialized junctions in, 16–18
Cellular accumulations, 76–81
Cellular adaptation, 47–50, 47f
and cell injury, 50–76. *See also* Cellular injury.
Cellular adhesion molecules (CAMs), examples of, in leukocyte interaction with endothelial cells, 199t
Cellular aging, 88–89. *See also* Aging.
Cellular biology, 1–45
altered, 46–95. *See also* Altered cellular biology.
cell-to-cell adhesions in, 15–18
communication and signal transduction in, 18–20
functional, 2
intracellular environment in, 96–125. *See also* Cellular environment.
membrane transport in, 25–33. *See also* Plasma membrane transport.
metabolic, 21–25
prokaryotes and eukaryotes in, 1–2
references on, 44

Cellular biology *(Continued)*
reproduction and cell cycle in, 33–35
structural and functional components in, 2–15
summary review of, 42b
and tissue formation, 35–44
Cellular communication, 18–20, 18f–19f
extracellular messengers and channel regulation in, 20
second messengers in, 20
signal transduction in, 19–20
Cellular components, structure and function of, 2–15, 3f
Cellular division, rates of, 35
Cellular environment, 96
acid-base balance in, 114–117
alterations in, 102–104
acid-base, 117. *See also* Acid-base balance.
calcium and phosphate, 111–112
magnesium, 114
potassium, 106–108
sodium and chloride, 102. *See also* Water balance.
water movement, 98–99
body fluid distribution and, 96–98
physiologic terminology of, 125b
references on, 125
sodium and chloride balance in, 101–102
summary review of, 123b
Cellular functions, 2
Cellular immunity
stress and, 344–346, 345f
tests evaluating, 287, 287t
Cellular injury, 50–76
asphyxial, 68–69
chemical, 55–62
common themes in, 52t
free radicals and reactive oxygen species in, 54–55
genetic factors in, 69
hypoxic, 52–62
immunologic and inflammatory, 69
infectious, 69
manifestations of, 76–81
mechanisms of, 52
nutritional imbalances causing, 69–71
progressive, and responses, 51t
reversible and irreversible, 50–51, 51f–52f
systemic manifestations of, 81, 81t
and tissue injury, 62–69
asphyxial, 68–69
blunt force in, 62–65
gunshot wounds in, 66–68
physical agents in, 71–76
sharp force in, 65–66
Cellular ion exchange buffering, 117
Cellular junctions, 16–18
Cellular mediation, of inflammatory response, 192–203
basophils in, 202
cellular receptors in, 192–195
eosinophils in, 202
mast cells in, 195–198
monocytes and macrophages in, 201–202
natural killer (NK) cells in, 202

Cellular mediation, of inflammatory response *(Continued)*
neutrophils in, 201
phagocytosis in, 198–201
platelets in, 202–203
products of, 203–205, 203f
Cellular metabolism, 21–25
adenosine triphosphate in, 22–23
altered, in shock, 1697–1699, 1698f
food and, 23–24
intermediary, 8
oxidative phosphorylation in, 24–25
Cellular receptors. *See* Plasma membrane receptors.
Cellular reproduction, 33–35
Cellular self-digestion, 5
Cellular swelling, 76
Cellulitis, 1663
Central canal, of spinal cord, 456
Central cervical cord syndrome, 594t
Central chemoreceptors, of pulmonary system, 1251
Central cyanosis, 1268–1269
Central lymphoid organs, 230
in B cell maturation, 233–235
in T cell maturation, 230–233
Central nervous system (CNS), 442–443, 449–465
afferent and efferent pathways of, 457–458
blood-brain barrier of, 465b
blood supply of, 462–465
cerebrospinal fluid and ventricular system of, 461
changes in aging of, 471–474, 474t
cellular, 471–474
functional, 474
structural, 471–474
divisions of, 449–456, 450t
forebrain, 452–455
hindbrain, 455–456
midbrain, 455
spinal cord, 456–458
embryonic development of, 665–668
imaging of, 474–480
angiographic, 476
computed tomographic, 474
echoencephalographic, 476
magnetic resonance, 474–475
magnetic resonance angiographic, 475
myelographic, 476
positron emission tomographic, 475
radionuclide, 475–476
roentgenographic, 474
motor pathways of, 458
nervous tissue organization in, 443
pain sensory pathways of, 483–486, 485f
plasticity of, 450–452
protective structures of, 459–462
references on, 480
sensory pathways of, 458–459
summary review of, 477b
testing of
cerebrospinal fluid, 476–480
electroencephalographic, 476
evoked potential, 476
thermal sensory pathways of, 485f

Central nervous system disorders, 583–591
causing visual dysfunction, 511–512
cerebrovascular, 600. *See also* Cerebrovascular disorders.
in children, 665–695
and adults, comparison of, 668
cerebrovascular disease, 684–685
encephalopathies, 675. *See also* Childhood encephalopathies.
structural malformations, 668–669. *See also* Congenital hydrocephalus; Cranial deformities; Neural tube defects.
tumors, 685. *See also* Childhood cancer.
demyelinating, 630. *See also* Multiple sclerosis.
genetic basis of selected, 526t
headache in, 609–611
infective and inflammatory, 620–623. *See also* Central nervous system infection / inflammation.
neurodegenerative, 633–634
pathophysiologic processes in cerebral hemodynamics, 557–560
cognitive function, 525–528
motor function, 561–570
references on, 643
sleep disorders associated with, 505–506
spinal degenerative, 596–598
summary review of, 641b
traumatic, 583–591
involving brain, 583–591. *See also* Traumatic brain injury.
involving spinal cord, 591. *See also* Spinal cord injury.
and temperature regulation disorders, 502
tumors in, 611–619. *See also* Brain cancer, and tumors; Nerve sheath tumors; Spinal cord tumors.
Central nervous system infection / inflammation, 620–623
in encephalitis, 625–626
in Lyme disease, 629–630
in meningitis, 620–623. *See also* Meningitis.
as neurologic complications of AIDS, 626–630. *See also under* AIDS.
in suppurative cerebral masses, 624. *See also* Brain abscess; Spinal cord abscess.
Central neurogenic hyperventilation, 529–531, 531f
Central pain, 494
Central reflex hyperpnea, 530t
Central sensitization, 488
Central stress response, 339–346, 340f
catecholamines in, 339–343, 342t
cortisol in, 343–344, 343t
Central sulcus, 452

Central tolerance, 222
 in bone marrow, 235
 breakdown of, in autoimmunity, 267–269
 in thymus, 233
Central transtentorial herniation, 559
Centriacinar emphysema, 1289–1290
Centriole, 9
Centromere, 34–35
Cephalic phase, of gastric secretion, 1427
Cerebellar (ataxic) gait, 576
Cerebellar memory, 543
Cerebellar motor syndromes, 577, 578t
Cerebellar multiple sclerosis, 632b, 633
Cerebellum, 450t, 455
Cerebral angiography, 476
Cerebral aqueduct, 455
Cerebral arteries, anterior, middle, posterior, 462
 areas of brain supplied by, **and occlusive conditions,** 463t, 464f
Cerebral blood flow, 557, 557b
Cerebral blood volume, 557, 557b
Cerebral concussion, classic, 590
Cerebral contusions, 585, 585f
 clinical manifestations of, 585–586
Cerebral cortex, 450–452, 450t
 pain processing in, 484
Cerebral death, 534–535
Cerebral edema, 559–560, 559f
Cerebral hemisphere(s), 450t
 midline cortical and deep areas of, 544f
 regions of, 451f
Cerebral hemodynamic alterations, 557–560
 edema in, 559–560
 herniation syndromes in, 559
 hydrocephalus in, 560
 increased intracranial pressure in, 557–559
 references on, 580
 summary review of, 578b
 treatment goals in, 554t
Cerebral hemodynamics, 557–559, 557b
Cerebral hemorrhage, 602
Cerebral infarctions, 602
Cerebral nuclei, 452–453
Cerebral palsy, 675, 1632
 associated neurologic disorders in, 676
 clinical manifestations of, 676
 diagnosis of, 1632–1633
 evaluation and treatment of, 676–679, 1633
 pathophysiology of, 675–676
 risk factors and known causes of, 676t
Cerebral peduncles, 450t
Cerebral perfusion pressure (CPP), 557, 557b
Cerebral thrombosis, 601
Cerebral vasospasm, 608
Cerebromedullary cistern, 460
Cerebrospinal fluid (CSF), 461
 analysis of, 476–480, 476t
 composition of, 461t

Cerebrovascular accidents (CVAs), 600–601
 in children, 600b
 clinical manifestations of, 602–603
 ethnicity and, 600
 evaluation and treatment of, 603–606
 incidence of, 600
 morbidity and mortality in, 600
 pathophysiology of, 602, 603f
 preventing recurrence of, 606
 risk factors for, 600–601
 secondary to occlusion or stenosis, 604t
 stroke syndromes caused by, 601
Cerebrovascular disorders, 600
 cerebrovascular accidents in, 600–601
 in children, 684–685
 intracranial aneurysms in, 606
 subarachnoid hemorrhage in, 608
 vascular malformations in, 607
Cerebrum, 452
Cervical cancer, 841
 clinical manifestations of, 842–844, 842b
 environmental factors associated with, 397t
 evaluation and treatment of, 844–846, 844t
 human papillomaviruses and, 425
 pathogenesis of, 841–842
 prognosis for, 844
 staging of, 842t
Cervical cancer prevention, humanpapilloma virus (HPV) vaccine in, 805b
Cervical cancer screening, recent recommendations for, 942t
Cervical carcinoma in situ, 841–842, 843f–844f
Cervical dysplasia, 841–842
Cervical epithelial cell abnormalities, 841, 841t
Cervical intraepithelial carcinoma, 841–842, 843f
Cervical mucus test, 808t
Cervical spondylosis, 598
Cervicitis, 832
 chlamydial, 936, 936f
 gonococcal, 925–926, 926f
Cervix, uterine, 787–789
cGMP. *See* Cyclic guanosine monophosphate.
Chalazion, 506
Chancre(s), 928
 penile and vulvar, 928, 929f
Chancroid, 932
 clinical manifestations of, 932, 933f
 evaluation and treatment of, 932–933
 pathophysiology of, 932
 penile and vulvar, 928, 932, 933f
Channel-linked plasma membrane receptors, 15, 15t
Channel regulation, 20, 21f
Charcot neuroarthropathy, 763
CHD. *See* Coronary heart disease.
Chédiak-Higashi syndrome, 283, 1049
Chemical agents, affecting heart rate, 1113

Chemical asphyxiants, 68
Chemical burns, 1742
Chemical carcinogens, 426
 and breast cancer risk, 893–895, 894t
 classification of, 427b
Chemical cell injury, 55–62
 agents causing, 56–62
Chemical reactions, of metabolism, 496
Chemical synapses, 18–19, 448–449
Chemical thermogenesis, heat production in, 496
Chemo brain, 390
Chemokines, 203, 203f, 205
Chemoreceptor reflex, 1126f
Chemoreceptors, 445b
 arterial, 1125
Chemotactic factor, 36, 189
Chemotaxis, 36, 196
Chemotherapy, 387–388. *See also* evaluation and treatment under specific malignancy.
 adjuvant, 388
 induction, 388
 molecular-era, 387–388, 387t
 neoadjuvant, 388
 and secondary immune deficiencies, 286
Chest radiography, 1262–1263
 in cardiac function evaluation, 1134
Chest wall, 1249
 in children, 1311–1312
 disorders of, 1271–1272
 elastic properties of, 1253
Chest wall compliance, 1253
 in children, 1311–1312
Chest wall restriction, 1271–1272
Cheyne-Stokes respiration, 530t, 531, 531f, 1268
Chickenpox, 1664, 1687–1688, 1687t
 clinical manifestations of, 1687–1688, 1688f
 complications of, 1688
 treatment of, 1688
Chief cells, 1426
Child abuse, 1640
 burn injuries in, 1741, 1742f
Childhood asthma, 1330–1331
 clinical manifestations of, 1333
 controller therapy in, 1334
 evaluation and treatment of, 1333–1334
 goal of therapy in, 1334
 pathophysiology of, 1331–1333, 1331f–1332f
Childhood cancer, 436–441, 685. *See also* Childhood leukemia(s).
 brain neoplasms in, 685
 drugs that increase risk of, 440t
 embryonal, 688
 environmental factors associated with, 401, 403–404, 427b, 436, 439
 etiology of, 437–439
 genetics of, 438–439, 438t
 incidence and types of, 436–437
 nutritional support in, 440b
 prognosis for, 440–441
 references on, 441
 summary review of, 440b

Childhood disorders
 burns in, 1741–1743. *See also* Pediatric burn injury.
 cancer in, 436–441, 685. *See also* Childhood cancer.
 cardiovascular, 1209
 acquired, 1234. *See also* Childhood obesity; Hypertension; Kawasaki disease.
 congenital, 1213–1214. *See also* Congenital heart defects.
 encephalopathic, 675. *See also* Childhood encephalopathies.
 gastrointestinal, 1516
 acquired, 1522–1523
 congenital, 1516
 diarrhea in, 1530–1531
 impaired nutrition in, 1524
 hematologic, 1062
 anemias, 1065, 1066t
 clotting factor and platelet disorders, 1078–1079
 erythrocyte disorders, 1065
 leukemias and lymphomas, 1083–1084
 mood disorders in, 657, 657b
 musculoskeletal, 1620–1621
 abnormal skeletal modeling in, 1624
 bone infection in, 1628
 cerebral palsy in, 1632
 congenital, 1620–1621
 juvenile rheumatoid arthritis in, 1630–1631
 muscular dystrophy in, 1633
 nonaccidental trauma in, 1640
 osteochondroses in, 1631
 tumors in, 1637
 neurologic, 665–695. *See also* Childhood neurologic disorders.
 renal and urinary, 1404–1408
 congenital, 1404–1407. *See also* Congenital renal and urinary tract disorders.
 glomerular, 1407–1408
 renal injury in, 1411
 Wilms tumor in, 1413
 respiratory, 1310–1343. *See also* Childhood respiratory disorders.
 shock and multiple organ dysfunction syndrome in, 1727. *See also* Multiple organ dysfunction syndrome; Shock.
 of skin, 1680–1695. *See also* Skin disorders.
 tumors in, 685
 of brain, 685
 embryonal, 688
Childhood encephalopathies, 675
 acute, 681
 drug induced, 682
 meningitis in, 682
 Reye syndrome in, 681
 viral meningitis in, 684
 HIV infection in, 684
 static, 675
 cerebral palsy in, 675
 inherited metabolic disorders in, 677–679
 seizure disorders in, 679

Childhood leukemia(s), 437,
1083–1084
classification of, 1083
clinical manifestations of,
1084–1085, 1085f
evaluation and treatment of,
1085–1087
immunologic classification of,
1084
pathogenesis of, 1084
prognosis in, 1086, 1086t
treatment phases in, 1086
types of, 1083–1084
Childhood lymphoma(s),
1086–1087
Hodgkin, 1088
non-Hodgkin, 1087
Childhood neurologic disorders,
665–695
adult and, comparison of, 668
cerebrovascular disease in,
684–685
encephalopathies in, 675. *See also*
Childhood encephalopathies.
references on, 693
structural malformations in,
668–669. *See also* Congenital
hydrocephalus; Cranial
deformities; Neural tube
defects.
summary review of, 691b
tumors in, 685. *See also* Brain
cancer, and tumors;
Embryonic tumors.
Childhood obesity, 1237–1238
incidence and epidemiology of,
1237
and nonalcoholic fatty liver,
1532–1533, 1533b
prevention of, 1238
Childhood respiratory disorders
diagnostic breathing sounds in,
1313–1314, 1313f–1314f
infectious, 1315–1316, 1315t, 1326
aspiration pneumonitis,
1329–1330
bronchiolitis, 1326
croup, 1316
epiglottitis, 1317
pneumonia, 1327
of lower airway, 1320–1321
acute respiratory distress
syndrome in, 1334
asthma in, 1330–1331
bronchiolitis obliterans in, 1330
bronchopulmonary dysplasia
in, 1323–1324
cystic fibrosis in, 1336
infectious, 1326
respiratory distress syndrome
in, 1321
protective strategies for
ventilation in, 1323, 1326
references on, 1341
summary review of, 1339b
of upper airway, 1313–1318,
1313b
angioedema, 1318
congenital malformations, 1320
foreign body aspiration,
1317–1318
infections, 1315–1316,
1315t. *See also* Croup;
Epiglottitis.

Childhood respiratory disorders
(Continued)
laryngomalacia and
tracheomalacia, 1319
obstructive sleep apnea, 1320
subglottic stenosis, 1318–1319
vocal cord paralysis, 1319
Children. *See also* Childhood
disorders; Infant(s);
Neonate(s).
cardiovascular development in,
1213
fever response in, 500
fluid and electrolyte balance in,
1404
hematologic assessment values in,
985t, 1063–1064, 1064t
hematologic development in, 982
immune response in, 251
innate immunity in, 213
nonaccidental trauma to, 1640
pain perception in, 495
sleep patterns in, 504
temperature regulation in, 498
urine output in, 1403–1404, 1404t
Chlamydia spp., 298, 299t
Chlamydia trachomatis, 298, 299t,
935
Chlamydiae, 298t
Chlamydial cervicitis, 936, 936f
Chlamydial conjunctivitis, 507
Chlamydial ophthalmia, 936–937,
937f
Chlamydial pneumonia, 1291
in children, 1328t, 1329
Chlamydial urogenital infections,
935
clinical manifestations of,
935–937
diagnostic tests for, 806t
evaluation and treatment of, 937
gonococcal infection and, 927
similarity of clinical syndromes,
936t
lymphogranuloma venereum
in, 937
pathophysiology of, 935
Chloride, extracellular, 102
alterations in, 102–104
Chlorination byproducts, in cancer
epidemiology, 397t
Choking asphyxiation, 68
Cholangiocellular carcinoma,
1503–1504
Cholecalciferol. *See* Vitamin D.
Cholecystitis, 1495
chronic, and associated cancer, 378t
in sickle cell disease, 1076
Cholecystokinin, 1425, 1425t, 1444,
1479
Cholelithiasis, 1494–1495
clinical manifestations of, 1495
evaluation and treatment of,
1495–1496
pathophysiology of, 1495
Cholera pandemic, 297t
Choleresis, 1440
Choleretic agent, 1440
Cholesterol esterase, 1432–1433
Cholesterol gallstones, 1495
Cholinergic crisis, 640
Cholinergic transmission, 467–469
and nicotinic and muscarinic
neuroreceptors, 472t

Chondroblasts, 1542f
Chondrocytes, 1550–1551
Chondrogenic tumors, 1591
Chondroid, 1591
Chondrosarcoma, 1591, 1591f
Chopping wounds, 66
Chordae tendinae, 1094
Chordee, 1404–1405, 1405f
Chorea, 568t, 570
in rheumatic fever, 1186
Choroid, 507
Choroid plexus tumor, 612t
Choroid plexuses, 460
functions of, 461
Christmas disease, 1078–1079
Christmas factor (clotting
factor IX), 977t
disorders associated with, 1079t
Chromaffin cells, 719
Chromatids, 34–35, 138f
Chromatin, 3f–4f, 126
changes in, during cell cycle, 34
Chromophils, 707
Chromophobes, 707
Chromosomal mosaics, 137
Chromosome(s), 34, 134–143
gene loci assigned to specific, 157
in metaphase spread, 134
structure of, 4f, 138f
Chromosome aberrations
numerical, and associated
diseases, 135–143
aneuploidy, 136–142
polyploidy, 135–136
prenatal diagnosis of, 139b
structural, and associated diseases,
142–143
Chromosome bands, 135, 138f
Chromosome breakage, 142
Chromosome instability, 375
Chromosome theory of inheritance,
146
Chromosome translocation
mutations, in oncogenes,
371–372
Chronic active hepatitis, 1490
Chronic alcoholic hepatitis, 1492
Chronic alcoholism, 60–61
Chronic bacterial prostatitis, 862
Chronic bronchitis, 1286
airway obstruction in, 1282,
1282f
clinical manifestations of,
1287–1288, 1288t
evaluation and treatment of,
1288–1289
pathophysiology of, 1286–1287,
1287f
Chronic conjunctivitis, 507
Chronic cough, 1266–1267
Chronic diarrhea, in children,
1530–1531
Chronic fatigue syndrome, 1608
clinical manifestations of, 1608
evaluation and treatment of,
1608–1611
pathophysiology of, 1608
Chronic gastritis, 1464
signs and symptoms of, 1464
Chronic glomerulonephritis, 1381t,
1383, 1384f
clinical manifestations of,
1383–1384
evaluation and treatment of, 1384

Chronic graft rejection, 275
Chronic granulomatous disease,
283–284
Chronic hepatitis, 1490
in children, 1532
Chronic (complicated)
hypertension, 1152–1154
pathophysiology of, 1152–1154,
1155t
Chronic inflammation, 206–208,
207f
and cancer, 377–378, 378t
lymphocyte and macrophage
action in, 207–208
Chronic kidney disease, 1389
clinical manifestations of,
1393–1396, 1393f
evaluation and treatment of,
1386t, 1396–1398
nutritional support in, 1396b
pathophysiology of, 1389–1393
progression of, 1392, 1392f
indicators of, 1391t–1392t,
1393–1396
stages of, 1390t
Chronic left heart failure,
management of, 1194. *See also*
Systolic heart failure.
Chronic leukemia(s), 1019, 1025
clinical manifestations of,
1027–1028
evaluation and treatment of,
1028–1029
pathophysiology of, 1025–1027
Chronic lung disease of infancy,
1323–1324
Chronic lymphocytic leukemia
(CLL), 1025
cellular morphology in, 1029f
clinical manifestations of,
1027–1028
Chronic lymphocytic thyroiditis,
741
Chronic mesenteric insufficiency,
1477
Chronic mucocutaneous
candidiasis, 279
Chronic myelogenous leukemia
(CML), 1025
cellular morphology in, 1029f
chromosome translocation in,
371–372
clinical manifestations of, 1028
Chronic myeloproliferative
disorders, 1009, 1027
clinical manifestations of, 1010
evaluation and treatment of,
1010–1012
pathophysiology of, 1009–1010
Chronic nonspecific diarrhea, 1530
Chronic obstructive pulmonary
disease (COPD), 1286
air trapping mechanism in, 1287,
1288f
chronic bronchitis in, 1286. *See
also* Chronic bronchitis.
clinical manifestations of, 1288t
emphysema in, 1288–1289. *See
also* Emphysema.
risk factors for, 1286
malnutrition in, 1286b
sleep disorders and, 506
upper and lower airway
inflammation in, 1283b

Chronic orthostatic hypotension, 1157
Chronic otitis media, 515
Chronic pain, 492–493
  acute pain and, comparison of, 491t
  behavioral and psychologic responses to, 492
  in cancer patients, 493
  in low back, 492
  in myofascial pain syndrome, 492
  neuromatrix theory of, 494b
  physiologic responses to, 492
  postoperative, 492–493
Chronic pancreatitis, 1497
Chronic paroxysmal hemicrania, 611
Chronic pericarditis, 1177–1178
Chronic pyelonephritis, 1377
  in children, 1411–1412
  clinical manifestations of, 1378
  evaluation and treatment of, 1378
Chronic renal failure. *See* Chronic kidney disease.
Chronic venous insufficiency, 1143
Chvostek sign, 112
Chylomicrons, 1161–1162, 1433
Chylothorax, 1273, 1274t
Chyme, 1423–1424
Chymotrypsin, 1430–1432
Cigar/pipe smoke, and cancer, 404
Cigarette smoking
  cancer and, 404
  coronary artery disease and, 1164
Cilia, 36
Ciliate protozoa, 310, 310t
Cingulate gyrus herniation, 559
Circadian rhythm, 496
Circadian rhythm sleep disorders, 505
Circle of Willis, 462, 463f
Circulating anticoagulants test, 983t
Circulatory system, 1091–1093, 1092f
  autonomic innervation of, 1100–1103, 1101f
  blood flow function in, 1117–1122
  blood pressure regulation in, 1122–1130. *See also* Blood pressure.
  cardiac anatomy and function in, 1093–1096. *See also* Heart.
  coronary, 1130–1131
  fetal, and fetal shunts, 1211–1213, 1212f
  great vessels of, 1095. *See also* Heart.
  lymphatic, 1131–1133
  neonatal, 1211–1213
  postnatal, 1213
  pulmonary, 1247–1249
  summary review of, 1137b
  transitional, 1211–1213
  vascular anatomy and function in, 1113–1131, 1114f. *See also* Blood vessels.
Circumflex artery, 1097
Cirrhosis, 77, 1491–1492
  in alcoholic hepatitis, 61f, 1491–1492
  ascites development in, 1483, 1484f
  in children, 1532–1533
  clinical manifestations of, 1492–1493, 1494f

Cirrhosis *(Continued)*
  etiologies of, 1492t
  evaluation and treatment of, 1493–1495
  pathophysiology of, 1492
  reversal of, cellular mechanisms of, 60–61, 60b
CIS (carcinoma in situ), 361, 362f
Cisterna magna, 460
Cisternae, 5
Citric acid cycle, 23–24
Cl⁻. *See* Chloride.
Clasp-knife phenomenon, 538, 634
Class I restriction, of CD8+ T cells, 243–244, 247–248
Class II restriction, of CD4+ T cells, 238–239
Class switch, immunoglobulin, 242, 242f
Classic cerebral concussion, 590
Classical pathway, of complement cascade activation, 188–189, 190f
Clastogens, 142
Clathrin, 5, 31
Clathrin coated vesicles, 5
Clear cell tumors, 1372
Clearance, 1360
  and glomerular filtration rate, 1360
  and renal blood flow, 1360
Cleft lip and/or cleft palate, 167, 1516, 1517f
  clinical manifestations of, 1517
  evaluation and treatment of, 1517–1518
  pathophysiology of, 1516–1517
  recurrence risks for, 170t
Clitoris, 785
Cloacal exstrophy, 1406
Clonal deletion, 233
Clonal diversity, generation of, 218, 219f, 229–235, 230t
Clonal expansion, 368
Clonal proliferations, 368, 369f
Clonal selection, 218–219, 219f, 230
  antigen processing and presentation in, 235–237
  pathways of, 236–237
  B cell activation in, 240–243, 241f
  in development of cancer, 368
  helper T cell subpopulations in, 237–240, 239f
  induction of, 230t, 235–244
  secondary lymphoid sites of, 235, 236f
Clonic phase, 538
Cloning
  gene, 159
    human, 160b
  lymphocyte, in immune response, 217–220, 219f
Closed angle glaucoma, 510t, 511f
Closed fracture, 1569
Closed head trauma, 583–584
Clostridium botulinum, 299t
Clostridium botulinum toxin, 305
Clostridium difficile, 299t
Clostridium difficile toxin, 305
Clostridium perfringens, 299t
Clostridium perfringens enterotoxin, 305
Clostridium tetani, 298, 299t
Clostridium tetani neurotoxin, 305

Clot retraction test, 983t
Clotting factor(s), 954
  antihemophilic (clotting factor VIII), 977t
  assays for, 1446t
  calcium, 977t
  Christmas (clotting factor IX), 977t
  clinical evaluation of, 983t
  fibrin-stabilizing (clotting factor XIII), 977t
  fibrinogen (clotting factor I), 953–954, 977t
  function of, 976–977
  Hageman (clotting factor XII), 192, 977t
  labile (clotting factor V), 977t
  plasma thromboplastin antecedent (clotting factor XI), 977t
  prothrombin (clotting factor II), 977t
  stable (clotting factor VII), 977t
  Stuart-Prower (clotting factor X), 977t
  synonyms for, 977t
  tissue, 976–977
Clotting factor disorders, 1049–1051
  in children, 1078–1079
  consumptive thrombohemorrhagic, 1050–1051
  disseminated intravascular coagulation in, 1050–1051
  liver disease and, 1049–1050
  thromboembolic, 1055–1059
  vitamin K deficiency and, 1049
Clotting (coagulation) system, 976, 978f
  in inflammatory response, 190–191
Clotting time(s), tests evaluating, 1079–1081
Clubbing, digital, 1269, 1269f
  paraneoplastic, 389t
Clubfoot (talipes), 167. *See also Equinovarus* entries.
  recurrence risks for, 170t
Cluster breathing, 530t, 531f
Cluster headache, 611
Coagulation cascade, 190, 191f, 1710
  activating pathways of, 190
Coagulation disorders, 1049–1051. *See also* Clotting factor disorders.
Coagulation factors. *See* Clotting factor(s).
Coagulation inhibitor levels, assays for, 1054
Coagulative necrosis, 82, 83f
Coal miner lung, 1278
Coal worker pneumoconiosis, 1278
Coarctation of aorta, 1226
  clinical manifestations of, 1226
  evaluation and treatment of, 1228
  pathophysiology of, 1226
  postductal and preductal, 1227f
  hemodynamics of, 1227f
Coated pits, 31
Cobalamin. *See* Vitamin B12.
Cocaine and crack use, biological effects of, 63t
Coccidioides immitis, 307, 308t

Cochlea, 514
Codominance, 145
Codon(s), 129
Cognitive competence, 525
Cognitive dysfunction, 525–528
  awareness alterations in, 542–544
  coma in, 528
  data processing deficits in, 546–548
  genetic basis of selected, 526t
  HIV associated, 628t
  key terminology of, 580b
  references on, 580
  seizures in, 536–537
  summary review of, 578b
Cognitive function, central neural areas mediating, 542, 542f–543f
Cogwheel rigidity, 573
Cold agglutinin autoimmune hemolytic anemia, 1005
Cold autoimmune hemolytic anemia, 274
Cold hemolysin autoimmune hemolytic anemia, 1005
Cold shock, 1735
Cold sores, 1663
Colipase, 1432–1433
Collagen, 16, 210
Collagen fibers
  in bone matrix, 1544–1545
  in musculoskeletal tissues, 1545t
Collagen fibril, heterotypic, 1550–1551, 1553f
Collagen matrix assembly, impaired, 211–212
Collagen synthesis, gene mutations affecting, 1624–1625
Collagen zones, 1550–1551, 1552f
Collagenic tumors, 1591–1592
Collagenous fibers, 36–38
Collateral arteries, 1097–1098
Collateral ganglia, 467
Collecting ducts, nephron, 1347
Collectins, 186
Colloid osmotic pressure, 27–28
Colloid replacement, in shock therapy, 1738, 1740, 1745–1746
Colon, 1435–1437, 1436f
Colon and rectal cancer, 175–176, 1498t, 1500
  clinical manifestations of, 1501
    by location of primary lesion, 1502f
  differential diagnosis of, 1502t
  evaluation and treatment of, 1501–1503
  metastasis of, 384t
  pathogenesis of, 1500–1501, 1500f–1501f
  staging of, 1502–1503
Colonic movement, 1436
Colonization, by infectious microorganisms, 296
Colony stimulating factors (CSFs), 961t, 963
  clinical uses of, 965
  physiologic effects of, 965, 966f
Color blindness, 511
Color vision dysfunction, 511
Colorectal cancer. *See* Colon and rectal cancer.
Columnar cells, 36

Coma, 528
  clinical manifestations of, 529t
    comparative, 536t
  differentiation of causes of, 529t
  evaluation of, 528, 529t
    breathing patterns in, 529–531
    level of consciousness in,
      528–535
    motor responses in, 532
    oculomotor responses in,
      531–532
    pupillary changes in, 531
  irreversible, 534–535
  outcomes of, 532–535
  pathophysiology of, 528
  prognosis for emergence from,
    535
**Combined T and B lymphocyte
  deficiencies,** 278–281
Combustion byproducts, in cancer
  epidemiology, 397t
Comedone, 1653t
Commensalism, 295b
Comminuted fracture, 1569
Commissural fibers, 452
Common bile duct, 1439
Common bundle, 1100–1101
**Common variable immune
  deficiency,** 279
Communicability, of pathogen, 297
Communicating hydrocephalus,
  560
**Community acquired methicillin-
  resistant _Staphylococcus
  aureus_ (C-MRSA) infection,
  cutaneous,** 1662–1663, 1662b
Community acquired pneumonia,
  1290–1291
  in children, 1327
Compact (cortical) bone,
  1545–1546, 1547f
Compartment disorders, 820
Compartment II disorders, 820
Compartment III disorders, 820
Compartment IV disorders, 820
Compartment syndrome, 1575–1576
  pathogenesis of, 1578f
**Compensated disseminated
  intravascular coagulation,**
  1053
Compensated maintenance,
  bicarbonate and carbonic acid,
  115–116, 116f
Compensated shock, 1727
Compensation, 166
Compensatory growth, 1367
Compensatory hyperplasia, 49, 210
Compensatory hypertrophy, 1367
Competence, 525
Competitive inhibitors, 28
Complement cascade, 188
Complement cascade activation,
  in inflammatory response,
  188–190, 1710
  most important result of, 189
  pathways of, 188, 190f
Complement deficiencies, 278, 281,
  282f
  gene defects in, 276t
Complement receptors, 194–195
Complementary base pairing, 129
Complementary-determining region
  (CDR), of antibody molecule,
  224–225

**Complete atrioventricular canal
  defect,** 1222
Complete blood count (CBC), in
  immune deficiency evaluation,
  287, 287t
Complete fracture, 1569
**Complex motor performance
  disorders,** 575–577
  expressive alterations in,
    576–577
  gait alterations in, 576
  postural alterations in,
    575–576
Complex regional pain syndromes,
  494
Complex sclerosing lesion, breast,
  874–875
Compliance, ventilatory, 1253
  in children, 1311–1312
Complicated plaque, 1159–1160
Compound fracture, of skull, 584,
  588
Compression atelectasis, 1275
Compressive syndrome, 619
Computed tomography (CT)
  in cardiac function testing,
    1134–1135
  of central nervous system, 474
  of gastrointestinal tract, 1444
  risks from ionizing radiation
    exposure in, 416, 417b
  in systemic vascular evaluation,
    1136
Concentration gradient, 26
Concordant traits, 170, 171t
Concussion(s)
  classic cerebral, 590
  mild, 590
  sports related, 590b
Conditional response, 339
Conducting airway(s), pulmonary,
  1242–1244, 1243f, 1246f
Conduction dysphasia, 549t
Conduction system, of heart,
  1099–1103, 1101f
  adrenergic receptors of, 1105
Conductive hearing loss, 515
Conductive heat loss, 497
Condylomata acuminata, 940–941,
  1664
  penile, 941f
  vulvar and perineal, 941f
Condylomata lata, 930f
Cones, 507
Confusion, differences between
  organic and functional,
  551–553, 552t
Confusional states, acute, 548
  clinical manifestations of, 551
  evaluation and treatment of,
    551–553, 552t
  pathophysiology of, 548–551
Congenital aganglionic megacolon,
  1521, 1521f
  clinical manifestations of, 1521
  evaluation and treatment of,
    1521–1523
  pathophysiology of, 1521
**Congenital conditions, and
  diseases,** 171
  associated with cancer in children,
    438–439, 438t
Congenital foot deformities,
  1622–1624

**Congenital gastrointestinal
  disorders,** 1516
  aganglionic megacolon in, 1521
  anorectal malformations in, 1522
  cleft lip and palate in, 1516
  distal intestinal obstruction
    syndrome in, 1520–1521
  duodenal, jejunal and ileal
    obstructions in, 1521
  esophageal malformations in,
    1518
  intestinal malrotation in, 1519
  meconium ileus in, 1520
  pyloric stenosis in, 1519
Congenital glaucoma, 510t
Congenital heart defects, 1213–1214
  classification of, 1215–1216, 1216t
  conditions resulting from
    decreasing pulmonary blood
      flow, 1223
    heart failure, 1216, 1216t
    hypoxemia, 1217–1218
    increasing pulmonary blood
      flow, 1218
    mixing hemodynamics,
      1230–1231
    obstructed hemodynamics,
      1226
  disorders coexistent with, 1215t
  environmental factors associated
    with, 1214t
  etiology of, 1214–1216, 1215t
  genetic factors associated with,
    1214, 1215t
  risk of endocarditis in children
    with, 1214b
Congenital hemolytic anemia, 1070
Congenital hydrocephalus,
  673–674, 675f
  clinical manifestations of, 674
  evaluation and treatment of, 675
  pathophysiology of, 674, 674f
Congenital hypothyroidism,
  741–742
Congenital immune deficiencies,
  275. _See also_ Primary immune
  deficiencies.
Congenital malformations
  and childhood cancers, 438
  genes and environmental
    interaction in, 171–172
  liability distribution of, 167
  prevalence of, in Caucasian
    population, 172t
  recurrence risks for relatives, 170t
**Congenital musculoskeletal
  disorders,** 1620–1621
  developmental dysplasia of hip
    in, 1621
  foot deformities in, 1622–1624
  syndactyly in, 1620–1621
Congenital myasthenic syndromes,
  638–639
Congenital nephrotic syndrome,
  1410
Congenital neutropenia, severe, 282
Congenital nipple inversion, 876t
**Congenital renal and urinary tract
  disorders,** 1404–1407
  bladder exstrophy in, 1405–1406
  bladder outlet obstruction in, 1406
  epispadias in, 1405
  hypoplastic and dysplastic kidneys
    in, 1406–1407

**Congenital renal and urinary tract
  disorders** (Continued)
  hypospadias in, 1404–1405
  polycystic kidneys in, 1407
  renal agenesis in, 1407
  robotic surgical repair of, 1406b
  ureteropelvic junction obstruction
    in, 1406
Congenital syphilis, 929–930
Congestive cardiomyopathy,
  1178–1180
Congestive heart failure. _See_ Left
  heart failure.
Congestive splenomegaly, 1043
Conjugated bile salts, 1471
Conjugated bilirubin, 1440
Conjunctivitis, 506–507
Conn disease, 768
Connective tissue, 16, 36–38
  types of, with location and
    function, 39t
Connective tissue disorders
  autoimmune, 257t
  congenital heart defects associated
    with, 1215t
  incidence of, in children, 1630t
Connexons, 16–18
Consanguinity, 151–152
Consciousness, 525–528
Consolidation, of lung tissue, 1294
Constipation, 1453
  clinical manifestations of, 1454
  evaluation and treatment of, 1454
  pathophysiology of, 1453–1454,
    1453b
  Rome III criteria for, 1454
Constrictive pericarditis,
  1177–1178, 1178f
**Consumptive thrombohemorrhagic
  disorders,** 1050–1051
Contact burns, 1741
Contact dermatitis, 267, 268f
  allergic, 1655–1656
  irritant, 1656
  substances causing, 1657b
Contact factor. _See_ Hageman factor.
Contact guidance, 36
Contact range entrance wounds, 66
Content of thought, 525–528
Continuous renal replacement therapy
  (hemodialysis), 1389, 1390b
Contraction, muscle fiber, 1561
Contracture(s), 212, 1606
  of burn scar, 1715f
Contralateral control, 452
contrecoup pattern of injury, 63
Contusion(s), 62–63, 64f
Conus, 1231
Conus medullaris, 456
Conus medullaris syndrome, 594t
Convalescent period, of infectious
  disease, 296
Convective heat loss, 497
Convergence, of axons, 443
Cooley anemia, 1077
Coping strategies, for stress, 354
Copper
  and effect on bone tissue
    physiology, 1580b
  in erythropoiesis, 969t
Cor pulmonale, 1298
  clinical manifestations of, 1298
  evaluation and treatment of, 1298
  pathophysiology of, 1297f

Core temperature, body, mechanisms of preserving, 497–498

Corner (metaphyseal) fracture, 1640, 1640f

Cornification, 795

Coronary angiography, 1135

Coronary arterial evaluation fluoroscopic, 1135
single-photon emission computed tomography in, 1134
stress testing in, 1134

Coronary arteries, 1096–1097, 1100f
collateral arteries and, 1097–1098
in oxygen supply to cardiac metabolism, 1108

Coronary arterioles, adrenergic receptors of, 1105

Coronary artery bypass graft (CABG), 1169

Coronary artery disease (CAD), 1160–1165
in chronic diabetes mellitus, 763–764
development of, 1160–1165
cigarette smoking in, 1164
diabetes mellitus in, 1164
dyslipidemia in, 1161–1164
hypertension in, 1164
obesity in, 1164
sedentary life style in, 1164
lipoprotein genes contributing to risk of, 175t
risk factors for, 1160–1161
modifiable, 1161
nonmodifiable, 1161
nontraditional, 1164–1165
serum markers as, 1164b
sleep disorders and, 506
in women, 1161b

Coronary artery evaluation, 1133–1135

Coronary capillaries, 1098

Coronary circulation, 1100f
autoregulation of, 1131
regulation of, 1130–1131
autonomic, 1131

Coronary heart disease (CHD)
familial hypercholesterolemia in development of, 172, 173b
genes and environmental interaction in, 172–174
psychosocial stress and progression to, 347, 347b

Coronary perfusion pressure, 1130

Coronary sulcus, 1097

Coronary veins, and lymphatics, 1099, 1100f

Coronary vessels, 1096–1099, 1100f
adrenergic receptors of, 1105

Corpora cavernosa, 798–799

Corpora quadrigemina, 450t, 455

Corpus, uterine, 787–788

Corpus callosum, 452

Corpus luteum, 789

Corpus luteum cyst, 837

Corpus spongiosum, 798–799

Corpus striatum, 452–453

Correction, of buffering system, 116, 116f

Cortex, somatic sensory and motor areas of, 453f

Corticobulbar tract, 458

Corticospinal tracts, 452

Corticosteroid-binding globulin, 343

Corticosteroid treatment, for nephrotic syndrome in children, 1375t

Corticotropin, 1706–1707

Corticotropin-dependent Cushing syndrome, 765

Corticotropin-independent Cushing syndrome, 765

Corticotropin-related hormones, 707, 708t

Corticotropin-releasing hormone (CRH), 339
hypothalamic release of, 703–704, 707t
indirect effect of, on immune response, 345, 346f
stress induced, and altered female reproductive physiology, 349, 350t

Cortisol, 717
in central stress response, 343–344
physiologic effects of, 343t
immune system and, 344–346
stress induced, 346
and development of type 2 diabetes, 343, 344b
and effect on female reproductive physiology, 349

Cortisol secretion
ACTH stimulation of, 717
aging and effects on, 722
regulation of, 717

Corynebacterium diphtheriae, 299t

Corynebacterium diphtheriae toxin, 305

Costal cartilage, 1549, 1551f

Cough, 1266–1267

Coughing up blood, 1268

Coumate, 667, 885, 908

Countercurrent exchange system, 1357

Coup and contrecoup mechanisms, of focal brain injury, 585, 585f

coup pattern of injury, 63

Coupling, in muscle fiber contraction, 1561

Cowper glands, 800

COX-1, COX-2 (cyclooxygenase enzymes), in breast cancer, 877b

COX-1 (cyclooxygenase-1), in platelet activation, 976

Coxsackievirus(es), 314t
and associated congenital heart defects, 1214t
in central nervous system infections, 621t

Crab louse, 945, 945f

Cracked-pot sign, 674

Cradle cap, 1656

Cranial deformities, 672
acrania, in 672
congenital hydrocephalus in, 673–674
craniosynostosis in, 672
microcephaly in, 673–674

Cranial meningocele, 669

Cranial nerve root tumors, 612t

Cranial nerves, 442–443, 465
origins, course, functions, and testing of, 468t
origins of, 466f, 467

Cranial tumors, 611–618

Craniopharyngioma, 686, 686t
clinical manifestations of, 687–688
treatment of, 687t, 688

Craniosacral division, of autonomic nervous system, 467

Craniosynostosis, 672
clinical manifestations of, 672f–673f, 673
evaluation and treatment of, 673–674

Cranium, 459

Creatine, 1560

Creatine kinase, 1560

Creatinine clearance, 1360
in chronic kidney disease, 1392t, 1393, 1393f

Crescentic glomerulonephritis, 1381t, 1383

Cretinism, 742, 742f

Creutzfeldt-Jakob disease
differential diagnosis of, 554t
molecular basis of, 553t

CRH. *See* Corticotropin releasing hormone.

Cri du chat syndrome, 142, 142f
congenital heart defects associated with, 1215t
genetic basis and pathophysiology of, 526t

Cricopharyngeal muscle, 1423

Crista ampullaris, 514

Crista supraventricularis, 1095–1096

Cristae, 7

Critical micelle concentration, 1439–1440, 1471

Crohn disease, 1473, 1474t, 1475f
and associated cancer, 378t
clinical manifestations of, 1473–1474
distribution patterns of, 1472f
evaluation and treatment of, 1474
pathophysiology of, 1473

Cross-bridge theory, of muscle contraction, 1108, 1108f, 1110, 1561

Cross-reactive antibody, 269

Crossing over, genetic exchange in, 155, 156f

Croup, 1315t, 1316
clinical manifestations of, 1316–1317, 1316f
evaluation and treatment of, 1317
pathophysiology of, 1316
spasmodic, 1316–1317
upper airway obstruction in, 1317f

Crush syndrome, 1575–1576
pathogenesis of, 1578f

Crusted scabies, 1689

Cryogenic epilepsy, 539–542

Cryogens, endogenous, 498

Cryoglobulins, 264

Cryptococcus neoformans, 308t, 629
capsule of, 308–309
immunosuppression by, 309

Cryptorchidism, 856
and associated childhood cancer, 438t

Cryptosporidium spp., 310t

Crypts of Lieberkühn, 1429

Crystal growth–inhibiting substances, 1368

Crystalline fragment (Fc), 224

Crystallization, in urine, 1368

Crystalloids, in shock therapy, 1738, 1740

Crystals, in urine analysis, 1361

CTLs. *See* Cytotoxic T cells.

Cuboidal bones, 1547

Cuboidal cells, 36

Cul-de-sac, 786

Culture, 805

Curling ulcer, 1467

Cushing disease, 765
clinical manifestations in, 766–767, 767f
evaluation and treatment of, 767–768
pathophysiology of, 765–766

Cushing syndrome, 343, 344b, 765
clinical manifestations in, 766–767, 767f
paraneoplastic, 389t

Cushing ulcer, 1467

Cutaneous vasculitis, 1665–1666, 1666f

CXC-chemokines, 205

Cyanide asphyxiation, 68

Cyanosis, 1217, 1268–1269

Cyclic adenosine monophosphate (cyclic AMP, cAMP), 20, 22f
in second messenger signaling pathways, 23t, 702, 702t

Cyclic guanosine monophosphate (cyclic GMP, cGMP), 20
as second messenger for atrial natriurctic peptide, 23t
in second messenger signaling pathways, 702, 702t

Cyclic neutropenia, 282

Cyclin dependent kinases, 369

Cyclooxygenase (COX 1), in platelet activation, 976

Cyclooxygenase enzymes (COX-1, COX 2), in breast cancer, 877b

Cylindrical bronchiectasis, 1276

Cylindromas, 1304

Cyst(s), 1648t
aneurysmal bone, 1637
Bartholin, 832
benign bone, 1637
benign ovarian, 836–837, 836f
breast, 873–874
corpus luteum, 837
dermoid, 837
epididymal, 855–856
follicular, 836–837
functional, 836
inflamed, 205
sebaceous, 1648t
simple bone, 1637

Cystatin C, plasma, 1361

Cystic acne, 1680–1681, 1681f

Cystic fibrosis, 1336, 1524
autosomal recessive inheritance of, 151–152, 152f
chronic endobronchial infection associated with, 1337
clinical manifestations of, 1337–1338, 1525t
complications of, 1525t
evaluation and treatment of, 1338–1339, 1524–1526
lung appearance in end-stage, 1336f

Cystic fibrosis *(Continued)*
   pathophysiology of, 1336–1337, 1337f, 1524, 1525t
      inflammatory, 1337
         mucus plugging in, 1336–1337
   prognosis for, 1338–1339
   screening newborns for, 1338b
   severity of, gene modification of, 1337–1338
Cystic fibrosis transmembrane conductance regulator (CFTCR) protein, 1336
Cystinuria, 1368–1369
Cystitis, 1374–1375
   and associated cancer, 378t
   in children, 1411
   clinical manifestations of, 1376
   evaluation and treatment of, 1376–1377
   pathophysiology of, 1375–1376
Cystocele, 833–834, 835f
Cystourethrocele, 835
Cytochromes, 24
Cytokine receptor superfamily, 701
Cytokines, 35, 49, 202–205, 203f. *See also* Interferon(s); Interleukin(s); Tumor necrosis factor-α.
   cancer associated release of, and clinical manifestations, 390, 390f
   effects of, in skeletal tissue, 1542–1543, 1544t
   hematopoietic, 961t, 963
   in immune response, 228–229, 229t
   inflammatory, 203f, 204
      and development of depression, 653b
      in pathophysiology of systolic heart failure, 1190
Cytokinesis, 33–34
Cytologic examination, 806–807
Cytomegalovirus (CMV), 314t
   and associated congenital heart defects, 1214t
   placental transmission of, 296
Cytomegalovirus (CMV) infection
   AIDS associated, 629
   central nervous system, 621t
   congenital, 948
   cutaneous, 1663
   sexually transmitted, 948
      clinical manifestations of, 948
      evaluation and treatment of, 948–950
      pathophysiology of, 948
Cytomegalovirus retinitis, in AIDS, 324f
Cytoplasm, 2
Cytoplasmic matrix, 4–5
Cytoplasmic organelles, 3f, 4–10
Cytosine, 129
Cytosine guanine dinucleotides, 405–406
Cytoskeleton, 8–10, 10f
Cytosol, 4–5, 8
Cytosolic receptors, 700t, 702–703
Cytotoxic cerebral edema, 560
Cytotoxic T cells (Tc cells, CTLs), 231–233, 231f
   in cell mediated hypersensitivity, 264
   clonal selection of, 243–244, 243f

Cytotoxic T cells (Tc cells, CTLs) *(Continued)*
   differentiation of, into memory T cells, 244
   functions of, 247–248
Cytotoxin necrotizing factor-1, 1375
Cytotropic antibody, 259

D
D cells, 1426
D-dimer, 1054
D2-receptor blockade, 651
DAG (diacylglycerol), 23t, 702
Dairy foods, and cancer risk, 410t
Dandy-Walker malformation, 674
Dark adaptation, changes in, 510
Data processing deficits, 546–548, 548t
   in acute confusional states, 548
   in agnosia, 546
   in dementia, 552–553
   in dysphasia, 546–548
Dawn phenomenon, 758
Deafferentation, 493–494
Deafferentation pain, 494
Deamination, 1442
Death receptor pathway, 85, 85f
Débridement, 208
Decerebrate posture, 575
Decerebrate posturing/rigidity, 533t, 536f
Declarative memory, 543, 545f
Declarative memory deficits, 543, 547t
Decompression sickness, 72
Decornification, 795
Decorticate posture, 575
Decorticate posturing/rigidity, 533t, 536f
Decreased libido, 848
Decreased pulmonary blood flow, congenital heart defects causing, 1223
Decubitus ulcer, 1647
Deep-ended hypothermia, 502t
Deep partial thickness burns, 1714–1715, 1715t, 1716f
Deep venous thrombosis, 1143
   embolism formation in, 1144
Defecation reflex, 1437
Defective class-switch, 278
Defense mechanisms, 184, 184t
   in aging, 213
   first line, 184–186
      bacteria-derived chemicals in, 186
      biochemical barriers in, 184–186
      epithelial-derived chemicals in, 185–186
      physical and mechanical barriers in, 184, 185f
   in neonates, 212
   references on, 215
   second line, 186–205. *See also* Inflammation; Inflammatory response.
   summary review of, 213b
   third line, 217. *See also* Immune response.
   in urinary tract infections, 1375–1376

Defensins, 185–186
Degenerative disk disease, 596–598
   pathophysiology of, 596–597
   spinal stenosis in, 598
   spondylolisthesis in, 598
   spondylolysis in, 598
Dehiscence, 212
Dehydration, 104
   in children, 1730, 1731t
Delayed cerebral ischemia, 608
Delayed hypersensitivity reactions, 258, 268f
Delayed hypersensitivity skin test, 264
Delayed puberty, 817
   causes of, 817, 817b
   incidence of, 817
Delayed union, of fractured bones, 1571–1572
Deletions, chromosome, 142
Delirium, 551
Delta cells, of pancreas, 714–715
Delusions, schizophrenic, 650
Dementia(s), 552–553
   Alzheimer, 553–554
   causative processes in, 552–553, 552b
   clinical manifestations of, 553, 553t
   degenerative, 553
      clinical differentiation of, 554t
      molecular basis of, 553t
   evaluation and treatment of, 553–554
   human immunodeficiency virus associated, 627–628
   pathophysiology of, 553
   WHO definition of, 552b
Dementia of Alzheimer type. *See* Alzheimer disease.
Dementia with Lewy bodies
   differential diagnosis of, 554t
   molecular basis of, 553t
Demyelinating disorders, 630. *See also* Multiple sclerosis.
Demyelinating neuropathy, 635
Dendrites, neuronal, 443
Dendritic cells, 957, 957t
   role of, in capturing antigen, 235, 237f
Dengue virus, 314t
Denosumab, 1584
Dense bodies, of platelets, 976
Dense connective tissue, 39t
Dental amalgams, safety of, 61
Denticulate ligaments, 460
Deoxyhemoglobin, 967–968
Deoxyribonucleic acid (DNA), 126. *See also* DNA.
Depolarization, 32–33, 1102
   diastolic, 1103
Depression, 652
   clinical manifestations of, 655–656, 656f
   major symptoms of, 652b
   monoamine hypothesis of, 653
   neuroendocrine dysfunction in, 653–654, 653b
   sleep disorders in, 506, 655–656
   treatment of, 657–658, 657b
Dermal appendages, 1646
Dermal ischemia, 1743

Dermatitis
   allergic contact, 1655–1656
   atopic, 1656, 1681–1682
   in children, 1681–1682
   diaper, 1682
   irritant contact, 1656, 1682
   seborrheic, 1656
   stasis, 1656
Dermatologic disorders. *See* Skin disorders.
Dermatomes, 467
Dermatomyositis, 1611
   clinical manifestations of, 1612, 1612f
   evaluation and treatment of, 1612–1615
   paraneoplastic, 389t
   pathophysiology of, 1611–1612, 1611f
Dermatophytes, 307, 308t, 1664
Dermis, 1645, 1645t
Dermoid cysts, 837
Descending colon, 1435–1436
Descending pathways. *See* Motor pathways.
Desensitization, to allergens, 267
Desire, disorders of, 848
Desmoplastic stroma, 820, 900
Desmosome(s), 16–18, 17f
Detection, 544, 545f
Detection deficits, 544, 547t
Detrusor areflexia, 1369
Detrusor hyperreflexia, 1369–1370
Detrusor hyperreflexia with vesicosphincter dyssynergia, 1370
Detrusor muscle, 1350
Detrusor overactivity, neurogenic, 1367f
Developing fetus, 781
Developmental dysplasia of hip, 1621, 1621f
   clinical manifestations of, 1622
   evaluation and treatment of, 1622–1624
   pathophysiology of, 1621–1622
   risk factors for, 1621
Developmental plasticity, 403
DHT (dihydrotestosterone), 801–802
Diabetes Control and Complications Trial (DCCT), 749–750
Diabetes insipidus, 730
   clinical manifestations of, 730
   evaluation and treatment of, 730–731
   nephrogenic, 730
   neurogenic, 730
   pathophysiology of, 730
Diabetes mellitus, 745
   acute complications of, 754–756, 757t
      dawn phenomenon in, 758
      diabetic ketoacidosis in, 755–756
      hyperosmolar hyperglycemic nonketotic syndrome in, 757
      hypoglycemia in, 754–755
      Somogyi effect in, 758
   and associated congenital heart defects, 1214t
   category(ies) of, 745, 746t

Diabetes mellitus (Continued)
gestational, 754
other specific, 753–754
type1, 745. See also Type 1 diabetes mellitus.
type2, 750. See also Type 2 diabetes mellitus.
chronic complications of, 758–765
hyperglycemia in, 758. See also Hyperglycemia.
infection in, 765
macrovascular disease in, 763–765. See also Coronary artery disease; Peripheral arterial disease; Stroke.
microvascular disease in, 759–763. See also Microvascular disease.
coronary artery disease and, 1164
diagnostic criteria for, 745, 747b
epidemiology and etiology of type 1 and type2, 747t
genes and environmental interaction in, 176–177
pancreatic islet cell transplantation in, 714b
sleep disorders in, 506
Diabetic ketoacidosis (DKA), 749, 751f, 755–756, 757t
clinical manifestations of, 756
evaluation and treatment of, 756–757
pathophysiology of, 756
Diabetic nephropathy, 760–761
pathogenesis of, 762f
Diabetic neuropathy(ies), 761–763
classification of, 763t
distal symmetric, 762
pathogenesis of, 762, 762f
Diabetic retinopathy, 759–760
pathogenesis of, 760f
pathologic findings in, 761t
Diacylglycerol (DAG), 702
in second messenger signaling pathways, 23t
Diapedesis, 198–199, 199t
Diaper dermatitis, 1682
Diaphragm, 1252
Diaphragmatic breathing, 1311–1312
Diaphysis, bone, 1546
Diarrhea, 1454
in children, 1530–1531
acute, 1530
chronic, 1530
chronic nonspecific, 1530
infectious, 1530
viral, 1530
clinical manifestations of, 1455
evaluation and treatment of, 1455–1456
infant, 1530
motility, 1455
osmotic, 1454
pathophysiology of, 1454–1455
in postgastrectomy syndromes, 1470
secretory, 1454–1455
Diarthrosis, 1549. See also Synovial joint(s).
Diascopy, 1647t
Diastole, 1095
Diastolic depolarization, 1103

Diastolic heart failure, 1194
clinical manifestations of, 1194
pathologic ventricular changes in, 1194
systolic and, comparison of, 1195t
Diastolic pressures, normal intracardiac, 1098t
Diencephalon, 450t, 453–455
Dietary factors
and associated cancer risks, 410t
studies of, 410t
in cancer epidemiology, 404–415, 407t
and risk for breast cancer, 891–893
Dietary fats, 1433b
Dietary insufficiencies
in cancer epidemiology, 406
essential fatty acids and inflammation in, 199b
immune competency and, 285
postmenopausal osteoporosis and, 1579
prevention of, in children with cancer, 440b
Diethylstilbestrol (DES), prenatal exposure to, 403, 439
Differential white cell count, 983t
pediatric, 985t
Differentiation, cell, 2
in cancer, 362–363, 363f
Diffuse axonal injury, 584, 590
mild, 590
moderate, 590
severe, 591
Diffuse brain injury, 588–591, 589f
categories of, 589
in cerebral concussion, 590
in mild concussion, 590
primary and secondary pathology of, 589
severity of, 589, 589f
Diffuse noxious inhibitory controls, 486
Diffusing capacity, 1262
Diffusion, 26, 27f
facilitated, 28–29
Diffusion rate, 26
DiGeorge syndrome, 279
facial anomalies associated with, 280f
Digestion, 23
Digestive enzymes, 1429–1430, 1430b
Digestive function
exocrine pancreatic secretions in, 1443–1444
gallbladder secretions in, 1439–1440, 1442
gastric acidity in, 1426–1427
gastric motility in, 1424–1425
gastric secretion in, 1425–1428
phases of, 1427–1428
hormones and neurotransmitters in, 1425t
intestinal motility in, 1434–1435
intestinal nutrient digestion and absorption in, 1429–1434. See also Small intestine.
liver secretions in, 1439–1440
mucus production in, 1427
pepsin activity in, 1427
salivation in, 1422
swallowing in, 1423

Digestive function (Continued)
tests of, 1444–1447, 1445t
water and electrolyte transport in, 1430
Digestive system, 1420, 1421f
accessory organs of, 1437–1444
disorders of, 1482. See also Gallbladder disorders; Liver disorders; Pancreatic disorders.
assessments of, 1444–1447
cancer of, 1498
gastrointestinal tract of, 1421–1437
disorders of, 1452–1453. See also Gastrointestinal disorders.
Digital clubbing, 1269, 1269f
paraneoplastic, 389t
Dihydrotestosterone (DHT), 801–802
Dilated cardiomyopathy, 1178–1180
pathophysiology of, and major symptoms, 1178f
treatment of, 1180
Diltiazem, calcium channel blocking activity of, 1108–1109
Dilutional hyponatremia, 105
Dimorphic fungi, 307
Dimorphism, 998
Dipeptidyl peptidase IV (DPP-IV), 752
Diphtheria, 1316
Diphtheria (D) vaccine, 329
adult, 329t
child, 330t
Diplegia, 564
Diploid cells, 134
Diplopia, 509
Dipsticks, urinalysis, 1362
Direct antiglobulin test, 983t
Direct Coombs test, 1068
Direct effects, of hormones, 699
Direct excitation, 487–488
Discoid (cutaneous) lupus erythematosus, 1659–1660, 1660f
categories of, and manifestations, 1660t
Discordant trait, 170
Disease of adaptation, 338
Dislocations, and subluxations, 1572, 1572f
clinical manifestations of, 1572–1573
evaluation and treatment of, 1573
pathophysiology of, 1572
Disorganized behavior, schizophrenic, 651
Disorganized speech, schizophrenic, 651
Disse space, 1438–1439
Dissecting aneurysms, 606–607
Disseminated gonococcal infection, 926
Disseminated intravascular coagulation (DIC), 1050–1051
clinical manifestations of, 1053, 1053b
compensated, 1053
etiologies of, 1050b
evaluation and treatment of, 1053–1059

Disseminated intravascular coagulation (Continued)
laboratory diagnostic criteria for, 1054b
pathophysiology of, 1051–1053, 1052f
other inflammatory pathways activated in, 1051
risk of hemorrhage in, 1051
as secondary to other conditions, 1050, 1050b
Distal axonal neuropathy, 635
Distal intestinal obstruction syndrome, 1520–1521
Distal symmetric polyneuropathy, 762
Distal tubule(s), 1347
transport within, 1356–1357
Distributive shock, 1728. See also Anaphylactic shock; Neurogenic shock; Septic shock.
pathogenesis of, 1728b, 1729
Disuse atrophy, 1609
Diuresis, postobstructive, 1367–1368
Diuretics, 1359t
and urine formation, 1358, 1359t
Diurnal enuresis, 1415
Divergence, of axons, 443
Diverticula, 1474
Diverticular disease of colon, 1474, 1475f
clinical manifestations of, 1474–1475
evaluation and treatment of, 1475
pathophysiology of, 1474, 1475b
Diverticulitis, 1474
Diverticulosis, 1461t, 1474
Dizygotic (DZ, fraternal) twins, 170
DNA (deoxyribonucleic acid), 126, 129–132
composition and structure of, 129, 130f
as genetic code, 129
methylation of, and epigenetic modification of gene expression, 149
mutation of, 129–132
replication of, 129, 131f
transcription of, in protein synthesis, 132–133
DNA dependent RNA polymerase, 132–133
DNA methylation, 373–374, 406f
in cancer epidemiology, 374–375, 403
chemotherapeutic drugs regulating, 374–375, 376f
in epigenetic modification of gene expression, 149, 403, 405–406
nutrition and, 405–406, 405f
DNA methyltransferases (DNMTs), 374–375, 376f, 405–406, 405f
DNA polymerase, 129
Dolichocephaly, 672f–673f
Doll's eye phenomenon, 534f
Dominant allele, 145
Donovan bodies, 934
Donovanosis, 933
Dopamine, 447–448, 455
functions of, 448t
hypothalamic release of, 707t
in shock therapy for children, 1740t

Dopamine hypothesis, of schizophrenic dysfunction, 648–649
Dopamine system, of brain, 649, 649f
Doppler ultrasonography, of vascular system, 1136
Dormancy, of cancer cells, 384
Dorsolateral prefrontal cortex, 648, 649f
Dorsolateral prefrontal cortex dysfunction, in schizophrenic brain, 648
Dorsolateral tract of Lissauer, 483–484
Double-helix model, 129
Down-regulation, of hormone receptors, 699
Down syndrome, 137
    childhood cancers associated with, 438–439, 438t
    congenital heart defects associated with, 1215t
    facial features of, 140f
    karyotype of, 140f
    risk of, with maternal age, 141f
Dressler postinfarction syndrome, 1176
Drowning, 68–69
Drug associated congenital heart defects, 1214t
Drug induced acute encephalopathies, 682
Drug induced hemolytic anemia, 1006
    models of, 1006f
Drug reactions, allergic immune response in, 267
Drug resistant microorganisms. *See* Antibiotic resistant microorganisms.
Drug use, social (street)
    cell injury in, 62
    effects of, 63t
Dry gangrene, 83–84
Dual-photon x-ray absorptiometry (DXA), 1583
Duchenne muscular dystrophy, 1633, 1634t
    clinical manifestations of, 1634, 1635f
    evaluation and treatment of, 1634–1637
    genetic basis and pathophysiology of, 526t
    genetic inheritance of, 154
    major syndromes of, 1634t
    pathophysiology of, 1633–1634
Ductal carcinoma in situ, 361, 898–905, 901f
Ductal hyperplasia, 875
    atypical, 876f
Ductus arteriosus, 1211
    closure of, 1213
Dumping syndrome, 1468–1469
Duodenal ulcers, 1465, 1466f, 1468t
    clinical manifestations of, 1465
    evaluation and treatment of, 1465–1467
    pathophysiology of, 1465
Duodenum, 1428
Duplications, chromosome, 142–143
Dura mater, 459–460
Dwarfism, hypopituitary, 731, 732f

DXA (dual-photon x-ray absorptiometry), 1583
Dynorphins, 489
    inhibition of pain transmission by, 488
Dysfunctional uterine bleeding (DUB), 822–823
    clinical manifestations of, 823–824
    evaluation and treatment of, 824
    pathophysiology of, 823, 823t
Dyskinesias, 568–570, 568t
Dyskinetic cerebral palsy, 676
Dyslipidemia, 1161–1164
    in chronic kidney disease, 1392t, 1395
    diagnostic criteria for, 1162t
    familial, 1163t
    treatment of, 1174–1175
Dyslipoproteinemia, 1162
Dysmenorrhea
    clinical manifestations of, 819
    evaluation and treatment of, 819–820
    pathophysiology of, 819
    primary, 819
    secondary, 819–821
Dysmnesia, 543
Dyspareunia, 849
Dysphagia, 1456
    clinical manifestations of, 1457–1458
    evaluation and treatment of, 1458
Dysphasias, 546–548
    examples of, 551t
    major types of, 549t
Dysphoric mood, 655–656
Dysplasia, 47f, 49–50, 361, 362f
    of uterine cervix, 50f
Dyspnea, 1267
    in pleural effusion, 1273–1274
Dyspnea on exertion, 1267
Dyspraxias, 576t, 577
    neural pathways disrupted in, 577f
Dysreflexia, 595
Dysrhythmias, 1175, 1196–1203
    as complication of myocardial infarction, 1175–1176
    impulse conduction disorders causing, 1199t
    impulse formation disorders causing, 1197t
    pediatric, 1738, 1738b
    in rewarming in accidental hypothermia, 502t
    sudden death resulting from, 1176
Dyssomnias, common, 504–505
Dyssynergia, 1369
Dystonia, 562t, 575
Dystonic movements, 575
Dystonic postures, 575
Dystonic posturing, 563, 563f
Dystrophic calcification, 79
Dystrophin, 154, 1633

E

Ear anatomy, 512–514, 513f
    inner, 513f, 514
Ear infections, 514–515
Early asthmatic response, 1331–1332, 1331f
Early dumping syndrome, 1468–1469

Eastern equine encephalitis, 625–626, 626t
Eating behavior. *See* Appetite, and satiety.
Ebb phase, of burn injury, 1744
Ebola virus, 314t
Eccrine sweat glands, 1646
ECF. *See* Extracellular fluid.
ECG. *See* Electrocardiogram.
Echinococcus spp., complement evasion by, 311
Echocardiography, in cardiac function evaluation, 1134
Echoencephalography, of central nervous system, 476
Ectopic testis, 856
Eczema, 1655, 1681
Edema, 98–99
    clinical manifestations of, 100–101
    evaluation and treatment of, 101
    pathophysiology of, 99–100, 100f
EEG. *See* Electroencephalogram.
Effective osmolality, 27
Effective renal blood flow (ERBF), 1360
Effective renal plasma flow (ERPF), 1360
Effector mechanisms, of immune response, 244–251
Effector organs, 442–443
Effector T cells, 243, 243f
Efferent lymphatic vessels, 1133
Efferent (motor) neurons, 444, 457, 567f
Efferent (descending) pathways, 442–443, 457–458, 457f
Efferent tubules, 797
EGF (epidermal growth factor), 36t, 49
Eisenmenger syndrome, 1217, 1221–1222
Ejaculatory duct, 800
Ejection fraction, 1109
Elastic arteries, 1113
Elastic connective tissue, 39t
Elastic fibers, 36–38
Elastic recoil, 1253
Elastin, 16
Electrical burns, 1742, 1742f
Electrocardiogram (ECG), 1133
    and myocardial infarction, 1174
    and myocardial ischemia, 1167, 1168f
    normal, 1103, 1104f
    serial 12-lead, 1133–1134
Electroconvulsive therapy, 658
Electroencephalogram (EEG), 476
    of seizure activity, 542f
    of wakefulness and NREM sleep, 503f
Electroencephalography, of central nervous system, 476
Electrolyte(s), 26
Electrolyte distribution
    in body compartments, 101–102, 101t
    in body fluids, 107t
    calcium and phosphate, 111–112
    magnesium, 114
    potassium, 106–108
    sodium and chloride, 101–102
    alterations in, 102–104. *See also* Water balance.

Electromagnetic radiation, cancer and, 424–425
Electromechanical dissociation, 1197t
Electromyogram (EMG), 1563–1564
Electron transport chain, 24
Electrophysiologic studies, of cardiac function evaluation, 1135
ELISA (enzyme-linked immunosorbent assay), 720
Elliptocytosis, hereditary, 992f
Ellis-van Creveld syndrome, congenital heart defects associated with, 1215t
Embolic stroke, 601
Embolism, 1147
    arterial, 1147–1148
Embolus, 1055, 1147
Embryo, 781, 1209, 1210f
Embryonic hemoglobins, 1063
Embryonic tumors, 437, 688
    neuroblastoma in, 688
    retinoblastoma in, 689–690
EMG (electromyogram), 1563–1564
Emission, 799
Emotional memory, 543
Emotional stress, and adverse heart effects, 337, 337b
Emphysema, 1288–1289
    airway obstruction in, 1282, 1282f
    clinical manifestations of, 1288t, 1290
    evaluation and treatment of, 1290–1291
    pathophysiology of, 1289–1290
    types of, 1289–1290, 1289f
Empirical risks, 167
Empyema, 1273–1274, 1274t
    bacterial causes of, 1274
Emulsification, of fats, 1432–1433
Encephalitis, 625–626, 625f
    arthropod borne, 625–626, 626t
    clinical manifestations of, 626
    evaluation and treatment of, 626–630
    pathophysiology of, 626
Encephalocele, 669, 669f
Encephalopathy(ies)
    childhood, 675. *See also* Childhood encephalopathies.
    definition of, 675
End-diastolic volume, 1109–1110
End-stage renal failure, 1386
Endemic, definition of, 297
Endemic goiter, 741
Endocardial cushions, 1209–1210
Endocardial disorders, 1181–1184. *See also* Infective endocarditis; Rheumatic heart disease; Valvular dysfunction.
Endocarditis, infective, 1187
    in children with congenital heart defects, 1214b
    clinical manifestations of, 1189
    evaluation and treatment of, 1189
    of mitral valve, 1189f
    pathophysiology of, 1187–1188, 1188f
Endocardium, 1093
Endocervical canal, 787–788
    columnar epithelium of, 789

Endochondral bone formation (ossification), 1541, 1618–1619, 1619f
Endochondroma, 1591
Endocrine disorders, 727–728
  adrenal cortical, 765
  adrenal medullary, 772
  anterior pituitary, 731
  autoimmune, 257t
  in female, 819. See also Menstrual disorders; Puberty.
  gland dysfunction in, 727–728
  hormone level alterations in, 727–728, 728t
  hypothalamic-pituitary, 728–729
  and metabolic muscle disease, 1610
  obesity and, 1478–1480, 1478b, 1479f
  pancreatic endocrine, 745
  paraneoplastic, 389t
  parathyroid, 742
  posterior pituitary, 728–729
  references on, 776
  secondary hypertension in, 1153t
  summary review of, 773b
  thyroid, 736
Endocrine disruptor chemicals, 818b
Endocrine function tests, 720
Endocrine gland(s), 697f, 703–720
  adrenal, 715–720
  pancreatic, 712–715
  pituitary, 703–708
  thyroid and parathyroid, 708–712
Endocrine system, 696–726, 697f
  in aging, 720–725
  chronic kidney disease and effects on, 1391t, 1396
  functions of, 696
  hormonal regulation within, 696–703
    altered0021. See also Hormonal disorders.
  hormone transport in, 698–699
  interaction of, with immune and nervous systems, 347, 348t, 720
  references on, 725
  summary review of, 723b
  and target cell receptors, 699–703
Endocrinopathies. See Endocrine disorders.
Endocytosis, 30–31, 31f
  receptor mediated, 31, 32f
Endogenous cryogens, 498
Endogenous opiates, 350. See also Endorphins; Enkephalins.
Endogenous opioids
  in behavior modification, 490
  inhibition of pain transmission by, 488
  in maintenance of feeding behavior, 490
Endogenous osteomyelitis, 1587
Endogenous pyrogens, 297, 498
Endogenous sex steroids, adiposity and, 409
Endolymph, 514
Endometrial biopsy, 808t
Endometrial cancer, 845–846, 845f
  adiposity and, 409
  screening and detection of, 846
  treatment of, 846
Endometrial polyps, 837, 837f

Endometriosis, 839–840, 839f
  classification of, 841t
  clinical manifestations of, 840
  evaluation and treatment of, 840–841
  pathophysiology of, 839–840, 840b
  pelvic sites of implantation in, 840f
Endometrium, 788–789
Endomitosis, 971–972
Endomorphins, 490
  inhibition of pain transmission by, 488
Endomysium, 1555
Endoneurium, 443
Endoplasmic reticulum, 5, 6f
Endorphins, 489
  functions of, 448t
  inhibition of pain transmission by, 488
  in pain modulation, 489f
  stress induced release of, 350
Endoscopy, of gastrointestinal tract, 1444, 1445t
Endosteal layer, 459–460
Endothelial cells, 1116
Endothelin, and effect on endothelium, 1119b
Endothelium, of blood vessels, 1116, 1118f. See also Vascular endothelium.
Endotoxic shock, 305
Endotoxins, bacterial, 301
  physiologic effects of, 302f
Energy metabolism diseases, 1610–1611
Energy production, cellular, 23–24
Enkephalins, 489
  functions of, 448t
  inhibition of pain transmission by, 488
  stress induced release of, 350
Enneking staging system, for malignant bone tumors, 1589, 1590t
Entamoeba histolytica, 310, 310t, 946
  evasion of phagocytosis by, 311
  immune suppression by, 312
Enteric plexus, 1421
Entero-oxyntin, 1425t, 1428
Enterobius vermicularis, 310t
Enterocele, 836
Enterochromaffin-like cells, 1426
Enterococcus spp., 299t
Enteroglucagon, 1425t
Enterohepatic circulation, 1439, 1440f
Enterokinase, 1444
Enthesis, 1600
Entrance inhibitors, viral, 323–324
Entrance wounds, 66–67
Enuresis, 1414
  clinical manifestations of, 1415
  evaluation and treatment of, 1415–1417
  genetic factors in, 1415
  pathogenesis of, 1414–1415
  secondary, 1415
Environmental antigens, 257t
Environmental factors
  in cancer epidemiology, 396–431, 397t, 401b, 893–895
  air pollution in, 426–431

Environmental factors (Continued)
  alcohol consumption in, 415–416
  chemical and occupational, 426
  in children, 439
  dietary intake in, 404–415, 407t, 410t
  electromagnetic radiation in, 424–425
  genetic and epigenetic, 401–404
  ionizing radiation in, 73–74, 416–422
  obesity in, 406–415
  prenatal, 401, 403–404, 439
  sexual and reproductive behaviors in, 425
  tobacco-related, 404
  ultraviolet radiation in, 422–424
  viral and microbial, 425
  in disease etiologies, 164, 169–171. See also Multifactorial disorder(s).
  adoption studies of, 170–171
  and secondary immune deficiencies, 285
  twin studies of, 170
Environmental tobacco smoke. See also Cigarette smoking.
  and cancer, 404
Enzyme-linked immunosorbent assay (ELISA), 720
Enzyme-linked plasma membrane receptors, 701
Eosinopenia, 1016t, 1017
Eosinophil cationic protein, 247
Eosinophil chemotactic factor of anaphylaxis (ECF-A), 196, 203f, 247
Eosinophil count, 983t
  pediatric, 985t
Eosinophilia, 1015–1017, 1016t
Eosinophilic esophagitis, 1459
  in children, 1524
Eosinophils, 956
  hematopoietic differentiation of, 964f
  in inflammatory response, 202, 203f
  pediatric values for, 1064t
Ependymal cells, 444–445, 445f
  functions of, 446t
Ependymoma, 612t, 616, 616f
  in children, 686, 686t
    clinical manifestations of, 687
    treatment strategies for, 687t, 688
  intramedullary spinal cord, 619
Epicardium, 1093
Epicondylitis, 1574, 1574f
Epicritic sensation, 458–459
Epidemic, definition of, 297
Epidermal growth factor (EGF), 36t, 49
Epidermis, 1644–1645, 1645t
Epididymal cyst, 855–856
Epididymis, 797
Epididymitis, 859, 859f
  clinical manifestations of, 860
  evaluation and treatment of, 860–861
  pathophysiology of, 860
Epidural hematoma, 62–63, 460–461, 586, 586f
Epidural space, 460–461

Epigenetic alteration, of gene expression, 149–150, 403
  and cancer etiology, 401–406, 403f
Epigenetic silencing, 149–150, 151f, 367, 373–377
  in cancer etiology, 373–375, 376f
  chemotherapeutic drugs regulating, 374–375, 376f
  nutrition and, 403, 405–406
Epigenome, 403
Epiglottitis, 1315t, 1317
Epilepsies, International Classification of, 538b
Epilepsy, 537, 539–542
  childhood, 679
    clinical manifestations of, 679–680
    evaluation and treatment of, 680
    ketogenic diet for, 680b
    pathophysiology of, 679
  definition of, 679
Epileptogenesis, 538–539
Epileptogenic focus, 538–539
Epimysium, 1555
Epinephrine. See also Catecholamines.
  in cardiac and metabolic regulation, 340–342
  cardiovascular effects of, 1125
  renal effects of, 1358
  in shock therapy for children, 1740t
Epiphyseal plate, 1546–1547
  bone growth and, 1619–1620
Epiphysis, bone, 1546–1547
Epispadias, 1405
Epithalamus, 450t, 453
Epithelial-derived chemicals, as human defense mechanisms, 185–186
Epithelial hyperplasia, of breast, 874
Epithelial-mesenchymal transition, in carcinogenesis, 382, 901, 903f
  signaling pathways of, 906f
Epithelial tissue, 36
  types of, with location and function, 37t
Epithelial tumors, 364t
Epithelialization, 208
  impaired, 212
Epithelioid cells, 207–208
Epitope, 221–222, 221f
Epstein-Barr virus (EBV), 314t
  in Burkitt lymphoma, 1035
  cancer and, 379–380, 381t, 439
  in central nervous system infections, 621t
  in childhood Hodgkin lymphoma, 1088
  in cutaneous infections, 1663
  sexually transmitted infection by, 947
Equatorial (metaphase) plate, 35
Equilibrium receptors, 514
Equine encephalitis virus, 621t
Equinovarus, teratologic, 1623
Equinovarus deformity, 1622–1624, 1623f
Erectile reflex, 799
  autonomic regulation of, 799
Erlotinib (Tarceva), 387t
Erosion, skin, 1648t
Erysipelas, 1663

Erythema marginatum, in rheumatic fever, 1186
Erythema multiforme, 1661–1662, 1661f
Erythema toxicum neonatorum, 1692
Erythroblast, 965–966
Erythroblastosis fetalis, 271, 1065, 1067
Erythrocyte appearance, in anemic disorders, 992f
Erythrocyte disorders, 989
   anemia(s) in, 989
      cancer associated, 391
      classification of
         etiologic (pathologic), 989, 990b
         morphologic, 991t
      clinical manifestations of, 989–993, 993f
      definition of, 989
      hemodynamic alterations in, 990
      macrocytic-normochromic, 990–993
      microcytic-hypochromic, 995–996
      normocytic-normochromic, 1000–1002
      paraneoplastic, 389t
      progression of, 993f
      secondary to drug effects, 1001t
   in children, 1065
   myeloproliferative, 1008–1009
   references on, 1012
   summary review of, 1011b
Erythrocyte hemoglobin content, terminology of, 991t
Erythrocyte osmotic fragility test, 983t
Erythrocyte progenitors, 971
Erythrocyte volume, terminology of, 991t
Erythrocytes, 954–955, 955f
   assessment of, terminology used in, 991t
   clinical evaluation of, 983t
   hematopoietic differentiation of, 964f
   in infants and children, 955–957
   normal smear, 992f
   oxygen-carrying protein of, 967–968, 967f. See also Hemoglobin.
   senescent, normal destruction of, 968–969
   vascular relaxation and, 968
Erythrodermic (exfoliative) psoriasis, 1658
Erythromelalgia, 611
Erythromyalgia, 1048
Erythropoiesis, 965–971, 966f
   in children, 1062–1063
   iron cycle in, 969–971
   nutritional requirements for, 968, 969t
   regulation of, 966–967, 967f
Erythropoietic hemochromatosis, 999
Erythropoietin (Epo), 1360
   development of clinical use of, 966–967, 967f, 1360
   physiologic functions of, 961t, 965, 1360
   renal synthesis of, 1360

Eschar, 1743
Escharotomy, 1715f
Escharotomy/fasciotomy, in severe burn injury, 1743, 1743f
Escherichia coli, 299t
   antigenic variation in, 304
   enterotoxins of, 305
   intracellular survival of, 302–303
   pathogenic, adhesion mechanisms of, 298, 301f
   uropathic strains of, 1375
Escherichia coli O157:H7, 299t
Esophageal atresia, 1518, 1518f
Esophageal cancer, 1498, 1498t
   clinical manifestations of, 1498–1499
   evaluation and treatment of, 1499
   pathogenesis of, 1498
Esophageal malformations, 1518, 1518f
   clinical manifestations of, 1518–1519
   evaluation and treatment of, 1519
   pathophysiology of, 1518
Esophageal phase, of swallowing, 1423
Esophageal sphincter(s), upper and lower, 1423
Esophageal varices, 1483
Esophagitis
   eosinophilic, 1459
   reflux, 1458
   ulcerations in, 1459f
Esophagus, 1421–1423
   and process of swallowing, 1423
Essential fatty acids, and inflammation, 199b
Essential (primary) thrombocythemia, 1047
Estradiol (E2), 790
Estradiol (E2) fertility test, 808t
Estrogen(s), 790–791
   adiposity and influence on, 409
   adrenal cortical secretion of, 718
   altered synthesis of, 791
   in breast cancer development, 883–886, 884f
   and effect on endothelium, 1119b
   elevated, and effects on reproductive physiology, 349–350
   physiologic effects of, 790
   in postmenopausal bone maintenance, 1579, 1582
   progesterone and, complementary and opposing effects, 792t
   synthesis of, 790
      in breast tissue, 884–885, 886f
Estrogen hypersecretion, adrenal, 771–772
Estrogen metabolites, carcinogenic effects of, 883–884, 885f
Estrogen-progestin therapy, and breast cancer risk, 887
Estrogen therapy, and breast cancer risk, 886–887
Ethacrynic acid, diuretic action of, 1359t
Ethanol associated cell injury, 59–61
Etiologic pain, 491b
Eukaryote(s), 2
Euploid cells, 135–136
Eustachian tube, 513–514

Evaporative heat loss, 497
Evaporative water loss, in burn injury, 1721, 1749
Evoked potentials (EPs), 476
Ewing sarcoma, 1635f, 1638
   clinical manifestations of, 1638
   environmental factors in, 397t, 401
   evaluation and treatment of, 1638–1639
   pathophysiology of, 1638
Exanthema subitum, 1687, 1687t
Excess scar formation, 211
Excitation, of neuromuscular junction, 1561
Excitation-contraction coupling, myocardial, 1108–1109
Excitatory interneurons, 484
Excitatory neurotransmitters, 488
Excitatory postsynaptic potentials (EPSPs), 448–449
Excoriation, 1648t
Excretion, 1352
Executive attention deficits, 544, 547t
Executive attention functions, 544
Exercise tolerance, in aging, 1263
Exfoliative toxin, 1683
Exhaustion stage, of general adaptation syndrome, 338
Exit wounds, gunshot, 67
Exocrine pancreas, 1443–1444
   and associated structures, 1443f
   secretions of, in digestive process, 1437–1444
Exocrine pancreas function tests, 1446–1447, 1447t
Exocytosis, 31, 31f
Exogenous osteomyelitis, 1587
Exogenous pyrogens, 297, 498
Exons, 134
Exophthalmos, 737
Exotoxins, 301
Expiration, mechanics of, 1254f
   in children, 1312f
Expressive disorders, 576–577, 576t
Expressive dysphasia, 549t
Expressivity, genetic, 148–149
External anal sphincter, 1435–1436
External auditory canal, 512
External fixation devices, 1571, 1571f
External urethral sphincter, 1350
Extinction, 542
Extracellular changes, in aging, 88
Extracellular fluid (ECF), 96, 97t
   electrolyte content of, 1718
   intracellular fluid and, water movement between, 97–98, 98f
Extracellular matrix, 15–16, 16f
Extracellular messengers, 20, 21f
   in activation of calcium second messenger system, 22f
   in activation of cAMP second messenger system, 22f
Extracellular signal regulated kinases (ERKs), 1582
Extracerebral brain tumors, 616–618
Extracerebral disorders, 528
Extradural brain abscess, 625
Extradural hematomas, 586, 586f
   temporal, 586

Extradural spinal tumors, 618
Extrafusal, 1555
Extrahepatic portal hypertension, 1533
Extramedullary invasion, by leukemic cells, 1085
Extramedullary spinal cord tumors, 618
   pathophysiology of, 619
Extraocular muscle paralysis, 509
Extraocular muscles, 508, 508f
Extrapyramidal motor syndromes, 577–580, 578t
Extrapyramidal/nonspastic cerebral palsy, 676
Extraventricular hydrocephalus, 560
Extrinsic pathway, of clotting cascade, 190, 191f, 202, 976–977
Exstrophy of bladder, 1405–1406, 1406f
Exudates, in inflammation, 205
Exudative effusion, 1273, 1274t
Eye anatomy
   disorders of, 509–512. *See also* Visual dysfunction.
   external, 506, 507f
   extrinsic muscles in, 508, 508f
   internal, 506–507f, 507–508
Eye infections
   bacterial agents causing, 299t, 506–507
   microbial agents causing, 506–507

F

F cells, of pancreas, 715
Fab (antigen binding fragment), 224
Facial nerve (CN VII), 466f
   origins, course, functions, and testing of, 468t
Facial nerve palsy syndromes, 568t
Facilitated diffusion, 28–29
Facilitation, of action potentials, 449
Factor H deficiency, 281
Factor I deficiency, 281
Factor V Leiden, 1055–1056
Factor XI deficiency, 1079
Failure to thrive, 1528
   clinical manifestations of, 1529
   evaluation and treatment of, 1529
   nonorganic, 1528
   pathophysiology of, 1528–1529
Fallopian tube(s), 788f, 789
False aneurysm, 1146
Falx cerebri, 460
Familial adenomatous polyposis, 175, 1500
   genetic expression in, 375–377
Familial Alzheimer disease, genetic basis and pathophysiology of, 526t
Familial dyslipidemia, 1163t
Familial hypercholesterolemia
   cellular physiology in, 174f
   in development of heart disease, 172, 173b
Familial hypocalciuric hypercalcemia, 743
Familial hypokalemic periodic paralysis, 108–109
Familial melanoma, 375t
Familial postural tremor, 568t
Fanconi anemia, 1002
   and associated childhood cancers, 438t, 439

Fas (CD95), 248
Fascia, 1555
Fascicle(s), 1555
    axon/dendrite bundling in, 443,
        444f, 465
Fasciola hepatica, 310t
**Fascioscapulohumeral muscular
    dystrophy,** 1634t, 1636
Fasting glucose, normal, 745
Fat(s), 1162, 1432
    and cancer risk, 410t
    dietary, 1432, 1433b
    digestion and absorption of,
        1431f, 1432–1433, 1434f
    metabolism of
        in chronic kidney disease,
            1394–1395
        in liver, 1441–1442
Fat embolism, 1148
Fat-free mass, 90
Fat necrosis, 83, 83f
    breast, 874t, 876t
Fatigue, cancer associated, 390
Fatigue fracture, 1569
Fatty change, 76–77
    in liver, 77f
Fatty streak, 1159
Fc (crystalline fragment), 224
Febrile response, 499f
Fecal mass, 1436
Feces, 1437
Female breast(s), 802–805
    anatomy of, 802–805, 803f, 898f
    changes in
        during menopause, 810–811
        during menstrual cycle, 803–804
    development of, 803
    examination of, 807
    function of, 804–805
    lymphatic drainage of, 803, 804f
Female breast disorders, 871
    benign breast disease in, 872–875
    breast cancer in, 880–896. *See also*
        Breast cancer.
    developmental, 876t
    dietary iodine and development
        of, 879b
    galactorrhea in, 871
    iatrogenic, 876t
    inflammatory, 876t
Female infertility, 849–850
Female pattern alopecia, 1674
Female reproductive disorders, 819
    benign growths and proliferative
        conditions in, 836–838
    cancer in, 841
    hormonal and menstrual
        alterations in, 819. *See
        also* Menstrual disorders;
        Polycystic ovary syndrome;
        Premenstrual disorders.
    impaired fertility in, 849–850
    infections and inflammation
        in, 828. *See also* Pelvic
        inflammatory disease.
    references on, 913
    sexual dysfunction in, 848–849
    sexually transmitted infections in,
        924–925
        bacterial, 299t, 924–925
        chlamydial, 935
        parasitic, 942–943
        viral, 938
    summary review of, 909b

Female reproductive physiology,
    stress induced alterations in,
    349–350, 351f
Female reproductive system,
    784–796
    aging and changes in, 807–814
    breast glands in, 802–805
    development of, 782–783,
        782f–783f
    external genitalia of, 784–786,
        786f
    internal genitalia of, 786–790,
        787f
    menstrual cycle in, 792–796
    sex hormones of, 790–792
Female sexual dysfunction, 848–849
    chronic disease and, 849t
Female urogenital system,
    menopausal changes in, 811
Feminization, 771
Fenestrations, 1113
Ferritin, 969, 1434
Ferritin determination, serum, 983t
Fertility tests, 807, 850
    normal values in, 808t
    serum hormone value, 809t
Fetal alcohol syndrome, 60–61
Fetal hemoglobin (HbF), 1063
Fetal immune function, 250
Fetal shunts, 1209–1211, 1212f
    closure of, 1212–1213
Fetus, 781
    cardiovascular development in,
        1209–1211
    circulation in, and fetal shunts,
        1211–1213, 1212f
    effects of exposure to ionizing
        radiation in, 417b
    hematopoiesis in, 1062–1063
Fever
    benefits of, 498–500
    chemical mediators of, 203f
    in inflammation, 206
    pathogenesis of, 498, 499f
    physiologic effect of, 297
Fever blisters, 1663
FGF. *See* Fibroblast growth factor.
Fiber, dietary, and cancer risk, 410t
Fibrils, of collagen, 1544
Fibrin, 190
Fibrin degradation products, 980,
    980f
    laboratory assays for, 983t, 1054
Fibrin-stabilizing factor (clotting
    factor XIII), 977t
    disorder(s) associated with, 1079t
Fibrinogen (clotting factor I),
    953–954, 977t
    disorder(s) associated with, 1079t
Fibrinogen assay, 983t
Fibrinolysis, 972, 979–980
    products of, 980
Fibrinolytic cascade, 1710
Fibrinolytic system, 979–980, 980f
    congenital defects in, 980
Fibrinous exudates, in inflammation,
    205
Fibroadenoma, breast, 874t, 875f
Fibroblast growth factor (FGF), 36t
    in maintaining serum phosphate
        levels, 1584–1585
Fibroblasts, 16, 1542f
    in wound healing, 210
Fibrocystic changes, 873–874

Fibromyalgia, 1606–1607
    clinical manifestations of, 1607,
        1607f
    concomitant conditions with,
        1608t
    differential diagnosis of, 1608t
    evaluation and treatment of, 1607
    and myofascial pain syndrome,
        1607, 1607t
    pathophysiology of, 1607
    patient education regarding, 1608,
        1608b
Fibronectin, 16
Fibrosarcoma, 1591–1592
Fibrous adhesions, 211
Fibrous cortical deficit, 1637
Fibrous dysplasia, 1637
Fibrous joints, 1549
Fibrous plaque, 1159
Filamentous bacteria, 297
Filtration, 26–27
Filtration forces, capillary, 98–99,
    99f
Filtration slits, 1345–1346
Filum terminale, 456
Fimbriae
    bacterial, 298, 301f
    of oviduct, 789
Fine needle biopsy, 807
First-degree block, 1199t
First degree burns, 1714, 1715t
First messenger(s), 20, 700–701, 701f
Fish consumption, safety of, 61–62
Fisher syndrome, 636, 637t
Fissure(s), 452
    skin, 1648t
Fissure of Rolando, 452
5-Hydroxytryptamine (5-HT). *See*
    Serotonin.
Flaccid paralysis, 566
Flaccid paresis, 566, 634
Flaccidity, 562t
Flagella, bacterial, 300
Flagellate protozoa, 310, 310t
Flail chest, 1272, 1272f
Flame burns, 1742
Flat bones, 1547
Flat foot, 1623–1624. *See also* Pes
    planus deformity.
Flat warts, 1648t
Flea bites, 1689, 1690f
Flight-or-flight response, 1103–1104
Florid hyperplasia, 874
Fluid and electrolyte balance, 102,
    102f
    alterations in, 102–104, 103t
        hypertonic, 103–104
        hypotonic, 104
        isotonic, 102–103
    in children, 1404
    in chronic kidney disease,
        1393–1394, 1394t
Fluid mosaic model, 13, 14f
Fluid resuscitation, in shock and
    burn injury, 1717, 1718t, 1718b
    in children, 1738, 1745–1750
Fluids, body, 96–98
    aging and distribution of, 97
    alterations in, 98–99. *See also*
        Edema.
    distribution of, 96–98, 97t
    electrolyte concentrations in,
        107t
    pH of, 114

Fluids, body *(Continued)*
    water movement between
        intracellular and extracellular
        compartments, 97–98
    water movement between·plasma
        and interstitial fluid, 98
Flukes (trematodes), 310, 310t
Fluoride, in bone tissue physiology,
    1580b
Fly bites, 1668
Foam cells, 1157–1159, 1159f
Focal brain injury, 584–588
    in cerebral contusions, 585, 585f
    coup and contrecoup mechanisms
        of, 585, 585f
    in extradural hematomas, 586,
        586f
    in intracerebral hematomas, 587
    in subdural hematomas, 586, 587f
Focal myopathy, 1613
Focal neuropathy, 635
Focal segmental glomerulosclerosis,
    1381t, 1409
Focal seizures, 536
Folate (folic acid)
    dietary, and cancer risk, 410t
    in erythropoiesis, 968, 969t
    in reducing risk of neural tube
        defects, 668b
Folate deficiency, and associated
    disorders, 70t
Folate deficiency anemia, 995
    clinical manifestations of, 995
    evaluation and treatment of,
        995–996
    laboratory findings in, 999t
    pathophysiology of, 995
Folate replacement therapy, 995
Folate therapy, in preventing
    megaloblastic crisis, 1007
Follicle(s)
    ovarian, 789, 790f
    thyroid, 709, 709f
Follicle stimulating hormone (FSH)
    anterior pituitary secretion of, 707
    in female reproductive
        development, 783–784
    physiologic effects of, 708t
    tests for levels of, 808t
    value of, 809t
**Follicle stimulating hormone (FSH)
    deficiency,** 732
Follicular cysts, 836–837
Follicular-proliferative phase, of
    menstrual cycle, 793–794
Folliculitis, 1662
Follistatin, 794
Fontan procedure, 1226, 1230
Fontanels, cranial, 666, 668f
Food poisoning, bacterial agents
    causing, 299t–300t
Foot deformities
    congenital, 1622–1624
    descriptive terminology of, 1622t
Foot lesions, in chronic diabetes
    mellitus, 765, 766f
Foramen of Monro, 461
Foramen ovale, 1210–1211
    closure of, 1212–1213
Foraminal herniation, 559
Forbidden clone(s), 269
Forced expiratory volume in one
    second (FEV₁), 1262t
Forced vital capacity (FVC), 1262t

Forebrain, 450t, 452–455
  diencephalon of, 453–455
  telencephalon of, 452–453
Foreign body aspiration, in
    children, 1317–1318, 1318f
Foreign matter embolism, 1148
Foreskin, 798
Formal thought disorder, 651
Fornix, vaginal, 786
Founder cells, 35–36
Fovea centralis, 507
Fracture(s), 65, 1568–1569
  clinical manifestations of,
    1570–1571
  corner (metaphyseal), 1640,
    1640f
  evaluation and treatment of,
    1571–1572
  pathophysiology of, 1570
  types and classification of, 1569,
    1569f
  definitions of, 1570t
Fragile sites, chromosomal, 143
Fragile X syndrome, 143
  inheritance of, 145f
Fragility fracture, 1569
Frailty, in aging, 90
Frameshift mutation, 132, 133f
Framework region, of antibody
    molecule, 224–225
Francisella tularensis, 299t
Frank-Starling law of heart,
    1109–1111, 1110f
FRAX (WHO Fracture Risk
    Assessment), 1583
Free fatty acids, elevated serum,
    750
Free radicals, 54–55. *See also*
    Reactive oxygen species.
  in aging theories, 88–89, 89f
  antioxidants active against, 57t
  biologically relevant, 57t
  diseases and disorders linked to
    oxygen-derived, 57t
  enzymes active against, 57t
  as indirect effects of ionizing
    radiation cellular damage,
    417–418, 418f
Freely movable joint, 1549
Freezing, 571–572
Fresh frozen plasma, 1080
Frontal lobe, 452
Frontotemporal dementia
  differential diagnosis of, 554t
  molecular basis of, 553t
Frostbite, 71–72, 1673
  treatment of, 1673
Fructosemia, 1534t
Fruits and vegetables, and cancer
    risk, 410t
FSH. *See* Follicle stimulating
    hormone.
Full thickness burns, 1715,
    1716f
Fulminant hepatitis, 1491
Functional cysts, 836
Functional hearing loss, 515
Functional incontinence, 1369t
Functional reserve (residual)
    capacity (FRC), 1262
  in children, 1312
Fundus
  gastric, 1423–1424, 1426
  uterine, 787–788

Fungal infections, 307–310. *See also*
    Fungal pathogens.
  cutaneous, 1664–1665
  in human immunodeficiency
    virus infection, 323b
  pathogenesis of, 309
Fungal meningitis, 622–623
  clinical manifestations of, 624
  pathophysiology of, 623
Fungal pathogens, 307–308, 308t
  evasion mechanisms of, 308–309
    antigenic variation, 309
    immunosuppression, 309
    intracellular survival, 308
    protection against phagocytosis,
      308–309
  tissue damage by, 309
  tissue invasion by, 308–309
  transmission and colonization by,
    307–308
Fungal skin infections, 1664–1665
  in children, 1684–1685
Fungal toxins, 309
Fungi, 298t, 307–310, 307f
Furosemide, diuretic action of, 1359t
Furuncle, 1662–1663, 1662f
Fusiform aneurysms, 606–607, 606f
Fusiform muscles, 1555

G

G cells, 1426
G-CSF. *See* Granulocyte colony
    stimulating factor.
G protein, 20
G protein coupled opioid receptors,
    488
G protein-coupled receptors, 15,
    15t, 23t, 701. *See also* Cyclic
    adenosine monophosphate.
G0 state, of cell cycle, 35
G6PD deficiency. *See* Glucose-6-
    phosphate dehydrogenase
    (G6PD) deficiency.
Gait disorders, 576
Galactorrhea, 871
  clinical manifestations of, 872
  evaluation and treatment of,
    872–875
  pathophysiology of, 871–872, 872b
Galactosemia, 1534t
Galea aponeurotica, 459
Gallbladder, 1437f, 1442
  and associated structures, 1443f
  secretions of, in digestive process,
    1437–1444
Gallbladder cancer, 1504
  clinical manifestations of, 1504
  evaluation and treatment of, 1504
  pathogenesis of, 1504
Gallbladder disorders, 1494–1495
Gallbladder function assessments,
    1446, 1447t
Gallstones, 1494, 1495f
Gametes, 134
Gamma-aminobutyric acid (GABA),
    447–448
  functions of, 448t
  in inhibitory neurotransmission,
    488
  and synaptic physiology in
    schizophrenic brain, 648
Gamma (γ) globulins, 953–954
  in immune deficiency therapies,
    287–288

Gamma neurons, 566
Gamma neuropathies, 566
Ganglia, neuronal, 443
Ganglioneuroblastoma, 688
Ganglioneuroma, 619, 688
Gangliosidosis, 678
Gangrenous necrosis, 83–84, 83f
Gap junction, 16–18, 17f–19f
Gap junction intercellular
    communication, 422
Gas emboli, 72
Gas exchange, pulmonary
    (respiratory), 1255–1260
  in aging, 1263
  airways of, 1244–1247, 1246f
  carbon dioxide, 1259–1260
  in children, 1310–1311
  effective, 1256
  oxygen, 1257–1259
Gas gangrene, 84
Gas pressure, measurement of,
    1254–1255, 1255f
Gasping breathing pattern, 530t
Gastric acid, 1426–1427
Gastric acid stimulation test, 1445t
Gastric cancer, 1498t, 1499
  clinical manifestations of, 1499
  evaluation and treatment of,
    1499–1500
  pathogenesis of, 1499
  typical sites of, 1499f
Gastric emptying, rate of, 1425
Gastric glands, 1426, 1426f
Gastric inhibitory peptide, 1425t
  activity of, in intestinal phase of
    gastric secretion, 1428
Gastric juice, 1426
  electrolyte composition and
    secretory rate of, 1426f
Gastric motility, 1424–1425
Gastric mucosa, 1427
Gastric phase, of gastric secretion,
    1427–1428
Gastric pit, 1426
Gastric secretion, 1425–1428, 1426f
  phases of, 1427–1428, 1427f
Gastric ulcers, 1467, 1468t
  benign, 1468f
  clinical manifestations of,
    1467–1471
  pathophysiology of, 1467, 1469f
Gastrin, 715, 1424, 1425t
Gastrin releasing peptide, 1425t
Gastritis, 1463–1464
  acute, 1463, 1464f
  alkaline reflux, 1469–1470
  and associated cancer, 378t
  chronic, 1464
Gastrocolic reflex, 1436
Gastroileal reflex, 1435
Gastrointestinal bleeding, 1456,
    1456f
  pathophysiology of, 1457f
Gastrointestinal cancers, 1498, 1498t
Gastrointestinal changes, cancer
    therapy associated, 391
Gastrointestinal disorders,
    1452–1453
  appendicitis in, 1475
  autoimmune, 257t
  in children, 1516
    acquired, 1522–1523
    congenital, 1516
    diarrhea in, 1530–1531

Gastrointestinal disorders
    (Continued)
  impaired nutrition in, 1524
  references on, 1536
  summary review of, 1535b
  clinical manifestations of,
    1452–1453
  gastritis in, 1463–1464
  inflammatory bowel disease in,
    1471
  malabsorption syndromes in,
    1470–1471
  motility dysfunction in, 1456
  in multiple organ dysfunction
    syndrome, 1712–1713
  nutritional disorders in,
    1477–1478
  peptic ulcer disease in, 1464–1465
  postgastrectomy syndromes in,
    1468–1470
  references on, 1509
  summary review of, 1505b
  vascular insufficiency in, 1477
Gastrointestinal infections
  bacterial agents causing, 299t
  sexually transmitted, 946
    giardiasis and amebiasis in, 946
    hepatitis B in, 946–947
    shigellosis and *Campylobacter*
      enteritis in, 946
Gastrointestinal reflux disease,
    1458
  in children, 1523
    clinical manifestations of, 1524
    evaluation and treatment of,
      1524
    pathophysiology of, 1523–1524
  clinical manifestations of, 1458
  evaluation and treatment of,
    1458–1459
  pathophysiology of, 1458
Gastrointestinal tract, 1421f
  in aging, 1447–1451
  bacterial flora of, 1437
  chronic kidney disease and effects
    on, 1391t, 1396
  disorders of, 1452–1515. *See also*
    Gastrointestinal disorders.
  function of, 1421. *See also*
    Digestive function.
  hormones and neurotransmitters
    in, 1425t
  large intestine of, 1435–1437
  mouth and esophagus of, 1421–1423
  references on, 1451
  salivary glands of, 1422
  small intestine of, 1428–1435
  stomach in, 1423–1428
  structural assessments of, 1444,
    1445t
  summary review of, 1448b
  wall and tissue layers of, 1421,
    1422f
Gate control theory, of pain, 482,
    486. *See also* Neuromodulation.
Gating, 18
GDP (guanosine diphosphate), 20
Gegenhalten, 562t, 563, 563f
Gene(s), 126
Gene amplification, 372, 374f
Gene cloning, 159
Gene-environment interaction, 171,
    171b, 396–431. *See also* Cancer
    epidemiology.

Gene expression, 148–149
  epigenetic alteration of, 149–150
Gene function, protein synthesis
  and, 132–134
Gene mapping, and linkage analysis,
  155–159
  prospects and benefits of, 157–159
Gene mutations, causing cancers,
  367–368. *See also* Cancer
    epidemiology.
  caretaker, 375–377
  clonal selection of, 368
  familial, 375–377, 377f
  hallmark, 370f
  oncogene and tumor suppressor,
    373t, 370–375
  types of, 368–370, 371b
    angiogenic, 369
    progrowth and antigrowth
      signaling, 368–369
    telomeric and unlimited
      growth, 369–370
Gene recombination, random
  in B cell receptor production,
    233–234, 235f
  in T cell receptor production,
    231–233, 232f
Gene silencing, 373–377
  chemotherapeutic drugs
    regulating, 374–375, 376f
  in development of cancer,
    374–375
Gene splicing, 133–134
Gene switching, 304
  in protozoans, 311
Gene therapy, 127b
  in immune deficiency treatment,
    288–290
General adaptations syndrome, 338
**Generalized acetylcholine receptor
  (AChR) myasthenia,** 639
Generalized anxiety disorder, 660
Generalized neuropathics, 635
Generalized seizures, 536, 537t, 679
  clinical manifestations of, 540t
**Generalized symmetric
  polyneuropathies,** 635
Generation of clonal diversity, 230.
  See also Clonal diversity.
Genetic cell injury, 69
Genetic code, 129
Genetic contribution, to disease,
  164–182. *See also* Multifactorial
    disorder(s).
Genetic disorders, 146–150
  autoimmune, 270
  gene mapping of specific,
    157–159, 158f, 158t
  inheritance of, 145–155
    autosomal dominant, 146–150
    autosomal recessive, 151–152
    consanguinity and, 152
    linkage analysis and gene
      mapping in, 155–159
    penetrance and expressivity in,
      148–149
    recurring risk for, 148
    X-linked, 152–155
  references on, 162
  and secondary immune
    deficiencies, 285
  summary review of, 160b
Genetic enhancement, 160b
Genetic instability, 419

Genetic lesions, cancer-causing,
  371b
Genetics, 126–163
  of cancer, 367–381
    in children, 438–439
    clonal selection in, 368
    familial, 375–377
    gene mutations in, 367–368
    oncogenes and tumor-
      suppressor genes in,
      370–375
  cancer epidemiology and,
    396–431
  chromosomal basis of, 134–143
  chromosomal number
    abnormalities in, 135–143
  chromosomal structural
    abnormalities in, 142–143
  dominance and recessiveness in,
    145
  environment and, interaction
    of, 164–182. *See also*
    Environmental factors;
    Multifactorial disorder(s).
  familial
    of cancer, 375–377
    and disease inheritance,
      145–155
  genomic imprinting in, 149–150
  inheritance of traits in, 143–145
  linkage analysis and gene mapping
    in, 155–159
  at molecular level, 129–134
  phenotype and genotype in, 145
  references on, 162
  summary review of, 160b
Genital herpes, 938, 1663
  clinical manifestations of,
    939–940, 939f
  evaluation and treatment of, 940
  pathophysiology of, 938–939
  penile and vulvar, 939, 939f
  primary, clinical course of, 940f
  primary and recurrent forms of,
    1664
Genital tubercle, 783
Genital ulceration, algorithm for
  diagnosis of, 931f
Genital warts. *See* Condylomata
  acuminata.
Genitourinary anomalies, and
  associated childhood cancer,
  438t
Genome, integral maintenance of,
  375–377
Genomic imprinting, 149–150
Genomic instability, 417–418,
  420–422, 421f
Genotype, 145
Genu valgum (knock knee), 1620
Genu varum (bow leg), 1620
Germ cell tumors, 612t
German measles, 1686, 1687t
Germinative layer, 1644–1645
Germline mosaicism, 148
Germline mutation, 375, 377f
Germline therapy, 160b
Gestational diabetes mellitus, 746t,
  754
GFR (glomerular filtration rate),
  1351, 1360
GH. *See* Growth hormone.
Ghrelin, 715, 752, 1479
  plasma, in obesity, 1479

GHRH. *See* Growth hormone
  releasing hormone.
Giant aneurysms, 606–607, 606f
Giant cell tumor, 1592, 1592f
Giant cells, 207–208, 207f
Giardia lamblia, 310, 310t, 946
Giardia spp., tissue damage caused
  by, 312
Giardiasis, sexually transmitted, 946
Gibbs-Donnan equilibrium, 27–28
Giemsa stain, 135
Gigantism, 733, 734f
Gilbert disease, 1486
Gingivitis, and associated cancer,
  378t
Gingivostomatitis, 1663
Glands of Montgomery, 803
Glans, 798
Glanzmann thrombasthenia,
  1048–1049
Glaucoma, 510
  structural causes of, 511f
  types of, 510t
Gleason score, 869, 869b
Glenn procedure, 1230
**Glioblastoma, intramedullary
  spinal cord,** 619
Glioblastoma multiforme, 612t,
  615f
Glioma(s), 612t, 613–616
  classification of, 613–614
  magnetic resonance imaging of,
    615f
Glisson capsule, 1438
Global dysphasia, 549t
Globins, 967
Globulins, 953–954
Glomerular capillaries, 1348, 1349f
Glomerular disorders, 1378–1383
  in children, 1407–1408
  glomerulonephritis and,
    1379–1383, 1381t,
    1407–1408. *See also*
    Glomerulonephritis.
  lesion classification in, 1378, 1380t
  in nephrotic syndrome, 1384,
    1409
  pathophysiology of, 1378, 1379f
  in sickle cell disease, 1075–1076
Glomerular endothelium,
  1345–1346
Glomerular filtration, 1354–1357,
  1354f
  rate of, 1354–1355
  tubular transport in, 1355–1357,
    1356b
Glomerular filtration membrane,
  1345–1346
Glomerular filtration pressures,
  1354, 1355f, 1356t
Glomerular filtration rate (GFR),
  1351
  clearance and, 1360
Glomerulonephritis, 267,
  1379–1383, 1381t
  acute postinfectious, 1380–1382
  acute poststreptococcal,
    1372–1373
  in children, 1407–1408, 1407t
  chronic, 1383
  crescentic or rapidly progressive,
    1383
  in Henoch-Schönlein purpura
    nephritis, 1408

Glomerulonephritis (*Continued*)
  in IgA nephropathy, 1382, 1408
  in lupus nephritis, 1382
  membranoproliferative, 1383
  in membranous nephropathy,
    1383
  mesangial proliferative, 1383
  pathophysiology of, 1380–1381t,
    1382f
Glomerulotubular balance, 1357
Glomerulus, 1345, 1349f
  vascular supply of, 1346–1347
Glossitis, in iron deficiency, 997f
Glossopharyngeal nerve (CN IX),
  466f
  origins, course, functions, and
    testing of, 468t
Glucagon, 714
Glucagon excess, in type 1 diabetes
  mellitus, 748–749
Glucagon-like peptide 1 (GLP-1),
  752, 1479
Glucocorticoid(s), 716–717. *See also*
  Cortisol.
  antenatal use of, in lessening
    severity of neonatal lung
    disease, 1322–1323
  cortisol, 717
  feedback control of synthesis and
    secretion of, 717, 718f
  permissive effects of, 717
  physiologic effects of, 716–717
**Glucocorticoid induced
  osteoporosis,** 1582
Gluconeogenesis, 1481
Glucose, and sodium transport,
  1430, 1432f
**Glucose-6-phosphate
  dehydrogenase (G6PD)
  deficiency,** in children, 1068
  clinical manifestations of, 1070,
    1531
  evaluation and treatment of, 1070
  pathophysiology of, 1068–1070
Glucose-6-phosphate dehydrogenase
  (G6PD) deficiency test, 983t
Glucose dependent insulinotropic
  polypeptide (GIP), 752
Glucose metabolic impairment, in
  shock, 1697–1699
Glucose tolerance, in chronic kidney
  disease, 1395
Glutamate
  in excitatory neurotransmission,
    488
  neurologic functions of, 448t
Glutamate deficits, in
  schizophrenia, 649–650
Gluten-sensitive arthropathy, 267
Gluten-sensitive enteropathy,
  1525–1526
  clinical manifestations of, 1527
  evaluation and treatment of,
    1527–1528
  pathophysiology of, 1526–1527,
    1526f–1527f
Glycerol, diuretic action of, 1359t
Glycine
  in inhibitory neurotransmission,
    488
  neurologic functions of, 448t
Glycogen accumulation, cellular,
  77–78
Glycogen storage diseases, 77–78

Glycogenolysis, 1481
Glycolysis, 23, 25f
Glycoprotein hormones, 697t, 707, 708t
receptors for, and mechanism of action, 700t
Glycoproteins, 12
in bone matrix, 1541t, 1545
in platelet-vascular adhesion, 1046, 1048
Glycosylated hemoglobin, 749
Glycosylation, nonenzymatic, 759
GM-CSF. *See* Granulocyte-macrophage colony stimulating factor.
Goblet cells, of bronchi, 1244
Golfer's elbow, 1574
Golgi complex (Golgi apparatus), 3f, 5, 7f
protein synthesis and transport in, 8f
Golgi tendon organs, 1556–1557
Gomphosis, 1549
Gonad(s), 781–782
hormonal stimulation of, 785f
Gonadal dysgenesis, and associated childhood cancer, 438t
Gonadarche, 784
Gonadostat, 784
Gonadotropic hormones, 708t
Gonadotropin releasing hormone (GnRH)
in embryonic and fetal development, 783–784
hypothalamic release of, 703–704, 707t
Gonococcal cervicitis, 925–926, 926f
Gonococcal ophthalmia neonatorum, 927, 927f
Gonococci, 924, 925f
Gonorrhea, 924–925. *See also Neisseria gonorrhoeae.*
clinical manifestations of, 925–927
diagnostic tests for, 806t
evaluation and treatment of, 927–928
outpatient treatment of uncomplicated, 928b
pathophysiology of, 925
Gonorrheal infection, and chlamydial infection, similarity of clinical syndromes, 936t
Goodpasture syndrome. *See* Antiglomerular basement membrane nephritis.
Gorlin syndrome, and associated childhood cancer, 438t
Gout, 1602
clinical manifestations of, 1605
pathophysiology of, 1602–1605, 1604f
treatment of, 1605–1606
Gouty arthritis, 1602, 1604f
acute, 1605
Gower hemoglobin, 1063
Gower sign, 1634
GPIIb-IIIa complex, 976
Graft rejection, 274–275
renal, 274f
Graft-versus-host disease, 286
Gram-negative bacteria, 297, 299t, 301f
endotoxins released by, 301

Gram-positive bacteria, 297, 299t, 301f
Granulation tissue, 208–210
Granulocyte colony stimulating factor (G-CSF), 961t, 963
Granulocyte-macrophage colony stimulating factor (GM-CSF), 961t, 963
Granulocyte progenitors, 971
Granulocytes, 955
hematopoietic differentiation of, 964f
quantitative alterations of, 1015–1017
Granulocytopenia, severe, 1015
Granulocytosis, 1015, 1016t
Granuloma, 207–208
tuberculous, 207f
Granuloma formation, in persistent bacterial infections, 305
Granuloma inguinale, 933
clinical manifestations of, 934
evaluation and treatment of, 934
Granulosa cells, 789
Graves dermopathy, 737
Graves disease, 736–737
clinical manifestations of, 737, 739f
maternal hypersensitivity in, 271
pathophysiology of, 737
treatment of, 737
Gray matter, 452–453
laminae of, 483–484
of spinal cord, 456
Great cardiac vein, 1099
Great vessels, of heart, 1095
Greenstick fracture, 1569
Ground substance, 36–38, 1540
Group A streptococci, 1185
in erysipelas, 1663
in impetigo, 1663
in pneumonia, 1328t
in tracheitis, 1315
Group B streptococci, 1185
in cellulitis, 1663
rapid division of, 302
in skin infections, 1662
in tracheitis, 1315
Growth factors, 35
examples of, and actions, 36t
Growth hormone (GH), 707–708
anterior pituitary secretion of, 707
hypothalamic regulation of, 707–708
physiologic effects of, 704f, 707–708, 708t
aging and, 721–722
anabolic, 708
stress induced, 350–351
receptors for, and mechanism of action, 700t
second messenger signaling pathways of, 23t
Growth hormone deficiency, 732
Growth hormone hypersecretion, 733
clinical manifestations of, 734–735
evaluation and treatment of, 735
pathophysiology of, 733–734
Growth hormone releasing hormone (GHRH), hypothalamic release of, 703–704, 707t
Growth hormones, 707, 708t

Growth plate, bone, 1546–1547
GTP (guanosine triphosphate), 20
Guanine, 129
Guanosine diphosphate (GDP), 20
Guanosine triphosphate (GTP), 20
Guillain-Barré syndrome, 636
classification of axonal subtypes in, 636, 637t
clinical manifestations of, 636
evaluation and treatment of, 636
pathophysiology of, 636
Gummas, 929
Gunshot wounds, 66–68
entrance, 66–67
indeterminate (distance) range, 67
intermediate range, 66–67
exit, 67
firearm potential in, 67–68
Gut hypothesis, 1711
Guttate psoriasis, 1658, 1658f
Gynecomastia, 141, 908

H

H1 and H2 receptors, 196, 196f
HAART (highly active antiretroviral therapy), 322–323
Haemophilus aegyptius, 299t
Haemophilus ducreyi, 932
Haemophilus influenzae, 299t
immune molecule degradation by, 304
type b, 298
Haemophilus influenzae **sepsis,** 1740
Haemophilus influenzae type b (Hib) immunization, 329, 1315, 1317
Hageman factor (clotting factor XII), 192, 977t
disorder(s) associated with, 1079t
Hair cells, 514
Hair disorders, 1673–1674
Hair follicles, 1646
Haldane effect, 1259–1260
Hallucinations, schizophrenic, 650
Halogen lamps, safety of, 74–75
Hamartoma, and associated childhood cancer, 438t
Hanging strangulation, 68
Hantavirus, 314t
Haploid cells, 134
Haplotype, 227–228
Hapten model, of drug induced hemolytic anemia, 1006
Haptens, 222
Hashimoto disease, 741
Hashimoto thyroiditis, and associated cancer, 378t
Haustra, 1436
Haversian system, 1546
HbF (fetal hemoglobin), 1063
HbO$_2$ (oxyhemoglobin), 967–968
association and dissociation of, 1259
HBsAg (hepatitis B surface antigen), 1489, 1532
hCG (human chorionic gonadotropin), in breast cancer treatment studies, 886
HDL (high density lipoprotein), 1161–1164
Head and neck cancer, metastasis of, 384t

Head trauma, 583–591
categories of, 583–584
causes of, 584–591
common types of, 584
diagnostic tools in, 591
diffuse, 588–591. *See also* Diffuse brain injury.
focal, 585–588. *See also* Focal brain injury.
genetics of, 484
incidence of, 583
penetrating focal, 588
primary and secondary, 584–585
severity of, and clinical manifestations, 584t
temperature regulation disorders in, 502
Headache, 609–611
chronic paroxysmal hemicranial, 611
classification of, 610t
cluster, 611
migraine, 609–611
tension-type, 611
Healing, wound, 208–213. *See also* Wound healing.
Hearing, 512–514
Hearing loss, 515
in aging, 514–516, 514t
associated with cell injury, 76
conductive, 515
functional, 515
mixed, 515
sensorineural, 515
Heart, 1093–1113
autonomic innervation of, 1101, 1101f, 1103–1105
adrenergic receptor function in, 1105
sympathetic and parasympathetic, 1104–1105
cardiac output of, 1109–1113
circulatory cycle of, 1095–1096. *See also* Cardiac cycle.
conduction system of, 1100–1103, 1101f. *See also* Cardiac cycle.
coronary vessels of, 1096–1099
development of, 1209–1213
embryologic, 1209
fetal, 1209–1211
in infant, 1213
in neonate, 1211–1213
functional anatomy of, 1093–1096, 1094f
atria and ventricles, 1093–1094, 1096f
fibrous skeleton, 1094
great vessels, 1095
heart valves, 1094, 1095f
mechanical function of, 1109–1110, 1110f. *See also* Cardiac output.
myocardium of, 1105–1108. *See also* Myocardium.
normal pressures within, 1096, 1097f
Heart attack, 1160. *See also* Myocardial infarction.
Heart disease, 1142, 1143t
aging and, 1136
AIDS associated, 629, 1189
in aldosteronism, 769b
arterial, 1144–1150
childhood, 1209

Heart disease (*Continued*)
acquired, 1234. *See also*
Childhood obesity;
Hypertension; Kawasaki
disease.
congenital, 1213–1214. *See also*
Congenital heart defects.
references on, 1240
heart wall disorders in, 1176–1184
manifestations of, 1189–1203
dysrhythmias in, 1196–1203.
See also Dysrhythmias.
heart failure in, 1189–1196. *See
also* Heart failure.
stress and, 337b, 347, 347b, 353
venous, 1142–1144
in women, 1161b
Heart failure, 1189–1196
in children, 1216
clinical manifestations of, 1217,
1217b
evaluation and treatment of,
1217–1218
pathophysiology of, 1216–1217,
1216t
high output, 1195–1196
incidence and etiologies of, 1189
left, 1190–1194
right, 1194–1195
systolic, 1190–1194
types of, 1190–1196
Heart health, stress and, 337b, 347,
347b, 353
Heart rate (HR), 1099, 1133t
atrial receptors affecting, 1112–1113
cardiac output and, 1111–1113
central nervous control of,
1111–1112
in children, 1730
hormonal and chemical effects
on, 1113
neural reflexes affecting, 1112
Heart valves, 1094, 1095f
Heart wall, 1093, 1093f
Heart wall disorders, 1176–1184
endocardial, 1181–1184. *See also*
Valvular dysfunction.
myocardial, 1178–1180. *See also*
Cardiomyopathy(ies).
pericardial, 1176–1178
Heat conservation, body,
mechanisms of, 497–498
Heat cramps, 72, 500
Heat exhaustion, 72, 500
Heat loss, body, mechanisms of,
496–497
Heat production
body, 496
in inflammation, 205
Heat stroke, 72, 500
Height, as multifactorial trait, 165,
166f
Helical CT angiography, 474
Helicobacter pylori, 299t
adhesion mechanisms of, 300
immune suppression induced
by, 305
Helicobacter pylori **infection,**
chronic. *See also* Duodenal
ulcers; Gastritis; Peptic ulcers.
and gastric carcinoma and
lymphoma, 380–381
pathogenesis of disease related to,
1464, 1465b

Helminthic infections, 310–313
in human immunodeficiency
virus infection, 323b
pathogenesis of, 312–313
Helminths, 298t, 310, 310t. *See also*
Parasitic pathogens.
Helper T cells. *See* T helper cells (Th
cells).
Hemangioblastoma(s), 612t, 619
Hemangiomas, 619, 1648t
in children, 1690–1691
Hematemesis, 1456, 1456t
Hematochezia, 1456, 1456t
Hematocrit, 983t
in chronic kidney disease, 1392t
pediatric, 985t, 1064t
Hematogenous osteomyelitis, 1587
Hematologic cancers,
environmental factors in, 397t
Hematologic disorders
autoimmune, 257t
in children, 1062
clotting factor and platelet
disorders, 1078–1079
erythrocyte disorders, 1065
leukemias and lymphomas,
1083–1084
references on, 1090
summary review of, 1088b
erythrocyte function alterations
in, 989–1013. *See also*
Erythrocyte disorders.
hemostatic alterations in,
1044. *See also* Hemostatic
disorders.
leukocyte function alterations
in, 1014–1018. *See also*
Leukocyte disorders.
lymphoid function alterations
in, 1030–1031. *See also*
Lymphoid disorders.
platelet alterations in, 1044. *See
also* Platelet disorders.
splenic function alterations in,
1042–1043
Hematologic lab values, in infancy
and childhood, 1064t
Hematologic system, 952
in aging, 982–987, 982t
blood components of, 952–957.
See also Blood.
in children, 982
chronic kidney disease and effects
on, 1391t, 1395
clinical evaluation of, 980–982
blood specimens in, 982, 983t
bone marrow aspirate in,
980–982
hematopoiesis in, 961–972
hemostasis in, 972–980. *See also*
Hemostasis.
lymphoid components of,
957–961. *See also* Lymphoid
organs.
references on, 987
summary review of, 986b
Hematoma, 62–63
Hematopoiesis, 961–965
bone marrow, components of,
962–963
cell differentiation in, 963–965,
964f
in depletion of circulating blood
cells, 965

Hematopoiesis (*Continued*)
erythrocyte development in, 965–
971. *See also* Erythropoiesis.
in health and illness, 1063f
leukocyte development in, 971
neonatal and fetal, 1062–1063
platelet development in, 971–972
postnatal changes in, 1063–1064
Hematopoietic growth factors, 36t,
961t, 963
Hematopoietic stem cells, 963–965,
964f
Hematuria, 1361, 1378
Heme, 967–968
Hemiagnosia pain, 494
Hemianopia, 511–512
Hemihypertrophy, and associated
childhood cancer, 438t
Hemiparesis, 564
Hemiplegia, 564
Hemiplegic posture, 575
Hemispheric breathing patterns,
530t
Hemizygous, 152–153
Hemoconcentration, 1743
Hemodialysis (continuous renal
replacement therapy), 1389,
1390b
Hemoglobin
fetal, 1063
Hemoglobin (Hb), 967–968, 967f
clinical determination of, 983t
fetal, 1063
intracellular buffering by, 116,
116f
normal values, 1262t
pediatric values of, 983t, 1064t
variants of, 967, 968t
Hemoglobin A, 143–145
Hemoglobin A1c, 749
Hemoglobin electrophoresis, 983t
Hemoglobin H disease, 1077
Hemoglobin metabolism, clinical
evaluation of, 983t
Hemoglobin oxygen saturation,
normal values, 1262t
Hemoglobin S (HbS), 143–145,
1071, 1072f
polymerization of, 1073
Hemolysins, 1375
Hemolytic anemia(s), 1003–1004
acquired, 1004t
causes of, 1003–1004, 1004t
in children, 1066t
clinical manifestations of, 1007
erythrocyte appearance in, 992f
evaluation and treatment of,
1007–1008
hereditary, 1004t
laboratory findings for, 999t
pathophysiology of, 1004–1006
secondary to drug effects, 1001t
Hemolytic disease of newborn,
1065–1067, 1066t
clinical manifestations of,
1067–1068, 1069f
evaluation and treatment of, 1068
pathophysiology of, 1067
Rh incompatibility in, 1067, 1067f
Hemolytic jaundice, 1486, 1487t
Hemolytic uremic syndrome, 1408
clinical manifestations of, 1409
evaluation and treatment of, 1409
pathophysiology of, 1408–1409

Hemophilia(s), 1078–1079
clinical manifestations of, 1079
evaluation and treatment of,
1079–1081
pathophysiology of, 1079
types of, 1078–1079
Hemophilia A, 1078–1079
pedigree of inheritance of, 150b
Hemophilia B, 1078–1079
Hemophilia C, 1079
Hemoproteins, 79
Hemoptysis, 1268
Hemorrhage, and delayed healing, 211
**Hemorrhagic cerebrovascular
disease,** 685
Hemorrhagic exudate, 205
Hemorrhagic infarcts, 602
Hemorrhagic shock
in children, 1730
classification of, 1733t
temperature regulation disorders
in, 502
Hemorrhagic stroke, 601
Hemosiderin, 79, 969
Hemosiderin accumulation, cellular,
64f
Hemosiderosis, 79
Hemostasis, 972–980
components of, 972
blood vessel, 972
clotting factor, 976–977
platelet, 972–976
definition of, 972
fibrinolysis in, 979–980
hepatic production of factors in,
1441
regulation of, 977–979
Hemostatic disorders, 1044
in children, 1078–1079
antibody mediated, 1081
inherited and congenital,
1078–1079
clotting factor dysfunction in,
1049–1051
consumptive
thrombohemorrhagic,
1050–1051
disseminated intravascular
coagulation in, 1050–1051
liver disease and, 1049–1050
thromboembolic, 1055–1059
vitamin K deficiency and, 1049
platelet dysfunction in, 1044
acquired and congenital, 1049
drug induced, 1049
immune thrombocytic purpura
in, 1045–1046
qualitative, 1048–1049
quantitative, 1044
systemic disorders and, 1049
thrombocythemia in, 1047
thrombocytopenia in, 1044
thrombotic thrombocytopenic
purpura in, 1046–1047
references on, 1059
summary review of, 1057b
Hemothorax, 1273, 1274t
Henderson-Hasselbalch equation,
115
**Henoch-Schönlein purpura
nephritis,** 1408
**Heparin-induced
thrombocytopenia,** 1044
pathophysiology of, 1045f

Hepatic artery, 1438
Hepatic encephalopathy, 1483, 1485
  in children, 1533
  clinical manifestations of, 1485
  evaluation and treatment of, 1485
  pathophysiology of, 1485
Hepatic portal circulation, 1438, 1439f
Hepatic portal vein, 1438
Hepatic vein, 1438–1439
Hepatitis
  in children, 1532
  fulminant, 1491
  viral, 1488–1490
    and associated cancer, 378t
    chronic, 1490
    clinical manifestations of, 1490
    evaluation and treatment of, 1490–1492
    icteric phase of, 1490
    incubation phase of, 1490
    pathophysiology of, 1490
    prodromal phase of, 1490
    recovery phase of, 1490
Hepatitis A (HAV) viral infection, 1488–1490, 1488f
  in children, 1532
Hepatitis A viral vaccine, 329
  adult, 329t
  child, 330t
Hepatitis A virus (HAV), 314t, 946–947, 1488t
Hepatitis B surface antigen (HBsAg), 1489, 1532
Hepatitis B (HBV) viral infection, 1489, 1489f
  in children, 1532
  sexually transmitted, 946–947
    clinical manifestations of, 947
    evaluation and treatment of, 947–948
    incidence of, 947
    pathophysiology of, 947
Hepatitis B viral vaccine, 329
  adult, 329t
  child, 330t
Hepatitis B virus (HBV), 314t, 946–947, 1488t
  in cancer, 378–379, 381t
Hepatitis C viral (HCV) infection, 1489
  in children, 1532
Hepatitis C virus (HCV), 314t, 946–947, 1488t
  in cancer, 378–379, 381t
Hepatitis D viral (HDV) infection, 1489
Hepatitis D virus (HDV), 1488t
Hepatitis delta agent, 947
Hepatitis E viral (HEV) infection, 1489–1490
Hepatitis E virus (HEV), 1488t
Hepatitis G viral (HGV) infection, 1490
Hepatitis G virus (HGV), 1488t
Hepatocellular carcinoma, 1503, 1503f, 1505f
Hepatocellular jaundice, 1485–1486, 1487t
Hepatocyte growth factor (HGF), 49
Hepatocytes, 1438–1439
Hepatopulmonary syndrome, 1483

Hepatorenal syndrome, 1487
  clinical manifestations of, 1487
  evaluation and treatment of, 1487–1490
  pathophysiology of, 1487
Hepcidin, 1434
HER-2/neu gene, 896
Herald patch, 1658, 1658f
Herd immunity, 332
Hereditary angioedema, genetic defect in, 192
Hereditary angioneurotic edema, 1318
Hereditary hemorrhagic telangiectasia, congenital heart defects associated with, 1215t
Hereditary nonpolyposis colorectal cancer, 175
  genetic basis of, 149
Hereditary sideroblastic anemia, 998
Hereditary spherocytosis, 1070
  clinical manifestations of, 1070–1071
  evaluation and treatment of, 1071
  pathophysiology of, 1070, 1070f
Hereditary thrombophilia, 1055–1056, 1056b
Heredity. *See* Genetics.
Hermansky-Pudlak syndrome, 1049
Herniated intervertebral disk, 599, 599f
  clinical manifestations of, 600
  evaluation and treatment of, 600–601
  pathophysiology of, 599
  risk factors for, 599
Herniation syndromes, 559
Heroin use, biological effects of, 63t
Herpes keratitis, 1663
Herpes simplex, 1663–1664
Herpes simplex encephalitis, 621t, 625–626, 625f
Herpes simplex labialis, 1663, 1663f
Herpes simplex virus type 1 (HSV-1), 314t
  in central nervous system infections, 621t
  in cutaneous infections, 1663
Herpes simplex virus type 2 (HSV-2), 314t
  in central nervous system infections, 621t
  in urogenital infections, 938, 1663. *See also* Genital herpes.
Herpes zoster, 1664, 1664f, 1688
Herpesviruses, 314t, 1663–1664
  Kaposi associated, 314t, 378–380, 381t
  types 6, 78, in cutaneous infections, 1663
Heterogeneous nuclear RNA (hnRNA), 133
Heterophagosome, 5–6
Heterophile antibodies, 1018
Heterosegmental control, of nociception, 486
Heterozygote, 145
Heterozygous inheritance, 145
Hexosamine pathway, in chronic hyperglycemia, 759

Hiatal hernia, 1459, 1459f
  clinical manifestations of, 1460
  evaluation and treatment of, 1460
  pathophysiology of, 1459–1460
Hibernating myocardium, 1172–1173
Hiccups, as sign of central nervous system dysfunction, 531
High altitude pulmonary edema, 72
High density lipoprotein (HDL), 1161–1162
  decreased, and risk for coronary artery disease, 1163–1164
High endothelial venules, 235
High output heart failure, 1195–1196, 1196f
High risk types of human papillomavirus, 425
Highly active antiretroviral therapy (HAART), 322–323
Highly sensitive C-reactive protein, 1164b, 1165, 1329
Hila, pulmonary, 1244
Hilum, renal, 1344–1345
Hindbrain, 450t, 455–456
Hinge region, of antibody molecule, 224
Hippocampal herniation, 559
Hippocampus, 453
Hirschsprung disease. *See* Congenital aganglionic megacolon.
Hirsutism, 1674
Histamine, 196, 203f, 447–448
  in digestive process, 1425t, 1426
  effects of, in type I hypersensitivity reactions, 265
  effects of, through H1 and H2 receptors, 196, 196f
  functions of, 448t
Histamine cephalalgia, 611
Histone deacetylation
  dietary inhibitors of, 406
  epigenetic gene modification in, 403, 406, 406f
Histones, 2
Histoplasma capsulatum, 307, 308t
HIV (human immunodeficiency virus), 314t, 318
  in central nervous system infections, 621t
  pathogenicity of, 319–321
  primary cellular targets of, 319
  tissues infected by, 319, 322f
  transmission of, 318–319
  vaccine development for infection prevention, 324
HIV-1 virion, 319, 320f
  life cycle of, and possible sites of therapeutic intervention, 319, 321f
HIV (human immunodeficiency virus) associated dementia, 627–628
HIV (human immunodeficiency virus) encephalopathy, 684
  evaluation and treatment of, 684
HIV (human immunodeficiency virus) infection
  cardiac complications in, 1189
  clinical manifestations of, 321–322
  diagnostic tests for, 806t
  neurologic complications in, 626–630, 627b

HIV (human immunodeficiency virus) infection *(Continued)*
  opportunistic infections and neoplasms development in, 323b
  pediatric
    classification system for, 326b
    encephalopathies in, 684
    progression of, to AIDS, in untreated persons, 323f
    treatment and prevention of, 322–324
HIV (human immunodeficiency virus) myelopathy, 628
HIV (human immunodeficiency virus) neuropathy, 628–629
HIV vaccine trials, 324, 325b
Hives, 265, 1666–1667
HLAs. *See* Human leukocyte antigens.
hnRNA (heterogeneous nuclear RNA), 133
Hodgkin lymphoma, 1031
  cervical, 1034f
  in children, 1088
  classification of, 1030b
  clinical differences between non-Hodgkin and, 1035t
  clinical manifestations of, 1031–1033, 1032b, 1032f
  Cotswold staging classification of, 1031–1032, 1033t
  evaluation and treatment of, 1033
  lymph node involvement in, 1031, 1033f
  pathophysiology of, 1031
  subtypes of, 1032t
  survival rate for, 1033
Holt-Oram syndrome, congenital heart defects associated with, 1215t
Homeostasis, 18
  immunologic, 258
Homocystinuria, congenital heart defects associated with, 1215t
Homologous chromosomes, 134
Homonymous hemianopia, 512
Homovanillic acid/vanillylmandelic acid (HVA/VMA), 368t
Homozygote, 145
Homozygous inheritance, 145
Homunculus, 452, 484
Hordeolum, 506
Horizontal transmission, of infections, 296
Hormesis, 419–420, 420t
Hormonal disorders, 727
  adrenal cortical, 765
  adrenal medullary, 772
  anterior pituitary, 731
  endocrine gland dysfunction in, 727–728
  in female, 819. *See also* Menstrual disorders; Puberty.
  hormone level alterations in, 727–728, 728t
  hypothalamic-pituitary, 728–729
  pancreatic endocrine, 745
  parathyroid, 742
  posterior pituitary, 728–729
  references on, 776
  summary review of, 773b–775b
  thyroid, 736
Hormonal hyperplasia, 49

Hormonal signal transduction, 18–19, 19f
cell surface receptor classification in, 701
first messenger ligands in, 700–701
second messenger pathways in, 702t, 702
by steroid (lipid soluble) hormones, 702–703, 703f
by water soluble hormones, 700–702, 701f
Hormonal therapies, and associated risk of breast cancer, 886–887
Hormone(s), 696
altered, 727–780. See also Hormonal disorders.
in appetite and satiety regulation, 1479
cardiovascular effects of, 1125–1130, 1127f
classification of, 697
general characteristics of, 696
heart rate and, interaction of, 1113
in immune response, 349
lipid soluble, 697t. See also Steroid hormones.
types of, receptors, and mechanisms of action, 700t
references on, 725
renal activation and synthesis of, 1358–1360
renal effects of, 1352, 1352f
stress induced, and physiologic alterations, 349–352
endorphin and enkephalin release, 350
female reproductive physiology, 349–350, 351f
growth hormone, 350–351
oxytocin, 351–352
prolactin, 351
testosterone, 352
structural categories of, 697t
summary review of, 723b–724b
water soluble, 697t
signal transduction by, 700–702, 701f
types of, receptors, and mechanisms of action, 700t
Hormone receptors, 699–700, 700f, 700t
Hormone release
by hypothalamus, 703–704, 707, 707t
by pineal gland, 704
by pituitary gland, 704–705, 704f. See also Anterior pituitary; Posterior pituitary.
regulation of, 697–698
negative feedback in, 697–698, 698f
neural, 698
Hormone transport, 698–699
factors and variables in, 699t
Horner syndrome, 594t
Horseshoe kidney, 1404
Horton syndrome, 611
Hospital acquired hyponatremia, 105b
Hot flashes, 810

Howell-Jolly bodies, 992f
HPA axis. See Hypothalamic-pituitary-adrenal (HPA) axis.
HPO4= or HPO42-. See Phosphate.
HPV. See Human papillomavirus.
HSV-1, HSV-2. See Herpes simplex virus type 1; Herpes simplex virus type 2.
HTLV. See Human T cell leukemia-lymphoma virus.
Human chorionic gonadotropin (hCG), in breast cancer treatment studies, 886
Human cloning, 160b
Human immunodeficiency virus. See HIV.
Human immunoglobulin, 332
Human leukocyte antigens (HLAs), 226–228
association of alleles of, and autoimmune disorders, 229t, 234–235
inheritance of, 228f
Human mammary epithelial cells (HMECs), 902–905
Human papillomavirus (HPV), 940
oncogenic, 379, 381t, 425
Human papillomavirus infection, 940, 1664
clinical manifestations of, 940–941
evaluation and treatment of, 941–943
pathophysiology of, 940
Human papillomavirus (HPV) vaccine
adult, 329t
in cervical cancer prevention, 805b, 940, 943b
child, 330t
Human T cell leukemia-lymphoma virus (HTLV), 380, 381t
in central nervous system infections, 621t
Humoral immunity, 219–220, 219f, 240–243. See also B lymphocytes (B cells), activation of.
tests evaluating, 287, 287t
Hunter syndrome, congenital heart defects associated with, 1215t
Huntington disease, 568t–569t, 570
clinical manifestations of, 570
evaluation and treatment of, 571–572
genetic basis of, 148, 526t–527t
molecular, 553t
polymorphisms in, 157
pathophysiology of, 526t–527t, 570, 570f
Hurler syndrome, congenital heart defects associated with, 1215t
Hyaline membrane disease, 1321
Hyaluronate, 1550
Hydrocele, 855, 855f
Hydrocephalus, 560, 561f
associated with myelomeningocele, 670–671
clinical manifestations of, 560
congenital, 673–674, 675f
clinical manifestations of, 674
evaluation and treatment of, 675
pathophysiology of, 674, 674f

Hydrocephalus (Continued)
course of, 560
evaluation and treatment of, 560–561
pathophysiology of, 560
types of, 560
Hydrocephalus ex vacuo, 560
Hydrocortisone, 343
Hydrogen ions, and pH, 114–117
Hydrogen sulfide asphyxiation, 68
Hydrolases, 5
Hydronephrosis, 1365–1367, 1366f
Hydrophilic pole, of molecule, 11
Hydrophobic pole, of molecule, 11
Hydrops fetalis, 1067
Hydrostatic pressure, 26–27, 99–100
Hydroureter, 1365–1367
Hydroxyapatite, 1545
Hymen, 785–786
Hyperactivity, 568t–569t
Hyperacute graft rejection, 274, 274f
Hyperaldosteronism, 768
clinical manifestations of, 769–770
evaluation and treatment of, 769–770
pathophysiology of, 768–769
primary, 768
secondary, 768
Hyperalgesia, 487–488
Hyperbaric oxygen therapy, 1588
Hyperbilirubinemia, 1067, 1485
Hypercalcemia, 113
and associated congenital heart defects, 1214t
in children, 1739
paraneoplastic, 389t
Hypercapnia, 120–121, 1269
Hyperchloremia, 104
Hyperchloremic metabolic acidosis, 118
Hypercoagulability, 1055
acquired, 1056–1059
congenital, 1080–1081
Hypercyanotic spell, 1223–1224
Hyperemia, and blood pressure, 1125
Hyperfunction, 1367
Hyperglycemia, 69
in children, 1729
effects of chronic, 758
hexosamine pathway in, 759
inappropriate protein kinase C activation in, 758–759
nonenzymatic glycosylation in, 759
oxidative stress in, 759
polyol pathway in, 758
in type 1 diabetes mellitus, 748–749
Hyperhemolytic crisis, in sickle cell disease, 1074
Hyperhomocysteinemia, and coronary artery disease, 1165
Hyperinsulinemia
in chronic kidney disease, 1395
compensatory, 751
Hyperkalemia, 110
in children, 1739
clinical manifestations of, 110–111
electrocardiogram in, 110f
evaluation and treatment of, 111–112

Hyperkalemia (Continued)
pathophysiology of, 110
prevention of, in acute kidney injury, 1389
Hyperkalemic periodic paralysis, 1609
Hyperketonemia, in type 1 diabetes mellitus, 748–749
Hyperkinesia, 568–570
Hyperkinesia syndromes, types of, 568t–569t
Hyperleptinemia, 1479
Hyperlipidemia, 69
Hypermagnesemia, 114
Hypermenorrhea, 823t
Hypermetabolic phase, of burn shock, 1744, 1747–1748
Hypermetabolism, 1711
Hypermimesis, 576–577
Hypernatremia, 103t, 104
Hyperopia, 511
Hyperosmolar hyperglycemic nonketotic syndrome (HHNKS), 757, 757t
clinical manifestations of, 757–758
evaluation and treatment of, 758
pathophysiology of, 757
Hyperparathyroidism, 742
in chronic kidney disease, 1394
clinical manifestations of, 743–744
evaluation and treatment of, 744
pathophysiology of, 742–743
primary, 742–743, 743t
pseudo-, 743
secondary, 743
Hyperphenylalaninemia, 677–678
Hyperphosphatemia, 113
Hyperpituitarism, 733
clinical manifestations of, 733
evaluation and treatment of, 733
pathophysiology of, 733
Hyperplasia, 47f, 48–49
atypical breast epithelial, 875
breast epithelial, 874
bronchial epithelial, 50f
Hyperpnea, 1268
Hyperpolarization, 1102
of cell membrane, 108–109, 109f
Hyperpolarized state, 33
Hyperprolactinemia, 735, 821–822
nonpuerperal, causes of, 871–872, 872b
Hypersensitivity, 256
initiation of, 256
mechanisms of, 258–264
Hypersensitivity reactions, 258–264
antigenic targets of, 264–271
immediate and delayed, 258
incidence of, and examples, 257t
Hypersomnia, 505
Hypersplenism, 1042
Hypertension, 1149–1150. See also Primary hypertension.
cerebral hemorrhage caused by, 602
in children, 1235
clinical manifestations of, 1236
evaluation and treatment of, 1236–1238, 1238t
pathophysiology of, 1235–1236, 1236f, 1237t
chronic (complicated), 1152–1154

Hypertension (Continued)
clinical manifestations of, 1154–1155
coronary artery disease and, 1164
evaluation and treatment of, 1155–1157, 1156f
genes and environmental interaction in, 174, 176f
malignant, 1154
obesity and, 1480
pathophysiology of, 1150–1154, 1151f
portal, 1482
primary, 1150–1152
in children, 1236
secondary, 1149
in children, conditions associated with, 1235b
systemic, in children, 1218
Hypertension reduction, in preventing stroke, 606
Hypertensive hemorrhage, 601, 602f
Hypertensive hypertrophic cardiomyopathy, 1180
Hyperthermic burn injury, 72
Hyperthermic disorders, 500–502
heat cramps, 500
heat exhaustion, 500
heat stroke, 500
hyperthermia, 500–501
malignant hyperthermia, 500–501
Hyperthyroidism, 736
clinical manifestations of, 737f
evaluation of, 738f
in Graves disease, 736–737
heart failure in, 1195
in nodular thyroid disease, 737–738
secondary, 736
systemic manifestations of, 738t
thyrotoxic crisis in, 738–739
thyrotoxicosis in, 736
Hypertonia, 562–564, 562t
Hypertonic alterations, in water balance, 103–104, 103t
causes and consequences of, 103t
Hypertonic hyponatremia, 105
Hypertonic solution, 28
Hypertrophic cardiomyopathy, 1180, 1180f
pathophysiology of, and major symptoms, 1178f
Hypertrophic muscle, 563–564, 563f
Hypertrophic obstructive cardiomyopathy, 1180
Hypertrophic osteoarthropathy, 1269
Hypertrophic scarring, 211–212, 1648t, 1654, 1721, 1721f
Hypertrophy, 47–48, 47f
of cardiac muscle, 49f
Hyperuricemia, asymptomatic, 1605
Hypervariable region, of antibody molecule, 224–225
Hyperventilation, 1268
Hyperviscosity syndrome, 1040
Hypervolemia, 103
Hyphae, 1665
Hypocalcemia, 112
in children, 1739
in chronic kidney disease, 1394–1396, 1394t

Hypocalcemia (Continued)
clinical manifestations of, 112–113
evaluation and treatment of, 113
pathophysiology of, 112
Hypocapnia, 122, 1268
Hypochloremia, 106
Hypochloremic metabolic alkalosis, 119, 120f
Hypocomplementemic, 263
Hypocortisolism, 770
secondary, 770
Hypoferremia, acquired, 996
Hypogammaglobulinemia, 278
Hypogammaglobulinemia of infancy, transient, 284
Hypogeusia, 516
Hypoglossal nerve (CN XII), 466f
origins, course, functions, and testing of, 468t
Hypoglossal nerve palsy syndromes, 568t
Hypoglycemia
in diabetes mellitus, 754–755, 757t
endogenous and exogenous causes of, 754t
functional causes of, 755t
treatment of, 755
in infants, 1729
paraneoplastic, 389t
Hypoglycemics, oral, 753, 753t
Hypokalemia, 108
in children, 1739
clinical manifestations of, 108–109
electrocardiogram in, 110f
evaluation and treatment of, 109–110
pathophysiology of, 108
Hypokalemic periodic paralysis, 1609
Hypokinesia, 571–572
in Parkinson disease, 573–574
Hypolipidemia, 69
Hypomagnesemia, 114
Hypomimesis, 576–577
Hyponatremia, 104, 105t
dilutional, 105
hospital acquired, 105b
hypertonic, 105
hypotonic, 105
Hypoparathyroidism, 744
clinical manifestations of, 744–745
evaluation and treatment of, 745
pathophysiology of, 744
Hypophosphatemia, 113
Hypophysial portal system, 706f
Hypophysiotropic hormones, 707t
Hypophysis, 704–705, 705f. See also Pituitary gland.
Hypopituitarism, 731
clinical manifestations of, 731–732
evaluation and treatment of, 732–733
pathophysiology of, 731
Hypoplastic anemia, 999
Hypoplastic kidney(s), 1406
Hypoplastic left heart syndrome, 1230, 1230f
clinical manifestations of, 1230
evaluation and treatment of, 1230–1231
pathophysiology of, 1230

Hypopolarization, of cell membrane, 110–111
Hypopolarized state, 33
Hypoproteinemia, 211
Hyposmia, 516
Hypospadias, 1404–1405, 1405f
Hypotensive shock, 1727
Hypothalamic-pituitary-adrenal (HPA) axis, 338, 338f
alterations in
and development of depression, 653–654, 653b–654b
and mood and behavior modulation, 654
cancer treatment and activation of, 353
in coping with stress, 653–654
influence of, on immune response, 348–349
Hypothalamic-pituitary axis, 703–708
alterations in, 728–729, 729f
anterior pituitary in, 707–708
hypothalamus in, 703–704
pituitary in, 704–705
posterior pituitary in, 705–707
Hypothalamic-pituitary cycle, of menstrual cycle, 793f, 794–795
Hypothalamic-pituitary-gonadal (HPG) axis, 784, 785f, 800–802
alterations of, in delayed puberty, 817
Hypothalamic-pituitary-testicular (HPT) axis, 802, 802f
Hypothalamohypophysial tract, 703, 706f
Hypothalamus, 450t, 453–455, 703–704
functions of, 455b
in sleep regulation, 503
in temperature regulation, 496–498
hormones released by, 703–704, 707, 707t
alterations in, 728, 729f
hypophysial nervous system and, 703, 706f
Hypothermia, 501–502
accidental, 501, 502t
therapeutic, 502
Hypothermic injury, 71
Hypothyroidism, 739
clinical manifestations of, 737f, 739–741
congenital, 741–742
evaluation and treatment of, 741–742
pathophysiology of, 739
primary, 741
primary and secondary, 739, 739f
subclinical, 741
systemic manifestations of, 740t
Hypotonia, 562, 562t, 634
Hypotonic disorders, 103t, 104
causes and consequences of, 105t
Hypotonic hyponatremia, 105
Hypotonic solution, 28
Hypoventilation, 1268
Hypovolemia, 103
in children, 1730, 1731t
assessment of, 1732, 1732t
dysfunctional inflammatory response and, 211

Hypovolemic shock, 1701–1702, 1717
in children, 1728–1729, 1745–1748
clinical manifestations of, 1729–1733
compensatory mechanisms in, 1729
pathophysiology of, 1701, 1701b, 1701f, 1728b
Hypoxemia
anemic, 990
caused by congenital heart defects, 1217–1218
clinical manifestations of, 1218
causes of, 1270t
pulmonary causes of, 1269–1271
Hypoxia, tissue, 52, 990, 1269
cell injury in, 52–62, 53f, 68
coronary, 1160
in shock, 1697, 1727
Hypoxia/hypothermia interaction, 72
Hypoxic pulmonary vasoconstriction, 1260–1261, 1261b
Hysterosalpingogram, 808t
Hysteroscopy, 808t

I

I bands, of myocardial muscle, 1106
Iatrogenic hypothyroidism, 741
ICF. See Intracellular fluid.
Icterus, 1485
Icterus gravis neonatorum, 1068
Icterus neonatorum, 1068
Idiojunctional rhythm, 1197t–1198t
Idiopathic congenital equinovarus, 1623
Idiopathic epilepsy, 539–542
Idiopathic equinovarus, 1623
Idiopathic pulmonary fibrosis, 1277
Idiopathic scoliosis, 1625
Idiopathic thrombocytopenic purpura, 1081
clinical manifestations of, 1081
evaluation and treatment of, 1081–1083, 1082b
pathophysiology of, 1081
Idioventricular rhythm, 1197t–1198t
IFN. See Interferon(s).
IgA, 223, 224f, 247
IgA deficiency
and associated childhood cancer, 438t
selective, 279
IgA nephropathy, 1381t, 1382
in children, 1408
IgA protease, bacterial, 304
IgD, 223–224, 224f
in B cell receptors, 234, 234f, 241–242, 241f
IgE, 224, 224f
function of, 247, 248f
serum, laboratory tests for, 267
IgE-mediated hypersensitivity reactions, 258–259, 259t
allergy and symptoms associated with, 265–267, 266f, 266t
mechanism of, 259, 260f
tests of, 265–267
IGF binding proteins, 414. See also Insulin-like growth factor.

IgG, 222, 224f, 247
IgG subclass deficiency, 279
IgM, 223, 224f, 247
  in B cell receptors, 234, 234f,
    241–242, 241f
IL. *See* Interleukin(s).
IL-7 receptor, 233, 234f
IL-7 receptor deficiency, 280
Ileocecal valve (sphincter), 1428,
    1435
Ileogastric reflex, 1435
Ileum, 1428
ILGF. *See* Insulin-like growth factor.
Illumination, in cell injury, 74–75
Image processing deficits, 547t
Imatinib (Gleevec), 387t
Immediate hypersensitivity
    reactions, 258
Immortality, of cancer cells, 362
Immovable joint, 1549
Immune competency, 284–285
Immune complex, 188–189
Immune complex deposition,
    glomerular, 1383
Immune complex disorders,
    263–264
Immune complex-mediated
    hypersensitivity reactions, 258,
    259t, 261–264, 263f
  allergy and symptoms associated
    with, 266t, 267
Immune complex model, of drug
    induced hemolytic anemia,
    1006
Immune corticotropin-releasing
    hormone, 339
Immune deficiency(ies), 275–290
  congenital and acquired, 275
  evaluation and treatment in,
    286–287, 287t
  initial clinical presentation in, 275
  primary, 275–284, 276t. *See*
    also Primary immune
    deficiencies.
    B lymphocyte deficiencies,
      278–279
    combined T and B lymphocyte
      deficiencies, 279–281
    complement deficiencies, 281
    phagocytic deficiencies, 281–284
    T lymphocyte deficiencies, 279
  replacement therapies for,
    287–290
    gamma globulins in, 287–288
    gene therapy in, 288–290
    immune modulator treatment
      in, 288
    transplantation and transfusion
      in, 288
  secondary, 284–286. *See also*
    Secondary immune
    deficiencies.
Immune modulator therapy, 288
Immune response (adaptive
    immunity), 217
  active and passive, 220
  in aging, 251
  antibody function in, 244–247
  clonal diversity in, 229–235. *See*
    also Clonal diversity.
  cortisol and, 344–346
  differentiating characteristics of,
    218
  fetal and neonatal, 250

Immune response (adaptive
    immunity) *(Continued)*
  general characteristics of, 217–220
  humoral and cell-mediated,
    219–220. *See also* B
    lymphocytes (B cells); T
    lymphocytes (T cells).
  key terminology of, 254b
  overview of, 219f
  primary and secondary, 240–241,
    240f
  recognition and, 220–229. *See also*
    Antibody(ies); B cell receptor
    (BCR) complex; T cell
    receptor (TCR) complex.
    adhesion molecule pairings in,
      228, 228b
    antigen presentation in, 226–228.
      See also CD1; Major
      histocompatibility complex.
    cytokines and receptors in,
      228–229, 229t
    induction of, 221–222. *See*
      also Antigen(s); Clonal
      selection; Immunogen(s).
  references on, 254
  secretory, 246–247
  summary review of, 252b–253b
  superantigen formation in, 244
Immune system, 246
  alteration(s) in, 256–275. *See also*
    Immune system disorders.
  chronic kidney disease and effects
    on, 1391t, 1395
  cortisol and, 344–346
  interaction of, with endocrine and
    nervous systems, 347, 348t
  secretory (mucosal), 246–247, 246f
  stress and, 347–352
Immune system disorders, 256–275
  alloimmune, 270–271. *See also*
    Alloimmune disorders;
    Alloimmunity.
  autoimmune, 267–270. *See also*
    Autoimmune disorders;
    Autoimmunity.
  and development of cancer, 378
  hypersensitivity, 258–264. *See*
    also Allergy; Hypersensitivity
    reactions.
  immune deficiency, 275–290. *See*
    also Immune deficiency(ies).
  stress and, 336–359 *See also*
    Stress.
Immune thrombocytic purpura,
    1045–1046
  clinical manifestations of, 1046
  evaluation and treatment of,
    1046–1047
  pathophysiology of, 1045
Immune thrombocytopenic
    purpura, maternal
    hypersensitivity in, 271
Immunity, 217–220. *See also*
    Immune response (adaptive
    immunity); Innate immunity.
  active and passive, 220
  alteration(s) in, 256–275. *See also*
    Immune system disorders.
  clinical evaluation of, 286–287, 287t
  key terminology of, 290b
  references on, 290
  summary review of, 289b–290b
  vaccine induced, 329–332

Immunization. *See* Infectious
    disease(s); Vaccines.
Immunocompetence, 218
  in children, 1312
Immunocompromised
    individuals. *See also* AIDS
    (acquired immunodeficiency
    syndrome); HIV (human
    immunodeficiency virus)
    infection.
  microorganisms causing
    pneumonia in, 1290
Immunocytes, 955
Immunogen(s), 221–222
Immunogenicity, 221–222
  pathogenic, 297
Immunoglobulin(s). *See also*
    Antibody(ies), *and specific*
    immunoglobulins., 217–218,
    222–225
  antigen binding by, 225
  antigen binding region of, 225,
    225f
  biological properties of, 225t
  classes of, 222–224
  in hypersensitivity reactions,
    258–264, 259t
  in passive immunotherapy, 332
  physicochemical properties of,
    224t
  secretory, 246–247
  structure of, 224–225, 224f
Immunologic and inflammatory cell
    injury, 69
Immunologic homeostasis, 258
Immunologically privileged sites,
    268–269
Immunosuppression
  bacterial induction of, 305
  fungal induction of, 309
Immunotherapy, passive, 332
Impaired hemostasis, 1049–1050.
    See also Hemostatic disorders.
Imperforate anus, 1522
Impetigo, 1663, 1683
  and herpes labialis, 1683f
Impetigo contagiosum, 1683
Implicit memory, 543
Inappropriate lactation, 871
Inbreeding, 141–142
Incidence of disease, in populations,
    164–165
  risk factors and, 165
Incidence rate, 164
Incident pain, 493–494
Incised wounds, 65, 65f
Incomplete fracture, 1569
Incontinence, types of, 1369t, 1415t
Increased intracranial pressure,
    557–559
  compensatory mechanisms in,
    558
  herniation resulting from,
    558–559, 558f. *See also*
    Herniation syndromes.
Increased pulmonary blood
    flow, congenital heart defects
    causing, 1218
Incretin hormones, in treating
    diabetes mellitus, 752b
Incretins, 752
Incubation period, of infectious
    disease, 296
Incus, 512–513

Independent assortment, principle
    of, 146
Indeterminate (distance) range
    gunshot wounds, 67, 67f
Indirect Coombs test, 983t–985t,
    1068
Individual carcinogens, 396
Induced ischemia, 1166–1167, 1167f
Induction chemotherapy, 388
Infant(s)
  blood pressure in, normal values,
    1237t
  cardiovascular development in,
    1209, 1213
  circulatory system of, 1213
  hematologic development in, 982
  hematologic test values in, 985t
  hemodynamics in, 1213
  pain perception in, 495, 495f
  recurrent seizures in, 539t
  reflexes in, 668, 668t
Infant diarrhea, 1530
Infantile autism
  liability distribution of, 167
  recurrence risks for, 170t
Infantile spasms, 679–680
Infarction, 1160
Infection(s), 293–335
  antibody protection against,
    244–246
  bacterial, 297–307. *See also*
    Bacterial infections.
  cancer associated, 391, 392t
  in chronic diabetes mellitus, 765
  congenital heart defects associated
    with, 1214t
  and coronary artery disease, 1165
  cutaneous, 1662–1665
  drug resistant, 294
  emergent, 294, 295t
  female reproductive system, 828
  fungal, 307–310. *See also* Fungal
    infections.
  increasing incidence of, 294
  infectious disease and, 293, 294t.
    See also Infectious disease(s).
  microorganisms causing, 295–318
  parasitic, 310–313. *See also*
    Parasitic infections.
  process of, 295–296
  protozoan, 310–313. *See also*
    Protozoan infections.
  recurrent, 275
  respiratory tract, 1290–1291.
    See also Acute bronchitis;
    Pneumonia; Pulmonary
    abscess; Tuberculosis.
  in children, 1315–1316, 1326.
    See also Childhood
    respiratory disorders.
  secondary immune deficiencies
    and, 286
  viral, 313–318. *See also* Viral
    infections.
Infection control measures, 326–327
Infectious arthritis, 1597t
Infectious bone disease, 1586–1587
  pathophysiology of, 1587–1588,
    1587f
Infectious cell injury, 69
Infectious disease(s), 293, 294t
  classification of, by prevalence and
    spread, 297
  clinical course of, 296–297

Infectious disease(s) (Continued)
countermeasures against, 326–332, 327t
antimicrobials, 327–329
infection control, 326–327
passive immunotherapy, 332
vaccination, 329–332
key terminology of, 334b
references on, 335
summary review of, 332b–334b
vaccine preventable, reductions in, 327t
Infectious microorganisms, 295–318. *See also* Pathogen(s).
classes of, 297–318, 298t
bacteria, 297–307. *See also* Bacterial infections.
fungi, 307–310. *See also* Fungal infections.
helminths, 310–313. *See also* Parasitic infections.
protozoa, 310–313. *See also* Protozoan infections.
viruses, 313–318. *See also* Viral infections.
colonization by, 296
in development of autoimmunity, 269
disease caused by, 296–297. *See also* Infectious disease(s).
emerging, 294
multiplication of, 296
pathogenicity of, 297
spread of, 296
tissue invasion by, 296
toxin production by, 245
used in bioterrorism, 294–295
Infectious mononucleosis, 1017–1018
clinical manifestations of, 1018
evaluation and treatment of, 1018–1020
peripheral blood smear in, 1019f
splenic rupture in, 1019
transmission of, 1018
Infective endocarditis, 1187
in children with congenital heart defects, 1214b
clinical manifestations of, 1189
evaluation and treatment of, 1189
of mitral valve, 1189f
pathophysiology of, 1187–1188, 1188f
Infectivity, of pathogen, 297
Inferior colliculi, 455
Inferior mesenteric ganglia, 467
Inferior vena cava, 1095
Infertility, 849–850
endometriosis and, 840
in female, 849–850
in male, 870–871, 871b
Infiltrating mammary carcinoma, 897t
Infiltrations, 76
Infiltrative splenomegaly, 1043
Inflammation, 183
acute phase, 186, 187f, 205–206, 209f. *See also* Inflammatory response.
chemical mediators of, 203f
plasma proteins circulating in, 206, 206t
cardinal signs of, 186, 205

Inflammation (Continued)
chronic, 206–208
and cancer, 377–378, 378t
essential fatty acids and, 199b
in human defense mechanisms, 184
limiting mediators of, 203f
local manifestations of, 205
maturation phase of, 210
resolution and repair phase of, 208–213. *See also* Wound healing.
sequence of events in, 187, 188–189f. *See also* Inflammatory response.
serum markers of, 1164b, 1165
systemic manifestations of, 205–206
Inflammatory acne, 1680–1681
Inflammatory bowel disease, 1471
and associated cancer, 378t
Crohn disease in, 1473, 1474t
diverticular disease of colon in, 1474
probiotics and, 1473b
ulcerative colitis in, 1471, 1474t
Inflammatory gastrointestinal infections, bacterial agents causing, 299t–300t
Inflammatory joint disease, 1596–1597
Inflammatory mediators, 487–488, 488b
Inflammatory muscle diseases, 1611
Inflammatory response, 184, 186–205
acute, 186, 187f
cellular mediators of, 192–203
basophils in, 202
cellular receptors in, 192–195
eosinophils in, 202
mast cells in, 195–198
monocytes and macrophages in, 201–202
natural killer (NK) cells in, 202
neutrophils in, 201
phagocytosis in, 198–201
platelets in, 202–203
products of, 203–205, 203f. *See also* Chemokines; Cytokines.
dysfunctional, 211
plasma protein systems in, 187–192
interactions among, 192, 193f
vascular, 186–187
Inflammatory skin disorders, 1655–1656
Inflammatory stromal component, 900–901
Inflow tract, 1094
Influenza, 1291
pathogenesis of, 316–318, 1291–1292. *See also* Viral pneumonia.
Influenza pandemic, of, 297t, 317–318, 1918–1919
Influenza vaccine, 329
adult, 329t
child, 330t
Influenza virus, 314t, 316
Infratentorial disorders, 528, 529t
Infratentorial herniation, 559

Infundibulum, of oviduct, 789
Inguinal canal, 796
formation of, 797f
Inheritance of traits
autosomal dominant, 146–150
autosomal recessive, 151–152
in consanguinity, 152
laws of, 146
multifactorial, 165–169. *See also* Multifactorial disorder(s).
sex-limited and sex-influenced, 155
X-linked, 152–155
Inherited metabolic disorders, of central nervous system, 677–679, 677t
Inherited myasthenic syndromes, 638–639
Inhibin, 794
Inhibited sexual desire, 848
Inhibitory interneurons, 484
Inhibitory neurotransmitters, 488b, 488–490
Inhibitory postsynaptic potentials (IPSPs), 448–449
INK4A, 902f
Innate immunity, 183–184, 184t, 345
in aging, 213
first line defenses in, 184–186, 345
bacteria-derived chemicals, 186
biochemical barriers, 184–186
epithelial-derived chemicals, 185–186
physical and mechanical barriers, 184, 185f
in neonates, 212
second line defense in, 186–205. *See also* Inflammation; Inflammatory response.
Inner dura, 459–460
Inner membrane, mitochondrial, 7
Inorganic ion transport systems, 30t
Inositol triphosphate (IP3), 702
in second messenger signaling pathways, 23t
Inotropic agents, 1111
calcium sensitizing, 1193–1194
for children in shock, 1740t
Insect bites, 1667–1668
in children, 1688–1690
Insomnia, 504–505
Inspiration, mechanics of, 1252, 1252f, 1254f
in children, 1311–1312, 1312f
Insufficiency fracture, 1569
Insula, 452
Insulin, 713–714
cardiovascular effects of, 1130, 1130b
endothelial response to, 1119b
increased plasma, and obesity, 1479
pancreatic cells secreting, 713
physiologic effects of, 713–714, 715t
and plasma potassium, 107
receptors for, and mechanism of action, 700t, 715f
second messengers in signal transduction by, 23t
Insulin deficiency, absolute, 745. *See also* Type 1 diabetes mellitus.

Insulin-like growth factor (ILGF), 36t, 409–414
aging and effects on secretion of, 721–722, 1579
in breast epithelial cell growth, 414–415, 885
Insulin-like growth factor II (ILGF-II), 36t
Insulin resistance, 750
adipocyte hormone release and, 713–714, 714b
and hypertension, 1152
in polycystic ovary syndrome, 824–825
and systolic heart failure, 1190
Insulin shock (insulin reaction), 754–755
Intact nephron hypothesis, 1390–1392
Integral membrane proteins, 11
Integrase, 319
Integrase inhibitors, 323–324
Integrins, 194–195, 198–199
osteoclasts binding to, 1544
in vascular endothelium, 972
Integumentary system, 1644
chronic kidney disease and effects on, 1391t, 1396
structure and function of, 1644–1646
Intentional tremor, 568t
Intercalated cells, of nephron collecting duct, 1347
Intercalated disks, 1105
Interdigestive myoelectric complex, 1435
Interferon(s) (IFN), 204–205
action of, 204–205
in immune response, 228–229, 229t–300t
in inflammatory response, 203f, 204–205
superantigen production of, 244
Interleukin(s) (ILs), 204
in inflammatory response, 203f
receptors of, in immune response, 228–229, 229t
Interleukin-1 (IL-1), 204, 228–229, 229t, 238–239, 239f, 349
Interleukin-2 (IL-2), 36t, 244, 961t
in immune response, 228–229, 229t, 239, 239f
Interleukin-3 (IL-3), 242, 961t
Interleukin-4 (IL-4), 228–229, 229t, 239f, 242, 961t
Interleukin-5 (IL-5), 228–229, 229t, 242, 961t
Interleukin-6 (IL-6), 49, 228–229, 229t, 239f
in pathogenesis of cardiogenic shock, 1700b
Interleukin-7 (IL-7), 228–229, 229t, 961t
Interleukin-8 (IL-8), 228–229, 229t
Interleukin-10 (IL-10), 204, 228–229, 229t
Interleukin-11 (IL-11), 961t
Interleukin-12 (IL-12), 228–229, 229t, 239f
Interleukin-13 (IL-13), 228–229, 229t
Interleukin-15 (IL-15), 961t
Interleukin-17 (IL-17), 228–229, 229t

Interleukin-22 (IL-22), 228–229, 229t
Interlobar arteries, renal, 1347–1348
Intermediary metabolism, 8
Intermediate range entrance wounds, 66–67, 66f
Intermediolateral gray (lateral horn), 456
Intermittent claudication, 1160
Internal anal sphincter, 1435–1436
Internal capsule, 452–453
Internal carotid arteries, 462
Internal carotid artery occlusion, stroke syndromes resulting from, 604t
Internal urethral sphincter, 1350
International Agency for Research on Cancer (IARC), 426
  classification of carcinogenic agents by, 427b
International classification of epilepsies, 538b
Interneurons, 444
Interphase, 33–34
Interstitial cell stimulating hormone (ICSH), target organs of, 704f
Interstitial cerebral edema, 560
Interstitial fluid, 96, 97t
  plasma and, water movement between, 98
Interstitial matrix. *See* Extracellular matrix.
Intervertebral disk, 461–462
  herniated, 599
Intestinal adhesions, 1461t, 1462f
Intestinal digestion and absorption in, 1429–1434
Intestinal herniation, 1461t, 1462f
Intestinal malrotation, 1519
  clinical manifestations of, 1520
  evaluation and treatment of, 1520
  pathophysiology of, 1519–1520
Intestinal motility, 1434–1435
Intestinal obstruction, 1460
  classification of, 1462t
  clinical manifestations of, 1461–1462
  evaluation and treatment of, 1462–1465
  pathophysiology of, 1460–1461, 1461t, 1463f
Intestinal peristalsis, 1435
Intestinal phase, of gastric secretion, 1428
Intestinal torsion, 1461t, 1462f
Intestinal transferrin, 1434
Intestinointestinal reflex, 1435
Intima, 1550
Intra-aortic balloon pump, 1193–1194
Intra-abdominal pressure, in burn injury, 1743–1744
Intracardiac pressures, normal, 1096, 1098f, 1099f
Intracellular bacteria, 302–303
Intracellular fluid (ICF), 96, 97t
  extracellular fluid and, water movement between, 97–98, 98f
Intracellular fungi, 308
Intracellular protozoa, 311
Intracellular signaling cascade, 20f
Intracellular viral cycle, 315, 315f
Intracerebral hematomas, 587

Intracerebral hemorrhage,
  pathophysiologic mechanisms in, 603f
Intracerebral tumors, 613–616
Intracranial aneurysms, 606
  clinical manifestations of, 607
  evaluation and treatment of, 607
  pathophysiology of, 606–607
  types of, 606–607, 606f
Intracranial hemorrhage, 601
Intracranial pressure (ICP), 557
  increased, 557–559
Intracranial tumors, 611–618
  clinical manifestations of, 613f
  common sites of, 613f
Intraductal papilloma, 874t
Intradural spinal tumors, 618
Intrahepatic portal hypertension, 1533
Intramedullary spinal cord abscess, 624
Intramedullary spinal cord tumors, 618
  clinical manifestations of, 620
  pathophysiology of, 619
Intramembranous bone formation, 1541, 1618
Intramuscular injections, repeated, myopathy resulting from, 1613
Intraosseous cannulation, 1746
Intraparenchymal hemorrhages, 587, 588f
  clinical manifestations of, 587–588
Intravascular fluid, 96, 97t
Intraventricular foramen, 461
Intraventricular hydrocephalus, 560
Intrinsic (intrarenal) acute kidney injury, 1386t, 1387
  in children, 1411
  urine characteristics in, 1389t
Intrinsic factor, in digestive process, 1427
Intrinsic factor deficiency, 993–994
  and development of pernicious anemia, 968, 1427
Intrinsic pathway, of clotting cascade, 187f, 190, 976–977
Introitus, 785–786
Introns, 134
Intussusception, 1461t, 1462f
  in children, 1522–1523
  clinical manifestations of, 1523
  evaluation and treatment of, 1523
  pathophysiology of, 1523, 1523f
Inulin clearance, 1360
Invariant chain, 236–237
Invasion period, of infectious disease, 296
Invasive breast carcinoma, 901–905
Invasive cancer, 361, 362f
Invasive carcinoma of cervix, 842
Invasive gastrointestinal infections, bacterial agents causing, 299t–300t
Inverse psoriasis, 603f
Inversions, chromosome, 143
Involucrum, 1587–1588, 1628–1629
Iodine, in bone tissue physiology, 1580b

Iodine deficiency, 741
  development of breast disorders and, 879b
Ion channel plasma membrane receptors, 701
Ion channels, 28
Ion exchange buffering, cellular, 117
Ionizing radiation. *See* Radiation exposure.
Ions, 12. *See also* Electrolyte(s).
IP3 pathway, 23t
Iris, 507
Iron
  in bone tissue physiology, 1580b
  in erythropoiesis, 969t
  intake and intestinal absorption of, 1434
  physiologic functions of, 996
Iron chelation therapy, for thalassemia, 1078
Iron cycle, 970f
  controlled iron absorption in, 969–971
  sources of iron introduced into, 971
Iron deficiency, and cognitive function, 666b
Iron deficiency anemia, 995–996
  in children, 1065
  clinical manifestations of, 1065–1066
  evaluation and treatment of, 1066–1067
  pathophysiology of, 1065
  clinical manifestations of, 996–997, 996–997f
  evaluation and treatment of, 997–998
  incidence and prevalence of, 996
  laboratory findings for, 999t
  pathophysiology of, 996
Iron depletion therapy, 999–1000
Iron dextran, 997–998
Iron replacement therapy, 997
Iron sucrose injection (Venofer), 997 998
Irregular bones, 1547
Irreversible coma, 534–535
Irritant contact dermatitis, 1656, 1682
Irritant receptors, pulmonary, 1251, 1267
Irritative syndrome, 619
Ischemia, 52, 990, 1269
  cell injury in, 52–62, 53f, 68
  coronary, 1160
  in shock, 1697, 1727
Ischemic preconditioning, 1171–1172
Ischemic ulcers, 1467
Islet cell transplantation, pancreatic, 714b
  in type 1 diabetes mellitus, 750b
Islets of Langerhans, 712
Isoflavones, and breast cancer risk, 893
Isohemagglutinins, 272
Isoimmunity, 256–258
Isolated systolic hypertension, 1149
Isometric contraction, 1562
Isotonic alterations, in water balance, 102–103, 103t
Isotonic contraction, 1562
Isotonic solution, 28

Isotonic volume depletion, 103
Isotonic volume excess, 103
Isotope cisternography, 476
Isotropic bands, of myocardial muscle, 1106
Isotype switch, immunoglobulin, 242
Isthmus, uterine, 787–788
Itching, 1654–1655

J

J receptors, pulmonary, 1251, 1267
JAK (Janus family of tyrosine kinases), 701
JAK/STAT pathway, 23t, 701, 702t
JAK3 deficiency, 280
Jaundice, 1485
  clinical manifestations of, 1486
  evaluation and treatment of, 1487
  hemolytic, 1486
  hepatocellular, 1485–1486
  neonatal, 1531
  obstructive, 1485
  pathophysiologic, 1531
  pathophysiology of, 1485–1486, 1486f, 1487t
JC virus, 621t
Jejunum, 1428
Jerk nystagmus, 509
Joint(s), 1548–1549, 1550f
  aging of, 1564
  cartilaginous, 1549
  classification of, 1549
  fibrous, 1549
  function testing of, 1563
  synovial, 1550–1554
  types of, 1551f
Joint capsule, 1550
Joint cavity, 1550
Joint disorders, 1592–1594
  ankylosing spondylitis in, 1600
  autoimmune, 257t–258t
  gout in, 1602
  inflammatory joint disease in, 1596–1597
  osteoarthritis in, 1592–1594
Joint effusion, 1595
Joint stiffness, 1595
Joint structure, and function, 1548–1554
Jones Criteria, for diagnosis of rheumatic fever, 1187t
Junctional bradycardia, 1197t–1198t
Junctional complex, 16–18
Junctional tachycardia, 1197t–1198t
Juvenile myoclonic epilepsy, 680
Juvenile rheumatoid arthritis, 1630–1631
Juxtaglomerular apparatus, 1346–1347, 1349f
Juxtaglomerular cells, 1346–1347
Juxtamedullary nephrons, 1345

K

K+. *See* Potassium.
Kallikrein-kinin cascade, 1710
Kaposi-associated herpesvirus, 378–380, 381t, 1663
Kaposi sarcoma, 1672–1673
  in AIDS patient, 324f, 1673f
Kartagener syndrome, congenital heart defects associated with, 1215t

Karyolysis, 81
Karyorrhexis, 81
Karyotype, 134, 138f
Kasai procedure, 1531–1532, 1532f
Kawasaki disease, 1234
  clinical manifestations of, 1234
  diagnostic criteria for, 1235b
  evaluation and treatment of,
    1234–1235
  pathological stages of, 1234
Keloids, 211–212, 212f, 1648t–1653t,
    1654, 1654f
  clawlike prolongations of, 1654,
    1654f
Keratin, 1644–1645
Keratinocytes, 1644–1645
Keratitis, 507
Keratoacanthoma, 1668, 1668f
Kernicterus, 1068, 1531
Kernig sign, 609
Ketogenic diet, for children with
    epilepsy, 680b
Ketosis prone diabetes, 755–756
Kidney(s). See also Renal entries.
  autoimmune disorders of,
    257t–258t
  blood flow within, 1351–1352,
    1353t
  hormone activation and synthesis
    in, 1358–1360
  nephron units of, 1345–1347
    glomerular filtration within,
      1352–1357, 1353t–1354f
    structure of, 1345, 1346f
    tubules of, 1347, 1347f
      transport within, 1355–1357,
        1356b
    types of, 1345
    vascular supply of, 1347–1350,
      1348f
  potassium balance regulation
    by, 107
  structure of, 1344–1350, 1345f
  urine formation within, 1354f,
    1357–1358, 1357f
    antidiuretic hormone and
      effects on, 1358
    catecholamines and effects on,
      1358
    concentration and dilution in,
      1357–1358
    decreased, 106
    diuretic effects on, 1358
    vascular supply of, 1347–1350
Kidney injury, classification of,
    1386, 1386t
Kidney stones, 1368, 1605
  clinical manifestations of, 1369
  evaluation and treatment of,
    1369–1371
  pathophysiology of, 1368–1369
Kidney tumors, 1372
Kinin system, in inflammatory
    response, 191
Kininases, 191
Klebsiella granulomatis, 933–934
Klebsiella pneumoniae, 299t
Klinefelter syndrome, 141, 141f
Knee joint, 1552f
Kohler disease, 1631
Koilonychia, in iron deficiency, 997f
Konno procedure, 1229
Koplik spots, 1686–1687
Krebs cycle, 23–24

Kupffer cells, 1438–1439, 1441
Kussmaul respiration, 1268
Kwashiorkor, 1481–1482. See also
    Protein energy malnutrition.
Kyphosis, 1582–1583, 1583f, 1601,
    1601f, 1620

L
Labia majora, 784–785
Labia minora, 785
Labile factor (clotting factor V), 977t
  disorder(s) associated with, 1079t
Labored breathing, 1268
Laceration(s), 64–65, 64f
Lacrimal apparatus, 506, 506f
Lactase deficiency, 1470–1471
Lacteal, 1429
Lactoferrin, 1008
Lactose intolerance, 1531
Lacuna, 1543
Lacunar stroke (lacunar infarct),
    601, 602f
Lafora disease, genetic basis and
    pathophysiology of, 526t–527t
Lambert-Eaton myasthenic
    syndrome, 638
Lamina propria, 1429
Laminae, in gray matter, 483–484
Laminar flow, 1121, 1124f
Langerhans cells, 1645
Langhans giant cell, 207–208, 207f
Language disturbances, 551t. See
    also Dysphasias.
Lanthanic (silent) disease,
    1154–1155
Laparoscopy, 808t
Laplace's law
  alveolar ventilation, 1252–1253
  and cardiac output, 1110
  and hemodynamics of aneurysm,
    1144–1145, 1145f
Large bowel obstruction, 1461,
    1461t
  clinical manifestations of, 1462
Large cell carcinoma,
    bronchogenic, 1301–1302,
    1302f
Large intestine, 1435–1437, 1436f
Laryngeal cancer, 1299
  clinical manifestations of, 1299,
    1299f
  evaluation and treatment of,
    1299–1303
  pathophysiology of, 1299
  risk factors for, 397t–400t, 401,
    1299
Laryngeal papillomas, 941
Laryngomalacia, in children, 1319,
    1319f
Laryngotracheobronchitis, 1315t,
    1316
  clinical manifestations of,
    1316–1317, 1316f
  evaluation and treatment of, 1317
  pathophysiology of, 1316
  spasmodic, 1316–1317
  upper airway obstruction in,
    1317f
Larynx, 1243–1244, 1245f
Lassa virus, 314t
Late asthma response, 1284
Late asthmatic response,
    1331–1332, 1331f
Late dumping syndrome, 1469

Latent syphilis, 928–929
  clinical manifestations of, 929
Latent TB infection, 1293
Lateral apertures (foramina of
    Luschka), 461
Lateral column, 456–457
Lateral corticospinal tract, 457f, 458
Lateral epicondylopathy, 1574
Lateral fissure, 452
Lateral mass herniation, 559
Lateral spinothalamic tract, 457f,
    458–459
Lateral sulcus, 452
Lawrence-Moon-Biedl syndrome,
    congenital heart defects
    associated with, 1215t
LDL (low density lipoprotein), 31,
    1161–1162
  elevated serum, and risk for
    coronary artery disease, 1162
  oxidation of, 1157–1159, 1159f
Lead, in chemical cell injury, 56–59
Lead poisoning, 682, 682b
  systemic effects of, 683f
Lean body mass, 1560
Lectin pathway, of complement
    cascade activation, 188–189,
    190f
Lectins, antimicrobial, 186
Lee-White coagulation time,
    983t–285t
Left anterior descending artery,
    1097
Left atrium, 1093
Left bundle branch, 1102
Left coronary artery, 1096
Left heart, 1091
Left heart failure, 1190–1194
  diastolic ventricular, 1194
  systolic ventricular, 1190–1194
Left pulmonary artery, 1095
Left ventricle, 1093
Left ventricular dysfunction, and
    stress, 337b
Left ventricular end-diastolic
    pressure, 1110–1111
Left ventricular end-diastolic
    volume, 1110–1111
Left ventricular hypertrophy, 1136
Legg-Calvé-Perthes disease, 1631
  clinical manifestations of, 1632
  evaluation and treatment of, 1632
  pathophysiology of, 1631–1632,
    1631f
Legionella pneumophila, 298–300,
    299t–300t
Legionella pneumophila
    pneumonia, community
    acquired, 1291
Leiomyomas, 837–838, 838f
  clinical manifestations of, 838
  evaluation and treatment of,
    838–840
  pathophysiology of, 838
Leishmania spp., 310t
  complement evasion by, 311
  intracellular survival of, 311
  transmission of, 311
Lennox-Gastaut syndrome, 680
Lens, 508
Lentiform nucleus, 452–453
Lentigo malignant melanoma, 1671,
    1672f, 1672t
Lepromatous leprosy, 202

Leptin, 1478b
  plasma, and obesity, 1479
  receptors of, mechanism of
    action, 700t
  in second messenger pathways,
    23t
Leptin resistance, 1479
Leptin secretion, in puberty, 350,
    784
Lesch-Nyhan syndrome, genetic
    basis and pathophysiology of,
    526t–257t
Lesions, caused by inflammation,
    205
Leucine enkephalin, 489
Leukemia(s), 364t, 1019–1020
  acute, 1019, 1021–1022
  cellular morphologic aspects of,
    1029f
  in children, 437, 1083–1084. See
    also Childhood leukemia(s).
  chronic, 1019, 1025
  clinical manifestations in, and
    related pathophysiology,
    1027t
  definition of, 361
  environmental factors in,
    397t–400t
  incidence of, 1019, 1020f
    in children, 1083
  and mortality rate, 1021t
  pathophysiology of, 1020–1022,
    1020f
Leukemic transformation, 1087
Leukemoid reaction, 1015
Leukocyte adhesion deficiencies,
    282
Leukocyte chemotaxis, induction
    of, 205
Leukocyte development, 971
Leukocyte disorders, 1014–1018,
    1016t
  leukemias in, 1019–1020. See also
    Leukemia(s).
  mononucleosis in, 1017–1018
  quantitative, 1014–1017
  references on, 1059
  summary review of, 1057b–1059b
Leukocytes, 955–957, 955f
  agranulocytic, 956–957
  classification of, 955
  clinical evaluation of, 983t–985t
  granulocytic, 955
  in human blood smear, 956f
  of infants and children, 955
  opioid producing, in pain control,
    489b
  pediatric values for, 1064t
Leukocytosis, 1014
  chemical mediators of, 203f
  in inflammation, 206
Leukopenia, 1014
  cancer associated, 391
Leukotrienes, 196–197, 203f
Level(s) of consciousness
  in brain dysfunction evaluation,
    528–535, 530t
  in children, 1729
Lewy bodies, 572
Leydig cells, 797
LFA-1, 228, 228b
LFA-3. See CD58.
LH. See Luteinizing hormone.
Lhermitte sign, 633

Li-Fraumeni syndrome, 369
and associated childhood cancer, 438t, 439
Liability distribution, 166, 167f
Libido, 800
Lice infestation, 1689
Lichen planus, 1658–1659
and associated cancer, 378t
hypertrophic, 1659f
Lichen sclerosis, and associated cancer, 378t
Lichenification, 1648t–1653t
Life expectancy, 86
changes in, in United States, 86–87, 86b
Life span, normal, 86–90
Ligament(s), 1573
Ligament sprain, 1573
Ligamentum venosum, formation of, 1212
Ligand(s), 13
Ligand-gated channels. See Channel-linked plasma membrane receptors.
Ligand internalization, 31. See also Receptor mediated endocytosis.
Ligature strangulation, 68
Limb girdle muscular dystrophy, 1634t, 1636–1637
Limbic system, 453, 659, 659f
pain sensory processing in, 485f, 486
Linear fracture, 1569
Linear no-threshold model, of dose-response, 419, 419f
Linear-quadratic model, of dose-response, 419, 419f
Linkage analysis, gene, 155–159
Lip cancer, 1298
clinical manifestations of, 1298, 1298f
evaluation and treatment of, 1299
pathophysiology of, 1298
Lipase(s), 83
action of, 1432–1433
Lipid(s)
plasma, 954
of plasma membrane, 11
Lipid absorption, in small intestine, 1434f. See also Fat(s).
Lipid-acceptor proteins, 55
Lipid hydrolysis, 1433, 1433f
Lipid metabolism disorders, 678–679, 1611
Lipid peroxidation, 54–55
Lipid soluble hormones, 697t. See also Steroid hormones.
types of, receptors, and mechanisms of action, 700t
Lipid vasoactive substances, mast cell production of, 198f
Lipocytes, 1438–1439
Lipofuscin, 6–7, 47
Lipoid nephrosis, 1381t
Lipolysis, 1432–1433
Lipopolysaccharides, bacterial, 301
physiologic effects of, 302f
Lipoprotein(s), 954, 1161, 1164
Lipoprotein genes, contributing to coronary artery disease, 175t
Lipoprotein metabolism, regulators of, 1478b
Liquefactive necrosis, 82, 83f
Listeria monocytogenes, 299t–300t
placental transmission of, 296

Listeria spp., intracellular survival of, 302–303
Lithium, and associated congential heart defects, 1214t
Lithium treatment, in bipolar disorder, 658
Liver, 1437f, 1438–1442
bilirubin metabolism in, 1440
gross anatomy of, 1438f
hematologic functions of, 1441
metabolic detoxification in, 1442
metabolic functions of, 1441–1442
mineral and vitamin storage in, 1442
secretions of, in digestive process, 1437–1444
Liver cancer, 1498t, 1503
clinical manifestations of, 1504
evaluation and treatment of, 1504
pathogenesis of, 397t–400t, 401, 1503–1504
risk factors for, 1503
Liver cell injury, by carbon tetrachloride, 58f
Liver disorders, 1482
in children, 1531
cirrhosis in, 1491–1492
clinical manifestations of, 1482
fulminant hepatitis in, 1491
and impaired hemostasis, 1049–1050
viral hepatitis in, 1488–1490
Liver fibrosis. See also Cirrhosis.
in alcoholic hepatitis, 61f
reversal of, cellular mechanisms of, 60–61, 60b
Liver function, artificial support of, 1491b
Liver function tests, 1446, 1446t
Liver lobules, 1438–1439, 1439f
Livor mortis, 90
Lobular carcinoma in situ (LCIS), 899–900
Lobular hyperplasia, 875
Local inflammation, 205
Locked-in syndrome, 535
Locus (loci), 143–145
assignation of, to specific chromosomes, 157
linkage of, 155
marker, 156–157
syntenic, 156
Locus ceruleus-norepinephrine dysfunction, in mood disorders, 654
Long-acting beta agonists, in treatment of asthma, 1285–1286, 1286b
Long bones, 1546
Long term starvation, 1481–1482
Longitudinal fissure, 452
Loop of Henle, 1347, 1357
transport within, 1356–1357
Loose connective tissue, 39t–40t
Lordosis, 1620
Loss of heterozygosity, of tumor suppressor genes, 373, 375–377
Lou Gehrig disease, 634
Low back pain, 492, 598
evaluation and treatment of, 493–495
pathophysiology of, 492–493
risk factors for, 495
Low bladder wall compliance, 1371

Low density lipoprotein (LDL), 31, 1161–1162
elevated serum, and risk for coronary artery disease, 1162
oxidation of, 1157–1159, 1159f
Low Dose Radiation Program, Dept. of Energy, 74, 74b
Low pressure adult hydrocephalus, 560
Low residue diet, 1454
Lower airway(s), 1244–1247, 1246f. See also Gas exchange, pulmonary.
in children, 1310–1311
Lower airway disease, childhood, 1320–1321
acute respiratory distress syndrome in, 1334
asthma in, 1330–1331
bronchiolitis obliterans in, 1330
bronchopulmonary dysplasia in, 1323–1324
cystic fibrosis in, 1336
protective strategies for ventilation in, 1323, 1326
respiratory distress syndrome in, 1321
respiratory infections in, 1326
aspiration pneumonitis, 1329–1330
bronchiolitis, 1326
pneumonia, 1327
Lower esophageal sphincter, 1423
Lower gastrointestinal bleeding, 1456
Lower motor neuron(s), 457–458, 565–566
Lower motor neuron syndromes, 564t, 565–567
amyotrophic, 567–568, 634
pathophysiology of, 565f
Lower motor neuron system, component structures of, 567f
Lower respiratory tract infections, bacterial agents causing, 299t–300t
Lower urinary tract obstruction, 1369–1371
anatomic causes of, 1371
evaluation and treatment of, 1371–1372
neurogenic bladder in, 1367f, 1369–1370
overactive bladder syndrome in, 1370–1371
Lown-Ganong-Levine syndrome, 1199t–1200t
Lumbar cistern, 460
Lumbar lordosis, 1601
Lumbar plexus, 465
Lumbar puncture, 461
Lumbar spine bone mass density, for females, by age, 1583f
Lumbar spondylosis, motor, sensory, and reflex changes in, 598, 598f
Lumbar vertebra, superior view, 462f
Lumbosacral disk disease, 598
Lumen, blood vessel, 1113
resistance to blood flow and, 1119, 1122f
Lung(s)
elastic properties of, 1253
zonal blood flow in, 1257, 1257f

Lung abscess, 1294
Lung cancer, 1299–1303
bronchial carcinoid, 1303–1304
causes of, and risk factors, 397t–400t, 401, 1300
characteristics of, 1300–1301, 1301f, 1302t
clinical manifestations of, 1303
evaluation and treatment of, 1303–1304
genetics of, 1300, 1300b
incidence and rates of, 401, 1300b
large cell, 1301–1302
metastasis of, 384t
non-small cell, 1301
pathogenesis of, 1303
primary, 1300–1301, 1301f, 1302t
TNM classification system of, 1303, 1304f
Lung capacities, 1261f, 1262
Lung disorders, 1266, 1271–1280
acute respiratory distress syndrome in, 1279–1280
autoimmune, 257t–258t
chest wall abnormalities in, 1271–1272
clinical manifestations of, 1266–1271
conditions caused by, 1269–1271
malignant, 1298. See also Lung cancer.
obstructive, 1282–1284. See also Asthma; Chronic obstructive pulmonary disease.
pleural abnormalities in, 1272–1274
respiratory tract infections in, 1290–1291. See also Acute bronchitis; Pneumonia; Pulmonary abscess; Tuberculosis.
restrictive, 1274–1280. See also Restrictive pulmonary disorders.
vascular disease in, 1294–1295. See also Pulmonary vascular disease.
Lung parenchyma, in children, 1310–1311
Lung receptors, 1251
Lung vasculature, 1247–1249, 1248f
Lupus erythematosus, 1659–1660
Lupus nephritis, 271, 271f, 1381t, 1382
Luteal-secretory phase, of menstrual cycle, 794
Luteinizing hormone (LH)
anterior pituitary secretion of, 707
in female reproductive development, 783–784
physiologic effects of, 704f, 708t, 791–792
value of, 809t
Luteinizing hormone deficiency, 732
Luxury perfusion syndrome, 602
Lycopene, and cancer risk, 410t–413t
Lyme disease, 1667
central nervous system, inflammation in, 629–630
Lymph, 1132

Lymph nodes, 1132f, 1133
  anatomic structure of, 959, 960f
  hematologic and immunologic
    functions of, 961
Lymphadenopathy, 1027–1028,
    1028f, 1030–1031
Lymphatic capillaries, 1132, 1132f
  pulmonary, 1249
Lymphatic system, 1131–1133
  anatomy of, 1132, 1132f
  fluid balance and, 1131–1132, 1131f
Lymphatic veins, 1132
Lymphatic venules, 1132
Lymphatic vessels, 1131–1133, 1132f
  of myocardium, 1099
Lymphedema, 100
  congenital heart defects associated
    with, 1215t
Lymphoblastic lymphoma, 1036
  clinical manifestations of,
    1036–1037
  evaluation and treatment of, 1037
  pathophysiology of, 1036
Lymphocyte count, 983t–985t
  pediatric, 985t
Lymphocytes, 217–218, 218f, 956
  autocrine or paracrine influence
    of, on immune response, 349
  pediatric values for, 1064t
  quantitative alterations of, 1017
  scanning electronmicrography
    of, 201f
  subsets of, in burn injury
    response, 1748, 1748b
Lymphocytic mastopathy, 876t
Lymphocytic meningitis, 620–622
Lymphocytopenia, 1016t, 1017
Lymphocytosis, 1016t, 1017
Lymphogranuloma venereum, 937
  clinical manifestations of, 937
  evaluation and treatment of,
    937–938
  pathophysiology of, 937
Lymphoid disorders, 1030–1031
  lymphadenopathy in, 1030
  malignant lymphomas in,
    1030–1031
  plasma cell malignancies in, 1037
  references on, 1059
  summary review of, 1057b–1059b
Lymphoid organs, 957–961. *See also*
    Lymph nodes; Spleen.
  B cell and T cell differentiation in,
    219–220, 220f, 230
  primary (central), 230
  secondary (peripheral), 235
  T cell maturation in, 230–233
Lymphoid stem cells, 230
Lymphoma(s), 364t
  Burkitt, 1035
  in children, 437, 1086–1087.
    See also Childhood
    lymphoma(s).
  classification of, 1030, 1030b
  definition of, 361
  differential diagnosis of, 1037
  environmental factors in, 184t
  Hodgkin, 1031
  incidence of, and deaths, 1021t,
    1030–1031
  lymphoblastic, 1036
  pathophysiology of, 1020f
Lymphoplasmacytic lymphoma,
    1042

Lys-bradykinin, 191
Lysosomal storage diseases, 678
Lysosome(s), 3f, 5–7, 8f
  within platelets, 976
Lytic lesions, in multiple myeloma,
    1038–1040, 1040f

M
M line, of myocardial muscle, 1106
M protein, 1038
  electrophoretic screening assay
    for, 1039f
MAC (membrane attack complex),
    189
Macewen sign, 674
**Macrocytic-normochromic
    anemias,** 990–993, 991t
Macromolecules, 15–16
Macrophage colony stimulating
    factor (M-CSF), 961t, 963
Macrophages, 957, 957t
  bone marrow, 963
  differentiation of, into epithelioid
    cells, 207–208
  hematopoietic differentiation of,
    964f
  in inflammatory response,
    201–202, 201f, 1710–1711
    activation of, 202
    chemokine production by, 205
  phagocytic activity of, in spleen,
    958
  T cell activation of, 250, 250f
  in wound healing, 208, 210
Macrovascular disease. *See also*
    Coronary artery disease;
    Peripheral arterial disease;
    Stroke.
  in diabetes mellitus, 763–765
Macular, 509
Macular densa, 1346–1347
Macule, 1648t–1653t
Maculopathy, in diabetes mellitus,
    759–760
Magnesium, 114
  in bone tissue physiology, 1580b
  intake and intestinal absorption
    of, 1434
  postmenopausal osteoporosis and
    intake of, 1584
Magnetic resonance angiography
    (MRA), of central nervous
    system, 475
Magnetic resonance imaging (MRI)
  in bone function and structural
    assessments, 1563
  in cardiac function testing,
    1134–1135
  of central nervous system,
    474–475
  of gastrointestinal tract, 1444
  in joint function evaluation, 1563
  in systemic vascular evaluation,
    1136
Magnetic resonance spectroscopy,
    474–475
Maintenance fluid, 1745–1746
Major basic protein, 247
Major calyx, 1345
Major (unipolar) depression, 652
  clinical manifestations of, 655–656
  genetic and environmental factors
    in, 652–653
  treatment of, 657–658, 657b

Major duodenal papilla, 1439
Major histocompatibility complex
    (MHC), 226–228. *See also*
    Human leukocyte antigens
    (HLAs).
  antigen processing and, 236–237
  diversity of, and organ
    transplantation, 226–228
Malabsorption syndromes,
    1470–1471
Malaria, pathogenesis of, 312–313,
    312f
Malassezia furfur, 308t
Maldigestion, 1470
Maldistribution of blood flow, 1711
Male breast, 805
Male breast cancer, 909
Male breast disorders, 908
Male infertility, 870–871
  evaluation of, 871b
Male pattern alopecia, 1673–1674
Male reproductive disorders,
    850–857
  balanitis in, 852
  cryptorchidism and ectopy in, 856
  epididymitis in, 859
  impaired sperm production and
    quality in, 870–871
  orchitis in, 857
  penile cancer in, 853–854
  penile disorders in, 850–854
  Peyronie disease in, 851–852
  priapism in, 852
  prostate disorders in, 860–861
  prostatitis in, 861–863
  references on, 913
  scrotal, testicular, epididymal
    disorders in, 854–857
  sexual dysfunction in, 869
  sexually transmitted infections in,
    924–925
    bacterial, 299t–300t, 924–925
    chlamydial, 935
    parasitic, 942–943
    viral, 938
  summary review of, 909b–912b
  testicular cancer in, 857
  testicular torsion in, 856–857
  urethral disorders in, 850
Male reproductive system, 796–802
  aging and changes in, 811–814
  development of, 782–783, 782f–783f
  external genitalia of, 796–799,
    796f
  internal genitalia of, 799–800, 799f
  sex hormones of, 800–802
  spermatogenesis in, 800
Male sexual dysfunction, 869
  evaluation and treatment of,
    870–871
  pathophysiology of, 869–870
Malignancies, and secondary
    immune deficiencies, 285
Malignant bone tumors, in
    children, 1637
Malignant hyperthermia, 500–501
Malignant melanoma, 1670–1671
  clinical characteristics of, 1672t
  environmental factors in,
    397t–400t, 401
  metastasis of, 384t
  staging of, 1671, 1672f–1673f
  ultraviolet radiation and,
    422–423, 1671b

Malignant tumor(s), 360–361
  characteristics of, 361t
  histology of, 362–363, 363f
  naming, 361
  nomenclature and classification
    of, 364t
Malleus, 512–513
Malnutrition
  in cancer epidemiology, 406
  essential fatty acids and
    inflammation in, 199b
  immune competency and, 285
  postmenopausal osteoporosis
    and, 1579
  prevention of, in children with
    cancer, 440b
  protein energy, 69, 1528
    clinical manifestations of, 1528
    evaluation and treatment of,
      1528
    pathophysiology of, 1528
**MALT (mucosa associated
    lymphoid tissue) lymphoma,**
    380–381, 1499
Malunion, of fractured bones,
    1571–1572
Mammary duct carcinoma, 897t
Mammary duct ectasia, 874t, 876t
Mammary lobule carcinoma, 897t
Mammographic breast density,
    888f
  and breast cancer risk, 887–888
Mammography, 807
  in diagnosis and staging of cancer,
    361
  false-positive rate for,
    386–387
  recommended screening with,
    387
  risk for breast cancer in, 888–891
Manganese, in bone tissue
    physiology, 1580b
Mania
  clinical manifestations of,
    656–657
  major symptoms of, 652b
Manic-depressive disorder (illness),
    652. *See also* Bipolar disorder.
Mannitol, diuretic action of, 1359t
Mannose-binding lectin (MBL), 189
**Mannose-binding lectin (MBL)
    deficiency,** 281
Mannose binding protein, and
    systemic inflammatory
    response syndrome in children,
    1741
Manometry, of gastrointestinal
    motility, 1445t
Manual strangulation, 68
MAOIs (monoamine oxidase
    inhibitors), 657–658, 657b
MAP kinase pathway, 23t
Map unit, 156
Maple syrup urine disease. *See*
    Branched chain ketoaciduria.
Marasmus, 1481–1482. *See also*
    Protein energy malnutrition.
Marburg virus, 314t
Marfan syndrome, congenital heart
    defects associated with, 1215t
Marginal layer, 483–484
Marginating storage pool, 963–965,
    965f
Margination, 198–199, 199t

Marijuana use, biological effects of, 63t
Marker locus, 156–157
Mass reflex, 595
Mast cell degranulation, 195, 195f, 196, 259, 260f
Mast cells, 956
  in inflammatory response, 195–198, 203f, 1710
  lipid vasoactive substances produced by, 198f
  synthesis of mediators in, 195f, 196–198
Mastalgia, 879t
Mastitis, 876t
Mastoid process, 512
Maternal age, and associated congenital heart defects, 1214t
Maternal immunologic hypersensitivity diseases, 271
Maternal microchimerism, and development of autoimmune disease, 269b
Matrix metalloproteinases (MMPs), 210
  in breast cancer development, 891, 905
Maturation phase, of healing, 208, 209f, 210
Maturity-onset diabetes of youth, 746t, 753–754
May-Hegglin syndrome, 1044
McArdle disease, 1610
  muscle tissue in, 1610f
Mean arterial pressure (MAP), 1122–1123, 1133t
  factors affecting, 1125t
Mean corpuscular hemoglobin, 983t–985t
Mean corpuscular hemoglobin concentration, 983t–985t
Mean corpuscular volume, 983t–985t
  pediatric, 1064t
Measles
  rash distribution in rubella, 1686f
  rubella, 1686
  rubeola, 1686–1687
Measles, mumps, rubella (MMR) vaccine, 329–330
  adult, 329t
  child, 330t
Measles, mumps (MM) vaccine, 329
Measles virus, 314t
  in central nervous system infections, 621t
Meat, and cancer risk, 410t–413t
Mechanical stresses, in cell injury, 75, 75t
Mechanics of breathing, 1251–1254, 1254f
Mechanism of action, of pathogen, 297
Mechanoporation, 75
Mechanoreceptors, 445b, 482–483
Mechanothermal nociceptors, 482–483
Meconium ileus, 1520
  clinical manifestations of, 1520
  evaluation and treatment of, 1520–1521
  pathophysiology of, 1520
Medial epicondylopathy, 1574

Median aperture (foramen of Magendie), 461
Median eminence, 705
Mediastinum, 1242
Mediated transport, 28–29, 29f
  active, 29
  channel model of, 28f
  conformational change model of, 28f
  passive, 28–29
Medical nutrition therapy (MNT), for prevention and treatment of diabetes, 753b
Medications. See also drug entries.
  secondary hypertension caused by, 1143t
  and secondary immune deficiencies, 286
Medulla, 454f
Medulla oblongata, 450t, 455
Medullary hematopoiesis, 965
Medulloblastoma, 612t
  in children, 686, 686t
    clinical manifestations of, 687
    treatment strategies for, 687t, 688
Megakaryocyte progenitors, 971
Megakaryocytes, 957, 958f
Megaloblastic anemia, 990–991
  in children, 1066t
  secondary to drug effects, 1001t
Meiosis, 134
  stages of, 137f
Meissner plexus, 1421
Melanin accumulation, cellular, 78–79
Melanocyte stimulating hormone (MSH)
  anterior pituitary secretion of, 707
  physiologic effects of, 704f, 708t
Melanocytes, 78, 1645
Melanoma, malignant, 1670–1671
  clinical characteristics of, 1672t
  environmental factors in, 397t–400t, 401
  metastasis of, 384t
  staging of, 1671, 1672t–1673f
  ultraviolet radiation and, 422–423, 1671b
Melatonin, 704
  in stress response, 348t
Melena, 1456, 1456t
Membrane attack complex (MAC), 189
Membrane excitability, potassium and calcium effects on, 108–109, 109f
Membrane potential(s), 32–33
  cardiac, 1102
Membrane transport, 25–33
  electrical impulses and, 32–33
  vesicle formation in, 30–32. See also Caveolae; Endocytosis; Exocytosis.
  water and solute movement in, 26–30. See also Active transport; Mediated transport; Passive transport.
  major systems in, 30t
Membranoproliferative glomerulonephritis, 1381t, 1383
Membranous glomerulonephritis, 1383

Membranous nephropathy, 1381t, 1383
Memory, 543
Memory deficits, 543, 547t
Memory T cells, 219–220, 243–244
Menarche, 792
Mendelian traits, 143–145
Ménière disease, 517
Meningeal layer, 459–460
Meninges, 459–461
  pathologic mechanisms involving, 460–461
Meningioma(s), 612t, 616–617, 617f, 619
Meningitis, 620–623, 682
  aseptic (viral), 620–622, 682
  bacterial, 620, 682
  clinical manifestations of, 623–624
    in children, 624, 684
  evaluation and treatment of, 624
    in children, 684
  fungal, 622–623
  pathogenesis of, 622f
  pathophysiology of, 623
  tubular, 623
Meningocele, 669, 670f
Meningococcal vaccine, 329, 1740
  adult, 329t
  pediatric, 330t
Menometrorrhagia, 823t
Menopause, 792. See also Perimenopause.
  physiologic changes in, and symptoms, 809–811, 810t
Menorrhagia, 823t
Menorrhea, 823t
Menstrual cycle, 792–796
  body temperature changes in, 796
  hormonal regulation of, 793f, 794–795
  phase(s) of, 792–794, 793f
    follicular-proliferative, 793–794
    luteal-secretory, 794
    uterine, 795
  vaginal changes in, 795
Menstrual disorders, 819
  abnormal uterine bleeding in, 822–823
  amenorrhea in, 820
  primary dysmenorrhea in, 819
Menstruation (menses), 793–794
  retrograde, 839
Mental disorders, 646–664
  anxiety disorders in, 658–662
  key terminology of, 663b
  mood disorders in, 652–658. See also Bipolar disorder; Depression.
  references on, 664
  schizophrenia in, 647–652
  sleep disorders associated with, 505–506
  summary review of, 662b–663b
Mental stress, silent ischemia and, 1166–1167. See also under Stress.
Mercury poisoning, 61–62
Merkel cells, 1645
Mesanephros, 1402
Mesangial cells, 1345
Mesangial matrix, 1345

Mesangial proliferative glomerulonephritis, 1381t, 1383
Mesencephalon, 450t, 455. See also Midbrain.
Mesenchymal stem cells, 963, 1541, 1542f
  lineages and differentiation of, 366f
Mesenchymal tumors, 364t
Mesenteric arterial occlusion, 1477
Mesenteric venous thrombosis, 1477
Mesentery, 1429
Meshed autografts, 1749, 1749f
Mesodermal germ layer, 437
Mesothelioma, 1304
Messenger RNA (mRNA), 132–133. See also mRNA.
Metabolic acidosis, 117
  clinical manifestations of, 118
  compensated and corrected, 119f
  evaluation and treatment of, 119
  pathophysiology of, 117–118, 118t
Metabolic alkalosis, 119
  clinical manifestations of, 120
  compensated and corrected, 121f
  evaluation and treatment of, 120–121
  pathophysiology of, 119–120
Metabolic bone diseases, 1576–1580
  osteomalacia in, 1584–1585
  osteoporosis in, 1576–1580
  Paget disease in, 1585–1586
Metabolic cerebral edema, 560
Metabolic cirrhosis, 1492t
Metabolic coma, 528
  clinical manifestations of, 529t
Metabolic detoxification, 1442
Metabolic disorders
  in children, 1534
  congenital heart defects associated with, 1214t
  energy metabolism diseases in, 1610–1611
  and secondary immune deficiencies, 285
Metabolic muscle diseases, 1610–1611
  endocrine disorders and, 1610
  energy metabolic dysfunction and, 1610–1611
Metabolic pathway(s), 21
Metabolic postural tremor, 568t–569t
Metabolic syndrome, 750, 1480
  clinical features of, 751b
Metabolism
  cellular, 21–25
    adenosine triphosphate in, 22–23
    altered, in shock, 1697–1699, 1708b. See also Shock.
    oxidative phosphorylation in, 24–25
  food and, 23–24
  heat production in, 496
  intermediary, 8
Metals, linked to cancers, 397t–400t
Metanephros, 1402
Metaphase, 35
Metaphase spread, 134
Metaphysis, of bone, 1546
Metaplasia, 47f, 50

Metarterioles, 1113
Metastasis, 381–384, 381f–382f
  cell detachment and invasion in,
    382
  cell survival and entrance into
    circulation in, 382
  common sites of, 384t
  genetic regulation of, 370
  heterogeneity and successful, 382
  microenvironment development
    in, 384
  patterns of, 383f
  selective adherence in, 382–384
  site determinants in, 383–384,
    385f
Metastatic calcification, 79–81
Metastatic cascade, 618
Metatarsus adductus, 1622
Metencephalon, 450t, 455
Methamphetamine (meth) use,
  biological effects of, 63t
Methemoglobin, 967–968
Methicillin-resistant *Staphylococcus
  aureus* (MRSA)
  antibiotic resistant mechanisms
    of, 306–307
  genetics in, 328
**Methicillin-resistant
  Staphylococcus aureus (MRSA)
  infection,** community acquired,
    1662–1663, 1662b
Methionine enkephalin, 489
Methylation. See DNA methylation.
Metrorrhagia, 823t
Mg++, Mg2+. *See* Magnesium.
MHC (major histocompatibility
  complex), 226–228. *See also*
  Human leukocyte antigens
  (HLAs).
  antigen processing and, 236–237
  diversity of, and organ
    transplantation, 226–228
MHC class I deficiency, 280–281
MHC class I genes, 226
MHC class II deficiency, 280–281
MHC class II genes, 226
Micelles, 1433, 1433f
Micro-ribonucleic acids (miRNAs),
  403
Microangiopathic anemia,
  erythrocyte appearance in, 992f
Microbodies, 7. *See also*
  Peroxisome(s).
Microcephaly, 672f, 673–674
  causes of, 673b
Microchimerism, maternal, and
  development of autoimmune
  disease, 269b
**Microcytic-hypochromic
  anemia(s),** 991t, 995–996
  in children, 1066t
  erythrocyte appearance in, 992f
Microdomains, 32
Microfilaments
  actin, 9–10
  of neurons, 443
Microglia, 444–445, 445f
  functions of, 446t
β2 Microglobulin, 226, 1041
Microorganisms, 295
  human relationship with, 295,
    295b
  infectious, 295–318. *See also*
    Pathogen(s).

Microorganisms *(Continued)*
  colonization by, 296
  in development of
    autoimmunity, 269
  diseases caused by, 296–297. *See
    also* Infectious disease(s).
  emerging, 294
  multiplication of, 296
  spread of, 296
  tissue invasion by, 296
  toxin production by, 245
  used in bioterrorism, 294–295
Microsomal ethanol oxidizing
  system (MEOS), 59
Microspherocytes, 1070f
Microsporum canis, 308t
Microtubules, 9
  of neurons, 443
Microvascular disease, in diabetes
  mellitus, 759–763
  nephropathic, 760–761
  neuropathic, 761–763
  retinopathic, 759–760
Microvascular thrombosis, 1048
Microvilli, 36, 1429
Micturition, 1350
Micturition reflex, 1350–1351
Midbrain, 450t, 454f, 455
Midcortical nephrons, 1345
Middle cerebral artery, 462, 463t,
  464f
Middle cerebral artery occlusion,
  stroke syndromes resulting
  from, 604t–605t
Middle fossa, 459
Middle internodal pathway, 1102
Migraine headache, 609–611
  classification of, 610
  evaluation and management of,
    610
  pathophysiology of, 610
  prophylaxis of, 611
Mild concussion, 590
Mild diffuse axonal injury, 590
Miliaria crystallina, 1692
Miliaria rubra, 1692, 1692f
Milk-line remnants, 876t
Milliequivalent, 26
Milroy disease, congenital heart
  defects associated with, 1215t
Mineralocorticoid(s), 717–718
Minerals
  in bone, 1541t, 1545
  dietary intake of, 1433–1434
  intestinal absorption of,
    1433–1434
  storage of, in liver, 1442
Minimal change disease, 1381t
Minimal change nephropathy, 1409
Minimally conscious state, 535
  comparative clinical
    manifestations of, 536t
Minimally invasive direct coronary
  artery bypass (MIDCAB),
  1169
Minor calyx, 1345
Minute volume, 1249
Mirror focus, 539
Mis-sense mutation, 129–132
Mitochondria (mitochondrion),
  3f, 7, 9f
  cellular aging and, 89, 89f
Mitochondrial pathway, of cell
  death, 85, 85f

Mitosis, 33–34
  phases of, 34–35
Mitral and tricuspid complex, 1094
Mitral regurgitation, 1183
  clinical manifestations of, 1182t
Mitral stenosis, 1181–1183, 1182f,
  1186f
  clinical manifestations of, 1182t
Mitral valve, 1094
Mitral valve infection, bacterial,
  1189f
Mitral valve prolapse, 1184f
Mitral valve prolapse syndrome,
  1183–1184
  treatment of, 1184
Mixed hearing loss, 515
Mixed hemodynamics, congenital
  cardiac defects causing,
  1230–1231
Mixed incontinence, 1369t
Mixed (general) multiple sclerosis,
  631–632, 632b
Mixed nerves, 465
Mixed venous blood gases, normal
  ranges in, 1262t
MMPs (matrix metalloproteinases),
  210
  in breast cancer development,
    891, 905
MMR (mumps, measles, rubella)
  vaccine, 1686
Mobitz I block, 1199t–1200t
Mobitz II block, 1199t–1200t
Mode of inheritance, 145
Moderate diffuse axonal injury, 590
Mold, 307
Molecular-era anticancer drugs,
  387–388, 387t
Molecular mimicry, 269
Molluscous bodies, 941–942
Molluscum contagiosum, 941–942,
  1685–1686, 1688f
  papules of, 943f
Mongolism, 137
**Monoamine hypothesis of
  depression,** 653
Monoamine oxidase inhibitors
  (MAOIs), 657–658, 657b
Monoamines, neurologic functions
  of, 448t–449t
**Monoclonal gammopathy of
  undetermined significance,**
  1040
Monocyte count, 983t–985t
  pediatric, 985t
Monocyte progenitors, 971
Monocytes, 957
  hematopoietic differentiation of,
    964f
  in inflammatory response,
    201–202, 201f, 203f
  pediatric values for, 1064t
  quantitative alterations of,
    1015–1017
Monocytopenia, 1016t, 1017
Monocytosis, 1016t, 1017
Mononuclear phagocyte system,
  957, 957t
Mononucleosis
  and associated cancer, 378t
  infectious, 1017–1018
    clinical manifestations of, 1018
    evaluation and treatment of,
      1018–1020

Mononucleosis *(Continued)*
  peripheral blood smear in,
    1019f
  splenic rupture in, 1019
  transmission of, 1018
Monosomy, 136–137
  chromosomal translocation in,
    144f
Monounsaturated fats, 1162b
Monozygotic (MZ, identical) twins,
  170
Mons pubis, 784
Mood, 652
Mood disorders, 652–658
  clinical manifestations of,
    655–657
  genetic and environmental factors
    in, 652–653
  neurochemical dysregulation in,
    653
  neuroendocrine dysregulation in,
    653–654
  neurologic and functional causes
    of, 654–655
  treatment of, 657–658
    in children, 657, 657b
    medical, 657b
Mood stabilizers, 658
Moraxella catarrhalis, 299t–300t
Mosquito bites, and disease
  transmission, 1668
Motilin, 1424, 1425t
Motility diarrhea, 1455
Motility dysfunction, 1456
  dysphagia in, 1456
  gastrointestinal reflux disease in,
    1458
  hiatal hernia in, 1459
  intestinal obstruction and ileus
    in, 1460
  pyloric obstruction in, 1460
Motor dysphasia, 549t–550t
Motor function alterations,
  561–570
  complex, 575–577
  extrapyramidal motor syndromes
    in, 577–580
  genetic basis of selected,
    526t–527t
  key terminology of, 580b
  movement alterations in,
    564–570, 565f
  muscle tone alterations in,
    562–564
  references on, 580
  summary review of, 578b–579b
Motor neuron disease, 633–634
Motor neuron syndromes, 564–568,
  564t
Motor neurons, 444, 457
Motor pathways, 454f, 457f, 458
Motor responses, in brain
  dysfunction evaluation, 532,
  533t, 535f
Motor unit(s), 458, 1556–1560,
  1557f
  contraction of, 1559–1560,
    1559f
    molecular level of, 1561
  muscle fibers of, 1557–1560
  recruitment of, in muscle
    contraction, 1562
  sensory receptors of, 1556–1557
Mouth, 1421–1423

Movement dysfunction, 564–570, 564t
amyotrophic, 567–568, 568t
associated movement loss in, 572
hyperkinetic, 568–570, 568t
hypokinetic, 571–572
partial and complete paralytic, 564–568, 564t
Moyamoya disease, 685
mRNA (messenger RNA), 132–133
translation of, 134, 136f
MTHFR mutation, 1056
Mucocutaneous candidiasis, chronic, 279
Mucoepidermoid carcinoma, 1304
Mucopurulent cervicitis, 832
Mucosa associated lymphoid tissue (MALT) lymphoma, 380–381, 1499
Mucosal barrier, 1427
Multichannel urodynamic testing, 1371
Multifactorial disorder(s), 165–169
in adult population, 172–180, 172t
basic model of, 165–166
general principles and conclusions regarding, 180
recurrence risks and transmission patterns in, 167–169
reduced or variably expressed single gene disease in, 168
references on, 182
specific
alcoholism, 178–179
Alzheimer disease, 178
cancer, 174–176
congenital malformations, 171–172
coronary heart disease, 172–174
diabetes mellitus, 176–177
hypertension, 174
obesity, 177–178
psychiatric disorders, 179–180
summary review of, 181b
threshold model of, 166–167
Multifactorial etiology, 437
Multifactorial inheritance, 1516
Multifactorial trait, 165
Multifocal neuropathies, 635
Multinucleated giant cells, 316
Multiple causation, 437
Multiple myeloma, 1037
clinical manifestations of, 1038–1040
diagnostic criteria for, 1042b
evaluation and treatment of, 1041–1042
myeloma cell proliferation in, 1037–1038, 1038f
pathophysiology of, 1037–1038
plasma cell appearance in, 1041f
prognosis in, 1041–1042
staging system for, 1041t
Multiple organ dysfunction syndrome, 1696, 1707
in children, 1727–1728
evaluation and treatment of, 1737–1741, 1737b
clinical manifestations of, 1711–1713, 1712b
evaluation and treatment of, 1713–1714, 1713b
pathophysiology of, 1707–1711, 1709f

Multiple organ dysfunction syndrome *(Continued)*
gut hypothesis in, 1711
hypermetabolism in, 1711
inflammatory leukocytes in, 1710
inflammatory mediators in, 1710
initiating causes in, 1707, 1708b
maldistribution of blood flow in, 1711
myocardial depression in, 1711
neuroendocrine, 1710
primary, 1707
references on, 1724
secondary, 1708
summary review of, 1722b–1723b
Multiple sclerosis, 630
clinical course of, 630b, 631–633
demyelinating plaque formation in, 631f–632f
evaluation and treatment of, 633–634, 633t
immunopathology of, 630
pathologic patterns of, 631, 632b
pathophysiology of, 630–631
syndromes of, 632b
cerebellar type, 633
mixed type, 631–632
spinal type, 632–633
Multipolar neurons, 444, 445f
Multipotent cells, 363–365
Mumps virus, 314t
in central nervous system infections, 621t
Muscle cell, 1557
Muscle contraction, 1559–1563, 1559f
mechanics of, 1562
molecular, 1561
types of, 1562
Muscle disorders, skeletal, 1606–1607
inflammatory, 1611
membrane abnormalities in, 1609
metabolic, 1610–1611
myopathies in, 1612–1613
paraneoplastic, 389t
secondary muscle dysfunction in, 1606–1607
tumors in, 1613–1615
Muscle fiber(s), 1557–1560
characteristics of, 1557–1558, 1558t
components of, 1557f, 1558
contraction of, 1559–1563, 1559f
mechanics of, 1562
molecular level of, 1561
diameter of, and muscle strength, 1558
metabolism in, 1561–1562
myofibrillar organization in, 1557–1560, 1557f
myofibrils of, 1559–1560, 1559f
nonprotein components of, 1560
Muscle fiber action potential, 1561
Muscle fiber function, testing, 1563–1564
Muscle groups, movement of, 1562–1563
Muscle growth, and development, 1620
Muscle membrane, 1558

Muscle membrane abnormalities, 1609
myotonia in, 1609
periodic paralysis in, 1609
Muscle power, United Kingdom Medical Research Council Classification, 563–564, 563t
Muscle proteins, 1560, 1560t
Muscle pump, 1117, 1122f
Muscle strains, 1575
types of, and treatment, 1576t
Muscle tissue, 38
types of, location and function, 41t
Muscle tone alterations, 562–564, 562t
Muscle tone decrease, in heat loss, 497
Muscle trauma, complications of, 1575–1576
Muscle tumors, 1613–1615
in children, 1639
Muscle wasting, in shock, 1699
Muscular arteries, 1113
Muscular dystrophy, 1633
Becker, 1636–1637
Duchenne, 1633
fascioscapulohumeral, 1636
limb girdle, 1636–1637
muscle groups involved in types of, 1633f
scapuloperoneal, 1636
Muscular hypertrophy, 47–48
Musculoskeletal disorders, 1568–1617. *See also* Musculoskeletal injuries.
bone disorders in, 1576–1580. *See also* Bone disorders.
in children, 1620–1621
abnormal skeletal modeling in, 1624
bone infection in, 1628
cerebral palsy in, 1632
congenital, 1620–1621
juvenile rheumatoid arthritis in, 1630–1631
muscular dystrophy in, 1633
nonaccidental trauma in, 1640
osteochondroses in, 1631
references on, 1642
summary review of, 1641b
tumors in, 1637
joint disorders in, 1592–1594
references on, 1615
skeletal muscle disorders in, 1606–1607. *See also* Skeletal muscle disorders.
summary review of, 1613b–1614b
Musculoskeletal injuries, 1568–1569
dislocations and subluxations in, 1572
fractures in, 1568–1569
muscle strains in, 1575
rhabdomyolysis in, 1575–1576
support structure injuries in, 1573. *See also* Tendon and ligament injuries.
Musculoskeletal system, 1540
in aging, 1564–1566
bone structure and function in, 1540–1548
in children, 1618–1643
development of, 1618–1620

Musculoskeletal system *(Continued)*
disorders of, 1568–1617. *See also* Bone disorders; Joint disorders; Musculoskeletal injuries; Skeletal muscle disorders.
references on, 1615
summary review of, 1613b–1614b
function testing of, 1563–1564
joint structure and function in, 1548–1554
references on, 1566
skeletal muscle structure and function in, 1554–1563
summary review of, 1565b
Mustard and Senning operations, 1232
Mutagens, 132
exposure to, 375
Mutation(s)
bacterial, 304
chromosome, 129–132, 132f–133f
structural, 142–143, 142f
gene, 367–368
viral, 316–317
Mutational hot spots, 132
Mutualism, 295f
Muzzle imprint, 66, 66f
Myasthenia, paraneoplastic, 389t
Myasthenia gravis, 639
antibodies and role in, 639t, 583–645, 638f
clinical manifestations of, 639–640
evaluation and treatment of, 640–643
maternal hypersensitivity in, 271
pathophysiology of, 639
Myasthenic crisis, 640
MYC protein, 371
Mycobacterium leprae, 297, 299t–300t
immune suppression induced by, 305
Mycobacterium spp., intracellular survival of, 302–303
Mycobacterium tuberculosis, 297–300, 299t–300t. *See also* Tuberculosis.
antibiotic resistance of, 327–328
capsule protection of, 304
immune suppression induced by, 305
Mycoplasma, 298t
Mycoplasma spp., 298, 299t–300t
Mycoplasmal pneumonia, 1291
in children, 1328t, 1329
Mycosis (mycoses), 307, 1664, 1684
Mycotic aneurysms, 606–607
Myelencephalon, 450t
Myelin, 443
physiologic effect of, 443
Myelin sheath, 443, 667
Myelodysplasia, 669–670
evaluation and treatment of, 671–672
functional alterations in, 670, 670t
Myelodysplastic syndrome, 998
Myelofibrosis, 992f
Myelogenic tumors, 1592, 1592f
Myelogram, 476
Myelography, 476
Myeloid progenitors, 971
Myeloid tissue, 962

Myelomeningocele, 669–670, 670f
  clinical manifestations of,
    670–671, 670t
  evaluation and treatment of,
    671–672
Myelopathy, 597–598
Myeloperoxidase deficiency, 283
Myeloproliferative disorders, 1025,
  1027
**Myeloproliferative red blood cell
  disorders,** 1008–1009
Myencephalon, 455–456
Myenteric plexus, 1421, 1436
MYH9 mutation, 1044
**Myoadenylate deaminase
  deficiency,** 1611
Myoblasts, 1557
Myocardial contractility, 1108
  and cardiac output, 1111
Myocardial depression, 1711, 1717
Myocardial disorders, 1178–1180.
    See also Cardiomyopathy(ies).
Myocardial hypertrophy, 48, 49f
Myocardial hypoxia, 53
Myocardial infarction (MI), 1169,
  1171
  cellular death in, 1172
  cellular injury in, 1171–1172
  clinical manifestations of, 1173
  complications of, 1175–1176
  definition of, universal, 1174b
  electrocardiographic alterations
    in, 1174, 1175f
  evaluation and treatment of,
    1173–1175
  pathophysiology of, 1171–1173
  plaque disruption and, 1170f–1171f
  repair of, 1173
  sites of, and vessel involvement,
    1175f
  structural and functional changes
    in, 1172–1173, 1172f, 1173t
Myocardial ischemia, 1165
  clinical manifestations of,
    1165–1167
  evaluation and treatment of,
    1167–1170
  pathophysiology of, 1165, 1166f
  and stress, 337b, 1166–1167,
    1167f–1168f
Myocardial necrosis, coagulative,
  83f
Myocardial oxygen consumption
  (MVO₂), 1107–1108
Myocardial remodeling, 1172–1173
Myocardial stunning, 1172–1173
Myocardium, 1093, 1093f
  action potential generation in,
    1099–1109. *See also* Cardiac
      action potential(s).
  adrenergic receptors of, 1105
  cells of, 1105–1108
    and skeletal muscle cells,
      comparisons, 1105
  contraction of, 1108–1109
    calcium in excitation and,
      1108–1109
    cross-bridge theory of, 1108
  disorders of, 1178–1180. *See also*
    Cardiomyopathy(ies).
  electrical impulse transmission
    through, 1105
  intracellular and extracellular ion
    concentration in, 1102t

Myocardium *(Continued)*
  mitochondrial metabolism in,
    1105–1108
  molecular basis of muscle
    contraction in, 1106, 1107f
  relaxation of, 1109
  T tubule system of, 1106
Myocyte(s), 38
  calcium transport, in
    pathophysiology of systolic
    heart failure, 1190
Myofascial pain syndrome, 492
Myofibrils, 1557, 1559–1560
  contractile proteins of, 1560,
    1560t
  molecular level of contraction
    in, 1561
  organization of, in muscle fiber,
    1557–1560, 1557f
Myofibroblasts, 210
  in keloid formation, 1654
Myofilaments, in cardiac muscle
    contraction, 1106, 1107f
Myogenic mechanism, 1351
Myoglobin, 1575–1576
  iron bound in, 969
  oxygen binding by, 1130–1131
  release of, in burn injury, 1744
Myoglobinuria, 1575–1576, 1613
Myomas, 837
Myometrium, 788–789
Myoneural junction, 458
Myopathy(ies), 1612–1613
  toxic, 1612–1613
Myopia, 511
Myosin, 1559, 1560t
  myocardial, 1106, 1106f
Myositis, 1611
  CD4+ and CD8+ lymphocyte
    distribution in, 1611f
Myositis ossificans, 1575
Myotonia, 562t, 1609
Myotonic dystrophy, 1634t
Myxedema, 739, 741f
Myxedema coma, 741

N
Na+. *See* Sodium.
Nail disorders, 1674–1676
Nail-patella syndrome, 156, 157f
Nails, 1646, 1646f
Narcolepsy, 505
Nasal and nasopharyngeal cancer,
    environmental factors in,
    397t–400t
Nasopharynx, 1242–1243, 1245f
Native immunity, 183
Natriuretic peptides, 102
  and cardiovascular function, 1128
  and hypertension, 1151–1152,
    1153f
  physiologic roles of, 1128b
  and renal function, 1352
  and systolic heart failure, 1190
Natural barriers, 184
Natural immunity, 183
Natural killer (NK) cell(s), 957
  function of, 248–250
  hematopoietic differentiation of,
    964f
  in inflammatory response, 202,
    203f
  in tissue specific hypersensitivity
    reactions, 261

Natural killer (NK) cell
    lymphoma(s), 1033
  classification of, 1030b
Nausea, 1453
Necator americanus, 310t
Necrosis, 81–84, 82f
  apoptosis and, differences
    between, 85
Necrotizing enterocolitis, 1529
  clinical manifestations of, 1529
  evaluation and treatment of,
    1529–1531
  pathophysiology of, 1529
Needle biopsy, 805–806
Negative dimensions, in
    schizophrenia, 651
Negative selection, 233
Neglect syndrome, 542
Neisseria gonorrhoeae, 298,
    299t–300t
  antigenic variation in, 304, 927
  drug resistant strains of, 927
  immune molecule degradation
    by, 304
  immune molecule neutralization
    by, 304–305
  immune suppression induced
    by, 305
  intracellular survival of, 302–303
Neisseria meningitidis, 298,
    299t–300t, 682
  immune molecule degradation
    by, 304
Neisseria meningitidis vaccine, 329
  adult, 329t
  child, 330t
Neisseria spp.
  adhesion mechanisms of, 298–300
  complement evasion by, 305
Neoadjuvant chemotherapy, 388
Neoantigen(s), 269
**Neonatal alloimmune
    thrombocytopenic purpura,**
  1082
Neonatal diabetes, 748
Neonatal herpes simplex infections,
  938
Neonatal jaundice, 1068, 1531
  clinical manifestations of, 1531
  pathophysiology of, 1531
Neonatal myasthenia, 639
Neonatal purpura fulminans,
  1080–1081
**Neonatal respiratory distress
    syndrome,** 1321, 1321b
  clinical manifestations of, 1322
  pathophysiology of, 1321–1322,
    1322f
  treatment of, 1322–1324
    antenatal, glucocorticoids in,
      1322
    exogenous surfactant in, 1322
    supportive care in, 1323
Neonatal thrombocytopenia,
    autoimmune, 1082
Neonate(s)
  cardiovascular development in,
    1209, 1211–1213
  hematologic development in, 982
  hematopoiesis in, 1062–1063
  immune function in, 250, 251f
  innate immunity in, 212
  protective strategies for
    ventilation in, 1323, 1326

Neonate(s) *(Continued)*
  pulmonary resuscitation of, and
    lung injury, 1323b
  recurrent seizures in, 539t
  reflexes in, 668, 668t
  transient alloimmunity in,
    270–271
Neoplasms
  benign and malignant,
    characteristics of, 361t
  cellular biology of, 362–366
  classification and nomenclature
    of, 361–362
  definition of, 360–361
  histology and genetics of, 361–362
  in HIV (human
    immunodeficiency virus)
    infection, 323b
  immune system and, interaction
    of, 378
  progression of, 361, 362f, 368,
    369f
  soft tissue, classification of, 1639t
Neovascularization, 383–384
Nephrin, 1345–1346
Nephritic sediment, 1378
Nephritic syndrome, glomerular
    disorders associated
    with, 1381t. *See also*
    Glomerulonephritis.
Nephroblastoma, 1413
Nephrogenic diabetes insipidus,
  730
Nephron(s), 1345–1347
  glomerular filtration in,
    1352–1357, 1353f–1354f
  structure of, 1345, 1346f
  tubules of
    epithelial cells of, 1347, 1347f
    Henle loop, 1347
    proximal, 1347
    transport within, 1355–1357,
      1356f
  types of, 1345
  vascular supply of, 1347–1350,
    1348f
Nephropathy, in diabetes mellitus,
    760–761
Nephrotic sediment, 1378
Nephrotic syndrome, 1384
  in children, 1409
    clinical manifestations of, 1410,
      1410f
    edema in, 1410, 1410f
    evaluation and treatment of,
      1410–1412
    hypercoagulation in, 1410
    hyperlipidemia in, 1410
    pathophysiology of, 1409–1410
  clinical manifestations of, 1385,
    1385t
  evaluation and treatment of,
    1375t, 1377t, 1385
  paraneoplastic, 389t
  pathophysiology of, 1381t,
    1384–1385, 1385f
Nerve growth factor (NGF), 36t
Nerve impulse, 446–449
Nerve sheath tumors, 617–618
Nerve tissue, injury and regeneration
    of, 445–446, 446f
Nerves, cranial and spinal, 465.
    See also Cranial nerves; Spinal
    nerves.

Nervous system, 442
in aging, 471–474, 474t
alterations in, 525–582. *See also*
Neurologic disorders.
cerebral hemodynamic,
557–560
cognitive, 525–528. *See also*
Cognitive dysfunction.
genetic basis of selected,
526t–527t
motor function, 561–570.
See also Motor function
alterations.
ascending (afferent) pathways of,
442–443
autonomic, 443, 467–471. *See also*
Autonomic nervous system.
cells of, 443–446. *See also*
Neuroglia; Neuron(s).
central, 442–443, 449–465. *See
also* Central nervous system
(CNS).
descending (efferent) pathways of,
442–443
effector organs of, 442–443
embryonic development of,
665–668
impulse transmission in, 446–449
interaction of, with immune and
endocrine systems, 347, 348t
key terminology of, 478
normal growth and development
of, 668, 668t
organization of, 442–443
peripheral, 442–443, 465–467.
See also Cranial nerves;
Peripheral nervous system
(PNS); Spinal nerves.
references on, 480
sensory and regulatory function
of, 481–524. *See also*
Neurologic function.
sensory receptors of, 445b
somatic, 443
summary review of, 477b–478b
tissue injury and regeneration in,
445–446
Nesiritide (recombinant BNP),
1193–1194
Net filtration, 98
Net filtration pressure, 1354
Neural crest, 665–666
Neural folds, 665
Neural groove, 665
Neural lobe, 704–705
Neural plate, 665
Neural tissue, 41–44
Neural tube, 665
at 3 weeks gestation, 666f
Neural tube defects, 167, 168b, 169f,
668–669
in anencephaly, 669
in encephalocele, 669
in meningocele, 669
in myelomeningocele, 669–670
reducing risk of, 668b
in spina bifida, 671–672
Neurilemma (Schwann sheath), 443,
444f. *See also* Myelin sheath.
Neuroblastoma, 688
clinical manifestations of, 689
evaluation and treatment of,
689–690
pathophysiology of, 688

Neurodegenerative disorders,
633–634
amyotrophic lateral sclerosis in,
633–634
Neuroendocrine system, 703, 706f
Neurofibrillary tangles, 471–474,
554–556
Neurofibrils, 443
Neurofibroma(s), 612t, 617, 619
Neurofibromatosis
congenital heart defects associated
with, 1215t
genetics and pathophysiology of,
526t–527t
Neurofibromatosis type1, 149f,
617–618
and associated childhood cancer,
438–439, 438t
diagnostic criteria for, 617b
genetic expression in, 148–149,
375–377
genetics and pathophysiology of,
526t–527t
Neurofibromatosis type2, 617–618
and associated childhood cancer,
438t
diagnostic criteria for, 617b
genetics and pathophysiology of,
526t–527t
Neurofibromin gene, 375t. *See also*
Neurofibromatosis.
Neurogenic bladder, 1369–1370
detrusor overactivity in, 1367f
pathophysiology of, 1369–1370,
1370f
Neurogenic diabetes insipidus, 730
Neurogenic pain, 491b
Neurogenic shock, 593, 1702, 1728
in children, 1732
pathophysiology of, 1702, 1702f,
1729
Neuroglia, 444–445, 445f
functions of, 446t, 446b
neurosteroid synthesis by, 446b
Neuroglial cells, 443
Neurohormonal signaling, 18–19, 19f
Neurohormones, 488
Neurohypophysis. *See* Posterior
pituitary.
Neurolemmocytes. *See* Schwann
cell(s).
Neurolemmoma, 612t, 617
Neuroleptics, 651–652, 651b
Neurologic disorders, 525–582
central, 583–591. *See also* Central
nervous system disorders.
cerebral hemodynamic,
557–560. *See also* Cerebral
hemodynamic alterations.
in children, 665–695
and adults, comparison of, 668
cerebrovascular disease,
684–685
encephalopathies, 675.
See also Childhood
encephalopathies.
structural malformations,
668–669. *See also*
Congenital hydrocephalus;
Cranial deformities;
Neural tube defects.
tumors, 685. *See also* Brain
cancer, and tumors;
Embryonic tumors.

Neurologic disorders *(Continued)*
cognitive, 525–528. *See also*
Cognitive dysfunction.
embryonic development and
associated, 665–668, 667f
genetic basis of selected, 526t–527t
mental, 646–664
anxiety disorders in, 658–662
mood disorders in, 652–658
schizophrenia in, 647–652
motor function, 561–570. *See also*
Motor function alterations.
neuromuscular junction, 638–639.
See also Neuromuscular
junction disorders.
paraneoplastic, 389t
peripheral, 635. *See also* Peripheral
nervous system disorders.
secondary hypertension in, 1143t
sensory and regulatory, 481–524
hearing loss, 515
olfactory dysfunction, 516
pain and pain perception,
482–495
somatosensory dysfunction,
517
taste dysfunction, 516
temperature regulatory
dysfunction, 500–502
visual dysfunction, 509–512
Neurologic function
in aging, 471–474, 474t
alterations in, 525–582. *See also*
Neurologic disorders.
cerebral hemodynamic,
557–560
cognitive, 525–528. *See also*
Cognitive dysfunction.
genetic basis of selected,
526t–527t
motor function, 561–570.
See also Motor function
alterations.
chronic kidney disease and effects
on, 1391t, 1396
imaging and testing, 474–480
immune and endocrine systems
in, 347, 348t
normal growth and development
of, 668, 668t
sensory and regulatory, 481–524
key terminology of, 520b
pain in, 482–495. *See also* Pain;
Pain perception.
references on, 521
sleep in, 502–505
somatosensation in, 517–520
special senses in, 481–482,
506–508
hearing, 512–514
olfaction and taste, 515–516
vision, 506–508
summary review of,
517b–520b
thermal, 496–498
Neuroma, 617
Neuromodulation, 486–490
neurotransmitters in, 487–490
pathways of, 486, 487f
Neuromodulators, 447–448
functions of, 448t–449t
**Neuromuscular autoimmune
disorders,** 257t–258t
Neuromuscular junction, 458, 459f

Neuromuscular junction disorders,
638–639
antibodies and mechanisms of
action in, 638f, 639t
references on, 643
summary review of, 641b–642b
Neuron(s), 41, 443–444
action potential of, 449
axons of, 443
classification of
by function, 444, 446b, 446t
by structural processes, 444,
445f
dendrites of, 443
grouping cell bodies of, 443
impulse transmission by, 446–449,
447f
injury and regeneration of,
445–446
structure of, 443, 444f
Neuronal cell tumors, 612t
Neuropathic pain, 490, 493–495
evaluation and management of,
494–495
Neuropathy(ies), 635. *See
also* Guillain-Barré
syndrome; Plexus injuries;
Radiculopathy(ies).
classification of, 635
clinical manifestations of,
635–636
in diabetes mellitus, 761–763
evaluation and treatment of, 636
pathophysiology of, 635
and proprioceptive dysfunction,
517
Neuropeptide Y (NPY), in stress
response, 348t
Neuropeptides
functions of, 448t–449t
influence of
on eating behavior, 1478–1479,
1478b
on immune response, 349
Neurophysiologic pain, 491b
Neuroreceptors, autonomic,
467–470
actions of, in adrenergic
and cholinergic
neurotransmission, 472t
Neuroregulin, 1556–1557
Neurosteroid synthesis, by
neuroglia, 446b
Neurosyphilis, 929
Neurotonia, 638
Neurotransmitter(s), 18–19, 41,
447–449, 447f
of autonomic nervous system,
467–470, 471f
definition of, 447–448
functions of, 448t–449t
pain modulating, 487–490, 488b
excitatory, 488
inhibitory, 488–490
physiology of, in synaptic cleft,
448–449
in schizophrenia, 648–650
in sleep mechanisms, 503–504
Neurotransmitter secretion, 19f
Neutralization, antigen, 244
Neutropenia, 1015, 1016t
due to phagocytic deficiencies, 282
Neutrophil count, 983t–985t
pediatric, 985t

Neutrophilia, 1015, 1016t
Neutrophils, 955
  hematopoietic differentiation of,
    964f
  in inflammatory response, 201,
    207–208, 1710
  pediatric values for, 1064t
Nevi (moles), 78, 1669, 1671f
  classification of, 1671t
Nevus flammeus, 1691
Newborn. See Neonate(s),
  and neonatal entries.
NGF (nerve growth factor), 36t
Niacin, in erythropoiesis, 969t
Niacin deficiency, and associated
  disorders, 70t
Nifedipine, calcium channel
  blocking activity of, 1108–1109
Nipple, breast, 803
Nipple retraction, in breast
  carcinoma, 906f
Nissl substance, in neurons, 443, 445
Nitrates
  and cancer risk, 410t–413t
  for myocardial ischemia,
    1168–1169
Nitric oxide (NO), 203f
  and effect on endothelium, 1119b
  in hemostasis, 972
  neurologic functions of, 448t–449t
  in vascular relaxation, 968
Nitric oxide (NO) system, in
  vascular endothelium, 973f
NK cells. See Natural killer (NK)
  cell(s).
NMDA (N-methyl-D-aspartate)
  receptors, 488
  in learning and memory, 649–650
Nocebo effect, 486
Nociception, 482
  central processing in, 484–486
  neuromodulation in, 486–490
  neurotransmitters in, 487–490,
    488b
    excitatory, 488
    inhibitory, 488–490
  pathways of, 483–484, 483f–484f
  receptors in, 482–483
  segmental inhibition of, 486
Nociceptive pain, 490
Nociceptors, 445b, 482–483
  categorization of, 482–483
  stimuli activating, 483t
Nocturnal enuresis, 1415
Nodes, myocardial, 1099
Nodes of Ranvier, 443
Nodular thyroid disease, 737–738
Nodule, skin, 1648t–1653t
Noise, in cell injury, 75–76
Non-Hodgkin lymphoma, 1033
  Ann Arbor staging for, 1035t
  in children, 1087
    clinical manifestations of, 1087
    evaluation and treatment of,
      1087–1088
    pathogenesis of, 1087
  classification of, 1034
  clinical differences between
    Hodgkin and, 1035t
  clinical manifestations of, 1034
  evaluation and treatment of,
    1034–1035
  incidence of, 1033
  pathophysiology of, 1033–1034

Non-nociceptive pain, 490
Non-small cell lung cancer, 1301
Non-ST elevation MI (non-STEMI),
  1169, 1174
Non-tyrosine kinase activated
  receptors, 23t
Nonaccidental trauma, to children,
  1640
  etiology of, 1640
  evaluation of, 1640, 1640f
  treatment of, 1640
Nonalcoholic fatty liver disease,
  1532–1533, 1554b
Nonbacterial infectious cystitis,
  1376
Nonbacterial prostatitis, 863
**Nonbacterial thrombotic
  endocarditis,** 1187
Noncardiogenic pulmonary edema,
  1280–1281
**Noncommunicating
  hydrocephalus,** 560
Nonconscious memory, 543
Nondeclarative memory, 543
Nondisjunction, of chromosomes,
  137, 140f
Nonenzymatic glycosylation, in
  chronic hyperglycemia, 759
Nongonococcal urethritis (NGU),
  937–938
  clinical manifestations of, 938
  evaluation and treatment of, 938
  pathophysiology of, 938
Nonheme iron, 997
Nonimmunologic urticaria, 265
Noninfectious cystitis, 1376
Noninflammatory acne, 1680–1681
Noninflammatory joint disease,
  1592–1594
Nonobstructive jaundice, 1486
Nonorganic failure to thrive, 1528
Nonossifying fibroma, 1637
Nonproliferative breast lesions,
  873–874
Nonpuerperal hyperprolactinemia,
  871
Nonpurulent meningitis, 620–622
Nonshivering thermogenesis, 496
Nonspecific urethritis. See
  Nongonococcal urethritis.
Nonstructural scoliosis, 1625
Nonsyndromic craniosynostosis, 672
Nonthermal burns, 1714
Nonunion, of fractured bones,
  1571–1572
Nonvolatile forms, of body acids,
  114
Norepinephrine, 447–448. See also
  Catecholamines.
  cardiovascular effects of, 340,
    1125
  functions of, 448t–449t
  in pain modulation, 488
  release in sympathetic
    neurotransmission, 467–469
  renal effects of, 1358
Norepinephrine system, 654, 656f
Normal bacterial flora, 186
Normal pressure hydrocephalus,
  560
Normoblast, 965–966
**Normocytic-normochromic
  anemia(s),** 991t, 1000–1002
  in children, 1066t

Norovirus, 314t
Norwegian scabies, 1689
Norwood procedure, 1230
Nosocomial infections, bacterial
  agents causing, 299t–300t
Nosocomial pneumonia, bacteria
  causing, 1290–1291
NREM (non-rapid eye movement)
  sleep phase, 502–503, 503f
Nuclear envelope, 2, 3–4f
Nuclear palsies, 567
Nuclear palsy syndromes, 568t
Nuclear receptors, 700t, 702–703
Nuclei, composed of neuron cell
  bodies, 443
Nucleolus, 2
Nucleoplasm, 4f
Nucleotide(s), 129, 133f
Nucleus, cell, 2–4, 4f
Nucleus accumbens, as
  reinforcement center, 475b
Nucleus proprius, 483–484
Nucleus pulposus, 461–462, 462f
Nutrients. See also Carbohydrates;
  Fat(s); Mineral(s); Protein(s);
  Vitamin(s).
  digestion and absorption of,
    1429–1434
  metabolism of, in liver,
    1441–1442
Nutrition
  in cancer epidemiology, 403–406.
    See also Dietary factors.
  disorders of, 1477–1478. See also
    Anorexia nervosa; Bulimia
    nervosa; Obesity; Starvation.
    in children, 1524
  DNA methylation and, 403,
    405–406, 405f
  essential fatty acids and
    inflammation in, 199b
  immune competency and, 285
Nutrition & Disease, 69–71, 70b. See
  also Dietary insufficiencies.
  Alzheimer disease and diet, 556b
  breast cancer risk and diet
    updates, 892b
  breast disease and iodine, 401
  cancer prevention diet, 413b
  chronic obstructive pulmonary
    disease, 1286b
  cognitive function and iron,
    666b
  diverticular disease and diet,
    1475b
  fats, basic facts, 1162b
  ketogenic diet for children with
    epilepsy, 680b
  kidney disease, acute and chronic,
    1396b
  medical nutrition therapy for
    diabetics, 753b
  nutrition and risk reduction for
    prostate cancer, 864b
  olive oil and immunologic
    function, 1713b
  pediatric cancer and prevention of
    malnutrition, 440b
  premenstrual syndrome and diet,
    828b
  skeletal tissue and trace elements,
    1580b
Nystagmus, 509
  vestibular, 517

O
Oat cell carcinoma, 1302–1303,
  1302t
O'Beirne sphincter, 1435–1436
Obesity, 1477–1478
  cancer and, 406–415, 414f, 1480
    biologic mechanisms of,
      409–415, 415f
    and cancer mortality risk, 408f
  in children, 1237–1238. See also
    Childhood obesity.
  clinical manifestations of, 1480
  coronary artery disease and, 1164
  evaluation and treatment of,
    1480–1482
  hypertension and, 1152, 1152b
  insulin resistance and, 1479–1480
  pathophysiology of, 1478–1480,
    1478b, 1479f
    endogenous hormones and,
      409–415, 415f, 1479, 1479f
    genes and environmental
      interaction in, 177–178,
      1477–1479
    glucocorticoids, insulin, and
      inflammation in, 344b,
      1479
    insulin resistance and, 750,
      1479–1480
Obligate carriers, 148
Obligatory growth, 1367
Oblique fracture, 1569
Obsessive-compulsive disorders,
  661–662
  pathophysiology of, 661–662
  treatment of, 662
Obstructed hemodynamics,
  congenital cardiac defects
  causing, 1226
Obstructive jaundice, 1485, 1487t
Obstructive pulmonary disease,
  1282–1284
  airway obstruction caused by,
    1282, 1282f
  asthma in, 1283–1284. See also
    Asthma.
  chronic, 1286. See also Chronic
    obstructive pulmonary
    disease.
Obstructive shock, 1728
  pathophysiology of, 1729
Obstructive sleep apnea syndrome,
  505
  childhood, 1320
    clinical manifestations of, 1320
    evaluation and treatment of,
      1320–1321
    pathophysiology of, 1320
  in obesity, 1480
Obstructive uropathy, 1365–1368.
  See also Urinary tract
  obstruction.
Occipital lobe, 452
Occlusive cerebrovascular disease,
  685
Occult bleeding, 1456, 1456t
Occult hydrocephalus, 560
Occupational carcinogens, 426
Ocular anatomy
  disorders of, 509–512. See also
    Visual dysfunction.
  external, 506, 507f
  extrinsic muscles in, 508, 508f
  internal, 506f–507f, 507–508

Ocular infections
 bacterial agents causing, 299t, 506–507
 microbial agents causing, 506–507
Ocular movement disorders, 509–512
Ocular myasthenia, 639
Ocular nerve palsy syndromes, 568t
Oculomotor nerve (CN III), 466f
 origins, course, functions, and testing of, 468t
Oculomotor response(s)
 in brain dysfunction evaluation, 531–532, 533t
 doll's eye, 534f
Oculovestibular reflex, 534f
Olfaction, and taste, 515–516, 516f
 in aging, 516
Olfactory dysfunction, 516
Olfactory hallucinations, 516
Olfactory nerve (CN I), 466f
 origins, course, functions, and testing of, 468t
Oligodendroglia (oligodendrocytes), 444–445, 445f
 functions of, 446t
Oligodendroglioma(s), 612t, 615–616
 intramedullary spinal cord, 619
Oligomenorrhea, 823t
Oliguria, 1358
 mechanisms of, 1387, 1388f
Olive oil, and immune physiology, 1713b
Omalizumab, 1285–1286
Omega-3 fatty acids, 1162b
Onchocerca volvulus, 310t
Oncogene(s), 373t, 370–375
 activation mechanisms for, 374f
 chromosome translocation mutations, 371–372
 gene amplification, 372, 374f
 point mutations, 370
 associated with childhood cancers, 438–439, 439t
Oncosis, 76, 77f
Oncotic pressure, 27–28
Onychomycosis, 1674–1676
Oophoritis, 828
Open-angle glaucoma, 510t, 511f
Open brain trauma, 583–584, 588
Open fracture, 1569
Open head injury, 588
Open (communicating) pneumothorax, 1273
OPG. *See* Osteoprotegerin.
OPG/RANKL/RANK system, 1580–1582, 1581f
Ophthalmia, chlamydial, 936–937, 937f
Ophthalmia neonatorum, 927, 927f
Opioid producing leukocytes, in pain control, 489b
Opioid receptors, 488
 agonist activity at, 488
Opisthorchis viverrini, 425
Opportunism, 295b
Opportunistic infections, in acquired immunodeficiency syndrome, 323b, 629
Opportunistic microorganisms, 295
Opsonin(s), 190, 246
Opsonization, 199–200, 246
Optic chiasm, 512

Optic disc, 507
Optic nerve (CN II), 466f
 image formation through, 507–508
 inflammation of, 510
 origins, course, functions, and testing of, 468t
Optic nerve glioma, 686, 686t
 clinical manifestations of, 687–688
 treatment strategies for, 687t, 688
Oral cavity, 1421–1423
Oral phase of swallowing, 1423
Orchitis, 857, 857f
Orexins, 1478–1479, 1478b
Organ of Corti, 514
Organ-specific autoimmune adrenalitis, 770
Organ transplantation
 and associated childhood cancer, 438t
 human leukocyte antigens and, 226–228
Organic brain syndrome, as complication of myocardial infarction, 1176
Organic molecular transport systems, 30t
Orgasmic dysfunction, 849
Orientation, 543, 545f
Orienting deficit, 543, 547t
Oropharynx, 1242–1243
Orthopnea, 1267
Orthostatic hypotension, 1156–1157
 acute, 1157
 chronic, 1157
 definition of, 1156–1157
 idiopathic or primary, 1157
Osgood-Schlatter disease, 1631–1632
 clinical manifestations of, 1632
 evaluation and treatment of, 1632
 pathophysiology of, 1632
Osler-Weber-Rendu disease, congenital heart defects associated with, 1215t
Osmolality, 27
 tonicity and, 28
Osmolarity, 27
Osmoreceptors, 102
Osmosis, 27–28
Osmotic diarrhea, 1454
Osmotic diuretics, 1359t
Osmotic pressure, 27
Osteitis deformans, 1585. *See also* Paget disease.
Osteoarthritis, 1592–1594, 1593f
 clinical manifestations of, 1594–1595, 1595f
 evaluation and treatment of, 1596–1597
 obesity and, 1480
 pathophysiology of, 1594
Osteoarthropathy, paraneoplastic hypertrophic, 389t
Osteoblasts, 1542–1543, 1542f
Osteocalcin, 1545
Osteochondroses, 1631
Osteoclasts, 1543–1544
Osteoclasts, precursors of, 963
Osteocytes, 1543

Osteogenesis imperfecta, 1618–1619
 classification of, 1624t
 clinical manifestations of, 1625
 congenital heart defects associated with, 1215t
 evaluation and treatment of, 1625, 1626f
 pathophysiology of, 1624–1625
Osteogenic tumors, 1590–1591
Osteoid osteoma, 1637
Osteoid synthesis, 1542–1543
Osteolytic lesions, in multiple myeloma, 1038–1040, 1040f
Osteomalacia, 1584–1585
 clinical manifestations of, 1585
 evaluation and treatment of, 1585–1586
 pathophysiology of, 1585
Osteomyelitis, 1587
 age related pathogenic differences in, 1628b, 1628f, 1630
 and associated cancer, 378t
 in children, 1628
 clinical manifestations of, 1629–1630
 evaluation and treatment of, 1630–1631
 pathophysiology of, 1628–1629, 1629f
 clinical manifestations of, 1588
 evaluation and treatment of, 1588–1592
 pathophysiology of, 1587–1588
Osteonectin, 1545
Osteopenia, 1576–1577, 1582f
Osteophytes, 1593
Osteopontin, 1545
Osteoporosis, 1576–1580
 age related, 1582, 1582–1583f
 clinical manifestations of, 1582–1583
 definition of, 1576–1577
 evaluation and treatment of, 1583–1585
 fracture risk in, 1577–1579, 1579b
 WHO assessment tool for, 1583
 glucocorticoid induced, 1582
 pathophysiology of, 1580–1582
 postmenopausal, 1579
 prevalence of, 1578
 regional, 1580
 secondary, 1580
 severe, 1577
 trace elements and effects in, 1579–1580, 1580b
 vertebral fractures in, 1578
Osteoprotegerin (OPG), 1542–1543, 1579
 in pathophysiology of osteoporosis, 1580–1582, 1581f
Osteosarcoma, 1590–1591, 1590f
 in children, 1637
 clinical manifestations of, 1638
 evaluation and treatment of, 1638
 pathophysiology of, 1637–1638
 clinical manifestations of, 1591
 treatment of, 1591
Ostium primum, 1210
Ostium secundum, 1210
Other specific types of diabetes mellitus, 746t, 753–754

Otitis externa, 514
Otitis media, 514–515
 bacterial agents causing, 299t–300t
Otoliths, 514
Outer membrane, mitochondrial, 7
Outflow tract, 1094
Oval window, 512–513
Ovarian ablation, in breast cancer treatment, 907–908
Ovarian cancer, 846, 847f
 clinical manifestations of, 847–848
 evaluation and treatment of, 848–850, 848t
 metastasis of, 381f, 384t, 847, 847f
 pathogenesis of, 846–847
Ovarian cycle, 789, 793f, 794–795
Ovarian cysts, benign, 836–837, 836f
Ovarian failure, premature, 807
Ovarian follicles, 789, 790f
 alterations in, 836–837
 development of, 791f
 in polycystic ovary syndrome, 825
 dynamic process of growth of, 795, 795b
 menopausal changes in, 807, 809b
Ovary(ies), 789–790
 anatomy of, 788f
 cross-section of, during reproductive years, 790f
 follicles of, 789, 790f
Overactive bladder syndrome, 1370–1371
Overflow incontinence, 1369t
Overwhelming postoperative infection, after splenectomy, 1019, 1043
Oviducts, 789
Ovulation, 789
Ovum, 781
Oxidation, 23
Oxidative cellular metabolism, 23
Oxidative phosphorylation, 24–25
Oxidative stress, 54
 in chronic hyperglycemia, 759
Oxygen consumption
 impaired, in shock, 1697
 supply-dependent, 1711
Oxygen consumption index, 1133t
Oxygen content, blood, 1258–1259
Oxygen debt, 1562
Oxygen-dependent killing mechanism, 201
Oxygen partial pressure, normal values, 1262t
Oxygen toxicity, 1277–1278
Oxygen transport, pulmonary, 1257–1259
Oxyhemoglobin (HbO$_2$), 967–968
 association and dissociation of, 1259
Oxyhemoglobin dissociation curve, 1259, 1260f
Oxyntic cells, 1426
Oxytocin, 705–707
 hypothalamic regulation of, 703–704, 707
 physiologic effects of, 707
 stress induced, 351–352, 707
 target organs of, 704f

P

P cells, cardiac, 1100
P wave, of electrocardiogram, 1103
p16 gene, 902–905
    in etiology of breast cancer,
        902–905
    in etiology of melanoma, 375t,
        422. *See also* Familial
        melanoma.
p53 gene, 369, 375t. *See also* Li-
    Fraumeni syndrome.
    in etiology of breast cancer, 896
    in etiology of skin cancer, 422
Pacemaker, of heart, 1100
PAF (platelet activating factor), 198,
    203f
Paget disease, 1585–1586
    clinical manifestations of, 1586,
        1586f
    evaluation and treatment of,
        1586–1587
    pathophysiology of, 1586
Pain, 481–495
    abdominal, 1455–1456
    acute, 490–491. *See also* Acute
        pain.
    cancer associated, 388–390
        treatment of, 389–390
    categories of, 491b
    central, 494
    chronic, 492–493. *See also*
        Chronic pain.
    classification of, 490
    deafferentation, 494
    of inflammation, 205
        chemical mediators of, 203f
    intensity of, and tissue damage,
        482
    neuroanatomy of, 482–486
    neuromatrix theory of, 494b
    neuropathic, 493–495
    perception of, 482. *See also* Pain
        perception.
    phantom limb, 494
    in pulmonary disorders, 1267
    sympathetically maintained, 494
    theories of, 482
Pain perception, 482. *See also*
    Nociception.
    in aging, 495–496
    central processing in, 484–486
    in children, 495
    gender and, 495b
    neural pathways in, 483–484,
        484f
    neuromodulation in, 486–490,
        488b
    neurotransmitters in, 488,
        487–490
        excitatory, 488
        inhibitory, 488–490
    nociceptors in, 482–483
    segmental inhibition of, 486
    threshold and tolerance of, 490
Pain threshold, 490
Pain tolerance, 490
Painful bladder syndrome/
    interstitial cystitis, 1376–1377
Painful intercourse, 849
Painless thyroiditis, 741
Pallor, in iron deficiency, 996f
PAMPs. *See* Pathogen-associated
    molecular patterns.
Panacinar emphysema, 1289–1290

Pancreas, 712, 713f, 1437f, 1443,
    1443f
    digestive enzymes of, 1430b
    endocrine, 712–715, 713f
        aging and effects on, 721
        amylin secretion by, 714
        gastrin, ghrelin, pancreatic
            polypeptide secretion by,
            715
        glucagon secretion by, 714
        hormonal alterations in, 704.
            See also Diabetes mellitus.
        hormonal secretion stimulated
            by, 712–713
        insulin secretion by, 713–714
        somatostatin secretion by,
            714–715
    exocrine, 713f, 1443–1444
        and associated structures, 1443f
        secretions of, in digestive
            process, 1437–1444
    fat necrosis of, 83f
Pancreatic α-amylase, 1444
Pancreatic cancer, 1498t, 1504
    clinical manifestations of, 1505
    evaluation and treatment of,
        1505–1509
    pathogenesis of, 1504–1505
Pancreatic disorders, 1495–1496
Pancreatic duct, 1443
Pancreatic enzymes, 1444
Pancreatic function assessments,
    1447t
Pancreatic insufficiency, 1470
Pancreatic lipases, 1444
Pancreatic polypeptide, 715, 1425t
Pancreatitis, 1495–1496
    acute, 1496
    chronic, 1497
    and associated cancer, 378t
Pancytopenia, 1000, 1021
Pandemic(s)
    definition of, 297
    historic examples of, 297t
Paneth cells, 1429
Panhypopituitarism, 731
Panic disorder, 659–660
    etiology of, 659
    pathophysiology of, 659
    treatment of, 659–660
Panner disease, 1631
Pannus, 1598
Pantothenic acid (vitamin B₅)
    deficiency, and associated
    disorders, 70t
Papanicolaou (Pap) test, 806–807
    efficiency of, in cervical cancer
        screening, 842b
Papez circuit, 453
Papillary capillaries, 1646
Papillary muscles, 1094
Papilledema, 510
Papilloma(s), 612t
    breast, 875
Papillomavirus, 314t
Papule, 1648t
Papulosquamous skin disorders,
    1657–1660
Paracrine secretion, 19f
Paracrine signaling, 18–19, 19f
Paradoxic breathing, 1311–1312
Paradoxic sleep, 503
Paraesophageal hiatal hernia,
    1459–1460, 1459f

Parageusia, 516
Paragonimus westermani, 310t
Parainfluenza virus, 314t
Paralysis, 564–568
    periodic, 1609
    upper and lower motor neuron
        syndromes in, 564–567, 564t
Paralytic ileus, 1460, 1461t
Paraneoplastic syndromes, 388,
    389t
Paraparesis, 564
Paraphimosis, 850–851, 851f
Paraplegia, 564, 594
Parasites, 310t
Parasitic infections, 310–313. *See*
    also Parasitic pathogens.
    AIDS associated, 629
    pathogenesis of, 312–313
    sexually transmitted, 942–943.
        See also Pediculosis pubis;
        Scabies; Trichomoniasis.
Parasitic myositis, 1611
Parasitic pathogens, 310–313, 310t
    evasion mechanisms of, 311–312
        antigenic variation, 311
        complement evasion, 311
        immune molecule degradation,
            311
        immune molecule
            neutralization, 311
        immune suppression, 311–312
        intracellular survival, 311
        protection against phagocytosis,
            311
        self-protein coatings, 311
    invasion of, 311–312
    tissue damage caused by, 312
    toxins released by, 312
    transmission and colonization
        by, 311
Parasitic worms, 298t, 310, 310t. *See*
    also Parasitic pathogens.
Parasomnias, common, 505
Parasympathetic nervous system,
    467–470, 470f
Paratenonitis, 1574t
Paratenonitis with tendinosis,
    1574t
Parathyroid(s), 708–712, 709f
    aging and effects on, 722
    hormone secretion by, 711, 711f
Parathyroid hormonal disorders,
    742
    hyperparathyroidism in, 742
    hypoparathyroidism in, 744
Parathyroid hormone (PTH), 111,
    711
    recombinant, 712b
    serum calcium level and, 711–712,
        712f
    aging and effects on, 722
Paratonia, 562t, 563
Paratope, 221–222
Paraurethral glands, 785–786
Parenchyma, 36–38
Paresis, 564–568
    upper and lower motor neuron
        syndromes in, 564–567, 564t
Parietal abdominal pain, 1455
Parietal cells, 1426
    hydrochloric acid secretion by,
        1426f
Parietal epithelium, 1345–1346
Parietal lobe, 452

Parietal pericardium, 1093
Parietal peritoneum, 1428–1429
Parkinson disease, 572
    autonomic and neuroendocrine
        symptoms in, 574
    clinical manifestations of,
        572–575
    cognitive-affective symptoms
        in, 574
    evaluation and treatment of,
        575–580
    genetic basis of, 526t–527t
    influence of symptoms in,
        574–575
    invasive treatments of, 455b
    pathophysiology of, 526t–527t,
        572, 572f
        dopaminergic
            neurodegeneration in,
            573f
    postural abnormalities in,
        574–575, 574f
Parkinson syndrome, 572
Parkinsonian bradykinesia, 573
Parkinsonian rigidity, 573
Parkinsonian syndrome, 572
Parkinsonian tremor, 568t–569t,
    573
Parkinsonism, 572
    etiologic classification of, 571b,
        572
    primary and secondary causes
        of, 571b
Paronychia, 1674
Parosmia, 516
Paroxysmal cold hemoglobinuria,
    1005
Paroxysmal dyskinesias, 569
Paroxysmal nocturnal dyspnea,
    1267
Paroxysmal nocturnal
    hemoglobinuria, 1005
Pars distalis, 704–705
Pars intermedia, 704–705
Pars nervosa, 704–705
Pars tuberalis, 704–705
Partial atrioventricular canal
    defect, 1222
Partial pressure(s), 1254–1255, 1255f
    of respiratory gases, 1257–1258,
        1258f
    normal values, 1262t
Partial seizures, 536, 537t, 679
    clinical manifestations of,
        540t–541t
Partial thickness burn injury, 1714
Partial thromboplastin time (PTT),
    983t–985t
Partial trisomy, 137
Passive acquired immunity, 220
Passive immunity, 220
Passive immunotherapy, 332
Passive mediated transport, 28–29
Passive transport, 25
    processes of, 26–28
Patch (skin lesion), 1648t–1653t
Patch and scratch tests, 1647t
Patched gene, in etiology of basal cell
    carcinoma, 422
Patent ductus arteriosus, 1218, 1219f
    clinical manifestations of, 1218
    evaluation and treatment of,
        1218–1219
    pathophysiology of, 1218

Pathogen(s)
bacterial, 297–307, 298t, 301f
countermeasures against, 326–332, 327t
antimicrobial, 327–329
infection control, 326–327
passive immunotherapy, 332
vaccination, 329–332
fungal, 307–308, 308t
processing of, by antigen presentation cells, 235–237
secondary immune deficiencies and, 286
true, 295
viral, 313–318, 314t
virulence of, 1375–1376
Pathogen-associated molecular patterns (PAMPs), 192–194, 204–205
Pathogenicity, 295b
definition of, 297
factors influencing, 297
Pathologic atrophy, 47
Pathologic fracture, 1569
Pathologic hyperplasia, 49
Pathophysiologic jaundice, 1531
Pattern recognition receptors (PRRs), 192–194
Pauci immune glomerulonephritis, 1383
Pavementing, 198–199
PDGF. *See* Platelet-derived growth factor.
Peak bone mass, 1577–1578
peau d'orange, 905
Pediatric AIDS. *See* AIDS (acquired immunodeficiency syndrome).
Pediatric burn injury, 1741–1743, 1742f, 1745t
biphasic physiologic response to, 1744, 1745t
clinical manifestations of, 1745–1748
evaluation and treatment of, 1748–1750
airway maintenance in, 1746–1747
comfort management in, 1750
fluid resuscitation in, 1745–1750
nutritional support in, 1750
pulmonary support in, 1749
scar and contracture management in, 1748
wound management in, 1748–1749, 1749f
hypermetabolic phase of, 1744, 1747–1748
pathophysiology of, 1743–1745
recovery from, 1750
references on, 1752
scar maturation in, 1745, 1746f, 1748
severity of, 1742–1743
summary review of, 1750b
Pediatric immune response, 251
Pediatric innate immunity, 213
Pediculosis, 1689
Pediculosis pubis, 945
clinical manifestations of, 945
evaluation and treatment of, 945–946
Pedigree analysis, classical, 155–157

Pedigree characteristics
in autosomal dominant inheritance, 146
in autosomal recessive inheritance, 151–152
in X-linked inheritance, 154
Pedigree chart, 146, 146f
for achondroplasia, 147f
evaluation of, 155
for hemophilia, 150b
Pelvic inflammation, chronic, and associated cancers, 378t
Pelvic inflammatory disease (PID), 828, 829f
CDC recommended treatment of acute, 831b–832b
clinical manifestations of, 829
complications of, 830
evaluation and treatment of, 829–838
pathophysiology of, 828–829
Pelvic nerve, 467
Pelvic organ prolapse, 833–836
evaluation of, 834b
obstructed urine flow in, 1371
physical examination terminology for, 834b
risk factors for, 833, 833b
symptoms and treatment of, 836t.
See also Cystocele; Rectocele.
Pelvic pain, diagnosis of, 829–830, 830f
Pemphigus, 1660–1661
Pendular nystagmus, 509
Penetrance, of trait, 148
age-dependent, 148
Penetrating brain injury, 584
types of, 588
Penetrating head trauma, 583–584
Penile cancer, 853–854
staging system for, 853, 853b
treatment of, 853–854
Penile carcinoma in situ, 853, 853f
Penis, 798–799
cross-section of, 798f
disorders of, 850–854
Pennate muscles, 1555
Pepsin, 1426
activity in digestive process, 1427
Pepsinogen, 1426
Peptic ulcers, 1464–1465
chronic, 1464, 1465f
duodenal, 1465, 1466f
gastric, 1467
stress related, 1467–1470
surgical treatment of, 1467–1468
Peptide hormones, 697t
receptors for, and mechanism of action, 700t
Peptide YY, 1425t, 1479
increased plasma, and obesity, 1479
Perceptual dominance, 490
Percutaneous coronary intervention (PCI), for myocardial ischemia, 1169
Perfusion, and ventilation, 1256–1257
Pericardial cavity, 1093
Pericardial effusion, 1177
Pericardial fluid, 1093
Pericarditis
acute, 1176–1177, 1177f
as complication of myocardial infarction, 1176
constrictive, 1177–1178

Pericardium, 1093
disorders of, 1176–1178
Perichondrium, 1618–1619
Periduodenal band, 1519
Perihepatitis, 926
Perilymph, 514
Perimenopause, 807
endocrine changes in, 809f, 809t, 810
ovarian follicle changes in, 807, 809, 809b
timeline of, and associated physiology and symptoms, 811t
Perimetrium, 788–789
Perimysium, 1555
Perineal body, 786
Perineum, 786
Periodic paralysis, 1609
Periosteal collar, 1618–1619
Periosteum, 459–460, 1546
Periosteal reaction, 1590
Peripheral arterial disease, 1148–1149, 1160
in chronic diabetes mellitus, 765, 766f
Peripheral blood, marginating storage pool in, 963–965, 965f
Peripheral blood stem cell transplantation, in aplastic anemia, 1002
Peripheral chemoreceptors, 1250
of pulmonary system, 1251
Peripheral corticotropin-releasing hormone, 339
Peripheral cyanosis, 1268–1269
Peripheral lymphoid system, 230
Peripheral membrane proteins, 11
Peripheral nerves, 466f
structural components of, 465, 466f
Peripheral nervous system (PNS), 442–443, 465–467
embryonic development of, 665–668
nervous tissue organization in, 443, 665–666
Peripheral nervous system disorders, 635
clinical manifestations of, 635–636
evaluation and treatment of, 636
Guillain-Barré syndrome in, 636
pathophysiology of, 635
plexus injuries in, 638
proprioceptive dysfunction in, 517
radiculopathies in, 636
references on, 643
summary review of, 641b–642b
Peripheral sensitization, 487–488
Peripheral tolerance, 222, 233
Peripheral tolerance dysfunction, and autoimmunity, 269
Peripheral vascular system, 1113
Peristalsis, 1423
intestinal, 1435
primary and secondary, 1423
Peristaltic movements, 1436
Peritoneal cavity, 1428–1429
Peritoneum, 1428–1429
Peritonitis, 1428–1429
Peritonsillar abscess, 1315t, 1316, 1316f

Peritubular capillaries, 1348–1350
Permeable membrane, 26
Permissive effects, of hormones, 699
Pernicious anemia, 991–993
bone marrow aspirate in, 994f
clinical manifestations of, 994
erythrocyte appearance in, 992f
evaluation and treatment of, 994–995
laboratory findings for, 999t
pathophysiology of, 993–994
Peroxisome(s), 7
Peroxisome proliferator activated receptors (PPARs), 23t
Personalized cancer therapy, 371–372
Personalized medicine, 361
Pertussis (aP) vaccine, 329, 329t–330t
Pes planus deformity, 1623–1624
Pessary, 833–834, 1372
Pesticides, in cancer epidemiology, 397t–400t
PET (positron emission tomography) scan, 475
Petechiae, 1653t
Petrochemicals, in cancer epidemiology, 397t–400t
Peyronie disease, 851–852, 852f
pH, and hydrogen ions, 114–117
Phage therapy, 328b
Phagocytes, 955
neutrophilic, 201
Phagocytic deficiencies, 278, 281–284, 283f
gene defects in, 276t
Phagocytosis, 30–31
bacterial protection against, 303–304
chemical mediators of, 203f
fungal protection against, 308–309
in inflammation, 198–201
process of, 197f
protozoan protection against, 311
scanning electronmicrography of, 200f
Phagolysosome, 200–201
Phagosome, 200–201
Phakomatosis, congenital heart defects associated with, 1215t
Phantom limb pain, 494
Pharmacogenetics, in treatment of asthma, 1285–1286, 1286b
Pharyngeal phase of swallowing, 1423
Pharyngitis, gonococcal, 926
Pharyngotympanic tube, 513–514
Pharynx, 1245f
Phase I activation enzymes, 404–405
Phase II detoxification enzymes, 404–405
Phenobarbital, and vitamin D deficiency, 1585
Phenotype, 145
expressivity and variability of, 148–149
Phenylketonuria (PKU), 145, 677–678
and associated congenital heart defects, 1214t
metabolism and central nervous function consequences in, 678f

Phenytoin
and associated congential heart
defects, 1214t
and vitamin D deficiency, 1585
Pheochromocytes, 719
Pheochromocytomas, 772, 772f
clinical manifestations of, 772
evaluation and treatment of,
772–776
pathophysiology of, 772
Philadelphia chromosome, 371–372,
438
and resulting disorder,
1020–1021, 1022f
Phimosis, 850–851, 851f
Phocomelia, 172
Phosphate, 111
absorption of, 1434
in bone, 1541t
in bone homeostasis, 1579–1580
Phosphate-calcium balance, in
chronic kidney disease, 1392t,
1394–1396, 1394t
Phosphate-calcium metabolism, in
chronic kidney disease, 1395t
Phosphatidylinositol, 11
Phosphatidylserine externalization,
failure of, 1049
Phospholipase, 1432–1433
Phospholipid molecule(s), 11, 12f
Photochemical receptors, 445b
Phyllodes tumor, 874t
Physeal closure, 1619–1620
Physical activity
cancer epidemiology and,
426–431
muscle metabolism in,
1561–1562, 1561t
protective effect of, against breast
cancer, 895
Physical agents, in cell injury, 71–76
atmospheric pressure changes, 72
illumination, 74–75
ionizing radiation, 73–74
mechanical stresses, 75
noise, 75–76
temperature extremes, 71–72
Physiologic atrophy, 47
Physiologic dead space, 1257
Physiologic jaundice of newborn,
1531
Physiologic reflux, 1458
Physiologic stress, 338
PI3 kinase pathway, 23t
Pia mater, 460
Pica, 682
Pigment accumulation, cellular,
78–79
Pigmented stones, 1495
Pili, bacterial, 298, 301f
Pineal gland, 704
hormones released by, 704
in immune response, 348
Pinkeye, 506–507
Pinna, 512
Pinocytosis, 30–31
Pit cells, 1438–1439
Pitting edema, 100–101
Pituitary adenoma, 733
Pituitary gland, 704–705
anatomical location of, 705f
anterior, 707–708
hormones released by, 704f, 705
posterior, 705–707

Pituitary stalk, 705
Pituitary tumors, 612t
Pityriasis rosea, 1658
pK value, 115
Placebo effect, 486
Plaque (skin lesion),
1648t–1653t
Plaque, atherosclerotic, 1157
complicated, 1159–1160
in coronary artery, 1161f
fibrous, 1159
formation of, 1158f, 1159
unstable, 1169–1171,
1170–1171f
Plaque psoriasis, 1657–1658,
1657f
Plasma, 952–954
arterial, organic and inorganic
components of, 953t
interstitial fluid and, water
movement between, 98
Plasma albumin decrease, 100
Plasma cell count, 983t–985t
Plasma cell malignancies, 1037
monoclonal gammopathies in,
1037, 1037f
multiple myeloma in, 1037
Waldenström macroglobulinemia
in, 1042
Plasma cells, 240. See also B
lymphocytes.
hematopoietic differentiation of,
964f
Plasma creatinine concentration,
1360–1361
Plasma cystatin C concentration,
1361
Plasma enzyme cascades, 1710
Plasma kinin cascade, 191, 191f
Plasma lipids, 954
Plasma membrane, 10–13
carbohydrates within, 13
cell receptors on, 13–15. See also
Plasma membrane
receptors.
cellular intake and output
through, 25–33. See also
Membrane transport.
composition and structure of,
10–13, 12f
fluidity of, 13
functions of, 10, 11f, 12t
lipids of, 11
proteins of, 11–12
proteolytic cascades within,
12–13
Plasma membrane receptors, 13–15,
15t, 18f
on B cell, 233–235
classification of, 701
G protein-coupled, 15, 15t, 23t,
701. See also Cyclic adenosine
monophosphate.
hormonal, 700–702, 700t
classification of, 701
first messenger activation of,
700–701, 701f
and second messenger
pathways, 701f, 702, 702t
in inflammatory response,
192–195
major types of, and signal
transduction pathways, 23t
on T cell, 231–233

Plasma membrane transport, 25–33
electrical impulses and, 32–33
vesicle formation in, 30–32. See
also Caveolae; Endocytosis;
Exocytosis.
water and solute movement
in, 26–30. See also Active
transport; Mediated
transport; Passive transport.
major systems in, 30t
Plasma protein(s), 952–954
Plasma protein synthesis
in inflammatory process, 206,
206t
in liver, 1442
Plasma protein systems, in
inflammatory response,
187–192
clotting components of, 190–191
complement components of,
188–190
interactions among, 192, 193f
kinin components of, 191
Plasma thromboplastin antecedent
(clotting factor XI), 977t
disorder(s) associated with, 1079t
Plasma transferrin, 1434
Plasma volume. See Total plasma
volume.
Plasmin, 192, 979
Plasminogen, 979–980
Plasminogen-plasmin system, 979
Plasmodium spp., 310, 310t, 312
pathogenesis of infection by,
312–313, 312f
transmission of, 311
Plastic rigidity, 573
Plasticity, of central nervous system,
450–452
Platelet(s), 957, 958f
active and moderately active,
micrograph of, 976f
clinical evaluation of, 983t–985t
granules within, 976
hematopoietic differentiation of,
964f
hemostatic function of, 972–976
of infants and children, 955
in inflammatory response,
202–203
Platelet activating factor (PAF), 198,
203f
Platelet activation, in damaged
vascular endothelium, 972–976,
974f–975f
Platelet adhesion, 973, 975f
in atherosclerosis, 1055
Platelet adhesion studies, 983t–985t
Platelet aggregation, 975f, 976
Platelet aggregation tests, 983t–985t
Platelet count, 983t–985t
pediatric, 985t
Platelet-derived growth factor
(PDGF), 35, 36t, 369
Platelet development, 971–972
Platelet disorders, 1044
acquired and congenital, 1049
in children, 1078–1079
drug induced, 1049
immune thrombocytic purpura
in, 1045–1046
qualitative, 1048–1049
quantitative, 1044
systemic disorders and, 1049

Platelet disorders (Continued)
thrombocythemia in, 1047
thrombocytopenia in, 1044
thrombotic thrombocytopenic
purpura in, 1046–1047
Platelet endothelial cell adhesion
molecule-1 (PECAM-1), 972
Platelet granule secretion, impaired,
1049
Platelet-platelet interaction,
impaired, 1048–1049
Platelet-release reaction, 973–976
Platelet-vascular adhesion,
aberrations of, 1048
Pleiotropic actions, of chemokines
(cytokines), 203–204, 203f
Pleomorphic cells, 362–363, 363f
Pleura, 1249
Pleural abnormalities, 1272–1274
Pleural cavity, 1249
Pleural effusion, 1273–1274
pathophysiology of, 1273, 1274t
Pleural friction rub, 1267
Pleural space, 1249
Plexus injuries, 638
Plexuses, neuronal, 443
PMN. See Polymorphonuclear
neutrophil.
Pneumococcal pneumonia, 1291,
1292f
in children, 1327–1329, 1328t
Pneumococcal vaccine, 324, 329
adult, 329t
child, 330t
Pneumoconiosis, pulmonary
fibrosis in, 1278
Pneumocystis carinii, 308
Pneumocystis jiroveci, 308, 308t
Pneumonia, 1290–1291
aspiration, 1275
in children, 1327
evaluation and treatment of,
1329–1331
pathophysiology and clinical
manifestations of,
1327–1329, 1328t
clinical manifestations of, 1292
evaluation and treatment of,
1292–1293
microorganisms causing, 1290
pathophysiology of, 1291–1292
pneumococcal, 1291
Pneumothorax, 1272–1273, 1272f
Podocin, 1345–1346
Podocytes, 1345–1346
Podosomes, 1543
Point mutation, of oncogenes, 370
Poiseuille's formula, 1119
Poison ivy, 1655f
Poisoning, acute encephalopathies
in, 682, 682b
Poisons, common, 682b
Polarity, electrolyte, 26
Polio pandemic, 297t
Polio vaccine(s), 330
effects of, on global reported polio
cases, 331f
Sabin and Salk, 331
Poliomyelitis, paralytic, 567
Poliovirus, 314t
in central nervous system
infections, 621t
Polyarthritis, in rheumatic fever,
1186

Polycystic kidney disease, 1407
Polycystic ovary syndrome, 824, 824f
  clinical manifestations of, 825, 826b
  evaluation and treatment of, 825–827
  insulin resistance and hyperinsulinemia in, 824–825, 825f
  pathophysiology of, 824–825, 825b
Polycythemia, 1008–1009. See also Myeloproliferative red blood cell disorders.
  paraneoplastic, 389t
Polycythemia vera, 1009
  clinical manifestations of, 1010
  diagnostic criteria for, 1010b
  evaluation and treatment of, 1010–1012
  pathophysiology of, 1009–1010
Polygenic traits, 165
Polymenorrhea, 823t
Polymorphic locus, 143–145
Polymorphism, 143–145
Polymorphonuclear neutrophil (PMN), 201, 955
  immune defense mechanisms of, 1291
Polymyositis, 1611
  clinical manifestations of, 1612
  evaluation and treatment of, 1612–1615
  paraneoplastic, 389t
  pathophysiology of, 1611–1612, 1611f
Polyol pathway complications, in chronic diabetes mellitus, 758
Polypeptide(s), 129
Polypeptide hormones, 697t
Polypeptide synthesis, 134, 136f
Polyploid cells, 135–136
Polyploidy, 135–136
Polyribosomes, 8
Polyunsaturated fats, 1162b
Polyunsaturated fatty acids, and cancer risk, 410t
Pompe disease, 5, 1610–1611
  congenital heart defects associated with, 1215t
Pons, 450t, 454f, 455
Ponseti casting, 1623, 1623b
Pores of Kohn, 1244, 1276f
Porphyrin analysis, 983t–985t
Porphyrin, reduction to bilirubin, 969
Port wine stain, 1691
Portal hypertension, 1482
  in children, 1533
    clinical manifestations of, 1533
    evaluation and treatment of, 1533–1534
  chronic, complications of, 1483
  clinical manifestations of, 1483
  complications of, 1483
  evaluation and treatment of, 1483
  pathophysiology of, 1482–1483
  varices related to, 1482, 1482f
Portal of entry, pathogen, 297
Portal vein, 1438
  major tributaries of, and shunts, 1482f
Portland hemoglobin, 1063

Portosystemic encephalopathy, 1483
Position effect, 143
Positional equinovarus, 1623
Positive selection process, 233
Positron emission tomography (PET) scan, 475
Post coital cervical mucus test, 808t
Post thrombotic syndrome, 1144
Post-transplant lymphoproliferative disorder, 379–380
Postcentral gyrus, 452
Postconcussive syndrome, 590
Posterior cerebral artery, 462, 463t, 464f
Posterior cerebral artery occlusion, stroke syndromes resulting from, 604t
Posterior column (dorsal column), 456–457
Posterior cord syndrome, 594t
Posterior fossa, 459
Posterior horn (dorsal horn), 456
Posterior internodal pathway, 1102
Posterior pituitary, 705–707
  disorders of, 728–729
    diabetes insipidus in, 730
    syndrome of inappropriate antidiuretic hormone in, 729
  hormone release by, 704f
    antidiuretic, 706–707
    oxytocin, 707
Posterior spinal arteries, 463–465
Posterior vein of left ventricle, 1099
Postganglionic neurons, 467
  functions of, 467
  neurotransmission by, 471f
Postgastrectomy syndromes, 1468–1470
Posthemorrhagic anemia, 1003
  laboratory findings for, 999t
Posthyperventilation apnea, 529–531, 530t
Postictal state, 536–537
Postmenopausal osteoporosis, 1579
  pathophysiology of, 1580–1582
Postmortem autolysis, 90
Postmortem changes, cellular, 90
Postnecrotic cirrhosis, 1492t
Postobstructive diuresis, 1367–1368
Postoperative pain, chronic, 492–493
Postpartum thyroiditis, 741
Postrenal acute kidney injury, 1386t, 1387
  in children, 1411
Postsynaptic neurons, 446–447, 447f
Posttraumatic hypermetabolic response, 1719
Posttraumatic stress disorder (PTSD), 339, 353, 660–661
  etiology of, 661
  pathophysiology of, 661
  treatment of, 661
Postural disorders, 575–576
Postural hypotension, 1156–1157
Postural tremor, 568t–569t
Potassium, in cellular environment, 106–108
  hyperkalemia and, 110
  hypokalemia and, 108
  pH changes and, 107
  regulation of, 107

Potassium adaptation, 107
Potassium imbalance. See also Hyperkalemia; Hypokalemia.
  in chronic kidney disease, 1392t, 1393–1394, 1394t
Potassium ion leak channels, 28
Potassium-sparing diuretics, 1359t
Potocytosis, 32
Potter syndrome, 1407
Poverty of content, 651
PPARs. See Peroxisome proliferator activated receptors.
PR interval, of electrocardiogram, 1103
Prader-Willi syndrome, 150
Precapillary sphincters, 1113
Precentral gyrus, 452
Precipitation, 244
Precocious puberty, 818–819
  causes of, 818b–819b
  central, 818
  complete, 818
  mixed, 819
  partial, 818–819
  primary forms of, 818b
  treatment of, 819
Prediabetes, 745
Predisposition-infection-response-organ dysfunction, 1708t
Preexcitation syndromes, 1199t–1200t
Prefrontal area, 452
Prefrontal cortex, 648, 649f
Preganglionic neurons, 467
  neurotransmission by, 471f
Pregnancy
  breast cancer risk in, 881–882
  erythrocyte appearance in, 992f
  ionizing radiation exposure in, effects of, 417b
  secondary hypertension risk in, 1153t
Prehepatic jaundice, 1486
Prehepatic portal hypertension, 1533
Preimplantation genetic diagnosis, 1076
Prekallikrein activator, 191
Preload, 1109
  cardiac output and, 1110–1111
Premature atrial contractions, 1197t–1198t
Premature infant, congenital heart defects in, 1214t
Premature junctional contractions, 1197t–1198t
Premature ovarian failure, 807
Premature ventricular contractions, 1197t–1198t
Premenstrual disorders, 826–827
  clinical manifestations of, 827
  evaluation and treatment of, 827–828
Premenstrual dysphoric disorder, 826
  diagnostic criteria for, 827b
Premenstrual syndrome (PMS), 826
  diet and symptoms of, 828b
Premotor area, 452
Prenatal diagnosis, of chromosome aberrations, 139b
Prenatal exposure, to environmental cancer risk factors, 401, 403–404, 427b, 436, 439

Prepregnancy sickle cell test, 1076, 1077f
Prerenal acute kidney injury, 1386–1387, 1386t
  in children, 1411
  urine characteristics in, 1389t
Presbycusis, 515
Presbyopia, 511
Pressure, in liquid system, 1117
Pressure ulcers, 1647–1654
  preventive measures for, 1654
  progression of, 1653f
  staging of, 1647–1653
  treatment of, 1654
Presynaptic neurons, 446–447, 447f
Preterm delivery, bacterial vaginosis as risk factor in, 934b
Pretibial myxedema, 737
Prevalence rate, 164
Priapism, 852, 852f, 870
Primary adrenal insufficiency, 770. See also Addison disease.
Primary aldosteronism, 768
  pathophysiology of, 768, 769f
Primary amenorrhea, 820
Primary bile acids, 1439
Primary biliary cirrhosis, 1492t, 1493
Primary brain tumors, 613–616
  classification of, 613–614
  treatment of, 614
Primary centers of ossification, 1618
Primary dysmenorrhea, 819
Primary enuresis, 1415
Primary extracerebral tumors, 616–618
Primary gout, 1602–1603
Primary hyperparathyroidism, 742–743
  clinical manifestations of, 743t
Primary hypertension, 1150–1152
  factors associated with, 1150
  genetic risk of, 1150, 1150b
  pathophysiology of, 1150–1152, 1151f
  treatment of, 1155–1156
Primary hypothyroidism, 741
  clinical manifestations of, 742, 742f
Primary immune deficiencies, 275–284
  classes of, 276t, 278
Primary immune response, 240–241, 240f
Primary intention, healing by, 208, 209f
Primary lactose intolerance, 1531
Primary lymphoid organ(s), 230
  in B cell maturation, 233–235
  in T cell maturation, 230–233
Primary lysosomal granules, 200–201
Primary lysosome, 5–6, 8f
Primary motor area, 452, 453f
Primary motor neurons. See Lower motor neuron(s).
Primary multiple organ dysfunction syndrome, 1707
Primary nephrotic syndrome, 1409
Primary order neurons, 483–484
Primary peristalsis, 1423
Primary (spontaneous) pneumothorax, 1272–1273
Primary polycythemia, 1009

Primary sensory area, of cortex, 453f
Primary spermatocytes, 800
Primary spinal cord tumors, 618, 618b
Primary syphilis, 928
  clinical manifestations of, 929–930, 929f
Primary thrombocytopenic purpura, 1081
Primary voluntary motor area, 452, 453f
Principal cells, of nephron collecting duct, 1347
Prinzmetal angina, 1165–1166
Pro-opiomelanocortin (POMC), 707
Proaccelerin. See Labile factor.
Proband, 167
  in recurrence risk in multifactorial inheritance, 168
Probiotics, and inflammatory bowel disease, 1473b, 1475
Procalcitonin, as indicator of first urinary tract infection, 1413b
Procallus, 1548
Procedural memory, 543
Proconvertin (clotting factor VII). See Stable factor.
Prodroma, 542
Prodromal stage, of infectious disease, 296
Proenzymes, 187–188
Proerythroblasts, 965–966
Progenitor cells, hematopoietic, 963, 964f
Progesterone, 791–792
  adiposity and influence on, 409
  effects of, in pregnancy, 792
  and estrogen, complementary and opposing effects of, 792t
  serum, 809t
Programmed cell death, 19, 81b, 84–85
Progressive bulbar palsy, 567–568
Progressive multifocal leukoencephalopathy, 629
Progressive myoclonus epilepsy, genetics and pathophysiology of, 526t
Progressive relaxation training, 1606
Progressive spinal muscular atrophy, 567–568
Progrowth signals, alterations in cellular, 368–369
Projectile vomiting, 1453
Projecting (nutrient) arteries, 462
Projection cells, 484
Prokaryote(s), 2
Prolactin, 708
  anterior pituitary secretion of, 707
  physiologic effects of, and 704f, 708t
  receptors for, and mechanism of action, 700t
  second messengers pathways of, 23t
  stress induced, 351
  in synthesis of testosterone, 801–802
Prolactin hypersecretion, 735
  clinical manifestations of, 735
  evaluation and treatment of, 735–736
  pathophysiology of, 735
Prolactin inhibiting factor (PIF), 703–704, 871

Prolactin releasing factor, hypothalamic release of, 707t
Prolactinoma, 735
Proliferative breast lesions
  with atypia, 875
  without atypia, 874–875, 874t
Promoter site, 132–133
Pronephros, 1402
Properdin deficiency, 281
Prophase, 34–35
Propionibacterium acnes, 1681
Proprioception, 517–520
Proprioceptive dysfunction, 517–520
Proprioceptors, 445b
Prosencephalon, 450t. See also Forebrain.
Prostacyclin, 972
  and effect on endothelium, 1119b
Prostacyclin production, in vascular endothelium, 973f
Prostaglandins, 197–198, 203f
  and effect on endothelium, 1119b
Prostate, 799f, 800, 866f
Prostate cancer, 863–865, 868f
  clinical manifestations of, 867
  dietary factors in risk for, 864–865, 864b
  evaluation and treatment of, 867–869
  genetic and epigenetic factors in, 865
  grading of, 869, 869b
  incidence of, and mortality rate, 863–864, 863f
  metastasis of, 384t, 868f
  pathogenesis of, 865–867
    hormones and, 865–867
    hypothetical model of, 867f
    stromal, 866–867
  treatment of, 869
  vasectomy as risk factor for, 865
Prostate disorders, 860–861
Prostate enlargement, obstructed urine flow in, 1371
Prostate screening, 868b
Prostate specific antigen (PSA), 367, 368t, 867–868
  in screening for prostate cancer, 868b
Prostatic intraepithelial neoplasia (PIN), 866
Prostatitis, 861–863, 862f
  bacterial, 862–863
  nonbacterial, 863
Prostatodynia, 861–862
Protease inhibitor, viral, 322–323
Proteasome, up-regulation of, 47
Protein(s), 1430–1432
  cellular accumulation of, 78
  dietary intake of, 1430
  digestion and absorption of, 1430–1432, 1431f
  metabolism of
    in chronic kidney disease, 1394–1395
    in liver, 1442
  plasma membrane, 11–12
  roles of, body function, 1442t
Protein buffering, 116, 116f
Protein C, 979, 1080
Protein C deficiency, 1080
Protein C/protein 5 pathway, in vascular endothelium, 973f

Protein depletion, in shock, 1699
Protein energy (calorie) malnutrition, 69, 1528
  clinical manifestations of, 1528
  evaluation and treatment of, 1528
  pathophysiology of, 1528
Protein kinase C (PKC) activation, inappropriate, 758–759
Protein-linked plasma membrane receptors, 701
Protein S, 979, 1080
Protein S deficiency, 1081
Protein synthesis, 132–133, 135f
  genes and, 132–134
  RNA transcription in, 132–133, 134f
  translation in, 134
Proteinuria, 1378
  in chronic kidney disease, 1392t, 1394–1395
Proteoglycans
  in bone matrix, 1545
  in cartilage, 1553
  in hypertrophic scarring, 1654
Proteolytic cascade(s), 12–13, 13f
Prothrombin (clotting factor II), 977t
  disorder(s) associated with, 1079t
Prothrombin consumption time, 1080
Prothrombin gene mutation, 1056
Prothrombin time, 983t
Prothrombin time (PT), 1080
Proto-oncogene(s), 370, 438
Protopathic sensation, 458–459
Protoporphyrin, 967–968
Protoporphyrin analysis, 983t
Protozoa, 298t, 310t
Protozoan infections, 310–313
  in HIV (human immunodeficiency virus) infection, 323b
Protozoan pathogens, 310–313, 310t
  evasion mechanisms of, 311–312
    antigenic variation, 311
    complement evasion, 311
    immune molecule degradation, 311
    immune molecule neutralization, 311
    immune suppression, 311–312
    intracellular survival, 311
    protection against phagocytosis, 311
    self-protein coatings, 311
  invasion of, 311–312
  tissue damage caused by, 312
  transmission and colonization by, 311
Proximal tubule(s), 1347
  transport within, 1355–1356
Pruritus, 1654–1655
Psammoma bodies, 79
Pseudo-hyperparathyroidism, 743
Pseudobuboes, 934
Pseudogout, 1602
Pseudomonas aeruginosa, 299t–300t
  protective mechanisms of, against phagocytes, 303–304
Pseudomonas aeruginosa **pneumonia,** nosocomial, 1291
Pseudostratified epithelium, 36
Pseudothrombocytopenia, differential diagnosis of thrombocytopenia and, 1044

Pseudounipolar neurons, 444, 445f
Psoriasis, 1657–1658
  treatment of, 1658
  types of, 1657
Psoriatic arthritis, 1658
Psoriatic nail disease, 1658
Psychiatric disorders
  genes and environmental interaction in, 179–180
  studies of, 179–180
Psychogenic polydipsia, 730
Psychogenic unresponsiveness, 528
Psychologic stress, and immune competency, 285
Psychoneuroimmunologic mediators, of stress, 339
Psychoneuroimmunology (PNI), 339
Psychotherapy, in bipolar disorder, 658
Psychotic dimension, 650
Psychotic episode, 650
PTH. See Parathyroid hormone.
Puberty, 784
  delayed, 817
  early onset of, 816–819
  precocious, 818–819
Pulmonary abscess, 1294
Pulmonary artery(ies), 1095, 1247
Pulmonary artery hypertension, 1296–1297
  classification of, 1297b
  clinical manifestations of, 1297–1298
  evaluation and treatment of, 1298
  pathophysiology of, 1297, 1297f
Pulmonary atresia, 1229
Pulmonary capillaries, 1247
Pulmonary circulation, 1091, 1092f, 1247–1249, 1248f
  blood flow in, 1256–1257, 1256f
  zones of, 1257, 1257f
  control of, 1260–1261
Pulmonary disorders, 1266, 1271–1280
  acute respiratory distress syndrome in, 1279–1280
  autoimmune, 257t–258t
  chest wall abnormalities in, 1271–1272
  in children, 1313–1316. See also Childhood respiratory disorders; Sudden infant death syndrome.
  clinical manifestations of, 1266–1271
  conditions caused by, 1269–1271
  malignant, 1298. See also Lung cancer.
  in obesity, 1480
  obstructive, 1282–1284. See also Asthma; Chronic obstructive pulmonary disease.
  pleural abnormalities in, 1272–1274
  references on, 1307
  respiratory tract infections in, 1290–1291. See also Acute bronchitis; Pneumonia; Pulmonary abscess; Tuberculosis.
  restrictive, 1274–1280. See also Restrictive pulmonary disorders.

Pulmonary disorders (Continued)
summary review of, 1304b
vascular disease in, 1294–1295.
See also Pulmonary vascular
disease.
Pulmonary edema, 1279
pathogenesis of, 1279f
Pulmonary embolism, 1294–1295
clinical manifestations of,
1295–1296
evaluation and treatment of,
1296–1297
pathophysiology of, 1295, 1296f
Pulmonary embolus (emboli),
1147, 1294–1295, 1295f
Pulmonary fibrosis, 1277–1278
in allergic alveolitis, 1278
idiopathic, 1277
in pneumoconiosis, 1278
in toxic gas exposure, 1277–1278
Pulmonary function(s), abbreviation
of, 1255t
Pulmonary function testing,
1261–1263
Pulmonary resuscitation, of newborn,
and lung injury, 1323b
Pulmonary stenosis, 1229, 1229f
clinical manifestations of, 1229
evaluation and treatment of,
1229–1230
pathophysiology of, 1229
Pulmonary (respiratory) system, 1242
in aging, 1263–1265, 1263f
autonomic innervation of, 1251
breathing mechanics of,
1251–1254, 1254f
chemoreceptors of, 1251
chest wall and pleura of, 1249
in children, 1310–1312
chronic kidney disease and effects
on, 1391t, 1395
circulation within, 1247–1249
control of, 1260–1261
conducting airways of,
1242–1244, 1243f
function testing of, 1261–1263.
See also Pulmonary function
testing.
gas exchange airways of,
1244–1247, 1246f
gas pressure measurement in,
1254–1255
gas transport in, 1255–1260
carbon dioxide, 1259–1260
oxygen, 1257–1259
immunologic defense mechanisms
of, 1244, 1244t
lymphatics of, 1249
references on, 1265
structures of, 1242–1249, 1243f
summary review of, 1264b
ventilatory and respiratory
functions of, 1249–1255, 1249f
neurochemical control of,
1249–1251, 1250f
Pulmonary thromboembolism, risk
factors for, 1295
Pulmonary vascular disease,
1294–1295
cor pulmonale in, 1298
pulmonary artery hypertension in,
1296–1297
pulmonary embolism in,
1294–1295

Pulmonary vascular resistance
(PVR), 1133t
Pulmonary vasoconstriction,
hypoxic, 1260–1261, 1261b
Pulmonary vein(s), 1095, 1247
Pulmonary ventilation, and lung
capacity, 1261f
Pulmonic semilunar valves, 1094
Pulse tracing, in vascular evaluation,
1135–1136, 1136f
Pulsus paradoxus, 1177, 1284
Puncture wounds, 66
Punnett square, 147f
Pupil, 507
Pupillary changes, in brainstem
dysfunction evaluation, 531,
532f
Pure red cell aplasia, 1001–1002
Pure sodium deficit, 105
Purine metabolism, 1602–1603
**Purine nucleoside phosphorylase
(PNP) deficiency,** 280
Purines, 129, 133f
Purkinje fibers, 1102
Purpura, 1044, 1653t
Purpura fulminans, neonatal,
1080–1081
Purulent exudates, in inflammation,
205
Pustular psoriasis, 1658
Pustule, 1648t
Pyelonephritis
acute, 1377
causes of, 1377t
chronic, 1377, 1377f
Pyelonephritis associated fimbriae,
1375
Pyknosis, 81
Pyloric obstruction, 1460
clinical manifestations of, 1460
evaluation and treatment of, 1460
pathophysiology of, 1460
Pyloric sphincter, 1423–1424
Pyloric stenosis
in children, 1519
genetics of, 166–167
recurrence risk for, 167, 167t
Pylorus, 1423–1424
Pyramidal motor syndrome, 564,
578t
Pyramidal/spastic cerebral palsy,
676
Pyramidal system, 452, 566f. *See also*
Upper motor neuron(s).
Pyridoxine. *See* Vitamin B$_6$.
Pyrimidines, 129, 133f
Pyrogenic bacteria, 301
Pyrogens, exogenous and
endogenous, 297, 498
Pyruvate oxidation, 25f
Pyuria, 1362

Q

QRS complex, of electrocardiogram,
1103
QT interval, of electrocardiogram,
1103
Quadriparesis, 564
Quadriplegia, 564, 594
Qualitative leukocyte disorders,
1014
Quantitative leukocyte disorders,
1014–1017
Quantitative traits, 165

R

Rabies virus, 314t
Radial scar, 874–875
Radial sclerosing lesion, 874–875
Radiation exposure, 73t
bystander effects of, 421–422
cancers caused by, 73–74, 397t,
888–891
cell injury caused by, 73–74, 73f,
416–420
in childhood, 417b
congenital heart defects associated
with, 1214t
dose-response relationships for,
416–420
estimated doses in, during
diagnostic procedures, 416,
416t
genomic instability induced by,
420–422
immunologic effects of, 74
low level, risks of, 74, 74b, 416
in pregnancy, infancy, and
childhood, 417b
Radiation induced genomic
instability (RIGI), 420, 421f,
889
Radiation therapy, 388. *See also*
Radiation exposure.
Radiational heat loss, 497
Radicular pain, 638
Radicular paresthesia, 638
Radicular syndrome, 619
Radiculitis (radiculoneuritis), 636
Radiculopathy(ies), 597–598, 636
clinical manifestations of, 638
evaluation and treatment of,
638–639
pathophysiology of, 637
Radioimmunoassay (RIA), 720
Radionuclide imaging, of brain,
475–476
Radon, 426
Rafts, 13, 14f
RAG-1, RAG-2 (recombination
activating genes), 231–232,
232f
***RAG-1* and *RAG-2* deficiencies,** 280
Raloxifene, 908, 1580–1582, 1584
RANK, 1580
RANKL (receptor activator of
nuclear factor κβ ligand),
1542–1543
in pathophysiology of
osteoporosis, 1580–1582,
1581f
Raphe nuclei, 654
Raphe nuclei-serotonin dysfunction,
in mood disorders, 654
Rapid orgasm, 849
**Rapidly progressive
glomerulonephritis,** 1381t,
1383
RAS, 368
in growth factor signaling, 371f
ras gene, point mutation in, 370,
371f
Rashkind procedure, 1226
Rastelli procedure, 1232
modified, 1234
Raynaud disease, 1149
diagnostic criteria for, 1149
Raynaud phenomenon, 264,
1148–1149

Rb gene. *See* Retinoblastoma (*Rb*)
gene.
Reactive chemicals, in cancer
epidemiology, 397t–400t
Reactive oxygen species, 54–55
antioxidants and, 56f, 57t
biologically relevant, 57t
cellular effect of, 54b
diseases and disorders linked to,
57t
enzymes and, 57t
functional effects of, depending
on cell type, 55f
generation of, 56f
Reactive response, 338
Reagent strips, urinalysis, 1362
Reagin, 259
Receptive dysphasia, 549t–550t
Receptor(s)
serum transferrin, 997–998
Receptor activator of nuclear factor
κβ ligand (RANKL), 1542–1543
in pathophysiology of
osteoporosis, 1580–1582,
1581f
Receptor mediated endocytosis,
31, 32f
Receptors
α-adrenergic, 469–470
in central stress response, 340
physiologic actions of,
342t, 469–470,
471f
specific, and physiologic actions
of neurotransmitters,
472t
AMPA/kinate, 488
auditory/positional, 445b
B cell, 222–226
production of, gene
recombination in,
233–234, 235f
baro-, 102
β-adrenergic, 469–470
in central stress response, 340
physiologic actions of,
342t, 469–470,
471f
specific, and physiologic actions
of neurotransmitters,
472t
catalytic plasma membrane, 15,
15t
channel-linked plasma
membrane, 15, 15t
chemo-, 445b
complement, 194–195
cytosolic, 700t, 702–703
death, 85, 85f
equilibrium, 514
G protein-coupled, 15, 15t, 23t,
701. *See also* Cyclic adenosine
monophosphate.
H1, 196, 196f
H2, 196, 196f
hormone, 699–700, 700t
IL-7, 233, 234f
mechano-, 445b
neuro-, autonomic, 467–470
actions of, in adrenergic
and cholinergic
neurotransmission, 472t
NMDA, 488
non-tyrosine kinase activated, 23t

Receptors (Continued)
nuclear, 700t, 702–703
opioid, 488
osmo-, 102
pain, 482–483, 483t. See also
Nociceptors.
pattern recognition, 192–194
peroxisome proliferator activated,
23t
photochemical, 445b
plasma membrane, 13–15,
15t, 18f. See also Plasma
membrane receptors.
on B cell, 233–235
hormonal, 700–702, 700t
in inflammatory response,
192–195
major types of, and signal
transduction pathways, 23t
on T cell, 231–233
pulmonary, 1251
scavenger, 195
sensory, 445b
steroid hormone, 23t
T cell, 222–226
production of, gene
recombination in,
231–233, 232f
thermo-, 445b
toll-like, 194, 205
cell, and microbial target, 194t
tyrosine kinase activated, 23t
volume sensitive, 102
Recessive allele, 145
Reciprocal translocations, 143
Recombinant alleles, 156, 156f
Recombinant antihemolytic factor
plasma/albumin free (Advate),
1080
Recombinant DNA technology, 127b
Recombination, bacterial, 304
Recombination activating genes
(RAG-1, RAG-2), 231–232, 232f
Reconstructive phase, of healing,
208–210, 209f
dysfunctional, 211–212
Rectal carcinoma, 1501
Rectal gonococcal infection, 926
Rectocele, 833, 835f, 836
Rectosphincteric reflex, 1437
Recurrence risk, 148
in autosomal recessive
inheritance, 152
transmission patterns and, in
multifactorial disease,
167–169
in X-linked inheritance, 154–155
Recurrent infections, 275
Recurrent seizures, in adults,
adolescents, 539t
Red blood cells (RBCs), 954. See also
Erythrocytes.
Red cell count, 983t–985t
Red measles, 1686–1687
Red nucleus, 455
Redness, in inflammation, 205
Reduction and immobilization, of
fractures, 1571–1572
Reed-Sternberg cells, 1031, 1031f
Referred abdominal pain, 1456
Referred pain, 491
origins of, 491, 492f
Reflex arc, 458f
structures necessary for, 457

Reflex sympathetic dystrophy, 494
Reflexes, in infancy, 668, 668t
Reflexive memory, 543
Reflux esophagitis, 1458
and associated cancer, 378t
Refractive visual dysfunction, 511,
511f
Regeneration, tissue, 208
Regional osteoporosis, 1580
Regional pain, 491b
Rehabilitation, after pediatric burn
injury, 1750
Relative polycythemia, 1008–1009
Relative refractory period, 33
Relative risk, 165
Relaxation, of muscle contraction,
1561
REM sleep behavior disorder, 506
REM (rapid eye movement) sleep
phase, 502–504
disorders associated with, 505
Remodeling, bone, 1547–1548
Renal adenoma, 1372
Renal agenesis, 1407
Renal and urinary systems, 1344
blood flow within, 1351–1352
autoregulation of, 1351
hormonal regulation of, 1352
neural regulation of, 1351–1352
in children, 1402–1404
disorders of. See also Renal
disorders; Urinary tract
disorders.
embryonic development of,
1402–1404, 1403f
kidney function in, 1352–1360.
See also Glomerular
filtration; Nephron(s).
references on, 1364
renal structure and anatomy in,
1344–1351, 1345f. See also
Kidney(s); Nephron(s).
summary review of, 1362b
urinary structure and anatomy in,
1350–1351. See also Bladder;
Ureter(s); Urethra.
urine formation in, 1357–1358
vascular supply of, 1347–1350
Renal aplasia, 1406
Renal artery(ies), 1347–1348
Renal blood flow, 1351–1352, 1353t
clearance and, 1360
Renal buffer system, 116–117, 117f
Renal cancer, environmental factors
in, 361t, 377
Renal capsule, 1344
Renal cell carcinoma, 1372, 1372f
clinical manifestations of, 1372
evaluation and treatment of,
1372–1373
pathogenesis of, 1372
staging of, 1373t
Renal colic, 1369
Renal columns, 1345
Renal corpuscle, 1345
Renal cortex, 1345
Renal disorders, 1365
acute kidney injury in, 1386
in aldosteronism, 769b
autoimmune, 257t–258t
in children, 1404–1408
congenital, 1404–1407. See
also Congenital renal and
urinary tract disorders.

Renal disorders (Continued)
glomerular, 1407–1408
references on, 1417
renal injury in, 1411
summary review of, 1416b
Wilms tumor in, 1413
chronic kidney disease in, 1389
glomerular disease in, 1378–1383.
See also Glomerular
disorders.
references on, 1398
secondary hypertension in, 1153t
summary review of, 1397b
Renal dysplasia, 1406–1407
Renal fascia, 1344
Renal failure, 1386
Renal function, 1344, 1352–1360.
See also Glomerular filtration;
Nephron(s).
in aging, 1362–1364
Renal function testing, 1360–1362
blood tests in, 1360–1361
blood urea nitrogen in, 1361
concept of clearance in, 1360
plasma creatinine concentration
in, 1360–1361
plasma cystatin C concentration
in, 1361
urinalysis in, 1361–1362
urine sediment in, 1361–1362
Renal injury
in children, 1411, 1411t
classification of, 1386, 1386t,
1411t
Renal insufficiency, 1386, 1389
Renal medulla, 1345
Renal papillae, 1350
Renal pelvis, 1345
Renal pyramids, 1345
Renal tubule therapy, 1390b
Renal tubules
distal, 1347
epithelial cells of, 1347, 1347f
Henle loop, 1347
proximal, 1347
transport within, 1355–1357, 1356b
Renal tumors, 1372
Renalase, 1358
Renin, 101–102
cardiovascular effects of, 1125
Renin-angiotensin-aldosterone
system, 101–102, 1352, 1352f
cardiovascular effects of,
1126–1127, 1128b
and hypertension, 174, 176f,
1150–1151
renal effects of, 1352
and systolic heart failure, 1190
Repair and healing, tissue, 208. See
also Wound healing.
chemical mediators of, 203f
Reperfusion (reoxygenation) injury,
54, 1711
in children, 1737
Repetitive discharge, 1562
Replication, DNA, 129
Repolarization, 33, 1102
Reproductive system, 781
in aging, 807–814
cancer therapy-associated changes
in, 391–392
chronic kidney disease and effects
on, 1391t, 1396
diagnostic tests of, 805–807

Reproductive system (Continued)
for infection and cancer,
805–807, 805b, 806t
for reproductive function
(fertility), 807, 808–809t
embryonic and fetal development
of, 781–784, 782–783f
female, 784–796. See also Female
reproductive system.
alterations of, 819. See also
Female reproductive
disorders; Sexually
transmitted infections.
male, 796–802. See also Male
reproductive system.
alterations of, 850–857. See
also Male reproductive
disorders; Sexually
transmitted infections.
in puberty, 784. See also Puberty.
altered, 816–819
references on, 815
sexually transmitted infections of,
924–925
bacterial, 924–925
chlamydial, 935
parasitic, 942–943
viral, 938
summary review of, 812b–814b
Reservoirs, of infectious agents, 296
Residual bodies, 6–7
Residual volume (RV), 1262
Resistance
to blood flow through blood
vessels, 1120, 1121f, 1123f
in fluid system, 1118
Poiseuille's formula for, 1119
Resistance (adaptation) stage, of
general adaptation syndrome,
338
Resistin, 1478b
Resistin-like molecule, 186
Resolution, of repair, 208
Resorption cavity, 1547–1548
Respiration, 1249–1255, 1249f
altered cellular, in shock, 1697
physiologic control of, 1249–1251,
1250f
in children, 1312
Respiratory acidosis, 120–121
clinical manifestations of, 121
compensated, 122f
evaluation and treatment of, 122
pathophysiology of, 120–121
Respiratory airway(s), 1244–1247,
1246f
Respiratory alkalosis, 122
clinical manifestations of, 122
compensated, 123f
evaluation and treatment of, 123–125
pathophysiology of, 122
Respiratory bronchioles, 1244, 1246f
Respiratory burst, 201
Respiratory center, 1250
Respiratory distress syndrome, of
the newborn, 1321, 1321b
clinical manifestations of, 1322
pathophysiology of, 1321–1322,
1322f, 1324f
treatment of, 1322–1324
antenatal, glucocorticoids in,
1322
exogenous surfactant in, 1322
supportive care in, 1323

Respiratory failure, acute, 1271
Respiratory syncytial virus (RSV), 314t
Respiratory tract disorders, 1266, 1271–1280
  acute respiratory distress syndrome in, 1279–1280
  autoimmune, 257t–258t
  chest wall abnormalities in, 1271–1272
  childhood, 1313–1316. *See also* Childhood respiratory disorders.
  clinical manifestations of, 1266–1271
  conditions caused by, 1269–1271
  infectious, 299t–300t, 1290–1291. *See also* Acute bronchitis; Lung abscess; Pneumonia; Tuberculosis.
  malignant, 1298. *See also* Laryngeal cancer; Lip cancer; Lung cancer.
  obstructive, 1282–1284. *See also* Asthma; Chronic obstructive pulmonary disease.
  pleural abnormalities in, 1272–1274
  restrictive, 1274–1280. *See also* Restrictive pulmonary disorders.
  vascular disease in, 1294–1295. *See also* Pulmonary vascular disease.
Resting membrane potential, 32
Restless leg syndrome (RLS), 505
Restricted breathing, 1268
Restrictive cardiomyopathy, 1180
  pathophysiology of, and major symptoms, 1178f
Restrictive pericarditis, 1177–1178
Restrictive pulmonary disorders, 1274–1280
  aspiration in, 1274–1275
  atelectasis in, 1275
  bronchiectasis in, 1275–1277
  bronchiolitis in, 1277
  pulmonary fibrosis in, 1277–1278
  in systemic diseases, 1278–1279
Retching, 1453
Rete testes, 797
Reticular activating system, 449–450, 450f
  pain sensory processing in, 485f, 486
Reticular connective tissue, 39t–40t
Reticular dysgenesis, 279–280
Reticular fibers, 36–38
Reticular formation, 449–450, 450f
Reticulocyte count, 983t–985t
  pediatric, 985t, 1064t
Reticuloendothelial system. *See* Mononuclear phagocyte system.
Retina, 507
  layers of, 507f
Retinal detachment, 510
Retinoblastoma, 689–690, 689f
  bilateral, 691f
  clinical manifestations of, 691
  evaluation and treatment of, 691–693
  pathophysiology of, 690–691
  two-mutation development model of, 690, 690f

Retinoblastoma *(Rb)* gene, 148, 148f, 369, 375–377, 375t, 690–691
  and associated childhood cancer, 438–439
Retinoids, 864–865
Retinopathy, in diabetes mellitus, 759–760, 760f
Retraction balls, 589
Retrograde menstruation, 839
Retropharyngeal abscess, 1315t, 1316
Retropulsion, 1424–1425
Rett syndrome, genetic basis and pathophysiology of, 526t–527t
Reverse transcriptase, 315, 319
Reverse transcriptase inhibitor, 322–323
Rewarming shock, 502t
Reye syndrome, 681
  clinical manifestations of, 681
  evaluation and treatment of, 681–682
  pathophysiology of, 681
Rh alloimmunization, maternal hypersensitivity in, 271
Rh blood group, 272–273
Rh immune globulin (Rho-GAM), 1068
Rh transfusion reactions, 272–274
Rhabdomyolysis, 1575–1576, 1613
  clinical manifestations of, 1576
  evaluation and treatment of, 1576
  pathophysiology of, 1576, 1577b
Rhabdomyoma, 1613
Rhabdomyosarcoma, 1613
  in children, 1639
  clinical manifestations of, 1639, 1639t
  evaluation and treatment of, 1639–1640
  pathophysiology of, 1639
  primary prognostic factor in, 1640
Rheumatic fever, 1185
Rheumatic heart disease, 1185
  clinical manifestations of, 1186
  evaluation and treatment of, 1186–1187, 1187t
  pathophysiology of, 1185–1186, 1185f
Rheumatoid arthritis, 1596–1597, 1596f
  clinical manifestations of, 1598–1600
  complications of chronic, 1599
  evaluation and treatment of, 1600
  joint lesions in, 1599f
  juvenile, 1630–1631
  pathophysiology of, 1597–1598, 1598f
Rheumatoid factors, 1597t
Rheumatoid nodules, 1599
Rhinencephalon, 450t
Rhinophyma, 1659
Rhinovirus, 314t
Rhombencephalon, 450t. *See also* Hindbrain.
Rhythmicity, of cardiac cycle, 1103
Riboflavin. *See* Vitamin B2.
Ribonucleic acid (RNA), 132–134. *See also* RNA.
Ribosomal RNA (rRNA), 134
Ribosome, 3f, 5, 6f, 134
  protein synthesis in, 8, 136f

Rickets, 1584–1585, 1625
Rickettsia spp., 298, 299t–300t
Rickettsiae, 298t
RIFLE criteria
  for chronic kidney disease, 1386t
  modified, for nephrotic syndrome in children, 1377t
Right atrium, 1093
Right bundle branch (RBB), 1101–1102
Right coronary artery (RCA), 1096
Right heart, 1091
Right heart failure, 1194–1195
  in lung disease, 1194–1195, 1195f
Right lymphatic duct, 1132
Right pulmonary artery, 1095
Right ventricle, 1093
Rigidity, 562t, 563
  cogwheel, 573
  four types of, 562t–563t, 563
  Parkinsonian, 529–531, 573
  plastic, 573
Rigor mortis, 90
Ringer lactate solution, electrolyte content of, 1718t
Ringworm, 1664–1665, 1684. *See also* Tinea entries.
Risedronate, and postmenopausal osteoporosis, 1584
Risk factors, for disease, 165
Rituximab, 387t, 1035
  for treatment of idiopathic thrombocytopenic purpura, 1081–1082, 1082b
RNA (ribonucleic acid), 132–134
  transcription of, 132–133, 134f
RNA polymerase, 132–133
Robertsonian translocations, 143, 144f
Robotic surgical repair, of pediatric urology disorders, 1406b
Rods, 507
Roentgenograms, 474
Roentgenography
  of central nervous system, 474
  of gastrointestinal tract, 1444, 1445f
Roseola, 1687, 1687t
Rotationplasty, 1591
Rotavirus, 314t, 1530
Rotavirus vaccine, 330
Rough endoplasmic reticulum, 5
Roundworms (nematodes), 310, 310t
rRNA (ribosomal RNA), 134
Rubella, 621t, 1686, 1687t
  and associated congenital heart defects, 1214t
Rubella in combination vaccine, 1686
Rubella (R) vaccine, 330, 330t
Rubella virus, 314t
Rubeola, 1686–1687, 1687t
Ruffled borders, 1543–1544
Rule of nines, 1716, 1716f

S

S-adenosylhomocysteine (SAM), 405–406
S cells, 1444
Saccular aneurysm(s), 606, 606f, 1146
Saccular bronchiectasis, 1276
Sacral plexus, 465
Salicylates, and development of Reye syndrome, 681

Saliva, 1422
  electrolyte concentration of, and flow rate, 1423f
Salivary α-amylase, 1422
Salivary glands, 1422, 1422f
  digestive enzymes of, 1430b
Salivation, 1422
Salmon patches, 1691–1692
Salmonella spp.
  adhesion mechanisms of, 300
  degradation of immune molecules by, 304
  enterotoxins of, 305
  intracellular survival of, 302–303
Salmonella typhi, 299t–300t
  intracellular survival of, 302
Salpingitis, 828, 829f
  as complication of gonorrhea, 926
Saltatory conduction, of ionic flow, 443
Sano modification, of Norwood procedure, 1230
Sarcolemma, 1558
Sarcoma(s), 364t
  definition of, 361
  metastasis of, 384t
Sarcomere, 1558–1559
  myocardial, 1105, 1106f
Sarcopenia, 90, 1564
Sarcoplasm, 1558
Sarcoplasmic reticulum, 1558–1559
Sarcotubular system, 1558–1559
Sarcotubules, 1558–1559
SARS virus, 314t
Saturated fats, 1162b
Saturated fatty acids, 1433b
Scabies, 944, 1688–1689, 1689f
  clinical manifestations of, 944, 944f–945f
  evaluation and treatment of, 944–945
  excoriation in, 1648t–1653t
  mite causing, 1689f
  pathophysiology of, 944
Scale, 1648t–1653t
Scapuloperoneal muscular dystrophy, 1636
Scar, hypertrophic, 211–212, 1648t–1653t, 1654
Scar maturation, in pediatric burn injury, 1745, 1746f, 1748
Scar tissue, 208, 1648t–1653t
Scavenger receptors, 195
Schistosoma haematobium, 425
Schistosoma mansoni, 310t
  antigenic variation in, 311
  tissue damage caused by, 312
Schizophrenia, 647–652
  clinical manifestations in, 650–651, 650b
  dorsolateral prefrontal cortex dysfunction in, 648
  genetic predisposition to, 179, 647, 647b
  negative dimensions in, 651
  neuroanatomic alterations in, 647–648, 648f
  neurotransmitters alterations in, 648–650
  prenatal and perinatal factors in development of, 179, 179t, 647
  psychotic dimension of, 650
  treatment of, 651–652

Schwann cell(s), 443–445, 444f, 667
functions of, 446t
Scissors gait, 576
Sclera, 507
Scleroderma, 1667, 1667f
Sclerosing adenosis, breast, 874
Sclerosing papillary proliferation,
874–875
Scoliosis, 1625
clinical manifestations of, 1627,
1627f
evaluation and treatment of,
1627–1628
pathophysiology of, 1626–1627
Scotoma, 509
Scott syndrome, 1049
Scrotal cancer, environmental
factors in, 375t, 377
Scrotal disorders, 854–856
selected, differential diagnosis of,
856–857, 857t
Scrotal mass, diagnostic algorithm
for, 854f
Scrotum, 797
Sebaceous cyst, 1648t–1653t
Sebaceous glands, 1646
Seborrheic dermatitis, 1656, 1657f
Seborrheic keratosis, 1668, 1668f
Second-degree block, 1199t–1200t
Second degree burns, 1714, 1715t,
1716f
Second-hand smoke, in
epidemiology of cancer, 404
Second messenger(s), 20, 701f, 702
Second messenger signaling
pathways
for specific hormones, 23t
Second order neurons, classes of,
484
Secondary aldosteronism, 768, 768t
pathophysiology of, 769
Secondary amenorrhea, 820–821
clinical manifestations of, 822
evaluation and treatment of,
822–823
pathophysiology of, 821–822, 822f
Secondary biliary cirrhosis, 1492t,
1493–1494
Secondary bone, 1548
Secondary centers of ossification,
1619
Secondary dysmenorrhea, 819
Secondary enuresis, 1415
Secondary generalization, 536
Secondary gout, 1602–1603
Secondary granules, 200–201
Secondary hyperparathyroidism,
743
clinical manifestations of, 744
Secondary hypertension, 1149
pathophysiology of, 1152, 1153t
Secondary hyperthyroidism, 736
Secondary hypocortisolism, 770
Secondary (central)
hypothyroidism, 739, 739f
Secondary immune deficiencies,
275, 284–286
AIDS (acquired
immunodeficiency
syndrome) in, 318–325
dietary insufficiencies and, 285
environmental factors in, 285
infections and, 286
malignancies and, 285

Secondary immune deficiencies
(Continued)
medical treatments and, 286
metabolic disease, genetic
syndromes and, 285
physical trauma to skin and,
285–286
psychologic stress and, 285
Secondary immune response,
240–241, 240f
Secondary intention, healing by,
208, 209f
Secondary (peripheral) lymphoid
organs, 235
histology of, 236f
Secondary lymphoid system, 230
Secondary lysosome, 5–6
Secondary multiple organ
dysfunction syndrome, 1708
Secondary muscle dysfunction,
1606–1607
chronic fatigue syndrome in, 1608
contractures in, 1606
disuse atrophy in, 1609
fibromyalgia in, 1606–1607
stress-induced muscle tension
in, 1606
Secondary nephrotic syndrome,
1409
Secondary osteoporosis, 1580
Secondary peristalsis, 1423
Secondary pneumothorax,
1272–1273
Secondary polycythemia, 1009
Secondary septic arthritis, 1629
Secondary spermatocytes, 800
Secondary spinal cord injury, 592
Secondary syphilis, 928–929
clinical manifestations of, 929,
930f
Secondary ureteropelvic junction
obstruction, 1406
Secretin, 1425t, 1444
Secretory diarrhea, 1454–1455
Secretory (mucosal) immune
system, 246–247, 246f
Secretory immunoglobulins,
246–247
Secretory vesicles, 5
Sedentary lifestyle, and coronary
artery disease, 1164
Segmental inhibition, of pain
perception, 486
Segmentation, 1435
Segregation, principle of, 146
Seizure initiation, 538
Seizure syndromes, 539–542
Seizures, 536–537
in children, 679
benign febrile, 680
epileptic, 679
clinical manifestations of,
540t–541t, 542
diseases and conditions associated
with, 537
evaluation and treatment of,
542–544
international classification of,
537t
pathophysiology of, 537–542
recurrent, in different age groups,
539t
terminology of, 537t
types of, 536–537

Selected serotonin reuptake
inhibitors (SSRIs), 657b
Selectins, 198–199, 199t
Selective attention deficit, 543, 547t
Selective estrogen receptor
modulators (SERMs),
1580–1582, 1584
Selective IgA deficiency, 279
Selenium, and cancer risk, 410t
Self-antigen(s), 222, 257t
central tolerance of, 233, 267–269
of specific autoimmune disorders,
257t–258t
Semantic processing deficits, 547t
Semen, 799
Semen analysis fertility test, 808t
Semicircular canals, 514
Semilunar valves, 1094
Seminal vesicles, 799f, 800
Seminiferous tubules, 797
spermatogenesis within, 800, 801f
Senile disease complex. See
Alzheimer disease.
Senile gait, 576
Senile plaques, 471–474, 554
Senile posture, 576
Sensorimotor syndrome, 619
Sensorineural hearing loss, 515
Sensory dysfunction, 481
Sensory dysphasia, 549t
Sensory ganglion (dorsal root
ganglion), 456
Sensory homunculus, 452, 484
Sensory inattentiveness, 542
Sensory neurons, 444, 457
Sensory neuropathies, 635
Sensory pathways, 454f, 457f,
458–459
Sensory receptors, 445b
of motor unit, 1556–1557
Sepsis, 300–301, 1733
in children, 1735
definitions and clinical criteria
for, 1736t
disseminated intravascular
coagulation and,
1050–1051
staging system in, 1708t
Septation, cardiac, 1209–1211,
1210–1211f
Septic shock, 305, 1703–1707, 1728
in children, 1733–1735
clinical manifestations of,
1735–1741
definitions and clinical criteria
for, 1736t
goals of therapy for, 1741
treatment of, 1738, 1740–1741
clinical manifestations of, 1706,
1706f
pathophysiology of, 1703–1706,
1704t, 1705f, 1728b, 1729
treatment of, 1706–1707
Septicemia, heart failure in, 1195
Septum primum, 1210
Septum secundum, 1210
Sequestered antigen, 268–269
Sequestration crisis, in sickle cell
disease, 1074
Sequestrum (sequestra), 1587–1588,
1628–1629
Serine kinase, 701
SERMs (selective estrogen receptor
modulators), 1580–1582, 1584

Serologic testing, 805
Serotonin, 447–448
functions of, 448t–449t
in pain modulation, 488
Serotonin system, 654, 656f
Serous exudates, in inflammation,
205
Sertoli cells, 800
Serum, 952
Serum alkaline phosphatase, in bone
tumor diagnosis, 1589–1590
Serum calcium levels, parathyroid
hormone and, 711–712, 712f
Serum enzyme assessments, 1446t
Serum ferritin determination,
983t–985t
Serum free fatty acids, elevated, 750
Serum IgE, laboratory tests for, 267
Serum markers, of cardiovascular
risk, 1164b, 1165
Serum progesterone, 809t
Serum protein assessments, 1446t
Serum sickness, 263–264
Serum testosterone, 809t
Serum transferrin receptor (sTfR),
997–998
Sever disease, 1631
Severe combined immune
deficiency (SCID), 279–280
X-linked, 280
Severe congenital neutropenia, 282
Severe diffuse axonal injury, 591
Severe sepsis, 1735
Sex chromosome(s), 134
Sex chromosome aneuploidy,
138–142
Sex hormone binding globulin,
801–802
Sex hormones, 697t, 702–703, 781
adipose tissue and, 409–415
adrenal cortical secretion of, 718
aging and effects on circulating,
722
female, 790–792. See also
Estrogen(s); Progesterone.
male, 800–802. See also
Testosterone.
in postmenopausal bone
maintenance, 1579, 1582
receptors for, 23t, 702–703
serum, evaluation of, 809t
signal transduction by, 702–703,
703f
types of, receptors, and
mechanisms of action, 700t
Sex-influenced trait, 155
Sex-limited trait, 155
Sex-linked inheritance, of disease,
152. See also X-linked
inheritance.
Sexual dysfunction
female, 848–849
chronic disease and, 849t
male, 869
Sexual maturation, 784
alterations of, 816–819, 909b
Sexually transmitted infections,
923–925, 924t
bacterial, 299t–300t, 924–925
Campylobacter enteritis in, 946
chancroid in, 932
gonorrhea in, 924–925
granuloma inguinale in, 933
shigellosis in, 946

Sexually transmitted infections (Continued)
  syphilis in, 927–928
  vaginosis in, 934
  chlamydial, 935
    and gonorrheal infection, similarity of clinical syndromes, 927, 936t
    lymphogranuloma venereum in, 937
  diagnostic tests for, 805–807, 806t
  in epidemiology of cancer, 425
  of gastrointestinal system, 946
  nongonococcal urethritis in, 937–938
  parasitic, 942–943
    pediculosis pubis in, 945
    scabies in, 944
    trichomoniasis in, 942–943
  protozoal, 946
  references on, 950
  summary review of, 948b
  systemic, 947–948
  in United States, CDC statistical summary, 925b
  of urogenital tracts, 924–925
  viral, 938
    genital herpes in, 938
    hepatitis in, 946–947
    human papillomavirus in, 940
    molluscum contagiosum in, 941–942
Shaken baby syndrome, 62–63
Sharp force injuries, 65–66
Shear stress, of blood flow, 1097
Sheehan syndrome, 731
Shift-to-the-left reaction, 1015, 1063
Shigella sonnei, 299t, 302–303
Shigella spp., enterotoxins of, 305
Shigellosis, sexually transmitted, 946
Shingles, 1664, 1688
Shivering, 501
Shock, 1696–1707
  anaphylactic, 1702–1703, 1728
  burn, 1717. See also Burn shock; Pediatric burn injury.
  cardiogenic, 1699–1701, 1728
    in children, 1732–1733
  cellular alterations in, 1697
  in children, 1727
    clinical manifestations of, 1728–1729
    developing therapies for, 1740–1741, 1740t
    evaluation and treatment of, 1737–1741
  classification of, by cause, 1728, 1728b
  clinical manifestations of, 1711–1713, 1712b
  distributive, 1728
  hypermetabolic response in, 1719, 1747–1748
  hypovolemic, 1701–1702
    in children, 1728–1729
  neurogenic, 1702, 1728
  obstructive, 1728
  pathophysiology of, 1697–1699
    in children, 1728–1729
  references on, 1724
  septic, 1703–1707, 1728
    in children, 1733–1735
  spinal, 565, 593

Shock (Continued)
    autonomic hyperreflexive syndrome after, 595
    clinical manifestations of, 594t–595t
    summary review of, 1722b
    treatment of, 1707
    types of, 1699–1707
  SHOCK trial, 1700b
  Shored exit wound, 67
  Short bones, 1547
Short bowel syndrome, 1474
Short term starvation, 1481
  Shunting, in ventilation-perfusion mismatch, 1270, 1270f
Sialadenitis, and associated cancer, 378t
  Sialoprotein, 1545
Sickle cell anemia, 1066t, 1071
    erythrocyte appearance in, 992f
Sickle cell disease, 1071
    clinical manifestations of, 1073–1076, 1075f
    evaluation and treatment of, 1076–1077
    inheritance of, 1073t
    pathophysiology of, 1071–1073, 1072t–1073f
Sickle cell HbC disease, 1071
  Sickle cell test, 983t–985t
Sickle cell thalassemia disease, 1071
  Sickle cell trait, 1071
  Sickled erythrocytes, 1071–1073, 1073f–1074f
Sideroblastic anemia(s), 998
    clinical manifestations of, 999
    erythrocyte appearance in, 992f
    evaluation and treatment of, 999–1002
    laboratory findings for, 999t
    pathophysiology of, 998–999
    secondary to drug effects, 998, 1001t
  Sideroblasts, ringed, 998
  Siderophores, 1375
  Sigmoid colon, 1435–1436
  Signal transducers and activators of transcription (STAT), 701
  Signal transduction, 18–19f, 19–20, 700–701
    first messenger in, 700–701
    hormonal, 700–702, 701f
    major cell receptors and pathways in, 23t
  Signaling cascades, 19
    intracellular, 20f
  Silence classification, of osteogenesis imperfecta syndromes, 1624, 1624t
  Silencing, gene, 373–374
Silent ischemia, 1165–1167, 1167f
    and mental stress, 1166
  Silent substitution, 129–132
Silicosis, 1278
    and associated cancer, 378t
Simple bone cyst, 1637
  Simple columnar epithelium, 37t–38t
  Simple cuboidal epithelium, 37t–38t
  Simple epithelium, 36
Simple sinus tachycardia, 1197t–1198t
  Simple squamous epithelium, 37t–38t

Sinding-Larsen-Johansson syndrome, 1631
Single gene diseases, 146
  Single photon emission computed tomography (SPECT), 1134
  Sinoatrial (SA, sinus) node, 1100
Sinus block, 1199t–1200t
Sinus bradycardia, 1197t–1198t
Sinus dysrhythmias, 1197t–1198t
Sinus tachycardia, 1197t–1198t
  Sinusoids, hepatic, 1438–1439
  SIRS. See Systemic inflammatory response syndrome.
  Sister chromatids, 34–35
Sjögren syndrome, and associated cancer, 378t
  Skeletal development, 1620
  Skeletal homeostasis, 1579–1580
  Skeletal muscle(s), 41t, 1555–1560, 1556f
    aging of, 1564–1566
    contraction of, 1559–1563, 1559f
      mechanics of, 1562
      molecular, 1561
    cross-sectional view of, 1556f
    development and growth of, 1620
    function testing of, 1563–1564
    groups of, in movement, 1562–1563
    metabolism of, 1561–1562, 1561t
    motor units of, 1556–1560
    myofibrillar organization of, 1557f
    structure and function of, 1554–1563
  Skeletal muscle contraction, heat production in, 496
Skeletal muscle disorders, 1606–1607
    inflammatory, 1611
    membrane abnormalities in, 1609
    metabolic, 1610–1611
    myopathies in, 1612–1613
    secondary muscle dysfunction in, 1606–1607
    tumors in, 1613–1615
  Skeletal muscle fiber(s), 1557–1560
    characteristics of, 1557–1558, 1558t
    components of, 1557f, 1558
    diameter of, and muscle strength, 1558
    myofibrillar organization in, 1557–1560, 1557f
    myofibrils of, 1559–1560, 1559f
    nonprotein components of, 1560
  Skeletal system, 1540–1548, 1548f
    bone structure and function in, 1540–1548
    bone tissue of, 1540–1545, 1541t
      types of, 1545–1546
    bones and bone characteristics of, 1546–1547
    chronic kidney disease and effects on, 1391t, 1394–1396, 1394t
Skeletal trauma, 1568–1569
    dislocations and subluxations in, 1572. See also Dislocations and subluxations.
    fractures in, 1568–1569. See also Fracture(s).
    support structure injuries in, 1573. See also Tendon and ligament injuries.
  Skene glands, 785–786

Skin
    in aging, 1646–1655
    blood supply and innervation of, 1646
    layers of, 1644–1645, 1645f, 1645t
  Skin biopsy, 1647t
Skin cancer, 1669–1673
    environmental factors in, 397t–400t, 401
    trends in incidence of, 1669b
    ultraviolet radiation in etiology of, 422–424
Skin disorders, 1655–1673. See also Burn injury.
    and associated cancer, 378t
    autoimmune, 257t–258t
    benign tumors in, 1668–1669
    in children, 1680
      acne vulgaris, 1680–1681
      dermatitis, 1681–1682
      infections, 1683–1688
      insect bites and parasitic infestations, 1688–1690
      other, 1692–1694
      references on, 1694
      summary review of, 1693b
      vascular malformations, 1690–1692
    clinical manifestations of, 1647–1655. See also Pruritus; Skin lesions.
    frostbite in, 1673
    infectious, 1662–1665
    inflammatory, 1655–1656
    insect bites in, 1667–1668
    papulosquamous, 1657–1660
    paraneoplastic, 389t
    references on, 1677
    summary review of, 1675b
    vascular abnormalities in, 1665–1667
    vesiculobullous, 1660–1662
  Skin function tests, 1647, 1647t
  Skin grafts, 1721–1722, 1721f
    improving, 1722b
Skin infections, 1662–1665
    bacterial, 1662–1663, 1683–1684
    in children, 1683–1688
    fungal, 1664–1665, 1684–1685
    viral, 1663–1664, 1685–1688
Skin lesions, 1647–1654
    of pressure ulcers, 1647–1654
    primary and secondary, 1648t–1653t
    special, 1653t
Skin trauma, and secondary immune deficiencies, 285–286
Skin tumors, 1648t–1653t
    benign, 1668–1669
    in children, 1690–1691
    malignant, 1669–1673
  Skull roentgenograms, 474
  Sleep, 481, 502–504
  Sleep cycles, normal, 504f
Sleep disorders, 504–505
    associated with mental, neurologic, and medical disorders, 505–506
  Sleep patterns
    in aging, 504–506
    in children, 504
Sleep-wake transition disorders, 505

Sliding filament theory, of muscle contraction, 1561
Sliding hiatal hernia, 1459, 1459f
Slightly movable joint, 1549
Slow wave sleep. *See* NREM (non-rapid eye movement) sleep phase.
Small cell carcinoma, bronchogenic, 1302–1303, 1302t
Small intestine, 1428–1435, 1428f
carbohydrate digestion and absorption in, 1430, 1431f
digestive enzymes of, 1430b
fat digestion and absorption in, 1431f, 1432–1433
mineral and vitamin absorption and transport in, 1433–1434
motility of, 1434–1435
protein digestion and absorption in, 1430–1432, 1431f
water and electrolyte transport in, 1430
Small intestine carcinoma, 1500
Small intestine obstruction, 1460–1461, 1461t
clinical manifestations of, 1461–1462
Small vessel disease, stroke syndromes resulting from, 604t–605t
Smallpox, 1688
Smallpox pandemic, 297t
Smell, sense of. *See* Olfaction.
Smoke, environmental and tobacco, in cancer epidemiology, 397t–400t
Smoldering myeloma, 1040
Smooth endoplasmic reticulum, 5
Smooth muscle, 41t
Social (street) drug use
cell injury in, 62
effects of, 63t
Sodium, and water balance
in chronic kidney failure, 1393–1394, 1394t
extracellular and intracellular, 101–102
alterations in, 102–104
low dietary intake of, 105
Sodium/chloride reabsorption, 1357–1358
inhibitors of, 1359t
Sodium ferric gluconate complex in sucrose (Ferrlecit), 997–998
Sodium-potassium pump
in active transport, 29–30, 29f
aldosterone regulation of, 717
and propagation of action potential, 32–33, 33f
Sodium transport, glucose and, 1430, 1432f
Soft tissue sarcoma, environmental factors in, 397t–400t, 401
Soft tissue tumors, classification of, 1639t
Solitary plasmacytoma, 1040
Solute movement, across plasma membrane, 26–30
Solutes, 26
Solvents, in cancer epidemiology, 397t–400t
Somatic cells, 134

Somatic death, 90
Somatic motor pathways, 454f
Somatic nervous system, 443
Somatic pain, 490
origins of, 491
Somatic recombination, 230
Somatic-sensory pathways, 454f
Somatosensory cortex, 484
Somatosensory dysfunction, 517
Somatosensory function, 517–520
Somatostatin
in digestive process, 1425t, 1426
hypothalamic release of, 703–704, 707t
pancreatic release of, 714–715
in stress response, 348t
Somatotropic hormones, 707, 708t
Somatotropin. *See* Growth hormone.
Somite, 665–666
Somogyi effect, 758
Spasmodic croup, 1316–1317
Spasmodic torticollis, 563, 563f
botulinum toxin therapy for, 575b
Spastic gait, 576
Spastic paresis, 634
Spasticity, 562t, 563, 563f
Spatial agnosia, 548t
Spatial summation, 449
Special senses, 481–482, 506–508
hearing in, 512–514
olfaction and taste in, 515–516
vision in, 506–508
Specialized cell junctions, 16–18, 17f
Specific gravity, 1361
Specificity theory, of pain, 482
SPECT (single photon emission computed tomography), 1134
Sperm motility, 871
Sperm production and quality, impaired, 870–871
Spermatic cord, 796
Spermatids, 800
Spermatocele, 855–856, 855f
Spermatogenesis, 797, 800, 801f
Spermatogenic dysfunction, 870–871
Spermatogonia, 800
Spermatozoon (sperm cell), 781, 802f
Spherocytes, 992f, 1070f
Spherocytosis, hereditary, 1070
Sphincter of Oddi, 1439, 1442
Spina bifida, 167, 168b, 169f, 671–672
Spina bifida occulta, 671–672
Spinal accessory nerve (CN XI)
origins, course, functions, and testing of, 468t
Spinal arteries, anterior and posterior, 463–465, 465f
Spinal cord, 450t, 456–458, 456f
anatomical structures of, 457f
blood supply of, 463–465, 465f
major tracts of, 457f
neural circuits of, 457
protective coverings of, 457f, 459–462, 461f
Spinal cord abscess, 624, 625f
clinical manifestations of, 625
evaluation and treatment of, 625–626
pathophysiology of, 624–625

Spinal cord injury, 591
clinical manifestations of, 593–596, 594t
comparison of, in children and adults, 594t
evaluation and treatment of, 596–598
incidence of, 591
pathophysiology of, 591–593, 591f–592f
primary, 591–592
secondary, 592
types of, 593t
Spinal cord tumors, 612t, 618–619
clinical manifestations of, 619–620
distribution of, 619f
evaluation and treatment of, 620–623
metastatic, 618–619
pathophysiology of, 619
primary, 618, 618b
staging of, 620, 620b
Spinal degenerative disorders, 596–598
disk degeneration in, 596–598
herniated intervertebral disk in, 599
low back pain and, 598
Spinal multiple sclerosis, 632–633, 632b
Spinal nerve root tumors, 612t
Spinal nerves, 442–443, 456f, 465
dermatomes innervated by, 467
mixed sensory and motor, 465
plexuses of, 465–467
Spinal shock, 565, 593
autonomic hyperreflexive syndrome after, 595
clinical manifestations of, 594t
Spinal stenosis, 598
Spinal tracts, 456–457, 457f
of motor pathways, 458
of sensory pathways, 458–459
Spindle fibers, 34–35
Spindles, 1556–1557
Spine roentgenograms, 474
Spinothalamic tract, 456–457
Spinous layer, 1644–1645
Spiral (helical) computed tomography, 474
Spirochetes, 298
Spirometry, 1261
ventilatory values measured in, 1262t
Spironolactone, diuretic action of, 1359t
Splanchnic nerves, 467
Spleen, 958
absence of, and physiologic effects, 958
anatomic features of, 958
blood circulation through, 958
macrophages and phagocytic activity in, 958, 959f, 968
Splenectomy
in hypersplenism, 1043
in immune thrombocytic purpura, 1046
laparoscopic, in sickle cell disease, 1076, 1076b
in thalassemia, 1078
Splenic dysfunction, 1042–1043
clinical manifestations of, 1043
evaluation and treatment of, 1043
pathophysiology of, 1043

Splenic sinus, blood cell movement in, 960f
Splenomegaly, 1042
in children, 1533
classification of, 1043b
clinical manifestations of, 1043
congestive, 1043
evaluation and treatment of, 1043
infiltrative, 1043
pathophysiology of, 1043
in portal hypertension, 1483
Splints, and casts, in fractured bone immobilization, 1571–1572
Split-thickness sheet grafts, 1749, 1749f
Spondyloarthritis. *See* Ankylosing spondylitis.
Spondylolisthesis, 598
Spondylosis, 598
cervical, 598
lumbar, 598, 598f
Spongy (cancellous) bone, 1545–1546, 1547f
Spontaneous mutation, 132
Sporadic motor neuron disease (sporadic motor system disease), 633–634
Sporothrix schenckii, 308t
Sporozoa, 310, 310t
Sports-related concussion, 590b
Sprained ligament, 1573
Sprains and strains, 1573
clinical manifestations of, 1573
evaluation and treatment of, 1573–1574
pathophysiology of, 1573
Sputum, abnormal, 1267
Squamous cell carcinoma, 1670, 1670f
bronchogenic, 1301, 1302t
Squamous cells, 36
Squamous-columnar junction, at cervical-vaginal junction, 789
SSRIs (selected serotonin reuptake inhibitors), 657b
warnings in treatment of children, 657, 657b
ST elevation MI (STEMI), 1169, 1174
ST interval, of electrocardiogram, 1103
St Louis encephalitis, 625–626, 626t
Stab wounds, 65–66, 65f
Stable angina, 1165–1166
Stable factor (clotting factor VII), 977t
disorder(s) associated with, 1079t
Stachybotrys chartarum, 308t
Stage, of cancer spread, 384, 386f, 387t
Staghorn calculi, 1368, 1605
Stapes, 512–513
Staphylococcal pneumonia, 1291
in children, 1327–1328, 1328t
Staphylococcal scalded skin syndrome, 1684, 1684f
Staphylococcus aureus, 299t–300t. *See also* Bacterial tracheitis.
antibiotic resistant mechanisms of, 306–307
antibiotic resistant strains of, 294
antigenic variation in, 304
enterotoxins of, 305

Staphylococcus aureus (Continued)
  immune molecule neutralization by, 304–305
  intracellular survival of, 302–303
  in nosocomial infections, 305, 327
  pathogenesis of infection by, 305–307, 306f
  in skin infections, 1662–1663
Staphylococcus spp., 299t–300t
  in cutaneous infections, 1662–1665
  protective mechanisms of, against phagocytes, 303–304
Starling hypothesis, 98
Starvation, 1481–1482
Stasis dermatitis, 1648t, 1656, 1656f
Static (holding) contraction, 1562
Static encephalopathies, 675
  cerebral palsy in, 675
  inherited metabolic disorders in, 677–679
  seizure disorders in, 679
Statins, in preventing cardiovascular events, 606, 1174–1175
Status asthmaticus, 1284, 1333
Status epilepticus, 536–537, 681
STC64, 908
Steel factor, 961t, 963
Stellate cells, 1438–1439
Stem cell factor, in hematopoiesis, 961t
Stem cell pool, 963–965, 965f
Stem cells, 363–366, 1429
  adult, 363–365
  asymmetric division of, 366f
  cancer, 365–366
  global epigenetic silencing and formation of, 373–374
  mesenchymal, lineages and differentiation of, 366f
Steroid hormones, 697t, 702–703
  adipose tissue and, 409–415
  receptors for, 23t, 702–703
  sex, adrenal cortical secretion of, 718
  signal transduction by, 702–703, 703f
  types of, receptors, and mechanisms of action, 700t
Steroids, in shock therapy for children, 1740t
Stevens-Johnson syndrome, 1661, 1692–1694
Stippling, in gunshot wounds, 66–67
Stomach, 1423–1428, 1424f
  digestive enzymes of, 1430b
Stomach cancer, 1498t, 1499
  clinical manifestations of, 1499
  evaluation and treatment of, 1499–1500
  pathogenesis of, 1499
  typical sites of, 1499f
Stomatocytes, 992t
Stool studies, 1445t
Stormoken syndrome, 1049
Strabismus, 509
Strain(s)
  muscle, 1575
  tendon, 1573
Strangulation, 68
Stratified epithelium, 36
Stratified squamous epithelium, 37t–38t
Stratum basale, 1644–1645

Stratum corneum, 1644–1645, 1645t
Stratum germinativum, 1644–1645
Stratum spinosum, 1644–1645
Strawberry hemangiomas, 1690, 1691f
Streptococcus pneumoniae, 298, 299t–300t, 682. *See also* Pneumococcal pneumonia.
  antibiotic resistant strains of, 294, 327
  capsule protection of, 304
  immune molecule degradation by, 304
  immune molecule neutralization by, 304–305
  vaccine for, 329, 329t–330t, 331
Streptococcus pyogenes, 298
  antigenic variation in, 304
  protective survival mechanisms of, 304
Streptococcus spp., 299t–300t
  adhesion mechanisms of, 300
  complement evasion by, 305
  in cutaneous infections, 1662–1665
Stress, 337
  aging and, 337, 355
  concepts of, 337–339
  coping strategies for, 354
  definition of, 337
  disease and conditions related to, 337t, 353
  general adaptation syndrome and, 338, 721
  immune system and, 347–353
  myocardial ischemia and, 337, 337b, 347b, 1166–1167, 1167f–1168f
  neuroendocrine response in, 720
  as precipitating factor in disease, 337
  psychoneuroimmunologic mediators of, 339
  references on, 356
  secondary hypertension in, 1143t
  specificity of, and psychologic mediators, 338–339
  summary review of, 355b
  systemic and local responses to, 346
  tumor growth and, 353
  wound healing and, 346
Stress fracture, 1569
Stress incontinence, 1369t
Stress induced muscle tension, 1606
Stress response, 339–352
  in central nervous system, 339–346
  and physiologic responses, 340f
  cortisol secretion during, 344–346
  reasons for, 346
  in healthy individuals, potential effects of, 352–356, 354f
  hormonal alterations in,
    349–352, 1710
    endorphin and enkephalin release, 350
    female, 349–350, 351f
    growth hormone, 350–351
    oxytocin, 351–352
    prolactin, 351
    testosterone, 352
  immune system and, 347–352
  in medical interventions, potential effects of, 353, 354f
  psychoneuroimmunologic interaction in, 347–352, 348t

Stress testing
  in aging, 1136–1137
  in cardiac function evaluation, 1134
Stress ulcers (stress related mucosal disease), 1467–1470
Stressors, 352–356
  physiologic, 352
  psychosocial, 352–353
Stretch receptors, pulmonary, 1251, 1267
Striated muscle, 1555
Stridor, 1313–1314
  diagnostic approach to, 1314f
Stroke rehabilitation, 603, 606
Stroke syndromes, 600–601. *See also* Cerebrovascular accidents.
  in chronic diabetes mellitus, 764–765
  clinical manifestations of, 602–603
  embolic, 601
  evaluation and treatment of, 603–606
  hemorrhagic, 601
  lacunar, 601
  pathophysiology of, 602, 603f
  secondary to occlusion or stenosis, 604t
  thrombotic, 601
Stroke volume (SV), 1109, 1133t
  in children, 1730
Stroke volume index (SVI), 1133t
Stroke work index (SWI), 1133t
Stromal cells, bone marrow, 963
Strongyloides stercoralis, 310t
Structural scoliosis, 1625
Structurally induced coma, 528
  clinical manifestations of, 529t
Struvite stones, 1368
Stuart-Prower factor (clotting factor X), 977t
  activation of, in disseminated intravascular coagulation, 1052
  disorder(s) associated with, 1079t
Sturge-Weber-Dimitri disease, congenital heart defects associated with, 1215t
Stye, 506
Subacute thyroiditis, 741
Subarachnoid hemorrhage, 460, 608, 608f
  classification of, 609t
  clinical manifestations of, 609
  evaluation and treatment of, 609–619
  pathophysiology of, 608–609
Subarachnoid space, 460
Subclinical hypothyroidism, 741
Subcutaneous layer, 1645–1646, 1645t
Subdural hematoma(s), 62–63, 586, 587f
  acute, 586
  chronic, 587, 587f
  clinical manifestations of, 586–587
Subdural space, 460
Subfalcine herniation, 559
Subglottic stenosis, 1318–1319
Subintima, 1550
Subluxation, 1572. *See also* Dislocations and subluxations.

Submucosal plexus, 1421
Subserosal plexus, 1421
Substance P
  functions of, 448t
  hypothalamic release of, 703–704, 707t
  in stress response, 348t
Substantia gelatinosa, 456, 483–484
Substantia nigra, 455
Substrate, 21
Substrate phosphorylation, 24
Subthalamic nucleus, 455
Subthalamus, 450t, 453
Succussion splash, 1460
Sudden infant death syndrome, 1339–1341
  etiologies of, 1339
  preventive measures against, 1339
  risk groups for, 1339
Suffocation, 68
Sugar transport systems, 30t
Sulci, 452
Sulcus limitans, 666, 666f
Sulfatase inhibitors, 884–885
Summation, of potentials, 449
Superantigens (SAGs), 244, 244f
Superficial (conducting) arteries, 462
Superficial cortical nephrons, 1345
Superficial partial thickness burns, 1714, 1715f, 1715t
Superior colliculi, 455
Superior mesenteric ganglia, 467
Superior sagittal sinus, 461
Superior vena cava, 1095
Superior vena cava syndrome, 1144
Supply-dependent oxygen consumption, 1711
Suppurative exudates, in inflammation, 205
Supra-linear model, of dose-response, 419, 419f
Suprachiasmatic nucleus, 502
Supratentorial disorders, 528, 529t
Supratentorial herniation, 559
Surfactant, pulmonary, 1244, 1311
  exogenous use of, in lessening severity of neonatal lung disease, 1322–1323
  and surface tension at alveolocapillary membrane, 1252–1253
  update on, 1253b
Surfactant impairment, causing atelectasis, 1275, 1321–1322
Surgery
  secondary immune deficiencies and, 286
  temperature regulation disorders and, 502
Surgical procedures
  Fontan procedure, 1226, 1230
  Glenn procedure, 1230
  Kasai procedure, 1531–1532, 1532f
  Konno procedure, 1229
  Norwood procedure, 1230
  Rashkind procedure, 1226
  Rastelli procedure, 1232
    modified, 1234
  Sano modification, of Norwood procedure, 1230
Surgical wounds, healing phases of, 208–210

Suture(s)
  cranial, 666, 668f
  of flat bones, 1549
Swallowing, process of, 1423
Swelling, in inflammation, 205
Sylvian fissure, 452
Symbiosis, 295, 295b
Sympathetic ganglia (paravertebral ganglia), 467
Sympathetic nervous system, 467, 469f
  functions of, 473f
  hypertension and, 1147, 1150
Sympathetically maintained pain, 494
Symphysis, 1549
Symport, 28
Symptomatic epilepsy, 539–542
Synapse(s), neuronal, 41, 446–447, 447f
  chemical, 448–449
  neurotransmitters of chemical, 447–448, 448t–449t
Synaptic boutons, 447, 447f
Synaptic cleft, 447, 447f
Synarthrosis, 1549
Synchondrosis, 1549
Syndactyly, 1620–1621, 1621f
Syndesmophyte, 1601
Syndesmosis, 1549
Syndrome of inappropriate antidiuretic hormone (SIADH), 106, 729
  clinical manifestations of, 729
  etiologies of, 729
  evaluation and treatment of, 729–730
  paraneoplastic, 389t
  pathophysiology of, 729
Syndrome of neuropraxia, 594t–595t
Syndromic craniosynostosis, 673
Synovial cavity, 1550
Synovial fluid, 1550
Synovial joint(s), 1550–1554, 1552f
  body movements using, 1555f
  movement of, 1554, 1554f
  structures of, 1550–1554
Synovial membrane, 1550
Synovium, 1550, 1552f
Syntenic loci, 156
Syphilis, 927–928. *See also* *Treponema pallidum.*
  clinical manifestations of, 929–930
    in primary stage, 929–930, 929f
    in secondary stage, 929, 930f
    in tertiary and latent stages, 929
  congenital, 929–930
  darkfield examination test for, 806t
  evaluation and treatment of, 930–932
    false positive test results in, 930, 932b
  pathophysiology of, 928–929
  primary, 928
  secondary, 928–929
  serologic tests for, 806t
  tertiary, 929
  untreated, progression of, 928, 928b
Syringomyelic syndrome, 620
Systemic circulation, 1091, 1092f

Systemic hypertension, in children, 1218
Systemic immune system, 246
Systemic inflammatory response, 1703
Systemic inflammatory response syndrome (SIRS), 1735, 1741
Systemic lupus erythematosus (SLE), 271–272
  clinical manifestations of, 272
  immunoglobulin G deposition in skin and kidneys in, 271, 271f, 1382
  maternal hypersensitivity in, 271
  treatment goals in, 272
Systemic manifestations, of inflammation, 205–206
Systemic mean arterial pressure, 1133t
Systemic scleroderma, 1667
Systemic vascular resistance (SVR), 1133t
Systole, 1095
Systolic compressive effect, 1130–1131
Systolic heart failure, 1190–1194
  clinical manifestations of, 1193
  diastolic and, comparison of, 1195t
  management of, 1193–1194
  pathophysiology of, 1190–1194
    initial insult in, 1190, 1192f
    metabolic changes in, 1190, 1193b
  progression of, 1192–1193, 1192f
Systolic pressures, normal intracardiac, 1098t

T

T cell lymphoma(s), 1033
  classification of, 1030b
T cell receptor (TCR) complex, 226
T cell receptors, 222–226
  gene recombination and, 231–233, 232f
T helper cells (Th cells), 218–219, 231–233, 231f, 237–240. *See also* Th1 cells; Th2 cells.
  interaction with antigen presenting cells, 238–239
  subpopulations of, 239–240, 239f. *See also* Th1 cells; Th2 cells; Th17 cells.
T-independent antigens, 242, 242f
T lymphocyte deficiencies, 278–279
  gene defects in, 276t, 277f
T lymphocytes (T cells), 218
  activation of, 243–244. *See also* Cytotoxic T cells; Memory T cells; T regulatory (Treg) cells.
  autoreactive, 233
  cell surface marker changes on, 233
  clonal selection of, 243–244
  cross-reactive, 269
  differentiation and maturation of, 219–220, 220f, 230–233, 231f
  functions of, 247–251
  helper, 237–240. *See also* T helper cells (Th cells).
  hematopoietic differentiation of, 964f
  macrophage activation by, 250, 250f

T regulatory (Treg) cells, 222, 239–240
  dysfunctional, and autoimmune disorders, 269
  functions of, 250–251
Tachycardia, 1197t–1198t
  in children, 1730
Tactile agnosia, 548t
Tactile sensory dysfunction, 517
Taenia solium, 310t
  tissue damage caused by, 312
Tamm-Horsfall glycoprotein, 1356–1357
Tamm-Horsfall protein, 1368, 1374
Tamoxifen, 1584
Tamponade, 1177
Tapeworms (cestodes), 310, 310t
TAR syndrome, 1044
Tardive dyskinesias, 569
Target cell(s), 699, 992f
  direct and permissive effects of hormones on, 699
  hormone binding at, 700f
  sensitivity of, 699, 699f
    altered, 728, 728t
Target cell receptors, 699, 699f
Taste, 515–516
Taste dysfunction, 516
Tattooing, in gunshot wounds, 66–67
Tay-Sachs disease, 5, 678–679
  genetics and pathophysiology of, 526t–527f
Tc cells. *See* Cytotoxic T cells.
TCAs (tricyclic antidepressants), 657–658, 657b
Technetium scanning, in cardiac function evaluation, 1135
Tectum, 455
Tegmentum, 450t, 455
Telangiectasia, 313, 1648t–1653t
Telencephalon, 450t, 452–453
Telomerase, 369–370, 373f
Telomere(s), 369–370, 373f
Telomere crisis model, of breast carcinogenesis, 898
Telophase, 35
Temperature extremes, in cell injury, 71–72
Temperature regulation, 496–498
  in aging, 498–502
  in children, 498
  hypothalamic control of, 496–498
Temperature regulatory dysfunction, 500–502
  hyperthermic, 500–501
  hypothermic, 501–502
  in trauma, 502
Template, 129
Temporal extradural hematoma, 586
Temporal fossa, 459
Temporal lobe, 452
Temporal pain, 491b
Temporal summation, 449
Tendinitis, 1574, 1574f, 1574t
Tendinopathy, 1574
  clinical manifestations of, 1575
  evaluation and treatment of, 1575–1576
  histopathologic classification of, 1574t
  pathophysiology of, 1574–1575
Tendinosis, 1574, 1574t

Tendon(s), 1555, 1573
Tendon and ligament injuries, 1573
  inflammatory, 1574
  sprains and strains in, 1573
Tendon strain, 1573
Teniae coli, 1436
Tennis elbow, 1574
Tension pneumothorax, 1273
Tension-type headache, 611
Tentorium cerebelli, 460
Teratologic equinovarus, 1623
Teriparatide, 1584
Termination (nonsense) codon, 129
Termination sequence, 137
Tertiary syphilis, 929
  clinical manifestations of, 929
Testes, 796–797
  descent of, 796, 797f
  interior anatomy of, 798f
Testicular cancer, 857, 858f
  clinical manifestations of, 858
  evaluation and treatment of, 858–859
  fetal diethylstilbestrol exposure and, 403
  metastasis of, 384t
  pathogenesis of, 858
Testicular torsion, 856–857, 856f
Testicular tumors, and germ cell origin, 859t
Testosterone, 800–802
  adiposity and, 409
  physiologic effects of, 352
  stress induced, 352
Tet spell, 1223–1224
Tetanus, 1562
Tetanus, diphtheria, pertussis (Td/Tdap, DTaP) vaccine, 329–330, 330t
  adult, 329t
  child, 330t
  in pregnancy, 330t
Tetanus (T) vaccine, 330
  adult, 329t
  child, 330t
Tethered cord syndrome, 671
Tetralogy of Fallot, 1223, 1224f
  clinical manifestations of, 1223–1225
  evaluation and treatment of, 1225
  pathophysiology of, 1223
Tetraploidy, 135–136
TGF. *See transforming growth factor* entries.
Th1 cells, 239–240, 345
  in cell mediated hypersensitivity, 264
  in cellular immunity, 345, 345f
Th1 to Th 2 shift, 345
Th2 cells, 239–240, 345
  in humoral immunity, 345, 345f
Th17 cells, 239–240
Thalamic pain, 494
Thalamus, 450t, 453
  as principal target of nociceptive afferents, 484
Thalassemia(s), 1066t, 1076–1077
  clinical manifestations of, 1077–1078
  evaluation and treatment of, 1078
  pathophysiology of, 1077
Theca cells, 789
Thelarche, 784, 803

Therapeutic hyperthermia, 500
Therapeutic hypothermia, 502
Thermal burns, 1714
    and temperature regulation
        disorders, 502
Thermoreceptors, 445b
Thermoregulatory response, after
    burn injury, 1747–1748
Thiamine (vitamin B₁) deficiency,
    and associated disorders, 70t
Thiazides, diuretic action of, 1359t
Thimerosol, 62
Third-degree block, 1199t–1200t
Third degree burns, 1715, 1715t,
    1716f
Third order neurons, 484
Third spacing, of fluids, 1729
Thoracic cavity, 1249, 1249f
Thoracic disk disease, 598
Thoracic duct, 1132
Thoracolumbar division, of
    autonomic nervous system, 467
Thought disorders, 647
3-day measles, 1686
Threshold model, of dose-response,
    419, 419f
Threshold of liability, 166
Threshold potential, 33
Thrombin activity markers, ELISAs
    for, 1054
Thrombin time, 983t, 1079–1080
Thromboangiitis obliterans, 1148
Thrombocytes, 957. *See also*
    Platelet(s).
Thrombocythemia, 1047
    clinical manifestations of, 1048
    essential (primary), 1047
    evaluation and treatment of,
        1048–1051
    pathophysiology of, 1047–1048
Thrombocytopenia, 1044
    autoimmune neonatal, 1082
    cancer associated, 391
    clinical manifestations of,
        1044–1045
    differential diagnosis of
        pseudothrombocytopenia
        and, 1044
    evaluation and treatment of,
        1045–1046
    heparin induced, 1044
    pathophysiology of, 1044
Thrombocytosis, 1047
Thromboembolic disease, 1044,
    1055–1059
    hereditary, 1055–1056
    risk factors for, 1055, 1056b
    treatment of, 1055
Thromboembolism, 1147
    as complication of myocardial
        infarction, 1176
Thromboembolization, 1144
Thromboembolus, 1143–1144
Thrombolytics, in stroke
    management, 603
Thrombomodulin, 973f, 979
Thrombophilia, 1055, 1080
Thromboplastin generation test,
    1080
Thrombopoietin, 971–972
    in hematopoiesis, 961t
Thrombosis
    congenital, 1080–1081
    serum markers of, 1164b, 1165

Thrombotic crisis, in sickle cell
    disease, 1074
Thrombotic endocarditis
    nonbacterial, 1187
    paraneoplastic, 389t
Thrombotic stroke, 601
**Thrombotic thrombocytopenic
    purpura,** 1046–1047
    acute idiopathic, 1047
    chronic relapsing, 1047
    clinical manifestations of, 1047
    evaluation and treatment of, 1047
    incidence of, 1046
    pathophysiology of, 1046–1047
Thromboxane, and effect on
    endothelium, 1119b
Thromboxane A2 (TXA2), 976
Thrombus, 1055, 1055f, 1143–1144
    venous, 1144f
Thrush, 1685
Thymine, 129
Thymus, T cell maturation in,
    230–233, 231f
Thyrocalcitonin, 709
Thyroid, 708–712, 709f
    aging and effects on, 721
    C cells of, 709
    follicular tissue of, 709, 709f
    isthmus of, 709
    thyroid hormone synthesis in,
        710–711
Thyroid cancer, environmental
    factors in, 397t–400t, 401
Thyroid carcinoma, 742
Thyroid hormonal disorders, 736
    hyperthyroidism in, 736
    hypothyroidism in, 739
Thyroid hormone(s), 697t, 709–710,
    710t
    direct physiologic effects of, 711
    permissive physiologic effects
        of, 711
    receptors for, and mechanism of
        action, 700t
    regulation of secretion of, 709
    synthesis of, 710–711
Thyroid stimulating hormone
    (TSH), 710
    anterior pituitary secretion of, 707
    physiologic effects of, 704f, 708t,
        710
**Thyroid stimulating hormone
    (TSH) deficiency,** 732
Thyroid storm, 738–739
Thyrotoxic crisis, 738–739
Thyrotoxicosis, 736
    clinical manifestations of, 736,
        739f
    evaluation and treatment of,
        736–739
    pathophysiology of, 736, 736f
Thyrotropin releasing hormone
    (TRH), hypothalamic release
    of, 703–704, 707t, 709
Thyroxine (T4), 710t, 711. *See also*
    Thyroid hormone(s).
Tick borne disease, 1667–1668
Tidemark, 1553
Tight junction(s), 16–18, 17f, 1429
Tinea, 1664–1665, 1684
    common sites of, 1665t
Tinea capitis, 1656f, 1664–1665,
    1684–1685
Tinea corporis, 1664–1665, 1685

Tinea pedis, 1664–1665, 1684
Tissue(s), 35–44
    cellular organization in, 35–36
    connective, 36–38
    epithelial, 36
    formation of, 35–36, 37f
    four primary types of, 35
    muscle, 38
    neural, 41–44
Tissue and systemic aging, 89–90
Tissue-based renin-angiotensin
    system, 1126–1127
Tissue biopsy, 385t, 805
Tissue factor
    in clotting mechanism, 976–977,
        977t
    and thrombus formation after
        atherosclerotic plaque
        rupture, 978f
    in vascular endothelial signaling
        pathways, 977, 979f
Tissue factor inhibitor (TFI) system,
    in vascular endothelium, 973f
Tissue factor pathway inhibitor
    (TFPI), 979
Tissue hypoxia, 990
Tissue injury, 62–69
    asphyxial, 68–69
    by bacterial pathogens, 305
    blunt force, 62–65
    example of, 305–307
    from gunshot, 66–68
    physical agents in, 71–76
    sharp force, 65–66
Tissue invasion
    by bacterial pathogens, 300–305
    by infectious microorganisms, 296
Tissue plasminogen activator (t-PA),
    979–980
Tissue regeneration, 208
Tissue-specific antigens, 259–260
**Tissue-specific hypersensitivity
    reactions,** 258–261, 259t
    allergy and symptoms associated
        with, 266t, 267
    mechanisms of, 260, 262f
Tissue thromboplastin, 976–977
Titratable acid, renal formation of,
    116–118, 117f
*TNF. See tumor necrosis factor
    entries.*
TNM cancer staging system, 384, 386f
    for non-small cell lung cancer,
        1303, 1304f
Tobacco use, in epidemiology of
    cancer, 404
Tolerance, immune, 222
Toll-like receptors (TLRs), 194, 205
    cell, and microbial target, 194t
Tonic phase, 538
Tonicity, 28
Tonsillar infections, 1316
Tophaceous gout, 1605
Tophi, 1602, 1605
Torsemide, diuretic action of, 1359t
Torsion of testes, 856–857, 856f
Torus fracture, 1569
**Total anomalous pulmonary
    venous connection,** 1232, 1232f
    clinical manifestations of,
        1232–1233
    evaluation and treatment of,
        1233–1234
    pathophysiology of, 1232

Total body surface area (TBSA),
    1716, 1742
Total body water (TBW), 97. *See also*
    Body fluids; Water balance.
    alterations in, 102–104
    distribution of, 97t
    normal gains and losses in, 97t
    in relation to body weight, 97t
Total iron-binding capacity,
    983t–985t
Total lung capacity (TLC), 1262
Total peripheral resistance
    blood pressure and, 1123–1130
    neural control of, 1124
Total plasma volume regulation,
    mechanisms of, 1125–1130,
    1127f
Touch, 517
Toxic adenoma, 737–738
Toxic epidermal necrolysis, 1661,
    1692–1694
Toxic gases, exposure to, 1277–1278
Toxic multinodular goiter, 737–738
Toxic myopathy, 1612–1613
Toxigenicity, of pathogen, 297
Toxoids, 331
Toxoplasma gondii, 310t
    placental transmission of, 296
Toxoplasmosis, AIDS-associated,
    629
Trabeculae, bone, 1546
Trabeculae carneae, 1095–1096
Trachea, 1244, 1245–1246f
**Tracheal malformations,
    congenital,** 1320
Tracheitis
    acute, 1315t
    bacterial, 1315
Tracheoesophageal fistulae, 1518,
    1518f
Tracheomalacia, in children, 1319,
    1319f
Trachoma, 507
Traction, for bone fractures, 1571,
    1571f
Trade-off hypothesis, 1390–1392
Traits. *See also* Allele(s).
    concordant and discordant, 170
    inheritance of
        autosomal dominant, 146–150
        autosomal recessive, 151–152
        in consanguinity, 152
        laws of, 146
        multifactorial, 165–169
        sex-limited and sex-influenced,
            155
        X-linked, 152–155
        penetrance and expressivity of,
            148–149
trans fats, 1162b
Transchondral fracture, 1569
Transcortical dysphasias, 548,
    549f
Transcortin, 343, 717
Transcription, RNA, 132–133, 134f
Transfalcial herniation, 559
Transfer reactions, 24
Transfer RNA (tRNA), 134. *See also*
    tRNA.
Transferrin, 971
Transferrin saturation, 983t–985t
Transformation, cellular, 362, 363f
Transforming growth factor-α,
    (TGF-α), 49

Transforming growth factor-β (TGF-β), 36t, 203f
and breast cancer risk, 889, 890f
in healing wounds, 210
in immune response, 228–229, 229t–300t, 242
Transfusion, blood, in immune deficiency therapies, 288
Transfusion reactions, blood, 272–274
agglutinated red blood cells in, 273f
Transgeneration effects, 417–418
Transient hypogammaglobulinemia of infancy, 284
Transient ischemic attack (TIA), 601
Transient osteoporosis of hip, 1580
Transient receptor linkup, 19f
Transient receptor potential (TRP) channels, 482
Transitional atrioventricular canal defect, 1222
Transitional cell carcinoma, 1372–1373
Transitional circulation, 1211–1213
Transitional connective tissue, 39t–40t
Translation, and polypeptide synthesis, 134
Translocations, chromosome, 143, 144f
Transmembrane proteins, 11
Transmission, of infectious agents, 296
Transplant rejection, 274–275
Transplantation, in immune deficiency therapies, 288
Transport maximum (Tm), 1355–1357
Transport protein(s), 28, 954
Transposition of the great arteries, 1231, 1231f
clinical manifestations of, 1231
evaluation and treatment of, 1231–1232
pathophysiology of, 1231
Transudative effusion, 1273, 1274t, 1483
Transverse colon, 1435–1436
Transverse fracture, 1569
Transverse tubules, 1558–1559
Trastuzumab (Herceptin), 387t, 907–908
Trauma. See Tissue injury.
Traumatic aneurysms, 606–607
Traumatic brain injury (TBI), 583–591
categories of, 583–584
causes of, 584–591
common types of, 584
diagnostic tools in, 591
diffuse, 588–591. See also Diffuse brain injury.
focal, 585–588. See also Focal brain injury.
genetics of, 484
incidence of, 583
penetrating focal, 588
primary and secondary, 584–585
severity of, and clinical manifestations, 584t
temperature regulation disorders in, 502

Treg cells. See T regulatory (Treg) cells.
Treitz ligament, 1428
Tremor at rest, 568t–569t
Treponema pallidum, 298, 299t–300t, 928
microscopic identification of, 930–932
placental transmission of, 296
protective survival mechanisms of, 304
TRH. See Thyrotropin releasing hormone.
Triamterene, diuretic action of, 1359t
Tricarboxylic acid cycle, 23–24
Trichinella spiralis, 310t
antigenic variation in, 311
immune suppression by, 311–312
Trichomonas vaginalis, 310t, 942
Trichomoniasis, 942–943
clinical manifestations of, 943
evaluation and treatment of, 943–944
pathophysiology of, 943
Trichophyton mentagrophytes, 308t
Trichophyton rubrum, 308t
Trichuris trichiura, 310t
Tricuspid atresia, 1225, 1225f
clinical manifestations of, 1226
evaluation and treatment of, 1226
pathophysiology of, 1225–1226
Tricuspid regurgitation, 1183
clinical manifestations of, 1182t
Tricuspid valve, 1094
Tricyclic antidepressants (TCAs), 657–658, 657b
Trigeminal nerve (CN V), 466f
origins, course, functions, and testing of, 468t
Trigone, 1350
Triiodothyronine (T3), 710t, 711. See also Thyroid hormone(s).
Triploidy, 135–136
Trisomy, 136–137
chromosomal translocation in, 144f
partial, 137
Trisomy13, congenital heart defects associated with, 1215t
Trisomy18, congenital heart defects associated with, 1215t
Trisomy21. See Down syndrome.
Trisomy X, 139
tRNA (transfer RNA), 134
Trochlear nerve (CN IV), 466f
origins, course, functions, and testing of, 468t
Trophozoites, 946
Tropomyosin, 1560t
Troponin(s), 1106, 1560t
cardiac, 1173–1174
Troponin C, 1106
Troponin T, 1106
Troponin-tropomyosin complex, myocardial, 1106
Trousseau sign, 112
True aneurysm, 1146
True bacteria, 297
Truncus arteriosus, 1211, 1233–1234, 1233f
clinical manifestations of, 1234
evaluation and treatment of, 1234
pathophysiology of, 1234

Trypanosoma brucei, 310t
tissue damage caused by, 312
Trypanosoma cruzi, 310t
intracellular survival of, 311
neurotoxin release by, 312
Trypanosoma spp., 310
transmission of, 311
Trypsin, 1430–1432
Trypsin inhibitor, 1444
TSH. See Thyroid stimulating hormone.
Tubercle, 1293
Tuberculin test, 1293
Tuberculosis, 1293
clinical manifestations of, 1293
evaluation and treatment of, 1293–1295
incidence of, 1293
pathophysiology of, 1293
preventive measures against, 1294
Tuberculous granuloma, 207f, 208
Tuberous sclerosis
and associated childhood cancer, 438t
genetic basis and pathophysiology of, 526t–527t
Tuberous sclerosis complex, 679–680
Tubular meningitis, 623
Tubular reabsorption, 1352, 1354f
Tubular secretion, 1352, 1354f
Tubular transport, in glomerular filtration, 1355–1357
Tubules, renal
distal, 1347
epithelial cells of, 1347, 1347f
Henle loop, 1347
proximal, 1347
transport within, 1355–1357, 1356b
Tubuloglomerular feedback, 1351
Tubulointerstitial fibrosis, 1365–1367
Tubulus rectus, 797
Tumor(s). See Neoplasms.
Tumor biology, 35
Tumor growth
stress and, 353
and wound healing, comparison of, 378, 379f
Tumor markers, 367, 368t
Tumor necrosis factor-α (TNF-α), 49, 203f, 205
in immune response, 228–229, 229t
superantigen production of, 244
Tumor necrosis factor-β (TNF-β)
in immune response, 228–229, 229t–300t
Tumor-related genes, 401–404, 896, 896f
Tumor suppressor gene(s), 365f, 148, 370–375
allelic inactivation of, 373, 376f
associated with childhood cancers, 438, 439t
dysfunctional, in familial cancer syndromes, 375–377, 375t. See also Epigenetic silencing.
Tunica albuginea, 797
Tunica dartos, 797
Tunica externa, 1113
Tunica intima, 1113
Tunica media, 1113

Tunica vaginalis, 796
Turbulent flow, 1121, 1124f
Turner syndrome, 139, 141f
congenital heart defects associated with, 1215t
Twins
and associated childhood cancer, 438t, 439
in studies of environmental factors in disease, 170, 171t
Tympanic cavity, 512–513
Tympanic membrane, 512
Type 1 diabetes mellitus, 745
acute complications of, 754–756, 757t
dawn phenomenon, 758
diabetic ketoacidosis, 755–756
hyperosmolar hyperglycemic nonketotic syndrome, 757
hypoglycemia, 754–755
Somogyi effect, 758
autoimmune destruction of beta cells in, 746–748
chronic complications of, 758–765
hyperglycemia, 758. See also Hyperglycemia.
infection, 765
macrovascular disease, 763–765. See also Coronary artery disease; Peripheral arterial disease; Stroke.
microvascular disease, 759–763. See also Microvascular disease.
clinical manifestations of, 749, 749t
environmental factors linked to, 746, 748b
epidemiology and etiology of, 747t
evaluation and treatment of, 749–750
genetic and environmental interaction in, 176–177, 746
genetic susceptibility to, 745–746
hormonal alterations in, 748–749
pathophysiology of, 745–749, 746t, 748f
and type 2 diabetes, comparison of, 177t
Type 2 diabetes mellitus, 750
acute complications of, 754–756, 757t
dawn phenomenon, 758
diabetic ketoacidosis, 755–756
hyperosmolar hyperglycemic nonketotic syndrome, 757
hypoglycemia, 754–755
Somogyi effect, 758
chronic complications of, 758–765
hyperglycemia, 758. See also Hyperglycemia.
infection, 765
macrovascular disease, 763–765. See also Coronary artery disease; Peripheral arterial disease; Stroke.
microvascular disease, 759–763. See also Microvascular disease.
clinical manifestations of, 752, 752t
dietary medical treatment of, 753, 753b

Type 2 diabetes mellitus (*Continued*)
environmental-genetic interaction in development of, 177, 750
epidemiology and etiology of, 747t
evaluation and treatment of, 752–756, 752b–753b
exercise in treatment of, 753
incidence of, 750
medications in treatment of, 753, 753t
pathophysiology of, 733, 746t, 756f
stress induced cortisol in development of, 343, 344b
type 1 diabetes and, comparison of, 177t
Type A synovial cells, 1550
Type B synovial cells, 1550
Type I hypersensitivity reactions, 258–259, 259t
allergy and symptoms associated with, 265–267, 266f, 266t
mechanism of, 259, 260f
tests of, 265–267
Type I muscle fibers, 1557
characteristics of, 1558t
Type II hypersensitivity reactions, 258–261, 259t
allergy and symptoms associated with, 266t, 267
mechanisms of, 260, 262f
Type II muscle fibers, 1557
characteristics of, 1558t
metabolism of, 1562
Type III hypersensitivity reactions, 258, 259t, 261–264, 263f
allergy and symptoms associated with, 266t, 267
Type IV hypersensitivity reactions, 258, 259t, 264, 264f
allergy and symptoms associated with, 266t, 267
Typhus pandemic, 297t
Tyrosine kinase activated receptors, 23t, 701, 702t
Tzanck test, 1647t

U

Ubiquitin-proteasome pathway, 47
Ulcer(s)
in colitis, 1471, 1474t
Curling, 1467
Cushing, 1467
decubitus, 1647
duodenal, 1465, 1466f, 1468t
in esophagitis, 1459f
gastric, 1467, 1468t
ischemic, 1467
peptic, 1464–1465
pressure, 1647–1654
skin, 1648t
stress, 1467–1470
venous stasis, 1143
Ulcerative colitis, 1471, 1474t
chronic, and associated cancer, 378t
clinical manifestations of, 1471–1472
distribution patterns of, 1472f
evaluation and treatment of, 1472–1473
pathophysiology of, 1471
Ultrafiltration, 1352

Ultrasonography, 807
of central nervous system, 476
of gastrointestinal tract, 1444, 1445t
Ultraviolet radiation, in cancer epidemiology, 422–424, 1671b
Uncal herniation, 559
Unclassified epileptic seizures, 679
Unconjugated bilirubin, 1440
Underactive bladder syndrome, 1370
Undescended testes, 856
Undifferentiated large cell anaplastic cancer, 1301–1302
Unilateral renal agenesis, 1407
Unipolar neurons, 444, 445f
Uniport, 28
Universal donor, 272
Universal recipient, 272
Unmyelinated axons, 443
Unmyelinated C polymodal nociceptors, 483, 483f
Unsaturated fats, 1162b
Unsaturated fatty acids, 1433b
Unstable angina, 1169–1170
clinical manifestations of, 1170
evaluation and treatment of, 1170–1171
pathophysiology of, 1170
three principal presentations of, 1171b
Unverricht-Lundborg disease, genetics and pathophysiology of, 526t–527t
Up-regulation
of hormone receptors, 699
of proteasome, 47
Upper airway, 1242–1243, 1243f, 1245f
in children, 1310
Upper airway obstruction, in children, 1313–1318, 1313b
breathing sounds in, 1313–1314, 1313f–1314f
causes of
angioedema, 1318
congenital malformations, 1320
foreign body aspiration, 1317–1318
infections, 1315–1316, 1315t. *See also* Croup; Epiglottitis.
laryngomalacia and tracheomalacia, 1319
obstructive sleep apnea, 1320
subglottic stenosis, 1318–1319
vocal cord paralysis, 1319
Upper esophageal sphincter, 1423
Upper gastrointestinal bleeding, 1456
Upper motor neuron(s), 457–458
Upper motor neuron dysfunction gait, 576
Upper motor neuron syndromes, 564–565, 564t
in amyotrophic lateral sclerosis, 634
pathophysiology of, 565f
Upper motor neuron system, component structures of, 566f
Upper respiratory tract infections, bacterial agents causing, 299t–300t

Upper urinary tract obstruction, 1365–1368, 1366f
compensatory mechanisms in, 1367
diuresis in, 1367–1368
kidney stones in, 1368
pathophysiology of, 1367
Urate accumulation, cellular, 81
Urate concentrations, mean, by age and gender, 1602t
Urate oxidase, 7
Urea
diuretic action of, 1359t
filtration and reabsorption of, 1358
Urea clearance, in chronic kidney disease, 1392t, 1393, 1393f
Ureaplasma urealyticum, 938
Uremia, 1386
systemic effects of, 1391t
Uremic syndrome, 1393, 1393f
Ureter(s), 1350
Ureteral orifices, normal and abnormal configurations of, 1412, 1413f
Ureterohydronephrosis, 1365–1367, 1366f
Ureteropelvic junction obstruction, 1406
Urethra, 1350
Urethral atresia, 1406
Urethral obstruction
in children, 1406
urine flow in, 1371
Urethral polyps, 1406
Urethral sphincters, 1350
Urethral stricture, 850, 1371–1372
Urethral syndrome, acute, 936
Urethral valve, 1406
Urethritis, 850
Urethrocele, 835
Urge incontinence, 1369t
Uric acid, 1368–1369
elimination of, 1602–1603, 1603f
Uric acid stones, 1368–1369
Uric acid-urate equilibrium, 1602–1603f
Urinary calculi (stones), 1368
Urinary meatus, 785–786
Urinary structures, 1350–1351
Urinary system. *See* Renal and urinary systems.
Urinary tract disorders, 1365. *See also* Urinary tract infections; Urinary tract obstruction.
in children, 1404–1408
bladder related, 1411–1412
congenital, 1404–1407. *See also* Congenital renal and urinary tract disorders.
enuresis and, 1414
references on, 1417
summary review of, 1416b
references on, 1398
summary review of, 1397b
Urinary tract infections, 1373–1376
acute pyelonephritis in, 1377
causes of, 1373–1375
in children, 1411–1412, 1413b
chronic pyelonephritis in, 1377
cystitis in, 1374–1375
host defense mechanisms in, 1375–1376

Urinary tract infections (*Continued*)
painful bladder syndrome/interstitial cystitis in, 1376–1377
resistance to antibiotics in, 1376b
types of, 1373
virulence of pathogens causing, 1375–1376
Urinary tract obstruction, 1365–1368
lower, 1369–1371
anatomic causes of, 1371
evaluation and treatment of, 1371–1372
neurogenic bladder in, 1367f, 1369–1370
overactive bladder syndrome in, 1370–1371
tumors in, 1372
upper, 1365–1368, 1366f
compensatory mechanisms in, 1367
diuresis in, 1367–1368
kidney stones in, 1368
pathophysiology of, 1367
Urine color, 1361
Urine formation, 1354f, 1357–1358, 1357f
antidiuretic hormone and effects on, 1358
catecholamines and effects on, 1358
concentration and dilution in, 1357–1358
urea, 1358
water, sodium, chloride, 1357–1358
decreased, 106
diuretic effects in, 1358
Urine output, in children, 1403–1404, 1404t
Urine pH, 1361
Urine sediment analysis, 1361–1362
Urine specific gravity, 1361
Urobilinogen, 1440
Urodilatin
cardiovascular effects of, 1128
physiologic roles of, 1128b
renal effects of, 1352
Uroflowmetry, 1371
Urogenital sexually transmitted infections, 924–925
bacterial, 924–925. *See also* Bacterial urogenital infections.
chlamydial, 935. *See also* Chlamydial urogenital infections.
parasitic, 942–943. *See also* Pediculosis pubis; Scabies; Trichomoniasis.
viral, 938. *See also* Viral urogenital infections.
Urogenital ulceration, algorithm for diagnosis of, 931f
Urokinase-like plasminogen activator (u-PA), 979–980
Urotensin II, and effect on endothelium, 1119b
Urothelial carcinoma, 1372–1373
Urticaria, 265, 1666–1667, 1666f
lesions in, 1666–1667
Urushiol, 267
Uterine fibroids, 837, 838f

Uterine phase, of menstrual cycle, 793f, 795
Uterine prolapse, 833–834
    degrees of, 834f
Uterine sarcoma, 846
Uterine tubes, 789
Uterus, 787–789
    anatomy of, 787–788, 788f
    positions of, 787, 788f

V
v wave, 1096
Vaccination programs
    compliance in, 332
    success of, in United States, 327t
    world-wide, 330, 331f
Vaccines, 329–332
    adult immunization schedule and, 329t
    against bacterial toxins, 331
    development of, 330–331
    pediatric immunization schedule and, 330t
    safety of, 62, 332
    used in United States, 329, 329–330t
Vacuolar degeneration, 76
Vacuolar myelopathy, 628
Vacuolation, 53–54
Vacuoles, 30–31
Vagal nerve palsy syndromes, 568t–569t
Vagina, 786–787
    epithelial changes in, from pre-puberty to menopause, 787
Vaginal cancer, 844–845
Vaginal scanning, ultrasound, 808t
Vaginismus, 848–849
Vaginitis, 830–832
Vagus nerve (CN X), 466f
    origins, course, functions, and testing of, 468t
Valence, antibody, 225
Valsalva maneuver, 1437
Valve(s), venous, 1116f, 1120, 1121f
Valvular dysfunction, 1181–1184
    clinical manifestations of, 1182t
    evaluation and treatment of, 1184–1185
    regurgitative, 1183
    stenotic, 1181–1183, 1182t
Valvular hypertrophic cardiomyopathy, 1180
Valvular regurgitation, 1181, 1181f
    clinical manifestations of, 1182t
Valvular stenosis, 1181, 1181f
    clinical manifestations of, 1182t
Variant HMECs (vHMECs), 902–905
Varicella, 1664, 1687–1688, 1687t
Varicella vaccine, 330
    adult, 329t
    child, 330t
Varicella-zoster virus (VZV; herpes simplex type 3), 314t, 1663
    in central nervous system infections, 621t
    in skin infections, 1663
Varicocele, 854, 855f
Varicose bronchiectasis, 1276
Varicose veins, 1142–1143, 1143f
    causes of, 1142
Variola, 1688
Vas deferens, 797

Vasa recta, 1347–1348
Vasa vasorum, 1113
Vascular anatomy, and function, 1113–1131, 1114f. *See also* Blood vessels.
Vascular compliance, 1122
    blood flow and, 1122
Vascular connective tissue, 39t–40t
Vascular dementia, differential diagnosis of, 554t
Vascular disorders
    pulmonary, 1294–1295
    secondary hypertension in, 1153t
    and skin disorders, 1665–1667
Vascular endothelial cell-specific cadherin (VE-cadherin), 972
Vascular endothelial growth factor (VEGF), 369
    in wound healing, 203f, 210
Vascular endothelial injury
    and atherosclerotic disease, 1157–1160
    and hypertension, 1152
    mechanisms of, 1055
Vascular endothelium, 1091, 1113, 1118f
    antithrombotic mechanisms of, 977t, 979–980
    cell growth and inhibition in, 1119b
    hemostatic function of, 972, 973f, 1119b, 1120f
    molecular movement facilitation by, 1119b
    nitrogen oxide release by, 199, 972
    vasomotive function of, 1119b, 1120–1121f
Vascular evaluation
    coronary, 1133–1135. *See also* Coronary arterial evaluation.
    systemic, 1135–1136
Vascular inflammatory response, 186–187
Vascular insufficiency, gastrointestinal, 1477
Vascular malformations, 607, 607f
    in children, 1691–1692, 1691f
    clinical manifestations of, 608
    congenital heart defects associated with, 1215t
    evaluation and treatment of, 608
    pathophysiology of, 607–608
    and skin disorders, 1665–1667
    types of, 607
Vascular permeability, chemical mediators of, 203f
Vascular remodeling, 1297
Vasculitis, 267
    in activation of coagulation cascade, 1049
Vasectomy, as risk factor for prostate cancer, 865
Vasoactive intestinal (poly)peptide (VIP), 1425t
    secretion of, in children, 689
    in stress response, 348t
Vasoconstriction, 1113, 1119b
    hypoxic pulmonary, 1260–1261, 1261b
    in preserving body core temperature, 498
Vasoconstrictors, 1119b
Vasodilation, 1113, 1119b
    chemical mediators of, 203f
    in heat loss, 497

Vasodilators, 1119b
    in shock therapy for children, 1740t
Vasodilatory shock, 1706, 1706f
Vasogenic cerebral edema, 560
Vasomotion, 1116
Vasomotor flush, 810
Vasoocclusive crisis, in sickle cell disease, 1074
Vasopressin. *See also* Antidiuretic hormone.
    in shock therapy for children, 1740t
Vasopressin blockers, diuretic effect of, 1359t
Vaspin, 1478b
Vaults, 7–8, 9f
VDJ genes
    in B cell receptor production, 233–234
    in T cell receptor production, 232, 232f
Vectors, of infectious agents, 296
Vegetative state, 535
    comparative clinical manifestations of, 536t
VEGF. *See* Vascular endothelial growth factor.
Vein(s), 1113, 1117. *See also* Venous blood vessels.
    diseases of, 1142–1144
    lymphatic, 1132
Velocardiofacial syndrome, 649
Venereal Disease Research Laboratory (VDRL), 805
    serologic tests of, for diagnosis of syphilis, 930
Venezuelan equine encephalitis, 625–626, 626t
Venography, 1136
Venous angioma, 607
Venous blood vessels, 1113, 1114f, 1117
    blood flow through, 1117, 1122f
    structure of, 1116f
    valves of, 1116f, 1120, 1121f
Venous insufficiency, chronic, 1143
Venous obstruction, 99–100
Venous pressure, maintenance of, 1130
Venous stasis ulcers, 1143
Venous system
    of brain, 462
    of head, 464f
Venous thrombi, 1055, 1144f
Venous thromboembolism, 1294–1295
Venous thrombosis, 1143–1144
    paraneoplastic, 389t
    pathogenesis of, 1144
Ventilation, 1249–1255, 1249f
    alveolar, 1249
    distribution of, 1256–1257
    increase in, and heat loss, 497
    mechanics of, 1251–1254, 1252f
    in neonates, protective strategies for, 1323, 1326
    neurochemical control of, 1249–1251, 1250f
Ventilation-perfusion ratio, 1257
    abnormalities of, 1270, 1270f
Ventricles
    brain, 461
    cardiac, 1093

Ventricular aneurysm, 1176
Ventricular block, 1199t–1200t
Ventricular bradycardia, 1197t–1198t
Ventricular dysrhythmias, and stress, 337b
Ventricular fibrillation, 1197t–1198t
Ventricular remodeling, 1190, 1191f
Ventricular septal defect, 1220, 1221f
    clinical manifestations of, 1222
    evaluation and treatment of, 1222
    pathophysiology of, 1220–1222
    recurrence risk for, 168
Ventricular septation, 1211
Ventricular tachycardia, 1197t–1198t
Ventricular wall aneurysm, 1145f, 1146
Venules, 1113
    lymphatic, 1132
Verapamil, calcium channel blocking activity of, 1108–1109
Vermiform appendix, 1435–1436
Vermis, 455
Verrucae, 1664, 1664f
Vertebra, lumbar, superior view, 462f
Vertebral arteries, 462, 465f
Vertebral artery occlusions, stroke syndromes resulting from, 604t–605t
Vertebral column, 461–462, 461f
Vertebral fracture(s)
    in osteoporosis, 1578, 1578f
    in spinal cord injuries, 591–592, 592f, 593t
Vertical transmission, of infections, 296
Vertigo, 517
Very low density lipoproteins (VLDL), 1161–1162
Vesicants, 1714
Vesicle, skin, 1648t–1653t
Vesicle formation, macromolecule transport by, 30–32
Vesicoureteral reflux, 1412
    clinical manifestations of, 1412–1413
    evaluation and treatment of, 1413
    grades of, 1412, 1412f
    pathophysiology of, 1412
Vesicular impetigo, 1683
Vesiculobullous skin disorders, 1660–1662
Vestibular dysfunction, 517
Vestibular nystagmus, 517
Vestibule
    labyrinthine, 514
    vaginal, 785–786
Vestibulocochlear nerve (CN VIII), 466f
    origins, course, functions, and testing of, 468t
Vestibulospinal tract, 457f, 458
Vestigial tabs, 1620–1621
Vibrio cholerae, 298, 299t–300t, 300
    antigenic variation in, 304
    enterotoxins of, 305
    intracellular survival of, 302
    rapid division of, 302

Vibrio parahaemolyticus, 299t–300t
Video-urodynamic recordings, 1371
Vigilance deficits, 544, 547t
Vigilance system, 544, 545f
Villi, intestinal, 1429
Viral central nervous system infections/inflammation, 621t
Viral conjunctivitis, 507
Viral hepatitis, 1488–1490
 types of, 1488t. *See also* Hepatitis A; Hepatitis B; Hepatitis C; Hepatitis D; Hepatitis E.
Viral infections, 313–318, 314t. *See also* Viral pathogens.
 and acquired immunodeficiency syndrome, 318–325
 and associated congenital heart defects, 1214t
 of central nervous system, 621t, 622f
 cutaneous, 1663–1664
 in HIV (human immunodeficiency virus) infection, 323b
 pathogenesis of, 316–318
 stages of, 315, 315f
 urogenital, 938. *See also* Viral urogenital infections.
 vaccination protection against, 244–245
Viral meningitis, 620–622, 682
 AIDS associated, 629
 in children, 684
 clinical manifestations of, 624
 evaluation and treatment of, 624
 infection of cells in, 621t, 622f
Viral myositis, 1611
Viral pathogens, 313–318, 314t
 evasion mechanisms of, 315–316
  antigenic variation, 315–316
  complement evasion, 316
  immune molecule neutralization, 316
  immune suppression, 316
  intracellular survival, 315
  rapid division, 315
  self-protein coating, 315
 tissue damage caused by, 316
 tissue invasion by, 315–316
 transmission and colonization by, 313–315
Viral pneumonia, 1291–1292
 in children, 1328–1329, 1328t
Viral skin infections, 1663–1664
 in children, 1685–1688, 1687t
Viral urogenital infections, 938
 diagnostic tests for, 806t
 genital herpes in, 938
 human papillomavirus in, 940
 molluscum contagiosum in, 941–942
Virchow triad, 1055, 1295
Virilization, 771, 771f
Virulence, of pathogen, 297
Viruses, 298t, 313–318
 attenuated, 244–245, 330–331
 cancer and, 378–380, 381t
Visceral abdominal pain, 1455
Visceral epithelium, 1345–1346
Visceral pain, 490
 origins of, 491
Visceral pericardium, 1093
Visceral peritoneum, 1428–1429

Viscosity, in fluid system, 1118
Visfatin, 1478b
Vision, 506–508
 in aging, 508–514, 509t
Visual acuity alterations, 509–511
Visual agnosia, 548t
Visual dysfunction, 509–512
 alterations causing
  accommodative, 511
  acuity, 509–511
  autoimmune, 257f
  color perceptive, 511
  neurologic, 511–512
  oculomotor, 509–512
  refractive, 511
Visual fields, and neuronal pathways, 508f
Visual pathway defects, 512, 512f
Vital signs, normal pediatric, 1729–1730, 1730t
Vitamin(s)
 in cell function, 69
 intestinal absorption of, 1434–1435, 1435t
 storage of, in liver, 1442
Vitamin A deficiency, and associated disorders, 70t
Vitamin B$_2$, in erythropoiesis, 969t
Vitamin B$_2$ deficiency, and associated disorders, 70t
Vitamin B$_6$, in erythropoiesis, 968, 969t
Vitamin B$_6$ deficiency, and associated disorders, 70t
Vitamin B$_{12}$, in erythropoiesis, 968, 969t
Vitamin B$_{12}$ deficiency, and associated disorders, 70t
Vitamin B$_{12}$ replacement therapy, 994
Vitamin C
 and cancer risk, 410t
 in erythropoiesis, 969t
Vitamin C deficiency, and associated disorders, 70t
Vitamin D, 111–112
 and cancer risk, 410t
 immunologic functions of, 1359b
 importance of, 70b, 71f
 physiologic functions of, 1359–1360, 1359b
 renal influence in activation of, 1358–1360
Vitamin D deficiency
 and associated disorders, 70t
 in autoimmune disease, 1359b
 in chronic kidney disease, 1394
 in osteomalacia and rickets, 1584–1585
Vitamin D$_3$, 1359, 1359b
 malignant melanoma prevention and, 1671b
Vitamin deficiencies, and associated disorders and diseases, 70t
Vitamin E
 and cancer risk, 410t
 in erythropoiesis, 969t
Vitamin E deficiency, and associated disorders, 70t
Vitamin K deficiency
 and associated disorders, 70t
 impaired hemostasis and, 1049
Vitiligo, 1648t–1653t

Vitreous humor, 508
VJ genes
 in B cell receptor production, 233–234
 in T cell receptor production, 231–232, 232f
Vocal cord paralysis, in children, 1319
Volatile forms, of body acids, 114
Volkmann ischemic contracture, 1575–1576
Volume restoration. *See* Fluid resuscitation.
Volume sensitive receptors, 102
Voluntary actions
 in preserving body core temperature, 498
 in producing heat loss, 497
Voluntary muscle, 1555
Volvulus, 1461t, 1462f, 1519–1520
Vomiting, 1452–1453
 projectile, 1453
 as sign of central nervous system dysfunction, 531
von Hippel-Lindau disease
 and associated childhood cancer, 438t
 congenital heart defects associated with, 1215t
von Recklinghausen disease. *See* Neurofibromatosis type 1.
von Willebrand disease, 1079
von Willebrand factor (vWF), 972–973
Vulva, 784
Vulvar cancer, 845
Vulvovaginal glands, 785–786
Vulvovaginitis, 1666t
Vulvovestibulitis, 832

W
Waldenström macroglobulinemia, 1042
 clinical manifestations of, 1042
 evaluation and treatment of, 1042
 pathophysiology of, 1042
Wallerian degeneration, 445
Wandering, 568t–569t
Warfarin, and associated congenital heart defects, 1214t
Warm autoimmune hemolytic anemia, 274, 1005
Warm shock, 1735
Warmer climate, adaptation to, 497
Warts, 1664, 1664f
Water balance, 102, 102f
 alterations in, 102–104, 103t
  hypertonic, 103–104
  hypotonic, 104
  isotonic, 102–103
 in chronic kidney disease, 1393–1394, 1394t
Water deficit, 104
Water diuresis, 1358
Water drinking, compulsive, 106
Water excess, 106
Water intoxication, 104, 105t, 106
Water movement, across plasma membrane, 26–30, 98
 alterations in, 98–99. *See also* Edema.
Water reabsorption, in urine formation, 1357–1358

Water soluble hormones, 697t
 signal transduction by, 700–702, 701f
 types of, receptors, and mechanisms of action, 700t
Water transport, 30t
Weight-bearing exercise, and postmenopausal osteoporosis, 1584
Weight loss, in postgastrectomy syndromes, 1470
Wenckebach block, 1199t–1200t
Wernicke area, 452
Wernicke dysphasia, 549t–550t
West Nile encephalitis, 621t, 625–626, 626t
West Nile virus, 314t
 emergence of, 627b
West syndrome, 679–680
Western equine encephalitis, 625–626, 626t
Wet gangrene, 83–84
Wheal, 1648t–1653t
Wheal and flare reaction, 265
White blood cells (WBCs), 954. *See also* Leukocytes.
White matter, 452–453
 of spinal cord, 456–457
WHO Fracture Risk Assessment, 1583
Whole-blood clotting time, 983t
Wilms tumor, 1413
 clinical manifestations of, 1414
 evaluation and treatment of, 1414
 pathogenesis of, 1413–1414
 prognosis for survival with, 1414, 1414t
 staging of, 1414t
Wilms tumor genes, 375–377, 438–439, 1413–1414
 kidney development and role of, 1402
Wilson disease, 1534, 1534t
 clinical manifestations of, 1535
 evaluation and treatment of, 1535–1536
 pathophysiology of, 1534–1535
Windchill factor, 497
Window period, 322
Wirsung duct, 1443
Wiskott-Aldrich syndrome, 281, 1044
 and associated childhood cancer, 438t
Wnt signaling, 1541
Wolff-Parkinson-White syndrome, 1199t–1200t
Wood lamp examination, 1647t
Word blindness, 548t
Work of breathing, 1254
 in children, 1312
Working memory, 544, 545f–546f
Working memory deficits, 544, 547t
 in schizophrenia, 648
Wound contraction, 208, 210
 impaired, 212. *See also* Contracture(s).
Wound disruption, 212–213
Wound healing, 208–213, 209f
 dysfunctional, 211–213
 phase(s) of, 208–213, 209f
  maturation, 210
  reconstructive, 208–210
 tumor growth and, comparison of, 378, 379f, 901, 902f

Wound infections
  after burn injury, 1748
  bacterial agents causing,
    299t–300t
Wound sepsis, 211
Wounding potential, of firearms,
  67–68
Woven bone, 1548
Wuchereria bancrofti, 310t
  tissue damage caused by, 312

X

X chromosome, 134
  in meiosis, 154f
x descent, 1096
X-linked hyper-IgM syndrome, 278

X-linked inheritance, 152–155
  pedigree characteristics in, 154
  Punnett squares in, 155f
  recurrence risks in, 154–155
  sex determination and, 153–154
  X inactivation in, 153
**X-linked lymphoproliferative
  syndrome,** 1019
**X-linked severe combined immune
  deficiency** (X-linked SCID),
  280
X-linked sideroblastic anemia, 998
X-ray films, 474
Xanthelasma, and dyslipidemia,
  1167
Xanthinuria, 1368–1369

Xanthomas, in familial
  hypercholesterolemia, 174f
Xenobiotics, 404–405
Xenoestrogens, 893–895
D-Xylose absorption assessment, 1445t

Y

Y chromosome, 134
  in meiosis, 154f
y descent, 1096
Yawning, as sign of central nervous
  system dysfunction, 531
Yeast, 307
Yellow fever virus, 314t
Yellow marrow, 1546
Yersinia pestis, 299t–300t, 302–303

Z

Z bands, of myocardial muscle, 1106
Zinc, in bone tissue physiology, 1580b
Zollinger-Ellison syndrome, 1467
Zona binding test, 808t
Zona fasciculata, 716
Zona glomerulosa, 716
Zona reticularis, 716
Zonula adherens, 17f
Zoonotic infections
  bacterial agents in, 299t–300t
  viral agents in, 313
Zoster, 1688
Zoster vaccine, 330
  adult, 329t
  child, 330t

Most Common Laboratory Values

Constituent	Normal Mean Value and Some Ranges	Normal Range in SI Units
ELECTROLYTES	Total, 1% of plasma weight	
Na^+	142 mEq/L (136-145)	136-145 mmol/L
K^+	3.5-5.0 mEq/L	3.5-5.0 mmol/L
Ca^{++}	8.8-10.5 mg/dl	2.25-2.75 mmol/L
Mg^{++}	1.8-3.0 mg/dl	1.25-1.75 mmol/L
Cl^-	95-105 mEq/L	95-105 mmol/L
HCO_3^-	24-28 mEq/L	24-28 mmol/L
Phosphate (mostly HPO_4^-)	2.5-5.0 mg/L	0.5-1.25 mmol/L
SO_4^-	1 mEq/L	0.25-0.75 mmol/L
PROTEINS	6-8 g/dl	60-80 g/L
Albumins	4-6 g/dl	40-60 g/L
Gamma globulin	0.5-1.6 g/dl	5-16 g/L
Globulins	2-4 g/dl	20-40 g/L
Fibrinogen	200-400 mg/dl	2-4 mmol/L
BLOOD GASES		
pH	7.35-7.45	
CO_2 content (arterial)	35-45 mm Hg	4.65-5.32 kPa
O_2 content (arterial)	75-100 mm Hg	9.97-13.30 kPa
Bicarbonate	24-28 mEq/L	24-28 mmol/L
NUTRIENTS		
Glucose (fasting)	75-110 mg/dl	3.85-6.05 mmol/L
Total proteins	6-8 g/dl	—
Total lipids	400-800 mg/dl	4.0-8.0 g/L
Cholesterol (total)	<200 mg/dl	<5.20 mmol/L
Triglycerides	<160 mg/dl	0.45-1.81 mmol/L (males)
		0.40-1.52 mmol/L (females)
Phospholipids	150-380 mg/dl	1.50-3.80 mol/L
Free fatty acids	9.0-15.0 mM/L	9.0-15.0 mM/L
WASTE PRODUCTS		
Urea (BUN)	7-18 mg/dl	2.9-8.2 mmol/L
Uric acid	2-6 mg/dl	0.110-0.360 mmol/L
Creatinine	0.6-1.2 mg/dl	53-106 μmol/L
Creatinine clearance	107-139 ml/min	1.78-2.32 mmol/L
Uric acid (from nucleic acids)	2-7 mg/dl	0.120-0.360 mmol/L
Bilirubin (direct)	Up to 0.3 mg/dl	Up to 5.1 μmol/L
Bilirubin (indirect)	0-1.0 mg/dl	1.7-17.1 μmol/L
INDIVIDUAL HORMONES		
Prolactin	<20 ng/ml	<869 pmol
Thyroid tests		
Thyroxine (T_4)	4-11 ng/dl	51-142 nmol/L
T_4 expressed as iodine	3.2-7.2 ng/dl	253-569 nmol/L
T_3	75-220 ng/dl	975.00 nmol/L
Free thyroxine (T_4)	0.8-2.4 ng/dl	10.4 nmol/L
T_3 resin uptake	25%-38% relative uptake	0.25%-0.38% relative uptake
TSH*	0.3-3.04 mlU/L	2-11 μU/L